Human Herpesviruses

This comprehensive account of the human herpesviruses provides an encyclopedic overview of their basic virology and clinical manifestations. This group of viruses includes human simplex type 1 and 2, Epstein–Barr virus, Kaposi's Sarcoma-associated herpesvirus, cytomegalovirus, HHV6A, 6B, and 7, and varicella-zoster virus. The viral diseases and cancers they cause are significant and often recurrent. Their prevalence in the developed world accounts for a major burden of disease, and as a result there is a great deal of research into the pathophysiology of infection and immunobiology. Another important area covered within this volume concerns antiviral therapy and the development of vaccines. All these aspects are covered in depth, both scientifically and in terms of clinical guidelines for patient care. The text is illustrated generously throughout and is fully referenced to the latest research and developments.

ANN ARVIN is Professor of Pediatrics, Microbiology, and Immunology at Stanford University.

GABRIELLA CAMPADELLI-FIUME is Professor of Microbiology and Virology at the University of Bologna, Italy.

EDWARD MOCARSKI is Professor of Microbiology and Immunology at Emory University.

PATRICK MOORE is Professor of Molecular Genetics and Biochemistry at the University of Pittsburgh.

BERNARD ROIZMAN is Professor of Molecular Genetics, Cell Biology, Biochemistry, and Molecular Biology at the University of Chicago.

RICHARD WHITLEY is Professor of Pediatrics, Microbiology, Medicine, and Neurosurgery at the University of Alabama Birmingham.

KOICHI YAMANISHI is Professor of Microbiology at Osaka University, Japan.

Human Herpesviruses

Biology, Therapy, and Immunoprophylaxis

Edited by

Ann Arvin
Stanford University, CA School of Medicine

Gabriella Campadelli-Fiume
University of Bologna, Italy

Edward Mocarski
Emory University School of Medicine, USA

Patrick S. Moore
University of Pittsburgh Cancer Institute, PA, USA

Bernard Roizman
The University of Chicago, IL, USA

Richard Whitley
University of Alabama at Birmingham, AL, USA

Koichi Yamanishi
Osaka University School of Medicine, Japan

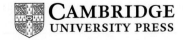

CAMBRIDGE UNIVERSITY PRESS

Cambridge, New York, Melbourne, Madrid, Cape Town, Singapore, São Paulo

Cambridge University Press
The Edinburgh Building, Cambridge CB2 8RU, UK

Published in the United States of America by Cambridge University Press, New York

www.cambridge.org
Information on this title: www.cambridge.org/9780521827140

© Cambridge University Press 2007

This publication is in copyright. Subject to statutory exception
and to the provisions of relevant collective licensing agreements,
no reproduction of any part may take place without
the written permission of Cambridge University Press.

First published 2007

Printed in the United Kingdom at the University Press, Cambridge

A catalog record for this publication is available from the British Library

ISBN-13 978-0-521-82714-0 hardback

Every effort has been made in preparing this Publication to provide accurate and up-to-date information which is in accord with accepted standards and practice at the time of publication. Although case histories are drawn from actual cases, every effort has been made to disguise the identities of the individuals involved. Nevertheless, the authors, editors and publishers can make no warranties that the information contained herein is totally free from error, not least because clinical standards are constantly changing through research and regulation. The authors, editors and publishers therefore disclaim all liability for direct or consequential damages resulting from the use of material contained in this publication. Readers are strongly advised to pay careful attention to information provided by the manufacturer of any drugs or equipment that they plan to use.

Cambridge University Press has no responsibility for the persistence or accuracy of URLs for external or third-party internet websites referred to in this publication, and does not guarantee that any content on such websites is, or will remain, accurate or appropriate.

Contents

List of contributors	*page* ix
Preface	xix

Part I Introduction: definition and classification of the human herpesviruses

Bernard Roizman

1	Overview of classification Andrew Davison	3
2	Comparative analysis of the genomes Andrew Davison	10
3	Comparative virion structures of human herpesviruses Fenyong Liu and Z. Hong Zhou	27
4	Comparative analysis of herpesvirus–common proteins Edward Mocarski, Jr.	44

Part II Basic virology and viral gene effects on host cell functions: alphaherpesviruses

Gabriella Campadelli-Fiume and Bernard Roizman

5	Genetic comparison of human alphaherpesvirus genomes Joel Baines and Philip Pellett	61
6	Alphaherpes viral genes and their functions Bernard Roizman and Gabriella Campadelli-Fiume	70
7	Entry of alphaherpesviruses into the cell Gabriella Campadelli-Fiume and Laura Menotti	93

8	Early events pre-initiation of alphaherpes viral gene expression Thomas Kristie	112		

8 Early events pre-initiation of alphaherpes viral gene expression 112
   Thomas Kristie

9 Initiation of transcription and RNA synthesis, processing, and transport in HSV and VZV infected cells 128
   Rozanne Sandri-Goldin

10 Alphaherpesvirus DNA replication 138
   John Hay and William Ruyechan

11 Envelopment of HSV nucleocapsids at the inner nuclear membrane 144
   Joel Baines

12 The egress of alphaherpesviruses from the cell 151
   Gabriella Campadelli-Fiume

13 The strategy of herpes simplex virus replication and takeover of the host cell 163
   Bernard Roizman and Brunella Taddeo

Part II Basic virology and viral gene effects on host cell functions: betaherpesviruses

Edward Mocarski

14 Comparative betaherpes viral genome and virion structure 177
   Andrew Davison and David Bhella

15 Betaherpes viral genes and their functions 204
   Edward Mocarski

16 Early events in human cytomegalovirus infection 231
   Teresa Compton and Adam Feire

17 Immediate–early CMV gene regulation and function 241
   Mark Stinski and Jeffrey Meier

18 Early CMV gene expression and function 264
   Elizabeth White and Deborah Spector

19 CMV DNA synthesis and late viral gene expression 295
   David Anders, Julie Kerry and Gregory Pari

20 CMV maturation and egress 311
   William Britt

21 CMV modulation of the host response to infection 324
   A. Louise McCormick and Edward Mocarski, Jr.

Part II Basic virology and viral gene effects on host cell functions: gammaherpesviruses

Patrick S. Moore

22 Introduction to the human γ-herpesviruses 341
   Richard Longnecker and Frank Neipel

23 Gammaherpesviruses entry and early events during infection 360
   Bala Chandran and Lindsey Hutt-Fletcher

24 Gammaherpesvirus maintenance and replication during latency 379
   Paul Lieberman, Jianhong Hu, and Rolf Renne

25 Reactivation and lytic replication of EBV 403
   Shannon Kenney

26 Reactivation and lytic replication of KSHV 434
   David Lukac and Yan Yuan

27 EBV gene expression and regulation 461
   Lawrence S. Young, John R. Arrand, and Paul G. Murray

28 KSHV gene expression and regulation 490
   Thomas Schultz and Yuan Chang

29 Effects on apoptosis, cell cycle and transformation, and comparative aspects of EBV with other DNA tumor viruses 514
   George Klein and Ingemar Ernberg

30 KSHV manipulation of the cell cycle and programmed cell death pathways 540
   Patrick Moore

31 Human gammaherpesvirus immune evasion strategies 559
   Robert Means, Sabine Lang, and Jae Jung

Part III Pathogenesis, clinical disease, host response, and epidemiology: HSV-1 and HSV-2

Ann Arvin and Richard Whitley

32 HSV-1 AND 2: pathogenesis and disease 589
   Richard Whitley, David Kimberlin, and Charles Prober

33 HSV-1 and 2: molecular basis of HSV latency and reactivation 602
   Christopher Preston and Stacey Efstathiou

34 HSV-1 and 2: immunobiology and host response 616
David Koelle

35 HSV: immunopathological aspects of HSV infection 642
Kaustuv Banerjee and Barry Rouse

36 HSV: persistence in the population: epidemiology, transmission 656
Anna Wald and Lawrence Corey

Part III Pathogenesis, clinical disease, host response, and epidemiology: VZU

Ann Arvin and Richard Whitley

37 VZV: pathogenesis and the disease consequences of primary infection 675
Jennifer Moffat, Chia-chi Ku, Leigh Zerboni, Marvin Sommer, and Ann Arvin

38 VZV: molecular basis of persistence (latency and reactivation) 689
Jeffrey Cohen

39 VZV: immunobiology and host response 700
Ann Arvin and Allison Abendroth

40 VZV: persistence in the population: transmission and epidemiology 713
Jane Seward and Aisha Jumaan

Part III Pathogenesis, clinical disease, host response, and epidemiology: HCMV

Ann Arvin and Richard Whitley

41 HCMV: pathogenesis and disease consequences 737
William Britt

42 HCMV: molecular basis of persistence and latency 765
Michael Jarvis and Jay Nelson

43 HCMV: immunobiology and host response 780
Mark Wills, Andrew Carmichael, J. H. Sinclair, and J. G. Patrick Sissons

44 HCMV: persistence in the population: epidemiology and transmission 795
Suresh Boppana and Karen Fowler

45 HCMV: persistence in the population: potential transplacental transmission 814
Lenore Peirera, Ekaterina Maidji, and Susan Fisher

Part III Pathogenesis, clinical disease, host response, and epidemiology: HHV- 6A, 6B, and 7

Ann Arvin and Richard Whitley

46 HHV-6A, 6B, and 7: pathogenesis, host response, and clinical disease 833
Yasuko Mori and Koichi Yamanishi

47 HHV-6A, 6B, and 7: molecular basis of latency and reactivation 843
Kaszuhiro Kondo and Koichi Yamanishi

48 HHV-6A, 6B, and 7: immunobiology and host response 850
Fu-Zhang Wang and Philip Pellet

49 HHV-6A, 6B, and 7: persistence in the population: epidemiology, transmission 875
Vincent Emery and Duncan Clark

Part III Pathogenesis, clinical disease, host response, and epidemiology: gammaherpesviruses

Patrick S. Moore

50 Clinical and pathological aspects of EBV And KSHV infection 885
Richard Ambinder and Ethel Cesarman

51 EBV: Immunobiology and host response 904
Denis Moss, Scott Burrows, and Rajiv Khanna

52 Immunobiology and host response to KSHV infection 915
Dimitrios Lagos and Chris Boshoff

53 The epidemiology of EBV and its association with malignant disease 929
Henrik Hjalgrim, Jeppe Friborg, and Mads Melbye

54 The epidemiology of KSHV and its association with malignant disease 960
Jeffrey Martin

55 EBV-induced oncogenesis 986
Nancy Raab-Traub

56 KSHV-induced oncogenesis 1007
Donald Ganem

Part IV Non-human primate herpesviruses

Ann Arvin, Patrick Moore, and Richard Whitley

57 Monkey B virus   1031
    Julia Hilliard

58 Simian varicella virus   1043
    Ravi Mahalingam and Donald Gilden

59 Primate betaherpesviruses   1051
    Peter Barry and William Chang

60 Gammaherpesviruses of New World primates   1076
    Armin Ensser and Bernhard Fleckenstein

61 EBV and KSHV-related herpesviruses in non-human primates   1093
    Blossom Damania

Part V Subversion of adaptive immunity

Richard Whitley and Ann Arvin

62 Herpesvirus evasion of T-cell immunity   1117
    Jatin Vyas, Benjamin Gewurz, and Hidde Ploegh

63 Subversion of innate and adaptive immunity: immune evasion from antibody and complement   1137
    Lauren Hook and Harvey Friedman

Part VI Antiviral therapy

Richard Whitley

64 Antiviral therapy of HSV-1 and -2   1153
    David Kimberlin and Richard Whitley

65 Antiviral therapy of varicella-zoster virus infections   1175
    John Gnann, Jr.

66 Antiviral therapy for human cytomegalovirus   1192
    Paul Griffiths and Michael Boeckh

67 New approaches to antiviral drug discovery (genomics/proteomics)   1211
    Mark Prichard

68 Candidate anti-herpesviral drugs; mechanisms of action and resistance   1219
    Karen Biron

Part VII Vaccines and immunothgerapy

Ann Arvin and Koichi Yamanishi

69 Herpes simplex vaccines   1253
    George Kemble and Richard Spaete

70 Varicella-zoster vaccine   1262
    Anne Gershon

71 Human cytomegalovirus vaccines   1274
    Thomas Heineman

72 Epstein–Barr virus vaccines   1292
    Andrew Morgan and Rajiv Khanna

73 DNA vaccines for humanherpesviruses   1306
    Thomas Evans and Mary Wloch

74 Adoptive immunotherapy for herpesviruses   1318
    Ann M. Leen, Uluhan Sili, Catherine Bollard, and Cliona Rooney

75 Immunotherapy of HSV infections – antibody delivery   1332
    David Kimberlin

Part VIII Herpes as therapeutic agents

Richard Whitley and Bernard Roizman

76 Herpesviruses as therapeutic agents   1341
    Frank Tufaro and James Markert

Index   1353

Contributors

Allison Abendroth
Centre for Virus Research
Westmead Millennium Institute and Research Centres
Westmead NSW 2145
Australia

Richard Ambinder
Johns Hopkins University School of Medicine
1650 Orleans Street, Room 389
Baltimore, MD 21231, USA

David Anders
Wadsworth Center
The David Axelrod Institute
PO Box 22002
Albany, NY 12201, USA

John Arrand
Cancer Research UK Institute for Cancer Studies
University of Birmingham
Edgbaston, Birmingham
B15 2TT, UK

Ann Arvin
Department of Pediatrics and Microbiology and Immunology
Stanford University School of Medicine
300 Pasteur Drive, Room G311
Stanford, CA 94305, USA

Joel Baines
Cornell University
Department of Microbiology and Immunology
C5169 Veterinary Education Ctr.
Ithaca, NY 14853, USA

Contributors

Kasstruf Banerjee
Department of Microbiology
College of Veterinary Medicine
University of Tennessee
1414 W. Cumberland Avenue
F403 Walters Life Sciences
Knoxville, TN 37996, USA

Peter Barry
Department of Pathology
Center for Comparative Medicine
University of California at Davis
One Shields Avenue
Davis, CA 95616, USA

David Bhella
Institute of Virology
MRC Virology Unit
Church Street
Glasgow, G11 5JR, UK

Karen Biron
Department of Clinical Virology
Glaxo Smith Kline
5 Moore Drive
Research Triangle Park, NC 27709, USA

Michael Boeckh
Fred Hutchinson Cancer Research Center
1100 Fairview Avenue, N.
Seattle, WA 98109, USA

Catherine M. Bollard
Center for Cell and Gene Therapy
Baylor College of Medicine
1102 Bates Street, BCM 320
Houston, TX 77030, USA

Suresh Boppana
University of Alabama at Birmingham
1600 7th Avenue, South. CHB 114
Birmingham, AL 35233, USA

Chris Boshoff
Cancer Research UK Viral Oncology Group
Wolfson Institute for Biomedical Research
University College London
Gower Street
London, WC1E 6BT, UK

William Britt
Department of Pediatrics
University of Alabama at Birmingham
CHB 107, 1600 7th Avenue South
Birmingham, AL, 35233, USA

Scott Burrows
Division of Infectious Diseases and Immunology
Queensland Institute of Medical Research
300 Herston Road
Herston (Qld) 4006
Australia

Gabriella Campadelli-Fiume
Department of Experimental Pathology
University of Bologna
Via San Giacomo 12, Bologna 40126,
Italy

Andrew Carmichael
Department of Medicine, University of Cambridge
Clinical School, Box 157, Addenbrooke's Hospital, Hills
Road, Cambridge CB2 2QQ, UK

Ethel Cesarman
Pathology Department
Weill Medical College of Cornell University
1300 York Avenue, Room C410
New York, NY 10021, USA

Bala Chandran
Department of Microbiology and Immunobiology
Rosalind Franklin University of Medicine and
Science
3333 Green Bay Road
North Chicago
IL 60064, USA

William Chang
Center for Comparative Medicine
University of California, Davis
County Road 98 & Hutchison Drive
Davis, CA 95616, USA

Yuan Chang
Department of Pathology
University of Pittsburgh Cancer Institute
Hillman Cancer Center, Research Pavilion, Suite 1.8
5117 Centre Avenue
Pittsburgh, PA 15213-1863, USA

Contributors

Duncan Clark
Virology
Royal Free University College Medical School
Rowland Hill Street,
London, NW3 2QG, UK

Jeffrey Cohen
Laboratory of Clinical Investigation,
National Institute of Health
10 Center Drive, MSC 1888
Bldg. 10, Rm 11N228
Bethesda, MD, 20892, USA

Teresa Compton
NIBRI (Novartis)
100 Technology
Square, Suite 4153,
Cambridge MA 02139, USA

Lawrence Corey
Virology Division, Laboratory Medicine
University of Washington
1100 Fairview Avenue N D3-100
Box 358080
Seattle, WA 98109, USA

Blossom Damania
University of North Carolina-Chapel Hill
Lineberger Cancer Center, CB#7295
Chapel Hill, NC 27599, USA

Andrew Davison
Institute of Virology
MRC Virology Unit
Church Street
Glasgow, G11 5JR, UK

Stacey Efstathiou
Division of Virology, Department of Pathology
University of Cambridge, Tennis Court Road
Cambridge, CB2, LQP, UK

Vincent Emery
Royal Free University College Medical School
Virology Department
Rowland Hill Street
London, NW3 2PF, UK

Armin Ensser
Institut für Klinische und Molekulare Virologie
der Friedrich-Alexander Universität Erlangen-Nürnberg
Schlossgarten 4
D-91054Erlangen
Germany

Thomas Evans
NIBRI (Novartis)
100 Technology Square
Suite 4153
Cambridge, MA 02139, USA

Adam Feire
McArdle Laboratory for Cancer Research, Room 610
University of Wisconsin
Madison, WI 53706, USA

Susan Fisher
Departments of Stomatology, Anatomy, Pharmaceutical
Chemistry and the Biomedical Sciences Graduate Program
and the Oral Biology Graduate Program
University of California, San Francisco
513 Parnassus Avenue MC 0512
San Francisco, CA 94143, USA

Bernhard Fleckenstein
Institut für Klinische und Molekulare Virologie
der Friedrich-Alexander Universität Erlangen-Nürnberg
Schlossgarten 4
D-91054Erlangen
Germany

Karen Fowler
Department of Pediatrics, Epidemiology and Maternal and
Child Health
University of Alabama
1530 3rd Avenue South, CHB 306
Birmingham, AL 35294-0011, USA

Jeppe Friborg
Department of Epidemiology Research
Statens Serum Institute
5 Artillerivej, DK-2300
Copenhagen S, Denmark

Harvey Friedman
Department of Medicine
University of Pennsylvania School of Medicine
502 Johnson Pavilion
Philadelphia, PA 19104-6073, USA

Contributors

Donald Ganem
Department of Medicine
University of California San Francisco
513 Parnassus Avenue
San Francisco, CA 94143, USA

Anne Gershon
College of Physicians and Surgeons
Columbia University
Pediatrics, BB4-427
650 W. 168th St.
New York, NY 10032, USA

Benjamin Gewurz
Harvard Medical School
200 Longwood Avenue
Department of Pathology
Boston, MA, USA

Donald Gilden
Department of Neurology
University of Colorado Health Sciences Center
4200 E. 9th Ave., B182
Denver, CO 80262, USA

John Gnann, Jr.
Department of Medicine
University of Alabama at Birmingham
845 19th St. S.
Birmingham, AL 35294, USA

Paul Griffiths
Royal Free University College Medical School
Virology Department
Rowland Hill Street,
London, NW3 2PF, UK

John Hay
State University of New York
Microbiology, Farber Hall, Rm. 138
3435 Main Street, Bldg. 26
Buffalo, NY, 14214, UK

Thomas Heineman
St. Louis University Health Sciences Center
3635 Vista Avenue at Grand Blvd.
PO Box 15250
St. Louis, MO 63110, USA

Julia Hilliard
Georgia State University
Biology, 424 Science Annex
29 Peachtree Center Avenue
Atlanta, GA 30303, USA

Henrik Hjalgrim
Department of Epidemiology Research
Statens Serum Institute
5 Artillerivej, DK-2300
Copenhagen S, Denmark

Lauren Hook
Department of Medicine
University of Pennsylvania School of Medicine
502 Johnson Pavilion

Jianhong Hu
Department of Molecular Genetics and Microbiology
University of Florida
1376 Mowry Road, Rm 375E
Gainesville, FL 32610, USA

Lindsey Hutt-Fletcher
Louisiana State University
Health Sciences Center
Feist-Weiller Cancer Center
1501 Kings Highway
PO Box 33932
Shreveport, LA 71130-3932, USA

Michael A. Jarvis
Vaccine and Gene Therapy Institute
Oregon Health Sciences University
3181 S. W. Sam Jackson Park Road
Portland, OR 97201, USA

Aisha Jumaan
Center for Disease Control
1600 Clifton Road., MS E-61
Atlanta, GA 30333, USA

Jae Jung
Division of Tumor Virology
New England Primate Research Center
Harvard Medical School
One Pine Hill Drive
Southborough, MA 01772, USA

George Kemble
MedImmune, Inc.
297 North Bernardo Avenue
Mt. View, CA 94043, USA

Shannon Kenney
Department of Medical Microbiology and Immunology
1400 University Avenue
Madison, WI 53706, USA
102 Mason Farm Road, Box 7295
Chapel Hill, NC 27599-7295, USA

Julie Kerry
Department of Microbiology and Molecular Cell Biology
Eastern Virginia Medical School
700 West Olney Road, Lewis Hall #3152
Norfolk, VA 23507, USA

Rajiv Khanna
Australian Centre for Vaccine Development
Division of Infectious Diseases and Immunology
Queensland Institute of Medical Research
300 Herston Road
Herston (Qld) 4006
Australia

David Kimberlin
Department of Pediatrics
University of Alabama at Birmingham
1600 7th Avenue South
CHB 303
Birmingham, AL 35233, USA

George Klein
Microbiology and Tumor Biology Center
Karolinska Institute
PO Box 280
S-171, 77 Stockholm, Sweden

David Koelle
Department of Medicine/Infectious Diseases
University of Washington
HMC Virology Division, M.S. 359690
325 9th Avenue
Seattle, WA 98104, USA

Kaszuhiro Kondo
Osaka University School of Medicine
2-2 Yamada-oka, Suita
Osaka 565-9871, Japan

Thomas Kristie
National Institute of Health
Building – 133
9000 Rockville Pike
Bethesda, MD, 20910, USA

Chia-chi Ku
Department of Pediatrics
Stanford University School of Medicine
300 Pasteur Drive, Room G312, MC 5208
Stanford, CA 94305, USA

Dimitrios Lagos
Cancer Research UK Viral Oncology Group
Wolfson Institute for Biomedical Research
Gower Street
University College London
WC1E 6BT, UK

Sabine Lang
Department of Pathology
Yale University School of Medicine, LH 304
New Haven, CT 06520, USA

Ann Leen
Baylor College of Medicine
Center for Cell and Gene Therapy
1102 Bates Street, Suite 760.01
Houston, TX 77030, USA

Paul Lieberman
The Wistar Institute
3601 Spruce Street
Philadelphia, PA 19104, USA

Fenyong Liu
University of California at Berkeley
School of Public Health
140 Warren Hall
Berkeley, CA 94720, USA

Richard Longnecker
Department of Microbiology-Immunology
Feinberg School of Medicine
Northestern University
303 East Chicago Avenue
Chicago, IL 60611, USA

David Lukac
UMDN/NJ Medical School
Department of Microbiology and Molecular Genetics
Int'l Center for Public Health
225 Warren Street, Room E350T
Newark, NJ 07103, USA

Louise McCormick
Department of Microbiology and Immunology
Emory University School of Medicine
1462 Clifton Road,
Suite 429
Atlanta, GA 30322, USA

Susan McDonagh
University of California San Francisco
513 Parnassus Avenue
HSW-604
San Francisco, CA 94143, USA

Ravi Mahalingam
Department of Neurology
University of Colorado Health Sciences Center
4200 East 9th Avenue, Mail Stop B182
Denver, CO 80262, USA

Ekaterina Maidji
University of California San Francisco
513 Parnassus Avenue
HSW-604
San Francisco, CA 94143, USA

James M. Markert
Department of Surgery
University of Alabama at Birmingham
FOT#1050
1530 3rd Avenue S.
Birmingham, AL 35294-3410, USA

Jeffrey Martin
University of California at San Francisco
185 Berry Street, Suite 5700
San Francisco, CA 94107, USA

Robert Means
Department of Pathology
Yale University School of Medicine
310 Cedar Street LH 315 B
New Haven, CT 065201, USA

Jeffrey Meier
Department Internal Medicine
University of Iowa
Iowa City, Iowa 52242, USA

Mads Melbye
Department of Epidemiology Research
Statens Serum Institute
5 Artillerivej, DK-2300
Copenhagen S, Denmark

Laura Menotti
Department of Experimental Pathology
University of Bologna
Via San Giacomo 12, Bologna 4016
Italy

Edward Mocarski
Department of Microbiology and Immunology
Emory University School of Medicine
Current address:
Emory Vaccine Center
1462 Clifton Road, Suite 429
Atlanta, GA 30322, USA

Jennifer Moffat
SUNY Upstate Medical University
Department of Microbiology and Immunology
750 E. Adams, Room 2215
Syracuse, NY 13210, USA

Patrick Moore
Molecular Virology Program
University of Pittsburgh Cancer Institute
Hillman Cancer Center
Research Pavilion, Suite 1.8
5117 Centre Avenue
Pttsburgh, PA 15213-1863, USA

Andrew Morgan
University of Bristol
School of Medical Sciences
Department of Pathology and Microbiology
University Walk, Clifton, Bristol
BS8 1TD, UK

Yasuko Mori
Department of Microbiology
Osaka University School of Medicine
2-2 Yamada-oka, Suita
Osaka, 565-0871, Japan

Denis Moss
EBV Biology Laboratory
Queensland Institute of Medical
Research
Post Office, Royal Brisbane Hospital
Brisbane 4029, Australia

Paul Murray
Cancer Research UK Institute for Cancer Studies
University of Birmingham
Edgbaston, Birmingham
B15 2TT, UK

Frank Neipel
Institute fur Klinische und Molekulare Virologie
SchloBgarten 4,
D-91054 Erlangen, Germany

Jay Nelson
Department of Molecular Microbiology and Immunology
Oregon Health Sciences Center
3181 S.W. Sam Jackson Park Road
Portland, OR 97201, USA

Gregory Pari
Department of Microbiology/320
University of Nevada, Reno
School of Medicine
Reno, NV 89557, USA

Lenore Peirera
University of California San Francisco
513 Parnassus Ave.
HSW-604
San Francisco, CA 94143, USA

Philip Pellett
Department of Virology
Lerner Research Institute, NN10, Cleveland Clinic
Foundation
9500 Euclid Avenue
Cleveland, OH 44195, USA

Hidde Ploegh
Whitehead Institute for Biomedical Research
Cambridge, MA 02142, USA

Christopher Preston
Medical Research Council Virology Unit
Church Street
Glasgow G11 5JR
UK

Mark Prichard
University of Alabama at Birmingham
Department of Pediatrics
1600 6th Avenue South
128 Children's Harbor Building
Birmingham, AL 35233, USA

Charles Prober
Department of Pediatrics and Microbiology and
Immunology
Stanford University School of Medicine
300 Pasteur Drive, G312, MC 5208
Stanford, CA 94305, USA

Nancy Raab-Traub
University of North Carolina
Lineberger Cancer Center
102 Mason Farm Road
Chapel Hill, NC 27599–7295, USA

Rolf Renne
Department of Molecular Genetics and Microbiology
University of Florida
1376 Mowry Road, Rm 361
Gainesville, FL 32610, USA

Bernard Roizman
The Marjorie B. Kovler Viral Oncology Laboratories
The University of Chicago
910 East 58th Street
Chicago, IL 60637, USA

Cliona Rooney
Center for Cell and Gene Therapy
Baylor College of Medicine
1102 Bates Street, BCM 320
Houston, TX 77030, USA

Barry Rouse
Department of Microbiology
College of Veterinary Medicine
University of Tennessee
1414 W. Cumberland Avenue
F403 Walters Life Sciences
Knoxville, TN 37996, USA

Contributors

William Ruyechan
State University of New York
Microbiology, Farber Hall, Rm. 138
3435 Main Street, Bldg. 26
Buffalo, NY, 14214, USA

Rozanne Sandri-Goldin
Department of Microbiology and Molecular
Genetics
College of Medicine
University of California at Irvine
C135 Medical Sciences Building
Irvine, CA, 92697, USA

Thomas Schulz
Institute fur Virologie, OE 5230
Medizinische Hochschule Hannover
Carl-Neuberg-Str. 1
D-30625 Hannover
Germany

Jane Seward
Centers for Disease Control
1600 Clifton Road
Atlanta, GA 30333, USA

Uluhan Sili Ph.D.
Center for Cell and Gene Therapy
Baylor College of Medicine
1102 Bates Street
Houston, TX 77030, USA

J. H. Sinclair
Department of Medicine, University of Cambridge
Clinical School, Box 157, Addenbrooke's Hospital, Hills Road,
Cambridge CB2 2QQ, UK

Patrick Sissons
Department of Medicine,
University of Cambridge Clinical School
Box 157
Aldenbrooke's Hospital, Hills Road
Cambridge, CB2 2QQ, UK

Marvin Sommer
Department of Pediatrics
Stanford University School of Medicine
300 Pasteur Drive, Room G312, MC 5208
Stanford, CA 94305, USA

Richard Spaete
MedImmune, Inc.
297 North Bernardo Avenue
Mt. View, CA 94043, USA

Deborah Spector
Department of Cellular and Molecular Medicine
Skaggs School of Pharmacy and Pharmacentical
Sciences, Center for Molecular Genetics
University of California San Diego
9500 Gilman Drive, MC 0366
La Jolla, CA 92093–0712, USA

Mark Stinski
University of Iowa
Department of Microbiology
University of Iowa
Iowa City, Iowa 52242, USA

Takako Tabata
University of California San Francisco
513 Parnassus Avenue
HSW-604
San Francisco, CA 94143, USA

Brunella Taddeo
The Marjorie B. Kovler Viral Oncology Labs.
The University of Chicago
910 East 58th Street
Chicago, IL 60637, USA

Frank Tufaro
Allera Health Products, Inc.
360 Central Avenue, Suite 1560
St. Petersburg, FL 33701, USA

Jatin Vyas
55 First St. GRJ 504
Massachusetts General Hospital
Division of Infections Diseases
Boston, MA 02114, USA

Anna Wald
Virology Research Clinic
600 Broadway, Suite 400
Seattle, WA 98122, USA

Fu-Zhang Wang
Cornell University
Department of Microbiology & Immunology
C5169 Veterinary Education Ctr.
Ithaca, NY 14853, USA

Elizabeth White
Department of Cellular and Molecular Medicine
Skaggs School of Pharmacy and Pharmacentical
Sciences Center for Molecular Genetic and Division of
Biological Science
University of California, San Diego
9500 Gilman Drive, MC 0366
La Jolla, CA 92095-0712, USA

Richard Whitley
Department of Pediatrics
University of Alabama at Birmingham
1600 7th Avenue, S. CHB 303
Birmingham, AL 35233, USA

Mark Wills
Department of Medicine, University of Cambridge
Clinical School, Box 157, Addenbrooke's Hospital, Hills
Road, Cambridge, CB2 2QQ, UK

Mary K. Wloch
Vical Incorporated
10390 Pacific Center Ct.
San Diego, CA 92121, USA

Koichi Yamanishi
Department of Microbiology
Osaka University School of Medicine
2-2 Yamada-oka, Suita
Osaka, 565-0871, Japan

Lawrence Young
Cancer Research UK Institute for Cancer Studies
University of Birmingham
Edgbaston, Birmingham
B15 2TT, UK

Yan Yuan
University of Pennsylvania
School of Dental Medicine
3451 Walnut Street
248 Levy/6002
Philadelphia, PA 19104, USA

Leigh Zerboni
Department of Pediatrics
Stanford University School of Medicine
300 Pasteur Drive, Room G312, MC 5208
Stanford, CA 94305, USA

Hong Zhou
Department of Pathology and Laboratory
Medicine
University of Texas
Houston Medical School
Houston, TX 77030, USA

Preface

Diseases caused by the human herpesviruses were recognized by the earliest practitioners of medicine. Hippocrates, Celsus, Herodotus, Galen, Avicenna and others described cutaneous lesions typical of infections caused by herpes simplex viruses (HSV) 1 and 2, and varicella-zoster virus (VZV). 'Herpes,' the family name of these viruses, is traced to the Greek term for lesions that appeared to creep or crawl over the skin. Among the duties of John Astruc, physician to King Louis XIV, was to understand the diseases of French prostitutes, in Latin, the '*Puellae publicae*', which led to his description of *herpes genitalis*. Distinguishing between genital herpes and syphilis was an obvious concern in this social context as it is now. The modern scientific investigation of HSV can be dated to the work of Gruter, who first isolated the virus and demonstrated its serial transmission in rabbits. During the 19th century, experiments in human subjects showed that HSV and VZV could be transmitted from fluid recovered from HSV and VZV lesions. Demonstrating that Koch's posulates were fulfilled was important but arguably the truly revolutionary discovery about the herpesviruses was made by Andrews and Carmichael in the 1930s who showed that recurrent *herpes labialis* occurred only in adults who already had neutralizing antibodies against HSV. Since our modern understanding of all of the human herpesviruses revolves around latency and reactivation as established facts of their biology, it is important to remember that these concepts are far from obvious and to appreciate the creative insights of Doerr who proposed that recurrent HSV was not an exogenous infection but resulted from stimuli to the cell that caused the endogenous production of a virus-like agent and of Burnet and Williams who perfected the notion that HSV persists for life and "*remains for the most part latent; but under the stimulus of trauma, fever, and so forth it may at any time be called into activity and provoke a visible herpetic lesion.*"

Although their relationships to HSV and VZV were by no means appreciated, the more subtle members of the herpesvirus family began to be discovered after an interval of many hundreds of years. The first of these was human cytomegalovirus (HCMV), which was initially associated with human disease through the detection of enlarged cells containing unusual cytoplasmic inclusions in the urine and organs of infants who were born with signs of intrauterine damage that had been attributed to syphilis. In the early 1950s, HCMV as well as VZV were the first human herpesviruses to be isolated in cultured cells. Within a decade, Epstein-Barr virus (EBV) particles were found in Burkitt's lymphoma cells and EBV was shown to be associated with mononucleosis. By the mid-1990s, three more human herpesviruses, HHV-6A, HHV-6B and HHV-7, which share a tropism for T lymphocytes, were discovered and the etiologic agent of the unusual vascular skin tumor called 'Kaposi's sarcoma, first described in 1872, was identified as "Kaposi's sarcoma-asscoiated herpesvirus (KSHV, HHV8). These four new human herpesviruses were identified during the early years of the human immunodeficiency virus (HIV) epidemic because these viruses caused aggressive disease in HIV-infected patients or were discovered during intensive research on human T cell biology. In each instance, discovery of the human herpesviruses paralleled technologic progress, illustrated by animal models for HSV, cell culture methods for VZV and CMV, the cultivation of B lymphocytes for the detection of EBV and of T lymphocytes for identification of HHV-6 and 7, and differential nucleic acid detection for revealing the existence of HHV8.

Molecular genetics methods demonstrate that the human herpesviruses share a common ancestor. However, each virus has evolved to occupy a particular niche during millions of years of co-evolution with their primate, and eventually human, host. Understanding the nuances of the adaptive strategies that have allowed all of these viruses to be transmitted efficiently and to persist so successfully in the human population, and often in the same individual, constitutes a fascinating enterprise. At the same time, infections caused by these ubiquitous viruses create a substantial global burden of disease affecting healthy and immunocompromised patients and among people living in developed and developing countries. Because of their serious and potentially life-threatening consequences, the human herpesviruses are medically important targets for basic and clinical research.

The goal of this book is to describe the remarkable recent progress towards elucidating the basic and clinical virology of these human pathogens, in conjunction with a summary of the many new insights about their epidemiology, mechanisms of pathogenesis and immune control, approaches to clinical diagnosis and the recognition of the clinical illnesses that result from primary and recurrent herpesvirus infections across the age spectrum. All of the herpesviruses have common genes, structures, replication strategies and mechanisms of defense against the host response but each virus also has unique properties that allow it to find its particular ecological refuge. An unexpected outcome of research over the past decade is the finding that the human herpesviruses have devised many different ways to achieve the same biologic effect, as illustrated by their unique strategies for down-regulation of major histocompatibility complex proteins. Functional similarities exist among these viruses even when they do not share similar genes or infect similar tissues. Each chapter of the book explores these viral themes and variations from the virologic and clinical perspectives. The contributions of the many distinguished authors highlight the basic science aspects of the field, emphasizing the comparative virology of the human herpesviruses and virus-host cell interactions, and the significant clinical developments, including antiviral drugs and vaccines, that are essential for the best practice of medicine in the 21st century. The concluding chapter illustrates how therapies for cancer may emerge from these advances in basic and clinical research, to create a fundamentally new era in the complex history of the relationship between the human herpesviruses and their hosts.

The editors are deeply grateful for the generosity of the authors who have shared their comprehensive knowledge of the human herpesviruses. We hope that this book will serve as a resource for investigators and physicians, and most importantly, that it will motivate a new generation of students and trainees to address the many unresolved questions about these herpesviruses as agents of human disease. Since the genomes of all of these viruses have been sequenced, it is obvious that many genes exist for which functions have not been identified and we now understand that most herpesviral proteins can be expected to have multiple functions. Basic research on the human herpesviruses also reveals fundamental facts about human cellular biology, including surface receptors, metabolic pathways, cell survival mechanisms, malignant transformation as well as innate antiviral defenses. In the clinical realm, every improvement in diagnostic methods expands the spectrum of clinical disorders that are recognized as being caused by these viruses. Clinical interventions exist that could not have been imagined fifty years ago but the need for better therapeutic and preventive measures has become even more apparent as the burden of herpesvirus disease is defined with precision. Given that four human herpesviruses have been discovered in the past 15 years, are there others?

Part I

Introduction: definition and classification of the human herpesviruses

Edited by Bernard Roizman

Part 1

1

Overview of classification

Andrew J. Davison

MRC Virology Unit, Institute of Virology, Glasgow, UK

Introduction

Taxonomy aims to structure relationships among diverse organisms in order to provide a broader understanding of Nature than is afforded by consideration of organisms in isolation. Since biological systems are shaped by evolution, which is not influenced by the human desire to impose order, any taxonomical scheme is bound to be incomplete and to some extent arbitrary. The criteria applied are necessarily confined to what is technically possible, and thus taxonomy has an important historical component. In addition, taxonomy develops conservatively, since striving for the ideal must be tempered by the need to maintain utility. It is also an unfortunate fact that taxonomy provides fertile soil for debate among a few but is of little interest to most. However, it is beyond dispute that the setting of herpesviruses in a taxonomical framework is vital for understanding the origins and behavior of this fascinating family of organisms.

Historically, herpesvirus taxonomy has been addressed since 1971 by the International Committee on Taxonomy of Viruses (ICTV) (Wildy, 1971). A provisional approach to endowing herpesviruses with formal names (Roizman *et al.*, 1973) was followed by grouping into subfamilies largely on the basis of biological criteria (Roizman *et al.*, 1981). This effort was rather successful, but not free from what turned out in hindsight to be a few misclassifications (Roizman *et al.*, 1992). Further division of the subfamilies into genera utilized molecular data to a greater extent than before, primarily in relation to genome characteristics such as size and structure (Roizman *et al.*, 1992). In the latest report of the ICTV Herpesvirus Study Group (Davison *et al.*, 2005), the family *Herpesviridae* consists of three subfamilies: *Alphaherpesvirinae* (containing the *Simplexvirus*, *Varicellovirus*, *Mardivirus* and *Iltovirus* genera), *Betaherpesvirinae* (containing the *Cytomegalovirus*, *Muromegalovirus* and *Roseolovirus* genera) and *Gammaherpesvirinae* (containing the *Lymphocryptovirus* and *Rhadinovirus* genera). In addition, there is a genus (*Ictalurivirus*) unattached to any subfamily and a large number of species not assigned to genera. The current list is given in Table 1.1. All but one of the viruses assigned to taxa infect mammals or birds, although a substantial number of unassigned herpesviruses have lower vertebrate (reptilian, amphibian and fish) or invertebrate (bivalve) hosts.

Morphological criteria

The primary criterion for inclusion of an agent in the family *Herpesviridae* is that of virion morphology. The virion is spherical, and comprises four major components: the core, the capsid, the tegument and the envelope (see Chapter 3). The diameter of the virion depends on the viral species, but is approximately 200 nm. The core consists of a single copy of a linear, double-stranded DNA molecule packaged at high density into the capsid. The capsid is an icosahedron, and has an external diameter of 125–130 nm. It consists of 162 capsomeres, 12 of which are pentons and 150 hexons, each containing five and six copies, respectively, of the major capsid protein. The capsomeres are joined via the triplexes, each of which contains two copies of one protein and one copy of another. The tegument, which surrounds the capsid, contains perhaps 30 or more viral protein species and is poorly defined structurally. In the tegument, structures positioned with symmetry corresponding to that of the capsid are detectable only in the region close to the capsid. The lipid envelope surrounds the exterior of the tegument, and is studded with at least ten viral membrane

Table 1.1. Herpesvirus taxonomy and nomenclature

Formal name[a]	Abbrev.	Common name[b]	Abbrev.[c]
Subfamily Alphaherpesvirinae			
Genus Simplexvirus			
Ateline herpesvirus 1	AtHV-1	Spider monkey herpesvirus	
Bovine herpesvirus 2	BoHV-2	Bovine mamillitis virus	
Cercopithecine herpesvirus 1	CeHV-1	B-virus	HVB
Cercopithecine herpesvirus 2	CeHV-2	SA8 virus	
Cercopithecine herpesvirus 16	CeHV-16	Herpesvirus papio 2	
Human herpesvirus 1	HHV-1	Herpes simplex virus [type] 1	HSV-1
Human herpesvirus 2	HHV-2	Herpes simplex virus [type] 2	HSV-2
Macropodid herpesvirus 1	MaHV-1	Parma wallaby herpesvirus	
Macropodid herpesvirus 2	MaHV-2	Dorcopsis wallaby herpesvirus	
Saimiriine herpesvirus 1	SaHV-1	Herpesvirus tamarinus	
Genus Varicellovirus			
Bovine herpesvirus 1	BoHV-1	Infectious bovine rhinotracheitis virus	BHV-1
Bovine herpesvirus 5	BoHV-5	Bovine encephalitis virus	BHV-5
Bubaline herpesvirus 1	BuHV-1	Water buffalo herpesvirus	
Canid herpesvirus 1	CaHV-1	Canine herpesvirus	
Caprine herpesvirus 1	CpHV-1	Goat herpesvirus	
Cercopithecine herpesvirus 9	CeHV-9	Simian varicella virus	SVV
Cervid herpesvirus 1	CvHV-1	Red deer herpesvirus	
Cervid herpesvirus 2	CvHV-2	Reindeer herpesvirus	
Equid herpesvirus 1	EHV-1	Equine abortion virus	
Equid herpesvirus 3	EHV-3	Equine coital exanthema virus	
Equid herpesvirus 4	EHV-4	Equine rhinopneumonitis virus	
Equid herpesvirus 8	EHV-8	Asinine herpesvirus 3	
Equid herpesvirus 9	EHV-9	Gazelle herpesvirus	
Felid herpesvirus 1	FeHV-1	Feline rhinotracheitis virus	
Human herpesvirus 3	HHV-3	Varicella-zoster virus	VZV
Phocid herpesvirus 1	PhoHV-1	Harbour seal herpesvirus	
Suid herpesvirus 1	SuHV-1	Pseudorabies virus	PRV
Tentative species in genus Varicellovirus			
Equid herpesvirus 6	EHV-6	Asinine herpesvirus 1	
Genus Mardivirus			
Gallid herpesvirus 2	GaHV-2	Marek's disease virus type 1	MDV-1
Gallid herpesvirus 3	GaHV-3	Marek's disease virus type 2	MDV-2
Meleagrid herpesvirus 1	MeHV-1	Turkey herpesvirus	HVT
Genus Iltovirus			
Gallid herpesvirus 1	GaHV-1	Infectious laryngotracheitis virus	ILTV
Unassigned species in subfamily Alphaherpesvirinae			
Psittacid herpesvirus 1	PsHV-1	Parrot herpesvirus	
Subfamily Betaherpesvirinae			
Genus Cytomegalovirus			
Cercopithecine herpesvirus 5	CeHV-5	African green monkey cytomegalovirus	SCMV
Cercopithecine herpesvirus 8	CeHV-8	Rhesus monkey cytomegalovirus	RhCMV
Human herpesvirus 5	HHV-5	Human cytomegalovirus	HCMV
Pongine herpesvirus 4	PoHV-4	Chimpanzee cytomegalovirus	CCMV
Tentative species in genus Cytomegalovirus			
Aotine herpesvirus 1	AoHV-1	Herpesvirus aotus 1	
Aotine herpesvirus 3	AoHV-3	Herpesvirus aotus 3	

Table 1.1. (*cont.*)

Formal name[a]	Abbrev.	Common name[b]	Abbrev.[c]
Genus *Muromegalovirus*			
Murid herpesvirus 1	MuHV-1	Mouse cytomegalovirus	MCMV
Murid herpesvirus 2	MuHV-2	Rat cytomegalovirus	RCMV
Genus *Roseolovirus*			
Human herpesvirus 6	HHV-6		
Human herpesvirus 7	HHV-7		
Unassigned species in subfamily *Betaherpesvirinae*			
Caviid herpesvirus 2	CavHV-2	Guinea pig cytomegalovirus	GPCMV
Tupaiid herpesvirus 1	TuHV-1	Tree shrew herpesvirus	THV
Subfamily *Gammaherpesvirinae*			
Genus *Lymphocryptovirus*			
Callitrichine herpesvirus 3	CalHV-3	Marmoset lymphocryptovirus	Marmoset LCV
Cercopithecine herpesvirus 12	CeHV-12	Herpesvirus papio	
Cercopithecine herpesvirus 14	CeHV-14	African green monkey EBV-like virus	
Cercopithecine herpesvirus 15	CeHV-15	Rhesus lymphocryptovirus	Rhesus LCV
Human herpesvirus 4	HHV-4	Epstein-Barr virus	EBV
Pongine herpesvirus 1	PoHV-1	Herpesvirus pan	
Pongine herpesvirus 2	PoHV-2	Orangutan herpesvirus	
Pongine herpesvirus 3	PoHV-3	Gorilla herpesvirus	
Genus *Rhadinovirus*			
Alcelaphine herpesvirus 1	AlHV-1	Malignant catarrhal fever virus	AHV-1
Alcelaphine herpesvirus 2	AlHV-2	Hartebeest malignant catarrhal fever virus	
Ateline herpesvirus 2	AtHV-2	Herpesvirus ateles	HVA
Bovine herpesvirus 4	BoHV-4	Movar virus	BHV-4
Cercopithecine herpesvirus 17	CeHV-17	Rhesus rhadinovirus	RRV
Equid herpesvirus 2	EHV-2		
Equid herpesvirus 5	EHV-5		
Equid herpesvirus 7	EHV-7	Asinine herpesvirus 2	
Hippotragine herpesvirus 1	HiHV-1	Roan antelope herpesvirus	
Human herpesvirus 8	HHV-8	Kaposi's sarcoma-associated herpesvirus	KSHV
Murid herpesvirus 4	MuHV-4	Murine gammaherpesvirus 68	MHV-68
Mustelid herpesvirus 1	MusHV-1	Badger herpesvirus	
Ovine herpesvirus 2	OvHV-2	Sheep-associated malignant catarrhal fever virus	
Saimiriine herpesvirus 2	SaHV-2	Herpesvirus saimiri	HVS
Tentative species in genus *Rhadinovirus*			
Leporid herpesvirus 1	LeHV-1	Cottontail rabbit herpesvirus	
Leporid herpesvirus 2	LeHV-2	Herpesvirus cuniculi	
Leporid herpesvirus 3	LeHV-3	Herpesvirus sylvilagus	
Marmodid herpesvirus 1	MarHV-1	Woodchuck herpesvirus	
Unassigned species in subfamily *Gammaherpesvirinae*			
Callitrichine herpesvirus 1	CalHV-1	Herpesvirus saguinus	
Unassigned genus *Ictalurivirus* in family *Herpesviridae*			
Ictalurid herpesvirus 1	IcHV-1	Channel catfish virus	CCV
Unassigned viruses in family *Herpesviridae*			
Acipenserid herpesvirus 1	AciHV-1	White sturgeon herpesvirus 1	
Acipenserid herpesvirus 2	AciHV-2	White sturgeon herpesvirus 2	
Acciptrid herpesvirus 1	AcHV-1	Bald eagle herpesvirus	
Anatid herpesvirus 1	AnHV-1	Duck plague herpesvirus	
Anguillid herpesvirus 1	AngHV-1	Japanese eel herpesvirus	

(*cont.*)

Table 1.1. (cont.)

Formal name[a]	Abbrev.	Common name[b]	Abbrev.[c]
Ateline herpesvirus 3	AtHV-3	Herpesvirus ateles strain 73	
Boid herpesvirus 1	BoiHV-1	Boa herpesvirus	
Callitrichine herpesvirus 2	CalHV-2	Marmoset cytomegalovirus	
Caviid herpesvirus 1	CavHV-1	Guinea pig herpesvirus	
Caviid herpesvirus 3	CavHV-3	Guinea pig herpesvirus 3	
Cebine herpesvirus 1	CbHV-1	Capuchin herpesvirus AL-5	
Cebine herpesvirus 2	CbHV-2	Capuchin herpesvirus AP-18	
Cercopithecine herpesvirus 3	CeHV-3	SA6 virus	
Cercopithecine herpesvirus 4	CeHV-4	SA15 virus	
Cercopithecine herpesvirus 10	CeHV-10	Rhesus leukocyte-associated herpesvirus strain 1	
Cercopithecine herpesvirus 13	CeHV-13	Herpesvirus cyclopis	
Chelonid herpesvirus 1	ChHV-1	Grey patch disease of turtles	
Chelonid herpesvirus 2	ChHV-2	Pacific pond turtle herpesvirus	
Chelonid herpesvirus 3	ChHV-3	Painted turtle herpesvirus	
Chelonid herpesvirus 4	ChHV-4	Argentine turtle herpesvirus	
Ciconiid herpesvirus 1	CiHV-1	Black stork herpesvirus	
Columbid herpesvirus 1	CoHV-1	Pigeon herpesvirus	
Cricetid herpesvirus	CrHV-1	Hamster herpesvirus	
Cyprinid herpesvirus 1	CyHV-1	Carp pox herpesvirus	
Cyprinid herpesvirus 2	CyHV-2	Goldfish herpesvirus	
Elapid herpesvirus 1	EpHV-1	Indian cobra herpesvirus	
Elephantid herpesvirus 1	ElHV-1	Elephant [loxodontal] herpesvirus	
Erinaceid herpesvirus 1	ErHV-1	European hedgehog herpesvirus	
Esocid herpesvirus 1	EsHV-1	Northern pike herpesvirus	
Falconid herpesvirus 1	FaHV-1	Falcon inclusion body diseases	
Gruid herpesvirus 1	GrHV-1	Crane herpesvirus	
Iguanid herpesvirus 1	IgHV-1	Green iguana herpesvirus	
Lacertid herpesvirus	LaHV-1	Green lizard herpesvirus	
Lorisine herpesvirus 1	LoHV-1	Kinkajou herpesvirus	
Murid herpesvirus 3	MuHV-3	Mouse thymic herpesvirus	
Murid herpesvirus 5	MuHV-5	Field mouse herpesvirus	
Murid herpesvirus 6	MuHV-6	Sand rat nuclear inclusion agents	
Ostreid herpesvirus 1	OsHV-1	Pacific oyster herpesvirus	OHV
Ovine herpesvirus 1	OvHV-1	Sheep pulmonary adenomatosis-associated herpesvirus	
Percid herpesvirus 1	PeHV-1	Walleye epidermal hyperplasia	
Perdicid herpesvirus 1	PdHV-1	Bobwhite quail herpesvirus	
Phalacrocoracid herpesvirus 1	PhHV-1	Cormorant herpesvirus	
Pleuronectid herpesvirus 1	PlHV-1	Turbot herpesvirus	
Ranid herpesvirus 1	RaHV-1	Lucké frog herpesvirus	
Ranid herpesvirus 2	RaHV-2	Frog herpesvirus 4	
Salmonid herpesvirus 1	SalHV-1	Herpesvirus salmonis	
Salmonid herpesvirus 2	SalHV-2	*Oncorhynchus masou* herpesvirus	
Sciurid herpesvirus 1	ScHV-2	European ground squirrel cytomegalovirus	
Sciurid herpesvirus 2	ScHV-2	American ground squirrel cytomegalovirus	
Sphenicid herpesvirus 1	SpHV-1	Black footed penguin herpesvirus	
Strigid herpesvirus 1	StHV-1	Owl hepatosplenitis herpesvirus	
Suid herpesvirus 2	SuHV-2	Swine cytomegalovirus	

[a] Type species of genera are in italics.
[b] Some viruses have several common names. Only one is given for each.
[c] The list is restricted to abbreviations used in this publication.
Adapted from Davison *et al.* (2005).

glycoproteins, in addition to some cellular proteins. The protein composition of the tegument and envelope varies widely across the family.

Serological criteria

In contrast to virion morphology, which operates as a criterion at the level of the family, serological relationships are useful only for detecting closely related viruses. Neutralizing antibodies form a subset of serological tools, and are directed against some of the envelope glycoproteins.

Biological criteria

The observation that several distinct herpesviruses have been found in the most extensively studied animals implies that the number of herpesvirus species in Nature must far exceed that catalogued to date. The natural host range of individual viruses is usually restricted to a single species. Occasional transfer to other species can occur, although it could be argued that the settings involved (farms, zoos and keeping pets) are the results of human activities. In experimental animal systems, some members of the *Alphaherpesvirinae* can infect a wide variety of species, whereas *Beta-* and *Gammaherpesvirinae* are very restricted. The same general observation characterizes growth in cell culture.

Herpesviruses are highly adapted to their hosts, and severe symptoms of infection are usually limited to very young or immunosuppressed individuals. Natural transmission routes range from aerosol spread to mucosal contact. Most herpesviruses establish a systemic infection associated with a cell-associated viraemia, although infection with some members of genus *Simplexvirus* is limited to the epithelium at the inoculation site and to innervating sensory neurons. Herpesviruses have elaborate means of modulating the host responses to infection, and are able to establish lifelong latent infections. In simplified, general terms, the cell types involved in latency are the neuron for the *Alphaherpesvirinae*, the monocyte lineage for the *Betaherpesvirinae*, and lymphocytes for the *Gammaherpesvirinae*.

Genomic criteria

Herpesvirus genomes studied to date range in size from about 125 to 240 kbp, and the most extensively characterized contain from about 70 to 165 genes. Prior to the generation of extensive sequence data, genome structures (see Chapter 2) were an aid to classification. However, the usefulness of this criterion is limited, since similar structures have evidently evolved more than once in the family. Nucleic acid hybridization data also provided input and, like serological data, are limited to demonstrating relationships between closely related viruses. As with other groups of organisms, data derived from nucleotide and amino acid sequences have gained increasing prominence and now dominate herpesvirus taxonomy. Figure 1.1 shows one example of such data, a phylogenetic tree based upon amino acid sequence alignments (McGeoch *et al.*, 1994, 1995, 2000). Another approach yielded different schemes of relationships, but was based on analytical criteria not widely accepted in depicting evolutionary relationships (Karlin *et al.*, 1994).

It has long been thought from the apparent adaptation of herpesviruses to their hosts that a substantial degree of co-evolution has occurred. Similarities between the phylogenetic relationships among the viruses and those among their hosts provide strong support for this model, and in some instances indicate that co-speciation has occurred. A number of possible exceptions have been noted and are discussed in further detail in Chapter 2.

Species definition

A virus species is defined as a polythetic class of viruses constituting a replicating lineage and occupying a particular ecological niche (Van Regenmortel, 1989, 1990). Members of a polythetic class share a subset of properties, with each property possessed by several members but no property possessed by all. Herpesviruses are defined as separate species if their nucleotide sequences differ in a readily assayable and distinctive manner across the entire genome and if they occupy different ecological niches by virtue of their distinct epidemiology and pathogenesis or their distinct natural hosts (Roizman *et al.*, 1992; Roizman and Pellett, 2001; Davison *et al.*, 2005). However, genomic data have come to dominate biological properties, with taxa corresponding to genetic lineages defined by sequence comparisons and identification of genes unique to certain lineages. An increasing number of herpesviruses in the tissues of various animals are being inferred from short PCR-derived sequences, usually from a single locus in the genome and often in the absence of any other information. These "virtual viruses" cannot readily be classified under the current species definition. However, their incorporation (perhaps in a special category) could be facilitated by

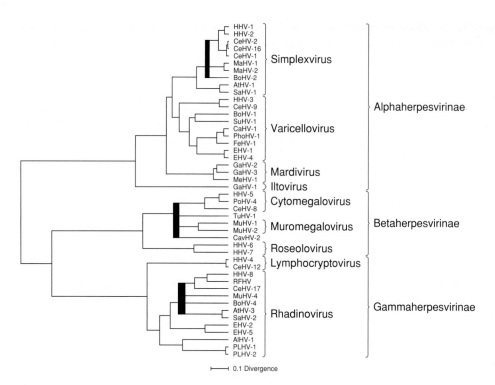

Fig. 1.1. Composite phylogenetic tree for herpesviruses. The tree is based on amino acid sequence alignments of eight sets of homologous genes, constructed from maximum-likelihood trees for subsets of these genes, with molecular clock imposed. Thick lines designate regions of uncertain branching. Formal species abbreviations and designations for genera and subfamilies are given on the right (see Table 1.1). Viruses that are not yet incorporated formally into genera are denoted in italics. Three unclassified viruses are included (RFHV, retroperitoneal fibromatosis herpesvirus of macaques; PLHV-1 and PLHV-2, porcine lymphotropic herpesviruses 1 and 2). Modified from McGeoch *et al.* (2000) with permission from the American Society for Microbiology.

addition to the species definition of a third criterion, that of phylogeny based on the relatedness of conserved genes. Recognition that taxonomy should reflect evolutionary history would also aid rational incorporation of herpesviruses of lower vertebrates and invertebrates into a taxonomy that is currently dominated by herpesviruses of higher vertebrates. Current problems in this area, and a suggested solution, are given in Chapter 2.

Acknowledgment

I am grateful to Duncan McGeoch for a critical reading of this chapter.

REFERENCES

Davison, A. J., Eberle, R., Hayward, G. S. *et al.* (2005). Family *Herpesviridae*. In *Virus Taxonomy, VIIIth Report of the International Committee on Taxonomy of Viruses*, ed. C. M. Fauquet, M. A. Mayo, J. Maniloff, U. Desselberger and L. A. Ball, pp. 193–212. London: Academic Press/Elsevier.

Karlin, S., Mocarski, E. S., and Schachtel, G. A. (1994). Molecular evolution of herpesviruses: genomic and protein sequence comparisons. *J. Virol.*, **68**, 1886–1902.

McGeoch, D. J. and Cook, S. (1994). Molecular phylogeny of the Alphaherpesvirinae subfamily and a proposed evolutionary timescale. *J. Mol. Biol.*, **238**, 9–22.

McGeoch, D. J., Cook, S., Dolan, A., Jamieson, F. E., and Telford, E. A. R. (1995). Molecular phylogeny and evolutionary timescale for the family of mammalian herpesviruses. *J. Mol. Biol.*, **247**, 443–458.

McGeoch, D. J., Dolan, A., and Ralph, A. C. (2000). Toward a comprehensive phylogeny for mammalian and avian herpesviruses. *J. Virol.*, **74**, 10401–10406.

Roizman, B. and Pellett, P. E. (2001). Herpes simplex viruses and their replication. In *Fields Virology*, 4th edn. ed. D. M. Knipe and P. M. Howley, pp. 2399–2459. Philadelphia: Lippincott, Williams and Wilkins.

Roizman, B., Bartha, A., Biggs, P. M. *et al.* (1973). Provisional labels for herpesviruses. *J. Gen. Virol.*, **20**, 417–419.

Roizman, B., Carmichael, L. E., Deinhardt, F. *et al.* (1981). Herpesviridae. Definition, provisional nomenclature, and taxonomy. *Intervirology*, **16**, 201–217.

Roizman, B., Desrosiers, R. C., Fleckenstein, B., Lopez, C., Minson, A. C., and Studdert, M. J. (1992). The *Herpesviridae*: an update. *Arch. Virol.*, **123**, 425–449.

Van Regenmortel, M. H. V. (1989). Applying the species concept to plant viruses. *Arch. Virol.*, **104**, 1–17.

Van Regenmortel, M. H. V. (1990). Virus species, a much overlooked but essential concept in virus classification. *Intervirology*, **31**, 241–254.

Wildy, P. (1971). Classification and nomenclature of viruses. In *Monographs in Virology*, vol. 5, ed. J. L. Melnick, ed., pp. 33–34. Basel: Karger.

2

Comparative analysis of the genomes

Andrew J. Davison

MRC Virology Unit, Institute of Virology, Glasgow, UK

Introduction

Members of the family *Herpesviridae* replicate their genomes in the infected cell nucleus and have a characteristic virion morphology, which consists of the envelope, tegument, capsid and core (Davison and Clements, 1997). An extensive description of virion structure is given in Chapter 3. The present chapter focuses on the viral genome, which occupies the core of the virus particle. Electron microscopy of negatively stained capsids gives the impression that the core consists of the viral DNA molecule wrapped toroidally around a protein spindle (Furlong *et al.*, 1972). Images reconstructed from electron micrographs of virions frozen in ice in the absence of stain, a technique by which morphology is better preserved, show that the core consists of the DNA packed at high density in liquid crystalline form, probably as a spool lacking a spindle (Booy *et al.*, 1991; Zhou *et al.*, 1999).

Herpesvirus genomes consist of linear, double-stranded DNA molecules that range in size from about 125 to 240 kbp and in nucleotide composition from 32 to 75% G+C, depending on the virus species (Honess, 1984). The genome termini are not covalently closed (as in the *Poxviridae*; Moss, 2001) or covalently linked to a protein (as in the *Adenoviridae*; Shenk, 2001). In those herpesvirus genomes that have been examined in sufficient detail, unpaired nucleotides are present at the termini; for example, HSV-1, VZV and HCMV have a single 3′-overhanging nucleotide at each terminus (Mocarski and Roizman, 1982; Davison, 1984; Tamashiro and Spector, 1986). Larger herpesvirus genomes are accommodated in larger capsids, but the relationship is not proportional, as the packing density of the DNA varies somewhat between species (Trus *et al.*, 1999; Bhella *et al.*, 2000). The reasons for the striking range in nucleotide composition of herpesvirus genomes are not clear, but a similar phenomenon is found in other virus families and in cellular organisms. In contrast to the *Alpha*- and *Betaherpesvirinae*, the genomes of most *Gammaherpesvirinae* are generally deficient in the CG dinucleotide (Table 2.1). In vertebrate genomes, this phenomenon is thought to be due to spontaneous deamination of 5-methylcytosine residues in DNA to thymidine residues, followed by fixation through DNA replication. CG depletion in herpesviruses, and concomitant enrichment in TG and CA, has been taken as indicative of latency in dividing cell populations, in which the latent genome is obliged to replicate as host cells divide (Honess *et al.*, 1989). Thus, HSV-1, which is resident in non-dividing neurons, has a CG content consistent with its nucleotide composition, whereas EBV, which latently infects dividing B cell populations, is depleted. Local CG suppression of the major immediate early gene locus of HCMV has also been noted (Honess *et al.*, 1989).

Genome structures

Herpesvirus genomes are not simple lengths of unique DNA, but characteristically contain direct or inverted repeats. The reasons for this are not known, but it is intriguing that similar structures appear to have arisen independently on several occasions during herpesvirus evolution. Herpesvirus genomes are thought to replicate by circularization, followed by production of concatemers and cleavage of unit-length genomes during packaging into capsids (Boehmer and Lehman, 1997). The explanation for the presence of repeats is probably connected in some way with the mode of DNA replication, rather than with any advantage gained by having multiple copies of certain genes. Although greater expression would be a consequence of repeated genes, this appears a simplistic explanation in an evolutionary context, since subtler processes of nucleotide

Table 2.1. Sequenced herpesvirus genomes

Common name	Strain[a]	Abbreviation Common	Abbreviation Formal	Accession	Size (bp)[b]	Composition[c] G+C	CG	Reference
Mammalian herpesvirus group[d]								
Alphaherpesvirinae								
Simplexvirus								
Herpes simplex virus type 1	17	HSV-1	HHV-1	X14112	152261	68.3	1.01	McGeoch *et al.* (1988)
Herpes simplex virus type 2	HG52	HSV-2	HHV-2	Z86099	154746	70.4	1.06	Dolan *et al.* (1998)
B virus	E2490	HVB	CeHV-1	AF533768	156789	74.5	1.09	Perelygina *et al.* (2003)
SA8	B264	SA8	CeHV-2	AY714813	150715	76.0	1.09	Tyler *et al.* (2005)
Herpes papio 2	X313	HVP2	CeHV-16	DQ149153	156487	76.1	1.08	Tyler and Severini (2006)
Varicellovirus								
Varicella-zoster virus	Dumas	VZV	HHV-3	X04370	124884	46.0	1.14	Davison and Scott (1986)
	Oka vaccine			AB097932	125078			Gomi *et al.* (2002)
	Oka parental			AB097933	125125			Gomi *et al.* (2002)
	MSP			AY548170	124883			Grose *et al.* (2004)
	BC			AY548171	125459			Grose *et al.* (2004)
	Varilrix			DQ008354	124821			Vassilev (2005)
	Varilrix			DQ008355	124815			Vassilev (2005)
	HJO			AJ871403	124928			Fickenscher *et al.* (unpublished)
Simian varicella virus	Delta	SVV	CeHV-9	AF275348	124138	40.4	1.12	Gray *et al.* (2001)
Bovine herpesvirus 1	[Cooper]	BHV-1	BoHV-1	AJ004801	135301	72.4	1.19	Schwyzer & Ackermann (1996)
Bovine herpesvirus 5	SSV507/99	BHV-5	BoHV-5	AY261359	138390	74.9	1.17	Delhon *et al.* (2003)
Pseudorabies virus	[Kaplan]	PRV	SuHV-1	BK001744	143461	73.6	1.12	Klupp *et al.* (2004)
Equine herpesvirus 1	Ab4	EHV-1	EHV-1	AY665713	150224	56.7	0.99	Telford *et al.* (1992)
	V592			AY464052	149430			Nugent *et al.* (2006)
Equine herpesvirus 4	NS80567	EHV-4	EHV-4	AF030027	145597	50.5	0.93	Telford *et al.* (1998)
Mardivirus								
Marek's disease virus type 1	Md5	MDV-1	GaHV-2	AF243438	177874	44.1	1.01	Tulman *et al.* (2000)
	GA			AF147806	174077			Lee *et al.* (2000)
	Md11			[AY510475]	170950			Niikura *et al.* (unpublished)
Marek's disease virus type 2	HPRS24	MDV-2	GaHV-3	AB049735	164270	53.6	1.23	Izumiya *et al.* (2001)
Turkey herpesvirus	FC126	HVT	MeHV-1	AF291866	159160	47.6	1.11	Afonso *et al.* (2001)
Iltovirus								
Infections laryngotracheitis virus	[SA-2]	ILTV	GaHV-1	NC006623	148687	48.2	1.01	Thureen and Keeler (2006)
Psittacid herpesvirus 1[e]	97-0001	PsHV-1	PsHV-1	AY372243	163025	60.9	1.21	Thureen and Keeler (2006)
Betaherpesvirinae								
Cytomegalovirus								
Human cytomegalovirus	Merlin	HCMV	HHV-5	AY446894	235645	57.5	1.19	Dolan *et al.* (2004)
	AD169			X17403	229354			Chee *et al.* (1990)
	AD169			BK000394	230287			Davison *et al.*(2003a)
	AD169			[AC146999]	[233739]			Murphy *et al.* (2003b)
	Towne			[AY315197]	[231236]			Dunn *et al.* (2003)
	Towne			[AC146851]	[229483]			Murphy *et al.* (2003b)
	Toledo			[AC146905]	[226889]			Murphy *et al.* (2003b)
	PH			[AC146904]	[229700]			Murphy *et al.* (2003b)
	TR			[AC146906]	[234881]			Murphy *et al.* (2003b)
	FIX			[AC146907]	[229209]			Murphy *et al.* (2003b)
Chimpanzee cytomegalovirus	–	CCMV	PoHV-4	AF480884	241087	61.7	1.11	Davison *et al.* (2003a)
Rhesus cytomegalovirus	68-1	RhCMV	CeHV-8	AY186194	221454	49.1	0.99	Hansen *et al.* (2003)
Unassigned								
Tupaiid herpesvirus	2	THV	TuHV-1	AF281817	195859	66.6	1.28	Bahr & Darai (2001)
Muromegalovirus								
Murine cytomegalovirus	Smith	MCMV	MuHV-1	U68299	230278	58.7	1.22	Rawlinson *et al.* (1996)
Rat cytomegalovirus	Maastricht	RCMV	MuHV-2	AF232689	230138	61.0	1.25	Vink *et al.* (2000)
Roseolovirus								
Human herpesvirus 6	U1102	HHV-6A	HHV-6	X83413	159321	42.4	1.13	Gompels *et al.* (1995)
	Z29	HHV-6B		AF157706	162114	42.8	1.10	Dominguez *et al.* (1999)
	HST			AB021506	161573			Isegawa *et al.* (1999)

(cont.)

Table 2.1. (cont.)

Common name	Strain[a]	Abbreviation Common	Abbreviation Formal	Accession	Size (bp)[b]	Composition[c] G+C	Composition[c] CG	Reference
Human herpesvirus 7	JI	HHV-7	HHV-7	U43400	144861	35.3	0.80	Nicholas (1996)
	RK			AF037218	153080			Megaw et al. (1998)
Gammaherpesvirinae								
Lymphocryptovirus								
Epstein–Barr virus	[B95-8]	EBV	HHV-4	AJ507799	171823	59.5	0.61	de Jesus et al. (2003)
	GD1			AY961628	171656			Zeng et al. (2005)
	AG876			DQ279927	172764			Dolan et al. (2006)
	B95-8			V01555	172281			Baer et al. (1984)
Marmoset lymphocryptovirus	CJ0149	marmoset LCV	CalHV-3	AF319782	149696	49.3	0.70	Rivailler et al. (2002a)
Rhesus lymphocryptovirus	LCL8664	rhesus LCV	CeHV-15	AY037858	171096	61.9	0.68	Rivailler et al. (2002b)
Rhadinovirus								
Human herpesvirus 8	BC-1	HHV-8	HHV-8	U75698	[137508]	53.5	0.81	
				U75699	801	84.5	0.92	Russo et al. (1996)
	–			U93872	[133661]			Neipel et al. (1997)
Rhesus rhadinovirus	17577	RRV	CeHV-17	AF083501	133719	52.2	1.11	Searles et al. (1999)
	26-95			AF210726	130733			Alexander et al. (2000)
Murine herpesvirus 68[f]	WUMS	MHV-68	MuHV-4	U97553	119450	47.2	0.43	Virgin et al. (1997)
	g2.4			AF105037	119550			Nash et al. (2001)
Bovine herpesvirus 4	66-p-347	BHV-4	BoHV-4	AF318573	108873	41.4	0.23	Zimmermann et al. (2001)
				AF092919	2267	71.2	0.42	
Herpesvirus ateles	73	HVA	AtHV-3	AF083424	108409	36.6	0.40	Albrecht (2000)
				AF126541	1582	77.1	0.79	
Herpesvirus saimiri	A11	HVS	SaHV-2	X64346	112930	34.5	0.33	Albrecht et al. (1992)
				K03361	1444	70.9	0.61	
	C488			AJ410493	113027			Ensser et al. (2003)
				AJ410494	1458			
Equine herpesvirus 2	86/67	EHV-2	EHV-2	U20824	184427	57.5	0.63	Telford et al. (1995)
Alcelaphine herpesvirus 1	C500	AHV-1	AlHV-1	AF005370	130608	46.2	0.42	Ensser et al. (1997)
				AF005368	1113	72.0	0.69	
Ovine herpesvirus 2	BJ1035	OvHV-2	OvHV-2	AY839756	135135	52.9	0.58	Stewart et al. (unpublished)
Fish herpesvirus group[d]								
Undefined subfamily								
Ictalurivirus								
Channel catfish virus	Auburn 1	CCV	IcHV-1	M75136	134226	56.2	1.1	Davison (1992)
Bivalve herpesvirus group[d]								
Undefined subfamily								
Undefined genus								
Ostreid herpesvirus 1	–	OHV	OsHV-1	AY509253	207439	38.7	0.68	Davison et al. (2005)

[a] Square brackets indicate the strain that was used most extensively in assembling a sequence combining data from several strains. A hyphen indicates that the strain was not specified.

[b] Sizes were obtained from the latest version of the accessions, and may differ from those in the references through correction of errors. Square brackets indicate sequences that fall marginally short of full length: for MDV-1 and HCMV strains, sequences are for bacterial artificial chromosomes, the sizes representing a deleted form of the genome plus the vector; for HHV-8 strains, the sequence at the right end of the unique region was not determined. For members of subfamily *Gammaherpesvirinae* other than EHV-2, actual genome sizes are larger than those listed (approximately 150–180 kbp), owing to the presence of variable copy numbers of terminal repeats at both ends of the genome. Where a single value is given, this represents either the unique region flanked by partial terminal repeats or the unique region only. Where two values are given, the first is for the unique region and the second is for the terminal repeat.

[c] G + C content is given as moles %, CG content is given as observed/expected frequency, taking into account overall nucleotide composition. Where multiple strains have been sequenced for a species, values are given for one strain only. For members of the *Gammaherpesvirinae*, values are given for the deposited sequences, which consist either of the unique region flanked by partial terminal repeat sequence, the unique region only, or separate accessions for the unique region and terminal repeat.

[d] This taxon is used for the purposes of discussion, and, unlike the others in the Table, has no formal standing.

[e] PsHV-1 is the closest relative of ILTV and is placed informally in this genus.

[f] MHV-68 strains g2.4 and WUMS are essentially identical, since the latter was derived from the former.

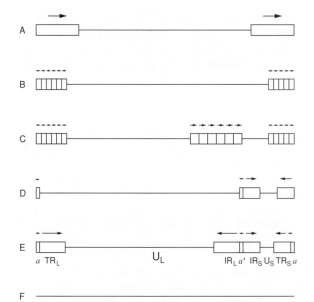

Fig. 2.1. Classes of herpesvirus genome structures (not to scale) as defined by Roizman and Pellett (2001). Unique and repeat regions are shown as horizontal lines and rectangles, respectively. The orientations of repeats are shown by arrows. The nomenclature of unique and repeat regions, including the terminal redundancy (*a*) and its internal, inverted copy (*a'*), is indicated for the class E genome.

substitution can readily alter transcriptional levels over a much greater range. In addition, repeats often do not contain protein-coding regions. As elaborated below, certain genomes exhibit a further structural complexity known as segment inversion, in which unique regions flanked by inverted repeats are found in both orientations in virion DNA. Thus, a genome with two such unique regions would produce either two or four isomers depending on whether one or both regions invert. This phenomenon is probably a consequence of recombination between repeats in concatemeric DNA. Isomers are functionally equivalent (Jenkins and Roizman, 1986), and segment inversion appears to be unrelated to the biology of the virus.

Figure 2.1 shows the major classes of genome structure found among the herpesviruses, as summarized by Roizman and Knipe (2001). The class A genome consists of a unique sequence flanked by a direct repeat. It was first described for CCV (Chousterman *et al.*, 1979), but is also represented among the *Betaherpesvirinae* (HHV-6: Lindquester and Pellett, 1991; Martin *et al.*, 1991; HHV-7: Dominguez *et al.*, 1996; Ruvolo *et al.*, 1996) and one member of the *Gammaherpesvirinae* (EHV-2; Browning and Studdert, 1989). In these examples, the direct repeat is several kbp in size. Other members of the *Betaherpesvirinae*

also have this arrangement, but the repeat is smaller, at 504 bp in RCMV (Vink *et al.*, 1996) and 30–31 bp in MCMV (Marks and Spector, 1988; Rawlinson *et al.*, 1996).

Class B genomes also have directly repeated sequences at the termini, but these consist of variable copy numbers of a tandemly repeated sequence of 0.8–2.3 kbp. This arrangement characterizes most *Gammaherpesvirinae* in the *Rhadinovirus* genus, such as HVS and HHV-8 (Bornkamm *et al.*, 1976; Russo *et al.*, 1996). The repeated regions may comprise up to 30% of the DNA molecule (Bornkamm *et al.*, 1976; Lagunoff and Ganem, 1997). The presence of additional terminal repeat sequences in inverse orientation internally in the genome gives rise to a related structure, which is present in another member of the *Gammaherpesvirinae*, cottontail rabbit herpesvirus (Cebrian *et al.*, 1989). The virion DNA of this virus exhibits segment inversion because the two unique regions are flanked by inverted repeats. The class C structure represents another derivative of class B, in which an internal set of direct repeats is present but is unrelated to the terminal set. EBV, a member of the *Gammaherpesvirinae* in the *Lymphocryptovirus* genus, has this arrangement (Given and Kieff, 1979). Segment inversion does not occur because the internal and terminal repeats are not related.

Class D genomes contain two unique regions (U_L and U_S), each flanked by inverted repeats (TR_L/IR_L and TR_S/IR_S). This structure is characteristic of *Alphaherpesvirinae* in the *Varicellovirus* genus, such as PRV and VZV (Rixon and Ben-Porat, 1979; Dumas *et al.*, 1981), and has also evolved separately in salmonid herpesvirus 1 (Davison, 1998). Segment inversion occurs inasmuch as equimolar amounts of genomes containing the two orientations of U_S are found in virion DNA, but U_L is present predominantly or completely in one orientation. The latter feature cannot be explained solely by recombination, and is probably due also to the presence of the cleavage signal solely or largely in the region comprising TR_L/IR_L and one end of U_L (Davison, 1984; Rall *et al.*, 1991).

Class E is the most complex genome structure, and was the first to be described, for HSV-1 (Sheldrick and Berthelot, 1975). It is similar to class D, except that TR_L/IR_L is much larger and segment inversion gives rise to four equimolar genome isomers (Wadsworth *et al.*, 1975; Hayward *et al.*, 1975; Delius and Clements, 1976; Clements *et al.*, 1976; Wilkie and Cortini, 1976). Also, class E genomes are terminally redundant, containing a sequence of a few hundred bp (termed the *a* sequence) that is repeated directly at the genome termini and inversely at the IR_L-IR_S junction (Sheldrick and Berthelot, 1975; Grafstrom *et al.*, 1975a,b; Wadsworth *et al.*, 1976; Hyman *et al.*, 1976).

Minor proportions of genomes contain multiple copies of the *a* sequence at the left terminus or the IR_L-IR_S junction (Wilkie, 1976; Wagner and Summers, 1978; Locker and Frenkel, 1979). The class E arrangement is characteristic of *Alphaherpesvirinae* in the *Simplexvirus* genus, and has evolved independently in the lineage giving rise to HCMV and CCMV, members of the *Betaherpesvirinae* (Weststrate *et al.*, 1980; DeMarchi, 1981; Davison *et al.*, 2003a). A structure similar to both class D and E genomes has also evolved in an invertebrate herpesvirus, OsHV-1 (Davison *et al.*, 2005). This contains two segments, each consisting of a unique region flanked by an substantial inverted repeat, linked via an additional small, non-inverting unique region. As in class E genomes, the two segments undergo inversion, but, like class D, the genome is not terminally redundant.

Class F is represented by a member of the *Betaherpesvirinae*, THV, which apparently lacks the types of inverted and direct repeats that characterize other herpesvirus genomes (Koch *et al.*, 1985; Albrecht *et al.*, 1985). However, since the genome ends of THV have not been analyzed directly, the existence of this unusual structure is considered tentative.

Genome sequences

Table 2.1 lists the 39 herpesvirus species for which genome sequences are currently available in the public databases. Additional strains have been sequenced for some species, yielding a total of 63 sequenced strains. The ease of generating data will continue to expand the number of herpesvirus species and strains sequenced in coming years. Indeed, substantial inroads have been made into large-scale studies of strain variation for certain of the human herpesviruses. It appears that the scale and extent of variation is lineage dependent, with *Betaherpesvirinae* more variable than *Gammaherpesvirinae*, and *Alphaherpesvirinae* the least variable (Murphy *et al.*, 2003b; Dolan *et al.*, 2004; Poole *et al.*, 1999; Midgley *et al.*, 2003; Muir *et al.*, 2002; Gomi *et al.*, 2002). The development of tools to study variation in increasing detail will enhance understanding of viral epidemiology, in terms both of its relation to human evolution and migration and of the changes that are occurring in human populations at the present time.

Gene content

Sequencing herpesvirus genomes is now routine, but the process of describing gene content (annotation) is not trivial. Thus, as with other groups of organisms, the quality of annotation of herpesvirus entries in the public databases varies widely. It is an unfortunate fact that no set of objective criteria is sufficient to interpret the gene content of a sequence completely. Although most genes can be catalogued relatively easily, there are genuine difficulties in identifying all of them, even in the best characterized herpesviruses.

A primary criterion in defining gene content involves identifying open reading frames (ORFs), usually those initiated by methionine (ATG) codons. A tendency to include ORFs that do not encode proteins may be reduced by setting a minimum size. Comparative genomics, which operates on the principle that genes are conserved in evolution, and algorithms that compare sequence patterns within ORFs to the protein-coding regions of known genes, are also useful. However, these tools yield results with least confidence when applied to small, spliced, overlapping or poorly conserved ORFs, and in instances where translation initiates from internal codons, alternative splicing occurs, or esoteric translational mechanisms are employed (e.g., suppression of termination codons and forms of translational editing). In addition to sequence analysis, experimental data on production of an RNA or protein from an ORF provides important imput, although even this falls short of proving functionality. Also, most approaches are aimed at identifying protein-coding genes, and cannot detect genes that encode functional transcripts that are not mRNAs.

The use of different criteria for gene identification may create a degree of uncertainty and debate, and lead to different pictures of gene layout. The case of HCMV provides a contemporary example. In the first analysis of the gene content of HCMV strain AD169, Chee *et al.* (1990) catalogued 189 protein-coding ORFs (counting duplicates once only). Later, the gene number was reduced to 147 by comparing the HCMV and CCMV genomes, allowing, where appropriate, for the presence of genes unique to either genome (Davison *et al.*, 2003a,b). As modified criteria were applied, this number rebounded in a series of increments, first to 157 (Yu *et al.*, 2003), next to 171 (Murphy *et al.*, 2003a), then to 220 (Murphy *et al.*, 2003b) and finally to 232 (Varnum *et al.*, 2004). Although the conservative numbers in this example are more supportable, the existence of unrecognized genes should not be ruled out even in well-characterized genomes, and candidates should be examined rigorously. For example, new genes were identified in previously analysed sequences for VZV (Kemble *et al.*, 2000) and HHV-8 (Glenn *et al.*, 1999).

The genes of HSV-1, presumably like those of all herpesviruses, are transcribed by host RNA polymerase II

(Wagner, 1985; Roizman and Knipe, 2001). Transcription of the first genes to be expressed, the immediate early genes, does not require ongoing protein synthesis, and is enhanced by a tegument protein at low multiplicities of infection (O'Hare, 1993). Some of the immediate early proteins regulate expression of early and late genes (Honess and Roizman, 1974). Early genes, defined as those expressed in the presence of immediate early proteins and before the onset of DNA replication, include enzymes involved in nucleotide metabolism and DNA replication and a number of envelope glycoproteins. Some late genes are expressed at low levels under early conditions, but full expression of "leaky" and "true" late genes is dependent on DNA replication; these genes encode mainly virion proteins. Although the details differ, a similar pattern of regulated gene expression is characteristic of all herpesviruses examined; for example, HCMV (Stinski, 1978), HHV-8 (Sarid et al., 1998) and CCV (Silverstein et al., 1995). In addition, herpesviruses express RNAs whose functions apparently do not involve translation. The best characterized are small RNAs probably transcribed by RNA polymerase III in *Gammaherpesvirinae* such as EBV (Rosa et al., 1981) and MHV-68 (Bowden et al., 1997). Larger noncoding RNAs transcribed by RNA polymerase II include the latency-associated transcripts in HSV-1 (Stevens et al., 1987) and several virion-associated RNAs in HCMV (Bresnahan and Shenk, 2000).

With the exception of a small number of genes that are expressed by splicing from a common 5'-leader, such as the EBNA genes of EBV (Bodescot et al., 1987) and the IE1 and IE2 genes of HCMV (Stenberg et al., 1985), herpesvirus genes have individual promoters. However, it is common for genes to share a polyadenylation site, leading to families of 3'-coterminal transcripts (Wagner, 1985). Apart from families of duplicated genes, there is no pronounced clustering of genes on the basis of function or kinetics of expression. Splicing is uncommon throughout the family, affecting no more than about 20% of the gene number in any genome. Most splicing involves genes that are relatively recent evolutionary developments, and *Beta-* and *Gammaherpesvirinae* have more spliced genes than *Alphaherpesvirinae*.

Genome comparisons and evolution

The availability of extensive sequence data for herpesviruses has facilitated detailed phylogenetic analyses of the family based on amino acid sequence comparisons of conserved genes, as described in Chapter 1. In this section, an overview is given of genetic relatedness at selected levels in the phylogenetic tree, starting with the three major groups that encompass all known herpesviruses, proceeding to the best characterized of these groups, and ending with one subfamily in this group. In chronological terms, this proceeds from earlier to more recent evolutionary events. Detailed information on the gene content of, and the relationships between, the human herpesviruses is available elsewhere in this book.

Three major groups

Three major groups of viruses possess the herpesvirus morphology, including closely similar capsid structures, but share very little genetic similarity (Davison, 1992; Booy et al., 1996; Davison et al., 2005). Viruses in the best characterized group infect mammals, birds and reptiles, viruses in the second group infect amphibians and fish, and the third group contains the single known herpesvirus of an invertebrate, the oyster. Currently, the family *Herpesviridae* comprises the first group classified into three subfamilies and component genera, one member (CCV) of the second group representing an unassigned genus, and the oyster virus is a floating species. The most logical means of accommodating all known herpesviruses taxonomically would be to establish three families under the umbrella of a new order (*Herpesvirales*), containing herpesviruses of mammals, birds and reptiles, of amphibians and fish, and of bivalves, respectively. Since these taxa are presently a proposal and lack any formal standing, the terms mammalian, fish and bivalve herpesvirus groups are used to denote the proposed families in the following discussion.

Only three genes have clear counterparts in all three groups that are detectable by amino acid sequence comparisons. The proteins encoded by two (DNA polymerase and dUTPase) have ubiquitous cellular relatives and could have been captured independently from the host repertoire. The third gene apparently lacks a counterpart in the host cell but has distant relatives in T4 and similar bacteriophages (Davison, 1992; Mitchell et al., 2002). The T4 gene is known to encode the ATPase subunit of a DNA packaging enzyme complex called the terminase (Rao and Black, 1988; Bhattacharyya and Rao, 1993), and the HSV-1 gene has properties that are consistent with a similar function (Yu and Weller, 1998).

The existence of groups of viruses that exhibit close morphological similarities but generally lack detectable genetic relationships is not unique to the herpesviruses, and may be explained as the result either of convergence from distinct evolutionary sources or as divergence from an ancestor so ancient that sequence similarities have been obliterated. The latter hypothesis is currently favored, but the existence of a common ancestor of all herpesviruses and any contingent dates for divergence of the groups must be viewed cautiously. More speculatively, apparent similarities in aspects of DNA packaging (Booy *et al.*, 1991) and capsid maturation (Newcomb *et al.*, 1996) could be interpreted as supporting an even earlier common evolutionary origin between herpesviruses and certain double-stranded DNA bacteriophages, including T4.

Phylogenetic analyses strongly support the view that herpesviruses have largely co-evolved with their hosts, often co-speciating with them. As would be expected of evolutionary phenomena, a number of problematic observations and exceptions have emerged as data have multiplied, especially in relation to early divergences. From comparisons between the phylogenies of the viruses and their hosts, McGeoch and Cook (1994) proposed an evolutionary timescale for the *Alphaherpesvirinae* in which the *Simplex-* and *Varicellovirus* genera diverged about 73 million years ago, roughly coincident with the period of the mammalian radiation. Even at this stage, potential exceptions to the co-evolution model were apparent. For example, the taxonomical position of avian herpesviruses among the *Alphaherpesvirinae* did not fit well, and prompted the suggestion of ancient interspecies transfers between mammals and birds. In this scheme, a similar argument may be necessary to explain the position of reptilian (turtle) herpesviruses in the same subfamily (Quackenbush *et al.*, 1998; Yu *et al.*, 2001; Coberley *et al.*, 2002), especially given their distance from amphibian herpesviruses (Davison *et al.*, 1999 and unpublished data). Assuming the constancy of the molecular clock derived for the *Alphaherpesvirinae*, McGeoch *et al.* (1995) tentatively dated the divergence of the *Alpha-*, *Beta-* and *Gammaherpesvirinae* at 180–220 million years ago. Given the contrasting lack of relationships between the groups and substantial relationships within them (see below), this date did not fit well qualitatively with a model in which the fish and mammalian herpesvirus groups co-speciated when teleosts separated from other vertebrates. In a recent analysis utilizing improved algorithms and the latest estimates for host divergence dates, McGeoch and Gatherer (2005) pushed back the common ancestor of the *Alpha-*, *Beta-* and *Gammaherpesvirinae* to about 400 million years ago, which permitted a greater degree of support for co-evolution of the *Alphaherpesvirinae*, including avian and reptilian members. In this scheme, a much earlier, non-co-speciative divergence may be indicated for the mammalian and fish herpesvirus groups (along with one of similar or greater antiquity for the bivalve herpesvirus group). However, this would lack the advantage of explaining the segregation of the viral groups to distinct parts of the animal kingdom and necessitate additional arguments involving viral extinction.

The mammalian herpesvirus group

In contrast to the lack of extensive relationships between the three groups, members of the mammalian herpesvirus group are clearly related to each other (Davison, 2002), as are those in the fish herpesvirus group (Bernard and Mercier, 1993; Davison, 1998; Davison *et al.*, 1999; Waltzek *et al.*, 2005, and unpublished data). Figure 2.2 shows the gene layout in representatives of two genera for each of the three subfamilies in the mammalian herpesvirus group. The subfamilies share 43 genes, termed "core genes," which were presumably inherited from a common ancestor (McGeoch and Davison, 1999). This number assumes a small degree of approximation, since amino acid sequence conservation among the set varies from substantial to marginal. The core genes are shaded grey in Fig. 2.2, and are largely confined to the central regions of the genomes, as is especially apparent with HCMV. Accumulation of more recently evolved genes near the termini is a feature of linear, double-stranded DNA genomes from other virus families, such as the *Poxviridae* (Upton *et al.*, 2003; McLysaght *et al.*, 2003; Gubser *et al.*, 2004) and the *Adenoviridae* (Davison *et al.*, 2003c), and also of eukaryotic chromosomes (Kellis *et al.*, 2003). The core genes are ordered similarly in the same subfamily, except for certain members of the *Alphaherpesvirinae* in which different arrangements are apparent: PRV in the *Varicellovirus* genus (Ben-Porat *et al.*, 1983; Davison and Wilkie 1983; Dezelee *et al.*, 1996; Bras *et al.*, 1999) and ILTV in the *Iltovirus* genus (Ziemann *et al.*, 1998). However, as shown in Fig. 2.2, the core genes are arranged differently in the different subfamilies, in the form of blocks, some of which are inverted (Davison and Taylor, 1987; Gompels *et al.*, 1995; Hannenhalli *et al.*, 1995). As indicated in Table 2.2, core genes are involved in vital aspects of herpesvirus growth, and many are involved directly or indirectly in DNA replication, in packaging of replicated DNA into capsids, and in capsid formation and structure. Most of the core genes are essential for growth of virus in cell culture (Ward and Roizman, 1994; Yu *et al.*, 2003; Dunn *et al.*, 2003).

Most core genes are present in all three subfamilies of the mammalian herpesvirus group, but three (encod-

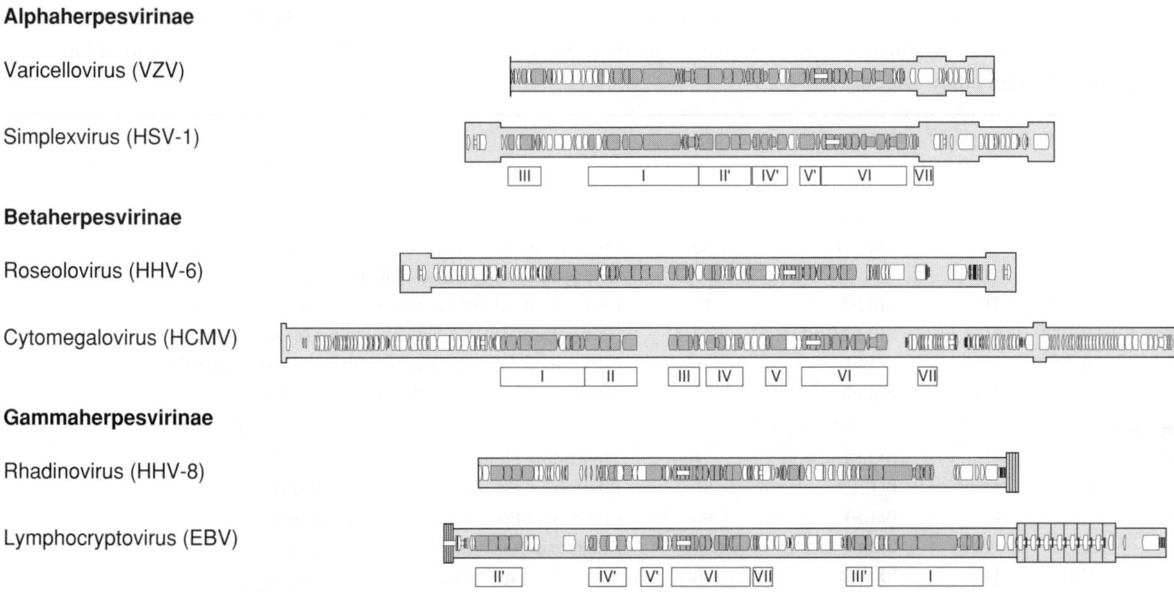

Alphaherpesvirinae

Varicellovirus (VZV)

Simplexvirus (HSV-1)

Betaherpesvirinae

Roseolovirus (HHV-6)

Cytomegalovirus (HCMV)

Gammaherpesvirinae

Rhadinovirus (HHV-8)

Lymphocryptovirus (EBV)

Fig. 2.2. Layout of genes in mammalian herpesvirus genomes. Repeat regions are shown in thicker format than unique regions. Protein-coding regions are shown as arrows shaded grey (core genes) or white (non-core genes), and introns as narrow white bars. Blocks of core genes that are rearranged between the subfamilies are indicated by rectangles I–VII for HSV-1, HCMV and EBV, with inverted blocks marked with a prime (Chee *et al.*, 1990). Block II also contains a local inversion and transposition of one gene (encoding DNA polymerase) that is not indicated. Genome coordinates and gene locations were obtained from accessions X04370 (VZV), X14112 (HSV-1), X83413 (HHV-6) as modified by Megaw *et al.* (1998), AY446894 (HCMV), U93872 (HHV-8) as extended at the right end of the unique region by Glenn *et al.* (1999), and AJ507799 (EBV). Variable numbers of terminal repeats are present in HHV-8 and EBV, but are shown at one end or the other other according to the accessions.

ing thymidine kinase, the small subunit of ribonucleotide reductase and the helicase that binds to the origin of DNA synthesis) have been lost from individual lineages. Thus, the origin-binding helicase gene has been retained in the *Roseolovirus* genus, but lost from other genera in the *Betaherpesvirinae*. This is mirrored in the presence of an origin of lytic DNA replication with similar structure in lineages that have retained this gene (Dewhurst *et al.*, 1993; Inoue *et al.*, 1994).

In addition to protein-coding regions, certain *cis*-acting sequences are conserved. These include the origin of lytic DNA replication, which is located similarly in each subfamily in comparison with adjacent genes, allowing for rearrangement of gene blocks. Certain members of the *Alpha-* and *Gammaherpesvirinae* contain additional lytic origins. Also, short elements near the genome termini that are involved in cleavage and packaging of unit-length genomes are conserved in all subfamilies (Broll *et al.*, 1999).

As well as the part played by the gradual processes of nucleotide substitution, insertion or deletion in generating diversity, acquisition of genes from the cell or from other viruses has played an important role throughout the evolution of the herpesviruses. There are examples of captured genes in all herpesvirus lineages. Among the mammalian herpesvirus group, the *Gammaherpesvirinae* exhibit a particularly impressive number of such genes, ranging from one encoding a product related to an enzyme involved in *de novo* purine biosynthesis (phosphoribosylformylglycineamide amidotransferase; FGARAT; Ensser *et al.*, 1997), which is present in all *Gammaherpesvirinae*, through a cyclin D gene (Nicholas *et al.*, 1992), which features in a subset of the *Rhadinovirus* genus, interferon regulatory factor genes (vIRFs), which are found only in HHV-8 and RRV (Russo *et al.*, 1996; Searles *et al.*, 1999), to a relatively recently captured core 2 β-1,6-*N*-acetylglucosaminyltransferase-mucin gene in BHV-4 (Markine-Goriaynoff *et al.*, 2003).

Duplication of genes, captured or otherwise, followed by divergence, is also apparent in all herpesvirus lineages. For example, up to three copies of the FGARAT gene are present in *Gammaherpesvirinae* (Virgin *et al.*, 1997), and HHV-8 and RRV contain four and eight vIRF genes, respectively (Searles *et al.*, 1999; Jenner *et al.*, 2001; Cunningham *et al.*, 2003). Examples of duplicated genes among other members of the mammalian herpesvirus group include

Table 2.2. Core genes in human herpesviruses, grouped according to functional class. HSV-2 and HHV-7 are not included, since their nomenclatures are the same as those for HSV-1 and HHV-6, respectively. HSV-1 and HCMV genes that are essential for growth in cell culture are marked by asterisks

HSV-1	VZV	HCMV	HHV-6	EBV	HHV-8	Function
DNA replication machinery						
UL30*	28	UL54*	U38	BALF5	9	Catalytic subunit of DNA polymerase complex
UL42*	16	UL44*	U27	BMRF1	59	Processivity subunit of DNA polymerase complex
UL9*	51	–	U73	–	–	Origin-binding protein; helicase
UL5*	55	UL105*	U77	BBLF4	44	Component of DNA helicase-primase complex; helicase
UL8*	52	UL102*	U74	BBLF2/BBLF3	40/41	Component of DNA helicase-primase complex
UL52*	6	UL70*	U43	BSLF1	56	Component of DNA helicase-primase complex; primase
UL29*	29	UL57*	U41	BALF2	6	Single-stranded DNA-binding protein
Peripheral enzymes						
UL23	36	–	–	BXLF1	21	Thymidine kinase
UL39	19	UL45[a]	U28[a]	BORF2	61	Ribonucleotide reductase; large subunit
UL40	18	–	–	BaRF1	60	Ribonucleotide reductase; small subunit
UL50	8	UL72[a]	U45[a]	BLLF3	54	Deoxyuridine triphosphatase
UL2	59	UL114	U81	BKRF3	46	Uracil-DNA glycosylase
Processing and packaging of DNA						
UL12	48	UL98*	U70	BGLF5	37	Deoxyribonuclease; role in DNA maturation and recombination
UL15*	42/45	UL89*	U66	BGRF1/BDRF1	29	Putative ATPase subunit of terminase; capsid-associated
UL28*	30	UL56*	U40	BALF3	7	Putative subunit of terminase; *pac* site-specific binding; capsid-associated
UL6*	54	UL104*	U76	BBRF1	43	Portal protein; forms dodecameric ring at capsid vertex; complexed with terminase
UL25*	34	UL77*	U50	BVRF1	19	Possibly caps the portal after DNA packaging is complete; tegument protein
UL32*	26	UL52*	U36	BFLF1	68	Involved in proper capsid localization in the nucleus
UL33*	25	UL51*	U35	BFRF1A	67A	Interacts with terminase
UL17*	43	UL93*	U64	BGLF1	32	Involved in proper capsid localization in the nucleus; tegument protein
Egress of capsids from nucleus						
UL31*	27	UL53*	U37	BFLF2	69	Nuclear matrix protein; component of capsid docking complex on nuclear lamina
UL34*	24	UL50*	U34	BFRF1	67	Inner nuclear membrane protein; component of capsid docking complex on nuclear lamina
Capsid assembly and structure						
UL19*	40	UL86*	U57	BcLF1	25	Major capsid protein; component of hexons and pentons
UL18*	41	UL85*	U56	BDLF1	26	Component of intercapsomeric triplex between hexons and pentons
UL38*	20	UL46*	U29	BORF1	62	Component of intercapsomeric triplex between hexons and pentons
UL35	23	UL48A*	U32	BFRF3	65	Small capsid protein located on tips of hexons; interacts with dynein and microtubules
UL26*	33	UL80*	U53	BVRF2	17	Maturational protease; generates mature forms of scaffolding proteins
UL26.5	33.5	UL80.5	U53.5	BdRF1	17.5	Scaffolding protein removed from capsid during DNA packaging
Tegument						
UL7	53	UL103	U75	BBRF2	42	Associated with intracellular capsids
UL11	49	UL99*	U71	BBLF1	38	Role in virion egress and secondary envelopment in the cytoplasm; myristylated and palmitylated protein; interacts with UL16 protein
UL14	46	UL95*	U67	BGLF3	34	Interacts with UL11 protein; regulates UL13 protein kinase
UL16	44	UL94*	U65	BGLF2	33	Interacts with UL11 protein; regulates UL13 protein kinase
UL21[b]	38	UL88	U59	BTRF1	23	
UL36*	22	UL48*	U31	BPLF1	64	Huge virion protein; interacts with UL37 protein; influences release of DNA from capsids during entry

Table 2.2. (cont.)

HSV-1	VZV	HCMV	HHV-6	EBV	HHV-8	Function
UL37*	21	UL47	U30	BOLF1	63	Interacts with UL36 protein
UL51	7	UL71*	U44	BSRF1	55	
Surface and membrane						
UL27*	31	UL55*	U39	BALF4	8	gB
UL1*	60	UL115*	U82	BKRF2	47	gL; complexed with gH
UL22*	37	UL75*	U48	BXLF2	22	gH; complexed with gL
UL10	50	UL100*	U72	BBRF3	39	gM; complexed with gN
UL49A[c]	9A	UL73*	U46	BLRF1	53	gN; complexed with gM; not glycosylated in some herpesviruses
Control and modulation						
UL13	47	UL97	U69	BGLF4	36	Serine–threonine protein kinase; tegument protein
UL54*	4	UL69	U42	BSLF1/BMLF1	57	Multifunctional regulator of gene expression
Unknown						
UL24	35	UL76*	U49	BXRF1	20	Nuclear protein

[a] Probably not an active enzyme, as catalytic residues are absent.
[b] This assignment is tentative and is excluded from the total of 43 core genes given in the text. It depends on positional, rather than sequence, conservation, and is compromised by that fact that UL21 is not flanked in each subfamily by clear homologues, unlike other core genes assigned on a positional basis.
[c] Also referred to as UL49.5.

a family of glycoprotein genes in the *Alphaherpesvirinae* (McGeoch, 1990) and 12 families, each containing up to 14 genes, in HCMV as a representative of the *Betaherpesvirinae* (Dolan et al., 2004). There are four gene families in the fish herpesvirus, CCV (Davison, 1992), and 12 in the bivalve herpesvirus, OsHV-1 (Davison et al., 2005). Given that gene duplication has been widely employed in host evolution (Prince and Pickett, 2002), and the greater evolutionary rates of herpesviruses, it seems likely that this means for generating diversity has played a greater part in herpesvirus evolution than can be detected by primary sequence comparisons.

The *Alphaherpesvirinae* subfamily

The employment of gene capture and duplication among the *Beta-* or *Gammaherpesvirinae* to generate diversity has received extensive attention in the literature (for details, see Chapters 15 and 22). In contrast, the *Alphaherpesvirinae* have evolved less adventurously in terms of gene content since their divergence from a common ancestor, and it is clear that gene loss has occurred. This mode of survival is considered in the following paragraphs.

The *Alphaherpesvirinae* contain four genera, plus the reptilian herpesviruses. Several complete genomes have been sequenced for the *Simplexvirus*, *Varicellovirus* and *Mardivirus* genera (Table 2.1). Data for the *Iltovirus* genus are more sparse. Limited sequence data are available for reptilian herpesviruses. Figure 2.3 illustrates the genetic content of members of the *Varicello-*, *Simplex-* and *Mardivirus* genera. Three examples (VZV, EHV-1 and BHV-1) were chosen to represent the major lineages in the *Varicellovirus* genus (see Chapter 1), plus SVV as a close relative of VZV. Core genes are shown in grey, and other genes that have counterparts in all three genera are shown in white. All of these genes were presumably present in the common ancestor, which is estimated to have existed 135 million years ago (McGeoch and Gatherer, 2005), and they comprise all or nearly all of the genes in extant *Alphaherpesvirinae*. It seems that only a few genes have developed since that era, and that the most of these are located near the genome termini.

Figure 2.4 shows a scheme of relationships between the genes at the left end of the genome, based on sequence conversation and the observation that two genes (UL56 and ORF1) encode potential membrane proteins. Also included are data for PRV (whose closest sequenced relative is BHV-1), MDV-2 and ILTV. Since U_L inverts in HSV-1, and U_L in the prototype genome orientation turned out to be inverted in comparison with the *Varicellovirus* genus (Hayward et al., 1975; Wadsworth et al., 1975), the genes at the left end of HSV-1 U_L are presented in the reverse order. In Fig. 2.4,

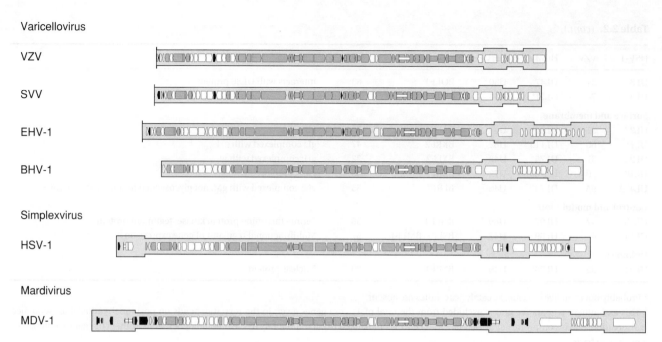

Fig. 2.3. Layout of genes in genomes of the *Alphaherpesvirinae*. Repeat regions are shown in thicker format than unique regions. Protein-coding regions are shown as arrows shaded grey (core genes), white (other genes shared by two or more genera) or black (other genus-specific genes that have presumably evolved more recently), and introns as narrow white bars. Genome coordinates and gene locations were obtained from accessions listed in the legend to Fig. 2.2, and from AF275348 (SVV), M86664 (EHV-1), AJ004801 (BHV-1) and AF243438 (MDV-1).

UL56 and UL55 thus precede UL54, which is a core gene. VZV has two extra genes (ORF1 and ORF2) sandwiched between UL55 and UL56, and the other viruses have between one and four genes in this region. For example, SVV lacks ORF2 and has a partial duplication of UL54 near the end of the genome. A parsimonious approach indicates that the ancestor preceding divergence of the *Iltovirus* genus had at least one of the genes at the left genome terminus (UL56; 180 million years ago; McGeoch and Gatherer, 2005), that the ancestor preceding divergence of the *Mardivirus* genus had at least three (UL56 (since lost), UL55 and ORF2; 135 million years ago), that the ancestor of the *Varicellovirus* and *Simplexvirus* genera had at least three (UL56, UL55 and ORF2; 120 million years ago) and that the ancestor of VZV and EHV-1 had all four genes (82 million years ago). Various of these genes have been lost during subsequent evolution of the mammalian viruses.

Gene loss is also apparent at the right genome terminus (Fig. 2.4), where, again, few genes are specific to one virus or a few closely related viruses. Even the more recently evolved genes may have substantial histories. Of the three HSV-1 genes in this category, two at the right end of U_S (US11 and US12) have counterparts in related viruses of monkeys (HVB and SA8; Ohsawa *et al.*, 2002; Tyler *et al.*, 2005). HSV-1 and HVB are considered to have co-speciated with their hosts about 23 million years ago (McGeoch *et al.*, 2000). The gene at the left genome terminus (RL1; repeated internally) has a counterpart at a similar location in a wallaby herpesvirus genome (Guliani *et al.*, 2002).

Outlook

Investigation of the genome structures, genetic contents and evolution of herpesviruses is a maturing field that undergirds the rest of herpesvirology. As with other complex analytical subjects, future advances will require incisive examination of both new data and the framework into which they are fitted. There is yet room for more surprises.

"It is a mistake to try to look too far ahead. The chain of destiny can only be grasped one link at a time." *Winston Churchill.*

Acknowledgment

I am grateful to Duncan McGeoch for many helpful discussions and for a critical reading of this chapter.

Comparative analysis of the genomes 21

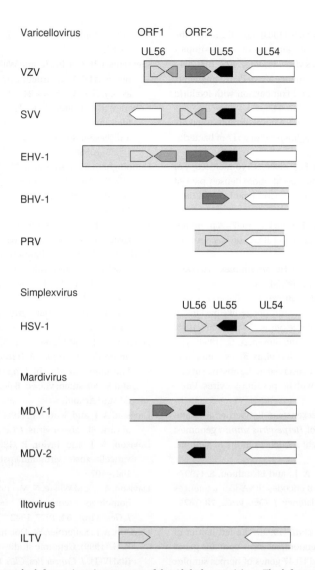

Fig. 2.4. Layout of genes at or near the left terminus in genomes of the *Alphaherpesvirinae*. The left terminus, where included, is shown by a vertical line. Homologous genes are shaded equivalently, and their nomenclature is indicated. An additional non-homologous gene is present in the *Mardi-* and *Iltovirus* genomes down stream from UL55, but is not shown. Gene locations were derived or deduced from accessions listed in the legend to Fig. 2.3, and from BK001744 (PRV), AB049735 (MDV-2) and U80762 (ILTV).

REFERENCES

Afonso, C. L., Tulman, E. R., Lu, Z., Zsak, L., Rock, D. L., and Kutish, G. F. (2001). The genome of turkey herpesvirus. *J. Virol.*, **75**, 971–978.

Albrecht, J. C. (2000). Primary structure of the *Herpesvirus ateles* genome. *J. Virol.*, **74**, 1033–1037.

Albrecht, M., Darai, G., and Flugel, R. M. (1985). Analysis of the genomic termini of tupaia herpesvirus DNA by restriction mapping and nucleotide sequencing. *J. Virol.*, **56**, 466–474.

Albrecht, J. C., Nicholas, J., Biller, D. *et al.* (1992). Primary structure of the herpesvirus saimiri genome. *J. Virol.*, **66**, 5047–5058.

Alexander, L., Denekamp, L., Knapp, A., Auerbach, M. R., Damania, B., and Desrosiers, R. C. (2000). The primary sequence of rhesus monkey rhadinovirus isolate 26–95: sequence similarities to Kaposi's sarcoma-associated herpesvirus and rhesus monkey rhadinovirus isolate 17577. *J. Virol.*, **74**, 3388–3398.

Baer, R., Bankier, A. T., Biggin, M. D. *et al.* (1984). DNA sequence and expression of the B95-8 Epstein–Barr virus genome. *Nature*, **310**, 207–211.

Bahr, U. and Darai, G. (2001). Analysis and characterization of the complete genome of tupaia (tree shrew) herpesvirus. *J. Virol.*, **75**, 4854–4870.

Ben-Porat, T., Veach, R. A., and Ihara, S. (1983). Localization of the regions of homology between the genomes of herpes simplex virus, type 1, and pseudorabies virus. *Virology*, **127**, 194–204.

Bernard, J. and Mercier, A. (1993). Sequence of two Eco RI fragments from salmonis herpesvirus 2 and comparison with ictalurid herpesvirus 1. *Arch. Virol.*, **132**, 437–442.

Bhattacharyya, S. P. and Rao, V. B. (1993). A novel terminase activity associated with the DNA packaging protein gp17 of bacteriophage T4. *Virology*, **196**, 34–44.

Bhella, D., Rixon, F. J., and Dargan, D. J. (2000). Cryomicroscopy of human cytomegalovirus virions reveals more densely packed genomic DNA than in herpes simplex virus type 1. *J. Mol. Biol.*, **295**, 155–161.

Bodescot, M., Perricaudet., M., and Farrell, P. J. (1987). A promoter for the highly spliced EBNA family of RNAs of Epstein–Barr virus. *J. Virol.*, **61**, 3424–3430.

Boehmer, P. E. and Lehman, I. R. (1997). Herpes simplex virus DNA replication. *Annu. Rev. Biochem.*, **66**, 347–384.

Booy, F. P., Newcomb, W. W., Trus, B. L., Brown, J. C., Baker, T. S., and Steven, A. C. (1991). Liquid-crystalline, phage-like packing of encapsidated DNA in herpes simplex virus. *Cell*, **64**, 1007–1015.

Booy, F. P., Trus, B. L., Davison, A. J., and Steven, A. C. (1996). The capsid architecture of channel catfish virus, an evolutionarily distant herpesvirus, is largely conserved in the absence of discernible sequence homology with herpes simplex virus. *Virology*, **215**, 134–141.

Bornkamm, G. W., Delius, H., Fleckenstein, B., Werner, F. J., and Mulder, C. (1976). Structure of *Herpesvirus saimiri* genomes: arrangement of heavy and light sequences in the M genome. *J. Virol.*, **19**, 154–161.

Bowden, R. J., Simas, J. P., Davis, A. J., and Efstathiou, S. (1997). Murine gammaherpesvirus 68 encodes tRNA-like sequences which are expressed during latency. *J. Gen. Virol.*, **78**, 1675–1687.

Bras, F., Dezelee, S., Simonet, B. *et al.* (1999). The left border of the genomic inversion of pseudorabies virus contains genes homologous to the UL46 and UL47 genes of herpes simplex virus type 1, but no UL45 gene. *Virus Res.*, **60**, 29–40.

Bresnahan, W. A. and Shenk, T. (2000). A subset of viral transcripts packaged within human cytomegalovirus particles. *Science*, **288**, 2373–2376.

Broll, H., Buhk, H.-J., Zimmermann, W., and Goltz, M. (1999). Structure and function of the prDNA and genomic termini of the γ_2-herpesvirus bovine herpesvirus type 4. *J. Gen. Virol.*, **80**, 979–986.

Browning, G. F. and Studdert, M. J. (1989). Physical mapping of a genome of equine herpesvirus 2 (equine cytomegalovirus). *Arch. Virol.*, **104**, 77–86.

Cebrian, J., Berthelot, N., and Laithier, M. (1989). Genome structure of cottontail rabbit herpesvirus. *J. Virol.*, **63**, 523–531.

Chee, M. S., Bankier, A. T., Beck, S. *et al.* (1990). Analysis of the protein coding content of the sequence of human cytomegalovirus strain AD169. *Curr. Top. Microbiol. Immunol.*, **154**, 125–169.

Chousterman, S., Lacasa, M., and Sheldrick, P. (1979). Physical map of the channel catfish virus genome: location of sites for restriction endonucleases *Eco*RI, *Hin*dIII, *Hpa*I and *Xba*I. *J. Virol.*, **31**, 73–85.

Clements, J. B., Cortini, R., and Wilkie, N. M. (1976). Analysis of herpesvirus DNA substructure by means of restriction endonucleases. *J. Gen. Virol.*, **30**, 243–256.

Coberley, S. S., Condit, R. C., Herbst, L. H., and Klein, P. A. (2002). Identification and expression of immunogenic proteins of a disease-associated marine turtle herpesvirus. *J. Virol.*, **76**, 10553–10558.

Cunningham, C., Barnard, S., Blackbourn, D. J., and Davison, A. J. (2003). Transcription mapping of human herpesvirus 8 genes encoding viral interferon regulatory factors. *J. Gen. Virol.*, **84**, 1471–1483.

Davison, A. J. (1984). Structure of the genome termini of varicella-zoster virus. *J. Gen. Virol.*, **65**, 1969–1977.

Davison, A. J. (1992). Channel catfish virus: a new type of herpesvirus. *Virology*, **186**, 9–14.

Davison, A. J. (1998). The genome of salmonid herpesvirus 1. *J. Virol.*, **72**, 1974–1982.

Davison, A. J. (2002). Evolution of the herpesviruses. *Vet. Microbiol.*, **86**, 69–88.

Davison, A. J. and Clements, J. B. (1997). Herpesviruses: general properties. In *Topley & Wilson's Microbiology and Microbial Infections*, 9th edn, vol. 1, pp. 309–323. ed. L. Collier, A. Balows and M. Sussman; vol. ed. B. W. J. Mahy and L. Collier. London: Edward Arnold.

Davison, A. J. and Scott, J. E. (1986). The complete DNA sequence of varicella-zoster virus. *J. Gen. Virol.*, **67**, 1759–1816.

Davison, A. J. and Taylor, P. (1987). Genetic relations between varicella-zoster virus and Epstein–Barr virus. *J. Gen. Virol.*, **68**, 1067–1079.

Davison, A. J. and Wilkie, N. M. (1983). Location and orientation of homologous sequences in the genomes of five herpesviruses. *J. Gen. Virol.*, **64**, 1927–1942.

Davison, A. J., Sauerbier, W., Dolan, A., Addison, C., and McKinnell, R. G. (1999). Genomic studies of the Lucké tumor herpesvirus (RaHV-1). *J. Cancer Res. Clin. Oncol.*, **125**, 232–238.

Davison, A. J., Dolan, A., Akter, P. *et al.* (2003a). The human cytomegalovirus genome revisited: comparison with the chimpanzee cytomegalovirus genome. *J. Gen. Virol.*, **84**, 17–28.

Davison, A. J., Akter, P., Cunningham, C. *et al.* (2003b). Homology between the human cytomegalovirus RL11 gene family and human adenovirus E3 genes. *J. Gen. Virol.*, **84**, 657–663.

Davison, A. J., Benko, M., and Harrach, B. (2003c). Genetic content and evolution of adenoviruses. *J. Gen. Virol.*, **84**, 2895–2908.

Davison, A. J., Trus, B. L., Cheng, N. *et al.* (2005). A novel class of herpesvirus with bivalve hosts. *J. Gen. Virol.*, **86**, 41–53.

de Jesus, O., Smith, P. R., Spender, L. C. *et al.* (2003). Updated Epstein-Barr virus (EBV) DNA sequence and analysis of a promoter for the BART (CST, BARF0) RNAs of EBV. *J. Gen. Virol.*, **84**, 1443–1450.

Delhon, G., Moraes, M. P., Lu, Z. *et al.* (2003). Genome of bovine herpesvirus 5. *J. Virol.*, **77**, 10339–10347.

Delius, H. and Clements, J. B. (1976). A partial denaturation map of herpes simplex virus type 1 DNA: evidence for inversions of the unique DNA regions. *J. Gen. Virol.*, **33**, 125–133.

DeMarchi, J. M. (1981). Human cytomegalovirus DNA: restriction enzyme cleavage maps and map locations for immediate–early, early, and late RNAs. *Virology*, **114**, 23–38.

Dewhurst, S., Dollard, S. C., Pellett, P. E., and Dambaugh, TR. (1993). Identification of a lytic-phase origin of DNA replication in human herpesvirus 6B strain Z29. *J. Virol.*, **67**, 7680–7683.

Dezelee, S., Bras, F., Vende, P. *et al.* (1996). The *Bam*HI fragment 9 of pseudorabies virus contains genes homologous to the UL24, UL25, UL26, and UL26.5 genes of herpes simplex virus type 1. *Virus Res.*, **42**, 27–39.

Dolan, A., Jamieson, F. E., Cunningham, C., Barnett, B. C., and McGeoch, D. J. (1998). The genome sequence of herpes simplex virus type 2. *J. Virol.*, **72**, 2010–2021.

Dolan, A., Cunningham, C., Hector, R. D. *et al.* (2004). Genetic content of wild type human cytomegalovirus. *J. Gen. Virol.*, **85**, 1301–1312.

Dolan, A., Addison, C., Gatherer, D., Davison, A. J., and McGeoch, D. J. (2006). The genome of Epstein–Barr virus type 2 strain AG876. *Virology*, **350**, 164–170.

Dominguez, G., Black, J. B., Stamey, F. R., Inoue, N., and Pellett, P. E. (1996). Physical and genetic maps of the human herpesvirus 7 strain SB genome. *Arch. Virol.*, **141**, 2387–2408.

Dominguez, G., Dambaugh, T. R., Stamey, F. R., Dewhurst, S., Inoue, N., and Pellett, P. E. (1999). Human herpesvirus 6B genome sequence: coding content and comparison with human herpesvirus 6A. *J. Virol.*, **73**, 8040–8052.

Dumas, A. M., Geelen, J. L., Weststrate, M. W., Wertheim, P., and van der Noordaa, J. (1981). *Xba*I, *Pst*I, and *Bgl*II restriction enzyme maps of the two orientations of the varicella-zoster virus genome. *J. Virol.*, **39**, 390–400.

Dunn, W., Chou, C., Li, H. *et al.* (2003). Functional profiling of a human cytomegalovirus genome. *Proc. Natl Acad. Sci. USA*, **100**, 14223–14228.

Ensser, A., Pflanz, R., and Fleckenstein, B. (1997). Primary structure of the alcelaphine herpesvirus 1 genome. *J. Virol.*, **71**, 6517–6525.

Ensser, A., Thurau, M., Wittmann, S., and Fickenscher, H. (2003). The genome of herpesvirus saimiri C488 which is capable of transforming human T cells. *Virology*, **314**, 471–487.

Furlong, D., Swift, H., and Roizman, B. (1972). Arrangement of herpesvirus deoxyribonucleic acid in the core. *J. Virol.*, **10**, 1071–1074.

Given, D. and Kieff, E. (1979). DNA of Epstein–Barr virus. VI. Mapping of the internal tandem reiteration. *J. Virol.*, **31**, 315–324.

Glenn, M., Rainbow, L., Aurade, F., Davison, A., and Schulz, T. F. (1999). Identification of a spliced gene from Kaposi's sarcoma-associated herpesvirus encoding a protein with similarities to latent membrane proteins 1 and 2A of Epstein–Barr virus. *J. Virol.*, **73**, 6953–6963.

Gomi, Y., Sunamachi, H., Mori, Y., Nagaike, K., Takahashi, M., and Yamanishi, K. (2002). Comparison of the complete DNA sequences of the Oka varicella vaccine and its parental virus. *J. Virol.*, **76**, 11447–11459.

Gompels, U. A., Nicholas, J., Lawrence, G. *et al.* (1995). The DNA sequence of human herpesvirus-6: structure, coding content, and genome evolution. *Virology*, **209**, 29–51.

Grafstrom, R. H., Alwine, J. C., Steinhart, W. L., and Hill, C. W. (1975a). Terminal repetitions in herpes simplex virus type 1 DNA. *Cold Spring Harb. Symp. Quant. Biol.*, **39**, 679–681.

Grafstrom, R. H., Alwine, J. C., Steinhart, W. L., Hill, C. W., and Hyman, R. W. (1975b). The terminal repetition of herpes simplex virus DNA. *Virology*, **67**, 144–157.

Gray, W. L., Starnes, B., White, M. W., and Mahalingam, R. (2001). The DNA sequence of the simian varicella virus genome. *Virology*, **284**, 123–130.

Grose, C., Tyler, S., Peters, G. *et al.* (2004). Complete DNA sequence analyses of the first two varicella-zoster virus glycoprotein E (D150N) mutant viruses found in North America: evolution of genotypes with an accelerated cell spread phenotype. *J. Virol.*, **78**, 6799–6807.

Gubser, C., Hue, S., Kellam P., and Smith, G. L. (2004). Poxvirus genomes: a phylogenetic analysis. *J. Gen. Virol.*, **85**, 105–117

Guliani, S., Polkinghorne, I., Smith, G. A., Young, P., Mattick, J. S., and Mahony, T. J. (2002). Macropodid herpesvirus 1 encodes genes for both thymidylate synthase and ICP34.5. *Virus Genes*, **24**, 207–213.

Hannenhalli, S., Chappey, C., Koonin, E. V., and Pevzner, P. A. (1995). Genome sequence comparison and scenarios for gene rearrangements: a test case. *Genomics*, **30**, 299–311.

Hansen, S. G., Strelow, L. I., Franchi, D. C., Anders, D. G., and Wong, S. W. (2003). Complete sequence and genomic analysis of rhesus cytomegalovirus. *J. Virol.*, **77**, 6620–6636.

Hayward, G. S., Jacob, R. J., Wadsworth, S. C., and Roizman, B. (1975). Anatomy of herpes simplex virus DNA: evidence for four populations of molecules that differ in the relative orientations of their long and short components. *Proc. Natl Acad. Sci. USA*, **72**, 4243–4247.

Honess, R. W. (1984). Herpes simplex and 'the herpes complex': diverse observations and a unifying hypothesis. The Eighth Fleming Lecture. *J. Gen. Virol.*, **65**, 2077–2107.

Honess, R. W. and Roizman, B. (1974). Regulation of herpesvirus macromolecular synthesis. I. Cascade regulation of the synthesis of three groups of viral proteins. *J. Virol.*, **14**, 8–19.

Honess, R. W., Gompels, U. A., Barrell, B. G. *et al.* (1989). Deviations from expected frequencies of CpG dinucleotides in herpesvirus DNAs may be diagnostic of differences in the states of their latent genomes. *J. Gen. Virol.*, **70**, 837–855.

Hyman, R. W., Burke, S., and Kudler, L. (1976). A nearby inverted repeat of the terminal sequence of herpes simplex virus DNA. *Biochem. Biophys. Res. Commun.*, **68**, 609–615.

Inoue, N., Dambaugh, T. R., Rapp, J. C., and Pellett, P. E. (1994). Alphaherpesvirus origin-binding protein homolog encoded by human herpesvirus 6B, a betaherpesvirus, binds to nucleotide sequences that are similar to *ori* regions of alphaherpesviruses. *J. Virol.*, **68**, 4126–4136.

Isegawa, Y., Mukai, T., Nakano, K. *et al.* (1999). Comparison of the complete DNA sequences of human herpesvirus 6 variants A and B. *J. Virol.*, **73**, 8053–8063.

Izumiya, Y., Jang, H. K., Ono, M., and Mikami, T. (2001). A complete genomic DNA sequence of Marek's disease virus type 2, strain HPRS24. *Curr. Top. Microbiol. Immunol.*, **255**, 191–221.

Jenkins, F. J., and Roizman, B. (1986). Herpes simplex virus 1 recombinants with noninverting genomes frozen in different isomeric arrangements are capable of independent replication. *J. Virol.*, **59**, 494–499.

Jenner, R. G., Albà, M. M., Boshoff, C., and Kellam, P. (2001). Kaposi's sarcoma-associated herpesvirus latent and lytic gene expression as revealed by DNA arrays. *J. Virol.*, **75**, 891–902.

Kellis, M., Patterson, N., Endrizzi, M., Birren, B., and Lander, E. S. (2003). Sequencing and comparison of yeast species to identify genes and regulatory elements. *Nature*, **423**, 241–254.

Kemble, G. W., Annunziato, P., Lungu, O. *et al.* (2000). Open reading frame S/L of varicella-zoster virus encodes a cytoplasmic protein expressed in infected cells. *J. Virol.*, **74**, 11311–11321.

Klupp, B. G., Hengartner, C. J., Mettenleiter, T. C., and Enquist, L. W. (2004). Complete, annotated sequence of the pseudorabies virus genome. *J. Virol.*, **78**, 424–440.

Koch, H. G., Delius, H., Matz, B., Flugel, R. M., Clarke, J., and Darai, G. (1985). Molecular cloning and physical mapping of the tupaia herpesvirus genome. *J. Virol.*, **55**, 86–95.

Lagunoff, M. and Ganem, D. (1997). The structure and coding organization of the genomic termini of Kaposi's sarcoma-associated herpesvirus. *Virology*, **236**, 147–154.

Lee, L. F., Wu, P., Sui, D. *et al.* (2000). The complete unique long sequence and the overall genomic organization of the GA strain of Marek's disease virus. *Proc. Natl Acad. Sci. USA*, **97**, 6091–6096.

Lindquester, G. J. and Pellett, P. E. (1991). Properties of the human herpesvirus 6 strain Z29 genome: G + C content, length, and presence of variable-length directly repeated terminal sequence elements. *Virology*, **182**, 102–110.

Locker, H. and Frenkel, N. (1979). *Bam*I, *Kpn*I, and *Sal*I restriction enzyme maps of the DNAs of herpes simplex virus strains Justin and F: occurrence of heterogeneities in defined regions of the viral DNA. *J. Virol.*, **32**, 429–441.

Markine-Goriaynoff, N., Georgin, J. P., Goltz, M. *et al.* (2003). The core 2 β-1,6-N-acetylglucosaminyltransferase-mucin encoded by bovine herpesvirus 4 was acquired from an ancestor of the African buffalo. *J. Virol.*, **77**, 1784–1792.

Marks, J. R. and Spector, D. H. (1988). Replication of the murine cytomegalovirus genome: structure and role of the termini in generation and cleavage of concatenates. *J. Virol.*, **162**, 98–107.

Martin, M. E., Thomson, B. J., Honess, R. W. *et al.* (1991). The genome of human herpesvirus 6: maps of unit-length and concatemeric genomes for nine restriction endonucleases. *J. Gen. Virol.*, **72**, 157–168.

McGeoch, D. J. (1990). Evolutionary relationships of virion glycoprotein genes in the S regions of alphaherpesvirus genomes. *J. Gen. Virol.*, **71**, 2361–2367.

McGeoch, D. J. and Cook, S. (1994). Molecular phylogeny of the Alphaherpesvirinae subfamily and a proposed evolutionary timescale. *J. Mol. Biol.*, **238**, 9–22.

McGeoch, D. J. and Davison, A. J. (1999). The molecular evolutionary history of the herpesviruses. In *Origin and Evolution of Viruses*, ed. E. Domingo, R. Webster, and J. Holland, pp. 441–465. London: Academic Press.

McGeoch, D. J. and Gatherer, D. (2005). Integrating reptilian herpesviruses into the family *Herpesviridae*. *J. Virol.*, **79**, 725–731.

McGeoch, D. J., Dalrymple, M. A., Davison, A. J. *et al.* (1988). The complete DNA sequence of the long unique region in the genome of herpes simplex virus type 1. *J. Gen. Virol.*, **69**, 1531–1574.

McGeoch, D. J., Cook, S., Dolan, A., Jamieson, F. E., and Telford, E. A. R. (1995). Molecular phylogeny and evolutionary timescale for the family of mammalian herpesviruses. *J. Mol. Biol.*, **247**, 443–458.

McGeoch, D. J., Dolan, A., and Ralph, A. C. (2000). Toward a comprehensive phylogeny for mammalian and avian herpesviruses. *J. Virol.*, **74**, 10401–10406.

McLysaght, A., Baldi, P. F., and Gaut, B. S. (2003). Extensive gene gain associated with adaptive evolution of poxviruses. *Proc. Natl Acad. Sci. USA*, **100**, 15655–15660.

Megaw, A. G., Rapaport, D., Avidor, B., Frenkel, N., and Davison A. J. (1998). The DNA sequence of the RK strain of human herpesvirus 7. *Virology*, **244**, 119–132.

Midgley, R. S., Bell, A. I., McGeoch, D. J., and Rickinson, A. B. (2003). Latent gene sequencing reveals familial relationships among Chinese Epstein–Barr virus strains and evidence for positive selection of A11 epitope changes. *J. Virol.*, **77**, 11517–11530.

Mitchell, M. S., Matsuzaki, S., Imai, S., and Rao, V. B. (2002). Sequence analysis of bacteriophage T4 DNA packaging/terminase genes 16 and 17 reveals a common ATPase center in the large subunit of viral terminases. *Nucleic Acids Res.*, **30**, 4009–4021.

Mocarski E. S. and Roizman, B. (1982). Structure and role of the herpes simplex virus DNA termini in inversion, circularization and generation of virion DNA. *Cell*, **31**, 89–97.

Moss, B. (2001). Poxviridae: the viruses and their replication. In *Fields Virology*, 4th edn., ed. D. M. Knipe, P. M. Howley, D. E. Griffin *et al.* vol. 2, pp. 2849–2883. Philadelphia: Lippincott, Williams and Wilkins.

Muir, W. B., Nichols, R., and Breuer, J. (2002). Phylogenetic analysis of varicella-zoster virus: evidence of intercontinental spread of genotypes and recombination. *J. Virol.*, **76**, 1971–1979.

Murphy, E., Rigoutsos, I., Shibuya, T., and Shenk, T. E. (2003a). Reevaluation of human cytomegalovirus coding potential. *Proc. Natl Acad. Sci. USA*, **100**, 13585–13590.

Murphy, E., Yu, D., Grimwood, J. *et al.* (2003b). Coding potential of laboratory and clinical strains of human cytomegalovirus. *Proc. Natl Acad. Sci. USA*, **100**, 14976–14981.

Nash, A. A., Dutia, B. M., Stewart, J. P., and Davison, A. J. (2001). Natural history of murine γ-herpesvirus infection. *Phil. Trans. Roy. Soc. Lond. B Biol. Sci.*, **356**, 569–579.

Neipel, F., Albrecht, J. C., and Fleckenstein, B. (1997). Cell-homologous genes in the Kaposi's sarcoma-associated rhadinovirus human herpesvirus 8: determinants of its pathogenicity? *J. Virol.*, **71**, 4187–4192.

Newcomb, W. W., Homa, F. L., Thomsen, D. R. *et al.* (1996). Assembly of the herpes simplex virus capsid: characterization of intermediates observed during cell-free capsid formation. *J. Mol. Biol.*, **263**, 432–446.

Nicholas, J. (1996). Determination and analysis of the complete nucleotide sequence of human herpesvirus 7. *J. Virol.*, **70**, 5975–5989.

Nicholas, J., Cameron, K. R., and Honess, R. W. (1992). Herpesvirus saimiri encodes homologues of G protein-coupled receptors and cyclins. *Nature*, **355**, 362–365.

Nugent, J., Birch-Machin, I., Smith, K. C. *et al.* (2006). Analysis of equid herpesvirus 1 strain variation reveals a point mutation of the DNA polymerase strongly associated with neuropathogenic versus nonneuropathogenic disease outbreaks. *J. Virol.*, **80**, 4047–4060.

O'Hare, P. (1993). The virion transactivator of herpes simplex virus. *Semin. Virol.*, **4**, 145–155.

Ohsawa, K., Black, D. H., Sato, H., and Eberle, R. (2002). Sequence and genetic arrangement of the U$_S$ region of the monkey B virus (*Cercopithecine herpesvirus 1*) genome and comparison with the U$_S$ regions of other primate herpesviruses. *J. Virol.*, **76**, 1516–1520.

Perelygina, L., Zhu, L., Zurkuhlen, H., Mills, R., Borodovsky, M., and Hilliard, J. K. (2003). Complete sequence and comparative analysis of the genome of herpes B virus (*Cercopithecine herpesvirus 1*) from a rhesus monkey. *J. Virol.*, **77**, 6167–6177.

Poole, L. J., Zong, J. C., Ciufo, D. M. *et al.* (1999). Comparison of genetic variability at multiple loci across the genomes of the major subtypes of Kaposi's sarcoma-associated herpesvirus reveals evidence for recombination and for two distinct types of open reading frame K15 alleles at the right-hand end. *J. Virol.*, **73**, 6646–6660.

Prince, V. E. and Pickett, F. B. (2002). Splitting pairs: the diverging fates of duplicated genes. *Nat. Rev. Genet.*, **3**, 827–837.

Quackenbush, S. L., Work, T. M., Balazs, G. H. *et al.* (1998). Three closely related herpesviruses are associated with fibropapillomatosis in marine turtles. *Virology*, **246**, 392–399.

Rall, G. F., Kupershmidt, S., Lu, X. Q., Mettenleiter, T. C., and Ben-Porat, T. (1991). Low-level inversion of the L component of pseudorabies virus is not dependent on sequence homology. *J. Virol.*, **65**, 7016–7019.

Rao, V. B. and Black, L. W. (1988). Cloning, overexpression and purification of the terminase proteins gp16 and gp17 of bacteriophage T4. Construction of a defined in-vitro DNA packaging system using purified terminase proteins. *J. Mol. Biol.*, **200**, 475–488.

Rawlinson, W. D., Farrell, H. E., and Barrell, B. G. (1996). Analysis of the complete DNA sequence of murine cytomegalovirus. *J. Virol.*, **70**, 8833–8849.

Rivailler, P., Cho, Y. G., and Wang, F. (2002a). Complete genomic sequence of an Epstein–Barr virus-related herpesvirus naturally infecting a new world primate: a defining point in the evolution of oncogenic lymphocryptoviruses. *J. Virol.*, **76**, 12055–12068.

Rivailler, P., Jiang, H., Cho, Y. G., Quink, C., and Wang, F. (2002b). Complete nucleotide sequence of the rhesus lymphocryptovirus: genetic validation for an Epstein–Barr virus animal model. *J. Virol.*, **76**, 421–426.

Rixon, F. J. and Ben-Porat, T. (1979). Structural evolution of the DNA of pseudorabies-defective viral particles. *Virology*, **97**, 151–163.

Roizman, B. and Knipe, D. M. (2001). Herpes simplex viruses and their replication. In *Fields Virology*, 4th edn., ed. D. M. Knipe, P. M. Howley, D. E. Griffin *et al.* vol. 2, pp. 2399–2459, Philadelphia: Lippincott, Williams and Wilkins.

Roizman, B. and Pellett, P. E. (2001). The family *Herpesviridae*: a brief introdution. In *Fields Virology*, 4th edn., ed. D. M. Knipe, P. M. Howley, D. E. Griffin *et al.* vol. 2, pp. 2381–2397, Philadelphia: Lippincott, Williams and Wilkins.

Rosa, M. D., Gottlieb, E., Lerner, M. R., and Steitz, J. A. (1981). Striking similarities are exhibited by two small Epstein–Barr virus-encoded ribonucleic acids and the adenovirus-associated ribonucleic acids VAI and VAII. *Mol. Cell. Biol.*, **1**, 785–796.

Russo, J. J., Bohenzky, R. A., Chien, M. C. *et al.* (1996). Nucleotide sequence of the Kaposi sarcoma-associated herpesvirus (HHV8). *Proc. Natl Acad. Sci. USA*, **93**, 14862–14867.

Ruvolo, V. R., Berneman, Z., Secchiero, P., and Nicholas, J. (1996). Cloning, restriction endonuclease mapping and partial sequence analysis of the genome of human herpesvirus 7 strain JI. *J. Gen. Virol.*, **77**, 1901–1912.

Sarid, R., Flore, O., Bohenzky, R. A., Chang, Y., and Moore, P. S. (1998). Transcription mapping of the Kaposi's sarcoma-associated herpesvirus (human herpesvirus 8) genome in a body cavity-based lymphoma cell line (BC-1). *J. Virol.*, **72**, 1005–1012.

Schwyzer, M. and Ackermann, M. (1996). Molecular virology of ruminant herpesviruses. *Vet. Microbiol.*, **53**, 17–29.

Searles, R. P., Bergquam, E. P., Axthelm, M. K., and Wong, S. W. (1999). Sequence and genomic analysis of a rhesus macaque rhadinovirus with similarity to Kaposi's sarcoma-associated herpesvirus/human herpesvirus 8. *J. Virol.*, **73**, 3040–3053.

Sheldrick, P. and Berthelot, N. (1975). Inverted repetitions in the chromosome of herpes simplex virus. *Cold Spring Harb. Symp. Quant. Biol.*, **39**, 667–678.

Shenk, T. (2001). Adenoviridae: the viruses and their replication. In *Fields Virology*, 4th edn., ed. D. M. Knipe, P. M. Howley, D. E. Griffin *et al.* vol. 2, pp. 2265–2300, Philadelphia: Lippincott, Williams & Wilkins.

Silverstein, P. S., Bird, R. C., van Santen, V. L., and Nusbaum, K. E. (1995). Immediate–early transcription from the channel catfish virus genome: characterization of two immediate–early transcripts. *J. Virol.*, **69**, 3161–3166.

Stenberg, R. M., Witte, P. R., and Stinski, M. F. (1985). Multiple spliced and unspliced transcripts from human cytomegalovirus immediate–early region 2 and evidence for a common initiation site within immediate–early region 1. *J. Virol.*, **56**, 665–675.

Stevens, J. G., Wagner, E. K., Devi-Rao, G. B., Cook, M. L., and Feldman, L. T. (1987). RNA complementary to a herpesvirus alpha gene mRNA is prominent in latently infected neurons. *Science*, **235**, 1056–1059.

Stinski, M. F. (1978). Sequence of protein synthesis in cells infected by human cytomegalovirus: early and late virus-induced polypeptides. *J. Virol.*, **26**, 686–701.

Tamashiro, J. C. and Spector, D. H. (1986). Terminal structure and heterogeneity in human cytomegalovirus strain AD169. *J. Virol.*, **59**, 591–594.

Telford, E. A. R., Watson, M. S., McBride, K., and Davison, A. J. (1992). The DNA sequence of equine herpesvirus-1. *Virology*, **189**, 304–316.

Telford, E. A. R., Watson, M. S., Aird, H. C., Perry, J., and Davison, A. J. (1995). The DNA sequence of equine herpesvirus 2. *J. Mol. Biol.*, **249**, 520–528.

Telford, E. A. R., Watson, M. S., Perry, J., Cullinane, A. A., and Davison, A. J. (1998). The DNA sequence of equine herpesvirus-4. *J. Gen. Virol.*, **79**, 1197–1203.

Thureen, D. R. and Keeler, C. L. Jr. (2006). Psittacid herpesvirus 1 and infectious laryngotracheitis virus: comparative genome sequence analysis of two avian alphaherpesviruses. *J. Virol.*, **80**, 7863–7872.

Trus, B. L., Gibson, W., Cheng, N., and Steven A. C. (1999). Capsid structure of simian cytomegalovirus from cryoelectron microscopy: evidence for tegument attachment sites. *J. Virol.*, **73**, 2181–2192.

Tulman, E. R., Afonso, C. L., Lu, Z., Zsak, L., Rock, D. L., and Kutish, G. F. (2000). The genome of a very virulent Marek's disease virus. *J. Virol.*, **74**, 7980–7988.

Tyler, S. D. and Severini, A. (2006). The complete genome sequence of herpesvirus papio 2 (*Cercopithecine herpesvirus 16*) shows evidence of recombination events among various progenitor herpesviruses. *J. Virol.*, **80**, 1214–1221.

Tyler, S. D., Peters, G. A., and Severini, A. (2005). Complete genome sequence of cercopithecine herpesvirus 2 (SA8) and comparison with other simplexviruses. *Virology*, **331**, 429–440.

Upton, C., Slack, S., Hunter, A. L., Ehlers, A., and Roper, R. L. (2003). Poxvirus orthologous clusters: toward defining the minimum essential poxvirus genome. *J. Virol.*, **77**, 7590–7600.

Varnum, S. M., Streblow, D. N., Monroe, M. E. *et al.* (2004). Identification of proteins in human cytomegalovirus (HCMV) particles: the HCMV proteome. *J. Virol.*, **78**, 10960–10966.

Vassilev, V. (2005). Stable and consistent genetic profile of Oka varicella vaccine virus is not linked with appearance of infrequent breakthrough cases postvaccination. *J. Clin. Microbiol.*, **43**, 5415–5416.

Vink, C., Beuken, E., and Bruggeman, C. A. (1996). Structure of the rat cytomegalovirus genome termini. *J. Virol.*, **70**, 5221–5229.

Vink, C., Beuken, E., and Bruggeman, C. A. (2000). Complete DNA sequence of the rat cytomegalovirus genome. *J. Virol.*, **74**, 7656–7665.

Virgin, H. W. 4th, Latreille, P., Wamsley, P. *et al.* (1997). Complete sequence and genomic analysis of murine gammaherpesvirus 68. *J. Virol.*, **71**, 5894–5904.

Wadsworth, S., Jacob, R. J., and Roizman, B. (1975). Anatomy of herpes simplex virus DNA. II. Size, composition, and arrangement of inverted terminal repetitions. *J. Virol.*, **15**, 1487–1497.

Wadsworth, S., Hayward, G. S., and Roizman, B. (1976). Anatomy of herpes simplex virus DNA. V. Terminally repetitive sequences. *J. Virol.*, **17**, 503–512.

Wagner, E. K. (1985). Individual HSV transcripts. In *The Herpesviruses*, ed. B. Roizman, vol. 3, pp. 45–104, New York: Plenum Press.

Wagner, M. J. and Summers, W. C. (1978). Structure of the joint region and the termini of the DNA of herpes simplex virus type 1. *J. Virol.*, **27**, 374–387.

Waltzek, T. B., Kelley, G. O., Stone, D. M. *et al.* (2005). Koi herpesvirus represents a third cyprinid herpesvirus (CyHV-3) in the family *Herpesviridae*. *J. Gen. Virol.*, **86**, 1659–1667.

Ward, P. L. and Roizman, B. (1994). Herpes simplex genes: the blueprint of a successful human pathogen. *Trends Genet.*, **10**, 267–274.

Weststrate, M. W., Geelen, J. L., and van der Noordaa, J. (1980). Human cytomegalovirus DNA: physical maps for restriction endonucleases *Bgl*II, *Hin*dIII and *Xba*I. *J. Gen. Virol.*, **49**, 1–21.

Wilkie, N. M. (1976). Physical maps for herpes simplex virus type 1 DNA for restriction endonucleases *Hind* III, *Hpa*-1, and *X. bad*. *J. Virol.*, **20**, 222–233.

Wilkie, N. M. and Cortini, R. (1976). Sequence arrangement in herpes simplex virus type 1 DNA: identification of terminal fragments in restriction endonuclease digests and evidence for inversions in redundant and unique sequences. *J. Virol.*, **20**, 211–221.

Yu, D. and Weller, S. K. (1998). Genetic analysis of the UL15 gene locus for the putative terminase of herpes simplex virus type 1. *Virology*, **243**, 32–44.

Yu, D., Silva, M. C., and Shenk, T. (2003). Functional map of human cytomegalovirus AD169 defined by global mutational analysis. *Proc. Natl Acad. Sci. USA*, **100**, 12396–12401.

Yu, Q., Hu, N., Lu, Y., Nerurkar, V. R., and Yanagihara, R. (2001). Rapid acquisition of entire DNA polymerase gene of a novel herpesvirus from green turtle fibropapilloma by a genomic walking technique. *J. Virol. Methods*, **91**, 183–195.

Zeng, M. S., Li, D. J., Liu, Q. L. *et al.* (2005). Genomic sequence analysis of Epstein–Barr virus strain GD1 from a nasopharyngeal carcinoma patient. *J. Virol.*, **79**, 15323–15330.

Zhou, Z. H., Chen, D. H., Jakana, J. Rixon F. J., and Chiu W. (1999). Visualization of tegument–capsid interactions and DNA in intact herpes simplex virus type 1 virions. *J. Virol.*, **73**, 3210–3218.

Ziemann, K., Mettenleiter, T. C., and Fuchs, W. (1998). Gene arrangement within the unique long genome region of infectious laryngotracheitis virus is distinct from that of other alphaherpesviruses. *J. Virol.*, **72**, 847–852.

Zimmermann, W., Broll, H., Ehlers, B., Buhk, H. J., Rosenthal, A., and Goltz, M. (2001). Genome sequence of bovine herpesvirus 4, a bovine *Rhadinovirus*, and identification of an origin of DNA replication. *J. Virol.*, **75**, 1186–1194.

Comparative virion structures of human herpesviruses

Fenyong Liu[1] and Z. Hong Zhou[2]

[1] Division of Infectious Diseases School of Public Health University of California Berkeley, CA, USA
[2] Department of Pathology and Laboratory Medicine University of Texas-Houston Medical School Houston, TX, USA

Introduction

The herpesvirus family consists of a group of viruses distinguished by the large size of their linear double-stranded DNA genomes (~130–250 kbp) and a common architecture of infectious particles (Fig. 3.1) (Chiu and Rixon, 2002; Gibson, 1996; Steven and Spear, 1997). Indeed, before the birth of molecular biology and the availability of genomic sequencing, the common hallmark structural features shared by these viruses were the most important criteria for the classification of a herpesvirus (Roizman and Pellett, 2001). All herpesviruses identified to date, which include eight different types that are known to infect human, and more than 170 other viruses that are found in animals as well as in fish and amphibians (Roizman and Pellett, 2001), exhibit identical structural design as illustrated using human cytomegalovirus shown in Fig. 3.1. These viruses have a highly ordered icosahedral-shape nucleocapsid of about 125–130 nm in diameter, which encases the viral DNA genome. The nucleocapsid is surrounded by a partially ordered proteinaceous layer called the tegument, which in turn is enclosed within the envelope, a polymorphic lipid bilayer containing multiple copies of more than 10 different kinds of viral glycoproteins that are responsible for viral attachment and entry to host cells.

Based on their biological properties such as growth characteristics and tissue tropism, herpesviruses can be further divided into three subfamilies. Among the eight human herpesviruses, the alpha subfamily includes neurotropic viruses and contains the herpes simplex virus (HSV) 1 and 2, and Varicella zoster virus (VZV). The members of the gamma subfamily are lymphotropic viruses and include Epstein–Barr virus (EBV) and Kaposi's sarcoma-associated herpesvirus (KSHV). The viruses of the beta subfamily appear to be able to establish infections in many different types of cells and tissues, and include human cytomegalovirus (HCMV), and human herpesvirus 6 and 7. This subfamily classification system is largely consistent with the extensive genomic information that is now available (McGeoch et al., 2000). While studies have been attempted to investigate the structure and architecture of each of the eight human herpesviruses, virion and virus-related particles of herpes simplex virus 1 (HSV-1), the prototype of all herpesviruses, have been subjected to the most extensive structural studies (Booy et al., 1991; Newcomb et al., 1993, 2000; Schrag et al., 1989; Trus et al., 1996; Zhou et al., 1999, 2000). During the last several years, significant progress has also been made in understanding the structure of cytomegaloviruses (Bhella et al., 2000; Chen et al., 1999; Trus et al., 1999), the prototype of the beta herpesvirus family, and KSHV, a representative of the gamma herpesvirus family (Lo et al., 2003; Nealon et al., 2001; Trus et al., 2001; Wu et al., 2000). Using HSV-1, HCMV, and KSHV as examples for each of the subfamilies, this chapter focuses primarily on the structures of these three viruses, and discusses the recent progress on understanding the structures of human herpesviruses.

Different virus-related particles found in infected cells

Summary of virion assembly pathway

Each of the herpesviruses encodes a specific set of proteins that form the different compartments of the virion (e.g. capsid, Table 3.1). Although many of the primary amino acid sequences of these proteins are not highly conserved among different viruses, the assembly pathway of the virus particles is highly similar (Fig. 3.2) (Gibson, 1996; Roizman and Knipe, 2001; Yu et al., 2003). The nucleocapsid

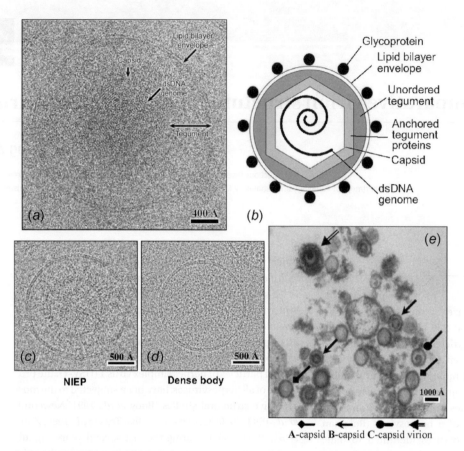

Fig. 3.1. Herpesvirus architecture. (*a*) Electron cryomicrograph of a human cytomegalovirus virion showing the different compartments of a herpes virion. (*b*) Schematic diagram illustrating the multilayer organization of human herpesviruses. Also shown are the electron cryomicrograph of a non-infectious enveloped particle (NIEP) (*c*) and a dense body (*d*) isolated from HCMV virion preparations. (*e*) Virions and different kinds of capsids observed in the thin sections of human foreskin fibroblasts infected with HCMV by negative stain electron microscopy.

is formed in the nucleus and follows a pathway that bears a marked resemblance to those of DNA bacteriophages (Casjens and Hendrix, 1988). First, a procapsid is assembled with the formation of the capsid shell and the internal scaffolding structure. Second, the procapsid is converted into mature nucleocapsid, during which time, the morphogenic internal scaffolding protein is released and replaced by the viral DNA genome, concomitant with a major conformation change of the capsid shell (Newcomb *et al.*, 1999; Yu *et al.*, 2005). Subsequent events, however, differ from the phage assembly pathway (Fig. 3.2). The mature nucleocapsid exits the nucleus and acquires its tegument and envelope, through repeated fusion with and detachment from nuclear membranes and other cellular membranous structures. Eventually, the mature infectious virion particles are released into the extracellular space via cellular secretory pathways. During this assembly process, different virus-related particles and structures, including the mature nucleocapsids and virions as well as the intermediate and aberrant products, can be found in the infected cells and the extracellular media (Figs. 3.1(*c*)–(*e*) and 3.2).

Different virus-like particles secreted from infected cells

Since the discovery of the herpesviruses, it has been long recognized that, in addition to producing infectious virus particles, the infected host cells also generate noninfectious particles such as noninfectious enveloped particles (NIEP, Fig. 3.1(*c*)) and dense bodies (DB) (Figs. 3.1(*d*) and 3.2) (Gibson, 1996; Steven and Spear, 1997). Both NIEP and DB are commonly found in the culture media of cells that are lytically infected with HSV-1 and HCMV. The ratio

Table 3.1. Major virion proteins present in HSV-1, HCMV and KSHV

Location	Common name	HSV-1			HCMV			KSHV			
		Protein name	ORF	Size (aa)	Protein name	ORF	Size (aa)	Protein name	ORF	Size (aa)	
inside the capsid	protease	protease	UL26	635	NP1c	UL80a	708	Pr	ORF17	553	~100
	Scaffolding	VP22a	UL26.5	329	AP	UL80.5	373	AP	ORF17.5	283	~1200 in B-capsid, 0 in A- & C-capsids
on the Capsid shell	MCP	VP5	UL19	1374	MCP	UL86	1370	MCP	ORF25	1376	960; penton & hexon subunit
	TRI-2	VP23	UL18	318	mCP	UL85	306	TRI-2	ORF26	305	640, dimer in triplex
	TRI-1	VP19c	UL38	465	mCBP	UL46	290	TRI-1	ORF62	331	320, monomer in triplex
	SCP	VP26	UL35	112	SCP	UL48.5	75	SCP	ORF65	170	900; hexon tip

Abbreviations: MCP, major capsid protein; TRI-2, triplex dimer protein; TRI-1, triplex monomer protein; SCP, smallest capsid protein; Pr, protease; AP, assembly protein.

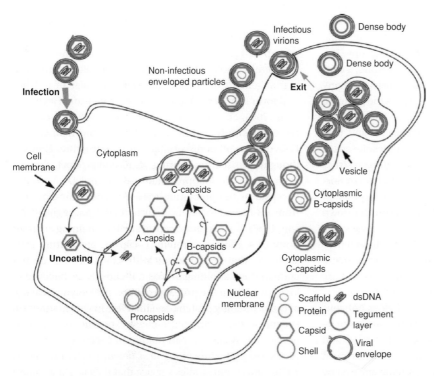

Fig. 3.2. Different virus-like particles and structures during lytic cycle of herpesvirus replication. The infectious virion initializes infection by either endocytosis or fusion with the cell membrane, which releases the nucleocapsid and some tegument proteins into the cytoplasm. The nucleocapsid is uncoated and transported across the cytoplasm (Sodeik *et al.*, 1997), allowing injection of the viral DNA through nuclear pores into the nucleus, where replication and capsid assembly take place. Procapsids mature into the C-capsid by encapsidating the viral dsDNA. Failure of DNA encapsidation results in the abortive A-capsid. Both B-capsid and C-capsid can acquire a layer of tegument proteins at the nuclear membrane of the host cell to become cytoplasmic capsids, and are enveloped and released by exocytosis to become non-infectious (NIEP) and infectious particles, respectively. Dense bodies, which contain a large amount of tegument proteins but no capsids or viral DNA, can also be found in the extracellular media.

of these particles to mature infectious virion particles can sometimes reach 20:1, suggesting that they are produced in great excess (Gibson, 1996; Steven and Spear, 1997). The exact function of these non-infectious particles in viral infection and replication is currently unknown, although they have been proposed to act as decoys that saturate and overwhelm the immune surveillance thereby facilitating the survival of the infectious virions in the hosts (Gibson, 1996; Steven and Spear, 1997).

Structurally, both the NIEP and DB are significantly different from the infectious virion (cf. Fig. 3.1(a), (c), (d)). They can be easily distinguished using electron cryo-microscopy (cryoEM) and separated from the mature infectious virions using ultracentrifugation approaches. As described above, all infectious herpesvirus virions share four common structural features (Fig. 3.1(b)). First, all herpesviruses contain a large double-stranded DNA (dsDNA) genome. The genomic DNA represents a dense core of ~90 nm in diameter, which can be stained with uranyl acetate and visualized using electron microscopy (Gibson, 1996; Steven and Spear, 1997) and appears as "fingerprint" patterns when examined by electron cryomicroscopy (Fig. 3.1(a)) (Booy et al., 1991; Zhou et al., 1999). Second, a capsid of icosahedral shape, which primarily consists of many copies of four different viral proteins, encases the genomic DNA. Third, a protein layer structure, named as the tegument first by Roizman and Furlong (Roizman and Furlong, 1974), surrounds the capsid and occupies the space between the capsid and the envelope. The tegument structure contains many virus-encoded factors that are important for initiating viral gene transcription and expression as well as modulating host metabolism and shutting down host antiviral defense mechanism (for a brief review, see Roizman and Sears, 1996). Finally, a lipid-bilayer envelope constitutes the outermost perimeters of the particles, and contains all the surface virion glycoproteins that are responsible for viral infectivity and entry (Fig. 3.1).

Unlike infectious virion particles, a NIEP does not contain a genomic DNA core and its capsid core appears to be B-capsid-like under electron microscopy (Figs. 3.1(c) and 3.2). In contrast, a dense body does not contain a capsid and appears as a cluster of tegument proteins encased by the lipid-bilayer membranous envelope (Fig. 3.1(d)). The presence of NIEP and DB indicates that neither packaging of viral genome nor capsid formation is required for viral envelopment.

Different capsid-like structures inside the infected cells

The capsid assembly is a continuous sequential process, leading to the synthesis of the highly ordered capsid structures. In cells that are lytically infected with herpesviruses, several kinds of virus capsid-like structures have been identified as representing stable endpoints or long-lived states (Figs. 3.1 and 3.2). Gibson and Roizman first introduced the terms A-, B-, and C-capsids to describe these intracellular capsid-like structures in HSV-1 infected cells (Gibson and Roizman, 1972). Similar capsid structures have been observed in cells infected with HCMV (Gibson, 1996; Irmiere and Gibson, 1985). Recent work has revealed A-, B- and C-capsids of comparable chemical composition and structural features in the nuclei of gammaherpesvirus infected cells and this suggests that the gammaherpesvirus capsid assembly probably also proceeds in a similar manner (O'Connor et al., 2003; Yu et al., 2003). These capsids all have a distinctive polyhedral shape when examined under electron microscope. Another capsid type, termed procapsid, can be obtained from in vitro assembly experiments using recombinant capsid proteins or from cells infected by a HSV-1 mutant containing a temperature sensitive mutation at the gene encoding the viral protease (Rixon and McNab, 1999; Trus et al., 1996). The procapsid has a distinctive spherical shape and is only transiently stable. They undergo spontaneous structural rearrangement to become the stable angular or polyhedral form similar to the other types of capsids (Heymann et al., 2003; Yu et al., 2005; Zhou et al., 1998b). A-capsids represent empty capsid shells that contain neither viral DNA nor any other discernible internal structure. They are thought to arise from abortive, dead-end products derived from either the inappropriate loss of viral DNA from a C-capsid or the premature release of scaffolding protein from a B-capsid without concurrent DNA packaging (Gibson, 1996). B-capsids are capsid shells containing an inner array of scaffolding protein. C-capsids are mature capsid shells that are packaged with viral DNA and do not contain the scaffolding proteins. B-capsids are believed to be derived from the procapsids upon proteolytic cleavage of the scaffolding protein, and their fate in viral maturation is controversial. Early pulse-chase experiments have suggested that B-capsids can mature to C-capsids, which in turn serve as the infectious virus precursors (Perdue et al., 1976), and recent studies suggest that they might also be a dead-end product in capsid assembly similar to A-capsids (Trus et al., 1996; Yu et al., 2004). It remains unclear whether the spherical procapsids first adapt to the stable angular form before or after the cleavage of its scaffolding protein. The C-capsid buds through the nuclear membrane using an envelopment and de-envelopment process and acquires an additional layer of proteins that forms the tegument in the cytoplasm (for review, see Mettenleiter, 2002). Enveloped virions are then released by exocytosis (Fig. 3.2).

Assembly of viral capsid

A-, B- and C-capsids represent the stable intermediates or the end products of the herpesvirus capsid assembly process (Figs. 3.1(e) and 3.2). In HSV-1, capsid assembly begins with the formation of the spherical procapsid through the association of the carboxyl terminus of the scaffolding protein with the amino terminus of the viral major capsid protein (MCP), similar to bacteriophage proheads (Conway et al., 1995; Jiang et al., 2003). Previous experiments have shown that the procapsid can be assembled in vitro from the capsid and scaffolding proteins, in the absence of the viral capsid maturation protease (Newcomb et al., 1999) or from cells infected with viruses containing a temperature-sensitive protease mutant (Heymann et al., 2003). These procapsids can spontaneously rearrange into a large-cored, angular particle resembling the B-capsid, but these large-cored particles do not encapsidate DNA or become mature virions. Past studies have also shown that cells infected with a HSV-1 mutant containing a temperature-sensitive mutation in the protease gene produced capsids that assemble at the non-permissive temperature, similar to the in vitro-assembled procapsids (Rixon and McNab, 1999). The capsids matured when protease activity was restored (Rixon and McNab, 1999), demonstrating that the procapsid is the precursor to the angular capsid (Fig. 3.2). The proteolytic cleavage of the intra-capsid scaffolding proteins at their C-termini by the viral protease (Hong et al., 1996; Liu and Roizman, 1991, 1992; Preston et al., 1992; Welch et al., 1991) interrupts the interactions between the scaffolding proteins and the major capsid proteins (Zhou et al., 1998b). The interactions between the scaffolding protein, the major capsid protein, and viral protease are important targets for antiviral drug design in treating and controlling herpesvirus infections (Flynn et al., 1997; Qiu et al., 1996; Shieh et al., 1996; Tong et al., 1996, 1998). Proteolytic cleavage of the scaffolding protein is followed by the recruitment of the smallest capsid protein, VP26, through an ATP-dependent process (Chi and Wilson, 2000), leading to the formation of the intermediate or B-capsids. The mature procapsids are believed to arise spontaneously by packaging the viral genome DNA, a process that is currently not completely understood (Yu et al., 2005).

Compositions and three-dimensional structural comparisons of alpha, beta and gammaherpesvirus capsids

A-, B-, and C-capsids (Yu et al., 2005) can be isolated from the nucleus of the host cells lytically infected by herpesviruses and they have been subjected to three-dimensional structure studies for HSV-1 (Zhou et al., 1998a, 1994), HCMV (Butcher et al., 1998; Chen et al., 1999; Trus et al., 1999), and KSHV (Nealon et al., 2001; Trus et al., 2001; Wu et al., 2000; Yu et al., 2003). While these three types of capsids have different composition (e.g., viral DNA and internal scaffolding protein), they all have a common shell structure that consists of 150 hexameric (hexon) and 12 pentameric (penton) capsomers, which are connected in groups of three by the triplexes, asymmetric structures that lie on the capsid floor (Fig. 3.3). During the last few years, considerable progress of the three-dimensional structure of the capsids and the assembly of the capsomers and triplexes has been made on the studies.

The capsid, approximately 1250–1300 Å in diameter, is a $T = 16$ icosahedron with 12 pentons forming the vertices, 150 hexons forming the faces and edges, and 320 triplexes interconnecting the pentons and hexons (Rixon, 1993; Steven and Spear, 1997). One of the 20 triangular faces of the icosahedral capsid is indicated by the dotted triangle in Fig. 3.3(a) with three fivefold ('5'), a twofold ('2') and threefold (through triplex Tf) symmetry axes labeled. The six fivefold axes pass through the vertices, the ten threefold (3f) axes pass through the centers of the faces, and the 15 twofold (2f) axes pass through the middle of the edges. The structural components in one asymmetric unit are labeled, including 1/5 of a penton ('5'), one P (peri-pentonal) hexon, one C (center) hexons a half E (edge) hexon (Steven et al., 1986), and one each of Ta, Tb, Tc, Td and Te triplex and 1/3 of Tf triplex (Fig. 3.3(a)) (Zhou et al., 1994).

HSV-1 is the easiest to grow among all human herpesviruses and has been subjected to the most thorough structural analyses, and its capsid has been reconstructed to 8.5 Å resolution (Fig. 3.3(a)) (adapted from Zhou et al., 2000 with permission from the publisher). The capsid shell has a total mass of about 200 MDa. The structural features of the capsid are built from four of the six capsid proteins: 960 copies of the major capsid protein (MCP), VP5; 320 copies of triplex monomer protein (TRI-1), VP19c; 640 copies of triplex dimer protein (TRI-2), VP23; and 900 copies of the smallest capsid protein (SCP), VP26. At this high resolution, details of secondary structure can be resolved that are not visible at lower resolution. Alpha-helices, for example, appear as extended, cylindrical rods of 5–7 Å diameter. The VP5 major capsid protein of HSV-1 was found to contain 24 helices. These assignments of helices to densities were corroborated by docking the cryoEM structure with X-ray crystallographic data which were subsequently obtained for the upper domain of VP5 (Fig. 3.3(c)) (Baker et al., 2003; Bowman et al., 2003). A group of seven helices is clustered near the area of the protein that forms the narrowest part of the

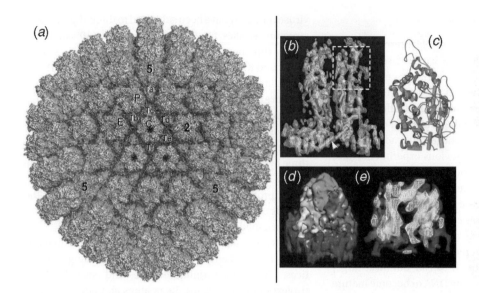

Fig. 3.3. HSV-1 capsid at 8 Å resolution (Zhou et al., 2000) and atomic model of upper domain of the major capsid protein (MCP), VP5 (Bowman et al., 2003). (a) Radially color-coded surface representation of the HSV-1 B capsid structure at 8.5 Å. One of the 20 triangular faces is denoted by dashed triangle. The penton and three types of hexons are indicated by '5', P, E and C. Also labeled are the six quasi-equivalent triplexes, Ta, Tb, Tc, Td, Te, Tf. (b) Two hexon subunits were shown in wire frame representation with α helices identified in one of the VP5 subunit illustrated by orange cylinders (5 Å in diameter). The red arrowhead points to the 7 helix bundle in the middle domain and the white arrow identifies the long helix in the floor domain that connects adjacent subunits.
(c) Ribbon representation of the atomic structure of the HSV-1 MCP upper domain determined by X-ray crystallography (Bowman et al., 2003). The helices identified in the hexon VP5 subunit in the 8.5 Å HSV1 capsid map (Zhou et al., 2000) are shown as cylinders: those in green match with helices present in the X-ray structure and those in yellow are absent in the X-ray model, suggesting possible structural differences of MCP packed in the crystal and inside the virion. (d) One single triplex is shown as shaded surface representation with individual subunits in different colors: VP19c in green and the two quasi-equivalent VP23 subunits in light and dark grey, all situated on the capsid shell domains of VP5 (blue). (e) α-helices identified in the two quasi-equivalent VP23 molecules (in red and yellow cylinders of 5 Å diameter, respectively). Adapted with permissions from publishers. (See color plate section.)

axial channel of the pentons and hexons (indicated by the red arrowhead in Fig. 3.3(b)). Shifts in these helices might be responsible for the constriction that closes off the channel to prevent release of packaged DNA. The floor domain of VP5 also contains several helices, including an unusually long one that interacts with the scaffolding core and may also interact with adjacent subunits to stabilize the capsid (arrow in Fig. 3.3(b)). Structural studies of in vitro assembled capsids that are representatives of capsid maturation stages suggest that substantial structural rearrangement at this region is directly related to the reinforcement of penton and hexons during morphogenesis (Heymann et al., 2003).

The higher resolution of this reconstruction also revealed the quaternary structure of the triplexes, which are composed of two molecules of VP23 and one molecule of VP19c (Fig. 3.3(d), (e)). The lower portion of the triplex, which interacts with the floor of the pentons and hexons, are threefold symmetric with all three subunits roughly equivalent. This arrangement alters through the middle of the triplex such that the upper portion is composed mostly of VP23 in a dimeric configuration. It appears that all three subunits of the triplex are required for the correct tertiary structure to form because VP23 in isolation exists only as a molten globule with no distinct tertiary structure (Kirkitadze et al., 1998).

The capsids of other human herpesviruses have also been studied by electron cryomicroscopy, including HCMV and simian cytomegalovirus (SCMV), and KSHV, members of the beta and gammaherpesviruses, respectively (Fig. 3.4) (Bhella et al., 2000; Chen et al., 1999; Trus et al., 1999, 2001; Wu et al., 2000). The HCMV capsid structure is very similar to HSV-1 in overall organization, with four homologous structural proteins at the same stoichiometries (Fig. 3.4(a) and (b)). The main difference is that the HCMV capsid had a larger diameter (650 Å) than HSV-1 (620 Å), resulting in a volume ratio of 1.17 (Bhella et al., 2000; Chen et al., 1999; Trus et al., 1999). The increased size of the HCMV

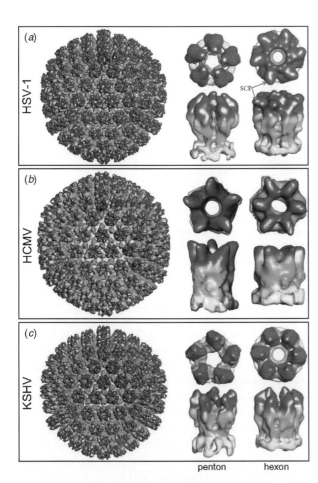

Fig. 3.4. Comparison of the three-dimensional structures of alpha, beta and gammaherpesvirus capsids. The capsid maps of HSV-1 (*a*), HCMV (*b*) and KSHV (*c*) are shown as shaded surfaces colored according to particle radius and viewed along an icosahedral three-fold axis. The resolution of the HSV-1 and KSHV capsid maps is 24 Å and that of the HCMV capsid (Butcher *et al.*, 1998) is 35 Å. The right two columns are detailed comparisons of a penton and an E hexon, which were extracted computationally from each map and shown in their top and side views. (See color plate section.)

capsid despite the similar molecular mass of its component proteins results in a greater center-to-center spacing of the capsomers compared to HSV-1 (Fig. 3.4(*b*)).

The structure of KSHV capsids was also determined by cryoEM to 24 Å resolution and exhibit structural features very similar to those of HSV-1 and HCMV capsids (Fig. 3.4(*c*)) (Trus *et al.*, 2001; Wu *et al.*, 2000). The KSHV and HSV-1 capsids are identical in size and capsomer organization. However, some notable differences are seen upon closer inspection. The KSHV capsid appears slightly more spherical than the HSV-1 capsid, which exhibits a somewhat angular, polyhedral shape. When viewed from the top, the hexons in the KSHV capsid appear flower-shaped, whereas those of HSV-1 have slightly tilted subunits and as a result appear more gear-shaped (see below). Also, the KSHV triplexes are slightly smaller and deviate less from threefold symmetry than the much-elongated triplexes in the HSV-1 capsid. The differences in the upper domains of HSV-1 and KSHV triplexes indicate that the HSV-1 triplexes are slightly taller. The radial density profiles show that the KSHV and HSV-1 capsids have identical inner radii of 460 Å (Wu *et al.*, 2000). Because both viruses also have similar genome sizes, their identical inner radii suggest that their DNA packing densities inside the capsids are similar. In contrast, betaherpesvirus capsids, such as those of HCMV, have a somewhat larger internal volume than HSV-1 or KSHV capsids (Bhella *et al.*, 2000; Chen *et al.*, 1999; Trus *et al.*, 1999). However, the increase in volume is disproportionate to the large increase in the size of the HCMV genome over the HSV-1 and KSHV genomes. This implies that the viral DNA is more densely packed into HCMV virions than into HSV-1 or KSHV virions.

In herpesvirus capsids, both the penton and hexon have a cylindrical shape (about 140-Å diameter, 160-Å height) with a central, axial channel approximately 25 Å in diameter (Fig. 3.4). The penton and hexon subunits both have an elongated shape with multiple domains, including upper, middle, lower, and floor domains. The middle domains of the subunits interact with the triplexes. The lower domains connect the subunits to each other and form the axial channels. While the upper domains of adjacent hexon subunits interact with one another, adjacent penton subunits are disconnected at their upper domains, resulting in the V-shaped side view of the pentons (Fig. 3.4). Another major difference between the penton and hexon concerns their floor domains. These domains play an essential role in maintaining capsid stability, as suggested by the higher-resolution structural studies of the HSV-1 capsid (Zhou *et al.*, 2000), where a long α-helix inserts into the floor domain of the adjacent subunit (Fig. 3.3(*b*)). The relative angle between the floor and lower domains is about 110° in the penton subunit and becomes less than 90° in the hexon subunit, making the penton to appear longer in its side view.

The HSV-1 penton and hexon subunits have the same basic shape as the HCMV and KSHV subunits (Fig. 3.4). Each consists of upper, middle, lower, and floor domains. However, the upper domains of the HSV-1 penton subunits point inward toward the channel, whereas those of the HCMV and KSHV penton subunits point outward. The upper domain of the KSHV subunit has a rectangular

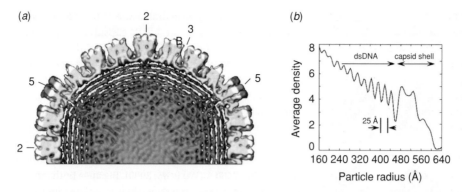

Fig. 3.5. Packing of dsDNA inside herpesvirus capsid (Yu *et al.*, 2003). (*a*) The upper half of a 100-Å thick central slice extracted from the 21 Å resolution reconstruction of the C-capsid of the rhesus rhadinovirus (RRV), a gammaherpesvirus and the closest KSHV homologue. The slice exhibits high-density features organized as multiple spherical shells inside the inner surface of the capsid floor. At least six concentric shells can be distinguished before the pattern becomes indistinct toward the center of the capsid. (*b*) Radial density distribution of the C-capsid obtained by spherically averaging the C-capsid reconstruction and plotted as a function of radius. It is evident that the distance between neighboring peaks is about 25 Å.

shape, while that of the HSV-1 penton subunit appears as a triangle. The most striking difference is that the HSV-1 hexon subunits contain an extra horn-shaped density which is not found in the HSV-1 penton (Fig. 3.4(*a*), arrow in right panel). This extra density binds to the top of each HSV-1 hexon subunit and has been shown to be the SCP, VP26, by difference imaging (Trus *et al.*, 1995; Zhou *et al.*, 1995), which associate with one another to form a hexameric ring around the hexon at a radius of approximately 600 Å. This accounts for the tilted or gear-like appearance of the HSV-1 hexon top view. The KSHV homolog of HSV-1 VP26 is ORF65. Difference map of anti-ORF65 antibody labeled and unlabeled KSHV capsids also showed that ORF65 binds only to the upper domain of the major capsid proteins in hexons but not to those in pentons (Lo *et al.*, 2003). The lack of horn-shaped densities on the hexons indicates that KSHV SCP exhibits substantially different structural features from HSV-1 SCP. The location of SCP at the outermost regions of the capsid suggests a possible role in mediating capsid interactions with the tegument and cytoskeleton proteins during infection.

Structure and packaging of viral genomic DNA

The sizes of the dsDNA genomes of different human herpesviruses vary substantially, e.g., the HCMV genome is 51% longer than HSV-1 (Davison *et al.*, 2003; McGeoch *et al.*, 2000). The major point of interest concerns the packing of their genomes within the capsids. The HCMV capsid is 117% larger than HSV-1. Besides the volume, factors such as DNA density, capsid capacity, and capsid expansion can also influence DNA packaging in viruses. The genome of HCMV might be more densely packed than that of HSV-1, or might induce expansion of the capsid upon packaging. Alternatively, the two viruses might have a similar capacity but differ in the amount of unoccupied space at the center of the capsids.

In HSV-1, the genomic DNA within the nucleocapsid is closely packed into multiple shells of regularly spaced densities, with 26 Å between adjacent DNA duplexes (Zhou *et al.*, 1999). The central slice and radial density plot in Fig. 3.5 indicate that the C-capsid of Rhesus rhadinovirus (RRV), a gammaherpesvirus, has an almost identical pattern of DNA organization to those observed in HSV-1, though slightly more compact, with a 25-Å inter-duplex distance (Yu *et al.*, 2003). Although the RRV capsid, like the KSHV capsid, has nearly the same diameter as the HSV-1 capsid (1250 Å), RRV has a slightly larger genome size than HSV-1, ~165 vs. 153 kb, respectively (Alexander *et al.*, 2000; Lagunoff and Ganem, 1997; Renne *et al.*, 1996; Searles *et al.*, 1999). Therefore, the smaller inter-duplex distance may merely reflect the need to compact this greater amount of DNA into the same volume within the capsid. HCMV has the largest genome (~230 kb) of all human herpesviruses but has a capsid that is only slightly larger (1300 Å diameter), and its DNA was shown to pack with an interduplex distance of only 23 Å (Bhella *et al.*, 2000). Based on the interduplex spacing and the genome sizes, we estimate that the closely packed DNA genomes of HSV-1, RRV, and HCMV would occupy a total volume of 3.52×10^8 Å^3, 3.51×10^8 Å^3, and 4.05×10^8 Å^3, respectively (Yu *et al.*, 2003). These volumes would measure approximately 92%, 92%, and 90% of the total available spaces inside the HSV-1, RRV, and

HCMV capsids, as estimated on the basis of their inner diameters of 900 Å, 900 Å and 950 Å, respectively. The 23–26 Å packing of strands of herpesvirus dsDNA is very close to the 20-Å diameter of B-type dsDNA, suggesting that herpesvirus genomes are packed as "naked" DNA without any bound histone-like basic proteins. In this regard, SDS-PAGE analyses demonstrated that the A-capsids and C-capsids have the same protein composition (Booy et al., 1991; O'Connor et al., 2003). In the absence of histone-like proteins, close packing of naked DNA would lead to a potentially strong electrostatic repulsion between the juxtaposed negatively charged DNA duplexes. This would make the packaging of DNA into procapsid energetically unfavorable, supporting the need for an energy-dependent DNA packaging machinery such as the bacteriophage-like connector recently reported in HSV-1 capsids (Newcomb et al., 2001). Even so, it is conceivable that the negative charge of DNA may at least be partially neutralized by binding polyamines (Gibson and Roizman, 1971) or some other undiscovered small basic molecules to reduce the strong electrostatic repulsion.

Structure and assembly of tegument

Composition of viral tegument

The tegument occupies the space between the capsid and the envelope. Since the capsid and virion are ∼125 nm and ∼220 nm in diameter, respectively, the tegument represents a significant part of the virion space and indeed, contains approximately 40% of the herpesvirus virion protein mass (Gibson, 1996;). Since they are components of virions, tegument proteins are delivered to cells at the very initial stage of infection and they have the potential to function even before the viral genome is activated. Extensive studies, including amino acid sequencing and mass spectrometric analyses, have been carried out to determine the protein content of the tegument. These results have revealed the compositions of the teguments of HSV and HCMV, and provided insight into its function.

The tegument of HSV-1 contains more than 20 virus-encoded proteins (Roizman and Knipe 2001). The most notable proteins include the α-trans-inducing factor (αTIF, VP16), the virion host shutoff (vhs) protein (UL41), and a very large protein (VP1–2). VP16 functions as a transcription activator to induce the transcription of viral immediate–early genes, and in addition, plays an essential function as a structural component in the tegument (McKnight et al., 1987; Preston et al., 1988; Weinheimer et al., 1992). The protein vhs is a non-sequence specific RNase that degrades most of the host mRNAs during the initial stage of viral infection, and facilitates the translation of viral mRNAs and viral gene expression (Everly et al., 2002; Read and Frenkel, 1983). VP1–2 is found to be associated with a complex that binds to the terminal a sequence of the viral genome, which contains the signal for packaging the genome into the capsid (Chou and Roizman, 1989).

At least 30 virus-encoded proteins have been found in the HCMV tegument (Gibson, 1996; Mocarski and Courcelle, 2001). Significant progress has been made to delineate the function of these HCMV-encoded tegument proteins. For example, the UL69 protein acts to block cell cycle progression, while the UL99-encoded pp28 protein is required for cytoplasmic envelopment of the nucleocapsids (Hayashi et al., 2000; Sanchez et al., 2000; Silva et al., 2003).

There are five predominant protein species found in the HCMV tegument: the high molecular weight protein (HMWP) encoded by UL48, the HMWP-binding protein encoded by UL47, the basic phosphoprotein (BPP or pp150) encoded by UL32, the upper matrix protein (UM or pp71) encoded by UL82, and the lower matrix protein (LM or pp83) encoded by UL83 (Gibson, 1996; Mocarski and Courcelle, 2001). Although their organization within the virion is not completely understood, these abundant proteins are believed to form the structural backbone of the tegument. UL48 and UL32 products, both of which are essential for viral replication (Dunn et al., 2003; Meyer et al., 1997), have been proposed to interact intimately with nucleocapsids (see below). Blocking UL32 expression resulted in accumulation of the nucleocapsid, suggesting that this protein is essential for tegument formation (Meyer et al., 1997).

UL82 is also believed to be involved in direct interaction with the newly synthesized nucleocapsid, and is important for initiation of tegument assembly (Trus et al., 1999). Moreover, the UL82-encoded pp71 protein is a transcriptional activator that helps to induce the transcription of the immediate-early genes within the infected cells (Liu and Stinski, 1992). UL83, the most abundant tegument protein, accounts for more than 15% of the virion protein mass (Gibson, 1996). The encoded pp65 protein has been reported to block major histocompatibility complex class I presentation of a viral immediate–early protein, and more recently, has been implicated to inhibit the induction of host interferon response (Browne and Shenk, 2003; Gilbert et al., 1996). Remarkably, pp65 is not essential for viral replication and infectious virion production (Schmolke et al., 1995). However, UL83 constitutes 90% of the protein mass in the noninfectious dense bodies, which have similar envelope structure, but lack a capsid core (Gibson, 1996). Non-infectious envelope particles, which contain B-capsid like core without the viral DNA genome, have a reduced amount (30–60% lower) amount of pp65, as do low passage clinical isolates, compared to the laboratory-adapted AD169 and Towne strains (Gibson, 1996; Klages et al., 1989). These observations suggest that UL83 serves as a nonstringent, volume-filling function in facilitating the assembly of virions, non-infectious enveloped particles, and dense bodies. Furthermore, the abundance of this protein in the viral particles and its function in blocking host immune response is believe to allow the virus to escape immune surveillance and significantly contributes to CMV survival (Browne and Shenk, 2003; Gilbert et al., 1996).

Comparative structure of viral tegument

Overview of tegument structure

While significant progress has been made during the last few years to identify tegument proteins and study their functions, little is currently known about the structure of the tegument and the organization of the proteins within the tegument. Equally elusive is the pathway of the assembly and formation of the tegument, which involves the packaging of all the tegument proteins and is certainly a highly regulated, ordered process.

Recent electron cryomicroscopy studies on the virus-related particles of HSV-1, HCMV, and simian CMV (SCMV) provide significant insight into the structure and organization of the herpesvirus tegument (Chen et al., 1999; Trus et al., 1999; Zhou et al., 1999). In these studies, the three-dimensional structures for the infectious virions or cytoplasmic tegumented capsids were reconstructed, and compared to the structures of the intranuclear capsids. The tegument can be seen in the virion as a region of relative low density covering an area in the 60–100 nm radius (Figs. 3.1(a), (c) and 3.6(a), (c)) (Chen et al., 1999; Zhou et al., 1999). Although the diameters of the nucleocapsids in different particles appear uniform, the sizes and shapes of the virus particles and the relative locations of nucleocapsids inside the particles vary. These observed variations suggest that most of the tegument proteins do not maintain rigid interactions with the enclosed nucleocapsids, and thus the bulk of the tegument layer does not possess icosahedral symmetry (Chen et al., 1999; Zhou et al., 1999).

The protein densities are also unevenly distributed across the tegument space. Studies on the localization of the tegument proteins have been reported using immunoelectron microscopy with antibodies specifically against tegument proteins and chemical treatment approaches for step-wise removal of layers of virion particles (Gibson, 1996; Steven and Spear, 1997). Several proteins have been found to be located at the tegument space distant to the nucleocapsids. For example, UL23 and UL24 are localized in the HCMV tegument space close to the inner side of the envelope membrane (Adair et al., 2002).

Detailed comparison of the electron cryomicroscopic images of the intact virion particles, the cytoplasmic tegumented capsids, and the nucleocapsids, revealed the unique tegument densities that are present in virion and tegumented capsids but not in capsid preparations. Some of these tegument densities, which are closely associated with nucleocapsid, also exhibit a certain degree of symmetry, and their structures were reconstructed to a resolution of 18–30 Å (Fig. 3.6) (Chen et al., 1999; Trus et al., 1999; Zhou et al., 1999). Since the surface of the nucleocapsid represents the starting site for tegument acquisition and envelopment, these tegument densities are believed to involve specific and direct interactions with capsid proteins and serve as anchors to recruit other tegument proteins for initiation of tegument formation. The tegument densities of HSV1 that are closely associated with the capsids exhibit a dramatic difference from those of HCMV and SCMV (Chen et al., 1999; Trus et al., 1999; Zhou et al., 1999) (Fig. 3.6). This may not be unexpected since there is little evolutionary conservation in the sequence of tegument proteins between HSV-1 and CMV, and many CMV tegument proteins do not have sequence homologues in HSV-1 (Davison et al., 2003; McGeoch et al., 2000).

Tegument structure of HSV-1

Comparison of the maps of HSV-1 intact virion particles and B capsids revealed the marked differences between the two maps in the region of the pentons, which are highlighted in color in the superposition of the difference map on the B-capsid map (Fig. 3.6(b)). The most obvious difference is the presence of additional material extending from the surface of the pentons. The extra material has a molecular mass of 170–200 kDa, extends from the interface between the upper domains of two adjacent VP5 subunits in the penton and connects to the nearby triplexes that are made up of VP19C and VP23 proteins (Fig. 3.6(b)). The restriction of the tegument contacts to the pentons is consistent with previous observations of tightly attached tegument material at the vertices of capsids in negative stain and freeze-etching images of detergent-treated equine herpevirus virions (Vernon et al., 1982). An identical pattern of tegument protein interaction was observed in a VP26-minus virion mutant (Chen et al., 2001). This result indicates that the lack of tegument association of the HSV-1 hexons is not due to the presence of VP26 on the hexon upper domain, but rather likely due to the inherent structural difference on the upper domains of penton and hexon VP5.

Comparative virion structures of human herpesviruses

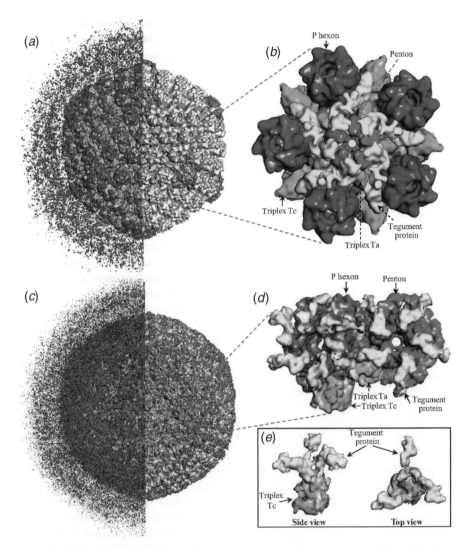

Fig. 3.6. Difference of the anchored tegument proteins between HSV-1 ((*a*) and (*b*)) and HCMV ((*c*)–(*e*)). ((*a*) and (*c*)) Radially color-coded shaded surface views of the three-dimensional reconstruction of HSV-1 (*a*) and HCMV (*c*) virions as viewed along an icosahedral three-fold axis. The bulk of the tegument components and the viral envelope are not icosahedrally ordered or polymorphic, thus appearing as disconnected low densities in the icosahedral reconstruction. These disconnected densities were masked out for the right hemisphere to better reveal the icosahedrally ordered tegument proteins, which are shown in blue to purple colors in (*a*) and in purple in (*c*). ((*b*) and (*d*)) Close-up views of the region indicated in (*a*) and (*c*), respectively, showing the molecular interactions of the tegument proteins (yellow) with the penton (red), P hexon (blue) and triplexes (green). In HSV-1, contrary to the extensive tegument association with all hexons, the tegument densities do not interact with any hexon. (*e*) Extracted triplex HCMV Tc with its attached tegument densities. Three tegument densities interact with the upper domain of each triplex (insert Table 3.1). (See color plate section.)

Based on its close association with the capsid and relative abundance in the tegument, the essential tegument protein VP1–3 has been proposed to constitute a major part of the protein complexes representing the tegument material (Zhou *et al.*, 1999). VP1–3 is an interesting yet poorly characterized protein. It has been shown that VP1–3 is associated with a complex that binds to the terminal *a* sequence of the viral genome, which contains the signal for genome packaging into the capsid (Chou and Roizman, 1989). A temperature-sensitive mutant (*ts* B7) with a mutation in VP1–3 fails to release viral DNA from the infecting capsids into the nucleus during viral decoating process (Batterson and Roizman, 1983). Since the penton has been suggested to be the route by which viral DNA leaves the capsid (Newcomb and Brown, 1994), an interaction between VP1–3 and the penton proteins would place it in an appropriate position to influence the passage of the viral genome. Further studies are needed to test these hypotheses and completely reveal the identity of the proteins coding for the tegument material.

Tegument structure of CMV

The tegument densities of HCMV that are closely associated with nucleocapsid are dramatically different from those of HSV-1 (cf. Fig. 3.6 (a) and (c)) (Chen et al., 1999). A difference map between the HCMV particles and B-capsids revealed a thin shell of loosely connected filamentous densities, representing the icosahedrally ordered, capsid-proximal portion of the tegument in HCMV (Fig. 3.6(c)–(e)). Unlike HSV-1, the tegument densities interact with all of the structural components of the nucleocapsid: penton (made up of major capsid protein UL86), hexon (consisted of UL86 and smallest capsid protein UL48.5), and triplex (composed of minor capsid protein UL85 and its binding protein UL46). Figure 3.6(d) shows the close-up views of a region from the intact virus reconstruction that includes one penton (red), one P hexon (blue), and two representative adjacent triplexes Ta and Tc (green). Superimposed on the penton and hexon are their associated tegument densities (yellow). Clusters of five and six tegument densities attach to the pentons and hexons, respectively. Moreover, neighboring clusters associate with each by bridging over the intercapsomer space, apparently using triplexes as piers. Each of the filamentous tegument densities, which is about 12 nm in length and 2–3 nm in diameter, acts as the bridge arch. Thus, the capsid appears to act as the scaffold of the ordered tegument protein layer. These results imply that the ordered tegument layer cannot form without the underlying capsid and are consistent with the observations that no such tegument layer was found in dense bodies (Chen et al., 1999).

Detailed examination of the interactions between triplexes and tegument densities further revealed minor differences between the structures of SCMV cytoplasmic tegumented capsids and HCMV particles (Chen et al., 1999; Trus et al., 1999). In SCMV cytoplasmic capsids, two tegument densities were found to be associated with each triplex. In contrast, three densities were shown to be attached to each triplex of the nucleocapsid of the HCMV particles (Fig. 3.6(e)). It is conceivable that the extra tegument densities observed in HCMV structure may represent those that were loosely associated with the capsids and probably lost during the purification of the SCMV capsids.

Based on their relative abundance and close association with the nucleocapsids, two CMV tegument proteins, UL32 and UL82, have been proposed to constitute the majority of the observed tegument material that attach to the capsids (Chen et al., 1999; Trus et al., 1999). UL82, which encodes a transcriptional activator (Liu and Stinski, 1992), has a molecular weight of ∼70 kDa, similar to the estimated molecule mass of the capsomer-capping tegument protein densities. UL32 has been suggested to be involved in the transport of DNA-containing capsids through nuclear membrane during envelopment or in the stabilization of capsids in the cytoplasm (Meyer et al., 1997). In recent experiments, CMV virion particles were subjected to different chemical conditions, which do not disrupt the integrity of the nucleocapsids, to selectively remove the components not tightly associated with the capsids. These experiments showed that most of the known tegument proteins, including UL99 and UL83, are removed, but UL32 is not affected (Yu, X., Lee, M., Lo, P., Liu, F., and Zhou, Z. H., unpublished results). Thus, these results further suggest that UL99 and UL83 are loosely and distantly associated with capsids and that UL32 is in close proximity and possibly involved in direct interactions with the capsids.

Structure and assembly of viral envelope

The envelope contains most, if not all, of the virion glycoproteins. Each of the herpesviruses encodes a set of 20–80 glycoproteins, very few of which are highly conserved among all the herpesviruses (Kieff and Rickinson, 2001; Mocarski and Courcelle, 2001; Roizman and Knipe, 2001). For example, HSV-1 encodes at least 20 glycoproteins, 11 of which are found in the virions (Roizman and Knipe, 2001). HCMV potentially encodes more than 75 membrane-associated proteins, at least 15 of which are found in the virions (Mocarski and Courcelle, 2001). The exact organization of viral surface glycoproteins in the envelope is not completely understood. Virion glycoproteins are found to aggregate into complexes on the surface of the virion. For example, HCMV glycoproteins gH, gL, and gO are associated to form a heterotrimeric envelope glycoprotein complex (Gibson, 1996; Mocarski and Courcelle, 2001). These proteins may form their complexes in the cellular membrane compartment before trafficking to the viral envelope. However, it remains possible that further higher-order complexes are assembled after these protein components are delivered in the viral envelope membrane.

In addition to the viral encoded glycoproteins, the envelope also contains numerous host proteins or constituents. For example, host proteins associated with HCMV envelope include β2-microglobumin, CD55 and CD59, and annexin II (Grundy et al., 1987a, b; Wright et al., 1995). These molecules may participate in the induction of host cellular responses. It is conceivable that these host proteins, in combination with the viral encoded G protein-coupled receptors associated with the HCMV envelop, play an important role in modulating host cell response during initial virus attachment, as observed in recent studies (Compton et al., 2003; Zhu et al., 1998).

Herpesvirus envelopment is believed to take place initially at the inner nuclear membrane, and then further proceeds with an envelopment/de-envelopment process that allows the capsid to cross the double nuclear membranes and other cytoplasmic membrane structures (Gibson, 1996; Steven and Spear, 1997). Cytoplasmic envelopment of HSV-1 and CMV capsids can also take place in endosomes as well as Golgi networks (Eggers et al., 1992). Thus, it is not surprising that the envelope contains diverse lipid components that are associated with different parts of the cytoplasmic membrane system in addition to the nuclear membrane. These components include the phosphatidylcholine, phosphatidylethanolamine, phosphatidylserine, and phosphatidylinositol (Roby and Gibson, 1986). Whether these lipid components may be important in maintaining the integrity of the viral envelope has not been determined and their functional role in stabilizing virion structure is unknown.

The envelopment process appears to be not affected in the absence of a mature capsid since noninfectious enveloped particles and dense bodies can be produced and contain similar envelop contents. In the case of HCMV, pp65 constitutes at least 90% of the dense body protein mass (Gibson, 1996). It is conceivable that this protein may contain signals that promote its own envelopment. There are presumably interactions between proteins of the tegument and envelope that promote the envelopment process. Indeed, recent results indicate that HCMV UL99, a tegument protein, facilitates the cytoplasmic envelopment of the nucleocapsid (Sanchez et al., 2000; Silva et al., 2003). Two HSV-1 membrane proteins, UL34 and UL31, are also implicated to be essential for viral envelopment (Reynolds et al., 2001). Further studies on the organization of the proteins in these particles and their potential interactions with envelope components will provide insight into the process of their assembly.

Other constituents in the virions

Recent studies indicated that viral mRNAs were found in HSV-1 and HCMV virions (Bresnahan and Shenk, 2000; Sciortino et al., 2001). These mRNAs appear to be packaged selectively into the infectious virion particles. They have been proposed to function to facilitate the initiation of viral infection upon viral entry. It is unknown whether these virion mRNAs play a role in maintaining the integrity of the virion structure, as ribosomal RNAs provide the backbone for ribosome assembly.

Depending on the approach of how the virions are prepared and the quality of the preparations being analyzed, numerous host constituents, including lipids, polyamines, and cellular enzyme and structural proteins, are also found to be associated with the viral particles. In particular, two of these host constituents, polyamines and actin-related protein (ARP), may play an important role in stabilizing and maintaining the intact structure of the infectious particles. Two kinds of polyamines, spermidine and spermine, have commonly been found in herpesvirus virions, including HSV-1 and HCMV (Gibson and Roizman, 1971; Gibson et al., 1984). In highly purified HSV-1 virion preparations, there are about 70 000 molecules of spermidine and 40 000 molecules of spermine per virion (Gibson and Roizman, 1971). The functions of these polyamines are believed to provide positive charges to neutralize the highly negatively charged viral DNA genome during the genome replication and packaging. This hypothesis is consistent with the observations that none of the herpesvirus capsid proteins are highly positive charged and addition of arginine facilitates capsid assembly and virion production (Mark and Kaplan, 1971). Spermidine appears to be in the tegument while spermine is localized in the nucleocapsid. It is estimated that the spermine contained in the virion has the capacity to neutralize about 40% of the DNA phosphate, consistent with its role in stabilizing the packed genomic DNA in the nucleocapsid core.

In analyzing highly purified HCMV virions as well as noninfectious enveloped particles and dense bodies, Baldick and Shenk first reported the presence of a substantial amount of a cellular actin-related protein (ARP) in the tegument compartment (Baldick and Shenk, 1996). The exact localization of the ARP is currently unknown, and preliminary studies using stepwise chemical treatment of HCMV virion for removal of different parts of the particles have suggested that ARP is localized in the tegument space distant from the nucleocapsid (Yu, X., Lee, M., Lo, P., Liu, F., and Zhou, Z. H., unpublished results). Based on their roles for providing cytoskeleton and maintaining cellular structure and morphology, it is conceivable that actin-related proteins stabilize the tegument structure. Meanwhile, some ARPs have been implicated in participating dynein-driven microtubule transport system (Lees-Miller et al., 1992; Schroer et al., 1994). Given the fact that viral capsid trafficking from cytoplasm to the nuclear pore complex is driven by the dynein-microtubule system (Dohner et al., 2002; Sodeik et al., 1997), it is possible that these ARPs are specifically incorporated into the teguments and facilitate the transport of the viral particles from the nucleus to the cytoplasmic membrane during viral envelopment and to the nucleus during post-penetration. Further studies are needed to completely elucidate the function of these proteins in assembly and maintenance of the virus structure.

Acknowledgments

We thank NIH for financial support; Pierrette Lo for assistance in preparing Figs. 3.1(*b*), 4; and Dr. Sarah Butcher for providing an HCMV capsid map.

REFERENCES

Adair, R., Douglas, E. R., Maclean, J. B. *et al.* (2002). The products of human cytomegalovirus genes UL23, UL24, UL43 and US22 are tegument components. *J. Gen. Virol.*, **83**, 1315–1324.

Alexander, L., Denekamp, L., Knapp, A., Auerbach, M. R., Damania, B., and Desrosiers, R. C. (2000). The primary sequence of rhesus monkey rhadinovirus isolate 26–95: sequence similarities to Kaposi's sarcoma-associated herpesvirus and rhesus monkey rhadinovirus isolate 17577. *J. Virol.*, **74**, 3388–3398.

Baker, M. L., Jiang, W., Bowman, B. R. *et al.* (2003). Architecture of the herpes simplex virus major capsid protein derived from structural bioinformatics. *J. Mol. Biol.*, **331**, 447–456.

Baldick, C. J., Jr. and Shenk, T. (1996). Proteins associated with purified human cytomegalovirus particles. *J. Virol.*, **70**, 6097–6105.

Batterson, W. and Roizman, B. (1983). Characterization of the herpes simplex virion-associated factor responsible for the induction of alpha genes. *J. Virol.*, **46**, 371–377.

Bhella, D., Rixon, F. J., and Dargan, D. J. (2000). Cryomicroscopy of human cytomegalovirus virions reveals more densely packed genomic DNA than in herpes simplex virus type 1. *J. Mol. Biol.*, **295**, 155–161.

Booy, F. P., Newcomb, W. W., Trus, B. L., Brown, J. C., Baker, T. S., and Steven, A. C. (1991). Liquid-crystalline, phage-like packing of encapsidated DNA in herpes simplex virus. *Cell*, **64**, 1007–1015.

Bowman, B. R., Baker, M. L., Rixon, F. J., Chiu, W., and Quiocho, F. A. (2003). Structure of the herpesvirus major capsid protein. *EMBO J.*, **22**, 757–765.

Bresnahan, W. A. and Shenk, T. (2000). A subset of viral transcripts packaged within human cytomegalovirus particles. *Science*, **288**, 2373–2376.

Browne, E. P. and Shenk, T. (2003). Human cytomegalovirus UL83-coded pp65 virion protein inhibits antiviral gene expression in infected cells. *Proc. Natl Acad. Sci., USA*, **100**, 11439–11444.

Butcher, S. J., Aitken, J., Mitchell, J., Gowen, B., and Dargan, D. J. (1998). Structure of the human cytomegalovirus B capsid by electron cryomicroscopy and image reconstruction. *J. Struct. Biol.*, **124**, 70–76.

Casjens, S. and Hendrix, R. (1988). Control mechanisms in dsDNA bacteriophage assembly. In *The Bacteriophages*, ed. R. Celander, New York: Plenum Publishing Corp, pp. 15–91.

Chen, D. H., Jiang, H., Lee, M., Liu, F., and Zhou, Z. H. (1999). Three-dimensional visualization of tegument/capsid interactions in the intact human cytomegalovirus. *Virology*, **260**, 10–16.

Chen, D. H., Jakana, J., and McNab, D. (2001). The pattern of tegument-capsid interaction in the herpes simplex virus type 1 virion is not influenced by the small hexon-associated protein VP26. *J. Virol.*, **75**, 11863–11867.

Chi, J. H. and Wilson, D. W. (2000). ATP-dependent localization of the herpes simplex virus capsid protein VP26 to sites of procapsid maturation. *J. Virol.*, **74**, 1468–1476.

Chiu, W. and Rixon, F. J. (2002). High resolution structural studies of complex icosahedral viruses: a brief overview. *Virus Res.*, **82**, 9–17.

Chou, J. and Roizman, B. (1989). Characterization of DNA sequence-common and sequence-specific proteins binding to cis-acting sites for cleavage of the terminal a sequence of the herpes simplex virus 1 genome. *J. Virol.*, **63**, 1059–1068.

Compton, T., Kurt-Jones, E. A., Boehme, K. W. *et al.* (2003). Human cytomegalovirus activates inflammatory cytokine responses via CD14 and Toll-like receptor 2. *J. Virol.*, **77**, 4588–4596.

Conway, J. F., Duda, R. L., Cheng, N., Hendrix, R. W., and Steven, A. C. (1995). Proteolytic and conformational control of virus capsid maturation: the bacteriophage HK97 system. *J. Mol. Biol.*, **253**, 86–99.

Davison, A. J., Dolan, A., Akter, P. *et al.* (2003). The human cytomegalovirus genome revisited: comparison with the chimpanzee cytomegalovirus genome. *J. Gen. Virol.*, **84**, 17–28.

Dohner, K., Wolfstein, A., Prank, U. *et al.* (2002). Function of dynein and dynactin in herpes simplex virus capsid transport. *Mol. Biol. Cell*, **13**, 2795–2809.

Dunn, W., Chou, C., Li, H. *et al.* (2003). Functional profiling of human cytomegalovirus genome. *Proc. Natl Acad. Sci. USA*, **100**, 14223–14228.

Eggers, M., Bogner, E., Agricola, B., Kern, H. F., and Radsak, K. (1992). Inhibition of human cytomegalovirus maturation by brefeldin A. *J. Gen. Virol.*, **73**(Pt 10), 2679–2692.

Everly, D. N., Jr., Feng, P., Mian, I. S., and Read, G. S. (2002). mRNA degradation by the virion host shutoff (Vhs) protein of herpes simplex virus: genetic and biochemical evidence that Vhs is a nuclease. *J. Virol.*, **76**, 8560–8571.

Flynn, D. L., Abood, N. A., and Howerda, B. C. (1997). Recent advances in antiviral research: identification of inhibitors of the herpesvirus proteases. *Curr. Opin. Chem. Biol.*, **1**, 190–196.

Gibson, W. (1996). Structure and assembly of the virion. *Intervirology*, **39**, 389–400.

Gibson, W. and Roizman, B. (1971). Compartmentalization of spermine and spermidine in the herpes simplex virion. *Proc. Natl Acad. Sci. USA*, **68**, 2818–2821.

Gibson, W. and Roizman, B. (1972). Proteins specified by herpes simplex virus. 8. Characterization and composition of multiple capsid forms of subtypes 1 and 2. *J. Virol.*, **10**, 1044–1052.

Gibson, W., van Breemen, R., Fields, A., LaFemina, R., and Irmiere, A. (1984). D,L-alpha-difluoromethylornithine inhibits human cytomegalovirus replication. *J. Virol.*, **50**, 145–154.

Gilbert, M. J., Riddell, S. R., Plachter, B., and Greenberg, P. D. (1996). Cytomegalovirus selectively blocks antigen processing and presentation of its immediate–early gene product. *Nature*, **383**, 720–722.

Grundy, J. E., McKeating, J. A., and Griffiths, P. D. (1987a). Cytomegalovirus strain AD169 binds beta 2 microglobulin in vitro after release from cells. *J. Gen. Virol.*, **68**(Pt 3), 777–784.

Grundy, J. E., McKeating, J. A., Ward, P. J., Sanderson, A. R., and Griffiths, P. D. (1987b). Beta 2 microglobulin enhances the infectivity of cytomegalovirus and when bound to the virus enables class I HLA molecules to be used as a virus receptor. *J. Gen. Virol.*, **68**(Pt 3), 793–803.

Hayashi, M. L., Blankenship, C., and Shenk, T. (2000). Human cytomegalovirus UL69 protein is required for efficient accumulation of infected cells in the G1 phase of the cell cycle. *Proc. Natl Acad. Sci. USA*, **97**, 2692–2696.

Heymann, J. B., Cheng, N., Newcomb, W. W., Trus, B. L., Brown, J. C., and Steven, A. C. (2003). Dynamics of herpes simplex virus capsid maturation visualized by time-lapse cryo-electron microscopy. *Nat. Struct. Biol.*, **10**, 334–341.

Hong, Z., Beaudet-Miller, M., Durkin, J., Zhang, R., and Kwong, A. D. (1996). Identification of a minimal hydrophobic domain in the herpes simplex virus type 1 scaffolding protein which is required for interaction with the major capsid protein. *J. Virol.*, **70**, 533–540.

Irmiere, A. and Gibson, W. (1985). Isolation of human cytomegalovirus intranuclear capsids, characterization of their protein constituents, and demonstration that the B-capsid assembly protein is also abundant in noninfectious enveloped particles. *J. Virol.*, **56**, 277–283.

Jiang, W., Li, Z., Zhang, Z., Baker, M. L., Prevelige, P. E., Jr., and Chiu, W. (2003). Coat protein fold and maturation transition of bacteriophage P22 seen at subnanometer resolutions. *Nat. Struct. Biol.*, **10**, 131–135.

Kieff, E. and Rickinson, A. B. (2001). Epstein–Barr virus and its replication. In *Fields Virology*, ed. D. M. Knipe and P. M. Howley, pp. 2511–2574. Lippincott, Williams & Wilkins, Philadelphia.

Kirkitadze, M. D., Barlow, P. N., Price, N. C. (1998). The herpes simplex virus triplex protein, VP23, exists as a molten globule. *J. Virol.*, **72**, 10066–10072.

Klages, S., Ruger, B., and Jahn, G. (1989). Multiplicity dependent expression of the predominant phosphoprotein pp65 of human cytomegalovirus. *Virus Res.*, **12**, 159–168.

Lagunoff, M. and Ganem, D. (1997). The structure and coding organization of the genomic termini of Kaposi's sarcoma-associated herpesvirus. *Virology*, **236**, 147–154.

Lees-Miller, J. P., Helfman, D. M., and Schroer, T. A. (1992). A vertebrate actin-related protein is a component of a multisubunit complex involved in microtubule-based vesicle motility. *Nature*, **359**, 244–246.

Liu, F. and Roizman, B. (1991). The herpes simplex virus 1 gene encoding a protease also contains within its coding domain the gene encoding the more abundant substrate. *J. Virol.*, **65**, 5149–5156.

Liu, F. and Roizman, B. (1992). Differentiation of multiple domains in the herpes simplex virus 1 protease encoded by the UL26 gene. *Proc. Natl Acad. Sci. USA*, **89**, 2076–2080.

Liu, B. and Stinski, M. F. (1992). Human cytomegalovirus contains a tegument protein that enhances transcription from promoters with upstream ATF and AP-1 cis-acting elements. *J. Virol.*, **66**, 4434–4444.

Lo, P., Yu, X., Atanasov, I., Chandran, B., and Zhou, Z. H. (2003). Three-dimensional localization of pORF65 in Kaposi's sarcoma-associated herpesvirus capsid. *J. Virol.*, **77**, 4291–4297.

Mark, G. E. and Kaplan, A. S. (1971). Synthesis of proteins in cells infected with herpesvirus. VII. Lack of migration of structural viral proteins to the nucleus of arginine-deprived cells. *Virology*, **45**, 53–60.

McGeoch, D. J., Dolan, A., and Ralph, A. C. (2000). Toward a comprehensive phylogeny for mammalian and avian herpesviruses. *J. Virol.*, **74**, 10401–10406.

McKnight, J. L., Kristie, T. M., and Roizman, B. (1987). Binding of the virion protein mediating alpha gene induction in herpes simplex virus 1-infected cells to its *cis* site requires cellular proteins. *Proc. Natl Acad. Sci. USA*, **84**, 7061–7065.

Mettenleiter, T. C. (2002). Herpesvirus assembly and egress. *J. Virol.*, **76**, 1537–1547.

Meyer, H. H., Ripalti, A., Landini, M. P., Radsak, K., Kern, H. F., and Hensel, G. M. (1997). Human cytomegalovirus late-phase maturation is blocked by stably expressed UL32 antisense mRNA in astrocytoma cells. *J. Gen. Virol.*, **78**(Pt 10), 2621–2631.

Mocarski, E. S. and Courcelle, C. T. (2001). Cytomegalovirus and their replication. In *Fields Virology*, ed. D. M. Knipe and P. M. Howley, pp. 2629–2673. Lippincott, Williams & Wilkins, Philadelphia.

Nealon, K., Newcomb, W. W., Pray, T. R., Craik, C. S., Brown, J. C., and Kedes, D. H. (2001). Lytic replication of Kaposi's sarcoma-associated herpesvirus results in the formation of multiple capsid species: isolation and molecular characterization of A, B, and C capsids from a gammaherpesvirus. *J. Virol.*, **75**, 2866–2878.

Newcomb, W. W. and Brown, J. C. (1994). Induced extrusion of DNA from the capsid of herpes simplex virus type 1. *J. Virol.*, **68**, 433–440.

Newcomb, W. W., Trus, B. L., Booy, F. P., Steven, A. C., Wall, J. S., and Brown, J. C. (1993). Structure of the herpes simplex virus capsid. Molecular composition of the pentons and the triplexes. *J. Mol. Biol.*, **232**, 499–511.

Newcomb, W. W., Homa, F. L., Thomsen, D. R. *et al.* (1999). Assembly of the herpes simplex virus procapsid from purified components and identification of small complexes containing the major capsid and scaffolding proteins. *J. Virol.*, **73**, 4239–4250.

Newcomb, W. W., Trus, B. L., Cheng, N. *et al.* (2000). Isolation of herpes simplex virus procapsids from cells infected with a protease-deficient mutant virus. *J. Virol.*, **74**, 1663–1673.

Newcomb, W. W., Juhas, R. M., Thomsen, D. R. *et al.* (2001). The UL6 gene product forms the portal for entry of DNA into the herpes simplex virus capsid. *J. Virol.*, **75**, 10923–10932.

O'Connor, C. M., Damania, B., and Kedes, D. H. (2003). Capsid and virion production in Rhesus monkey rhadinovirus: a model for structure and assembly of Kaposi's sarcoma-associated herpesvirus. *Submitted*.

Perdue, M. L., Cohen, J. C., Randall, C. C., and O'Callaghan, D. J. (1976). Biochemical studies of the maturation of herpesvirus nucleocapsid species. *Virology*, **74**, UNKNOWN.

Preston, C. M., Frame, M. C., and Campbell, M. E. (1988). A complex formed between cell components and an HSV structural polypeptide binds to a viral immediate early gene regulatory DNA sequence. *Cell*, **52**, 425–434.

Preston, V. G., Rixon, F. J., McDougall, I. M., McGregor, M., and Al-Kobaisi, M. F. (1992). Processing of the herpes simplex virus assembly protein ICP35 near its carboxy terminal end requires the product of the whole of the UL26 reading frame. *Virology*, **186**, 87–98.

Qiu, X., Culp, J. S., DeLilla, A. G. *et al.* (1996). Unique fold and active site in cytomegalovirus protease. *Nature (London)*, **383**, 275–279.

Read, G. S. and Frenkel, N. (1983). Herpes simplex virus mutants defective in the virion-associated shutoff of host polypeptide synthesis and exhibiting abnormal synthesis of alpha (immediate early) viral polypeptides. *J. Virol.*, **46**, 498–512.

Renne, R., Lagunoff, M., Zhong, W., and Ganem, D. (1996). The size and conformation of Kaposi's sarcoma-associated herpesvirus (human herpesvirus 8) DNA in infected cells and virions. *J. Virol.*, **70**, 8151–8154.

Reynolds, A. E., Ryckman, B. J., Baines, J. D., Zhou, Y., Liang, L., and Roller, R. J. (2001). U(L)31 and U(L)34 proteins of herpes simplex virus type 1 form a complex that accumulates at the nuclear rim and is required for envelopment of nucleocapsids. *J. Virol.*, **75**, 8803–8817.

Rixon, F. J. (1993). Structure and assembly of herpesviruses. *Seminars in Virology*, **4**, 135–144.

Rixon, F. J. and McNab, D. (1999). Packaging-competent capsids of a herpes simplex virus temperature-sensitive mutant have properties similar to those of in vitro-assembled procapsids. *J. Virol.*, **73**, 5714–5721.

Roby, C. and Gibson, W. (1986). Characterization of phosphoproteins and protein kinase activity of virions, noninfectious enveloped particles, and dense bodies of human cytomegalovirus. *J. Virol.*, **59**, 714–727.

Roizman, B. and Furlong, D. (1974). The replication of herpes viruses. In *Comprehensive Virology*, ed. H. Fraenkel-Conrat, H., and R. R. Wagner, pp. 229–403. New York, NY: Plenum Press.

Roizman, B. and Knipe, D. M. (2001). Herpes simplex viruses and their replication. In *Fields Virology*, ed. D. M. Knipe and P. M. Howley, vol. 2, pp. 2399–2460. Philadelphia, PA: Lippincott, Williams & Wilkins.

Roizman, B. and Pellett, P. E. (2001). The family herpesviridae: a brief introduction. In *Fields Virology*, ed. D. M. Knipe and P. M. Howley, vol. 2, pp. 2381–2398. Philadelphia, PA. Lippincott, Williams & Wilkins.

Roizman, B. and Sears, A. E. (1996). Herpes simplex viruses and their replication. In Fields, B. N., Knipe, D. M. and Howley, P. M. (eds.), *Fields Virology*, ed. B. N. Fields, D. M. Knipe, and P. M. Howley, vol. 2, pp. 2231–2295. Philadelphia, PA: Lippincott–Raven Publishers.

Sanchez, V., Sztul, E., and Britt, W. J. (2000). Human cytomegalovirus pp28 (UL99) localizes to a cytoplasmic compartment which overlaps the endoplasmic reticulum–golgi–intermediate compartment. *J. Virol.*, **74**, 3842–3851.

Schmolke, S., Kern, H. F., Drescher, P., Jahn, G., and Plachter, B. (1995). The dominant phosphoprotein pp65 (UL83) of human cytomegalovirus is dispensable for growth in cell culture. *J. Virol.*, **69**, 5959–5968.

Schrag, J. D., Prasad, B. V., Rixon, F. J., and Chiu, W. (1989). Three-dimensional structure of the HSV1 nucleocapsid. *Cell*, **56**, 651–660.

Schroer, T. A., Fyrberg, E., Cooper, J. A. *et al.* (1994). Actin-related protein nomenclature and classification. *J. Cell Biol.*, **127**, 1777–1778.

Sciortino, M. T., Suzuki, M., Taddeo, B., and Roizman, B. (2001). RNAs extracted from herpes simplex virus 1 virions: apparent selectivity of viral but not cellular RNAs packaged in virions. *J. Virol.*, **75**, 8105–8116.

Searles, R. P., Bergquam, E. P., Axthelm, M. K., and Wong, S. W. (1999). Sequence and genomic analysis of a Rhesus macaque rhadinovirus with similarity to Kaposi's sarcoma-associated herpesvirus/human herpesvirus 8. *J. Virol.*, **73**, 3040–3053.

Shieh, H.-S., Kurumbail, R. G., Stevens, A. M. *et al.* (1996). Three-dimensional structure of human cytomegalovirus protease. *Nature (London)*, **383**, 279–282.

Silva, M. C., Yu, Q. C., Enquist, L., and Shenk, T. (2003). Human cytomegalovirus UL99encoded pp28 is required for the cytoplasmic envelopment of tegument-associated capsids. *J. Virol.*, **77**, 10594–10605.

Sodeik, B., Ebersold, M. W., and Helenius, A. (1997). Microtubule-mediated transport of incoming herpes simplex virus 1 capsids to the nucleus. *J. Cell Biol.*, **136**, 1007–1021.

Steven, A. C. and Spear, P. G. (1997). Herpesvirus capsid assembly and envelopment. In *Structural Biology of Viruses*, ed. W. Chiu, R. M. Burnett, and R. L. Garcea, pp. 312–351. New York: Oxford University Press.

Steven, A. C., Roberts, C. R., Hay, J., Bisher, M. E., Pun, T., and Trus, B. L. (1986). Hexavalent capsomers of herpes simplex virus type 2: symmetry, shape, dimensions, and oligomeric status. *J. Virol.*, **57**, 578–584.

Tong, L., Qian, C., Massariol, M.-J., Bonneau, P. R., Cordingley, M. G., and Lagace, L. (1996). A new serine-protease fold revealed by the crystal structure of human cytomegalovirus protease. *Nature (London)*, **383**, 272–275.

Tong, L., Qian, C., Massariol, M. J., Deziel, R., Yoakim, C., and Lagace, L. (1998). Conserved mode of peptidomimetic inhibition and substrate recognition of human cytomegalovirus protease. *Nature Struct. Biol.*, **5**, 819–826.

Trus, B. L., Homa, F. L., Booy, F. P. *et al.* (1995). Herpes simplex virus capsids assembled in insect cells infected with recombinant baculoviruses: structural authenticity and localization of VP26. *J. Virol.*, **69**, 7362–7366.

Trus, B. L., Booy, F. P., Newcomb, W. W. *et al.* (1996). The herpes simplex virus procapsid: structure, conformational changes upon maturation, and roles of the triplex proteins VP19c and VP23 in assembly. *J. Mol. Biol.*, **263**, 447–462.

Trus, B. L., Gibson, W., Cheng, N., and Steven, A. C. (1999). Capsid structure of simian cytomegalovirus from cryoelectron microscopy: evidence for tegument attachment sites. *J. Virol.*, **73**, 2181–2192.

Trus, B. L., Heymann, J. B., Nealon, K. *et al.* (2001). Capsid structure of Kaposi's sarcoma-associated herpesvirus, a gammaherpesvirus, compared to those of an alphaherpesvirus, herpes simplex virus type 1, and a betaherpesvirus, cytomegalovirus. *J. Virol.*, **75**, 2879–2890.

Vernon, S. K., Lawrence, W. C., Long, C. A., Rubin, B. A., and Sheffield, J. B. (1982). Morphological components of herpesvirus. IV. Ultrastructural features of the envelope and tegument. *J. Ultrastruct. Res.*, **81**, 163–171.

Weinheimer, S. P., Boyd, B. A., Durham, S. K., Resnick, J. L., and O'Boyle, D. R., 2nd. (1992). Deletion of the VP16 open reading frame of herpes simplex virus type 1. *J. Virol.*, **66**, 258–269.

Welch, A. R., Woods, A. S., McNally, L. M., Cotter, R. J., and Gibson, W. (1991). A herpesvirus maturational proteinase, assemblin: identification of its gene, putative active site domain, and cleavage site. *Proc. Natl Acad. Sci. USA*, **88**, 10792–10796.

Wright, J. F., Kurosky, A., Pryzdial, E. L., and Wasi, S. (1995). Host cellular annexin II is associated with cytomegalovirus particles isolated from cultured human fibroblasts. *J. Virol.*, **69**, 4784–4791.

Wu, L., Lo, P., Yu, X., Stoops, J. K., Forghani, B., and Zhou, Z. H. (2000). Three-dimensional structure of the human herpesvirus 8 capsid. *J. Virol.*, **74**, 9646–9654.

Yu, X.-K., O'Connor, C. M., Atanasov, I., Damania, B., Kedes, D. H., and Zhou, Z. H. (2003). Three-dimensional structures of the A, B and C capsids of Rhesus monkey rhadinovirus: insights into gammaherpesvirus capsid assembly, maturation and DNA packing. *J. Virol.*, **77**, 14182–14193.

Yu, X., Trang, P., Shah, S. *et al.* (2005). Dissecting human cytomegalovirus gene function and capsid maturation by ribozyme targeting and electron cryomicroscopy. *Proc. Natl Acad. Sci. USA*, **102**, 7103–7108.

Zhou, Z. H., Prasad, B. V., Jakana, J., Rixon, F. J., and Chiu, W. (1994). Protein subunit structures in the herpes simplex virus A-capsid determined from 400 kV spot-scan electron cryomicroscopy. *J. Mol. Biol.*, **242**, 456–469.

Zhou, Z. H., He, J., Jakana, J., Tatman, J. D., Rixon, F. J., and Chiu, W. (1995). Assembly of VP26 in herpes simplex virus-1 inferred from structures of wild-type and recombinant capsids. *Nat. Struct. Biol.*, **2**, 1026–1030.

Zhou, Z. H., Chiu, W., Haskell, K. *et al.* (1998a). Refinement of herpesvirus B-capsid structure on parallel supercomputers. *Biophys. J.*, **74**, 576–588.

Zhou, Z. H., Macnab, S. J., Jakana, J., Scott, L. R., Chiu, W., and Rixon, F. J. (1998b). Identification of the sites of interaction between the scaffold and outer shell in herpes simplex virus-1 capsids by difference electron imaging. *Proc. Natl Acad. Sci. USA*, **95**, 2778–2783.

Zhou, Z. H., Chen, D. H., Jakana, J., Rixon, F. J., and Chiu, W. (1999). Visualization of tegument–capsid interactions and DNA in intact herpes simplex virus type 1 virions. *J. Virol.*, **73**, 3210–3218.

Zhou, Z. H., Dougherty, M., Jakana, J., He, J., Rixon, F. J., and Chiu, W. (2000). Seeing the herpesvirus capsid at 8.5 Å. *Science*, **288**, 877–880.

Zhu, H., Cong, J. P., Mamtora, G., Gingeras, T., and Shenk, T. (1998). Cellular gene expression altered by human cytomegalovirus: global monitoring with oligonucleotide arrays. *Proc. Natl Acad. Sci. USA*, **95**, 14470–14475.

4

Comparative analysis of herpesvirus-common proteins

Edward S. Mocarski, Jr.

Department of Microbiology & Immunology, Stanford University School of Medicine, CA, USA

Introduction

Despite the evolutionary and biological divergence represented by the nine human herpesviruses that have been classified into three broad subgroups, a large number of herpesvirus-common (core) gene products are evolutionarily conserved (Table 4.1 see chapter 2). These appear to carry out functions upon which every herpesvirus relies because all exhibit a common virion structure, a core genome replication process, and similar entry and egress pathways. These herpesvirus common functions are most often recognized through deduced protein sequence similarity that extends throughout alpha-, beta-, and gammaherpesviruses subfamilies infecting mammals, reptiles and birds (see Chapter 2, Table 2.2). These herpesviruses exhibit conservation that suggests a shared common ancestor at least 50 million years ago. Other evolutionarily distant herpesviruses infecting fish, amphibians, and invertebrates share less similarity with these better-studied herpesviruses, suggesting a common evolutionary origin dating back over 150 million years. In the more distant relatives, a common virion structure, genome organization and similarity across a small subset herpesvirus-common gene products provide the evidence of a common origin.

A few herpesvirus-common gene products have been recognized via a common enzymatic or binding activity long before any systematic genome sequence analysis became available. The homologous function of envelope glycoprotein B, DNA polymerase, alkaline exonuclease and single strand DNA binding protein, to give a few examples, emerged from biochemical studies in a number of herpesvirus systems. Given the high level of conservation and the importance of DNA synthesis as a target for antiviral inhibitors, these remain among the most broadly studied and best understood of the core gene products. DNA synthesis functions and virion structural components are also among the most highly conserved based on sequence comparisons. Importantly, however, common activity of well-recognized core functions, such as the DNA polymerase processivity factor, the smallest capsid protein or a capsid triplex component, is not based on the level of primary amino acid sequence identity, but rather is supported by a common role in several herpesviruses. Additional core functions initially recognized based on activity have undergone evolutionary divergence to take on new functions. For example, the large subunit of ribonucleotide reductase (HSV-1 *UL39* gene product), which associates with a small subunit to form an active enzyme in the alphaherpesviruses and gammaherpesviruses, is expressed without small subunit in the betaherpesviruses (HCMV, HHV-6, HHV-7) and completely lacks enzymatic activity. This leaves a question as to its true role. Thus, herpesvirus-common proteins may preserve common function as well as sequence homology, function with only limited sequence homology, or sequence homology with distinct function. Homologs may therefore be predicted to carry out similar functions in most situations, but will certainly not behave identically in all settings.

Herpesvirus-common gene products have been recognized as key proteins that form the characteristic herpesvirus virion structure and provide key common functions for the replicative cycle, beginning with entry into cells, continuing through the process of viral DNA synthesis and nucleic acid metabolism and concluding with capsid maturation and egress of virions. The presence of herpesvirus-common genes (see Chapter 2) allows predictions about functional conservation; however, most functional information has been derived from studies in a single or at most two herpesvirus subfamilies. The requirement for herpesvirus-common functions varies considerably with cell type, as well as between viruses of the same

Table 4.1. Identity, function and proposed nomenclature for known and putative functions of herpesvirus-common gene products of human herpesviruses

Common name[a]	Abbrev. name	HSV	VZV	HCMV	HHV 6/7	EBV	KSHV	Key function
Capsid								
major capsid protein[c]	MCP	UL19	40	UL86	U57	BcLF1	ORF25	hexon, penton, capsid structure
triplex monomer[c]	TRI1	UL38	20	UL46	U29	BORF1	ORF62	TRI1 and TRI2 assoc to form TRI complex, capsid structure
triplex dimer[c]	TRI2	UL18	41	UL85	U56	BDLF1	ORF26	
small capsid protein[b]	SCP	UL35	23	UL48A	U32	BFRF3	ORF65	capsid transport
portal protein	PORT	UL6	54	UL104	U76	BBRF1	ORF43	penton for DNA encapsidation
portal capping protein[c]	PCP	UL25	34	UL77	U50	BVRF1	ORF19	covers portal in mature virions
Tegument and cytoplasmic egress								
virion protein kinase	VPK	UL13	47	UL97	U69	BGLF4	ORF36	phosphorylation, regulation
largest tegument protein[c]	LTP	UL36	22	UL48	U31	BPLF1	ORF64	uncoating, secondary envelopment
LTP binding protein[b]	LTPbp	UL37	21	UL47	U30	BOLF1	ORF63	
encapsidation and egress protein[c]	EEP	UL7	53	UL103	U75	BBRF2	ORF42	nuclear egress
cytoplamsic egress tegument protein[b]	CETP	UL11	49	UL99	U71	BBLF1	ORF38	secondary envelopment, cytoplasmic egress
CETP binding protein[b]	CETPbp	UL16	44	UL94	U65	BGLF2	ORF33	
cytoplasmic egress facilitator-1[b]	CEF1	UL51	7	UL71	U44	BSRF1	ORF55	cytoplasmic egress
encapsidation chaperone protein[b]	ECP	UL14	46	UL95	U67	BGLF3	ORF34	TERbp chaperone
capsid transport tegument protein[c]	CTTP	UL17	43	UL93	U64	BGLF1	ORF32	capsid transport in the nucleus
cytoplasmic egress facilitator-2[b]	CEF2	UL21	38	UL88	U59	BTRF1	ORF23	egress, interact with CETPbp
		UL24	35	UL76	U49	BXRF1	ORF20	putative membrane or tegument
Envelope								
glycoprotein B[c]	gB	UL27	31	UL55	U39	BALF4	ORF8	heparan-binding, fusion
glycoprotein H[c]	gH	UL22	60	UL75	U48	BXLF2	ORF22	gH assoc, fusion
glycoprotein L[c]	gL	UL1	37	UL115	U82	BKRF2	ORF47	gL assoc, fusion
glycoprotein M[b]	gM	UL10	50	UL100	U72	BBRF3	ORF39	gN assoc
glycoprotein N[b]	gN	UL49A	9A	UL73	U46	BLRF1	ORF53	gM assoc
Regulation								
multifunctional regulator of expression[c]	MRE	UL54	4	UL69	U42	BSLF1 BMLF1	ORF57	transcriptional, RNA transport regulation
DNA Replication, recombination and metabolism								
DNA polymerase[c]	POL	UL30	28	UL54	U38	BALF5	ORF9	DNA synthesis
DNA polymerase processivity subunit[c]	PPS	UL42	16	UL44	U27	BMRF1	ORF59	POL processivity
helicase-primase ATPase subunit[c]	HP1	UL5	55	UL105	U77	BBLF4	ORF44	HP1, HP2 and HP3 assoc to form HP, unwinding and primer synthesis
helicase-primase RNA pol subunit B[c]	HP2	UL52	6	UL70	U43	BSLF1	ORF56	
helicase-primase subunit C[c]	HP3	UL8	52	UL102	U74	BBLF2 BBLF3	ORF40 ORF41	
single strand DNA binding protein[c]	SSB	UL29	29	UL57	U41	BALF2	ORF6	DNA fork, recombination
alkaline deoxyribonuclease[b]	NUC	UL12	48	UL98	U70	BGLF5	ORF37	recombination
deoxyuridine triphosphatase[b]	dUTPase	UL50	8	UL72	U45	BLLF3	ORF54	reduce dUTP
uracil-DNA glycosidase[b]	UNG	UL2	59	UL114	U81	BKRF3	ORF46	remove uracil from DNA
ribonucleotide reductase large subunit[b]	RR1	UL39	19	UL45	U28	BORF2	ORF61	active enzyme only in viruses with RR2
Capsid assembly, DNA encapsidation and nuclear egress								
maturational protease[c]	PR	UL26	33	UL80	U53	BVRF2	ORF17	capsid assembly, scaffolding, DNA encapsidation
assembly protein[c]	AP (NP)[d]	UL26.5 (UL26)	33.5 (33)	UL80.5 (UL80)	U53.5 (U53)	BdRF1 (BVRF2)	ORF17.5 (ORF17)	

(cont.)

Table 4.1. (cont.)

Common name[a]	Abbrev. name[a]	HSV	VZV	HCMV	HHV 6/7	EBV	KSHV	Key function
capsid **t**ransport **n**uclear **p**rotein[c]	CTNP	UL32	26	UL52	U36	BFLF1	ORF68	capsid transport to sites of DNA replication
terminase ATPase subunit 1[c]	TER1	UL15	42 45	UL89	U66	BGRF1 BDRF1	ORF29	TER1 and TER2 form TER, packaging machinery
terminase DNA binding subunit 2[c]	TER2	UL28	30	UL56	U40	BALF3	ORF7	
terminase **b**inding **p**rotein[c]	TERbp	UL33	25	UL51	U35	BFRF1A	ORF67	TER assoc
nuclear **e**gress **m**embrane **p**rotein[c]	NEMP	UL34	24	UL50	U34	BFRF2	ORF66	nuclear egress, primary envelopment
nuclear **e**gress **l**amina **p**rotein[c]	NELP	UL31	27	UL53	U37	BFLF2	ORF69	

[a] proposed.
[b] required for replication in some viruses or some settings.
[c] required for replication in all viruses and settings tested.
[d] AP and NP are related proteins derived from different primary translation products.

or different subfamilies. Currently, 36 of the 40 core functions have an impact on replication in at least one herpesvirus and in at least some experimental setting (Table 4.1), although many are not absolutely essential for replication in any of the herpesviruses where they have been studied. The striking cell type dependence of so many herpesvirus functions suggests that many of these proteins carry out activities that are redundant with other viral or cellular functions. This chapter will seek to deduce the general role of each core function based on data available in different systems. The phenotype of mutants showing even a modest growth defect under any conditions will be an important component for consideration. All core functions are likely to be important for viral replication and pathogenesis in the host even when considered dispensable for replication in cultured cells. While even limited information is useful, experimental confirmation across several distinct viruses builds confidence in the common role of homologs, but this information is limited in many cases.

All herpesviruses form particles that have a characteristic 125–130 nm icosohedral capsid containing a linear DNA genome, surrounded by a protein-containing tegument enclosed in a host-membrane derived lipid bilayer envelope modified by virus-encoded glycoproteins. The overall virion particle size ranges from 200 to 300 nm, depending on the particular virus. This common structure provides the strongest evidence for evolutionary conservation in the replication and maturation processes. The set of core, homologous open reading frames (ORFs) are predominantly involved in the processes of DNA replication through maturation and egress from cells (Fig. 4.1). These also facilitate estimations of the evolutionary relatedness of the three major subfamilies (alpha-, beta-, and gammaherpesviruses) comprising mammalian and avian herpesviruses (see Chapter 2). Recognizable sequence homologs of only three of these proteins (DNA polymerase, DUT and a terminase subunit are conserved in the genomes of every known herpesviruses, including those infecting amphibians, fish, and invertebrates. Of these, the gene for the terminase subunit is remarkable, producing a conserved spliced mRNA that remains a key genomic feature (Davison, 2002) of every herpesvirus genome that has been annotated. The nine distinct human herpesviruses, including three members of alphaherpesviruses (HSV-1, HSV-2 and VZV), four members of the betaherpesviruses (CMV, HHV-6A, HHV-6B and HHV-7) and two members of the gammaherpesviruses (EBV and KSHV/HHV-8) share 40 of the 43 ORFs that have been included in the core set (see Chapter 2 Table 2.2). Although widely distributed amongst alpha- and gammaherpesviruses characterized to date, a thymidine kinase (TK) and a small subunit of ribonuclease (RR2) are absent from all betaherpesviruses. Although all herpesviruses appear to use sequence-specific DNA binding proteins to initiate DNA replication, a homolog of DNA replication origin binding protein (OBP) is not conserved in cytomegaloviruses or gammaherpesviruses.

This chapter stresses common features, while evolution has clearly provided the herpesviruses with a broad canvas on which to evolve the remarkable range of biological properties that characterize individual members. Genome annotation and comparison has suggested a higher level of similarity within subfamilies than between biologically distinct subfamilies. Even though biological properties of the individual subfamily members are distinct, they retain a recognizable evolutionary link.

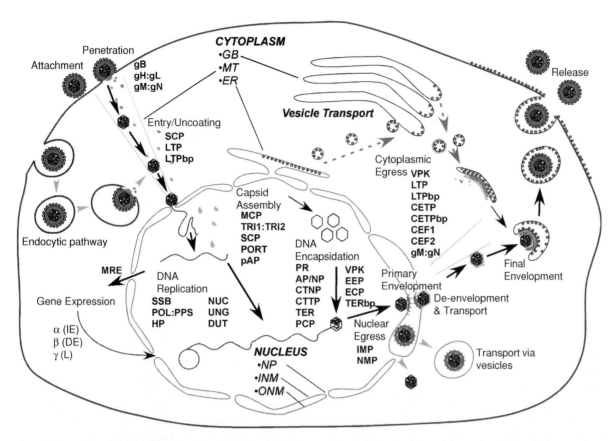

Fig. 4.1. Summary of replication functions carried out by herpesvirus-conserved gene products. Major steps in productive replication are indicated in larger font style and core functions contributing to each step are listed by their proposed abbreviated designations (see Table 4.1). The major entry pathway (black arrows) employs direct fusion at the cell surface (attachment and penetration), which is dependent upon gB and the gH:gL complex, followed by nucleocapsid transport along microtubules to nuclear pores where viral DNA is released into the nucleus. Alternatively, in certain cell types, entry follows the endocytic pathway and virion fusion with an endocytic vesicle (grey arrowheads). Uncoating requires the envelope fusion machinery (gB, gH:gL and in some cases gM:gN) as well as the LTP:LTPbp to direct docking at nuclear pores and release of virion DNA into the nucleus. Following entry and uncoating, one core regulatory protein (MRE) is involved in transcriptional and post-transcriptional regulation. DNA replication depends on several core replication fork proteins (SSB, POL:PPS, HP) as well as accessory functions (NUC, UNG, DUT). Capsid assembly uses MCP, TRI1:TRI2, SCP, and PORT. Pre-formed capsids translocate to sites of DNA replication where PRO, AP/NP (AP and NP are related proteins), CTNP, TER, TERbp and PCP, with possible accessory functions EEP, ECP and CTTP complete the encapsidation of viral DNA. Nuclear egress is controlled by NEMP and NELP. The main pathway of cytoplasmic egress (black arrows) and secondary (final) envelopment is controlled VPK, LTP:LTPbp, CETP, and CETPbp, with possible accessory proteins CEF1, CEF2 and gM:gN. Nucleocapsids are transported on MT and virion envelope glycoproteins follow vesicle transport to sites of final envelopment. Alternative maturation pathways of vesicle formation at the outer nuclear membrane with the mature virion following vesicle transport pathways or release of nucleocapsids directly through nuclear pores into the cytoplasm for transport to sites of final envelopment remain possible (grey arrowheads). Golgi body (GB), microtubules (MT) and endoplasmic reticulum (ER) are identified in the cytoplasm, and nuclear pores (NP), inner nuclear membrane (INM) and outer nuclear membrane (ONM) are identified in the nucleus. The cellular vesicle transport pathway from the ER to GB is also designated (dashed grey arrows).

There is little doubt that herpesviruses encode additional structurally related, functionally similar proteins that are not recognized as sequence homologs and all herpesvirus-common components cannot be recognized through sequence information alone. Other structural and functional properties complement sequence information and may constitute an independent set of criteria on which comparisons can be based. Relative position in a cluster of conserved ORFs, biological activity and the phenotype of mutant viruses all provide important comparative information. The existence of ORFs that fail to show sequence identity but are included in the list of core proteins due to other information, such as the functional information on DNA polymerase processivity subunit already mentioned, suggests future work will require consideration of a broader set of characteristics. Additional structural and functional homologs will likely emerge as viral proteins are studied in greater detail by X-ray diffraction as by well as computer programs that model primary amino acid sequence on known protein structures.

Available information on the activities of core functions has often been generated in only one of the nine human herpesviruses, sometimes using herpesviruses of veterinary interest (e.g., PRV) and sometimes using rodent herpesviruses (e.g., MCMV). The remarkable diversity in functional organization, replication, latency and disease patterns exhibited by diverse human herpesviruses contrast the common activities of core functions which are key to viral replication. Functions will therefore be presented in relationship to the virus replicative cycle, starting with virion structure and entry, proceeding through regulation of gene expression, DNA synthesis, processing, and packaging and, finally, maturation and egress. Some of the functions involved in entry are structural components that are also involved with maturation and release of progeny virus, but most of the core functions can be implicated in at least one step in the replication pathway, and this is sometimes dependent on cell type. These core replication processes, including entry into cells and viral DNA synthesis, as well as the overall scheme of assembly, maturation and egress occur via evolutionarily conserved proteins and mechanisms. The role of core functions is best understood where they have been subjected to study by a combination of genetics and cell biology, this is often in alphaherpesviruses such as HSV-1 and PRV or in betaherpesviruses such as HCMV and MCMV. There have been many reviews dealing with herpesvirus-common features and evolutionarily common themes that have emerged over the years, both from a biological perspective (Roizman, 1999; Roizman and Pellett, 2001) as well as from a variety of analyses derived from genomic sequence (Davison, 2002; Karlin *et al.*, 1994; McGeoch *et al.*, 2000).

There are several common genome features described in Chapter 2 beyond the ultrastructural appearance of capsids and core proteins described in Chapter 3. All herpesviruses have a linear DNA genome that is cleaved from concatemers formed during replication, which where known, uses a conserved recognition sequence and leaves single base 3 overhanging nucleotide at each genomic terminus (Mocarski and Roizman, 1982). The position of origins of DNA replication that control DNA synthesis during the replicative cycle is conserved in most herpesviruses with a common location adjacent to the conserved single stranded DNA binding protein gene. While exceptions exist, the common evolutionary origin of these viruses is very clear from the range of conserved *cis*-acting elements as well as proteins.

Virion structural proteins

The virion particle of herpesviruses consists of a DNA-containing nucleocapsid with 162 regularly arranged capsomeres arranged in a $T = 16$ icosohedral lattice forming the protein shell. Detailed structural information has been derived from cryo-electron micrograph (cryo-EM) reconstructions involving studies on several different herpesviruses (Chapter 3). In the virion, the nucleocapsid is covered by a protein matrix or tegument that is surrounded by a lipid bilayer envelope derived from host cell membranes into which at least a dozen viral envelope proteins are inserted. Human herpesviruses have been estimated to have as few as 37 (e.g., alphaherpesviruses) and to well over 50 (e.g., cytomegaloviruses) virion proteins (Bortz *et al.*, 2003; Johannsen *et al.*, 2004; Kattenhorn *et al.*, 2004; Varnum *et al.*, 2004; Zhu *et al.*, 2005). About half (22) of the herpesvirus-conserved proteins are components of the virion, providing a genetic basis for the common ultrastructural appearance of all herpesviruses. Additional core proteins collaborate with structural proteins during maturation and egress (see below). Although similar in size, herpesvirus nucleocapsids package double-stranded DNA genomes range from a low of 125 kilobase pairs (VZV) to a high of 240 kilobase pairs (CCMV), which is remarkable given such a uniform capsid shell. The virion provides protection of the viral genome during transmission and mediates a two-stage entry process, first a fusion event between the envelope and cellular membranes that leads to release of the nucleocapsid into the cytoplasm and second a trafficking event that delivers the viral nucleocapsid to the nucleus where the genome is released.

Icosohedral herpesvirus capsids are composed of five herpesvirus-conserved proteins, the major capsid protein (MCP, HSV-1 *UL19* gene product), triplex monomer and dimer proteins (TRI1 and TRI2, HSV-1 *UL38* and *UL18* gene products, respectively), the smallest capsid protein (SCP, HSV-1 *UL35* gene product) and the portal protein (PORT, HSV-1 *UL6* gene product). The 150 hexons that make up the bulk of the capsid consist of six MCP molecules together with six molecules of SCP. Eleven of the 12 capsid pentons consist of five MCP molecules without SCP. One specialized penton consists of 12 molecules of PORT and has an axial channel for entry and exit of viral

DNA. The 125–130 nm diameter capsid has a wall that is 15 nm thick. Although different in shape, each hexon and penton appears cylindrical. Based on cryo-EM studies of HSV-1, HCMV, and KSHV (Chapter 3), the hexons and pentons are held in place by interactions between their bases on the inner side as well as by interconnections via triplexes located midway through the capsid shell. Detailed analyses suggests that beta- and gammaherpesvirus capsids resemble one another more closely than either resembles alphaherpesvirus capsids. Although the least conserved of the structural proteins, SCP is located at hexon tips, and absent from penton tips, in all herpesviruses (Yu et al., 2005). There is a discernible SCP ring around hexons in HSV-1 where this structure contributes to the shape of the outermost capsid surface. Although widely conserved, the SCP is not universally essential for virion maturation and is, for example, dispensable for HSV-1 replication in cell lines (Desai et al., 1998) but essential for HCMV replication (Borst et al., 2001). Thus, the nucleocapsid of every human herpesvirus consists entirely of herpesvirus-conserved proteins, but the functional requirements for capsid maturation vary to some extent.

A large number of tegument proteins are located between the capsid and envelope in herpesviruses. Tegument proteins carry out a remarkably diverse range of activities during infection, although the most well-characterized functions and the most abundant tegument proteins in any herpesvirus are often not in the core set. Eleven proteins are conserved (see Chapter 2). Many are essential for replication in those viruses that have been subjected to systematic study, HSV-1 (Roizman and Knipe, 2001), PRV (Mettenleiter, 2004) and HCMV (Dunn et al., 2003; Yu et al., 2003). In HSV-1, five of the conserved tegument proteins are essential for replication (HSV-1 *UL7*, *UL17*, *UL25*, *UL36*, and *UL37* gene products), including a largest tegument protein (LTP, HSV-1 *UL36* gene product) and the protein that binds to the largest tegument protein (LTPbp) encoded by the adjacent (*UL37*) gene. These play roles in entry as well as in egress. The viral serine–threonine protein kinase (VPK, HSV-1 *UL13* gene product), and five additional tegument proteins (homologues of HSV-1 *UL11*, *UL14*, *UL16*, *UL21*, and *UL51* gene products) exhibit compromised growth, sometimes in specific cell types or under certain growth conditions. In contrast, HCMV requires an overlapping, but distinct set of seven homologs to replicate, without an absolute need for some that are essential in HSV-1. In HCMV, the LTP (UL48), UL77 and UL93 (homologs of HSV-1 *UL36*, *UL25*, and *UL17*, respectively) as well as UL99, UL95, UL94, and UL71 (homologs of HSV-1 *UL11*, *UL14*, *UL16*, and *UL51*, respectively) are required for replication when the entire ORF is eliminated (Dunn et al., 2003). Mutants in the LTPbp (UL47) and UL103 (homologs of HSV-1 *UL37*, and *UL7*, respectively) as well as mutants in VPK and UL88 genes exhibit a reduced level of growth. While it is possible that some of these differences stem from experimental variability or the choice of different host cells in which to study mutants, evolutionary differences are likely to dictate the extent to which each virus relies on overlapping functions as well as the extent to which functional redundancy occurs. HSV-1 UL11 and HCMV UL99 proteins are known as small myristolated tegument proteins, localize to cytoplasm of infected cells, and are involved in the latter stages of virion egress. The HSV-1, *UL11* protein interacts with two other conserved tegument proteins, *UL14* and *UL16* as well as with the envelope glycoprotein, gM, which is part of the gM/gN glycoprotein complex. Although ultrastructural analysis does not provide much information on tegument organization, an association between the LTP:LTPbp complex with the SCP ring or with triplexes in the region of the capsid vertices has been suggested with HSV-1. Investigation of tegument protein activities and capsid : tegument interactions remain important areas for experimental investigation.

One additional protein is conserved amongst herpesviruses, represented by the *UL24* gene of HSV-1 about which little is known. The HCMV homologue (UL76), a minor tegument constituent that is essential for replication (Dunn et al., 2003), localizes in a pattern that suggests it may be involved in regulating events immediately following infection or during maturation (Wang et al., 2004).

One enzyme contained in this set of conserved proteins, VPK apparently acts in tandem with host cell cycle kinases to regulate a variety of replication events. VPK ensures efficient phosphorylation of other viral proteins, some of which have been reported to increase the efficiency of the host translation machinery as well as other events in gene expression and DNA replication extending from early times during infection to egress. This enzyme is dispensable for replication in alphaherpesviruses as well as in rapidly dividing host cells infected with HCMV where its role is presumably redundant with host protein kinases, possibly including Cdk2. A requirement for VPK is most readily demonstrated in primary, non-dividing host cells that have lower levels of host cell kinases. VPK is also critical for efficient replication in host animals. Interestingly, the homologue in HCMV (UL97) as well as in HHV-6B is a nucleoside kinase required for phosphorylation of the antiviral drug ganciclovir, in addition to being a protein kinase. The UL97-encoded VPK is also the primary target of a candidate antiviral compound, maribavir, which is specifically active against HCMV and EBV, but not other herpesviruses.

Human herpesvirus envelopes are estimated to carry between 12 (HSV-1) and 20 (HCMV) viral integral membrane proteins. Many envelope proteins are specific to each herpesvirus type. Five, gB, gH, gL, gM, and gN, are conserved broadly amongst herpesviruses. Sequence conservation resulted in the adaptation of a common nomenclature for structural glycoproteins, using names originally applied to HSV-1 envelope constituents. Although these names do not imply function, they are now widely used by investigators in the field. One gene product that is an O-glycosylated glycoprotein in some herpesviruses, gN, does not undergo glycosylation in some alphaherpesviruses, such as HSV-1 and VZV. Furthermore, the specific interaction between gH and gL drives stable expression of these proteins, suggesting that they are molecular chaperones as well as functional partners. A similar relationship also appears to occur with gM and gN. Although gB does not form a complex with other viral proteins, complexes of gH:gL and gM:gN form in cells and associate with cellular membranes to be incorporated into the viral envelope of progeny virions during egress. In betaherpesviruses and gammaherpesviruses, gH:gL complexes may be further modified by additional viral glycoproteins that influence cell tropism.

Entry into host cells

Attachment and entry, which typically occurs by fusion with the plasma membrane is followed by translocation of the nucleocapsid through the cytoplasm and delivery of viral genome to the cell nucleus (Fig. 4.1). This process involves a series of distinct steps that have each received varying amounts of attention in different human herpesviruses: (i) binding to specific cell surface receptors, (ii) fusion of envelope with the cellular membrane to release nucleocapsids into the cytoplasm, (iii) nucleocapsid association with cytoskeletal elements and translocation towards the nucleus, (iv) nucleocapsid interaction with nuclear pores and (v) release of the viral genome into the nucleus (see Fig. 4.1). These steps are controlled by unique as well as herpesvirus-common functions. The first step in this process involves multiple cell surface components interacting with viral envelope glycoproteins in a stepwise process that leads to membrane fusion and delivery of the nucleocapsid to the cytoplasm of host cells (Spear, 2004; Spear and Longnecker, 2003) (see specific chapters on individual viruses). Attachment to cells has been studied in most human herpesviruses and usually requires both unique and conserved, sometimes functionally redundant, viral envelope glycoproteins. With the apparent exception of EBV, cell surface proteoglycans such as heparan sulfate play a role for initial contact with cells. Heparan sulfate-dependent entry has been demonstrated in alpha- (HSV-1, VZV), beta- (HCMV, HHV-6A, HHV-6B, HHV-7) and gammaherpesvirus (KSHV/HHV-8) subfamily members (Spear, 2004; Spear and Longnecker, 2003). As a result, many herpesviruses exhibit a broad cell tropism for attachment and entry steps. In these eight human herpesviruses, gB and typically other unique viral envelope proteins exhibit heparan sulfate binding activity and direct the first attachment step in entry. Binding appears to be part of the essential role of gB in the viruses where the process has been dissected. In EBV, gB lacks the domain that controls interaction with the glycosaminoglycan and this step does not seem to be required for entry. In addition to the initial binding step, viruses where entry has been studied in detail engage additional receptors using herpesvirus-conserved as well as unique viral envelope proteins. Attachment steps may rely on unique viral envelope proteins such as EBV gp350/220, which interacts with host CD21 and EBV gH:gL:gp42 complex which interacts with MHC class II protein, KSHV K8.1A which interacts with proteoglycan, or HSV-1 gD, which interacts with nectins as well as a TNF receptor family member. In some herpesviruses conserved envelope glycoproteins are responsible for subsequent steps, such as the role of KSHV gB in binding to integin $\alpha3\beta1$ or the role of HCMV gB in binding to the EGF receptor, although these may be more important in the fusion step (Spear and Longnecker, 2003). Thus, except for initial contact with proteoglycan, herpesvirus attachment mechanisms appear unique to each type of virus.

In most cells that have been studied, binding through specific cellular receptors leads to fusion of the viral envelope and plasma membrane, releasing the viral nucleocapsid into the cytoplasm. Fusion typically occurs at the plasma membrane and is under the control of the herpesvirus-conserved envelope glycoproteins, gB and gH:gL which are essential for this step in all studied herpesviruses. In HCMV gH:gL may associate with additional unique proteins that provide receptor specificity, either gO encoded by UL74 or a complex of glycoproteins encoded by UL128, UL130. In HHV-6, either gO encoded by V47 or gQ encoded by U100 provide specificity. There are parallels in human beta- and gammaherpesviruses. In EBV, the presence of gp42-containing complexes reduces epithelial cell tropism, whereas the presence of gp42-free complexes reduces tropism for B lymphocytes (Borza and Hutt-Fletcher, 2002). gM:gN complex is required for entry in some settings, a feature that suggests this complex may also contribute to host cell specificity. Although entry by fusion at the plasma membrane is the most common entry mechanism, entry via endocytosis has been characterized in some systems (Fig. 4.1). EBV entry into epithelial cells occurs by fusion directly at the cell surface whereas entry into B lymphocytes involves endocytosis (see Chapter 24). The viral functional requirements for different entry processes are still incompletely understood. Thus, both major modes of virus entry may be employed by herpesviruses depending on the setting. Signaling that results from gB or gH:gL binding to cellular receptors has also been implicated as a step in replication but no common themes have emerged from such studies. Essential core glycoproteins seem to play key roles for entry, rather than later in the replication cycle or during egress. All core glycoproteins are incorporated into infected cell membranes as well as into the virion envelope. The evolutionarily conserved manner in which gB and gH:gL control membrane fusion between the viral envelope and plasma membrane has been studied most extensively in the alphaherpesviruses where mutations in each of these gives rise to syncytial viral strains that have provided initial clues to gene products controlling this step.

Herpesviruses exploit normal cytoplasmic transport systems that control cell shape and vesicular traffic, making use of tubulin-containing microtubules and actin-containing microfilaments (Dohner and Sodeik, 2004) to control nucleocapsid transit through the cytoplasm. Like many viruses that traverse the cytoplasm, herpesviruses rely on microtubules to gain access to the nucleus and nuclear pores where uncoating is completed and the viral genome is released into the nucleoplasm. This process was suspected long ago, initially in studies with adenoviruses and herpesviruses (Dales, 1973) and has been the focus of growing attention. Microtubule-destabilizing drugs such as nocadazole and colchacine block transport and entry (Mabit et al., 2002). Net transport proceeds towards microtubule minus ends that terminate at the microtubule organizing center, which is located adjacent to the nucleus. The bidirectional nature of microtubule-directed transport (Welte, 2004) allows these filaments to act as the major highways of virus particle translocation during entry as well as egress (Fig. 4.1). Microfilaments do not play as direct a role during entry; however, evidence suggests depolymerization of the actin-containing cortex may be a requisite event during entry (Jones et al., 1986). Intracellular transport mechanisms that have been intensively studied in neurotropic alphaherpesviruses, predominantly HSV-1, HSV-2 and PRV, because of the requirement to translocate across long expanses of cytoplasm. Herpesvirus-conserved capsid proteins appear to rely on common cellular pathways for movement in neurons as well as all other cell types. Nucleocapsid movement occurs in both directions on microtubules (Smith and Enquist, 2002) and is likely to be regulated in ways similar to vesicle transport (Welte, 2004). Minus-end-directed transport during entry depends on the dynein:dynactin motor complex (Dohner et al., 2002), which is the same motor used for directional vesicle transport. Although still controversial, contact between the SCP of HSV-1 and the cellular constituent of the dynein complex, RP3 (and possibly other proteins) has been implicated in transport (Douglas et al., 2004), suggesting that this herpesvirus-conserved protein may play a similar role in other viruses. Thus, a common bridge may be built between the nucleocapsid and the microtubule to allow an appropriate direction of movement to initiate infection. Thereafter, capsid and tegument proteins act in concert to release viral DNA into the nucleus at nuclear pores although the exact process that occurs once the nucleocapsid reaches the nucleus remains largely unexplored. A conditional, temperature sensitive HSV-1 mutant together with biochemical studies have long implicated the herpesvirus-common LTP in the uncoating process (Chapter 7). The LTP of HSV-1 is needed for uncoating and release of viral DNA at nuclear pores. Studies of other tegument proteins have employed null mutants propagated on cells that complement function in egress, and result in virions that contain the protein. This approach generally masks any role tegument proteins play during entry, leaving this an important area for future exploration.

Regulation of gene expression and replication

Most regulatory proteins encoded by herpesviruses are unique. Only one core protein is purely regulatory, acting as a multifunctional regulator of expression (MRE). MRE has been most extensively studied in HSV-1 (see Chapter 9) where it is the product of *UL54* called ICP27, and EBV (Hiriart et al., 2003) where it is the product of BMLF1 called EB2. MRE binds RNA and localizes to sites of transcription in the nucleus and interacts with components of the RNA polymerase II transcription machinery, the spliceosome complex and pre-mRNA export machinery. MRE stimulates late gene transcription (Jean et al., 2001) and dictates the location of viral transcripts in infected cells (Pearson et al., 2004). MRE is best known for impeding cellular mRNA splicing to allow the mostly intronless viral transcripts to be preferentially exported from the nucleus (Sandri-Goldin, 2001). During the early phase of infection, MRE causes splicing to stall by recruiting host cell kinases to the nucleus to inactivate splicing factors through phosphorylation. In alphaherpesvirus and gammaherpesvirus systems, MRE also recruits an export adaptor protein (Aly/REF) to sites of viral transcription to facilitate export. This inhibition is relieved during the late phase of infection when splicing and export of host and viral transcripts resumes. Based on studies in HCMV (Lischka et al., 2006; Toth et al., 2006), the function of betaherpesvirus MRE interacts with an RNA helicase, UAP56 to promote cytoplasmic accumulation of unspliced mRNA, and this process is independent of an RNA-binding motif. The MRE may also influence shut-off of the host cell and transcriptional events through a mechanism(s) that remains to be elucidated. Although the level of sequence conservation among MRE homologs is quite limited, others appear to carry out regulatory activities and are sometimes incorporated into the virion tegument, such as in HCMV (Mocarski and Courcelle, 2001).

Viral DNA synthesis and nucleotide metabolism

All herpesviruses encode a core set of six DNA synthesis enzymes that direct the synthesis of viral DNA during productive (lytic) infection. Herpesviruses initiate lytic DNA replication at defined sites on the viral genome that are readily assayed as virus-infection-dependent autonomously replicating sequences. Some herpesviruses have a single origin of DNA replication (ori_{Lyt}), such as in the betaherpesviruses (HCMV, HHV-6A, HHV-6B, HHV-7). Others have either two (VZV, EBV, KSHV) or three (HSV-1, HSV-2) ori_{Lyt} sites that retain sequence homology, although the reason for multiple origins in the biology of viruses that carry them remains a mystery. The relative position of one copy of ori_{Lyt} adjacent to the single stranded DNA binding protein (SSB) gene is conserved in many alpha-, beta- and gammaherpesviruses, even though the primary DNA sequence of ori_{Lyt} is not conserved in all of these settings. All herpesviruses appear to rely on virus-encoded DNA binding proteins to control initiation at ori_{Lyt}. In alphaherpesviruses and the reseolavirus subgroup of betaherpesviruses, a dedicated *ori* binding protein (OBP, HSV-1 *UL9* gene product) is essential for replication. Gammaherpesviruses and cytomegaloviruses rely on DNA binding regulatory proteins that control gene expression and also function during initiation of replication.

In general, DNA replication of herpesviruses, as in other DNA viruses, starts near nuclear structures, called nuclear domain 10, which become disrupted in the course of viral infection. This process overtakes the nucleus and leads to the formation of large, distinct replication compartments where viral replication proteins and DNA accumulate (Wilkinson and Weller, 2003). Viral DNA levels can equal cellular DNA content at late times of infection. Herpesvirus DNA replication proceeds through either of two potential mechanisms that have continued to be the focus of experimental investigation. Initial models of herpesvirus DNA replication have been analogous to bacteriophage lambda (Kornberg and Baker, 1992), starting with genome circularization and theta form replication for which evidence is scant and proceeding to a rolling circle form which has been experimentally well documented (Boehmer and Lehman, 1997; Boehmer and Nimonkar, 2003; Lehman and Boehmer, 1999). This model is based on the existence of ori_{Lyt} sites and site-specific DNA binding proteins and the expectation that the viral genome circularizes upon entry into cells. More recently, a recombination-dependent branching mechanism has been proposed (Wilkinson and Weller, 2003) and supported by the failure to detect circular intermediates during infection as well as by the behavior of HSV-1 mutants that exhibit increased accumulation of circular genomes early after infection (Jackson and DeLuca, 2003). This model has been reinforced by the observation that circular forms of HSV-1 DNA do not correlate with productive replication, but rather with latency. A mechanism analogous to that in the T even bacteriophages (Kornberg and Baker, 1992) has been suggested (Wilkinson and Weller, 2003). Either mechanism of synthesis results in the production of multi-genomic length concatemers that are the substrate for progeny genome packaging using conserved viral gene products. Distinct DNA replication origins separate from ori_{Lyt} sites that are responsible for the synthesis of viral DNA during latent infection have been identified in gammaherpesviruses but not in other subfamilies.

There are two structural categories of ori_{Lyt}. In alphaherpesviruses and non-CMV betaherpesviruses that rely on OBP, the initiation of DNA replication involves a targeted unwinding to enable the assembly of a replication fork complex. This process is best understood in HSV-1. An OBP complex with the viral single stranded DNA binding protein (SSB; HSV-1 *UL29* gene product also called ICP8) unwinds DNA and binds specific sequence motifs (called Box I and Box II in HSV-1) that are symmetrically arranged within ori_{Lyt} (Macao et al., 2004). This allows a more dramatic unwinding at an AT-rich region that is located between Box I and Box II followed by replication fork machinery initiating uni- or bidirectional replication (Boehmer and Lehman, 1997). Beta- and gammaherpesviruses rely on DNA-binding transactivators that are not conserved between subfamilies but act in an analogous fashion to increase transcription across the ori_{Lyt} region which opens the DNA and allows interaction with replication machinery (Xu et al., 2004). Studies in HCMV, EBV and KSHV have all provided evidence for a transcriptional activator-dependent initiation that appears to be distinct from OBP-dependent initiation in alphaherpesviruses and the betaherpesviruses like HHV-6. The betaherpesvirus HCMV encodes a virion-associated transcript that associates with ori_{Lyt} to form a three-stranded structure whose precise role in DNA synthesis is still under investigation (Prichard et al., 1998). The replication fork machinery includes a highly conserved set of six herpesvirus gene products: SSB, a viral catalytic subunit of DNA polymerase (POL; HSV-1 *UL30* gene product) and associated polymerase processivity subunit (PPS; HSV-1 *UL42* gene product) and a heterotrimeric helicase-primase (HP) consisting of an ATPase subunit (HP1; HSV-1 *UL5* gene product), a primase subunit (HP2; HSV-1 *UL52* gene product) and an accessory subunit (HP3; HSV-1 *UL8* gene product). These proteins direct continuous, leading strand viral DNA replication in a rolling circle mode when used in cell-free assays (Boehmer and Lehman, 1997; Boehmer and Nimonkar, 2003; Lehman and Boehmer, 1999). Following OBP binding to specific sites in ori_{Lyt}, an interaction with single stranded DNA binding protein (SSB) leads to localized unwinding and access of replication fork proteins. Specific interaction of the HP complex with the OBP and synthesis of RNA primers may be an intermediary step leading to DNA replication mediated by the POL–PPS complex. Recombination-directed initiation may be the consequence of SSB and HP activities (Boehmer and Nimonkar, 2003) and may underlie continued viral DNA synthesis (Wilkinson and Weller, 2003; Wilkinson and Weller, 2004). Thus, these six functions provide the core DNA synthesis machinery and mediate homologous recombination during viral replication. Cellular enzymes such as ligase and topoisomerases are highly likely to be required for replication; however, a complete understanding of the steps of herpesvirus DNA replication awaits the development of defined cell-free assay conditions.

Although a high level of recombination has long been associated with herpesvirus replication (Wilkinson and Weller, 2003) and with the isolated biochemical properties of replication proteins (Boehmer and Nimonkar, 2003), only recently has this process received some support as a component of DNA replication (Jackson and DeLuca, 2003). Under conditions where replication is blocked, the HSV-1 genome circularizes more efficiently, suggesting an association of circularization with latency rather than productive replication. Though provocative, this work provides little insight into the steps required for herpesvirus replication. The circumstantial evidence that recombination plays some role either early or late in replication remains strong. In addition to its role in coating single stranded DNA at the replication fork, SSB of HSV-1 appears to direct recombination in a manner similar to *E. coli* RecA (Kornberg and Baker, 1992). Homologous recombination requires SSB as well as another herpesvirus-conserved gene product, alkaline deoxyribonuclease (NUC, HSV-1 *UL12* gene product) (Wilkinson and Weller, 2003; Wilkinson and Weller, 2004). Interestingly, this DNase is absolutely required for HCMV replication (Dunn et al., 2003). In addition to the contribution of sequence specific recombination to DNA replication, circularization of the genome may itself be dependent on recombination and number of herpesviruses that undergo genome isomerization via a recombination event mediated by the *a* sequence which is located at genomic ends and at an internal junction (Mocarski and Roizman, 1982).

Two different nucleotide metabolism enzymes are also broadly conserved, deoxyuridine triphosphatase (DUT; HSV-1 *UL50* gene product) and uracil-DNA glycosidase (UNG; HSV-1 *UL2* gene product). These seem to play accessory roles in replication that are redundant with cellular enzymes. The DUT eliminates pools of dUTP, preventing the incorporation of deoxyuridine into viral DNA and produces dUMP which can be converted to TTP through cellular pathways. The DUT appears to be inactive as an enzyme in betaherpesviruses. UNG cleaves deaminated cytosines (uracil) from the sugar backbone of DNA, leading to base excision and the activation of cellular DNA repair synthesis. In cytomegalovirus, where UNG is required for replication in quiescent cells, the process of uracil incorporation and excision has been proposed to introduce strand breaks that facilitate DNA replication (Courcelle et al., 2001). Functions that are important for replication in nondividing cells where cellular nucleotide metabolism enzymes would be low or absent appear to be critical for replication in the host where differentiated cells lack cellular DNA metabolism enzymes.

Finally, the large subunit of ribonucleotide reductase (RR1, HSV-1 *UL39* gene product) is conserved in all herpesviruses; however, RR1 only forms an active enzyme with a small subunit (RR2, HSV-1 *UL40* gene product) in alphaherpesviruses and gammaherpesviruses. Somewhat surprisingly, betaherpesviruses retain an RR1 that lacks enzymatic activity and do not carry a homolog of RR2 at all. RR1 may have role in cell death suppression in the betaherpesviruses as well as in some alphaherpesviruses.

Capsid assembly and DNA encapsidation

The basic features of herpesvirus capsid maturation common to all herpesviruses have been established through a combination of work with HSV-1 infected cells, recombinant baculovirus-infected cells (Thomsen et al., 1994) and, importantly, cell-free systems (Newcomb et al., 1996). Assembly employs the herpesvirus-conserved components of the capsid shell (MCP, SCP, TRI1 and TRI2) working in conjunction with a precursor of the assembly protein (pAP, HSV-1 *UL26.5* gene product). Assembly of HSV-1 capsids can proceed without SCP, but at a lower efficiency. A protease (PR, also called assemblin) is required to mature the capsid. This protein is made as a precursor consisting of PR as its amino terminus fused to a longer polypeptide that contains the pAP sequence as its carboxyl end (together called prePR, e.g., HSV-1 UL26 gene product). PR is a serine protease that processes both pAP and prePR. The protease domain self-cleaves in prePR to release PR as well as a variant of pAP, and also processes the carboxyl terminus of PR, pAP, and all variants of pAP (Gibson, 1996). This processing leads to the production of multiple forms of pAP, all colinear at the carboxyl terminus. The presence of pAP is sufficient for capsid assembly, but the presence of prePR, its self-cleavage to PR and variant pAP, and its cleavage of pAP to AP are all necessary for DNA encapsidation to proceed following capsid assembly. In addition, PORT is completely dispensable for the formation of normal appearing capsids, however, this protein is absolutely required for encapsidation of viral DNA. PORT associates with pAP in order to be incorporated into capsids (Newcomb et al., 2003; Singer et al., 2005). During infection, pNP must be cleaved into PR and variant AP for encapsidation to follow capsid formation but both of these proteins, as well as AP, are absent from capsids once encapsidation has occurred. Phosphorylation by VPK has been implicated in the encapsidation step (Wolf et al., 2001).

Once herpesvirus DNA has replicated, encapsidation is controlled by a conserved *cis*-acting element (cleavage/packaging or *pac* site) and a series of seven herpesvirus conserved *trans*-acting functions (Yu and Weller, 1998). Encapsidation has been most extensively studied in alphaherpesviruses but these studies have implications for all herpesviruses. Although initially assigned roles in viral DNA packaging, two of the conserved proteins play roles in transporting preformed capsids to DNA replication compartments, the sites of viral DNA synthesis where packaging also occurs. These two proteins, capsid transport tegument protein (CTTP, HSV-1 *UL17* gene product) and capsid transport nuclear protein (CTNP, HSV-1 *UL32* gene product) are necessary for packaging to proceed. Little is known about the way that these proteins work, except that CTTP is a virion tegument protein and may bind to the capsid (Thurlow et al., 2005). CTNP is a non-structural protein and remains in the nucleus.

Packaging of progeny viral genomes follows a modified head full packaging process reminiscent of bacteriophage λ (Campbell, 1994). Capsid localization, packaging and cleavage of viral DNA are regulated by the conserved VPK as well as by cellular kinases. VPK and cellular kinases may be redundant. The packaging machinery includes a heterodimeric terminase (TER) consisting of an ATPase subunit (TER1; HSV-1 *UL15* gene product) encoded by a conserved spliced gene and a DNA recognition subunit (TER2; HSV-1 *UL28* gene product). This machinery associates with the vertex of the specialized portal penton for the introduction of a free end of a viral DNA concatemer. The PORT protein interacts with TER and brings the packaging machinery and viral DNA to the capsid vertex. This machinery controls the threading of one genome length of DNA into the capsid before scanning for a *pac* site and determining the position of DNA cleavage and therefore the genomic ends. Thus, packaging and cleavage reactions are triggered by *pac* elements located near genomic termini, typically within terminal repeats (*a* sequences). The *pac* signal is composed of at least two elements, referred to as *pac* 1 and *pac* 2, and is broadly conserved among herpesviruses such that the *pac* from HCMV can direct packaging into HSV-1 virions (Spaete and Mocarski, 1985). All studies thus far have suggested that packaging yields single base 3′ extensions at both genomic ends and that packaging proceeds directionally with regard to the viral genome orientation as originally determined for HSV-1 (Mocarski and Roizman, 1982). The conservation of signals, functions and structure strongly suggests that this process is similar across all herpesviruses.

The heterodimeric TER, which is non-structural, and the portal complex, which takes the place of one penton of the capsid, associate with two additional conserved proteins, a TER binding protein (TERbp, HSV-1 *UL33* gene product) that interacts with capsids independent of PORT and a portal capping protein (PCP; HSV-1 *UL25* gene product). PCP remains associated with the nucleocapsid after packaging and thus appears as a minor capsid protein in mature virions. These five proteins are sufficient for recognition of a *pac* site on multi-genome DNA concatamers, docking with the appropriate site on a capsid, threading viral DNA into the caspid, cleavage at a *pac* site and sealing the genome into the progeny nucleocapsid (Fig. 4.1). As such they define a set of viral functions that are likely to be required for genome packaging in all herpesviruses. Once DNA has been packaged and PCP has covered the portal, the packaging stage of replication is completed and the nucleocapsid undergoes initial envelopment at the inner nuclear membrane (Fig. 4.1).

Two additional nuclear proteins, HSV-1 *UL7* and *UL14* gene products contribute to events in capsid maturation or DNA packaging. The *UL14* gene product is a minor tegument protein that appears to act as an encapsidation chaperone protein (ECP) to bring SCP and TERbp into the nucleus (Nishiyama, 2004). The *UL7* gene product appears to act as an encapsidation and egress protein (EEP), colocalizing with capsids in patterns that suggest a role in DNA encapsidation or egress from the nucleus.

Maturation

Following the formation of the nucleocapsid, the best evidence from several systems suggests that tegument proteins function together with non-structural proteins to control a complex two-stage envelopment and egress process that starts in the nucleus and leads to virion release by exocytosis at the plasma membrane. This two-stage envelopment process has been controversial but strong evidence has accumulated in favor of this pathway in all three herpesvirus subfamilies. The alphaherpesviruses HSV-1 and PRV have been extensively studied, along with the betaherpesviruses HCMV and MCMV (Mettenleiter, 2002; Mettenleiter, 2004). Evidence suggests that nuclear egress starts with primary envelopment at the inner nuclear membrane followed by a de-envelopment event at the outer nuclear membrane, a process that releases the nucleocapsid into the cytoplasm (Fig. 4.1). Secondary envelopment occurs in the cytoplasm at endosomal (or possibly Golgi complex) membranes with resulting vesicles carrying the fully mature virions to the cell surface using the cellular exocytic pathway. Alternatively, the older model of egress has the enveloped viral particle itself following a vesicle transport pathway without deenvelopment (Roizman and Knipe, 2001) (see Chapter 10). These steps, like the initial entry process, rely on membrane fusion events; however, envelopment and egress are relatively independent of viral envelope glycoproteins that play critical roles during entry. Non-replicating mutants in gB or the gH:gL complex mature normally but show defects in entry. Only the gM:gN complex may contribute to secondary, or final, envelopment.

Initial envelopment event occurs at the inner nuclear membrane, following and dependent upon genome packaging that produces nucleocapsids. Capsids lacking DNA do not mature efficiently and nucleocapsids must localize correctly in the nucleus to properly egress. Studies in alphaherpesviruses and betaherpesviruses have shown that two conserved proteins form a nuclear egress complex on the inner nuclear membrane to control egress from the nucleus (Mettenleiter, 2004) and disruption of the nuclear lamina. The nuclear egress membrane protein (NEMP, HSV-1 *UL34* gene product) acts as a type II membrane-spanning protein to anchor the nuclear egress lamina protein (NELP, HSV-1 *UL31* gene product), a phosphoprotein that interacts with the nuclear lamina as well as with membrane-associated NEMP. NEMP and NELP are dependent on one another for proper transport and localization to the inner nuclear membrane. Additional viral proteins or the process of viral maturation itself appear to be necessary for the formation of the nuclear egress complex. Direct binding to nucleocapsids has not been observed, however, the complex recruits viral and/or cellular protein kinases that appear to be important for phosphorylation and disruption of the nuclear lamina to allow egress. Viral mutants in NEMP or NELP are debilitated for egress, likely unable to bud through the inner nuclear membrane (primary envelopment) and so accumulate nucleocapsids inside nuclei. The nuclear egress complex may also participate in membrane fusion events at the outer nuclear membrane that are required to deposit the nucleocapsid in the cytoplasm (de-envelopment). Although NEMP, as a primary envelope protein, and NELP, as a primary tegument protein, are important components of primary virions, neither is retained in fully mature virions.

Primary envelopment delivers viral particles to the perinuclear space between the inner and outer nuclear membranes, a compartment contiguous with the endoplasmic reticulum. Over the past 10 years evidence has accumulated in several different herpesviruses that final herpesvirus envelopment occurs in the cytoplasm at late endosomal or Golgi body membranes. It is likely that primary envelopment is followed by a de-envelopment step that releases the nucleocapsid into the cytoplasm. It remains possible, but topologically unlikely that nucleocapsids move to the cytoplasm without any envelopment step through modified nuclear pores. Either way, movement of nucleocapsids to sites of final envelopment appears to be a microtubule-dependent process. Protein kinases appear to play regulatory roles in primary envelopment as well as de-envelopment occurring at the outer nuclear membrane or endoplasmic reticulum. In alphaherpesvirus, viral US3 kinase facilitates these processes by facilitating phosphorylation of NEMP or other proteins. Primary envelopment and de-envelopment may also rely on cellular kinases. In HCMV, the conserved VPK contributes to nuclear egress (Krosky et al., 2003) whereas in other betaherpesviruses such as MCMV, host protein kinase C has been implicated in nuclear egress (Muranyi *et al.*, 2002). All of this data suggests that there is redundancy and possible interplay between viral and host kinases (presumably in conjunction with host phosphatases) in establishing the appropriate phosphorylation state for egress from the nucleus.

While some virion tegument proteins are associated with nucleocapsids during nuclear egress, many are added in the cytoplasm. Major tegument proteins, though not conserved, localize to the cytoplasm in all herpesviruses that have been studied and it now appears that the bulk of tegument proteins found in mature herpesvirus virions are added to the nucleocapsid as it traverses the cytoplasm or at sites of final envelopment. There is currently little precise understanding of how nucleocapsids engage microtubules to traverse the cytoplasm, how final envelopment at endosomal (or Golgi complex) membranes occurs or how tegument proteins might be added prior to final envelopment. There is growing suspicion that addition may be nucleated by the conserved, very large LTP:LTPbp protein complex (Mettenleiter, 2004). This and a number of additional interactions between tegument proteins (Vittone et al., 2005) may be important in function. Current evidence on alphaherpesviruses and betaherpesviruses suggests that a conserved cytoplasmic egress tegument protein (CETP, HSV-1 *UL11* gene product) plays a central role in the secondary, or final, envelopment process. In alphaherpesviruses and betaherpesviruses, CETP is a myrisoylated and pamitoylated protein that localizes to the cytoplasmic face of cellular membranes and is known to interact with another herpesvirus-conserved tegument protein, the CETP binding protein (CETPbp, HSV-1 *UL16* gene product). Together, these may form a complex involved in transport. An additional tegument protein called cytoplasmic egress facilitator 1 (CEF1, HSV-1 *UL51* gene product) is a palmitated protein that is conserved amongst herpesviruses and also associates with cytoplasmic membranes (Nishiyama, 2004). In PRV, mutants in CEF1 fail to egress properly. One final tegument protein, called cytoplasmic egress facilitator 2 (CEF2, HSV-1 *UL21* gene product) enhanced maturation and interacts with CETPbp. Limited evidence supports a role for the gM:gN complex in secondary envelopment, particularly when disrupted together with *UL11*(Kopp et al., 2004; Tischer et al., 2002), although this complex is dispensable for replication in a number of other alphaherpesviruses, including HSV-1. Both gM and gN are essential for HCMV replication (Dunn et al., 2003) as well as for assembly in EBV (Lake and Hutt-Fletcher, 2000). gM:gN is a major EBV structural component and has recently been recognized as the major glycoprotein complex on the HCMV envelope (Varnum et al., 2004).

Thus, final envelopment occurs in the cytoplasm and, as a consequence the tegument of virions includes small amounts of cellular proteins, in particular actin (Bortz et al., 2003; Johannsen et al., 2004; Kattenhorn et al., 2004; Varnum et al., 2004; Zhu et al., 2005), as well as RNAs (Sciortino et al., 2001; Terhune et al., 2004) that may represent a quantitative sampling of the cytosol, although a role for any virion component in replication cannot be discounted as yet. Once final envelopment has occurred, exocytosis is believed to carry the mature virion inside of a vesicle to the cell surface for release. Thus, the final step in egress is fusion of an exocytic vesicle with the plasma membrane, a process that is likely to follow cellular vesicle trafficking pathways (Fig. 4.1).

This analysis of the role of herpesvirus-conserved gene products has attempted to evaluate data generated in a wide variety of systems. As a result, some data will certainly have been generalized inappropriately as further investigation reveals unique characteristics or distinguishing activities. While many common names are already in use across the different herpesviruses, the hope is that a common nomenclature for herpesvirus-common functions should emerge to facilitate comprehension of work in otherwise diverse systems. This presentation is intended to provide a starting point for evaluation of data on herpesvirus core functions no matter what virus system is being studied or discussed.

REFERENCES

Boehmer, P. E., and Lehman, I. R. (1997). Herpes simplex virus DNA replication. *Annu. Rev. Biochem.*, **66**, 347–384.

Boehmer, P. E. and Nimonkar, A. V. (2003). Herpes virus replication. *IUBMB Life*, **55**(1), 13–22.

Borst, E. M., Mathys, S., Wagner, M., Muranyi, W., and Messerle, M. (2001). Genetic evidence of an essential role for cytomegalovirus small capsid protein in viral growth. *J. Virol.* **75**(3), 1450–1458.

Bortz, E., Whitelegge, J. P., Jia, Q. et al. (2003). Identification of proteins associated with murine gammaherpesvirus 68 virions. *J. Virol.*, **77**(24), 13425–13432.

Borza, C. M. and Hutt-Fletcher, L. M. (2002). Alternate replication in B cells and epithelial cells switches tropism of Epstein–Barr virus. *Nat. Med.*, **8**(6), 594–599.

Campbell, A. (1994). Comparative molecular biology of lambdoid phages. *Annu. Rev. Microbiol.*, **48**, 193–222.

Courcelle, C. T., Courcelle, J., Prichard, M. N., and Mocarski, E. S. (2001). Requirement for uracil-DNA glycosylase during the transition to late-phase cytomegalovirus DNA replication. *J. Virol.*, **75**(16), 7592–7601.

Dales, S. (1973). Early events in cell-animal virus interactions. *Bacteriol. Rev.*, **37**(2), 103–135.

Davison, A. J. (2002). Evolution of the herpesviruses. *Vet. Microbiol.*, **86**(1–2), 69–88.

Desai, P., DeLuca, N. A., and Person, S. (1998). Herpes simplex virus type 1 VP26 is not essential for replication in cell culture but influences production of infectious virus in the nervous system of infected mice. *Virology*, **247**(1), 115–124.

Dohner, K. and Sodeik, B. (2004). The role of the cytoplasm during viral infection. *Curr. Top. Microbiol. Immunol.*, **285**, 67–108.

Dohner, K., Wolfstein, A., Prank, U. et al. (2002). Function of dynein and dynactin in herpes simplex virus capsid transport. *Mol. Biol. Cell*, **13**(8), 2795–2809.

Douglas, M. W., Diefenbach, R. J., Homa, F. L. *et al.* (2004). Herpes simplex virus type 1 capsid protein VP26 interacts with dynein light chains RP3 and Tctex1 and plays a role in retrograde cellular transport. *J. Biol. Chem.*, **279**(27), 28522–28530.

Dunn, W., Chou, C., Li, H. *et al.* (2003). Functional profiling of a human cytomegalovirus genome. *Proc. Natl Acad. Sci. USA*, **100**(24), 14223–14228.

Gibson, W. (1996). Structure and assembly of the virion. *Intervirology*, **39**(5–6), 389–400.

Hiriart, E., Bardouillet, L., Manet, E. *et al.* (2003). A region of the Epstein-Barr virus (EBV) mRNA export factor EB2 containing an arginine-rich motif mediates direct binding to RNA. *J. Biol. Chem.*, **278**(39), 37790–37798.

Jackson, S. A. and DeLuca, N. A. (2003). Relationship of herpes simplex virus genome configuration to productive and persistent infections. *Proc. Natl Acad. Sci. USA*, **100**(13), 7871–7876.

Jean, S., LeVan, K. M., Song, B., Levine, M., and Knipe, D. M. (2001). Herpes simplex virus 1 ICP27 is required for transcription of two viral late (gamma 2) genes in infected cells. *Virology*, **283**(2), 273–284.

Johannsen, E., Luftig, M., Chase, M. R. *et al.* (2004). Proteins of purified Epstein–Barr virus. *Proc. Natl Acad. Sci. USA*, **101**(46), 16286–16291.

Jones, N. L., Lewis, J. C., and Kilpatrick, B. A. (1986). Cytoskeletal disruption during human cytomegalovirus infection of human lung fibroblasts. *Eur. J. Cell Biol.*, **41**(2), 304–312.

Karlin, S., Mocarski, E. S., and Schachtel, G. A. (1994). Molecular evolution of herpesviruses: genomic and protein sequence comparisons. *J. Virol.* **68**(3), 1886–1902.

Kattenhorn, L. M., Mills, R., Wagner, M. *et al.* (2004). Identification of proteins associated with murine cytomegalovirus virions. *J. Virol.*, **78**(20), 11187–11197.

Kopp, M., Granzow, H., Fuchs, W., Klupp, B., and Mettenleiter, T. C. (2004). Simultaneous deletion of pseudorabies virus tegument protein UL11 and glycoprotein M severely impairs secondary envelopment. *J. Virol.*, **78**(6), 3024–3034.

Kornberg, A. and Baker, T. A. (1992). *DNA Replication*. 2nd edn. New York: W. H. Freeman and Company.

Krosky, P. M., Baek, M. C., and Coen, D. M. (2003). The human cytomegalovirus UL97 protein kinase, an antiviral drug target, is required at the stage of nuclear egress. *J. Virol.*, **77**(2), 905–914.

Lake, C. M. and Hutt-Fletcher, L. M. (2000). Epstein–Barr virus that lacks glycoprotein gN is impaired in assembly and infection. *J. Virol.*, **74**(23), 11162–11172.

Lehman, I. R. and Boehmer, P. E. (1999). Replication of herpes simplex virus DNA. *J. Biol. Chem.*, **274**(40), 28059–28062.

Lischka, P., Toth, Z., Thomas. M., Mueller, R., and Stamminger, T. (2006). The UL69 transactivator protein of human cytomegalovirus interacts with DEXD&H-Box RNA helicase UAP56 to promote cytoplasmic accumulation of unspliced RNA. *Mol. Cell. Biol.* **26**(5), 1631–1643.

Mabit, H., Nakano, M. Y., Prank, U. *et al.* (2002). Intact microtubules support adenovirus and herpes simplex virus infections. *J. Virol.*, **76**(19), 9962–9971.

Macao, B., Olsson, M., and Elias, P. (2004). Functional properties of the herpes simplex virus type I origin-binding protein are controlled by precise interactions with the activated form of the origin of DNA replication. *J. Biol. Chem.*, **279**(28), 29211–29217.

McGeoch, D. J., Dolan, A., and Ralph, A. C. (2000). Toward a comprehensive phylogeny for mammalian and avian herpesviruses. *J. Virol.*, **74**(22), 10401–10406.

Mettenleiter, T. C. (2002). Herpesvirus assembly and egress. *J. Virol.*, **76**(4), 1537–1547.

Mettenleiter, T. C. (2004). Budding events in herpesvirus morphogenesis. *Virus Res.* **106**(2), 167–180.

Mocarski, E. S., Jr., and Courcelle, C. T. (2001). Cytomegaloviruses and their replication. In *Fields Virology*, 4th edn., ed. D. M. Knipe, P. M. Howley, D. E. Griffin *et al.*, Vol. 2, pp. 2629–2673. Philadelphia: Lippincott, Williams & Wilkins.

Mocarski, E. S. and Roizman, B. (1982). Structure and role of the herpes simplex virus DNA termini in inversion, circularization and generation of virion DNA. *Cell*, **31**(1), 89–97.

Muranyi, W., Haas, J., Wagner, M., Krohne, G., and Koszinowski, U. H. (2002). Cytomegalovirus recruitment of cellular kinases to dissolve the nuclear lamina. *Science*, **297**(5582), 854–857.

Newcomb, W. W., Homa, F. L., Thomsen, D. R. *et al.* (1996). Assembly of the herpes simplex virus capsid: characterization of intermediates observed during cell-free capsid formation. *J. Mol. Biol.*, **263**(3), 432–446.

Newcomb, W. W., Thomsen, D. R., Homa, F. L., and Brown, J. C. (2003). Assembly of the herpes simplex virus capsid: identification of soluble scaffold-portal complexes and their role in formation of portal-containing capsids. *J. Virol.*, **77**(18), 9862–9871.

Nishiyama, Y. (2004). Herpes simplex virus gene products: the accessories reflect her lifestyle well. *Rev. Med. Virol.* **14**(1), 33–46.

Pearson, A., Knipe, D. M., and Coen, D. M. (2004). ICP27 selectively regulates the cytoplasmic localization of a subset of viral transcripts in herpes simplex virus type 1-infected cells. *J. Virol.*, **78**(1), 23–32.

Prichard, M. N., Jairath, S., Penfold, M. E., St Jeor, S., Bohlman, M. C., and Pari, G. S. (1998). Identification of persistent RNA–DNA hybrid structures within the origin of replication of human cytomegalovirus. *J. Virol.*, **72**(9), 6997–7004.

Roizman, B. (1999). HSV gene functions: what have we learned that could be generally applicable to its near and distant cousins? *Acta Virol.* **43**(2–3), 75–80.

Roizman, B., and Knipe, D. M. (2001). Herpes simplex viruses and their replication. In *Fields Virology*, 4th edn., ed. D. M. Knipe, P. M. Howley, D. E. Griffin *et al.*, Vol. 2, pp. 2399–2459. 2 vols. Philadelphia: Lippincott, Williams and Wilkins.

Roizman, B. and Pellett, P. E. (2001). The family Herpesviridae: A Brief Introduction. In *Fields Virology*, 4th edn., ed. D. M. Knipe, P. M. Howley, D. E. Griffin *et al.*, Vol. 2, pp. 2221–2230. 2 vols. Philadelphia: Lippincott, Williams & Wilkins.

Sandri-Goldin, R. M. (2001). Nuclear export of herpes virus RNA. *Curr. Top. Microbiol. Immunol.*, **259**, 2–23.

Sciortino, M. T., Suzuki, M., Taddeo, B., and Roizman, B. (2001). RNAs extracted from herpes simplex virus 1 virions: apparent selectivity of viral but not cellular RNAs packaged in virions. *J. Virol.*, **75**(17), 8105–8116.

Singer, G. P., Newcomb, W. W., Thomsen, D. R., Homa, F. L., and Brown, J. C. (2005). Identification of a region in the herpes simplex virus scaffolding protein required for interaction with the portal. *J. Virol.*, **79**(1), 132–139.

Smith, G. A. and Enquist, L. W. (2002). Break ins and break outs: viral interactions with the cytoskeleton of Mammalian cells. *Annu Rev Cell Dev. Biol.*, **18**, 135–161.

Spaete, R. R. and Mocarski, E. S. (1985). The a sequence of the cytomegalovirus genome functions as a cleavage/packaging signal for herpes simplex virus defective genomes. *J. Virol.*, **54**, 817–824.

Spear, P. G. (2004). Herpes simplex virus: receptors and ligands for cell entry. *Cell Microbiol* **6**(5), 401–410.

Spear, P. G. and Longnecker, R. (2003). Herpesvirus entry: an update. *J. Virol.*, **77**(19), 10179–10185.

Terhune, S. S., Schroer, J., and Shenk, T. (2004). RNAs are packaged into human cytomegalovirus virions in proportion to their intracellular concentration. *J. Virol.*, **78**(19), 10390–10398.

Thomsen, D. R., Roof, L. L., and Homa, F. L. (1994). Assembly of herpes simplex virus (HSV) intermediate capsids in insect cells infected with recombinant baculoviruses expressing HSV capsid proteins. *J. Virol.*, **68**(4), 2442–2457.

Thurlow, J. K., Rixon, F. J., Murphy, M., Targett-Adams, P., Hughes, M., and Preston, V. G. (2005). The herpes simplex virus type 1 DNA packaging protein UL17 is a virion protein that is present in both the capsid and the tegument compartments. *J. Virol.*, **79**(1), 150–158.

Tischer, B. K., Schumacher, D., Messerle, M., Wagner, M., and Osterrieder, N. (2002). The products of the UL10 (gM) and the UL49.5 genes of Marek's disease virus serotype 1 are essential for virus growth in cultured cells. *J. Gen. Virol.*, **83**(Pt 5), 997–1003.

Toth, Z., Lischka, P., and Stamminger, T. (2006). RNA-binding of the human cytomegalovirus transactivator protein UL69, mediated by arginine-rich motifs, is not required for nuclear export of unspliced RNA. *Nucleic Acids Res.* **34**(4), 1237–1249.

Varnum, S. M., Streblow, D. N., Monroe, M. E. *et al.* (2004). Identification of proteins in human cytomegalovirus (HCMV) particles: the HCMV proteome. *J. Virol.*, **78**(20), 10960–10966.

Vittone, V., Diefenbach, E., Triffett, D., Douglas, M. W., Cunningham, A. L., Diefenbach, R. J. (2005). Determination of interactions between tegument proteins of herpes simplex virus type 1. *J. Virol.* **79**(15), 9566–9571.

Wang, S. K., Duh, C. Y., and Wu, C. W. (2004). Human cytomegalovirus UL76 encodes a novel virion-associated protein that is able to inhibit viral replication. *J. Virol.*, **78**(18), 9750–9762.

Welte, M. A. (2004). Bidirectional transport along microtubules. *Curr. Biol.*, **14**(13), R525–R537.

Wilkinson, D. E. and Weller, S. K. (2003). The role of DNA recombination in herpes simplex virus DNA replication. *IUBMB Life*, **55**(8), 451–458.

Wilkinson, D. E., and Weller, S. K. (2004). Recruitment of cellular recombination and repair proteins to sites of herpes simplex virus type 1 DNA replication is dependent on the composition of viral proteins within prereplicative sites and correlates with the induction of the DNA damage response. *J. Virol.*, **78**(9), 4783–4796.

Wolf, D. G., Courcelle, C. T., Prichard, M. N., and Mocarski, E. S. (2001). Distinct and separate roles for herpesvirus-conserved UL97 kinase in cytomegalovirus DNA synthesis and encapsidation. *Proc. Natl Acad. Sci. USA*, **98**(4), 1895–1900.

Xu, Y., Cei, S. A., Rodriguez Huete, A., Colletti, K. S., and Pari, G. S. (2004). Human cytomegalovirus DNA replication requires transcriptional activation via an IE2- and UL84-responsive bidirectional promoter element within oriLyt. *J. Virol.*, **78**(21), 11664–11677.

Yu, D. and Weller, S. K. (1998). Herpes simplex virus type 1 cleavage and packaging proteins UL15 and UL28 are associated with B but not C capsids during packaging. *J. Virol.*, **72**(9), 7428–7439.

Yu, D., Silva, M. C., and Shenk, T. (2003). Functional map of human cytomegalovirus AD169 defined by global mutational analysis. *Proc. Natl Acad. Sci. USA*, **100**(21), 12396–12401.

Yu, X., Shah, S., Atanasov, I. *et al.* (2005). Three-dimensional localization of the smallest capsid protein in the human cytomegalovirus capsid. *J. Virol.*, **79**(2), 1327–1332.

Zhu, F. X., Chong, J. M., Wu, L., and Yuan, Y. (2005). Virion proteins of Kaposi's sarcoma-associated herpesvirus. *J. Virol.*, **79**(2), 800–811.

Part II

Basic virology and viral gene effects on host cell functions: alphaherpesviruses

Edited by Gabriella Campadelli-Fiume and Bernard Roizman

part II

5

Genetic comparison of human alphaherpesvirus genomes

Joel D. Baines[1] and Philip E. Pellett[2]

[1]College of Veterinary Medicine, Cornell University, Ithaca, NY, USA
[2]Lerner Research Institute, The Cleveland Clinic, Cleveland, OH, USA

Human herpesviruses 1, 2, and *3* (herpes simplex virus 1 (HSV-1), herpes simplex virus 2 (HSV-2), and varicella-zoster virus (VZV)) have been classified as alphaherpesviruses based originally upon their biological properties, and subsequently on the sequences of their respective genomes (Minson *et al.*, 2000; Pellett and Roizman, in press). All of these viruses maintain latent infections in sensory ganglia, and can productively infect a variety of human cells, including the living cells of mucous membranes and skin. These epithelial sites also provide exit points for the virus to infect other individuals.

The structure of the genomes of the alphaherpesviruses that infect humans are quite similar at first glance (Fig. 5.1). All have two unique segments that are flanked by repeats of different lengths. The unique segments are designated short (S) and long (L) and the repeats designated as internal (IR) or terminal (TR). Members of the genus simplexvirus (HSV-1 and HSV-2) exist as four roughly equimolar isomers, each isomer differing in the relative orientations of the long and short components. The orientation of one of the HSV isomers has been designated prototypical, and could therefore be designated TRL-U_L-IRL-IRS-U_S-TRS. VZV also produces 4 genomic isomers, but those in which the long component is inverted are significantly reduced in frequency, to about 5% of total genomes. It is tempting to speculate that this is a consequence of the shorter repeats flanking the VZV long component (88.5 bp) as compared to the repeats flanking U_S in human alphaherpesviruses (6000–7400 bp) and U_L in HSV-1 and HSV-2 (around 9,000 bp). The shorter repeat region would be expected to reduce the frequency of homologous recombination events leading to less frequent inversion of the long component in VZV genomes.

The 129 kbp VZV genome is the smallest genome of the human herpesviruses, whereas the HSV-1 and HSV-2 genomes are over 152 kbp in length. The G + C content of the human simplexviruses is around 68% whereas the VZV genome is only 46% G + C. Thus, considerable numbers of mutations have occurred since the two lineages arose from a common progenitor. All three viruses encode well-conserved sequences that guide lytic replication (oriLyt) and genome cleavage and packaging (Frenkel & Roffman 1996). Copies of oriLyt are present in IRS and TRS of all three viruses, and near the center of L for HSV-1 and HSV-2.

Several features are apparent in the global sequence comparisons shown in Fig. 5.2. HSV-1 and HSV-2 are much more closely related to each other than is either to VZV. HSV-1 and HSV-2 genomes are most similar in their U_L components, and least similar in the inverted repeats that bound U_L (TRL and IRL). The VZV sequence is most closely related to HSV in their U_L components. These observations can be extended by measuring the level of sequence identity along the dot plot diagonal, as shown in the nucleotide sequence similarity plot for HSV-1 vs. HSV-2 (Fig. 5.3). As can be seen, the similarity is highest across U_L, with most of the peaks corresponding to protein coding regions, and the valleys to intergenic regions, the exceptions being U_L 42 through U_L 44, and U_L 49. The L component repeats are much less well conserved, with the peak of similarity being in the region encoding ICP0 (RL2). The most highly conserved region in the S component repeats is the ICP4 gene (RS1). Overall, U_S is less well conserved than U_L. This region includes the U_S 4 (gG) gene, which is approximately 1500 bp longer in HSV-2 than in HSV-1 and represents the region of greatest dissimilarity between HSV-1 and HSV-2.

The gene arrangement in the long component of the most common isomer of the VZV genome is inverted relative to the U_L of the prototypical isomer of HSV (Fig. 5.1). With this inversion in mind, the genes in the HSV-1 and HSV-2 U_L segments are mostly collinear with VZV U_L (Fig. 5.2), and all but a few U_L genes are conserved across all human alphaherpesviruses. This consideration also underscores the significance of the overall similarity of the genes,

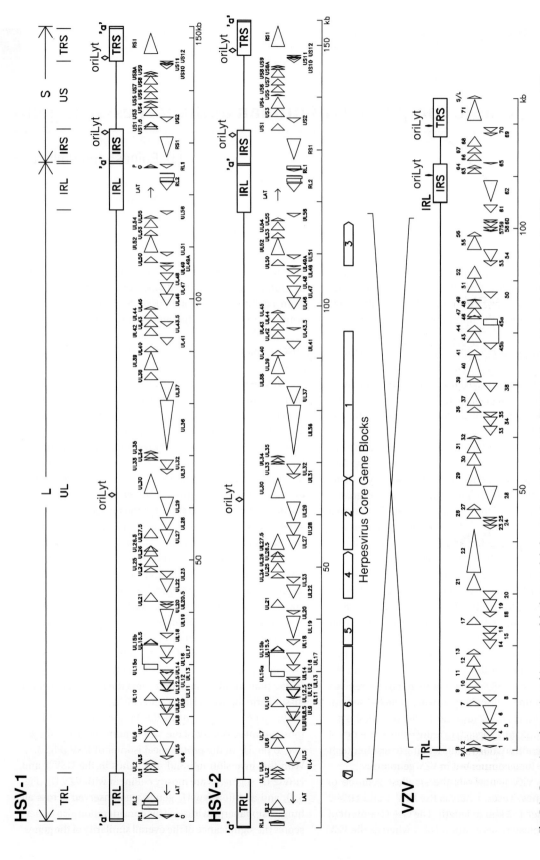

Fig. 5.1. Genomic and genetic architectures of the human alphaherpesviruses. Note that the VZV L component is inverted relative to the HSV prototypic arrangement. The representations are based primarily on annotations in Genbank Accession numbers X14112 (HSV-1 strain 17), Z86099 (HSV-2 strain HG52), and X04370 (VZV strain Dumas), and information in references cited in the text. L, long component; S, short component; TRL, long component terminal repeat; IRS, short component internal repeat; TRS, short component terminal repeat.

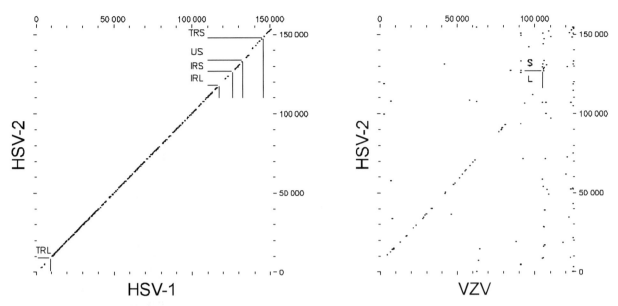

Fig. 5.2. Global genome sequence similarity comparisons among the human alphaherpesviruses. Dot similarity plots were constructed from comparisons of complete genome sequences. For HSV-1 vs. HSV-2, the window was 50 and the stringency was 45 identical residues. For HSV-2 vs. VZV, the window was 50 and the stringency was 25 identical residues. This reduced stringency was needed, because there were no dots when the HSV-2 and VZV were compared at the same stringency used for the HSV-1/HSV-2 comparison. Because the prototypic genomes of HSV-2 and VZV have relatively inverted L components, the HSV-2/VZV comparison was done with a VZV sequence in which the L component was inverted. Sequence sources and abbreviations are the same as for Fig. 5.1.

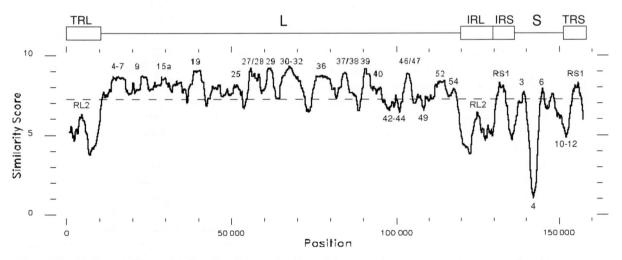

Fig. 5.3. Nucleotide sequence similarity between HSV-1 and HSV-2. HSV-1 and HSV-2 nucleotide sequences were aligned in approximately 20 kb segments, the aligned segments were joined to generate genome-length alignments, and then the similarity along the aligned genomes was plotted as a running percentage of identity in windows of 2000 residues. x-axis positions do not correspond precisely to genomic coordinates because of spaces inserted during the alignment. Boundaries of major architectural features are indicated, as are the locations of various genes along the plot. Sequence sources and abbreviations are the same as for Fig. 5.1.

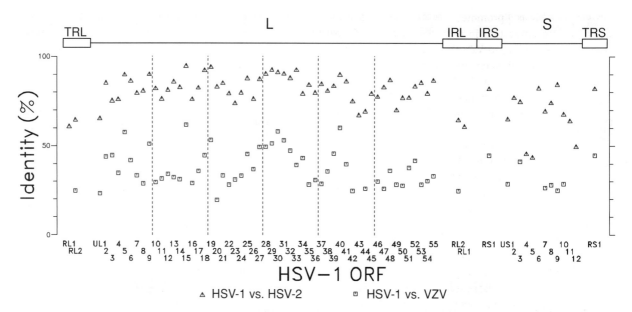

Fig. 5.4. Amino acid sequence identities between proteins encoded by the human alphaherpesviruses. Homologous protein sequences were aligned, and the percentage of identical residues determined in comparisons between HSV-1 and HSV-2 (triangles), and between HSV-1 and VZV (squares). Identity scores were plotted as a function of their location in the HSV-1 genome, relative to the major genomic architectural features. As detailed in the text, some HSV genes do not have identified homologues in VZV, and vice versa, and some genes are encoded within and in frame with others (and are thus not represented individually in this figure). Sequence sources and abbreviations are the same as for Fig. 5.1.

suggesting that they are considerably constrained by their respective functions. The most highly conserved genes between VZV and HSV-1 (HSV U_L 5, U_L 15, U_L 30, and U_L 40) are among the most highly conserved between HSV-1 and HSV-2 (Fig. 5.4). Their encoded proteins are enzymes involved in DNA replication and metabolism. This suggests that there is both little external pressure for these genes to change and little tolerance for accepting the products of random mutation. The least conserved genes between HSV-1 and HSV-2 are encoded in the S component and TRL/IRL; as detailed below, many of these genes do not have homologues between HSV and VZV. These gene products are likely to be important in defining the precise biological niche occupied by each virus.

VZV genes that are absent from HSV genomes

Although homologues of most long component genes exist in HSV-1, HSV-2 and VZV, there are some notable exceptions. Six VZV U_L genes have no homologue in the HSV U_L (ORF1, ORF2, ORF13, ORF32, ORF57 and ORF S/L). All of these genes are dispensable for replication in cell culture in at least some cell types.

ORF1 encodes an integral membrane protein of approximate M_r 17 000 with a C-terminal hydrophobic domain. Its function is not known, but it is completely dispensable for growth of the virus in MeWo cells (Cohen and Seidel, 1995). Equine herpesvirus 1 (EHV-1) and EHV-4 are both members of the genus *Varicellovirus* in the subfamily *Alphaherpesvirinae* (Telford *et al.*, 1992, 1995). Although these viruses encode a gene (termed EHV gene 2) in a position that corresponds to VZV ORF1, it has no obvious similarity with the VZV counterpart.

VZV ORF2 also encodes a phosphorylated membrane-associated protein that is dispensable for growth in cell culture and establishment of latency in dorsal root ganglia of cotton rats (Sato *et al.*, 2002). Genes with very limited homology with VZV ORF2 are present in other Varicelloviruses including gene 3 of EHV-1 and EHV-4. The functions of these genes are not known.

VZV ORF13 encodes thymidylate synthetase. Interestingly, homologues are not present in other alphaherpesviruses, but the genomes of several gammaherpesviruses, including human herpesvirus 8, herpesvirus saimiri, herpesvirus ateles, and equine herpesvirus 2 contain functional homologues. Moreover, human cytomegalovirus upregulates cellular thymidine synthetase (Gribaudo *et al.*, 2002). Thus, incorporation into the viral genome, or other means of upregulation of thymidylate synthetase in the host cell likely confers a selective advantage to these viruses, possibly as it promotes availability of nucleotides for viral DNA replication in quiescent cells. Within the region corresponding to VZV ORF13, HSV-1 and HSV-2 encode U_L 45, which is encoded on the opposite strand and has no homologue in VZV. The U_L 45 gene encodes a type II membrane protein that is dispensable for replication in cell culture (Cockrell and Muggeridge 1998; Visalli and Brandt 1991).

VZV ORF32 is homologous to gene 34 of EHV-1 and EHV-4, but has no counterparts in other herpesvirus genera. The encoded protein of 16,000–18,000 M_r is posttranslationally modified by the ORF47 protein kinase and is dispensable for change replication in cell culture and the establishment of latency (Reddy et al., 1998; Sato et al., 2003).

VZV ORF57 is located in a region of unusually high diversity among the U_L segments of alphaherpesvirus genomes. VZV ORF57 has no sequence similarity to genes in herpesviridae for which DNA sequence data are available. In HSV, the corresponding region encodes no obvious open reading frame, and in fact has served as an insertion site for the expression of exogenous genes and bacterial artificial chromosome vector sequences without obvious detriment to the virus in cultured cells or animals (Baines and Roizman, 1991; Tanaka et al., 2003). On the other hand, the region between U_L 3 and U_L 4 in the Suid herpesvirus 1 (Pseudorabies virus or PRV) genome encodes gene U_L 3.5 that is necessary for viral egress (Fuchs et al., 1996). Like VZV ORF57, the PRV U_L 3.5 has no obvious homologue in any other herpesvirus.

ORF S/L is also unique to VZV. The encoded protein is located in the cytoplasm of infected cells and varies in size from about 21 000–30 000 apparent M_r among different VZV strains (Kemble et al., 2000). The initiation codon of ORF S/L lies at the right end of TRS with translation crossing into the L component (this requires genome circularization or concatemerization). VZV ORF B is translated from within the same ORF, but initiates within the L component, terminating at the same stop codon as ORF S/L (Mahalingam et al., 2000). The functions of either protein are unknown.

L component genes unique to the simplexviruses

Unless otherwise noted, it should be assumed that the following genes are encoded by HSV-1 and HSV-2, but not VZV.

The 248 residue ORF P lies in the repeats bordering U_L (TRL and IRL). The associated transcript is antisense to the RL1 gene encoding γ_1 34.5, and ends where the full length latency associated transcript (LAT) terminates. The gene is expressed primarily under conditions where other HSV genes, including those of the immediate early or alpha class, are not expressed (Lagunoff and Roizman, 1994). Deletion of an ICP4 binding site in the ORF P promoter augments expression, suggesting that ICP4 normally acts to repress ORF P (Lagunoff et al., 1996). Because HSV alpha genes are not expressed during latent infection, it has been speculated that ORF P might be expressed preferentially in latently infected neurons, although this has not been demonstrated. The predicted HSV-2 counterpart of ORF P is 130 amino acids in length and has substantial similarity over the first 49 codons, after which the similarity drops off significantly at a site corresponding to an intron in HSV-2 RL1, which is encoded on the opposite strand (Dolan et al., 1998). It has not been determined if the HSV-2 counterpart to ORF P is expressed.

ORF O of HSV-1 is shorter than, and entirely contained within, ORF P. The protein is regulated in a similar fashion to ORF P, and appears to be translated from the same inititation codon, but shifts frame by an unknown mechanism after codon 35 to a different reading frame, resulting in translation of a 20 000 apparent M_r protein. The protein can interact with ICP4 and preclude the latter's binding to DNA (Randall et al., 1997). Similar to ORF P, the homology to an HSV-2 counterpart is only convincing at the extreme N-terminus and it is not known if the HSV-2 protein is expressed.

The γ_1 34.5 protein is encoded by RL1 in the repeat region, with the promoter located in the a sequence, and the open reading frame in the b sequence. The protein is a major determinant of neurovirulence and has a number of interesting functions including the recruitment of phosphatase alpha to dephosphorylate elongation initiation factor alpha and thus preserve translation of viral proteins, even in the presence of PKR (He et al., 1997). The HSV-2 counterpart contains an intron, but is otherwise conserved. There is no obvious homologue in VZV or in herpes B virus (Perelygina et al., 2003).

The U_L 8.5 gene is present in both HSV-1 and HSV-2. The gene product, designated OBPC, represents the C terminal 438 amino acids of the U_L 9 gene that encodes the origin binding protein (OBP). OBPC can bind origin sequences and can interfere with DNA replication in vitro (Baradaran et al., 1996; Baradaran et al., 1994).

The U_L 12.5 open reading frame is translated in frame with U_L 12 to yield a 60 000 M_r protein. It retains some of the nuclease activity of U_L 12, but lacks a nuclear localization signal at the N-terminus, perhaps explaining why U_L 12.5 cannot complement a U_L 12 null mutant. The precise function of U_L 12.5 is not known (Martinez et al., 1996; Reuven et al., 2004).

The U_L 15.5 open reading frame is present in VZV, but in contrast to the case with HSV-1, it is not known if the VZV protein is expressed. The open reading frame constitutes most of exon II of U_L 15 and the protein is in frame with U_L 15. The function is not known (Baines et al., 1994, 1997; Yu et al., 1997).

The U_L 20.5 open reading frame is located upstream of U_L 20. The gene product is expressed in infected cells and localizes in discrete sites in the nucleus. The open reading frame is not conserved in HSV-2 or VZV and the function is not known (Ward et al., 2000).

U_L 27.5 is encoded in opposite sense to U_L 27, which encodes glycoprotein B. The 43 000 apparent M_r protein identified in infected cells is much smaller than the 575 codon open reading frame would predict. An HSV-2 protein of similar size that shares epitopes with the HSV-1 gene product is derived from an open reading frame of 985 codons (Chang et al., 1998). The mechanism by which these large open reading frames lead to production of smaller than expected proteins is unknown.

U_L 43.5 is a 311 aa ORF that is encoded completely within U_L 43 coding sequences but is translated in opposite sense to that of U_L 43 (Ward et al., 1996). The genomic region encoding these open reading frames is dispensable for viral growth in cell culture (MacLean et al., 1991). The protein localizes in assemblons, discrete sites within infected cell nuclei that contain a variety of capsid and tegument proteins. The U_L 43.5 open reading frame is not conserved in HSV-2 (Dolan et al., 1998).

The U_L 56 gene is unique to the simplexviruses of humans. The gene lies in a region that is necessary for a virulent phenotype of certain HSV-1 strains, but the gene itself does not contribute substantially to this virulence, at least in mice (Nash and Spivack, 1994). The gene product is associated with virions and is not essential for growth in cultured cells (Rosen-Wolff et al., 1991).

The unspliced latency associated transcript or LAT is around 7–9 kbp in length, and this is extensively spliced. The introns of approximately 1.5 and 2.0 kbp are presumably very stable and accumulate to high levels in the nuclei of latently infected sensory neurons. Both the large and small transcripts are derived from transcriptional units within IRL and TRL and are transcribed in a sense opposite to that of RL1 (encoding ICP0) with which they overlap. Transcription through the repeat regions and antisense to ICP0 is a common theme among many alphaherpesviruses including bovine herpesvirus 1 and PRV, but these transcripts are not greatly similar to HSV LAT, other than in regions that overlap conserved open reading frames (Cheung, 1991; Rock et al., 1987). More extensive discussions of the latency associated transcripts are included elsewhere in this volume.

S component genes unique to the human simplexviruses

The short components of the human alphaherpesviruses are considerably less well conserved than the long components (Figs. 5.1 to 5.4). Perhaps the most striking difference is that homologues of six HSV genes, including U_S 6 encoding the essential glycoprotein D, are not present in the VZV genome (Dolan et al., 1998; McGeoch et al., 1988). In addition, the order of the existing homologues of U_S is considerably rearranged (Davison and McGeoch, 1986).

The U_S1 gene of 420 codon encodes ICP22 whereas the U_S1.5 open reading frame of 273 codons is contained within the U_S 1 gene, and is translated in the same reading frame as ICP22 but from a different initiation codon (Carter and Roizman, 1996). A homologous, but highly diverged gene to that encoded by U_S 1.5 is present in HSV-2, but this lacks an obvious start codon. The VZV counterpart is ORF 63/70 (the gene is duplicated at the ends of the short component of VZV); the region of highest similarity with HSV-1 is limited to the C-terminus which includes US1.5.

The U_S2 gene of HSV is present in many other alphaherpesviruses, but is conspicuously absent from the VZV genome. The function of the gene is not known but the gene product is found in HSV-2 virions and can associate with cytokeratin 18 in vitro and in infected cells (Goshima et al., 2001). U_S2 is not essential for growth in cell culture and the HSV-2 gene is dispensable for virulence in mice inoculated by the footpad route (Jiang et al., 1998; Longnecker and Roizman, 1987). The homologous gene product of pseudorabies virus (PRV) is prenylated, a modification that changes its localization from association with membranes to punctate regions in the cytoplasm (Clase et al., 2003). The gene product is associated with virions and this association may be regulated by postranslation modification, inasmuch as the virion-associated gene product is not prenylated.

The U_S 4 gene encodes glycoprotein G (gG). The gene is dispensable for growth in cell culture and differs significantly in sequence such that the HSV-2 gene is approximately 1500 bp larger (Ackermann et al., 1986; Dolan et al., 1998; Longnecker et al., 1987; McGeoch et al., 1988). This difference is exploited in serologic assays to distinguish HSV-2 specific antibodies from those induced by HSV-1

(Lee et al., 1985). The function of gG is not known, but speculation that it has something to do with tropism unique to HSV-2 vs. HSV-1 seems warranted.

$U_S 5$ encodes glycoprotein J (gJ) (Ghiasi et al., 1998). gJ prevents apoptosis in cells infected with HSV-1 gD null mutants, and precludes apoptosis induced by granzyme B and Fas ligation, such as would be expected upon attack of an infected cell by cytotoxic T-lymphocytes (Jerome et al., 2001; Zhou et al., 2000). Interestingly, HSV-2 does not preclude apoptosis induced by ultraviolet radiation or Fas antibody, whereas HSV-1 blocks apoptosis through these stimuli, suggesting a difference in function of anti-apoptotic mechanisms mediated at least partly through gJ (Jerome et al., 1999).

$U_S 6$ encodes gD that is necessary for HSV entry and has been shown to bind a variety of proteinaceous viral receptors (Spear, 2004). The fact that a gene essential for entry of HSV is absent from the VZV genome suggests that the essential steps mediated by gD must be mediated by different VZV proteins. This issue is treated extensively in chapters dealing with herpesvirus entry.

$U_S 8.5$ encodes a phosphoprotein that localizes to nucleoli (Georgopoulou et al., 1995). The gene is dispensable for replication in cultured cells and the function is not known. Although $U_S 8.5$ is a late gene, the mRNA is packaged into virions and presumably delivered to infected cells upon entry (Sciortino et al., 2002).

The 161 codon $U_S 11$ of HSV-1 is an RNA binding protein that is unique to the simplexviruses of humans. If expressed as an alpha gene, the protein can dephosphorylate $EIF2\alpha$ and thereby rescue the ability of a $\gamma_1 34.5$ deletion mutant to replicate in neuronal cell lines (Mohr and Gluzman, 1996; Roller et al., 1996).

$U_S 12$ encodes ICP47, an 88 amino acid immediate early protein. ICP47 can block the transporter associated with antigen transport (TAP) and thus preclude loading of antigenic peptides onto class 1 molecules in the ER (York et al., 1994). Although ICP47 may be unique to human simplexviruses, it can be viewed as functionally conserved inasmuch as interference with antigen presentation is a function common to many viral proteins, including a number from both gamma- and betaherpesviruses (Vossen et al., 2002).

In considering the information outlined herein, the authors would like to include a note of caution. While comparison of the sequences of the human alphaherpesviruses with one another and with other herpesviruses leads to a series of hypotheses regarding functions of individual genes, such an analysis is at once both potentially valuable and misleading. Fortunately, such hypotheses are experimentally testable in the context of the most relevant viral genome. It is anticipated that some surprises will result from these studies. Perhaps this is best illustrated by studies of herpesvirus glycoproteins, as various sequence homologues may have markedly different functions depending on the viral system studied. At the least, the preceding analyses of similarities in the genetic content of the human alphaherpesviruses should be considered with this caveat in mind.

REFERENCES

Ackermann, M., Longnecker, R., Roizman, B., and Pereira, L. (1986). Identification and gene location of a novel glycoprotein specified by herpes simplex virus 1. Virology, **150**, 207–220.

Baines, J. D. and Roizman, B. (1991). The open reading frames UL3, UL4, UL10 and UL16 are dispensable for the growth of herpes simplex virus 1 in cell culture. J. Virol., **65**, 938–944.

Baines, J. D., Poon, A. P. W., Rovnak, J., and Roizman, B. (1994). The $U_L 15$ gene of herpes simplex virus encodes two proteins and is required for cleavage of viral DNA. J. Virol., **68**, 8118–8124.

Baines, J. D., Cunningham, C., Nalwanga, D., and Davison, A. J. (1997). The $U_L 15$ gene of herpes simplex virus type 1 contains within its second exon a novel open reading frame that is translated in frame with the $U_L 15$ gene product. J. Virol., **71**, 2666–2673.

Baradaran, K., Dabrowski, C. E., and Schaffer, P. A. (1994). Transcriptional analysis of the region of the herpes simplex virus type 1 genome containing the UL8, UL9, and UL10 genes and identification of a novel delayed-early gene product, OBPC. J. Virol., **68**(7), 4251–4261.

Baradaran, K., Hardwicke, M. A., Dabrowski, C. E., and Schaffer, P. A. (1996). Properties of the novel herpes simplex virus type 1 origin binding protein, OBPC. J. Virol., **70**(8), 5673–5679.

Carter, K. L. and Roizman, B. (1996). The promoter and transcriptional unit of a novel herpes simplex virus 1 alpha gene are contained in, and encode a protein in frame with, the open reading frame of the alpha 22 gene. J. Virol., **70**(1), 172–178.

Chang, Y. E., Menotti, L., Filatov, F., Campadelli-Fiume, G., and Roizman, B. (1998). UL27.5 is a novel gamma2 gene antisense to the herpes simplex virus 1 gene encoding glycoprotein B. J. Virol., **72**(7), 6056–6064.

Cheung, A. K. (1991). Cloning of the latency gene and the early protein 0 gene of pseudorabies virus. J. Virol., **65**(10), 5260–5271.

Clase, A. C., Lyman, M. G., del Rio, T. et al. (2003). The pseudorabies virus Us2 protein, a virion tegument component, is prenylated in infected cells. J. Virol., **77**, 12285–12298.

Cockrell, A. S. and Muggeridge, M. I. (1998). Herpes simplex virus 2 UL45 is a type II membrane protein. J. Virol., **72**(5), 4430–4433.

Cohen, J. I. and Seidel, K. E. (1993). Generation of varicella-zoster virus (VZV) and viral mutants from cosmid DNAs: VZV thymidylate synthetase is not essential for replication in vitro. *Proc. Natl Acad. Sci. USA*, **90**(15), 7376–7380.

Cohen, J. I. and Seidel, K. E. (1995). Varicella-zoster virus open reading frame 1 encodes a membrane protein that is dispensable for growth of VZV in vitro. *Virology*, **206**(2), 835–842.

Cox, E., Reddy, S., Iofin, I., and Cohen, J. I. (1998). Varicella-zoster virus ORF57, unlike its pseudorabies virus UL3.5 homolog, is dispensable for viral replication in cell culture. *Virology*, **250**(1), 205–209.

Davison, A. J. and McGeoch, D. J. (1986). Evolutionary comparisons of the S segments in the genomes of herpes simplex virus type 1 and varicella-zoster virus. *J. Gen. Virol.*, **67**, 597–611.

Dolan, A., Jamieson, F. E., Cunningham, C., Barnett, B. C., and McGeoch, D. J. (1998). The genome of herpes simplex virus type 2. *J. Virol.*, **72**, 2010–2021.

Frenkel, N. and Roffman, E. (1996). Human Herpesvirus 7. In *Fields Virology*, 3rd edn, ed. B. N. Fields *et al.*, pp. 2609–2622. Philadelphia: Lippincott-Raven.

Fuchs, W., Klupp, B. G., Granzow, H., Rziha, H.-J., and Mettenleiter, T. C. (1996). Identification and characterization of the pseudorabies virus UL3.5 protein, which is involved in virus egress. *J. Virol.*, **70**, 3517–3527.

Georgopoulou, U., Kakkanas, A., Miriagou, V., Michaelidou, A., and Mavromara, P. (1995). Characterization of the US8.5 protein of herpes simplex virus. *Arch. Virol.*, **140**(12), 2227–2241.

Ghiasi, H., Nesburn, A. B., Cai, S., and Wechsler, S. L. (1998). The US5 open reading frame of herpes simplex virus type 1 does encode a glycoprotein (gJ). *Intervirology*, **41**(2–3), 91–97.

Goshima, F., Watanabe, D., Suzuki, H., Takakuwa, H., Yamada, H., and Nishiyama, Y. (2001). The US2 gene product of herpes simplex virus type 2 interacts with cytokeratin 18. *Arch. Virol.*, **146**(11), 2201–2209.

Gribaudo, G., Riera, L., Rudge, T. L., Caposio, P., Johnson, L. F., and Landolfo, S. (2002). Human cytomegalovirus infection induces cellular thymidylate synthase gene expression in quiescent fibroblasts. *J. Gen. Virol.*, **83**(Pt 12), 2983–2993.

He, B., Gross, M., and Roizman, B. (1997). The gamma(1)34.5 protein of herpes simplex virus 1 complexes with protein phosphatase 1 alpha to dephosphorylate the alpha subunit of the eukaryotic translation initiation factor 2 and preclude the shutoff of protein synthesis by double-stranded RNA-activated protein kinase. *Proc. Natl Acad. Sci. USA*, **94**(3), 843–848.

Jerome, K. R., Fox, R., Chen, Z., Sears, A. E., Lee, H., and Corey, L. (1999). Herpes simplex virus inhibits apoptosis through the action of two genes, Us5 and Us3. *J. Virol.*, **73**(11), 8950–8957.

Jerome, K. R., Chen, Z., Lang, R. *et al.* (2001). HSV and glycoprotein J inhibit caspase activation and apoptosis induced by granzyme B or Fas. *J. Immunol.*, **167**(7), 3928–3935.

Jiang, Y. M., Yamada, H., Goshima, F. *et al.* (1998). Characterization of the herpes simplex virus type 2 (HSV-2) US2 gene product and a US2-deficient HSV-2 mutant. *J. Gen. Virol.*, **79**, 2777–2784.

Kemble, G. W., Annunziato, P., Lungu, O. *et al.* (2000). Open reading frame S/L of varicella-zoster virus encodes a cytoplasmic protein expressed in infected cells. *J. Virol.*, **74**(23), 11311–11321.

Lagunoff, M. and Roizman, B. (1994). Expression of a herpes simplex virus 1 open reading frame antisense to the gamma(1)34.5 gene and transcribed by an RNA 3 coterminal with the unspliced latency-associated transcript. *J. Virol.*, **68**, 6021–6028.

Lagunoff, M., Randall, G., and Roizman, B. (1996). Phenotypic properties of herpes simplex virus 1 containing a derepressed open reading frame P gene. *J. Virol.*, **70**(3), 1810–1817.

Lee, F. K., Coleman, R. M., Pereira, L., Bailey, P. D., Tatsuno, M., and Nahmias, A. J. (1985). Detection of herpes simplex virus type 2-specific antibody with glycoprotein G. *J. Clin. Microbiol.*, **22**(4), 641–644.

Longnecker, R. and Roizman, B. (1987). Clustering of genes dispensable for growth in culture in the S component of the HSV-1 genome. *Science*, **236**, 573–576.

Longnecker, R., Chatterjee, S., Whitley, R., and Roizman, B. (1987). Identification of a herpes simplex virus 1 glycoprotein gene within a gene cluster dispensable for growth in tissue culture. *Proc. Natl Acad. Sci. USA*, **84**, 4303–4307.

MacLean, C. A., Efstathiou, S., Elliott, M. L., Jamieson, F. E., and McGeoch, D. J. (1991). Investigation of herpes simplex virus type 1 genes encoding multiply inserted membrane proteins. *J. Gen. Virol.*, **72**, 897–906.

Mahalingam, R., White, T., Wellish, M., Gilden, D. H., Soike, K., and Gray, W. L. (2000). Sequence analysis of the leftward end of simian varicella virus (EcoRI-I fragment) reveals the presence of an 8-bp repeat flanking the unique long segment and an 881-bp open-reading frame that is absent in the varicella zoster virus genome. *Virology*, **274**(2), 420–428.

Martinez, R., Shao, L., Bronstein, J. C., Weber, P. C., and Weller, S. K. (1996). The product of a 1.9-kb mRNA which overlaps the HSV-1 alkaline nuclease gene (UL12) cannot relieve the growth defects of a null mutant. *Virology*, **215**(2), 152–164.

McGeoch, D. J., Dalrymple, M. A., Davison, A. J. (1988). The complete DNA sequence of the long unique region in the genome of herpes simplex virus type 1. *J. Gen. Virol.*, **69**, 1531–1574.

Minson, A., Davidson, A., Eberle, R. *et al.* (2000). Family *herpesviridae*. In *Virus Taxonomy. Seventh report of the International Committee on Taxonomy of Viruses*, ed. M. Van Regenmortel *et al.*, pp. 203–225. New York/San Diego: Academic Press.

Mohr, I. and Gluzman, Y. (1996). A herpesvirus genetic element which affects translation in the absence of the viral GADD34 function. *Europ. Molec. Biol. Org. J.*, **15**(17), 4759–4766.

Nash, T. C. and Spivack, J. G. (1994). The UL55 and UL56 genes of herpes simplex virus type 1 are not required for viral replication, intraperitoneal virulence, or establishment of latency in mice. *Virology*, **204**(2), 794–798.

Pellett, P. E. and Roizman, B. (in press). The Herpesviridae: a brief introduction. In *Fields Virology*, 5th edn, ed. D. M. Knipe *et al.*, vol. 2, chapter 66, Philadelphia: Lippincott, Williams, & Wilkins.

Perelygina, L., Zhu, L., Zurkuhlen, H., Mills, R., Borodovsky, M., and Hilliard, J. K. (2003). Complete sequence and comparative analysis of the genome of herpes B virus (Cercopithecine herpesvirus 1) from a rhesus monkey. *J. Virol.*, **77**(11), 6167–6177.

Randall, G., Lagunoff, M., and Roizman, B. (1997). The product of ORF O located within the domain of herpes simplex virus 1 genome transcribed during latent infection binds to and inhibits in vitro binding of infected cell protein 4 to its cognate DNA site. *Proc. Natl Acad. Sci. USA*, **94**(19), 10379–10384.

Reddy, S. M., Cox, E., Iofin, I., Soong, W., and Cohen, J. I. (1998). Varicella-zoster virus (VZV) ORF32 encodes a phosphoprotein that is posttranslationally modified by the VZV ORF47 protein kinase. *J. Virol.*, **72**(10), 8083–8088.

Reuven, N. B., Antoku, S., and Weller, S. K. (2004). The UL12.5 gene product of herpes simplex virus type 1 exhibits nuclease and strand exchange activities but does not localize to the nucleus. *J. Virol.*, **78**(9), 4599–4608.

Rock, D. L., Beam, S. L., and Mayfield, J. E. (1987). Mapping bovine herpesvirus type 1 latency-related RNA in trigeminal ganglia of latently infected rabbits. *J. Virol.*, **61**(12), 3827–3831.

Roller, R. J., Monk, L. L., Stuart, D., and Roizman, B. (1996). Structure and function in the herpes simplex virus 1 RNA-binding protein U(s)11: mapping of the domain required for ribosomal and nucleolar association and RNA binding in vitro. *J. Virol.*, **70**, 2842–2851.

Rosen-Wolff, A., Lamade, W., Berkowitz, C., Becker, Y., and Darai, G. (1991). Elimination of UL56 gene by insertion of LacZ cassette between nucleotide position 116030 to 121753 of the herpes simplex virus type 1 genome abrogates intraperitoneal pathogenicity in tree shrews and mice. *Virus Res.*, **20**(3), 205–221.

Sato, H., Pesnicak, L., and Cohen, J. I. (2002). Varicella-zoster virus open reading frame 2 encodes a membrane phosphoprotein that is dispensable for viral replication and for establishment of latency. *J. Virol.*, **76**(7), 3575–3578.

Sato, H., Pesnicak, L., and Cohen, J. I. (2003). Varicella-zoster virus ORF47 protein kinase, which is required for replication in human T cells, and ORF66 protein kinase, which is expressed during latency, are dispensable for establishment of latency. *J. Virol.*, **77**(20), 11180–11185.

Sciortino, M. T., Taddeo, B., Poon, A. P., Mastino, A., and Roizman, B. (2002). Of the three tegument proteins that package mRNA in herpes simplex virions, one (VP22) transports the mRNA to uninfected cells for expression prior to viral infection. *Proc. Natl Acad. Sci. USA*, **99**(12), 8318–8323.

Spear, P. G. (2004). Herpes simplex virus: receptors and ligands for cell entry. *Cell Microbiol.*, **6**(5), 401–410.

Tanaka, M., Kagawa, H., Yamanashi, Y., Sata, T., and Kawaguchi, Y. (2003). Construction of an excisable bacterial artificial chromosome containing a full-length infectious clone of herpes simplex virus type 1: viruses reconstituted from the clone exhibit wild-type properties in vitro and in vivo. *J. Virol.*, **77**(2), 1382–1391.

Telford, E. A., Watson, M. S., McBride, K., and Davison, A. J. (1992). The DNA sequence of equine herpesvirus-1. *Virology*, **189**(1), 304–316.

Telford, E. A., Watson, M. S., Aird, H. C., Perry, J., and Davison, A. J. (1995). The DNA sequence of equine herpesvirus 2. *J. Mol. Biol.*, **249**(3), 520–528.

Visalli, R. J. and Brandt, C. R. (1991). The HSV-1 UL45 gene product is not required for growth in Vero cells. *Virology*, **185**(1), 419–423.

Vossen, M. T., Westerhout, E. M., Soderberg-Naucler, C., and Wiertz, E. J. (2002). Viral immune evasion: a masterpiece of evolution. *Immunogenetics*, **54**(8), 527–542.

Ward, P. L., Barker, D. E., and Roizman, B. (1996). A novel herpes simplex virus 1 gene, $U_L 43.5$, maps antisense to the $U_L 43$ gene and encodes a protein which colocalizes in nuclear structures with capsid proteins. *J. Virol.*, **70**, 2684–2690.

Ward, P. L., Taddeo, B., Markovitz, N. S., and Roizman, B. (2000). Identification of a novel expressed open reading frame situated between genes $U_{(L)}20$ and $U_{(L)}21$ of the herpes simplex virus 1 genome. *Virology*, **266**(2), 275–285.

York, I. A., Roop, C., Andrews, D. W., Riddell, S. R., Graham, F. L., and Johnson, D. C. (1994). A cytosolic herpes simpelx virus protein inhibits antigen presentation to CD8+ T lymphocytes. *Cell*, **77**, 525–535.

Zhou, G., Galvan, V., Campadelli-Fiume, G., and Roizman, B. (2000). Glycoprotein D or J delivered in *trans* blocks apoptosis in SK-N-SH cells induced by a herpes simplex virus 1 mutant lacking intact genes expressing both glycoproteins. *J. Virol.*, **74**(24), 11782–11791.

Alphaherpes viral genes and their functions

Bernard Roizman[1] and Gabriella Campadelli-Fiume[2]

[1]The Marjorie B. Kovler Viral Oncology Labs. The University of Chicago, IL, USA
[2]Department of Experimental Pathology, University of Bologna, Italy

Introduction

In this chapter the emphasis is on viral replication and on the viral gene products that define the outcome of the interaction of the alphaherpesviruses with their host. Viral replicative and host management functions account for some of the RNAs and a large number of proteins encoded by the viruses. There are, however, numerous viral gene products whose functions have not been identified or which do not play a prominent role in viral replication in the systems in which these have been tested. The objective of the table contained in this section is to summarize the functions of all known gene products and provide at least a few references for each product. It should be noted however that: of the three human alphaherpesviruses, we know more about the functions of herpes simplex virus-1 and -2 (HSV-1 and HSV-2) genes than about those of varicella zoster virus (VZV). We have identified in this table the VZV genes that are related to HSV by amino acid sequence homology. We note that partial sequence conservation does not necessarily mean that the homologous HSV and VZV gene products perform identical functions.

The list understates both the number of the products and their functions. The problem is twofold. The HSV genome encodes a large number of open reading frames (ORFs) with 50 or more codons and not all of the ORFs have been probed for to determine whether they are expressed. In addition, standard annotations exclude ORFs that are antisense to known ORFs or that do not have TATA boxes or other motifs that indicate that they encode proteins. HSV encodes several proteins whose ORFs are antisense to each other. An additional problem is that transcripts arising late in infection frequently do not terminate at predicted termination signals. In addition, several viral RNAs either do not encode a protein or the protein is made in undetectable amounts. In several instances, ORFs contain within their domain a transcriptional unit encoding proteins identical to the C terminal domain of the protein encoded by the larger ORF. In essence, we do not know the absolute number of transcripts or proteins encoded by the viral genome.

The third limitation of the table stems from the observation that virtually all viral proteins studied in detail appear to perform multiple functions. Not all of the functions are known and, in some instances, the table lists the most prominent functions of the gene product.

We further note that (i) some alphaherpesvirus genes are found only in HSV-1 (ORF-O and ORF-P), some in HSV-1 and HSV-2 ($\gamma_1$34.5), some in HSV-1, HSV-2 and B virus (the simplexviruses), some in the simplexviruses plus pseudorabies virus, and some are in all of the above, plus VZV. This is annotated in the "Conservation" column. (ii) Some genes have positional homologues (conserved size, orientation, and conserved surrounding genes) for which no functional data are available. We included positional homologues, in cases in which good candidates are present in members of all three herpesviruses subfamilies.

Gene designation	Alternative name	Main properties	Conservation[b]	Gene Block[c]	Homologues[d] VZV	γ-HV	HCMV	HHV-6	Ref.
$\gamma_1 34.5$		This ORF encodes a 248-residue γ_1 protein consisting of two unequal domains linked by a variable number of alanine-proline-threonione repeats. The C-terminal domain is homologous to the C-terminal domain of GADD34 and functions as a phosphatase accessory factor which binds phosphatase 1α and redirects it to dephosphorylate the α subunit of the translation initiation factor 2 (eIF-2). In the absence of $\gamma_1 34.5$ gene, protein kinase R is activated, eIF-2α is phosphorylated and all protein synthesis ceases. The loss of this function is responsible for the loss of the capacity of mutants to replicate in experimental animal systems (loss of neurovirulence). $\gamma_1 34.5$ protein is also involved in the evasion of MHC class 2 responses and encodes other, as yet poorly defined functions. γ_1.[a]	HSV-2, Gadd34 (MyD116)						(100, 101, 230)
ORF-P		A 233-residue ORF encoded on the strand complementary to $\gamma_1 34.5$. The transcription of ORF-P is blocked by ICP4 bound to a high affinity transcription initiation site of the ORF. Derepression of ORF-P results in decreased expression of the $\gamma_1 34.5$ ORF. ORF-P protein binds p32 and localizes in spliceosomes. Overexpression of ORF-P results in decreased expression of spliced RNAs. Pre-α.	not in HSV-2 or B virus						(128, 129)
ORF-O		The product of ORF-O is made of 117 residues. The amino terminus is identical to that of ORF-P. The amino acid sequence beyond residue 35 is in an alternate reading frame. Expression of ORF-O is repressed by ICP4. In vitro ORF-O blocks the binding of ICP4 to its cognate high affinity DNA binding sites. Viral gene products encoded by these ORFs have not been detected in murine ganglia harboring latent virus. Pre-α.	not in HSV-2 or B virus						(198)
$\alpha 0$	ICP0	The 3 exons encode a 775-residue protein containing a RING finger domain. ICP0 is dispensable for viral replication in cultured cells. In transfected cells it acts as a promiscuous transactivator of genes introduced by transfection or infection although activation of resident genes has been reported. ICP0 expresses multiple functions, including those of a double ubiquitin ligase targeting promyelocytic leukemia protein to block exogenous interferon, cdc34 to block turnover of cyclin D3, CNP-C, CNP-A, and DNA dependent protein kinase. ICP0 is also associated with the restructuring of chromatin. Additional functions have been described. α	α-HV		ORF61				(99, 171, 222)
$U_L 1$	gL	224 residue soluble glycoprotein. It interacts with and serves as the chaperone of gH. In its absence gH is not transported to plasma membrane and is not fully glycosylated. Essential glycoprotein for virion infectivity and cell-cell fusion. Locus of syncytial mutation. Stimulates neutralizing antibody. γ_1.	α-HV, β-HV, γ-HV	7	ORF60	ORF47	UL115	U82	(78, 106, 203)

(cont.)

Gene designation	Alternative name	Main properties	Conservation[b]	Gene Block[c]	Homologues[d] VZV	γ-HV	HCMV	HHV-6	Ref.
U_L2		U_L2 encodes uracil-DNA glycosylase, a highly conserved enzyme associated with the base excision repair pathway. Uracil-DNA glycosylase replaces uracil in G:U base pairs resulting from deamination of cytosine residues in DNA. U_L2 is highly conserved and no other functions have been ascribed it. 334 aa. β or γ$_1$.	α-HV, β-HV, γ-HV.	7	ORF59	ORF46	UL114	U81	(41, 244)
U_L3		U_L3 is a 235 residue phosphoprotein forming multiple bands in denaturing polyacrylamide gels due in part to phosphorylation mediated by U_L13 protein kinase. It co-localizes with ICP22-$U_S1.5$ proteins in small dense nuclear structures. In the absence of ICP22 or $U_S1.5$ it is diffuse throughout the nucleus. The function is unknown: the gene can be deleted without impairment of viral replication in cultured cells. The protein is transcribed predominantly from the second methionine of its reading frame. γ$_2$.	α-HV Possible positional homologue in γ-HV		ORF58	ORF45			(10, 152, 245)
U_L4		U_L4 is a 199-residue virion protein. In infected cells it localizes in small dense nuclear structures formed prior to the onset of viral DNA synthesis together with ICP22/$U_S1.5$. In the absence of other viral proteins it remains in the cytoplasm. U_L4 and is dispensable for viral replication in cultured cells. γ$_2$.	α-HV		ORF56				(110, 113, 249)
U_L5		U_L5 is a component of the helicase – primase complex. The 882-residue protein contains sequence motifs shared by members of the superfamily of RNA and DNA helicases ranging from bacteria to mammals. Stable U_L5-U_L52, complex has DNA-dependent ATPase and GTPase, DNA primase and DNA helicase activities. A viral mutant in U_L5 exhibiting a neuron specific restriction was shown to produce lower levels of viral DNA in restricted cells. β.	α-HV, β-HV, γ-HV	6	ORF55	ORF44	UL105	U77	(28, 76)
U_L6		The 676-residue protein forms a dodecameric ring located at the vertices of the HSV capsid. The ring structure is similar to the portal for the entry of DNA in bacteriophages. U_L6 has been reported interact with U_L15 and U_L28 (the putative terminase) proteins. Resistance of a class of thiourea drugs that blocks cleavage and packaging of DNA was mapped to U_L6 ORF: Unknown.	α-HV, β-HV, γ-HV	6	ORF54	ORF43	UL104	U76	(176, 232, 242)
U_L7		The 296-residue protein is well conserved among herpesvirus families and may be a component of the tegument. Its function is not known. It is not essential for replication in cell culture. γ$_1$.	α-HV, β-HV, γ-HV	6	ORF53	ORF42	UL103	U75	(181)
U_L8		The 750-residue U_L8 protein is required for the transport of U_L52 and U_L5 to the nucleus. It interacts with both U_L9 and U_L30. One likely function of U_L8 protein is to facilitate the synthesis of RNA primers on the DNA template. β.	α-HV, β-HV, γ-HV	6	ORF52	ORF41	UL102	U74	(18, 40, 153, 159, 229)

(cont.)

Gene designation	Alternative name	Main properties	Conservation[b]	Gene Block[c]	VZV	γ-HV	HCMV	HHV-6	Ref.
$U_L8.5$		The 487-residue $U_L8.5$ protein corresponds to the C-terminal domain of U_L9 protein. $U_L8.5$ was reported to be synthesized both early and late in infection and to bind to the origin of DNA synthesis. In transient assays the $U_L8.5$ protein inhibited DNA synthesis. It may play a role in shifting the pattern of synthesis for de novo initiation at origins to a rolling circle model of viral DNA synthesis. γ_1.	α-HV						(15, 16)
U_L9		U_L9, a 851-residue protein, binds to two specific sites flanking the origin of viral DNA synthesis. ICP8 (U_L29) which binds and separates the DNA strands, enables the unwinding of the DNA at the site of the origin by U_L9 protein and allows the entry of the machinery that replicates the DNA. U_L9 is conserved in α-herpesviruses and except for HHV6 and HHV7 it is absent from the genomes of β- or γ-herpesviruses. The function of U_L9 after the initiation of viral DNA synthesis has not been demonstrated. U_L9 protein was reported to interact with two proteins. hTid-1 enhances the binding of a multimer of U_L9 to the origin of DNA synthesis. NFB42, a F box component of the SCF ubiquitin ligase, binds phosphorylated U_L9 protein and targets it for ubiquitin-proteasomal degradation. The phosphorylation and degradation of U_L9 may be a mechanism by which the virus favors a rolling circle type of DNA replication instead of de novo initiation of DNA synthesis at the origins or replication. β.	α-HV, Roseoloviruses	6	ORF51			U73	(50, 81, 126, 132, 148, 224, 238)
$U_L9.5$		The transcript of $U_L9.5$ is coterminal with those of U_L8, $U_L8.5$, and U_L9. 472 aa. γ_2.							(16)
U_L10	gM	Abundant virion glycoprotein of 473 residues, with apparent M_r 53–63,000. Topology predicts six to eight transmembrane segments. A deletion mutant virus has no major phenotype. In other herpesviruses, gM forms a complex with gN, or gN-gO. Based on phenotype of ΔgM-gE-gI PrV and ΔgM EBV viral mutants, gM is thought to play a role in virion maturation and exocytosis, but this function may be redundant. However, a ΔgMgE HSV mutant shows no defect. γ.	α-HV, β-HV, γ-HV	6	ORF50	ORF39	UL100	U72	(11, 35)
U_L11		U_L11 is a 96-residue tegument protein that is both myristoylated and palmitoylated. ΔU_L11 mutants exhibit reduced levels of envelopment and egress of virus from infected cells. The protein binds the cytoplasmic face of cellular membranes and is particularly abundant in Golgi. U_L11 protein interacts with and directs U_L16 to the Golgi. The precise function of U_L11 is not known. γ.	α-HV, β-HV, γ-HV	6	ORF49	ORF38	UL99	U71	(12, 140, 141, 143, 144)
U_L12	Alkaline nuclease	U_L12 is a 626-residue alkaline nuclease that functions as a resolvase, an enzyme required for processing of replication intermediates-structures defined by their inability to enter pulse field gels and that would interfere with the packaging of viral DNA into capsids. β.	α-HV, β-HV, γ-HV	6	ORF48	ORF37	UL98	U70	(93, 154, 241)

(cont.)

Gene designation	Alternative name	Main properties	Conservation[b]	Gene Block[c]	Homologues[d]				Ref.
					VZV	γ-HV	HCMV	HHV-6	
$U_L12.5$	No VZV	The ORF encodes a 500-residue product from a 1.9 kb RNA and corresponds to the C-terminal portion of the U_L12 alkaline nuclease. The protein does not have nuclease activity, does not complement U_L12-null mutants and does not appear to be a structural component of capsids. Its function is not known. Unknown							(154)
U_L13	Protein kinase	U_L13 encodes a 518-residue (M_r 56,000) serine/tyrosine protein kinase for viral and cellular proteins. Its function as a tegument protein is unknown. The gene is essential for viral replication in experimental animal systems but not in cells in culture. U_L13 appears to regulate multifunctional proteins. The substrate specificity of U_L13 protein kinase is similar to that of the mitotic cyclin dependent kinase cdc2. (Y. Kawaguchi, personal communication). γ.	α-HV, β-HV, γ-HV	6	ORF47	ORF36	UL97	U69	(25, 67, 116, 117, 196, 217)
U_L14		The ORF encodes a tegument protein of 219 residues. $ΔU_L14$ mutants replicate well in cell culture but are highly attenuated in the mouse. The only function attributed to U_L14 protein is enhancement of nuclear localization of U_L17 and U_L26. Co-expression of U_L14 enhances nuclear import of the U_L35 (VP26) and U_L33 proteins and increases luciferase expression suggesting that it may facilitate folding of a variety of proteins. $γ_2$.	α-HV, β-HV, γ-HV	6	ORF46	ORF34	UL96	U67	(65, 250)
U_L15		The ORF consists of two exons. The intron encodes a sequence antisense to U_L16 and U_L17 proteins. U_L15 is a 735-residue (M_r of 83,000) protein that binds U_L28 protein. U_L15 is required for cleavage and packaging of viral DNA and with U_L28 may function as a terminase. U_L15 is cleaved near the amino terminus, a reaction coupled with maturation of viral DNA into unit length molecules. γ.	α-HV, β-HV, γ-HV	6	ORF 42/45	ORF29a	UL89ex1	U66 ex1	(9, 64, 206, 208)
$U_L15.5$		$U_L15.5$ Exon 2 or U_L15 encodes a M_r 55,000 protein associated with capsids. 293 aa. Unknown	α-HV, β-HV, γ-HV	6		ORF29b	UL89ex2	U66ex2	(9)
U_L16		The 373-residue U_L16 protein is encoded in the intron located between exon 1 and 2 of U_L15. It is a virion component not essential for viral replication. γ.	α-HV, β-HV, γ-HV <positional>	6	ORF44	ORF33	UL94	U65	(174, 208)
UL17		The U_L17 ORF is contained in the intron located between exon 1 and 2 of U_L15, and encodes a 703-residue protein essential for DNA cleavage and packaging. In productive infection U_L17 localizes preformed capsid to the replication compartment. U_L17 has also been reported to be a tegument protein. γ.	α-HV, β-HV, γ-HV <positional>	6	ORF43	ORF32	UL93	U64	(206, 207, 227)
U_L18	VP23	The 318-residue (M_r 34,000) protein encoded by U_L18 is a capsid protein designated VP23. Together with the VP19C encoded by U_L38 it forms triplexes consisting of two copies of VP23 and one copy of VP19C. The 320 triplexes connect adjacent hexons (150) and pentons (12). $γ_1$.	α-HV, β-HV, γ-HV	5	ORF41	ORF26	UL85	U56	(124, 231)

(cont.)

Gene designation	Alternative name	Main properties	Conservation[b]	Gene Block[c]	VZV	γ-HV	HCMV	HHV-6	Ref.
U_L19	ICP5	Major capsid protein made of 1311 residues (M_r 149,000). Capsid hexons appear as tower like complexes containing 6 copies of the protein whereas pentons contain 5 copies. γ_1.	α-HV, β-HV, γ-HV	5	ORF40	ORF25	UL86	U57	(32, 175, 177, 243)
U_L20		U_L20 is a 222 residue polytopic membrane protein, with four predicted transmembrane segments. It localizes to virions, nuclear membranes and Golgi but is absent from plasma membranes. When expressed singly, it localizes mainly to endoplasmic reticulum. Coexpressed with gK, It localizes to the Golgi. Dispensable in cell culture. A deletion mutant in UL20 gene is defective in transport of the virions out of the perinuclear space, particularly in cells with fragmented Golgi. The ΔUL20 mutant is syncytial. Together with gK, inhibits cell-cell fusion. Its postulated role is to prevent fusion of the infected cells with adjacent cells. γ.	α-HV		ORF39				(5, 6, 13, 86)
$U_L20.5$		The $U_L20.5$ ORF is located 5' to U_L20. The 160-residue protein localizes at small dense nuclear structures containing ICP22, $U_S1.5$, U_L3, and U_L4 proteins and is dispensable for viral replication. Its function is not known. γ_2.	None						(237)
U_L21		The 535-residue U_L21 protein is in tegument and may be weakly associated with capsids. U_L21 binds to microtubules but not to purified tubulin. In overexpressed cells it induces the formation of long cytoplasmic projections possibly due to its interaction with microtubules. It is not required for viral replication in cultured cells. γ_1.	α-HV		ORF38				(8, 226)
U_L22	gH	The 838-residues glycoprotein is essential for virion infectivity and cell-cell fusion. In cells infected with a deletion mutant virus in gH or a ts mutant at non permissive temperature, viruses lacking gH egress from the cell but are non infectious. Transport of gH from the endoplasmic reticulum to the Golgi and plasma membranes requires the interaction with the soluble gL. gH is an essential component of the complex enabling cell-cell fusion and induces neutralizing antibodies. VZV gH carries an endocytosis motif in the C-tail, absent from HSV gH. γ. Carries elements typical of viral fusion proteins. Possible fusogen.	α-HV, β-HV, γ-HV	4	ORF37	ORF22	UL75	U48	(36, 73, 79, 85, 94, 184)
U_L23	Thymidine kinase	Although known primarily as a thymidine kinase, it is a wide spectrum nucleoside kinase capable of phosphorylating both purine and pyrimidine nucleosides and their analogues. 376 aa. β.	α-HV, γ-HV		ORF36	ORF21			(63, 89, 158, 170)
U_L24		A 269-residue membrane-associated nuclear protein with an apparent M_r of 30,000. Mutations or deletions result in formation of small polykaryocytes in cell culture, somewhat diminished virus yields and decreased virulence in mice. The bulk of the protein is translated from the first AUG. A shorter transcript containing the second in frame AUG is also translated but the translation of 2 additional 3' co-terminal transcripts encoding C-terminal portions of U_L24 protein is uncertain. The UL24 ORF partly overlaps the TK gene in antisense direction. UL24 is dispensable in cell culture. γ_1.	α-HV, β-HV, γ-HV	4	ORF35	ORF20	UL76	U49	(185)

(cont.)

Gene designation	Alternative name	Main properties	Conservation[b]	Gene Block[c]	VZV	γ-HV	HCMV	HHV-6	Ref.
U_L25		The 580 residue product of the U_L25 ORF encodes a capsid protein involved in packaging of viral DNA into capsids. Dispensable for generation of the S terminus but required for correct generation of the L-terminus and possibly for retention of DNA in the capsid. γ_2.	α-HV, β-HV, γ-HV	4	ORF34	ORF19	UL77	U50	(161, 223)
U_L26	capsid scaffolding protein and protease	This ORF encodes a protein of 635 residues that is cleaved in *cis*- or *trans*- by itself at two sites. The N-terminal polypeptide is a protease required for assembly of a scaffolding within capsids for DNA packaging. The larger, middle cleavage product is a component of the scaffolding. γ.	α-HV, β-HV, γ-HV	4	ORF33	ORF17	UL80	U53	(90, 136, 137)
$U_L26.5$		The promoter and coding domain of $U_L26.5$ is contained in its entirety within the U_L26 ORF: The protein product of 328 residues is identical to the corresponding sequence of the U_L26 protein. It is cleaved by the protease at its C-terminus at the same site as the U_L26 protein. γ.	α-HV	4	ORF 33.5			U53.5	(137)
U_L27	gB	A 904-residue glycoprotein with apparent M_r of 110.000. It carries two, or three trasmembrane segments. Essential for virion infectivity and cell-cell fusion. Virions lacking gB egress the cell but are non infectious. The protein binds heparan sulfate and is a component of the cell-cell fusion complex. The cytoplasmic tail carries syncytial mutations, and endocytosis motifs, which mediate gB endocytosis into large vacuoles. Down modulation of gB at cell surfaces may be responsible for negative control of the cell-cell fusion. A *ts* mutation in ectodomain affects virus entry into the cell (*ts* B5). Induces neutralizing antibodies. γ_1. Crystal structure shows a trimer. Possible fusogen.	α-HV, β-HV, γ-HV	2	ORF31	ORF8	UL55	U39	(37–39, 109, 151, 186)
$U_L27.5$		The $U_L27.5$ ORF maps antisense to U_L27 and yields a γ_2 protein with an apparent M_r of 43,000. The predicted size of the coding capacity of the ORF is much larger. The protein accumulates in the cytoplasm. Its function is unknown. 575 aa. γ_2.	HSV-2						(46)
U_L28		A component of cleavage and packaging complex. See Functions of U_L15 and U_L6. 785 aa. Binds *pac1* sequences and is required for correct generation of the L-terminus. See functions of U_L6, U_L14 and U_L33. γ.	α-HV, β-HV, γ-HV	2	ORF30	ORF7	UL56	U40	(23)
U_L29	ICP8, single-stranded DNA binding protein	ICP8 is an essential 1196 residue single stranded DNA binding protein made very early in infection. ICP8 is required for viral DNA synthesis. β.	α-HV, β-HV, γ-HV	2	ORF29	ORF6	UL57	U41	(150, 253)
U_L30	DNA pol.	DNA polymerase. 1235 aa. γ.	α-HV, β-HV, γ-HV	2	ORF28	ORF9	UL54	U38	(29, 114, 234, 239, 240)
U_L31		Nuclear phosphoprotein that requires U_L34 protein for localization at the inner nuclear membrane. Binds lamin A/C in the nuclear lamina and directs envelopment at inner nuclear membrane. Carries a nucleotidylation recognition sequence. 306 aa. γ.	α-HV, β-HV, γ-HV	1	ORF27	ORF69	UL53	U37	(27, 48, 49, 147, 200, 201)
U_L32		U_L32 is 596-residue protein required for cleavage and packaging of viral DNA. The predominant localization of U_L32 in the cytoplasm suggests that either it shuttles between the nucleus and cytoplasm, or that it encodes additional functions. γ_2.	α-HV, β-HV, γ-HV	1	ORF26	ORF68	UL52	U36	(47, 130)

(cont.)

Gene designation	Alternative name	Main properties	Conservation[b]	Gene Block[c]	Homologues[d] VZV	Homologues[d] γ-HV	Homologues[d] HCMV	Homologues[d] HHV-6	Ref.
U_L33		A 130-residue capsid associated protein that forms a complex with the U_L15 and U_L28 proteins. Required for packaging of viral DNA into preformed capsids. γ_2.	α-HV, β-HV, γ-HV	1	ORF25	ORF67A	UL51	U35	(22, 199)
U_L34		An essential membrane-associated virion protein of 275 residues was reported to be a type 2 membrane protein phosphorylated by U_S3 kinase. Required for virion envelopment at inner nuclear membrane. Exclusive localization of UL34 protein at the nuclear membrane requires U_L31 protein. Extracellular virions do not contain UL31–UL34 proteins. The U_L34 homologue in murine cytomegalovirus recruits cellular protein kinase C to the nuclear lamina and induces lamin phosphorylation. γ_1.	α-HV, β-HV, γ-HV	1	ORF24	ORF67	UL50	U34	(200, 201, 215)
U_L35	VP26, capsid protein NC7	The 112-residue (M_r 12,000) protein forms a hexameric structure located on the outer surface of each hexon. Previously know as NC7. Dispensable for growth in cell culture but not in vivo. γ_2.	α-HV, β-HV, γ-HV	1	ORF23	ORF65	UL49	U32	(57, 71)
U_L36	VP1/2	The 3165-residue (M_r 270,000) protein essential for viral replication is located in the tegument essential for egress of virions through the cytoplasm. A ts mutation in UL36 blocks release of viral DNA into the nucleus at the non permissive temperature. γ_2.	α-HV, β-HV, γ-HV	1	ORF22	ORF64	UL48	U31	(20, 72)
U_L37	tegument protein	A 1123-residue (M_r 120,000) tegument phosphoprotein binds to DNA in the presence of ICP8. It is essential for viral replication. In its absence, nucleocapsids accumulate aberrantly in the nucleus and unenveloped capsids accumulate in the cytoplasm. γ_1.	α-HV, β-HV, γ-HV	1	ORF21	ORF63	UL47	U30	(146, 213, 247)
U_L38	VP19C Capsid protein	This 465-residue protein forms triplexes together with VP23, consisting of two copies of VP23 and one copy of VP19C. The 320 triplexes connect adjacent hexons (150) and pentons. γ_2.	α-HV	1	ORF20	ORF62	UL46	U29	(219, 231)
U_L39	Ribonucleotide reductase, large subunit	This ORF encodes a 1137-residue protein of M_r of 136,000. The protein is anchored in membranes and has protein kinase activity mapping to the N terminus but not required for ribonucleotide kinase activity. U_L39 may play a role in maintaining dTTP pools in infected cells. β.	α-HV, β-HV, γ-HV	1	ORF19	ORF61	UL45	U28	(54, 68, 189)
U_L40	Ribonucleotide-reductase small subunit	This ORF encodes the 340-residue small subunit of ribonucleotide kinase. β.	α-HV, γ-HV		ORF18	ORF60			(108)
U_L41	vhs, virion host shutoff protein	vhs (virion host shutoff protein) is a 489-residue protein packaged in the tegument and mediates the degradation of RNA early in infection. The degradation appears to be selective for viral RNAs. At late times after infection it is associated with VP16 (product of U_L48) and no longer exhibits this function. γ_1.	α-HV		ORF17				(82, 83, 211, 216, 225)
U_L42		DNA polymerase accessory protein. Binds double stranded DNA. It also associates with cdc2 and topoisomerase IIa. 488 aa. β.	α-HV, β-HV, γ-HV	1	ORF16	ORF59	UL44	U27	(3, 96)
U_L43		Non-essential protein. Sequence suggests that it is a hydrophobic, myristylated integral membrane protein. 434 residues. γ.	α-HV		ORF15				(44, 144, 145)

(cont.)

Gene designation	Alternative name	Main properties	Conservation[b]	Gene Block[c]	VZV	Homologues[d] γ-HV	HCMV	HHV-6	Ref.
$U_L43.5$		This ORF is located antisense to U_L43. Tagged epitope revealed the synthesis of a M_r 32,000 γ_2 protein, dispensable for growth in cell culture. Its function is not known. γ.	HSV-2						(44, 236)
U_L44	gC	A 511 residue glycoprotein heavily N- and O-glycosylated. Some gC-minus mutants arise in culture, but all primary isolates express gC. A deletion gC mutant attaches to cells with reduced efficiency, but is viable. gC mediates attachment of virions to glycosaminoglycans of heparan sulphate, or chondroitin sulphate. The heparan sulphate binding site on gC maps to the N-terminus of the ectodomain. gC is part of the immune evasion strategy of HSV, as it carries two domains involved in modulating complement activation; one binds C3, and the other is required for blocking C5 and properdin binding to C3. Each region contributes to virulence, as viruses lacking these domains are less virulent than wt-virus. γ_2.	α-HV		ORF14				(88, 103, 122, 142)
U_L45		The 172 residue type 2 membrane protein is dispensable for viral replication in cultured cells. U_L45 is required for herpes simplex virus type 1 glycoprotein B-induced fusion. It is dispensable for growth in cell culture. γ_2.	HSV-2, B virus						(98, 233)
U_L46	VP11/12 tegument protein,	The ORF encodes the 718-residue tegument proteins VP11 and VP12, differentiated solely by their migration in denaturing gels. The ORF is dispensable in cultured cells. Available data suggests that it is a γ_1 protein present along with U_L47 in stechiometric amounts with U_L48 gene product and capable of enhancing its activity. In the absence of U_L48 protein, U_L46 protein inhibits activation of α promoters. γ.	α-HV		ORF12				(157, 252)
U_L47	VP13/14 tegument protein	The two products of the ORF have apparent M_r of 82000 and 81000. They are abundant glycosylated, phosphorylated components of the tegument, dispensable for viral replication in cells in culture. U_L47 binds RNA and is reported to shuttle between the cytoplasm and nucleus. 693 aa. γ_1.	α-HV		ORF11				(77, 123, 164)
U_L48	α-TIF; VP16, ICP25	α-TIF (α-trans-inducing factor), a 491 residue protein, is a multifunctional tegument protein. It induces α-genes by interacting with two cellular proteins, HCF and Oct-1. The complex binds to specific sequences with the consensus GyATGnTAATGArATTCyTTGnGGG-NC. It is also required for virion assembly. Essential for growth in cell culture and has gamma expression regulation. Crystal structure of the conserved core has been solved. γ.	α-HV		ORF10				(59, 138, 172, 187)
U_L49	VP22	Encodes the nonessential tegument protein VP22. VP22 translocates into cells exposed to the protein. Prior to cell division it localizes to microtubules in the cytoplasm. After cell division it is bound to chromatin. VP22 binds RNA and is thought to translocate mRNA from infected to uninfected cells. It has also been reported to bind membranes, and to induce the stabilization and hyperacetylation of microtubules (putative microtubule-associated protein). It is not required for tegument assembly and its role in viral replication is unclear. γ.	α-HV		ORF 9				(33, 80, 194, 214)

(cont.)

Gene designation	Alternative name	Main properties	Conservation[b]	Gene Block[c]	Homologues[d] VZV	Homologues[d] γ-HV	Homologues[d] HCMV	Homologues[d] HHV-6	Ref.
$U_L49.5$	gN	This 91 residues membrane-associated protein with apparent M_r of 6700 is abundant in virions. The PrV homologue is gN, which forms a complex with gM. In other herpesviruses the complex is gM-gN-gO. PrV gN is not accessible in the infected cell plasma membrane. In other herpesviruses, it forms a complex with gM that inhibits fusion. In PrV, gN may be disulphide-linked to the tegument, and gN was absent from virions in the absence of gN. Thus, gM appears to be required for virion localization of gN. UL49.5 is dispensable for viral replication in cultured cells. γ2.	α-HV, β-HV, γ-HV						(2, 17, 19, 134)
U_L50	deoxyuridine triphosphatase, dUTPase	U_L50 encodes a dUTPase. The ORF is not essential for viral replication in cells in culture. 371 aa. β.	α-HV, β-HV, γ-HV		ORF 8				(14, 17, 205)
U_L51		The 244 residue protein is a component of the virion tegument. Dispensable for growth in cell culture. γ1.	α-HV, β-HV, γ-HV		ORF 7				(17, 66)
U_L52		U_L52 is a component of the helicase-primase complex. It strongest affinity appears to be for ICP8, but both U_L52 an U_L5 proteins are required for DNA binding. 1058 aa. β.	α-HV, β-HV, γ-HV		ORF6				(26, 62)
U_L53	gK	The 338 amino acid protein encoded by this ORF is a low abundance glycoprotein with M_r 40000. Sequence predicts three or four transmembrane segments. Topology, investigated by epitope mapping, shows an extracellular N-terminus and intracellular C-terminus. In infected cells gK localizes to Golgi apparatus. Plasma membrane localization is debated. gK is the most frequent locus of syncytial (syn) mutations. A deletion mutant in gK is defective in exocytosis of virions, and is syncytial. When expressed singly, gK localizes mainly at ER. Its transport to the Golgi apparatus requires the UL20 protein. gK inhibits fusion in the cell-cell fusion assay. Inhibition is augmented by coexpression with UL20 protein. gK role appears to prevent infected cells from fusing with adjacent cells. γ.	α-HV		ORF5				(4, 5, 70, 87, 107, 167, 193)
U_L54 α27	ICP27	ICP27 is a multifunctional 512-residue protein with two well defined functions. Early in infection it blocks splicing of RNA, thereby enabling the transport of unspliced RNA into the cytoplasm. At late times it acts as an RNA transporter and shuttles between the nucleus and cytoplasm. α.	α-HV, β-HV, γ-HV		ORF4	ORF57	UL69	U42	(21, 51, 52, 173, 210, 220)
U_L55		This ORF encodes a nonstructural 186-residue protein associated with sites of virion assembly. It is dispensable for viral replication in cultured cells. γ2.	α-HV (not PrV)		ORF 3				

(cont.)

Gene designation	Alternative name	Main properties	Conservation[b]	Gene Block[c]	Homologues[d] VZV	γ-HV	HCMV	HHV-6	Ref.
U_L56		This ORF encodes a phosphorylated 234-residue, type II membrane protein associated with virions. The protein is essential for pathogenesis in experimental animal systems but is not required for viral replication in cultured cells. γ2.	HSV-2						(127, 204)
α4	ICP4	ICP4 is an essential regulatory 1298-residue protein. It acts as a transactivator and a repressor of viral gene functions. As a repressor it binds to high affinity sites overlapping the transcription initiation sites of its own ORF and that of ORF P and ORF O. The interaction of ICP4 together with transcriptional factors to low affinity sites - some significantly divergent from the high affinity sites — may account for the trans activating function of ICP4. While the interaction of ICP4 with transcriptional factors has been well documented, the role of low affinity sites remains unclear. α.	α-HV		ORF62/71				(61, 97, 121, 183, 188)
α22 U_S1	ICP22	This ORF encodes a 420-residue regulatory protein of 420 residues essential in some cells and in experimental animal systems but not in human or primate cells in continuous cultivation. See $U_S1.5$ for details regarding its functions. The protein is extensively phosphorylated by viral and cellular kinases and nucleotidylylated by casein kinase II. α.	α-HV		ORF63/70				(3, 7, 31, 118, 139, 165, 195, 209)
$U_S1.5$		The promoter and coding domain of $U_S1.5$ is contained within the α22 ORF and the α22 met 14 acts as the initiator methionine of $U_S1.5$ protein. Most of the known functions of ICP22 map to the $U_S1.5$ ORF. Thus in the absence of ICP22 or U_L13 a set of late proteins (U_L41, U_S11 and U_L38) accumulates in smaller amounts. The results of two studies may account for this observation. Thus, both ICP22 and U_L13 are required for the activation of cdc2 and degradation of the partners, cyclin A and B. cdc2 partners with U_L42 and together bind and mediate posttranscriptional modification of topoisomerase IIα. In other studies the two proteins have been shown to mediate an "intermediate" phopshorylation of RNA Polymerase II. ICP22 also affects the accumulation of α0 mRNA. 274 aa. VZV ORF63/70 appears to correspond to Us1.5 rather than to ORF Us1. α.	α-HV		ORF63/70				(3, 43)
U_S2		The ORF encodes a 291 residue tegument protein not essential for viral replication in culture or in experimental animals. It is conserved among most α-HV. Its function is not known. The PrV homologue is prenylated. γ2.	HSV-2 and B virus, but not PrV or VZV						(55, 112, 163)
U_S3	Serine/threonine protein kinase	A multifunctional protein kinase that phosphorylates a large number of both cellular and viral proteins. The kinase is not essential for viral replication. U_S3 protein kinase blocks apoptosis induced by viral mutants or exogenous agents. 481 aa. γ1.	α-HV		ORF66				(24, 102, 119, 120, 133, 197)

(cont.)

Gene designation	Alternative name	Main properties	Conservation[b]	Gene Block[c]	Homologues[d] VZV	γ-HV	HCMV	HHV-6	Ref.
U_S4	gG	A 238 residue envelope glycoprotein of unknown function used in serologic assays to differentiate HSV-1 from HSV-2 antibody responses. The HSV-2 gG is larger that HSV-1 gG. γ1.	α-HV except VZV						(1, 131)
U_S5	gJ	This 92-residue glycoprotein protects the cells from apoptosis induced by gD−/+ and gD−/− virions. Dispensable in cell cultures. γ.	HSV-2, B virus, not PrV or VZV						(111, 254)
U_S6	gD	gD is a virion glycoprotein of 394 residues, with apparent M_r of 56000, essential for virus entry into the cell, and cell-cell fusion. gD is the receptor-binding glycoprotein, and interacts with three alternative receptors, named HVEM, nectin, and modified heparan sulphate. Major determinant of HSV tropism. Crystal structure shows an Ig-folded core with N- and C-terminal extensions. Upon receptor binding, a change in conformation ensues. A deletion gD mutant produces virions that exit the cell, but are non infectious. Soluble gD blocks infectivity. Ectopic expression of full length gD induces in the cell restriction to infection, by sequestering the gD receptor. Mutations at N-terminus allow usage of an alternative receptor. gD protects the cell from apoptosis induced by gD−/+ and gD−/− virions. Antiapoptotic activity is mediated by mannose-phosphate receptor. β-γ.	α-HV except VZV						(42, 53, 56, 92, 135, 180, 254)
U_S7	gI	gI is a 390-residue virion glycoprotein. It forms a heterodimer with gE. The gI-gE complex constitutes a viral Fc receptor for monomeric IgG. The gE-gI complex has basolateral localization in epithelial cells and facilitates basolateral spread of progeny virus in polarized cells. Dispensable in transformed cells, but critical in non transformed cells. γ1.	α-HV		ORF67				(74, 75, 149, 168, 235)
U_S8	gE	gE is a 550-residue virion glycoprotein. It forms a heterodimer with gI. See, gI. gE is phosphorylated by UL13 protein kinase. γ1.	α-HV		ORF68				(74, 75, 166, 182, 255)
$U_S8.5$		The 159-residue (M_r 19,000) protein localizes to nucleoli and is dispensable for viral replication. Its mRNA is among the most abundant species packaged in virions. γ1.	HSV-2, B virus, not PrV or VZV						(91, 214)
U_S9		A dispensable type II membrane-associated protein of 90 residues, reported to play no role in neurovirulence or latency. May be involved in anterograde axonal transport of virions. γ.	α-HV		ORF65				(34, 58, 178, 179)
U_S10		A dispensable tegument phosphoprotein made of 312 residues. Reported to play no role in neurovirulence or latency and to copurify with the nuclear matrix. γ.	α-HV		ORF 64/69				(179, 218, 248)
U_S11		This ORF encodes an abundant 161-residues protein expressing multiple functions. Virion associated U_S11 localizes to polyribosomes. Late in infection U_S11 is also found in nucleoli. U_S11 synthesized under an α promoter blocks phosphorylation of eIF-2α. U_S11 binds RNA in sequence and conformation dependent fashion and is in part responsible for the packaging of RNA in virions. γ2.	HSV-2						(45, 202, 214)

(cont.)

Gene designation	Alternative name	Main properties	Conservation[b]	Gene Block[c]	Homologues[d] VZV	γ-HV	HCMV	HHV-6	Ref.
U_S12, $\alpha47$	ICP47	The small 88-residues ORF encodes a M_r 9776 protein that binds to TAP1/TAP2 and blocks the transport of antigenic peptides to ER for presentation by MHC class 2 proteins. α.	HSV-2, B virus, not PrV or VZV						(104, 155, 156, 251)
LAT		The primary latency associated transcript is a low abundance transcript 8.5 to 9 kb in size and extends through the length of the ab and b'a' sequences flanking the unique long sequences. Both productively infected and latently infected cells accumulate transcripts 2.0 and 1.5 kb in size thought to be stable introns of the primary transcript. The smaller LAT sequences terminate antisense to and within the coding sequences of α0 gene. Deletion of the sequences encoding LAT reduces the mortality and morbidity in experimental animal systems and the number of neurons harboring latent virus. The decrease in the number of neurons in LAT minus mutants has been linked to pro-apoptotic manifestations of latent virus. Pre-α.							(191, 221, 246)
ORI_S RNA		This RNA originates in the c sequences flanking the unique short sequences at or near the transcription initiation sites of α22 or α47 genes, extends across the ORI_S sequence and co-terminates with the transcript encoding ICP4. The RNA is detected after the onset of viral DNA synthesis. Its function is not known.							(105)
αX and βX RNAs		These overlapping RNAs 0.9 and 4.9 Kb in size originate upstream of ORF P and extend across the L-S junction. Their function is not known.							(30)
AL-RNA		RNA reported to be antisense to the 5' sequence of LAT							(192)
VZV ORF1		Membrane protein			ORF1				(60)
VZV ORF 2					ORF2				(212)
VZV ORF 13		Thymidylate synthetase			ORF 13				
VZV ORF 32					ORF 32				
VZV ORF 57					ORF 57				
VZV ORFS/L					ORF S/L				(115)

[a] kinetic class: α, β, γ, Unknown.
[b] Abbreviations: alphaherpesvirinae or α-HV, betaherpesvirinae or β-HV, gammaherpesvirinae or γ-HV
[c] Conserved gene block to which the sequences belongs
[d] Identification of homologues in other herperviruses was based on informations contained in ref.s 69, 95, 125, 162, 169, 190, 228

Acknowledgments

We thank Drs. Ann Arvin, Joel Baines, Laura Menotti and Phil Pellett for invaluable help in reviewing the table.

REFERENCES

The numbers for each reference refer to the reference numbers in Table 6.1.

1. Ackermann, M., Longnecker, R., Roizman, B., and Pereira, L. (1986). Identification, properties, and gene location of a novel glycoprotein specified by herpes simplex virus 1. *Virology*, **150**, 207–220.
2. Adams, R., Cunningham, C., Davison, M. D., MacLean, C. A., and Davison, A. J. (1998). Characterization of the protein encoded by gene UL49A of herpes simplex virus type 1. *J. Gen. Virol.*, **79**(4), 813–823.
3. Advani, S. J., Weichselbaum, R. R., and Roizman, B. (2003). Herpes simplex virus 1 activates cdc2 to recruit topoisomerase II alpha for post-DNA synthesis expression of late genes. *Proc. Natl Acad. Sci. USA*, **100**, 4825–4830.
4. Avitabile, E., Lombardi, G., and Campadelli-Fiume, G. (2003). Herpes simplex virus glycoprotein K, but not its syncytial allele, inhibits cell–cell fusion mediated by the four fusogenic glycoproteins, gD, gB, gH and gL. *J. Virol.*, **77**, 6836–6844.
5. Avitabile, E., Lombardi, G., Gianni, T., Capri, M., and Campadelli-Fiume, G. (2004). Coexpression of UL20p and gK inhibits cell–cell fusion mediated by herpes simplex virus glycoproteins gD, gH-gL, and wt- gB or an endocytosis-defective gB mutant, and downmodulates their cell surface expression. *J. Virol.*
6. Avitabile, E., Ward, P. L., Di Lazzaro, C., Torrisi, M. R., Roizman, B., and Campadelli-Fiume, G. (1994). The herpes simplex virus UL20 protein compensates for the differential disruption of exocytosis of virions and membrane glycoproteins associated with fragmentation of the Golgi apparatus. *J. Virol.*, **68**, 7397–7405.
7. Baiker, A., Bagowski, C., Ito, H. *et al.* (2004). The immediate-early 63 protein of varicella-zoster virus: analysis of functional domains required for replication in vitro and for T-cell and skin tropism in the SCIDhu model in vivo. *J. Virol.*, **78**, 1181–1194.
8. Baines, J. D., Koyama, A. H., Huang, T., and Roizman, B. (1994). The UL21 gene products of herpes simplex virus 1 are dispensable for growth in cultured cells. *J. Virol.*, **68**, 2929–2936.
9. Baines, J. D., Poon, A. P., Rovnak, J., and Roizman, B. (1994). The herpes simplex virus 1 UL15 gene encodes two proteins and is required for cleavage of genomic viral DNA. *J. Virol.*, **68**, 8118–8124.
10. Baines, J. D. and Roizman, B. (1991). The open reading frames UL3, UL4, UL10, and UL16 are dispensable for the replication of herpes simplex virus 1 in cell culture. *J. Virol.*, **65**, 938–944.
11. Baines, J. D. and Roizman, B. (1993). The UL10 gene of herpes simplex virus 1 encodes a novel viral glycoprotein, gM, which is present in the virion and in the plasma membrane of infected cells. *J. Virol.*, **67**, 1441–1452.
12. Baines, J. D. and Roizman, B. (1992). The UL11 gene of herpes simplex virus 1 encodes a function that facilitates nucleocapsid envelopment and egress from cells. *J. Virol.*, **66**, 5168–5174.
13. Baines, J. D., Ward, P. L., Campadelli-Fiume, G., and Roizman, B. (1991). The UL20 gene of herpes simplex virus 1 encodes a function necessary for viral egress. *J. Virol.*, **65**, 6414–6424.
14. Baldo, A. M. and McClure, M. A. (1999). Evolution and horizontal transfer of dUTPase-encoding genes in viruses and their hosts. *J. Virol.*, **73**, 7710–7721.
15. Baradaran, K., Dabrowski, C. E., and Schaffer, P. A. (1994). Transcriptional analysis of the region of the herpes simplex virus type 1 genome containing the UL8, UL9, and UL10 genes and identification of a novel delayed-early gene product, OBPC. *J. Virol.*, **68**, 4251–4261.
16. Baradaran, K., Hardwicke, M. A., Dabrowski, C. E., and Schaffer, P. A. (1996). Properties of the novel herpes simplex virus type 1 origin binding protein, OBPC. *J. Virol.*, **70**, 5673–5679.
17. Barker, D. E. and Roizman, B. (1990). Identification of three genes nonessential for growth in cell culture near the right terminus of the unique sequences of long component of herpes simplex virus 1. *Virology*, **177**, 684–691.
18. Barnard, E. C., Brown, G., and Stow, N. D. (1997). Deletion mutants of the herpes simplex virus type 1 UL8 protein: effect on DNA synthesis and ability to interact with and influence the intracellular localization of the UL5 and UL52 proteins. *Virology*, **237**, 97–106.
19. Barnett, B. C., Dolan, A., Telford, E. A., Davison, A. J., and McGeoch, D. J. (1992). A novel herpes simplex virus gene (UL49A) encodes a putative membrane protein with counterparts in other herpesviruses. *J. Gen. Virol.*, **73**(8), 2167–2171.
20. Batterson, W. and Roizman, B. (1983). Characterization of the herpes simplex virion-associated factor responsible for the induction of alpha genes. *J. Virol.*, **46**, 371–377.
21. Baudoux, L., Defechereux, P., Rentier, B., and Piette, J. (2000). Gene activation by Varicella-zoster virus IE4 protein requires its dimerization and involves both the arginine-rich sequence, the central part, and the carboxyl-terminal cysteine-rich region. *J. Biol. Chem.*, **275**, 32822–32831.
22. Beard, P. M. and Baines, J. D. (2004). The DNA cleavage and packaging protein encoded by the UL33 gene of herpes simplex virus 1 associates with capsids. *Virology*.
23. Beard, P. M., Taus, N. S., and Baines, J. D. (2002). DNA cleavage and packaging proteins encoded by genes U(L)28, U(L)15, and U(L)33 of herpes simplex virus type 1 form a complex in infected cells. *J. Virol.*, **76**, 4785–4791.
24. Benetti, L., Munger, J., and Roizman, B. (2003). The herpes simplex virus 1 US3 protein kinase blocks caspase-dependent double cleavage and activation of the proapoptotic protein BAD. *J. Virol.*, **77**, 6567–6573.

25. Besser, J., Sommer, M. H., Zerboni, L. (2003). Differentiation of varicella-zoster virus ORF47 protein kinase and IE62 protein binding domains and their contributions to replication in human skin xenografts in the SCID-hu mouse. *J. Virol.*, **77**, 5964–5974.
26. Biswas, N. and Weller, S. K. (2001). The UL5 and UL52 subunits of the herpes simplex virus type 1 helicase-primase subcomplex exhibit a complex interdependence for DNA binding. *J. Biol. Chem.*, **276**, 17610–17619.
27. Blaho, J. A., Mitchell, C., and Roizman, B. (1994). An amino acid sequence shared by the herpes simplex virus 1 alpha regulatory proteins 0, 4, 22, and 27 predicts the nucleotidylylation of the UL21, UL31, UL47, and UL49 gene products. *J. Biol. Chem.*, **269**, 17401–17410.
28. Bloom, D. C. and Stevens, J. G. (1994). Neuron-specific restriction of a herpes simplex virus recombinant maps to the UL5 gene. *J. Virol.*, **68**, 3761–3772.
29. Bludau, H. and Freese, U. K. (1991). Analysis of the HSV-1 strain 17 DNA polymerase gene reveals the expression of four different classes of pol transcripts. *Virology*, **183**, 505–518.
30. Bohenzky, R. A., Lagunoff, M., Roizman, B., Wagner, E. K., and Silverstein, S. (1995). Two overlapping transcription units which extend across the L-S junction of herpes simplex virus type 1. *J. Virol.*, **69**, 2889–2897.
31. Bontems, S., Di Valentin, E., Baudoux, L., Rentier, B., Sadzot-Delvaux, C., and Piette, J. (2002). Phosphorylation of varicella-zoster virus IE63 protein by casein kinases influences its cellular localization and gene regulation activity. *J. Biol. Chem.*, **277**, 21050–21060.
32. Bowman, B. R., Baker, M. L., Rixon, F. J., Chiu, W., and Quiocho, F. A. (2003). Structure of the herpesvirus major capsid protein. *EMBO J.*, **22**, 757–765.
33. Brewis, N., Phelan, A., Webb, J., Drew, J., Elliott, G., and O'Hare, P. (2000). Evaluation of VP22 spread in tissue culture. *J. Virol.*, **74**, 1051–1056.
34. Brideau, A. D., Banfield, B. W., and Enquist, L. W. (1998). The Us9 gene product of pseudorabies virus, an alphaherpesvirus, is a phosphorylated, tail-anchored type II membrane protein. *J. Virol.*, **72**, 4560–4570.
35. Browne, H., Bell, S., and Minson, T. (2004). Analysis of the requirement for glycoprotein m in herpes simplex virus type 1 morphogenesis. *J. Virol.*, **78**, 1039–1041.
36. Buckmaster, E. A., Gompels, U., and Minson, A. (1984). Characterisation and physical mapping of an HSV-1 glycoprotein of approximately 115 X 10(3) molecular weight. *Virology*, **139**, 408–413.
37. Bzik, D. J., Fox, B. A., DeLuca, N. A., and Person, S. (1984). Nucleotide sequence of a region of the herpes simplex virus type 1 gB glycoprotein gene: mutations affecting rate of virus entry and cell fusion. *Virology*, **137**, 185–190.
38. Cai, W. Z., Person, S., DebRoy, C., and Gu, B. H. (1988). Functional regions and structural features of the gB glycoprotein of herpes simplex virus type 1. An analysis of linker insertion mutants. *J. Mol. Biol.*, **201**, 575–588.
39. Cai, W. Z., Person, S., Warner, S. C., Zhou, J. H., and DeLuca, N. A. (1987). Linker-insertion nonsense and restriction-site deletion mutations of the gB glycoprotein gene of herpes simplex virus type 1. *J. Virol.*, **61**, 714–721.
40. Calder, J. M., Stow, E. C., and Stow, N. D. (1992). On the cellular localization of the components of the herpes simplex virus type 1 helicase-primase complex and the viral origin-binding protein. *J. Gen. Virol.*, **73**(3), 531–538.
41. Caradonna, S., Worrad, D., and Lirette, R. (1987). Isolation of a herpes simplex virus cDNA encoding the DNA repair enzyme uracil-DNA glycosylase. *J. Virol.*, **61**, 3040–3047.
42. Carfi, A., Willis, S. H., Whitbeck, J. C. *et al.* (2001). Herpes simplex virus glycoprotein D bound to the human receptor HveA. *Mol. Cell.*, **8**, 169–179.
43. Carter, K. L. and Roizman, B. (1996). The promoter and transcriptional unit of a novel herpes simplex virus 1 alpha gene are contained in, and encode a protein in frame with, the open reading frame of the alpha 22 gene. *J. Virol.*, **70**, 172–178.
44. Carter, K. L., Ward, P. L., and Roizman, B. (1996). Characterization of the products of the U(L)43 gene of herpes simplex virus 1: potential implications for regulation of gene expression by antisense transcription. *J. Virol.*, **70**, 7663–7668.
45. Cassady, K. A., Gross, M., and Roizman, B. (1998). The herpes simplex virus US11 protein effectively compensates for the gamma1(34.5) gene if present before activation of protein kinase R by precluding its phosphorylation and that of the alpha subunit of eukaryotic translation initiation factor 2. *J. Virol.*, **72**, 8620–8626.
46. Chang, Y. E., Menotti, L., Filatov, F., Campadelli-Fiume, G., and Roizman, B. (1998). UL27.5 is a novel gamma2 gene antisense to the herpes simplex virus 1 gene encoding glycoprotein B. *J. Virol.*, **72**, 6056–6064.
47. Chang, Y. E., Poon, A. P., and Roizman, B. (1996). Properties of the protein encoded by the UL32 open reading frame of herpes simplex virus 1. *J. Virol.*, **70**, 3938–3946.
48. Chang, Y. E. and Roizman, B. (1993). The product of the UL31 gene of herpes simplex virus 1 is a nuclear phosphoprotein which partitions with the nuclear matrix. *J. Virol.*, **67**, 6348–6356.
49. Chang, Y. E., Van Sant, C., Krug, P. W., Sears, A. E., and Roizman, B. (1997). The null mutant of the U(L)31 gene of herpes simplex virus 1: construction and phenotype in infected cells. *J. Virol.*, **71**, 8307–8315.
50. Chen, D., Stabell, E. C., and Olivo, P. D. (1995). Varicella-zoster virus gene 51 complements a herpes simplex virus type 1 UL9 null mutant. *J. Virol.*, **69**, 4515–4518.
51. Chen, I. H., Sciabica, K. S., and Sandri-Goldin, R. M. (2002). ICP27 interacts with the RNA export factor Aly/REF to direct herpes simplex virus type 1 intronless mRNAs to the TAP export pathway. *J. Virol.*, **76**, 12877–12889.
52. Cheung, P., Ellison, K. S., Verity, R., and Smiley, J. R. (2000). Herpes simplex virus ICP27 induces cytoplasmic accumulation of unspliced polyadenylated alpha-globin pre-mRNA in infected HeLa cells. *J. Virol.*, **74**, 2913–2919.

53. Chiang, H. Y., Cohen, G. H., and Eisenberg, R. J. (1994). Identification of functional regions of herpes simplex virus glycoprotein gD by using linker-insertion mutagenesis. *J. Virol.*, **68**, 2529–2543.
54. Chung, T. D., Wymer, J. P., Smith, C. C., Kulka, M., and Aurelian, L. (1989). Protein kinase activity associated with the large subunit of herpes simplex virus type 2 ribonucleotide reductase (ICP10). *J. Virol.*, **63**, 3389–3398.
55. Clase, A. C., Lyman, M. G., del Rio, T. *et al.* (2003). The pseudorabies virus Us2 protein, a virion tegument component, is prenylated in infected cells. *J. Virol.*, **77**, 12285–12298.
56. Cocchi, F., Menotti, L., Mirandola, P., Lopez, M., and Campadelli-Fiume, G. (1998). The ectodomain of a novel member of the immunoglobulin superfamily related to the poliovirus receptor has the attributes of a *bonafide* receptor for herpes simplex viruses 1 and 2 in human cells. *J. Virol.*, **72**, 9992–10002.
57. Cohen, G. H., Ponce de Leon, M., Diggelmann, H., Lawrence, W. C., Vernon, S. K., and Eisenberg, R. J. (1980). Structural analysis of the capsid polypeptides of herpes simplex virus types 1 and 2. *J. Virol.*, **34**, 521–531.
58. Cohen, J. I., Sato, H., Srinivas, S., and Lekstrom, K. (2001). Varicella-zoster virus (VZV) ORF65 virion protein is dispensable for replication in cell culture and is phosphorylated by casein kinase II, but not by the VZV protein kinases. *Virology*, **280**, 62–71.
59. Cohen, J. I. and Seidel, K. (1994). Varicella-zoster virus (VZV) open reading frame 10 protein, the homolog of the essential herpes simplex virus protein VP16, is dispensable for VZV replication in vitro. *J. Virol.*, **68**, 7850–7858.
60. Cohen, J. I. and Seidel, K. E. (1995). Varicella-zoster virus open reading frame 1 encodes a membrane protein that is dispensable for growth of VZV in vitro. *Virology*, **206**, 835–842.
61. Compel, P. and DeLuca, N. A. (2003). Temperature-dependent conformational changes in herpes simplex virus ICP4 that affect transcription activation. *J. Virol.*, **77**, 3257–3268.
62. Constantin, N. and Dodson, M. S. (1999). Two-hybrid analysis of the interaction between the UL52 and UL8 subunits of the herpes simplex virus type 1 helicase-primase. *J. Gen. Virol.*, **80**(9), 2411–2415.
63. Cook, W. J., Lin, S. M., DeLuca, N. A., and Coen, D. M. (1995). Initiator elements and regulated expression of the herpes simplex virus thymidine kinase gene. *J. Virol.*, **69**, 7291–7294.
64. Costa, R. H., Draper, K. G., Kelly, T. J., and Wagner, E. K. (1985). An unusual spliced herpes simplex virus type 1 transcript with sequence homology to Epstein-Barr virus DNA. *J. Virol.*, **54**, 317–328.
65. Cunningham, C., Davison, A. J., MacLean, A. R., Taus, N. S., and Baines, J. D. (2000). Herpes simplex virus type 1 gene UL14: phenotype of a null mutant and identification of the encoded protein. *J. Virol.*, **74**, 33–41.
66. Daikoku, T., Ikenoya, K., Yamada, H., Goshima, F., and Nishiyama, Y. (1998). Identification and characterization of the herpes simplex virus type 1 UL51 gene product. *J. Gen. Virol.*, **79**(12), 3027–3031.
67. Daikoku, T., Shibata, S., Goshima, F. *et al.* (1997). Purification and characterization of the protein kinase encoded by the UL13 gene of herpes simplex virus type 2. *Virology*, **235**, 82–93.
68. Daikoku, T., Yamamoto, N., Maeno, K., and Nishiyama, Y. (1991). Role of viral ribonucleotide reductase in the increase of dTTP pool size in herpes simplex virus-infected Vero cells. *J. Gen. Virol.*, **72**(6), 1441–1444.
69. Davison, A. (1983). DNA sequence of the US component of the varicella-zoster virus genome. *EMBO J.*, **2**, 2203–2209.
70. Debroy, C., Pederson, N., and Person, S. (1985). Nucleotide sequence of a herpes simplex virus type 1 gene that causes cell fusion. *Virology*, **145**, 36–48.
71. Desai, P., DeLuca, N. A., and Person, S. (1998). Herpes simplex virus type 1 VP26 is not essential for replication in cell culture but influences production of infectious virus in the nervous system of infected mice. *Virology*, **247**, 115–124.
72. Desai, P. J. (2000). A null mutation in the UL36 gene of herpes simplex virus type 1 results in accumulation of unenveloped DNA-filled capsids in the cytoplasm of infected cells. *J. Virol.*, **74**, 11608–11618.
73. Desai, P. J., Schaffer, P. A., and Minson, A. C. (1988). Excretion of non-infectious virus particles lacking glycoprotein H by a temperature-sensitive mutant of herpes simplex virus type 1: evidence that gH is essential for virion infectivity. *J. Gen. Virol.*, **69**(6), 1147–1156.
74. Dingwell, K. S., Brunetti, C. R., Hendricks, R. L. *et al.* (1994). Herpes simplex virus glycoproteins E and I facilitate cell-to-cell spread in vivo and across junctions of cultured cells. *J. Virol.*, **68**, 834–845.
75. Dingwell, K. S. and Johnson, D. C. (1998). The herpes simplex virus gE-gI complex facilitates cell-to-cell spread and binds to components of cell junctions. *J. Virol.*, **72**, 8933–8942.
76. Dodson, M. S. and Lehman, I. R. (1991). Association of DNA helicase and primase activities with a subassembly of the herpes simplex virus 1 helicase-primase composed of the UL5 and UL52 gene products. *Proc. Natl Acad. Sci. USA*, **88**, 1105–1109.
77. Donnelly, M. and Elliott, G. (2001). Nuclear localization and shuttling of herpes simplex virus tegument protein VP13/14. *J. Virol.*, **75**, 2566–2574.
78. Duus, K. M. and Grose, C. (1996). Multiple regulatory effects of varicella-zoster virus (VZV) gL on trafficking patterns and fusogenic properties of VZV gH. *J. Virol.*, **70**, 8961–8971.
79. Duus, K. M., Hatfield, C., and Grose, C. (1995). Cell surface expression and fusion by the varicella-zoster virus gH:gL glycoprotein complex: analysis by laser scanning confocal microscopy. *Virology*, **210**, 429–440.
80. Elliott, G. and O'Hare, P. (1997). Intercellular trafficking and protein delivery by a herpesvirus structural protein. *Cell*, **88**, 223–233.
81. Eom, C. Y. and Lehman, I. R. (2003). Replication-initiator protein (UL9) of the herpes simplex virus 1 binds NFB42 and is degraded via the ubiquitin-proteasome pathway. *Proc. Natl Acad. Sci. USA*, **100**, 9803–9807.

82. Esclatine, A., Taddeo, B., Evans, L., and Roizman, B. (2004a). The herpes simplex virus 1 UL41 gene-dependent destabilization of cellular RNAs is selective and may be sequence-specific. *Proc. Natl Acad. Sci. USA*, **101**, 3603–3608.
83. Esclatine, A., Taddeo, B., and Roizman, B. (2004b). The UL41 protein of herpes simplex virus mediates selective stabilization or degradation of cellular mRNAs. *Proc. Natl Acad. Sci. USA*, **101**, 18165–18170.
84. Farrell, M. J., Dobson, A. T., and Feldman, L. T. (1991). Herpes simplex virus latency-associated transcript is a stable intron. *Proc. Natl Acad. Sci. USA*, **88**, 790–794.
85. Forrester, A., Farrell, H., Wilkinson, G., Kaye, J., Davis Poynter, N., and Minson, T. (1992). Construction and properties of a mutant of herpes simplex virus type 1 with glycoprotein H coding sequences deleted. *J. Virol.*, **66**, 341–348.
86. Foster, T. P., Alvarez, X., and Kousoulas, K. G. (2003). Plasma membrane topology of syncytial domains of herpes simplex virus type 1 glycoprotein K (gK): the UL20 protein enables cell surface localization of gK but not gK-mediated cell-to-cell fusion. *J. Virol.*, **77**, 499–510.
87. Foster, T. P. and Kousoulas, K. G. (1999). Genetic analysis of the role of herpes simplex virus type 1 glycoprotein K in infectious virus production and egress. *J. Virol.*, **73**, 8457–8468.
88. Frink, R. J., Eisenberg, R., Cohen, G., and Wagner, E. K. (1983). Detailed analysis of the portion of the herpes simplex virus type 1 genome encoding glycoprotein C. *J. Virol.*, **45**, 634–647.
89. Gambhir, S. S., Bauer, E., Black, M. E. *et al.* (2000). A mutant herpes simplex virus type 1 thymidine kinase reporter gene shows improved sensitivity for imaging reporter gene expression with positron emission tomography. *Proc. Natl Acad. Sci. USA*, **97**, 2785–2790.
90. Garcia-Valcarcel, M., Fowler, W. J., Harper, D. R., Jeffries, D. J., and Layton, G. T. (1997). Cloning, expression, and immunogenicity of the assembly protein of varicella-zoster virus and detection of the products of open reading frame 33. *J. Med. Virol.*, **53**, 332–339.
91. Georgopoulou, U., Kakkanas, A., Miriagou, V., Michaelidou, A., and Mavromara, P. (1995). Characterization of the US8.5 protein of herpes simplex virus. *Arch. Virol.*, **140**, 2227–2241.
92. Geraghty, R. J., Krummenacher, C., Cohen, G. H., Eisenberg, R. J., and Spear, P. G. (1998). Entry of alphaherpesviruses mediated by poliovirus receptor-related protein 1 and poliovirus receptor. *Science*, **280**, 1618–1620.
93. Goldstein, J. N. and Weller, S. K. (1998). In vitro processing of herpes simplex virus type 1 DNA replication intermediates by the viral alkaline nuclease, UL12. *J. Virol.*, **72**, 8772–8781.
94. Gompels, U. and Minson, A. (1986). The properties and sequence of glycoprotein H of herpes simplex virus type 1. *Virology*, **153**, 230–247.
95. Gompels, U. A., Nicholas, J., Lawrence, G. *et al.* (1995). The DNA sequence of human herpesvirus-6: structure, coding content, and genome evolution. *Virology*, **209**, 29–51.
96. Gottlieb, J., Marcy, A. I., Coen, D. M., and Challberg, M. D. (1990). The herpes simplex virus type 1 UL42 gene product: a subunit of DNA polymerase that functions to increase processivity. *J. Virol.*, **64**, 5976–5987.
97. Grondin, B. and DeLuca, N. (2000). Herpes simplex virus type 1 ICP4 promotes transcription preinitiation complex formation by enhancing the binding of TFIID to DNA. *J. Virol.*, **74**, 11504–11510.
98. Haanes, E. J., Nelson, C. M., Soule, C. L., and Goodman, J. L. (1994). The UL45 gene product is required for herpes simplex virus type 1 glycoprotein B-induced fusion. *J. Virol.*, **68**, 5825–5834.
99. Hagglund, R. and Roizman, B. (2004). Role of ICP0 in the strategy of conquest of the host cell by herpes simplex virus 1. *J. Virol.*, **78**, 2169–2178.
100. He, B., Gross, M., and Roizman, B. (1998). The gamma1 34.5 protein of herpes simplex virus 1 has the structural and functional attributes of a protein phosphatase 1 regulatory subunit and is present in a high molecular weight complex with the enzyme in infected cells. *J. Biol. Chem.*, **273**, 20737–20743.
101. He, B., Gross, M., and Roizman, B. (1997). The gamma(1)34.5 protein of herpes simplex virus 1 complexes with protein phosphatase 1alpha to dephosphorylate the alpha subunit of the eukaryotic translation initiation factor 2 and preclude the shutoff of protein synthesis by double-stranded RNA-activated protein kinase. *Proc. Natl Acad. Sci. USA*, **94**, 843–848.
102. Heineman, T. C., Seidel, K., and Cohen, J. I. (1996). The varicella-zoster virus ORF66 protein induces kinase activity and is dispensable for viral replication. *J. Virol.*, **70**, 7312–7317.
103. Herold, B. C., WuDunn, D., Soltys, N., and Spear, P. G. (1991). Glycoprotein C of herpes simplex virus type 1 plays a principal role in the adsorption of virus to cells and in infectivity. *J. Virol.*, **65**, 1090–1098.
104. Hill, A., Jugovic, P., York, I. *et al.* (1995). Herpes simplex virus turns off the TAP to evade host immunity. *Nature*, **375**, 411–415.
105. Hubenthal-Voss, J., Starr, L., and Roizman, B. (1987). The herpes simplex virus origins of DNA synthesis in the S component are each contained in a transcribed open reading frame. *J. Virol.*, **61**, 3349–3355.
106. Hutchinson, L., Browne, H., Wargent, V. *et al.* (1992). A novel herpes simplex virus glycoprotein, gL, forms a complex with glycoprotein H (gH) and affects normal folding and surface expression of gH. *J. Virol.*, **66**, 2240–2250.
107. Hutchinson, L., Goldsmith, K., Snoddy, D., Ghosh, H., Graham, F. L., and Johnson, D. C. (1992). Identification and characterization of a novel herpes simplex virus glycoprotein, gK, involved in cell fusion. *J. Virol.*, **66**, 5603–5609.
108. Ingemarson, R., Graslund, A., Darling, A., and Thelander, L. (1989). Herpes simplex virus ribonucleotide reductase: expression in Escherichia coli and purification to homogeneity of a tyrosyl free radical-containing, enzymatically active form of the 38-kilodalton subunit. *J. Virol.*, **63**, 3769–3776.

109. Jacquet, A., Haumont, M., Chellun, D. *et al.* (1998). The varicella zoster virus glycoprotein B (gB) plays a role in virus binding to cell surface heparan sulfate proteoglycans. *Virus Res.*, **53**, 197–207.
110. Jahedi, S., Markovitz, N. S., Filatov, F., and Roizman, B. (1999). Colocalization of the herpes simplex virus 1 UL4 protein with infected cell protein 22 in small, dense nuclear structures formed prior to onset of DNA synthesis. *J. Virol.*, **73**, 5132–5138.
111. Jerome, K. R., Fox, R., Chen, Z., Sears, A. E., Lee, H., and Corey, L. (1999). Herpes simplex virus inhibits apoptosis through the action of two genes, Us5 and Us3. *J. Virol.*, **73**, 8950–8957.
112. Jiang, Y. M., Yamada, H., Goshima, F. *et al.* (1998). Characterization of the herpes simplex virus type 2 (HSV-2) US2 gene product and a US2-deficient HSV-2 mutant. *J. Gen. Virol.*, **79**(11), 2777–2784.
113. Jun, P. Y., Strelow, L. I., Herman, R. C. *et al.* (1998). The UL4 gene of herpes simplex virus type 1 is dispensable for latency, reactivation and pathogenesis in mice. *J. Gen. Virol.*, **79**(7), 1603–1611.
114. Kamiyama, T., Kurokawa, M., and Shiraki, K. (2001). Characterization of the DNA polymerase gene of varicella-zoster viruses resistant to acyclovir. *J. Gen. Virol.*, **82**, 2761–2765.
115. Kemble, G. W., Annunziato, P., Lungu, O. *et al.* (2000). Open reading frame S/L of varicella-zoster virus encodes a cytoplasmic protein expressed in infected cells. *J. Virol.*, **74**, 11311–11321.
116. Kenyon, T. K., Cohen, J. I., and Grose, C. (2002). Phosphorylation by the varicella-zoster virus ORF47 protein serine kinase determines whether endocytosed viral gE traffics to the trans-Golgi network or recycles to the cell membrane. *J. Virol.*, **76**, 10980–10993.
117. Kenyon, T. K., Lynch, J., Hay, J., Ruyechan, W., and Grose, C. (2001). Varicella-zoster virus ORF47 protein serine kinase: characterization of a cloned, biologically active phosphotransferase and two viral substrates, ORF62 and ORF63. *J. Virol.*, **75**, 8854–8858.
118. Kinchington, P. R., Bookey, D., and Turse, S. E. (1995). The transcriptional regulatory proteins encoded by varicella-zoster virus open reading frames (ORFs) 4 and 63, but not ORF 61, are associated with purified virus particles. *J. Virol.*, **69**, 4274–4282.
119. Kinchington, P. R., Fite, K., Seman, A., and Turse, S. E. (2001). Virion association of IE62, the varicella-zoster virus (VZV) major transcriptional regulatory protein, requires expression of the VZV open reading frame 66 protein kinase. *J. Virol.*, **75**, 9106–9113.
120. Kinchington, P. R., Fite, K., and Turse, S. E. (2000). Nuclear accumulation of IE62, the varicella-zoster virus (VZV) major transcriptional regulatory protein, is inhibited by phosphorylation mediated by the VZV open reading frame 66 protein kinase. *J. Virol.*, **74**, 2265–2277.
121. Kinchington, P. R., Hougland, J. K., Arvin, A. M., Ruyechan, W. T., and Hay, J. (1992). The varicella-zoster virus immediate-early protein IE62 is a major component of virus particles. *J. Virol.*, **66**, 359–366.
122. Kinchington, P. R., Ling, P., Pensiero, M., Moss, B., Ruyechan, W. T., and Hay, J. (1990). The glycoprotein products of varicella-zoster virus gene 14 and their defective accumulation in a vaccine strain (Oka). *J. Virol.*, **64**, 4540–4548.
123. Kinoshita, H., Hondo, R., Taguchi, F., and Yogo, Y. (1988). Variation of R1 repeated sequence present in open reading frame 11 of varicella-zoster virus strains. *J. Virol.*, **62**, 1097–1100.
124. Kirkitadze, M. D., Barlow, P. N., Price, N. C. *et al.* (1998). The herpes simplex virus triplex protein, VP23, exists as a molten globule. *J. Virol.*, **72**, 10066–10072.
125. Klupp, B. G., Hengartner, C. J., Mettenleiter, T. C., and Enquist, L. W. (2004). Complete, annotated sequence of the pseudorabies virus genome. *J. Virol.*, **78**, 424–440.
126. Koff, A., Schwedes, J. F., and Tegtmeyer, P. (1991). Herpes simplex virus origin-binding protein (UL9) loops and distorts the viral replication origin. *J. Virol.*, **65**, 3284–3292.
127. Koshizuka, T., Goshima, F., Takakuwa, H. *et al.* (2002). Identification and characterization of the UL56 gene product of herpes simplex virus type 2. *J. Virol.*, **76**, 6718–6728.
128. Lagunoff, M., Randall, G., and Roizman, B. (1996). Phenotypic properties of herpes simplex virus 1 containing a derepressed open reading frame P gene. *J. Virol.*, **70**, 1810–1817.
129. Lagunoff, M. and Roizman, B. (1995). The regulation of synthesis and properties of the protein product of open reading frame P of the herpes simplex virus 1 genome. *J. Virol.*, **69**, 3615–3623.
130. Lamberti, C. and Weller, S. K. (1998). The herpes simplex virus type 1 cleavage/packaging protein, UL32, is involved in efficient localization of capsids to replication compartments. *J. Virol.*, **72**, 2463–2473.
131. Lee, F. K., Coleman, R. M., Pereira, L., Bailey, P. D., Tatsuno, M., and Nahmias, A. J. (1985). Detection of herpes simplex virus type 2-specific antibody with glycoprotein G. *J. Clin. Microbiol.*, **22**, 641–644.
132. Lee, S. S. and Lehman, I. R. (1997). Unwinding of the box I element of a herpes simplex virus type 1 origin by a complex of the viral origin binding protein, single-strand DNA binding protein, and single-stranded DNA. *Proc. Natl Acad. Sci. USA*, **94**, 2838–2842.
133. Leopardi, R., Van Sant, C., and Roizman, B. (1997). The herpes simplex virus 1 protein kinase US3 is required for protection from apoptosis induced by the virus. *Proc. Natl Acad. Sci. USA*, **94**, 7891–7896.
134. Liang, X., Tang, M., Manns, B., Babiuk, L. A., and Zamb, T. J. (1993). Identification and deletion mutagenesis of the bovine herpesvirus 1 dUTPase gene and a gene homologous to herpes simplex virus UL49.5. *Virology*, **195**, 42–50.
135. Ligas, M. W. and Johnson, D. C. (1988). A herpes simplex virus mutant in which glycoprotein D sequences are replaced by beta-galactosidase sequences binds to but is unable to penetrate into cells. *J. Virol.*, **62**, 1486–1494.

136. Liu, F. Y. and Roizman, B. (1991). The herpes simplex virus 1 gene encoding a protease also contains within its coding domain the gene encoding the more abundant substrate. *J. Virol.*, **65**, 5149–5156.
137. Liu, F. Y. and Roizman, B. (1991). The promoter, transcriptional unit, and coding sequence of herpes simplex virus 1 family 35 proteins are contained within and in frame with the UL26 open reading frame. *J. Virol.*, **65**, 206–212.
138. Liu, Y., Gong, W., Huang, C. C., Herr, W., and Cheng, X. (1999). Crystal structure of the conserved core of the herpes simplex virus transcriptional regulatory protein VP16. *Genes Dev.*, **13**, 1692–1703.
139. Long, M. C., Leong, V., Schaffer, P. A., Spencer, C. A., and Rice, S. A. (1999). ICP22 and the UL13 protein kinase are both required for herpes simplex virus-induced modification of the large subunit of RNA polymerase II. *J. Virol.*, **73**, 5593–5604.
140. Loomis, J. S., Bowzard, J. B., Courtney, R. J., and Wills, J. W. (2001). Intracellular trafficking of the UL11 tegument protein of herpes simplex virus type 1. *J. Virol.*, **75**, 12209–12219.
141. Loomis, J. S., Courtney, R. J., and Wills, J. W. (2003). Binding partners for the UL11 tegument protein of herpes simplex virus type 1. *J. Virol.*, **77**, 11417–11424.
142. Lubinski, J., Wang, L., Mastellos, D., Sahu, A., Lambris, J. D., and Friedman, H. M. (1999). In vivo role of complement-interacting domains of herpes simplex virus type 1 glycoprotein gC. *J. Exp. Med.*, **190**, 1637–1646.
143. MacLean, C. A., Clark, B., and McGeoch, D. J. (1989). Gene UL11 of herpes simplex virus type 1 encodes a virion protein which is myristylated. *J. Gen. Virol.*, **70**(12), 3147–3157.
144. MacLean, C. A., Dolan, A., Jamieson, F. E., and McGeoch, D. J. (1992). The myristylated virion proteins of herpes simplex virus type 1: investigation of their role in the virus life cycle. *J. Gen. Virol.*, **73**, 539–547.
145. MacLean, C. A., Efstathiou, S., Elliott, M. L., Jamieson, F. E., and McGeoch, D. J. (1991). Investigation of herpes simplex virus type 1 genes encoding multiply inserted membrane proteins. *J. Gen. Virol.*, **72**(4), 897–906.
146. Mahalingam, R., Lasher, R., Wellish, M., Cohrs, R. J., and Gilden, D. H. (1998). Localization of varicella-zoster virus gene 21 protein in virus-infected cells in culture. *J. Virol.*, **72**, 6832–6837.
147. Mahalingam, R., Wellish, M., Cabirac, G., Gilden, D., and Vafai, A. (1988). Regulation of varicella zoster virus gene 27 translation in vitro by upstream sequences. *Virus Res.*, **10**, 193–204.
148. Makhov, A. M., Lee, S. S., Lehman, I. R., and Griffith, J. D. (2003). Origin-specific unwinding of herpes simplex virus 1 DNA by the viral UL9 and ICP8 proteins: visualization of a specific preunwinding complex. *Proc. Natl Acad. Sci. USA*, **100**, 898–903.
149. Mallory, S., Sommer, M., and Arvin, A. M. (1997). Mutational analysis of the role of glycoprotein I in varicella-zoster virus replication and its effects on glycoprotein E conformation and trafficking. *J. Virol.*, **71**, 8279–8288.
150. Mapelli, M., Muhleisen, M., Persico, G., van Der Zandt, H., and Tucker, P. A. (2000). The 60-residue C-terminal region of the single-stranded DNA binding protein of herpes simplex virus type 1 is required for cooperative DNA binding. *J. Virol.*, **74**, 8812–8822.
151. Maresova, L., Pasieka, T., Wagenaar, T., Jackson, W., and Grose, C. (2003). Identification of the authentic varicella-zoster virus gB (gene 31) initiating methionine overlapping the 3' end of gene 30. *J. Med. Virol.*, **70** Suppl 1, S64–S70.
152. Markovitz, N. S., Filatov, F., and Roizman, B. (1999). The U(L)3 protein of herpes simplex virus 1 is translated predominantly from the second in-frame methionine codon and is subject to at least two posttranslational modifications. *J. Virol.*, **73**, 8010–8018.
153. Marsden, H. S., McLean, G. W., Barnard, E. C. *et al.* (1997). The catalytic subunit of the DNA polymerase of herpes simplex virus type 1 interacts specifically with the C terminus of the UL8 component of the viral helicase-primase complex. *J. Virol.*, **71**, 6390–6397.
154. Martinez, R., Sarisky, R. T., Weber, P. C., and Weller, S. K. (1996). Herpes simplex virus type 1 alkaline nuclease is required for efficient processing of viral DNA replication intermediates. *J. Virol.*, **70**, 2075–2085.
155. Mavromara-Nazos, P., Ackermann, M., and Roizman, B. (1986). Construction and properties of a viable herpes simplex virus 1 recombinant lacking coding sequences of the alpha 47 gene. *J. Virol.*, **60**, 807–812.
156. Mavromara-Nazos, P., Silver, S., Hubenthal-Voss, J., McKnight, J. L., and Roizman, B. (1986). Regulation of herpes simplex virus 1 genes: alpha gene sequence requirements for transient induction of indicator genes regulated by beta or late (gamma 2) promoters. *Virology*, **149**, 152–164.
157. McKnight, J. L., Pellett, P. E., Jenkins, F. J., and Roizman, B. (1987). Characterization and nucleotide sequence of two herpes simplex virus 1 genes whose products modulate alpha-trans-inducing factor-dependent activation of alpha genes. *J. Virol.*, **61**, 992–1001.
158. McKnight, S. L. (1980). The nucleotide sequence and transcript map of the herpes simplex virus thymidine kinase gene. *Nucl. Acids Res.*, **8**, 5949–5964.
159. McLean, G. W., Abbotts, A. P., Parry, M. E., Marsden, H. S., and Stow, N. D. (1994). The herpes simplex virus type 1 origin-binding protein interacts specifically with the viral UL8 protein. *J. Gen. Virol.*, **75**(10), 2699–2706.
160. McMillan, D. J., Kay, J., and Mills, J. S. (1997). Characterization of the proteinase specified by varicella-zoster virus gene 33. *J. Gen. Virol.*, **78**(9), 2153–2157.
161. McNab, A. R., Desai, P., Person, S. *et al.* (1998). The product of the herpes simplex virus type 1 UL25 gene is required for encapsidation but not for cleavage of replicated viral DNA. *J. Virol.*, **72**, 1060–1070.
162. Megaw, A. G., Rapaport, D., Avidor, B., Frenkel, N., and Davison, A. J. (1998). The DNA sequence of the RK strain of human herpesvirus 7. *Virology*, **244**, 119–132.
163. Meindl, A. and Osterrieder, N. (1999). The equine herpesvirus 1 Us2 homolog encodes a nonessential membrane-associated virion component. *J. Virol.*, **73**, 3430–3437.

164. Meredith, D. M., Lindsay, J. A., Halliburton, I. W., and Whittaker, G. R. (1991). Post-translational modification of the tegument proteins (VP13 and VP14) of herpes simplex virus type 1 by glycosylation and phosphorylation. *J. Gen. Virol.*, **72**(11), 2771–2775.
165. Mitchell, C., Blaho, J. A., McCormick, A. L., and Roizman, B. (1997). The nucleotidylylation of herpes simplex virus 1 regulatory protein alpha22 by human casein kinase II. *J. Biol. Chem.*, **272**, 25394–25400.
166. Mo, C., Lee, J., Sommer, M., Grose, C., and Arvin, A. M. (2002). The requirement of varicella zoster virus glycoprotein E (gE) for viral replication and effects of glycoprotein I on gE in melanoma cells. *Virology*, **304**, 176–186.
167. Mo, C., Suen, J., Sommer, M., and Arvin, A. (1999). Characterization of Varicella-Zoster virus glycoprotein K (open reading frame 5) and its role in virus growth. *J. Virol.*, **73**, 4197–4207.
168. Moffat, J., Ito, H., Sommer, M., Taylor, S., and Arvin, A. M. (2002). Glycoprotein I of varicella-zoster virus is required for viral replication in skin and T cells. *J. Virol.*, **76**, 8468–8471.
169. Montague, M. G. and Hutchison, C. A., 3rd (2000). Gene content phylogeny of herpesviruses. *Proc. Natl Acad. Sci. USA*, **97**, 5334–5339.
170. Mori, H., Shiraki, K., Kato, T., Hayakawa, Y., Yamanishi, K., and Takahashi, M. (1988). Molecular analysis of the thymidine kinase gene of thymidine kinase-deficient mutants of varicella-zoster virus. *Intervirology*, **29**, 301–310.
171. Moriuchi, H., Moriuchi, M., and Cohen, J. I. (1994). The RING finger domain of the varicella-zoster virus open reading frame 61 protein is required for its transregulatory functions. *Virology*, **205**, 238–246.
172. Moriuchi, H., Moriuchi, M., Pichyangkura, R., Triezenberg, S. J., Straus, S. E., and Cohen, J. I. (1995). Hydrophobic cluster analysis predicts an amino-terminal domain of varicella-zoster virus open reading frame 10 required for transcriptional activation. *Proc. Natl Acad. Sci. USA*, **92**, 9333–9337.
173. Moriuchi, M., Moriuchi, H., Debrus, S., Piette, J., and Cohen, J. I. (1995). The acidic amino-terminal region of varicella-zoster virus open reading frame 4 protein is required for transactivation and can functionally replace the corresponding region of herpes simplex virus ICP27. *Virology*, **208**, 376–382.
174. Nalwanga, D., Rempel, S., Roizman, B., and Baines, J. D. (1996). The UL 16 gene product of herpes simplex virus 1 is a virion protein that colocalizes with intranuclear capsid proteins. *Virology*, **226**, 236–242.
175. Newcomb, W. W. and Brown, J. C. (1989). Use of Ar+ plasma etching to localize structural proteins in the capsid of herpes simplex virus type 1. *J. Virol.*, **63**, 4697–4702.
176. Newcomb, W. W., Juhas, R. M., Thomsen, D. R. *et al.* (2001). The UL6 gene product forms the portal for entry of DNA into the herpes simplex virus capsid. *J. Virol.*, **75**, 10923–10932.
177. Newcomb, W. W., Trus, B. L., Booy, F. P., Steven, A. C., Wall, J. S., and Brown, J. C. (1993). Structure of the herpes simplex virus capsid. Molecular composition of the pentons and the triplexes. *J. Mol. Biol.*, **232**, 499–511.
178. Niizuma, T., Zerboni, L., Sommer, M. H., Ito, H., Hinchliffe, S., and Arvin, A. M. (2003). Construction of varicella-zoster virus recombinants from parent Oka cosmids and demonstration that ORF65 protein is dispensable for infection of human skin and T cells in the SCID-hu mouse model. *J. Virol.*, **77**, 6062–6065.
179. Nishiyama, Y., Kurachi, R., Daikoku, T., and Umene, K. (1993). The US 9, 10, 11, and 12 genes of herpes simplex virus type 1 are of no importance for its neurovirulence and latency in mice. *Virology*, **194**, 419–423.
180. Noble, A. G., Lee, G. T., Sprague, R., Parish, M. L., and Spear, P. G. (1983). Anti-gD monoclonal antibodies inhibit cell fusion induced by herpes simplex virus type 1. *Virology*, **129**, 218–224.
181. Nozawa, N., Daikoku, T., Yamauchi, Y. *et al.* (2002). Identification and characterization of the UL7 gene product of herpes simplex virus type 2. *Virus Genes*, **24**, 257–266.
182. Olson, J. K. and Grose, C. (1997). Endocytosis and recycling of varicella-zoster virus Fc receptor glycoprotein gE: internalization mediated by a YXXL motif in the cytoplasmic tail. *J. Virol.*, **71**, 4042–4054.
183. Papavassiliou, A. G., Wilcox, K. W., and Silverstein, S. J. (1991). The interaction of ICP4 with cell/infected-cell factors and its state of phosphorylation modulate differential recognition of leader sequences in herpes simplex virus DNA. *EMBO J.*, **10**, 397–406.
184. Pasieka, T. J., Maresova, L., and Grose, C. (2003). A functional YNKI motif in the short cytoplasmic tail of varicella-zoster virus glycoprotein gH mediates clathrin-dependent and antibody-independent endocytosis. *J. Virol.*, **77**, 4191–4204.
185. Pearson, A. and Coen, D. M. (2002). Identification, localization, and regulation of expression of the UL24 protein of herpes simplex virus type 1. *J. Virol.*, **76**, 10821–10828.
186. Pellett, P. E., Kousoulas, K. G., Pereira, L., and Roizman, B. (1985). Anatomy of the herpes simplex virus 1 strain F glycoprotein B gene: primary sequence and predicted protein structure of the wild type and of monoclonal antibody-resistant mutants. *J. Virol.*, **53**, 243–253.
187. Pellett, P. E., McKnight, J. L., Jenkins, F. J., and Roizman, B. (1985). Nucleotide sequence and predicted amino acid sequence of a protein encoded in a small herpes simplex virus DNA fragment capable of trans-inducing alpha genes. *Proc. Natl Acad. Sci. USA*, **82**, 5870–5874.
188. Peng, H., He, H., Hay, J., and Ruyechan, W. T. (2003). Interaction between the varicella zoster virus IE62 major transactivator and cellular transcription factor Sp1. *J. Biol. Chem.*, **278**, 38068–38075.
189. Peng, T., Hunter, J. R., and Nelson, J. W. (1996). The novel protein kinase of the RR1 subunit of herpes simplex virus has autophosphorylation and transphosphorylation activity that differs in its ATP requirements for HSV-1 and HSV-2. *Virology*, **216**, 184–196.
190. Perelygina, L., Zhu, L., Zurkuhlen, H., Mills, R., Borodovsky, M., and Hilliard, J. K. (2003). Complete sequence and comparative

190. analysis of the genome of herpes B virus (Cercopithecine herpesvirus 1) from a rhesus monkey. *J. Virol.*, **77**, 6167–6177.
191. Perng, G. C., Jones, C., Ciacci-Zanella, J. *et al.* (2000). Virus-induced neuronal apoptosis blocked by the herpes simplex virus latency-associated transcript. *Science*, **287**, 1500–1503.
192. Perng, G. C., Maguen, B., Jin, L. *et al.* (2002). A gene capable of blocking apoptosis can substitute for the herpes simplex virus type 1 latency-associated transcript gene and restore wild-type reactivation levels. *J. Virol.*, **76**, 1224–1235.
193. Pogue-Geile, K. L., Lee, G. T., Shapira, S. K., and Spear, P. G. (1984). Fine mapping of mutations in the fusion-inducing MP strain of herpes simplex virus type 1. *Virology*, **136**, 100–109.
194. Pomeranz, L. E. and Blaho, J. A. (1999). Modified VP22 localizes to the cell nucleus during synchronized herpes simplex virus type 1 infection. *J. Virol.*, **73**, 6769–6781.
195. Post, L. E., Mackem, S., and Roizman, B. (1981). Regulation of alpha genes of herpes simplex virus: expression of chimeric genes produced by fusion of thymidine kinase with alpha gene promoters. *Cell*, **24**, 555–565.
196. Purves, F. C. and Roizman, B. (1992). The UL13 gene of herpes simplex virus 1 encodes the functions for posttranslational processing associated with phosphorylation of the regulatory protein alpha 22. *Proc. Natl Acad. Sci. USA*, **89**, 7310–7314.
197. Purves, F. C., Spector, D., and Roizman, B. (1991). The herpes simplex virus 1 protein kinase encoded by the US3 gene mediates posttranslational modification of the phosphoprotein encoded by the UL34 gene. *J. Virol.*, **65**, 5757–5764.
198. Randall, G., Lagunoff, M., and Roizman, B. (1997). The product of ORF O located within the domain of herpes simplex virus 1 genome transcribed during latent infection binds to and inhibits in vitro binding of infected cell protein 4 to its cognate DNA site. *Proc. Natl Acad. Sci. USA*, **94**, 10379–10384.
199. Reynolds, A. E., Fan, Y., and Baines, J. D. (2000). Characterization of the U(L)33 gene product of herpes simplex virus 1. *Virology*, **266**, 310–318.
200. Reynolds, A. E., Ryckman, B. J., Baines, J. D., Zhou, Y., Liang, L., and Roller, R. J. (2001). U(L)31 and U(L)34 proteins of herpes simplex virus type 1 form a complex that accumulates at the nuclear rim and is required for envelopment of nucleocapsids. *J. Virol.*, **75**, 8803–8817.
201. Reynolds, A. E., Wills, E. G., Roller, R. J., Ryckman, B. J., and Baines, J. D. (2002). Ultrastructural localization of the herpes simplex virus type 1 UL31, UL34, and US3 proteins suggests specific roles in primary envelopment and egress of nucleocapsids. *J. Virol.*, **76**, 8939–8952.
202. Roller, R. J., Monk, L. L., Stuart, D., and Roizman, B. (1996). Structure and function in the herpes simplex virus 1 RNA-binding protein U(s)11: mapping of the domain required for ribosomal and nucleolar association and RNA binding in vitro. *J. Virol.*, **70**, 2842–2851.
203. Roop, C., Hutchinson, L., and Johnson, D. C. (1993). A mutant herpes simplex virus type 1 unable to express glycoprotein L cannot enter cells, and its particles lack glycoprotein H. *J. Virol.*, **67**, 2285–2297.
204. Rosen-Wolff, A., Lamade, W., Berkowitz, C., Becker, Y., and Darai, G. (1991). Elimination of UL56 gene by insertion of LacZ cassette between nucleotide position 116030 to 121753 of the herpes simplex virus type 1 genome abrogates intraperitoneal pathogenicity in tree shrews and mice. *Virus Res.*, **20**, 205–221.
205. Ross, J., Williams, M., and Cohen, J. I. (1997). Disruption of the varicella-zoster virus dUTPase and the adjacent ORF9A gene results in impaired growth and reduced syncytia formation in vitro. *Virology*, **234**, 186–195.
206. Salmon, B. and Baines, J. D. (1998). Herpes simplex virus DNA cleavage and packaging: association of multiple forms of U(L)15-encoded proteins with B capsids requires at least the U(L)6, U(L)17, and U(L)28 genes. *J. Virol.*, **72**, 3045–3050.
207. Salmon, B., Cunningham, C., Davison, A. J., Harris, W. J., and Baines, J. D. (1998). The herpes simplex virus type 1 U(L)17 gene encodes virion tegument proteins that are required for cleavage and packaging of viral DNA. *J. Virol.*, **72**, 3779–3788.
208. Salmon, B., Nalwanga, D., Fan, Y., and Baines, J. D. (1999). Proteolytic cleavage of the amino terminus of the U(L)15 gene product of herpes simplex virus type 1 is coupled with maturation of viral DNA into unit-length genomes. *J. Virol.*, **73**, 8338–8348.
209. Sato, B., Ito, H., Hinchliffe, S., Sommer, M. H., Zerboni, L., and Arvin, A. M. (2003). Mutational analysis of open reading frames 62 and 71, encoding the varicella-zoster virus immediate-early transactivating protein, IE62, and effects on replication in vitro and in skin xenografts in the SCID-hu mouse in vivo. *J. Virol.*, **77**, 5607–5620.
210. Sato, B., Sommer, M., Ito, H., and Arvin, A. M. (2003). Requirement of varicella-zoster virus immediate-early 4 protein for viral replication. *J. Virol.*, **77**, 12369–12372.
211. Sato, H., Callanan, L. D., Pesnicak, L., Krogmann, T., and Cohen, J. I. (2002). Varicella-zoster virus (VZV) ORF17 protein induces RNA cleavage and is critical for replication of VZV at 37 degrees C but not 33 degrees C. *J. Virol.*, **76**, 11012–11023.
212. Sato, H., Pesnicak, L., and Cohen, J. I. (2002). Varicella-zoster virus open reading frame 2 encodes a membrane phosphoprotein that is dispensable for viral replication and for establishment of latency. *J. Virol.*, **76**, 3575–3578.
213. Schmitz, J. B., Albright, A. G., Kinchington, P. R., and Jenkins, F. J. (1995). The UL37 protein of herpes simplex virus type 1 is associated with the tegument of purified virions. *Virology*, **206**, 1055–1065.
214. Sciortino, M. T., Taddeo, B., Poon, A. P., Mastino, A., and Roizman, B. (2002). Of the three tegument proteins that package mRNA in herpes simplex virions, one (VP22) transports the mRNA to uninfected cells for expression prior to viral infection. *Proc. Natl Acad. Sci. USA*, **99**, 8318–8323.
215. Shiba, C., Daikoku, T., Goshima, F. *et al.* (2000). The UL34 gene product of herpes simplex virus type 2 is a tail-anchored type II membrane protein that is significant for virus envelopment. *J. Gen. Virol.*, **81**, 2397–2405.

216. Smiley, J. R. (2004). Herpes simplex virus virion host shutoff protein: immune evasion mediated by a viral RNase γ *J. Virol.*, **78**, 1063–1068.
217. Smith, R. F. and Smith, T. F. (1989). Identification of new protein kinase-related genes in three herpesviruses, herpes simplex virus, varicella-zoster virus, and Epstein–Barr virus. *J. Virol.*, **63**, 450–455.
218. Sommer, M. H., Zagha, E., Serrano, O. K. *et al.* (2001). Mutational analysis of the repeated open reading frames, ORFs 63 and 70 and ORFs 64 and 69, of varicella-zoster virus. *J. Virol.*, **75**, 8224–8239.
219. Spencer, J. V., Newcomb, W. W., Thomsen, D. R., Homa, F. L., and Brown, J. C. (1998). Assembly of the herpes simplex virus capsid: preformed triplexes bind to the nascent capsid. *J. Virol.*, **72**, 3944–3951.
220. Spengler, M. L., Ruyechan, W. T., and Hay, J. (2000). Physical interaction between two varicella zoster virus gene regulatory proteins, IE4 and IE62. *Virology*, **272**, 375–381.
221. Stevens, J. G., Wagner, E. K., Devi-Rao, G. B., Cook, M. L., and Feldman, L. T. (1987). RNA complementary to a herpesvirus alpha gene mRNA is prominent in latently infected neurons. *Science*, **235**, 1056–1059.
222. Stevenson, D., Colman, K. L., and Davison, A. J. (1994). Delineation of a sequence required for nuclear localization of the protein encoded by varicella-zoster virus gene 61. *J. Gen. Virol.*, **75**(11), 3229–3233.
223. Stow, N. D. (2001). Packaging of genomic and amplicon DNA by the herpes simplex virus type 1 UL25-null mutant KUL25NS. *J. Virol.*, **75**, 10755–10765.
224. Stow, N. D., Weir, H. M., and Stow, E. C. (1990). Analysis of the binding sites for the varicella-zoster virus gene 51 product within the viral origin of DNA replication. *Virology*, **177**, 570–577.
225. Strom, T. and Frenkel, N. (1987). Effects of herpes simplex virus on mRNA stability. *J. Virol.*, **61**, 2198–2207.
226. Takakuwa, H., Goshima, F., Koshizuka, T., Murata, T., Daikoku, T., and Nishiyama, Y. (2001). Herpes simplex virus encodes a virion-associated protein which promotes long cellular processes in over-expressing cells. *Genes Cells*, **6**, 955–966.
227. Taus, N. S., Salmon, B., and Baines, J. D. (1998). The herpes simplex virus 1 UL 17 gene is required for localization of capsids and major and minor capsid proteins to intranuclear sites where viral DNA is cleaved and packaged. *Virology*, **252**, 115–125.
228. Telford, E. A., Watson, M. S., Aird, H. C., Perry, J., and Davison, A. J. (1995). The DNA sequence of equine herpesvirus 2. *J. Mol. Biol.*, **249**, 520–528.
229. Tenney, D. J., Hurlburt, W. W., Micheletti, P. A., Bifano, M., and Hamatake, R. K. (1994). The UL8 component of the herpes simplex virus helicase-primase complex stimulates primer synthesis by a subassembly of the UL5 and UL52 components. *J. Biol. Chem.*, **269**, 5030–5035.
230. Trgovcich, J., Johnson, D., and Roizman, B. (2002). Cell surface major histocompatibility complex class II proteins are regulated by the products of the gamma(1)34.5 and U(L)41 genes of herpes simplex virus 1. *J. Virol.*, **76**, 6974–6986.
231. Trus, B. L., Booy, F. P., Newcomb, W. W. *et al.* (1996). The herpes simplex virus procapsid: structure, conformational changes upon maturation, and roles of the triplex proteins VP19c and VP23 in assembly. *J. Mol. Biol.*, **263**, 447–462.
232. van Zeijl, M., Fairhurst, J., Jones, T. R. *et al.* (2000). Novel class of thiourea compounds that inhibit herpes simplex virus type 1 DNA cleavage and encapsidation: resistance maps to the UL6 gene. *J. Virol.*, **74**, 9054–9061.
233. Visalli, R. J. and Brandt, C. R. (1991). The HSV-1 UL45 gene product is not required for growth in Vero cells. *Virology*, **185**, 419–423.
234. Visse, B., Huraux, J. M., and Fillet, A. M. (1999). Point mutations in the varicella-zoster virus DNA polymerase gene confers resistance to foscarnet and slow growth phenotype. *J. Med. Virol.*, **59**, 84–90.
235. Wang, Z. H., Gershon, M. D., Lungu, O., Zhu, Z., Mallory, S., Arvin, A. M., and Gershon, A. A. (2001). Essential role played by the C-terminal domain of glycoprotein I in envelopment of varicella-zoster virus in the trans-Golgi network: interactions of glycoproteins with tegument. *J. Virol.*, **75**, 323–340.
236. Ward, P. L., Barker, D. E., and Roizman, B. (1996). A novel herpes simplex virus 1 gene, UL43.5, maps antisense to the UL43 gene and encodes a protein which colocalizes in nuclear structures with capsid proteins. *J. Virol.*, **70**, 2684–2690.
237. Ward, P. L., Taddeo, B., Markovitz, N. S., and Roizman, B. (2000). Identification of a novel expressed open reading frame situated between genes U(L)20 and U(L)21 of the herpes simplex virus 1 genome. *Virology*, **266**, 275–285.
238. Weir, H. M. and Stow, N. D. (1990). Two binding sites for the herpes simplex virus type 1 UL9 protein are required for efficient activity of the oriS replication origin. *J. Gen. Virol.*, **71**(6), 1379–1385.
239. Weisshart, K., Kuo, A. A., Hwang, C. B., Kumura, K., and Coen, D. M. (1994). Structural and functional organization of herpes simplex virus DNA polymerase investigated by limited proteolysis. *J. Biol. Chem.*, **269**, 22788–22796.
240. Weisshart, K., Kuo, A. A., Painter, G. R., Wright, L. L., Furman, P. A., and Coen, D. M. (1993). Conformational changes induced in herpes simplex virus DNA polymerase upon DNA binding. *Proc. Natl Acad. Sci. USA*, **90**, 1028–1032.
241. Weller, S. K., Seghatoleslami, M. R., Shao, L., Rowse, D., and Carmichael, E. P. (1990). The herpes simplex virus type 1 alkaline nuclease is not essential for viral DNA synthesis: isolation and characterization of a lacZ insertion mutant. *J. Gen. Virol.*, **71**(12), 2941–2952.
242. White, C. A., Stow, N. D., Patel, A. H., Hughes, M., and Preston, V. G. (2003). Herpes simplex virus type 1 portal protein UL6 interacts with the putative terminase subunits UL15 and UL28. *J. Virol.*, **77**, 6351–6358.
243. Wingfield, P. T., Stahl, S. J., Thomsen, D. R. *et al.* (1997). Hexon-only binding of VP26 reflects differences between the hexon

and penton conformations of VP5, the major capsid protein of herpes simplex virus. *J. Virol.*, **71**, 8955–8961.
244. Winters, T. A. and Williams, M. V. (1993). Purification and characterization of the herpes simplex virus type 2-encoded uracil-DNA glycosylase. *Virology*, **195**, 315–326.
245. Worrad, D. M. and Caradonna, S. (1993). The herpes simplex virus type 2 UL3 open reading frame encodes a nuclear localizing phosphoprotein. *Virology*, **195**, 364–376.
246. Wu, T. T., Su, Y. H., Block, T. M., and Taylor, J. M. (1996). Evidence that two latency-associated transcripts of herpes simplex virus type 1 are nonlinear. *J. Virol.*, **70**, 5962–5967.
247. Xia, D. and Straus, S. E. (1999). Transcript mapping and transregulatory behavior of varicella-zoster virus gene 21, a latency-associated gene. *Virology*, **258**, 304–313.
248. Yamada, H., Daikoku, T., Yamashita, Y., Jiang, Y. M., Tsurumi, T., and Nishiyama, Y. (1997). The product of the US10 gene of herpes simplex virus type 1 is a capsid/tegument-associated phosphoprotein which copurifies with the nuclear matrix. *J. Gen. Virol.*, **78**(11), 2923–2931.
249. Yamada, H., Jiang, Y. M., Oshima, S. *et al.* (1998). Characterization of the UL4 gene product of herpes simplex virus type 2. *Arch. Virol.*, **143**, 1199–1207.
250. Yamauchi, Y., Wada, K., Goshima, F. *et al.* (2001). The UL14 protein of herpes simplex virus type 2 translocates the minor capsid protein VP26 and the DNA cleavage and packaging UL33 protein into the nucleus of coexpressing cells. *J. Gen. Virol.*, **82**, 321–330.
251. York, I. A., Roop, C., Andrews, D. W., Riddell, S. R., Graham, F. L., and Johnson, D. C. (1994). A cytosolic herpes simplex virus protein inhibits antigen presentation to CD8+ T lymphocytes. *Cell*, **77**, 525–535.
252. Zhang, Y. and McKnight, J. L. (1993). Herpes simplex virus type 1 UL46 and UL47 deletion mutants lack VP11 and VP12 or VP13 and VP14, respectively, and exhibit altered viral thymidine kinase expression. *J. Virol.*, **67**, 1482–1492.
253. Zhou, C. and Knipe, D. M. (2002). Association of herpes simplex virus type 1 ICP8 and ICP27 proteins with cellular RNA polymerase II holoenzyme. *J. Virol.*, **76**, 5893–5904.
254. Zhou, G., Galvan, V., Campadelli-Fiume, G., and Roizman, B. (2000). Glycoprotein D or J delivered in trans blocks apoptosis in SK-N-SH cells induced by a herpes simplex virus 1 mutant lacking intact genes expressing both glycoproteins. *J. Virol.*, **74**, 11782–11791.
255. Zhu, Z., Hao, Y., Gershon, M. D., Ambron, R. T., and Gershon, A. A. (1996). Targeting of glycoprotein I (gE) of varicella-zoster virus to the trans-Golgi network by an AYRV sequence and an acidic amino acid-rich patch in the cytosolic domain of the molecule. *J. Virol.*, **70**, 6563–6575.

Entry of alphaherpesviruses into the cell

Gabriella Campadelli-Fiume and Laura Menotti

Department of Experimental Pathology, Alma Mater Studiorum-University of Bologna, Italy

Introduction

Herpes simplex virus (HSV) represents the most comprehensive example of virus-receptor interaction in the *Herpesviridae* family, and the prototype virus encoding multipartite entry genes. Whereas small enveloped viruses package the functions required for entry and fusion into one or two fusion glycoproteins, in HSV the same functions are distributed over several distinct glycoproteins, each with a specialized activity. In addition, HSV encodes a highly sophisticated system for promoting and blocking fusion between the viral envelope and cell membrane. Because the most obvious models of virus entry into the cell do not fit with the HSV complexity, and despite our detailed knowledge of the HSV receptors and of the crystal structure of glycoprotein D (gD), the receptor-binding glycoprotein, and of gB, HSV entry is still, in part, a puzzle (WuDunn and Spear, 1989; Cocchi *et al.*, 1998b; Geraghty *et al.*, 1998; Carfi *et al.*, 2001).

The current model of HSV entry envisions that, first, the virus attaches to cell membranes by the interaction of gC, and possibly gB, to glycosaminoglycans (GAGs) (Herold *et al.*, 1991). This binding likely creates multiple points of adhesion, is reversible, and the detached virus maintains its infectivity, indicating that fusion has yet to take place. Penetration requires gD, whose ectodomain contains two physically separate and functionally distinct regions, i.e., the region made of the N-terminus that carries the receptor-binding sites, and the C-terminus that carries the profusion domain (Ligas and Johnson, 1988; Cocchi *et al.*, 2004). The role of gD in entry is to interact with one of the entry receptors, to signal receptor-recognition and thus trigger fusion, by recruiting three additional glycoproteins – gB, gH, gL. The trio of gB, gH, gL execute fusion with the plasma membrane or endocytic vesicle of the target cell (Fig. 7.1) (Cai, W. H. *et al.*, 1988; Forrester *et al.*, 1992; Roop *et al.*, 1993; Campadelli-Fiume *et al.*, 2000; Spear *et al.*, 2000; Nicola *et al.*, 2003). Of these, gH carries elements characteristic of viral fusion glycoproteins, i.e., a hydrophobic α-helix with attributes of an internal fusion peptide, and two heptad repeats with propensity to form coiled coils (Gianni *et al.*, 2005a,b). gB is a trimer with a coiled coil core; its structure closely resembles that of viral fusion proteins (Heldwein *et al.*, 2006; Roche *et al.*, 2006). Following fusion, the released tegumented nucleocapsid travels along microtubules to the nuclear pore, where the viral DNA is released into the nucleus (Sodeik *et al.*, 1997).

Much less is known about varicella zoster virus (VZV) entry. The process may be very different from that of HSV inasmuch as virion-to-cell infection is inefficient in the VZV system, and the viral genome presents a striking difference from that of HSV, namely the lack of gD (Davison and Scott, 1986).

The membrane proteins

The HSV envelope contains at least eleven glycoproteins (gB, gC, gD, gE, gG, gH, gI, gJ, gK, gL, and gM). Additional membrane proteins not detected in the extracellular virion envelope are UL20, UL34, UL45 and possibly US9. The transcripts for UL24, UL43, and UL49.5 ORFs have been recognized, but the proteins have yet to be identified. A summary list with references is presented in Chapter 6.

From a structural point of view, the majority of HSV glycoproteins are type I glycoproteins. Variants include gL, which is soluble (Hutchinson *et al.*, 1992a); gB, which may carry two or three α-helices in the transmembrane (TM) region (Pellett *et al.*, 1985) and gK, gM, and UL20, which carry information for multiple transmembrane segments

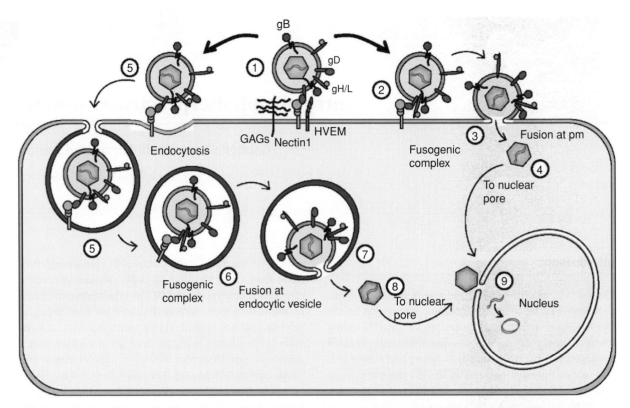

Fig. 7.1. Schematic drawing of HSV entry. Entry can occur either by endocytosis (pathway at the left), or by fusion at the plasma membrane (pathway at the right). Following attachment to cells, gD binds to a cellular receptor (frame 1), and presumably following a conformational change it recruits the glycoproteins B, H and L in an active fusogenic complex (frame 2), triggering the fusion between viral envelope and cellular plasma membrane (frame 3). The naked nucleocapsids are transported to the nucleus (frames 4 and 9). In a cell line-dependent manner or with modified forms of the receptor (see text for details) bound virions can enter cells by endocytosis (frame 5). It is conceivable that at this stage the four fusogenic glycoproteins are in a non-fusion-active form. Following acidification/maturation of the endocytic vesicles, a fusogenic complex may form (frame 6) and fusion ensue between the virion envelope and the vesicle membrane (frame 7). Nucleocapsids delivered to the cytoplasm are transported to the nucleus (frames 8 and 9).

(McGeoch *et al.*, 1988). US9 and HSV-2 UL45 are type II glycoproteins with a C-terminal ectodomain.

At the ultrastructural level, HSV glycoproteins form long thin spikes, each made of a single species. As visualized in cryo-electron tomograms of isolated virions, the envelope contains 600–750 glycoprotein spikes that vary in length, spacings, and in the angle at which they emerge from the membrane. Their distribution in the envelope suggests functional clustering (Grunewald *et al.*, 2003). In contrast, slender spikes have not been seen in varicella zoster virions (VZV) grown in cultured cells. Instead, the virion appears to be covered by an envelope studded with protrusions rather than spikes. An example is shown in Fig. 7.2. Further studies at even higher resolution will be required to determine differences between HSV and VZV envelopes.

HSV

Attachment to cells

Attachment of HSV to cells occurs upon binding of gC to GAGs that decorate heparan sulphate or chondroitin sulphate (Spear *et al.*, 1992) (Fig. 7.1). This step enhances HSV infectivity, but is not an absolute requirement, as cells defective in heparan sulphate and chondroitin sulphate exhibit a 100-fold reduced susceptibility to infection, yet can be infected (Gruenheid *et al.*, 1993). A large variety of viruses use heparan sulphate proteoglycans as receptors; their broad expression argues that they can not be responsible for any specific viral tropism.

The major actor during attachment is gC, a non essential glycoprotein encoded by the UL44 gene. gC is a

Entry of alphaherpesviruses into the cell

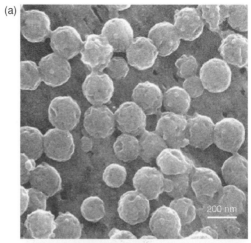

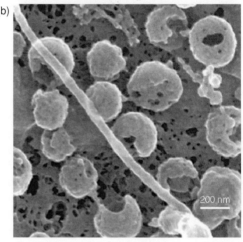

Fig. 7.2. Scanning electron micrographs of HSV-1 and VZV. Images of both viruses were taken by SEM after infection of cultured cells. HSV-1 virions have a more uniform appearance although indentations are seen in an occasional virion envelope (a). In contrast, VZV virions are more aberrant (b). Several of the virions have indentations, while other virions have incomplete envelopes. Since both viruses were examined under the same SEM conditions, it is unlikely that the aberrant nature of the VZV envelope is due to fixation artifacts. Micrographs kindly provided by Dr. Charles Grose.

mucin-type glycoprotein because of its high content in N-linked and O-linked oligosaccharides. Its ectodomain structure is provided in part by 8 cysteines, and harbors two physically separate antigenic regions, antigenic sites I and II, that map at the C- and N-termini of the molecule, respectively (Dolter *et al.*, 1992). Evidence for the role of gC in attachment rests on several lines of evidence. Initially, it was observed that the polycations neomycin and polylysine inhibit attachment of HSV-1, but not HSV-2 to cells, and this differential effect was mapped to gC (Campadelli-Fiume *et al.*, 1990). gC and gB bind heparin-Sepharose columns (Herold *et al.*, 1991). The affinity of binding to heparan sulphate is on the order of 10^{-8} M (Rux *et al.*, 2002). The region important for the interaction with heparan sulphate maps to the N-terminus of gC (Tal-Singer *et al.*, 1995). Virion binding to cells is reduced in HSV-1 mutants lacking gC-type1 gene, but not in HSV-2 mutants lacking gC-type2 (Herold *et al.*, 1991; Gerber *et al.*, 1995). The majority of these studies were performed with mutants constructed in the background of the HSV-1(KOS) strain. In contrast, deletion of gC gene in the genetic background of Sc16 and HFEM strains yielded viruses with unimpaired attachment activity, suggesting that in different virus strains, attachment may be carried out by different proteins (Griffiths *et al.*, 1998). gC has also been implicated in virus attachment to the baso-lateral domain of MDCK polarized epithelial cells, and to the apical domain of polarized human CaCo2 cells.

Interaction of gD with its receptors

gD

The ectodomain of gD is required and sufficient to enable HSV entry into cells. It is made of two separate and distinct regions, i.e., the N-terminus, carrying the receptor-binding sites (approximately contained between residues 1 and 250–260), and the C-terminus carrying the profusion domain (residues 250–260 to 305) (Cocchi *et al.*, 2004).

A breakthrough in our understanding of HSV entry came from resolution of the crystal structure of a soluble form of gD, initially up to amino acid residue 259 (Carfi *et al.*, 2001), and later on up to residue 306 (Krummenacher *et al.*, 2005). The initial structure was determined for gD alone and for gD in complex with one of the gD receptors, HVEM (herpesvirus entry mediator) (Fig. 7.3). The N-terminus consists of three portions, an Ig-folded central core (residues 56–184) made of β-strands forming two antiparallel β-sheets, and two extensions, one N-terminal (residues 1–37) and one C-terminal (Fig. 7.3). The N-terminus, which harbors all the contact residues to HVEM, is disordered in the crystal of gD alone, but forms a hairpin when gD is complexed with HVEM. gD and HVEM thereby form an intermolecular β-sheet, which is believed to stabilize the complex. Formation of the N-terminal hairpin documents a conformational change to gD when it binds HVEM.

The crystal structure of gD in complex with nectin1 has not yet been solved. The nectin1-binding site on gD, determined by means of insertion-deletion or substitution mutants, appears to be more widespread than the HVEM interaction region, (Milne *et al.*, 2003; Yoon *et al.*, 2003; Zhou

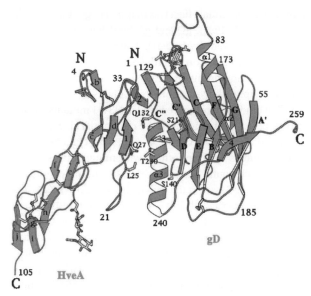

Fig. 7.3. Ribbon diagram of the 3D structure of a soluble truncated form of gD (gD285t, colored in orange) bound to HVEM receptor (HveA, colored in green) as determined by X-ray crystallography. The N-terminus (residues 1–37) of gD is devoid of a specific structure when in the unbound state, but folds into a hairpin when bound to HVEM receptor. The β-strand formed by residues 27–29 (indicated with number 1) forms an intermolecular β-sheet with HVEM residues 35–37 (letter d). The core of gD (residues 56–184) has a V-type immunglobulin domain structure, composed of 9 parallel and antiparallel β-strands (letters A to G) that form two opposing β-sheets, and carries an additional α-helix (α1). The residues 185–259 form two α-helices that fold back to the N-ter (α2 and α3), and two β-strands (numbered 3 and 4). The α3 helix supports gD's N-terminal hairpin. An additional β-strand (number 2) is located in the connector sequence (residues 33–55) that precedes the Ig-like core. Reprinted from (Carfi *et al.*, 2001), with permission. (See color plate section.)

et al., 2003; Jogger *et al.*, 2004; Manoj *et al.*, 2004; Connolly *et al.*, 2005). The only recombinant described so far debilitated for interaction with nectin1 carries the V34S substitution (Zhou and Roizman, 2006).

Receptors

Entry receptors interact with gD. This notion was established long before the actual receptors were identified, and rests on two lines of evidence. First, soluble gD binds in a saturable manner to cells and prevents infection (Johnson, D. C. *et al.*, 1990; Nicola *et al.*, 1997). Second, expression of gD from a transgene renders cells resistant to infection, because of its ability to sequester the receptor, a phenomenon designated restriction to infection or gD-mediated interference (Campadelli-Fiume *et al.*, 1988; Johnson, R. M. and Spear, 1989).

The search for HSV receptors was an active field in the 1990s, and a number of molecules were described as potential receptors. A breakthrough came from Spear and coworkers, who made use of HSV-resistant CHO cells, and identified a HeLa cell cDNA clone that encoded HVEM (Montgomery *et al.*, 1996). However, three observations in that study suggested the existence of additional receptors. First, HVEM appeared to be expressed by a limited number of cell lines. Second, antibodies to HVEM failed to completely block HSV infection. Third, several virus strains were unable to enter CHO cells expressing HVEM but were otherwise viable. This boosted further efforts in the field, which quickly led to the discovery of nectins, and, later on, of modified heparan sulphate. Altogether, the receptors known to date belong to three unrelated molecular families. Their present and past nomenclature, and the viruses for which they serve as receptors are reported in the table.

Nectins are intercellular adhesion molecules

Research in the field of nectins has proceeded in parallel with their characterization as HSV receptors (Takai *et al.*, 2003). Nectins 1–4 form a subfamily of Ca^{2+}-independent immunoglobulin (Ig)-type intercellular adhesion molecules. Together with nectin-like molecules and poliovirus receptor, they share the same overall structure consisting of three Ig-type domains. Splice variant isoforms are designated with Greek letters. Nectins form homo *cis*-dimers on the plasma membranes and *trans*-dimers with nectins present on the adjacent cell. Each nectin has a specialized pattern of *trans*-dimer formation with itself or other nectins (Reymond *et al.*, 2000; Takai *et al.*, 2003). Their main attribute is the formation, together with cadherins, of the adherens junctions of epithelial cells, and in cooperation or not with cadherins, the organization of claudin-based tight junctions. In addition, they are involved in the formation of synapses in neurons and the organization of heterotypic junctions between Sertoli cells and spermatids in the testis (Takai *et al.*, 2003).

Most nectins carry a C-terminal conserved motif that binds afadin, thus anchoring the adhesion molecules to the cytoskeleton (Takai *et al.*, 2003). This domain is absent from nectin1β which is not restricted to adherens junctions. Nectin-mediated signalling activity leads to activation of a variety of extracellular and intracellular molecules, such as scatter factor/hepatocyte growth factor, Ras, Cdc42 and Rac small G proteins (Takai *et al.*, 2003).

Table 7.1. Human HSV receptors and the viral strains for which they serve

| | | Human α-herpesvirus | | | Animal α-herpesvirus | |
| | | | Unrestricted/*rid* | | | |
Receptor name	Alternative name	HSV-1	HSV-2	mutants	PrV	BHV-1
HVEM	HveA	+	+	−	−	−
Nectin1	PRR1, HIgR, HveC	+	+	+	+	+
Nectin2	PRR2, HveB	−	+/−	+	+	−

Nectin1

Human nectin1 is a broad spectrum receptor for human and animal alphaherpesviruses (Table 7.1). Three isoforms are known, two of which: -α and -β are membrane-bound (Cocchi *et al.*, 1998a,b; Geraghty *et al.*, 1998; Krummenacher *et al.*, 1998; Krummenacher *et al.*, 1999; Campadelli-Fiume *et al.*, 2000). Their main properties as HSV receptors are as follows.

(i) Nectin1 is broadly expressed in human tissues, including tissues and organs targeted by HSV, like CNS, ganglia and muco-epithelia (Cocchi *et al.*, 1998b; Haarr *et al.*, 2001; Matsushima *et al.*, 2003; Richart *et al.*, 2003; Linehan *et al.*, 2004). It is expressed in virtually all human cell lines, including epithelial cells, neurons and fibroblasts (Campadelli-Fiume *et al.*, 2000; Spear *et al.*, 2000). Some of these cells simultaneously express HVEM (Krummenacher *et al.*, 2004).

When HSV initially infects mucosal epithelium, the apical domain of polarized epithelial cells are targeted initially, whereas basolateral domains of epithelial cells are available to the virus only if a lesion disrupts the integrity of the lining. It was therefore of interest to know whether nectin1 can serve as an HSV receptor in polarized epithelial cells. Human CaCo2 cells can be infected with HSV from the apical domain (Griffiths *et al.*, 1998), whereas MDCK cells and primary human keratinocytes are preferentially infected from the basolateral domain (Schelhaas *et al.*, 2003; Marozin *et al.*, 2004). These differences may reflect cell line-dependent differences in the pattern of polarization of a same molecule, or distribution of receptors like nectin1-β and HVEM, which do not appear to be restricted to adherens junctions.

(ii) Nectin1 interacts physically with gD (Krummenacher *et al.*, 1999). The interaction requires the first 250 residues of gD and the V domain of nectin1. The affinity ranges from 10^{-6} to 10^{-8} molar, with the highest affinity observed with forms of gD that were truncated at or after residue 250. Affinity decreases by 100-fold with gD$_{306t}$, reflecting a folding of the most C-terminal portion of gD towards the core (Whitbeck *et al.*, 1999; Krummenacher *et al.*, 2005).

Insertion mutations alter the binding affinity; insertions at the N-terminus (e.g., at residues 34, and 43) modify the binding to HVEM but not to nectin1 (Milne *et al.*, 2003; Jogger *et al.*, 2004). Remarkably, even when the binding affinities are low, or undetectable, the mutant forms of gD maintain the ability to mediate HSV entry and cell–cell fusion, implying that gD functions in virus entry and cell fusion regardless of its receptor-binding affinity and kinetics, and that as long as interaction with a functional receptor occurs, entry takes place (Milne *et al.*, 2003; Zhou *et al.*, 2003).

Human nectin1 also binds isoforms of gD from animal α-herpesviruses. The affinity may be even higher than for HSV-1 gD (in the case of PrV), or very low (in the case of BHV-1) (Connolly *et al.*, 2001). Even when the affinity is very low, human nectin1 is capable of mediating entry (Cocchi *et al.*, 1998b; Geraghty *et al.*, 1998).

(iii) The domain of nectin1 functional in HSV entry and in binding to gD was initially mapped to the N-terminal V domain, and subsequently to the C-C'-C'' ridge (Krummenacher *et al.*, 2000; Cocchi *et al.*, 2001; Menotti *et al.*, 2002b). Critical residues that may be part of the interface with gD are amino acids 77 and 85 (Martinez and Spear, 2002).

(iv) Nectin1-γ is a natural soluble isoform of nectin1 generated by alternative splicing. Although it contains the three Ig domains, it has a narrow distribution in human tissues, unlike nectin1-α and -β. Like soluble recombinant forms of nectin1, it has the capacity to bind to virions and block infectivity. An unexpected property was that the soluble nectin1-γ molecules suffices to mediate virus entry into receptor-negative cells. This may be consequent either to an association to endogenous nectins, or to a direct binding of the soluble receptor to virions (Lopez *et al.*, 2001).

Nectin 2 and the unrestricted or rid *mutations*

The remarkable feature about nectin2 is that a single amino acid substitution in gD confers to HSV the ability to use nectin2 as an alternative receptor, without hampering its ability to use nectin1 (Table 7.1). At the same time, this mutation abolishes the interaction with HVEM (Connolly *et al.*, 2003; Yoon *et al.*, 2003). The end result is that the host range of the virus is modified. The mutations are L25P, Q27P, or Q27R, and are present in the unrestricted, or *rid* HSV-1 mutants. Nectin2 also serves as a weak receptor for some strains of HSV-2, but is inactive for wt-HSV-1 (Warner *et al.*, 1998; Lopez *et al.*, 2000; Krummenacher *et al.*, 2004). Physical interaction studies were in agreement with these properties (Warner *et al.*, 1998; Lopez *et al.*, 2000; Yoon *et al.*, 2003). The nectin2 residues critical for HSV entry were identified as amino acids 75–81 and 89, which lie adjacent to the predicted C'C" β-strands, i.e., the region corresponding to the nectin1 region involved in interaction with wild-type gD.

The TNF receptor family
TNFRs (tumor necrosis factor receptors) form a family of signal transduction molecules involved in regulation of cell proliferation, differentiation and apoptotic death. Structurally, their ectodomain is composed of four typical cysteine-rich domains (CRDs). The family includes twenty nine human members, classified into three groups according to their cytoplasmic sequences and signaling properties. Members of the first group (exemplified by Fas) contain a death domain (DD) in the cytoplasmic tail. After binding to their ligands they interact with intracellular adaptors, which, in turn, induce apoptosis by activation of the caspase cascade. Members of the second group (exemplified by TNFR2 and HVEM) lack a death domain, and instead contain one or more TRAF (TNFR-associated factor) interacting motifs (TIMs), which trigger a variety of signal transduction pathways, including those for activation of nuclear factor κB (NF-κB), Jun N-terminal kinase (JNK), p38, extracellular signal-related kinase (ERK) and phosphoinositide 3-kinase (PI3K). Members of the third group (e.g., TNFR3, TNFR4, etc.) lack intracellular signaling motifs, and act as decoy receptors.

The natural ligands of the TNFRs are a family of cytokines whose prototype is TNF, and include lymphotoxin (LT)α, LTβ, and LIGHT. They are biologically active as trimers: their binding to the receptors causes the trimerization of the intracellular domains, which, in turn, interact with high affinity with trimeric cellular adaptors (e.g., TRAFs). Each cytokine interacts with more than one receptor.

HVEM
HVEM was first identified as a HSV receptor and was classified as a novel member of the TNFR family based on structural motifs (Montgomery *et al.*, 1996). The cytoplasmic tail interacts with several members of the TRAF family, leading to the activation of targets like NF-κB, Jun N-terminal kinase, and AP-1, and the consequent induction of T cell activation, proliferation, cytokine release, and expression of cell surface activation markers (Harrop *et al.*, 1998). Its ligands are LTα$_3$ and LIGHT (Mauri *et al.*, 1998). LIGHT–HVEM interactions contribute to the cytotoxic T-lymphocyte-mediated immune response.

The main properties of HVEM as an HSV receptor are as follows.
(i) In early studies HVEM was found to be expressed mainly in cells of the immune system, and in a number of non-hematopoietic tissues and organs. Expression was not observed in brain or skeletal muscle (Montgomery *et al.*, 1996; Kwon *et al.*, 1997).
(ii) HVEM serves as receptor for HSV-1 and HSV-2, as a weak receptor for the U10 HSV mutant (L25P substitution), but not for HSV *rid*-1 and *rid*-2 unrestricted mutants (Connolly *et al.*, 2003; Yoon *et al.*, 2003).
(iii) HVEM binds wild-type gD. The affinity of the binding is of the same order of magnitude as that of nectin1/gD binding, and the interaction requires the same region of gD, i.e., the first 250 residues, or longer (Willis *et al.*, 1998). gD and LIGHT compete with each other for the binding to HVEM; accordingly, LIGHT interferes with HSV entry in HVEM-expressing cells (Mauri *et al.*, 1998).
(iv) The gD contact site on HVEM involves CRD1 and 2, with the majority of contacts lying in CRD1. Residues 35–37 form the intermolecular antiparallel β-sheet with gD (Carfi *et al.*, 2001; Connolly *et al.*, 2003). A systematic structure-based mutagenesis approach revealed that 17 residues in CRD1 and 4 in CRD2 are directly involved in the HVEM-gD interface. Some mutations completely abolish the HVEM binding to gD and its function as an HSV-1 receptor (Connolly *et al.*, 2002).

Modified heparan sulphate
3-O-sulphated heparan sulphate represents the third identified HSV receptor, structurally unrelated to nectins and HVEM (Shukla *et al.*, 1999). It serves as receptor for HSV-1, but not for unrestricted *rid* mutants or HSV-2. Thus, HSV-1 can use heparan sulphate GAGs not only for the initial step of attachment to the target cell, but it also recognizes some specifically modified sites on heparan sulphate (Shukla and Spear, 2001). The physical interaction with gD is in the range of 10^{-6} M, as measured by affinity co-electrophoresis, and was not detectable by ELISA.

The sites on heparan sulphate recognized by gD are generated by heparan sulphate D-glucosaminyl 3-O-sulfotransferases (3-OSTs). 3-O-sulphates are rare substitutions in heparan sulphate, generated by at least six 3-OSTs isoforms identified in humans and mice, 3-OST-3$_A$ and 3-OST-3$_B$, 3-OST-2, 3-OST-4 and 3-OST-5 (Shukla and

Spear, 2001). Of note, 3-OST-3s are not receptors *per se*, consistent with the finding that gD does not bind to the purified enzymes; rather, they catalyze the substitutions, which, in turn, generate the receptors and render CHO cells susceptible to HSV.

The relevance of this potential receptor to HSV infection in human cell lines and in humans remains to be ascertained. In terms of distribution, the 3-OST-3s are broadly expressed isoforms in cells of different origins and tissues; 3-OST-2 and 3-OST-4 expression is mainly in the brain. 3-OST-5 expression is limited to the skeletal muscle.

Receptor preference and usage

The availability of multiple alternative receptors raises a number of questions, such as: What receptor is preferred in cells that coexpress both molecules? Do both serve as *bona fide* receptors in humans? Are they differentially distributed, or employed in different tissues? Limited information is available on these topics.

Two parameters that may guide receptor preference in cell cultures are the affinity of the binding and the cell surface density of the receptors. Neither appears to be relevant in the case of gD, since gD affinity to nectin1 and to HVEM is of the same order of magnitude (Krummenacher *et al.*, 1998). Moreover, cells that appear to be nectin1-negative by fluorescent antibody cell sorting (e.g., EA-1 cells) can be infected and entry is inhibited by antibody to nectin1 (our unpublished result), implying that low density receptors suffice to mediate entry. The same phenomenon is observed with HVEM (Krummenacher *et al.*, 2004).

As far as infection of animal and human tissues is concerned, nectin1 is expressed in nearly every neuron of adult mice, in rat sensory neurons, in some synapses, and serves as the primary receptor for HSV-1 infection in sensory neurons (Haarr *et al.*, 2001; Mata *et al.*, 2001; Richart *et al.*, 2003). Nectin1 is also expressed in the epithelium of the human and murine vagina where it mediates HSV-1 and -2 entry in the genital mucosa of female hosts (Linehan *et al.*, 2004). Nectin1-α is detected at the cell–cell adherens junctions in human skin (Matsushima *et al.*, 2003). Cumulatively, these data are compatible with a major role of nectin1 in the infection of sensory neurons and mucoepithelia in vivo. The tissue distribution of HVEM suggests that it serves as the principal receptor for HSV in activated T lymphocytes, or in lymphoid organs (spleen and thymus), in liver and lung. However, these organs are not target of HSV in the natural history of infection, except in the rare cases of disseminated infection. Recent data show that several clinical/primary isolates can use both receptors, as laboratory strains do (Krummenacher *et al.*, 2004). The fact that viruses of different origin retain the ability to use both receptors suggests that this is a requirement for successful infection and spread in the host (Krummenacher *et al.*, 2004). The interaction with HVEM in particular may have a role in immune evasion (La *et al.*, 2002).

For other viruses, formal proof that a given receptor plays a critical role in humans has rested on correlations between genetic defects in the locus encoding the receptor and a diminished susceptibility to viral infection. A rare truncation of the nectin1 gene has been identified. The phenotypes associated with loss of both alleles include cleft lip/palate, hidrotic ectodermal dysplasia (CLPED1), hair abnormalities, developmental defects of the hands and, in some cases, mental retardation. Studies on the serostatus of these patients for evidence of HSV infection have not been published. A few studies investigated nectin1, nectin2 and HVEM gene polymorphisms and correlations with HSV infection. At present, no relatively common polymorphism has been found to correlate with HSV serostatus or symptoms (Patera *et al.*, 2002; Struyf *et al.*, 2002; Krummenacher *et al.*, 2004). Wild-type HSV can infect CLPED1 fibroblasts through HVEM in vitro, indicating that the ability to exploit redundant receptors may be favorable to the virus in vivo as well (Krummenacher *et al.*, 2004).

The animal orthologues of nectin and HVEM

HSV infects numerous mammalian species, some of which – mice, rabbits and primates – are extensively employed as animal models. The question arises whether they are faithful models in terms of receptor usage.

Porcine and bovine alphaherpesviruses promiscuously use human nectin1, implying that animal orthologs of nectins serve as receptors of these viruses in their hosts (Cocchi *et al.*, 1998b; Geraghty *et al.*, 1998; Warner *et al.*, 1998). Indeed, nectins are conserved among mammals, and nectin1 orthologs have been found in cells derived from mice, hamsters, pigs, cows and monkeys, and nectin2 has a mouse ortholog, suggesting a conserved function in the evolution of these proteins (Milne *et al.*, 2001). A HVEM ortholog is expressed in mice (Yoon *et al.*, 2003). In turn, the murine orthologs of nectin1, nectin2, HVEM, and the porcine and bovine hortologs of human nectin1 can serve as species non-specific HSV receptors when transfected into receptor-negative cells (Menotti *et al.*, 2000; Shukla *et al.*, 2000; Menotti *et al.*, 2001; Milne *et al.*, 2001; Menotti *et al.*, 2002a). The affinity of these potential receptors for gD ranges from as high as that of human nectin1, to very low or undetectable. Because the animal orthologs of nectin, and perhaps also of HVEM serve as receptors of HSV in mice and other animal species, these systems appear to relatively faithfully model HSV receptor usage in humans.

Site of HSV entry into the cell
It has been a long held paradigm that HSV enters cells by fusion at the plasma membrane. Recent evidence indicates that in some cells entry is through an endocytic pathway, and that both the cell type, and the structural features of the receptors are determinants that control the site of entry. Specifically, in cells like HeLa and CHO expressing nectin1 or HVEM, entry is inhibited by drugs that modify the pH of the endosomal compartment (low pH-sensitive entry) (Nicola *et al.*, 2003). However, when nectin1 or HVEM are expressed in J cells, they mediate entry at the plasma membrane. Furthermore, when nectin1 is retargeted to endosomes, by means of a chimeric nectin1-EGFR (epidermal growth factor receptor) chimera, or is sorted to lipid rafts, by means of a nectin1-glycosylphosphatidylinositol anchor chimera, the pathway of entry into J cells becomes endocytic (Gianni *et al.*, 2004). Of note, when HSV infects cells carrying wt-nectin1, neither nectin nor gD localize at lipid rafts, but gB does (Bender *et al.*, 2003). All in all, HSV fusion glycoproteins are well suited to perform two quite different pathways of entry.

Role of gD-receptor interaction in triggering fusion
Crucial to our understanding of how HSV enters cells is the comprehension of how gD binding to its receptor triggers fusion. A hint has come from the unexpected observation that the soluble gD ectodomain is both necessary and sufficient to rescue the infectivity of the non infectious gDnull HSV mutant (Cocchi *et al.*, 2004). Entry mediated by soluble gD requires not only the N-terminus, carrying the receptor-binding sites, but also the C-terminus carrying the pro-fusion domain, required to trigger fusion but not for receptor binding. These findings, together with the observation that a glycosylphosphatidylinositol-anchored form of gD, or substitution of the transmembrane and cytoplasmic tail with heterologous regions leave gD function unaltered (Browne *et al.*, 2003) demonstrate that the transmembrane region and cytoplasmic tail do not play any demonstrable function, except to ensure that gD is delivered to the gD receptor along with the virion, and argue that the role of gD in HSV entry is to signal receptor-recognition to the downstream glycoproteins and to trigger fusion (Cocchi *et al.*, 2004).

Biochemical and structural studies indicate that the receptor-mediated activation of gD takes the form of a conformational change (Cocchi *et al.*, 2004; Fusco *et al.*, 2005; Krummenacher *et al.*, 2005). In the unliganded state the virion gD adopts a conformation in which the flexible C terminus folds back, wraps the N-terminus and masks the receptor binding sites. At receptor binding, the C-terminus is displaced from its binding site on the N-terminus, the receptor binding sites are unmasked and become occupied by the receptor. The binary complex made of receptor plus gD with the displaced C-terminus must create a surface suitable for gB and gH-gL recruitment.

Execution of membrane fusion and its control

gB, gH, gL are essential for entry of all herpesviruses, since they are conserved among all human herpesviruses, with the highest extent of sequence conservation seen in gB. Heterodimer formation between gH and gL is also a conserved feature amongst herpesviruses. Altogether, gB, gH and gL appear to be the executors of fusion and constitute the conserved fusion machinery across the herpesvirus family.

Critical properties of gH and gB have been elucidated recently, and provide an intriguing scenario. On one hand, molecular and biochemical analyses of gH highlighted properties typical of class 1 fusion glycoproteins. Because the gH structure has not yet been solved, these properties wait for confirmation at the structural level. On the other hand, the crystal structure of gB has been solved, it exhibits a remarkable similarity to that of vesicular stomatitis G protein, and to viral fusion glycoproteins in general. Biochemical and mutational confirmation are still to be provided. At present, a most likely scenario is that both gB and gH·gL are fusion executors. How the two glycoproteins cooperate to execute fusion, and why two, and not one, fusion executors are required in the herpesviridae family is unclear. It is worthwhile to note that entry by fusion at plasma membrane, and entry by fusion in endocytic vesicles require all four glycoproteins (gD, gB, gH and gL) (Nicola *et al.*, 2003; Nicola and Straus, 2004). These requirements rule out the possibility that gB serves as fusion executor in one cellular compartment, and gH·gL serves as fusion executor in another cell compartment.

The glycoproteins that execute fusion
gH –gL
gH is a type-1 virion glycoprotein encoded by the UL22 gene (Gompels and Minson, 1986). Soon after its discovery, it was recognized as an essential glycoprotein for virion infectivity, as its deletion produced non infectious progeny and abolished cell–cell fusion (Forrester *et al.*, 1992). Neutralizing antibodies to gH block virus entry but permit attachment, indicating a role at a post-attachment step (Fuller *et al.*, 1989). gH appears to contain elements associated with fusion of membranes, i.e. a hydrophobic α-helix 1 (residues 377-397) with properties typical of a fusion peptide and two heptad repeats with propensity to form a coiled coil. α-Helix 1 is positionally conserved in all the

gH orthologs across the herpesviridae family; in HSV-2 it is located in a loop made of two cysteines. α-Helix 1 is able to interact with biological membranes, can convert a soluble glycoprotein (gD amino acid residues 1-260) into a membrane-bound glycoprotein, and can be functionally replaced by fusion peptides derived from glycoproteins of other, unrelated viruses (Gianni et al., 2005a). A peptide with the sequence of α-helix 1 induces fusion of liposomes and exhibits a strong flexibility documented as ability to adopt an α-helical conformation (Galdiero, S. et al., 2006; Gianni et al., 2006a). These properties strongly argue in favor of α-helix 1 as a candidate fusion peptide loop. Two heptad repeats, capable to form coiled coils and to interact with each other, form a structure of increased α-helical content and are potentially suitable to form a six-helix bundle (Gianni et al., 2005b; Galdiero, S. et al., 2006; Gianni et al., 2006b). Additional elements in gH are a second predicted α-helical domain of lower hydrophobicity than the candidate fusion peptide (aa 513-531), and a pre-transmembrane sequence (aa 626-644) with predicted propensity to partition at membrane interface (Galdiero, S. et al., 2006; Gianni et al., 2006a).

Synthetic peptides corresponding to the heptad repeats inhibit virus infection if present at the time of virus entry into the cell (Gianni et al., 2005b; Galdiero, S. et al., 2006; Gianni et al., 2006b). The presence of coiled coil motifs predicts that gH must undergo profound conformational changes at fusion. Because fusion peptides and coiled coil heptad repeats represent characteristic functional domains in type 1 viral fusion glycoproteins, gH is a candidate fusion executor in HSV.

It remains to be determined whether gH interacts with cellular receptors. The interaction with an integrin is not critical given that mutagenesis of a RGD motif did not reduce virus entry and cell fusion (Galdiero, M. et al., 1997). It is of interest that the transmembrane and C-terminal tail regions of gH can not be exchanged with those of heterologous proteins, in contrast with what happens with gD (Harman et al., 2002; Jones and Geraghty, 2004).

A ts mutant, tsQ26, exhibited a phenotype characterized by the production of non-infectious extracellular virions, along with the intracellular retention of gH and of infectious virions (Desai et al., 1988). This phenotype suggested a peculiar mechanism of intracellular retention of gH. A clue to understanding the intracellular trafficking of gH came from the observations that, when expressed from a transgene, gH had a M_r lower than that of mature gH, was not transported to the cell surface, and was retained in the ER unless the cells were superinfected (Gompels and Minson, 1986; Foà-Tomasi et al., 1991; Roberts et al., 1991). The gene product required for gH trafficking and maturation, identified by Johnson and coworkers, is gL (Hutchinson et al., 1992a); gL is required for proper folding and trafficking of gH in all human Herpesviruses (Kaye et al., 1992; Liu et al., 1993).

gL is a soluble glycoprotein encoded by UL1 gene; its presence in the virion envelope is ensured by complex formation with gH (Hutchinson et al., 1992a). In accordance with gH attributes, an HSV mutant unable to express gL could not enter cells, and its particles lacked glycoprotein H (Roop et al., 1993). Both gH and gL are required for fusion in the cell–cell fusion assay (Turner et al., 1998). The first 323 amino acids of gH and the first 161 amino acids of gL can form a stable secreted hetero-oligomer, while the first 648 amino acids of gH are required for reactivity to conformation-dependent antibodies, indicative of correct conformation and oligomerization (Peng et al., 1998). gL is a locus of a *syn* mutation, confirming a role of the gH-gL hetero-oligomer in HSV fusion. The exact role of gL in fusion remains to be elucidated. Because its binding site on gH maps both upstream and downstream of the hydrophobic α-helix, it has been proposed that its role may be to shield the gH hydrophobic sequence, and thus to enable gH water solubility and solvent interface (Gianni et al., 2005a).

gB

gB plays two opposite roles in fusion, i.e. it participates in fusion execution, and it exerts anti-fusion activity. The two functions are physically separated and reside in the ectodomain and the cytoplasmic tail, respectively. gB is a type-1 virion glycoprotein encoded by the UL27 gene (Bzik et al., 1984; Pellett et al., 1985). Its crystal structure reveals a trimer with a coiled coil core. Remarkably, its structure resembles closely that of vesicular stomatitis virus G protein (Heldwein et al., 2006; Roche et al., 2006). Despite the facts that a canonical fusion peptide has not been detected by biochemical, molecular or structural analyses, and that the region homologous to the fusion peptide loop in vesicular stomatitis virus G protein appears to be suboptimal for membrane insertion, the structural similarity between gB and vesicular stomatitis virus G protein strongly relates gB to viral fusion glycoproteins. It has been proposed that the two glycoproteins may represent a novel class of fusion glycoproteins (Heldwein et al., 2006; Roche et al., 2006).

From a structural point of view, gB is a trimeric spike. Each of the three protomers (residues 103–730) appears to be composed of five distinct domains (named I-V), displaying multiple contact sites (Heldwein et al., 2006). Domain I, the "base", is a continous chain with a fold typical of pleckstrin homology domains. Domain II, the "middle", is made of two discontinuous segments, forming a structure reminiscent of a pleckstrin homology superfold. Domain III, the "core", comprises three discontinuous segments: its prominent feature is a 44-residue α-helix that forms the central coiled coil with its trimeric counterparts. Domain IV, the "crown", adopts a novel structure, and is fully exposed on top of the trimeric spike. Domain V, the "arm", is a long extension spanning the full length of the protomer. Of note, its residues do not contact residues of the same protomer, but instead accommodate into the groove formed by the "cores" of the other two protomers.

The role of gB in virion infectivity and cell–cell fusion is inferred by numerous lines of evidence, including (i) the phenotype of a gB deletion mutant virus which produces non-infectious particles, (ii) the neutralizing activity of antibodies to gB, (iii) gB as a genetic locus of syncytial mutations, and (iv) the requirement for gB in the cell-cell fusion assay (Manservigi et al., 1977; Cai, W. Z. et al., 1987; Turner et al., 1998). Functional domains in the ectodomain were identified by means of two sets of mutations: temperature sensitive mutations for viral growth, and resistance to antibodies with potent neutralizing activity. The first ones, exemplified by the mutants tsB5 and tsJ12, reside in the gB ectodomain, confer a temperature-sensitive phenotype, and affect the rate of virus entry (Bzik et al., 1984). Likely, these mutations affect the gB domain involved in execution of fusion. Following the determination of gB crystal structure, it was recognized that the epitopes of potent neutralizing antibodies, either centered around single amino acid residues or formed by continuous regions, reside on the trimer surface, on the lateral faces of the spike or on the tip of the crown (Pellett et al., 1985; Kousoulas et al., 1988; Highlander et al., 1989; Pereira et al., 1989; Qadri et al., 1991; Heldwein et al., 2006).

The quartet of gD, gB, gH and gL assemble into a complex at virus entry

The nature of the interactions between the complex formed by gD plus its receptor and the executors of fusion is critical to understand the mechanisms by which HSV (and by extension all other herpesviruses) enter cells.

The quartet of glycoproteins essential for HSV entry and fusion (gD, gB, gH and gL) assemble into a complex at virus entry and in infected cells. Complex assembly strictly requires one of the gD receptors, either nectin1 or HVEM. The same complex is assembled also in cells transfected with the quartet, implying that no additional viral protein other than those that participate in the complex itself is required. Because the complex is assembled at virus entry and in transfected cells committed to form polykaryocytes, and fails to be assembled in the absence of either a receptor to gD or of gD, complex assembly appears to be a critical step in the process of virus entry and fusion.

The proteins that negatively control fusion

Cells infected with wt-virus do not form syncytia, despite the fact that they express the fusion glycoproteins at their surface. Syncytia are only formed when the virus carries one of the syncytial (*syn*) mutations, which map to genes encoding gB, gL, gK, UL24, or UL20. By contrast, cells expressing the quartet of gB, gD, gH and gL readily form syncytia (Turner et al., 1998). The paradox may be explained by assuming that the wt-alleles of proteins that are target of *syn* mutations exert a negative control on fusion. This has, in fact, been verified for gB, gK, and UL20 (Fan et al., 2002; Avitabile et al., 2003; Avitabile et al., 2004). As outlined below, HSV has evolved at least two mechanisms by which it blocks fusion. One is exerted through downmodulation of gB cell surface expression, the other is exerted through the concerted action of gK and UL20p. Still other proteins (UL24 and UL45) are likely to exert anti-fusion activity. The evolution of functional redundancy implies that uncontrolled fusion is inimical to HSV-1 replication and spread in nature, and therefore the virus needs to exert a tight control on it.

gB

The anti-fusion activity of gB is located in the cytoplasmic tail, which carries at least two physically distinct functional domains: the *syn* mutation and the endocytosis motifs. Each of them, separately, appears to reduce fusion. Structurally, the cytoplasmic tail carries two predicted α-helices. The *syn* mutations are located immediately downstream of the most N-terminal α-helix. Embedded in the region of the C-terminal α-helix is one, and possibly two functional endocytosis motifs (YTQV889–892 and LL871 (Fan et al., 2002; Avitabile et al., 2004; Beitia Ortiz de Zarate et al., 2004). Deletion of the membrane-proximal α-helix abrogates virus infectivity, implying that this region is critical. Its role, and the molecular mechanism of the *syn3* mutation remain to be elucidated. The membrane-distal α-helix is also implicated in the negative control of fusion, since its deletion increases fusion in the cell fusion assay, and confers a syncytial phenotype upon virus-infected cells (Foster, et al., 2001a; Avitabile et al., 2004). Its antifusion activity is mainly exerted through endocytosis, which acts to decrease the steady state amounts of gB from the cell surface, such that gB becomes a limiting factor in fusion. Of note, the gB-decorated endocytosis vesicles-vacuoles represent the hallmark of gB localization in infected cells.

gK

gK is a polytopic glycoprotein encoded by the UL53 gene, whose topology is still debated (Hutchinson et al., 1992b; Foster, et al., 2001b). It carries an N-terminal extracellular domain, and two or three TM regions connected by loops (Foster, et al., 2003b). Its hydrophobicity, poor immunogenicity and overall problems in its detection have made this glycoprotein a difficult one to study. In infected cells, gK localizes mainly to the Golgi apparatus. One controversial aspect is whether it localizes to the plasma membranes and to virions. When expressed from a transgene, gK is primarily located is at the ER (Hutchinson et al., 1992b; Avitabile et al., 2003; Foster, et al., 2003a). When coexpressed with UL20, both proteins localize to the Golgi apparatus (Avitabile et al., 2004).

gK exerts anti-fusion activity in the cell–cell fusion assay (Avitabile et al., 2003). Mutant viruses carrying a partial or a complete deletion in the gK gene have two major phenotypes (Hutchinson and Johnson, 1995; Foster, and Kousoulas, 1999). First, they form syncytia, arguing that the anti-fusion activity is exerted also in the context of infected cells. Second, they are defective in virus egress, arguing that the anti-fusion activity of gK is exerted not only at the plasma membrane, but also in the membranes of the exocytic compartment. This would provide an explanation as to why these membranes are heavily decorated with fusion glycoproteins, yet do not fuse one with the other. According to this model, the gK role in virion egress may be exerted by maintaining a functional exocytic pathway. It should be stressed that, if indeed gK is also a virion constituent, then, at virus entry into the cell, the trigger to fusion must simultaneously relieve the block to fusion exerted by gK (Avitabile et al., 2004).

UL20

UL20p is a polytopic unglycosylated protein with several analogies to gK. Its hydrophobicity and scarce immunogenicity have hampered its characterization. UL20p is predicted to carry 4 transmembrane segments (McGeoch et al., 1988; Melancon et al., 2004). In the infected cells UL20p localizes at the Golgi apparatus and the nuclear membranes, and is not detectable at the plasma membrane. It has not been detected in virions. When expressed from a transgene, UL20p predominant localization is at the ER (Avitabile et al., 1994; Ward et al., 1994). It relocalizes to the Golgi apparatus, when coexpressed with gK (Foster, et al., 2003b; Avitabile et al., 2004).

Two mutant viruses deleted in UL20 gene have been constructed, both of which are highly defective in secretion of virions to the extracellular space (Baines et al., 1991; Foster, et al., 2004). The first deletion virus was subsequently reported to carry an in-frame fusion between UL20.5 (not known at the time the deletion virus was constructed) and the C-terminus of UL20 gene, and was characterized by syncytia formation and by the entrapping of virions in the perinuclear space (i.e., the space between the inner and outer nuclear membranes) – a phenotype particularly evident in cells whose Golgi apparatus became fragmented following infection (Baines et al., 1991). This phenotype can be interpreted as indication that the UL20p exerts a negative control on fusion. Cells infected with the second deletion virus showed enveloped virions as well as unenveloped nucleocapsids accumulating in the cytoplasm, and occasionally virion envelopes containing multiple capsids within intracytoplasmic vacuoles. These phenotypes were also interpreted to mean that UL20p acts as an inhibitor of membrane fusion, and, interestingly, that UL20p may act to maintain a single nucleocapsid for each envelope and to prevent fusion of enveloped virions among themselves (Foster, et al., 2004). The complexity of these phenotypes reflects both direct and indirect effects of UL20p, including the role of UL20p in the intracellular transport of gK and possibly of the fusion glycoproteins.

The possibility that UL20p exerts an anti-fusion activity was probed in the cell–cell fusion assay, which showed a block to fusion in cells coexpressing UL20p and gK, but not in cells expressing UL20 alone. The block was cell line dependent (Avitabile et al., 2004). The similar behavior of gK and UL20p, their colocalization, their mutual ability to influence each other localization, and their concerted anti-fusion activity make it likely that the two proteins act in a complex, and that they share a common target.

Nucleocapsid transport to the nuclear pore

Virus entry culminates in the release of capsids and approximately twenty tegument proteins into the cytosol. The capsids and some of the tegument proteins, e.g., αTIF, travel to the nuclear pore. Since diffusion of molecules larger than 500 kDa is restricted in the cytoplasm, viruses and nucleocapsids require a transport system. This is particularly true for neurotropic viruses that travel long distances in the axon during retrograde or anterograde transport (Enquist et al., 1998). It has been calculated that in the absence of an active transport mechanism, it would take a herpes virus capsid 231 years to diffuse 10 mm in the axonal cytoplasm (Sodeik, 2000).

Microtubules represent the cytoplasmic highways on which HSV is transported (reviewed in Döhner and Sodeik, 2005). At virus entry, capsids co-localize with microtubules, and their depolymerization reduces capsid transport to the nucleus (Sodeik *et al.*, 1997; Mabit *et al.*, 2002). Microtubules are polar structures with fast growing plus-ends typically localized in the cell periphery, and less dynamic minus-ends that are usually anchored in close proximity of the nucleus at the microtubule organizing centre (MTOC). Molecular motors use ATP-driven conformational changes to transport cargo along microtubules. Transport to the plus-ends is catalyzed by kinesins and that to minus-end by cytoplasmic dynein and dynactin (Döhner and Sodeik, 2005). Dynein and dynactin mediate capsid transport to the cell centre, since incoming capsids colocalize with these motors (Sodeik *et al.*, 1997; Döhner *et al.*, 2002), and overexpression of dynamitin, a subunit of the dynactin complex, inhibits capsid transport (Döhner *et al.*, 2002). How capsids move further from MTOC to the nuclear pore complex is unclear.

Analysis of HSV-1 entry by digital time-lapse fluorescence microscopy showed that GFP-tagged capsids can move along microtubules both towards and away from the nucleus, with maximal speeds of 1.1 μm/s. The transport is saltatory and bidirectional, but in neuronal processes it shows a retrograde bias towards the cell body (Smith *et al.*, 2001). Efforts are underway to identify the virion proteins that may interact with kinesins as well as dynein or dynactin. Two candidates are UL34p, which, however, is absent from mature virions, and US11, which appears to bind the heavy chain of conventional kinesin (Diefenbach *et al.*, 2002). Once the capsids have reached the proximity of the nucleus, they seem to bind to filaments emanating from the nuclear pores (Batterson *et al.*, 1983; Sodeik *et al.*, 1997). This docking is believed to induce capsid destabilization, release of the viral DNA, and its translocation through the nuclear pore into the nucleoplasm (Ojala *et al.*, 2000). Temperature-sensitive mutants in the UL36 gene accumulate filled viral capsids at the nuclear pore complexes at the non-permissive temperature, suggesting that the large tegument protein VP1–3 is involved in uncoating of the viral genome (Batterson *et al.*, 1983; Ojala *et al.*, 2000).

VZV

There are several remarkable differences between VZV and HSV entry. Because the respective viral glycoproteins undoubtedly influence these differences, the VZV gene products will be briefly summarized.

Is VZV gE a substitute for functions of HSV gD?

All but one of the proteins that have been illustrated above for HSV have a counterpart in VZV. For those glycoproteins for which sufficient information is available, a substantial functional similarity is observed. The single most notable difference between VZV and HSV in terms of the glycoproteins is the absence of gD in the VZV genome. At the same time, VZV is well suited for cell-to-cell spread, which takes place by fusion of the infected cell with an adjacent uninfected cell, whereas HSV is better suited for virion-to-cell infection (at least in cultured cells). So, it is tempting to speculate that the absence of a VZV gD gene may contribute to these differences.

Despite the fact that gD plays such a pivotal role in HSV entry, gD is not conserved throughout the alphaherpesviruses. In the porcine herpesvirus PrV, gD is required for virion-to cell infectivity but not for cell-to-cell spread of the virus. Consistently, gD is not a requirement for the PrV cell-cell fusion assay, although its presence greatly enhances fusion efficiency. Assuming that common basic mechanisms are shared by all of the alphaherpesviruses and given that the triplet gH-gL-gB is conserved, the question then arises: which VZV glycoprotein substitutes for the functions encoded in HSV gD, i.e., receptor recognition and triggering of fusion. The two functions might well be distributed over different entities, but a trigger to fusion consequent to virion interaction with a receptor appears to be essential.

In VZV, four glycoproteins are known to be essential. They are gB, gH, gL and gE (Keller *et al.*, 1984; Montalvo and Grose, 1986; Forghani *et al.*, 1994; Duus *et al.*, 1995; Mallory *et al.*, 1997; Mo *et al.*, 2002). Of note, the HSV gE gene lies in the S component of the genome, proximal to gD; as stated above, VZV lacks the gD gene. Instrumental to our understanding of the role of gE are the results of VZV glycoprotein cell–cell fusion assays. In transfected cells, fusion is induced by coexpression of either gH-gL or of gB-gE (Duus *et al.*, 1995; Duus and Grose, 1996; Maresova *et al.*, 2001). With regard to genome stability, VZV is considered to be one of the more genetically stable herpesviruses. However, viral mutants carrying missense mutations in the gE ectodomain are being isolated from humans; one of them is more fusogenic in cell cultures and in the SCID-hu mice (Santos *et al.*, 1998, 2000). Cumulatively, both circumstantial and genetic evidence supports the possibility that VZV gE subsumes at least some of roles of HSV gD.

Endocytosis of the VZV glycoproteins gE, gB, gH, and the negative regulation of fusion

Three VZV glycoproteins carry functional tyrosine-based endocytosis motifs; they are gE, gB and gH.

The gE cytoplasmic tail has a YAGL sequence beginning with a tyrosine residue 582. As determined by mutagenesis studies, the tyrosine residue is part of a conserved YXXL endocytosis motif. The internalized gE trafficks to the trans-Golgi or is recycled to the cell surface. In addition, the C-tail also contains phosphorylation sites (Kenyon et al., 2002). It has been suggested that serine/threonine and tyrosine phosphorylation of gE may serve as sorting signals for internalized receptors and that formation of a gE–gI complex facilitates gE endocytosis (Olson and Grose, 1997; Olson et al., 1998).

VZV gB contains three predicted endocytosis motifs within its cytoplasmic domain: YMTL (aa 818–821), YSRV (aa 857–860), and LL (aa 841–842). Both tyrosine-based motifs mediate gB internalization, but only the YSRV motif is absolutely required for endocytosis. The YMTL motif functions in trafficking of internalized gB to its subsequent localization in the trans Golgi. The third potential endocytosis motif is a dileucine sequence, whose function is under study (Heineman and Hall, 2001). Of note, VZV gI, the partner of VZV gE, also contains a dileucine endocytosis motif in its C-tail (Olson and Grose, 1998).

Like VZV gE and gB, VZV gH contains a functional but previously unrecognized tyrosine based YNKI motif in its short cytoplasmic tail, which mediates clathrin-dependent and antibody-independent endocytosis. Alignment analysis of the VZV gH cytoplasmic tail with other herpesvirus gH homologues reveals two interesting features: (i) herpes simplex virus types 1 and 2 homologues lack an endocytosis motif while all other alphaherpesvirus gH homologues contain a potential motif, and (ii) the VZV gH C-tail is actually longer than predicted in the original sequence analysis and thus can provide the proper context for a functional endocytosis motif (Pasieka et al., 2003). Surprisingly, the endocytosis-deficient VZV gH mutant plasmid effects greater cell-cell fusion than the wild-type gH plasmid. This result leads to the conclusion that VZV gH endocytosis represents a mechanism through which cell–cell fusion is negatively regulated, i.e., by modulating the amount of fusogenic gH on the cell surface (Pasieka et al., 2004). In this respect, therefore, VZV gH shares a basic mechanism of negative regulation of fusion with HSV gB.

Cumulatively, this comparison of the VZV and HSV-1 systems is very instructive as it highlights that both viruses have evolved an essentially similar mechanism of control of fusion, based on endocytosis and consequent limitation of cell surface expression of the fusion executors themselves. A notable difference between the two viruses is that this type of control appears to be is exerted in HSV-1 mainly by gB and in VZV mainly by gH.

Acknowledgments

We are grateful to Drs. Roselyn Eisenberg, Joel Baines, Charles Grose, and Beate Sodeik for critical reading of this chapter.

REFERENCES

Avitabile, E., Ward, P. L., Di Lazzaro, C., Torrisi, M. R., Roizman, B., and Campadelli-Fiume, G. (1994). The herpes simplex virus UL20 protein compensates for the differential disruption of exocytosis of virions and membrane glycoproteins associated with fragmentation of the Golgi apparatus. *J. Virol.*, **68**, 7397–7405.

Avitabile, E., Lombardi, G., and Campadelli-Fiume, G. (2003). Herpes simplex virus glycoprotein K, but not its syncytial allele, inhibits cell–cell fusion mediated by the four fusogenic glycoproteins, gD, gB, gH and gL. *J. Virol.*, **77**, 6836–6844.

Avitabile, E., Lombardi, G., Gianni, T., Capri, M., and Campadelli-Fiume, G. (2004). Coexpression of UL20p and gK inhibits cell–cell fusion mediated by herpes simplex virus glycoproteins gD, gH-gL, and wt-gB or an endocytosis-defective gB mutant, and downmodulates their cell surface expression. *J. Virol.*, **78**, 8015–8025.

Baines, J. D., Ward, P. L., Campadelli-Fiume, G., and Roizman, B. (1991). The UL20 gene of herpes simplex virus 1 encodes a function necessary for viral egress. *J. Virol.*, **65**, 6414–6424.

Batterson, W., Furlong, D., and Roizman, B. (1983). Molecular genetics of herpes simplex virus. VIII. Further characterization of a temperature-sensitive mutant defective in release of viral DNA and in other stages of the viral reproductive cycle. *J. Virol.*, **45**, 397–407.

Beitia Ortiz de Zarate, I., Kaelin, K., and Rozenberg, F. (2004). Effects of mutations in the cytoplasmic domain of herpes simplex virus type 1 glycoprotein B on intracellular transport and infectivity. *J. Virol.*, **78**, 1540–1551.

Bender, F. C., Whitbeck, J. C., Ponce de Leon, M., Lou, H., Eisenberg, R. J., and Cohen, G. H. (2003). Specific association of glycoprotein B with lipid rafts during herpes simplex virus entry. *J. Virol.*, **77**, 9542–9552.

Browne, H., Bruun, B., Whiteley, A., and Minson, T. (2003). Analysis of the role of the membrane-spanning and cytoplasmic tail domains of herpes simplex virus type 1 glycoprotein D in membrane fusion. *J. Gen. Virol.*, **84**, 1085–1089.

Bzik, D. J., Fox, B. A., DeLuca, N. A., and Person, S. (1984). Nucleotide sequence of a region of the herpes simplex virus type 1 gB glycoprotein gene: mutations affecting rate of virus entry and cell fusion. *Virology*, **137**, 185–190.

Cai, W. Z., Person, S., Warner, S. C., Zhou, J. H., and DeLuca, N. A. (1987). Linker-insertion nonsense and restriction-site deletion mutations of the gB glycoprotein gene of herpes simplex virus type 1. *J. Virol.*, **61**, 714–721.

Cai, W. Z., Gu, B., and Person, S. (1988). Role of glycoprotein B of herpes simplex virus type 1 in viral entry and cell fusion [published erratum appears in *J. Virol.* 1988 Nov;**62**(11):4438]. *J. Virol.*, **62**, 2596–2604.

Campadelli-Fiume, G., Arsenakis, M., Farabegoli, F., and Roizman, B. (1988). Entry of herpes simplex virus 1 in BJ cells that constitutively express viral glycoprotein D is by endocytosis and results in degradation of the virus. *J. Virol.*, **62**, 159–167.

Campadelli-Fiume, G., Stirpe, D., Boscaro, A. *et al.* (1990). Glycoprotein C-dependent attachment of herpes simplex virus to susceptible cells leading to productive infection. *Virology*, **178**, 213–222.

Campadelli-Fiume, G., Cocchi, F., Menotti, L., and Lopez, M. (2000). The novel receptors that mediate the entry of herpes simplex viruses and animal alphaherpesviruses into cells. *Rev. Med. Virol.*, **10**, 305–319.

Carfi, A., Willis, S. H., Whitbeck, J. C. *et al.* (2001). Herpes simplex virus glycoprotein D bound to the human receptor HveA. *Mol. Cell*, **8**, 169–179.

Cocchi, F., Lopez, M., Menotti, L., Aoubala, M., Dubreuil, P., and Campadelli-Fiume, G. (1998a). The V domain of herpesvirus Ig-like receptor (HIgR) contains a major functional region in herpes simplex virus-1 entry into cells and interacts physically with the viral glycoprotein D. *Proc. Natl Acad. Sci. USA*, **95**, 15700–15705.

Cocchi, F., Menotti, L., Mirandola, P., Lopez, M., and Campadelli-Fiume, G. (1998b). The ectodomain of a novel member of the immunoglobulin superfamily related to the poliovirus receptor has the attributes of a *bonafide* receptor for herpes simplex viruses 1 and 2 in human cells. *J. Virol.*, **72**, 9992–10002.

Cocchi, F., Lopez, M., Dubreuil, P., Campadelli-Fiume, G., and Menotti, L. (2001). Chimeric nectin1-poliovirus receptor molecules identify a nectin1 region functional in herpes simplex virus entry. *J. Virol.*, **75**, 7987–7994.

Cocchi, F., Fusco, D., Menotti, L. *et al.* (2004). The soluble ectodomain of herpes simplex virus gD contains a membrane-proximal pro-fusion domain and suffices to mediate virus entry. *Proc. Natl Acad. Sci. USA*, **101**, 7445–7450.

Connolly, S. A., Whitbeck, J. J., Rux, A. H. *et al.* (2001). Glycoprotein D homologs in herpes simplex virus type 1, pseudorabies virus, and bovine herpes virus type 1 bind directly to human HveC(nectin-1) with different affinities. *Virology*, **280**, 7–18.

Connolly, S. A., Landsburg, D. J., Carfi, A., Wiley, D. C., Eisenberg, R. J., and Cohen, G. H. (2002). Structure-based analysis of the herpes simplex virus glycoprotein D binding site present on herpesvirus entry mediator HveA (HVEM). *J. Virol.*, **76**, 10894–10904.

Connolly, S. A., Landsburg, D. J., Carfi, A., Wiley, D. C., Cohen, G. H., and Eisenberg, R. J. (2003). Structure-based mutagenesis of herpes simplex virus glycoprotein D defines three critical regions at the gD-HveA/ HVEM binding interface. *J. Virol.*, **77**, 8127–8140.

Connolly, S. A., Landsburg, D. J., Carfi, A. *et al.* (2005). Potential nectin-1 binding site on herpes simplex virus glycoprotein D. *J. Virol.*, **79**, 1282–1295.

Davison, A. J. and Scott, J. E. (1986). The complete DNA sequence of varicella-zoster virus. *J. Gen. Virol.*, **67**(9), 1759–1816.

Desai, P. J., Schaffer, P. A., and Minson, A. C. (1988). Excretion of non-infectious virus particles lacking glycoprotein H by a temperature-sensitive mutant of herpes simplex virus type 1: evidence that gH is essential for virion infectivity. *J. Gen. Virol.*, **69**(6), 1147–1156.

Diefenbach, R. J., Miranda-Saksena, M., Diefenbach, E. *et al.* (2002). Herpes simplex virus tegument protein US11 interacts with conventional kinesin heavy chain. *J. Virol.*, **76**, 3282–3291.

Döhner, K. and Sodeik, B. (2005). The role of the cytoskeleton during viral infection. *Curr. Top. Microbiol. Immunol.*, **285**, 67–108.

Döhner, K., Wolfstein, A., Prank, U. *et al.* (2002). Function of dynein and dynactin in herpes simplex virus capsid transport. *Mol. Biol. Cell*, **13**, 2795–2809.

Dolter, K. E., Goins, W. F., Levine, M., and Glorioso, J. C. (1992). Genetic analysis of type-specific antigenic determinants of herpes simplex virus glycoprotein C. *J. Virol.*, **66**, 4864–4873.

Duus, K. M. and Grose, C. (1996). Multiple regulatory effects of varicella-zoster virus (VZV) gL on trafficking patterns and fusogenic properties of VZV gH. *J. Virol.*, **70**, 8961–8971.

Duus, K. M., Hatfield, C., and Grose, C. (1995). Cell surface expression and fusion by the varicella-zoster virus gH:gL glycoprotein complex: analysis by laser scanning confocal microscopy. *Virology*, **210**, 429–440.

Enquist, L. W., Husak, P. J., Banfield, B. W., and Smith, G. A. (1998). Infection and spread of alphaherpesviruses in the nervous system. *Adv. Virus Res.*, **51**, 237–247.

Fan, Z., Grantham, M. L., Smith, M. S., Anderson, E. S., Cardelli, J. A., and Muggeridge, M. I. (2002). Truncation of herpes simplex virus type 2 glycoprotein B increases its cell surface expression and activity in cell–cell fusion, but these properties are unrelated. *J. Virol.*, **76**, 9271–9283.

Foà-Tomasi, L., Avitabile, E., Boscaro, A. *et al.* (1991). Herpes simplex virus (HSV) glycoprotein H is partially processed in a cell line that expresses the glycoprotein and fully processed in cells infected with deletion or ts mutants in the known HSV glycoproteins. *Virology*, **180**, 474–482.

Forghani, B., Ni, L., and Grose, C. (1994). Neutralization epitope of the varicella-zoster virus gH:gL glycoprotein complex. *Virology*, **199**, 458–462.

Forrester, A., Farrell, H., Wilkinson, G., Kaye, J., Davis Poynter, N., and Minson, T. (1992). Construction and properties of a mutant of herpes simplex virus type 1 with glycoprotein H coding sequences deleted. *J. Virol.*, **66**, 341–348.

Foster, T. P. and Kousoulas, K. G. (1999). Genetic analysis of the role of herpes simplex virus type 1 glycoprotein K in infectious virus production and egress. *J. Virol.*, **73**, 8457–8468.

Foster, T. P., Melancon, J., and Kousoulas, K. (2001a). An alpha-helical domain within the carboxyl terminus of herpes simplex virus type 1 (HSV-1) glycoprotein B (gB) is associated with cell fusion and resistance to heparin inhibition of cell fusion. *Virology*, **287**, 18–29.

Foster, T. P., Rybachuk, G. V., and Kousoulas, K. G. (2001b). Glycoprotein K specified by herpes simplex virus type 1 is expressed on virions as a Golgi complex-dependent glycosylated species and functions in virion entry. *J. Virol.*, **75**, 12431–12438.

Foster, T. P., Alvarez, X., and Kousoulas, K. G. (2003a). Plasma membrane topology of syncytial domains of herpes simplex virus type 1 glycoprotein K (gK): the UL20 protein enables cell surface localization of gK but not gK-mediated cell-to-cell fusion. *J. Virol.*, **77**, 499–510.

Foster, T. P., Rybachuk, G. V., Alvarez, X., Borkhsenious, O., and Kousoulas, K. G. (2003b). Overexpression of gK in gK-transformed cells collapses the Golgi apparatus into the endoplasmic reticulum inhibiting virion egress, glycoprotein transport, and virus-induced cell fusion. *Virology*, **317**, 237–252.

Foster, T. P., Melancon, J. M., Baines, J. D., and Kousoulas, K. G. (2004). The herpes simplex virus type 1 UL20 protein modulates membrane fusion events during cytoplasmic virion morphogenesis and virus-induced cell fusion. *J. Virol.*, **78**, 5347–5357.

Fuller, A. O., Santos, R. E., and Spear, P. G. (1989). Neutralizing antibodies specific for glycoprotein H of herpes simplex virus permit viral attachment to cells but prevent penetration. *J. Virol.*, **63**, 3435–3443.

Fusco, D., Forghieri, C., and Campadelli-Fiume, G. (2005). The profusion domain of herpes simplex virus glycoprotein D (gD) interacts with the gD N terminus and is displaced by soluble forms of viral receptors. *Proc. Natl Acad. Sci. USA*, **102**, 9323–9328.

Galdiero, M., Whiteley, A., Bruun, B., Bell, S., Minson, T., and Browne, H. (1997). Site-directed and linker insertion mutagenesis of herpes simplex virus type 1 glycoprotein H. *J. Virol.*, **71**, 2163–2170.

Galdiero, S., Vitiello, M., D'Isanto, M. *et al.* (2006). Analysis of synthetic peptides from heptad-repeat domains of herpes simplex virus type 1 glycoproteins H and B. *J. Gen. Virol.*, **87**, 1085–1097.

Geraghty, R. J., Krummenacher, C., Cohen, G. H., Eisenberg, R. J., and Spear, P. G. (1998). Entry of alphaherpesviruses mediated by poliovirus receptor-related protein 1 and poliovirus receptor. *Science*, **280**, 1618–1620.

Gerber, S. I., Belval, B. J., and Herold, B. C. (1995). Differences in the role of glycoprotein C of HSV-1 and HSV-2 in viral binding may contribute to serotype differences in cell tropism. *Virology*, **214**, 29–39.

Gianni, T., Campadelli-Fiume, G., and Menotti, L. (2004). Entry of herpes simplex virus mediated by chimeric forms of nectin1 retargeted to endosomes or to lipid rafts occurs through acidic endosomes. *J. Virol.*, **78**, 12268–12276.

Gianni, T., Martelli, P. L., Casadio, R., and Campadelli-Fiume, G. (2005a). The ectodomain of herpes simpex virus glycoprotein H contains a membrane alpha-helix with attributes of an internal fusion peptide, positionally conserved in the Herpesviridae family. *J. Virol.*, **79**, 2931–2940.

Gianni, T., Menotti, L., and Campadelli-Fiume, G. (2005b). A heptad repeat in herpes simplex virus gH, located downstream of the alpha-helix with attributes of a fusion peptide, is critical for virus entry and fusion. *J. Virol.*, **79**, 7042–7049.

Gianni, T., Fato, R., Bergamini, C., Lenaz, G., and Campadelli-Fiume, G. (2006a). Hydrophobic alpha-helices 1 and 2 of herpes simplex virus gH interact with lipids, and their mimetic peptides enhance virus infection and fusion. *J. Virol.*, **80**, 8190–8198.

Gianni, T., Piccoli, A., Bertucci, C., and Campadelli-Fiume, G. (2006b). Heptad repeat 2 in herpes simplex virus-1 gH interacts with heptad repeat 1 and is critical for virus entry and fusion. *J. Virol.*, **80**, 2216–2224.

Gompels, U. and Minson, A. (1986). The properties and sequence of glycoprotein H of herpes simplex virus type 1. *Virology*, **153**, 230–247.

Griffiths, A., Renfrey, S., and Minson, T. (1998). Glycoprotein C-deficient mutants of two strains of herpes simplex virus type 1 exhibit unaltered adsorption characteristics on polarized or non-polarized cells. *J. Gen. Virol.*, **79**(4), 807–812.

Gruenheid, S., Gatzke, L., Meadows, H., and Tufaro, F. (1993). Herpes simplex virus infection and propagation in a mouse L cell mutant lacking heparan sulfate proteoglycans. *J. Virol.*, **67**, 93–100.

Grunewald, K., Desai, P., Winkler, D. C. *et al.* (2003). Three-dimensional structure of herpes simplex virus from cryo-electron tomography. *Science*, **302**, 1396–1398.

Haarr, L., Shukla, D., Rodahl, E., Dal Canto, M. C., and Spear, P. G. (2001). Transcription from the gene encoding the herpesvirus entry receptor nectin-1 (HveC) in nervous tissue of adult mouse. *Virology*, **287**, 301–309.

Harman, A., Browne, H., and Minson, T. (2002). The transmembrane domain and cytoplasmic tail of herpes simplex virus type 1 glycoprotein H play a role in membrane fusion. *J. Virol.*, **76**, 10708–10716.

Harrop, J. A., Reddy, M., Dede, K. *et al.* (1998). Antibodies to TR2 (herpesvirus entry mediator), a new member of the TNF receptor superfamily, block T cell proliferation, expression of activation markers, and production of cytokines. *J. Immunol.*, **161**, 1786–1794.

Heineman, T. C. and Hall, S. L. (2001). VZV gB endocytosis and Golgi localization are mediated by YXXphi motifs in its cytoplasmic domain. *Virology*, **285**, 42–49.

Heldwein, E. E., Lou, H., Bender, F. C., Cohen, G. H., Eisenberg, R. J., and Harrison, S. C. (2006). Crystal structure of glycoprotein B from herpes simplex virus 1. *Science*, **313**, 217–220.

Herold, B. C., WuDunn, D., Soltys, N., and Spear, P. G. (1991). Glycoprotein C of herpes simplex virus type 1 plays a principal role in the adsorption of virus to cells and in infectivity. *J. Virol.*, **65**, 1090–1098.

Highlander, S. L., Dorney, D. J., Gage, P. J. *et al.* (1989). Identification of mar mutations in herpes simplex virus type 1 glycoprotein B which alter antigenic structure and function in virus penetration. *J. Virol.*, **63**, 730–738.

Hutchinson, L. and Johnson, D. C. (1995). Herpes simplex virus glycoprotein K promotes egress of virus particles. *J. Virol.*, **69**, 5401–5413.

Hutchinson, L., Browne, H., Wargent, V. *et al.* (1992a). A novel herpes simplex virus glycoprotein, gL, forms a complex with glycoprotein H (gH) and affects normal folding and surface expression of gH. *J. Virol.*, **66**, 2240–2250.

Hutchinson, L., Goldsmith, K., Snoddy, D., Ghosh, H., Graham, F. L., and Johnson, D. C. (1992b). Identification and characterization of a novel herpes simplex virus glycoprotein, gK, involved in cell fusion. *J. Virol.*, **66**, 5603–5609.

Jogger, C. R., Montgomery, R. I., and Spear, P. G. (2004). Effects of linker-insertion mutations in herpes simplex virus 1 gD on glycoprotein-induced fusion with cells expressing HVEM or nectin-1. *Virology*, **318**, 318–326.

Johnson, D. C., Burke, R. L., and Gregory, T. (1990). Soluble forms of herpes simplex virus glycoprotein D bind to a limited number of cell surface receptors and inhibit virus entry into cells. *J. Virol.*, **64**, 2569–2576.

Johnson, R. M. and Spear, P. G. (1989). Herpes simplex virus glycoprotein D mediates interference with herpes simplex virus infection. *J. Virol.*, **63**, 819–827.

Jones, N. A. and Geraghty, R. J. (2004). Fusion activity of lipid-anchored envelope glycoproteins of herpes simplex virus type 1. *Virology*, **324**, 213–228.

Kaye, J. F., Gompels, U. A., and Minson, A. C. (1992). Glycoprotein H of human cytomegalovirus (HCMV) forms a stable complex with the HCMV UL115 gene product. *J. Gen. Virol.*, **73**(10), 2693–2698.

Keller, P. M., Neff, B. J., and Ellis, R. W. (1984). Three major glycoprotein genes of varicella-zoster virus whose products have neutralization epitopes. *J. Virol.*, **52**, 293–297.

Kenyon, T. K., Cohen, J. I., and Grose, C. (2002). Phosphorylation by the varicella-zoster virus ORF47 protein serine kinase determines whether endocytosed viral gE traffics to the trans-Golgi network or recycles to the cell membrane. *J. Virol.*, **76**, 10980–10993.

Kousoulas, K. G., Huo, B., and Pereira, L. (1988). Antibody-resistant mutations in cross-reactive and type-specific epitopes of herpes simplex virus 1 glycoprotein B map in separate domains. *Virology*, **166**, 423–431.

Krummenacher, C., Nicola, A. V., Whitbeck, J. C. *et al.* (1998). Herpes simplex virus glycoprotein D can bind to poliovirus receptor-related protein 1 or herpesvirus entry mediator, two structurally unrelated mediators of virus entry. *J. Virol.*, **72**, 7064–7074.

Krummenacher, C., Rux, A. H., Whitbeck, J. C. *et al.* (1999). The first immunoglobulin-like domain of HveC is sufficient to bind herpes simplex virus gD with full affinity, while the third domain is involved in oligomerization of HveC. *J. Virol.*, **73**, 8127–8137.

Krummenacher, C., Baribaud, I., Ponce De Leon, M. *et al.* (2000). Localization of a binding site for herpes simplex virus glycoprotein D on herpesvirus entry mediator C by using antireceptor monoclonal antibodies. *J. Virol.*, **74**, 10863–10872.

Krummenacher, C., Baribaud, I., Ponce De Leon, M. *et al.* (2004). Comparative usage of herpesvirus entry mediator A and nectin-1 by laboratory strains and clinical isolates of herpes simplex virus. *Virology*, **322**, 286–299.

Krummenacher, C., Supekar, V. M., Whitbeck, J. C. *et al.* (2005). Structure of unliganded HSV gD reveals a mechanism for receptor-mediated activation of virus entry. *EMBO J.*, **24**, 4144–4153.

Kwon, B. S., Tan, K. B., Ni, J. *et al.* (1997). A newly identified member of the tumor necrosis factor receptor superfamily with a wide tissue distribution and involvement in lymphocyte activation. *J. Biol. Chem.*, **272**, 14272–14276.

La, S., Kim, J., Kwon, B. S., and Kwon, B. (2002). Herpes simplex virus type 1 glycoprotein D inhibits T-cell proliferation. *Mol. Cells*, **14**, 398–403.

Ligas, M. W. and Johnson, D. C. (1988). A herpes simplex virus mutant in which glycoprotein D sequences are replaced by beta-galactosidase sequences binds to but is unable to penetrate into cells. *J. Virol.*, **62**, 1486–1494.

Linehan, M. M., Richman, S., Krummenacher, C., Eisenberg, R. J., Cohen, G. H., and Iwasaki, A. (2004). In vivo role of nectin-1 in entry of herpes simplex virus type 1 (HSV-1) and HSV-2 through the vaginal mucosa. *J. Virol.*, **78**, 2530–2536.

Liu, D. X., Gompels, U. A., Foà-Tomasi, L., and Campadelli-Fiume, G. (1993). Human herpesvirus-6 glycoprotein H and L homologs are components of the gp100 complex and the gH external domain is the target for neutralizing monoclonal antibodies. *Virology*, **197**, 12–22.

Lopez, M., Cocchi, F., Menotti, L., Avitabile, E., Dubreuil, P., and Campadelli-Fiume, G. (2000). Nectin2a (PRR2a or HveB) and nectin2d are low-efficiency mediators for entry of herpes simplex virus mutants carrying the Leu25Pro substitution in glycoprotein D. *J. Virol.*, **74**, 1267–1274.

Lopez, M., Cocchi, F., Avitabile, E. *et al.* (2001). Novel, soluble isoform of the herpes simplex virus (HSV) receptor nectin1 (or PRR1-HIgR-HveC) modulates positively and negatively susceptibility to HSV infection. *J. Virol.*, **75**, 5684–5691.

Mabit, H., Nakano, M. Y., Prank, U. *et al.* (2002). Intact microtubules support adenovirus and herpes simplex virus infections. *J. Virol.*, **76**, 9962–9971.

Mallory, S., Sommer, M., and Arvin, A. M. (1997). Mutational analysis of the role of glycoprotein I in varicella-zoster virus replication and its effects on glycoprotein E conformation and trafficking. *J. Virol.*, **71**, 8279–8288.

Manoj, S., Jogger, C. R., Myscofski, D., Yoon, M., and Spear, P. G. (2004). Mutations in herpes simplex virus glycoprotein D that prevent cell entry via nectins and alter cell tropism. *Proc. Natl Acad. Sci. USA*, **101**, 12414–12421.

Manservigi, R., Spear, P. G., and Buchan, A. (1977). Cell fusion induced by herpes simplex virus is promoted and suppressed by different viral glycoproteins. *Proc. Natl Acad. Sci. USA*, **74**, 3913–3917.

Maresova, L., Pasieka, T. J., and Grose, C. (2001). Varicella-zoster Virus gB and gE coexpression, but not gB or gE alone, leads to abundant fusion and syncytium formation equivalent to those from gH and gL coexpression. *J. Virol.*, **75**, 9483–9492.

Marozin, S., Prank, U., and Sodeik, B. (2004). Herpes simplex virus type 1 infection of polarized epithelial cells requires microtubules and access to receptors at cell–cell contact sites. *J. Gen. Virol.*, **85**, 775–786.

Martinez, W. M. and Spear, P. G. (2002). Amino acid substitutions in the V domain of nectin-1 (HveC) that impair entry activity for herpes simplex virus types 1 and 2 but not for Pseudorabies virus or bovine herpesvirus 1. *J. Virol.*, **76**, 7255–7262.

Mata, M., Zhang, M., Hu, X., and Fink, D. J. (2001). HveC (nectin-1) is expressed at high levels in sensory neurons, but not in motor neurons, of the rat peripheral nervous system. *J. Neurovirol.*, **7**, 476–480.

Matsushima, H., Utani, A., Endo, H. *et al.* (2003). The expression of nectin-1alpha in normal human skin and various skin tumours. *Br. J. Dermatol.*, **148**, 755–762.

Mauri, D. N., Ebner, R., Montgomery, R. I. *et al.* (1998). LIGHT, a new member of the TNF superfamily, and lymphotoxin alpha are ligands for herpesvirus entry mediator. *Immunity*, **8**, 21–30.

McGeoch, D. J., Dalrymple, M. A., Davison, A. J. *et al.* (1988). The complete DNA sequence of the long unique region in the genome of herpes simplex virus type 1. *J. Gen. Virol.*, **69**, 1531–1574.

Melancon, J. M., Foster, T. P., and Kousoulas, K. G. (2004). Genetic analysis of the herpes simplex virus type 1 UL20 protein domains involved in cytoplasmic virion envelopment and virus-induced cell fusion. *J. Virol.*, **78**, 7329–7343.

Menotti, L., Lopez, M., Avitabile, E. *et al.* (2000). The murine homolog of human-Nectin1d serves as a species non-specific mediator for entry of human and animal aherpesviruses in a pathway independent of a detectable binding to gD. *Proc. Natl Acad. Sci. USA*, **97**, 4867–4872.

Menotti, L., Avitabile, E., Dubreuil, P., Lopez, M., and Campadelli-Fiume, G. (2001). Comparison of murine and human nectin1 binding to herpes simplex virus glycoprotein D (gD) reveals a weak interaction of murine nectin1 to gD and a gD-dependent pathway of entry. *Virology*, **282**, 256–266.

Menotti, L., Casadio, R., Bertucci, C., Lopez, M., and Campadelli-Fiume, G. (2002a). Substitution in the murine nectin1 receptor of a single conserved amino acid at a position distal from herpes simplex virus gD binding site confers high affinity binding to gD. *J. Virol.*, **76**, 5463–5471.

Menotti, L., Cocchi, F., and Campadelli-Fiume, G. (2002b). Critical residues in the CC' ridge of the human nectin1 receptor V domain enable herpes simplex virus entry into the cell and act synergistically with the downstream region. *Virology*, **301**, 6–12.

Milne, R. S., Connolly, S. A., Krummenacher, C., Eisenberg, R. J., and Cohen, G. H. (2001). Porcine HveC, a member of the highly conserved HveC/nectin 1 family, is a functional alphaherpesvirus receptor. *Virology*, **281**, 315–328.

Milne, R. S., Hanna, S. L., Rux, A. H., Willis, S. H., Cohen, G. H., and Eisenberg, R. J. (2003). Function of herpes simplex virus type 1 gD mutants with different receptor-binding affinities in virus entry and fusion. *J. Virol.*, **77**, 8962–8972.

Mo, C., Lee, J., Sommer, M., Grose, C., and Arvin, A. M. (2002). The requirement of varicella zoster virus glycoprotein E (gE) for viral replication and effects of glycoprotein I on gE in melanoma cells. *Virology*, **304**, 176–186.

Montalvo, E. A. and Grose, C. (1986). Neutralization epitope of varicella zoster virus on native viral glycoprotein gp118 (VZV glycoprotein gpIII). *Virology*, **149**, 230–241.

Montgomery, R. I., Warner, M. S., Lum, B. J., and Spear, P. G. (1996). Herpes simplex virus-1 entry into cells mediated by a novel member of the TNF/NGF receptor family. *Cell*, **87**, 427–436.

Nicola, A. V. and Straus, S. E. (2004). Cellular and viral requirements for rapid endocytic entry of herpes simplex virus. *J. Virol.*, **78**, 7508–7517.

Nicola, A. V., Peng, C., Lou, H., Cohen, G. H., and Eisenberg, R. J. (1997). Antigenic structure of soluble herpes simplex virus (HSV) glycoprotein D correlates with inhibition of HSV infection. *J. Virol.*, **71**, 2940–2946.

Nicola, A. V., McEvoy, A. M., and Straus, S. E. (2003). Roles for endocytosis and low pH in herpes simplex virus entry into HeLa and Chinese hamster ovary cells. *J. Virol.*, **77**, 5324–5332.

Ojala, P. M., Sodeik, B., Ebersold, M. W., Kutay, U., and Helenius, A. (2000). Herpes simplex virus type 1 entry into host cells: reconstitution of capsid binding and uncoating at the nuclear pore complex in vitro. *Mol. Cell Biol.*, **20**, 4922–4931.

Olson, J. K. and Grose, C. (1997). Endocytosis and recycling of varicella-zoster virus Fc receptor glycoprotein gE: internalization mediated by a YXXL motif in the cytoplasmic tail. *J. Virol.*, **71**, 4042–4054.

Olson, J. K. and Grose, C. (1998). Complex formation facilitates endocytosis of the varicella-zoster virus gE:gI Fc receptor. *J. Virol.*, **72**, 1542–1551.

Olson, J. K., Santos, R. A., and Grose, C. (1998). Varicella-zoster virus glycoprotein gE: endocytosis and trafficking of the Fc receptor. *J. Infect. Dis.*, **178** Suppl 1, S2–S6.

Pasieka, T. J., Maresova, L., and Grose, C. (2003). A functional YNKI motif in the short cytoplasmic tail of varicella-zoster virus glycoprotein gH mediates clathrin-dependent and antibody-independent endocytosis. *J. Virol.*, **77**, 4191–4204.

Pasieka, T. J., Maresova, L., Shiraki, K., and Grose, C. (2004). Regulation of varicella-zoster virus-induced cell-to-cell fusion by the endocytosis-competent glycoproteins gH and gE. *J. Virol.*, **78**, 2884–2896.

Patera, A., Ali, M. A., Tyring, S. *et al.* (2002). Polymorphisms in the genes for herpesvirus entry. *J. Infect. Dis.*, **186**, 444–445.

Pellett, P. E., Kousoulas, K. G., Pereira, L., and Roizman, B. (1985). Anatomy of the herpes simplex virus 1 strain F glycoprotein

B gene: primary sequence and predicted protein structure of the wild type and of monoclonal antibody-resistant mutants. *J. Virol.*, **53**, 243–253.

Peng, T., Ponce de Leon, M., Novotny, M. J. *et al.* (1998). Structural and antigenic analysis of a truncated form of the herpes simplex virus glycoprotein gH-gL complex. *J. Virol.*, **72**, 6092–6103.

Pereira, L., Ali, M., Kousoulas, K., Huo, B., and Banks, T. (1989). Domain structure of herpes simplex virus 1 glycoprotein B: neutralizing epitopes map in regions of continuous and discontinuous residues. *Virology*, **172**, 11–24.

Qadri, I., Gimeno, C., Navarro, D., and Pereira, L. (1991). Mutations in conformation-dependent domains of herpes simplex virus 1 glycoprotein B affect the antigenic properties, dimerization, and transport of the molecule. *Virology*, **180**, 135–152.

Reymond, N., Borg, J., Lecocq, E. *et al.* (2000). Human nectin3/PRR3: a novel member of the PVR/PRR/nectin family that interacts with afadin. *Gene*, **255**, 347–355.

Richart, S., Simpson, S., Krummenacher, C. *et al.* (2003). Entry of herpes simplex virus type 1 into primary sensory neurons in vitro is mediated by Nectin-1/HveC. *J. Virol.*, **77**, 3307–3311.

Roberts, S. R., Ponce de Leon, M., Cohen, G. H., and Eisenberg, R. J. (1991). Analysis of the intracellular maturation of the herpes simplex virus type 1 glycoprotein gH in infected and transfected cells. *Virology*, **184**, 609–624.

Roche, S., Bressanelli, S., Rey, F. A., and Gaudin, Y. (2006). Crystal structure of the low-pH form of the vesicular stomatitis virus glycoprotein G. *Science*, **313**, 187–191.

Roop, C., Hutchinson, L., and Johnson, D. C. (1993). A mutant herpes simplex virus type 1 unable to express glycoprotein L cannot enter cells, and its particles lack glycoprotein H. *J. Virol.*, **67**, 2285–2297.

Rux, A. H., Lou, H., Lambris, J. D., Friedman, H. M., Eisenberg, R. J., and Cohen, G. H. (2002). Kinetic analysis of glycoprotein C of herpes simplex virus types 1 and 2 binding to heparin, heparan sulfate, and complement component C3b. *Virology*, **294**, 324–332.

Santos, R. A., Padilla, J. A., Hatfield, C., and Grose, C. (1998). Antigenic variation of varicella zoster virus Fc receptor gE: loss of a major B cell epitope in the ectodomain. *Virology*, **249**, 21–31.

Santos, R. A., Hatfield, C. C., Cole, N. L. *et al.* (2000). Varicella-zoster virus gE escape mutant VZV-MSP exhibits an accelerated cell-to-cell spread phenotype in both infected cell cultures and SCID-hu mice. *Virology*, **275**, 306–317.

Schelhaas, M., Jansen, M., Haase, I., and Knebel-Morsdorf, D. (2003). Herpes simplex virus type 1 exhibits a tropism for basal entry in polarized epithelial cells. *J. Gen. Virol.*, **84**, 2473–2484.

Shukla, D. and Spear, P. G. (2001). Herpesviruses and heparan sulfate: an intimate relationship in aid of viral entry. *J. Clin. Invest.*, **108**, 503–510.

Shukla, D., Liu, J., Blaiklock, P. *et al.* (1999). A novel role for 3-O-sulfated heparan sulfate in herpes simplex virus 1 entry. *Cell*, **99**, 13–22.

Shukla, D. Dal Canto, M. C., Rowe, C. L., and Spear, P. G. (2000). Striking Similarity of murine nectin-1alpha to human nectin-1alpha (HveC) in sequence and activity as a glycoprotein D receptor for alphaherpesvirus entry. *J. Virol.*, **74**, 11773–11781.

Smith, G. A., Gross, S. P., and Enquist, L. W. (2001). Herpesviruses use bidirectional fast-axonal transport to spread in sensory neurons. *Proc. Natl Acad. Sci. USA*, **98**, 3466–3470.

Sodeik, B. (2000). Mechanisms of viral transport in the cytoplasm. *Trends Microbiol*, **8**, 465–472.

Sodeik, B., Ebersold, M. W., and Helenius, A. (1997). Microtubule-mediated transport of incoming herpes simplex virus 1 capsids to the nucleus. *J. Cell Biol.*, **136**, 1007–1021.

Spear, P. G., Shieh, M. T., Herold, B. C., WuDunn, D., and Koshy, T. I. (1992). Heparan sulfate glycosaminoglycans as primary cell surface receptors for herpes simplex virus. *Adv. Exp. Med. Biol.*, **313**, 341–353.

Spear, P. G., Eisenberg, R. J., and Cohen, G. H. (2000). Three classes of cell surface receptors for alphaherpesvirus entry. *Virology*, **275**, 1–8.

Struyf, F., Posavad, C. M., Keyaerts, E., Van Ranst, M., Corey, L., and Spear, P. G. (2002). Search for polymorphisms in the genes for herpesvirus entry mediator, nectin-1, and nectin-2 in immune seronegative individuals. *J. Infect. Dis.*, **185**, 36–44.

Takai, Y., Irie, K., Shimizu, K., Sakisaka, T., and Ikeda, W. (2003). Nectins and nectin-like molecules: roles in cell adhesion, migration, and polarization. *Cancer Sci.*, **94**, 655–667.

Tal-Singer, R., Peng, C., Ponce De Leon, M. *et al.* (1995). Interaction of herpes simplex virus glycoprotein gC with mammalian cell surface molecules. *J. Virol.*, **69**, 4471–4483.

Turner, A., Bruun, B., Minson, T., and Browne, H. (1998). Glycoproteins gB, gD, and gHgL of herpes simplex virus type 1 are necessary and sufficient to mediate membrane fusion in a Cos cell transfection system. *J. Virol.*, **72**, 873–875.

Ward, P. L., Campadelli-Fiume, G., Avitabile, E., and Roizman, B. (1994). Localization and putative function of the UL20 membrane protein in cells infected with herpes simplex virus 1. *J. Virol.*, **68**, 7406–7417.

Warner, M. S., Geraghty, R. J., Martinez, W. M. *et al.* (1998). A cell surface protein with herpesvirus entry activity (HveB) confers susceptibility to infection by mutants of herpes simplex virus type 1, herpes simplex virus type 2, and pseudorabies virus. *Virology*, **246**, 179–189.

Whitbeck, J. C., Muggeridge, M. I., Rux, A. H. *et al.* (1999). The major neutralizing antigenic site on herpes simplex virus glycoprotein D overlaps a receptor-binding domain. *J. Virol.*, **73**, 9879–9890.

Willis, S. H., Rux, A. H., Peng, C. *et al.* (1998). Examination of the kinetics of herpes simplex virus glycoprotein D binding to the herpesvirus entry mediator, using surface plasmon resonance. *J. Virol.*, **72**, 5937–5947.

WuDunn, D. and Spear, P. G. (1989). Initial interaction of herpes simplex virus with cells is binding to heparan sulfate. *J. Virol.*, **63**, 52–58.

Yoon, M., Zago, A., Shukla, D., and Spear, P. G. (2003). Mutations in the N termini of herpes simplex virus type 1 and 2 gDs alter functional interactions with the entry/fusion receptors HVEM, nectin-2, and 3-O-sulfated heparan sulfate but not with nectin-1. *J. Virol.*, **77**, 9221–9231.

Zhou, G. and Roizman, B. (2006). Construction and properties of a herpes simplex virus 1 designed to enter cells solely via the IL-13alpha2 receptor. *Proc. Natl Acad. Sci. USA*, **103**, 5508–5513.

Zhou, G., Avitabile, E., Campadelli-Fiume, G., and Roizman, B. (2003). The domains of glycoprotein D required to block apoptosis induced by herpes simplex virus 1 are largely distinct from those involved in cell-cell fusion and binding to nectin1. *J. Virol.*, **77**, 3759–3767.

8

Early events pre-initiation of alphaherpes viral gene expression

Thomas M. Kristie

National Institute of Allergy and Infectious Diseases, National Institutes of Health, Bethesda, MD, USA

The regulated transcription of the HSV IE (immediate–early, α) genes has been a model system for elucidating principles and mechanisms of combinatorial-differential regulation, basic RNAPII-directed transcription, and multiprotein assembly specificities. The regulation exemplifies viral mechanisms dedicated to the recruitment of cellular components into complex viral–host interactions that illustrate general parameters of protein–protein, DNA–protein, RNA transcription, and protein complex assembly. Continued studies hold promise of advancing the understanding of the complexities of biochemical interactions in gene expression as well as complex cellular response pathways. The regulation of the IE genes within specific contexts may also lead to the understanding of signals and pathways which modulate viral infection and determine the extent of lytic-latent infection. While HSV has been extensively studied and will represent the focus of this review, the regulatory domain of the VZV IE gene (IE62) contains similar elements and is regulated by similar mechanisms.

The HSV IE regulatory domains: multiple sites for differential regulation

The regulatory domains of the HSV IE genes have been the focus of numerous studies that have defined the sequence elements and their contributions to the basal and induced levels of transcription. These IE domains typically consist of a reiterated inducible enhancer core element (consensus: TAATGARAT) that is flanked by binding sites for members of the ets and kruppel transcription family (Fig. 8.1, left) (Roizman and Sears, 1996; Vogel and Kristie, 2001).

The primary focus has been on the regulated induction of the expression of the IE genes by the HSV IE transactivator (VP16, αTIF, ICP25) via the enhancer core element (Phillips and Luisi, 2000; Roizman and Sears, 1996; Roizman and Sears, 1996; Vogel and Kristie, 2001; Vogel et al., 2001; Wysocka and Herr, 2003). This focus led to the identification of cellular proteins (Oct-1 and HCF-1) that are required for the stable enhancer complex assembly and the induction of the IE gene transcription (Kristie et al., 1989, 1995; Kristie and Sharp, 1993; Roizman and Sears, 1996; Vogel and Kristie, 2001; Vogel et al., 2001; Wilson et al., 1993; Wysocka and Herr, 2003). Extensive characterization of these components illustrates the multiple levels of complex regulatory interactions inherent in this process.

The assembly of the HSV IE enhancer core complex

The assembly of the HSV IE enhancer core complex illustrates the basic elements of the specificities governing the regulatory process. The stages of the assembly are modeled upon in vitro studies of protein–DNA recognition, protein-protein interactions, selective recognition, affinities, and cooperative interactions. As shown in Fig. 8.1 (Right), the cellular Oct-1 POU domain protein recognizes the divergent octamer element in the IE core and provides a nucleation point for the association of the heterodimeric protein complex consisting of VP16 and HCF-1. Specificity for the HSV IE element is determined by selective recognition of the Oct-1 POU-homeobox and the enhancer core DNA sequences by VP16 while the complex is stabilized by HCF-1 interactions. The full enhancer domain complex contains additional cellular transcription factors such as GABP and Sp1. The activation potential is dependent upon the core complex, likely through additional protein–protein interactions. The complexity of the regulatory complex provides for multiple levels of regulation dictated by various protein combinations, interactions, and the specific regulation of the individual components. Therefore, each component

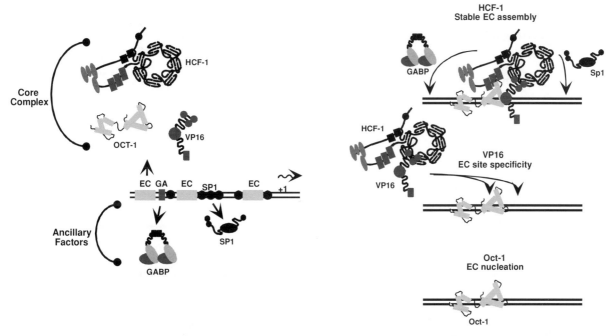

Fig. 8.1. The HSV IE enhancer domain elements, components, and assembly process. (Left) Representation of a typical HSV IE enhancer-promoter domain containing the reiterated enhancer core (EC), GABP (GA), and Sp1 (Sp1) binding sites. The enhancer core components (HCF-1, Oct-1, VP16) and ancillary transcription factors (GABP, Sp1) are represented. (Right) Specificities and interactions in the assembly of the multiprotein enhancer core complex. Oct-1 binds to the octamer element in the 5′ end of the ATGCTAATGARAT enhancer core and nucleates the association of the heteromeric HCF-1/VP16 protein complex. VP16 cooperatively interacts with the Oct-1 POU-homeobox and recognized the 3′ sequences of the core element. The stable enhancer core complex may recruit or interact with the additional factors to form the fully assembled enhancer complex.

will be described with respect to its defined structure, function, interactions, and regulatory mechanisms.

Oct-1

Oct-1 is a representative of the POU family of proteins (Pit, Oct, unc86) containing bipartite DNA binding domains (POU-specific box, POUs and POU-homeobox, POUh) consisting of helix-turn-helix structures that cooperate to recognize the consensus element (ATGCAAAT) (Clerc et al., 1988; Phillips and Luisi, 2000; Sturm et al., 1988). The structure and DNA contacts of the POU-specific box are analogous to the λ repressor in which all four helices make significant network DNA backbone contacts while DNA recognition by the POU-homeobox is characteristic of homeodomains in which helix 3 lies in the major groove and provides sequence recognition. The two DNA binding units recognize bases (POUs, ATGC; POUh, AAAT) in the major groove on opposite sides of the helix and are separated by a flexible and disordered linker region (Fig. 8.2-Oct-1) (Klemm et al., 1994).

In the case of the HSV IE domains, Oct-1 nucleates the enhancer core assembly by binding the divergent octamer sequences of the core consensus (ATGCTAAT). Selective recognition of the Oct-1 POU-homeobox by VP16 was elucidated by comparative analysis of Oct-1 and the highly related Oct-2 protein. While only seven amino acids differ between the exposed homeodomain surfaces of these two proteins, VP16 selectively interacts with Oct-1 (Lai et al., 1992; Pomerantz et al., 1992). As shown (Fig. 8.2-Oct-1), four amino acids (K18, S19, E22, E30) in helixes 1 and 2 are required for high affinity recognition by VP16. Strikingly, only the single position 22 (Oct-1, E22) determines the specificity that accounts for the affinity difference in the recognition of Oct-1 over Oct-2 by VP16. This selective recognition by VP16 elucidated a principle of homeobox protein interaction and specificity that has been reflected in multiple Oct-1 interactions in differential positive, negative, and inducible regulatory events. Studies addressing these contextual interactions elucidate the functions of the protein and illustrate the various diverse mechanisms used to regulate these processes:

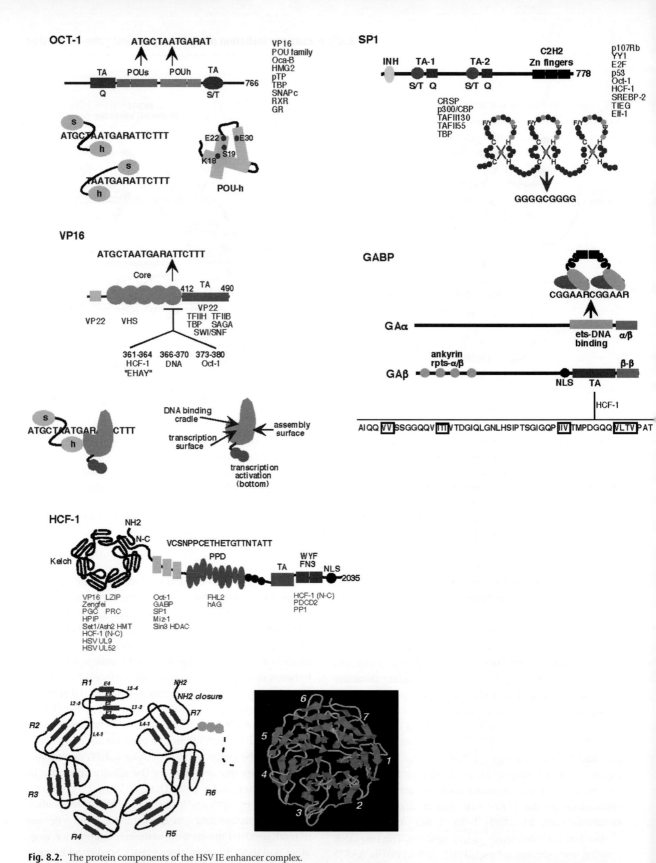

Fig. 8.2. The protein components of the HSV IE enhancer complex.
Oct-1: The transactivation (TA-Q and TA-S/T) and POU (POUs and POUh) domains are shown. The POU-specific box recognizes ATGC while the POU-homeobox recognizes TAAT within the enhancer core element (ATGCTAATGARAT). Proteins that bind to the Oct-1 POU domain are listed. The inherent flexibility of the POU domain and the potential orientations of the POUs box in recognition of the core element are depicted. In the schematic representation of the Oct-1 POU-homeobox, the residues which are important for the recognition by VP16 are indicated. *(cont.)*

(i) The stimulation of transcription preinitiation complex formation via the interaction of the Oct-1 POU domain with TBP in a non-DNA dependent manner has suggested that the interaction enhances TBP-TATA box binding by alleviating TBP autorepression, thus resulting in synergistic activation of octamer containing promoters (Mittal et al., 1999; Zwilling et al., 1994). Similarly, snRNA transcription is regulated via Oct-1/SNAPc interaction in which SNAPc is recruited to the snRNA proximal element via interactions that relieve SNAPc autorepression (Mittal et al., 1999). The interaction of Oct-1 POU with SNAPc utilizes the same POU interaction surface as is bound by specific Oct-1 coactivators illustrating that the DNA site context is a determining factor in the selection of cofactors and coactivators (Hovde et al., 2002).

(ii) Oct-1 stimulates transcription from TATA-less promoters via recruitment of TFIIB, functioning in lieu of TBP to orient the basal factor for RNAPII positioning (Phillips and Luisi, 2000).

(iii) Numerous synergistic interactions with other transcription factors also determine the roles of Oct-1 in positive, negative, and inducible regulation of gene expression. This regulation may be DNA dependent, promoter context dependent, or via DNA-independent protein-protein interactions. At the mouse mammary tumor virus (MMTV) promoter, interaction of the glucocorticoid receptor with the Oct-1 POU domain mediates glucocorticoid induction. Similarly, interaction with the androgen receptor promotes SRC-1 coactivator recruitment and transcription enhancement (Phillips and Luisi, 2000). In contrast, Oct-1 POU-homeobox interaction with the zinc finger domain of RXR disrupts the thyroid hormone receptor TR/RXR heterodimer, leading to repression of TR-dependent transcription (Gonzalez and Robins, 2001).

At the cyclin D1 promoter, interaction of CREB with the Oct-1 POU domain occurs independently of an octamer element and results in CBP coactivator recruitment in the absence of the normally responsive mechanism that depends upon CREB phosphorylation (Boulon et al., 2002). Induction of GADD45 following UV-induced DNA damage is a second example of Oct-1 mediated regulation that is distinct from the defined primary p53 dependent regulatory mechanism (Jin et al., 2001).

(iv) Another level of regulation is exemplified by Oct-1 interactions with cell-type or process-specific coactivators (Phillips and Luisi, 2000; Wysocka and Herr, 2003). The stimulation of immunoglobulin gene transcription by Oct-1 is mediated by binding of the B-cell specific coactivator OCA-B that interacts in a hydrophobic pocket with both subdomains of the Oct-1-POU domain. This interaction requires the Oct-1-DNA assembly, preferentially interacting with Oct-1 bound to the consensus ATGCAAAT vs. the HSV ATGCTAAT. The selection of site-specific Oct-1-DNA complexes by OCA-B is determined by binding a different surface of the Oct-1 POUs/POUh subdomains than VP16 that is positioned to the center of the consensus octamer element and includes OCA-B-DNA contacts (Babb et al., 1997; Chasman et al., 1999). Recent studies have identified a second process-specific coactivator, OCA-S that is involved in the S-phase, cell-cycle dependent stimulation of the histone H2B promoter by Oct-1. Strikingly, this coactivator contains the enzyme GAPDH that may link cellular metabolism to cell growth and division (Zheng et al., 2003). These differential interactions illustrate the structural versatility in Oct-1 protein interactions.

(v) Oct-1 also plays a role in the stimulation of DNA replication as exemplified by the binding of the adenovirus pTP-Pol to the POU-homeobox (Coenjaerts et al., 1994; Phillips and Luisi, 2000). The interaction enhances the association of the pTP-pol with the origin-binding complex. In this case, the interactions are via the DNA binding surface of the

Fig. 8.2. (*continued*) *VP16*: The structure and protein interactions of VP16 are represented. The core structure contains the clustered residues that are critical for the assembly of the IE enhancer complex (HCF-1, Oct-1, DNA) while the transactivation domain (TA, aa 412–490) interacts with a number of basal factors and chromatin modifying components. A schematic representation of the VP16 protein structure is shown (left) indicating the various protein interaction surfaces oriented in recognition of the Oct-1 POU-homeobox/ DNA complex.
HCF-1: The amino-terminal kelch, mid-aminoterminal, proteolytic processing (PPD), autocatalytic (Auto), transactivation (TA), WYF-rich, FN3 repeat, and nuclear localization signal (NLS) regions are represented. The proteins that interact with each region are listed below the appropriate domain. The PPD is represented as a series of consensus (large oval) and divergent (small oval) reiterations of the HCF-1 cleavage sequence shown above. (Bottom left) A stylized representation of the HCF-1 kelch domain is shown illustrating the seven predicted blades (antiparallel sheets, E1 through E4; loops, L1–2 through L4–1). For HCF-1, the predicted ring closure utilizes E4 from the animoterminus and E1-2-3 from the carboxyterminus of the domain (NH2 closure). (Bottom right) The derived molecular model of the HCF-1 kelch domain structure is depicted.
Sp1: The inhibitory domain (INH), transactivation domains (TA-1, TA-2), and DNA binding domains (C2H2, Zn fingers) are represented. Proteins or protein complexes that interact with Sp1 are listed. The structure of the C2H2 Zn finger domain is schematically represented: C, cysteine; H, histadine; F/Y, phenylalanine or tyrosine; y, hydrophobic residue. Light circles represent amino acids that are predicted to make DNA contacts.
GABP: The α subunit contains the ets DNA binding domain recognizing the GA box and the heterodimerization domain (α/β). The β subunit contains ankyrin repeats (α/β heterodimerization region), nuclear localization signals (NLS), transactivation domain (TA), and tetramerization sequences (β–β). The sequence of the transactivation domain is shown and the residues that are critical for both transactivation and interaction with HCF-1 are boxed. (See color plate section.)

POU-homeobox and are distinct from those of the VP16-Oct homeobox complex (de Jong et al., 2002).

Clearly there are a number of distinct mechanisms by which Oct-1 may regulate the basal level expression, induction, or repression of target genes via interactions with specific sites, transcription factors, and coactivators that are mediated through the POU domain. In addition, the protein contains two transactivation domains (Fig. 8.2-Oct-1) that flank the POU domain and function in a promoter context dependent manner, suggesting that additional protein interactions at a given promoter further modulate the regulatory process (Tanaka et al., 1992). The multitude of promoter targets and protein interactions and the diverse regulatory mechanisms involving Oct-1 is reflective of an innate flexibility of the protein conferred by the linker segment separating the POU subdomains (Phillips and Luisi, 2000; Wysocka and Herr, 2003). This flexibility allows for the recognition of sequences and contexts that are divergent from the consensus octamer element. As illustrated by binding to both octamer + and octamer − TAATGARAT elements, the flexibility of the Oct-1 POU domain allows for alternative configurations or positions of the POU-specific box relative to the POU-homeobox (Fig. 8.2-Oct-1). This ability allows for interaction of these domains with proteins in nonconsensus configurations. The configuration is dictated by the sequence of the DNA element and can provide distinct interfaces for various coregulators that are promoter dependent.

The activity of Oct-1 is also regulated by a number of post-transcriptional mechanisms including: (i) enhancement of DNA-binding activity following UV-induced DNA damage (Zhao et al., 2000); (ii) phosphorylation by PKA, PKC, and CKII (Grenfell et al., 1996); (iii) interaction with HMG2 which may function to order the DNA-binding domain for high affinity recognition (Zwilling et al., 1995) and (iv) enhanced phosphorylation of Oct-1 via interaction with MAT1 cyclin dependent kinase activating kinase (Inamoto et al., 1997). Similarly additional levels of regulation exist which impact the function of Oct-1 as illustrated by the modulation of the levels of the OCA-B coactivator by the ring finger protein Siah-1 (Tiedt et al., 2001). The various types of interactions and levels of regulation that impinge on the function of Oct-1 will clearly have implications for the function of the protein in the stimulation of the HSV IE genes in different cellular contexts.

VP16

Vp16 (ICP25, VMW65, αTIF) is the HSV-encoded component of the enhancer core complex that determines the specificity for the HSV elements. Approximately 900 molecules of the protein are packaged within the tegument structure of a virion and are released into the cytoplasm of the cell upon infection (Roizman, 1996). The protein is transported to the nucleus and assembled into the stable enhancer core complex. VP16 is a critical component of the complex as it determines the specificity of the HSV IE core complex by direct recognition of the TAATGARAT DNA element and by selective recognition of the DNA bound Oct-1 (Figs. 8.1 and 8.2) (Kristie and Sharp, 1990; Lai et al., 1992; Pomerantz et al., 1992).

The 490 amino acid protein consists of a conserved structural core (aa 49–403) that contains the specificity surfaces for interaction with Oct-1, DNA, and HCF-1 (Lai and Herr, 1997; Simmen et al., 1997; Wysocka and Herr, 2003) as well as a highly characterized transcription activation domain (aa 412–490) that interacts with both basal transcription factors and chromatin remodeling/nucleosome modification factors (Fig. 8.2-VP16). Surprisingly, the protein lacks a nuclear localization signal and nuclear transport is provided by protein interaction with HCF-1 (La Boissiere et al., 1999). As HCF-1 is a key cell-cycle component, this interaction may play a significant role in the initial "sensing" of the cell state for viral replication.

Advances in the determination of the structure of VP16 have provided an understanding of the protein–protein and protein–DNA interactions that are critical for the protein's selective induction of the HSV IE genes. The highly structured core domain consists of internal symmetry that is dominated by two-stranded antiparallel coiled coils. The resulting structure resembles a "seat" complete with bottom, back, and headrest regions (Fig. 8.2-VP16). Interestingly, the region representing the interaction domain for Oct-1, HCF-1, and DNA (aa 350–394) is disordered in the crystal, suggesting that this domain adopts a structure upon binding these components (Babb et al., 2001; Liu et al., 1999). Correlation of the structure with numerous mutagenesis studies clearly indicates that there are distinct surfaces for interaction with components involved in virion assembly (right surface) vs. transcription (left surface) while the DNA recognition surface is formed by a cleft in the seat structure (Fig. 8.2-VP16, bottom right) (Babb et al., 2001; Liu et al., 1999). As different VP16 orthologs such as those encoded by VZV and BHV recognize different TAATGARAT elements dependent upon the 3′ sequences, the VP16 structure presents a model by which the unstructured region may also contribute to DNA binding by adopting a structure to specifically recognize the GARAT sequences while the "seat" recognizes the 3′ portion of the element. Furthermore, the DNA binding model predicts that the Oct-1 POU-specific box may lie to either side of the TAAT in the enhancer complex (refer to Fig. 8.2 -VP16) and may modulate the VP16-DNA interaction.

The specific residues that are important for the interactions of VP16 in the IE enhancer core complex have been defined by numerous mutagenesis and peptide inhibition studies (Vogel and Kristie, 2001; Wysocka and Herr, 2003). This work elucidated a clustered core of residues for interaction with HCF-1 (E361, H362, Y364) that is now recognized as the HCF-1 interaction (D/E HXY) motif in a number of cellular proteins that interact with this coactivator protein (Freiman and Herr, 1997; Lu et al., 1998; Wysocka and Herr, 2003). Mutations in residues (Y373, G374, S375) affect the VP16- Oct1 interaction while mutations in residues (R360, R366, R368, K370) affect DNA binding (Lai and Herr, 1997). Interestingly, S375 is a target for CKII-dependent phosphorylation. This residue is normally modified in cell extracts and is required for efficient complex formation, suggesting post-transcriptional modulation of the VP16 interactions required for the IE complex assembly (O'Reilly et al., 1997).

The second unstructured region in the crystal determination is the transcription activation domain (TA, aa 412–490) that is located at the "bottom" of the determined structure (Liu et al., 1999). The VP16 TA domain has been perhaps the most utilized tool in studies of the mechanisms involved in transcription activation. Initially, mutagenesis studies defined the TA domain and determined that this region consisted of two distinct subdomains containing important aromatic and hydrophobic residues (Regier et al., 1993). The effects of substitutions at these positions also suggested that the structure of these subdomains were distinct and were likely to be involved in different stages of transcription stimulation. The unstructured nature of the domain both in solution and in the crystal determination suggests that this region also becomes structurally constrained upon protein-protein interactions (Shen et al., 1996).

Many studies on the mechanisms of transcription activation have utilized the VP16 TA domain, generally in the context of a DNA binding domain fusion protein. These studies have elucidated protein interactions and general principles or mechanisms in the regulation of transcription activation. While early studies demonstrated that activators promote "open complex" formation by enhancing the formation of the RNAPII preinitiation complex and promoter assemblies; later analyses addressed the rate limiting stages, protein interactions, and stepwise activation stages that were affected by the TA domain in given promoter contexts. The data from many such studies have resulted in general models for promoter activation via multiple steps which are not necessarily strictly ordered but can be affected by activators including: activator access and binding, histone modification and chromatin remodeling, binding and assembly of the basal factor-RNAPII complexes, open complex formation, RNAPII promoter escape, RNAPII pausing, transcription elongation, coupled transcription-mRNA splicing, and transcription reinitiation (Cosma, 2002).

Studies that focus upon protein interactions of the VP16 TA domain have suggested that the unstructured domain adopts conformations upon binding specific targets. This flexibility allows for numerous conformations and sequential interactions with factors involved in different stages of promoter activation (basal factors TFIIB, TFIIH, TBP; histone modification SAGA; and chromatin remodeling SWI2/SNF2) (Gold et al., 1996; Hall and Struhl, 2002; Herrmann et al., 1996; Herrera and Triezenberg, 2004; Krumm et al., 1995; Memedula and Belmont, 2003; Nishikawa et al., 1997; Vignali et al., 2000; Walker et al., 1993; Xiao et al., 1994; Yudkovsky et al., 2000). Consistent with early studies, the two subregions of the TA domain interact with distinct factors and function in multiple steps or activation stages including: (i) the ATP-dependent chromatin remodeling and histone modifications that allow factor access and promoter targeting (SWI, SAGA, p300) as demonstrated by the ability of the TA domain to mediate large scale chromatin remodeling; (ii) the assembly of the RNAPII preinitiation complex by alleviating TBP autorepression or by direct recruitment of the protein followed by competition with TBP-basal TAFs interactions to promote enhanced activation; (iii) recruitment of TFIIB leading to RNAPII positioning and open complex formation; (iv) recruitment of TFIIH and CTD kinases that mediate RNAPII promoter escape; (v) regulation of the efficiency of the initiation complex formation that functions to increase the elongation competency of the complexes, thereby affecting the coupled mRNA splicing efficiency; and (vi) stabilization of the reinitiation scaffold (TFIID, TFIIA, TFIIE, mediator and TFIIH) via interactions with TFIIH, leading to efficient reassembly and reinitiation.

These studies have resulted in significant advances in the understanding of general transcription initiation and promoter activation and have suggested mechanisms by which the VP16 TA domain may participate in the activation of the IE gene transcription. It remains, however, to be determined exactly what the inherent rate-limiting steps are for the activation of the IE genes and what the contribution(s) of the VP16 TA domain are within this context. In addition, clearly the contributions of all of the core and ancillary factors will be affected by the interplay of the regulatory proteins and signals within a given cellular milieu.

HCF-1

The last required component for the stable assembly of the core enhancer protein complex is the cellular coactivator HCF-1. Originally identified as a required component derived from extracts of insect or mammalian cells for the formation of a stable core complex in vitro, HCF-1 was subsequently biochemically purified and the gene encoding it was cloned (Kristie et al., 1989, 1995; Kristie and Sharp, 1993; Vogel et al., 2001; Wilson et al., 1993; Wysocka et al., 2003). Interestingly, rather than a single polypeptide, the protein is actually a family of polypeptides ranging from 68–230 kD that are derived from a common precursor via site-specific proteolysis (Kristie et al., 1995; Vogel and Kristie, 2000a; Wilson et al., 1993). The protein is ubiquitously expressed and localized in the nucleus of all cell types with a notable exception (discussed below). Numerous studies in recent years have illuminated both the functions of the protein in HSV IE gene expression as well as its functions in basic cellular processes. The importance of both lies in the strict requirement for HCF-1 in the initiation of HSV lytic cycle as well as the importance of the protein in several basic cellular processes that may impact the viral cycle.

As shown in Fig. 8.2, multiple functional domains and protein interactions have been defined which have identified HCF-1 as a critical component of processes such as cell-cycle control, positive and negative transcription regulation, chromatin modulation, DNA replication, and mRNA splicing. Many studies have focused upon the amino terminal domain of the protein as this region is required for the formation of the HSV IE enhancer core complex as well as for cell cycle progression (Goto et al., 1997; Hughes et al., 1999; LaBoissiere et al., 1997; Wilson et al., 1997). The predicted structure of the amino-terminus of HCF-1 is based upon structural alignments to related "kelch" domain proteins (Adams et al., 2000; Wilson et al., 1997) and a molecular model has been derived based upon the crystal structure of galactose oxidase "kelch" domain (Fig. 8.2 -HCF-1, bottom right) (J.L. Vogel and T.M. Kristie, unpublished data). The domain model consists of seven reiterations of four antiparallel β sheets that form the blades of a propeller-type structure. The ring is closed via the E4 sheet of the aminoterminus with the E1-E2-E3 sheets at the carboxyterminus of the domain to form the 7th blade (Fig. 8.2-HCF-1, bottom left). Kelch domain proteins are involved in a broad range of functions from structural assemblies to signal transduction and the domain presents several distinct protein interaction surfaces formed by the seven L2-3 loops, the L4-1 loops, and the E4 sheets (Adams et al., 2000).

As defined in numerous studies, the kelch domain mediates the high affinity interaction of HCF-1 with VP16 in the assembly of the HSV IE enhancer complex. The analysis of this interaction led to the elucidation of the HCF-1 interaction motif (D/E HXY) recognized in VP16 and subsequently determined to be a common motif found in cellular proteins that interact with the HCF-1 kelch domain (Freiman and Herr, 1997; Lu et al., 1998; Simmen et al., 1997). However, selective mutagenesis has suggested that distinct surfaces within the reiterated kelch structure are involved in the interactions that are mediated by this short common motif (Mahajan and Wilson, 2000). Differences between HCF-1 and the highly related HCF-2 in blades 5 and 6 encode part of the specificity for the preferential binding of VP16 to HCF-1 in a manner analogous to the discrimination between Oct-1 and Oct-2 (Johnson et al., 1999). While the kelch domain is the minimal domain required for the assembly of the VP16 enhancer core complex, it is unlikely to represent the only domain involved in this assembly. Some studies have suggested that additional domains are required, perhaps to constrain or alter the positioning of the VP16 activation domain for stable assembly into the complex (La Boissiere et al., 1997). Notably, multiple other cellular proteins that interact with the kelch domain have also been isolated including transcription factors (LZIP, Zhangfei) E2F1, E2F4, Krox 20 (Freiman and Herr, 1997; Knez et al., 2006; Lu and Misra, 2000b; Lu et al., 1997; Luciano and Wilson, 2002, 2003), transcription coactivators (PGC, PRC) (Lin et al., 2002), a nuclear export protein (HPIP) that may control the nucleo-cytoplasmic pool of HCF-1 (Mahajan et al., 2002), and chromatin modification components (set1/Ash HMT) (Wysocka et al., 2003); suggesting that the protein is involved in numerous or global cellular transcription functions.

In its role during the initial stages of the HSV lytic cycle, the protein is described as the coordinator of the HSV IE enhancer complex assembly as it has interactions with each of the enhancer components (VP16, Oct-1, Sp1, GABP) and may orient the assembled factors for effective activation of the IE gene transcription (Vogel and Kristie, 2000b; Vogel et al., 2001). The interactions may also reflect a central role in the activation of the IE transcription in response to multiple distinct regulatory signals that are mediated by the various factors involved (see below). An additional function of the protein in the regulation of the IE genes is evidenced by its activity as a mediator or coactivator of transcription via interaction with various transcription factors, chromatin modification components and other coactivators (Fig. 8.2 -HCF-1). Several lines of evidence support the proposal that HCF-1 can function as a general coactivator and mediates transcription activation of the assembled IE complex including: (i) an activation domain in the carboxyterminus of HCF-1 functions synergistically with the VP16 TA domain and may affect a distinct rate-limiting stage (Luciano and Wilson, 2002); (ii) HCF-1 is required to mediate the transcriptional activation potential of LZIP at CRE sites (Lu et al., 1997); (iii) HCF-1 interacts directly with the TA domain of GABP where mutations which affect the transactivation potential correlate directly with affects upon the GABP-HCF-1 interaction (Vogel and Kristie, 2000b); (iv) HCF-1 interacts with chromatin modifying proteins presumably to recruit these enzymes in early stages of transcription activation (Wysocka et al., 2003); and (v) depletion of HCF-1 results in ablation of HSV 1E expression (Narayanan et al., 2005). Significantly, HCF-1 dependent transcription events such as defined for GABP can provide a VP16-independent alternative mechanism for the induction of the HSV IE gene expression outside of the TAATGARAT element core.

In addition to its role in the direct assembly of the IE enhancer core complex, studies delineating the HCF-1 NLS (aa 2015–2035) have demonstrated that HCF-1 is required for the nuclear transport of VP16 during productive infection (La Boissiere et al., 1999). These results suggest that the pool of HCF-1 that is utilized by HSV is likely to be free cytoplasmic protein and that preassociation with VP16 is a critical stage in the enhancer complex assembly. Proteins such as the nuclear export factor HPIP, which interacts with the kelch domain of HCF-1, may play a role in regulating the nucleo-cytoplasmic shuttling of the protein, can therefore have a significant regulatory impact on the availability of cytoplasmic HCF-1 for the HCF-1/VP16 interaction and transport.

HCF-1 is also a critical control component of the cell-cycle as initially demonstrated by the isolation of a ts mutant (P134S) that resulted in G0-G1 cell cycle arrest (Goto et al., 1997). While the exact mechanism(s) of HCF-1 dependent cell-cycle progression remain unclear, studies indicate that the protein has multiple roles in promoting several cell-cycle stages: (i) the dissociation of ts-HCF-1 from cell chromatin at the non-permissive temperature suggests a global effect on cellular transcription (Wysocka et al., 2001); (ii) the interaction of HCF-1 with the TA domain of Miz-1 results in repression of Miz-1 activation of cdk $p15^{INK4b}$ expression, potentiating cell cycle progression (Piluso et al., 2002); (iii) the WYF domain (aa 1793–2005) in the carboxyterminus of HCF-1 interacts with PDCD2 which can suppress complementation of growth arrested ts-HCF-1 cells suggesting that PDCD2 may negatively regulate HCF-1 functions possibly through the association with additional transcription repression components such as NcoR (Scarr and Sharp, 2002); (iv) RNAi-mediated depletion of HCF-1 results in defects in both G_0–G_1 progression and cytokinesis/exit from mitosis which can be rescued by expression of the HCF-1 aminoterminus or carboxyterminus, respectively (Julien and Herr, 2003; and (iv) array studies have implicated HCF-1 in the expression of critical cellular proteins involved in general transcription, cell cycle progression, DNA replication-repair, and signal transduction (Khurana and Kristie, 2004). These studies collectively suggest that HCF-1 regulates cell cycle progression through its multiple roles in the regulation of gene expression. Interestingly, observations that novel HCF-1 aminoterminal polypeptides accumulate in the cytoplasm of cells arrested in G_0 may indicate that specific subdomains of the protein are localized in a regulated manner to control cell-cycle progression (Scarr et al., 2000).

Located in the central region of the 230 kD HCF-1 precursor is one of the more unusual domains consisting of a series of 20 amino acid reiterations that are sites of the specific proteolytic cleavages that results in the family of HCF-1 amino and carboxyterminal polypeptides (PPD domain, Fig. 8.2 -HCF-1). However, the amino and carboxyterminal proteins do not segregate but remain tightly associated via interactions between fibronectin type II repeats in the carboxyterminus (aa 1800–2000) and the 7th blade of the kelch domain (Kristie et al., 1995; Kristie and Sharp, 1993; Wilson et al., 2000). The processing of the protein has been determined to be autocatalytic and requires the PPD and residues carboxyterminal to this domain for efficient processing in vitro (Vogel and Kristie, 2000a). The functional role of the processing remains elusive but may represent a regulatory mechanism for controlling HCF-1-protein interactions and amino-carboxyterminal cooperativity. A novel regulatory function is proposed by the identification of a series of protein-protein interactions within the PPD in which specific reiterations encode an inherent specificity for particular protein binding partners. This model predicts that processing of HCF-1 would regulate the ability of the resulting cleavage products to interact with a specific subset of cofactors, thereby determining the activity of the particular HCF-1 cleavage product (Vogel and Kristie, 2006). Ultimately, the processing may control the protein's nuclear transport, cell-cycle functions, and/or determine its transcription activation or repression potential.

While the emphases of HCF-1 studies have been the roles of the protein in transcriptional regulation and cell cycle progression, the protein has also been implicated in mRNA splicing where it may be a general cofactor (Ajuh *et al.*, 2002) and in protein modification complexes (HCF-1-Protein Phosphatase 1) (Ajuh *et al.*, 2000) where it may regulate the activity of the phosphatase or determine it's targets. In addition, HCF-1 may play roles in the later stages of HSV lytic replication as suggested by the interaction of the kelch domain with HSV DNA replication proteins (Peng M.L., Nogueira, and T.M. Kristie 2006, unpublished data).

Clearly HCF represents one of the more complex components of the HSV IE regulatory assembly and has diverse and essential cellular functions. This protein may also be the component that is most critical for viral IE expression suggesting that the evolution of the virus to usurp the functions of this factor has more implications for the regulation of the HSV lytic cycle than is initially readily apparent.

Ancillary factors: Sp1 and GABP

In addition to the enhancer core complex, each IE regulatory domain contains a number of binding sites for cellular transcription factors such as Sp1 and GABP. The expression of the IE genes, even in the absence of VP16, attests to the significance of these components. However, the potential of these elements are dependent upon and enhanced by the presence of the assembled IE enhancer core complex, reflecting an interdependence of the elements.

Sp1

Sp1 is a member of the Zn finger/krupple family and was the first transcription factor to be purified and cloned (Black *et al.*, 2001; Kaczynski *et al.*, 2003; Suske, 1999). The protein recognizes the element GGGCGG (GC box) that is present in multiple copies in the HSV IE regulatory domains (Fig. 8.1) and has been determined to contribute to the basal expression level (Jones and Tjian, 1985). Originally considered to be a ubiquitously expressed, housekeeping factor, the protein is now known to be a member of a large family of related proteins that are subject to and involved in distinct regulatory pathways. Sp1 through Sp6 are highly related proteins which all interact with the GC element although there is some variability in specific binding affinity.

Sp1 is a 778 amino acid protein consisting of a three C2H2 Zn-finger DNA binding domain (C-X_{2-5} C-X_3-(F/Y)-X_5-ψ-X_2-H-X_{3-5}-H) located in the carboxyterminus with an embedded nuclear localization signal (NLS, Fig. 8.2-Sp1). Models that predict the DNA binding contacts are based upon similar structures and suggest that key residues in the various Sp family members determine the specificity for the GC box (Kaczynski *et al.*, 2003). The protein also contains two TA domains [(S/T) and Q-rich] that function in a promoter-dependent context, conceptually similar to those in Oct-1 (Black *et al.*, 2001; Suske, 1999).

Sp1 interacts with a number of known transcription activators (e.g., Oct-1), transcription coactivators (e.g., HCF-1, p300/CBP), and basal transcription factors (e.g., TBP)(Gunther *et al.*, 2000; Kaczynski *et al.*, 2003; Suske, 1999). In a manner analogous to Oct-1, the protein interactions and functional significance can largely be determined by the promoter context. Most significantly, the accumulating data illustrates that this family of proteins is subject to several regulatory signals and pathways in which specific GC boxes mediate responses to particular stimuli via binding proteins involved in those pathways. In addition, the particular regulatory response of a given GC box can also vary depending upon the particular cell context. These proteins interact with factors such as Rb-p107, p53, E2F, and Oct-1 and respond to signals as diverse as growth stimuli, NGF, TGFb, hormones, DNA damage, and apoptosis (Black *et al.*, 2001; Gunther *et al.*, 2000; Kaczynski *et al.*, 2003; Ryu *et al.*, 2003; Suske, 1999; Yan and Ziff, 1997). An additional level of regulation is provided by varying levels of the Sp family within a given cell type and under specific response conditions. As Sp1 and Sp3 are expressed in the same cell types, bind with equal affinity to the GC box, and have distinct functions; the ratio of the proteins can determine the activation vs. repression of given target genes. This regulatory mechanism is exemplified by alterations in the ratios of these proteins during cell differentiation or specific signaling pathways (Black *et al.*, 2001; Gunther *et al.*, 2000; Kaczynski *et al.*, 2003; Suske, 1999). The activation and repression functions of the Sp family are hypothesized to be mediated via interactions with HAT or HDAC complexes, respectively.

Finally, as expected by the involvement of these proteins in response to environmental signals, modifications of the factors also modulate that activity of the family. For example, acetylation of Sp1 in response to neuronal oxidative stress plays a role in neuronal survival pathways (Ryu *et al.*, 2003). In an HSV infection, phosphorylation of Sp1 later in infection decreases the protein's TA potential and may contribute to the down regulation of the IE gene expression (Kim and DeLuca, 2002).

GABP

GA rich sequences adjacent to at least one TAATGARAT element in each of the HSV IE regulatory domains were originally identified in mutagenesis studies and reporter assays where these elements contributed to the VP16-dependent induction of IE expression (Triezenberg *et al.*, 1988). In vitro transcription assays further demonstrated the significance of the elements for VP16-mediated transcription and suggested that the sites functioned synergistically with the enhancer core (Wu et al., 1994).

The factors binding to these elements (GABP) are related to the ets and notch protein families and consist of an α-subunit containing a carboxyterminal ets DNA binding domain and a β subunit containing the TA domain, NLS, and series of ankyrin repeats that mediate dimerization with the α subunit as well as contributes to DNA binding (Fig. 8.2-GABP) (LaMarco et al., 1991; Thompson et al., 1991). The proteins also form tetrameric structures via carboxyterminal sequences in the β subunits forming helical intertwined coiled coils (de la Brousse et al., 1994). In the β-subunit, the TA domain consists of a series of hydrophobic clusters which are critical for the TA potential (Gugneja et al., 1996; Gugneja et al., 1995). These regions correlate with the ability of the domain to interact with the enhancer core coactivator HCF-1, indicating that HCF-1 mediates the activation potential of the factor (Vogel and Kristie, 2000b).

The focus of many GABP studies has been in elucidating the role of the protein in the activation of nuclear encoded mitochondrial respiration component and assembly genes (Puigserver and Spiegelman, 2003; Scarpulla, 2002). These studies have delineated multiple levels of regulation and have indicated that an important mechanism for regulation of these factors is via regulation of the coactivators which respond to a variety of stimuli resulting in phosphorylation, induction, activation, and stabilization of these coactivators. The coactivators subsequently recruit additional cofactors, coactivators, and histone modification complexes. Two coactivators have been intensely studied in this context: PRC that mediates activation in proliferative responses and PGC that mediates thermogenic effector responses (Scarpulla, 2002). Interestingly, PGC has not been shown to directly interact and modulate GABP activity but may, in fact, do so via its interaction with the kelch domain of HCF-1 (Fig. 8.2-HCF-1). The activity of GABP and its cofactors are modulated by several signaling pathways such as p38 MAPK. For PGC, p38 mediated phosphorylation results in stabilization of the cofactor (Puigserver and Spiegelman, 2003). The phosphorylated PGC is also involved in direct induction of the expression of GABP.

Numerous regulatory response pathways are mediated by GABP including (i) induction of neuregulin expression (Fromm and Burden, 1998); (ii) insulin dependent prolactin gene expression via MAP pathway phosphorylation of GABP (Ouyang et al., 1996); (iii) TPA stimulated IL2 induction which is mediated via JNK activation of GABP (Hoffmeyer et al., 1998); (iv) the HIV LTR induction mediated via Raf-1 kinase activation of GABP (Flory et al., 1996)

and (v) the MMTV LTR which is synergistically activated by GABP in the presence of glucocorticoids (Aurrekoetxea-Hernandez and Buetti, 2000). The protein is also involved in numerous regulatory events by synergistic interactions with other transcription factors such as Sp1 and the cAMP responsive proteins CREB and ATF (Bannert et al., 1999; Sawada et al., 1999).

VZV IE gene expression: parallels and divergence

This review has focused on the regulation of HSV IE genes as a representative model of the mechanisms involved in the IE expression of an alpha herpesvirus due to the focus of studies in this area. In contrast, little has been elucidated concerning the mechanisms involved in the regulation of VZV IE gene expression. What has been determined, however, shows striking parallels to the HSV model. In VZV, the expression of the IE gene (IE62) is controlled by an enhancer domain (Fig. 8.3) consisting of multiple defined elements (Bannert et al., 1999; McKee and Preston, 1991; Moriuchi et al., 1995; Sawada et al., 1999).

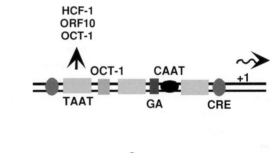

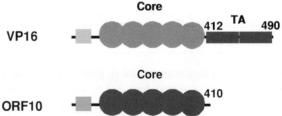

Fig. 8.3. The VZV IE62 regulatory domain. (Top) The arrangement of elements that have been delineated in the VZV IE62 regulatory region are indicated (TAAT, enhancer core element TAATGARAT; Oct, Octamer element; GA, GABP binding site; CAAT, CAT box; CRE, c-AMP responsive element). The assembly of the components HCF-1, Oct-1, and the VZV VP16 ortholog ORF-10 on the TAAT element is indicated. (Bottom) Comparison of the domain structure of HSV VP16 and VZV ORF-10 illustrates conservation of the aminoterminus and core domain and the absence of an ORF-10 transactivation domain.

Similar to HSV, the domain contains reiterations of a TAAT-GARAT element that is important for induction via the VZV virion component ORF10, the ortholog of the HSV VP16 (Moriuchi et al., 1995). Additional elements include a GABP binding site and c-AMP responsive sites (CRE) that also contribute to the ORF10-mediated stimulation of the IE62 gene expression. As has been demonstrated for HSV, the VZV IE62 TAATGARAT elements can nucleate the assembly of enhancer core complexes that contain Oct-1 and HCF-1 in concert with the ORF10 protein (Moriuchi et al., 1995).

The VZV ORF10 transactivator, while sharing significant homology to VP16, exhibits a striking difference that impacts the regulatory process. In contrast to VP16, ORF10 does not contain a transactivation domain, indicating that the interaction of the protein with other factors and coactivator components (e.g., Oct-1, HCF-1) must provide this function. A second significant difference between the regulatory mechanisms involved in the induction of HSV IE and the VZV IE genes is the autoregulatory response mediated by the major IE gene products (Perera et al., 1992). In HSV, α4/ICP4 functions to down regulate the IE genes in the transition from IE to E gene expression (Roizman, 1996). In VZV, IE62 functions to induce or enhance its own transcription. Interestingly, IE62 is also a component of the virion tegument structure (Kinchington et al., 1992) and may be a significant component of the IE induction response, thus compensating for the lack of the transactivation potential of the ORF10 activator. However, despite minor variations, data on the regulation of the VZV IE62 gene closely parallels the components and mechanisms defined in the regulation of HSV IE genes.

Regulation of the IE genes: multiple levels and response potentials

Studies on the regulation of the IE genes and the various components involved have led to advances in the understanding of enhancer complexes, ordered assembly processes, protein surfaces and interactions, mechanisms of transcriptional activation, and orders of interplay regulation. In addition to the modulation of DNA site recognition, the various transcription factors themselves are subject to modifications, alterations in turnover rates, subcellular localization, and signaling response pathways. Transcription factor synergy (activation or repression) is also dependent upon the cellular milieu and the balance of factors including the availability, competition, activator/repressor ratios, and cell-specific cofactors and coactivators. Additional higher orders of regulation are dependent upon the regulation of the coactivator levels, interactions, and functions. The ability and efficiency of the various assembled complexes to circumvent or alter rate limiting stages in the transcriptional assembly, initiation, elongation, and reinitiation is also likely to depend upon the cell type and state as the consequences of chromatin/nucleosomal structure, available factors, and signal environment will impinge upon a given rate limiting stage and determine the requirements for efficient transcription.

Most strikingly, the complex interactions of the components involved in the regulation of the IE enhancer complexes (e.g., Oct-1, Sp1, GABP, HCF-1) and the ability of these components to respond differentially to multiple environmental signals point to the evolution of the IE regulatory domains to respond to diverse signals.

The regulation of the IE genes: reactivation of HSV from the latent state

The components expressed in specific cell types may impact the normal lytic cycle regulation as suggested by the low levels of Oct-1 expression in sensory neurons. In this situation, other POU proteins such as Oct-2 or members of the Brn family may play a role in suppression or inefficient activation of the IE gene (Brownlees et al., 1999; Latchman, 1996; Latchman, 1999; Lillycrop et al., 1994). For the Brn family, Brn3a functions as an activator while Brn3b functions as a transcriptional repressor and the relative levels of these proteins change upon differentiation or neuronal stimulation (Latchman, 1999). Similarly, the levels of Sp1/Sp3 provide potential for repressor assemblies that may play a role in modulating IE expression in neuronal cells.

The potential of the IE gene domains to respond to diverse environmental stimuli suggests that these domains may respond to latency-reactivation stimuli by targeting distinct elements or components. Significantly, each of the identified IE regulatory factors is commonly linked by its interaction with the HCF-1 coactivator. Therefore, while distinct signals and factors may respond to distinct stimuli, the critical response component may be represented by the common coactivator. Interestingly, HCF-1 itself is uniquely sequestered in the cytoplasm of sensory neurons and is rapidly transported to the nucleus in response to reactivation signals (Fig. 8.4, Top) (Kristie et al., 1999). This regulated transport may well reflect an important element of the activation of the IE genes during the reactivation process. Furthermore, this provides a mechanism for the induction of the IE gene expression in response to signaling events in a VP16-independent manner, utilizing com-

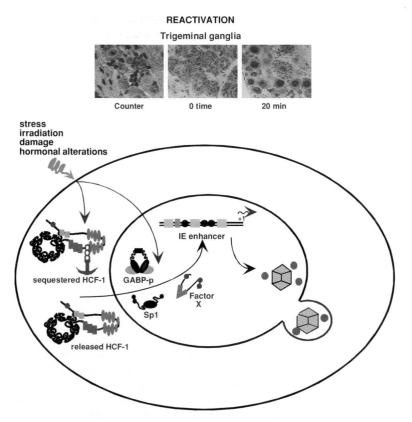

Fig. 8.4. Model of the induction of the IE genes during HSV reactivation from latency. (Top) Immunohistochemistry studies of HCF-1 demonstrate that the protein is specifically sequestered in the cytoplasm of sensory neurons (0 time, middle panel) and rapidly transported to the nucleus under experimental conditions that reactivate HSV from latency (explant reactivation stimuli, right panel). (Bottom) Schematic depiction of the activation of IE enhancer components during the initiation of reactivation. Environmental signal(s) result in the release of cytoplasmically sequestered HCF-1 and the activation of DNA binding factors such as GABP, Sp1, or other factors which function in concert with HCF-1 to activate the IE genes and initiate the viral lytic cycle. (See color plate section.)

plexes such as GABP-HCF-1 and Sp1-HCF-1. In support of these potential mechanisms, studies in Oct-1 knock-out cells have demonstrated that the protein is important but not essential for IE expression, thereby suggesting that alternative complexes and factors can initiate the cycle (Nogueira *et al.*, 2004). In contrast, IE expression is not detected in cells depleted of HCF-1 (Narayanan *et al.*, 2005). As proposed in Fig. 8.4, Sp1 or GABP may be involved in the activation of the IE genes during the reactivation process. However, other factors may be involved as suggested by the activation of ICP0 transcription via L-ZIP. L-ZIP, like HCF-1 exhibits a cytoplasmic sequestering and may also respond to signals that result in reactivation (Lu and Misra, 2000a). It is interesting to speculate that multiple reactivation pathways are possible utilizing distinct subsets of factors that respond to distinct signals.

Questions and future directions

Much has been learned in recent years and as is often the case, new information leads to many new questions and directions. Future studies certainly will extend the work established by the identification of the critical components of the HSV IE transcription complexes. Continuing assessment of the functions of these components in chromatin modulation, alteration of rate limiting stages and transcriptional mechanisms will provide additional basic process information. Determination of the regulation of each component within varying cellular contexts as well as the development of genetic animal models can delineate the response and impact of the factors subject to various signal pathways and stimuli. Protein modifications, localization dynamics, regulation of turnover, and the relationship of the components within a given context are key areas for the determination of the components which may play central roles in the HSV lytic, latent, and reactivation processes.

Acknowledgments

We thank J. Vogel, M. Nogueria, and A. McBride for their critical reading of this manuscript. We thank all of the laboratories who have made such significant contributions to the field and regret that all primary references could not be included in this section.

REFERENCES

Adams, J., Kelso, R., and Cooley, L. (2000). The kelch repeat superfamily of proteins: propellers of cell function. *Trends Cell Biol.*, **10**, 17–24.

Ajuh, P. M., Browne, G. J., Hawkes, N. A., Cohen, P. T., Roberts, S. G., and Lamond, A. I. (2000). Association of a protein phosphatase 1 activity with the human factor C1 (HCF) complex. *Nucl. Acids Res.*, **28**, 678–686.

Ajuh, P., Chusainow, J., Ryder, U., and Lamond, A. I. (2002). A novel function for human factor C1 (HCF-1), a host protein required for herpes simplex virus infection, in pre-mRNA splicing. *EMBO J.*, **21**, 6590–6602.

Aurrekoetxea-Hernandez, K., and Buetti, E. (2000). Synergistic action of GA-binding protein and glucocorticoid receptor in transcription from the mouse mammary tumor virus promoter. *J. Virol.*, **74**, 4988–4998.

Babb, R., Cleary, M. A., and Herr, W. (1997). OCA-B is a functional analog of VP16 but targets a separate surface of the Oct-1 POU domain. *Mol. Cell Biol.*, **17**, 7295–7305.

Babb, R., Huang, C. C., Aufiero, D. J., and Herr, W. (2001). DNA recognition by the herpes simplex virus transactivator VP16: a novel DNA-binding structure. *Mol. Cell Biol.*, **21**, 4700–4712.

Bannert, N., Avots, A., Baier, M., Serfling, E., and Kurth, R. (1999). GA-binding protein factors, in concert with the coactivator CREB binding protein/p300, control the induction of the interleukin 16 promoter in T lymphocytes. *Proc. Natl Acad. Sci. USA*, **96**, 1541–1546.

Black, A. R., Black, J. D., and Azizkhan-Clifford, J. (2001). Sp1 and kruppel-like factor family of transcription factors in cell growth regulation and cancer. *J. Cell Physiol.*, **188**, 143–160.

Boulon, S., Dantonel, J. C., Binet, V. *et al.* (2002). Oct-1 potentiates CREB-driven cyclin D1 promoter activation via a phospho-CREB- and CREB binding protein-independent mechanism. *Mol. Cell Biol.*, **22**, 7769–7779.

Brownlees, J., Gough, G., Thomas, S. *et al.* (1999). Distinct responses of the herpes simplex virus and varicella zoster virus immediate early promoters to the cellular transcription factors Brn-3a and Brn-3b. *Int. J. Biochem. Cell Biol.*, **31**, 451–461.

Chasman, D., Cepek, K., Sharp, P. A., and Pabo, C. O. (1999). Crystal structure of an OCA-B peptide bound to an Oct-1 POU domain/octamer DNA complex: specific recognition of a protein–DNA interface. *Genes Dev.*, **13**, 2650–2657.

Clerc, R. G., Corcoran, L. M., LeBowitz, J. H., Baltimore, D., and Sharp, P. A. (1988). The B-cell-specific Oct-2 protein contains POU box- and homeo box-type domains. *Genes Dev.*, **2**, 1570–1581.

Coenjaerts, F. E., van Oosterhout, J. A., and van der Vliet, P. C. (1994). The Oct-1 POU domain stimulates adenovirus DNA replication by a direct interaction between the viral precursor terminal protein-DNA polymerase complex and the POU homeodomain. *EMBO J.*, **13**, 5401–5409.

Cosma, M. P. (2002). Ordered recruitment: gene-specific mechanism of transcription activation. *Mol. Cell*, **10**, 227–236.

de Jong, R. N., Mysiak, M. E., Meijer, L. A., van der Linden, M., and van der Vliet, P. C. (2002). Recruitment of the priming protein pTP and DNA binding occur by overlapping Oct-1 POU homeodomain surfaces. *EMBO J.*, **21**, 725–735.

de la Brousse, F. C., Birkenmeier, E. H., King, D. S., Rowe, L. B., and McKnight, S. L. (1994). Molecular and genetic characterization of GABP beta. *Genes Dev.*, **8**, 1853–1865.

Flory, E., Hoffmeyer, A., Smola, U., Rapp, U. R., and Bruder, J. T. (1996). Raf-1 kinase targets GA-binding protein in transcriptional regulation of the human immunodeficiency virus type 1 promoter. *J. Virol.*, **70**, 2260–2268.

Freiman, R. N. and Herr, W. (1997). Viral mimicry: common mode of association with HCF by VP16 and the cellular protein LZIP. *Genes Dev.*, **11**, 3122–3127.

Fromm, L. and Burden, S. J. (1998). Synapse-specific and neuregulin-induced transcription require an ets site that binds GABPalpha/GABPbeta. *Genes Dev.*, **12**, 3074–3083.

Gold, M. O., Tassan, J. P., Nigg, E. A., Rice, A. P., and Herrmann, C. H. (1996). Viral transactivators E1A and VP16 interact with a large complex that is associated with CTD kinase activity and contains CDK8. *Nucl. Acids Res.*, **24**, 3771–3777.

Gonzalez, M. I. and Robins, D. M. (2001). Oct-1 preferentially interacts with androgen receptor in a DNA-dependent manner that facilitates recruitment of SRC-1. *J. Biol. Chem.*, **276**, 6420–6428.

Goto, H., Motomura, S., Wilson, A. C. *et al.* (1997). A single-point mutation in HCF causes temperature-sensitive cell-cycle arrest and disrupts VP16 function. *Genes Dev.*, **11**, 726–737.

Grenfell, S. J., Latchman, D. S., and Thomas, N. S. (1996). Oct-1 [corrected] and Oct-2 DNA-binding site specificity is regulated in vitro by different kinases. *Biochem J.*, **315**(3), 889–893.

Gugneja, S., Virbasius, J. V., and Scarpulla, R. C. (1995). Four structurally distinct, non-DNA-binding subunits of human nuclear respiratory factor 2 share a conserved transcriptional activation domain. *Mol. Cell Biol.*, **15**, 102–111.

Gugneja, S., Virbasius, C. M., and Scarpulla, R. C. (1996). Nuclear respiratory factors 1 and 2 utilize similar glutamine-containing clusters of hydrophobic residues to activate transcription. *Mol. Cell Biol.*, **16**, 5708–5716.

Gunther, M., Laithier, M., and Brison, O. (2000). A set of proteins interacting with transcription factor Sp1 identified in a two-hybrid screening. *Mol. Cell Biochem.*, **210**, 131–142.

Hall, D. B. and Struhl, K. (2002). The VP16 activation domain interacts with multiple transcriptional components as determined by protein-protein cross-linking in vivo. *J. Biol. Chem.*, **277**, 46043–46050.

Herrera, F. J. and Triezenberg, S. J. (2004). VP16-dependent association of chromatin-modifying coactivators and underrpresentation of histones at immediate-early gene promoters during herpes simplex virus infection. *J. Virol.*, **78**(18), 9689–9696.

Herrmann, C. H., Gold, M. O., and Rice, A. P. (1996). Viral transactivators specifically target distinct cellular protein kinases that phosphorylate the RNA polymerase II C-terminal domain. *Nucl. Acids Res.*, **24**, 501–508.

Hoffmeyer, A., Avots, A., Flory, E., Weber, C. K., Serfling, E., and Rapp, U. R. (1998). The GABP-responsive element of the interleukin-2 enhancer is regulated by JNK/SAPK-activating pathways in T lymphocytes. *J. Biol. Chem.*, **273**, 10112–10119.

Hovde, S., Hinkley, C. S., Strong, K. et al. (2002). Activator recruitment by the general transcription machinery: X-ray structural analysis of the Oct-1 POU domain/human U1 octamer/SNAP190 peptide ternary complex. *Genes Dev.*, **16**, 2772–2777.

Hughes, T. A., La Boissiere, S., and O'Hare, P. (1999). Analysis of functional domains of the host cell factor involved in VP16 complex formation. *J. Biol. Chem.*, **274**, 16437–16443.

Inamoto, S., Segil, N., Pan, Z. Q., Kimura, M., and Roeder, R. G. (1997). The cyclin-dependent kinase-activating kinase (CAK) assembly factor, MAT1, targets and enhances CAK activity on the POU domains of octamer transcription factors. *J. Biol. Chem.*, **272**, 29852–29858.

Jin, S., Fan, F., Fan, W. et al. (2001). Transcription factors Oct-1 and NF-YA regulate the p53-independent induction of the GADD45 following DNA damage. *Oncogene*, **20**, 2683–2690.

Johnson, K. M., Mahajan, S. S., and Wilson, A. C. (1999). Herpes simplex virus transactivator VP16 discriminates between HCF-1 and a novel family member, HCF-2. *J. Virol.*, **73**, 3930–3940.

Jones, K. A. and Tjian, R. (1985). Sp1 binds to promoter sequences and activates herpes simplex virus 'immediate-early' gene transcription in vitro. *Nature*, **317**, 179–182.

Julien, E. and Herr, W. (2003). Proteolytic processing is necessary to separate and ensure proper cell growth and cytokinesis functions of HCF-1. *Embo J.*, **22**, 2360–2369.

Kaczynski, J., Cook, T., and Urrutia, R. (2003). Sp1- and Kruppel-like transcription factors. *Genome Biol.*, **4**, 206.

Khurana, B. and Kristie, T. M. (2004). A protein sequestering system reveals control of cellular programs by the transcriptional coactivator HCF-1. *J. Biol. Chem.*, **279**(32), 33673–33683.

Kim, D. B. and DeLuca, N. A. (2002). Phosphorylation of transcription factor Sp1 during herpes simplex virus type 1 infection. *J. Virol.*, **76**, 6473–6479.

Kinchington, P. R., Hougland, J. K., Arvin, A. M., Ruyechan, W. T., and Hay, J. (1992). The varicella-zoster virus immediate–early protein IE62 is a major component of virus particles. *J. Virol.*, **66**, 359–366.

Klemm, J. D., Rould, M. A., Aurora, R., Herr, W., and Pabo, C. O. (1994). Crystal structure of the Oct-1 POU domain bound to an octamer site: DNA recognition with tethered DNA-binding modules. *Cell*, **77**, 21–32.

Knez, J., Piluso, D. et al. (2006). Host cell factor-1 and E2F4 intract via multiple determinants in each protein. *Mol. Cell Biochem.* Apr 22; [Epub ahead of print].

Kristie, T. M. and Sharp, P. A. (1990). Interactions of the Oct-1 POU subdomains with specific DNA sequences and with the HSV alpha-trans-activator protein. *Genes Dev.*, **4**, 2383–2396.

Kristie, T. M. and Sharp, P. A. (1993). Purification of the cellular C1 factor required for the stable recognition of the Oct-1 homeodomain by the herpes simplex virus alpha-trans-induction factor (VP16). *J. Biol. Chem.*, **268**, 6525–6534.

Kristie, T. M., LeBowitz, J. H., and Sharp, P. A. (1989). The octamer-binding proteins form multi-protein–DNA complexes with the HSV alpha TIF regulatory protein. *Embo J.*, **8**, 4229–4238.

Kristie, T. M., Pomerantz, J. L., Twomey, T. C., Parent, S. A., and Sharp, P. A. (1995). The cellular C1 factor of the herpes simplex virus enhancer complex is a family of polypeptides. *J. Biol. Chem.*, **270**, 4387–4394.

Kristie, T. M., Vogel, J. L., and Sears, A. E. (1999). Nuclear localization of the C1 factor (host cell factor) in sensory neurons correlates with reactivation of herpes simplex virus from latency. *Proc. Natl Acad. Sci. USA*, **96**, 1229–1233.

Krumm, A., Hickey, L. B., and Groudine, M. (1995). Promoter-proximal pausing of RNA polymerase II defines a general rate-limiting step after transcription initiation. *Genes Dev.*, **9**, 559–572.

La Boissiere, S., Walker, S., and O'Hare, P. (1997). Concerted activity of host cell factor subregions in promoting stable VP16 complex assembly and preventing interference by the acidic activation domain. *Mol. Cell Biol.*, **17**, 7108–7118.

La Boissiere, S., Hughes, T., and O'Hare, P. (1999). HCF-dependent nuclear import of VP16. *EMBO J.*, **18**, 480–489.

Lai, J. S. and Herr, W. (1997). Interdigitated residues within a small region of VP16 interact with Oct-1, HCF, and DNA. *Mol. Cell Biol.*, **17**, 3937–3946.

Lai, J. S., Cleary, M. A., and Herr, W. (1992). A single amino acid exchange transfers VP16-induced positive control from the Oct-1 to the Oct-2 homeo domain. *Genes Dev.*, **6**, 2058–2065.

LaMarco, K., Thompson, C. C., Byers, B. P., Walton, E. M., and McKnight, S. L. (1991). Identification of Ets- and notch-related subunits in GA binding protein. *Science*, **253**, 789–792.

Latchman, D. S. (1996). The Oct-2 transcription factor. *Int. J. Biochem. Cell Biol.*, **28**, 1081–1083.

Latchman, D. S. (1999). POU family transcription factors in the nervous system. *J. Cell Physiol.*, **179**, 126–133.

Lillycrop, K. A., Dawson, S. J., Estridge, J. K., Gerster, T., Matthias, P., and Latchman, D. S. (1994). Repression of a herpes simplex virus immediate–early promoter by the Oct-2 transcription factor is dependent on an inhibitory region at the N terminus of the protein. *Mol. Cell Biol.*, **14**, 7633–7642.

Lin, J., Puigserver, P., Donovan, J., Tarr, P., and Spiegelman, B. M. (2002). Peroxisome proliferator-activated receptor gamma coactivator 1beta (PGC-1beta), a novel PGC-1-related transcription coactivator associated with host cell factor. *J. Biol. Chem.*, **277**, 1645–1648.

Liu, Y., Gong, W., Huang, C. C., Herr, W., and Cheng, X. (1999). Crystal structure of the conserved core of the herpes simplex virus transcriptional regulatory protein VP16. *Genes Dev.*, **13**, 1692–1703.

Lu, R. and Misra, V. (2000a). Potential role for luman, the cellular homologue of herpes simplex virus VP16 (alpha gene trans-inducing factor), in herpesvirus latency. *J. Virol.*, **74**, 934–943.

Lu, R. and Misra, V. (2000b). Zhangfei: a second cellular protein interacts with herpes simplex virus accessory factor HCF in a manner similar to Luman and VP16. *Nucl. Acids Res.*, **28**, 2446–2454.

Lu, R., Yang, P., O'Hare, P., and Misra, V. (1997). Luman, a new member of the CREB/ATF family, binds to herpes simplex virus VP16-associated host cellular factor. *Mol. Cell Biol.*, **17**, 5117–5126.

Lu, R., Yang, P., Padmakumar, S., and Misra, V. (1998). The herpesvirus transactivator VP16 mimics a human basic domain leucine zipper protein, luman, in its interaction with HCF. *J. Virol.*, **72**, 6291–6297.

Luciano, R. L. and Wilson, A. C. (2002). An activation domain in the C-terminal subunit of HCF-1 is important for transactivation by VP16 and LZIP. *Proc. Natl Acad. Sci. USA*, **99**, 13403–13408.

Luciano, R. L. and Wilson, A. C. (2003). HCF-1 function as a coactivator for the zinc finger protein Krox20. *J. Biol. Chem.*, **278**(51), 51116–51124.

Mahajan, S. S. and Wilson, A. C. (2000). Mutations in host cell factor 1 separate its role in cell proliferation from recruitment of VP16 and LZIP. *Mol. Cell Biol.*, **20**, 919–928.

Mahajan, S. S. Little, M. M., Vazquez, R., and Wilson, A. C. (2002). Interaction of HCF-1 with a cellular nuclear export factor. *J. Biol. Chem.*, **277**, 44292–44299.

McKee, T. A. and Preston, C. M. (1991). Identification of two protein binding sites within the varicella-zoster virus major immediate early gene promoter. *Virus Res.*, **20**, 59–69.

Memedula, S. and Belmont, A. S. (2003). Sequential recruitment of HAT and SWI/SNF components to condensed chromatin by VP16. *Curr. Biol.*, **13**, 241–246.

Mittal, V., Ma, B., and Hernandez, N. (1999). SNAP(c): a core promoter factor with a built-in DNA-binding damper that is deactivated by the Oct-1 POU domain. *Genes Dev.*, **13**, 1807–1821.

Moriuchi, H., Moriuchi, M., and Cohen, J. I. (1995). Proteins and cis-acting elements associated with transactivation of the varicella-zoster virus (VZV) immediate–early gene 62 promoter by VZV open reading frame 10 protein. *J. Virol.*, **69**, 4693–4701.

Narayanan, A., Nogueira, M. L., and Kristie, T. M. (2005). Combinatorial transcription of herpes simplex virus and varicella zoster virus immediate early genes is strictly determined by the cellular co-activator HCF-1. *J. Biol. Chem.*, **280**, 1369–1375.

Nishikawa, J., Kokubo, T., Horikoshi, M., Roeder, R. G., and Nakatani, Y. (1997). Drosophila TAF(II)230 and the transcriptional activator VP16 bind competitively to the TATA box-binding domain of the TATA box-binding protein. *Proc. Natl Acad. Sci. USA*, **94**, 85–90.

Nogueira, M. L., Wang, V. E. H., Tantin, D., Sharp, P. A., and Kristie, T. M. (2004). Herpes simplex virus infections are arrested in Oct-1 deficient cells. *Proc. Natl Acad. Sci. USA*, **101**, 1473–1478.

O'Reilly, D., Hanscombe, O., and O'Hare, P. (1997). A single serine residue at position 375 of VP16 is critical for complex assembly with Oct-1 and HCF and is a target of phosphorylation by casein kinase II. *Embo J.*, **16**, 2420–2430.

Ouyang, L., Jacob, K. K., and Stanley, F. M. (1996). GABP mediates insulin-increased prolactin gene transcription. *J. Biol. Chem.*, **271**, 10425–10428.

Perera, L. P., Mosca, J. D., Sadeghi-Zadeh, M., Ruyechan, W. T., and Hay, J. (1992). The varicella-zoster virus immediate early protein, IE62, can positively regulate its cognate promoter. *Virology*, **191**, 346–354.

Phillips, K. and Luisi, B. (2000). The virtuoso of versatility: POU proteins that flex to fit. *J. Mol. Biol.*, **302**, 1023–1039.

Piluso, D., Bilan, P., and Capone, J. P. (2002). Host cell factor-1 interacts with and antagonizes transactivation by the cell cycle regulatory factor Miz-1. *J. Biol. Chem.*, **277**, 46799–46808.

Pomerantz, J. L., Kristie, T. M., and Sharp, P. A. (1992). Recognition of the surface of a homeo domain protein. *Genes Dev.*, **6**, 2047–2057.

Puigserver, P. and Spiegelman, B. M. (2003). Peroxisome proliferator-activated receptor-gamma coactivator 1 alpha (PGC-1 alpha): transcriptional coactivator and metabolic regulator. *Endocr. Rev.*, **24**, 78–90.

Regier, J. L., Shen, F., and Triezenberg, S. J. (1993). Pattern of aromatic and hydrophobic amino acids critical for one of two subdomains of the VP16 transcriptional activator. *Proc. Natl Acad. Sci. USA*, **90**, 883–887.

Roizman, B. and Sears, A. E. (1996). Herpes simplex viruses and their replication. In *Fundamental Virology*, ed. B. N. Fields, Knipe, D. M., and Howley, P. M., Philadelphia: Lippincott-Raven Publishers: 1043–1107.

Ryu, H., Lee, J., Zaman, K. *et al.* (2003). Sp1 and Sp3 are oxidative stress-inducible, antideath transcription factors in cortical neurons. *J. Neurosci.*, **23**, 3597–3606.

Sawada, J., Simizu, N., Suzuki, F. *et al.* (1999). Synergistic transcriptional activation by hGABP and select members of the activation transcription factor/cAMP response element-binding protein family. *J. Biol. Chem.*, **274**, 35475–35482.

Scarpulla, R. C. (2002). Nuclear activators and coactivators in mammalian mitochondrial biogenesis. *Biochim. Biophys. Acta.*, **1576**, 1–14.

Scarr, R. B. and Sharp, P. A. (2002). PDCD2 is a negative regulator of HCF-1 (C1). *Oncogene*, **21**, 5245–5254.

Scarr, R. B., Smith, M. R., Beddall, M., and Sharp, P. A. (2000). A novel 50-kilodalton fragment of host cell factor 1 (C1) in G(0) cells. *Mol. Cell Biol.*, **20**, 3568–3575.

Shen, F., Triezenberg, S. J., Hensley, P., Porter, D., and Knutson, J. R. (1996). Transcriptional activation domain of the herpesvirus protein VP16 becomes conformationally constrained upon interaction with basal transcription factors. *J. Biol. Chem.*, **271**, 4827–4837.

Simmen, K. A., Newell, A., Robinson, M. *et al.* (1997). Protein interactions in the herpes simplex virus type 1 VP16-induced complex: VP16 peptide inhibition and mutational analysis of host cell factor requirements. *J. Virol.*, **71**, 3886–3894.

Sturm, R. A., Das, G., and Herr, W. (1988). The ubiquitous octamer-binding protein Oct-1 contains a POU domain with a homeo box subdomain. *Genes Dev.*, **2**, 1582–1599.

Suske, G. (1999). The Sp-family of transcription factors. *Gene*, **238**, 291–300.

Tanaka, M., Lai, J. S., and Herr, W. (1992). Promoter-selective activation domains in Oct-1 and Oct-2 direct differential activation of an snRNA and mRNA promoter. *Cell*, **68**, 755–767.

Thompson, C. C., Brown, T. A., and McKnight, S. L. (1991). Convergence of Ets- and notch-related structural motifs in a heteromeric DNA binding complex. *Science*, **253**, 762–768.

Tiedt, R., Bartholdy, B. A., Matthias, G., Newell, J. W., and Matthias, P. (2001). The RING finger protein Siah-1 regulates the level of the transcriptional coactivator OBF-1. *EMBO J.*, **20**, 4143–4152.

Triezenberg, S. J., LaMarco, K. L., and McKnight, S. L. (1988). Evidence of DNA: protein interactions that mediate HSV-1 immediate early gene activation by VP16. *Genes Dev.*, **2**, 730–742.

Vignali, M., Steger, D. J., Neely, K. E., and Workman, J. L. (2000). Distribution of acetylated histones resulting from Gal4-VP16 recruitment of SAGA and NuA4 complexes. *EMBO J.*, **19**, 2629–2640.

Vogel, J. L. and Kristie, T. M. (2000a). Autocatalytic proteolysis of the transcription factor-coactivator C1 (HCF): a potential role for proteolytic regulation of coactivator function. *Proc. Natl Acad. Sci. USA*, **97**, 9425–9430.

Vogel, J. L. and Kristie, T. M. (2000b). The novel coactivator C1 (HCF) coordinates multiprotein enhancer formation and mediates transcription activation by GABP. *EMBO J.*, **19**, 683–690.

Vogel, J. L. and Kristie, T. M. (2001). The C1 factor (HCF). In *The Encyclopedia of Molecular Medicine*, ed. T. E. Creighton, New York: John Wiley and Sons, Inc.: 732–735.

Vogel, J. L. and Kristie, T. M. (2006). Site-specific proteolysis of the transcriptional coactivator HCF-1 can regulate its interaction with protein cofactors. *Proc. Natl Acad. Sci. USA*, **103**(18), 6817–6822.

Walker, S., Greaves, R., and O'Hare, P. (1993). Transcriptional activation by the acidic domain of Vmw65 requires the integrity of the domain and involves additional determinants distinct from those necessary for TFIIB binding. *Mol. Cell Biol.*, **13**, 5233–5244.

Wilson, A. C., LaMarco, K., Peterson, M. G., and Herr, W. (1993). The VP16 accessory protein HCF is a family of polypeptides processed from a large precursor protein. *Cell*, **74**, 115–125.

Wilson, A. C., Freiman, R. N., Goto, H., Nishimoto, T., and Herr, W. (1997). VP16 targets an amino-terminal domain of HCF involved in cell cycle progression. *Mol. Cell Biol.*, **17**, 6139–6146.

Wilson, A. C., Boutros, M., Johnson, K. M., and Herr, W. (2000). HCF-1 amino- and carboxy-terminal subunit association through two separate sets of interaction modules: involvement of fibronectin type 3 repeats. *Mol. Cell Biol.*, **20**, 6721–6730.

Wu, T. J., Monokian, G., Mark, D. F., and Wobbe, C. R. (1994). Transcriptional activation by herpes simplex virus type 1 VP16 in vitro and its inhibition by oligopeptides. *Mol. Cell Biol.*, **14**, 3484–3493.

Wysocka, J. and Herr, W. (2003). The herpes simplex virus VP16-induced complex: the makings of a regulatory switch. *Trends Biochem. Sci.*, **28**, 294–304.

Wysocka, J., Reilly, P. T., and Herr, W. (2001). Loss of HCF-1-chromatin association precedes temperature-induced growth arrest of tsBN67 cells. *Mol. Cell Biol.*, **21**, 3820–3829.

Wysocka, J., Myers, M. P., Laherty, C. D., Eisenman, R. N., and Herr, W. (2003). Human Sin3 deacetylase and trithorax-related Set1/Ash2 histone H3-K4 methyltransferase are tethered together selectively by the cell-proliferation factor HCF-1. *Genes Dev.*, **17**, 896–911.

Xiao, H., Pearson, A., Coulombe, B. *et al.* (1994). Binding of basal transcription factor TFIIH to the acidic activation domains of VP16 and p53. *Mol. Cell Biol.*, **14**, 7013–7024.

Yan, G. Z. and Ziff, E. B. (1997). Nerve growth factor induces transcription of the p21 WAF1/CIP1 and cyclin D1 genes in PC12 cells by activating the Sp1 transcription factor. *J. Neurosci.*, **17**, 6122–6132.

Yudkovsky, N., Ranish, J. A., and Hahn, S. (2000). A transcription reinitiation intermediate that is stabilized by activator. *Nature*, **408**, 225–229.

Zhao, H., Jin, S., Fan, F., Fan, W., Tong, T., and Zhan, Q. (2000). Activation of the transcription factor Oct-1 in response to DNA damage. *Cancer* Res., **60**, 6276–6280.

Zheng, L., Roeder, R. G., and Luo, Y. (2003). S phase activation of the histone H2B promoter by OCA-S, a coactivator complex that contains GAPDH as a key component. *Cell*, **114**, 255–266.

Zwilling, S., Annweiler, A., and Wirth, T. (1994). The POU domains of the Oct1 and Oct2 transcription factors mediate specific interaction with TBP. *Nucl. Acids Res.*, **22**, 1655–1662.

Zwilling, S., Konig, H., and Wirth, T. (1995). High mobility group protein 2 functionally interacts with the POU domains of octamer transcription factors. *Embo J.*, **14**, 1198–1208.

9

Initiation of transcription and RNA synthesis, processing and transport in HSV and VZV infected cells

Rozanne M. Sandri-Goldin

Department of Microbiology & Molecular Genetics University of California, Irvine, CA, USA

Initiation of transcription and RNA synthesis

The alphaherpesviruses, HSV-1 and VZV encode TATA-box containing promoters that are transcribed by the cellular RNA polymerase II

During productive infection by herpes simplex virus type 1 (HSV-1), approximately 80 genes encoded within the linear 152-kbp viral genome are expressed in three sequential phases that are termed immediate early (IE; α), early (E; β) and late (L; γ) (Honess and Roizman, 1974; McGeoch, 1991). The smaller, 125-kbp varicella zoster virus (VZV) genome encodes around 70 genes, which are also expressed as IE, E and L products (Davison and Scott, 1986). HSV-1 and VZV genes are transcribed by the cellular RNA Polymerase II and each viral promoter has a TATA box homology about 25 nucleotides upstream of the start site of transcription (for review, see Wagner et al., 1995). In HSV-1infections, the first genes to be transcribed are the five IE genes, which are distinguished from E and L genes by specific sequence elements termed TAATGARAT sequences in the upstream regions of IE promoters. These elements are recognized by a virion tegument protein, VP16, which binds as part of a protein complex that contains two cellular factors, Oct-1 and HCF, to transcriptionally activate expression of IE genes (Wysocka and Herr, 2003). VZV IE genes do not appear to encode upstream promoter elements similar to the TAATGARAT sequence, however VZV does encode a protein, ORF10 that exhibits similarities with VP16, although its activity has been much less well characterized than that of VP16 (Piette et al., 1995).

HSV-1 E promoters, unlike the IE promoters, do not contain VP16-responsive sequence elements, however they do contain a number of cis-acting elements upstream of the TATA box that have been shown to bind cellular transcriptional activators, including Sp1 (Kim and DeLuca, 2002; Wagner et al., 1995). In contrast, HSV-1 late promoters lack upstream cis-acting sequence elements, and instead the region downstream of the TATA box has been shown to play an important role in regulating the expression of several late genes (Guzowski and Wagner, 1993; Kim et al., 2002; Pederson et al., 1992). The architecture of VZV promoters appears similar to that of HSV-1 promoters, however, binding sites for the cellular transcription factors Sp1 and USF have been found in a large number of potential promoters for VZV genes from all three kinetic classes (Ruyechan et al., 2003).

Viral factors required for the initiation of transcription on HSV-1 and VZV promoters

Like HSV-1 IE genes, which are activated by VP16, the E and L genes also require a virally-encoded transcription factor to induce expression. The factor that is required is one of the IE proteins, termed infected cell polypeptide 4 (ICP4). ICP4 is a nuclear phosphoprotein that acts as a homodimer to activate or repress transcription depending upon the promoter (Shepard et al., 1990). ICP4 is absolutely required for abundant expression of all E and L gene products, and thus it is essential for productive infection (DeLuca et al., 1985). In the absence of functional ICP4, not only are early genes poorly expressed, but some IE genes are overexpressed. The overexpression of IE genes in the absence of functional ICP4 reflects the ability of ICP4 to repress transcription from its own promoter in an autoregulatory fashion, as well as from other IE promoters (Gu et al., 1995; Leopardi et al., 1995). Genetic and biochemical studies have shown that ICP4 binds to DNA. ICP4 represses transcription from specific viral promoters that have a high-affinity ICP4 binding site spanning the transcription initiation site, and it does so by interacting with the basal transcription factors TATA-binding protein (TBP) and TFIIB (Faber and Wilcox, 1988; Gu et al., 1995; Leopardi et al., 1995). ICP4 also stimulates transcription from early and late viral promoters through interactions with viral DNA and cellular basal transcription factors. However, despite extensive analyses, specific sequences that bind ICP4 with high affinity that are common to all promoters activated by ICP4 have not been uncovered, although the ICP4 DNA binding domain is essential for activation of transcription (Shepard et al., 1989; Smiley et al., 1992). The minimal cis-acting elements required for stimulation of transcription by ICP4 are a TATA box and in some late promoters, an initiator element (Cook et al., 1995; Kim et al., 2002). ICP4 facilitates formation of the preinitiation complex through interactions with one or more components of the cellular transcription machinery. ICP4 forms a tripartite complex with TFIIB and TBP on DNA, enhancing the binding of TFIID to DNA (Grondin and DeLuca, 2000). ICP4 also interacts with TBP-associated factor 250 (TAF250), and promotes the formation of transcription preinitiation complexes on promoters (Carrozza and DeLuca, 1996).

A number of genetic and biochemical analyses have been conducted to determine which of the observed interactions between ICP4, viral DNA, and cellular proteins are relevant to the function of ICP4 as an activator. ICP4 is comprised of 1,298 amino acids. It has been found that ICP4 residues 1 to 315 function as a transactivation domain (Xiao et al., 1997); further, this region binds to the cellular EAP protein (EBV EBER-associated protein) (Leopardi et al., 1997), and is required for formation of a complex with DNA that contains TBP and TFIIB (Smith et al., 1993). ICP4 amino acids 316 to 490 are necessary for homodimerization (Everett et al., 1991a; Gallinari et al., 1994) and DNA binding (Everett et al., 1990; Kristie and Roizman, 1986; Wu and Wilcox, 1990), whereas residues 491 to 796 encompass a nuclear localization signal (Paterson and Everett, 1988). ICP4 residues 797 to 1298 are involved in the interaction with TAF250 (Carrozza and DeLuca, 1996; Yao and Schaffer, 1994), and with the HSV-1 IE proteins ICP0 (Yao and Schaffer, 1994), and ICP27 (Panagiotidis et al., 1997), and are required for efficient transcriptional activation (Bruce and Wilcox, 2002; DeLuca and Schaffer, 1988; Paterson and Everett, 1988). ICP4 is highly phosphorylated during infection by at least three cellular kinases, Protein Kinase A (PKA), PKC and cdc2 (Advani et al., 2001; Xia et al., 1996a,b), however the specific role of phosphorylation in regulating the transcriptional activities of ICP4 has not been fully elucidated.

The homologue of ICP4 in VZV is termed IE62 and is encoded by the duplicated genes ORF62 and ORF71, which map to the internal repeats (Piette et al., 1995). IE62 has been shown to induce transcription of all classes of VZV genes, although it has only been recently demonstrated by genetic analysis that IE62 is essential for VZV infection (Sato et al., 2003). IE62 is to a large extent functionally conserved with HSV-1 ICP4, and in fact ICP4 mutants can be complemented by IE62 (Felser et al., 1988). However, there are several important differences. A substantial amount of IE62 is found in the virion tegument (Kinchington et al., 1992), and this appears to require phosphorylation by a VZV encoded protein kinase, ORF 66, which is required for the cytoplasmic localization of IE62 late in infection and the subsequent incorporation of IE62 into virions (Kinchington et al., 2001). Another VZV encoded kinase, ORF 47, which is also a component of the virion, interacts with IE62 and disrupting either the kinase function of ORF47 or its ability to bind to IE62 blocked infectivity of VZV in vivo (Besser et al., 2003). Further, IE62 encodes a potent acidic activation domain in the N-terminus, which is similar to the acidic activation domain of VP16 (Perera et al., 1993). Thus, IE62 also bears some similarity to the HSV-1 transactivator VP16, which is also a component of the virion tegument. Like ICP4, IE62 has been found to interact with other VZV IE proteins. IE62 interacts with IE63 (Lynch et al., 2002), the VZV homologue of HSV-1 ICP22, and with IE4 (Spengler et al., 2000), the homologue of ICP27. The functional importance of these interactions for transcriptional activation of VZV genes during infection remains poorly understood. It has been demonstrated that, in the context of a minimal promoter, a TATA element is sufficient and essential for IE62 activation of transcription, and like its HSV-1 counterpart, IE62 also binds the basal transcription factors TBP and TFIIB in vitro (Perera, 2000). However, upstream binding sites for the cellular transcription factors USF and Sp1 have also been found to be important for the regulation of a number of VZV genes and numerous Sp1 and USF sites have been identified in VZV promoters from all kinetic classes (Ruyechan et al., 2003). USF is a basic-helix-loop-helix-leucine zipper (bHLH-zip) transcription factor that was shown to cooperate with IE62 in the regulation of an early bidirectional promoter driving both the DNA polymerase and DNA-binding protein genes (Meier et al., 1994), and in the regulation of the IE promoter driving IE4 (Michael et al., 1998). Sp1 sites were reported to be important for the regulation of the gE and gI genes (He et al., 2001; Rahaus and Wolff, 2000), and IE62 has been shown to interact with Sp1 in vitro and in vivo (Peng et al., 2003).

Viral IE proteins that contribute to the induced expression of viral genes

In addition to ICP4, HSV-1 encodes three other IE proteins that have regulatory functions. ICP0, a 775 amino acid nuclear phosphoprotein was first described as a promiscuous transactivator in transient transfection studies because it can transactivate HSV-1 IE, E and L promoters as well as heterologous promoters (for a review, see Everett, 2000). Activation of gene expression by ICP0 was shown to occur at the level of mRNA synthesis (Jordan and Schaffer, 1997). ICP0 does not bind DNA directly (Everett et al., 1991b), and therefore is likely to activate gene expression through interactions with proteins. A large number of interactions have in fact been reported. ICP0 was found to interact with a ubiquitin specific protease, USP7 (Everett et al., 1997), cyclin D3 (Van Sant et al., 1999), elongation factor EF-1δ (Kawaguchi et al., 1997), transcription factor BMAL1 (Kawaguchi et al., 2001), and the HSV-1 transactivator ICP4 (Yao and Schaffer, 1994). ICP0 has also been shown to activate cdk4 and to stabilize cyclins D1 and D3 (Van Sant et al., 2001). However, the mechanism by which ICP0 activates gene expression remains obscure. A major biological activity of ICP0 is the disruption of nuclear structures, termed ND10 or promyelocytic leukemia (PML) bodies. ICP0 encodes two E3 ubiquitin ligase domains, one of which is specified by a RING-finger motif also found in other U3 ubiquitin ligases (Boutell et al., 2002; Hagglund et al., 2002; Hagglund and Roizman, 2002). ICP0 has been linked to the proteasome-dependent degradation of several proteins including the catalytic subunit of DNA protein kinase (Parkinson et al., 1999), the centromere proteins CENP-C and CENP-A (Lomonte et al., 2001), and two components of ND10, PML and Sp100 (Everett et al., 1998a). Because the proteasome inhibitor MG132 interferes with the ability of ICP0 to stimulate viral infection (Everett et al., 1998b), and mutations in the RING finger correlate with ICP0's ability to transactivate (Everett et al., 1991c), it has been thought the destruction of ND10 by ICP0 is an integral event in viral replication. This is supported by evidence from other viruses that also disrupt ND10 structures (reviewed in (Everett, 2001)). However, it has been shown recently that overexpression of PML protein precludes the dispersal of ND10 structures and yet there was no effect on HSV-1 replication (Lopez et al., 2002). Therefore, the mechanism(s) by which ICP0 acts to contribute to virus expression during lytic infection remains to be elucidated.

VZV also encodes a RING-finger protein termed IE61. The N-terminal RING finger domain is the only obvious similarity to ICP0. IE61 does not contain a USP7 binding domain and does not affect the distribution of USP7 (Parkinson and Everett, 2000). IE61 does induce colocalizing conjugated ubiquitin, suggesting that it may also act as an ubiquitin ligase (Parkinson and Everett, 2001). Little else has been reported on the activity of VZV IE 61.

Another HSV-1 IE protein that has been implicated in the regulation of viral IE and L gene expression is ICP22. ICP22 is not essential for virus infection in cultured cells, and mutants grow as well as wild-type virus in Vero and HEp-2 cells, but ICP22 mutants do exhibit a host range and replicate much less efficiently in primary human, rabbit and rodent cells. In these latter cells the expression of a subset of late genes is greatly reduced (Ogle and Roizman, 1999). Further, phosphorylation of ICP22 by an HSV-1 encoded kinase, UL13, is required for the accumulation of a subset of both IE and L genes in primary human, rodent and rabbit cells (Purves et al., 1993) and this appears to be mediated by the activation of the cdc2 cyclin-dependent kinase (Advani et al., 2000). A possible mechanism for the requirement for ICP22 and UL13 for appropriate expression of L transcripts is the intriguing finding that ICP22 and UL13 are both required for an HSV-1 induced modification of RNA polymerase II (Long et al., 1999). Specifically, infection with HSV-1 results in the depletion of both the hypo- and hyperphosphorylated forms of RNA polymerase II, known as the IIa and IIo forms, which represent the initiating and elongating forms of RNA polymerase II. Instead, early in HSV-1 infection, an intermediately phosphorylated form appears (Rice et al., 1995). Infection of human primary embryonic lungs cells with mutants defective in ICP22 or UL13 led to significantly reduced viral gene transcription at late times after infection (Long et al., 1999). These results suggest that the modification in the phosphorylation of RNA polymerase by ICP22 and UL13 promotes HSV-1 transcription over transcription of cellular genes. However, despite the attractiveness of this model, there are findings that cannot be explained solely by the modification of the phosphorylation of RNA polymerase II. First, ICP22 is not required for L gene expression in many cell lines, and the modification of RNA polymerase II to the intermediate form is not seen in infections with ICP22 or UL13 mutants. Thus, this modification is not absolutely required for transcription of HSV-1 genes. Second, RNA polymerase II is still recruited to viral transcription/replication compartments, whether or not it is modified, thus altered phosphorylation is not a prerequisite for its nuclear relocalization (Rice et al., 1995). Third, an additional change to the RNA polymerase II holoenzyme was reported that depends on HSV-1 IE proteins, but not specifically on ICP22. That is, the loss of the general transcription factor TFIIE from the holoenzyme was found to require HSV-1 IE proteins, which may be redundant because no single IE deletion mutant eliminated this change (Jenkins and Spencer, 2001). TFIIE is necessary for activated transcription initiation in uninfected cells, and thus the loss of this general transcription factor from the complex may result in the repression of transcription of cellular genes that has been reported following HSV-1 infection (Spencer et al., 1997).

It has been shown recently that the phosphoserine-2 form of the RNA polymerase C-terminal terminal domain, which is found in elongating transcription complexes, is decreased during HSV-1 infection (Fraser and Rice, 2005; Dai-Ju et al., 2006). Furthermore, total levels of RNA polymerase were decreased indicating that this was due to a loss of protein, indicating protein degradation rather than dephosphorylation, and proteasome inhibitors prevented the degradation (Dai-Ju et al., 2006). The degradation appeared to be due to robust HSV-1 transcription because in infections with viral mutants in which viral transcription was greatly reduced, or in which viral transcription was blocked by inhibitors, degradation was prevented. By contrast preventing the degradation of the elongating serine-2 phosphorylated RNA polymerase II decreased late viral gene expression and viral yields (Dai-Ju et al., 2006). These findings suggest that during periods of robust viral transcription in HSV-1 infected cells, elongating polymerase complexes may become arrested or stalled because of a pile-up of transcribing complexes on families of co-linear transcripts, or because of collisions of transcribing complexes on opposite strands that are being transcribed at the same time. Resolution of these stalled complexes by proteasomal degradation may thus be required to allow transcription to resume and proceed through the gene.

Interestingly, the VZV homologue of ICP22, termed IE63 has been shown to be essential for VZV infection (Sommer et al., 2001), although it does not appear to play a major role in gene regulation on its own. IE63 was reported to be able to repress two VZV promoters in an activity assay and this repression was regulated by phosphorylation by two cellular casein kinases (Bontems et al., 2002b). However, in another report, IE63 was found to have no transcriptional activating or repressing activity within the context of a minimal VZV glycoprotein promoter, however, the presence of IE63 upregulated IE62 transactivation of the promoter (Lynch et al., 2002). Further, IE63 protein was shown to interact with IE62 through the N-terminal 142 amino acids, and a portion of the IE63 and IE62 proteins colocalized in VZV-infected cells (Lynch et al., 2002). IE63 is phosphorylated in infected cells and can be phosphorylated in vitro by casein kinase II (Bontems et al., 2002a; Stevenson et al., 1996). Further, IE63 has been found to be heavily phosphorylated by, and tightly bound to, the VZV ORF47 kinase (Kenyon et al., 2003), a homologue of HSV-1 UL13, which phosphorylates ICP22. Intriguingly, IE63 protein can be coimmunoprecipitated with the cellular RNA polymerase II from infected cell extracts, indicating that it is present in a complex with that enzyme (Lynch et al., 2002). It has not been demonstrated whether or not the IE63-ORF47 complex can alter the phosphorylation of RNA polymerase II in VZV-infected cells. See Fig. 9.1.

RNA processing and transport

Following synthesis of transcripts in eukaryotic cells, the nascent pre-mRNAs are processed by capping at the 5′ end, cleavage and polyadenylation to form the 3′ end, and splicing to remove intervening sequences. After processing, mRNAs must be exported through the nuclear pore complex to the cytoplasm for translation. Export of mRNAs requires binding by RNA export adaptor proteins, recognition by export factors and translocation through the nuclear pore complex (NPC). Three classes of factors appear to be required for mRNA export: adaptor proteins that bind directly to the mRNA, receptor proteins that recognize and bind to adaptor proteins, and nuclear pore complex components termed nucleoporins that mediate export across the nuclear membrane (for review see (Komeili and O'Shea, 2001; Zenklusen and Stutz, 2001). In metazoan cells, the processing events occur co-transcriptionally because the processing factors are recruited to the sites on the nascent transcripts where their activities are required by binding to the highly conserved C-terminal domain (CTD) of RNA polymerase II (for review see Reed, 2003). In addition, RNA export is closely coupled to splicing (Luo and Reed, 1999). This occurs because a complex of proteins that includes one or more export adaptor proteins binds to the pre-mRNA at a specific site just upstream of what will become exon–exon junctions in the spliced product. This so-called exon junction complex or EJC remains bound to the spliced RNA and escorts the mRNA to the cellular mRNA export receptor, termed TAP or NXF1, with which the export adaptor proteins interact directly. The mRNP complex is then exported through the nuclear pore (for review see Reed and Magni, 2001).

In HSV-1 infected cells, viral transcripts are processed by 5′ capping and 3′ end formation by the cellular machinery. However, it has been reported that some polyadenylation sites present primarily on late transcripts are utilized inefficiently by cellular polyadenylation factors and these sites were operationally defined as weak. The activity of an HSV-1 IE protein, ICP27 stimulated the use of these sites in vitro (McLauchlan et al., 1992). Further analysis suggested that ICP27 recruits the cleavage stimulation factor, Cst64, which is required for poly(A) site recognition, to weak HSV-1 poly(A) sites (McGregor et al., 1996). However, a study investigating differential polyadenylation of two transcripts that arise from the UL24 gene by the use of two different poly(A) sites, one weak and one strong, found that the accumulation of transcripts during infection from the weak poly(A) site did not require ICP27 (Hann et al., 1998). In addition, a recent study using various HSV-1 gC gene plasmid constructs showed that the stimulatory effect of ICP27 occurred post-transcriptionally but was independent of the inserted polyadenylation site (Perkins et al., 2003). Thus, the role of ICP27 in enhancing the use of weak poly(A) sites has not been firmly established.

The role of ICP27 in another RNA processing event has been defined to a significant extent, namely the effect of ICP27 on pre-mRNA splicing. Although most metazoan mRNAs are multiply spliced, the majority of HSV-1 transcripts are intronless. This presents an interesting paradox for the virus because cellular RNA export is intimately coupled to splicing through the deposition of the exon junction complex on the spliced mRNAs, which marks mRNAs for export by TAP/NXF1 (Cullen, 2000). Although there are cellular transcripts that are intronless, these transcripts have been found to contain specific recognition elements that allows their export via TAP/NXF1 (Huang et al., 2003). Following infection with HSV-1, the cell is presented with thousands of viral intronless transcripts that would compete poorly with cellular transcripts for export. ICP27 shifts the balance by shutting down the cellular splicing machinery, albeit temporarily, thus cellular pre-mRNAs are not fully processed and exported (Bryant et al., 2001; Sciabica et al., 2003). Further, ICP27 recruits an export adaptor protein, termed Aly/REF, which is part of the EJC, to sites of HSV-1 transcription (Chen et al., 2002). Thus, HSV-1 mRNAs are given access to the TAP/NXF1 pathway (Chen et al., 2002; Koffa et al., 2001). ICP27 inhibits cellular splicing at early times after infection by recruiting a predominantly cellular kinase, SRPK1, to the nucleus of infected cells where it inappropriately phosphorylates a family of splicing factors, termed SR proteins, which are required for splicesome assembly (Sciabica et al., 2003). Proper phosphorylation is required for SR proteins to perform their roles in splicing and consequently, spliceosome complex formation is stalled. ICP27 interacts with SR proteins and other spliceosomal components (Bryant et al., 2001; Sciabica et al., 2003), and most likely then encounters Aly/REF, the export adaptor, which is part of the EJC (Chen et al., 2002; Koffa et al., 2001). ICP27 recruits Aly/REF to sites of HSV-1 transcription, marked by staining with an antibody to ICP4 (Chen et al., 2005), and ICP27 then binds to HSV-1 intronless transcripts through its RGG box RNA binding motif (Sandri-Goldin, 1998). The RNA-ICP27-Aly/REF complex binds to TAP/NFX1 through the interaction of both ICP27 and Aly/REF with TAP/NXF1 (Chen et al., 2002), and HSV-1 transcripts are exported through the NPC. Splicing is restored at later times of infection, when ICP27 is actively shuttling and exporting viral mRNA. The nature of the switch between these early and late activities of ICP27 has not been defined but could involve post-translational modifications. ICP27 is phosphorylated by several cellular kinases (Zhi and Sandri-Goldin, 1999) and it undergoes arginine-methylation in the RGG box (Mears and Rice, 1996). A recent report suggests that ICP27 may be directed initially to sites of cellular transcription and splicing, similar to cellular RNA processing factors, by interacting with RNA polymerase II. ICP27 was found to co-immunoprecipitate with RNA polymerase II in HSV-1-infected cells (Zhou and Knipe, 2001). Further, ICP27 was found to interact directly with the CTD of RNA polymerase II in vitro and in virus-infected cells (Dai-Ju et al., 2006).

The homologue of ICP27 in VZV is IE4. The IE4 protein is a transactivator of gene expression whose regulatory properties are not fully understood. IE4 stimulates VZV gene expression and it also is capable of heterologous transactivation (Defechereux et al., 1997; Perera et al., 1994), and IE4 has been suggested to exert its function through both transcriptional and post-transcriptional mechanisms (Defechereux et al., 1993; Defechereux et al., 1997; Perera et al., 1994). IE4 shares considerable amino acid sequence homology with HSV-1 ICP27, especially in the carboxyl terminus and in the central part of the protein (Davison and Scott, 1986). The carboxyl-terminal region of ICP27 that is rich in cysteine and histidine residues has been shown to bind zinc (Vaughan et al., 1992) and to be required for multimerization (Zhi et al., 1999). Whereas the carboxyl-terminal region of IE4 also contains cysteine and histidine residues, it is not known whether this region binds zinc, and dimerization of IE4 was found to require the C-terminal cysteine-rich domain and the central region of the protein (Baudoux et al., 2000). The amino-terminal regions of the two proteins have a more limited amino acid homology; however, both are highly acidic. In transfection assays, it was demonstrated that the IE4 N-terminal acidic region was required for its trans-activating function and that it could be replaced in part by substituting the corresponding region of ICP27 (Moriuchi et al., 1995). While IE4 is not a potent transactivator on its own, it can act as a major coactivator of transactivation mediated by IE62, and was found to interact with IE62 in infected cells and in vitro (Spengler et al., 2000). The interaction depended on the phosphorylation state of IE62. The nature of the post-transcriptional activation seen with IE4 has not been defined, and it is not known if IE4 is involved in the regulation of splicing or viral RNA export. Many VZV transcripts are also intronless, and IE4 was reported to shuttle between the nucleus and

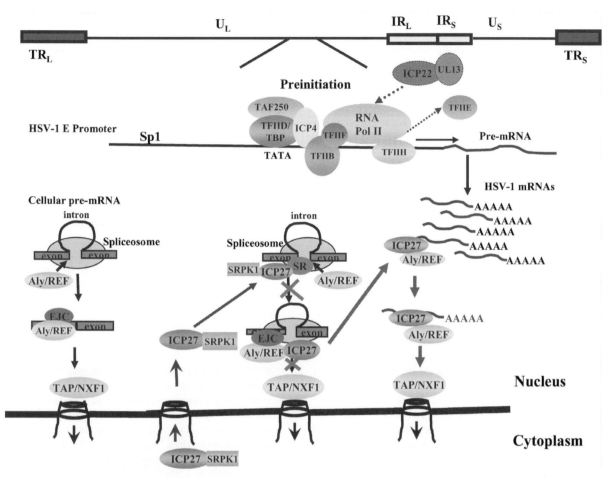

Fig. 9.1. Model of HSV-1 early (E) gene expression showing the initiation of transcription, RNA synthesis and export. The HSV-1 genome is depicted in schematic form. An E gene promoter from the U_L region is blown up to illustrate the upstream Sp1 site and the TATA box. The HSV-1 modified preinitiation complex includes ICP4, which forms a tripartite complex with TBP, a component of TFIID, and TFIIB (Grondin and DeLuca, 2000). ICP4 also interacts with TAF250, which stabilizes the interaction of TFIID with DNA (Carrozza and DeLuca, 1996). In VZV infected cells, IE62 has also been shown to bind TBP and TFIIB (Perera, 2000). The altered phosphorylation of RNA polymerase II by ICP22 and U_L13 (Long et al., 1999) is shown by a dashed line, as is the release of TFIIE from RNA polymerase holoenzyme (Jenkins and Spencer, 2001). The pathway for mRNA export in uninfected cells is disrupted during HSV-1 infection. ICP27 recruits SRPK1 to the nucleus where it inappropriately phosphorylates the splicing SR proteins and splicesome assembly is stalled (Sciabica et al., 2003). ICP27 encounters the export adaptor Aly/REF, which is part of the EJC and directs it to HSV-1 intronless transcripts (Chen et al., 2002; Koffa et al., 2001). ICP27 binds viral intronless RNA and the ICP27-RNA-Aly/Ref complex interacts with the export receptor TAP/NXF1 to export viral RNAs to the cytoplasm. It has not been demonstrated whether VZV IE4 affects splicing or is involved in viral RNA export.

cytoplasm, however, this activity was not further delineated (Baudoux et al., 2000). See Fig. 9.1.

Concluding remarks

Both HSV-1 and VZV have evolved mechanisms for usurping the cellular machinery to produce viral transcripts to insure the successful generation of viral progeny. The viral regulatory proteins that are involved in the initiation of transcription, RNA processing and export are the IE proteins in both viruses. These proteins all have unique roles in the expression of viral gene products. While the HSV-1 and VZV IE proteins share homology, they have clearly diverged to meet the unique requirements of their parent viruses. For example, HSV-1 IE proteins are not significant components of the virion tegument, whereas, VZV IE62, IE4 and IE63 are. Further, HSV-1 IE proteins are not expressed in latently infected cells; however, VZV IE63 is expressed as a major protein during latency along with IE4 (Kenyon *et al.*, 2003). Both HSV-1 and VZV encode essential IE proteins, ICP4 and IE62, that transactivate viral gene expression, and both encode IE proteins, ICP22 and IE63, that interact with or modify RNA polymerase II, although the functional repercussions of this are not yet fully appreciated. The roles of the RING finger proteins, ICP0 and IE61 have not been fully elucidated despite the fact that we now know a great about what these proteins do in the infected cell. While HSV-1 hijacks the cellular export machinery via ICP27 to facilitate translation of its transcripts, little is known about how the switch from an early splicing inhibitor to a late viral export factor is controlled. It remains to be seen if VZV IE4 functions in this manner. Thus, there is still much to learn about gene regulation in the alphaherpesviruses.

REFERENCES

Advani, S. J., Weichselbaum, R. R., and Roizman, B. (2000). The role of cdc2 in the expression of herpes simplex virus genes. *Proc. Natl Acad. Sci. USA*, **97**, 10996–11001.

Advani, S. J., Hagglund, R., Weichselbaum, R. R., and Roizman, B. (2001). Posttranslational processing of infected cell proteins 0 and 4 of herpes simplex virus 1 is sequential and reflects the subcellular compartment in which the proteins localize. *J. Virol.*, **75**, 7904–7912.

Baudoux, L., Defechereux, P., Rentier, B., and Piette, J. (2000). Gene activation by Varicella-zoster virus IE4 protein requires its dimerization and involves both the arginine-rich sequence, the central part, and the carboxyl-terminal cysteine-rich region. *J. Biol. Chem.*, **275**, 32822–32831.

Besser, J., Sommer, M. H., Zerboni, L., Bagowski, C. P., Ito, H., Moffat, J., Ku, C. C., and Arvin, A. M. (2003). Differentiation of varicella-zoster virus ORF47 protein kinase and IE62 protein binding domains and their contribution to replication in human skin xenografts in the SCID-hu mouse. *J. Virol.*, **77**, 5964–5974.

Bontems, S., De Valentin, E., Baudoux, L., Rentier, B., Sadzot-Delvaux, C., and Piette, J. (2002a). Phosphorylation of varicella-zoster virus IE63 protein by casein kinases influences its cellular localization and gene regulation activity. *J. Biol. Chem.*, **277**, 21050–21060.

Bontems, S., De Valentin, E., Baudoux, L., Rentier, B., Sadzot-Delvaux, C., and Piette, J. (2002b). Phosphorylation of varicella-zoster virus IE63 protein by casein kinases influences its cellular localization and gene regulation activity. *J. Biol. Chem.*, **277**, 21050–21060.

Boutell, C., Sadis, S., and Everett, R. D. (2002). Herpes simplex virus type 1 immediate-early protein ICP0 and its isolated RING finger domain act as ubiquitin E3 ligases in vitro. *J. Virol.*, **76**, 841–850.

Bruce, J. W. and Wilcox, K. W. (2002). Identification of a motif in the C terminus of herpes simplex virus regulatory protein ICP4 that contributes to activation of transcription. *J. Virol.*, **76**, 195–207.

Bryant, H. E., Wadd, S., Lamond, A. I., Silverstein, S. J., and Clements, J. B. (2001). Herpes simplex virus IE63 (ICP27) protein interacts with spliceosome-associated protein 145 and inhibits splicing prior to the first catalytic step. *J. Virol.*, **75**, 4376–4385.

Carrozza, M. J. and DeLuca, N. A. (1996). Interaction of the viral activator protein ICP4 with TFIID through TAF250. *Mol. Cell. Biol.*, **16**, 3085–3093.

Chen, I. B., Sciabica, K. S., and Sandri-Goldin, R. M. (2002). ICP27 interacts with the export factor Aly/REF to direct herpes simplex virus 1 intronless RNAs to the TAP export pathway. *J. Virol.*, **76**, 12877–12889.

Chen, I. B., Li, L., Silva, L., and Sandri-Golden, R. M. (2005). ICP27 recruits Aly/REF but not TAP/NXF1 to herpes simplex Virus type 1 transcription sites although TAP/NXF1 is required for ICP27 export. *J. Virol.*, **79**, 3949–3961.

Cook, W. J., Gu, B., DeLuca, N. A., Moynihan, E. B., and Coen, D. M. (1995). Induction of transcription by a viral regulatory protein depends on the relative strengths of functional TATA boxes. *Mol. Cell. Biol.*, **15**, 4998–5006.

Cullen, B. R. (2000). Connections between the processing and nuclear export of mRNA: evidence for an export license? *Proc. Natl Acad. Sci. USA*, **97**, 4–6.

Dai-Ju, J. Q., Li, L., Johnson, L. A., and Sandri-Goldin, R. M. (2006). ICP27 interacts with the C-terminal domain of RNA polymerase II and facilitates its recruitment to herpes simplex virus-1 transcription sites, where it undergoes proteasomal degradation during infection. *J. Virol.*, **80**, 3567–3581.

Davison, A. J. and Scott, J. E. (1986). The complete DNA sequence of varicella-zoster virus. *J. Gen. Virol.*, **67**, 1759–1816.

Defechereux, P., Melen, L., Baudoux, L., Merville-Louis, M. P., Rentier, B., and Piette, J. (1993). Characterization of the regulatory functions of varicella-zoster virus open reading frame 4 gene product. *J. Virol.*, **67**, 4379–4385.

Defechereux, P., Debrus, S., Baudoux, L., Rentier, B., and Piette, J. (1997). Varicella-zoster virus open readinig frame 4 encodes an immediate-early protein with posttranscriptional regulatory properties. *J. Virol.*, **71**, 7073–7079.

DeLuca, N. A. and Schaffer, P. A. (1988). Physical and functional domains of the herpes simplex virus transcriptional regulatory protein ICP4. *J. Virol.*, **62**, 732–743.

DeLuca, N. A., McCarthy, A. M., and Schaffer, P. A. (1985). Isolation and characterization of deletion mutants of herpes simplex virus type 1 in the gene encoding immediate–early regulatory protein ICP4. *J. Virol.*, **56**, 558–570.

Everett, R. D. (2000). ICP0, a regulator of herpes simplex virus during lytic and latent infection. *Bioessays*, **22**, 761–770.

Everett, R. D. (2001). DNA viruses and viral proteins that interact with PML nuclear bodies. *Oncogene*, **20**, 7266–7273.

Everett, R. D., Paterson, T., and Elliot, M. (1990). The major transcriptional regulatory protein of herpes simplex virus type 1 includes a protease resistant DNA binding domain. *Nucl. Acids Res.*, **18**, 4579–4585.

Everett, R. D., Elliot, R. M., Hope, G., and Orr, A. (1991a). Purification of the DNA binding domain of herpes simplex virus type 1 immediate-early protein Vmw175 as a homodimer and extensive mutagenesis of its DNA recognition site. *Nucl. Acids Res.*, **19**, 4901–4908.

Everett, R. D., Orr, A., and Elliot, M. (1991b). High level expression and purification of herpes simplex virus type 1 immediate early polypeptide Vmw110. *Nucl. Acids Res.*, **19**, 6155–6161.

Everett, R. D., Preston, C. M., and Stow, N. D. (1991c). Functional and genetic analysis of the role of Vmw110 in herpes simplex virus replication. In *Herpesvirus Transcription and Its Regulation*, ed. E. K. Wagner, pp. 49–73. Boca Ratan: CRC Press.

Everett, R. D., Meredith, D. M., Orr, A., Cross, A., Kathoria, M., and Parkinson, J. (1997). A novel ubiquitin-specific protease is dynamically associated with the PML nuclear domain and binds to a herpesvirus regulatory protein. *EMBO J.*, **16**, 1519–1530.

Everett, R. D., Freemont, P., Saitoh, H. *et al.* (1998a). The disruption of ND10 during herpes simplex virus infection correlates with the Vmw110- and proteasome-dependent loss of several PML isoforms. *J. Virol.*, **72**, 6581–6591.

Everett, R. D., Orr, A., and Preston, C. M. (1998b). A viral activator of gene expression functions via the ubiquitin-proteasome pathway. *EMBO J.*, **17**, 7169.

Faber, S. W. and Wilcox, K. W. (1988). Association of herpes simplex virus regulatory protein ICP4 with sequences spanning the ICP4 gene transcription initiation site. *Nucl. Acids Res.*, **16**, 555–570.

Felser, J. M., Kinchington, P. R., Inchauspe, G., Straus, S. E., and Ostrove, J. M. (1988). Cell lines containing varicella-zoster virus open reading frame 62 and expressing the "IE"175 protein complement ICP4 mutants of herpes simplex virus type 1. *J. Virol.*, **62**, 2076–2082.

Fraser, K. A. and Rice, S. A. (2005). Herpes simplex virus type 1 infection leads to loss of Serine-2 phosphorylation on the carboxyl-terminal domain of RNA polymerase II. *J. Virol.* **79**, 11323–11334.

Gallinari, P., Wiebauer, K., Nardi, M. C., and Jiricny, J. (1994). Localization of a 34-amino-acid segment implicated in dimerization of the herpes simplex virus type 1 ICP4 polypeptide by a dimerization trap. *J. Virol.*, **68**, 3809–3820.

Grondin, B. and DeLuca, N. A. (2000). Herpes simplex virus type 1 ICP4 promotes transcription preinitiation complex formation by enhancing the binding of TFIID to DNA. *J. Virol.*, **74**, 11504–11510.

Gu, B., Kuddus, R., and DeLuca, N. A. (1995). Repression of activator-mediated transcription by herpes simplex virus ICP4 via a mechanism involving interactions with the basal transcription factors TATA-binding protein and TFIIB. *Mol. Cell. Biol.*, **15**, 3618–3626.

Guzowski, J. F. and Wagner, E. K. (1993). Mutational analysis of the herpes simplex virus type 1 strict late UL38 promoter/leader reveals two regions critical in transcriptional regulation. *J. Virol.*, **67**, 5098–5108.

Hagglund, R. and Roizman, B. (2002). Characterization of the novel E3 ubiquitin ligase encoded in exon 3 of herpes simplex virus-1-infected cell protein 0. *Proc. Natl Acad. Sci. USA*, **99**, 7889–7894.

Hagglund, R., Van Sant, C., Lopez, P., and Roizman, B. (2002). Herpes simplex virus 1-infected cell protein 0 contains two E3 ubiquitin ligase sites for different E2 ubiquitn-conjugating enzymes. *Proc. Natl Acad. Sci. USA*, **99**, 631–636.

Hann, L. E., Cook, W. J., Uprichard, S. L., Knipe, D. M., and Coen, D. M. (1998). The role of herpes simplex virus ICP27 in the regulation of UL24 gene expression by differential polyadenylation. *J. Virol.*, **72**, 7709–7714.

He, H., Boucaud, D., Hay, J., and Ruyechan, W. T. (2001). Cis and trans elements regulating expression of the varicella zoster gI gene. *Arch. Virol.*, **17**, 57–70.

Honess, R. W. and Roizman, B. (1974). Regulation of herpesvirus macromolecular synthesis. I. Cascade regulation of the synthesis of three groups of viral proteins. *J. Virol.*, **41**, 8–19.

Huang, Y., Gattoni, R., Stevenin, J., and Steitz, J. A. (2003). SR splicing factors serve as adaptor proteins for TAP-dependent mRNA export. *Mol. Cell*, **11**, 837–843.

Jenkins, H. L. and Spencer, C. A. (2001). RNA polymerase II holoenzyme modifications accompany transcription reprogramming in herpes simplex virus type 1-infected cells. *J. Virol.*, **75**, 9872–9884.

Jordan, R. and Schaffer, P. A. (1997). Activation of gene expression by herpes simplex virus type 1 ICP0 occurs at the level of mRNA synthesis. *J. Virol.*, **71**, 6850–6862.

Kawaguchi, Y., Bruni, R., and Roizman, B. (1997). Interaction of herpes simplex virus 1 regulatory protein ICP0 with elongation factor 1δ: ICP0 affects translational machinery. *J. Virol.*, **71**, 1019–1024.

Kawaguchi, Y., Tanaka, M., Yokoymama, A. *et al.* (2001). Herpes simplex virus 1 alpha regulatory protein ICP0 functionally interacts with cellular transcription factor BMAL 1. *Proc. Natl Acad. Sci. USA*, **98**, 1877–1882.

Kenyon, T. K., Lynch, J., Hay, J., Ruyechan, W., and Grose, C. (2003). Varicella-zoster virus ORF47 protein serine kinase: characterization of a cloned, biologically active phosphotransferase and two viral substrates, ORF62 and ORF63. *J. Virol.*, **75**, 8854–8858.

Kim, D. and DeLuca, N. A. (2002). Phosphorylation of transcription factor Sp1 during herpes simplex virus type 1 infection. *J. Virol.*, **76**, 6473–6479.

Kim, D., Zabierowski, S., and DeLuca, N. A. (2002). The initiator element in a herpes simplex virus type 1 late-gene promoter enhances activation by ICP4, resulting in abundant late gene expression. *J. Virol.*, **76**, 1548–1558.

Kinchington, P. R., Fite, K., Seman, A., and Turse, S. E. (2001). Virion association of IE62, the varicella-zoster virus (VZV) major transcriptional regulatory protein, requires expression of the VZV open reading frame 66 protein kinase. *J. Virol.*, **75**, 9106–9113.

Kinchington, P. R., Hougland, J. K., Arvin, A. M., Ruyechan, W. T., and Hay, J. (1992). The varicella-zoster virus immediate-early protein IE62 is a major component of virus particles. *J. Virol.*, **66**, 359–366.

Koffa, M. D., Clements, J. B., Izaurralde, E. *et al.* (2001). Herpes simplex virus ICP27 protein provides viral mRNAs with access to the cellular mRNA export pathway. *EMBO J.*, **20**, 5769–5778.

Komeili, A. and O'Shea, E. K. (2001). New perspectives on nuclear transport. *Annu. Rev. Genet.*, **35**, 341–364.

Kristie, T. M. and Roizman, B. (1986). Site of the major regulatory protein alpha 4 specifically associated with promoter-regulatory domains of alpha genes of herpes simplex virus type 1. *Proc. Natl Acad. Sci. USA*, **83**, 4700–4704.

Leopardi, R., Michael, N., and Roizman, B. (1995). Repression of the herpes simplex virus 1 alpha 4 gene by its gene product (ICP4) within the context of the viral genome is conditioned by the distance and stereoaxial alignment of the ICP4 DNA binding site relative to the TATA box. *J. Virol.*, **69**, 3042–3048.

Leopardi, R., Ward, P. L., and Roizman, B. (1997). Association of herpes simplex virus regulatory protein ICP22 with transcriptional complexes containing EAP, ICP4, RNA Polymerase II, and viral DNA requires posttranslational modification by the U_L 13 protein kinase. *J. Virol.*, **71**, 1133–1139.

Lomonte, P., Sullivan, K. F., and Everett, R. D. (2001). Degradation of nucleosome-associated centromeric histone H3-like protein CENP-A induced by herpes simplex virus type 1 protein ICP0. *J. Biol. Chem.*, **276**, 5829–5835.

Long, M. C., Leong, V., Schaffer, P. A., Spencer, C. A., and Rice, S. A. (1999). ICP22 and the UL13 protein kinase are both required for herpes simplex virus-induced modification of the large subunit of RNA polymerase II. *J. Virol.*, **73**, 5593–5604.

Lopez, P., Jacob, R. T., and Roizman, B. (2002). Overexpression of promyelocytic leukemia protein precludes the dispersal of ND10 structures and has no effect on accumulation of infectious herpes simplex virus 1 or its proteins. *J. Virol.*, **76**, 9355–9367.

Luo, M. J. and Reed, R. (1999). Splicing is required for rapid and efficient mRNA export in metazoans. *Proc. Natl Acad. Sci. USA*, **96**, 14937–14942.

Lynch, J. M., Kenyon, T. K., Grose, C., Hay, J., and Ruyechan, W. T. (2002). Physical and functional interaction between the varicella zoster virus IE63 and IE62 proteins. *Virology*, **302**, 71–82.

McGeoch, D. J. (1991). Correlation between HSV-1 DNA sequence and viral transcription maps. In *Herpesvirus Transcription and Its Regulation*, ed. E. K. Wagner, pp. 29–47. Boca Ratan: CRC Press, Inc.

McGregor, F., Phelan, A., Dunlop, J., and Clements, J. B. (1996). Regulation of herpes simplex virus poly(A) site usage and the action of immediate-early protein IE63 in the early-late switch. *J. Virol.*, **70**, 1931–1940.

McLauchlan, J., Phelan, A., Loney, C., Sandri-Goldin, R. M., and Clements, J. B. (1992). Herpes simplex virus IE63 acts at the posttranscriptional level to stimulate viral mRNA 3' processing. *J. Virol.*, **66**, 6939–6945.

Mears, W. E. and Rice, S. A. (1996). The RGG box motif of the herpes simplex virus ICP27 protein mediates an RNA-binding activity and determines in vivo methylation. *J. Virol.*, **70**, 7445–7453.

Meier, J. L., Luo, X., Sawadogo, M., and Straus, S. E. (1994). The cellular transcription factor USF cooperates with varicella-zoster virus immediate–early protein 62 to symmetrically activate a bidirectional promoter. *Mol. Cell. Biol.*, **14**, 6896–6906.

Michael, E., Kuck, K., and Kinchington, P. R. (1998). Anatomy of the varicella zoster virus open reading frame 4 promoter. *J. Infect. Dis.*, **178**, S27–S33.

Moriuchi, M., Moriuchi, H., Debrus, S., Piette, J., and Cohen, J. I. (1995). The acidic amino-terminal region of varicella-zoster virus open reading frame 4 protein is required for transactivatioin and can functionally replace the corresponding region of herpes simplex virus ICP27. *Virology*, **208**, 376–382.

Ogle, W. O. and Roizman, B. (1999). Functional anatomy of herpes simplex virus 1 overlapping genes encoding infected-cell protein 22 and US1.5 protein. *J. Virol.*, **73**, 4305–4315.

Panagiotidis, C. A., Lium, E. K., and Silverstein, S. (1997). Physical and functional interactions between herpes simplex virus immediate-early proteins ICP4 and ICP27. *J. Virol.*, **71**, 1547–1557.

Parkinson, J. and Everett, R. D. (2000). Alphaherpesvirus proteins related to herpes simplex type 1 ICP0 affect cellular structures and proteins. *J. Virol.*, **74**, 10006–10017.

Parkinson, J. and Everett, R. D. (2001). Alphaherpesvirus proteins related to herpes simplex virus type 1 ICP0 induce the formation of colocalizing, conjugated ubiquitin. *J. Virol.*, **75**, 5357–5362.

Parkinson, J., Lees-Miller, S. P., and Everett, R. D. (1999). Herpes simplex virus type 1 immediate-early protein vmw110 induces the proteasome-dependent degradation of the catalytic subunit of DNA-dependent protein kinase. *J. Virol.*, **73**, 650–657.

Paterson, T. and Everett, R. D. (1988). Mutational dissection of the HSV-1 immediate-early protein Vmw175 involved in transcriptional transactivation and repression. *Virology*, **166**, 186–196.

Pederson, N. E., Person, S., and Homa, F. L. (1992). Analysis of the gB promoter of herpes simplex virus type 1: high-level expression requires both an 89-base-pair promoter fragment and a nontranslated leader sequence. *J. Virol.*, **66**, 6226–6236.

Peng, H., He, H., Hay, J., and Ruyechan, W. T. (2003). Interaction between varicella zoster virus IE62 major transactivator and cellular transcription factor Sp1. *J. Biol. Chem.*, **278**, 38068–38075.

Perera, L. P. (2000). The TATA motif specifies the differential activation of minimal promoters by varicella zoster virus immediate-early regulatory protein IE62. *J. Biol. Chem.*, **275**, 487–496.

Perera, L. P., Mosca, J. D., Ruyechan, W. T., Hayward, G. S., Straus, S. E., and Hay, J. (1993). A major transactivator of varicella-zoster virus, the immediate-early protein IE62, contains a potent N-terminal activation domain. *J. Virol.*, **67**, 4474–4483.

Perera, L. P., Kaushal, S., Kinchington, P. R., Mosca, J. D., Hayward, G. S., and Straus, S. E. (1994). Varicella-zoster virus open reading frame 4 encodes a transcriptional activator that is functionally distinct from that of herpes simplex virus homology ICP27. *J. Virol.*, **68**, 2468–2477.

Perkins, K. D., Gregonis, J., Borge, S., and Rice, S. A. (2003). Transactivation of a viral target gene by herpes simplex virus ICP27 is posttranscriptional and does not require the endogenous promoter or polyadeylation site. *J. Virol.*, **77**, 9872–9884.

Piette, J., Defechereux, P., Baudoux, L., Debrus, S., Merville, M. P., and Rentier, B. (1995). Varicella-zoster virus gene regulation. *Neurology*, **45**, S23–S27.

Purves, F. C., Ogle, W. O., and Roizman, B. (1993). Processing of the herpes virus regulatory protein alpha 22 mediated by the UL13 protein kinase determines the accumulation of a subset of alpha and gamma mRNAs and proteins in infected cells. *Proc. Natl Acad. Sci. USA*, **90**, 6701–6705.

Rahaus, M. and Wolff, M. (2000). Transcription factor Sp1 is involved in the regulation of varicella zoster virus glycoprotein E. *Virus Res.*, **69**, 69–81.

Reed, R. (2003). Coupling transcription, splicing and mRNA export. *Curr. Opin. Cell Biol.*, **15**, 326–331.

Reed, R. and Magni, K. (2001). A new view of mRNA export: separating the wheat from the chaff. *Nature Cell Biol.*, **3**, 201–204.

Rice, S. A., Long, M. C., Lam, V., Schaffer, P. A., and Spencer, C. A. (1995). Herpes simplex virus immediate-early protein ICP22 is required for viral modification of host RNA polymerase II and establishment of the normal viral transcription program. *J. Virol.*, **69**, 5550–5559.

Ruyechan, W. T., Peng, H., Yang, M., and Hay, J. (2003). Cellular factors and IE62 activation of VZV promoters. *J. Med. Virol.*, **70**, S90–S94.

Sandri-Goldin, R. M. (1998). ICP27 mediates herpes simplex virus RNA export by shuttling through a leucine-rich nuclear export signal and binding viral intronless RNAs through an RGG motif. *Genes Dev.*, **12**, 868–879.

Sato, B., Ito, H., Hinchliffe, S., Sommer, M. H., Zerboni, L., and Arvin, A. M. (2003). Mutational analysis of open reading frame 62 and 71, encoding the varicella-zoster virus immediate–early transactivating protein, IE62, and effects on replication in vitro and in skin xenografts in the SCID-hu mouse in vivo. *J. Virol.*, **77**, 5607–5620.

Sciabica, K. S., Dai, Q. J., and Sandri-Goldin, R. M. (2003). ICP27 interacts with SRPK1 to mediate HSV-1 inhibtion of pre-mRNA splicing by altering SR protein phosphorylation. *EMBO J.*, **22**, 1608–1619.

Shepard, A. A., Imbalzano, A. N., and DeLuca, N. A. (1989). Separation of primary structural components conferring autoregulation, transactivation, and DNA-binding properties to the herpes simplex virus transcriptional regulatory protein ICP4. *J. Virol.*, **63**, 3714–3728.

Shepard, A. A., Tolentino, P., and DeLuca, N. A. (1990). Transdominant inhibition of herpes simplex virus transcriptional regulatory protein ICP4 by heterodimer formation. *J. Virol.*, **64**, 3916–3926.

Smiley, J. R., Johnson, D. C., Pizer, L. I., and Everett, R. D. (1992). The ICP4 binding sites in the herpes simplex virus type 1 glycoprotein D (gD) promoter are not essential for efficient gD transcription during virus infection. *J. Virol.*, **66**, 623–631.

Smith, C. A., Bates, P., Rivera-Gonzolos, R., Gu, B., and DeLuca, N. A. (1993). ICP4, the major transcriptional regulatory protein of herpes simplex virus type 1 forms tripartite complex with TATA-binding protein and TFIIB. *J. Virol.*, **67**, 4676–4687.

Sommer, M. H., Zagha, E., Serrano, O. K. *et al.* (2001). Mutational analysis of the repeated open reading frames, ORFs 63 and 70 and ORFs 64 and 69, of varicella zoster virus. *J. Virol.*, **75**, 8224–8239.

Spencer, C. A., Dahmus, M. E., and Rice, S. A. (1997). Repression of host RNA polymerase II transcription by herpes simplex virus type 1. *J. Virol.*, **71**, 2031–2040.

Spengler, M. L., Ruyechan, W. T., and Hay, J. (2000). Physical interaction between two varicella zoster virus gene regulatory proteins, IE4 and IE62. *Virology*, **272**, 375–381.

Stevenson, D., Xue, M., Hay, J., and Ruyechan, W. T. (1996). Phosphorylation and nuclear localization of the varicella zoster virus gene 63 protein. *J. Virol.*, **70**, 658–662.

Van Sant, C., Kawaguchi, Y., and Roizman, B. (1999). A single amino acid substitution in the cyclin D binding domain of the infected cell protein no. 0 abrogates the neuroinvasiveness of herpes simplex virus without affecting its ability to replicate. *Proc. Natl Acad. Sci. USA*, **96**, 8184–8189.

Van Sant, C., Lopez, P., Advani, S. J., and Roizman, B. (2001). Role of cyclin D3 in the biology of herpes simplex virus 1 ICP0. *J. Virol.*, **75**, 1888–1898.

Vaughan, P. J., Thibault, K. J., Hardwicke, M. A., and Sandri-Goldin, R. M. (1992). The herpes simpex virus type 1 immediate early protein ICP27 encodes a potential metal binding domain and is able to bind to zinc. *Virology*, **189**, 377–384.

Wagner, E. K., Guzowski, J. F., and Singh, J. (1995). Transcription of the herpes simplex virus genome during productive and latent infection. *Progr. Nucl. Acid Res. Mol. Biol.*, **51**, 123–165.

Wu, C.-L. and Wilcox, K. W. (1990). Codons 262 to 490 from the herpes simplex virus ICP4 gene are sufficient to encode a sequence-specific DNA binding protein. *Nucl. Acids Res.*, **18**, 531–538.

Wysocka, J. and Herr, W. (2003). The herpes simplex virus VP16-induced complex: the makings of a regulatory switch. *Trends Biochem. Sci.*, **28**, 294–304.

Xia, K., DeLuca, N. A., and Knipe, D. M. (1996a). Analysis of phosphorylation sites of herpes simplex virus type 1 ICP4. *J. Virol.*, **70**, 1061–1071.

Xia, K., Knipe, D. M., and DeLuca, N. A. (1996b). Role of protein kinase A and the serine-rich region of herpes simplex virus type ICP4 in viral replication. *J. Virol.*, **70**, 1050–1060.

Xiao, W., Pizer, L. I., and Wilcox, K. W. (1997). Identification of a promoter specific transactivation domain in the herpes simplex virus regulatory protein ICP4. *J. Virol.*, **71**, 1757–1765.

Yao, F. and Schaffer, P. A. (1994). Physical interaction between the herpes simplex virus type 1 immediate–early regulatory proteins ICP0 and ICP4. *J. Virol.*, **68**, 8158–8168.

Zenklusen, D. and Stutz, F. (2001). Nuclear export of mRNA. *FEBS Lett.* **498**, 150–156.

Zhi, Y. and Sandri-Goldin, R. M. (1999). Analysis of the phosphorylation sites of the herpes simplex virus type 1 regulatory protein ICP27. *J. Virol.*, **73**, 3246–3257.

Zhi, Y., Sciabica, K. S., and Sandri-Goldin, R. M. (1999). Self interaction of the herpes simplex virus type 1 regulatory protein ICP27. *Virology*, **257**, 341–351.

Zhou, C. and Knipe, D. M. (2001). Association of herpes simplex virus 1 ICP8 and ICP27 with cellular RNA polymerase II holoenzyme. *J. Virol.*, **76**, 5893–5904.

10

Alphaherpesvirus DNA replication

John Hay and William T. Ruyechan

Witebsky Center for Microbial Pathogenesis and Immunology, SUNY at Buffalo School of Medicine, NY, USA

DNA replication in alphaherpesviruses has been the subject of study in bursts over the years. Interest in the subject depends not just on simple curiosity about this central feature of the viral growth cycle, but also because DNA replication is a potentially useful target for antiviral therapy, as has already been shown with agents such as acyclovir. The viral contributions to the mechanism of genome replication are quite well understood but we still are unable to duplicate the in vivo situation in an in vitro assay. Much of the recent interesting work involves the host cell's contribution to the process, and this seems likely to remain a focus for the future.

Structure of the genome

There are over 30 alphaherpesviruses that infect a wide range of host species. Their genomes fall into two general categories, either herpes simplex (HSV) – like or varicella zoster (VZV) – like, with four or two, respectively, isomeric forms (Fig. 10.1). There is a wide range of G + C content (32%–75%), with a bias towards higher (>50%) numbers. There is also size heterogeneity (125–180 kbp) which, although quantitatively less than the nucleotide composition variation, may be much more significant for the lifestyle of the virus. All alphaherpesvirus genomes contain four general structural components: unique long and short (U_L, U_S) sequences that encode single-copy genes and inverted repeat regions that bound the unique regions; these may contain diploid genes and sequences required for cleavage and packaging of viral DNA (Fig. 10.1). DNA replication initiates at origin sequences (*ori*), and there are two or three of these in each genome, depending on the virus. Evidence suggests that only one *ori* is required for viral DNA replication, however, and the importance of multiple origins, if any, remains to be discovered (Roizman and Knipe, 2001; Balliet *et al.*, 2005). Only a few of the alphaherpesviruses have been studied at the molecular level regarding DNA replication (e.g., HSV, VZV, equine herpesvirus type 1 (EHV-1), pseudorabies virus (SuHV-1), and infectious bovine rhinotracheitis virus (BoHV-1). Most of the work, however, has been carried out with HSV, reviewed by Boehmer and Lehman (1997) and Lehman and Boehmer, (1999); the majority of the information presented here will be that gathered for HSV.

The origins of DNA replication

For those viruses with an ori_L, this is found in the middle of the U_L segment, in the region lying between DNA polymerase and the major DNA-binding protein for HSV, but not necessarily for other viruses (Telford *et al.*, 1992). The ori_S sequences sit in the repeat regions bounding the

$a_1\ a_n\ b$------------ ori_L-------------- $b'a_n'c'\ ori_S$ -------- $ori_S\ c\ a_S$

<TR_L>< U_L >< $IR_L\ IR_S$>< U_S><TR_S>

Fig. 10.1. The structure of alphaherpesvirus genomes. The upper diagram shows the sequence organization of the herpes simplex virus genome, with the origins of DNA replication shown as ori_L or ori_S. The lower diagram shows the general layout of the regions of the genome, with TR = terminal repeat, IR = internal repeat and the subscripts $_L$ and $_S$ denoting long and short regions, respectively. This is the scheme for the simplexviruses, that invert the U_L and U_S regions relative to each other, to yield four isomeric forms of the genome. For the varicelloviruses, the TR_L and TR_S sequences are so short that U_L does not invert, and there are only two isomeric genome forms, resulting from inversion of U_S. In addition, the varicelloviruses have no ori_L but do have two copies of ori_S.

```
                              BOX I >
5'-GGGTAAAAGAAGTGAGAACGCGAAGCGTTCGCACTTCGTCCCAATATATATATATTATTAGGGCGAAGTGCGAGC-3'

3'-CCCATTTTCTTCACTCTTGCGCTTCGCAAGCGTGAAGCAGGGTTATATATATATAATAATCCCGCTTCACGCTCG-5'
        < BOX III                                                    < BOX II
```

Fig. 10.2. The structure of alphaherpesvirus origins of replication. Shown above is the HSV-1 ori_S sequence. Box III is a low-affinity UL9 recognition site, Box I is a high affinity UL9 binding site and Box II has a ten-fold lower affinity for UL9 than Box I. The ori_S has a large dyad symmetry element (45 bp) centered around an AT region of 18 bp. The ori_L is similar but has a larger symmetry element (144 bp) and AT region (20 bp); in addition, it has a second copy of Box III and, instead of Box II, has a second copy of Box I. Other viral origins have analagous structural elements.

U_S region. The two origins in HSV are very similar but not identical (Fig. 10.2), and other alphaherpesvirus origins also have the same general structural features (Telford *et al.*, 1992; Kuperschmidt *et al.*, 1991), to the extent that HSV infection can support limited replication of a VZV *ori*-containing plasmid (Stow and Davison, 1986), for example. These herpesvirus origins are not dissimilar to other origins in other mammalian viruses, with a dyad symmetry element adjacent to an AT-rich sequence, flanked by binding sites for the origin recognition protein and possibly other factors (Fig. 10.2), implying similar general mechanisms for initiation of genome replication.

Location of DNA synthesis

Viral DNA replication takes place in the nucleus. Prereplicative sites form as DNA-protein complexes that appear as punctuate elements by immunofluorescence microscopy, in association with nuclear domain 10 (ND10) (Ishov and Maul, 1996). As synthesis proceeds, larger areas of the nucleus become involved, and are visualized as globular replication compartments (Quinlan *et al.*, 1984). Recently, it has been demonstrated that active viral transcription assists in the association of viral DNA with ND10 (Sourvinos and Everett, 2002), implying that assembly of transcription and/or replication complexes promote this association. The authors suggest that a critical step in initiating DNA synthesis is ND10 association, and this idea is supported by work with Epstein–Barr virus, in which postreactivation, but not latent, genomes are ND10-associated (Bell *et al.*, 2000).

Proteins involved in DNA synthesis

It is generally accepted that, prior to replication, the linear viral DNA initially circularizes; then synthesis initiates at an origin(s) and proceeds bidirectionally to form theta structures. Soon after, synthesis switches to a rolling circle mode, in which genome-sized pieces are cleaved and packaged as they are produced. This all takes place in the presence of UL9, the origin-binding protein; UL29 (ICP8), a single-strand DNA-binding protein; UL30 and UL42, the DNA polymerase and DNA polymerase processivity factor, which make up the DNA polymerase complex; and UL5, 52 and 8 which make up the DNA helicase/primase complex. These constitute, at present, the essential alphaherpesvirus replication proteins. The assembly of the viral replication complex appears to be an ordered process, in which UL9, ICP8 and the helicase-primase heterotrimer first form replication foci, and the polymerase holoenzyme (UL30 and UL42) are then recruited; this recruitment process seems to require primer synthesis (Carrington-Lawrence and Weller, 2003). Despite our knowledge of the viral polypeptides required for origin-dependent DNA synthesis in vivo, it has still not been possible to reconstitute this theta mode of replication in vitro. Instead, work has focused on rolling circle replication, which can be demonstrated using a replisome containing ori_S and the two viral protein complexes – DNA polymerase/UL42 and the heterotrimeric helicase-primase; the viral SSB (UL29) is not required (Falkenberg *et al.*, 2000).

The origin-binding protein dimerizes and binds to the CGTTCGCACTT *ori* sequence; it also has ATP-binding and helicase functions. Opening the viral *ori* appears to involve several viral and cellular proteins; on a superhelical template in the presence of ATP, UL9 and ICP8 allowed about half of the *ori* s to unwind, and following addition of the cellular topoisomerase I, the extent of unwinding was augmented to >1 kb.

ICP8, the UL29 gene product, is a classical single-stranded DNA binding protein (SSB), with helix-destabilizing activity. It has been shown to interact with all the other replication proteins (above) and seems likely to be the principal scaffold for the generation of prereplication complexes adjacent to ND10 sites. Recent work shows that a C-terminal alpha helix is important in binding viral and/or cellular factors, allowing targeting of ICP8 to specific nuclear sites (Taylor and Knipe, 2003). In addition, it seems to operate in concert with the alkaline endo-exonuclease activity of the virus to constitute a viral recombinase activity similar to that of the bacteriophage lambda (Reuven *et al.*, 2003). In that context, it has recently been shown to stimulate, and regulate, the processivity of, the pseudorabies virus DNase (Hsiang, 2002).

DNA polymerase is a heterodimer, with the UL30 gene product as the typical polymerase/3′–5′ exonuclease (proofreading) activities, and UL42 as the processivity factor. The holoenzyme has a broad substrate specificity that allows it to be a useful target for antiviral therapy, as discussed elsewhere in this volume. The UL42 protein stimulates polymerase activity and increases the fidelity of replication (Chaudhuri et al., 2003); it has been hypothesized to function by interdigitation of its termini, using a hinge region at aa241–261 (Thornton et al., 2000). C-terminal residues in the polymerase polypeptide are important for UL42 interaction and interference with this may be a useful antiviral tool (Bridges et al., 2000). UL42 is an unusual processivity factor, in that it binds directly to DNA, unlike the "sliding clamps" such as PCNA and the E. coli β protein. Nevertheless, it seems to resemble PCNA both in its interaction with polymerase (Zuccola et al., 2000) and its ability to slide downstream with polymerase during replication (Randell and Coen, 2001).

The UL5 and UL52 polypeptides constitute the core of the helicase–primase complex, with DNA helicase, primase and ATPase activities. UL5 and UL52 also demonstrate DNA-binding activity when they form complexes, and this DNA-binding activity is preferentially to forked substrates, as opposed to single-stranded or duplex molecules (Biswas and Weller, 2001). The contribution of UL8 to the complex is to work with ICP8 to promote unwinding activity and to catalyze nuclear localization of the complex. An HSV-1/HSV-2 recombinant, in which UL5 is the only HSV-2 gene, is non-neurovirulent and defective in DNA replication in neurons. The primary defect was in primase activity, suggesting that interactions between subunits in the complex are vital in ensuring its full catalytic activity (Barrera et al., 1998). Inhibitors of helicase–primase activity have recently been investigated as potential antiviral agents. The most powerful compounds inhibited primase, helicase and ATPase activities and, as expected, were active against viral mutants resistant to nucleoside-based therapies (Crute et al., 2002).

A second set of proteins with links to DNA synthesis are considered non-essential for replication in cultured cells, but several appear to be essential for "normal" behavior of virus in animal models. These include: pyrimidine deoxynucleoside kinase; alkaline endo-exonuclease; ribonucleotide reductase; uracil N-glycosylase and deoxyuridine triphosphatase.

The pyrimidine deoxynucleoside kinase, popularly known as thymidine kinase (TK) phosphorylates a wide range of nucleoside substrates, as well as TMP, and is responsible for the rise in the TTP pool that is characteristic of HSV-infected cells. The enzyme, because of its broad specificity, also acts on the acyclovir family of antivirals, and has been used extensively in gene therapy in combination with ganciclovir and acyclovir (Hayashi et al., 2002). This broad specificity has recently been analysed and seems to depend on the electric dipole moment of ligands interacting with a negatively charged residue at aa 225 (Glu) (Sulpizi et al., 2001). TK-deletion mutants will establish latency in mouse ganglia but do not reactivate, presumably owing to a lack of an equivalent cellular activity. However, viral strains that only produce small quantities of enzyme are able to reactivate with wild-type efficiency (Griffiths et al., 2003).

The UL12 ORF encodes an endo-exonuclease that is most active between pH 9 and 10; the significance of this is uncertain. This protein interacts with ICP8 and plays a role in the maturation and packaging of viral DNA; this is consistent with the behavior of UL12 null mutants, which make DNA and late proteins, but do not produce infectious virus particles efficiently. The hypothesis is that the enzyme acts on gaps and/or nicks in progeny DNA, either to process or repair it on its way towards encapsidation. The UL12 phosphoprotein and ICP8 can also work in concert to promote strand exchange, similar to recombination events in lambda phage (Reuven et al., 2003).

Ribonucleotide reductase allows formation of deoxynucleoside diphosphates from ribonucleoside substrates and is not negatively regulated by the high TTP pools in HSV-infected cells, as would be the cellular equivalent. It is made up from the products of two ORFs (UL39, R1 and UL40, R2) to form a symmetric heterotetramer, and seems to be necessary for viral growth in "resting" cells. There are reports of protein kinase activity associated with the R1 polypeptide of HSV-2, but there is also evidence that, while HSV-2 R1 is itself a substrate for protein kinase activity, the polypeptide does not itself possess intrinsic protein kinase activity (Langelier et al., 1998). Recently it has been shown that an accessory function of the reductase may be to protect HSV-1 infected cells against cytokine-induced apoptosis.

Uracil N-glycosylase (encoded in UL2) is a repair enzyme that cleaves mutated U residues from the DNA sugar backbone resulting from a cytosine deamination event, subsequent to repair by viral and cellular enzymes. It is curious that the virus should encode an enzyme that is ubiquitous in host cells, but activities may be low in non-dividing cells that the virus encounters in vivo. This may also be the explanation for reduction in neurovirulence and a poor ability to reactivate from latency that is characteristic of UL2-deletion mutants.

Deoxyuridine triphosphatase (dUTPase), the product of the UL50 gene, breaks down dUTP, preventing dU incorporation into viral DNA. At the same time, the product of its action, dUMP, is a substrate for the pathway that leads to TTP synthesis. UL50 null mutants are impaired in their ability to replicate in the central nervous system in mice, although they seem capable of normal growth in peripheral tissues. They also fail to reactivate effectively.

In addition to the viral proteins described above, there are cellular proteins that contribute both essential and/or accessory roles in viral DNA replication. Among the obvious examples of the former are DNA ligase and topoisomerase activities, as well as repair endonuclease activity and an endonuclease G, that may contribute to maturation of the viral genome (Huang et al., 2002). Among the latter are the numerous cellular enzymes that contribute substrates for DNA synthesis, and that are found in all dividing cells. There will likely be additional cellular proteins found, however, such as the promyelocytic leukemia protein (PML) that is recruited to replication foci following the arrival of the polymerase complex (Carrington-Lawrence et al., 2003), and the OF-1 protein that has a function in initiation of replication (Baker et al., 2000). It also contains the Ku70/Ku80 heterodimer which is present in origin-specific DNA-binding complexes in primates and yeast (Murata et al., 2004).

DNA replication and the cell cycle

HSV downregulates host cell DNA synthesis during lytic infection, implying that the normal cell cycle is dysregulated by the virus. The reason for this, presumably, is to allow the virus maximum access to DNA precursors, replication sites and replication proteins that would otherwise be involved in cellular genome synthesis. In a parallel scenario, it has been shown that, using the inhibitor roscovitine, cyclin-dependent kinases are required for HSV DNA replication, even although the early viral proteins required for synthesis are all present (Schang et al., 2000). Cell cycle arrest has been shown to involve the viral ICP0 protein, using mechanisms that appear to be both p53-dependent and p53-independent. One mechanism whereby ICP0 is effective, is through arresting the cycle at the G1->S stage, blocking cells at the pseudo-prometaphase stage of mitosis (Lomonte and Everett, 1999). The data suggest that viral factors other than ICP0 may be involved in this cell cycle block but that ICP0 alone may be responsible for the mitotic block. The authors make the point that ICP0 expression is incompatible with the growth of a cell population. One additional viral protein that affects the cell cycle is ICP27; it blocks the cycle at S phase, through inhibiting the phosphorylation of pRb (Song et al., 2001). Thus, the virus has evolved a number of different mechanisms to interfere with normal cell cycle progression, emphasizing the potential importance of this step in the viral growth cycle.

Maturation and packaging of viral DNA

The a sequences of the HSV genome (Fig. 10.1) constitute the *cis*-acting signals for cleavage of the newly synthesized DNA, resulting from rolling circle replication, into genome-sized pieces for packaging into capsids. The DR1 repeat sequences that flank the a sequences contain the actual cleavage site, and two unique regions, Uc and Ub, are next to the genomic ends. A fragment, Uc/DR1/Ub, is sufficient to constitute a minimal packaging signal, and elements inside the U sequences can be found in other herpesvirus genomes; these are the pac elements. Data suggest that these pac sequences contain signals for both initiation and termination of packaging (White et al., 2003). The proteins involved in the process are UL6, UL15 and UL28 in HSV-1, and these are sufficient for cleavage of the concatameric DNA, as well as their packaging into procapsids. UL6 likely constitutes the gateway on the preformed capsid for entry of the genome and is present at one vertex, while a UL15/UL28 complex has the properties of the engine that drives the genome into the procapsid. UL6 is capable of specific interaction with both UL15 and UL28 (Hodge and Stow, 2001). A fourth protein, UL25, seems to play a final role in the packaging process, prior to the movement of nucleocapsids into the cytoplasm.

Recombination

Homologous recombination is a frequent event in herpesvirus infected cells, and it has been used experimentally to investigate gene functions, for example, by generation of HSV-1/HSV-2 intertypic recombinants. Viral DNA molecules that are undergoing replication are the best substrates for recombination and the genomic inversions that give rise to the different isoforms of the HSV genome are generated through recombination involving the repeat regions. While it seems likely that cellular enzymes or other proteins will be important in the process, there are clearly roles for viral gene products. For example, ICP8, as outlined earlier, appears potentially to be a key player in the recombination process. In in vitro assays, it promotes strand exchange in conjunction with the viral helicase-primase and catalyzes single-strand invasion in an ATP-independent manner (Nimonkar and Boehmer, 2003). It also may be involved in single-strand transfer, in collaboration with the HSV endo-exonuclease activity, UL12. The 5'-3' exonuclease activity of this protein shares homology with the lambda exonuclease (Redalpha) that is known to be essential for homologous recombination in the phage. It is proposed that the two viral proteins work in concert to promote strand exchange, shown experimentally by generating a gapped circle and a displaced strand from an M13 duplex DNA molecule and an M13 single-stranded circular DNA molecule. Interestingly, UL12 polypeptide that lacked nuclease activity was incapable of catalyzing this experimental recombination (Reuven *et al.*, 2003). In addition to the various roles that recombination might play in the virus life cycle, it has been proposed that recombination may also be important for the switch that occurs between the early theta mode of replication of viral DNA and the mainstream rolling circle mode, in a way reminiscent of the mechanisms occurring in the lytic phase of lambda replication (Boehmer and Lehman, 1997).

Latency

Alphaherpesvirus latency, as typified by HSV, is characterized by a lack of infectious virus in latently infected neural tissue and expression of specific LATs (latency-associated transcripts). VZV, on the other hand, has no LATs, and expresses a restricted set of transcripts and proteins seen in the early phases of normal lytic infection. Calculations of the numbers of viral genomes present in latently-infected neurons have shown a small but significant number to be present; in HSV, a recent estimate gives a mean of 178 per LAT-positive neuron using laser capture microdissection (Chen *et al.*, 2002). This number is not dramatically different from less sophisticated measurements on VZV-infected ganglia. This raises the issue of how this number of genomes arises, and the simplest explanation is that initial infection of the neuron proceeds by the normal lytic route, initiates some DNA replication (only through a theta-like mode?) but is quickly curtailed by factors within the cell. At present, we have no clues as to what constitutes this inhibitory mechanism. Reactivation must involve renewed viral DNA synthesis and, indeed, the presence of several viral proteins of the "non-essential-in-cell-culture" variety is necessary to allow the process to proceed. In addition, there is a proposal that the cellular C1 factor, responsible for assembly of transcriptional enhancer complexes, is normally missing from neuronal nuclei but present soon after reactivation (Kristie *et al.*, 1999). Thus, as with other herpesvirus systems (e.g., EBV), it is likely that the HSV reactivation is initiated through production of gene regulatory viral proteins.

Future directions

Future investigation is likely increasingly to focus on the host cell's contribution to viral genome replication. The recent interest in nuclear structures will provide the field with a new set of findings that may provide the clues necessary to allow faithful replication of the in vivo situation in an in vitro environment. Aside from replication, the host cell also plays a role in the repair/recombination events that characterize the viral growth cycle, and these contributions also remain to be precisely defined. Finally, the issue of latent vs. lytic viral behavior has focused primarily on transcription and its control; perhaps it is now time to look more closely at viral DNA replication in latently infected cells.

REFERENCES

Baker, R. O., Murata, L. B., Dodson, M. S., and Hall, J. D. (2000). Purification and characterization of OF-1, a host factor implicated in herpes simplex replication. *J. Biol. Chem.*, **275**, 30050–30057.

Balliet, J. W., Min, J. C., Cabatingan, M. S., and Schaffer, P. A. (2005). Site-directed mutagenesis of large DNA palindromes: construction and in vitro characterization of herpes simplex virus type 1 mutants containing point mutations that eliminate the oriL or oriS function. *J. Virol.*, **79**, 12783–12797.

Barrera, I., Bloom, D., and Challberg, M. (1998). An intertypic herpes simplex virus helicase–primase complex associated with a defect in neurovirulence has reduced primase activity. *J. Virol.*, **72**, 1203–1209.

Bell, P., Lieberman, P. M., and Maul, G. G. (2000). Lytic but not latent replication of Epstein–Barr virus is associated with PML and induces sequential release of nuclear domain 10 proteins. *J. Virol.*, **74**, 11800–11810.

Biswas, N. and Weller, S. K. (2001). The UL5 and UL52 subunits of the herpes simplex virus type 1 helicase–primase subcomplex exhibit a complex interdependence for DNA binding. *J. Biol. Chem.*, **276**, 17610–17619.

Boehmer, P. E. and Lehman, I. R. (1997). Herpes simplex virus DNA replication. *Ann. Rev. Biochem.*, **66**, 147–184.

Bridges, K. G., Hua, Q., Brigham-Burke, M. R. *et al.* (2000). Secondary structure and structure–activity relationships of peptides corresponding to the subunit interface of herpes simplex virus DNA polymerase. *J. Biol. Chem.*, **275**, 472–478.

Carrington-Lawrence, S. D., and Weller, S. K. (2003). Recruitment of polymerase to herpes simplex virus type 1 replication foci in cells expressing mutant primase (UL52) proteins. *J. Virol.*, **77**, 4237–4247.

Chaudhuri, M., Song, L., and Parris, D. S. (2003) The herpes simplex virus type 1 DNA polymerase processivity factor increases fidelity without altering pre-steady-state rate constants for polymerization or excision. *J. Biol. Chem.*, **278**, 8996–9004.

Chen, X. P., Mata, M., Kelley, M., Glorioso, J. C., and Fink, D. J. (2002) The relationship of herpes simplex virus latency associated transcript expression to genome copy number: a quantitative study using laser capture microdissection. *J. Neurovirol.*, **8**, 204–210.

Crute, J. J., Grygon, C. A., Hargarce, K. D. *et al.* (2002). Herpes simplex virus helicase-primase inhibitors are active in animal models of human disease. *Nature Med.*, **8**, 386–391.

Falkenberg, M., Lehman, I. R., and Elias, P. (2000). Leading and lagging strand DNA synthesis in vitro by a reconstituted herpes simplex virus type 1 replisome. *Proc. Natl Acad. Sci. USA*, **97**, 3896–3900.

Griffiths, A., Chen, S. H., Horsburgh, B. C., and Coen, D. M. (2003). Translational compensation of a frameshift mutation affecting herpes simplex virus thymidine kinase is sufficient to permit reactivation from latency. *J. Virol.*, **77**, 4703–4709.

Hayashi, K., Hayashi, T., Sun, H. D., and Takeda, Y. (2002). Contribution of a combination of ponicidin and acyclovir/ganciclovir to the antitumor afficacy of the herpes simplex virus thymidine kinase gene therapy system. *Hum. Gene Therapy*, **13**, 415–423.

Hodge, P. D. and Stow, N. D. (2001). Effects of mutations within the herpes simplex virus type 1 DNA encapsidation signal on packaging efficiency. *J. Virol.*, **65**, 8977–8986.

Hsiang, C. Y. (2002). Pseudorabies virus DNA-binding protein stimulates the exonuclease activity and regulates the processivity of pseudorabies virus DNase. *Biochem. Biophys. Res. Commun.*, **293**, 1301–1308.

Huang, K. J., Zemelman, B. V., and Lehman, I. R. (2002). Endonuclease G, a candidate human enzyme for the initiation of genomic inversion in herpes simplex type 1 virus. *J. Biol. Chem.*, **277**, 21071–21079.

Ishov, A. M. and Maul, G. G. (1996). The periphery of nuclear domain 10 (ND10) as a site of DNA virus deposition. *J. Cell Biol.*, **134**, 815–826.

Komatsu, T., Ballestas, M. E., Barbera, A. J., Kelly-Clarke, B., and Kaye, K. M. (2004). KSHV LANA-1 binds DNA as an oligomer and residues N-terminal to the oligomerization domain are essential for DNA binding, replication and episome persistence. *Virology*, **319**, 225–236.

Kristie, T. M., Vogel, J. L., and Sears, A. (1999). Nuclear localization of the C1 factor (host cell factor) in sensory neurons correlates with reactivation of herpes simplex virus from latency. *Proc. Natl Acad. Sci, USA*, **96**, 1229–1233.

Kuperschmidt, S., DeMarchi, J. M., Lu, Z., and Ben-Porat, T. (1991). Analysis of an origin of DNA replication located at the L terminus of the genome of pseudorabies virus. *J. Virol.*, **65**, 6283–6291.

Langelier, Y., Champoux, L., Hamel, M. *et al.* (1998). The R1 subunit of herpes simplex virus ribonucleotide reductase is a good substrate for host cell protein kinases but is not itself a protein kinase. *J. Biol. Chem.*, **273**, 1435–1443.

Lehman, I. R. and Boehmer, P. E. (1999). Replication of herpes simplex virus DNA. *J. Biol. Chem.*, **274**, 28059–28062.

Lomonte, P. and Everett, R. (1999). Herpes simplex virus type 1 immediate early protein Vmw110 inhibits progression of cells through mitosis and from G(1) into S phase of the cell cycle. *J. Virol.*, **73**, 9456–9467.

Murata, L. B., Dodson, M. S., and Hall, J. D. (2004). A human cellular protein activity (OF-1), which binds herpes simplex type 1 origins, contains the Ku70/Ku80 heterodimer. *J. Virol.*, **78**, 7839–7842.

Nimonkar, A. V. and Boehman, P. E. (2003). The herpess implex virus type 1 single-strand DNA-binding protein (ICP8) promotes strand invasion. *J. Biol. Chem.*, **278**, 9678–9682.

Quinlan, M. P., Chen, L. B., and Knipe, D. M. (1984). The intranuclear location of a herpes simplex virus DNA-binding protein is determined by the status of viral DNA replication. *Cell*, **36**, 857–868.

Randell, J. C. and Coen, D. M. (2001). Linear diffusion on DNA despite high-affinity binding by a DNA polymerase processivity factor. *Mol. Cell*, **8**, 911–920.

Reuven, N. B., Staire, A. E., Myers, R. S., and Weller, S. K. (2003). The herpes simplex virus type 1 alkaline nuclease and single stranded DNA binding protein mediate strand exchange in vitro. *J. Virol.*, **77**, 7425–7433.

Roizman, B. and Knipe D. (2001). Herpes simplex viruses and their replication. In *Fields Virology*, ed. D. M. Knipe and P. M. Howley, pp. 2399–2459. Philadelphia, PA: Lippincott, Williams and Wilkins.

Schang, L. M., Rosenberg, A., and Schaffer, P. A. (2000). Roscovitine, a specific inhibitor of cellular cyclin-dependent kinases inhibits herpes simplex virus DNA synthesis in the presence of viral early proteins. *J. Virol.*, **74**, 2107–2120.

Song, B., Yeh, K. C., Liu, J., and Knipe, D. M. (2001). Herpes simplex virus gene products required for viral inhibition of expression of G1-phase functions. *Virology*, **290**, 320–328.

Sourvinos, G. and Everett, R. D. (2002). Visualization of parental HSV-1 genomes and replication compartments in association with ND10 in live infected cells. *EMBO J.*, **21**, 4989–4997.

Stow N. D. and Davison A. J. (1986). Identification of a varicella-zoster virus origin of DNA replication and its activation by herpes simplex virus type 1 gene products. *J. Gen. Virol.*, **67**, 1613–1623.

Sulpizi, M., Schelling, P., Folkers, G. Carloni, P., and Scapozza, L. (2001). The rationale of catalytic activity of herpes simplex virus thymidine kinase: a combined biochemical and quantum chemical study. *J. Biol. Chem.*, **276**, 21692–21697.

Taylor, T. J. and Knipe, D. M. (2003). C-terminal region of herpes simplex virus ICP8 protein needed for intranuclear localization. *Virology*, **309**, 219–231.

Telford, E. A. R., Watson, M. S., McBride, K., and Davison, A. (1992). The DNA sequence of equine herpesvirus-1. *Virology*, **189**, 304–316.

Thornton, K. E., Chaudhuri, M., Monahan, S. J., Grinstead, L. A., and Parris, D. S. (2000). Analysis of in vitro activities of herpes simplex virus type 1 UL42 mutant proteins: correlation with in vivo function. *Virology*, **275**, 373–390.

White, C. A., Stow, N. D., Patel, A. H., Hughes, M., and Preston, V. G. (2003). Herpes simplex virus type 1 portal protein UL6 interacts with the putative terminase subunits UL15 and UL28. *J. Virol.*, **77**, 6351–6358.

Zuccola, H. J., Filman, D. J., Coen, D. M., and Hogle, J. M. (2000). The crystal structure of an unusual processivity factor, herpes simplex virus UL42, bound to the C terminus of its cognate polymerase. *Mol. Cell*, **5**, 267–278.

11

Envelopment of herpes simplex virus nucleocapsids at the inner nuclear membrane

Joel D. Baines

Cornell University Department of Microbiology and Immunology, Ithaca, NY, USA

Introduction

As in all herpesviruses, Herpes simplex nucleocapsids assembled in the nucleoplasm obtain an initial envelope by budding through the inner nuclear membrane of infected cells. This chapter will focus on the proteins responsible for nucleocapsid budding in the herpes simplex virus system. Of interest is the observation that orthologs of at least the UL31 and UL34 genes of herpes simplex virus genes likely mediate similar functions in members of both the beta- and gamma herpesvirinae (Muranyi *et al.*, 2002; Gonnella *et al.*, 2005). Thus, it is expected that this information will be relevant to the study of nucleocapsid envelopment of all herpesviruses.

Anatomy of the nuclear membrane: it's all connected

The nuclear envelope consists of two leaflets: the inner leaflet or inner nuclear membrane (INM) partitions the nucleoplasm from the lumen of the nuclear envelope, whereas the outer leaflet (ONM) contacts the cytoplasm. The space between the leaflets is ultimately continuous with the lumen of the endoplasmic reticulum. Both leaflets are continuous with the nuclear pore membrane that serves as an anchoring point for nuclear pore complexes (NPCs), which serve as conduits to mediate protein and RNA transport between the nucleus and cytoplasm.

The nuclear lamina lines the inner surface of the INM and is maintained in this orientation by interaction with both chromatin in the nucleoplasm, and integral membrane proteins specifically concentrated in the INM. How proteins are targeted to the INM has been the focus of active research for several years (Ellenberg *et al.*, 1997; Ostlund *et al.*, 1999; Soullam and Worman, 1993). The leading "diffusion and retention" model proposes that proteins destined for the nuclear membrane are translated by membrane-bound ribosomes, and become integrated into the ER membrane. Proteins then migrate laterally towards the nuclear pore membrane. Those with extraluminal domains greater than 60–70 kD are excluded from the inner nuclear membrane, presumably because the bulky domain interferes with migration past the nuclear pore membrane (Soullam and Worman, 1995). Upon passing the nuclear pore membrane, the nucleoplasmic (or extraluminal) domain is in a position to interact with components of the nuclear lamina. For proteins such as lamin B receptor, emerin, and lamin associated proteins 1 and 2, interaction with lamina components essentially anchors the proteins at the INM, completing the targeting mechanism. For most proteins, however, a nucleoplasmic ligand to retain them at the inner nuclear membrane does not exist, so the proteins eventually migrate anterograde past the nuclear pore membrane into the ONM. Such proteins presumably continue in an anterograde direction to the ER, Golgi and beyond. Thus, most integral membrane proteins do not accumulate to high levels within the inner nuclear membrane, although they would be expected to localize there at least transiently.

The nuclear lamina is required for maintaining the structure of the nucleus and has been shown to line the entire inner surface of the nuclear membrane (Belmont *et al.*, 1993). The lamina is also required for functions normally associated with chromatin such as transcription and DNA replication (Gruenbaum *et al.*, 2000). The precise structure of the nuclear lamina is not well understood. Although many components of the lamina have been identified, understanding how these proteins interact to form higher order structures is complicated by the molecular complexity and redundancy of many of the interactions. What is clear is that most of the integral proteins within the INM that have been studied (such as lamin B receptor and emerin) have been shown to bind lamins. Lamins are type V intermediate filaments and the nuclear lamina contains polymers of lamins A, B and C (McKeon et al., 1986; Stuurman et al., 1998). Lamins A and C are derived from splice variants of *LmnA* transcripts, whereas lamin B1 and lamin B2 are derived from different genes (Fisher et al., 1986; Hoger et al., 1988, 1990; Lin and Worman, 1993). As a result of RNA splicing, the C-terminus of Lamin C contains 6 unique amino acids that replace an isoprenylation motif and the C-terminal 90 amino acids of lamin A.

Lamins, like most intermediate filaments, contain globular head and tail domains separated by a coiled-coil helical rod-like domain that contributes the rigidity and most of the length of the filament. Lamins dimerize as a result of the intertwining of the rod domains, and larger filaments are produced upon multimerization of lamin dimers through the interactions of the rod domains of different protomers. The tail domain can form an immunoglobulin-like fold that likely interacts with chromatin (Dhe-Paganon et al., 2002; Stierle et al., 2003; Taniura et al., 1995).

Envelopment at the nuclear membrane

Herpesvirus nucleocapsids are unique in virology because their nucleocapsids bud through the inner nuclear membrane (INM) to obtain a virion envelope. As a result of the envelopment reaction, the nascent virions accumulate between the inner and outer leaflets of the nuclear membrane. The nuclear membrane in sites that accommodate budding are more electron dense than other regions of the nuclear membrane, suggesting they bear a high density of proteins. Such envelopment sites are readily observed by electron microscopy along the inner nuclear membranes of HSV infected cells. While only a small subset of HSV proteins has been examined in this regard, at least proteins encoded by U_L11 (a peripheral membrane protein), U_L31, U_L34, and glycoproteins B, D and M become incorporated into perinuclear virions and are present at the INM (Baines et al., 1995; Jensen and Norrild, 1998; Reynolds et al., 2002; Torrisi et al., 1992; J. D. Baines, Jacob and B. Roizman, unpublished data). Because no HSV integral membrane protein is predicted to contain an extraluminal domain that exceeds the size that can preclude migration past the nuclear pore membrane (McGeoch et al., 1988), it is likely that additional HSV integral membrane proteins will be discovered along the inner nuclear membrane. It is also likely that at least some tegument proteins are present at the INM, and that some associate with the nucleocapsid before they engage envelopment sites at the INM. Which of the many tegument proteins become targeted to virions in this manner has not been defined.

A critical question is whether the virions that accumulate in the perinuclear space are infectious. If so, it would seem advantageous to the virus because virions are often abundant in the perinuclear space late in infection, and would therefore represent a source of infectious virus upon immune-mediated cytolysis. The critical experiment to determine whether these virions are infectious has not been performed. Two seemingly disparate pieces of evidence argue both for and against: (i) cells infected with a virus encoding a truncated U_L20 gene fused to $U_L20.5$ contain abundant particles that appear to accumulate in the perinuclear space and these virions are infectious (Baines et al., 1991); (ii) cells infected with a virus lacking U_S3 accumulate virions aberrantly in the perinuclear space, and there is a delay in the onset of infectious virus production (Reynolds et al., 2002). Thus, it would seem that, unless an unforeseen defect in INM envelopment is also mediated by U_S3, these virions are not infectious until they exit the perinuclear space.

Studies of viral mutants lacking the U_L11, U_L31, U_L34, U_L37, and U_L53 (gK) proteins have shown that these proteins either facilitate or are required for nucleocapsid envelopment at the INM (Baines and Roizman, 1992; Desai et al., 2001; Jayachandra et al., 1997; Roller et al., 2000). Except for U_L11 and U_L37 which are always dispensable, these proteins are essential for envelopment in different circumstances. Glycoprotein K is especially important for envelopment in quiescent cells (Jayachandra et al., 1997). While U_L31 and U_L34 are essential for envelopment in Vero and Hep2 cells, U_L31 is dispensable for viral replication in rabbit skin cells (Chang et al., 1997; Liang et al., 2004; Roller et al., 2000). Thus it seems likely that functions of the host cell can sometimes complement the functions of gK, and U_L31.

The U_L31/U_L34 protein complex and the nuclear lamina

The U_L31 protein of HSV-1 is a phosphoprotein that contains a bipartite nuclear localization signal at codons 8–25 and is predominantly intranuclear when transiently expressed in the absence of other viral proteins; in infected cells, however, the protein associates with the nuclear rim (McGeoch et al., 1988; Reynolds et al., 2001; Zhu et al., 1999). Immunogold electron microscopy has revealed that the U_L31 protein associates with both leaflets of the nuclear membrane and that this association is dependent on U_L34 protein (Chang and Roizman, 1993; Reynolds et al., 2001; Reynolds et al., 2002). It was noted that U_L31 protein, like other components of the nuclear matrix, is resistant to extraction with detergent, DNAse and high salt (Chang and Roizman, 1993). Association with the nuclear matrix, coupled with the distribution at the nuclear rim, strongly suggest that U_L31 protein integrates into the nuclear lamina of infected cells, components of which display similar resistance to extraction (Chang and Roizman, 1993; Reynolds et al., 2001).

In vitro, U_L31 protein binds GST fusion proteins containing U_L34, and lamin A amino acids 369 to 633 (Reynolds et al., 2004). The solubility of U_L31 protein under various extraction conditions strongly parallels the solubilization of lamin A/C, further supporting an in vivo interaction between these proteins. The presence of U_L31 protein in HSV-infected Vero cells reduces immunoreactivity of an epitope located between amino acids 369–519 of lamin A/C, suggesting that U_L31 directly or indirectly induces a conformational change in lamin A/C that masks the epitope. This region of lamin A/C includes the globular tail domain that has been shown to form an immunoglobulin-like fold that may interact with chromatin (Dhe-Paganon et al., 2002; Stierle et al., 2003). Thus, it is possible that U_L31 may compete for sites on lamin A/C that normally interact with chromatin. Such an interaction could conceivably play a a role in the U_L31-dependent HSV-mediated displacement of chromatin from regions of the INM (Simpson-Holley et al., 2004).

Remarkably, overexpression of the U_L31 protein is sufficient to completely displace lamin A/C from the nuclear rim and cause it to colocalize with U_L31 protein within nucleoplasmic aggregates (Reynolds et al., 2003). Similar lamina – disrupting activity has been seen upon overexpression of lamin A head or tail domains (Izumi et al., 2000). The mechanism by which overexpressed U_L31 mediates lamin displacement is unclear. It is possible that this displacement reflects a competition between domains of U_L31 protein and lamin A/C that mediate: (i) anchoring of the lamina to the nuclear membrane or (ii) polymerization of lamin A/C filaments. However, such dramatic lamin A/C displacement is not observed in infected cells. Reasons include the possibilities that: (i) the distribution of U_L31 protein is restricted to the nuclear rim by its association with the U_L34 protein within the nuclear membrane, thus limiting its diffusion within the nucleus (Reynolds et al., 2001), and (ii) the levels of U_L31 protein in infected cells are lower when expression is driven by the U_L31 promoter as opposed to the CMV early promoter/enhancer used to drive transient expression. If the ability of U_L31 to displace lamins reflects its utility as a lamin depolymerizing agent during infection, it seems more likely that in infected cells the U_L31 protein would serve to act within discrete regions of the nuclear membrane rather than globally. Limiting the destructive capacity of U_L31 protein to a local region may thus avoid more global nuclear disruption and preserve nuclear functions for optimal virus production.

U_L34 protein is likely a type II integral membrane protein, with the bulk of its 275 residue protein protruding into the nucleoplasm. Only the last five amino acids are predicted to reside between the lamella of the nuclear membrane or lumen of the endoplasmic reticulum (i.e., the perinuclear space). The U_L34 protein is necessary for nucleocapsid envelopment at the inner nuclear membrane in most cells tested including Vero and Hep2 cells. The U_L34 protein directly interacts with the U_L31 protein, and is essential for proper targeting of the latter to the nuclear membrane (Reynolds et al., 2001). Changes in various charged clusters of U_L34 do not disrupt the interaction with U_L31 protein suggesting a hydrophobic region of the U_L34 protein may be responsible for the interaction or multiple areas interact (Bjerke et al., 2003). Further work has indicated that amino acids 137–181 of UL34 protein are necessary and sufficient to interact with UL31 protein in the context of the infected cell (Liang and Baines, 2005). In the absence of U_L34, the U_L31 protein is more susceptible to degradation by the proteosome, and U_L31-specific epitopes localize mostly in the nucleoplasm (Ye and Roizman, 2000). In the reverse situation, the U_L31 protein is necessary for exclusive localization of U_L34 protein to the nuclear rim (Reynolds et al., 2001).

Taken together, it is likely that the U_L31 and U_L34 proteins form a complex that is targeted to the nuclear rim. In many cell types, this targeting requires expression of both proteins. In rabbit skin cells, however, U_L34 protein localizes to the NM of infected cells even in the absence of U_L31 (Liang et al., 2004). Thus, in certain situations, host cell functions are sufficient to properly target U_L34 protein to the NM.

The similarity of the U_L31/U_L34 protein complex to coupled pairs of lamin receptors and lamins is striking. For example, emerin, like U_L34 protein, is a type II integral membrane protein that interacts with lamin A/C (Clements et al., 2000). Like lamin A/C, U_L31 integrates into the nuclear lamina and becomes associated with the nuclear membrane via binding its cognate lamin receptor (in this case U_L34 protein) at the nuclear membrane. Thus the U_L31/U_L34 protein protein complex is retained efficiently and invariantly at the nucleoplasmic surface of the INM.

Budding from the nuclear membrane

A promininent hypothesis is that the U_L31 and U_L34 proteins are retained at the inner nuclear membrane to engage nucleocapsids during envelopment. Support for this hypothesis includes the observations that (i) U_L34 protein can interact with ICP5, the major capsid protein (Ye *et al.*, 2000), and (ii) both the U_L31 and U_L34 proteins are incorporated into virions that accumulate between the lamellae of the nuclear membrane. The latter indicates that the U_L31 and U_L34 proteins, directly or indirectly, interact with nucleocapsids in vivo (Reynolds *et al.*, 2002). Neither the U_L31 or U_L34 proteins are detectable in extracellular virions by electron microscopic immunogold staining. Thus, previous observations that the U_L34 protein was present in immunoblots of virions prepared from cytoplasmic lysates probably reflects the presence of at least some perinuclear virions in the cytoplasmic virion preparations (Purves *et al.*, 1992). It is presumed that the U_L31 and U_L34 proteins are released from the nascent virion envelope when this fuses with the outer nuclear membrane and the de-enveloped nucleocapsid is released into the cytoplasm. More detailed information on the cytoplasmic egress pathways of alphaherpesviruses is indicated in Chapter 12 of this volume.

US3: a kinase that phosphorylates U_L34 and U_L31 proteins

The U_L34 and U_L31 proteins are phosphorylated by the protein encoded by U_S3 (Purves *et al.*, 1991; Kato *et al.*, 2005; Poon and Roizman 2005). The U_S3 protein is not essential for growth of HSV in cell culture, but in the absence of U_S3, the onset of production of infectious virus is slightly delayed, and peak infectious titers are reduced about 30-fold, depending on the cell line (Purves *et al.*, 1987; Reynolds *et al.*, 2002). In the absence of U_S3, the architecture of the nuclear membrane is altered such that the membrane contains enveloped virions within round punctate extensions of the nuclear membrane. The virions in these regions also contain U_L31 and U_L34 proteins. It has been speculated that the presence of virions in these punctate nuclear membrane extensions (for simplicity of discussion, here termed NM evaginations) reflects a delay in egress from the perinuclear space (Klupp *et al.*, 2001; Reynolds *et al.*, 2002). The formation of NM evaginations is precluded by U_S3-encoded protein kinase activity (Ryckman and Roller, 2004). Interestingly, NM evaginations do not occur in cells infected with viruses bearing mutations that obviate U_L34 phosphorylation by U_S3. Thus, substrate(s) of the U_S3 kinase other than U_L34 protein are relevant to these particular NM perturbations. The identity of these novel substrate(s) is of considerable interest, and U_L31 is a lead candidate to explain the effects of U_S3 on virion envelopment at the INM.

gK

The localization of gK at the ultrastructural level has yet to be determined, largely because few epitopes in this mostly hydrophobic protein are recognized by available antibodies. In monolayers of tightly packed Vero cells infected with a U_L53 deletion mutant, nucleocapsids accumulate in the nucleus and few are detected in the cytoplasm, suggesting that at least under some conditions, gK plays an important role in nucleocapsid envelopment at the INM (Jayachandra *et al.*, 1997). How the protein facilitates nucleocapsid envelopment is not known.

U_L11

The U_L11 protein, composed of 96-residues, is both myristoylated and palmitoylated (Loomis *et al.*, 2001; MacLean *et al.*, 1989). Both modifications contribute to the association with membranes whereas an acidic cluster mediates trafficking from the plasma membrane to the Golgi apparatus in uninfected cells (Loomis *et al.*, 2001). Cells infected with the U_L11 deletion virus produce infectious virus at levels 100–1000-fold below those of wild-type viruses (Baines and Roizman, 1992). The most striking abnormalities in cells infected with this mutant are abundant unenveloped nucleocapsids in the cytoplasm and abutting the INM. These observations suggest roles in nucleocapsid envelopment at the nuclear membrane or completion of the envelopment reaction, and a second defect in cytoplasmic egress. The latter could reflect a defect that causes de-envelopment or one that precludes re-envelopment at cytoplasmic membranes. Although the U_L11 protein is targeted to the INM and cytoplasmic membranes of infected cells, the protein localizes primarily to the Golgi apparatus in uninfected cells (Baines *et al.*, 1995; Loomis *et al.*, 2001). The disparity between localization in infected and uninfected cells suggests that other infected cell proteins, or alteration of membranes or membrane trafficking by HSV helps mediate trafficking of the U_L11 protein to the nuclear membrane.

U_L37

Unlike many tegument proteins, the low U_L37 protein copy number in the virion tegument is invariant (McLaughlin, 1997), suggesting that it binds a repetitive structure on the nucleocapsid, and might serve as a limiting factor for tegument formation. A likely repetitive feature of nucleocapsids, and possible binding point of UL37 protein, would include capsid pentons which are structurally distinct from hexons and are believed to serve as anchor points for the tegument (Zhou et al., 1999). In pseudorabies virus, the ortholog of U_L37 has been termed a primary tegument protein to indicate its presence in the tegument layer most intimately associated with the surface of the nucleocapsid (Mettenleiter, 2002). Deletion of U_L37 does not greatly affect production of nucleocapsides, but causes most of these to remain in the nucleus at time after infection when large amounts of cytoplasmic particles would be expected (Desai et al., 2001). Thus U_L37 is ultimately dispensable for nucleocapsid envelopment, but greatly facilitates the process. Taken together, the data suggest the (perhaps oversimplified) hypothesis that U_L37 protein association with intranuclear capsids serves to bridge the nucleocapsid to a U_L37-interacting protein in the envelopment apparatus at the INM, but how pU_L37 becomes incorporated into the tegument, or whether it interacts with appropriate envelopment proteins to accomplish a bridging function have yet to be determined.

Model of nucleocapsid envelopment at the INM

A model for nucleocapsid envelopment at the nuclear membrane that is consistent with the above data is as follows. (i) The U_L31 protein is imported through the nuclear pores via its N-terminal nuclear localization signal. The protein interacts with the globular tail domain of lamin A/C and thereby becomes incorporated into the nuclear lamina. (ii) The U_L34 protein becomes incorporated into the ER membrane via its C-terminal transmembrane domain with the bulk of the protein located in the cytoplasm. The protein migrates past the nuclear pore complex and into the INM where it engages U_L31 protein located in the lamina, causing it to become anchored in the INM. (iii) Chromatin and associated lamins are displaced from regions containing U_L31 and U_L34 proteins and the conformation of lamins is significantly altered directly or indirectly by the U_L31/U_L34 protein complex, resulting in localized thinning of the lamina. (iv) several other viral proteins including gD, gB, gM, gK, and U_L11 protein are recruited to patches on the nuclear membrane that correspond to areas of lamin thinning. These regions also contain the U_L31 and U_L34 protein complex. (v) Nucleocapsids engage at least the U_L34 protein to initiate nucleocapsid budding at the INM. As a result of the budding reaction, the U_L31, U_L34, and U_L11 proteins, along with gB, gD, gK, and gM (as well as other unidentified proteins) become incorporated into nascent virions (vi) The envelopes of virions within the perinuclear space fuse with the outer nuclear membrane (ONM). The U_L31 and U_L34 proteins are left at the ONM, and the de-enveloped nucleocapsid proceeds into the cytoplasm to receive another membrane from a cytoplasmic organelle.

Although the above model is consistent with current observations, it is likely that certain aspects (and future surprises) will invite revision as more data accumulates. The usefulness of the model lies in its many testable predictions, and it is hoped that such a paradigm will invite vigorous experimentation in the future.

REFERENCES

Baines, J. D. and Roizman, B. (1992). The U_L11 gene of herpes simplex virus 1 encodes a function that facilitates nucleocapsid envelopment and egress from cells. *J. Virol.*, **66**, 5168–5174.

Baines, J. D., Ward, P. L., Campadelli-Fiume, G., and Roizman, B. (1991). The U_L20 gene of herpes simplex virus 1 encodes a function necessary for viral egress. *J. Virol.*, **65**, 6414–6424.

Baines, J. D., Jacob, R. J., Simmerman, L., and Roizman, B. (1995). The U_L11 gene products of herpes simplex virus 1 are present in the nuclear and cytoplasmic membranes, and intranuclear dense bodies of infected cells. *J. Virol.*, **69**, 825–833.

Belmont, A. S., Zhai, Y., and Thilenius, A. (1993). Lamin B distribution and association with peripheral chromatin revealed by optical sectioning and electron microscopy tomography. *J. Cell Biol.*, **123**, 1671–1685.

Bjerke, S. L., Cowan, J. M., Kerr, J. K., Reynolds, A. E., Baines, J. D., and Roller, R. J. (2003). Effects of charged cluster mutations on the function of herpes simplex virus type 1 UL34 protein. *J. Virol.*, **77**(13), 7601–7610.

Chang, Y. E. and Roizman, B. (1993). The product of the U_L31 gene of herpes simplex virus 1 is a nuclear phosphoprotein which partitions with the nuclear matrix. *J. Virol.*, **67**, 6348–6356.

Chang, Y. E., Van Sant, C., Krug, P. W., Sears, A. E., and Roizman, B. (1997). The null mutant of the U_L31 gene of herpes simplex virus 1: construction and phenotype of infected cells. *J. Virol.*, **71**, 8307–8315.

Clements, L., Manilal, S., Love, D. R., and Morris, G. E. (2000). Direct interaction between emerin and lamin A. *Biochem. Biophys. Res. Commun.*, **267**, 709–714.

Desai, P. Sexton, G. L. McCaffery, J. M., and Person S. (2001). A null mutation in the gene encoding the herpes simplex virus type 1 UL37 polypeptide abrogates virus maturation. *J. Virol.*, **75**(21), 10259–10271.

Dhe-Paganon, S., Werner, E. D., Chi, Y. I., and Shoelson, S. E. (2002). Structure of the globular tail of nuclear lamin. *J. Biol. Chem.*, **277**(20), 17381–17384.

Ellenberg, J., Siggia, E. D., Moreira, J. E. et al. (1997). Nuclear membrane dynamics and reassembly in living cells: targeting of an inner nuclear membrane protein in interphase and mitosis. *J. Cell Biol.*, **138**(6), 1193–1206.

Fisher, D. Z., Chaudhary, N., and Blobel, G. (1986). cDNA sequencing of nuclear lamins A and C reveals primary and secondary structural homology to intermediate filament proteins. *Proc. Natl Acad. Sci. USA*, **83**(17), 6450–6454.

Gonnella, R., Farina, A., Santarelli, R. et al. (2005). Characterization and intracellular localization of the Epstein–Barr virus protein BFLF2: interactions with BFRF1 and with the nuclear lamina. *J. Virol.*, **79**(6), 3713–3727.

Gruenbaum, Y., Wilson, K. L., Harel, A., Goldberg, M., and Cohen, M. (2000). Review: nuclear lamins–structural proteins with fundamental functions. *J. Struct. Biol.*, **129**(2–3), 313–323.

Hoger, T. H., Krohne, G., and Franke, W. W. (1988). Amino acid sequence and molecular characterization of murine lamin B as deduced from cDNA clones. *Europ. J. Cell Biol.*, **47**(2), 283–290.

Hoger, T. H., Zatloukal, K., Waizenegger, I., and Krohne, G. (1990). Characterization of a second highly conserved B-type lamin present in cells previously thought to contain only a single B-type lamin. *Chromosoma*, **100**(1), 67–69.

Izumi, M., Vaughan, O. A., Hutchison, C. J., and Gilbert, D. M. (2000). Head and/or CaaX domain deletions of lamin proteins disrupt preformed lamin A and C but not lamin B structure in mammalian cells. *Mol. Biol. Cell*, **11**(12), 4323–4337.

Jayachandra, S., Baghian, A., and Kousoulas, K. G. (1997). Herpes simplex virus type 1 glycoprotein K is not essential for infectious virus production in actively replicating cells but is required for efficient envelopment and translocation of infectious virions from the cytoplasm to the extracellular space. *J. Virol.*, **71**, 5012–5024.

Jensen, H. L. and Norrild, B. (1998). Herpes simplex virus type 1-infected human embryonic lung cells studied by optimized immunogold cryosection electron microscopy. *J. Histochem. Cytochem.*, **46**(4), 487–496.

Kato, A., Yamamoto, M., Ohno, T., Kodaira, H., Nishiyama, Y., and Kawaguchi, Y. (2005). Identification of proteins phosphorylated directly by the Us3 protein kinase encoded by herpes simplex virus 1. *J. Virol.*, **79** (14), 9325–9331.

Klupp, B. G., Granzow, H., and Mettenleiter, T. C. (2001). Effect of the pseudorabies virus US3 protein on nuclear membrane localization of the UL34 protein and virus egress from the nucleus. *J. Gen. Virol.*, **82**(10), 2363–2371.

Liang, L. and Baines, J. D. (2005). Identification of an essential domain in the Herpes Simplex Virus 1 U(L)34 protein that is necessary and sufficient to interact with U(L)31 protein. *J. Virol.*, **79**, 3797–3806.

Lin, F. and Worman, H. J. (1993). Structural organization of the human gene encoding nuclear lamin A and nuclear lamin C. *J. Biol. Chem.*, **268**(22), 16321–16326.

Loomis, J. S., Bowzard, J. B., Courtney, R. J., and Wills, J. W. (2001). Intracellular trafficking of the UL11 tegument protein of herpes simplex virus type 1. *J. Virol.*, **75**(24), 12209–12219.

MacLean, C. A., Clark, B., and McGeoch, D. J. (1989). Gene UL11 of herpes simplex virus type 1 encodes a virion protein which is myristylated. *J. Gen. Virol.* **70**, 3147–3157.

McGeoch, D. J., Dalrymple, M. A., Davison, A. J. et al. (1988). The complete DNA sequence of the long unique region in the genome of herpes simplex virus type 1. *J. Gen. Virol.*, **69**, 1531–1574.

McKeon, F. D., Kirschner, M. W., and Caput, D. (1986). Homologies in both primary and secondary structure between nuclear envelope and intermediate filament proteins. *Nature*, **319**(6053), 463–468.

McLauchlan, J. (1997). The abundance of the herpes simplex virus type 1 UL37 tegument protein in virus particles in closely controlled. *J. Gen. Virol.*, 189–194.

Mettenleiter, T. C. Herpesvirus assembly and egress. *J. Virol.*, **76**: 1537–1540.

Muranyi, W., Haas, J., Wagner, M., Krohne, G., and Koszinowski, U. H. (2002). Cytomegalovirus recruitment of cellular kinases to dissolve the nuclear lamina. *Science*, **297**(5582); 854–857.

Ostlund, C., Ellenberg, J., Hallberg, E., Lippincott-Schwartz, J., and Worman, H. J. (1999). Intracellular trafficking of emerin, the Emery–Dreifuss muscular dystrophy protein. *J. Cell Sci.*, **112**(11), 1709–1719.

Poon, A. P. and Roizman, B. (2005). Herpes simplex virus 1 ICP22 regulates the accumulation of a shorter mRNA and of a truncated US3 protein kinase that exhibits altered fuctions. *J. Virol.*, **79** (13), 8470–8479.

Purves, F. C., Longnecker, R. M., Leader, D. P., and Roizman, B. (1987). The herpes simplex virus 1 protein kinase is encoded by open reading frame US3 which is not essential for virus growth in cell culture. *J. Virology*, **61**, 2896–2901.

Purves, F. C., Spector, D., and Roizman, B. (1991). The herpes simplex virus protein kinase encoded by the U_S3 gene mediates posttranslational modification of the phosphoprotein encoded by the U_L34 gene. *J. Virol.*, **65**, 5757–5764.

Purves, F. C., Spector, D., and Roizman, B. (1992). U_L34, the target gene of the herpes simplex virus U_S3 protein kinase, is a membrane protein which in its unphosphorylated state associates with novel phosphoproteins. *J. Virol.*, **66**, 4295–4303.

Reynolds, A. E., Ryckman, B., Baines, J. D., Zhou, Y., Liang, L., and Roller, R. J. (2001). U_L31 and U_L34 proteins of herpes simplex virus type 1 form a complex that accumulates at the nuclear rim and is required for envelopment of nucleocapsids. *J. Virol.*, **75**, 8803–8817.

Reynolds, A. E., Wills, E. G., Roller, R. J., Ryckman, B. J., and Baines, J. D. (2002). Ultrastructural localization of the HSV-1 U_L31, U_L34, and U_S3 proteins suggests specific roles in primary envelopment and egress of nucleocapsids. *J. Virol.*, **76**, 8939–8952.

Reynolds, A. E., Liang, L., and Baines, J. D. (2003). Primary envelopment of nucleocapsids is facilitated by physical interaction of HSV-1 UL31 protein with lamin A/C in the nuclear lamina.

Reynolds, A. E., Liang, L., and Baines, J. D. (2004). Confomational changes in the nuclear lamina of cells infected with herpes simplex virus 1 requires genes UL31 and UL34. *J. Virol.*, **78**, 5564–5575.

Roller, R., Zhou, Y., Schnetzer, R., Ferguson, J., and Desalvo, D. (2000). Herpes simplex virus type 1 U_L34 gene product is required for viral envelopment. *J. Virol.*, **74**, 117–129.

Ryckman, B. J. and Roller, R. J. (2004). Herpes simplex virus type 1 primary envelopment: UL34 protein modification and the US3-UL34 catalytic relationship. *J. Virol.*, **78**(1), 399–412.

Simpson-Holley, M., Baines, J., Roller, R., and Knipe, D. M. (2004). Herpes simplex virus 1 U(L)31 and U(L)34 gene products promote the late maturation of viral replication compartments to the nuclear periphery. *J. Virol.*, **78**(11), 5591–5600.

Soullam, B. and Worman, H. J. (1993). The amino-terminal domain of the lamin B receptor is a nuclear envelope targeting signal. *J. Cell Biol.*, **120**(5), 1093–1100.

Soullam, B. and Worman, H. J. (1995). Signals and structural features involved in integral membrane protein targeting to the inner nuclear membrane. *J. Cell Biol.*, **130**(1), 15–27.

Stierle, V., Couprie, J., Ostlund, C. *et al.* (2003). The carboxyl-terminal region common to lamins A and C contains a DNA binding domain. *Biochemistry*, **42**(17), 4819–4828.

Stuurman, N., Heins, S., and Aebi, U. (1998). Nuclear lamins: their structure, assembly, and interactions. *J. Struct. Biol.*, **122**(1–2), 42–66.

Taniura, H., Glass, C., and Gerace, L. (1995). A chromatin binding site in the tail domain of nuclear lamins that interacts with core histones. *J. Cell Biol.*, **131**(1), 33–44.

Torrisi, M. R., Di Lazzaro, C., Pavan, A., Pereira, L., and Campadelli-Fiume, G. (1992). Herpes simplex virus envelopment and maturation studies by fracture label. *J. Virol.*, **66**, 554–561.

Ye, G. J. and Roizman, B. (2000). The essential protein encoded by the UL31 gene of herpes simplex virus 1 depends for its stability on the presence of the UL34 protein. *Proc. Natl Acad. Sci. USA*, **97**(20), 11002–11007.

Ye, G. J., Vaughan, K. T., Vallee, R. B., and Roizman, B. (2000). The herpes simplex virus 1 UL34 protein interacts with a cytoplasmic dynein intermediate chain and targets nuclear membrane. *J. Virol.*, **74**, 1355–1363.

Zhou, Z. H., Chen, D. H., Jakana, J., Rixon, F. J., and Chiu, W. (1999). Visualization of tegument-capsid interactions and DNA in intact herpes simplex virus type 1 virions. *J. Virol.*, **73**, 3210–3218.

Zhu, H. Y., Yamada, H., Jiang, Y. M., Yamada, M., and Nishiyama, Y. (1999). Intracellular localization of the UL31 protein of herpes simplex virus type 2. *Arch. Virol.*, **144**, 1923–1935.

12

The egress of alphaherpesviruses from the cell

Gabriella Campadelli-Fiume

Department of Experimental Pathology, Studiorum-University of Bologna, Italy

A commonly accepted concept in herpesvirology holds that herpesvirions are formed by budding of nucleocapsids at the inner nuclear membrane and the enveloped virions are released into the perinuclear space (see Chapter 13). This is a closed compartment that virions need to exit, in order to reach the extracellular space and start a new infection cycle. How alphaherpesviruses accomplish this goal is a controversial issue. Of the two pathways of virus exit proposed, the single envelopment and the double envelopment, also referred to as de-envelopment–re-envelopment, each has evidence and supporters in the literature (the topic has been covered in excellent reviews and papers (Enquist *et al.*, 1998; Skepper *et al.*, 2001; Johnson and Huber, 2002; Mettenleiter, 2002). Part of the uncertainties that still dominate this topic comes from the difficulties in interpreting static electron microscopy images. Thus cytoplasmic virions juxtaposed to curved vesicles were interpreted in some studies as budding virions, i.e., as evidence for secondary envelopment and for the deenvelopment-reenvelopment pathway. In other studies they were interpreted as virions undergoing fusion with encasing vesicles, i.e., as evidence of de-envelopment (Campadelli-Fiume *et al*, 1991: Roizman and Knipe, 2001). To solve these ambiguities, several approaches have been undertaken in recent years, including the generation of genetically modified mutants and cytochemistry.

In the single envelopment pathway, credited to a study by Johnson and Spear (Johnson and Spear, 1982) in which monensin was observed to block herpes simplex virus (HSV) glycoprotein maturation and to induce the accumulation of virions in large cytoplasmic vacuoles, virions leave the perinuclear space by becoming encased in vesicles–vacuoles formed by the outer nuclear membrane (Fig. 12.1, left pathway). At this stage they carry immature oligosaccharides in their glycoproteins and glycolipids. The virion-encasing vesicles then travel along the exocytic or secretory pathway, and interact with membranes of the exocytic pathway, mainly the Golgi apparatus, leading to a modification in their content of glycosyl transferases and glycosidases that results in the *in situ* maturation of the oligosaccharides of viral glycoproteins. The mature virions are then released in the extracellular space by fusion of the virion-encasing vesicle with the cytoplasmic face of the plasma membrane. In this pathway the virion maintains the tegument acquired in the nucleus as well as the envelope acquired at the inner nuclear membrane, hence the glycoprotein species present in the initial envelope do not change, but their oligosaccharidic moieties are subject to maturation.

In the de-envelopment–re-envelopment pathway, originally proposed by Stackpole in a study of frog herpesvirus (Stackpole, 1969), the envelope of the virions present in the perinuclear space fuses with the outer nuclear membrane (de-envelopment), thus releasing the nucleocapsids into the cytoplasm. The de-enveloped nucleocapsids acquire a tegument in the cytoplasm and undergo a secondary envelopment (re-envelopment) by nucleocapsid budding into a *trans*-Golgi compartment or *trans*-Golgi network (TGN), or, into an endosomal compartment (Harley *et al.*, 2001) (Fig. 12.1, right pathway). As the virus buds from these membranes, the membrane gives rise simultaneously to the envelope and to a vesicle that surrounds the enveloped virion. The final release of the virions into the extracellular space takes place by fusion of the virion-encasing vesicle with the cytoplasmic face of the plasma membranes, just as it occurs in the single envelopment pathway. In this pathway the virus acquires in the cytoplasm a tegument and a secondary envelope, both of which may differ in protein composition from the ones acquired at the primary envelopment.

The key differences between the two routes are (i) the number of envelopes that the virus acquires: one

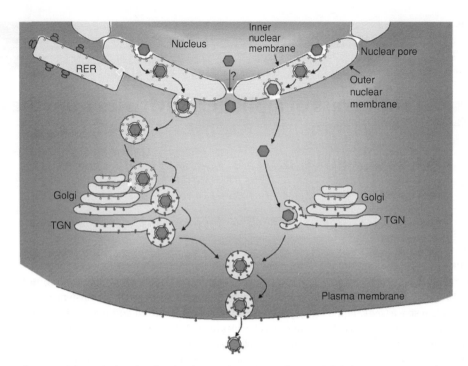

Fig. 12.1. Schematic drawing showing the two alternative pathways of alphaherpesvirus egress from infected cells. The single envelopment pathway is depicted to the left, and the double envelopment, or de-envelopment-re-envelopment is depicted to the right of the illustration. The schematic drawing does not shows the gross ultrastructural modifications of the Golgi apparatus and TGN. Perinuclear virions and nuclear membranes are decorated with glycoproteins of different color than virions at the level of the Golgi apparatus and TGN, as well as extracellular virions, to emphasize that the oligosaccharide moieties of the viral glycoproteins are of the immature type in early exocytic compartment, but are of the mature type in the late exocytic compartments and in extracellular virions. The drawing considers also the possibility that nucleocapsids exit the nucleoplasm through modified nuclear pores, without transiting through the perinuclear lumen. (Drawing by courtesy of L. Menotti.) (See color plate section.)

in the single envelopment, two in the de-envelopment-re-envelopment pathway; the composition of the two envelopes may well differ one from the other; (ii) The significance of the capsids in the cytoplasm. In the single envelopment pathway, the cytoplasmic nucleocapsids are dead-ends that result from fusion of the envelope with the membrane of the virion-encasing vesicles (Campadelli-Fiume *et al.*, 1991). In the de-envelopment–re-envelopment pathway, they are the key players for the secondary envelopment. (iii) The site of tegument assembly, which is necessarily the nucleus in the single envelopment pathway, and can be either the nucleus or the cytoplasm in the double envelopment egress. In the latter case, the tegument may even be absent from perinuclear virions.

In recent years there has been a growing consensus in favour of the de-envelopment–re-envelopment pathway for egress of both HSV and varicella zoster virus (VZV) (Jones and Grose, 1988; Enquist *et al.*, 1998; Wang *et al.*, 2001; Mettenleiter, 2002). As some crucial questions concerning this route remain unsolved, both models are presented here, along with the evidence in favour of or against each of the pathways. For an elegant and in-depth analysis of both pathways, and of strengths and weaknesses of the lines of evidence, also see Enquist *et al.* (1998).

HSV

Single envelopment pathway

Evidence and arguments in favor
A major virtue of this pathway is its simplicity. It became widely accepted some years ago, and was supported by three lines of evidence.

(i) When analyzing the types of oligosaccharides that are present in the glycoproteins and in the glycolipds of the virion envelope, the model predicts that the perinuclear virions carry immature glycomoieties, the extracellular virions carry mature glycomoieties, and the cytoplasmic virions carry both intermediate and mature glycomoieties. This intermediate type of glycomoieties cannot be present in virions formed in the de-envelopment–re-envelopment pathway, unless the secondary envelopment takes place at the *cis*- or *medial*-Golgi. If this is the case, then the question arises "how does the virion travel from *cis*- or *medial*-Golgi to farther compartments of the exocytic pathway in order to obtain its final envelope with mature oligosaccharides?" When the HSV oligosaccharides were characterized in a cytochemical study, it was found that perinuclear virions carry immature oligosaccharides, the intracytoplasmic virions carry both intermediate and mature types of oligosaccharides, and extracellular virions carry exclusively mature oligosaccharides (Di Lazzaro *et al.*, 1995).

(ii) A similar line of reasoning applies to the significance of the markers of the *cis*- and *medial*-Golgi in extracellular virions. It is a well-known phenomenon that viral envelopes carry cellular proteins that are constituents of the membranes where budding of virions occurred, or of the compartments which the virus transited. As a consequence, the cellular proteins that are present in the envelope of extracellular virions are indicators of the cellular membranes from which the envelope was derived, or through which the viruses transited. Specifically, if virions undergo a secondary envelopment at *trans*-Golgi or TGN, the extracellular virions are not expected to carry proteins typical of *cis*- or *medial*-Golgi. By contrast, if these markers are present in the extracellular virions, two mutually exclusive implications are possible, i.e., either the virions transited through *cis*- or *medial*-Golgi, as is the case for the single envelopment pathway, or budding took place at *cis*- or *medial*-Golgi. As discussed above, if this is the case, the same question as above arises: "How does the virion move from *cis*- *medial*-Golgi to *trans*-Golgi or TGN?" A detailed immunocytochemical study, summarized below, has been conducted in neurons, and showed that extracellular virions carry giantin and mannosidase II, two markers typical of *cis*- and *medial*-Golgi, respectively (Miranda-Saksena *et al.*, 2002).

(iii) A further issue centers on the glycoprotein composition of the perinuclear virions, and particularly whether the glycoproteins required for virion infectivity are acquired during envelopment at the inner nuclear membrane. It is a well established notion that HSV infectivity requires the four glycoproteins gB, gD, gH, gL (see Chapter 7). Perinuclear virions were isolated from cells infected with a UL20-deletion virus, which induces the accumulation of virions in the perinuclear space. They are infectious, implying that they carry the four glycoproteins gB, gD, gH, gL (Baines *et al.*, 1991; Avitabile *et al.*, 1994a). The actual presence of the essential glycoproteins at nuclear membranes and at the perinuclear virions was established in *in situ* experiments for the two glycoproteins that were analyzed: gD and gB (Torrisi *et al.*, 1992; Skepper *et al.*, 2001; Miranda-Saksena *et al.*, 2002). All in all, the essential glycoproteins that were searched for have been detected in perinuclear virions, suggesting that, if the de-envelopment–re-envelopment takes places, it is not a requirement in order for the virus to obtain its asset of essential glycoproteins.

Evidence and arguments against

There are two major lines of evidence against the single envelopment model. They are: the presence of the UL31 and UL34 proteins at the nuclear membranes and at the perinuclear virions, and their concomitant absence from extracellular virions, and the lipid composition of the virion envelope (van Genderen *et al.*, 1994; Reynolds *et al.*, 2001, 2002). Both rest on the notion that the chemical composition of the virion envelope reflects the composition of the membrane where nucleocapsid budding took place.

(i) The UL31 protein is a matrix-associated phosphoprotein that localizes to the nuclear membranes in the infected cells, and when coexpressed with the UL34 protein (see Chapter 13). The UL34 protein is a predicted type-2 membrane-bound phosphoprotein with the bulk of the protein constituting the endodomain exposed to the interior of the nucleus. It requires the UL31 protein for localization at the nuclear envelope. The two proteins are required for virus envelopment. Specifically, electron microscopic analyses show that morphogenesis of a UL34 gene deletion virus proceeds to the point of formation of DNA-containing nuclear capsids, but enveloped virus particles in the cytoplasm or at the surface of infected cells are absent, suggesting that the UL34 protein is essential for efficient envelopment of capsids. The phenotype of the UL31 gene deletion virus is similar (Roller *et al.*, 2000; Ye and Roizman, 2000). Remarkably, both proteins are present at perinuclear virions but absent from the extracellular virions, providing evidence that the primary envelope differs in composition from the envelope of extracellular virions. This strongly argues in favour of the de-envelopment-re-envelopment pathway (Reynolds *et al.*, 2001, 2002). The same localization is observed with pseudorabies virus (PrV) UL31 and UL34 proteins (Fuchs *et al.*, 2002). An alternative explanation for the absence of UL31 and UL34 proteins from the extracellular virions would be that a specific protease degrades these two proteins during virus maturation, in analogy to what happens for the scaffolding protein VP26, or, less likely, that epitopes become masked.

(ii) The phospholipid composition was determined in infected cells fractionated into three fractions: a nuclear fraction (which contains nuclei and virions at perinuclear space), a cytoplasmic fraction (which contains the cytoplasmic membranes, the intracytoplasmic virions and the plasma membranes), and a fraction consisting of extracellular virions. It was found that the phospholipid composition of extracellular Herpes Simplex virions and of the cytoplasmic fraction differs from that of nuclei, in that the former contains threefold higher concentrations of sphingomyelin and phosphatidylserine, lipids that are typically enriched in the Golgi apparatus and plasma membrane (van Genderen et al., 1994). This difference implies that the lipid composition of the envelope acquired at the inner nuclear membrane differs from that of extracellular virions. It has been interpreted as evidence in favour of the de-envelopment–re-envelopment pathway (Enquist et al., 1998), even though alternative mechanisms for the modification in lipid composition may be envisioned, e.g., exchange of lipids between the virion envelope and the Golgi membranes during exocytosis in the single envelopment pathway (van Genderen et al., 1994).

De-envelopment–re-envelopment pathway

Evidence and arguments in favor

A major virtue of the double envelopment route of egress is that the separate transport of nucleocapsids and glycoproteins, and their assembly into virions at the cell periphery seems a rational way of transport in the neuron: a key host cell for HSV. In addition to the localization of the UL31 and UL34 proteins, and to the lipid composition of the virion envelope, discussed above, three lines of evidence argue in favour of a double envelopment process, namely the separate transport of nucleocapsids and glycoproteins in neuronal axons, the phenotype of mutants carrying deletions in tegument genes or multiple deletions in glycoprotein genes with accumulation of unenveloped nucleocapsids in the cytoplasm, and the differential distribution of a form of gD retargeted to the endoplasmic reticulum.

(i) A first line of evidence for separate transport of capsids and viral glycoproteins was provided in an electron microscope study of HSV assembly in neurons. Capsids were observed migrating in anterograde direction within axons, whereas the viral glycoproteins (gD) were observed in vesicles which do not colocalize with nucleocapsids, suggesting that virion assembly in axons represents a final step that occurs at the axon end (Penfold et al., 1994).

(ii) Tegument assembly: the tegument is one of the most complex and least understood components of the virion, in terms of structure, assembly and role in virus entry and in virion morphogenesis. Functionally, it is analogous to the matrix layer of other viruses, as it connects the capsid to the intravirion tails of the envelope glycoproteins. Its role is twofold. First, it delivers into the cytosol of the infected cell virion components which are immediately available to the viral metabolism, before the onset of viral protein synthesis. These components facilitate the initiation of infection. Two such examples are *alpha*-TIF (α-*trans*-inducing factor), also named VP16, and *vhs* (virion host shut off), the product of UL41 gene (Batterson et al., 1983; Read and Frenkel, 1983; Campbell et al., 1984). The second function is structural (Mossman et al., 2000). In terms of composition, it is made of almost 20 proteins (see Chapter 7). Despite its amorphous appearance, the tegument appears to contain an inner and an outer layer, of different composition. For both HSV and PrV, the inner layer contains the products of the UL36 (VP1/2) and UL37 genes. The UL36 protein interacts with the major capsid protein, ICP5, which forms both pentons and exons. The outer layer includes major components, UL48-αTIF-VP16, UL49-VP22, *vhs*, and minor components, UL11, UL13-PK (protein kinase), UL14, UL21, UL46-Vp11/12, UL47-VP13/14, UL51, UL56, US3-PK, US10, US11.

Studies of tegument assembly were interpreted as evidence that the site of assembly is the cytoplasm. They fall into two series: electron microscopic analysis and the phenotype of mutant viruses deleted in the tegument-encoding genes.

Work performed mainly with PrV indicates that intranuclear nucleocapsids do not contain a well-defined tegument, detected as an electrondense layer surrounding the capsid, whereas extracellular virions and cytoplasmic nucleocapsids contain an electrondense tegument (Mettenleiter, 2002). In line with these observations, in live virus-infected cells the tegument protein VP22 is observed almost exclusively in the cytoplasm, favoring the cytoplasm as the site of tegument assembly (Elliott and O'Hare, 1999).

In terms of deletion mutant viruses, the UL36 protein appears to play a critical role in tegument assembly, since in its absence capsids acquire the envelope at the inner nuclear membrane, are subsequently translocated into the cytoplasm, but do not mature into enveped virus and do not exit the cell. Also the deletion of HSV UL37 gene abrogates virus maturation and induces a phenotype similar to that induced by the UL36 gene deletion (Desai, P. J., 2000; Desai, P. et al., 2001). The physical interaction between UL36 and UL37 proteins has been demonstrated in PrV (Klupp et al., 2002). These phenotypes have been interpreted to mean that a defect in tegument assembly hampers the secondary envelopment with consequent accumulation of cytoplasmic nucleocapsids, although they do not formally prove it (Desai, P. J., 2000).

In contrast to the effect of UL36 and UL37 deletions, virion morphogenesis is not hampered in a VP22 deletion mutant HSV, nor in a number of deletion mutant viruses in the genes encoding other tegument proteins (Pomeranz and Blaho, 2000; Mettenleiter, 2002). A defective phenotype is however observed in the deletion mutant virus of α-TIF, a phenotype complicated by the fact that the protein has two functions, i.e., it is a potent transactivator of α-genes and is required for the structural integrity of the tegument (Batterson et al., 1983; Campbell et al., 1984; Ace et al., 1988; Mossman et al., 2000). The observation that most of the deletion mutants in tegument genes fail to induce a defect in virus assembly and production has been interpreted as evidence that tegument proteins play redundant functions, and that the absence of a single tegument protein does not hamper tegument assembly (Mettenleiter, 2002).

An immunocytochemical study of tegument assembly and envelope acquisition in rat dorsal neurons showed that the site of HSV tegument assembly is the cytoplasm of the neuronal cell body and that major sites of envelope acquisition are the vesicles of the Golgi and TGN. Evidence rested on the finding that the tegument proteins VP13/14, VP16, VP22, and US9 were readily detected in the nucleus, but almost absent from the budding virions at the nuclear membranes and from virions in the perinuclear space. By contrast, they were abundant on cytoplasmic unenveloped and enveloped nucleocapsids and in extracellular virions (Miranda-Saksena et al., 2002). Of note, the same pattern of labelling was observed for gD. Altogether, the results of this study were interpreted as evidence that the pathway of virion egress from the cell body of neurons does not differ from the pathway of egress from axons during anterograde transport, and follows the de-envelopment–re-envelopment pathway. As mentioned above, in this same study the extracellular virions and the cytoplasmic vesicles also labelled for markers of *cis*- and *medial*-Golgi and of TGN. The significance of this finding was not discussed (Miranda-Saksena et al., 2002).

(iii) Multiple deletion of glycoprotein genes, especially non essential glycoproteins. Practically all HSV glycoproteins, both essential and non-essential, have been deleted singly or in groups, and none of the deletion viruses is defective in virus transport out of the perinuclear space (Longnecker et al., 1987; Longnecker and Roizman, 1987; Cai et al., 1988; Ligas and Johnson, 1988; Forrester et al., 1992; Baines and Roizman, 1993; Roop et al., 1993; Dingwell et al., 1994), suggesting that no single glycoprotein plays a critical role in virus exocytosis. The exceptions are the gK- and UL20-deletion mutant viruses discussed below. In contrast, viruses carrying multiple deletions in glycoprotein genes exhibited defects in virus morphogenesis, cumulatively suggesting that gE, gI and gD participate in secondary envelopment and that they act in a redundant manner, such that viruses carrying single or double deletions do not exhibit a marked phenotype, whereas viruses carrying a triple deletion do (Farnsworth et al., 2003). Specifically, gE and gI play a role in the cell-to-cell spread of HSV, visible in untransformed cells (see below). gM is an abundant glycoprotein conserved in all human herpesviruses. While its conservation argues for a role of the glycoprotein, a deletion mutant virus has no phenotype in cell culture. In PrV the simultaneous deletion of gE–gI and gM drastically inhibits plaque formation and replication, and induces the accumulation of nucleocapsids in cytoplasmic areas where tegument proteins accumulate (Brack et al., 1999). This phenotype indicates that the deleted glycoproteins are cumulatively responsible for secondary envelopment. Following these observations, HSV deletion viruses in gE–gI or gE–gI–gM have been constructed. Remarkably, they exhibit no defect in growth, plaque formation, particle to PFU ratio, hence they carry none of the defects of the triple deletion PrV mutant (Browne et al., 2004). In an independent work, HSV mutants carrying a double or a triple deletion in gD–gE or gD–gE–gI, respectively, exhibited severe defects in envelopment, detected as accumulation of a large number of unenveloped nucleocapsids in the cytoplasm (Farnsworth et al., 2003). These aggregated capsids were immersed in an electron-dense layer that appeared to be tegument. Because none of the glycoproteins, when deleted singly, produced this phenotype, it was proposed that gD and the gE–gI act in a redundant fashion to enable the interaction of the virion envelope with tegument-coated capsids. In the absence of either one of these HSV glycoproteins, envelopment proceeds; however, without both gD and gE, or gE/gI, an inhibition of cytoplasmic envelopment is observed (Farnsworth et al., 2003).

(iv) A form of gD carrying an endoplasmic reticulum (ER) retrieval motif. The rational of this study was to engineer into HSV a form of gD carrying an ER-retrieval motif. The ER-retrieved gD was expected to be present at the ER and the nuclear membranes, which are continuous with the ER, but not to travel along the exocytic pathway. Virions at the perinuclear space were expected to be decorated with gD; virions undergoing de-envelopment–re-envelopment were expected to exchange this envelope, so that extracellular virions would be devoid of gD (Whiteley et al., 1999; Skepper et al., 2001). When analyzed by immunocytochemistry, the perinuclear virions and the nuclear membranes were indeed decorated with the ER-retargeted gD, whereas the extracellular virions and the plasma membrane were not (Whiteley et al., 1999; Skepper et al., 2001). These results are consistent with a double envelopment route of egress. However, in the same study quantification of the distribution of gD in wild-type virus-infected cells showed that the plasma membranes contained 20-fold less, or even lower amount of gD than the nuclear and cytoplasmic membranes (Skepper *et al.*, 2001). This contrasts with the detection of gD in approximately the same amounts at the nuclear membranes and at the plasma membranes in a fracture-label study, with the abundant detection of gD at the plasma membrane by immunofluorescence, and with the detection of gD more abundantly at the plasma membrane than at the nuclear membranes in neurons and raises the possibility that the degree of detection may be affected by the specific reactivity of the antibodies employed (Torrisi *et al.*, 1992; Miranda-Saksena *et al.*, 2002).

Evidence and arguments against
(i) The major weakness of the de-envelopment–re-envelopment pathway is the inability to explain how virions leave the perinuclear space (Campadelli-Fiume and Roizman, 2006). The pathway envisions that perinuclear virions fuse with the luminal face of the outer nuclear membrane, thus releasing the de-enveloped nucleocapsids in the cytoplasm. The glycoproteins necessary for the HSV fusion that leads to virus entry are the quartet of gB, gD, gH, gL (Cai *et al.*, 1988; Ligas and Johnson, 1988; Forrester *et al.*, 1992; Roop *et al.*, 1993). These same glycoproteins are necessary and sufficient to induce cell–cell fusion when transiently expressed in transfected cells (Turner *et al.*, 1998) (see Chapter 7). Absence of each member of the quartet abolishes virion infectivity and fusion in the cell–cell fusion assay, but does not cause any defect in the release of (non-infectious) virions to the extracellular space. Paradoxically therefore, the perinuclear virions of the deleted viruses are able to carry out fusion with the outer nuclear membrane in the absence of each one of the known viral fusion glycoproteins.

To solve this conundrum, three alternative possibilities can be envisioned. First, some of the non-essential glycoproteins or membrane proteins which form the envelope of the perinuclear virions substitute for the fusion activity of the quartet. As a corollary, deletion mutants in these putative fusion proteins are expected to accumulate in the perinuclear space and be defective in the release of extracellular virus. Apart from the fact that a fusion activity has not been observed with ensembles of HSV glycoproteins other than the quartet (Turner *et al.*, 1998), deletion viruses have been produced for almost all of the non essential glycoproteins (gC, gE, gI, gJ, gG, gM), and they are not defective in the release of virions to the extracellular space (Longnecker *et al.*, 1987; Longnecker and Roizman, 1987; Cai *et al.*, 1988; Ligas and Johnson, 1988; Forrester *et al.*, 1992; Baines and Roizman, 1993; Roop *et al.*, 1993; Dingwell *et al.*, 1994). This makes it unlikely that the non-essential envelope proteins carry out fusion with the outer nuclear membrane. The phenotype of two deletion viruses is interesting under this respect. They are a gK-minus and a UL20-minus virus (Baines *et al.*, 1991; Avitabile *et al.*, 1994b; Hutchinson and Johnson, 1995). The first-generation deletion viruses exhibit an accumulation of virions at the perinuclear space. The second-generation deletion mutants are still defective in virus egress, but the unenveloped nucleocapsids appear to accumulate in the cytoplasm rather than in the perinuclear space (Foster and Kousoulas, 1999; Foster *et al.*, 2004). This phenotype is consistent with the hypothesis that gK and/or UL20 proteins, singly or in association, enable fusion. Because these proteins accumulate at the ER, or in the Golgi, but only in minimal quantity, or not at all, in the plasma membrane, when expressed by transgenes (Avitabile *et al.*, 2003, 2004; Foster *et al.*, 2003), the possibility that they induce fusion at the nuclear membranes can not be tested.

Secondly, it can be envisioned that fusion of perinuclear virions with the outer nuclear membranes is carried out by cellular proteins, e.g. members of the v-SNARE and t-SNARE family. This possibility appears untenable because of the topology of these proteins, whose functional domains are located in the cytoplasmic face of the cytoplasmic vesicles. They would need to flip–flop to the luminal face, while maintaining their activity, and travel all the way to the outer and then to the inner nuclear membrane, in order for perinuclear virions to carry them in their envelope. Further yet, these proteins need a number of membrane-bound and soluble factors, all of which are absent from the perinuclear space.

All in all, the virus has to rely on viral fusion proteins other than those known to date in order to exit the perinuclear space, and an unconventional and so far totally elusive mechanism of fusion must be hypothesized in order to explain how virions leave the perinuclear space in the deenvelopment and re-envelopment pathway.

A third possibility is raised by the recent finding that in HSV-and BHV-infected cells the nuclear pores appear to be enlarged such that they allow the exit of nucleocapsids directly from the nucleoplasm to the cytoplasm (Wild and Engels, 2004; Leuzinger *et al.*, 2005).

(ii) A second weakness of the double envelopment pathway is the failure to explain how the de-enveloped nucleocapsids travel from the cytoplasmic face of the outer nuclear membrane to the Golgi or TGN. As discussed in Chapter 7, nucleocapsids that do not travel along microtubules move very slowly (see the calculations that have been present for incoming nucleocapsids), and therefore the de-enveloped nucleocapsids need to travel along some kind of cellular routes for efficient transport. Transport along microtubules seems untenable since the microtubule architecture is dramatically modified in the course of infection, a modification that appears to be conserved in herpesviruses (Avitabile *et al.*, 1995). The infected cell microtubules form circular rings at the periphery of the cell, and seem rather unsuitable to export nucleocapsids from outside the outer nuclear membrane to the TGN.

Finally, as mentioned above, the presence of *cis*- and *medial*-Golgi markers in extracellular virions produced by neurons suggests that either these membranes were the site of secondary envelopment, or that virions have transited through these compartments, with exchange of components, as may happen in the single envelopment route of egress (Miranda-Saksena *et al.*, 2002).

Cell-to-cell spread

The prominent route by which HSV infection spreads in human tissues is cell-to-cell spread, i.e., the direct passage of progeny virus from an infected cell to an adjacent cell. This occurs at primary infection when progeny virus spreads from the primary infected cell to adjacent cells in the mucocutaneous tissue and then to axonal termini of sensory neurons (retrograde transport). It also occurs at reactivation from latency, when newly replicated virus spreads from the sensory neuron to the mucocutaneous tissue (anterograde transport). It is generally assumed that this mechanism of spread represents an immune evasion strategy, as it shields the virus from antibodies and cells of the immune system. The simplest models of cell-to-cell transmission in cell cultures are plaque formation and the infectious center assay. Some of requirements are relatively well characterized, and coincide with those for virus entry, i.e., the quartet of gD, gB, gH, gL and the presence of a gD receptor on target cells. In addition, gE and gI play a critical role.

gE–gI

gE and gI form a functional heterodimer (gE–gI), found both in infected cell membranes and in virion envelopes (Johnson *et al.*, 1988), an attribute conserved in VZV and PrV (Zuckermann *et al.*, 1988; Yao *et al.*, 1993). The role of the gE–gI complex was not recognized in early studies because single deletion mutants are not hampered in their replication, or in the rate at which extracellular virus particles enter cells, whether the virus is applied to the apical or basolateral surfaces of the cells (Dingwell *et al.*, 1994).

The lack of phenotype of the single deletion mutants has been later ascribed to the transformed cells in which they were characterized; in cells that form extensive cell junctions, like normal human fibroblasts and epithelial cells, the mutants are compromised (Collins and Johnson, 2003). The deleted viruses are also severely attenuated in vivo, and fail to spread efficiently into and within specialized circuits of the nervous system (Dingwell and Johnson, 1998). Several mechanisms appear to regulate the gE–gI-mediated cell-to-cell spread. Thus, gE–gI facilitate the movement of HSV across the extensive junctions formed between epithelial cells, fibroblasts, and neurons in vivo, likely by sorting the newly assembled virions to lateral surfaces and cell junctions (Johnson *et al.*, 2001), and by promoting envelopment into vesicles that are sorted to epithelial cells of junctions (Johnson and Huber, 2002).

US9

Although PrV is beyond the scope of this chapter, the role of US9 protein is better illustrated in this system. US9 protein is critical in axonal transport and in interneuronal spread of PrV (Enquist *et al.*, 1998; Brideau *et al.*, 2000). Structurally, it is a phosphorylated type II membrane glycoprotein present in the lipid envelope of viral particles and in the infected cell *trans*-Golgi network in a unique tail-anchored topology. Its maintenance in the TGN region is a dynamic process involving retrieval of molecules from the cell surface, mediated by an acidic cluster containing putative phosphorylation sites and by a dileucine endocytosis signal (Brideau *et al.*, 1999). The role of US9 protein in transneuronal spread of PrV was inferred by the phenotype of US9-null mutants, which exhibited a defect in anterograde spread in the visual and cortical circuitry of the rat. Hence, the US9 protein functions together with gE, and gI to promote efficient anterograde transneuronal infection and in the directional spread in the rat central nervous system (Brideau *et al.*, 2000; Tomishima and Enquist, 2001). The phenotype of the US9-null virus is consequent to the ability of the protein to regulate the intracellular traffic of viral proteins in axons. Specifically, in US9-null mutant infections the viral membrane proteins fail to enter axons, while the capsids and tegument proteins do enter axons. These findings have been interpreted as evidence that virion subassemblies, but not complete virions, are transported in the axon, and consequently that the final assembly of virions takes place at the axon periphery (Tomishima and Enquist, 2001). Although a detailed characterization of HSV US9 is missing, the PrV and HSV proteins are likely to behave in a similar manner.

VZV

As compared to HSV, there have been relatively few studies dealing with the topic of VZV egress; they were performed mainly by transmission electron microscopy and immunocytochemistry and made use of a limited number of viral mutants. Indeed, the wealth of deletion and genetically modified viruses that characterizes the studies of HSV egress has no match in VZV. Cumulatively, these studies led to the conclusion that the pathway of VZV egress involves envelopment at the TGN, thus favouring the idea that the virus undergoes a de-envelopement–re-envelopment process.

Three glycoproteins, gE, gI, and gB, play a role in VZV egress. A major focus has been on gE, the most abundant envelope glycoprotein. By contrast with HSV gE, VZV gE is essential (Jones and Grose, 1988; Mo et al., 2000, 2002; Moffat et al., 2004). Electron microscopy showed that gE is absent from perinuclear virions, but present in TGN-derived membranes, and in the cytoplasmic and extracellular virions. The TGN membranes acquire a flattened "C" shape and are decorated with the tegument proteins on the concave face, which appears to serve as a budding site for envelopment (Gershon et al., 1994). gE carries several structural motifs. A tyrosine-based motif in the C-tail acts as a determinant for TGN-targeting, and was interpreted as a driving element for secondary envelopment at TGN (Zhu et al., 1996). A detailed mutational analysis of this domain indicates that proper subcellular localization and cycling of gE depend not only on the tyrosine-containing tetrapeptide related to endocytosis sorting signals, but also on a cluster of acidic amino acids containing casein kinase II phosphorylatable residues (Alconada et al., 1996). gE is phosphorylated by the tegument ORF47 protein kinase; phosphorylation is critical for gE trafficking to the TGN and for its recycling from the plasma membrane (Kenyon et al., 2002). As mentioned above, in the UL47(PK) deletion mutant the lack of gE phosphorylation results in a recycling back to the plasma membrane (Kenyon et al., 2002).

As in HSV, gE forms a complex with gI, and the gE–gI complex is a determinant of VZV cell-to-cell spread, as well as of the maturation, endocytosis and recycling from the plasma membrane of both glycoproteins (Alconada et al., 1998, 1999; Olson and Grose, 1998; Mo et al., 2002); The role of gI in virion morphogenesis was investigated in cells infected with VZV mutants lacking gI, or a portion of gI ectodomain. It was observed that the TGN loses the ability to bind tegument proteins, a property correlated with an overall reduction in cytoplasmic envelopment, and interpreted as confirmation that the TGN acts as site of envelopment (Wang et al., 2001).

The key contribution of VZV gE to cell-to-cell spread is seen not only in cell cultures, but also in an elegant in vivo model developed by the Arvin laboratory, consisting of T-cells or skin cell xenografts in the SCHID-hu mice system (Santos et al., 2000). Of note, in the same system, gI is necessary, despite the fact that it is dispensable in cell culture (Moffat, et al., 2002).

Recent studies with VZV gE have greatly expanded the role of this glycoprotein in replication in general and egress in particular. As part of a larger project to produce recombinant VZV genomes, several mutations were introduced in the cytoplasmic tail of gE, and the mutated gE was inserted back into an otherwise complete VZV genome (Moffat et al., 2004). A single mutation in the YAGL endocytosis motif was lethal, whereas other mutations were not. Shortly thereafter, endocytosis of gE was documented to be an important trafficking mechanism for the delivery of this glycoprotein to the site of virion assembly in the cytoplasm of infected cells (Maresova et al., 2005). Altogether the properties of gE, its role in fusion, as well as the location of its gene next to that of gD in HSV genome (discussed in Chapter 7) make VZV gE the analogue of HSV gD.

A third protein that plays a role in VZV egress is gB, particularly its endodomain. As is the case with gB from HSV and other herpesviruses, the endodomain contains determinants for the intracellular transport and localization of gB, including an ER to Golgi transport signal, and two tyrosine-based internalization signals for trafficking from the plasma membrane to the Golgi. Deletion of the portion of gB endodomain encoding these motifs alters gB localization at the Golgi apparatus and drastically reduces the transport of VZ virions to the extracellular space (Heineman and Hall, 2001, 2002). VZV gB endocytosis, as it relates to fusion activity, has been reviewed in Cole and Grose (2003), and dealt with in Chapter 7.

Thus, in addition to gE, endocytosis of gB and also that of gH have been documented to be a means for their delivery from the surface of the infected cells to the cytoplasmic site of virion assembly (Pasieka et al., 2003, 2004). These studies were performed by first biotinylating cell surface proteins, and then demonstrating that they were subsequently transported to purified virions isolated from infected cells by density gradient sedimentation (Maresova et al., 2004). The results were confirmed by immunolabeling and transmission electron microscopy. Cumulatively, these findings highlight that endocytosis must be added to the trafficking pathways by which glycoproteins can be transported to the cytoplasmic site of envelopment, as part of the de-envelopment–re-envelopment model.

It should be noted that PrV gE does not follow the same trafficking pathways as VZV gE. Also PrV gE is endocytosed.

However, trafficking studies with PrV gE demonstrated that little or no gE from the cell surface is subsequently carried to and incorporated within the virion (Tirabassi and Enquist, 1999). These differences may be related to the fact that gE is an essential glycoprotein in VZV, but not in PrV.

A peculiar morphological feature of VZV egress, not observed with HSV or other herpesviruses, is the exit from the infected cell surface in a distinctive pattern designated as "viral highways." By scanning electron microscopy, these consist of thousands of particles arranged in a linear pathway across the syncytial surfaces. gE is a determinant of this polarized egress (Santos et al., 2000).

Concluding remarks

A growing support to the de-envelopment-re-envelopment pathway of alphaherpesviruses exit has been provided in recent years. In some cases, the evidence rests on conclusions that are not unique, and alternative interpretations of data are possible. As outlined by Enquist and collaborators a few years ago, "evidence supporting both models of herpesvirus exit can be found, and neither model has been disproved conclusively" (Enquist et al., 1998). This remark still holds true.

We also note that most of the attention has been paid to elucidate the role of viral gene products in virus exocytosis, while the contribution of cellular proteins, and of the exocytic compartment in general, has been largely neglected. Studies of the role of cellular functions is complicated by the fact that the cell is deeply modified following HSV infection, e.g., the Golgi apparatus is fragmented into small, but functional pieces, the TGN is redistributed, the architecture of nuclear and cytoplasmic cytoskeleton are altered (Campadelli-Fiume et al., 1993; Avitabile et al., 1995; Scott and O'Hare, 2001; Reynolds et al., 2004; Wisner and Johnson, 2004), phenomena which contribute to mislocalization of cellular markers. These changes are strongly cell line dependent, and may contribute, in part, to apparent discrepancies between different studies. Finally, it is worth noting that most of the studies on alphaherpesviruses' exocytosis have been carried out in cultures of epithelial cells or fibroblasts. Exit from the neuronal cells may well be different.

Acknowledgments

I am grateful to A. Arvin, J. Baines and C. Grose for critical reading, and to L. Menotti for helpful discussion and artwork.

REFERENCES

Ace, C. I., Dalrymple, M. A., Ramsay, F. H., Preston, V. G., and Preston, C. M. (1988). Mutational analysis of the herpes simplex virus type 1 *trans*-inducing factor Vmw65. *J. Gen. Virol.*, **69** (10), 2595–2605.

Alconada, A., Bauer, U., and Hoflack, B. (1996). A tyrosine-based motif and a casein kinase II phosphorylation site regulate the intracellular trafficking of the varicella-zoster virus glycoprotein I, a protein localized in the *trans*-Golgi network. *EMBO J.* **15**, 6096–6110.

Alconada, A., Bauer, U., Baudoux, L., Piette, J., and Hoflack, B. (1998). Intracellular transport of the glycoproteins gE and gI of the varicella-zoster virus. gE accelerates the maturation of gI and determines its accumulation in the *trans*-Golgi network. *J. Biol. Chem.*, **273**, 13430–13436.

Alconada, A., Bauer, U., Sodeik, B., and Hoflack, B. (1999). Intracellular traffic of herpes simplex virus glycoprotein gE: characterization of the sorting signals required for its *trans*-Golgi network localization. *J. Virol.*, **73**, 377–387.

Avitabile, E., Ward, P. L., Di Lazzaro, C., Torrisi, M. R., Roizman, B., and Campadelli-Fiume, G. (1994a). The herpes simplex virus UL20 protein compensates for the differential disruption of exocytosis of virions and membrane glycoproteins associated with fragmentation of the Golgi apparatus. *J. Virol.*, **68**, 7397–7405.

Avitabile, E., Ward, P. L., Di Lazzaro, C., Torrisi, M. R., Roizman, B., and Campadelli-Fiume, G. (1994b). The herpes simplex virus UL20 protein compensates for the differential disruption of exocytosis of virions and viral membrane glycoproteins associated with fragmentation of the Golgi apparatus. *J. Virol.*, **68**, 7397–7405.

Avitabile, E., Di Gaeta, S., Torrisi, M. R., Ward, P. L., Roizman, B., and Campadelli-Fiume, G. (1995). Redistribution of microtubules and Golgi apparatus in herpes simplex virus-infected cells and their role in viral exocytosis. *J. Virol.*, **69**, 7472–7482.

Avitabile, E., Lombardi, G., and Campadelli-Fiume, G. (2003). Herpes simplex virus glycoprotein K, but not its syncytial allele, inhibits cell–cell fusion mediated by the four fusogenic glycoproteins, gD, gB, gH and gL. *J. Virol.*, **77**, 6836–6844.

Avitabile, E., Lombardi, G., Gianni, T., Capri, M., and Campadelli-Fiume, G. (2004). Coexpression of UL20p and gK inhibits cell-cell fusion mediated by herpes simplex virus glycoproteins gD, gH-gL, and wt- gB or an endocytosis-defective gB mutant, and downmodulates their cell surface expression. *J. Virol.* In press.

Baines, J. D. and Roizman, B. (1993). The UL10 gene of herpes simplex virus 1 encodes a novel viral glycoprotein, gM, which is present in the virion and in the plasma membrane of infected cells. *J. Virol.*, **67**, 1441–1452.

Baines, J. D., Ward, P. L., Campadelli-Fiume, G., and Roizman, B. (1991). The UL20 gene of herpes simplex virus 1 encodes a function necessary for viral egress. *J. Virol.*, **65**, 6414–6424.

Batterson, W., Furlong, D., and Roizman, B. (1983). Molecular genetics of herpes simplex virus. VIII. further characterization of a temperature-sensitive mutant defective in release of viral DNA and in other stages of the viral reproductive cycle. *J. Virol.*, **45**, 397–407.

Brack, A. R., Dijkstra, J. M., Granzow, H., Klupp, B. G., and Mettenleiter, T. C. (1999). Inhibition of virion maturation by simultaneous deletion of glycoproteins E, I, and M of pseudorabies virus. *J. Virol.*, **73**, 5364–5372.

Brideau, A. D., del Rio, T., Wolffe, E. J., and Enquist, L. W. (1999). Intracellular trafficking and localization of the pseudorabies virus Us9 type II envelope protein to host and viral membranes. *J. Virol.*, **73**, 4372–4384.

Brideau, A. D., Card, J. P., and Enquist, L. W. (2000). Role of pseudorabies virus Us9, a type II membrane protein, in infection of tissue culture cells and the rat nervous system. *J. Virol.*, **74**, 834–845.

Browne, H., Bell, S., and Minson, T. (2004). Analysis of the requirement for glycoprotein m in herpes simplex virus type 1 morphogenesis. *J. Virol.*, **78**, 1039–1041.

Cai, W. H., Gu, B., and Person, S. (1988). Role of glycoprotein B of herpes simplex virus type 1 in viral entry and cell fusion [published erratum appears in *J. Virol.* 1988 Nov;**62**(11):4438]. *J. Virol.*, **62**, 2596–2604.

Campadelli-Fiume, G., Farabegoli, F., Di Gaeta, S., and Roizman, B. (1991). Origin of unenveloped capsids in the cytoplasm of cells infected with herpes simplex virus 1. *J. Virol.*, **65**, 1589–1595.

Campadelli-Fiume, G., Brandimarti, R., Di Lazzaro, C., Ward, P. L., Roizman, B., and Torrisi, M. R. (1993). Fragmentation and dispersal of Golgi proteins and redistribution of glycoproteins and glycolipids processed through the Golgi apparatus after infection with herpes simplex virus 1. *Proc. Natl Acad. Sci. USA*, **90**, 2798–2802.

Campadelli-Fiume, G. and Roizman, B. (2006), The egress of herpesviruses from cells: the unanswered questions. *J. Virol.* **80**, 6716–6717.

Campbell, M. E., Palfreyman, J. W., and Preston, C. M. (1984). Identification of herpes simplex virus DNA sequences which encode a trans-acting polypeptide responsible for stimulation of immediate early transcription. *J. Mol. Biol.*, **180**, 1–19.

Cole, N. L. and Grose, C. (2003). Membrane fusion mediated by herpesvirus glycoproteins: the paradigm of varicella-zoster virus. *Rev. Med. Virol.*, **13**, 207–222.

Collins, W. J. and Johnson, D. C. (2003). Herpes simplex virus gE/gI expressed in epithelial cells interferes with cell-to-cell spread. *J. Virol.*, **77**, 2686–2695.

Desai, P., Sexton, G. L., McCaffery, J. M., and Person, S. (2001). A null mutation in the gene encoding the herpes simplex virus type 1 UL37 polypeptide abrogates virus maturation. *J. Virol.*, **75**, 10259–10271.

Desai, P. J. (2000). A null mutation in the UL36 gene of herpes simplex virus type 1 results in accumulation of unenveloped DNA-filled capsids in the cytoplasm of infected cells. *J. Virol.*, **74**, 11608–11618.

Di Lazzaro, C., Campadelli-Fiume, G., and Torrisi, M. R. (1995). Intermediate forms of glycoconjugates are present in the envelope of herpes simplex virions during their transport along the exocytic pathway. *Virology*, **214**, 619–623.

Dingwell, K. S. and Johnson, D. C. (1998). The herpes simplex virus gE-gI complex facilitates cell-to-cell spread and binds to components of cell junctions. *J. Virol.*, **72**, 8933–8942.

Dingwell, K. S., Brunetti, C. R., Hendricks, R. L. *et al*. (1994). Herpes simplex virus glycoproteins E and I facilitate cell-to-cell spread in vivo and across junctions of cultured cells. *J. Virol.*, **68**, 834–845.

Elliott, G. and O'Hare, P. (1999). Live-cell analysis of a green fluorescent protein-tagged herpes simplex virus infection. *J. Virol.*, **73**, 4110–4119.

Enquist, L. W., Husak, P. J., Banfield, B. W., and Smith, G. A. (1998). Infection and spread of alphaherpesviruses in the nervous system. *Adv. Virus Res.*, **51**, 237–347.

Farnsworth, A., Goldsmith, K., and Johnson, D. C. (2003). Herpes simplex virus glycoproteins gD and gE/gI serve essential but redundant functions during acquisition of the virion envelope in the cytoplasm. *J. Virol.*, **77**, 8481–8494.

Forrester, A., Farrell, H., Wilkinson, G., Kaye, J., Davis Poynter, N., and Minson, T. (1992). Construction and properties of a mutant of herpes simplex virus type 1 with glycoprotein H coding sequences deleted. *J. Virol.*, **66**, 341–348.

Foster, T. P., Alvarez, X., and Kousoulas, K. G. (2003). Plasma membrane topology of syncytial domains of herpes simplex virus type 1 glycoprotein K (gK): the UL20 protein enables cell surface localization of gK but not gK-mediated cell-to-cell fusion. *J. Virol.*, **77**, 499–510.

Foster, T. P. and Kousoulas, K. G. (1999). Genetic analysis of the role of herpes simplex virus type 1 glycoprotein K in infectious virus production and egress. *J. Virol.*, **73**, 8457–8468.

Foster, T. P., Melancon, J. M., Baines, J. D., and Kousoulas, K. G. (2004). The herpes simplex virus type 1 UL20 protein modulates membrane fusion events during cytoplasmic virion morphogenesis and virus-induced cell fusion. *J. Virol.*, **78**, 5347–5357.

Fuchs, W., Klupp, B. G., Granzow, H., Osterrieder, N., and Mettenleiter, T. C. (2002). The interacting UL31 and UL34 gene products of pseudorabies virus are involved in egress from the host-cell nucleus and represent components of primary enveloped but not mature virions. *J. Virol.*, **76**, 364–378.

Gershon, A. A., Sherman, D. L., Zhu, Z., Gabel, C. A., Ambron, R. T., and Gershon, M. D. (1994). Intracellular transport of newly synthesized varicella-zoster virus: final envelopment in the trans-Golgi network. *J. Virol.*, **68**, 6372–6390.

Harley, C. A., Dasgupta, A., and Wilson, D. W. (2001). Characterization of herpes simplex virus-containing organelles by subcellular fractionation: role for organelle acidification in assembly of infectious particles. *J. Virol.*, **75**, 1236–1251.

Heineman, T. C. and Hall, S. L. (2001). VZV gB endocytosis and Golgi localization are mediated by YXXphi motifs in its cytoplasmic domain. *Virology*, **285**, 42–49.

Heineman, T. C. and Hall, S. L. (2002). Role of the varicella-zoster virus gB cytoplasmic domain in gB transport and viral egress. *J. Virol.*, **76**, 591–599.

Hutchinson, L. and Johnson, D. C. (1995). Herpes simplex virus glycoprotein K promotes egress of virus particles. *J. Virol.*, **69**, 5401–5413.

Johnson, D. C. and Spear, P. G. (1982). Monensin inhibits the processing of herpes simplex virus glycoproteins, their transport to the cell surface, and the egress of virions from infected cells. *J. Virol.*, 43, 1102–1112.

Johnson, D. C. and Huber, M. T. (2002). Directed egress of animal viruses promotes cell-to-cell spread. *J. Virol.*, **76**, 1–8.

Johnson, D. C., Frame, M. C., Ligas, M. W., Cross, A. M., and Stow, N. D. (1988). Herpes simplex virus immunoglobulin G Fc receptor activity depends on a complex of two viral glycoproteins, gE and gI. *J. Virol.*, **62**, 1347–1354.

Johnson, D. C., Webb, M., Wisner, T. W., and Brunetti, C. (2001). Herpes simplex virus gE/gI sorts nascent virions to epithelial cell junctions, promoting virus spread. *J. Virol.*, **75**, 821–833.

Jones, F. and Grose, C. (1988). Role of cytoplasmic vacuoles in varicella-zoster virus glycoprotein trafficking and virion envelopment. *J. Virol.*, **62**, 2701–2711.

Kenyon, T. K., Cohen, J. I., and Grose, C. (2002). Phosphorylation by the varicella-zoster virus ORF47 protein serine kinase determines whether endocytosed viral gE traffics to the *trans*-Golgi network or recycles to the cell membrane. *J. Virol.*, **76**, 10980–10993.

Klupp, B. G., Fuchs, W., Granzow, H., Nixdorf, R., and Mettenleiter, T. C. (2002). Pseudorabies virus UL36 tegument protein physically interacts with the UL37 protein. *J. Virol.*, **76**, 3065–3071.

Leuzinger, H., Ziegler, U., Schraner, E. M. *et al.* (2005). Herpes simplex virus 1 envelopment follows two diverse pathways. *J. Virol.*, **79**, 13047–13059.

Ligas, M. W. and Johnson, D. C. (1988). A herpes simplex virus mutant in which glycoprotein D sequences are replaced by beta-galactosidase sequences binds to but is unable to penetrate into cells. *J. Virol.*, **62**, 1486–1494.

Longnecker, R. and Roizman, B. (1987). Clustering of genes dispensable for growth in culture in the S component of the HSV-1 genome. *Science*, **236**, 573–576.

Longnecker, R., Chatterjee, S., Whitley, R. J., and Roizman, B. (1987). Identification of a herpes simplex virus 1 glycoprotein gene within a gene cluster dispensable for growth in cell culture. *Proc. Natl Acad. Sci. USA*, **84**, 4303–4307.

Maresova, L., Pasieka, T. J., Homan, E., Gerday, E., and Grose, C. (2004). Incorporation of three endocytosed varicella-zoster virus glycoproteins gE, gH and gB into the virion envelope. *J. Virol.*, **79**, 997–1007.

Mettenleiter, T. C. (2002). Herpesvirus assembly and egress. *J. Virol.*, **76**, 1537–1547.

Miranda-Saksena, M., Boadle, R. A., Armati, P., and Cunningham, A. L. (2002). In rat dorsal root ganglion neurons, herpes simplex virus type 1 tegument forms in the cytoplasm of the cell body. *J. Virol.*, **76**, 9934–9951.

Mo, C., Schneeberger, E. E., and Arvin, A. M. (2000). Glycoprotein E of varicella-zoster virus enhances cell–cell contact in polarized epithelial cells. *J. Virol.*, **74**, 11377–11387.

Mo, C., Lee, J., Sommer, M., Grose, C., and Arvin, A. M. (2002). The requirement of varicella zoster virus glycoprotein E (gE) for viral replication and effects of glycoprotein I on gE in melanoma cells. *Virology*, **304**, 176–186.

Moffat, J., Ito, H., Sommer, M., Taylor, S., and Arvin, A. M. (2002). Glycoprotein I of varicella-zoster virus is required for viral replication in skin and T cells. *J. Virol.*, **76**, 8468–8471.

Moffat, J., Mo, C., Cheng, J. *et al.* (2004). Functions of the C-terminal domain of varicella-zoster virus glycoprotein E in viral replication in vitro and skin and T-cell tropism in vivo. *J. Virol.*, **78**, 12406–12415.

Mossman, K. L., Sherburne, R., Lavery, C., Duncan, J., and Smiley, J. R. (2000). Evidence that herpes simplex virus VP16 is required for viral egress downstream of the initial envelopment event. *J. Virol.*, **74**, 6287–6299.

Olson, J. K. and Grose, C. (1998). Complex formation facilitates endocytosis of the varicella-zoster virus gE:gI Fc receptor. *J. Virol.*, **72**, 1542–1551.

Pasieka, T. J., Maresova, L., and Grose, C. (2003). A functional YNKI motif in the short cytoplasmic tail of varicella-zoster virus glycoprotein gH mediates clathrin-dependent and antibody-independent endocytosis. *J. Virol.*, **77**, 4191–4204.

Pasieka, T. J., Maresova, L., Shiraki, K., and Grose, C. (2004). Regulation of varicella-zoster virus-induced cell-to-cell fusion by the endocytosis-competent glycoproteins gH and gE. *J. Virol.*, **78**, 2884–2896.

Penfold, M. E., Armati, P., and Cunningham, A. L. (1994). Axonal transport of herpes simplex virions to epidermal cells: evidence for a specialized mode of virus transport and assembly. *Proc. Natl Acad. Sci., USA*, **91**, 6529–6533.

Pomeranz, L. E. and Blaho, J. A. (2000). Assembly of infectious herpes simplex virus type 1 virions in the absence of full-length VP22. *J. Virol.*, **74**, 10041–10054.

Read, G. S. and Frenkel, N. (1983). Herpes simplex virus mutants defective in the virion-associated shutoff of host polypeptide synthesis and exhibiting abnormal synthesis of alpha (immediate early) viral polypeptides. *J. Virol.*, **46**, 498–512.

Reynolds, A. E., Ryckman, B. J., Baines, J. D., Zhou, Y., Liang, L., and Roller, R. J. (2001). U(L)31 and U(L)34 proteins of herpes simplex virus type 1 form a complex that accumulates at the nuclear rim and is required for envelopment of nucleocapsids. *J. Virol.*, **75**, 8803–8817.

Reynolds, A. E., Wills, E. G., Roller, R. J., Ryckman, B. J., and Baines, J. D. (2002). Ultrastructural localization of the herpes simplex virus type 1 UL31, UL34, and US3 proteins suggests specific roles in primary envelopment and egress of nucleocapsids. *J. Virol.*, **76**, 8939–8952.

Reynolds, A. E., Liang, L., and Baines, J. D. (2004). Conformational changes in the nuclear lamina induced by herpes simplex virus type 1 require genes U(L)31 and U(L)34. *J. Virol.*, **78**, 5564–5575.

Roizman, B. and Knipe, D. M. (2001). Herpes simplex viruses and their replication. In *Fields Virology*, 4th edn, vol. 2, ed. D. M. Knipe, P. Howley, D. Griffin, R. *et al.* pp. 2399–2459. Philadelphia: Lippincott, Williams & Wilkins.

Roller, R. J., Zhou, Y., Schnetzer, R., Ferguson, J., and DeSalvo, D. (2000). Herpes simplex virus type 1 U(L)34 gene product is required for viral envelopment. *J. Virol.*, **74**, 117–129.

Roop, C., Hutchinson, L., and Johnson, D. C. (1993). A mutant herpes simplex virus type 1 unable to express glycoprotein L cannot enter cells, and its particles lack glycoprotein H. *J. Virol.*, **67**, 2285–2297.

Santos, R. A., Hatfield, C. C., Cole, N. L. *et al.* (2000). Varicella-zoster virus gE escape mutant VZV-MSP exhibits an accelerated cell-to-cell spread phenotype in both infected cell cultures and SCID-hu mice. *Virology*, **275**, 306–317.

Scott, E. S. and O'Hare, P. (2001). Fate of the inner nuclear membrane protein lamin B receptor and nuclear lamins in herpes simplex virus type 1 infection. *J. Virol.*, **75**, 8818–8830.

Skepper, J. N., Whiteley, A., Browne, H., and Minson, A. (2001). Herpes simplex virus nucleocapsids mature to progeny virions by an envelopment –> deenvelopment –> reenvelopment pathway. *J. Virol.*, **75**, 5697–5702.

Stackpole, C. W. (1969). Herpes-type virus of the frog renal adenocarcinoma. I. Virus development in tumor transplants maintained at low temperature. *J. Virol.*, **4**, 75–93.

Tirabassi, R. S. and Enquist, L. W. (1999). Mutation of the YXXL endocytosis motif in the cytoplasmic tail of pseudorabies virus gE. *J. Virol.*, **73**, 2717–2728.

Tomishima, M. J. and Enquist, L. W. (2001). A conserved alphaherpesvirus protein necessary for axonal localization of viral membrane proteins. *J. Cell Biol.*, **154**, 741–752.

Torrisi, M. R., Di Lazzaro, C., Pavan, A., Pereira, L., and Campadelli-Fiume, G. (1992). Herpes simplex virus envelopment and maturation studied by fracture label. *J. Virol.*, **66**, 554–561.

Turner, A., Bruun, B., Minson, T., and Browne, H. (1998). Glycoproteins gB, gD, and gHgL of herpes simplex virus type 1 are necessary and sufficient to mediate membrane fusion in a Cos cell transfection system. *J. Virol.*, **72**, 873–875.

van Genderen, I. L., Brandimarti, R., Torrisi, M. R., Campadelli, G., and van Meer, G. (1994). The phospholipid composition of extracellular herpes simplex virions differs from that of host cell nuclei. *Virology*, **200**, 831–6.

Wang, Z. H., Gershon, M. D., Lungu, O. *et al.* (2001). Essential role played by the C-terminal domain of glycoprotein I in envelopment of varicella-zoster virus in the *trans*-Golgi network: interactions of glycoproteins with tegument. *J. Virol.*, **75**, 323–340.

Whiteley, A., Bruun, B., Minson, T., and Browne, H. (1999). Effects of targeting herpes simplex virus type 1 gD to the endoplasmic reticulum and *trans*-Golgi network. *J. Virol.*, **73**, 9515–9520.

Wild, P. and Engels, M. (2004). Impairment of nuclear pores in bovine herpesvirus 1 infected MDBK cells. *J. Virol.*, xx, xx.

Wisner, T. W. and Johnson, D. C. (2004). Redistribution of cellular and herpes simplex virus proteins from the *trans*-Golgi network to cell junctions without enveloped capsids. *J. Virol.*, **78**, 11519–11535.

Yao, Z., Jackson, W., Forghani, B., and Grose, C. (1993). Varicella-zoster virus glycoprotein gpI/gpIV receptor: expression, complex formation, and antigenicity within the vaccinia virus-T7 RNA polymerase transfection system. *J. Virol.*, **67**, 305–314.

Ye, G. J. and Roizman, B. (2000). The essential protein encoded by the UL31 gene of herpes simplex virus 1 depends for its stability on the presence of UL34 protein. *Proc. Natl Acad. Sci. USA*, **97**, 11002–11007.

Zhu, Z., Hao, Y., Gershon, M. D., Ambron, R. T., and Gershon, A. A. (1996). Targeting of glycoprotein I (gE) of varicella-zoster virus to the *trans*-Golgi network by an AYRV sequence and an acidic amino acid-rich patch in the cytosolic domain of the molecule. *J. Virol.*, **70**, 6563–6575.

Zuckermann, F. A., Mettenleiter, T. C., Schreurs, C., Sugg, N., and Ben-Porat, T. (1988). Complex between glycoproteins gI and gp63 of pseudorabies virus: its effect on virus replication. *J. Virol.*, **62**, 4622–4626.

The strategy of herpes simplex virus replication and takeover of the host cell

Bernard Roizman and Brunella Taddeo

The Marjorie B. Kovler Viral Oncology Laboratories, The University of Chicago, USA

Introduction

The fundamental mission of all viruses is to replicate and spread, and above all, to persist in the host environment to which they have become adapted. Viruses vary with respect to the mechanisms by which they attain their objectives. This variation is reflected not only in the basic mechanisms of viral entry into cells, synthesis of viral proteins, viral nuclei acid synthesis, virion assembly, and egress but also with respect to the basic strategies by which they preclude the enormous resources of the host cell and of the multicellular organism from totally blocking viral replication. The terminology used: "totally blocking" is appropriate; in essence the evolution of functions encoded in the viral genome reflects a fundamental accommodation between replication and spread as well as persistence in the human population. A replication and spread that kills the host will not permit the survival of the virus. The objective of this chapter is to examine the basic strategies evolved by HSV to replicate in its cellular environment.

Gene content, organization, and fundamental design of the viral genome

Several aspects of the structure, content and function of the viral genome are worthy of note. They are as follows.

(i) We do not know with any degree of certainty the exact number of transcriptional units or proteins encoded by the viral genome. The problem stems from several considerations. The initial enumeration of open reading frames (ORFs) excluded sequences that lacked a TATA box, a canonical methionine intiation codon, a suitable length, or that situated antisense to a known or readily demonstrable ORF. The current list of HSV sequences that are expressed (see section on gene content) includes RNAs that do not appear to encode proteins (e.g., Oris RNAs), TATA-less ORFs (e.g., $\gamma_1 34.5$), and ORFs that are antisense to each other (e.g., ORF P and ORF O vs. $\gamma_1 34.5$, $U_L 43.5$ vs. $U_L 43$, $U_L 27.5$ vs. $U_L 27$, $U_L 9.5$ vs. $U_L 10$).

(ii) Viral proteins can express multiple functions. The order of expression of these functions may be regulated by post-translational modification of the proteins or by interacting proteins present within various compartments of the cell. For example, the interaction of ICP22 with cellular proteins is determined by the status of post-translational phosphorylation by viral kinases (Leopardi et al., 1997b; Purves and Roizman, 1992; Purves et al., 1993). Post-translational modification of ICP0 is also required for its ubiquitin-ligase activities (Boutell et al., 2002; Hagglund et al., 2002) but is not necessary for other functions required for optimal replication of the virus such as its interactions with CoREST (Gu et al., 2005).

A powerful mechanism for regulation of specific functions encoded in a single protein is the synthesis from an independent transcriptional unit of a truncated protein whose sequence is colinear with the carboxyl-terminal domain of the larger protein. The functions encoded by the truncated proteins could enhance (e.g., $U_S 1.5$ vs. $\alpha 22$) (Carter and Roizman, 1996; Purves et al., 1993) or inhibit ($U_L 8.5$ vs. $U_L 9$) (Baradaran et al., 1994) the function of the larger protein.

(iii) There is little doubt that herpes simplex virions contain at least three proteins ($U_S 11$, $U_L 47$ and $U_L 49$) that bind RNA from the infected cell and translocate it into the newly infected cell (Roller and Roizman, 1990; Sciortino et al., 2002). Evidence has been reported that this RNA can be expressed (Sciortino et al., 2002). A central issue is the impact of this RNA on the outcome of infection. A fundamental unanswered question is why HSV would carry RNA rather than more tegument proteins. One argument presented by Shenk (2002) is that proteins destined to membranes or secretory pathway would have to be made *de novo* and cannot be brought as components of the tegument.

(iv) The presence and function of the inverted repeats has been a long-standing puzzle. The repeats are present in many, but not in all herpesvirus genomes. Mutants lacking the inverted repeats replicate well in cultured cells but tend to be avirulent in experimental animals. The loss of virulence has been attributed to the loss of one copy of the $\gamma_1 34.5$ genes but in fact one copy of the $\gamma_1 34.5$ gene is sufficient to block the shut off of protein synthesis by activated protein kinase R (PKR) (He *et al.*, 1997a).

(v) As detailed in the section on gene content, more than half of the transcriptional units contained in the viral genome are not essential for viral replication at least in cultured cells. The functions encoded by many of these genes are unknown. Preliminary studies suggest that some genes may play a role in viral maturation or spread. Those that have been studied in detail (e.g., ICP0, $U_L 41$, $\gamma_1 34.5$, $U_S 3$, $U_L 47$, etc.) as well as some of the essential genes (e.g., $\alpha 27$) appear to encode function designed to block host responses to infection. The key observation relevant to this section is that viruses lacking non-essential genes do not circulate in nature and that in most instances mutants lacking one or more of these genes tend to be either incapable of replication or are less virulent than wild-type viruses in experimental animals.

In essence, the functional content of the HSV genome is not fully understood. We do not know the total number of diverse functions encoded by the viral genome. What is readily apparent is that many of the known functions encoded by the virus are directed toward total control of the infected cell. Some of these functions are redundant: they are expressed by different proteins but ultimately have the same objective. Since the functions of many "dispensable" proteins are not yet identified, there may be additional anti-host functions yet to be discovered.

Mobilization of cellular proteins for enhanced replication of HSV

There are three examples that illustrate recruitment and post-translational modifications that benefit viral replication. Current wisdom is that, on discharge of the viral DNA into the nucleoplasm, it is confronted by a wide range of cellular proteins that assemble around it and, if allowed to prevail, are likely to either enable minimal transcription or silence it, and viral transcriptional factors (e.g., α-transinducing factor or VP16) that activate transcription and ultimately enable its replication. Recent studies from several laboratories indicated the presence of histones associated with viral DNA but it is unclear whether the histones are associated with a small fraction or the vast majority of the DNA (Poon *et al.*, 2003). One perennial candidate for restructuring of DNA protein complexes to enable efficient transcription is ICP0, a product of the $\alpha 0$ gene (for review, see Hagglund and Roizman, 2004). ICP0 is a promiscuous transactivator of genes introduced into cells by infection or transfection, that is presumably of genes associated with cellular proteins but which have not yet assumed a tight chromatin structure. In recent studies unmodified ICP0, i.e., ICP0 made before significant accumulation of viral protein kinases, interacts with CoREST/REST and HDAC1 complexes and disrupts the interaction of HDAC1 with CoREST/REST complex (Gu *et al.*, 2005). Ultimately, late viral functions promote the export of CoREST and HDAC1 to the cytoplasm. This function of ICP0 is consistent with the hypothesis that activation of transcription of the viral genome is essential for efficient expression of viral genes and for denuding the DNA from cellular proteins that impede transcription and ultimately replication of viral DNA.

The second example centers on the observation that, early in infection, HSV-1 $U_L 13$ kinase mediates the hyperphosphorylation of the translation elongation factor EF-1δ, an event associated with more efficient protein synthesis (Kawaguchi *et al.*, 1998). The $U_L 13$ protein kinase is highly conserved among members of all three subfamilies of herpesviruses and studies on representative members indicate that this function of the $U_L 13$ orthologs is also conserved (Kawaguchi *et al.*, 1999).

The third example relates to the function of ICP22, a product of the $\alpha 22$ gene. Mutants lacking this gene grow poorly and synthesize suboptimal amounts of a subset of late (γ_2) proteins exemplified by the $U_S 11$, $U_L 38$ and $U_L 41$ proteins in primary human cell cultures and in some non-human cell lines (Purves *et al.*, 1993). ICP22 is a multifunctional protein. The functions enabling optimal synthesis of the subset of late proteins map to the carboxyl-terminal domain of ICP22 (Ogle and Roizman, 1999). At least two functions of ICP22 may account for the optimal synthesis of this subset of late viral proteins. First, ICP22 and $U_L 13$ stabilize and activate the cyclin-dependent kinase cdc2 but enable the degradation of its partners, cyclins A and B (Advani *et al.*, 2000). cdc2 acquires a new partner, the HSV-1 DNA polymerase accessory protein encoded by $U_L 42$ ORF (Advani *et al.*, 2001). The cdc2-$U_L 42$ complex binds topoisomerase IIα – all in an ICP22-dependent manner (Advani *et al.*, 2003). It has been postulated that the mRNA encoding the subset of late proteins is transcribed off progeny DNA contained in massive tangles of concatemeric DNA and that the presence of the topoisomerase enables more efficient transcription of the DNA. A second function of ICP22 and U_L13 protein kinase reported initially by Spencer and colleagues is to mediate the post-translational modification of the carboxyl-terminal domain of RNA polymerase II (RNA POL II) (Long et al., 1999; Rice et al., 1994, 1995). The modified RNA POL II acquires an "intermediate electrophoretic mobility" (RNA POL IIi). Recent studies in this laboratory indicate ICP22 interacts with the U_S3 protein kinase to recruit cdk9, a cyclin-dependent kinase involved in transcription (Durand et al., 2005). The cdk9–ICP22 complex can phosphorylate the carboxyl-terminal domain of RNA POL II in vitro. This interaction appears to be independent of the posttranslational modification of RNA POL IIi. The presumption is that these modifications of RNA POL II enable more efficient elongation in the course of mRNA synthesis.

These are but three examples of modification of cellular structures designed to enhance the synthesis of viral gene products. Additional modifications are likely to emerge.

The objectives and general strategy of anti-host functions

A cursory review of the anti-host functions expressed by HSV indicates that they fall into four categories. In essence HSV (i) selectively blocks the synthesis of new proteins, (ii) blocks the function of preexisting cellular proteins activated after infection, (iii) selectively degrades cellular proteins (iv) blocks signaling to the host immune system indicating that the cell is infected. These functions are also expressed by other alphaherpesviruses and to a lesser extent by members of the beta- and gamma- herpesviruses. The fundamental strategy of HSV as opposed to that of members of the beta- and gamma- herpesviruses is to encode proteins that bind and subvert the function of cellular proteins. Unlike beta- and gamma-herpesviruses, HSV does not make extensive use of cellular orthologs to reinforce, substitute or block the function of cellular genes. At most, HSV encodes a short amino acid sequence related to that of a cellular protein such as the one present at the carboxyl terminal of the $\gamma_134.5$ protein. This sequence is homologous to that of the corresponding domain of the GADD34 gene (Mohr and Gluzman, 1996).

The activation of NF-κB

On the basis of viral efforts to suppress its activation, NF-κB may well be viewed as a nemesis of viral replication and spread. Activation of NF-κB results in the synthesis of cytokines and growth factors that would lead to a potentially undesirable host response to infection (for review, see Santoro et al., 2003). In HSV-1 infected cells NF-κB is activated (Amici et al., 2001, Patel et al., 1998), although studies on just a few products induced by activated NF-κB suggest that synthesis of NF-κB-dependent proteins may be selective (Esclatine et al., 2004a,c).

In human and mouse cells tested to date, stable activation of NF-κB requires activated PKR (Taddeo et al., 2003b). This protein is resident in cells and is activated by interferon and double stranded RNAs (for review, see Williams, 2001). Activated PKR phosphorylates the α subunit of the translation initiation factor 2 (eIF-2α). In turn, eIF-2α-P shuts off protein synthesis. Activated PKR could be viewed as an ancient response to infection and viruses have evolved many and diverse strategies to block its activation. Indeed HSV-1 contains a late gene: U_S11 which, when expressed early, blocks activation of PKR (Cassady et al., 1998). HSV has evolved a very different but puzzling strategy to deal with PKR. Instead of blocking its activation, HSV encodes a protein, $\gamma_134.5$, which binds the protein phosphatase 1α and redirects it to dephosphorylate eIF-2α (He et al., 1997a,b, 1998). This strategy makes little sense in light of the observation that HSV-1 yields are 10- to 50-fold higher in PKR−/− cells than in sibling PKR+/+ cells (Taddeo et al., 2004a). HSV requires activated PKR for some of its functions. Several lines of evidence indicate that activation of NF-κB is tied to activation of PKR. Thus, NF-κB is not activated by wild-type virus in infected PKR−/− cells. The HSV-1 mutant virus R5104 in which U_S11 was converted from a γ_2 to an early gene replicates as well as the wild-type virus but does not induce NF-κB (Taddeo et al., 2003b).

A central question is why NF-κB is induced. As indicated above, wild-type HSV-1 replicated better in PKR−/− cells than in the sibling, PKR+/+ cells. In contrast, the yields of wild-type virus were at least 10-fold lower in NF-κB knockout fibroblasts, i.e. p50−/−, p65−/− and p50/p65−/− cells than in wild-type cells derived from NF-κB+/+ siblings (Taddeo et al., 2004a). Currently, two hypotheses prevail. One hypothesis holds that NF-κB induces the synthesis of proteins that are required to block apoptosis (Goodkin et al., 2003; Gregory et al., 2004). The other hypothesis is that HSV-1 requires NF-κB-dependent proteins for its replication. This laboratory failed to find support for the first hypothesis. Indeed, HSV-1 encodes at least three proteins known to block apoptosis (see below) and p50−/−, p65−/− and p50/p65−/− cells appear to be resistant to apoptosis induced by defective HSV-1 viruses, although they are sensitive to exogenous pro-apoptotic agents

(Taddeo et al., 2004a). The second hypothesis remains unproven.

Degradation of mRNA in infected cells

Studies carried out several decades ago (Roizman et al., 1965; Sydiskis and Roizman, 1966, 1968) showed that cellular protein synthesis is downregulated, but the mechanisms did not become apparent until Frenkel and associates (Kwong et al., 1988; Strom and Frenkel, 1987) described the role of U_L41 protein, dubbed *vhs* for virion host shutoff, in degrading mRNA (for review, see Smiley, 2004). The typical experiment designed to show the degradation involved a short labeled amino acid pulse at a time after infection. The results of these experiments showed that incorporation of amino acids into both viral and cellular proteins was diminished in wild-type virus infected cells but not in ΔU_L41 mutant infected cells. Other studies demonstrated that both viral and cellular mRNAs were degraded but that viral RNA transcripts nevertheless accumulated in infected cells, possibly as a consequence of higher rates of transcription of viral genes.

Subsequent studies reported that U_L41 interacted with the translation elongation factors eIF-4H and eIF-4B to degrade mRNA beginning at or near its 5′ terminus (Doepker et al., 2004; Everly et al., 2002; Karr and Read, 1999; Perez-Parada et al., 2004). Moreover, consistent with the observation that U_L41 is a γ_2 structural protein made late in infection and hence if active would preclude the synthesis of viral protein, it was shown that the degradation of RNA ablated several hours after infection very likely as a consequence of the interaction of U_L41 protein with VP16 encoded by the U_L48 ORF (Smibert et al., 1994). Other studies demonstrated that the shut-off of cellular protein synthesis was also the consequence of the function of ICP27. Early in infection ICP27 blocks the splicing of mRNA (Hardwicke and Sandri-Goldin, 1994). Late in infection, defined in reference to the initiation of synthesis of viral DNA, ICP27 shuttles between the nucleus and cytoplasm (Sandri-Goldin, 1998). The anti-RNA splicing functions of ICP27 do not appear to affect viral gene expression since, of the four transcriptional units that yield spliced mRNAs, three ($\alpha 0$, $\alpha 22$, $\alpha 47$) are expressed before the effect of ICP27 becomes apparent whereas the fourth (U_L15) is expressed at a time when ICP27 shuttles RNA. The net effect of blocking splicing is that unspliced mRNA is transported into the cytoplasm.

More recent studies (Esclatine et al., 2004a,c; Taddeo et al., 2003a) indicate that the degradation of cellular mRNA is a consequence of a process far more complex than that deduced from earlier studies. In essence, the degradation of mRNA and the mechanism by which this degradation is achieved appears to vary. In the case of housekeeping and constitutively expressed mRNAs (e.g., GAPDH and β-actin) the mRNAs are rapidly degraded very early after infection by an unknown mechanism in a U_L41-dependent fashion (Esclatine et al., 2004c). In contrast, several mRNAs induced after infection and which normally have a relatively short half-life appear to linger even though the translation products may or may not accumulate. For example, IEX-1 mRNA is induced after infection (Taddeo et al., 2002, 2003b). This mRNA contains AU-rich pentameric elements (AREs) in its 3′ untranslated region (UTR) that signal a short half-life (Bakheet et al., 2003; Chen and Shyu, 1995). In mock-infected cells subject to stress this mRNA is made and then sequestered in exosomes (for review, see Butler, 2002) by members of the tristetraprolin (TTP) family (Chen et al., 2001) and rapidly degraded in a 3′ to 5′ direction (Wilusz et al., 2001). IEX-1 mRNA induced in ΔU_L41-infected cells is subject to a similar rapid degradation process (Esclatine et al., 2004c). Unlike the situation in mock-infected cells, the mRNA appears to be stable in wild-type virus infected cells (Esclatine et al., 2004c). However, a more detailed examination of the mRNA accumulating in the cytoplasm of wild-type virus infected cells indicated that this mRNA consists of full-length processed mRNA, mRNA containing the single intron of IEX-1, and finally, truncated forms of the mRNAs (Esclatine et al., 2004a; Taddeo et al., 2003a). The bulk of full-length mRNAs appear to be deadenylated. The truncated forms arise by 3′ to 5′ degradation and endonucleolytic cleavage at or near AREs (Esclatine et al., 2004a). It is thus not surprising that IEX-1 protein is not detected beyond the first hour after infection. A similar picture is presented by mRNAs encoding IκBα and c-*fos* (Esclatine et al., 2004a). Although all of these mRNAs contain AREs, not all AREs-containing mRNAs are subject to a similar fate. Thus TTP mRNA, which contains AREs in the 3′ UTR (Brooks et al., 2004), is upregulated and translated to yield relatively large amounts of protein (Esclatine et al., 2004a,b; Taddeo et al., 2004b). Another mRNA, that of GADD45β, is also upregulated and translated (Esclatine et al., 2004a). This mRNA does not contain AREs.

The model that best takes into account the available data is that HSV attempts to counter the multiple pathways of activation of stress responses by insuring that they are fully activated (e.g., specific activation of NF-κB) and then blocking those that are inimical to viral replication. Among these are responses that signal to the environment that the cell is infected or that activate pro-apoptotic pathways. A key cellular gene activated in the course of infection and which may be the basis of discrimination between mRNAs that are degraded and those that are not is TTP. As noted above, members of the TTP family regulate the life span of AREs mRNAs (for review, see Blackshear, 2002). As yet, preliminary studies indicate that U_L41 protein interacts with components of the exosome (Esclatine et al., 2004b; B. Taddeo and B. Roizman, unpublished data). Of the many issues yet unresolved is the mechanism by which some mRNAs containing AREs (e.g., TTP mRNA) are less rapidly degraded than those encoding IEX-1 or the molecular basis for the U_L41-dependent rapid degradation of GAPDH or β-actin mRNAs as compared to those of mRNAs containing AREs (Esclatine et al., 2004c).

Specific degradation of cellular proteins in wild-type virus-infected cells

It could be expected that proteins with a relatively short half-life and whose mRNA is degraded after infection, as described above, would disappear and not be replenished in the wild-type virus infected cells. An example of just such a protein is Jak1, described later in the text. Analyses of a relatively small number of cellular proteins led to the discovery of several proteins that turn over in infected cells in a manner dependent on α0 rather than on U_L41 and α27 genes. The cellular proteins degraded in an ICP0-dependent manner include the promyelocytic leukemia protein (PML) SP100, the centromeric proteins (CNP) A and C, and the DNA-dependent protein kinase. In contrast to the disappearance of the proteins listed above, cyclins D3 and D1 turned over at a much slower rate or were stabilized over many hours after infection (for review, see Hagglund and Roizman, 2004).

ICP0 is a 775-residue protein translated from a spliced mRNA. The coding sequences are derived from 3 exons containing 19, 241, and 515 residues, respectively. The protein contains a RING finger located between residues 116 and 156 of exon 2. The protein was shown to interact physically with a ubiquitin specific protease (USP7), EF-1δ, the transcriptional factor BMAL and a protein of unknown function designated as p60 (for review, see Hagglund and Roizman, 2004). Early in infection ICP0 localizes in nuclear structures known as PODs, ND10, etc. Within a few hours after infection, ICP0 mediates the degradation of ND10 structures and becomes dispersed throughout the cytoplasm. After the onset of viral DNA synthesis, ICP0 is translocated into the cytoplasm. The available data indicate that ICP0 is actually retained in the cytoplasm by a β or γ_1 function until viral DNA synthesis inasmuch as in cells infected with the d120 (Δα4) mutant, ICP0 is translocated to the cytoplasm and aggregated with proteasomes after the degradation of ND10 but within a very short time after infection (Lopez et al., 2001).

Three lines of investigation led to the realization that ICP0 acts as a two-sited ubiquitin ligase (for review, see Hagglund and Roizman, 2004). First, ICP0 has many features similar to that of ubiquitin ligases. Thus the RING finger is characteristic of many ubiquitin ligases and ICP0 dynamically interacts with proteasomal components. Second, the dispersal of ND10 could be directly related to the ICP0 domain encoding the RING finger. The third line of evidence emerged from studies of the interaction of ICP0 with cyclins D3 and D1. Thus, it has been shown that ICP0 could interact physically and genetically with cyclin D3, but not with cyclin D1, and independently that cdc34 was degraded in infected cells in a proteasome- and ICP0-dependent manner. The observations that both proteins did not turn over as rapidly as expected and that no new transcripts were detected suggested that ICP0 blocks their turnover possibly by degrading the ubiquitin conjugating enzyme (cdc34 or UbcH3) responsible for the degradation of cyclin D1 in uninfected cells. In vitro substrate-independent assays showed that cdc34 was polyubiquitylated in an ATP-dependent manner by sequences encoded by exon 3 rather than the expected exon 2 (Hagglund and Roizman, 2002; Hagglund et al., 2002). The ubiquitylation activity was mapped to residues 621 to 624 and indeed viral mutant carrying ICP0 gene lacking these sequences did not bind or mediate the degradation of cdc34 or the stabilization of the D cyclins (Hagglund and Roizman, 2002). In addition, RING domain mutants did not affect the degradation of cdc34. The ubiquitin conjugating enzymatic site mapping in the sequences encoded by exon 3 was designated herpesvirus ubiquitin ligase 1 (HUL-1), does not resemble in sequence any of the known ubiquitin ligases and may therefore represent a new class of these enzymes.

The in vitro substrate-independent ubiquitylation assays indicated that the sequences encoded by exon 2 polyubiquitylated UbcH5A and UbcH6 ubiquitin conjugating enzymes but not a large number of others. This observation indicated that exon 2 encodes a second ubiquitin conjugating enzyme (HUL-2) (for review, see Hagglund and Roizman, 2004) and further assays using dominant negative ubiquitin conjugating enzymes established that HUL-2 employs UbcH5A to degrade PML, SP100, and the DNA-dependent protein kinase (Gu and Roizman, 2003). The context of the interaction of ICP0 with UbcH6 or the mechanism by which ICP0 mediates the degradation of CENP-C and CENP-A are not known. It is conceivable that ICP0 targets other protein for degradation.

The objectives attained by the degradation of cdc34 and PML are at least in part apparent. By degrading cdc34,

HSV precludes the degradation of cyclin D3. This protein appears to mediate the transport of ICP0 to the ND10 structure and later to the cytoplasm. A mutation that affects the binding of ICP0 to cyclin D3 affects viral replication in stationary cells and reduces the viability of the virus administered at a peripheral site from invading the central nervous system (Hagglund and Roizman, 2003). Stabilization of cyclin D3 does not drive the cell into the S phase.

PML is the organizing protein of the ND10 structures. An extensive literature attributes to ND10 numerous functions related to transactivation or repression of cellular genes (for review, see Everett, 2001; Regad and Chelbi-Alix, 2001). Ectopic overexpression of PML did not affect viral replication, although it resulted in the formation of highly enlarged ND10 structures that were not dispersed in the course of HSV-1 infection (Lopez et al., 2002). Similarly, wild-type virus replicated equally well in both PML−/− and PML+/+ cells. However, on pretreatment of cells with either interferon α or γ resulted in a significantly higher decrease in viral replication in PML+/+ cells as compared to PML−/− cells (Chee et al., 2003). The necessary conclusion derived from these studies is that the activation of the antiviral state is mediated through ND10 and that the objective of degrading PML and dispersal of ND10 is to preclude the potential inhibition of viral replication by exogenous interferon.

Shut down of the interferon pathways to host resistance to infection

The preceding sections cited several mechanisms by which HSV blocks interferon-mediated pathways of host resistance to infection.

(i) Both $\gamma_1 34.5$ and, to a lesser, degree $U_S 11$ proteins circumvent the consequences of phosphorylatation of eIF-2α, the former by sequestering and redirecting phosphatase 1α to dephosphorylate eIF-2α (He et al., 1997a,b, 1998). The effect on the interferon pathway is apparent from the observation that $\Delta \gamma_1 34.5$ mutants are highly attenuated in wild-type mice but not in mice lacking interferon receptors (Leib et al., 1999, 2000).

(ii) Some of the proteins in the interferon pathways have a relatively short half life (e.g., Jak1). The $U_L 41$-dependent RNase activity blocks the replenishment of Jak1 and possibly other proteins in the pathway (Chee and Roizman, 2004).

(iii) As noted above, absence or overexpression of PML has no effect on viral replication. The role of PML and the objective of insuring its degradation are readily apparent in interferon-treated cells. In absence of PML, the infected cells are insensitive to either α- or γ-interferon (Chee et al., 2003). Thus the interferon-based activation of antiviral genes is mediated via the ND10 structures. By targeting PML for degradation, HSV pre-empts antiviral activity of exogenously produced interferon.

Consistent with the overall strategy of viral interference with host defense mechanisms, the pathways by which the HSV blocks the interferon pathways of host defense are redundant but the above list may not be exhaustive. For example, in recent studies it has been observed that the cells surface receptor for interferon γ is rapidly reduced after infection (Y. Liang and B. Roizman, unpublished data). The mechanism by which HSV causes a reduction in the amount of this receptor is not yet known. It is conceivable that as yet other anti-interferon pathways are encoded by the viral genome.

HSV blocks pro-apoptotic cellular functions

Programmed cell death or apoptosis is a mechanism by which a multicellular organism rids itself of unwanted cells. External or internal stimuli activate a cascade of proteases that degrade essential proteins and ultimately the cellular DNA. In the context of infection, apoptosis is a supreme sacrifice by cells to diminish the impact of the infection and enable the survival of the organism. While earlier studies on other viruses and human cytomegalovirus (Shen and Shenk, 1995; Zhu et al., 1995) anticipated that HSV-1 would regulate apoptosis, three fundamental reports initiated an exciting excursion into the control of pro-apoptotic pathways by HSV. Thus, within a short time, three laboratories reported that HSV blocked apoptosis induced by FAS ligand (Galvan and Roizman, 1998; Jerome et al., 1999, 2001; Sieg et al., 1996), osmotic shock, thermal shock (Galvan and Roizman, 1998; Galvan et al., 1999; Koyama and Miwa, 1997; Leopardi and Roizman, 1996), and a defective viral mutant lacking the genes encoding ICP4 (Galvan and Roizman, 1998; Sieg et al., 1996; Munger et al., 2001). Subsequent studies identified at least two other viral mutants capable of inducing apoptosis and at least four genes whose products block programmed cell death induced by viral gene products or by a variety of exogenous agents (Aubert and Blaho, 1999; Benetti et al., 2003; Jerome et al., 1999, 2001; Leopardi et al., 1997a; Munger and Roizman 2001; Munger et al., 2001; Murata et al., 2002; Perkins et al., 2002; Zhou and Roizman, 2001; Zhou et al., 2000). The key issues are the mechanisms by which viral or exogenous biologic agents induced programmed cell death and the mechanisms by which the virus blocks apoptosis. The current literature may be summarized as follows.

(i) Wild-type HSV-1 does not induce apoptosis in cultured cells in the course of productive infection. Viral mutants reported to induce apoptosis are those lacking α4 (Galvan and Roizman, 1998; Leopardi and Roizman, 1996; Munger et al., 2001), α27 (Aubert and Blaho, 1999) or U_L39, the gene encoding the major subunit of ribonucleotide reductase (Perkins et al., 2002). The mechanism by which these mutants induce apoptosis is not clear. There is no compelling evidence to support the argument that all viral mutants induce apoptosis by a similar mechanism. For example, the mutant lacking the α4 genes induces apoptosis in virtually all cell lines tested to date including Vero cells, whereas the mutant lacking the α27 gene induces apoptosis in some cell lines but not in Vero cells (Aubert and Blaho, 1999). Overexpression of ICP22, ICP0 or ICP27 did not lead to apoptosis in several of the cell lines tested.

(ii) Of the four viral proteins shown to block apoptosis, i.e., ribonucleotide reductase, the U_S3 protein kinase, and the glycoproteins D and J (gD and gJ), only three have been studied in some detail. Nothing is known of the mechanism of action of the U_L39 gene product other than the observation that ΔU_L39 mutants complemented by U_L39 protein do not induce apoptosis (Perkins et al., 2002). It should be noted that the HSV-2 U_L39 protein encodes a kinase but the substrates of the kinase other than itself are not known.

(iii) Ectopic expression of the U_S3 protein kinase was initially reported to block apoptosis induced by the Δα4 mutant (Leopardi and Roizman, 1996). Subsequently, this protein was shown to block apoptosis induced by a variety of agents including sorbitol, ectopic expression of several pro-apoptotic genes including BAD, Bax, Bid (Benetti et al., 2003; Munger and Roizman, 2001; Ogg et al., 2004). Curiously, U_S3 does not appear to phosphorylate BAD contrary to the published report inasmuch as BAD protein lacking the known phosphorylation sites induces apoptosis that is blocked by the U_S3 protein kinase (Benetti et al., 2003). ΔU_S3 mutants induce apoptosis albeit weakly and only in some cell lines (e.g., rabbit skin cells) but not in human or primate cells susceptible to apoptosis induction by other viral mutants. More recent studies have shown that the substrate specificity of U_S3 protein kinase is very similar to that of cyclic AMP dependent protein kinase A (PKA) (Benetti and Roizman, 2003). Thus forskolin, an inducer of PKA, blocks apoptosis induced by the Δα4 mutants, and that a specific inhibitory peptide that blocks activation of PKA reverses the effect of forskolin. U_S3 also mediates the phosphorylation of the regulatory subunit of PKA in in vitro studies. Still more recent studies place U_S3 in mitochondria (Van Minnebruggen et al., 2003). The data suggest that the anti-apoptotic substrates of U_S3 protein kinase are mitochondrial proteins and that activated PKA may substitute for the U_S3 protein kinase in blocking apoptosis.

(iv) The role of gD and gJ in blocking apoptosis emerged from the observation that viral mutant stocks lacking gD in both the gene and the protein in the virion envelope (gD−/−) or viral stocks lacking the gD gene but containing the glycoprotein provided by cells ectopically expressing the protein (gD−/+) induced apoptosis that was blocked by ectopic expression of gD or gJ (Zhou and Roizman, 2001; Zhou et al., 2000). The mechanisms by which the two stocks induce apoptosis differ. The model that best fits the results of the studies on gD as the blocker of apoptosis is as follows. In cells exposed to high rations of gD−/− mutant per cell, the virus enters the cells by endocytosis and triggers massive lysosomal discharge that causes cell death. Consistent with these events, chloroquine blocks apoptosis induced by gD−/− mutants (Zhou and Roizman, 2002a). To block apoptosis, gD must be either intact or consist of ectodomain and transmembrane domain linked by disulfate bonds to a transmembrane domain and a cytoplasmic domain (Zhou and Roizman, 2002b). In contrast, gD−/+ mutant stocks induce apoptosis even after infection of cells at low multiplicities of infection, chloroquine does not block apoptosis and the evidence suggests that apoptosis is induced late rather than early in infection. In this instance the etcodomain of gD is the only component of gD essential for blocking apoptosis induced by gD−/+ stocks. One hypothesis that remains to be explored in greater detail rests on an earlier report that gD interacts and colocalizes with the cation-independent mannose-6-phosphate receptor, a regulator of lysosomal enzyme transport (Zhou and Roizman, 2002a). The hypothesis predicts that, to block apoptosis induced by gD−/− mutant, the ectopically expressed gD must be translocated to the lysosomal vesicles and interact with the mannose-6-phosphate receptor. In contrast, the gD−/+ virus does not trigger apoptosis by lysosomal discharge but rather infects cells, replicates, and it is the gD−/− progeny of the gD−/+ virus that triggers apoposis during its transport through the exocytic pathway. The target of gD in this instance could be mannose-6-phosphate receptor or another as yet unidentified protein.

(v) gJ is the smallest of the glycoproteins encoded by HSV and its function until recently was largely unknown. Studies by Jerome and colleagues indicate that gJ blocks Fas ligand- or granzyme B-induced apoptosis and more important, it is involved in the protection of infected cells from CTL-induced apoptosis (Jerome et al., 1998, 2001).

Conclusions

As indicated earlier in the text, the strategic objective underlying the evolution of HSV is total control of the biosynthetic and defensive pathway of the cell. This is achieved though physical interaction between viral and cellular proteins and results in the modification and diversion of the host protein to fulfill the needs of the virus. The three fundamental conclusions of the studies carried out so far are that (i) viral proteins are largely multifunctional, the function at any given time most likely determined either by the partner to which they are bound or the post-translational modification to which they are subjected; (ii) the full complement of viral protein functions remains to be discovered and (iii) HSV exhibits a functional but not sequence driven redundancy. In essence, numerous functions expressed by different viral proteins aim to modify or suppress a specific metabolic pathway, although the targeted aspects of the pathway are not identical. If HSV had the arrogance (and capacity) to express it, its motto would be "we take no chances."

Acknowledgments

When not writing chapters or reviews, our studies are supported by grants from the National Cancer Institute (CA78766, CA71933, CA83939, CA87661, and CA88860), the United States Public Service.

REFERENCES

Advani, S. J., Brandimarti, R., Weichselbaum, R. R., and Roizman, B. (2000). The disappearance of cyclins A and B and the increase in activity of the G2/M-phase cellular kinase cdc2 in herpes simplex virus 1-infected cells require expression of the $\alpha 22/Us1.5$ and $U_L 13$ viral genes. *J. Virol.*, **74**, 8–15.

Advani, S. J., Weichselbaum, R. R., and Roizman, B. (2001). cdc2 cyclin-dependent kinase binds and phosphorylates herpes simplex virus 1 $U_L 42$ DNA synthesis processivity factor. *J. Virol.*, **75**, 10326–10333.

Advani, S. J., Weichselbaum, R. R., and Roizman, B. (2003). Herpes simplex virus 1 activates cdc2 to recruit topoisomerase IIα for post-DNA synthesis expression of late genes. *Proc. Natl Acad. Sci. USA*, **100**, 4825–4830.

Amici, C., Belardo, G., Rossi, A., and Santoro, M. G. (2001). Activation of IκB kinase by herpes simplex virus type 1. A novel target for anti-herpetic therapy. *J. Biol. Chem.*, **276**, 28759–28766.

Aubert, M. and Blaho, J. A. (1999). The Herpes simplex virus type 1 regulatory protein ICP27 is required for the prevention of apoptosis in infected human cells. *J. Virol.*, **73**, 2803–2813.

Bakheet, T., Williams, B. R., and Khabar, K. S. (2003). ARED 2.0: an update of AU-rich element mRNA database. *Nucl. Acids Res.*, **31**, 421–423.

Baradaran, K., Dabrowski, C. E., and Schaffer, P. A. (1994). Transcriptional analysis of the region of the herpes simplex virus type 1 genome containing the $U_L 8$, $U_L 9$, and $U_L 10$ genes and identification of a novel delayed-early gene product, OBPC. *J. Virol.*, **68**, 4251–4261.

Benetti, L. and Roizman, B. (2003). Herpes simplex virus protein kinase $U_S 3$ activates and functionally overlaps protein kinase A to block apoptosis. *Proc. Natl Acad. Sci. USA*, **101**, 9411–9416.

Benetti, L., Munger, J., and Roizman, B. (2003). The herpes simplex virus 1 $U_S 3$ protein kinase blocks caspase-dependent double cleavage and activation of the proapoptotic protein BAD. *J. Virol.*, **77**, 6567–6573.

Blackshear, P. J. (2002). Tristetraprolin and other CCCH tandem zinc-finger proteins in the regulation of mRNA turnover. *Biochem. Soc. Trans.*, **30**, 945–952.

Boutell, C., Sadis, S., and Everett, R. D. (2002). Herpes simplex virus type 1 immediate-early protein ICP0 and is isolated RING finger domain act as ubiquitin E3 ligases in vitro. *J. Virol.*, **76**, 841–850.

Brooks, S. A., Connolly, J. E., and Rigby, W. F. (2004). The role of mRNA turnover in the regulation of tristetraprolin expression: evidence for an extracellular signal-regulated kinase-specific, AU-rich element-dependent, autoregulatory pathway. *J. Immunol.*, **172**, 7263–7271.

Butler, J. S. (2002). The yin and yang of the exosome. *Trends Cell Biol.*, **12**, 90–96.

Carter, K. L. and Roizman, B. (1996). The promoter and transcriptional unit of a novel herpes simplex virus 1α gene are contained in, and encode a protein in frame with, the open reading frame of the $\alpha 22$ gene. *J. Virol.*, **70**, 172–178.

Cassady, K. A., Gross, M., and Roizman, B. (1998). The herpes simplex virus $U_S 11$ protein effectively compensates for the $\gamma_1 34.5$ gene if present before activation of protein kinase R by precluding its phosphorylation and that of the alpha subunit of eukaryotic translation initiation factor 2. *J. Virol.*, **72**, 8620–8626.

Chee, A. V. and Roizman, B. (2004). Herpes simplex virus 1 gene products occlude the interferon signaling pathway at multiple sites. *J. Virol.*, **78**, 4185–4196.

Chee, A. V., Lopez, P., Pandolfi, P. P., and Roizman, B. (2003). Promyelocytic leukemia protein mediates interferon-based anti-herpes simplex virus 1 effects. *J. Virol.*, **77**, 7101–7105.

Chen, C. Y. and Shyu, A. B (1995). AU-rich elements: characterization and importance in mRNA degradation. *Trends Biochem. Sci.*, **20**, 465–470.

Chen, C. Y., Gherzi, R., Ong, S. E. *et al.* (2001). AU binding proteins recruit the exosome to degrade ARE-containing mRNAs. *Cell*, **107**, 451–464.

Doepker, R. C., Hsu, W. L., Saffran, H. A., and Smiley, J. R. (2004). Herpes simplex virus virion host shutoff protein is stimulated by translation initiation factors eIF4B and eIF4H. *J. Virol.*, **78**, 4684–4699.

Durand, L. O., Advani, S. J. Poon, A. P., and Roizman B. (2005). The carboxyl-terminal domain of RNA polymerase II is phosphorylated by a complex containing cdk9 and infected-cell protein 22 of herpes simplex virus 1. *J. Virol.*, **79**, 6757–6762.

Esclatine, A., Taddeo, B., Evans, L., and Roizman, B. (2004a). The herpes simplex virus 1 U_L41 gene-dependent destabilization of cellular RNAs is selective and may be sequence-specific. *Proc. Natl Acad. Sci. USA*, **101**, 3603–3608.

Esclatine, A., Taddeo, B., and Roizman, B. (2004b). Herpes simplex virus 1 induces cytoplasmic accumulation of TIA-1/TIAR and both synthesis and cytoplasmic accumulation of tristetraprolin, two cellular proteins that bind and destabilize AU-rich RNAs. *J. Virol.*, **78**, 8582–8592.

Esclatine, A., Taddeo, B., and Roizman, B. (2004c). The U_L41 protein of herpes simplex virus mediates selective stabilization or degradation of cellular mRNAs. *Proc. Natl Acad. Sci. USA*, **101**, 18165–18170.

Everett, R. D. (2001). DNA viruses and viral proteins that interact with PML nuclear bodies. *Oncogene*, **20**, 7266–7273.

Everly, D. N. Jr., Feng, P., Mian, I. S., and Read, G. S. (2002). mRNA degradation by the virion host shutoff (Vhs) protein of herpes simplex virus: genetic and biochemical evidence that Vhs is a nuclease. *J. Virol.*, **76**, 8560–8571.

Galvan, V. and Roizman, B. (1998). Herpes simplex virus 1 induces and blocks apoptosis at multiple steps during infection and protects cells from exogenous inducers in a cell-type-dependent manner. *Proc. Natl Acad. Sci. USA*, **95**, 3931–3936.

Galvan, V., Brandimarti, R., and Roizman, B. (1999). Herpes simplex virus 1 blocks caspase-3-independent and caspase-dependent pathways to cell death. *J. Virol.*, **73**, 3219–3226.

Goodkin, M. L., Ting, A. T., and Blaho, J. A. (2003). NF-κB is required for apoptosis prevention during herpes simplex virus type 1 infection. *J. Virol.*, **77**, 7261–7280.

Gregory, D., Hargett, D., Holmes, D., Money, E., and Bachenheimer, S. L. (2004). Efficient replication by herpes simplex virus type 1 involves activation of the IκB kinase-IκB-p65 pathway. *J. Virol.*, **78**, 13582–13590.

Gu, H. and Roizman, B. (2003). The degradation of promyelocytic leukemia and Sp100 proteins by herpes simplex virus 1 is mediated by the ubiquitin-conjugating enzyme UbcH5a. *Proc. Natl Acad. Sci. USA*, **100**, 8963–8968.

Gu, H., Liang, Y., Mandel, G., and Roizman, B. (2005). Components of the REST/CoREST/histone deacetylase repressor complex are disrupted, modified, and translocated in HSV-1-infected cells. *Proc. Natl Acad. Sci. USA*, **102**, 7571–7576.

Hagglund, R. and Roizman, B. (2002). Characterization of the novel E3 ubiquitin ligase encoded in exon 3 of herpes simplex virus-1-infected cell protein 0. *Proc. Natl Acad. Sci. USA*, **99**, 7889–7894.

Hagglund, R. and Roizman, B. (2003). Herpes simplex virus 1 mutant in which the ICP0 HUL-1 E3 ubiquitin ligase site is disrupted stabilizes cdc34 but degrades D-type cyclins and exhibits diminished neurotoxicity. *J. Virol.*, **77**, 13194–13202.

Hagglund, R. and Roizman, B. (2004). Role of ICP0 in the strategy of conquest of the host cell by herpes simplex virus 1. *J. Virol.*, **78**, 2169–2178.

Hagglund, R., Van Sant, C., Lopez, P., and Roizman, B. (2002). Herpes simplex virus 1-infected cell protein 0 contains two E3 ubiquitin ligase sites specific for different E2 ubiquitin-conjugating enzymes. *Proc. Natl Acad. Sci. USA*, **99**, 631–636.

Hardwicke, M. A. and Sandri-Goldin, R. M. (1994). The herpes simplex virus regulatory protein ICP27 contributes to the decrease in cellular mRNA levels during infection. *J. Virol.*, **68**, 4797–4810.

He, B., Chou, J., Brandimarti, R., Mohr, I., Gluzman, Y., and Roizman, B. (1997a). Suppression of the phenotype of $\gamma_1 34.5$- herpes simplex virus 1: failure of activated RNA-dependent protein kinase to shut off protein synthesis is associated with a deletion in the domain of the α47 gene. *J. Virol.*, **71**, 6049–6054.

He, B., Gross, M., and Roizman, B. (1997b). The $\gamma_1 34.5$ protein of herpes simplex virus 1 complexes with protein phosphatase 1 α to dephosphorylate the α subunit of the eukaryotic translation initiation factor 2 and preclude the shutoff of protein synthesis by double-stranded RNA-activated protein kinase. *Proc. Natl Acad. Sci. USA*, **94**, 843–848.

He, B., Gross, M., and Roizman, B. (1998). The $\gamma_1 34.5$ protein of herpes simplex virus 1 has the structural and functional attributes of a protein phosphatase 1 regulatory subunit and is present in a high molecular weight complex with the enzyme in infected cells. *J. Biol. Chem.*, **273**, 20737–20743.

Jerome, K. R., Tait, J. F., Koelle, D. M., and Corey, L. (1998). Herpes simplex virus type 1 renders infected cells resistant to cytotoxic T-lymphocyte-induced apoptosis. *J. Virol.*, **72**, 436–441.

Jerome, K. R., Fox, R., Chen, Z., Sears, A. E., Lee, H.-Y., and Corey, L. (1999). Herpes simplex virus inhibits apoptosis through the action of two genes, U_S5 and U_S3. *J. Virol.*, **73**, 8950–8957.

Jerome, K. R., Chen, Z., Lang, R. *et al.* (2001). HSV and glycoprotein J inhibit caspase activation and apoptosis induced by granzyme B or Fas. *J. Immunol.*, **167**, 3928–3935.

Karr, B. M. and Read, G. S. (1999). The virion host shutoff function of herpes simplex virus degrades the 5 end of a target mRNA before the 3 end. *Virology*, **264**, 195–204.

Kawaguchi, Y., Van Sant, C., and Roizman, B. (1998). Eukaryotic elongation factor 1δ is hyperphosphorylated by the protein kinase encoded by the U_L13 gene of herpes simplex virus 1. *J. Virol.*, **72**, 1731–1736.

Kawaguchi, Y., Matsumura, T., Roizman, B., and Hirai, K. (1999). Cellular elongation factor 1 δ is modified in cells infected with representative alpha-, beta-, or gamma-herpesviruses. *J. Virol.*, **73**, 4456–4460.

Koyama, A. H. and Miwa, Y. (1997). Suppression of apoptotic DNA fragmentation in herpes simplex virus type 1-infected cells. *J. Virol.*, **71**, 2567–2571.

Kwong, A. D., Kruper, J. A., and Frenkel, N. (1988). Herpes simplex virus virion host shutoff function. *J. Virol.*, **62**, 912–921.

Leib, D. A., Harrison, T. E., Laslo, K. M., Machalek, M. A., Moorman, N. J., and Virgin, H. W. (1999). Interferons regulate the phenotype of wild-type and mutant herpes simplex viruses in vivo. *J. Exp. Med.*, **189**, 663–672.

Leib, D. A., Machalek, M. A., Williams, B. R., Silverman, R. H., and Virgin, H. W. (2000). Specific phenotypic restoration of an attenuated virus by knockout of a host resistance gene. *Proc. Natl Acad. Sci. USA*, **97**, 6097–6101.

Leopardi, R. and Roizman, B. (1996). The herpes simplex virus major regulatory protein ICP4 blocks apoptosis induced by the virus or by hyperthermia. *Proc. Natl Acad. Sci. USA*, **93**, 9583–9587.

Leopardi, R., Van Sant, C., and Roizman, B. (1997a). The herpes simplex virus 1 protein kinase U_S3 is required for protection from apoptosis induced by the virus. *Proc. Natl Acad. Sci. USA*, **94**, 7891–7896.

Leopardi, R., Ward, P. L., Ogle, W. O., and Roizman, B. (1997b). Association of herpes simplex virus regulatory protein ICP22 with transcriptional complexes containing EAP, ICP4, RNA polymerase II, and viral DNA requires posttranslational modification by the U_L13 protein kinase. *J. Virol.*, **71**, 1133–1139.

Long, M. C., Leong, V., Schaffer, P. A., Spencer, C. A., and Rice, S. A. (1999). ICP22 and the U_L13 protein kinase are both required for herpes simplex virus-induced modification of the large subunit of RNA polymerase II. *J. Virol.*, **73**, 5593–5604.

Lopez, P., Van Sant, C., and Roizman, B. (2001). Requirements for the nuclear-cytoplasmic translocation of infected-cell protein 0 of herpes simplex virus 1. *J. Virol.*, **75**, 3832–3840.

Lopez, P., Jacob, R. J., and Roizman, B. (2002). Overexpression of promyelocytic leukemia protein precludes the dispersal of ND10 structures and has no effect on accumulation of infectious herpes simplex virus 1 or its proteins. *J. Virol.*, **76**, 9355–9367.

Mohr, I. and Gluzman, Y. (1996). A herpesvirus genetic element which affects translation in the absence of the viral GADD34 function. *EMBO J.*, **15**, 4759–4766.

Munger, J. and Roizman, B. (2001). The U_S3 protein kinase of herpes simplex virus 1 mediates the posttranslational modification of BAD and prevents BAD-induced programmed cell death in the absence of other viral proteins. *Proc. Natl Acad. Sci. USA*, **98**, 10410–10415.

Munger, J., Chee, A. V., and Roizman, B. (2001). The U_S3 protein kinase blocks apoptosis induced by the d120 mutant of herpes simplex virus 1 at a premitochondrial stage. *J. Virol.*, **75**, 5491–5497.

Murata, T., Goshima, F., Yamauchi, Y., Koshizuka, T., Takakuwa, H., and Nishiyama, Y. (2002). Herpes simplex virus type 2 U_S3 blocks apoptosis induced by sorbitol treatment. *Microbes Infect.*, **4**, 707–712.

Ogg, P. D., McDonell, P. J., Ryckman, B. J., Knudson, C. M., and Roller R. J. (2004). The HSV-1 U_S3 protein kinase is sufficient to block apoptosis induced by overexpression of a variety of Bcl-2 family members. *Virology*, **319**, 212–224.

Ogle, W. O. and Roizman, B. (1999). Functional anatomy of herpes simplex virus 1 overlapping genes encoding infected-cell protein 22 and $U_S1.5$ protein. *J. Virol.*, **73**, 4305–4315.

Patel, A., Hanson, J., McLean, T. I. *et al.* (1998). Herpes simplex type 1 induction of persistent NF-κB nuclear translocation increases the efficiency of virus replication. *Virology*, 247, 212–222.

Perez-Parada, J., Saffran, H. A., and Smiley, J. R. (2004). RNA degradation induced by the herpes simplex virus vhs protein proceeds 5′ to 3′ in vitro. *J. Virol.*, **78**, 13391–13394.

Perkins, D., Pereira, E. F. R., Gober, M., Yarowsky, P. J., and Aurelian, L. (2002). The Herpes Simplex virus type 2 R1 protein kinase (ICP10 PK) blocks apoptosis in hippocampal neurons, involving activation of the MEK/MAPK survival pathway. *J. Virol.*, **76**, 1435–1449.

Poon, A. P., Liang, Y., and Roizman, B. (2003) Herpes simplex virus 1 gene expression is accelerated by inhibitors of histone deacetylases in rabbit skin cells infected with a mutant carrying a cDNA copy of the infected-cell protein no. 0. *J. Virol.*, **77**, 12671–12678.

Purves, F. P. and Roizman, B. (1992). The U_L13 gene of herpes simplex virus 1 encodes the functions for posttranslational processing associated with phosphorylation of the regulatory protein 22. *Proc. Natl Acad. Sci. USA*, **89**, 7310–7314.

Purves, F. P., Ogle, W. O., and Roizman, B. (1993) Processing of the herpes simplex virus regulatory protein 22 mediated by the U_L13 protein kinase determines the accumulation of a subset of α and γ mRNAs and proteins in infected cells. *Proc. Natl Acad. Sci. USA*, **90**, 6701–6705.

Regad, T. and Chelbi-Alix, M. K. (2001). Role and fate of PML nuclear bodies in response to interferon and viral infections. *Oncogene*, **20**, 7274–7286.

Rice, S. A., Long, M. C., Lam, V., and Spencer, C. A. (1994). RNA polymerase II is aberrantly phosphorylated and localized to viral replication compartments following herpes simplex virus infection. *J. Virol.*, **68**, 988–1001.

Rice S. A., Long, M. C., Lam, V., Schaffer, P. A., and Spencer, C. A. (1995). Herpes simplex virus immediate-early protein ICP22 is required for viral modification of host RNA polymerase II and establishment of the normal viral transcription program. *J. Virol.*, **69**, 5550–5559.

Roizman, B., Borman, G. S., and Kamali-Rousta, M. (1965). Macromolecular synthesis in cells infected with herpes simplex virus. *Nature*, **206**, 374–1375.

Roller, R. J. and Roizman, B. (1990). The herpes simplex virus U_S11 open reading frame encodes a sequence specific RNA-binding protein. *J. Virol.*, **64**, 3463–3470.

Sandri-Goldin, R. M. (1998). ICP27 mediates HSV RNA export by shuttling through a leucine-rich nuclear export signal and binding viral intronless RNAs through an RGG motif. *Genes Dev.*, **12**, 868–879.

Santoro, M. G., Rossi, A., and Amici, C. (2003). NF-κB and virus infection: who controls whom. *EMBO J.*, **22**, 2552–2260.

Sciortino, M. T., Taddeo, B., Poon, A. P., Mastino, A., and Roizman, B. (2002). Of the three tegument proteins that package mRNA in herpes simplex virions, one (VP22) transports the mRNA to uninfected cells for expression prior to viral infection. *Proc. Natl Acad. Sci. USA*, **99**, 8318–8323.

Shen, Y. and Shenk, T. (1995). Viruses and apoptosis. *Curr. Opin. Genet. Dev.*, **5**, 105–111.

Shenk, T. (2002). Might a vanguard of mRNAs prepare cells for the arrival of herpes simplex virus? *Proc. Natl Acad. Sci. USA*, **99**, 8465–8466.

Sieg, S., Yildirim, Z., Smith, D. *et al.* (1996). Herpes simplex virus type 2 inhibition of Fas ligand expression. *J. Virol.*, **70**, 8747–8751.

Smibert, C. A., Popova, B., Xiao, P., Capone, J. P., and Smiley, J. R. (1994). Herpes simplex virus VP16 forms a complex with the virion host shutoff protein vhs. *J. Virol.*, **68**, 2339–2346.

Smiley, J. R. (2004). Herpes simplex virus virion host shutoff protein: immune evasion mediated by a viral RNase? *J. Virol.*, **78**, 1063–1068.

Strom, T. and Frenkel, N. (1987). Effects of herpes simplex virus on mRNA stability. *J. Virol.*, **61**, 2198–2207.

Sydiskis, R. J. and Roizman, B. (1966). Polysomes and protein synthesis in cells infected with a DNA virus. *Science*, **153**, 76–78.

Sydiskis, R. J. and Roizman, B. (1968). The disaggregation of host polyribosomes in productive and abortive infection with herpes simplex virus. *Virology*, **32**, 678–686.

Taddeo, B., Esclatine, A., and Roizman, B. (2002). The patterns of accumulation of cellular RNAs in cells infected with a wild-type and a mutant herpes simplex virus 1 lacking the virion host shutoff gene. *Proc. Natl Acad. Sci. USA*, **99**, 17031–17036.

Taddeo, B., Esclatine, A., Zhang, W., and Roizman, B. (2003a). The stress-inducible immediate-early responsive gene IEX-1 is activated in cells infected with herpes simplex virus 1, but several viral mechanisms, including 3' degradation of its RNA, preclude expression of the gene. *J. Virol.*, **77**, 6178–6187.

Taddeo, B., Luo, T. R., Zhang, W., and Roizman, B. (2003b). Activation of NF-κB in cells productively infected with HSV-1 depends on activated protein kinase R and plays no apparent role in blocking apoptosis. *Proc. Natl Acad. Sci. USA*, **100**, 12408–12413.

Taddeo, B., Zhang, W., Lakeman, F., and Roizman, B. (2004a). Cells lacking NF-κB or in which NF-κB is not activated vary with respect to ability to sustain herpes simplex virus 1 replication and are not susceptible to apoptosis induced by a replication-incompetent mutant virus. *J. Virol.*, **78**, 11615–11621.

Taddeo, B., Esclatine, A., and Roizman, B. (2004b). Post-transcriptional processing of cellular RNAs in herpes simplex virus-infected cells. *Biochem. Soc. Trans.*, **32**, 697–701.

Van Minnebruggen, G., Favoreel, H. W., Jacobs, L., and Nauwynck, H. J. (2003). Pseudorabies virus U_S3 protein kinase mediates actin stress fiber breakdown. *J. Virol.*, **77**, 9074–9080.

Williams, B. R. (2001). Signal integration via PKR. *Sci STKE*, **89**, RE2, 1–10.

Wilusz, C. J., Wormington, M., and Peltz, S. W. (2001). The cap-to-tail guide to mRNA turnover. *Nat. Rev. Mol. Cell Biol.*, **2**, 237–246.

Zhou, G. and Roizman, B. (2001). The domains of glycoprotein D required to block apoptosis depend on whether glycoprotein D is present in the virions carrying herpes simplex virus 1 genome lacking the gene encoding the glycoprotein. *J. Virol.*, **75**, 6166–6172.

Zhou, G. and Roizman, B. (2002a). Cation-independent mannose 6-phosphate receptor blocks apoptosis induced by herpes simplex virus 1 mutants lacking glycoprotein D and is likely the target of antiapoptotic activity of the glycoprotein. *J. Virol.*, **76**, 6197–6204.

Zhou, G. and Roizman, B. (2002b). Truncated forms of glycoprotein D of herpes simplex virus 1 capable of blocking apoptosis and of low-efficiency entry into cells form a heterodimer dependent on the presence of a cysteine located in the shared transmembrane domains. *J. Virol.*, **76**, 11469–11475.

Zhou, G., Galvan, V., Campadelli-Fiume, G., and Roizman, B. (2000). Glycoprotein D or J delivered in trans blocks apoptosis in SK-N-SH cells induced by a herpes simplex virus 1 mutant lacking intact genes expressing both glycoproteins. *J. Virol.*, **74**, 11782–11791.

Zhu, H., Shen, Y., and Shenk, T. (1995). Human cytomegalovirus IE1 and IE2 proteins block apoptosis. *J. Virol.*, **69**, 7960–7970.

Part II

Basic virology and viral gene effects on host cell functions: betaherpesviruses

Edited by Edward Mocarski

14

Comparative genome and virion structure

Andrew J. Davison and David Bhella

MRC Virology Unit, Institute of Virology, Glasgow, UK

Introduction

The two major lineages in the *Betaherpesvirinae* are the cytomegaloviruses (the *Cytomegalovirus* and *Muromegalovirus* genera, plus a number of other viruses whose taxonomy is only partially defined) and the *Roseolovirus* genus (see Chapter 1). The best characterized members of these lineages are HCMV (the prototype of the subfamily) and HHV-6, respectively. Cytomegaloviruses are present in a wide range of mammalian species, and have been termed "salivary gland viruses" because of their ease of isolation from explanted tissue. An earlier divergence of the *Betaherpesvirinae* may be represented by a herpesvirus of elephants (Richman et al., 1999; Ehlers et al., 2001). This chapter starts by describing the genome structures of *Betaherpesvirinae*, then examines the genetic content of HCMV and HHV-6, and finally focuses on the virion structure of HCMV.

Genome structures

The genomes of viruses in the *Roseolovirus* genus are significantly smaller, at 145–162 kbp, than those of other *Betaherpesvirinae*, at 196–241 kbp. Indeed, HCMV has the largest genome among the human herpesviruses, and thus far its closest relative, CCMV, has the largest genome of all sequenced herpesviruses. It seems likely that the ancestor of the *Betaherpesvirinae* had a genome consisting of a unique region flanked by a direct repeat (the class A genome described in Chapter 2), since this structure is characteristic of most extant members of the subfamily. Earlier studies ruled out the presence of large repeats in the genomes of MCMV (Ebeling et al., 1983a; Mercer et al., 1983; Marks and Spector, 1984), THV (Koch et al., 1985) and RCMV (Meijer et al., 1986). Later work confirmed that MCMV and RCMV have terminal direct repeats of 30 and 504 bp, respectively (Marks and Spector, 1988; Vink et al., 1996). A corresponding repeat has not been detected in THV, but the genome termini have not been examined directly. GPCMV has a terminal direct repeat of about 1 kbp, and a proportion of genomes lacks one copy (Gao and Isom, 1984; McVoy et al., 1997; Nixon and McVoy, 2002). RhCMV has a terminal repeat of about 500 bp that may be present in multiple copies in some genomes (Hansen et al., 2003). Interestingly, this resembles the class B genome structure found in many *Gammaherpesvirinae*. Information on the genome of another monkey cytomegalovirus, SCMV, is also available (Huang et al., 1978; Jeang and Hayward, 1983), but the termini have not been characterized. The most commonly studied strain of SCMV, Colburn, was isolated ostensibly from a human (Huang et al., 1978). Sequences from an agent dubbed "stealth virus," which was also suggested to be of human origin, have shown that this virus is SCMV (Martin, 1999).

Cytomegaloviruses of higher primates, HCMV and CCMV, have the class E genome structure, in which two unique regions (U_L and U_S) are flanked by direct repeats (TR_L and IR_L; TR_S and IR_S) (Weststrate et al., 1980; Davison et al., 2003a). A copy of the terminal direct repeat of approximately 300–600 bp (the *a* sequence) is present in inverted orientation at the junction between IR_L and IR_S (Spaete and Mocarski, 1985; Tamashiro and Spector, 1986). The genomes exhibit segment inversion, which results in virions containing equimolar amounts of four genome isomers differing in the relative orientations of U_L and U_S. The genomes of two closely related herpesviruses of New World monkeys (aotine herpesviruses 1 and 3) appear to have a similar structure (Ebeling et al., 1983b). However, as mentioned above, RhCMV, a virus of an Old World monkey, does not. This suggests that the class E genome structure arose in an ancestral primate cytomegalovirus from a class

A genome by duplication of fused terminal sequences at a location internally in the genome, but that this duplication was lost in the lineage represented by RhCMV. The biological reason for a class E genome structure, which is also characteristic of certain alphaherpesviruses such as HSV-1 and HSV-2 (see Chapter 5), remains unknown.

The genomes of both variants of HHV-6 (referred to as HHV-6A and HHV-6B; Martin et al., 1991b; Lindquester and Pellett, 1991) and HHV-7 (Dominguez et al., 1996) contain a substantial terminal direct repeat, whose size was determined by sequencing as 8.1–8.8 kbp in the former and 5.8–10.0 kbp in the latter. The ranges are due to the presence in the direct repeat of regions of variable size consisting of reiterated short sequences.

Genes

Genome sequences

Complete genome sequences are available for eight species in the *Betaherpesvirinae*, as listed in Table 2.1. These include HCMV (Chee et al., 1990; Murphy et al., 2003b; Dunn et al., 2003b; Dolan et al., 2004), MCMV (Rawlinson et al., 1996), RCMV (Vink et al., 2000), THV (Bahr and Darai, 2001), RhCMV (Hansen et al., 2003), CCMV (Davison et al., 2003a), HHV-6A (Gompels et al., 1995), HHV-6B (Dominguez et al., 1999; Isegawa et al., 1999) and HHV-7 (Nicholas, 1996; Megaw et al., 1998). Partial sequence data are also available in the literature or public sequence databases for *Betaherpesvirinae* that infect Old World primates, such as the baboon (Blewett et al., 2001), drill (Blewett et al., 2003), colobus monkey and orangutan, the New World primate, aotine herpesvirus 1, and members of the *Suidae* including the domestic pig (Ehlers et al., 1999; Rupasinghe et al., 2001; Widen et al., 2001) and the warthog (Ehlers and Lowden, 2004).

Genetic content

The remainder of this section focuses on a genetic comparison of HCMV, as the most extensively characterized cytomegalovirus, with HHV-6, in the *Roseolovirus* genus. Derivation of the genetic content of HCMV has been a protracted process, because strain AD169, which was sequenced first (Chee et al., 1990), lacks 15 kbp at the right end of U_L in comparison with wild-type strains (Cha et al., 1996), having in place of the deleted sequence an inverted duplication of a 10 kbp region from the left end of U_L. AD169 also bears several additional mutations (Davison et al., 2003a) that can vary with respect to the strain variant being used and have important functional consequences (Skaletskaya et al., 2001). Also, all passaged strains examined to date are compromised in one or more genes by mutations that introduce deletions, frameshifts or termination codons (Akter et al., 2003; Dolan et al., 2004). The deduced gene layout in wild-type HCMV is shown in Fig. 14.1, and that of HHV-6 is shown in Fig. 14.2. The genetic content of HHV-6B appears to be the same as that of HHV-6A; nine additional small ORFs were listed by Dominguez et al. (1999) as unique to HHV-6B, but their protein-coding status remains unknown. HCMV and HHV-6 are currently estimated to contain 165 and 86 genes, respectively, counting duplicated genes only once. The gene content of HHV-7 is similar to that of HHV-6: all HHV-7 genes but one (U55B, which is related to U55) have HHV-6 counterparts, and all but three HHV-6 genes (U22, U83 and U94) have HHV-7 counterparts. The HHV-6 genome contains several regions consisting of complex and simple repeats (T1, T2, R1, R2 and R3 in Fig. 14.3), only one which encodes protein. In contrast, HCMV lacks such repeats, but many proteins contain quasi-repetitive regions of one or a few amino acid residues. Although infrequent in all herpesviruses, mRNA splicing is involved in transcription of at least 12 HCMV genes (7% of the total) and at least 14 HHV-6 genes (16%).

Table 14.1 details the correspondence between HCMV and HHV-6 genes, alongside functional information. HCMV and HHV-6, respectively, possess 40 and 41 of the 43 core genes inherited by the *Alpha-*, *Beta-* and *Gammaherpesvirinae* from their common ancestor (see Chapter 2), located centrally in the genomes. Both lack homologues to the genes encoding thymidine kinase and the small subunit of ribonucleotide reductase, and HCMV lacks the core gene encoding a homologue of a protein that binds to ori_{Lyt}, the origin of DNA synthesis used during productive replication. In addition, four genes common to HCMV and HHV-6 have clear homologues in the *Gamma-* but not the *Alphaherpesvirinae*. These are UL49 (related to BFRF2 and ORF66 in the *Lymphocryptovirus* and *Rhadinovirus* genera, respectively), UL79 (BVLF1 and ORF18), UL87 (BcRF1 and ORF24) and UL92 (BDLF4 and ORF31). A fifth gene, UL88, is distantly related to BTRF1 and ORF23 and positionally equivalent to a gene in the *Alphaherpesvirinae* (UL21 in HSV-1). A sixth gene, UL91, is positionally equivalent to BDLF3.5 and ORF30 in the *Lymphocryptovirus* and *Rhadinovirus* genera, respectively. These six genes are considered at present to have arisen after the lineage that led to the *Beta-* and *Gammaherpesvirinae* diverged from the *Alphaherpesvirinae*, but it is also possible that the ancestral core set included UL88 along with one or more of the others, which were lost at an early stage from the lineage giving rise to *Alphaherpesvirinae*.

Table 14.1. Proteins encoded by HCMV and HHV-6 genes

HCMV[a]	HHV-6[a]	Function[b]	Selected references[c]
RL1			
RL5A		RL11 family	Davison et al. (2003b)
RL6		RL11 family	Davison et al. (2003b)
RL10		Virion envelope glycoprotein	Spaderna et al. (2002)
RL11		RL11 family; IgG Fc-binding membrane glycoprotein	Lilley et al. (2001); Atalay et al. (2002)
RL12		RL11 family; putative membrane glycoprotein	
RL13		RL11 family; putative membrane glycoprotein	Yu et al. (2002)
UL1		RL11 family; putative membrane glycoprotein	
UL2		Putative membrane protein	
UL4		RL11 family; virion glycoprotein	Chang et al. (1989)
UL5		RL11 family; putative membrane protein	
UL6		RL11 family; putative membrane glycoprotein	
UL7		RL11 family; putative membrane glycoprotein	
UL8		RL11 family; putative membrane glycoprotein	
UL9		RL11 family; putative membrane glycoprotein	
UL10		RL11 family; putative membrane glycoprotein	
UL11		RL11 family; membrane glycoprotein	Hitomi et al. (1997)
UL13		Putative secreted protein	
UL14		UL14 family; putative membrane glycoprotein	
UL15A		Putative membrane protein	
UL16		Membrane glycoprotein; inhibits NK cell cytotoxicity	Kaye et al. (1992a); Cosman et al. (2001); Odeberg et al. (2003); Dunn et al. (2003b)
UL17			
UL18		UL18 family; putative membrane glycoprotein; MHC-I homologue; possibly inhibits NK cell cytotoxicity	Browne et al. (1990); Cosman et al. (1997)
UL19			
UL20		Putative membrane glycoprotein	
UL21A			
UL22A		Putative secreted glycoprotein	Rawlinson and Barrell (1993)
UL23	U2	US22 family; tegument protein	Adair et al. (2002)
UL24	U3	US22 family; tegument protein	Adair et al. (2002); [Mori et al. (1998)]
UL25		UL25 family; tegument phosphoprotein	Baldick and Shenk (1996)
UL26		US22 family; tegument protein; transcriptional activator of major immediate early promoter	Baldick and Shenk (1996); Stamminger et al. (2002)
UL27	U4, U7	Locus of resistance to maribavir	Komazin et al. (2003); Chou et al. (2004)
UL28	U7	US22 family (spliced to an unidentified upstream exon)	
UL29	U8	US22 family	
UL30			
UL31	U10	DURP family	Davison and Stow (2005)
UL32	U11	Major tegument phosphoglycoprotein (pp150); highly immunogenic; binds to capsids	Jahn et al., (1987); Benko et al. (1988); Baxter and Gibson (2001); [Neipel et al. (1992)]
UL33	U12	GPCR family; membrane protein; putative chemokine receptor; virion protein	Margulies et al. (1996); Fraile-Ramos et al. (2002); [Isegawa et al. (1998)]
UL34		Represses US3 transcription	LaPierre et al. (2001)
	U13		
UL35	U14	UL25 family; tegument phosphoprotein; interacts with UL82 protein	Liu and Biegalke (2002); Schierling et al. (2004); [Stefan et al. (1997)]
	U15		
UL36	U17	US22 family; immediate early tegument protein; inhibitor of caspase-8-induced apoptosis (vICA)	Smith and Pari (1995b); Patterson and Shenk (1999); Skaletskaya et al. (2001)
UL37	U18	Immediate early envelope glycoprotein; possible auxiliary role in DNA replication; exon 1 product is mitochondrial inhibitor of apoptosis (vMIA)	Smith and Pari (1995b); Sarisky and Hayward (1996); Al-Barazi and Colberg-Poley (1996); Goldmacher et al. (1999)
UL38	U19		

(cont.)

Table 14.1. (cont.)

HCMV[a]	HHV-6[a]	Function[b]	Selected references[c]
UL40		Putative membrane glycoprotein; inhibits NK cell cytotoxicity	Tomasec et al. (2000)
	U20	Putative membrane glycoprotein	
	U21	Putative membrane glycoprotein	
	U22	Putative membrane glycoprotein	
	U23	Putative membrane glycoprotein	
	U24	Putative membrane protein	
	U24A	Putative membrane protein	
UL41A		Putative membrane protein	Dargan et al. (1997)
UL42		Putative membrane protein	Dargan et al. (1997); Mocarski et al. (1997)
UL43	U25	US22 family; tegument protein	Adair et al. (2002)
	U26	Putative multiple transmembrane protein	
UL44	U27	Processivity subunit of DNA polymerase (ICP36)	Mocarski et al. (1985); Ertl and Powell (1992); Weiland et al. (1994); Appleton et al. (2004); [Agulnick et al. (1993); Lin and Ricciardi (1998)]
UL45	U28	Large subunit of ribonucleotide reductase; lacks catalytic residues and is probably enzymatically inactive; tegument protein	McGeoch and Davison (1999); Patrone et al. (2003); [Sun and Conner (1999)]
UL46	U29	Component of intercapsomeric triplexes in capsids (mC-BP)	Gibson et al. (1996a)
UL47	U30	Tegument protein; possible role in intracellular transport; binds to UL48 protein	Baldick and Shenk (1996); Bechtel and Shenk (2002)
UL48	U31	High molecular weight tegument protein; binds to UL47 protein	Bradshaw et al. (1994); Gibson (1996); Ogawa-Goto et al. (2002)
UL48A	U32	Located on tips of hexons in capsids (SCP)	Gibson et al. (1996b); Baldick and Shenk (1996); Yu et al. (2005)
UL49	U33	Conserved in *Gammaherpesvirinae*	
UL50	U34	Inner nuclear membrane protein; role in egress of capsids from nucleus	Muranyi et al. (2002)
UL51	U35	Role in DNA packaging	
UL52	U36	Role in DNA packaging	
UL53	U37	Nuclear matrix protein; tegument protein; role in egress of capsids from nucleus	Muranyi et al. (2002); Dal Monte et al. (2002)
UL54	U38	Catalytic subunit of DNA polymerase; inhibited by pyrophosphate (e.g. foscarnet), nucleoside (e.g. ganciclovir) and certain non-nucleoside compounds	Heilbronn et al. (1987); Kouzarides et al. (1987); D'Aquila et al. (1989); [Teo et al. (1991)]
UL55	U39	Virion glycoprotein B (gB); component of gCI; involved in virus entry	Cranage et al. (1986); Boyle and Compton (1998); Boehme et al. (2004); [Ellinger et al. (1993)]
UL56	U40	Putative subunit of terminase; virion protein; binds to DNA packaging motif and exhibits nuclease activity; involved in inhibition by benzimidazole ribonucleosides and certain non-nucleoside compounds	Bogner et al. (1993); Bogner et al. (1998); Bradshaw et al. (1994); Krosky et al. (1998); Buerger et al. (2001); Scheffczik et al. (2002)
UL57	U41	Single-stranded DNA-binding protein	Kemble et al. (1987); Anders and Gibson (1988)
UL69	U42	Regulatory protein; tegument protein; contributes to cell cycle block; exhibits nucleocytoplasmic shuttling	Winkler et al. (1994); Winkler and Stamminger (1996); Hayashi et al. (2000); Lischka et al. (2001)
UL70	U43	Component of DNA helicase-primase complex; primase	McMahon and Anders (2002)
UL71	U44	Putative tegument protein	
UL72	U45	DURP family; derived from deoxyuridine triphosphatase; lacks catalytic residues and is enzymatically inactive	McGeoch and Davison (1999); McGeehan et al. (2001); Caposio et al. (2004); Davison and Stow (2005)
UL73	U46	Virion glycoprotein N (gN); component of gCII	Mach et al. (2000)
UL74	U47	Virion glycoprotein O (gO); component of gCIII	Huber and Compton (1997); Li et al. (1997); Huber and Compton (1998)
UL75	U48	Virion glycoprotein H (gH); component of gCIII; involved in entry	Cranage et al. (1988); Milne et al. (1998); [Liu et al. (1993); Mori et al. (2003b); Santoro et al. (2003)]
UL76	U49	Virion-associated regulatory protein	Wang et al. (2000); Wang et al. (2004)
UL77	U50	Role in DNA packaging	
UL78	U51	GPCR family; putative chemokine receptor	[Milne et al. (2000)]

Table 14.1. (*cont.*)

HCMV[a]	HHV-6[a]	Function[b]	Selected references[c]
UL79	U52	Conserved in *Gammaherpesvirinae*	
UL80	U53	Protease (N terminus) and minor capsid scaffold protein (C terminus)	Welch *et al.* (1991); Welch *et al.* (1993); Chen *et al.* (1996); Tong *et al.* (1996); Qiu *et al.* (1996); Shieh *et al.* (1996); [(Tigue *et al.* (1996)]
UL80.5	U53.5	Major capsid scaffold protein	Robson and Gibson (1989); Wood *et al.* (1997); Oien *et al.* (1997)
UL82	U54	DURP family; tegument phosphoprotein (pp71; upper matrix protein); transcriptional activator; targeted to ND10; targets Rb proteins for ubiquitin-independent proteosomal degradation	Ruger *et al.* (1987); Liu and Stinski (1992); Homer *et al.* (1999); Bresnahan and Shenk (2000b); Hofmann *et al.* (2002); Ishov *et al.* (2002); Kalejta and Shenk (2003); Davison and Stow (2005)
UL83	U55	DURP family; tegument phosphoprotein (pp65; lower matrix protein); suppresses interferon response	Ruger *et al.* (1987); Browne and Shenk (2003); Davison and Stow (2005)
UL84		DURP family; role in DNA replication; exhibits nucleocytoplasmic shuttling; binds to IE2 protein; transdominant inhibitor of IE transcription	He *et al.* (1992); Sarisky and Hayward (1996); Gebert *et al.* (1997); Lischka *et al.* (2003); Reid *et al.* (2003); Xu *et al.* (2004); Davison and Stow (2005)
UL85	U56	Component of intercapsomeric triplexes in capsids (mCP)	Baldick and Shenk (1996)
UL86	U57	Major capsid protein; component of hexons and pentons (MCP)	Chee *et al.* (1989); [Littler *et al.* (1990)]
UL87	U58	Conserved in *Gammaherpesvirinae*	
UL88	U59	Conserved in *Gammaherpesvirinae*; tegument protein	Baldick and Shenk (1996)
UL89	U66	Putative ATPase subunit of terminase; involved in inhibition by benzimidazole ribonucleosides and certain non-nucleoside compounds	Krosky *et al.* (1998); Buerger *et al.* (2001); Scheffczik *et al.* (2002)
UL91	U62	Positionally conserved in *Gammaherpesvirinae*	
UL92	U63	Conserved in *Gammaherpesvirinae*	
UL93	U64	Role in DNA packaging; tegument protein	
UL94	U65	Tegument protein; binds single-stranded DNA	Wing *et al.* (1996)
UL95	U67	Positionally conserved in *Gammaherpesvirinae*	
UL96	U68	Tegument protein	
UL97	U69	Serine-threonine protein kinase; tegument protein; phosphorylates ganciclovir; inhibited by maribavir; roles in DNA synthesis, DNA packaging and nuclear egress; phosphorylates UL44 protein	Littler *et al.* (1992); Sullivan *et al.* (1992); van Zeijl *et al.* (1997); Talarico *et al.* (1999); Wolf *et al.* (2001); Biron *et al.* (2002); Krosky *et al.* (2003a); Krosky *et al.* (2003b); Marschall *et al.* (2003); [Ansari and Emery (1999)]
UL98	U70	Deoxyribonuclease	Sheaffer *et al.* (1997); Gao *et al.* (1998)
UL99	U71	Myristylated tegument phosphoprotein (pp28)	Landini *et al.* (1987); Meyer *et al.* (1988); Sanchez *et al.* (2000)
UL100	U72	Virion envelope glycoprotein M (gM); component of gCII	Lehner *et al.* (1989); Kari *et al.* (1994)
	U73	Binds to origin of DNA synthesis; helicase	Inoue *et al.* (1994); Inoue and Pellett (1995)
UL102	U74	Component of DNA helicase-primase complex	Smith and Pari (1995a); McMahon and Anders (2002)
UL103	U75	Tegument protein	
UL104	U76	Portal protein; possibly interacts with terminase	Komazin *et al.* (2004); Dittmer and Bogner (2005)
UL105	U77	Component of DNA helicase-primase complex; helicase	Smith *et al.* (1996); McMahon and Anders (2002)
UL111A		Viral interleukin 10 (vIL-10)	Kotenko *et al.* (2000); Lockridge *et al.* (2000); Jones *et al.* (2002)
UL112	U79	Role in transcriptional activation or orchestrating DNA replication proteins	Penfold and Mocarski (1997); Ahn *et al.* (1999); Li *et al.* (1999)
UL114	U81	Uracil-DNA glycosylase; roles in excision of uracil from DNA and temporal regulation of DNA replication	Prichard *et al.* (1996); Courcelle *et al.* (2001)
UL115	U82	Virion envelope glycoprotein L (gL); component of gCIII; involved in entry	Kaye *et al.* (1992b); Milne *et al.* (1998); [Liu *et al.* (1993)]
UL116		Putative membrane glycoprotein	
	U83	CC chemokine	Zou *et al.* (1999); French *et al.* (1999); Lüttichau *et al.* (2003)

(*cont.*)

Table 14.1. (*cont.*)

HCMV[a]	HHV-6[a]	Function[b]	Selected references[c]
UL117	U84		
UL119	U85	IgG Fc-binding membrane glycoprotein related to OX-2	Atalay *et al.* (2002)
UL120		UL120 family; putative membrane glycoprotein	
UL121		UL120 family; putative membrane glycoprotein	
UL122	U86	Immediate early transcriptional activator (IE2); interacts with basal transcriptional machinery and cellular transcription factors; specific DNA-binding protein	Hermiston *et al.* (1987); Hagemeier *et al.* (1992); Arlt *et al.* (1994); Marchini *et al.* (2001); Heider *et al.* (2002); [Papanikolaou *et al.* (2002); Gravel *et al.* (2003)]
UL123	U90[d]	Immediate early transcriptional activator (IE1); enhances activation by IE2; interacts with basal transcriptional machinery and a cellular transcription factor; disrupts ND10	Hermiston *et al.* (1987); Greaves and Mocarski (1998); Ahn and Hayward (2000); Xu *et al.* (2001); Gawn and Greaves (2002); Lee *et al.* (2004); Nevels *et al.* (2004); [Martin *et al.*, 1991a); Gravel *et al.* (2002); Nikolauo *et al.* (2003)]
UL124	U91[d]	Putative membrane glycoprotein	
	U94	Parvovirus Rep protein homologue; binds to a transcription factor and single-stranded DNA; possible transcriptional regulator and involvement in latency	Thomson *et al.* (1991); Rotola *et al.* (1998); Mori *et al.* (2000); Dhepakson *et al.* (2002)
	U95	US22 family; immediate early gene	Takemoto *et al.* (2001)
	U100	Virion glycoprotein Q; complexed with gH and gL	Pfeiffer *et al.* (1995); Mori *et al.* (2003a)
	DR1	US22 family	
	DR6	US22 family; possible transactivator	Kashanchi *et al.* (1997)
UL128		Virion protein with role in endotheliotropism; putative CC chemokine motifs; associated with gH and gL	Akter *et al.* (2003); Hahn *et al.* (2004); Wang and Shenk (2005)
UL130		Virion glycoprotein with role in endotheliotropism; associated with gH and gL	Akter *et al.* (2003); Hahn *et al.* (2004); Patrone *et al.* (2005); Wang and Shenk (2005)
UL131A		Virion protein with role in endotheliotropism; associated with gH and gL	Akter *et al.* (2003); Hahn *et al.* (2004); Adler *et al.* (2006)
UL132		Putative membrane glycoprotein	
UL148		Putative membrane glycoprotein	
UL147A		Putative membrane protein	
UL147		UL146 family; putative secreted glycoprotein; putative CXC chemokine	Prichard *et al.* (2001)
UL146		UL146 family; secreted glycoprotein; CXC chemokine	Penfold *et al.* (1999); Prichard *et al.* (2001)
UL145			
UL144		Putative membrane glycoprotein; TNF receptor homologue	Benedict *et al.* (1999)
UL142		UL18 family; putative membrane glycoprotein; MHC-I homologue; inhibits NK cell cytotoxicity	Davison *et al.* (2003a); Wills *et al.* (2005)
UL141		UL14 family; membrane glycoprotein; inhibits NK cell cytotoxicity by downregulating CD155	Davison *et al.* (2003a); Tomasec *et al.* (2005)
UL140		Putative membrane protein	
UL139		Putative membrane glycoprotein	
UL138		Putative membrane protein	
UL136		Putative membrane protein	
UL135		Putative secreted protein	
UL133		Putative membrane protein	
UL148A		Putative membrane protein	
UL148B		Putative membrane protein	
UL148C		Putative membrane protein	
UL148D		Putative membrane protein	
UL150		Putative secreted protein	
IRS1		US22 family; immediate early transcriptional activator; tegument protein; involved in shutoff of host protein synthesis	Stasiak and Mocarski (1992); Romanowski and Shenk (1997); Romanowski *et al.* (1997); Child *et al.* (2004)
US1		US1 family; duplicated TT virus ORF2 motif	
US2		US2 family; membrane glycoprotein; causes selective degradation of MHC-I and MHC-II	Jones *et al.* (1995); Wiertz *et al.* (1996b); Jones and Sun (1997); Machold *et al.* (1997); Tomazin *et al.* (1999); Gewurz *et al.* (2001); Gewurz *et al.* (2002)

Table 14.1. (*cont.*)

HCMV[a]	HHV-6[a]	Function[b]	Selected references[c]
US3		US2 family; immediate early gene; membrane glycoprotein; inhibits processing and transport of MHC-I and MHC-II	Jones *et al.* (1996); Ahn *et al.* (1996); Hegde *et al.* (2002); Zhao and Biegalke (2003); Misaghi *et al.* (2004)
US6		US6 family; putative membrane glycoprotein; inhibits TAP-mediated peptide transport	Ahn *et al.* (1997); Lehner *et al.* (1997); Hewitt *et al.* (2001)
US7		US6 family; membrane glycoprotein	Huber *et al.* (2002)
US8		US6 family; membrane glycoprotein; binds to MHC-I	Huber *et al.* (2002); Tirabassi and Ploegh (2002)
US9		US6 family; membrane glycoprotein	Huber *et al.* (2002)
US10		US6 family; membrane glycoprotein; delays trafficking of MHC-I	Huber *et al.* (2002); Furman *et al.* (2002)
US11		US6 family; membrane glycoprotein; causes selective degradation of MHC-I	Jones *et al.* (1995); Wiertz *et al.* (1996a); Machold *et al.* (1997); Lilley and Ploegh (2004)
US12		US12 family; putative multiple transmembrane protein	
US13		US12 family; putative multiple transmembrane protein	
US14		US12 family; putative multiple transmembrane protein	
US15		US12 family; putative multiple transmembrane protein	
US16		US12 family; putative multiple transmembrane protein	
US17		US12 family; putative multiple transmembrane protein	
US18		US12 family; putative multiple transmembrane protein	Guo *et al.* (1993)
US19		US12 family; putative multiple transmembrane protein	Guo *et al.* (1993)
US20		US12 family; putative multiple transmembrane protein	Guo *et al.* (1993)
US21		US12 family; putative multiple transmembrane protein	
US22		US22 family; tegument protein; released from cells	Mocarski *et al.* (1988); Adair *et al.* (2002)
US23		US22 family	
US24		US22 family	
US26		US22 family	
US27		GPCR family; membrane protein	Fraile-Ramos *et al.* (2002)
US28		GPCR family; membrane protein; broad spectrum CC chemokine receptor; mediates cellular migration	Neote *et al.* (1993); Gao and Murphy (1994); Streblow *et al.* (1999)
US29		Putative membrane glycoprotein	
US30		Putative membrane glycoprotein	
US31		US1 family; duplicated TT virus ORF2 motif	
US32		US1 family; duplicated TT virus ORF2 motif	
US34		Putative secreted protein	
US34A		Putative membrane protein	
TRS1		US22 family; immediate early transcriptional activator; tegument protein; involved in shutoff of host protein synthesis and capsid assembly	Stasiak and Mocarski (1992); Romanowski and Shenk (1997); Romanowski *et al.* (1997); Child *et al.* (2004); Adamo *et al.* (2004)

[a] The layout here and in Fig. 14.1 is that derived by Davison *et al.* (2003a,b) and Dolan *et al.* (2004) for genes encoding functional proteins in wild type HCMV. A substantial number of additional protein-coding regions have been proposed (Chee *et al.*, 1990; Yu *et al.*, 2003; Murphy *et al.*, 2003a,b; Varnum *et al.*, 2004), and are not included because their status is considered generally less secure. The region between UL74 and UL75 may contain a small, rightward-oriented protein-coding exon (Scalzo *et al.*, 2004), and is also omitted. Homologous genes are in the same row. Blanks indicate the absence of detectable homologues. Bold font indicates HCMV genes that proved essential for growth in fibroblast cell lines in the study of Yu *et al.* (2003). Dunn *et al.* (2003b) also found that UL48, UL71, UL76, UL94 and UL96 are essential.

[b] Core genes (those inherited from the common ancestor of *Alpha-*, *Beta-* and *Gammaherpesvirinae*) are shaded, and functions take into account what is known about the homologue in the best characterized herpesvirus, which is often HSV-1 (see Chapter 2, Table 2.2). For genes conserved between HCMV and HHV-6, the information almost exclusively concerns the former. A blank indicates the absence of functional information.

[c] References primarily concern published data on gene identification and protein characterization, and are not exhaustive. Information on other aspects (e.g. dispensability, sequence variation or transcription) is generally not included. References to HHV-6 data (or, failing this, HHV-7 data) are denoted by square brackets.

[d] Positional homologue with similar functional characteristics.

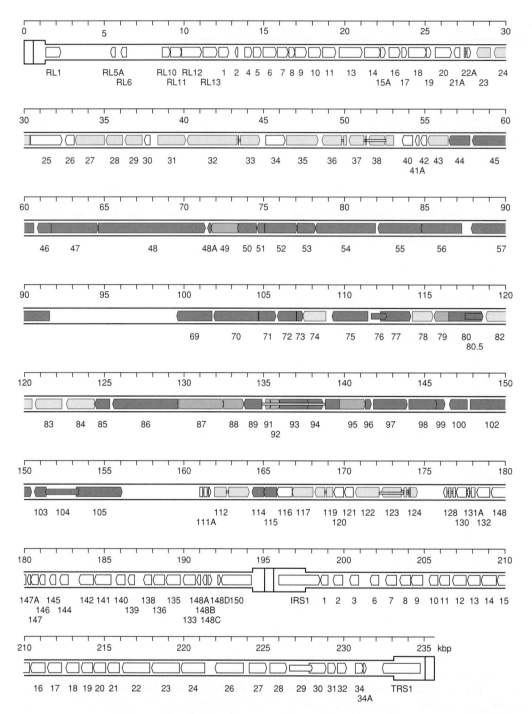

Fig. 14.1. Genetic content of wild-type HCMV, based on an interpretation of the genome sequence of strain Merlin (Dolan *et al.*, 2004), which in turn depended on analyses carried out by Chee *et al.* (1990), Cha *et al.* (1996) and Davison *et al.* (2003a, b). The inverted repeats TR_L/IR_L and TR_S/IR_S (which contain the *a* sequence depicted by a rectangle) are shown in a thicker format than U_L and U_S. Protein-coding regions are indicated by arrows, with gene nomenclature below. Introns are shown as narrow white bars. Genes corresponding to those in TR_L/IR_L and TR_S/IR_S of strain AD169 are given their full nomenclature, but the UL and US prefixes have been omitted from UL1–UL150 and US1–US34A. Core genes derived from the ancestor of *Alpha*, *Beta*- and *Gammaherpesvirinae* are shaded dark grey, additional genes derived from the ancestor of the *Beta*- and *Gammaherpesvirinae* are shaded mid grey, and other genes conserved between HCMV and HHV-6 are shaded light grey. White genes are unique to HCMV TRS1, US26 and US22 may be the counterparts of HHV-6 U95, DR1 and DR6, respectively, but are shown as unique.

Comparative genome and virion structure 185

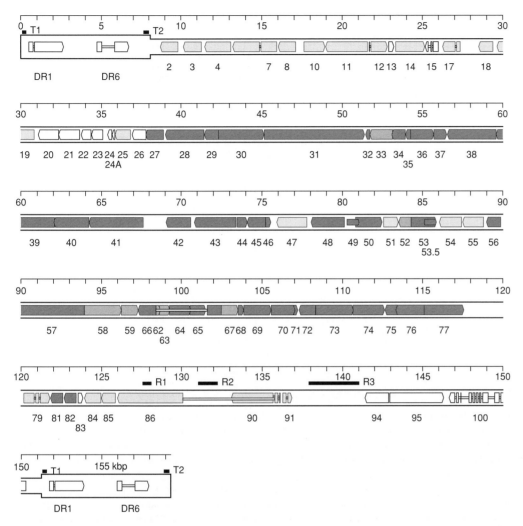

Fig. 14.2. Genetic content of HHV-6, based on strain U1102 of variant A (Gompels *et al.*, 1995) as modified by Megaw *et al.* (1998) and updated by the reintroduction of one gene (U83) and the incorporation of the splicing pattern for another (U86). The terminal direct repeat is shown in a thicker format than the unique region. Protein-coding regions are indicated by arrows, with gene nomenclature below. Introns are shown as narrow white bars. Genes in the direct repeat are given their full nomenclature, but the U prefix has been omitted from genes in the unique region. Core genes derived from the ancestor of *Alpha-, Beta-* and *Gammaherpesvirinae* are shaded dark grey, additional genes derived from the ancestor of the *Beta-* and *Gammaherpesvirinae* are shaded light grey, and other genes conserved between HCMV and HHV-6 are shaded light grey. White genes are specific to HHV-6. U95, DR1 and DR6 may be the counterparts of HCMV TRS1, US26 and US22, respectively, but are shown as unique. Reiterated sequences T1, T2, R1, R2 and R3 are indicated by black bars.

The genes shared by HCMV and HHV-6 are collinear, probably as a result of being inherited from a common ancestor, but it is difficult to specify their number precisely. The best estimate, 73 genes, consists of 40 herpesvirus core genes, six genes inherited by the *Beta-* and *Gammaherpesvirinae*, and 27 genes specific to HCMV and HHV-6 (and HHV-7). The last class can be subdivided into 22 genes whose predicted amino acid sequences are detectably conserved (albeit weakly in some cases) in both genomes, along with the major immediate early gene (HCMV UL123) and the adjacent UL124 which lack amino acid similarity but correspond in position and orientation to HHV-6 genes (U90 and U91) with which they share properties, and three members of the US22 gene family (see below) that lack positional counterparts but have amino acid sequence counterparts elsewhere in the genome. HHV-6 U95, DR1 and

```
    MCMV UL119    NHILNASHSAVAPGVTFFKCHFYHIARTRDGGPDWKEATWKVTAYPLI.SLTTGF.QVKDLFVRVTYKNRTDLKPKPK
    RCMV UL119    NNIFSINHTRCPLGYTEYMCNFTHYQGKRPPS.....FHWWLTGYPLM.KLQIGI.WIRHLKISIVLPQANVSQSTVL
    TCMV UL119    RHQLNVSRQQPQFAVEDYRCQFIFTGQYVAIA......FWTFYAYPSL.SATYTE.YRSTVRVNAIVSRNTSVLLELK
    RhCMV UL119   TTQTFFTMYRQAPNVTTQYSCRFIATGQTLNKS.......WEFLVMPIK.AVFASP.TNDSMIQLRVLVNDHPCTNETV
    CCMV UL119    TGQALSVVGPVPRTTVEYNCSFISLWRTVHTS.......WNFFTYPIY.AVYGTH.LNATTMQIRVLLKNHTHCLLNG
    HCMV UL119    TAQELLISGLRPQETTEYTCSFFSWGRHHNAT......WDLFTYPIY.AVYGTR.LNATTMRVRVLLQEHEHCLLNG
    HHV-6 U85     TTSLLKIKAKSAYDATCLTCTFTVDNEKTSAT.....SCLKLFMKPIV.VLYFRY.LDNFLDVTCTVTSYPKPNVVIK
    HHV-7 U85     TA.LLKFKSRTINDAGCLTCAFFAKTLSTMS......CVHLSMKPII.ALYYRH.LQNFLDVTCSVTSYPKPLVAIL
    OX-2          QNSTITFWNITLEDEGCYMCLFNTFGFGKISG....TACLTVYVQPIV.SLHYKF.SEDHLNITCSATARPAPMVFWK
                                    C F                        P  :            :   :
                                    :                         :  :            :   :
                                    :                         :  :            :   :

    HCMV UL120    MYRAGVTLLVVAVVSFGRWDSVTVATTIRVGWWYEPQVKMAYIYEHNDTNLTIFCNTTAYDSPFLASG
    CCMV UL120    MQRVRVTVVLVSVAAALRYAVTAGGEAAVAQVHDRTGEPGVNISYLYK.NDTNLTILCNTTALQSPFLASG
    RhCMV UL120   MLRFYHAIYLGIVCMVIIMTVVYSLPFYSGDPFAPHVKVAYIYY.NASNLTIYCNTSARYSRFLAGG
    SCMV UL120    MLRFSDVVWLSLGLGLLIVTVVYGIPFYKGDRYAPTVKMAYIYY.NASNLTIYCNTSSRRSRFLAAG
    HCMV UL121                     MWGCGWSRILVLLLLMCMALMARGTYGAYICSPNPGRLRISCALSVLDQRLWWEI
    CCMV UL121                      MMVAWWYLVCTVLLWMTVGGSGAVYICSPNTGMVKISCYLPKLDRRLWWSL
    RhCMV UL121                      MLLGLAIVLLTSVVVSVCGVQTPDMCWDRN.HMKVKCLLRQLDTRLYWFM
    SCMV UL121                      MLGLSVVWILMSVMMNVCAGMDTPQMCVDDKHQVKVKCSLLRLNTELYWFV

    HCMV UL120    MMIV.LPHRTQFLTRKVNYSEDMENIKQNYTHQLTHMLTGEPGTYVNGSVTCWGSNGTFGAGTFI.........VRS
    CCMV UL120    IMVS.TKRNTTIVAGKVNYTADNE..KKDYHHYLNVTLRAEYGTYLNAGVTCWGSNGTWGAKTFE.........VHS
    RhCMV UL120   IMIT.TNHNTTFLKG..GYYEYTRHPKPFYLQFVKVLDTAPYGFYLNSTVTCWGSNGTYGVRSFMVTKITNTSNKDA
    SCMV UL120    MMIT.TKYNTTIVKG..GYKIAKR.PRPIYLKFVKVLDKASYKFYMNSTVTCWGSNGTYGIHSFRVRKITCPSSINV
    HCMV UL121    QYSS......GRLTRVLVFHDEGEEGDDV.HLTDTHHCTSCTHPYVISLVTPLTINATLRLLIRD....GMYGRGEK
    CCMV UL121    RDGETRVPVFSPEDEEEGGEQKSGHEERGLHSVSVRHCKSCVRPHVVSLVTPLLLNRTVSLLLVD.....REQNEEK
    RhCMV UL121   NDTK..........RVWAFDYDSQTPLSVPYRVEVRGSLWSSESAVILRMPPYPMTTVGLLLKMD........EDREG
    SCMV UL121    NDSQ..........RIWAFDFETQLPYRVE..VHPSMMQPSEFEMILRIPLSPQTTVGILLDMG........ENRQD

    HCMV UL120    MVNKTAGNTNTFIHFVEDSELVENPAYFRRSDHRAFMIVILTQVVFVVFIINASFIWSWTFRRHKR
    CCMV UL120    MANQTDNATEISFHRVTEQELIDNPEYFRRSNKKLVMIVIVSQLVFVMLIINASFVWSWKFRRHR
    RhCMV UL120   I.......VLVNDTDLVETPDAALNWWPRSQQNRVVMIVLLAQLVFVVFIINACLIWSCKFKRHN
    SCMV UL120    SADAYETPNIVNDTDLVETPDVALRWWPQNQQNQIVMGVLLTQLV...FIINACLIWSCKFRRHK
    HCMV UL121    ELCIAHLPTLRDIRTCRVDADLGLLYAVCLILSFSIVTAALWKVDYDRSVAVVSKSYKS
    CCMV UL121    LLCFTRLTTLEGIRTCRIDPDLGLLYAMCLILSLSIVTAALWKLDCDR....RARGYKS
    RhCMV UL121   VLCVGVVPKKRYLNPCGWDSDLSLWYCVCVLLTVGVMIAGILKLDYDT..TRHLTDYKSWLSRRTRYFEPAVKRW
    SCMV UL121    LLCTGVVPHRKHMSDCGPEIDVYILCSVCVMLSLSVVVAGILKMDYDT..SRHLTGYKSWLSRRTRYFEPAVKRW
```

Fig. 14.3. Amino acid sequence alignments of proteins encoded by HCMV and HHV-6 genes putatively derived from a cellular OX-2 gene. (A) Conserved region in the ectodomains of human OX-2 (accession P41217), the HHV-6 and HHV-7 U85 proteins and cytomegalovirus UL119 proteins. The region includes residues 150–208 and 106–176 of the HCMV and HHV-6 proteins, respectively. Bold residues are conserved between OX-2 and one or both of the U85 proteins, or between both U85 proteins and at least two UL119 proteins. Three residues conserved throughout are indicated at the foot of the alignment. (B) Conserved residues in two regions of the primate cytomegalovirus UL120 and UL121 proteins. The entire sequence of each protein is shown. Bold residues are conserved in at least three orthologous proteins and at least one non-orthologous protein. Predicted signal and transmembrane sequences are indicated in grey and by underlining, respectively. The SCMV sequences are derived from Chang et al. (1995). Residues that are partially conserved between the OX-2-related proteins in (A) and the UL120 or UL121 proteins are indicated by colons.

DR6 may be the counterparts of HCMV TRS1, US26 and US22, respectively (Gompels et al., 1995), but are not indicated as conserved in Figs. 14.1 and 14.2 or Table 14.1 because the precise correspondence is unclear. With these three exceptions, all of the genes inherited by HCMV and HHV-6 from their common ancestor are located between UL23 and UL124 in HCMV and U2 and U91 in HHV-6. Genes flanking this betaherpesvirus-common set are unique to each virus. Nonetheless, each virus possesses a number of genes within the conserved region that appear to be unique. These include genes lacking sequence and positional counterparts (e.g., HCMV UL116 and HHV-6 U83), genes whose positional counterparts lack sequence or functional similarities (e.g., HCMV UL34 and HHV-6 U13), and genes that are related to others and probably arose by duplication (e.g., HCMV UL25).

Gene duplication

Gene duplication has been employed widely by large eukaryotic DNA viruses and their hosts as a means of generating diversity (Prince and Pickett, 2002). Table 14.2 lists the 13 gene families that appear to have arisen in HCMV. Only four or five families have representatives, and each has fewer members, in HHV-6. The genes that have arisen by duplication appear to function in various specific aspects of the host response to infection. It is interesting to note evidence for duplication in the more recent evolution of these lineages, in the form of additional family members. For example, HHV-7 has two counterparts of HHV-6 U55 (termed U55A and U55B; Nicholas, 1996), CCMV lacks a counterpart to HCMV UL1 and has two additional counterparts of UL146 (Davison et al., 2003a), and RhCMV and

Table 14.2. Gene families in HCMV and HHV-6

Family	HCMV	HHV-6	Features and putative functions
RL11	RL5A, RL6, RL11, RL12, RL13, UL1, UL4, UL5, UL6, UL7, UL8, UL9, UL10, UL11	None	Most are membrane glycoproteins; most share a putative immunoglobulin domain with certain human adenovirus E3 proteins
UL14	UL14, UL141	None	Membrane glycoproteins containing an immunoglobulin domain; UL141 is involved in NK cell evasion
UL18	UL18, UL142	None	MHC-I-related membrane glycoproteins; involved in immune evasion
US22	UL23, UL24, UL26, UL28, UL29, UL36, UL43, US22, US23, US24, US26, IRS1, TRS1	U2, U3, U7, U8, U17, U25, U95, DR1, DR6	Tegument proteins; involved in modulation of the cellular response
UL25	UL25, UL35	U14	Tegument proteins
GPCR	UL33, UL78, US27, US28	U12, U51	Chemokine receptors; some may have been captured independently
DURP	UL31, UL72, UL82, UL83, UL84	U10, U45, U54, U55 (U55A, U55B in HHV-7)	Derived from dUTPase; some are tegument proteins; multiple roles in modulating cellular responses
UL120	UL120, UL121, possibly UL119	Possibly U85	Membrane glycoproteins; possibly derived from OX-2
UL146	UL146, UL147	None	CXC chemokines
US1	US1, US31, US32	None	Related to TT virus ORF2
US2	US2, US3	None	Membrane glycoproteins; roles in immune evasion
US6	US6, US7, US8, US9, US10, US11	None	Membrane glycoproteins; roles in immune evasion
US12	US12, US13, US14, US15, US16, US17, US18, US19, US20, US21	None	Multiple transmembrane proteins

SCMV have additional members of the GPCR family corresponding to the US27 and US28 subset (Martin, 2000; Penfold et al., 2003; Hansen et al., 2003; Sahagun-Ruiz et al., 2004). The potential for rapid evolution of gene family members is illustrated by the observation that certain examples (e.g., UL146 and some of the RL11 family) are among the most variable HCMV genes (Murphy et al., 2003b; Dolan et al., 2004).

It is likely that gene duplication in *Betaherpesvirinae* is more common than can be detected by amino acid sequence similarity, since it is possible for duplicated genes to diverge so extensively that similarity is obliterated. Consideration of two regions potentially in this category exemplifies the difficulties of defining evolutionary origins in such cases. In the first region, the three genes UL40-UL42 in HCMV are positionally equivalent to the six genes U20-U24A in HHV-6. Although the proteins encoded by these genes share no sequence similarity, the fact that all are predicted to be membrane-associated raises the possibility that the genes that encode them are derived from a single ancestor. It is interesting to note that one of the three HHV-6 genes (U22, U83 and U94) lacking counterparts in HHV-7 is located in this region. The analysis summarized in Fig. 14.3 sheds light on a second region, which contains the three genes UL119-UL121 in HCMV and the single gene U85 in HHV-6, all encoding putative membrane glycoproteins. The U85 protein is related to the cellular OX-2 surface glycoprotein, with greatest similarity apparent in an immunoglobulin domain (Gompels et al., 1995). Atalay et al. (2002) also noted that an HCMV Fc-receptor encoded by HCMV UL119 contains an immunoglobulin domain. The alignment in Fig. 14.3(a) draws on data from several *Betaherpesvirinae* to support the view that U85 and UL119 are related, but with the latter diverging from OX-2 to a greater extent than the former. The alignment in Fig. 14.3(b) shows that the pair of genes adjacent to UL119 (UL120 and UL121) are distantly related to each other, and thus comprise a novel HCMV gene family. The colons between residues in Fig. 14.3(a) and Fig. 14.3(b) hint that UL120 and UL121 may be related to UL119 via the C-terminal portion of the immunoglobulin domain, although the degree of conservation is marginal. Thus, it appears that U85 and UL119 are both derived from a cellular OX-2 gene, and it is possible that UL120 and UL121 may also have arisen via duplication events involving the ancestor of UL119.

Gene capture

The simplest explanation for the presence in HCMV of genes that have counterparts in the cellular genome is that of gene capture, a process which appears to involve insertion into the viral genome of a cDNA copy of a cellular mRNA or pre-mRNA, since most such genes lack introns. Recombination events of this sort probably occur commonly on an evolutionary scale, but few would result in viable virus, even fewer would provide a growth advantage, and even fewer still would become fixed in viral populations. The advantages of gene capture are illustrated in the case of cellular cyclo-oxygenase-2, which is involved in prostaglandin synthesis. Expression of this gene facilitates growth of HCMV (Speir *et al.*, 1998; Zhu *et al.*, 2002; Mocarski, 2002), and, unlike HCMV and CCMV, RhCMV has a copy in its genome (Hansen *et al.*, 2003). Gene capture has occurred throughout herpesvirus evolution, with ancient examples such as the dUTPase and uracil-DNA glycosylase genes common to the *Alpha-, Beta-* and *Gammaherpesvirinae*, more recent examples in certain of the GPCR family common to the *Betaherpesvirinae*, and even more recent examples such as the UL146 chemokine gene in primate cytomegaloviruses. Some, perhaps all, of the gene families have arisen from captured genes.

In addition to incorporating cellular genes, *Betaherpesvirinae* appear to have exchanged genetic information with other viruses. Thus, HHV-6 U94 is related to the Rep gene of *Parvoviridae*, but lacks a counterpart in HHV-7 (Thomson *et al.*, 1991). The RL11 family proteins of primate cytomegaloviruses share a putative immunoglobulin domain with a glycoprotein family encoded in the E3 region of primate *Adenoviridae* (Davison *et al.*, 2003b). A previously unreported finding concerns the primate cytomegalovirus US1 gene family, whose functions are unknown. Hijikata *et al.* (1999) noted a motif ($WX_7 HX_3 CXCX_5 H$) that is conserved near the N terminus of VP2 in a small, single-stranded DNA virus, chicken anaemia virus (CAV; *Circoviridae*). The N-terminal region of the ORF2 protein in the related TT viruses (TTVs) and TT-like viruses, which are common in humans, also contain this motif. Figure 14.4 shows that the N-terminal regions of proteins specified by the primate cytomegalovirus US1 gene family contain two copies of this motif, each of which, as suggested from the nature of the conserved residues, might coordinate a metal ion. Parenthetically, it is interesting to note that the motif is located within an extended region identified by Peters *et al.* (2002) as conserved between CAV VP2 and cellular protein-tyrosine phosphatases (PTPases). However, the significance of the relationship to PTPases is dubious, since most of the PTPase residues conserved in CAV VP2 are not conserved in the TTV ORF2 protein, and proposed catalytic residues are significantly diverged in VP2 and essentially absent from the ORF2 protein. In any case, the known PTPase catalytic residues are C-terminal to the region aligned with the proposed catalytic residues in VP2, and well outside the conserved region. It is surprising, therefore, that Peters *et al.* (2002) were able to show that VP2 and the ORF2 protein of a TT-like virus have PTPase activity.

Variation

HCMV isolates exhibit a high degree of variation in a wide range of genes (Murphy *et al.*, 2003b; Dolan *et al.*, 2004; Pignatelli *et al.*, 2004). The most variable genes potentially encode proteins that are secreted or associated with membranes, and therefore most exposed to selection by the immune system. Attempts to associate certain alleles with particular pathogenic properties have been largely unsuccessful. This may reflect the multifactorial nature of such properties, and the fact that recombination has played a part in HCMV evolution (Arav-Boger *et al.*, 2002; Rasmussen *et al.*, 2003). Limited studies of variation have also been carried out in HHV-6 (Dominguez *et al.*, 1996; Stanton *et al.*, 2003) and HHV-7 (Chan *et al.*, 2003).

Gene function

Most effort on gene function has been carried out on HCMV, but advances with other cytomegaloviruses have been substantial. Indeed, the use of the powerful bacterial articificial chromosome technology for generating mutants was innovated for MCMV (Messerle *et al.*, 1997) before it was applied to other cytomegaloviruses, including HCMV (Borst *et al.*, 1999; McGregor and Schleiss, 2001; Yu *et al.*, 2002; Chang and Barry, 2003; Murphy *et al.*, 2003b). Studies on non-human cytomegaloviruses form a vital basis for assessing the functions of genes in pathogenesis by means that cannot be applied for HCMV. The parallels are incomplete, however, as even the closest relative of HCMV that could be used practically as an animal model, RhCMV, exhibits genetic differences in comparison with HCMV. With regard to the effects of infection with *Betaherpesvirinae* on cellular transcription, several microarray analyses have been carried out (Zhu *et al.*, 1998; Kenzelmann and Muhlemann, 2000; Simmen *et al.*, 2001; Browne *et al.*, 2001). Further details on HCMV gene function are given in Chapter 15.

Virion structure

In all *Herpesviridae*, the genome is packaged within the icosahedral capsid, which is embedded in a dense proteinaceous matrix termed the tegument, and in turn surrounded by a lipid envelope extensively decorated with viral

```
HCMV   US1-1       MASGLGDLSVGVSSLPMRELAWRRVADDSHDLWCCCMDWKAHVEYAHPASELRPGSGG.
CCMV   US1-1    MASDCGHPPVVGMPVMSSAVSSLPMRELAWRRVADDSHDLWCACMDWKAHVEYVGVSAELRPGSGA.
RhCMV  US1-1        MEPVVSCGLVGHMPMRELAWRRVADDSHDLWCACMDWKAHIEYVVPLAEDILPRPES
HCMV   US31-1                 MSLLEREESWRRVVDYSHNLWCTCGNWQSHVEIQDEEPNCEQPEPAH
CCMV   US31-1                  MSLLEREERWRRVIDYSHELWCDCGNWQTHVEIQDDGPNSQEPEPAH
RhCMV  US31-1                    MEKEETWRGLMVYSHSLWCICGHWKAHIIMSDEANSEEVACSN.
HCMV   US32-1                MAMYTSESERDWRRVIHDSHGLWCDCGDWREHLYCVYDSHFQRRPTT..
CCMV   US32-1                  MVIATTDSERDWRRVMVESHALWCDCDEWQSHLYRVFDSDFHRRARN..
RhCMV  US32-1         MNRPRDLIPTLHDSCTQTELRWRRVLTESHALWCNCGDWTPHVECVDDAYFQLRWRS..

HCMV   US1-2              WPEHAEAQWRQQVHAAHDVWCNCGDWQGHALRS>
CCMV   US1-2              WPEQVEAQWRHQVHVAHDVWCDCGDWQGHALRS>
RhCMV  US1-2              WPAQVEAQWRLQIKGAHDVWCQCGDWRGHALRS>
HCMV   US31-2             WLEYVAVQWQARVRDSHDRWCLCNAWRDHALRG>
CCMV   US31-2             WLQYVECQWQLRVRDSHDRWCLCNGWRDHALRG>
RhCMV  US31-2             WMEDATMRWIRNARETHDKWCRCTDWRGHALSL>
HCMV   US32-2             RAERRAANWRRQMRRLHRLWCFCQDWKCHALYA>
CCMV   US32-2             REERRAANWRRQMRRLHRLWCFCRDWKSHALFT>
RhCMV  US32-2             RQERTALRWRRQMHRLHNLWCMCGNWREHALYR>


Human  TTV 1              >LNWQWYSSILSSHAAMCGCPDAVAHFNHL>
Human  TTV 2              >QERQFYEACLHAHDAFCGCGDFVAHINSV>
Human  TTV 3              >REQQWFESTLRSHHSFCGCGDPVLHFTNL>
Human  TTV 4              >RENQWFAAVFHSHASWCGCGDFVGHLNSI>
Human  TTV 5              >IQRLWYESFHRGHAAFCGCGDPILHITAL>
Human  TLMV 1             >LENQWMNTIFNTHDLMCGCNDTIKHLFAI>
Human  TLMV 2             >KQTQWINDIHCTHDLWCSCDHVLKHLLLS>
Chimp  TTV 1              >KGKALLNSVAHSHDLLCHCDHPLKHLCEI>
Chimp  TTV 2              >LERNWYESCLRSHAAFCGCGDFVSHLNNL>
Macaque TTV 1             >RELDWWRGTWWNHAAFCGCGDPSFHLALL>
Macaque TTV 2             >REEAWLRSVVDSHQSFCGCNDPGFHLGLL>
Tamarin TTV               >QELIWKELVDNSHKLFCNCMDPQNHYRLI>
Owl monkey TTV            >QEDRWLKAVESCHQLFCSCSSAWDHLRNI>
Tupaia TTV                >PAKIWWHSCLLSHKSWCNCTEPRNHLPGW>
Pig    TTV                >WEEAWLTSCTSIHDHHCDCGSWRDHLWTL>
Dog    TTV                >HEAAWKQHCSWSHGLWCHCHDWTRHLKKE>
Cat    TTV                >QEALWKQLVSAEHRKFCSCGDYTQHFRFP>
CAV                       >SIAVWLRECSRSHAKICNCGQFRKHWFQE>
                           W       H  C C         H
```

Fig. 14.4. Amino acid sequence alignments of the WX$_7$HX$_3$CXCX$_5$H motif near the N termini of primate cytomegalovirus proteins encoded by the US1 gene family (US1, US31 and US32), the ORF2 proteins of TT viruses (TTV) of various hosts (five, two and two types for humans, chimpanzees and macaques, respectively) and TTV-like miniviruses (TLMV) of humans (two types), and VP2 of chicken anaemia virus (CAV). The cytomegalovirus sequences in the upper two panels commence at the N-terminus and proceed continuously for each virus, so that the two copies of the motif are aligned sequentially. The TTV, TLMV and CAV proteins contain a single copy of the motif. Sequences were derived via the information given in Fig. 2 in Okamoto *et al.* (2002). Arrowheads indicate that the sequences extend further towards the C terminus (cytomegalovirus proteins) or both termini (TTV, TLMV and CAV proteins). The motif is shown at the foot of the alignment.

glycoproteins (see Chapter 3). Virion morphogenesis commences in the host cell nucleus, beginning with assembly of the spherical procapsid by condensation of the capsid and scaffold proteins (see Chapter 20). By analogy with HSV-1 (Newcomb *et al.*, 1996), proteolytic maturation of the HCMV procapsid separates the scaffold from the inside surface of the capsid, giving rise to a more angular particle, while packaging of the viral genome leads to egress of the scaffold component and formation of mature C-capsids (Irmiere and Gibson, 1985). A-capsids and B-capsids are also found in great abundance in the nucleus and in mature virions (Irmiere and Gibson, 1983). A-capsids are devoid of scaffold or DNA, and are thought to be the product of aborted packaging. B-capsids are mature particles containing large or small scaffold cores that are thought to be either precursors of DNA packaging or byproducts of failed packaging (Fig. 14.5(a)). Mature capsids (A, B and C) bud out of the nucleus, and are thought to undergo a process of envelopment and de-envelopment as they traverse the nuclear membrane (see Chapter 20). The maturing virion then acquires its tegument in perinuclear compartments termed tegusomes. Finally, capsids bud into Golgi-derived cytoplasmic compartments, gaining their lipid membrane and envelope glycoproteins in the process, and exit the cell by the exocytotic pathway.

The genome

HCMV has a larger genome than members of the *Alpha-* and *Gammaherpesvirinae*, and it is consequently more tightly packaged within the capsid. However, this is not a generalized feature of the *Betaherpesvirinae*, as the genomes of HHV-6 and HHV-7 are smaller. Nonetheless, the requirement for orderly ingress and egress of the genome, through

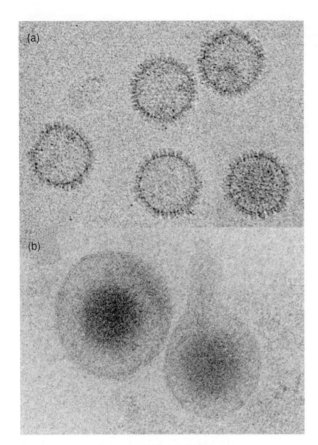

Fig. 14.5. Cryo-micrographs of (a) purified HCMV B-capsids and (b) purified HCMV virions showing the characteristic swirling pattern of the packaged genomic DNA (from Bhella et al., 2000; with permission from Academic Press).

a portal complex, suggests a high degree of organization in genome packaging.

Imaging of HCMV virions by cryo-microscopy allows the packaged DNA molecule to be visualized (Fig. 14.5(b)), revealing the characteristic swirled, striated and punctate array patterns seen in many *Herpesviridae*, as well as in the double-stranded DNA bacteriophages T4, T7, λ and p22 (Bhella et al., 2000). These patterns suggest a mode of packaging in which DNA enters the capsid and spools around the inner surface, winding inwards, towards the centre, in successive layers (Booy et al., 1991; Zhou et al., 1999). Measurements indicate that the HCMV genome is packaged in layers approximately 23 Å apart. Assuming hexagonal packing, which is the preferred conformation of DNA fibres at this packing density, this corresponds to an average interhelix spacing of 26 Å. HSV-1 virions show an interlayer spacing of 26 Å, corresponding to an interhelix distance of 30 Å. At such packing densities, the DNA would be expected to be in a liquid-crystalline state, with possible

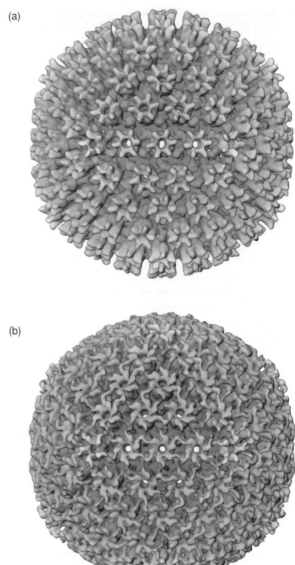

Fig. 14.6. Three-dimensional reconstructions of (a) the HCMV B-capsid (adapted from Butcher et al., 1998; with permission from Academic Press), and (b) the HCMV virion (adapted from Zhou et al., 1999; with permission from the American Society for Microbiology). Both structures are viewed along the icosahedral twofold symmetry axes and are radially depth-cued so that darker regions are closer to the center of the particle and lighter regions are further away. (See color plate section.)

local transitions to three-dimensional hexagonal packing in those viruses with a tighter packing density. However, curvature of the packaged DNA would prevent extensive transition to a crystalline state, suggesting that 26 Å is the upper limit of packing density achievable. In order to package its genome, HCMV has evolved to produce a larger capsid, with a diameter of 130 nm rather than 125 nm (Butcher et al., 1998).

The capsid

Investigation of B-capsid structure in HCMV strain AD169 by cryo-microscopy and image reconstruction (Fig. 14.5(a)) has revealed an architecture very similar to that of HSV-1, consisting of a hexamer-pentamer clustered T=16 icosadeltahedral shell (Butcher et al., 1998). The capsid is complex, consisting of four structural proteins: the major capsid protein (MCP; encoded by UL86), the minor capsid protein (mCP; UL85), the minor capsid protein-binding protein (mC-BP; UL46) and the smallest capsid protein (SCP; UL48A) (Gibson, 1983; Irmiere and Gibson, 1985; Sedarati and Rosenthal, 1988; Gibson, 1996; Gibson et al., 1996a; Gibson et al., 1996b). In addition, the portal complex, which is presumed to occupy one of the fivefold vertices, is considered a capsid component.

The major structural components of the capsid are the capsomeres, termed pentons and hexons. These large, turret-like structures are composed primarily of five or six copies of the MCP, respectively. In total, there are 150 hexons occupying positions of local six-fold symmetry, and 12 pentons, located at the icosahedral five-fold symmetry axes (Fig. 14.6(a)). The hexons and pentons are 15 nm tall and have a central channel running through them that is constricted some 7.4 nm from the capsid floor, which is also composed of the MCP and appears thicker in HCMV than in HSV-1. The tips of each hexon are decorated with six copies of SCP (Yu et al., 2005), a feature also found in HSV-1, in which the hexons are capped by the homologous protein, VP26 (Booy et al., 1994; Trus et al., 1995; Zhou et al., 1995). A small capsid protein is also associated with the tips of hexons in HHV-8, but is also present at the tips of pentons (Trus et al., 2001). Between the HCMV capsomeres, lying on the capsid floor at positions of local threefold symmetry, are the triplexes. These heterotrimeric structures are composed of two copies of the mCP and one copy of the mC-BP. The triplexes are critical for capsid morphogenesis, most likely linking together the capsomeres in the procapsid, directing assembly, and stabilizing the structure prior to maturation.

The tegument

Perhaps the most striking morphological difference between HCMV and HSV-1 is the extent of icosahedrally ordered tegument in the virion. Cryomicroscopy and image reconstruction have shown that in HSV-1 the only additional, icosahedrally ordered protein that is present in the virion but not the B-capsid is located at the fivefold vertices, where a single rod-like structure connects the tips of each penton MCP (VP5) subunit with the adjacent triplex and its nearest neighboring triplex (Zhou et al., 1999). However, HCMV has an extensive network of icosahedral tegument that, while appearing similar to that found at the HSV-1 penton, also decorates the hexons (Fig. 14.6(b)) (Chen et al., 1999). Appearing as a bridge of density, approximately 120 Å in length and 20–30 Å in diameter, the icosahedrally ordered tegument is anchored to the tip of the hexons and pentons and the top of the adjacent triplex. Investigation of the cytoplasmic B-capsids of SCMV revealed a similar pattern of tegumentation (Trus et al., 1999), although independent reconstruction of lightly, moderately and heavily tegumented capsids suggests that this density is composed of at least two protein species. The first is a capsomere capping protein, which is found at the tips of both the hexons and pentons and therefore binds to the MCP rather than the SCP, which is not present on the penton. The second protein is attached to the capsomere capping protein and the adjacent triplex. The rest of the tegument appears to not be rigidly icosahedral in distribution, but this does not preclude the existence of further order.

Many tegument proteins play roles in the early stages of virus infection and are therefore packaged within the virion to ensure their presence upon infection of a new host, and many are phosphorylated (Roby and Gibson, 1986). The most abundant proteins are the basic phosphoprotein (pp150; encoded by UL32), which is O-glycosylated (Benko et al., 1988) and binds directly to the capsid through its N-terminal one-third (Baxter and Gibson, 2001), the lower matrix protein (pp65; UL83), the upper matrix protein (pp71; UL82), the membrane-associated myristylated protein (pp28; UL99; Sanchez et al., 2000), and the high molecular weight tegument protein (UL48) and its binding protein (UL47). The requirement to incorporate specific proteins suggests that tegument morphogenesis may involve specific interactions between individual components, leading to the formation of a structure that is at least partially ordered. This hypothesis is borne out by the finding that HCMV infections in cell culture give rise to production of many particles composed of enveloped tegument lacking a capsid (dense bodies), suggesting that the tegument can spontaneously self-assemble, possibly around aggregates of pp65 (Irmiere and Gibson, 1983). Moreover, immuno-gold labelling experiments on thin sections of virus-infected cells can reproducibly locate tegument proteins to the outer or inner regions of the tegument (Landini et al., 1987). Logically, specific proteins might be expected to be located at the outer edge of the tegument, since in most enveloped viruses there is a requirement for a specific interaction between viral matrix proteins and the cytoplasmic tail of envelope glycoproteins. Indeed, pp28 has been shown to be essential for envelopment, and may well serve this function (Silva *et al.*, 2003).

Envelope glycoproteins

Many HCMV genes encode putative membrane glycoproteins. However, few thus far have been identified as components of the virion. The most abundant protein species in the viral envelope have homologues throughout the *Herpesviridae*. These are distributed among three complexes: gCI, gCII and gCIII (Gretch *et al.*, 1988). gCI is composed of homodimers of glycoprotein B (gB; UL55), a type I integral membrane protein (Cranage *et al.*, 1986). gB is cleaved by furin into two fragments (gp55 and gp116), which remain covalently associated (Vey *et al.*, 1995). Dimerization of gB is disulfide bond dependent, and mass spectrometric analysis of proteolytic fragments of recombinant gB has revealed extensive disulfide bond formation, both between gB monomers and also between gp55 and gp116 (Eickmann *et al.*, 1998; Lopper and Compton, 2002). Along with gCII, gCI mediates cell attachment, a two-step process involving initial attachment to heparan sulfate, followed by a stabilizing interaction with another receptor (Boyle and Compton, 1998; see Chapter 16). gCII comprises two proteins: gM (UL100), a type III membrane protein, and gN (UL73), a type I membrane protein (Kari *et al.*, 1994; Mach *et al.*, 2000). gCII components are also heavily disulfide linked, although the presence of monomeric forms of these glycoproteins in the virion suggests that these bonds may not be essential for formation and function of the gCII complex (Kari *et al.*, 1990). gCIII includes a heterotrimer of gH (UL75) as well as a heterotrimer of these proteins plus a third component, gO (UL74), which lacks counterparts in *Alpha-* and *Gammaherpesvirinae* (Kaye *et al.*, 1992b; Spaete *et al.*, 1993; Huber and Compton, 1998; Li *et al.*, 1997). gCIII is involved in mediating fusion of viral and host cell membranes, in concert with gCI. In HHV-6, the third component of gCIII is gQ (U100) rather than gO (Mori *et al.*, 2003a).

In addition to glycoproteins that have counterparts throughout the *Herpesviridae*, HCMV-specific glycoproteins encoded by UL4 and RL10 have been identified as virion components (Chang *et al.*, 1989; Spaderna *et al.*, 2002). Analysis of the trafficking in cells of the RL10 protein in isolation from other HCMV proteins indicates that it may be necessary for this glycoprotein to form complexes with other membrane glycoproteins in order to facilitate incorporation into nascent virions. Similarly to the glycoproteins common to the *Herpesviridae*, the RL10 protein forms high molecular weight complexes in mature virions, possibly by disulfide bond formation.

Additional virion components

In addition to the genome, two small RNA molecules are present in the core of the virion, hybridized to the origin of DNA replication (Prichard *et al.*, 1998). These molecules may play a role in initiating DNA replication by providing a point of action for an RNase H-like enzyme, and digestion of the DNA:RNA hybrid could lead to formation of a primer in the form of the opened DNA or possibly a small fragment of the RNA. A number of mRNAs are also associated with virions, most likely located in the tegument (Bresnahan and Shenk, 2000a). The RNAs detected are specified by UL22A (also termed UL21.5) and RL13, and putative non-protein-coding regions encompassing ORFs UL106-UL109, RL2-RL5 and RL7 as defined by Chee *et al.* (1990). Translation of certain of these RNAs could ensure targeting of encoded proteins to the endoplasmic reticulum and Golgi network, before the viral genome becomes transcriptionally active. Alternatively, these molecules may be modulators of cellular immunity or structural components of the tegument. However, the biological significance of virion RNAs is questionable, since it is now known that incorporation of viral and cellular mRNAs occurs non-specifically, with the abundance of RNAs associated with the virion reflecting that in infected cells (Greijer *et al.*, 2000; Terhune *et al.*, 2004).

As there are no histone-like proteins present in herpesvirions to neutralize the charge of the packaged DNA molecule, some other mechanism must be employed. Detection of the polyamines spermine and spermidine in HCMV virions, and the finding that inhibition of polyamine biosynthesis inhibits virus growth at the level of virion assembly, has led to the suggestion that these molecules may fulfil this role (Gibson *et al.*, 1984). Other virion components contributed by the host cell include annexin II (Wright *et al.*, 1995), phospholipase A2 (Allal *et al.*, 2004), the complement control proteins CD55 and CD59 (Spear *et al.*, 1995) and β-2-microglobulin (McKeating *et al.*, 1987), which are associated with the virion envelope. β-2-microglobulin has also been detected in the tegument (Stannard, 1989), as has an actin-like protein (Baldick and Shenk, 1996). Mass spectrometric methods have recently enabled the proteins present in HCMV virions to be catalogued, including a number of viral proteins not detected hitherto and an impressive number of cellular proteins (Varnum *et al.*, 2004). However, caution needs to be exercised in assessing the biological relevance of proteins detected in low abundance by sensitive immunological or physical methods, since proving the absence of contamination with non-virion material is problematic.

REFERENCES

Adair, R., Douglas, E. R., Maclean, J. B. *et al.* (2002). The products of human cytomegalovirus genes UL23, UL24, UL43 and US22 are tegument components. *J. Gen. Virol.*, **83**, 1315–1324.

Adamo, J. E., Schroer, J., and Shenk, T. (2004). Human cytomegalovirus TRS1 protein is required for efficient assembly of DNA-containing capsids. *J. Virol.*, **78**, 10221–10229.

Adler, B., Scrivano, L., Ruzcics, Z., Rupp, B., Sinzger, C., and Koszinowski, U. (2006). Role of human cytomegalovirus UL131A in cell type-specific virus entry and release. *J. Gen. Virol.*, **87**, 2451–2460.

Agulnick, A. D., Thompson, J. R., Iyengar, S., Pearson, G., Ablashi, D., and Ricciardi, R. P. (1993). Identification of a DNA-binding protein of human herpesvirus 6, a putative DNA polymerase stimulatory factor. *J. Gen. Virol.*, **74**, 1003–1009.

Ahn, J. H. and Hayward, G. S. (2000). Disruption of PML-associated nuclear bodies by IE1 correlates with efficient early stages of viral gene expression and DNA replication in human cytomegalovirus infection. *Virology*, **274**, 39–55.

Ahn, K., Angulo, A., Ghazal, P., Peterson, P. A., Yang, Y., and Fruh, K. (1996). Human cytomegalovirus inhibits antigen presentation by a sequential multistep process. *Proc. Natl Acad. Sci. USA*, **93**, 10990–10995.

Ahn, K., Gruhler, A., Galocha, B. *et al.* (1997). The ER-luminal domain of the HCMV glycoprotein US6 inhibits peptide translocation by TAP. *Immunity* 6, 613–621.

Ahn, J. H., Jang, W. J., and Hayward, G. S. (1999). The human cytomegalovirus IE2 and UL112–113 proteins accumulate in viral DNA replication compartments that initiate from the periphery of promyelocytic leukemia protein-associated nuclear bodies (PODs or ND10). *J. Virol.*, **73**, 10458–10471.

Akter, P., Cunningham, C., McSharry, B. P. *et al.* (2003). Two novel spliced genes in human cytomegalovirus. *J. Gen. Virol.*, **84**, 1117–1122.

Al-Barazi, H. O. and Colberg-Poley, A. M. (1996). The human cytomegalovirus UL37 immediate-early regulatory protein is an integral membrane N-glycoprotein which traffics through the endoplasmic reticulum and Golgi apparatus. *J. Virol.*, **70**, 7198–7208.

Allal, C., Buisson-Brenac, C., Marion, V. *et al.* (2004). Human cytomegalovirus carries a cell-derived phospholipase A2 required for infectivity. *J. Virol.*, **78**, 7717–7726.

Anders, D. G. and Gibson, W. (1988). Location, transcript analysis, and partial nucleotide sequence of the cytomegalovirus gene encoding an early DNA-binding protein with similarities to ICP8 of herpes simplex virus type 1. *J. Virol.*, **62**, 1364–1372.

Ansari, A. and Emery, V. C. (1999). The U69 gene of human herpesvirus 6 encodes a protein kinase which can confer ganciclovir sensitivity to baculoviruses. *J. Virol.*, **73**, 3284–3291.

Appleton, B. A., Loregian, A., Filman, D. J., Coen, D. M., and Hogle, J. M. (2004). The cytomegalovirus DNA polymerase subunit UL44 forms a C clamp-shaped dimer. *Mol. Cell.*, **15**, 233–244.

Arav-Boger, R., Willoughby, R. E., Pass, R. F. *et al.* (2002). Polymorphisms of the cytomegalovirus (CMV)-encoded tumor necrosis factor-α and β-chemokine receptors in congenital CMV disease. *J. Infect. Dis.*, **186**, 1057–1064.

Arlt, H., Lang, D., Gebert, S., and Stamminger, T. (1994). Identification of binding sites for the 86-kilodalton IE2 protein of human cytomegalovirus within an IE2-responsive viral early promoter. *J. Virol.*, **68**, 4117–4125.

Atalay, R., Zimmermann, A., Wagner, M. *et al.* (2002). Identification and expression of human cytomegalovirus transcription units coding for two distinct Fcγ receptor homologs. *J. Virol.*, **76**, 8596–8608.

Bahr, U. and Darai, G. (2001). Analysis and characterization of the complete genome of tupaia (tree shrew) herpesvirus. *J. Virol.*, **75**, 4854–4870.

Baldick, C. J. Jr. and Shenk, T. (1996). Proteins associated with purified human cytomegalovirus particles. *J. Virol.*, **70**, 6097–6105.

Baxter, M. K. and Gibson, W. (2001). Cytomegalovirus basic phosphoprotein (pUL32) binds to capsids in vitro through its amino one-third. *J. Virol.*, **75**, 6865–6873.

Bechtel, J. T. and Shenk, T. (2002). Human cytomegalovirus UL47 tegument protein functions after entry and before immediate-early gene expression. *J. Virol.*, **76**, 1043–1050.

Benedict, C. A., Butrovich, K. D., Lurain, N. S. *et al.* (1999). Cutting edge: a novel viral TNF receptor superfamily member in virulent strains of human cytomegalovirus. *J. Immunol.*, **162**, 6967–6970.

Benko, D. M., Haltiwanger, R. S., Hart, G. W., and Gibson, W. (1988). Virion basic phosphoprotein from human cytomegalovirus contains O-linked N-acetylglucosamine. *Proc. Natl Acad. Sci. USA*, **85**, 2573–2577.

Bhella, D., Rixon, F. J., and Dargan, D. J. (2000). Cryomicroscopy of human cytomegalovirus virions reveals more densely packed genomic DNA than in herpes simplex virus type 1. *J. Mol. Biol.*, **295**, 155–161.

Biron, K. K., Harvey, R. J., Chamberlain, S. C. *et al.* (2002). Potent and selective inhibition of human cytomegalovirus replication by 1263W94, a benzimidazole L-riboside with a unique mode of action. *Antimicrob. Agents Chemother.*, **46**, 2365–2372.

Blewett, E. L., White, G., Saliki, J. T., and Eberle, R. (2001). Isolation and characterization of an endogenous cytomegalovirus (BaCMV) from baboons. *Arch. Virol.*, **146**, 1723–1738.

Blewett, E. L., Lewis, J., Gadsby, E. L., Neubauer, S. R., and Eberle, R. (2003). Isolation of cytomegalovirus and foamy virus from the drill monkey (*Mandrillus leucophaeus*) and prevalence of antibodies to these viruses amongst wild-born and captive-bred individuals. *Arch. Virol.*, **148**, 423–433.

Boehme, K. W., Singh, J., Perry, S. T., and Compton, T. (2004). Human cytomegalovirus elicits a coordinated cellular antiviral response via envelope glycoprotein B. *J. Virol.*, **78**, 1202–1211.

Bogner, E,. Reschke, M., Reis, B., Mockenhaupt, T., and Radsak, K. (1993). Identification of the gene product encoded by ORF UL56 of the human cytomegalovirus genome. *Virology*, **196**, 290–293.

Bogner, E., Radsak, K., and Stinski, M. F. (1998). The gene product of human cytomegalovirus open reading frame UL56 binds the pac motif and has specific nuclease activity. *J. Virol.*, **72**, 2259–2264.

Booy, F. P., Newcomb, W. W., Trus, B. L., Brown, J. C., Baker, T. S., and Steven, A. C. (1991). Liquid-crystalline, phage-like packing of encapsidated DNA in herpes simplex virus. *Cell*, **64**, 1007–1015.

Booy, F. P., Trus, B. L., Newcomb, W. W., Brown, J. C., Conway, J. F., and Steven, A. C. (1994). Finding a needle in a haystack: detection of a small protein (the 12-kDa VP26) in a large complex (the 200-MDa capsid of herpes simplex virus). *Proc. Natl Acad. Sci. USA*, **91**, 5652–5656.

Borst, E. M., Hahn, G., Koszinowski, U. H., and Messerle, M. (1999). Cloning of the human cytomegalovirus (HCMV) genome as an infectious bacterial artificial chromosome in *Escherichia coli*: a new approach for construction of HCMV mutants. *J. Virol.*, **73**, 8320–8329.

Boyle, K. A. and Compton, T. (1998). Receptor-binding properties of a soluble form of human cytomegalovirus glycoprotein B. *J. Virol.*, 72, 1826–1833.

Bradshaw, P. A., Duran-Guarino, M. R., Perkins, S. *et al.* (1994). Localization of antigenic sites on human cytomegalovirus virion structural proteins encoded by UL48 and UL56. *Virology*, **205**, 321–328.

Bresnahan, W. A. and Shenk, T. (2000a). A subset of viral transcripts packaged within human cytomegalovirus particles. *Science*, **288**, 2373–2376.

Bresnahan, W. A. and Shenk, T. E. (2000b). UL82 virion protein activates expression of immediate early viral genes in human cytomegalovirus-infected cells. *Proc. Natl Acad. Sci. USA*, **97**, 14506–14511.

Browne, E. P. and Shenk, T. (2003). Human cytomegalovirus UL83-coded pp65 virion protein inhibits antiviral gene expression in infected cells. *Proc. Natl Acad. Sci. USA*, **100**, 11439–11444.

Browne, E. P., Wing, B., Coleman, D. and Shenk, T. (2001). Altered cellular mRNA levels in human cytomegalovirus-infected fibroblasts: viral block to the accumulation of antiviral mRNAs. *J. Virol.*, **75**, 12319–12330.

Browne, H., Smith, G., Beck, S., and Minson, T. (1990). A complex between the MHC class I homologue encoded by human cytomegalovirus and β-2 microglobulin. *Nature*, **347**, 770–772.

Buerger, I., Reefschlaeger, J., Bender, W. *et al.* (2001). A novel non-nucleoside inhibitor specifically targets cytomegalovirus DNA maturation via the UL89 and UL56 gene products. *J. Virol.*, **75**, 9077–9086.

Butcher, S. J., Aitken, J., Mitchell, J., Gowen, B., and Dargan, D. J. (1998). Structure of the human cytomegalovirus B capsid by electron cryomicroscopy and image reconstruction. *J. Struct. Biol.*, **124**, 70–76.

Caposio, P., Riera, L., Hahn, G., Landolfo, S., and Gribaudo, G. (2004). Evidence that the human cytomegalovirus 46-kDa UL72 protein is not an active dUTPase but a late protein dispensable for replication in fibroblasts. *Virology*, **325**, 264–276.

Cha, T. A., Tom, E., Kemble, G. W., Duke, G. M., Mocarski, E. S., and Spaete, R. R. (1996). Human cytomegalovirus clinical isolates carry at least 19 genes not found in laboratory strains. *J. Virol.*, **70**, 78–83.

Chan, P. K., Li, C. K., Chik, K. W. *et al.* (2003). Genetic variation of glycoproteins B and H of human herpesvirus 7 in Hong Kong. *J. Med. Virol.*, **71**, 429–433.

Chang, C. P., Vesole, D. H., Nelson, J., Oldstone, M. B., and Stinski, M. F. (1989). Identification and expression of a human cytomegalovirus early glycoprotein. *J. Virol.*, **63**, 3330–3337.

Chang, W. L. and Barry, P. A. (2003). Cloning of the full-length rhesus cytomegalovirus genome as an infectious and self-excisable bacterial artificial chromosome for analysis of viral pathogenesis. *J. Virol.*, **77**, 5073–5083.

Chang, Y. N., Jeang, K. T., Lietman, T., and Hayward, G. S. (1995). Structural organization of the spliced immediate-early gene complex that encodes the major acidic nuclear (IE1) and transactivator (IE2) proteins of African green monkey cytomegalovirus. *J. Biomed. Sci.*, **2**, 105–130.

Chee, M., Rudolph, S. A., Plachter, B., Barrell, B., and Jahn, G. (1989). Identification of the major capsid protein gene of human cytomegalovirus. *J. Virol.*, **63**, 1345–1353.

Chee, M. S., Bankier, A. T., Beck, S. *et al.* (1990). Analysis of the protein coding content of the sequence of human cytomegalovirus strain AD169. *Curr. Top. Microbiol. Immunol.*, **154**, 125–169.

Chen, D. H., Jiang, H., Lee, M., Liu, F., and Zhou, Z. H. (1999). Three-dimensional visualization of tegument/capsid interactions in the intact human cytomegalovirus. *Virology*, **260**, 10–16.

Chen, P., Tsuge, H., Almassy, R. J. *et al.* (1996). Structure of the human cytomegalovirus protease catalytic domain reveals a novel serine protease fold and catalytic triad. *Cell*, **86**, 835–843.

Child, S. J., Hakki, M., DeNiro, K. L., and Geballe, A. P. (2004). Evasion of cellular antiviral responses by human cytomegalovirus TRS1 and IRS1. *J. Virol.*, **78**, 197–205.

Chou, S., Marousek, G. I., Senters, A. E., Davis, M. G., and Biron, KK. (2004). Mutations in the human cytomegalovirus UL27 gene that confer resistance to maribavir. *J. Virol.*, **78**, 7124–7130.

Cosman, D., Fanger, N., Borges, L. *et al.* (1997). A novel immunoglobulin superfamily receptor for cellular and viral MHC class I molecules. *Immunity*, **7**, 273–282.

Cosman, D., Mullberg, J., Sutherland, C. L. *et al.* (2001). ULBPs, novel MHC class I-related molecules, bind to CMV glycoprotein UL16 and stimulate NK cytotoxicity through the NKG2D receptor. *Immunity*, **14**, 123–133.

Courcelle, C. T., Courcelle, J., Prichard, M. N., and Mocarski, E. S. (2001). Requirement for uracil-DNA glycosylase during the transition to late-phase cytomegalovirus DNA replication. *J. Virol.*, **75**, 7592–7601.

Cranage, M. P., Kouzarides, T., Bankier, A. T. *et al.* (1986). Identification of the human cytomegalovirus glycoprotein B gene and induction of neutralizing antibodies via its expression in recombinant vaccinia virus. *EMBO J.*, **5**, 3057–3063.

Cranage, M. P., Smith, G. L., Bell, S. E. *et al.* (1988). Identification and expression of a human cytomegalovirus glycoprotein with homology to the Epstein–Barr virus BXLF2 product, varicella-zoster virus gpIII, and herpes simplex virus type 1 glycoprotein H. *J. Virol.*, **62**, 1416–1422.

Dal Monte, P., Pignatelli, S., Zini, N. *et al.* (2002). Analysis of intracellular and intraviral localization of the human cytomegalovirus UL53 protein. *J. Gen. Virol.*, **83**, 1005–1012.

D'Aquila, R. T., Hayward, G. S., and Summers, W. C. (1989). Physical mapping of the human cytomegalovirus (HCMV) (Towne) DNA polymerase gene: DNA-mediated transfer of a genetic marker for an HCMV gene. *Virology*, **171**, 312–316.

Dargan, D. J., Jamieson, F. E., MacLean, J., Dolan, A., Addison, C., and McGeoch, D. J. (1997). The published DNA sequence of human cytomegalovirus strain AD169 lacks 929 base pairs affecting genes UL42 and UL43. *J. Virol.*, **71**, 9833–9836.

Davison, A. J. and Stow, N. D. (2005). New genes from old: redeployment of dUTPase by herpesviruses. *J. Virol.*, **79**, 12880–12892.

Davison, A. J., Dolan, A., Akter, P. *et al.* (2003a). The human cytomegalovirus genome revisited: comparison with the chimpanzee cytomegalovirus genome. *J. Gen. Virol.*, **84**, 17–28.

Davison, A. J., Akter, P., Cunningham, C. *et al.* (2003b). Homology between the human cytomegalovirus RL11 gene family and human adenovirus E3 genes. *J. Gen. Virol.*, **84**, 657–663.

Dhepakson, P., Mori, Y., Jiang, Y. B. *et al.* (2002). Human herpesvirus-6 rep/U94 gene product has single-stranded DNA-binding activity. *J. Gen. Virol.*, **83**, 847–854.

Dittmer, A. and Bogner, E. (2005). Analysis of the quaternary structure of the putative HCMV portal protein pUL104. *Biochemistry*, **44**, 759–765.

Dolan, A., Cunningham, C., Hector, R. D. *et al.* (2004). Genetic content of wild type human cytomegalovirus. *J. Gen. Virol.*, **85**, 1301–1312.

Dominguez, G., Black, J. B., Stamey, F. R., Inoue, N., and Pellett, P. E. (1996). Physical and genetic maps of the human herpesvirus 7 strain SB genome. *Arch. Virol.*, **141**, 2387–2408.

Dominguez, G., Dambaugh, T. R., Stamey, F. R., Dewhurst, S., Inoue, N., and Pellett, P. E. (1999). Human herpesvirus 6B genome sequence: coding content and comparison with human herpesvirus 6A. *J. Virol.*, **73**, 8040–8052.

Dunn, C., Chalupny, N. J., Sutherland, C. L. *et al.* (2003a). Human cytomegalovirus glycoprotein UL16 causes intracellular sequestration of NKG2D ligands, protecting against natural killer cell cytotoxicity. *J. Exp. Med.*, **197**, 1427–1439.

Dunn, W., Chou, C., Li, H. *et al.* (2003b). Functional profiling of a human cytomegalovirus genome. *Proc. Natl Acad. Sci. USA*, **100**, 14223–14228.

Ebeling, A., Keil, G. M., Knust, E. and Koszinowski, U. H. (1983a). Molecular cloning and physical mapping of murine cytomegalovirus DNA. *J. Virol.*, **47**, 421–433.

Ebeling, A., Keil, G., Nowak, B., Fleckenstein, B., Berthelot, N., and Sheldrick, P. (1983b). Genome structure and virion polypeptides of the primate herpesviruses *Herpesvirus aotus* types 1 and 3: comparison with human cytomegalovirus. *J. Virol.*, **45**, 715–726.

Ehlers, B. and Lowden, S. (2004). Novel herpesviruses of *Suidae*: indicators for a second genogroup of artiodactyl gammaherpesviruses. *J. Gen. Virol.*, **85**, 857–862.

Ehlers, B., Ulrich, S., and Goltz, M. (1999). Detection of two novel porcine herpesviruses with high similarity to gammaherpesviruses. *J. Gen. Virol.*, **80**, 971–978.

Ehlers, B., Burkhardt, S., Goltz, M. *et al.* (2001). Genetic and ultrastructural characterization of a European isolate of the fatal endotheliotropic elephant herpesvirus. *J. Gen. Virol.*, **82**, 475–482.

Eickmann, M., Lange, R., Ohlin, M., Reschke, M., and Radsak, K. (1998). Effect of cysteine substitutions on dimerization and interfragment linkage of human cytomegalovirus glycoprotein B (gp UL55). *Arch. Virol.*, **143**, 1865–1880.

Ellinger, K., Neipel, F., Foa-Tomasi, L., Campadelli-Fiume, G., and Fleckenstein, B. (1993). The glycoprotein B homologue of human herpesvirus 6. *J. Gen. Virol.*, **74**, 495–500.

Ertl, P. F. and Powell, K. L. (1992). Physical and functional interaction of human cytomegalovirus DNA polymerase and its accessory protein (ICP36) expressed in insect cells. *J. Virol.*, **66**, 4126–4133.

Fraile-Ramos, A., Pelchen-Matthews, A., Kledal, T. N., Browne, H., Schwartz, T. W., and Marsh, M. (2002). Localization of HCMV UL33 and US27 in endocytic compartments and viral membranes. *Traffic*, **3**, 218–232.

French, C., Menegazzi, P., Nicholson, L., Macaulay, H., DiLuca, D., and Gompels U. A. (1999). Novel, nonconsensus cellular splicing regulates expression of a gene encoding a chemokine-like protein that shows high variation and is specific for human herpesvirus 6 *Virology*, **262**, 139–151.

Furman, M. H., Dey, N., Tortorella, D., and Ploegh, H. L. (2002). The human cytomegalovirus US10 gene product delays trafficking of major histocompatibility complex class I molecules. *J. Virol.*, **76**, 11753–11756.

Gao, M. and Isom, H. C. (1984). Characterization of the guinea pig cytomegalovirus genome by molecular cloning and physical mapping. *J. Virol.*, **52**, 436–447.

Gao, J. L. and Murphy, P. M. (1994). Human cytomegalovirus open reading frame *US28* encodes a functional β chemokine receptor. *J. Biol. Chem.*, **269**, 28539–28542.

Gao, M., Robertson, B. J., McCann, P. J. *et al.* (1998). Functional conservations of the alkaline nuclease of herpes simplex type 1 and human cytomegalovirus. *Virology*, **249**, 460–470.

Gawn, J. M. and Greaves, R. F. (2002). Absence of IE1 p72 protein function during low-multiplicity infection by human cytomegalovirus results in a broad block to viral delayed-early gene expression. *J. Virol.*, **76**, 4441–4455.

Gebert, S., Schmolke, S., Sorg, G., Floss, S., Plachter, B., and Stamminger, T. (1997). The UL84 protein of human cytomegalovirus acts as a transdominant inhibitor of immediate–early-mediated transactivation that is able to prevent viral replication. *J. Virol.*, **71**, 7048–7060.

Gewurz, B. E., Gaudet, R., Tortorella, D., Wang, E. W., Ploegh, H. L., and Wiley, D. C. (2001). Antigen presentation subverted: Structure of the human cytomegalovirus protein US2 bound to the class I molecule HLA-A2. *Proc. Natl Acad. Sci. USA*, **98**, 6794–6799.

Gewurz, B. E., Ploegh, H. L., and Tortorella, D. (2002). US2, a human cytomegalovirus-encoded type I membrane protein, contains a non-cleavable amino-terminal signal peptide. *J. Biol. Chem.*, **277**, 11306–11313.

Gibson, W. (1983). Protein counterparts of human and simian cytomegaloviruses. *Virology*, **128**, 391–406.

Gibson, W. (1996). Structure and assembly of the virion. *Intervirology* 39, 389–400.

Gibson, W., van Breemen, R., Fields, A., LaFemina, R., and Irmiere, A. (1984). D,L-α-difluoromethylornithine inhibits human cytomegalovirus replication. *J. Virol.*, **50**, 145–154.

Gibson, W., Baxter, M. K., and Clopper, K. S. (1996a). Cytomegalovirus "missing" capsid protein identified as heat-aggregable product of human cytomegalovirus UL46. *J. Virol.*, **70**, 7454–7461.

Gibson, W., Clopper, K. S., Britt, W. J. and Baxter, M. K. (1996b). Human cytomegalovirus (HCMV) smallest capsid protein identified as product of short open reading frame located between HCMV UL48 and UL49. *J. Virol.*, **70**, 5680–5683.

Goldmacher, V. S., Bartle, L. M., Skaletskaya, A. *et al.* (1999). A cytomegalovirus-encoded mitochondria-localized inhibitor of apoptosis structurally unrelated to Bcl-2. *Proc. Natl Acad. Sci. USA*, **96**, 12536–12541.

Gompels, U. A., Nicholas, J., Lawrence, G. *et al.* (1995). The DNA sequence of human herpesvirus-6: structure, coding content, and genome evolution. *Virology*, **209**, 29–51.

Gravel, A., Gosselin, J., and Flamand, L. (2002). Human herpesvirus 6 immediate-early 1 protein is a sumoylated nuclear phosphoprotein colocalizing with promyelocytic leukemia protein-associated nuclear bodies. *J. Biol. Chem.*, **277**, 19679–19687.

Gravel, A., Tomoiu, A., Cloutier, N., Gosselin, J., and Flamand, L. (2003). Characterization of the immediate-early 2 protein of human herpesvirus 6, a promiscuous transcriptional activator. *Virology*, **308**, 340–353.

Greaves, R. F. and Mocarski, E. S. (1998). Defective growth correlates with reduced accumulation of a viral DNA replication protein after low-multiplicity infection by a human cytomegalovirus *ie1* mutant. *J. Virol.*, **72**, 366–379.

Greijer, A. E., Dekkers, C. A., and Middeldorp, J. M. (2000). Human cytomegalovirus virions differentially incorporate viral and host cell RNA during the assembly process. *J. Virol.*, **74**, 9078–9082.

Gretch, D. R., Kari, B., Rasmussen, L., Gehrz, R. C., and Stinski, M. F. (1988). Identification and characterization of three distinct families of glycoprotein complexes in the envelopes of human cytomegalovirus. *J. Virol.*, **62**, 875–881.

Guo, Y. W. and Huang, E. S. (1993). Characterization of a structurally tricistronic gene of human cytomegalovirus composed of U_S18, U_S19, and U_S20. *J. Virol.*, **67**, 2043–2054.

Hagemeier, C., Walker, S., Caswell, R., Kouzarides, T., and Sinclair, J. (1992). The human cytomegalovirus 80-kilodalton but not the 72-kilodalton immediate–early protein transactivates heterologous promoters in a TATA box-dependent mechanism and interacts directly with TFIID. *J. Virol.*, **66**, 4452–4456.

Hahn, G., Revello, M. G., Patrone, M. *et al.* (2004). Human cytomegalovirus UL131–128 genes are indispensable for virus growth in endothelial cells and virus transfer to leukocytes. *J. Virol.*, **78**, 10023–10033

Hansen, S. G., Strelow, L. I., Franchi, D. C., Anders, D. G., and Wong, S. W. (2003). Complete sequence and genomic analysis of rhesus cytomegalovirus. *J. Virol.*, **77**, 6620–6636.

Hayashi, M. L., Blankenship, C., and Shenk, T. (2000). Human cytomegalovirus UL69 protein is required for efficient accumulation of infected cells in the G1 phase of the cell cycle. *Proc. Natl Acad. Sci. USA*, **97**, 2692–2696.

He, Y. S., Xu, L. and Huang, E. S. (1992). Characterization of human cytomegalovirus UL84 early gene and identification of its putative protein product. *J. Virol.*, **66**, 1098–1108.

Hegde, N. R., Tomazin, R. A., Wisner, T. W. *et al.* (2002). Inhibition of HLA-DR assembly, transport, and loading by human cytomegalovirus glycoprotein US3: a novel mechanism for evading major histocompatibility complex class II antigen presentation. *J. Virol.*, **76**, 10929–10941.

Heider, J. A., Bresnahan, W. A., and Shenk, T. E. (2002). Construction of a rationally designed human cytomegalovirus variant encoding a temperature-sensitive immediate-early 2 protein. *Proc. Natl Acad. Sci. USA*, **99**, 3141–3146.

Heilbronn, R., Jahn, G., Burkle, A., Freese, U. K., Fleckenstein, B., and zur Hausen, H. (1987). Genomic localization, sequence analysis, and transcription of the putative human cytomegalovirus DNA polymerase gene. *J. Virol.*, **61**, 119–124.

Hermiston, T. W., Malone, C. L., Witte, P. R., and Stinski, M. F. (1987). Identification and characterization of the human cytomegalovirus immediate–early region 2 gene that stimulates gene expression from an inducible promoter. *J. Virol.*, **61**, 3214–3221.

Hewitt, E. W., Gupta, S. S., and Lehner, P. J. (2001). The human cytomegalovirus gene product US6 inhibits ATP binding by TAP. *EMBO J.*, **20**, 387–396.

Hijikata, M., Takahashi, K., and Mishiro, S. (1999). Complete circular DNA genome of a TT virus variant (isolate name SANBAN) and 44 partial ORF2 sequences implicating a great degree of diversity beyond genotypes. *Virology*, **260**, 17–22.

Hitomi, S., Kozuka-Hata, H., Chen, Z., Sugano, S., Yamaguchi, N., and Watanabe, S. (1997). Human cytomegalovirus open reading frame UL11 encodes a highly polymorphic protein expressed on the infected cell surface. *Arch. Virol.*, **142**, 1407–1427.

Hofmann, H., Sindre, H., and Stamminger, T. (2002). Functional interaction between the pp71 protein of human cytomegalovirus and the PML-interacting protein human Daxx. *J. Virol.*, **76**, 5769–5783.

Homer, E. G., Rinaldi, A., Nicholl, M. J., and Preston, C. M. (1999). Activation of herpesvirus gene expression by the human cytomegalovirus protein pp71. *J. Virol.*, **73**, 8512–8518.

Huang, E. S., Kilpatrick, B., Lakeman, A., and Alford C. A. (1978). Genetic analysis of a cytomegalovirus-like agent isolated from human brain. *J. Virol.*, **26**, 718–723.

Huber, M. T. and Compton, T. (1997). Characterization of a novel third member of the human cytomegalovirus glycoprotein H-glycoprotein L complex. *J. Virol.*, **71**, 5391–5398.

Huber, M. T. and Compton, T. (1998). The human cytomegalovirus UL74 gene encodes the third component of the glycoprotein H-glycoprotein L-containing envelope complex. *J. Virol.*, **72**, 8191–8197.

Huber, M. T., Tomazin, R., Wisner, T., Boname, J., and Johnson, D. C. (2002). Human cytomegalovirus US7, US8, US9, and US10 are cytoplasmic glycoproteins, not found at cell surfaces, and US9 does not mediate cell-to-cell spread. *J. Virol.*, **76**, 5748–5758.

Inoue, N., and Pellett, P. E. (1995). Human herpesvirus 6B origin-binding protein: DNA-binding domain and consensus binding sequence. *J. Virol.*, **69**, 4619–4627.

Inoue, N., Dambaugh, T. R., Rapp, J. C., and Pellett, P. E. (1994). Alphaherpesvirus origin-binding protein homolog encoded by human herpesvirus 6B, a betaherpesvirus, binds to nucleotide sequences that are similar to *ori* regions of alphaherpesviruses. *J. Virol.*, **68**, 4126–4136.

Irmiere, A. and Gibson, W. (1983). Isolation and characterization of a noninfectious virion-like particle released from cells infected with human strains of cytomegalovirus. *Virology*, **130**, 118–133.

Irmiere, A. and Gibson, W. (1985). Isolation of human cytomegalovirus intranuclear capsids, characterization of their protein constituents, and demonstration that the B-capsid assembly protein is also abundant in noninfectious enveloped particles. *J. Virol.*, **56**, 277–283.

Isegawa, Y., Ping, Z., Nakano, K., Sugimoto, N., and Yamanishi, K. (1998). Human herpesvirus 6 open reading frame U12 encodes a functional β-chemokine receptor. *J. Virol.*, **72**, 6104–6112.

Isegawa, Y., Mukai, T., Nakano, K. et al. (1999). Comparison of the complete DNA sequences of human herpesvirus 6 variants A and B. *J. Virol.*, **73**, 8053–8063.

Ishov, A. M., Vladimirova, O. V., and Maul, G. G. (2002). Daxx-mediated accumulation of human cytomegalovirus tegument protein pp71 at ND10 facilitates initiation of viral infection at these nuclear domains. *J. Virol.*, **76**, 7705–7712.

Jahn, G., Kouzarides, T., Mach, M. et al. (1987). Map position and nucleotide sequence of the gene for the large structural phosphoprotein of human cytomegalovirus. *J. Virol.*, **61**, 1358–1367.

Jeang, K. T. and Hayward, G. S. (1983). A cytomegalovirus DNA sequence containing tracts of tandemly repeated CA dinucleotides hybridizes to highly repetitive dispersed elements in mammalian cell genomes. *Mol. Cell. Biol.*, **3**, 1389–1402.

Jones, B. C., Logsdon, N. J., Josephson, K., Cook, J., Barry, P. A., and Walter, M. R. (2002). Crystal structure of human cytomegalovirus IL-10 bound to soluble human IL-10R1. *Proc. Natl Acad. Sci. USA*, **99**, 9404–9409.

Jones, T. R. and Sun, L. (1997). Human cytomegalovirus US2 destabilizes major histocompatibility complex class I heavy chains. *J. Virol.*, **71**, 2970–2979.

Jones, T. R., Hanson, L. K., Sun, L., Slater, J. S., Stenberg, R. M., and Campbell, A. E. (1995). Multiple independent loci within the human cytomegalovirus unique short region down-regulate expression of major histocompatibility complex class I heavy chains. *J. Virol.*, **69**, 4830–4841.

Jones, T. R., Wiertz, E. J., Sun, L., Fish, K. N., Nelson, J. A., and Ploegh, H. L. (1996). Human cytomegalovirus US3 impairs transport and maturation of major histocompatibility complex class I heavy chains. *Proc. Natl Acad. Sci. USA*, **93**, 11327–11333.

Kalejta, R. F. and Shenk, T. (2003). Proteasome-dependent, ubiquitin-independent degradation of the Rb family of tumor suppressors by the human cytomegalovirus pp71 protein. *Proc. Natl Acad. Sci. USA*, **100**, 3263–3268.

Kari, B., Goertz, R., and Gehrz, R. (1990). Characterization of cytomegalovirus glycoproteins in a family of complexes designated gC-II with murine monoclonal antibodies. *Arch. Virol.*, **112**, 55–65.

Kari, B., Li, W., Cooper, J., Goertz, R., and Radeke, B. (1994). The human cytomegalovirus UL100 gene encodes the gC-II glycoproteins recognized by group 2 monoclonal antibodies. *J. Gen. Virol.*, **75**, 3081–3086.

Kashanchi, F., Araujo, J., Doniger, J. (1997). Human herpesvirus 6 (HHV-6) ORF-1 transactivating gene exhibits malignant transforming activity and its protein binds to p53. *Oncogene*, **14**, 359–367.

Kaye, J., Browne, H., Stoffel, M., and Minson, T. (1992a). The UL16 gene of human cytomegalovirus encodes a glycoprotein that is dispensable for growth in vitro. *J. Virol.*, **66**, 6609–6615.

Kaye, J. F., Gompels, U. A., and Minson, A. C. (1992b). Glycoprotein H of human cytomegalovirus (HCMV) forms a stable complex with the HCMV UL115 gene product. *J. Gen. Virol.*, **73**, 2693–2698.

Kemble, G. W., McCormick, A. L., Pereira, L., and Mocarski, E. S. (1987). A cytomegalovirus protein with properties of herpes simplex virus ICP8: partial purification of the polypeptide and map position of the gene. *J. Virol.*, **61**, 3143–3151.

Kenzelmann, M. and Muhlemann, K. (2000). Transcriptome analysis of fibroblast cells immediate-early after human cytomegalovirus infection. *J. Mol. Biol.*, **304**, 741–751.

Koch, H. G., Delius, H., Matz, B., Flügel, R. M., Clarke, J., and Darai, G. (1985). Molecular cloning and physical mapping of the tupaia herpesvirus genome. *J. Virol.*, **55**, 86–95.

Komazin, G., Ptak, R. G., Emmer, B. T., Townsend, L. B., and Drach, J. C. (2003). Resistance of human cytomegalovirus to the benzimidazole L-ribonucleoside maribavir maps to UL27. *J. Virol.*, **77**, 11499–11506.

Komazin, G., Townsend, L. B., and Drach, J. C. (2004). Role of a mutation in human cytomegalovirus gene UL104 in resistance to benzimidazole ribonucleosides. *J. Virol.*, **78**, 710–715.

Kotenko, S. V., Saccani, S., Izotova, L. S., Mirochnitchenko, O. V., and Pestka, S. (2000). Human cytomegalovirus harbors its own unique IL-10 homolog (cmvIL-10). *Proc. Natl Acad. Sci. USA*, **97**, 1695–1700.

Kouzarides, T., Bankier, A. T., Satchwell, S. C., Weston, K., Tomlinson, P., and Barrell, B. G. (1987). Sequence and transcription analysis of the human cytomegalovirus DNA polymerase gene. *J. Virol.*, **61**, 125–133.

Krosky, P. M., Underwood, M. R., Turk, S. R. *et al.* (1998). Resistance of human cytomegalovirus to benzimidazole ribonucleosides maps to two open reading frames: UL89 and UL56. *J. Virol.*, **72**, 4721–4728.

Krosky, P. M., Baek, M. C., and Coen, D. M. (2003a). The human cytomegalovirus UL97 protein kinase, an antiviral drug target, is required at the stage of nuclear egress. *J. Virol.*, **77**, 905–914.

Krosky, P. M., Baek, M. C., Jahng, W. J. *et al.* (2003b). The human cytomegalovirus UL44 protein is a substrate for the UL97 protein kinase. *J. Virol.*, **77**, 7720–7727.

Landini, M. P., Severi, B., Furlini, G., and Badiali De Giorgi, L. (1987). Human cytomegalovirus structural components: intracellular and intraviral localization of p28 and p65–69 by immunoelectron microscopy. *Virus Res.*, **8**, 15–23.

LaPierre, L. A. and Biegalke, B. J. (2001). Identification of a novel transcriptional repressor encoded by human cytomegalovirus. *J. Virol.*, **75**, 6062–6069.

Lee, H. R., Kim, D. J., Lee, J. M. *et al.* (2004). Ability of the human cytomegalovirus IE1 protein to modulate sumoylation of PML correlates with its functional activities in transcriptional regulation and infectivity in cultured fibroblast cells. *J. Virol.*, **78**, 6527–6542.

Lehner, P. J., Karttunen, J. T., Wilkinson, G. W. G., and Cresswell, P. (1997). The human cytomegalovirus US6 glycoprotein inhibits transporter associated with antigen processing-dependent peptide translocation. *Proc. Natl Acad. Sci. USA*, **94**, 6904–6909.

Lehner, R., Meyer, H., and Mach, M. (1989). Identification and characterization of a human cytomegalovirus gene coding for a membrane protein that is conserved among human herpesviruses. *J. Virol.*, **63**, 3792–3800.

Li, L., Nelson, J. A., and Britt, W. J. (1997). Glycoprotein H-related complexes of human cytomegalovirus: identification of a third protein in the gCIII complex. *J. Virol.*, **71**, 3090–3097.

Li, J., Yamamoto, T., Ohtsubo, K., Shirakata, M., and Hirai, K. (1999). Major product pp43 of human cytomegalovirus U_L112–113 gene is a transcriptional coactivator with two functionally distinct domains. *Virology*, **260**, 89–97.

Lilley, B. N. and Ploegh, H. L. (2004). A membrane protein required for dislocation of misfolded proteins from the ER. *Nature*, **429**, 834–840.

Lilley, B. N., Ploegh, H. L., and Tirabassi, R. S. (2001). Human cytomegalovirus open reading frame TRL11/IRL11 encodes an immunoglobulin G Fc-binding protein. *J. Virol.*, **75**, 11218–11221.

Lin, K. and Ricciardi, R. P. (1998). The 41-kDa protein of human herpesvirus 6 specifically binds to viral DNA polymerase and greatly increases DNA synthesis. *Virology*, **250**, 210–219.

Lindquester, G. J. and Pellett, P. E. (1991). Properties of the human herpesvirus 6 strain Z29 genome: G + C content, length, and presence of variable-length directly repeated terminal sequence elements. *Virology*, **182**, 102–110.

Lischka, P., Rosorius, O., Trommer, E. and Stamminger, T. (2001). A novel transferable nuclear export signal mediates CRM1-independent nucleocytoplasmic shuttling of the human cytomegalovirus transactivator protein pUL69. *EMBO J.*, **20**, 7271–7283.

Lischka, P., Sorg, G., Kann, M., Winkler, M., and Stamminger, T. (2003). A nonconventional nuclear localization signal within the UL84 protein of human cytomegalovirus mediates nuclear import via the importin α/β pathway. *J. Virol.*, **77**, 3734–3748.

Littler, E., Lawrence, G., Liu, M. Y., Barrell, B. G., and Arrand, J. R. (1990). Identification, cloning, and expression of the major capsid protein gene of human herpesvirus 6. *J. Virol.*, **64**, 714–722.

Littler, E., Stuart, A. D., and Chee, M. S. (1992). Human cytomegalovirus UL97 open reading frame encodes a protein that phosphorylates the antiviral nucleoside analogue ganciclovir. *Nature*, **358**, 160–162.

Liu, B. and Stinski, M. F. (1992). Human cytomegalovirus contains a tegument protein that enhances transcription from promoters with upstream ATF and AP-1 *cis*-acting elements. *J. Virol.*, **66**, 4434–4444.

Liu, D. X., Gompels, U. A., Nicholas, J., and Lelliott, C. (1993). Identification and expression of the human herpesvirus 6 glycoprotein H and interaction with an accessory 40K glycoprotein. *J. Gen. Virol.*, **74**, 1847–1857.

Liu, Y. and Biegalke, B. J. (2002). The human cytomegalovirus UL35 gene encodes two proteins with different functions. *J. Virol.*, **76**, 2460–2468.

Lockridge, K. M., Zhou, S. S., Kravitz, R. H. *et al.* (2000). Primate cytomegaloviruses encode and express an IL-10-like protein. *Virology*, **268**, 272–280.

Lopper, M. and Compton, T. (2002). Disulfide bond configuration of human cytomegalovirus glycoprotein B. *J. Virol.*, **76**, 6073–6082.

Lüttichau, H. R., Clark-Lewis, I., Jensen, P. O., Moser, C., Gerstoft, J., and Schwartz, T. (2003). A highly selective CCR2 chemokine agonist encoded by human herpesvirus 6. *J. Biol. Chem.*, **278**, 10928–10933.

Mach, M., Kropff, B., Dal Monte, P., and Britt, W. (2000). Complex formation by human cytomegalovirus glycoproteins M (gpUL100) and N (gpUL73). *J. Virol.*, **74**, 11881–11892.

Machold, R. P., Wiertz, E. J., Jones, T. R., and Ploegh, H. L. (1997). The HCMV gene products US11 and US2 differ in their ability to attack allelic forms of murine major histocompatibility complex (MHC) class I heavy chains. *J. Exp. Med.*, **185**, 363–366.

Marchini, A., Liu, H., and Zhu, H. (2001). Human cytomegalovirus with IE-2 (UL122) deleted fails to express early lytic genes. *J. Virol.*, **75**, 1870–1878.

Margulies, B. J., Browne, H., and Gibson, W. (1996). Identification of the human cytomegalovirus G protein-coupled receptor homologue encoded by UL33 in infected cells and enveloped virus particles. *Virology*, **225**, 111–125.

Marks, J. R. and Spector D. H. (1984). Fusion of the termini of the murine cytomegalovirus genome after infection. *J. Virol.*, **52**, 24–28.

Marks, J. R. and Spector, D. H. (1988). Replication of the murine cytomegalovirus genome: structure and role of the termini in the generation and cleavage of concatenates. *Virology*, **162**, 98–107.

Marschall, M., Freitag, M., Suchy, P. *et al.* (2003). The protein kinase pUL97 of human cytomegalovirus interacts with and phosphorylates the DNA polymerase processivity factor pUL44. *Virology*, **311**, 60–71.

Martin, M. E., Nicholas, J., Thomson, B. J., Newman, C., and Honess, R. W. (1991a). Identification of a transactivating function mapping to the putative immediate–early locus of human herpesvirus 6. *J. Virol.*, **65**, 5381–5390.

Martin, M. E., Thomson, B. J., Honess, R. W. *et al.* (1991b). The genome of human herpesvirus 6: maps of unit-length and concatemeric genomes for nine restriction endonucleases. *J. Gen. Virol.*, **72**, 157–168.

Martin, W. J. (1999). Stealth adaptation of an African green monkey simian cytomegalovirus. *Exp. Mol. Pathol.*, **66**, 3–7.

Martin, W. J. (2000). Chemokine receptor-related genetic sequences in an african green monkey simian cytomegalovirus-derived stealth virus. *Exp. Mol. Pathol.*, **69**, 10–16.

McGeehan, J. E., Depledge, N. W., and McGeoch, D. J. (2001). Evolution of the dUTPase gene of mammalian and avian herpesviruses. *Curr. Protein Pept. Sci.*, **2**, 325–333.

McGeoch, D. J. and Davison, A. J. (1999). The molecular evolutionary history of the herpesviruses. In *Origin and Evolution of Viruses*, pp. 441–465, ed E. Domingo, R. Webster and J. Holland. London: Academic Press.

McGregor, A. and Schleiss, M. R. (2001). Molecular cloning of the guinea pig cytomegalovirus (GPCMV) genome as an infectious bacterial artificial chromosome (BAC) in *Escherichia coli*. *Mol. Genet. Metab.*, **72**, 15–26.

McKeating, J. A., Griffiths, P. D., and Grundy, J. E. (1987). Cytomegalovirus in urine specimens has host β_2 microglobulin bound to the viral envelope: a mechanism of evading the host immune response? *J. Gen. Virol.*, **68**, 785–792.

McMahon, T. P. and Anders, D. G. (2002). Interactions between human cytomegalovirus helicase-primase proteins. *Virus Res.*, **86**, 39–52.

McVoy, M. A., Nixon, D. E., and Adler, S. P. (1997). Circularization and cleavage of guinea pig cytomegalovirus genomes. *J. Virol.*, **71**, 4209–4217.

Megaw, A. G., Rapaport, D., Avidor, B., Frenkel, N., and Davison, A. J. (1998). The DNA sequence of the RK strain of human herpesvirus 7. *Virology*, **244**, 119–132.

Meijer, H., Dreesen, J. C., and Van Boven, C. P. (1986). Molecular cloning and restriction endonuclease mapping of the rat cytomegalovirus genome. *J. Gen. Virol.*, **67**, 1327–1342.

Mercer, J. A., Marks, J. R., and Spector, D. H. (1983). Molecular cloning and restriction endonuclease mapping of the murine cytomegalovirus genome (Smith strain). *Virology*, **129**, 94–106.

Messerle, M., Crnkovic, I., Hammerschmidt, W., Ziegler, H., and Koszinowski, U. H. (1997). Cloning and mutagenesis of a herpesvirus genome as an infectious bacterial artificial chromosome. *Proc. Natl Acad. Sci. USA*, **94**, 14759–14763.

Meyer, H., Bankier, A. T., and Landini, M. P. (1988). Identification and procaryotic expression of the gene coding for the highly immunogenic 28-kilodalton structural phosphoprotein (pp28) of human cytomegalovirus. *J. Virol.*, **62**, 2243–2250.

Milne, R. S. B, Paterson, D. A., and Booth, J. C. (1998). Human cytomegalovirus glycoprotein H/glycoprotein L complex modulates fusion-from-without. *J. Gen. Virol.*, **79**, 855–865.

Milne, R. S. B., Mattick, C., Nicholson, L., Devaraj, P., Alcami, A., and Gompels, U. A. (2000). RANTES binding and down-regulation by a novel human herpesvirus-6 β chemokine receptor. *J. Immunol.*, **164**, 2396–2404.

Misaghi, S., Sun, Z. Y., Stern, P., Gaudet, R., Wagner, G., and Ploegh, H. (2004). Structural and functional analysis of human cytomegalovirus US3 protein. *J. Virol.*, **78**, 413–423.

Mocarski, E. S. (2002). Virus self-improvement through inflammation: no pain, no gain. *Proc. Natl Acad. Sci. USA*, **99**, 3362–3364.

Mocarski, E. S., Pereira, L. and Michael, N. (1985). Precise localization of genes on large animal virus genomes: use of λ gt11 and monoclonal antibodies to map the gene for a cytomegalovirus protein family. *Proc. Natl Acad. Sci. USA*, **82**, 1266–1270.

Mocarski, E. S., Pereira, L., and McCormick, L. A. (1988). Human cytomegalovirus ICP22, the product of the HWLF1 reading frame, is an early nuclear protein that is released from cells. *J. Gen. Virol.*, **69**, 2613–2621.

Mocarski, E. S., Prichard, M. N., Tan, C. S., and Brown J. M. (1997). Reassessing the organization of the UL42-UL43 region of the human cytomegalovirus strain AD169 genome. *Virology*, **239**, 169–175.

Mori, Y., Yagi, H., Shimamoto, T. *et al.* (1998). Analysis of human herpesvirus 6 U3 gene, which is a positional homolog of human cytomegalovirus UL 24 gene. *Virology*, **249**, 129–139.

Mori, Y., Dhepakson, P., and Shimamoto, T. (2000). Expression of human herpesvirus 6B rep within infected cells and binding of its gene product to the TATA-binding protein in vitro and in vivo. *J. Virol.*, **74**, 6096–6104.

Mori, Y., Akkapaiboon, P., Yang, X., and Yamanishi, K. (2003a). The human herpesvirus 6 U100 gene product is the third component of the gH-gL glycoprotein complex on the viral envelope. *J. Virol.*, **77**, 2452–2458.

Mori, Y., Yang, X., Akkapaiboon, P., Okuno, T., and Yamanishi, K. (2003b). Human herpesvirus 6 variant A glycoprotein H-glycoprotein L-glycoprotein Q complex associates with human CD46. *J. Virol.*, **77**, 4992–4999.

Muranyi, W., Haas, J., Wagner, M., Krohne, G., and Koszinowski, U. H. (2002). Cytomegalovirus recruitment of cellular kinases to dissolve the nuclear lamina. *Science*, **297**, 854–857.

Murphy, E., Rigoutsos, I., Shibuya, T., and Shenk, T. E. (2003a). Reevaluation of human cytomegalovirus coding potential. *Proc. Natl Acad. Sci. USA*, **100**, 13585–13590.

Murphy, E., Yu, D., Grimwood, J. *et al.* (2003b). Coding potential of laboratory and clinical strains of human cytomegalovirus. *Proc. Natl Acad. Sci. USA*, **100**, 14976–14981.

Neipel, F., Ellinger, K., and Fleckenstein, B. (1992). Gene for the major antigenic structural protein (p100) of human herpesvirus 6. *J. Virol.*, **66**, 3918–3924.

Neote, K., DiGregorio, D., Mak, J. Y., Horuk, R., and Schall, T. J. (1993). Molecular cloning, functional expression, and signaling characteristics of a CC chemokine receptor. *Cell*, **72**, 415–425.

Nevels, M., Paulus, C., and Shenk, T. (2004). Human cytomegalovirus immediate-early 1 protein facilitates viral replication by antagonizing histone deacetylation. *Proc. Natl Acad. Sci. USA*, **101**, 17234–17239.

Newcomb, W. W., Homa, F. L., Thomsen, D. R. et al. (1996). Assembly of the herpes simplex virus capsid: characterization of intermediates observed during cell-free capsid formation. *J. Mol. Biol.*, **263**, 432–446.

Nicholas, J. (1996). Determination and analysis of the complete nucleotide sequence of human herpesvirus 7. *J. Virol.*, **70**, 5975–5989.

Nikolaou, K., Varinou, L., Inoue, N. and Arsenakis, M. (2003). Identification and characterization of gene products of ORF U90/89 of human herpesvirus 6. *Acta Virol.*, **47**, 17–26.

Nixon, D. E. and McVoy, M. A. (2002). Terminally repeated sequences on a herpesvirus genome are deleted following circularization but are reconstituted by duplication during cleavage and packaging of concatemeric DNA. *J. Virol.*, **76**, 2009–2013.

Odeberg, J., Browne, H., Metkar, S. et al. (2003). The human cytomegalovirus protein UL16 mediates increased resistance to natural killer cell cytotoxicity through resistance to cytolytic proteins. *J. Virol.*, **77**, 4539–4545.

Ogawa-Goto, K., Irie, S., Omori, A. et al. (2002). An endoplasmic reticulum protein, p180, is highly expressed in human cytomegalovirus-permissive cells and interacts with the tegument protein encoded by UL48. *J. Virol.*, **76**, 2350–2362.

Oien, N. L., Thomsen, D. R., Wathen, M. W., Newcomb, W. W., Brown, J. C., and Homa, F. L. (1997). Assembly of herpes simplex virus capsids using the human cytomegalovirus scaffold protein: critical role of the C terminus. *J. Virol.*, **71**, 1281–1291.

Okamoto, H., Takahashi, M., Nishizawa, T. et al. (2002). Genomic characterization of TT viruses (TTVs) in pigs, cats and dogs and their relatedness with species-specific TTVs in primates and tupaias. *J. Gen. Virol.*, **83**, 1291–1297.

Papanikolaou, E., Kouvatsis, V., Dimitriadis, G., Inoue, N., and Arsenakis, M. (2002). Identification and characterization of the gene products of open reading frame U86/87 of human herpesvirus 6. *Virus. Res.*, **89**, 89–101.

Patrone, M., Percivalle, E., Secchi, M. et al. (2003). The human cytomegalovirus UL45 gene product is a late, virion-associated protein and influences virus growth at low multiplicities of infection. *J. Gen. Virol.*, **84**, 3359–3370.

Patrone, M., Secchi, M., Fiorina, L., Ierardi, M., Milanesi, G., and Gallina, A. (2005). Human cytomegalovirus UL130 protein promotes endothelial cell infection through a producer cell modification of the virion. *J. Virol.*, **79**, 8361–8373.

Patterson, C. E. and Shenk, T. (1999). Human cytomegalovirus UL36 protein is dispensable for viral replication in cultured cells. *J. Virol.*, **73**, 7126–7131.

Penfold, M. E. and Mocarski, E. S. (1997). Formation of cytomegalovirus DNA replication compartments defined by localization of viral proteins and DNA synthesis. *Virology*, **239**, 46–61.

Penfold, M. E., Dairaghi, D. J., Duke, G. M. et al. (1999). Cytomegalovirus encodes a potent α chemokine. *Proc. Natl Acad. Sci. USA*, **96**, 9839–9844.

Penfold, M. E., Schmidt, T. L., Dairaghi, D. J., Barry, P. A., and Schall, T. J. (2003). Characterization of the rhesus cytomegalovirus US28 locus. *J. Virol.*, **77**, 10404–10413.

Peters, M. A., Jackson, D. C., Crabb, B. S., and Browning, G. F. (2002). Chicken anemia virus VP2 is a novel dual specificity protein phosphatase. *J. Biol. Chem.*, **277**, 39566–39573.

Pfeiffer, B., Thomson, B., and Chandran, B. (1995). Identification and characterization of a cDNA derived from multiple splicing that encodes envelope glycoprotein gp105 of human herpesvirus 6. *J. Virol.*, **69**, 3490–3500.

Pignatelli, S., Dal Monte, P., Rossini, G. and Landini, M. P. (2004). Genetic polymorphisms among human cytomegalovirus (HCMV) wild-type strains. *Rev. Med. Virol.*, **14**, 383–410.

Prichard, M. N., Duke, G. M., and Mocarski, E. S. (1996). Human cytomegalovirus uracil DNA glycosylase is required for the normal temporal regulation of both DNA synthesis and viral replication. *J. Virol.*, **70**, 3018–3025.

Prichard, M. N., Jairath, S., Penfold, M. E., St. Jeor, S., Bohlman, M. C., and Pari, G. S. (1998). Identification of persistent RNA-DNA hybrid structures within the origin of replication of human cytomegalovirus. *J. Virol.*, **72**, 6997–7004.

Prichard, M. N., Penfold, M. E., Duke, G. M., Spaete, R. R., and Kemble, G. W. (2001). A review of genetic differences between limited and extensively passaged human cytomegalovirus strains. *Rev. Med. Virol.*, **11**, 191–200.

Prince, V. E. and Pickett, F. B. (2002). Splitting pairs: the diverging fates of duplicated genes. *Nat. Rev. Genet.*, **3**, 827–837.

Qiu, X., Culp, J. S., DiLella, A. G. et al. (1996). Unique fold and active site in cytomegalovirus protease. *Nature*, **383**, 275–279.

Rasmussen, L., Geissler, A., and Winters, M. (2003). Inter- and intragenic variations complicate the molecular epidemiology of human cytomegalovirus. *J. Infect. Dis.*, **187**, 809–819.

Rawlinson, W. D. and Barrell, B. G. (1993). Spliced transcripts of human cytomegalovirus. *J. Virol.*, **67**, 5502–5513.

Rawlinson, W. D., Farrell, H. E., and Barrell, B. G. (1996). Analysis of the complete DNA sequence of murine cytomegalovirus. *J. Virol.*, **70**, 8833–8849.

Reid, G. G., Ellsmore, V., and Stow, N. D. (2003). An analysis of the requirements for human cytomegalovirus *ori*Lyt-dependent DNA synthesis in the presence of the herpes simplex virus type 1 replication fork proteins. *Virology*, **308**, 303–316.

Richman, L. K., Montali, R. J., Garber, R. L. et al. (1999). Novel endotheliotropic herpesviruses fatal for Asian and African elephants. *Science*, **283**, 1171–1176.

Robson, L. and Gibson, W. (1989). Primate cytomegalovirus assembly protein: genome location and nucleotide sequence. *J. Virol.*, **63**, 669–676.

Roby, C. and Gibson, W. (1986). Characterization of phosphoproteins and protein kinase activity of virions, noninfectious enveloped particles, and dense bodies of human cytomegalovirus. *J. Virol.*, **59**, 714–727.

Romanowski, M. J. and Shenk, T. (1997). Characterization of the human cytomegalovirus *irs1* and *trs1* genes: a second immediate–early transcription unit within *irs1* whose product antagonizes transcriptional activation. *J. Virol.*, **71**, 1485–1496.

Romanowski, M. J., Garrido-Guerrero, E., and Shenk, T. (1997). pIRS1 and pTRS1 are present in human cytomegalovirus virions. *J. Virol.*, **71**, 5703–5705.

Rotola, A., Ravaioli, T., Gonelli, A., Dewhurst, S., Cassai, E., and Di Luca, D. (1998). U94 of human herpesvirus 6 is expressed in latently infected peripheral blood mononuclear cells and blocks viral gene expression in transformed lymphocytes in culture. *Proc. Natl Acad. Sci. USA*, **95**, 13911–13916.

Ruger, B., Klages, S., Walla, B. *et al.* (1987). Primary structure and transcription of the genes coding for the two virion phosphoproteins pp65 and pp71 of human cytomegalovirus. *J. Virol.*, **61**, 446–453.

Rupasinghe, V., Iwatsuki-Horimoto, K., Sugii, S., and Horimoto, T. (2001). Identification of the porcine cytomegalovirus major capsid protein gene. *J. Vet. Med. Sci.*, **63**, 609–618.

Sahagun-Ruiz, A., Sierra-Honigmann, A. M., Krause, P., and Murphy, P. M. (2004). Simian cytomegalovirus encodes five rapidly evolving chemokine receptor homologues. *Virus Genes*, **28**, 71–83.

Sanchez, V., Sztul, E., and Britt, W. J. (2000). Human cytomegalovirus pp28 (UL99) localizes to a cytoplasmic compartment which overlaps the endoplasmic reticulum-Golgi-intermediate compartment. *J. Virol.*, **74**, 3842–3851.

Santoro, F., Greenstone, H. L., Insinga, A. *et al.* (2003). Interaction of glycoprotein H of human herpesvirus 6 with the cellular receptor CD46. *J. Biol. Chem.*, **278**, 25964–25969.

Sarisky, R. T. and Hayward, G. S. (1996). Evidence that the UL84 gene product of human cytomegalovirus is essential for promoting *ori*Lyt-dependent DNA replication and formation of replication compartments in cotransfection assays. *J. Virol.*, **70**, 7398–7413.

Scalzo, A. A., Dallas, P. B., Forbes, C. A. *et al.* (2004). The murine cytomegalovirus M73.5 gene, a member of a 3' co-terminal alternatively spliced gene family, encodes the gp24 virion glycoprotein. *Virology*, **329**, 234–250.

Scheffczik, H., Savva, C. G., Holzenburg, A., Kolesnikova, L., and Bogner, E. (2002). The terminase subunits pUL56 and pUL89 of human cytomegalovirus are DNA-metabolizing proteins with toroidal structure. *Nucl. Acids Res.*, **30**, 1695–1703.

Schierling, K., Stamminger, T., Mertens, T., and Winkler, M. (2004). Human cytomegalovirus tegument proteins ppUL82 (pp71) and ppUL35 interact and cooperatively activate the major immediate-early enhancer. *J. Virol.*, **78**, 9512–9523.

Sedarati, F. and Rosenthal, L. J. (1988). Isolation and partial characterization of nucleocapsid forms from cells infected with human cytomegalovirus strains AD169 and Towne. *Intervirology*, **29**, 86–100.

Sheaffer, A. K., Weinheimer, S. P., and Tenney, D. J. (1997). The human cytomegalovirus UL98 gene encodes the conserved herpesvirus alkaline nuclease. *J. Gen. Virol.*, **78**, 2953–2961.

Shieh, H. S., Kurumbail, R. G., Stevens, A. M. *et al.* (1996). Three-dimensional structure of human cytomegalovirus protease. *Nature*, **383**, 279–282.

Silva, M. C., Yu, Q. C., Enquist, L., and Shenk, T. (2003). Human cytomegalovirus UL99-encoded pp28 is required for the cytoplasmic envelopment of tegument-associated capsids. *J. Virol.*, **77**, 10594–10605.

Simmen, K. A., Singh, J., Luukkonen, B. G. *et al.* (2001). Global modulation of cellular transcription by human cytomegalovirus is initiated by viral glycoprotein B. *Proc. Natl Acad. Sci. USA*, **98**, 7140–7145.

Skaletskaya, A., Bartle, L. M., Chittenden, T., McCormick, A. L., Mocarski, E. S., and Goldmacher, V. S. (2001). A cytomegalovirus-encoded inhibitor of apoptosis that suppresses caspase-8 activation. *Proc. Natl Acad. Sci. USA*, **98**, 7829–7834.

Smith, J. A. and Pari, G. S. (1995a). Human cytomegalovirus UL102 gene. *J. Virol.*, **69**, 1734–1740.

Smith, J. A. and Pari, G. S. (1995b). Expression of human cytomegalovirus UL36 and UL37 genes is required for viral DNA replication. *J. Virol.*, **69**, 1925–1931.

Smith, J. A., Jairath, S., Crute, J. J., and Pari, G. S. (1996). Characterization of the human cytomegalovirus UL105 gene and identification of the putative helicase protein. *Virology*, **220**, 251–255.

Spaderna, S., Blessing, H., Bogner, E., Britt, W., and Mach, M. (2002). Identification of glycoprotein gpTRL10 as a structural component of human cytomegalovirus. *J. Virol.*, **76**, 1450–1460.

Spaete, R. R. and Mocarski, E. S. (1985). The *a* sequence of the cytomegalovirus genome functions as a cleavage/packaging signal for herpes simplex virus defective genomes. *J. Virol.*, **54**, 817–824.

Spaete, R. R., Perot, K., Scott, P. I., Nelson, J. A., Stinski, M. F., and Pachl, C. (1993). Coexpression of truncated human cytomegalovirus gH with the UL115 gene product or the truncated human fibroblast growth factor receptor results in transport of gH to the cell surface. *Virology*, **193**, 853–861.

Spear, G. T., Lurain, N. S., Parker, C. J., Ghassemi, M., Payne, G. H., and Saifuddin, M. (1995). Host cell-derived complement control proteins CD55 and CD59 are incorporated into the virions of two unrelated enveloped viruses. Human T cell leukemia/lymphoma virus type I (HTLV-I) and human cytomegalovirus (HCMV). *J. Immunol.*, **155**, 4376–4381.

Speir, E., Yu, Z. X., Ferrans, V. J., Huang, E. S., and Epstein, S. E. (1998). Aspirin attenuates cytomegalovirus infectivity and gene expression mediated by cyclooxygenase-2 in coronary artery smooth muscle cells. *Circ. Res.*, **83**, 210–216.

Stamminger, T., Gstaiger, M., Weinzierl, K., Lorz, K., Winkler, M., and Schaffner, W. (2002). Open reading frame UL26 of human cytomegalovirus encodes a novel tegument protein that contains a strong transcriptional activation domain. *J. Virol.*, **76**, 4836–4847.

Stannard, L. M. (1989). β_2 microglobulin binds to the tegument of cytomegalovirus: an immunogold study. *J. Gen. Virol.*, **70**, 2179–2184.

Stanton, R., Wilkinson, G. W. G., and Fox, J. D. (2003). Analysis of human herpesvirus-6 IE1 sequence variation in clinical samples. *J. Med. Virol.*, **71**, 578–584.

Stasiak, P. C. and Mocarski, E. S. (1992). Transactivation of the cytomegalovirus ICP36 gene promoter requires the α gene product TRS1 in addition to IE1 and IE2. *J. Virol.*, **66**, 1050–1058.

Stefan, A., Secchiero, P., Baechi, T., Kempf, W., and Campadelli-Fiume, G. (1997). The 85-kilodalton phosphoprotein (pp85) of human herpesvirus 7 is encoded by open reading frame U14 and localizes to a tegument substructure in virion particles. *J. Virol.*, **71**, 5758–5763.

Streblow, D. N., Soderberg-Naucler, C., Vieira, J. et al. (1999). The human cytomegalovirus chemokine receptor US28 mediates vascular smooth muscle cell migration. *Cell*, **99**, 511–520.

Sullivan, V., Talarico, C. L., Stanat, S. C., Davis, M., Coen, D. M., and Biron, K. K. (1992). A protein kinase homologue controls phosphorylation of ganciclovir in human cytomegalovirus-infected cells. *Nature*, **358**, 162–164.

Sun, Y. and Conner, J. (1999). The U28 ORF of human herpesvirus-7 does not encode a functional ribonucleotide reductase R1 subunit. *J. Gen. Virol.*, **80**, 2713–2718.

Takemoto, M., Shimamoto, T., Isegawa, Y., and Yamanishi, K. (2001). The R3 region, one of three major repetitive regions of human herpesvirus 6, is a strong enhancer of immediate-early gene U95. *J. Virol.*, **75**, 10149–10160.

Talarico, C. L., Burnette, T. C., Miller, W. H. et al. (1999). Acyclovir is phosphorylated by the human cytomegalovirus UL97 protein. *Antimicrob. Agents Chemother.*, **43**, 1941–1946.

Tamashiro, J. C. and Spector, D. H. (1986). Terminal structure and heterogeneity in human cytomegalovirus strain AD169. *J. Virol.*, **59**, 591–604.

Teo, I. A., Griffin, B. E., and Jones, M. D. (1991). Characterization of the DNA polymerase gene of human herpesvirus 6. *J. Virol.*, **65**, 4670–4680.

Terhune, S. S., Schroer, J., and Shenk, T. (2004). RNAs are packaged into human cytomegalovirus virions in proportion to their intracellular concentration. *J. Virol.*, **78**, 10390–10398.

Thomson, B. J., Efstathiou, S., and Honess, R. W. (1991). Acquisition of the human adeno-associated virus type-2 *rep* gene by human herpesvirus type-6. *Nature*, **351**, 78–80.

Tigue, N. J., Matharu, P. J., Roberts, N. A., Mills, J. S., Kay, J., and Jupp, R. (1996). Cloning, expression and characterization of the proteinase from human herpesvirus 6. *J. Virol.*, **70**, 4136–4141.

Tirabassi, R. S. and Ploegh, H. L. (2002). The human cytomegalovirus US8 glycoprotein binds to major histocompatibility complex class I products. *J. Virol.*, **76**, 6832–6835.

Tomasec, P., Braud, V. M., Rickards, C. et al. (2000). Surface expression of HLA-E, an inhibitor of natural killer cells, enhanced by human cytomegalovirus gpUL40. *Science*, **287**, 1031.

Tomasec, P., Wang, E. C., Davison, A. J. et al. (2005). Downregulation of natural killer cell-activating ligand CD155 by human cytomegalovirus UL141. *Nat. Immunol.*, **6**, 181–188.

Tomazin, R., Boname, J., Hegde, N. R. et al. (1999). Cytomegalovirus US2 destroys two components of the MHC class II pathway, preventing recognition by CD4+ T cells. *Nat. Med.*, **5**, 1039–1043.

Tong, L., Qian, C., Massariol, M. J., Bonneau, P. R., Cordingley, M. G., and Lagace, L. (1996). A new serine-protease fold revealed by the crystal structure of human cytomegalovirus protease. *Nature*, **383**, 272–275.

Trus, B. L., Homa, F. L., Booy, F. P. et al. (1995). Herpes simplex virus capsids assembled in insect cells infected with recombinant baculoviruses: structural authenticity and localization of VP26. *J. Virol.*, **69**, 7362–7366.

Trus, B. L., Gibson, W., Cheng, N., and Steven, A. C. (1999). Capsid structure of simian cytomegalovirus from cryoelectron microscopy: evidence for tegument attachment sites. *J. Virol.*, **73**, 2181–2192.

Trus, B. L., Heymann, J. B., Nealon, K. et al. (2001). Capsid structure of Kaposi's sarcoma-associated herpesvirus, a gammaherpesvirus, compared to those of an alphaherpesvirus, herpes simplex virus type 1, and a betaherpesvirus, cytomegalovirus. *J. Virol.*, **75**, 2879–2890.

van Zeijl, M., Fairhurst, J., Baum, E. Z., Sun, L., and Jones, T. R. (1997). The human cytomegalovirus UL97 protein is phosphorylated and a component of virions. *Virology*, **231**, 72–80.

Varnum, S. M., Streblow, D. N., Monroe, M. E. et al. (2004). Identification of proteins in human cytomegalovirus (HCMV) particles: the HCMV proteome. *J. Virol.*, **78**, 10960–10966.

Vey, M., Schafer, W., Reis, B. et al. (1995). Proteolytic processing of human cytomegalovirus glycoprotein B (gpUL55) is mediated by the human endoprotease furin. *Virology*, **206**, 746–749.

Vink, C., Beuken, E., and Bruggeman, C. A. (1996). Structure of the rat cytomegalovirus genome termini. *J. Virol.*, **70**, 5221–5229.

Vink, C., Beuken, E., and Bruggeman, C. A. (2000). Complete DNA sequence of the rat cytomegalovirus genome. *J. Virol.*, **74**, 7656–7665.

Wang, D. and Shenk, T. (2005). Human cytomegalovirus virion protein complex required for epithelial and endothelial cell tropism. *Proc. Natl Acad. Sci. USA*, **102**, 18153–18158.

Wang, S. K., Duh, C. Y., and Chang, T. T. (2000). Cloning and identification of regulatory gene UL76 of human cytomegalovirus. *J. Gen. Virol.*, **81**, 2407–2416.

Wang, S. K., Duh, C. Y., and Wu, C. W. (2004). Human cytomegalovirus UL76 encodes a novel virion-associated protein that is able to inhibit viral replication. *J. Virol.*, **78**, 9750–9762.

Weiland, K. L, Oien, N. L., Homa, F., and Wathen, M. W. (1994). Functional analysis of human cytomegalovirus polymerase accessory protein. *Virus. Res.*, **34**, 191–206.

Welch, A. R., Woods, A. S., McNally, L. M., Cotter, R. J., and Gibson, W. (1991). A herpesvirus maturational proteinase, assemblin: identification of its gene, putative active site domain, and cleavage site. *Proc. Natl Acad. Sci. USA*, **88**, 10792–10796.

Welch, A. R., McNally, L. M., Hall, M. R., and Gibson, W. (1993). Herpesvirus proteinase: site-directed mutagenesis used to study maturational, release, and inactivation cleavage sites of precursor and to identify a possible catalytic site serine and histidine. *J. Virol.*, **67**, 7360–7372.

Weststrate, M. W., Geelen, J. L., and van der Noordaa, J. (1980). Human cytomegalovirus DNA: physical maps for restriction endonucleases *Bgl*II, *Hin*dIII and *Xba*I. *J. Gen. Virol.*, **49**, 1–21.

Widen, F., Goltz, M., Wittenbrink, N., Ehlers, B., Banks, M., and Belak, S. (2001). Identification and sequence analysis of the glycoprotein B gene of porcine cytomegalovirus. *Virus Genes*, **23**, 339–346.

Wiertz, E. J., Jones, T. R., Sun, L., Bogyo, M., Geuze, H. J., and Ploegh, H. L. (1996a). The human cytomegalovirus US11 gene product dislocates MHC class I heavy chains from the endoplasmic reticulum to the cytosol. *Cell*, **84**, 769–779.

Wiertz, E. J., Tortorella, D., Bogyo, M. *et al.* (1996b). Sec61-mediated transfer of a membrane protein from the endoplasmic reticulum to the proteasome for destruction. *Nature*, **384**, 432–438.

Wills, M. R., Ashiru, O., Reeves, M. B. *et al.* (2005). Human cytomegalovirus encodes an MHC class I-like molecule (UL142) that functions to inhibit NK cell lysis. *J. Immunol.*, **175**, 7457–7465.

Wing, B. A., Lee, G. C., and Huang, E. S. (1996). The human cytomegalovirus UL94 open reading frame encodes a conserved herpesvirus capsid/tegument-associated virion protein that is expressed with true late kinetics. *J. Virol.*, **70**, 3339–3345.

Winkler, M. and Stamminger, T. (1996). A specific subform of the human cytomegalovirus transactivator protein pUL69 is contained within the tegument of virus particles. *J. Virol.*, **70**, 8984–8987.

Winkler, M., Rice, S. A., and Stamminger, T. (1994). UL69 of human cytomegalovirus, an open reading frame with homology to ICP27 of herpes simplex virus, encodes a transactivator of gene expression. *J. Virol.*, **68**, 3943–3954.

Wolf, D. G., Courcelle, C. T., Prichard, M. N. and Mocarski, E. S. (2001). Distinct and separate roles for herpesvirus-conserved UL97 kinase in cytomegalovirus DNA synthesis and encapsidation. *Proc. Natl Acad. Sci. USA*, **98**, 1895–1900.

Wood, L. J., Baxter, M. K., Plafker, S. M., and Gibson, W. (1997). Human cytomegalovirus capsid assembly protein precursor (pUL80.5) interacts with itself and with the major capsid protein (pUL86) through two different domains. *J. Virol.*, **71**, 179–190.

Wright, J. F., Kurosky, A., Pryzdial, E. L., and Wasi, S. (1995). Host cellular annexin II is associated with cytomegalovirus particles isolated from cultured human fibroblasts. *J. Virol.*, **69**, 4784–4791.

Xu, Y., Ahn, J. H., Cheng, M. *et al.* (2001). Proteasome-independent disruption of PML oncogenic domains (PODs), but not covalent modification by SUMO-1, is required for human cytomegalovirus immediate-early protein IE1 to inhibit PML-mediated transcriptional repression. *J. Virol.*, **75**, 10683–10695.

Xu, Y., Cei, S. A., Huete, A. R., and Pari, G. S. (2004). Human cytomegalovirus UL84 insertion mutant defective for viral DNA synthesis and growth. *J. Virol.*, **78**, 10360–10369.

Yu, D., Smith, G. A., Enquist, L. W., and Shenk, T. (2002). Construction of a self-excisable bacterial artificial chromosome containing the human cytomegalovirus genome and mutagenesis of the diploid TRL/IRL13 gene. *J. Virol.*, **76**, 2316–2328.

Yu, D., Silva, M. C., and Shenk, T. (2003). Functional map of human cytomegalovirus AD169 defined by global mutational analysis. *Proc. Natl Acad. Sci. USA*, **100**, 12396–12401.

Yu, X., Shah, S., Atanasov, I. *et al.* (2005). Three-dimensional localization of the smallest capsid protein in the human cytomegalovirus capsid. *J. Virol.*, **79**, 1327–1332.

Zhao, Y. and Biegalke, B. J. (2003). Functional analysis of the human cytomegalovirus immune evasion protein, pUS3(22kDa). *Virology*, **315**, 353–361.

Zhou, Z. H., He, J., Jakana, J., Tatman, J. D., Rixon, F. J., and Chiu, W. (1995). Assembly of VP26 in herpes simplex virus-1 inferred from structures of wild-type and recombinant capsids. *Nat. Struct. Biol.*, **2**, 1026–1030.

Zhou, Z. H., Chen, D. H., Jakana, J., Rixon, F. J., and Chiu, W. (1999). Visualization of tegument-capsid interactions and DNA in intact herpes simplex virus type 1 virions. *J. Virol.*, **73**, 3210–3218.

Zhu, H., Cong, J. P., Mamtora, G., Gingeras, T., and Shenk, T. (1998). Cellular gene expression altered by human cytomegalovirus: global monitoring with oligonucleotide arrays. *Proc. Natl Acad. Sci. USA*, **95**, 14470–14475.

Zhu, H., Cong, J. P., Yu, D., Bresnahan, W. A., and Shenk, T. E. (2002). Inhibition of cyclooxygenase 2 blocks human cytomegalovirus replication. *Proc. Natl Acad. Sci. USA*, **99**, 3932–3937.

Zou, P., Isegawa, Y., Nakano, K., Haque, M., Horiguchi, Y., and Yamanishi, K. (1999). Human herpesvirus 6 open reading frame U83 encodes a functional chemokine. *J. Virol.*, **73**, 5926–5933.

15

Betaherpes viral genes and their functions

Edward S. Mocarski, Jr.

Department of Microbiology and Immunology, Stanford University School of Medicine, Stanford, CA, USA

Introduction

Despite biological divergence, human cytomegalovirus (HCMV, HHV-5), on the one hand, and the three human roseolaviruses (HHV-6A, HHV-6B, HHV-7), on the other hand, share approximately 70 evolutionarily conserved and collinear genes (italics, Table 15.1). Mammalian betaherpesviruses probably have a common ancestor dating back over 50 million years. The genomes of all betaherpesviruses vary in the regions flanking a large conserved block of genes spanning UL23 to UL124 in HCMV. There appear to be two distinct evolutionary lineages represented by cytomegaloviruses and roseolaviruses infecting primates (Chapter 14). These lineages are not preserved in lower mammals such as rodents where divergence within the cytomegaloviruses is striking. Similarity between rodent cytomegaloviruses and either primate cytomegaloviruses or roseolaviruses is about the same, and includes the same set of 70 conserved genes. Thus, despite the fact that this subgroup of herpesviruses is the most highly distributed amongst mammals, evolutionary divergence is dramatic. The betaherpesvirus-common genes are composed of 41 herpesvirus core functions discussed in Chapters 3, 4 and 14 plus approximately 30 betaherpesvirus-specific gene products that are involved in replication and cell tropism. Biological similarities include tropism for hematopoietic cells in the myeloid lineage (Kondo et al., 2002a; Sissons et al., 2002). In addition to the 70 conserved replication genes human betaherpesviruses HCMV and HHV-6B also have latent genes with a common structure and genomic location (Kondo et al., 1996, 2002b 2003b) suggesting evolutionary conservation in this important process as well. Although little is known about their functions, homologues of several betaherpesvirus-specific genes (UL49, UL79, UL87, UL88, UL91, UL92, and possibly UL95) are common to gammaherpesviruses (see Table 14.1). Thus these two groups are more closely related to each other than to any alphaherpesviruses. Outside of the betaherpesvirus-common genes, there is considerable diversity in this virus group, including the presence of an alphaherpesvirus-like DNA replication origin and origin binding protein in roseolaviruses as well as genes that have been retained only in certain lineages, such as the presence of an adeno-associated virus *rep* gene homologue in closely related HHV-6A and HHV-6B, but not HHV-7, a gene that is conserved as well in the distant rodent betaherpesvirus, rat cytomegalovirus. The presence of specific immunomodulatory genes in only a subset of cytomegaloviruses is also striking (Mocarski, 2002, 2004). How such an array of distinct gene products entered the betaherpesvirus lineage and why they have been retained remain unresolved questions.

As discussed in Chapters 14, the betaherpesvirus-conserved genes include the herpesvirus core set. These genes are clustered towards the center of viral genomes within the unique long (U_L) genomic component of HCMV (Table 15.1). The role of HCMV genes in replication has been systematically studied in variants (*var*) of two laboratory strains Towne*var*ATCC (Dunn et al., 2003b) or AD169*var*ATCC (Yu et al., 2003), and five categories of growth relative to wild-type (parental) virus, have been described: (1) replication better than wild-type (temperance), (2) replication the same as wild-type, (3) complete replication deficiency, (4) severely reduced replication efficiency, (5) slightly reduced replication efficiency (Table 15.1). The host cell type dictates the category for some genes (Dunn et al., 2003b; Hahn et al., 2004) and varying behavior has been observed when viral mutants are studied in fibroblasts, endothelial cells and retinal pigment epithelial cells. In addition to varying behavior in different cell types, HCMV exhibits sensitivity to the cell cycle state at the time of infection (Fortunato et al., 2002) and some

Table 15.1. Summary information on human betaherpesvirus gene products

HCMV[a]	HHV-6[a]	HHV-7[a]	HCMV gene family or function[b]	Selected references[c]
RL1				
RL5A			RL11 family	
RL6			RL11 family	
RL10			Virion envelope glycoprotein	(Spaderna et al., 2002; Spaderna et al., 2004)
RL11			RL11 family; IgG Fc-binding glycoprotein	(Atalay et al., 2002; Lilley et al., 2001)
RL12			RL11 family; putative membrane glycoprotein	
RL13			RL11 family; putative membrane glycoprotein	(Yu et al., 2002)
UL1			RL11 family	
UL2			Putative membrane protein	
UL4			RL11 family; translationally regulated virion glycoprotein	(Alderete et al., 2001; Janzen et al., 2002)
UL5			RL11 family; virion membrane protein?	(Varnum et al., 2004)
UL6			RL11 family; putative membrane glycoprotein	
UL7			RL11 family; putative membrane glycoprotein	
UL8			RL11 family; putative membrane glycoprotein	
UL9*			RL11 family; putative membrane glycoprotein; temperance for fibroblasts	
UL10*			RL11 family; putative membrane glycoprotein temperance for RPE	
UL11			RL11 family; membrane glycoprotein	(Hitomi et al., 1997)
UL13			Putative secreted protein	
UL14			UL14 family; putative membrane glycoprotein	
UL15A			Putative membrane protein	
UL16*			Membrane glycoprotein; inhibits NK cell cytotoxicity; MICA-ULBP ligand; temperance for RPE	(Dunn et al., 2003a; Vales-Gomez et al., 2003)
UL17				
UL18			UL18 family; putative membrane glycoprotein; MHC-I homologue; LIR-1 ligand	(Saverino et al., 2004; Vales-Gomez et al., 2005; Willcox et al., 2003))
UL19				
UL20			T cell receptor γ chain homologue	
UL21A*¥			CC chemokine binding protein (also called UL20A and UL21.5); temperance for fibroblasts	(Wang et al., 2004a)
UL22A¥			Virion protein, secreted glycoprotein (also called UL22.5)	(Varnum et al., 2004)
UL23*	U2	U2	US22 family; tegument protein; temperance for fibroblasts	(Adair et al., 2002)
UL24	U3	U3	US22 family; tegument protein, necessary in HMVECs.	(Adair et al., 2002) [(Kondo et al., 2003a)]
UL25			UL25 family; tegument phosphoprotein	(Battista et al., 1999; Zini et al., 1999; Zini et al., 2000)
UL26¥			US22 family; tegument protein; transcriptional activator of major immediate early promoter	(Stamminger et al., 2002)
UL27	U4	U4	Maribavir resistance	(Chou et al., 2004; Komazin et al., 2003)[(Kondo et al., 2003a)]
UL28¥	U7 × 2U7 × 1	U5 U7	US22 family	[(Kondo et al., 2003a)]
UL29¶	U8	U8	US22 family, growth efficiency in RPE cells	
UL30¥	U9[d]			
UL31¶	U10	U10	[HHV-7 IE gene]	[(Menegazzi et al., 1999)]

(cont.)

Table 15.1. (*cont.*)

HCMV[a]	HHV-6[a]	HHV-7[a]	HCMV gene family or function[b]	Selected references[c]
UL32[†]	U11	U11	Major tegument phosphoprotein (pp150); highly immunogenic; binds to capsids [HHV-6 p100]	(Baxter and Gibson, 2001; Sampaio *et al.*, 2005) [(Neipel *et al.*, 1992; Stefan *et al.*, 1997)]
UL33 × 1 UL33 × 2	U12 × 1 U12 × 2	U12 × 1 U12 × 2	GPCR-7TM family; constitutive signaling, envelope protein [HHV-6A, HHV-6B, HHV-7 are chemokine receptors]	(Casarosa *et al.*, 2003; Fraile-Ramos *et al.*, 2002); [(Isegawa *et al.*, 1998; Milne *et al.*, 2000; Nakano *et al.*, 2003)]
UL34[†]	U13[d]	U13[d]	Represses US3 transcription	(Biegalke *et al.*, 2004; LaPierre and Biegalke, 2001)
UL35[¶]	U14	U14	UL25 family; tegument phosphoprotein; interacts with UL82 protein [HHV-7 IE gene]	(Liu and Biegalke, 2002; Schierling *et al.*, 2005; Schierling *et al.*, 2004) [(Menegazzi *et al.*, 1999; Stefan *et al.*, 1997)]
	U15	U15		
UL36 × 1 UL36 × 2	U17 × 1 U17 × 2	U17 × 1 U17 × 2	US22 family; immediate early protein, tegument protein; inhibitor of caspase-8-induced apoptosis (vICA). [HHV-6 IE gene]	(McCormick *et al.*, 2003; Patterson and Shenk, 1999; Skaletskaya *et al.*, 2001) [(Flebbe-Rehwaldt *et al.*, 2000; Mirandola *et al.*, 1998)]
UL37 × 1[¶]			mitochondrial inhibitor of apoptosis (vMIA) protein.	(Goldmacher *et al.*, 1999; Hayajneh *et al.*, 2001a; McCormick *et al.*, 2003; Reboredo *et al.*, 2004; McCormick *et al.* 2005)
UL37 × 3	U18	U18	Immediate early glycoprotein. [HHV-6. HHV-7 IE gene]	(Adair *et al.*, 2003; Hayajneh *et al.*, 2001b) [(Menegazzi *et al.*, 1999; Mirandola *et al.*, 1998)]
UL38[¶]	U19	U19	virion glycoprotein	(Varnum *et al.*, 2004) [(Flebbe-Rehwaldt *et al.*, 2000; Menegazzi *et al.*, 1999; Mirandola *et al.*, 1998)]
UL40			Membrane glycoprotein; signal peptide binds HLA-E to inhibit NK cell cytotoxicity	(Tomasec *et al.*, 2000; Ulbrecht *et al.*, 2000; Wang *et al.*, 2002)
	U20	U20	Putative membrane glycoprotein	[(Mirandola *et al.*, 1998)]
	U21	U21	Putative membrane glycoprotein [directs MHC class I to lysosomes]	[(Hudson *et al.*, 2001)]
	U22	U22	Putative membrane glycoprotein	
	U23	U23	Putative membrane glycoprotein	
	U24	U24	Putative membrane protein	
	U24A	U24A	Putative membrane protein	
UL41A			Virion membrane protein (also called UL41.5)	(Varnum *et al.*, 2004)
UL42			Putative membrane protein	(Dargan *et al.*, 1997; Mocarski *et al.*, 1997)
UL43	U25	U25	US22 family; tegument protein	(Adair *et al.*, 2002)
	U26	U26	Putative multiple transmembrane protein	
UL44[†]	U27	U27	(core) DNA polymerase processivity subunit (PPS)	(Appleton *et al.*, 2004; Loregian *et al.*, 2004a; Loregian *et al.*, 2004b) [(Agulnick *et al.*, 1993; Lin and Ricciardi, 1998)]
UL45	U28	U28	(core) Tegument; Large subunit of ribonucleotide reductase homologue (enzymatically inactive); virion protein (RR1)	(Hahn *et al.*, 2002; Patrone *et al.*, 2003) [(Sun and Conner, 1999)]
UL46[†]	U29	U29	(core) Component of capsid triplexes (minor capsid binding protein; TRI1)	(Gibson *et al.*, 1996)
UL47[¶]	U30	U30	(core) Tegument; intracellular capsid transport; binds to UL48 protein? (LTPbp)	(Bechtel and Shenk, 2002)
UL48[†]	U31	U31	(core) Largest tegument protein; binds to UL47 protein?; intracellular capsid transport? (LTP) [HHV-7 IE gene]	(Ogawa-Goto *et al.*, 2002) [(Menegazzi *et al.*, 1999)]
UL48A[†]	U32	U32	(core) Located on tips of hexons in capsids; capsid transport? (SCP) (also called UL48.5)	(Lai and Britt, 2003; Yu *et al.*, 2005)

Table 15.1. (cont.)

HCMV[a]	HHV-6[a]	HHV-7[a]	HCMV gene family or function[b]	Selected references[c]
UL49[†]	U33	U33		
UL50[†]	U34	U34	(core) Inner nuclear membrane protein; nuclear egress of capsids in MCMV; virion protein? (NEMP)	(Muranyi et al., 2002; Varnum et al., 2004)
UL51[†]	U35	U35	(core) DNA packaging; terminase-binding? (TERbp)	(Krosky et al., 2000)
UL52[†]	U36	U36	(core) Capsid transport? (CNTP)	(Krosky et al., 2000)
UL53[†]	U37	U37	(core) Nuclear matrix protein; nuclear egress of capsids in MCMV (NELP)	(Dal Monte et al., 2002; Muranyi et al., 2002)
UL54[†]	U38	U38	(core) DNA polymerase catalytic subunit (POL)	(Ihara et al., 1994; Loregian et al., 2004a; Loregian et al., 2004b) [(Yoon et al., 2004)]
UL55[†]	U39	U39	(core) Virion glycoprotein B (gB); homomultimers; heparan-binding, entry and signaling. [roseolavirus IE gene]	(Jarvis et al., 2004; Lopper and Compton, 2004; Strive et al., 2004; Wang et al., 2003) [(Menegazzi et al., 1999; Mirandola et al., 1998)]
UL56[†]	U40	U40	(core) Terminase subunit?; binds to DNA packaging motif, exhibits nuclease activity (TER2).	(Bogner, 2002; Krosky et al., 1998; Scheffczik et al., 2002; Scholz et al., 2003)
UL57[†]	U41	U41	(core) Single-stranded DNA-binding protein (SSB) [roseolavirus IE gene]	(Anders and Gibson, 1988; Kemble et al., 1987) [(Menegazzi et al., 1999; Rotola et al., 1998)]
oriLyt[†]	oriLyt	oriLyt	*DNA replication origin for productive infection (cis-acting) Position conserved, sequence diverged between HCMV and roseolaviruses.*	(Anders et al., 1992; Masse et al., 1992; Prichard et al., 1998) [(Dewhurst et al., 1993; Dykes et al., 1997; Krug et al., 2001; Stamey et al., 1995; van Loon et al., 1997)]
UL69[¥]	U42	U42	(core) Regulatory protein; tegument protein; contributes to cell cycle block; exhibits nucleocytoplasmic shuttling; tegument protein [roseolavirus IE gene]	(Hayashi et al., 2000; Lischka et al., 2001) [(Menegazzi et al., 1999; Mirandola et al., 1998)]
UL70[†]	U43	U43	(core) Component of DNA helicase-primase; primase homology (HP2)	(McMahon and Anders, 2002)
UL71[†]	U44	U44	(core) Tegument protein; cytoplasmic egress? (CEF1)	
UL72	U45	U45	(core) Deoxyuridine triphosphatase homologue (enzymatically inactive), virion protein (dUTPase);	(Caposio et al., 2004; Varnum et al., 2004)
UL73[†]	U46	U46	(core) Virion glycoprotein N (gN); complexes with gM; entry	(Dal Monte et al., 2004; Mach et al., 2000; Mach et al., 2005)
UL74[¶]	U47	U47	Virion glycoprotein O (gO); complexes with gH and gL in HCMV and roseolaviruses	(Hobom et al., 2000; Huber and Compton, 1998; Theiler and Compton, 2002) [(Mori et al., 2004)]
UL75[†]	U48	U48	(core) Virion glycoprotein H (gH); complexes with gL and gO; entry	(Baldwin et al., 2000; Hobom et al., 2000) [(Santoro et al., 2003)]
UL76[†]	U49	U49	(core) Virion-associated regulatory protein	(Wang et al., 2004b)
UL77[†]	U50	U50	(core) Portal capping protein; role in DNA packaging (PCP)	
UL78	U51	U51	GPCR family; putative chemokine receptor	(Michel et al., 2005) [(Menotti et al., 1999; Milne et al., 2000)]
UL79[†]	U52	U52		
UL80[†]	U53	U53	(core) Protease (N terminus) and capsid assembly (scaffold) protein (C terminus) (PR) [HHV-7 IE gene]	(Gibson, 1996; Kim et al., 2004; Plafker and Gibson, 1998) [(Menegazzi et al., 1999; Tigue et al., 1996)]
UL80.5[†]	U53.5	U53.5	(core) Capsid assembly (scaffold) protein (AP)	(Casaday et al., 2004; Oien et al., 1997; Wood et al., 1997)

(cont.)

Table 15.1. (cont.)

HCMV[a]	HHV-6[a]	HHV-7[a]	HCMV gene family or function[b]	Selected references[c]
UL82[¥]	U54	U54	UL82 family; tegument phosphoprotein (pp71; upper matrix protein); virion transactivator; ND10 localized; degrades Rb	(Bresnahan and Shenk, 2000; Hofmann et al., 2002; Ishov et al., 2002; Kalejta and Shenk, 2003)
UL83			UL82 family; major tegument phosphoprotein (pp65; lower matrix protein); suppresses interferon response	(Abate et al., 2004)
UL84[†]	U55	U55	Role in organizing DNA replication; exhibits nucleocytoplasmic shuttling; binds IE2	(Colletti et al., 2004; Colletti et al., 2005; Xu et al., 2004a; Xu et al., 2004b)
UL85[†]	U56	U56	(core) Component of capsid triplexes (minor capsid protein; TRI2)	
UL86[†]	U57	U57	(core) Major capsid protein; component of hexons and pentons (MCP)	(Lai and Britt, 2003; Wood et al., 1997) [(Littler et al., 1990; Mukai et al., 1995)]
UL87[†]	U58	U58		
UL88[¶]	U59	U59	(core) Tegument protein; cytoplasmic egress? (CEF2)	
UL89 × *1*[†]	U66 × 1	U66 × 1	(core) Terminase ATPase subunit; inhibition by antiviral compounds (TER1)	(Bogner, 2002; Buerger et al., 2001; Krosky et al., 1998; Scheffczik et al., 2002)
UL89 × 2	U66 × 2	U66 × 2		
UL90[†]				
UL91[†]	U62	U62		
UL92[†]	U63	U63		
UL93[†]	U64	U64	(core) Tegument protein; capsid transport? (CTTP)	(Wing and Huang, 1995)
UL94[†]	U65	U65	(core) Tegument protein; binds single-stranded DNA; cytoplasmic egress? (CETPbp) [HHV-6 IE gene]	(Wing and Huang, 1995; Wing et al., 1998; Wing et al., 1996) [(Mirandola et al., 1998)]
UL95[†]	U67	U67	(core) encapsidation chaperone protein? (ECP)	(Wing and Huang, 1995)
UL96[†]	U68	U68	Tegument protein	(Wing and Huang, 1995)
UL97[¶]	U69	U69	(core) Viral serine-threonine protein kinase; tegument protein; phosphorylates ganciclovir; inhibited by maribavir; roles in DNA synthesis, DNA packaging and nuclear egress; mimics cdc2/CDK1 (VPK)	(Baek et al., 2004; Kawaguchi et al., 2003; Krosky et al., 2003a; Krosky et al., 2003b; Talarico et al., 1999; Wolf et al., 2001; Wolf et al., 1998) [(Ansari and Emery, 1999; Manichanh et al., 2001; Michel and Mertens, 2004)]
UL98[†]	U70	U70	(core) Deoxyribonuclease (NUC)	(Gao et al., 1998; Wing and Huang, 1995)
UL99[†]	U71	U71	(core) Myristylated tegument phosphoprotein pp28; cytoplasmic egress tegument protein CETP)	(Britt et al., 2004; Jones and Lee, 2004; Sanchez et al., 2000b; Silva et al., 2005; Silva et al., 2003; Wing and Huang, 1995)
UL100[†]	U72	U72	(core) Virion glycoprotein M (gM); complexes with gN; entry	(Mach et al., 2000; Mach et al., 2005)
	U73	U73	oriBP, binds to roseolavirus oriLyt; helicase [roseolavirus IE gene]	[(Inoue and Pellett, 1995; Krug et al., 2001; Menegazzi et al., 1999; Mirandola et al., 1998)]
UL102[†]	U74	U74	(core) Component of DNA helicase-primase (HP3)	(McMahon and Anders, 2002)
UL103[¶]	U75	U75	(core) Tegument protein; nuclear egress? (EEP)	
UL104[†]	U76	U76	(core) Portal protein; DNA encapsidation (PORT)	(Dittmer and Bogner, 2005; Komazin et al., 2004)
UL105[†]	U77	U77	(core) Component of DNA helicase-primase; helicase homology (HP1)	(McMahon and Anders, 2002; Smith et al., 1996)
UL108[¶]				
UL111A			Viral interleukin 10 (vIL-10)	(Chang et al., 2004; Kotenko et al., 2000; Lockridge et al., 2000; Spencer et al., 2002)
UL112[¥]	U79 × 1–2	U79 × 1–2	Transcriptional activation, orchestration of DNA replication	(Ahn et al., 1999; Li et al., 1999; Penfold and Mocarski, 1997) [(Taniguchi et al., 2000)]
UL113[¥]	U79 × 3	U79 × 3		

Table 15.1. (cont.)

HCMV[a]	HHV-6[a]	HHV-7[a]	HCMV gene family or function[b]	Selected references[c]
UL114¶	U81	U81	(core) Uracil-DNA glycosylase; roles in excision of uracil from DNA and temporal regulation of DNA replication (UNG) [HHV-6 IE gene]	(Courcelle et al., 2001; Prichard et al., 1996) [(Rotola et al., 1998)]
UL115†	U82	U82	(core) Virion glycoprotein L (gL); complexes with gH and gO; entry	(Britt and Mach, 1996; Huber and Compton, 1999; Kaye et al., 1992; Milne et al., 1998) [(Mori et al., 2004; Mori et al., 2003b)]
UL116			Putative membrane glycoprotein	
	U83		CC chemokine	(French et al., 1999; Luttichau et al., 2003; Zou et al., 1999)
UL117¥	U84	U84		
UL119		U85[d]	IgG Fc-binding membrane glycoprotein related to OX-2; virion glycoprotein	(Atalay et al., 2002; Varnum et al., 2004)
UL120			UL120 family; putative membrane glycoprotein	
UL121			UL120 family; putative membrane glycoprotein	
UL122†	U86	U86	Immediate early transactivator (IE2); interacts with transcriptional machinery; repression via specific DNA-binding activity	(Barrasa et al., 2005; Heider et al., 2002; Lee and Ahn, 2004; Marchini et al., 2001; Sanchez et al., 2002) [(Gravel et al., 2003; Papanikolaou et al., 2002)]
UL123¥	U90[d]	U90[d]	Immediate early transactivator (IE1); enhances activation by IE2; indirect effect on transcription machinery; disrupts ND10 [roseolavirus IE gene]	(Ahn and Hayward, 2000; Gawn and Greaves, 2002; Greaves and Mocarski, 1998; Lee and Ahn, 2004; Mocarski et al., 1996; Nevels et al., 2004; Reinhardt et al., 2005) [(Gravel et al., 2003; Menegazzi et al., 1999; Mirandola et al., 1998; Nikolaou et al., 2003)]
UL124	U91[d]	U91[d]	Membrane glycoprotein, latent protein [HHV-6 IE gene]	(Kondo et al., 1996; Landini et al., 2000) [(Rotola et al., 1998)]
	U94	U94	Parvovirus Rep protein homologue; binds to a transcription factor and single-stranded DNA; latent protein	[(Dhepakson et al., 2002; Rotola et al., 1998);]
	U95	U95	US22 family; HHV-6 IE gene related to MCMV IE2; positional to HCMV IRS1/TRS1	(Takemoto et al., 2001)
	U100	U100	Virion glycoprotein Q; complexed with gH and gL	(Mori et al., 2003a; Mori et al., 2003b)
UL128			Putative secreted protein; putative CC chemokine; endothelial cell tropism	(Akter et al., 2003; Hahn et al., 2004)
UL129¶				
UL130			Putative secreted protein	(Akter et al., 2003; Hahn et al., 2004)
UL131A			Putative secreted protein	(Akter et al., 2003; Hahn et al., 2004)
UL132¶			Virion glycoprotein	(Varnum et al., 2004)
UL148			Putative membrane glycoprotein	
UL147A			Putative membrane protein	
UL147			UL146 family; putative secreted glycoprotein; putative CXC chemokine	(Penfold et al., 1999; Prichard et al., 2001)
UL146			UL146 family; secreted glycoprotein; CXC chemokine	(Penfold et al., 1999; Prichard et al., 2001
UL145				
UL144			Membrane glycoprotein; TNF receptor homologue; Regulate lymphocytes via BTLA	(Sedy et al., 2005) (Ware, personal communication)
UL142			UL18 family; putative membrane glycoprotein; MHC-I homologue	(Davison et al., 2003)

(cont.)

Table 15.1. (*cont.*)

HCMV[a]	HHV-6[a]	HHV-7[a]	HCMV gene family or function[b]	Selected references[c]
UL141			UL14 family; membrane glycoprotein; inhibits NK cell cytotoxicity by downregulating CD155	(Tomasec *et al.*, 2005)
UL140			Putative membrane protein	
UL139			Putative membrane glycoprotein	
UL138			Putative membrane protein	
UL136			Putative membrane protein	
UL135			Putative secreted protein	
UL133			Putative membrane protein	
UL148A			Putative membrane protein	
UL148B			Putative membrane protein	
UL148C			Putative membrane protein	
UL148D			Putative membrane protein	
UL150			Putative secreted protein	
IRS1			US22 family; immediate early transcriptional activator; tegument protein; blocks shut-off of host protein synthesis; virion protein [positional to roseolavirus U95]	(Child *et al.*, 2002; Romanowski *et al.*, 1997; Romanowski and Shenk, 1997; Stasiak and Mocarski, 1992); Child *et al.*, 2004
US1			US1 family	
US2			US2 family; membrane glycoprotein; degradation of MHC-I and, possibly, MHC-II	(Gewurz *et al.*, 2001; Tortorella *et al.*, 2000)
US3			US2 family; immediate early gene; membrane glycoprotein; inhibits processing and transport of MHC-I and MHC-II	(Gewurz *et al.*, 2001; Hegde *et al.*, 2002; Misaghi *et al.*, 2004; Tortorella *et al.*, 2000; Zhao and Biegalke, 2003)
US6			US6 family; putative membrane glycoprotein; inhibits TAP-mediated ER peptide transport	(Gewurz *et al.*, 2001; Hewitt *et al.*, 2001; Tortorella *et al.*, 2000; Ulbrecht *et al.*, 2003)
US7			US6 family; membrane glycoprotein	(Huber *et al.*, 2002)
US8			US6 family; membrane glycoprotein; binds to MHC-I	(Tirabassi and Ploegh, 2002)
US9			US6 family; membrane glycoprotein; cell-to-cell spread	(Huber *et al.*, 2002; Maidji *et al.*, 1998)
US10			US6 family; membrane glycoprotein; delays trafficking of MHC-I	(Furman *et al.*, 2002)
US11			US6 family; membrane glycoprotein; selective degradation of MHC-I	(Gewurz *et al.*, 2001; Tirosh *et al.*, 2005; Tortorella *et al.*, 2000)
US12			US12 family; putative multiple transmembrane protein	
US13¶			US12 family; putative multiple transmembrane protein	
US14			US12 family; putative multiple transmembrane protein	
US15			US12 family; putative multiple transmembrane protein	
US16*			US12 family; putative multiple transmembrane protein; temperance for ECs	
US17			US12 family; putative multiple transmembrane protein	
US18			US12 family; putative multiple transmembrane protein	(Guo and Huang, 1993)
US19*			US12 family; putative multiple transmembrane protein; temperance for ECs	(Guo and Huang, 1993)
US20			US12 family; putative multiple transmembrane protein	(Guo and Huang, 1993)

Table 15.1. (*cont.*)

HCMV[a]	HHV-6[a]	HHV-7[a]	HCMV gene family or function[b]	Selected references[c]
US21			US12 family; putative multiple transmembrane protein	
US22	DR1 × 1 DR1 × 2	DR1 DR2	US22 family; tegument protein; released from cells (HHV-6 DR1 homologue)	(Adair *et al.*, 2002)
US23¶			US22 family; tegument protein	(Varnum *et al.*, 2004)
US24			US22 family; tegument protein	(Varnum *et al.*, 2004)
US26¥	DR6 × 1 DR6 × 2	DR6 DR7	US22 family (HHV-6 DR-6 homologue)	[(Doniger *et al.*, 1999)]
US27			GPCR family; virion glycoprotein	(Fraile-Ramos *et al.*, 2002; Varnum *et al.*, 2004)
US28			GPCR family; membrane protein; broad spectrum CC and CX3C chemokine receptor; mediates cellular activation and migration	(Billstrom *et al.*, 1999; Casarosa *et al.*, 2001; Gao and Murphy, 1994; Hertel and Mocarski, 2004; Kledal *et al.*, 1998; Melnychuk *et al.*, 2004; Neote *et al.*, 1993; Streblow *et al.*, 1999; Vieira *et al.*, 1998)
US29			Putative membrane glycoprotein, necessary in RPE cells.	
US30*			Putative membrane glycoprotein; temperance for fibroblasts	
US31			US1 family	
US32			US1 family	
US34			Putative secreted protein	
US34A			Putative membrane protein	
TRS1¶			US22 family; immediate early transcriptional activator; tegument protein involved in capsid assembly; blocks shut-off of translation [positional to roseolavirus U95]	(Child *et al.*, 2002; Romanowski *et al.*, 1997; Romanowski and Shenk, 1997; Stasiak and Mocarski, 1992); Child *et al.*, 2004

[a] Commonly annotated ORFs of HCMV, together with selected ORFs of HHV-6 (A or B) and HHV-7. Emphasis is on ORFs that are conserved between these viruses. General references to gene mapping, homologies and annotation (Cha *et al.*, 1996; Chee *et al.*, 1990; Davison *et al.*, 2003; Dolan *et al.*, 2004; Dominguez *et al.*, 1999b; Gompels *et al.*, 1995; Nicholas, 1996). Functional dissection of HCMV (Dunn *et al.*, 2003b; Yu *et al.*, 2003) by mutagenesis showing replication better than wild type (*), indistinguishable from wild type (normal type) or one of three broad growth deficient phenotypes: failure to replicate (bold †), very poor replication (bold ¥), slight replication defect (bold ¶) when viruses are assayed in human fibroblasts. Mutations of putative HCMV ORFs UL60 and UL61 are interpreted as disruption of HCMV oriLyt (Masse *et al.*, 1992) rather than a protein-coding ORF.

[b] Betaherpesvirus-common genes in italics, and include 40 herpesvirus core functions (see Chapters 2 and 3). Gene family, characteristics and functional information are provided for HCMV where a blank indicates the absence of functional information.

[c] References listed are to gene function where known in HCMV, with those specific to HHV-6 indicated within []; see Chapter 14 for additional references to mapping and physical characteristics. General reference for HCMV structural proteins is (Baldick and Shenk, 1996).

[d] Positional homologue.

viral mutants accentuate these effects. The herpesvirus core gene products, discussed elsewhere (Chapter 4), play roles in replication. A majority, 33, core genes (UL44, UL46, UL48, UL48A, UL50–UL57, UL70, UL71, UL73, UL75–UL77, UL80, UL80.5, UL85, UL86, UL89, UL93–UL95, UL98, UL99, UL100, UL102, UL104, UL105, UL115) are absolutely essential for HCMV replication. Mutants deficient in one (UL69) exhibit severely reduced replication efficiency (Hayashi *et al.*, 2000) and mutants in five (UL47, UL88, UL97, UL103, UL114) exhibit slightly reduced replication efficiency (Table 15.1) that for UL97 or UL114 can be dependent on the fibroblast cell cycle state (Courcelle *et al.*, 2001; Prichard *et al.*, 1996, 1999; Wolf *et al.*, 2001). Only two core genes, the ribonucleotide reductase homologue (HCMV UL45) and the dUTPase homologue (HCMV UL72), lack any detectable role in replication (Hahn *et al.*, 2002, 2003). Neither of these betaherpesvirus homologues conserve key motifs for enzymatic activity that are found in other herpesviruses leaving an open question as to function.

Many of the 30-odd betaherpesvirus-specific genes investigated individually (Bresnahan and Shenk, 2000;

Greaves and Mocarski, 1998; Marchini et al., 2001) or systematically (Dunn et al., 2003b; Yu et al., 2003) have been found to play some role in viral replication. Ten are essential for HCMV replication in fibroblasts (UL32, UL34, UL49, UL79, UL84, UL87, UL91, UL92, UL96, UL122), six (UL28, UL82, UL112–113, UL117, UL123, US26) have a strong impact on growth and six (UL29, UL31, UL35, UL38, UL74, TRS1) have only a slight impact on growth. While the two systematic mutagenesis efforts (Dunn et al., 2003b; Yu et al., 2003) did not completely agree on the phenotype associated with each gene, there was a remarkable consistency given that different laboratory strains of virus were analyzed and each was completed independently. Although characterization has not continued for most genes, 11 betaherpesvirus-specific genes (UL23, UL24, UL27, UL33, UL36, UL37 × 3, UL43, UL78, UL124, IRS1, US22) play no detectable role in fibroblasts (Dunn et al., 2003b). These include a tropism factor encoded by UL24, which is necessary for replication in endothelial cells (Dunn et al., 2003b), as well as UL36, which encodes the viral inhibitor of caspase 8 activation (vICA), a potent cell death suppressor (McCormick et al., 2003; Skaletskaya et al., 2001) that influences infected cell survival in the presence of inducers of cell death. The role of the two cell death suppressors encoded by HCMV, vICA and viral mitochondrial inhibitor of apoptosis (vMIA), appear to overlap in protection from cell death during infection (McCormick et al., 2005) despite evidence that only vMIA was important in strain AD169 var ATCC (Reboredo et al., 2004).

Genetic analysis has only begun in the roseolaviruses due to the relative intractability of these viruses to molecular genetic manipulation. The one insertion mutant of HHV-6B that has been reported, disrupting betaherpesvirus-specific U3-U7 (homologues of HCMV UL24, UL27 and UL28), replicates normally (Kondo et al., 2003a), consistent with the behavior of individual gene mutants in HCMV homologues (Dunn et al., 2003b).

One long-standing unique characteristic of the HCMV genome is the presence of gene families (Chee et al., 1990; Dolan et al., 2004), as described in Chapter 14, which extend to all betaherpesviruses (Dominguez et al., 1999a; Gompels and Macaulay, 1995; Nicholas, 1996). The US22 family is the largest and most highly conserved of these families, and includes a great many genes that are dispensable for replication but that play roles in cell survival, cell tropism and pathogenesis (Dunn et al., 2003b; McCormick et al., 2003; Menard et al., 2003; Skaletskaya et al., 2001). HCMV encodes 13 US22 family members (Chee et al., 1990) whereas roseolaviruses encode ten, nine of which are conserved in sequence or genomic location (Table 15.1). Cell tropism appears to be influenced by different members of the US22 family in different viruses. In HCMV, these are involved in tropism for particular cell types or in tempering viral replication in certain cell types (Dunn et al., 2003b). For example, US22 family member UL23 has been implicated as a temperance factor for HCMV growth in fibroblasts. Other identified temperance genes (Table 15.1) are not in the US22 family and are not conserved in betaherpesviruses. The US22 family member UL24 has been implicated as a tropism factor in endothelial cells (Dunn et al., 2003b) and TRS1 protein blocks activation of protein kinase R in the interferon response (Child et al., 2004). Many additional genomic regions have been implicated in the control of cell tropism (Bolovan-Fritts and Wiedeman, 2002; Brown et al., 1995; Cha et al., 1996; Dunn et al., 2003b; Gerna et al., 2003; Hahn et al., 2004; Hertel et al., 2003; Jahn et al., 1999; Kahl et al., 2000; Mocarski et al., 1993; Riegler et al., 2000; Sinzger and Jahn, 1996; Sinzger et al., 2000) but none of these has been associated with specific betaherpesvirus-conserved genes or US22 family members. Insights into tropism have been derived from studies on animal models, primarily MCMV (Brune et al., 2001; Cavanaugh et al., 1996; Grzimek et al., 1999; Manning et al., 1992; Menard et al., 2003; Morello et al., 1999), where evaluation in cell culture as well as in the natural host is experimentally tractable. Using MCMV, tropism for endothelial cells and macrophages has been studied in cultured cells as well as in mice and is influenced by herpesvirus core (RR1) as well as by betaherpesvirus-common (US22 family) gene products (Brune et al., 2001; Hanson et al., 2001; Menard et al., 2003). Betaherpesvirus-conserved tegument-associated US22 family member M36, which encodes vICA similar to HCMV UL36 (McCormick et al., 2003), as well as other US22 family members whose precise homologues cannot be assigned, is a specific determinant of cell tropism for macrophages but not for fibroblasts or endothelial cells (Hanson et al., 2001; Menard et al., 2003). The US22 family member M43 appears to influence viral growth in macrophage-like cells as well as immortalized fibroblasts, but not in primary cells of either cell type (Menard et al., 2003). Unfortunately, the two US22 family members contributing to HCMV endothelial cell tropism (UL24) or temperance (UL23) (Dunn et al., 2003b) have not been found to play a role in tropism for endothelial cells or macrophages when MCMV has been studied (Menard et al., 2003). Also, MCMV studies have thus far not given insights into HCMV (Dunn et al., 2003b; Hahn et al., 2002) such that HCMV RR1 and particular US22 family members implicated in MCMV cell tropism do not exhibit a similar impact on HCMV tropism. Thus, betaherpesvirus-conserved genes have not yet been implicated in common pathways of tropism even though a large proportion of the gene products in betaherpesviruses such as HCMV as well as MCMV appear to be involved in modulating the host response to infection (Mocarski, 2002; 2004). All betaherpesviruses encode homologues of HCMV UL33 and UL78, seven transmembrane spanning receptors as well as chemokine receptor homologues. Viruses like HCMV and MCMV immunomodulate similar cellular processes, however, these viruses often rely on evolutionarily distinct gene products to do so. Important immunomodulatory functions are therefore largely not reflected in the betaherpesvirus-conserved set of genes.

Discussion here will focus on HCMV, with presentation of betaherpesvirus-common functions in virion structure and entry, proceeding through regulation of gene expression, DNA synthesis, processing and packaging and, finally, maturation and egress. Because of apparent similarity in the genomic location and structure latent transcripts that have been mapped in HCMV (Kondo et al., 1996) and HHV-6B (Kondo et al., 2002b, 2003b), the chapter will conclude with a brief discussion of the molecular basis of betaherpesvirus latency.

Virion structural proteins

Virion structure is highly conserved among betaherpesviruses such that over half the betaherpesvirus-common genes encode structural proteins. As shown in Table 15.1, 23 herpesvirus core genes encode HCMV structural proteins as components of the capsid (UL46, UL48A, UL85, UL86, UL104 gene products), tegument (UL45, UL47, UL48, UL69, UL71, UL72, UL76, UL77, UL88, UL93, UL94, UL95, UL97, UL99, UL103 gene products) or envelope (UL55, UL73, UL75, UL100, UL115 gene products). Many additional core genes are involved in assembly and maturation of virions (Chapter 4). Fifteen betaherpesvirus-specific genes (UL23, UL24, UL32, UL33, UL35, UL36, UL38, UL43, UL74, UL78, UL82, UL96, IRS1, US22, TRS1) encode structural proteins, localizing to the tegument or envelope.

Betaherpesvirus capsids are composed of four major and two minor herpesvirus-conserved proteins (Chapter 4). The major capsid protein (MCP, HCMV UL86 gene product), triplex monomer and dimer proteins (TRI1 and TRI2, HCMV UL46 and UL85 gene products, respectively), and the smallest capsid protein (SCP, HCMV UL48A gene product) are prominent capsid constituents, along with the portal protein (PORT, HCMV UL104 gene product), which likely constitutes one penton used for encapsidation of viral DNA as it does in alphaherpesviruses.

Most herpesvirus core structural proteins localize to the tegument. In HCMV, all core tegument proteins (HCMV UL47, UL48, UL71, UL76, UL77, UL88, UL93–UL97, UL99, UL103 gene products) play some role in replication (Table 15.1), although four, including a protein that likely binds to the largest tegument protein, the homologue of a cytoplasmic egress facilitator, the viral serine-threonine protein kinase (VPK) and a homologue of an encapsidation and egress protein (HCMV UL47, UL88, UL97 and UL103 gene products, respectively), have only a slight impact on viral growth. VPK apparently acts in tandem with host cell cycle kinases to regulate replication events across a spectrum depending on the state of the host cell (Krosky et al., 2003a; Prichard et al., 1999; Wolf et al., 2001) and is dispensable for replication in rapidly dividing host cells where its role is presumably redundant with host protein kinases, possibly as a cdk1 or cdk2 analogue (Kawaguchi et al., 2003). The portal capping protein (HCMV UL77 gene product) is considered part of the tegument and is essential for replication. By analogy with HSV-1, UL48 may be involved in entry (Ogawa-Goto et al., 2002) and others may be involved in egress (Chapter 4). UL76 protein localizes in a pattern that suggests it may be involved in regulating events immediately following infection or during maturation (Wang et al., 2004b). HCMV UL99 protein (pp28) is an abundant, small myristolated tegument protein that localizes to the cytoplasm and is involved in the late stages of virion egress (Jones and Lee, 2004; Silva et al., 2003). If information from alphaherpesviruses is predictive, UL99 protein may be expected to interact with other tegument proteins, such as the UL94 and UL95 gene products, as well as with the gM:gN glycoprotein complex. Investigation of tegument protein activities and capsid–tegument or tegument–envelope interactions remain important areas for experimental investigation.

A bulk of betaherpesvirus-specific structural proteins also localize to the virion tegument (Table 15.1). The most abundant include two UL82 family members, pp65 (lower matrix protein), the UL83 gene product and is the most abundant HCMV tegument protein, and pp71 (upper matrix protein), UK82 gene product, as well as pp150 (large matrix phosphoprotein), UL32 gene product, and pp28 (myristylated tegument phosphoprotein), the UL99 gene product pp65 is a major constituent of dense bodies that are produced during HCMV replication. The abundance of UL82 family members varies in other betaherpesviruses. (Gibson, 1996) as well as several minor tegument proteins. The most abundant HCMV tegument protein (pp65, upper matrix protein, UL83 gene product), a UL82 family member, is not conserved in roseolaviruses. HCMV UL82 encodes pp71, the virion transactivator (Liu and Stinski, 1992) that exhibits an MOI-dependent role in replication (Bresnahan and Shenk, 2000). A minor HCMV tegument protein encoded by UL35 interacts with the pp71 and co-stimulates transcription (Liu and Biegalke, 2002; Schierling et al., 2004, 2005). HCMV UL32 encodes pp150, an essential tegument protein (Dunn et al., 2003b) that interacts with capsids (Baxter and Gibson, 2001) and localizes to nuclear and cytoplasmic compartments (Sampaio et al., 2005) where it may be involved in virion assembly, maturation or egress. Conserved US22 family members (HCMV genes UL23, UL24, UL36, UL43, IRS1, US22, TRS1) all encode tegument proteins (Table 15.1). These include the UL24 tropism factor as well as UL36, cell death suppressor (McCormick et al., 2003; Skaletskaya et al., 2001), as discussed in Chapter 21.

The most abundant, and functionally important envelope glycoproteins found in HCMV virions, gB, gH:gL and gM:gN, are all herpesvirus core functions. Betaherpesviruses have not yet been found to encode any unique glycoproteins that control viral attachment or entry such as gD in HSV-1 or gp220/350 in EBV. In betaherpesviruses, as well as gammaherpesviruses, the gH:gL complex may be modified by a third component. These variants may influence cell type specificity as has been characterized best in the gammaherpesvirus EBV (Chapter 23). In both HCMV and roseolaviruses, a betaherpesvirus-specific protein, gO, may associate with this complex (Huber and Compton, 1998; Mori et al., 2004), and, in roseolaviruses a separate glycoprotein that is not conserved in HCMV, gQ, may be a component of gH:gL complexes (Mori et al., 2003b). Functional studies on gM:gN have been reported (Mach et al., 2005), suggesting that this most abundant complex in virion envelopes (Varnum et al., 2004) is critical for being involved in some step in entry. Other membrane proteins such as UL33, a ligand-independent seven-transmembrane-spanning signaling protein (Casarosa et al., 2003), UL78, and UL38 may be associated with the virion envelope (Varnum et al., 2004), but viral replication in fibroblasts is not influenced in their absence (Dunn et al., 2003b).

Entry into host cells

The mechanisms of betaherpesvirus binding to the cell surface and of fusion-mediated penetration have been extensively studied but the details of these processes are still incomplete (Chapters 16 and 46). Herpesvirus core glycoproteins appear to play the critical roles in entry (Fig. 15.1), relying on gB, gH:gL and gM:gN (Chapter 4). HCMV entry into fibroblasts is via direct fusion at the cell surface (Compton et al., 1992) and possibly via endocytosis in other cell types (see Chapter 16). Roseolaviruses employ direct penetration as well as endocytic pathways of entry (Mori et al., 2002). Entry of betaherpesviruses appears to involve the interaction of these envelope glycoproteins with a number of distinct receptors, and is initiated by a common use of the cell surface proteoglycan heparan sulfate (Compton et al., 1993; Conti et al., 2000; Neyts et al., 1992). The core protein gB from both HCMV (Compton et al., 1993; Kari and Gehrz, 1993) and roseolaviruses (Conti et al., 2000; Secchiero et al., 1997) binds heparan sulfate. This initial contact is followed by interactions with additional receptors. In HCMV, a variety of cell surface proteins have been proposed to play roles in the subsequent steps in attachment (Chapter 16), although none is yet widely accepted. In addition to the role of receptors as entry mediators, HCMV binding to cells induces signaling cascades (Evers et al., 2004) that activate NF-κB (Yurochko and Huang, 1999; Yurochko et al., 1995), mitogen-activated protein kinase (Johnson et al., 2000), phosphotidylinositol 3 kinase (Johnson et al., 2001), and toll-like pathways (Compton et al., 2003). gB binding seems sufficient for induction of some pathways (Boehme et al., 2004; Boyle et al., 1999; Wang et al., 2003; Yurochko et al., 1997). HCMV gB has been shown to utilize the EGF receptor as well as integrins as entry mediators (Feire et al., 2004; Wang et al., 2003). Signaling may play a critical role in conditioning the cell for viral replication following entry (Wang et al., 2003). In HHV-6A or HHV-6B, CD46 (Santoro et al., 1999) is a critical cellular receptor and interacts with gH-containing glycoprotein complexes (Mori et al., 2004; Mori et al., 2003b; Santoro et al., 2003). Entry of HHV-7 into T cells relies on CD4 (Lusso et al., 1994). Thus, except for initial contact with proteoglycan and the apparent use of core glycoproteins, betaherpesvirus attachment and entry mechanisms appear diverse at the level of current knowledge.

The same set of envelope glycoproteins (gB, gH:gL and gM:gN) have been implicated in fusion between the envelope and the cell membrane (Compton, 2004). HCMV gB and gH have been the most extensively studied for fusion (Baldwin et al., 2000; Feire et al., 2004; Lopper and Compton, 2004; Navarro et al., 1993; Tugizov et al., 1994; Wang et al., 2003). HHV-6A gB is also relatively well studied (Santoro et al., 2003). Recent evidence suggests core envelope glycoproteins gM and gN (gM:gN) may also be important for entry of betaherpesviruses (Mach et al., 2005) despite the fact that their involvement in alphaherpesvirus entry is variable (Chapter 4). The best evidence suggests that the core envelope glycoprotein complexes formed by gB (also called gCI) or gH:gL (also called gCIII) are essential for replication in HCMV (Hobom et al., 2000) because of the role these conserved glycoproteins play in fusion. The role of gH:gL modification by betaherpesvirus-specific UL74 gene product, gO (Hobom et al., 2000; Huber and Compton, 1998; Theiler and Compton, 2002) remains unknown due to its relatively minor impact on viral replication (Dunn et al., 2003b). In HHV-6B, gH:gL modified by either the U47 gene product gO (Mori et al., 2004) or the U100 gene product gQ (Mori et al., 2003a) (Table 15.1) facilitate entry into cells via CD46 (Mori et al., 2003b).

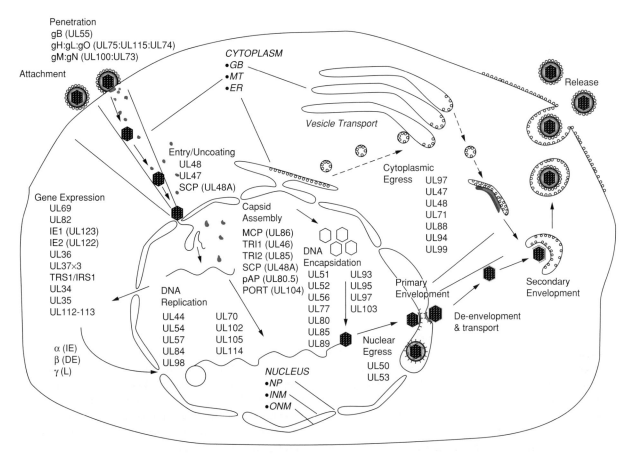

Fig. 15.1. Summary of replication functions carried out by betaherpesvirus-conserved gene products using HCMV gene designations. Major steps in productive replication are indicated along with functions (see Table 15.1) contributing to each step are listed in plain font. The entry pathway shown (black arrows) employs direct fusion at the cell surface (attachment and penetration). Entry may also follow an endocytic pathway and virion fusion with an endocytic vesicle in some betaherpesviruses (see text). Entry requires gB, gH:gL, possibly with gO, and gM:gN. HCMV UL47, UL48 and SCP gene products may mediate transport on microtubules, docking at nuclear pores and release of virion DNA into the nucleus based on work with alphaherpesviruses. One core regulatory protein (UL69) and several betaherpesvirus-specific proteins in the virion (HCMV UL82, UL36, TRS1/IRS1 gene products). expressed as IE genes (HCMV IE1, IE2, UL37 × 3 gene products) or expressed as DE genes (HCMV UL34, UL35 UL112–113 gene products) are involved in transcriptional regulation. DNA replication depends on several core proteins (HCMV UL44, UL54, UL57, UL70, UL102, UL105, UL98, UL114 gene products) as well as one betaherpesvirus-specific protein (UL84 gene product). Capsid assembly uses core functions MCP, TRI1:TRI2, SCP, PORT and pAP. Pre-formed capsids likely translocate to sites of DNA replication where several core proteins (HCMV UL51, UL56, UL77, UL80.5, UL85, UL89, UL93, UL95, UL97, UL103 gene products) are likely to be involved in encapsidation of viral DNA. Nuclear egress is likely to be controlled by HCMV UL50 and UL53 gene products, which are core proteins. Cytoplasmic egress (black arrows) and secondary (final) envelopment are controlled by core functions (HCMV UL47, UL48, UL71, UL88, UL94, UL97, UL99 gene products). Nucleocapsids are likely transported on MT and virion envelope glycoproteins follow vesicle transport to sites of final envelopment in the cytoplasm. Golgi body (GB), microtubules (MT) and endoplasmic reticulum (ER) are identified in the cytoplasm, and nuclear pores (NP), inner nuclear membrane (INM) and outer nuclear membrane (ONM) are identified in the nucleus. The cellular vesicle transport pathway from the ER to GB is also designated (dashed grey arrow). The core functions UL45 (RR1 homologue) and UL72 (dUTPase homologue) are not assigned. Functions for the betherpesvirus-common genes UL28, UL29, UL31, UL32, UL38, UL49, UL76, UL79, UL87, UL91, UL92, UL96, UL117 and US26, all of which have measurable roles in HCMV replication (Table 15.1) are not known.

The importance of the nocadozole-sensitive microtubule network in transport of HCMV nucleocapsids through the cytoplasm to the nucleus (Ogawa-Goto et al., 2003) suggests that betaherpesviruses exploit normal cytoplasmic transport systems to control nucleocapsid transit through the cytoplasm. The bidirectional nature of microtubule-directed transport may allow these filaments to act as the major highways of virus particle translocation during entry as well as egress of all herpesviruses (Chapter 4). It is likely that capsid or proximal tegument proteins that are exposed following fusion mediate trafficking as well as release of the viral genome into the nucleus.

Regulation of gene expression and replication

One of the largest categories of betaherpesvirus-conserved genes encode regulatory proteins. The core homologue of the multifunctional regulator of expression found in all herpesviruses, HCMV UL69, encodes a late gene product incorporated into the tegument. This gene product regulates cell cycle progression (Hayashi et al., 2000) and exhibits similarities to other herpesvirus homologues such as the capacity to shuttle between the nucleus and cytoplasm (Lischka et al., 2001). In the roseolaviruses, this gene (U42) is expressed with immediate early characteristics similar to the alpha-and gammaherpesviruses (Menegazzi et al., 1999; Mirandola et al., 1998), although its function has not been elucidated. Although only this one regulatory protein is included in the herpesvirus core set, a number of additional virion-associated, immediate early and delayed early gene products common to all betaherpesvirus appear to carry out regulatory processes critical to replication.

HCMV UL82 encodes pp71, a virion structural protein that localizes to the nucleus soon after infection and controls transactivation of the immediate early genes (Liu and Stinski, 1992), impacting the levels of viral infection (Bresnahan and Shenk, 2000) as well as the efficiency of viral DNA transfection (Baldick et al., 1997). This gene product facilitates the interaction of viral regulatory and DNA replication proteins with nuclear domain (ND) 10 regions at the start of infection (Hofmann et al., 2002; Ishov et al., 2002), and may possibly control cell cycle regulation via Rb degradation (Kalejta and Shenk, 2003). The UL82 gene product interacts with another betaherpesvirus-conserved tegument protein encoded by the UL35 gene, and appears to cooperate in transactivation as well as play an accessory role in maturation (Schierling et al., 2004, 2005). The roseolaviruses have only a single copy of this gene and this is most closely related to HCMV UL82. Additional UL82 family members are present in many betaherpesviruses where they encode major tegument proteins, such as the UL83 gene product (major tegument phosphoprotein) of HCMV that modulates the host cell response to infection (Abate et al., 2004).

HCMV and roseolaviruses encode major immediate early nuclear proteins that have been designated IE1 and IE2 (Chapter 17). This gene cluster exhibits positional, structural and functional similarities across the betaherpesviruses although the primary amino acid sequence of these two proteins diverges dramatically. These multiply spliced gene products are abundantly made in infected cells where they are the major transactivators of viral gene expression during productive infection. In HCMV, where these gene products have been studied extensively, IE2, an 86 kDa protein, is a critical regulatory gene product responsible for activation of delayed early and late genes (Heider et al., 2002; Marchini et al., 2001; Pizzorno et al., 1991), and IE1, a 72 kDa protein, increases the potency of IE2 in the activation of viral genes and is critical for viral replication following low MOI infection (Gawn and Greaves, 2002; Greaves and Mocarski, 1998). HCMV IE2 interacts with a variety of cellular transcription factors as an adapter or modulator of the host transcription complex to activate gene expression. IE2 is a site-specific DNA binding protein that mediates autoregulatory shut-off of IE1/IE2 region transcription at late times of infection via a specific promoter element (Chapters 17 and 18). IE1 interacts with host chromatin and cellular proteins but has not been found to directly bind DNA. IE1 (Reinhardt et al., 2005) and IE2 (Pizzorno et al., 1991; White et al., 2004) contain distinct acidic activation domains that appear to be crucial for transactivation as well as for their critical role in viral replication.

Minor immediate early proteins are also conserved as betaherpesvirus-specific gene products (Chapter 21). HCMV immediate early proteins TRS1 and IRS1 were initially recognized as regulatory proteins working in conjunction with IE1 and IE2 in activation of delayed early and late gene expression (Iskenderian et al., 1996; Stasiak and Mocarski, 1992), and although virus replication is more highly dependent on TRS1 than IRS1, neither gene product is crucial for virus replication (Blankenship and Shenk, 2002; Dunn et al., 2003b). Mechanistically, the function of these proteins seems focused on the interferon response (Child et al., 2004), which possibly underlies all phenotypes that have been reported.

HCMV also encodes two cell death suppressors (HCMV vICA encoded by UL36 and vMIA encoded by UL37 × 1), one of which (UL36) is more obviously conserved in all betaherpesviruses examined (McCormick et al., 2003), is mutated in some strains of HCMV (Skaletskaya et al., 2001) and is dispensable for replication (Patterson and Shenk,

Betaherpes viral genes and their functions

1999). HCMV UL37 × 1 is a potent inhibitor of apoptosis (Goldmacher et al., 1999) also dispensable (McCormick et al., 2005), that was first thought to only be conserved amongst primate cytomegaloviruses (McCormick et al., 2003). It is now clear that the MCMVm 38.5 gene functions like vMIA (McCormick et al., 2005). HCMV UL37×3, which was originally designated UL37 (Chee et al., 1990), is an immediate early gene product that is spliced to UL37×1 to produce a number of related gene products (Adair et al., 2003). An upstream exon has not been detected in other betaherpesviruses (Table 15.1). HCMV UL37×3 does not block apoptosis when expressed without UL37×1. UL37×3 and UL37×1 are dispensable for replication (Borst et al., 1999; McCormick et al., 2005) UL37×3 may play some role as a transactivator of viral or cellular gene expression (Hayajneh et al., 2001b), possibly in conjunction with the expression of DNA replication genes (Colberg-Poley et al., 1998).

Several delayed early regulatory HCMV genes are also conserved and betaherpesvirus-specific. UL112-UL113 gene products are multiply spliced and abundant delayed early nuclear proteins (Chapter 18) critical for replication (Dunn et al., 2003b; Yu et al., 2003) playing roles in regulation of gene expression as well as in the initial formation of viral DNA replication compartments together with IE2 (Ahn et al., 1999; Penfold and Mocarski, 1997). The conserved HCMV gene UL34 encodes a number of related regulatory gene products at early and late times during infection (Biegalke et al., 2004) and is an essential replication function (Dunn et al., 2003b). One activity of UL34 that has been characterized is repression of US3 expression; however, the function of UL34 that is important for viral replication must lie elsewhere because US3 is itself an immediate early immunomodulatory gene that is dispensable for replication (Chapter 62). UL84 is another nuclear delayed early protein that, in HCMV, interacts with IE2 and appears crucial for viral DNA replication (Sarisky and Hayward, 1996; Xu et al., 2004a) as well as in the possible modulation of IE2 transactivation activity (Gebert et al., 1997).

Viral DNA synthesis and nucleotide metabolism

Betaherpesviruses have conserved the herpesvirus core set of six DNA synthesis enzymes necessary for lytic (productive) infection as well as a number of functions that, in HCMV, play roles in the initiation of DNA replication (Chapter 19). HCMV and the roseolaviruses replicate DNA in the nucleus of the cell and have a single, positionally conserved, lytic replication origin (oriLyt), located between the genes encoding homologues of HCMV UL57 and UL69. These viruses, however, have very different cis- as well as trans-acting functions involved in the initiation of DNA replication. On the one hand, HCMV has a large, complex origin region (Anders et al., 1992; Masse et al., 1992) with an embedded RNA transcript (Prichard et al., 1998) that apparently requires transcriptional transactivators IE2 and ppUL84 for initiation (Xu et al., 2004b). The dependence of HCMV oriLyt dependent replication on UL84 or IE2 varies with assay used (Sarisky and Hayward, 1996; Reid et al., 2003). Other cytomegaloviruses such as MCMV share the complex origin in a similar genomic position, but do not share any obvious sequence elements that define oriLyt functional domains (Masse et al., 1992). On the other hand, HHV-6A, HHV-6B and HHV-7 have a less complex oriLyt arranged as an inverted repeat region that interacts with a viral oriBP (Table 15.1) to initiate replication (Dewhurst et al., 1993; Inoue and Pellett, 1995; Krug et al., 2001; Stamey et al., 1995; van Loon et al., 1997). Roseolavirus DNA replication likely occurs in ways analogous to alphaherpesviruses (Boehmer and Nimonkar, 2003).

UL84, together with IE2, plays an essential role in HCMV DNA replication (Pari and Anders, 1993; Sarisky and Hayward, 1996) and is conserved in other betaherpesviruses. In HCMV, an UL84:IE2 complex (Spector and Tevethia, 1994) may orchestrate the sequential association of viral proteins with ND10 regions to promotes both transcription of viral genes and development of replication centers. The stepwise addition of UL112-UL113 gene products and the six core replication proteins is likely controlled by UL84 (Ahn et al., 1999; Colletti et al., 2004; Penfold and Mocarski, 1997; Xu et al., 2004a,b). The phenotype of a UL84 mutant is consistent with a crucial role in the intermediate events of DNA replication in a way that may be similar to the established role of IE transactivators in gammaherpesvirus lytic DNA replication (Chapter 26). One poorly understood aspect of HCMV DNA replication is the function of RNA incorporated as a triple-stranded complex associated within oriLyt (Prichard et al., 1998). Active transcription from this region during infection seems to be associated with DNA replication (Huang et al., 1996), although transcripts arise from several different regions across the oriLyt region.

One unexplained, but interesting twist is that, despite their genome complexity, betaherpesviruses lack ancillary nucleotide metabolism functions to the extent found in most other herpesviruses. The betaherpesviruses lack a widely conserved thymidine kinase gene. Instead, VPK (HCMV UL97 gene product) acts as the nucleoside kinase for antiviral drugs such as ganciclovir. Herpesvirus core genes with homology to ribonucleotide reductase (RR1, the HCMV UL45 gene product) or deoxyuridine triphosphatase (dUTPase, the HCMV UL72 gene product) encode enzymatically inactive proteins, based on studies of the

RR1 homologue in HHV-7 (Sun and Conner, 1999), MCMV (Lembo *et al.*, 2004), HCMV (Hahn *et al.*, 2002; Patrone *et al.*, 2003) and the dUTPase homologue in HCMV (Caposio *et al.*, 2004). In HCMV, UL84 has been assigned UTPase activity (Colletti *et al.*, 2005) although it is not yet clear how this may be related to dUTPase or other activities of this gene product in viral replication.

Capsid assembly and DNA encapsidation

The basic features of capsid maturation common to all herpesviruses appear to be preserved in the betaherpesviruses based on the conservation of genes known to be involved in this process in alphaherpesviruses (Chapter 4). Capsid assembly in the nucleus of the host cell employs the herpesvirus-conserved components of the capsid shell (MCP, SCP, TRI1 and TRI2) working in conjunction with a precursor of the assembly protein (pAP, HCMV UL80.5 gene product). A protease (PR, also called assemblin,) is also required for maturation. This protein is made as a precursor (pre-PR) consisting of PR as its amino terminus fused to a longer polypeptide that contains a region that includes the pAP sequence as its carboxyl end (HCMV UL80 gene product). PR is a serine protease that self-cleaves in prePR to release PR as well as a variant of pAP, and also processes the PR, pAP, as well as all variants of pAP (Gibson, 1996). This processing results in the production of multiple forms of pAP with identical carboxyl termini. In addition, PORT (HCMV UL104 gene product) is incorporated as one penton likely to be necessary for DNA encapsidation. During infection, pre-PR must be cleaved into PR and variant AP for encapsidation to follow capsid formation but both of these proteins, as well as AP, are absent from mature, DNA-containing capsids. Maturation is regulated by phosphorylation of the participating proteins.

Once betaherpesvirus DNA has replicated in the nucleus, encapsidation is controlled by a conserved *cis*-acting element (cleavage/packaging or *pac* site) and a series of seven herpesvirus conserved *trans*-acting functions. Functional herpesvirus-conserved *pac*1 and *pac*2 signals are located near the genomic ends of HCMV, although their arrangement appears to be unique (Bogner *et al.*, 1998; Kemble and Mocarski, 1989; Mocarski *et al.*, 1987). The processes of DNA recognition, encapsidation and cleavage are all carried out by herpesvirus core functions (Fig. 15.1). Based on systematic mutagenesis (Dunn *et al.*, 2003b; Yu *et al.*, 2003) but limited functional investigation, encapsidation of viral DNA in HCMV is likely to involve the core gene products encoded by the essential UL51, UL52, UL56, UL77, UL80, UL89, UL93 and UL95 genes (Table 15.1; Fig. 15.1), with the UL56 and UL89 gene products forming the heterodimeric, benzimidizole-sensitive terminase (TER) (Krosky *et al.*, 1998; Scheffczik *et al.*, 2002). This complex probably interacts with the PORT (UL104 gene product) penton of the capsid (Dittmer and Bogner, 2005), likely in combination with a TER-associated protein (UL51 gene product) and portal capping protein (UL77 gene product). Based on studies in other herpesviruses (Chapter 4), these five proteins mediate recognition of a *pac* site on multi-genome DNA concatamers, docking with the appropriate site on a capsid, threading viral DNA into the caspid, cleavage at a *pac* site and sealing the genome into the nucleocapsid (Fig. 15.1). Also the herpesvirus core HCMV UL52 gene product may play a role in capsid transport and the UL80 gene product, which contains the maturational protease and assembly protein, are likely to be involved in encapsidation. Phosphorylation by the VPK influences encapsidation efficiency (Wolf *et al.*, 2001), although cellular enzymes may also play a role because the requirement for VPK is relaxed in dividing cells (Prichard *et al.*, 1999; Wolf *et al.*, 2001).

Maturation

Once viral DNA has been packaged, the nucleocapsid interacts with tegument proteins together with non-structural proteins in a complex, two-stage envelopment and egress process that starts in the nucleus and leads to virion release by exocytosis at the plasma membrane (Fig. 15.1). Insights into how this process proceeds are coming from studies in HCMV and MCMV, and the functions that have thus far been implicated are encoded by herpesvirus core genes (Chapter 4). The initial envelopment event occurs at the inner nuclear membrane and favors DNA-containing nucleocapsids. In betaherpesviruses, capsids lacking DNA mature, appear in the cytoplasm and accumulate as non-infectious enveloped particles (Gibson, 1996). Correct localization in the nucleus appears critical to proper egress. Based on studies on the MCMV homologues (Muranyi *et al.*, 2002), two proteins (HCMV UL50 and UL53 gene products) appear to form a nuclear egress complex on the inner nuclear membrane to control egress from the nucleus as well as disruption of the nuclear lamina. Based on studies in alphaherpesviruruses, the nuclear egress membrane protein (HCMV UL50 gene product), likely to be a type II membrane-spanning protein, would anchor the nuclear egress lamina protein (HCMV UL53 gene product), a phosphoprotein that interacts with the nuclear lamina (Mettenleiter, 2004). Protein kinases appear to play regulatory roles in nuclear egress. In HCMV, the conserved VPK influences nuclear egress (Krosky *et al.*, 2003a), and, in MCMV, host protein kinase C has been implicated in disruption of the nuclear lamina to allow egress (Muranyi et al., 2002). The nuclear egress complex may also participate in membrane fusion events at the outer nuclear membrane that are required to deposit the nucleocapsid in the cytoplasm (de-envelopment).

Evidence for final betaherpesvirus envelopment in the cytoplasm at late endosomal or Golgi body membranes has been suspected for many years (Tooze et al., 1993). Certain virion tegument proteins associate with nucleocapsids during nuclear egress, but many are added in the cytoplasm where they play essential roles in maturation (Sanchez et al., 2000a). Current evidence on alphaherpesviruses and betaherpesviruses suggests that a conserved cytoplasmic egress tegument protein (HCMV UL99 gene product, pp28) plays a critical role in the secondary, or final, envelopment at cytoplasmic membranes (Britt et al., 2004; Jones and Lee, 2004; Silva et al., 2003). This protein is modified by myristylation and palmitylation and localizes to the cytoplasmic face of cellular membranes. In alphaherpesviruses, this homologue interacts with another herpesvirus-conserved tegument protein, a homologue of the HCMV UL94 gene product, to form a complex involved in transport (Mettenleiter, 2004). Two additional tegument proteins conserved amongst herpesviruses (HCMV UL71 and UL88 gene products) may associate with cytoplasmic membranes and be involved in egress.

A critical role in final envelopment has recently been ascribed to the major tegument phosphoprotein pp150 (encoded by UL32), a betaherpesvirus-conserved function (Aucoin et al., 2006).

Thus, final envelopment occurs in the cytoplasm and, as a consequence the tegument of virions includes small amounts of cellular proteins, in particular actin (Kattenhorn et al., 2004; Varnum et al., 2004), as well as RNAs (Greijer et al., 2003; Terhune et al., 2004) that appear to represent a quantitative sampling of the cytosol. Once final envelopment has occurred, the mature virion is transported inside of a vesicle to the cell surface for release by fusion of an exocytic vesicle with the plasma membrane, a process that is likely to follow cellular vesicle trafficking pathways (Fig. 15.1).

Latency

Although there are biological differences in the pathogenesis of betaherpesviruses, infections with cytomegaloviruses and roseolaviruses appear to share a common involvement of myeloid cells, particularly in the monocyte-macrophage lineage (Kondo et al., 2002a; Sissons et al., 2002; Mocarski et al., 2005). Persistence, latency and reactivation of these viruses exhibit similarities as well as clear differences (Chapters 42 and 47). In HCMV as well as HHV-6B, latent transcripts with a common structure and genomic location have been mapped to the major IE locus (Chapter 47). These transcripts are found in bone marrow-derived granulocyte–macrophage progenitors naturally infected with HCMV (Kondo et al., 1996) or in peripheral blood monocytes naturally infected with HHV-6B (Kondo et al., 2002a,b). Although the genomic region encoding these transcripts also encodes the productive phase IE1 and IE2 gene products, and IE1 is a chromatin tethering protein similar to genome maintenance functions encoded by gammaherpesviruses (Reinhardt et al., 2005), the major IE gene products are not encoded during natural or experimental latent infection. In both HCMV and HHV-6B, a number of novel gene products are associated with latent transcripts (Chapter 47). In HHV-6B, these transcripts may control a stage when IE1 is needed to facilitate reactivation (Kondo, 2003). Thus far, the function of novel latent gene products has not emerged from studies using cell culture models.

This analysis of the role of betaherpesvirus-conserved gene products has attempted to evaluate data generated in a wide variety of systems such that some predictions will certainly be clarified by further investigation. This chapter is intended to provide a starting point for evaluation of data on additional betaherpesvirus-conserved functions by providing a perspective on what is known about better-studied homologues.

REFERENCES

Abate, D. A., Watanabe, S., and Mocarski, E. S. (2004). Major human cytomegalovirus structural protein pp65 (ppUL83) prevents interferon response factor 3 activation in the interferon response. *J. Virol.*, **78**, 10995–11006.

Adair, R., Douglas, E. R., Maclean, J. B. et al. (2002). The products of human cytomegalovirus genes UL23, UL24, UL43 and US22 are tegument components. *J. Gen. Virol.*, **83**, 1315–1324.

Adair, R., Liebisch, G. W., and Colberg-Poley, A. M. (2003). Complex alternative processing of human cytomegalovirus UL37 pre-mRNA. *J. Gen. Virol.*, **84**, 3353–3358.

Agulnick, A. D., Thompson, J. R., Iyengar, S., Pearson, G., Ablashi, D., and Ricciardi, R. P. (1993). Identification of a DNA-binding protein of human herpesvirus 6, a putative DNA polymerase stimulatory factor. *J. Gen. Virol.*, **74**(6), 1003–1009.

Ahn, J. H. and Hayward, G. S. (2000). Disruption of PML-associated nuclear bodies by IE1 correlates with efficient early stages of viral gene expression and DNA replication in human cytomegalovirus infection. *Virology*, **274**, 39–55.

Ahn, J. H., Jang, W. J., and Hayward, G. S. (1999). The human cytomegalovirus IE2 and UL112–113 proteins accumulate in viral DNA replication compartments that initiate from the periphery of promyelocytic leukemia protein-associated nuclear bodies (PODs or ND10). *J. Virol.*, **73**, 10458–10471.

Akter, P., Cunningham, C., McSharry, B. P. *et al.* (2003). Two novel spliced genes in human cytomegalovirus. *J. Gen. Virol.*, **84**, 1117–1122.

Alderete, J. P., Child, S. J., and Geballe, A. P. (2001). Abundant early expression of gpUL4 from a human cytomegalovirus mutant lacking a repressive upstream open reading frame. *J. Virol.*, **75**, 7188–7192.

Anders, D. G. and Gibson, W. (1988). Location, transcript analysis, and partial nucleotide sequence of the cytomegalovirus gene encoding an early DNA-binding protein with similarities to ICP8 of herpes simplex virus type 1. *J. Virol.*, **62**, 1364–1372.

Anders, D. G., Kacica, M. A., Pari, G., and Punturieri, S. M. (1992). Boundaries and structure of human cytomegalovirus oriLyt, a complex origin for lytic-phase DNA replication. *J. Virol.*, **66**, 3373–3384.

Ansari, A. and Emery, V. C. (1999). The U69 gene of human herpesvirus 6 encodes a protein kinase which can confer ganciclovir sensitivity to baculoviruses. *J. Virol.*, **73**, 3284–3291.

Appleton, B. A., Loregian, A., Filman, D. J., Coen, D. M., and Hogle, J. M. (2004). The cytomegalovirus DNA polymerase subunit UL44 forms a C clamp-shaped dimer. *Mol. Cell*, **15**, 233–244.

Atalay, R., Zimmermann, A., Wagner, M. *et al.* (2002). Identification and expression of human cytomegalovirus transcription units coding for two distinct Fcgamma receptor homologs. *J. Virol.*, **76**, 8596–8608.

AuCoin, D. P., Smith, G. B., Meiering, C. D., and Mocarski, E. S. (2006). Betaherpesvirus-conserved cytomegalovirus tegument protein ppUL32 (pp150) controls cytoplasmic events during virion maturation. *J. Virol.*, **80**, 8199–8821.

Baek, M. C., Krosky, P. M., Pearson, A., and Coen, D. M. (2004). Phosphorylation of the RNA polymerase II carboxyl-terminal domain in human cytomegalovirus-infected cells and in vitro by the viral UL97 protein kinase. *Virology*, **324**, 184–193.

Baldick, C. J., Jr. and Shenk, T. (1996). Proteins associated with purified human cytomegalovirus particles. *J. Virol.*, **70**, 6097–6105.

Baldick, C. J., Jr., Marchini, A., Patterson, C. E., and Shenk, T. (1997). Human cytomegalovirus tegument protein pp71 (ppUL82) enhances the infectivity of viral DNA and accelerates the infectious cycle. *J. Virol.*, **71**, 4400–4408.

Baldwin, B. R., Zhang, C. O., and Keay, S. (2000). Cloning and epitope mapping of a functional partial fusion receptor for human cytomegalovirus gH. *J. Gen. Virol.*, **81**, 27–35.

Barrasa, M. I., Harel, N. Y., and Alwine, J. C. (2005). The phosphorylation status of the serine-rich region of the human cytomegalovirus 86-kilodalton major immediate–early protein IE2/IEP86 affects temporal viral gene expression. *J. Virol.*, **79**, 1428–1437.

Battista, M. C., Bergamini, G., Boccuni, M. C., Campanini, F., Ripalti, A., and Landini, M. P. (1999). Expression and characterization of a novel structural protein of human cytomegalovirus, pUL25. *J. Virol.*, **73**, 3800–3809.

Baxter, M. K. and Gibson, W. (2001). Cytomegalovirus basic phosphoprotein (pUL32) binds to capsids in vitro through its amino one-third. *J. Virol.*, **75**, 6865–6873.

Bechtel, J. T. and Shenk, T. (2002). Human cytomegalovirus UL47 tegument protein functions after entry and before immediate-early gene expression. *J. Virol.*, **76**, 1043–1050.

Biegalke, B. J., Lester, E., Branda, A., and Rana, R. (2004). Characterization of the human cytomegalovirus UL34 gene. *J. Virol.*, **78**, 9579–9583.

Billstrom, M. A., Lehman, L. A., and Worthen, S. G. (1999). Depletion of extracellular RANTES during human cytomegalovirus infection of endothelial cells. *Am. J. Respir. Cell. Mol. Biol.*, **21**, 163–167.

Blankenship, C. A. and Shenk, T. (2002). Mutant human cytomegalovirus lacking the immediate-early TRS1 coding region exhibits a late defect. *J. Virol.*, **76**, 12290–12299.

Boehme, K. W., Singh, J., Perry, S. T., and Compton, T. (2004). Human cytomegalovirus elicits a coordinated cellular antiviral response via envelope glycoprotein B. *J. Virol.*, **78**, 1202–1211.

Boehmer, P. E. and Nimonkar, A. V. (2003). Herpes virus replication. *IUBMB Life*, **55**, 13–22.

Bogner, E. (2002). Human cytomegalovirus terminase as a target for antiviral chemotherapy. *Rev. Med. Virol.*, **12**, 115–127.

Bogner, E., Radsak, K., and Stinski, M. F. (1998). The gene product of human cytomegalovirus open reading frame UL56 binds the pac motif and has specific nuclease activity. *J. Virol.*, **72**, 2259–2264.

Bolovan-Fritts, C. A., and Wiedeman, J. A. (2002). Mapping the viral genetic determinants of endothelial cell tropism in human cytomegalovirus. *J. Clin. Virol.*, **25** Suppl 2, S97–109.

Borst, E. M., Hahn, G., Koszinowski, U. H., and Messerle, M. (1999). Cloning of the human cytomegalovirus (HCMV) genome as an infectious bacterial artificial chromosome in Escherichia coli: a new approach for construction of HCMV mutants. *J. Virol.*, **73**, 8320–8329.

Boyle, K. A., Pietropaolo, R. L., and Compton, T. (1999). Engagement of the cellular receptor for glycoprotein B of human cytomegalovirus activates the interferon-responsive pathway. *Mol. Cell Biol.*, **19**, 3607–3613.

Bresnahan, W. A. and Shenk, T. E. (2000). UL82 virion protein activates expression of immediate early viral genes in human cytomegalovirus-infected cells *Proc. Natl Acad. Sci. USA*, **97**, 14506–14511.

Britt, W. J. and Mach, M. (1996). Human cytomegalovirus glycoproteins. *Intervirology*, **39**, 401–412.

Britt, W. J., Jarvis, M., Seo, J. Y., Drummond, D., and Nelson, J. (2004). Rapid genetic engineering of human cytomegalovirus by using a lambda phage linear recombination system: demonstration that pp28 (UL99) is essential for production of infectious virus. *J. Virol.*, **78**, 539–543.

Brown, J. M., Kaneshima, H., and Mocarski, E. S. (1995). Dramatic interstrain differences in the replication of human cytomegalovirus in SCID-hu mice. *J. Infect. Dis.*, **171**, 1599–1603.

Brune, W., Menard, C., Heesemann, J., and Koszinowski, U. H. (2001). A ribonucleotide reductase homolog of cytomegalovirus and endothelial cell tropism. *Science*, **291**, 303–305.

Buerger, I., Reefschlaeger, J., Bender, W. *et al.* (2001). A novel non-nucleoside inhibitor specifically targets cytomegalovirus DNA maturation via the UL89 and UL56 gene products. *J. Virol.*, **75**, 9077–9086.

Caposio, P., Riera, L., Hahn, G., Landolfo, S., and Gribaudo, G. (2004). Evidence that the human cytomegalovirus 46-kDa UL72 protein is not an active dUTPase but a late protein dispensable for replication in fibroblasts. *Virology*, **325**, 264–276.

Casaday, R. J., Bailey, J. R., Kalb, S. R. *et al.* (2004). Assembly protein precursor (pUL80.5 homolog) of simian cytomegalovirus is phosphorylated at a glycogen synthase kinase 3 site and its downstream "priming" site: phosphorylation affects interactions of protein with itself and with major capsid protein. *J. Virol.*, **78**, 13501–13511.

Casarosa, P., Bakker, R. A., Verzijl, D. *et al.* (2001). Constitutive signaling of the human cytomegalovirus-encoded chemokine receptor US28. *J. Biol. Chem.*, **276**, 1133–1137.

Casarosa, P., Gruijthuijsen, Y. K., Michel, D. *et al.* (2003). Constitutive signaling of the human cytomegalovirus-encoded receptor UL33 differs from that of its rat cytomegalovirus homolog R33 by promiscuous activation of G proteins of the Gq, Gi, and Gs classes. *J. Biol. Chem.*, **278**, 50010–50023.

Cavanaugh, V. J., Stenberg, R. M., Staley, T. L. *et al.* (1996). Murine cytomegalovirus with a deletion of genes spanning HindIII-J and -I displays altered cell and tissue tropism. *J. Virol.*, **70**, 1365–1374.

Cha, T. A., Tom, E., Kemble, G. W., Duke, G. M., Mocarski, E. S., and Spaete, R. R. (1996). Human cytomegalovirus clinical isolates carry at least 19 genes not found in laboratory strains. *J. Virol.*, **70**, 78–83.

Chang, W. L., Baumgarth, N., Yu, D., and Barry, P. A. (2004). Human cytomegalovirus-encoded interleukin-10 homolog inhibits maturation of dendritic cells and alters their functionality. *J. Virol.*, **78**, 8720–8731.

Chee, M. S., Bankier, A. T., Beck, S. *et al.* (1990). Analysis of the protein-coding content of the sequence of human cytomegalovirus strain AD169. *Curr. Top. Microbiol. Immunol.*, **154**, 125–170.

Child, S. J., Jarrahian, S., Harper, V. M., and Geballe, A. P. (2002). Complementation of vaccinia virus lacking the double-stranded RNA-binding protein gene E3L by human cytomegalovirus. *J. Virol.*, **76**, 4912–4918.

Child, S. J., Hakki, M., De Niro, K. L., and Geballe, A. P. (2004). Evasion of cellular antiviral responses by human cytomegalovirus TRS1 and IRS1. *J. Virol.*, **78**, 197–205.

Chou, S., Marousek, G. I., Senters, A. E., Davis, M. G., and Biron, K. K. (2004). Mutations in the human cytomegalovirus UL27 gene that confer resistance to maribavir. *J. Virol.*, **78**, 7124–7130.

Colberg-Poley, A. M., Huang, L., Soltero, V. E., Iskenderian, A. C., Schumacher, R. F., and Anders, D. G. (1998). The acidic domain of pUL37 × 1 and gpUL37 plays a key role in transactivation of HCMV DNA replication gene promoter constructions *Virology*, **246**, 400–408.

Colletti, K. S., Xu, Y., Cei, S. A., Tarrant, M., and Pari, G. S. (2004). Human cytomegalovirus UL84 oligomerization and heterodimerization domains act as transdominant inhibitors of oriLyt-dependent DNA replication: evidence that IE2-UL84 and UL84-UL84 interactions are required for lytic DNA replication. *J. Virol.*, **78**, 9203–9214.

Colletti, K. S., Xu, Y., Yamboliev, I., and Pari, G. S. (2005). Human cytomegalovirus UL84 Is a phosphoprotein that exhibits UTPase activity and is a putative member of the DExD/H box family of proteins. *J. Biol. Chem.*, **280**, 11955–11960.

Compton, T. (2004). Receptors and immune sensors: the complex entry path of human cytomegalovirus. *Trends Cell Biol.*, **14**, 5–8.

Compton, T., Nepomuceno, R. R., and Nowlin, D. M. (1992). Human cytomegalovirus penetrates host cells by pH-independent fusion at the cell surface. *Virology*, **191**, 387–395.

Compton, T., Nowlin, D. M., and Cooper, N. R. (1993). Initiation of human cytomegalovirus infection requires initial interaction with cell surface heparan sulfate. *Virology*, **193**, 834–841.

Compton, T., Kurt-Jones, E. A., Boehme, K. W. *et al.* (2003). Human cytomegalovirus activates inflammatory cytokine responses via CD14 and toll-like receptor 2. *J. Virol.*, **77**, 4588–4596.

Conti, C., Cirone, M., Sgro, R., Altieri, F., Zompetta, C., and Faggioni, A. (2000). Early interactions of human herpesvirus 6 with lymphoid cells: role of membrane protein components and glycosaminoglycans in virus binding. *J. Med. Virol.*, **62**, 487–497.

Courcelle, C. T., Courcelle, J., Prichard, M. N., and Mocarski, E. S. (2001). Requirement for uracil-DNA glycosylase during the transition to late-phase cytomegalovirus DNA replication. *J. Virol.*, **75**, 7592–7601.

Dal Monte, P., Pignatelli, S., Zini, N. *et al.* (2002). Analysis of intracellular and intraviral localization of the human cytomegalovirus UL53 protein. *J. Gen. Virol.*, **83**, 1005–1012.

Dal Monte, P., Pignatelli, S., Rossini, G., and Landini, M. P. (2004). Genomic variants among human cytomegalovirus (HCMV) clinical isolates: the glycoprotein n (gN) paradigm. *Hum. Immunol.*, **65**, 387–394.

Dargan, D. J., Jamieson, F. E., MacLean, J., Dolan, A., Addison, C., and McGeoch, D. J. (1997). The published DNA sequence of human cytomegalovirus strain AD169 lacks 929 base pairs affecting genes UL42 and UL43. *J. Virol.*, **71**, 9833–9836.

Davison, A. J., Dolan, A., Akter, P. *et al.* (2003). The human cytomegalovirus genome revisited: comparison with the chimpanzee cytomegalovirus genome. *J. Gen. Virol.*, **84**, 17–28.

Dewhurst, S., Dollard, S. C., Pellett, P. E., and Dambaugh, T. R. (1993). Identification of a lytic-phase origin of DNA replication in human herpesvirus 6B strain Z29. *J. Virol.*, **67**, 7680–7683.

Dhepakson, P., Mori, Y., Jiang, Y. B. *et al.* (2002). Human herpesvirus-6 rep/U94 gene product has single-stranded DNA-binding activity. *J. Gen. Virol.*, **83**, 847–854.

Dittmer, A. and Bogner, E. (2005). Analysis of the quaternary structure of the putative HCMV portal protein pUL104. *Biochemistry*, **44**, 759–765.

Dolan, A., Cunningham, C., Hector, R. D. *et al.* (2004). Genetic content of wild-type human cytomegalovirus. *J. Gen. Virol.*, **85**, 1301–1312.

Dominguez, G., Dambaugh, T. R., Stamey, F. R., Dewhurst, S., Inoue, N., and Pellett, P. E. (1999a). Human herpesvirus 6B genome sequence: coding content and comparison with human herpesvirus 6A. *J. Virol.*, **73**, 8040–8052.

Dominguez, G., Dambaugh, T. R., Stamey, F. R., Dewhurst, S., Inoue, N., and Pellett, P. E. (1999b). Human herpesvirus 6B genome sequence: coding content and comparison with human herpesvirus 6A. *J. Virol.*, **73**, 8040–8052.

Doniger, J., Muralidhar, S., and Rosenthal, L. J. (1999). Human cytomegalovirus and human herpesvirus 6 genes that transform and transactivate. *Clin. Microbiol. Rev.*, **12**, 367–382.

Dunn, C., Chalupny, N. J., Sutherland C. L. *et al.* (2003a). Human cytomegalovirus glycoprotein UL16 causes intracellular sequestration of NKG2D ligands, protecting against natural killer cell cytotoxicity. *J. Exp. Med.*, **197**, 1427–1439.

Dunn, W., Chou, C., Li, H. *et al.* (2003b). Functional profiling of a human cytomegalovirus genome. *Proc. Natl Acad. Sci. USA*, **100**, 14223–14228.

Dykes, C., Chan, H., Krenitsky, D. M., and Dewhurst, S. (1997). Stringent structural and sequence requirements of the human herpesvirus 6B lytic-phase origin of DNA replication. *J. Gen. Virol.*, **78**(5), 1125–1129.

Evers, D. L., Wang, X., and Huang, E. S. (2004). Cellular stress and signal transduction responses to human cytomegalovirus infection. *Microbes Infect.* **6**, 1084–1093.

Feire, A. L., Koss, H., and Compton, T. (2004). Cellular integrins function as entry receptors for human cytomegalovirus via a highly conserved disintegrin-like domain. *Proc. Natl Acad. Sci. USA*, **101**, 15470–15475.

Flebbe-Rehwaldt, L. M., Wood, C., and Chandran, B. (2000). Characterization of transcripts expressed from human herpesvirus 6A strain GS immediate-early region B U16–U17 open reading frames. *J. Virol.*, **74**, 11040–11054.

Fortunato, E. A., Sanchez, V., Yen, J. Y., and Spector, D. H. (2002). Infection of cells with human cytomegalovirus during S phase results in a blockade to immediate-early gene expression that can be overcome by inhibition of the proteasome. *J. Virol.*, **76**, 5369–5379.

Fraile-Ramos, A., Pelchen-Matthews, A., Kledal, T. N., Browne, H., Schwartz, T. W., and Marsh, M. (2002). Localization of HCMV UL33 and US27 in endocytic compartments and viral membranes. *Traffic*, **3**, 218–232.

French, C., Menegazzi, P., Nicholson, L., Macaulay, H., DiLuca, D., and Gompels, U. A. (1999). Novel, nonconsensus cellular splicing regulates expression of a gene encoding a chemokine-like protein that shows high variation and is specific for human herpesvirus 6. *Virology*, **262**, 139–151.

Furman, M. H., Dey, N., Tortorella, D., and Ploegh, H. L. (2002). The human cytomegalovirus US10 gene product delays trafficking of major histocompatibility complex class I molecules. *J. Virol.*, **76**, 11753–11756.

Gao, J. L. and Murphy, P. M. (1994). Human cytomegalovirus open reading frame US28 encodes a functional beta chemokine receptor. *J. Biol. Chem.*, **269**, 28539–28542.

Gao, M., Robertson, B. J., McCann, P. J. *et al.* (1998). Functional conservations of the alkaline nuclease of herpes simplex type 1 and human cytomegalovirus. *Virology*, **249**, 460–470.

Gawn, J. M. and Greaves, R. F. (2002). Absence of IE1 p72 protein function during low-multiplicity infection by human cytomegalovirus results in a broad block to viral delayed–early gene expression. *J. Virol.*, **76**, 4441–4455.

Gebert, S., Schmolke, S., Sorg, G., Floss, S., Plachter, B., and Stamminger, T. (1997). The UL84 protein of human cytomegalovirus acts as a transdominant inhibitor of immediate-early-mediated transactivation that is able to prevent viral replication. *J. Virol.*, **71**, 7048–7060.

Gerna, G., Percivalle, E., Sarasini, A., Baldanti, F., Campanini, G., and Revello, M. G. (2003). Rescue of human cytomegalovirus strain AD169 tropism for both leukocytes and human endothelial cells. *J. Gen. Virol.*, **84**, 1431–1436.

Gewurz, B. E., Gaudet, R., Tortorella, D., Wang, E. W., and Ploegh, H. L. (2001). Virus subversion of immunity: a structural perspective. *Curr. Opin. Immunol.*, **13**, 442–450.

Gibson, W. (1996). Structure and assembly of the virion. *Intervirology*, **39**, 389–400.

Gibson, W., Baxter, M. K., and Clopper, K. S. (1996). Cytomegalovirus "missing" capsid protein identified as heat-aggregable product of human cytomegalovirus UL46. *J. Virol.*, **70**, 7454–7461.

Goldmacher, V. S., Bartle, L. M., Skaletskaya, A. *et al.* (1999). A cytomegalovirus-encoded mitochondria-localized inhibitor of apoptosis structurally unrelated to Bcl-2. *Proc. Natl Acad. Sci. USA*, **96**, 12536–12541.

Gompels, U. A. and Macaulay, H. A. (1995). Characterization of human telomeric repeat sequences from human herpesvirus 6 and relationship to replication. *J. Gen. Virol.*, **76**, 451–458.

Gompels, U. A., Nicholas, J., Lawrence, G. *et al.* (1995). The DNA sequence of human herpesvirus-6: structure, coding content, and genome evolution. *Virology*, **209**, 29–51.

Gravel, A., Tomoiu, A., Cloutier, N., Gosselin, J., and Flamand, L. (2003). Characterization of the immediate-early 2 protein of human herpesvirus 6, a promiscuous transcriptional activator. *Virology*, **308**, 340–353.

Greaves, R. F. and Mocarski, E. S. (1998). Defective growth correlates with reduced accumulation of a viral DNA replication protein after low multiplicity infection by a human cytomegalovirus *ie1* mutant. *J. Virol.*, **72**, 366–379.

Greijer, A. E., Dekkers, C. A., and Middeldrop, J. M. (2000). Human cytomegalovirus virions differentially incorporate viral and host cell RNA during the assembly process. *J. Virol.*, **74**, 9078–9082.

Grzimek, N. K., Podlech, J., Steffens, H. P., Holtappels, R., Schmalz, S., and Reddehase, M. J. (1999). In vivo replication of recombinant murine cytomegalovirus driven by the paralogous major immediate-early promoter-enhancer of human cytomegalovirus. *J. Virol.*, **73**, 5043–5055.

Guo, Y. W. and Huang, E. S. (1993). Characterization of a structurally tricistronic gene of human cytomegalovirus composed of U(s)18, U(s)19, and U(s)20. *J. Virol.*, **67**, 2043–2054.

Hahn, G., Khan, H., Baldanti, F., Koszinowski, U. H., Revello, M. G., and Gerna, G. (2002). The human cytomegalovirus ribonucleotide reductase homolog UL45 is dispensable for growth in endothelial cells, as determined by a BAC-cloned clinical isolate of human cytomegalovirus with preserved wild-type characteristics. *J. Virol.*, **76**, 9551–9555.

Hahn, G., Jarosch, M., Wang, J. B., Berbes, C., and McVoy, M. A. (2003). Tn7-mediated introduction of DNA sequences into bacmid-cloned cytomegalovirus genomes for rapid recombinant virus construction. *J. Virol. Methods*, **107**, 185–194.

Hahn, G., Revello, M. G., Patrone, M. *et al.* (2004). Human cytomegalovirus UL131–128 genes are indispensable for virus growth in endothelial cells and virus transfer to leukocytes. *J. Virol.*, **78**, 10023–10033.

Hanson, L. K., Slater, J. S., Karabekian, Z., Ciocco-Schmitt, G., and Campbell, A. E. (2001). Products of US22 genes M140 and M141 confer efficient replication of murine cytomegalovirus in macrophages and spleen. *J. Virol.*, **75**, 6292–6302.

Hayajneh, W. A., Colberg-Poley, A. M., Skaletskaya, A. *et al.* (2001a). The sequence and antiapoptotic functional domains of the human cytomegalovirus UL37 exon 1 immediate early protein are conserved in multiple primary strains. *Virology*, **279**, 233–240.

Hayajneh, W. A., Contopoulos-Ioannidis, D. G., Lesperance, M. M., Venegas, A. M., and Colberg-Poley, A. M. (2001b). The carboxyl terminus of the human cytomegalovirus UL37 immediate-early glycoprotein is conserved in primary strains and is important for transactivation. *J. Gen. Virol.*, **82**, 1569–1579.

Hayashi, M. L., Blankenship, C., and Shenk, T. (2000). Human cytomegalovirus UL69 protein is required for efficient accumulation of infected cells in the G1 phase of the cell cycle *Proc. Natl Acad. Sci. USA*, **97**, 2692–2696.

Hegde, N. R., Tomazin, R. A., Wisner, T. W. *et al.* (2002). Inhibition of HLA-DR assembly, transport, and loading by human cytomegalovirus glycoprotein US3: a novel mechanism for evading major histocompatibility complex class II antigen presentation. *J. Virol.*, **76**, 10929–10941.

Heider, J. A., Bresnahan, W. A., and Shenk, T. E. (2002). Construction of a rationally designed human cytomegalovirus variant encoding a temperature-sensitive immediate-early 2 protein. *Proc. Natl Acad. Sci. USA*, **99**, 3141–3146.

Hertel, L. and Mocarski, E. S. (2004). Global analysis of host cell gene expression late during cytomegalovirus infection reveals extensive dysregulation of cell cycle gene expression and induction of Pseudomitosis independent of US28 function. *J. Virol.*, **78**, 11988–12011.

Hertel, L., Lacaille, V. G., Strobl, H., Mellins, E. D., and Mocarski, E. S. (2003). Susceptibility of immature and mature Langerhans cell-type dendritic cells to infection and immunomodulation by human cytomegalovirus. *J. Virol.*, **77**, 7563–7574.

Hewitt, E. W., Gupta, S. S., and Lehner, P. J. (2001). The human cytomegalovirus gene product US6 inhibits ATP binding by TAP. *EMBO J.*, **20**, 387–396.

Hitomi, S., Kozuka-Hata, H., Chen, Z., Sugano, S., Yamaguchi, N., and Watanabe, S. (1997). Human cytomegalovirus open reading frame UL11 encodes a highly polymorphic protein expressed on the infected cell surface. *Arch. Virol.*, **142**, 1407–1427.

Hobom, U., Brune, W., Messerle, M., Hahn, G., and Koszinowski, U. H. (2000). Fast screening procedures for random transposon libraries of cloned herpesvirus genomes: mutational analysis of human cytomegalovirus envelope glycoprotein genes. *J. Virol.*, **74**, 7720–7729.

Hofmann, H., Sindre, H., and Stamminger, T. (2002). Functional interaction between the pp71 protein of human cytomegalovirus and the PML-interacting protein human daxx. *J. Virol.*, **76**, 5769–5783.

Huang, L., Zhu, Y., and Anders, D. G. (1996). The variable 3 ends of a human cytomegalovirus *ori*Lyt transcript (SRT) overlap an essential, conserved replicator element. *J. Virol.*, **70**, 5272–5281.

Huber, M. T. and Compton, T. (1998). The human cytomegalovirus UL74 gene encodes the third component of the glycoprotein H-glycoprotein L-containing envelope complex. *J. Virol.*, **72**, 8191–8197.

Huber, M. T. and Compton T. (1999). Intracellular formation and processing of the heterotrimeric gH-gL-gO (gCIII) glycoprotein envelope complex of human cytomegalovirus. *J. Virol.*, **73**, 3886–3892.

Huber, M. T., Tomazin, R., Wisner, T., Boname, J., and Johnson, D. C. (2002). Human cytomegalovirus US7, US8, US9, and US10 are cytoplasmic glycoproteins, not found at cell surfaces, and US9 does not mediate cell-to-cell spread. *J. Virol.*, **76**, 5748–5758.

Hudson, A. W., Howley, P. M., and Ploegh, H. L. (2001). A human herpesvirus 7 glycoprotein, U21, diverts major histocompatibility complex class I molecules to lysosomes. *J. Virol.*, **75**, 12347–12358.

Ihara, S., Takekoshi, M., Mori, N., Sakuma, S., Hashimoto, J., and Watanabe, Y. (1994). Identification of mutation sites of a temperature-sensitive mutant of HCMV DNA polymerase activity. *Arch. Virol.*, **137**, 263–275.

Inoue, N. and Pellett, P. E. (1995). Human herpesvirus 6B origin-binding protein: DNA-binding domain and consensus binding sequence. *J. Virol.*, **69**, 4619–4627.

Isegawa, Y., Ping, Z., Nakano, K., Sugimoto, N., and Yamanishi, K. (1998). Human herpesvirus 6 open reading frame U12 encodes a functional beta- chemokine receptor. *J. Virol.*, **72**, 6104–6112.

Ishov, A. M., Vladimirova, O. V., and Maul, G. G. (2002). Daxx-mediated accumulation of human cytomegalovirus tegument protein pp71 at ND10 facilitates initiation of viral infection at these nuclear domains. *J. Virol.*, **76**, 7705–7712.

Iskenderian, A. C., Huang, L., Reilly, A., Stenberg, R. M., and Anders, D. G. (1996). Four of eleven loci required for transient complementation of human cytomegalovirus DNA replication cooperate to activate expression of replication genes. *J. Virol.*, **70**, 383–392.

Jahn, G., Stenglein, S., Riegler, S., Einsele, H., and Sinzger, C. (1999). Human cytomegalovirus infection of immature dendritic cells and macrophages. *Intervirology*, **42**, 365–372.

Janzen, D. M., Frolova, L., and Geballe, A. P. (2002). Inhibition of translation termination mediated by an interaction of eukaryotic release factor 1 with a nascent peptidyl-tRNA. *Mol. Cell Biol.*, **22**, 8562–8570.

Jarvis, M. A., Jones, T. R., Drummond, D. D. *et al.* (2004). Phosphorylation of human cytomegalovirus glycoprotein B (gB) at the acidic cluster casein kinase 2 site (Ser900) is required for localization of gB to the *trans*-Golgi network and efficient virus replication. *J. Virol.*, **78**, 285–293.

Johnson, R. A., Huong, S. M., and Huang, E. S. (2000). Activation of the mitogen-activated protein kinase p38 by human cytomegalovirus infection through two distinct pathways: a novel mechanism for activation of p38. *J. Virol.*, **74**, 1158–1167.

Johnson, R. A., Wang, X., Ma, X. L., Huong, S. M., and Huang, E. S. (2001). Human cytomegalovirus up-regulates the phosphatidylinositol 3-kinase (PI3-K) pathway: inhibition of PI3-K activity inhibits viral replication and virus-induced signaling. *J. Virol.*, **75**, 6022–6032.

Jones, T. R. and Lee, S. W. (2004). An acidic cluster of human cytomegalovirus UL99 tegument protein is required for trafficking and function. *J. Virol.*, **78**, 1488–1502.

Kahl, M., Siegel-Axel, D., Stenglein, S., Jahn, G., and Sinzger, C. (2000). Efficient lytic infection of human arterial endothelial cells by human cytomegalovirus strains. *J. Virol.*, **74**, 7628–7635.

Kalejta, R. F. and Shenk, T. (2003). Proteasome-dependent, ubiquitin-independent degradation of the Rb family of tumor suppressors by the human cytomegalovirus pp71 protein. *Proc. Natl Acad. Sci. USA*, **100**, 3263–3268.

Kari, B. and Gehrz, R. (1993). Structure, composition and heparin binding properties of a human cytomegalovirus glycoprotein complex designated gC-II. *J. Gen. Virol.*, **74**, 255–264.

Kattenhorn, L. M., Mills, R., Wagner, M. *et al.* (2004). Identification of proteins associated with murine cytomegalovirus virions. *J. Virol.*, **78**, 1187–1197.

Kawaguchi, Y., Kato, K., Tanaka, M., Kanamori, M., Nishiyama, Y., and Yamanashi, Y. (2003). Conserved protein kinases encoded by herpesviruses and cellular protein kinase cdc2 target the same phosphorylation site in eukaryotic elongation factor 1delta. *J. Virol.*, **77**, 2359–2368.

Kaye, J. F., Gompels, U. A., and Minson, A. C. (1992). Glycoprotein H of human cytomegalovirus (HCMV) forms a stable complex with the HCMV UL115 gene product. *J. Gen. Virol.*, **73**, 2693–2698.

Kemble, G. W., and Mocarski, E. S. (1989). A host cell protein binds to a highly conserved sequence element (pac-2) within the cytomegalovirus *a* sequence. *J. Virol.*, **63**, 4715–4728.

Kemble, G. W., McCormick, A. L., Pereira, L., and Mocarski, E. S. (1987). A cytomegalovirus protein with properties of herpes simplex virus ICP8: partial purification of the polypeptide and map position of the gene. *J. Virol.*, **61**, 3143–3151.

Kim, K., Trang, P., Umamoto, S., Hai, R., and Liu, F. (2004). RNase P ribozyme inhibits cytomegalovirus replication by blocking the expression of viral capsid proteins. *Nucl. Acids Res.*, **32**, 3427–3434.

Kledal, T. N., Rosenkilde, M. M., and Schwartz, T. W. (1998). Selective recognition of the membrane-bound CX3C chemokine, fractalkine, by the human cytomegalovirus-encoded broad-spectrum receptor US28. *FEBS Lett.*, **441**, 209–214.

Komazin, G., Ptak, R. G., Emmer, B. T., Townsend, L. B., and Drach, J. C. (2003). Resistance of human cytomegalovirus to the benzimidazole L-ribonucleoside maribavir maps to UL27. *J. Virol.*, **77**, 11499–11506.

Komazin, G., Townsend, L. B., and Drach, J. C. (2004). Role of a mutation in human cytomegalovirus gene UL104 in resistance to benzimidazole ribonucleosides. *J. Virol.*, **78**, 710–715.

Kondo, K., Xu, J., and Mocarski, E. S. (1996). Human cytomegalovirus latent gene expression in granulocyte–macrophage progenitors in culture and in seropositive individuals. *Proc. Natl Acad. Sci. USA*, **93**, 11137–11142.

Kondo, K., Kondo, T., Shimada, K., Amo, K., Miyagawa, H., and Yamanishi, K. (2002a). Strong interaction between human herpesvirus 6 and peripheral blood monocytes/macrophages during acute infection. *J. Med. Virol.*, **67**, 364–369.

Kondo, K., Shimada, K., Sashihara, J., Tanaka-Taya, K., and Yamanishi, K. (2002b). Identification of human herpesvirus 6 latency-associated transcripts. *J. Virol.*, **76**, 4145–4151.

Kondo, K., Nozaki, H., Shimada, K., and Yamanishi, K. (2003a). Detection of a gene cluster that is dispensable for human herpesvirus 6 replication and latency. *J. Virol.*, **77**, 10719–10724.

Kondo, K., Sashihara, J., Shimada, K. *et al.* (2003b). Recognition of a novel stage of betaherpesvirus latency in human herpesvirus 6. *J. Virol.*, **77**, 2258–2264.

Kotenko, S. V., Saccani, S., Izotova, L. S., Mirochnitchenko, O. V., and Pestka, S. (2000). Human cytomegalovirus harbors its own unique IL-10 homolog (cmvIL-10). *Proc. Natl Acad. Sci. USA*, **97**, 1695–1700.

Krosky, P. M., Underwood, M. R., Turk, S. R. *et al.* (1998). Resistance of human cytomegalovirus to benzimidazole ribonucleosides maps to two open reading frames: UL89 and UL56. *J. Virol.*, **72**, 4721–4728.

Krosky, P. M., Ptak, R. G., Underwood, M. R., Biron, K. K., Townsend, L. B., and Drach, J. C. (2000). Differences in DNA packaging genes and sensitivity to benzimidazole ribonucleosides between human cytomegalovirus strains AD169 and Towne. *Antivir Chem Chemother*, **11**, 349–352.

Krosky, P. M., Baek, M. C., and Coen, D. M. (2003a). The human cytomegalovirus UL97 protein kinase, an antiviral drug target, is required at the stage of nuclear egress. *J. Virol.*, **77**, 905–914.

Krosky, P. M., Baek, M. C., Jahng, W. J. *et al.* (2003b). The human cytomegalovirus UL44 protein is a substrate for the UL97 protein kinase. *J. Virol.*, **77**, 7720–7727.

Krug, L. T., Inoue, N., and Pellett, P. E. (2001). Differences in DNA binding specificity among Roseolovirus origin binding proteins. *Virology*, **288**, 145–153.

Lai, L. and Britt, W. J. (2003). The interaction between the major capsid protein and the smallest capsid protein of human cytomegalovirus is dependent on two linear sequences in the smallest capsid protein. *J. Virol.*, **77**, 2730–2735.

Landini, M. P., Lazzarotto, T., Xu, J., Geballe, A. P., and Mocarski, E. S. (2000). Humoral immune response to proteins of human cytomegalovirus latency-associated transcripts *Biol. Blood Marrow Transpl.*, **6**, 100–108.

LaPierre, L. A. and Biegalke, B. J. (2001). Identification of a novel transcriptional repressor encoded by human cytomegalovirus. *J. Virol.*, **75**, 6062–6069.

Lee, H. R. and Ahn, J. H. (2004). Sumoylation of the major immediate-early IE2 protein of human cytomegalovirus Towne strain is not required for virus growth in cultured human fibroblasts. *J. Gen. Virol.*, **85**, 2149–2154.

Lembo, D., Donalisio, M., Hofer, A. *et al.* (2004). The ribonucleotide reductase R1 homolog of murine cytomegalovirus is not a functional enzyme subunit but is required for pathogenesis. *J. Virol.*, **78**, 4278–4288.

Li, J., Yamamoto, T., Ohtsubo, K., Shirakata, M., and Hirai, K. (1999). Major product pp43 of human cytomegalovirus U(L)112–113 gene is a transcriptional coactivator with two functionally distinct domains. *Virology*, **260**, 89–97.

Lilley, B. N., Ploegh, H. L., and Tirabassi, R. S. (2001). Human cytomegalovirus open reading frame TRL11/IRL11 encodes an immunoglobulin G Fc-binding protein. *J. Virol.*, **75**, 11218–11221.

Lin, K. and Ricciardi, R. P. (1998). The 41-kDa protein of human herpesvirus 6 specifically binds to viral DNA polymerase and greatly increases DNA synthesis. *Virology*, **250**, 210–219.

Lischka, P., Rosorius, O., Trommer, E., and Stamminger, T. (2001). A novel transferable nuclear export signal mediates CRM1-independent nucleocytoplasmic shuttling of the human cytomegalovirus transactivator protein pUL69. *EMBO J.*, **20**, 7271–7283.

Littler, E., Lawrence, G., Liu, M. Y., Barrell, B. G., and Arrand, J. R. (1990). Identification, cloning, and expression of the major capsid protein gene of human herpesvirus 6. *J. Virol.*, **64**, 714–722.

Liu, B. and Stinski, M. F. (1992). Human cytomegalovirus contains a tegument protein that enhances transcription from promoters with upstream ATF and AP-1 *cis*-acting elements. *J. Virol.*, **66**, 4434–4444.

Liu, Y. and Biegalke, B. J. (2002). The human cytomegalovirus UL35 gene encodes two proteins with different functions. *J. Virol.*, **76**, 2460–2468.

Lockridge, K. M., Zhou, S. S., Kravitz, R. H. *et al.* (2000). Primate cytomegaloviruses encode and express an IL-10-like protein *Virology*, **268**, 272–280.

Lopper, M. and Compton, T. (2004). Coiled-coil domains in glycoproteins B and H are involved in human cytomegalovirus membrane fusion. *J. Virol.*, **78**, 8333–8341.

Loregian, A., Appleton, B. A., Hogle, J. M., and Coen, D. M. (2004a). Residues of human cytomegalovirus DNA polymerase catalytic subunit UL54 that are necessary and sufficient for interaction with the accessory protein UL44. *J. Virol.*, **78**, 158–167.

Loregian, A., Appleton, B. A., Hogle, J. M., and Coen, D. M. (2004b). Specific residues in the connector loop of the human cytomegalovirus DNA polymerase accessory protein UL44 are crucial for interaction with the UL54 catalytic subunit. *J. Virol.*, **78**, 9084–9092.

Lusso, P., Secchiero, P., Crowley, R. W., Garzino-Demo, A., Berneman, Z. N., and Gallo, R. C. (1994). CD4 is a critical component of the receptor for human herpesvirus 7: interference with human immunodeficiency virus. *Proc. Natl Acad. Sci. USA*, **91**, 3872–3876.

Luttichau, H. R., Clark-Lewis, I., Jensen, P. O., Moser, C., Gerstoft, J., and Schwartz, T. W. (2003). A highly selective CCR2 chemokine agonist encoded by human herpesvirus 6. *J. Biol. Chem.*, **278**, 10928–10933.

Mach, M., Kropff, B., Dal Monte, P., and Britt, W. (2000). Complex formation by human cytomegalovirus glycoproteins M (gpUL100) and N (gpUL73) *J. Virol.*, **74**, 11881–11892.

Mach, M., Kropff, B., Kryzaniak, M., and Britt, W. (2005). Complex formation by glycoproteins M and N of human cytomegalovirus: structural and functional aspects. *J. Virol.*, **79**, 2160–2170.

Maidji, E., Tugizov, S., Abenes, G., Jones, T., and Pereira, L. (1998). A novel human cytomegalovirus glycoprotein, gpUS9, which promotes cell- to-cell spread in polarized epithelial cells, colocalizes with the cytoskeletal proteins E-cadherin and F-actin. *J. Virol.*, **72**, 5717–5727.

Manichanh, C., Olivier-Aubron, C., Lagarde, J. P. *et al.* (2001). Selection of the same mutation in the U69 protein kinase gene of human herpesvirus-6 after prolonged exposure to ganciclovir in vitro and in vivo. *J. Gen. Virol.*, **82**, 2767–2776.

Manning, W. C., Stoddart, C. A., Lagenaur, L. A., Abenes, G. B., and Mocarski, E. S. (1992). Cytomegalovirus determinant of replication in salivary glands. *J. Virol.*, **66**, 3794–3802.

Marchini, A., Liu, H., and Zhu, H. (2001). Human cytomegalovirus with IE-2 (UL122) deleted fails to express early lytic genes. *J. Virol.*, **75**, 1870–1878.

Masse, M. J., Karlin, S., Schachtel, G. A., and Mocarski, E. S. (1992). Human cytomegalovirus origin of DNA replication (oriLyt) resides within a highly complex repetitive region. *Proc. Natl Acad. Sci. USA*, **89**, 5246–5250.

Masse, M. J., Messerle, M., and Mocarski, E. S. (1997). The location and sequence composition of the replicator (orilyst) murine cytomegalovirus. *Virology*, **230**, 350–360.

McCormick, A. L., Skaletskaya, A., Barry, P. A., Mocarski, E. S., and Goldmacher, V. S. (2003). Differential function and expression of the viral inhibitor of caspase 8-induced apoptosis (vICA) and the viral mitochondria-localized inhibitor of apoptosis (vMIA) cell death suppressors conserved in primate and rodent cytomegaloviruses. *Virology*, **316**, 221–233.

McCormick, A. L., Meiring, C. D., Smith, G. D., and Mocarskhi, E. S. (2005). Mitochondrial cell death supprenors carried by human and murine cytomegalovirus confer resistance to proteasome inhibitor-induced apoptosis. *J. Virol.*, **79**, 12205–12217.

McMahon, T. P. and Anders, D. G. (2002). Interactions between human cytomegalovirus helicase-primase proteins. *Virus Res.*, **86**, 39–52.

Melnychuk, R. M., Streblow, D. N., Smith, P. P., Hirsch, A. J., Pancheva, D., and Nelson, J. A. (2004). Human cytomegalovirus-encoded G protein-coupled receptor US28 mediates smooth muscle cell migration through Galpha12. *J. Virol.*, **78**, 8382–8391.

Menard, C., Wagner, M., Ruzsics, Z. *et al.* (2003). Role of murine cytomegalovirus US22 gene family members in replication in macrophages. *J. Virol.*, **77**, 5557–5570.

Menegazzi, P., Galvan, M., Rotola, A., Ravaioli, T., Gonelli, A., Cassai, E., and Di Luca, D. (1999). Temporal mapping of transcripts in human herpesvirus-7. *J. Gen. Virol.*, **80**(10), 2705–2712.

Menotti, L., Mirandola, P., Locati, M., and Campadelli-Fiume, G. (1999). Trafficking to the plasma membrane of the seven-transmembrane protein encoded by human herpesvirus 6 U51 gene involves a cell-specific function present in T lymphocytes. *J. Virol.*, **73**, 325–333.

Mettenleiter, T. C. (2004). Budding events in herpesvirus morphogenesis. *Virus Res.*, **106**, 167–180.

Michel, D. and Mertens, T. (2004). The UL97 protein kinase of human cytomegalovirus and homologues in other herpesviruses: impact on virus and host. *Biochim. Biophys. Acta*, **1697**, 169–180.

Michel, D., Milotic, I., Wagner, M. *et al.* (2005). The human cytomegalovirus UL78 gene is highly conserved among clinical isolates, but is dispensable for replication in fibroblasts and a renal artery organ-culture system. *J. Gen. Virol.*, **86**, 297–306.

Milne, R. S., Paterson, D. A., and Booth, J. C. (1998). Human cytomegalovirus glycoprotein H/glycoprotein L complex modulates fusion-from-without. *J. Gen. Virol.*, **79**, 855–865.

Milne, R. S., Mattick, C., Nicholson, L., Devaraj, P., Alcami, A., and Gompels, U. A. (2000). RANTES binding and down-regulation by a novel human herpesvirus-6 beta chemokine receptor. *J. Immunol.*, **164**, 2396–2404.

Mirandola, P., Menegazzi, P., Merighi, S., Ravaioli, T., Cassai, E., and Di Luca, D. (1998). Temporal mapping of transcripts in herpesvirus 6 variants. *J. Virol.*, **72**, 3837–3844.

Misaghi, S., Sun, Z. Y., Stern, P., Gaudet, R., Wagner, G., and Ploegh, H. (2004). Structural and functional analysis of human cytomegalovirus US3 protein. *J. Virol.*, **78**, 413–423.

Mocarski, E. S. (2002). Immunomodulation by cytomegaloviruses: manipulative strategies beyond evasion. *Trends Microbiol.*, **10**, 332–339.

Mocarski, E. S., Jr. (2004). Immune escape and exploitation strategies of cytomegaloviruses: impact on and imitation of the major histocompatibility system. *Cell Microbiol.*, **6**, 707–717.

Mocarski, E. S., Liu, A. C., and Spaete, R. R. (1987). Structure and variability of the a sequence in the genome of human cytomegalovirus (Towne strain). *J. Gen. Virol.*, **68**, 2223–2230.

Mocarski, E. S., Bonyhadi, M., Salimi, S., McCune, J. M., and Kaneshima, H. (1993). Human cytomegalovirus in a SCID-hu mouse: thymic epithelial cells are prominent targets of viral replication. *Proc. Natl Acad. Sci. USA*, **90**, 104–108.

Mocarski, E. S., Kemble, G. W., Lyle, J. M., and Greaves, R. F. (1996). A deletion mutant in the human cytomegalovirus gene encoding IE1(491aa) is replication defective due to a failure in autoregulation. *Proc. Natl Acad. Sci. USA*, **93**, 11321–11326.

Mocarski, E. S., Prichard, M. N., Tan, C. S., and Brown, J. M. (1997). Reassessing the organization of the UL42–UL43 region of the human cytomegalovirus strain AD169 genome. *Virology*, **239**, 169–175.

Mocarski, E.S., Hahn, G., White, K.L., Xu, J. *et al.* (2005) Myeloid cell recruitment and function in pathogenesis and latency. In *Cytomegaloviruses: Molecular Biology and Immunology*, ed. M. J. Reddehase, Hethersett, Norfolk. UK: Horizon Scientific Press. (in press)

Morello, C. S., Cranmer, L. D., and Spector, D. H. (1999). In vivo replication, latency, and immunogenicity of murine cytomegalovirus mutants with deletions in the M83 and M84 genes, the putative homologs of human cytomegalovirus pp65 (UL83). *J. Virol.*, **73**, 7678–7693.

Mori, Y., Seya, T., Huang, H. L., Akkapaiboon, P., Dhepakson, P., and Yamanishi, K. (2002). Human herpesvirus 6 variant A, but not variant B induces fusion from without in a variety of human cells through a human herpesvirus 6 entry receptor, C046. *J. Virol.*, **76**, 6750–6761.

Mori, Y., Akkapaiboon, P., Yang, X., and Yamanishi, K. (2003a). The human herpesvirus 6 U100 gene product is the third component of the gH–gL glycoprotein complex on the viral envelope. *J. Virol.*, **77**, 2452–2458.

Mori, Y., Yang, X., Akkapaiboon, P., Okuno, T., and Yamanishi, K. (2003b). Human herpesvirus 6 variant A glycoprotein H-glycoprotein L-glycoprotein Q complex associates with human CD46. *J. Virol.*, **77**, 4992–4999.

Mori, Y., Akkapaiboon, P., Yonemoto, S. *et al.* (2004). Discovery of a second form of tripartite complex containing gH–gL of human herpesvirus 6 and observations on CD46. *J. Virol.*, **78**, 4609–4616.

Mukai, T., Isegawa, Y., and Yamanishi, K. (1995). Identification of the major capsid protein gene of human herpesvirus 7. *Virus Res.*, **37**, 55–62.

Muranyi, W., Haas, J., Wagner, M., Krohne, G., and Koszinowski, U. H. (2002). Cytomegalovirus recruitment of cellular kinases to dissolve the nuclear lamina. *Science*, **297**, 854–857.

Nakano, K., Tadagaki, K., Isegawa, Y., Aye, M. M., Zou, P., and Yamanishi, K. (2003). Human herpesvirus 7 open reading frame U12 encodes a functional beta-chemokine receptor. *J. Virol.*, **77**, 8108–8115.

Navarro, D., Paz, P., Tugizov, S., Topp, K., La Vail, J., and Pereira, L. (1993). Glycoprotein B of human cytomegalovirus promotes virion penetration into cells, transmission of infection from cell to cell, and fusion of infected cells. *Virology*, **197**, 143–158.

Neipel, F., Ellinger, K., and Fleckenstein, B. (1992). Gene for the major antigenic structural protein (p100) of human herpesvirus 6. *J. Virol.*, **66**, 3918–3924.

Neote, K., DiGregorio, D., Mak, J. Y., Horuk, R., and Schall, T. J. (1993). Molecular cloning, functional expression, and signaling characteristics of a C-C chemokine receptor. *Cell*, **72**, 415–425.

Nevels, M., Paulus, C., and Shenk, T. (2004). Human cytomegalovirus immediate-early 1 protein facilitates viral replication by antagonizing histone deacetylation. *Proc. Natl Acad. Sci. USA*, **101**, 17234–17239.

Neyts, J., Snoeck, R., Schols, D. *et al.* (1992). Sulfated polymers inhibit the interaction of human cytomegalovirus with cell surface heparan sulfate. *Virology*, **189**, 48–58.

Nicholas, J. (1996). Determination and analysis of the complete nucleotide sequence of human herpesvirus 7. *J. Virol.*, **70**, 5975–5989.

Nikolaou, K., Varinou, L., Inoue, N., and Arsenakis, M. (2003). Identification and characterization of gene products of ORF U90/89 of human herpesvirus 6. *Acta Virol.*, **47**, 17–26.

Ogawa-Goto, K., Irie, S., Omori, A. et al. (2002). An endoplasmic reticulum protein, p180, is highly expressed in human cytomegalovirus-permissive cells and interacts with the tegument protein encoded by UL48. *J. Virol.*, **76**, 2350–2362.

Ogawa-Goto, K., Tanaka, K., Gibson, W. et al. (2003). Microtubule network facilitates nuclear targeting of human cytomegalovirus capsid. *J. Virol.*, **77**, 8541–8547.

Oien, N. L., Thomsen, D. R., Wathen, M. W., Newcomb, W. W., Brown, J. C., and Homa, F. L. (1997). Assembly of herpes simplex virus capsids using the human cytomegalovirus scaffold protein: critical role of the C terminus. *J. Virol.*, **71**, 1281–1291.

Papanikolaou, E., Kouvatsis, V., Dimitriadis, G., Inoue, N., and Arsenakis, M. (2002). Identification and characterization of the gene products of open reading frame U86/87 of human herpesvirus 6. *Virus Res.*, **89**, 89–101.

Pari, G. S. and Anders, D. G. (1993). Eleven loci encoding trans-acting factors are required for transient complementation of human cytomegalovirus oriLyt-dependent DNA replication. *J. Virol.*, **67**, 6979–6988.

Patrone, M., Percivalle, E., Secchi, M. et al. (2003). The human cytomegalovirus UL45 gene product is a late, virion-associated protein and influences virus growth at low multiplicities of infection. *J. Gen. Virol.*, **84**, 3359–3370.

Patterson, C. E. and Shenk, T. (1999). Human cytomegalovirus UL36 protein is dispensable for viral replication in cultured cells. *J. Virol.*, **73**, 7126–7131.

Penfold, M. E. and Mocarski, E. S. (1997). Formation of cytomegalovirus DNA replication compartments defined by localization of viral proteins and DNA synthesis. *Virology*, **239**, 46–61.

Penfold, M. E., Dairaghi, D. J., Duke, G. M. et al. (1999). Cytomegalovirus encodes a potent alpha chemokine. *Proc. Natl Acad. Sci. USA*, **96**, 9839–9844.

Pizzorno, M. C., Mullen, M. A., Chang, Y. N., and Hayward, G. S. (1991). The functionally active IE2 immediate-early regulatory protein of human cytomegalovirus is an 80-kilodalton polypeptide that contains two distinct activator domains and a duplicated nuclear localization signal. *J. Virol.*, **65**, 3839–3852.

Plafker, S. M. and Gibson, W. (1998). Cytomegalovirus assembly protein precursor and proteinase precursor contain two nuclear localization signals that mediate their own nuclear translocation and that of the major capsid protein. *J. Virol.*, **72**, 7722–7732.

Prichard, M. N., Duke, G. M., and Mocarski, E. S. (1996). Human cytomegalovirus uracil DNA glycosylase is required for the normal temporal regulation of both DNA synthesis and viral replication. *J. Virol.*, **70**, 3018–3025.

Prichard, M. N., Jairath, S., Penfold, M. E., St Jeor, S., Bohlman, M. C., and Pari, G. S. (1998). Identification of persistent RNA-DNA hybrid structures within the origin of replication of human cytomegalovirus. *J. Virol.*, **72**, 6997–7004.

Prichard, M. N., Gao, N., Jairath, S. et al. (1999). A recombinant human cytomegalovirus with a large deletion in UL97 has a severe replication deficiency. *J. Virol.*, **73**, 5663–5670.

Prichard, M. N., Penfold, M. E., Duke, G. M., Spaete, R. R., and Kemble, G. W. (2001). A review of genetic differences between limited and extensively passaged human cytomegalovirus strains. *Rev. Med. Virol.*, **11**, 191–200.

Reboredo, M., Greaves, R. F., and Hahn, G. (2004). Human cytomegalovirus proteins encoded by UL37 exon 1 protect infected fibroblasts against virus-induced apoptosis and are required for efficient virus replication. *J. Gen. Virol.*, **85**, 3555–3567.

Reid, G. G., Ellsmore, V., and Stow, N. D. (2003). An analysis of the requirements for human cytomegalovirus oriLyt-dependent DNA synthesis in the presence of the herpes simplex virus type 1 replication fork proteins. *Virology*, **308**, 303–316.

Reinhardt, J., Smith, G. B., Himmelheber, C. T., Azizkhan-Clifford, J., and Mocarski, E. S. (2005). The carboxyl-terminal region of human cytomegalovirus IE1$_{491aa}$ contains an acidic domain that plays a regulatory role and a chromatin-tethering domain that is dispensable during viral replication. *J. Virol.*, **79**, 225–233.

Riegler, S., Hebart, H., Einsele, H., Brossart, P., Jahn, G., and Sinzger, C. (2000). Monocyte-derived dendritic cells are permissive to the complete replicative cycle of human cytomegalovirus. *J. Gen. Virol.*, **81**, 393–399.

Romanowski, M. J. and Shenk, T. (1997). Characterization of the human cytomegalovirus irs1 and trs1 genes: a second immediate-early transcription unit within irs1 whose product antagonizes transcriptional activation. *J. Virol.*, **71**, 1485–1496.

Romanowski, M. J., Garrido-Guerrero, E., and Shenk, T. (1997). pIRS1 and pTRS1 are present in human cytomegalovirus virions. *J. Virol.*, **71**, 5703–5705.

Rotola, A., Ravaioli, T., Gonelli, A., Dewhurst, S., Cassai, E., and Di Luca, D. (1998). U94 of human herpesvirus 6 is expressed in latently infected peripheral blood mononuclear cells and blocks viral gene expression in transformed lymphocytes in culture. *Proc. Natl Acad. Sci. USA*, **95**, 13911–13916.

Sampaio, K. L., Cavignac, Y., Stierhof, Y. D., and Sinzger, C. (2005). Human cytomegalovirus labeled with green fluorescent protein for live analysis of intracellular particle movements. *J. Virol.*, **79**, 2754–2767.

Sanchez, V., Greis, K. D., Sztul, E., and Britt, W. J. (2000a). Accumulation of virion tegument and envelope proteins in a stable cytoplasmic compartment during human cytomegalovirus replication: characterization of a potential site of virus assembly *J. Virol.*, **74**, 975–986.

Sanchez, V., Sztul, E., and Britt, W. J. (2000b). Human cytomegalovirus pp28 (UL99) localizes to a cytoplasmic compartment which overlaps the endoplasmic reticulum-Golgi-intermediate compartment. *J. Virol.*, **74**, 3842–3851.

Sanchez, V., Clark, C. L., Yen, J. Y., Dwarakanath, R., and Spector, D. H. (2002). Viable human cytomegalovirus recombinant virus with an internal deletion of the IE2 86 gene affects late stages of viral replication. *J. Virol.*, **76**, 2973–2989.

Santoro, F., Kennedy, P. E., Locatelli, G., Malnati, M. S., Berger, E. A., and Lusso, P. (1999). CD46 is a cellular receptor for human herpesvirus 6. *Cell*, **99**, 817–827.

Santoro, F., Greenstone, H. L., Insinga, A. *et al.* (2003). Interaction of glycoprotein H of human herpesvirus 6 with the cellular receptor CD46. *J. Biol. Chem.*, **278**, 25964–25969.

Sarisky, R. T. and Hayward, G. S. (1996). Evidence that the UL84 gene product of human cytomegalovirus is essential for promoting oriLyt-dependent DNA replication and formation of replication compartments in cotransfection assays. *J. Virol.*, **70**, 7398–7413.

Saverino, D., Ghiotto, F., Merlo, A. *et al.* (2004). Specific recognition of the viral protein UL18 by CD85j/LIR-1/ILT2 on CD8+ T cells mediates the non-MHC-restricted lysis of human cytomegalovirus-infected cells. *J. Immunol.*, **172**, 5629–5637.

Scheffczik, H., Savva, C. G., Holzenburg, A., Kolesnikova, L., and Bogner, E. (2002). The terminase subunits pUL56 and pUL89 of human cytomegalovirus are DNA-metabolizing proteins with toroidal structure. *Nucl. Acids Res.*, **30**, 1695–1703.

Schierling, K., Stamminger, T., Mertens, T., and Winkler, M. (2004). Human cytomegalovirus tegument proteins ppUL82 (pp71) and ppUL35 interact and cooperatively activate the major immediate-early enhancer. *J. Virol.*, **78**, 9512–9523.

Schierling, K., Buser, C., Mertens, T., and Winkler, M. (2005). Human cytomegalovirus tegument protein ppUL35 is important for viral replication and particle formation. *J. Virol.*, **79**, 3084–3096.

Scholz, B., Rechter, S., Drach, J. C., Townsend, L. B., and Bogner, E. (2003). Identification of the ATP-binding site in the terminase subunit pUL56 of human cytomegalovirus. *Nucl. Acids Res.*, **31**, 1426–1433.

Secchiero, P., Sun, D., De Vico, A. L. *et al.* (1997). Role of the extracellular domain of human herpesvirus 7 glycoprotein B in virus binding to cell surface heparan sulfate proteoglycans. *J. Virol.*, **71**, 4571–4580.

Sedy, J. R., Gavrieli, M., Potter, K. G. *et al.* (2005). B and T lymphocyte attenuator regulates T cell activation through interaction with herpesvirus entry mediator. *Nat. Immunol.*, **6**, 90–98.

Silva, M. C., Yu, Q. C., Enquist, L., and Shenk, T. (2003). Human cytomegalovirus UL99-encoded pp28 is required for the cytoplasmic envelopment of tegument-associated capsids. *J. Virol.*, **77**, 10594–10605.

Silva, M. C., Schroer, J., and Shenk, T. (2005). Human cytomegalovirus cell-to-cell spread in the absence of an essential assembly protein. *Proc. Natl Acad. Sci. USA*, **102**, 2081–2086.

Sinzger, C. and Jahn, G. (1996). Human cytomegalovirus cell tropism and pathogenesis. *Intervirology*, **39**, 302–319.

Sinzger, C., Kahl, M., Laib, K. *et al.* (2000). Tropism of human cytomegalovirus for endothelial cells is determined by a post-entry step dependent on efficient translocation to the nucleus. *J. Gen. Virol.*, **81**, 3021–3035.

Sissons, J. G., Bain, M., and Wills, M. R. (2002). Latency and reactivation of human cytomegalovirus. *J. Infect.*, **44**, 73–77.

Skaletskaya, A., Bartle, L. M., Chittenden, T., McCormick, A. L., Mocarski, E. S., and Goldmacher, V. S. (2001). A cytomegalovirus-encoded inhibitor of apoptosis that suppresses caspase-8 activation. *Proc. Natl Acad. Sci. USA*, **98**, 7829–7834.

Smith, J. A., Jairath, S., Crute, J. J., and Pari, G. S. (1996). Characterization of the human cytomegalovirus UL105 gene and identification of the putative helicase protein. *Virology*, **220**, 251–255.

Spaderna, S., Blessing, H., Bogner, E., Britt, W., and Mach, M. (2002). Identification of glycoprotein gpTRL10 as a structural component of human cytomegalovirus. *J. Virol.*, **76**, 1450–1460.

Spaderna, S., Hahn, G., and Mach, M. (2004). Glycoprotein gpTRL10 of human cytomegalovirus is dispensable for virus replication in human fibroblasts. *Arch. Virol.*, **149**, 495–506.

Spector, D. J. and Tevethia, M. J. (1994). Protein-protein interactions between human cytomegalovirus IE2-580aa and pUL84 in lytically infected cells. *J. Virol.*, **68**, 7549–7553.

Spencer, J. V., Lockridge, K. M., Barry, P. A. *et al.* (2002). Potent immunosuppressive activities of cytomegalovirus-encoded interleukin-10. *J. Virol.*, **76**, 1285–1292.

Stamey, F. R., Dominguez, G., Black, J. B., Dambaugh, T. R., and Pellett, P. E. (1995). Intragenomic linear amplification of human herpesvirus 6B oriLyt suggests acquisition of oriLyt by transposition. *J. Virol.*, **69**, 589–596.

Stamminger, T., Gstaiger, M., Weinzierl, K., Lorz, K., Winkler, M., and Schaffner, W. (2002). Open reading frame UL26 of human cytomegalovirus encodes a novel tegument protein that contains a strong transcriptional activation domain. *J. Virol.*, **76**, 4836–4847.

Stasiak, P. C. and Mocarski, E. S. (1992). Transactivation of the cytomegalovirus ICP36 gene promoter requires the α gene product TRS1 in addition to IE1 and IE2. *J. Virol.*, **66**, 1050–1058.

Stefan, A., Secchiero, P., Baechi, T., Kempf, W., and Campadelli-Fiume, G. (1997). The 85-kilodalton phosphoprotein (pp85) of human herpesvirus 7 is encoded by open reading frame U14 and localizes to a tegument substructure in virion particles. *J. Virol.*, **71**, 5758–5763.

Streblow, D. N., Soderberg-Naucler, C., Vieira, J. *et al.* (1999). The human cytomegalovirus chemokine receptor US28 mediates vascular smooth muscle cell migration. *Cell*, **99**, 511–520.

Strive, T., Gicklhorn, D., Wohlfahrt, M. *et al.* (2004). Site directed mutagenesis of the carboxyl terminus of human cytomegalovirus glycoprotein B leads to attenuation of viral growth in cell culture. *Arch. Virol.*

Sun, Y. and Conner, J. (1999). The U28 ORF of human herpesvirus-7 does not encode a functional ribonucleotide reductase R1 subunit. *J. Gen. Virol.*, **80**(10), 2713–2718.

Takemoto, M., Shimamoto, T., Isegawa, Y., and Yamanishi, K. (2001). The R3 region, one of three major repetitive regions of human herpesvirus 6, is a strong enhancer of immediate-early gene U95. *J. Virol.*, **75**, 10149–10160.

Talarico, C. L., Burnette, T. C., Miller, W. H. *et al.* (1999). Acyclovir is phosphorylated by the human cytomegalovirus UL97 protein. *Antimicrob. Agents Chemother.*, **43**, 1941–1946.

Taniguchi, T., Shimamoto, T., Isegawa, Y., Kondo, K., and Yamanishi, K. (2000). Structure of transcripts and proteins encoded by U79–80 of human herpesvirus 6 and its subcellular localization in infected cells. *Virology*, **271**, 307–320.

Terhune, S. S., Schroer, J., and Shenk, T. (2004). RNAs are packaged into human cytomegalovirus virions in proportion to their intracellular concentration. *J. Virol.*, **78**, 10390–10398.

Theiler, R. N. and Compton, T. (2002). Distinct glycoprotein O complexes arise in a post-Golgi compartment of cytomegalovirus-infected cells. *J. Virol.*, **76**, 2890–2898.

Tigue, N. J., Matharu, P. J., Roberts, N. A., Mills, J. S., Kay, J., and Jupp, R. (1996). Cloning, expression and characterization of the proteinase from human herpesvirus 6. *J. Virol.*, **70**, 4136–4141.

Tirabassi, R. S. and Ploegh, H. L. (2002). The human cytomegalovirus US8 glycoprotein binds to major histocompatibility complex class I products. *J. Virol.*, **76**, 6832–6835.

Tirosh, B., Iwakoshi, N. N., Lilley, B. N., Lee, A. H., Glimcher, L. H., and Ploegh, H. L. (2005). Human cytomegalovirus protein US11 provokes an unfolded protein response that may facilitate the degradation of class I major histocompatibility complex products. *J. Virol.*, **79**, 2768–2779.

Tomasec, P., Braud, V. M., Rickards, C. *et al.* (2000). Surface expression of HLA-E, an inhibitor of natural killer cells, enhanced by human cytomegalovirus gpUL40. *Science*, **287**, 1031–1033.

Tomasec, P., Wang, E. C., Davison, A. J. *et al.* (2005). Downregulation of natural killer cell-activating ligand CD155 by human cytomegalovirus UL141. *Nat. Immunol.*, **6**, 181–188.

Tooze, J., Hollinshead, M., Reis, B., Radsak, K., and Kern, H. (1993). Progeny vaccinia and human cytomegalovirus particles utilize early endosomal cisternae for their envelopes. *Eur. J. Cell Biol.*, **60**, 163–178.

Tortorella, D., Gewurz, B. E., Furman, M. H., Schust, D. J., and Ploegh, H. L. (2000). Viral subversion of the immune system. *Annu. Rev. Immunol.*, **18**, 861–926.

Tugizov, S., Navarro, D., Paz, P., Wang, Y., Qadri, I., and Pereira, L. (1994). Function of human cytomegalovirus glycoprotein B: syncytium formation in cells constitutively expressing gB is blocked by virus-neutralizing antibodies. *Virology*, **201**, 263–276.

Ulbrecht, M., Martinozzi, S., Grzeschik, M. *et al.* (2000). Cutting edge: the human cytomegalovirus UL40 gene product contains a ligand for HLA-E and prevents NK cell-mediated lysis. *J. Immunol.*, **164**, 5019–5022.

Ulbrecht, M., Hofmeister, V., Yuksekdag, G. *et al.* (2003). HCMV glycoprotein US6 mediated inhibition of TAP does not affect HLA-E dependent protection of K-562 cells from NK cell lysis. *Hum. Immunol.*, **64**, 231–237.

Vales-Gomez, M., Browne, H., and Reyburn, H. T. (2003). Expression of the UL16 glycoprotein of Human Cytomegalovirus protects the virus-infected cell from attack by natural killer cells. *BMC Immunol.*, **4**, 4.

Vales-Gomez, M., Shiroishi, M., Maenaka, K., and Reyburn, H. T. (2005). Genetic variability of the major histocompatibility complex class I homologue encoded by human cytomegalovirus leads to differential binding to the inhibitory receptor ILT2. *J. Virol.*, **79**, 2251–2260.

van Loon, N., Dykes, C., Deng, H., Dominguez, G., Nicholas, J., and Dewhurst, S. (1997). Identification and analysis of a lytic-phase origin of DNA replication in human herpesvirus 7. *J. Virol.*, **71**, 3279–3284.

Varnum, S. M., Streblow, D. N., Monroe, M. E. *et al.* (2004). Identification of proteins in human cytomegalovirus (HCMV) particles: the HCMV proteome. *J. Virol.*, **78**, 10960–10966.

Vieira, J., Schall, T. J., Corey, L., and Geballe, A. P. (1998). Functional analysis of the human cytomegalovirus US28 gene by insertion mutagenesis with the green fluorescent protein gene. *J. Virol.*, **72**, 8158–8165.

Wang, D., Bresnahan, W., and Shenk, T. (2004a). Human cytomegalovirus encodes a highly specific RANTES decoy receptor. *Proc. Natl Acad. Sci. USA*, **101**, 16642–16647.

Wang, E. C., McSharry, B., Retiere, C. *et al.* (2002). UL40-mediated NK evasion during productive infection with human cytomegalovirus. *Proc. Natl Acad. Sci. USA*, **99**, 7570–7575.

Wang, S. K., Duh, C. Y., and Wu, C. W. (2004b). Human cytomegalovirus UL76 encodes a novel virion-associated protein that is able to inhibit viral replication. *J. Virol.*, **78**, 9750–9762.

Wang, X., Huong, S. M., Chiu, M. L., Raab-Traub, N., and Huang, E. S. (2003). Epidermal growth factor receptor is a cellular receptor for human cytomegalovirus. *Nature*, **424**, 456–461.

White, E. A., Clark, C. L., Sanchez, V., and Spector, D. H. (2004). Small internal deletions in the human cytomegalovirus IE2 gene result in nonviable recombinant viruses with differential defects in viral gene expression. *J. Virol.*, **78**, 1817–1830.

Willcox, B. E., Thomas, L. M., and Bjorkman, P. J. (2003). Crystal structure of HLA-A2 bound to LIR-1, a host and viral major histocompatibility complex receptor. *Nat. Immunol.*, **4**, 913–919.

Wing, B. A. and Huang, E. S. (1995). Analysis and mapping of a family of 3′-coterminal transcripts containing coding sequences for human cytomegalovirus open reading frames UL93 through UL99. *J. Virol.*, **69**, 1521–1531.

Wing, B. A., Lee, G. C., and Huang, E. S. (1996). The human cytomegalovirus UL94 open reading frame encodes a conserved herpesvirus capsid/tegument-associated virion protein that is expressed with true late kinetics. *J. Virol.*, **70**, 3339–3345.

Wing, B. A., Johnson, R. A., and Huang, E. S. (1998). Identification of positive and negative regulatory regions involved in regulating expression of the human cytomegalovirus UL94 late promoter: role of IE2-86 and cellular p53 in mediating negative regulatory function. *J. Virol.*, **72**, 1814–1825.

Wolf, D. G., Honigman, A., Lazarovits, J., Tavor, E., and Panet, A. (1998). Characterization of the human cytomegalovirus UL97 gene product as a virion-associated protein kinase. *Arch. Virol.*, **143**, 1223–1232.

Wolf, D. G., Courcelle, C. T., Prichard, M. N., and Mocarski, E. S. (2001). Distinct and separate roles for herpesvirus-conserved UL97 kinase in cytomegalovirus DNA synthesis and encapsidation. *Proc. Natl Acad. Sci. USA*, **98**, 1895–1900.

Wood, L. J., Baxter, M. K., Plafker, S. M., and Gibson, W. (1997). Human cytomegalovirus capsid assembly protein precursor (pUL80.5) interacts with itself and with the major capsid protein (pUL86) through two different domains. *J. Virol.*, **71**, 179–190.

Xu, Y., Cei, S. A., Huete, A. R., and Pari, G. S. (2004a). Human cytomegalovirus UL84 insertion mutant defective for viral DNA synthesis and growth. *J. Virol.*, **78**, 10360–10369.

Xu, Y., Cei, S. A., Rodriguez Huete, A., Colletti, K. S., and Pari, G. S. (2004b). Human cytomegalovirus DNA replication requires transcriptional activation via an IE2- and UL84-responsive bidirectional promoter element within oriLyt. *J. Virol.*, **78**, 11664–11677.

Yoon, J. S., Kim, S. H., Shin, M. C. *et al.* (2004). Inhibition of herpesvirus-6B RNA replication by short interference RNAs. *J. Biochem. Mol. Biol.*, **37**, 383–385.

Yu, D., Smith, G. A., Enquist, L. W., and Shenk, T. (2002). Construction of a self-excisable bacterial artificial chromosome containing the human cytomegalovirus genome and mutagenesis of the diploid TRL/IRL13 gene. *J. Virol.*, **76**, 2316–2328.

Yu, D., Silva, M. C., and Shenk, T. (2003). Functional map of human cytomegalovirus AD169 defined by global mutational analysis. *Proc. Natl Acad. Sci. USA*, **100**, 12396–12401.

Yu, X., Shah, S., Atanasov, I., Lo, P., Liu, F., Britt, W. J., and Zhou, Z. H. (2005). Three-dimensional localization of the smallest capsid protein in the human cytomegalovirus capsid. *J. Virol.*, **79**, 1327–1332.

Yurochko, A. D. and Huang, E. S. (1999). Human cytomegalovirus binding to human monocytes induces immunoregulatory gene expression. *J. Immunol.*, **162**, 4806–4816.

Yurochko, A. D., Kowalik, T. F., Huong, S. M., and Huang, E. S. (1995). Human cytomegalovirus upregulates NF-kappa B activity by transactivating the NF-kappa B p105/p50 and p65 promoters. *J. Virol.*, **69**, 5391–5400.

Yurochko, A. D., Hwang, E. S., Rasmussen, L., Keay, S., Pereira, L., and Huang, E. S. (1997). The human cytomegalovirus UL55 (gB) and UL75 (gH) glycoprotein ligands initiate the rapid activation of Sp1 and NF-kappaB during infection. *J. Virol.*, **71**, 5051–5059.

Zhao, Y. and Biegalke, B. J. (2003). Functional analysis of the human cytomegalovirus immune evasion protein, pUS3(22kDa). *Virology*, **315**, 353–361.

Zini, N., Battista, M. C., Santi, S. *et al.* (1999). The novel structural protein of human cytomegalovirus, pUL25, is localized in the viral tegument. *J. Virol.*, **73**, 6073–6075.

Zini, N., Santi, S., Riccio, M., Landini, M. P., Battista, M. C., and Maraldi, N. M. (2000). pUL25 immunolocalization in human cytomegalovirus-infected and gene-transfected cells. *Arch. Virol.*, **145**, 795–803.

Zou, P., Isegawa, Y., Nakano, K., Haque, M., Horiguchi, Y., and Yamanishi, K. (1999). Human herpesvirus 6 open reading frame U83 encodes a functional chemokine. *J. Virol.*, **73**, 5926–5933.

16

Early events in human cytomegalovirus infection

Teresa Compton and Adam Feire

McArdle Laboratory for Cancer Research, University of Wisconsin, Madison, WI, USA

Introduction

All viruses must deliver their genomes to host cells to initiate infection. The plasma membrane together with cell surface constituents serve as initial barriers to entry as well as the mediators that facilitate the process. This chapter will summarize what is known about the entry pathway of human cytomegalovirus, noting certain parallels and commonalities between human cytomegalovirus (HCMV) and other betaherpesviruses (see Chapter 46 for specific pathways of HHV-6 and HHV-7 entry). The roles of HCMV envelope glycoproteins and cellular receptors that control virion attachment and membrane fusion will be summarized. This chapter will also discuss the emerging role of signaling pathways in the early events in infection and examine how virus entry and innate immune activation may be coordinated.

In the simplest context, entry requires that enveloped viruses, including HCMV, HHV-6A or B and HHV-7, use virion envelope proteins to facilitate adherence to the cell surface and fusion between the virus envelope and a cellular membrane that results in the deposition of virion components into the cytoplasm. Following delivery to the cytoplasm, capsid or tegument proteins facilitate transport through the cytoplasm to and delivery of the viral genome to the nucleus in a process known as uncoating. Tegument proteins also translocate independent of the capsid to cytoplasmic or nuclear sites. For structurally complex viruses whose envelopes contain as many as 20 proteins and glycoproteins, attachment is a multi-step process typically involving more than one envelope glycoprotein interacting with a series of cell surface receptors that serve as primary receptors and coreceptors. One consequence of these virus-cell interactions based largely on information from negative strand RNA viruses is that predicted receptor-activated conformational changes in envelope glycoproteins play roles in membrane fusion. Multiple HCMV envelope glycoproteins are required to fuse membranes. Another consequence of these initial virus-host interactions may be the formation and/or delivery of bound virions to specialized membrane domains or compartments that are optimal for fusion and for activation of signal transduction into the cell. We have also recently learned that HCMV entry is accompanied by innate immune activation. This considerably heightens the complexity of the molecular events occurring during the early events in HCMV infection.

To begin a discussion of virus entry at the cellular level, one must first consider the basis of cellular tropism since receptors involved in entry are expressed on permissive cells. In the human host, HCMV causes systemic infection and exhibits a tropism for fibroblasts, endothelial cells, epithelial cells, monocytes/macrophages, smooth muscle cells, stromal cells, neuronal cells, neutrophils, and hepatocytes (Myerson et al., 1984; Sinzger et al., 2000). This exceptionally broad cellular tropism in the infected host is the basis of HCMV disease manifestation by this opportunist in a variety of organ systems and tissue types in the immunocompromised host. HCMV is considered to have a restricted cell tropism in vitro, however, entry into target cells is very promiscuous, since HCMV is able to bind, fuse and initiate replication in all tested vertebrate cell types. Productive in vitro replication is supported by primary fibroblast, endothelial and certain differentiated myeloid cells as well as some astrocytoma lines (Ibanez et al., 1991; Nowlin et al., 1991). The ability of HCMV to enter such a wide range of cells is consistent with either one broad common receptor or a number of cell-specific multiple cell specific receptors or a complex entry pathway in which a combination of both cell specific and broadly expressed cellular receptors are utilized. By contrast, both major variants of HHV-6 and HHV-7 are predominately T-lymphotropic although HHV-6 can infect certain cells of myeloid lineage as well. HHV-7 uses CD4, a strictly T-lymphocyte expressed molecule as a receptor while HHV-6A and B use a more broadly distributed molecule CD46 as a receptor (Lusso et al., 1994; Santoro et al., 1999).

Cellular receptors for HCMV

It has been known for some time that HCMV initiates infection by binding to cell surface heparan sulfate proteoglycans (HSPGs) (Compton et al., 1991). Engagement of HSPGs is one relatively conserved feature of herpesvirus entry pathways and is also thought to play a role in HHV-6 and HHV-7 interactions with lymphoid cells (Conti et al., 2000). At least in cell culture systems, HCMV engagement of HSPGs is thought to play a crucial role in initial stage of entry by enhancing the engagement of subsequent receptors in a cascade that ultimately leads to fusion (Compton et al., 1993). This hypothesis is further supported by biochemical analysis of HCMV binding, which indicates biphasic binding properties with multiple distinct affinities (Boyle and Compton, 1998).

The ability of HCMV to bind a broad range of cell types in culture has hampered efforts to identify cellular receptors using modern molecular approaches such as expression cloning. Over the past 20 years, numerous receptor candidates have been proposed, but none has been found to be absolutely necessary for infection of all susceptible cell types. These candidate receptor molecules have been selected on the basis of solid initial criteria but none have turned out to be a general entry mediator following further investigation. It is possible that each is important only in certain cell types or tissues. It also remains possible that functional redundancy masks their individual roles.

HCMV virions were initially shown to bind β_2 microglobulin (β_2m) in urine samples (Grundy et al., 1988; McKeating et al., 1987; McKeating et al., 1986). This observation led to binding studies showing that HCMV tegument, not envelope, binds β_2m during release from cells (Grundy et al., 1987a,b; McKeating et al., 1987; Stannard, 1989). This β_2m–HCMV complex was then thought to associate with the alpha chain of host cell major histocompatibility complex (MHC) class I antigens (Beersma et al., 1990; 1991; Browne et al., 1990; Grundy et al., 1987a,b). These data led to a model in which β_2m-coated HCMV bound MHC class I molecules, displacing β_2m. However, it was later determined that β_2m expression had no correlation with in vitro entry of HCMV or in vivo spread of MCMV infectivity (Beersma et al., 1991; Polic et al., 1996; Wu et al., 1994). The demonstration that β_2m-deficient and MHC class I-deficient mice maintain full susceptiblity to MCMV infection (Polic et al., 1996) provided the last piece of evidence confounding this hypothesis.

Virus-cell overlay blots identified a cell surface protein of approximately 30 kDa whose expression correlated with cells permissive for entry, suggesting that this cellular protein may be involved in HCMV entry (Nowlin et al., 1991; Taylor and Cooper, 1990). This protein was later identified as annexin II, a protein that normally binds phospholipids and calcium and has membrane bridging capabilities (Wright et al., 1993, 1995). Annexin II found associated with HCMV virions (Wright et al., 1994, 1995). Although annexin II binds gB and enhances HCMV binding and fusion to phospholipid-containing membranes (Pietropaolo and Compton, 1997; Raynor et al., 1999), cells devoid of annexin II are fully permissive for entry and initiation of infection (Pietropaolo and Compton, 1999). The role, if any, for annexin II in HCMV entry remains unknown but this protein's membrane bridging activity may enhance entry, cell–cell spread and/or maturation and egress.

CD13, or human aminopeptidase N, is a glycosylphosphatidylinositol-linked membrane protein that has also been implicated as a receptor. This hypothesis was based on that fact only human peripheral blood mononuclear cells (PBMCs) that were CD13 positive supported productive infection (Larsson et al., 1998; Soderberg et al., 1993a,b). This led to a more thorough study of this possibility in which CD13-specific antibodies, and chemical inhibitors of CD13 activity were both shown to inhibit HCMV binding and entry (Soderberg et al., 1993a). Excitement from this report was dampened by later reports that CD13 antibodies bind to and neutralize virus before contact with cells and by the fact that entry of HCMV into CD13 depleted cells remains normal (Giugni et al., 1996). More recently, an interaction between HCMV and CD13 was shown to be important in inhibition of differentiation of monocytes into macrophages suggesting this may be a strategy for interference with cellular differentiation pathways (Gredmark et al., 2004).

A consideration of HCMV-induced signaling cascades led Huang and colleagues to hypothesize a role for epidermal growth factor receptor (EGFR) as a HCMV receptor (Wang et al., 2003). EGFR was reported to be phosphorylated in response to HCMV and this phosphorylation event correlated with the activation of phosphatidylinositol 3-kinase (PI-3 kinase) and Akt, as well as the mobilization of intracellular Ca^{2+}. These signaling events were blocked in the presence of EGFR antibodies. In addition, chemically cross-linked virus provided evidence for a gB–EGFR interaction. A limitation of the study, however was that there was no experimental evidence that EGFR functioned in entry *per se* nor was it determined whether EGFR was required for the delivery of virion components across the plasma membrane. Also, conflicting results exist in the literature. Fairley and colleagues demonstrated that HCMV promoted inactivation of EGFR phosphorylation and signaling (Fairley *et al.*, 2002). In these experiments, EGFR polyclonal antibodies had no effect on HCMV entry (Soderberg *et al.*, 1993a). It is important to note that EGFR is not expressed on all HCMV susceptible cells, such as those of a hematopoeitic lineage.

Finally, an anti-idiotype antibody to viral envelope glycoprotein H (gH), identified a phosphorylated 92.5kDa cell surface glycoprotein that may be involved in the steps that follow attachment (Keay and Baldwin, 1991, 1992, 1996; Keay *et al.*, 1989, 1995). Combined, the study of HCMV entry receptors, like studies aimed at identifying entry mediators in other herpesviruses, include reports that cannot be reconciled with the ability of this virus to enter and uncoat in a broad range of cell types without invoking functional redundancy. There is continued need for data confirmation as well as further functional investigation of all receptor candidates.

Entry activated cell signaling

The first and foremost observation about HCMV biology was its namesake characteristic, cytomegaly, or cell enlargement. In vitro studies initially demonstrated a unique cytopathogenic effect (CPE) of infected cells, with HCMV infected cells appearing rounded and developing an enlarged appearance with both intracellular and intranuclear inclusion bodies late during infection (Albrecht and Weller, 1980). Infection proceeded with two waves of cell rounding, the first beginning as early as a few hours postinfection and corresponding to the impact of entry, and another starting at approximately 24 hours postinfection, when there is a distinct peak in cellular transcription and translation. The cause of this phenomenon was widely speculated upon however, and theories for HCMV-induced cell rounding included cation influx, suppression of fibronectin synthesis and integrin down-regulation (Albrecht *et al.*, 1983; Albrecht and Weller, 1980; Ihara *et al.*, 1982; Warren *et al.*, 1994).

It has been apparent for many years that cells respond to HCMV virions by activation of numerous cell signaling pathways including changes in Ca^{2+} homeostasis, activation of phospholipases C and A2, as well as increased release of arachidonic acid and its metabolites (for review, see Fortunato *et al.*, 2000). All of these changes can be triggered by UV-inactivated virions (Boldogh *et al.*, 1990, 1991b), suggesting that structural components of the virus are responsible for activation during virus–cell contact and/or virus entry. Virus–cell contact also results in the activation of transcription factors such as cfos/jun, myc, NF-κB, SP-1, as well as phosphatidylinositol 3-kinase (PI3-kinase) and mitogen-activated protein (MAP) kinases ERK1/2 and p38 (Boyle *et al.*, 1999; Kowalik *et al.*, 1993; Yurochko *et al.*, 1995, 1997; Boldogh *et al.*, 1991a; Johnson *et al.*, 2001)). These virally induced cellular physiological changes are associated with a profound effect on host cell gene expression. The levels of hundreds of host cell transcripts are altered within a few hours after exposure to virus, virus particles or soluble gB (Browne *et al.*, 2001; Simmen *et al.*, 2001; Zhu *et al.*, 1998). Thus, transcriptional changes immediately after infection do not reflect viral gene expression. These data are consistent with the interpretation that HCMV engages a cellular receptor(s) that activate signal transduction pathways culminating in reprogramming of cellular transcription.

Cellular integrins may serve as coreceptors for betaherpesviruses

Cellular integrins are ubiquitously expressed cell surface receptors that, when activated, lead to major reorganization of the cytoskeleton. Integrins exist on the plasma membrane as non-covalently linked heterodimers consisting of an α- and a β-subunit, which convey specificity in cell–cell and cell–ECM (extracellular matrix) attachment, immune cell recruitment, extravasation, and signaling (Berman and Kozlova, 2000; Berman *et al.*, 2003; Cary *et al.*, 1999). In addition, integrins have emerged as receptors for a broad range of pathogens and mediate binding of plant spores, bacteria and viruses. Feire *et al.* (2004) investigated the role that integrins play in the HCMV entry pathway. Analysis of the effects of various neutralizing antibodies implicated α2β1, α6β1, and αVβ3 integrins in entry (Feire *et al.*, 2004). Furthermore, cells devoid of β1 integrin exhibited dramatically reduced susceptibility to infection with HCMV or MCMV while entry and spread were restored when the expression of β1 integrin was re-introduced into cells. Integrin-blocking antibodies did not prevent virus attachment but specifically inhibited the delivery of a virion component, pp65, into cells suggesting that integrins function at a post-attachment stage of infection, possibly at the level of membrane fusion. The involvement of multiple integrin heterodimers is consistent with integrin biology in that many natural integrin ligands, such as extracellular matrix proteins, bind to a variety of heterodimers. Furthermore, other integrin-binding viruses are characterizd by binding to a number of different integrin heterodimers (Stewart et al., 2003).

Integrins are capable of engaging ligands through a number of identified ECM protein motifs, the most common of which contain the amino acid sequence RGD. However, there are a number of RGD-independent integrin binding motifs, including the disintegrin domain proteins of the A Disintegrin and A Metalloprotease (ADAM) family of proteins. After inspection of all HCMV structural glycoproteins, the strongest homology to an integrin-binding domain was a disintegrin-like consensus sequence (RX_{5-7} DLXXF/L) (Eto et al., 2002; Stone et al., 1999; Wolfsberg et al., 1995) on the amino-terminus of gB. Sequence alignments confirmed that the gB disintegrin loop was more than 98% identical among 44 clinical isolates analyzed. The role of this sequence in entry was confirmed through the use of synthetic peptides that inhibited both HCMV and MCMV entry, but had no impact on entry of HSV, correlating with the lack of a disintegrin-loop in gB of this virus. Furthermore, the HCMV gB disintegrin-loop was conserved throughout much of the gamma and all of the betaherpesvirus subfamilies, but not in the alphaherpesvirus subfamily where previously identified RGD sequences appear to carry out interactions with integrins. The presence of integrin-binding sequences among conserved herpesvirus glycoproteins strongly suggests that integrins may be important for entry and signaling throughout this medically important family. EGFR has also been shown to become phosphorylated and signal indirectly, as a result of integrin activation through src family kinases or focal adhesion kinase (FAK) (Jones et al., 1997; Miyamoto et al., 1996; Moro et al., 1998). Future work will no doubt be aimed at an analysis of the integrin-triggered signaling events and defining their roles in entry and infection.

Activation of innate immunity during entry

The cellular response to HCMV particles includes dramatic upregulation of interferon stimulated genes, including interferon β itself and inflammatory cytokines; indicators of host innate immunity (Browne et al., 2001; Simmen et al., 2001; Zhu et al., 1998; Yurochko and Huang, 1999). Toll-like receptors (TLRs) are ancient, conserved, pathogen sensors now well appreciated to activate signal transduction pathways that lead to induction of antimicrobial/antiviral genes and inflammatory cytokines (Akira, 2001). Until recently, however, TLRs were not known to recognize virus particles. To date, members of the herpesvirus, retrovirus and paramyxovirus families have been shown to be subject to innate sensing by TLRs (Compton et al., 2003; Haynes et al., 2001; Kurt-Jones et al., 2000; Rassa et al., 2002). In particular, TLR2 on PBMCs recognize HCMV particles or virus in a comparable manner, suggesting that binding and/or entry events involve the activation of this receptor. Soluble gB is able to induce a similar pattern of innate immune gene expression and can induce an antiviral state in cells (Boehme et al., 2004; Boyle, Pietropaolo and Compton, 1999). Another envelope glycoprotein (gH) activates cells (Yurochko et al., 1997) and the gH/gI/gO complex may contribute to a pattern of innate immune activation as a component of entry (Netterwald et al., 2004), Guerrero M. and T. Compton, unpublished observations). TLR2 stimulation results in activation of NF-κB and stimulation of inflammatory cytokine production (Compton et al., 2003). A common theme has emerged implicating viral envelope glycoprotein as a specific molecular trigger for TLR activation and that viral gene expression is not required (Boehme and Compton, 2004). These studies suggest a heretofore-unknown host cell response that detects viruses during entry, prior to the onset of replication events and products such as double stranded RNA that have long been recognized as TLR ligands (Boehme and Compton, 2004). Innate sensing of viruses during entry does not result in signaling that is essential to viral replication and appears more important as a determinant of the host cell response. The interaction of envelope glycoprotein and TLR suggests that entry and innate sensing may be coordinated in some manner.

Roles of betaherpesvirus envelope glycoproteins in virus entry

The HCMV envelope is exceedingly complex and currently incompletely defined. The HCMV genome encodes ORFs to at least 57 putative glycoproteins; far more than other herpesviruses, however, the extent of transcription, translation and function of the majority of these glycoproteins remains unknown. Biochemical studies of HCMV virions have revealed that 14 structural glycoproteins; eight of which have been experimentally shown to reside in the envelope (Britt et al., 2004). HCMV appears to rely on herpesvirus-common homologues for entry. These include herpesvirus-common gene products gB and gH as well as glycoproteins L (gL), O (gO), M (gM), and N (gN). A number of other structural glycoproteins (gpTRL10, gpTRL11, gpTRL12 and gpUL132, gpUS28) are HCMV-specific (Table 16.1) but so far have no role in entry.

For years, the large genome and complicated reverse genetics system have made the creation of HCMV knockout and mutant viruses difficult. Recently, a system capable of such mutations was developed whereby HCMV is

Table 16.1. Envelope proteins of CMV

ORF	Protein name	Essential	Complex partner	Role in entry
UL4	gpUL4; gp48	No	None known	None known
UL33	UL33	No	None known	None known
UL55	gB	Yes	None known	Receptor binding, fusion, Signal transduction Innate immune activation
UL73	gN	Yes	UL100; gM	None known
UL74	gO	Moderate defect in cell to cell spread	UL75;gH UL115; gL	Enhancer of cell–cell spread
UL75	gH	Yes	UL74;gO UL115;gL	Fusion, receptor binding (?)Innate immune activation
UL100	gM	Yes	UL73;gN	HSPG binding
UL115	gL	Yes	UL75;gH UL74;gO	Required for gH activity
TRL10	gpTRL10	Not determined	None known	None known
TLR12	gpTRL12	Not determined	None known	None known
US27	gpUS27	No	None known	None known
US28	gpUS28	No	None known	None known

maintained as an infectious bacterial artificial chromosome (BAC) within *Escherichia coli* (Borst *et al.*, 1999). This development has greatly hastened the process of mutating individual ORFs and will generate much information regarding both the structure and function of many envelope glycoproteins. In fact, the BAC system has demonstrated the requirement for several glycoprotein genes in the production of replication competent virus (Dunn *et al.*, 2003; Hobom *et al.*, 2000; Yu *et al.*, 2002). The HCMV glycoprotein homologues gB, gM, gN, gH, gL, have been shown to be essential for growth, while gO knockout virus remained viable with a small plaque phenotype (Hobom *et al.*, 2000). Genes for all the currently identified HCMV-specific envelope glycoproteins, including UL4 (gp48), TRL10 (gpTRL10), TRL11 (gpTRL11), TRL12 (gpTRL12), US27, UL33, UL132, have been shown to be dispensable for replication and therefore are not critical for entry (Dunn *et al.*, 2003). The HCMV-encoded chemokine receptor US28 is present in the virion envelope and has been shown to promote cell–cell fusion mediated by HIV and VSV viral proteins, however the gene has been shown to be non-essential and there is no evidence for a role for gpUS28 in either HCMV–cell or cell–cell fusion events (Dunn *et al.*, 2003; Pleskoff *et al.*, 1997, 1998).

Essential and abundant HCMV envelope glycoproteins conserved throughout the herpesviruses (including gB and gH:gL) were classified as distinct disulfide-linked high molecular weight complexes (gCI and gCIII) in HCMV-infected cells (Gretch *et al.*, 1988). The gCI complex is composed of homodimers of gB (Britt, 1984; Britt and Auger, 1986) and the gCIII complex is a heterotrimeric complex composed of gH, gL, and gO (Huber and Compton, 1997, 1998; Li *et al.*, 1997). The designation gCII has been applied to a heterodimeric complex composed of gM and gN (Mach *et al.*, 2000).

At least two glycoprotein complexes have heparan sulfate proteoglycan (HSPG) binding ability, gB and the gM component of the gM:gN complex, suggesting a critical role for cell surface proteoglycan in initial virus:cell contact (Carlson *et al.*, 1997; Kari and Gehrz, 1993). Heparin binding is a property that HCMV shares with other herpesviruses, and gB is the common glycoprotein involved in this activity. HCMV gB also appears to be the primary receptor binding protein. Soluble forms of gB exhibit biphasic binding properties and cells treated with gB are refractory to infection suggesting that gB ties up critical receptor sites used by the virus (Boyle and Compton, 1998). One of the binding sites for gB is HSPGs in that cells lacking HSPGs had a single component Scatchard plot as compared to a biphasic plot for HSPG bearing cells. As noted above, it now seems clear that a second binding partner is an integrin (Feire *et al.*, 2004) but much work remains to formally prove the disintegrin hypothesis and confirm the role of this domain in receptor engagement. The gB protein may also engage EGFR (Wang *et al.*, 2003), at least in certain cell types, however it is not yet known if this interaction requires initial interaction with integrin. The gH complex may also have a distinct receptor. Syngeneic monoclonal anti-idiotypic antibodies were created that bear the "image" of this glycoprotein complex (Keay *et al.*, 1988) and led to a putative gH receptor (Keay and Baldwin, 1989, 1991, 1992, 1996). These investigations relied heavily on a single reagent (anti-idiotypic antibodies) and has led to only a partially sequenced receptor clone, lacking homology to known human proteins (Baldwin et al., 2000; Keay and Baldwin, 1996). Thus, the identity of a HCMV gH/gL/gO receptor remains unknown. Since HCMV gH and gL are essential and infectivity can be neutralized with gH antibodies, anti-idiotypic antibodies can neutralize infectivity and the closest relative of HCMV, HHV-6, contains an analogous complex consisting of the herpesvirus-common gH and gL with the product of U100 (gQ), a complex that has been shown to interact with a candidate receptor (Santoro et al., 1999). HHV-6 U47 is the homolog of HCMV UL74 (gO), and is also involved in complex formation.

Membrane fusion remains a poorly understood component of entry for any of the herpesviruses. Unlike orthomyxoviruses, paramyxoviruses, filoviruses and retroviruses that employ a single envelope glycoprotein for membrane fusion, herpesviruses appear to employ multicomponent fusion machines, with evidence that these consist of gB, gH and gL (Spear and Longnecker, 2003). Both the HCMV gB- and gH-dependent entry processes are susceptible to inhibition by neutralizing antibodies that block infection at a postattachment stage of entry, presumably at the level fusion (Bold et al., 1996; Britt, 1984; Keay and Baldwin, 1991; Tugizov et al., 1994; Utz et al., 1989). One limitation of these conclusions, however, is the lack of a direct fusion assay and thus a role for these glycoproteins in fusion is inferred. Despite the complexity of multicomponent fusion machines, it is very likely that there are strong parallels to single component fusion proteins. Alpha helical coiled-coils critical structural domains involved in fusion that function to drive the energetic folding of membranes together. Conformational changes in fusogenic proteins bearing these coiled-coils are also a defining paradigm. Using an algorithm to detect potential structural motifs, Lopper and Compton identified heptad repeat regions in gB and gH that were predicted to form alpha helical coiled coils (Lopper and Compton, 2004). Synthetic peptides to these motifs substantially inhibit HCMV entry including virion content delivery suggesting that these motifs play a fundamental role in membrane fusion. Genetic analysis of these motifs in the context of HCMV virions will be required to further analyze the importance of alpha helical coiled coils in HCMV entry. Another fundamental question will be to determine if the gB integrin interaction is a trigger of conformational change that leads to exposure of membrane fusion domains. Intriguingly, disintegrin-bearing cellular proteins in the ADAM family are known to trigger fusion via integrin interaction in a variety of processes including sperm–egg fusion and myoblast fusion (White, 2003). Development of a reliable fusion assay is also greatly needed to begin a dissection of the biophysical properties of HCMV fusion glycoproteins.

Coordination of entry and innate immune activation

We are left with an apparent dichotomy. As HCMV enters cells to establish infection, the host recognizes the virions and activates innate immune responses. How are the two processes coordinated, or are they coordinated at all? At this time, there is no apparent role for TLRs in entry in that cell stimulation that follows this event does not contribute to replication efficiency in any observable way. It seems more likely that this is a component of the entry process where the host cell senses a pathogen-associated molecular pattern displayed on HCMV envelope glycoproteins and uses this activatation to initiate a host innate defense response. One possibility is that entry receptors such as EGFR, integrins and signaling machinery, and innate immunity sensors such as TRLs, cytoplasmic adaptors and signaling machinery, coalesce into specialized membrane microdomains with integrins playing a central ligating role. Concentration of all of these cell surface receptors into a defined platform likely facilitates cell signaling events, some of which are optimal for replication and others of which are clearly hostile to the virus. Intriguingly integrins associate with TLR2 and partition into cholesterol rich lipid rafts (Ogawa et al., 2002; Triantafilou et al., 2002). The complexity of events at the cell surface during the initial encounter of HCMV and cells represents an exciting opportunity to better understand the molecular underpinnings of the early virus-host interactions. The recent identification of cell surface molecules involved in the early steps in infection has greatly enhanced our knowledge of entry events in infection. Yet much remains to be done to elucidate aspects of mechanism of entry events and the corresponding innate immune activation.

REFERENCES

Akira, S. (2001). Toll-like receptors and innate immunity. *Adv. Immunol.*, **78**, 1–56.

Albrecht, T. and Weller, T. H. (1980). Heterogeneous morphologic features of plaques induced by five strains of human cytomegalovirus. *Am. J. Clin. Pathol.*, **73**(5), 648–654.

Albrecht, T., Speelman, D. J., and Steinsland, O. S. (1983). Similarities between cytomegalovirus-induced cell rounding and contraction of smooth muscle cells. *Life Sci.*, **32**(19), 2273–2278.

Baldwin, B. R., Zhang, C., and Keay, S. (2000). Cloning and epitope mapping of a functional partial fusion receptor for human cytomegalovirus gH. *J. Gen. Virol.*, **81**, 27–35.

Beersma, M. F., Wertheim, van, D. P., and Feltkamp, T. E. (1990). The influence of HLA-B27 on the infectivity of cytomegalovirus for mouse fibroblasts. *Scand. J. Rheumatol. Suppl.*, **87**(102), 102–103.

Beersma, M. F., Wertheim, van, D. P., Geelen, J. L., and Feltkamp, T. E. (1991). Expression of HLA class I heavy chains and beta 2-microglobulin does not affect human cytomegalovirus infectivity. *J. Gen. Virol.*, **72**, 2757–2764.

Berman, A. E. and Kozlova, N. I. (2000). Integrins: structure and functions. *Membr. Cell Biol.*, **13**(2), 207–244.

Berman, A. E., Kozlova, N. I., and Morozevich, G. E. (2003). Integrins: structure and signaling. *Biochemistry (Mosc).*, **68**(12), 1284–1299.

Boehme, K. and Compton, T. (2004). Innate sensing of viruses by toll-like receptors. *J. Virol.*, **78**, 7867–7873.

Boehme, K. W., Singh, J., Perry, S. T., and Compton, T. (2004). Human cytomegalovirus elicits a coordinated cellular antiviral response via envelope glycoprotein B. *J. Virol.*, **78**(3), 1202–1211.

Bold, S., Ohlin, M., Garten, W., and Radsak, K. (1996). Structural domains involved in human cytomegalovirus glycoprotein B-mediated cell–cell fusion. *J. Gen. Virol.*, **77**, 2297–2302.

Boldogh, I., AbuBakar, S., and Albrecht, T. (1990). Activation of proto-oncogenes: an immediate early event in human cytomegalovirus infection. *Science*, **247**, 561–564.

Boldogh, I., AbuBakar, S., Deng, C. Z., and Albrecht, T. (1991a). Transcriptional activation of cellular oncogenes fos, jun, and myc by human cytomegalovirus. *J. Virol.*, **65**(3), 1568–1571.

Boldogh, I., AbuBakar, S., Millinoff, D., Deng, C. Z., and Albrecht, T. (1991b). Cellular oncogene activation by human cytomegalovirus. Lack of correlation with virus infectivity and immediate early gene expression. *Arch. Virol.*, **118**, 163–177.

Borst, E. M., Hahn, G., Koszinowski, U. H., and Messerle, M. (1999). Cloning of the human cytomegalovirus (HCMV) genome as an infectious bacterial artificial chromosome in *Escherichia coli*: a new approach for construction of HCMV mutants. *J. Virol.*, **73**(10), 8320–8329.

Boyle, K. A. and Compton, T. (1998). Receptor-binding properties of a soluble form of human cytomegalovirus glycoprotein B. *J. Virol.*, **72**, 1826–1833.

Boyle, K. A., Pietropaolo, R. L., and Compton, T. (1999). Engagement of the cellular receptor for glycoprotein B of human cytomegalovirus activates the interferon-responsive pathway. *Mol. Cell Biol.* **19**, 3607–3713.

Britt, W. J. (1984). Neutralizing antibodies detect a disulfide-linked glycoprotein complex within the envelope of human cytomegalovirus. *Virology*, **135**, 369–378.

Britt, W. J. and Auger, D. (1986). Human cytomegalovirus virion-associated protein with kinase activity. *J. Virol.*, **59**(1), 185–188.

Britt, W. J., Jarvis, M., Seo, J. Y., Drummond, D., and Nelson, J. (2004). Rapid genetic engineering of human cytomegalovirus by using a lambda phage linear recombination system: demonstration that pp28 (UL99) is essential for production of infectious virus. *J. Virol.*, **78**(1), 539–543.

Browne, E. P., Wing, B., Coleman, D., and Shenk, T. (2001). Altered cellular mRNA levels in human cytomegalovirus-infected fibroblasts: viral block to the accumulation of antiviral mRNAs. *J. Virol.*, **75**(24), 12319–12330.

Browne, H., Smith, G., Beck, S., and Minson, T. (1990). A complex between the MHC class I homologue encoded by human cytomegalovirus and beta 2 microglobulin. *Nature*, **347**(6295), 770–772.

Carlson, C., Britt, W. J., and Compton, T. (1997). Expression, purification and characterization of a soluble form of human cytomegalovirus glycoprotein B. *Virology*, **239**, 198–205.

Cary, L. A., Han, D. C., and Guan, J. L. (1999). Integrin-mediated signal transduction pathways. *Histol. Histopathol.*, **14**(3), 1001–1009.

Compton, T., Nowlin, D. M., and Cooper, N. R. (1993). Initiation of human cytomegalovirus infection requires initial interaction with cell surface heparan sulfate. *Virology*, **193**(2), 834–841.

Compton, T., Kurt-Jones, E. A., Boehme, K. W. *et al.* (2003). Human cytomegalovirus activates inflammatory cytokine responses via CD14 and Toll-like receptor 2. *J. Virol.*, **77**(8), 4588–4596.

Conti, C., Cirone, M., Sgro, R., Altieri, F., Zompetta, C., and Faggioni, A. (2000). Early interactions of human herpesvirus 6 with lymphoid cells: role of membrane protein components and glycosaminoglycans in virus binding. *J. Med. Virol.*, **62**(4), 487–497.

Dunn, W., Chou, C., Li, H., Hai, R., Patterson, D., Stolc, V., Zhu, H., and Liu, F. (2003). Functional profiling of a human cytomegalovirus genome. *Proc. Natl Acad. Sci. USA*, **100**(24), 14223–14228.

Eto, K., Huet, C., Tarui, T. *et al.* (2002). Functional classification of ADAMs based on a conserved motif for binding to integrin alpha 9beta 1: implications for sperm–egg binding and other cell interactions. *J. Biol. Chem.*, **277**(20), 17804–17810.

Fairley, J. A., Baillie, J., Bain, M., and Sinclair, J. H. (2002). Human cytomegalovirus infection inhibits epidermal growth factor (EGF) signalling by targeting EGF receptors. *J. Gen. Virol.*, **83**(11), 2803–2810.

Feire, A. L., Koss, H., and Compton, T. (2004). Cellular integrins function as entry receptors for human cytomegalovirus via a highly conserved disintegrin-like domain. *Proc. Natl Acad. Sci. USA*, **101**(43), 15470–15475.

Fortunato, E. A., McElroy, A. K., Sanchez, I., and Spector, D. H. (2000). Exploitation of cellular signaling and regulatory pathways by human cytomegalovirus. *Trends Microbiol.*, **8**(3), 111–119.

Giugni, T. D., Soderberg, C., Ham, D. J. *et al.* (1996). Neutralization of human cytomegalovirus by human CD13-specific antibodies. *J. Infect. Dis.*, **173**(5), 1062–1071.

Gredmark, S., Britt, W. B., Xie, X., Lindbom, L., and Soderberg-Naucler, C. (2004). Human cytomegalovirus induces inhibition of macrophage differentiation by binding to human aminopeptidase N/CD13. *J. Immunol.*, **173**(8), 4897–4907.

Gretch, D. R., Kari, B., Rasmussen, L., Gehrz, R. C., and Stinski, M. F. (1988). Identification and characterization of three distinct families of glycoprotein complexes in the envelopes of human cytomegalovirus. *J. Virol.*, **62**(3), 875–881.

Grundy, J. E., McKeating, J. A., and Griffiths, P. D. (1987a). Cytomegalovirus strain AD169 binds beta 2 microglobulin in vitro after release from cells. *J. Gen. Virol.*, **68**, 777–784.

Grundy, J. E., McKeating, J. A., Ward, P. J., Sanderson, A. R., and Griffiths, P. D. (1987b). Beta 2 microglobulin enhances the infectivity of cytomegalovirus and when bound to the virus enables class I HLA molecules to be used as a virus receptor. *J. Gen. Virol.*, **68**, 793–803.

Grundy, J. E., McKeating, J. A., Sanderson, A. R., and Griffiths, P. D. (1988). Cytomegalovirus and beta 2 microglobulin in urine specimens. Reciprocal interference in their detection is responsible for artifactually high levels of urinary beta 2 microglobulin in infected transplant recipients. *Transplantation*, **45**(6), 1075–1079.

Haynes, L. M., Moore, D. D., Kurt-Jones, E. A., Finberg, R. W., Anderson, L. J., and Tripp, R. A. (2001). Involvement of toll-like receptor 4 in innate immunity to respiratory syncytial virus. *J. Virol.*, **75**(22), 10730–10737.

Hobom, U., Brune, W., Messerle, M., Hahn., G., and Koszinowski, U. (2000). Fast screening procedures for random transposon libraries of cloned herpesvirus genomes: mutational analysis of human cytomegalovirus envelope glycoprotein genes. *J. Virol.*, **74**(17), 7720–7729.

Huber, M. T. and Compton, T. (1997). Characterization of a novel third member of the human cytomegalovirus glycoprotein H-glycoprotein L complex. *J. Virol.*, **71**, 5391–5398.

Huber, M. T. and Compton, T. (1998). The human cytomegalovirus UL74 gene encodes the third component of the glycoprotein H-glycoprotein L-containing envelope complex. *J. Virol.*, **72**(10), 8191–8197.

Ibanez, C. E., Schrier, R., Ghazal, P., Wiley, C., and Nelson, J. A. (1991). Human cytomegalovirus productively infects primary differentiated macrophages. *J. Virol.*, **65**(12), 6581–6588.

Ihara, S., Saito, S., and Watanabe, Y. (1982). Suppression of fibronectin synthesis by an early function(s) of human cytomegalovirus. *J. Gen. Virol.*, **59**(2), 409–413.

Johnson, R. A., Wang, X., Ma, X. L., Huong, S. M., and Huang, E. S. (2001) Human cytomegalovirus upregulates the phosphatidylinositol 3-kinase (PI3-K) pathway: inhibition of PI3-K activity inhibits replication and virus-induced signalling. *J. Virol.*, **75**, 6022–6032,

Jones, P. L., Crack, J., and Rabinovitch, M. (1997). Regulation of tenascin-C, a vascular smooth muscle cell survival factor that interacts with the alpha v beta 3 integrin to promote epidermal growth factor receptor phosphorylation and growth. *J. Cell Biol.*, **139**(1), 279–293.

Kari, B. and Gehrz, R. (1993). Structure, composition and heparin binding properties of a human cytomegalovirus glycoprotein complex designated gC-II. *J. Gen. Virol.*, **74**(2), 255–264.

Keay, S. and Baldwin, B. (1991). Anti-idiotype antibodies that mimic gp86 of human cytomegalovirus inhibit viral fusion but not attachment. *J. Virol.*, **65**(9), 5124–5128.

Keay, S. and Baldwin, B. (1992). The human fibroblast receptor for gp86 of human cytomegalovirus is a phosphorylated glycoprotein. *J. Virol.*, **66**(8), 4834–4838.

Keay, S. and Baldwin, B. R. (1996). Evidence for the role of cell protein phosphorylation in human cytomegalovirus/host cell fusion. *J. Gen. Virol.*, **77**(10), 2597–2604.

Keay, S., Rasmussen, L., and Merigan, T. C. (1988). Syngeneic monoclonal anti-idiotype antibodies that bear the internal image of a human cytomegalovirus neutralization epitope. *J. Immunol.*, **140**(3), 944–948.

Keay, S., Merigan, T. C., and Rasmussen, L. (1989). Identification of cell surface receptors for the 86-kilodalton glycoprotein of human cytomegalovirus. *Proc. Natl Acad. Sci. USA*, **86**(24), 10100–10103.

Keay, S., Baldwin, B. R., Smith, M. W., Wasserman, S. S., and Goldman, W. F. (1995). Increases in $[Ca^{2+}]_i$ mediated by the 92.5-kDa putative cell membrane receptor for HCMV gp86. *Am. J. Physiol.*, **269**(1 Pt 1), C11–21.

Kowalik, T. F., Wing, B., Haskill, J. S., Azizkhan, J. C., Baldwin, A. S., Jr., and Huang, E. S. (1993). Multiple mechanisms are implicated in the regulation of NF-kappa B activity during human cytomegalovirus infection. *Proc. Natl Acad. Sci. USA*, **90**(3), 1107–1111.

Kurt-Jones, E. A., Popova, L., Kwinn, L. *et al.* (2000). Pattern recognition receptors TLR4 and CD14 mediate response to respiratory syncytial virus. *Nat. Immunol.*, **1**(5), 398–401.

Larsson, S., Soderberg-Naucler, C., Wang, F. Z., and Moller, E. (1998). Cytomegalovirus DNA can be detected in peripheral blood mononuclear cells from all seropositive and most seronegative healthy blood donors over time. *Transfusion*, **38**(3), 271–278.

Li, L., Nelson, J. A., and Britt, W. J. (1997). Glycoprotein H-related complexes of human cytomegalovirus: identification of a third protein in the gCIII complex. *J. Virol.*, **71**, 3090–3097.

Lopper, M. and Compton, T. (2004). Coiled-coil domains in glycoproteins B and H are involved in human cytomegalovirus membrane fusion. *J. Virol.*, **78**(15), 8333–8341.

Lusso, P., Secchiero, P., Crowley, R. W., Garzino-Demo, A., Berneman, Z. N., and Gallo, R. C. (1994). CD4 is a critical component of the receptor for human herpesvirus 7: interference with human immunodeficiency virus. *Proc. Natl Acad. Sci. USA*, **91**(9), 3872–3876.

Mach, M., Kropff, B., Dal Monte, P., and Britt, W. (2000). Complex formation by human cytomegalovirus glycoproteins M (gpUL100) and N (gpUL73). *J. Virol.*, **74**(24), 11881–11892.

McKeating, J. A., Grundy, J. E., Varghese, Z., and Griffiths, P. D. (1986). Detection of cytomegalovirus by ELISA in urine samples is inhibited by beta 2 microglobulin. *J. Med. Virol.*, **18**(4), 341–348.

McKeating, J. A., Griffiths, P. D., and Grundy, J. E. (1987). Cytomegalovirus in urine specimens has host beta 2 microglobulin bound to the viral envelope: a mechanism of evading the host immune response? *J. Gen. Virol.*, **68**, 785–792.

Miyamoto, S., Teramoto, H., Gutkind, J. S., and Yamada, K. M. (1996). Integrins can collaborate with growth factors for phosphorylation of receptor tyrosine kinases and MAP kinase activation: roles of integrin aggregation and occupancy of receptors. *J. Cell Biol.*, **135**(6 Pt 1), 1633–1642.

Moro, L., Venturino, M., Bozzo, C. *et al.* (1998). Integrins induce activation of EGF receptor: role in MAP kinase induction and adhesion-dependent cell survival. *EMBO J.*, **17**(22), 6622–6632.

Myerson, D., Hackman, R. C., Nelson, J. A., Ward, D. C., and McDougall, J. K. (1984). Widespread presence of histologically occult cytomegalovirus. *Hum. Pathol.*, **15**(5), 430–439.

Netterwald, J. R., Jones, T. R., Britt, W. J., Yang, S. J., McCrone, I. P., and Zhu, H. (2004). Postattachment events associated with viral entry are necessary for induction of interferon-stimulated genes by human cytomegalovirus. *J. Virol.*, **78**(12), 6688–6691.

Nowlin, D. M., Cooper, N. R., and Compton, T. (1991). Expression of a human cytomegalovirus receptor correlates with infectibility of cells. *J. Virol.*, **65**(6), 3114–3121.

Ogawa, T., Asai, Y., Hashimoto, M., and Uchida, H. (2002). Bacterial fimbriae activate human peripheral blood monocytes utilizing TLR2, CD14 and CD11a/CD18 as cellular receptors. *Eur. J. Immunol.*, **32**(9), 2543–2550.

Pietropaolo, R. and Compton, T. (1997). Direct interaction between human cytomegalovirus glycoprotein B and cellular annexin II. *J. Virol.*, **71**, 9803–9807.

Pietropaolo, R. and Compton, T. (1999). Interference with annexin II has no effect on entry of human cytomegalovirus into fibroblast cells. *J. Gen. Virol.*, **80**(7), 1807–1816.

Pleskoff, O., Treboute, C., Brelot, A., Heveker, N., Seman, M., and Alizon, M. (1997). Identification of a chemokine receptor encoded by human cytomegalovirus as a cofactor for HIV-1 entry. *Science*, **276**(5320), 1874–1878.

Pleskoff, O., Treboute, C., and Alizon, M. (1998). The cytomegalovirus-encoded chemokine receptor US28 can enhance cell–cell fusion mediated by different viral proteins. *J. Virol.*, **72**(8), 6389–6397.

Polic, B., Jonjic, S., Pavic, I. *et al.* (1996). Lack of MHC class I complex expression has no effect on spread and control of cytomegalovirus infection in vivo. *J. Gen. Virol.*, **77**(2), 217–225.

Rassa, J. C., Meyers, J. L., Zhang, Y., Kudaravalli, R., and Ross, S. R. (2002). Murine retroviruses activate B cells via interaction with toll-like receptor 4. *Proc. Natl Acad. Sci. USA*, **99**(4), 2281–2286.

Raynor, C. M., Wright, J. F., Waisman, D. M., and Pryzdial, E. L. (1999). Annexin II enhances cytomegalovirus binding and fusion to phospholipid membranes. *Biochemistry*, **38**(16), 5089–5095.

Santoro, F., Kennedy, P. E., Locatelli, G., Malnati, M. S., Berger, E. A., and Lusso, P. (1999). CD46 is a cellular receptor for human herpesvirus 6. *Cell*, **99**(7), 817–827.

Simmen, K. A., Singh, J., Luukkonen, B. G., Lopper, M., Bittner, A., Miller, N. E., Jackson, M. R., Compton, T., and Fruh, K. (2001). Global modulation of cellular transcription by human cytomegalovirus is initiated by viral glycoprotein B. *Proc. Natl Acad. Sci. USA*, **98**(13), 7140–7145.

Sinzger, C., Kahl, M., Laib, K. *et al.* (2000). Tropism of human cytomegalovirus for endothelial cells is determined by a postentry step dependent on efficient translocation to the nucleus. *J. Gen. Virol.*, **81**(12), 3021–3035.

Soderberg, C., Giugni, T. D., Zaia, J. A., Larsson, S., Wahlberg, J. M., and Moller, E. (1993a). CD13 (human aminopeptidase-N) mediates human cytomegalovirus infection. *J. Virol.*, **67**(11), 6576–6585.

Soderberg, C., Larsson, S., Bergstedtlindqvist, S., and Moller, E. (1993b). Definition of a subset of human peripheral blood mononuclear cells that are permissive to human cytomegalovirus infection. *J. Virol.*, **67**(6), 3166–3175.

Spear, P. G. and Longnecker, R. (2003). Herpesvirus entry: an update. *J. Virol.*, **77**(19), 10179–10185.

Stannard, L. M. (1989). Beta 2 microglobulin binds to the tegument of cytomegalovirus: an immunogold study. *J. Gen. Virol.*, **70**, 2179–2184.

Stewart, P. L., Dermody, T. S., and Nemerow, G. R. (2003). Structural basis for nonenveloped virus entry. *Adv. Protein Chem.*, **64**, 455–491.

Stone, A. L., Kroeger, M., and Sang, Q. X. (1999). Structure–function analysis of the ADAM family of disintegrin-like and metalloproteinase-containing proteins (review). *J. Protein Chem.*, **18**(4), 447–465.

Taylor, H. P. and Cooper, N. R. (1990). The human cytomegalovirus receptor on fibroblasts is a 30-kilodalton membrane protein. *J. Virol.*, **64**(6), 2484–2490.

Triantafilou, M., Miyake, K., Golenbock, D. T., and Triantafilou, K. (2002). Mediators of innate immune recognition of bacteria concentrate in lipid rafts and facilitate lipopolysaccharide-induced cell activation. *J. Cell Sci.*, **115**(12), 2603–2611.

Tugizov, S., Navarro, D., Paz, P., Wang, Y. L., Qadri, I., and Pereira, L. (1994). Function of human cytomegalovirus glycoprotein B: syncytium formation in cells constitutively expressing gB is blocked by virus-neutralizing antibodies. *Virology*, **201**(2), 263–276.

Utz, U., Britt, W., Vugler, L., and Mach, M. (1989). Identification of a neutralizing epitope on glycoprotein gp58 of human cytomegalovirus. *J. Virol.*, **63**, 1995–2001.

Wang, X., Huong, S. M., Chiu, M. L., Raab-Traub, N., and Huang, E. S. (2003). Epidermal growth factor receptor is a cellular receptor for human cytomegalovirus. *Nature*, **424**(6947), 456–461.

Warren, A. P., Owens, C. N., Borysiewicz, L. K., and Patel, K. (1994). Down-regulation of integrin alpha 1/beta 1 expression and association with cell rounding in human cytomegalovirus-infected fibroblasts. *J. Gen. Virol.*, **75**(12), 3319–3325.

White, J. M. (2003). ADAMs: modulators of cell-cell and cell-matrix interactions. *Curr. Opin. Cell Biol.*, **15**(5), 598–606.

Wolfsberg, T. G., Primakoff, P., Myles, D. G., and White, J. M. (1995). ADAM, a novel family of membrane proteins containing a disintegrin and metalloprotease domain: multipotential functions in cell-cell and cell-matrix interactions. *J. Cell Biol.*, **131**(2), 275–278.

Wright, R., Kurosky, A., and Wasi, S. (1993). Annexin II associated with human cytomegalovirus particles: possible implications for cell infectivity. *FASEB J.*, **7**, A1301.

Wright, J. F., Kurosky, A., and Wasi, S. (1994). An endothelial cell-surface form of annexin II binds human cytomegalovirus. *Biochem. Biophys. Res. Commun.*, **198**(3), 983–989.

Wright, J. F., Kurosky, A., Pryzdial, E. L., and Wasi, S. (1995). Host cellular annexin II is associated with cytomegalovirus particles isolated from cultured human fibroblasts. *J. Virol.*, **69**, 4784–4791.

Wu, Q. H., Trymbulak, W., Tatake, R. J., Forman, S. J., Zeff, R. A., and Shanley, J. D. (1994). Replication of human cytomegalovirus in cells deficient in beta(2)-microglobulin gene expression. *J. Gen. Virol.*, **75**(10), 2755–2759.

Yu, D., Smith, G. A., Enquist, L. W., and Shenk, T. (2002). Construction of a self-excisable bacterial artificial chromosome containing the human cytomegalovirus genome and mutagenesis of the diploid TRL/IRL13 gene. *J. Virol.*, **76**(5), 2316–2328.

Yurochko, A. D. and Huang, E. S. (1999). Human cytomegalovirus binding to human monocytes induces immunoregulatory gene expression. *J. Immunol.*, **162**, 4806–4816.

Yurochko, A. D., Kowalik, T. F., Huong, S. M., and Huang, E. S. (1995). Human cytomegalovirus upregulates NF-kappa B activity by transactivating the NF-kappa B p105/p50 and p65 promoters. *J. Virol.*, **69**(9), 5391–5400.

Yurochko, A. D., Hwang, E. S., Rasmussen, L., Keay, S., Pereira, L., and Huang, E. S. (1997). The human cytomegalovirus UL55 (gB) and UL75 (gH) glycoprotein ligands initiate the rapid activation of Sp1 and NF-kappaB during infection. *J. Virol.*, **71**, 5051–5059.

Zhu, H., Cong, J. P., Mamtora, G., Gingeras, T., and Shenk, T. (1998). Cellular gene expression altered by human cytomegalovirus: global monitoring with oligonucleotide arrays. *Proc. Natl Acad. Sci. USA*, **95**(24), 14470–14475.

Immediate-early viral gene regulation and function

Mark F. Stinski[1] and Jeffery L. Meier[2]

[1]Department of Microbiology, [2]Department of Internal Medicine
Carver College of Medicine, University of Iowa, Iowa City, IA, USA

Introduction

Betaherpesviruses such as human cytomegalovirus (HCMV), human herpesvirus-6A and 6B (HHV-6), and human herpesvirus-7 (HHV-7) replicate more slowly than alphaherpesviruses, are highly species-specific for infection, and establish latency in progenitor cells of the bone marrow and monocytes of the blood. HCMV has been the prototype of the betaherpesviruses for studies of gene expression and regulation. In cell culture, HCMV strains have been adapted to preferentially infect and replicate in fibroblasts. However, low passage isolates replicate well in other cell types, such as endothelial cells, macrophages and dendritic cells. In the host, HCMV replicates in macrophages, dendritic cells, colonic and retinal pigmented epithelial cells, endothelial cells, fibroblasts, smooth muscle cells, neuronal cells, glial cells, hepatocytes, and trophoblasts (Fish et al., 1995, 1996; Hertel et al., 2003; Ibanez et al., 1991; Lathey and Spector, 1991; Maidji et al., 2002; Schmidbauer et al., 1989; Sinzger et al., 1993, 1995, 1996). In contrast, HHV-6 and HHV-7 infect CD4+ lymphocytes (Takahashi et al., 1989) as well as monocyte/macrophages. Although HCMV can be transferred into and out of polymorphonuclear leukocytes via cell-to-cell contact, these cells do not permit viral replication (Grundy et al., 1998; Sinclair and Sissons, 1996; Sinzger and Jahn, 1996).

Various animal betaherpesviruses have been used as models for HCMV infection. CMVs infecting seven different mammalian hosts (humans, chimpanzees, African green monkeys, rhesus macaques, guinea pigs, rats and mice) have been investigated in some level of detail. Murine CMV (MCMV) infection of mice has been the most widely used animal model. MCMV tissue tropism, virulence, latency, and reactivation exhibit similarities to those of HCMV infections (Hudson, 1979; Jordan, 1983) and many important insights have emerged from this model despite the fact that rodent and primate CMVs are evolutionarily distant relatives. Between 75 and 80 open reading frames (ORFs) of MCMV have significant sequence homology to the predicted ORFs of HCMV (Chee et al., 1990; Davison et al., 2003; Murphy et al., 2003a,b; Rawlinson et al., 1996). Rhesus CMV (RhCMV) and chimpanzee CMV (CCMV) have approximately 138 and 166 ORFs with significant homology to HCMV, respectively (Davison et al., 2003; Hanson et al., 2003). Current estimates suggest that HCMV has at least 165 genes, but estimates of over 190 genes have been reported, depending on the method of prediction. HCMV has 45 essential genes and 15 of them have an unknown function. The majority of the non-essential genes also have unknown functions (Dunn et al., 2003). For replication in human fibroblast, 68 ORFs are completely dispensable (Dunn et al., 2003). Some of the viral genes that are dispensable for replication in human fibroblast cells are required for replication in human microvascular endothelial cells or in retinal pigment epithelial cells (Dunn et al., 2003). Although many of the HCMV genes are dispensable for viral growth in cell culture, studies with MCMV or RhCMV suggest that many dispensable genes are important for modulating the virus–host interaction. Approximately two-thirds of the genes of HHV-6 are collinear with the unique long (U_L) region of the HCMV genome (Chee et al., 1990; Gompels et al., 1995; Neipel et al., 1991).

This chapter will review viral replication events, with emphasis on expression and function of the betaherpesvirus immediate early (IE) genes. Understanding betaherpesvirus replication is important for the development of better strategies to prevent and treat virus-induced disease.

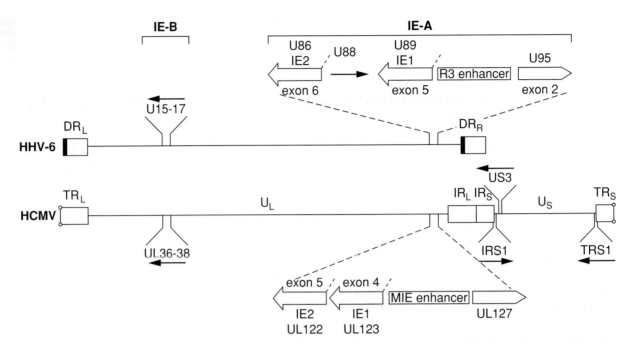

Fig. 17.1. Diagram of the immediate early (IE) genes of human cytomegalovirus (HCMV) and human herpesvirus-6 (HHV-6). The genes of the unique long (UL) components are colinear and designated alpha numerically. The unique short (US) component containing the TRS1/IRS1 and US3 genes is unique to HCMV. The unique components are flanked by either left (L) or right (R) direct repeats (DR), terminal repeats (TR), and internal repeats (IR) of the long (L) or short (S) components. Two genetically related IE loci are designated IE-A and IE-B. The major exons of the IE1 and IE2 genes in loci IE-A are designated as well as the enhancers and divergent viral gene.

Betaherpesvirus immediate early genes

The IE genes are the first viral genes transcribed after infection, and their transcription does not require *de novo* viral protein synthesis. These gene products optimize the cell for viral gene expression and replication. Figure 17.1 depicts the location of the IE gene loci on the HCMV and HHV-6 genomes. The HCMV long (L) genomic component encodes two betaherpesvirus-conserved transcription loci, the major IE genes (IE-A locus) and the IE-B locus as well as UL119-115 locus. The UL119–115 genes are not known to be involved in regulation of cellular or viral gene expression, and are not discussed in this chapter. The HCMV short (S) genomic component encodes US3 and the TRS1/IRS1 IE genes. HHV-6 lacks a region analogous to the S component of HCMV and so does not encode homologues of these HCMV genes.

The IE-A locus of HCMV encodes the major immediate early (MIE) genes and is collinear with a homologous region in HHV-6. In both viruses there is a strong transcriptional enhancer between two divergent genes (Fig. 17.1), with regulatory genes transcribed in the leftward direction designated IE1 and IE2. The function of the viral genes tran- scribed to the right is unknown. These viral genes and their enhancers have a major effect on productive viral replication for all betaherpesviruses where they have been studied and, consequently, they will be the focus of a majority of this chapter. For both MCMV (m128) and HCMV (UL127), the rightward transcribed viral genes in this locus are dispensable for replication in cell culture.

The IE-B locus is located in the L-component of the HCMV genome and exhibits homologous protein coding regions to HHV-6 (Flebbe-Rehwaldt *et al.*, 2000; Nicholas and Martin, 1994) (Fig. 17.1), as well as to other betaherpesviruses. The HCMV UL36–38 genes in the IE-B locus encode proteins that are required for viral growth. There are at least five transcripts from three different promoters in this region (Colberg-Poley, 1996). The products of the HCMV UL36–37 gene locus (e.g., UL37 exon 1, gpUL37, gpUL37m, and UL36) are expressed with IE kinetics and presumably serve to quickly thwart the cellular anti-viral response of apoptosis (see Chapter 21). The UL37 exon 1 unspliced RNA is abundant at IE times and remains abundant until late times after infection (Su *et al.*, 2003). HCMV oriLyt-mediated DNA replication assays are also enhanced by the UL36–38 gene products (Pari *et al.*, 1993). The HHV-6

U15–17 genes are multiply spliced in a pattern reminiscent of UL36–38 and have regulatory activities. For example, U16/17 spliced gene product activates expression from the HIV LTR promoter (Geng et al., 1992).

The US3 gene is transcribed at IE times to yield three alternatively spliced transcripts (Colberg-Poley, 1996). IE gene expression is controlled at multiple levels. Upstream of the US3 promoter is two sequence repeats designated R2 and R1 (Weston, 1988). R2 is a NF-κB containing enhancer that promotes a high level of US3 transcription. R1 has 19 repetitions of a 5'-TRTCG-3' pentanucleotide arranged as direct repeats, inverted repeats, and variably spaced single pentanucleotides. Although R1 was reported to silence expression from the US3 promoter in transient transfection assays (Chan et al., 1996; Thrower et al., 1996), R1 enhances expression of the flanking US3 and US6 genes by an unknown mechanism when assayed in the context of viral infection (Bullock et al., 2001, 2002). The US3 and US6 viral gene products disrupt the process of cellular HLA presentation of viral antigens at the cell surface and, consequently, they likely contribute to evasion of the host immune response (see Chapter 62). Between the start site of transcription and the TATA box of the US3 promoter is a *cis*-acting repressor element that binds the viral protein encoded by the essential HCMV UL34 gene (Dunn et al., 2003; LaPierre and Biegalke, 2001). Mutation of the *cis*-acting element causes a high level of expression of the US3 gene at early and late times after infection (Lashmit et al., 1998). The positive regulation of US3 gene expression may trap viral antigens introduced into the cell upon virus entry or expressed *de novo*. The negative regulation may prevent the toxic consequences of continued trapping of cellular HLA molecules on the membranes of the endoplasmic reticulum. US3 expression is repressed at late times after infection when the viral proteins encoded by US2, US6, and US11 contribute to immune evasion (see Chapter 62).

Because their transcription initiates in repeats flanking the U_S region, the TRS1/IRS1 genes are controlled by identical promoter elements. This arrangement results in proteins with identical N-terminal domains and divergent C-terminal domains, given the 3'-end, of their transcripts arise from different unique sequences in the U_S region (Fig. 17.1). TRS1 and IRS1 proteins are packaged into the virion as tegument components and, therefore, these viral proteins are introduced into cells in advance of IE gene expression (Romanowski et al., 1997). Viruses lacking IRS1 replicate normally. However, mutation of TRS1 together with IRS diminishes the yield of infectious virus and the mutant viral particles sediment abnormally in gradients, suggesting defective viral assembly (Blankenship and Shenk, 2002). In transient assays, TRS1/IRS1 gene products activate expression of early viral promoters in cooperation with the viral MIE gene products (Romanowski and Shenk, 1997) and are necessary components for HCMV oriLyt-dependent DNA replication (Pari et al., 1993). An amino terminal truncated IRS1 gene product (pIRS1^{263}) controlled by a downstream promoter in the unique region antagonizes the activation function of the IRS1 and TRS1 viral proteins (Romanowski and Shenk, 1997). Recent work has suggested that both TRS1 and IRS1 encode functions that evade interferon response in HCMV-infected cells (Child et al., 2004). These HCMV gene products appear to be RNA-binding proteins that prevent activation of host cell protein kinase R (PKR) pathways, thereby averting shut off of protein synthesis (Hakki and Geballe, 2005). It remains possible that all of the activities previously ascribed to these IE proteins are due to this central control of the cellular response to infection as has been found for PKR inhibitors encoded by other DNA viruses.

Betaherpesvirus transcriptional enhancers upstream of the MIE genes

Transient transfection and transgenic mouse experiments with the HCMV enhancer-containing MIE promoter driving expression of an indicator gene suggest that the activity of this enhancer is influenced by the cell type and the state of cell differentiation (Baskar et al., 1996a,b). However, additional transgenic mice studies yielded different data failing to show such correlation expression patterns. During infection, viral IE gene expression is first affected by attachment and entry requirements, and then, by cellular signal transduction pathways induced by the virus or other external stimuli. Serum and virion components increase MIE promoter activity at low multiplicity of infection (MOI). The relative importance of individual enhancer *cis*-acting sites may vary depending on the type of cell and external stimulus. In addition, it is not known which *cis*-acting elements in the MIE enhancer are important in a given cell type. For example, the NF-κB sites may be important in the hepatocytes under conditions of inflammation, when pro-inflammatory factors activate the transcription factor NF-κB (Prosch et al., 1995). The function of the MIE enhancers of betaherpesviruses is important to understand because the enhancers likely play a pivotal role in regulating viral latency, reactivation, and pathogenesis.

Figure 17.2 compares the known consensus binding sites for eukaryotic transcription factors in enhancer elements upstream of the MIE genes of human, chimpanzee, simian, murine, and rat (England and Maastricht strains) CMVs. Uncharacterized *cis*-acting elements may emerge from

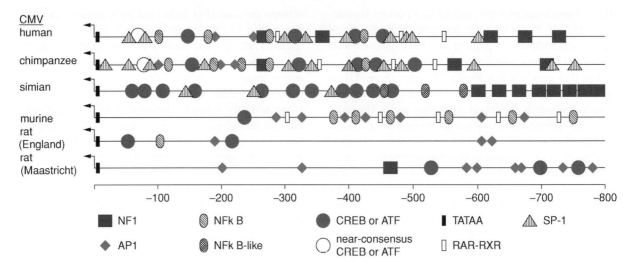

Fig. 17.2. Comparison of the enhancers of cytomegaloviruses. The known consensus binding sites of cellular transcription factors in the major immediate early enhancers are designated.

further studies seeking an impact on viral replication. CMV MIE enhancer elements have an array of *cis*-acting sites that bind cellular transcription factors (Angulo *et al.*, 1996, 1998a; Beisser *et al.*, 1998; Chang *et al.*, 1990; Davison *et al.*, 2003; Dorsch-Hasler *et al.*, 1985; Meier and Stinski, 1996; Sandford and Burns, 1996; Stinski, 1999; Thomsen *et al.*, 1984; Vink *et al.*, 2000; Meier and Stinski, 2006). Many of these binding sites are repetitive, but their arrangement and numbers vary among the different species-specific viruses. HCMV, ChCMV, SCMV, and MCMV share common regulatory elements that are functional binding sites for NF-κB, CREB/ATF, AP-1, and RAR-RXR (Angulo *et al.*, 1995, 1996, 1998a). RCMV (England strain) is unusual in that it contains fewer *cis*-acting elements than other viruses. The HCMV enhancer also has functional binding sites for serum response factor, Elk-1, Sp-1, CAAT/enhancer binding protein and gamma-interferon activating sequence (Meier and Stinski, 1996; Netterwald *et al.*, 2005). Binding sites for other cellular transcription activators are also present in this enhancer, but their significance is unknown. In transient transfection assays, the different *cis*-acting elements act individually or cooperatively to attract the RNA polymerase II transcription initiation complex to the MIE promoter (Hunninghake *et al.*, 1989).

The betaherpesvirus MIE enhancer elements are considered important because they may also serve as a target for reactivation from latency. The original hypothesis was that the MIE enhancer contributed to a quick and robust expression of the MIE genes, and evidence supporting this remains strong when expression of viruses carrying mutations in this region are studied in cell culture (Meier and Pruessner, 2000). Substitution of the enhancer of HCMV with the MCMV IE enhancer generates a virus with reduced expression and growth in culture (Isomura and Stinski, 2003), whereas subsitution of the MCMV with the HCMV MIE enhancer generates a virus that can replicate in culture or in mice (Grzimek *et al.*, 1999) with characteristics that indicated a role for the enhancer in increasing the number of cells expressing IE gene products in specific infected host tissues.

Figure 17.3 compares the enhancers of HCMV and HHV-6. Although these viruses share little common sequence, the enhancers are positioned similarly between divergent promoters upstream of the IE1 and IE2 genes (Lashmit *et al.*, 2004; Lundquist *et al.*, 1999; Takemoto *et al.*, 2001). The HHV-6 enhancer is characterized by repeat elements of 104 to 107-bp which contain polyomavirus enhancer A binding protein (PEA3) sites, NF-κB binding sites, some AP-2 binding sites (not identified in Fig. 17.3). The only obvious common elements shared by the two enhancers are NF-κB sites. The HHV-6 enhancer cannot substitute for the HCMV enhancer (H. Isomura and M. F. Stinski, unpublished data). While the HCMV enhancer influences IE1 and IE2 gene transcription, the HHV-6 enhancer has an effect on the divergent IE U95 gene transcription and is only speculated to have an effect on transcription of the IE1 and IE2 genes (Takemoto *et al.*, 2001). The HCMV MIE region has two repressor elements, one that binds IE2 proteins located immediately upstream of the IE1/IE2 transcription start site that likely represses gene expression when IE2 levels rise at early times of infection (Cherrington *et al.*, 1991; Liu *et al.*, 1991; Pizzorno and Hayward, 1990) and one that binds a cellular protein immediately upstream of the TATA box of the divergent UL127 gene and blocks expression

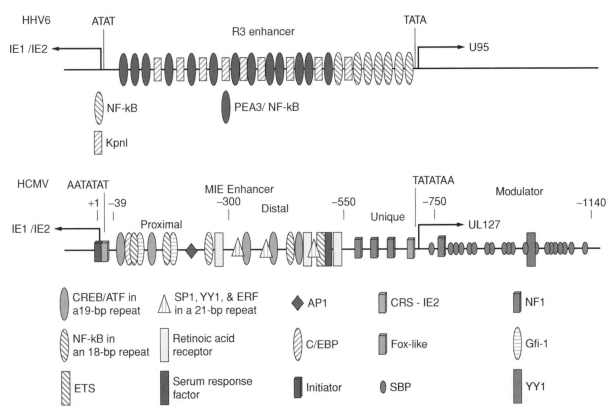

Fig. 17.3. Comparison between the HCMV major immediate early (MIE) and the HHV-6 R3 enhancer. Viral genes and promoter/transcription start sites are designated by an arrow. The HCMV also has a unique region and a modulator discussed in the text. The various transcription factor binding sites identified for HCMV and HHV-6 are designated. The AP-2 sites in the R3 enhancer are not identified. (See color plate section.)

throughout infection (Angulo et al., 2000b; Lashmit et al., 2004; Lundquist et al., 1999). Additionally, silencing of the MIE enhancer appears to occur through a variety of cellular transcription factors in certain cell types, particularly when the cells are undifferentiated. Murine CMV has a similar arrangement of enhancer, MIE gene and divergent gene, but transcriptional repression signals have not been found. As far as has been determined, the IE1 and IE2 homologues are important in replication but the divergent genes of the betaherpesviruses are non-essential for replication in cell culture and their function is not known. The U94 gene of HHV-6, of interest because it is similar to the *rep* gene of adeno-associated virus (AAV), is located in the intron of the viral U95 gene and is transcribed in the opposite direction of U95 (Takemoto et al., 2001). The AAV *rep* gene product is a DNA binding protein with ATPase and helicase activity and is required for AAV DNA replication. The HHV-6 U94 gene product is found in very low abundance during productive HHV-6 infection but shares some of these properties (see Chapter 47).

Function of the betaherpesvirus major immediate-early enhancers

Thus far, two approaches have been used to study the function of betaherpesvirus MIE enhancers during viral infection: (i) mutation of enhancer components, and (ii) substitution of the enhancer from one species with that from a different species. Mutational analysis in the context of the viral genome demonstrated that the HCMV enhancer has two functional components referred to as the distal enhancer (−580 to −300) and the proximal enhancer (−300 to −39) relative to the transcription start site (+1) (Fig. 17.3). The distal enhancer is dispensable at high MOIs in cultured cells but has a significant effect on the efficiency of viral replication at low MOIs (Meier and Pruessner, 2000). Without the distal enhancer, the virus has a small plaque phenotype. The distal enhancer is composed of multiple *cis*-acting elements. Deletion of −300 to −347 or −347 to −579 has little to no effect on MIE promoter-dependent transcription, but deletion of the entire region (−580 to −300) has a significant effect (Meier et al., 2002). The distal enhancer functions in cis and is orientation-independent relative to the transcription start site. The hypothetical ORFs in the distal enhancer are not important for viral replication in cell culture because insertion of stop codons at −300 or −345 had no effect on IE gene expression or virus titer (Meier et al., 2002). The proximal enhancer upstream of −39 also determines the efficiency of virus replication in cell culture (Isomura et al., 2004). Deletion of the proximal enhancer affects IE and early viral gene expression, viral DNA synthesis, and the rate of viral growth (Isomura et al., 2004). Which elements in the distal or proximal enhancer are required for virus replication in various cell types is currently unknown. Despite the commonality of NF-κB sites in betaherpesvirus enhancers, the minimal enhancer element for HCMV appears to be an Sp-1 binding site (Isomura et al., 2004, 2005).

Mutation of the CREB/ATF binding sites in the entire enhancer had little to no effect on HCMV replication in human fibroblast (HF) or in NTera2-derived neuronal cells at high or low MOIs (Keller et al., 2003). Likewise, mutation of the NF-κB sites in the entire enhancer had little to no effect on viral replication at high or low MOIs in HF cells (Benedict et al., 2004). Since MCMV and HCMV replicate efficiently in cells where the NF-κB activation pathway has been inhibited (Benedict et al., 2004; Melnychuk et al., 2003), the NF-κB transcription factor may not always be necessary for replication in cell culture. The requirement for particular HCMV MIE enhancer elements has not yet been assessed using viral mutants.

Enhancer substitution experiments have also demonstrated that CMV MIE enhancers affect viral replication. Recombinant with the rat CMV (England) MIE enhancer substituted with the MCMV MIE enhancer was deficient in replication in rat fibroblasts and in the infected rat, with greatly reduced levels of viral replication in the salivary glands (Sandford and Burns, 1996). While recombinant HCMV with the MIE enhancer substituted by the SCMV (Colburn) MIE enhancer replicated as well as wild-type virus (H. Isomura and M. F. Stinski, unpublished data), recombinant HCMV with the enhancer substituted with the MCMV enhancer replicated slower and to lower levels in HF cells (Isomura and Stinski, 2003). Consistent with this, the plaques of the enhancer substituted HCMV recombinant virus had a small plaque phenotype. When a recombinant MCMV substituted with the HCMV MIE enhancer was made, the recombinant MCMV replicated in mouse fibroblast (Angulo et al., 1998b) and in mouse liver at levels similar to wild-type virus, but there was a decrease in the infection at other sites in the mouse (Grzimek et al., 2001). While the MCMV enhancer is not essential for replication in cultured murine fibroblasts at high MOI, this region is required for cytopathic effects in culture and disease in the mouse (Angulo et al., 1998b). Taken together, these observations suggest that CMV enhancers are not always functionally equivalent and suggest one role they play is to optimize the efficiency of viral replication in various cell types with which the virus normally interacts. The cis-acting elements in the betaherpesvirus enhancers have evolved over millions of years for each of the species-specific viruses.

Silencing of the immediate-early genes

Betaherpesvirus MIE genes are regulated in a cell type- and differentiation-dependent manner. The viral genomes may be organized into a nucleosome-array like latent genomes of herpesviruses in other subfamilies (Deshmane and Fraser, 1989; Dyson and Farrell, 1985). Conditionally permissive cell lines have been used to investigate silencing and reactivation of HCMV. In the undifferentiated cell, the MIE enhancer-containing promoter is silent, and the cells are non-permissive for viral replication. In the differentiated cell, the MIE enhancer-containing promoter is active, and the cells are permissive for viral replication. For example, HCMV fails to replicate after penetration into NTera2 cells, an undifferentiated embryonic carcinoma line (Gonczol et al., 1984). This postentry block corresponds to silencing of the MIE promoter-dependent transcription (LaFemina and Hayward, 1986; Meier, 2001; Nelson and Groudine, 1986). Inactivity of the MIE promoter appears to be a feature of natural HCMV latency (Taylor-Wiedeman et al., 1994; Kondo et al., 1994, 1996; Slobedman and Mocarski, 1999). The MIE promoter of MCMV is generally inactive during viral latency, except in a rare subset of cells where spontaneous reactivation appears to be occurring (Grzimek et al., 2001; Hummel et al., 2001; Koffron et al., 1998; Kurz et al., 1999; Kurz and Reddehase, 1999).

Transient transfection studies identified the HCMV 21-bp-repeats, the unique region, and the modulator as cis-acting sites that confer repression of transcription in the undifferentiated monocytic THP-1 and embryonal NTera2 cell lines (Fig. 17.3) (Huang et al., 1996; Kothari et al., 1991; Liu et al., 1994; Nelson et al., 1987; Shelbourn et al., 1989; Sinclair et al., 1992). Three copies of the 21-bp-repeats are located in the distal MIE enhancer, whereas the unique region and modulator forms the 5′-extent of the MIE regulatory region. The following cellular repressors of transcription have also been proposed to act through one or more elements in the modulator, the unique region, or the enhancer: silencing binding protein (SBP) (Thrower et al., 1996), modulator recognition factor (Huang et al., 1996),

PDX1 (Chao et al., 2004), Yin Yang-1 (YY1) (Liu et al., 1994), methylated DNA-binding protein (Zhang et al., 1995), growth factor independence-1 (Gfi-1) (Zweidler-McKay et al., 1996), and the ETS2-repressor factor (ERF) (Wright et al., 2002). While eliminating any one of these sets of negative cis-acting elements increases the MIE promoter activity in transient transfection experiments, their selective removal from the HCMV genome results in a completely different outcome. Silencing in the context of the viral genome is not alleviated by removal of the 21-bp-repeats, the modulator, the unique region, or both 21-bp-repeats and modulator in either undifferentiated monocytic THP-1 or embryonal NTera2 cells (Meier, 2001). Site-specific mutation of the Gfi-1 sites has no effect in undifferentiated monocytic THP-1 cells (R. Schnetzer and M. F. Stinski, unpublished data). Thus, silencing occurs in the context of viral infection, and its regulatory mechanism differs quantitatively from that observed in transfected cells. It remains possible that redundancy of negative cis-acting elements explains these differences, but studies have not yet provided any evidence of this. Nonetheless, the findings suggest that the HCMV MIE promoter becomes silenced in undifferentiated cells, but this process depends on factors that remain to be identified.

In the embryonal NTera2 cell culture model, a portion of quiescent HCMV genomes have a super-coiled structure (Meier, 2001), which appears similar to CMV latency in blood monocytes of healthy subjects (Bolovan-Fritts et al., 1999). The super-coiled structure would be expected to package into nucleosomes as is the case for gammaherpesviruses. The HCMV MIE enhancer of the quiescent viral genomes is inactive even when positive-acting transcription factors NF-κB and RAR-RXR are activated (Meier, 2001). However, inhibition of cellular histone deacetylase (HDAC) reactivates transcription from the MIE promoter. These data suggest that betaherpesvirus MIE promoter silencing may involve HDAC-based modification of viral chromatin. Murphy et al. (2002) showed that the silent HCMV MIE promoter is associated with less acetylated histone H4 as compared to an active MIE promoter. Acetylated H4 was also less abundant on silent MIE promoters in experimentally infected blood monocytes compared to active MIE promoters in permissive monocyte-derived macrophages (Murphy et al., 2002). In addition, the cellular HP1 protein, which selectively binds methylated histone H3 at lysine 9 in cellular heterochromatin (Jenuwein and Allis, 2001), is preferentially associated with the repressed MIE promoters (Murphy et al., 2002). While MCMV MIE promoter reactivation can also be achieved in latently infected murine tissue (Hummel et al., 2003), direct evidence for CMV DNA silencing via chromatin components is lacking at this time. The combined findings imply that chromatin may condense on the betaherpesvirus genomes in non-permissive and undifferentiated cells to restrict MIE promoter activity.

Reactivation of the immediate-early genes

Reactivation of betaherpesviruses is observed commonly in the setting of immunosuppression, particularly where allogeneic stimulation and proinflammatory cytokines are present and stimulate monocyte differentiation (Cook et al., 2002; Fietze et al., 1994; Hahn et al., 1998; Hummel et al., 2001; Mutimer et al., 1997; Soderberg-Naucler et al., 1997b; Soderberg-Naucler et al., 2001). Proinflammatory cytokines, such as those released during allogeneic transplantation, AIDS, sepsis, or myelosuppressive chemotherapy, induce the MIE promoter-dependent transcription.

For MCMV, the effect of MIE promoter reactivation can be dampened by a mechanism that prohibits the production of the alternatively spliced ie3 RNA (Grzimek et al., 2001; Kurz et al., 1999), which is the functional equivalent of the HCMV IE2 gene. HCMV MIE promoter reactivation may also be subjected to further regulation in infected monocytes, as certain stimuli only reactivate production of spliced RNA for IE1, but not IE2 (Taylor-Wiedeman et al., 1994). Stimuli sufficient to induce differentiation of these cells into a monocyte-derived macrophage or dendritic cell phenotype, enables completion of the HCMV reactivation program (Soderberg-Naucler et al., 1997b 2001).

The molecular mechanisms that trigger and sustain CMV reactivation are largely unknown. Transgenic mice and transient transfection experiments implicate NF-κB and CREB/ATF as important mediators in stimulus-induced MIE promoter reactivation (Hummel et al., 2001; Prosch et al., 1995; Stein et al., 1993). TNF-α potently induces NF-κB activity and reactivates MCMV's MIE promoter in latently infected lung tissue, but is not alone sufficient to sustain the reactivation process (Hummel et al., 2001). HCMV reactivation from monocytes in cell culture induced by allogeneic stimulation does not require TNF-α, but instead, depends on the combination of interferon-γ and other unidentified factors (Soderberg-Naucler et al., 2001). The mechanism(s) by which these cytokines or other factors stimulate HCMV reactivation is unknown. In the embryonal NTera2 cell model, forskolin stimulation of the cyclic AMP signaling pathway and inhibition of HDAC induce HCMV MIE promoter reactivation. The reactivation is dependent on CREB/ATF-binding sites within the enhancer (M. Keller and J. Meier, unpublished data). Taken together, it appears that betaherpesvirus reactivation from

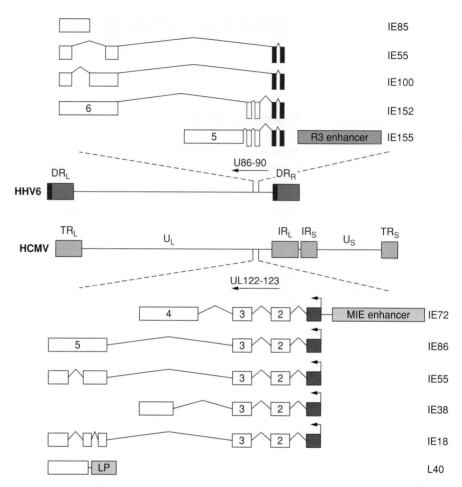

Fig. 17.4. Comparison of the IE1 and IE2 genes and their isomers for HCMV and HHV-6. The exons with ORFs for the IE1 and IE2 genes are designated as open boxes. The isomers of the IE1 and IE2 genes are designated according to apparent molecular weight. A HCMV late (L) isomer and late promoter (LP) are designated.

latency may entail multiple regulatory mechanisms for orchestrating both derepression and activation of the viral IE gene expression.

Betaherpesvirus major immediate-early genes

All betaherpesviruses have CpG dinucleotide suppression in the major immediate early (MIE) locus. The significance of CpG dinucleotide suppression is unknown, but it suggests that these genes are regulated by host methylation in a certain setting such as latency. Downstream of the betaherpesvirus enhancer-containing MIE promoter are two regulatory genes designated IE1 and IE2 in HCMV and HHV-6 as well as most other betaherpesviruses. Importantly, in MCMV, they are designated ie1 and ie3, respectively. In all betaherpesviruses, multiple gene products are encoded by these two genes through differential mRNA spicing and promoter usage throughout infection. For the CMVs, the single MIE promoter directs transcription of three small exons that are spliced alternatively to either exon 4 or exon 5 of the precursor IE RNA followed by cleavage and polyadenylation (Fig. 17.4) (Nicholas, 1994 Stenberg et al., 1984, 1985). An initiation codon in exon 2 and a termination codon in either exon 4 or exon 5 gives rise to the major proteins encoded by IE1 and IE2, respectively, at IE times (Fig. 17.4). In HHV-6, the first four exons of a precursor RNA are spliced alternatively to either exon 5 or exon 6 (Fig. 17.4) (Nicholas, 1994; Schiewe et al., 1994). An initiation codon in exon 3 and a termination codon in either exon 5 or exon 6 give rise to the proteins encoded by IE1 and IE2, respectively. The viral proteins encoded by HCMV are designated according to their apparent molecular weight and have amino acids in common at the amino terminus, with the exception of a late viral protein, designated L40 that arises from a unique promoter element within the exon 5 region (Fig. 17.4). HHV-6 also generates multiple forms of the IE1 and IE2 proteins by alternate splicing between and within exons. The HHV-6 MIE proteins are also designated according to their apparent molecular weight (Fig. 17.4) (Papanikolaou et al., 2002).

Functions of the major immediate–early viral proteins

While it is assumed that the proteins encoded by betaherpesvirus IE1 and IE2 genes have similar functions, these proteins exhibit dramatic evolutionary divergence in amino acid sequence. These differences may have evolved to meet the regulatory needs for broadly different species-specific and cell-specific herpesviruses represented by this subgroup. The functions of the major HCMV IE1 and IE2 gene products, IE72 and IE86, have been investigated extensively, and minor products IE38, IE55, and IE18 isomers have received less attention. During the two hours after HCMV infection of HFs, the mRNA for the IE2 gene is expressed predominantly, and this is followed by a period when the mRNA for the IE1 gene predominates (Stamminger et al., 1991). In contrast, the expression of HHV-6 IE1 precedes that of IE2 (Papanikolaou et al., 2002). Relative to the mRNAs for HCMV IE72 and IE86 proteins, the amount of mRNA for IE55 or IE38 is low in fibroblasts. The mRNA for IE18 is lower in HFs than in macrophages (Stenberg, 1996). The IE2 protein of HCMV negatively autoregulates the expression of the IE1 and IE2 genes, but there is no evidence to date that HHV-6 IE2 protein negatively autoregulates (Cherrington et al., 1991; Liu et al., 1991; Pizzorno and Hayward, 1990). The IE86 protein of HCMV binds to the minor groove of the MIE promoter that contains a *cis*-repression sequence (crs) between −13 and −1 relative to the transcription start site (+1) (Lang and Stamminger, 1994). The late 40 kDa protein (L40) of the IE2 gene can also bind to the crs and negatively autoregulate transcription of the MIE genes (Plachter et al., 1993; Puchtler and Stamminger, 1991; Stenberg et al., 1989). While the IE1 and IE2 gene products are discussed separately below, they seem to work synergistically in executing their functions during viral infection.

The IE1 proteins

The IE1 proteins of CMVs have only a few regions of homology and a characteristic acidic acid residue cluster towards the C-termini. The IE1 genes of human and MCMV are dispensable for viral replication at high MOIs (1 to 5 PFU/cell). When the IE1 gene is deleted, the efficiency of viral replication is reduced at low MOIs (0.001 to 0.05 PFU/cell) (Greaves and Mocarski, 1998; Mocarski et al., 1996). After infection at low MOI with recombinant HCMV containing an IE1 gene deletion, there are insufficient levels of early viral gene expression required for viral DNA replication (Gawn and Greaves, 2002). At high MOIs, virion-associated proteins present in infectious and non-infectious particles may compensate for the absence of functional IE1.

After synthesis in the cytoplasm, IE72 is transported to the nucleus and targeted to nuclear bodies known as promyelocytic leukemia (PML) oncogenic domains (PODs) or nuclear domain 10 (ND10). The viral protein is modified by conjugation of SUMO-1 or SUMO-2 (small ubiquitin-like modifier) at lysine residue 450. The apparent molecular weight of IE72 following modification is approximately 92 kDa (Spengler et al., 2002; Xu et al., 2001). Although sumoylation may be important for the efficiency of viral replication, a recombinant virus with lysine residue 450 mutated is replication competent in HFs (Lee et al., 2004). Recombinant virus with lysine residue 450 mutated expresses lower levels of IE2 RNA and IE86 protein (Nevels et al., 2004). With or without SUMO conjugation, IE72 displaces the ND10 presumably by binding to its associated proteins, such as PML, SP100, and hDaxx. The central hydrophobic region of IE72 binds to PML (Lee et al., 2004) and inhibits the accumulation of sumoylated forms of PML. A PML-associated transcriptional repressor, HDAC-2, is inactivated (Ahn and Hayward, 1997; Ahn et al., 1998a; Wilkinson et al., 1998) and, consequently, the basal transcription initiation complex is activated (Muller and Dejean, 1999; Tang and Maul, 2003; Xu et al., 2001). Early after infection, the viral DNA and transcripts are detected in the nucleus, and RNA polymerase and mRNA spliceosome assembly factors are juxtaposed to the ND10 (Ishov et al., 1997). HHV-6 IE1 protein is also localized to ND10 and modified by SUMO-1 at lysine residue 802, but the IE1 protein does not dispense PML (Gravel et al., 2002). The reason for this significant difference in the function of these betaherpesvirus IE1 proteins is not known; however, disruption of ND10 is not a requisite for HCMV replication. The multiple functions of the betaherpesvirus IE1 proteins are not fully understood. One function of the HCMV IE72 protein may be to counter the innate immune response in cells by down-regulation of virus-induced interferon-like response (Singh and Compton, 2004) and another may block apoptosis (Zhu et al., 1995), promoting conditions for viral replication in the host cell.

IE38 (IE19) is reported to be an HCMV IE1 gene product that lacks amino acids 88 to 404 of IE72 (Fig. 17.4). A radioactive probe to the 5 end of IE1 detected a cDNA of 0.65 kb that could code for IE38 (Shirakata et al., 2002). An antibody to a peptide between amino acids 383 and 420 detected both IE72 and IE38 (Kerry et al., 1995). Others have not detected IE38 and suggest it may represent an

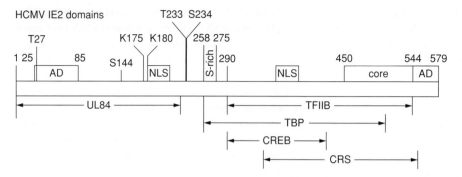

Fig. 17.5. Domains of HCMV IE86 encoded by the IE2 gene. The domains are demarcated according to amino acid residue. Transcription activation domains (AD) are located at the amino and carboxyl termini. There are serine-rich (S-rich) domains and two nuclear localization signals (NLS). There is an essential region designated the core domain. Regions of the viral protein that interact with another viral gene product (UL84), cellular transcription factors, or the *cis* repression sequence (crs) of the MIE promoter are designated.

N-terminal cleavage product of IE72 (Awasthi *et al.*, 2004). Transient transfection experiments suggested that IE38 functions synergistically with IE72 (Shirakata *et al.*, 2002). Whether or not these functions of IE38 occur in the virus-infected cell remains to be determined.

It is unclear how IE72 (or IE38) activates cellular promoters, but an association of IE72 with TATA box-associated factors (TAFs) and transcription factors (Sp-1, E2F-1, CTF-1) has been proposed (Hayhurst *et al.*, 1995; Lukac *et al.*, 1997; Margolis *et al.*, 1995). In transient transfection experiments, IE72 moderately activates the viral MIE promoter and the cellular DNA polymerase α, c-fos, c-myc and dihydrofolate reductase promoters (Cherrington and Mocarski, 1989; Hagemeier *et al.*, 1992b; Sambucetti *et al.*, 1989; Wade *et al.*, 1992). The mechanism by which IE72 protein activates promoters may be related to inhibition of HDAC-2 activity (Tang and Maul, 2003).

It has been proposed that HCMV IE72 has intrinsic protein kinase activity (Pajovic *et al.*, 1997). The related protein, IE38 does not have the proposed protein kinase domain. The Rb family members p107 and p130, the E2F transcription factor family members, and PML are phosphorylated by the IE72 protein (Ippolito *et al.*, 2003; Pajovic *et al.*, 1997). Phosphorylation of the Rb family members would dissociate the repressor from E2F and activate the E2F cellular transcription factor. The leucine zipper region of IE72 can bind the N-terminus of p107, alleviate the repressive effect of p107 and, consequently, activate cyclin dependent kinase-2 (cdk2)/cyclin E activity (Zhang *et al.*, 2003). Therefore, IE72 induces cycle cell progression, but the effect of the viral protein is more demonstrable in a p53 negative cell than in a p53 positive cell (Castillo *et al.*, 2000). An active p53 pathway should increase levels of p21 cyclin-dependent kinase inhibitor even in the presence of activated E2F transcription factors, but p21 is decreased in the HCMV-infected cell (Chen *et al.*, 2001; Noris *et al.*, 2002).

HCMV infection affects p53 because the cellular protein is sequestered in the nucleus in viral replication centers (Fortunato and Spector, 1998).

The IE2 proteins

The betaherpesvirus proteins encoded by the IE2 gene exhibit amino acid similarity across their C-terminal regions. The HCMV IE2 gene and its functional homologue in MCMV (ie3) are absolutely essential for the cascade of viral gene expression (Angulo *et al.*, 2000a; Marchini *et al.*, 2001). Recombinant viruses with deletion of the HCMV IE2 gene or the MCMV ie3 gene are unable to activate early viral gene expression, and, consequently, viral DNA synthesis and late gene expression are also affected. The betaherpesvirus IE2 proteins have N- and/or C-terminal domains that activate viral gene expression and are considered a master regulator of productive infection. The IE2 gene of HCMV has been studied in detail. It regulates activation of transcription from viral and cellular promoters, negatively auto-regulates the MIE promoter, and induces cell cycle progression. Figure 17.5 is a diagram of the functional domains of the HCMV IE2 protein IE86. IE86 is also targeted to ND10 in the nucleus and modified by conjugation with SUMO-1 or SUMO-2 at lysine (K) residues 175 or 180. The apparent molecular weight of the modified protein is 105 kDa (Ahn *et al.*, 2001; Hofmann *et al.*, 2000); however, sumoylation of IE86 is not required for viral growth (Lee and Ahn, 2004).

Unlike IE72, IE86 does not disperse ND10. However, IE86 remains adjacent to ND10 where a portion of the input viral DNA is also located (Ishov *et al.*, 1997). Modification of IE86 by SUMO may facilitate interaction with the basal transcription machinery and/or with cellular or viral transcription factors. In transient transfection experiments, IE86 mutated at lysine residues 175 and 180 autoregulates the

MIE promoter, but fails to efficiently activate early viral promoters (Hofmann et al., 2000). A recombinant virus with deletion of amino acid residues 136 to 290 still down-regulates transcription from the MIE promoter, but the mutant exhibited lower levels of late gene (UL83 and UL99) expression (Sanchez et al., 2002). Late gene expression is also disrupted by deletion of four amino acids from 356 to 359 (White et al., 2004). This mutation would disrupt a region where IE86 interacts with the basal transcription factors TFIIB and TBP (Fig. 17.5). IE86 has a serine-rich region from amino acids residues 258 to 275. Mutation of the serine residues from 258 to 264 or 266 to 269 delays viral growth, but mutation from 271 to 275 accelerates viral growth (Barrasa et al., 2005). These serine residues are in a region of the protein that can bind TBP (Fig. 17.5). IE86 is also modified by phosphorylation at amino acid residues T27, S144, T233, and S234 (Harel and Alwine, 1998) (Fig. 17.5). Differences in phosphorylation may have significant effects on the function of the viral protein.

Data indicate that mutation of amino acids between 427 to 435 and 505 to 511 caused a loss of auto-regulation of the MIE promoter by IE86 (White et al., 2004). Mutation of histidines 446 and 452 generates a protein that cannot bind to the crs and negatively autoregulates the MIE promoter in an in vitro transcription assay (Macias and Stinski, 1993). Therefore, the carboxyl region of the IE86 protein is critical for auto-regulation of the MIE promoter (Fig. 17.5). Autoregulation of the MIE promoter by the IE86 protein at early times is likely due to the blockage of RNA polymerase II and transcription initiation factors at the transcription start site (Macias et al., 1996). At late times after infection the IE86 protein was found to be associated with repressive chromatin (Reeves et al., 2006). With murine CMV, the M112/113 gene product co-localizes with and binds ie3 protein (the equivalent of human CMV IE86) to inhibit the repressive effect on the MIE promoter and promotes continued MIE gene expression (Tang et al., 2005).

In transient transfection assays, multiple regions of IE86 are reported to be important for promoter activation. Two activation domains (AD) are located at amino acid 25 to 85 and 544 to 579 (Fig. 17.5). Amino acid residues 1 to 98, 169 to 194, 175 to 180, and multiple regions in the carboxyl terminal half of the protein are also important for viral promoter activation (Malone et al., 1990; Pizzorno et al., 1991; Sommer et al., 1994; Stenberg, 1996; Yeung et al., 1993). Other important regions of IE86 are amino acid residues 388 to 542, and 463 to 513, which encompass a dimerization region and a helix–loop–helix region, respectively (Ahn et al., 1998b; Macias et al., 1996; Macias and Stinski, 1993; Waheed et al., 1998). There is a core region between amino acids 450 and 544. Mutations in this region affect most of the activities of this protein (Fig. 17.5) (Asmar et al., 2004).

IE86 interacts with a wide variety of cellular transcription factors (Bryant et al., 2000; Lang et al., 1995; Lukac et al., 1994; Yoo et al., 1996). These factors include TBP, TFIIB, and TAF4 as well as histone acetyl-transferase (Bryant et al., 2000; Caswell et al., 1993; Fortunato and Spector, 1999; Hagemeier et al., 1992a; Lukac and Alwine, 1997; Spector, 1996). IE86 may serve as a link between various upstream sequence-specific DNA binding regulators of transcription and the basal transcription initiation complex. The protein also interacts with an early viral protein encoded by the UL84 gene of HCMV (Colletti et al., 2004; Samaniego et al., 1994; Spector and Tevethia, 1994). Over-expression of UL84 prior to viral infection will antagonize activation of early viral promoters by IE86 protein (Gebert et al., 1997). The UL84 gene is essential for viral DNA synthesis and growth (Xu et al., 2004b). The UL84 protein interacts with itself and with the IE86 protein which is essential for oriLyt-dependent viral DNA synthesis (Colletti et al., 2004; Sarisky and Hayward, 1996). DNA synthesis is initiated by the activation of a oriLyt bidirectional promoter by IE86 and UL84 viral proteins (Xu et al., 2004a). The other HCMV IE genes, IE1, UL36–38, and IRS1/TRS1, have a stimulatory effect on ori-Lyt-mediated DNA replication in HF cells (Anders and McCue, 1996).

The IE86 protein also interacts with cellular proteins that control cell cycle progression. Several types of biological assays indicate that IE86 physically binds Rb (Fortunato et al., 1997; Hagemeier et al., 1994; Sommer et al., 1994). The release of the cellular E2F transcription factor from Rb, as a consequence of this interaction, is considered to be one of the key HCMV mechanisms for induction of cell cycle progression. As many as 4-fold more serum-starved glioblastoma U373 or 293T cells are induced into S phase by wild type IE86 compared to a mutant protein (Murphy et al., 2000). IE86 blocks cell division by arresting p53 wild type cells at G_1/S (Murphy et al., 2000; Song and Stinski, 2002; Wiebusch and Hagemeier, 1999; Wiebusch et al., 2003). In p53 mutant U373 cells or p53 null Saos-2 cells, IE86 does not inhibit cell cycle progression at G_1/S (Song and Stinski, 2005). These cells synthesize cellular DNA and cell cycle progression stops at the S phase for U373 cells or the G2/M-phase for Saos-2 cells (Murphy et al., 2000; Song and Stinski, 2005). In p53 null Saos-2 cells, a block in cell cycle progression at the G_2/M-phase by the IE86 protein correlates with an aberrant increase in cyclin B and cdk1 levels (Song and Stinski, 2002). IE86 likely prepares the cell for DNA synthesis by activating cellular genes that regulate the cell cycle, enzymes for DNA precursor synthesis, and proteins for initiation of cellular DNA synthesis (Song and Stinski, 2002). For example, production of mRNAs for cyclin E, cdk-2, E2F-1, DNA polymerase α, and MCMs is significantly increased by IE86 (Song and Stinski, 2002). Preparation for DNA synthesis is critical for the virus because CMVs typically infect terminally differentiated cells in the G_0/G_1 phase of the cell cycle when the pool of dideoxynucleotide triphosphates and biosynthetic enzyme levels are low. HCMV IE86 is an unusual regulatory protein in comparison to regulatory proteins of adenovirus, SV40, or papilloma DNA viruses because it pushes the p53 wild type cell from G_0/G_1 to the G_1/S transition, yet blocks further cell cycle progression (Murphy et al., 2000; Wiebusch and Hagemeier, 2001). Both of the IE 72 and IE86 proteins stabilize p53, which is associated with phosphorylation of p53 at serine residue 15 (Castillo et al., 2005; Song and Stinski, 2005). The IE86 protein induces the degradation of cellular mdm2 and thereby prevents ubiquitination and proteasome degradation of p53 (Zhang et al., 2006). Recombinant virus with a mutant IE86 protein that fails to block cell cycle progression at the G1/S interface and allows for cellular DNA synthesis, replicates slowly relative to wild type virus (Petrik et al., 2006). The IE86 protein may block rather than promote apoptosis (Zhu et al., 1995).

One of the functions of cellular p53 tumor suppressor protein is to ensure termination of cells that have lost the ability to regulate growth. Even though the HCMV IE86 protein binds to p53 (Bonin and McDougall, 1997; Speir et al., 1994), p53 is not inactivated by the IE86 protein and, as a result, cdk inhibitor p21 increases in relative amount (Shen et al., 2004; Song and Stinski, 2002). However, in the HCMV infected cell the levels of p21 decrease (Chen et al., 2001; Noris et al., 2002). In the p53 wild type HF cell, IE86 induces senescence that is manifested in continued cellular metabolism, production of plasminogen activator inhibitor type I, and neutral β-galactosidase activity (Noris et al., 2002).

While the viral IE86 protein acts by a different mechanism to activate cellular gene expression, it acts to favor virus survival by inhibiting cellular beta-interferon, cytokine, and pro-inflammatory chemokine expression by an unknown mechanism (Taylor and Bresnahan, 2005, 2006).

Factors that stimulate betaherpesvirus immediate-early gene expression

Cellular signal transduction events

Infection of HF cells with HCMV triggers activation of multiple signal transduction pathways. There is an activation of the phosphatidylinositol 3-kinase (PI3K), the mitogen-activated protein kinase/extracellular signal-regulated kinase (MAPK/ERK), and the p38 MAPK signal transduction pathways (Johnson et al., 2000, 2001; Rodems and Spector, 1998). Inhibitors of these signal transduction pathways suppress HCMV replication, which implies that the signal transduction pathways are necessary for efficient viral replication. The PI3K pathway is activated by virion components immediately upon entry. An activated PI3K pathway induces production of secondary messengers like phosphotidyl inositol and diacylglycerol (Albrecht et al., 1990, 1991; Wang et al., 2003) and increases in cyclic AMP, GMP, and intracellular stores of calcium. The MAPK/ERK and p38 MAPK pathways are activated early after infection and sustained until late times (Johnson et al., 2000; Rodems and Spector, 1998). The PI3K, MAPK/ERK, and p38 MAPK pathways have major effects on the activation of a variety of cellular transcription factors. This activation often results from phosphorylation of the transcription factors and, consequently, up-regulates both cellular and viral gene expression. HCMV early promoters are suppressed by inhibitors of signal transduction pathways (Chen and Stinski, 2002). Therefore, activation of signal transduction pathways is an important step in the efficient replication of betaherpesviruses.

Prostaglandins and reactive oxygen species (ROS) also serve as secondary messengers that elicit multiple responses in betaherpesvirus-infected cells (Zhu et al., 2002). Virions of HCMV up-regulate cellular cyclooxygenase-2 (cCOX-2) (Zhu et al., 2002). The rhesus CMV encodes a viral COX-2 (vCOX-2), which is required for efficient viral replication in endothelial cells (Hanson et al., 2003; Rue et al., 2004). Prostaglandin E2, a product of COX-2, activates the HCMV MIE enhancer-containing promoter (Kline et al., 1998). HCMV infection generates ROS partly through a COX-2-dependent pathway. ROS also activates the HCMV MIE promoter and augments viral replication. Inhibition of cCOX-2 or scavenging of ROS decreases HCMV IE gene expression and viral replication (Speir et al., 1998; Zhu et al., 2002). Treatment with prostaglandin E2 reverses the inhibitory effects on HCMV replication.

Lastly, proinflammatory cytokines induce various signaling pathways that stimulate MIE gene expression and viral replication. This outcome is observed, for example, in HCMV-infected macrophages or granulocyte–macrophage progenitors treated with tumor necrosis factor-α or interferon-γ (Soderberg-Naucler et al., 1997a; Hahn et al., 1998).

Virion components

A wide variety of virion components are involved in activating betaherpesvirus IE gene expression. Engagement of HCMV or viral glycoprotein gB with epidermal growth factor receptor activates the PI3K-mediated signaling pathway (Wang et al., 2003). HCMV glycoproteins also have a role in stimulating the release of pro-inflammatory cytokines mediated by the CD14 and Toll-like receptor 2 molecules on the cell surface (Compton et al., 2003). These cytokines may act on signaling pathways, which in turn, activate cellular transcription factors.

HHV-6 U54 is similar in amino acid sequence to HCMV UL82. The HCMV UL82 gene and the UL35 gene, which encode viral tegument proteins, have a profound positive impact on the efficiency of viral replication (Bresnahan and Shenk, 2000; Dunn et al., 2003; Schierling et al., 2004). These viral tegument proteins are transported to the nucleus of the infected cell where they are targeted to the ND10 (Schierling et al., 2004). UL82 (pp71) protein interacts with a cellular repressor of transcription, hDaxx, and may disrupt or inactivate the hDaxx-histone deacetylase (HDAC) complex (Cantrell and Bresnahan, 2006; Hensel et al., 1996; Hofmann et al., 2002; Ishov et al., 1997, 2002). The viral pp71 tegument protein induces proteasome dependent degradation of hDaxx and thereby neutralizes an intrinsic immune defense mechanism of the cell (Saffert and Kalejta, 2006). In cells deficient in hDaxx, UL82 protein is not targeted to the ND10. The viral MIE promoter and early promoters are activated by UL82 protein (Baldick et al., 1997; Bresnahan and Shenk, 2000; Liu and Stinski, 1992). Heterologous promoters, like herpes simplex virus IE promoters, are also activated by UL82 protein (Homer et al., 1999). The mechanism involves interaction with cellular repressors of transcription and reduction of HDAC activity. The UL82 protein also has effects on cell cycle progression. It stimulates quiescent cells to re-enter the cell cycle and accelerates cells through G_1 (Kalejta and Shenk, 2003a). The UL82 protein binds to members of the retinoblastoma (Rb) protein family and induces proteosome-dependent Rb family degradation (Kalejta and Shenk, 2002, 2003b). A release of the Rb family of repressors from E2F responsive cellular promoters increases cellular cyclins, cdks, and biosynthetic enzymes for DNA synthesis. UL82 protein increases the infectivity of HCMV in HF cells (Baldick et al., 1997).

HHV-6 U42 is the homologue of HCMV UL69. Deletion of the HCMV UL69 gene, which also encodes a tegument protein, causes a delay in viral DNA replication and late gene expression (Lu Hayashi et al., 2000). At low MOI, virus mutated in the UL69 gene replicate slower and take longer to reach peak levels of infectious virus (Lu Hayashi et al., 2000). The UL69 protein is transported to the nucleus where it may interact with proteins that regulate chromatin structure such as hSPT6 (Winkler et al., 1994). The UL69 protein enhances transcription from the viral MIE promoter in transient transfection assays (Winkler et al., 1994). It also affects cell cycle progression by blocking G_1/S transition (Lu Hayashi et al., 2000).

Members of the betaherpesvirus family also have structural homologues of seven transmembrane G-protein-coupled receptors (GPCRs) (Chee et al., 1990; Gompels et al., 1995; Gruijthuijsen et al., 2002; Nicholas, 1996; Rawlinson et al., 1996; Vink et al., 2000; Waldhoer et al., 2002). Recombinant viruses with deletions of the GPCR genes replicate less efficiently in certain cell types. For example, recombinant murine or rat CMV with M33, R33, or M78 genes deleted replicate less efficiently in macrophages and are unable to disseminate to the salivary gland of the animal (Beisser et al., 1999; Davis-Poynter et al., 1997). Several of the viral GPCRs have been shown to initiate ligand-independent constitutive signaling through the G protein phospholipase C (PLC) pathway. Human and rhesus CMV US28 GPCRs induce intracellular signaling following binding of ligands such as fractalkine and CC chemokines. Although HCMV has a sequence homologue (UL33), US28 has been proposed to act in a manner similar to MCMV M33 in that both result in activation of the PLC pathway and activation of CREB and NF-κB. Betaherpesvirus GPCRs are postulated to have a role in the early re-programming of the host cell to favor viral replication. Their activation of cellular transcription factors may enhance IE and early gene transcription.

Infection and dysregulation of the cell cycle by betaherpesviruses

Although betaherpesviruses encode a viral DNA polymerase, processivity factor, single-stranded DNA binding protein and helicase/primase complex for viral DNA synthesis, the viruses depend on many host cell enzymes for this process. The betaherpesviruses do not encode many of the enzymes for synthesis of DNA precursors. Permissive HF cells are typically in the G_0/G_1 phase of the cell cycle and have low amounts of dideoxynucleotide triphosphates and biosynthetic enzymes of DNA precursors at the time of infection. Infection of mouse fibroblasts by MCMV or HF cells by HCMV stimulates production of cellular enzymes of DNA precursor synthesis, e.g., thymidylate synthetase, ribonucleotide reductase, deoxycytidylate deaminase, and dihydrofolate reductase (Gribaudo et al., 2000; Hertel and Mocarski, 2004; Song and Stinski, 2002). Upon HCMV infection, there is a 30-fold increase in the size of the thymidylate triphosphate pool (Biron et al., 1986). In addition, cells are primed for cellular DNA synthesis when the virus induces production or activities of select cellular cyclins and cdks, which are required for cell cycle progression. For example, cyclin E and cdk2, which are necessary for the G_1/S transition, are highly activated after HCMV infection of HF cells

(Bresnahan et al., 1997; Jault et al., 1995; McElroy et al., 2000; Salvant et al., 1998). In contrast, cyclin D, which is necessary for G_1 phase, and cyclin A, which is necessary for the S phase, are not induced by HCMV in HF cells (Zhu et al., 1998). Betaherpesviruses appear to activate the cell differently from that of mitogenic stimulation where the cyclins are activated in a cascade fashion.

The cdks phosphorylate Rb family members and activate the E2F family of transcription factors (Nevins, 1992; Weinberg, 1995). E2F expression is increased after HCMV infection (Salvant et al., 1998; Song and Stinski, 2002), which, along with cyclin E, comprises a feed-forward loop allowing amplification of signals that promote cell cycle progression from G_1 to S phase. However, with HCMV-infected HF cells, the majority of the cells are blocked at the G_1/S transition point (Bresnahan et al., 1996; Dittmer and Mocarski, 1997; Lu and Shenk, 1996). Progression into S phase interferes with efficient HCMV replication because there is little to no IE gene expression during S phase (Fortunato et al., 2002; Salvant et al., 1998). Cellular proteins might be involved in suppressing IE gene expression during S phase, because an inhibitor of cellular proteosome activity allows for a higher level of IE gene expression (Fortunato et al., 2002). In general, the G_1/S compartment of the cell cycle is the most favorable environment for betaherpesvirus gene expression, but the S phase is unfavorable.

An increase in cyclins and cdk activity is likely important for HCMV because cdk inhibitors like roscovitine and olomoucine affect splicing of the IE mRNAs (Sanchez et al., 2004) and inhibit infectious virus production (Bresnahan et al., 1997). In addition, inhibitors of cellular enzymes involved in DNA precursor synthesis (e.g., thymidylate synthetase and deoxycytidylate deaminase) can block HCMV and MCMV replication (Gribaudo et al., 2000). The combination of inactivation of the repressor proteins such as Rb and the activation of proteins involved in movement of the cell cycle such as cyclin E and cdk2 induce an environment most favorable for betaherpesvirus DNA replication. IE proteins of betaherpesviruses play an important role in this stage of the viral replication cycle.

Summary

Betaherpesviruses infect multiple cell types in the host. In general, the productive infection ensues in cells that are terminally differentiated and in the G_0/G_1 phase of the cell cycle. Expression of the IE genes is tightly regulated because these gene products are required for viral replication and have a potential detrimental impact on viral latency. The virions contain components that stimulate both cellular and viral genes. Viral glycoproteins, tegument proteins, and GPCRs can stimulate signal transduction pathways that activate cellular transcription factors and enhance the efficiency of viral replication. The MIE gene products directly activate early viral genes and further stimulate the cell for efficient early and late viral gene expression. Both viral tegument proteins and the MIE proteins cause dysregulation of the cell cycle. The cell is pushed from the G_0/G_1 phase to the G_1/S transition point, with concomitant activation of cellular proteins for DNA precursor synthesis, cell cycle progression, and DNA initiation and synthesis. In the HCMV-infected cell, the level of phospho-serine15-p53 is increased, which stabilizes p53. In p53 wild type cells, the cell cycle stops at the G_1/S transition. The HCMV UL69 tegument protein also prevents transition into S phase. Replication of betaherpesviruses appears to be best in a cell that progresses to the G_1/S transition point, but is prevented from entering the S phase. The betaherpesviruses include both human and animal pathogens for which there are no vaccines, and the available antiviral therapies are fraught with limited efficacy and high rates of adverse effects. A better understanding of betaherpesvirus replication and pathogenesis is needed for developing novel strategies to prevent disease by these opportunists.

Acknowledgments

Because of page and reference limitations, the authors regret that they were unable to acknowledge all important details and contributions. We thank members of the Stinski laboratory and anonymous reviewers for helpful comments on the manuscript. Our work is supported by grants AI-13562 (MFS) and AI-40130 (JLM) from the National Institutes of Health and a grant from the Department of Veterans Affairs (JLM).

REFERENCES

Ahn, J.-H. and Hayward, G. S. (1997). The major immediate-early proteins IE1 and IE2 of human cytomegalovirus colocalize with and disrupt PML-associated nuclear bodies at very early times in infected permissive cells. *J. Virol.*, **71**, 4599–4613.

Ahn, J.-H., Chiou, C.-J., and Hayward, G. S. (1998a). Evaluation and mapping of the DNA binding and oligomerization domains of the IE2 regulatory protein of human cytomegalovirus using yeast one and two hybrid interaction assays. *Gene*, **210**, 25–36.

Ahn, J.-H., Xu, Y., Jang, W.-J., Matunis, M., and Hayward, G. S. (1998b). Disruption of PML subnuclear domains by the acidic IE1 protein of human cytomegalovirus is mediated through interaction with PML and may modulate a RING finger-dependent cryptic transactivator function of PML. *Mol. Cell. Biol.*, **18**, 4899–4913.

Ahn, J.-H., Xu, Y., Jang, W.-J., Matunis, M. J., and Hayward, G. S. (2001). Evaluation of interactions of human cytomegalovirus immediate-early IE2 regulatory protein with small ubiquitin-like modifiers and their conjugation enzyme Ubc9. *J. Virol.*, **75**, 3859–3872.

Albrecht, T., Boldogh, I., Fons, M., Abubakar, S., and Deng, C. Z. (1990). Cell activation signals and the pathogenesis of human cytomegalovirus infection. *Intervirology*, **31**, 68–75.

Albrecht, T., Fons, M. P., Boldogh, I., Deng, S., and Millinoff, D. (1991). Metabolic and cellular effects of human cytomegalovirus infection. *Transplant. Proc.*, **23**, 48–55.

Anders, D. G. and McCue, L. A. (1996). The human cytomegalovirus genes and proteins required for DNA synthesis. *Intervirology*, **39**, 378–388.

Angulo, A., Suto, C., Boehm, M. F., Heyman, R. A., and Ghazal, P. (1995). Retinoid activation of retinoic acid receptors but not of retinoid X receptors promotes cellular differentiation and replication of human cytomegalovirus in embryonal cells. *J. Virol.*, **69**, 3831–3837.

Angulo, A., Suto, C., Heyman, R. A., and Ghazal, P. (1996). Characterization of the sequences of the human cytomegalovirus enhancer that mediate differential regulation by natural and synthetic retinoids. *Mol. Endocrinol.*, **10**, 781–793.

Angulo, A., Chandraratna, R. A. S., LeBlanc, J. F., and Ghazal, P. (1998a). Ligand induction of retinoic acid receptors alters an acute infection by murine cytomegalovirus. *J. Virol.*, **72**, 4589–4600.

Angulo, A., Messerle, M., Koszinowski, U. H., and Ghazal, P. (1998b). Enhancer requirement for murine cytomegalovirus growth and genetic complementation by the human cytomegalovirus enhancer. *J. Virol.*, **72**, 8502–8509.

Angulo, A., Ghazal, P., and Messerle, M. (2000a). The major immediate-early gene ie3 of mouse cytomegalovirus is essential for viral growth. *J. Virol.*, **74**, 11129–11136.

Angulo, A., Kerry, D., Huang, H. *et al.* (2000b). Identification of a boundary domain adjacent to the potent human cytomegalovirus enhancer that represses transcription of the divergent UL127 promoter. *J. Virol.*, **74**, 2826–2839.

Asmar, J., Wiebusch, L., Truss, M., and Hagemeier, C. (2004). The putative zinc-finger of the human cytomegalovirus IE2 86-kilodalton protein is dispensable for DNA-binding and autorepression thereby demarcating a concise core domain in the C-terminus of the protein. *J.Virol.*, **78**, 11853–11864.

Awasthi, S., Isler, J. A., and Alwine, J. C. (2004). Analysis of splice variants of the immediate-early 1 region of human cytomegalovirus. *J. Virol.*, **78**, 8191–8200.

Baldick, C. J., Marchini, A., Patterson, C. E., and Shenk, T. (1997). Human cytomegalovirus tegument protein pp71 (ppUL82) enhances the infectivity of viral DNA and accelerates the infectious cycle. *J. Virol.*, **71**, 4400–4408.

Barrasa, M. I., Harel, N. Y., and Alwine, J. C. (2005). The phosphorylation status of the serine-rich region of the human cytomegalovirus 86 kDa major immediate early protein IE2/IE86 affects temporal viral gene expression. *J. Virol.*, **79**, 1428–1437.

Baskar, J. F., Smith, P. P., Ciment, G. S. *et al.* (1996a). Developmental analysis of the cytomegalovirus enhancer in transgenic animals. *J. Virol.*, **70**, 3215–3226.

Baskar, J. F., Smith, P. P., Nilauer, G. *et al.* (1996b). The enhancer domain of the human cytomegalovirus major immediate-early promoter determines cell type-specific expression in transgenic mice. *J. Virol.*, **70**, 3207–3214.

Beisser, P. S., Kaptein, S. J., Beuken, E., Bruggeman, C. A., and Vink, C. (1998). The Maastricht strain and England strain of rat cytomegalovirus represent different betaherpesvirus species rather than strains. *Virology*, **246**, 341–351.

Beisser, P. S., Grauls, G., Bruggeman, C. A., and Vink, C. (1999). The R33 G protein-coupled receptor gene from rat cytomegalovirus plays an essential role in the pathogenesis of viral infection. *J. Virol.*, **72**, 2352–2363.

Benedict, C. A., Angulo, A., Patterson, G. *et al.* (2004). Neutrality of the canonical NF-kB-dependent pathway for human and murine cytomegalovirus transcription and replication in vitro. *J. Virol.*, **78**, 741–750.

Biron, K. K., Fyfe, J. A., Stanat, S. C., Leslie, K., Sorrell, J. A., and Lambe, C. U. (1986). A human cytomegalovirus mutant resistant to the nucleoside analog 9-[2-hydroxy-1-(hydroxymethyl)ethoxy] methylguanine (BW B759U) induces reduced levels of BW B759U triphosphate. *Proc. Natl. Acad. Sci. USA*, **83**, 8769–8773.

Blankenship, C. A. and Shenk, T. (2002). Mutant human cytomegalovirus lacking the immediate-early TRS1 coding region exhibits a late defect. *J. Virol.*, **76**, 12290–12299.

Bolovan-Fritts, C. A., Mocarski, E. S., and Wiedeman, J. A. (1999). Peripheral blood CD14+ cells from healthy subjects carry a circular conformation of latent cytomegalovirus genome. *Blood*, **93**, 394–398.

Bonin, L. R. and McDougall, J. K. (1997). Human cytomegalovirus IE2 86-kilodalton protein binds p53 but does not abrogate G1 checkpoint function. *J. Virol.*, **71**, 5861–5870.

Bresnahan, W. A. and Shenk, T. E. (2000). UL82 virion protein activates expression of immediate early viral genes in human cytomegalovirus-infected cells. *Proc. Natl Acad. Sci. USA*, **97**, 14506–14511.

Bresnahan, W. A., Boldogh, I., Thompson, E. A., and Albrecht, T. (1996). Human cytomegalovirus inhibits cellular DNA synthesis and arrests productively infected cells in late G1. *Virology*, **224**, 150–160.

Bresnahan, W. A., Boldogh, I., Chi, P., Thompson, E. A., and Albrecht, T. (1997). Inhibition of cellular Cdk2 activity blocks human cytomegalovirus replication. *Virology*, **231**, 239–247.

Bryant, L. A., Mixon, P., Davidson, M., Bannister, A. J., Kouzarides, T., and Sinclair, J. H. (2000). The human cytomegalovirus 86-kilodalton major immediate–early protein interacts physically and functionally with histone acetyltransferase P/CAF. *J. Virol.*, **74**, 7230–7237.

Bullock, G. C., Lashmit, P. E., and Stinski, M. F. (2001). Effect of the R1 element on expression of the US3 and US6 immune evasion genes of human cytomegalovirus. *Virology*, **288**, 164–174.

Bullock, G. C., Thrower, A. R., and Stinski, M. F. (2002). Cellular proteins bind to sequence motifs in the R1 element between the HCMV immune evasion genes. *Exp. Mol. Pathol.*, **72**, 196–206.

Cantrell, S. R. and Bresnahan, W. A. (2005). Interaction between the human cytomegalovirus UL82 gene product (pp71) and hDaxx regulates immediate-early gene expression and viral replication. *J. Virol.*, **79**, 7792–7802.

Castillo, J. P., Yurochko, A. D., and Kowalik, T. F. (2000). Role of human cytomegalovirus immediate-early proteins in cell growth control. *J. Virol.*, **74**, 8028–8037.

Castillo, J. P., Frame, F. M., Rogoff, H. A., Pickering, M. T., Yurochko, A. D., and Kowalik, T. F. (2005). Human cytomegalovirus IE1-72 activates ataxia telangiectsia mutated kinase and a p53/p21-mediated growth arrest response. *J. Virol.*, **79**, 11467–11475.

Caswell, R., Hagemeier, C., Chiou, C.-J., Hayward, G., Kouzarides, T., and Sinclair, J. (1993). The human cytomegalovirus 86K immediate early (IE2) protein requires the basic region of the TATA-box binding protein (TBP) for binding, and interacts with TBP and transcription factor TFIIB via regions of IE2 required for transcriptional regulation. *J. Gen. Virol.*, **74**, 2691–2698.

Chan, Y.-J., Tseng, W.-P., and Hayward, G. S. (1996). Two distinct upstream regulatory domains containing multicopy cellular transcription factor binding sites provide basal repression and inducible enhancer characteristics to the immediate-early IE (US3) promoter from human cytomegalovirus. *J. Virol.*, **70**, 5312–5328.

Chang, Y. N., Crawford, S., Stall, J., Rawlins, D. R., Jeang, K. T., and Hayward, G. S. (1990). The palindromic series I repeats in the simian cytomegalovirus major immediate-early promoter behave as both strong basal enhancers and cyclic-AMP response elements. *J. Virol.*, **64**, 264–277.

Chao, S.-H., Harada, J. N., Hyndman, F. *et al.* (2004). PDX1, a cellular homeoprotein, binds to and regulates the activity of human cytomegalovirus immediate early promoter. *J. Biol. Chem.*, **279**, 16111–16120.

Chee, M. A., Bankier, A. T., Beck, S. *et al.* (1990). Analysis of the protein-coding content of the sequence of human cytomegalovirus strain AD169. *Curr. Top. Microbiol. Immun.*, **154**, 125–169.

Chen, J. and Stinski, M. F. (2002). Role of regulatory elements and the MAPK/ERK or p38 MAPK pathways for activation of human cytomegalovirus gene expression. *J. Virol.*, **76**, 4873–4885.

Chen, Z., Knutson, E., Kurosky, A., and Albrecht, T. (2001). Degradation of p21cip1 in cells productively infected with human cytomegalovirus. *J. Virol.*, **75**(8), 3613–3625.

Cherrington, J. M. and Mocarski, E. S. (1989). Human cytomegalovirus ie1 transactivates the α promoter-enhancer via an 18-base pair repeat element. *J. Virol.*, **63**, 1435–1440.

Cherrington, J. M., Khoury, E. L., and Mocarski, E. S. (1991). Human cytomegalovirus ie2 negatively regulates α gene expression via a short target sequence near the transcription start site. *J. Virol.*, **65**, 887–896.

Child, S. J., Child, S. J., Hakki, M., De Niro, K. L., and Geballe, A. P. (2004). Evasion of cellular antiviral responses by human cytomegalovirus TRS1 and IRS1. *J. Virol.*, **78**, 197–205.

Colberg-Poley, A. M. (1996). Functional roles of immediate early proteins encoded by the human cytomegalovirus UL36–38, UL115–119, TRS1/IRS1 and US3 loci. *Intervirology*, **39**, 350–360.

Colletti, K. S., Xu, Y., Cei, S. A., Tarrant, M., and Pari, G. S. (2004). Expression of human cytomegalovirus UL84 homodimerization and heterodimerization domains act as transdominant inhibitors of OriLyt-dependent DNA replication: Evidence that IE2-UL84 and UL84-UL84 interactions are required for lytic DNA replication. *J. Virol.*, **78**, 9203–9214.

Compton, T., Kurt-Jones, E. A., Boehme, K. W. *et al.* (2003). Human cytomegalovirus activates inflammatory cytokine responses via CD14 and toll-like receptor 2. *J. Virol.*, **77**, 4588–4596.

Cook, C. H., Zhang, Y., McGuinness, B. J., Lahm, M. C., Sedmak, D. D., and Ferguson, R. M. (2002). Intra-abdominal bacterial infection reactivates latent pulmonary cytomegalovirus in immunocompetent mice. *J. Infect. Dis.*, **185**, 1395–1400.

Davis-Poynter, N. J., Lynch, D. M., Vally, H. *et al.* (1997). Identification and characterization of a G protein coupled receptor homolog encoded by murine cytomegalovirus. *J. Virol.*, **71**, 1521–1529.

Davison, A. J., Dolan, A., Akter, P. *et al.* (2003). The human cytomegalovirus genome revisited: comparison with the chimpanzee cytomegalovirus genome. *J. Gen. Virol.*, **84**, 17–28.

Deshmane, S. L. and Fraser, N. W. (1989). During latency, herpes simplex virus type 1 DNA is associated with nucleosomes in a chromatin structure. *J. Virol.*, **63**, 943–947.

Dittmer, D. and Mocarski, E. S. (1997). Human cytomegalovirus infection inhibits G1/S transition. *J. Virol.*, **71**, 1629–1634.

Dorsch-Hasler, K., Keil, G. M., Weber, F., Schaffner, J. M., and Koszinowski, U. H. (1985). A long and complex enhancer activates transcription of the gene coding for the highly abundant immediate early mRNA in murine cytomegalovirus. *Proc. Natl Acad. Sci. USA*, **82**, 8325–8329.

Dunn, W., Chou, C., Hong, L. *et al.* (2003). Functional profiling of a human cytomegalovirus genome. *Proc. Natl Acad. Sci. USA*, **100**, 14223–14228.

Dyson, P. J. and Farrell, P. J. (1985). Chromatin structure of Epstein Barr virus. *J. Gen. Virol.*, **66**, 1931–1940.

Fietze, E., Prosch, S., Reinke, P. *et al.* (1994). Cytomegalovirus infection in transplant recipients: the role of tumor necrosis factor. *Transplantation*, **58**, 675–680.

Fish, K. N., Britt, W., and Nelson, J. A. (1996). A novel mechanism for persistence of human cytomegalovirus in macrophages. *J. Virol.*, **70**, 1855–1862.

Fish, K. N., Depto, A. S., Moses, A. V., Britt, W., and Nelson, J. A. (1995). Growth kinetics of human cytomegalovirus are altered in monocyte-derived macrophages. *J. Virol.*, **69**, 3737–3743.

Flebbe-Rehwaldt, L. M., Wood, C., and Chandran, B. (2000). Characterization of transcripts expressed from human herpesvirus 6A strain GS immediate–early region B U16-U17 open reading frames. *J. Virol.*, **74**, 11040–11054.

Fortunato, E. A. and Spector, D. H. (1998). p53 and RPA are sequestered in viral replication centers in the nuclei of cells infected with human cytomegalovirus. *J. Virol.*, **72**, 2033–2039.

Fortunato, E. A. and Spector, D. H. (1999). Regulation of human cytomegalovirus gene expression. *Adv. Virus Res.*, **54**, 61–128.

Fortunato, E. A., Sommer, M. H., Yoder, K., and Spector, D. H. (1997). Identification of domains within the human cytomegalovirus major immediate–early 86-kilodalton protein and the retinoblastoma protein required for physical and functional interaction with each other. *J. Virol.*, **71**, 8176–8185.

Fortunato, E., Sanchez, V., Yen, J. Y., and Spector, D. H. (2002). Infection of cells with human cytomegalovirus during S phase results in a blockade to immediate–early gene expression that can be overcome by inhibition of the proteasome. *J. Virol.*, **76**, 5369–5379.

Gawn, J. M. and Greaves, R. F. (2002). Absence of IE1 p72 protein function during low-multiplicity infection by human cytomegalovirus results in a broad block to viral delayed-early gene expression. *J. Virol.*, **76**, 4441–4455.

Gebert, S., Schmolke, S., Sorg, G., Floss, S., Plachter, B., and Stamminger, T. (1997). The UL84 protein of human cytomegalovirus acts as a transdominant inhibitor of immediate-early-mediated transactivation that is able to prevent viral replication. *J. Virol.*, **71**, 7048–7060.

Geng, Y., Chandran, B., Josephs, S. F., and Wood, C. (1992). Identification and characterization of a human herpesvirus 6 gene segment that trans activates the human immunodeficiency virus type 1 promoter. *J. Virol.*, **66**, 1564–1570.

Gompels, U. A., Nicholas, J., Lawrence, G. *et al.* (1995). The DNA sequence of human herpesvirus-6: structure, coding content, and genome evolution. *Virology*, **209**, 29–51.

Gonczol, E., Andrews, P. W., and Plotkin, S. A. (1984). Cytomegalovirus replicates in differentiated but not in undifferentiated human embryonal carcinoma cells. *Science*, **224**, 159–161.

Gravel, A., Gosselin, J., and Flamand, L. (2002). Human herpesvirus 6 immediate-early 1 protein is a sumoylated nuclear phosphoprotein colocalizing with promyelocytic leukemia protein-associated nuclear bodies. *J. Biol. Chem.*, **277**, 19679–19687.

Greaves, R. F. and Mocarski, E. S. (1998). Defective growth correlates with reduced accumulation of viral DNA replication protein after low-multiplicity infection by a human cytomegalovirus ie1 mutant. *J. Virol.*, **72**, 366–379.

Gribaudo, F., Riera, L., Lembo, D. *et al.* (2000). Murine cytomegalovirus stimulates cellular thymidylate synthetase gene expression in quiescent cells and requires the enzyme for replication. *J. Virol.*, **74**, 4979–4987.

Gruijthuijsen, Y. K., Casarosa, P., Kaptein, S. J. F. *et al.* (2002). The rat cytomegalovirus R33-encoded G protein-coupled receptor signals in a constitutive fashion. *J. Virol.*, **76**, 1328–1338.

Grundy, J. E., Lawson, K. M., MacCormac, L. P., Fletcher, J. M., and Yong, K. L. (1998). Cytomegalovirus-infected endothelial cells recruit neutrophils by the secretion of C-X-C chemokines and transmit virus by direct neutrophil- endothelial cell contact and during neutrophil transendothelial migration. *J. Infect. Dis.*, **177**, 1465–1474.

Grzimek, N. K. A., Podlech, J., Steffens, H.-P., Holtappels, R., Schmalz, S., and Reddehase, M. J. (1999). In vivo replication of recombinant murine cytomegalovirus driven by the paralogous major immediate-early promoter-enhancer of human cytomegalovirus. *J. Virol.*, **73**, 5043–5055.

Grzimek, N. K. A., Dreis, D., Schmalz, S., and Reddehase, M. J. (2001). Random, asynchronous, and asymetric transcriptional activity of enhancer-flanking major immediate-early genes ie1/3 and ie2 during murine cytomegalovirus latency in the lungs. *J. Virol.*, **75**, 2692–2705.

Hagemeier, C., Walker, S., Caswell, R., Kouzarides, T., and Sinclair, J. (1992a). The human cytomegalovirus 80-kilodalton but not the 72-kilodalton immediate–early protein transactivates heterologous promoters in a TATA box-dependent mechanism and interacts directly with TFIID. *J. Virol.*, **66**, 4452–4456.

Hagemeier, C., Walker, S. M., Sissons, P. J., and Sinclair, J. H. (1992b). The 72K IE1 and 80K IE2 proteins of human cytomegalovirus independently trans-activate the c-fos, c-myc and hsp70 promoters via basal promoter elements. *J. Gen. Virol.*, **73**(9), 2385–2393.

Hagemeier, C., Caswell, R., Hayhurst, G., Sinclair, J., and Kouzarides, T. (1994). Functional interaction between the HCMV IE2 transactivator and the retinoblastoma protein. *EMBO J.*, **13**, 2897–2903.

Hahn, G., Jores, R. and Mocarski, E. S. (1998). Cytomegalovirus remains latent in a common precursor of dendritic and myeloid cells. *Proc. Natl Acad. Sci.*, **95**, 3937–3942.

Hakki, M. and Geballe, A. P. (2005). Double-stranded RNA binding by human cytomegalovirus pTRS1. *J. Virol.*, **79**, 7311–7318.

Hanson, S. G., Strelow, L. I., Franchi, D. C., Anders, D. G., and Wong, S. W. (2003). Complete sequence and genomic analysis of rhesus cytomegalovirus. *J. Virol.*, **77**, 6620–6636.

Harel, N. Y. and Alwine, J. C. (1998). Phosphorylation of the human cytomegalovirus 86-kilodalton immediate-early protein IE2. *J. Virol.*, **72**, 5481–5492.

Hayhurst, G. P., Bryant, L. A., Caswell, R. C., Walker, S. M., and Sinclair, J. H. (1995). CCAAT box-dependent activation of the TATA-less human DNA polymerase alpha promoter by the human cytomegalovirus 72-kilodalton major immediate-early protein. *J. Virol.*, **69**, 182–188.

Hensel, G. M., Meyer, H. H., Buchman, I. *et al.* (1996). Intracellular localization and expression of the human cytomegalovirus matrix protein pp71 (UL82). *J. Gen. Virol.*, **77**, 3087–3097.

Hertel, L. and Mocarski, E. S. (2004). Global analysis of host cell gene expression late during cytomegalovirus infection reveals extensive dysregulation of cell cycle expression and induction of pseudomitosis independent of US28 function. *J. Virol.*, **78**, 11988–12011.

Hertel, L., Lacaille, V. G., Strobl, H., Mellins, E. D., and Mocarski, E. S. (2003). Susceptibility of immature and mature Langerhans cell-type dendritic cells to infection and immunomodulation by human cytomegalovirus. *J. Virol.*, **77**, 7563–7574.

Hofmann, H., Floss, S., and Stamminger, T. (2000). Covalent modification of the transactivator protein IE2-p86 of human cytomegalovirus by conjugation to the ubiquitin-homologous proteins SUMO-1 and hSMT3b. *J. Virol.*, **74**, 2510–2524.

Hofmann, H., Sindre, H., and Stamminger, T. (2002). Functional interaction between the pp71 protein of human cytomegalovirus and the PML-interacting protein human Daxx. *J. Virol.*, **76**, 5769–5783.

Homer, E. G., Rinaldi, A., Nicholi, M. J., and Preston, C. M. (1999). Activation of herpesvirus gene expression by the human cytomegalovirus protein pp71. *J. Virol.*, **73**, 8512–8518.

Huang, T. H., Oka, T., Asai, T. *et al.* (1996). Repression by a differentiation-specific factor of the human cytomegalovirus enhancer. *Nucl. Acids Res.*, **24**, 1695–1701.

Hudson, J. B. (1979). The murine cytomegalovirus as a model for the study of viral pathogenesis and persistent infections. *Arch. Virol.*, **62**, 1–29.

Hummel, M., Zheng, Z., Yan, S. *et al.* (2001). Allogeneic transplantation induces expression of cytomegalovirus immediate–early genes in vivo: a model for reactivation from latency. *J. Virol.*, **75**, 4814–4822.

Hummel, M., Yan, S., Varghese, T. K., Li, Z., and Abecassis, M. (2003). Transcriptional activation of MCMV IE gene expression by 5-axa-2′-deoxycytidine in latently infected spleen explants. *28th International Herpesvirus Workshop, Madison, WI.*

Hunninghake, G. W., Monick, M. M., Liu, B., and Stinski, M. F. (1989). The promoter-regulatory region of the major immediate–early gene of human cytomegalovirus responds to T-lymphocyte stimulation and contains functional cyclic AMP-response elements. *J. Virol.*, **63**, 3026–3033.

Ibanez, C. E., Schrier, R., Ghazal, P., Wiley, C., and Nelson, J. A. (1991). Human cytomegalovirus productively infects primary differentiated macrophages. *J. Virol.*, **65**, 6581–6588.

Ippolito, A. J., Spengler, M. L., Chang, K. S., Berkowitz, J. L., and Azizkhan-Clifford, J. (2003). Kinase activity of human cytomegalovirus protein IE1/IE72 correlates with POD disruption and desumoylation of PML. *28th International Herpesvirus Workshop, Madison, WI.*

Ishov, A. M., Stenberg, R. M., and Maul, G. G. (1997). Human cytomegalovirus immediate early interaction with host nuclear structures: definition of an immediate transcript environment. *J. Cell Biol.*, **138**, 5–16.

Ishov, A. M., Vladimirova, O. V., and Maul, G. G. (2002). Daxx-mediated accumulation of human cytomegalovirus tegument protein pp71 at ND10 facilitates initiation of viral infection at these nuclear domains. *J. Virol.*, **76**, 7705–7712.

Isomura, H. and Stinski, M. F. (2003). Effect of substitution of the human cytomegalovirus enhancer or promoter with the murine cytomegalovirus enhancer or promoter on replication in human fibroblasts. *J. Virol.*, **77**, 3602–3614.

Isomura, H., Tatsuya, T., and Stinski, M. F. (2004). The role of the proximal enhancer of the major immediate early promoter in human cytomegalovirus replication. *J. Virol.*, **78**, 12788–12799.

Isomura, H., Stinski, M. F., Kudoh, A., Daikoku, T., Shirata, N., and Tatsuya, T. (2005). Two Sp1/Sp3 binding sites in the major immediate-early proximal enhancer of human cytomegalovirus have a significant role in viral replication. *J. Virol.*, **79**, 9597–9607.

Jault, F. M., Jault, J.-M., Ruchti, F. *et al.* (1995). Cytomegalovirus infection induces high levels of cyclins, phosphorylated RB, and p53, leading to cell cycle arrest. *J. Virol.*, **69**, 6697–6704.

Jenuwein, T. and Allis, C. D. (2001). Translating the histone code. *Science*, **293**, 1074–1080.

Johnson, R. A., Huong, S. M., and Huang, E. S. (2000). Activation of the mitogen-activated protein kinase p38 by human cytomegalovirus infection through two distinct pathways: a novel mechanism for activation of p38. *J. Virol.*, **74**, 1158–1167.

Johnson, R. A., Wang, X., Ma, X. L., Huong, S. M., and Huang, E. S. (2001). Human cytomegalovirus up-regulates the phosphatidylinositol 3-kinase (PI3-K) pathway: inhibition of PI3-K activity inhibits viral replication and virus-induced signaling. *J. Virol.*, **75**, 6022–6032.

Jordan, M. C. (1983). Latent infection and the elusive cytomegalovirus. *Rev. Infect. Dis.*, **5**, 205–215.

Kalejta, R. F. and Shenk, T. (2002). Manipulation of the cell cycle by human cytomegalovirus. *Frontiers in Biosci.*, **7**, 295–306.

Kalejta, R. F. and Shenk, T. (2003a). The human cytomegalovirus UL82 gene product (pp71) accelerates progression through the G1 phase of the cell cycle. *J. Virol.*, **77**, 3451–3459.

Kalejta, R. F. and Shenk, T. (2003b). Proteasome-dependent, ubiquitin-independent degradation of the Rb family of tumor suppressors by the human cytomegalovirus pp71 protein. *Proc. Natl Acad. Sci. USA*, **100**, 3263–3268.

Keller, M. J., Wheeler, D. G., Cooper, E., and Meier, J. L. (2003). Role of the human cytomegalovirus major immediate-early promoter's 19-base-pair-repeat cyclic AMP-response element in acutely infected cells. *J. Virol.*, **77**, 6666–6675.

Kerry, J. A., Sehgal, A., Barlow, S. W., Gavanaugh, V. J., Fish, K., and Nelson, J. A. (1995). Isolation and characterization of a low-abundance splice variant from the human cytomegalovirus major immediate-early gene region. *J. Virol.*, **69**, 3868–3872.

Kline, J. N., Hunninghake, G. M., He, B., and Monick, M. M. (1998). Synergistic activation of the human cytomegalovirus major immediate early promoter by prostaglandin E2 and cytokines. *Exp. Lung Res.*, **1**, 3–14.

Koffron, A. J., Hummel, M., Patterson, B. K. *et al.* (1998). Cellular localization of latent murine cytomegalovirus. *J. Virol.*, **72**, 95–103.

Kondo, K., Kaneshima, H., and Mocarski, E. S. (1994). Human cytomegalovirus latent infection of granulocyte-macrophage progenitors. *Proc. Natl Acad. Sci. USA*, **91**, 11879–11883.

Kondo, K., Xu, J., and Mocarski, E. S. (1996). Human cytomegalovirus latent gene expression in granulocyte–macrophage progenitors in culture and in seropositive individuals. *Proc. Natl Acad. Sci. USA*, **93**, 11137–11142.

Kothari, S. K., Baillie, J., Sissons, J. G. P., and Sinclair, J. H. (1991). The 21 bp repeat element of the human cytomegalovirus major immediate early enhancer is a negative regulator of gene expression in undifferentiated cells. *Nucl. Acids Res.*, **19**, 1767–1771.

Kurz, S. K. and Reddehase, M. J. (1999). Patchwork pattern of transcriptional reactivation in the lungs indicates sequential checkpoints in the transition from murine cytomegalovirus latency to recurrence. *J. Virol.*, **73**, 8612–8622.

Kurz, S. K., Rapp, M., Steffens, H.-P., Grzimek, N. K. A., Schmalz, S., and Reddehase, M. J. (1999). Focal transcriptional activity of murine cytomegalovirus during latency in the lungs. *J. Virol.*, **73**, 482–494.

LaFemina, R. and Hayward, G. S. (1986). Constitutive and retinoic acid-inducible expression of cytomegalovirus immediate-early genes in human teratocarcinoma cells. *J. Virol.*, **58**, 434–440.

Lang, D. and Stamminger, T. (1994). Minor groove contacts are essential for an interaction of the human cytomegalovirus IE2 protein with its DNA target. *Nucl. Acids Res.*, **22**, 3331–3338.

Lang, D., Gebert, S., Arlt, H., and Stamminger, T. (1995). Functional interaction between the human cytomegalovirus 86-kilodalton IE2 protein and the cellular transcription factor CREB. *J. Virol.*, **69**, 6030–6037.

LaPierre, L. A. and Biegalke, B. J. (2001). Identification of a novel transcriptional repressor encoded by human cytomegalovirus. *J. Virol.*, **75**, 6062–6069.

Lashmit, P. E., Stinski, M. F., Murphy, E. A., and Bullock, G. C. (1998). A cis-repression sequence adjacent to the transcription start site of the human cytomegalovirus US3 gene is required to down regulate gene expression at early and late times after infection. *J. Virol.*, **72**, 9575–9584.

Lashmit, P. E., Lundquist, C. A., Meier, J. L., and Stinski, M. F. (2004). A cellular repressor inhibits human cytomegaloviurs transcription from the UL127 promoter. *J. Virol.*, **78**, 5113–5123.

Lathey, J. L. and Spector, S. A. (1991). Unrestricted replication of human cytomegalovirus in hydrocortisone-treated macrophages. *J. Virol.*, **65**, 6371–6375.

Lee, H. and Ahn, J. (2004). The sumoylation of HCMV (Towne) IE2 is not required for viral growth in cultured human fibroblast. *29th International Herpesvirus Workshop, Reno, Nevada.*

Lee, H.-R., Kim, D.-J., Lee, J.-M. *et al.* (2004). Ability of the human cytomegalovirus IE1 protein to modulate sumoylation of PML correlates with its functional activities in transcriptional regulation and infectivity in cultured fibroblast cells. *J. Virol.*, **78**, 6527–6542.

Liu, B. and Stinski, M. F. (1992). Human cytomegalovirus contains a tegument protein that enhances transcription from promoters with upstream ATF and AP-1 cis-acting elements. *J. Virol.*, **66**, 4434–4444.

Liu, B., Hermiston, T. W., and Stinski, M. F. (1991). A cis-acting element in the major immediate early (IE) promoter of human cytomegalovirus is required for negative regulation by IE2. *J. Virol.*, **65**, 897–903.

Liu, R., Baillie, J., Sissons, J. G. P., and Sinclair, J. H. (1994). The transcription factor YY1 binds to negative regulatory elements in the human cytomegalovirus major immediate early enhancer/promoter and mediates repression in nonpermissive cells. *Nucl. Acids Res.*, **22**, 2453–2459.

Lu Hayashi, M., Blankenship, C., and Shenk, T. (2000). Human cytomegalovirus UL69 protein is required for efficient accumulation of infected cells in the G1 phase of the cell cycle. *Proc. Natl Acad. Sci. USA*, **97**, 2692–2696.

Lu, M. and Shenk, T. (1996). Human cytomegalovirus infection inhibits cell cycle progression at multiple points including the transition from G1 to S. *J. Virol.*, **70**, 8850–8857.

Lukac, D. M. and Alwine, J. C. (1997). Effects of the human cytomegalovirus major immediate–early proteins in controlling the cell cycle and inhibiting apoptosis: studies with ts13 cells. *J. Virol.*, **73**, 2825–2831.

Lukac, D. M., Manuppello, J. R., and Alwine, J. C. (1994). Transcriptional activation by the human cytomegalovirus immediate–early proteins: Requirements for simple promoter structures and interactions with multiple components of the transcription complex. *J. Virol.*, **68**, 5184–5193.

Lukac, D. M., Harel, N. Y., Tanese, N., and Alwine, J. C. (1997). TAF-like functions of human cytomegalovirus immediate–early proteins. *J. Virol.*, **71**, 7227–7239.

Lundquist, C. A., Meier, J. L., and Stinski, M. F. (1999). A strong negative transcriptional regulatory region between the human cytomegalovirus UL127 gene and the major immediate early enhancer. *J. Virol.*, **73**, 9039–9052.

Macias, M. P. and Stinski, M. F. (1993). An in vitro system for human cytomegalovirus immediate early 2 protein (IE2)-mediated site-dependent repression of transcription and direct binding of IE2 to the major immediate early promoter. *Proc. Natl Acad. Sci. USA*, **90**, 707–711.

Macias, M. P. Huang, L., Lashmit, P. E., and Stinski, M. F. (1996). Cellular and viral protein binding to a cytomegalovirus promoter transcription initiation site: Effects on transcription. *J. Virol.*, **70**, 3628–3635.

Maidji, E., Percivalle, E., Gerna, G., Fisher, S., and Pereira, L. (2002). Transmission of human cytomegalovirus from infected uterine microvascular endothelial cells to differentiating placental cytotrophoblasts. *Virology*, **304**, 53–69.

Malone, C. L., Vesole, D. H., and Stinski, M. F. (1990). Transactivation of a human cytomegalovirus early promoter by gene products from the immediate–early gene IE2 and augmentation by IE1: mutational analysis of the viral proteins. *J. Virol.*, **64**, 1498–1506.

Marchini, A., Liu, H., and Ahu, H. (2001). Human cytomegalovirus with IE-2 (UL122) deleted fails to express early lytic genes. *J. Virol.*, **75**, 1870–1878.

Margolis, M. J., Pajovic, S., Wong, E. L. *et al.* (1995). Interaction of the 72-kilodalton human cytomegalovirus IE1 gene product with E2F, coincides with E2F-dependent activation of dihrofolate reductase transcription. *J. Virol.*, **69**, 7759–7767.

McElroy, A. K., Dwarakanath, R. S., and Spector, D. H. (2000). Dysregulation of cyclin E gene expression in human cytomegalovirus-infected cells requires viral early gene expression and is associated with changes in the Rb-related protein p130. *J. Virol.*, **74**, 4192–4206.

Meier, J. L. (2001). Reactivation of the human cytomegalovirus major immediate-early regulatory region and viral replication in embryonal NTera2 cells: role of trichostatin A, retinoic acid, and deletion of the 21-base-pair repeats and modulator. *J. Virol.*, **75**, 1581–1593.

Meier, J. L. and Pruessner, J. A. (2000). The human cytomegalovirus major immediate–early distal enhancer region is required for efficient viral replication and immediate–early expression. *J. Virol.*, **74**, 1602–1613.

Meier, J. L. and Stinski, M. F. (1996). Regulation of human cytomegalovirus immediate-early gene expression. *Intervirology*, **39**, 331–342.

Meier, J. L. and Stinski, M. F. (2006). Major immediate–early enhancer and its gene products. In *Cytomegalovirus Molecular Biology and Immunology*, ed. M. J. Reddehase, pp. 151–166. Norfolk, UK: Caister Academic Press.

Meier, J. L., Keller, M. J., and McCoy, J. J. (2002). Requirement of multiple *cis*-acting elements in the human cytomegalovirus major immediate–early distal enhancer for viral gene expression and replication. *J. Virol.*, **76**, 313–326.

Melnychuk, R. M., Streblow, D. N., Lordanov, M., and Nelson, J. A. (2003). Efficient replication of MCMV is dependent on AP-1. *28th International Herpesvirus Workshop, Madison, WI.*

Mocarski, E. S., Kemble, G., Lyle, J., and Greaves, R. F. (1996). A deletion mutant in the human cytomegalovirus gene encoding IE1 491aa is replication defective due to a failure in autoregulation. *Proc. Natl Acad. Sci. USA*, **93**, 11321–11326.

Muller, S. and Dejean, A. (1999). Viral immediate-early proteins abrogate the modification by SUMO-1 of PML and Sp100 proteins, correlating with nuclear body disruption. *J. Virol.*, **73**, 5137–5143.

Murphy, E., Dong, Y., Grimwood, J., Schmutz, J. *et al.* (2003a). Coding potential of laboratory and clinical stains of human cytomegalovirus. *Proc. Natl Acad. Sci. USA*, **100**, 14976–14981.

Murphy, E., Rigoutsos, I., Shibuya, T., and Shenk, T. (2003b). Reevaluation of human cytomegalovirus coding potential. *Proc. Natl Acad. Sci. USA*, **100**, 13585–13590.

Murphy, E. A., Streblow, D. N., Nelson, J. A., and Stinski, M. F. (2000). The human cytomegalovirus IE86 protein can block cell cycle progression after inducing transition into the S-phase of permissive cells. *J. Virol.*, **74**, 7108–7118.

Murphy, J., Fischle, W., Verdin, E., and Sinclair, J. (2002). Control of cytomegalovirus lytic gene expression by histone acetylation. *EMBO J.*, **21**, 1112–1120.

Mutimer, D., Mirza, D., Shaw, J., O'Donnell, K., and Elias, E. (1997). Enhanced (cytomegalovirus) viral replication associated with septic bacterial complications in liver transplant recipients. *Transplantation*, **63**, 1411–1415.

Neipel, F., Ellinger, K., and Fleckenstein, B. (1991). The unique region of the human herpesvirus 6 genome is essentially collinear with the UL segment of human cytomegalovirus. *J. Gen. Virol.*, **72**, 2293–2297.

Nelson, J. A. and Groudine, M. (1986). Transcriptional regulation of the human cytomegalovirus major immediate–early gene is associated with induction of DNase I-hypersensitive sites. *Mol. Cell. Biol.*, **6**, 452–461.

Nelson, J. A., Reynolds-Kohler, C., and Smith, B. (1987). Negative and positive regulation by a short segment in the 5′-flanking region of the human cytomegalovirus major immediate–early gene. *Mol. Cell. Biol.*, **7**, 4125–4129.

Netterwald, J., Yang, S., Wang, W. *et al.* (2005). Two gamma interferon-activated site-like elements in the human cytomegalovirus major immediate-early promoter/enhancer are important for virus replication. *J. Virol.*, **79**, 5035–5046.

Nevels, M., Brune, W., and Shenk, T. (2004). SUMOylation of the human cytomegalovirus 72-kilodalton IE1 protein facilitates expression of the 86-kilodalton IE2 protein and promotes viral replication. *J. Virol.*, **78**, 7803–7812.

Nevins, J. R. (1992). E2F: a link between the Rb tumor suppressor and viral oncoproteins. *Science*, **258**, 424–429.

Nicholas, J. (1994). Nucleotide sequence analysis of a 21-kbp region of the genome of human herpesvirus-6 containing homologues of human cytomegalovirus major immediate–early and replication genes. *Virology*, **204**, 738–750.

Nicholas, J. (1996). Determination and analysis of the complete nucleotide sequence of human herpesvirus 7. *J. Virol.*, **70**, 5975–5989.

Nicholas, J. and Martin, M. (1994). Nucleotide sequence analysis of a 38.5-kilobase-pair region of the genome of human herpesvirus 6 encoding human cytomegalovirus immediate–early gene homologs and transactivating functions. *J. Virol.*, **68**, 597–610.

Noris, E., Zannetti, C., Demurtas, A. *et al.* (2002). Cell cycle arrest by human cytomegalovirus 86-kDa IE2 protein resembles premature senescence. *J. Virol.*, **76**, 12135–12148.

Pajovic, S., Wong, E. L., Black, A. R., and Azizkhan, J. C. (1997). Identification of a viral kinase that phosphorylates specific E2Fs and pocket proteins. *Mol. Cell. Biol.*, **17**, 6459–6464.

Papanikolaou, E., Kouvatsis, V., Dimitriadis, G., Inoue, N., and Arsenakis, M. (2002). Identification and characterization of the gene products of open reading frame U86/87 of human herpesvirus 6. *Virus Res.*, **89**, 89–101.

Pari, G. S. and Anders, D. G. (1993). Eleven loci encoding trans-acting factors are required for transient complementation of human cytomegalovirus oriLyt-dependent DNA replication. *J. Virol.*, **67**, 6979–6988.

Pari, G. S., Kacica, M. A., and Anders, D. G. (1993). Open reading frames UL44, IRS1/TRS1, and UL36–38 are required for transient complementation of human cytomegalovirus oriLyt-dependent DNA synthesis. *J. Virol.*, **67**, 2575–2582.

Petrik, D. T., Schmitt, K. P., and Stinski, M. F. (2006). Recombinant human cytomegalovirus containing a site specific mutation in the IE86 protein is unable to inhibit cellular DNA synthesis or arrest cell cycle progression. *J. Virol.*, **80**, 3872–3883.

Pizzorno, M. C. and Hayward, G. S. (1990). The IE2 gene products of human cytomegalovirus specifically down-regulate expression from the major immediate–early promoter through a target located near the cap site. *J. Virol.*, **64**, 6154–6165.

Pizzorno, M. C., Mullen, M. A., Chang, Y. N., and Hayward, G. S. (1991). The functionally active IE2 immediate–early regulatory protein of human cytomegalovirus is an 80-kilodalton polypeptide that contains two distinct activator domains and a duplicated nuclear localization signal. *J. Virol.*, **65**(7), 3839–3852.

Plachter, B., Britt, W., Vornhagen, R., Stamminger, T., and Jahn, G. (1993). Analysis of proteins encoded by IE regions 1 and 2 of human cytomegalovirus using monoclonal antibodies generated against recombinant antigens. *Virology*, **193**, 642–652.

Prosch, S., Staak, K., Stein, J. *et al.* (1995). Stimulation of the human cytomegalovirus IE enhancer/promoter in HL-60 cells by TNFalpha is mediated via induction of NF-kappaB. *Virology*, **208**(1), 197–206.

Puchtler, E. and Stamminger, T. (1991). An inducible promoter mediates abundant expression from the immediate-early 2 gene region of human cytomegalovirus at late times after infection. *J. Virol.*, **65**, 6301–6303.

Rawlinson, W. D., Farrell, H. E., and Barrell, B. G. (1996). Analysis of the complete DNA sequence of murine cytomegalovirus. *J. Virol.*, **70**, 8833–8849.

Reeves, M., Murphy, J. Greaves, R., Fairly, J. Brehm, A., and Sinclair, J. (2006). Auto-repression of the HCMV major immediate early promoter/enhancer at late times of infection is mediated by the recruitment of chromatin remodeling enzymes by IE86. *J. Virol.* (In press).

Rodems, S. M. and Spector, D. H. (1998). Extracellular signal-regulated kinase activity is sustained early during human cytomegalovirus infection. *J. Virol.*, **72**, 9173–9180.

Romanowski, M. J. and Shenk, T. (1997). Characterization of the human cytomegalovirus irs1 and trs1 genes: a second immediate–early transcription unit within irs1 whose product antagonizes transcription activation. *J. Virol.*, **71**, 1485–1496.

Romanowski, M. J., Garrido-Guerrero, E., and Shenk, T. (1997). pIRS1 and pTRS1 are present in human cytomegalovirus virions. *J. Virol.*, **71**, 5703–5705.

Rue, C. A., Jarvis, A., Knocke, A. J. *et al.* (2004). A cyclooxygenase-2 homologue encoded by rhesus cytomegalovirus is a determinant for endothelial cell tropism. *J. Virol.*, **78**, 12529–12536.

Saffert, R. T. and Kalejta, R. F. (2006). Inactivating a cellular intrinsic immune defense mediated by Daxx is the mechanism through which the human cytomegalovirus pp71 protein stimulates viral immediate–early gene expression. *J. Virol.*, **80**, 3863–3871.

Salvant, B. S., Fortunato, E. A., and Spector, D. H. (1998). Cell cycle dysregulation by human cytomegalovirus: Influence of the cell cycle phase at the time of infection and effects on cyclin transcription. *J. Virol.*, **72**, 3729–3741.

Samaniego, L. A., Tevethia, M. J., and Spector, D. J. (1994). The human cytomegalovirus 86-kilodalton immediate-early 2 protein: Synthesis as a precursor polypeptide and interaction with a 75-kilodalton protein of probable viral origin. *J. Virol.*, **68**, 720–729.

Sambucetti, L. C., Cherrington, J. M., Wilkinson, G. W. G., and Mocarski, E. S. (1989). NF-kappa B activation of the cytomegalovirus enhancer is mediated by a viral transactivator and by T cell stimulation. *EMBO J.*, **8**, 4251–4258.

Sanchez, V., Clark, C. L., Yen, J. Y., Dwarakanath, R., and Spector, D. H. (2002). Viable human cytomegalovirus recombinant virus with an internal deletion of the IE2 86 gene affects late stages of viral replication. *J. Virol.*, **76**, 2973–2989.

Sanchez, V., Mc Elroy, A. K., Yen, J. *et al.* (2004). Cyclin-dependent kinase activity is required at early times for accurate processing and accumulation of the human cytomegalovirus UL122–123 and UL37 immediate–early transcripts and at later times for virus production. *J. Virol.*, **78**, 11219–11232.

Sandford, G. R. and Burns, W. H. (1996). Rat cytomegalovirus has a unique immediate early gene enhancer. *Virology*, **222**, 310–317.

Sarisky, R. T. and Hayward, G. S. (1996). Evidence that the UL84 gene product of human cytomegalvorus is essential for promoting oriLyt-dependent DNA replication and formation of replication compartments in cotransfection assays. *J. Virol.*, **70**, 7398–7413.

Schierling, K., Stamminger, T., Mertens, T., and Winkler, M. (2004). Human cytomegalovirus tegument proteins ppUL82(pp71) and ppUL35 interact and co-operatively activate the major immediate-early enhancer. *J. Virol.*, **78**, 9512–9523.

Schiewe, U., Neipel, F., Schreiner, D., and Fleckenstein, B. (1994). Structure and transcription of an immediate–early region in the human herpesvirus 6 genome. *J. Virol.*, **68**, 2978–2985.

Schmidbauer, M., Budka, H., Ulrich, W., and Ambros, P. (1989). Cytomegalovirus (CMV) disease of the brain in AIDS and connatal infection: a comparative study by histology, immunocytochemistry, and in situ DNA hybridization. *Acta Neuropathol. Berlin*, **79**, 286–293.

Shelbourn, S. L., Kothari, S. K., Sissons, J. G. P., and Sinclair, J. H. (1989). Repression of human cytomegalovirus gene espression associated with a novel immediate early regulatory region binding factor. *Nucl. Acid Res.*, **17**, 9165–9171.

Shen, Y. H., Utama, B., Wang, J. *et al.* (2004). Human cytomegalovirus causes endothelial injury through the ataxia telangiectasia mutant and p53 DNA damage signaling pathways. *Circ. Res.*, **94**, 1310–1317.

Shirakata, M., Terauchi, M., Ablikim, M. *et al.* (2002). Novel immediate–early protein IE19 of human cytomegalovirus activates the origin recognition complex I promoter in a cooperative manner with IE72. *J. Virol.*, **76**, 3158–3167.

Sinclair, J. and Sissons, P. (1996). Latent and persistent infections of monocytes and macrophages. *Intervirology*, **39**, 293–301.

Sinclair, J. H., Baillie, J., Bryant, L. A., Taylor-Wiedeman, J. A., and Sissons, J. G. P. (1992). Repression of human cytomegalovirus major immediate early gene expression in a monocytic cell line. *J. Gen. Virol.*, **73**, 433–435.

Singh, J. and Compton, T. (2004). The IE1 protein of human cytomegalovirus is a key component of host innate immune repression. *29th International Herpesvirus Workshop, Reno, Nevada*.

Sinzger, C. and Jahn, G. (1996). Human cytomegalovirus cell tropisim and pathogenesis. *Intervirology*, **39**, 302–319.

Sinzger, C., Muntefering, H., Loning, T., Stoss, H., Placther, B., and Jahn, G. (1993). Cell types infected in human cytomegalovirus placentitis identified by immunohistochemical double staining. *Virchows Arch. A. Pathol. Anat. Histopathol.*, **4233**, 249–256.

Sinzger, C., Grefte, A., Plachter, B., Gouw, A. S. H., Hauw The, T., and Jahn, G. (1995). Fibroblasts, epithelial cells, endothelial cells, and smooth muscle cells are the major targets of human cytomegalovirus infection in lung and gastrointestinal tissues. *J. Gen. Virol.*, **76**, 741–750.

Sinzger, C., Plachter, B., Grefte, A., Gouw, A. S. H., The, T. H., and Jahn, G. (1996). Tissue macrophages are infected by human cytomegalovirus. *J. Infect. Dis.*, **173**, 240–245.

Slobedman, B. and Mocarski, E. S. (1999). Quantitative analysis of latent human cytomegalovirus. *J. Virol.*, **73**, 4806–4812.

Soderberg-Naucler, C., Fish, K. N., and Nelson, J. A. (1997a). Interferon-gamma and tumor necrosis factor-alpha specifically induce formation of cytomegalovirus-permissive monocyte-derived macrophages that are refractory to the antiviral activity of these cytokines. *J. Clin. Invest.*, **100**, 3154–3163.

Soderberg-Naucler, C., Fish, K. N., and Nelson, J. A. (1997b). Reactivation of latent human cytomegalovirus by allogeneic stimulation of blood cells from healthy donors. *Cell*, **91**, 119–126.

Soderberg-Naucler, C., Streblow, D. N., Fish, K. N., Allan-Yorke, J., Smith, P. P., and Nelson, J. A. (2001). Reactivation of latent human cytomegalovirus in CD14+ monocytes is differentiation dependent. *J. Virol.*, **75**, 7543–7554.

Sommer, M. H., Scully, A. L., and Spector, D. H. (1994). Transactivation by the human cytomegalovirus IE2 86-kilodalton protein requires a domain that binds to both the TATA box-binding protein and the retinoblastoma protein. *J. Virol.*, **68**, 6223–6231.

Song, Y.-J. and Stinski, M. F. (2002). Effect of the human cytomegalovirus IE86 protein on expression of E2F-responsive genes: A DNA microarray analysis. *Proc. Natl Acad. of Sci. USA*, **99**, 2836–2841.

Song, Y.-J. and Stinski, M. F. (2005). Inhibition of cell division by the human cytomegalovirus IE86 protein: Role of the p53 pathway or cdk1/cyclin B1. *J. Virol.*, **79**, 2597–2603.

Spector, D. H. (1996). Activation and regulation of human cytomegalovirus early genes. *Intervirology*, **39**, 361–377.

Spector, D. J. and Tevethia, M. J. (1994). Protein–protein interactions between human cytomegalovirus IE2–580aa and pUL84 in lytically infected cells. *J. Virol.*, **68**, 7549–7553.

Speir, E., Modali, R., Huang, E.-S., Leon, M. B., Shawl, F., Finkel, T., and Epstein, S. E. (1994). Potential role of human cytomegalovirus and p53 interaction in coronary restenosis. *Science*, **265**, 391–394.

Speir, E., Yu, Z.-X., Ferrans, V. J., Huang, E.-S., and Epstein, S. E. (1998). Aspirin attenuates cytomegalovirus infectivity and gene expression mediated by cyclooxygenase-2 in coronary artery smooth muscle cells. *Circ. Res.*, **83**, 210–216.

Spengler, M. L., Kurapatwinski, K., Black, A. R., and Azizkhan-Clifford, J. (2002). SUMO-1 modification of human cytomegalovirus IE1/IE72. *J. Virol.*, **76**, 2990–2996.

Stamminger, T., Puchtler, E., and Fleckenstein, B. (1991). Discordant expression of the immediate-early 1 and 2 gene regions of human cytomegalovirus at early times after infection involves posttranscriptional processing events. *J. Virol.*, **65**, 2273–2282.

Stein, J., Volk, H., Liebenthal, C., Kruger, D. H., and Prosch, S. (1993). Tumour necrosis factor α stimulates the activity of the human cytomegalovirus major immediate early enhancer/promoter in immature monocytic cells. *J. Gen. Virol.*, **74**, 2333–2338.

Stenberg, R. M. (1996). The human cytomegalovirus major immediate-early gene. *Intervirology*, **39**, 343–349.

Stenberg, R. M., Thomsen, D. R., and Stinski, M. F. (1984). Structural analysis of the major immediate early gene of human cytomegalovirus. *J. Virol.*, **49**, 190–199.

Stenberg, R. M., Witte, P. R., and Stinski, M. F. (1985). Multiple spliced and unspliced transcripts from human cytomegalovirus immediate-early region 2 and evidence for a common initiation site within immediate-early region 1. *J. Virol.*, **56**, 665–675.

Stenberg, R. M., Depto, A. S., Fortney, J., and Nelson, J. (1989). Regulated expression of early and late RNAs and proteins from the human cytomegalovirus immediate-early gene region. *J. Virol.*, **63**, 2699–2708.

Stinski, M. F. (1999). Cytomegalovirus promoter for expression in mammalian cells. In *Gene Expression Systems: Using Nature for the Art of Expression*, San Diego, CA: ed. J. M. Ferandez and J. P. Hoeffler, pp. 211–233 Academic Press.

Su, Y., Adair, R., Davis, C. N., DiFronzo, N. L., and Colberg-Poley, A. M. (2003). Convergence of RNA cis elemets and cellular polyadenylation factors in the regulation of human cytomegalovirus UL37 exon 1 unspliced RNA production. *J. Virol.*, **77**, 12729–12741.

Takahashi, K., Sonoda, S., Higashi, K. *et al.* (1989). Predominant CD4 T-lymphocyte tropism of human herpesvirus 6-related virus. *J. Virol.*, **63**, 3161–3163.

Takemoto, M., Shimamoto, T., Isegawa, Y., and Yamanishi, K. (2001). The R3 region, one of three major repetitive regions of human herpesvirus 6, is a strong enhancer of immediate-early gene U95. *J. Virol.*, **75**, 10149–10160.

Tang, Q. and Maul, G. G. (2003). Mouse cytomegalovirus immediate-early protein 1 binds with host cell repressors to relieve suppressive effects on viral transcription and replication during lytic infection. *J. Virol.*, **77**, 1357–1367.

Tang, Q., Li, L., and Maul, G. G. (2005). Mouse cytomegalovirus early M112/113 proteins control the repressive effect of IE3 on the major immediate-early promoter. *J. Virol.*, **79**, 257–263.

Taylor, R. T. and Bresnahan, W. A. (2005). Human cytomegalovirus immediate-early 2 gene expression blocks virus-induced beta interferon production. *J. Virol.*, **79**, 3873–3877.

Taylor, R. T. and Bresnahan, W. A. (2006). Human cytomegalovirus immediate-early 2 protein IE86 blocks virus-induced chemokine expression. *J. Virol.* **80**, 920–928.

Taylor-Wiedeman, J. A., Sissons, J. G. P., and Sinclair, J. H. (1994). Induction of endogenous human cytomegalovirus gene expression after differentiation of monocytes from healthy carriers. *J. Virol.*, **68**, 1597–1604.

Thomsen, D. R., Stenberg, R. M., Goins, W. F., and Stinski, M. F. (1984). Promoter-regulatory region of the major immediate early gene of human cytomegalovirus. *Proc. Natl Acad. Sci. USA*, **81**, 659–663.

Thrower, A. R., Bullock, G. C., Bissell, J. E., and Stinski, M. F. (1996). Regulation of a human cytomegalovirus immediate early gene (US3) by a silencer/enhancer combination. *J. Virol.*, **70**, 91–100.

Vink, C., Beuken, E., and Bruggeman, C. A. (2000). Complete DNA sequence of the rat cytomegalovirus genome. *J. Virol.*, **74**, 7656–7665.

Wade, M., Kowalik, T. F., Mudryj, M., Huang, E. S., and Asiskhan, J. C. (1992). E2F mediates dihydrofolate reductase promoter activation and multiprotein complex formation in human cytomegalovirus infection. *Mol. Cell. Biol.*, **12**, 4364–4374.

Waheed, I., Chiou, C., Ahn, J., and Hayward, G. S. (1998). Binding of the human cytomegalovirus 80-kDa immediate–early protein (IE2) to minor groove A/T-rich sequences bounded by CG dinucleotides is regulated by protein oligomerization and phosphorylation. *Virology*, **252**, 235–257.

Waldhoer, M., Kledal, T. N., Farrell, H., and Schwartz, T. W. (2002). Murine cytomegalovirus (CMV) M33 and human CMV US28 receptors exhibit similar constitutive signaling activities. *J. Virol.*, **76**, 8161–8168.

Wang, X. L., Huong, S. M., Chiu, M. L., Raab-Traub, N., and Huang, E. S. (2003). Epidermal growth factor receptor is a cellular receptor for human cytomegalovirus. *Nature*, **424**, 456–461.

Weinberg, R. A. (1995). The retinoblastoma protein and cell cycle control. *Cell*, **81**(3), 323–330.

Weston, K. (1988). An enhancer element in the short unique region of human cytomegalovirus regulates the production of a group of abundant immediate early transcripts. *Virology*, **162**, 406–416.

White, E. A., Clark, C. L., Sanchez, V., and Spector, D. H. (2004). Small internal deletions in the human cytomegalovirus IE2 gene result in nonviable recombinant viruses with differential defects in viral gene expression. *J. Virol.*, **78**, 1817–1830.

Wiebusch, L., Asmar, J., Uecker, R., and Hagemeier, C. (2003). Human cytomegalovirus immediate-early protein 2 (IE2)-mediated activation of cyclin E is cell-cycle-independent and forces S-phase entry in IE2-arrested cells. *J. Gen. Virol.*, **84**, 51–60.

Wiebusch, L. and Hagemeier, C. (1999). Human cytomegalovirus 86-kiodalton IE2 protein blocks cell cycle progression in G1. *J. Virol.*, **73**, 9274–9283.

Wiebusch, L. and Hagemeier, C. (2001). The human cytomegalovirus immediate early 2 protein dissociates cellular DNA synthesis from cyclin-dependent kinase activation. *EMBO J.*, **20**, 1086–1098.

Wilkinson, G. W., Kelly, C., Sinclair, J. H., and Richards, C. (1998). Disruption of PML-associated nuclear bodies mediated by the human cytomegalovirus major immediate early gene product. *J. Gen. Virol.*, **79**, 1233–1245.

Winkler, M., Rice, S. A., and Stamminger, T. (1994). UL69 of human cytomegalovirus, an open reading frame with homology to ICP27 of herpes simplex virus, encodes a transactivator of gene expression. *J. Virol.*, **68**, 3943–3954.

Wright, E., Bain, M., Teague, L., Murphy, J., and Sinclair, J. (2005). Ets-2 repressor factor recruits deacetylases to silence human cytomegalovirus immediate-early gene expression in non-permissive cells. *J. Gen. Virol.*, **86**, 535–544.

Xu, Y., Ahn, J.-H., Cheng, M. *et al.* (2001). Proteasome-independent disruption of PML oncogenic domains (PODS), but not covalent modification by SUMO-1, is required for human cytomegalovirus immediate-early protein IE1 to inhibit PML-mediated transcriptional repression. *J. Virol.*, **75**, 10683–10695.

Xu, Y., Cei, S. A., Huete, A. R., Colletti, K. S., and Pari, G. S. (2004a). Human cytomegalovirus DNA replication requires transcriptional activation via an IE2- and UL84-responsive bidirectional promoter element within oriLyt. *J. Virol.*, **78**, 11664–11677.

Xu, Y., Cei, S. A., Huete, A. R., and Pari, G. S. (2004b). Human cytomegalovirus UL84 insertion mutant defective for viral DNA synthesis and growth. *J. Virol.*, **78**, 10360–10369.

Yeung, K. C., Stoltzfus, C. M., and Stinski, M. F. (1993). Mutations of the cytomegalovirus immediate–early 2 protein defines regions and amino acid motifs important in transactivation of transcription from the HIV-1 LTR promoter. *Virology*, **195**, 786–792.

Yoo, Y. D., Chiou, C.-J., Choi, K. S. *et al.* (1996). The IE2 regulatory protein of human cytomegalovirus induces expression of the human transforming growth factor beta 1 gene through an Egr-1 binding site. *J. Virol.*, **70**, 7062–7070.

Zhang, X. Y., Ni, Y. S., Saifudeen, Z., Asiedu, C. K., Supakar, P. C., and Ehrlich, M. (1995). Increasing binding of a transcription factor immediately downstream of the cap site of a cytomegalovirus gene represses expression. *Nucl. Acids Res.*, **23**, 3026–3033.

Zhang, Z., Evers, D. L., McCarville, J. F., Dantonel, J-C., Huong, S-M., and Huang, E-S. (2006). Evidence that the human cytomegalovirus IE2-86 protein binds mdm2 and facilitates mdm2 degradation. *J. Virol.*, **80**, 3833–3843.

Zhang, Z., Huong, S.-M., Wang, X., Huang, D. Y., and Huang, E.-S. (2003). Interactions between human cytomegalovirus IE1–72 and cellular p107: functional domains and mechanisms of up-regulation of cyclin E/cdk2 kinase activity. *J. Virol.*, **77**, 12660–12670.

Zhu, H., Shen, Y., and Shenk, T. (1995). Human cytomegalovirus IE1 and IE2 proteins block apoptosis. *J. Virol.*, **69**, 7960–7970.

Zhu, H., Cong, J. P., Mamtora, G., Gingeras, T., and Shenk, T. (1998). Cellular gene expression altered by human cytomegalovirus: global monitoring with oligonucleotide arrays. *Proc. Natl Acad. Sci. USA*, **95**, 14470–14475.

Zhu, H., Cong, J. P., Yu, D., Bresnahan, W. A., and Shenk, T. E. (2002). Inhibition of cyclooxygenase 2 blocks human cytomegalovirus replication. *Proc. Natl Acad. Sci. USA*, **99**, 3932–3937.

Zweidler-McKay, P. A., Grimes, H. L., Flubacher, M. M., and Tsichlis, P. N. (1996). Gfi-1 encodes a nuclear zinc finger protein that binds DNA and functions as a transcriptional repressor. *Mol. Cell. Biol.*, **16**, 4024–4034.

Early viral gene expression and function

Elizabeth A. White and Deborah H. Spector

Department of Cellular and Molecular Medicine and Center for Molecular Genetics, University of California, San Diego, La Jolla, CA, USA

Introduction

Viral early genes are defined by two criteria: they require prior *de novo* synthesis of viral immediate-early (IE) and cellular proteins for their transcription, and this expression is insensitive to inhibitors of viral DNA synthesis such as phosphonoformate, ganciclovir, cidofovir, and phosphonoacetate. Close inspection of the kinetics of synthesis of this class of genes reveals multiple subgroups (for review, see Fortunato and Spector, 1999). The earliest of the early gene transcripts appear and accumulate to their highest levels by 8 hours postinfection (h p.i.) (e.g., the HCMV 2.2 kb family of transcripts – UL112–113), while the latest of the early transcripts cannot be detected until just prior to the onset of viral DNA replication (e.g., the HCMV 2.7 kb major early transcript – $\beta_{2.7}$ or TRL4) and accumulate to highest levels much later during infection when viral DNA replication is allowed to proceed. (Mocarski and Courcelle, 2001) Levels of a third subgroup increase at late times (e.g., the abundant HCMV 1.2 kb RNA – TRL7) and are partially blocked by inhibitors of viral DNA synthesis. This subgroup may be further divided into genes that are referred to as early–late or leaky–late.

This review will describe the viral factors and cellular environment required for the expression of the viral early genes, the function of the early genes with respect to viral replication, and the subversion of host cellular processes and modulation of host immune responses that are associated with the expression of these genes. Selected examples of early genes will be used to illustrate different mechanisms controlling this complex class of genes. The focus is on human cytomegalovirus (HCMV) and its replication in fibroblasts, the most extensively studied betaherpesvirus. A separate section at the end of the review is devoted to human herpesvirus 6 (HHV-6) and human herpesvirus 7 (HHV-7).

The host cell range of HCMV permissivity in vivo is broad. The major targets of infection are cell types such as epithelial and endothelial cells as well as peripheral blood leukocytes in the myelomonocytic lineage. Infection also extends to specialized parenchymal cells such as neurons and astrocytes in the brain and retina, smooth muscle cells, and hepatocytes (Sinzger and Jahn, 1996). Infection is restricted, however, when the virus is grown in tissue culture cells. Primary human fibroblasts have been used for virus isolation as well as for most studies on the cellular and molecular biology of HCMV. Fresh clinical isolates of this virus retain the ability to replicate in cultured epithelial cells and macrophages. This is not a property of laboratory propagated strains. It should be kept in mind that the rules governing early gene expression and the functional importance of the gene products might be quite different in other cell types than in fibroblasts.

Identification of HCMV early genes

The initial identification of HCMV early genes was based on studies that measured the rate of accumulation of viral transcripts. Pulse-labeled whole cell, nuclear, or cytoplasmic RNA was hybridized to cloned subgenomic fragments or viral DNA cleaved with restriction endonucleases and fractionated by gel electrophoresis (DeMarchi, 1981; DeMarchi, 1983; DeMarchi *et al.*, 1980; McDonough and Spector, 1983; Wathen and Stinski, 1982; Wathen *et al.*, 1981). In complementary experiments, the size and abundance of various RNAs were determined by hybridization of radiolabeled viral DNA or cloned subgenomic fragments to dot blots or Northern blots of RNA isolated at various times in the infection (DeMarchi, 1983; McDonough and Spector, 1983; Wathen and Stinski, 1982). Two important points emerged from these studies. First, there is no clustering of

RNA transcripts in the genome according to their temporal expression. Furthermore, some HCMV early expression appeared to be subject to post-transcriptional controls that governed either the transport of RNA from the nucleus to the cytoplasm or the stability of the RNA in the cytoplasm. These early studies provided information on the relative abundance, size, and temporal expression of about 30% of the RNAs (Chambers *et al.*, 1999; Mocarski and Courcelle, 2001) and served as the framework for more detailed analysis of individual transcription units.

More recently, additional studies have used PCR analysis, gene arrays, and large-scale mutagenesis to classify each of the predicted HCMV ORFs as IE, early, or late and to characterize these as essential or dispensable for growth in tissue culture cells (Chambers *et al.*, 1999; Dunn *et al.*, 2003; Yu *et al.*, 2003). In one study (Chambers *et al.*, 1999), infected cell RNA was hybridized to a DNA microarray carrying oligonucleotides corresponding to the majority of the strain AD169 ORFs and four ORFs present in the Towne strain. IE transcripts were isolated from cells infected in the presence of the protein synthesis inhibitor cycloheximide and harvested at 13 h p.i., while cells treated with ganciclovir for 72 h were the source of RNAs transcribed with early kinetics. Late RNA was isolated from untreated cells at 72 h p.i., and differential sensitivity to ganciclovir was the basis for further characterization of these transcripts as early–late or late. The expression of selected transcripts not previously characterized was confirmed by further hybridization analysis. In agreement with the initial studies, there was no clear correlation of kinetic class with location or polarity of the ORF in the genome, although the majority of the US region ORFs were expressed with early kinetics.

HCMV-mediated changes in the cellular environment prior to early gene expression

Examination of the viral growth cycle reveals intricate interactions between HCMV and the host cellular machinery that optimize the environment for viral replication and prevent recognition of the infected cell by the immune system. The details of these events are discussed in depth in Chapters 16, 19, 20, 21, 58, and 59. Because early gene products are important in many aspects of infection, a brief summary is provided here.

Events triggered by the binding of the virus to the host cell

The initial contact of the virus with the cell membrane triggers physiological changes and activates signaling pathways that in many ways resemble the interferon response or the second messenger-type response that occurs during regulation via hormones and growth factors (for review, see Chapter 16 and Fortunato *et al.*, 2000). For example, there is hydrolysis of phosphatidylinositol(4,5)-biphosphate, stimulation of arachidonic acid metabolism, a transient influx of calcium, upregulation of the transcription factors Sp1 and NF-κB, and activation of the mitogen activated protein kinases (ERK1/2 and pp38) and the phosphatidylinositol 3-kinase pathways (Albrecht *et al.*, 1991; Johnson *et al.* 2000, 2001a,b; Rodems and Spector, 1998). Also associated with this immediate activation of the host cell is the induction of a subset of RNAs encoding genes induced by alpha or beta interferon (IFN-α/β) in uninfected cells (Boyle *et al.*, 1999; Browne *et al.*, 2001; Navarro *et al.*, 1998; Zhu *et al.*, 1997, 1998). The HCMV-associated induction occurs in the absence of any detectable IFN-α/β or *de novo* protein synthesis and appears to require simply the exposure of the cell to virions, non-infectious enveloped particles, or dense bodies. The up-regulation of the interferon-responsive genes, however, is tempered by the viral matrix protein pp65 as well as by one or more viral gene products or cellular factors that are expressed during the first few hours of the infection (Abate *et al.*, 2004; Browne and Shenk, 2003; Browne *et al.*, 2001). It has recently been shown that the IE1 and IE2 genes encode at least two of the proteins responsible for the downregulation of this IFN-α/β-mediated signaling response. IE2 86 kDa protein blocks the production of IFN-β and several chemokines (Taylor and Bresnahan, 2005; Taylor and Bresnahan, 2006), while IE1 72 acts further downstream to block type I interferon-mediated signaling and the induction of multiple interferon-responsive genes (Paulus *et al.*, 2006).

ND10 are sites of genome deposition and IE transcription

Upon infection of cells with a variety of DNA viruses, the morphology of nuclear structures referred to variously as ND10 (nuclear domain 10), PODs (PML oncogenic domains), or PML bodies is rapidly altered (for review, see Chapter 17). While infection with adenovirus 5 (Ad5) results in these punctate structures acquiring a reticular appearance, both HCMV and herpes simplex virus type 1 (HSV-1) infections disrupt ND10 sites and disperse associated proteins. In uninfected cells, a number of proteins including the growth suppressors promyelocytic leukemia protein (PML), Sp100, HP1, and Daxx are localized to ND10 domains, and many of these are interferon inducible. As is the case for Ad5 and HSV-1, a subset of HCMV genomes are deposited at ND10 sites immediately following infection, and it is these genomes that provide the template for early transcription (Ishov and Maul, 1996; Ishov et al., 1997). Transcripts produced at these sites are consequently in close proximity to spliceosome assembly factor SC35 domains, which may further aid in rapid expression of IE genes following infection.

Once the major HCMV IE proteins, IE1 72 and IE2 86, are expressed during the infection, these first localize to ND10 sites. While the punctate pattern of IE2 86 expression persists for a longer time, between 3 and 6 h p.i. both IE1 72 and ND10-associated proteins, including PML, become completely dispersed throughout the nucleus (Ahn and Hayward, 1997; Ishov et al., 1997; Kelly et al., 1995; Korioth et al., 1996). Further studies involving either transfection of IE1 or IE2 expression vectors or infection with a recombinant virus unable to express IE1 72 indicate that IE2 86 protein is able to localize to ND10 sites in the absence of IE1 72, but disruption does not occur (Ahn et al., 1998a; Ahn and Hayward, 1997; Ishov et al., 1997). IE1 72 is required for disruption of the ND10 sites, but since the IE1 deletion mutant virus replicates well under high multiplicity conditions, this event appears not to be required for the infection to proceed. Modification of IE1 by SUMO-1 is also not required for HCMV-mediated ND10 dispersal or for viral replication, although a virus with a mutation in the IE1 sumoylation site grows more slowly (Lee et al., 2004; Nevels et al., 2004; Xu et al., 2001). The observation that IE1 abrogates sumoylation of PML and Sp100 suggests that this is at least one element of the mechanism by which ND10 associated proteins are dispersed during the infection (Muller and Dejean, 1999).

A growing body of evidence suggests that even after IE1 72 has caused dispersal of ND10 sites, these locations remain important for viral replication. Between 3 and 8 hours p.i., aggregates of cyclin dependent kinase (cdk) 9 and cdk 7 appear in the nuclei of HCMV-infected cells. Input viral genomes and IE1 and IE2 proteins are also present at some, but not all, of these sites (Tamrakar et al., 2005). When cells are infected with the IE1 72 deletion mutant virus, ND10 structures are maintained and the cdk 9 aggregates can be visualized at the periphery of the PML-containing ND10 sites. In addition, the UL112–113 early gene proteins appear to colocalize with IE2 86 at the periphery of the original ND10 sites beginning about 6 h p.i., and these nucleate viral DNA replication compartments that form later during infection (Ahn et al., 1999a).

Finally, a series of studies suggest that an interaction between the HCMV tegument protein pp71 and the ND10-associated Daxx is the basis of a mechanism by which early events in the viral life cycle are initiated at ND10 sites (Hofmann et al., 2002; Ishov et al., 2002; Marshall et al., 2002). Work using recombinant viruses has shown that the Daxx-binding ability of pp71 is required for efficient HCMV replication and IE gene expression during low, but not high, multiplicity infections (Cantrell and Bresnahan, 2005; Cantrell and Bresnahan, 2006; Saffert and Kalejta, 2006). When Daxx expression is reduced, the activity of the major IE promoter increases in transient transfection assays. Knockdown of Daxx expression also alleviates the reduced IE gene expression observed in pp71 deletion mutant virus-infected cells (Cantrell and Bresnahan, 2006; Preston and Nicholl, 2006). These findings are further explained by the observation that pp71 is required for the proteasome-mediated degradation of Daxx that begins 2 h p.i. in HCMV-infected cells. This degradation is required for efficient IE gene expression and is thought to increase gene activity by eliminating Daxx-mediated histone deacetylase recruitment to promoters (Saffert and Kalejta, 2006).

Inhibition of apoptosis

Two viral IE proteins from the UL36–38 region of the genome serve to prevent the host cell from undergoing apoptosis (for review see Chapter 21). One (vMIA) is the protein product of UL37 exon 1, and the second (vICA) is encoded by UL36. vMIA, which is essential for viral replication, travels from the endoplasmic reticulum (ER) to the Golgi and finally to mitochondria. Its expression in transiently transfected HeLa cells blocks apoptosis induced by either anti-Fas antibody plus cycloheximide or by TNF-α, and in stably transfected HeLa clones, it appears to act at a stage between activation of caspase 8 and cytochrome c release into the cytoplasm (Goldmacher et al., 1999; McCormick et al., 2003b). Recently, it was found that vMIA sequesters the pro-apoptotic protein Bax in the mitochondria, thus suppressing mitochondrial permeabilization (Arnoult et al., 2004). The half-life and localization pattern of vICA in infected cells vary depending on the strain of virus used in the infection (Patterson and Shenk, 1999). Like vMIA, vICA is involved in preventing apoptosis in infected cells, but it acts further upstream to block cleavage of procaspase 8 and its subsequent activation (Skaletskaya et al., 2001). Either protein appears to be dispensable for growth in culture so long as the other is retained. Many laboratory-adapted viral strains express non-functional UL36 (Skaletskaya et al., 2001). The high degree of UL36 and UL37 exon 1 conservation across the cytomegalovirus family indicates that both contribute critical functions to replication of the virus in the host organism (McCormick et al., 2003a; McCormick et al., 2005).

Functions of viral early genes

Many early gene products are required for successful viral replication. In libraries of HCMV BACs constructed to disrupt each unique ORF (Dunn et al., 2003; Yu et al., 2003) 41–45 of the ORFs examined appear essential for replication in fibroblasts; 117 are not required but when deleted, give rise to phenotypes ranging from growth like wild type to severe impairment of viral replication. Interestingly, some of these dispensable ORFs (UL24, UL64, and US29) are required for viral growth in cell types other than fibroblasts. In addition, four of the mutants with non-essential genes deleted (UL10, UL16, US16, and US19) grow significantly better than the wild type in cell types other than fibroblasts. Early gene products constitute a significant proportion of essential loci, given that 23 to 25 essential and augmenting genes were characterized as early or early–late in the study by Chambers et al. (1999).

Most of the viral early genes function in one of two ways. A subset of the early products required for growth in tissue culture are directly involved in viral DNA synthesis, cleavage and packaging of the viral genome, and assembly of the virus particles (see Chapters 19 and 20). A second group of genes functions to create a cellular and extracellular environment that is optimal for viral gene expression and replication, either by modulating factors involved in the control of cellular DNA synthesis or by altering the host organism's immune response to the virus.

Genes involved directly in viral replication

The majority of the proteins required for synthesis and processing of the viral DNA are expressed with early kinetics, as are many of the factors involved in the initial stages of viral particle assembly. In conjunction with some of the IE and late viral proteins, these products provide the central functions of the viral life cycle.

Initial studies on the replication of the viral DNA identified 11 loci required for origin of lytic replication (oriLyt)-dependent DNA replication (Pari and Anders, 1993; Pari et al., 1993) (Chapter 19). These were conducted as complementation assays in which cloned fragments of the HCMV genome were tested for their ability to support replication of a vector containing oriLyt sequences. Six of the required genes are predicted to function directly in DNA replication and are homologous to factors required for herpes simplex virus type 1 (HSV-1) DNA replication. The products of these genes are pUL54, the viral DNA polymerase; ppUL44, the polymerase processivity factor; ppUL57, a single-stranded DNA binding protein; and three proteins that comprise a helicase-primase complex: pUL70, pUL102, and pUL105.

Each of these genes is expressed with early or delayed early kinetics (Chambers et al., 1999; Smith and Pari, 1995). Two additional early loci, UL112–113 and UL84, were identified in the complementation assays and are required together with UL122–123, IRS/TRS1, and UL36–38, three IE loci with regulatory functions that are discussed elsewhere in this chapter.

The functions of several viral early proteins have been closely examined in subsequent work. Viable viruses with point mutations in the UL54 gene, selected on the basis of reduced sensitivity to ganciclovir and cidofovir, tend to grow more slowly than parental virus (Cihlar et al., 1998; Smith et al., 1997). The DNA polymerase processivity factor encoded by UL44 forms a complex with the viral polymerase and binds to double-stranded DNA, thereby stabilizing interactions with the template (Ertl and Powell, 1992; Hwang et al., 2000; Weiland et al., 1994). Recently, residues in the C-terminus of the polymerase have been shown to be required for the ppUL44–pUL54 interaction (Loregian et al., 2004; Loregian et al., 2003). The function of the UL57 gene product has not been examined directly, but by analogy to its homologous HSV-1 counterpart ICP8, this protein is predicted to bind the single-stranded DNA unwound by the helicase–primase complex (Kiehl et al., 2003). The UL102 and UL105 genes have been characterized (Smith et al., 1996; Smith and Pari, 1995), and biochemical studies demonstrating interactions between their protein products and the product of the UL70 gene further support the idea that, as in HSV-1, these three factors function together as the HCMV helicase-primase (McMahon and Anders, 2002).

The product of the UL84 gene is essential for viral DNA synthesis and productive infection (Dunn et al., 2003; Xu et al., 2003, 2004; Yu et al., 2003). The protein localizes to replication centers in the nuclei of infected cells (Lischka et al., 2003; Xu et al., 2002), interacts with IE2 86 (Spector and Tevethia, 1994), and can promote oriLyt-dependent DNA replication when core replication proteins from Epstein-Barr virus are supplied (Sarisky and Hayward, 1996). Recent studies with a BAC defective for the expression of UL84 suggest that it may regulate some of the functions of IE2 86 as well as contribute to the early formation of the replication centers. Interpretation of the results with this mutant BAC, however, is complicated by the observation that the UL84 protein provided in trans does not complement viral growth (Xu et al., 2004). There is also evidence that the UL112–113 proteins localize to viral replication centers early in their formation and may play a role in the recruitment of additional factors to these sites (Ahn et al., 1999b; Iwayama et al., 1994; Penfold and Mocarski, 1997).

UL114 is an early gene that, although not identified in these complementation assays, appears to contribute to efficient replication of viral DNA (Courcelle et al., 2001; Prichard et al., 1996). The UL114-encoded uracil-DNA glycosylase is not strictly required for growth in fibroblasts, but a mutant lacking this gene is delayed in the initiation of DNA replication.

Following synthesis, viral DNA is cleaved into genome-length segments and packaged into preformed capsids (Chapter 19). Early proteins involved are introduced only briefly here. Four early–late products (major capsid protein, minor capsid protein, minor capsid binding protein, and small capsid protein) contribute to capsid formation and are the products of the UL86, UL85, UL46, and UL48.5 genes, respectively (Gibson, 1996). Capsid formation also relies on the assemblin precursor UL80.5 and the proteinase precursor UL80a. UL89 and UL56 early gene products play roles in DNA cleavage (Buerger et al., 2001; Krosky et al., 2003; Underwood et al., 1998), and by homology to HSV-1 proteins at least four HCMV products, most expressed with early kinetics, are predicted to be involved in packaging cleaved DNA into progeny capsids. These four proteins are encoded by the HCMV UL51, UL52, UL77, and UL104 genes and are predicted to have functions including transport of the capsids to sites of DNA packaging and formation of a structure through which DNA enters the capsid. Recently, it has been shown that the TRS1 protein also may be involved in packaging at a step that occurs after the cleavage of the DNA (Adamo et al., 2004).

Preparing the cell for viral DNA replication

In a cell that is permissive for the viral infection, the expression of the early genes is associated with a cascade of events that results in the stimulation of host cell genes, particularly those encoding proteins that are required for host cell DNA synthesis and proliferation. Early studies revealed a marked increase in the levels of the enzymes ornithine decarboxylase, thymidine kinase, DNA polymerase alpha, and dihydrofolate reductase following HCMV infection (Boldogh et al., 1991; Estes and Huang, 1977; Hirai and Watanabe, 1976; Isom, 1979; Wade et al., 1992). More recent DNA microarray analyses show that the viral infection leads to upregulation of multiple DNA synthesis and cell cycle genes at the level of transcription (Browne et al., 2001). In part, this may follow HCMV-induced hyperphosphorylation of the retinoblastoma family of proteins (Jault et al., 1995; McElroy et al., 2000), which likely releases the inhibition that these proteins confer to the E2F/DP transcription factors that regulate the transcription of many of these same genes (Dyson, 1998). The tumor suppressor protein p53 is stabilized in HCMV-infected cells and is sequestered in viral replication centers (Fortunato and Spector, 1998; Jault et al., 1995). Other proteins that are sequestered in the viral replication centers are PCNA and RPA, which are both essential for the elongation phase of host cell DNA synthesis and may play some role in viral DNA synthesis (Dittmer and Mocarski, 1997; Jault et al., 1995).

HCMV also induces elevated levels of cyclin E and cyclin B and their associated kinase activities (Bresnahan et al., 1996; Jault et al., 1995; McElroy et al., 2000; Salvant et al., 1998; Sanchez et al., 2003). Cyclin E transcription is induced, and this up-regulation requires the expression of viral early genes (McElroy et al., 2000; Salvant et al., 1998). In contrast, multiple posttranscriptional pathways are used in the activation of Cdk1/cyclin B1 complexes (Sanchez et al., 2003). The accumulation of the cyclin B1 subunit is the result of increased synthesis and reduced degradation of the protein via the ubiquitin-proteasome pathway. In addition, the active catalytic subunit of the complex, Cdk1, accumulates in virus-infected cells. This is due partially to the down-regulation of the expression and activity of the Cdk1 inhibitory kinases Myt1 and Wee1 and the accumulation of the Cdc25 phosphatases that remove the inhibitory phosphates from Cdk1. Modulation of these pathways appears to require at least some early gene expression (Sanchez et al., 2003).

During this early period in the infection, HCMV also inhibits selective host cell functions, presumably to ensure that viral replication is favored over that of the host. These events lead the cell to a fully "activated" state, but it is clear that the virus primes the cell for its own DNA replication at the host's expense and has sufficiently dysregulated the cell cycle and signaling pathways to ensure that cellular DNA synthesis and cell division is blocked (Bresnahan et al., 1996; Dittmer and Mocarski, 1997; Jault et al., 1995; Lu and Shenk, 1996; Salvant et al., 1998). In contrast to the activation of cyclins E and B, the expression of cyclin A and its associated kinase activity is inhibited by infection with HCMV (Jault et al., 1995). Although the failure to induce cyclin A in the virus-infected cells probably plays a role in the blockage of cellular DNA synthesis, it has recently been found that viral early gene products also affect key steps in this process prior to the requirement for cyclin A. Briefly, DNA synthesis in eukaryotic cells is precisely regulated such that genomic DNA doubles only once during each cell cycle (Diffley, 2001; Fujita, 1999; Lei and Tye, 2001). The first step involves the assembly of prereplication complexes (pre-RC) at the replication origins. The origin recognition complex (Orc), a multisubunit complex, binds to the origins of cellular DNA replication and remains bound during most of the cell cycle (Quintana and Dutta, 1999; Tatsumi et al., 2000; Vashee et al., 2001). Cdc6 and Cdt1 are recruited to the complex and facilitate the loading of the family of six Mcm proteins on to DNA (Maiorano et al., 2000; Nishitani et al., 2000, 2001; Rialland et al., 2002). Cdt1 itself is regulated by a protein called geminin that normally accumulates during S-phase and ensures that each origin is used only once. Analysis of this process has revealed that there is a delay in the expression of the Mcm proteins in infected cells. The greatest effect is observed with Mcm5, whose levels remain low until after 32 h p.i. The loading of the Mcm proteins onto the DNA pre-RC complex is also defective in the virus-infected cells and is associated with the premature accumulation of geminin (Biswas et al., 2003; Wiebusch et al., 2003b). Interestingly, as is the case with cyclin B, the increased levels of geminin results from decreased levels of proteasome-mediated degradation (J. W. Choi and D. H. Spector, unpublished results).

Although there is evidence from transient expression systems that the IE1 and IE2 proteins and the virion constituent proteins UL69 and UL82 contribute to the virus-mediated alteration in cell growth control (Bresnahan et al., 1998; Castillo et al., 2000; Kalejta et al., 2003; Kalejta and Shenk, 2003; Lu and Shenk, 1999; Murphy et al., 2000; Sinclair et al., 2000; Song and Stinski, 2002; Wiebusch et al., 2003a; Wiebusch and Hagemeier, 1999, 2001), studies in the context of viral infection show that early gene products are also required (McElroy et al., 2000; Sanchez et al., 2003). A challenge remains to determine which viral genes are involved and elucidate the mechanisms governing their activity. Given the large number of early genes, most of which have not yet been studied, the task is not trivial.

Modulation of host immune responses

In addition to subversion of the intracellular machinery, HCMV needs to deal early in the infection with its survival in its human host and evasion of the immune response. This topic is discussed in detail in Chapters 58 and 59, and so is only briefly summarized here (for other reviews, see (Mocarski, 2002, 2004)). Optimization of in vivo pathogenesis and viral persistence is accomplished by effects on intracellular processes, the release of soluble factors, and regulation of cellular receptors that are involved in modulation of innate, inflammatory, and adaptive immune responses. The number of viral genes that are known to play a role in these processes is still small, and all of these have proven to be dispensable for productive infection in tissue culture. The general consensus, however, is that the large block of "non-essential" early genes in the U_S region whose functions have yet to be determined are key players in viral pathogenesis.

One well-studied mechanism of viral immune evasion involves interference with MHC class I antigen presentation by at least four gene products (US2, US3, US6, and US11) (Ploegh, 1998) (Chapter 58). At early times in the infection, HCMV also disarms the interferon-mediated branch of the host's antiviral defense. The cells become refractory to IFN-α/β-mediated stimulation of MHC class I, IRF-1, MxA, and $2'$–$5'$-oligoadenylate synthetase gene expression, transcription factor activation, and signaling (Miller et al., 1999). Viral genes that have been implicated in these events include UL83 and TRS1/IRS1 (Abate et al., 2004; Browne and Shenk, 2003; Child et al., 2004). In addition, there is repression of IFN-γ-mediated signal transduction, and thus cells do not respond to the presence of IFN-γ by upregulating the expression of MHC class II genes (Miller et al., 1998; Sedmak et al., 1994). The viral US2, and possibly US3, proteins can also downregulate HLA-DRα and DMα, two proteins that are involved in MHC class II antigen presentation (Tomazin et al., 1999).

Another mechanism that HCMV uses to interfere with immune surveillance is modulation of extracellular host factors (i.e., interleukins and chemokines) that are involved in inflammatory reactions and function to activate and recruit T cells, NK cells, neutrophils, and monocytes to the sites of infection. HCMV also encodes several chemokines, cytokines, and receptors that likely play a role in the inflammatory response and in the dissemination of the virus. One factor, cmvIL-10 (UL111A), is a functional homologue of IL-10 that has been proposed to downregulate macrophage and T cell responses and hence have an anti-inflammatory role (Kotenko et al., 2000; Spencer et al., 2002). Another is a functional alpha chemokine, vCXCL-1 (UL146), that attracts neutrophils via CXCR2 (Penfold et al., 1999). HCMV also encodes four glycoproteins with homology to G-protein-coupled seven-TM receptor proteins (UL33, UL78, US27, and US28) (Chee et al., 1990a). One of these (US28) serves as a specific receptor for the CX3C chemokine fractalkine and can also bind many other CC chemokines (Gao and Murphy, 1994; Kuhn et al., 1995; Mizoue et al., 2001). The observation that expression of US28 in vascular smooth muscle cells causes the cells to exhibit enhanced migration towards inflammatory cytokines has led to the hypothesis that US28 may not only facilitate viral dissemination, but also contribute to the progression of vascular diseases. (Streblow et al., 1999).

Transactivating functions of the major IE proteins

Since viral immediate–early (IE) gene products are the primary regulators of HCMV early gene expression, it is important to introduce these proteins and their functions. This topic is covered in detail in Chapters 17, and only the salient points are discussed here. The main sites of IE transcription are the UL122–123 (major immediate early, MIE), UL36–38, US3, and IRS1/TRS1 open reading frames (Fig. 18.1).

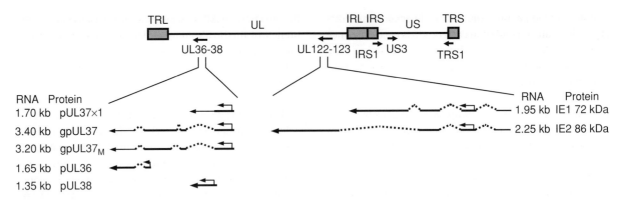

Fig. 18.1. Sites of IE transcription in the HCMV genome. Relative positions in the genome of the IE loci encoding regulatory proteins are shown. The splice patterns of the four IE transcripts expressed from the UL36–38 region and of the two major IE transcripts expressed from the UL122–123 region are indicated. Also shown is the early UL38 transcript.

The predominant and best-characterized members of this group are the products of the major IE region: the IE1 72 and IE2 86 kDa proteins and related products.

Structure and function of the IE1 72 and IE2 86 kDa proteins

The tight control and remarkably strong transactivating capacity of IE1 and IE2 proteins have caused significant effort to be directed towards understanding how they control the progression of the infection. A single, five-exon transcript from the major IE region is differentially spliced to give two predominant products the IE1 72 kDa protein (exons 1–4) and IE2 86 kDa protein (exons 1–3 and 5). Translation of each mRNA initiates in exon 2, and the two proteins share 85 amino acids (aa) at their amino termini (Stenberg et al., 1984, 1985; Stinski et al., 1983). IE1 72 has modest transactivating effects, including the ability to transactivate the major immediate early promoter (MIEP). Both the regions unique to IE1 and to IE2 encode additional, minor transcripts, some of which are cell-type specific (Awasthi et al., 2004; Jenkins et al., 1994; Kerry et al., 1995; Puchtler and Stamminger, 1991; Shirakata et al., 2002; Stenberg et al., 1989).

IE2 86 is thought to transactivate and repress transcription via protein-protein and protein-DNA interactions. IE2 86 binds to itself, to the UL84 gene product, and to a number of cellular proteins. These host factors include components of the basal transcription complex TBP, TFIIB, and multiple TBP-associated factors (TAFs), Rb, p53, and transcription factors including Sp1, Tef-1, c-Jun, JunB, ATF-2, NF-κB, protein kinase A-phosphorylated delta CREB, p300, CBP, P/CAF, Nil-2A, CHD-1, Egr-1, and UBF (Bonin and McDougall, 1997; Bryant et al., 2000; Caswell et al., 1993; Chiou et al., 1993; Choi et al., 1995; Fortunato et al., 1997; Furnari et al., 1993; Gebert et al., 1997; Hagemeier et al., 1992, 1994; Jupp et al., 1993; Lang et al., 1995; Lukac et al., 1994, 1997; Schwartz et al., 1994, 1996; Scully et al., 1995; Sommer et al., 1994; Spector and Tevethia, 1994; Speir et al., 1994; Wara-Aswapati et al., 1999; Wu et al., 1998; Yoo et al., 1996) (F. Ruchti and D. H. Spector, unpublished results). While interactions between IE1 72 and cellular proteins including p107 (Johnson et al., 1999) have also been demonstrated, the IE1 product does not bind to DNA. IE2 86 binds to specific DNA sequences through interactions that are thought to involve the minor groove (Lang and Stamminger, 1994; Waheed et al., 1998), a notable example being its site-specific binding to the 14 bp cis-repression signal (crs) located between the TATA box and transcription start site in the major immediate–early promoter (MIEP). It has been shown that this interaction with DNA is the mechanism by which IE2 86 negatively regulates its own transcription (Cherrington et al., 1991; Huang and Stinski, 1995; Lang and Stamminger, 1994; Liu et al., 1991; Macias and Stinski, 1993; Pizzorno and Hayward, 1990). In addition, IE2 86 binds to similar 14 bp sites upstream of the TATA box in early promoters including the UL112–113 (2.2kb RNA), TRL7 (1.2 kb RNA), and UL4 promoters (Arlt et al., 1994; Chang et al., 1989; Huang and Stinski, 1995; Schwartz et al., 1994; Scully et al., 1995).

Multiple studies have aimed to define motifs and domains of IE2 86 that are required for both protein–protein and protein–DNA interactions as well as to identify amino acids that are likely to be post-translationally modified. The ability of IE2 86 to interact with other proteins maps broadly to the region not shared with IE1 72, amino acids 86–542 (Chiou et al., 1993; Sommer et al., 1994). A subset of this region, aa 388–542, is required for IE2 86 dimerization (Ahn et al., 1998b; Chiou et al., 1993; Furnari et al., 1993). The DNA-binding capability of IE2, which controls regulation of early promoters and autoregulation, is also the result of sequences present in the C-terminal half of the protein between residues 290–579 (Chiou et al., 1993; Lang and Stamminger, 1993; Schwartz et al., 1994). Regions spanning the full length of the protein appear to be important for IE2 86 transactivation of promoters, including HCMV early promoters, with the critical regions located between aa 1–98 and 170–579 (Hermiston et al., 1990; Malone et al., 1990; Pizzorno et al., 1991; Scully et al., 1995; Sommer et al., 1994; Stenberg et al., 1990; Yeung et al., 1993). Activation of different viral promoters may require different IE2 86 domains, such as the requirement of sequences from aa 26–85 and aa 290–579 to transactivate the UL112–113 promoter and the additional requirement for aa 86–135 for activation of the 1.2 kb RNA promoter (Scully et al., 1995; Sommer et al., 1994).

The extensive posttranslational modifications of the major IE products suggest that they may be important for the functions of the proteins. Both IE1 72 and IE2 86 are phosphorylated and modified by sumoylation (Ahn et al., 2001; Heider et al., 2002a, b; Hofmann et al., 2000; Spengler et al., 2002; Xu et al., 2001). Although a virus with a mutation in the IE1 sumoylation site grows slightly more slowly than the wild type, mutation of the IE2 sumoylation sites has no effect on viral replication (Lee and Ahn, 2004; Nevels et al., 2004). In vitro and in vivo studies show that IE2 86 is phosphorylated on multiple residues (Harel and Alwine, 1998). When the consensus MAP kinase motifs at amino acids 27, 144, 233–234, and 555 are mutated to alanine, some of the resulting proteins have a stronger capacity to transactivate in transient expression assays than wild type IE2 86. However, in the context of the viral genome, these mutations have no effect on viral replication in fibroblasts (Heider et al., 2002b). In contrast, mutations of the multiple serines in the region between amino acids 258 and 275 have complex effects on viral growth, with some mutations accelerating and others inhibiting the infection (Barrasa et al., 2005). The fact that these major differences in growth rate are associated with only modest effects of the mutations on the transactivation function of IE2 86 in transient expression assays underscores the difficulty of extrapolating results from transient expression assays to events that occur in the context of viral infection.

In vitro and transient expression assays demonstrating the transactivating functions of the major IE proteins

Numerous studies have shown that the major IE proteins function together and separately to activate their own promoter as well as a wide range of heterologous viral and cellular promoters. Studies have been conducted primarily using transient transfection of effector plasmids expressing IE proteins and target plasmids expressing reporters driven by a range of viral promoters. In particular, these include the 1.2 and 2.7 kb RNA and UL112–113 (2.2 kb RNA) early promoters and sequences driving expression of genes involved in viral DNA replication (Colberg-Poley et al., 1992; Klucher et al., 1993; Schwartz et al., 1994; Scully et al., 1995). The results of these studies indicate that IE2 86 makes the greatest contribution to activation and in some cases, increases the level of reporter expression 40- to 80-fold over expression in the absence of IE1 72 or IE2 86. IE1 72 alone is a relatively weak transactivator, and only affects a limited number of promoters that have been tested. The transient assay function that best accounts for the growth defects exhibited by mutant viruses lacking IE1 72 is cooperation with IE2 86 in the activation of early promoters (Gawn and Greaves, 2002; Greaves and Mocarski, 1998).

Mutational analysis of the major IE products in the viral genome

The above studies laid the groundwork for elucidating the critical domains and functions of the major IE products. The recent studies that have used recombinant viruses with mutations in the UL122–123 ORFs, however, are more biologically relevant. A human fibroblast cell line expressing IE1 72 allowed the propagation of a mutant virus lacking UL123 exon 4 that was unable to express full-length IE1 72 (Mocarski et al., 1996). While our laboratory and others have attempted the construction of a similar cell line expressing the IE2 86 protein, to date none has been isolated. In the absence of a complementing cell line, it is difficult to propagate recombinant viruses with mutations in essential genes like IE2 86; however, the advent of bacterial artificial chromosomes (BACs) as vectors for the cloning of herpesvirus genomes has largely allowed this problem to be circumvented (for review see Adler et al., 2003). Since the majority of the viral genome is present in the BAC, mutations can be made and characterized entirely in bacteria regardless of the viability of the resulting virus. Reconstitution of virus from the clone is achieved by transfecting the altered genome and a construct expressing pp71 into cells permissive for HCMV infection (Baldick et al., 1997).

Several groups have since used this approach to construct HCMV IE2 86 mutants. A recombinant virus with most of the unique region of the IE2 gene (ORF UL122) deleted is defective in early gene expression and does not produce infectious progeny, providing additional evidence that IE2 86 is required for the activation of early genes and for viral replication (Marchini et al., 2001). Members of our group generated a viable mutant with a deletion spanning IE2 86 residues 136–290 and showed that this virus expresses IE and early genes and replicates its DNA comparably to the wild type but is delayed in expression of a subset of late genes (Sanchez *et al.*, 2002).

Smaller mutations introduced into the IE2 86 gene in the viral genome have also been used to define specific regions of the protein required for the activation of early promoters. Members of our laboratory have constructed recombinants with internal deletions of amino acids 356–359, 427–435, or 505–511 (White *et al.*, 2004). These mutations were selected on the basis of the IE2 86 domain mapping and functional studies discussed above and are located in the C-terminal region important for protein–protein interactions and DNA binding. Each deletion results in a non-viable virus. The IE2 86Δ356–359 mutation removes amino acids implicated in the activation of the UL112–113 and UL54 promoters (Stenberg *et al.*, 1990) and results in a clone that is able to support limited early gene expression but not replication of viral DNA. The IE2 86Δ427–435 and IE2 86Δ505–511 mutations disrupt the zinc finger and helix-loop-helix motifs present in the protein, and the resulting recombinants do not support early gene expression. All are defective in *crs*-mediated autorepression of the major IE promoter, although the degree of this defect varies with the mutant. Similarly, a temperature-sensitive IE2 86 mutant virus that contains the point mutation C509G (C510G in AD169) is able to transactivate the UL112–113 promoter at 32.5°C, but not at 39.5°C (Heider *et al.*, 2002a). This mutant also exhibits increased transcription from immediate early loci consistent with a defect in autoregulation.

The use of other recombinant viruses has helped elucidate the contributions of IE2 86 to host cell cycle dysregulation during HCMV infection. A virus with a deletion of the majority of exon 3 of the major IE region expresses altered forms of both IE1 72 and IE2 86 proteins and is viable, but severely growth impaired (White and Spector, 2005). It is defective both in the activation of viral early promoters and in altering the expression of certain cellular proteins including cyclin E. Neither of these defects can be fully complemented by growth in the presence of wild type IE1 72 protein. C-terminal sequences of IE2 86 are also required for host cell cycle dysregulation, as infection with a virus carrying a glutamine-to-arginine point mutation at aa 548 does not arrest the host cell cycle and does allow host DNA replication to proceed (Petrik *et al.*, 2006).

Fewer HCMV mutants with disruptions in the IE1 72 coding region have been isolated and characterized, but an existing mutant constructed by deleting exon 4 of the major IE region gives important information about the role of this protein in regulation of the infection. The recombinant is viable, exhibiting minimal growth defects in cells infected at a high multiplicity but exhibits striking replication deficiency at low MOIs (Gawn and Greaves, 2002; Greaves and Mocarski, 1998; Mocarski *et al.*, 1996). Fibroblasts infected with 0.4 pfu/cell of IE1 mutant virus express IE2 86 about as frequently, and to similar levels, as wild-type infected cells, but by immunostaining, deletion mutant-infected cells express delayed early proteins, including ppUL44, ppUL57, and pUL69, much less frequently or to lower levels than wild-type infected cells. This effect on protein expression is apparent at the transcriptional level as well, with decreased accumulation of delayed early RNAs in cells infected at low multiplicity with the mutant. UL112–113 expression is supported to an intermediate degree, with fewer mutant-infected cells staining positively for these proteins than for IE2 86, but more than stained positive for ppUL44. Apparently, while high levels of IE2 86 or another factor are able to compensate for the loss of IE1 72 during a high multiplicity infection, efficient activation of early genes in cells infected at low multiplicity requires IE1 72. A further study used constructs expressing wild type or mutant forms of IE1 72 to complement the IE1 deletion mutant virus in *trans* (Reinhardt *et al.*, 2005). This work showed that aa 476–491 tether IE1 72 to chromatin but are not required for complementation, while aa 421–475 comprise an acidic domain necessary for complementation and restoration of wild type titers during low multiplicity growth.

Additional immediate early proteins have regulatory roles

In addition to UL122–123, the UL36–38 and IRS1/TRS1 families and the US3 locus encode IE proteins with regulatory functions. Knockout mutants constructed to date suggest that either UL37 exon 1 or UL36 are necessary for progression of the infection (Blankenship and Shenk, 2002; Borst *et al.*, 1999; Dunn *et al.*, 2003; Patterson and Shenk, 1999; Yu *et al.*, 2003; McCormick *et al.*, 2005). The IRS1 and TRS1 ORFs encode three proteins: two expressed from a promoter located in the repeated region flanking the US segment of the genome with an ORF continuing into the unique region, and a third, smaller, protein designated pIRS1[263] which is expressed from an internal promoter in the unique region of the IRS1 gene (Romanowski and Shenk, 1997). In transient expression assays, either the IRS1 or TRS1 protein can complement HCMV origin-dependent DNA replication and modestly upregulate transcription from the MIEP or cooperate with IE1 72 and IE2 86 in activation of other viral promoters (Pari and Anders, 1993; Romanowski and Shenk, 1997). None of these three gene products is essential for viral replication in tissue culture, since recombinant viruses lacking the unique regions of the IRS or TRS1 open reading frames are viable (Blankenship and Shenk, 2002; Jones and Muzithras, 1992). The mutant lacking the IRS1 products grows normally, whereas the TRS1 deletion mutant exhibits a multiplicity-dependent growth phenotype. The amount of virus released from cells infected with the TRS1 deletion mutant at a low MOI is reduced drastically compared to that released from wild-type infected cells, but cells infected at a high MOI produce only slightly less virus than the wild type. TRS1 mutant virus replication proceeds normally through DNA replication, and appears to be defective in packaging the viral DNA at a step that occurs after the cleavage of the DNA (Adamo et al., 2004). Two studies have investigated TRS1 and IRS1 protein function using recombinant vaccinia or herpes simplex type 1 viruses that lack the normal ability to block host cell protein synthesis shutoff upon infection (Child et al., 2004; Cassady, 2005; Hakki and Geballe, 2005). TRS1 and IRS1 proteins were able to restore this ability in both cases, either after transient expression in the vaccinia virus-infected cell or from the HSV-1 recombinant. TRS1 protein also binds dsRNA via an N-terminal domain distinct from the C-terminal region that contributes to the evasion of the shutoff of translation (Hakki and Geballe, 2005).

The UL36–38 gene products were also identified in the study that identified eleven loci required for complementation of DNA replication (Pari and Anders, 1993), and are individually dispensable for growth in culture (Dunn et al., 2003; Yu et al., 2003; McCormick et al., 2005). Four of five transcripts from this region are expressed with IE kinetics, three from the UL37 promoter and one coding for the UL36 product (Fig. 18.1) (Chee et al., 1990b; Goldmacher et al., 1999; Kouzarides et al., 1988). The 3.4 kb spliced transcript from the UL37 promoter is present only at IE times and encodes an integral membrane glycoprotein, gpUL37 (Kouzarides et al., 1988; Tenney and Colberg-Poley, 1991a,b). An alternative splice of this transcript generates the 3.2 kb mRNA coding for gpUL37$_M$ (Goldmacher et al., 1999; Colberg-Poley et al., 2000), and these proteins traffic from the ER to mitochondria. While gpUL37 is able to transactivate the hsp70 promoter in transient assays, and UL37 exon 2 or exon 3 sequences are required for this activity, deletion of these exons does not affect the ability of the virus to replicate in culture (Borst et al., 1999; Colberg-Poley et al., 1998; Goldmacher et al., 1999; Tenney et al., 1993; Zhang et al., 1996). The conservation of the UL37 exon 1 sequence in clinical isolates and high-passage laboratory strains, as well as in other primate CMVs, and in rodent CMVs (McCormick et al., 2003b, 2005) suggest that the anti-apoptotic functions of vMIA homologues are important in response to the stress of infection. In transient transfection assays, a construct expressing UL37 exon 1 can also activate the UL54, UL44, and other early viral promoters. Although this activation is observed when constructs expressing IE1 72 and IE2 86 are used in this assay (Colberg-Poley et al., 1998), adding UL37 exon 1 and IE1/IE2 expression vectors together results in a synergistic activation effect. The final IE transcript from the UL36–38 region is the UL36 RNA, which encodes a protein (vICA) that is also involved in preventing apoptosis in infected cells (Skaletskaya et al., 2001). The fifth transcript from this region is the product of the UL38 gene and is expressed with early kinetics.

A third region transcribed with IE kinetics is the US3 gene, which specifies at least three alternatively spliced RNAs coding for related proteins. It is the target of complex positive and negative regulatory control (Biegalke, 1995, 1997, 1998, 1999; Chan et al., 1996; Thrower et al., 1996) and like much of UL36–38, is dispensable for growth in culture (Jones and Muzithras, 1992). Proteins generated from this region help the virus to evade the host immune response by keeping MHC class I molecules retained in the ER and unable to traffic to the plasma membrane (Ahn et al., 1996; Jones et al., 1996). US3 transcripts are abundant during the first three hours of infection and decrease by five h p.i. Transcription is regulated by a combination of elements located near the promoter including a silencer, enhancer, and transcriptional repressive element (tre) which shares sequence similarity with the crs element involved in control of major IE region expression (Biegalke, 1998; Bullock et al., 2001, 2002; Chan et al., 1996; Lashmit et al., 1998; Thrower et al., 1996). The product of the UL34 gene binds the tre element and represses transcription of US3 (LaPierre and Biegalke, 2001). The US3 proteins seem to possess limited intrinsic transactivating capability, as they have only been shown to induce the cellular hsp70 promoter in transient assays (Colberg-Poley et al., 1992; Tenney et al., 1993; Zhang et al., 1996).

UL112–113 transcription is differentially controlled at early and late times

Many of our current views on the regulation of early gene expression are derived from studies on the UL112–113 region of the HCMV genome (Fig. 18.2). The UL112–113 ORFs encode a family of phosphoproteins of 84, 50, 43, and 34 kDa that share a common amino terminal domain. The initial evidence for the importance of these gene products came from the studies of Pari and Anders, who identified the locus encoding them as one of the eleven required for the replication of a plasmid containing the HCMV origin of DNA replication oriLyt (Pari and Anders, 1993). As noted above, the UL112–113 proteins were found to be among

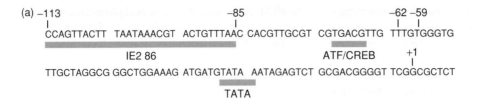

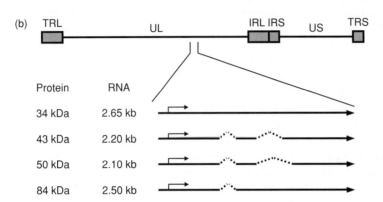

Fig. 18.2. Structure of the HCMV UL112–113 region. (a) The UL112–113 promoter from nt −113 to +7 relative to the early transcription start site, +1. The IE2 86 binding site located between −113 and −85, the consensus ATF/CREB site, and the late transcription start site at −62 are indicated. Sequences between −84 and −59 are required for IE2 86-mediated activation of the UL112–113 promoter. (b) Four transcripts from the UL112–113 region encode phosphoproteins with common N-termini. Splice patterns and sizes of the transcripts and corresponding proteins are indicated. The 2.1 and 2.2 kb RNAs are expressed by 8 h p.i., while the 2.5 and 2.65 species increase in abundance later.

the first to colocalize with IE2 86 at the periphery of the original ND10 sites and appeared to form the initial nucleation sites for subsequent viral DNA replication (Ahn et al., 1999a). Transient expression assays also have shown that they can cooperate with the UL36–38 and IRS1/TRS1 ORFs to augment the stimulation of several early gene promoters by the IE1 and IE2 proteins. Although the recent studies with mutant recombinant viruses that do not express these proteins indicate that the gene products are not absolutely essential for the viral infection, the resulting viruses are severely debilitated in their ability to replicate (Dunn et al., 2003; Yu et al., 2003). The molecular and cellular mechanisms underlying their function, however, are still unknown.

Transcription from the UL112–113 locus begins as early as 8 h p.i. and continues for the duration of the infection, although the relative abundance of members of the family changes as the infection progresses (Staprans et al., 1988; Staprans and Spector, 1986). Two spliced RNAs of 2.1 and 2.2 kb are expressed by 8 h p.i. and encode 50 kDa and 43 kDa phosphoproteins, respectively (Staprans et al., 1988; Staprans and Spector, 1986; Wright and Spector, 1989; Wright et al., 1988). These transcripts are coterminal at both 5′ and 3′ ends and share identical 5′ and internal exons, but use different splice acceptor sites in the 3′ exon to generate the two species, which encode proteins with different carboxyl termini. Later in the infection, transcription from the early start site decreases and initiation of transcription occurs at a site further upstream at nt −62. Two RNAs of 2.5 and 2.65 kb also increase in abundance as the infection proceeds, with the 2.5 kb transcript having spliced out only the first intron and encoding an 84 kDa phosphoprotein and the unspliced 2.65 kb transcript specifying a 34 kDa phosphoprotein (Staprans and Spector, 1986; Wright and Spector, 1989; Wright et al., 1988).

In initial studies, transiently transfected UL112–113 promoter-CAT reporter constructs were used to determine that the region located at −113 to −59 relative to the transcription start site is required for activation of this promoter during the infection. These assays utilized 5′ and internal promoter deletion mutants to show that these sequences were required for activation by IE2 86; this region also contained one of four binding sites for IE2 86, at −113 to −85 (Schwartz et al., 1994; Staprans et al., 1988). Further work indicated that although this IE2 86 binding site contributes to full activation of the UL112–113 promoter, it is in fact sequences between −84 and −59 that are strictly required for full activation of this promoter by IE2 86 (Arlt et al., 1994; Schwartz et al., 1996). A consensus ATF/CREB site is located between nt −71 to −66, suggesting that a member of the ATF/CREB family of transcription factors contributes significantly to IE2 86-mediated promoter activation

(Staprans et al., 1988). Additional mutational analyses of the region indicate that this contribution is modulated by interactions with factors bound to other regions of the promoter.

Further work used a series of gel shift analyses to establish that CREB is the major ATF-related protein in uninfected U373 MG cells that binds to this site (Schwartz et al., 1996). Three bands were observed following incubation of wild-type UL112–113 promoter sequences from −84 to −59 with nuclear extracts from U373 MG cells, and two of these were reduced or eliminated when wild type sequences from −72 to −61 were mutated. A complex comigrating with one of the bands also formed when a DNA fragment containing a consensus ATF/CREB site was used as the probe instead of the UL112–113 promoter. The majority of this consensus probe-protein complex was supershifted by the addition of anti-CREB antibody, as was most of the corresponding band in the UL112–113 promoter-protein complexes. The other two bands were less affected by the addition of anti-CREB antibody, but also were not supershifted in the presence of either anti-ATF-2 or anti-ATF-4.

Subsequent studies from our laboratory have used recombinant viruses to define the promoter elements controlling UL112–113 expression in the infected cell (Rodems et al., 1998). In these viruses, a cassette containing the UL112–113 promoter driving expression of the CAT reporter was inserted between the US9 and US10 loci in the viral genome. Reporter expression from this ectopic location authentically reproduced the kinetics of UL112–113 expression, in particular the switch from the +1 to the −62 transcription start site late in the infection (Staprans and Spector, 1986). The family of viruses was constructed based on the observations discussed above and comprised recombinants containing the wild type UL112–113 promoter or one of a series of IE2 86 and/or ATF/CREB binding site mutations in the promoter. As in transient assays, deletion of the ATF/CREB site in the virus resulted in a severe reduction in reporter activity early in the infection, but by 72 h p.i. wild type and ATF/CREB deletion mutants differed in reporter activity by less than twofold. Deletion of the ATF/CREB site also resulted in a shift of the late transcription start site downstream by the number of residues deleted. Consistent with data from transient transfection assays, when the IE2 86 binding site between −113 and −85 was deleted, the level of transcription from the mutant promoter was reduced to half of wild-type promoter levels at early times. Later in the infection, this level was not sustained, and extracts from IE2 86 binding site mutant-infected cells exhibited 15-fold less CAT activity than extracts from wild-type promoter virus-infected cells. These results support a model in which transcription from the UL112–113 promoter is differentially controlled at early and late times postinfection, with the ATF/CREB site providing significant regulatory control at early times and little to none at late times. The IE2 86 binding site, in contrast, modulates UL112–113 transcription at early times but is even more important for the maintenance of elevated transcript levels late in the infection.

Further mutational analysis of the UL112–113 promoter was used to define the sequences between −113 and −85 involved in the control of late transcription. Insertion of 5- or 10-nt sequences into the promoter and a corresponding shift in the late transcription start site suggest that sequences in this region direct late transcription from the UL112–113 promoter with distance-dependent characteristics (D. Kim and D. H. Spector, unpublished results). This complex control of transcription from the UL112–113 region reinforces the idea that, while overall expression of a given viral gene may appear to change little as the infection progresses, this steady-state level is achieved through a series of temporally distinct regulatory mechanisms.

In addition to the above controls operating at the level of transcription, analysis of the pattern of expression of the four RNAs and their corresponding proteins revealed that there were additional mechanisms being used to regulate the level of the proteins (Wright and Spector, 1989). The high levels of the 43 kDa UL112–113 protein at early times correlated well with the abundance of the 2.2 kb RNA at this time. The kinetics of synthesis of the 84- and 34-kDa proteins also correlated well with those of their corresponding RNAs. In contrast, the level of the 2.1 kb RNA was only slightly lower than that of the 2.2 kb RNA at all times during the infection, but the 50 kDa protein did not accumulate until later in the infection. Interestingly, the level of the 50 kDa protein was most sensitive to inhibition of viral DNA replication, suggesting that its accumulation at late times might be coupled to ongoing viral DNA replication. The mechanism for this post-transcriptional regulation is still unknown. It does not appear to be related to stability of the full-length protein, as in pulse-chase experiments at early times in the infection, the 50 kDa protein showed similar kinetics of decay as the 43 kDa protein. Other possibilities are that there is some block to efficient translation of the RNA or that the protein is transiently unstable during translation.

Multiple *cis*-acting sequences regulate UL54 expression

UL54, the ORF encoding the HCMV DNA polymerase, is a prototypical early–late gene whose regulation has been studied both in the context of the viral genome and in numerous transient expression and in vitro assays

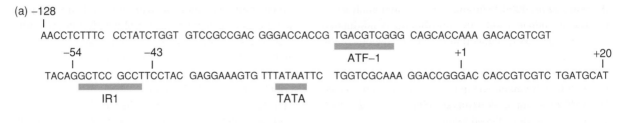

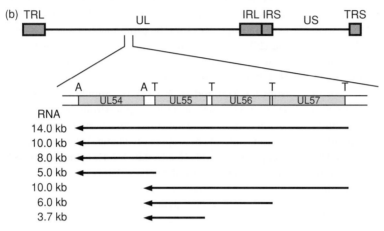

Fig. 18.3. Structure of the HCMV UL54 region. (a) The minimal UL54 promoter from nt −128 to +20 relative to the transcription start site, +1. The IR1 element located between −53 and −45 and the ATF-1 binding site from −88 to −80 are indicated. Sequences between nt −54 and −43 are required for IE protein-mediated promoter activation. (b) Transcripts expressed from the UL54-UL57 region. At least seven RNAs resulting from transcription from four start sites (predominant TATA elements, T) and polyadenylation at two sites (predominant poly A sites, A) are expressed from this region.

(Fig. 18.3). Seven transcripts resulting from initiation at four sites and polyadenylation at two sites in the UL54–57 region are expressed from this cluster of genes. The first RNA transcripts containing UL54 sequences are detectable as early as 8–12 h p.i., but in contrast to the UL112–113 family of transcripts, their level increases significantly at later times (Smuda et al., 1997).

Initial transient expression studies on the regulation of the UL54 promoter indicated that IE2 86 was required for its activation and that other IE and early products including IE1 72, TRS/IRS1, and the UL112–113 proteins cooperated to further activate transcription from the promoter (Kerry et al., 1996). These experiments also identified promoter elements required for activation in transient and in vitro assays, defining the minimal polymerase promoter as the region from −128 to +20 relative to the transcription start site and demonstrating that an 8 bp inverted repeat element at −53 to −45, IR1, was required for activation of the polymerase promoter by viral IE proteins in transient transfection assays (Kerry et al., 1994, 1996). A second copy of the IR1 element is present at −225, but did not contribute significantly to activation of the polymerase promoter in these assays (Kerry et al., 1996). IR1 was found to bind cellular factors found in nuclear extracts prepared from infected cells. If the IR1 element was mutated, the cellular factors failed to bind and activation of the promoter by IE proteins was decreased threefold (Kerry et al., 1994). A pair of studies identified the transcription factor Sp1 as one of the cellular proteins that could bind the IR1 element. In one study (Luu and Flores, 1997), scanning mutagenesis of the promoter from −270 to +200 confirmed the requirement of the −54 to −43 region for IE mediated activation of the promoter. Using a 30 bp DNA probe and uninfected HeLa cell extracts, the authors demonstrated that Sp1 bound to this region. In the other study (Wu et al., 1998), a shorter IR1-containing DNA probe also bound Sp1 in extracts of U373 cells overexpressing IE2 86, but not in parental U373MG cells or in HeLa cells. The complex could be supershifted by the addition of antibody specific to IE2 86, but the presence of IE2 86 in this complex did not seem to require DNA binding activity since addition of an unlabeled DNA probe containing the *crs* did not reduce complex formation. In addition, an Sp1 binding oligonucleotide competed away this complex in the IE2 86-expressing U373 cells. Based on these results, the authors proposed that an inhibitory factor present in HeLa cells prevents the Sp1-UL54 promoter interaction from occurring.

Numerous differences in experimental design prevent further direct comparison of these studies, and the role of Sp1 in control of UL54 expression in infected cells has not yet been examined.

Another regulatory domain in the UL54 promoter was localized to between nt −88 to −80 (Kerry et al., 1994, 1997). A 40 bp DNA probe from this region bound nuclear proteins from infected human fibroblasts, with DNA binding activity particularly strong in 48–72 h p.i. extracts and weaker at earlier times or when DNA replication was inhibited by the addition of phosphonoacetate (PAA). Supershift analyses confirmed that one protein present in this complex is ATF-1. Since recombinant ATF-1/DNA complexes migrate differently than those present in infected cell nuclear extracts, it is possible that an additional protein is involved in this interaction or that ATF-1 is differentially modified during the infection.

Analysis of the UL54 promoter in the context of the viral genome began with the characterization of this promoter driving a CAT reporter in a construct inserted between ORFs US9 and US10 (Kohler et al., 1994). Subsequent studies used similar recombinant viruses to better define the role of the IR1 element in UL54 promoter activation. A family of viruses was constructed in which either the full-length polymerase promoter (−425 to +20), the full length promoter with a mutation in the IR1 site, or the minimal activation domain (−128 to +20) drove expression of the CAT reporter (Kerry et al., 1996). Based on CAT activity and RNA levels by Northern blot, UL54 promoter activity at early times was three- to fourfold lower than the wildtype when the IR1 element was mutated. In contrast, deleting the upstream promoter region and including only the minimal promoter resulted in a slight increase in promoter activity. This was consistent with the increase in promoter activity observed in transient assays when the −425 to −128 region was deleted, but the effect was smaller in the context of the viral genome. At late times, the IR1 element appears to be less important to the activation of this promoter, since the virus carrying the IR1 mutation exhibited only a slight reduction in both RNA levels and CAT activity by 72 to 96 h p.i. The ATF site in the UL54 promoter was similarly examined by constructing recombinant viruses (Kerry et al., 1997). In contrast to the IR1 element, the ATF binding site appears to control UL54 promoter activity both at early and late times p.i. Mutation of the ATF site in a UL54 promoter-CAT reporter virus resulted in five- to sixfold decreases in both mRNA expression and CAT activity over a range of times, from 24–96 h p.i.

Finally, recent work has attempted to use regulation of the UL54 promoter to understand the species specificity of HCMV (Garcia-Ramirez et al., 2001). These experiments examined the activity of the HCMV polymerase promoter following HCMV infection of murine NIH 3T3 cells transiently or stably transfected with a yeast artificial chromosome (YAC) clone containing much of the HCMV genome. The authors found that mutating the IR1 element in this context reduced reporter activity and interpreted these results to invoke similar cellular factors in both 3T3 and human cells, suggesting that species specific cellular factors do not underlie activation of the UL54 promoter. Given the many differences between murine and human fibroblasts, it is difficult to put these findings in context. A complete characterization of the UL54 promoter-reporter YAC construct in human cells to understand the consequences of promoter mutations in the natural context might help understand any work across species barriers.

UL4 expression is controlled at the transcriptional and translational levels

UL4 is an example of an early gene whose expression is regulated by unique mechanisms operating at both the transcriptional and translational levels (Fig. 18.4). Three unspliced transcripts are expressed from the UL4 locus, with 1.4 and 1.5 kb RNAs present at early times and a 1.7 kb product detectable later. These encode an incompletely characterized membrane glycoprotein, gp48, which is a virion component that is completely dispensable for viral growth in tissue culture (Hobom et al., 2000).

Transcriptional control of the UL4 gene was first analyzed in a series of transient transfection assays demonstrating that the UL4 promoter is responsive to IE2 86 and that there are two cis-acting sites in the UL4 promoter upstream of the TATA box (Chang et al., 1989; Huang et al., 1994). The first site, a CCAAT box with inverted dyad symmetry between −88 and −98 relative to the transcription start site, appeared to be a positive regulatory element that could bind the transcription factor NF-Y in vitro (Huang et al., 1994). Gel shift analyses demonstrated the formation of two complexes that were inhibited by the addition of a competing oligonucleotide containing the NF-Y target sequence or supershifted by the addition of antibody to NF-Y. Neither could be supershifted by the addition of IE2 86-specific antibody. One complex was present in both uninfected and infected cells; the second was only detected in infected cells. When phosphatase was added, the second complex decreased in abundance while the first increased, suggesting that NF-Y may be differentially phosphorylated in HCMV-infected cells.

A second regulatory region located between −169 and −139 in the UL4 promoter, site 2, bound a cellular factor in

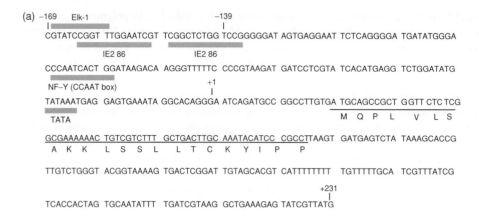

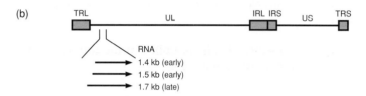

Fig. 18.4. Structure of the HCMV UL4 region. (a) The UL4 promoter and transcript leader sequences from nt −169 to the start site of gp48 (pUL4) translation. Sequences are representative of HCMV Towne strain and are numbered relative to the start site of 1.5 kb RNA transcription, +1. Site 2 is located between −169 and −139 and contains two putative IE2 86 binding sites and the Elk-1 site. The CCAAT box binds NF-Y. uORF2, which encodes the *cis*-acting repressor of UL4 transcription, is underlined, and the sequence of the 22 aa peptide is indicated. (b) Transcripts expressed from the UL4 region. Three 3′ coterminal transcripts with different 5′ ends are produced. Two RNAs of 1.4 and 1.5 kb are present at early times, with the 1.5 kb transcript expressed more abundantly. The 1.7 kb transcript is present later in the infection.

vitro, as indicated by DNA footprinting and gel shift assays, and negatively influenced transcription (Huang *et al.*, 1994; Huang and Stinski, 1995). The importance of IE2 86 in the activation of this promoter was suggested by the following observations: first, the negative effect on the promoter was relieved when an IE2 86 expression vector was cotransfected with the UL4 promoter–CAT reporter construct; second, a truncated version of IE2 86 containing amino acids 290 to 579 bound site 2 in vitro (Huang and Stinski, 1995). These results led to the hypothesis that IE2 86 binds to a specific negative regulatory region (which is 65% homologous to the *crs* element in the major IE promoter) and in the process displaces a bound cellular factor, thus allowing activation of the UL4 promoter. Mutation of the putative zinc finger region of IE2 86 resulted in a protein that could no longer interact with the promoter, lending further support to this idea.

Recent studies examining transcriptional control of the UL4 promoter in the context of the viral genome confirm some, but not all, of these initial findings and demonstrate important differences between control of viral gene expression in transient assays and in the infected cell. A series of HCMV recombinants containing the CAT reporter cassette driven by a wild type or mutant UL4 promoter inserted into the viral genome between US7 and US12 were derived (Chen and Stinski, 2000). In this ectopic location, the CAT transcript was expressed with kinetics much like those of the native UL4 transcript, but to slightly lower overall levels. Here, a mutation in the UL4 promoter NF-Y binding site did not alter CAT transcript levels, leading to the conclusion that in the virus, the NF-Y binding site contributes little or nothing to control of UL4 transcription. In contrast, site 2 mutants displayed altered reporter expression. Site 2 contains two putative (but non-consensus) IE2 86 binding sites and a predicted Elk-1 binding site that together appeared to be required for maximal expression in the context of viral infection (Chen and Stinski, 2000). In a later study, however, disruption of the Elk-1 site alone was sufficient for the effect, indicating that it is likely Elk-1 or a related cellular factor and not the IE2 86 binding sites that play the critical regulatory role (Chen and Stinski, 2002). Elk-1 binding to this site is supported by EMSA data in which a consensus Elk-1 site competes for cellular factor binding and an Elk-1 antibody partially supershifts the UL4 promoter-cellular factor complex (Chen and Stinski, 2000).

Transcriptional upregulation of UL4 expression has been used to demonstrate the importance of the MAPK/ERK and p38 MAPK pathways in HCMV replication. Peak activation of these signal transduction cascades occur at 4 and 8 h p.i., respectively, and appears to be important to the progression of productive infection via efficient expression of early and late genes (Johnson et al., 2001a; Rodems and Spector, 1998). In one study (Chen and Stinski, 2002), the requirement for these pathways was analyzed in the context of UL4 transcription using the MAPK/ERK kinase (MEK) inhibitor UO126 and the p38 MAPK inhibitor FHPI. Cells infected with one of the recombinant viruses expressing the CAT gene from wild-type or mutant UL4 promoters were treated with an inhibitor and assayed for CAT activity. Strikingly, inhibition of MEK with the chemical inhibitor UO126 caused UL4 promoter activity to drop by 70%–80% for all promoters tested, with approximately equivalent loss of expression when the wild-type UL4 promoter was used as well as when site 2 or the NF-Y or Elk-1 binding sites were disrupted. The effect of the inhibitor FHPI was very similar, with no effect on UL4 promoter constructs when used at a low concentration and a 50%–80% reduction of both wild type and mutant promoter activity at a higher concentration. These data suggest that the UL4 promoter is responsive to both MAPK/ERK and p38 MAPK pathways and that the minimal responsive element is the TATA, not one of the other transcription factor binding sites that have been analyzed. This effect, however, was less prominent when endogenous UL4 RNA expression was examined, and the possibility of general inhibition of viral transcription or downregulation of other upstream factors in the presence of these inhibitors has not yet been addressed.

Novel post-transcriptional controls also distinguish the regulation of UL4 expression. Three small ORFs are located in the UL4 transcript upstream of the gp48 transcription start site. The largest of these, uORF2, encodes a 22 aa product which acts in *cis* to repress translation of the authentic UL4 transcript (Degnin et al., 1993). Interestingly, this repression is amino acid- (but not nucleotide-) sequence dependent and is particularly sensitive to mutations in codons near the C-terminus of uORF2. In transient transfection-superinfection assays, missense mutation or deletion of the terminal amino acid, a proline, resulted in significantly elevated expression of reporter protein while the level of UL4 promoter-driven transcript remained unchanged. Changes in the N-terminal leader sequence also had an effect, with missense mutations at codons 7 and 8 reducing the ability of uORF2 to block translation. A further series of modified primer extension assays showed that ribosomes are stalled on the RNA at the uORF2 termination codon. These data have led to the following hypothesis regarding the mechanism of inhibition of downstream translation by uORF2. A ribosome translates through the uORF2 sequence until it reaches the final proline codon. Here, the nascent uORF2 peptide remains covalently linked to the peptidyl-tRNA and bound to the ribosome on the transcript. A possible interaction between this complex and the release factor eRF1, mediated by C-terminal prolines at positions 21 and 22 in the uORF2 peptide and a GGQ motif in eRF1, stabilizes the intermediate and prevents hydrolysis of the peptidyl-tRNA bond (Cao and Geballe, 1996, 1998; Janzen et al., 2002). Ribosomes stall before they are able to reach the gp48 translation start site, resulting in uORF2-dependent repression of gp48 translation.

The above model is supported by results from recombinant viruses as well. When the uORF2 initiation codon in the UL4 region was mutated, there was a significant upregulation of gp48 protein expression by the mutant relative to the wild-type virus (Alderete et al., 2001). In vivo, ribosomes were also stalled at the uORF2 termination codon in wild-type but not mutant-infected cells. The relatively normal expression of other early proteins indicates that it is not a general upregulation of translation in mutant-infected cells that accounts for this phenotype. Curiously, it appears that there is a slight delay in the accumulation of the UL4 transcript in mutant infected cells, with the UL4 RNA detectable by Northern blot 24 h p.i. in cells infected with the parental wild-type virus, but not until 48 h p.i. in uORF2 mutant-infected cells.

Since neither loss of nor overexpression of UL4 appears detrimental to viral replication in cultured fibroblasts (Alderete et al., 2001; Hobom et al., 2000), it seems likely that this complex regulation is important in the infected host where gp48 may have a cell type-specific role. Control of its transcription and translation remain interesting illustrations of the diverse methods used by the virus to regulate gene expression.

Human herpesviruses 6 and 7

Human herpesvirus 6 is distinguished by its ability to grow in T-lymphocytes. There are two variants: HHV-6A (GS and U1102-like isolates) and HHV-6B (Z-29 and HST-like isolates). Although the variants have approximately 90% nucleotide sequence identity and share many properties, they differ with respect to their epidemiology, cell tropism, interaction with the host cell, and in vivo pathogenesis. HHV-6B infection is very common in early childhood and is associated with exanthem subitum (roseola infantum), a mild illness that lasts only a few days (Yamanishi

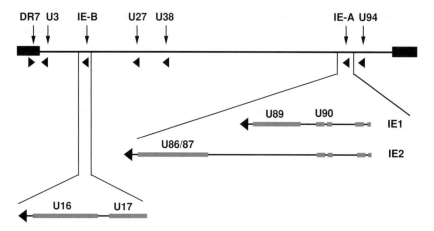

Fig. 18.5. HHV-6A Genome. The HHV-6 gene products with regulatory activities – DR7, U3, IE-B, U27 (DNA polymerase processivity factor), IE-A, and U94 – are shown on the map. The location of the U38 (DNA polymerase) ORF is also shown. The solid arrowheads indicate the direction of transcription. An expanded view of the IE transcripts encoded by the IE-A and IE-B loci is shown below the genome. The dark boxes are coding exons, the lighter boxes are non-coding exons, and the thin lines between the boxes are introns.

et al., 1988). HHV-7 is biologically similar to the two HHV-6 variants and is less frequently associated with this illness (Dominguez *et al.*, 1999; Isegawa *et al.*, 1999; Megaw *et al.*, 1998; Nicholas, 1996; Tanaka *et al.*, 1994). The DNA genomes of HHV-6 and HHV-7 are smaller than that of HCMV, with the length 159 kbp for HHV-6A, 161–170 kbp for HHV-6B, and 145–153 kbp for HHV-7 DNA. The genome of all of these viruses consists of a long unique segment bounded by direct repeats (Dominguez *et al.*, 1999; Gompels *et al.*, 1995; Isegawa *et al.*, 1999; Lindquester and Pellett, 1991; Martin *et al.*, 1991b; Megaw *et al.*, 1998; Nicholas, 1996)). In general, the genes of these viruses are collinear with those of human cytomegalovirus U_L region (see Chapter 14).

Analysis of the molecular biology of HHV-6 and HHV-7 has been limited by poor growth and low yields in cultured cells. Thus, the elucidation of the regulation of gene expression is not well advanced and has relied almost exclusively on transient assays that are known to be relatively poor predictors of behavior in the context of viral infection. The overall pattern of gene expression (IE, early, and late) resembles that of HCMV and other herpesviruses, but the assignment of many of the individual genes to a particular class is still tentative and has been influenced by the sensitivity of the assay applied, the specific strain of virus, and cell line used in the analysis. The reader is referred to Chapters 42 and 43 as well as the following papers for the details: Menegazzi *et al.* (1999); Mirandola *et al.* (1998); Oster and Hollsberg (2002); Rapp *et al.* (2000). For the purposes of this review, only HHV-6 IE genes that appear to have some regulatory functions and two early genes whose regulation has been studied in greatest depth – the HHV-6 DNA polymerase (U38) and the DNA polymerase processivity factor (U27) (Fig. 18.5) – will be discussed.

HHV-6 IE gene products with regulatory activities

The HHV-6 regulatory proteins that have been studied are encoded by the IE-A and IE-B loci, DR7, U3, U27, and U94. The IE-A and IE-B loci of both HHV-6 and HHV-7 are the major sites of IE gene expression (Fig. 18.5). The IE-A region (U86 to U90) is collinear with the major immediate early region of HCMV that encodes the IE1 and IE2 proteins (UL122–123), and the IE-B region (U16 to U19) is collinear with the HCMV IE ORFs UL36 to UL38 (see Chapter 17).

These putative viral regulatory proteins have only been studied with promoters from cellular genes and genes from heterologous viruses. Because HHV-6 has been proposed to be a cofactor in the progression of AIDS, many of these studies have used the HIV-1 LTR promoter (for review, see Lusso and Gallo, 1995). The HIV-1 LTR has been found to be activated by regions of the HHV-6A genome corresponding to the IE-B locus (Chen *et al.*, 1994; Garzino-Demo *et al.*, 1996; Geng *et al.*, 1992; Horvat *et al.*, 1991), the IE-A locus (Gravel *et al.*, 2003; Martin *et al.*, 1991a; Papanikolaou *et al.*, 2002; Stanton *et al.*, 2002), DR7 (Kashanchi *et al.*, 1994; Thompson *et al.*, 1994a), U3 (Mori *et al.*, 1998), and U27 (Zhou *et al.*, 1994). The IE-A locus also transactivates the CD4 promoter (Flamand *et al.*, 1998) and adenovirus E3 and E4 promoters (Martin *et al.*, 1991a), and the IE-B locus activates HPV 16 and 18 promoters (Chen *et al.*, 1994). Some of the regulatory proteins also appear to have negative effects. For example, U94 negatively regulates HIV-1 and H-ras promoters (Araujo *et al.*, 1995), and DR7 negatively regulates promoters that are responsive to p53 (Kashanchi et al., 1997).

IE-A

HHV-6A and HHV-6B exhibit a different organization in the IE-A region (Dominguez et al., 1999; Isegawa et al., 1999). The HHV-6A IE-A locus consists of two genetic units that are referred to as IE1 and IE2 (Chapter 17). Although this region is collinear with the HCMV major IE locus UL123 (IE1 72) and UL122 (IE2 86), it shares no nucleotide or protein sequence homology. The IE1 region encodes a 3.5 kb transcript that consists of 4 small 5' exons and a large 3' exon (Fig. 18.5) (Schiewe et al., 1994). Translation begins in exon 3, yielding a major protein of approximately 150 to 170 kDa that contains ORFs U90 and U89 (Papanikolaou et al., 2002). The corresponding region of HHV-6B shares only 62% identity at the amino acid level and encodes a major IE protein of approximately 150 kDa (Gravel et al., 2002; Takeda et al., 1996). The proteins are phosphorylated and conjugated to the ubiquitin-like protein SUMO-1 (Chang and Balachandran, 1991; Gravel et al., 2002). The sequence divergence of the HHV-6A and HHV-6B IE1 protein is reflected in their function in that the HHV-6A IE1 protein is a stronger activator of heterologous promoters in transient expression assays than the corresponding HHV-6B protein (Flamand et al., 1998; Gravel et al., 2002; Martin et al., 1991a).

Both HHV-6A and HHV-6B IE1 proteins are able to traffic to the ND10 sites (PODs). However, in contrast to other herpesviruses, interaction of the ND10 domains with IE1 does not lead to their dispersal, and IE1 maintains a stable interaction with ND10 throughout the infection (Gravel et al., 2002; Stanton et al., 2002). By immunostaining, the highest number of individual IE1 bodies can be detected at 12 h p.i., when they begin to coalesce into 1–3 larger bodies. It is likely that other viral proteins are needed to generate the larger bodies, since when the IE1 proteins were individually expressed, they colocalized with PML and SUMO-1 but the ND10 sites did not coalesce. Thus as is the case for HCMV, dispersal of ND10 domains is not a prerequisite for productive infection.

Recently, a full-length cDNA encoding the HHV-6A IE2 protein was isolated (Gravel et al., 2003); it contains ORFs U90 and U86/87, the positional homologues of the HCMV ORF encoding IE2 86 (Fig. 18.5). The 5.5 kb IE2 mRNA is expressed in the absence of de novo protein synthesis with kinetics that are somewhat delayed relative to the IE1 transcript. The IE2 mRNA is also less abundant, but it continues to increase throughout the infection while the IE1 mRNA reaches maximal levels by 12 h p.i. At later times, larger transcripts that have not been characterized and may initiate from upstream sites appear. The processed IE2 mRNA consists of 5 exons; 4 small exons located upstream of U89 are shared with IE1 and the fifth exon corresponds to the IE2 specific ORF U86/87. The sequence of the HHV-6A IE2 transcript diverges from that encoded by the HHV-6B variant, with only 64% identity at the amino acid level. The HHV-6A IE2 protein is also 167 amino acids shorter. By Western blot analysis with an antibody specific for the IE2 region, it appears that the major IE2 protein is approximately 220 kDa. At later times in the infection, additional smaller proteins of 100, 85 and 55 kDa have also been observed (Gravel et al., 2003; Papanikolaou et al., 2002). Analogous to the HCMV IE2 86 protein, the full-length HHV-6A IE2 protein functions in transient expression assays as a promiscuous activator of multiple promoters, including minimal promoters containing only a TATA box (Gravel et al., 2003; Papanikolaou et al., 2002). Recently, deletion analysis showed that both the N- and C-terminal domains of this protein are required for full function (Tomoiu et al., 2006). Interestingly, the HHV-6A IE2 protein does not appear to downregulate its own promoter, possibly because it does not contain the HCMV cis-repression signal.

IE-B

The HHV-6 IE-B region consists of the ORFs U16, U17, U18, and U19 and is collinear with the HCMV region containing the UL36–38 ORFs. As shown for the HCMV UL36–38 region, transcription from the HHV-6 IE-B region is complex (Flebbe-Rehwaldt et al., 2000; Mirandola et al., 1998). In HHV-6A (GS strain), the U17 and U16 ORFs are positional homologues of HCMV UL36 and yield a spliced IE RNA (Fig. 18.5) (Flebbe-Rehwaldt et al., 2000; Mirandola et al., 1998). HCMV UL36 also consists of 2 exons, with exon 2 corresponding to HHV-6A U16 (Tenney and Colberg-Poley, 1991a, b). In addition to the HHV-6 transcripts that contain the U17/U16 ORFs, there are also transcripts that include the U16 and U15 ORFs (U15 is unique to HHV-6). The HHV-6A and HHV-6B U17/U16 RNAs first appear at IE times and are maintained throughout the infection. The other U16 containing transcripts are expressed primarily as early RNAs, although a low level of transcription can be detected at IE times.

The HHV-6 U18 and U19 ORFs are transcribed as multiply spliced early RNAs. These are positional homologues of the HCMV UL37 and UL38 genes, respectively, but may not be functional homologues. With the caveat that all of the functional assays have been performed with transient assays and plasmid constructs, the ORFs do not correspond to their HCMV homologues with respect to their potential role as transactivators. In HHV-6, the ORFs that can

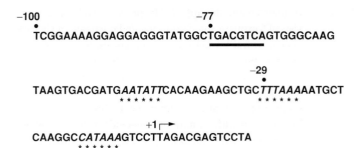

Fig. 18.6. HHV-6A DNA polymerase (U38) promoter. Sequences that could potentially serve as TATA boxes are italicized and marked with asterisks. The arrow at position +1 shows the transcription start site. The consensus ATF/CREB binding site is underlined.

transactivate the HIV-1 LTR promoter are U17/U16, not U18/U19 (Chen et al., 1994; Garzino-Demo et al., 1996; Geng et al., 1992; Horvat et al., 1991). UL37 exon 1, which has no apparent homologue in HHV-6 or HHV-7, serves as a cell death suppressor and transactivator of HCMV early gene promoters in transient assays (Colberg-Poley et al., 1998; Patterson and Shenk, 1999; Goldmacher et al., 1999).

U94

U94 is encoded by HHV-6A and HHV-6B and is a homologue of the adenovirus associated virus 2 (AAV-2) rep gene (Thomson et al., 1991). Although not conserved in primate CMVs, a homologue is found in rat CMV (Vink et al., 2000). In AAV-2, the rep68 gene encodes a site-specific ATP-dependent endonuclease and helicase that is involved in the site-specific integration of AAV into chromosome 19. U94 can serve as a helper for AAV-2 replication and can complement an AAV-2 virus with a mutation in the rep gene (Thomson et al., 1994). The role of the U94 protein is yet to be elucidated, but it may play a role in latency and modulation of the infection. Relevant to this are the data showing that cell lines expressing HHV-6B U94 cannot be infected by HHV-6A and that the U94 transcript can be detected during latency in PBMC (Rotola et al., 1998). U94 was also found to suppress H-ras and BPV-1 transformation (Araujo et al., 1997) and transcription from H-ras and HIV-1 LTR promoters (Araujo et al., 1995). HHV-7 does not encode a U94 homologue.

cis-acting sequences within HHV-6 early promoters

DNA polymerase (U38)

Analogous to HCMV, the HHV-6 DNA polymerase gene has been used as a prototypical early gene for examining cis-acting regulatory sequences on the promoter (Fig. 18.6). Based on the position of the RNA start site, standard transient expression assays with promoter-CAT reporter genes have been used to identify and characterize the major regulatory region for transcription (Agulnick et al., 1994). The data showed that expression of CAT from a construct containing sequences −524 to +115 relative to the transcription start site was below the limit of detection in uninfected HSB-2 human T cells, but was highly up-regulated in infected cells. By mutational analysis, the cis-acting sequences for activation were localized to the sequences between −78 and +13. The major regulatory element within this region was a consensus ATF/CREB binding site located at nt −77 to −70. Further support for this domain serving a regulatory role was the observation that in gel shift assays, this site bound to two protein complexes in both infected and uninfected nuclear extracts. The ATF/CREB site, however, is not required for activation of this promoter by the HHV-6A IE2 protein in transient assays (Tomoiu et al., 2006).

The U38 promoter does not contain a consensus TATA element in the −30 region, although there are several AT-rich domains located at positions −48 to −43, −29 to −24, and −11 to −6. When point mutations were introduced into each of the domains individually, there was no effect on the promoter, leading the authors to conclude that the promoter is TATA-less (Agulnick et al., 1994). However, the start site for transcription was not identified for any of the mutants in the transient expression assays, and thus the possibility that the elements might be able to compensate for one another, albeit with a change in start site, cannot be excluded. As has been the case for all herpesvirus promoters, conclusions cannot be drawn from transient assays alone and each promoter must be assessed in the context of the viral genome. It would seem likely that the ATF/CREB site is the major regulatory element, as this sequence is located in a similar position in the promoter of the HCMV DNA polymerase gene and its function has been confirmed in the context of the HCMV genome (Kerry et al., 1994, 1996, 1997).

Early viral gene expression and function

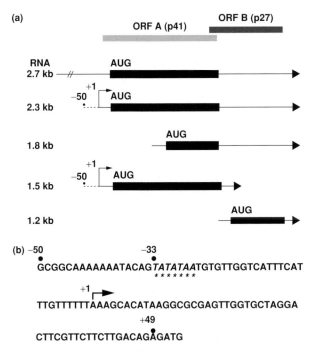

Fig. 18.7. HHV-6A DNA polymerase processivity factor (U27). (a) The early–late transcripts from the U27 region are shown. ORF A encodes the 41-kDa DNA polymerase processivity factor. The dark boxes represent the putative protein product. (b) Promoter for the 1.5 kb and 2.3 kb U27 RNAs. The sequence that could potentially serve as a TATA box is italicized and marked with asterisks. The arrow at position +1 shows the transcription start site. The translation initiation codon at nt +49 is also indicated.

DNA polymerase processivity factor (U27)

U27 encodes a 41 kDa nuclear phosphoprotein that is the homologue of the HCMV UL44 gene encoding DNA polymerase processivity factor (Fig. 18.7) (Agulnick *et al.*, 1993; Chang and Balachandran, 1991). The U27 region actually includes two ORFs, ORF A and ORF B. ORF A corresponds to a 41 kDa protein, and the downstream ORF B could encode a 27 kDa protein (Zhou *et al.*, 1997). The transcription pattern of this gene is similar for both the variant A HHV-6 GS strain and the variant B HHV-6 Z29 strain. At least five early–late unspliced RNA species ranging in size from 1.2 to 2.7 kb (1.2, 1.5, 1.8, 2.3, and 2.7 kb) map to this locus, with the 2.3 kb RNA being the most abundant (Agulnick *et al.*, 1993; Zhou *et al.*, 1997). Four of the RNAs (2.7, 2.3, 1.8, and 1.2 kb RNAs) are 3′ co-terminal. The 1.5 kb RNA utilizes the same start site as the 2.3 kb RNA but terminates upstream of the other four RNAs. The 2.3 kb and 1.5 kb RNAs have the potential to encode the p41 protein in ORF A, and the 1.2 kb RNA could specify a protein of about 17 kDa within ORF B. Although the 2.7 kb RNA includes ORF A, the presence of several AUGs before ORF A makes it unlikely that it encodes p41. Likewise, the 1.8 kb RNA has several AUGs with short ORFs before ORF B, but it could be translated into a truncated version of ORF A.

Regulation of the promoter for the 1.5 kb and 2.3 kb U27 RNAs was studied for the HHV-6A GS strain in HSB-2 human T-cell line (Thompson *et al.*, 1994b). The transcription start site, which is 48 bp upstream of the translation initiation codon AUG, is preceded by a TATA sequence starting at nt −33 relative to the RNA start site. Using mutant promoter-CAT constructs in transient expression assays, an essential regulatory element that was activated in the infected cells was localized between nt −73 and −52. Within this region were a putative binding site for the transcription factor C/EBP (CAAT enhancer-binding protein) and two other repeat sequences. The activity of this site was both distance and orientation dependent relative to the TATA sequence.

Mobility shift assays indicated that there were four complexes that bound to this region. The two that were present in both uninfected and infected cells (C1 and C2) did not appear to contain C/EBP factors. Point mutations within these sites that eliminated binding also inactivated the promoter. Two of the binding complexes were only present in uninfected cells (C3 and C4) and they could be competed by an oligonucleotide containing a consensus C/EBP site. The construction and use of a HHV-6 BAC will greatly facilitate further studies on the regulation of this and other promoters during the viral life cycle.

Conclusions

The studies presented here highlight the central role that early gene expression plays in the viral life cycle. It is the middleman in the relay race leading to the production of infectious virus. Events precipitated by the initial contact of the virus with the host cell and the synthesis of IE gene products set the stage for early gene expression. The products of these early genes not only provide the component parts for the factories devoted to viral DNA synthesis, cleavage and packaging of the viral genome, and assembly of the virus particles, but also serve to commandeer the host cell machinery and signaling pathways to create a cellular environment that is optimal for viral gene expression and DNA replication. Although dispensable for growth in tissue culture, a cadre of the early genes must also establish a blockade to the host's immune response and prepare routes of escape for viral dissemination. Analogous to the control of host cell genes, viral early gene expression is regulated at multiple levels by mechanisms operating at the initiation of transcription, RNA processing and transport, translation, and mRNA and protein stability. The development of BACs as vectors for the cloning of herpesvirus genomes has revolutionized the field so that the function of viral genes and the regulation of their expression can be studied in the biologically relevant context of the viral infection. These techniques coupled with the rapidly moving fields of genomics and proteomics will greatly enhance our ability to elucidate the cellular and molecular mechanisms governing the interaction of the virus with its host.

REFERENCES

Abate, D. A., Watanabe, S., and Mocarski, E. S. (2004). Major human cytomegalovirus structural protein pp65 (ppUL83) prevents interferon response factor 3 activation in the interferon response. *J. Virol.*, **78**, 10995–11106.

Adamo, J. E., Schroer, J., and Shenk, T. (2004). Human cytomegalovirus TRS1 protein is required for efficient assembly of DNA-containing capsids. *J. Virol.*, **78**, 10221–10229.

Adler, H., Messerle, M., and Koszinowski, U. H. (2003). Cloning of herpesvirus genomes as bacterial artificial chromsomes. *Rev. Med. Virol.*, **13**, 111–121.

Agulnick, A. D., Thompson, J. R., Iyengar, S., Pearson, G., Ablashi, D., and Ricciardi, R. P. (1993). Identification of a DNA-binding protein of human herpesvirus 6, a putative DNA polymerase stimulatory factor. *J. Gen. Virol.*, **74**, 1003–1009.

Agulnick, A. D., Thompson, J. R., and Ricciardi, R. P. (1994). An ATF/CREB site is the major regulatory element in the human herpesvirus 6 DNA polymerase promoter. *J. Virol.*, **68**, 2970–2977.

Ahn, J. H. and Hayward, G. S. (1997). The major immediate-early proteins IE1 and IE2 of human cytomegalovirus colocalize with the disrupt PML-associated nuclear bodies at very early times in infected permissive cells. *J. Virol.*, **71**, 4599–4613.

Ahn, K., Angulo, A., Ghazal, P., Peterson, P. A., Yang, Y., and Fruh, K. (1996). Human cytomegalovirus inhibits antigen presentation by a sequential multistep process. *Proc. Natl Acad. Sci. USA*, **93**, 10990–10995.

Ahn, J. H., Brignole, E. R., and Hayward, G. S. (1998a). Disruption of PML subnuclear domains by the acidic IE1 protein of human cytomegalovirus is mediated through interaction with PML and may modulate a RING finger-dependent cryptic transactivator function of PML. *Mol. Cell. Biol.*, **18**, 4899–4913.

Ahn, J. H., Chiou, C. J., and Hayward, G. S. (1998b). Evaluation and mapping of the DNA binding and oligomerization domains of the IE2 regulatory protein of human cytomegalovirus using yeast one and two hybrid interaction assays. *Gene*, **210**, 25–36.

Ahn, J.-H., Jang, W.-J., and Hayward, G. S. (1999a). The human cytomegalovirus IE2 and UL112–113 proteins accumulate in viral DNA replication compartments that initiate from the periphery of promyelocytic leukemia protein-associated nuclear bodies (PODs or ND10). *J. Virol.*, **73**, 10458–10471.

Ahn, J. H., Jang, W. J., and Hayward, G. S. (1999b). The human cytomegalovirus IE2 and UL112–113 proteins accumulate in viral DNA replication compartments that initiate from the periphery of promyelocytic leukemia protein-associated nuclear bodies (PODs or ND10). *J. Virol.*, **73**, 10458–10471.

Ahn, J. H., Xu, Y., Jang, W. J., Matunis, M. J., and Hayward, G. S. (2001). Evaluation of interactions of human cytomegalovirus immediate-early IE2 regulatory protein with small ubiquitin-like modifiers and their conjugation enzyme Ubc9. *J. Virol.*, **75**, 3859–3872.

Albrecht, T., Fons, M. P., Bologh, I., AbuBakar, S., Deng, C. Z., and Millinoff, D. (1991). Metabolic and cellular effects of human cytomegalovirus infection. *Transpl. Proc.*, **23**, 48–55.

Alderete, J. P., Child, S. J., and Geballe, A. P. (2001). Abundant early expression of gpUL4 from a human cytomegalovirus mutant lacking a repressive upstream open reading frame. *J. Virol.*, **75**, 7188–7192.

Araujo, J. C., Doniger, J., Kashanchi, F., Hermonat, P. L., Thompson, J., and Rosenthal, L. J. (1995). Human herpesvirus 6A ts suppresses both transformation by H-ras and transcription by the H-ras and human immunodeficiency virus type 1 promoters. *J. Virol.*, **69**, 4933–4940.

Araujo, J. C., Doniger, J., Stoppler, H., Sadaie, M. R., and Rosenthal, L. J. (1997). Cell lines containing and expressing the human herpesvirus 6A ts gene are protected from both H-ras and BPV-1 transformation. *Oncogene*, **14**, 937–943.

Arlt, H., Lang, D., Gebert, S., and Stamminger, T. (1994). Identification of binding sites for the 86-kilodalton IE2 protein of human cytomegalovirus within an IE2-responsive viral early promoter. *J. Virol.*, **68**, 4117–4125.

Arnoult, D., Bartle, L. M., Skaletskaya, A. *et al.* (2004). Cytomegalovirus cell death suppressor vMIA blocks Bax- but not Bak-mediated apoptosis by binding and sequestering Bax at mitochondria. *Proc. Natl Acad. Sci. USA*, **101**, 7988–7993.

Awasthi, S., Isler, J. A., and Alwine, J. C. (2004). Analysis of splice variants of the immediate-early 1 region of human cytomegalovirus. *J. Virol.*, **78**, 8191–8200.

Baldick, C., Jr., Marchini, A., Patterson, C. E., and Shenk, T. (1997). Human cytomegalovirus tegument protein pp71 (ppUL82) enhances the infectivity of viral DNA and accelerates the infectious cycle. *J. Virol.*, **71**, 4400–4408.

Barrasa, M. I., Harel, N. Y., and Alwine, J. C. (2005). The phosphorylation status of the serine-rich region of the human cytomegalovirus 86-kilodalton major immediate–early protein IE2/IEP86 affects temporal gene expression. *J. Virol.*, **79**, 1428–1437.

Biegalke, B. J. (1995). Regulation of human cytomegalovirus US3 gene transcription by a cis-repressive sequence. *J. Virol.*, **69**, 5362–5367.

Biegalke, B. J. (1997). IE2 protein is insufficient for transcriptional repression of the human cytomegalovirus US3 promoter. *J. Virol.*, **71**, 8056–8060.

Biegalke, B. J. (1998). Characterization of the transcriptional repressive element of the human cytomegalovirus immediate–early US3 gene. *J. Virol.*, **72**, 5457–5463.

Biegalke, B. J. (1999). Human cytomegalovirus US3 gene expression is regulated by a complex network of positive and negative regulators. *Virology*, **261**, 155–164.

Biswas, N., Sanchez, V., and Spector, D. H. (2003). Human cytomegalovirus infection leads to accumulation of geminin and inhibition of the licensing of cellular DNA replication. *J. Virol.*, **77**, 2369–2376.

Blankenship, C. A. and Shenk, T. (2002). Mutant human cytomegalovirus lacking the immediate–early TRS1 coding region exhibits a late defect. *J. Virol.*, **76**, 12290–12299.

Boldogh, I., AbuBakar, S., Deng, C. Z., and Albrecht, T., 1991. Transcriptional activation of cellular oncogenes *fos*, *jun* and *myc* by human cytomegalovirus. *J. Virol.*, **65**, 1568–1571.

Bonin, L. R. and McDougall, J. K. (1997). Human cytomegalovirus IE2 86-kilodalton protein binds p53 but does not abrogate G1 checkpoint function. *J. Virol.*, **71**, 5831–5870.

Borst, E. M., Hahn, G., Koszinowski, U. H., and Messerle, M. (1999). Cloning of the human cytomegalovirus (HCMV) genome as an infectious bacterial artificial chromosome in *Escherichia coli*: a new approach for construction of HCMV mutants. *J. Virol.*, **73**, 8320–8329.

Boyle, K. A., Pietropaolo, R. L., and Compton, T. (1999). Engagement of the cellular receptor for glycoprotein B of human cytomegalovirus activites the interferon-responsive pathway. *Mol. Cell. Biol.*, **19**, 3607–3613.

Bresnahan, W. A., Boldogh, I., Thompson, E. A., and Albrecht, T. (1996). Human cytomegalovirus inhibits cellular DNA synthesis and arrests productively infected cells in late G1. *Virology*, **224**, 156–160.

Bresnahan, W. A., Albrecht, T., and Thompson, E. A. (1998). The cyclin E promoter is activated by human cytomegalovirus 86-kDa immediate early protein. *J. Biol. Chem.*, **273**, 22075–22082.

Browne, E. P. and Shenk, T. (2003). Human cytomegalovirus UL83-coded pp65 virion protein inhibits antiviral gene expression in infected cells. *Proc. Natl Acad. Sci. USA*, **100**, 11439–11444.

Browne, E. P., Wing, B., Coleman, D., and Shenk, T. (2001). Altered cellular mRNA levels in human cytomegalovirus-infected fibroblasts: viral block to the accumulation of antiviral mRNAs. *J. Virol.*, **75**, 12319–12330.

Bryant, L. A., Mixon, P., Davidson, M., Bannister, A. J., Kouzarides, T., and Sinclair, J. H. (2000). The human cytomegalovirus 86-kilodalton major immediate–early protein interacts physically and functionally with histone acetyltransferase P/CAF. *J. Virol.*, **74**, 7230–7237.

Buerger, I., Reefschlaeger, J., Bender, W. *et al.* (2001). A novel non-nucleoside inhibitor specifically targets cytomegalovirus DNA maturation via the UL89 and UL56 gene products. *J. Virol.*, **75**, 9077–9086.

Bullock, G. C., Lashmit, P. E., and Stinski, M. F. (2001). Effect of the R1 element on expression of the US3 and US6 immune evasion genes of human cytomegalovirus. *Virology*, **288**, 164–174.

Bullock, G. C., Thrower, A. R., and Stinski, M. F. (2002). Cellular proteins bind to sequence motifs in the R1 element between the HCMV immune evasion genes. *Exp. Mol. Pathol.*, **72**, 196–206.

Cantrell, S. R. and Bresnahan, W. A. (2005). Interaction between the human cytomegalovirus UL82 gene product (pp71) and hDaxx regulates immediate-early gene expression and viral replication. *J. Virol.*, **79**(12), 7792–7802.

Cantrell, S. R. and Bresnahan, W. A. (2006). Human cytomegalovirus (HCMV) UL82 gene product (pp71) relieves hDaxx-mediated repression of HCMV replication. *J. Virol.*, **80**(12), 6188–6191.

Cao, J. and Geballe, A. P. (1998). Ribosomal release without peptidyl tRNA hydrolysis at translation termination in a eukaryotic system. *RNA*, **4**, 181–188.

Cao, J. and Geballe, A. P. (1996). Coding sequence-dependent ribosomal arrest at termination of translation. *Mol. Cell. Biol.*, **16**, 603–608.

Cassady, K. A. (2005). Human cytomegalovirus TRS1 and IRS1 gene products block the double-stranded-RNA-activated host protein shutoff response induced by herpes simplex virus type 1 infection. *J. Virol.*, **79**(14), 8707–8715.

Castillo, J. P., Yurochko, A., and Kowalik, T. F. (2000). Role of human cytomegalovirus immediate–early proteins in cell growth control. *J. Virol.*, **74**, 8028–8037.

Caswell, R., Hagemeier, C., Chiou, C.-J., Hayward, G., Kouzarides, T., and Sinclair, J. (1993). The human cytomegalovirus 86K immediate early (IE) 2 protein requires the basic region of the TATA-box binding protein (TBP) for binding, and interacts with TBP and transcription factor TFIIB via regions of IE2 required for transcriptional regulation. *J. Gen. Virol.*, **74**, 2691–2698.

Chambers, J., Angulo, A., Amaratunga, D. (1999). DNA microarrays of the complex human cytomegalovirus genome: profiling kinetic class with drug sensitivity of viral gene expression. *J. Virol.*, **73**, 5757–5766.

Chan, Y. J., Tseng, W. P. and Hayward, G. S. (1996). Two distinct upstream regulatory domains containing multicopy cellular transcription factor binding sites provide basal repression and inducible enhancer characteristics to the immediate–early IES (US3) promoter from human cytomegalovirus. *J. Virol.*, **70**, 5312–5328.

Chang, C. K. and Balachandran, N. (1991). Identification, characterization, and sequence analysis of a cDNA encoding a phosphoprotein of human herpesvirus 6. *J. Virol.*, **65**, 2884–2894.

Chang, C.-P., Malone, C. L., and Stinski, M. F., 1989. A human cytomegalovirus early gene has three inducible promoters that are regulated differentially at various times after infection. *J. Virol.*, **63**, 281–290.

Chee, M., Satchwell, S., Preddie, E., Weston, K., and Barrell, B. (1990a). Human cytomegalovirus encodes three G protein-coupled receptor homologues. *Nature*, **344**, 774–777.

Chee, M. S., Bankier, A. T., Beck, S. *et al.* (1990b). Analysis of the protein-coding content of the sequence of human cytomegalovirus strain AD169. *Curr. Top. Microbiol. Immunol.*, **154**, 125–169.

Chen, J. and Stinski, M. F. (2000). Activation of transcription of the human cytomegalovirus early UL4 promoter by the Ets transcription factor binding element. *J. Virol.*, **74**, 9845–9857.

Chen, J. and Stinski, M. F. (2002). Role of regulatory elements and the MAPK/ERK or p38 MAPK pathways for activation of human cytomegalovirus gene expression. *J. Virol.*, **76**, 4873–4885.

Chen, M., Popescu, N., Woodworth, C. (1994). Human herpesvirus 6 infects cervical epithelial cells and transactivates human papillomavirus gene expression. *J. Virol.*, **68**, 1173–1178.

Cherrington, J. M., Khoury, E. L., and Mocarski, E. S. (1991). Human cytomegalovirus IE2 negatively regulates α gene expression via a short target sequence near the transcription start site. *J. Virol.*, **65**, 887–896.

Child, S. J., Hakki, M., DeNiro, K. L., and Geballe, A. P. (2004). Evasion of cellular antiviral responses by human cytomegalovirus TRS1/IRS1. *J. Virol.*, **78**, 197–205.

Chiou, C.-J., Zong, J., Waheed, I., and Hayward, G. S. (1993). Identification and mapping of dimerization and DNA-binding domains in the C terminus of the IE2 regulatory protein of human cytomegalovirus. *J. Virol.*, **67**, 6201–6214.

Choi, K. S., Kim, and S.-J., Kim, S. (1995). The retinoblastoma gene product negatively regulates transcriptional activation mediated by the human cytomegalovirus IE2 protein. *Virology*, **208**, 450–456.

Cihlar, T., Fuller, M. D., Mulato, A. S., and Cherrington, J. M. (1998). A point mutation in the human cytomegalovirus DNA polymerase gene selected in vitro by cidofovir confers a slow replication phenotype in cell culture. *Virology*, **248**, 382–393.

Colberg-Poley, A. M., Santomenna, L. D., Harlow, P. P., Benfield, P. A., and Tenney, D. J. (1992). Human cytomegalovirus US3 and UL36-38 immediate-early proteins regulate gene expression. *J. Virol.*, **66**, 95–105.

Colberg-Poley, A. M., Huang, L., Soltero, V. E., Iskenderian, A. C., Schumacher, R. F., and Anders, D. G. (1998). The acidic domain of pUL37x1 and gpUL37 plays a key role in transactivation of HCMV DNA replication gene promoter constructions. *Virology*, **246**, 400–408.

Colberg-Poley, A. M., Patel, M. B., Erezo, D. P., and Slater, J. E. (2000). Human cytomegalovirus UL37 immediate–early regulatory proteins traffic through the secretory apparatus and to mitochondria. *J. Gen. Virol.*, **81**, 1779–1789.

Courcelle, C. T., Courcelle, J., Prichard, M. N., and Mocarski, E. S. (2001). Requirement for uracil-DNA glycosylase during the transition to late-phase cytomegalovirus DNA replication. *J. Virol.*, **75**, 7592–7601.

Degnin, C. R., Schleiss, M. R., Cao, J., and Geballe, A. P. (1993). Translational inhibition mediated by a short upstream open reading frame in the human cytomegalovirus gpUL4 (gp48) transcript. *J. Virol.*, **67**, 5514–5521.

DeMarchi, J. M. (1981). Human cytomegalovirus DNA: restriction enzyme cleavage maps and map locations for immediate–early, early, and late RNAs. *Virology*, **114**, 23–28.

DeMarchi, J. M. (1983). Posttranscriptional control of human cytomegalovirus gene expression. *Virology*, **124**, 390–402.

DeMarchi, J. M., Schmidt, C. A., and Kaplan, A. S. (1980). Patterns of transcription of human cytomegalovirus in permissively infected cells. *J. Virol.*, **35**, 277–286.

Diffley, J. F. (2001). DNA replication: building the perfect switch. *Curr. Biol.*, **11**, R367–R370.

Dittmer, D. and Mocarski, E. S. (1997). Human cytomegalovirus infection inhibits G1/S transition. *J. Virol.*, **71**, 1629–1634.

Dominguez, G., Dambaugh, T. R., Stamey, F. R., Dewhurst, S., Inoue, N., and Pellett, P. E. (1999). Human herpesvirus 6B sequence: coding content and comparison with human herpesvirus 6A. *J. Virol.*, **73**, 8040–8052.

Dunn, W., Chou, C., Li, H. et al. (2003). Functional profiling of a human cytomegalovirus genome. *Proc. Natl Acad. Sci. USA*, **100**, 14223–14228.

Dyson, N. (1998). The regulation of E2F by pRB-family proteins. *Genes Dev.*, **12**, 2245–2262.

Ertl, P. F. and Powell, K. L. (1992). Physical and functional interaction of human cytomegalovirus DNA polymerase and its accessory protein (ICP36) expressed in insect cells. *J. Virol.*, **66**, 4126–4133.

Estes, J. E. and Huang, E.-S. (1977). Stimulation of cellular thymidine kinases by human cytomegalovirus. *J. Virol.*, **24**, 13–21.

Flamand, L., Romerio, F., Reitz, M. S., and Gallo, R. C. (1998). CD4 promoter transactivation by human herpesvirus 6. *J. Virol.*, **72**, 8797–8805.

Flebbe-Rehwaldt, L. M., Wood, C., and Chandran, B. (2000). Characterization of transcripts expressed from human herpesvirus 6A strain GS immediate–early region B U16-U17 open reading frames. *J. Virol.*, **74**, 11040–11054.

Fortunato, E. A. and Spector, D. H. (1999). Regulation of human cytomegalovirus gene expression. *Adv. Virus Res.*, **54**, 61–128.

Fortunato, E. A., Sommer, M. H., Yoder, K., and Spector, D. H. (1997). Identification of domains within the human cytomegalovirus major immediate–early 86-kilodalton protein and the retinoblastoma protein required for physical and functional interaction with each other. *J. Virol.*, **71**, 8176–8185.

Fortunato, E. A. and Spector, D. H. (1998). p53 and RPA are sequestered in viral replication centers in the nuclei of cells infected with human cytomegalovirus. *J. Virol.*, **72**, 2033–2039.

Fortunato, E. A., McElroy, A. K., Sanchez, V., and Spector, D. H. (2000). Exploitation of cellular signaling and regulatory pathways by human cytomegalovirus. *Trends Microbiol.*, **8**, 111–119.

Fujita, M. (1999). Cell cycle regulation of DNA replication initiation proteins in mammalian cells. *Front. Biosci.*, **4**, D816–D823.

Furnari, B. A., Poma, E., Kowalik, T. F., Huong, S.-M., and Huang, E.-S. (1993). Human cytomegalovirus immediate–early gene 2 protein interacts with itself and with several novel cellular proteins. *J. Virol.*, **67**, 4981–4991.

Gao, J. L. and Murphy, P. M. (1994). Human cytomegalovirus open reading frame US28 encodes a functional β chemokine receptor. *J. Biol. Chem.*, **269**, 28539–28542.

Garcia-Ramirez, J. J., Ruchti, F., Huang, H., Simmen, K., Angulo, A., and Ghazal, P. (2001). Dominance of virus over host factors in cross-species activation of human cytomegalovirus early gene expression. *J. Virol.*, **75**, 26–35.

Garzino-Demo, A., Chen, M., Lusso, P., Berneman, Z., and DiPaolo, J. A. (1996). Enhancement of TAT-induced transactivation of the HIV-1 LTR by two genomic fragments of HHV-6. *J. Med. Virol.*, **50**, 20–24.

Gawn, J. M. and Greaves, R. F. (2002). Absence of IE1 p72 protein function during low-multiplicity infection by human cytomegalovirus results in a broad block to viral delayed–early gene expression. *J. Virol.*, **76**, 4441–4455.

Gebert, S., Schmolke, S., Sorg, G., Floss, S., Plachter, B., and Stamminger, T. (1997). The UL84 protein of human cytomegalovirus acts as a transdominant inhibitor of immediate–early-mediated transactivation that is able to prevent viral replication. *J. Virol.*, **71**, 7048–7060.

Geng, Y. Q., Chandran, B., Josephs, S. F., and Wood, C. (1992). Identification and characterization of a human herpesvirus 6 gene segment that *trans* activates the human immunodeficiency virus type 1 promoter. *J. Virol.*, **66**, 1564–1570.

Gibson, W. (1996). Structure and assembly of the virion. *Intervirology*, **39**, 389–400.

Goldmacher, V. S., Bartle, L. M., Skaletskaya, A. *et al.* (1999). A cytomegalovirus-encoded mitochondria-localized inhibitor of apoptosis structurally unrelated to Bcl-2. *Proc. Natl Acad. Sci. USA*, **96**, 12536–12541.

Gompels, U. A., Nicholas, J., Lawrence, G. *et al.* (1995). The DNA sequence of human herpesvirus-6: structure, coding content, and genome evolution. *Virology*, **209**, 29–51.

Gravel, A., Gosselin, J. and Flamand, L. (2002). Human herpesvirus 6 immediate-early 1 protein is a sumoylated nuclear phosphoprotein colocalizing with promyelocytic leukemia protein-associated nuclear bodies. *J. Biol. Chem.*, **277**, 19679–19687.

Gravel, A., Tomoiu, A., Cloutier, N., Gosselin, J., and Flamand, L. (2003). Characterization of the immediate–early 2 protein of human herpesvirus 6, a promiscuous transcriptional activator. *Virology*, **308**, 340–353.

Greaves, R. F. and Mocarski, E. S. (1998). Defective growth correlates with reduced accumulation of a viral DNA replication protein after low-multiplicity infection by a human cytomegalovirus *ie1* mutant. *J. Virol.*, **72**, 366–379.

Hagemeier, C., Walker, S., Caswell, R., Kouzarides, T., and Sinclair, J. (1992). The human cytomegalovirus 80-kilodalton but not the 72-kilodalton immediate–early protein transactivates heterologous promoters in a TATA box-dependent mechanism and interacts directly with TFIID. *J. Virol.*, **66**, 4452–4456.

Hagemeier, C., Caswell, R., Hayhurst, G., Sinclair, J., and Kouzarides, T. (1994). Functional interaction between the HCMV IE2 transactivator and the retinoblastoma protein. *EMBO J.*, **13**, 2897–2903.

Hakki, M. and Geballe, A. P. (2005). Double-stranded RNA binding by human cytomegalovirus pTRS1. *J. Virol.*, **79**(12), 7311–7318.

Harel, N. Y. and Alwine, J. C. (1998). Phosphorylation of the human cytomegalovirus 86-kilodalton immediate–early protein IE2. *J. Virol.*, **72**, 5481–5492.

Hayajneh, W. A., Colberg-Poley, A. M., Skaletskaya, A. *et al.* (2001). The sequence and antiapoptotic functional domains of the human cytomegalovirus UL37 exon 1 immediate early protein are conserved in multiple primary strains. *Virology*, **279**, 233–240.

Heider, J. A., Bresnahan, W. A., and Shenk, T. E. (2002a). Construction of a rationally designed human cytomegalovirus variant encoding a temperature-sensitive immediate–early 2 protein. *Proc. Natl Acad. Sci. USA*, **99**, 3141–3146.

Heider, J. A., Yu, Y., Shenk, T., and Alwine, J. C. (2002b). Characterization of a human cytomegalovirus with phosphorylation site mutations in the immediate–early 2 protein. *J. Virol.*, **76**, 928–932.

Hermiston, T. W., Malone, C. L., and Stinski, M. F. (1990). Human cytomegalovirus immediate–early two-protein region involved in negative regulation of the major immediate–early promoter. *J. Virol.*, **64**, 3532–3536.

Hirai, K. and Watanabe, Y. (1976). Induction of α-type DNA polymerases in human cytomegalovirus-infected WI-38 cells. *Biochim. Biophys. Acta*, **447**, 328–339.

Hobom, U., Brune, W., Messerle, M., Hahn, G., and Koszinowski, U. H. (2000). Fast screening procedures for random transposon libraries of cloned herpesvirus genomes: mutational analysis of human cytomegalovirus envelope glycoprotein genes. *J. Virol.*, **74**, 7720–7729.

Hofmann, H., Floss, S., and Stamminger, T. (2000). Covalent modification of the transactivator protein IE2-p86 of human cytomegalovirus by conjugation to the ubiquitin-homologous proteins SUMO-1 and hSMT3b. *J. Virol.*, **74**, 2510–2524.

Hofmann, H., Sindre, H., and Stamminger, T. (2002). Functional interaction between the pp71 protein of human cytomegalovirus and the PML-interacting protein human Daxx. *J. Virol.*, **76**, 5769–5783.

Horvat, R. T., Wood, C., Josephs, S. F., and Balachandran, N. (1991). Transactivation of human immunodeficiency virus promoter by human herpesvirus 6 (HHV6) strains GS and Z-29 in primary human T lymphocytes and identification of transactivating HHV-6 (GS) gene fragments. *J. Virol.*, **65**, 2895–2902.

Huang, L. and Stinski, M. F. (1995). Binding of cellular repressor protein or the IE2 protein to a *cis*-acting negative regulatory element upstream of a human cytomegalovirus early promoter. *J. Virol.*, **69**, 7612–7621.

Huang, L., Malone, C. L., and Stinski, M. F. (1994). A human cytomegalovirus early promoter with upstream negative and positive *cis*-acting elements: IE2 negates the effect of the negative element, and NF-Y binds to the positive element. *J. Virol.*, **68**, 2108–2117.

Hwang, E. S., Kim, J., Jong, H. S., Park, J. W., Park, C. G., and Cha, C. Y. (2000). Characteristics of DNA-binding activity of human cytomegalovirus ppUL44. *Microbiol. Immunol.*, **44**, 827–832.

Isegawa, Y., Mukai, T., Nakano, K. *et al.* (1999). Comparison of the complete DNA sequences of human herpesvirus 6 variants A and B. *J. Virol.*, **73**, 8053–8063.

Ishov, A. M. and Maul, G. G. (1996). The periphery of nuclear domain 10 (ND10) as site of DNA virus deposition. *J. Cell Biol.*, **134**, 815–826.

Ishov, A. M., Stenberg, R. M., and Maul, G. G. (1997). Human cytomegalovirus immediate early interaction with host nuclear structures: Definition of an immediate transcript environment. *J. Cell Biol.*, **138**, 5–16.

Ishov, A. M., Vladimirova, O. V., and Maul, G. G. (2002). Daxx-mediated accumulation of human cytomegalovirus tegument protein pp71 at ND10 facilitates initiation of viral infection at these nuclear domains. *J. Virol.*, **76**, 7705–7712.

Isom, H. C. (1979). Stimulation of ornithine decarboxylase by human cytomegalovirus. *J. Gen. Virol.*, **42**, 265–278.

Iwayama, S., Yamamoto, T., Furuya, T., Kobayashi, R., Ikuta, K., and Hirai, K. (1994). Intracellular localization and DNA-binding activity of a class of viral early phosphoproteins in human fibroblasts infected with human cytomegalovirus (Towne strain). *J. Gen. Virol.*, **75**, 3309–3318.

Janzen, D. M., Frolova, L., and Geballe, A. P. (2002). Inhibition of translation termination mediated by an interaction of eukaryotic release factor 1 with a nascent peptidyl-tRNA. *Mol. Cell. Biol.*, **22**, 8562–8570.

Jault, F. M., Jault, J.-M., Ruchti, F. *et al.* (1995). Cytomegalovirus infection induces high levels of cyclins, phosphorylated RB, and p53, leading to cell cycle arrest. *J. Virol.*, **69**, 6697–6704.

Jenkins, D. E., Martens, C. L., and Mocarski, E. S. (1994). Human cytomegalovirus late protein encoded by ie2: a transactivator as well as a repressor of gene expression. *J. Gen. Virol.*, **75**, 2337–2348.

Johnson, R. A., Yurochko, A. D., Poma, E. E., Zhu, L., and Huang, E. S. (1999). Domain mapping of the human cytomegalovirus IE1-72 and cellular p107 protein–protein interaction and the possible functional consequences. *J. Gen. Virol.*, **80**, 1293–1303.

Johnson, R. A., Huong, S.-M., and Huang, E.-S. (2000). Activation of the mitogen-activated protein kinase p38 by human cytomegalovirus infection through two distinct pathways: a novel mechanism for activation of p38. *J. Virol.*, **74**, 1158–1167.

Johnson, R. A., Ma, X. L., Yurochko, A. D., and Huang, E. S. (2001a). The role of MKK1/2 kinase activity in human cytomegalovirus infection. *J. Gen. Virol.*, **82**, 493–497.

Johnson, R. A., Wang, X., Ma, X.-L., Huong, S.-M., and Huang, E.-S. (2001b). Human cytomegalovirus up-regulates the phosphatidylinositol 3-kinase (PI3-K) pathway: inhibition of PI3-K activity inhibits viral replication and virus-induced signaling. *J. Virol.*, **75**, 6022–6032.

Jones, T. R. and Muzithras, V. P. (1992). A cluster of dispensable genes within the human cytomegalovirus genome short component: IRS1, US1 through US5, and the US6 family. *J. Virol.*, **66**, 2541–2546.

Jones, T. R., Wiertz, E. J., Sun, L., Fish, K. N., Nelson, J. A., and Ploegh, H. L. (1996). Human cytomegalovirus US3 impairs transport and maturation of major histocompatibility complex class I heavy chains. *Proc. Natl Acad. Sci. USA*, **93**, 11327–11333.

Jupp, R., Hoffmann, S., Stenberg, R. M., Nelson, J. A., and Ghazal, P. (1993). Human cytomegalovirus IE86 protein interacts with promoter-bound TATA-binding protein via a specific region distinct from the autorepression domain. *J. Virol.*, **67**, 7539–7546.

Kalejta, R. F. and Shenk, T. (2003). The human cytomegalovirus UL82 gene product (pp71) accelerates progression through the G1 phase of the cell cycle. *J. Virol.*, **77**, 3451–3459.

Kalejta, R. F., Bechtel, J. T., and Shenk, T. (2003). Human cytomegalovirus pp71 stimulates cell cycle progression by inducing the proteasome-dependent degradation of the retinoblastoma family of tumor suppressors. *Mol. Cell. Biol.*, **23**, 1885–1895.

Kashanchi, F., Thompson, J., Sadaie, M. R. *et al.* (1994). Transcriptional activation of minimal HIV-1 promoter by ORF-1 protein expressed from the SalI-L fragment of human herpesvirus 6. *Virology*, **201**, 95–106.

Kashanchi, F., Araujo, J., Doniger, J. *et al.* (1997). Human herpesvirus 6 (HHV-6) ORF-1 transactivating gene exhibits malignant transforming activity and its protein binds to p53. *Oncogene*, **14**, 359–367.

Kelly, C., Driel, R. V., and Wilkinson, G. W. (1995). Disruption of PML-associated nuclear bodies during human cytomegalovirus infection. *J. Gen. Virol.*, **76**, 2887–2893.

Kerry, J. A., Priddy, M. A., and Stenberg, R. M. (1994). Identification of sequence elements in the human cytomegalovirus DNA polymerase gene promoter required for activation by viral gene products. *J. Virol.*, **68**, 4167–4176.

Kerry, J. A., Sehgal, A., Barlow, S. W., Cavanaugh, V. J., Fish, K., Nelson, J. A., and Stenberg, R. M. (1995). Isolation and characterization of a low-abundance splice variant from the human cytomegalovirus major immediate–early gene region. *J. Virol.*, **69**, 3868–3872.

Kerry, J. A., Priddy, M. A., Jervey, T. Y. *et al.* (1996). Multiple regulatory events influence expression of human cytomegalovirus DNA polymerase (UL54) expression during viral infection. *J. Virol.*, **70**, 373–382.

Kerry, J. A., Priddy, M. A., Staley, T. L., Jones, T. R., and Stenberg, R. M. (1997). The role of ATF in regulating the human cytomegalovirus DNA polymerase (UL54) promoter during viral infection. *J. Virol.*, **71**, 2120–2126.

Kiehl, A., Huang, L., Franchi, D., and Anders, D. G. (2003). Multiple 5′ ends of human cytomegalovirus UL57 transcripts identify a complex, cycloheximide-resistant promoter region that activates oriLyt. *Virology*, **314**, 410–422.

Klucher, K. M., Sommer, M., Kadonaga, J. T., and Spector, D. H. (1993). In vivo and in vitro analysis of transcriptional activation mediated by the human cytomegalovirus major immediate–early proteins. *Mol. Cell. Biol.*, **13**, 1238–1250.

Kohler, C. P., Kerry, J. A., Carter, M., Muzithras, V. Z., Jones, T. R., and Stenberg, R. M. (1994). Use of recombinant virus to assess human cytomegalovirus early and late promoters in the context of the viral genome. *J. Virol.*, **68**, 6589–6597.

Korioth, F., Maul, G. G., Plachter, B., Stamminger, T., and Frey, J. (1996). The nuclear domain 10 (ND10) is disrupted by the human cytomegalovirus gene product IE1. *Exp. Cell Res.*, **229**, 155–158.

Kotenko, S. V., Saccani, S., Izotova, L. S., Mirochnitchenko, O. V., and Pestka, S. (2000). Human cytomegalovirus harbors its own unique IL-10 homolog (cmvIL-10). *Proc. Natl Acad. Sci. USA*, **97**, 1695–1700.

Kouzarides, T., Bankier, A. T., Satchwell, A. C., Preddy, E., Barrell, B. G. (1988). An immediate early gene of human cytomegalovirus encodes a potential membrane glycoprotein. *Virology*, **165**, 151–164.

Krosky, P. M., Baek, M. C., Jahng, W. J. (2003). The human cytomegalovirus UL44 protein is a substrate for the UL97 protein kinase. *J. Virol.*, **77**, 7720–7727.

Kuhn, D., Beall, C., and Kolattukudy, P. (1995). The cytomegalovirus US28 protein binds multiple CC chemokines with high affinity. *Biochem. Biophys. Res. Comm.*, **211**, 325–330.

Lang, D. and Stamminger, T. (1993). The 86-kilodalton IE-2 protein of human cytomegalovirus is a sequence-specific DNA-binding protein that interacts directly with the negative autoregulatory response element located near the cap site of the IE-1/2 enhancer-promoter. *J. Virol.*, **67**, 323–331.

Lang, D., and Stamminger, T. (1994). Minor groove contacts are essential for an interaction of the human cytomegalovirus IE2 protein with its DNA target. *Nucl. Acids Res.*, **22**, 3331–3338.

Lang, D., Gebert, S., Arlt, H., and Stamminger, T. (1995). Functional interaction between the human cytomegalovirus 86-kilodalton IE2 protein and the cellular transcription factor CREB. *J. Virol.*, **69**, 6030–6037.

LaPierre, L. A. and Biegalke, B. J. (2001). Identification of a novel transcriptional repressor encoded by human cytomegalovirus. *J. Virol.*, **75**, 6062–6069.

Lashmit, P. E., Stinski, M. F., Murphy, E. A., and Bullock, G. C. (1998). A *cis* repression sequence adjacent to the transcription start site of the human cytomegalovirus US3 gene is required to down-regulate gene expression at early and late times after infection. *J. Virol.*, **72**, 9575–9584.

Lee, H.-R. and Ahn, J.-H. (2004). Sumoylation of the major immediate-early IE2 protein of human cytomegalovirus Towne strain is not required for virus growth in cultured human fibroblasts. *J. Gen. Virol.*, **85**, 2149–2154.

Lee, H.-R., Kim, D.-J., Lee, J.-M. *et al.* (2004). Ability of the human cytomegalvirus IE1 protein to modulate sumoylation of PML correlates with its functional activities in transcriptional regulation and infectivity in cultured fibroblast cells. *J. Virol.*, **78**, 8527–8542.

Lei, M. and Tye, B. K. (2001). Initiating DNA synthesis: from recruiting to activating the MCM complex. *J. Cell. Sci.*, **114**, 1447–1454.

Lindquester, G. J. and Pellett, P. E. (1991). Properties of the human herpesvirus 6 strain Z29 genome: G + C content, length, and presence of variable-length directly repeated terminal sequence elements. *Virology*, **182**, 102–110.

Lischka, P., Sorg, G., Kann, M., Winkler, M., and Stamminger, T. (2003). A nonconventional nuclear localization signal within the UL84 protein of human cytomegalovirus mediates nuclear import via the importin alpha/beta pathway. *J. Virol.*, **77**, 3734–3748.

Liu, B., Hermiston, T. W., and Stinski, M. F. (1991). A *cis*-acting element in the major immediate–early (IE) promoter of human cytomegalovirus is required for negative regulation by IE2. *J. Virol.*, **65**, 897–903.

Loregian, A., Rigatti, R., Murphy, M., Schievano, E., Palu, G., and Marsden, H. S. (2003). Inhibition of human cytomegalovirus DNA polymerase by C-terminal peptides from the UL54 subunit. *J. Virol.*, **77**, 8336–8344.

Loregian, A., Appleton, B. A., Hogle, J. M., and Coen, D. M. (2004). Residues of human cytomegalovirus DNA polymerase catalytic subunit UL54 that are necessary and sufficient for interaction with the accessory protein UL44. *J. Virol.*, **78**, 158–167.

Lu, M. and Shenk, T. (1996). Human cytomegalovirus infection inhibits cell cycle progression at multiple points, including the transition from G1 to S. *J. Virol.*, **70**, 8850–8857.

Lu, M. and Shenk, T. (1999). Human cytomegalovirus UL69 protein induces cells to accumulate in G_1 phase of the cell cycle. *J. Virol.*, **73**, 676–683.

Lukac, D. M., Manuppello, J. R., and Alwine, J. C. (1994). Transcriptional activation by the human cytomegalovirus immediate–early proteins: requirements for simple promoter structures and interactions with multiple components of the transcription complex. *J. Virol.*, **68**, 5184–5193.

Lukac, D. M., Harel, N. Y., Tanese, N., and Alwine, J. C. (1997). TAF-like functions of human cytomegalovirus immediate early proteins. *J. Virol.*, **71**, 7227–7239.

Lusso, P. and Gallo, R. C. (1995). Human herpesvirus 6 in AIDS. *Immunol. Today*, **16**, 67–71.

Luu, P. and Flores, O. (1997). Binding of SP1 to the immediate–early protein-responsive element of the human cytomegalovirus DNA polymerase promoter. *J. Virol.*, **71**, 6683–6691.

Macias, M. P. and Stinski, M. F. (1993). An *in vitro* system for human cytomegalovirus immediate early 2 protein (IE-2)-mediated site-dependent repression of transcription and direct binding of IE2 to the major immediate–early promoter. *Proc. Natl Acad. Sci. USA*, **90**, 707–711.

Maiorano, D., Moreau, J., and Mechali, M. (2000). XCDT1 is required for the assembly of pre-replicative complexes in *Xenopus laevis*. *Nature*, **404**, 622–625.

Malone, C. L., Vesole, D. H., and Stinski, M. F. (1990). Transactivation of a human cytomegalovirus early promoter by gene products from the immediate–early gene IE2 and augmentation by IE1: mutational analysis of the viral proteins. *J. Virol.*, **64**, 1498–1506.

Marchini, A., Liu, H., and Zhu, H. (2001). Human cytomegalovirus with IE-2 (UL122) deleted fails to express early lytic genes. *J. Virol.*, **75**, 1870–1888.

Marshall, K. R., Rowley, K. V., Rinaldi, A. *et al.* (2002). Activity and intracellular localization of the human cytomegalovirus protein pp71. *J. Gen. Virol.*, **83**, 1601–1612.

Martin, M. E., Nicholas, J., Thomson, B. J., Newman, C., and Honess, R. W. (1991a). Identification of a transactivating function mapping to the putative immediate–early locus of human herpesvirus 6. *J. Virol.*, **65**, 5381–5390.

Martin, M. E., Thomson, B. J., Honess, R. W. *et al.* (1991b). The genome of human herpesvirus 6: maps of unit-length and concatemeric genomes for nine restriction endonucleases. *J. Gen. Virol.*, **72**, 157–168.

McCormick, A. L., Skaletskaya, A., Barry, P. A., Mocarski, E. S., and Goldmacher, V. S. (2003a). Differential function and expression of the viral inhibitor of caspase 8-induced apoptosis (vICA) and the viral mitochondria-localized inhibitor of apoptosis (vMIA) cell death suppressors conserved in primate and rodent cytomegaloviruses. *Virology*, **316**, 221–233.

McCormick, A. L., Smith, V. L., Chow, D., and Mocarski, E. S. (2003b). Disruption of mitochondrial networks by the human cytomegalovirus UL37 gene product viral mitochondrion-localized inhibitor of apoptosis. *J. Virol.*, **77**, 631–641.

McCormick, A. L., Meiering, C. D., Smith, G. B., and Mocarski, E. S. (2005). Mitochondrial cell death suppressors carried by human and murine cytomegalovirus confer resistance to proteasome inhibitor-induced apoptosis. *J. Virol.*, **79**, 12205–12217.

McDonough, S. H., and Spector, D. H. (1983). RNA transcription in human fibroblasts permissively infected by human cytomegalovirus strain AD169. *Virology*, **125**, 31–46.

McElroy, A. K., Dwarakanath, R. S., and Spector, D. H. (2000). Dysregulation of cyclin E gene expression in human cytomegalovirus-infected cells requires viral early gene expression and is associated with changes in the Rb-related protein p130. *J. Virol.*, **74**, 4192–4206.

McMahon, T. P. and Anders, D. G. (2002). Interactions between human cytomegalovirus helicase-primase proteins. *Virus Res.*, **86**, 39–52.

Megaw, A. G., Rapaport, D., Avidor, B., Frenkel, N., and Davison, A. J. (1998). The DNA sequence of the RK strain of human herpesvirus 7. *Virology*, **244**, 119–132.

Menegazzi, P., Galvan, M., Rotola, A. *et al.* (1999). Temporal mapping of transcripts in human herpesvirus-7. *J. Gen. Virol.*, **80**, 2705–2712.

Miller, D., Rahill, B., Boss, J. *et al.* (1998). Human cytomegalovirus inhibits major histocompatibility complex class II expression by disruption of the JAK/STAT pathway. *J. Exp. Med.*, **187**, 675–683.

Miller, D., Zhang, Y., Rahill, B., Waldman, W., and Sedmak, D. (1999). Human cytomegalovirus inhibits IFN α-stimulated antiviral and immunoregulatory responses by blocking multiple levels of IFN-α signal transduction. *J. Immunol.*, **162**, 6107–6113.

Mirandola, P., Menegazzi, P., Merighi, S., Ravaioli, T., Cassai, E., and Luca, D. D. (1998). Temporal mapping of transcripts in herpesvirus 6 variants. *J. Virol.*, **72**, 3837–3844.

Mizoue, L. S., Sullivan, S. K., King, D. S. (2001). Molecular determinants of receptor binding and signaling by the CX3C chemokine fractalkine. *J. Biol. Chem.*, **276**, 33906–33914.

Mocarski, E. S. (2002). Immunomodulation by cytomegaloviruses: manipulative strategies beyond evasion. *Trends Microbiol.*, **10**, 332–339.

Mocarski, E. S. (2004). Immune escape and exploitation strategies of cytomegaloviruses: impact on and imitation of the major histocompatibility system. *Cell. Microbiol.*, **6**, 707–717.

Mocarski, E. S. and Courcelle, C. T. (2001). Cytomegaloviruses and their replication. In *Fields Virology* 4th edn., ed. D. M. Knipe, and P. M. Howley, Vol. 2, pp. 2629–2673. 2 vols. Philadelphia: Lippincott, Williams & Wilkins.

Mocarski, E. S., Kemble, G. W., Lyle, J. M., and Greaves, R. F. (1996). A deletion mutant in the human cytomegalovirus gene encoding *ie1* (491aa) is replication defective due to a failure in autoregulation. *Proc. Natl Acad. Sci. USA*, **93**, 11321–11326.

Mori, Y., Yagi, H., Shimamoto, T. *et al.* (1998). Analysis of human herpesvirus 6 U3 gene, which is a positional homolog of human cytomegalovirus UL24 gene. *Virology*, **249**, 129–139.

Muller, S. and Dejean, A. (1999). Viral immediate-early proteins abrogate the modification by SUMO-1 of PML and Sp100 proteins, correlating with nuclear body disruption. *J. Virol.*, **73**, 5137–5143.

Murphy, E. A., Streblow, D. N., Nelson, J. A., and Stinski, M. F. (2000). The human cytomegalovirus IE86 protein can block cell cycle progression after inducing transition into the S phase of the cell cycle. *J. Virol.*, **74**, 7108–7118.

Navarro, L., Mowen, K., Rodems, S. *et al.* (1998). Cytomegalovirus activates interferon immediate–early response gene expression and an interferon regulatory factor 3-containing interferon-stimulated response element-binding complex. *Mol. Cell. Biol.*, **18**, 3796–3802.

Nevels, M., Brune, W., and Shenk, T. (2004). SUMOylation of human cytomegalovirus 72-kilodalton IE1 protein facilitates expression of the 86-kilodalton IE2 protein and promotes viral replication. *J. Virol.*, **78**, 7803–7812.

Nicholas, J. (1996). Determination and analysis of the complete nucleotide sequence of human herpesvirus 7. *J. Virol.*, **70**, 5975–5989.

Nishitani, H., Lygerou, Z., Nishimoto, T., and Nurse, P. (2000). The Cdt1 protein is required to license DNA for replication in fission yeast. *Nature*, **404**, 625–628.

Nishitani, H., Taraviras, S., Lygerou, Z., and Nishimoto, T. (2001). The human licensing factor or DNA replication cdt1 accumulates in G1 and is destabilized after initiation of S-phase. *J. Biol. Chem.*, **276**, 44905–44911.

Oster, B. and Hollsberg, P. (2002). Viral gene expression patterns in human herpesvirus 6B-infected cells. *J. Virol.*, **76**, 7578–7586.

Papanikolaou, E., Kouvatsis, V., Dimitriadis, G., Inoue, N., and Arsenakis, M. (2002). Identification and characterization of the gene products of open reading frame U86/87 of human herpesvirus 6. *Virus Res.*, **89**, 89–101.

Pari, G. S. and Anders, D. G. (1993). Eleven loci encoding transacting factors are required for transient complementation of human cytomegalovirus oriLyt-dependent DNA replication. *J. Virol.*, **67**, 6979–6988.

Pari, G. S., Kacica, M. A., and Anders, D. G. (1993). Open reading frames UL44, IRS1/TRS1, and UL36–38 are required for transient complementation of human cytomegalovirus oriLyt-dependent DNA synthesis. *J. Virol.*, **67**, 2575–2582.

Patterson, C. E. and Shenk, T. (1999). Human cytomegalovirus UL36 protein is dispensable for viral replication in cultured cells. *J. Virol.*, **73**, 7126–7131.

Paulus, C., Krauss S., and Nevels, M. (2006). A human cytomegalovirus antagonist of type I IFN-dependent signal transducer and activator of transcription signaling. *Proc. Natl. Acad. Sci. USA*, **103**(10), 3840–3845.

Penfold, M. E. and Mocarski, E. S. (1997). Formation of cytomegalovirus DNA replication compartments defined by localization of viral proteins and DNA synthesis. *Virology*, **239**, 46–61.

Penfold, M., Dairaghi, D., Duke, G. *et al.* (1999). Cytomegalovirus encodes a potent α chemokine. *Proc. Natl Acad. Sci. USA*, **96**, 9839–9844.

Petrik, D. T., Schmitt, K. P., and Stinski, M. F. (2006). Inhibition of cellular DNA synthesis by the human cytomegalovirus IE86 protein is necessary for efficient virus replication. *J. Virol.*, **80**(8), 3872–3883.

Pizzorno, M. C. and Hayward, G. S. (1990). The IE2 gene products of human cytomegalovirus specifically down-regulate expression from the major immediate–early promoter through a target sequence located near the cap site. *J. Virol.*, **64**, 6154–6165.

Pizzorno, M. C., Mullen, M.-A., Chang, Y.-N., and Hayward, G. S. (1991). The functionally active IE2 immediate–early regulatory protein of human cytomegalovirus is an 80-kilodalton polypeptide that contains two distinct activator domains and a duplicated nuclear localization signal. *J. Virol.*, **65**, 3839–3852.

Ploegh, H. L. (1998). Viral strategies of immune evasion. *Science*, **280**, 248–253.

Preston, C. M. and Nicholl, M. J. (2006). Role of the cellular protein hDaxx in human cytomegalovirus immediate-early gene expression. *J. Gen. Virol.*, **87**(Pt 5), 1113–1121.

Prichard, M. N., Duke, G. M., and Mocarski, E. S. (1996). Human cytomegalovirus uracil DNA glycosylase is required for the normal temporal regulation of both DNA synthesis and viral replication. *J. Virol.*, **70**, 3018–3025.

Puchtler, E. and Stamminger, T. (1991). An inducible promoter mediates abundant expression from the immediate–early 2 gene region of human cytomegalovirus at late times after infection. *J. Virol.*, **65**, 6301–6303.

Quintana, D. G. and Dutta, A. (1999). The metazoan origin recognition complex. *Front. Biosci.*, **4**, D805-D815.

Rapp, J. C., Krug, L. T., Inoue, N., Dambaugh, T. R., and Pellet, P. E. (2000). U94, the human herpesvirus 6 homolog of the parvovirus nonstructural gene, is highly conserved among isolates and is expressed at low mRNA levels as a spliced transcript. *Virology*, **268**, 504–516.

Reinhardt, J., Smith, G. B., Himmelheber, C. T., Azizkhan-Clifford, J., and Mocarski, E. S. (2005). The carboxyl-terminal region of human cytomegalovirus IE1491aa contains an acidic domain that plays a regulatory role and a chromatin-tethering domain that is dispensable during viral replication. *J. Virol.*, **79**(1), 225–233.

Rialland, M., Sola, F., and Santocanale, C. (2002). Essential role of human CDT1 in DNA replication and chromatin licensing. *J. Cell Sci.*, **115**, 1435–1440.

Rodems, S. M. and Spector, D. H. (1998). Extracellular signal-regulated kinase activity is sustained early during human cytomegalovirus infection. *J. Virol.*, **72**, 9173–9180.

Rodems, S. M., Clark, C. L., and Spector, D. H. (1998). Separate DNA elements containing ATF/CREB and IE86 binding sites differentially regulate the human cytomegalovirus UL112–113 promoter at early and late times in the infection. *J. Virol.*, **72**, 2697–2707.

Romanowski, M. J. and Shenk, T. (1997). Characterization of the human cytomegalovirus irs1 and trs1 genes: A second immediate-early transcription unit within irs1 whose product antagonizes transcriptional activation. *J. Virol.*, **71**, 1485–1496.

Rotola, A., Ravaioli, T., Gonelli, A., Dewhurst, S., Cassai, E., and Di Luca, D. (1998). U94 of human herpesvirus 6 is expressed in latently infected peripheral blood mononuclear cells and blocks viral gene expression in transformed lymphocytes in culture. *Proc. Natl Acad. Sci. USA*, **95**, 13911–13916.

Saffert, R. T. and Kalejta, R. F. (2006). Inactivating a cellular intrinsic immune defense mediated by Daxx is the mechanism through which the human cytomegalovirus pp71 protein stimulates viral immediate-early gene expression. *J. Virol.*, **80**(8), 3863–3871.

Salvant, B. S., Fortunato, E. A., and Spector, D. H. (1998). Cell cycle dysregulation by human cytomegalovirus: Influence of the cell cycle phase at the time of infection and effects on cyclin transcription. *J. Virol.*, **72**, 3729–3741.

Sanchez, V., Clark, C. L., Yen, J. Y., Dwarakanath, R., and Spector, D. H. (2002). Viable human cytomegalovirus recombinant virus with an internal deletion of the IE2 86 gene affects late stages of viral replication. *J. Virol.*, **76**, 2973–2989.

Sanchez, V., McElroy, A. K., and Spector, D. H. (2003). Mechanisms governing maintenance of cdk1/cyclin B1 kinase activity in cells infected with human cytomegalovirus. *J. Virol.*, **77**, 13214–13224.

Sarisky, R. T. and Hayward, G. S. (1996). Evidence that the UL84 gene product of human cytomegalovirus is essential for promoting oriLyt-dependent DNA replication and formation of replication compartments in cotransfection assays. *J. Virol.*, **70**, 7398–7413.

Schiewe, U., Neipel, F., Schreiger, D., and Fleckenstein, B. (1994). Structure and transcription of an immediate early region in the human herpesvirus 6 genome. *J. Virol.*, **68**, 2978–2985.

Schwartz, R., Sommer, M. H., Scully, A., and Spector, D. H. (1994). Site-specific binding of the human cytomegalovirus IE2 86-kilodalton protein to an early gene promoter. *J. Virol.*, **68**, 5613–5622.

Schwartz, R., Helmich, B., and Spector, D. H. (1996). CREB and CREB-binding proteins play an important role in the IE2 86-kilodalton protein-mediated transactivation of the human cytomegalovirus 2.2-kilobase RNA promoter. *J. Virol.*, **70**, 6955–6966.

Scully, A. L., Sommer, M. H., Schwartz, R., and Spector, D. H. (1995). The human cytomegalovirus IE2 86 kDa protein interacts with an early gene promoter via site-specific DNA binding and protein–protein associations. *J. Virol.*, **69**, 6533–6540.

Sedmak, D. D., Guglielmo, A. M., Knight, D. A., Birmingham, D. J., Huang, E.-H., and Waldman, W. J. (1994). Cytomegalovirus inhibits major histocompatibility class II expression on infected endothelial cells. *Am. J. Pathol.*, **144**, 683–692.

Shirakata, M., Terauchi, M., Ablikim, M. *et al.* (2002). Novel immediate–early protein IE19 of human cytomegalovirus activates the origin recognition complex I promoter in a cooperative manner with IE72. *J. Virol.*, **76**, 3158–3167.

Sinclair, J., Baillie, J., Bryant, L., and Caswell, R. (2000). Human cytomegalovirus mediates cell cycle progression through G(1) into early S phase in terminally differentiated cells. *J. Gen. Virol.*, **81**, 1553–1565.

Sinzger, C. and Jahn, G. (1996). Human cytomegalovirus cell tropism and pathogenesis. *InterVirology*, **39**, 302–319.

Skaletskaya, A., Bartle, L. M., Chittenden, T., McCormick, A. L., Mocarski, E. S., and Goldmacher, V. S. (2001). A cytomegalovirus-encoded inhibitor of apoptosis that suppresses caspase-8 activation. *Proc. Natl Acad. Sci. USA*, **98**, 7829–7834.

Smith, I. L., Cherrington, J. M., Jiles, R. E., Fuller, M. D., Freeman, W. R., and Spector, S. A. (1997). High-level resistance of cytomegalovirus to ganciclovir is associated with alterations in both the UL97 and DNA polymerase genes. *J. Infect. Dis.*, **176**, 69–77.

Smith, J. A. and Pari, G. S. (1995). Human cytomegalovirus UL102 gene. *J. Virol.*, **69**, 1734–1740.

Smith, J. A., Jairath, S., Crute, J. J., and Pari, G. S. (1996). Characterization of the human cytomegalovirus UL105 gene and identification of the putative helicase protein. *Virology*, **220**, 251–255.

Smuda, C., Bogner, E., and Radsak, K. (1997). The human cytomegalovirus glycoprotein B gene (ORF UL55) is expressed early in the infectious cycle. *J. Gen. Virol.*, **78**, 1981–1992.

Sommer, M. H., Scully, A. L., and Spector, D. H. (1994). Transactivation by the human cytomegalovirus IE2 86 kDa protein requires a domain that binds to both TBP and RB. *J. Virol.*, **68**, 6223–6231.

Song, Y.-J., and Stinski, M. F. (2002). Effect of the human cytomegalovirus IE86 protein on expression of E2F responsive genes: a DNA microarray analysis. *Proc. Natl Acad. Sci. USA*, **99**, 2836–2841.

Spector, D. J. and Tevethia, M. J. (1994). protein–protein interactions between human cytomegalovirus IE2-580aa and pUL84 in lytically infected cells. *J. Virol.*, **68**, 7549–7553.

Speir, E., Modali, R., Huang, E. S. *et al.* (1994). Potential role of human cytomegalovirus and p53 interaction in coronary restenosis. *Science*, **265**, 391–394.

Spencer, J. V., Lockridge, K. M., Berry, P. A. *et al.* (2002). Potent immunosuppressive activities of cytomegalovirus-encoded interleukin-10. *J. Virol.*, **76**, 1285–1292.

Spengler, M. L., Kurapatwinski, K., Black, A. R., and Azizkhan-Clifford, J. (2002). SUMO-1 modification of human cytomegalovirus IE1/IE72. *J. Virol.*, **76**, 2990–2996.

Stanton, R., Fox, J. D., Caswell, R., Sherratt, E., and Wilkinson, G. W. (2002). Analysis of the human herpesvirus-6 immediate-early 1 protein. *J. Gen. Virol.*, **83**, 2811–2820.

Staprans, S. I. and Spector, D. H. (1986). 2.2-kilobase class of early transcripts encoded by cell-related sequences in human cytomegalovirus strain AD169. *J. Virol.*, **57**, 591–602.

Staprans, S. I., Rabert, D. K., and Spector, D. H. (1988). Identification of sequence requirements and *trans*-acting functions necessary for regulated expression of a human cytomegalovirus early gene. *J. Virol.*, **62**, 3463–3473.

Stenberg, R. M., Thomsen, D. R., and Stinski, M. F. (1984). Structural analysis of the major immediate early gene of human cytomegalovirus. *J. Virol.*, **49**, 190–199.

Stenberg, R. M., Witte, P. R., and Stinski, M. F. (1985). Multiple spliced and unspliced transcripts from human cytomegalovirus immediate-early region 2 and evidence for a common initiation site within immediate-early region 1. *J. Virol.*, **56**, 665–675.

Stenberg, R. M., Depto, A. S., Fortney, J., and Nelson, J. A. (1989). Regulated expression of early and late RNAs and proteins from the human cytomegalovirus immediate–early gene region. *J. Virol.*, **63**, 2699–2708.

Stenberg, R. M., Fortney, J., Barlow, S. W., Magrane, B. P., Nelson, J. A., and Ghazal, P. (1990). Promoter-specific *trans* activation and repression by human cytomegalovirus immediate–early proteins involves common and unique protein domains. *J. Virol.*, **64**, 1556–1565.

Stinski, M. F., Thomsen, D. R., Stenberg, R. M., and Goldstein, L. C. (1983). Organization and expression of the immediate–early genes of human cytomegalovirus. *J. Virol.*, **46**, 1–14.

Streblow, D. N., Soderberg-Naucler, C., Vieira, J., Smith, P. *et al.* (1999). The human cytomegalovirus chemokine receptor US28 mediates vascular smooth muscle cell migration. *Cell*, **99**, 511–520.

Tamrakar, S., Kapasi, A. J. and Spector, D. H. (2005). Human cytomegalovirus infection induces specific hyperphosphorylation of the carboxyl-terminal domain of the large subunit of RNA polymerase II that is associated with changes in the abundance, activity, and localization of cdk9 and cdk7. *J. Virol.*, **79**(24), 15477–15493.

Takeda, K., Nakagawa, N., Yamamoto, T. *et al.* (1996). Prokaryotic expression of an immediate early gene of human herpesvirus 6 and analysis of its viral antigen expression in human cells. *Virus Res.*, **41**, 193–200.

Tanaka, K., Kondo, T., Torigoe, S., Okada, S., Mukai, T., and Yamanishi, K. (1994). Human herpesvirus 7: another causal agent for roseola (exanthum subitum). *J. Pediatr.*, **125**, 1–5.

Tatsumi, Y., Tsurimoto, T., Shirahige, K., Yoshikawa, H., and Obuse, C. (2000). Association of human origin recognition complex 1 with chromatin DNA and nuclease-resistant nuclear structures. *J. Biol. Chem.*, **275**, 5904–5910.

Taylor, R. T. and Bresnahan, W. A. (2005). Human cytomegalovirus immediate-early 2 gene expression blocks virus-induced beta interferon production. *J. Virol.*, **79**(6), 3873–3877.

Taylor, R. T. and Bresnahan, W. A. (2006). Human cytomegalovirus immediate-early 2 protein IE86 blocks virus-induced chemokine expression. *J. Virol.*, **80**(2), 920–928.

Tenney, D. J. and Colberg-Poley, A. M. (1991a). Expression of the human cytomegalovirus UL36-38 immediate early region during permissive infection. *Virology*, **182**, 199–210.

Tenney, D. J. and Colberg-Poley, A. M. (1991b). Human cytomegalovirus UL36-38 and US3 immediate–early genes: temporally regulated expression of nuclear, cytoplasmic, and polysome-associated transcripts during infection. *J. Virol.*, **65**, 6724–6734.

Tenney, D. J., Santomenna, L. D., Goudie, K. B., and Colberg-Poley, A. M. (1993). The human cytomegalovirus US3 immediate–early protein lacking the putative transmembrane domain regulates gene expression. *Nucl. Acids Res.*, **21**, 2931–2937.

Thompson, J., Choudhury, S., Kashanchi, F. *et al.* (1994a). A transforming fragment within the direct repeat region of human herpesvirus type 6 that transactivates HIV-1. *Oncogene*, **9**, 1167–1175.

Thompson, J. R., Agulnick, A. D., and Ricciardi, R. P. (1994b). A novel cis element essential for stimulated transcription of the p41 promoter of human herpesvirus 6. *J. Virol.*, **68**, 4478–4485.

Thomson, B. J., Efstathiou, S., and Honess, R. W. (1991). Acquisition of the human adeno-associated virus type-2 rep gene by human herpesvirus type-6. *Nature*, **351**, 78–80.

Thomson, B. J., Weindler, F. W., Gray, D., Schwaab, V., and Heilbronn, R. (1994). Human herpesvirus 6 (HHV-6) is a helper virus for adeno-associated virus type 2 (AAV-2) and the AAV-2 rep gene homologue in HHV-6 can mediate AAV-2 DNA replication and regulate gene expression. *Virology*, **204**, 304–311.

Thrower, A. R., Bullock, G. C., Bissell, J. E., and Stinski, M. F. (1996). Regulation of a human cytomegalovirus immediate–early gene (US3) by a silencer-enhancer combination. *J. Virol.*, **70**, 91–100.

Tomazin, R., Boname, J., Hegde, N. R. *et al.* (1999). Cytomegalovirus US2 destroys two components of the MHC class II pathway, preventing recognition of CD4+ T cells. *Nat. Med.*, **5**, 1039–1043.

Tomoiu, A., Gravel, A. and Flamand, L. (2006). Mapping of human herpesvirus 6 immediate-early 2 protein transactivation domains. *Virology*.

Underwood, M. R., Harvey, R. J., Stanat, S. C. *et al.* (1998). Inhibition of human cytomegalovirus DNA maturation by a benzimidazole ribonucleoside is mediated through the UL89 gene product. *J. Virol.*, **72**, 717–725.

Vashee, S., Simancek, P., Challberg, M. D., and Kelly, T. J. (2001). Assembly of the human origin recognition complex. *J. Biol. Chem.*, **276**, 26666–26673.

Vink, C., Beuken, E., and Bruggeman, C. A. (2000). Complete DNA sequence of the rat cytomegalovirus genome. *J. Virol.*, **74**, 7656–7665.

Wade, M., Kowalik, T. F., Mudryj, M., Huang, E. S., and Azizkhan, J. C. (1992). E2F mediates dihydrofolate reductase promoter activation and multiprotein complex formation in human cytomegalovirus infection. *Mol. Cell. Biol.*, **12**, 4364–4374.

Waheed, I., Chiou, C. J., Ahn, J. H., and Hayward, G. S. (1998). Binding of the human cytomegalovirus 80-kDa immediate–early protein (IE2) to minor groove A/T-rich sequences bounded by CG dinucleotides is regulated by protein oligomerization and phosphorylation. *Virology*, **252**, 235–257.

Wara-Aswapati, N., Yang, Z., Waterman, W. R. *et al.* (1999). Cytomegalovirus IE2 protein stimulates interleukin 1 beta gene transcription via tethering to Spi-1/PU.1. *Mol. Cell. Biol.*, **19**, 6803–6814.

Wathen, M. W. and Stinski, M. F. (1982). Temporal patterns of human cytomegalovirus transcription: mapping the viral RNAs synthesized at immediate early, early, and late times after infection. *J. Virol.*, **41**, 462–477.

Wathen, M. W., Thomsen, D. R., and Stinski, M. F. (1981). Temporal regulation of human cytomegalovirus transcription at immediate early and early times after infection. *J. Virol.*, **38**, 446–459.

Weiland, K. L., Oien, N. L., Homa, F., and Wathen, M. W. (1994). Functional analysis of human cytomegalovirus polymerase accessory protein. *Virus Res.*, **34**, 191–206.

White, E. A. and Spector, D. H. (2005). Exon 3 of the human cytomegalovirus major immediate-early region is required for efficient viral gene expression and for cellular cyclin modulation. *J. Virol.*, **79**(12), 7438–7452.

White, E. A., Clark, C. L., Sanchez, V., and Spector, D. H. (2004). Small internal deletions in the human cytomegalovirus IE2 gene result in non-viable recombinant viruses with differential defects in viral gene expression. *J. Virol.*, **78**, 1817–1830.

Wiebusch, L. and Hagemeier, C. (1999). Human cytomegalovirus 86-kilodalton IE2 protein blocks cell cycle progression in G_1. *J. Virol.*, **73**, 9274–9283.

Wiebusch, L., and Hagemeier, C. (2001). The human cytomegalovirus immediate early 2 protein dissociates cellular DNA synthesis from cyclin dependent kinase activation. *EMBO J.*, **20**, 1086–1098.

Wiebusch, L., Asmar, J., Uecker, R., and Hagemeier, C. (2003a). Human cytomegalovirus immediate–early over protein 2 (IE2)-mediated activation of cyclin E is cell-cycle-independent and forces S-phase entry in IE2-arrested cells. *J. Gen. Virol.*, **84**, 51–60.

Wiebusch, L., Uecker, R., and Hagemeier, C. (2003b). Human cytomegalovirus prevents replication licensing by inhibiting MCM loading onto chromatin. *EMBO Rep.*, **4**, 42–46.

Wright, D. A. and Spector, D. H. (1989). Posttranscriptional regulation of a class of human cytomegalovirus phosphoproteins encoded by an early transcription unit. *J. Virol.*, **63**, 3117–3127.

Wright, D. A., Staprans, S. I., and Spector, D. H. (1988). Four phosphoproteins with common amino termini are encoded by human cytomegalovirus AD169. *J. Virol.*, **62**, 331–340.

Wu, J., O'Neill, J., and Barbosa, M. S. (1998). Transcription factor Sp1 mediates cell-specific *trans*-activation of the human cytomegalovirus DNA polymerase gene promoter by immediate–early protein IE86 in glioblastoma U373MG cells. *J. Virol.*, **72**, 236–244.

Xu, Y., Ahn, J. H., Cheng, M. *et al.* (2001). Proteasome-independent disruption of PML oncogenic domains (PODs), but not covalent modification by SUMO-1, is required for human cytomegalovirus immediate–early protein IE1 to inhibit PML-mediated transcriptional repression. *J. Virol.*, **75**, 10683–10695.

Xu, Y., Colletti, K. S., and Pari, G. S. (2002). Human cytomegalovirus UL84 localizes to the cell nucleus via a nuclear localization signal and is a component of viral replication compartments. *J. Virol.*, **76**, 8931–8938.

Xu, Y., Cei, S. A., Huete, A. R., and Pari, G. S. (2004). Human cytomegalovirus UL84 insertion mutant defective for viral DNA synthesis and growth. *J. Virol.*, **78**, 10360–10369.

Yamanishi, K., Okuno, T., Shiraki, K. *et al.* (1988). Identification of human herpesvirus 6 as a causal agent for exanthem subitum. *Lancet*, **1**, 1065–1067.

Yeung, K. C., Stoltzfus, C. M., and Stinski, M. F. (1993). Mutations of the human cytomegalovirus immediate–early 2 protein defines regions and amino acid motifs important in transactivation of transcription from the HIV-1 LTR promoter. *Virology*, **195**, 786–792.

Yoo, Y. D., Chiou, C.-J., Choi, K. S. *et al.* (1996). The IE2 regulatory protein of human cytomagalovirus induces expression of the human transforming growth factor B1 gene through an Egr-1 binding site. *J. Virol.*, **70**, 7062–7070.

Yu, D., Silva, M. C., and Shenk, T. (2003). Functional map of human cytomegalovirus AD169 defined by global mutational analysis. *Proc. Natl Acad. Sci. USA*, **100**, 12396–12401.

Zhang, H., al-Barazi, H. O., and Colberg-Poley, A. M. (1996). The acidic domain of the human cytomegalovirus UL37 immediate early glycoprotein is dispensable for its transactivating activity and localization but is not for its synergism. *Virology*, **223**, 292–302.

Zhou, Y., Chandran, B., and Wood, C. (1997). Transcriptional patterns of the pCD41 (U27) locus of human herpesvirus 6. *J. Virol.*, **71**, 3420–3430.

Zhou, Y., Chang, C. K., Qian, G., Chandran, B., and Wood, C. (1994). *trans*-activation of the HIV promoter by a cDNA and its genomic clones of human herpesvirus-6. *Virology*, **199**, 311–322.

Zhu, H., Cong, J. P., and Shenk, T. (1997). Use of differential display analysis to assess the effect of human cytomegalovirus infection on the accumulation of cellular RNAs: induction of interferon-responsive RNAs. *Proc. Natl Acad. Sci. USA*, **94**, 13985–13990.

Zhu, H., Cong, J. P., Mamtora, G., Gingeras, T., and Shenk, T. (1998). Cellular gene expression altered by human cytomegalovirus: global monitoring with oligonucleotide arrays. *Proc. Natl Acad. Sci. USA*, **95**, 14470–14475.

19

DNA synthesis and late viral gene expression

David G. Anders[1], Julie A. Kerry,[2] and Gregory S. Pari[3]

[1]Division of Infectious Diseases, Wadsworth Center, NYSDOH, Albany, NY, USA
[2]Department of Microbiology and Molecular Cell Biology, Eastern Virginia Medical School, Norfolk, VA, USA
[3]Department of Microbiology and Immunology, University of Nevada-Reno, Reno, NV, USA

Overview

Much of the current understanding of betaherpesvirus DNA synthesis is based on studies with the cytomegaloviruses and is further shaped by comparison with prototypic alpha- and gammaherpesviruses. As for all herpesviruses, betaherpesvirus DNA synthesis occurs in the nucleus and relies on a core set of virus-coded proteins composing the replication fork machinery (detailed later) working together with *trans*-acting functions that promote initiation on a genetically defined, *cis*-acting replicator, called *ori*Lyt. DNA synthesis initiates in the vicinity of *ori*Lyt as soon as essential virus coded proteins appear, producing high molecular weight replication intermediates whose structure has not been fully characterized. Onset of viral DNA synthesis licenses transcription of a subset of the late class of viral genes, many of which encode proteins that assemble and constitute the complex virion. Subsequently, replication intermediates are resolved, and the progeny genomes are packaged into preformed capsids and mature ends are formed by the encapsidation machinery. Because these replication functions are essential for viral replication and pathogenesis, and differ from host counterparts, they have been candidate targets for the development of antiviral drugs. Moreover, further study of DNA replication and encapsidation may provide new insights about cellular components that contribute to these processes. Our goals in this chapter are to provide an up-to-date summary of betaherpesvirus lytic-phase replication machinery, to highlight emerging contrasts to other herpesviruses, and to consider how DNA synthesis-dependent late gene expression is regulated.

Soon after nuclear entry, a fraction of the input linear cytomegalovirus genomes circularizes by a process that does not require *de novo* protein synthesis, and these circular forms have been considered the likely template for subsequent transcription and replication events. In this model concatemeric products are generated from a rolling circle intermediate in much the same way this process is envisioned for other herpesviruses (Chapter 4). Unfortunately, the lack of any cell-free replication systems has left the process of DNA replication in any of the herpesviruses poorly understood. Consistent with a rolling circle model is the finding that *ori*Lyt-containing circular plasmids are replicated in virus-infected cells to form head-to-tail concatemers. Some models posit an initial theta form mode, but evidence is scant and there is no published evidence to support this possibility for any betaherpesvirus. Authentic HCMV replication intermediates contain very few circles and have structural characteristics consistent with the rolling circle model, but the majority are not readily resolved in monomeric form by digestion with unique-cutting restriction enzymes, arguing that more complex – probably branched – structures predominate, rather than simple concatemers or circles (McVoy and Adler, 1994). The observed abundance of apparently complex products might arise from redundant initiation, from the presence of recombination intermediates, or from strand invasion; however, unambiguous evidence for any of these mechanisms is lacking. Interestingly, HHV-6 produces concatemers with relatively little branching (Severini *et al.*, 2003), suggesting that whatever event(s) contributes to the complex replication intermediates seen in cytomegaloviruses and many other herpesviruses are not a requisite component of roseolovirus replication.

Recent, well-received evidence employing HSV-1 regulatory gene mutants supports a model for viral DNA synthesis beginning on linear genomes, and proceeding via branched intermediates rather than via circularization and rolling circle mechanisms. This work implies that circularization may actually suppress replication and promote establishment of latency (Jackson and DeLuca, 2003).

Available data do not exclude such a model for HCMV, because the inhibition of DNA synthesis by drug treatment from the time of infection results in the persistence of both circular and nuclease-sensitive linear HCMV genomes (McVoy and Adler, 1994). Given that circular genomes are associated with HCMV latency (Bolovan-Fritts et al., 1999), these certainly appear to serve as templates for initiation of DNA synthesis upon reactivation. The extent to which the high molecular weight cytomegalovirus replication intermediates observed following infection of permissive cells arise preferentially by a rolling circle mechanism from circular templates or by some other mechanism will require further study.

Despite biological similarities between cytomegaloviruses and roseolaviruses, initiation of DNA replication proceeds with distinct mechanisms. The genomic location of the *cis*-acting element, *ori*Lyt is similar, being positioned between genes encoding the homologues of HCMV UL57 and UL69; however the sequence elements are very different. HCMV has a highly complex *ori*Lyt region that spans over a kilobase of DNA, whereas roseolaviruses rely on a simpler *ori*Lyt with structural similarities to alphaherpesviruses DNA replication origins (Chapter 10). Likewise, the *trans*-acting functions are distinct, with HCMV relying on transcriptional transactivators and roseolaviruses relying on an origin binding protein homologous to those encoded by alphaherpesviruses.

Betaherpesvirus replication proteins

A cotransfection–replication assay has enabled the identification of the subset of betaherpesvirus proteins required for origin-dependent DNA replication. In this assay, cloned viral genes are transfected along with a plasmid containing *ori*Lyt. When all *trans*-acting functions are included, amplification of the *ori*Lyt-containing plasmid occurs. Amplification of *ori*Lyt is detected using the restriction enzyme *Dpn* I, which removes bacterially propagated plasmid DNA due to cleavage specificity for methylated adenine. Input, non-replicated DNA, is thereby removed and subsequent DNA blot hybridization detects specifically replicated DNA. This assay identified HSV-1 replication proteins (Wu et al., 1988) and eleven essential loci contributing to the amplification of HCMV *ori*Lyt (Pari and Anders, 1993). The genes and their protein designations are listed in Table 19.1. HCMV DNA replication requires the same set of core replication proteins as HSV-1. Later studies, performing cotransfections using plasmids encoding the replication proteins under the control of strong constitutively active promoters, showed that one subset of these genes was directly involved in the enzymatic activity of DNA synthesis whereas other

Table 19.1. HCMV genes required for *ori*Lyt-dependent DNA replication

HCMV genes	HHV6 genes	Proposed function
UL44	U27	Polymerase accessory protein
UL54	U38	Polymerase
UL57	U41	Single-stranded DNA binding protein
UL70	U43	Primase
UL84		Early protein with UTPase and nucleic and binding activity
UL102	U74	Primase-associated factor
UL105	U77	Helicase
IE2		Transactivator; along with UL84 activates *ori*Lyt promoter
UL36–38		Auxiliary functions
UL112–113		Auxiliary functions
IRS1/TRS1		Auxiliary functions

genes had roles in gene regulation or cell death suppression (Sarisky and Hayward, 1996). It was determined that one protein, UL84, appeared to be unique among the HCMV replication proteins together with a requirement IE2 in human fibroblast cells (Pari and Anders, 1993; Sarisky and Hayward, 1996).

HCMV DNA replication has characteristics that distinguish it from HSV-1, as well as from the roseolaviruses. Divergence includes a distinct type of origin binding protein (OBP) for each type of virus. HSV-1 encodes an OBP (Olivo et al., 1988; Wu et al., 1988) that initiates DNA synthesis by interacting with specific DNA sequences within *ori*Lyt (Chapter 10) and has associated enzymatic activities consistent with a role in initiation such as helicase activity (Bruckner et al., 1991; Hazuda et al., 1991). Both HHV-6B and HHV-7 encode an OBP that may function similar to that encoded by the alphaherpesvirus HSV-1. Roseolaviruses have *ori*Lyt sequences with OBP sites and other apparent similarities (Dewhurst et al., 1994; Krug et al., 2001) to HSV-1, including a role in transient replication (Dewhurst et al., 1994; Dykes et al., 1997). These origins are not similar in any way to HCMV *ori*Lyt or replication origins of other cytomegaloviruses. HCMV relies on IE2 and UL84 as apparent OBPs and both are betaherpesvirus-conserved proteins (Chapter 15); however, testing a role in cytomegalovirus replication awaits development of a suitable assay. What follows is a description of each HCMV replication protein and the current status with respect to proposed function.

Helicase–primase complex (UL105, UL70 and UL102)

As in all herpesviruses the HCMV helicase–primase is a heterotrimeric complex composed of a helicase subunit

(UL105), a primase subunit (UL70) and a linking subunit (UL102). In vitro assays determined that the three proteins interact as a complex (McMahon and Anders, 2002). The proposed helicase for HCMV was first identified as the homologue for HSV-1 UL5. The UL105 gene encodes a 3.4 kb transcript that is present in infected cells as early as 24 hours post-infection and a 110 kDa protein was detected using UL105 specific antiserum (Smith et al., 1996). With respect to UL102, initial controversy regarding sequence data suggested that UL102 was a spliced transcript. Subsequent studies involving the identification of the UL102 mRNA isolated from an HCMV cDNA library indicated that UL102 is an unspliced 2.7 kb transcript which encodes an 873 codon ORF (Smith and Pari, 1995). The UL70 ORF encodes a 945 amino acid protein that is the proposed homologue for HSV-1 UL52. Like the HSV-1 primase, pUL70 contains a putative DXD motif that is common to the metal binding site found in prokaryotic primases and family B DNA polymerases (Dracheva et al., 1995; Ilyina et al., 1992; Li et al., 1993). To date, no published study has demonstrated helicase or primase activity using recombinant HCMV proteins or betaherpesvirus homologues.

DNA polymerase (UL54) and polymerase accessory protein (UL44)

The HCMV polymerase and the polymerase accessory protein are among the most well-characterized HCMV proteins. Contrary to many herpesvirus proteins, the polymerase and its accessory protein appear to be easily purified as recombinant proteins and retain native function in in vitro assays. Using purified UL54 from insect cells, this protein was shown to synthesize DNA from a variety of templates. In addition, the polymerase accessory protein, the gene product of UL44, stimulated DNA polymerase activity in a template dependent manner (Ertl and Powell, 1992). In infected cells the HCMV DNA polymerase associates with the UL44 gene product (Ertl and Powell, 1992). UL54 along with UL44 were efficiently expressed in an in vitro-coupled transcription/translation reticulocyte lysate system and the activity of the enzymes was comparable to what was observed from the native infected cell purified proteins (Cihlar et al., 1997). This method established a simple protocol for the expression and purification of the recombinant proteins. Homologous domains of ppUL54, with significantly conserved sequences and similar enzymatic properties in HSV and other herpesviruses have been identified (Coen, 1996). The expression of ppUL54 is controlled by multiple regulatory elements during viral infection. ppUL54 is resistant to high salt concentrations and is sensitive to particular deoxyribonucleoside and pyrophosphate analogue antiviral agents (Freitas et al., 1985; Huang, 1975; Wahren et al., 1985). Proteins expressed from both UL112–113 and IRS1/TRS1 loci in association with the major immediate–early (MIE) proteins, were implicated as transactivators of UL54 expression (Kerry et al., 1996, 1997). These studies implicated cellular factors as one of the major factors involved in control of UL54 expression. Since UL54, along with the product of another conserved gene, UL97 (viral protein kinase), are targets of many antiviral compounds, many studies have focused on the genetic changes occurring in these genes in drug-resistant HCMV isolates. Several of these studies have shown that the main mechanism conferring drug resistance is through point mutations within the DNA polymerase gene locus (Cihlar et al., 1998 a,b; Eckle et al., 2000; Eizuru, 1998; Mousavi-Jazi et al., 2001). One drug in particular, foscarnet (PFA), induced specific point mutations in a conserved region of the polymerase gene likely to be associated with pyrophospate release (Mousavi-Jazi et al., 2003). Studies involving the use of siRNA demonstrated that UL54 inhibition by this method can be as efficient as conventional drug therapies (Wiebusch et al., 2004).

The polymerase accessory protein, ppUL44 (originally designated ICP36) (Mocarski et al., 1985), is an abundant, nuclear phosphorylated DNA-binding protein with an approximate molecular weight of 52 kDa that partitions into viral replication compartments (Anders and McCue, 1996; Gibson, 1983, 1984; Gibson et al., 1981; Ho, 1991; Mocarski et al., 1985). UL44 protein can be detected in infected cells during the early phase of viral infection and accumulates in the nuclei of infected cells until, and throughout, the late phase (Ho, 1991). UL44 was shown to be a substrate for UL97 protein kinase demonstrating that the phosphorylation of UL44 may be controlled by both viral encoded and cellular kinases (Krosky et al., 2003). In addition, the requirement for UL44 in the transient replication assay, studies using the expression of antisense RNA to the UL44 transcript also demonstrated UL44 as being an essential protein in the context of the viral genome in virus infected cells (Ripalti et al., 1995). It was shown that transactivation of the UL44 promoter depends on a gene product(s) encoded by the TRS1 segment of the genome in conjunction with IE1 and IE2 immediate–early proteins (Stasiak and Mocarski, 1992).

Because UL54 and UL44 represent significant drug targets recent studies have focused on the interaction of these two proteins. In vitro analysis determined that the C-terminal end of UL54 was essential for interaction with UL44. A small peptide, corresponding to residues 1161–1242 of UL54, effectively interfered with the interaction of the two proteins (Loregian et al., 2003). Further studies indicated that specific point mutations within the UL54 protein in amino acid residues Leu1227 and Phe1231, were sufficient to impede the interaction of UL54 with UL44, as well as affecting the ability of the enzyme complex to synthesis long chain DNA (Loregian et al., 2004).

Single-stranded DNA binding protein (UL57)

The single-stranded DNA (ssDNA) binding protein has similar size and biochemical properties to the HSV-1 single-stranded DNA binding protein encoded by the UL29 gene (Anders and Gibson, 1988; Anders et al., 1986, 1987; Kemble et al., 1987). The HSV-1 ssDNA binding activity is essential for viral DNA replication (Lee and Knipe, 1985; Ruyechan, 1983) and exhibits a helix-destabilizing activity but can also catalyze the renaturation of complementary single strands of DNA (Dutch and Lehman, 1993). Recent studies indicate that this protein exhibits RNA binding and R-loop formation in addition to functioning as a recombinase (Boehmer, 2004; Reuven et al., 2004). HSV ssDNA binding protein interacts with several other viral DNA replication proteins including DNA polymerase and the OBP, and binding may stimulate the activities of DNA polymerase, OBP helicase, and helicase–primase (Boehmer et al., 1993; Boehmer and Lehman, 1993a,b; Chiou et al., 1985; Falkenberg et al., 1997; Hamatake et al., 1997; Hernandez and Lehman, 1990; Tanguy LeGac et al., 1998).

HCMV ssDNA binding protein is encoded by UL57 as a 140 kDa protein that localizes to intranuclear DNA replication compartments by 48 h post-infection and accumulates in characteristic prereplicative sites when DNA synthesis is inhibited by treatment with drugs that inhibit viral DNA synthesis (Anders et al., 1987; Penfold and Mocarski, 1997).

UL84

The requirement for the core replication proteins: polymerase, polymerase processivity factor, trimeric helicase-primase and ssDNA binding protein is common among all herpesviruses. One additional protein, the UL84 gene product (ppUL84) is necessary for replication. ppUL84 is a 586aa polypeptide present in infected cells as early as 2.5 hpi (He et al., 1992) and is a nuclear-localizing phosphoprotein. UL84 colocalizes with UL44 and IE2 (580 aa) in the nucleus and is a component of viral replication compartments in infected and transfected cells (Xu et al., 2002). UL84 stably interacts with IE2 in infected cells (Samaniego et al., 1994; Spector and Tevethia, 1994) and overexpression of UL84 decreases IE2-mediated transient transactivation (Gebert et al., 1997). ppUL84 nuclear localization can either use a signal similar to the SV40 T antigen nuclear localization signal (Xu et al., 2002) or a non-conventional importin alpha protein-dependent process (Lischka et al., 2003). ppUL84 probably dimerizes (Colletti et al., 2004). The self-interaction domain is localized to a highly charged region of the protein. UL84 is the only HCMV function needed to facilitate replication of HCMV oriLyt by the six Epstein–Barr virus replication-fork proteins in Vero cells (Sarisky and Hayward, 1996). Although there were different HCMV-encoded factors required in human fibroblasts versus Vero cells, UL84 was the only auxiliary component that could not be omitted (Sarisky and Hayward, 1996). Other laboratories have observed cell type dependent requirements for HCMV replication proteins, indicating that replication may proceed by different mechanisms depending on cellular factors present (Reid et al., 2003). The UL84 ORF is essential for virus growth as evidenced by the generation of recombinant viruses with insertions or replacement in UL84 (Dunn et al., 2003; Xu et al., 2004). Interestingly, all kinetic classes of viral transcripts are made in cells transfected with recombinant UL84 deficient viral bacmid DNA (Xu et al., 2004), despite the fact that UL84-defective BACs fail to accumulate any viral DNA.

Recent evidence showed that ppUL84 acts in concert with IE2-p86 to activate a cis-acting element within oriLyt suggesting that a ppUL84-IE2-p86 interaction may supply a "trigger" for viral DNA synthesis. Therefore, ppUL84 appears to have a dual function in HCMV DNA replication. The first is either as a coactivator of transcription along with IE2 or a repressor of IE2-mediated transcriptional activation. Activation of a promoter within oriLyt may provide an essential signal for initiation of DNA synthesis. The second function may involve an as yet undefined enzymatic activity such as a helicase. This is based on the observation that the amino acid sequence of UL84 has a significant homology to the DExD/H box family of RNA helicases. Consistent with this possibility, HCMV UL84 shows UTPase activity (Colletti et al., 2005). These proteins may act as either coactivators or repressors of transcription in a promoter-specific manner (Wilson et al., 2004). New electromobility shift assay (EMSA) data from the Pari laboratory show that UL84 can interact with both DNA and RNA in vitro. This interaction appears to be non-specific but a higher affinity for RNA sequences that form a stem-loop suggests that UL84 may bind to these structures within oriLyt. Moreover, chromatin immunoprecipitation (ChIP) assays using either infected-cell DNA or DNA contained within purified virus showed that UL84 is associated with the HCMV genome. UL84 binding was localized to three distinct regions within oriLyt.

HCMV UL84 homologues are found in all betaherpesviruses (Chapter 15) but have highest DNA sequence similarity in closely related chimpanzee or baboon CMV (Davison et al., 2003). This is in contrast to UL84 homologues found within MCMV and GPCMV, or in the roseolaviruses where the UL84 ORF retains little similarity to the HCMV counterpart. This lack of sequence homology also appears to translate to a functional distinction between primate CMVs and other species since it was demonstrated that the UL84 ORF is non-essential for virus growth in both MCMV and GPCMV (Morello et al., 2002) (M. Schleiss and A. McGregor, personal communication).

Origin binding proteins in roseoloviruses

Initiator proteins for HHV6 and HHV7 appear to have close homology to OBP of HSV-1. These proteins, the gene product of U73 for both HHV6 and HHV7, each interact with two sites within the *ori*Lyt for both viruses. These sequences are equivalent to Box I and Box II of HSV-1 *ori*Lyt, flank AT-rich sequences and exhibit other similar sequence characteristics. Other DNA replication proteins within HHV6 and HHV7 have been assumed based on nucleotide sequence homology to the HSV-1 and HCMV functions. They include: U38 (DNA polymerase), U27 (polymerase accessory protein), U43, U74 and U77 (helicase–primase complex) and U41 (ssDNA binding protein).

Immediate–early protein IE2–580aa

As is summarized in Chapter 17, IE2 encodes an 86-kDa nuclear immediate–early phosphoprotein that is essential for lytic replication in tissue culture (Heider et al., 2002; Marchini et al., 2001). IE2-p86 is thought to be the major transcription-activating protein of HCMV and is also responsible for negative autoregulation of the major immediate–early promoter (MIEP) (Mocarski, 2001). IE2 has been implicated in multiple protein–protein interactions including the formation of dimers, association with ppUL84 and several transcription factors, for example CREB, CBP, SP-1, and c-Jun (Chiou et al., 1993; Furnari et al., 1993; Lang et al., 1995; Lukac et al., 1994; Schwartz et al., 1996; Scully et al., 1995; Wara-aswapati et al., 1999).

The role of IE2 with respect to DNA replication is less well understood. It has been shown that IE2-p86 interacts with ppUL84 to activate a responsive promoter within *ori*Lyt (Xu et al., 2004). However, the requirement for IE2 in origin-dependent DNA replication is apparently cell type dependent. The *ori*Lyt promoter is constitutively active in Vero cells, thereby enabling amplification of *ori*Lyt in the absence of IE2 (Xu et al., 2004).

UL36–38

Although these genes were identified as being required for DNA replication (Pari and Anders, 1993), they appear to play an auxiliary role (Sarisky and Hayward, 1996). In addition, in a human fibroblast cell line immortalized with the catalytic subunit for telomerase (hTERT), the gene products of UL36–38 are no longer necessary for origin-dependent DNA replication (Xu et al., 2004). These proteins may function to facilitate a more favorable cellular environment for transient DNA replication. The UL36–38 locus encodes at least five transcripts from three different transcriptional promoters: the UL36, UL37, UL37$_M$, UL37×1 and UL38 RNAs (Goldmacher et al., 1999; Kouzarides et al., 1988; Tenney and Colberg-Poley, 1991a,b; Wilkinson et al., 1984). Despite being initiated at the same IE promoter, three UL37 RNAs, UL37×1, UL37, UL37$_M$, are generated by differential RNA splicing and polyadenylation and show dramatically different temporal expression during HCMV infection. The UL37×1 unspliced RNA is expressed abundantly at IE times and remains abundant until late times of infection. In contrast, the other two UL37 RNAs, which are spliced, are expressed at low abundance during IE times and encoding two UL37 glycoproteins (gpUL37 and gpUL37$_M$) that are dispensable for replication. Only pUL37×1 is required for viral replication (Reboredo et al., 2004) possibly via its anti-apoptotic activity (Goldmacher et al., 1999; Hayajneh et al., 2001).

Betaherpesvirus replication origins

Cytomegalovirus *ori*Lyt

Several lines of evidence show that a unique HCMV origin of lytic DNA synthesis, called *ori*Lyt, lies near the middle of U_L, between the UL57 and UL69 ORFs. First, this region directs virus-mediated replication of plasmids in transient replication assays (Anders and Punturieri, 1991). Such assays allowed the mapping of functional replicator sequences (Anders et al., 1992; Masse et al., 1992; Zhu et al., 1998); see below). Second, evidence from an inhibitor study indicates that DNA synthesis initiates in or near this region of the virus genome during productive infection of permissive cells (Hamzeh et al., 1990). Third, although poorly conserved at the nucleotide sequence level, the position of *ori*Lyt next to the single-stranded DNA binding protein gene is conserved in all other cytomegaloviruses studied to date, and the corresponding regions confer replication competence in the transient assay (Masse et al., 1997; Vink et al., 1997). Finally, in contrast to the lytic replicators of many other herpesviruses, cytomegalovirus *ori*Lyt appears to be single-copy, because it is not duplicated in the genomes of either laboratory or clinical isolates, and recombinant HCMV BACs deleted for *ori*Lyt fail to produce virus or replicate their genomes (Dunn et al., 2003; D. G. Anders, unpublished results; Borst and Messerle, 2005). This is consistent with previous findings that no other segment of the viral genome has replicator activity in the transient assay. Therefore, *ori*Lyt is thought to be essential for lytic replication in the host. Because it is essential and may play an important regulatory role in the virus–host relationship, we provide a complete summary of work-to-date.

Cytomegalovirus *ori*Lyt structure

Cytomegalovirus *ori*Lyt is distinguished from most other herpesvirus replicators, including those of the roseoloviruses, in that it is large and complex. Some structural features are shared with gammaherpesvirus *ori*Lyt sequences. Deletions to define the external borders established a minimal *ori*Lyt region containing essential elements, and showed that sequences spanning more than 2.5 kbp can contribute to replicator activity in transient assays (Anders *et al.*, 1992; Masse *et al.*, 1992). Kanamycin cassette insertion studies defined a similar core region, roughly nt 91 750 to 93 300, within which the insertions either eliminated or greatly impaired replicator function (Zhu *et al.*, 1998). This minimal oriLyt core region does not support efficient replicator activity, at least in transient assays, in the absence of left or right flanking sequences. The flanking sequences independently contribute to *ori*Lyt activity with relaxed position dependence, in that insertions do not significantly compromise activation of the *ori*Lyt core, and therefore they have been referred to as "auxiliary" sequences.

Two notable features characterize the cytomegalovirus *ori*Lyt region. First, it contains a high density of direct and inverted repeats (Masse *et al.*, 1992). Several of these appear virus specific, including multiple copies of a 10-bp motif similar to the known binding site for the UL34 protein clustered in the left auxiliary region, and 13- (also known as FspI/SphI) and 19-bp directly repeated sequences within the core region. Reiterated sequences similar to the 10-bp and 13-bp motifs are present at corresponding positions in other cytomegaloviruses. Two large, but imperfect inverted repeats are present on the right side of the *ori*Lyt core region; similar structures are present at the corresponding positions of all known CMV *ori*Lyt sequences. Interestingly, these can be variably reiterated in laboratory strains (Prichard *et al.*, 1998). Other repeated elements include a variety of consensus host transcription factor recognition sequences, most notably clusters of potential Sp1 and CREB sites. Which of these reiterated motifs contribute to replicator activity, how and under what circumstances, remains to be determined. A second characteristic feature of CMV *ori*Lyt is its overall base composition asymmetry. Most of the *ori*Lyt region approximates the overall GC content of the viral genome, but AT-rich segments lie on the left side, and a very GC-rich region on the right. The imperfect inverted repeats lie in the GC-rich region. EBV *ori*Lyt shows a similar organization. The roles of AT-rich and GC-rich segments are not understood, but the AT-rich segment in the leftward minimal activating sequence contributes to activation of the core replicator in transient assays (Kiehl *et al.*, 2003).

A series of overlapping 200-bp deletions spanning the *ori*Lyt core region were made and tested for activity in the transient replication assay to search for essential elements (Zhu *et al.*, 1998). All except one of the core deletions reduced replicator activity from about 20- to greater than 100-fold, suggesting that elements contributing to replicator activity are scattered throughout the core region, or that spatial relationships of distant elements are important. Two regions critical for replicator activity were identified by this approach. One of these, extending from nt 92 400 to 92 573, includes the only known individually essential element, a pyrimidine (Y)-rich tract followed by a purine (R)-rich tract of nucleotides, referred to as a "Y-block." Y·R elements are present in all other CMV *ori*Lyt sequences as well as in EBV *ori*Lyt, but are absent from origins that characterize HHV-6, HHV-7 and alphaherpesviruses that interact with an origin binding protein (Huang *et al.*, 1996). Nucleotide substitutions in this element eliminate replicator activity in the transient assay. The other essential segment spans nt 92 887 to 93 145, and contains the cluster of Sp1 consensus sites and overlaps the vRNA-2 region. A 405 bp deletion starting at starting at 92 574, which was less than threefold reduced in activity relative to the wild type in the transient replication assay, identified the only dispensable sequence in the *ori*Lyt core region. Lastly, because the core region alone has minimal activity in the transient assay, auxiliary sequences probably play an important role in activating *ori*Lyt. A minimal *ori*Lyt activating sequence overlapping the UL57 promoter was defined by reconstitution, providing a model to study how auxiliary sequences enhance core replicator function (Kiehl *et al.*, 2003).

Finally, there are two important caveats to conclusions regarding functional elements of CMV *ori*Lyt. First, they were drawn on the basis of transient assays. Specific sequence requirements for *ori*Lyt function in the context of the virus genome have yet to be investigated. Second, most of this work was done in permissive fibroblasts; comparative studies in other cell types important in the infected host, in which different sets of cellular regulatory proteins predominate, may reveal distinct sequence requirements. Indeed, the HCMV *ori*Lyt bidirectional promoter *ori*Lyt$_{PM}$ is constitutively active in Vero cells, but requires both IE2 and UL84 for activity in fibroblasts (Xu *et al.*, 2004).

*ori*Lyt open reading frames and transcripts

The HCMV *ori*Lyt region includes predicted ORFs UL58-UL61, and a newly described ORF 3 lies at the right boundary (Murphy et al., 2003a). In addition, the *ori*Lyt region is actively transcribed and several transcripts have been characterized. However, the predicted proteins are not conserved in other cytomegaloviruses including chimpanzee CMV and moreover, with the exceptions of UL59 and to a lesser extent ORF3, the *ori*Lyt ORFs are not conserved amongst clinical isolates, suggesting that they may not represent authentic protein-coding genes (Murphy et al., 2003b; see Chapter 14).

The UL59 ORF is interesting in that it is absent in other other CMV genomes sequenced to date, and appears to have been recently acquired as an insertion between the organizationally conserved *ori*Lyt core and leftward auxiliary regions. It is better conserved among clinical isolates than the other potential *ori*Lyt coding sequences, and a corresponding late transcript of 0.4–0.7 kb is made. However, it is not known whether the predicted protein is expressed. The segment upstream of UL59, extending about 900 bp to Y·R element, is rich in consensus transcription factor binding site sequences, and contains an apparently bidirectional promoter, *ori*Lyt$_{PM}$, that is regulated by IE2 and UL84 (Xu et al., 2004). Transcripts spanning UL59 initiate from several sites in this region. Deletion of the UL59 ORF does not affect HCMV growth in fibroblasts, but tests of growth in other cell types have not been reported (Dunn et al., 2003).

Recombinant HCMV BACs carrying an insertion in either the UL60 or UL61 ORF or a deletion of the UL60 ORF failed to replicate, but these mutations would be predicted on the basis of previous findings to inactivate *ori*Lyt, and therefore more subtle mutations would be needed to determine whether these ORFs are essential (Dunn et al., 2003; Yu et al., 2003). A second, late transcript of around 6.5 kb that has the same orientation and is 3 co-terminal with the UL59 transcript crosses *ori*Lyt from right-to-left, but the complete structure of that transcript is not known.

Three other *ori*Lyt RNA species have been described. The first, called the small replicator transcript, is a roughly 250 nt early, non-polyadenylated species with a single 5′ end and a variable 3′ end that overlaps the essential "Y-block" element (Huang et al., 1996). It lies within the UL60 ORF. An upstream promoter for the small replicator transcript is active in transient assays, but studies to confirm this in the genome context have yet to be done. Two other RNAs, called virus-associated or "vRNAs," were found to be covalently associated with progeny DNA at least partly in RNA–DNA hybrid form, and present in virions (Prichard et al., 1998).

vRNA-1 localizes between nt 93 799 and 94 631, and vRNA-2 between nt 92 636 and 93 513. Nothing is known about how these transcripts are expressed or how they function. The apparently non-coding nature of the small replicator transcript and the vRNAs, the timing of their expression, their unusual properties and their association with genetically defined segments essential for *ori*Lyt activity have led to suggestions that they may participate in initiation of DNA synthesis.

The mechanism of initiation

Initiation of CMV DNA synthesis is not understood. Based on the information available from a variety of DNA replication systems that have been studied, initiation can be predicted to require several steps, including (i) an initial strand separation followed by unwinding, and (ii) assembly of replication fork proteins to form an active complex at the site of initiation. In SV40, T-antigen binds to specific origin sequences to form a complex that, in cooperation with certain structural features of the origin, untwists and subsequently, with an intrinsic helicase activity, unwinds the origin duplex. In addition, it directs polymerase alpha/primase association. The alpha-herpesviruses origin-binding protein (e.g., HSV-1 UL9), as well as the homologous HHV-6 and HHV-7 proteins, are thought to play an analogous role, using an essential intrinsic helicase activity to provide the initial unwinding in cooperation with the single-strand DNA binding protein. However, as noted above, the cytomegaloviruses lack a UL9 homologue. Therefore, it is not clear how initial unwinding occurs or how the replication fork proteins may be directed to load. One frequently discussed possibility is that RNA–DNA hybrids formed during transcription may produce open regions that could be used to load the helicase–primase complex. This suggestion is supported by the synthesis of candidate RNAs and the observation of residual RNA-DNA hybrids, the vRNAs, in replicated viral DNA at sites critical to *ori*Lyt activity. This could explain, at least in part, the complexity of CMV *ori*Lyt, as this mechanism requires not only the transcript itself, but also control regions for transcription and elements to direct assembly to the replication fork complex. However, there are many other possibilities including co-opting the cellular initiation machinery, as EBV does for latent phase DNA synthesis. Initiation remains one of the most interesting areas for investigation of CMV DNA synthesis.

Roseolovirus replication origins

Human herpesviruses 6 and 7 lytic-phase replicators were identified using a transient replication assay (Dewhurst et al., 1993; van Loon et al., 1997). The roseolovirus lytic origins are located adjacent to the single-stranded DNA binding protein gene, U41, a position that is similar to CMV oriLyt; however, the structure of roseolovirus oriLyt exhibits similarity to that of the alphaherpesviruses. As is the case for cytomegalovirus, HHV-6 and HHV-7 oriLyt sequences are thought to be unique, although this has not been fully tested. The HHV-6 oriLyt region is unusually AT rich, and includes a large, imperfect directly repeated (IDR) sequence. In contrast, HHV-7 oriLyt is more compact and is missing the IDR region and adjacent sequences that contribute to HHV-6 replicator activity. Both are smaller and less structurally complex than cytomegalovirus oriLyt, and include comparatively fewer potential transcription factor recognition sequences. Plasmids carrying HHV-6 oriLyt were replicated following introduction into either HHV-6- or HHV-7-infected cells, although HHV-7 oriLyt was only replicated in HHV-7-infected cells (van Loon et al., 1997).

In striking contrast to HCMV oriLyt, the roseolovirus replicators are characterized by the presence of at least two binding sites for a virus-coded protein, U73, homologous to the alphaherpesvirus OBP. As noted above (see Chapter 15), OBP homologues are not found in the cytomegaloviruses. As detailed earlier, the roseolovirus OBP homologues bind specifically to defined oriLyt sites in vitro (Inoue et al., 1994; Inoue and Pellett, 1995; Krug et al., 2001), and mutation of either site, or of the spacer region separating them, inactivates the replicator when tested in the transient assay (Dewhurst et al., 1994; Dykes et al., 1997). Therefore, OBP binding to the oriLyt sites is probably essential for lytic viral replication, and mechanistically the roseolovirus replicators appear to resemble alphaherpesvirus counterparts rather than those of the cytomegaloviruses. Nevertheless, it is noteworthy that, although the HHV-6 minimal replicator spans only about 400 bp including the OBP sites, flanking sequences boost replicator activity in the transient assay suggesting that they may play an important role in regulating activity in the context of the virus genome. The minimal efficient origin includes the IDR region, which greatly enhances activity by an unknown mechanism (Dewhurst et al., 1993). The IDR spans the most A+T rich segment, which may serve as a "DNA unwinding element." Comparison of the HHV-6A and B strain oriLyt sequences revealed that they are more than 95% identical over the minimal essential region including the OBP binding sites, but considerably divergent in the auxiliary flanking regions, particularly beyond the IDR sequences. HHV-6A strains contain three copies of the imperfect direct repeat, whereas HHV-6B carries two copies. Interestingly, a sequence similar to the experimentally defined HHV-6 minimal efficient origin was reiterated in some cultured lineages of HHV6B, presumably by homologous recombination, and the reiterated oriLyt enhanced replicator activity in the transient assay (Dewhurst et al., 1994; Stamey et al., 1995). This is reminiscent of the reiterations seen in HCMV oriLyt laboratory strains. Specific elements within the auxiliary regions contributing to replicator activity have not been identified and, aside from the OBP binding sequences, little is known about the functional elements regulating the roseolovirus replicator.

Latent phase replication

EBV and other herpesviruses that establish latency in replicating cell types have a separate origin (oriP) that is responsible for maintenance and replication of the viral genome during latency. However, no latent phase origin has been identified in the cytomegalovirus genome. Indeed, a latent origin may not be required if the primary sites of latency are in non-dividing cells, particularly if the latency reservoir is replenished by cycles of reactivation as the latency hosts are stimulated to differentiate and divide. Nevertheless, little is known about the molecular aspects of betaherpesvirus latency, and the existence of a latency maintenance element cannot be excluded.

Late gene expression

Replication of the viral genome provides an essential activating event for the expression of high levels of the betaherpesvirus late genes. It is widely understood that late genes encode for proteins required for virus assembly and egress. These genes can be divided into two broad classes. The gamma 1 or leaky-late class are expressed at very low levels at early times after infection and are dramatically upregulated at late times. In contrast, the gamma 2 or "true" late genes are expressed exclusively after and are dependent upon viral DNA replication. The mechanism that restricts late gene activation to after DNA replication has not yet been determined, although at least two general possibilities have been considered. First, the restriction may be related to DNA structure, or possibly DNA modifications that are altered immediately post replication. Alternatively, binding of viral or cellular proteins to repressor elements within late promoters may inhibit late gene expression, with subsequent displacement or titration of the repressors being accomplished by DNA replication.

Our understanding of late gene regulation in the betaherpesviruses lags far behind that of early gene regulation (Chapter 17). Only a handful of late gene promoters have been analyzed in detail. One of the primary reasons for this has been the difficulty in recapitulating the appropriate kinetic regulation of late genes in transient transfection/superinfection assays. Initial studies of betaherpesviruses late promoters in this type of assay system revealed that upon superinfection, promoter activity could be detected at early times after infection (Depto and Stenberg, 1992; Rudolph et al., 1990). Thus, it was assumed that transient assays would not provide complete information regarding the necessary promoter components required to restrict viral gene expression to late times, requiring the assessment of these promoters in the context of the viral genome. In this respect, the recent development of the bacterial artificial chromosome (BAC) system to rapidly generate viral mutants will likely facilitate the analysis of late gene regulation.

However, even though a limited subset of late genes have been analyzed to date, some general features associated with their regulation have been identified. Typically, late promoters seem to require a TATA element but no further upstream sequences for transcriptional activation (Depto and Stenberg, 1989, 1992; Kohler et al., 1994; McWatters et al., 2002; Wing et al., 1998). Similar findings have been observed for late gene promoters of herpes simplex virus, where the TATA box and downstream elements are sufficient to direct late gene activation (Flanagan et al., 1991; Homa et al., 1986; Weir, 2001). This is in contrast to the betaherpesviruses early promoters, where specific upstream sequence elements capable of binding to cellular transcription factors are critical for promoter activation. The most extensive studies on late gene regulation published to date have examined the human cytomegalovirus UL99 gene encoding the virion tegument protein pp28 (Depto and Stenberg, 1992; Kerry et al., 1997; Kohler et al., 1994). This gene, which is expressed as a gamma 2 late gene, requires only sequences from -40 relative to the cap site to restrict expression to late times (Kohler et al., 1994). In order to accurately replicate appropriate promoter kinetics, these studies were performed by introducing the promoter construct regulating the CAT reporter gene into an alternate, transcriptionally inert site in the HCMV genome. This type of study led to the hypothesis that late promoters are relatively simple promoters consisting primarily of a TATA element and downstream sequences and lacking a requirement for multiple transcriptional regulatory elements.

Despite some limitations, transient assays have yielded important information about the minimal promoters of a number of late genes. (Depto and Stenberg, 1989; McWatters et al., 2002; Wing et al., 1998). For example, in the analysis of the HCMV UL75 promoter, which controls expression of the envelope glycoprotein gH, sequences from −38 to +15 relative to the cap site were sufficient to activate this promoter (McWatters et al., 2002). However, although additional regions of the promoter were not essential for activation, closer examination of those sequences revealed a much more complex mode of regulation (McWatters et al., 2002). Specifically, sequences downstream of the UL75 cap site appeared to function as a dominant regulatory element. In the absence of this region, both activation and repressor elements were identified in the upstream sequences. (McWatters et al., 2002). Similarly, analysis of the HCMV UL94 late promoter identified a dominant regulatory element downstream of the cap site that functioned as a derepressor (Wing et al., 1998). In the absence of this downstream element, deletion of the upstream sequences enhanced promoter activity, suggesting the presence of an upstream negative regulatory element. This negative regulatory element contained two p53 binding sites that were important, although not sufficient for the repressive effects (Wing et al., 1998). These studies suggest that the regulation of late gene expression may be more complex than previously thought, with additional sequences allowing the binding of viral and/or cellular proteins that may influence the regulation of late promoters. However, it remains to be determined if these elements truly play a role in late gene regulation in the context of a normal viral infection, or if these are artifacts resulting from the assay system.

Studies suggesting a more complex model for late promoter activation are intriguing, given that a number of HCMV late promoters have been identified in the midst of both immediate early and early gene regions (Leach and Mocarski, 1989; Leatham et al., 1991; Puchtler and Stamminger, 1991). In fact, in some cases, specific late transcripts with alternate TATA elements and start sites have been identified within HCMV early promoters (Jones and Muzithras, 1991; Leach and Mocarski, 1989). Thus it might be expected that adjacent regulatory elements or enhancers within the promoter context could influence the activation or kinetics of expression of such late transcriptional units. In this context, it is important to note that analyses of late promoter regulation in the context of the viral genome have been performed in a transcriptionally inert region (Kohler et al., 1994), and the association of repressors and activators may be critical for restricting viral late gene expression within their natural genomic context. Thus, a more complex model of late promoter regulation emerges, with a possible role for multiple repressor and activator proteins influencing the kinetics of gene expression.

Some efforts have been made to identify specific regulatory proteins that are involved in the activation of HCMV late promoters. With respect to cellular transcription factors, analysis of the UL75 promoter indicated a role for a cellular PEA3-related protein in transcriptional activation (McWatters et al., 2002). Inversely, a role for p53 in transcriptional repression of the UL94 promoter has been identified (Wing et al., 1998). Some recent studies suggest that the NF-κB transcription factor may also be involved in activating viral late gene expression (DeMeritt et al., 2006). Other studies have identified sequence elements involved in late promoter activation, although the specific proteins required for activation remain to be identified (Depto and Stenberg, 1989, 1992). Intriguingly, a more global analysis of the putative promoter regions of HCMV late genes revealed a palindromic GC-rich sequence (CCGCGGGCGCGG) in the promoters of 17% of viral late genes (Chambers et al., 1999). The significance of this sequence element in late gene regulation remains to be determined.

In addition to cellular proteins, there is evidence for the role of viral factors in the activation of late promoters. The fact that late kinetics are not conserved when the promoters are relieved of the constraints of the viral genome suggests that the viral factors required for activation are present at early times of infection. Indeed, the HCMV immediate–early proteins can activate some late promoters, although to minimal extents (Depto and Stenberg, 1989, 1992; Wu et al., 2001). Other HCMV proteins, such as trs1 may also play a role in activating late promoters (Romanowski and Shenk, 1997; Stasiak and Mocarski, 1992). The finding that the IE proteins of HCMV may be involved in regulating viral late gene expression is interesting in the light of recent studies examining the role of IE2 during viral infection (Sanchez et al., 2002; White et al., 2004). Deletion of IE2 sequences from amino acids 136 to 290 resulted in reduced amounts of IE2 in infected cells but had minimal impact on viral DNA replication (Sanchez et al., 2002). Interestingly, two viral late proteins, pp65 and pp28 were found to be expressed at reduced levels. Likewise, UL83 mRNA levels that encode the pp65 gamma 1 late protein were reduced (Sanchez et al., 2002). Small internal deletions in IE2 from amino acids 356–359, 427–435, and 505–511 and one substitution mutant of IE2 were also assessed using the same strategy (White et al., 2004). The deletion of amino acids 356–359 and the substitution mutant were both defective in late gene expression. In contrast, deletion of amino acids 427–435 and 505–511 resulted in an IE2 protein that did not activate early gene expression, but expressed certain gamma 1 and gamma 2 genes at early times after infection. Sequence analysis located a potential IE2-binding site within the promoter region of one of these genes, suggesting that IE2 may be involved in transcriptional repression of late genes (White et al., 2004). These findings suggest that IE2 plays a hitherto unrecognized role in directly regulating late gene expression in both a positive and a negative manner.

A role for IE2 in late promoter regulation would appear to be in conflict with the kinetics of expression of this protein. One possibility is that IE2 is differentially modified at late times after viral infection. IE2 can be modified by both phosphorylation and sumoylation, and differential modification through the course of infection could influence the ability of IE2 to regulate gene expression (Heider et al., 2002; Hofmann et al., 2000; Lee et al., 2003). Alternatively, an IE2-related protein, p40 corresponding to amino acids 242–580 of IE2 (Plachter et al., 1993) has been characterized that is expressed via an alternate promoter at late times. This protein has been demonstrated to function as a transactivator, but its specific role during infection has not been defined (Jenkins et al., 1994). The possibility exists that the p40 protein is involved in the activation of late promoters. Indeed, the IE2 deletion from amino acids 136 to 290 that exhibits defects in late gene expression removes the start codon for the p40 late gene product from the IE2 region (Sanchez et al., 2002). Thus, IE2 or IE2-related proteins may play a differential role in transcriptional activation of viral promoters at multiple stages of viral infection. Recent studies have identified a gammaherpesvirus gene, ORF18 that is essential for late gene expression (Arumugaswami et al., 2006). While a direct role for the betaherpesvirus homolog of ORF18, UL79 in late gene activation has yet to be assessed, it is highly likely that additional viral proteins will be found to be important for the regulation of late promoters.

To date, there has been only one study addressing the direct role of DNA replication in stimulating late gene transcription. In this analysis, the HCMV TRL7 gene that is expressed with gamma 1 kinetics was assessed in the context of a plasmid containing the HCMV oriLyt region (Wade and Spector, 1994). This approach restored the dependence on DNA replication for high levels of the TRL7 promoter-directed transcript in transient assays. While the plasmid itself did replicate upon superinfection with HCMV, the level of replication appeared to be insufficient to explain the increased transcription rates. In addition, enhanced transcription of the gamma 1 gene at late times did not appear to be related to methylation differences, or dependent on specific upstream promoter elements. One intriguing possibility discussed by the authors is that factors required for replication may play a dual role in both replication and transcriptional activation, with replication providing a mechanism for bringing such factors into proximity of the promoter, and thereby providing for enhanced transcription, based on a model originally identified in the bacteriophage T4 (Herendeen et al., 1989, 1992).

In addition to transcriptional events, there is evidence that post-transcriptional regulation may play a critical role in controlling the appearance of viral late gene products. Analysis of the HCMV UL99 5' untranslated region revealed that these sequences influenced translational regulation, via a putative stem–loop structure (Kerry et al., 1997). While the mechanism of this regulation has not yet been characterized, recent analysis of IE2 mutants revealed that this protein may be involved, suggesting that the influence of IE2 on late gene expression is at multiple levels (White et al., 2004). Post-transcriptional regulation has also been identified as a potential influence on the expression of late genes in the other betaherpesviruses, HHV-6 and -7. For these two viruses, specific splice variants that are restricted to the late phase of viral infection have been identified (Menegazzi et al., 1999; Mirandola et al., 1998). Thus, post-transcriptional control of gene expression at the late stages of viral infection may be a common mechanism in the betaherpesviruses to control the function and time of appearance of viral proteins. Post-transcriptional mechanisms also play an important role in the regulation of late gene expression during herpes simplex virus infection (McCormick et al., 1999; Perkins et al., 2003), suggesting that this may represent a common theme in the control of late gene expression throughout the herpesviruses.

In summary, although minimal sequences may be sufficient to restrict expression to late times in a transcriptionally inactive environment, a more accurate picture of the complexity of betaherpesvirus late gene regulation is now emerging. A role for viral and cellular transcriptional regulators, both positive and negative, has been identified, although definitive studies to truly assess late promoter requirements in a natural genomic environment remain to be performed. In addition, post-transcriptional events likely play a critical role in controlling the time of appearance of viral late proteins. Such strict control over the expression of late proteins is likely to be key for the appropriate assembly and egress of new virion particles.

REFERENCES

Anders, D. G. and Gibson, W. (1988). Location, transcript analysis, and partial nucleotide sequence of the cytomegalovirus gene encoding an early DNA-binding protein with similarities to ICP8 of herpes simplex virus type 1. *J. Virol.*, **62**(4), 1364–1372.

Anders, D. G. and McCue, L. A. (1996). The human cytomegalovirus genes and proteins required for DNA synthesis. *Intervirology*, **39**(5–6), 378–388.

Anders, D. G. and Punturieri, S. M. (1991). Multicomponent origin of cytomegalovirus lytic-phase DNA replication. *J. Virol.*, **65**(2), 931–937.

Anders, D. G., Irmiere, A., and Gibson, W. (1986). Identification and characterization of na major early cytomegalovirus DNA-binding protein. *J. Virol.*, **58**(2), 253–262.

Anders, D. G., Kidd, J. R., and Gibson, W. (1987). Immunological characterization of an early cytomegalovirus single-strand DNA-binding protein with similarities to the HSV major DNA-binding protein. *Virology*, **161**(2), 579–588.

Anders, D. G., Kacica, M. A., Pari, G. S., and Punturieri, S. M. (1992). Boundaries and structure of human cytomegalovirus *ori*Lyt, a complex origin for lytic-phase DNA replication. *J. Virol.*, **66**(6), 3373–3384.

Arumugaswami, V., Wu, T. T., Martinez-Guzman, D. et al. (2006). ORF18 is a transfactor that is essential for late gene transcription of a gammaherpesvirus. *J. Virol.*, **80**(19), 9730–9740.

Boehmer, P. E. (2004). RNA binding and R-loop formation by the herpes single-stranded DNA-binding protein (ICP8). *Nucl. Acids Res*, **32**(15), 4576–4584.

Boehmer, P. E. and Lehman, I. R. (1993a). Herpes simplex virus type 1 ICP8: helix-destabilizing properties. *J. Virol.*, **67**(2), 711–5.

(1993b). Physical interaction between the herpes simplex virus 1 origin-binding protein and single-stranded DNA-binding protein ICP8. *Proc. Natl Acad. Sci. USA*, **90**(18), 8444–8448.

Boehmer, P. E., Dodson, M. S., and Lehman, I. R. (1993). The herpes simplex virus type-1 origin binding protein. DNA helicase activity. *J. Biol. Chem.*, **268**(2), 1220–5.

Bolovan-Fritts, C. A., Mocarski, E. S., and Wiedeman, J. A. (1999). Peripheral blood CD14(+) cells from healthy subjects carry a circular conformation of latent cytomegalovirus genome. *Blood*, **93**(1), 394–398.

Borst, E. M. and Messerle, M. (2005). Analysis of human cytomegalovirus *ori*Lyt sequence requirements in the context of the viral genome. *J. Virol.*, **79**(6), 3615–3626.

Bruckner, R. C., Crute, J. J., Dodson, M. S., and Lehman, I. R. (1991). The herpes simplex virus 1 origin binding protein: a DNA helicase. *J. Biol. Chem.*, **266**, 2669–2674.

Chambers, J., Angulo, A., Amaratunga, D. et al. (1999). DNA microarrays of the complex human cytomegalovirus genome: profiling kinetic class with drug sensitivity of viral gene expression. *J. Virol.*, **73**(7), 5757–5766.

Chiou, C. J., Zong, J., Waheed, I., and Hayward, G. S. (1993). Identification and mapping of dimerization and DNA-binding domains in the C terminus of the IE2 regulatory protein of human cytomegalovirus. *J. Virol.*, **67**(10), 6201–6214.

Chiou, H. C., Weller, S. K., and Coen, D. M. (1985). Mutations in the herpes simplex virus major DNA-binding protein gene leading to altered sensitivity to DNA polymerase inhibitors. *Virology*, **145**(2), 213–226.

Cihlar, T., Fuller, M. D., and Cherrington, J. M. (1997). Expression of the catalytic subunit (UL54) and the accessory protein (UL44) of human cytomegalovirus DNA polymerase in a coupled in vitro transcription/translation system. *Protein Expr. Purif.*, **11**(2), 209–218.

Cihlar, T., Fuller, M. D., and Cherrington, J. M. (1998a). Characterization of drug resistance-associated mutations in the human cytomegalovirus DNA polymerase gene by using recombinant mutant viruses generated from overlapping DNA fragments. *J. Virol.*, **72**(7), 5927–5936.

Cihlar, T., Fuller, M. D., Mulato, A. S., and Cherrington, J. M. (1998b). A point mutation in the human cytomegalovirus DNA polymerase gene selected in vitro by cidofovir confers a slow replication phenotype in cell culture. *Virology*, **248**(2), 382–393.

Coen, D. M. (1996). Viral DNA polymerases. In 'DNA Replication in Eukaryotic Cells' ed. (D. ML, Ed.), pp. 495–523. Cold Spring Harbor: Cold Spring Harbor Press.

Colberg-Poley, A. M. (1996). Functional roles of immediate early proteins encoded by the human cytomegalovirus UL36–38, UL115–119, TRS1/IRS1 and US3 loci. *Intervirology*, **39**(5–6), 350–360.

Colberg-Poley, A. M., Santomenna, L. D., Harlow, P. P., Benfield, P. A., and Tenney, D. J. (1992). Human cytomegalovirus US3 and UL36–38 immediate–early proteins regulate gene expression. *J. Virol.*, **66**(1), 95–105.

Colberg-Poley, A. M., Huang, L., Soltero, V. E., Iskenderian, A. C., Schumacher, R. F. and Anders, D. G. (1998). The acidic domain of pUL37×1 and gpUL37 plays a key role in transactivation of HCMV DNA replication gene promoter constructions. *Virology*, **246**(2), 400–408.

Colletti, K. S., Xu, Y., Cei, S. A., Tarrant, M., and Pari, G. S. (2004). Human cytomegalovirus UL84 oligomerization and act as transdominant inhibitors of oriLyt- evidence that IE2-UL84 and UL84-UL84 interactions DNA replication. *J. Virol.*, **78**(17), 9203–9214.

Colletti, K. S., Yu, Y., Yamboliev, I., and Pari, G. S. (2005). Human cytomegalovirus UL84 is a phosphoprotein that exhibits UTPase activity and is a putative member of the DExD/H Box family of proteins. *J. Biol. Chem.* (in press)

Davison, A. J., Dolan, A., Akter, P. et al. (2003). The human cytomegalovirus genome revisited: comparison with the chimpanzee cytomegalovirus genome. *J. Gen. Virol.*, **84**(1), 17–28.

DeMeritt, I. B., Podduturi, J. P., Tilley, A. M., Nogalski, M. T., and Yurochko, A. D. (2006). Prolonged activation of NF-κB by human cytomegalovirus promotes efficient viral replication and late gene expression. *Virology*, **346**(1), 15–31.

Depto, A. S. and Stenberg, R. M. (1989). Regulated expression of the human cytomegalovirus pp65 gene: octamer sequence in the promoter is required for activation by viral gene products. *J. Virol.*, **63**(3), 1232–1238.

Depto, A. S. and Stenberg, R. M. (1992). Functional analysis of the true late human cytomegalovirus pp28 upstream promoter: *cis*-acting elements and viral *trans*-acting proteins necessary for promoter activation. *J. Virol.*, **66**(5), 3241–3246.

Dewhurst, S., Dollard, S. C., Pellett, P. E., and Dambaugh, T. R. (1993). Identification of a lytic-phase origin of DNA replication in human herpesvirus 6B strain Z29. *J. Virol.*, **67**(12), 7680–7683.

Dewhurst, S., Krenitsky, D. M., and Dykes, C. (1994). Human herpesvirus 6B origin: sequence diversity, requirement for two binding sites for origin-binding protein, and enhanced replication from origin multimers. *J. Virol.*, **68**(10), 6799–6803.

Dracheva, S., Koonin, E. V., and Crute, J. J. (1995). Identification of the primase active site of the herpes simplex virus type 1 helicase–primase. *J. Biol. Chem.*, **270**(23), 14148–14153.

Dunn, W., Chou, C., Li, H. et al. (2003). Functional profiling of a human cytomegalovirus genome. *Proc. Natl Acad. Sci. USA*, **100**(24), 14223–14228. Epub 2003 Nov 17.

Dutch, R. E. and Lehman, I. R. (1993). Renaturation of complementary DNA strands by herpes simplex virus type 1 ICP8. *J. Virol.*, **67**(12), 6945–9.

Dykes, C., Chan, H., Krenitsky, D. M., and Dewhurst, S. (1997). Stringent structural and sequence requirements of the human herpesvirus 6B lytic-phase origin of DNA replication. *J. Gen. Virol.*, **78**(5), 1125–1129.

Eckle, T., Prix, L., Jahn, G. et al. (2000). Drug-resistant human cytomegalovirus infection in children after allogeneic stem cell transplantation may have different clinical outcomes. *Blood*, **96**(9), 3286–3289.

Eizuru, Y. (1998). [Analysis of ganciclovir-resistant cytomegalovirus]. *Nippon Rinsho*, **56**(1), 151–155.

Ertl, P. F. and Powell, K. L. (1992). Physical and functional interaction of human cytomegalovirus DNA polymerase and its accessory protein (ICP36) expressed in insect cells. *J. Virol.*, **66**(7), 4126–4133.

Falkenberg, M., Bushnell, D. A., Elias, P., and Lehman, I. R. (1997). The UL8 subunit of the heterotrimeric herpes simplex virus type 1 helicase-primase is required for the unwinding of single strand DNA-binding protein (ICP8)-coated DNA substrates. *J. Biol. Chem.*, **272**(36), 22766–22770.

Fierer, D. S. and Challberg, M. D. (1992). Purification and characterization of UL9, the herpes simplex virus type 1 origin-binding protein. *J. Virol.*, **66**, 3986–3995.

Flanagan, W. M., Papavassiliou, A. G., Rice, M., Hecht, L. B., Silverstein, S., and Wagner, E. K. (1991). Analysis of the herpes simplex virus type 1 promoter controlling the expression of UL38, a true late gene involved in capsid assembly. *J. Virol.*, **65**(2), 769–786.

Freitas, V. R., Smee, D. F., Chernow, M., Boehme, R., and Matthews, T. R. (1985). Activity of 9-(1,3-dihydroxy-2-propoxymethyl)guanine compared with that of acyclovir against human, monkey, and rodent cytomegaloviruses. *Antimicrob. Agents Chemother.*, **28**(2), 240–245.

Furnari, B. A., Poma, E., Kowalik, T. F., Huong, S. M., and Huang, E. S. (1993). Human cytomegalovirus immediate–early gene 2 protein interacts with itself and with several novel cellular proteins. *J. Virol.*, **67**(8), 4981–4991.

Gebert, S., Schmolke, S., Sorg, G., Floss, S., Plachter, B., and Stamminger, T. (1997). The UL84 protein of human cytomegalovirus acts as a transdominant inhibitor of immediate–early-mediated transactivation that is able to prevent viral replication. *J. Virol.*, **71**(9), 7048–7060.

Gibson, W. (1983). Protein counterparts of human and simian cytomegaloviruses. *Virology*, **128**(2), 391–406.

Gibson, W. (1984). Synthesis, structure and function of cytomegalovirus major nonvirion nuclear protein. In *Herpesvirus* ed. F. Rapp, pp. 423–440. New York: Liss.

Gibson, W., Murphy, T. L., and Roby, C. (1981). Cytomegalovirus-infected cells contain a DNA-binding protein. *Virology*, **111**(1), 251–262.

Goldmacher, V. S., Bartle, L. M., Skaletskaya, A. (1999). A cytomegalovirus-encoded mitochondria-localized inhibitor of apoptosis structurally unrelated to Bcl-2. *Proc. Natl Acad. Sci. USA*, **96**(22), 12536–12541.

Hamatake, R. K., Bifano, M., Hurlburt, W. W., and Tenney, D. J. (1997). A functional interaction of ICP8, the herpes simplex virus single-stranded DNA-binding protein, and the helicase–primase complex that is dependent on the presence of the UL8 subunit. *J. Gen. Virol.*, **78**(4), 857–865.

Hamzeh, F. M., Lietman, P. S., Gibson, W., and Hayward, G. S. (1990). Identification of the lytic origin of DNA replication in human cytomegalovirus by a novel approach utilizing ganciclovir-induced chain termination. *J. Virol.*, **64**(12), 6184–6195.

Hayajneh, W. A. *et al.* (2001). The sequence and antiapoptotic functional domains of the human cytomegalovirus UL37 exon 1 immediate early protein are conserved in multiple primary strains. *Virology*, **279**(1), 233–240.

Hazuda, D. J., Perry, H. C., Naylor, A. M., and McClements, W. L. (1991). Characterization of the herpes simplex virus origin binding protein interaction with ori$_s$. *J. Biol. Chem.*, **266**(36), 24621–24626.

He, Y. S., Xu, L., and Huang, E. S. (1992). Characterization of human cytomegalovirus UL84 early gene and identification of its putative protein product. *J. Virol.*, **66**(2), 1098–1108.

Heider, J. A., Bresnahan, W. A., and Shenk, T. E. (2002). Construction of a rationally designed human cytomegalovirus variant encoding a temperature-sensitive immediate–early 2 protein. *Proc. Natl Acad. Sci. USA*, **99**(5), 3141–3146.

Herendeen, D. R., Kassavetis, G. A., Barry, J., Alberts, B. M., and Geiduschek, E. P. (1989). Enhancement of bacteriophage T4 late transcription by components of the T4 DNA replication apparatus. *Science*, **245**(4921), 952–958.

Herendeen, D. R., Kassavetis, G. A., and Geiduschek, E. P. (1992). A transcriptional enhancer whose function imposes a requirement that proteins track along DNA. *Science*, **256**(5061), 1298–1303.

Hernandez, T. R. and Lehman, I. R. (1990). Functional interaction between the herpes simplex-1 DNA polymerase and UL42 protein. *J. Biol. Chem.*, **265**(19), 11227–11232.

Ho, M. (1991). *Cytomegalovirus: Biology and Infection*. 2nd edn. New York: Plenum Publishing Corporation.

Hofmann, H., Floss, S., and Stamminger, T. (2000). Covalent modification of the transactivator protein IE2-p86 of human cytomegalovirus by conjugation to the ubiquitin-homologous proteins SUMO-1 and hSMT3b. *J. Virol.*, **74**(6), 2510–2524.

Homa, F. L., Otal, T. M., Glorioso, J. C., and Levine, M. (1986). Transcriptional control signals of a herpes simplex virus type 1 late (gamma 2) gene lie within bases -34 to +124 relative to the 5′ terminus of the mRNA. *Mol. Cell Biol.*, **6**(11), 3652–3666.

Huang, E. S. (1975). Human cytomegalovirus. III. Virus-induced DNA polymerase. *J. Virol.*, **16**(2), 298–310.

Huang, L., Zhu, Y., and Anders, D. G. (1996). The variable 3′ ends of a human cytomegalovirus oriLyt transcript (SRT) overlap an essential, conserved replicator element. *J. Virol.*, **70**(8), 5272–5281.

Ilyina, T. V., Gorbalenya, A. E., and Koonin, E. V. (1992). Organization and evolution of bacterial and bacteriophage primase–helicase systems. *J. Mol. Evol.*, **34**(4), 351–357.

Inoue, N. and Pellett, P. E. (1995). Human herpesvirus 6B origin-binding protein: DNA-binding domain and consensus binding sequence. *J. Virol.*, **69**(8), 4619–4627.

Inoue, N., Dambaugh, T. R., Rapp, J. C., and Pellett, P. E. (1994). Alphaherpesvirus origin-binding protein homolog encoded by human herpesvirus 6B, a betaherpesvirus, binds to nucleotide sequences that are similar to ori regions of alphaherpesviruses. *J. Virol.*, **68**(7), 4126–4136.

Jackson, S. A. and DeLuca, N. A. (2003). Relationship of herpes simplex virus genome configuration to productive and persistent infections. *Proc. Natl Acad. Sci. USA*, **100**(13), 7871–7876. Epub 2003 Jun 9.

Jenkins, D. E., Martens, C. L., and Mocarski, E. S. (1994). Human cytomegalovirus late protein encoded by ie2: a trans-activator as well as a repressor of gene expression. *J. Gen. Virol.*, **75**(9), 2337–2348.

Jones, T. R. and Muzithras, V. P. (1991). Fine mapping of transcripts expressed from the cytomegalovirus strain AD169. *J. Virol.*, **65**(4), 2024–2036.

Kemble, G. W., McCormick, A. L., Pereira, L., and Mocarski, E. S. (1987). A cytomegalovirus protein with properties of herpes simplex virus ICP8: partial purification of the polypeptide and map position of the gene. *J. Virol.*, **61**(10), 3143–3151.

Kerry, J. A., Priddy, M. A., Jervey, T. Y. *et al.* (1996). Multiple regulatory events influence human cytomegalovirus DNA polymerase (UL54) expression during viral infection. *J. Virol.*, **70**(1), 373–382.

Kerry, J. A., Priddy, M. A., Kohler, C. P. *et al.* (1997). Translational regulation of the human cytomegalovirus pp28 (UL99) late gene. *J. Virol.*, **71**(2), 981–987.

Kiehl, A., Huang, L., Franchi, D., and Anders, D. G. (2003). Multiple 5′ ends of human cytomegalovirus UL57 transcripts identify a complex, cycloheximide-resistant promoter region that activates oriLyt. *Virology*, **314**(1), 410–422.

Kohler, C. P., Kerry, J. A., Carter, M., Muzithras, V. P., Jones, T. R., and Stenberg, R. M. (1994). Use of recombinant virus to assess human cytomegalovirus early and late promoters in the context of the viral genome. *J. Virol.*, **68**(10), 6589–6597.

Kouzarides, T., Bankier, A. T., Satchwell, S. C., Preddy, E., and Barrell, B. G. (1988). An immediate early gene of human cytomegalovirus encodes a potential membrane glycoprotein. *Virology*, **165**(1), 151–164.

Krosky, P. M., Baek, M. C., Jahng, W. J. *et al.* (2003). The human cytomegalovirus UL44 protein is a substrate for the UL97 protein kinase. *J. Virol.*, **77**(14), 7720–7727.

Krug, L. T., Inoue, N., and Pellett, P. E. (2001). Sequence requirements for interaction of human herpesvirus 7 origin binding protein with the origin of lytic replication. *J. Virol.*, **75**(8), 3925–3936.

Lang, D., Gebert, S., Arlt, H., and Stamminger, T. (1995). Functional interaction between the human cytomegalovirus 86-

kilodalton IE2 protein and the cellular transcription factor CREB. *J. Virol.*, **69**(10), 6030–6037.

Leach, F. S. and Mocarski, E. S. (1989). Regulation of cytomegalovirus late-gene expression: differential use of three start sites in the transcriptional activation of ICP36 gene expression. *J. Virol.*, **63**(4), 1783–1791.

Leatham, M. P., Witte, P. R., and Stinski, M. F. (1991). Alternate promoter selection within a human cytomegalovirus immediate–early and early transcription unit (UL119–115) defines true late transcripts containing open reading frames for putative viral glycoproteins. *J. Virol.*, **65**(11), 6144–6153.

Lee, C. K. and Knipe, D. M. (1985). An immunoassay for the study of DNA-binding activities of herpes simplex virus protein ICP8. *J. Virol.*, **54**(3), 731–738.

Lee, J. M., Kang, H. J., Lee, H. R., Choi, C. Y., Jang, W. J., and Ahn, J. H. (2003). PIAS1 enhances SUMO-1 modification and the major immediate-early IE2 protein of human. *FEBS Lett.*, **555**(2), 322–328.

Li, R., Yang, L., Fouts, E., and Botchan, M. R. (1993). Site-specific DNA-binding proteins important for replication and transcription have multiple activities. *Cold Spring Harb. Symp. Quant. Biol.*, **58**, 403–413.

Lischka, P., Sorg, G., Kann, M., Winkler, M., and Stamminger, T. (2003). A nonconventional nuclear localization signal within the UL84 protein of human cytomegalovirus mediates nuclear import via the importin alpha/beta pathway. *J. Virol.*, **77**(6), 3734–3748.

Loregian, A., Rigatti, R., Murphy, M., Schievano, E., Palu, G., and Marsden, H. S. (2003). Inhibition of human cytomegalovirus DNA polymerase by C-terminal peptides from the UL54 subunit. *J. Virol.*, **77**(15), 8336–8344.

Loregian, A., Appleton, B. A., Hogle, J. M., and Coen, D. M. (2004). Residues of human cytomegalovirus DNA polymerase catalytic subunit UL54 that are necessary and sufficient for interaction with the accessory protein UL44. *J. Virol.*, **78**(1), 158–167.

Lukac, D. M., Manuppello, J. R., and Alwine, J. C. (1994). Transcriptional activation by the human cytomegalovirus immediate–early proteins: requirements for simple promoter structures and interactions with multiple components of the transcription complex. *J. Virol.*, **68**(8), 5184–5193.

Marchini, A., Liu, H., and Zhu, H. (2001). Human cytomegalovirus with IE-2 (UL122) deleted fails to express early lytic genes. *J. Virol.*, **75**(4), 1870–1878.

Masse, M. J., Karlin, S., Schachtel, G. A., and Mocarski, E. S. (1992). Human cytomegalovirus origin of DNA replication (oriLyt) resides within a highly complex repetitive region. *Proc. Natl Acad. Sci. USA*, **89**(12), 5246–5250.

Masse, M. J., Messerle, M., and Mocarski, E. S. (1997). The location and sequence composition of the murine cytomegalovirus replicator (oriLyt). *Virology*, **230**(2), 350–360.

McCormick, L., Igarashi, K., and Roizman, B. (1999). Posttranscriptional regulation of US11 in cells infected with a herpes simplex virus 1 recombinant lacking both 222-bp domains containing S-component origins of DNA synthesis. *Virology*, **259**(2), 286–298.

McMahon, T. P. and Anders, D. G. (2002). Interactions between human cytomegalovirus helicase–primase proteins. *Virus Res.*, **86**(1–2), 39–52.

McVoy, M. A. and Adler, S. P. (1994). Human cytomegalovirus DNA replicates after early circularization by concatemer formation, and inversion occurs within the concatemer. *J. Virol.*, **68**(2), 1040–1051.

McWatters, B. J., Stenberg, R. M., and Kerry, J. A. (2002). Characterization of the human cytomegalovirus UL75 (glycoprotein H) late gene promoter. *Virology*, **303**(2), 309–316.

Menegazzi, P., Galvan, M., Rotola, A. *et al.* (1999). Temporal mapping of transcripts in human herpesvirus-7. *J. Gen. Virol.*, **80**(10), 2705–2712.

Mirandola, P., Menegazzi, P., Merighi, S., Ravaioli, T., Cassai, E., and Di Luca, D. (1998). Temporal mapping of transcripts in herpesvirus 6 variants. *J. Virol.*, **72**(5), 3837–3844.

Mocarski, E. J. and Courcelle, CT., (2001). Cytomegaloviruses and their replication. In *Fields Virology* 4th edn. ed. D. M. Knipe, P. M. Howley, D. E. Griffin *et al.* Vol. 2, pp. 2629–2673. 2 vols. Philadelphia, PA: Lippincott Williams & Wilkins.

Mocarski, E. S., Pereira, L., and Michael, N. (1985). Precise localization of genes on large animal virus genomes: use of lambda gt11 and monoclonal antibodies to map the gene for a cytomegalovirus protein family. *Proc. Natl Acad. Sci. USA*, **82**(4), 1266–1270.

Morello, C. S., Ye, M., and Spector, D. H. (2002). Development of a vaccine against murine cytomegalovirus (MCMV), consisting of plasmid DNA and formalin-inactivated MCMV, that provides long-term, complete protection against viral replication. *J. Virol.*, **76**, 4822–4835.

Mousavi-Jazi, M., Hokeberg, I., Schloss, L. *et al.* (2001). Sequence analysis of UL54 and UL97 genes and evaluation of antiviral susceptibility of human cytomegalovirus isolates obtained from kidney allograft recipients before and after treatment. *Transpl. Infect. Dis.*, **3**(4), 195–202.

Mousavi-Jazi, M., Schloss, L., Wahren, B., and Brytting, M. (2003). Point mutations induced by foscarnet (PFA) in the human cytomegalovirus DNA polymerase. *J. Clin. Virol.*, **26**(3), 301–306.

Murphy, E., Rigoutsos, I., Shibuya, T., and Shenk, T. E. (2003a). Reevaluation of human cytomegalovirus coding potential. *Proc. Natl Acad. Sci. USA*, **100**(23), 13585–13590. Epub 2003 Oct 30.

Murphy, E., Yu, D., Grimwood, J. *et al.* (2003b). Coding potential of laboratory and clinical strains of human cytomegalovirus. *Proc. Natl Acad. Sci. USA*, **100**(25), 14976–14981. Epub 2003 Dec 1.

Olivo, P. D., Nelson, N. J., and Challberg, M. D. (1988). Herpes simplex virus DNA replication: the UL9 gene encodes an origin-binding protein. *Proc. Natl Acad. Sci. USA*, **85**(15), 5414–5418.

Pari, G. S. and Anders, D. G. (1993). Eleven loci encoding trans-acting factors are required for transient complementation of human cytomegalovirus oriLyt-dependent DNA replication. *J. Virol.*, **67**(12), 6979–6988.

Penfold, M. E. and Mocarski, E. S. (1997). Formation of cytomegalovirus DNA replication compartments defined by localization of viral proteins and DNA synthesis. *Virology*, **239**(1), 46–61.

Perkins, K. D., Gregonis, J., Borge, S., and Rice, S. A. (2003). Transactivation of a viral target gene by herpes simplex virus ICP27 is posttranscriptional and does not require the endogenous promoter or polyadenylation site. *J. Virol.*, **77**(18), 9872–9884.

Plachter, B., Britt, W., Vornhagen, R., Stamminger, T., and Jahn, G. (1993). Analysis of proteins encoded by IE regions 1 and 2 of human cytomegalovirus using monoclonal antibodies generated against recombinant antigens. *Virology*, **193**(2), 642–652.

Prichard, M. N., Jairath, S., Penfold, M. E., St Jeor, S., Bohlman, M. C., and Pari, G. S. (1998). Identification of persistent RNA-DNA hybrid structures within the origin of replication of human cytomegalovirus. *J. Virol.*, **72**(9), 6997–7004.

Puchtler, E. and Stamminger, T. (1991). An inducible promoter mediates abundant expression from the immediate–early 2 gene region of human cytomegalovirus at late times after infection. *J. Virol.*, **65**(11), 6301–6306.

Reboredo, M., Greaves, R. F., and Hahn, G. (2004). Human cytomegalovirus proteins encoded by UL37 exon 1 protect infected fibroblasts against virus-induced apoptosis and are required for efficient virus replication. *J. Gen. Virol.*, **85**, 3555–3567.

Reid, G. G., Ellsmore, V., and Stow, N. D. (2003). An analysis of the requirements for human cytomegalovirus oriLyt-dependent DNA synthesis in the presence of the herpes simplex virus type 1 replication fork proteins. *Virology*, **308**(2), 303–316.

Reuven, N. B., Willcox, S., Griffith, J. D., and Weller, S. K. (2004). Catalysis of strand exchange by the HSV-1 UL12 ICP8 recombinase activity is revealed upon nuclease. *J. Mol. Biol.*, **342**(1), 57–71.

Ripalti, A., Boccuni, M. C., Campanini, F., and Landini, M. P. (1995). Cytomegalovirus-mediated induction of antisense mRNA expression to UL44 inhibits virus replication in an astrocytoma cell line: identification of an essential gene. *J. Virol.*, **69**, 2047–2057.

Romanowski, M. J. and Shenk, T. (1997). Characterization of the human cytomegalovirus irs1 and trs1 genes: a second immediate–early transcription unit within irs1 whose product antagonizes transcriptional activation. *J. Virol.*, **71**(2), 1485–1496.

Rudolph, S. A., Stamminger, T., and Jahn, G. (1990). Transcriptional analysis of the eight-kilobase mRNA encoding the major capsid protein of human cytomegalovirus. *J. Virol.*, **64**(10), 5167–5172.

Ruyechan, W. T. (1983). The major herpes simplex virus DNA-binding protein holds single-stranded DNA in an extended configuration. *J. Virol.*, **46**(2), 661–666.

Samaniego, L. A., Tevethia, M. J., and Spector, D. J. (1994). The human cytomegalovirus 86-kilodalton immediate–early 2 protein: synthesis as a precursor polypeptide and interaction with a 75-kilodalton protein of probable viral origin. *J. Virol.*, **68**(2), 720–729.

Sanchez, V., Clark, C. L., Yen, J. Y., Dwarakanath, R., and Spector, D. H. (2002). Viable human cytomegalovirus recombinant virus with an internal deletion of the IE2 86 gene affects late stages of viral replication. *J. Virol.*, **76**(6), 2973–2989.

Sarisky, R. T. and Hayward, G. S. (1996). Evidence that the UL84 gene product of human cytomegalovirus is essential for promoting oriLyt-dependent DNA replication and formation of replication compartments in cotransfection assays. *J. Virol.*, **70**(11), 7398–7413.

Schwartz, R., Helmich, B., and Spector, D. H. (1996). CREB and CREB-binding proteins play an important role in the IE2 86-kilodalton protein-mediated transactivation of the human cytomegalovirus 2.2-kilobase RNA promoter. *J. Virol.*, **70**(10), 6955–6966.

Scully, A. L., Sommer, M. H., Schwartz, R., and Spector, D. H. (1995). The human cytomegalovirus IE2 86-kilodalton protein interacts with an early gene promoter via site-specific DNA binding and protein–protein associations. *J. Virol.*, **69**(10), 6533–6540.

Severini, A., Sevenhuysen, C., Garbutt, M., and Tipples, G. A. (2003). Structure of replicating intermediates of human herpesvirus type 6. *Virology*, **314**(1), 443–450.

Smith, J. A. and Pari, G. S. (1995). Human cytomegalovirus UL102 gene. *J. Virol.*, **69**(3), 1734–1740.

Smith, J. A., Jairath, S., Crute, J. J., and Pari, G. S. (1996). Characterization of the human cytomegalovirus UL105 gene and identification of the putative helicase protein. *Virology*, **220**(1), 251–255.

Spector, D. J. and Tevethia, M. J. (1994). Protein-protein interactions between human cytomegalovirus IE2–580aa and pUL84 in lytically infected cells. *J. Virol.*, **68**(11), 7549–7553.

Stamey, F. R., Dominguez, G., Black, J. B., Dambaugh, T. R., and Pellett, P. E. (1995). Intragenomic linear amplification of human herpesvirus 6B oriLyt suggests acquisition of oriLyt by transposition. *J. Virol.*, **69**(1), 589–596.

Stasiak, P. C. and Mocarski, E. S. (1992). Transactivation of the cytomegalovirus ICP36 gene promoter requires the alpha gene product TRS1 in addition to IE1 and IE2. *J. Virol.*, **66**(2), 1050–1058.

Tanguy LeGac, N., Villani, G., and Boehmer, P. E. (1998). Herpes simplex virus type-1 single-strand DNA-binding protein (ICP8) enhances the ability of the viral DNA helicase–primase to unwind cisplatin-modified DNA. *J. Biol. Chem.*, **273**(22), 13801–13807.

Tenney, D. J. and Colberg-Poley, A. M. (1991a). Expression of the human cytomegalovirus UL36–38 immediate early region during permissive infection. *Virology*, **182**(1), 199–210.

Tenney, D. J., and Colberg-Poley, A. M. (1991b). Human cytomegalovirus UL36–38 and US3 immediate–early genes: temporally regulated expression of nuclear, cytoplasmic, and polysome-associated transcripts during infection. *J. Virol.*, **65**(12), 6724–6734.

van Loon, N., Dykes, C., Deng, H., Dominguez, G., Nicholas, J., and Dewhurst, S. (1997). Identification and analysis of a lytic-phase origin of DNA replication in human herpesvirus 7. *J. Virol.*, **71**(4), 3279–3284.

Vink, C., Beuken, E., and Bruggeman, C. A. (1997). Cloning and functional characterization of the origin of lytic-phase DNA replication of rat cytomegalovirus. *J. Gen. Virol.*, **78**(11), 2963–2973.

Wade, E. J. and Spector, D. H. (1994). The human cytomegalovirus origin of DNA replication (oriLyt) is the critical *cis*-acting sequence regulating replication-dependent late induction of the viral 1.2-kilobase RNA promoter. *J. Virol.*, **68**(10), 6567–6577.

Wahren, B., Ruden, U., Gadler, H., Oberg, B., and Eriksson, B. (1985). Activity of the cytomegalovirus genome in the presence of PPi analogs. *J. Virol.*, **56**(3), 996–1001.

Wara-aswapati, N., Yang, Z., Waterman, W. R. *et al.* (1999). Cytomegalovirus IE2 protein stimulates interleukin 1beta gene transcription via tethering to Spi-1/PU.1. *Mol. Cell Biol.*, **19**(10), 6803–6814.

Weir, J. P. (2001). Regulation of herpes simplex virus gene expression. *Gene*, **271**(2), 117–130.

White, E. A., Clark, C. L., Sanchez, V., and Spector, D. H. (2004). Small internal deletions in the human cytomegalovirus IE2 gene result in nonviable recombinant viruses with differential defects in viral gene expression. *J. Virol.*, **78**(4), 1817–1830.

Wiebusch, L., Truss, M., and Hagemeier, C. (2004). Inhibition of human cytomegalovirus replication by small interfering RNAs. *J. Gen. Virol.*, **85**(1), 179–184.

Wilkinson, G. W., Akrigg, A., and Greenaway, P. J. (1984). Transcription of the immediate early genes of human cytomegalovirus strain AD169. *Virus Res.*, **1**(2), 101–106.

Wilson, B. J., Bates, G. J., Nicol, S. M., Gregory, D. J., Perkins, N. D., and Fuller-Pace, F. V. (2004). The p68 and p72 DEAD box RNA helicases interact transcription in a promoter-specific manner. *BMC Mol. Biol.*, **5**(1), 11.

Wing, B. A., Johnson, R. A., and Huang, E. S. (1998). Identification of positive and negative regulatory regions involved in regulating expression of the human cytomegalovirus UL94 late promoter: role of IE2–86 and cellular p53 in mediating negative regulatory function. *J. Virol.*, **72**(3), 1814–1825.

Wu, C. A., Nelson, N. J., McGeoch, D. J., and Challberg, M. D. (1988). Identification of herpes simplex virus type 1 genes required for origin-dependent DNA synthesis. *J. Virol.*, **62**(2), 435–443.

Wu, J., O'Neill, J., and Barbosa, M. S. (2001). Late temporal gene expression from the human cytomegalovirus pp28US (UL99) promoter when integrated into the host cell chromosome. *J. Gen. Virol.*, **82**(5), 1147–1155.

Xu, Y., Colletti, K. S., and Pari, G. S. (2002). Human cytomegalovirus UL84 localizes to the cell nucleus via a nuclear localization signal and is a component of viral replication compartments. *J. Virol.*, **76**(17), 8931–8938.

Xu, Y., Cei, S. A., Rodriguez Huete, A., Colletti, K. S., and Pari, G. S. (2004). Human cytomegalovirus DNA replication requires transcriptional activation via an IE2- and UL84-responsive bidirectional promoter element within oriLyt. *J. Virol.*, **78**(21), 11664–11677.

Yu, D., Silva, M. C., and Shenk, T. (2003). Functional map of human cytomegalovirus AD169 defined by global mutational analysis. *Proc. Natl Acad. Sci. USA*, **100**(21), 12396–12401. Epub 2003 Sep 30.

Zhang, H., al-Barazi, H. O., and Colberg-Poley, A. M. (1996). The acidic domain of the human cytomegalovirus UL37 immediate early glycoprotein is dispensable for its transactivating activity and localization but is not for its synergism. *Virology*, **223**(2), 292–302.

Zhu, Y., Huang, L., and Anders, D. G. (1998). Human cytomegalovirus oriLyt sequence requirements. *J. Virol.*, **72**(6), 4989–4996.

20

Maturation and egress

William J. Britt

Department of Pediatrics, University of Alabama at Birmingham, AL, USA

Introduction

The assembly of betaherpesviruses, specifically cytomegaloviruses, is a topic of considerable interest to virologists and structural biologists. These viruses are among the largest and most complex animal viruses and encode a large number of proteins. Some clinical isolates of human cytomegalovirus (HCMV) have been predicted to contain as many as 250 ORFs (Chee et al., 1990; Murphy et al., 2003), while other authors have suggested that the coding capacity of HCMV may actually be on the order of 165 ORFs (see Chapter 14). Although the number of virus-encoded proteins that are incorporated into the infectious particle is unknown, estimates from several laboratories suggest that it could approach 100 proteins (Varnum et al., 2004). In addition, the particle also contains an unknown number of host cell proteins, some that may have functional significance in the replicative cycle of these viruses (Varnum et al., 2004). Thus, the complexity of virus assembly rivals that of some cellular organelles. Furthermore, CMVs do not arrest host cell protein synthesis even at late phases of replication as do the alphaherpesviruses and therefore during their assembly can either compete with host cell protein synthetic and targeting pathways or more likely, express viral specific functions that modulate host cellular pathways to optimize viral protein synthesis and transport. Identification of these virus-specified host cell modifications together with their interactions with virion proteins will aid in the understanding of the assembly of this virus. Similar approaches have provided a reasonably detailed view of the assembly pathways of bacteriophages and eukaryotic RNA viruses, including HIV-1, and these studies have in some instances served as templates for investigations of DNA virus assembly. However, herpesviruses encode vastly more virion proteins compared to RNA viruses, and assembly takes place in both nuclear and cytoplasmic compartments. Definitive studies of capsid assembly have been carried out in alphaherpesviruses and have been extended to include in vitro, cell free assembly of the herpes simplex viral (HSV) capsid (Newcomb et al., 1994). Many of the capsid proteins of CMVs and other betaherpesviruses share extensive structural and functional homology with HSV capsid proteins and cryoelectron microscopic analysis of the HCMV capsid suggests similar, but not identical, capsid structure (Butcher et al., 1998; Chen et al., 1999; Trus et al., 1999; Zhou et al., 1999, 2000). The most structurally diverse region of the herpesvirus virion appears to be the tegument which is composed of a great many betaherpesvirus- and CMV-unique proteins. Although proteins with homologous functions localized to this region of the virus can be readily identified for many different herpesviruses, only a limited number of these proteins exhibit significant structural homologies (Mocarski and Tan Courcelle, C., 2001). Despite these similarities, a large number of structural proteins appear to be unique for each subfamily of herpesviruses and in some cases, such as HCMV, several tegument proteins have no counterparts in alphaherpesviruses (Mocarski and Tan Courcelle, C., 2001). Together, these findings suggest that, although common themes likely exist for herpesvirus assembly, it is almost certain that distinct aspects of the assembly pathway of each of these viruses will be identified and these differences in the assembly of different herpes viruses could point to key features of the infectious cycle of these viruses.

Early studies of the assembly of alphaherpesviruses including HSV suggested that virion envelopment occurred at the nuclear membrane (Campadelli-Fiume et al., 1991; Johnson and Spear, 1982). This concept was extended to other herpesviruses including HCMV, even though early studies utilizing electron microscopy suggested major differences between the morphogenesis of these two viruses, both within the infected cell and in the overall appearance of extracellular virions (Smith and DeHarven, E., 1973). Subsequent studies of alphaherpesviruses provided evidence for nuclear envelopment–de-envelopment followed by envelopment at cytoplasmic membranes (Granzow et al., 1997; Jones et al., 1988; Whealy et al., 1991). These reports provided clear evidence that perinuclear virions contained a different subset of tegument and envelope proteins than mature virions, findings that support acquisition and then loss of an immature envelope by perinuclear virions (Brack et al., 1999; Granzow et al., 1997, 2001; Klupp et al., 2000). These results have been further supported by more recent studies of viruses with deletion mutations in genes encoding both virion envelope and tegument proteins (Brack et al., 1999; Fuchs et al., 2002; Kopp et al., 2003). The elegant studies of pseudorabies virus (PRV) have provided definitive evidence of cytoplasmic virion envelopment and served as a guide for studies of the envelopment of β-herpesviruses (Mettenleiter, 2002). The envelopment of CMVs, specifically HCMV, also appears to take place within a cytoplasmic compartment based on studies of tegument protein trafficking and incorporation into the virion particle (Britt et al., 2004; Sanchez et al., 2000a; Silva et al., 2003). Major gaps remain in the understanding of capsid tegumentation, capsid egress from the nucleus, and cytoplasmic assembly of the mature, infectious HCMV particle. The development of bacterial artificial chromosome (BAC) technology that allows the maintenance of HCMV as infectious clones coupled with the application of techniques of recombinant prokaryotic genetic manipulation has accelerated experimental studies in HCMV assembly (Adler et al., 2003; Borst et al., 1999; Messerle et al., 2000; Smith and Enquist, L. W., 1999). Together with other technologies such as mass spectrometry and cryoelectron microscopy, current studies should provide more definitive understanding of this complex process. In the following review, the focus will be on the assembly of HCMV as a model for betaherpesvirus assembly because the majority of studies have been carried out in systems utilizing HCMV or the related virus, murine CMV (MCMV). When possible, studies of other betaherpesvirus will be discussed.

Assembly of the capsid

Structural studies of the HSV capsid have indicated that structural and functional protein homologues of HSV capsid proteins are present in the capsid of HCMV, HHV-6, and HHV-7 (Table 20.1). Cryoelectron microscopic analysis of the capsids of HCMV and HSV have revealed near identical structures, albeit with slight differences in the floor of the capsid, perhaps because of the larger size of the HCMV genome (Butcher et al., 1998; Chen et al., 1999; Trus et al., 1999; Zhou et al., 2000). Because of this structural conservation, it has been assumed that the assembly of the HCMV capsid as well as capsids of other β-herpesviruses follow a very similar assembly pathway as that of HSV (Steven et al., 1997; Grunewald et al., 2003). The size of the HCMV particle is approximately 2000 angstroms. The nucleocapsid is approximately 1300 angstroms and is of iscosahedral $T = 16$ symmetry (Butcher et al., 1998; Chen et al., 1999). As noted in Table 20.1, there are six identified protein components of the mature HCMV capsid present in the infectious particle (Gibson, 1996). Interestingly, the capsid proteins from both HSV and HCMV share considerable structural and biochemical characteristics and, in the case of MCP, even express cross-reactive antibody binding sites (Rudolph et al., 1990).

The HCMV capsid is composed of 162 capsomeres consisting of 150 hexons and 12 pentons (Butcher et al., 1998; Chen et al., 1999). The most abundant protein components of the capsid is the major capsid protein (MCP, UL86) and the smallest capsid protein (SCP, UL48–49), with 960 and 900 copies respectively present in each capsid. Two copies of the minor capsid protein (MnCP, UL85; triplex dimer or TR-2) combined with a single copy of the minor capsid binding protein (MnCP-bp; triplex monomer or TR-1) UL46 form the triplexes that are located between adjacent pentons and hexons (Fig. 20.1) (Butcher et al., 1998; Chen et al., 1999; Gibson, 1996; Gibson et al., 1996; Trus et al., 1999). The capsid pentons and hexons are assembled entirely from the major capsid protein. Each hexon is decorated on each vertex with the smallest capsid protein (Yu et al., 2005). The smallest capsid protein of HSV, Vp26, has been shown to be dispensable for capsid assembly in cell culture, whereas deletion of the HCMV homologue results in the loss of infectivity, presumably by preventing the assembly of infectious virions (Borst et al., 2001). A cartoon depicting the assembly pathway is detailed in Fig. 20.1.

Protein interactions and capsid assembly

As noted above, evidence from transmission electron microscopy and cryo-EM, combined with the conservation of capsid protein function, suggests that the capsid assembly of HCMV and other betaherpesviruses closely follows that of HSV (Beaudet-Miller et al., 1996; Gibson, 1996, Gibson et al., 1996, 1990, 1993; Welch et al., 1991a,b; Wood et al., 1997; Grunewald et al., 2003). Yet several unique features of the HCMV capsid such as the role of the smallest capsid protein in production of infectious virions suggest that there are differences in the assembly of capsids of these two viruses. Although the atomic structure of HCMV capsid proteins has not been determined, several reports have characterized some of the more relevant protein–protein

Table 20.1. Proteins of the capsid of β-herpesviruses: comparison with HSV

Protein	HSV	HCMV[1]	HHV-6; HHV-7[2]
Major capsid protein	Vp5 (UL119)	MCP (UL86)*	U57
Small capsid protein	Vp26 (UL35)	SCP (UL48A)*	U32
Minor capsid protein[3]	Vp 23(UL18)	MnCP (UL85)*	U56
Minor capsid protein[3]	Vp19c (UL38)	MnCP-bp (UL46)*	U29
Assembly protein	Vp 22a (UL26.5)	Assembly protein (UL80.5)	–
Assembly protein precursor	Vp21(UL26)	Assemblin precursor$_{COOH}$ (UL80a)	U53
Assembly protein precursor	Vp24 (UL26)	Assemblin (UL80a)*	–
Portal protein	Vp (UL6)	UL104	U76

[1] The * indicates capsid proteins that have been demonstrated in infectious virions. Pre-B capsids are thought to contain products of both the UL80a and UL80.5 orfs, mature virions have also been shown to contain products of the UL80a orf, but not UL80.5. Modified from Gibson (Gibson, 1996)

[2] Homologous orf from HHV-6 and HHV-7 based on published nucleotide sequence (Dominguez et al., 1999; Gompels et al., 1995; Nicholas, 1996)

[3] The MnCP (UL85) is also referred to as the triplex dimer protein or TR-2 and the MnCP-bp is referred to as the triplex monomer protein or TR-1.

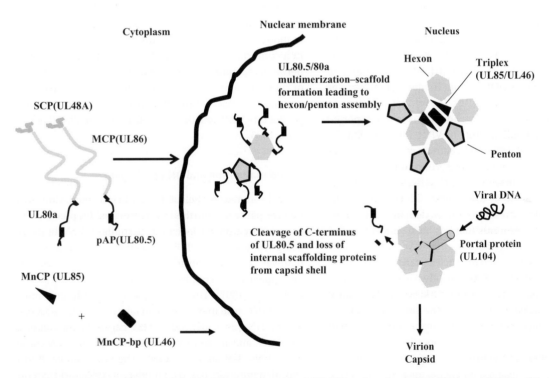

Fig. 20.1. Model of HCMV encapsidation. (1) The capsid proteins MCP, SCP, and products of the UL80a and UL80.5 orf that contain a MCP binding domain are thought to interact in the cytoplasm and are then translocated into the nucleus of the infected cell. The MnCP (UL85) and MnCP-bp (UL46) are also translocated into the nucleus but not as part of the SCP/MCP/UL80a,80.5 complex. (2) Once in the nucleus, self-interaction domains in the products of the UL80a (assemblin precursor) or the UL80.5 (assembly protein) lead to formation of pentons and hexons and the generation of the capsid scaffold. These structures then interact with the triplex formed between MnCP and MnCP-bp and pre-capsid shells form. (3) Unit length viral DNA is inserted into the capsid shell by proteins of the packaging/terminase complex including the proteins encoded by the UL89 and UL56 orfs through the capsid portal formed by the products of the UL104 orf. Coupled with the entry of viral DNA is the extrusion of the assembly protein (and forms of the assembling precursor secondary to cleavage at the carboxyl domain of these proteins). Nomenclature and model adapted from Gibson (Gibson 1996).

interactions that appear to be required for HCMV capsid assembly. The identity of participating cellular proteins and in many cases the temporal order of protein–protein interactions that lead to capsid formation remain undefined. The template for HCMV capsid assembly can be derived from the pioneering studies of HSV capsid assembly from several laboratories (Heymann et al., 2003; Newcomb et al., 1994, 1996, 1999, 2001; Oien et al., 1997; Tatman et al., 1994; Zhou et al., 2000).

The initial steps of capsid assembly involve formation of a scaffold for the generation of the capsid subunit and the pre-capsid structures, protein interactions between the MCP and UL80a and UL80.5, and possible interactions between MCP and SCP. The scaffolding protein(s) of HCMV has been identified as gene products of UL80a and UL80.5 ORFs (Welch et al., 1991a, b). These genes are organized as nested, in-frame 3-coterminal genes that give rise to four transcripts and four gene products with common carboxyl termini (Welch et al., 1991a). The largest transcript is derived from UL80a and encodes the proteinase precursor which includes the HCMV proteinase in the amino terminal half of the precursor and the assembly protein in the carboxyl terminal half (Welch et al., 1991a,b). Self-cleavage of UL80a by the proteinase function leads to generation of the assemblin and a COOH terminal fragment that overlaps with UL80.5 (Welch et al., 1991b). The role of this protein in capsid assembly appears to be analogous to that reported for the HSV scaffolding protein, VP24 (Liu and Stinski, 1992b; Preston et al., 1992, 1994; Tatman et al., 1994). A second protein, the assembly protein, is the product of UL80.5, a nested ORF collinear with the carboxyl terminus of UL80a. The proteins encoded by the longest ORF, UL80a, and the UL80.5 ORF both express a conserved domain (CCD) at the extreme carboxyl terminus that has been shown to interact with the HCMV MCP (Gibson, 1996; Wood et al., 1997). This interaction is required for nuclear translocation of the MCP (and presumably SCP) because the MCP lack a nuclear localization signal and its mass of 150 kDa would exclude it from passive nuclear entry. Consistent with this prediction is the finding that expression of MCP in the absence of other viral proteins results in cytoplasmic localization (Beaudet-Miller et al., 1996; Lai and Britt, W. J., 2003; Nicholson et al., 1994). Because a conserved functional nuclear localization signal is present in the C-terminal domain of UL80.5 as well as some forms of UL80a, interaction between these proteins and MCP results in the nuclear translocation of MCP (Beaudet-Miller et al., 1996) as depicted in Fig. 20.1. An amino-terminal conserved domain (ACD) can be found in the amino terminal domain of UL80.5 and the corresponding cleavage product of UL80a. This domain promotes self-interaction and has been suggested to lead to the generation of UL80a and UL80.5 multimers (Beaudet-Miller et al., 1996; Gibson, 1996; Wood et al., 1997). The self-interaction, together with interactions with MCP, is thought to catalyze the association of MCP into multimers leading to the formation of intranuclear hexons and pentons (Fig. 20.1) (Gibson, 1996). Interestingly, the SCP has also been shown to interact with the MCP in the absence of other viral proteins (Lai and Britt, W. J., 2003). The sequences of SCP that are responsible for this interaction have been mapped but the functional significance of this interaction has not been studied in the context of replicating virus (Lai and Britt, W. J., 2003). The interaction between these two abundant and essential components of the capsid raises several important questions, including if the observed interaction between the SCP and MCP is critical for structural events leading to capsid assembly or for a downstream event in virion assembly such as capsid/tegument interactions required for capsid tegumentation and virion assembly. Interactions between the products of the UL85 and UL46 have also been demonstrated by two-hybrid systems (Gibson et al., 1996). This interaction is required for the formation of the triplexes of the capsid and presumably results in a conformational change that allows their positioning between capsomeres. The interacting sequences of this set of capsid proteins have not been unequivocally mapped, perhaps as a result of the limited solubility of the protein products of UL46 and their aggregation by heating (Gibson et al., 1996).

Capsid maturation and DNA packaging

Once the immature shell of the capsid is formed, viral DNA must be packaged into this immature capsid or precapsid to generate a mature nucleocapsid. In studies of HSV the packaging of unit length viral DNA takes place in a well described pathway in which capsid maturation and DNA packaging appear to be coupled (Heymann et al., 2003; Steven and Spear, 1997). However, capsid assembly and most aspects of capsid maturation can take place in the absence of viral DNA as evidenced by HSV capsid formation in a virus-free and in an in vitro cell free system (Newcomb et al., 1994; Tatman et al., 1994). The final step in HCMV capsid maturation, based on models of HSV capsid assembly, involve proteolytic cleavage of the carboxyl terminal MCP binding domain (M domain) of UL80.5 and M domain containing forms of UL80a in the shells of the immature B-capsids and including any full length UL80a that may be present in these precapsid forms (Gibson, 1996). The loss of the UL80 encoded scaffolding structures appears to be coupled to viral DNA packaging (Gibson, 1996; Lee et al., 1988). Unit length viral DNA enters the maturing capsid presumably through an asymmetric site of the capsid structure that based on the HSV model, contains a portal protein. In the case of HCMV, the portal protein has been proposed to be encoded by the UL104 product (Komazin et al., 2004). Entering viral DNA is thought to lead to extrusion of the cleavage products of the UL80 from the virion capsid (Gibson, 1996). It is likely that fragments of UL80a or 80.5 remain in the capsid; however, their role in the maintenance of the structure of the virion capsid is unclear.

The packaging of viral DNA is mediated through virus-encoded protein recognition of two conserved sequence motifs, the *pac-1* and *pac-2* sequences, that are located in the *a* sequence at each end of the viral genome (Mocarski and Tan Courcelle C., 2001). The virus proteins mediating packaging comprise the viral terminase complex that consists of at least two proteins, the products of the UL56 and UL89 orfs, that function together with the UL104 portal protein (Bogner et al., 1998; Giesen et al., 2000; Scheffczik et al., 2002; Scholz et al., 2003). The product of UL56 is a 130 kDa protein that has been shown to bind to AT rich sequences in the *pac* sequences and also to have nuclease activity, both activities that suggest its role in packaging as well as cleavage of viral DNA (Bogner et al., 1998; Scholz et al., 2003). More recently, studies from this same laboratory have suggested that the product of the UL89 ORF, a 75 kDa protein, is actually responsible for the DNA cleavage activity that has been assigned to the terminase complex (Scheffczik et al., 2002). Interestingly, the activity of several members of a group of antiviral drugs that have in common a benzimidazole core structure has been shown to map to UL89 and UL56 (Krosky et al., 1998). Although these two proteins are essential for the recognition and packaging of unit length viral DNA, several unexpected findings in studies of the mechanism of action of the benzimidazole antiviral drugs, including maribavir, have suggested that other virus-encoded proteins could be present in this cleavage-packaging complex.

Nuclear tegumentation and nuclear egress

Reports from several laboratories in the early 1990s resolved several inconsistencies in the literature of alphaherpesvirus envelopment. These studies lead to a model in which virion capsids are initially enveloped at the nuclear envelope and following a de-envelopment step at the outer nuclear membrane are delivered to the cytoplasm for final envelopment at cytoplasmic membranes (Brack et al., 1999; Jones and Grose, C., 1988; Skeppner et al., 2001; Wang et al., 2000; Whealy et al., 1991; Zhu et al., 1995). These studies of capsid egress from the nucleus of HSV (or PRV, VZV) infected cells have been illuminating, but differences in cellular tropism, replication, virion protein composition and virion morphology between betaherpesviruses and alphaherpesviruses suggest that virion assembly distal to the nuclear events of encapsidation could be significantly different. Furthermore, more recent studies have demonstrated that a significant number of tegument proteins encoded by HCMV lack sequence homologues in HSV, and in some cases virion tegument proteins of one betaherpesvirus (HCMV) do not have homologues in other betaherpesviruses, including other cytomegaloviruses. Finally, the changes in the size and morphology of the nucleus that are observed in HCMV infected primary fibroblasts are characteristic of the cytopathic effect of this virus and distinct from changes in cells infected with HSV or PRV. As a result, investigators studying the assembly of HCMV and other betaherpesviruses have postulated models for nuclear egress and envelopment that could be specific to this group of viruses.

Perhaps the most poorly understood aspect of the assembly of herpesviruses is the tegumentation of virion particle. In addition to the undefined number of proteins in the tegument, it remains to be determined whether the essential function of individual tegument proteins is regulatory such as pp71 (UL82), interference with host responses such as pp65 (UL83), structural such as pp28 (UL99), or in some cases multifunctional (Baldick et al., 1997; Browne et al., 2003; Kalejta and Shenk, T., 2003; Liu and Stinski, 1992a; Silva et al., 2003). Thus, genetic deletions affecting ORFs encoding tegument proteins that result in loss of infectivity could be ascribed to several possible mechanisms other than a block in the assembly of an infectious particle secondary to the loss of an essential structural protein. Furthermore, the trafficking of nuclear tegument proteins that eventually are incorporated into the infectious particle remains almost completely unstudied. Examples of the different distribution of HCMV tegument proteins are illustrated in Table 20.2. The most striking aspect of the differing cellular localization of this subset of tegument proteins is that virus assembly presumably requires organization of the tegument to insure ordered incorporation of tegument proteins as well as maintenance of essential protein–protein interactions.

This can be readily explained by a radial distribution of tegument proteins in the particle and by the sequential addition of these proteins during nucleocapsid transit from the nucleus through cellular compartments that are used for final assembly. However, cryoelectron microscopic analysis of the virion structure, although consistent with the sequential acquisition of tegument proteins, has not provided definitive evidence for such a pathway leading to tegument assembly (Chen et al., 1999; Trus et al., 1999).

Table 20.2. Cellular localization of a subset of HCMV tegument proteins

		Cellular localization in productive infection		
ORF	Protein	Nucleus	Cytoplasm	Nucleus and cytoplasm
UL25	ppUL25	−	+	−
UL26	ppUL26	+	−	−
UL32	pp150	+[2]	+	−
UL48	pp200	+	−	−
UL50	p35	+	−	−
UL53	pp38	+	−	+[1]
UL69	ppUL69	+	−	−
UL82	pp71	+	−	?
UL83	pp65	+	−	+[1]
UL94	pp36	+	−	−
UL99	pp28	−	+	−

[1] This set of tegument proteins remains localized exclusively to the nucleus until late in the replication cycle and then can be found in both the nucleus and cytoplasm.

[2] Nuclear localization of pp150 can be demonstrated with different conditions of fixation.

Thus, the assembly of the tegument layer of HCMV remains unclear and may involve nuclear tegumentation and detegumentation as has been proposed for PRV (Fuchs *et al.*, 2002; Granzow *et al.*, 1997, 2001). Studies of the alphaherpesvirus PRV have demonstrated that nuclear viral capsids are essentially free of detectable tegument proteins and acquire tegument entirely in the cytoplasm (Granzow *et al.*, 1997, 2001). From a combination of elegant electron microscopic analyses and studies of viral deletion mutants, Mittenleiter and colleagues have proposed compelling arguments that the PRV capsid interacts with non-structural virus-encoded nuclear proteins that facilitate capsid envelopment and de-envelopment at the nuclear envelope (Fig. 20.2) (Mettenleiter, 2002). The virus-encoded proteins UL31 and UL34 of PRV are thought to be essential for nuclear egress and have been shown to be localized to the nucleus of infected cells but cannot be detected in the virion (Fuchs *et al.*, 2002). The viral and/or cellular proteins that participate in these nuclear fusion events, other than UL31 and UL 34, have not been identified. Although this model of PRV nuclear egress is consistent with a number of observations from these and other investigators, other examples of tegument protein trafficking fail to fit precisely with this model. An example is the HSV tegument

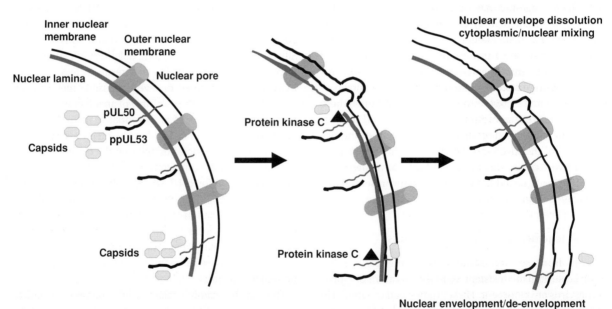

Fig. 20.2. Two models of nuclear egress of the HCMV capsid. The structure of the bi-leaflet nuclear envelope and underlying nuclear lamina is shown. Nuclear pore complexes are depicted as cylinders. Focal accumulation of intranuclear capsids adjacent to inner nuclear membrane domains containing viral proteins encoded by UL50 and UL53, with UL50 shown inserting into inner nuclear membrane. In the top model, nuclear lamina dissolution secondary to lamin phosphorylation associated with localization of protein kinase C activity leads to nuclear envelope herniation, nuclear cytoplasmic mixing and eventual capsid release into the cytoplasm (Muranyi *et al.*, 2002). The nuclear envelope rapidly reseals resulting in only transient nuclear/cytoplasmic mixing. In the bottom model, the focal accumulation of capsids and their interaction with as yet unidentified cellular or virus-encoded proteins leads to a fusion with the inner nuclear envelope protein, translocation into intranuclear space and a second event leading to budding into the cytoplasm. Note the second mechanism of capsid egress is also postulated to require nuclear lamina dissolution.

protein Vp22 (UL49) that has been shown localized to the nucleus of the infected cell and cannot be detected on immature perinuclear capsids, yet it is eventually incorporated into the virion as a tegument protein, presumably during cytoplasmic tegumentation (del Rio et al., 2002). Early electron microscopic findings indicated that the cytoplasmic forms of HCMV contained a considerably thicker tegument as compared to HSV (and presumably PRV) and it is well known that numerous HCMV nuclear tegument proteins are present in the virion. Thus, it is likely that nuclear egress of the HCMV capsid is more complex than the models proposed for alphaherpesviruses. This HCMV pathway of nuclear egress could involve nuclear tegumentation, de-tegumentation, and a final tegumentation that would incorporate virion tegument proteins that localize to the nucleus, or even more simply, both nuclear and cytoplasmic tegumentation.

Early studies of HCMV egress noted that virion structural proteins could be localized to the nuclear matrix of virus infected cells (Sanchez et al., 1998). The nuclear matrix of eukaryotic cells can be viewed as the cytoskeleton of the nucleus. This nuclear structure has been shown to be a site of transcription and DNA replication, including for DNA viruses (Pombo et al., 1994; Schirmbeck et al., 1989). Major components of the nuclear matrix include the nuclear lamins, a group of cellular proteins that represent the intermediate filaments of the nucleus (Stuurman et al., 1998). Nuclear lamins are known to play an important role in the integrity of the nuclear envelope and have been shown to link the nuclear matrix with the inner membrane of the nuclear envelope through their interactions with a number of integral membrane proteins in the inner nuclear membrane, thus creating what is referred to as the nuclear lamina. The finding of a specific interaction of HCMV virion tegument proteins with the nuclear matrix, and in particular lamin B, raised the possibility that this interaction could represent a pathway of nuclear egress of tegumented capsids (Sanchez et al., 1998). Studies have demonstrated that nuclear lamin phosphorylation and dephosphorylation can be coupled with loss of lamin structure and, in some cases, the disruption of the nuclear envelope (Steen et al., 2000; Stuurman et al., 1998). Lamin phosphorylation has been demonstrated in HCMV infected cells and it was initially suggested that either an intrinsic kinase activity of an HCMV encoded protein or a cellular kinase activity localized to regions adjacent to the nuclear envelope could account for phosphorylation of nuclear lamins (Muranyi et al., 2002; Radsak et al., 1991). The focal loss of nuclear envelope integrity has been suggested to contribute to the nuclear egress of the HCMV capsid (Gallina et al., 1999; Sanchez et al., 1998). However, it should be noted that loss of lamin structure alone cannot account for loss of nuclear membrane integrity.

Consistent with proposed mechanisms of egress of HCMV that include a focal loss of nuclear membrane integrity have been studies of the Vpr protein of HIV-1. Expression of this virus-encoded protein has been shown to be associated with the focal loss of nuclear membrane integrity and mixing of cytoplasmic and nuclear proteins (de Noronha et al., 2001). A recent study utilizing murine CMV as a model system reported similar findings by demonstrating that two non-structural nuclear proteins encoded by m50 and m53 could localize host protein kinase C activity to an area adjacent to the nuclear envelope (Muranyi et al., 2002). The redistribution of protein kinase C activity resulted in the phosphorylation of lamins A and C at levels that could be associated with loss of structural integrity of the inner nuclear membrane (Muranyi et al., 2002). The m50 and m53 are sequence homologues of the alphaherpesvirus UL34 and UL31, respectively, and are believed to represent the functional homologues of these proteins. Similar to the alphaherpesvirus UL34 protein, the m50 product is a type II membrane protein that contains motifs with limited homology with known integral membrane proteins of the nuclear envelope (Muranyi et al., 2002). Because both m50 and m53 encode essential functions for virus replication, this finding suggests that nuclear egress of CMVs could require focal disruption of the nuclear lamins leading to the loss of the integrity of the inner nuclear membrane. The homologous proteins of HCMV, pUL50 and ppUL53, have also been shown to be essential for virus replication and interestingly, ppUL53 can be detected in the virion tegument, suggesting that it has an additional role in virus assembly other than its proposed function in facilitating nuclear egress (Dal Monte et al., 2002). Studies of ppUL53 trafficking indicate that, in the absence of other virus-encoded proteins, it is expressed only in the nucleus but that it can be detected in both the nucleus and the virus assembly compartment in virus infected cells late in infection (Dal Monte et al., 2002) (W. Britt, unpublished data). Thus, in contrast to findings in the PRV, one of the essential nuclear virus-encoded proteins that is thought to be required for modification of the nuclear envelope is also found within the tegument of the mature virion. It is unclear if HCMV pUL50 is present in the virion tegument. Expression of the abundant HCMV virion tegument protein pp65 (UL83) is also restricted to the nucleus of infected cells secondary to a functional bipartite nuclear localization signal until late in infection when it is distributed in the cytoplasm and can be detected predominantly in the assembly compartment (Sanchez et al., 2000a). These findings would indicate that either HCMV virions are partially tegumented in the nucleus or that nuclear tegument proteins have trafficking pathways to sites of tegument assembly in the cytoplasm.

Other models of nuclear egress have been proposed yet insufficient data is available to determine their validity. In studies of HHV-7, Frenkel and co-workers described an intranuclear, cytoplasmic vacuole or invagination that appeared to be a site of nuclear budding of the mature capsid (Roffman et al., 1990). This structure designated a tegusome and was identified by electron microscopic analysis of infected cells (Roffman et al., 1990). This structure provided an explanation consistent with the incorporation of virus-encoded nuclear proteins into the tegument of the mature particle. Similar structures have not been identified in other betaherpesviruses.

A pathway of egress of herpesvirus capsids from nucleus that unifies available data has yet to be described. However, it is clear that these viruses have devoted at least some of their genomic information to encode proteins that can either directly modify key structures of the nuclear envelope or recruit cellular functions to the nuclear membrane. These findings would suggest that immature capsids (and possibly tegumented capsids) could exit the nucleus through focal herniations of nuclear membrane as proposed for the function of Vpr of HIV. Alternatively, translocation of the capsid across the nuclear envelope into the cytoplasm of the infected cell could require a membrane fusion event, a mechanism that is favored by the bulk of the literature describing alphaherpesvirus assembly.

Cytoplasmic tegumentation and envelopment

Final tegumentation and envelopment of the infectious betaherpesvirus particle appear to occur exclusively in the cytoplasm of the infected cell. Studies that have described the trafficking of virion tegument and envelope proteins have led to several proposed models of cytoplasmic assembly of the infectious virion. Two studies of HCMV utilizing cryoelectron microscopy indicated that the tegument layer adjacent to the capsid exhibited aspects of iscosahedral symmetry and, from estimates of the mass of the presumed tegument protein that occupied this layer, one group of investigators argued that the protein adjacent to the capsid was pp150 (UL32) (Trus et al., 1999); however, the identity of the protein was not pursued either biochemically or immunologically. The suggestion that the tegument protein pp150 was adjacent to the capsid raised the possibility that this virion protein was acquired during nuclear egress of the capsid. The distribution of pp150 within infected cells was initially proposed to be nuclear and cytoplasmic, although a subsequent study that employed a larger number of viral and cell markers suggested that pp150 was expressed only in the cytoplasm of infected cells (Hensel et al., 1995; Sanchez et al., 2000a). In this latter study, pp150 was used to define an isolable cellular compartment that was designated as the assembly compartment (Sanchez et al., 2000a). This compartment was shown to be localized to a juxtanuclear site that was in close proximity to the microtubular organizing center (MTOC) of infected cells (Sanchez et al., 2000a). Subsequent studies from other laboratories have also identified this cytoplasmic structure (Dal Monte et al., 2002; Silva et al., 2003). A number of both nuclear and cytoplasmic localized tegument proteins have been shown to localize to the assembly compartment, including many of the proteins listed in Tables 20.2 and 20.3. Isolation of this compartment by centrifugation of cell lysates over density gradients allowed the identification of both tegument and envelope proteins, including processed glycoprotein B (gB, UL55) within in this compartment, consistent with this compartment being a site of virus envelopment and assembly. The trafficking and accumulation of virion proteins and subviral structures to this site is not understood; however, recent studies of tegument protein trafficking coupled with a greater understanding of glycoprotein trafficking are beginning to suggest model pathways for its formation within infected cells and may represent a cytoplasmic inclusion identified in early studies of HCMV morphogenesis.

Tegument protein trafficking and incorporation into the particle

Although it is likely that understanding the trafficking of virion tegument proteins will be key to understanding the assembly of the infectious particle, little is known about the localization of these proteins to the assembly compartment. One structural tegument protein for which some features of its intracellular trafficking are known is pp28 (UL99). Studies demonstrated that this small (191 amino acid) myristylated protein is membrane associated and when expressed in the absence of other viral proteins, is retained in the ER/Golgi intermediate compartment (ERGIC) (Sanchez et al., 2000b). In virus infected cells, pp28 is transported to the assembly compartment, where it localizes with envelope glycoproteins and with other tegument proteins including pp150 (Sanchez et al., 2000a; Silva et al., 2003). Recombinant viruses in which the gene encoding UL99 has been deleted, the reading frame has been interrupted, or the protein mistargeted in the infected cell by deletion of the myristylation site are non-infectious and non-enveloped particles were observed in the cytoplasm of cells infected with the mutant pp28 deletion virus (Britt

Table 20.3. HCMV envelope glycoproteins

Glycoprotein	Orf[1]	Complex formation	Essential for infectivity	Proposed function
gB	UL55(U39)	oligomer	Yes	Attachment/fusion
gH	UL75 (U48)	gH/gL/gO	Yes	Fusion/penetration
gL	UL115(U82)	gH/gL/gO	Yes	Fusion/penetration
gO	UL74(U100[2])	gH/gL/gO	Yes	Fusion/penetration
gM	UL100(U72)	gM/gN	Yes	Unknown
gN	UL73(U46)	gM/gN	Yes	Unknown
gpTRL10	TRL10	Unknown	No	Unknown
gpUL132	UL132	Unknown	No	Unknown

[1] Homologous orf from HHV-6 and HHV-7 based on published nucleotide sequence are shown in parentheses (Dominguez *et al.*, 1999; Gompels *et al.*, 1995; Nicholas, 1996).
[2] Note the HHV-6 functional homologue of HCMV gO has been identified as the glycoprotein encoded by HHV-6 orf U100 and has been designated gQ (Mori *et al.*, 2003).

et al., 2004; Jones and Lee, 2004; Silva *et al.*, 2003). Interestingly, the virion assembly compartment was formed in cells infected with the UL99 deletion mutant, indicating that this protein was not required for trafficking of other tegument and presumably envelope proteins to this cytoplasmic compartment. The trafficking of other tegument proteins, including nuclear tegument proteins, to the assembly compartment has not been studied in sufficient detail to allow investigators to develop a model of HCMV tegument assembly.

Envelope glycoprotein trafficking and envelopment of the particle

Similar to the uncertainties that surround the structure and composition of the tegument, the envelope of HCMV remains poorly defined. Although the analysis of the coding sequence of HCMVs suggest that as many as 50 ORFs could encode proteins with N-linked carbohydrate modification, to date, some eight experimentally defined virus specific glycoproteins have been shown to be present in the virion envelope (Table 20.3). At least six of these have been shown to exist as disulfide-linked oligomers (gB, gH/gL/gO; gM/gN) in the virion, a characteristic of CMVs that at first glance appears unique in the herpesvirus family. Formation of these disulfide-linked oligomers takes place in the ER prior to transport of these complexes through the secretory pathway. When expressed in the absence of other viral proteins, glycoproteins (gB) or complexes of glycoproteins (gH/gL/gO; gM/gN) listed in Table 20.3, with the exception of gpTRL10, traffic to Golgi and post-Golgi compartments.

Many of these glycoproteins have been shown to contain well-described signals within their cytoplasmic domains that enable them to utilize the cellular secretory pathway for intracellular trafficking. Examples of these signals include phosphorylated amino acid residues and acidic amino acid clusters that are recognized by cellular adaptor proteins including PACS-1 that localize proteins to the TGN, tyrosine and di-leucine signals that promote glycoprotein retrieval from the cell surface and possibly from other cellular membranes through their interactions with cellular adaptor proteins, and likely other motifs that facilitate interactions with tegument proteins (Crump *et al.*, 2003; Jarvis *et al.*, 2002, Tugizov *et al.*, 1999). Although the role of these various signals on individual glycoproteins has been shown in many cases to function in intracellular trafficking as predicted based on studies of similar signals on other viral glycoproteins, it remains unclear what role these signals play in the assembly and infectivity of the mature virion. As an example, it has been argued that gB in the envelope of infectious virus was derived from cell surface gB retrieved from the cell surface by endocytosis and targeted to the TGN, a presumed site of virus assembly (Radsak *et al.*, 1996; Tugizov *et al.*, 1999). Yet recent studies have shown that mutation of this targeting signal in gB has no effect on the phenotype of the mutant virus when compared to wild-type virus (Jarvis *et al.*, 2002). This latter finding raises several possible interpretations such as a redundancy of targeting signals in the cytoplasmic domain of HCMV virion glycoproteins or that additional intracellular pathways are operative in cells infected with this virus that enable the virion glycoproteins to localize in the assembly compartment. However, it is important to note that several of these glycoproteins have very conventional targeting motifs that are conserved in their cytoplasmic domains, a finding that suggests that well-described cellular pathways of viral glycoprotein localization are utilized during virion assembly. A complete discussion of the intracellular trafficking of these proteins is beyond the scope of this section but, because of the potential cooperativity between proteins and redundancy of function, many of the observations made in the study of individual HCMV glycoproteins in isolation from virus infection could be of limited value in definition of their role in assembly and function in the mature virion. The development of recombinant systems that enable investigators to insert specific mutations should help address these aspects of HCMV envelopment.

The mechanisms leading to final envelopment of the infectious HCMV or other betaherpesvirus particles have not been described. In fact, localizing the virion tegument proteins and envelope glycoproteins to an isolable cellular compartment suggests that envelopment takes place after tegumentation of the nucleocapsid. The recent findings that described unenveloped particles in the cytoplasm of cells infected with the UL99 (pp28) deletion virus supports a working model of envelopment that includes budding of a tegumented capsid through a membrane that contains viral envelope glycoproteins (Silva et al., 2003). The source of the membrane structure and the mechanisms that localize the large number of glycoproteins to this single membrane have not been well described but recent studies of the trafficking of HCMV UL33 and UL27 have suggested that virions were wrapped in membrane tubules as well as budding into multivesicular bodies, structures connected with the endosomal system (Fraile-Ramos et al., 2001). The location of these membranous structures in a juxtanuclear compartment and the differentiation of this compartment from Golgi and TGN are consistent with previous studies of the virus assembly compartment identified in virus infected cells (Fraile-Ramos et al., 2001; Sanchez et al., 2000a; Homman-Londiyi et al., 2003). Previous studies also suggested that HCMV was enveloped in an endosomal compartment (Tooze et al., 1993). Other enveloped viruses, most notably retroviruses, have been shown to utilize a pathway that includes budding into late endosomal compartments during their assembly (Amara et al., 2003; Pelchen-Matthews et al., 2003). If such cellular structures are ultimately shown to be a site of HCMV envelopment (budding), it could follow that HCMV exits the infected cell by a similar exocytic pathway (Gould et al., 2003).

REFERENCES

Adler, H., Messerle, M., and Koszinowski, U. H. (2003). Cloning of herpesviral genomes as bacterial artificial chromosomes. *Rev. Med. Virol.*, **13** (2), 111–121.

Amara, A. and Littman, D. R. (2003). After Hrs with HIV. *J. Cell Biol.*, **162** (3), 371–375.

Baldick, C. J., Jr., Marchini, A., Patterson, C. E., and Shenk, T. (1997). Human cytomegalovirus tegument protein pp71 (ppUL82) enhances the infectivity of viral DNA and accelerates the infectious cycle. *J. Virol.*, **71**(6), 4400–4408.

Beaudet-Miller, M., Zhang, R., Durkin, J., Gibson, W., Kwong, A. D., and Hong, Z. (1996). Virus-specific interaction between the human cytomegalovirus major capsid protein and the C terminus of the assembly protein precursor. *J. Virol.*, **70**(11), 8081–8088.

Bogner, E., Radsak, K., and Stinski, M. F. (1998). The gene product of human cytomegalovirus open reading frame UL56 binds the pac motif and has specific nuclease activity. *J. Virol.*, **72** (3), 2259–2264.

Borst, E. M., Hahn, G., Koszinowski, U. H., and Messerle, M. (1999). Cloning of the human cytomegalovirus (HCMV) genome as an infectious bacterial artificial chromosome in *Escherichia coli*: a new approach for construction of HCMV mutants. *J. Virol.*, **73** (10), 8320–8329.

Borst, E. M., Mathys, S., Wagner, M., Muranyi, W., and Messerle, M. (2001). Genetic evidence of an essential role for cytomegalovirus small capsid protein in viral growth. *J. Virol.*, **75**(3), 1450–1458.

Brack, A. R., Dijkstra, J. M., Granzow, H., Klupp, B. G., and Mettenleiter, T. C. (1999). Inhibition of virion maturation by simultaneous deletion of glycoproteins E, I, and M of pseudorabies virus. *J. Virol.*, **73**(7), 5364–5372.

Britt, W., Jarvis, M., Seo, J.Y., Drummond, D., and Nelson, J. (2004). Rapid genetic engineering of human cytomegalovirus using a lambda phage based linear recombination system: demonstration that pp28 (UL99) is essential for production of infectious virus. *J. Virol.*, **78**(1), 539–543.

Browne, E. P. and Shenk, T. (2003). Human cytomegalovirus UL83-coded pp65 virion protein inhibits antiviral gene expression in infected cells. *Proc. Natl Acad. Sci. USA*, **100**(20), 11439–11444.

Butcher, S. J., Aitken, J., Mitchell, J., Gowen, B., and Dargan, D. J. (1998). Structure of the human cytomegalovirus B capsid by electron cryomicroscopy and image reconstruction. *J. Struct. Biol.*, **124**(1), 70–76.

Campadelli-Fiume, G., Farabegoli, F., Di Gaeta, S., and Roizman, B. (1991). Origin of unenveloped capsids in the cytoplasm of cells infected with herpes simplex virus 1. *J. Virol.*, **65**(3), 1589–1595.

Chee, M. S., Bankier, A. T. Beck, S. *et al.* (1990). Analysis of the protein-coding content of the sequence of human cytomegalovirus strain AD169. *Curr. Top. Microbiol. Immunol.*, **154**, 125–170.

Chen, D. H., Jiang, H., Lee, M., Liu, F., and Zhou, Z. H. (1999). Three-dimensional visualization of tegument/capsid interactions in the intact human cytomegalovirus. *Virology*, **260**, 10–16.

Crump, C. M., Hung, C. H., Thomas, L., Wan, L., and Thomas, G. (2003). Role of PACS-1 in trafficking of human cytomegalovirus glycoprotein B and virus production. *J. Virol.*, **77**(20), 11105–11113.

Dal Monte, P., Pignatelli, S., Zini, N. *et al.* (2002). Analysis of intracellular and intraviral localization of the human cytomegalovirus UL53 protein. *J. Gen. Virol.*, **83**(5), 1005–1012.

de Noronha, C. M., Sherman, M. P., Lin, H. W. *et al.* (2001). Dynamic disruptions in nuclear envelope architecture and integrity induced by HIV-1 Vpr.[see comment]. *Science*, **294** (5544), 1105–1108.

del Rio, T., Werner, H. C., and Enquist, L. W. (2002). The pseudorabies virus VP22 homologue (UL49) is dispensable for virus growth in vitro and has no effect on virulence and neuronal spread in rodents. *J. Virol.*, **76**(2), 774–782.

Dominguez, G., Dambaugh, T. R., Stamey, F. R., Dewhurst, S., Inoue, N., and Pellett, P. E. (1999). Human herpesvirus 6B genome sequence: coding content and comparison with human herpesvirus 6A. *J. Virol.*, **73** (10), 8040–8052.

Fraile-Ramos, A., Kledal, T. N., Pelchen-Matthews, A., Bowers, K., Schwartz, T. W., and Marsh, M. (2001). The human cytomegalovirus US28 protein is located in endocytic vesicles and undergoes constitutive endocytosis and recycling. *Mol. Biol. Cell*, **12** (6), 1737–1749.

Fuchs, W., Klupp, B. G., Granzow, H., Osterrieder, N., and Mettenleiter, T. C. (2002). The interacting UL31 and UL34 gene products of pseudorabies virus are involved in egress from the host-cell nucleus and represent components of primary enveloped but not mature virions. *J. Virol.*, **76** (1), 364–378.

Gallina, A., Simoncini, L., Garbelli, S. *et al.* (1999). Polo-like kinase 1 as a target for human cytomegalovirus pp65 lower matrix protein. *J. Virol.*, **73** (2), 1468–1478.

Gibson, W. (1996). Structure and assembly of the virion. *Intervirology*, **39** (5–6), 389–400.

Gibson, W., Marcy, A. I., Comolli, J. C., and Lee, J. (1990). Identification of precursor to cytomegalovirus capsid assembly protein and evidence that processing results in loss of its carboxy-terminal end. *J. Virol.*, **64**, 1241–1249.

Gibson, W., McNally, L. M., Welch, A. R. *et al.* (1993). Cytomegalovirus maturational proteinase: site-directed mutagenesis used to probe enzymatic and substrate domains. In *Multidisciplinary Approach to Understanding Cytomegalovirus Disease* ed. S. Michelson, and S. A. Plotkin, pp. 21–25. Amsterdam: Elsevier.

Gibson, W., Baxter, M. K., and Clopper, K. S. (1996). Cytomegalovirus "missing" capsid protein identified as heat-aggregable product of human cytomegalovirus UL46. *J. Virol.*, **70**(11), 7454–7461.

Giesen, K., Radsak, K., and Bogner, E. (2000). The potential terminase subunit of human cytomegalovirus, pUL56, is translocated into the nucleus by its own nuclear localization signal and interacts with importin alpha. *J. Gen. Virol.*, **81**(9), 2231–2244.

Gompels, U. A., Nicholas, J., Lawrence, G. *et al.* (1995). The DNA sequence of human herpesvirus 6: structure, coding content, and genome evolution. *Virology*, **209**, 29–51.

Gould, S. J., Booth, A. M., and Hildreth, J. E. (2003). The Trojan exosome hypothesis. *Proc. Natl Acad. Sci. USA*, **100**(19), 10592–10597.

Granzow, H., Weiland, F., Jons, A., Klupp, B. G., Karger, A., and Mettenleiter, T. C. (1997). Ultrastructural analysis of the replication cycle of pseudorabies virus in cell culture: a reassessment. *J. Virol.*, **71**(3), 2072–2082.

Granzow, H., Klupp, B. G., Fuchs, W., Veits, J., Osterrieder, N., and Mettenleiter, T. C. (2001). Egress of alphaherpesviruses: comparative ultrastructural study. *J. Virol.*, **75**(8), 3675–3684.

Grunewald, K., Desai, P., Winkler, D. C. *et al.* (2003). Three-dimensional structure of herpes simplex virus from cryo-electron tomography. *Science*, **302**, 1396–1398.

Hensel, G., Meyer, H., Gartner, S., Brand, G., and Kern, H. F. (1995). Nuclear localization of the human cytomegalovirus tegument protein pp150 (ppUL32). *J. Gen. Virol.*, **76**, 1591–1601.

Heymann, J. B., Cheng, N., Newcomb, W. W., Trus, B. L., Brown, J. C., and Steven, A. C. (2003). Dynamics of herpes simplex virus capsid maturation visualized by time-lapse cryo-electron microscopy [comment]. *Nat. Struct. Biol.*, **10**(5), 334–341.

Homman-Loudiyi, M., Hultenby, K., Britt, W., and Soderberg-Naucler, C. (2003). Envelopment of human cytomegalovirus occurs by budding into Golgi-derived vacuole compartments positive for gB, Rab 3, trans-golgi network 46, and mannosidase II. *J. Virol.*, **77**, 3191–3203.

Jarvis, M. A., Fish, K. N., Soderberg-Naucler, C. *et al.* (2002). Retrieval of human cytomegalovirus glycoprotein B from cell surface is not required for virus envelopment in astrocytoma cells. *J. Virol.*, **76**(10), 5147–5155.

Jarvis, M. A., Jones, T. R., Drummond, D. D. *et al.* (2004). Phosphorylation of human cytomegalovirus glycoprotein B (gB) at the acidic cluster casein kinase 2 site (Ser900) is required for localization of gB to the trans-Golgi network and efficient virus replication. *J. Virol.*, **78**(1), 285–293.

Johnson, D. C. and Spear, P. G. (1982). Monesin inhibits the processing of herpes simplex virus glycoproteins, their transport to the cell surface, and egress of virions from infected cells. *J. Virol.*, **43**, 1102–1112.

Jones, F. and Grose, C. (1988). Role of cytoplasmic vacuoles in varicella-zoster virus glycoprotein trafficking and virion envelopment. *J. Virol.*, **62**(8), 2701–2711.

Jones, T. R. and Lee, S. W. (2004). An acidic cluster of human cytomegalovirus UL99 tegument protein is required for trafficking and function. *J. Virol.*, **78**, 1488–1502.

Kalejta, R. F. and Shenk, T. (2003). The human cytomegalovirus UL82 gene product (pp71) accelerates progression through the G1 phase of the cell cycle. *J. Virol.*, **77**(6), 3451–3459.

Klupp, B. G., Granzow, H., and Mettenleiter, T. C. (2000). Primary envelopment of pseudorabies virus at the nuclear membrane requires the UL34 gene product. *J. Virol.*, **74**(21), 10063–10073.

Komazin, G., Townsend, L. B., and Drach, J. C. (2004). Role of a mutation in human cytomegalovirus gene UL104 in resistance to benzimidazole ribonucleosides. *J. Virol.*, **78**(2), 710–715.

Kopp, M., Granzow, H., Fuchs, W. *et al.* (2003). The pseudorabies virus UL11 protein is a virion component involved in secondary envelopment in the cytoplasm. *J. Virol.*, **77**(9), 5339–5351.

Krosky, P. M., Underwood, M. R., Turk, S. R. *et al.* (1998). Resistance of human cytomegalovirus to benzimidazole ribonucleosides maps to two open reading frames: UL89 and UL56. *J. Virol.*, **72**(6), 4721–4728.

Lai, L. and Britt, W. J. (2003). The interaction between the major capsid protein and the smallest capsid protein of human cytomegalovirus is dependent on two linear sequences in the smallest capsid protein. *J. Virol.*, **77**(4), 2730–2735.

Lee, J. Y., Irmiere, A., and Gibson, W. (1988). Primate cytomegalovirus assembly: evidence that DNA packaging occurs subsequent to B capsid assembly. *Virology*, **167**(1), 87–96.

Liu, B. and Stinski, M. F. (1992). Human cytomegalovirus contains a tegument protein that enhances transcription from promoters with upstream ATF and AP-1 *cis*-acting elements. *J. Virol.*, **66**, 4434–4444.

Liu, F. and Roizman, B. (1992). Differentiation of multiple domains in the herpes simplex virus 1 protease encoded by the UL26 gene. *Proce. Natl Acad. Sci. USA*, **89**(6), 2076–2080.

Messerle, M., Hahn, G., Brune, W., and Koszinowski, U. H. (2000). Cytomegalovirus bacterial artificial chromosomes: a new herpesvirus vector approach. *Adv. Virus Res.*, **55**, 463–478.

Mettenleiter, T. C. (2002). Herpesvirus assembly and egress. *J. Virol.*, **76**(4), 1537–1547.

Mocarski, E. S. and TanCourcelle, C. (2001). Cytomegaloviruses and their replication. 4th ed. In *Fields Virology* 4th edn., ed. D. M. K. a. P. M. Howley, Vol. 2, pp. 2629–2673. Philadelphia: Lippincott, Williams and Wilkins.

Mori, Y., Yang, X., Akkapaiboon, P., Okuno, T., and Yamanishi, K. (2003). Human herpesvirus 6 variant A glycoprotein H-glycoprotein L-glycoprotein Q complex associates with human CD46. *J. Virol.*, **77**(8), 4992–4999.

Muranyi, W., Haas, J., Wagner, M., Krohne, G., and Koszinowski, U. H. (2002). Cytomegalovirus recruitment of cellular kinases to dissolve the nuclear lamina.[comment]. *Science*, **297**(5582), 854–857.

Murphy, E., Yu, D., Grimwood, J. *et al.* (2003). Coding capacity of laboratory and clinical strains of human cytomegalovirus. *Proc. Natl Acad. Sci. USA*, **100**(25), 14976–14981.

Newcomb, W. W., Homa, F. L., Thomsen, D. R., Ye, Z., and Brown, J. C. (1994). Cell-free assembly of the herpes simplex virus capsid. *J. Virol.*, **68**, 6059–6063.

Newcomb, W. W., Homa, F. L., Thomsen, D. R. *et al.* (1996). Assembly of the herpes simplex virus capsid: characterization of intermediates observed during cell-free capsid formation. *J. Mol. Biol.*, **263**(3), 432–446.

Newcomb, W. W., Homa, F. L., Thomsen, D. R. *et al.* (1999). Assembly of the herpes simplex virus procapsid from purified components and identification of small complexes containing the major capsid and scaffolding proteins. *J. Virol.*, **73**(5), 4239–4250.

Newcomb, W. W., Homa, F. L., Thomsen, D. R., and Brown, J. C. (2001). In vitro assembly of the herpes simplex virus procapsid: formation of small procapsids at reduced scaffolding protein concentration. *J. Struct. Biol.*, **133**(1), 23–31.

Nicholas, J. (1996). Determination and analysis of the complete nucleotide sequence of human herpesvirus. *J. Virol.*, **70**(9), 5975–5989.

Nicholson, P., Addison, C., Cross, A. M., Kennard, J., Preston, V. G., and Rixon, F. J. (1994). Localization of the herpes simplex virus type 1 major capsid protein VP5 to the cell nucleus requires the abundant scaffolding protein VP22a. *J. Gen. Virol.*, **75**(5), 1091–1099.

Oien, N. L., Thomsen, D. R., Wathen, M. W., Newcomb, W. W., Brown, J. C., and Homa, F. L. (1997). Assembly of herpes simplex virus capsids using the human cytomegalovirus scaffold protein: critical role of the C terminus. *J. Virol.*, **71**(2), 1281–1291.

Pelchen-Matthews, A., Kramer, B., and Marsh, M. (2003). Infectious HIV-1 assembles in late endosomes in primary macrophages. *J. Cell Biol.*, **162**(3), 443–455.

Pombo, A., Ferreira, J., Bridge, E., and Carmo-Fonseca, M. (1994). Adenovirus replication and transcription sites are spatially separated in the nucleus of infected cells. *EMBO J.*, **13**(21), 5075–5085.

Preston, V. G., Rixon, F. J., McDougall, I. M., McGregor, M., and al-Kobaisi, M. F. (1992). Processing of the herpes simplex virus assembly protein ICP35 near its carboxy terminal end requires the product of the whole of the UL26 reading frame. *Virology*, **186**(1), 87–98.

Preston, V. G., al-Kobaisi, M. F., McDougall, I. M., and Rixon, F. J. (1994). The herpes simplex virus gene UL26 proteinase in the presence of the UL26.5 gene product promotes the formation of scaffold-like structures. *J. Gen. Virol.*, **75**(9), 2355–2366.

Radsak, K. D., Brucher, K. H., and Georgatos, S. D. (1991). Focal nuclear envelope lesions and specific nuclear lamin A/C dephosphorylation during infection with human cytomegalovirus. *Eur. J. Cell Biol.*, **54**, 299–304.

Radsak, K., Eickmann, M., Mockenhaupt, T. *et al.* (1996). Retrieval of human cytomegalovirus glycoprotein B from the infected cell surface for virus envelopment. *Arch. Virol.*, **141**, 557–572.

Roffman, E., Albert, J. P., Goff, J. P., and Frenkel, N. (1990). Putative site for the acquisition of human herpesvirus 6 virion tegument. *J. Virol.*, **64**(12), 6308–6313.

Rudolph, S. A., Kuhn, J. E., Korn, K., Braun, R. W., and Jahn, G. (1990). Prokaryotic expression of the major capsid protein of human cytomegalovirus and antigenic cross-reactions with herpes simplex virus type 1. *J. Gen. Virol.*, **71**, 2023–2031.

Sanchez, V., Angeletti, P. C., Engler, J. A., and Britt, W. J. (1998). Localization of human cytomegalovirus structural proteins to the nuclear matrix of infected human fibroblasts. *J. Virol.*, **72**, 3321–3329.

Sanchez, V., Greis, K. D., Sztul, E., and Britt, W. J. (2000a). Accumulation of virion tegument and envelope proteins in a stable cytoplasmic compartment during human cytomegalovirus replication. Characterization of a potential site of virus assembly. *J. Virol.*, **74**, 975–986.

Sanchez, V., Sztul, E., and Britt, W. J. (2000b). Human cytomegalovirus pp28 (UL99) localizes to a cytoplasmic compartment which overlaps the endoplasmic reticulum-golgi-intermediate compartment. *J. Virol.*, **74**(8), 3842–3851.

Scheffczik, H., Savva, C. G., Holzenburg, A., Kolesnikova, L., and Bogner, E. (2002). The terminase subunits pUL56 and pUL89 of human cytomegalovirus are DNA-metabolizing proteins with toroidal structure. *Nucl. Acids Res.*, **30**(7), 1695–1703.

Schirmbeck, R. and Deppert, W. (1989). Nuclear subcompartmentalization of simian virus 40 large T antigen: evidence for in vivo regulation of biochemical activities. *J. Virol.*, **63**(5), 2308–2316.

Scholz, B., Rechter, S., Drach, J. C., Townsend, L. B., and Bogner, E. (2003). Identification of the ATP-binding site in the terminase subunit pUL56 of human cytomegalovirus. *Nucl. Acids Res.*, **31**(5), 1426–1433.

Silva, M. C., Yu, Q. C., Enquist, L., and Shenk, T. (2003). Human cytomegalovirus UL99-encoded pp28 is required for the cytoplasmic envelopment of tegument-associated capsids. *J. Virol.*, **77**(19), 10594–10605.

Skeppner J. N., Browne, H. and Minson, A. (2001). Herpes simplex virus nucleocapsids mature to progeny virus by an envelopment–deenvelopment–reenvelopment pathway. *J. Virol.*, **75**(12), 5697–5702.

Smith, G. A. and Enquist, L. W. (1999). Construction and transposon mutagenesis in *Escherichia coli* of a full-length infectious clone of pseudorabies virus, an alphaherpesvirus. *J. Virol.*, **73**(8), 6405–6414.

Smith, J. D. and DeHarven, E. (1973). Herpes simplex virus and human cytomegalovirus replication in WI-38 cells. I. Sequence of viral replication. *J. Virol.*, **12**, 919–930.

Steen, R. L., Martins, S. B., Tasken, K., and Collas, P. (2000). Recruitment of protein phosphatase 1 to the nuclear envelope by A-kinase anchoring protein AKAP149 is a prerequisite for nuclear lamina assembly. *J. Cell Biol.*, **150**(6), 1251–1262.

Steven, A. C. and Spear, P. G. (1997). Herpes capsid assembly and envelopment. In *Structural Biology of Viruses* ed. W. Chiu, R. M. Burnett, and R. L. Garcea, pp. 312–351. New York: Oxford University Press.

Stuurman, N., Heins, S., and Aebi, U. (1998). Nuclear lamins: their structure, assembly, and interactions. *J. Struct. Biol.*, **122**(1–2), 42–66.

Tatman, J. D., Preston, V. G., Nicholson, P., Elliott, R. M., and Rixon, F. J. (1994). Assembly of herpes simplex virus type 1 capsids using a panel of recombinant baculoviruses. *J. Gen. Virol.*, **75**(5), 1101–1113.

Tooze, J., Hollinshead, M., Reis, B., Radsak, K., and Kern, H. (1993). Progeny vaccinia and human cytomegalovirus particles utilize early endosomal cisternae for their envelopes. *Eur. J. Cell. Biol.*, **601**(1), 163–178.

Trus, B. L., Gibson, W., Cheng, N., and Steven, A. C. (1999). Capsid structure of simian cytomegalovirus from cryoelectron microscopy: evidence for tegument attachment sites [erratum appears in *J. Virol.* 1999 May;73(5):4530]. *J. Virol.*, **73**(3), 2181–2192.

Tugizov, S., Maidji, E., Xiao, J., and Pereira, L. (1999). An acidic cluster in the cytosolic domain of human cytomegalovirus glycoprotein B is a signal for endocytosis from the plasma membrane. *J. Virol.*, **73**(10), 8677–8688.

Varnum, S. M., Streblow, D. N., Monroe, M. E. *et al.* (2004). Identification of proteins in human cytomegalovirus (HCMV) particles: the HCMV proteome. *J. Virol.*, **78**, 10960–10966.

Wang, Z. H., Gershon, M. D., Lungu, O., Zhu, Z., and Gershon, A. A. (2000). Trafficking of varicella-zoster virus glycoprotein gI: T(338)-dependent retention in the *trans*-Golgi network, secretion, and mannose 6-phosphate-inhibitable uptake of the ectodomain. *J. Virol.*, **74**(14), 6600–6613.

Welch, A. R., McNally, L. M., and Gibson, W. (1991a). Cytomegalovirus assembly protein nested gene family: four 3′-coterminal transcripts encode four in-frame, overlapping proteins. *J. Virol.*, **65**(8), 4091–4100.

Welch, A. R., Woods, A. S., McNally, L. M., Cotter, R. J., and Gibson, W. (1991b). A herpesvirus maturational proteinase, assemblin: identification of its gene, putative active site domain, and cleavage site. *Proc. Natl Acad. Sci. USA*, **88**, 10792–10796.

Whealy, M. E., Card, J. P., Meade, R. P., Robbins, A. K., and Enquist, L. W. (1991). Effect of Brefeldin A on alphaherpesvirus membrane protein glycosylation and virus egress. *J. Virol.*, **65**, 1066–1081.

Wood, L. J., Baxter, M. K., Plafker, S. M., and Gibson, W. (1997). Human cytomegalovirus capsid assembly protein precursor (pUL80.5) interacts with itself and with the major capsid protein (pUL86) through two different domains. *J. Virol.*, **71**(1), 179–190.

Yu, X., Shah, S., Atanasov, I. *et al.* (2005). Three-dimensional localization of the smallest capsid protein in the human cytomegalovirus capsid. *J. Virol.*, **79**(2), 1327–1332.

Zhu, Z., Gershon, M. D., Hao, Y., Ambron, R. T., Gabel, C. A., and Gershon, A. A. (1995). Envelopment of varicella-zoster virus: targeting of viral gylcoproteins to the *trans*-Golgi network. *J. Virol.*, **69**, 7951–7959.

Zhou, Z. H., Chen, D. H., Jakana, J., Rixon, F. J., and Chiu, W. (1999). Visualization of tegument-capsid interactions and DNA in intact herpes simplex virus type 1 virions. *J. Virol.*, **73**(4), 3210–3218.

Zhou, Z. H., Dougherty, M., Jakana, J., He, J., Rixon, F. J., and Chiu, W. (2000). Seeing the herpesvirus capsid at 8.5 A. *Science*, **288**(5467), 877–880.

21

Viral modulation of the host response to infection

A. Louise McCormick and Edward S. Mocarski, Jr.

Department of Microbiology and Immunology, Stanford University School of Medicine, Stanford CA

Betaherpesviruses such as HCMV dramatically affect host cell physiology and encode a wide variety of functions that modulate the infected host cell as well as the immune response (Mocarski, 2002, 2004). Major structural and nonstructural proteins modulate host cell transcriptional repression (Saffert and Kalejta, 2006, Tavalai et al., 2006), cell-intrinsic responses (Abate et al., 2004; Goldmacher, 2004), responses to interferon (Child et al., 2004; Khan et al., 2004) and natural killer (NK) lymphocytes (Lodoen and Lanier, 2005), and adaptive antibody or T-lymphocyte immunity (Chapter 62). The host immune components that are targets of modulation by HCMV are the same host functions that are important in suppressing virus infection, suggesting that the balance between host clearance and viral escape mechanisms dictates many aspects of viral pathogenesis. By reducing the overall impact of antiviral defenses, HCMV seems to be able to escape the full brunt of host innate and adaptive immunity, thereby allowing the virus to persist. It now appears that an overwhelming majority of viral gene products are dedicated to modulation of host cell and immune modulation (Chapter 15). The overwhelming majority (∼100 gene products) may be implicated in modulation because they are dispensable for replication in cultured fibroblasts (Dunn et al., 2003; Yu et al., 2003).

During infection, HCMV and other cytomegaloviruses have a striking impact on cellular gene expression, cell cycle progression, and cellular behavior. More limited information suggests that roseolaviruses, HHV-6A, HHV-6B, and HHV-7 have a similar impact on cells (Chapters 18 and 47). In HCMV several major phases of cellular modulation occur. An interferon-like stimulation of host cells immediately follows virus entry due to the effect of virus particles (see Chapter 16) even though cellular alarm systems involved in IRF-3 and apoptosis are defused. Activation of viral gene transcription by derepression of histone deacetylase activity underlies expression of viral gene products (see Chapters 17 and 18). A dysregulation of cell cycle progression follows early viral gene expression (see Chapter 18) and extends through a pseudo-S phase, and can culminate in pseudomitosis (a property that varies among viral) (Hertel and Mocarski, 2004). A poorly understood process results in the death of the host cell following several days of productive replication. All of these likely vary with host cell type and susceptibility, and all of these may impact replication efficiency. Modulation of host cell and host cell behavior is also a factor in pathogenesis, possibly mediating important stages and cell type specific events during acute and chronic disease in the infected host. Thus, specific HCMV-encoded proteins have been shown to modulate interferon regulated factor (IRF)-3, host cell susceptibility to apoptosis, induction and activity of host cytokines and interferons, stability and cell surface expression of both classical and non-classical major histocompatibility complex (MHC) proteins, and many key processes involved in host cell signaling, gene expression, and metabolism (Mocarski, 2002, 2004; Mocarski and Courcelle, 2001). Together, these broad modulatory capabilities likely contribute to the success of the betaherpesviruses as ubiquitous pathogens. Although many interface with known cellular growth control points in ways that are better studied in the gammaherpesviruses, little evidence supports an oncogenic role for this group of viruses. The impact of HCMV on cells has reinforced the notion that the virus may be involved in acute and chronic diseases affecting the vasculature, and is supported by experiments with rodent cytomegaloviruses. This chapter will focus on viral modulation of the cellular response to betaherpesvirus infection, focusing primarily on HCMV due to the information available.

Modulation of histone deacetylase activity

HCMV replication is stimulated when permissive cells are treated with inhibitors of histone deacetylases (Murphy et al., 2002) or when virus is propagated in cells in which expression of histone deacetylases has been inhibited (Tavalai et al., 2006). Two viral gene products have been implicated in derepression. One major tegument protein, ppUL82 (pp71), also known as the virion transactivator, appears to inactivate Daxx (Cantrell et al., 2005; Everett, 2006; Hofmann et al., 2002; Ishov et al., 2002; Staffert and Kalejta, 2006). The major immediate early protein, IE1-p72, long known to disrupt nuclear domain 10 (ND-10) sites early after infection (Korioth et al., 1996), has been ascribed a role in inactivate a family of promyelocytic leukemia protein (PML) proteins, that also act as repressors of viral gene expression (tavalai et al., 2006).

Modulation of IRF-3

HCMV entry into cells is associated with a dramatic induction of NF-κB (Yurochko et al., 1997a) that is likely to drive the interferon-like response of cells exposed to infectious virus, viral particles, or soluble envelope glycoprotein gB (Simmen et al., 2001; Yurochko et al., 1997a; Zhu et al., 1997, 1998). Although the interferon β transcript is induced in virus-infected cells, even following high MOI infection, interferon itself is only produced in cell cultures subjected to low MOI infection (Rodriguez et al., 1987; Zhu et al., 1997). Several investigators, have described the induction of IRF-3 immediately after infection of permissive fibroblasts (Boehme et al., 2004; Browne and Shenk, 2003; Navarro et al., 1998; Preston et al., 2001), using a variety of viral strains and infection conditions. Induction has been associated with the appearance of a novel IRF-3 complex (Navarro et al., 1998). In contrast, experiments that included both uniform high MOI and use of a monoclonal antibody to detect IRF-3 demonstrated that wild type strains of HCMV fail to induce IRF-3 (Abate et al., 2004), a property that may be shared by rhesus CMV (DeFilippis and Fruh, 2005). Experimental differences in MOI and time post infection, as well as in choice of viral strains and strain variants, may contribute to differences in IRF-3 activation and level of inhibition by pp65 (ppUL83) during infection. Virion pp65 reduces the level of activation of IRF-3 immediately following infection and pp65 expression independent of viral infection is sufficient to inhibit IRF-3 activation by a variety of signals (Abate et al., 2004). In the presence of pp65, there appears to be a transient activation of IRF-3 (Yang et al., 2005) that does not exhibit kinetics consistent with the dramatic impact of virus infection on cells. NF-kB, which has been a topic of study for many years (see below), may also be a target of pp65 depending on experimental conditions (Browne et al., 2003). Even though IRF-3 activation that occurs within 2 h postinfection is likely to be dependent on preformed cytoplasmic protein, the ability of IRF-3 siRNA to increase expression of certain IRF-3 responsive genes and decrease HCMV replication levels has been reported (DeFilippis et al., 2006). The mechanism of IRF-3 regulation over the first few hours of infection will emerge from further mechanistic studies.

Activation of NK-κB and interferon response genes

A classical NF-κB response occurs in two distinct phases following HCMV infection of fibroblasts (Johnson et al., 2001a; Kowalik et al., 1993; Sambucetti et al., 1989; Yurochko et al., 1995). The first phase follows as early as 5 minutes after exposure of cells to virus or virus particles and apparently results from the release of preformed NF-κB mediated by the binding and postattachment events (Boyle et al., 1999; Yurochko et al., 1997a; Netterwald et al., 2004). This initial NF-κB activation may underlie the virion-induced interferon-like response (Browne et al., 2001; Zhu et al., 1997, 1998) and enhance expression of immediate early (IE) genes through the enhancer (DeMeritt et al., 2004). Based on studies with MCMV, the NF-κB sites in the enhancer region may not be essential in all settings (Benedict et al., 2004). NF-κB activation requires phosphorylation-dependent degradation of an inhibitor of NF-κB (IκB), and this degradation is activated in response to infection and continues throughout the infection cycle (Kowalik et al., 1993). Phosphorylation is dependent on a three subunit IκB kinase (IKK) that is both activated and, based solely on the use of chemical inhibitors, required for initiation of viral replication (Caposio et al., 2004) in quiescent fibroblasts. Activation is not critical in actively growing astrocytoma cells (Eickhoff and Cotten, 2005). Deletions made through the enhancer reduce viral replication efficiency in a pattern that suggests a possible role of NF-κB as well as other transcription factor binding sites (Isomura et al., 2004). Another phase of NF-κB activation due to the initiation of NF-κB transcription, allowing continued expression throughout infection (Kowalik et al., 1993; Yurochko et al., 1997b). A physiological role for activation is masked by the relative complexity of events as well as the activities of viral regulatory gene products (Castillo et al., 2000).

The interferon-like and likely NF-kB-dependent activation of cellular gene expression begins within a few hours after virus particle contact with cells (Browne et al., 2001; Simmen et al., 2001) and the response includes a wide range of signaling pathways in addition to those that activate NF-κB (Albrecht et al., 1992; Boldogh et al., 1990, 1991, 1997; Evers et al., 2004; Wang et al., 2003). The production of interferon β itself during HCMV infection is inversely associated with MOI (Rodriguez et al., 1987). Levels of this interferon sufficient to influence the behavior of cells is only induced following exposure of cells to low MOIs or to inactive virus particles (Boehme et al., 2004; Compton, 2004). There is little detectable interferon in the medium or associated with virus particles following high MOI infection (Abate et al., 2004; Rodriguez et al., 1987; Zhu et al., 1997). Interferon has long been known to be relatively ineffective against this group of viruses, whether tested in culture (Holmes et al., 1978) or in patients (Cheeseman et al., 1977). HCMV infected cells do not support interferon receptor signaling or the translation of interferon β transcripts but viral functions that carry out these activities remain to be identified. HCMV deflects major interferon regulated pathways through the action of the closely related viral TRS1 and IRS1 gene products (Child et al., 2002, 2004; Cassady, 2005). These can replace either the vaccinia dsRNA binding protein E3L or the herpes simplex virus-1 (HSV-1) γ34.5 gene product and suppress both protein kinase R (PKR) and the 2–5 oligoadenylate (2–5OAS) synthetase/RNase L system. Despite the lack of obvious motifs, pTRS1 binds dsRNA and includes an unconventional dsRNA-binding domain conserved in pIRS1; however, this domain is not sufficient to rescue E3L mutant virus (Hakki and Geballe, 2005). Thus, TRS1 primarily, but IRS1 secondarily, impede PKR-mediated inactivation of eukaryotic intiation factor 2 as well as the activation of RNase L by products of 2–5A synthetases and the resultant degradation of mRNA and rRNA. IRS1 mutants are fully growth proficient, but growth of TRS1 mutants is reduced (Blankenship and Shenk, 2002; Dunn et al., 2003) and impacts virion assembly (Adamo, et al., 2004).

Impact on the host cell cycle

Betaherpesvirus genomes are transcribed and replicated within the nucleus, the same cellular compartment that regulates the cell cycle and controls apoptosis following DNA damage or aberrant protooncogene expression. Cellular DNA is damaged, the cell cycle is dysregulated, and protooncogene expression is increased following cytomegalovirus infection. DNA damage induced by HCMV includes both randomly distributed and specific chromosomal breaks and gaps (AbuBakar et al., 1988; Deng et al., 1992; Fortunato et al., 2000a). It is not evident that any of these processes requires viral replication.

Cell cycle dysregulation occurs during HCMV productive infection and gives the impression of progression into S phase and mitosis, although cellular DNA synthesis and cell division are blocked. Initial reports of a G2/M arrest, defined by presence of what appeared to be a 4N chromosomal peak (Jault et al., 1995; Lu and Shenk, 1996) were clarified by further work showing host cell DNA content does not increase in infected cells (Bresnahan et al., 1996; Dittmer and Mocarski, 1997; Salvant et al., 1998). Specific inhibition of viral and cellular DNA replication showed that this increase was due to the accumulation of viral DNA (Dittmer and Mocarski, 1997]. Interestingly, viral replication is delayed in cells infected during S phase until after the cell cycle has progressed at least to G2/M, and the majority of cells must apparently cycle to G1 prior to the initiation of viral gene expression (Salvant et al., 1998; Fortunato et al., 2002). It remains possible that the CMV-induced block to cellular DNA synthesis and dysregulation of the cell cycle will vary with each differentiated cell type tested, as detailed studies have not been undertaken in relevant cell types such as endothelial cells, myeloid cells, or epithelial cells. It is notable that studies in MCMV have suggested that induction of apoptosis as a result of viral infection is cell type dependent and that viral inhibitors of apoptosis show cell type specificity (Brune et al., 2001, 2003; Menard et al., 2003).

The structural proteins that modulate host cells most dramatically include two relatively abundant viral tegument proteins, ppUL82 (pp71) (Bresnahan and Shenk, 2000; Kalejta and Shenk, 2002) and pUL69 (Hayashi et al., 2000; Lu and Shenk, 1999). Both are introduced into cells during viral entry. In addition, the IE2 p86 regulatory protein encoded immediately following entry (Murphy et al., 2000; Song and Stinski, 2002) has a dramatic impact on the cell. All three have been characterized for their impact on cell cycle independent of viral replication. pUL69 and IE2 p86 inhibit cell progression past G1 and S, respectively, and pUL82 (pp71) induces quiescent cells to enter the cell cycle. The impact of any of these during viral infection remains poorly understood, but ppUL82 (pp71) may act through derepression of HDACs (Cantrell et al., 2005; Hofmann et al., 2002; Ishov et al., 2002; Saffert and Kalejta, 2006). The situation is complicated by the fact that virus-infected cells do not remain at any distinct stage of the cell cycle but can have characteristics that extend from resting, Go-like to a pseudomitotic state (Hertel and Mocarski, 2004). HHV-7 infection apparently promotes accumulation of polyploid cells with enlarged single cells that have a polylobated nucleus and >4N genome content (Secchiero et al., 1998).

HCMV and HHV-7 grossly alter cyclin and other cell cycle regulatory protein expression patterns (Fortunato et al., 2000b; Hertel and Mocarski, 2004), as described in Chapter 18. Cell cycle dysregulation is accompanied by increases in cyclin E and cdk2 (Bresnahan et al., 1996; Jault et al., 1995) as well as cdk2 translocation to the nucleus (Bresnahan et al., 1997). Additionally, infected cells accumulate hyperphosphorylated pRB (Jault et al., 1995), consistent with induced E2F-specific gene transcription (Song and Stinski, 2002). Proteins that are normally involved in cellular DNA replication, including PCNA (Dittmer and Mocarski, 1997; Mate et al., 1998) and RPA (Fortunato and Spector, 1998), increase and accumulate within sites of viral DNA replication in the nucleus. Increases in cyclin B and cdc2 activity were first demonstrated in infected cells that appeared to have progressed to the G2/M boundary based on DNA content (Jault et al., 1995), but cyclin B levels clearly increase in fibroblasts arrested by CMV at a G1/S-like boundary (Dittmer and Mocarski, 1997). Despite the presence of regulatory factors required for transition through S phase, cellular DNA synthesis is restricted through virus-specific inhibition of licensing factors (Biswas et al., 2003; Wiebusch et al., 2003). All of these studies provide clear evidence of severe dysregulation by HCMV. Although less well characterized, HHV-7 will likely differ from CMV since cdc2 activity decreases after HHV-7 infection. Similar to CMV, cyclin B increases in HHV-7 infected cells despite a G1/S-like arrest. In conjunction with cell cycle alterations, HCMV infection increases expression of the protooncogenes c-jun, c-fos, c-myc (Boldogh et al., 1990), and the tumor suppressor p53 (Jault et al., 1995; Speir et al., 1994). p53 is a transcription factor that promotes growth arrest or apoptosis in response to cell stress (Haupt et al., 2003) or other regulators of intrinsic cell death such as oncogene activation, nucleotide depletion, hypoxia, redox modulation, and loss of normal cell contacts (Giaccia and Kastan, 1998). p53-induced cell death is primarily due to *trans*-activation of specific apoptosis regulators including several proapototic Bcl-2 family members that promote mitochondria membrane permeability transition. The outcome of p53 activity, growth arrest or induction of apoptosis, depends on many factors including p53 expression levels, p53 co-activators, cell type, and type of stress (Haupt et al., 2003). p53 levels are controlled via Mdm2 (mice) or Hdm2 (humans), which direct degradation via the proteasome. Early during HCMV infection, p53 levels increase due to a decrease in protein turnover (Jault et al., 1995; Muganda et al., 1998; Speir et al., 1994). Further, specific coactivators of p53, such as myc, are induced but apoptosis is not induced, possibly due to accumulation in discrete subnuclear regions colocalizing with the viral DNA polymerase processivity factor, ppUL44 (Fortunato and Spector, 1998), a marker of viral DNA replication compartments (Penfold and Mocarski, 1997). A direct physical interaction with IE2 p86 may inhibit p53-mediated transactivation (Speir et al., 1994). One reported interaction of IE2 p86 and p53 (Bonin and McDougall, 1997), however, was carried out in cells that expressed a non-functional IE2 p86 (Murphy et al., 2000), such that this area needs additional investigation. IE2 p86-deficient viruses fail to replicate at all (Heider et al., 2002; Marchini et al., 2001), and a variety of deletions have been made within the protein coding sequences to delineate regions that are necessary for viral replication (Sanchez et al., 2002; White et al., 2004), as described in Chapter 18. In addition to sequestration of the protein, HCMV may have additional means of negating p53 activity, including the increased expression of inhibitory proteins in the p53-family. p53-mediated transcription of apoptotic genes is influenced by the presence of p73 (Flores et al., 2002). In p53 deficient astrocytoma cells, the presence of p73 confers sensitivity to DNA damaging agents such as cisplatin, and HCMV infection alters sensitivity to such agents (Allart et al., 2002) and increases the expression of a cellular dominant negative isoform of p73 that may interfere with both p53- and p73-dependent activities.

Suppression of apoptosis

Apoptosis is an evolutionarily conserved cellular process that removes cells during infection, development, or homeostasis. Apoptosis is initiated by intrinsic stress or DNA damage within the cell that accompanies infection by obligate intracellular parasites and viruses (Ferri and Kroemer, 2001; Polster et al., 2004). Death of the cell early after viral infection prevents the production of progeny, and such mechanisms would exert a strong impact on the slow growing betaherpesviruses. This evolutionarily ancient host defense strategy may be induced in mammals through intrinsic signals, as a consequence of cell stress induced by virus infection, or extrinsic signals through the engagement of death receptors on the cell surface or other immune effector mechanisms. Apoptotic bodies and cellular debris from dead cells are cleared by professional phagocytic cells, such as MΦ and DCs, which carry out critical roles priming the adaptive immune response. A wide range of cellular sensors may be triggered by viral infection, including alterations of the cellular tumor-suppressor p53 or other cell cycle regulators, alterations in mitochondrial function, nuclear changes resulting from DNA damage and repair, modification of endoplasmic reticulum, and activation of PKR (Everett and McFadden, 1999, 2001). A wide range of antiapoptotic proteins encoded by DNA and RNA viruses have been recognized (Cuconati and White, 2002; Polster et al., 2004), and many target the mitochondrion (Boya et al., 2004). These inhibitors suppress cell death resulting from the intrinsic impact of virus infection or from extrinsic inducers or stimuli that accompany the host immune response. The consequence of keeping cells alive is enhancement of viral replication levels that increase the chances of a virus gaining a foothold in the host.

Betaherpesviruses rely on a variety of virus-encoded regulators that prevent cells from showing molecular or morphological hallmarks of apoptosis (Allart et al., 2002; Brune et al., 2003; Goldmacher et al., 1999; Reboredo et al., 2004; Skaletskaya et al., 2001), as depicted in Fig. 21.1. Two HCMV genes, UL37x1 (Goldmacher et al., 1999; Reboredo et al., 2004), which encodes the viral mitochondrial localized inhibitor of apoptosis (vMIA), and UL36 (Skaletskaya et al., 2001), which encodes the viral inhibitor of caspase 8 activation (vICA), inhibit apoptosis through clearly defined mechanisms. The major IE gene products have also been suspected of blocking apoptosis but little mechanistic insights have been gained. Four MCMV gene products inhibit apoptosis, with one (M36) being homologous to HCMV UL36 (McCormick et al., 2003a; Menard et al., 2003), one (m38.5) being a positional and functional homolog of vMIA (McCormick, 2005) and two (m41 and M45) functioning differently than any known HCMV gene product (Brune et al., 2001, 2003; Hahn et al., 2002; Patrone et al., 2003). HHV-6B infected CD4+ cultures include apoptotic cells and virus-positive cells are more resistant to apoptosis than neighboring cells (Inoue et al., 1997), suggesting that this virus also encoded genes that are antiapoptotic. The homologue of UL36 is the most likely candidate. There is also evidence that apoptosis may occur following exposure of nonpermissive cells to betaherpes-viruses or in non-infected cells in productively infected cultures. Thus, all evidence is consistent with a role for betaherpesvirus gene products regulating apoptosis to prolong the life of the infected cell or make it resistant to host immune defense mechanisms. A role for suppression of apoptosis in species specificity of MCMV replication has also been demonstrated by converting human cells to a susceptible state using HCMV vMIA (Jurak and Brune, 2006).

vMIA (pUL37x1)

The genomic region of HCMV encoding the ORFs UL36, UL37, and UL38 is transcriptionally complex (Fig. 21.2). Sequence analysis combined with transcription and in vitro translation studies (Kouzarides et al., 1988; Tenney and Colberg-Poley, 1990, 1991a, 1991b) indicated the presence of two immediate–early transcripts that include UL37x1. The larger transcript, 3.2–3.4 kb in length, is present only at immediate early times, encodes the glycoprotein gpUL37, and terminates at a polyadenylation signal located between UL36 and UL35. The more abundant, 1.7kb transcript, encoding pUL37x1, is present at immediate early times as well as throughout the remainder of infection. This transcript terminates at a polyadenylation signal located between UL38 and UL37x2. A splice variant encoding gpUL37$_M$ includes UL37x1, UL37x2, and a portion of UL37x3 (Goldmacher et al., 1999). Transcription and translation in vitro predicted apparent molecular weights of 58 kDa and 24 kDa, respectively for gpUL37 and pUL37x1 (Tenney and Colberg-Poley, 1990). More recently, cDNA cloning has revealed that transcription through this region may produce as many as 11 spliced and unspliced transcripts (Adair et al., 2003), including all those that had been previously identified. HCMV-induced alterations to the cellular splicing machinery apparently ensures the continued production of the unspliced transcript encoding pUL37x1 throughout infection (Su et al., 2003).

The fact that UL37x1-containing gene products provide antiapoptotic activity emerged from transient expression of viral DNA fragments and functional analyses of pUL37x1, gpUL37 and gpUL37M clones in a cell death suppression assay (Goldmacher et al., 1999). The name vMIA is reserved for the most potent of these, pUL37x1. vMIA prevents cell death induced by TNF, Fas ligand (Goldmacher et al., 1999), TRAIL (Skaletskaya et al., 2001), E1B19K deficient adenovirus (Goldmacher et al., 1999), HIV Vpr (Roumier et al., 2002), doxorubicin (Goldmacher et al., 1999), nitric oxide, peroxynitrite, 4-hydroxynonenal (Vieira et al., 2001), hydroxychloroquine (Boya et al., 2003a), ionidamine, arsenite, the retinoid derivative CD437 (Belzacq et al., 2001), propionibacterial short chain fatty acids (Jan et al., 2002), N-(4-hydroxyphenyl)retinamide (Boya et al., 2003b), and macroautophagy (Boya, 2005). vMIA increases the susceptibility of human cells to MCMV productive infection (Jurak and Brune, 2006). vMIA mediates protection at the level of the mitochondria and prevents release of cytochrome c and subsequent downstream events (Fig. 21.1), but does not prevent upstream events including cleavage of either procaspase-8 or Bid (Goldmacher, 1999). vMIA can be immunoprecipitated with adenine nucleotide transporter, a component of the mitochondria membrane pore that interacts with Bax and other Bcl-2 family members but for vMIA, this interaction is non-specific. vMIA also interacts with Bax in cells (Arnoult et al., 2004; Poncet et al., 2004), and Bax also localizes to mitochondria during MCMV infection (Andoniou et al., 2004). More recently an interaction with growth arrest and DNA damage 45 alpha (GADD45α) was established

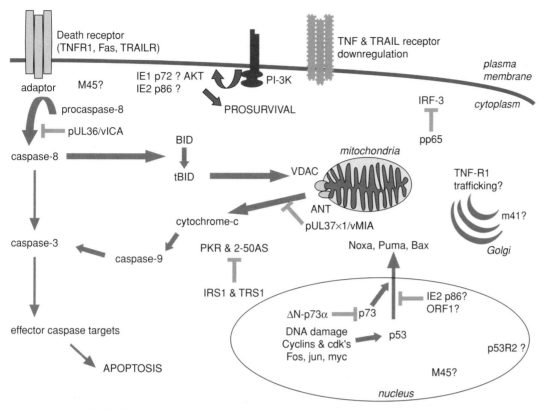

Fig. 21.1. Betaherpesvirus inhibition of apoptosis and interferon response. Grey arrows represent proapoptotic pathways while black arrows indicate prosurvival pathways and black lines indicate interruption of proapoptotic pathways. Cellular functions are listed in grey font and viral functions are indicated in black font. Plasma membrane, cytoplasm, nucleus, mitochondria, and Golgi, are depicted in italics. Bold black text indicates viral inhibitors with known or suspected mechanisms. Question marks indicate possible points of interference by viral proteins.

through yeast two hybrid and significantly, this interaction was shown to be critical for cell-death protection since addition of any GADD45 family member (alpha, beta, or gamma) enhanced survival and function was impaired by siRNA-mediated GADD45 family reduction. vMIA lacks the BH domains that characterize Bcl-2 family members and Bax also localizes to mitochondria during MCMV infection (Andoniou *et al.*, 2004). Rather this, protein is composed of an amino terminal region, aa 5–34, that is important for localization to mitochondria and a carboxyl terminal region, aa 118–147, that is critical for anti-apoptotic activity (Hayajneh *et al.*, 2001). This domain also mediates the interaction with GADD45 family members that facilitates vMIA activity (Smith *et al.*, 2005).

vMIA does not exhibit sequence variation in HCMV (Hayajneh *et al.*, 2001) and sequence homologs can only be found in primate CMVs. The regions of highest sequence conservation are coincident with regions defined by mutational studies to be required for vMIA activity (McCormick *et al.*, 2003b). "In fact, a minimal 69 aa protein that includes amino acids 1–34 and 112–147 of vMIA retains full activity (Hayajneh *et al.*, 2001) and is very similar to homologues in monkey CMVs (McCormick *et al.*, 2003b)." At a positionally conserved location in the viral genome, MCMV and rat CMV retain a functional homolog which despite limited sequence homology, functions in cell death assays (McCormick *et al.*, 2005). A UL37x1 homolog has not been identified in other betaherpesviruses, although all betaherpesviruses carry a gene homologous to UL37x3, which as the largest exon, has been annotated as UL37 in most betaherpesviruses but that lacks independent anti-apoptotic activity (Chapter 15; McCormick *et al.*, 2003b). UL37x1 is not essential for viral replication in Towne*var*ATCC, a strain carrying a functional vICA (McCormick *et al.*, 2005). In contrast, transposon mutants disrupting HCMV UL37x1 fail to produce infectious virus, in AD169*var*ATCC, a strain carrying a mutant UL36 (Reboredo *et al.*, 2004). Other, independently derived UL37x1 deletion mutants made in AD169*var*ATCC had also suggested that vMIA is required for viral replication (Brune *et al.*, 2003; Dunn *et al.*, 2003; Yu *et al.*, 2003). Thus, vMIA is dispensable unless other mutations are present which render the virus

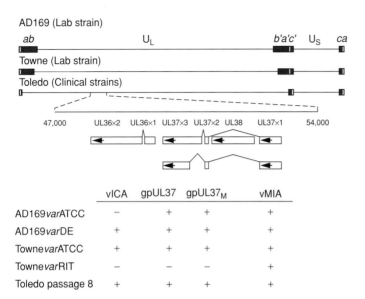

Fig. 21.2. Presence of functional antiapoptotic genes in HCMV strains. (top) Depiction of the commonly used laboratory strains AD169, Towne, and Toledo genomes. Rectangles represent repeated ab - $b'a'$ sequence flanking the unique long (U_L) and the $c'a$ - ac sequences flanking the short (U_S) genome components. An expansion of the region including nucleotides 47,000–54,000 is depicted with a representation of ORFs (open rectangles) in the UL36-UL37 region. Splicing patterns relevant to proteins with demonstrated antiapoptotic function are indicated by lines connecting ORFs and polyadenylation sites are indicated by arrowheads. The presence (+) or absence (–) of vICA, gpUL37, gpUL37$_M$, and vMIA in AD169var ATCC, AD169var DE, Townevar ATCC, Townevar RIT and Toledo (passage 8) is indicated below the ORF diagram (Dunn et al., 2003; Skaletskaya et al., 2001).

similar to the viral and cellular FLICE inhibitory proteins (v-FLIP and c-FLIP), but lacks any sequence similar to death effector domains typical of this class of protein. Like FLIPs, vICA prevents cleavage by binding to the pro-domain of procaspase-8 and provides protection from apoptosis initiated by death receptors TNFR, TRAILR, or Fas that require caspase 8 activation. vICA only slightly delays cell death induced by E1B19K deficient adenovirus or doxorubicin. The presence of vICA correlates with an increased resistance of HCMV to inducers of extrinsic cell death (Skaletskaya et al., 2001). Mutants of the MCMV homologue M36 show a reduced growth phenotype in macrophages (IC-21, J774-A1, and peritoneal exudate cells) but not in fibroblasts or endothelial cells, but this behavior does not appear to extend to the HCMV gene product (Dunn et al., 2003). M36 mutant infected cells are, however, more susceptible to induction of apoptosis by the Fas pathway similar to HCMV viruses defective in UL36 (Skaletskaya et al., 2001).

UL36 homologs and vICA function are widely conserved among betaherpesviruses and sequence conservation includes regions outside the boundaries of the US22-family domains (McCormick et al., 2003a). The homolog is an immediate early gene in MCMV, while the rhesus macaque CMV homolog is an early gene similar to vMIA in that virus. The homologs of UL36 in HHV-6A and HHV-7 are each encoded by a spliced transcript. The HHV-6A is regulated as an immediate–early gene (Flebbe-Rehwaldt et al., 2000), whereas the HHV-7 spliced RNA seems to be regulated as an early gene (Menegazzi et al., 1999).

Other cell death suppressors

Ribonucleotide reductases convert ribonucleoside diphosphates to deoxyribonucleoside diphosphates and are generally important for DNA synthesis and repair. While alphaherpesviruses and gammaherpesviruses encode both ribonucleotide subunits RR1 and RR2 and make an active enzyme, the betaherpesviruses only encode a homolog of the RR1 subunit that lacks enzymatic activity (Chapter 15). Viral mutants of MCMV M45, but not the HCMV homolog UL45, show cell-type dependent growth properties (Brune et al., 2001; Hahn et al., 2002). Insertional mutants of M45 grow similar to wild-type viruses in cultured fibroblasts, bone marrow stromal cells, and hepatocytes but fail to grow in either endothelial cells or macrophages (Brune et al., 2001), which enter apoptosis by about 1 day postinfection. Cell to cell spread is thus severely restricted. The alphaherpesvirus HSV-2 RR1 subunit prevents cell death upstream of caspase 8 activation due to an amino-terminal extention relative to other RR1 homologs (Langelier et al.,

dependent on the gene to prevent apoptosis. (Dunn et al., 2003; Brune et al., 2003; Reboredo et al., 2004; Yu et al., 2003; Skaletskaya et al., 2001). Consistent with this conclusion and in contrast to the caspase-dependent cell death noted for strains that require vMIA, premature death in TownevarATCC mutant virus is caspase-independent (McCormick et al., 2005).

vICA (pUL36)

This betaherpesvirus-conserved anti-apoptotic gene product is dispensable for HCMV replication in cultured fibroblasts and is mutated in many common laboratory strains (Patterson and Shenk, 1999; Skaletskaya et al., 2001), as depicted in Fig. 21.2. Evidence that UL36 encodes the antiapoptotic protein vICA first emerged from transient expression of viral DNA fragments in a cell death suppression assay (Skaletskaya et al., 2001). Caspase 8, the target of pUL36, is also known as FLICE. vICA is mechanistically

2002) in addition to being a component of an active ribonucleoside reductase enzyme. It is possible that M45 has preserved such an antiapoptotic function, although there is little sequence similarity to guide how the two may be related. Cell-type restricted growth and induced apoptosis are not observed in HCMV UL45 mutants, which grow poorly and are less efficient at cell-to-cell spread (Patrone et al., 2003), but do not exhibit cell type specific defects in fibroblasts, macrophages, or endothelial when used at high MOIs (Hahn et al., 2002). Mutant HCMV is somewhat reduced compared to wt in ability to withstand Fas-induced apoptosis (26% survival vs. 50% survival), however; HCMV UL45 is unable to independently block cell death in the absence of viral infection.

MCMV mutant defective in m41 prematurely kills cells and replicates to reduced levels compared to parental virus (Brune et al., 2003). Caspase inhibition reduces but does not eliminate cell death, suggesting that apoptosis may underlie the process. Expression of epitope-tagged m41 during viral infection shows localization to Golgi. The mechanism of protection remains to be elucidated.

HCMV IE1 p72 and IE2 p86 are nuclear proteins that regulate transcription of cellular and viral genes (Chapters 17 and 18) and each can associate with cellular proteins. Cellular transcription factor E2F is modulated by IE1 p72 interaction with the Rb-pocket protein p107 (Poma et al., 1996) or by IE2 p86 interaction with pRB (Hagemeier et al., 1994). Regulation of E2F1 is mediated by binding to IE1 p72 (Margolis et al., 1995). IE1 p72 and IE2 p86 suppress apoptosis induced by TNF or E1B19K defective adenovirus (Zhu et al., 1995) and anti-apoptotic activity maps to disparate sequences without any hint of mechanism. Importantly, fibroblasts constitutively expressing IE1 p72 that have been used to complement growth of IE1 p72 mutant viruses do not exhibit any obvious altered cell cycle progression or susceptibility to apoptosis. In transient assays, a genomic clone including IE1 p72 and IE2 p86 rescues a temperature sensitive derivative of $TAF_{II}250$ mutant cells (ts 13) from transcriptional repression and apoptosis but not cell cycle arrest (Lukac et al., 1997). Further analysis indicated either IE2 p86 or IE1 p72 activates the PI3 kinase pathway and AKT as a consequence (Yu and Alwine, 2002) similar to the response of these prosurvival pathways to infection (Johnson et al., 2001b), but the role of IE1 p72 and IE2 p86 as suggested by the $TAF_{II}250$ mutant cells has not been extended to natural infection. IE2 p86 but not IE1 p72 protects from overexpression of p53 in smooth muscle cells (Tanaka et al., 1999). In contrast IE2 p86 but not IE1 p72 expression in endothelial cells induces apoptosis (Wang et al., 2000). Control of cell-intrinsic responses is the suggested mechanism for HCMV IE1 facilitation of MCMV replication in human cells (Tang and Maul, 2006). These data may suggest that any potential protective role includes both an induction-specific and a cell-type specific component.

Alteration of extrinsic cell death pathways during infection

TNF-R1 surface expression levels decrease following HCMV infection of macrophage or astrocytoma cell lines (Baillie et al., 2003) as well as following MCMV infection of bone marrow derived macrophages (Popkin and Virgin, 2003). Although the viral factors required for the down-regulation have not been identified, either virus seems to employ a post-transcriptional mechanism. Uninfected fibroblasts insensitive to TRAIL mediated apoptosis become sensitive to TRAIL following HCMV infection (Sedger et al., 1999). Infection increases expression of death-inducing TRAIL-R1 and TRAIL-R2, but not decoy receptors TRAIL-R3 and TRAIL-R4. Analysis of HHV-7 revealed downregulation of TRAIL-R1 but not TRAIL-R2, TNF-R1, TNF-R2, or Fas during infection of CD4 cells (Secchiero et al., 2001). Infections by other betaherpesviruses maintain the Fas receptor available for activation. Fibroblasts infected by HCMV and MCMV are susceptible to Fas-mediated apoptosis (Chaudhuri et al., 1999; Goldmacher et al., 1999; Menard et al., 2003; Skaletskaya et al., 2001) and some, but not all, strains of HCMV may increase Fas receptor surface expression (Chaudhuri et al., 1999; Chiou et al., 2001).

HCMV encodes a potential TNF-receptor homolog (Benedict et al., 1999), although this protein has not been assigned any role in blocking apoptosis. UL144 encodes a glycoprotein consisting of a leader peptide, cysteine-rich domains (CRD), membrane extension region, transmembrane domain, and a short cytoplasmic tail. UL144 exhibits dramatic strain-to-strain sequence variability (Bale, 2001; Lurain, 1999), although the protein has highly conserved transmembrane and cytoplasmic domains. UL144 is the closest known relative of the cell surface herpesvirus entry mediator (HVEM; Chapter 7) protein, whose normal function is as a cognate ligand for the B- and T-lymphocyte attenuator (Sedy et al., 2005). UL144 binds B and T lymphocyte attenuator (BTLA) and inhibits T-cell proliferation.

Summary

The betaherpesviruses all appear to alter cell cycle and to block rather than promote apoptosis during infection. Cytomegaloviruses prevent cellular DNA synthesis whereas roseolaviruses allow continued cellular DNA synthesis during productive infection, although cell division is blocked in all of these viruses. While none of the betaherpesviruses has been implicated in malignancy, such an impact on the host cell has raised interest of persistent betaherpesvirus infection in certain chronic diseases. These viruses encode a wide variety of functions that modulate the cellular environment, including functions that modulate cell cycle progression and that derail apoptosis induced by either intrinsic or extrinsic mediators.

REFERENCES

Abate, D. A., Watanabe, S., and Mocarski, E. S. (2004). Major human cytomegalovirus structural protein pp65 (ppUL83) prevents interferon response factor 3 activation in the interferon response. *J. Virol.*, **78**, 10995–11006.

AbuBakar, S., Au, W. W., Legator, M. S., and Albrecht, T. (1988). Induction of chromosome aberrations and mitotic arrest by cytomegalovirus in human cells. *Environ. Mol. Mutagen.*, **12**, 409–420.

Adair, R., Liebisch, G. W., and Colberg-Poley, A. M. (2003). Complex alternative processing of human cytomegalovirus UL37 pre-mRNA. *J. Gen. Virol.*, **84**, 3353–3358.

Adamo, J. E., Schroer, J., and Shenk, T. (2004). Human cytomegalovirus TRS1 protein is required for efficient assembly of DNA-containing capsids. *J. Virol.*, **78**, 10221–10229.

Albrecht, T., Boldogh, I., and Fons, M. P. (1992). Receptor-initiated activation of cells and their oncogenes by herpes-family viruses. *J. Invest. Dermatol.*, **98**(6 Suppl), 29S–35S.

Allart, S., Martin, H., Detraves, C., Terrasson, J., Caput, D., and Davrinche, C. (2002). Human cytomegalovirus induces drug resistance and alteration of programmed cell death by accumulation of deltaN-p73alpha. *J. Biol. Chem.*, **277**, 29063–29068.

Andoniou, C. E., Andrews, D. M., Manzur, M., Ricciardi-Castagnoli, P., and Degli-Esposti, M. A. (2004). A novel checkpoint in the Bcl-2-regulated apoptotic pathway revealed by murine cytomegalovirus infection of dendritic cells. *J. Cell Bio.*, **166**, 827–837.

Arnoult, D., Bartle, L. M., Skaletskaya, A. *et al.* (2004). Cytomegalovirus cell death suppressor vMIA blocks Bax- but not Bak-mediated apoptosis by binding and sequestering Bax at mitochondria. *Proc. Natl Acad. Sci. USA*, **101**, 7988–7993.

Baillie, J., Sahlender, D. A., and Sinclair, J. H. (2003). Human cytomegalovirus infection inhibits tumor necrosis factor alpha (TNF-alpha) signaling by targeting the 55-kilodalton TNF-alpha receptor. *J. Virol.*, **77**, 7007–7016.

Belzacq, A. S., El Hamel, C., Vieira, H. L. *et al.* (2001). Adenine nucleotide translocator mediates the mitochondrial membrane permeabilization induced by lonidamine, arsenite and CD437. *Oncogene*, **20**, 7579–7587.

Benedict, C. A., Butrovich, K. D., Lurain, N. S. *et al.* (1999). Cutting edge: a novel viral TNF receptor superfamily member in virulent strains of human cytomegalovirus. *J. Immunol.*, **162**, 6967–6970.

Benedict, C. A., Angulo, A., Patterson, G. *et al.* (2004). Neutrality of the canonical NF-kappaB-dependent pathway for human and murine cytomegalovirus transcription and replication in vitro. *J. Virol.*, **78**, 741–750.

Biswas, N., Sanchez, V., and Spector, D. H. (2003). Human cytomegalovirus infection leads to accumulation of geminin and inhibition of the licensing of cellular DNA replication. *J. Virol.*, **77**, 2369–2376.

Blankenship, C. A., and Shenk, T. (2002). Mutant human cytomegalovirus lacking the immediate-early TRS1 coding region exhibits a late defect. *J. Virol.*, **76**, 12290–12299.

Boehme, K. W., Singh, J., Perry, S. T., and Compton, T. (2004). Human cytomegalovirus elicits a coordinated cellular antiviral response via envelope glycoprotein B. *J. Virol.*, **78**, 1202–1211.

Boldogh, I., AbuBakar, S., and Albrecht, T. (1990). Activation of proto-oncogenes: an immediate early event in human cytomegalovirus infection. *Science*, **247**, 561–564.

Boldogh, I., AbuBakar, S., Millinoff, D., Deng, C. Z., and Albrecht, T. (1991). Cellular oncogene activation by human cytomegalovirus. Lack of correlation with virus infectivity and immediate early gene expression. *Arch. Virol.*, **118**, 163–177.

Boldogh, I., Bui, T. K., Szaniszlo, P., Bresnahan, W. A., Albrecht, T., and Hughes, T. K. (1997). Novel activation of gamma-interferon in nonimmune cells during human cytomegalovirus replication. *Proc. Soc. Exp. Biol. Med.*, **215**, 66–73.

Bonin, L. R. and McDougall, J. K. (1997). Human cytomegalovirus IE2 86-kilodalton protein binds p53 but does not abrogate G1 checkpoint function. *J. Virol.*, **71**, 5861–5870.

Boya, P., Gonzalez-Polo, R. A., Poncet, D. *et al.* (2003a). Mitochondrial membrane permeabilization is a critical step of lysosome-initiated apoptosis induced by hydroxychloroquine. *Oncogene*, **22**, 3927–3936.

Boya, P., Morales, M. C., Gonzalez-Polo, R. A. *et al.* (2003b). The chemopreventive agent N-(4-hydroxyphenyl)retinamide induces apoptosis through a mitochondrial pathway regulated by proteins from the Bcl-2 family. *Oncogene*, **22**, 6220–6230.

Boya, P., Pauleau, A. L., Poncet, D., Gonzalez-Polo, R. A., Zamzami, N., and Kroemer, G. (2004). Viral proteins targeting mitochondria: controlling cell death. *Biochim. Biophys. Acta*, **1659**, 178–189.

Boyle, K. A., Pietropaolo, R. L., and Compton, T. (1999). Engagement of the cellular receptor for glycoprotein B of human cytomegalovirus activates the interferon-responsive pathway. *Mol. Cell. Biol.*, **19**, 3607–3613.

Bresnahan, W. A. and Shenk, T. E. (2000). UL82 virion protein activates expression of immediate early viral genes in human cytomegalovirus-infected cells *Proc. Natl Acad. Sci. USA*, **97**, 14506–14511.

Bresnahan, W. A., Boldogh, I., Thompson, E. A., and Albrecht, T. (1996). Human cytomegalovirus inhibits cellular DNA synthesis and arrests productively infected cells in late G1. *Virology*, **224**, 150–160.

Bresnahan, W. A., Thompson, E. A., and Albrecht, T. (1997). Human cytomegalovirus infection results in altered Cdk2 subcellular localization. *J. Gen. Virol.*, **78**, 1993–1997.

Browne, E. P. and Shenk, T. (2003). Human cytomegalovirus UL83-coded pp65 virion protein inhibits antiviral gene expression in infected cells. *Proc. Natl Acad. Sci. USA*, **100**, 11439–11444.

Browne, E. P., Wing, B., Coleman, D., and Shenk, T. (2001). Altered cellular mRNA levels in human cytomegalovirus-infected fibroblasts: viral block to the accumulation of antiviral mRNAs. *J. Virol.*, **75**, 12319–12330.

Brune, W., Menard, C., Heesemann, J., and Koszinowski, U. H. (2001). A ribonucleotide reductase homologue of cytomegalovirus and endothelial cell tropism. *Science*, **291**, 303–305.

Brune, W., Nevels, M., and Shenk, T. (2003). Murine cytomegalovirus m41 open reading frame encodes a Golgi-localized antiapoptotic protein. *J. Virol.*, **77**, 11633–11643.

Cantrell, S. R., and Bresnahan, W. A. (2005). Interaction between the human cytomegalovirus UL82 gene product (pp71) and hDaxx regulates immediate-early gene expression and viral replication. *J. Virol.*, **79**, 7792–7802.

Caposio, P., Dreano, M., Garotta, G., Gribaudo, G., and Landolfo, S. (2004). Human cytomegalovirus stimulates cellular IKK2 activity and requires the enzyme for productive replication. *J. Virol.*, **78**, 3190–3195.

Cassady, K. A. (2005). Human cytomegalovirus TRS1 and IRS1 gene products block the double-stranded-RNA-activated host protein shutoff response induced by herpes simplex virus type 1 infection. *J. Virol.*, **79**, 8707–8715.

Castillo, J. P., Yurochko, A. D., and Kowalik, T. F. (2000). Role of human cytomegalovirus immediate–early proteins in cell growth control. *J. Virol.*, **74**, 8028–8037.

Chaudhuri, A. R., St. Jeor, S., and Maciejewski, J. P. (1999). Apoptosis induced by human cytomegalovirus infection can be enhanced by cytokines to limit the spread of virus. *Exp. Hematol.*, **27**, 1194–1203.

Cheeseman, S. H., Rinaldo, C. J., and Hirsch, M. S. (1977). Use of interferon in cytomegalovirus infections in man. *Tex. Rep. Biol. Med.*, **35**, 523–527.

Child, S. J., Jarrahian, S., Harper, V. M., and Geballe, A. P. (2002). Complementation of vaccinia virus lacking the double-stranded RNA-binding protein gene E3L by human cytomegalovirus. *J. Virol.*, **76**, 4912–4918.

Child, S. J., Hakki, M., De Niro, K. L., and Geballe, A. P. (2004). Evasion of cellular antiviral responses by human cytomegalovirus TRS1 and IRS1. *J. Virol.*, **78**, 197–205.

Chiou, S. H., Liu, J. H., Hsu, W. M. *et al.* (2001). Up-regulation of Fas ligand expression by human cytomegalovirus immediate-early gene product 2: a novel mechanism in cytomegalovirus-induced apoptosis in human retina. *J. Immunol.*, **167**, 4098–4103.

Compton, T. (2004). Receptors and immune sensors: the complex entry path of human cytomegalovirus. *Trends Cell Biol.*, **14**, 5–8.

Cuconati, A. and White, E. (2002). Viral homologs of BCL-2: role of apoptosis in the regulation of virus infection. *Genes Dev.*, **16**, 2465–2478.

DeMeritt, I. B., Milford, L. E., and Yurochko, A. D. (2004). Activation of the NF-kappaB pathway in human cytomegalovirus-infected cells is necessary for efficient transactivation of the major immediate–early promoter. *J. Virol.*, **78**, 4498–4507.

DeFilippis, V. and Fruh, K. (2005). Rhesus cytomegalovirus particles prevent activation of interferon regulatory factor 3. *J. Virol.*, **79**, 6419–6431.

DeFilippis, V. R., Robinson, B., Keck, T. M., Hansen, S. G., Nelson, J. A., and Fruh, K. J. (2006). Interferon regulatory factor 3 is necessary for induction of antiviral genes during human cytomegalovirus infection. *J. Virol.*, **80**, 1032–1037.

DeFilippis, V., and Fruh, K. (2005). Rhesus cytomegalovirus particles prevent activation of interferon regulatory factor 3. *J. Virol.*, **79**(10), 6419–31.

Deng, C. Z., AbuBakar, S., Fons, M. P. *et al.* (1992). Cytomegalovirus-enhanced induction of chromosome aberrations in human peripheral blood lymphocytes treated with potent genotoxic agents. *Environ. Mol. Mutagen*, **19**, 304–310.

Dittmer, D. and Mocarski, E. S. (1997). Human cytomegalovirus infection inhibits G1/S transition. *J. Virol.*, **71**, 1629–1634.

Dunn, W., Chou, C., Li, H. *et al.* (2003). Functional profiling of a human cytomegalovirus genome. *Proc. Natl Acad. Sci. USA*, **100**, 14223–14228.

Eickhoff, J. E. and Cotten, M. (2005). NF-kappaB activation can mediate inhibition of human cytomegalovirus replication. *J. Gen. Virol.*, **86**, 285–295.

Everett, R. D. (2006). Interactions between DNA viruses, ND10 and the DNA damage response. *Cell Microbiol*, **8**, 365–374.

Everett, H. and McFadden, G. (1999). Apoptosis: an innate immune response to virus infection. *Trends Microbiol.*, **7**, 160–165.

Everett, H. and McFadden, G. (2001). Viral proteins and the mitochondrial apoptotic checkpoint. *Cytokine Growth Factor Rev.*, **12**, 181–188.

Evers, D. L., Wang, X., and Huang, E. S. (2004). Cellular stress and signal transduction responses to human cytomegalovirus infection. *Microbes. Infect.*, **6**, 1084–1093.

Ferri, K. F. and Kroemer, G. (2001). Organelle-specific initiation of cell death pathways. *Nat. Cell Biol.*, **3**, E255–E263.

Flebbe-Rehwaldt, L. M., Wood, C., and Chandran, B. (2000). Characterization of transcripts expressed from human herpesvirus 6A strain GS immediate-early region B U16–U17 open reading frames. *J. Virol.*, **74**, 11040–11054.

Flores, E. R., Tsai, K. Y., Crowley, D. *et al.* (2002). p63 and p73 are required for p53-dependent apoptosis in response to DNA damage. *Nature*, **416**, 560–564.

Fortunato, E. A. and Spector, D. H. (1998). p53 and RPA are sequestered in viral replication centers in the nuclei of cells infected with human cytomegalovirus. *J. Virol.*, **72**, 2033–2039.

Fortunato, E. A., Dell'Aquila, M. L., and Spector, D. H. (2000a). Specific chromosome 1 breaks induced by human cytomegalovirus. *Proc. Natl Acad. Sci. USA*, **97**, 853–858.

Fortunato, E. A., McElroy, A. K., Sanchez, I., and Spector, D. H. (2000b). Exploitation of cellular signaling and regulatory pathways by human cytomegalovirus. *Trends Microbiol*, **8**, 111–119.

Fortunato, E. A., Sanchez, V., Yen, J. Y., and Spector, D. H. (2002). Infection of cells with human cytomegalovirus during S phase results in a blockade to immediate–early gene expression that can be overcome by inhibition of the proteasome. *J. Virol.*, **76**, 5369–5379.

Giaccia, A. J. and Kastan, M. B. (1998). The complexity of p53 modulation: emerging patterns from divergent signals. *Genes Dev.*, **12**, 2973–2983.

Goldmacher, V. S. (2004). Cell death suppressors encoded by cytomegalovirus. *Prog. Mol. Subcell Biol.*, **36**, 1–18.

Goldmacher, V. S., Bartle, L. M., Skaletskaya, A. *et al.* (1999). A cytomegalovirus-encoded mitochondria-localized inhibitor of apoptosis structurally unrelated to Bcl-2. *Proc. Natl Acad. Sci. USA*, **96**, 12536–12541.

Hagemeier, C., Caswell, R., Hayhurst, G., Sinclair, J., and Kouzarides, T. (1994). Functional interaction between the HCMV IE2 transactivator and the retinoblastoma protein. *EMBO J.*, **13**, 2897–2903.

Hahn, G., Khan, H., Baldanti, F., Koszinowski, U. H., Revello, M. G., and Gerna, G. (2002). The human cytomegalovirus ribonucleotide reductase homologue UL45 is dispensable for growth in endothelial cells, as determined by a BAC-cloned clinical isolate of human cytomegalovirus with preserved wild-type characteristics. *J. Virol.*, **76**, 9551–9555.

Hakki, M., and Geballe, A. P. (2005). Double-stranded RNA binding by human cytomegalovirus pTRS1. *J. Virol.*, **79**, 7311–7318.

Haupt, S., Berger, M., Goldberg, Z., and Haupt, Y. (2003). Apoptosis – the p53 network. *J. Cell Sci.*, **116**, 4077–4085.

Hayajneh, W. A., Colberg-Poley, A. M., Skaletskaya, A. *et al.* (2001). The sequence and antiapoptotic functional domains of the human cytomegalovirus UL37 exon 1 immediate early protein are conserved in multiple primary strains. *Virology*, **279**, 233–240.

Hayashi, M. L., Blankenship, C., and Shenk, T. (2000). Human cytomegalovirus UL69 protein is required for efficient accumulation of infected cells in the G1 phase of the cell cycle *Proc. Natl Acad. Sci. USA*, **97**, 2692–2696.

Heider, J. A., Bresnahan, W. A., and Shenk, T. E. (2002). Construction of a rationally designed human cytomegalovirus variant encoding a temperature-sensitive immediate-early 2 protein. *Proc. Natl Acad. Sci. USA*, **99**, 3141–3146.

Hertel, L. and Mocarski, E. S. (2004). Global analysis of host cell gene expression late during cytomegalovirus infection reveals extensive dysregulation of cell cycle gene expression and induction of Pseudomitosis independent of US28 function. *J. Virol.*, **78**, 11988–12011.

Hofmann, H., Sindre, H., and Stamminger, T. (2002). Functional Interaction between the pp71 Protein of Human Cytomegalovirus and the PML-Interacting Protein Human Daxx. *J. Virol.*, **76**, 5769–5783.

Holmes, A. R., Rasmussen, L., and Merigan, T. C. (1978). Factors affecting the interferon sensitivity of human cytomegalovirus. *Intervirology*, **9**, 48–55.

Inoue, Y., Yasukawa, M., and Fujita, S. (1997). Induction of T-cell apoptosis by human herpesvirus 6. *J. Virol.*, **71**, 3751–3759.

Ishov, A. M., Vladimirova, O. V., and Maul, G. G. (2002). Daxx-mediated accumulation of human cytomegalovirus tegument protein pp71 at ND10 facilitates initiation of viral infection at these nuclear domains. *J. Virol.*, **76**, 7705–7712.

Isomura, H., Tsurumi, T., and Stinski, M. F. (2004). Role of the proximal enhancer of the major immediate-early promoter in human cytomegalovirus replication. *J. Virol.*, **78**, 12788–12799.

Jan, G., Belzacq, A. S., Haouzi, D. *et al.* (2002). Propionibacteria induce apoptosis of colorectal carcinoma cells via short-chain fatty acids acting on mitochondria. *Cell Death Differ.*, **9**, 179–188.

Jault, F. M., Jault, J. M., Ruchti, F. *et al.* (1995). Cytomegalovirus infection induces high levels of cyclins, phosphorylated Rb, and p53, leading to cell cycle arrest. *J. Virol.*, **69**, 6697–6704.

Johnson, R. A., Ma, X. L., Yurochko, A. D., and Huang, E. S. (2001a). The role of MKK1/2 kinase activity in human cytomegalovirus infection. *J. Gen. Virol.*, **82**, 493–497.

Johnson, R. A., Wang, X., Ma, X. L., Huong, S. M., and Huang, E. S. (2001b). Human cytomegalovirus up-regulates the phosphatidylinositol 3-kinase (PI3-K) pathway: inhibition of PI3-K activity inhibits viral replication and virus-induced signaling. *J. Virol.*, **75**, 6022–6032.

Jurak, I., and Brune, W. (2006). Induction of apoptosis limits cytomegalovirus cross-species infection. *EMBO J.*, **25**, 2634–2642.

Kalejta, R. F. and Shenk, T. (2002). Manipulation of the cell cycle by human cytomegalovirus. *Front Biosci.*, **7**, D295–D306.

Khan, S., Zimmermann, A., Basler, M., Groettrup, M., and Hengel, H. (2004). A cytomegalovirus inhibitor of gamma interferon signaling controls immunoproteasome induction. *J. Virol.*, **78**, 1831–1842.

Korioth, F., Maul, G. G., Plachter, B., Stamminger, T., and Frey, J. (1996). The nuclear domain 10 (ND10) is disrupted by the human cytomegalovirus gene product IE1. *Exp. Cell. Res.*, **229**, 155–158.

Kouzarides, T., Bankier, A. T., Satchwell, S. C., Preddy, E., and Barrell, B. G. (1988). An immediate early gene of human cytomegalovirus encodes a potential membrane glycoprotein. *Virology*, **165**, 151–164.

Kowalik, T. F., Wing, B., Haskill, J. S., Azizkhan, J. C., Baldwin, A. J., and Huang, E. S. (1993). Multiple mechanisms are implicated in the regulation of NF-kappa B activity during human cytomegalovirus infection. *Proc. Natl Acad. Sci. USA*, **90**, 1107–1111.

Langelier, Y., Bergeron, S., Chabaud, S. *et al.* (2002). The R1 subunit of herpes simplex virus ribonucleotide reductase protects cells against apoptosis at, or upstream of, caspase-8 activation. *J. Gen. Virol.*, **83**, 2779–2789.

Lodoen, M. B. and Lanier, L. L. (2005). Viral modulation of NK cell immunity. *Nat. Rev. Microbiol.*, **3**, 59–69.

Lu, M. and Shenk, T. (1996). Human cytomegalovirus infection inhibits cell cycle progression at multiple points, including the transition from G1 to S. *J. Virol.*, **70**, 8850–8857.

Lu, M. and Shenk, T. (1999). Human cytomegalovirus UL69 protein induces cells to accumulate in G1 phase of the cell cycle. *J. Virol.*, **73**, 676–683.

Lukac, D. M., Harel, N. Y., Tanese, N., and Alwine, J. C. (1997). TAF-like functions of human cytomegalovirus immediate-early proteins. *J. Virol.*, **71**, 7227–7239.

Marchini, A., Liu, H., and Zhu, H. (2001). Human cytomegalovirus with IE-2 (UL122) deleted fails to express early lytic genes. *J. Virol.*, **75**, 1870–1878.

Margolis, M. J., Pajovic, S., Wong, E. L. *et al.* (1995). Interaction of the 72-kilodalton human cytomegalovirus IE1 gene product with E2F1 coincides with E2F-dependent activation of dihydrofolate reductase transcription. *J. Virol.*, **69**, 7759–7767.

Mate, J. L., Ariza, A., Munoz, A., Molinero, J. L., Lopez, D., and Navas-Palacios, J. J. (1998). Induction of proliferating cell nuclear antigen and Ki-67 expression by cytomegalovirus infection. *J. Pathol.*, **184**, 279–282.

McCormick, A. L., Skaletskaya, A., Barry, P. A., Mocarski, E. S., and Goldmacher, V. S. (2003a). Differential function and expression of the viral inhibitor of caspase 8-induced apoptosis (vICA) and the viral mitochondria-localized inhibitor of apoptosis (vMIA) cell death suppressors conserved in primate and rodent cytomegaloviruses. *Virology*, **316**, 221–233.

McCormick, A. L., Smith, V. L., Chow, D., and Mocarski, E. S. (2003b). Disruption of mitochondrial networks by the human cytomegalovirus UL37 gene product viral mitochondrion-localized inhibitor of apoptosis. *J. Virol.*, **77**, 631–641.

McCormick, A. L., Meiering, C. D., Smith, G. B., and Mocarski, E. S. (2005). Mitochondrial cell death suppressors carried by human and murine cytomegalovirus confer resistance to proteasome inhibitor-induced apoptosis. *J. Virol.*, **79**, 12205–12217.

Menard, C., Wagner, M., Ruzsics, Z. *et al.* (2003). Role of murine cytomegalovirus US22 gene family members in replication in macrophages. *J. Virol.*, **77**, 5557–5570.

Menegazzi, P., Galvan, M., Rotola, A. *et al.* (1999). Temporal mapping of transcripts in human herpesvirus-7. *J. Gen. Virol.*, **80**, 2705–2712.

Mocarski, E. S. (2002). Immunomodulation by cytomegaloviruses: manipulative strategies beyond evasion. *Trends Microbiol.*, **10**, 332–339.

Mocarski, E. S., Jr. (2004). Immune escape and exploitation strategies of cytomegaloviruses: impact on and imitation of the major histocompatibility system. *Cell Microbiol.*, **6**, 707–717.

Mocarski, E. S., Jr. and Courcelle, C. T. (2001). Cytomegaloviruses and their replication. ed. In *Fields Virology* 4th edn., ed. D. M. Knipe, P. M. Howley, D. E. Griffin *et al.* Vol. 2, pp. 2629–2673. Philadelphia: Lippincott, Williams & Wilkins.

Muganda, P., Carrasco, R., and Qian, Q. (1998). The human cytomegalovirus IE2 86 kDa protein elevates p53 levels and transactivates the p53 promoter in human fibroblasts. *Cell Mol. Biol., (Noisy-le-grand)*, **44**, 321–331.

Murphy, E. A., Streblow, D. N., Nelson, J. A., and Stinski, M. F. (2000). The human cytomegalovirus IE86 protein can block cell cycle progression after inducing transition into the S phase of permissive cells. *J. Virol.*, **74**, 7108–7118.

Navarro, L., Mowen, K., Rodems, S. *et al.* (1998). Cytomegalovirus activates interferon immediate-early response gene expression and an interferon regulatory factor 3-containing interferon- stimulated response element-binding complex. *Mol. Cell Biol.*, **18**, 3796–3802.

Netterwald, J. R., Jones, T. R., Britt, W. J., Yang, S. J., McCrone, I. P., and Zhu, H. (2004). Postattachment events associated with viral entry are necessary for induction of interferon-stimulated genes by human cytomegalovirus. *J. Virol.*, **78**, 6688–6691.

Patrone, M., Percivalle, E., Secchi, M. *et al.* (2003). The human cytomegalovirus UL45 gene product is a late, virion-associated protein and influences virus growth at low multiplicities of infection. *J. Gen. Virol.*, **84**, 3359–3370.

Patterson, C. E. and Shenk, T. (1999). Human cytomegalovirus UL36 protein is dispensable for viral replication in cultured cells. *J. Virol.*, **73**, 7126–7131.

Penfold, M. E. and Mocarski, E. S. (1997). Formation of cytomegalovirus DNA replication compartments defined by localization of viral proteins and DNA synthesis. *Virology*, **239**, 46–61.

Polster, B. M., Pevsner, J., and Hardwick, J. M. (2004). Viral Bcl-2 homologues and their role in virus replication and associated diseases. *Biochim. Biophys. Acta*, **1644**, 211–227.

Poma, E. E., Kowalik, T. F., Zhu, L., Sinclair, J. H., and Huang, E. S. (1996). The human cytomegalovirus IE1-72 protein interacts with the cellular p107 protein and relieves p107-mediated transcriptional repression of an E2F-responsive promoter. *J. Virol.*, **70**, 7867–7877.

Poncet, D., Larochette, N., Pauleau, A. L. *et al.* (2004). An anti-apoptotic viral protein that recruits Bax to mitochondria. *J. Biol. Chem.*, **279**, 22605–22614.

Popkin, D. L. and Virgin, H. W. (2003). Murine cytomegalovirus infection inhibits tumor necrosis factor alpha responses in primary macrophages. *J. Virol.*, **77**, 10125–10130.

Preston, C. M., Harman, A. N., and Nicholl, M. J. (2001). Activation of interferon response factor-3 in human cells infected with herpes simplex virus type 1 or human cytomegalovirus. *J. Virol.*, **75**, 8909–8916.

Reboredo, M., Greaves, R. F., and Hahn, G. (2004). Human cytomegalovirus proteins encoded by UL37 exon 1 protect infected fibroblasts against virus-induced apoptosis and are required for efficient virus replication. *J. Gen. Virol.*, **85**, 3555–3567.

Rodriguez, J. E., Loepfe, T. R., and Swack, N. S. (1987). Beta interferon production in primed and unprimed cells infected with human cytomegalovirus. *Arch. Virol.*, **94**, 177–189.

Roumier, T., Vieira, H. L., Castedo, M. *et al.* (2002). The C-terminal moiety of HIV-1 Vpr induces cell death via a caspase-independent mitochondrial pathway. *Cell Death Differ.*, **9**, 1212–1219.

Saffert, R. T., and Kalejta, R. F. (2006). Inactivating a cellular intrinsic immune defense mediated by Daxx is the mechanism through which the human cytomegalovirus pp71 protein stimulates viral immediate-early gene expression. *J. Virol.*, **80**, 3863–3871.

Salvant, B. S., Fortunato, E. A., and Spector, D. H. (1998). Cell cycle dysregulation by human cytomegalovirus: influence of the cell cycle phase at the time of infection and effects on cyclin transcription. *J. Virol.*, **72**, 3729–3741.

Sambucetti, L. C., Cherrington, J. M., Wilkinson, G. W. G., and Mocarski, E. S. (1989). NF-kB activation of the cytomegalovirus enhancer is mediated by a viral transactivator and by T cell stimulation. *EMBO J.*, **8**, 4251–4258.

Sanchez, V., McElroy, A. K., and Spector, D. H. (2003). Mechanisms governing maintenance of Cdk1/cyclin B1 kinase activity in cells infected with human cytomegalovirus. *J. Virol.*, **77**, 13214–13224.

Sanchez, V., Clark, C. L., Yen, J. Y., Dwarakanath, R., and Spector, D. H. (2002). Viable human cytomegalovirus recombinant virus with an internal deletion of the IE2 86 gene affects late stages of viral replication. *J. Virol.*, **76**, 2973–2989.

Secchiero, P., Bertolaso, L., Casareto, L. et al. (1998). Human herpesvirus 7 infection induces profound cell cycle perturbations coupled to disregulation of cdc2 and cyclin B and polyploidization of CD4(+) T cells. *Blood*, **92**, 1685–1696.

Secchiero, P., Mirandola, P., Zella, D. et al. (2001). Human herpesvirus 7 induces the functional up-regulation of tumor necrosis factor-related apoptosis-inducing ligand (TRAIL) coupled to TRAIL-R1 down-modulation in CD4(+) T cells. *Blood*, **98**, 2474–2481.

Sedger, L. M., Shows, D. M., Blanton, R. A. et al. (1999). IFN-gamma mediates a novel antiviral activity through dynamic modulation of TRAIL and TRAIL receptor expression. *J. Immunol.*, **163**, 920–926.

Sedy, J. R., Gavrieli, M., Potter, K. G. et al. (2005). B and T lymphocyte attenuator regulates T cell activation through interaction with herpesvirus entry mediator. *Nat. Immunol.*, **6**, 90–98.

Simmen, K. A., Singh, J., Luukkonen, B. G. et al. (2001). Global modulation of cellular transcription by human cytomegalovirus is initiated by viral glycoprotein B. *Proc. Natl Acad. Sci. USA*, **98**, 7140–7145.

Skaletskaya, A., Bartle, L. M., Chittenden, T., McCormick, A. L., Mocarski, E. S., and Goldmacher, V. S. (2001). A cytomegalovirus-encoded inhibitor of apoptosis that suppresses caspase-8 activation. *Proc. Natl Acad. Sci. USA*, **98**, 7829–7834.

Smith, G. B. and Mocarski, E. S. (2005). GADD45a directly enhances the mitochondrial apoptosis inhibitors Bcl-xL and vMIA. *Nat. Cell Biol.* (submitted for publication).

Song, Y. J. and Stinski, M. F. (2002). Effect of the human cytomegalovirus IE86 protein on expression of E2F-responsive genes: A DNA microarray analysis. *Proc. Natl Acad. Sci. USA*, **99**, 2836–2841.

Speir, E., Modali, R., Huang, E. S. et al. (1994). Potential role of human cytomegalovirus and p53 interaction in coronary restenosis. *Science*, **265**, 391–394.

Su, Y., Adair, R., Davis, C. N., DiFronzo, N. L., and Colberg-Poley, A. M. (2003). Convergence of RNA cis elements and cellular polyadenylation factors in the regulation of human cytomegalovirus UL37 exon 1 unspliced RNA production. *J. Virol.*, **77**, 12729–12741.

Tanaka, K., Zou, J. P., Takeda, K. et al. (1999). Effects of human cytomegalovirus immediate-early proteins on p53- mediated apoptosis in coronary artery smooth muscle cells *Circulation*, **99**, 1656–1659.

Tavalai, N., Papior, P., Rechter, S., Leis, M., and Stamminger, T. (2006). Evidence for a role of the cellular ND10 protein PML in mediating intrinsic immunity against human cytomegalovirus infections. *J. Virol.*, **80**, 8006–8018.

Tang, Q. and Maul, G. G. (2006). Mouse cytomegalovirus crosses the species barrier with help from a few human cytomegalovirus proteins. *J. Virol.*, **80**, 7510–7521.

Tenney, D. J. and Colberg-Poley, A. M. (1990). RNA analysis and isolation of cDNAs derived from the human cytomegalovirus immediate-early region at 0.24 map units. *Intervirology*, **31**, 203–214.

Tenney, D. J. and Colberg-Poley, A. M. (1991a). Expression of the human cytomegalovirus UL36–38 immediate early region during permissive infection. *Virology*, **182**, 199–210.

Tenney, D. J. and Colberg-Poley, A. M. (1991b). Human cytomegalovirus UL36–38 and US3 immediate-early genes: temporally regulated expression of nuclear, cytoplasmic, and polysome-associated transcripts during infection. *J. Virol.*, **65**, 6724–6734.

Vieira, H. L., Belzacq, A. S., Haouzi, D. et al. (2001). The adenine nucleotide translocator: a target of nitric oxide, peroxynitrite, and 4-hydroxynonenal. *Oncogene*, **20**, 4305–4316.

Wang, J., Marker, P. H., Belcher, J. D. et al. (2000). Human cytomegalovirus immediate early proteins upregulate endothelial p53 function. *FEBS Lett.*, **474**, 213–216.

Wang, X., Huong, S. M., Chiu, M. L., Raab-Traub, N., and Huang, E. S. (2003). Epidermal growth factor receptor is a cellular receptor for human cytomegalovirus. *Nature*, **424**, 456–461.

White, E. A., Clark, C. L., Sanchez, V., and Spector, D. H. (2004). Small internal deletions in the human cytomegalovirus IE2 gene result in nonviable recombinant viruses with differential defects in viral gene expression. *J. Virol.*, **78**, 1817–1830.

Wiebusch, L., Asmar, J., Uecker, R., and Hagemeier, C. (2003a). Human cytomegalovirus immediate-early protein 2 (IE2)-mediated activation of cyclin E is cell-cycle-independent and forces S-phase entry in IE2-arrested cells. *J. Gen. Virol.*, **84**, 51–60.

Wiebusch, L., and Hagemeier, C. (1999). Human cytomegalovirus 86-kilodalton IE2 protein blocks cell cycle progression in G(1). *J. Virol.*, **73**, 9274–9283.

Wiebusch, L., and Hagemeier, C. (2001). The human cytomegalovirus immediate early 2 protein dissociates cellular DNA synthesis from cyclin-dependent kinase activation. *Embo. J.*, **20**, 1086–1098.

Wiebusch, L., Uecker, R., and Hagemeier, C. (2003). Human cytomegalovirus prevents replication licensing by inhibiting MCM loading onto chromatin. *EMBO Rep.*, **4**, 42–46.

Yang, S., Netterwald, J., Wang, W., and Zhu, H. (2005). Characterization of the elements and proteins responsible for interferon-stimulated gene induction by human cytomegalovirus. *J. Virol.*, **79**, 5027–5034.

Yu, D., Silva, M. C., and Shenk, T. (2003). Functional map of human cytomegalovirus AD169 defined by global mutational analysis. *Proc. Natl Acad. Sci. USA*, **100**, 12396–12401.

Yu, Y. and Alwine, J. C. (2002). Human cytomegalovirus major immediate–early proteins and simian virus 40 large T antigen can inhibit apoptosis through activation of the phosphatidylinositide 3'-OH kinase pathway and the cellular kinase Akt. *J. Virol.*, **76**, 3731–3738.

Yurochko, A. D., Kowalik, T. F., Huong, S. M., and Huang, E. S. (1995). Human cytomegalovirus upregulates NF-kappa B activity by transactivating the NF-kappa B p105/p50 and p65 promoters. *J. Virol.*, **69**, 5391–5400.

Yurochko, A. D., Hwang, E. S., Rasmussen, L., Keay, S., Pereira, L., and Huang, E. S. (1997a). The human cytomegalovirus UL55 (gB) and UL75 (gH) glycoprotein ligands initiate the rapid activation of Sp1 and NF-kappaB during infection. *J. Virol.*, **71**, 5051–5059.

Yurochko, A. D., Mayo, M. W., Poma, E. E., Baldwin, A. S., Jr., and Huang, E. S. (1997b). Induction of the transcription factor Sp1 during human cytomegalovirus infection mediates upregulation of the p65 and p105/p50 NF-kappaB promoters. *J. Virol.*, **71**, 4638–4648.

Zhu, H., Shen, Y., and Shenk, T. (1995). Human cytomegalovirus IE1 and IE2 proteins block apoptosis. *J. Virol.*, **69**, 7960–7970.

Zhu, H., Cong, J. P., and Shenk, T. (1997). Use of differential display analysis to assess the effect of human cytomegalovirus infection on the accumulation of cellular RNAs: induction of interferon-responsive RNAs. *Proc. Natl Acad. Sci. USA*, **94**, 13985–13990.

Zhu, H., Cong, J. P., Mamtora, G., Gingeras, T., and Shenk, T. (1998). Cellular gene expression altered by human cytomegalovirus: global monitoring with oligonucleotide arrays. *Proc. Natl Acad. Sci. USA*, **95**, 14470–14475.

Part II

Basic virology and viral gene effects on host cell functions: gammaherpesviruses

Edited by Patrick Moore

Part III

Basic virology and viral gene effects on host cell functions: gammaherpesviruses

edited by Patrick Moore

Introduction to the human γ-herpesviruses

Richard Longnecker[1] and Frank Neipel[2]

[1]Feinberg School of Medicine, Northwestern University Medical School, Chicago, IL, USA
[2]Institute for Clinical and Molecular Virology, University of Erlangen, Germany

Introduction

This chapter will provide a brief background into the γ-herpesviruses family in comparison to other members of the herpesvirus family; but the primary focus of this chapter will be to recount the discovery of the two human γ-herpesviruses (EBV and KSHV) and the diseases associated with infection of each virus, a brief introduction into their life cycles, and finally a description of the genome characteristics of the viruses including a description of their respective genomes. In many ways, the discovery and association with human diseases for both EBV and KSHV have many parallels despite almost three decades separating their discoveries and association with human disease.

The γ-herpesvirus family

The γ-herpesviruses are a subfamily of herpesviruses that were first distinguished by their cellular tropism for lymphocytes. Subsequent molecular phylogenetic analyses have confirmed the close relationship among these viruses that is distinct from the α- and β-herpesviruses subfamilies (Fig. 22.1). *Gammaherpesvirinae* is currently divided into two genera, *Lymphocryptoviridae* which includes human Epstein–Barr virus (EBV or HHV4) and *Rhadinoviridae*, which includes human Kaposi's sarcoma-associated herpesvirus (KSHV or HHV8). Recent studies suggest that primate rhadinoviruses can be further subdivided in KSHV-like viruses, a second closely related but distinct lineage of Old World primate viruses related to the rhesus rhadinovirus (RRV), and the New World monkey rhadinoviruses represented by herpesvirus saimiri (HVS). A more detailed analysis of the non-human γ-herpesviruses will be discussed in Chapters 60 and 61.

Although the best-studied members of the γ-herpesviruses are EBV and KSHV, γ-herpesviruses are parasites of a broad range of mammals from mice (murine herpesvirus-68 and related viruses) to cows and horses (bovine herpesvirus 4 and equine herpesvirus 2), as well as primates. Surprisingly, γ-herpesviruses of lower mammals most closely resemble the rhadinoviruses, and exhibit extensive molecular piracy of host regulatory genes that is not found in EBV and related viruses. Interestingly, the lymphocryptoviruses have been found only in primates and humans. The γ-herpesviruses share a similar genomic structure that the 172 kilobase pair, linear double-stranded DNA genome of the B95–8 EBV strain serves as the prototype since it was the first γ-herpesvirus that was sequenced (Baer *et al.*, 1984). The large central region of the genome contains most of the coding capacity for the viruses, including blocks of highly conserved genes that are shared among the herpesviruses (Fig. 22.2). The ends of the molecule are capped by variable numbers of direct repeat sequences that are the sites for genome circularization during latency. Unlike the α-herpesviruses (Chapter 10), the γ-herpesviruses do not undergo genomic isomerization and only linearize and recircularize in their terminal repeat regions, although the numbers of terminal repeats can be highly variable.

The γ-herpesviruses also share a number of characteristics in common with the α- and β-herpesviruses, particularly related to lytic viral replication. During lytic replication, the γ-herpesviruses genome is packaged as a linear molecule in a proteinaceous capsid, which is then enveloped by a lipid bilayer prior to release from the cell. This process starts when viral transactivators initiate viral genome-wide transcription through a series of orderly transcriptional cascades. Different classes of viral genes (immediate–early, early and late) are transcribed resulting in the production of infectious virions. As with other

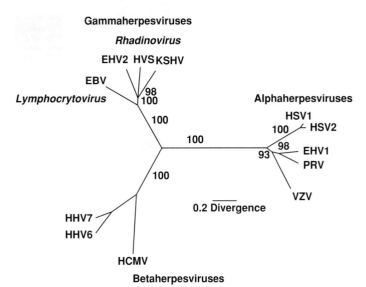

Fig. 22.1. Phylogenetic tree for selected herpesviruses. Phylogenetic trees are based on comparison of aligned amino acid sequences between herpesviruses for the MCP gene. The comparison of MCP sequences was obtained by the NJ method and is shown in unrooted form, with branch lengths proportional to divergence (mean number of substitution events per site) between the nodes bounding each branch. The number of times (of 100 bootstrap samplings) that the division indicated by each internal branch was obtained is shown next to each branch; bootstrap values below 75 are not shown. Figure adapted from Fig. 2A from reference (Moore et al., 1996). Used with permission of American Society of Microbiology.

herpesviruses, γ-herpesviruses lytic replication is thought generally to cause cell death. While specific mechanisms for lytic replication differ between the herpesviruses, and even among the γ-herpesviruses, they all broadly share similar capsid structures and have similar overall mechanisms for lytic replication. As would be expected, genes involved in lytic replication and viral capsid production tend to be highly conserved across the herpesvirus subfamilies, including the γ-herpesviruses.

The γ-herpesviruses differ the most dramatically from each other and from other herpesviruses during the latent portion of their lifecycle. Unlike the other human herpesviruses, both EBV and KSHV latency can be established and manipulated in vitro, providing an important experimental system that is unavailable for other viruses. Latency occurs after infection of a cell and transport of the capsid to the nucleus where the genome is released. The viral genome, still a linear DNA fragment, then circularizes by ligation of terminal repeat sequences and replicates as an episome using the host cell replication machinery.

A key feature of the γ-herpesviruses is their common capacity to induce lymphoproliferation and cancers. Tumors caused by EBV and KSHV include lymphoproliferative diseases and lymphomas, but also include tumors from other tissue-types, such as smooth muscle cells and endothelial cell origin. In some cases, tumorigenesis occurs when viruses cross species such as bovine infection by the wildebeest γ-herpesviruses, alcelaphine herpesvirus 1, in Africa (Ensser et al., 1997). In other cases, tumorigenesis is a rare occurrence among infected individuals, except when the host is specifically susceptible through immunosuppression or through a rare familial mutation altering normal immune function.

EBV was the first human tumor virus discovered and has been a rich source of information for tumor biologists as well as a tool for immortalizing cell lines for use as reagents. As shown by the Henles in 1967, EBV has the unusual property of immortalizing primary B lymphocytes in culture (Henle et al., 1967). Continuous cell lines that result from this immortalization are termed lymphoblastoid cell lines (LCLs) reflecting their activated phenotype. These LCLs contain EBV episomes and express a very limited number of viral genes and have served as an important model of EBV latent infection and transformation as will be further discussed in Chapter 24. These latently infected cell lines, as shown in 1978 by zur Hausen and colleagues can be induced to lytic replication by treatment with phorbol esters (zur Hausen et al., 1978). Interestingly, similar treatment of cell lines harboring KSHV causes induction of lytic replication (Arvanitakis et al., 1996; Renne et al., 1996).

KSHV, more recently discovered, provides a unique tumor virus model since it has incorporated cellular proto-oncogenes and serves as a rosetta stone between cancer biology and tumor virology. The natural lifecycles of EBV and KSHV are well studied and experimentally tractable allowing for the careful examination of oncogenes from these viruses not only in terms of their capacity to induce cell transformation but also in terms of their roles in the natural viral life cycle.

The discovery of Epstein–Barr virus (EBV)

Although there was considerable evidence to indicate the role of viruses in human cancers from animal studies dating from the early 1900s, it was not until the identification of Burkitt's lymphoma and the subsequent identification of EBV in this unusual tumor that a clear role of viruses in human cancers became apparent. The first key to the puzzle of a human virus being associated with a human

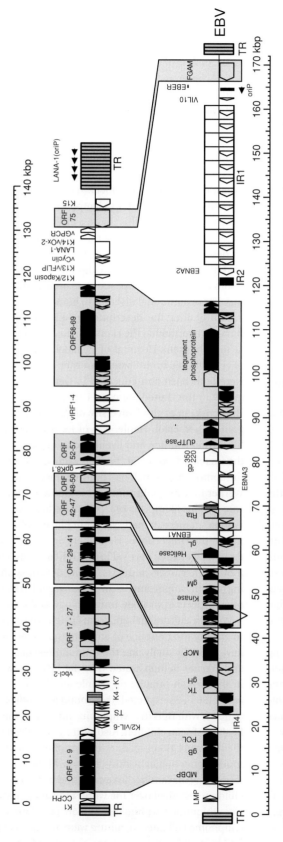

Fig. 22.2. Colinearity of the genetic maps of KSHV (top) and EBV (bottom). Schematic representation of the genomes of KSHV and EBV were drawn to scale based on the sequences by Russo et al. (PNAS 93, 14862–14867, 1996; Genbank acc. no. U75698) and the inverted sequence of EBV strain B95-8 (Baer et al., Nature **310** (5974), 207–211 (1984), Genbank acc. no. NC001345), respectively. According to Russo et al., protein coding regions (open reading frames, ORF) of KSHV that are conserved amongst KSHV and herpesvirus saimiri are numbered from 1 to 75. KSHV ORFS without detectable homology to herpesvirus saimiri genes are numbered with the prefix "K" or from K1 to K15. Open arrows symbolize herpesvirus genes not conserved amongst all human herpesvirus groups (alpha, beta, and gamma), whereas "core" herpesvirus genes that share homology detectable by BLAST amongst all groups of human herpesviruses are represented by arrows filled in black. The names of a few hallmark-genes are given above the EBV genome. Essentially, conserved genes are localized in five (seven) major blocks on the genomes of KSHV and EBV, linked here by trapezoid boxes. Most genes of the lytic replication cycle (virion proteins, DNA-replication proteins) are found here. These blocks of core herpesvirus genes are interspersed by areas coding for more strain- or virus-specific genes. In the case of KSHV, these are usually the "K" genes that are frequently homologous to genes of the host cell. In the case of EBV, the Epstein-Barr virus nuclear antigens (EBNA 1–3) and latent membrane proteins (LMP1–2) are present at these positions. In addition, two major envelope glycoproteins of KSHV and EBV, gpK8.1 and gp350–220, respectively, are not conserved amongst the viruses. However, both genes are located at comparable positions close to the center of the coding regions.

Abbreviations: CCPH, complement control protein homologue; MDBP, major DNA binding protein; gB, glycoprotein B; pol, DNA polymerase; vIL-6, viral IL-6 homologue; vbcl-2, viral bcl-2; TK, thymidine kinase; gH, glycoprotein H; MCP, major capsid protein; gM, glycoprotein M; gL, glycoprotein L; Rta: R-transactivator of transcription; vIRF1–4: interferon regulatory factors 1–4; vFLIP: viral flice-inhibitory protein; vCyclin: viral cyclin-D homologue; vOx-2: viral Ox-2 (CD200) homologue; LANA-1: latent nuclear antigen 1; vGPCR: viral G-protein coupled receptor homologue; FGAM: formyl-glycin-amid transferase homologue; vIL10: viral interleukin 10 homologue; EBER: EBV-encoded small RNAs; TR, terminal repeat; IR: internal repeat; oriP: plasmid origin of replication.

tumor resulted from the interest of Denis Burkitt with a malignancy in children in Africa.

Denis Burkitt was born in 1911 and lived in Lawnkilla near Enniskillen, County Fermanagh, Ireland. He received his medical training at Trinity College in Dublin with his clinical training at Adelaide Hospital. Following graduation and after working in hospitals in his native Ireland and military service as army surgeon in the Royal Army Medical Corps, Burkitt embarked on a career of medical service in Africa due in part to his strong religious convictions and interest in service in the third world. In 1957, after being in Kampala, Uganda, for 10 years, he was asked by Hugh Trowell, a colleague in Kampala, to see a young boy with swellings on both sides of his upper and lower jaws that proved to be a lymphoma. The tumor was a very common cancer in African children, was fast growing causing grotesque disfigurement, and was fatal upon metastasis to other parts of the body.

Burkitt's fascination and interest in the tumor led him to carefully examine hospital records and to send out a questionnaire to government and mission hospitals throughout Africa. He also embarked on what he would call his long safari to document the incidence of this lymphoma. From this trip, which took 10 weeks, covered 10 thousand miles, journeyed through 12 countries, and stopped at 57 hospitals; Burkitt found a definite pattern of distribution with the lymphoma confined to a region 10 degrees north and 10 degrees south of the equator following closely the pattern of distribution of mosquito borne diseases such as malaria and yellow fever. These initial results were published in the *British Journal of Surgery* in 1958 (Burkitt, 1958). But it was not until 1961 after publication of a more detailed version in *Cancer* with a pathologist Greg O'Conor (Burkitt and O'Conor, 1961) and an invitation to give a lecture at Middlesex Hospital in London in March of 1961 that allowed the next step in the identification of EBV to fall into place.

In the audience of Burkitt's talk at Middlesex Hospital was Anthony Epstein who immediately developed an interest in the Burkitt's tumor. Epstein, who had worked on the Rous sarcoma virus, had developed an interest in the role of viruses in cancer and he was fascinated with Burkitt's description of his findings. Rous sarcoma virus was shown in 1911 by Peyton Rous at the Rockefeller Institute in New York to be responsible for a sarcoma that was transmissible in chickens. Epstein and Burkitt immediately began to collaborate. Biopsies were flown from Kampala to Epstein's laboratory in London, but it was not until 1963 after Yvonne Barr and Bert Achong joined the hunt that herpesvirus-like particles were observed in February 1964 from a cell line established from a biopsy delivered from Africa early in December of 1963 (Epstein *et al.*, 1964). Interestingly, both Achong and Barr were graduates of schools in Ireland. Achong graduated from University College Dublin and Yvonne Barr was a graduate of Trinity College Dublin.

Human disease associated with EBV infection

Considerable interest has focused on EBV since its discovery and its link with Burkitt's lymphoma. Along with KSHV, as we will learn also in this chapter, EBV is the only other herpesvirus with an etiological role in human malignancies. As described above, EBV is a causative agent in endemic Burkitt's lymphoma, but since the link of EBV with this lymphoma, EBV has also been shown to be important for a large number of additional diseases in humans.

Shortly after the description of EBV association with Burkitt's lymphoma, the Henles, a husband and wife team at the Children's Hospital of Philadelphia obtained a set of cell cultures from Epstein. Werner and Gertrude Henle were both born and educated in Germany. Werner emigrated to the United States in 1936 finding an instructorship position at the University of Pennsylvania. Werner's grandfather, Jacob Henle, was of Jewish descent, making his further training and livelihood in question because of the increased power of the Nazi regime in Germany and the approaching war. It had become "increasingly clear" to Werner that he could "not stay in Germany and pursue a career to his liking." In 1937, Gertrude Szpingier, who was Werner's fiancée, joined Werner in Philadelphia. They had met at the University of Heidelberg and were married the day after Gertrude's arrival in the United States. They spent their entire careers at the University of Pennsylvania making not only important discoveries in regard to EBV, but also other aspects of virology, immunology, and viral oncology.

With the cultures in hand from Epstein, the Henles began to explore the presence of antibodies directed against the new virus. By analyzing the immune response, Gertrude and Werner demonstrated that the EBV was widespread in the human population (Henle and Henle 1966; Henle *et al.*, 1969). As expected, they found antibodies to EBV in children with Burkitt's lymphoma, but also in the serum of healthy African children. Also, as may have been expected, the antibody titers in Burkitt's lymphoma patients were much higher that in healthy children. More surprising, was the finding that antibodies were found in most serums from children tested all over the world indicating that the virus was ubiquitous within the human population. Burkitt's lymphoma cell lines in culture were also used at this time by Lloyd Old and his colleagues at the Memorial Sloan–Kettering Cancer Center in New York to make the initial connection of EBV infection and nasopharyngeal carcinoma (Old *et al.*, 1966).

Because antibodies to EBV were so ubiquitous, the Henles suspected that infections with EBV were common and were generally self-limited in nature. Interestingly, this has been a common observation in regard to most of the herpesviruses that were subsequently discovered. At the time of the discovery of EBV, only three other human herpesviruses were known. These were herpes simplex virus (HSV), varicella-zoster virus (VZV), and cytomegalovirus (CMV). All of these viruses caused overt symptoms as in the case for HSV and VZV, or were associated with serious congenital defects. As will be discussed in other chapters and this chapter, HHV6, HHV7, and KSHV cause little disease in immune competent individuals. It is only when the immune host immune system is compromised that overt symptoms typically appear with infection of these viruses.

As is the case for many discoveries, serendipity led to the discovery of the association of EBV with infectious mononucleosis. Late in 1967, a technician working in the Henle laboratory developed classical symptoms of infectious mononucleosis (Henle *et al.*, 1968). Prior to her symptoms, she had shown no antibodies to EBV, but with her symptoms, antibodies appeared to EBV. As will be reviewed in the later chapters, we will learn that, along with the association of EBV with Burkitt's lymphoma, NPC, and infectious mononucleosis, EBV has now been found to be involved in a much wider range of human disease. It is generally accepted that EBV is involved with several other malignancies of lymphocyte origin such as some types of Hodgkin's lymphoma, and epithelial origin such as gastric carcinoma. Table 22.1 contains a list of diseases with known EBV etiology. Each of these disease associations will be expanded in later chapters and specific references can be found in these chapters. EBV is also a factor in a variety of other human malignancies including some T and NK cell lymphomas.

The association of EBV with other diseases, such as breast carcinoma and hepatocellular carcinoma, remain controversial and will likely only be resolved in the coming years with additional research. In immunosuppressed patients, EBV causes a variety of proliferative disorders including oral hairy leukoplakia in AIDS patients, immunoblastic lymphomas, and an unusual tumor of muscle origin in children with AIDS or who are under immune suppression for liver transplantation. In young boys with X-linked immunodeficiencies, EBV causes severe mononucleosis that results in death.

Evidence is accumulating that the EBV may also be associated with immune mediated diseases. In particular, there is a variety of auto-immune diseases that appear to have an infectious agent as a cofactor such as multiple sclerosis, rheumatoid arthritis, and diabetes. For each of these autoimmune diseases, it has been suggested that EBV may have an involvement in causing deregulation of the normal immune response to self-antigens. But, since EBV is so ubiquitous, many of these studies are also controversial. The linking of EBV infection to autoimmune disease and controversial malignancies such as breast carcinoma and hepatocellular carcinoma may await the development of an effective vaccine against EBV which will be discussed in Chapter 72. By preventing primary infection, an effective vaccine would offer convincing proof of a disease association due to absence of a particular disease or malignancy in those vaccinated for EBV. This may allow the true appreciation of the wide variety of disease associated with EBV infection in humans.

EBV life cycle

Infection with EBV usually occurs early in childhood, resulting in an asymptomatic infection. The virus is spread through saliva. If primary infection occurs later, B-cell proliferation and the resulting immune response results in infectious mononucleosis. After primary infection, most individuals will harbor the virus for the remainder of their life, and carriers develop cellular immunity against a variety of both lytic and latency associated proteins that will be more discussed later in this chapter as well as in Chapter 51. By adulthood, the majority of the human population (upwards of 90%) is infected with EBV. Periodically, virus is shed from latently infected individuals by the induction of lytic replication in B lymphocytes. The true site of latent infection has not been determined, but the virus likely resides in B lymphocytes. Recent studies have shown that EBV can be detected in circulating peripheral blood lymphocytes in carriers of EBV latent infections by PCR (both for viral DNA and viral mRNA) (Tierney *et al.*, 1994; Chen *et al.*, 1995; Babcock *et al.*, 1999; Qu *et al.*, 2000) and virus isolation and outgrowth of immortalized cell lines by culturing peripheral lymphocytes (Yao *et al.*, 1985). It has not been determined if this is the true site of latency. Other potential sites of EBV latency may include bone marrow, lymph nodes, or other lymphoid organs.

Early experiments suggested that latency is not maintained by constant re-infection of circulating B-lymphocytes as evidenced in patients treated with acyclovir (Yao *et al.*, 1989). Acyclovir, a nucleoside analogue that can inhibit lytic replication in the oral epithelium had no effect on the number of B-cells in the peripheral blood population that harbor the virus. More recent experiments have shown

Table 22.1. EBV associated pathologies in the human host

Pathology	Sub-type	Percent EBV +	Notes
Burkitt's lymphoma			
	Endemic	95–100%	Africa and New Guinea
	Sporadic	20–30%	Outside endemic region
Infectious mononucleosis		100%	
Chronic active EBV infection		100%	
Nasopharyngeal carcinoma		100%	Near 100% association with Type II and Type III, Type I frequently associated with EBV in endemic regions (South East Asia and North Africa)
Hodgkin's disease			90% in children in Latin America
	Mixed cell, lymphocyte depleted	60–80%	
	Nodular schlerozing	20–40%	
Fatal IM/X-linked lymphoproliferative syndrome		100%	
Immunocompromised disorders			
	Post-transplant Lymphoproliferative disorder	80%	
	Burkitt's lymphoma	30–50%	
	Diffuse large cell lymphoma – Centroblastic	30%	
	Diffuse large cell lymphoma – Immunoblastic	90%	
	Primary CNS lymphoma	100%	
	Non-Hodgkin's lymphoma	30–50%	
	Leiomyosarcoma	100%	Unusual muscle tumor found primarily in children
	Oral Hairy leukoplakia	100%	
T-Cell lymphoma			
	Nasal T/NK lymphomas	100%	EBV Infected B cells detected along with the lymphoma. T/NK cells can be infected with EBV.
	Angioimmunoblastic lymphadenopathy with dysproteinemia	30%	
Gastic carcinoma			
	Undifferentiated carcinoma of nasopharyngeal type	100%	
	adenocarcinoma	5–15%	

that viral gene expression may be greater than may have previously been thought in lymphoid organs such as the tonsil suggesting that the virus may manipulate normal B-cell development and survival to insure continued latency by the expansion of infected cells without lytic replication (Miyashita et al., 1997; Babcock et al., 1998, 2000; Babcock and Thorley-Lawson, 2000; Joseph et al., 2000a,b; Thorley-Lawson, 2001; Hochberg et al., 2004a,b). This will be more fully discussed in later chapters.

Further evidence of the hematopoetic site of EBV latency comes from engraftment of bone marrow cells that can result in the loss of the resident virus or the appearance of a new virus strain from donor lymphocytes (Gratama et al., 1989). Lytic replication is presumed to occur when EBV infected B lymphocytes traffic through and transmit infection to oral epithelium providing a source for infection of other individuals. Interestingly, recent studies have suggested different virus strains are present within different compartments in humans with EBV latent infection such as peripheral blood and the oral cavity suggesting that epithelial infection may be more important than previously thought (Sitki-Green et al., 2003). Understanding the complex interplay in EBV latency in the human host and the importance of viral gene expression requires the careful analysis of EBV gene function which will be the topic of other chapters.

The discovery of Kaposi's sarcoma-associated herpesvirus (KSHV)

The discovery of KSHV or human herpesvirus 8 (HHV8), has many parallels with the discovery of Epstein–Barr virus. Like Dennis Burkitt, Patrick Moore and Yuan Chang, were intrigued by the appearance of a new cancer in the United States, but rather than appearing in very young children, the disorder was appearing in young healthy gay men (Jaffe et al., 1983). This disorder was Kaposi's sarcoma (KS). KS was originally described as idiopathic purplish pigmented sarcoma of the skin by Moriz Kaposi in 1872 (Kaposi, 1872). Kaposi, born Moriz Kohn in Kaposvar, Hungary, obtained his MD in Vienna in 1861 and worked with Ferdinand Hebra, the founder of a renowned School of Viennese Dermatology. He would later become Hebra's son-in-law in 1869 and his successor in 1881. Also in 1869, Kaposi wrote the initial description of lupus erythematosus with a more comprehensive description published in 1872. He also described xeroderma pigmentosum. In 1871, two years after converting from Judaism to Roman Catholic and marrying Hebra's daughter, he changed his name to reflect his birthplace. In contrast to the frequent surname Kohn, Kaposi was certainly unique in Vienna, thus avoiding being mixed-up with others. In addition, this name change may have guarded against the harsh anti-semitism during the rule of Emperor Franz-Josef. Like his more comprehensive description of lupus erythematosus, it was also in 1872 that Kaposi published his description of the sarcoma that now bears his name. KS was a relatively rare, indolent, pigmented growth typically found on the skin of elderly men. Initially, Kaposi reported on the clinical features of six cases, including one of a young boy, but the remaining cases were all in men over 40 years of age. He reported that the disease was incurable and often resulted in death within two years after the disease appeared. In the 1960s, before the AIDS epidemic, it was realized that KS was not as rare as initially thought. The incidence in equatorial tropical Africa or sub-Sarahan African is much greater as will be more fully discussed below.

Following the outbreak of AIDS in the 1980s, in which there was a dramatic increase of KS in AIDS patients, there was considerable interest in the further study of this unusual malignancy and in particular the association of KS with infection with a human pathogen. Like Burkitt's lymphoma, a role for a virus was suspected in KS lesions long before the onset of HIV infection and the resulting AIDS epidemic. As early as 1972, herpesvirus-like particles were found in electron microscopic analysis of KS biopsies (Giraldo et al., 1972). This virus was determined to be cytomegalovirus (CMV), a herpesvirus that is ubiquitous in the human population. By the early 1990s, a number of other pathogens had also been found in KS lesions by a variety of investigators. Typically, these agents were not found in all the lesions and in many cases they were ubiquitous agents in the human population and were subsequently dismissed as having a role in KS. Like Burkitt's lymphoma, there was epidemiological data that suggested the role of an infectious agent in the development of KSHV. But before the identification of KSHV, it was thought that HIV may be the critical factor in the development of AIDS-associated KS. However, the uneven distribution of KS among different transmission groups for the human immunodeficiency virus (HIV) resulted in the hypothesis that an environmental factor or a transmissible agent other than HIV was involved in KS pathogenesis (Beral et al., 1990). Most notably, whereas more than 20% of homosexual and bisexual AIDS patients developed KS, only 1% of age- and sex-matched men with hemophilia suffered from this uncommon tumor, suggesting transmission of a KS-related virus by sexual practice.

The first real break that led to the discovery that a herpesvirus was linked to KS came in 1993 when Yuan Chang moved to Columbia University to take up a position in neuropathology. Chang received her medical degree from the University of Utah College of Medicine. Patrick Moore married Yuan Chang and in 1989 he left his job at the Centers for Disease Control to follow Chang to New York. Moore received a MS from Stanford in 1980, his MD from the University of Utah School of Medicine in 1985, and his MPH from the University of California, Berkeley in 1990. Once in New York, Moore was unable to find an appropriate academic position, so he joined the New York City Health Department. Both Moore and Chang were interested in identifying new pathogens without in vitro culture since this was a question that Moore was interested in from his work at the Centers for Disease Control. A recent publication from Michael Wiglers' laboratory at Cold Spring Harbor detailed a new technique called representational difference analysis (RDA). This technique, which was developed by the Lisitsyns, used PCR to identify DNA sequences present in one sample but not a control sample. On the surface, this looked ideal for the identification of unique infectious agents. The paper describing this technique was published in *Science* (Lisitsyn et al., 1993). It was not used to detect unique pathogen, but only the feasibility of using this technique was demonstrated using lambda or adenovirus DNA. Barry Miller, a colleague of Patrick Moore at the Centers for Disease Control, suggested that Moore and Chang apply this technique in their pathogen discovery.

With a single KSHV lesion and control tissue, the husband and wife team began to perform RDA. The initial experiments were performed by Chang and Melissa Pessin. Pessin was a pathology resident on a research rotation at Columbia. Moore helped in the evenings after finishing his duties at the New York City Health Department. The initial amplifications resulted in four prominent bands. Two KS lesions were positive for two of the four bands by Southern hybridization, but surprisingly, a control tissue from an AIDS patient was also positive. The control tissue was from an unusual lymphoma found in AIDS patients. This lymphoma, characterized by pleural, pericardial, or peritoneal lymphomatous effusions, is referred to as primary effusion lymphoma (PEL) or body-cavity based lymphoma and would also be shown to be positive for the new herpesvirus that Chang and Moore identified as will be detailed later.

Testing a larger panel tissue, Moore and Chang found that virtually all of the KS lesions were positive while none of the controls showed the same number of positives. From sequencing the RDA products, they developed internal PCR primers for one of the sequences that allowed a simple PCR based screen for analysis of additional tissues. Surprisingly, when the initial sequences were compared to sequences available in the current databases, no homologous sequences were identified. This suggested an unknown pathogen. Moore quit the Health Department in January 1994 so that he could devote his efforts full-time to the project at Columbia. Chang made an important contact working in the spring of 1994 with Frank Lee and Janice Culpepper at the DNAX Institute for molecular biology. Lee, working with newly developed BLAST sequence alignment algorithms, was able to show that DNA fragments isolated by RDA from KS lesions unambiguously belonged to a new herpesvirus, similar to but distinct from known herpesviruses. With this data in hand, a paper was submitted to *Science* and was accepted for publication in December of 1994, identifying a new herpesvirus (Chang *et al.*, 1994). Both Moore and Chang have recently moved to the University of Pittsburgh School of Medicine, where Chang is a Professor of Pathology and Moore is a Professor of Molecular Genetics and Biochemistry and Director of the Molecular Virology Program at the University of Pittsburgh Cancer Institute.

KSHV life cycle

Like EBV, KSHV requires intimate contact for transmission. At least in regions endemic for KS, all evidence points to similar modes of transmission in young children as has been described for EBV (Mayama *et al.*, 1998; Martro *et al.*, 2004). Primary infection likely occurs from contact via saliva with parents, siblings, playmates, and close relatives at a very early age. Similarly, in adult populations close intimate contact is also required. Interestingly, in comparison to EBV the infection rates of KSHV within the human population can vary dramatically throughout the world population based on serology. In endemic regions such as Africa, infections rates are well over 50%, whereas in Northern Europe and the United States, infection rates range from 1–6% (Gao *et al.*, 1996; Kedes *et al.*, 1996; Simpson *et al.*, 1996). Southern Europe, which like Africa, has a higher incidence of KS, also has a higher rate ranging from 10%–30% when compared to infection rates in the United States and Northern Europe (Schatz *et al.*, 2001). As might be expected, infection rates measured by serology are higher in homosexual men than in the general population in western countries, ranging from 20%–40% in homosexual men not suffering from KS (Martin *et al.*, 1998). In immunocompromised KSHV infected individuals, a wide assortment of cells and tissues has been shown to harbor KSHV. Most frequently, peripheral B cells have been reported to carry the KSHV genome (Ambroziak *et al.*, 1995). But T-cells, monocytes, and endothelial cells have also been found positive for KSHV DNA (Henry *et al.*, 1999; Blackbourn *et al.*, 2000). In contrast, the site of latency in immunocompetent individuals is essentially unknown. Difficulties in detecting viral DNA in seropositive, healthy individuals may reflect a low frequency of spontaneous KSHV reactivation, which would in turn result in the scarceness of KSHV positive cells and relatively low KSHV transmission rates at least in North America, Northern Europe and most parts of Asia. As a consequence, sites of persistence and the overall strategy of KSHV latency in the human host have been difficult to determine as of this date. The supposedly low rate of spontaneous reactivation in immunocompetent individuals is also reflected by low and declining antibody titers (Martro *et al.*, 2004). The latter has made it difficult initially to estimate the seroprevalence of KSHV in the general population (Pellett *et al.*, 2003), as will be detailed in Chapter 54.

Human disease associated with KSHV infection

Symptoms related to primary infection with KSHV have only recently been described (Andreoni *et al.*, 2002). Like EBV, it would appear that symptoms in immunocompetent individuals are very modest with primary infection being largely asymptomatic. In children, this primary infection may be associated with a febrile maculopapular skin rash (Andreoni *et al.*, 2002). Reports have indicated that primary infection in adults undergoing immune suppression for organ transplantation have experienced bone marrow failure, splenomegaly, and fever (Luppi *et al.*, 2002). There is also evidence that KSHV may be transmitted by solid organ transplants, eventually resulting in the development of rapidly progressing KS (Barozzi et al., 2003; Marcelin et al., 2004). However, at present it is not clear whether screening of organ donors for KSHV infection is beneficial.

Despite the only recent identification of KSHV, remarkable progress has been made in the identification of pathological consequences of infection with KSHV. Along with EBV, as described above, KSHV is also associated with proliferative disorders in both immune competent and immune deficient humans. In endemic regions of Africa, KS is a common debilitating cancer among men, women, and children. Following the establishment of this link, KSHV has also been shown to be important for a number of other diseases in the human population as will be described.

Classical KS, as originally identified by Kaposi, was typically seen in elderly Mediterranean patients, was indolent in nature, and affected the skin of the lower limbs. In endemic KSHV infection in Africa, before the HIV epidemic hit, KSHV infection presents as four distinct clinical syndromes: relatively benign, nodular cutaneous disease which is very similar to classical KS, aggressive cutaneous disease which invades both bone and localized soft tissue, florid visceral and mucocutaneous disease, and finally lymphadenopathic disease that can rapidly disseminate to lymph nodes and visceral organs (quite often in the absence of cutaneous disease). The final syndrome typically occurs in children. KS associated with immune suppression either from HIV infection or organ transplantation commonly presents multifocally and symmetrically and may arise quickly. These lesions will often undergo spontaneous remission with improving immune status.

As discussed earlier, there were early indications that another proliferative disorder observed in HIV patients might also be related to KSHV infection. Early work by Chang and Moore found that an unusual lymphoma in patients with AIDS was also positive for KSHV DNA (Chang et al., 1994). The lymphoma was confined primarily to body cavities and grows as an effusion. Hence the names primary effusion lymphoma (PEL) or body-cavity based lymphoma. Daniel Knowles and Ethel Ceserman working with Moore and Chang established that these tumors are also uniformly positive for KSHV (Cesarman et al., 1995). Interestingly, the vast majority of these tumors are also positive for EBV.

The final disease in human associated with KSHV infection is multicentric Castleman's disease (MCD). MCD was first described by Castleman in 1956 and is an unusual lymphoproliferative disorder that is characterized by lymphadenopathy, fever, and splenic infiltration (Castleman et al., 1956). KSHV is present in nearly all the cases of MCD in AIDS patients as originally shown by Soulier and colleagues in 1995 and about half of the cases in HIV-negative patients (Soulier et al., 1995). MCD is considered to be a semi-malignant lymphoproliferative disorder, associated with IL-6 hyperproduction and inflammatory symptoms. In the context of MCS, however, a highly aggressive plasmablastic non-Hodgkin-lymphoma may arise which is also KSHV positive and likely to have arisen from monoclonal "microlymphomas" detectable in some MCD lesions (Dupin et al., 2000).

Finally, there have been reports of the potential association of KSHV infection with sarcoidosis (Di Alberti et al., 1997) and multiple myeloma (Rettig et al., 1997), but as is the case with EBV association with liver and breast cancer, the linkage of KSHV infection with these two pathologies requires additional confirmation before a definitive link is established. In 2003, C. D. Cool et al. detected DNA and antigen of KSHV in lung tissues of 10 out of 16 patients with severe primary pulmonary hypertension (Cool et al., 2003). It is fascinating to note that, like MCD, PEL, and KS, primary pulmonary hypertension is frequently associated with HIV-1 infection. However, several follow-up studies were not able to confirm this intriguing finding (Henke-Gendo et al., 2004 and reviewed in D. Rimar et al., July 2006). But C. D. Cool and coworkers argue, that in contrast to their initial work most follow-up studies were based on serological assays. In fact, only two of the studies used DNA-PCR and/or histochemistry Katano et al., 2005; Daibata et al., 2004), and these were performed on patients from Japan, were KSHV prevalence is very low. Thus, further work is needed before a link between PPH and KSHV infection can be considered shown.

Phylogenetic relationship between EBV, KSHV, and non-human γ-herpesvirus genomes

The γ-herpesviruses are split into two subfamilies: the γ1-herpesviruses and the γ2-herpesviruses. The two human γ-herpesviruses include the recently identified KSHV, and EBV, which are distinguished by their latent infection of lymphoblastoid cell lines either of T- or B-cell origin. EBV is the only human member of the genus γ1-herpesvirus also termed lymphocryptovirus. A number of related viruses have been identified that infect both New World and Old World primates (Wang, 2001; Wang et al., 2001). These viruses serve as important models to investigate the pathogenesis of the lymphocryptoviruses in vivo (see Chapters 60 and 61). KSHV is a member of the γ2-herpesviruses or rhadinoviridae and like EBV has important related viruses that infect New and Old World primates. Herpesvirus saimiri (HVS), which infects squirrel monkeys, has been well studied and also provides an important model of KSHV in vivo pathogenesis (Fickenscher and Fleckenstein, 2001).

Following the discovery of KSHV in man, several studies were undertaken to detect additional Old-World primate rhadinoviruses. By searching for antibodies cross-reactive with KSHV, the group of Ronald Desrosiers at the New England Primate Research Centre isolated the rhesus monkey rhadinovirus (RRV) (Desrosiers et al., 1997). The complete genomic sequence of RRV clearly showed that this virus is more closely related to KSHV than herpesvirus saimiri (Searles et al., 1999). In particular, most genes not conserved between KSHV and herpesvirus saimiri, the so-called "K" genes, do have homologues in RRV. In contrast to HHV-8, RRV can be readily propagated in cell culture. While RRV was discovered at the East Coast, Timothy M. Rose and Marnix Bosch were sleepless in Seattle. They studied tissue specimens from rhesus monkeys suffering from retroperitoneal fibromatosis (RF) at the Washington Regional Primate Research Centre. RF has been identified as an infrequent disease syndrome occurring in immunosuppressed macaques (Giddens et al., 1985). RF lesions somewhat resemble KS: they consist of an aggressively proliferating fibrous tissue with a high degree of vascularization, and transmission studies indicated that an infectious agent may be involved in RF pathogenesis. By using a degenerated PCR technique, fragments of a herpesvirus DNA polymerase gene were identified in RF tissues from two macaque species, *Macaca nemestrina* and *Macaca mulatta* (Rose et al., 1997). Sequence comparisons indicated that, at least the DNA polymerase genes of these two novel rhadinoviruses, tentatively termed RFHVMm and RFHVMn, are more closely related to KSHV than the DNA polymerase genes of RRV. In addition, the LANA gene of RVHVmn is closely related to KSHV in structure and sequence. A role of RFHVMn in the pathogenesis of RF is suggested by the finding that RF spindle cells are highly positive for RFHVMn LANA (Burnside et al., 2006). However, attempts to isolate these viruses on cultured cells have not been successful so far. Several rhadinoviruses have been discovered since then in various Old World primates, including chimpanzees, gorillas and orang-utans. Phylogenetic analysis clearly showed that these Old Word primate rhadinoviruses form two clades. KSHV is the prototype of one clade, and RRV the prototype of the second clade. The thrilling point here is: most Old World primate species seem to harbor representatives of both clades. The search for a second rhadinovirus in man has not been successful to date, however.

Human γ-herpesviruses genomes

At least two EBV types have been identified in human populations and these were formerly designated EBV type A and type B (Zimber et al., 1986) but have recently been designated EBV-1 and EBV-2 to parallel the HSV-1 and HSV-2 nomenclature. The majority of EBV isolates in western communities are type 1, while type 2 EBV isolates appear to be largely restricted to equatorial Africa and Papua New Guinea. Unlike HSV-1 and HSV-2, there is extensive nucleotide homology and restriction endonuclease site conservation throughout most of the EBV-1 and EBV-2 genomes. However, there are important differences in the sequence of key EBV genes such as EBNA2 and the EBNA3 family of genes (Dambaugh et al., 1984; Sample et al., 1990). But, overall, the two types of EBV are considerably more closely related to each other than are HSV-1 and HSV-2 (Lees et al., 1993). Related to the differences in key EBV genes, the EBV-1 strains transform lymphocytes more readily and to faster growing cell lines than do EBV-2 strains (Rickinson et al., 1987).

EBV has a linear double-stranded genome of approximately 172 kilobase pairs (kb) and has a base composition of 59% guanine plus cytosine. It was the first large DNA virus whose complete sequence was determined (Baer et al., 1984). Subsequent to the sequencing of the EBV genome, the VZV, HSV, CMV, HHV6, and KSHV genomes were cloned and sequenced. The EBV genome sequenced, designated B95–8, was from an EBV-infected marmoset cell line partially permissive for lytic replication (Miller et al., 1972). Upon further analysis, it was determined that this virus isolate contained a deletion of approximately 12 kb relative to other EBV strains. Sequence analysis of Raji EBV strain revealed the 12 kb region deleted from B95–8 contained three potential open reading frames (Parker et al., 1990). The sequence analysis to date predicts around 85 to 95 open reading frames (Table 22.3, Fig. 22.2). The nomenclature for each identified gene in the sequence is based on the BamHI fragment in which the reading begins. This is followed by an "L" or an "R," depending on the whether the reading frame is leftward or rightward. The reading frames in each BamHI fragment are then numbered. As is apparent from the Table 22.2, many of the reading frames also have another name based on the prior identification of the gene product or homology to well described genes or gene products described in other herpesviruses.

The KSHV genome is a linear, double-stranded DNA of approximately 160 kbp and has the overall structure typical for rhadinoviruses (Fig. 22.2) (Russo et al., 1996). A complete rhadinovirus genome is usually termed M genome, as it is of intermediate density (M-DNA). The γ2-herpesviruses were termed "rhadino" viruses utilizing the ancient greek word for fragile, because this M-DNA tends to split into two fractions of DNA molecules with highly different density, the L-DNA containing genes (low density, low G+C content) and the terminal repetitive H-DNA (high density, high G+C content). The latter is, as far as

Table 22.2. KSHV associated pathologies in the human host

Pathology	Sub-type	Percent KSHV Positive	Notes
Kaposi's sarcoma	Classical	100%	
	African endemic	100%	
	iatrogenic immunosuppression	100%	
	AIDS-associated	100%	
Primary effusion lymphoma		~100%	50% of PEL are also positive for EBV
Multifocal Castleman disease	HIV-associated	90%–100%	
	Non-HIV associated	~40%	
	Plasma cell variant	50–100%	50% in HIV-negative, up to 100% in HIV positive patients
	Hyaline vascular variant	Usually negative	
Primary pulmonary hypertension		60%	unconfirmed report

known until today, without coding capacity. The L-DNA contains at least 89 open reading frames, 67 of which have homologues in the closely related γ2-herpesvirus prototype herpesvirus saimiri. The overall amino acid sequence identity of these 67 KSHV reading frames to homologues identified in herpesvirus saimiri ranges from 22.4 to 66% (average: 42%). Conserved genes are usually found in a comparable genomic position and orientation. Thus, KSHV genes that share homology with herpesvirus saimiri are numbered from left to right according to their position on the herpesvirus saimiri genome. Open reading frames which do not share recognizable amino acid homology with genes in herpesvirus saimiri are numbered with the prefix "K" (Table 22.4). Until today, 19 genes have been identified which are not clearly homologous to genes identified in herpesvirus saimiri (K1 – K15, K4.1, K4.2, K8.1, K10.5). Frequently, these "K" genes are strikingly homologous to known cellular genes. They code for proteins interfering with the immune system, for enzymes of the nucleotide metabolism, and for putative regulators of cell growth (Table 22.4).

Despite enormous differences in base composition, it is apparent that herpesvirus genomes have many open reading frames in common. Many products of EBV genes can be predicted on the basis of their amino acid homology with HSV genes and genes from other herpesvirus genes such as KSHV. The predictions and known functions are shown in Tables 22.3 and 22.4. These similarities between proteins encoded by the different herpesviruses, such as HSV-1, KSHV, and EBV underscores the relationships between the various herpesviruses. The homologous genes are primarily limited to genes required for the cleavage and packaging of the viral genome and infection of susceptible host cells. Included among the conserved genes are virion structural proteins, enzymes involved in DNA replication, some regulators of gene expression, and glycoprotein genes. Lytic gene function has been primarily described in HSV, because lytic replication is easily observed in tissue culture systems allowing gene function studies. In contrast, EBV and KSHV, which are largely latent in tissue culture systems, have been less amenable to studies of lytic gene function.

Characteristics of the γ-herpesvirus virion

Morphologically, the EBV and KSHV virions are very similar to other herpesvirus virions, consisting of an envelope containing viral glycoproteins (Epstein *et al.*, 1964, 1965). A tegument layer is found between envelope and nucleocapsid. The envelope contains viral transmembrane glycoproteins that mediate attachment and entry, either via fusion or endocytosis. Most glycoproteins of EBV and KSHV are conserved amongst the different herpesvirus families (gB, gH, gL, gM and gN). However, the most abundant envelope glycoproteins of EBV and KSHV are not found in more distant herpesviruses. These are termed gp350/220 and gpK8.1, respectively (Hutt-Fletcher, 1995; Raab *et al.*, 1998). The EBV and KSHV capsids are similar to those of other herpesviruses. The icosahedral capsid shells are composed of 162 capsomers (12 pentons, 150 hexons). It contains the linear, double stranded DNA molecule wrapped around a toroid-like protein core. The three-dimensional structure of the KSHV capsid has been determined by cryo electron-microscopy using viral particles produced from cultured primary effusion lymphoma (PEL) cells at a resolution of 22 – 24A (Wu *et al.*, 2000).

Conclusions

There has been dramatic progress in the understanding the molecular biology and disease associations of oncogenic

Table 22.3. EBV genes

EBV gene	HSV gene	KSHV gene	EBV Name	Known or proposed function
BNRF1		ORF75		Tegument protein, putative phosphoribosylformylglycinamidine synthase
EBER1,2				*Cell survial factor*
BCRF1				IL-10 homologue – host immune modulator
BCRF2				
BWRF1			*EBNALP*	*Regulator of latent viral gene Transcription (EBNA5)*
BYRF1			*EBNA2*	*Major regulator of viral gene Transcription*
BHRF1		ORF16		Bcl-2 homologue
BHLF1				
BFLF2	UL31	ORF69		Associates with nuclear matrix
BFLF1	UL32	ORF68		Virion protein – DNA cleavage/packaging
BFRF1	UL34	ORF67		Virion protein – capsid assembly
BFRF2		ORF66		
BFRF3	UL35	ORF65		Capsid protein
BPLF1	UL36	ORF64		Virion phosphoprotein – DNA release
BOLF1	UL37	ORF63		Cytoplasmic phosphoprotein
BORF1	UL38	ORF62		Capsid assembly – binds DNA
BORF2	UL39	ORF61		Ribonucleotide reductase (large subunit)
BaRF1	UL40	ORF60		Ribonucleotide reductase (small subunit)
BMRF1	UL42	ORF59		Polymerase associated processivity factor
BMRF2	*UL43*	ORF58		Transmembrane glycoprotein, 53/55kDa
BSLF2/ BMLF1	UL54	ORF57		Post-transcriptional regulator of viral gene expression
BSLF1	UL52	ORF56		DNA replication – helicase/primase complex
BSRF1	*UL51*	ORF55		
BLRF1		ORF53		gN
BLRF2		ORF52		p23 capsid antigen
BLLF1a			gp350	Virion binding to CR2 (CD21)
BLLF1b			gp220	Virion binding to CR2 (CD21)
BLLF3	UL50	ORF54		dUTPase
BLRF3-BERF1			*EBNA3C*	*Regulator of latent viral gene Transcription (EBNA6)*
BERF2a,b			*EBNA3B*	*Regulator of latent viral gene Transcription (EBNA4)*
BERF3-BERF4			*EBNA3A*	*Regulator of latent viral gene Transcription (EBNA3)*
BZLF2			gp42	Complexes with gp25 and gp85 – binds HLA Class II
BZLF1				Z transactivator
RAZ				Z regulator
BRLF1		ORF50		R transactivator
BRRF1		ORF49		Transcription factor
BRRF2		ORF48		
BKRF1			*EBNA1*	*Maintenance of viral episome*
BRKF2	UL1	ORF47	gp25	gL – complexes with gp42 and gp85
BKRF3	UL2	ORF46		Uracil-DNA glycosylase
BKRF4	*UL3*	ORF45		Nuclear phosphoprotein
BBLF4	UL5	ORF44		DNA replication – helicase/primase complex
BBRF1	UL6	ORF43		Virion protein – DNA packaging
BBRF2	UL7	ORF42		
BBLF3	UL8	ORF41		DNA replication – helicase/primase complex
BBLF2	UL9	ORF40		DNA replication – helicase
BBRF3	UL10	ORF39		gM
BBLF1	UL11	ORF38		Myristylated virion protein
BGLF5	UL12	ORF37		exonuclease
BGLF4	UL13	ORF36		Virion protein kinase

Table 22.3. (cont.)

EBV gene	HSV gene	KSHV gene	EBV Name	Known or proposed function
BGLF3	UL14	ORF34		Putative virion tegument protein, anti-apoptotic
BGLF3.5		ORF35		
BGRF1	UL15	ORF29a		DNA packaging protein
BGLF2	UL16	ORF33		Capsid maturation/assembly protein
BGLF1	UL17	ORF32		Capsid maturation/DNA packaging
BDLF4		ORF31		
BDRF1	UL15	ORF29b		DNA packaging protein
BDLF3		*ORF28*	gp150	Enhances epithelial infection
BDLF3.5		*ORF30*		
BDLF2		ORF27		
BDLF1	UL18	ORF26		Minor capsid protein
BcLF1	UL19	ORF25		Major capsid protein
BcRF1		ORF24		
BTRF1	*UL21*	ORF23		
BXLF2	UL22	ORF22	gp85	gH – complexes with gp25 and gp42
BXLF1	UL23	ORF21		Thymidine kinase
BXRF1	UL24	ORF20		Membrane protein – fusion
BVRF1	UL25	ORF19		Virion protein
BVRF2	UL26	ORF17		Serine protease
BILF2			gp78/55	
BILF1				GPCR
BALF5	UL30	ORF9		DNA polymerase
BALF4	UL27	ORF8	gp110	gB – virus maturation
BALF3	UL28	ORF7		DNA cleavage/packaging
BALF2	UL29	ORF6		ssDNA binding protein
BALF1				
BARF0/RK-BARF0				*Regulator of notch pathway*
BARTS				*Various functions?*
BARF1				Growth factor
BNLF1a,b,c			*LMP1*	*Constitutive CD40 mimic – oncoprotein*
			LMP2A	*Constitutive B Cell receptor mimic (TP1)*
			LMP2B	*Regulator of LMP2A and LMP1 function? (TP2)*
Raji LF3				
Raji LF2		ORF11		
Raji LF1				Part of BILF1

Note: Genes in italics in the "EBV" column are expressed in EBV latent infections. In the "HSV" and "KSHV" columns, the homology of the genes in italics with EBV is statistically not significant when standard blast comparisons are made. However, due to positional analogy, it is likely that the genes are evolutionary related. Based on the sequence data published in references (Baer *et al.*, 1984; McGeoch *et al.*, 1985, 1988; Parker *et al.*, 1990; Russo *et al.*, 1996).

γ-herpesviruses like EBV and KSHV. Many years of research on lymphomas induced by EBV and herpesvirus saimiri have identified viral factors that are critical for the proliferative disorders observed with these viruses. Upon infection of naïve B- or T-cells, respectively, differentiation and proliferation are induced in an antigen-independent manner, most likely to expand the pool of virus-infected or -infectable cells. To achieve this goal, both EBV and herpesvirus saimiri make use of transmembrane proteins mimicking constitutively active signaling receptors. In the case of EBV, the latent membrane proteins 1 and 2A are likely essential for the differentiation and expansion of latently infected cells observed in vivo. In herpesvirus saimiri, these latent transmembrane proteins are STP (saimiri transforming protein) and a second protein termed TIP (tyrosine kinase interacting protein) that is found in some strains of herpesvirus saimiri. Usually, this process does not result in the development of malignant disease, but is likely important for the establishment of latency. However, other circumstances can occur which may result

Table 22.4. KHSV genes

KSHV gene	HSV gene	EBV gene	KHSV name	Known or proposed properties and function
K1			K1	Transmembrane glycoprotein, signaling protein
ORF04			CCPH	Complement binding protein
ORF06	UL29	BALF2		ssDNA binding protein
ORF07	UL28	BALF3		DNA cleavage/packaging
ORF08	UL27	BALF4		gB – virus maturation
ORF09	UL30	BALF5		DNA polymerase
ORF10				
ORF11		Raji LF2		
K2			*vIL-6*	*viral interleukin-6, direct binding to gp130*
ORF02			DHFR	Dihydrofolate reductase
K3			IE-1B	Downregulates MHC I
ORF70				Thymidylate synthase
K4			vMIP-II / vMIP-1a	Viral macrophage inflammatory protein (chemokine)
K4.1			vMIP-III / vMIP-1b	Viral macrophage inflammatory protein (chemokine)
K4.2				
K5			IE-1A	Downregulates MHC I
K6			vMIP-I / vMIP-1a	Viral macrophage inflammatory protein (chemokine)
K7				partially overlaps w. non-translated T1.1RNA (=Nut-1, PAN RNA)
ORF16		BHRF1		Bcl-2 homologue
ORF17	UL26	BVRF2		Serine protease
ORF18				
ORF19	UL25	BVRF1		Virion protein
ORF20	UL24	BXRF1		Membrane protein – fusion
ORF21	UL23	BXLF1		Thymidine kinase
ORF22	UL22	BXLF2		gH – complexes with gp25 and gp42
ORF23	*UL21*	BTRF1		
ORF24		BcRF1		
ORF25	UL19	BcLF1		Major capsid protein
ORF26	UL18	BDLF1		Minor capsid protein
ORF27		BDLF2		
ORF28		*BDLF3*		
ORF29a	UL15	BGRF1		DNA packaging protein
ORF29b	UL15	BDRF1		DNA packaging protein
ORF30		*BDLF3.5*		
ORF31		BDLF4		
ORF32	UL17	BGLF1		Capsid maturation/DNA packaging
ORF33	UL16	BGLF2		Capsid maturation/assembly protein
ORF34	UL14	BGLF3		Putative virion tegument protein, anti-apoptotic
ORF35		BGLF3.5		
ORF36	UL13	BGLF4		Virion protein kinase
ORF37	UL12	BGLF5		Exonuclease
ORF38	UL11	BBLF1		Myristylated virion protein
ORF39	UL10	BBRF3		gM
ORF40	UL9	BBLF2		DNA replication – helicase
ORF41	UL8	BBLF3		DNA replication – helicase/primase complex
ORF42	UL7	BBRF2		
ORF43	UL6	BBRF1		Virion protein – DNA packaging
ORF44	UL5	BBLF4		DNA replication – helicase/primase complex
ORF45	UL3	BKRF4		Nuclear phosphoprotein
ORF46	UL2	BKRF3		Uracil-DNA glycosylase

Table 22.4. (cont.)

KSHV gene	HSV gene	EBV gene	KHSV name	Known or proposed properties and function
ORF47	UL1	BRKF2		gL – complexes with gp42 and gp85
ORF48		BRRF2		
ORF49		BRRF1		Na transcription factor
ORF50		BRLF1	Rta, art, lyt-a	KSHV Rta transactivator
K8			K-bZip, RAP	Represses Rta, required for viral DNA replication
K8.1			gpK8.1, gp35–57	Viral envelope glycoprotein, antigenic, binds to heparan sulfate
ORF52		BLRF2		p23 capsid antigen
ORF53		BLRF1		gN
ORF54	UL50	BLLF3		dUTPase
ORF55	*UL51*	BSRF1		
ORF56	UL52	BSLF1		DNA replication – helicase/primase complex
ORF57	UL54	BSLF2/ BMLF1		Transactivator/repressor
K9			vIRF-1	Viral interferon regulatory factor
K10			vIRF-4	Viral interferon regulatory factor
K10.5			*vIRF-3, LANA-2*	*Viral interferon regulatory factor, latent nuclear Antigen 2*
K11			vIRF-2	Viral interferon regulatory factor
ORF58	*UL43*	BMRF2		Putative integral membrane glycoprotein
ORF59	UL42	BMRF1		Polymerase associated processivity factor
ORF60	UL40	BaRF1		Ribonucleotide reductase (small subunit)
ORF61	UL39	BORF2		Ribonucleotide reductase (large subunit)
ORF62	UL38	BORF1		Capsid assembly – binds DNA
ORF63	UL37	BOLF1		Cytoplasmic phosphoprotein
ORF64	UL36	BPLF1		Virion phosphoprotein – DNA release
ORF65	UL35	BFRF3		Capsid protein
ORF66		BFRF2		
ORF67	UL34	BFRF1		Virion protein – capsid assembly
ORF67.5	UL33	BFRF4		DNA packaging
ORF68	UL32	BFLF1		Virion protein – DNA cleavage/packaging
ORF69	UL31	BFLF2		Associates with nuclear matrix
K12			*Kaposin A,B,C*	
K13			*vFLIP*	*Anti-apoptotic viral flice inhibitory protein*
K14			*vCyclin*	*Cyclin-D homologue*
ORF73			*LANA*	*Latent nuclear antigen, maintenance of latent viral genome, functional analogue to EBV EBNA 1*
K14			vOx-2	Viral Ox-2 homologue, immunomodulatory protein
ORF74			vIL8R, vGPCR	viral interleukin-8 receptor, viral G-protein coupled receptor; constitutively active, KS-like lesions in transgenic mice
ORF75		BNRF1		Tegument protein, putative Phosphoribosylformylglycinamidine synthase
K15				Signaling protein

Note: Genes in italics in the "KSHV" column are expressed in KSHV latent infections. In the "HSV" and "EBV" columns, the homology of the genes in italics with KSHV is statistically not significant when standard blast comparisons are made. However, due to positional analogy, it is likely that the genes are evolutionary related. Based on sequence data published in references (McGeoh *et al.*, 1985, 1988; Parker *et al.*, 1990; Russo *et al.*, 1996).

in overt malignant disease such as accidental infection of a foreign host, immunosuppression, or infection with malaria. Each of these increases the risk of development of disease associated with viral infection. In addition, genetic changes may occur in infected cells within the host that may also be important for the development of malignant disease. This may be quite rapid as seen in Burkitt's lymphoma or have a lengthy latency period as seen in Hodgkin's lymphoma. Besides the latent membrane proteins, other EBV viral proteins such as EBNA1 (Wilson *et al.*, 1996; Drotar *et al.*, 2003) and the virally encoded small RNAs called the EBERs (Komano *et al.*, 1999; Ruf *et al.*, 2000) may also have a role in EBV-associated malignant diseases in the human host. This will be more fully covered in later chapters.

Several lines of evidence indicate that KSHV plays an essential role in KS pathogenesis: the virus is invariably present in KS, KSHV infection precedes KS-development, the virus is present in the tumor cells themselves, and it is rather infrequently found outside the population at risk of KS (see Chapters 50 and 54). Research on KSHV pathogenesis is hampered by the lack of a cell culture system for transformation and animal models for KSHV proliferative diseases. Studies using rodents transgenic for single KSHV genes have been more successful, but results from such experiments should still be interpreted with caution, no matter how tempting the resemblance of lesions in mice transgenic for vIL8R to KS may be (Yang *et al.*, 2000).

At least two concurring models exist for the role of KSHV in oncogenesis. The "cytokine model" emphasizes the role of inflammatory cytokines induced or produced by KSHV. A closer look at clinical course and histopathology of KS raises doubts about the relevance of "classical," transforming genes for the pathogenesis of this peculiar tumor. The peculiar pathology of KS hints at a more complex, indirect mechanism of pathogenesis. Based on clinical observations and data derived from cell culture systems, models of KS pathogenesis were developed before KSHV was discovered. Several groups agreed upon the notion that KS develops as an interplay of inflammatory cytokines and angiogenic factors (Ensoli and Stürzl, 1998), although the cytokines focused on varied in different reports. Interestingly, KSHV encodes or induces several cytokines with intriguing similarity to the cellular factors shown to be required for in vitro models of KS. An example is VEGF that is secreted by cells expressing the constitutively active vIL-8R. This leads to a model of KS pathogenesis, where increased secretion of both viral and cellular cytokines, the latter in part induced by KSHV, promote inflammatory infiltrates (vMIP, vIL-6), angiogenesis (vMIP, vIL-8R), and enhance spindle cell proliferation (vIL-6, vIL-8R via VEGF).

The reliable presence of KSHV in the spindle cells may point to additional factors beyond those induced through the 1%–3% productively infected cells, voting for a role more compatible with a typical "oncogenic transformation" model by latently expressed viral genes. Starting from the close relationship to EBV and herpesvirus saimiri, it is intriguing to assume that transmembrane proteins mimicking constitutively active receptors mechanisms, similar to those identified in EBV and herpesvirus saimiri, might be relevant for KSHV pathogenesis. At first sight, KSHV genes K1 and K15 might fall into this category. However, attempts to detect expression of these genes in latently infected tumor cells remain unsuccessful.

Thus, KS may result from a complex interplay of both viral and cellular cytokines and angiogenic factors, induced by a sustained inflammatory reaction initiated by up to 3% productively infected cells. Perhaps the viral cyclin and other latency-associated proteins such as LANA-1 might further enhance the proliferation of KS cells and favor the development of truly malignant cells by indirect means, e.g., the reduced control of accidental DNA damage. As KS is an unusual malignancy, resembling hyperplastic, angioproliferative inflammatory changes rather than true sarcoma, such a multistep/multifactorial model might be more compatible with KS pathogenesis than classical transformation models by viral oncogenes, as described for EBV, herpesvirus saimiri, and possibly for KSHV-associated B-cell malignancies (PEL).

Acknowledgments

R. L. is a Stohlman Scholar of the Leukemia and Lymphoma Society of America and supported by the Public Health Service grants CA62234, CA73507, and CA93444 from the National Cancer Institute and DE13127 from the National Institute of Dental and Craniofacial Research. F.N. is supported by the German Research Foundation (SFB466 and SFB643) and the "Mainzer Akademie der Wissenschaften und der Literatur." We would like to thank current and former members of the Longnecker, and Neipel laboratories for their contributions to the work described, as well as our many colleagues throughout the world whose work we were unable to formally cite in this chapter.

GENERAL HISTORICAL READING

Coakley, D. (1992). Irish masters of medicine. *Town House Publishing*, 333–344.

Epstein, A. (1994). Thirty years of Epstein–Barr virus. *Epstein–Barr Virus Report*, **1**(1), 3–4.

Epstein, A. (1999). On the discovery of Esptein–Barr virus: a memoir. *Epstein–Barr Virus Report*, **6**(3), 58–63.

Glermser, B. (1970). *Mr. Burkitt and Africa*. New York and Cleveland: The World Publishing Company.

Henle, W., Henle, G., and Lennette, E. T. (1979). The Epstein–Barr virus. *Sci. Am.*, **241**(1), 48–59.

Moore, P. S. and Chang, Y. (1998). The discovery of KSHV (HHV8). *Epstein–Barr Virus Report*, **5**(1), 1–2.

REFERENCES

Ambroziak, J. A., Blackbourn, D. J., Harndier, B. G. *et al.* (1995). Herpes-like sequences in HIV-infected and uninfected Kaposi's sarcoma patients. *Science*, **268**(5210), 582–583.

Andreoni, M., Sarmati, L., Nicastri, E. *et al.* (2002). Primary human herpesvirus 8 infection in immunocompetent children. **287**(10), 1295–1300.

Arvanitakis, L., Mesri, E. A., Nador, R. G. *et al.* (1996). Establishment and characterization of a primary effusion (body cavity-based) lymphoma cell line (BC-3) harboring kaposi's sarcoma-associated herpesvirus (KSHV/HHV-8) in the absence of Epstein–Barr virus. *Blood*, **88**(7), 2648–2654.

Babcock, G. J. and Thorley-Lawson, D. A. (2000). Tonsillar memory B cells, latently infected with Epstein–Barr virus, express the restricted pattern of latent genes previously found only in Epstein-Barr virus-associated tumors. *Proc. Natl Acad. Sci. USA*, **97**(22), 12250–12255.

Babcock, G. J., Decker, L. L., Volk, M., and Thorley-Lawson, D. A. (1998). EBV persistence in memory B cells in vivo. *Immunity*, **9**(3), 395–404.

Babcock, G. J., Decker, L. L., Freeman, R. B., and Thorley-Lawson, D. A. (1999). Epstein–Barr virus-infected resting memory B cells, not proliferating lymphoblasts, accumulate in the peripheral blood of immunosuppressed patients. *J. Exp. Med.*, **190**(4), 567–576.

Babcock, G. J., Hochberg, D., and Thorley-Lawson, D. A. (2000). The expression pattern of Epstein-Barr virus latent genes in vivo is dependent upon the differentiation stage of the infected B cell. *Immunity*, **13**(4), 497–506.

Baer, R., Bankier, A. T., Biggin, M. D. *et al.* (1984). DNA sequence and expression of the B95-8 Epstein–Barr virus genome. *Nature*, **310**(5974), 207–211.

Barozzi, P., Luppi, M., Facchetti, F. *et al.* (2003). Post-transplant Kaposi sarcoma originates from the seeding of donor-derived progenitors. *Nat. Med.*, **9**(5), 554–561.

Beral, V., Peterman, T. A., Berkelman, R. L., and Jaffe, H. W. (1990). Kaposi's sarcoma among persons with AIDS: a sexually transmitted infection? *Lancet*, **335**, 123–128.

Blackbourn, D. J., Lennette, E., Klencke, B. *et al.* (2000). The restricted cellular host range of human herpesvirus 8. *Aids*, **14**(9), 1123–1133.

Burkitt, D. (1958). A sarcoma involving the jaws in African children. *Br. J. Surg.*, **46**(197), 218–223.

Burkitt, D. and O'Conor, G. T. (1961). Malignant lymphoma in African children. I. A clinical syndrome. *Cancer*, **14**, 258–269.

Burnside, K. L., Ryan, J. T., Bielefeldt-Ohmann, H. (2006). RFHVMn ORF73 is structurally related to the KSHV ORF73 latency-associated nuclear antigen (LANA) and is expressed in retroperitoneal fibromatosis (RF) tumor cells. *Virology*, July 29.

Castleman, B., Iverson, L., and Menendez, V. P. (1956). Localized mediastinal lymphnode hyperplasia resembling thymoma. *Cancer*, **9**(4), 822–830.

Cesarman, E., Chang, Y., Moore, P. S., and Knowles, D. M. (1995). Kaposi's sarcoma-associated herpesvirus-like DNA sequences in AIDS-related body-cavity-based lymphomas. *N. Engl. J. Med.*, **332**, 1186–1191.

Chang, Y., Cesarman, E., Pessin, M. S. *et al.* (1994). Identification of herpesvirus-like DNA sequences in AIDS- associated Kaposi's sarcoma. *Science*, **266**, 1865–1869.

Chen, F., Zou, J. Z., di Renzol L. *et al.* (1995). A subpopulation of normal B cells latently infected with Epstein–Barr virus resembles Burkitt lymphoma cells in expressing EBNA-1 but not EBNA-2 or LMP1. *J. Virol.* **69**(6), 3752–3758.

Cool, C. D., Rai, P. R., Jeager, M. E. *et al.* (2003). Expression of human herpesvirus 8 in primary pulmonary hypertension. *N.Engl. J. Med.*, **349**(12), 1113–1122.

Daibata, M., Miyoshi, I., Taguchi, H. *et al.* (2004). Absence of human herpesvirus 8 in lung tissues from Japanese patients with primary pulmonary hypertension. *Respir. Med.*, **98**(12), 1231–1232.

Dambaugh, T., Hennessy, K., Chanmankit, L., and Kieff, E. (1984). U2 region of Epstein–Barr virus DNA may encode Epstein–Barr nuclear antigen 2. *Proc. Natl Acad. Sci. USA*, **81**(23), 7632–7636.

Desrosiers, R. C., Sasseville, V. G., Czajak, S. C. *et al.* (1997). A herpesvirus of rhesus monkeys related to the human Kaposi's sarcoma-associated herpesvirus. *J. Virol.*, **71**(12), 9764–9769.

Di Alberti, L., Piattelli, A., Artese, L. *et al.* (1997). Human herpesvirus 8 variants in sarcoid tissues. *Lancet*, **350**(9092), 1655–1661.

Drotar, M. E., Silva, S., Barone, E. *et al.* (2003). Epstein–Barr virus nuclear antigen-1 and Myc cooperate in lymphomagenesis. *Int. J. Cancer*, **106**(3), 388–395.

Dupin, N., Diss, T. L., Kellam, P. *et al.* (2000). HHV-8 is associated with a plasmablastic variant of Castleman disease that is linked to HHV-8-positive plasmablastic lymphoma. *Blood*, **95**(4), 1406–1412.

Ensoli, B. and St∞rzl, M. (1998). Kaposi's sarcoma: a result of the interplay among inflammatory cytokines, angiogenic factors and viral agents. **9**(1), 63–83.

Ensser, A., Pflanz, R., and Fleckenstein, B. (1997). Primary structure of the alcelaphine herpesvirus 1 genome. *J. Virol.*, **71**(9), 6517–6525.

Epstein, M. A., Achong, B. G., and Barr, Y. M. (1964). Virus particles in cultured lymphoblasts from Burkitt's lymphoma. *Lancet*, **15**, 702–703.

Epstein, M. A., Henle, G., Achong, B. G., and Barr, Y. M. (1965). Morphological and biological studies on a virus in cultured lymphoblasts from Burkitt's lymphoma. *J. Exp. Med.*, **121**, 761–770.

Fickenscher, H. and Fleckenstein, B. (2001). Herpesvirus saimiri. **356**(1408), 545–567.

Gao, S. J., Kingsley, L., Li, M. *et al.* (1996). KSHV antibodies among Americans, Italians and Ugandans with and without Kaposi's sarcoma. **2**, 925–928.

Giddens, W. E., Jr., Tsai, C. C., Morton, W. R. *et al.* (1985). Retroperitoneal fibromatosis and acquired immunodeficiency syndrome in macaques. Pathologic observations and transmission studies. **119**(2), 253–263.

Giraldo, G., Beth, E., and Haguenau, F. (1972). Herpes-type virus particles in tissue culture of Kaposi's sarcoma from different geographic regions. **49**(6), 1509–1526.

Gratama, J. W., Oosterveer, M. A., Lepoutre, J. et al. (1989). Persistence and transfer of Epstein–Barr virus after allogeneic bone marrow transplantation. *Transpl. Proc.*, **21**(1 Pt 3), 3097–3098.

Henke-Gendo, C., Schulz, T. F., Hoeper, M. M. et al. (2004). HHV-8 in pulmonary hypertension. *N. Engl. J. Med.*, **350**(2), 194–195.

Henle, G. and Henle, W. (1966). Immunofluorescence in cells derived from Burkitt's lymphoma. *J. Bacteriol.*, **91**(3), 1248–1256.

Henle, W., Diehl, V., Kohn, G., Zur Hausen, H., and Henle, G. (1967). Herpes-type virus and chromosome marker in normal leukocytes after growth with irradiated Burkitt cells. *Science*, **157**(792), 1064–1065.

Henle, G., Henle, W., and Diehl, V. (1968). Relation of Burkitt's tumor-associated herpes-type virus to infectious mononucleosis. *Proc. Natl Acad. Sci. USA*, **59**(1), 94–101.

Henle, G., Henle, W., Clifford, P. et al. (1969). Antibodies to Epstein–Barr virus in Burkitt's lymphoma and control groups. *J. Natl Cancer Inst.*, **43**(5), 1147–1157.

Henry, M., Uthman, A., Geusan, A. et al. (1999). Infection of circulating CD34+ cells by HHV-8 in patients with Kaposi's sarcoma. **113**(4), 613–616.

Hochberg, D., Middeldorp, J. M., Catalina, M. et al. (2004a). Demonstration of the Burkitt's lymphoma Epstein–Barr virus phenotype in dividing latently infected memory cells in vivo. *Proc. Natl Acad. Sci. USA*, **101**(1), 239–244.

Hochberg, D., Souza, T., Catalina, M. et al. (2004b). Acute infection with Epstein–Barr virus targets and overwhelms the peripheral memory B-cell compartment with resting, latently infected cells. *J. Virol.*, **78**(10), 5194–5204.

Hutt-Fletcher, L. M. (1995). Epstein–Barr virus glycoproteins – beyond gp350/220. *Epstein–Barr Virus Rep.*, **2**(3), 49–53.

Jaffe, H. W., Choi, K., Thomas, P. A. et al. (1983). National case-control study of Kaposi's sarcoma and *Pneumocystis carinii* pneumonia in homosexual men: Part 1. Epidemiologic results. *Ann. Intern. Med.*, **99**(2), 145–151.

Joseph, A. M., Babcock, G. J., and Thorley-Lawson, D. A. (2000a). Cells expressing the Epstein–Barr virus growth program are present in and restricted to the naive B-cell subset of healthy tonsils. *J. Virol.*, **74**(21), 9964–9971.

Joseph, A. M., Babcock, G. J., and Thorley-Lawson, D. A. (2000b). EBV persistence involves strict selection of latently infected B cells. *J. Immunol.*, **165**(6), 2975–2981.

Kaposi, M. (1872). Idiopathisches multiples Pigment-Sarcom der Haut. *Archiv für Dermatol. Syphilis*, **4**, 265–273.

Katano, H., Ito, K., Shibuya, K., Saji, T., Sato, Y., and Sata. T. (2005). Lack of human herpesvirus 8 infection in lungs of Japanese patients with primary pulmonary hypertension. *J. Infect. Dis.*, **191**(5), 743–745.

Kedes, D. H., Operskalski, E., Busch, M. et al. (1996). The seroepidemiology of human herpesvirus 8 (Kaposi's sarcoma-associated herpesvirus): distribution of infection in KS risk groups and evidence for sexual transmission. *Nat. Med.*, **2**(8), 918–924.

Komano, J., Maruo, S., Kurozumi, K., Oda, T., and Takada, K. (1999). Oncogenic role of Epstein–Barr virus-encoded RNAs in Burkitt's lymphoma cell line Akata. *J. Virol.*, **73**(12), 9827–9831.

Lees, J. F., Arrand, J. E., Pepper, S. D. et al. (1993). The Epstein–Barr virus candidate vaccine antigen gp340/220 is highly conserved between virus types A and B. *Virology*, **195**(2), 578–586.

Lisitsyn, N. A., Lisitsyn, N. M., and Wigler, M. (1993). Cloning the differences between to complex genomes. *Science*, **259**(5097), 946–951.

Luppi, M., Barozzi, P., Rasini, V. et al. (2002). Severe pancytopenia and hemophagocytosis after HHV-8 primary infection in a renal transplant patient successfully treated with foscarnet. *Transplantation*, **74**(1), 131–132.

Marcelin, A. G., Roque-Afonso, A. M., Hurbova, M. et al. (2004). Fatal disseminated Kaposi's sarcoma following human herpesvirus 8 primary infections in liver-transplant recipients. *Liver Transpl.*, **10**(2), 295–300.

Martin, J. N., Ganem, D. E., Osmond, D. H. et al. (1998). Sexual transmission and the natural history of human herpesvirus 8 infection. *N. Engl. J. Med.*, **338**(14), 948–954.

Martro, E., Bulterys, M., Stewart, J. A. et al. (2004). Comparison of human herpesvirus 8 and Epstein–Barr virus seropositivity among children in areas endemic and non-endemic for Kaposi's sarcoma. *J. Med. Virol.*, **72**(1), 126–131.

Mayama, S., Cuevas, L. E., Sheidon, J. et al. (1998). Prevalence and transmission of Kaposi's sarcoma-associated herpesvirus (human herpesvirus 8) in Ugandan children and adolescents. **77**(6), 817–820.

McGeoch, D. J., Dolan, A., Donald, S., and Rixon, F. J. (1985). Sequence determination and genetic content of the short unique region in the genome of herpes simplex virus type 1. *J. Mol. Biol.*, **181**(1), 1–13.

McGeoch, D. J., Dalrymple, M. A., Davison, A. J. et al. (1988). The complete DNA sequence of the long unique region in the genome of herpes simplex virus type 1. *J. Gen. Virol.*, **69** (7), 1531–1574.

Miller, G., Shope, T., Lisco, H., Stitt, D., and Lipman, M. (1972). Epstein–Barr virus: transformation, cytopathic changes, and viral antigens in squirrel monkey and marmoset leukocytes. *Proc. Natl Acad. Sci. USA*, **69**(2), 383–387.

Miyashita, E. M., Yang, B., Babcock, G. J., and Thorley-Lawson, D. A. (1997). Identification of the site of Epstein–Barr virus persistence in vivo as a resting B cell. *J. Virol.*, **71**(7), 4882–4891.

Moore, P. S., Gao, S. J., Dominguez, G. et al. (1996). Primary characterization of a herpesvirus agent associated with Kaposi's sarcomae. *J. Virol.*, **70**(1), 549–558.

Old, L. L., Boyse, E. A., and Oettgen, H. F. (1966). Precipitating antibody in human serum to an an antigen present in cultured Burkitt's lymphoma cells. *Proc. Natl Acad. Sci. USA*, **56**, 1678–1699.

Parker, B. D., Bankier, A., Satchwell, S., Barrell, B., and Farrell, P. J. (1990). Sequence and transcription of Raji Epstein-Barr virus DNA spanning the B95–8 deletion region. *Virology*, **179**(1), 339–346.

Pellett, P. E., Wright, D. J., Engels, E. A. *et al.* (2003). Multicenter comparison of serologic assays and estimation of human herpesvirus 8 seroprevalence among US blood donors. **43**(9), 1260–1268.

Qu, L., Green, M., Webber, S. *et al.* (2000). Epstein–Barr virus gene expression in the peripheral blood of transplant recipients with persistent circulating virus loads. *J. Infect. Dis.*, **182**(4), 1013–1021.

Raab, M. S., Albrecht, J. C., Birkmann, A. *et al.* (1998). The immunogenic glycoprotein gp35–37 of human herpesvirus 8 is encoded by open reading frame K8.1. *J. Virol.*, **72**(8), 6725–6731.

Renne, R., Zhong, W., Hemdier, B. *et al.* (1996). Lytic growth of Kaposi's sarcoma-associated herpesvirus (human herpesvirus 8) in culture. *Nat. Med.*, **2**(3), 342–346.

Rettig, M. B., Ma, H. J., Vescio, R. A. *et al.* (1997). Kaposi's sarcoma-associated herpesvirus infection of bone marrow dendritic cells from multiple myeloma patients. *Science*, **276**(5320), 1851–1854.

Rickinson, A. B., Young, L. S., and Rowe, M. (1987). Influence of the Epstein–Barr virus nuclear antigen EBNA 2 on the growth phenotype of virus-transformed B cells. *J. Virol.*, **61**(5), 1310–1317.

Rimar, D., Rimar, Y., and Keynan, Y. (2006). Human herpesvirus-8: beyond Kaposi's. *Isr. Med. Assoc. J.*, **8**(7), 489–493.

Rose, T. M., Strand, K. B., Schultz, E. R. *et al.* (1997). Identification of two homologs of the Kaposi's sarcoma-associated herpesvirus (human herpesvirus 8) in retroperitoneal fibromatosis of different macaque species. *J. Virol.*, **71**(5), 4138–4144.

Ruf, I. K., Rhyne, P. W., Yang, C., Cleveland, J. L., and Sample, J. T. (2000). Epstein–Barr virus small RNAs potentiate tumorigenicity of Burkitt lymphoma cells independently of an effect on apoptosis. *J. Virol.*, **74**(21), 10223–10228.

Russo, J. J., Bohenzky, R. A., Chen, M. C. *et al.* (1996). Nucleotide sequence of the Kaposi's sarcoma-accociated herpesvirus (HHV8). *Proc. Natl Acad. Sci. USA*, **93**, 14862–14867.

Sample, J., Young, L., Martin, B. *et al.* (1990). Epstein–Barr virus types 1 and 2 differ in their EBNA-3A, EBNA-3B, and EBNA-3C genes. *J. Virol.*, **64**(9), 4084–4092.

Schatz, O., Monini, P., Bugarini, R. *et al.* (2001). Kaposi's sarcoma-associated herpesvirus serology in Europe and Uganda: multicentre study with multiple and novel assays, **65**(1), 123–132.

Searles, R. P., Bergquam, E. P. Axthelm, M. K., and Wong, S. W. (1999). Sequence and genomic analysis of a rhesus macaque rhadinovirus with similarity to Kaposi's sarcoma-associated herpesvirus/human herpesvirus 8. *J. Virol.*, **73**(4), 3040–3053.

Simpson, G. R., Schulz, T. F., Whitby, D. *et al.* (1996). Prevalence of Kaposi's sarcoma associated herpesvirus infection measured by antibodies to recombinant capsid protein and latent immunofluorescence antigen. *Lancet*, **348**(9035), 1133–1138.

Sitki-Green, D., Covington, M., and Raab-Traub, N. (2003). Compartmentalization and transmission of multiple epstein-barr virus strains in asymptomatic carriers. *J. Virol.*, **77**(3), 1840–1847.

Soulier, J., Grollet, L., Oksenhendler, E. *et al.* (1995). Kaposi's sarcoma-associated herpesvirus-like DNA sequences in multicentric Castleman's disease. *Blood*, **86**, 1276–1280.

Thorley-Lawson, D. A. (2001). Epstein–Barr virus: exploiting the immune system. *Nat. Rev. Immunol.*, **1**(1), 75–82.

Tierney, R. J., Steven, N., Young, L. S., and Rickinson, A. B. (1994). Epstein–Barr virus latency in blood mononuclear cells: analysis of viral gene transcription during primary infection and in the carrier state. *J. Virol.*, **68**(11), 7374–7385.

Wang, F. (2001). A new animal model for Epstein–Barr virus pathogenesis. *Curr. Top. Microbiol. Immunol.*, **258**, 201–219.

Wang, F., Rivailler, P., Rao, P. *et al.* (2001). Simian homologues of Epstein–Barr virus. *Phil. Trans. R. Soc. Lond. B Biol. Sci.*, **356**(1408), 489–497.

Wilson, J. B., Bell, J. L., and Levine, A. J. (1996). Expression of Epstein–Barr virus nuclear antigen-1 induces B cell neoplasia in transgenic mice. *EMBO J.*, **15**(12), 3117–3126.

Wu, L., Lo, P., Yu, X. *et al.* (2000). Three-dimensional structure of the human herpesvirus 8 capsid., **74**(20), 9646–9654.

Yang, B. T., Chen, S. C., Leach, M. W. *et al.* (2000). Transgenic expression of the chemokine receptor encoded by human herpesvirus 8 induces an angioproliferative disease resembling Kaposi's sarcoma, *J. Exp. Med.*, **191**(3), 445–454.

Yao, Q. Y., Rickinson, A. B., and Epstein, M. A. (1985). A re-examination of the Epstein–Barr virus carrier state in healthy seropositive individuals. *Int. J. Cancer*, **35**(1), 35–42.

Yao, Q. Y., Ogan, P., Rowe, M., Wood, M., and Rickinson, A. B. (1989). Epstein–Barr virus-infected B cells persist in the circulation of acyclovir-treated virus carriers. *Int. J. Cancer*, **43**(1), 67–71.

Zimber, U., Addlinger, H. K., Lenoir, G. M. *et al.* (1986). Geographical prevalence of two types of Epstein-Barr virus. *Virology*, **154**(1), 56–66.

zur Hausen, H., O'Neill, F. J., Freese, U. K., and Hecker, E. (1978). Persisting oncogenic herpesvirus induced by the tumour promotor TPA. *Nature*, **272**(5651), 373–375.

23

Gammaherpesviruses entry and early events during infection

Bala Chandran[1] and Lindsey Hutt-Fletcher[2]

[1]Rosalind Franklin University, North Chicago, IL, USA
[2]Louisiana State University, Shreveport, LA, USA

The two human gammaherpesviruses, Epstein–Barr virus (EBV), a gamma 1 lymphocryptovirus and Kaposi's sarcoma associated virus (KSHV), a gamma 2 rhadinovirus, have many features in common. They share an architecture that is typical of all members of the herpesvirus family, they share an ability to establish latency in lymphocytes, and they are both initiators or potentiators of human tumors. For the virologist some of the challenges they present are the same, in particular the relative dearth of fully permissive, easily manipulated cell culture systems for study. In this respect the many years of work on EBV provided an initial roadmap to accelerate study of KSHV. However, the strategies that the viruses use for cell infection and replication provide not only interesting reflections of common ancestry, but also interesting contrasts in adaptation to unique cellular niches in their human hosts.

Target cells for EBV

EBV can infect a variety of cell types under different circumstances, including T-cells, NK-cells, smooth muscle cells and possibly follicular dendritic cells (Rickinson and Kieff, 2001). However, B-lymphocytes and epithelial cells are its two major targets. B-cells are the primary reservoir of virus in persistently infected individuals and it is likely, although not certain, that the first cell infected in vivo is an epithelial cell. There has been some controversy over whether EBV normally infects epithelial cells during the courses of a primary infection or whether the virus infects epithelial cells only in the context of oncogenesis (nasopharyngeal carcinoma) or extreme immune dysfunction (oral hairy leukoplakia). Detection of EBV in epithelial tissue of healthy donors or patients with acute infectious mononucleosis has not always been consistent (Anagnostopoulos et al., 1995: Frangou et al., 2005; Lemon et al., 1977; Niedobitek et al., 1989; Pegtel et al., 2004; Sixbey et al., 1984; Venables et al., 1989). However, the preponderance of findings and the characteristics of virus shed in saliva of healthy carriers support a role for epithelial cells in amplification of virus during primary and persistent infection (Jiang et al., 2006). The clear association of the virus with significant epithelial pathology and its ability to infect epithelial cells in vitro either as free virus (Tugizov et al., 2003; Turk et al., 2006) or as B-cell associated virus (Imai et al., 1998, Shannon-Rowe et al., 2006) also reinforce the position that failures to detect virus may represent technical difficulties rather than reality.

B cells have been most extensively studied because the immortalizing effects of virus are so striking in this cell type, because B-cells are easier to isolate and because, after EBV infection, they are extremely easy to grow as latently infected cells. They retain episomes well in culture and are the best source of cell-free virus. Reactivation occurs spontaneously in a small subpopulation of some semipermissive B cell lines and can be induced in larger numbers of cells by agents such as phorbol esters, sodium butyrate or by cross-linking of immunoglobulin on the cell surface (Kieff and Rickinson, 2001). Epithelial cells typically lose episomes in vitro, but recent derivation of recombinant viruses that carry drug resistant markers has allowed selection of cells that can support episomal maintenance. The degree of lytic replication that occurs in epithelial cells varies from cell line to cell line. In many cell lines virus remains latent unless reactivated by treatment with inducing agents, but there is a recent report of extensive lytic replication in two polarized cell lines (Tugizov et al., 2003).

Target cells for KSHV

The in vivo host cell range of KSHV is not yet fully characterized, but appears to be broad in that KSHV viral DNA and transcripts have been detected in B-cells from the peripheral blood, B-cells in primary effusion lymphomas (PEL) or body-cavity based B-cell lymphomas (BCBL) and multicentric Castleman's disease (MCD), flat endothelial cells lining the vascular spaces of Kaposi's sarcoma (KS) lesions, typical KS spindle cells, CD45+/CD68+ monocytes in KS lesions, keratinocytes, and epithelial cells (Antman and Chang, 2000; Dourmishev et al., 2003; Ganem, 1998; Sarid et al., 1999; Schulz et al., 2002). KSHV DNA is present in a latent form in the vascular endothelial and spindle cells of KS tissues and expresses the latency associated LANA1 (ORF 73), cyclin D (ORF72), vFLIP (ORF 71) and K12 genes. However, virus DNA is lost within a few passages of cells cultured from the KS lesions. This is reminiscent of the loss of EBV episomes from nasopharyngeal carcinoma cells in tissue culture and the reason for it is not currently known. KSHV DNA is found in the CD19+ peripheral blood B cells of KSHV seropositive individuals and the detection of both lytic and latent forms in B- cells of KS patients suggests that CD19+ B-cells may be a primary reservoir for persistent infection (Antman and Chang, 2000; Dourmishev et al., 2003; Schulz et al., 2002).

Cell lines with B-cell characteristics such as BC-1, HBL-6, JSC, BCBL-1 and BC-3 have been established from PEL tumors (Dourmishev et al., 2003). The BC-1, HBL-6 and JSC cells carry KSHV and EBV genomes, while BCBL-1 and BC-3 cells carry only KSHV genome. KSHV exists in a latent state in these BCBL cells and expresses the latency associated ORF73, ORF72, K13, K12, K15 and ORF 10.5 genes. In parallel with EBV, spontaneous reactivation and expression of lytic cycle proteins occurs in 1% to 5% of BCBL cells. The lytic cycle can also be induced in about 20% to 30% of cells by phorbol esters, sodium butyrate and the lytic cycle switch protein known as RTA encoded by KSHV ORF 50 (Antman and Chang, 2000; Dourmishev et al., 2003; Liao et al., 2003; Schulz et al., 2002)

KSHV also has a much broader in vitro tropism than EBV. The virus can infect human B, lymphocytes, endothelial, epithelial, and fibroblast cells, as well as a variety of animal cells such as owl monkey kidney cells, baby hamster kidney fibroblast cells, Chinese hamster ovary (CHO) cells, and mouse fibroblasts (Akula et al., 2001b; Bechtel et al., 2003; Blackbourn et al., 2000; Ciufo et al., 2001; Dezube et al., 2002; Lagunoff et al., 2002; Moses et al., 1999; Naranatt et al., 2003; Renne et al., 1998; Vieira et al., 2001). Unlike EBV, infection of primary B-cells by KSHV does not result in immortalization. However, like EBV in vitro infection by KSHV is characterized by the expression of latency associated genes and the absence of productive lytic replication. After activation with phorbol esters or ORF 50 protein, lytic replication is supported by many cells including primary human microvascular dermal endothelial cells (HMVEC-d), human umbilical vein endothelial cells (HUVEC), human foreskin fibroblast cells (HFF), human endothelial cells immortalized by telomerase (TIME) or the E6/E7 proteins of human papilloma virus, monkey kidney cells and mouse fibroblasts (Bechtel et al., 2003).

Detection of KSHV latency associated nuclear antigen (LANA-1) encoded by ORF 73 after 2 days post-infection has led to the notion that the establishment of latency is the default pathway of infection (Bechtel et al., 2003; Lagunoff et al., 2002; Schulz et al., 2002; Tomescu et al., 2003). However, in vitro KSHV latent infection in primary fibroblasts, endothelial cells, or non-adherent B-cells is unstable, and viral DNA is not efficiently maintained (Tomescu et al., 2003). Even during primary infection of endothelial and other cells, the proportion of KSHV-infected cells decreases over time (Grundhoff and Ganem, 2004). Loss of genomes begins approximately 4 days after infection and by 3 weeks fewer than 15% of the cells remain positive for LANA1 (Tomescu et al., 2003). Whether the wild-type KSHV from the saliva of infected individuals or KSHV isolates from Africa have similar properties and tropisms remains unknown at the present time.

Virion structure

The virions of EBV and KSHV are at least superficially very similar to those of other herpesviruses. Each consists of a linear double stranded genome, an icosahedral capsid surrounded by an amorphous layer of tegument proteins and a lipid envelope carrying multiple unique glycoprotein species.

The KSHV genome is made up of a unique long region (LUR) of about 145kb flanked by varying numbers of terminal repeats. A large region of the KSHV genome is conserved among herpesviruses, and is colinear with both the gamma 1 EBV and the gamma 2 herpesvirus saimiri (HVS) (Neipel et al., 1997; Russo et al., 1996). It encodes more than 90 open reading frames (ORFs), designated ORFs 4 to 75 for their homology to those of HVS (Neipel et al. 1997; Russo et al., 1996). Divergent regions in-between the conserved gene blocks contain more than 20 KSHV unique genes which are designated with the prefix K.

The EBV genome is slightly larger than that of KSHV at approximately 180 kb. However, it includes a large, internal, tandemly reiterated 300 kb repeat known as IR1, a number of smaller internal repeats (IR2-IR4) and 500 bp terminal repeats arranged in tandem, all of which can vary in number in different strains of viruses. The more than 90 ORFs of

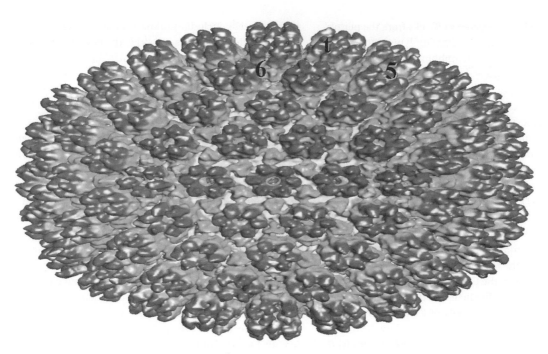

Fig. 23.1. 3D structure of the KSHV capsid at 24-Å resolution by electron cryomicroscopy. The capsid is shown as shaded surface color-coded according to particle radius. The three structural components of the capsid are indicated, including 12 pentons ("5"), 150 hexons ("6") and 320 triplexes ("t"). (Wu *et al.*, 2000 with permission). (See color plate section.)

EBV are named for the fragment within the original *Bam*H 1 restriction map of the B95–8 genome (Baer *et al.*, 1984) in which they originate and their direction of transcription. The BALF4 ORF, for example, is the fourth leftward reading ORF originating in the *Bam*H 1 A fragment.

Cryoelectron microscopy analyses reveal that KSHV capsid has the same $T = 16$ triangulation number, capsid architecture, structural organization and size as herpes simplex virus (HSV) and the human cytomegalovirus (HCMV) (Lo *et al.*, 2003; Trus *et al.*, 2001; Wu *et al.*, 2000) (Fig. 23.1). As in other herpesviruses, the capsids have a typical icosahedral shell and are composed of four structural proteins encoded by KSHV ORFs 25, 26, 62 and 65. The major capsid protein encoded by ORF 25 forms the hexameric and pentameric capsomers. The capsid floor between the hexons and pentons is formed by the heterotrimeric complexes composed of one molecule of the ORF62 protein and two molecules of the ORF26 protein. Both these proteins show significant amino acid sequence homology to the capsid proteins of alpha- and betaherpesviruses. The fourth protein, ORF65, is a small basic and highly antigenic protein, lacks significant sequence homology with its structural counterparts from the other subfamilies; however, similar to the small basic capsid protein VP26 of HSV, KSHV ORF 65 decorates the surface of the capsids. Lytic replication of KSHV leads to the formation of at least three capsid species, A, B, and C, and the A capsids are empty, B capsids contain an inner array of a fifth structural protein, ORF17.5, and C capsids contain the viral genome (Lo *et al.*, 2003; Trus *et al.*, 2001; Wu *et al.*, 2000).

No similar detailed analyses of the EBV capsid have yet been done, although transmission electron microscopy reveals a structural organization and size similar to other herpesviruses. Very little is known about the individual capsid proteins and assignments of ORFs as encoding capsid proteins have been made until recently only by homology with known HSV capsid proteins. Even less has been hypothesized about the composition of the tegument as few EBV ORFs have homology to any of the known HSV tegument proteins. The only EBV protein, which has been consistently described as a tegument protein is p140, which is thought to be encoded by the BNRF1 ORF (Hummel and Kieff, 1982). This ORF is described as having homology with *N*-formylglycinamide ribotide amidotransferases of *Eschericia coli* and *Drosophila melanogaster* (Russo *et al.*, 1996), but the significance of the homology is unknown. The first proteomic analysis of the proteins in the virion particle promises to stimulate new research in this under-studied area (Johannsen *et al.*, 2004).

Virus structural proteins involved in entry

In contrast, considerable effort has been expended on analysis of the biochemistry and function of the envelope

Table 23.1. Genes encoding membrane proteins that are expressed only in the lytic cycle

EBV protein/gene	KSHV protein/gene	EBV function	KSHV function
gp350/220/BLLF1	—	attachment to B cell receptor CR2	—
gH/BXLF2	gH/ORF22	virus cell fusion; attachment to epithelial cell receptor/coreceptor; complexes with gL	virus entry; complexes with gL
gL/BKRF2	gL/ORF47	chaperone for gH	chaperone for gH
gp42/BZLF2	—	interaction with B cell coreceptor HLA class II	—
gB/BALF4	gB/ORF8	assembly/exit/fusion	attachment to cells via heparan sulfate; interacts with integrins; virus entry; egress
gN/BLRF1	gN/ORF53	codependent on gM for processing; complex of gNgM required for production of enveloped virions	complexes with gM
gM/BBRF3	gM/ORF39	complexes with gN; complex required for production of enveloped virions	codependent on gN for processing; complex inhibits cell fusion
BMRF2	—	interacts with integrins; important to infection of polarized epithelial cell lines	—
gp150/BDLF3	—	unknown	—
p38/BFRF1		homologue of alphaherpesvirus UL34 proteins	
	?ORF67	interacts with BFLF2 protein (UL31 homologue) localizes to the nuclear rim, facilitates nuclear egress	?
gp78/BILF2	—	unknown	—
BILF1	—	constitutively active G protein-coupled receptor	—
—	gpK8.1A/K8.1	—	attachment to cells via heparan sulfate; virus entry
—	gpK8.1B/K8.1	—	unknown
—	OX-2/K14	—	adhesion of infected cells
—	K1/K1	—	signal induction
—	K15/K15	—	signal induction

proteins. These are the proteins that are critically needed to mediate attachment, entry, assembly and egress of virus and the majority of them are glycoproteins. The different tropisms of herpesviruses are potentially due to unique complements of these glycoproteins as well as subtle differences among those that are conserved.

The precise number of EBV membrane proteins that are exclusively expressed during the lytic cycle is not yet known, but there is evidence for at least twelve (Table 23.1). Five of these are glycoproteins that have homologues in all herpesvirus studied to date and are now commonly referred to by the naming system originally developed for the prototype alphaherpesvirus, herpes simplex virus. They are gB gH, gL, gM, and gN (Hutt-Fletcher, 2002). The remaining seven proteins are named for their apparent mass or referred to by the name of the open reading frame (ORF) that encodes them. One, p38, the product of the BFRF1 gene (Farina et al., 2000) is also conserved among all the herpesvirus families and is the homolog of the most widely studied alphaherpesvirus UL34. It is not glycosylated and is not found in the virion particle (Farina, 2004; Johannsen et al., 2004). It interacts with the BFLF2 gene product, the homolog of alphaherpesvirus UL31 (Gonella et al., 2005; Lake and Hutt-Fletcher, 2004) and like its homologs in other herpesviruses its major role is probably to facilitate exit of the newly formed EBV nucleocapsid from the nucleus (Farina et al., 2005). The remaining six are glycoproteins that are unique to the gammaherpesviruses. Glycoproteins gp150 (Kurilla et al., 1995; Nolan and Morgan, 1995), gp78 (Mackett et al., 1990) and the product of the BILF1 gene, which is glycoprotein with an apparent mass of approximately 50 kDa (Paulson et al., 2005), have counterparts only in lymphocryptoviruses (Rivailler et al., 2002). Glycoproteins gp350/220 (Hummel et al., 1984), gp42 (Li et al., 1995) and the BMRF2 protein (Tugizov et al., 2003) have counterparts in lymphocryptoviruses (Rivailler et al., 2002) and in certain of the rhadinoviruses (Russo et al., 1996; Telford et al., 1995; Virgin et al., 1997). Glycoproteins gp350/220, gp42 and the BMRF2 protein, together with the conserved glycoproteins gB, gH and gL, are all involved in virus entry as described below. It also is possible that complexes of gN and gM may play a role in this process although their major role is probably in envelopment and egress of newly made virus as described in Chapter 25 (Lake and Hutt-Fletcher, 2000). The phenotype of a virus that lacks gp150 is little changed from wild type virus, except that its ability to infect epithelial cells is very slightly enhanced (Borza and Hutt-Fletcher, 1998). The BILF1 gene product functions as a constitutively active G protein-coupled receptor. It is not found in the virion (Johannsen et al., 2004), but may play a role in modulating intracellular signaling pathways (Beisser et al., 2005). Nothing is known about possible functions of gp78.

KSHV also expresses the five conserved herpesvirus glycoproteins. (Table 23.1). Open reading frames 8, 22, 47, 39 and 53 encode glycoproteins gB, gH, gL, gM and gN, respectively (Akula et al., 2001a; Baghian et al., 2000; Naranatt et al., 2002; Neipel et al., 1997; Russo et al., 1996). HHV-8 also encodes for additional glycoproteins such as gpK8.1A, gpK8.1B, K1, K14 and K15 that are expressed during lytic replication (Birkmann et al., 2001; Chandran et al., 1998; Neipel et al., 1997; Russo et al., 1996). Studies have shown that gB, gH/ gL, gM/gN and gpK8.1A are virion-envelope associated glycoproteins (Akula et al., 2001a; Baghian et al., 2000; Koyano et al., 2003; Naranatt et al., 2002; Neipel et al., 1997; Russo et al., 1996; Zhu et al., 1999).

Virus attachment

Entry of enveloped viruses into cells involves at least two events, attachment to the cell surface and penetration through the cell membrane. Herpesviruses, not unexpectedly given the large number of different proteins found in a herpesvirus envelope, use multiple different proteins to complete the entry process. Increasingly, in recent years it has also become apparent not only that multiple proteins are involved in entry, but also that the complement of proteins that is used can vary considerably when different cells are the target of infection and different molecules are available for interaction with the virus.

Attachment of EBV

Attachment of EBV to B-cells has been known for many years to be mediated by a high affinity (Moore et al., 1989) protein–protein interaction between the virus glycoprotein gp350/220 and the complement receptor type 2, CR2 or CD21 (Fingeroth et al., 1984; Frade et al., 1985; Nemerow et al., 1985). Glycoprotein gp350/220 is an abundant, highly glycosylated type 1 membrane protein and has a dual nomenclature because its gene is expressed in two alternatively spliced forms with masses of approximately 350 and 220 kDa (Beisel et al., 1985; Hummel et al., 1984). The splice maintains the reading frame of the protein and results in the loss of residues 500 to 757 of the full-length 907 amino acid form which contain three repeats of a 21 amino acid motif with amphipathic characteristics. The splice does, however, retain the CR2 binding domain at the amino terminus of the molecule. Although not definitively mapped, this binding site is thought to include a short sequence of 21 amino acids that is very similar to the proposed binding sequence of the natural ligand of CR2, the C3d component of complement (Lambris et al., 1985; Nemerow et al., 1989; Tanner et al., 1988). The functional significance of the existence of the two spliced forms of the EBV protein, if any, is unclear. However, the initial interaction between gp350/220 and CR2 tethers the virus approximately 50 nm from the B -cell surface (Nemerow and Cooper, 1984) so one possibility is that exchange of the larger for the smaller form might bring the virus a little closer to the cell membrane.

CR2 is a type 1 membrane protein and a member of a large family of proteins involved in tissue repair, inflammation and the immune response that is characterized by structural modules known as short consensus repeats (SCR). The EBV binding site has been very precisely mapped to the amino terminal SCR-1 and SCR-2 (Martin et al., 1991). The tandem repeats, which comprise the entire extracellular domain of CR2, are 60–75 amino acids in length each forming discrete structural units (Moore et al., 1989) that probably provide some segmental flexibility to the molecule (Weisman et al., 1990) and that may also be important to positioning the virus for entry.

The ligand/receptor pair that is responsible for attachment of EBV to an epithelial cell is much less clear. Early models proposed that epithelial cells were infected when B-cells fused with epithelial membranes, but there are no data that either refute or confirm this possibility (Bayliss and Wolf, 1980). Some epithelial cell lines express at least low levels of CR2 (Fingeroth et al., 1999; Imai et al., 1998) and stable expression from a cDNA clone of CR2 renders a significant proportion of the cells permissive to infection (Li et al., 1992). However, the physiological relevance of this is uncertain. Identification of CR2-expressing epithelial cells in vivo has been confounded by the fact that the monoclonal antibodies used to make the determinations cross-react with an unrelated epithelial cell protein (Young et al., 1989). Cells that carry the polymorphic IgA receptor can be infected with virus that is coated with IgA specific for gp350/220 (Sixbey and Yao, 1992). This may be particularly relevant to infection of cells at the basolateral surface in an immune host, although in polarized cells virus was transported intact from the basolateral to the apical surface so it may be more important for virus shedding than virus infection (Gan et al., 1997).

Epithelial lines also express an as yet unidentified molecule that facilitates virus binding via a complex of gH and gL (Molesworth et al., 2000; Oda et al., 2000). Virus lacking gHgL loses the ability to bind to these lines and soluble forms of gHgL can be shown to attach specifically (Borza et al., 2004). However, infection rates are low and it is possible that this interaction represents inefficient use, in the absence of a primary attachment receptor, of a coreceptor that is more important for penetration (see below). Most recently, an interaction between the BMRF2 protein and α5β1 integrins on the basolateral surfaces of polarized epithelial cells has been reported to lead to high levels of infection and lytic replication in vitro (Tugizov et al., 2003). This observation is particularly compelling since polarized epithelial cells are probably closer to the environment encountered by virus in vivo. The BMRF2 protein is predicted to span the membrane many times and one of the predicted extracellular loops contains an RGD motif. Further work will be necessary to determine whether use of this motif is most relevant to attachment or penetration of virus, but it may provide parallel to the use of an RGD sequence in KSHV gB (see below) for entry. Unlike KSHV and many other herpesviruses, discussed in the next section, EBV is not known to encode any heparan sulfate binding proteins.

Attachment of KSHV

The broad cellular tropism of KSHV which binds to a variety of target cells such as human B, endothelial and epithelial cells, and monocytes (but not T and NK cells), as well as a variety of animal cells (Akula et al., 2001b; Dezube et al., 2002) may be in part due to its interaction with the ubiquitous cell surface heparan sulfate (HS) (Akula et al., 2001b). The initial virus–cell interactions of many other herpesviruses including herpes simplex types 1 and 2, pseudorabies virus, bovine herpesvirus 1, human cytomegalovirus, human herpesvirus 7 and bovine herpesvirus 4 also involve binding to HS. The first indication that HS might be involved in KSHV infection of target cells came from the serendipitous observation that infection of primary HMVEC cells was difficult in the presence of the heparin that is used in the growth medium of these cells. Further analyses showed that KSHV infection can be inhibited in a dose-dependent manner by soluble heparin, a glycosaminoglycan closely related to HS, but not by chondroitin sulfates A and C (Akula et al., 2001b). Infectivity is reduced by enzymatic removal of cell surface HS with heparinase I and III, virus binding is blocked or displaced by soluble heparin and binding is drastically reduced on CHO cells that are deficient in HS (Akula et al., 2001b). The interaction with HS may be the first set of ligand-receptor interactions that concentrates KSHV on the cell surface where it can subsequently bind to one or more additional host cell molecules that are essential to the entry process.

Two consensus motifs for the heparin binding domain (HBD) of polypeptides have been proposed, XBBXBX and XBBBXXBX, where B is a positively charged basic amino acid (lysine, arginine or histidine) flanked by an additional positively charged residue separated by hydrophobic amino acids "X" (Akula et al., 2001a). Heparin-binding proteins often contain more than one of these sequences, and analysis of HBD of several proteins suggest that the negatively charged sulfate or carboxylate groups on heparin may interact via electrostatic interactions with positively charged cationic residues in a protein or peptide (Akula et al., 2001a). Predictive analysis of KSHV sequences revealed putative HBD in the extracellular domains of HHV-8 gB and gpK8.1A. KSHV-gB contains the BXXBXB-BXBB (^{108}HIFKVRRYRK^{117}) type HBD, which is conserved throughout the γ2 herpesviruses (Akula, 2001a), and gpK8.1A possess two possible, although atypical heparin-binding motifs, gpK8.1A-H1 (^{150}SRTTRIRV^{157}, XBXXBXBX) and gpK8.1A-H2 (^{182}TRGRDAHY^{189}, XBXBXXBX) (Wang et al., 2001).

The KSHV K8.1 gene is positionally colinear to glycoprotein genes in other members of the gammaherpesvirus subfamily including the EBV gene encoding gp350/gp220, the gp150 gene of murine gamma herpesvirus 68, the ORF 51 gene of HVS, and the BORFD1 gene of bovine herpesvirus 4 (Neipel et al., 1997; Russo et al., 1996). The K8.1 gene (genomic nucleotide position 76 214 bp – 76 808 bp) encodes a 197-aa long ORF with a predicted molecular weight of about 22 kDa, with a N-terminal signal sequence and five putative N-glycosylation sites, but without any transmembrane sequence. Screening of a cDNA library from TPA induced BCBL-1 library with a HIV+KS+ serum identified two cDNAs encoded by the gpK8.1 gene (Chandran et al., 1998). Analyses of these cDNAs show that the gpK8.1 gene encodes two ORFs, designated gpK8.1A and gpK8.1B, from spliced messages. The larger cDNA is 752 bp long (76 214 – 76 941 bp) and utilizes the polyadenylation signal sequence (AATAAA) at position 77 013 bp. The 228-aa long encoded protein is designated gpK8.1.A which contains a signal sequence, transmembrane domain, and four N-glycosylation sites.

The first 142 amino acids encoded by the gpK8.1A cDNA are identical to the genomic gpK8.1 ORF sequence. This cDNA is derived from a transcript with a 95bp sequence spliced out [CAG/(GT)GTAT donor site and TCTAC(AG)/G acceptor site] and ends at the genomic nucleotide position 76 941 bp, which is 187bp beyond the end of genomic gpK8.1 ORF. This has resulted in the generation of a transmembrane domain not seen in the genomic gpK8.1 ORF. The smaller 569 bp long cDNA encodes the gpK8.1B, with a 183-bp sequence spliced out. The splice acceptor site for the ORF gpK8.1B transcript is the same as the gpK8.1A ORF; however, the splice donor site [CGA/(GT)GAGT] for the gpK8.1B cDNA is upstream of the splice donor site of the gpK8.1.A cDNA resulting in frame deletion of 61 amino acids in the smaller ORF. The resulting 167 aa long ORF is a typical class I glycoprotein with a cleavable signal sequence, a transmembrane domain, three putative N-glycosylation sites and is predicted to code for a protein of about 18.5 kDa. Except for an amino acid change near the splice site (S to R), the gpK8.1B shares identical amino acid sequences with the gpK8.1.A. Both gpK8.1A and gpK8.1B contain N- and O-linked sugars, and gpK8.1A is the predominant form detected within the infected cells and the virion envelopes (Chandran et al., 1998; Neipel et al., 1997; Zhu et al., 1999). Both are immunogenic proteins (Zhu et al., 1999).

The 845 amino acid KSHV-gB ORF includes a predicted signal sequence between residues 1–23, a predicted transmembrane domain between amino acids 710–729 and 13 potential N-glycosylation sites. There is a potential proteolytic cleavage site (RKRR/S) at amino acid position 440–441, and cleavage at this site would result in two proteins with predicted masses of about 48 and 45 kDa (Akula et al., 2001a; Baghian et al., 2000). Experimentally the protein has been shown to be expressed on the surface of the infected cell and in virion envelopes (Akula et al., 2001a; Baghian et al., 2000). It is synthesized as a 110 kDa precursor protein, undergoes cleavage and processing, and the envelope-associated form consists of 75 and 54 kDa polypeptides that form disulfide-linked heterodimers and multimers (Akula et al., 2001a).

Several lines of evidence indicate that KSHV-gB and gpK8.1A bind to cell surface HS molecules (Akula et al., 2001a; Birkmann et al., 2001; Wang et al., 2001). Binding of soluble forms of the proteins made in baculovirus is saturable and can be blocked by soluble heparin (Wang et al., 2001, 2003). Full-length gB and gpK8.1A in the virion envelope specifically bind heparin-agarose, and can be eluted by high concentrations of soluble heparin, but not by chondroitin sulfates (Akula et al., 2001a; Wang et al., 2001). KSHV-gpK8.1A binds to heparin with an affinity comparable to that of glycoproteins B and C of herpes simplex virus (Birkmann et al., 2001) and the gpK1A binds more strongly than gB (Wang et al., 2003). Even though the involvement of KSHV-gB residues 108–117 and gpK8.1A residues 150–157 in binding to HS-like moieties has been convincingly demonstrated, it is also possible that other weak and/or high affinity HBDs may appear in HHV-8 gB and gpK8.1A in their native quaternary structures if basic amino acids separated linearly are juxtaposed, forming a typical HBD. The presence of two or more heparin-binding glycoproteins within a single virus is not unprecedented, since the well-studied human α-and β-herpesviruses contain at least two HS binding glycoproteins e.g. gB and gC for herpes simplex 1 and 2, gB and gCII for human cytomegalovirus, and gB and gp65 for human herpesvirus 7. The presence of two-HS binding proteins in KSHV re-emphasizes the importance of cell surface HS for attachment of many, although not all, herpesviruses.

Penetration

Penetration of any enveloped virus into a cell involves fusion of the virion envelope with the membrane of the cell and can occur either at the cell surface or after endocytosis. Endocytosis affords a convenient and often rapid system of transit across the plasma membrane and through the cytoplasm for delivery of viral cargo to the vicinity of the nucleus (Sieczkarski and Whittaker, 2002; Whittaker, 2003). The best understood paradigm for virus cell fusion is provided by the RNA viruses such as the human immunodeficiency virus, which fuses at the cell surface, and influenza virus, which fuses with the endocytic vesicle. The virus glycoproteins that mediate fusion are made as single type 1 membrane proteins, but are cleaved during processing to create two species which reassociate in a metastable state (Colman and Lawrence, 2003). The fragment that retains the transmembrane domain includes a hydrophobic sequence or "fusion peptide" that can be triggered by conformational changes to insert into an opposing cell membrane and initiate formation of a fusion pore. The conformational change in the human immunodeficiency virus is triggered by interaction with coreceptors, the conformational change in the influenza virus fusion protein is triggered by exposure to the low pH of the endosome. However, no clear-cut paradigm has yet been identified for any herpesvirus. Fusion appears to require cooperation between several unique protein species, none of which include readily identifiable "fusion peptides" and the site at which fusion occurs varies from virus to virus and even cell type to cell type.

Penetration by EBV

Penetration of EBV into B cells and epithelial cells is significantly different both in terms of the virus and cell proteins involved and in terms of the routes that are used. Attachment of EBV to the B cell surface via CR2 stimulates endocytosis of virus into thin-walled non-clathrin coated vesicles (Nemerow and Cooper, 1984; Tanner et al., 1987) and fusion occurs in a low pH environment. Exposure to low pH is not an essential requirement, but endocytosis does appear to be necessary as virus fails to fuse with B cells treated with the endocytosis inhibitors chlorpromazine and sodium azide. In contrast, fusion with an epithelial cell occurs at neutral pH and is resistant to treatment with either chlorpromazine or sodium azide (Miller and Hutt-Fletcher, 1992).

Fusion of the EBV envelope with the B cell requires at least three and probably four virus glycoproteins, gB, gH, gL and gp42. EBV gB is a 857-residue protein that shares some structural, although little sequence homology with its counterparts in other herpes viruses (Gong et al., 1987). The positions of many of the cysteine residues in gB are conserved. Like gB of HHV-8 it undergoes cleavage to produce two polypeptides of approximately 56 and 80 kDa that are linked by disulfide bonds (Johannsen et al., 2004; C. M. Lake and L. M. Hutt-Fletcher, unpublished data). Although some strains of EBV carry very little gB in the virion (Gong and Kieff, 1990) and, as discussed in Chapter 25, EBV gB plays a very important role in virus assembly (Lee and Longnecker, 1997), recent work in which different combinations of virus proteins were expressed and examined for their abilities to fuse cell membranes indicates that EBV gB is also an essential part of the fusion machinery (Haan et al., 2001).

The remaining three proteins that are known to be required for fusion with B cells, gH, gL and gp42, form a non-covalently linked complex in virus (Li et al., 1995). Liposomes that contain all virus envelope proteins, except gH, gL and gp42, bind to receptor positive cells but fail to fuse (Haddad and Hutt-Fletcher, 1989) and recombinant virus that lacks all three can bind to but cannot penetrate B cells (Molesworth et al., 2000). Glycoprotein gH, the largest of the three is a 708 residue type 1 membrane protein with five potential N-linked glycosylation sites and it carries about 10 kDa of N-linked sugar (Baer et al., 1984; Heineman et al., 1988; Oba and Hutt-Fletcher, 1988). Although members of the gH family of proteins share little sequence homology, if aligned at a conserved N-linked glycosylation site at the carboxyterminus they show a co-linearity of cysteine residues that suggests a conservation of secondary structure (Klupp and Mettenleiter, 1991). Each member is also dependent on the smaller membrane protein, gL, for folding and transport through the cell. The EBV gL is a 137-residue glycoprotein of approximately 25 kDa that remains anchored in the envelope by an uncleaved signal sequence (Li et al., 1995; Yaswen et al., 1993). Because of the dependence of gH on gL and because EBV in which expression of the gH gene is interrupted phenotypically lacks gL as well (Molesworth et al., 2000), there are only few instances in which the functions of the two proteins can be separated.

Glycoprotein gp42, the third member of the complex required for penetration of a B cell, is not dependent on gHgL for processing and does not have counterparts in most herpesviruses (Li et al., 1995). The gHgL complex in both human cytomegalovirus and human herpes virus 6 also include a third component known, respectively, as gO and gQ (Huber and Compton, 1998; Mori et al., 2003), but these latter proteins, have no obvious homology to gp42. Only in the gammaherpesviruses are similar proteins predicted (Rivailler et al., 2002; Telford et al., 1995). EBV gp42 is a 223 residue type 2 membrane glycoprotein that has weak similarity to a C-type lectin (Spriggs et al., 1996). The predicted signal sequence and transmembrane anchor lie between residues 7 and 28, the region of the molecule that is responsible for the interaction with gHgL lies between residues 40 and 58 (Wang et al., 1998; Ressing et al., 2005) and the carboxyterminal domain of the protein interacts with the variable region of the β chain of HLA class II (Spriggs et al., 1996).

Several lines of evidence indicate that the interaction between gp42 and HLA class II is essential to B-cell infection. A monoclonal antibody to gp42 that blocks the interaction with HLA class II inhibits virus cell fusion (Miller and Hutt-Fletcher, 1988) and a monoclonal antibody to HLA class II that blocks gp42 binding neutralizes virus infection (Li et al., 1997). A soluble form of gp42 in which the transmembrane domain is replaced with the Fc domain of human immunoglobulin competes with gp42 in virus for binding to HLA class II and blocks infection and B-cells that lack HLA class II cannot be infected unless HLA class II expression is restored (Li et al., 1997). Finally, a recombinant virus that lacks gp42 fails to infect B-cells unless cells and bound virus are fused with polyethylene glycol (Wang and Hutt-Fletcher, 1998), or a soluble form of gp42 which lacks a transmembrane domain but which retains the ability to bind to gH and gL is added in trans (Wang et al., 1998). Binding shows some allelic specificity (Haan and Longnecker, 2000) and the crystal structure of HLA class II bound to gp42 reveals that gp42 binds peripherally to the variable domain of the β-chain (Mullen et al., 2002). A current minimalist model of B cell penetration would then suggest that, following attachment of virus via gp350 and CR2, gp42 interacts with HLA class II and that this event leads to triggering of the fusion machinery, gHgL and gB.

Fusion of virus with epithelial cells requires only gB and gHgL (McShane and Longnecker, 2004) and residues required for fusion can be distinguished from those required for fusion with B cells (Omerovic et al., 2005; Wu et al., 2005). However, epithelial cells do not express HLA class II constitutively, and recombinant virus that lacks gp42 infects epithelial cells as well as wild-type virus. Not only is gp42 dispensable for infection of epithelial cells, its presence is also inhibitory. Stoichiometric analysis of wild-type virus demonstrates the presence of much larger amounts of gHgL than gp42 in the virion, implying that some complexes naturally lack or are low in gp42. Saturation of the complexes by addition of soluble gp42 in *trans* blocks epithelial infection. In addition infection of epithelial cells, but not B cells, can be blocked by antibodies that interact with gHgL or gH alone (Wang et al., 1998). These findings have been interpreted to mean that there is a coreceptor on epithelial cells that can substitute for HLA class II and with which gHgL interacts in the absence of gp42. Soluble forms of gHgL bind saturably to epithelial cells. Scatchard analysis indicates the presence of as many as 200 000 high affinity receptors per cell with a K_D of approximately 5×10^{-9} M (L. Chesnokova, A. Morgan and L. Hutt-Fletcher, unpublished data). Whether or not this receptor is the same as that which can be used to attach virus to epithelial cells is not yet known. However, a minimal model of penetration of an epithelial cell suggests that following attachment an interaction of gHgL alone with a coreceptor triggers the activity of the fusion machinery.

The observation that gp42 is essential for B-cell infection but dispensable for epithelial infection suggested that changes in the stoichiometry of the gHgLgp42 complex would influence tropism of EBV for the two cell types and comparisons of virus made in HLA class II positive B-cells and HLA class II negative epithelial cells support the hypothesis that such changes might occur in vivo (Borza and Hutt-Fletcher, 2002). Virus made in HLA class II-negative epithelial cells can be as much as two logs more infectious for B-lymphocytes than the same amount of virus produced by an HLA class II-positive B-cell. Virus originating from either cell type binds equally well to CR2 on the B-cell surface, but virus made in the B-cell enters less efficiently. This appears to reflect the fact that in a class II-positive virus-producing cell some complexes containing gp42 interact with class II during biosynthesis and are targeted to the class II trafficking pathway where they are vulnerable to degradation. The resulting loss of three-part complexes from virus reduces the efficiency of class II-dependent entry. Such a loss does not occur in a class II-negative epithelial cell where virus has a relative increase in gp42 and an increased efficiency for class II-dependent entry and induction of HLA class II expression can reverse the phenotype. The levels of gp42 in virus also impact infec-

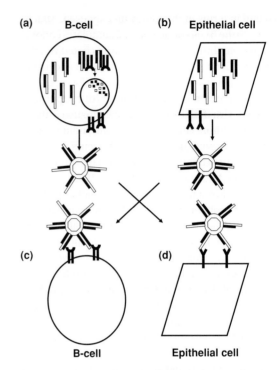

Fig. 23.2. Glycoprotein gp42 can function as a switch of EBV tropism. (a) EBV makes both three part gHgLgp42 complexes and two part gHgL complexes. When virus is made in a B-cell, some of the three-part gHgLgp42 complexes bind to HLA class II within the cell and as a result traffic along the same exocytic pathway as that followed by HLA class II. This includes passage through a vesicle rich in proteolytic enzymes which normally digests exogenous protein for presentation by HLA class II. The gHgLgp42 complexes bound to HLA class II are proteolytically digested in this compartment and as a result fewer of the three-part complexes are available for incorporation into virus. (b) In an epithelial cell which does not express HLA class II a larger number of three part complexes are available for incorporation into virus. (c) Entry into a B-cell requires an interaction between gp42 and HLA class II. The relative increase of gp42 in virus derived from an epithelial cell thus increases the ability of virus to infect a B-cell. (d) Infection of an epithelial cell requires an interaction with a gHgL coreceptor. Interaction of the gHgL complex with this coreceptor is blocked by gp42. The relative reduction of gp42 in virus derived from an HLA class II positive B-cell thus increases the ability of this virus to infect an epithelial cell. ∥ gHgL; ∥ gHgLgp42; ᴎ HLA class II; Y gHgLR.

tion of epithelial cells via the class II-independent pathway. B cell virus is on average fivefold better at infecting epithelial cells than epithelial virus. These findings suggest that gp42 may function as a switch of virus tropism that might be relevant to spread of virus between tissues in vivo (Borza and Hutt-Fletcher, 2002) (Fig. 23.2). However, since the effects on B-cell infection are by far the most striking, the biological effects may primarily be to drive into the B-cell pool any virus that initiates infection by replicating in an epithelial cell.

The events that occur concurrent with, and following, fusion of the virus and cell membrane that are necessary to facilitate transport, uncoating and delivery of the genome to the nucleus are largely unknown and currently can only be guessed at, based on what little is understood for other herpesviruses. There are, however, hints that additional envelope proteins may be involved in efficient delivery of infectious virus. Loss of the complex of gM and gN not only severely compromises envelopment and egress of EBV, as described in Chapter 25, but also leads to a defect in infection that cannot be rescued by treating bound virus with exogenous mediators of fusion. One possible explanation for this finding is that there is a defect in dissociation of envelope and tegument necessary for movement of virus toward the nucleus (Lake and Hutt-Fletcher, 2000).

Penetration by KSHV

KSHV enters the B-cell line BJAB (Akula *et al.*, 2001a), HFF (Akula *et al.*, 2003), the human epithelial line 293 (Inoue *et al.*, 2003; Liao *et al.*, 2003) and endothelial cells (Akula *et al.*, 2002) by endocytosis. HHV-8 virions can be visualized in endocytic vesicles of BJAB (Akula *et al.*, 2001b, 2003) within 5 min of infection where they fuse with the vesicle wall (Akula *et al.*, 2003), and viral capsids are found in the vicinity of nuclear membranes by 15 minutes after infection. Anti-KSHV- gB antibodies colocalize with virus-containing endocytic vesicles. In HFF cells, KSHV infection is significantly inhibited by the preincubation of cells with chlorpromazine HCl, which blocks endocytosis via clathrin-coated pits, but not by nystatin and cholera toxin B, which block endocytosis via caveolae and induce the dissociation of lipid rafts, respectively. Infection is also inhibited by blocking the acidification of endosomes by NH_4 Cl and bafilomycin A in HFF and 293 cells (Akula *et al.*, 2003; Liao *et al.*, 2003). These findings suggest that penetration of KSHV occurs in and requires a low pH intracellular environment. Further work is required to determine if virus takes the same route into other cell types.

The KSHV gHgL complex consists of a 120 kDa protein (gH) and a 41–42 kDa protein (gL) linked by non-covalent bonds and found both on the surface of the cell and in virions (Naranatt *et al.*, 2002). As in other herpesviruses, KSHV-gL is required for gH processing and intracellular transport and the complex is required for entry. Anti-gH and anti-gL antibodies neutralize KSHV infectivity, individually and more efficiently together, without having any effect on virus binding to target cells (Naranatt *et al.*, 2002). Deletion of 58 amino acids in the cytoplasmic tail of KSHV-gB removed the putative endocytosis signals (YXXΦ). Expression of this truncated KSHV-gB (gBMUT), but not the full length gB, can be detected on the surface of CHO cells (Pertel, 2002). Co-expression of KSHV- gBMUT, gH, and gL resulted in the fusion of CHO cells with 293 cells (Pertel, 2002). Further work is necessary to determine the role of KSHV gB, gH and gL mediated fusion in entry of target cells, but at this point it seems likely that the minimal fusion machinery of both KSHV and EBV comprises gB, gH and gL.

Much more is known about the involvement of KSHV gpK8.1 and gB in post binding events. Although these proteins are involved in the interaction with the cell surface HS molecules, even high concentrations of rabbit polyclonal and monoclonal anti-gB and anti-gpK8.1A antibodies which neutralize infection do not block the binding of KSHV to target cells (Akula *et al.*, 2001a; Zhu *et al.*, 1999). This implies a role for the proteins after attachment has occurred; possibly as a result of interaction with additional cell surface molecules. Among all the gB homologues sequenced to date, only KSHV-gB possesses an integrin-binding RGD motif at amino acids 27 to 29 which is predicted to be immediately adjacent to the putative signal sequence of the protein (Akula *et al.*, 2002). The RGD motif is the minimal peptide region of many extracellular matrix (ECM) proteins known to interact with subsets of host cell surface integrins. KSHV infectivity of fibroblasts and endothelial cells is neutralized by RGD peptides, by antibodies to α3 and β1 integrins, and by soluble α3β1 integrin (Akula *et al.*, 2002) and anti-gB antibodies immunoprecipitate a complex of virus and α3β1. At the same time, RGD peptides, anti-integrin antibodies and soluble integrins fail to block virus binding to adherent target cells such as human endothelial and fibroblast cells suggesting that KSHV uses the α3β1 integrin as one of the cell receptors or coreceptors for entry (Akula *et al.*, 2002). Expression of human α3 integrin also increases the infectivity of virus for CHO cells (Akula *et al.*, 2002).

Additional studies suggest that infection of fibroblasts or endothelial cells can also be neutralized by soluble αVβ3 and αVβ5 integrins with higher levels of neutralization with soluble α3β1 integrin. Virus binding and viral DNA internalization studies suggest that αVβ3 and αVβ5 integrins also play roles in KSHV entry and may expand the in vivo target cells for KSHV. Using an RTA-dependent reporter 293-T cell line (Inoue *et al.*, 2003) reported the inability of soluble α3β1 integrin and RGD peptides to block the infectivity of KSHV. However, in this study virus was centrifuged with cell in the presence of polybrene which may account for the apparent discrepancy. Polybrene is a positively charged cation which can complex with the virus envelope and may bypass the need for a receptor. This property of polybrene is the basis for its use to increase the infectivity of many viruses and to deliver nucleic acid for gene therapy. The nature of other receptor(s) recognized by KSHV and the glycoproteins involved need to be evaluated further.

KSHV also utilizes the dendtric cell-specific ICAM-3 grabbing nonintegrin (DC-SIGN; CD209) as a receptor for infection of myeloid DCs and macrophages (Rappocciolo et al., 2006). DC-SIGN was required for virus attachment to these cells and DC-SIGN-expressing cell lines. KSHV binding and infection were blocked by anti-DC-SIGN monoclonal antibody and soluble DC-SIGN, and mannan, a natural ligand for DC-SIGN. The residual level of KSHV binding and infection in cells pretreated with anti-DC-SIGN antibodies in these studies were attributed to additional receptors for KSHV on these cells. Expression of DC-SIGN on B-lymphoblastoid cell lines (LCL) and K562 cells which are normally resistant to KSHV rendered them susceptible to KSHV infection (Rappocciolo et al., 2006). Since neither of these cells expressed α3β1 on their surface, this suggested that other molecules such as DC-SIGN may be involved in infection of these target cells.

Another recent study showed that KSHV also utilizes the 12-transmembrane transporter protein xCT for entry into adherent cells (Kaleeba and Berger, 2006). The xCT molecule is part of the cell surface 125 kDa disulfide linked heterodimeric membrane glycoprotein CD98 (4F2 antigen) complex containing a common glycosylated heavy chain (80kDa) and a group of 45 kDa light chains. The xCT molecule involved in glutamate/cystine exchange is one of the light chain (Kaleeba and Berger, 2006). Expression of recombinant xCT rendered otherwise not susceptible target cells permissive for both KSHV cell fusion and virion entry. Antibodies against xCT blocked KSHV fusion and entry with naturally permissive target cells such as the adherent target cells of human and nonhuman cell types. However, xCT mRNA was not detected in human CD19 primary B cells isolated from fresh peripheral blood mononuclear cells (Kaleeba and Berger, 2006). These studies further suggest that like EBV, KSHV may possess alternative receptor(s) in adherent and non-adherent cells and other molecules besides xCT may be involved in infection of B cells. It is interesting to note that the CD98 complex usually associates with β1 integrin and has been shown to be involved in membrane clustering and β1 integrin-mediated signal cascades (Fenczik et al,. 2001; Feral et al., 2005).

Cell surface signaling during entry

The interactions of eukaryotic cells with their extracellular environments are largely mediated by ligand-induced signaling molecules exposed at the cell surface. The ensuing multitudes of biological processes are mediated by highly inter-linked networks of signaling pathways. Ligand mimicry is an opportunistic mechanism by which microbes, including viruses, subvert host signaling molecules for their benefit (Virji, 1996). By evolving to use cell surface molecules for attachment or entry into a cell, viruses have also evolved to take advantage of the events triggered by signaling to facilitate intracellular transport, to manipulate cell defense mechanisms, or to induce the pattern of cellular gene expression that is most conducive to establishment of latent or productive infection. Understanding virus induced signaling and its consequence is emerging as an important area of virology.

Signaling by EBV during the early stages of infection

The B cell receptor for EBV, CR2, can function as a signal transducer both independently and as a part of a signal transduction complex. This complex, composed of CR2, CD19 and CD81, modifies cell surface immunoglobulin-mediated signaling. CR2-transduced signaling is not required for infection of tumor derived cell lines by EBV (Martin et al., 1994), which suggests that it is not required for intracellular transport or uncoating of virus, but several studies suggest that it may be critical for transformation of a resting B cell. Binding of EBV to CR2 stimulates capping of both CR2 and immunoglobulin and leads to increased blast formation, cell adhesion, surface CD23 expression and increased RNA synthesis (Gordon et al., 1986; Tanner and Tosato, 1992). Interleukin 6, which is a paracrine or autocrine growth factor for EBV immortalized B cells (Tanner and Tosato, 1992), is activated by purified gp350/220 by a pathway that is sensitive to inhibitors of protein kinase C and tyrosine kinases and probably occurs as a result of downstream activity of NFκB (D'Addario et al., 2001). Activation of NFκB increases transcription from the EBV Wp promoter which is responsible for initiation of latent gene expression and inhibition of NFκB inhibits transformation (Sugano et al., 1997). Interaction of gp350/220 with CR2 also induces tyrosine phosphorylation of CD19 and activation of phosphatidylinositol 3-kinase (PI 3-K). Inhibition of these pathways inhibits expression of essential transforming genes (Sinclair and Farrell, 1995).

It is unlikely that signal transduction by EBV structural components and cell proteins is limited to the interaction between gp350/220 and its effects on gene expression, but potential effects of other virus proteins have yet to be studied. The interactions between gp42 and HLA class II and between the BMRF2 protein and integrins, which, as discussed in detail below, play important roles in HHV-8 infection, appear to be very promising avenues for future exploration.

Signaling by KSHV during the early stages of infection

The integrins with which KSHV gB interacts are part of a large family of heterodimeric receptors containing noncovalently associated transmembrane α and β glycoprotein subunits (Giancotti, 2000; Giancotti and Ruoslahti, 1999; Sastry and Burridge, 2000). There are 17 α and 9 β subunits, generating more than 24 known combinations of αβ cell surface receptors. Each cell expresses several combinations of αβ integrins, and each αβ combination has its own binding specificity and signaling properties (Giancotti, 2000; Giancotti and Ruoslahti, 1999; Sastry and Burridge, 2000). Integrin interactions with ECM proteins provide robust signals for host-cell gene expression and mediate a variety of cell functions such as activation of cytoskeleton elements, endocytosis, attachment, cell cycle progression, cell growth, apoptosis, and differentiation (Giancotti, 2000; Giancotti and Ruoslahti, 1999; Sastry and Burridge, 2000). FAK is a non-receptor protein-tyrosine kinase that localizes in focal adhesions with vinculin, and FAK activation is the first step necessary for the outside–in signaling of integrins (Calderwood et al., 2000; Giancotti, 2000; Sastry and Burridge, 2000). Within 5 minutes of infection, KSHV induces the integrin-mediated activation of FAK in endothelial and fibroblast cells, and co-localizes with the focal adhesion component vinculin (Akula et al., 2002). Soluble gB, but not soluble gpK8.1A, induces FAK, which also colocalizes with pakillin (Wang et al., 2003). FAK activation is inhibited by the pre-incubation of virus or gB with soluble α3β1 integrin or anti-gB antibodies, and is not activated by a soluble form of gB in which the RGD sequence had been mutated (Akula et al., 2002; Wang et al., 2003). The ability of anti-integrin antibodies and soluble integrin to neutralize virus infection without affecting virus entry suggests that integrin and the associated signaling pathways have a role to play in KSHV entry and infection of target cells.

Studies with FAK knockout mouse fibroblasts Du3 (FAK$^{-/-}$) and parental Du17 (FAK$^{+/+}$) cells confirm that FAK plays a key role in HHV-8 infection (Naranatt et al., 2003). Since activation of FAK is central to many paradigms of outside-in signaling by integrins, actin assembly, and endocytosis, KSHV may be taking advantage of these signaling pathways both to promote entry and to produce a cellular state that facilitates infection.

KSHV induced the phosphorylation of FAK in FAK-positive Du17 mouse embryonic fibroblasts early during infection. The absence of FAK in Du3 (FAK$^{-/-}$) cells resulted in about 70% reduction in the internalization of KSHV DNA, suggesting that FAK plays a role in KSHV entry. Expression of FAK in Du3 (FAK$^{-/-}$) cells via an adenovirus vector augmented the internalization of viral DNA. Expression of the FAK dominant-negative mutant FAK-related non kinase (FRNK) in Du17 cells significantly reduced the entry of virus. Reduced quantity of virus entry in Du3 cells, delivery of viral DNA to the infected cell nuclei (Krishnan et al., 2006), and expression of KSHV genes suggested that in the absence of FAK, another molecule(s) may be partially compensating for FAK function. Infection of Du3 cells induced the phosphorylation of the FAK-related proline-rich tyrosine kinase (Pyk2) molecule, which has been shown to complement some of the functions of FAK. Expression of an autophosphorylation site mutant of Pyk2 in which Y402 is mutated to F (F402 Pyk2) reduced viral entry in Du3 cells, suggesting that Pyk2 facilitates viral entry moderately in the absence of FAK. These results suggest a critical role for KSHV infection-induced FAK in the internalization of viral DNA into target cells (Krishnan et al., 2006). One of the important downstream effectors of FAK that is activated directly or through Src kinase via Ras is PI 3-K, a member of a family of lipid kinases (Giancotti and Ruoslahti, 1999; Sastry and Burridge, 2000) that act as second messengers for a number of cell functions including the activation of Rho-GTPases and anti-apoptotic pathway Akt molecule (Giancotti and Ruoslahti, 1999; Sastry and Burridge, 2000). KSHV induces PI 3-K within 5 min of infection which decreased after 15 min (Naranatt et al., 2003). The response can be inhibited by pre-incubating KSHV with integrin and by the PI 3-K inhibitors wortmannin and LY294002. Another hallmark of integrin interaction with ligands is the reorganization and remodeling of actin cytoskeleton. This is controlled by the Rho family of small GTPases, such as Rho, Rac, and Cdc42, and the morphological changes induced by Rho, Rac and Cdc42 activation are downstream effects of PI 3-K activation (Hall and Nobes, 2000). Immediately following KSHV infection, target cells exhibit morphological changes and cytoskeletal rearrangements such as filopodia, lamellipodia and stress fibers. This together with the phosphorylation of PI 3-K by KSHV at early time infection suggests the induction of RHo-GTPases and the associated signal pathways (Naranatt et al., 2003).

FAK represents a point of convergence from activated integrins and initiates a cascade of intracellular signals that eventually activate the mitogen activated protein kinase (MAPK) pathways (Giancotti and Ruoslahti, 1999;

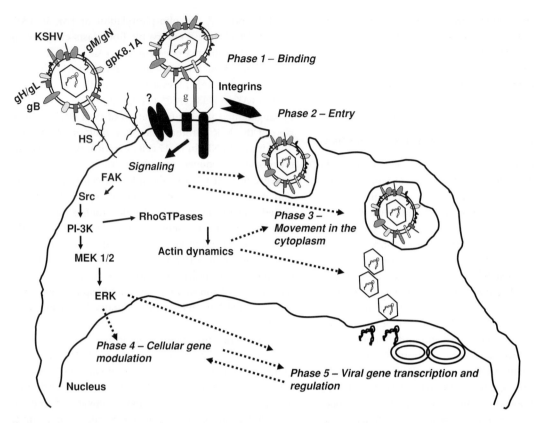

Fig. 23.3. Model for early events of KSHV infection of target cells. Early events of KSHV infection are depicted in overlapping dynamic phases. In phase 1, KSHV binds to the cell surface via its interactions with heparan sulfate proteoglycans (HSPGs) and integrins and possibly to other yet to be identified molecule(s). In phase 2, virus enters into the target cells, overlapping with the induction of host cell signal pathways. In phase 3, viral capsid/tegument moves in the cytoplasm, probably facilitated by the induced signal pathways, and probably overlaps with phase 4, the induced host cell gene transcription and expression. In phase 5, viral DNA enters into the nucleus followed by the viral gene expression. Solid arrows depict the KSHV-induced host cell signaling events that have been so far characterized. The dotted lines depict the potential stages of virus entry and infection at which the induced signaling events may have a role based on the known functions of these signaling events.

Sastry and Burridge, 2000). MAPK pathways exist in all eukaryotes and control fundamental cellular processes such as proliferation, differentiation, survival and apoptosis (Giancotti and Ruoslahti, 1999; Sastry and Burridge, 2000). As early as 5 minutes postinfection, KSHV activates the MEK (MAPK/ERK kinase) and extracellular-signal-regulated kinase (ERK) (Naranatt et al., 2003) (Fig. 23.3). Focal adhesion components PI 3-K and protein kinase C-ζ (PKC-ζ) are recruited as upstream mediators of the HHV-8 induced ERK pathway.

Antibodies to KSHV-gB that neutralize infection and soluble α3β1 integrin inhibit the virus-induced ERK signaling pathways. Early kinetics of the cellular signaling pathway and its activation by UV-inactivated KSHV suggest a role for virus binding or entry, but not viral gene expression, in this induction. Studies with human α3 integrin transfected CHO cells, and FAK negative mouse DU 3 cells suggest that the α3β1 integrin and FAK play critical roles in the KSHV mediated signal induction (Naranatt et al., 2003). Inhibitors specific for PI 3-K, PKC-ζ, MEK and ERK significantly reduce virus infectivity without affecting virus binding to the target cells. Examination of entry of viral DNA supports a role for PI 3-K in KSHV entry and a role for PKC-ζ, MEK and ERK at a stage after entry (Naranatt et al., 2003). PI 3-K is involved in the activation of Rho-GTPases. These in turn are critical for the activation of Rac, Rho, Cdc42 and Rab5 which are involved in the modulation of actin dynamics, formation of endocytic vesicles and the fission of endocytic vesicles. Furthermore, viral capsid movement in the cytoplasm probably depends upon the microfilaments and microtubules, which are controlled by the RhoGTPases. Since KSHV induces the RhoGTPases, it is reasonable to speculate that these inductions serve a vital role in the infectious process. The interaction of KSHV with cells induces the polymerization of cortical actin filaments (Naranatt et al., 2003). Further detailed analyses are essential to decipher the link between these pathways and their potential roles not only in KSHV entry into target cells but also the release and movement of capsids in the cytoplasm and delivery of viral DNA into the nucleus.

Besides playing an important role in the entry of viral nucleic acid into the nucleus of the infected cells, KSHV interactions with HS, integrins and other host cell surface molecules may also dictate the outcome of an infection by creating an appropriate intracellular environment facilitating infection. For example, there are many obstacles that viruses have to overcome during the early and late stages of infection of target cells in the host. They include external threats to infected cells from the innate and adaptive immune systems as well as internal obstacles such as transcriptional blocks and cellular apoptosis that may be triggered by virus binding and entry. To establish a successful infection, herpesviruses must have developed many ways to manipulate and overcome these obstacles early during infection. In this respect, stimulation of PI 3-K by KSHV, which may influence the Akt induced anti-apoptotic pathway, and modulation of interferon response factors by the virion associated tegument protein ORF 45 protein (Zhu and Yuan, 2003) are of considerable interest.

Cytoplasmic trafficking, delivery of viral genome into the nucleus

After release into the cytoplasm, the EBV and KSHV capsid/tegument must traffic through the cell in order for viral DNA to be delivered into the nucleus. HSV-1 utilizes dynein motors and microtubules for this purpose and the activation by KSHV of RhoGTPases, which are important to control of microtubules, is consistent with a similar mechanism of transport for this virus.

Similar to HSV, KSHV utilizes the dynein motors in the cytoplasmic trafficking and delivery of viral DNA to the nucleus (Narranat et al., 2005). Microtubules play important roles in KSHV infection since depolymerization of microtubules even though did not affect KSHV binding and internalization, it inhibited the nuclear delivery of viral DNA and infection (Narranat et al., 2005). The interesting aspect is that KSHV induced the acetylation of microtubules, an essential step for the microtubule aggregation, which are mediated by the host cell pre-existing signals induced by KSHV binding an entry steps. The inactivation of Rho GTPases by Clostridium difficile toxin B significantly reduced the microtubular acetylation and the delivery of viral DNA to the nucleus (Narranat et al., 2005). Activation of Rho GTPases by *Escherichia coli* cytotoxic necrotizing factor significantly augmented the nuclear delivery of viral DNA. Activation of RhoA-GTP-dependent diaphanous 2 was observed, with no significant activation in the Rac- and Cdc42-dependent PAK1/2 and stathmin molecules. The nuclear delivery of viral DNA increased in cells expressing a constitutively active RhoA mutant and decreased in cells expressing a dominant-negative mutant of RhoA. Like in HSV-1, KSHV capsids colocalized with the microtubules, and the colocalization was abolished by the destabilization of microtubules with nocodazole and by the PI-3K inhibitor affecting the Rho GTPases. These results suggest that KSHV induces Rho GTPases, modulates microtubules and promotes the trafficking of viral capsids and the establishment of infection (Narranat et al., 2005). These studies demonstrated for the first time modulation of the microtubule dynamics by virus-induced host cell signaling pathways to aid in the trafficking of viral DNA to the infected cell nucleus. These data strongly suggest that KSHV manipulates the host cell signaling pathway to create an appropriate intracellular environment that is conducive to the establishment of a successful infection.

No studies of EBV have directly addressed this issue, although the observation that at least in epithelial cells the EBV BMRF2 protein interacts with integrins is provocative (Tugizov et al., 2003). In primary B cells transcription from incoming EBV DNA can be detected within 10–12 h post infection and since circularization of the genome requires host protein synthesis (Sinclair and Farrell, 1995), whereas initiation of transcription from the viral genome does not (Hurley and Thorley-Lawson, 1988), it can be inferred that transcription initiates from the incoming linear genome. Transcription is unaffected by inhibitors of tyrosine kinases and PI 3-K, but synthesis of virus proteins is reduced implying that stimulation of kinases is not required for transport of virus to the nucleus, as it may be for KSHV, but for a later stage in the infection process (Sinclair and Farrell, 1995). Circular episomes have been detected by 16 h post infection and their formation may require that the cell move from G0 to G1 (Alfieri et al., 1991; Hurley and Thorley-Lawson, 1988). De novo protein synthesis is probably necessary for circularization and a cellular protein complex that includes Sp1 and binds to the recombination junctions within the terminal repeats of the genome may be involved in the process (Sun et al., 1997). Early studies have suggested that amplification of the first formed episome does not occur in primary B cells until more than one week after infection (Hurley and Thorley-Lawson, 1988). No similar studies have yet been reported for KSHV, although the virus is found in episomal form in PEL cells (Ballestas et al., 1999). Clearly much more needs to be known about the events between entry and early transcription from the incoming genome for both KSHV and EBV.

Summary

The importance of EBV and KSHV as oncogenic viruses has appropriately focused efforts on understanding the ways in which they influence cell survival and growth. An unintended consequence has been that information about productive replication of both viruses has been less forthcoming. Recent progress, particularly in understanding the early events that initiate entry, has been promising, but many important gaps remain to be filled. The determinants of tropism remain incompletely defined for both EBV and KSHV and although the perennial problem of how herpesviruses mediate virus cell fusion is not unique to either EBV or KSHV, it is still largely unsolved. The effect of entry on cell signaling pathways is proving to be an extremely fertile area of study, not just for understanding how viruses establish a suitable intracellular milieu for gene expression and DNA replication, but also for understanding how viruses are transported to the nucleus after the cell membrane has crossed. Progress with KSHV has been particularly interesting in this regard. It already appears likely that infection of endothelial cells by KSHV and infection of B cells by EBV may follow different pathways. However, whether this reflects fundamental differences in virus strategy, or adaptation to different host cells will require study of the viruses in more than one of the cell types that each infects. As important as a comprehensive understanding of lytic replication is to understanding the pathogenesis of disease as a whole, for EBV and KSHV it remains a distant goal.

REFERENCES

Akula, S. M., Pramod, N. P., Wang, F. Z., and Chandran, B. (2001a). Human herpesvirus 8 envelope-associated glycoprotein B interacts with heparan sulfate-like moieties. *Virology*, **284**(2), 235–249.

Akula, S. M., Wang, F. Z., Vieira, J., and Chandran, B. (2001b). Human herpesvirus 8 interaction with target cells involves heparan sulfate. *Virology*, **282**(2), 245–255.

Akula, S. M., Pramod, N. P., Wang, F. Z., and Chandran, B. (2002). Integrin a3b1 (CD49c/29) is a cellular receptor for Kaposi's sarcoma-associated herpesvirus (KSHV/HHV8) entry into target cells. *Cell*, **108**, 407–419.

Akula, S. M., Naranatt, P. P., Walia, N. S., Wang, F. Z., Fegley, B., and Chandran, B. (2003). Kaposi's sarcoma-associated herpesvirus (human herpesvirus 8) infection of human fibroblast cells occurs through endocytosis. *J. Virol.*, **77**(14), 7978–7990.

Alfieri, C., Birkenbach, M., and Kieff, E. (1991). Early events in Epstein–Barr virus infection of human B lymphocytes. *Virology*, **181**, 595–608.

Anagnostopoulos, I., Hummel, M., Kreschel, C., and Stein, H. (1995). Morphology, immunophenotype and distribution of latently and/or productively Epstein–Barr virus-infected cells in acute infectious mononucleosis: implications for the interindividual individual infection route of Epstein–Barr virus. *Blood*, **5**, 744–750.

Antman, K. and Chang, Y. (2000). Kaposi's sarcoma. *N. Engl. J. Med.*, **342**(14), 1027–1038.

Baer, R., Bankier, A. T., Biggin, M. D. *et al.* (1984). DNA sequence and expression of the B95–8 Epstein–Barr virus genome. *Nature*, **310**, 207–211.

Baghian, A., Luftig, M., Black, J. B. *et al.* (2000). Glycoprotein B of human herpesvirus 8 is a component of the virion in a cleaved form composed of amino- and carboxyl-terminal fragments. *Virology*, **269**(1), 18–25.

Ballestas, M. E., Chatis, P. A., and Kaye, K. M. (1999). Efficient persistence of extrachromosomal KSHV DNA mediated by latency-associated nuclear antigen. *Science*, **282**, 641–644.

Bayliss, G. J. and Wolf, H. (1980). Epstein–Barr virus induced cell fusion. *Nature*, **287**, 164–165.

Bechtel, J. T., Liang, Y., Hvidding, J., and Ganem, D. (2003). Host range of Kaposi's sarcoma-associated herpesvirus in cultured cells. *J. Virol.*, **77**(11), 6474–6481.

Beisel, C., Tanner, J., Matsuo, T. *et al.* (1985). Two major outer envelope glycoproteins of Epstein–Barr virus are encoded by the same gene. *J. Virol.*, **54**, 665–674.

Beisser, P. S., Versijl, D., Gruijthuijsen, Y. K. *et al.* (2005). The Epstein–Barr virus BILF1 gene encodes a G protein-coupled receptor that inhibits phosphorylation of RNA-dependent protein kinase. *J. Virol.*, **79**, 441–449.

Birkmann, A., Mahr, K., Ensser, A. *et al.* (2001). Cell surface heparan sulfate is a receptor for human herpesvirus 8 and interacts with envelope glycoprotein K8.1. *J. Virol.*, **75**(23), 11583–11593.

Blackbourn, D. J., Lennette, E., Klencke, B. *et al.* (2000). The restricted cellular host range of human herpesvirus 8. *AIDS*, **14**(9), 1123–1133.

Borza, C. and Hutt-Fletcher, L. M. (1998). Epstein–Barr virus recombinant lacking expression of glycoprotein gp150 infects B cells normally but is enhanced for infection of the epithelial line SVKCR2. *J. Virol.*, **72**, 7577–7582.

Borza, C. M. and Hutt-Fletcher, L. M. (2002). Alternate replication in B cells and epithelial cells switches tropism of Epstein–Barr virus. *Nature Med.*, **8**, 594–599.

Borza, C. M., Morgan, A. J., Turk, S. M., and Hutt-Fletcher, L. M. (2004). Use of gHgL for attachment of Epstein–Barr virus to epithelial cells compromises infection. *J. Virol.*, **78**, 5007–5014.

Calderwood, D. A., Shattil, S. J., and Ginsberg, M. H. (2000). Integrins and actin filaments: reciprocal regulation of cell adhesion and signaling. *J. Biol. Chem.*, **275**(30), 22607–22610.

Chandran, B., Bloomer, C., Chan, S. R., Zhu, L., Goldstein, E., and Horvat, R. (1998). Human herpesvirus-8 ORF K8.1 gene encodes immunogenic glycoproteins generated by spliced transcripts. *Virology*, **249**(1), 140–149.

Ciufo, D. M., Cannon, J. S., Poole, L. J. *et al.* (2001). Spindle cell conversion by Kaposi's sarcoma-associated herpesvirus: formation of colonies and plaques with mixed lytic and latent gene expression in infected primary dermal microvascular endothelial cell cultures. *J. Virol.*, **75**(12), 5614–5626.

Colman, P. M. and Lawrence, M. C. (2003). The structural biology of type 1 viral membrane fusion. *Nat. Rev. Mol. Cell Biol.*, **4**, 309–319.

D'Addario, M. D., Libermann, T. A., Xu, J., Ahmad, A., and Menezes, J. (2001). Epstein–Barr virus and its glycoprotein-350 upregulate IL-6 in human B-lymphocytes via CD21, involving activation of NF-kB and different signaling pathways. *J. Mol. Biol.*, **308**, 501–504.

Dezube, B. J., Zambela, M., Sage, D. R., Wang, J. F., and Fingeroth, J. D. (2002). Characterization of Kaposi sarcoma-associated herpesvirus/human herpesvirus-8 infection of human vascular endothelial cells: early events. *Blood*, **100**(3), 888–896.

Dourmishev, L. A., Dourmishev, A. L., Palmeri, D., Schwartz, R. A., and Lukac, D. M. (2003). Molecular genetics of Kaposi's sarcoma-associated herpesvirus (human herpesvirus-8) epidemiology and pathogenesis. *Microbiol. Mol. Biol. Rev.*, **67**(2), 175–212.

Farina, A., Santarello, R., Gonnella, R. *et al.* (2000). The BFRF1 gene of Epstein–Barr virus encodes a novel protein. *J. Virol.*, **74**, 3235–3244.

Farina, A., Cardinale, G., Santarella, R. *et al.* (2004). Intracellular localization of the Epstein–Barr virus BFRF1 gene product in lymphoid cell lines and oral hairy leukoplakis lesions. *J. Med. Virol.*, **72**, 102–111.

Farina, A., Feederle, R., Raffa, S. *et al.* (2005). BFRF1 of Epstein–Barr virus is essential fro efficient primary envelopment and egress. *J. Virol.*, **79**, 3703–3712.

Feral, C. C., Nishiya, N., Fenczik, C. A., Stuhlmann, H., Slepak, M., and Ginsberg, M. H. (2005). CD98hc (SLC3A2) mediates integrin signaling. *Proc. Natl Acad. Sci. USA*, **102**, 355–360.

Fenczik, C. A., Zent, R., Dellos, M. *et al.* (2001). Distinct domains of CD98hc regulate integrins and amino acid transport. *J. Biol. Chem.*, **276**, 8746–8752.

Fingeroth, J. D., Weis, J. J., Tedder, T. F., Strominger, J. L., Biro, P. A., and Fearon, D. T. (1984). Epstein–Barr virus receptor of human B lymphocytes is the C3d complement CR2. *Proc. Natl Acad. Sci. USA*, **81**, 4510–4516.

Fingeroth, J. D., Diamond, M. E., Sage, D. R., Hayman, J., and Yates, J. L. (1999). CD-21 dependent infection of an epithelial cell line, 293, by Epstein–Barr virus. *J. Virol.*, **73**, 2115–2125.

Frade, R., Barel, M., Ehlin-Henricksson, B., and Klein, G. (1985). gp140 the C3d receptor of human B lymphocytes is also the Epstein–Barr virus receptor. *Proc. Natl Acad. Sci. USA*, **82**, 1490–1493.

Frangou, P., Buettner, M., and Niedobitek, G. (2005). Epstein–Barr virus (EBV) infection in epithelial cells in vivo; rare detection of EBV replication in tongue mucosa but not in salivary glands. *J. Infect. Dis.*, **191**, 238–242.

Gan, Y., Chodosh, J., Morgan, A., and Sixbey, J. W. (1997). Epithelial cell polarization is a determinant in the infectious outcome of immunoglobulin A-mediated entry by Epstein–Barr virus. *J. Virol.*, **71**, 519–526.

Ganem, D. (1998). Human herpesvirus 8 and its role in the genesis of Kaposi's sarcoma. *Curr. Clin. Top. Infect. Dis.*, **18**, 237–251.

Giancotti, F. G. (2000). Complexity and specificity of integrin signalling. *Nat. Cell Biol.*, **2**(1), E13–E14.

Giancotti, F. G. and Ruoslahti, E. (1999). Integrin signaling. *Science*, **285**(5430), 1028–1032.

Gong, M. and Kieff, E. (1990). Intracellular trafficking of two major Epstein–Barr virus glycoproteins, gp350/220 and gp110. *J. Virol.*, **64**, 1507–1516.

Gong, M., Ooka, T., Matsuo, T., and Kieff, E. (1987). Epstein-Barr virus glycoprotein homologous to herpes simplex virus gB. *J. Virol.*, **61**, 499–508.

Gonnella, R., Farina, A., Santarella, R. *et al.* (2005). Characterization and intracellular localization of the Epstein-Barr virus protein BFLF2: interactions with BFRF1 and with the nuclear lamina. *J. Virol.*, **49**, 3713–3237.

Gordon, J. S., Walker, L., Guy, G., Brown, G., Rowe, M., and Rickinson, A. (1986). Control of human B-lymphocyte transformation. II. Transforming Epstein-Barr virus exploits three distinct viral signals to undermine three separate control points in B cell growth. *Immunology*, **58**, 591–595.

Grundhoff, A. and Ganem, D. (2004). Inefficient establishment of KSHV latency suggests an additional role for continued lytic replication in Kaposi sarcoma pathogenesis. *J. Clin. Invest.*, **113**, 124–136.

Haan, K. M. and Longnecker, R. (2000). Coreceptor restriction within the HLA-DQ locus for Epstein-Barr virus infection. *Proc. Natl Acad. Sci. USA*, **97**, 9252–9257.

Haan, K. M., Lee, S. K., and Longnecker, R. (2001). Different functional domains in the cytoplasmic tail of glycoprotein gB are involved in Epstein–Barr virus induced membrane fusion. *Virology*, **290**, 106–114.

Haddad, R. S. and Hutt-Fletcher, L. M. (1989). Depletion of glycoprotein gp85 from virosomes made with Epstein–Barr virus proteins abolishes their ability to fuse with virus receptor-bearing cells. *J. Virol.*, **63**, 4998–5005.

Hall, A. and Nobes, C. D. (2000). Rho GTPases: molecular switches that control the organization and dynamics of the actin cytoskeleton. *Phil. Trans. R. Soc. Lond. B Biol. Sci.*, **355**(1399), 965–970.

Heineman, T., Gong, M., Sample, J., and Kieff, E. (1988). Identification of the Epstein-Barr virus gp85 gene. *J. Virol.*, **62**, 1101–1107.

Huber, M. T. and Compton, T. (1998). The human cytomegalovirus UL74 gene encodes the third component of the glycoprotein H-glycoprotein L-containing envelope complex. *J. Virol.*, **72**, 8191–8197.

Hummel, M. and Kieff, E. (1982). Epstein-Barr virus RNA. VIII. Viral RNA in permissively infected B95-8 cells. *J. Virol.*, **43**, 262–272.

Hummel, M., Thorley-Lawson, D., and Kieff, E. (1984). An Epstein-Barr virus DNA fragment encodes messages for the two major envelope glycoproteins (gp350/300 and gp220/200). *J. Virol.*, **49**, 413–417.

Hurley, E. A. and Thorley-Lawson, D. A. (1988). B cell activation and the establishment of Epstein–Barr virus latency. *J. Exp. Med.*, **168**, 2059–2075.

Hutt-Fletcher, L. M. (2002). Epstein–Barr virus glycoproteins and their roles in virus entry and egress. In *Structure–function Relationships of Human Pathogenic Viruses*, ed. A. Holzenburg and E. Bogner. New York: Kluwer Academic/Plenum.

Imai, S., Nishikawa, J., and Takada, K. (1998). Cell-to-cell contact as an efficient mode of Epstein-Barr virus infection of diverse human epithelial cells. *J. Virol.*, **72**, 4371–4378.

Inoue, N., Winter, J., Lal, R. B., Offermann, M. K., and Koyano, S. (2003). Characterization of entry mechanisms of human herpesvirus 8 by using an Rta-dependent reporter cell line. *J. Virol.*, **77**, 8143–8152.

Jiang, R., Scott, R. S., and Hutt-Fletcher, L. M. (2006). Epstein–Barr virus shed in saliva is high in B cell tropic gp42. *J. Virol.*, **80**, 7281–7283.

Johannsen, E., Luftig, M., Weicksel, S. et al. (2004). Proteins of purified Epstein–Barr virus. *Proc. Natl Acade. Sci. USA*, **101**, 16286–16291.

Kaleeba, J. A. R and Berger, E. A. (2006). Kaposi's Sarcoma–associated herpesvirus fusion-entry receptor: cystine transporter xCT. *Science*, **311**, 1921–1924.

Kieff, E. and Rickinson, A. B. (2001). Epstein–Barr virus and its replication. In *Fields Virology* ed. D. M. Knipe, and P. M. Howley, Vol. 2, pp. 2511–2573. 2 vols. Philadelphia: Lippincott Williams and Wilkins.

Klupp, B. and Mettenleiter, T. C. (1991). Sequence and expression of the glycoprotein gH gene of pseudorabies virus. *Virology*, **182**, 732–741.

Koyano, S., Mar, E. C., Stamey, F. R., and Inoue, N. (2003). Glycoproteins M and N of human herpesvirus 8 form a complex and inhibit cell fusion. *J. Gen. Virol.*, **84**, 1485–1491.

Krishnan, H. H., Walia, N. S., Streblow, D. N., Naranatt, P. P., and Chandran, B. (2006). Focal adhesion kinase (FAK) is critical for Kaposi's Sarcoma-associated herpesvirus (KSHV/HHV-8) entry into the target cells. *J. Virol.*, **80**, 1167–1180.

Kurilla, M. G., Heineman, T., Davenport, L. C., Kieff, E., and Hutt-Fletcher, L. M. (1995). A novel Epstein–Barr virus glycoprotein gp150 expressed from the BDLF3 open reading frame. *Virology*, **209**, 108–121.

Lagunoff, M., Bechtel, J., Venetsanakos, E. et al. (2002). De novo infection and serial transmission of Kaposi's sarcoma-associated herpesvirus in cultured endothelial cells. *J. Virol.*, **76**(5), 2440–2448.

Lake, C. M. and Hutt-Fletcher, L. M. (2000). Epstein–Barr virus that lacks glycoprotein gN is impaired in assembly and infection. *J. Virol.*, **74**, 11162–11172.

Lake, C. M. and Hutt-Fletcher, L. M. (2004). The Epstein–Barr virus BFRF1 and BFLF2 proteins interact and coexpression alters their cellular localization. *Virology*, **320**, 99–106.

Lambris, J. D., Ganu, V. S., Hirani, S., and Muller-Eberhard, H. J. (1985). Mapping of the C3d receptor (CR2) binding site and a neoantigenic site in the C3d domain of the third component of complement. *Proc. Natl Acad. Sci. USA*, **82**, 4235–4239.

Lee, S. K. and Longnecker, R. (1997). The Epstein–Barr virus glycoprotein 110 carboxy-terminal tail domain is essential for lytic virus replication. *J. Virol.*, **71**, 4092–4097.

Lemon, S. M., Hutt, L. M., Shaw, J. E., Li, J.-L. H., and Pagano, J. S. (1977). Replication of EBV in epithelial cells during infectious mononucleosis. *Nature*, **268**, 268–270.

Li, Q. X., Young, L. S., Niedobitek, G. et al. (1992). Epstein–Barr virus infection and replication in a human epithelial system. *Nature*, **356**, 347–350.

Li, Q. X., Turk, S. M., and Hutt-Fletcher, L. M. (1995). The Epstein–Barr virus (EBV) BZLF2 gene product associates with the gH and gL homologs of EBV and carries an epitope critical to infection of B cells but not of epithelial cells. *J. Virol.*, **69**, 3987–3994.

Li, Q. X., Spriggs, M. K., Kovats, S. et al. (1997). Epstein–Barr virus uses HLA class II as a cofactor for infection of B lymphocytes. *J. Virol.*, **71**(6), 4657–4662.

Liao, W., Tang, Y., Kuo, Y. L., Liu, B. Y., Xu, C. J., and Giam, C. Z. (2003). Kaposi's sarcoma-associated herpesvirus/human herpesvirus 8 transcriptional activator Rta is an oligomeric DNA-binding protein that interacts with tandem arrays of phased A/T-trinucleotide motifs. *J. Virol.*, **77**(17), 9399–9411.

Lo, P., Yu, X., Atanasov, I., Chandran, B., and Zhou, Z. H. (2003). Three-dimensional localization of pORF65 in Kaposi's sarcoma-associated herpesvirus capsid. *J. Virol.*, **77**(7), 4291–4297.

McShane, M. P. and Longnecker, R. (2004). Cell-surface expression of a mutated Epstein–Barr virus glycoprotein B allows fusion independent of other viral glycoproteins. *Proc. Natl Acad. Sci. USA*, **101**, 17474–17479.

Mackett, M., Conway, M. J., Arrand, J. R., Haddad, R. S., and Hutt-Fletcher, L. M. (1990). Characterization and expression of a glycoprotein encoded by the Epstein–Barr virus BamHI 1 fragment. *J. Virol.*, **64**, 2545–2552.

Martin, D. R., Yuryev, A., Kalli, K. R., Fearon, D. T., and Ahearn, J. M. (1991). Determination of the structural basis for selective binding of Epstein-Barr virus to human complement receptor type 2. *J. Exp. Med.*, **174**, 1299–1311.

Martin, D. R., Marlowe, R. L., and Ahearn, J. M. (1994). Determination of the role for CD21 during Epstein–Barr virus infection of B lymphoblastoid cells. *J. Virol.*, **68**, 4716–4726.

Miller, N. and Hutt-Fletcher, L. M. (1988). A monoclonal antibody to glycoprotein gp85 inhibits fusion but not attachment of Epstein–Barr virus. *J. Virol.*, **62**, 2366–2372.

Miller, N. and Hutt-Fletcher, L. M. (1992). Epstein–Barr virus enters B cells and epithelial cells by different routes. *J. Virol.*, **66**(6), 3409–3414.

Molesworth, S. J., Lake, C. M., Borza, C. M., Turk, S. M., and Hutt-Fletcher, L. M. (2000). Epstein–Barr virus gH is essential for penetration of B cell but also plays a role in attachment of virus to epithelial cells. *J. Virol.*, **74**, 6324–6332.

Moore, M. D., DiScipio, R. G., Cooper, N. R., and Nemerow, G. R. (1989). Hydrodynamic, electron microscopic and ligand binding analysis of the Epstein–Barr virus/C3dg receptor (CR2). *J. Biol. Chem.*, **34**, 20576–20582.

Mori, Y., Akkapaiboon, P., Yang, X., and Yamanishi, K. (2003). The human herpesvirus 6 U100 gene product is the third component of the gH–gL glycoprotein complex on the viral envelope. *J. Virol.*, **77**, 2452–2458.

Moses, A. V., Fish, K. N., Ruhl, R. *et al.* (1999). Long-term infection and transformation of dermal microvascular endothelial cells by human herpesvirus 8. *J. Virol.*, **73**(8), 6892–6902.

Mullen, M. M., Haan, K. M., Longnecker, R., and Jardetzky, T. S. (2002). Structure of the Epstein–Barr virus gp42 protein bound to the MHC class II receptor HLA-DR1. *Mol. Cell*, **9**, 375–385.

Naranatt, P. P., Akula, S. M., and Chandran, B. (2002). Characterization of gamma2-human herpesvirus-8 glycoproteins gH and gL. *Arch. Virol.*, **147**(7), 1349–1370.

Naranatt, P. P., Akula, S. M., Zien, C. A., Krishnan, H. H., and Chandran, B. (2003). Kaposi's sarcoma-associated herpesvirus induces the phosphatidylinositol 3-kinase-PKC-zeta-MEK-ERK signaling pathway in target cells early during infection: implications for infectivity. *J. Virol.*, **77**(2), 1524–1539.

Naranatt, P. P., Krishnan, H. H., Smith, M. S., and Chandran, B. (2005). Kaposi's sarcoma-associated herpesvirus (KSHV/HHV-8) modulates the microtubule dynamics via RhoA-GTP-Diaphenous-2 signaling and utilizes the dynein motors to deliver its DNA to the nucleus. *J. Virol.*, **79**, 1191–1206.

Neipel, F., Albrecht, J. C., and Fleckenstein, B. (1997). Cell-homologous genes in the Kaposi's sarcoma-associated rhadinovirus human herpesvirus 8: determinants of its pathogenicity? *J. Virol.*, **71**(6), 4187–4192.

Nemerow, G. R. and Cooper, N. R. (1984). Early events in the infection of human B lymphocytes by Epstein-Barr virus. *Virology*, **132**, 186–198.

Nemerow, G. R., Wolfert, R., McNaughton, M., and Cooper, N. R. (1985). Identification and characterization of the Epstein–Barr virus receptor on human B lymphocytes and its relationship to the C3d complement receptor (CR2). *J. Virol.*, **55**, 347–351.

Nemerow, G. R., Houghton, R. A., Moore, M. D., and Cooper, N. R. (1989). Identification of the epitope in the major envelope proteins of Epstein-Barr virus that mediates viral binding to the B lymphocyte EBV receptor (CR2). *Cell*, **56**, 369–377.

Niedobitek, G., Hamilton-Dutoit, S., Herbst, H. *et al.* (1989). Identification of Epstein–Barr virus-infected cells in tonsils of acute infectious mononucleosis by in situ hybridization. *Hum. Pathol.*, **20**, 796–799.

Nolan, L. A. and Morgan, A. J. (1995). The Epstein–Barr virus open reading frame BDLF3 codes for a 100–150 kDa glycoprotein. *J. Gen. Virol.*, **76**, 1381–1392.

Oba, D. E. and Hutt-Fletcher, L. M. (1988). Induction of antibodies to the Epstein–Barr virus glycoprotein gp85 with a synthetic peptide corresponding to a sequence in the BXLF2 open reading frame. *J. Virol.*, **62**, 1108–1114.

Oda, T., Imai, S., Chiba, S., and Takada, K. (2000). Epstein–Barr virus lacking glycoprotein gp85 cannot infect B cells and epithelial cells. *Virology*, **276**, 52–58.

Omerovic, J., Lev, L., and Longnecker, R. (2005). The amino terminus of Epstein–Barr virus glycoprotein gH is important for fusion with B cells and epithelial cells. *J. Virol.*, **79**, 12408–12415.

Paulsen, S. J., Rosenkilde, M. M., Eugen-Olsen, J., and Kledal, T. N. (2005). Epstein–Barr virus-encoded BILF1 is a constitutively active G protein-coupled receptor. *J. Virol.*, **79**, 536–546.

Pegtel, D. M., Middledorp, J., and Thorley-Lawson, D. A. (2004). Epstein–Barr virus infection in ex-vivo tonsil epithelial cultures of asymptomatic carriers. *J. Virol.*, **78**, 12613–12624.

Pertel, P. E. (2002). Human herpesvirus 8 glycoprotein B (gB), gH, and gL can mediate cell fusion. *J. Virol.*, **76**, 4390–4400.

Rappocciolo, G., Jenkins, F. L., Hensler, H. R. *et al.* (2006). DC-SIGN is a receptor for human herpesvirus 8 on dendritic cells and macrophages. *J. Immunol.*, **176**, 1741–1749.

Renne, R., Blackbourn, D., Whitby, D., Levy, J., and Ganem, D. (1998). Limited transmission of Kaposi's sarcoma-associated herpesvirus in cultured cells. *J. Virol.*, **72**(6), 5182–5188.

Ressing, M. E., van Leeuwen, D., Verreck, F. A. W. *et al.* (2005). Epstein–Barr virus gp42 is postranslationally modified to produce s-gp42 that mediates class II immune evasion. *J. Virol.*, **79**, 841–852.

Rickinson, A. B. and Kieff, E. (2001). Epstein–Barr virus. In *fields virology* ed. D. M. Knipe, and P. M. Howley, Vol. 2, pp. 2575–2627. 2 vols. Philadelphia: Lippincott, Williams and Wilkins.

Rivailler, P., Jiang, H., Cho, Y.-G., Quink, C., and Wang, F. (2002). Complete nucleotide sequence of the rhesus lymphocryptovirus: genetic validation for an Epstein–Barr virus animal model. *J. Virol.*, **76**, 421–426.

Russo, J. J., Bohenzky, R. A., Chien, M. C. *et al.* (1996). Nucleotide sequence of the Kaposi sarcoma-associated herpesvirus (HHV8). *Proc. Natl Acad. Sci. USA*, **93**, 14862–14867.

Sarid, R., Olsen, S. J., and Moore, P. S. (1999). Kaposi's sarcoma-associated herpesvirus: epidemiology, virology, and molecular biology. *Adv. Virus Res.*, **52**, 139–232.

Sastry, S. K. and Burridge, K. (2000). Focal adhesions: a nexus for intracellular signaling and cytoskeletal dynamics. *Exp. Cell Res.*, **261**(1), 25–36.

Schulz, T. F., Sheldon, J., and Greensill, J. (2002). Kaposi's sarcoma associated herpesvirus (KSHV) or human herpesvirus 8 (HHV8). *Virus Res.*, **82**(1–2), 115–126.

Shannon-Rowe, C. D., Neuhierl, B., Baldwin, G., Rickinson, A. B., and Delecluse, H. -J. (2006). Resting B cells as a transfer vehicle for Epstein–Barr virus infection of epithelial cells. *Proc. Natl Acad. Sci. USA*, **103**, 7065–7070

Sieczkarski, S. B. and Whittaker, G. R. (2002). Dissecting virus entry via endocytosis. *J. Gen. Virol.*, **83**(7), 1535–1545.

Sinclair, A. J. and Farrell, P. J. (1995). Host cell requirements for efficient infection of quiescent primary B lymphocytes by Epstein–Barr virus. *J. Virol.*, **69**, 5461–5468.

Sixbey, J. W. and Yao, Q.-Y. (1992). Immunoglobulin A-induced shift of Epstein–Barr virus tissue tropism. *Science*, **255**, 1578–1580.

Sixbey, J. W., Nedrud, J. G., Raab-Traub, N., Hanes, R. A., and Pagano, J. S. (1984). Epstein–Barr virus replication in oropharyngeal epithelial cells. *N. Engl. J. Med.*, **310**, 1225–1230.

Spriggs, M. K., Armitage, R. J., Comeau, M. R. et al. (1996). The extracellular domain of the Epstein–Barr virus BZLF2 protein binds the HLA-DR beta chain and inhibits antigen presentation. *J. Virol.*, **70**, 5557–5563.

Sugano, N., Chen, W., Roberts, M. L., and Cooper, N. R. (1997). Epstein–Barr virus binding to CD21 activates the initial viral promoter via NFkB induction. *J. Exp. Med.*, **186**, 731–737.

Sun, R., Spain, T. A., Lin, S.-F., and Miller, G. (1997). Sp1 binds to the precise locus of end processing within the terminal repeats of Epstein–Barr virus DNA. *J. Virol.*, **71**, 6136–6143.

Tanner, J., Weis, J., Fearon, D., Whang, Y., and Kieff, E. (1987). Epstein–Barr virus gp350/220 binding to the B lymphocyte C3d receptor mediates adsorption, capping and endocytosis. *Cell*, **50**, 203–213.

Tanner, J., Whang, Y., Sample, J., Sears, A., and Kieff, E. (1988). Soluble gp350/220 and deletion mutant glycoproteins block Epstein–Barr virus adsorption to lymphocytes. *J. Virol.*, **62**, 4452–4464.

Tanner, J. E. and Tosato, G. (1992). Regulation of B-cell growth and immunoglobulin gene transcription by interleukin-6. *Blood*, **79**, 452–459.

Telford, E. A., Watson, M. S., Aird, H. C., Perry, J., and Davison, A. J. (1995). The DNA sequence of equine herpesvirus 2. *J. Mol. Biol.*, **249**, 520–528.

Tomescu, C., Law, W. K., and Kedes, D. H. (2003). Surface downregulation of major histocompatibility complex class I, PE-CAM, and ICAM-1 following de novo infection of endothelial cells with Kaposi's sarcoma-associated herpesvirus. *J. Virol.*, **77**(17), 9669–9684.

Trus, B. L., Heymann, J. B., Nealon, K. et al. (2001). Capsid structure of Kaposi's sarcoma-associated herpesvirus, a gammaherpesvirus, compared to those of an alphaherpesvirus, herpes simplex virus type 1, and a betaherpesvirus, cytomegalovirus. *J. Virol.*, **75**(6), 2879–2890.

Tugizov, S. M., Berline, J. W., and Palefsky, J. M. (2003). Epstein–Barr virus infection of polarized tongue and nasopharyngeal epithelial cells. *Nature Med.*, **9**, 307–314.

Turk, S. M., Jiang, R., Chesnokova, L. S., and Hutt-Fletcher, L. M. (2006). Antibodies to gp350/220 enhance the ability of Epstein–Barr virus to infect epithelial cells. *J. Virol.*, **80**, 9628–9633.

Venables, P. J. W., Teo, C. G., Baboonian, C., Griffin, B. E., and Hughes, R. A. (1989). Persistence of Epstein–Barr virus in salivary gland biopsies from healthy individuals and patients with Sjogren's syndrome. *Clin. Exp. Immunol.*, **75**, 359–364.

Vieira, J., O'Hearn, P., Kimball, L., Chandran, B., and Corey, L. (2001). Activation of Kaposi's sarcoma-associated herpesvirus (human herpesvirus 8) lytic replication by human cytomegalovirus. *J. Virol.*, **75**(3), 1378–1386.

Virgin, H. W. I., Latreille, P., Wamsley, P. et al. (1997). Complete sequence and analysis of murine gammaherpesvirus 68. *J. Virol.*, **71**, 5894–5904.

Virji, M. (1996). Microbial utilization of human signalling molecules. *Microbiology*, **142**(12), 3319–3336.

Wang, F. Z., Akula, S. M., Pramod, N. P., Zeng, L., and Chandran, B. (2001). Human herpesvirus 8 envelope glycoprotein K8.1A interaction with the target cells involves heparan sulfate. *J. Virol.*, **75**(16), 7517–7527.

Wang, F. Z., Akula, S. M., Sharma-Walia, N., Zeng, L., and Chandran, B. (2003). Human herpesvirus 8 envelope glycoprotein B mediates cell adhesion via its RGD sequence. *J. Virol.*, **77**(5), 3131–3147.

Wang, X. and Hutt-Fletcher, L. M. (1998). Epstein–Barr virus lacking glycoprotein gp42 can bind to B cells but is not able to infect. *J. Virol.*, **72**, 158–163.

Wang, X., Kenyon, W. J., Li, Q. X., Mullberg, J., and Hutt-Fletcher, L. M. (1998). Epstein–Barr virus uses different complexes of glycoproteins gH and gL to infect B lymphocytes and epithelial cells. *J. Virol.*, **72**, 5552–5558.

Weisman, H. F., Bartow, T., Leppo, M. K. et al. (1990). Soluble human complement receptor type 1: in vivo inhibitor of complement suppressing post-ischemic myocardial inflammation and necrosis. *Science*, **249**, 146–151.

Whittaker, G. R. (2003). Virus nuclear import. *Adv. Drug Deliv. Rev.*, **55**(6), 733–747.

Wu, L., Lo, P., Yu, X., Stoops, J. K., Forghani, B., and Zhou, Z. H. (2000). Three-dimensional structure of the human herpesvirus 8 capsid. *J. Virol.*, **74**, 9646–9654.

Wu, L., Borza, C. M., and Hutt-Fletcher, L. M. (2005). Mutations of Epstein–Barr virus gH that are differentially able to support fusion with B cells or epithelial cells. *J. Virol.*, **79**, 10923–10930.

Yaswen, L. R., Stephens, E. B., Davenport, L. C., and Hutt-Fletcher, L. M. (1993). Epstein-Barr virus glycoprotein gp85 associates with the BKRF2 gene product and is incompletely processed as a recombinant protein. *Virology*, **195**, 387–396.

Young, L. S., Dawson, C. W., Brown, K. W., and Rickinson, A. B. (1989). Identification of a human epithelial cell surface protein sharing an epitope with the C3d/Epstein-Barr virus receptor molecule of B lymphocytes. *Int. J. Cancer*, **43**, 786–794.

Zhu, F. X. and Yuan, Y. (2003). The ORF45 protein of Kaposi's sarcoma-associated herpesvirus is associated with purified virions. *J. Virol.*, **77**(7), 4221–4230.

Zhu, L., Puri, V., and Chandran, B. (1999). Characterization of human herpesvirus-8 K8.1A/B glycoproteins by monoclonal antibodies. *Virology*, **262**(1), 237–249.

Zhu, L., Wang, R., Sweat, A., Goldstein, E., Horvat, R., and Chandran, B. (1999). Comparison of human sera reactivities in immunoblots with recombinant human herpesvirus (HHV)-8 proteins associated with the latent (ORF73) and lytic (ORFs 65, K8.1A, and K8.1B) replicative cycles and in immunofluorescence assays with HHV-8-infected BCBL-1 cells. *Virology*, **256**(2), 381–392.

Maintenance and replication during latency

Paul M. Lieberman[1], Jianhong Hu[2] and Rolf Renne[2]

[1]The Wistar Institute, Philadelphia, PA
[2]University of Florida, Gainesville, FL

Introduction

The human gammaherpesviruses Epstein–Barr Virus (EBV) and Kaposi's sarcoma-associated herpesvirus (KSHV) are associated with a variety of malignancies involving cells of various lineages.

After primary infection and initial viral propagation in epithelial and lymphoid cells, both viruses establish latency in a subset of CD19 positive B-cells. In this often lifelong asymptomatic stage, in which EBV genomes are detectable primarily in resting memory B-cells, the number of infected cells is extremely low and virus load is tightly controlled by the host cellular and humoral immune response.

Loss of this balance leads to an increase in viral load, which often precedes the onset of malignant diseases. Both tissue involvement and histopathology are highly variable between EBV- and KSHV-associated malignancies and involve either lymphoid (Burkitt's lymphoma and primary effusion lymphoma), epithelial (nasopharyngeal carcinoma), or endothelial (Kaposi's sarcoma) tissues.

However, common to all gammaherpesvirus-associated tumors is that the majority of tumor cells are latently infected, and harbor extrachromosomal circularized viral genomes called episomes that are replicated and segregated by the host cellular replication machinery indefinitely. This ability to maintain long-term latent infection in quiescent and proliferating cells may be a defining property shared by both the lymphocryptoviruses (LCV, represented by EBV) and the rhadinoviruses (RDV, represented by KSHV).

This chapter aims to summarize our current understanding of the underlying mechanisms by which EBV and KSHV achieve long-term episomal maintenance in latently infected cells, which conceptually can be viewed as a two step process: replication of the viral genome and faithful segregation to daughter cells (Fig. 24.1).

Before going into the details about viral DNA replication, episomal maintenance and their *cis*- and *trans*-requirements, it is important to note that much less is known about the molecular events that precede the establishment of stable latency after primary infection. Initially, KSHV, like most herpesvirus virions, attaches to heparin sulfate prior to interactions with its receptor. On B-cells KSHV binds to members of the alpha integrin family which may serve as receptor or coreceptor (Akula *et al.*, 2001, 2002). However, EBV does not encode a heparin binding protein and directly binds to the high affinity receptor CD21 which is highly expressed on B-cells (Ahearn *et al.*, 1988; Li *et al.*, 1992). Attachment, binding and internalization, which for both viruses are believed to be dependent on endocytosis, are discussed in detail in Chapter 23. Virion binding to cell surface receptors also triggers signal transduction pathways, which may facilitate viral entry. The concurrent steps: transport of capsids through the cytoplasm and delivery of the linear viral genome to the nucleus have not been studied in great detail for either EBV, or KSHV. It is believed that circularization of viral genomes occurs early after infection prior or concurrent with the onset of viral mRNA synthesis (Hurley and Thorley-Lawson, 1988; Alfieri *et al.*, 1991). Recent studies on KSHV show that DNA is detectable in infected cells as early as 5 min post-inoculation. Furthermore, first viral transcripts are detectable by 30 min post-infection. Surprisingly, one study on KSHV found that many of the genes expressed after *de novo* infection were early lytic genes rather than latency-associated genes. However, after latency-associated genes were detectable, a marked down-regulation of lytic gene expression was noted (Naranatt *et al.*, 2004). This new finding suggests that early lytic genes contribute the establishment of latency by providing auxiliary functions such as perturbing immune recognition of infected cells. The

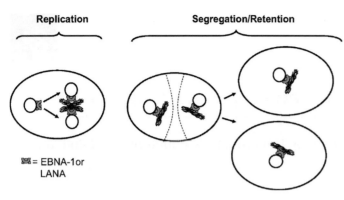

Fig. 24.1. Plasmid maintenance model for EBV and KSHV. EBNA1 and LANA tether viral genomes to cellular chromosomes. This tethering can occur through numerous chromosome-associated proteins and appears to be sufficient for stable plasmid maintenance.

question about how latency is established is also discussed in Chapter 23 which is specifically focused on early events after infection. The focus of this chapter, however, is how the viral episome is maintained in cells in which latency has been established.

During latency, viral gene expression is limited to a small subset of genes dedicated to viral genome maintenance and host-cell accommodation. Although many genes required for lytic replication and virion structure are highly conserved among the herpesvirus family, those genes required for the establishment and maintenance of latency are quite distinct even within the gammaherpesviruses. EBV encodes a total of eight different latency-associated genes whose expression differences among lymphoid malignancies gave rise to the classification of three latency programs. While some Burkitt's lymphomas express only a single latent antigen (Epstein–Barr virus nuclear antigen 1, EBNA1), rare immunoblastic lymphomas may express all EBNAs in addition to the latent membrane proteins (LMP 1 and 2). For KSHV, gene expression analysis showed that tumor cells in KS lesions and PEL-derived cell lines also express only a small number of genes. Although viral gene expression during latency may differ between KS and PEL, PEL-derived cell lines have been instrumental for the identification and characterization of so far five KSHV latency-associated genes. These are the latency-associated nuclear antigens (LANA and LANA2), vCyclin, vFLIP, and Kaposin A and B.

With the exception of LANA and EBNA1, which both play an important role in viral DNA replication and genome maintenance during latency, there is little conservation between the latency-associated genes of lymphocryptoviruses and rhadinoviruses. The functions and roles of these gene products in the biology of KSHV and EBV will be discussed elsewhere in this volume and have recently been subject to a number of excellent review articles (Boshoff and Weiss, 2002; Herndier and Ganem, 2001).

Both LCV and RDV family members encode origin binding proteins (EBNA1 and LANA) and possess genetic elements (origins) dedicated to viral genome maintenance and replication during latent infection in proliferating cells. The specific protein interactions and detailed mechanisms used by LCV and RDV have evolutionarily diverged, but many of the underlying strategies of viral persistence are quite similar. A review of the properties of the latent viral genome and the mechanisms of DNA replication, maintenance, and segregation during latency should highlight important differences and essential similarities among the gammaherpesviruses.

EBV (Lymphocryptovirus)

A number of excellent reviews address the biology of EBV replication and plasmid maintenance during latency (Leight and Sugden, 2000; Sugden and Leight, 2001). Most of this section will focus on the molecular biology of Epstein–Barr nuclear antigen 1 (EBNA1) and its interactions with the origin of plasmid replication (*OriP*). It is this interaction that is primarily responsible for EBV genome stability during latency. However, other aspects of the viral chromosome will be considered, including the importance of DNA methylation status, chromatin organization, and nuclear matrix attachment.

Properties of the episomal latent viral genome

The prototypical latent gammaherpesvirus exists as multicopy (5–100) covalently closed circular genomes that can be separated from chromosomal DNA by density gradient centrifugation (Adams and Lindahl, 1975; Nonoyama and Tanaka, 1975) and by gel electrophoresis using the Gardella gel system (Gardella *et al.*, 1984). However, integrated forms of the virus can be detected, and numerous cell lines have been described that have complete and partial EBV genomes integrated into the cellular chromosome (Adams and Lindahl, 1975; Nonoyama and Tanaka, 1975; Andersson-Anvret and Lindahl, 1978; Lindahl *et al.*, 1978; Koliais, 1979; Anvret *et al.*, 1984; Lawrence *et al.*, 1988; Popescu *et al.*, 1993; Kripalani-Joshi and Law, 1994; Wuu *et al.*, 1996; Ohshima *et al.*, 1998; Chang *et al.*, 2002). In the prototypical latent infection, EBV circularizes rapidly after initial infection through an annealing event at the terminal repeats (Kintner and Sugden, 1979; Laux et al., 1989; Cheung et al., 1993; Zimmermann and Hammerschmidt, 1995). The circular form is thought to be essential for reactivation of the lytic cycle and production of progeny virus. Circularization is also required for the expression of the terminal repeat transcript LMP2a that may contribute to the stability of the latent state by inhibiting B-cell receptor mediated reactivation signals (Laux et al., 1989; Miller et al., 1994).

Chromatin organization of the latent episome

Packaging of cellular DNA into nucleosomal chromatin is essential for its protection and stability throughout much of the cell cycle. This holds true for viral episomal DNA, as well. During latency, the viral episome is associated with nucleosomes in arrays that are indistinguishable from bulk cellular DNA (Shaw et al., 1979; Dyson and Farrell, 1985). Micrococcal nuclease laddering assays revealed that the majority of the EBV latent genome is organized in nucleosome arrays (Dyson and Farrell, 1985), with the exception of the region covering *OriP* (Wensing et al., 2001). Nucleosomes were also disorganized in the adjacent sequences encompassing the EBERs, which are two genes constitutively transcribed by RNA polymerase III during most forms of latency (Sexton and Pagano, 1989; Wensing et al., 2001). Consistent with these findings, biochemical studies revealed that EBNA1 can displace a mononucleosome positioned over an EBNA1-binding site in vitro, suggesting that EBNA1 binding to *OriP* is sufficient for displacing an ordered array of nucleosomes from this region of the latent genome (Avolio-Hunter et al., 2001).

In contrast to the latent genome, EBV DNA found in the virion or after lytic replication appears to be nucleosome free (Shaw et al., 1979; Dyson and Farrell, 1985). Nucleosome assembly on newly synthesized lytic DNA might inhibit DNA insertion into the nucleocapsid, and thus might inhibit infectious virion production. It is not clear what mechanism prevents nucleosome assembly during lytic infection; nucleosome assembly on newly synthesized cellular DNA is coupled to DNA replication proteins, and these cellular enzymes do not participate in viral lytic replication. Alternatively, viral encoded proteins may actively prevent nucleosome assembly on the viral genome during lytic replication by an as yet unknown mechanism.

Nucleosome positioning and histone modification may also contribute to the gene regulation during latent infection. Lytic gene promoters are transcriptionally repressed during latent infection. Inhibitors of histone deacetylases, like sodium butyrate and trichostatin A, are potent activators of lytic cycle gene expression (Saemundsen et al., 1980; Jenkins et al., 2000). The positioned nucleosome contributes to transcriptional repression of the immediate early gene, but it is not clear how the nucleosome is positioned in the viral genome. Nucleosome positioning may be affected by at least two mechanisms including nucleosome positioning elements inherent in DNA sequence, and sequence specific binding proteins that recruit nucleosome modifying activities. Histone deacetylases associated with DNA binding proteins MEF2D and RBP-Jk are known to maintain repressive chromatin at the EBV BZLF1 (Liu et al., 1997; Speck et al., 1997; Gruffat et al., 2002) and EBNA2 Cp (Hsieh et al., 1999; Alazard et al., 2003) promoters. In addition to restricting gene expression, chromatin structure and histone modifications may protect the viral genome from DNA damage during latency. Nucleosome position and remodeling may also play a role in the regulation of plasmid replication during latency of both EBV and KSHV (Stedman et al., 2004; Zhou et al., 2005).

DNA methylation of latent EBV

DNA methylation is an epigenetic mark associated with transcriptional silence (Bird, 1986; Jones and Wolffe, 1999). The EBV genome is highly methylated during latency (Saemundsen et al., 1983) and there is evidence that virion DNA is also hypermethylated (Diala and Hoffman, 1983). DNA methylase inhibiting drugs, like 5-aza-cytidine, can induce lytic gene expression from latently infected cells (Ben-Sasson and Klein, 1981). DNA methylation has also been found to play a critical role in regulating LMP1 and EBNA2-6 transcription (Ernberg et al., 1989; Masucci et al., 1989; Allday et al., 1990; Hu et al., 1991; Minarovits et al., 1994; Robertson et al., 1996; Robertson and Ambinder, 1997; Schaefer et al., 1997; Falk et al., 1998; Ambinder et al., 1999; Robertson, 2000) and thus contributes to the transition between various latency programs.

Like nucleosome phasing, DNA methylation is not uniform throughout the viral genome. DNA methylation is generally spared from sequence elements of *OriP* (Falk and Ernberg, 1993; Salamon et al., 2001). EBNA1 binding to *OriP* contributes to the sparing of DNA methylation, but the mechanism preventing DNA methylation is not known (Hsieh, 1999; Lin et al., 2000; Salamon et al., 2000). EBNA1 bound to *OriP* can also affect transcription of LMP1p (Gahn and Sugden, 1995) and Cp (Reisman and Sugden, 1986; Puglielli et al., 1996; Nilsson et al., 2001), and it is possible that effects on DNA methylation and chromatin structure

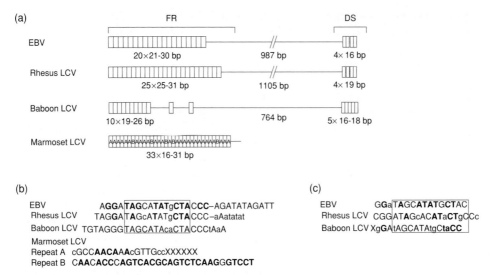

Fig. 24.2. Comparative *OriP* structure of lymphocryptoviruses. (a) Family of repeat (FR) and dyad symmetry elements of human and primate viruses. (b) and (c) Alignment of EBNA1 binding sites within FR and DS elements (courtesy of Rivaillier *et al.* (2002).

at *OriP* contribute to latent cycle transcription. In this respect, *OriP* may be a significant control element determining gene expression patterns in the various types of EBV latency.

Molecular biology of *OriP*

The genetic elements responsible for plasmid maintenance and DNA replication were identified through the elegant experiments of Yates and Sugden (Yates *et al.*, 1984, 1985; Reisman *et al.*, 1985). In these experiments, plasmid subclones of the B95-8 genome were tested for their stable maintenance in EBV positive cell lines and only one region (nucleotides 7000 and 9258 in EBV coordinates) possessed clear plasmid maintenance and DNA replication activity (Yates *et al.*, 1984). This region is referred to as the origin of plasmid replication (*OriP*) and consists of two functional domains, the family of repeats (FR) and the Dyad symmetry (DS) region (Fig. 24.2) (Lupton and Levine, 1985; Reisman *et al.*, 1985; Yates *et al.*, 1985; Chittenden *et al.*, 1989; Wysokenski and Yates, 1989). The Epstein–Barr virus nuclear antigen 1 (EBNA1), which is expressed in most forms of viral latency, binds directly to the 30 bp repeat elements found in FR and DS in *OriP* (Rawlins *et al.*, 1985). EBNA1 is the only viral protein required for episomal maintenance and replication of *OriP*-containing plasmids (Yates and Camiolo, 1988; Wysokenski and Yates, 1989).

OriP consists of at least two functional elements that are separated by a non-essential 1 kb spacer region (Fig. 24.2). The family of repeats (FR) consists of 20×30 bp repeats each containing a 16 bp EBNA1 binding site. The DS element consists of four lower affinity EBNA1 binding sites that are organized as two functional pairs. The minimal replicator for *OriP* consists of one functional pair of EBNA1 binding sites spaced precisely 21 nucleotides from the center of each site (Yates *et al.*, 2000). The DS element of EBV consists of two minimal replicators, and mutagenesis shows that at least one intact pair is essential for replication function (Harrison *et al.*, 1994; Koons *et al.*, 2001). DS also consists of three nine base pair repeat elements, referred to as nonamer repeats, which are positioned adjacent to each pair of EBNA1 sites (Niller *et al.*, 1995; Vogel *et al.*, 1998). Mutations of the nonamer sites have 2–5 fold effects on replication and plasmid maintenance, but appear not to be absolutely essential for minimal replicator activity (Vogel *et al.*, 1998; Yates *et al.*, 2000; Koons *et al.*, 2001; Deng *et al.*, 2002, 2003). The nonamer sites are identical to telomere repeats, and were found to interact directly with the telomere repeat binding factors TRF1 and TRF2 (Deng *et al.*, 2002).

An *OriP*-like structure is conserved in sequence and position in all lymphocryptovirus family members, although there is considerable variation in the number, spacing, and sequence of EBNA1 binding sites (Rivailler *et al.*, 2002) (Fig. 24.2). The rhesus EBV (CalHV-3) contains an unusual family of repeats that consists of two repetitive sequences that diverge considerably from consensus EBNA1 sites. This observation is surprising since the DNA binding domain of the rhesus EBNA1 protein is strongly conserved.

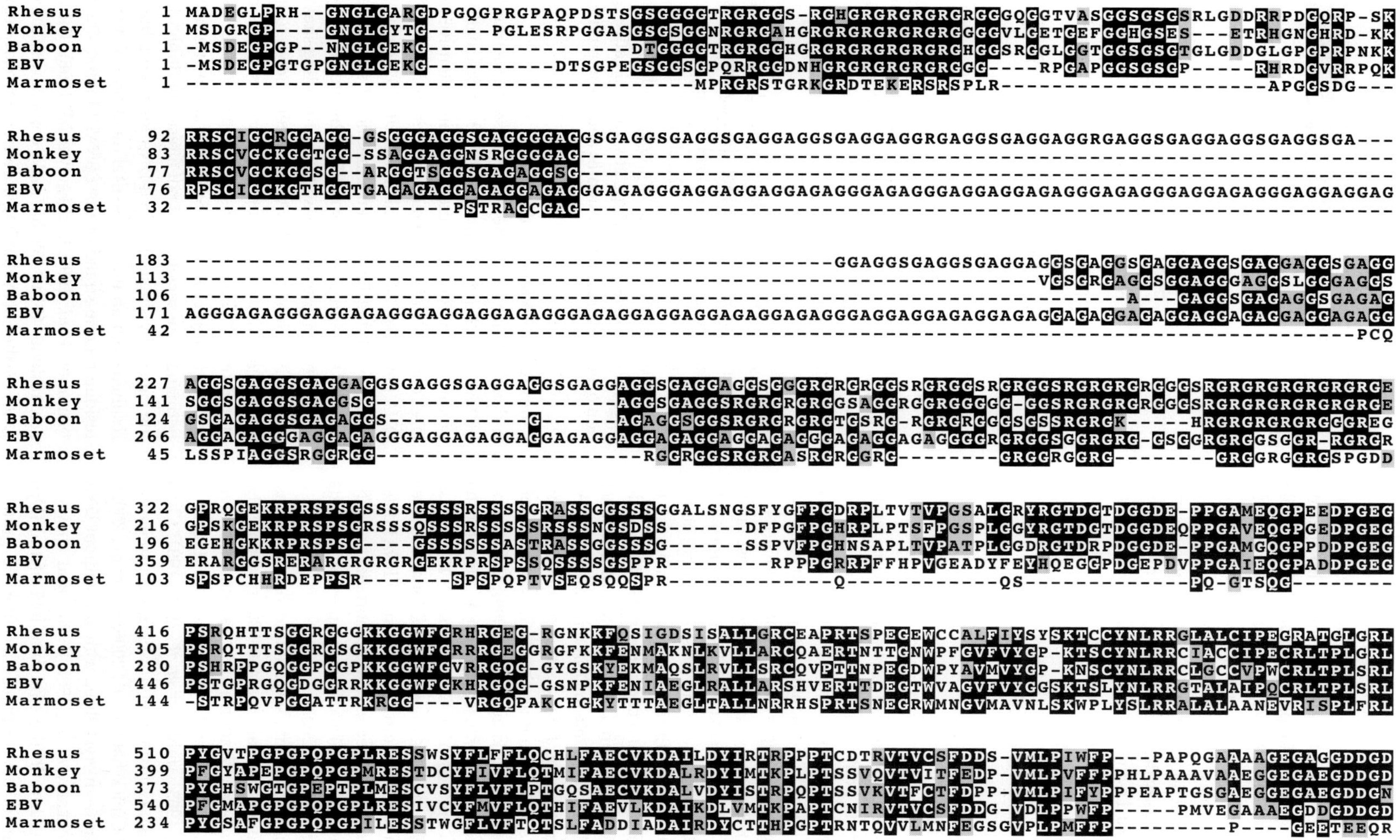

```
Rhesus    1  MADEGLPRH--GNGLGARGDPGQGPRGPAQPDSTSGSGGGTRGGS-RGHGRGRGRGRGGGTVASGGSGSRLGDDRRPDGQRP-SK
Monkey    1  MSDGRGP---GNGLGYTG------PGLESRPGGASGSGSGNRGRGRGRGGGVLGETGEFGGHGSES-ETHGNGHRD-KK
Baboon    1  -MSDEGP---NNGLGEKG-------DTGGGTRGRGGHGRGRGHGGSGGTGGGSGSGLGPGPRPNKK
EBV       1  -MSDEGPTGPGNGLGEKG--------DTSGPESGGSGPQRRGGDNHGRGRGRGGG--RPGAPGGSGSGP--APGSDG--
Marmoset  1  ------------------------MPRGRSTGRKGRDTEKERSRSPLR----------RHRDGVRRPQK--

Rhesus    92  RRSCIGRGGAGG--GSGGGAGGSGAGGGSGAGGSGAGGGAG-GAGGSGAGGSGAGGSGAGGAGGSGAGG--
Monkey    83  RRSCVGCKKGGTGG--SSAGGAGGNSRGGGAG--------------VGSGRGAGGSGAGGSLGGGAGGS
Baboon    77  RRSCVGCKKGGSG--ARGGTSGGSGAGAGGSG---------------A--GAGGSGAGAG
EBV       76  RPSCIGCKKGTHGGTGAGAGGAGAGGAGGAGGAGGAGGAGGAGGAGGAGGAG--AGGAGGAGGAGGAGGAGGAGGAGGAG
Marmoset  32  ----PSTRAGCGAG--------------------------------------------PCQ

Rhesus    183 --------------------------GGAGGSGAGGSGAGGSGAGG-GAGGSGAGG--
Monkey    113 ---------------------------------------------VGSCRGAGGSGAGGSLGGGAGGS
Baboon    106 ---------------------------------------------------A----GAGGSGAGAG
EBV       171 AGGAGAGGAGAGGAGAGGAGAGGAGAGGAGAGGAGAGGAGAGGAGAGGAGAGGAGAGGAGAGGAG--
Marmoset  42  -----

Rhesus    227 AGGSGAGGSGAGGSGAGGAGGAGGAGGAGGSGAGGAGGSGAGGSRGRGRGRGGS-RGRGRGRGRGRGRGE
Monkey    141 SGSGAGGSGAGGSGAGGSG-----AGGSGAGGSRGRGRGSAGGG-RGSSRGRGGGRGSGRGRGRGRGRGCE
Baboon    124 GSGAGGSGAGGSGAGGS-------G-----AGGSGAGGSRGRGRGRGRGS-RGRGRGRGRGRGRGREG
EBV       266 AGGAGAGGAGAGGAGAGGAGAGGAGAGGAGAGGAGAGGAG--G-AGAGGGRGRGGGGSGRGRGRGRGRGRGGRGR
Marmoset  45  LSSPIAGGSRGRGRG--------------RGGRGGSRGRGASRGRGGG----GRGGRGRGSPGDD

Rhesus    322 GPRQGEKRPRSPSGSSSGSSSRSPSPSGSSSGSSSGRA-SSGGSSG-----DFPGFPGHRPLPTSFPGSPLGGYRGTDGDPPGAMEQGPEEDPGEG
Monkey    216 GPSKGEKRPRSPSGRGSS-QSSSRSSSSS-----GSSSSSSASTRASSGGSSSG-----SSPVFPGHNSAPLTVPATPLGGDRGTDRPPGDE
Baboon    196 EGEHCKKRPRSPSG-----GSSSGSSSSS-----GSSSSSSASTRASSGGSSSG-----SSPVFPGHNSAPLTVPATPLGGDRGTDRPPGDE
EBV       359 ERARGGSRERARGRGRGEKRPSPSS-QSSSGSSPR-----RPPPGRPFFHPVGEADYFEYHQEGGPDGEPDVPPGAIEQGPADDPGEG
Marmoset  103 SPSPCHHRDEPPSR-------------------SPSPQPTVSEQSQQSPR------QS----PQ-GTSQG--

Rhesus    416 PSRQHTTSGRGGKKGWFGRHREG--RGNKKFQSIGDSISALLGRCEAPRTSPEGEWCCALFIVSYSKTCCYNLRRGLALCIPEGRATGLGRL
Monkey    305 PSRQTTTSGGRGSGKKGGWFGRHRRGEG-GKKFKFENMAKNLKVLLARCQAERTNTGNWPFGVFVYGP-KTSCYNLRRCIACCIPECRLTPL
Baboon    280 PSHRPGQGGPGCGPKKGWFGVRRGQG-GYGSKVEKMAQSLRVLISRCQVPFTNPEGDWPYAVMVYGP-KNSCYNLRRCLGCCVPWCRLTPLSRL
EBV       446 PSTGPRGQDGRGRKKGGWFGKHRGQG-GSNPKFENIAEGLRALLARSHVERTTDEGTWVAGVFVYGGSKTSLYNLRRGTALAIPQCRLTPLSRL
Marmoset  144 -STRPQVPGGATTRKRGG----VRGQPAKCHGKYTTAEGLTALINRRHSPRTSNEGRWMNGVMAVNLSKWPLYSLRRALALAANEVRISPLFRL

Rhesus    510 PYGVTPGPGPGPQPGPLRESSWSYFLFFLQCHLFAECVKDAILDYIRTRPPTCDTRVTVCSFDDS--VMLPIWFP---PAPQGVAPAAAGEGAGGDDGD
Monkey    399 PFGYAPEPGPQPGPMRESTDCYFLVFLQTMIFAECVKDALRDYIMFRPLPTSSVQVVITFEDP--VMLPIFVFPPPHLPAAAVAVAEGGEAGDDGD
Baboon    373 PIGHSWGTGPEPTPLMESCVSYFLFPGTPGQSAECVKDALVDYISTRPQPTSSVKVTCFTDPP--VMLPIFYPPPEAPTGSGAEGGEACGDDGD
EBV       540 PFGMAPGPGPQPGPLRESIVCYFMVFLQTHIFAEVLKDAIKDLVMTKPAPTCNIRVTVCSFDDG--VDLPWFP---PMVEGAAAEGDDGDDGD
Marmoset  234 PYGSAFGPGPQPGPILESSTWGFLVFTQISLFADDIADAIRDYCTTHPGPIRNTQVVLMNFEGSGVFLPMFFP---P--GEETEEQR
```

Fig. 24.3. EBNA1 proteins are highly conserved among lymphocryptoviruses. Amino acid alignment demonstrating that the N- and C-terminus of EBNA1 from all five viruses are conserved. Only Rhesus and EBV contain the immune modulatory GA repeats.

Interestingly, no apparent DS element could be identified at the correct position in the rhesus genome (Rivailler *et al.*, 2002). A recent study has shown that the 14 bp spacing (found in EBV) is optimal for plasmid maintenance, while the 10 bp spacing (found in HVP) functions better in transcription enhancement (Hebner *et al.*, 2003). Earlier studies indicated that at least 7-8 EBNA1 binding sites were required for FR function in plasmid maintenance assays, and this seems to vary depending on the spacing of these sites (Lupton and Levine, 1985; Chittenden *et al.*, 1989; Hebner *et al.*, 2003). The spacing between EBNA1 sites in the DS appear to be more highly conserved, and these spacing constraints are likely to be critical for replication initiation function (Bashaw and Yates, 2001).

Properties of EBNA1

All of the known members of the lymphocryptovirus family have a protein with homology to EBNA1, including those found in the rhesus (cercopithicine HV 15), marmoset (callitrichine herpesvirus 3), baboon (herpesvirus papio), and squirrel monkey (cynomolgus herpesvirus A4) (Fig. 24.3). Human Epstein–Barr virus EBNA1 has been most intensively studied, and is necessary and sufficient for *OriP*-dependent DNA replication and plasmid maintenance (Yates *et al.*, 1984, 1985). EBNA1 deletion mutants fail to establish episomal latent infection (Lee *et al.*, 1999) indicating that EBNA1 is required in the context of the intact genome. In addition to its role in DNA replication, EBNA1 can activate transcription from a synthetic plasmid containing multiple EBNA1 binding sites upstream of simple viral promoter (Wysokenski and Yates, 1989). *OriP* bound EBNA1 can function as a transcriptional enhancer for the LMP1 promoter and EBNA2–6 Cp promoter 2–10 kilobase pair away. EBNA1 may also possess additional activities associated with B-cell immortalization since EBNA1 deletion leads to a dramatic decrease in immortalization efficiency (Humme *et al.*, 2003) and its overexpression inhibits apoptosis (Kennedy *et al.*, 2003).

EBNA1 can be divided into several functional domains, with the C-terminal domain (aa 450–620) encoding the DNA binding and dimerization activity essential for interaction with DS, FR, and BamHI Q binding sites (Fig. 24.4) (Rawlins *et al.*, 1985; Ambinder *et al.*, 1990, 1991; Chen *et al.*, 1993, 1994; Goldsmith *et al.*, 1993; Ceccarelli and Frappier, 2000; Cruickshank *et al.*, 2000; Wu *et al.*, 2002). This domain has been crystallized with and without DNA (Fig. 24.5) (Bochkarev *et al.*, 1995, 1996), and shows a remarkable similarity to the structural fold of the DNA binding domain of bovine papilloma virus E2 protein, suggesting that these viral proteins share common ances-

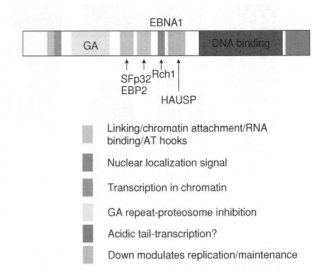

Fig. 24.4. Functional protein domains of EBNA1. Amino acid residues are indicated for the boundaries of protein domains for DNA binding, dimerization, chromosome binding sites (CBS), nuclear localization (NLS), or protein–protein interactions (as indicated). (See color plate section.)

tral precursor involved in plasmid-based replication. The papillomavirus E2 protein binds the papillomavirus DNA replication origin and helps to load the viral encoded helicase, E1 (Edwards *et al.*, 1998). E2 also has important function in papillomavirus transcription regulation and, like EBNA1, is involved in both positive and negative regulation of gene expression (Desaintes and Demeret, 1996).

C-terminal DNA binding domain

A detailed analysis of the X-ray crystal structure of the EBNA1 DNA binding domain reveals a fascinating and unique DNA interaction interface, with extensive protein DNA contacts in both the major and minor grooves of the DNA helix (Fig. 24.5) (Bochkarev *et al.*, 1996). The structures reveal that EBNA1 can introduce a strong bend in bound DNA, and provides some insight into the likely contacts between critically phased dimer binding sites in the DS minimal replicon. EBNA1 has been shown to induce permanganate sensitivity upon thymine residues of one strand on the two outermost binding sites in DS (sites 1 and 4) (Hearing *et al.*, 1992). Structural studies revealed that permanganate sensitivity is not a result of duplex breathing caused by single stranded DNA formation, but rather resulted from an unusual helical distortion of a thymine residue on one strand of the EBNA1 binding sites in DS (Summers *et al.*, 1997; Bochkarev *et al.*, 1998). The amino acid residues 461 to 469 that make contact with the minor groove of the EBNA1 binding site were shown to be essential for inducing the permanganate sensitivity (Summers *et al.*,

1997). The functional significance of this distorted thymine structure on DNA replication function remains unclear.

N- terminal domain linking activity

The amino terminal domains of EBNA1 possess genetically distinct activities essential for DNA replication, plasmid maintenance and transcription (Yates and Camiolo, 1988; Wu et al., 2002). Multiple regions amino terminal to the DNA binding domain contribute to DNA replication and plasmid maintenance activity (Fig. 24.4). The amino terminal regions of EBNA1 have no obvious sequence homology to other known proteins, but do contain three RGG-rich domains that were first recognized for their similarity to RGG-elements found in hnRNP RNA binding proteins (Burd and Dreyfuss, 1994). The RGG motifs (aa 34–56, and 339–377) were found to confer some RNA binding ability on EBNA1, but the biological significance of EBNA1 RNA binding has not been elucidated (Snudden et al., 1994). These RGG-rich regions in the amino terminal domain also confer intramolecular "linking" between EBNA1-DNA complexes as revealed by the formation of large non-resolved complexes in electrophoresis mobility shift assay (EMSA) (Frappier et al., 1994; Mackey et al., 1995). Electron microscopy revealed that EBNA1 can induce DNA looping between FR and DS (Su et al., 1991; Middleton and Sugden, 1992), and the aa 350–361 were shown to be responsible for DNA looping in both electron microscopy studies and ligation enhancement assays (Frappier et al., 1994). The linking domains (aa 40–89, 331–361, and 372–391) were also found to be important for EBNA1 replication and transcription activity (Mackey and Sugden, 1999). The precise mechanistic contribution of these RGG-rich linking domains remains unclear, but are likely to be involved in the protein-protein interactions and metaphase chromosome binding properties of EBNA1.

Metaphase chromosome attachment

EBNA1 can also associate with metaphase chromosomes through amino acids that appear to overlap the linking domains, and are essential for plasmid maintenance function (Marechal et al., 1999). EBNA1 attachment to metaphase chromosome has been mapped to three domains that correlate well with the ability of EBNA1 to confer plasmid maintenance (Marechal et al., 1999; Kanda et al., 2001; Wu et al., 2002). EBNA1 has also been shown to colocalize with DNA replication compartments even in the absence of viral DNA (Ito and Yanagi, 2003), suggesting that the association with interphase chromatin is independent of viral DNA sequences. Intriguingly, substitution of the amino terminal domain of EBNA1 with the HMG I/Y or histone H1 chromatin binding folds was sufficient to reconstitute efficient plasmid maintenance (Hung et al., 2001),

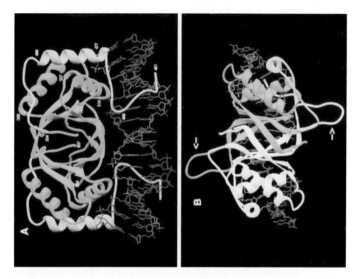

Fig. 24.5. X-ray crystal structure of EBNA1 dimer bound to a consensus DNA recognition site (courtesy of Bocharev et al., Cell in press). (a) Ribbon diagram showing the core domain (residues 504–607) from each monomer, in blue. Flanking domains are shown in yellow. (b) View down the non-crystallographic axis showing one monomer in white and the other in the same color scheme as used in (a). Proline loops are indicated by arrows. (See color plate section.)

suggesting that chromosome attachment is both necessary and sufficient for plasmid maintenance. One recent finding indicates that the chromosomal attachment sites of EBNA1 have AT-hook activity, and can bind to AT-rich DNA (Sears et al., 2003, 2004). This suggests that the linking-activity involves weak DNA binding through the amino terminal domain of EBNA1. These data would also account for why this region of EBNA1 can be substituted with HMG I/Y and histone H1, which have AT-hook domains and DNA binding activity.

Transcription regulation

The transcription regulatory properties of EBNA1 have also been investigated. As mentioned above, EBNA1 can stimulate transcription of Cp and LMP1 during latency (Sugden and Warren, 1989; Wysokenski and Yates, 1989; Puglielli et al., 1996; Nilsson et al., 2001). The amino terminal domain of EBNA1 is required for this activity, and can be distinguished from the DNA replication and plasmid maintenance properties by mutational analysis (Yates and Camiolo, 1988; Wu et al., 2002). Transcription activation of chromatin integrated templates required the conserved amino terminal sequence (aa 65–89), which was not essential for activation of transient plasmid based genes (Kennedy and Sugden, 2003). EBNA1 can also function as a transcription repressor, and can down-regulate transcription of its own mRNA initiating at the F promoter (Sung et al., 1994). In this autoregulatory loop, EBNA1 competes with E2F binding sites necessary for the cell cycle regulation of EBNA1. The detailed mechanisms of EBNA1 transcription activation and repression have not yet been characterized.

Proteosome inhibition by GA repeats

EBNA1 also has a variable length ~200 residue glycine-alanine repeat from aa 100 to 325 using the B95-8 strain. Deletion of the GA repeat has no apparent effect on DNA replication, plasmid maintenance, or transcription regulation. However, the GA repeats inhibit ubiquitin-dependent/proteosomal processing of EBNA1 (Levitskaya et al., 1995, 1997). The GA repeats reduce peptide processing and HLA class I presentation, and are responsible for the limited cytotoxic T-cell response to EBNA1 protein in latently infected cells (Blake et al., 1997). The GA repeats can also inhibit proteosome processing on foreign molecules, and may represent a general strategy for viral proteins to escape immune cell recognition (Levitskaya et al., 1997; Leonchiks et al., 2002). In addition to the effect on protein stability, the GA repeats inhibit EBNA1 translational efficiency, thus contributing to the low, but stable EBNA1 protein expression levels in latently infected cells (Yin et al., 2003).

Cellular proteins that interact with EBNA1

Yeast two hybrid assays and biochemical isolation have identified several cellular proteins that interact with EBNA1. The two hybrid assay isolated SFp32/TAP/hyaluronectin (Wang et al., 1997), importins α and β (Fischer et al., 1997; Kim et al., 1997; Ito et al., 2000), and EBP2 (Shire et al., 1999), while biochemical purifications isolated SFp32 (Chen et al., 1998; Van Scoy et al., 2000), and HAUSP (Holowaty et al., 2003). SFp32/TAP binds to two independent regions of EBNA1, aa 40–60 and aa 325–376, which overlaps the RGG motifs and linking domains (Wang et al., 1997) (Fig. 24.4). Overexpression of SFp32 inhibited EBNA1 transcription activation (Wang et al., 1997), and interacts with OriP by chromatin immunoprecipitation assay (Van Scoy et al., 2000). SFp32 has also been isolated as a binding partner with the herpesvirus simiri ORF73 LANA protein (Hall et al., 2002) and HIV-1 Tat (Fridell et al., 1995; Yu et al., 1995). SFp32 is thought to have a primary function in oxidative phosphorylation at the mitochondrial membrane (Muta et al., 1997), but may also have a role in the nucleus when shuttled with nuclear binding partners, like EBNA1 (Matthews and Russell, 1998).

EBP2 was also isolated in a two hybrid assay (Shire et al., 1999) and the interaction domain was mapped to the aa 325–376 which overlap with the DNA linking activity that is essential for plasmid maintenance. The yeast EBP2 orthologue has a role in ribosome biogenesis, and has a nucleolar localization (Huber et al., 2000). The most compelling evidence for a role of EBP2 has been in the reconstitution of OriP plasmid maintenance in budding yeast (Kapoor et al., 2001). In this system, OriP confers centromeric plasmid segregation activity only when EBNA1 is coexpressed with human EBP2. EBP2 and EBNA1 colocalize when expressed in yeast and human cell lines, and EBP2 has been shown to bind to metaphase chromosomes (Wu et al., 2000). EBP2 has been proposed to function in mediating EBNA1 interaction with metaphase chromosomes, and provide EBNA1 with a chromosome attachment and plasmid partitioning function required for stable plasmid maintenance (Wu et al., 2000, 2002).

HAUSP/USP7, along with nucleosome assembly protein (Nap1), template activating factor Ib/SET, protein-kinase CKII, and protein arginine methylase PRMT5, were identified by mass spectrometry analysis of EBNA1 associated proteins (Holowaty et al., 2003). HAUSP/USP7 has also been found to associate with HSV-1 ICP0 (Everett et al., 1999) and this binding correlates with ICP0 transcription activation function. Mutations in EBNA1 that disrupt HAUSP/USP7 binding caused a fourfold increase in plasmid maintenance activity of EBNA1, although no change in EBNA1 protein stability could be detected. EBNA1 binding to HAUSP/USP7 did affect the stability of p53 by blocking its binding and deubiquitylation by HAUSP/USP7. These studies are especially exciting since they provide a mechanism for the anti-apoptotic function of EBNA1 during B-cell immortalization (Saridakis et al., 2005). The functional characterization of other EBNA1-associated proteins has not yet been reported.

Cellular proteins that interact with *OriP*

Cellular factors that interact with OriP have also been characterized. A cellular factor, OBP-1/Kid, binds to and competes for the EBNA1 binding sites in OriP (Wen et al., 1990; Zhang and Nonoyama, 1994). OBP-1/Kid has kinesin-like motor activity and localizes to metaphase chromosomes and the mitotic spindle (Tokai et al., 1996). A specific role for OBP-1/Kid in OriP function has not been apparent, especially since OBP-1 competes for EBNA1 and EBNA1 is thought to bind OriP constitutively through most of the cell cycle (Hsieh et al., 1993). The region of EBV encompassing OriP and the EBERs associates with the nuclear matrix

(Jankelevich *et al.*, 1992), and it is likely that this binding is dependent upon EBNA1.

Telomere repeat binding factors also bind to *OriP* in association with EBNA1 (Deng *et al.*, 2002). These host-cell proteins include TRF1 and TRF2, as well as hRap1, tankyrase, and poly-ADP ribose polymerase (PARP1). Both tankyrase and PARP1 have poly-ADP ribose polymerase activity, and EBNA1 can be poly-ADP ribosylated in vitro. TRF1 and TRF2 have identical binding specificity for the nonamer repeats in DS, but have opposing activities in DNA replication assays (Deng *et al.*, 2003). TRF2 associates with DS throughout most of the cell cycle, while TRF1 binding peaks in G2/M and its overexpression inhibits *OriP* replication (Deng *et al.*, 2003). The precise function of these telomeric factors and their potential role in EBNA1 modification is under investigation.

Mechanism of *OriP*- DNA replication

OriP can function as a plasmid origin of replication, and the initiation site for replication has been mapped by a two-dimensional gel electrophoresis assay to a region within or quite close to DS (Gahn and Schildkraut, 1989). In contrast, DNA replication pauses or arrests at FR, suggesting that the bulk of DNA replication occurs in a rightward direction initiating at DS (Gahn and Schildkraut, 1989). Earlier studies also demonstrated that *OriP* is subject to cell cycle restricted replication using heavy-light and heavy-heavy strand density gradient isolation (Adams, 1987; Yates and Guan, 1991), as well as by using Mbo1 and Dpn1 restriction enzyme analysis (Shirakata *et al.*, 1999; Hirai and Shirakata, 2001). Early studies demonstrated that EBV genomes replicate once and only once in the early S phase of the cell cycle (Adams, 1987). Subsequently, it was shown that plasmids carrying *OriP* also replicate only once per cell division cycle in EBNA1 positive cells (Yates and Guan, 1991).

DNA replication at cellular origins requires the assembly of pre-replication licensing factors that include the origin recognition complex (ORC), the minichromosome maintenance (MCM) complex, CDC6, Geminin, and CDT1 (Bell and Dutta, 2002). Components of the ORC complex were shown to associate with *OriP* in vivo using chromatin immunoprecipitation assays (Chaudhuri *et al.*, 2001; Dhar *et al.*, 2001; Schepers *et al.*, 2001). Further genetic evidence that *OriP* is regulated by cellular origin components was demonstrated by a failure of *OriP* to replicate in cells haploinsufficient for ORC2 (Dhar *et al.*, 2001). Futhermore, EBNA1 coimmunoprecipitates with ORC2 and overexpression of geminin inhibited *OriP* replication (Dhar *et al.*, 2001). EBNA1 can also interact with purified replication protein A, the cellular single stranded DNA binding protein required for stabilizing the replication fork (Zhang *et al.*, 1998). From these studies, it is apparent that cellular proteins involved in the regulation of chromosomal replication also control *OriP* replication (Fig. 24.6). A recent study demonstrated that TRF2 can bind a subunit of ORC, and stimulate OriP replication (Atanasiu *et al.*, 2006). Despite these many protein interactions, the precise mechanism of ORC recruitment and DNA polymerase loading at OriP remain to be elucidated.

Mechanism of viral chromosome replication

In the context of the complete genome (Little and Schildkraut, 1995; Norio and Schildkraut, 2001) or plasmid containing large chromosomal DNA inserts (Krysan *et al.*, 1989; Krysan and Calos, 1991), replication may initiate at locations other than DS. Consistent with this, DS can be deleted from EBV genomes without disrupting episomal maintenance of the viral genome (Norio *et al.*, 2000). An alternative replicator sequence, referred to as Rep*, was identified between nt 9370 and 9668 in the EBV genome (Kirchmaier and Sugden, 1998). The Rep* can partially restore plasmid maintenance and DNA replication activity to FR plasmids lacking DS. Rep* does not contain any detectable EBNA1 binding sites by sequence analysis or by direct DNA binding assays, suggesting cellular initiation factors may bind to this region in the absence of EBNA1.

OriP and EBNA1 suffice for the reconstitution of DNA replication and plasmid maintenance on transfected plasmid DNA. However, in the context of the episomal viral genome, it appears as if *OriP* is only used a fraction of the time to initiate DNA synthesis during latency (Little and Schildkraut, 1995). Single molecule analysis of replicated DNA (SMARD) also indicated that *OriP* was not the primary site for initiation of DNA replication in Raji Burkitt

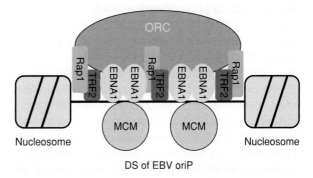

Fig. 24.6. Model for *OriP* of EBV. Indicated are protein–protein and protein DNA interactions that are required for the initiation of DNA synthesis at *OriP*. (See color plate section.)

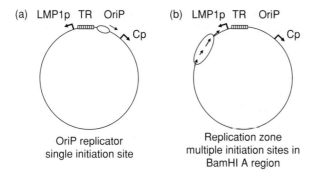

Fig. 24.7. Replication zone versus *OriP*. While in plasmid-based assays DNA synthesis starts at a discrete site near *OriP* (a) in EBV infected cells ori activity is dispersed over a replication zone (b).

lymphoma cell lines, and that the majority of replication initiated from a diffuse zone centered near a PAC1 site in the Bam HI A region (B95-8 coordinates 153, 637) (Little and Schildkraut, 1995; Norio *et al.*, 2000; Norio and Schildkraut, 2001). Initiation of replication in higher eukaryotes may be determined by higher order chromatin domains, rather than discrete replicators, like DS (Gilbert, 2001). EBV appears to have at least two mechanisms for initiating DNA replication, from the discrete DS replicator, or from the broader Bam HI A centered domain of the genome (Fig. 24.7). The possibility that Bam HI A has a replication initiation zone function is particularly intriguing since this region of the genome is transcriptionally active in most forms of EBV latency, and encodes a number of small RNA transcripts (Sadler and Raab-Traub, 1995). The alternative use of replication zones would explain why DS is dispensable for episomal maintenance of the EBV genomes during latency (Norio *et al.*, 2000). It is also likely that the large fragments of cellular DNA that substituted for DS in cosmids also possessed replication initiation zone activity (Krysan *et al.*, 1989; Krysan and Calos, 1991).

Mechanisms of plasmid segregation

Regardless of the flexibility in the site of replication intiation, EBNA1, and presumably FR, are essential for stable episomal maintenance (Lee *et al.*, 1999). EBV lacking EBNA1 can not establish latent episomal genomes (Lee *et al.*, 1999; Humme *et al.*, 2003). Tethering of *OriP* to metaphase chromosomes is thought to be the primary mechanism of plasmid maintenance (Fig. 24.1). The interactions with metaphase chromosome components appears to be highly flexible since substitution of the HMG I/Y and histone H1 chromosome binding regions with EBNA1 linking domains can rescue plasmid maintenance (Hung *et al.*, 2001). Chromosome tethering appears to be mediated by several factors, including the chromatin associated-EBP2 and the AT-hook activity found in the EBNA1 linking domains. Additionally, telomeric factors that bind adjacent to and cooperatively with EBNA1 at DS, contribute to *OriP* plasmid maintenance (Deng *et al.*, 2002). Although the precise role of telomere repeat factors at DS is unclear, recent studies suggest that they contribute to the establishment of a replication and maintenance competent plasmid, perhaps by contributing to the organization of chromatin structure on *OriP*-containing plasmids and facilitating metaphase chromosome attachment.

KSHV (Rhadinovirus)

Shortly after the discovery of KSHV DNA by representational display analysis in KS lesions (Chang *et al.*, 1994), gene expression analysis by *in situ* hybridization and RT-PCR showed that KSHV in KS-lesions are predominantly latently infected (Zhong *et al.*, 1996). Similarly, PEL-derived cell lines are latently infected and, analogous to EBV-infected Burkitt's lymphoma lines, can be induced to enter the lytic replication cycle (Cesarman *et al.*, 1995; Renne *et al.*, 1996a,b). Like BL cell lines for EBV, PEL-derived cell lines have been instrumental for cloning and characterization of the KSHV genome and for the identification of the latency-associated genes.

The KSHV episome in latently infected cells

KSHV episomal viral genomes have been detected by Gardella gel analysis in KS lesions and PEL-derived cell lines (Renne *et al.*, 1996a). Different PEL cell lines contain varying copy numbers (25 to several 100) that are stably maintained over time (Cesarman *et al.*, 1995; Renne *et al.*, 1996b; Cannon *et al.*, 2000). While deletions and duplications have been detected in PEL cells, no integration events have been reported for KSHV. The fact that sodium butyrate, a potent histone deacetylase inhibitor induces lytic replication in PEL cells suggests that nucleosome organization limits lytic cycle gene expression. Lu *et al.* demonstrated that a deacetylated nucleosome positioned over the transcriptional initiation sites of the ORF50 immediate early promoter and its acetylation and remodeling correlated with transcriptional activation and initiation of lytic cycle gene expression (Lu *et al.*, 2003). Similar to EBV, DNA methylation might play a role in the regulation of latency; recent studies suggest methylation of the ORF50 promoter during latency (Chen *et al.*, 2001).

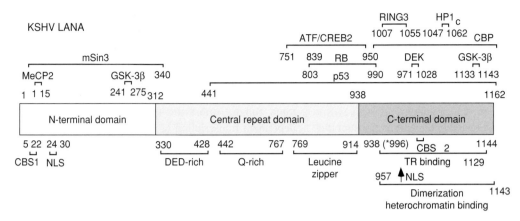

Fig. 24.8. Functional domains of LANA. Amino acid residues are indicated for the boundaries of protein domains for DNA binding, dimerization, chromosome binding sites (CBS), nuclear localization (NLS), or protein-protein interactions (as indicated). LANA amino acid numbering is based on the sequence published by Russo *et al.*, 1996. (* 996 denotes the N-terminus of the core DNA binding domain mapped by Komatsu *et al.*, 2004).

Further evidence that KS lesions harbor episomal DNA comes from the finding that KS spindle cells upon explantation lose viral genomes after only few passages in culture (Dictor *et al.*, 1996). Telomerase-immortalized microvascular endothelial cells can be infected with PEL-derived cell-free virions but lose the viral genome upon cultivation; similar results have recently been shown for a variety of cell lines. These data suggest that the establishment of stable latency at least in the context of *de novo* infection in vitro occurs with low frequency (Lagunoff *et al.*, 2002; Grundhoff and Ganem, 2004). In contrast to cultured cells from KS lesions, PEL cells cultivated in vitro, efficiently maintain KSHV genomes over a long time at a stable copy number (Renne *et al.*, 1996b; Cannon *et al.*, 2000; Cesarman *et al.*, 1995).

Properties of the latency-associated nuclear antigen (LANA)

The first evidence of a latency-associated gene product came from the fact that sera from KS patients contain antibodies that stain PEL cells in a specific nuclear speckled pattern by immunofluourescence assay. This then "unknown" antigen was termed LANA for latency-associated nuclear antigen (Gao *et al.*, 1996; Kedes *et al.*, 1996). Using Northern blot analysis and expression cloning it was subsequently shown that LANA is encoded by ORF73 of KSHV (Kedes *et al.*, 1997; Kellam *et al.*, 1997; Rainbow *et al.*, 1997). *In situ* hybridization studies revealed that nearly all cells in KS lesions express ORF73 mRNA (Dittmer *et al.*, 1998; Talbot *et al.*, 1999) and LANA protein is consistently detected by immunohistochemistry in all malignancies associated with KSHV (Rainbow *et al.*, 1997; Dupin *et al.*, 1999). The ORF73 gene is located in a cluster of four latency-associated genes and is expressed from a poly-cistronic singly spliced mRNA of 5.7 kb that also encodes ORF72, a viral cyclinD homologue, and ORF71, a v-Flip protein (Dittmer *et al.*, 1998; Talbot *et al.*, 1999). Furthermore, this latency-associated region of KSHV contains the Kaposin gene (Zhong *et al.*, 1996; Sadler *et al.*, 1999). The functions and roles of these additional latency-associated gene products in the biology of KS will be discussed elsewhere in this volume and have recently been subject to a number of excellent review articles (Ganem, 1997; Schulz, 1998; Herndier and Ganem, 2001; Boshoff and Weiss, 2002). Adding to the complexity of this region, a cluster of microRNAs, that may modulate host cellular and/or viral gene expression, was recently identified between ORF71 and the Kaposin gene (Cai *et al.*, 2005; Pfeffer *et al.*, 2005; Samols *et al.*, 2005).

Modular domain structure of LANA

LANA can be divided into three major domains: a proline- and serine-rich N-terminal region (312 aa), a central region variable in length between viral isolates (Gao *et al.*, 1999) that is composed of several acidic repeats including a leucine zipper motif, and a conserved C-terminal domain, containing both a proline-rich region and a region rich in charged and hydrophobic amino acids (Fig. 24.8). A comparison of LANA proteins across the rhadinovirus family revealed significant sequence homologies only within the C-terminal domain. While there is some limited homology within the N-termini, which differ dramatically in size between proteins, there is no conservation for the central domain – indeed this domain is often missing or reduced to a small number of acidic residues (Russo et al., 1996; Grundhoff and Ganem 2003; Alexander et al., 2000; Searles et al., 1999). Although there is only limited amino acid sequence homology between LANA and EBNA1, computer-assisted folding predictions for the LANA C-terminus revealed structural relatedness to the DNA binding domains of EBNA1 and the papillomavirus E2 protein whose structures have been solved (Bochkarev et al., 1996; Grossman and Laimins, 1996; Grundhoff and Ganem, 2003).

Transcriptional regulation and signaling properties of LANA

Two hybrid screens have identified LANA interactions with transcriptional coactivators RING 3 and ATF/CREB (Platt et al., 1999; Lim et al., 2000) and co-repressor mSin3 (Krithivas et al., 2000). Gene expression profiling and transient transcription assays have identified cellular and viral genes that are modulated by LANA (Krithivas et al., 2000; Hyun et al., 2001; Knight et al., 2001; Renne et al., 2001; An et al., 2005). LANA, like EBNA1, transcriptionally activates its own synthesis in part by binding to a low affinity site in its promoter LANAp (Jeong et al., 2001; Renne et al., 2001). On the other hand, Gal4/LANA fusion proteins can repress expression from a Gal4 binding site-containing reporter (Krithivas et al., 2000; Schwam et al., 2000). These results indicate that LANA is a complex transcription regulatory protein that can both activate and repress transcription, by direct DNA binding or indirectly through protein interactions, perhaps also depending on cellular and chromosomal environment. More recently, LANA has also been implicated in early steps that lead to the establishment of latency after de novo infection. First, Krishnan et al. analyzed viral transcription pattern at very early time points post entry and showed that the earliest gene detectable was ORF50, the viral transactivator which regulates the switch from latent to lytic replication (Krishnan et al., 2004). Next, the expression of LANA was detectable and there was an inverse relation between LANA expression and ORF50 expression. Subsequently, it was demonstrated that LANA inhibits ORF50-dependent transactivation (Lan et al., 2004) and furthermore this inhibitory effect appears to be disrupted by the acetylation of LANA (Lu et al., 2006). These data strongly suggest that LANA expression levels determine the outcome of de novo infection. This novel aspect of LANA-dependent regulation of latency and other signaling events that occur early after virus entry are discussed in Chapter 23 of this volume.

LANA also has profound effects on cellular growth regulation and cell cycle control. LANA interacts with p53, and down-regulates p53-dependent transcription (Friborg et al., 2000). LANA was also shown to bind the retinoblastoma tumor suppressor (pRB), and modulates E2F-dependent transcription of cell cycle control genes. Furthermore, ectopic LANA expression can transform RF cells in combination with H-ras (Radkov et al., 2000). Recently, LANA has been shown to promote S-phase entry by targeting the APC/wnt/β-catenin signaling pathway through inactivation with GSK3-beta in primary effusion lymphomas. This pathway is altered in many human malignancies (Fujimuro and Hayward, 2003; Fujimuro et al., 2003). Consistent with these findings, LANA prolongs the passage number of primary human umbilical vein endothelial cells (HUVEC) when introduced by retroviral transduction (Watanabe et al., 2003). However, no experimental system could demonstrate that LANA alone can transform primary cells. In summary, LANA targets key signaling pathways including cell cycle, apoptosis, and chromatin re-modeling and it is, therefore, intriguing to speculate that LANA may contribute to immortalization and/or transformation.

Latent DNA replication and segregation

Ballestas et al. first demonstrated through long-term maintenance assays that LANA plays a role in episomal maintenance. Cosmid clones spanning the entire KSHV genome were assayed for their ability to establish plasmid maintenance in BJAB cells in a LANA-dependent manner. Using a selectable marker, resistant cell clones were analyzed for the presence of episomal DNA by Gardella gel analysis. In these assays, a cosmid containing the left end of the genome including terminal repeat (TR) sequences was maintained only in LANA expressing cells. These data unambiguously identified LANA as the only viral protein required in trans for episomal long-term maintenance (Ballestas et al., 1999); these data demonstrated that with respect to its role in episomal maintenance, KSHV LANA is a functional homologue of the EBV origin binding protein EBNA1.

Mechanism of episomal segregation and chromosome tethering

Confocal microscopy demonstrated colocalization of LANA with both viral episomes and mitotic chromosomes suggesting that LANA, like EBNA1, contributes to long-term maintenance by tethering viral genomes to chromosomes (Ballestas *et al.*, 1999). The association of LANA with heterochromatin during interphase, and mitotic chromosomes during mitosis, has since been demonstrated by several laboratories, and data from Cotter et al demonstrating LANA/Histone H1 interaction first suggested protein-protein interaction as the underlying mechanism for chromosome tethering (Cotter and Robertson, 1999; Szekely *et al.*, 1999; Schwam *et al.*, 2000; Viejo-Borbolla *et al.*, 2003). By preparing a panel of LANA/GFP fusion proteins, Piolot *et al.* identified an 18 amino acid long chromosome binding site (CBS) within the N-terminus of LANA (aa 5 to 22) that confers chromatin association to GFP (Piolot *et al.*, 2001). Most recently, Barbera *et al.* reported a detailed analysis of the N-terminal CBS and provided biochemical and elegant genetic evidence that LANA tethers episomes to mitotic chromosomes through direct interactions with core histones H2A/B. The N-terminal chromosome attachment domain was found to be both critical and sufficient for the histone interaction, which was confirmed further by structural analysis and modeling (Barbera *et al.*, 2006).

Krithivas *et al.* further proved that LANA attaches to chromatin via protein-protein interactions by identifying two chromatin-associated cellular proteins that interact with LANA by two-hybrid screen and immunoprecipitation. MeCP2 is a methyl CpG binding protein and interacts with LANA through the N-terminal chromosome binding domain, referred to as CBS1. The second protein, DEK, interacts with CBS2 located in the C-terminus of LANA (aa 971–1028) (Fig. 24.8). Convincing evidence that two LANA domains are mediating chromosome attachment, binding to MeCP2 and DEK respectively, came from the observation that LANA does not bind to chromosomes in murine cells which are negative for both proteins. However, transfection of MeCP2 and/or DEK encoding cDNAs restored LANA/chromatin co-localization in mouse cells (Krithivas *et al.*, 2002). Although LANA interactions with MeCP2 and/or DEK are highly specific, it is important to note that for episomal maintenance the association of viral episomes and chromatin is sufficient. This was demonstrated by Shinohara et al who replaced the N-terminus of LANA, containing CBS1, with histone H1. The resulting fusion protein was able to co-localize with mitotic chromosomes and, moreover, as shown for a similar EBNA-1/HMG-Y fusion protein, functions in long-term maintenance assays (Hung *et al.*, 2001; Shinohara *et al.*, 2002; Sears *et al.*, 2003). Together, these data strongly suggest that LANA contributes to episomal long-term maintenance by tethering the viral genomes to chromatin (Fig. 24.1).

Mapping LANA's DNA binding motif and DNA binding domain

The long unique region (LUR) of KSHV is flanked on both sides by about 40 copies of terminal repeats which are believed to be important for circularization of the linear virion DNA after viral entry. Each TR unit of KSHV is 801 bp and 89% GC-rich (Lagunoff and Ganem, 1997). Scanning of the 140 kbp LUR did not reveal any repeats or sequence elements reminiscent of homology to the *OriP* of EBV. Instead, Cotter *et al.* provided the first evidence that LANA binds to the TR sequences of the viral genome. Radio-labeled cosmid clones harboring sequences from both ends of the genome were immunoprecipitated with LANA specific antibodies after DNA was incubated with lysates from LANA expressing cells (Cotter and Robertson, 1999).

Direct evidence that LANA could bind to TR DNA was generated with in vitro translated (Ballestas, 2001) or vaccinia virus expressed LANA proteins (Garber *et al.*, 2001, 2002). Electrophoresis mobility shift assays (EMSA) identified a 18 bp long GC rich sequence motif within TR that is bound by LANA (Ballestas, 2001; Garber *et al.*, 2001). Weaker binding sites within TR and one site outside of TR at the left end of the genome have been described but no further functional data for these sites have been reported (Cotter *et al.*, 2001).

Mutational analysis in combination with EMSA mapped the DNA binding domain to the C-terminus of LANA (residues 938 to 1144) (Cotter *et al.*, 2001; Garber *et al.*, 2001). Recently, additional studies have suggested a core DNA binding domain to a 143 amino acid long peptide that encompass residues 996 to 1129 (Komatsu *et al.*, 2004) (Fig. 24.8).

Identification of a DS-like element within TR

After identifying the DNA binding domain within the LANA C-terminus, quantitative EMSA in combination with DNA footprinting revealed that LANA binds to two adjacent sites within TR. When increasing amounts of purified LANA-C protein were incubated with a radio-labeled probe, a second complex with slower mobility was observed at high protein concentrations and its intensity further increased while the first complex seemed unchanged. In vitro DNaseI footprinting assays verified the presence of a second binding site. A re-examination of the TR sequence revealed that the 17 bp imperfect palindrome of LANA binding site 1 (LBS1) is separated by a 5 bp spacer from a second site (LBS2) with only three nucleotide changes, compared to LBS1. Mutation analysis revealed a cooperative binding mechanism by which the high affinity LBS1 permits

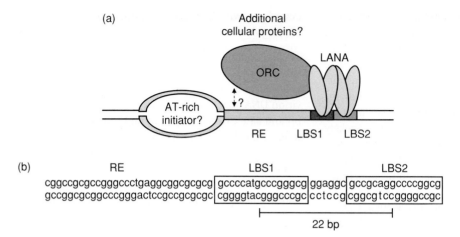

Fig. 24.9. Functional elements of KSHV origin within TR. (a) Model of latent KSHV ori. LBS1/2 and the RE element. LANA binds as dimmers to both sites and the RE element is required for function. ORC LANA and/or TR interaction have been shown both in vitro and in vivo. The AT-rich region may function as initiator element. (b) High (LBS1) and low affinity site (LBS2) are spaced by 22 bps. While this spacing is conserved to DS element of EBV *OriP* there is no sequence homology in binding sites.

loading of LANA onto LBS2 (the Kd for LBS1 was determined to be 1.4 nM) (Garber *et al.*, 2002) (Fig. 24.9).

The presence of both a high and low affinity site and the spacing of 22 bp from center to center within the TR of KSHV is reminiscent of the dyad symmetry element in the EBV *OriP* (21 bp spacing) which is bound by EBNA1 in a cooperative manner. Based on these data and the observation by Schwam et al that the C-terminal DNA binding domain of LANA forms dimers in solution (Schwam *et al.*, 2000), a model is proposed in which two LANA dimers bind to LBS1 and LBS2 in a cooperative fashion, comparable in stoichiometry and affinity to EBNA1 binding to *OriP* (Yates *et al.*, 2000).

The TR functions as LANA-dependent plasmid origin

Long-term maintenance of viral DNA in latently infected cells can be divided into two different steps. First, viral DNA needs to be replicated by the cellular replication machinery; second, viral genomes have to be faithfully segregated during mitosis. Ballestas *et al.* showed that plasmids containing two copies of TR sustain LANA-dependent long-term maintenance in lymphoid cell lines (Ballestas *et al.*, 1999)

Short-term replication assays allow the detection of newly synthesized DNA 48 to 72 hours post transfection by its resistance to DpnI digestion, a restriction enzyme that digests only dam methylated DNA. Using this assay several laboratories tested TR-containing plasmids for their ability to replicate in the presence and absence of LANA in primate cells of epithelial, endothelial, and lymphoid lineage. These data established that LANA, in addition to its role in epi-some segregation, also supports viral DNA replication during latency and that, at least in the context of plasmid replication, all necessary cis-elements are located within the TR sequences (Hu *et al.*, 2002; Lim *et al.*, 2002; Grundhoff and Ganem, 2003). Furthermore, deletion analysis yielded a TR subfragment of 105 bp that replicates as well as plasmids containing one or two copies of TR in the presence of LANA (Hu *et al.*, 2002). Within a TR element, both LANA binding sites contribute to DNA replication since the replication efficiency of mutant TR sequences is directly proportional to their affinity to LANA (Garber *et al.*, 2002).

Further detailed deletion mapping of the minimal replicator within TR revealed that the origin requires LBS1 and LBS2, reminiscent of a dyad symmetry element, and a 29 to 32 bp long GC-rich element upstream. This novel sequence element was termed replication element (RE) since a TR deletion mutant lacking RE does not replicate in the presence of LANA (Hu and Renne, 2005) (Fig. 24.9).

Trans-requirements for LANA and interaction with cellular ORC proteins

Mutational analysis of LANA revealed that the DNA binding domain is required for DNA replication of TR-containing plasmids (Hu *et al.*, 2002) while removal of the central domain has no effect. The C-terminal DNA binding domain of LANA (215 aa) has residual replication activity (25%), and its activity is greatly increased when fused to the N-terminus. This observation is consistent with a model by which the chromosome binding sites located in the N- and C-terminus of LANA contribute to both DNA replication and segregation (Piolot *et al.*, 2001; Krithivas *et al.*, 2002; Mattsson *et al.*, 2002).

Lim *et al.* has recently demonstrated that the C-terminus of LANA interacts with ORC 2, 3, 4, and 5 in an ATP dependent manner (Lim *et al.*, 2002). These promising in vitro GST pull-down results have been confirmed by in vivo interaction studies demonstrating ORC2 binding to TR in a LANA-dependent manner (Stedman *et al.*, 2004). Thus, in order to support DNA replication both EBNA1 and LANA bind to DS elements in their respective origin and recruit cellular licensing factors (Figs. 24.6 and 24.9).

Summary

All the reported data strongly suggests that the KSHV origin of latent replication is located within the TR sequences of KSHV – as a result, KSHV has many putative origins of replication. However, no genetic studies on KSHV have been reported that address the role of the TR sequences and LANA in the context of the viral genome. For HVS, a related rhadinovirus, it was shown that both the TR sequences and a functional ORF73 gene are required for the establishment of long-term episomal maintenance (Collins *et al.*, 2002). These results further suggest that rhadinoviruses do not contain an *OriP* element within the LUR.

Considerable progress has been made to analyze KSHV latent DNA replication and segregation in plasmid-based assays – many more studies are required to address the question of where DNA replication initiates within the context of the viral episome in vivo.

EBV and KSHV origins and origin binding proteins: conserved and diverged?

EBNA1 and LANA are functional homologues. Both proteins support latent DNA replication by specifically binding to their respective origins of replication and by recruiting host cellular ORC proteins (Figs. 24.6 and 24.9). In addition, EBNA1 and LANA promote long-term episomal maintenance by tethering viral genomes to chromatin.

There is no sequence homology between EBNA1 and LANA binding sites within the DS element of *OriP* and the TR of KSHV. However, there is significant similarity in the structural organization of the minimal replicator elements. Both proteins bind as dimers in a cooperative manner to two sites that have nearly identical spacing from center to center (21 bp for EBV and 22 bp for KSHV). This conserved binding mechanism induces structural changes on DNA such as bending towards the major groove that may directly contribute to origin activity and the formation of pre-replication complexes. LANA binding to TR bends DNA by 57 degrees and 110 degrees when both LBS1 and LBS2 are occupied (Bashew and Yates, 2001; Wong and Wilson, 2005). While for EBV a minimal replicator consists of only two EBNA1 binding sites, the KSHV origin requires a second GC-rich element outside of the LANA binding sites (Fig. 24.10). Additionally, EBNA1 and LANA can both interact with ORC proteins that are likely to be essential for the initiation of DNA replication. It is also likely that EBNA1 and LANA DNA binding domains are structurally similar, and share features with the papillomavirus E2 replication protein.

To facilitate genome segregation and maintenance, both proteins tether episomal viral DNA to cellular chromosomes through protein–protein interactions via multiple domains that target a variety of cellular proteins. Surprisingly, there is little overlap in the set of cellular interacting proteins that mediate attachments to cellular chromosomes for EBNA1 and LANA. The simplest interpretation, that chromosomal attachment can occur in a non-specific manner, has experimentally been supported by the observation that EBNA1 and LANA fusion proteins with known chromatin binding proteins support genome maintenance.

The genomic organization of the maintenance elements in EBV and KSHV appear to have diverged considerably (Fig. 24.10). The 1.2 kbp *OriP* is located within the unique long region of the EBV genome. *OriP* has evolved into two functionally different sequence elements that each contain multiple EBNA-1 binding sites: (i) the dyad symmetry (DS) element, required for EBNA1-dependent DNA replication and (ii) the family of repeats (FR), which are required for long-term maintenance. All lymphocryptoviruses have some *OriP*-like element with conserved genome positioning, although even among the lymphocryptoviruses there is considerable variation on the number and spacing of EBNA1 binding sites, and the requirement for a DS-like element may not exist in the cynomolgous herpesvirus (Fig. 24.2).

The structure of the origin of latent replication within the TRs of the rhadinovirus family is different in that each TR represents a putative origin that contains two LANA binding sites but no distinguishable elements comparable to DS and FR in *OriP*. The repetitive nature of the TRs may reflect some aspects of the EBV FR element; this notion is supported by the observation that more than one copy of TR is necessary for efficient long-term maintenance while a single TR is sufficient for DNA replication. Notably, the EBNA1 repetitive sites within FR are spaced 14 bp, while the LANA binding sites between TR are spaced ~800 bp. Whether this reflects an inherent difference in their mechanism of plasmid maintenance will be interesting to determine.

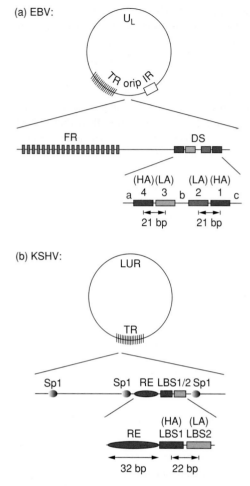

Fig. 24.10. Comparison between genomic structure and positioning of EBV and KSHV. (a) EBV: one *OriP* which contains two functionally different elements that are bound by EBNA1. The DS element contains four EBNA1 binding sites, two sites serve as minimal replicator. To ensure long-term maintenance the FR confer EBNA1-dependent chromatin tethering. (b) KSHV: many putative origins located within TR. Two LANA binding sites resemble DS-like element and together with RE compromise the minimal replicator. The array of TRs may provide tethering function analogous to FR.

in detail. Nor is it known if the repetitive origins found in the TRs of KSHV function coordinately or selectively to ensure cell cycle restricted genome duplication.

The transcription regulatory properties of EBNA1 and LANA may also be related to their ability to establish replication origins and maintenance elements. Both EBNA1 and LANA may have effects on local chromatin structure which may contribute to the transcription and replication activity at adjacent and distal regions of the genome. The association of LANA with histone modifying complexes and chromatin-associated proteins suggests that much of its activity is directed to altering the chromatin environment.

Some of the growth stimulating activities of LANA, that are not seen in EBNA1, may be attributed to its transcription regulatory and chromatin modulating activities. A similar genomic study of cellular gene expression changes induced by EBNA1 has not been reported, and may reveal unanticipated properties of EBNA1 that are reminiscent of LANA. LANA effects on cell cycle control that can be attributed to the interactions with cellular checkpoint proteins like p53 and Rb, are almost definitely lacking in EBNA1, but perhaps equivalent to the EBNA3 family of interactions. Similarly, LANA's interaction and alteration of the GSK-3β kinase activity and β-catenin signaling pathway may be more equivalent to the activities of EBV transforming proteins encoded by LMP1 and BARTs. This suggests that in addition to their similar but not identical mechanisms for latent DNA replication and genome maintenance, both EBV and KSHV have evolved common strategies to modulate cellular environment in latently infected cells. While in EBV these functions are distributed over an entire family of EBNA proteins, KSHV has evolved a multifunctional protein that has acquired many of the described EBNA activities.

It may also be important to note that both LANA and EBNA1 have a non-essential central linker domain characterized by stretches of copolymeric amino acids. The Gly–Ala repeats in EBNA1 have been shown to have an important function in reducing proteosomal processing and therefore limiting presentation of viral peptide on HLA surface molecules. Recently, a similar immune evasion mechanism was revealed for the highly acidic ED and QP repeats within the central domain of LANA. LANA-GFP fusion proteins containing an ovalbumin epitope are not efficiently presented to cytotoxic T cells. Like the EBNA1 Gly-Ala repeats the LANA central domain conveys reduced antigen presentation in cis (Zaldumbide *et al.*, 2006). Hence, although the sequences of these repeats are not related, this represents yet another example of functional homology between the origin binding proteins of lymphocrypto- and rhadinoviruses.

The maintenance elements created by repetitive EBNA1 and LANA binding sites are also efficient origins of replication, but these may not be the only replication origins in the large genomes of these viruses. Based on DS deletion studies and single molecule replication data from EBV (Norio *et al.*, 2000; Norio and Schildkraut, 2001), it is likely that both viruses can utilize alternative DNA replication initiation zones in the intact viral genome (Fig. 24.7). The mechanisms governing the utilization of alternative replication initiation sites in EBV or KSHV has not been explored

REFERENCES

Adams, A. (1987). Replication of latent Epstein–Barr virus genomes in Raji cells. *J. Virol.*, **61**(5): 1743–1746.

Adams, A. and Lindahl, T. (1975). Epstein–Barr virus genomes with properties of circular DNA molecules in carrier cells. *Proc. Natl Acad. Sci. USA*, **72**(4): 1477–1481.

Ahearn, J. M., Hayward, S. D., Hickey, J. C., and Fearon, D. T. (1988). Epstein–Barr virus (EBV) infection of murine L cells expressing recombinant human EBV/C3d receptor. *Proc. Natl Acad. Sci. USA*, **85**(23), 9307–9311.

Akula, S. M., Pramod, N. P., Wang, F. Z., and Chandran, B. (2001). Human herpesvirus 8 envelope-associated glycoprotein B interacts with heparan sulfate-like moieties. *Virology*, **284**(2), 235–249.

Akula, S. M., Pramod, N. P., Wang, F. Z. et al. (2002). Integrin alpha3beta1 (CD 49c/29) is a cellular receptor for Kaposi's sarcoma-associated herpesvirus (KSHV/HHV-8) entry into the target cells. *Cell*, **108**(3), 407–419.

Alazard, N., Gruffat, H., Hiriart, E., Sergeant, A., and Manet, E. (2003). Differential hyperacetylation of histones H3 and H4 upon promoter-specific recruitment of EBNA2 in Epstein-Barr virus chromatin. *J. Virol.*, **77**(14), 8166–8172.

Alexander, L., Denekamp, L., Knapp, A., Auerbach, M. R., Damania, B., and Desrosiers, R. C. (2000). The primary sequence of rhesus monkey rhadinovirus isolate 26–95: sequence similarities to Kaposi's sarcoma-associated herpesvirus and rhesus monkey rhadinovirus isolate 17577. *J. Virol.*, **74**, 3388–3398.

Alfieri, C., Birkenbach, M., and Kieff, E. (1991). Early events in Epstein-Barr virus infection of human B lymphocytes. *Virology*, **181**(2), 595–608.

Allday, M. J., Kundu, D., Finerty, S., and Griffin, B. E. (1990). CpG methylation of viral DNA in EBV-associated tumours. *Int. J. Cancer*, **45**(6), 1125–1130.

Ambinder, R. F., Lambe, B. C., Mann, R. B. et al. (1990). Oligonucleotides for polymerase chain reaction amplification and hybridization detection of Epstein–Barr virus DNA in clinical specimens. *Mol. Cell Probes*, **4**(5), 397–407.

Ambinder, R. F., Mullen, M. A., Chang, Y. N., Hayward, G. S., and Hayward, S. D. (1991). Functional domains of Epstein–Barr virus nuclear antigen EBNA-1. *J. Virol.*, **65**(3), 1466–1478.

Ambinder, R. F., Robertson, K. D., and Tao, Q. (1999). DNA methylation and the Epstein–Barr virus. *Semin. Cancer Biol.*, **9**(5), 369–375.

An, F. Q., Compitello, N., Horwitz, E., Sramkoski, M., Knudsen, E. S., and Renne, R. (2005). The latency-associated nuclear antigen of Kaposi's sarcoma-associated herpesvirus modulates cellular gene expression and protects lymphoid cells from p16 INK4A-induced cell cycle arrest. *J. Biol. Chem.*, **280**, 3862–3874.

Andersson-Anvret, M. and Lindahl, T. (1978). Integrated viral DNA sequences in Epstein–Barr virus-converted human lymphoma lines. *J. Virol.*, **25**(3), 710–718.

Anvret, M., Karlsson, A., and Bjursell, G. (1984). Evidence for integrated EBV genomes in Raji cellular DNA. *Nucl. Acids Res.*, **12**(2), 1149–1161.

Atanasiu, C., Deng, Z., Wiedmer, A., Norseen, J., and Lieberman, P. M., (2006). ORC binding to TRF2 stimulates OriP relplication. *EMBO Rep.*, **7**, 716–721.

Avolio-Hunter, T. M., Lewis, P. N., and Frappier, L. (2001). Epstein–Barr nuclear antigen 1 binds and destabilizes nucleosomes at the viral origin of latent DNA replication. *Nucl. Acids Res.*, **29**(17), 3520–3528.

Ballestas, M. (2001). Kaposi's sarcoma associated herpesvirus latency assoicieted nuclear antigen 1 mediates episome persistence through *cis*-acting terminal repeat (tr) sequence and specifically binds DNA. *J. Virol.*, **75**, 3250–3258.

Ballestas, M. E., Chatis, P. A., and Kaye, K. M. (1999). Efficient persistence of extrachromosomal KSHV DNA mediated by latency-associated nuclear antigen. *Science*, **284**(5414), 641–644.

Barbera, A. J., Chodaparambil, J. V., Kelley-Clarke, B. et al. (2006). The nucleosomal surface as a docking station for Kaposi's sarcoma herpesvirus LANA. *Science*, **311**, 856–861.

Bashaw, J. M. and Yates, J. L. (2001). OriP of Epstein–Barr virus requires exact spacing of two bound dimers of EBNA1 which bend DNA. *J. Virol.*, **75**, 10603–10611.

Bell, S. P. and Dutta, A. (2002). DNA replication in eukaryotic cells. *Annu. Rev. Biochem.*, **71**, 333–374.

Ben-Sasson, S. A. and Klein, G. (1981). Activation of the Epstein–Barr virus genome by 5-aza-cytidine in latently infected human lymphoid lines. *Int. J. Cancer*, **28**, 131–135.

Bird, A. P. (1986). CpG-rich islands and the function of DNA methylation. *Nature*, **321**, 209–213.

Blake, N., Lee, S., Redchenko, I. et al. (1997). Human CD8+ T cell responses to EBV EBNA1: HLA class I presentation of the (Gly–Ala)-containing protein requires exogenous processing. *Immunity*, **7**(6), 791–802.

Bochkarev, A., Barwell, J. A., Pfuetzner, R. A., Furey, W. J., Edwards, A. M., and Frappier, L. (1995). Crystal structure of the DNA binding domain of the Epstein-Barr virus origin binding protein EBNA-1. *Cell*, **83**, 39–46.

Bochkarev, A., Pfuetzner, R. A., Bochkareva, E., Frappier, L., and Edwards, A. M. (1996). Crystal structure of the DNA-binding domain of the Epstein–Barr virus origin-binding protein, EBNA1, bound to DNA. *Cell*, **84**, 791–800.

Bochkarev, A., Bochkareva, E., Frappier, L., and Edwards, A. M. (1998). The 2.2 A structure of a permanganate-sensitive DNA site bound by the Epstein-Barr virus origin binding protein, EBNA1. *J. Mol. Biol.*, **284**(5), 1273–1278.

Boshoff, C. and Weiss, R. (2002). AIDS-related malignancies. *Nature Reviews. Cancer*, **2**(5), 373–382.

Burd, C. G. and Dreyfuss, G. (1994). Conserved structures and diversity of functions of RNA-binding proteins. *Science*, **265**(5172), 615–621.

Cai, X., Lu, S., Zhang, Z., Gonzalez, C. M., Damania, B., and Cullen, B. R. (2005). Kaposi's sarcoma-associated herpesvirus expresses an array of viral microRNAs in latently infected cells. *Proc. Natl Acad. Sci. USA*, **102**, 5570–5575.

Cannon, J. S., Ciufo, D., Hawkins, A. L. et al. (2000). A new primary effusion lymphoma-derived cell line yields a highly infectious Kaposi's sarcoma herpesvirus-containing supernatant. *J. Virol.*, **74**, 10187–10193.

Ceccarelli, D. F. and Frappier, L. (2000). Functional analyses of the EBNA1 origin DNA binding protein of Epstein–Barr virus. *J. Virol.*, **74**, 4939–4948.

Cesarman, E., Moore, P. S., Rao, P. H., Inghirami, G., Knowles, D. M., and Chang, Y. (1995). In vitro establishment and characterization of two acquired immunodeficiency syndrome-related lymphoma cell lines (BC-1 and BC-2) containing Kaposi's sarcoma-associated herpesvirus (KSHV) DNA sequences. *Blood*, **86**, 2708–2714.

Chang, Y., Cheng, S. D., and Tsai, C. H. (2002). Chromosomal integration of Epstein–Barr virus genomes in nasopharyngeal carcinoma cells. *Head Neck*, **24**(2), 143–150.

Chang, Y. E., Cesarman, E., Pessin, M. S. *et al.* (1994). Identification of herpesvirus-like DNA sequences in AIDS-associated kaposis sarcoma. *Science*, **266**(5192), 1865–1869.

Chaudhuri, B., Xu, H., Todorov, I., Dutta, A., and Yates, T. L. (2001). Human DNA replication initiation factors, ORC and MCM, associate with *OriP* of Epstein–Barr virus. *Proc. Natl Acad. Sci. USA*, **98**, 10085–10089.

Chen, J., Ueda, K., Sakakibara, S. *et al.* (2001). Activation of latent Kaposi's sarcoma-associated herpesvirus by demethylation of the promoter of the lytic transactivator. *Proc. Natl Acad. Sci. USA*, **98**, 4119–4124.

Chen, M. R., Middeldorp, J. M., and Hayward, S. D. (1993). Separation of the complex DNA binding domain of EBNA-1 into DNA recognition and dimerization subdomains of novel structure. *J. Virol.*, **67**(8), 4875–4885.

Chen, M. R., Zong, J., and Hayward, S. D. (1994). Delineation of a 16 amino acid sequence that forms a core DNA recognition motif in the Epstein–Barr virus EBNA-1 protein. *Virology*, **205**(2), 486–495.

Chen, M. R., Yang, J. F., Wu, C. W., Middeldorp, J. M., and Chen, J. Y. (1998). Physical association between the EBV protein EBNA-1 and P32/TAP/hyaluronectin. *J. Biomed. Sci.*, **5**(3), 173–179.

Cheung, R. K., Miyazaki, I., and Dosch, H. M. (1993). Unexpected patterns of Epstein–Barr virus gene expression during early stages of B cell transformation. *Int. Immunol.*, **5**(7), 707–716.

Chittenden, T., Lupton, S., and Levine, A. J. (1989). Functional limits of *OriP*, the Epstein–Barr virus plasmid origin of replication. *J. Virol.*, **63**, 3016–3025.

Collins, C. M., Medveczky, M. M., Lund, T., and Medveczky, P. E. (2002). The terminal repeats and latency-associated nuclear antigen of herpesvirus saimiri are essential for episomal persistence of the viral genome. *J. Gen. Virol.*, **83**(9), 2269–2278.

Cotter, M. A., 2nd and Robertson, E. S. (1999). The latency-associated nuclear antigen tethers the Kaposi's sarcoma-associated herpesvirus genome to host chromosomes in body cavity-based lymphoma cells [In Process Citation]. *Virology*, **264**(2), 254–264.

Cotter, M. A., 2nd, Subramanian, C., and Robertson, E. S. (2001). The Kaposi's sarcoma-associated herpesvirus latency-associated nuclear antigen binds to specific sequences at the left end of the viral genome through its carboxy-terminus. *Virology*, **291**(2), 241–259.

Cruickshank, J., Shire, K., Davidson, A. R., Edwards, A. M., and Frappier, L. (2000). Two domains of the epstein-barr virus origin DNA-binding protein, EBNA1, orchestrate sequence-specific DNA binding. *J. Biol. Chem.*, **275**(29), 22273–22277.

Deng, Z., Lezina, L., Chen, C., Shtivelband, S., So, W., and Lieberman, P. M. (2002). Telomeric proteins regulate maintenance of Epstein–Barr Virus origin of plasmid replication. *Mol. Cell*, **9**, 493–503.

Deng, Z., Atanasiu, C., Burg, J. S., Broccoli, D., and Lieberman, P. M. (2003). Telomere repeat binding factors TRF1, TRF2, and hRAP1 modulate replication of Epstein–Barr virus *OriP*. *J. Virol.*, **77**(22), 11992–12001.

Desaintes, C. and Demeret, C. (1996). Control of papillomavirus DNA replication and transcription. *Semin. Cancer Biol.*, **7**(6), 339–347.

Dhar, S. K., Yoshida, K., Machida, Y. *et al.* (2001). Replication from *OriP* of Epstein–Barr virus requires human ORC and is inhibited by geminin. *Cell*, **106**, 287–296.

Diala, E. S. and Hoffman, R. M. (1983). Epstein–Barr HR-1 virion DNA is very highly methylated. *J. Virol.*, **45**(1), 482–483.

Dictor, M., Rambech, E., Way, D., Witte, M., and Bendsoe, N. (1996). Human herpesvirus 8 (Kaposi's sarcoma-associated herpesvirus) DNA in Kaposi's sarcoma lesions, AIDS Kaposi's sarcoma cell lines, endothelial Kaposi's sarcoma simulators, and the skin of immunosuppressed patients. *Am. J. Pathol.*, **148**, 2009–2016.

Dittmer, D., Lagunoff, M., Renne, R., Staskus, K., Haase, A., and Ganem, D. (1998). A cluster of latently expressed genes in Kaposi's sarcoma-associated herpesvirus. *J. Virol.*, **72**(10), 8309–8315.

Dupin, N., Fisher, C., Kellam, P. *et al.* (1999). Distribution of human herpesvirus-8 latently infected cells in Kaposi's sarcoma, multicentric Castleman's disease, and primary effusion lymphoma. *Proc. Natl Acad. Sci. USA*, **96**(8), 4546–4551.

Dyson, P. J. and Farrell, P. J. (1985). Chromatin structure of Esptein-Barr virus. *J. Gen. Virol.*, **66**, 1931–1940.

Edwards, A. M., Bochkarev, A., and Frappier, L. (1998). Origin DNA-binding proteins. *Curr. Opin. Struct. Biol.*, **8**(1), 49–53.

Ernberg, I., Falk, K., Miraovits, J. *et al.* (1989). The role of methylation in the phenotype-dependent modulation of Epstein-Barr nuclear antigen 2 and latent membrane protein genes in cells latently infected with Epstein–Barr virus. *J. Gen. Virol.*, **70**(11), 2989–3002.

Everett, R. D., Meredith, M., and Orr, A. (1999). The ability of herpes simplex virus type 1 immediate-early protein Vmw110 to bind to a ubiquitin-specific protease contributes to its roles in the activation of gene expression and stimulation of virus replication. *J. Virol.*, **73**(1), 417–426.

Falk, K. and Ernberg, I. (1993). An origin of DNA replication (*OriP*) in highly methylated episomal Epstein–Barr virus DNA localizes to a 4.5-kb unmethylated region. *Virology*, **195**(2), 608–615.

Falk, K. I., Szekely, L., Aleman, A., and Ernberg, I. (1998). Specific methylation patterns in two control regions of Epstein–Barr virus latency: the LMP-1-coding upstream regulatory region and an origin of DNA replication (*OriP*). *J. Virol.*, **72**(4), 2969–2974.

Fischer, N., Kremmer, E., Lavtshcam, G., Mueller-Lantzsch, N., and Grasser, F. A. (1997). α2. *J. Biol. Chem.*, **272**, 3999–4005.

Frappier, L., Goldsmith, K., and Bendell, L. (1994). Stabilization of the EBNA1 protein on the Epstein–Barr virus latent origin of DNA replication by a DNA looping mechanism. *J. Biol. Chem.*, **269**(2), 1057–1062.

Friborg, J., Kong, W., Hottiger, M. O., and Nabel, G. J. (2000). p53 inhibition by the LANA protein of KSHV protects against cell death. *Nature*, **402**(6764), 889–894.

Fridell, R. A., Harding, L. S., Bogerd, H. P., and Cullen, B. R. (1995). Identification of a novel human zinc finger protein that specifically interacts with the activation domain of lentiviral Tat proteins. *Virology*, **209**(2), 347–357.

Fujimuro, M. and Hayward, S. D. (2003). The latency-associated nuclear antigen of Kaposi's sarcoma-associated herpesvirus manipulates the activity of glycogen synthase kinase-3beta. *J. Virol.*, **77**(14), 8019–8030.

Fujimuro, M., Wu, F. Y., Ap Rhys, C. *et al.* (2003). A novel viral mechanism for dysregulation of beta-catenin in Kaposi's sarcoma-associated herpesvirus latency. *Nat. Med.*, **9**(3), 300–306.

Gahn, T. A. and Schildkraut, C. L. (1989). The Epstein–Barr virus origin of plasmid replication, *OriP*, contains both the initiation and termination sites of DNA replication. *Cell*, **58**, 527–535.

Gahn, T. A. and Sugden, B. (1995). An EBNA-1-dependent enhancer acts from a distance of 10 kilobase pairs to increase expression of the Esptein-Barr virus LMP Gene. *J. Virol.*, **69**, 2633–2636.

Ganem, D. (1997). KSHV and Kaposi'2 sarcoma. The end of the beginning? *Cell*, **91**, 157–160.

Gao, S. J., Kingsley, L., Li, M. *et al.* (1996). KSHV antibodies among Americans, Italians and Ugandans with and without Kaposi's sarcoma [see comments]. *Nat. Med.*, **2**(8), 925–928.

Gao, S. J., Zhang, Y. J., Deng, J. H., Rabkin, C. S., Flore, O., and Henson, H. B. (1999). Molecular polymorphism of Kaposi's sarcoma-associated herpesvirus (Human herpesvirus 8) latent nuclear antigen: evidence for a large repertoire of viral genotypes and dual infection with different viral genotypes [In Process Citation]. *J. Infect. Dis.*, **180**(5), 1466–1476.

Garber, A. C., Shu, M. A., Hu, J., and Renne, R. (2001). DNA binding and modulation of gene expression by the latency-associated nuclear antigen of Kaposi's sarcoma-associated herpesvirus. *J. Virol.*, **75**(17), 7882–7892.

Garber, A. C., Hu, J., and Renne, R. (2002). Latency-associated nuclear antigen (LANA) cooperatively binds to two sites within the terminal repeat, and both sites contribute to the ability of LANA to suppress transcription and to facilitate DNA replication. *J. Biol. Chem.*, **277**(30), 27401–27411.

Gardella, T., Medveczky, P., Saironji, T., and Mulder, C. (1984). Detection of circular and linear herpesvirus DNA molecules in mammalian cells by gel electrophoresis. *J. Virol.*, **50**(1), 248–254.

Gilbert, D. M. (2001). Making sense of eukaryotic DNA replication origins. *Science*, **294**(5540), 96–100.

Goldsmith, K., Bendell, L., and Frappier, L. (1993). Identification of EBNA1 amino acid sequences required for the interaction of the functional elements of the Epstein–Barr virus latent origin of DNA replication. *J. Virol.*, **67**(6), 3418–3426.

Grossman, S. R. and Laimins, L. A. (1996). EBNA1 and E2: a new paradigm for origin-binding proteins? *Trends Microbiol.*, **4**(3), 87–89.

Gruffat, H., Manet, E., and Sargeant, A. (2002). MEF2-mediated recruitment of class II HDAC at the EBV immediate early gene BZLF1 links latency and chromatin remodeling. *EMBO Rep.*, **3**(2), 141–146.

Grundhoff, A. and Ganem, D. (2003). The latency-associated nuclear antigen of Kaposi's sarcoma-associated herpesesvirus permits replication of terminal repeat-containing plasmids. *J. Virol.*, **77**(4), 2779–2783.

Grundhoff, A., and Ganem, D. (2004). Inefficient establishment of KSHV latency suggests an additional role for continued lytic replication in Kaposi sarcoma pathogenesis. *J. Clin. Invest.*, **113**, 124–136.

Hall, K. T., Giles, M. S., Calderwood, M. A., Goodwin, D. J., Mathews, D. A., and Witehouse, A. (2002). The Herpesvirus Saimiri open reading frame 73 gene product interacts with the cellular protein p32. *J. Virol.*, **76**(22), 11612–11622.

Harrison, S., Fisenne, K., and Hearing, J. (1994). Sequence requirements of the Epstein–Barr virus latent origin of DNA replication. *J. Virol.*, **68**(3), 1913–1925.

Hearing, J., Mulhaupt, Y., and Harper, S. (1992). Interaction of Epstein–Barr virus nuclear antigen 1 with the viral latent origin of replication. *J. Virol.*, **66**, 694–705.

Hebner, C., Lasanen, J., Battle, S., and Aiyar, A. (2003). The spacing between adjacent binding sites in the family of repeats affects the functions of Epstein–Barr nuclear antigen 1 in transcription activation and stable plasmid maintenance. *Virology*, **311**(2), 263–274.

Herndier, B. and Ganem, D. (2001). The biology of Kaposi's sarcoma. *Cancer Treat. Res.*, **104**, 89–126.

Hirai, K. and Shirakata, M. (2001). *OriP* Minichromosome. In *Epstein–Barr Virus and Human Cancer*, ed. K. Takada. Heidelberg, Springer, **258**.

Holowaty, M. N., Zeghouf, M., Wu, H. *et al.* (2003). Protein profiling with Epstein–Barr nuclear antigen-1 reveals an interaction with the herpesvirus-associated ubiquitin-specific protease HAUSP/USP7. *J. Biol. Chem.*, **278**(32), 29987–29994.

Hsieh, C. L. (1999). Evidence that protein binding specifies sites of DNA demethylation. *Mol. Cell Biol.*, **19**(1), 46–56.

Hsieh, D. J., Camiolo, S. M., and Yates, J. L. (1993). Constitutive binding of EBNA1 protein to the Epstein–Barr virus replication origin, *OriP*, with distortion of DNA structure during latent infection. *EMBO J.*, **12**(13), 4933–4944.

Hsieh, J. J., Zhou, S., Chen, L., Young, D. B., and Hayward, S. D. (1999). CIR, a corepressor linking the DNA binding factor CBF1 to the histone deacetylase complex. *Proc. Natl Acad. Sci. USA*, **96**(1), 23–28.

Hu, J. and Renne, R. (2005). Characterization of the minimal replicator of Kaposi's sarcoma-associated herpesvirus latent origin. *J. Virol.*, **79**, 2637–2642.

Hu, L. F., Minarovits, J., Cao, S. L. *et al.* (1991). Variable expression of latent membrane protein in nasopharyngeal carcinoma can be related to methylation status of the Epstein–Barr virus BNLF-1 5′-flanking region. *J. Virol.*, **65**(3), 1558–1567.

Hu, J., Garber, A. C., and Renne, R. (2002). The latency-associated nuclear antigen of Kaposi's sarcoma-associated herpesvirus supports latent DNA replication in dividing cells. *J. Virol.*, **76**(22), 11677–11687.

Huber, M. D., Dworet, J. H., Shire, K., Frappier, L., and McAlean, M. A. (2000). The budding yeast homolog of the human EBNA1-binding protein 2 (Ebp2p) is an essential nucleolar protein required for pre-rRNA processing. *J. Biol. Chem.*, **275**, 28764–28770.

Humme, S., Reisbach, G., Feederle, R. *et al.* (2003). The EBV nuclear antigen 1 (EBNA1) enhances B cell immortalization several thousandfold. *Proc. Natl Acad. Sci. USA*, **100**(19), 10989–10994.

Hung, S. C., Kang, M. S., and Kieff, E. (2001). Maintenance of Epstein–Barr virus (EBV) *OriP*-based episomes requires EBV-encoded nuclear antigen-1 chromosome-binding domains, which can be replaced by high-mobility group-I or histone H1. *Proc. Natl. Acad. Sci. USA*, **98**, 1865–1870.

Hurley, E. A. and Thorley-Lawson, D. A. (1988). B cell activation and the establishment of Epstein–Barr virus latency. *J. Exp. Med.*, **168**(6), 2059–2075.

Hyun, T. S., Subramanian, C., Cotter, M. A., 2nd, Thomas, R. A., and Robertson, E. S. (2001). Latency-associated nuclear antigen encoded by Kaposi's sarcoma-associated herpesvirus interacts with Tat and activates the long terminal repeat of human immunodeficiency virus type 1 in human cells. *J. Virol.*, **75**(18), 8761–8771.

Ito, S., Ikeda, M., Kato, N. *et al.* (2000). Epstein–Barr virus nuclear antigen-1 binds to nuclear transporter karyopherin alpha1/NPI-1 in addition to karyopherin alpha2/Rch1. *Virology*, **266**(1), 110–119.

Ito, S. and Yanagi, K. (2003). Epstein–Barr virus (EBV) nuclear antigen 1 colocalizes with cellular replication foci in the absence of EBV plasmids. *J. Virol.*, **77**(6), 3824–3831.

Jankelevich, S., Kolman, J. L., Bodnar, J. W., and Miller, G. (1992). A nuclear matrix attachment region organizes the Epstein–Barr viral plasmid in Raji cells into a single DNA domain. *EMBO J.*, **11**(3), 1165–1176.

Jenkins, P. J., Binne, U. K., and Farrel, P. J. (2000). Histone acetylation and reactivation of Epstein–Barr virus from latency. *J. Virol.*, **74**, 710–720.

Jeong, J., Papin, J., and Dittmer, D. (2001). Differential regulation of the overlapping Kaposi's sarcoma-associated herpesvirus vGCR (orf74) and LANA (orf73) promoters. *J. Virol.*, **75**(4), 1798–1807.

Jones, P. L. and Wolffe, A. P. (1999). Relationships between chromatin organization and DNA methylation in determining gene expression. *Semin. Cancer Biol.*, **9**(5), 339–347.

Kanda, T., Otter, M., and Wahl, G. M. (2001). Coupling of mitotic chromosome tethering and replication competence in epstein-barr virus-based plasmids. *Mol. Cell. Biol.*, **21**, 3576–3588.

Kapoor, P., Shire, K., and Frappier, L. (2001). Reconstitution of Epstein-Barr virus-based plasmid partitioning in budding yeast. *EMBO J.*, **15**, 222–230.

Kedes, D. H., Operskalski, E., Busch, M., Kohn, R., Flood, J., and Ganem, D. (1996). The seroepidemiology of human herpesvirus 8 (Kaposi's sarcoma-associated herpesvirus), distribution of infection in KS risk groups and evidence for sexual transmission [see comments] [published erratum appears in *Nat. Med.* 1996 Sep;**2**(9),1041]. *Nat. Med.*, **2**(8), 918–924.

Kedes, D. H., Lagunoff, M., Renne, R., and Ganem, D. (1997). Identification of the gene encoding the major latency-associated nuclear antigen of the Kaposi's sarcoma-associated herpesvirus. *J. Clin. Invest.*, **100**(10), 2606–2610.

Kellam, P., Boshoff, C., Whitby, D., Matthews, S., Weiss, R. A., and Talbot, S. J. (1997). Identification of a major latent nuclear antigen, LNA-1, in the human herpesvirus 8 genome. *J. Hum. Virol.*, **1**(1), 19–29.

Kennedy, G. and Sugden, B. (2003). EBNA-1, a bifunctional transcriptional activator. *Mol. Cell. Biol.*, **23**(19), 6901–6908.

Kennedy, G., Komano, J., and Sugden, B. (2003). Epstein–Barr virus provides a survival factor to Burkitt's lymphomas. *Proc. Natl Acad. Sci. USA*, **4**.

Kim, A. L., Maher, M., Hayman, J. B. *et al.* (1997). An imperfect correlation between the DNA replication activity of Epstein–Barr virus nuclear antigen 1 (EBNA1) and the binding to the nuclear import receptor, Rch1/importin alpha. *Virology*, **239**, 340–351.

Kintner, C. R. and Sugden, B. (1979). The structure of the termini of the DNA of Epstein–Barr virus. *Cell*, **17**(3), 661–671.

Kirchmaier, A. L. and Sugden, B. (1998). Rep*: a viral element that can partially replace the origin of plasmid DNA synthesis of Epstein–Barr virus. *J. Virol.*, **72**(6), 4657–4666.

Knight, J. S., Cotter, 2nd, M. A., and Robertson, E. S. (2001). The latency-associated nuclear antigen of Kaposi's sarcoma-associated herpesvirus transactivates the telomerase reverse transcriptase promoter. *J. Biol. Chem.*, **276**(25), 22971–22978.

Koliais, S. I. (1979). Mode of integration of Epstein–Barr virus genome into host DNA in Burkitt lymphoma cells. *J. Gen. Virol.*, **44**(2), 573–576.

Koons, M. D., Scoy, S. V., and Hearing, J. (2001). OriP, is composed of multiple functional elements. *J. Virol.*, **75**, 10582–10592.

Kripalani-Joshi, S. and Law, H. Y. (1994). Identification of integrated Epstein-Barr virus in nasopharyngeal carcinoma using pulse field gel electrophoresis. *Int. J. Cancer*, **56**(2), 187–192.

Krishnan, H. H., Naranatt, P. P., Smith, M. S., Zeng, L., Bloomer, C., and Chandran B. (2004). Concurrent expression of latent and a limited number of lytic genes with immune modulation and antiapoptotic function by Kaposi's sarcoma-associated herpesvirus early during infection of primary endothelial and fibroblast cells and subsequent decline of lytic gene expression. *J. Virol.*, **78**, 3601–3620.

Krithivas, A., Young, D. B. *et al.* (2000). Human herpesvirus 8 LANA interacts with proteins of the mSin3 corepressor complex and negatively regulates Epstein–Barr virus gene expression in dually infected PEL cells. *J. Virol.*, **74**(20), 9637–9645.

Krithivas, A., Fujimoro, M. *et al.* (2002). Protein interactions targeting the latency-associated nuclear antigen of Kaposi's sarcoma-associated herpesvirus to cell chromosomes. *J. Virol.*, **76**(22), 11596–11604.

Krysan, P. J. and Calos, M. P. (1991). Replication initiates at multiple locations on an autonomously replicating plasmid in human cells. *Mol. Cell. Biol.*, **11**(3), 1464–1472.

Krysan, P. J., Haase, S. B., and Calos, M. D. (1989). Isolation of human sequences that replicate autonomously in human cells. *Mol. Cell. Biol.*, **9**, 1026–1033.

Lagunoff, M. and Ganem, D. (1997). The structure and coding organization of the genomic termini of Kaposi's sarcoma-associated herpesvirus. *Virology*, **236**(1), 147–154.

Lagunoff, M., Bechtel, J., Venetsanakos, E. *et al.* (2002). De novo infection and serial transmission of Kaposi's sarcoma-associated herpesvirus in cultured endothelial cells. *J. Virol.*, **76**, 2440–2448.

Lan, K., Kuppers, D. A., Verma, S. C., and Robertson, E. S., (2004). Kaposi's sarcoma-associated herpesvirus-encoded latency-associated nuclear antigen inhibits lytic replication by targeting Rta: a protential mechanism for virus-mediated control of latency. *J. Virol.*, **78**, 6585–6594.

Laux, G., Economou, A., and Farrell, P. J. (1989). The terminal protein gene 2 of Epstein–Barr virus is transcribed from a bidirectional latent promoter region. *J. Gen. Virol.*, **70**(11), 3079–3084.

Lawrence, J. B., Villnave, C. A., and Singer, R. H. (1988). Sensitive, high-resolution chromatin and chromosome mapping in situ: presence and orientation of two closely integrated copies of EBV in a lymphoma line. *Cell*, **52**(1), 51–61.

Lee, M. A., Diamond, M. E., and Yates, J. L. (1999). Genetic evidence that EBNA-1 is needed for efficient, stable latent infection by Epstein–Barr virus. *J. Virol.*, **73**, 2974–2982.

Leight, E. R. and Sugden, B. (2000). EBNA-1: a protein pivotal to latent infection by Epstein–Barr virus. *Rev. Med. Virol.*, **10**(2), 83–100.

Leonchiks, A., Stavropoulou, V., Sharipo, A., and Massucci, G. (2002). Inhibition of ubiquitin-dependent proteolysis by a synthetic glycine-alanine repeat peptide that mimics an inhibitory viral sequence. *FEBS Lett.*, **522**(1–3), 93–98.

Levitskaya, J., Coram, M., Levitsky, V. *et al.* (1995). Inhibition of antigen processing by the internal repeat region of the Epstein–Barr virus nuclear antigen-1. *Nature*, **375**(6533), 685–688.

Levitskaya, J., Sharipo, A., Leonchiks, A., Ciechanover, A., and Masucci, M. G. (1997). Inhibition of ubiquitin/proteasome-dependent degradation by the Gly-Ala repeat domain of Epstein–Barr virus nuclear antigen 1. *Proc. Natl Acad. Sci. USA*, **94**, 12616–12621.

Li, Q. X., Young, L. S., Niedobitek, G. *et al.* (1992). Epstein–Barr virus infection and replication in a human epithelial cell system. *Nature*, **356**(6367), 347–350.

Lim, C., Sohn, H., Gwack, Y., and Choe, J. (2000). Latency-associated nuclear antigen of Kaposi's sarcoma-associated herpesvirus (human herpesvirus-8) binds ATF4/CREB2 and inhibits its transcriptional activation activity. *J. Gen. Virol.*, **81**(11), 2645–2652.

Lim, C., Sohn, H., Lee, D., Gwack, Y., and Choe, J. (2002). Functional dissection of LANA1 of Kaposi's sarcoma-associated herpesvirus involved in latent DNA replication and transcription of terminal repeats of the viral geneome. *J. Virol.*, **76**, 10320–10331.

Lin, I. G., Tomzynski, T. J., Ou, Q., and Hsieh, C. L. (2000). Modulation of DNA binding protein affinity directly affects target site demethylation. *Mol. Cell. Biol.*, **20**(7), 2343–2349.

Lindahl, T., Adams, A., Andersson-Anvret, M., and Falk, L. (1978). Integration of Epstein–Barr virus DNA. *IARC Sci. Publ.* (24, 1), 113–123.

Little, R. D. and Schildkraut, C. L. (1995). Initiation of latent DNA replication in the Epstein–Barr virus genome can occur at sites other than the genetically defined origin. *Mol. Cell. Biol.*, **15**, 2893–2903.

Liu, S., Liu, P., Borras, A., Chatila, T., and Speck, S. H. (1997). Cyclosporin A-sensitive induction of the Epstein–Barr virus lytic switch is mediated via a novel pathway involving a MEF2 family member. *EMBO J.*, **16**, 143–153.

Lu, F., Zhou, J., Wiedmer, A., Madden, K., Yuan, Y., and Lieberman, P. M. (2003). Chromatin remodeling of the Kaposi's sarcoma-associated herpesvirus ORF50 promoter correlates with reactivation from latency. *J. Virol.*, **77**(21), 11425–11435.

Lu, F., Day, L., Gao, S. J., and Lieberman, P. M. (2006). Acetylation of the latency-associated nuclear antigen regulates repression of Kaposi's sarcoma-associated herpesvirus lytic transcription. *J. Virol.*, **80**, 5273–5282.

Lupton, S. and Levine, A. (1985). Mapping genetic elements of Epstein–Barr virus that facilitate extrachromasomal persistence of Epstein–Barr virus-derived plasmids in human cells. *Mol. Cell. Biol.*, **5**, 2533–2542.

Mackey, D. and Sugden, B. (1999). The linking regions of EBNA1 are essential for its support of replication and transcription. *Mol. Cell. Biol.*, **19**, 3349–3359.

Mackey, D., Middleton, T., and Sugden, B. (1995). Multiple regions within EBNA1 can link DNAs. *J. Virol.*, **69**, 6199–6208.

Marechal, V., Dehee, A., Chikhi-Brachet, R., Piolot, T., and Coppey-Moisan, M. (1999). Mapping EBNA-1 domains involved in binding to metaphase chromosomes. *J., Virol.*, **73**, 4385–4392.

Masucci, M. G., Contreras-Salazar, B., Ragnar, E. *et al.* (1989). 5-Azacytidine up regulates the expression of Epstein–Barr virus nuclear antigen 2 (EBNA-2) through EBNA-6 and latent membrane protein in the Burkitt's lymphoma line real. *J. Virol.*, **63**(7), 3135–3141.

Matthews, D. A. and Russell, W. C. (1998). Adenovirus core protein V interacts with p32–a protein which is associated with both the mitochondria and the nucleus. *J. Gen. Virol.*, **79**(7), 1677–1685.

Mattsson, K., Kiss, C., Platt, G. M. *et al.* (2002). Latent nuclear antigen of Kaposi's sarcoma herpesvirus/human herpesvirus-8 induces and relocates RING3 to nuclear heterochromatin regions. *J. Gen. Virol.*, **83**(1), 179–188.

Middleton, T. and Sugden, B. (1992). EBNA1 can link the enhancer element to the initiator element of the Epstein–Barr virus plasmid origin of DNA replication. *J. Virol.*, **66**(1), 489–495.

Miller, C. L., Lee, J. H., Kieff, E., and Longnecker, R. (1994). An integral membrane protein (LMP2) blocks reactivation of Epstein–Barr virus from latency following surface immunoglobulin crosslinking. *Proc. Natl Acad. Sci. USA*, **91**(2), 772–776.

Minarovits, J., Hu, L. F., Minarorits-Kormata, S., Klein, G., and Ernberg, I. (1994). Sequence-specific methylation inhibits the activity of the Epstein–Barr virus LMP 1 and BCR2 enhancer-promoter regions. *Virology*, **200**(2), 661–667.

Muta, T., Kang, D., Kitajima, S., Fujiwara, T., and Hamasaki, N. (1997). p32 protein, a splicing factor 2-associated protein, is localized in mitochondrial matrix and is functionally important in maintaining oxidative phosphorylation. *J. Biol. Chem.*, **272**(39), 24363–24370.

Naranatt, P. P., Krishnan, H. H., Srojanovsky, S. R., Bloomer, C., Mathur, S., and Chandran, B. (2004). Host gene induction and transcriptional reprogramming in Kaposi's sarcoma-associated herpesvirus (KSHV/HHV-8)-infected endothelial, fibroblast, and B cells: insights into modulation events early during infection. *Cancer Res.*, **64**(1), 72–84.

Niller, H. H., Glaser, G., Knuchel, R., and Wolf, H. (1995). Nucleoprotein complexes and DNA 5-ends at *OriP* of Epstein–Barr virus. *J. Biol. Chem.*, **270**, 12864–12868.

Nilsson, T., Zetterberg, H., Wang, J. C., and Rymo, L. (2001). Promoter-proximal regulatory elements involved in *OriP*-EBNA1-independent and -dependent activation of the Epstein–Barr virus C promoter in B-lymphoid cell lines. *J. Virol.*, **75**(13), 5796–5811.

Nonoyama, M. and Tanaka, A. (1975). Plasmid DNA as a possible state of Epstein–Barr virus genomes in nonproductive cells. *Cold Spring Harb. Symp. Quant. Biol.*, **39**(2), 807–810.

Norio, P. and Schildkraut, C. L. (2001). Visualization of DNA replication on individual Epstein–Barr virus episomes. *Science*, **294**(5550), 2361–2364.

Norio, P., Schildkraut, C. L., and Yates, J. L. (2000). Initiation of DNA replication within *OriP* is dispensable for stable replication of the latent Epstein-Barr virus chromosome after infection of established cell lines. *J. Virol.*, **74**, 8563–8574.

Ohshima, K., Suzumiya, J., Kanda, M., Kato, A., and Kikuchi, M. (1998). Integrated and episomal forms of Epstein–Barr virus (EBV) in EBV associated disease. *Cancer Lett.*, **122**(1–2), 43–50.

Pfeffer, S., Sewer, A., Lagos-Quintana, M. et al. (2005). Identification of microRNAs of the herpesvirus family. *Nat. Methods*, **2**, 269–276.

Piolot, T., Tramier, M., Coppey, M., Nicolas, J. C., and Marechal, V. (2001). Close but distinct regions of human herpesvirus 8 latency-associated nuclear antigen 1 are responsible for nuclear targeting and binding to human mitotic chromosomes. *J. Virol.*, **75**(8), 3948–3959.

Platt, G. M., Simpson, G. R., Mittnacht, S., and Schule, T. F. (1999). Latent nuclear antigen of Kaposi's sarcoma-associated herpesvirus interacts with RING3, a homolog of the drosophila female sterile homeotic (fsh) gene [In Process Citation]. *J. Virol.*, **73**(12), 9789–9795.

Popescu, N. C., Chen, M. C., Simpson, S., Solinas, S., and D. Paolo, J. A. (1993). A Burkitt lymphoma cell line with integrated Epstein–Barr virus at a stable chromosome modification site. *Virology*, **195**(1), 248–251.

Puglielli, M. T., Woisetschlaeger, M., and Speck, S. H. (1996). *OriP* is essential for EBNA gene promoter activity in Epstein-Barr virus immortalized lymphoblastoid cell lines. *J. Virol.*, **70**, 5758–5768.

Radkov, S. A., Kellam, P., and Boshoff, C. (2000). The latent nuclear antigen of Kaposi sarcoma-associated herpesvirus targets the retinoblastoma-E2F pathway and with the oncogene Hras transforms primary rat cells. *Nat. Med.*, **6**(10), 1121–1127.

Rainbow, L., Platt, G. M., Simpson, G. R. et al. (1997). The 222- to 234-kilodalton latent nuclear protein (LNA) of Kaposi's sarcoma-associated herpesvirus (human herpesvirus 8) is encoded by orf73 and is a component of the latency-associated nuclear antigen. *J. Virol.*, **71**(8), 5915–5921.

Rawlins, D. R., Milman, G., Hayward, S. D., and Hayward, G. S. (1985). Sequence-specific DNA binding of the Epstein–Barr virus nuclear antigen (EBNA-1) to clustered sites in the plamid maintenance region. *Cell*, **42**, 859–868.

Reisman, D. and Sugden, B. (1986). *Trans*-activation of an Epstein–Barr viral transcriptional enhancer by the Epstein–Barr viral nuclear antigen 1. *Mol. Cell. Biol.*, **5**, 3838–3846.

Reisman, D., Yates, J., and Sugden, B. (1985). A putative origin of replication of plasmids derived from Epstein–Barr virus is composed of two *cis*-acting components. *Mol. Cell. Biol.*, **5**, 1822–1832.

Renne, R., Lagunoff, M., Zhong, W., and Ganem, D. (1996a). The size and conformation of Kaposi's sarcoma-associated herpesvirus (human herpesvirus 8) DNA in infected cells and virions. *J. Virol.*, **70**(11), 8151–8154.

Renne, R., Zhong, W., Herndier, B. et al. (1996b). Lytic growth of Kaposi's sarcoma-associated herpesvirus (human herpesvirus 8) in culture. *Nat. Med.*, **2**, 342–346.

Renne, R., Barry, C., Dittmer, D., Compitello, N., Brown, P., and Ganem, D. (2001). Modulation of cellular and viral transcription by the latency-associated nuclears antigen (LANA/ORF73) of KSHV. *J. Virol.*, **75**, 458–468.

Rivailler, P., Cho, Y. G., and Wang, F. (2002). Complete genomic sequence of an Epstein–Barr virus-related herpesvirus naturally infecting a new world primate: a defining point in the evolution of oncogenic lymphocryptoviruses. *J. Virol.*, **76**(23), 12055–12068.

Robertson, K. D. (2000). The role of DNA methylation in modulating Epstein–Barr virus gene expression. *Curr. Top. Microbiol. Immunol.*, **249**, 21–34.

Robertson, K. D. and Ambinder, R. F. (1997). Methylation of the Epstein–Barr virus genome in normal lymphocytes. *Blood*, **90**(11), 4480–4484.

Robertson, K. D., Manns, A., Swinnen, L. J., Zong, J. C., Gulley, M. L., and Ambinder, R. F. (1996). CpG methylation of the major Epstein–Barr virus latency promoter in Burkitt's lymphoma and Hodgkin's disease. *Blood*, **88**(8), 3129–3136.

Russo, J. J., Bohenzky, R. A., Chien, M. C. et al. (1996). Nucleotide sequence of the Kaposi sarcoma-associated herpesvirus (HHV8). *Proc. Natl Acad. Sci. USA*, **93**, 14862–14867.

Sadler, R., Wu, L., Forghani, B. et al. (1999). A complex translational program generates multiple novel proteins from the latently expressed kaposin (K12) locus of Kaposi's sarcoma-associated herpesvirus. *J. Virol.*, **73**(7), 5722–5730.

Sadler, R. H. and Raab-Traub, N. (1995). Structural analyses of the Epstein–Barr virus BamHI A transcripts. *J. Virol.*, **69**(2), 1132–1141.

Saemundsen, A. K., Kallin, B., and Klein, G. (1980). Effect of n-butyrate on cellular and viral DNA synthesis in cells latently infected with Epstein–Barr virus. *Virology*, **107**, 557–561.

Saemundsen, A. K., Perlmann, C., and Klein, G. (1983). Intracellular Epstein–Barr virus DNA is methylated in and around the EcoRI-J fragment in both producer and nonproducer cell lines. *Virology*, **126**(2), 701–706.

Salamon, D., Takacs, M., Myohanen, S., Marcsek, Z., Berencsi, G., and Minarovits, J. (2000). De novo DNA methylation at nonrandom founder sites 5′ from an unmethylated minimal origin of DNA replication in latent Epstein–Barr virus genomes. *Biol. Chem.*, **381**(2), 95–105.

Salamon, D., Takacs, M., Vjvari, D. et al. (2001). Protein–DNA binding and CpG methylation at nucleotide resolution of latency-associated promoters Qp, Cp, and LMP1p of Epstein–Barr virus. *J. Virol.*, **75**(6), 2584–2596.

Samols, M. A., Hu, J., Skalsky, R. L., and Renne, R. (2005). Cloning and identification of a microRNA cluster within the latency-associated region of Kaposi's sarcoma-associated herpesvirus. *J. Virol.*, **79**, 9301–9305.

Saridakis, V., Sheng, Y., Sarkari, F. et al. (2005). Structure of the p53 binding domain of HAUSP/USP7 bound to Epstein–Barr nuclear antigen 1 implications for EBV-mediated immortalization. *Mol. Cell.*, **18**, 25–36.

Schaefer, B. C., Strominger, J. L., and Speck, S. H. (1997). Host-cell-determined methylation of specific Epstein–Barr virus promoters regulates the choice between distinct viral latency programs. *Mol. Cell. Biol.*, **17**(1), 364–377.

Schepers, A., Ritzi, M., Bousset, K. et al. (2001). Human origin recognition complex binds to the region of the latent origin of DNA replication of Epstein–Barr virus. *EMBO J.*, **20**, 4588–4602.

Schulz, T. F. (1998). Kaposi's sarcoma-associated herpesvirus (human herpesvirus-8). *J. Gen. Virol.*, **79**(7), 1573–1591.

Schwam, D. R., Luciano, R. L., Mahajan, S. S., Wong, L., and Wilson, A. C. (2000). Carboxy terminus of human herpesvirus 8 latency-associated nuclear antigen mediates dimerization, transcriptional repression, and targeting to nuclear bodies. *J. Virol.*, **74**(18), 8532–8540.

Searles, R. P., Bergquam, E. P., Axthelm, M. K., and Wong, S. W. (1999). Sequence and genomic analysis of a Rhesus macaque rhadinovirus with similarity to Kaposi's sarcoma-associated herpesvirus/human herpesvirus 8. *J. Virol.*, **73**, 3040–3053.

Sears, J., Kolman, J., Wahl, G. M., and Aiyar, A. (2003). Metaphase chromosome tethering is necessary for the DNA synthesis and maintenance of *OriP* plasmids but is insufficient for transcription activation by EBNA1. *J. Virol.*, in press.

Sears, J., Ujihara, M., Wong, S., Ott, C., Middeldorp, J., and Aiyar, A. (2004). The amino terminus of Epstein–Barr Virus (EBV) nuclear antigen 1 contains AT hooks that facilitate the replication and partitioning of latent EBV genomes by tethering them to cellular chromosomes. *J. Virol.*, **78**, 11487–11505.

Sexton, C. J. and Pagano, J. S. (1989). Analysis of the Epstein–Barr virus origin of plasmid replication (*OriP*) reveals an area of nucleosome sparing that spans the 3′ dyad. *J. Virol.*, **63**(12), 5505–5508.

Shaw, J. E., Levinger, L. F., and Carter, C. W. (1979). Nucleosomal structure of Epstein–Barr virus DNA in transformed cell lines. *J. Virol.*, **29**, 657–665.

Shinohara, H., Fukushi, M., Higuchi, M. et al. (2002). Chromosome binding site of latency-associated nuclear antigen of Kaposi's sarcoma-associated herpesvirus is essential for persistent episome maintenance and is functionally replaced by histone H1. *J. Virol.*, **76**(24), 12917–12924.

Shirakata, M., Imadome, K. I., and Hirai, K. (1999). Requirement of replication licensing for the dyad symmetry element-dependent replication of the Epstein–Barr virus *OriP* minichromosome. *Virology*, **263**(1), 42–54.

Shire, K., Ceccarelli, D. F., Avolio-Hunter, T. M., and Frappier, L. (1999). EBP2, a human protein that interacts with sequences of the Epstein–Barr virus nuclear antigen 1 important for plasmid maintenance. *J. Virol.*, **73**, 2587–2595.

Snudden, D. K., Hearing, J., Smith, P. R., Grasser, F. A., and Griffin, B. E. (1994). EBNA-1, the major nuclear antigen of Epstein–Barr virus, resembles "RGG" RNA binding proteins. *EMBO J.*, **13**(20), 4840–4847.

Speck, S. H., Chatila, T., and Flemington, E. (1997). Reactivation of Epstein–Barr virus: regulation and function of the BZLF1 gene. *Trends Microbiol*, **5**, 399–405.

Stedman, W., Deng, Z., Lu, F., and Lieberman, P. M. (2004). ORC, MCM, and histone hyperacetylation at the Kaposi's sarcoma-associated herpesvirus latent replication origin. *J. Virol.*, **78**(22), 12566–12575.

Su, W., Middleton, T., Sugden, B., and Echols, H. (1991). DNA looping between the origin of replication of Epstein–Barr virus and its enhancer site: stabilization of an origin complex with Epstein–Barr nuclear antigen 1. *Proc. Natl Acad. Sci. USA*, **88**, 10870–10874.

Sugden, B. and Leight, E. R. (2001). EBV's plasmid replicon: an enigma in *cis* and *trans*. *Curr. Top. Microbiol. Immunol.*, **258**, 3–11.

Sugden, B. and Warren, N. (1989). A promoter of Esptein-Barr virus that can function during latent infection can be transactivated by EBNA-1, a viral protein required for viral DNA replication during latent infection. *J. Virol.*, **63**, 2644–2649.

Summers, H., Fleming, A., and Frappier, L. (1997). Requirements for Epstein-Barr nuclear antigen 1 (EBNA1)-induced permanganate sensitivity of the epstein–barr virus latent origin of DNA replication. *J. Biol. Chem.*, **272**(42), 26434–26440.

Sung, N. S., Wilson, J., Davenport, M., Sista, N. D., and Pagano, J. S. (1994). Reciprocal regulation of the Epstein–Barr virus BamHI-F promoter by EBNA-1 and an E2F transcription factor. *Mol. Cell. Biol.*, **14**(11), 7144–7152.

Szekely, L., Kiss, C., Mattson, K. et al. (1999). Human herpesvirus-8-encoded LNA-1 accumulates in heterochromatin-associated nuclear bodies. *J. Gen. Virol.*, **80** (11), 2889–2900.

Talbot, S. J., Weiss, R. A., Kellam, P., and Boshoff, C. (1999). Transcriptional analysis of human herpesvirus-8 open reading frames 71, 72, 73, K14, and 74 in a primary effusion lymphoma cell line. *Virology*, **257**(1), 84–94.

Tokai, N., Fujimoto-Nishiyama, A., Toyoshima, Y. et al. (1996). Kid, a novel kinesin-like DNA binding protein, is localized to chromosomes and the mitotic spindle. *EMBO J.*, **15**(3), 457–467.

Van Scoy, S., Watakabe, I., Krainer, A. R., and Hearing, J. (2000). Human p32: A coactivator for Epstein–Barr virus nuclear antigen-1-mediated transcriptional activation and possible role in viral latent cycle DNA replication. *Virology*, **275**, 145–157.

Viejo-Borbolla, A., Kati, E., Sheldon, J. A. et al. (2003). A domain in the C-terminal region of latency-associated nuclear antigen 1 of Kaposi's sarcoma-associated Herpesvirus affects transcriptional activation and binding to nuclear heterochromatin. *J. Virol.*, **77**(12), 7093–7100.

Vogel, M., Wittmann, K., Endl, E. et al. (1998). Plasmid maintenance assay based on green fluorescent protein and FACS of mammalian cells. *BioTechniques*, **24**, 540–544.

Wang, Y., Finan, J. E., Middledorp, J. M., and Hayward, S. D. (1997). P32/TAP, a cellular protein that interacts with EBNA-1 of Epstein–Barr virus. *Virology*, **236**, 18–29.

Watanabe, T., Sugaya, M., Atkins, A. M. et al. (2003). Kaposi's sarcoma-associated herpesvirus latency-associated nuclear antigen prolongs the life span of primary human umbilical vein endothelial cells. *J. Virol.*, **77**(11), 6188–6196.

Wen, L. T., Lai, P. K., Bradley, G., Tanaka, A., and Nonoyama, M. (1990). Interaction of Epstein–Barr viral (EBV) origin of replication (*OriP*) with EBNA-1 and cellular anti-EBNA-1 proteins. *Virology*, **178**(1), 293–296.

Wensing, B., Stuher, A., Jenkins, P., Hollyoake, M., Karstegl, C. E., and Farrell, P. J. (2001). Variant chromatin structure of the *OriP* region of Epstein–Barr virus and regulation of EBER1 expression by upstream sequences and *OriP*. *J. Virol.*, **75**, 6235–6241.

Wu, H., Ceccarelli, D. F., and Frappier, L. (2000). The DNA segregation mechanism of Epstein–Barr virus nuclear antigen 1. *EMBO Rep.*, **1**, 140–144.

Wu, H., Kapoor, P., and Frappier, L. (2002). Separation of the DNA replication, segregation, and transcriptional activation functions of Epstein–Barr nuclear antigen 1. *J. Virol.*, **76**(5), 2480–2490.

Wuu, K. D., Chen, Y. J., and Wuu, S. W. (1996). Frequency and distribution of chromosomal integration sites of the Epstein–Barr virus genome. *J. Formos. Med. Assoc.*, **95**(12), 911–916.

Wysokenski, D. A. and Yates, J. L. (1989). Multiple EBNA1-binding sites are required to form an EBNA1-dependent enhancer and to activate a minimal replicative origin within *OriP* of Epstein–Barr virus. *J. Virol.*, **63**(6), 2657–2666.

Yates, J. and Camiolo, S. M. (1988). Dissection of DNA replication and enhancer activation funcitons of Epstein–Barr virus nuclear antigen 1. *Cancer Cells*, **6**, 197–205.

Yates, J. L., and Guan, N. (1991). Epstein–Barr virus-derived plasmids replicate only once per cell cycle and are not amplified after entry into cells. *J. Virol.*, **65**(1), 483–488.

Yates, J. L., Warren, N., Reisman, P., and Sugden, B. (1984). *cis*-acting element from Epstein–Barr viral genome that permits stable replication of recombinant plasmids in latently infected cells. *Proc. Natl Acad. Sci. USA*, **81**, 3806–3810.

Yates, J. L., Warren, N., and Sugden, B. (1985). Stable replication of plasmids derived from Epstein–Barr virus in various mammalian cells. *Nature*, **313**, 812–815.

Yates, J. L., Camiolo, S. M., and Bashaw, J. D. (2000). The minimal replicator of Epstein–Barr virus *OriP*. *J. Virol.*, **74**, 4512–4522.

Yin, Y., Manoury, B., and Fahraeus, R. (2003). Self-inhibition of synthesis and antigen presentation by Epstein–Barr virus-endoded EBNA1. *Science*, **301**, 1334–1335.

Yu, L., Zhang, Z., Lowenstein, P. M. et al. (1995). Molecular cloning and characterization of a cellular protein that interacts with the human immunodeficiency virus type 1 Tat transactivator and encodes a strong transcriptional activation domain. *J. Virol.*, **69**(5), 3007–3016.

Zaldumbide, A., Ossevoort, M., Wiertz, E. J., and Hoeben, R. C. (2006). *In cis* inhibition of antigen processing by the latency-associated nuclear antigen I of Kaposi sarcoma Herpes virus. *Mol Immunol.*, in press.

Zhang, D., Frappier, L., Gibbs, E., Hurwitz, J., and O'Donnell, M. (1998). Human RPA (hSSB) interacts with EBNA1, the latent origin binding protein of Epstein–Barr virus. *Nucl. Acids Res.*, **26**, 631–637.

Zhang, S. and Nonoyama, M. (1994). The cellular proteins that bind specifically to the Epstein–Barr virus origin of plasmid DNA replication belong to a gene family. *Proc. Natl Acad. Sci. USA*, **91**(7), 2843–2847.

Zhong, W., Wang, H., Herndier, B., and Ganem, D. (1996). Restricted expression of Kaposi sarcoma-associated herpesvirus (human herpesvirus 8) genes in Kaposi sarcoma. *Proc. Natl Acad. Sci. USA*, **93**(13), 6641–6646.

Zimmermann, J. and Hammerschmidt, W. (1995). Structure and role of the terminal repeats of Epstein–Barr virus in processing and packaging of virion DNA. *J. Virol.*, **69**(5), 3147–3155.

Zhou, J., Chau, C. M., Deng, Z. et al. (2005). Cell cycle regulation of chromatin at an origin of DNA replication. *Embo J.*, **24**, 1406–1417.

Reactivation and lytic replication of EBV

Shannon C. Kenney

University of Wisconsin,
Madison, WI, USA

Viral pathogenesis

The lytic form of EBV infection is required for the production of progeny virus, and is thus essential for cell-to-cell spread of the virus, as well as transmission from host to host. Unfortunately, there is currently no cell culture system in vitro that is permissive for efficient primary lytic EBV infection. Although a recent report suggests that allowing the virus to first attach to the surface of primary B cells greatly facilitates EBV infection of epithelial cells in vitro (Shannon-Lowe et al., 2006), even this system of infection still does not result in efficient horizontal spread of virus from cell to cell. Thus, lytic EBV infection in vitro has been studied by reactivating the lytic form of infection from latently infected cell lines using a variety of inducing agents, including phorbol esters, butyrate, calcium ionophores, and B-cell receptor stimulation.

During primary infection, EBV probably initially infects oral epithelial cells in a lytic form, and then subsequently infects B-cells, where the virus usually assumes one of the latent forms of infection. In contrast to alpha and beta herpesviruses, which cause human diseases during the lytic form of viral infection but are essentially innocuous while in the latent form of infection, most illnesses attributable to EBV infection are associated with the latent forms of infection. During primary EBV infection, some individuals, particularly adolescents, develop the syndrome infectious mononucleosis (IM) approximately 1 month after being infected (Cohen, 2000; Jenson, 2000). The EBV-positive B-cells in patients with IM contain primarily the latent form(s) of infection, and the symptoms associated with this illness are attributable to the onset of a vigorous cytotoxic T-cell response against the virally infected B-cells (Cohen, 1999; Jenson, 2000; Andersson et al., 1987; Cohen, 2000). Lytic EBV infection (in either oral epithelial cells or B-cells) presumably precedes the onset of clinical IM, as IM patients have an extremely robust CD8 T-cell response directed against lytic viral protein epitopes (Steven et al., 1997; Hislop et al., 2002). Nevertheless, it has been difficult to document primary lytic EBV infection in patients, presumably due to the long asymptomatic incubation period for IM (Cohen, 1999, 2000).

Following recovery from IM, it is often difficult or impossible to find any lytically-infected cells in immunocompetent individuals (Herrmann et al., 2002), although the preponderance of evidence suggests that reactivated lytic EBV infection most commonly occurs in tonsillar plasma cells as well as in tonsillar B-cells (Laichalk et al., 2005; Pegtel et al., 2004; Niedobitek et al., 1997, 2000; Faulkner et al., 2000). Nevertheless, the only human disease that is unequivocally due to lytic EBV infection, oral hairy leukoplakia (OHL), occurs in epithelial cells on the lateral aspect of the tongue (Lau et al., 1993; Walling et al., 2001, 2003b; Greenspan et al., 1985; Resnick et al., 1990). This hyperproliferative lesion is observed only in highly immunocompromised patients and is easily treated by antiviral agents such as acyclovir that inhibit the lytic form of EBV infection. Interestingly, the lytic (but not latent) form of EBV infection was also recently found in the malignant breast epithelial cells, as well as normal breast cells, in some cases of breast cancer (Huang et al., 2003), suggesting that the breast may also be a site for lytic EBV replication.

The lytic form of EBV infection is clearly required for transmission of the virus from host to host, and thus is an essential aspect of viral pathogenesis. The saliva from immunocompetent hosts often contains infectious EBV (Shu et al., 1992; Lucht et al., 1995; Ikuta et al., 2000; Ling et al., 2003; Walling et al., 2003a), indicating that lytically infected cells in or near the oral cavity must exist, even if they are difficult to detect in the presence of a vigorous cytotoxic T-cell response (Tao et al., 1995). Thus it is not surprising that the great majority (90% or more) of the human population ultimately becomes infected with this virus. EBV has also been reported to be present in both male and female genital secretions, suggesting that this virus could in some instances be sexually transmitted (Israele *et al.*, 1991; Sixbey *et al.*, 1986).

Activation of lytic EBV infection

Lytic viral gene cascade

EBV lytic genes are expressed in a temporally regulated manner. In many cell lines the two immediate–early genes, BZLF1 and BRLF1, are the first viral genes expressed following lytic induction stimuli, and both BZLF1 and BRLF1 transcription occurs even in the presence of protein synthesis inhibitors (Biggin *et al.*, 1987; Flemington *et al.*, 1991; Takada and Ono, 1989). In some cell lines, such as the Burkitt lymphoma line, Akata, BZLF1 expression may precede BRLF1 expression (Yuan *et al.*, 2006). Once activated, the IE gene products function as transcription factors and together activate transcription of the early viral genes. Early viral genes are defined as genes that are transcribed prior to lytic viral replication (and thus are not inhibited by viral replication inhibitors), but are not transcribed in the presence of protein synthesis inhibitors. Early viral genes encode the viral replication proteins, including the virally encoded DNA polymerase. Following viral replication, the late viral genes are transcribed; late gene transcription is repressed by viral replication inhibitors. Many late genes encode structural proteins that make up the virion particle.

Stimuli that induce lytic EBV infection

In the human host, it is likely that differentiation of B cells into plasma following B-cell receptor stimulation by antigen (Laichalk and Thorley-Lawson, 2005) as well as differentiation in epithelial cells, both activate the lytic form of EBV infection (Tovey *et al.*, 1978; Young *et al.*, 1991). In cell culture systems in vitro, agents such as the phorbol ester, 12-0-tetradecanoyl phorbol-13-acetate (TPA), sodium butyrate, and calcium ionophores are commonly used to induce the lytic form of EBV infection (Faggioni *et al.*, 1986; zur Hausen *et al.*, 1978). Ultimately, what each of these various lytic EBV inducing stimuli shares is the ability to activate transcription of the two EBV IE genes, BZLF1 and BRLF1, from the latent viral genome. Lytic induction stimuli induce BZLF1 and BRLF1 transcription with similar kinetics (Biggin *et al.*, 1987; Flemington *et al.*, 1991; Takada and Ono, 1989), and many stimuli activate both the BZLF1 and BRLF1 promoters in EBV-negative cells (Zalani *et al.*, 1995; Shimizu and Takada, 1993; Feng *et al.*, 2004; Flemington and Speck, 1990d). Thus, other than possibly Akata cells, there is no firm evidence that one IE promoter is more important than the other for mediating lytic induction, and it may be that simultaneous activation of both promoters is required for efficient lytic induction. Once made, the BZLF1 and BRLF1 proteins function as transcription factors which activate their own promoters, as well as one another's promoters (Liu and Speck, 2003; Adamson *et al.*, 2000; Flemington *et al.*, 1991; Ragoczy and Miller, 2001; Sinclair *et al.*, 1991; Speck *et al.*, 1997; Zalani *et al.*, 1996), and thus greatly amplify the inducing effect of the initial lytic stimulus.

Of the various methods used in the lab to induce lytic EBV gene transcription, engagement of the B-cell receptor may be the most physiologic. B-cell receptor activation is accomplished using antibody directed against human IgG or IgM, depending upon which immunoglobulin is produced by the B-cell line. Akata Burkitt lymphoma cells are particularly responsive to this treatment, with up to 50% of cells converting to the lytic form of infection in a synchronous manner. Viral IE gene expression occurs very rapidly (30 minutes or less) after B-cell receptor engagement, followed a few hours later by early gene transcription (Takada and Ono, 1989; Mellinghoff *et al.*, 1991; Flemington *et al.*, 1991). Induction of lytic EBV infection by B-cell receptor engagement requires the activation of calcium-dependent signaling pathways (Chatila *et al.*, 1997; Liu *et al.*, 1997b), as well as the activation of numerous other signaling pathways (Adamson *et al.*, 2000; Bryant and Farrell, 2002; Darr *et al.*, 2001; Iwakiri and Takada, 2004; Mellinghoff *et al.*, 1991). The potential mechanism(s) leading from B-cell receptor engagement to EBV IE gene activation are outlined in Fig. 25.1. The LMP-2A viral latency protein helps to maintain viral latency by preventing the ability of antigen to activate B-cell receptor stimulated signaling pathways (Miller *et al.*, 1994a,b, 1995).

Certain cytokines, particularly TGF-beta, can also induce lytic viral infection in a subset of Burkitt lymphoma lines in vitro, and could potentially reactivate EBV in vivo (Fahmi *et al.*, 2000; Adler *et al.*, 2002). The interaction between CD4 T cells and EBV-infected B cells has also been reported to induce lytic infection (Fu and Cannon, 2000). Finally, there is increasing evidence that severe host cell stress in response to many different toxic stimuli (including chemotherapy and irradiation) can induce lytic EBV infection (Feng *et al.*, 2002a, 2004; Westphal *et al.*, 2000; Roychowdhury *et al.*, 2003).

In oral epithelial cells, lytic EBV infection is normally confined to differentiated cells. In OHL lesions, the EBV genome, and expression of lytic viral proteins, are only found in the more differentiated epithelial cell layers

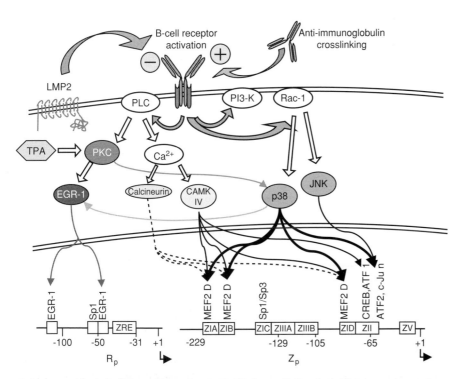

Fig. 25.1. Pathways leading to EBV reactivation in the host cell. Signal transduction pathways that are activated by B-cell receptor (BCR) engagement at the surface of the B-cell, or by phorbol ester (TPA) treatment of cells, are indicated. Promoter motifs in the two EBV IE promoters (Rp and Zp) that are activated by the signaling pathways are shown, as well as the transcription factors that bind to these motifs. Anti-immunoglobulin cross-links and activates the BCR, leading to activation of phosphotidylinositol 3-kinase (PI3K), Ras-family GTPases including Rac1, and phospholipase C gamma-2 (PLC). This is followed by activation of additional downstream pathways as indicated, including protein kinase C (PKC), calcium-dependent factors calcineurin and calcium/calmodulin-dependent kinase type IV (CAMK-IV), and stress MAP kinases (p38 and c-jun N-terminal kinase (JNK)). The EBV LMP-2 protein inhibits activation through the BCR. TPA activates PKC.

(Greenspan et al., 1985; Young et al., 1991). In vitro, differentiation of at least some EBV-positive epithelial lines induces the lytic form of EBV infection (Karimi et al., 1995; Li et al., 1992).

Many of the stimuli used to activate lytic EBV infection in vitro share the ability to activate a variety of signal transduction pathways, including PI3 kinase, p38 kinase, ERK kinase, and protein kinase C, and these kinases have been shown to be essential for induction of lytic EBV transcription by a number of different stimuli (Hayakawa et al., 2003; Mansouri et al., 2003; Fahmi et al., 2000; Fan and Chambers, 2001; Dent et al., 2003; Iwakiri and Takada, 2004; Furukawa et al., 2003; Ionescu et al., 2003; Gao et al., 2001; Satoh et al., 1999; Mellinghoff et al., 1991). In the case of anti-immunoglobulin treatment, activation of calcium-dependent signaling pathways also plays an essential role in lytic viral induction. Two different calcium-dependent proteins activated by B-cell receptor engagement, the calcium/calmodulin-dependent phosphatase, calcineurin, and the calcium/calmodulin-dependent protein kinase type IV/Gr, are required for lytic EBV induction by anti-IgG in Akata cells (Goldfeld et al., 1995; Chatila et al., 1997). Cyclosporin, an immunosuppressive drug that inhibits calcineurin, prevents anti-IgG induction of lytic EBV (Bryant and Farrell, 2002; Goldfeld et al., 1995). The relative importance of each particular signal transduction pathway may vary somewhat depending upon the nature of the stimulus and the cell type.

Organization of the IE gene region of EBV

The organization of the various transcripts and proteins derived from the EBV IE gene region is shown in Fig. 25.2. The immediate–early transcripts that encode BZLF1 and BRLF1 are derived from two different immediate–early promoters, Zp and Rp. The BRLF1 protein is encoded by messages initiating from Rp. These transcripts are bicistronic and could potentially make both the BRLF1 and BZLF1 gene products (Manet et al., 1989). There is some evidence that translation of the BZLF1 protein from the Rp-derived

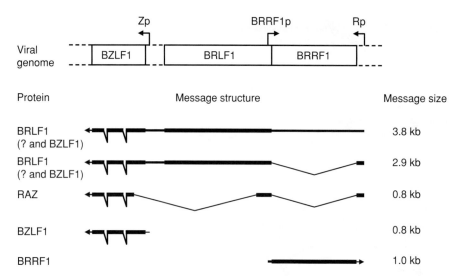

Fig. 25.2. Transcription of the EBV immediate-early gene region. The location of the two immediate-early (IE) genes, BZLF1 and BRLF1, the two IE promoters, Zp and Rp, and the BRRF1 early gene and promoter is shown. Rp directs transcription of a bicistronic message that encodes the BRLF1 and BZLF1 proteins. An alternatively spliced message encodes the RAZ protein, which may function as a negative regulator of BZLF1. The Zp-derived message is the major source of the BZLF1 protein. The BRRF1 promoter directs transcription of the early BRRF1 gene from the opposite DNA strand.

transcripts occurs in vivo, and that the BRLF1 protein is required for this process (Chang et al., 1998; Chang and Liu, 2001). However, the great majority of BZLF1 protein is probably derived from the BZLF1 transcript that initiates from the Zp promoter. A spliced message which contains parts of both BRLF1 and BZLF1 (referred to as RAZ), initiated from Rp, is transcribed later in infection and its gene product may serve as a negative regulator of BZLF1 transcriptional function (Furnari et al., 1994; Manet et al., 1989; Segouffin et al., 1996). The BRRF1 transcript, derived from the BRRF1 promoter and encoded by the opposite strand of the BRLF1 intron (Manet et al., 1989; Segouffin-Cariou et al., 2000), produces an early protein that was recently shown to be a transcriptional activator (Hong et al., 2004) important for efficient lytic EBV gene expression under certain circumstances.

Initial steps in viral reactivation

The promoters driving BZLF1 and BRLF1 transcription, Zp and Rp, are inactive in B-cells containing the latent form of EBV infection (Flemington et al., 1991; Zalani et al., 1992; Biggin et al., 1987; Takada and Ono, 1989; Mellinghoff et al., 1991). Epigenetic modifications such as DNA methylation and histone deacetylation likely contribute to inhibition of IE gene transcription in the context of the intact viral genome (Szyf et al., 1985; Paulson and Speck, 1999; Nonkwelo and Long, 1993; Falk and Ernberg, 1999; Ambinder et al., 1999; Paulson et al., 2002; Bhende et al., 2004; Jenkins et al., 2000; Gruffat et al., 2002b). Nevertheless, even "naked" DNA reporter gene constructs driven by the Zp and Rp promoters are essentially inactive in many EBV-negative B-cell lines (Feng et al., 2004; Kenney et al., 1989b; Sinclair et al., 1991; Zalani et al., 1995), but can be activated by lytic inducing stimuli such as TPA and B-cell receptor stimulation. Thus, the inactivity of the Zp and Rp promoters in unstimulated B cells must reflect the lack of trans-acting transcription factors, which positively regulate the two IE promoters, and/or the relative excess of cellular factors which negatively regulate the two IE promoters.

Cellular factors which activate Zp

Cellular transcription factors that positively and negatively regulate the Zp and Rp promoters are shown in Figs. 25.3 and 25.4. Regulation of the Zp promoter has been much more extensively studied than regulation of the Rp promoter. The region of Zp between −233 and +12 contains the cis-acting sequences required for Zp activation by lytic-inducing agents. Two types of cis-acting motifs, the "ZI" and "ZII" motifs, are critical for activation of Zp by a variety of different lytic-inducing stimuli. The four ZI motifs (ZIA, ZIB, ZIC, and ZID) are AT-rich sequences that have dual roles as both negative, as well as positive, regulators of Zp transcription (Borras et al., 1996; Daibata et al., 1994, Flemington and Speck, 1990a,b; Binne et al., 2002). In the absence of lytic-inducing agents, these elements down-regulate constitutive Zp activity in B cells. However,

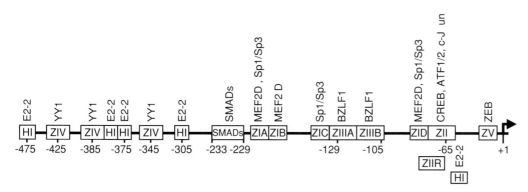

Fig. 25.3. Regulation of the EBV immediate–early BZLF1 promoter. Regulatory motifs in the BZLF1 (Zp) promoter are shown. Cellular and viral proteins known to bind to each motif are indicated.

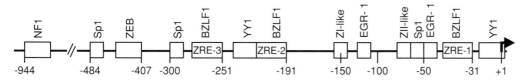

Fig. 25.4. Regulation of the EBV immediate–early BRLF1 promoter. Regulatory motifs in the BRLF1 (Rp) promoter are shown. Cellular and viral proteins known to bind to each motif are indicated.

the ZI elements are also essential for Zp activation by a variety of different inducing stimuli, including TPA, anti-immunoglobulin, calcium ionophores, and chemotherapy (Feng et al., 2004; Binne et al., 2002). Three of the four ZI motifs (ZIA, ZIB, ZID) bind to the transcription factor, MEF2D (Liu et al., 1997b). ZIA, ZIC and ZID also bind weakly to Sp1 and Sp3 (Liu et al., 1997a). This dual role of the ZI motifs as both negative, as well as positive, regulators of Zp transcription may reflect a preferential interaction of MEF2D with histone deacetylating complexes during viral latency (hence acting to inhibit Zp transcription), which is switched to a preferential interaction with acetylating complexes by lytic inducing stimuli (Gruffat et al., 2002b). The phosphorylation status of MEF2D may play an essential role in determining if it represses, versus activates, Zp transcription. Interestingly, calcium/calmodulin-dependent protein kinase type IV/Gr indirectly activates MEF2D by preventing the association between MEF2D and HDAC proteins, whereas MAP kinases directly activate MEF2D by phosphorylating the transcriptional activator domain and enhancing its function (McKinsey et al., 2000). Nevertheless, phosphorylation of other sites in MEF2D may inhibit its function (Li et al., 2001). Cross-linking the B-cell receptor in Akata Burkitt lymphoma cells results in rapid dephosphorylation of the MEF2D in a cyclosporine-sensitive manner, suggesting that calcineurin is involved in dephosphorylating (and perhaps activating) MEF2D (Bryant and Farrell, 2002).

The "ZII" motif is also essential for induction of BZLF1 transcription by most stimuli (Binne et al., 2002; Flamand and Menezes, 1996; Feng et al., 2004; Flemington and Speck, 1990d; Daibata et al., 1994; Chatila et al., 1997). The "ZII" motif is a slightly atypical CREB-responsive element (CRE) that binds CREB, ATF-1, the ATF-2/c-jun heterodimer, and possibly the c-jun/c-fos ("AP1") heterodimer as well (Flamand and Menezes, 1996; Flemington and Speck, 1990d; Liu et al., 1998; Adamson et al., 2000; Wang et al., 1997). The cellular factors which bind to CRE motifs are constitutively expressed in many cell lines, but cannot function as efficient transcriptional activators unless they are phosphorylated over specific residues by certain kinases. The c-jun N-terminal kinase (JNK) is the major activator of c-jun transcriptional function, while the stress Map kinase p38 phosphorylates and activates ATF-2. Many of the stimuli that induce lytic EBV infection in vitro (including B-cell receptor engagement, BRLF1-mediated induction, and certain chemotherapy agents) are known to activate the p38 and JNK kinases, and conversely, inhibitors of p38 and JNK kinases reduce the effectiveness of a number of lytic-inducing stimuli (Adamson et al., 2000; Feng et al., 2002a, 2004). Thus, the activated (phosphorylated) form of an ATF-2/c-jun heterodimer appears to be important for activation of BZLF1 transcription by a number of different stimuli.

Lytic induction may also be mediated through ATF-1 or CREB binding to the ZII motif (Wang et al., 1997), as the activated (phosphorylated) forms of these transcription factors activate Zp in reporter gene assays. Consistent with a role for ATF-1 and CREB in at least some cell types, activation of the Zp promoter induced by epithelial cell differentiation is associated with increased binding of ATF-1 and CREB to the Zp CRE motif (Karimi et al., 1995; MacCallum et al., 1999). In addition, engagement of the B-cell receptor results in calcium mobilization and activation of the calcium/calmodulin-dependent protein kinase type IV/Gr, which phosphorylates and activates CREB (Matthews et al., 1994). Both ATF-1 and CREB phosphorylation are observed transiently following anti-IgG treatment of Akata cells (Bryant and Farrell, 2002).

The BZLF1 promoter sequences –233 to –229 bind to Smad3/Smad4, which mediate signaling by the TGF-beta cytokine, and this region of the promoter is required for the TGF-beta activation of Zp that occurs in certain BL lines (Fahmi et al., 2000; Liang et al., 2002). In addition, TGF-beta activation of Zp requires the ZII motif (Liang et al., 2002). C-jun bound to the ZII motif interacts directly with Smad3/4 bound to the Smad binding site in Zp, perhaps explaining the need for both elements (Liang et al., 2002).

BZLF1 autoregulation

There are two ZRE sites in Zp (ZIIIA and ZIIIB), and BZLF1 activates Zp transcription in reporter gene assays (Binne et al., 2002; Flemington and Speck, 1990a). The Zp promoter (in the context of a stable oriP-containing episomal vector) cannot be efficiently activated by anti-IgG signaling in Akata cells when the ZIIIA site of Zp is deleted (Binne et al., 2002). These results suggest that the ability of Z to autoactivate its own transcription may be an essential component for induction of lytic EBV infection. However, it has been suggested that the ZIIIA site in Zp may also bind cellular factors required for induction of BZLF1 transcription by anti-Ig prior to the onset of BZLF1 binding to this site. Since BZLF1 activates TGF-beta transcription (Cayrol and Flemington, 1995), and TGF-beta activates the BZLF1 promoter in at least some cell lines, the TGF-beta pathway may serve as another potential mechanism by which BZLF1 activates its own promoter. Nevertheless, whether BZLF1 actually activates the Zp promoter in the context of the intact genome during viral reactivation remains controversial. A number of published reports suggest that it may not (Binne et al., 2002; Zalani et al., 1996; Le Roux et al., 1996).

Negative regulatory elements in Zp

Negative regulation of BZLF1 transcription may play a critical role in promoting viral latency in B cells. A number of different negative regulatory elements in the BZLF1 promoter have been identified. Of particular importance is the "ZV" motif located near the TATA box that binds to the zinc-finger protein, ZEB (Kraus et al., 2001, 2003). Deletion of this site significantly enhances activation of Zp induced by B-cell receptor engagement in Akata cells (Binne et al., 2002). Binding sites for the cellular YY-1 transcription factor have also been mapped (the "ZIV" elements), and shown to function as negative regulators of BZLF1 transcription (Montalvo et al., 1991, 1995). A cis-acting sequence, ZIIR, which overlaps the ZII motif, also reportedly inhibits Zp (Liu et al., 1998), although the cellular factor(s) binding to this repressor have not been identified. The cellular protein, smubp-2, binds to Zp ZI motifs and reportedly functions as a negative regulator, although it is not yet clear whether this negative regulation is mediated by direct binding of smubp-2 to Zp or acts more generally to disrupt formation of a stable TBP-TFIIA-DNA complex (Zhang et al., 1999b). Finally, a series of "H-box" elements, that are similar to E-box motifs and bind to the transcription factor E2–2, have been reported to function as negative regulators of Zp in B-cells, but positive regulators in epithelial cells (Thomas et al., 2003).

Regulation of Rp

Less is known about the regulation of the BRLF1 promoter (Rp) than the BZLF1 promoter. Both the BZLF1 and BRLF1 gene products activate this promoter in EBV-negative cells (Sinclair et al., 1991; Ragoczy and Miller, 2001; Zalani et al., 1992), and the combination of BZLF1 and BRLF1 together is more effective than either protein alone (Liu and Speck, 2003). The Rp promoter, like Zp, is activated by B-cell receptor stimulation, phorbol ester agents, and chemotherapy agents (Zalani et al., 1995; Sinclair et al., 1991; Feng et al., 2004). There are two EGR-1 (Zif-268) binding motifs in Rp, and activation of Rp by TPA and chemotherapy requires these sites in at least some cell types (Zalani et al., 1995; Feng et al., 2004). Phorbol esters, chemotherapy, and B-cell receptor engagement have all been shown to increase the level of cellular EGR-1, suggesting a common mechanism by which these inducing agents might activate BRLF1 transcription. There are also several Sp1 sites in Rp (Zalani et al., 1992), which are required for constitutive promoter activity as well as efficient autoactivation of Rp by its own gene product (Ragoczy and Miller, 2001; Liu and Speck, 2003). A binding site for NF1 has been reported to be a positive regulatory element in HeLa cells but not lymphoid cells (Glaser et al., 1998). There are at least three BZLF1 binding sites (ZREs) in Rp, and BZLF1 activation of Rp is mediated by direct binding of BZLF1 to these ZRE sites (Sinclair et al.,

1991; Liu and Speck, 2003; Bhende *et al.*, 2004). Like Zp, the Rp promoter also contains binding sites for the negative regulators, YY-1 and ZEB. The two YY-1 binding motifs function as negative regulators (Zalani *et al.*, 1997) of Rp; the role of the ZEB site, if any, has not yet been defined. Potential ZI-like and ZII-like motifs in Rp exist, but their function has not been studied.

Mechanisms by which TPA and Butyrate activate IE gene transcription

TPA treatment induces lytic EBV gene transcription in some cell lines, and this effect is at least partially mediated through TPA activation of protein kinase C (Gao *et al.*, 2001; Gradoville *et al.*, 2002). Why PKC activation leads to IE gene transcription is not totally clear, but it has been shown to require both the ZI and ZII motifs in Zp (Flemington and Speck, 1990d). In the case of the ZII motif, this may reflect the ability of TPA to activate the stress map kinases (p38 and c-jun N-terminal kinase) in a PKC-dependent manner (Grab *et al.*, 2004; Krappmann *et al.*, 2001), thus leading to phosphorylation of the ATF-2 and c-jun transcription factors which bind to the ZII site. TPA increases the level of EGR-1 in cells (Krappmann *et al.*, 2001), and the Rp EGR-1 binding sites are required for TPA activation of this promoter (Zalani *et al.*, 1995).

Agents that increase histone acetylation by inhibiting histone deacetylase (HDAC) activity, including sodium butyrate, trichostatin A, and valproic acid (Davie, 2003), also induce lytic EBV gene transcription in some cell lines. These agents presumably act by increasing the histone acetylation state of the two viral IE gene promoters (Jenkins *et al.*, 2000). Butyrate-responsive cellular genes (only 2% of all genes), like Zp and Rp, often have Sp1/Sp3 binding sites (Davie, 2003). Sp1 and Sp3 interact with HDAC proteins, as does MEF2D. Thus, in the absence of HDAC inhibitors, Sp1/Sp3 and MEF2D bound to the ZI motifs in Zp may act to inhibit Zp transcription by tethering HDAC complexes to the promoter, whereas in the presence of HDAC inhibitors these transcription factors instead interact with histone acetylases and activate Zp (Gruffat *et al.*, 2002b; Davie, 2003). Unlike the inducing effect of TPA, which requires PKC, the inducing effect of histone deacetylase inhibitors is PKC-independent (Gradoville *et al.*, 2002). HDAC inhibitors alone are insufficient to induce lytic EBV infection in many cell lines (Gradoville *et al.*, 2002), presumably because additional *trans*-acting factors are required to activate BZLF1 or BRLF1 transcription, and the combination of TPA and sodium butyrate is thus required for efficient induction of lytic viral gene expression in many cell lines.

Host cell and viral factors which influence stringency of viral latency

Of note, even in the most susceptible cell lines (generally BL lines), fewer than 50% of cells ever enter the lytic form of infection even when a combination of inducing agents is used. Why a portion of cells always remain in the latent form of viral infection (Gradoville *et al.*, 1990), while others switch to the lytic form of infection, is not currently well understood. In general, we have found that lymphoblastoid cell lines (LCLs) that have been extensively passaged are much more resistant to a variety of different inducing agents than newly derived lines, which often contain a portion of cells in the lytic form of infection even in the absence of inducing agents. In contrast to extensively passaged LCLs, BL lines often retain the ability to respond to one or more lytic-inducing agents.

The tendency of certain cell lines to remain tightly latent even in the face of multiple different inducing agents may be due to either viral and/or cellular factors. Viral factors that promote EBV latency include LMP-2A expression (since LMP-2A inhibits B-cell receptor mediated activation of Zp and Rp), as well as epigenetic modifications of Zp and Rp (including DNA methylation and/or chromatin deacetylation) (Gradoville *et al.*, 1990, 2002; Paulson and Speck, 1999; Nonkwelo and Long, 1993; Szyf *et al.*, 1985). Complete resistance to lytic inducing agents occasionally reflects an integrated viral genome. In some cell lines, such as the Raji BL line, inducing agents cause an abortive lytic infection, with expression of IE and early genes but no lytic viral replication, due to the deletion of one or more essential viral replication genes. In contrast, cell lines containing a defective rearranged form of the EBV genome, dHet, as well as wild-type virus, often have particularly high levels of lytic viral replication (Taylor *et al.*, 1989). This is because the defective rearranged viral genome contains the BZLF1 gene product under the control of the constitutively active EBNA-2 latency promoter, Wp (Countryman *et al.*, 1987; Rooney *et al.*, 1988; Grogan *et al.*, 1987). There is some evidence that similar defective rearranged viral genomes occur during natural infection in humans (Gan *et al.*, 2002; Walling *et al.*, 1992).

Cellular factors contributing to EBV latency include the activated (nuclear) form of NF-κB, which directly interacts with BZLF1 and inhibits its transcriptional function (Morrison and Kenney, 2004, Gutsch *et al.*, 1994). Likewise, the retinoic acid receptor also directly interacts with BZLF1 and inhibits its function (Sista *et al.*, 1993). Nitric oxide also potently down-regulates the lytic form of EBV infection (Gao *et al.*, 1999; Kawanishi, 1995). The cellular level of ZEB, which binds to the ZV motif and inhibits Zp activity

(Krauss et al., 2001, 2003), presumably also influences the stringency of EBV latency.

EBV immediate-early proteins

Introduction

Transcription of the BZLF1 and BRLF1 genes results in expression of the BZLF1 (also known at ZEBRA, Z, EB1 and Zta) and BRLF1 (R, Rta) proteins. Both BZLF1 and BRLF1 are transcription factors, and high-level expression of either BZLF1 or BRLF1 (under the control of a strong heterologous promoter) is sufficient to induce the switch from the latent to lytic form of EBV infection in some latently infected cell lines (Chevallier-Greco et al., 1986; Countryman and Miller, 1985; Rooney et al., 1989; Takada et al., 1986; Zalani et al., 1996; Westphal et al., 1999; Ragoczy et al., 1998). However, in many cell lines, BZLF1 is much more effective than BRLF1 for inducing lytic EBV gene expression, and in some cell lines (such as Raji cells and some lymphoblastoid lines) only BZLF1, and not BRLF1, can disrupt viral latency (Ragoczy and Miller, 1999; Zalani et al., 1996; Hong et al., 2004). Thus, activation of BZLF1 expression (and hence regulation of the Zp promoter) may be relatively more important in vivo for inducing lytic EBV infection than activation of BRLF1 expression. In contrast, only the BRLF1 homologue (and not the BZLF1 homologue) can induce lytic infection in latently infected KSHV cell lines.

BZLF1 transcriptional effects

BZLF1 is a homologue to c-jun and c-fos, and binds as a homodimer to AP-1 like motifs (including the consensus AP-1 site) known as Z-responsive elements (ZREs) (Chang et al., 1990; Packham et al., 1990; Lieberman et al., 1990; Lieberman and Berk, 1990; Farrell et al., 1989; Flemington and Speck, 1990a). BZLF1 transcriptionally activates immediate-early, and early, lytic EBV promoters (Urier et al., 1989; Lieberman et al., 1989; Rooney et al., 1989; Kenney et al., 1989b; Holley-Guthrie et al., 1990; Zetterberg et al., 2002). As shown in Fig. 25.5, the amino-terminus of BZLF1 encodes the transactivator domain (Flemington et al., 1992; Deng et al., 2001), as well as a region required for replication but not transcription (Sarisky et al., 1996). DNA binding is mediated through a domain that is highly homologous to the basic DNA binding domains of c-jun and c-fos (Flemington et al., 1994; Farrell et al., 1989). Homodimerization is mediated through a bZIP domain in the carboxy-terminal portion of the protein (Flemington and Speck, 1990c; Kouzarides et al., 1991). BZLF1 does

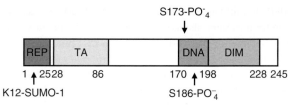

Fig. 25.5. EBV BZLF1 Immediate–early protein. Domains in the BZLF1 protein that mediate dimerization, DNA-binding and transactivation functions are shown, as well as certain phosphorylation and sumo-1 modification sites.

not heterodimerize efficiently with either c-fos or c-jun, but heterodimerizes with another cellular bZIP protein, C/EBP-alpha (Wu et al., 2003), and can activate at least some promoters through C/EBP-alpha binding sites. The crystal structure of BZLF1 was recently published (Petosa et al., 2006) and indicates that the bZIP domain in BZLF1 is somewhat unusual in that the carboxy-terminal region of the protein is also required to form a stable dimer.

BZLF1 activation of early lytic EBV promoters is generally mediated through direct binding of BZLF1 to ZRE motifs within the promoters (Flemington and Speck, 1990a; Urier et al., 1989). BZLF1 may also activate certain cellular promoters through a non-DNA binding mechanism (Flemington et al., 1994). In general, at least two ZRE sites are required for efficient activation of early viral promoters (Carey et al., 1992), and these sites are usually located within a few hundred basepairs of the transcriptional start site. Once bound to DNA, the ability of BZLF1 to interact directly with histone acetylating complexes (including CBP and p300) results in acetylation of chromatin, converting it to a conformation favorable for transcription (Adamson and Kenney, 1999; Chen et al., 2001a; Deng et al., 2003; Zerby et al., 1999). BZLF1 also interacts directly with a number of basic transcription factors, including TFIID and TFIIA (Chi and Carey, 1993; Chi et al., 1995; Lieberman and Berk, 1991, 1994; Lieberman et al., 1997; Mikaelian et al., 1993).

In the context of the intact viral genome, all evidence to date suggests that BZLF1 activation of the BRLF1 IE promoter precedes activation of the early lytic promoters, and that both the BZLF1 and BRLF1 gene products are required for activation of most early lytic genes (Feederle et al., 2000). BZLF1 may bind to the atypical ZRE sites in the BRLF1 promoter in a somewhat different manner (or perhaps conformation) than it binds to the consensus AP-1 site (El-Guindy et al., 2002). This point is perhaps most clearly indicated by the phenotype of a mutant BZLF1 protein in which serine 186 in the basic DNA binding domain is altered to alanine (the residue encoded by the analogous region in c-jun and c-fos). The Z(S186A) mutant cannot bind efficiently to either of the two ZRE sites in the BRLF1 promoter, although it binds efficiently to the consensus AP-1 site and a variety of ZRE sites within early EBV gene promoters (Adamson and Kenney, 1998; Francis et al., 1997). When transfected into latently infected cells, Z(S186A) cannot induce BRLF1 transcription, and consequently is completely defective for inducing early lytic EBV gene transcription, but its lytic defect is rescued by co-transfection with a BRLF1 expression vector (Francis et al., 1999; Adamson and Kenney, 1998). Serine residue 186 is phosphorylated by PKC in vitro, but whether this phosphorylation actually occurs in vivo remains controversial (El-Guindy et al., 2002; Baumann et al., 1998; Gradoville et al., 2002; Daibata et al., 1992). In lytically-infected B95–8 cells, BZLF1 is phosphorylated at residues Thr 14, Ser167, Ser173 and Ser186, and may be weakly phosphorylated at additional residues (El-Guindy et al., 2004, 2006). Phosphorylation of BZLF1 residues Ser167 and Ser173 by casein Kinase II, while not required for Z activation of early lytic genes, is required for efficient viral replication and modulates the ability of BRLF1 to regulate late gene transcription (El-Guindy and Miller, 2004).

BZLF1 activation of methylated ZRE motifs

The EBV genome is highly methylated during the latent form of viral infection, and DNA methylation of promoters generally acts as a potent inhibitor of cellular gene transcription. However, BZLF1 was recently shown to preferentially bind to the methylated vs. unmethylated, forms of two ZRE sites in Rp (Bhende et al., 2004). BZLF1 binding to the ZRE-2 site in Rp, which contains the sequence TGAGCGA, is much enhanced when the cytosine in this motif is methylated, and a previously unrecognized ZRE site in Rp, ZRE-3, which contains the sequence TTCGCGA, can only be bound by BZLF1 in the methylated form. Furthermore, BZLF1 preferentially activates the methylated form of the BRLF1 promoter in reporter-gene assays, and preferentially induces lytic EBV transcription from a methylated versus unmethylated, viral genome (Bhende et al., 2004). Thus, BZLF1 is the first example of a transcription factor that preferentially activates the methylated form of a downstream target gene. This unexpected ability of BZLF1 to activate methylated lytic viral promoters reveals a novel mechanism by which EBV circumvents the inhibitory effects of viral genome methylation.

BZLF1 activation of cellular genes

Not surprisingly, BZLF1 also transcriptionally activates certain cellular genes, some of which may be important for EBV pathogenesis. The cellular genes known to be activated by BZLF1 include TGF-beta (Cayrol and Flemington, 1995), c-fos (Flemington and Speck, 1990b), the tyrosine kinase TKT (Lu et al., 2000), matrix metalloproteinases 1 and 9 (Lu et al., 2003; Yoshizaki et al., 1999), and cellular IL-10 (Mahot et al., 2003). BZLF1 activation of the immunosuppressive cytokines, TGF-beta and IL-10, could potentially dampen the host immune response during the lytic form of virus infection, whereas induction of the matrix metalloproteinases could potentially enhance metastasis of EBV-positive tumors cells expressing BZLF1. In addition, cellular IL-10 is a potent B-cell growth factor, suggesting a mechanism by which lytic EBV gene expression in a small percentage of cells could promote B-cell malignancies in a paracrine manner.

BZLF1 replication function

In addition to its essential role as a transcription factor, BZLF1 also plays a direct role in lytic viral replication. BZLF1 binds directly to a number of ZRE sites in the lytic origin of replication, oriLyt, and this binding is required for oriLyt replication (Fixman et al., 1992, 1995; Hammerschmidt and Sugden, 1988; Schepers et al., 1993a,b). Furthermore, a BZLF1 mutant altered at residues 12/13 is transcriptionally competent, but completely defective for mediating viral replication (Sarisky et al., 1996). BZLF1 also interacts directly with some of the core viral replication proteins (Zhang et al., 1996; Takagi et al., 1991; Gao et al., 1998). Together, these results suggest that BZLF1 acts as an essential oriLyt binding protein during lytic EBV replication, and that this binding may promote formation of the initial replication complex.

The BZLF1-knockout virus is less efficient in promoting lymphoproliferative disease in SCID mice

The phenotype of a BZLF1-deleted EBV has been recently described (Feederle et al., 2000) in 293 cells and primary B cells. As expected, this mutant cannot undergo the lytic form of EBV replication unless the BZLF1 gene product is expressed in trans. In 293 cells infected with the BZLF1-knockout virus, expression of the BZLF1 gene product induces expression of the IE protein, BRLF1, as well as the complete complement of early and late lytic genes. In contrast, expression of the BRLF1 gene product in 293 cells infected with BZLF1-knockout virus does not result in expression of the majority of early or late genes. The BZLF1-knockout virus is not reported to be defective in immortalizing B cells. The phenotype of the BZLF1-knockout virus confirms that both BZLF1 and BRLF1 transcriptional functions are required for the induction of many (but not all) lytic EBV genes in the context of the intact viral genome.

Surprisingly, however, recent findings suggest that early-passage lymphoblastoid cell lines (LCLs) derived from either BZLF1-deleted, or BRLF1-deleted, viruses are less efficient than lines derived using wild-type virus in regard to their ability to form lymphoproliferative disease in SCID mice (Hong et al., 2005a,b). LCLs containing the BZLF1-deleted virus secrets less of the two B-cell growth factors, cellular IL-6 and cellular IL-10, and less of the potent angiogenesis factor, VEGF, than LCLs from the same donor containing wild-type EBV. These results suggest that a small number of lytically infected cells may contribute to the growth of some EBV-associated tumors in vivo through the release of paracrine growth factors or angiogenesis factors.

BZLF1 effects on the host cell environment

In addition to its essential roles as a transcription factor and viral replication protein, BZLF1 alters the host cell environment in numerous different ways that presumably act together to enhance the efficiency of lytic viral replication. As the first viral protein expressed during lytic reactivation (and primary lytic infection), BZLF1 is ideally situated to protect the virus from a variety of different host defenses, including cellular apoptosis and the host innate immunity, and to regulate the host cell cycle.

BZLF1 cell cycle effects

There is increasing evidence that herpesviruses usurp the host cell cycle control mechanisms to assure adequate substrates for lytic viral DNA replication. However, the cell cycle effects of BZLF1 appear to be cell-type dependent. BZLF1 produces a profound G1/S block in some cell types, including primary fibroblasts (Rodriguez et al., 1999, 2001a; Cayrol and Flemington, 1995, 1996a,b; Mauser et al., 2002b; Wu et al., 2003). In cell types susceptible to this G1/S block, BZLF1 decreases expression of cyclin A and c-myc (Mauser et al., 2002b; Rodriguez et al., 2001b), and increases p21 expression (Wu et al., 2003; Cayrol and Flemington, 1996b). BZLF1 activates p21 expression through a C/EBP-alpha binding site in the p21 promoter, an effect that involves the direct interaction between BZLF1 and C/EBP-alpha (Wu et al., 2003). In other cell types, such as HeLa cells, BZLF1 induces both a G2 and mitotic block (Mauser et al., 2002a; Cayrol and Flemington, 1996a). The G2 block results from decreased cyclin B, while the mitotic block is associated with a defect in chromosome condensation (Mauser et al., 2002a).

Nevertheless, the cell types in which BZLF1 induces cell cycle blocks are either not normally infected by EBV (fibroblasts), and/or are likely to be deficient in normal cell cycle regulation controls (tumor cells). In sharp contrast to the results in fibroblasts and tumor cell lines, in telomerase-immortalized, as well as primary, keratinocytes, BZLF1 actually enhances expression of a number of S-phase dependent cellular proteins, and increases the level of E2F-1, cyclin E and cyclin A (Mauser et al., 2002b). Likewise, inducible BZLF1 expression in the EBV-immortalized marmoset B-cell line, B95-8, results in enhanced activity of cyclin-dependent kinases, although cellular DNA replication is blocked (Kudoh et al., 2003). Most importantly, agents that inhibit the activity of cyclin-dependent kinases also inhibit lytic EBV gene expression (Kudoh et al., 2004), although it is not currently understood why cyclin-dependent kinases are required for efficient lytic EBV replication. These results suggest that a "pseudo-lateG1/S-phase" environment, in which certain late G1/S-phase restricted cellular proteins are expressed, but cellular DNA does not actually replicate, may be the ideal host cell environment for lytic EBV replication. Inhibition of cellular DNA replication presumably decreases competition between the virus and host cell DNA for limiting substrates involved in DNA replication, while the expression of certain G1/S-phase restricted cellular proteins, such as E2F-1, may be required for viral replication.

BZLF1 effects on p53

Activation of p53 in host cells serves as an important host defense mechanism, since p53 induces cellular apoptosis and hence limits viral replication. Not surprisingly, therefore, many viruses, including herpesviruses, encode proteins that inhibit various aspects of p53 function. The effects of BZLF1 on p53 in the host cell are quite complex. Somewhat paradoxically, in some (but not all) cell types, the presence of BZLF1 results in a rather dramatic increase in the level of total p53, and induces a number of post-translation modifications of p53 (including a series of activating phosphorylations and acetylations) that are usually associated with enhanced p53 transcriptional function (Mauser et al., 2002c). BZLF1 also increases the amount of p53 binding in some cell types (Mauser et al., 2002c). This activation of p53 that occurs in BZLF1-expressing cells may represent an attempt by the host cell to limit EBV replication. Nevertheless, the majority of evidence suggests that BZLF1 quite efficiently inhibits p53 transcriptional function (Zhang et al., 1994; Mauser et al., 2002c). BZLF1 inhibition of p53 may be due in part to the previously observed direct interaction between the BZLF1 and p53 proteins (Zhang et al., 1994). In addition, BZLF1 significantly reduces the level of the basic transcription factor, TATA-binding protein (TBP), in host cells, and restoration of this protein partially reverses the ability of BZLF1 to inhibit p53 transcriptional function (Mauser et al., 2002c). Finally, as discussed below, BZLF1-mediated dispersion of nuclear PML bodies in host cells may also decrease p53 function, since optimal p53 transcriptional function requires PML bodies. In any event, given that p53 is an important cellular mediator of apoptosis, the ability of BZLF1 to inhibit p53 function likely plays a crucial role in protecting the virus from apoptosis during the earliest timepoints of lytic infection.

BZLF1 dispersion of PML bodies

Promyelocytic leukemia (PML) bodies, also known as nuclear domain 10 (ND-10) bodies, are nuclear structures which contain a number of different cellular proteins, including CREB-binding protein (CBP), Sp100, Rb, Daxx, ISG20, and the small ubiquitin-related modifier, sumo-1 (Bernardi and Pandolfi, 2003; Salomoni and Pandolfi, 2002). Only the PML protein is absolutely essential for formation of PML bodies, and the PML protein must be covalently modified by sumo-1 in order to form these bodies. Although the exact function(s) of PML bodies is somewhat mysterious, the fact that the formation of these bodies is dramatically enhanced by both type I and type II interferons, and that a number of different viruses encode proteins capable of dispersing PML bodies, suggests that these bodies have an antiviral function (Chee et al., 2003; Bernardi and Pandolfi, 2003; Salomoni and Pandolfi, 2002). PML bodies have been proposed to be important for certain types of apoptosis, MHC class I presentation, efficient acetylation of p53, interferon effects, and for the stability and function of an important cellular DNA repair complex, Mre11/Rad50/NBS1 (Bernardi and Pandolfi, 2003; Salomoni and Pandolfi, 2002; Chee et al., 2003). As each of these proposed functions would be expected to reduce viral replication, it is perhaps not surprising that many viruses attempt to inhibit the formation of PML bodies.

High level BZLF1 expression in EBV-negative cells is sufficient to disperse PML bodies, and this effect is correlated with the ability of BZLF1 to inhibit sumo-1 modification of the PML protein (Bell et al., 2000; Adamson and Kenney, 2001). BZLF1 itself is efficiently modified by sumo-1 over lysine 12, and the ability of BZLF1 to inhibit PML protein sumo-1 modification may be at least partially due to competition between BZLF1 and PML for limiting amounts of sumo-1 in the host cell (Adamson and Kenney, 2001). A BZLF1 mutant altered at residues 12 and 13 is transcriptionally competent, but defective in mediating lytic replication (Sarisky et al., 1996). Thus, sumo-1 modification of BZLF1 may be primarily important for its replicative, rather than transcriptional, function.

In the context of the intact virus, lytic EBV infection in cells results in the release of proteins such as Sp100 and Daxx from ND10 bodies, followed by the release of PML (Bell et al., 2000). Lytic viral replication commences after dispersion of the Sp100 and Daxx proteins, but prior to the onset of PML dispersion, and lytic viral replication complexes are often closely associated with dispersed PML protein aggregates (Bell et al., 2000). These findings suggest that reorganized PML complexes may play a role in promoting lytic EBV replication.

BZLF1 effects on the host immune response

BZLF1 plays a key role in attenuating the host immune response to lytic viral infection. PML bodies are required for an efficient antiviral effect of interferon alpha in herpes simplex virus 1 infection (Chee et al., 2003), suggesting that BZLF1-mediated dispersion of PML bodies may protect lytic EBV infection from interferon alpha. BZLF1 also strongly inhibits transcription of the gene encoding an essential component of the interferon gamma receptor, and thereby abrogates interferon gamma signaling in host cells (Morrison et al., 2001). This ability of BZLF1 to inhibit interferon gamma signaling is likely important not only for protecting the virus from the immunostimulatory effects of interferon gamma (including induction of MHC class II and IRF-1), but may also be required for epithelial cell-derived virus to efficiently infect B cells. Virus produced in cells expressing MHC class II, which would normally be induced by gamma interferon in infected epithelial cells if BZLF1 did not prevent this, preferentially infects epithelial cells, whereas virus produced in cells not expressing MHC class II preferentially infects B cells (Borza and Hutt-Fletcher, 2002). In addition to preventing interferon gamma signaling, BZLF1 was recently shown to directly interact with, and inhibit the function of, IRF7 (Hahn et al., 2005). AS IRF7 augments production of type I interferons, the interaction between BZLF1 and IRF7 no doubt helps the virus to attenuate the antiviral effects of interferon alpha and beta in lytically infected cells.

Tumor necrosis factor alpha (TNF-alpha) is another important antiviral cytokine inhibited by BZLF1 expression in host cells. TNF-alpha not only activates expression of a number of important inflammatory genes (through its effects on NF-KB), but also induces cellular apoptosis. As TNF-alpha production is an immediate, and important component of the host immune response to viral infection, not surprisingly many viruses encode proteins that limit the effects of TNF-alpha in the infected host cell. In the case of lytic EBV infection, BZLF1 dramatically inhibits the activity of the promoter for the gene encoding the major

TNF-alpha receptor (TNF-R1) (Morrison et al., 2004). Since TNF-R1 is a fairly short-lived protein, this reduction in TNF-R1 transcription results in dramatically decreased expression of the TNF-R1 protein. Thus, TNF-alpha cannot activate transcription of important downstream target genes such as ICAM-1 in BZLF1-expressing cells, and is also unable to induce cellular apoptosis (Morrison et al., 2004). The exact mechanism(s) by which BZLF1 inhibits transcription of the genes encoding the TNF-R1 and interferon gamma receptors has not yet been defined.

Complex interactions between BZLF1 and the NF-KB transcription factor are also involved in inhibiting expression of many different NF-KB dependent cellular genes involved in the host immune response. BZLF1 interacts directly with the p65 component of NF-KB, and this interaction inhibits the transcriptional function of BZLF1 (Gutsch et al., 1994; Hong et al., 1997). However, recent evidence suggests that BZLF1 also potently inhibits NF-KB-dependent activation of promoters (Keating et al., 2002; Morrison and Kenney, 2004), and decreases NF-KB binding to promoters in the context of the intact cellular genome (Morrison and Kenney, 2004). Thus, the IL-1 cytokine cannot activate NF-KB-responsive cellular genes in the presence of BZLF1, even though the upstream components of the IL-1 signaling pathway appear to be unaffected by BZLF1 (Morrison and Kenney, 2004). Somewhat paradoxically, however, since one of the NF-KB responsive genes inhibited by BZLF1 is I-kappa B (IK-B) (Morrison and Kenney, 2004), and the IK-B protein normally acts to retain NF-KB in the cytoplasm in an inactive form, BZLF1-expressing cells actually have a very high level of nuclear NF-KB (Morrison and Kenney, 2004). This BZLF1-mediated translocation of NF-KB into the nucleus may act to negatively regulate BZLF1 transcriptional function and hence promote viral latency in situations where BZLF1 expression is limiting relative to the amount of nuclear NF-KB.

Finally, BZLF1 also regulates cellular cytokine expression in ways that would be anticipated to protect the virus. As discussed previously, BZLF1 stimulates expression of both TGF-beta, and IL-10 (Cayrol and Flemington, 1995). Both TGF-beta and IL-10 have immunomodulatory effects that would be expected to attenuate the cytotoxic T cell response directed against the virus. In addition, BZLF1 inhibits expression of MHC class I on cells (Keating et al., 2002; Mahot et al., 2003). This latter effect may be at least partially mediated through BZLF1 effects on NF-KB, although other pathways appear to be involved, as well (Keating et al., 2002). The immunomodulatory effects of BZLF1 are summarized in Fig. 25.6.

The role of BRLF1 in lytic induction

Expression of the EBV immediate–early protein, BRLF1, also induces lytic EBV infection in a subset of latently infected cell lines (Feederle et al., 2000; Ragoczy et al., 1998; Zalani et al., 1996; Westphal et al., 1999). Interestingly, the BRLF1 homologue in KSHV (ORF50) is the major inducer of lytic infection for this virus. Even in cell lines (such as the Raji Burkitt lymphoma line) where BRLF1 expression by itself is not sufficient to disrupt viral latency, it is clear that BRLF1 expression is required (in concert with BZLF1) to activate many early lytic genes, including BMRF1 (Feederle et al., 2000; Ragoczy and Miller, 1999). Consistent with this, the BRLF1 gene product is essential for lytic viral replication (Feederle et al., 2000). Like BZLF1, BRLF1 also binds directly to the EBV oriLyt (Gruffat and Sergeant, 1994; Hammerschmidt and Sugden, 1988). In contrast to the importance of certain oriLyt ZRE sites, the BRLF1 binding sites in oriLyt are not absolutely essential for oriLyt replication, at least in plasmid-based replication assays (Fixman et al., 1992).

The primarily nuclear BRLF1 gene product is a transcriptional activator that contains an amino-terminus DNA binding domain and homodimerization domain (Manet et al., 1991) and a carboxy-terminal transcriptional activation domain (Hardwick et al., 1988, 1992)(Fig. 25.7). The transcriptional activator domain of BRLF1 interacts directly with TBP and TFIIB (Manet et al., 1993). BRLF1 also interacts directly with the histone acetylase, CREB-binding protein (CBP) (Swenson et al., 2001). BRLF1 activates lytic EBV gene promoters through at least two different mechanisms. BRLF1 binds directly to a GC-rich motif (consensus GGCCN$_7$GTGGTG) which is present in the promoters of at least three early EBV genes, SM (formerly called BMLF1), BHRF1, and BMRF1 (Gruffat et al., 1990; Gruffat et al., 1992; Gruffat and Sergeant, 1994; Kenney et al., 1989a; Quinlivan et al., 1993). In the case of the BHRF1 and SM promoters, the BRLF1-binding motifs function as powerful enhancer elements in the presence of the BRLF1 protein (Kenney et al., 1989a; Cox et al., 1990; Chevallier-Greco et al., 1989). In the case of the BMRF1 promoter, BRLF1 by itself induces little activation, but cooperates with BZLF1 to produce efficient activation of this promoter (Holley-Guthrie et al., 1990; Quinlivan et al., 1993).

In contrast, BRLF1 activates its own promoter (Rp) and the BZLF1 promoter (Zp) through mechanisms that do not involve direct DNA binding of BRLF1 to these promoters. BRLF1 stimulation of its own promoter requires the Rp Sp1 motifs (Ragoczy and Miller, 2001; Liu and Speck, 2003), although it is not yet known exactly how (or if) BRLF1 regulates cellular factors binding to the Sp1 motif. BRLF1

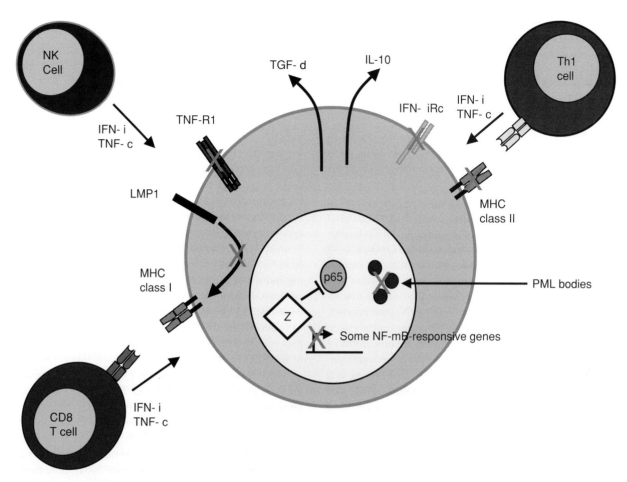

Fig. 25.6. Inhibitory effects of BZLF1 on host immunity. BZLF1 activates transcription of the immunosuppressive cytokines, TGF-beta and IL-10, while decreasing transcription of the receptors for interferon gamma and TNF-alpha. BZLF1 inhibits the transcriptional activity of the p65 component of NF-kappa B and abrogates MHC class I induction by LMP1. BZLF1 also mediates dispersion of PML bodies, which are important for MHC class I expression and response to alpha interferon.

stimulation of the Zp promoter requires the ZII motif, and is likely mediated by BRLF1 activation of the c-jun and ATF-2 transcription factors (Adamson et al., 2000). BRLF1 expression in cells activates the stress Map kinases (p38 and c-jun N-terminal kinase) (Adamson et al., 2000), as well as PI3 kinase (Darr et al., 2001), and inhibition of either p38 stress Map kinase, or PI3 kinase, activity abolishes the ability of BRLF1 to activate BZLF1 transcription, or disrupt viral latency (Adamson et al., 2000; Darr et al., 2001). BRLF1 stimulation of the viral DNA polymerase promoter is also mediated through an indirect mechanism, involving USF and E2F-1 binding motifs (Liu et al., 1996).

The inability of BRLF1 expression by itself to induce fully lytic gene expression in certain cell lines, such as Raji, primarily reflects the inability of BRLF1 to activate BZLF1 transcription in these cell lines (Zalani et al., 1996). In Raji cells, BRLF1 by itself efficiently activates an early promoter (SM promoter) that is directly bound by BRLF1, but cannot activate Zp, or an early viral promoter, BMRF1, which requires the combination of BZLF1 and BRLF1 for activation (Ragoczy and Miller, 1999). Why BRLF1 induces BZLF1 transcription in some latently infected cell lines, but not others, is not currently understood.

BRLF1-knockout virus phenotype

A BRLF1-deleted knockout virus has been made and its phenotype studied in 293 cells as well as primary B cells (Feederle et al., 2000). As is the case for the BZLF1-knockout virus, the BRLF1-knockout virus immortalizes primary B cells with efficiency similar to wild-type virus, but early-passage B cell lines obtained with BRLF1-deleted virus

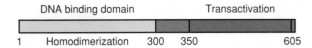

Fig. 25.7. EBV BRLF1 immediate–early protein. Domains in the BRLF1 protein that mediate dimerization, DNA-binding and *trans*-activation functions are shown.

are impaired for producing lymphoproliferative disease in SCID mice (Feederle et al., 2000; Hong et al., 2005a,b). In 293 cells, the BRLF1-knockout virus is unable to enter the lytic form of infection, or express the BZLF1 immediate–early gene, unless the BRLF1 gene product is supplied in trans. These results confirm that the BRLF1 gene product is an important and essential activator of the Zp IE promoter, and that many early viral promoters require both BZLF1 and BRLF1 functions for activation in the context of the intact viral genome. As discussed later, this particular BRLF1-knockout virus was subsequently discovered to be unable to express an early EBV gene product, BRRF1. The phenotype of the "BRLF1-knockout" virus in certain cell types is also partially due to the loss of BRRF1 expression, which cooperates with BRLF1 to activate transcription of BZLF1 (Hong et al., 2004). Nevertheless, it is clear that the BRLF1 gene product is essential for fully lytic EBV gene expression, as well as lytic viral replication, in all cell lines tested to date (Feederle et al., 2000; Hong et al., 2004).

There is emerging evidence that BRLF1 may be able to activate transcription of a subset of late viral genes even in the absence of viral replication. In 293 cells containing the BZLF1-knockout virus, BRLF1 induces expression of a subset of "late" genes, although the virus cannot replicate due to the lack of BZLF1 expression (Feederle et al., 2000). BRLF1 also activates some late genes in Raji cells, in which the viral genome is unable to replicate (Ragoczy and Miller, 1999). The exact mechanism by which BRLF1 activates late genes has not been well defined. Assuming that BRLF1 also activates certain late genes when expressed at a physiologic level in the context of the intact viral genome, the regulation of EBV late gene transcription may be fundamentally different from that of late viral genes in the alpha herpesviruses. The ability of BRLF1 to activate certain viral late genes is modulated by the BZLF1 protein (El-Guindy and Miller, 2004).

BRLF1 activation of the cellular fatty acid synthase gene

Recent evidence suggests that BRLF1 activation of the cellular gene, fatty acid synthase (FAS), may be an essential component in BRLF1-mediated induction of lytic EBV infection (Li et al., 2004). The FAS enzyme is required for the synthesis of many different lipids, including palmitate, and high-level expression of FAS is normally restricted to fat cells and liver cells. BRLF1 robustly activates FAS gene expression in host cells, and this effect is lost in the presence of p38 kinase inhibitors. Of potential therapeutic interest, agents known to specifically inhibit the FAS enzyme (cerulenin and C75) also inhibit the ability of transfected BRLF1 to induce the lytic form of EBV gene expression, including induction of BZLF1 transcription (Li et al., 2004). In contrast, FAS inhibitors do not affect the ability of transfected BZLF1 (driven by a strong heterologous promoter) to induce lytic EBV gene expression. These results suggest cellular FAS activity is required for BRLF1 activation of the BZLF1 promoter (Zp). Exactly why this is the case remains unknown, but may reflect the fact that palmitoylation of proteins is often required for entry of these proteins into lipid rafts, and the ability of these proteins to initiate signal transduction cascades. Since FAS inhibitors also repress anti-IgG induction of lytic EBV in Akata cells, and the constitutively lytic EBV infection which occurs in AGS (gastric carcinoma) cells (Li et al., 2004), they could potentially be developed as a completely novel approach for inhibiting the earliest aspects of lytic EBV infection in patients.

BRLF1 cell cycle effects

Like BZLF1, BRLF1 also profoundly affects the regulation of the host cell cycle. BRLF1 expression results in an increased number of cells in S-phase in both primary human fibroblasts and HeLa cells, and this effect is associated with dramatically increased E2F-1 expression (Swenson et al., 1999). In addition, since BRLF1 activates the promoter of the viral DNA polymerase gene through an E2F-1 site (rather than a direct binding mechanism) (Liu et al., 1996), the ability of BRLF1 to increase the level of E2F-1 in the host cell may be required for efficient transcription of the viral DNA polymerase (and consequently efficient lytic viral replication). BRLF1 also interacts directly with the tumor suppressor protein, Rb (Zacny et al., 1998). Since Rb plays an essential role in regulating the host cell cycle, the interaction between Rb and BRLF1 may be a mechanism by which BRLF1 activates cell cycle progression.

Early lytic EBV gene regulation

The expression of the two immediate–early proteins, BZLF1 and BRLF1, allows the subsequent expression of viral early genes. In the context of the intact viral genome, transcriptional activation of many early promoters, such as BMRF1, requires that both the BZLF1 and the BRLF1 gene products be expressed (Feederle et al., 2000; Cox et al., 1990). The most extensively studied early lytic EBV promoter is the BMRF1 gene promoter. This promoter contains two BZLF1 binding motifs, as well as one BRLF1 binding site (Holley-Guthrie et al., 1990; Quinlivan et al., 1993). In reporter gene assays in EBV-negative cells, BZLF1 alone efficiently activates the BMRF1 promoter (an effect which requires that both of the ZRE sites be present), whereas the BRLF1 gene product by itself at most modestly activates the BMRF1 promoter. In some cell types, but not others, the combination of BZLF1 and BRLF1 together is significantly more effective than BZLF1 alone at activating BMRF1 reporter gene plasmids (Holley-Guthrie et al., 1990). In cells containing the latent form of EBV infection, all data to date suggest that the combination of both BZLF1 and BRLF1 is required for significant activation of BMRF1 transcription, regardless of cell type (Adamson and Kenney, 1998; Feederle et al., 2000; Ragoczy and Miller, 1999; Zalani et al., 1996).

Nevertheless, the relative importance of the BZLF1 versus BRLF1 gene products for activation of early gene transcription in the context of the intact viral genome appears to be promoter-specific. The early SM promoter, which contains at least one BZLF1 binding motif, as well as a BRLF1 binding site, can be activated by transfected BRLF1 in a cell line (Raji) where BRLF1 cannot induce BZLF1 expression from the endogenous viral genome (Ragoczy and Miller, 1999; Swenson et al., 2001). Thus the SM early promoter can be activated by BRLF1 alone, even in the context of the intact viral genome. Two other early promoters, BHLF1 and BHRF1, which are divergent promoters contained within the lytic EBV origin of replication, oriLyt, have been extensively studied in vitro, but much less so in the context of the intact virus. There are two strong BRLF1 binding sites located between the BHLF1 and BHRF1 promoters in oriLyt (Gruffat and Sergeant, 1994); in reporter gene assays, the BHRF1 promoter appears to be more responsive to BRLF1 than the BHLF1 promoter (Hardwick et al., 1988; Cox et al., 1990). Both the BHLF1 and BHRF1 promoters have two or more BZLF1 sites and are activated by BZLF1 alone in reporter gene assays (Hardwick et al., 1988). The relative importance of BZLF1 vs. BRLF1 for BHLF1 vs. BHRF1 transcriptional activation in the context of the intact virus has not been well studied.

Early lytic EBV gene products

Replication proteins

Many of the early lytic EBV gene products are directly involved in mediating the lytic form of viral replication. The six core viral replication proteins which mediate lytic viral replication include the catalytic component of the viral DNA polymerase (BALF5), the DNA polymerase processivity factor (BMRF1), the single-stranded DNA binding protein (BALF2), helicase (BBLF4), primase (BSLF1), and primase-associated protein (BBLF2/3)(Fixman et al., 1992). In addition, some early EBV genes encode enzymes involved in deoxynucleotide metabolism, including the viral thymidine kinase gene (BXLF1) (Littler et al., 1986), the viral dUTPase gene (Fleischmann et al., 2002) and viral ribonucleotide reductase (BORF2 and BARF1). From the results of studies performed on the analogous genes in HSV-1, it is likely that these early EBV gene products are required for efficient production of nucleotide substrates in non-replicating cells. In addition, the EBV-encoded thymidine kinase (TK) function may be required for the therapeutic effect of the antiviral drug, acyclovir, as the EBV TK is a deoxypyrimidine kinase that phosphorylates a broad range of nucleoside analogues (such as acyclovir) not recognized efficiently by the cellular TK (Littler and Arrand, 1988).

Transcription factors

There are at least two viral transcription factors encoded by early lytic EBV genes. Interestingly, the BMRF1 gene product (Cho et al., 1985) functions not only as the viral DNA polymerase-processivity factor (Tsurumi et al., 1993, 1994), but also as a transcription factor (Zhang et al., 1997, 1999a). BMRF1 activates transcription of the oriLyt promoter, BHLF1, and the BMRF1-responsive region of this promoter is contained within a GC-rich domain (the downstream essential domain) that is also essential in cis for oriLyt replication (Zhang et al., 1997). The exact mechanism by which BMRF1 activates oriLyt transcription is not yet known. The transcriptional function of BMRF1 requires its carboxy-terminal domain (Zhang et al., 1999a), which is not required for DNA polymerase-processivity function in vitro (Kiehl and Dorsky, 1991; 1995).

Another early lytic viral transcription factor is the BRRF1 gene product (Hong et al., 2004). The BRRF1 gene is encoded by the opposite strand of the first intron of the BRLF1 immediate–early gene (Segouffin-Cariou et al., 2000). BRRF1 enhances the transcriptional function of c-jun, and activates the BZLF1 immediate–early promoter through the CRE ("ZII") motif (Hong et al., 2004). BRRF1 activation of c-jun transcriptional function is associated with increased c-jun phosphorylation, although the precise mechanism for this effect is not yet known. Although BRRF1 expression alone is not sufficient to activate BZLF1 transcription from the latent viral genome, BRRF1 function is required for efficient BRLF1-mediated activation of Zp in some latently infected cell lines (Hong et al., 2004). A knockout virus originally thought to specifically delete the BRLF1 gene product (Feederle et al., 2000) was subsequently shown to be defective in BRRF1 transcription, and rescue of the fully lytic phenotype of this virus requires both the BRLF1 and BRRF1 gene products in trans (Hong et al., 2004). KSHV contains a gene that is homologous to BRRF1 in the analogous position of the viral genome and has a similar function (Gonzalez et al., 2005).

SM: a protein that regulates RNA transport and stability

In contrast to the latent and IE genes of EBV, the early and late genes often contain no introns. RNA derived from intronless genes is often unstable in cells. The early lytic gene product, SM (previously known as BMLF1) (Cook et al., 1994), is an RNA-binding protein which plays an important role in increasing the stability of intronless lytic viral transcripts, as well as promoting the transport of such messages from the nucleus to the cytoplasm (Kenney et al., 1989c; Gruffat et al., 2002a; Hiriart et al., 2003a,b; Boyle et al., 1999, 2002; Buisson et al., 1989, 1999; Chen et al., 2001b; Farjot et al., 2000; Ruvolo et al., 1998, 2001, 2004; Semmes et al., 1998). The SM protein thus acts to create a cellular environment in which viral lytic (intronless) messages are preferentially expressed over cellular (intron-containing) messages. Recent studies of an SM-knockout virus confirm that the SM gene product is essential for efficient viral replication and virion production (Gruffat et al., 2002a). Another recently described function of the SM protein is its ability to inhibit PKR activation (Poppers et al., 2003), which appears to be distinct from its effect on RNA. PKR inhibition by SM would presumably allow the virus to escape the inhibitory effect of PKR activation on protein translation. In contrast, SM actually enhances the expression of STAT1 (Ruvolo et al., 2003); it is as yet unclear how this activation benefits the virus.

Proteins that inhibit cellular apoptosis and immune evasion

EBV also encodes an early lytic gene product, BHRF1, which inhibits cellular apoptosis. BHRF1 is a homologue of the cellular anti-apoptosis gene, BCL-2, and like BCL-2 inhibits apoptosis in response to a number of different stimuli (Henderson et al., 1993; Tarodi et al., 1994). The ability of BHRF1 to prevent cellular apoptosis very likely increases the efficiency of lytic EBV viral replication by preventing the death of the host cell prior to the completion of replication.

The BARF1 early gene encodes a soluble receptor for colony-stimulating factor 1 (Strockbine et al., 1998). BARF1 inhibits the differentiating and proliferative effects of this cytokine on monocytes/macrophages (Strockbine et al., 1998), and decreases alpha-interferon secretion from monocytes/macrophages (Cohen and Lekstrom, 1999). Thus, BARF1 may be important for protecting the virus from antiviral effects mediated through monocytes and macrophages.

A viral kinase

The BGLF4 early gene encodes a viral kinase (EBV-PK) which is homologous to the UL97 gene product of cytomegalovirus. In addition to autophosphorylation, at least two other EBV proteins, BMRF1 and the EBNA Leader protein, are phosphorylated by the BGLF4 kinase (Kato et al., 2001, 2003; Chen et al., 2000; Gershburg and Pagano, 2002), although the effect of this phosphorylation on BMRF1 and EBNA Leader protein function is not currently defined. In addition, like the CMV (UL97) and HSV (UL13) homologues, BGLF4 also phosphorylates the cellular protein, translation elongation factor 1 delta (Kato et al., 2001). To date the kinase motifs recognized by the BGLF4 and homologous proteins encoded by CMV and HSV appear to be similar to cdc2 kinase motifs (Kawaguchi et al., 2003). Although the exact function of the BGLF4 kinase during lytic EBV replication has not yet been clearly defined, as is the case with the CMV (but not HSV) homologue, BGLF4 expression in cells results in phosphorylation of the antiviral nucleoside analogue, ganciclovir, converting it to the active form (Marschall et al., 2002). Thus, ganciclovir (as well as acyclovir) can be used to inhibit lytic EBV replication.

Viral replication

Lytic EBV replication probably occurs through a rolling-circle mechanism and involves the formation of head-to-tail concatamers of the genome. Lytic EBV replication requires the lytic origin of replication (oriLyt) in cis, and the viral core replication proteins (BALF5, BMRF1, BBLF2, BBLF4, BSLF1, and BBLF2/3) in trans (Fixman et al., 1992,

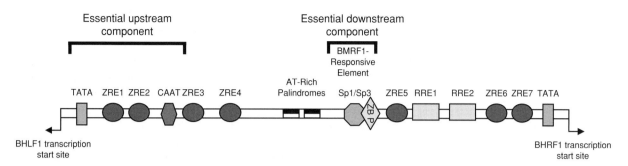

Fig. 25.8. *Cis*-acting elements of oriLyt. OriLyt overlaps the divergent promoters of two early genes, BHLF1 and BHRF1. The locations of BZLF1 (ZRE) and BRLF1 (RRE) binding sites, as well as the binding sites of cellular transcription factors ZBP-89, Sp1, and Sp3, are shown. The localization of two essential elements in oriLyt that are absolutely required for replication in indicated.

1995). Each of these core replication proteins is absolutely essential for the lytic form of replication, and a number of these core replication proteins directly interact with one another, presumably allowing formation of a large replication initiation complex (Daibata and Sairenji, 1993; Fujii *et al.*, 2000; Gao *et al.*, 1998; Liao *et al.*, 2001). In addition, the BZLF1 IE protein is absolutely required for replication, even when the core replication proteins are expressed under strong constitutive heterologous promoters. BZLF1 interacts directly with the core replication proteins, BMRF1 and BBLF4 (Zhang *et al.*, 1996; Liao *et al.*, 2001).

EBV DNA polymerase activity is mediated by the catalytic component of the enzyme (BALF5) in conjunction with the polymerase processivity factor (BMRF1). The catalytic component of the polymerase also has 3′-to 5′ proofreading exonuclease activity (Tsurumi *et al.*, 1993). The EBV polymerase, in contrast to cellular polymerase, is active in high-salt (100 mM ammonium sulfate) (Tsurumi *et al.*, 1993).

There are usually two copies of oriLyt in the EBV genome, although viral strains that contain only one copy of ori-Lyt (such as B95–8) seem to replicate equally well. The minimal oriLyt contains the divergent promoters of two EBV early genes, BHRF1 and BHLF1, as well as binding sites for the two EBV immediate-early proteins, BZLF1 and BRLF1 (Hammerschmidt and Sugden, 1988) (Fig. 25.8). Two domains of oriLyt are absolutely essential for replication. The "upstream" essential domain contains two binding sites for BZLF1, and BZLF1 binding to these sites is required for replication (Schepers *et al.*, 1993a,b, 1996). The "downstream" essential domain is a GC-rich sequence bound by the Sp1, Sp3 and ZBP-89 cellular transcription factors (Baumann *et al.*, 1999; Gruffat *et al.*, 1995; Schepers *et al.*, 1993b), and this region also mediates BMRF1 transcriptional effects (Zhang *et al.*, 1997). ZBP-89 binding appears to be particularly important for oriLyt replication, and ZBP-89 over-expression in cells enhances replication of an oriLyt containing plasmid (Baumann *et al.*, 1999). In addition, the ability of the downstream essential domain to form a triple helix DNA structure may be required for oriLyt replication (Portes-Sentis *et al.*, 1997).

Once replication is completed, the virus is clipped within the terminal repeat region of the genome into a linear, unit-length genome and then packaged into virion particles. The EBV terminal repeats are sufficient to allow packaging of plasmids in *cis* (Zimmermann and Hammerschmidt, 1995); however, the viral proteins that mediate the cleavage and packaging functions have not been identified.

Late viral gene regulation

Late EBV genes are traditionally defined as genes that are expressed after the onset of viral replication; expression of late genes is inhibited by agents that prevent viral DNA replication. Relatively little is known about the regulation of late EBV promoters. Unlike the early viral promoters, the late promoters do not usually contain BZLF1 or BRLF1 binding sites. Assuming that EBV late viral gene promoters are regulated in a similar manner as the late viral gene promoters in herpes simplex virus, it would be anticipated that EBV late promoters are primarily activated in cis by viral replication, and that this effect requires only a small region of the upstream promoter sequences. However, recent studies using the BZLF1- and BRLF1- knockout viruses have indicated that the requirement for viral replication may not be as absolute for late gene expression in gamma herpesviruses as it appears to be the case for alpha herpesviruses. For example, expression of the BRLF1 immediate-early protein in cells containing the BZLF1- knockout virus induces expression of a subset of "late" genes in the absence of viral replication (Feederle *et al.*, 2000). BRLF1 can also activate some late genes in Raji cells in the absence of viral replication (Ragoczy and Miller, 1999). In reporter gene assays, certain late promoters are also activated in a replication-independent manner (Serio *et al.*, 1997, 1998).

Late viral proteins

Many late genes encode structural viral proteins, including the nucleocapsid proteins that make up the virion particle. The viral glycoproteins which mediate EBV binding and fusion to the cellular receptor and co-receptor (gp350/220, gp85, gp42, gp25) are also encoded by late genes and are further discussed in Chapter 23. In addition, EBV encodes at least one late viral gene product, vIL-10 (BCLF1), that is likely important for protecting the virus from the host immune response. The vIL-10 gene product is a homologue of cellular IL-10 (Hsu *et al.*, 1990) and shares its ability to potently repress the cytotoxic T-cell response. Therefore, secretion of viral IL-10 from lytically infected cells would be expected to protect the virus from this response (Salek-Ardakani *et al.*, 2002). In addition, as both cellular and viral IL-10 function as B-cell growth factors, the lytically infected pool of EBV-positive B cells could potentially support the growth of the latently infected pool through a paracrine mechanism involving the release of viral IL-10 (Miyazaki *et al.*, 1993; Stuart *et al.*, 1995; Rousset *et al.*, 1992). An EBV mutant virus deleted in the viral IL-10 gene was not found to be defective in B-cell transformation in vitro or lymphoma formation in mice (Swaminathan *et al.*, 1993); however, the lack of an obvious phenotype in this mutant virus may reflect the finding that BZLF1 induces cellular IL-10, and that the functions of cellular and viral IL-10 are redundant. Perhaps not surprisingly, one or more late viral gene products also appear to inhibit apoptosis, suggesting that prevention of cellular apoptosis is important for efficient EBV infection throughout the lytic replication cycle (Inman *et al.*, 2001). A late viral protein which has homology to the anti-apoptotic cellular Bcl-2 protein is encoded by the BALF1 gene, but whether this protein inhibits or activates apoptosis remains controversial (Marshall *et al.*, 1999; Bellows *et al.*, 2002).

Viral assembly and egress

At the end of the lytic replication cycle, the structural proteins involved in initiation of infection must be reassembled into the mature virion. Current models of herpesvirus assembly and egress propose that capsids are first built around a scaffold in the nucleus, that the scaffold is then lost to make room for packaging of the genome, and that the completed nucleocapsids, associated with at least some of the tegument proteins, bud through the inner nuclear membrane into the perinuclear space, acquiring a first envelope in the process. De-enveloped nucleocapsids are then delivered to the cytoplasm by fusion with the outer nuclear membrane or that of the endoplasmic reticulum. The final envelope and additional or different tegument proteins are acquired during rebudding into a cytoplasmic compartment, probably the trans-golgi network, that puts the virus back into a later stage of the exocytic pathway for release by exocytosis (for review see Mettenleiter, 2002). This model has been developed primarily from the study of alphaherpesviruses. However, the probability that EBV follows a similar envelopment, de-envelopment, reenvelopment pathway is supported by observations of the B-958 strain of EBV where higher levels of glycoprotein gB are seen in the nuclear membrane of cells producing virus than in mature enveloped virions and there is a reverse distribution of the major virion glycoprotein gp350/220 (Gong and Kieff, 1990). This is, in turn, dependent on a second soluble nuclear protein, BFLF2 (Gonella *et al.*, 2005; Lake and Hutt-Fletcher, 2004). These two proteins are conserved throughout the herpesvirus family and appear to have similar functions in each. In addition, however, the EBV glycoprotein gB also plays a role in nuclear egress (Herrold *et al.*, 1995). This function is not shared by the gB homologs of the alpha and betaherpesviruses. One possibility is that gB, known to be essential for glycoprotein-mediated cell fusion (Haan *et al.*, 2001), is required for the fusion of the first virus envelope with the outer nuclear membrane. Acquisition of the second and final envelope requires a complex of glycoproteins gN and gM (Lake and Hutt-Fletcher, 2000), but little more is known about the process aside from the provocative finding that loss of the transforming protein LMP1 severely impairs virus release (Ahsan *et al.*, 2005). These final and critical stages in EBV replication remain poorly understood.

Treatment of lytic EBV infection

Lytic EBV infection is inhibited by both acyclovir and ganciclovir (Lin and Machida, 1988; Datta *et al.*, 1980; Lin *et al.*, 1987; Meerbach *et al.*, 1998). The nucleoside analogues, acyclovir and ganciclovir, are phosphorylated to their active forms in lytically infected cells, presumably due to the effects of the two viral kinases, EBV thymidine kinase and BGLF4 (Lin *et al.*, 1986; Moore *et al.*, 2001; Marschall *et al.*, 2002). As acyclovir is less toxic than ganciclovir in patients, acyclovir is the preferred agent for treating the one disease that is definitely due to lytic EBV infection, oral hairy leukoplakia. The antiviral drug foscarnet, which inhibits the viral DNA polymerases of all known herpesviruses and effectively inhibits lytic EBV replication in vitro (Datta and

Hood, 1981), could also theoretically be used to treat lytic EBV infection in patients. However, as foscarnet is quite toxic, and there is no evidence to date that EBV strains resistant to acyclovir or ganciclovir are a clinical problem, foscarnet is not currently used to treat lytic EBV infection in patients. There is no convincing evidence that inhibition of lytic EBV infection in immunocompetent patients with infectious mononucleosis shortens or ameliorates this illness (Torre and Tambini, 1999). Whether acyclovir or ganciclovir treatment is useful in treating early polyclonal EBV-associated lymphoproliferative disease in post-transplant patients is somewhat controversial (Cohen, 2000; Oertel et al., 1999). As lytic EBV gene products are not currently thought to be required for immortalization and growth of B cells in vitro (Feederle et al., 2000), it is not clear that preventing this form of infection in vivo would slow the growth of EBV-immortalized B cells in patients. There is more convincing evidence suggesting that anti-viral prophylaxis reduces the subsequent development of EBV-associated lymphoproliferative disease in transplant recipients (Farmer et al., 2002; Malouf et al., 2002; Green et al., 2001; Fong et al., 2000; McDiarmid et al., 1998; Darenkov et al., 1997). In this case, inhibition of lytic EBV infection presumably reduces the pool of latently infected B cells, thereby decreasing the probability that one or more of these cells eventually becomes malignant.

Lytic induction as a strategy for treating EBV-positive tumors

Finally, the purposeful induction of lytic EBV infection in EBV-positive tumor cells is increasingly being explored as a potential way to selectively kill EBV-infected tumor cells (Gutierrez et al., 1996; Israel and Kenney, 2003; Westphal et al., 1999). Theoretically, EBV-positive tumors containing the latent forms of viral infection could be switched to the lytic form of infection by either inducing expression of the EBV immediate–early genes from the endogenous viral genome in tumors, or by using gene delivery methods to express either of the EBV immediate–early proteins in tumor cells. When adenovirus vectors expressing either the BZLF1 or BRLF1 gene products are injected directly into EBV-positive nasopharyngeal carcinoma tumors grown in nude mice, tumor growth is inhibited, whereas control adenovirus vectors have no effect (Feng et al., 2002b). In addition, certain cytotoxic therapies, including some chemotherapy agents and gamma irradiation, have been found to induce lytic EBV gene transcription in at least a portion of tumor cells (Feng et al., 2002a, 2004; Roychowdhury et al., 2003; Westphal et al., 2000). Lytic induction by cytotoxic agents is mediated through activation of the two EBV immediate-early promoters and requires the PI3 kinase, p38 kinase, and MAP kinase pathways (Feng et al., 2002a, 2004). Specific transcription factor binding sites in both the BZLF1 promoter (ZI and ZII), and the BRLF1 promoter (EGR-1) are also required (Feng et al., 2004). Agents that inhibit histone deacetylases (such as butyrate compounds) have also been shown to enhance the amount of lytic EBV infection in some mouse tumor models (Westphal et al., 2000).

Lytic induction strategies are most effective for inhibiting tumor growth when combined with the antiviral drug, ganciclovir (Mentzer et al., 1998; Feng et al., 2002a, 2004; Faller et al., 2001; Roychowdhury et al., 2003; Westphal et al., 2000). In cells containing the lytic (but not latent) type of EBV infection, virally encoded kinases (BGLF4 and the viral thymidine kinase) are expressed which phosphorylate the nucleoside analogue, ganciclovir, converting it to its active cytotoxic form (Moore et al., 2001). Phosphorylated ganciclovir inhibits not only viral DNA replication, but also inhibits the host cell DNA replication, and is thus cytotoxic. Furthermore, phosphorylated ganciclovir can be transferred into nearby cells that are unable to phosphorylate ganciclovir (i.e., tumor cells with latent EBV infection), and thus induce "bystander" killing. As chemotherapy and irradiation induce lytic infection in only a portion of tumor cells, the combination of these agents with ganciclovir is much more effective than either agent alone for treating EBV-positive tumors in mouse models (Feng et al., 2002a, 2004). Whether ganciclovir will be effective in combination with lytic induction strategies for treating EBV-positive human tumors is currently being investigated (Faller et al., 2001; Mentzer et al., 2001).

Unresolved issues for the future

The discovery in 1985 that BZLF1 activates lytic EBV expression in latently infected cells was a true milestone in our understanding of lytic EBV gene regulation. Since then, many further advances have been made. However, many questions remain. For example, numerous EBV-encoded microRNAs were recently discovered, including microRNAs which overlap the lytic BHRF1 (anti-apoptosis) and BALF5 (viral DNA polymerase) genes (Shen and Goodman, 2004; Pfeffer et al., 2004) as well as multiple microRNAs located in the introns of the latent BART gene (Cai et al., 2006). Since microRNAs generally promote gene silencing by targeting homologous mRNAs for degradation, the EBV-encoded microRNAs may serve to promote the latent form of viral infection. However, at this point relatively little is known regarding the regulation of microRNA formation during EBV infection, and whether these microRNAs do indeed regulate viral gene expression. Furthermore, will EBV, like a growing list of other viruses, encode a mechanism for preventing the effect of host genome-derived, antiviral microRNAs?

We still know very little about the nature of the proteins comprising the viral tegument. Does EBV, like other herpesviruses, have a viral tegument protein which serves to transcriptionally activate the viral IE promoters during primary lytic infection? The availability of modern proteomic techniques should allow us to determine the cellular and viral protein composition of the virion, as well as how lytic EBV infection affects cellular proteins. A proteomic analysis of the virion particle was recently published (Johannsen et al., 2004).

It remains unclear which viral proteins confer sensitivity to commonly used antiviral drugs, including acyclovir and ganciclovir. Are these drugs activated primarily by the viral thymidine kinase, or the viral protein kinase (BGLF4)? Alternatively, is the combination of both of these viral proteins required for nucleoside analogue activation in EBV-infected cells? Can we develop new drugs (potentially fatty acid synthase inhibitors) that would inhibit lytic EBV infection at its earliest step, i.e., expression of the viral immediate-early proteins. If we could completely prevent lytic EBV infection in patients (such as organ transplant recipients) who are highly prone to the development of EBV-associated malignancies, would this reduce the number of EBV-induced tumors?

These are only a few of the many questions that will need to be answered by future investigators. What remains certain is that EBV will remain an important and fascinating pathogen for many years to come.

Acknowledgment

Many thanks to Lindsey Hutt-Fletcher, who wrote the "Viral assembly and egress" section in this chapter.

REFERENCES

Adamson, A. L. and Kenney, S. C. (1998). Rescue of the Epstein–Barr virus BZLF1 mutant, Z(S186A), early gene activation defect by the BRLF1 gene product. *Virology*, **251**(1), 187–197.

Adamson, A. L. and Kenney, S. (1999). The Epstein–Barr virus BZLF1 protein interacts physically and functionally with the histone acetylase CREB-binding protein. *J. Virol.*, **73**(8), 6551–6558.

Adamson, A. L. and Kenney, S. (2001). Epstein–Barr virus immediate-early protein BZLF1 is SUMO-1 modified and disrupts promyelocytic leukemia bodies. *J. Virol.*, **75**(5), 2388–2399.

Adamson, A. L., Darr, D., Holley-Guthrie, E. et al. (2000). Epstein–Barr virus immediate-early proteins BZLF1 and BRLF1 activate the ATF2 transcription factor by increasing the levels of phosphorylated p38 and c-Jun N-terminal kinases. *J. Virol.*, **74**(3), 1224–1233.

Adler, B., Schaadt, E., Kempkes, B., Zimber-Strobl, U., Baier, B., and Bornkamm, G. W. (2002). Control of Epstein–Barr virus reactivation by activated CD40 and viral latent membrane protein 1. *Proc. Natl Acad. Sci. USA*, **99**(1), 437–442.

Ahsan, N., Kanda, T., Nagashima, K., and Takada, K. (2005). Epstein–Barr virus transforming protein LMP1 plays a critical role in virus production. *J. Virol.*, **79**, 4415–4424.

Ambinder, R. F., Robertson, K. D., and Tao, Q. (1999). DNA methylation and the Epstein–Barr virus. *Semin. Cancer Biol.*, **9**(5), 369–375.

Andersson, J., Skoldenberg, B., Henle, W. et al. (1987). Acyclovir treatment in infectious mononucleosis: a clinical and virological study. *Infection*, **15 Suppl 1**, S14–S20.

Baumann, M., Mischak, H., Dammeier, S. et al. (1998). Activation of the Epstein–Barr virus transcription factor BZLF1 by 12-O-tetradecanoylphorbol-13-acetate-induced phosphorylation. *J. Virol.*, **72**(10), 8105–8114.

Baumann, M., Feederle, R., Kremmer, E., and Hammerschmidt, W. (1999). Cellular transcription factors recruit viral replication proteins to activate the Epstein–Barr virus origin of lytic DNA replication, oriLyt. *EMBO J.*, **18**(21), 6095–6105.

Bell, P., Lieberman, P. M., and Maul, G. G. (2000). Lytic but not latent replication of epstein–barr virus is associated with PML and induces sequential release of nuclear domain 10 proteins. *J. Virol.*, **74**(24), 11800–11810.

Bellows, D. S., Howell, M., Pearson, C., Hazlewood, S. A., and Hardwick, J. M. (2002). Epstein–Barr virus BALF1 is a BCL-2-like antagonist of the herpesvirus antiapoptotic BCL-2 proteins. *J. Virol.*, **76**(5), 2469–2479.

Bernardi, R. and Pandolfi, P. P. (2003). Role of PML and the PML-nuclear body in the control of programmed cell death. *Oncogene*, **22**(56), 9048–9057.

Bhende, P. M., Seaman, W. T., Delecluse, H. J., and Kenney, S. C. (2004). The EBV lytic switch protein, Z, preferentially binds to and activates the methylated viral genome. *Nat. Genet.*, **36**(10), 1099–1104.

Biggin, M., Bodescot, M., Perricaudet, M., and Farrell, P. (1987). Epstein–Barr virus gene expression in P3HR1-superinfected Raji cells. *J. Virol.*, **61**(10), 3120–3132.

Binne, U. K., Amon, W., and Farrell, P. J. (2002). Promoter sequences required for reactivation of Epstein-Barr virus from latency. *J. Virol.*, **76**(20), 10282–10289.

Borras, A. M., Strominger, J. L., and Speck, S. H. (1996). Characterization of the ZI domains in the Epstein–Barr virus BZLF1 gene promoter: role in phorbol ester induction. *J. Virol.*, **70**(6), 3894–3901.

Borza, C. M. and Hutt-Fletcher, L. M. (2002). Alternate replication in B cells and epithelial cells switches tropism of Epstein–Barr virus. *Nat. Med.*, **8**(6), 594–599.

Boyer, J. L., Swaminathan, S., and Silverstein, S. J. (2002). The Epstein–Barr virus SM protein is functionally similar to ICP27 from herpes simplex virus in viral infections. *J. Virol.*, **76**(18), 9420–9433.

Boyle, S. M., Ruvolo, V., Gupta, A. K., and Swaminathan, S. (1999). Association with the cellular export receptor CRM 1 mediates function and intracellular localization of Epstein–Barr virus SM protein, a regulator of gene expression. *J. Virol.*, **73**(8), 6872–6881.

Bryant, H. and Farrell, P. J. (2002). Signal transduction and transcription factor modification during reactivation of Epstein–Barr virus from latency. *J. Virol.*, **76**(20), 10290–10298.

Buisson, M., Manet, E., Trescol-Biemont, M. C., Gruffat, H., Durand, B., and Sergeant, A. (1989). The Epstein–Barr virus (EBV) early protein EB2 is a posttranscriptional activator expressed under the control of EBV transcription factors EB1 and R. *J. Virol.*, **63**(12), 5276–5284.

Buisson, M., Hans, F., Kusters, I., Duran, N., and Sergeant, A. (1999). The C-terminal region but not the Arg-X-Pro repeat of Epstein–Barr virus protein EB2 is required for its effect on RNA splicing and transport. *J. Virol.*, **73**(5), 4090–4100.

Cai, X., Schafer, A., Lu, S. et al. (2006). Epstein–Barr virus microRNAs are evolutionarily conserved and differentially expressed. *PLoS Pathog.* **2**(3), 236–247.

Carey, M., Kolman, J., Katz, D. A., Gradoville, L., Barberis, L., and Miller, G. (1992). Transcriptional synergy by the Epstein–Barr virus transactivator ZEBRA. *J. Virol.*, **66**(8), 4803–4813.

Cayrol, C. and Flemington, E. K. (1995). Identification of cellular target genes of the Epstein-Barr virus transactivator Zta: activation of transforming growth factor beta igh3 (TGF-beta igh3) and TGF-beta 1. *J. Virol.*, **69**(7), 4206–4212.

Cayrol, C. and Flemington, E. (1996a). G0/G1 growth arrest mediated by a region encompassing the basic leucine zipper (bZIP) domain of the Epstein–Barr virus transactivator Zta. *J. Biol. Chem.*, **271**(50), 31799–31802.

Cayrol, C. and Flemington, E. K. (1996b). The Epstein–Barr virus bZIP transcription factor Zta causes G0/G1 cell cycle arrest through induction of cyclin-dependent kinase inhibitors. *EMBO J.*, **15**(11), 2748–2759.

Chang, P. J., Chang, Y. S., and Liu, S. T. (1998). Role of Rta in the translation of bicistronic BZLF1 of Epstein–Barr virus. *J. Virol.*, **72**(6), 5128–5136.

Chang, P. J. and Liu, S. T. (2001). Function of the intercistronic region of BRLF1-BZLF1 bicistronic mRNA in translating the zta protein of Epstein–Barr virus. *J. Virol.*, **75**(3), 1142–1151.

Chang, Y. N., Dong, D. L., Hayward, G. S., and Hayward, S. D. (1990). The Epstein–Barr virus Zta transactivator: a member of the bZIP family with unique DNA-binding specificity and a dimerization domain that lacks the characteristic heptad leucine zipper motif. *J. Virol.*, **64**(7), 3358–3369.

Chatila, T., Ho, N., Liu, P. et al. (1997). The Epstein–Barr virus-induced Ca^{2+}-/calmodulin-dependent kinase type IV/Gr promotes a $Ca2(+)$-dependent switch from latency to viral replication. *J. Virol.*, **71**(9), 6560–6567.

Chee, A. V., Lopez, P., Pandolfi, P. P., and Roizman, B. (2003). Promyelocytic leukemia protein mediates interferon-based anti-herpes simplex virus 1 effects. *J. Virol.*, **77**(12), 7101–7105.

Chen, C. J., Deng, Z., Kim, A. Y., Blobel, G. A., and Lieberman, P. M. (2001a). Stimulation of CREB binding protein nucleosomal histone acetyltransferase activity by a class of transcriptional activators. *Mol. Cell. Biol.*, **21**(2), 476–487.

Chen, L., Liao, G., Fujimuro, M., Semmes, O. J., and Hayward, S. D. (2001b). Properties of two EBV Mta nuclear export signal sequences. *Virology*, **288**(1), 119–128.

Chen, M. R., Chang, S. J., Huang, H., and Chen, J. Y. (2000). A protein kinase activity associated with Epstein–Barr virus BGLF4 phosphorylates the viral early antigen EA-D in vitro. *J. Virol.*, **74**(7), 3093–3104.

Chevallier-Greco, A., Gruffat, H., Manet, E., Calender, A., and Sergeant, A. (1989). The Epstein–Barr virus (EBV) DR enhancer contains two functionally different domains: domain A is constitutive and cell specific, domain B is transactivated by the EBV early protein R. *J. Virol.*, **63**(2), 615–623.

Chi, T. and Carey, M. (1993). The ZEBRA activation domain: modular organization and mechanism of action. *Mol. Cell. Biol.*, **13**(11), 7045–7055.

Chi, T., Lieberman, P., Ellwood, K., and Carey, M. (1995). A general mechanism for transcriptional synergy by eukaryotic activators. *Nature*, **377**(6546), 254–257.

Cho, M. S., Milman, G., and Hayward, S. D. (1985). A second Epstein–Barr virus early antigen gene in BamHI fragment M encodes a 48- to 50-kilodalton nuclear protein. *J. Virol.*, **56**(3), 860–866.

Cohen, J. I. (1999). The biology of Epstein–Barr virus: lessons learned from the virus and the host. *Curr. Opin. Immunol.*, **11**(4), 365–370.

Cohen, J. I. (2000). Epstein–Barr virus infection. *N. Engl. J. Med.*, **343**(7), 481–492.

Cohen, J. I. and Lekstrom, K. (1999). Epstein–Barr virus BARF1 protein is dispensable for B-cell transformation and inhibits alpha interferon secretion from mononuclear cells. *J. Virol.*, **73**(9), 7627–7632.

Cook, I. D., Shanahan, F., and Farrell, P. J. (1994). Epstein–Barr virus SM protein. *Virology*, **205**(1), 217–227.

Countryman, J. and Miller, G. (1985). Activation of expression of latent Epstein–Barr herpesvirus after gene transfer with a small cloned subfragment of heterogeneous viral DNA. *Proc. Natl Acad. Sci. USA*, **82**(12), 4085–4089.

Countryman, J., Jenson, H., Seibl, R., Wolf, H., and Miller, G. (1987). Polymorphic proteins encoded within BZLF1 of defective and standard Epstein–Barr viruses disrupt latency. *J. Virol.*, **61**(12), 3672–3679.

Cox, M. A., Leahy, J., and Hardwick, J. M. (1990). An enhancer within the divergent promoter of Epstein–Barr virus responds synergistically to the R and Z transactivators. *J. Virol.*, **64**(1), 313–321.

Daibata, M. and Sairenji, T. (1993). Epstein–Barr virus (EBV) replication and expressions of EA-D (BMRF1 gene product), virus-specific deoxyribonuclese, and DNA polymerase in EBV-activated Akata cells. *Virology*, **196**(2), 900–904.

Daibata, M., Humphreys, R. E., and Sairenji, T. (1992). Phosphorylation of the Epstein–Barr virus BZLF1 immediate-early gene product ZEBRA. *Virology*, **188**(2), 916–920.

Daibata, M., Speck, S. H., Mulder, C., and Sairenji, T. (1994). Regulation of the BZLF1 promoter of Epstein–Barr virus by second messengers in anti-immunoglobulintreated B cells. *Virology*, **198**(2), 446–454.

Darenkov, I. A., Marcarelli, M. A., Basadonna, G. P. et al. (1997). Reduced incidence of Epstein–Barr virus-associated post-transplant lymphoproliferative disorder using preemptive antiviral therapy. *Transplantation*, **64**(6), 848–852.

Darr, C. D., Mauser, A., and Kenney, S. (2001). Epstein–Barr virus immediate-early protein BRLF1 induces the lytic form of viral replication through a mechanims involving phosphatidylinositol-3 kinase activation. *J. Virol.*, **75**(13), 6135–6142.

Datta, A. K. and Hood, R. E. (1981). Mechanism of inhibition of Epstein–Barr virus replication by phosphonoformic acid. *Virology*, **114**(1), 52–59.

Datta, A. K., Colby, B. M., Shaw, J. E., and Pagano, J. S. (1980). Acyclovir inhibition of Epstein–Barr virus replication. *Proc. Natl Acad. Sci. USA*, **77**(9), 5163–5166.

Davie, J. R. (2003). Inhibition of histone deacetylase activity by butyrate. *J. Nutr.*, **133**(7 Suppl), 2485S–2493S.

Deng, Z., Chen, C. J., Zerby, D., Delecluse, H. J., and Lieberman, P. M. (2001). Identification of acidic and aromatic residues in the Zta activation domain essential for Epstein–Barr virus reactivation. *J. Virol.*, **75**(21), 10334–10347.

Deng, Z., Chen, C. J., Chamberlin, M. et al. (2003). The CBP bromodomain and nucleosome targeting are required for Zta-directed nucleosome acetylation and transcription activation. *Mol. Cell. Biol.*, **23**(8), 2633–2644.

Dent, P., Yacoub, A., Fisher, P. B., Hagan, M. P., and Grant, S. (2003). MAPK pathways in radiation responses. *Oncogene*, **22**(37), 5885–5896.

El-Guindy, A. S., Heston, L., Endo, Y., Cho, M. S., and Miller, G. (2002). Disruption of Epstein–Barr virus latency in the absence of phosphorylation of ZEBRA by protein kinase C. *J. Virol.*, **76**(22), 11199–11208.

El-Guindy, A. S. and Miller, G. (2004). Phosphorylation of Epstein–Barr virus ZEBRA protein at its casein kinase 2 sites mediates its ability to repress activation of a viral lytic cycle late gene by Rta. *J. Virol.*, **78**(14):7634–7644.

El-Guindy, A. S., Paek, S. Y., Countryman, J., and Miller, G. (2006). Identification of constitutive phosphorylation sites on the Epstein–Barr virus ZEBRA protein. *J. Biol. Chem.*, **281**(6), 3085–3095.

Faggioni, A., Zompetta, C., Grimaldi, S., Barile, G., Frati, L., and Lazdins, J. (1986). Calcium modulation activates Epstein–Barr virus genome in latently infected cells. *Science*, **232**(4757), 1554–1556.

Fahmi, H., Cochet, C., Hmama, Z., Opolon, P., and Joab, I. (2000). Transforming growth factor beta 1 stimulates expression of the Epstein–Barr virus BZLF1 immediate-early gene product ZEBRA by an indirect mechanism which requires the MAPK kinase pathway. *J. Virol.*, **74**(13), 5810–5818.

Falk, K. I. and Ernberg, I. (1999). Demethylation of the Epstein–Barr virus origin of lytic replication and of the immediate early gene BZLF1 is DNA replication independent. Brief report. *Arch. Virol.*, **144**(11), 2219–2227.

Faller, D. V., Mentzer, S. J., and Perrine, S. P. (2001). Induction of the Epstein–Barr virus thymidine kinase gene with concomitant nucleoside antivirals as a therapeutic strategy for Epstein–Barr virus-associated malignancies. *Curr. Opin. Oncol.*, **13**(5), 360–367.

Fan, M. and Chambers, T. C. (2001). Role of mitogen-activated protein kinases in the response of tumor cells to chemotherapy. *Drug Resist. Updat.*, **4**(4), 253–267.

Farina, A., Feederle, R., Raffa, S. et al. (2005). BFRF1 of Epstein-Barr virus is essential for efficient primary viral envelopment and egress. *J. Virol.*, 3703–3712.

Farjot, G., Buisson, M., Duc Dodon, M., Gazzolo, L., Sergeant, A., and Mikaelian, I. (2000). Epstein–Barr virus EB2 protein exports unspliced RNA via a Crm-1-independent pathway. *J. Virol.*, **74**(13), 6068–6076.

Farmer, D. G., McDiarmid, S. V., Winston, D. et al. (2002). Effectiveness of aggressive prophylatic and preemptive therapies targeted against cytomegaloviral and Epstein–Barr viral disease after human intestinal transplantation. *Transpl. Proc.*, **34**(3), 948–949.

Farrell, P. J., Rowe, D. T., Rooney, C. M., and Kouzarides, T. (1989). Epstein–Barr virus BZLF1 trans-activator specifically binds to a consensus AP-1 site and is related to c-fos. *EMBO. J.*, **8**(1), 127–132.

Faulkner, G. C., Krajewski, A. S., and Crawford, D. H. (2000). The ins and outs of EBV infection. *Trends Microbiol.* **8**(4), 185–189.

Feederle, R., Kost, M., Baumann, M. et al. (2000). The Epstein–Barr virus lytic program is controlled by the co-operative functions of two transactivators. *EMBO J.* **19**(12), 3080–3089.

Feng, W. H., Israel, B., Raab-Traub, N., Busson, P., and Kenney, S. C. (2002a). Chemotherapy induces lytic EBV replication and confers ganciclovir susceptibility to EBV-positive epithelial cell tumors. *Cancer Res.*, **62**(6), 1920–1926.

Feng, W. H., Westphal, E., Mauser, A. et al. (2002b). Use of adenovirus vectors expressing Epstein–Barr virus (EBV) immediate-early protein BZLF1 or BRLF1 to treat EBV-positive tumors. *J. Virol.*, **76**(21), 10951–10959.

Feng, W. H., Hong, G., Delecluse, H. J., and Kenney, S. C. (2004). Lytic Induction therapy for Epstein–Barr virus-positive B-cell lymphomas. *J. Virol.*, **78**(4), 1893–1902.

Fixman, E. D., Hayward, G. S., and Hayward, S. D. (1992). trans-acting requirements for replication of Epstein–Barr virus ori-Lyt. *J. Virol.*, **66**(8), 5030–5039.

Fixman, E. D., Hayward, G. S., and Hayward, S. D. (1995). Replication of Epstein–Barr virus oriLyt: lack of a dedicated virally encoded origin-binding protein and dependence on Zta in cotransfection assays. *J. Virol.*, **69**(5), 2998–3006.

Flamand, L. and Menezes, J. (1996). Cyclic AMP-responsive element-dependent activation of Epstein–Barr virus zebra promoter by human herpesvirus 6. *J. Virol.*, **70**(3), 1784–1791.

Fleischmann, J., Kremmer, E., Greenspan, J. S., Grasser, F. A., and Niedobitek, G. (2002). Expression of viral and human dUTPase in Epstein–Barr virus-associated diseases. *J. Med. Virol.*, **68**(4), 568–573.

Flemington, E. and Speck, S. H. (1990a). Autoregulation of Epstein–Barr virus putative lytic switch gene BZLF1. *J. Virol.*, **64**(3), 1227–1232.

Flemington, E. and Speck, S. H. (1990b). Epstein–Barr virus BZLF1 trans activator induces the promoter of a cellular cognate gene, c-fos. *J. Virol.*, **64**(9), 4549–4552.

Flemington, E. and Speck, S. H. (1990c). Evidence for coiled-coil dimer formation by an Epstein–Barr virus transactivator that lacks a heptad repeat of leucine residues. *Proc. Natl Acad. Sci. USA*, **87**(23), 9459–9463.

Flemington, E. and Speck, S. H. (1990d). Identification of phorbol ester response elements in the promoter of Epstein–Barr virus putative lytic switch gene BZLF1. *J. Virol.*, **64**(3), 1217–1226.

Flemington, E. K., Goldfeld, A. E., and Speck, S. H. (1991). Efficient transcription of the Epstein–Barr virus immediate-early BZLF1 and BRLF1 genes requires protein synthesis. *J. Virol.*, **65**(12), 7073–7077.

Flemington, E. K., Borras, A. M., Lytle, J. P., and Speck, S. H. (1992). Characterization of the Epstein–Barr virus BZLF1 protein transactivation domain. *J. Virol.*, **66**(2), 922–929.

Flemington, E. K., Lytle, J. P., Cayrol, C., Borras, A. M., and Speck, S. H. (1994). DNA-binding-defective mutants of the Epstein–Barr virus lytic switch activator Zta transactivate with altered specificities. *Mol. Cell. Biol.*, **14**(5), 3041–3052.

Fong, I. W., Ho, J., Toy, C., Lo, B., and Fong, M. W. (2000). Value of long-term administration of acyclovir and similar agents for protecting against AIDS-related lymphoma: case-control and historical cohort studies. *Clin. Infect. Dis.*, **30**(5), 757–761.

Francis, A. L., Gradoville, L., and Miller, G. (1997). Alteration of a single serine in the basic domain of the Epstein–Barr virus ZEBRA protein separates its functions of transcriptional activation and disruption of latency. *J. Virol.*, **71**(4), 3054–3061.

Francis, A., Ragoczy, T., Gradoville, L., Heston, L., El-Guindy, A., Endo, Y., and Miller, G. (1999). Amino acid substitutions reveal distinct functions of serine 186 of the ZEBRA protein in activation of early lytic cycle genes and synergy with the Epstein–Barr virus R transactivator. *J. Virol.*, **73**(6), 4543–4551.

Fu, Z. and Cannon, M. J. (2000). Functional analysis of the CD4(+) T-cell response to Epstein–Barr virus: T-cell-mediated activation of resting B cells and induction of viral BZLF1 expression. *J. Virol.*, **74**(14), 6675–6679.

Fujii, K., Yokoyama, N., Kiyono, T. *et al.* (2000). The Epstein–Barr virus pol catalytic subunit physically interacts with the BBLF4-BSLF1-BBLF2/3 complex. *J. Virol.*, **74**(6), 2550–2557.

Furnari, F. B., Zacny, V., Quinlivan, E. B., Kenney, S., and Pagano, J. S. (1994). RAZ, an Epstein–Barr virus transdominant repressor that modulates the viral reactivation mechanism. *J. Virol.*, **68**(3), 1827–1836.

Furukawa, F., Matsuzaki, K., Mori, S. *et al.* (2003). p38 MAPK mediates fibrogenic signal through Smad3 phosphorylation in rat myofibroblasts. *Hepatology*, **38**(4), 879–889.

Gan, Y. J., Razzouk, B. I., Su, T., and Sixbey, J. W. (2002). A defective, rearranged Epstein–Barr virus genome in EBER-negative and EBER-positive Hodgkin's disease. *Am. J. Pathol.*, **160**(3), 781–786.

Gao, X., Tajima, M., and Sairenji, T. (1999). Nitric oxide down-regulates Epstein–Barr virus reactivation in epithelial cell lines. *Virology*, **258**(2), 375–381.

Gao, X., Ikuta, K., Tajima, M., and Sairenji, T. (2001). 12-O-tetradecanoylphorbol-13-acetate induces Epstein–Barr virus reactivation via NF-kappaB and AP-1 as regulated by protein kinase C and mitogen-activated protein kinase. *Virology*, **286**(1), 91–99.

Gao, Z., Krithivas, A., Finan, J. E., Semmes, O. J., Zhou, S., Wang, Y., and Hayward, S. D. (1998). The Epstein–Barr virus lytic transactivator Zta interacts with the helicase-primase replication proteins. *J. Virol.*, **72**(11), 8559–8567.

Gershburg, E. and Pagano, J. S. (2002). Phosphorylation of the Epstein–Barr virus (EBV) DNA polymerase processivity factor EA-D by the EBV-encoded protein kinase and effects of the L-riboside benzimidazole 1263W94. *J. Virol.*, **76**(3), 998–1003.

Glaser, G., Vogel, M., Wolf, H., and Niller, H. H. (1998). Regulation of the Epstein-Barr viral immediate early BRLF1 promoter through a distal NF1 site. *Arch. Virol.*, **143**(10), 1967–1983.

Goldfeld, A. E., Liu, P., Liu, S., Flemington, E. K., Strominger, J. L., and Speck, S. H. (1995). Cyclosporin A and FK506 block induction of the Epstein–Barr virus lytic cycle by anti-immunoglobulin. *Virology*, **209**(1), 225–229.

Gonella, R., Farina, A., Santarelli, R. *et al.* (2005). Characterization and intracellular localization of the Epstein-Barr virus protein BFLF2: interactions with BFRF1 and with the nuclear lamina. *J. Virol.*, **79**, 3713–3727.

Gong, M. and Kieff, E. (1990). Intracellular trafficking of two major Epstein-Barr virus glycoproteins, gp350/220 and gp110. *J. Virol.*, **64**, 1507–1516.

Gonzalez, C. M., Wong, E. L., Bowser, B. S., Hong, G. K., Kenney, S., and Damania, B. (2006). Identification and characterization of the Orf49 protein of Kaposi's sarcoma-associated herpesvirus. *J. Virol.*, **80**(6), 3062–3070.

Grab, L. T., Kearns, M. W., Morris, A. J., and Daniel, L. W. (2004). Differential role for phospholipase D1 and phospholipase D2 in 12-O-tetradecanoyl-13-phorbol acetate-stimulated MAPK activation, Cox-2 and IL-8 expression. *Biochim. Biophys. Acta*, **1636**(1), 29–39.

Gradoville, L., Grogan, E., Taylor, N., and Miller, G. (1990). Differences in the extent of activation of Epstein–Barr virus replicative gene expression among four nonproducer cell lines stably transformed by oriP/BZLF1 plasmids. *Virology*, **178**(2), 345–354.

Gradoville, L., Kwa, D., El-Guindy, A., and Miller, G. (2002). Protein kinase C-independent activation of the Epstein–Barr virus lytic cycle. *J. Virol.*, **76**(11), 5612–5626.

Green, M., Reyes, J., Webber, S., and Rowe, D. (2001). The role of antiviral and immunoglobulin therapy in the prevention of Epstein–Barr virus infection and post-transplant lymphoproliferative disease following solid organ transplantation. *Transpl. Infect. Dis.*, **3**(2), 97–103.

Greenspan, J. S., Greenspan, D., Lennette, E. T. *et al.* (1985). Replication of Epstein–Barr virus within the epithelial cells of oral "hairy" leukoplakia, an AIDS-associated lesion. *N. Engl. J. Med.*, **313**(25), 1564–1571.

Grogan, E., Jenson, H., Countryman, J., Heston, L., Gradoville, L., and Miller, G. (1987). Transfection of a rearranged viral DNA fragment, WZhet, stably converts latent Epstein–Barr viral infection to productive infection in lymphoid cells. *Proc. Natl Acad. Sci. USA*, **84**(5), 1332–1336.

Gruffat, H. and Sergeant, A. (1994). Characterization of the DNA-binding site repertoire for the Epstein–Barr virus transcription factor R. *Nucl. Acids Res.*, **22**(7), 1172–1178.

Gruffat, H., Manet, E., Rigolet, A., and Sergeant, A. (1990). The enhancer factor R of Epstein–Barr virus (EBV) is a sequence-specific DNA binding protein. *Nucl. Acids Res.*, **18**(23), 6835–6843.

Gruffat, H., Duran, N., Buisson, M., Wild, F., Buckland, R., and Sergeant, A. (1992). Characterization of an R-binding site mediating the R-induced activation of the Epstein–Barr virus BMLF1 promoter. *J. Virol.*, **66**(1), 46–52.

Gruffat, H., Renner, O., Pich, D., and Hammerschmidt, W. (1995). Cellular proteins bind to the downstream component of the lytic origin of DNA replication of Epstein–Barr virus. *J. Virol.*, **69**(3), 1878–1886.

Gruffat, H., Batisse, J., Pich, D. *et al.* (2002a). Epstein–Barr virus mRNA export factor EB2 is essential for production of infectious virus. *J. Virol.*, **76**(19), 9635–9644.

Gruffat, H., Manet, E., and Sergeant, A. (2002b). MEF2-mediated recruitment of class II HDAC at the EBV immediate early gene BZLF1 links latency and chromatin remodeling. *EMBO Rep.*, **3**(2), 141–146.

Gutierrez, M. I., Judde, J. G., Magrath, I. T., and Bhatia, K. G. (1996). Switching viral latency to viral lysis: a novel therapeutic approach for Epstein–Barr virus-associated neoplasia. *Cancer Res.*, **56**(5), 969–972.

Gutsch, D. E., Holley-Guthrie, E. A., Zhang, Q. *et al.* (1994). The bZIP transactivator of Epstein–Barr virus, BZLF1, functionally and physically interacts with the p65 subunit of NF-kappa B. *Mol. Cell. Biol.*, **14**(3), 1939–1948.

Haan, K. M., Lee, S. K., and Longnecker, R. (2001). Different functional domains in the cytoplasmic tail of glycoprotein gB are involved in Epstein–Barr virus induced membrane fusion. *Virology*, **290**, 106–114.

Hahn, A. M., Huye, L. E., Ning, S., Webster-Cyriaque, J., and Pagano, J. S. (2005). Interferon regulatory factor 7 is negatively regulated by the Epstein–Barr virus immediate-early gene, BZLF1. *J. Virol.*, **79**(15), 10040–10052.

Hammerschmidt, W. and Sugden, B. (1988). Identification and characterization of oriLyt, a lytic origin of DNA replication of Epstein–Barr virus. *Cell*, **55**(3), 427–433.

Hardwick, J. M., Lieberman, P. M., and Hayward, S. D. (1988). A new Epstein–Barr virus transactivator, R, induces expression of a cytoplasmic early antigen. *J. Virol.*, **62**(7), 2274–2284.

Hardwick, J. M., Tse, L., Applegren, N., Nicholas, J., and Veliuona, M. A. (1992). The Epstein–Barr virus R transactivator (Rta) contains a complex, potent activation domain with properties different from those of VP16. *J. Virol.*, **66**(9), 5500–5508.

Hayakawa, J., Depatie, C., Ohmichi, M., and Mercola, D. (2003). The activation of c-Jun NH2-terminal kinase (JNK) by DNA-damaging agents serves to promote drug resistance via activating transcription factor 2 (ATF2)-dependent enhanced DNA repair. *J. Biol. Chem.*, **278**(23), 20582–20592.

Henderson, S., Huen, D., Rowe, M., Dawson, C., Johnson, G., and Rickinson, A. (1993). Epstein–Barr virus-coded BHRF1 protein, a viral homologue of Bcl-2, protects human B cells from programmed cell death. *Proc. Natl Acad. Sci. USA*, **90**(18), 8479–8483.

Herrmann, K., Frangou, P., Middeldorp, J., and Niedobitek, G. (2002). Epstein–Barr virus replication in tongue epithelial cells. *J. Gen. Virol.*, **83**(12), 2995–2998.

Herrold, R. E., Marchini, A., Frueling, S., and Longnecker, R. (1995). Glycoprotein 110, the Epstein–Barr virus homolog of herpes simplex virus glycoprotein B, is essential for Epstein–Barr virus replication in vivo. *J. Virol.*, **70**, 2049–2054.

Hiriart, E., Bardouillet, L., Manet, E. *et al.* (2003a). A region of the Epstein–Barr virus (EBV) mRNA export factor EB2 containing an arginine-rich motif mediates direct binding to RNA. *J. Biol. Chem.*, **278**(39), 37790–37798.

Hiriart, E., Farjot, G., Gruffat, H., Nguyen, M. V., Sergeant, A., and Manet, E. (2003b). A novel nuclear export signal and a REF interaction domain both promote mRNA export by the Epstein–Barr virus EB2 protein. *J. Biol. Chem.*, **278**(1), 335–342.

Hislop, A. D., Annels, N. E., Gudgeon, N. H., Leese, A. M., and Rickinson, A. B. (2002). Epitope-specific evolution of human CD8(+) T cell responses from primary to persistent phases of Epstein–Barr virus infection. *J. Exp. Med.*, **195**(7), 893–905.

Holley-Guthrie, E. A., Quinlivan, E. B., Mar, E. C., and Kenney, S. (1990). The Epstein–Barr virus (EBV) BMRF1 promoter for early antigen (EA-D) is regulated by the EBV transactivators, BRLF1 and BZLF1, in a cell-specific manner. *J. Virol.*, **64**(8), 3753–3759.

Hong, G. K., Kumar, P., Damania, B. *et al.* (2005). Epstein–Barr virus lytic infection is required for efficient production of the angiogenesis factor vascular endothelial growth factor in lymphoblastoid cell lines. *J. Virol.*, **79**(22), 13984–13992.

Hong, G. K., Gulley, M. L., Feng, W. H., Delecluse, H. J., Holley-Guthrie, E., and Kenney, S.C. (2005). Epstein-Barr virus lytic infection contributes to lymphoproliferative disease in a SCID mouse model. *J. Virol.*, **79**(22), 13993–14003.

Hong, G. K., Delecluse, H.-J., Gruffat, H., Morrison, T. E., Feng, W., and Kenney, S. C. (2004). The BRRF1 early gene of Epstein–Barr virus encodes a transcription factor that enhances induction of lytic infection by BRLF1. *J. Virol.*, **78**(10), in press.

Hong, Y., Holley-Guthrie, E., and Kenney, S. (1997). The bZip dimerization domain of the Epstein–Barr virus BZLF1 (Z) protein mediates lymphoid-specific negative regulation. *Virology*, **229**(1), 36–48.

Hsu, D. H., de Waal Malefyt, R., Fiorentino, D. F. *et al.* (1990). Expression of interleukin-10 activity by Epstein–Barr virus protein BCRF1. *Science*, **250**(4982), 830–832.

Huang, J., Chen, H., Hutt-Fletcher, L., Ambinder, R. F., and Hayward, S. D. (2003). Lytic viral replication as a contributor to the detection of Epstein–Barr virus in breast cancer. *J. Virol.*, **77**(24), 13267–13274.

Ikuta, K., Satoh, Y., Hoshikawa, Y., and Sairenji, T. (2000). Detection of Epstein–Barr virus in salivas and throat washings in healthy adults and children. *Microbes Infect.*, **2**(2), 115–120.

Inman, G. J., Binne, U. K., Parker, G. A., Farrell, P. J., and Allday, M. J. (2001). Activators of the Epstein–Barr virus lytic program concomitantly induce apoptosis, but lytic gene expression protects from cell death. *J. Virol.*, **75**(5), 2400–2410.

Ionescu, A. M., Schwarz, E. M., Zuscik, M. J. *et al.* (2003). ATF-2 cooperates with Smad3 to mediate TGF-beta effects on chondrocyte maturation. *Exp. Cell. Res.*, **288**(1), 198–207.

Israel, B. F. and Kenney, S. C. (2003). Virally targeted therapies for EBV-associated malignancies. *Oncogene*, **22**(33), 5122–5130.

Israele, V., Shirley, P., and Sixbey, J. W. (1991). Excretion of the Epstein–Barr virus from the genital tract of men. *J. Infect. Dis.*, **163**(6), 1341–1343.

Iwakiri, D. and Takada, K. (2004). Phosphatidylinositol 3-kinase is a determinant of responsiveness to B cell antigen receptor-mediated Epstein–Barr virus activation. *J. Immunol.*, **172**(3), 1561–1566.

Jenkins, P. J., Binne, U. K., and Farrell, P. J. (2000). Histone acetylation and reactivation of Epstein–Barr virus from latency. *J. Virol.*, **74**(2), 710–720.

Jenson, H. B. (2000). Acute complications of Epstein–Barr virus infectious mononucleosis. *Curr. Opin. Pediatr.*, **12**(3), 263–268.

Johannsen, E., Luftig, M., Chase, M. R. *et al.* (2004). Proteins of purified EBV. *Proc. Natl Acad. Sci. USA*, **101**(46), 16286–16291.

Karimi, L., Crawford, D. H., Speck, S., and Nicholson, L. J. (1995). Identification of an epithelial cell differentiation responsive region within the BZLF1 promoter of the Epstein–Barr virus. *J. Gen. Virol.*, **76**(4), 759–765.

Kato, K., Kawaguchi, Y., Tanaka, M. *et al.* (2001). Epstein–Barr virus-encoded protein kinase BGLF4 mediates hyperphosphorylation of cellular elongation factor 1delta (EF-1delta): EF-1delta is universally modified by conserved protein kinases of herpesviruses in mammalian cells. *J. Gen. Virol.*, **82**(6), 1457–1463.

Kato, K., Yokoyama, A., Tohya, Y., Akashi, H., Nishiyama, Y., and Kawaguchi, Y. (2003). Identification of protein kinases responsible for phosphorylation of Epstein–Barr virus nuclear antigen leader protein at serine-35, which regulates its coactivator function. *J. Gen. Virol.*, **84**(12), 3381–3392.

Kawaguchi, Y., Kato, K., Tanaka, M., Kanamori, M., Nishiyama, Y., and Yamanashi, Y. (2003). Conserved protein kinases encoded by herpesviruses and cellular protein kinase cdc2 target the same phosphorylation site in eukaryotic elongation factor 1delta. *J. Virol.*, **77**(4), 2359–2368.

Kawanishi, M. (1995). Nitric oxide inhibits Epstein–Barr virus DNA replication and activation of latent EBV. *Intervirology*, **38**(3–4), 206–213.

Keating, S., Prince, S., Jones, M., and Rowe, M. (2002). The lytic cycle of Epstein–Barr virus is associated with decreased expression of cell surface major histocompatibility complex class I and class II molecules. *J. Virol.*, **76**(16), 8179–8188.

Kenney, S., Holley-Guthrie, E., Mar, E. C., and Smith, M. (1989a). The Epstein–Barr virus BMLF1 promoter contains an enhancer element that is responsive to the BZLF1 and BRLF1 transactivators. *J. Virol.*, **63**(9), 3878–3883.

Kenney, S., Kamine, J., Holley-Guthrie, E., Lin, J. C., Mar, E. C., and Pagano, J. (1989b). The Epstein–Barr virus (EBV) BZLF1 immediate-early gene product differentially affects latent versus productive EBV promoters. *J. Virol.*, **63**(4), 1729–1736.

Kenney, S., Kamine, J., Holley-Guthrie, E. *et al.* (1989c). The Epstein–Barr virus immediate-early gene product, BMLF1, acts in trans by a posttranscriptional mechanism which is reporter gene dependent. *J. Virol.*, **63**(9), 3870–3877.

Kiehl, A., and Dorsky, D. I. (1991). Cooperation of EBV DNA polymerase and EAD(BMRF1) in vitro and colocalization in nuclei of infected cells. *Virology*, **184**(1), 330–340.

Kiehl, A., and Dorsky, D. I. (1995). Bipartite DNA-binding region of the Epstein–Barr virus BMRF1 product essential for DNA polymerase accessory function. *J. Virol.*, **69**(3), 1669–1677.

Kouzarides, T., Packham, G., Cook, A., and Farrell, P. J. (1991). The BZLF1 protein of EBV has a coiled coil dimerisation domain without a heptad leucine repeat but with homology to the C/EBP leucine zipper. *Oncogene*, **6**(2), 195–204.

Krappmann, D., Patke, A., Heissmeyer, V., and Scheidereit, C. (2001). B-cell receptor- and phorbol ester-induced NF-kappaB and c-Jun N-terminal kinase activation in B cells requires novel protein kinase C's. *Mol. Cell. Biol.*, **21**(19), 6640–6650.

Kraus, R. J., Mirocha, S. J., Stephany, H. M., Puchalski, J. R., and Mertz, J. E. (2001). Identification of a novel element involved in regulation of the lytic switch BZLF1 gene promoter of Epstein–Barr virus. *J. Virol.*, **75**(2), 867–877.

Kraus, R. J., Perrigoue, J. G., and Mertz, J. E. (2003). ZEB negatively regulates the lytic-switch BZLF1 gene promoter of Epstein–Barr virus. *J. Virol.*, **77**(1), 199–207.

Kudoh, A., Fujita, M., Kiyono, T. *et al.* (2003). Reactivation of lytic replication from B cells latently infected with Epstein–Barr virus occurs with high S-phase cyclin-dependent kinase activity while inhibiting cellular DNA replication. *J. Virol.*, **77**(2), 851–861.

Kudoh, A., Daikoku, T., Sugaya, Y. *et al.* (2004). Inhibition of S-phase cyclin-dependent kinase activity blocks expression of Epstein–Barr virus immediate-early and early genes, preventing viral lytic replication. *J. Virol.*, **78**(1), 104–115.

Laichalk, L. L. and Thorley-Lawson, D. A. (2005). Terminal differentiation into plasma cells initiates the replicative cycle of Epstein–Barr virus in vivo. *J. Virol.*, **79**(2), 1296–307

Lake, C. M. and Hutt-Fletcher, L. M. (2000). Epstein–Barr virus that lacks glycoprotein gN is impaired in assembly and infection. *J. Virol.*, **74**, 11162–11172.

Lake, C. M. and Hutt-Fletcher, L. M. (2004). The Epstein–Barr virus BFRF1 and BFLF2 proteins interact and coexpression alters their cellular localization. *Virology*, **320**, 99–106.

Lau, R., Middeldorp, J., and Farrell, P. J. (1993). Epstein–Barr virus gene expression in oral hairy leukoplakia. *Virology*, **195**(2), 463–474.

Le Roux, F., Sergeant, A., and Corbo, L. (1996). Epstein–Barr virus (EBV) EB1/Zta protein provided in trans and competent for the activation of productive cycle genes does not activate the BZLF1 gene in the EBV genome. *J. Gen. Virol.*, **77**, 501–509.

Li, M., Linseman, D. A., Allen, M. P. *et al*. (2001). Myocyte enhancer factor 2A and 2D undergo phosphorylation and caspase-mediated degradation during apoptosis of rat cerebellar granule neurons. *J. Neurosci.*, **21**(17), 6544–6552.

Li, Q. X., Young, L. S., Niedobitek, G. *et al*. (1992). Epstein–Barr virus infection and replication in a human epithelial cell system. *Nature*, **356**(6367), 347–350.

Li, Y., Webster-Cyriaque, J., Tomlinson, C. C., Yohe, M., and Kenney, S. (2004). Fatty acid synthase expression is induced by the Epstein–Barr virus immediate-early protein BRLF1 and required for lytic viral gene expression. *J. Virol.*, **78**(8), in press.

Liang, C. L., Chen, J. L., Hsu, Y. P., Ou, J. T., and Chang, Y. S. (2002). Epstein–Barr virus BZLF1 gene is activated by transforming growth factor-beta through cooperativity of Smads and c-Jun/c-Fos proteins. *J. Biol. Chem.*, **277**(26), 23345–23357.

Liao, G., Wu, F. Y., and Hayward, S. D. (2001). Interaction with the Epstein–Barr virus helicase targets Zta to DNA replication compartments. *J. Virol.*, **75**(18), 8792–8802.

Lieberman, P. M. and Berk, A. J. (1990). In vitro transcriptional activation, dimerization, and DNA-binding specificity of the Epstein–Barr virus Zta protein. *J. Virol.*, **64**(6), 2560–2568.

Lieberman, P. M. and Berk, A. J. (1991). The Zta trans-activator protein stabilizes TFIID association with promoter DNA by direct protein-protein interaction. *Genes Dev.*, **5**(12B), 2441–2454.

Lieberman, P. M. and Berk, A. J. (1994). A mechanism for TAFs in transcriptional activation: activation domain enhancement of TFIID-TFIIA – promoter DNA complex formation. *Genes Dev.*, **8**(9), 995–1006.

Lieberman, P. M., Hardwick, J. M., and Hayward, S. D. (1989). Responsiveness of the Epstein–Barr virus NotI repeat promoter to the Z transactivator is mediated in a cell-type-specific manner by two independent signal regions. *J. Virol.*, **63**(7), 3040–3050.

Lieberman, P. M., Hardwick, J. M., Sample, J., Hayward, G. S., and Hayward, S. D. (1990). The zta transactivator involved in induction of lytic cycle gene expression in Epstein–Barr virus-infected lymphocytes binds to both AP-1 and ZRE sites in target promoter and enhancer regions. *J. Virol.*, **64**(3), 1143–1155.

Lieberman, P. M., Ozer, J., and Gursel, D. B. (1997). Requirement for transcription factor IIA (TFIIA)-TFIID recruitment by an activator depends on promoter structure and template competition. *Mol. Cell. Biol.*, **17**(11), 6624–6632.

Lin, J. C. and Machida, H. (1988). Comparison of two bromovinyl nucleoside analogs, 1-beta-D-arabinofuranosyl-E-5-(2-bromovinyl)uracil and E-5-(2-bromovinyl)-2-deoxyuridine, with acyclovir in inhibition of Epstein–Barr virus replication. *Antimicrob. Agents Chemother.*, **32**(7), 1068–1072.

Lin, J. C., Nelson, D. J., Lambe, C. U., and Choi, E. I. (1986). Metabolic activation of 9([2-hydroxy-1-(hydroxymethyl) ethoxy]methyl)guanine in human lymphoblastoid cell lines infected with Epstein–Barr virus. *J. Virol.*, **60**(2), 569–573.

Lin, J. C., DeClercq, E., and Pagano, J. S. (1987). Novel acyclic adenosine analogs inhibit Epstein–Barr virus replication. *Antimicrob. Agents Chemother.*, **31**(9), 1431–1433.

Ling, P. D., Lednicky, J. A., Keitel, W. A. *et al*. (2003). The dynamics of herpesvirus and polyomavirus reactivation and shedding in healthy adults: a 14-month longitudinal study. *J. Infect. Dis.*, **187**(10), 1571–1580.

Littler, E., and Arrand, J. R. (1988). Characterization of the Epstein–Barr virus-encoded thymidine kinase expressed in heterologous eucaryotic and procaryotic systems. *J. Virol.*, **62**(10), 3892–3895.

Littler, E., Zeuthen, J., McBride, A. A. *et al*. (1986). Identification of an Epstein–Barr virus-coded thymidine kinase. *EMBO J.*, **5**(8), 1959–1966.

Liu, C., Sista, N. D., and Pagano, J. S. (1996). Activation of the Epstein–Barr virus DNA polymerase promoter by the BRLF1 immediate-early protein is mediated through USF and E2F. *J. Virol.*, **70**(4), 2545–2555.

Liu, P. and Speck, S. H. (2003). Synergistic autoactivation of the Epstein–Barr virus immediate-early BRLF1 promoter by Rta and Zta. *Virology*, **310**(2), 199–206.

Liu, P., Liu, S., and Speck, S. H. (1998). Identification of a negative cis element within the ZII domain of the Epstein–Barr virus lytic switch BZLF1 gene promoter. *J. Virol.*, **72**(10), 8230–8239.

Liu, S., Borras, A. M., Liu, P., Suske, G., and Speck, S. H. (1997a). Binding of the ubiquitous cellular transcription factors Sp1 and Sp3 to the ZI domains in the Epstein–Barr virus lytic switch BZLF1 gene promoter. *Virology*, **228**(1), 11–18.

Liu, S., Liu, P., Borras, A., Chatila, T., and Speck, S. H. (1997b). Cyclosporin A-sensitive induction of the Epstein–Barr virus lytic switch is mediated via a novel pathway involving a MEF2 family member. *EMBO J.*, **16**(1), 143–153.

Lu, J., Chen, S. Y., Chua, H. H. *et al*. (2000). Upregulation of tyrosine kinase TKT by the Epstein–Barr virus transactivator Zta. *J. Virol.*, **74**(16), 7391–7399.

Lu, J., Chua, H. H., Chen, S. Y., Chen, J. Y., and Tsai, C. H. (2003). Regulation of matrix metalloproteinase-1 by Epstein–Barr virus proteins. *Cancer Res.*, **63**(1), 256–262.

Lucht, E., Biberfeld, P., and Linde, A. (1995). Epstein–Barr virus (EBV) DNA in saliva and EBV serology of HIV-1-infected persons with and without hairy leukoplakia. *J. Infect.*, **31**(3), 189–194.

MacCallum, P., Karimi, L., and Nicholson, L. J. (1999). Definition of the transcription factors which bind the differentiation responsive element of the Epstein–Barr virus BZLF1 Z promoter in human epithelial cells. *J. Gen. Virol.*, **80**(6), 1501–1512.

Mahot, S., Sergeant, A., Drouet, E., and Gruffat, H. (2003). A novel function for the Epstein–Barr virus transcription factor EB1/Zta: induction of transcription of the hIL-10 gene. *J. Gen. Virol.*, **84**(4), 965–974.

Malouf, M. A., Chhajed, P. N., Hopkins, P., Plit, M., Turner, J., and Glanville, A. R. (2002). Anti-viral prophylaxis reduces the incidence of lymphoproliferative disease in lung transplant recipients. *J. Heart Lung Transpl.*, **21**(5), 547–554.

Manet, E., Gruffat, H., Trescol-Biemont, M. C. *et al.* (1989). Epstein–Barr virus bicistronic mRNAs generated by facultative splicing code for two transcriptional trans-activators. *EMBO J.*, **8**(6), 1819–1826.

Manet, E., Rigolet, A., Gruffat, H., Giot, J. F., and Sergeant, A. (1991). Domains of the Epstein–Barr virus (EBV) transcription factor R required for dimerization, DNA binding and activation. *Nucl. Acids Res.*, **19**(10), 2661–2667.

Manet, E., Allera, C., Gruffat, H., Mikaelian, I., Rigolet, A., and Sergeant, A. (1993). The acidic activation domain of the Epstein–Barr virus transcription factor R interacts in vitro with both TBP and TFIIB and is cell-specifically potentiated by a prolinerich region. *Gene Expr.*, **3**(1), 49–59.

Mansouri, A., Ridgway, L. D., Korapati, A. L. *et al.* (2003). Sustained activation of JNK/p38 MAPK pathways in response to cisplatin leads to Fas ligand induction and cell death in ovarian carcinoma cells. *J. Biol. Chem.*, **278**(21), 19245–19256.

Marschall, M., Stein-Gerlach, M., Freitag, M., Kupfer, R., van den Bogaard, M., and Stamminger, T. (2002). Direct targeting of human cytomegalovirus protein kinase pUL97 by kinase inhibitors is a novel principle for antiviral therapy. *J. Gen. Virol.*, **83**(5), 1013–1023.

Marshall, W. L., Yim, C., Gustafson, E. *et al.* (1999). Epstein–Barr virus encodes a novel homolog of the bcl-2 oncogene that inhibits apoptosis and associates with Bax and Bak. *J. Virol.*, **73**(6), 5181–5185.

Matthews, R. P., Guthrie, C. R., Wailes, L. M., Zhao, X., Means, A. R., and McKnight, G. S. (1994). Calcium/calmodulin-dependent protein kinase types II and IV differentially regulate CREB-dependent gene expression. *Mol. Cell. Biol.*, **14**(9), 6107–6116.

Mauser, A., Holley-Guthrie, E., Simpson, D., Kaufmann, W., and Kenney, S. (2002a). The Epstein–Barr virus immediate-early protein BZLF1 induces both a G(2) and a mitotic block. *J. Virol.*, **76**(19), 10030–10037.

Mauser, A., Holley-Guthrie, E., Zanation, A. *et al.* (2002b). The Epstein–Barr virus immediate-early protein BZLF1 induces expression of E2F-1 and other proteins involved in cell cycle progression in primary keratinocytes and gastric carcinoma cells. *J. Virol.*, **76**(24), 12543–12552.

Mauser, A., Saito, S., Appella, E., Anderson, C. W., Seaman, W. T., and Kenney, S. (2002c). The Epstein–Barr virus immediate-early protein BZLF1 regulates p53 function through multiple mechanisms. *J. Virol.*, **76**(24), 12503–12512.

McDiarmid, S. V., Jordan, S., Kim, G. S. *et al.* (1998). Prevention and preemptive therapy of postransplant lymphoproliferative disease in pediatric liver recipients. *Transplantation*, **66**(12), 1604–1611.

McKinsey, T. A., Zhang, C. L., Lu, J., and Olson, E. N. (2000). Signal-dependent nuclear export of a histone deacetylase regulates muscle differentiation. *Nature*, **408**(6808), 106–111.

Meerbach, A., Holy, A., Wutzler, P., De Clercq, E., and Neyts, J. (1998). Inhibitory effects of novel nucleoside and nucleotide analogues on Epstein–Barr virus replication. *Antivir. Chem. Chemother.* **9**(3), 275–282.

Mellinghoff, I., Daibata, M., Humphreys, R. E., Mulder, C., Takada, K., and Sairenji, T. (1991). Early events in Epstein–Barr virus genome expression after activation: regulation by second messengers of B cell activation. *Virology*, **185**(2), 922–928.

Mentzer, S. J., Fingeroth, J., Reilly, J. J., Perrine, S. P., and Faller, D. V. (1998). Arginine butyrate-induced susceptibility to ganciclovir in an Epstein–Barr-virus-associated lymphoma. *Blood Cells Mol. Dis.*, **24**(2), 114–119.

Mentzer, S. J., Perrine, S. P., and Faller, D. V. (2001). Epstein–Barr virus post-transplant lymphoproliferative disease and virus-specific therapy: pharmacological reactivation of viral target genes with arginine butyrate. *Transpl. Infect. Dis.*, **3**(3), 177–185.

Mettenleiter, T. C. (2002). Herpesvirus assembly and egress. *J. Virol.*, **76**(4), 1537–1547.

Mikaelian, I., Manet, E., and Sergeant, A. (1993). The bZIP motif of the Epstein–Barr virus (EBV) transcription factor EB1 mediates a direct interaction with TBP. *C R Acad. Sci. III*, **316**(12), 1424–1432.

Miller, C. L., Lee, J. H., Kieff, E., Burkhardt, A. L., Bolen, J. B., and Longnecker, R. (1994a). Epstein–Barr virus protein LMP2A regulates reactivation from latency by negatively regulating tyrosine kinases involved in sIg-mediated signal transduction. *Infect. Agents. Dis.*, **3**(2–3), 128–136.

Miller, C. L., Lee, J. H., Kieff, E., and Longnecker, R. (1994b). An integral membrane protein (LMP2) blocks reactivation of Epstein–Barr virus from latency following surface immunoglobulin crosslinking. *Proc. Natl Acad. Sci. USA*, **91**(2), 772–776.

Miller, C. L., Burkhardt, A. L., Lee, J. H. *et al.* (1995). Integral membrane protein 2 of Epstein–Barr virus regulates reactivation from latency through dominant negative effects on protein-tyrosine kinases. *Immunity*, **2**(2), 155–166.

Miyazaki, I., Cheung, R. K., and Dosch, H. M. (1993). Viral interleukin 10 is critical for the induction of B cell growth transformation by Epstein–Barr virus. *J. Exp. Med.*, **178**(2), 439–447.

Montalvo, E. A., Shi, Y., Shenk, T. E., and Levine, A. J. (1991). Negative regulation of the BZLF1 promoter of Epstein–Barr virus. *J. Virol.*, **65**(7), 3647–3655.

Montalvo, E. A., Cottam, M., Hill, S., and Wang, Y. J. (1995). YY1 binds to and regulates cis-acting negative elements in the Epstein–Barr virus BZLF1 promoter. *J. Virol.*, **69**(7), 4158–4165.

Moore, S. M., Cannon, J. S., Tanhehco, Y. C., Hamzeh, F. M., and Ambinder, R. F. (2001). Induction of Epstein–Barr virus kinases to sensitize tumor cells to nucleoside analogues. *Antimicrob. Agents Chemother.*, **45**(7), 2082–2091.

Morrison, T. E. and Kenney, S. C. (2004). BZLF1, an Epstein–Barr virus immediate-early protein, induces p65 nuclear translocation while inhibiting p65 transcriptional function. *Virology*, **328**(2), 219–232.

Morrison, T. E., Mauser, A., Wong, A., Ting, J. P., and Kenney, S. C. (2001). Inhibition of IFN-gamma signaling by an Epstein–Barr virus immediate-early protein. *Immunity* **15**(5), 787–799.

Morrison, T. E., Mauser, A., Klingelhutz, A., and Kenney, S. C. (2004). Epstein–Barr virus immediate-early protein BZLF1 inhibits tumor necrosis factor alpha-induced signaling and apoptosis by downregulating tumor necrosis factor receptor 1. *J. Virol.*, **78**(1), 544–549.

Niedobitek, G., Agathanggelou, A., Herbst, H., Whitehead, L., Wright, D. H., and Young, L. S. (1997). Epstein–Barr virus (EBV) infection in infectious mononucleosis: virus latency, replication and phenotype of EBV-infected cells. *J. Pathol.*, **182**(2), 151–159.

Niedobitek, G., Agathanggelou, A., Steven, N., and Young, L. S. (2000). Epstein–Barr virus (EBV) in infectious mononucleosis: detection of the virus in tonsillar B lymphocytes but not in desquamated oropharyngeal epithelial cells. *Mol. Pathol.*, **53**(1), 37–42.

Nonkwelo, C. B. and Long, W. K. (1993). Regulation of Epstein–Barr virus BamHI-H divergent promoter by DNA methylation. *Virology*, **197**(1), 205–215.

Oertel, S. H., Ruhnke, M. S., Anagnostopoulos, I. *et al.* (1999). Treatment of Epstein–Barr virus-induced posttransplantation lymphoproliferative disorder with foscarnet alone in an adult after simultaneous heart and renal transplantation. *Transplantation*, **67**(5), 765–767.

Packham, G., Economou, A., Rooney, C. M., Rowe, D. T., and Farrell, P. J. (1990). Structure and function of the Epstein–Barr virus BZLF1 protein. *J. Virol.*, **64**(5), 2110–2116.

Paulson, E. J. and Speck, S. H. (1999). Differential methylation of Epstein–Barr virus latency promoters facilitates viral persistence in healthy seropositive individuals. *J. Virol.*, **73**(12), 9959–9968.

Paulson, E. J., Fingeroth, J. D., Yates, J. L., and Speck, S. H. (2002). Methylation of the EBV genome and establishment of restricted latency in low-passage EBV-infected 293 epithelial cells. *Virology*, **299**(1), 109–121.

Pegtel, D. M., Middeldorp, J., and Thorley-Lawson, D. A. (2004). Epstein–Barr virus infection in ex vivo tonsil epithelial cell cultures of asymptomatic carriers. *J. Virol.*, **78**(22), 12613–12624.

Petosa, C., Morand, P., Baudin, F., Moulin, M., Artero, J. B., and Muller, C. W. (2006). Structural basis of lytic cycle activation by the Epstein–Barr virus ZEBRA protein. *Mol. Cell*, **21**(4), 565–572.

Pfeffer, S., Zavolan, M., Grasser, F. A. *et al.* (2004). Identification of virus-encoded microRNAs. *Science*, **304**(5671), 734–736.

Poppers, J., Mulvey, M., Perez, C., Khoo, D., and Mohr, I. (2003). Identification of a lytic-cycle Epstein–Barr virus gene product that can regulate PKR activation. *J. Virol.*, **77**(1), 228–236.

Portes-Sentis, S., Sergeant, A., and Gruffat, H. (1997). A particular DNA structure is required for the function of a cis-acting component of the Epstein–Barr virus OriLyt origin of replication. *Nucl. Acids Res.*, **25**(7), 1347–1354.

Quinlivan, E. B., Holley-Guthrie, E. A., Norris, M., Gutsch, D., Bachenheimer, S. L., and Kenney, S. C. (1993). Direct BRLF1 binding is required for cooperative BZLF1/BRLF1 activation of the Epstein–Barr virus early promoter, BMRF1. *Nucl. Acids Res.*, **21**(14), 1999–2007.

Ragoczy, T. and Miller, G. (1999). Role of the Epstein–Barr virus RTA protein in activation of distinct classes of viral lytic cycle genes. *J. Virol.*, **73**(12), 9858–9866.

Ragoczy, T. and Miller, G. (2001). Autostimulation of the Epstein–Barr virus BRLF1 promoter is mediated through consensus Sp1 and Sp3 binding sites. *J. Virol.*, **75**(11), 5240–5251.

Ragoczy, T., Heston, L., and Miller, G. (1998). The Epstein–Barr virus Rta protein activates lytic cycle genes and can disrupt latency in B lymphocytes. *J. Virol.*, **72**(10), 7978–7984.

Resnick, L., Herbst, J. S., and Raab-Traub, N. (1990). Oral hairy leukoplakia. *J. Am. Acad. Dermatol.*, **22**(6 Pt 2), 1278–1282.

Rodriguez, A., Armstrong, M., Dwyer, D., and Flemington, E. (1999). Genetic dissection of cell growth arrest functions mediated by the Epstein–Barr virus lytic gene product, Zta. *J. Virol.*, **73**(11), 9029–9038.

Rodriguez, A., Jung, E. J., and Flemington, E. K. (2001a). Cell cycle analysis of Epstein–Barr virus-infected cells following treatment with lytic cycle-inducing agents. *J. Virol.*, **75**(10), 4482–4489.

Rodriguez, A., Jung, E. J., Yin, Q., Cayrol, C., and Flemington, E. K. (2001b). Role of cmyc regulation in Zta-mediated induction of the cyclin-dependent kinase inhibitors p21 and p27 and cell growth arrest. *Virology*, **284**(2), 159–169.

Rooney, C., Taylor, N., Countryman, J., Jenson, H., Kolman, J., and Miller, G. (1988). Genome rearrangements activate the Epstein–Barr virus gene whose product disrupts latency. *Proc. Natl Acad. Sci. USA*, **85**(24), 9801–9805.

Rooney, C. M., Rowe, D. T., Ragot, T., and Farrell, P. J. (1989). The spliced BZLF1 gene of Epstein–Barr virus (EBV) transactivates an early EBV promoter and induces the virus productive cycle. *J. Virol.*, **63**(7), 3109–3116.

Rousset, F., Garcia, E., Defrance, T. *et al.* (1992). Interleukin 10 is a potent growth and differentiation factor for activated human B lymphocytes. *Proc. Natl Acad. Sci. USA*, **89**(5), 1890–1893.

Roychowdhury, S., Peng, R., Baiocchi, R. A. *et al.* (2003). Experimental treatment of Epstein–Barr virus-associated primary central nervous system lymphoma. *Cancer Res.*, **63**(5), 965–971.

Ruvolo, V., Wang, E., Boyle, S., and Swaminathan, S. (1998). The Epstein–Barr virus nuclear protein SM is both a post-transcriptional inhibitor and activator of gene expression. *Proc. Natl Acad. Sci. USA*, **95**(15), 8852–8857.

Ruvolo, V., Gupta, A. K., and Swaminathan, S. (2001). Epstein–Barr virus SM protein interacts with mRNA in vivo and mediates a gene-specific increase in cytoplasmic mRNA. *J. Virol.*, **75**(13), 6033–6041.

Ruvolo, V., Navarro, L., Sample, C. E., David, M., Sung, S., and Swaminathan, S. (2003). The Epstein–Barr virus SM protein induces STAT1 and interferon-stimulated gene expression. *J. Virol.*, **77**(6), 3690–3701.

Ruvolo, V., Sun, L., Howard, K. *et al.* (2004). Functional analysis of Epstein–Barr virus SM protein: identification of amino acids essential for structure, transactivation, splicing inhibition, and virion production. *J. Virol.*, **78**(1), 340–352.

Salek-Ardakani, S., Arrand, J. R., and Mackett, M. (2002). Epstein–Barr virus encoded interleukin-10 inhibits HLA-class I, ICAM-1, and B7 expression on human monocytes: implications for immune evasion by EBV. *Virology*, **304**(2), 342–351.

Salomoni, P. and Pandolfi, P. P. (2002). The role of PML in tumor suppression. *Cell*, **108**(2), 165–170.

Sarisky, R. T., Gao, Z., Lieberman, P. M., Fixman, E. D., Hayward, G. S., and Hayward, S. D. (1996). A replication function associated with the activation domain of the Epstein–Barr virus Zta transactivator. *J. Virol.*, **70**(12), 8340–8347.

Satoh, T., Hoshikawa, Y., Satoh, Y., Kurata, T., and Sairenji, T. (1999). The interaction of mitogen-activated protein kinases to Epstein–Barr virus activation in Akata cells. *Virus Genes*, **18**(1), 57–64.

Schepers, A., Pich, D., and Hammerschmidt, W. (1993a). A transcription factor with homology to the AP-1 family links RNA transcription and DNA replication in the lytic cycle of Epstein–Barr virus. *EMBO J.*, **12**(10), 3921–3929.

Schepers, A., Pich, D., Mankertz, J., and Hammerschmidt, W. (1993b). Cis-acting elements in the lytic origin of DNA replication of Epstein–Barr virus. *J. Virol.*, **67**(7), 4237–4245.

Schepers, A., Pich, D., and Hammerschmidt, W. (1996). Activation of oriLyt, the lytic origin of DNA replication of Epstein–Barr virus, by BZLF1. *Virology*, **220**(2), 367–376.

Segouffin, C., Gruffat, H., and Sergeant, A. (1996). Repression by RAZ of Epstein–Barr virus bZIP transcription factor EB1 is dimerization independent. *J. Gen. Virol.*, **77**(7), 1529–1536.

Segouffin-Cariou, C., Farjot, G., Sergeant, A., and Gruffat, H. (2000). Characterization of the Epstein–Barr virus BRRF1 gene, located between early genes BZLF1 and BRLF1. *J. Gen. Virol.*, **81**(7), 1791–1799.

Semmes, O. J., Chen, L., Sarisky, R. T., Gao, Z., Zhong, L., and Hayward, S. D. (1998). Mta has properties of an RNA export protein and increases cytoplasmic accumulation of Epstein–Barr virus replication gene mRNA. *J. Virol.*, **72**(12), 9526–9534.

Serio, T. R., Cahill, N., Prout, M. E., and Miller, G. (1998). A functionally distinct TATA box required for late progression through the Epstein–Barr virus life cycle. *J. Virol.*, **72**(10), 8338–8343.

Serio, T. R., Kolman, J. L., and Miller, G. (1997). Late gene expression from the Epstein–Barr virus BcLF1 and BFRF3 promoters does not require DNA replication in cis. *J. Virol.*, **71**(11), 8726–8734.

Shannon-Lowe, C. D., Neuhierl, B., Baldwin, G., Rickinson, A. B., and Delecluse, H. J. (2006). Resting B cells as a transfer vehicle for Epstein–Barr virus infection of epithelial cells. *Proc. Natl Acad. Sci. USA*, **103**(18), 7065–7070.

Shen, B. and Goodman, H. M. (2004). Uridine addition after microRNA-directed cleavage. *Science*, **306**(5698), 997.

Shimizu, N. and Takada, K. (1993). Analysis of the BZLF1 promoter of Epstein–Barr virus: identification of an anti-immunoglobulin response sequence. *J. Virol.*, **67**(6), 3240–3245.

Shu, C. H., Chang, Y. S., Liang, C. L., Liu, S. T., Lin, C. Z., and Chang, P. (1992). Distribution of type A and type B EBV in normal individuals and patients with head and neck carcinomas in Taiwan. *J. Virol. Methods*, **38**(1), 123–130.

Sinclair, A. J., Brimmell, M., Shanahan, F., and Farrell, P. J. (1991). Pathways of activation of the Epstein–Barr virus productive cycle. *J. Virol.*, **65**(5), 2237–2244.

Sista, N. D., Pagano, J. S., Liao, W., and Kenney, S. (1993). Retinoic acid is a negative regulator of the Epstein–Barr virus protein (BZLF1) that mediates disruption of latent infection. *Proc. Natl Acad. Sci. USA*, **90**(9), 3894–3898.

Sixbey, J. W., Lemon, S. M., and Pagano, J. S. (1986). A second site for Epstein–Barr virus shedding: the uterine cervix. *Lancet*, **2**(8516), 1122–1124.

Speck, S. H., Chatila, T., and Flemington, E. (1997). Reactivation of Epstein–Barr virus: regulation and function of the BZLF1 gene. *Trends Microbiol.*, **5**(10), 399–405.

Steven, N. M., Annels, N. E., Kumar, A., Leese, A. M., Kurilla, M. G., and Rickinson, A. B. (1997). Immediate early and early lytic cycle proteins are frequent targets of the Epstein–Barr virus-induced cytotoxic T cell response. *J. Exp. Med.*, **185**(9), 1605–1617.

Strockbine, L. D., Cohen, J. I., Farrah, T. *et al.* (1998). The Epstein–Barr virus BARF1 gene encodes a novel, soluble colony-stimulating factor-1 receptor. *J. Virol.*, **72**(5), 4015–4021.

Stuart, A. D., Stewart, J. P., Arrand, J. R., and Mackett, M. (1995). The Epstein–Barr virus encoded cytokine viral interleukin-10 enhances transformation of human B lymphocytes. *Oncogene*, **11**(9), 1711–1719.

Swaminathan, S., Hesselton, R., Sullivan, J., and Kieff, E. (1993). Epstein–Barr virus recombinants with specifically mutated BCRF1 genes. *J. Virol.*, **67**(12), 7406–7413.

Swenson, J. J., Mauser, A. E., Kaufmann, W. K., and Kenney, S. C. (1999). The Epstein–Barr virus protein BRLF1 activates S phase entry through E2F1 induction. *J. Virol.*, **73**(8), 6540–6550.

Swenson, J. J., Holley-Guthrie, E., and Kenney, S. C. (2001). Epstein–Barr virus immediate-early protein BRLF1 interacts with CBP, promoting enhanced BRLF1 transactivation. *J. Virol.*, **75**(13), 6228–6234.

Szyf, M., Eliasson, L., Mann, V., Klein, G., and Razin, A. (1985). Cellular and viral DNA hypomethylation associated with induction of Epstein–Barr virus lytic cycle. *Proc. Natl Acad. Sci. USA*, **82**(23), 8090–8094.

Takada, K. and Ono, Y. (1989). Synchronous and sequential activation of latently infected Epstein–Barr virus genomes. *J. Virol.*, **63**(1), 445–449.

Takada, K., Shimizu, N., Sakuma, S., and Ono, Y. (1986). Trans activation of the latent Epstein–Barr virus (EBV) genome after transfection of the EBV DNA fragment. *J. Virol.*, **57**(3), 1016–1022.

Takagi, S., Takada, K., and Sairenji, T. (1991). Formation of intranuclear replication compartments of Epstein–Barr virus with redistribution of BZLF1 and BMRF1 gene products. *Virology*, **185**(1), 309–315.

Tao, Q., Srivastava, G., Chan, A. C., Chung, L. P., Loke, S. L., and Ho, F. C. (1995). Evidence for lytic infection by Epstein–Barr virus in mucosal lymphocytes instead of nasopharyngeal epithelial cells in normal individuals. *J. Med. Virol.*, **45**(1), 71–77.

Tarodi, B., Subramanian, T., and Chinnadurai, G. (1994). Epstein–Barr virus BHRF1 protein protects against cell death induced by DNA-damaging agents and heterologous viral infection. *Virology*, **201**(2), 404–407.

Taylor, N., Countryman, J., Rooney, C., Katz, D., and Miller, G. (1989). Expression of the BZLF1 latency-disrupting gene differs in standard and defective Epstein–Barr viruses. *J. Virol.*, **63**(4), 1721–1728.

Thomas, C., Dankesreiter, A., Wolf, H., and Schwarzmann, F. (2003). The BZLF1 promoter of Epstein–Barr virus is controlled by E box-/HI-motif-binding factors during virus latency. *J. Gen. Virol.*, **84**(4), 959–964.

Torre, D. and Tambini, R. (1999). Acyclovir for treatment of infectious mononucleosis: a meta-analysis. *Scand. J. Infect. Dis.*, **31**(6), 543–547.

Tovey, M. G., Lenoir, G., and Begon-Lours, J. (1978). Activation of latent Epstein–Barr virus by antibody to human IgM. *Nature*, **276**(5685), 270–272.

Tsurumi, T., Daikoku, T., Kurachi, R., and Nishiyama, Y. (1993). Functional interaction between Epstein–Barr virus DNA polymerase catalytic subunit and its accessory subunit in vitro. *J. Virol.*, **67**(12), 7648–7653.

Tsurumi, T., Daikoku, T., and Nishiyama, Y. (1994). Further characterization of the interaction between the Epstein–Barr virus DNA polymerase catalytic subunit and its accessory subunit with regard to the 3′-to-5′ exonucleolytic activity and stability of initiation complex at primer terminus. *J. Virol.*, **68**(5), 3354–3363.

Urier, G., Buisson, M., Chambard, P., and Sergeant, A. (1989). The Epstein–Barr virus early protein EBI activates transcription from different responsive elements including AP-1 binding sites. *EMBO J.*, **8**(5), 1447–1453.

Walling, D. M., Edmiston, S. N., Sixbey, J. W., Abdel-Hamid, M., Resnick, L., and Raab-Traub, N. (1992). Coinfection with multiple strains of the Epstein–Barr virus in human immunodeficiency virus-associated hairy leukoplakia. *Proc. Natl Acad. Sci. USA*, **89**(14), 6560–6564.

Walling, D. M., Flaitz, C. M., Nichols, C. M., Hudnall, S. D., and Adler-Storthz, K. (2001). Persistent productive Epstein–Barr virus replication in normal epithelial cells in vivo. *J. Infect. Dis.*, **184**(12), 1499–1507.

Walling, D. M., Brown, A. L., Etienne, W., Keitel, W. A., and Ling, P. D. (2003a). Multiple Epstein–Barr virus infections in healthy individuals. *J. Virol.*, **77**(11), 6546–6550.

Walling, D. M., Flaitz, C. M., and Nichols, C. M. (2003b). Epstein–Barr virus replication in oral hairy leukoplakia: response, persistence, and resistance to treatment with valacyclovir. *J. Infect. Dis.*, **188**(6), 883–890.

Wang, Y. C., Huang, J. M., and Montalvo, E. A. (1997). Characterization of proteins binding to the ZII element in the Epstein–Barr virus BZLF1 promoter: transactivation by ATF1. *Virology*, **227**(2), 323–330.

Westphal, E. M., Mauser, A., Swenson, J., Davis, M. G., Talarico, C. L., and Kenney, S. C. (1999). Induction of lytic Epstein–Barr virus (EBV) infection in EBV-associated malignancies using adenovirus vectors in vitro and in vivo. *Cancer Res.*, **59**(7), 1485–1491.

Westphal, E. M., Blackstock, W., Feng, W., Israel, B., and Kenney, S. C. (2000). Activation of lytic Epstein–Barr virus (EBV) infection by radiation and sodium butyrate in vitro and in vivo: a potential method for treating EBV-positive malignancies. *Cancer Res.*, **60**(20), 5781–5788.

Wu, F. Y., Chen, H., Wang, S. E. *et al.* (2003). CCAAT/enhancer binding protein alpha interacts with ZTA and mediates ZTA-induced p21(CIP-1) accumulation and G(1) cell cycle arrest during the Epstein–Barr virus lytic cycle. *J. Virol.*, **77**(2), 1481–1500.

Yoshizaki, T., Sato, H., Murono, S., Pagano, J. S., and Furukawa, M. (1999). Matrix metalloproteinase 9 is induced by the Epstein–Barr virus BZLF1 transactivator. *Clin. Exp. Metastasis*, **17**(5), 431–436.

Young, L. S., Lau, R., Rowe, M. *et al.* (1991). Differentiation-associated expression of the Epstein–Barr virus BZLF1 transactivator protein in oral hairy leukoplakia. *J. Virol.*, **65**(6), 2868–2874.

Yuan, J., Cahir-McFarland, E., Zhao, B., and Kieff, E. (2006). Virus and cell RNAs expressed during Epstein–Barr virus replication *J. Virol.*, **80**(5), 2548–2565.

Zacny, V. L., Wilson, J., and Pagano, J. S. (1998). The Epstein–Barr virus immediate-early gene product, BRLF1, interacts with the retinoblastoma protein during the viral lytic cycle. *J. Virol.*, **72**(10), 8043–8051.

Zalani, S., Holley-Guthrie, E. A., Gutsch, D. E., and Kenney, S. C. (1992). The Epstein–Barr virus immediate-early promoter BRLF1 can be activated by the cellular Sp1 transcription factor. *J. Virol.*, **66**(12), 7282–7292.

Zalani, S., Holley-Guthrie, E., and Kenney, S. (1995). The Zif268 cellular transcription factor activates expression of the Epstein–Barr virus immediate-early BRLF1 promoter. *J. Virol.*, **69**(6), 3816–3823.

Zalani, S., Holley-Guthrie, E., and Kenney, S. (1996). Epstein–Barr viral latency is disrupted by the immediate-early BRLF1 protein through a cell-specific mechanism. *Proc. Natl Acad. Sci. USA*, **93**(17), 9194–9199.

Zalani, S., Coppage, A., Holley-Guthrie, E., and Kenney, S. (1997). The cellular YY1 transcription factor binds a *cis*-acting, negatively regulating element in the Epstein–Barr virus BRLF1 promoter. *J. Virol.*, **71**(4), 3268–3274.

Zerby, D., Chen, C. J., Poon, E., Lee, D., Shiekhattar, R., and Lieberman, P. M. (1999). The amino-terminal C/H1 domain of CREB binding protein mediates zta transcriptional activation of latent Epstein–Barr virus. *Mol. Cell. Biol.*, **19**(3), 1617–1626.

Zetterberg, H., Jansson, A., Rymo, L. *et al.* (2002). The Epstein–Barr virus ZEBRA protein activates transcription from the early lytic F promoter by binding to a promoter-proximal AP-1-like site. *J. Gen. Virol.*, **83**(8), 2007–2014.

Zhang, Q., Gutsch, D., and Kenney, S. (1994). Functional and physical interaction between p53 and BZLF1: implications for Epstein–Barr virus latency. *Mol. Cell. Biol.*, **14**(3), 1929–1938.

Zhang, Q., Hong, Y., Dorsky, D. *et al.* (1996). Functional and physical interactions between the Epstein–Barr virus (EBV) proteins BZLF1 and BMRF1: Effects on EBV transcription and lytic replication. *J. Virol.*, **70**(8), 5131–5142.

Zhang, Q., Holley-Guthrie, E., Ge, J. Q., Dorsky, D., and Kenney, S. (1997). The Epstein–Barr virus (EBV) DNA polymerase accessory protein, BMRF1, activates the essential downstream component of the EBV oriLyt. *Virology*, **230**(1), 22–34.

Zhang, Q., Holley-Guthrie, E., Dorsky, D., and Kenney, S. (1999a). Identification of transactivator and nuclear localization domains in the Epstein–Barr virus DNA polymerase accessory protein, BMRF1. *J. Gen. Virol.*, **80**(1), 69–74.

Zhang, Q., Wang, Y. C., and Montalvo, E. A. (1999b). Smubp-2 represses the Epstein–Barr virus lytic switch promoter. *Virology*, **255**(1), 160–170.

Zimmermann, J. and Hammerschmidt, W. (1995). Structure and role of the terminal repeats of Epstein–Barr virus in processing and packaging of virion DNA. *J. Virol.*, **69**(5), 3147–3155.

zur Hausen, H., O'Neill, F. J., Freese, U. K., and Hecker, E. (1978). Persisting oncogenic herpesvirus induced by the tumour promotor TPA. *Nature*, **272**(5651), 373–375.

26

Reactivation and lytic replication of KSHV

David M. Lukac[1] and Yan Yuan[2]

[1]UMDNJ/NJ Medical School, Dept. of Microbiology and Molecular Genetics, Newark, NJ, USA
[2]University of Pennsylvania School of Dental Medicine, Dept. of Microbiology, Philadelphia, PA, USA

Overview: goals of lytic replication

Herpesviruses are extremely successful pathogens that have coevolved with their mammalian hosts over the past 60–80 million years (McGeoch and Davison, 1999). This success likely is attributable to the ability of the Herpesviridae to establish lifelong latent infections of their host. Latently infected cells provide a perpetual reservoir from which progeny viruses can be amplified for dissemination within the host and transmission between hosts. Herpesvirologists have traditionally used the term "lytic reactivation" to describe the biological events that begin with emergence of a virus from latency and end with lysis of the host cell and release of progeny virions. Clinicoepidemiologic studies suggest that lytic reactivation of KSHV is an essential pathogenic step in multiple human diseases. The goal of this chapter is to review the host–virus interactions that are critical for regulating induction of KSHV from latency, subsequent progression through the lytic cycle, replication of the viral genome, and assembly of mature viral particles.

Lytic reactivation of KSHV is a critical pathogenic step in development of KS and other human diseases

Numerous epidemiologic studies unanimously agree that reactivation of KSHV from latency is a critical pathogenic step during the progression to KS. Serologic assays (Gao et al., 1996a; Kedes et al., 1996; Martin et al., 1998; Simpson et al., 1996) demonstrate that primary infection by KSHV typically occurs at least 10 years prior to clinically apparent KS in AIDS patients (Martin et al., 1998). During progression of AIDS-KS, seroconversion precedes the first occurrence of detectable viral DNA in peripheral blood (Gao et al., 1996b; Martin et al., 1998; Moore et al., 1996; Whitby et al., 1995), and detection of viral DNA is associated with the appearance of new KS lesions (Cannon et al., 2003). The incidence of KS is tenfold higher in KSHV seropositive patients who have PBMC viremia vs. those without virus in the peripheral blood (Engels et al., 2003; Keller et al., 2001; Moore et al., 1996; Whitby et al., 1995). Furthermore, following KS diagnosis, the amount of KSHV DNA in PBMCs increases with the increased severity of KS staging (Campbell et al., 2000), while lower viral burden in the peripheral blood is associated with a more positive clinical prognosis (Quinlivan et al., 2002). Individual studies of HIV-negative forms of KS (African, Classic or iatrogenic) also concur that KSHV reactivation precedes KS, and viral replication increases during the progression to more severe KS stages (Beyari et al., 2003; Campbell et al., 2003; Cattani et al., 1999; Vitale et al., 2000; Mantina et al., 2001; Boneschi et al., 2001). During KS development, the infection of endothelial cells in skin appears to temporally follow the rise in peripheral blood virus, suggesting that the dermal lymphatics are not a major reservoir for the virus prior to KS (discussed further below).

Lytic replication of KSHV has also been implicated in the pathogenesis of a number of Human diseases other than KS. In AIDS patients with multicentric Castleman's disease (MCD), KSHV viremia in PBMCs fluctuates over a 1 to 2 log range, with peaks corresponding to symptomatic episodes (Oksenhendler et al., 2000; Grandadam et al., 1997). In patients with hemophagocytic lymphohistiocytosis (HL), the peripheral blood load of KSHV is increased at least one order of magnitude during HL events, and frequently precedes these events (Fardet et al., 2003). Methylation of the viral genome that represses the lytic cycle during latency seems to be relieved in patients with KS, MCD, or primary effusion lymphoma (PEL; described below) (Chen et al., 2001).

The successful treatment of KS patients with drugs that block herpesviral DNA replication suggests that ongoing viral replication is required not only for initiation of KS but for maintenance of the disease. Two such antivirals are: Ganciclovir, a nucleoside analogue that slows the elongation of nascent DNA chains by competitive inhibition of herpesviral DNA polymerase proteins (Field et al., 1983), and Foscarnet, a pyrophosphate analogue that interferes with pyrophosphate exchange between the herpesviral polymerases and deoxynucleoside triphosphates (Wahren et al., 1985). Both drugs reduce KSHV replication in PEL models of infection (Kedes and Ganem, 1997). Independent clinical studies have demonstrated that treatment of high-risk patients with either Ganciclovir (Martin et al., 1999) or Foscarnet (Jones et al., 1995) reduces KS risk, and both drugs slow KS progression if administered subsequent to diagnosis (Robles et al., 1999). Ganciclovir and Foscarnet may cause regression of AIDS-KS without clearance of detectable KSHV from blood (Humphrey et al., 1996), suggesting that viral persistence in the absence of lytic replication is not sufficient to promote KS; however, other treatments have been reported that lead to KS regression accompanied by clearance of peripheral blood viremia (Monini et al., 2001). MCD has also been treated successfully with Ganciclovir, with accompanying reductions in KSHV viremia (Casper et al., 2004a).

The immune system tempers lytic reactivation of KSHV and KS development

The inverse relationship between immunocompetence and the development of KS is most clearly observed in studies of solid organ transplant recipients. More than 50% of KSHV-positive, immunosuppressed organ recipients develop tumors (Farge et al., 1999), and post-transplant KS typically regresses upon cessation of immunosuppression (for review see Hengge et al., 2002). The majority of post-transplant KS patients are KSHV seropositive prior to transplantation, suggesting that reactivation of latent virus is etiologically responsible for the disease (Weigert et al., 2004; Parravicini et al., 1997; Cattani et al., 2001; Andreoni et al., 2001).

Similarly, AIDS-related immunosuppression appears to be a key facet of the contribution of HIV coinfection to KS development and progression. Although KSHV prevalence was 24.6% in 1978 prior to the emergence of HIV infection in San Francisco (Osmond et al., 2002), KS incidence remained low until the AIDS epidemic took hold (Eltom et al., 2002). Detection of KSHV DNA increases, and KS severity worsens, as CD4+ cell counts drop (Keller et al., 2001; Martin, et al., 1998; Min and Katzenstein, 1999; Tedeschi et al., 2001; Whitby et al., 1995). T-cell proliferative responses to KSHV are also reduced, in HIV-1+ and not HIV-1-men and may decrease prior to reduction in CD4+ cell numbers (Strickler et al., 1999). Independent of CD4+ cell count (or HIV-1 infection), antibodies that neutralize KSHV infection are also reduced in KSHV+ people who have KS, as compared to those who are KSHV+ but do not have KS (Kimball et al., 2004). Immune suppression also appears to play a critical role in development of Classic KS (Iscovich et al., 2000; Brenner et al., 2002); however, such patients may live many decades with latent KSHV before KS strikes (if at all) (Cerimele et al., 2000). For example, 13.2% of Sardinian (Italian) children between the ages of 6 and 14 were seropositive for KSHV (Serraino et al., 2000), yet Classic KS is associated with advanced age, with the highest risk for those at least 50 years old (Santarelli et al., 2001).

Immune restoration in AIDS patients treated with highly active antiretroviral therapy (HAART) also implicates the control of KSHV replication by the immune system as a key factor in KS incidence. The introduction of HAART has resulted in recent annual declines of KS of 8.8% to 39% in the USA and Europe (Jones et al., 2000; Mocroft et al., 2004). HAART also decreases progression of AIDS-KS to visceral disease (Nasti et al., 2003), and increases the median time of survival (Tam et al., 2002). During successful HAART, regression of KS and decreasing KSHV detection is accompanied by restoration of numbers and functions of CD4+ cells (Casper et al., 2004b; Lebbe et al., 1998; Mocroft et al., 2004; Wilkinson et al., 2002; Jones et al., 2000; Cattelan et al., 2001; Pellet et al., 2001), CD8+ cells (Bourboulia et al., 2004; Wilkinson et al., 2002), or NK cells (Sirianni et al., 2002). Conversely, HAART non-responders fail to clear KSHV from PBMCs (Sirianni et al., 2002; Cattelan et al., 2001).

However, the success of HAART in ameliorating KS likely is attributable not only to immune restoration, but also to the concomitant reduction in HIV-1 load (Cattelan et al., 2001; Lebbe et al., 1998; Wilkinson et al., 2002). Many studies have documented an increased risk of KS (Cannon et al., 2001; Jacobson et al., 2000) and increased detection of KSHV viremia (Gill et al., 2002; Mantina et al., 2001; Tedeschi et al., 2001) with higher viral loads of HIV-1. Some HAART-treated populations show regression of AIDS-KS that corresponds with decreased HIV-1 loads independently of CD4+ levels (Gill et al., 2002). HIV-1-infected cells produce a soluble factor that induces reactivation of latent KSHV in culture (Varthakavi et al., 1999; Mercader et al., 2000), and

HIV-1 infection of cultured PEL cells also reactivates KSHV (Merat et al., 2002; Varthakavi et al., 1999; Huang et al., 2001). The HIV-1 Tat and Vpr proteins can independently promote lytic cycle induction and replication of KSHV in culture (Huang et al., 2001; Harrington et al., 1997; Merat et al., 2002). HIV protease inhibitors may also block KS independently of the immune system by inhibiting KS cell invasion of the extracellular matrix, in part by blocking matrix metalloproteinase-2 activity (Sgadari et al., 2002).

MHV-68 is a model for immune control of gamma-herpesvirus reactivation from latency

There is currently no small animal model for KSHV infection that recapitulates KS, so it is not possible to scientifically test the host immune response to KSHV infection and the pathogenic consequences in a disease-specific fashion. However, murine gammaherpesvirus (MHV)-68 provides the most compelling experimental evidence of the requirement for a functioning immune system in controlling gammaherpesviral replication, reactivation, and pathogenesis. MHV-68 shares extensive colinearity and conserves many genes with KSHV (Virgin et al., 1997). Intranasal infection of immunocompetent mice leads to primary replicaton in alveolar epithelial cells, followed by establishment of latency in splenic B-cells (Sunil-Chandra et al., 1992a,b). The B-cell reservoir for MHV-68 is CD19+ (Weck et al., 1999a), as is a reservoir of KSHV infection (Dittmer et al., 1999; Ambroziak et al., 1995). A small fraction of latently infected immunocompetent mice proceed to develop lymphoproliferative disease (LPD), but the incidence of LPD can be strongly amplified by treatment of the mice with cyclosporine A (Sunil-Chandra et al., 1994), a calcineurin inhibitor commonly used in humans as an immunosuppressant to prevent rejection of solid organ transplants (for review see Kaufman et al., 2004). This observation has provided the basis for experimental evaluation of MHV-68 pathogenesis in mice with underlying immunodeficiencies generated by various gene-specific knockouts of critical immune effectors.

Mice from many of the respective immunodeficient lines, notably type I interferon null mice (Weck et al., 1997), die during primary, acute MHV-68 infection, before pathogenic analyses of latency and reactivation can be assessed (for review see Simas and Efstathiou, 1998; Speck and Virgin, 1999). However, in mouse lines that do not succumb to the initial viral challenge, both cellular and humoral immunity have been implicated in controlling various characteristics of MHV-68 latency and reactivation. In CD8+ deficient mice, the pool of latently infected cells in the spleen and peritoneum is enlarged, and reactivation efficiency is increased (Tibbetts et al., 2002; Weck et al., 1996; Cardin et al., 1996). Among effector molecules that can be produced by CD8+ T cells, IFNγ and perforin control reactivation efficiency, and the number of latently infected cells, in the peritoneum and in the spleen, respectively (Tibbetts et al., 2002). In mice deficient for major histocompatibility class (MHC) II, MHV-68 establishes a progressive, productive infection, suggesting that CD4+ cells may steer the early infection towards latency (Cardin et al., 1996). Repression of latency can be rescued in this model by treatment of mice with an agonistic antibody to CD40, whose ligand is normally expressed by CD4+ cells in providing help to the antiviral CD8+ cytolytic function (Sarawar et al., 2001). CD4+ cells can also function later during MHV-68 pathogenesis to cause regression of MHV-68 induced B-cell tumors when prestimulated and adoptively transferred to nude mice (Robertson et al., 2001).

Mice that are B-cell deficient as a result of the μ-immunoglobulin knockout (μ-MT) can nonetheless be infected by MHV-68, with latency established most prominently in non-B-cells in the peritoneum (Weck et al., 1999b). In this model, the virus reactivates more efficiently than in healthy mice, and sustains reactivation for greater than 100 days following initial infection, escaping the control of reactivation that normally occurs in healthy mice at 3–4 weeks postinfection (Stewart et al., 1998; Weck et al., 1996, 1999b). The ability of MHV-68 to establish latency in B-cell-depleted mice led to the discovery of a second major reservoir for the virus in macrophages, and therefore to the suggestion that bone marrow may be a source of latently infected macrophages continually available to replenish the periphery (Weck et al., 1999b).

The humoral response to MHV-68 infection also influences latency and reactivation of the virus. CD28-null mice have normal levels of CD4+ and CD8+ T-cells, and B-cells, but their humoral immunity is deficient due to defective T/B-cell collaboration (Shahinian et al., 1993). T-cell depletion by injection of anti-T-cell antibodies in these mice results in reactivation of latent MHV-68, which can be prevented by the prior passive transfer of antiviral immune serum (Kim et al., 2002). In B-cell deficient mice, passive transfer of antilytic cycle antibody, but not antilatent cycle antibody, reduces the frequency of cells harboring latent virus, and the frequency of lytic reactivation of the virus (Gangappa et al., 2002). Combined with the finding that the antiviral drug cidofavir also reduces the frequency of latently infected cells, this suggests that lytic reactivation is required for maintenance of viral persistence (Gangappa et al., 2002).

Experimental infection by MHV-68 has also proven powerful for differentiation of true latent infection from chronic/persistent infection, a distinction that is very difficult to ascertain in natural Human infections by gammaherpesviruses. MHV-68-specific immunoglobulin (Ig) G remains elevated after peaking 2 weeks following infection (Stevenson and Doherty, 1998), perhaps as a result of intermittent reactivation of latent virus (Simas et al., 1999). A similar elevation of virus-specific antibodies has been described for KSHV that is sustained for many years following seroconversion in HIV+ and HIV− men (Gao et al., 1996a; Biggar et al., 2003), suggesting that intermittent reactivation from latency, or persistent replication of KSHV, may occur in certain hosts. Chronic replication of MHV-68 primarily leads to smooth muscle infection of large vessels and arteritis, which occurs with different frequencies in mice lacking an interferon gamma response (type II interferon), functional B-cells, functional CD4+ cells, or MHC II (Dal Canto et al., 2002; Weck et al., 1997).

Sites of latency and reservoirs for viral amplification in vivo

All of the gammaherpesviruses can infect lymphoid cells, and all can produce disease in that lineage. KSHV can also establish latency in non-lymphoid cells, but each site appears to make unique contributions to KSHV pathogenesis, and not all sites appear to be significant long-term reservoirs of amplifiable virus.

As described earlier in this chapter, after a KSHV-infected individual seroconverts, the titer of viral DNA in peripheral blood varies in direct proportion to the speed of progress to KS and severity of subsequent disease. The peripheral blood reservoir for KSHV has been unanimously identified as CD19+ B-cells, both prior to, or during, KS and in MCD patients. (Ambroziak et al., 1995; Bigoni et al., 1996; Blackbourn et al., 1997; Harrington et al., 1996; Kikuta et al., 1997; Whitby et al., 1995). Infected B-cells have also been localized to lymph nodes (Dupin et al., 1999; Schalling et al., 1995), and can support both latent and lytic gene expression (Polstra et al., 2003). Virus has also occasionally been detected in peripheral T-cells and other monocytes (Blasig et al., 1997; Harrington et al., 1996; Kikuta et al., 1997; Sirianni et al., 1997), and monocytes can maintain the viral infection if cultured in vitro in the presence of inflammatory cytokines (Monini et al., 1999b). CD19 negative, cultured PEL specimens also support latent and lytic infection; moreover, PEL cells release mature virus that can infect primary CD19+ cells in culture (Renne et al., 1998), and that can establish long-term latency in CD19+ B-cells in human thymus/liver (thy/liv) tissue implanted into mice with severe-combined immunodeficiency (SCID) (Dittmer et al., 1999). Thus B-cells are regarded as one site of long-term KSHV latency that can serve as a reservoir of virus for subsequent dissemination throughout the body.

Endothelial cells are a second site of latency for KSHV, and are associated with a much higher frequency of pathology than other cells infected by the virus. In KS tumors, the KSHV-infected cell is a CD34+ endothelial cell with characteristic spindloid morphology (Boshoff et al., 1995; Staskus et al., 1997). However, endothelial cells do not appear to be a long-term latent reservoir for the virus that can provide a significant source of progeny virions. KSHV DNA is infrequently detected in non-diseased skin of KS patients (Nuovo and Nuovo, 2001; Boshoff et al., 1995; Chang et al., 1994; Moore and Chang, 1995) and the virus is usually not detected in skin following regression of lesions (Aluigi et al., 1996; Ambroziak et al., 1995). Furthermore, the number of viral copies per cell appears to be at least one order of magnitude lower in endothelial cells than in other latently infected cells (Boshoff et al., 1995; Chang et al., 1994). Although the dermal endothelium is probably not a long-term latent reservoir, infected spindle cells may release progeny virus that can subsequently infect local keratinocytes and eccrine epithelium in the tumor (Reed et al., 1998).

A significant question for KSHV reactivation and pathogenesis concerns the mechanism by which the virus disseminates from the peripheral blood reservoir to sites of KS development. A strong argument for direct seeding of putative tumor sites by infected B-cells comes from tissue culture studies that show: (i) promotion of specific arrest and transendothelial migration of KSHV-infected B-cells in response to the chemoattractant stromal derived factor (SDF)-1 (Yao et al., 2003), and (ii) transmission of virus from stimulated B (PEL) cells to primary endothelial cells (Sakurada et al., 2001). However, KSHV-infected mononuclear cells have only been detected in some (Blasig et al., 1997; Aluigi et al., 1996; Reed et al., 1998; Sirianni et al., 1998) but not all (Pyakurel et al., 2004; Staskus et al., 1997), histopathologic samples of KS tissue. Furthermore, among the studies that have detected KSHV-infected mononuclear cells in tumors, the immunophenotype of the cells has been described variably as either lymphocytic (Reed et al., 1998), or monocytic/macrophagic (Blasig et al., 1997; Pyakurel et al., 2004; Sirianni et al., 1998). Therefore, although early KS lesions contain readily detectible lymphocytic and plasma cell infiltrates (Niedt et al., 1990), the peripheral blood reservoir of the virus may not directly, or continually, seed the tumor. An alternative mechanism may be that KSHV-infected, CD34+ spindle cells circulating in peripheral blood (Henry et al., 1999; Browning et al., 1994; Sirianni et al., 1997, 1998) may be endothelial precursor cells (Asahara et al., 1997) that subsequently populate the tumors.

While the peripheral blood probably maintains the long-term cellular reservoir of KSHV that can serve as a source of progeny virus for dissemination within an individual, a second, oral/salivary reservoir appears to be critical for producing high titer virus that can be transmitted between individuals. In fact, the titer in saliva is higher than in PBMCs (LaDuca et al., 1998; Koelle et al., 1997; Pauk et al., 2000), and viral DNA can be detected in saliva in individuals with undetectable PBMC virus (Blackbourn et al., 1998). The virus appears to maintain latency in oral epithelium (Triantos et al., 2004; Pauk et al., 2000), but significant amounts of encapsidated KSHV can be found free of cells in salivary fluid (Vieira et al., 1997; Blackbourn et al., 1998), and are transmissible to cultured cells (Duus et al., 2004; Vieira et al., 1997). Thus, reactivation of virus from latently infected cells in the oral cavity may provide the natural source of KSHV for inter-personal transmission. However, direct transmission of cells infected by KSHV cannot be excluded, as this mechanism has been reported in some cases of post-transplant KS (Barozzi et al., 2003; Luppi et al., 2003).

Primary effusion lymphoma (PEL) cells: a tissue culture model for KSHV latency and reactivation

Within the family *Herpesviridae*, the most robust systems for understanding molecular events in latency and reactivation are tissue culture models of infection by the gamma-2-herpesviruses like KSHV (Cesarman et al., 1995, 1996; Nador et al., 1996; Renne et al., 1996a,b). The first model systems for understanding KSHV latency and reactivation have been cells cultured from clinical specimens of primary effusion lymphoma (PEL). PEL is the only B-cell lymphoma conclusively associated with KSHV infection (Drexler et al., 1998; Cesarman et al., 1995; Uphoff et al., 1998), and is pathologically and phenotypically unique among all non-Hodgkin's lymphomas (Nador et al., 1996). Comparison of all HIV-associated lymphomas shows that PELs are BCL-6-/MUM1+/syn-1+, an immunophenotype that is unique to PEL among all serous effusions (Carbone et al., 2000, 2001) but is shared with EBV-transformed cells that express LMP-1 (Carbone et al., 2001).

Cytogenetic and gene expression analyses classify PEL cells as preterminally differentiated, postgerminal center B-cells, with overall similarities to plasma cells. Although PELs are immunophenotypically non-B/non-T-cells, their B-cell origin is revealed by clonal rearrangements of heavy and light chain immunoglobulin (Ig) genes that contain mutations suggestive of antigen selection (Fais et al., 1999). Genome-wide expression profiling using microarrays has confirmed that PELs cluster phenotypically with transformed plasma cells, EBV lymphoblastoid cell lines, and multiple myeloma cells, but nonetheless remain a distinct NHL subset (Jenner et al., 2003; Klein et al., 2003). PEL cell lines are transformed (Picchio et al., 1997; Strauchen et al., 1996; Gaidano et al., 1996; Boshoff et al., 1998), and most PELs are coinfected with KSHV and EBV (Drexler et al., 1998); however, the existence of EBV-negative PEL lines suggests that KSHV infection is sufficient for transformation of B cells. In fact, the cellular gene expression profiles of PELs singly infected with KSHV, or doubly infected with KSHV and EBV, are indistinguishable (Jenner et al., 2003; Klein et al., 2003).

During normal maintenance and passage, the PEL cells are infected uniformly with 40–150 episomal copies of clonal virus per cell genome (a characteristic of each line (for review see Drexler et al., 1998), with the virus remaining circularized and nuclear (Renne et al., 1996a). Latency is distinguished by highly restricted viral gene expression and lack of mature virus production (although a characteristic 1–5% of each cell line's population undergoes spontaneous reactivation). Upon treatment with various stimuli, including phorbol ester (i.e., TPA) or histone deacetylase inhibitors (i.e., sodium butyrate or trichostatin A), viral lytic genes are induced in a cascade fashion, leading to viral replication and progeny virus production (Renne et al., 1996a,b; Zhong et al., 1996; Miller et al., 1997). As in the other gamma-herpesviruses, viral DNA is packaged into enveloped virions as a 160–170 kilo-basepair (kbp) linear molecule (Renne et al., 1996a).

Kinetic classification of KHSV lytic gene expression

In tissue culture and clinical samples, KSHV exhibits both latent (non-productive) and lytic (productive) replication, which are characterized by virtually distinct gene expression programs (Renne et al., 1996b; Zhong et al., 1996; Miller et al., 1997; Staskus et al., 1997). The formal classification of the kinetics of expression of the lytic genes following treatment of latent virus with inducing agents has been defined for immediate–early (IE) and late genes.

Transcription of IE genes requires no previous protein expression, as evidenced by resistance to protein synthesis inhibitors like cycloheximide (CHX). In herpesviral reactivation systems, the IE genes are the prime candidates to

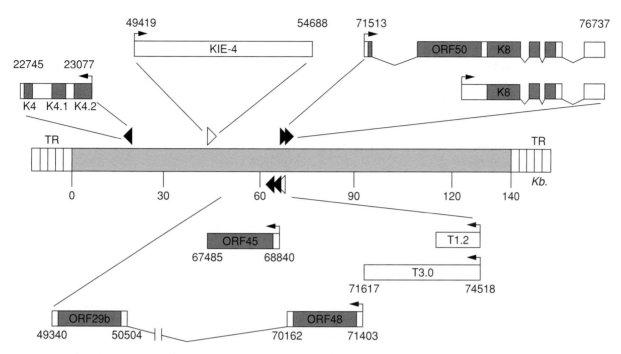

Fig. 26.1. The immediate–early (IE) loci of KSHV. This schematic represents the genome of KSHV. Arrowheads depict the relative locations and directions of IE gene expression. Each is expanded to show the details of transcript architecture. Each box represents a transcript, shading indicates open reading frames, non-shaded indicates untranslated regions, lines indicate introns. Names of each transcript and corresponding ORF are indicated. K8 is expressed in alternatively spliced, mono- and bi-cistronic transcripts; only one of K8's alternatively spliced products is shown here, for simplicity. "TR" = terminal repeat of virus. Numbering refers to nucleotide position on genome (as in Russo et al., 1996). References can be found in the text.

function as master controllers of the latent-to-lytic switch, a characteristic conserved in KSHV (discussed below). Eight distinct transcripts that are expressed in an IE fashion during KSHV reactivation encode ORF50/K8α/K8.2, K8α, ORF45, K4.2/K4.1/K4, ORF48 and ORF29b, K3 and ORF70, and two with no apparent coding potential (Fig. 26.1) (Wang et al., 2004b; Zhu et al., 1999a; Saveliev et al., 2002; Rimessi et al., 2001). Transcription of the L genes requires prior viral DNA replication, and the L transcriptome has been defined using the replication inhibitor cidofovir (CDV), a nucleoside analog (Lu et al., 2004). The study showed that expression of all of the known virion structural genes was inhibited by prior treatment of PEL cells with CDV. However, only about 25% of the viral membrane glycoproteins were inhibited by CDV. Most of the lytic cycle homologs of cellular genes were insensitive to CDV, except for the viral interferon regulatory factors vIRF-2 and vIRF-3/LANA2, viral macrophage inflammatory protein (vMIP)-III, and the viral FLICE inhibitory protein (vFLIP). Also insensitive to CDV were the IE transactivators and all of the known viral replication proteins. By default, lytic genes that have not been classified as IE or L fall into the delayed early (DE) class.

Genome-wide approaches have been used to classify KSHV transcription based on (i) quantity of expression in the presence or absence of TPA (Sarid et al., 1998), or (ii) time of first appearance and peak level of expression (Fakhari and Dittmer, 2002; Jenner et al., 2001; Paulose-Murphy et al., 2001). These studies have generally agreed that (i) the latent genes are typically expressed regardless of TPA addition, (ii) putative regulatory genes are expressed weakly prior to TPA addition, but strongly within 10 hours postinduction (pi), (iii) genes for putative DNA repair and nucleotide metabolism proteins are only expressed 10–24 hours pi, and (iv) genes for virion formation and structural proteins are expressed 48–72 hours pi. The mechanisms regulating coordinate induction of expression of most of the lytic genes during reactivation have not been evaluated in a systematic fashion.

ORF50/Rta is the viral lytic switch protein

Among a number of candidate KSHV genes, only transfection of Rta (the product of the ORF50 gene) can induce lytic reactivation of the virus in PEL cells, as detected by

Northern and Western blotting, and immunofluorescence (Lukac et al., 1998; Sun et al., 1998). Induction of the ORF59 (DE) and K8.1 (L) proteins by Rta transfection is quantitatively equivalent to TPA treatment, and K8.1 induction is blocked by PFA treatment, suggesting that Rta induces authentic viral DNA replication (Lukac et al., 1998; Polson et al., 2001). Productive release of encapsidated KSHV virions in response to forced expression of Rta confirms that Rta induces the entire lytic gene cascade (Gradoville et al., 2000; Nakamura et al., 2003).

ORF50 encodes a 691 amino acid protein that is a direct and selective transcriptional transactivator of DE promoters in uninfected cells (Lukac et al., 1998). Rta shares with its homologues in the gamma-herpesviruses two regions of relatively high primary amino acid homology, in the far N- and C-termini (Lukac et al., 1998). The N-terminal 272 amino acids can bind independently to KSHV promoter DNA (Lukac et al., 2001; Song et al., 2002), and the C-terminus is a potent transactivator when targeted to promoters by fusion to heterologous DNA binding domains (Lukac et al., 1999; Seaman et al., 1999; Wang et al., 2001). Deletion of the activation domain generates a mutant of Rta that forms mixed multimers with wild-type Rta and functions as an ORF50-specific dominant negative inhibitor of transactivation (Lukac et al., 1999). Expression of this dominant negative Rta mutant in PEL cells suppresses viral reactivation induced by TPA, sodium butyrate, and ionomycin (Lukac et al., 1999). Therefore, transcriptional transactivation by Rta is both sufficient and necessary for viral reactivation, and multiple reactivation signals that function using different biochemical mechanisms all converge at ORF50/Rta to successfully reactivate the virus (Lukac et al., 1999).

ORF50/Rta binds directly to the DNA of several KSHV promoters (Fig. 26.2) with varying affinity and sequence-specificity. The relative binding strengths for Rta to these promoter elements have been estimated as PAN>kaposin>ORF57>vIL-6 (Song et al., 2003), with a dissociation constant (K_d) for binding to the PAN element in the nanomolar range (Song et al., 2002). The PAN and kaposin promoters share a 16-bp core sequence that is also found in ori-Lyt (L) (Wang et al., 2004b; Kirshner et al., 2000; Song et al., 2002; Chang et al., 2002), but differs significantly from a second DNA element shared by the ORF57/Mta and K8 promoters (Lukac et al., 2001), and a third element in the viral IL-6 promoter (Deng et al., 2002).

However, direct DNA binding by Rta to all of these promoters is insufficient to specify them as targets for transactivation; instead, Rta requires combinatorial interactions with cellular proteins. Scanning mutagenesis of the Rta-responsive elements of both the PAN and Mta promoters demonstrated incomplete concordance between DNA binding by Rta and transactivation, i.e., some mutants that failed to bind Rta remained strongly transactivated by Rta, and vice versa (Song et al., 2002; Lukac et al., 2001). Furthermore, fusion of Rta's minimal DNA binding domain (Song et al., 2002; Lukac et al., 2001) to a heterologous activation domain is insufficient to transactivate the PAN promoter in vivo, but requires additional Rta amino acids that likely interact with heterologous proteins (Chang et al., 2002).

To this end, Rta transactivation requires cooperative interactions with various cellular transcription factors (Fig. 26.2). Genetic and biochemical experiments demonstrate that trans-activation of the ORF57/Mta promoter by Rta requires a direct interaction with the sequence-specific DNA binding protein RBP-Jk (aka CBF-1 and CSL). RBP-Jk-binding sites also mediate Rta-driven activation of the promoters of KSHV ORF6/single-stranded DNA binding (SSB) protein, the viral GPCR, and of Rta itself (auto-activation) (Liang and Ganem, 2003, 2004; Liang et al., 2002). A central regulatory role of the RBP-Jk/Rta interaction was demonstrated by the inhibition of KSHV reactivation in murine embryo fibroblasts null for RBP-Jk (Liang and Ganem, 2003). Rta promotes DNA binding of RBP-Jk, a mechanism that is fundamentally different from that established for the RBP-Jk-activating proteins, Notch intracellular domain (NICD) and EBV EBNA-2 (Carroll et al., 2006). Cooperation between RBP-Jk and Rta requires intact DNA binding sites for both proteins, and trimeric complex formation between the three molecules in vitro. In infected cells, chromatin immunoprecipitations reveal that RBP-Jk is virtually undetectable on the viral ORF57, K-bZIP, vGPCR, and cellular IL-6 and hairy/enhancer of split (HES)-1 promoters (Carroll et al., 2006). These data provide one explanation for the ability of KSHV to establish latency in RBP-Jk null cells (Liang and Ganem, 2003). However, during viral reactivation. RBP-Jk is significantly enriched on all of those promoters in an Rta-dependent fashion. Accordingly, Rta, but not EBNA2 and NICD, reactivates the complete viral lytic cycle. KSHV might have evolved this mechanism to ensure that only Rta efficiently reactivates the virus in environments of consititutive Notch activity.

Rta also participates in complex, combinatorial interactions with the cellular protein C/EBPα for transient transactivation of various KSHV promoters (Fig. 26.2). Rta and C/EBPα cooperate to activate transcription of the K8, ORF57/Mta, ORF50/Rta, and nut-1/PAN promoters, each of which contains at least one binding site for C/EBPα (Wang et al., 2003a,b). A direct interaction between C/EBPα and Rta is required for transcriptional cooperation (Wang

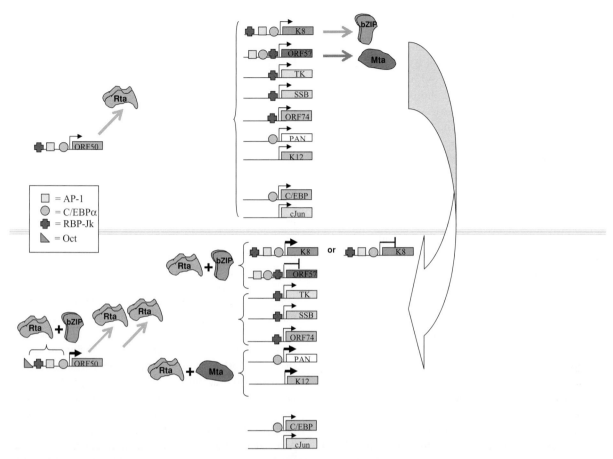

Fig. 26.2. Rta is the KSHV lytic switch protein. The viral and cellular promoters transactivated by Rta. *Cis* elements are indicated by symbols placed on each promoter, and *trans*-acting factors are indicated by the colored arrows. The size of the arrow at the transcriptional start site reflects relative amounts of transcription. See text for details.

et al., 2003a,b), and the C/EBPα binding sites overlap the Rta binding sites in the Mta and K8 promoters (Lukac *et al.*, 2001). In infected PEL cells, C/EBPα and Rta are found associated with the Rta, PAN, or Mta promoters only following viral reactivation (Wang *et al.*, 2003b); immunodepletion of C/EBPα prior to chromatin immunoprecipitation (ChIP) eliminates Rta's association with the Rta promoter, and reduces its association with the K8 promoter. Data also suggest that Rta cooperates with C/EBPα in auto-activation of the C/EBPα promoter, such that Rta and C/EBPα mutually participate in a positive autoregulatory loop during reactivation of KSHV from latency (Wang *et al.*, 2003a,b).

Rta and the cellular protein interferon regulatory factor (IRF)-7 participate in another regulatory loop. An IRF-7 binding site overlaps the Rta-responsive element in the ORF57 promoter, and IRF-7 inhibits Rta transactivation by competitive DNA binding to the element (Wang *et al.*, 2005). Rta contains intrinsic E3 ubiquitin ligase activity that targets IRF-7 for degradation by the host proteasome (Yu *et al.*, 2005). Interestingly, Rta also autoregulates its own degradation by self-ubiquitination (Yu *et al.*, 2005).

Rta also cooperates with other cellular proteins in promoter association and transactivation. cJun and cFos interact directly with each other and Rta, and all three cooperate to transiently transactivate the K8, Mta, and Rta promoters in uninfected cells (Wang *et al.*, 2004). Exogenous expression of Rta induces expression of cJun in BCBL-1 cells, and cJun coprecipitates with the K8, Mta, and Rta promoters in TPA-treated, but not untreated, BCBL-1 cells (Wang *et al.*, 2004). Rta and cJun may also cooperate through a mutual interaction with the coactivator CBP (Gwack *et al.*, 2001a). Rta can also be directed to autoactivate its own promoter through interactions with the cellular protein Octamer-1, but not Octamer-2, and an Octamer DNA element near the ORF50 transcription start site (Sakakibara *et al.*, 2001). Activation of the K9/vIRF promoter by Rta appears to depend exclusively upon unknown cellular DNA binding factors and not by direct Rta binding (Ueda *et al.*, 2002).

Nonetheless, DNA binding by Rta is obligatory for transactivation of the Rta-responsive elements of the PAN and Kaposin promoters (Chang et al., 2005b).

The promoter association of Rta is also regulated by post-translational modifications and homotypic interactions. Poly-ADP-ribosylation and phosphorylation of Rta's serine–threonine (ST)-rich region (AAs 505–520) decreases Rta's interactions with the Rta and Mta promoters in reactivating BCBL-1 cells (Gwack et al., 2003b). The cellular proteins poly(ADP-ribose) polymerase-(PARP)-1, and the human homologue of kinase from chicken (KFC), interact directly with the ST-rich region of Rta to add these modifications, elimination of which enhances Rta-mediated transactivation and viral reactivation (Gwack et al., 2003b). Other data show that Rta oligomerizes to bind the K8 promoter in vitro (Liao et al., 2003). All of the above data suggest that Rta expression alone may not be sufficient to reactivate KSHV, but additional levels of control following Rta expression are also essential. Indeed, in single cell reactivation assays, less than 10% of Rta-transfected PEL cells express viral lytic proteins (Lukac et al., 1998, 1999). Progression down the lytic gene cascade may therefore be inefficient, an observation reported, as well, in infection of cultured endothelial cells (Ciufo et al., 2001).

After Rta associates with lytic KSHV promoters, its ability to reactivate the virus from latency depends upon successful recruitment of the cellular SWI/SNF chromatin remodeling complex, and the TRAP/mediator coactivator (Gwack et al., 2003a). Direct contacts of Rta to individual proteins in both complexes is required for Rta-mediated transactivation, and Rta presumably recruits the remaining members in stoichiometric complexes to mediate these effects (Gwack et al., 2003a). In the case of promoters that require interactions of Rta with RBP-Jk (Liang et al., 2002; Liang and Ganem, 2004; Lukac et al., 2001), this suggests that Rta can replace the role of the activated cellular Notch protein in recruiting histone acetyl-transferase (HAT) complexes to RBP-Jk dependent promoters.

Rta's activity is also modulated by complex interactions with a second KSHV IE protein, K8/KbZIP (also known as RAP). Unlike its homologue in EBV, the Zta protein, KSHV KbZIP is unable to reactivate the KSHV lytic cycle (Polson et al., 2001). Instead, stable expression of the K8/KbZIP protein in BCBL-1 cells inhibits replication of KSHV in response to TPA induction (Izumiya et al., 2003a). This function may be due to the ability of K8/KbZIP to inhibit Rta-mediated transactivation of the ORF57/Mta and K8 promoters (Liao et al., 2003; Izumiya et al., 2003a). The K8/KbZIP protein directly targets the transcriptional coactivator CREB-binding protein (CBP) to transcriptionally repress signaling induced by either TPA or TGFβ, as well as the cFos promoter (Hwang et al., 2001; Tomita et al., 2004). However, the ability of K8/KbZIP to repress Rta-mediated activation requires a direct interaction between itself and Rta, and is not relieved by overexpressing transcriptional coactivators (Liao et al., 2003).

There are also conditions in which K8/KbZIP activates transcription. K8/KbZIP can cooperate with Rta to transactivate the K8 and Rta promoters (Wang et al., 2003a), but does not affect Rta-mediated activation of the nut-1/PAN promoter (Izumiya et al., 2003a). Collectively, these data suggest that K8/KbZIP may cooperate with Rta to ensure strong induction of Rta expression, but then tempers lytic cycle progression by inhibiting Rta's ability to activate downstream promoters, like that of ORF57 and K8. As described below, K8/KbZIP also inhibits cell cycling, so the mechanisms by which K8/KbZIP influences Rta function are likely to be complex.

Other viral proteins exert both positive and negative effects on Rta. A DE target of ORF50/Rta transactivation, ORF57/Mta, is essential for infectious virion production from latently infected cells (Han and Swaminathan, 2006). The Mta ORF encodes protein domains with putative transcriptional and post-transcriptional functions, and stimulates the accumulation of viral lytic mRNAs (Han and Swaminathan, 2006). Mta uses an un-characterized mechanism to synergize with Rta in a promoter-specific fashion (Kirshner et al., 2000). The ORF73 protein, Latency-Associated Nuclear Antigen (LANA)-1, represses both Rta-mediated transactivation and reactivation, as well as Rta expression, through interactions with the cellular protein RBP-Jk (Lan et al., 2005).

Signals that control lytic reactivation of KSHV

Various laboratory chemicals are the strongest inducers of the KSHV lytic cascade in PEL cells, and have provided important clues regarding the intracellular pathways that control viral reactivation. Since these chemicals function by divergent mechanisms, it suggests that more than one pathway is sufficient to reactivate KSHV. However, the candidate physiologic ligands that stimulate these pathways are virtually unknown (Fig. 26.3).

TPA has been the standard reagent that induces the entire lytic gene cascade and release of mature progeny virus from PEL cells (Renne et al., 1996b; Miller et al., 1997). TPA added to PEL cells rapidly induces the DNA binding of the cellular proteins C/EBPα and cJun to the Rta promoter; in the absence of TPA, transfection of expression vectors for C/EBPα or the AP-1 constituents cFos and cJun induce Rta expression (Wang et al., 2003a,b, 2004). Newly

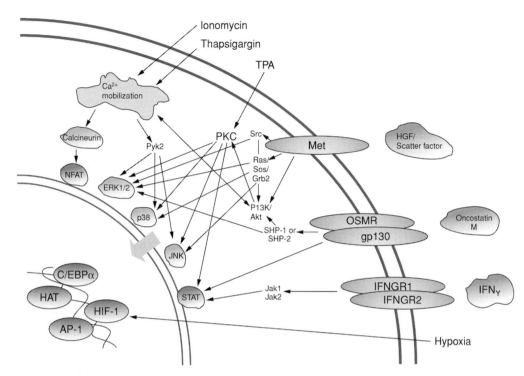

Fig. 26.3. Signals that reactivate KSHV in PEL models of latency. Published or hypothetical pathways that induce KSHV reactivation in PEL cells; see text for details and citations (for review see Maulik et al., 2002; Taga and Kishimoto, 1997; Ernst and Jenkins, 2004; Leonard and O'Shea, 1998; Feske et al., 2003; Yang and Kazanietz, 2003). Abbreviations: "NFAT" = nuclear factor of activated T cells, "TPA" = 12-O-tetradecanoyl-phorbol-13-acetate, "PKC" = protein kinase C, "HGF" = hepatocyte growth factor, "PI3K" = phospho-inositol-3-kinase, "JNK" = jun N-terminal kinase, "OSMR" = oncostatin M receptor, "SHP" = src homology domain-2 domain-containing protein tyrosine phosphatase, "IFN" = interferon, "IFNGR" = interferon gamma receptor, "Jak" = janus kinase, "STAT" = signal transducer and activator of transcription, "C/EBP" = CCAAT/enhancer binding protein, "HAT" = histone acetyl-transferase, "HIF" = hypoxia induced factor.

expressed Rta subsequently induces additional C/EBPα and cJun expression, and both proteins are detected in increasing amounts on DE promoters (Wang et al., 2003a,b, 2004). Chemical inhibitors of protein kinase C (PKC) reduce TPA-induced lytic reaction of KSHV in PELs by 70–75% (Zoeteweij et al., 2001). Collectively, these data suggest that TPA reactivates KSHV primarily by activating AP-1 and C/EBPα in the nucleus through induction of protein kinase C activity. As shown in Fig 26.3, PKC sits at the crossroads of many candidate physiologic ligands and downstream effectors (for review see Yang and Kazanietz, 2003), suggesting that it probably plays a prominent role in controlling KSHV reactivation in vivo.

Although stimulation of PKC can also lead to activation of the NF-kB family of transcription factors (Yang and Kazanietz, 2003), NF-kB is constitutively active in PELs in the absence of TPA. Rta and other lytic proteins are induced if NF-kB is inhibited, resulting in reactivation of KSHV (Brown et al., 2003). Transfection of an expression vector for p65, a transcriptionally active subunit of NF-kB, inhibits the ability of Rta to transactivate its own promoter, and that of nut-1/PAN. This effect is overcome by overexpression of a dominant negative inhibitor of NF-kB (Brown et al., 2003). The latently expressed KSHV protein, vFLIP (viral fas-ligand IL-1 β-converting enzyme inhitibory protein), maintains constitutive activity of NF-kB in PELs, inhibition of which induces apoptosis (Ghosh et al., 2003; Keller et al., 2000). Evolutionary pressure might thus have selected this function of vFLIP to enhance the stable maintenance of KSHV latency.

Calcium ionophores also reactivate KSHV from latency in PEL cells (Renne et al., 1996b; Chang et al., 2000), but are blocked by chemical inhibitors of calcineurin, suggesting a PKC-independent pathway downstream of Ca^{2+} (Yang and Kazanietz, 2003; Zoeteweij et al., 2001). Typically, calcineurin stimulation activates the nuclear factor of activated T cells (NFAT) growth control pathway (for review see Feske et al., 2003). However, NFAT signaling alone is apparently insufficient to reactivate KSHV: the viral K1 protein, a constitutive activator of NFAT (Lagunoff et al., 1999; Lee et al., 1998), is incapable of inducing reactivation when ectopically overexpressed in PEL cells (Lukac et al., 1998). A mutant of K1 unable to stimulate NFAT blocks reactivation of KSHV induced by Rta, suggesting that NFAT stimulation is essential for events downstream of Rta (Lagunoff et al., 2001). Overexpression of wild-type K1 can also inhibit reactivation without altering Rta expression (Lee et al., 2002), suggesting that NFAT activation must be "fine-tuned" during lytic cycle progression.

Many of the inflammatory cytokines and other soluble factors found in KS lesions (for review see Ensoli et al., 2001) can reactivate the virus if added to the growth media of PEL cells. These include oncostatin M, hepatocyte growth factor, interferon γ, HIV-1 Tat, and an unidentified soluble factor released from HIV-1 infected cells (Blackbourn et al., 2000; Chang et al., 2000; Huang et al., 2001; Mercader et al., 2000; Monini et al., 1999b; Varthakavi et al., 1999). Furthermore, many of these factors are required for growth of uninfected, explanted KS spindle cells (Cai et al., 1994; Ensoli et al., 1989; Miles et al., 1992; Naidu et al., 1994), suggesting that reactivation of KSHV may be co-regulated with stimulation of putative target cells. Supporting this hypothesis, the persistence of KSHV in explanted PBLs from infected humans requires the addition of inflammatory cytokines to the culture (Ensoli et al., 2000; Monini et al., 1999b; Sirianni et al., 1998). Similarly, MHV-68 infection induces the pro-inflammatory cyclooxygenase (COX)-2 protein, and COX-2 inhibitors globally suppress MHV-68 gene expression and virion production (Symensma et al., 2003). However, not all inflammatory cytokines augment KSHV replication: interferon α inhibits reactivation of KSHV in PELs, and reduces the viral load in cultured PBLs (Monini et al., 1999a).

Growth of PELs in hypoxia (limited O_2) results in the accumulation of the cellular transcription factor HIF-1 and also reactivates KSHV (Davis et al., 2001). The messages for Rta and ORF34 are induced in hypoxia, and both contain putative hypoxia response elements (HREs) in their promoters (Haque et al., 2003). Using reporter plasmids for the two viral promoters, the effect of hypoxia is also seen in uninfected cells, and can be reproduced by transfection of expression vectors for HIF-1 and HIF-2 (Haque et al., 2003). These data are provocative considering that (i) classic KS has a predilection to affect the lower extremities of elderly men (Hengge et al., 2002), which often have relatively low tissue oxygen concentrations (Ubbink et al., 1997), and (ii) endemic KS is highly prevalent in areas of the world with concurrent malaria or common hereditary anemias (Sarid et al., 1999), which also lead to tissue hypoxia. Thus, hypoxia may favor reactivation of latent virus, increased viral titer, and consequently, increased KS or increased transmission of KSHV.

Many studies suggest that KSHV reactivation signals ultimately lead to relief of transcriptionally repressive chromatin architecture by increasing acetylation and chromatin remodeling of viral promoters, especially that of Rta. Histone deacetylase (HDAC) inhibitors, like sodium butyrate, trichostatin A, and valproic acid (Lu et al., 2003; Miller et al., 1997; Renne et al., 1996b; Shaw et al., 2000; Vieira and O'Hearn, 2004), all reactivate KSHV from latency, and can directly activate Rta's promoter (Lu et al., 2003). ChIP experiments show that HDACs 1, 5, and 7 are associated with the Rta promoter in latently infected cells, and nuclease mapping shows that a nucleosome is stably positioned over the Rta start site under these conditions (Lu et al., 2003). Treatment with an HDAC inhibitor releases the positioned nucleosome, recruits the Ini1/Sn5 subunit of the BRG1 chromatin remodeling complex, and induces Rta expression (Lu et al., 2003). These data suggest that chromatin remodeling of the Rta promoter, specifically at its start site, may be the molecular mechanism that is critical for a reactivation signal to be effective. The relief of repressive chromatin by recruitment of histone acetyltransferases (HATs) to critical DNA elements of the EBV genome also appears to be a crucial regulatory event (Jenkins et al., 2000).

How are HDACs recruited to the Rta promoter to repress its expression and maintain KSHV latency? Bisulfite genomic sequencing demonstrates that the Rta promoter is highly methylated at CpG dinucleotides during latency; premethylation of the Rta promoter prior to transfection severely represses its activity in transient reporter assays (Chen et al., 2001). These data suggest that the methyl CpG binding protein MeCP2 might bind to methylated bases, and recruit HDAC complexes that promote latency. Indeed, treatment of BCBL-1 cells with 5-azacytidine, a DNA methyltransferase inhibitor, reactivates the virus from latency (Chen et al., 2001). Remarkably, even TPA treatment of BCBL-1 cells seems to relieve the repressive effects of methylation of the Rta promoter (Chen et al., 2001), suggesting that regulation of the methylation status of the promoter might be a general mechanism to regulate the latent-to-lytic transition of KSHV. Concordant with the orchestration of the KSHV lytic cycle by Rta and pathogenic progression, the ORF50/Rta promoter in a latent KSHV carrier was highly methylated, while it was virtually unmethylated in most patients with MCD, PEL, and KS (Chen et al., 2001).

However, there are also examples in which lytic cycle genes can be induced independently of Rta expression.

IFNα treatment of BCP-1 cells directly induces vIL-6 from latent KSHV in an IE fashion in the absence of any other viral gene expression (Chatterjee et al., 2002). Twenty-four KSHV genes are induced by forced over-expression of constitutively active Notch in PEL cells, in the absence of induction of Rta (Chang et al., 2005) or productive reactivation of the virus (Carroll et al., 2006). These data suggest that pathways of lytic gene induction that are independent of Rta expression can develop in latently infected cells.

Lytic replication and interactions with the host cell

G1 arrest

It is postulated that many herpesviruses actively promote G1 arrest to favor efficient lytic replication (for review see Flemington, 2001), a function that appears to have been conserved by KSHV. Induction of the lytic cycle by TPA in JSC-1 or BCP-1 (PEL) cells arrests them in G1, as measured by an increase in the 2N DNA content and lack of BrdU incorporation (Wu et al., 2002; Izumiya et al., 2003b). Stable expression of K8/KbZIP in BCBL-1 cells can further delay G1 progression after TPA induction (Izumiya et al., 2003b). The G1 arrest is reproduced by expression of the K8/KbZIP protein in KSHV-negative cells (Wu et al., 2002), in which K8/KbZIP cooperates with C/EBPα to transcriptionally activate the p21 cyclin-dependent kinase inhibitor WAF1/CIP in a p53-independent manner (Wu et al., 2002). These effects require a direct interaction of both proteins through their respective leucine zippers, and do not occur if K8/KbZIP is expressed in C/EBPα null cells (Wu et al., 2002). K8/KbZIP also regulates both C/EBPα and p21 post-translationally; in in vitro proteosomal degradation assays using BCBL-1 extracts, K8/KbZIP stabilizes both the C/EBPα and p21 proteins in a leucine-zipper dependent manner (Wu et al., 2002). K8/KbZIP can also inhibit the kinase activities of the cdk2/cyclinA and cdk2/cyclin E complexes by directly binding to them through the KbZIP basic domain (Izumiya et al., 2003b). Nonetheless, the K8/KbZIP protein itself is phosphorylated by cdk/cyclinA in complexes immunoprecipitated from induced BCBL-1 cells (Polson et al., 2001).

Expression of a second lytic cycle protein, the vGPCR, also promotes a G1 arrest in reactivating PEL cells (Cannon et al., 2006). vGPCR mediates this effect by inducing expression of the cdk inhibitor protein p21 to block cdk 2 activity. Interestingly, this results in counteracting the TPA-induced expression of viral lytic cycle proteins including the lytic switch Rta, and ORF26.

Apoptosis

Expression of Rta in uninfected BJAB cells results in apoptosis, but stable, tetracycline-regulated induction of Rta in BCBL-1 (PEL) cells does not lead to cell death, even up to 13 days following initial expression. These data suggest that, in the absence of viral infection, Rta is proapoptotic, but that a protein(s) expressed in infected cells counteracts cell death induction (Nishimura et al., 2003). KSHV encodes various lytic cycle proteins that are candidates for inhibiting Rta-induced programmed cell death, and use remarkably different mechanisms. Rta itself can inhibit p53-mediated cell death (Gwack et al., 2001b), and can also function as a ligand-independent inducer of the antiapoptotic STAT3 protein (Gwack et al., 2002). K8/KbZIP binds to p53 to repress its transcriptional activity (Park et al., 2000). KSHV ORF16 encodes vBcl-2, which partially reverses cell death induced by Bax (Cheng et al., 1997; Sarid et al., 1997), and counteracts the ability of the pro-apoptotic protein Diva to inhibit Bcl-XL. The K7/viral inhibitor of apoptosis protein (IAP) is a mitochondrial membrane protein that employs at least three different strategies: (i) it helps target cellular Bcl-2 to activated caspase-3 to inhibit its function (Wang et al., 2002); (ii) it binds a cellular cyclophilin ligand to enhance Ca^{2+} flow and protect cells from mitochrondrial damage (Feng et al., 2002); and (iii) it promotes degradation of IkB and p53 by preventing the cellular PLIC1 protein from protectively binding to them (Feng et al., 2004). K9 encodes vIRF-1, a homologue of cellular IRFs, that inhibits apoptosis induced by various means and is required for reactivation of KSHV and expression of lytic genes (Burysek et al., 1999; Flowers et al., 1998; Gao et al., 1997; Jayachandra et al., 1999; Kirchhoff et al., 2002; Li et al., 1998; Lin et al., 2001; Nakamura et al., 2001; Seo et al., 2001). K9 can inhibit p53-dependent transcription (Seo et al., 2001; Nakamura et al., 2001), and blocks transcriptional activation by the cellular proteins IRF-1 and IRF-3 (Burysek et al., 1999; Flowers et al., 1998; Kirchhoff et al., 2002; Li et al., 1998; Lin et al., 2001).

Shut-off of host gene expression

At early times during reactivation of KSHV (10–12 hours post-induction), global mRNA turnover is accelerated in KSHV infected endothelial cells (Glaunsinger and Ganem, 2004). Overexpression of the KSHV ORF37 gene reproduces this effect, so has been termed the SOX protein (for shut-off and exonuclease). Viral transcripts seem to be largely unaffected by the SOX protein, while only a limited number of host transcripts can escape the shut-off. These host transcripts include those encoding HIF-1α and IL-6, both of which play prominent roles in KSHV pathogenesis.

Regulation of lytic DNA replication

A subset of KSHV delayed–early RNAs encode enzymes required for lytic replication of the viral genome, and regulatory factors that initiate and control the DNA replication process. Viral DNA synthesis begins shortly after the appearance of the delayed–early proteins. As in other herpesviruses, KSHV lytic phase replication proceeds via a mechanism that is distinct from latent viral DNA replication (discussed in detail in the Chapter 24). First, latent DNA replication initiates at *ori-P* and proceeds bidirectionally, while viral lytic replication initiates from a distinct origin (*ori-Lyt*) and proceeds via a rolling-circle mechanism. Second, latent DNA replication depends on host cellular DNA polymerase and accessory factors, while viral lytic replication utilizes a DNA polymerase and other factors encoded by KSHV. Third, latent viral replication occurs in synchrony with the host cell to maintain a stable number of viral episomes per host genome, while viral lytic replication amplifies the viral DNA by one-hundred- or even one-thousand-fold.

Origins of lytic DNA replication

Lytic cycle DNA replication of KSHV initiates from two lytic origins (*ori-Lyt-L and ori-Lyt-R*), located in the genome between K4.2 and K5, and between K12 and ORF71, respectively (AuCoin *et al.*, 2002; Lin *et al.*, 2003). Both *ori-Lyt*s share an almost identical 1.1 kb core sequence, juxtaposed to 600 bp GC-rich repeats (Fig. 26.4).

Each 1.7 kb *ori-Lyt* sequence is necessary and sufficient as a *cis*-acting signal for KSHV lytic replication in transient replication assays (Lin *et al.*, 2003). However, in the context of the viral genome, *ori-Lyt-L* appears to be sufficient to propagate the viral genome whereas *ori-Lyt-R* alone seems inert to direct amplification of viral DNA, as suggested by an investigation using recombinant KSHVs that removed one or both of the *ori-Lyt*s in the genome (Xu *et al.*, 2006). Three essential sequence motifs are conserved in the 1.1 kb. region: (i) an 18-bp AT-palindromic sequence, (ii) eight C/EBP binding motifs, arranged as four spaced palindromes, and (iii) an ORF50/Rta responsive element (RRE) linked to a TATA box (Wang *et al.*, 2004b). Substitution or deletion of any of these three core elements abolishes *ori-Lyt* function (Wu *et al.*, 2003; Wang *et al.*, 2004b), while the 600-bp GC-rich tandem repeats are also required for efficient DNA replication (Lin *et al.*, 2003; Wang *et al.*, 2006).

The AT-palindromic sequence (Fig. 26.5) is also present in the core loop structures of HSV-1 *ori-L* and *ori-S*, as well as in the HHV6 and HHV-7 lytic origins. In fact, an AT-rich palindrome is a common feature of both cellular and viral DNA replication origins (Challberg and Kelly, 1989; DePamphilis, 1993). It is believed that an AT-rich palindrome facilitates DNA unwinding and enhances helicase activity during DNA replication.

The eight C/EBP binding motifs are organized as four spaced C/EBP palindromic pairs within a 240-bp sequence (Wu *et al.*, 2003; Wang *et al.*, 2004b). Each palindrome contains two head-to-head CCAAT consensus motifs that are separated by a 13- or 12-bp spacer sequence. One of the KSHV origin binding proteins (OBPs), the K8/KbZIP protein, associates with *ori-Lyt* at the CCAAT motifs (discussed below) (Wang *et al.*, 2004b, 2006).

The RRE/TATA box motif functions as a cis-acting transcriptional promoter whose activity is required for replication from *ori-Lyt*. The KSHV ORF50/Rta protein binds directly to the RRE to activate transcription at *ori-Lyt*. The promoter in *ori-Lyt-L* normally directs transcription of a 1.4 kb RNA containing the GC-rich repeats and a putative open reading frame of 75 amino acids, and the promoter in *ori-Lyt-R* controls the synthesis of the 2.3-kb mRNA encoding K12 (Wang *et al.*, 2004b). Transcription events controlled by these promoters are essential for DNA replication from the *ori-Lyt*, as prematurely termination of the transcription by inserting an SV40 polyadenylation sequence upstream of the GC-rich repeats completely abolished the transcription activity as well as DNA replication (Wang *et al.*, 2006). The EBV *ori-Lyt* also contains a promoter whose transcriptional activity is required for replication (Hammerschmidt and Sugden, 1988), but the role of these promoters and transcripts in gamma-herpesviral lytic replication are unknown.

The 600-bp GC-rich tandem repeat sequences adjacent to the *ori-Lyt* core sequences are represented as both 20-bp and 30-bp tandem arrays in the *ori-lyt-L*, and two types of 23-bp tandem repeats in the *ori-Lyt-R*. Such GC-rich tandem repeats are also found in the *ori-Lyt*s of EBV and RRV (Hammerschmidt and Sugden, 1988; Pari *et al.*, 2001).

K8/KbZIP and ORF50/Rta are origin-binding proteins that are responsible for recruiting pre-replication complexes to *ori-Lyt* DNA

Initiation of herpesviral lytic replication requires binding of OBPs to *ori-Lyt* elements. Subsequently, the OBPs recruit DNA replication enzymes and accessory factors to the origins. The recruitment of replication proteins by OBPs is dictated by specific protein–protein interactions, and facilitated by linking and distortion of the origin DNA by the OBPs.

All four of the C/EBP palindromes in *ori-Lyt* are indispensable for replication, and mutagenesis studies have

Goals of lytic replication 447

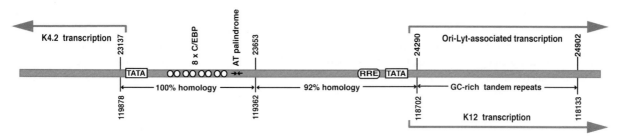

Fig. 26.4. Structure of the KSHV origin of DNA replication (*ori-Lyt*). The positions of various characteristic motifs (TATA boxes, C/EBP binding motifs, AT palindrome, RRE and GC tandem repeats) are as indicated. The homologies of subregions between two *ori-Lyts* are compared and shown on the bottom.

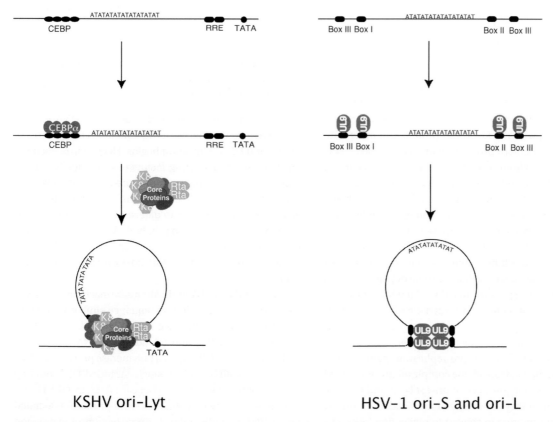

Fig. 26.5. Model for recruitment of core replication proteins to KSHV *ori-Lyt* DNA through ORF50/Rta and K8/KbZIP. Six core replication machinery proteins (referred to as core proteins for simplicity), ORF50/Rta and K8/KbZIP (referred to as Rta and K8, respectively, for simplicity) form a pre-replication complex regardless of the presence of *ori-Lyt* DNA. The pre-replication complex is loaded at a KSHV *ori-Lyt* by a two-point-contact through RTA and K8, each of which interacts with their binding motifs in the *ori-Lyt*. The interaction may lead to looping and distortion of the *ori-Lyt* DNA (left panel), which resembles the binding and looping of HSV-1 *ori-S* and *ori-L* by UL9 proteins (right panel)

shown that three of the individual C/EBP sites C/EBP 1, 2, and 6 are essential for *ori-Lyt* function. Although deletion or mutation of these C/EBP motifs also impairs the association of K8/KbZIP with the *ori-Lyt*, subsequent EMSA experiments have failed to demonstrate direct protein-DNA interactions between the two (Wang *et al.*, 2004b). However, the observation that (i) C/EBP α binds directly to four of the C/EBP sites, and (ii) C/EBP α binds specifically to the K8/KbZIP protein (Wu *et al.*, 2003), implies that K8/KbZIP binds to KSHV *ori-Lyt* through interacting with DNA-bound C/EBP α (Fig. 26.5) (Wang *et al.*, 2004b).

Binding of the ORF50/Rta protein to the RRE in *ori-Lyt* is absolutely essential for *ori-Lyt*-dependent DNA replication, suggesting that Rta is a second critical OBP. The RRE closely resembles the RRE sequence in the nut-1/PAN promoter (Wang *et al.*, 2004b; AuCoin *et al.*, 2004), and deletion of the RRE or the downstream TATA box abolishes transcription and replication at *ori-Lyt*. If the RRE is replaced by a binding site for the heterologous Gal4 protein, a Gal4-ORF50 fusion protein can rescue replication, suggesting that Rta-mediated transactivation is required for replication. In addition to the transcriptional activation Rta also participates in replication complex formation on *ori-Lyt* by interacting with the K8/KbZIP protein and other core replication machinery proteins (Wang *et al.*, 2006). This notion is derived from several lines of evidence as follows: (i) Rta was found to be a component of viral replication compartments in the nuclei of infected cells, and shown to interact with core replication machinery complexes (or pre-replication complexes) composed of at least six core replication proteins and K8/KbZIP, (ii) The loading of the core replication machinery complexes on the *ori-Lyt* DNA appears to be mediated by Rta and to be dependent upon the RRE in the *ori-Lyt*, as the deletion of the RRE abolished the association of replication proteins with *ori-Lyt* DNA. This suggests that Rta plays a role in recruiting the core replication machinery complexes to the *ori-Lyt* DNA, (iii) The association of Rta with pre-replication complexes is not DNA-mediated. Instead, the complexes are assembled independent of the presence of *ori-Lyt* DNA and become less stable once they are recruited and loaded on *ori-Lyt* DNA, perhaps in order to convert to replication fork complexes (Wang *et al.*, 2006).

K8/KbZIP also interacts with core replication machinery proteins and has a similar function as Rta in recruiting and loading pre-replication complexes to the *ori-Lyt* DNA. Thus, formation of a functional DNA replication initiation complex on an *ori-Lyt* requires the efforts of both RTA and K8/KbZIP in loading pre-replication complexes on *ori-Lyt* (Wang *et al.*, 2006). Based on these data, a model of K8/KbZIP and ORF50/Rta recruiting pre-replication complexes to *ori-Lyt* is proposed in Fig. 26.5. In this model, a pre-replication complex apparently binds to an *ori-Lyt* DNA through two contact points, one at the K8 binding region (the C/EBP cluster) near one end of the *ori-Lyt* and the other at the RRE near the opposite end. The two-contact-point binding may bring the two ends of the *ori-Lyt* element together, looping the DNA between the K8 and Rta binding sites. An 18-bp AT palindrome sequence is located in the looped region (Fig 26.5). A similar loop structure has been seen in the HSV-1 DNA replication system, in which two UL9 protein dimers (OBP) bind to two binding sites (Boxes I and II) in *ori-S* and *ori-L* and the protein-protein interactions between the UL9 molecules loops the *ori-Lyt* DNA centered by an AT-palindrome sequence (reviewed in Boehmer and Lehman, 1997). The looping leads to bending and distortion of *ori-Lyt* DNA, facilitating unwinding of the DNA sequence.

Viral enzymes and accessory factors essential for KSHV ori-Lyt-specific DNA replication and DNA replication machinery

Following binding of the OBPs to an origin, DNA replication enzymes and accessory factors are recruited to the origin, and DNA replication begins. Herpesvirus-encoded enzymes and trans-acting factors essential for lytic DNA replication are referred to as the core replication machinery. Homologues of the core proteins have been found in all herpesviruses studied to date, and are structurally and functionally conserved. In fact, both the HSV-1 and KSHV-encoded replication proteins can replicate the EBV *ori-Lyt* in the presence of the EBV OBP *Zta* (Fixman *et al.*, 1995; Wu *et al.*, 2001).

The candidate KSHV replication core machinery proteins were originally identified by sequence similarity to HSV-1 and EBV homologues (see Table 26.1) (Wu *et al.*, 2001; AuCoin *et al.*, 2004), and include (i) a DNA polymerase (POL encoded by ORF9), (ii) a polymerase processivity factor (PPF by ORF59), (iii) a single-stranded DNA binding protein (SSB by ORF6), (iv) a helicase (HEL by ORF44), (v) a primase (PRI by ORF56), and (vi) a primase-associated factor (PAF by ORF40/41). Co-transfection of expression vectors for these proteins and the OBPs (K8/KbZIP and ORF50/Rta) is necessary and sufficient to support DNA replication of a plasmid containing a KSHV *ori-Lyt* in mammalian cells. If any of the core replication proteins are omitted in the system, no replicated KSHV *ori-Lyt* plasmid DNA is detected (AuCoin *et al.*, 2004). In these crucial transient co-transfection-replication assays, replicated *ori-Lyt*-containing DNA becomes resistant to methylation-sensitive restriction enzymes that can only digest the input

Table 26.1. KSHV DNA replication proteins and their analogues in other herpesviruses

Protein and enzyme	Gene	Size (aa)	KSHV vs. HSV-1			KSHV vs. EBV			Activities
			Name	Sim(%)	Iden(%)	Name	Sim(%)	Iden(%)	
K8/KbZIP	K8	237				BZLF1		–	*Ori-Lyt binding protein*
ORF50/Rta	ORF50	691				BRLF1	32.2	20.6	Transcription activator, *ori-Lyt* binding protein
SSB	ORF6	1133	UL29	36.1	27.1	BALF2	65.5	42.1	Single-stranded DNA binding
HEL	ORF44	788	UL5	49.6	37.7	BBLF4	67.8	51.1	Helicase subunit
PRI	ORF56	843	UL52	39.5	29.0	BSLF1	56.6	35.4	Primase subunit
PAF	ORF40/41	670	UL8	—		BBLF2/3	47.1	23.3	Primase-associated factor
POL	ORF9	1012	UL30	60.0	41.7	BALF5	70.9	55.6	DNA polymerase subunit
PPF	ORF59	396	UL42	—		BMRF1	50.7	28.3	Double-stranded DNA binding protein, DNA polymerase processivity factor subunit

aa: amino acid; Sim%: percent similarity; Iden%: percent identity.

plasmid; the replication products are then detected by Southern blotting. The six core replication proteins can form a large globular shaped replication compartment even in the absence of an *ori-Lyt* DNA (Wu *et al.*, 2001), suggesting that they spontaneously assemble a pseudo-replication compartment (without DNA) in solution, then land on with the *ori-Lyt* DNA aid of OBPs. The biochemical properties of the individual KSHV DNA replication proteins are reviewed as follows:

Single-stranded DNA binding protein (SSB)

Among the core replication proteins, SSB is one of two intrinsic nuclear proteins (the other is PPF) that contributes to the nuclear translocation of the other core proteins, especially the primase-helicase tripartite subcomplex proteins PAF, HEL and PRI (Wu *et al.*, 2001; AuCoin *et al.*, 2004). The mechanism of KSHV SSB has not been studied in detail, but is probably similar to that of its HSV-1 counterpart (for review see Boehmer and Lehman, 1997). SSB rapidly and cooperatively binds to single-stranded *ori-Lyt* DNA formed as a result of binding of OBP proteins, and unwinds short regions of duplex DNA to further destabilize the DNA helix. These functions of SSB promote viral DNA replication by enhancing subsequent DNA polymerase and DNA helicase-primase activities.

DNA helicase–primase complex

The KSHV proteins HEL, PRI, and PAF form a tripartite primase/helicase complex, similar to their homologues in HSV-1 and EBV. Unlike its counterparts, efficient translocation of the KSHV complex to the nucleus requires co-expression of the three other core replication proteins (Wu *et al.*, 2001). High homologies between the KSHV and the HSV-1 proteins (or subunits if the tripartite complex is considered a holo-enzyme) suggest similar modes of action. The HSV-1 holoenzyme consists of a 1:1:1 association of UL5 (HEL), UL52 (PRI) and UL8 (PAF) proteins, and has a native molecular mass of 270 kDa. However, the UL5/UL52 sub-assembly displays DNA-dependent ATPase, 5′–3′ helicase, and primase activities, as well as a primer synthesis function that is stimulataed by the UL8 protein (reviewed in Boehmer and Lehman, 1997).

DNA polymerase and processivity factor

As in other herpesviruses, the KSHV DNA polymerase consists of two subunits, POL (polymerase) and PPF (polymerase processivity factor). KSHV POL not only shares a high homology with its HSV-1 counterpart, but also with DNA polymerases from mammals, yeast, *E. coli*, and bacteriophage. In the absence of the PPF subunit, the KSHV POL incorporates only several nucleotides from a primer template. However, association with the PPF enables POL to incorporate thousands of nucleotides continuously without dissociation from the template (Lin *et al.*, 1998).

Association with a processivity factor is an evolutionarily-conserved mechanism by which DNA polymerases achieve catalytic efficiency. The most conserved processivity factors are the ring-shaped sliding clamps, which encircle DNA templates and enable the associated DNA polymerases to slide along the template without dissociating. However, the HSV-1 processivity factor is of insufficient size to form an encircling sliding clamp; instead, it tethers the DNA polymerase to the DNA template by double stranded DNA binding. The KSHV and HSV-1 PPF subunits display only limited sequence similarity, ~40 amino acids near their carboxy termini, so the mechanism of KSHV PPF remains elusive (Chen et al., 2004). Since processivity factors adopt divergent states during DNA replication, they may serve as good targets for the design of novel and specific anti-herpesviral therapies.

In addition to these essential DNA replication proteins, KSHV also encodes several other enzymes for its DNA replication, including thymidine kinase, ribonucleotide reductase, alkaline exonuclease, uracil N-glycosylase and deoxyuridine triphosphatase. However, the functions of these enzymes are not essential for viral DNA replication.

Late genes and KSHV virion structure

The KSHV virion conserves the major structural elements of herpesviruses, including the genomic DNA, the capsid, the tegument, and the envelope. Proteins required for assembly and structure of DNA viruses have traditionally been regarded as viral late genes that require prior viral DNA replication for expression. This is likely true for the KSHV proteins that comprise the capsid and are inserted into the envelope, although there are exceptions (as discussed above and in Chapter 23). Proteins that comprise the tegument, however, are likely to be expressed from all kinetic classes of lytic replication; as discussed below, the ORF45 protein is an IE protein that is packaged into the KSHV tegument (Zhu and Yuan, 2003).

Virions released from induced PEL cells have provided the first detailed understanding of virion structures for the γ-herpesviruses. When PELs are treated with TPA and sodium butyrate, purified virions contain three types of capsid, named A, B, and C, respectively (Nealon et al., 2001). Fully mature C capsids have a total mass of 300 Mda, and in declining order of abundance, contain the proteins ORF25/MCP (Major capsid protein), ORF65/SCIP (small capsomer-interacting protein), ORF26/TRI-2 (triplex-2), ORF62/TRI-1, and the 160–170 kb (unique region plus repeats) viral genome (Nealon et al., 2001). A capsids contain the four proteins listed above, but lack viral genomic DNA. B capsids, the most abundant category released from lytic PEL cells, have the identical constituents as A capsids but also contain the scaffolding protein encoded by ORF17.5 (Nealon et al., 2001). The capsid components are organized into a discrete series of capsomers containing hexons, pentons, and triplexes of one or two proteins each. The hexons and pentons contain six and five copies of the MCP, respectively, and the triplexes contain a dimer of TRI-2 protein and a monomer of TRI-1 (Trus et al., 2001; Wu et al., 2000). SCIP associates with MCP on hexamers, but not pentamers, and its location at the outermost portions of the capsid suggests that it might directly contact the tegument (Lo et al., 2003). This localization of SCIP to the outer capsid region is conserved in virions of Rhesus monkey rhadinovirus, but not with α-herpesviruses, suggesting a potential unique function for γ-herpesvirus teguments (Yu et al., 2003).

Cryoelectron microscopy at 24-Ångström resolution and digital reconstruction demonstrate that the mature capsid is icosahedral with a diameter of approximately 1140–1300-Ångström (Wu et al., 2000; Trus et al., 2001). The $T=16$ icosahedral structure of the KSHV capsid is similar to that of the γ-herpesvirus herpes simplex virus-1, and the β-herpesvirus, Human cytomegalovirus, but the overall sizes of each capsid are proportional to the sizes of each virus's genome (Wu et al., 2000; Trus et al., 2001). Phylogenetic comparisons of the MCP protein reveal that the β- and γ-herpesviruses are more closely related to each other than to the α-herpesviruses (Trus et al., 2001).

When protein lysates of purified virions are displayed on SDS-PAGE gradient gels, approximately 30 proteins can be differentiated (Zhu and Yuan, 2003); 24 of these have been identified by proteomic analyses (Zhu et al., 2005). Those that are not capsid proteins are predicted to be parts of the tegument or envelope layers characteristic of mature herpesviral virions, which are presumably added to KSHV capsids during cellular egress. Various glycoproteins of KSHV, including K8.1, glycoprotein (g) B, gH, gL, gM, and gN, have been identified by sequence analysis and/or have been demonstrated to be membrane components of KSHV virions (Akula et al., 2001; Baghian et al., 2000; Pertel, 2002; Birkmann et al., 2001; Wang et al., 2001; Zhu et al., 1999). Detergent treatment of virions releases membrane glycoproteins, but not tegument proteins, which are sandwiched between the capsid and membrane (Zhu et al., 2005). Although the tegument of HSV-1 contains the well-characterized virion protein (VP)16, a transcriptional transactivator essential for expression of HSV-1 IE genes during de novo infection (reviewed in (Roizman and Sears, 1996)), the functions of KSHV tegument proteins are virtually unknown. The first tegument protein of KSHV to be identified is the product of ORF45 (Zhu and Yuan, 2003), a protein that counteracts the cellular α-interferon response by blocking the phosphorylation and nuclear accumulation of interferon regulatory factor (IRF)-7 (Zhu et al., 2002). This suggests that ORF45 is packaged into the tegument so that it can function at the earliest stages of de novo KSHV infection. Eleven KSHV RNAs are also found packaged in the virion, and may get translated after infection (Bechtel *et al.*, 2005).

Perspectives

KSHV has conserved the hallmark of herpesvirus pathogenesis: latent infection that persists for the lifetime of the host, requiring successful establishment and maintenance of latency in long-lived or self-perpetuating cellular reservoirs. Selective pressure exerted for millions of years on herpesviruses would not be expected to favor an increase in virulence unless it allowed greater replication and transmission of the virus. The obvious contribution of lytic genes to KS pathogenesis, therefore, is to facilitate dissemination of the virus from its long-term reservoir to sites of disease or of shedding. However, as highlighted in other chapters of this book, twelve viral open reading frames (ORFs) that have independent transforming, pro-angiogenic, pro-growth, anti-apoptotic, or immunomodulatory functions, are expressed following lytic reactivation of the virus. Therefore, it is likely that the pathogenic requirement for KSHV lytic reactivation and replication, as observed in epidemiologic studies, reflects both a necessity for increased viral titers to facilitate viral dissemination, as well as a contribution of viral lytic cycle proteins as direct effectors of the disease phenotypes. Lytically infected cells may thus serve not only as reservoirs of infectious virus but also as reservoirs of pathogenic viral proteins. Translated to the clinical setting, this may represent a pathogenic mechanism by which KSHV initiates or maintains the aggressive inflammatory infiltrate that characterizes KS lesions.

REFERENCES

Akula, S. M., Pramod, N. P., Wang, F. Z., and Chandran, B. (2001). Human herpesvirus 8 envelope-associated glycoprotein B interacts with heparan sulfate-like moieties. *Virology*, **284**(2), 235–249.

Aluigi, M. G., Albini, A., Carlone, S. *et al.* (1996). KSHV sequences in biopsies and cultured spindle cells of epidemic, iatrogenic and Mediterranean forms of Kaposi's sarcoma. *Res. Virol.*, **147**(5), 267–275.

Ambroziak, J., Blackbourn, D., Herndier, B. *et al.* (1995). Herpesvirus-like sequenes in HIV-infected and uninfected Kaposi's sarcoma patients. *Science*, **268**, 582–583.

Andreoni, M., Goletti, D., Pezzotti, P. *et al.* (2001). Prevalence, incidence and correlates of HHV-8/KSHV infection and Kaposi's sarcoma in renal and liver transplant recipients. *J. Infect.*, **43**(3), 195–199.

Asahara, T., Murohara, T., Sullivan, A. *et al.* (1997). Isolation of putative progenitor endothelial cells for angiogenesis. *Science*, **275**(5302), 964–967.

AuCoin, D. P., Colletti, K. S., Xu, Y. *et al.* (2002). Kaposi's sarcoma-associated herpesvirus (human herpesvirus 8) contains two functional lytic origins of DNA replication. *J. Virol.*, **76**(15), 7890–7896.

AuCoin, D. P., Colletti, K. S., Cei, S. A., Papouskova, I., Tarrant, M., and Pari, G. S. (2004). Amplification of the Kaposi's sarcoma-associated herpesvirus/human herpesvirus 8 lytic origin of DNA replication is dependent upon a cis-acting AT-rich region and an ORF50 response element and the trans-acting factors ORF50 (K-Rta) and K8 (K-bZIP). *Virology*, **318**, 542–555.

Baghian, A., Luftig, M., Black, J. B. *et al.* (2000). Glycoprotein B of human herpesvirus 8 is a component of the virion in a cleaved form composed of amino- and carboxyl-terminal fragments. *Virology*, **269**(1), 18–25.

Barozzi, P., Luppi, M., Facchetti, F. *et al.* (2003). Post-transplant Kaposi sarcoma originates from the seeding of donor-derived progenitors. *Nat. Med.*, **9**(5), 554–561.

Bechtel, J., Grundhoff, A., and Ganem, D. (2005). RNAs in the virion of Kaposi's sarcoma-associated herpesvirus. *J. Virol.*, **79**(16), 10138–10146.

Beyari, M. M., Hodgson, T. A., Cook, R. D. *et al.* (2003). Multiple human herpesvirus-8 infection. *J. Infect. Dis.*, **188**(5), 678–689.

Biggar, R. J., Engels, E. A., Whitby, D. Kedes, D. H., and Goederr, J. J. (2003). Antibody reactivity to latent and lytic antigens to human herpesvirus-8 in longitudinally followed homosexual men. *J. Infect. Dis.*, **187**(1), 12–18.

Bigoni, B., Dolcetti, R., de Lellis, L. *et al.* (1996). Human Herpesvirus 8 is present in the lymphoid system of healthy persons and can reactivate in the course of AIDS. *J. Infect. Dis.*, **173**, 542–549.

Birkmann, A., Mahr, K., Ensser, A. *et al.* (2001). Cell surface heparan sulfate is a receptor for human herpesvirus 8 and interacts with envelope glycoprotein K8.1. *J. Virol.*, **75**(23), 11583–11593.

Blackbourn, D. J., Ambroziak, J., Lennette, E., Adams, M., Ramachandran, B., and Levy, J. A. (1997). Infectious human herpesvirus 8 in a healthy North American blood donor [see comments]. *Lancet*, **349**(9052), 609–611.

Blackbourn, D. J., Lennette, E. T., Ambroziak, J., Mourich, D. V., and Levy, J. A. (1998). Human herpesvirus 8 detection in nasal secretions and saliva. *J. Infect. Dis.*, **177**(1), 213–216.

Blackbourn, D., Fujimura, S., Kutzkey, T., and Levy, J. (2000). Induction of human herpesvirus-8 gene expression by recombinant interferon gamma. *AIDS*, **14**, 98–99.

Blasig, C., Zietz, C., Haar, B. *et al.* (1997). Monocytes in Kaposi's sarcoma lesions are productively infected by human herpesvirus 8. *J. Virol.*, **71**, 7963–7968.

Boehmer, P. E. and Lehman, I. R. (1997). Herpes simplex virus DNA replication. *Annu. Rev. Biochem.*, **66**, 347–384.

Boneschi, V., Brambilla, L., Berti, E. *et al.* (2001). Human herpesvirus 8 DNA in the skin and blood of patients with Mediterranean Kaposi's sarcoma: clinical correlations. *Dermatology*, **203**(1), 19–23.

Boshoff, C., Schulz, T. F., Kennedy, M. M. et al. (1995). Kaposi's sarcoma-associated herpesvirus infects endothelial and spindle cells. *Nat. Med.*, **1**(12), 1274–1278.

Boshoff, C., Gao, S.-J., Healy, L. et al. (1998). Establishing a KSHV+ cell line (BCP-1) from peripheral blood and characterizing its growth in Nod/SCID mice. *Blood*, **91**, 1671–1679.

Bourboulia, D., Aldam, D., Lagos, D. et al. (2004). Short- and long-term effects of highly active antiretroviral therapy on Kaposi sarcoma-associated herpesvirus immune responses and viraemia. *AIDS*, **18**(3), 485–493.

Brenner, B., Weissmann-Brenner, A., Rakowsky, E. et al. (2002). Classical Kaposi sarcoma. *Cancer*, **95**(9), 1982–1987.

Brown, H. J., Song, M. J., Deng, H., Wu, T. T., Cheng, G., and Sun, R. (2003). NF-kappaB inhibits gammaherpesvirus lytic replication. *J. Virol.*, **77**(15), 8532–8540.

Browning, P., Sechler, J., Kaplan, M. et al. (1994). Identification and culture of Kaposi's sarcoma-like spindle cells from the peripheral blood of human immunodeficiency virus-1-infected individuals and normal controls. *Blood*, **84**, 2711–2720.

Burysek, L., Yeow, W. S., Lubyova, B. et al. (1999). Functional analysis of human herpesvirus 8-encoded viral interferon regulatory factor 1 and its association with cellular interferon regulatory factors and p300. *J. Virol.*, **73**, 7334–7342.

Cai, J., Gill, P. S., Masood, R. et al. (1994). Oncostatin-M is an autocrine growth factor in Kaposi's sarcoma. *Am. J. Pathol.*, **145**(1), 74–79.

Campbell, T. B., Borok, M., Gwanzura, L. et al. (2000). Relationship of human herpesvirus 8 peripheral blood virus load and Kaposi's sarcoma clinical stage. *AIDS*, **14**(14), 2109–2116.

Cannon, M. J., Dollard, S. C., Smith, D. K. et al. (2001). Blood-borne and sexual transmission of human herpesvirus 8 in women with or at risk for human immunodeficiency virus infection. *N. Engl. J. Med.*, **344**(9), 637–643.

Cannon, M. J., Dollard, S. C., Black, J. B. et al. (2003). Risk factors for Kaposi's sarcoma in men seropositive for both human herpesvirus 8 and human immunodeficiency virus. *AIDS*, **17**(2), 215–222.

Cannon, M., Cesarman, E., and Boshoff, C. (2006). KSHV G protein-coupled receptor inhibits lytic gene transcription in primary-effusion lymphoma cells via p21-mediated inhibition of Cdk2. *Blood*, **107**(1), 277–284.

Carbone, A., Gloghini, A., Cozzi, M. R. et al. (2000). Expression of MUM1/IRF4 selectively clusters with primary effusion lymphoma among lymphomatous effusions: implications for disease histogenesis and pathogenesis. *Br. J. Haematol.*, **111**(1), 247–257.

Carbone, A., Gloghini, A., Larocca, L. et al. (2001). Expression profile of MUM1/IRF4, BCL-6, and CD138/syndecan-1 defines novel histogenetic subsets of human immunodeficiency virus-related lymphomas. *Blood*, **97**, 744–751.

Cardin, R. D., Brooks, J. W., Sarawar, S. R., and Doherty, P. C. (1996). Progressive loss of CD8+ T cell-mediated control of a gammaherpesvirus in the absence of CD4+ T cells. *J. Exp. Med.*, **184**(3), 863–871.

Carroll, K. D., Bu, W., Palmeri, D. et al. (2006). The KSHV lytic switch protein stimulates DNA binding of RBP-Jk/CSL to activate the notch pathway. *J. Virol.*, **80**(19).

Casper, C., Nichols, W. G., Huang, M. L., Corey, L., and Wald, A. (2004). Remission of HHV-8 and HIV-associated multicentric Castleman disease with ganciclovir treatment. *Blood*, **103**(5), 1632–1634.

Casper, C., Redman, M., Huang, M. L. et al. (2004b). HIV infection and human herpesvirus-8 oral shedding among men who have sex with men. *J. Acquir. Immune Defic. Syndr.*, **35**(3), 233–238.

Cattani, P., Capuano, M., Cerimele, F. et al. (2001). Kaposi's sarcoma associated with previous human herpesvirus 8 infection in kidney transplant recipients. *J. Clin. Microbiol.*, **39**(2), 506–508.

Cattani, P., Capuano, M., Cerimele, F. et al. (1999). Human herpesvirus 8 seroprevalence and evaluation of nonsexual transmission routes by detection of DNA in clinical specimens from human immunodeficiency virus-seronegative patients from central and southern Italy, with and without Kaposi's sarcoma. *J. Clin. Microbiol.*, **37**(4), 1150–1153.

Cattelan, A., Calabro, M., Gasperini, P. et al. (2001). Acquired immunodeficiency syndrome-related kaposi's sarcoma regression after highly active antiretroviral therapy: biologic correlates of clinical outcome. *J. Natl Cancer Inst. Monogr.*, **28**, 44–49.

Cerimele, D., Cottoni, F., and Masala, M. V. (2000). Long latency of human herpesvirus type 8 infection and the appearance of classic Kaposi's sarcoma. *J. Am. Acad. Dermatol.*, **43**(4), 731–732.

Cesarman, E., Chang, Y., Moore, P. S., Said, J. W., and Knowles, D. M. (1995). Kaposi's sarcoma-associated herpesvirus-like DNA sequences in AIDS-related body-cavity-based lymphomas. *N. Engl. J. Med.*, **332**(18), 1186–1191.

Cesarman, E., Nador, R. G., Aozasa, K., Delsol, G., Said, J. W., and Knowles, D. M. (1996). Kaposi's sarcoma-associated herpesvirus in non-AIDS related lymphomas occurring in body cavities. *Am. J. Pathol.*, **149**(1), 53–57.

Challberg, M. D. and Kelly, T. J. (1989). Animal virus DNA replication. *Annu. Rev. Biochem.*, **58**, 671–717.

Chang, J., Renne, R., Dittmer, D., and Ganem, D. (2000). Inflammatory cytokines and the reactivation of Kaposi's sarcoma-associated herpesvirus lytic replication. *Virology*, **266**, 17–25.

Chang, P. J., Shedd, D., Gradoville, L. et al. (2002). Open reading frame 50 protein of Kaposi's sarcoma-associated herpesvirus directly activates the viral PAN and K12 genes by binding to related response elements. *J. Virol.*, **76**(7), 3168–3178.

Chang, Y., Cesarman, E., Pessin, M. S. et al. (1994). Identification of herpesvirus-like DNA sequences in AIDS-associated Kaposi's sarcoma [see comments]. *Science*, **266**(5192), 1865–1869.

Chang, H., Dittmer, D. P., Chul, S.-Y., Hong, Y., and Jung, J. U. (2005a). Role of notch signal transduction in Kaposi's sarcoma-associated herpesvirus gene Expression. *J. Virol.*, **79**(22), 14371–14382.

Chang, P.-J., Shedd, D., and Miller, G. (2005b). Two subclasses of Kaposi's sarcoma-associated herpesvirus lytic cycle promoters distinguished by open reading frame 50 mutant proteins that are deficient in binding to DNA. *J. Virol.*, **79**(14), 8750–8763.

Chatterjee, M., Osborne, J., Bestetti, G., Chang, Y., and Moore, P. S. (2002). Viral IL-6-induced cell proliferation and immune evasion of interferon activity. *Science*, **298**(5597), 1432–1435.

Chen, J., Ueda, K., Sakakibara, S. *et al.* (2001). Activation of latent Kaposi's sarcoma-associated herpesvirus by demethylation of the promoter of the lytic transactivator. *Proc. Natl Acad. Sci. USA*, **98**(7), 4119–4124.

Chen, X., Lin, K., and Ricciardi, R. P. (2004). Human Kaposi's sarcoma herpesvirus processivity factor-8 functions as a dimer in DNA synthesis. *J. Biol. Chem.*, **279**(27), 28375–28386.

Cheng, E. H., Nicholas, J., Bellows, D. S. *et al.* (1997). A Bcl-2 homolog encoded by Kaposi sarcoma-associated virus, human herpesvirus 8, inhibits apoptosis but does not heterodimerize with Bax or Bak. *Proc. Natl Acad. Sci. USA*, **94**(2), 690–694.

Ciufo, D. M., Cannon, J. S., Poole, L. J. *et al.* (2001). Spindle cell conversion by Kaposi's sarcoma-associated herpesvirus: formation of colonies and plaques with mixed lytic and latent gene expression in infected primary dermal microvascular endothelial cell cultures. *J. Virol.*, **75**(12), 5614–5626.

Dal Canto, A., Virgin, H. I., and Speck, S. (2002). Ongoing viral replication is required for gammaherpesvirus 68-induced vascular damage. *J. Virol.*, **74**, 11035–11310.

Davis, D. A., Rinderknecht, A. S., Zoeteweij, J. P. *et al.* (2001). Hypoxia induces lytic replication of Kaposi sarcoma-associated herpesvirus. *Blood*, **97**(10), 3244–3250.

Deng, H., Song, M. J., Chu, J. T., and Sun, R. (2002). Transcriptional regulation of the interleukin-6 gene of human herpesvirus 8 (Kaposi's sarcoma-associated herpesvirus). *J. Virol.*, **76**(16), 8252–8264.

DePamphilis, M. L. (1993). Origins of DNA replication that function in eukaryotic cells. *Curr. Opin. Cell. Biol.*, **5**(3), 434–441.

Dittmer, D., Stoddart, C., Renne, R. *et al.* (1999). Experimental transmission of Kaposi's sarcoma-associated herpesvirus (KSHV/HHV-8) to SCID-hu Thy/Liv mice. *J. Exp. Med.*, **190**(12), 1857–1868.

Drexler, H., Uphoff, C., Gaidano, G., and Carbone, E. (1998). Lymphoma cell lines: in vitro models for the study of HHV-8+ primary effusion lymphomas (body cavity-based lymphomas). *Leukemia*, **12**, 1507–1517.

Dupin, N., Fisher, C., Kellam, P. *et al.* (1999). Distribution of human herpesvirus-8 latently infected cells in Kaposi's sarcoma, multicentric Castleman's disease, and primary effusion lymphoma. *Proc. Natl Acad. Sci. USA*, **96**, 4546–4551.

Duus, K. M., Lentchitsky, V., Wagenaar, T., Grose, C., and Webster-Cyriaque (2004). Wild-type Kaposi's sarcoma-associated herpesvirus isolated from the oropharynx of immune-competent individuals has tropism for cultured oral epithelial cells. *J. Virol.*, **78**(8), 4074–4084.

Eltom, M. A., Jemal, A., and Mbulaiteye, S. M. (2002). Trends in Kaposi's sarcoma and non-Hodgkin's lymphoma incidence in the United States from 1973 through 1998. *J. Natl Cancer Inst.*, **94**(16), 1204–1210.

Engels, E. A., Biggar, R. J., Marshall, V. A. *et al.* (2003). Detection and quantification of Kaposi's sarcoma-associated herpesvirus to predict AIDS-associated Kaposi's sarcoma. *J. AIDS*, **17**(12), 1847–1851.

Ensoli, B., Nakamura, S., Salahuddin, S. *et al.* (1989). AIDS-Kaposi's Sarcoma-derived cells express cytokines with autocrine and paracrine growth effects. *Science*, **243**, 223–226.

Ensoli, B., Sturzl, M., and Monini, P. (2000). Cytokine-mediated growth promotion of Kaposi's sarcoma and primary effusion lymphoma. *Semin. Cancer Biol.*, **10**, 367–381.

Ensoli, B., Sgadari, C., Barillari, G., Sirianni, M. C., Sturzl, M., and Monini, P. (2001). Biology of Kaposi's sarcoma. *Eur. J. Cancer*, **37**(10), 1251–1269.

Ernst, M. and Jenkins, B. J. (2004). Acquiring signalling specificity from the cytokine receptor gp130. *Trends Genet.*, **20**(1), 23–32.

Fais, F., Gaidano, G., Capello, D. *et al.* (1999). Immunoglobulin V region gene use and structure suggest antigen selection in AIDS-related primary effusion lymphomas. *Leukemia*, **13**(7), 1093–1099.

Fakhari, F. D. and Dittmer, D. P. (2002). Charting latency transcripts in Kaposi's sarcoma-associated herpesvirus by whole-genome real-time quantitative PCR. *J. Virol.*, **76**(12), 6213–6223.

Fardet, L., Blum, L., Kerob, D. *et al.* (2003). Human herpesvirus 8-associated hemophagocytic lymphohistiocytosis in human immunodeficiency virus-infected patients. *Clin. Infect. Dis.*, **37**(2), 285–291.

Farge, D., Lebbe, C., Marjanovic, Z. *et al.* (1999). Human herpes virus-8 and other risk factors for Kaposi's sarcoma in kidney transplant recipients. Groupe Cooperatif de Transplantation d' Ile de France (GCIF). *Transplantation*, **67**(9), 1236–1242.

Feng, P., Park, J., Lee, B. S. *et al.* (2002). Kaposi's sarcoma-associated herpesvirus mitochondrial K7 protein targets a cellular calcium-modulating cyclophilin ligand to modulate intracellular calcium concentration and inhibit apoptosis. *J. Virol.*, **76**(22), 11491–11504.

Feng, P., Scott, C. W., Cho, N. H. *et al.* (2004). Kaposi's sarcoma-associated herpesvirus K7 protein targets a ubiquitin-like/ubiquitin-associated domain-containing protien to promote protein degradation. *Mol. Cell. Biol.*, **24**(9), 3938–3948.

Feske, S., Okamura, H., Hogan, P. G., and Rao, A. (2003). Ca^{2+}/calcineurin signalling in cells of the immune system. *Biochem. Biophys. Res. Commun.*, **311**(4), 1117–1132.

Field, A. K., Davies, M. E., DeWitt, C. *et al.* (1983). 9-([2-hydroxy-1-(hydroxymethyl)ethoxy]methyl)guanine: a selective inhibitor of herpes group virus replication. *Proc. Natl Acad. Sci. USA*, **80**(13), 4139–4143.

Fixman, E. D., Hayward, G. S., and Hayward, S. D. (1995). Replication of Epstein–Barr virus oriLyt: lack of a dedicated virally encoded origin-binding protein and dependence on Zta in cotransfection assays. *J. Virol.*, **69**(5), 2998–3006.

Flemington, E. K. (2001). Herpesvirus lytic replication and the cell cycle: arresting new developments. *J. Virol.*, **75**(10), 4475–4481.

Flowers, C. C., Flowers, S. P., and Nabel, G. J. (1998). Kaposi's sarcoma-associated herpesvirus viral interferon regulatory factor confers resistance to the antiproliferative effect of interferon-alpha. *Mol. Med.*, **4**(6), 402–412.

Gaidano, G., Cechova, K., Chang, Y., Moore, P. S., Knowles, D. M., and Dalla-Favera, R. (1996). Establishment of AIDS-related lymphoma cell lines from lymphomatous effusions. *Leukemia*, **10**(7), 1237–1240.

Gangappa, S., Kapadia, S. B., Speck, S. H., and Virgin, H. W. T. (2002). Antibody to a lytic cycle viral protein decreases gamma-herpesvirus latency in B-cell-deficient mice. *J. Virol.*, **76**(22), 11460–11468.

Gao, S. J., Kingsley, L., Hoover, D. R. *et al.* (1996a). Seroconversion to antibodies against Kaposi's sarcoma-associated herpesvirus-related latent nuclear antigens before the development of Kaposi's sarcoma. *N. Engl. J. Med.*, **335**(4), 233–241.

Gao, S. J., Kingsley, L., Li, M. *et al.* (1996b). KSHV antibodies among Americans, Italians and Ugandans with and without Kaposi's sarcoma. *Nat. Med.*, **2**(8), 925–928.

Gao, S. J., Boshoff, C., Jayachandra, S., Weiss, R. A., Chang, Y., and Moore, P. S. (1997). KSHV ORF K9 (vIRF) is an oncogene which inhibits the interferon signaling pathway. *Oncogene*, **15**(16), 1979–1985.

Ghosh, S. K., Wood, C., Boise, L. H. *et al.* (2003). Potentiation of TRAIL-induced apoptosis in primary effusion lymphoma through azidothymidine-mediated inhibition of NF-kappa B. *Blood*, **101**(6), 2321–2327.

Gill, J., Bourboulia, D., Wilkinson, J. *et al.* (2002). Prospective study of the effects of antiretroviral therapy on Kaposi sarcoma – associated herpesvirus infection in patients with and without Kaposi sarcoma. *J. Acquir. Immune Defic. Syndr.*, **31**(4), 384–390.

Glaunsinger, B. and Ganem, D. (2004). Highly selective escape from KSHV-mediated host mRNA shutoff and its implications for viral pathogenesis. *J. Exp. Med.*, **200**(3), 391.

Gradoville, L., Gerlach, J., Grogan, E. *et al.* (2000). Kaposi's sarcoma-associated herpesvirus open reading frame 50/Rta protein activates the entire lytic cycle in the HH-B2 primary effusion lymphoma cell line. *J. Virol.*, **74**, 6207–6212.

Grandadam, M., Dupin, N., Calvez, V. *et al.* (1997). Exacerbations of clinical symptoms in human immunodeficinecy virus type 1-infected patients with multicentric Castleman's disease are associated with a high increase in Kaposi's sarcoma herpesvirus DNA load in peripheral blood mononuclear cells. *J. Infect. Dis.*, **175**(5), 1198–1201.

Gwack, Y., Byun, H., Hwang, S., Lim, C., and Choe, J. (2001a). CREB-binding protein and histone deacetylase regulate the transcriptional activity of Kaposi's sarcoma-associated herpesvirus open reading frame 50. *J. Virol.*, **75**(4), 1909–1917.

Gwack, Y., Hwang, S., Byun, H. *et al.* (2001b). Kaposi's sarcoma-associated herpesvirus open reading frame 50 represses p53-induced transcriptional activity and apoptosis. *J. Virol.*, **75**(13), 6245–6248.

Gwack, Y., Hwang, S., Lim, C., Won, Y. S., Lee, C. H., and Choe, J. (2002). Kaposi's Sarcoma-associated Herpesvirus Open Reading Frame 50 Stimulates the Transcriptional Activity of STAT3. *J. Biol. Chem.*, **277**(8), 6438–6442.

Gwack, Y., Baek, H. J., Nakamura, H. *et al.* (2003a). Principal role of TRAP/mediator and SWI/SNF complexes in Kaposi's sarcoma-associated herpesvirus RTA-mediated lytic reactivation. *Mol. Cell. Biol.*, **23**(6), 2055–2067.

Gwack, Y., Nakamura, H., Lee, S. H. *et al.* (2003b). Poly(ADP-ribose) polymerase 1 and Ste20-like kinase hKFC act as transcriptional repressors for gamma-2 herpesvirus lytic replication. *Mol. Cell. Biol.*, **23**(22), 8282–8294.

Hammerschmidt, W. and Sugden, B. (1988). Identification and characterization of oriLyt, a lytic origin of DNA replication of Epstein–Barr virus. *Cell*, **55**(3), 427–433.

Haque, M., Davis, D. A., Wang, V., Widmer, I., and Yarchoan, R. (2003). Kaposi's sarcoma-associated herpesvirus (human herpesvirus 8) contains hypoxia response elements: relevance to lytic induction by hypoxia. *J. Virol.*, **77**(12), 6761–6768.

Han, Z. and Swaminathan, S. (2006). Kaposi's sarcoma-associated herpesvirus lytic gene ORF57 is essential for infectious virion production. *J. Virol.*, **80**(11), 5251–5260.

Harrington, W. J., Jr., Bagasra, O., Sosa, C. *et al.* (1996). Human herpesvirus type 8 DNA sequences in cell-free plasma and mononuclear cells of Kaposi's sarcoma patients. *J. Infect. Dis.*, **174**(5), 1101–1105.

Harrington, W., Jr., Sieczkowski, L., Sosa, C. *et al.* (1997). Activation of HHV-8 by HIV-1 tat. *Lancet*, **349**(9054), 774–775.

Hengge, U. R., Ruzicka, T., Tyring, S. K. *et al.* (2002). Update on Kaposi's sarcoma and other HHV8 associated diseases. Part 1: epidemiology, environmental predispositions, clinical manifestations, and therapy. *Lancet Infect. Dis.*, **2**(5), 281–292.

Henry, M., Uthman, A., Geusau, A. *et al.* (1999). Infection of circulating CD34+ cells by HHV-8 in patients with Kaposi's sarcoma. *J. Invest. Dermatol.*, **113**(4), 613–616.

Huang, L. M., Chao, M. F., Chen, M. F. *et al.* (2001). Reciprocal regulatory interaction between human herpesvirus 8 and human immunodeficiency virus type 1. *J. Biol. Chem.*, **276**(16), 13427–13432.

Humphrey, R. W., O'Brien, T. R., Newcomb, F. M. *et al.* (1996). Kaposi's sarcoma (KS)-associated herpesvirus-like DNA sequences in peripheral blood mononuclear cells: association with KS and persistence in patients receiving antiherpesvirus drugs. *Blood*, **88**(1), 297–301.

Inohara, N., Gourley, T. S., Carrio, R. *et al.* (1998). Diva, a Bcl-2 homologue that binds directly to Apaf-1 and induces BH3-independent cell death. *J. Biol. Chem.*, **273**(49), 32479–32486.

Iscovich, J., Boffetta, P., Franceschi, S., Azizi, E., and Sarid, R. (2000). Classic Kaposi sarcoma. *Cancer*, **88**, 500–517.

Izumiya, Y., Lin, S. F., Ellison, T. *et al.* (2003a). Kaposi's sarcoma-associated herpesvirus K-bZIP is a coregulator of K-Rta: physical association and promoter-dependent transcriptional repression. *J. Virol.*, **77**(2), 1441–1451.

Izumiya, Y., Lin, S. F., Ellison, T. J. *et al.* (2003b). Cell cycle regulation by Kaposi's sarcoma-associated herpesvirus K-bZIP: direct interaction with cyclin-CDK2 and induction of G1 growth arrest. *J. Virol.*, **77**(17), 9652–9661.

Jacobson, L. P., Jenkins, F. J., Springer, G. *et al.* (2000). Interaction of human immunodeficiency virus type 1 and human herpesvirus type 8 infections on the incidence of Kaposi's sarcoma. *J. Infect. Dis.*, **181**(16), 1940–1949.

Jayachandra, S., Low, K. G., Thick, A. E. *et al.* (1999). Three unrelated viral transforming proteins (vIRF, EBNA2, and E1A) induce the MYC oncogene through the interferon-responsive PRF element by using different transcription coadaptors. *Proc. Natl Acad. Sci. USA*, **96**(20), 11566–11571.

Jenkins, P., Binne, U., and Farrell, P. (2000). Histone acetylation and reactivation of Epstein-Barr virus from latency. *J. Virol.*, **74**, 710–720.

Jenner, R., Alba, M., Boshoff, C., and Kellam, P. (2001). Kaposi's sarcoma-associated herpesvirus latent and lytic gene expression as revealed by DNA arrays. *J. Virol*, **75**, 891–902.

Jenner, R. G., Maillard, K., Cattini, N. *et al.* (2003). Kaposi's sarcoma-associated herpesvirus-infected primary effusion lymphoma has a plasma cell gene expression profile. *Proc. Natl Acad. Sci. USA*, **100**(18), 10399–10404.

Jones, J. L., Hanson, D. L., Chu, S. Y., Ward, J. W., and Jaffe, H. W. (1995). AIDS-associated Kaposi's sarcoma. *Science*, **267**(5201), 1078–1079.

Jones, J. L., Hanson, D. L., Dworkin, M. S., and Jaffe, H. W. (2000). Incidence and trends in Kaposi's sarcoma in the era of effective antiretroviral therapy. *J. Acquir. Immune Defic. Syndr.*, **24**(3), 270–274.

Kaufman, D. B., Shapiro, R., Lucey, M. R. *et al.* (2004). Immunosuppression: practice and trends. *Am. J. Transpl.*, **4** Suppl 9, 38–53.

Kedes, D. H. and Ganem, D. (1997). Sensitivity of Kaposi's sarcoma-associated herpesvirus replication to antiviral drugs. Implications for potential therapy. *J. Clin. Invest.*, **99**(9), 2082–2086.

Kedes, D., Operskalski, E., Busch, M., Kohn, R., Flood, J., and Ganem, D. (1996). The seroepidemiology of human herpesvirus 8 (Kaposi's sarcoma-associated herpesvirus): distribution of infection in KS risk groups and evidence for sexual transmission. *Nat. Med.*, **2**, 918–924.

Keller, S. A., Schattner, E. J., and Cesarman, E. (2000). Inhibition of NF-kappaB induces apoptosis of KSHV-infected primary effusion lymphoma cells. *Blood*, **96**(7), 2537–2542.

Keller, R., Zago, A., Viana, M. C. *et al.* (2001). HHV-8 infection in patients with AIDS-related Kaposi's sarcoma in Brazil. *Braz. J. Med. Biol. Res.*, **34**(7), 879–886.

Kikuta, H., Itakura, O., Taneichi, K., and Kohno, M. (1997). Tropism of human herpesvirus 8 for peripheral blood lymphocytes in patients with Castleman's disease. *Br. J. Haematol.*, **99**(4), 790–793.

Kim, I. J., Flano, E., Woodland, D. L., and Blackman, M. A. (2002). Antibody-mediated control of persistent gamma-herpesvirus infection. *J. Immunol.*, **168**(8), 3958–3964.

Kimball, L. E., Casper, C., Koelle, D. M., Morrow, R., Corey, L., and Vieira, J. (2004). Reduced levels of neutralizing antibodies to Kaposi sarcoma-associated herpesvirus in persons with a history of Kaposi sarcoma. *J. Infect. Dis.*, **189**(11), 2016–2022.

Kirchhoff, S., Sebens, T., Baumann, S. *et al.* (2002). Viral IFN-regulatory factors inhibit activation-induced cell death via two positive regulatory IFN-regulatory factor 1-dependent domains in the CD95 ligand promoter. *J. Immunol.*, **168**(3), 1226–1234.

Kirshner, J. R., Lukac, D. M., Chang, J., and Ganem, D. (2000). Kaposi's sarcoma-associated herpesvirus open reading frame 57 encodes a posttranscriptional regulator with multiple distinct activities. *J. Virol.*, **74**, 3586–3597.

Klein, U., Gloghini, A., Gaidano, G. *et al.* (2003). Gene expression profile analysis of AIDS-related primary effusion lymphoma (PEL) suggests a plasmablastic derivation and identifies PEL-specific transcripts. *Blood*, **101**(10), 4115–4121.

Koelle, D. M., Huang, M. L., Chandran, B., Vieira, J., Piepkorn, M., and Corey, L. (1997). Frequent detection of Kaposi's sarcoma-associated herpesvirus (human herpesvirus 8) DNA in saliva of human immunodeficiency virus-infected men: clinical and immunologic correlates. *J. Infect. Dis.*, **176**(1), 94–102.

LaDuca, J. R., Love, J. L., Abbott, L. Z., Dube, S., Freidman-Kien, A. E., and Poiesz, B. J. (1998). Detection of human herpesvirus 8 DNA sequences in tissues and bodily fluids. *J. Infect. Dis.*, **178**(6), 1610–1615.

Lagunoff, M., Majeti, R., Weiss, A., and Ganem, D. (1999). Deregulated signal transduction by the K1 gene product of Kaposi's sarcoma-associated herpesvirus. *Proc. Natl Acad. Sci. USA*, **96**(10), 5704–5709.

Lagunoff, M., Lukac, D., and Ganem, D. (2001). Immunoreceptor tyrosine-based activation motif-dependent signaling by Kaposi's sarcoma-associated herpesvirus (KSHV) K1 protein: effects on lytic viral replication. *J. Virol.*, **75**, 5891–5898.

Lan, K., Kuppers, D. A., and Robertson, E. S. (2005). Kaposi's sarcoma-associated herpesvirus reactivation is regulated by interaction of latency-associated nuclear antigen with recombination signal sequence-binding protein Jk, the major downstream effector of the notch signaling pathway. *J. Virol.*, **79**(6), 3468–3478.

Lebbe, C., Blum, L., Pellet, C. *et al.* (1998). Clinical and biological impact of antiretroviral therapy with protease inhibitors on HIV-related Kaposi's sarcoma. *AIDS*, **12**(7), F45–F49.

Lee, B. S., Paulose-Murphy, M., Chung, Y. H. *et al.* (2002). Suppression of tetradecanoyl phorbol acetate-induced lytic reactivation of Kaposi's sarcoma-associated herpesvirus by K1 signal transduction. *J. Virol.*, **76**(23), 12185–12199.

Lee, H., Guo, J., Li, M. *et al.* (1998). Identification of an immunoreceptor tyrosine-based activation motif of K1 transforming protein of Kaposi's sarcoma-associated herpesvirus. *Mol. Cell. Biol.*, **18**(9), 5219–5228.

Leonard, W. J. and O'Shea, J. J. (1998). Jaks and STATs: biological implications. *Annu. Rev. Immunol.*, **16**, 293–322.

Li, M., Lee, H., Guo, J. *et al.* (1998). Kaposi's sarcoma-associated herpesvirus viral interferon regulatory factor. *J. Virol.*, **72**, 5433–5440.

Liang, Y. and Ganem, D. (2003). Lytic but not latent infection by Kaposi's sarcoma-associated herpesvirus requires host CSL protein, the mediator of Notch signaling. *Proc. Natl Acad. Sci. USA*, **100**(14), 8490–8495.

Liang, Y. and Ganem, D. (2004). RBP-J (CSL) is essential for activation of the K14/vGPCR promoter of Kaposi's sarcoma-associated herpesvirus by the lytic switch protein RTA. *J. Virol.*, **78**(13), 6818–6826.

Liang, Y., Chang, J., Lynch, S., Lukac, D. M., and Ganem, D. (2002). The lytic switch protein of KSHV activates gene expression via functional interaction with RBP-Jk, the target of the Notch signaling pathway. *Genes Dev.*, **16**, 1977–1989.

Liao, W., Tang, Y., Kuo, Y. L. *et al.* (2003). Kaposi's sarcoma-associated herpesvirus/human herpesvirus 8 transcriptional activator Rta is an oligomeric DNA-binding protein that interacts with tandem arrays of phased A/T-trinucleotide motifs. *J. Virol.*, **77**(17), 9399–9411.

Lin, C. L., Li, H., Wang, Y., Zhu, F. X., Kudchodkar, S., and Yuan, Y. (2003). Kaposi's sarcoma-associated herpesvirus lytic origin (ori-Lyt)-dependent DNA replication: identification of the ori-Lyt and association of K8 bZip protein with the origin. *J. Virol.*, **77**(10), 5578–5588.

Lin, K., Dai, C. Y., and Ricciardi, R. P. (1998). Cloning and functional analysis of Kaposi's sarcoma-associated herpesvirus DNA polymerase and its processivity factor. *J. Virol.*, **72**, 6228–6232.

Lin, R., Genin, P., Mamane, Y. *et al.* (2001). HHV-8 encoded vIRF-1 represses the interferon antiviral response by blocking IRF-3 recruitment of the CBP/p300 coactivators. *Oncogene*, **20**(7), 800–811.

Lo, P., Yu, X., Atanasov, I., Chandran, B., and Zhou, Z. H. (2003). Three-dimensional localization of pORF65 in Kaposi's sarcoma-associated herpesvirus capsid. *J. Virol.*, **77**(7), 4291–4297.

Lu, F., Zhou, J., Wiedmer, A., Madden, K., Yuan, Y., and Lieberman, P. M. (2003). Chromatin remodeling of the Kaposi's sarcoma-associated herpesvirus ORF50 promoter correlates with reactivation from latency. *J. Virol.*, **77**(21), 11425–11435.

Lu, M., Suen, J., Frias, C. *et al.* (2004). Dissection of the Kaposi's sarcoma-associated gene expression program using the viral DNA replication inhibitor cidofovir. *J. Virol.*, **78**(24), 13637–13652.

Lukac, D. M., Renne, R., Kirshner, J. R., and Ganem, D. (1998). Reactivation of Kaposi's sarcoma-associated herpesvirus infection from latency by expression of the ORF 50 transactivator, a homolog of the EBV R protein. *Virology*, **252**, 304–312.

Lukac, D. M., Kirshner, J. R., and Ganem, D. (1999). Transcriptional activation by the product of the open reading frame 50 of Kaposi's-associated herpesvirus is required for lytic viral reactivation in B cells. *J. Virol.*, **73**, 9348–9361.

Lukac, D., Garibyan, L., Kirshner, J., Palmeri, D., and Ganem, D. (2001). DNA binding by the Kaposi's sarcoma-associated herpesvirus lytic switch protein is necessary for transcriptional activation of two viral delayed early promoters. *J. Virol.*, **75**, 6786–6799.

Luppi, M., Barozzi, P., Guaraldi, G. *et al.* (2003). Human herpesvirus 8-associated diseases in solid-organ transplantation: importance of viral transmission from the donor. *Clin. Infect. Dis.*, **37**(4), 606–607; author reply 607.

Mantina, H., Kankasa, C., Klaskala, W. *et al.* (2001). Vertical transmission of Kaposi's sarcoma-associated herpesvirus. *Int. J. Cancer*, **94**(5), 749–752.

Martin, D. F., Kuppermann, B. D., Wolitz, R. A., Palestine, A. G., Li, H., and Robinson, C. A. (1999). Oral ganciclovir for patients with cytomegalovirus retinitis treated with a ganciclovir implant. Roche Ganciclovir Study Group. *N. Engl. J. Med.*, **340**, 1063–1070.

Martin, J. N., Ganem, D. E., Osmond, D. H. *et al.* (1998). Sexual transmission and the natural history of human herpesvirus 8 infection. *N. Engl. J. Med.*, **338**, 948–954.

Maulik, G., Shrikhande, A., Kijima, T., Ma, P. C., Morrison, P. T., and Salgia, R. (2002). Role of the hepatocyte growth factor receptor, c-Met, in oncogenesis and potential for therapeutic inhibition. *Cytokine Growth Factor Rev.*, **13**(1), 41–59.

McGeoch, D. J. and Davison, A. J. (1999). The descent of human herpesvirus 8. *Semin. Cancer Biol.*, **9**(3), 201–209.

Merat, R., Amara, A., de The, H., Morel, P., and Saib, A. (2002). HIV-1 infection of primary effusion lymphoma cell line triggers Kaposi's sarcoma-associated herpesvirus (KSHV) reactivation. *Int. J. Cancer*, **97**(6), 791–795.

Mercader, M., Taddeo, B., Panella, J., Chandran, B., Nickoloff, B., and Foreman, K. (2000). Induction of HHV-8 lytic cycle replication by inflammatory cytokines produced by HIV-1-infected T cells. *Am. J. Pathol.*, **156**, 1961–1971.

Miles, S. A., Martinez-Maza, O., Rezai, A. *et al.* (1992). Oncostatin M as a potent mitogen for AIDS-Kaposi's sarcoma-derived cells. *Science*, **255**(5050), 1432–1434.

Miller, G., Heston, L., Grogan, E. *et al.* (1997). Selective switch between latency and lytic replication of Kaposi's sarcoma herpesvirus and Epstein–Barr virus in dually infected body cavity lymphoma cells. *J. Virol.*, **71**(1), 314–324.

Min, J. and Katzenstein, D. A. (1999). Detection of Kaposi's sarcoma-associated herpesvirus in peripheral blood cells in human immunodeficiency virus infection: association with Kaposi's sarcoma, CD4 cell count, and HIV RNA levels. *AIDS Res. Hum. Retroviruses*, **15**(1), 51–55.

Mocroft, A., Kirk, O., Clumeck, N. *et al.* (2004). The changing pattern of Kaposi sarcoma in patients with HIV, 1994–2003: the EuroSIDA Study. *Cancer*, **100**(12), 2644–2654.

Monini, P., Carlini, F., Sturzl, M. *et al.* (1999a). Alpha interferon inhibits human herpesvirus 8 (HHV-8) reactivation in primary effusion lymphoma cells and reduces HHV-8 load in cultured peripheral blood mononuclear cells. *J. Virol.*, **73**(5), 4029–4041.

Monini, P., Colombini, S., Sturzl, M. *et al.* (1999b). Reactivation and persistence of human herpesvirus-8 infection in B cells and monocytes by Th-1 cytokines increased in Kaposi's sarcoma. *Blood*, **93**(12), 4044–4058.

Monini, P., Sirianni, M. C., Franco, M. *et al.* (2001). Clearance of human herpesvirus 8 from blood and regression of leukopenia-associated aggressive classic Kaposi's sarcoma during interferon-alpha therapy: a case report. *Clin. Infect. Dis.*, **33**(10), 1782–1785.

Moore, P. S. and Chang, Y. (1995). Detection of herpesvirus-like DNA sequences in Kaposi's sarcoma in patients with and without HIV infection. *N. Engl. J. Med.*, **332**(18), 1181–1185.

Moore, P. S., Kingsley, L. A., Holmberg, S. D. et al. (1996). Kaposi's sarcoma-associated herpesvirus infection prior to onset of Kaposi's sarcoma. *AIDS*, **10**, 175–180.

Nador, R. G., Cesarman, E., Chadburn, A. et al. (1996). Primary effusion lymphoma: a distinct clinicopathologic entity associated with the Kaposi's sarcoma-associated herpes virus. *Blood*, **88**(2), 645–656.

Naidu, Y. M., Rosen, E. M., Zitnick, R. et al. (1994). Role of scatter factor in the pathogenesis of AIDS-related Kaposi sarcoma. *Proc. Natl Acad. Sci. USA*, **91**(12), 5281–5285.

Nakamura, H., Li, M., Zarycki, J., and Jung, J. U. (2001). Inhibition of p53 tumor suppressor by viral interferon regulatory factor. *J. Virol.*, **75**(16), 7572–7582.

Nakamura, H., Lu, M., Gwack, Y., Souvlis, J., Zeichner, S. L., and Jung, J. U. (2003). Global changes in Kaposi's sarcoma-associated virus gene expression patterns following expression of a tetracycline-inducible Rta transactivator. *J Virol.*, **77**(7), 4205–4220.

Nasti, G., Martellotta, F., Berretta, M. et al. (2003). Impact of highly active antiretroviral therapy on the presenting features and outcome of patients with acquired immunodeficiency syndrome-related Kaposi sarcoma. *Cancer*, **98**(11), 2440–2446.

Nealon, K., Newcomb, W. W., Pray, T. R. et al. (2001). Lytic replication of Kaposi's sarcoma-associated herpesvirus results in the formation of multiple capsid species: isolation and molecular characterization of A, B, and C capsids from a gammaherpesvirus. *J. Virol.*, **75**(6), 2866–2878.

Niedt, G. W., Myskowski, P. L., Urmacher, C., Niedzwiecki, D., Chapman, D., and Safai, B. (1990). Histology of early lesions of AIDS-associated Kaposi's sarcoma. *Mod. Pathol.*, **3**(1), 64–70.

Nishimura, K., Ueda, K., Sakakibara, S. et al. (2003). A viral transcriptional activator of Kaposi's sarcoma-associated herpesvirus (KSHV) induces apoptosis, which is blocked in KSHV-infected cells. *Virology*, **316**(1), 64–74.

Nuovo, M. and Nuovo, G. (2001). Utility of HHV8 RNA detection for differentiating Kaposi's sarcoma from its mimics. *J. Cutan. Pathol.*, **28**(5), 248–255.

Oksenhendler, E., Carcelain, G., Aoki, Y. et al. (2000). High levels of human herpesvirus 8 viral load, human interleukin-6, interleukin-10, and C reactive protein correlate with exacerbation of multicentric castleman disease in HIV-infected patients. *Blood*, **96**(6), 2069–2073.

Osmond, D. H., Buchbinder, S., Cheng, A. et al. (2002). Prevalence of Kaposi sarcoma-associated herpesvirus infection in homosexual men at beginning of and during the HIV epidemic. *J. Am. Med. Assoc.*, **287**(2), 221–225.

Parravicini, C., Olsen, S. J., Capra, M. et al. (1997). Risk of Kaposi's sarcoma herpesvirus transmission from donor allografts among Italian posttransplant Kaposi's sarcoma patients. *Blood*, **90**, 2826–2829.

Pauk, J., Huang, M. L., Brodie, S. J. et al. (2000). Mucosal shedding of human herpesvirus 8 in men. *N. Engl. J. Med.*, **343**(19), 1369–1377.

Paulose-Murphy, M., Ha, N.-K., Xiang, C. et al. (2001). Transcription program of Human herpesvirus 8 (Kaposi's Sarcoma-associated herpesvirus). *J. Virol.*, **75**, 4843–4853.

Pellet, C., Chevret, S., Blum, L. et al. (2001). Virologic and immunologic parameters that predict clinical response of AIDS-associated Kaposi's sarcoma to highly active antiretroviral therapy. *J. Invest. Dermatol.*, **117**(4), 858–863.

Pertel, P. E. (2002). Human herpesvirus 8 glycoprotein B (gB), gH, and gL can mediate cell fusion. *J. Virol.*, **76**(9), 4390–4400.

Picchio, G. R., Sabbe, R. E., Gulizia, R. J. et al. (1997). The KSHV/HHV8-infected BCBL-1 lymphoma line causes tumors in SCID mice but fails to transmit virus to a human peripheral blood mononuclear cell graft. *Virology*, **238**(1), 22–29.

Polson, A., Huang, L., Lukac, D. et al. (2001). Kaposi's sarcoma-associated herpesvirus K-bZIP protein is phosphorylated by cyclin-dependent kinases. *J. Virol.*, **75**, 3175–3184.

Polstra, A. M., Goudsmit, J., and Cornelissen, M. (2003). Latent and lytic HHV-8 mRNA expression in PBMCs and Kaposi's sarcoma skin biopsies of AIDS Kaposi's sarcoma patients. *J. Med. Virol.*, **70**(4), 624–627.

Pyakurel, P., Massambu, C., Castanos-Velez, E. et al. (2004). Human herpesvirus 8/Kaposi sarcoma herpesvirus cell association during evolution of Kaposi sarcoma. *J. Acquir. Immune Defic. Syndr.*, **36**(2), 678–683.

Quinlivan, E. B., Zhang, C., Stewart, P. W., Komoltri, C., Davis, M. G., and Wehbie, R. S. (2002). Elevated virus loads of Kaposi's sarcoma-associated human herpesvirus 8 predict Kaposi's sarcoma disease progression, but elevated levels of human immunodeficiency virus type 1 do not. *J. Infect. Dis.*, **185**(12), 1736–1744.

Reed, J. A., Nador, R. G., Spaulding, D., Tani, Y., Cesarman, E., and Knowles, D. M. (1998). Demonstration of Kaposi's sarcoma-associated herpesvirus cyclin D homolog in cutaneous Kaposi's sarcoma by colorimetric in situ hybridization using a catalyzed signal amplification system. *Blood*, **91**(10), 3825–3832.

Renne, R., Lagunoff, M., Zhong, W., and Ganem, D. (1996a). The size and conformation of Kaposi's sarcoma-associated herpesvirus (human herpesvirus 8) DNA in infected cells and virions. *J. Virol.*, **70**(11), 8151–8154.

Renne, R., Zhong, W., Herndier, B. et al. (1996b). Lytic growth of Kaposi's sarcoma-associated herpesvirus (human herpesvirus 8) in culture. *Nat. Med.*, **2**(3), 342–346.

Renne, R., Blackbourn, D., Whitby, D., Levy, J., and Ganem, D. (1998). Limited transmission of Kaposi's sarcoma-associated herpesvirus in cultured cells. *J. Virol.*, **72**, 5182–5188.

Rimessi, P., Bonaccorsi, A., Sturzl, M. et al. (2001). Transcription pattern of human herpesvirus 8 open reading frame K3 in primary effusion lymphoma and Kaposi's sarcoma. *J. Virol.*, **75**(15), 7161–7174.

Robertson, K. A., Usherwood, E. J., and Nash, A. A. (2001). Regression of a murine gammaherpesvirus 68-positive b-cell lymphoma mediated by CD4 T lymphocytes. *J. Virol.*, **75**(7), 3480–3482.

Robles, R., Lugo, D., Gee, L., and Jacobson, M. A. (1999). Effect of antiviral drugs used to treat cytomegalovirus end-organ disease on subsequent course of previously diagnosed Kaposi's sarcoma in patients with AIDS. *J. Acquir. Immune Defic. Syndr. Hum. Retrovirol.*, **20**(1), 34–38.

Roizman, B. and Sears, A. E. (1996). Herpes simplex viruses and their replication. In Fields, B. N., Knipe, D. M., Howley, P. M. *et al.* eds *Fields Virology.* Philadelphia, Lippincott-Raven Publishers, pp. 2231–2295.

Sakakibara, S., Ueda, K., Chen, J., Okuno, T., and Yamanishi, K. (2001). Octamer-binding sequence is a key element for the autoregulation of Kaposi's sarcoma-associated herpesvirus ORF50/Lyta gene expression. *J. Virol.,* **75,** 6894–6900.

Sakurada, S., Katano, H., Sata, T., Ohkuni, H., Watanabe, T., and Mori, S. (2001). Effective human herpesvirus 8 infection of human umbilical vein endothelial cells by cell-mediated transmission. *J. Virol.,* **75**(16), 7717–7722.

Santarelli, R., DeMarco, R., Masala, M. *et al.* (2001). Direct correlation between human herpesvirus-8 seroprevalence and classic Kaposi's sarcoma incidence in Northern Sardinia. *J. Med. Virol.,* **65,** 368–372.

Sarawar, S. R., Lee, B. J., Reiter, S. K., and Schoenberger, S. P. (2001). Stimulation via CD40 can substitute for CD4 T cell function in preventing reactivation of a latent herpesvirus. *Proc. Natl Acad. Sci. USA,* **98**(11), 6325–6329.

Sarid, R., Sato, T., Bohenzky, R. A., Russo, J. J., and Chang, Y. (1997). Kaposi's sarcoma-associated herpesvirus encodes a functional bcl-2 homologue. *Nat. Med.,* **3**(3), 293–298.

Sarid, R., Flore, O., Bohenzky, R. A., Chang, Y., and Moore, P. S. (1998). Transcription mapping of the Kaposi's sarcoma-associated herpesvirus (Human Herpesvirus 8) genome in a body cavity-based lymphoma cell line (BC-1). *J. Virol.,* **72,** 1005–1012.

Sarid, R., Olsen, S. J., and Moore, P. S. (1999). Kaposi's sarcoma-associated herpesvirus: epidemiology, virology, and molecular biology. *Adv. Virus Res.,* **52,** 139–232.

Saveliev, A., Zhu, F., and Yuan, Y. (2002). Transcription mapping and expression patterns of genes in the major immediate-early region of Kaposi's sarcoma-associated herpesvirus. *Virology,* **299**(2), 301–314.

Schalling, M., Ekman, M., Kaaya, E. E., Linde, A., and Biberfield, P. (1995). A role for a new herpes virus (KSHV) in different forms of Kaposi's sarcoma. *Nat. Med.,* **1**(7), 707–708.

Seaman, W., Ye, D., Wang, R., Hale, E., Weisse, M., and Quinlivan, E. (1999). Gene expression from the ORF50/K8 region of Kaposi's sarcoma-associated herpesvirus. *Virology,* **263,** 436–449.

Seo, T., Park, J., Lee, D., Hwang, S. G., and Choe, J. (2001). Viral interferon regulatory factor 1 of Kaposi's sarcoma-associated herpesvirus binds to p53 and represses p53-dependent transcription and apoptosis. *J. Virol.,* **75**(13), 6193–6198.

Serraino, D., Tedeschi, R. M., Songini, M. *et al.* (2000). Prevalence of antibodies to human herpesvirus 8 in children from Sardinia and Croatia. *Infection,* **28**(5), 336–338.

Sgadari, C., Barillari, G., Toschi, E. *et al.* (2002). HIV protease inhibitors are potent anti-angiogenic molecules and promote regression of Kaposi sarcoma. *Nat. Med.,* **8**(3), 225–232.

Shahinian, A., Pfeffer, K., Lee, K. P. *et al.* (1993). Differential T cell costimulatory requirements in CD28-deficient mice. *Science,* **261**(5121), 609–612.

Shaw, R., Arbiser, J., and Offermann, M. K. (2000). Valproic acid induced human herpesvirus 8 lytic gene expression in BCBL-1 cells. *AIDS,* **14,** 899–.

Simas, J. and Efstathiou, S. (1998). Murine gammaherpesvirus 68: a model for the study of gammaherpesvirus pathogenesis. *Trend Microbiol.,* **6,** 276–282.

Simas, J. P., Swann, D., Bowden, R., and Efstathiou, S. (1999). Analysis of murine gammaherpesvirus-68 transcription during lytic and latent infection. *J. Gen. Virol.,* **80**(1), 75–82.

Sirianni, M. C., Uccini, S., Angeloni, A., Faggioni, A., Cottoni, F., and Ensoli, B. (1997). Circulating spindle cells: correlation with human herpesvirus-8 (HHV-8) infection and Kaposi's sarcoma [letter]. *Lancet,* **349**(9047), 255.

Sirianni, M. C., Vincenzi, L., Fiorelli, V. *et al.* (1998). Gamma-Interferon production in peripherala blood mononuclear cells and tumor infiltrating lymphocytes from Kaposi's sarcoma patients: correlation with the presence of human herpesvirus-8 in peripheral blood mononuclear cells and lesional macrophages. *Blood,* **91**(3), 968–976.

Sirianni, M. C., Vincenzi, L., Topino, S. *et al.* (2002). NK cell activity controls human herpesvirus 8 latent infection and is restored upon highly active antiretroviral therapy in AIDS patients with regressing Kaposi's sarcoma. *Eur. J. Immunol.,* **32**(10), 2711–2720.

Song, M. J., Li, X., Brown, H. J., and Sun, R. (2002). Characterization of interactions between RTA and the promoter of polyadenylated nuclear RNA in Kaposi's sarcoma-associated herpesvirus/human herpesvirus 8. *J. Virol.,* **76**(10), 5000–5013.

Song, M. J., Deng, H., and, Sun, R. (2003). Comparative study of regulation of RTA-responsive genes in Kaposi's sarcoma-associated herpesvirus/human herpesvirus 8. *J. Virol.,* **77**(17), 9451–9462.

Speck, S. and Virgin, H. I. (1999). Host and viral genetics of chronic infection: a mouse model of gamma-herpesvirus pathogenesis. *Curr. Opin. Microbiol.,* **2,** 403–409.

Staskus, K. A., Zhong, W., Gebhard, K. *et al.* (1997). Kaposi's sarcoma-associated herpesvirus gene expression in endothelial (spindle) tumor cells. *J. Virol.,* **71**(1), 715–719.

Stevenson, P. G. and Doherty, P. C. (1998). Kinetic analysis of the specific host response to a murine gammaherpesvirus. *J. Virol.,* **72**(2), 943–949.

Stewart, J. P., Usherwood, E. J., Ross, A., Dyson, H., and Nash, T. (1998). Lung epithelial cells are a major site of murine gammaherpesvirus persistence. *J. Exp. Med.,* **187**(12), 1941–1951.

Strauchen, J. A., Hauser, A. D., Burstein, D., Jimenez, R., Moore, P. S., and Chang, Y. (1996). Body cavity-based malignant lymphoma containing Kaposi sarcoma-associated herpesvirus in an HIV-negative man with previous Kaposi sarcoma. *Ann. Intern. Med.,* **125**(10), 822–825.

Strickler, H. D., Goedert, J. J., Bethke, F. R. *et al.* (1999). Human herpesvirus 8 cellular immune responses in homosexual men. *J. Infect. Dis.,* **180**(5), 1682–1685.

Sun, R., Lin, S. F., Staskus, K. *et al.* (1998). A viral gene that activates lytic cycle expression of Kaposi's sarcoma-associated herpesvirus. *Proc. Natl Acad. Sci. USA,* **95,** 10866–10871.

Sunil-Chandra, N., Efstathiou, S., Arno, J., and Nash, A. (1992a). Virological and pathological features of mice infected with murine gammaherpesvirus 68. *J. Gen. Virol.,* **73,** 2347–2356.

Sunil-Chandra, N., Efstathiou, S., and Nash, A. (1992b). Murine gammaherpesvirus 68 establishes a latent infection in mouse B lymphocytes in vivo. *J. Gen. Virol.*, **73**, 3275–3279.

Sunil-Chandra, N., Arno, J., Fazakerley, J., and Nash, A. (1994). Lymphoproliferative disease in mice infected with murine gammaherpesvirus 68. *Am. J. Pathol.*, **145**, 818–826.

Symensma, T. L., Martinez-Guzman, D., Jia, Q. et al. (2003). COX-2 induction during murine gammaherpesvirus 68 infection leads to enhancement of viral gene expression. *J. Virol.*, **77**(23), 12753–12763.

Taga, T. and Kishimoto, T. (1997). Gp130 and the interleukin-6 family of cytokines. *Annu. Rev. Immunol.*, **15**, 797–819.

Tam, H. K., Zhang, Z. F., Jacobson, L. P. et al. (2002). Effect of highly active antiretroviral therapy on survival among HIV-infected men with Kaposi and sarcoma or non-Hodgkin lymphoma. *Int. J. Cancer*, **98**(6), 916–922.

Tedeschi, R., Enbom, M., Bidoli, E., Linde, A., De Pauli, P., and Dillner, J. (2001). Viral load of human herpesvirus 8 in peripheral blood of human immunodeficiency virus-infected patients with Kaposi's sarcoma. *J. Clin. Microbiol.*, **39**(12), 4269–4273.

Tibbetts, S. A., van Dyk, L. F. et al. (2002). Immune control of the number and reactivation phenotype of cells latently infected with a gammaherpesvirus. *J. Virol.*, **76**(14), 7125–7132.

Triantos, D., Horefti, E., Paximadi, E. et al. (2004). Presence of human herpes virus-8 in salvia and non-lesional oral mucosa in HIV-infected and oncologic immunocompromised patients. *Oral Microbiol. Immunol.*, **19**(3), 201–204.

Trus, B. L., Heymann, J. B., Nealon, K. et al. (2001). Capsid structure of Kaposi's sarcoma-associated herpesvirus, a gammaherpesvirus, compared to those of an alphaherpesvirus, herpes simplex virus type 1, and a betaherpesvirus, cytomegalovirus. *J. Virol.*, **75**(6), 2879–2890.

Ubbink, D. T., II, Tulevski, den Hartog, D. et al. (1997). The value of non-invasive techniques for the assessment of critical limb ischaemia. *Eur. J. Vasc. Endovasc. Surg.*, **13**(3), 296–300.

Ueda, K., Ishikawa, K., Nishimura, K., Sakakibara, S., Do, E., and Yamanishi, K. (2002). Kaposi's sarcoma-associated herpesvirus (human herpesvirus 8) replication and transcription factor activates the K9 (vIRF) gene through two distinct *cis* elements by a non-DNA-binding mechanism. *J. Virol.*, **76**(23), 12044–12054.

Uphoff, C., Carbone, A., Gaidano, G., and Drexler, H. (1998). HHV-8 infection is specific for cell lines derived from primary effusion (body cavity-based) lymphomas. *Leukemia*, **12**, 1806–1809.

Varthakavi, V., Browning, P. J., and Spearman, P. (1999). Human immunodeficiency virus replication in a primary effusion lymphoma cell line stimulates lytic-phase replication of Kaposi's sarcoma-associated herpesvirus. *J. Virol.*, **73**(12), 10329–10338.

Vieira, J. and O'Hearn, P. M. (2004). Use of the red fluorescent protein as a marker of Kaposi's sarcoma-associated herpesvirus lytic gene expression. *Virology*, **325**(2), 225–240.

Vieira, J., Huang, M. L., Koelle, D. M., and Corey, L. (1997). Transmissible Kaposi's sarcoma-associated herpesvirus (human herpesvirus 8) in saliva of men with a history of Kaposi's sarcoma [In Process Citation]. *J. Virol.*, **71**(9), 7083–7087.

Virgin, H. W. t., Latreille, P., Wamsley, P. et al. (1997). Complete sequence and genomic analysis of murine gammaherpesvirus 68. *J. Virol.*, **71**(8), 5894–5904.

Vitale, F., Viviano, E., Perna, A. et al. (2000). Serological and virological evidence of non-sexual transmission of human herpesvirus type 8 (HHV8). *Epidemiol. Infect.*, **125**, 671–675.

Wahren, B., Ruden, U., Gadler, H., Oberg, B., and Eriksson, B. (1985). Activity of the cytomegalovirus genome in the presence of PPi analogs. *J. Virol.*, **56**(3), 996–1001.

Wang, F. Z., Akula, S. M., Pramod, N. P., Zeng, L., and Chandran, B. (2001). Human herpesvirus 8 envelope glycoprotein K8.1A interaction with the target cells involves heparan sulfate. *J. Virol.*, **75**(16), 7517–7527.

Wang, H. W., Sharp, T. V., Kuomi, A., Koentges, G., and Boshoff, C. (2002). Characterization of an anti-apoptotic glycoprotein encoded by Kaposi's sarcoma-associated herpesvirus which resembles a spliced variant of human survivin. *EMBO J.*, **21**(11), 2602–2615.

Wang, S., Liu, S., Wu, M., Geng, Y., and Wood, C. (2001a). Kaposi's sarcoma-associated herpesvirus/human herpesvirus-8 ORF50 gene product contains a potent C-terminal activation domain which activates gene expression via a specific target sequence. *Arch. Virol.*, **146**(7), 1415–1426.

Wang, J., Zhang, J., Zhang, L., Harrington, Jr., W., West, J. T., and Wood, C. (2005). Modulation of human herpesvirus 8/Kaposi's sarcoma-associated herpesvirus replication and transcription activator transactivation by interferon regulatory factor 7. *J. Virol.*, **79**(4), 2420–2431.

Wang, Y., Tang, Q., Maul, G. G., and Yuan, Y. (2006). Kaposi's sarcoma-associated herpesvirus *ori-Lyt*-dependent DNA replication: dual roles of RTA in the replication. *J. Virol.*, **80**(24), 12171–12186.

Wang, S. E., Wu, F. Y., Fujimuro, M., Zong, J., Hayward, S. D., and Hayward, G. S. (2003a). Role of CCAAT/enhancer-binding protein alpha (C/EBPalpha) in activation of the Kaposi's sarcoma-associated herpesvirus (KSHV) lytic-cycle replication-associated protein (RAP) promoter in cooperation with the KSHV replication and transcription activator (RTA) and RAP. *J. Virol.*, **77**(1), 600–623.

Wang, S. E., Wu, F. Y., Yu, Y., and Hayward, G. S. (2003b). CCAAT/enhancer-binding protein-alpha is induced during the early stages of Kaposi's sarcoma-associated herpesvirus (KSHV) lytic cycle reactivation and together with the KSHV replication and transcription activator (RTA) cooperatively stimulates the viral RTA, MTA, and PAN promoters. *J. Virol.*, **77**(17), 9590–9612.

Wang, S. E., Wu, F. Y., Chen, H., Shamay, M., Zheng, Q., and Hayward, G. (2004). Early activation of the Kaposi's sarcoma-associated herpesvirus RTA, RAP, and MTA promoters by the tetradecanoyl phorbol acetate-induced AP1 pathway. *J. Virol.*, **78**(8), 4248–4267.

Wang, Y., Chong, O. T., and Yuan, Y. (2004a). Differential regulation of K8 gene expression in immediate-early and delayed-early stages of Kaposi's sarcoma-associated herpesvirus. *Virology*, **325**(1), 149–163.

Wang, Y., Li, H., Chan, M. Y. *et al.* (2004b). Kaposi's sarcoma-associated herpesvirus ori-Lyt-dependent DNA replication: cis-acting requirements for replication and ori-Lyt-associated RNA transcription. *J. Virol.*, **78**(16), 8615–8629.

Weck, K., Barkon, M., Yoo, L., Speck, S., and Virgin, H. I. (1996). Mature B cells are required for acute splenic infection, but not for establishment of latency, by murine gammaherpesvirus 68. *J. Virol*, **70**, 6775–6780.

Weck, K. E., Dal Canto, A. J., Gould, J. D. *et al.* (1997). Murine gamma-herpesvirus 68 causes severe large-vessel arteritis in mice lacking interferon-gamma responsiveness: a new model for virus-induced vascular disease. *Nat. Med.*, **3**(12), 1346–1353.

Weck, K. E., Kim, S. S., Virgin, H. I., and Speck, S. H. (1999a). B cells regulate murine gammaherpesvirus 68 latency. *J. Virol.*, **73**(6), 4651–4661.

Weck, K. E., Kim, S. S., Virgin, H. I., and Speck, S. H. (1999b). Macrophages are the major reservoir of latent murine gamma-herpesvirus 68 in peritoneal cells. *J. Virol.*, **73**(4), 3273–3783.

Weigert, A. L., Pires, A., Adragao, T. *et al.* (2004). Human herpes virus-8 serology and DNA analysis in recipients of renal allografts showing Kaposi's sarcoma and their respective donors. *Transpl. Proc.*, **36**(4), 902–904.

Whitby, D., Howard, M. R., Tenant-Flowers, M. *et al.* (1995). Detection of Kaposi sarcoma associated herpesvirus in peripheral blood of HIV-infected individuals and progression to Kaposi's sarcoma [see comments]. *Lancet*, **346**(8978), 799–802.

Wilkinson, J., Cope, A., Gill, J. *et al.* (2002). Identification of Kaposi's sarcoma-associated herpesvirus (KSHV)-specific cytotoxic T-lymphocyte epitopes and evaluation of reconstitution of KSHV-specific responses in human immunodeficiency virus type 1-infected patients receiving highly active antiretroviral therapy. *J. Virol.*, **76**(6), 2634–2640.

Wu, F. Y., Ahn, J. H., Alcendor, D. J. *et al.* (2001). Origin-independent assembly of Kaposi's sarcoma-associated herpesvirus DNA replication compartments in transient cotransfection assays and association with the ORF-K8 protein and cellular PML. *J. Virol.*, **75**(3), 1487–1506.

Wu, F. Y., Tang, Q. Q., Chen, H. *et al.* (2002). Lytic replication-associated protein (RAP) encoded by Kaposi sarcoma-associated herpesvirus causes p21CIP-1-mediated G1 cell cycle arrest through CCAAT/enhancer-binding protein-alpha. *Proc. Natl Acad. Sci. USA*, **99**(16), 10683–10688.

Wu, F. Y., Wang, S. E., Tang, Q. Q. *et al.* (2003). Cell cycle arrest by Kaposi's sarcoma-associated herpesvirus replication-associated protein is mediated at both the transcriptional and posttranslational levels by binding to CCAAT/enhancer-binding protein alpha and p21(CIP-1). *J. Virol.*, **77**(16), 8893–8914.

Wu, L., Lo, P., Yu, X., Stoops, J. K., Forghani, B., and Zhou, Z. H. (2000). Three-dimensional structure of the human herpesvirus 8 capsid. *J. Virol.*, **74**(20), 9646–9654.

Xu, Y., Rodriguez-Huete, A., and Pari, G. S. (2006). Evaluation of lytic origins of replication of Kaposi's Sarcoma – associated Herpesvirus/Human herpesvirus 8 in the context of the viral genome. *J. Virol.*, **80**(19), 9905–9909.

Yang, C. and Kazanietz, M. G. (2003). Divergence and complexities in DAG signaling: looking beyond PKC. *Trends Pharmacol. Sci.*, **24**(11), 602–608.

Yao, L., Salvucci, O., Cardones, A. R. *et al.* (2003). Selective expression of stromal-derived factor-1 in the capillary vascular endothelium plays a role in Kaposi sarcoma pathogenesis. *Blood*, **102**(12), 3900–3905.

Yu, X. K., O'Connor, C. M., Atanasov, I., Damania, B., Kedes, D. H., and Zhou, Z. H. (2003). Three-dimensional structures of the A, B, and C capsids of rhesus monkey rhadinovirus: insights into gammaherpesvirus capsid assembly, maturation, and DNA packaging. *J. Virol.*, **77**(24), 13182–13193.

Yu, Y., Wang, S. E., and Hayward, G. S. (2005). The KSHV immediate–early transcription factor RTA encodes ubiquitin E3 ligase activity that targets IRF7 for proteasome-mediated degradation. *Immunity*, **22**, 59–70.

Zhong, W., Wang, H., Herndier, B., and Ganem, D. (1996). Restricted expression of Kaposi sarcoma-associated herpesvirus (human herpesvirus 8) genes in Kaposi sarcoma. *Proc. Natl Acad. Sci. USA*, **93**(13), 6641–6646.

Zhu, F., Cusano, T., and Yuan, Y. (1999). Identification of the immediate-early transcripts of Kaposi's sarcoma-associated herpesvirus. *J. Virol.*, **73**, 5556–5567.

Zhu, F. X. and Yuan, Y. (2003). The ORF45 protein of Kaposi's sarcoma-associated herpesvirus is associated with purified virions. *J. Virol.*, **77**(7), 4221–4230.

Zhu, F. X., King, S. M., Smith, E. J., Levy, D. E., and Yuan, Y. (2002). A Kaposi's sarcoma-associated herpesviral protein inhibits virus-mediated induction of type I interferon by blocking IRF-7 phosphorylation and nuclear accumulation. *Proc. Natl Acad. Sci. USA*, **99**(8), 5573–5578.

Zhu, L., Wang, R., Sweat, A., Goldstein, E., Horvat, R., and Chandran, B. (1999b). Comparison of human sera reactivities in immunoblots with recombinant human herpesvirus (HHV)-8 proteins associated with the latent (ORF73) and lytic (ORFs 65, K8.1A, and K8.1B) replicative cycles and in immunofluorescence assays with HHV-8-infected BCBL-1 cells. *Virology*, **256**(2), 381–392.

Zhu, F. X., Chong, J. M., Wu, L., and Yuan, Y. (2005). Virion proteins of Kaposi's sarcoma-associated herpesvirus. *J. Virol.*, **79**(2), 800–811.

Zoeteweij, J. P., Moses, A. V., Rinderknecht, A. S. *et al.* (2001). Targeted inhibition of calcineurin signaling blocks calcium-dependent reactivation of Kaposi sarcoma-associated herpesvirus. *Blood*, **97**(8), 2374–2380.

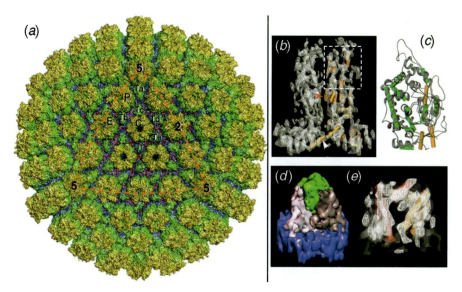

Figure 3.3. Herpesvirus capsid at 8 Å resolution (Zhou *et al.*, 2000) and atomic model of upper domain of the HSV-1 major capsid protein (MCP), VP5 (Bowman *et al.*, 2003). (*a*) Radially color-coded surface representation of the herpes simplex virus type 1 B capsid structure at 8.5 Å. One of the 20 triangular faces is denoted by dashed triangle. The penton and three types of hexons are indicated by '5', P, E and C. Also labeled are the six quasi-equivalent triplexes, Ta, Tb, Tc, Td, Te, Tf. (*b*) Two hexon subunits were shown in wire frame representation with α helices identified in one of the VP5 subunit illustrated by orange cylinders (5 Å in diameter). The red arrowhead points to the 7 helix bundle in the middle domain and the white arrow identifies the long helix in the floor domain that connects adjacent subunits. (*c*) Ribbon representation of the atomic structure of the HSV-1 MCP upper domain determined by X-ray crystallography (Bowman *et al.*, 2003). The helices identified in the hexon VP5 subunit in the 8.5 Å HSV1 capsid map (Zhou *et al.*, 2000) are shown as cylinders: those in green match with helices present in the X-ray structure and those in yellow are absent in the X-ray model, suggesting possible structural differences of MCP packed in the crystal and inside the virion. (*d*) One single triplex is shown as shaded surface representation with individual subunits in different colors: VP19c in green and the two quasi-equivalent VP23 subunits in light and dark grey, all situated on the capsid shell domains of VP5 (blue). (*e*) α-helices identified in the two quasi-equivalent VP23 molecules (in red and yellow cylinders of 5 Å diameter, respectively). Adapted with permissions from publishers.

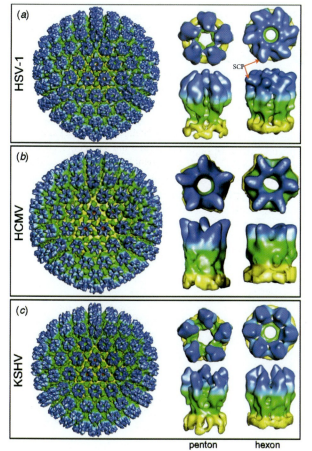

Figure 3.4. Comparison of the three-dimensional structures of alpha, beta and gammaherpesvirus capsids. The capsid maps of HSV-1 (*a*), HCMV (*b*) and KSHV (*c*) are shown as shaded surfaces colored according to particle radius and viewed along an icosahedral three-fold axis. The resolution of the HSV-1 and KSHV capsid maps is 24 Å and that of the HCMV capsid (Butcher *et al.*, 1998) is 35 Å. The right two columns are detailed comparisons of a penton and an E hexon, which were extracted computationally from each map and shown in their top and side views.

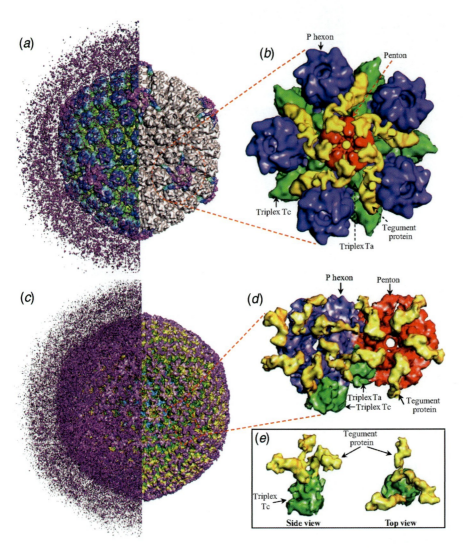

Figure 3.6. Difference of the anchored tegument proteins between HSV-1 ((*a*) and (*b*)) and HCMV ((*c*)–(*e*)). ((*a*) and (*c*)) Radially color-coded shaded surface views of the three-dimensional reconstruction of HSV-1 (*a*) and HCMV (*c*) virions as viewed along an icosahedral three-fold axis. The bulk of the tegument components and the viral envelope are not icosahedrally ordered or polymorphic, thus appearing as disconnected low densities in the icosahedral reconstruction. These disconnected densities were masked out for the right hemisphere to better reveal the icosahedrally ordered tegument proteins, which are shown in blue to purple colors in (*a*) and in purple in (*c*). ((*b*) and (*d*)) Close-up views of the region indicated in (*a*) and (*c*), respectively, showing the molecular interactions of the tegument proteins (yellow) with the penton (red), P hexon (blue) and triplexes (green). In HSV-1, contrary to the extensive tegument association with all hexons, the tegument densities do not interact with any hexon. (*e*) Extracted triplex HCMV Tc with its attached tegument densities. Three tegument densities interact with the upper domain of each triplex (insert Table 3.1).

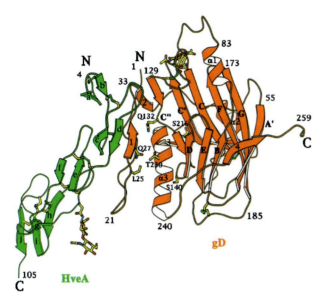

Figure 7.3. Ribbon diagram of the 3D structure of a soluble truncated form of gD (gD285t, colored in orange) bound to HVEM receptor (HveA, colored in green) as determined by X-ray crystallography. The N-terminus (residues 1–37) of gD is devoid of a specific structure when in the unbound state, but folds into a hairpin when bound to HVEM receptor. The β-strand formed by residues 27–29 (indicated with number 1) forms an intermolecular β-sheet with HVEM residues 35–37 (letter d). The core of gD (residues 56–184) has a V-type immunglobulin domain structure, composed of 9 parallel and antiparallel β-strands (letters A to G) that form two opposing β-sheets, and carries an additional α-helix (α1). The residues 185–259 form two α-helices that fold back to the N-ter (α2 and α3), and two β-strands (numbered 3 and 4). The α3 helix supports gD's N-terminal hairpin. An additional β-strand (number 2) is located in the connector sequence (residues 33–55) that precedes the Ig-like core. Reprinted from (Carfi et al., 2001), with permission.

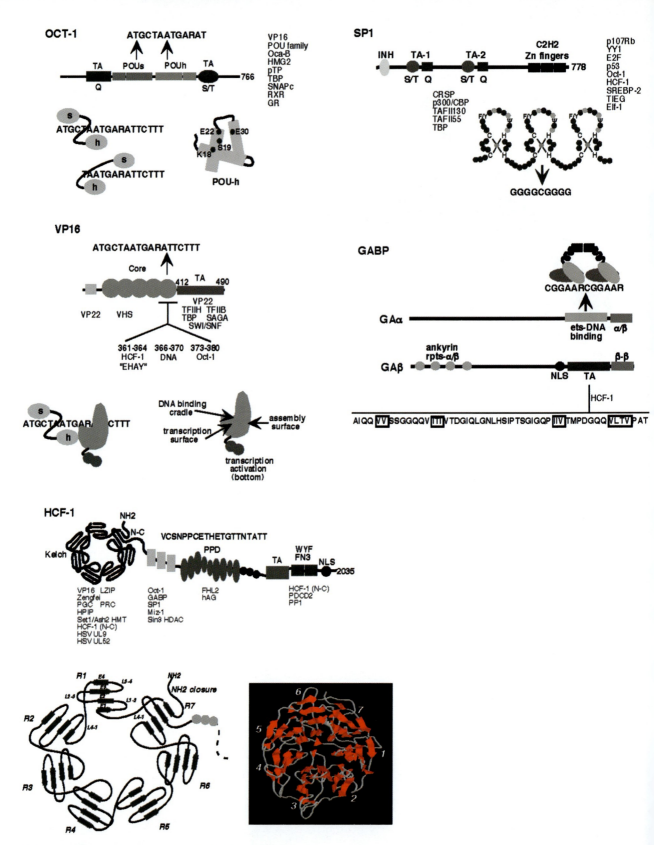

Figure 8.2. The protein components of the HSV IE enhancer complex.
Oct-1: The transactivation (TA-Q and TA-S/T) and POU (POUs and POUh) domains are shown. The POU-specific box recognizes ATGC while the POU-homeobox recognizes TAAT within the enhancer core element (ATGCTAATGARAT). Proteins that bind to the Oct-1 POU domain are listed. The inherent flexibility of the POU domain and the potential orientations of the POUs box in recognition of the core element are depicted. In the schematic representation of the Oct-1 POU-homeobox, the residues which are important for the recognition by VP16 are indicated. (*cont.*)

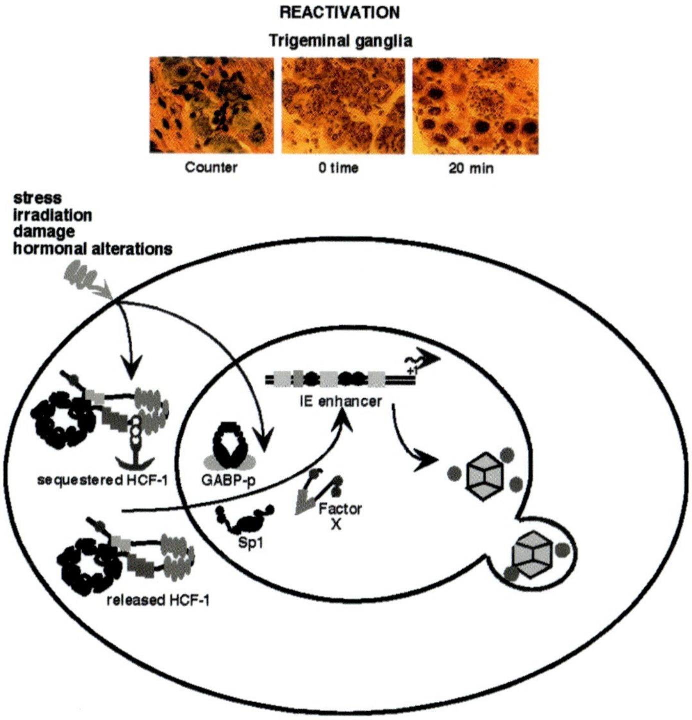

Figure 8.4. Model of the induction of the IE genes during HSV reactivation from latency. (Top) Immunohistochemistry studies of HCF-1 demonstrate that the protein is specifically sequestered in the cytoplasm of sensory neurons (0 time, middle panel) and rapidly transported to the nucleus under experimental conditions that reactivate HSV from latency (explant reactivation stimuli, right panel). (Bottom) Schematic depiction of the activation of IE enhancer components during the initiation of reactivation. Environmental signal(s) result in the release of cytoplasmically sequestered HCF-1 and the activation of DNA binding factors such as GABP, Sp1, or other factors which function in concert with HCF-1 to activate the IE genes and initiate the viral lytic cycle. (see colour plate section)

Figure 8.2. (*continued*) VP16: The structure and protein interactions of VP16 are represented. The core structure contains the clustered residues that are critical for the assembly of the IE enhancer complex (HCF-1, Oct-1, DNA) while the transactivation domain (TA, aa 412–490) interacts with a number of basal factors and chromatin modifying components. A schematic representation of the VP16 protein structure is shown (left) indicating the various protein interaction surfaces oriented in recognition of the Oct-1 POU-homeobox/ DNA complex.
HCF-1: The amino-terminal kelch, mid-aminoterminal, proteolytic processing (PPD), autocatalytic (Auto), transactivation (TA), WYF-rich, FN3 repeat, and nuclear localization signal (NLS) regions are represented. The proteins that interact with each region are listed below the appropriate domain. The PPD is represented as a series of consensus (large oval) and divergent (small oval) reiterations of the HCF-1 cleavage sequence shown above. (Bottom left) A stylized representation of the HCF-1 kelch domain is shown illustrating the seven predicted blades (antiparallel sheets, E1 through E4; loops, L1–2 through L4–1). For HCF-1, the predicted ring closure utilizes E4 from the animoterminus and E1-2-3 from the carboxyterminus of the domain (NH2 closure). (Bottom right) The derived molecular model of the HCF-1 kelch domain structure is depicted.
Sp1: The inhibitory domain (INH), transactivation domains (TA-1, TA-2), and DNA binding domains (C2H2, Zn fingers) are represented. Proteins or protein complexes that interact with Sp1 are listed. The structure of the C2H2 Zn finger domain is schematically represented: C, cysteine; H, histadine; F/Y, phenylalanine or tyrosine; y, hydrophobic residue. Light circles represent amino acids that are predicted to make DNA contacts.
GABP: The α subunit contains the ets DNA binding domain recognizing the GA box and the heterodimerization domain (α/β). The β subunit contains ankyrin repeats (α/β heterodimerization region), nuclear localization signals (NLS), transactivation domain (TA), and tetramerization sequences (β–β). The sequence of the transactivation domain is shown and the residues that are critical for both transactivation and interaction with HCF-1 are boxed. (see colour plate section)

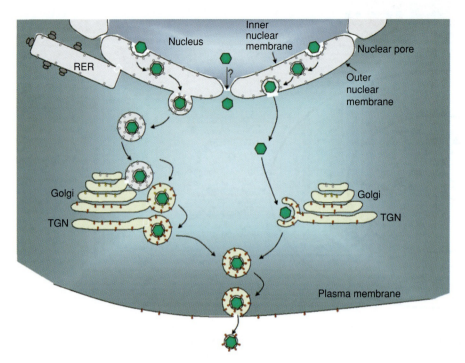

Figure 12.1. Schematic drawing showing the two alternative pathways of alphaherpesvirus egress from infected cells. The single envelopment pathway is depicted to the left, and the double envelopment, or de-envelopment-re-envelopment is depicted to the right of the illustration. The schematic drawing does not shows the gross ultrastructural modifications of the Golgi apparatus and TGN. Perinuclear virions and nuclear membranes are decorated with glycoproteins of different color than virions at the level of the Golgi apparatus and TGN, as well as extracellular virions, to emphasize that the oligosaccharide moieties of the viral glycoproteins are of the immature type in early exocytic compartment, but are of the mature type in the late exocytic compartments and in extracellular virions. The drawing considers also the possibility that nucleocapsids exit the nucleoplasm through modified nuclear pores, without transiting through the perinuclear lumen. (Drawing by courtesy of L. Menotti.)

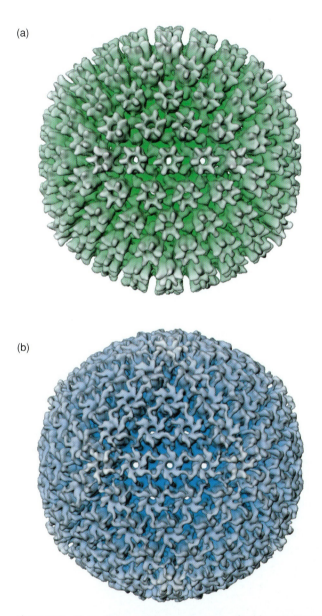

Figure 14.6. Three-dimensional reconstructions of (a) the HCMV B-capsid (adapted from Butcher *et al.*, 1998; with permission from Academic Press), and (b) the HCMV virion (adapted from Zhou *et al.*, 1999; with permission from the American Society for Microbiology). Both structures are viewed along the icosahedral twofold symmetry axes and are radially depth-cued so that darker regions are closer to the centre of the particle and lighter regions are further away.

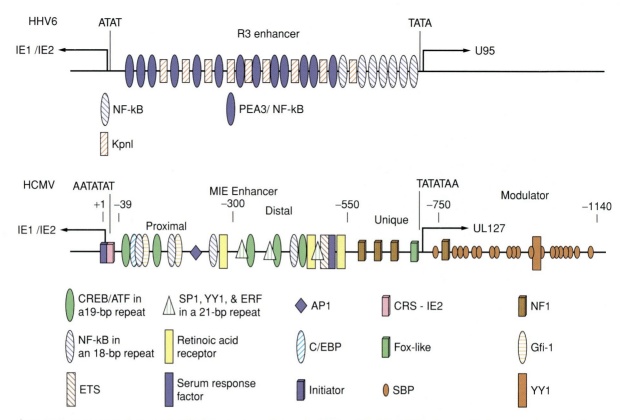

Figure 17.3. Comparison between the HCMV major immediate early (MIE) and the HHV-6 R3 enhancer. Viral genes and promoter/transcription start sites are designated by an arrow. The HCMV also has a unique region and a modulator discussed in the text. The various transcription factor binding sites identified for HCMV and HHV-6 are designated. The AP-2 sites in the R3 enhancer are not identified.

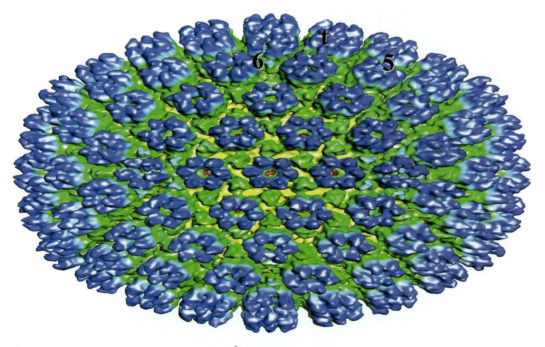

Figure 23.1. 3D structure of the KSHV capsid at 24-Å resolution by electron cryomicroscopy. The capsid is shown as shaded surface color-coded according to particle radius. The three structural component of the capsid are indicated, including 12 pentons ("5"), 150 hexons ("6") and 320 triplexes ("t"). (Wu *et al.*, 2000 with permission).

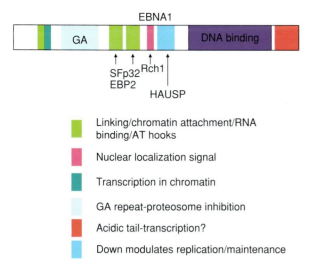

Figure 24.4. Functional protein domains of EBNA1. Amino acid residues are indicated for the boundaries of protein domains for DNA binding, dimerization, chromosome binding sites (CBS), nuclear localization (NLS), or protein–protein interactions (as indicated).

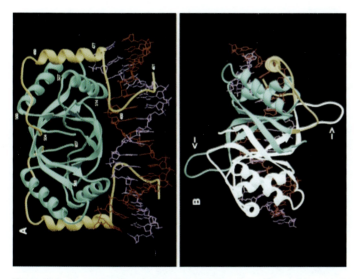

Figure 24.5. X-ray crystal structure of EBNA1 dimer bound to a consensus DNA recognition site (courtesy of Bocharev et al., Cell in press). (a) Ribbon diagram showing the core domain (residues 504–607) from each monomer, in blue. Flanking domains are shown in yellow. (b) View down the non-crystallographic axis showing one monomer in white and the other in the same color scheme as used in (a). Proline loops are indicated by arrows.

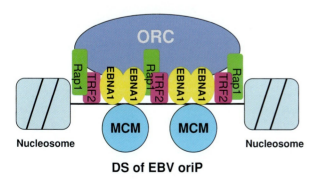

Figure 24.6. Model for *OriP* of EBV. Indicated are protein–protein and protein DNA interactions that are required for the initiation of DNA synthesis at *OriP*.

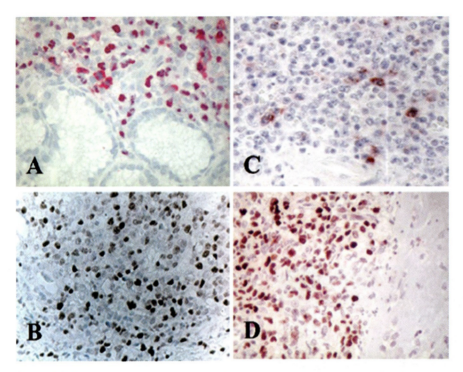

Figure 27.2. Latency III pattern characteristic of the majority of cases of post-transplant lymphoproliferative disease. All known EBV latent genes are expressed in this form of latency: (a) EBERs, (b) EBNA1, (c) LMP1, (d) EBNA2.

(a)

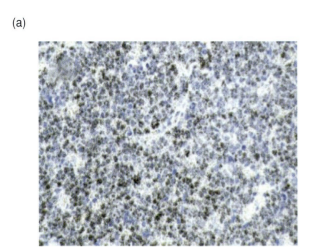

(b)

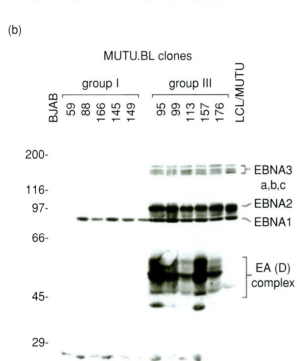

Figure 27.3. Latency pattern characteristic of Burkitt's lymphoma (BL). (a) Expression of EBERs in the tumor cells of BL tissue shown by isotopic *in* situ hybridization and (b) Immunoblotting demonstrating protein expression limited to EBNA1 in so-called 'group I' BL cell lines which recapitulate the in vivo expression profile. 'Group III' BL lines have an expression pattern similar to that of LCLs (Latency III) and represent cell lines that have 'drifted' from a latency I pattern in vitro.

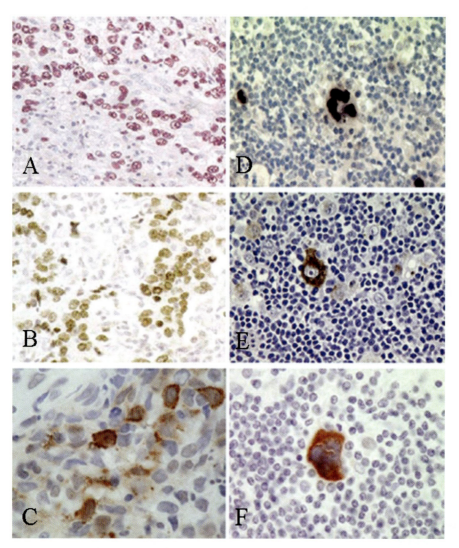

Figure 27.4. EBV latency type II. Left panel shows (a) Expression of EBERs, (b) EBNA1 and (c) LMP1, in the tumor cells of nasopharyngeal carcinoma (NPC). LMP1 expression is not a regular feature of these tumors. LMP2 protein has not yet been reported in NPC tumors, despite the detection of LMP2 RNA. Right panel shows EBV gene expression in the rare tumor cells of (HRS cells) Hodgkin's lymphoma. (d) EBERs, (e) LMP1 and (f) LMP2. EBNA1 protein is also detectable in the majority of cases (not shown). In contrast to NPC, both LMP1 and LMP2 protein are almost always detectable in EBV-infected HRS cells.

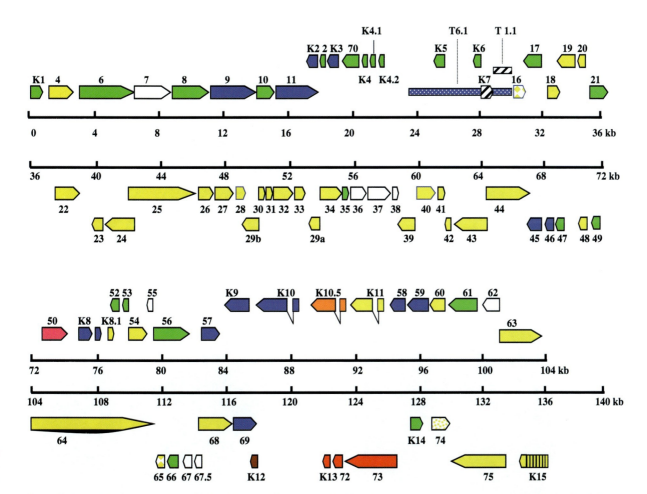

Figure 28.1. KSHV gene expression in PEL cell lines and biopsy samples. This Figure summarizes the expression of individual KSHV genes in PEL cells during latency and following reactivation of the lytic cycle by treatment with TPA, Na-butyrate or heterologous expression of RTA by transfection or transduction. Also included are results from in situ hybridization or immunohistochemistry studies on biopsy samples of KS, MCD or PEL tumors. As discussed in the text, the color-coding is based on a comparison of several reports that studied KSHV genes by Northern blot, real time PCR or DNA array. (See colour plate section)

▬ Latent gene
▬ Latent gene in B cells only
▬ Latent gene in KS spindle cells in vivo; early (in some studies delayed) expression kinetics in PEL cells in vitro
▬ Immediate–early gene as judged by cycloheximide resistance
▬ Very rapid onset of gene expression in at least 2 studies
▒ Early lytic transcript: TPA inducible, unaffected by PFA
▬ Delayed onset of gene expression
▬ Late gene expression profile
▢ Late gene expression profile confirmed by PAA sensitivity
▨ Discrepant results in different gene array studies

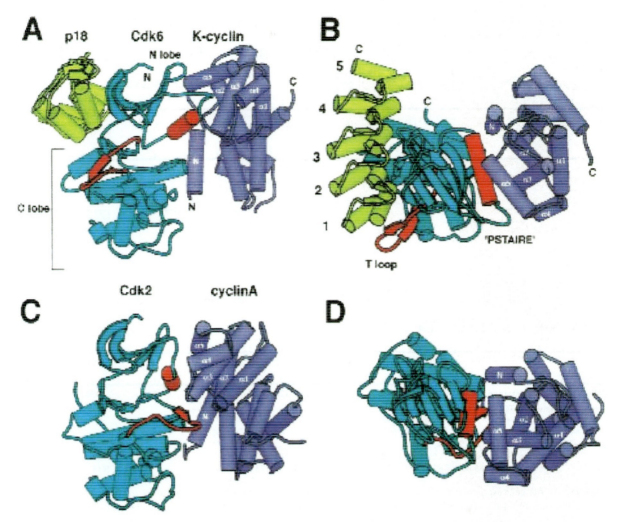

Figure 30.3. The structure of the vCYC (purple), CDK6 (cyan), p18Inkb (yellow) complex from side (a) and top (b) views, compared to cellular cyclin A (purple), CDK2 (cyan) side (c) and top (d) views. Unlike cellular cyclins, the regulatory T-loop of CDK6 is excluded from interaction with vCYC but the PSTAIRE regulatory helix of CDK6 still forms an interface with vCYC, The PSTAIRE helix forms part of the ATP binding domain required for kinase activity while the T loop acts as a negative regulator of kinase activity and must be phosphorylated by cyclin-activating kinases (CAK) in cellular cyclin–CDK complexes. While CAK phosphorylation may enhance vCYC-CDK6 stability, displacement of the T loop by vCYC allows this complex to be active in the absence of CAK activity. The structure of vCYC-CDK6 also reveals loss of the binding pocket used by cyclin-dependent kinase inhibitors (CDKI) of the CIP1/KIP1 family. These and other features support experimental data showing the vCYC-CDK6 not only have a broader target range than cellular D-type cyclins but also escape many normal negative regulatory controls imposed on the cellular cyclin machinery. Reprinted with permission (Jeffrey *et al.*, 2000).

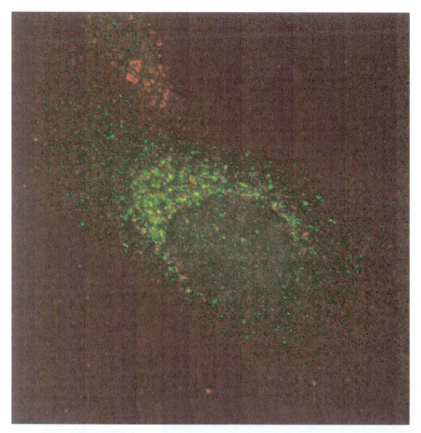

Figure 42.1. Immunofluorescent micrograph of HCMV-infected AEC. Telomerase life-extended human AEC were infected with HCMV. Cells were fixed and stained for the presence of HCMV protein, glycoprotein B (a late product; green) and a cellular marker of the *trans*-Golgi network (TGN46; red).

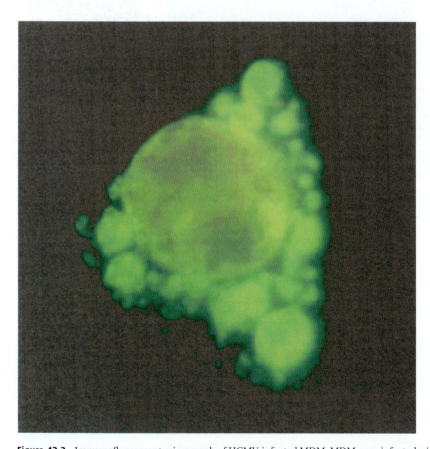

Figure 42.2. Immunofluorescent micrograph of HCMV-infected MDM. MDM were infected with HCMV. Cells were fixed and stained for the presence of HCMV proteins, pp65 (an early product; green) and IE-2 (an immediate-early productl; red).

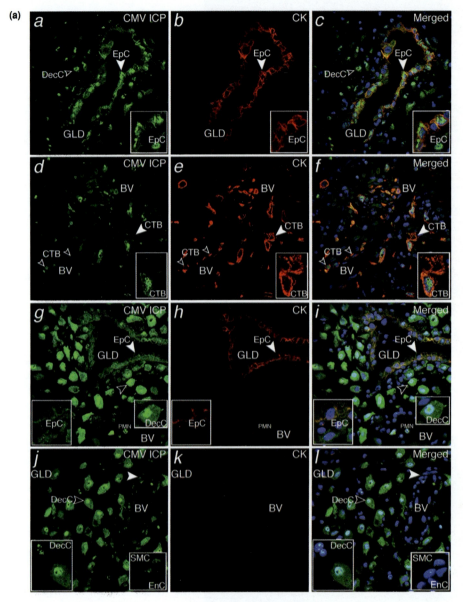

Figure 45.4a. Panel A: CMV replicates in diverse cell types in uterine decidua. CMV infects endometrial glands (GLD), uterine blood vessels (BV), resident decidual cells (DecC) and cytotrophoblasts (CTB) in the decidua. (*a*)–(*c*), Decidual biopsy specimens stained for CMV-infected-cell proteins (ICP, green) and cytokeratin (CK, red), which identified epithelial cells (EpC). (*d*)–(*i*), CMV-infected interstitial and endovascular CTB and DecC. (*j*)–(*l*), Endothelial cells (EnC) and smooth muscle cells (SMC) of uterine blood vessels (BV) are infected. Panel (*b*): Abundant innate immune cells infiltrating the decidua contain CMV proteins. (*a*)–(*c*) CMV gB (green), macrophages (Mφ/DC, CD68, red). (*d*)–(*f*) DC-SIGN+ (green) macrophage/dendritic cells (Mφ/DC) take up CMV gB (red). (*g* (and) *h*) CD56+ (green) natural killer (NK) cells target infection sites. (*i*) DC-SIGN+ cells containing gB. (*j*)–(*l*) Neutrophils (PMN) with phagocytosed proteins from virus-infected cells and endothelial cells (EnC) positive for von Willebrand factor (vWF) in blood vessels (BV). "Merged" indicates colocalized proteins (yellow). Large arrowheads indicate area shown in insets.

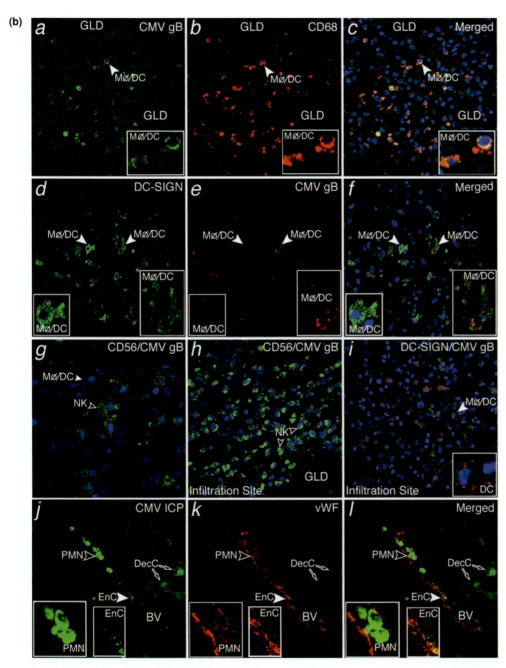

Figure 45.4b. (cont.)

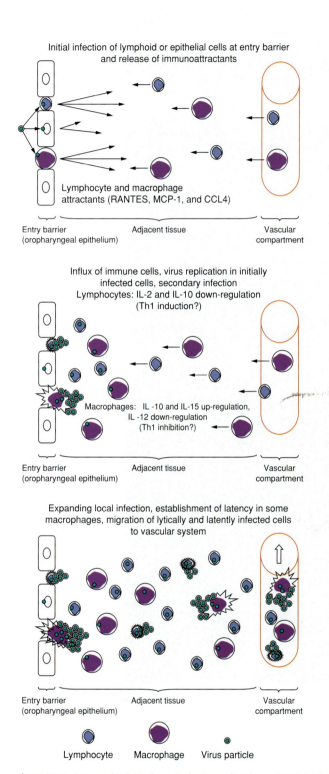

Figure 48.3. Immunobiological events during early primary HHV-6 infection and establishment of latency.

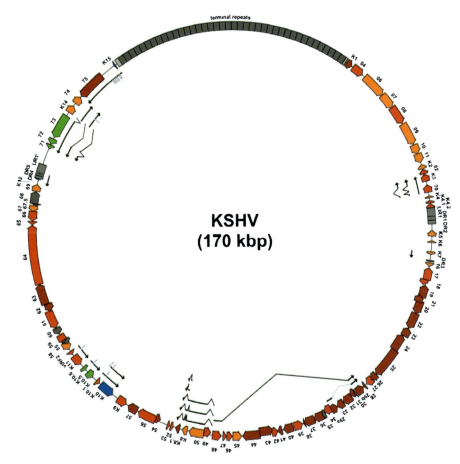

Figure 56.1. Latency genes of KSHV. Transcripts of latent genes are depicted as arrows, superimposed on the physical map of the circular latent viral genome.

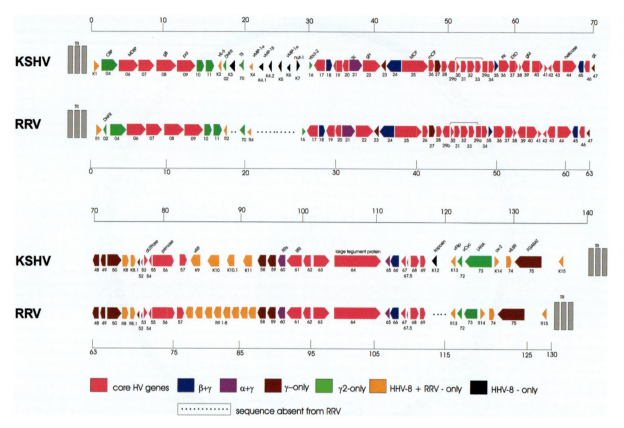

Figure 61.3. Alignment of the KSHV and RRV genomes. The different colors signify ORFs contained in KSHV and RRV 26–95 that are conserved in the indicated herpesvirus subfamilies or subgroups. The square side of the symbol signifies the 5′ end and the pointed side of the symbol signifies the 3′ end of the depicted ORFs. The ORFs are not drawn to scale. (Taken from Alexander *et al.*, 2000, with permission from the *Journal of Virology*.) (see colour plate section)

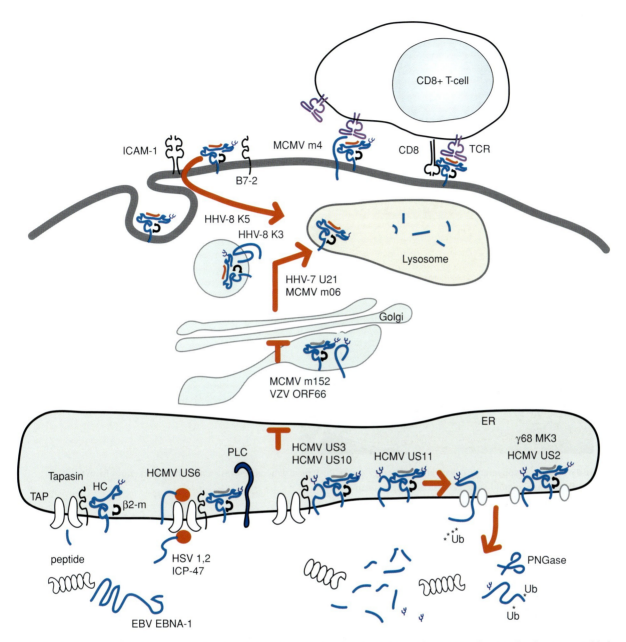

Figure 62.1. Herpesvirus immunoevasins that directly interfere with class I molecule biosynthesis. MHC class I molecules are assembled from free MHC class I HC and β-2 microgobulin within the ER, along with antigenic peptide. Peptides are produced by cytosolic 4m proteasome degradation via its GAr domain. Tapasin and the PLC facilitate loading of peptide cargo onto empty class I molecules. HSV ICP47 and HCMV US6 block TAP peptide transport, while HCMV US3 inhibits tapasin and retains class I complexes in the ER. Following receipt of peptide, the loaded class I molecules travel through the secretory pathway to the cell surface. HCMV US10 delays transport of class I molecules from the ER, while VZV ORF66 and MCMV m152 retain class I in the Golgi complex. HCMV US2, US11 and MHV γ68 MK3 dislocate class I molecules via an unidentified ER membrane pore to the cytosol. The dislocated class I heavy chains are ubiquinated (Ub) and deglycolylated by cellular PNGase prior to proteasomal cleavage. HHV-7 U21, MCMV m6, and HHV-8 K3 redirect class I molecules from the secretory to the endolysosomal pathway for degradation. HHV-8 K5 likewise targets MHC class I, B7-2 and ICAM-1 molecules to the endolysosmal pathway for destruction. MCMV m4 disrupts recognition of cell surface-disposed MHC class I-peptide complexes by the TCR 8of CD8+ T-cells.

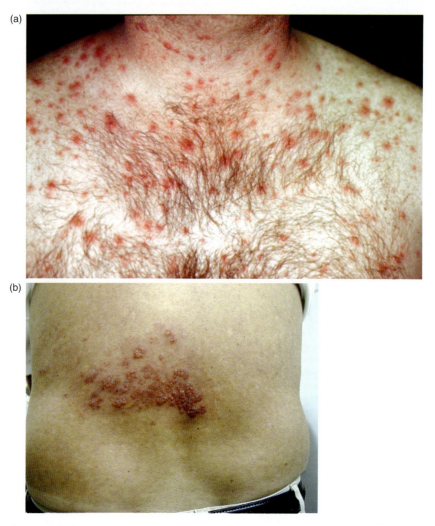

Figure 65.1. Clinical appearance of varicella and herpes zoster. (a) Typical generalized vesicular rash of chickenpox in an adult. (b) Typical dermatomal papulo-vesicular rash of shingles in an adult.

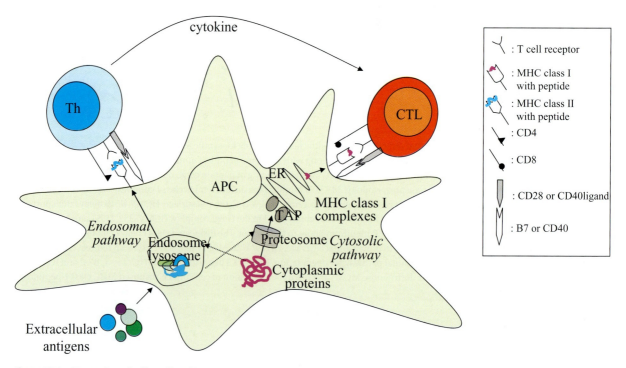

Figure 74.1. Generation of cell-mediated immune response.

27

EBV gene expression and regulation

Lawrence S. Young, John R. Arrand, and Paul G. Murray

Cancer Research UK Institute for Cancer Studies, University of Birmingham Edgbaston, UK

Introduction

Epstein–Barr virus (EBV) is an extremely efficient virus infecting the majority of the world's adult population (Rickinson and Kieff, 2001). Following primary infection, EBV persists in the infected host as a lifelong asymptomatic infection. Early in the course of primary infection, EBV infects B-lymphocytes, although it is not known where B-lymphocytes are infected and whether this involves epithelial cells of the upper respiratory tract. To achieve long-term persistence in vivo, EBV colonizes the memory B-cell pool where it establishes latent infection, which is characterized by the expression of a limited subset of virus genes, known as the "latent" genes (Thorley-Lawson, 2001). There are several well-described forms of EBV latency, each of which is utilized by the virus at different stages of the virus life cycle and which are also reflected in the patterns of latency observed in the various EBV-associated malignancies (Rickinson and Kieff, 2001; Young and Murray, 2003). Furthermore, during its life cycle EBV must periodically enter the replicative cycle in order to generate infectious virus for transmission to other susceptible hosts, although it is also not clear whether this occurs in B-lymphocytes or in other cell types of the oropharynx (Rickinson and Kieff, 2001).

This chapter describes the EBV latency and replicative programs utilized by the virus as a means to understand how the virus infects and then establishes persistence in the host. The function of each of the key latent and lytic genes will be described in detail and will provide the foundation for later chapters which describe the contribution of some of these EBV genes to the pathogenesis of the EBV-associated malignancies.

Virus and genome structure

EBV is a gammaherpesvirus of the *Lymphocryptovirus* (LCV) genus and is closely related to other LCVs present in Old World non-human primates, including EBV-like viruses of chimpanzees and rhesus monkeys. In fact, the rhesus monkey LCV and EBV share similar sequences and genetic organization, and are both capable of maintaining infection in the oropharynx and in B cells (Moghaddam *et al.*, 1997). Recently, a transforming, EBV-related virus has also been isolated from spontaneous B cell lymphomas of common marmosets and is thus the first EBV-like virus to be identified in a New World monkey species (Cho *et al.*, 2001; Rivailler *et al.*, 2002). Sequencing of the genome of the marmoset LCV revealed considerable divergence from the genomes of EBV and Old World primate EBV-related viruses.

The EBV genome is composed of linear double-stranded DNA, approximately 172 kilobase pairs (kb) in length. EBV has a series of 0.5 kb terminal direct repeats (TRs) and internal repeat sequences (IRs) that divide the genome into short and long, largely unique sequence domains (Fig. 27.1(a)). The infectious mononucleosis-derived, B95-8 strain of EBV was the first herpesvirus to have its genome completely cloned and sequenced (Baer *et al.*, 1984; Accession number V01555). This prototype B95-8 strain of EBV is atypical of the majority of isolates, in particular it is missing an 11.8 kb segment of the genome (Fig. 27.1). In order to present a sequence more representative of the majority of isolates, a "hybrid" sequence has been assembled (accession number NC_007605) in which the 11.8 kb sequence determined from the Raji strain of EBV (Parker *et al.*, 1990) has been

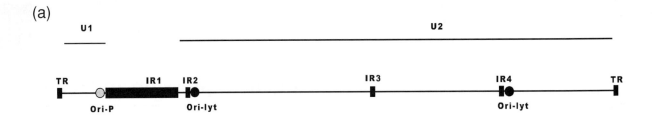

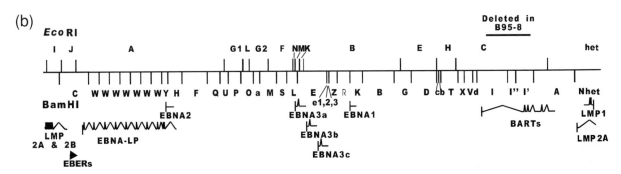

Fig. 27.1. The Epstein–Barr virus (EBV) genome. (a) General organization of linear, EBV virion DNA. U1 and U2 are the short and long unique regions of the genome, respectively. These are interspersed with the four internal repeat regions IR1–4. TR represent the terminal repeats. The origin of replication (Ori-P) of the intracellular, circular, episomal form of the genome is indicated by the grey circle whilst the lytic origins of replication (Ori-lyt) are shown as black circles. (b) *Eco*RI and *Bam*HI restriction endonuclease maps of EBV DNA and the positions of the genes expressed in latency. The *Bam*HI fragments are named according to the well-established B95–8 designations with the exception of I (which is larger than its B95–8 counterpart), I' and I'' (which are absent in the B95–8 strain). The splicing patterns of the latent RNAs through the coding regions are indicated. EBNA-LP is transcribed from variable numbers of repetitive exons. The full transcriptional patterns of the remaining EBNA genes are more complex than shown here (see text) and the BARTs consist of a number of differently spliced RNA species emanating from the same promoter (Smith *et al.*, 2000; de Jesus *et al.*, 2003). Note that the LMP2 proteins are produced from mRNAs that splice across the terminal repeats in the intracellular, circularised EBV genome. This region has often been referred to as Nhet to denote the heterogeneity in this region according to the number of terminal repeats within different virus isolates.

inserted into the B95–8 sequence to make good the deletion. Recently the complete sequences of two more strains of EBV have been determined: GD1, derived from a Chinese nasopharyngeal carcinoma patient (Zeng *et al.*, 2005; accession number AY961628) and AG876 (Dolan *et al.*, 2006; accession number DQ279927), derived from a Ghanaian Burkitt lymphoma (Pizzo *et al.*, 1978). Since the prototype B95–8 genome was sequenced from an EBV DNA *Bam*HI fragment cloned library, open reading frames (ORFs), genes and sites for transcription or RNA processing are frequently referenced to specific *Bam*HI fragments, from A to Z, in descending order of fragment size (Fig. 27.1(b)). The virus has the coding potential for around 80 proteins, not all of which have been identified or characterized. Characterized gene products are listed in Table 27.1. Analysis of the sequences of GD1 and AG876 together with correction of the B95–8 sequence has led to the identification of four previously unrecognized open reading frames: BVLF1 and BDLF3.5 whose functions are unknown, BFRF1A which by homology with other Herpesviruses probably has a role in DNA packaging, and BGLF3.5 which is likely to be a tegument protein (Dolan *et al.*, 2006).

EBV latency in vitro and in vivo

The lymphoblastoid cell line LCL

When peripheral blood lymphocytes from healthy EBV sero-positives are placed in culture, the few EBV-infected B-lymphocytes that are present regularly give rise to spontaneous outgrowth of EBV-transformed, immortalized cell lines, known as lymphoblastoid cell lines (LCLs), provided that immune T-lymphocytes are either removed or inhibited by the addition of cyclosporin A to the culture (Rickinson *et al.*, 1984). LCLs can also be generated by direct infection of resting B-lymphocytes with EBV derived from producer B-cell lines.

Table 27.1. List of characterised genes. References pertain to genes that are not considered further in the text. Open reading frames within the EBV genome are named sequentially after the *Bam*HI fragment within which they begin and the direction in which they are read. Thus, for example, BZLF1 refers to *Bam*HI-**Z** **l**eftward reading **f**rame number **1**.

ORF	Gene product	Reference
Latent genes		
BKRF1	EBNA1	
BYRF1	EBNA2	
BLRF3/BERF1	EBNA3A (EBNA3)	
BERF2a/b	EBNA3B (EBNA4)	
BERF3/4	EBNA3C (EBNA6)	
*Bam*HI-W (repeated multiple splices)	EBNA-LP (EBNA5)	
BNLF1	LMP1	
Fused TRs (multiple splices)	LMP2A/B	
BARTs	A73, RPMS1	
EBER1/2	small RNAs	
Early genes		
BZLF1	ZEBRA/Zta/EB1	
BRLF1	Rta	
BRRF1	transcription factor	
BORF2	ribonucleotide reductase large subunit	
BaRF1	ribonucleotide reductase small subunit	
BXLF1	thymidine kinase	
BGLF5	alkaline exonuclease	
BLLF3	dUTPase	Sommer *et al.*, 1996
BKRF3	uracil DNA glycosylase	Olsen *et al.*, 1989
BALF5	DNA polymerase	
BMRF1	polymerase accessory protein	
BALF2	DNA binding protein	
BSLF1	primase	
BBLF2/3	primase accessory protein	
BBLF4	helicase	
BMLF1	mRNA export factor	
BSLF2	spliced to BMLF1	Cook *et al.*, 1994
BHRF1	bcl-2 homologue	
BALF1	viral-bcl-2 antagonist	
BARF1	transformation-associated?	
BGLF4	protein kinase	Chen *et al.*, 2000; Kato *et al.*, 2001
BFRF1	37kDa membrane/virion protein	Farina *et al.*, 2000
BHLF1	ss-DNA binding protein	Nuebling and Mueller-Lantzsch, 1989
BHLF2	envelopment protein	Gonnella et al., 2005
BNLF2a	immune evasion	
Late genes		
BNRF1	major tegument protein p143	
BPLF1	large tegument protein	
BOLF1	tegument protein	
BVRF1	tegument protein	
BBLF1	tegument protein	
BGLF1	tegument protein	
BSRF1	tegument protein	
BRRF2	tegument protein	
BDLF2	tegument protein	
BKRF4	tegument protein	
BcLF1	major capsid protein	
BDLF1	minor capsid protein	
BFRF3	capsid protein p18	
BLRF2	capsid protein p23	
BdRF1	capsid protein p40	
BBRF1	capsid protein	
BVRF2	protease	
BGLF2	38Kd protein	
BORF1	may be needed for capsid assembly	Pertuiset *et al.*, 1989
BLRF1	glycoprotein gN	
BLLF1	glycoprotein gp350/220	
BZLF2	glycoprotein gp42	
BKRF2	glycoprotein gL (gp25)	
BBRF3	glycoprotein gM	
BXLF2	glycoprotein gH (gp85)	
BILF1	glycoprotein gp60	
BILF2	glycoprotein gp78/55	
BALF4	glycoprotein B (gp110)	
BDLF3	glycoprotein gp150	
BMRF2	53/55Kd membrane protein	
BALF3	glycoprotein transport?	Pellett *et al.*, 1986
BCRF1	viral IL-10	

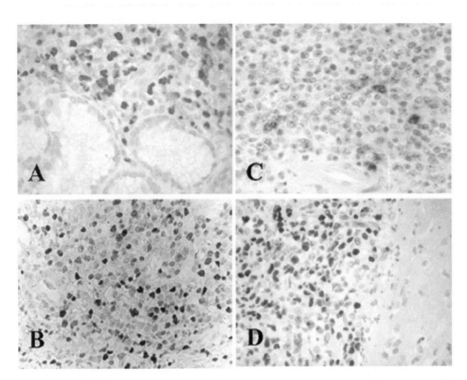

Fig. 27.2. Latency III pattern characteristic of the majority of cases of post-transplant lymphoproliferative disease. All known EBV latent genes are expressed in this form of latency: (a) EBERs, (b) EBNA1, (c) LMP1, (d) EBNA2. (See color plate section.)

Every cell in an LCL carries multiple copies of circular extra-chromosomal viral DNA (episomes) and produces a number of latent proteins, including six nuclear antigens (EBNAs 1, 2, 3A, 3B, 3C and -LP) and three latent membrane proteins (LMPs 1, 2A and 2B) (Fig. 27.1(b)). Transcripts, referred to as BARTs (BamHI A rightward transcripts), from the *Bam*HI A region (Bam A) of the viral genome are also detected, although whether these encode proteins remains controversial (Kieff and Rickinson, 2001). In addition to the latent proteins, LCLs also show abundant expression of the small non-polyadenylated RNAs, EBERs 1 and 2; the function of these transcripts is not clear but they are believed to be expressed in all forms of latent EBV infection and have served as excellent targets to detect EBV in tumors (see later chapters). The relative positions and orientations of these viral genes are illustrated in (Fig. 27.1(b)) under a linearized restriction map of the viral genome. The different EBNAs are encoded by individual mRNAs generated by differential splicing of the same long (over 100 kb) "rightward" primary transcript expressed from one of two promotors (Cp or Wp) located close together in the *Bam*HI C and W region of the genome (Speck and Strominger, 1989). A switch from Wp to Cp occurs early in B cell infection as a consequence of the transactivating effects of both EBNA1 and EBNA2 on Cp. The LMP transcripts are expressed from separate promoters in the *Bam*HI N region of the EBV genome, with the leftward LMP1 and rightward LMP2B mRNAs apparently controlled by the same bidirectional promoter sequence (ED-L1) which also responds to transactivation by EBNA2 (Hofelmayr *et al.*, 1999; Kieff and Rickinson, 2001; Speck and Strominger, 1989). The LMP2A promoter is also regulated by EBNA2. Both LMP2A and LMP2B transcripts cross the TRs into the U1 region thus requiring the circularization of the genome for transcription. Circularization occurs by homologous recombination of the TRs resulting in fused termini of unique length and this has been used as a measure of EBV clonality on the assumption that fused TRs with an identical number of repeats denote expansions of a single infected progenitor cell (Raab-Traub and Flynn, 1986). This contention has recently been challenged by the observation that EBV clonality post-infection may be a consequence of the selective growth advantage achieved by optimal LMP2A expression over a minimal number of TRs (Moody *et al.*, 2003). The pattern of latent EBV gene expression observed in LCLs is referred to as the "latency III" (Lat III) form of EBV infection and is characteristic of the majority of post-transplant lymphomas (Fig. 27.2).

The Lat III pattern of EBV gene expression seen in LCLs is matched by an equally consistent and characteristic cellular phenotype with high-level expression of the B-cell activation markers CD23, CD30, CD39 and CD70 and of the cellular adhesion molecules, leukocyte function associated molecule-1 (LFA-1; CD11a/18), LFA-3 (CD58) and intercellular adhesion molecule-1 (ICAM-1; CD54) (Rowe et al., 1987). These markers are usually absent or expressed at low levels on resting B cells, but are transiently induced to high levels when these cells are activated into short-term growth by antigenic or mitogenic stimulation, suggesting that EBV-induced immortalization can be elicited through the constitutive activation of the same cellular pathways that drive physiological B cell proliferation. The ability of EBNA2, EBNA3C and LMP1 to induce LCL-like phenotypic changes when expressed individually in human B cell lines implicates these viral proteins as key effectors of the immortalisation process (Kieff and Rickinson, 2001; Rickinson and Kieff, 2001; Wang et al., 1990).

Other forms of EBV latency

The examination of EBV latent gene expression in virus-associated tumors and in cell lines derived from Burkitt lymphoma (BL) biopsies identified at least two additional forms of EBV latency. EBNA1 is the only EBV protein consistently observed in EBV-positive BL tumors along with the EBER and BamHIA transcripts; this form of latency is referred to latency I or Lat I (Fig. 27.3) (Gregory et al., 1990; Rickinson and Kieff, 2001; Rowe et al., 1987). Some reports have documented expression of LMP1 and EBNA2 in small numbers of cells in a few cases of endemic BL (Niedobitek et al., 1995), and LMP1 in several cases of sporadic BL (Carbone et al., 1995). In BL biopsies and representative BL cell lines EBNA1 is transcribed from the Qp promoter rather than Wp or Cp (Nonkwelo et al., 1996). Qp, a TATA-less promoter, has many features of the promoters driving expression of housekeeping genes and a downstream element, the Q locus, binds EBNA1 resulting in the repression of Qp transcription (Sample et al., 1992). Recent studies indicate that Qp is also positively regulated by the JAK/STAT pathway (Chen et al., 1999).

BL cells exhibit high level expression of CD10 and CD77, a phenotype most closely resembling that of centroblasts in germinal centers. When cells from some EBV-positive BL tumors are passaged in culture, the other EBNAs and LMPs are expressed, and the EBNA2 and LMP1-induced cell surface antigens, such as CD23, CD30, CD39, LFA1, LFA3, and ICAM1, also are up-regulated (Gregory et al., 1990). EBNA2 and LMP1 are the major mediators of EBV-induced B lymphocyte growth in vitro and the lack of expression of these proteins in tumor cells suggests that they are not required for BL growth (Rickinson and Kieff, 2001).

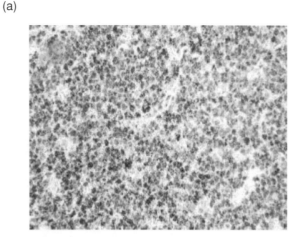

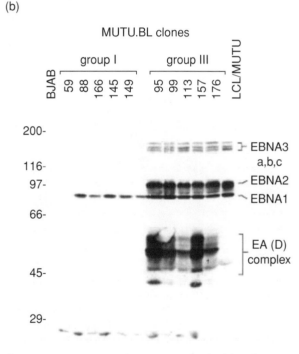

Fig. 27.3. Latency pattern characteristic of Burkitt's lymphoma (BL). (a) Expression of EBERs in the tumor cells of BL tissue shown by isotopic in situ hybridization and (b) Immunoblotting demonstrating protein expression limited to EBNA1 in so-called 'group I' BL cell lines which recapitulate the in vivo expression profile. 'Group III' BL lines have an expression pattern similar to that of LCLs (Latency III) and represent cell lines that have 'drifted' from a latency I pattern in vitro. (See color plate section.)

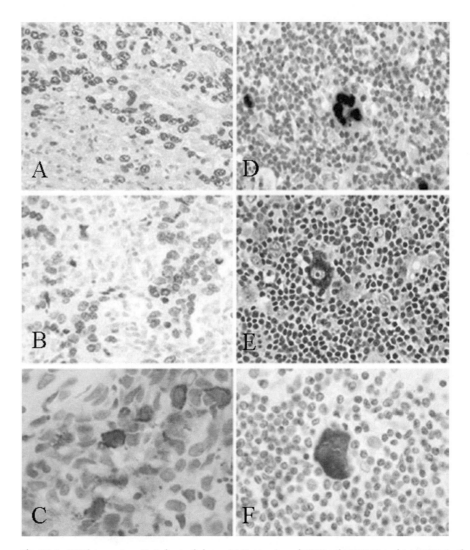

Fig. 27.4. EBV latency type II. Left panel shows (a) Expression of EBERs, (b) EBNA1 and (c) LMP1, in the tumor cells of nasopharyngeal carcinoma (NPC). LMP1 expression is not a regular feature of these tumors. LMP2 protein has not yet been reported in NPC tumors, despite the detection of LMP2 RNA. Right panel shows EBV gene expression in the rare tumor cells of (HRS cells) Hodgkin's lymphoma. (d) EBERs, (e) LMP1 and (f) LMP2. EBNA1 protein is also detectable in the majority of cases (not shown). In contrast to NPC, both LMP1 and LMP2 protein are almost always detectable in EBV-infected HRS cells. (See color plate section.)

Another form of EBV latency, Lat II, was originally identified in biopsies of nasopharyngeal carcinoma (NPC) and subsequently found in cases of EBV-associated Hodgkin's lymphoma (HL) (Brooks et al., 1992; Deacon et al., 1993; Pallesen et al., 1991; Young et al., 1988). Here, expression of the EBERs, Qp-driven EBNA1 and BamHI A transcripts is accompanied by expression of LMP1 and LMP2A/B (Fig. 27.4). Transcription of LMP1 is controlled by an EBNA2-independent promoter located within the viral terminal repeats (L1-TR) and is regulated by the JAK/STAT signaling pathway (Chen et al., 2001, 2003). The factors responsible for LMP2A and LMP2B expression in the absence of EBNA2 in NPC and HL have yet to be defined. Whilst this Lat II pattern of EBV latent gene expression is a consistent feature of virus-associated HL, LMP1 expression in NPC is variable with only around 20% of biopsies being unequivocally positive for LMP1 at the protein level (Niedobitek et al., 1992). The mechanisms underlying differential LMP1 expression in NPC and the consequent effects on the NPC phenotype remain unknown.

The observation that the majority of NPC tumors do not express the Lat II form of EBV latent infection and that EBNA2 can occasionally be detected in BL tumour cells emphasizes the limitations of the operational categorization of virus latency into three distinct forms. It is clear that in vivo there is often a spectrum of EBV latent and lytic gene expression within the same infected tissue. The need for caution in the rigid application of these forms of EBV latency is highlighted by a recent study in which expression of the EBNA3 family through Wp-driven transcription has been identified in a subset of BL biopsies (Kelly et al., 2002). It appears that in these tumors the selective pressure to down-regulate EBNA2 expression has occurred via deletion of the EBNA2 gene rather than through the switch to Qp usage observed in the conventional BL scenario. Other forms of EBV latency in which the EBERs are not expressed have been reported in breast carcinoma and hepatocellular carcinoma but here the association of EBV with these tumors remains controversial (Bonnet et al., 1999; Murray et al., 2003; Sugawara et al., 1999).

EBV replication/the lytic cascade

The cascade of events in the lytic phase of the EBV life cycle is divided into three phases of regulated gene expression: immediate–early, early and late. The immediate–early gene products are transactivator proteins that trigger the expression of the early genes, the products of which include enzymes that are required for viral DNA replication. In turn, amplification of EBV DNA defines the boundary between early and late gene expression. During the late phase of the cycle viral structural proteins are expressed and assembled into virus particles into which the DNA is packaged prior to release of infectious virions.

The principal switch from latency to productive infection involves activation of the immediate–early genes BZLF1 and BRLF1 (Biggin et al., 1987; Countryman and Miller, 1985; Hardwick et al., 1988; Rooney et al., 1989). On induction of the lytic cycle these two genes are expressed simultaneously (Sinclair et al., 1991) and respectively encode the transactivator proteins known as ZEBRA (Countryman et al., 1987), EB1 (Chevallier-Greco et al., 1986) or Zta (Lieberman et al., 1990) (BZLF1) and Rta (BRLF1). The two proteins can be expressed from a major 2.9 kb and a minor 3.8 kb bicistronic R-Z RNA transcribed from the R-promoter (Rp) whilst ZEBRA is also expressed from a smaller 0.9 kb mRNA initiated at the downstream Z-promoter (Zp). In addition, another 0.9kb message encoding a putative fusion protein known as RAZ and consisting of parts of both Rta and ZEBRA is transcribed at low level (Fig. 27.5) (Manet et al., 1989). The in vivo significance, if any, of the putative RAZ protein is unclear although it appears to be able to act as an inhibitor of ZEBRA (Furnari et al., 1994; Segouffin et al., 1996). Both Zp and Rp are activated by ZEBRA whilst Rta can up-regulate Zp and autoactivate its own synthesis. However, maximum activation of the upstream Rp promoter for the bicistronic messenger is obtained by the synergistic effects of ZEBRA and Rta (Liu and Speck, 2003). This synergism suggests that low levels of the two proteins are sufficient to trigger the lytic cascade. Transcription of the immediate–early genes does not require de novo protein synthesis (Biggin et al., 1987) implying that physiological signals from the host cell are involved in triggering activation of the lytic cycle. Lytic inducers activate intracellular signaling pathways that culminate in the dephosphorylation of the Zp-binding myocyte enhancer factor 2D (MEF-2D, see Fig. 27.5) which recruits histone acetylase leading to hyperacetylation of histones within the chromatin structure of Zp and promoter activation (Bryant and Farrell, 2002; Deng et al., 2003; Gruffat et al., 2002b; Jenkins et al., 2000; Speck et al., 1997). It has recently been shown that the BRRF1 gene product is a transcription factor that activates Zp and also cooperate with Rta to induce lytic infection (Hong et al., 2004).

ZEBRA is a member of the basic-zipper family of transcription factors and binds as a homodimer to ZEBRA response elements (ZREs) within early gene promoters. Whilst ZEBRA alone activates some early genes, others are maximally stimulated by the synergistic effects of ZEBRA and Rta, whereas a third class is maximally induced by Rta alone (Feederle et al., 2000; Ragoczy and Miller, 1999).

In common with other herpesviruses, EBV encodes several early genes that are involved in nucleotide metabolism e.g. thymidine kinase (BXLF1) and in DNA replication, e.g., DNA polymerase. Studies of herpes simplex virus (HSV) suggest that many genes of the former class are non-essential for replication of the virus, at least in cell culture, since their functions are duplicated by host cell enzymes (Roizman and Knipe, 2001). Conversely six of the latter, BMRF1 (polymerase-associated factor), BALF2 (single-stranded DNA binding protein), BALF5 (DNA polymerase), BSLF1 (primase), BBLF4 (helicase) and BBLF2/3 (primase accessory protein) have been referred to as core replication genes (Fixman et al., 1992) and are obligatory for viral DNA replication and the progression from the early to late phase of the life cycle.

The lytic origin of replication that is employed in the synthesis of virion DNA, ori-lyt (Hammerschmidt and Sugden, 1988), is distinct from the plasmid DNA replication origin, ori-P, that is used to maintain the episomal virus DNA in synchrony with host cell division during latency. Ori-lyt lies within the BamHI H region of EBV DNA and contains two essential cis-acting regions: the BHLF1 promoter and a second region about 0.5 kb distant that is required for

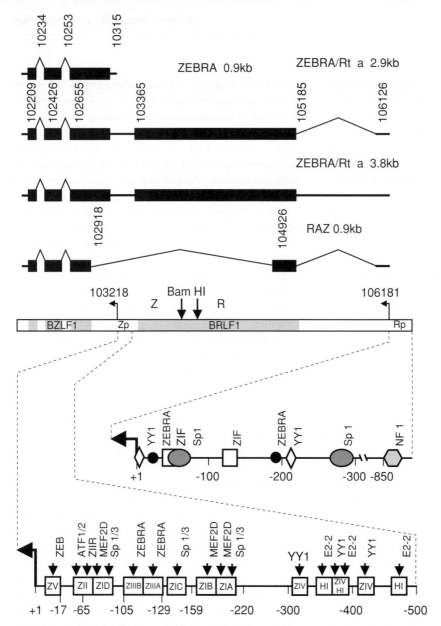

Fig. 27.5. Schematic organization of the immediate–early transactivator genes. The open box in the center represents the BamHI Z-R region of EBV DNA. The BZLF1 and BRLF1 open reading frames and their respective promoters Zp and Rp are indicated with their transcriptional initiation points represented by raised arrows. The four immediate–early transcripts are shown at the top. Horizontal lines represent exons with the coding regions indicated by thicker portions. Genome coordinates are numbered with reference to the B95–8 sequence (Genbank accession number V01555). The organization of the Rp and Zp promoters is illustrated below: +1 refers to the site of transcription initiation. Although Rp contains two ZREs the proximal site is dominant in mediating transcriptional activation by ZEBRA (Liu and Speck, 2003). The NF1 site appears to be a positive regulator in epithelial but not lymphoid cells (Glaser *et al.*, 1998) whilst the Sp1 sites may be involved in the autoactivation of Rp by Rta (Ragoczy and Miller, 2001). The Zif site is a positive trancriptional regulator (Zalani *et al.*, 1995) whereas the YY1 sites are negative regulatory elements that may be involved in the maintenance of latency (Zalani *et al.*, 1997). The Zp promoter (bottom) has been shown to contain multiple regulatory domains (for review see Speck *et al.*, 1997) indicated by the open boxes. Transcription factors that bind to the various domains are marked by the down arrows. The four ZI domains (ZIA – D) are A+T-rich sequences that bind MEF2 transcription factors, principally MEF2D, and seem to play a critical role in the latent to lytic switch (see text). With the exception of ZIB, the ZI domains also bind Sp1 and Sp3 factors. The ZII domain is also potentially responsive to extracellular stimuli by virtue of its affinity for cAMP response element binding (CREB) factors, e.g., ATF1 and 2. In addition, the ZII domain contains a *cis*-acting negative regulatory element (ZIIR) whose putative cellular binding-factor remains unknown (Liu *et al.*, 1998). The ZIII domains bind ZEBRA and are likely involved in autoactivation. The ZIV, ZV and HI domains are negative regulatory elements that bind YY1, zinc finger E-box binding factor (ZEB) and E2-2, respectively (Montalvo *et al.*, 1995; Kraus *et al.*, 2003; Thomas *et al.*, 2003).

replication but not needed for BHLF1 transcription. The BHLF1 promoter contains ZREs that, if mutated, eliminate ori-lyt-directed replication (Schepers *et al.*, 1993). These and other data have demonstrated that ZEBRA is an essential component of lytic DNA replication and it has recently been shown that physical interaction with the EBV helicase targets ZEBRA to viral DNA replication compartments within the nucleus (Liao *et al.*, 2001).

Several herpesviruses replicate their DNA only in G1-arrested host cells (Flemington, 2001); a situation that has been suggested as being advantageous to the virus due to lack of competition with cellular DNA replication. Again ZEBRA has been implicated as a key regulatory element in the EBV lytic cycle. In this instance ZEBRA interacts with C/EBPa leading to accumulation of p21^{CIP-1} and G1 cell cycle arrest (Wu *et al.*, 2003). Further studies suggest that whilst inhibiting cellular DNA synthesis, EBV induces an S-phase-like cellular environment during lytic replication (Kudoh *et al.*, 2003, 2004).

The checkpoint between early and late gene expression involves productive viral DNA replication. How is this linked to the induction of late gene expression? Methylation of promoter sequences can lead to gene repression (Jansson *et al.*, 1992) and thus newly replicated, unmethylated promoter sequences may be activated. However, this mechanism does not appear to be involved since inhibitors of DNA methyltransferase do not activate EBV late genes (Fronko *et al.*, 1989; Szyf *et al.*, 1985). A transient transfection-based reporter assay using EBV early and late promoters within non-replicating plasmids faithfully reproduced the early/late promoter expression profile during different phases of the virus life cycle (Serio *et al.*, 1997). This result demonstrates that a *trans*-relationship exists between viral DNA replication and late gene expression. The steps in the chain of events leading to the activation of late promoters remain to be elucidated. However, Serio *et al.* (1998) provide evidence that a variant TATA element within the core promoter region of the late genes is located within a transcriptionally inert environment and is a critical effector in their regulation. In addition, *cis*-regulatory elements appear to operate in the immediate vicinity of this core to activate late gene expression.

Functions and associated properties of lytic cycle gene products

Lytic cycle gene products were originally identified immunologically as distinct fluorescent antigen complexes referred to as virus capsid antigen (VCA), early antigen (EA) and membrane antigen (MA) (Ernberg and Klein, 1979).

These descriptions survive to this day but we now know that these antigens consist of a number of viral structural proteins, replicative enzymes and membrane proteins, respectively. Examination of the sequence of the EBV genome reveals a coding potential for around 80 proteins. Our knowledge of the properties of these gene products encompasses a spectrum of characterization ranging from genes that have been analyzed in minute detail to those that still remain hypothetical. Some aspects of the properties of lytic gene products are summarized below.

Early gene products, early antigens, and diagnostic tests

The early proteins constitute the serologically defined EA complex. More than 20 years ago Henle and colleagues showed that IgA antibodies to EA in the sera of NPC patients were indicative of the disease (Henle *et al.*, 1970). This work was extended as a potential diagnostic and prognostic test for NPC (Zeng *et al.*, 1983) and individual early gene products have now been identified as antigenic determinants and proposed as being potentially useful as more objective diagnostics (Baylis *et al.*, 1989; Connolly *et al.*, 2001; Dardari *et al.*, 2000; Feng *et al.*, 2001; Fones-Tan *et al.*, 1994; Liu *et al.*, 1994; Stolzenberg *et al.*, 1996). More recently, combination assays using more than one target antigen have been evaluated (Chan *et al.*, 2003; Cheng *et al.*, 2002). Whilst several assays appear promising, none has yet been routinely adopted.

DNA replicative enzymes

The six "core replication proteins" together with ZEBRA are absolutely required for the amplification and replication of the viral genome from ori-lyt. The intermediate replication product is a concatemeric structure consisting of several genome units linked head to tail (Hammerschmidt and Sugden, 1988). The enzymatic mechanism involved in cleavage of the concatemers is uncertain (Zimmermann and Hammerschmidt, 1995). The replication proteins have been shown to function as (a) complex(es). The helicase, primase and primase accessory protein physically associate as a nuclear complex (Yokoyama *et al.*, 1999). This heterotrimeric complex interacts (a) with ZEBRA via a helicase association (Gao *et al.*, 1998; Liao *et al.*, 2001) and (b) with the DNA polymerase (Fujii *et al.*, 2000) which itself binds the polymerase accessory protein (Zeng *et al.*, 1997). The DNA binding protein can interact with this tetrameric complex (Gao *et al.*, 1998) and also significantly stimulates DNA synthesis by the core polymerase suggesting an association between these molecules (Tsurumi *et al.*, 1996). These and other data suggest the following partial scenario for EBV lytic cycle DNA replication: ZEBRA interacts with the helicase/primase/accessory protein complex and recruits this to the ZEBRA binding sites on ori-lyt to form a pre-priming complex to which the DNA binding protein attaches. This complex opens the DNA helix at the origin and synthesizes RNA primers. The DNA polymerase and its accessory protein subsequently attach to the complex allowing DNA replication to proceed (Fujii et al., 2000).

In addition, the ori-lyt-binding host cell encoded transcription factors ZBP-89 and Sp1 interact with the polymerase/accessory protein complex and stimulate viral DNA replication (Baumann et al., 2000). These data suggest an additional, complementary mechanism whereby cellular transcription factors tether the viral replication proteins to ori-lyt.

The mRNA export factor, BMLF1

The early gene product from the BMLF1 ORF is referred to as EB2 (Chevallier-Greco et al., 1986), Mta (Fixman et al., 1992) or SM (Cook et al., 1994). It was originally thought to be a transcriptional transactivator that in conjunction with ZEBRA and Rta regulates lytic cycle activation. It is a heterogeneous, nuclear phosphoprotein with a major species of about 60 kDa.

The export of mRNA from the nucleus to the cytoplasm is significantly enhanced by splicing and requires the action of a multiprotein exon junction complex. However, since the majority of EBV lytic cycle mRNAs are unspliced, an alternative export mechanism such as an mRNA-bound adaptor protein needs to be invoked. The properties of the BMLF1 product are consistent with such a role since it shuttles between nucleus and cytoplasm, contains two nuclear export signals, is an RNA-binding protein in vivo and promotes the cytoplasmic accumulation of unspliced EBV mRNA, notably including some of the core replication genes (Gruffat et al., 2002a; Semmes et al., 1998).

Using a mutant EBV deleted for BMLF1 Gruffat et al., 2002a) showed that EB2/Mta is essential for virion production. The HSV protein homologue of EB2/Mta, ICP27, has been shown to be a viral adaptor molecule that is involved in the nuclear export of intronless viral mRNA (Koffa et al., 2001). ICP27 can partially complement the defect in the BMLF1negative EBV (Gruffat et al., 2002a).

Bcl-2-related proteins

Different members of the bcl-2 family of proteins either induce or repress apoptosis. EBV encodes two bcl-2 homologues; BHRF1 and BALF1. The BHLF1 gene product is a 17 kDa putative membrane protein that is highly conserved in all EBV isolates (Khanim et al., 1997) and is non-essential for virus replication or virus-mediated cellular transformation in vitro (Lee and Yates, 1992; Marchini et al., 1991).

Expression of BHRF1 in a number of cell types in vitro enhances their apoptosis resistance to a variety of appropriate stimuli (Henderson et al., 1993; Kawanishi, 1997; Tarodi et al., 1994). In addition to its anti-apoptotic function BHRF1 promotes rapid transit through the cell cycle (Dawson et al., 1998). These and other data suggest that in vivo the primary role of BHRF1 may be to delay host cell apoptosis during the EBV lytic cycle thereby facilitating complete virus replication and assembly (Dawson et al., 1995, 1998).

The second bcl-2 homologue, BALF1, is a 182 amino-acid polypeptide that has counterparts in the EBV-related viruses of other primates (Bellows et al., 2002). This protein appears to act as an antagonist of the anti-apoptotic effects of BHRF1; a situation reminiscent of cellular bcl-2 family members that can counteract each other's functions. How these two proteins interact in the virus's life cycle remains to be determined.

BNLF2a

The $CD8^+$ T-cell response to EBV lytic cycle antigens is markedly skewed towards immediate-early and early proteins whilst late proteins are recognised only rarely (Pudney et al., 2005). Nevertheless, in vivo EBV replicates successfully in spite of this robust immune reponse to lytic antigens. Ressing et al. (2005) demonstrated that cells undergoing lytic infection have reduced TAP-mediated transport of peptides to the endoplasmic reticulum and impaired presentation at the cell surface. It has recently been shown that the BNLF2a gene product is the mediator of this immune evasion mechanism by blocking the interaction of peptides with the TAP transporter and likely explains the bias of immune response towards early proteins, i.e. prior to BNLF2a function (A. D. Hislop, personal communication).

BARF1

The BARF1 ORF encodes a product of about 33 kDa that is secreted into the medium of cultured cells (Strockbine et al., 1998). It may be post-translationally modified by N-linked glycosylation, myristylation and phosphorylation (Sheng et al., 2001). It binds to and inhibits the proliferative effects of human colony-stimulating factor 1 (CSF-1). It was proposed that by blocking CSF-1 activity the BARF1 protein might impair cytokine release from mononuclear cells thereby modulating host immune responses to EBV infection (Cohen and Lekstrom, 1999; Strockbine et al.,

1998). In addition, a BARF1-negative EBV has revealed a second effect of the BARF1 protein on innate immunity; the deletant was impaired in its ability to inhibit α-interferon production by mononuclear cells (Cohen and Lekstrom, 1999).

Although BARF1 appears temporally as an early gene in the viral life cycle it can act as an oncogene when stably expressed in cultured murine, human or simian cells (Wei et al., 1994, 1997; Wei and Ooka, 1989). In addition, Akata BL cells that had lost their tumorigenic phenotype through loss of the EBV genome regained the ability to form tumors in SCID mice following transfection with BARF1 (Sheng et al., 2003). The N-terminal 49 a.a. appear to be essential for the transforming ability (Sheng et al., 2001). However, a BARF1deleted virus was not defective in its capacity to immortalize B cells in vitro indicating that in the context of the whole virus BARF1 is not essential for this function (Cohen and Lekstrom, 1999).

Nevertheless, observations of the EBV-positive epithelial tumors NPC and gastric carcinoma are provocative. Analysis of BARF1 transcription using RT-PCR or of protein expression by Western blot and immunohistochemistry detected the presence of this antigen in around 85% of NPCs and 100% of gastric carcinomas (Decaussin et al., 2000; zur Hausen et al., 2000). EBV-positive gastric carcinomas and the majority of NPCs do not express LMP1. It has been suggested that in these cases BARF1 may be acting as the viral oncogene in the absence of LMP1. These data also suggest that in epithelial tumors BARF1 is a latent, rather than early, gene.

Late gene products

Glycoproteins

EBV encodes a number of glycoproteins of which eleven have been described. The glycoproteins present in the classical MA complex are gp350/220 (BLLF1) and gH (gp85, BXLF2) (Edson and Thorley-Lawson, 1981). The BLLF1 ORF is transcribed as two mRNA species, the smaller of which is generated by an in-frame splice such that gp220 is effectively an internally deleted version of gp340 (Biggin et al., 1984). These products are highly glycosylated; around 50% of their mass is carbohydrate. The region that is spliced out of gp350 to generate gp220 contains a repetitive region consisting of a basic 21-amino-acid unit composed of three 7-amino-acid subunits. In some units, the third subunit is missing. In common with other repetitive regions of the EBV genome, the length varies between strains and has been observed to range from 56 to 126 a.a. (Lees et al., 1993).

The N-terminal region of gp350/220 mediates binding of EBV to its B-cell receptor, CD21 (also known as CR2) (Fingeroth et al., 1984; Nemerow et al., 1989). This interaction induces capping of the receptor, endocytosis of the virus into the cell (Tanner et al., 1987) and triggers tyrosine/PI kinase and NF-κB-dependent intracellular signaling pathways that activate the Wp promoter (Sinclair and Farrell, 1995; Sugano et al., 1997). However, a BLLF1 deletant was able to infect B-cells and epithelial cells indicating that the gp350/220-CD21 interaction is not exclusively required for infection and that other viral proteins can mediate cellular attachment (Janz et al., 2000). This function could be performed by the gH/gL/gp42 complex (see below).

gp350/220 is the major EBV neutralizing-antibody determinant (Thorley-Lawson and Poodry, 1982) and for this reason has been the focus of efforts to develop an anti-EBV vaccine (Arrand, 1992). Following encouraging human trials using a recombinant vaccinia-based delivery system (Gu et al., 1991) a subunit gp340 vaccine (Jackman et al., 1999) has progressed through phase 1 clinical trials and is now in phase 2 (http://www.medimmune.com/pipeline/EpsteinBarrVirusvaccine.asp).

The third component of MA, gH (BXLF2), forms a heterotrimeric complex with two more glycoproteins, gL (BKRF2) and gp42 (BZLF2). This complex is involved in the penetration of B-cells by EBV and uses cell-surface HLA class II molecules as coreceptor. It is proposed that primary binding of EBV to the B cell is mediated by the gp350/220–CD21 interaction. This is subsequently augmented by gp42 binding to HLA class II followed by virus–cell fusion mediated by the gH/gL complex (Hutt-Fletcher and Lake, 2001).

Infection of epithelial cells is somewhat different since they do not express surface HLA class II. In this case EBV uses a dimeric complex of gH-gL (without gp42) to bind to an unidentified receptor. EBV carries both dimeric and trimeric complexes in order to infect both types of host. The presence or absence of HLA class II in the virus-producing cell alters the ratio of these complexes such that epithelial cell-derived virus efficiently infects B cells and vice versa (Borza and Hutt-Fletcher, 2002).

A second EBV glycoprotein complex consists of gN (BLRF1) and gM (BBRF3). Co-expression of gM with gN is required for processing of the latter to its mature form (Lake et al., 1998). Recombinant EBV in which the gN gene is inactivated fails to accumulate gM. In cells infected with this virus many of the capsids remain trapped in the nucleus and the majority of the virions are non-enveloped (Lake and Hutt-Fletcher, 2000).

The BALF4 ORF encodes gp110, a highly conserved homologue of the abundant envelope protein gB of other herpesviruses which is involved in virus–cell fusion. In contrast, EBV gB appeared to be virtually absent from the virion and to be localized to the nuclear membrane and endoplasmic reticulum (Gong and Kieff, 1990; Gong et al., 1987; Papworth et al., 1997). A recombinant EBV lacking gp110 was not released from the cell (Herrold et al., 1996). These data led to the notion that the EBV gB is involved in the egress of virions from the lytically infected cell.

Recent data (Neuhierl et al., 2002) indicate that B95–8 cells and virions are unusual and that in other virus strains gB is present both in the virion and on the plasma membrane of the host cell. Virions that contain gB have an enhanced infectivity and a wider cell tropism, consistent with a role in virus–cell fusion and viral entry similar to other herpesviral gBs. In keeping with this, a virus-free assay has shown that gB can mediate membrane fusion (Haan et al., 2001).

EBV also encodes four poorly characterized membrane proteins; gp78 (BILF2), a highly glycosylated virion envelope glycoprotein of unknown function (Mackett et al., 1990), gp150 (BDLF3), gp60 (BILF1) and BMRF2.

gp150 is an envelope glycoprotein that is ~75% carbohydrate and is non-essential for growth in B cells in vitro. A gp150-negative virus was fully competent for binding, infectivity, assembly and egress of both B cells and epithelial cells. Mysteriously, it had an enhanced infectivity for epithelial cells (Borza and Hutt-Fletcher, 1998).

gp60 and BMRF2 are both predicted to have multiple membrane-spanning domains and gp60 appears to be glycosylated (Hutt-Fletcher and Lake, 2001). BMRF2 is a 55 kD membrane protein (Modrow et al., 1992) that can interact with integrins to facilitate the infection of basolateral surfaces of epithelial cells by EBV (Tugizov et al., 2003).

Structural proteins

In addition to the virion glycoproteins described above, some members of the immunologically defined VCA complex have been characterized as products of specific ORFs. The major capsid protein is p160 (BcLF1) and three small capsid proteins, p18, p23 and p40 (BFRF3, BLRF2 and BdRF1) have been identified (Reischl et al., 1996; van Grunsven et al., 1993). The BVRF2 ORF overlaps BdRF1 and appears to encode a protease that is involved in the maturation of p40 (Donaghy and Jupp, 1995).

Studies on the protein composition of purified virions (Johannsen et al., 2004) reveal that the tegument contains several late proteins including BNRF1, the major 143kD tegument component (Cameron et al., 1987) and the large, 3149 a.a. tegument protein BPLF1 (Schmaus et al., 2004). Interestingly a number of host cell proteins including β-actin, cofilin, tubulin, Hsp70 and Hsp90 were also present in the tegument. It is suggested that inclusion of these host cell proteins within the virion may indicate that they have a role as "mediators of morphogenesis" (Johannsen et al., 2004).

Immunofluorescent assays for VCA are still used in EBV diagnosis and, as with EA, the immunological utility of individual, purified VCA components as more objective targets has been examined. Immunogenic determinants have been associated with p160, p143, p38, p40, p18 and gB (Chen et al., 1991; Hinderer et al., 1999). As with novel ELISA assays using EA components, late proteins showed excellent performance in initial tests but the classical immunofluorescence assays remain in clinical use.

Viral interleukin-10

The BCRF1 ORF of EBV is highly conserved between strains (Stuart et al., 1995) and exhibits extensive sequence and functional homology with the human cytokine interleukin-10 (hIL-10) (Moore et al., 1990). It is therefore termed viral IL-10 (vIL-10). The mature protein sequences share 83% identity and most of their divergence is found in the N-terminal 20 amino acids. Functional activities, involving cells of the immune system, include deactivation of macrophages and dendritic cells, inhibition of cytokine synthesis by $CD4^+$ T cells and proliferation and differentiation of activated B-cells (Moore et al., 2001). However, some differences between hIL-10 and vIL-10 have been noted (Salek-Ardakani et al., 2001).

In terms of the effects of vIL-10 on the life cycle of EBV, it has been shown that whilst vIL-10 is not absolutely required for B-cell transformation addition of exogenous vIL-10 significantly enhanced the efficiency of viral transformation of B-cells, increased cell viability and inhibited the production of antiviral interferon-γ (Stuart et al., 1995; Swaminathan et al., 1993). In addition, vIL-10 has been shown to counteract the inhibitory effect of T-cells on EBV-induced B cell transformation (Bejarano and Masucci, 1998). Since vIL-10 is a late gene product these observations suggest a model whereby lytically infected cells produce both virions and vIL-10. The latter acts on the surrounding cellular environment to facilitate propagation of EBV both by enhancing the susceptibility of B-cells to be transformed by the virus and by inhibiting the host's immunological defences against such action.

EBV persistence in vivo

Several lines of evidence support a role for the B lymphocyte as the site of EBV persistence in vivo. Indeed, therapy aimed at eliminating virus replication using long-term acyclovir treatment (which following conversion to

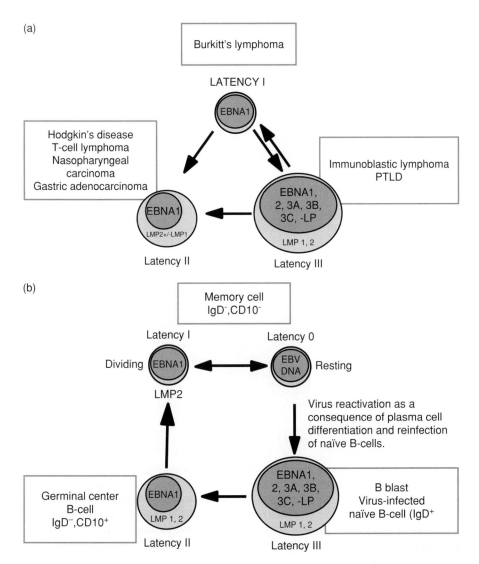

Fig. 27.6. The different forms of EBV latency manifest in virus-associated tumors (a) and during infection of normal differentiating B-cells (b). Arrows depict the interchangeable forms of latency observed by various manipulations in vitro (a) which are believed to recapitulate those occurring during B-cell differentiation in vivo (b).

acyclovir triphosphate interferes with viral replication by competing with deoxyguanosine triphosphate for viral DNA polymerase) eliminates virus excretion from the oropharnyx but does not affect the level of latent infection in B-cells (Ernberg and Andersson, 1986). As soon as treatment is halted, virus can be detected in the oropharyngeal secretions at pre-treatment levels (Yao et al., 1989). In addition, studies of EBV strains in donor–recipient pairs before and after bone marrow transplantation (BMT) have shown that the recipient's strain disappeared from the oropharynx and was replaced by the donor's strain, indicating that the bone marrow B-cells harbor EBV (Gratama et al., 1990).

Furthermore, patients with X-linked agammaglobulinemia (XLA), who are deficient in mature B-cells, are found to be free of EBV infection, suggesting they are not able to maintain a persistent infection (Faulkner et al., 1999).

EBV exists in the peripheral blood within the IgD memory B cell pool; EBV gene expression in these cells being restricted to LMP2A and possibly EBNA1 (Fig. 27.6) (Babcock et al., 1998). Recent work has shown that a subset of healthy tonsils contains EBV+ naïve (IgD+) B-cells and that these cells express the Lat III programme and show an activated phenotype, suggesting they have been directly infected (Joseph et al., 2000). These cells are presumably either eliminated by virus-specific cytotoxic T-lymphocytes (CTLs) or differentiate to IgD memory B-cells, which then leave the tonsil. Some of these memory B-cells will pass through mucosal lymphoid tissues and terminally differentiate into plasma cells, whereupon they might enter the lytic cycle. However, a proportion also exits the cell cycle and will replenish the peripheral pool of infected memory cells. Recent work suggests that the majority of resting EBV-infected memory B-cells in vivo do not express virus latent genes and that EBNA1 expression only occurs when these cells divide (Hochberg et al., 2004). The Lat II pattern of EBV gene expression has also been detected in tonsillar memory B-cells and germinal center B-cells (Babcock and Thorley-Lawson, 2000). LMP1 can provide surrogate T cell help via mimicry of an activated CD40 receptor and LMP2A can substitute for B cell receptor engagement (see later). Thus, the virus might enter a germinal center reaction and re-express LMP1 and LMP2A, providing a mechanism for the antigen-independent expansion of EBV-infected B-cells (Babcock and Thorley-Lawson, 2000; Thorley-Lawson, 2001). However, these data are not supported by studies of CD40 null mice, which are defective for isotype switching and germinal center formation. When LMP1 is constitutively expressed from a transgene in the B-cells of these mice, they are still not able to form germinal centers or produce high-affinity antibodies (Uchida et al., 1999). Furthermore, germinal centers are also not formed when LMP1 is expressed in a wild-type (CD40+) background suggesting that, rather than facilitating a germinal centre reaction, LMP1 actively inhibits this process. These conflicts remain to be resolved.

Although much of the evidence described above implicates the B cell compartment as the site of persistence, a role for infection of squamous epithelial cells is suggested by the detection of EBV in oral hairy leukoplakia (Fig. 27.7), a benign lesion of the oral epithelia observed in immunosuppressed patients characterized by intense lytic infection of these tissues (De Souza et al., 1989). However, EBV is not usually detectable in normal epithelial tissues, including desquamated oropharyngeal cells and tonsilar epithelium from IM patients (Karajannis et al., 1997; Niedobitek et al., 1989, 2000) and normal epithelium adjacent to EBV-positive UNPCs (Sam et al., 1993) and gastric carcinomas (Gulley et al., 1996). Therefore, it is still not clear what role, if any, epithelial cells play in the normal life cycle of the virus. It may be that epithelial infection acts to amplify EBV via virus replication during primary infection or occasionally during asymptomatic persistence and that this effect is exaggerated in hairy leukoplakia as a consequence of immunosuppression. The establishment of EBV latent infection in epithelial cells is likely to be an unusual

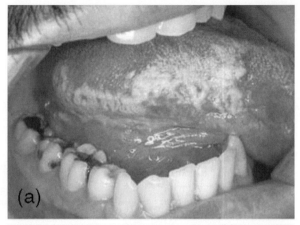

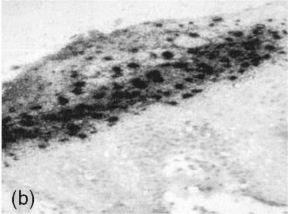

Fig. 27.7. Oral hairy leukoplakia (OHL) is a benign condition of the oral tissues that is characterized by white plaque-like lesions on the lateral tongue, as shown in (a). (b) *In situ* hybridization demonstrates the presence of abundant EBV DNA in the upper layers of the squamous epithelium of an OHL lesions consistent with virus replication.

event dependent on underlying changes within the cell that permit the stable maintenance of the virus genome (Jones et al., 2003; Knox et al., 1996). This latter scenario is consistent with recent studies on the genetics of NPC that demonstrate that loss of heterozygosity of certain key loci occurs as an initiating event prior to EBV infection (Lo and Huang, 2002).

EBV strain variation

The discovery of genetic differences between EBV carried in the Burkitt's lymphoma cell lines of West African origin, Jijoye and AG876, and the prototype B95.8 virus has led to the study of EBV strain differences. EBV isolates are characterized as type 1 (B95.8-like) or type 2 (Jijoye-and

AG876-like); these were originally referred to as A and B, respectively. EBV-1 and EBV-2 are mostly identical over the bulk of the EBV genome (Dolan et al., 2006) but show allelic polymorphism (with 50–80% sequence homology depending on the locus) in a subset of latent genes, namely those encoding EBNA-LP, EBNA2, EBNA3A, EBNA3B and EBNA3C (Dambaugh et al., 1984; Sample et al., 1990). A combination of virus isolation and sero-epidemiological studies suggest that type 1 virus isolates are predominant (but not exclusively so) in many Western countries, whereas both types are widespread in equatorial Africa, New Guinea and perhaps certain other regions (Young et al., 1987). In vitro studies show that type 1 isolates are more potent than type 2 in achieving B-cell transformation in vitro; the type 2 virus-transformed LCLs characteristically show much slower growth especially in early passage (Rickinson and Kieff, 2001). In addition to this broad distinction between EBV types 1 and 2, there is also minor heterogeneity within each virus type. Individual strains have been identified on the basis of changes, compared with B95.8, ranging from single base mutations to extensive deletions. Of particular note is the 11.8 kb deletion in the BamHIA region of the B95.8 strain (Fig. 27.1) which further emphasizes that this strain is not generally representative of the majority of naturally occurring isolates.

It was originally believed that in contrast to most immunologically compromised patients, who were shown to be infected with multiple EBV strains (Yao et al., 1996b, 1998), the majority of healthy individuals are only infected with one virus type (Yao et al., 1991). This led to the suggestion that the immune response to an existing EBV strain may protect the immunocompetent host from infection with additional exogenous viral strains. However, there is increasing evidence that immunocompetent carriers may also be infected with two or more separate EBV strains. For example, in one recent study that utilized the host cytotoxic T-lymphocyte response to a polymorphic EBV epitope as an indicator of the resident virus strains, 3/15 EBV-seropositive donors harbored more than one virus strain (Brooks et al., 2000). A further study, which examined EBV strain variation in collections of peripheral blood mononuclear cells and multiple lymphoid and epithelial tissues of EBV-positive carriers, also demonstrated that immunocompetent individuals frequently harbor at least two strains (Srivastava et al., 2000). More recent work using novel genotyping techniques confirmed that many healthy individuals harbor multiple EBV isolates and that their relative abundance and presence appears to vary over time (Sitki-Green et al., 2003; Walling et al., 2003).

An interpretation of the more recent data is that both immunocompromised persons and immunocompetent normal carriers are infected with multiple EBV strains, but that the rarer strains are more readily detectable in immunosuppressed individuals probably because of a higher viral load. This also implies that the immune response to an existing infection might not protect the host from subsequent infection with additional exogenous viral strains. Coinfection of the host with multiple virus strains could have evolutionary benefit to EBV enabling the generation of diversity by genetic recombination. Such intertypic recombination has been demonstrated in HIV-infected patients and appears to arise via recombination of multiple EBV strains during the intense EBV replication that occurs as a consequence of immunosuppression (Walling and Raab-Traub, 1994; Yao et al., 1996a).

More contentious is the possible contribution of EBV strain variation to virus-associated tumors. Many studies have failed to establish an epidemiological association between EBV strains and disease and suggest that the specific EBV gene polymorphisms detected in virus-associated tumors occur with similar frequencies in EBV isolates from healthy virus carriers from the same geographic region (Edwards et al., 1999; Khanim et al., 1996). However, this does not exclude the possibility that variation in specific EBV genes is responsible for the distinct geographic distribution of virus-associated malignancies. In this regard, an LMP1 variant containing a 10 amino acid deletion (residues 343 to 352) was originally identified in Chinese NPC biopsies and has oncogenic and other functional properties distinct from those of the B95.8 LMP1 gene (Dawson et al., 2000; Fielding et al., 2001; Li et al., 1996; Miller et al., 1998). It is therefore likely that variation in LMP1 and other EBV genes can contribute to the risk of developing virus-associated tumors but more biological studies using well-defined EBV variants are required.

Function of the EBV latent genes: from persistence to pathology

An understanding of EBV latent gene function is relevant both to the factors contributing to the establishment of persistent infection in the memory B-cell pool and to the role of the virus in the oncogenic process. The advent of recombinant EBV technology has confirmed the absolute requirement for EBNA2 and LMP1 in the in vitro transformation of B-cells and highlighted a role for EBNA-LP, EBNA3A, EBNA3C and LMP2A in this process (Kieff and Rickinson, 2001). These studies confirm that EBV-induced B cell transformation requires the coordinate action of several latent genes but do not address the consequences of the more restricted patterns of EBV latent gene expression observed in persistent infection and in certain EBV-associated tumors. More recent studies using recombinant EBV to infect either virus-negative BL cell lines or epithelial cell lines are beginning to define the contribution of more limited EBV latent gene expression to the cell phenotype and to dissect the mechanisms responsible for regulating virus gene expression in different cellular environments. A brief description of EBV latent gene function follows but other Chapters will provide a more comprehensive review of this area.

EBNA1

EBNA1 is a DNA-binding protein that is required for the replication and maintenance of the episomal EBV genome; a function that is achieved through the binding of EBNA1 to oriP, the plasmid origin of viral replication (Kieff and Rickinson, 2001). EBNA1 also interacts with two sites downstream of Qp to negatively regulate its own expression (Nonkwelo et al., 1996). EBNA1 also acts as a transcriptional transactivator and up-regulates Cp and the LMP1 promoter (Kieff and Rickinson, 2001). The EBNA1 protein contains a glycine–glycine–alanine (gly–gly–ala) repeat sequence, which varies in size in different EBV isolates. This gly–gly–ala repeat domain is a cis-acting inhibitor of MHC class I-restricted presentation and appears to function by inhibiting antigen processing via the ubiquitin-proteosome pathway (Levitskaya et al., 1995). Failure to present EBNA1-derived peptides results in ineffective CD8+ T-cell responses to EBNA1 when expressed in target cells. Directing EBNA1 expression to B-cells in transgenic mice results in B-cell lymphomas suggesting that EBNA1 might also have a direct role in oncogenesis (Wilson et al., 1996). On the contrary, similar experiments using a different strain of mice failed to reveal any EBNA1-induced lymphomagenesis (Kang et al., 2005). Furthermore, experiments using an EBNA1-negative EBV are also consistent with EBNA1 not being oncogenic: EBNA1 is not essential for the immortalisation of B cells by EBV and such immortalised cells have similar tumourigenic properties in SCID mice as do B-cells immortalised with wild-type, EBNA1-positive EBV (Humme et al., 2003). However, a previous study demonstrates that EBNA1 is toxic in certain epithelial cell environments and that this is associated with the processing and presentation of EBNA1 to specific CTLs (Jones et al., 2003). This suggests that the establishment of EBV latency is dependent on the cell background and that CTL responses to EBNA1 may contribute to the control of latent infection. EBNA1 has recently been shown to interact with an ubiquitin-specific protease called USP7 or HAUSP that has been previously implicated in the stabilisation of p53 and this may account for the ability of EBNA1 to protect B cells from apoptosis (Kennedy et al., 2003; Saridakis et al., 2005). Given these effects and the ability of EBNA1 to function as a transcriptional activator of several viral genes, it is likely that EBNA1 will also be able to influence cellular gene expression.

EBNA2

The inability of an EBV strain, P3HR-1, carrying a deletion of the gene encoding EBNA2 and the last two exons of EBNA-LP, to transform B cells in vitro was the first indication of the crucial role of the EBNA2 protein in the transformation process (Kieff and Rickinson, 2001). Restoration of the EBNA2 gene into P3HR-1 has unequivocally confirmed the importance of EBNA2 in B-cell transformation and has allowed the functionally relevant domains of the EBNA2 protein to be identified (Hammerschmidt and Sugden, 1989; Rabson et al., 1982). EBNA2 is a transcriptional activator of both cellular and viral genes, and up-regulates the expression of certain B-cell antigens, including CD21 and CD23, as well as LMP1 and LMP2 (Kieff and Rickinson, 2001; Wang et al., 1990). EBNA2 also transactivates the Cp promoter thereby inducing the switch from Wp to Cp observed early in B-cell infection. EBNA2 interacts with a ubiquitous DNA-binding protein, RBP-Jκ, and this is partly responsible for targeting EBNA2 to promoters that contain the RBP-Jκ sequence (Grossman et al., 1994). The RBP-Jκ homologue in Drosophila is involved in signal transduction from the Notch receptor, a pathway that is important in cell fate determination in Drosophila and has also been implicated in the development of T-cell tumors in humans (Artavanis-Tsakonas et al., 1995). Recent work demonstrates that EBNA2 can functionally replace the intracellular region of Notch (Hofelmayr et al., 2001; Sakai et al., 1998; Strobl et al., 2000). The c-myc oncogene is also a transcriptional target of EBNA2; an effect that is likely to be important for EBV-induced B-cell proliferation (Kaiser et al., 1999).

EBNA3 family

Studies with EBV recombinants have demonstrated that EBNA3A and EBNA3C are essential for B-cell transformation in vitro, whereas EBNA3B is dispensable (Robertson, 1997). EBNA3C can induce the up-regulation of both cellular (CD21) and viral (LMP1) gene expression (Allday and Farrell, 1994), repress the Cp promoter (Radkov et al.,

1997), and might interact with the retinoblastoma protein, pRb, to promote transformation (Parker *et al.*, 1996). While not essential for transformation, EBNA3B has been shown to induce expression of vimentin and CD40 (Silins and Sculley, 1994). The EBNA3 proteins associate with the RBP-Jκ transcription factor and disrupt its binding to the cognate Jκ sequence and to EBNA2, thus repressing EBNA2-mediated transactivation (Robertson, 1997). Thus, EBNA2 and the EBNA3 proteins work together to precisely control RBP-Jκ activity, thereby regulating the expression of cellular and viral promoters containing Jκ cognate sequence. EBNA3C has been shown to interact with human histone deacetylase 1, which, in turn, contributes to the transcriptional repression of Cp, by RBP-Jκ (Radkov *et al.*, 1999).

EBNA-LP

EBNA-LP is encoded by the leader of each of the EBNA mRNAs and encodes a protein of variable size depending on the number of *Bam*HI W repeats contained by a particular EBV isolate. The precise role of EBNA-LP in B-cell transformation *in* vitro is not clear but EBNA-LP is required for the efficient outgrowth of LCLs (Allan *et al.*, 1992). Transient transfection of EBNA-LP and EBNA2 into primary B-cells induces G0 to G1 transition as measured by the up-regulation of cyclin D2 expression (Sinclair *et al.*, 1994). EBNA-LP can also cooperate with EBNA2 in up-regulating transcriptional targets of EBNA2, including LMP1 (Harada and Kieff, 1997; Nitsche *et al.*, 1997). EBNA-LP has been shown to colocalize with pRb in LCLs and in vitro biochemical studies have demonstrated an interaction of EBNA-LP with both pRb and p53 (Jiang *et al.*, 1991; Szekely *et al.*, 1993). However, this interaction has not been verified in LCLs and, unlike the situation with the human papillomavirus (HPV)-encoded E6/E7 and adenovirus E1 proteins, EBNA-LP expression appears to have no effect on the regulation of the pRb and p53 pathways.

LMP1

LMP1 is the major transforming protein of EBV behaving as a classical oncogene in rodent fibroblast transformation assays and being essential for EBV-induced B-cell transformation in vitro (Kieff and Rickinson, 2001). LMP1 has pleiotropic effects when expressed in cells resulting in induction of cell surface adhesion molecules and activation antigens (Wang *et al.*, 1990), up-regulation of anti-apoptotic proteins (Bcl-2, A20) (Henderson *et al.*, 1991; Laherty *et al.*, 1992) and stimulation of cytokine production (IL-6, IL-8) (Eliopoulos *et al.*, 1997, 1999). Recent studies have demonstrated that LMP1 functions as a constitutively activated member of the tumor necrosis factor receptor (TNFR) superfamily activating a number of signaling pathways in a ligand-independent manner (Gires *et al.*, 1997; Kilger *et al.*, 1998). Functionally, LMP1 resembles CD40, a member of the TNFR, and can partially substitute for CD40 in vivo providing both growth and differentiation responses in B-cells (Uchida *et al.*, 1999). The LMP1 protein is an integral membrane protein of 63 kD and can be subdivided into three domains: (a) a N-terminal cytoplasmic tail (amino acids 1–23) which tethers and orientates the LMP1 protein to the plasma membrane, (b) six hydrophobic transmembrane loops which are involved in self aggregation and oligomerization (amino acids 24–186); (c) a long C-terminal cytoplasmic region (amino acids 187–386) which possesses most of the molecule's signaling activity. Two distinct functional domains referred to as C-terminal activation regions 1 and 2 (CTAR1 and CTAR2) have been identified on the basis of their ability to activate the NF-κB transcription factor pathway (Huen *et al.*, 1995). This effect contributes to the many phenotypic consequences of LMP1 expression including the induction of various anti-apoptotic and cytokine genes. More recent work demonstrates that LMP1 can also regulate the processing of p100 NF-κB2 to p52 and that this is independent of the pathways responsible for controlling the canonical NF-κB pathway (Eliopoulos *et al.*, 2003). LMP1 is also able to engage the MAP kinase cascade resulting in activation of ERK, JNK and p38 and to stimulate the JAK/STAT pathway (Eliopoulos *et al.*, 1999; Eliopoulos and Young, 1998; Gires *et al.*, 1999; Kieser *et al.*, 1997; Roberts and Cooper, 1998). Many of these effects result from the ability of TNFR-associated factors (TRAFs) to interact either directly with CTAR1 or indirectly via the death domain protein TRADD to CTAR2. The binding of TRAFs to the multimerized cytoplasmic tails of LMP1 provides a platform for the assembly and activation of upstream signaling molecules including the NIK and Tpl-2 MAPK kinase kinases (Eliopoulos *et al.*, 2002; Sylla *et al.*, 1998). The precise mechanisms responsible for signal initiation from these multiprotein complexes remain unknown. The region between CTAR1 and CTAR2 (so-called CTAR3) has been suggested to be responsible for the JAK/STAT pathway, although other data refute this finding and deletion of this region has no effect on the efficiency of B-cell transformation (Gires *et al.*, 1999; Higuchi *et al.*, 2002; Izumi *et al.*, 1999). Recent work has also demonstrated that LMP1 can also activate the phosphatidylinositol 3-kinase (PI3-K) pathway resulting in a variety of effects including cell survival mediated through the Akt (PKB) kinase, actin polymerisation and cell motility (Dawson et al., 2003).

LMP2

The gene encoding LMP2 yields two distinct proteins, LMP2A and LMP2B. The structures of LMP2A and LMP2B are similar; both have 12 transmembrane domains and a 27 amino acid cytoplasmic C-terminus (Kieff and Rickinson, 2001). In addition, LMP2A has a 119 amino acid cytoplasmic amino-terminal domain. LMP2A aggregates in patches within the plasma membrane of latently infected B-cells (Longnecker and Kieff, 1990). Neither LMP2A nor LMP2B are essential for B-cell transformation (Longnecker, 2000). The LMP2A amino-terminal domain contains eight tyrosine residues, two of which (Y74 and Y85) form an immunoreceptor tyrosine-based activation motif (ITAM) (Fruehling and Longnecker, 1997). When phosphorylated, the ITAM present in the B-cell receptor (BCR) plays a central role in mediating lymphocyte proliferation and differentiation by the recruitment and activation of the *src* family of protein tyrosine kinases (PTKs) and the *syk* PTK. LMP2A also interacts with these PTKs through its phosphorylated ITAM and this association appears to negatively regulate PTK activity (Fruehling and Longnecker, 1997). Thus, the LMP2A ITAM has been shown to be responsible for blocking BCR-stimulated calcium mobilization, tyrosine phosphorylation and activation of the EBV lytic cycle in B cells (Miller et al., 1995).

Expression of LMP2A in the B cells of transgenic mice abrogates normal B cell development allowing immunoglobulin-negative cells to colonize peripheral lymphoid organs (Caldwell et al., 1998). This suggests that LMP2A can drive the proliferation and survival of B-cells in the absence of signaling through the BCR. Taken together, these data support a role for LMP2 in modifying the normal programme of B-cell development to favor the maintenance of EBV latency and to prevent inappropriate activation of the EBV lytic cycle. A modulatory role for LMP2B in regulating LMP2A function has been suggested (Longnecker, 2000). The consistent expression of LMP2A in HD and NPC suggests an important function for this protein in oncogenesis but this remains to be shown. LMP2A also recruits Nedd4-like ubiquitin protein ligases; this might promote *lyn* and *syk* ubiquitination in a fashion that contributes to a block in B-cell signaling (Ikeda et al., 2000). Furthermore, a recent report shows that LMP2A can transform epithelial cells and that this effect is mediated, at least in part, by activation of the PI3-kinase/Akt pathway (Scholle et al., 2000). This suggests that LMP2A-induced activation of the Akt pathway may be relevant to the long-term survival of persistently infected memory B-cells.

EBERs

In addition to the latent proteins, two small non-polyadenylated (non-coding) RNAs, EBERs 1 and 2 are probably expressed in all forms of latency. However, the EBERs are not essential for EBV-induced transformation of primary B-lymphocytes (Swaminathan et al., 1991).

The EBERs assemble into stable ribonucleoprotein particles with the auto-antigen La (Lerner et al., 1981), with ribosomal protein L22 (Toczyski et al., 1994) and bind the interferon-inducible, double-stranded RNA-activated protein kinase PKR (Clemens et al., 1994). PKR has a role in mediating the antiviral effects of the interferons and it has been suggested that EBER-mediated inhibition of PKR function could be important for viral persistence perhaps by protecting cells from interferon induced apoptosis (Nanbo et al., 2002). Studies in transfected NIH 3T3 cells demonstrated that EBER1 can enhance protein synthesis by a PKR-independent mechanism (Laing et al., 2002).

Reintroduction of the EBERs into EBV-negative Akata BL cells restores their capacity for growth in soft agar, tumorigenicity in SCID mice and resistance to apoptotic inducers; features identical to those observed in the parental EBV-positive Akata cells (Komano et al., 1999). The detection of IL-10 expression in EBV-positive, but not in EBV negative, BL tumors and the observation that the EBERs can induce IL-10 expression in BL cell lines, suggests that IL-10 may be an important component in the pathogenesis of EBV-positive BL (Kitagawa et al., 2000). Recently, it has been shown that stable expression of bcl-2 or the EBERs in EBV-negative Akata cells significantly enhanced the tumourigenic potential of these cells, but neither bcl-2 nor the EBERs restored tumorigenicity to the same extent as EBV (Ruf et al., 2000). Overall, these studies suggest that EBV genes previously shown to be dispensable for transformation in B-cell systems (e.g., EBERs) might make more important contributions to the pathogenesis of some EBV-associated malignancies and to EBV persistence than was previously appreciated.

BARTs

The BARTs were first identified in NPC tissue (Hitt et al., 1989) and subsequently in other EBV-associated malignancies such as BL (Tao et al., 1998), HD (Deacon et al., 1993) and nasal T-cell lymphoma (Chiang et al., 1996) as well as in the peripheral blood of healthy individuals (Chen et al., 1999). The BARTs encode a number of potential open reading frames (ORFs) including BARF0, RK-BARF0, A73 and RPMS1. The protein products of these ORFs have not be identified and remain controversial (van Beek et al., 2003). However, in vitro studies have suggested potential functions including the negative regulation of EBNA2 and Notch activity (RPMS1) and the modulation of kinase signaling (A73) (Smith et al., 2000).

MicroRNAs

Micro RNAs (miRs) are small, noncoding RNA molecules of only 21–24 nucleotides in length and have been shown to play a role in the posttranscriptional downregulation of target mRNAs (Bartel, 2004; Du and Zamore, 2005; Kim and Nam, 2006). Eukaryotic cells express large numbers of miRs, often in a cell- or tissue-specific manner; indeed the July 2006 release of the microRNA database, miRBase, (Griffiths-Jones et al., 2006; http://microrna.sanger.ac.uk) lists 462 human miRs. Cellular miRs are transcribed by RNA polymerase II into a long precursor molecule (primary miRNA) containing one or a cluster of several miRs. This primary transcript is then processed and transported to the cytoplasm by a series of enzymatic mechanisms (Bartel, 2004; Du and Zamore, 2005). The resulting active complex containing the mature miR is called an RNA-induced silencing complex (RISC) (Bartel, 2004; Du and Zamore, 2005; Kim and Nam, 2006). If the RISC encounters an mRNA containing extensive homology to the miR within the complex then the mRNA is degraded. Alternatively, and probably more commonly, the RISC will bind to an mRNA with only partial complementarity in which case translational repression ensues (Bartel, 2004; Du and Zamore, 2005).

Herpesviruses also enode miRs: HSV1, MHV68, hCMV, KSHV, rLCV and EBV each encode at least 2, 9, 11, 12, 16 and 23 species respectively (Cullen, 2006; Gupta et al., 2006; Cui et al., 2006). The EBV miRs are arranged in two clusters within the viral genome: three adjacent to the BHRF1 gene (the BHRF1 cluster) and the BART cluster which comprises the remaining 20 miRs located in the introns of the BART transcripts. (Pfeffer et al., 2004; Cai et al., 2006; Grundhoff et al., 2006).

Intriguingly, the two clusters of EBV-encoded miRs are differentially expressed in cells exhibiting different forms of EBV latency. The BART cluster is expressed predominantly in latency I or II whereas the BHRF1 miRs are associated with latency III and Cp/Wp promoter usage. This suggests that the BHRF1 miRs may be processed from an intron in the large EBNA primary transcripts (Cai et al., 2006; Cullen, 2006). The expression levels of several miRs from both clusters are enhanced following induction of lytic infection (Cai et al., 2006). The significance of all these differential expression profiles is currently unclear.

The function of EBV-encoded miRs is also unclear. miR-BART2 is antisense to the BALF5 open reading frame and has been proposed to have a role in the regulation of viral DNA polymerase expression via the degradative mechanism (Pfeffer et al., 2004). The rest of the miRs do not exhibit such extensive homology with EBV genes leading to the hypothesis that they are more likely to target cellular genes by translational inhibition.

Conclusions

Compelling evidence implicates EBV in the pathogenesis of tumors arising in both lymphoid and epithelial tissues. The virus adopts different forms of latent infection in different tumor types recapitulating the forms of EBV latency used to establish long-term persistence in the memory B-cell pool. These forms of latency reflect the complex interplay between EBV and the host cell environment involving differential regulation by both viral and cellular factors of the promoters driving latent gene transcription. Superimposed on this intrinsic regulation of EBV latency are extrinsic factors such as the immune response and the local milieu that may influence the growth and survival of EBV-infected cells as well as govern their entry into the virus lytic cycle. Studies of the function of individual EBV latent and lytic genes have highlighted the ability of these proteins to target specific cellular pathways and more detailed analysis using recombinant forms of EBV offers the possibility of precisely defining the role of these viral genes in the EBV life cycle. Thus, as clearly evidenced by work with proteins encoded by other viruses, an understanding of the functions of EBV proteins will not only be relevant to the role of the virus in health and disease but will also help to elucidate the fundamental mechanisms regulating cell growth, survival and differentiation. It is hoped that this work will also provide novel approaches to the therapy of EBV-associated diseases. Adoptive transfer of EBV-specific CTLs has already proved useful in the treatment of immunoblastic B-cell lymphomas and this approach as well as other vaccine strategies are currently being evaluated in patients with HD or NPC. The possibility of more direct therapeutic intervention targeting the function of essential EBV latent genes such as EBNA1 and LMP1 is also a possibility. Thus, drugs that prevent the ability of EBNA1 to bind to oriP or of the TRAFs to interact with LMP1 are likely to be developed. Finally, gene therapy strategies which exploit either the transcriptional regulation of the EBV genome or target the functional effects of EBV latent genes offer exciting possibilities for the development of both therapeutic and preventative strategies.

REFERENCES

Allan, G. J., Inman, G. J., Parker, B. D., Rowe, D. T., and Farrell, P. J. (1992). Cell growth effects of Epstein–Barr virus leader protein. *J. Gen. Virol.*, **73**, 1547–1551.

Allday, M. J. and Farrell, P. J. (1994). Epstein–Barr virus nuclear antigen EBNA3C/6 expression maintains the level of latent membrane protein 1 in G1-arrested cells. *J. Virol.*, **68**, 3491–3498.

Arrand, J. R. (1992). Prospects for a vaccine against Epstein–Barr virus. *Cancer J.*, **5**, 188–193.

Artavanis-Tsakonas, S., Matsuno, K., and Fortini, M. E. (1995). Notch signaling. *Science*, **268**, 225–232.

Babcock, G. J. and Thorley-Lawson, D. A. (2000). Tonsillar memory B cells, latently infected with Epstein–Barr virus, express the restricted pattern of latent genes previously found only in Epstein–Barr virus-associated tumours. *Proc. Natl Acad. Sci. USA*, **97**, 12250–12255.

Babcock, G. J., Decker, L. L., Volk, M., and Thorley-Lawson, D. A. (1998). EBV persistence in memory B cells *in vivo*. *Immunity*, **9**, 395–404.

Baer, R., Bankier, A. T., Biggin, M. D. *et al.* (1984). DNA sequence and expression of the B95–8 Epstein–Barr virus genome. *Nature*, **310**, 207–211.

Bartel, D. P. (2004). MicroRNAs: genomics, biogenesis, mechanism and function. *Cell*, 116, 281–297.

Baumann, M., Feederle, R., Kremmer, E., and Hammerschmidt, W. (2000). Cellular transcription factors recruit viral replication proteins to activate the Epstein–Barr virus origin of lytic DNA replication, oriLyt. *EMBO J.*, **18**, 6095–6105.

Baylis, S. A., Purifoy, D. J., and Littler, E. (1989). The characterisation of the EBV alkaline deoxyribonuclease cloned and expressed in E. coli. *Nucl Acids Res.*, **17**, 7609–7622.

Bejarano, M. T. and Masucci, M. G. (1998). Interleukin-10 abrogates the inhibition of Epstein–Barr virus-induced B-cell transformation by memory T-cell responses. *Blood*, **92**, 4256–4262.

Bellows, D. S., Howell, M., Pearson, C., Hazlewood, S. A., and Hardwick, J. M. (2002). Epstein–Barr virus BALF1 is a BCL-2-like antagonist of the herpesvirus antiapoptotic BCL-2 proteins. *J. Virol.*, **76**, 2469–2479.

Biggin, M. D., Farrell, P. J., and Barrell, B. (1984). Transcription and DNA sequence of the BamHI L fragment of B95–8 Epstein–Barr virus. *EMBO J.*, **3**, 1083–1090.

Biggin, M. D., Bodescot, M., Perricaudet, M., and Farrell, P. J. (1987). Epstein–Barr virus gene expression in P3HR-1-superinfected Raji cells. *J. Virol.*, **61**, 3120–3132.

Bonnet, M., Guinebretiere, J. M., Kremmer, E. *et al.* (1999). Detection of Epstein-Barr virus in invasive breast cancers. *J. Natl Cancer Inst.*, **91**, 1376–1381.

Borza, C. M. and Hutt-Fletcher, L. M. (1998). Epstein–Barr virus recombinant lacking expression of glycoprotein gp150 infects B cells normally but is enhanced for infection of epithelial cells. *J. Virol.*, **72**, 7577–7582.

Borza, C. M. and Hutt-Fletcher, L. M. (2002). Alternate replication in B-cells and epithelial cells switches tropism of Epstein–Barr virus. *Nat. Med.*, **8**, 594–599.

Brooks, J. M., Croom-Carter, D., Leese, A., Tierney, R. J., Habeshaw, G., and Rickinson, A. B. (2000). Cytotoxic T-lymphocyte responses to a polymorphic Epstein–Barr virus epitope identify healthy carriers with co-resident viral strains. *J. Virol.*, **74**, 1801–1809.

Brooks, L., Yao, Q. Y., Rickinson, A. B., and Young, L. S. (1992). Epstein-Barr virus latent gene transcription in nasopharyngeal carcinoma cells: coexpression of EBNA1, LMP1, and LMP2 transcripts. *J. Virol.*, **66**, 2689–2697.

Bryant, H. and Farrell, P. J. (2002). Signal transduction and transcription factor modification during reactivation of Epstein–Barr virus from latency. *J. Virol.*, **76**, 10290–10298.

Cai, X., Schäfer, A., Lu, S. *et al.* (2006). Epstein–Barr virus microRNAs are evolutionarily conserved and differentially expressed. *PloS Pathogens*, **2**, e23.

Caldwell, R. G., Wilson, J. B., Anderson, S. J., and Longnecker, R. (1998). Epstein–Barr virus LMP2A drives B cell development and survival in the absence of normal B cell receptor signals. *Immunity*, **9**, 405–411.

Cameron, K. R., Stamminger, T., Craxton, M., Bodemer, W., Honess, R. W., and Fleckenstein, B. (1987). The 160,000-M_r virion protein encoded at the right end of the herpesvirus saimiri genome is homologous to the 140,000-Mr membrane antigen encoded at the left end of the Epstein–Barr virus genome. *J. Virol.*, **61**, 2063–2070.

Carbone, A., Gloghini, A., Zagonel, V. *et al.* (1995). The expression of CD26 and CD40 ligand is mutually exclusive in human T-cell non-Hodgkin's lymphomas/leukaemias. *Blood*, **86**, 4617–4626.

Chan, K. H., Gu, Y. L., Ng, F. *et al.* (2003). EBV specific antibody-based and DNA-based assays in serologic diagnosis of nasopharyngeal carcinoma. *Int. J. Cancer*, **105**, 706–709.

Chen, H., Smith, P., Ambinder, R. F., and Hayward, S. D. (1999). Expression of Epstein–Barr virus BamHI-A rightward transcripts in latently infected B cells from peripheral blood. *Blood*, **93**, 3026–3032.

Chen, H., Lee, J. M., Zong, Y. S. *et al.* (2001). Linkage between STAT regulation and Epstein–Barr virus gene expression in tumours. *J. Virol.*, **75**, 2929–2937.

Chen, H., Hutt-Fletcher, L. M., Cao, L., and Hayward, S. D. (2003). A positive autoregulatory loop of LMP1 expression and STAT activation in epithelial cells latently infected with Epstein–Barr virus. *J. Virol.*, **77**, 4139–4148.

Chen, M. R., Hsu, T. Y., Lin, S. W., Chen, J. Y., and Yang, C. S. (1991). Cloning and characterisation of cDNA clones corresponding to transcripts from the BamHI G region of the Epstein–Barr virus genome and expression of BGLF2. *J. Gen. Virol.*, **72**, 3047–3055.

Chen, M. R., Chang, S. J., Huang, H., and Chen, J. Y. (2000). A protein kinase activity associated with Epstein–Barr virus BGLF4 phosphorylates the viral early antigen EA-D *in vitro*. *J. Virol.*, **74**, 3093–3104.

Cheng, W. M., Chan, K. H., Chen, H. L. *et al.* (2002). Assessing the risk of nasopharyngeal carcinoma on the basis of EBV antibody spectrum. *Int. J. Cancer*, **97**, 489–492.

Chevallier-Greco, A., Manet, E., Chavrier, P., Mosnier, C., Daillie, J., and Sergeant, A. (1986). Both Epstein–Barr virus (EBV)-encoded trans-acting factors, EB1 and EB2, are required to activate transcription from an EBV early promoter. *EMBO J.*, **5**, 3241–3249.

Chiang, A. K., Tao, Q., Srivastava, G., and Ho, F. C. (1996). Nasal NK- and T-cell lymphomas share the same type of Epstein–Barr virus latency as nasopharyngeal carcinoma and Hodgkin's disease. *Int. J. Cancer*, **68**, 285–290.

Cho, Y., Ramer, J., Rivailler, P. *et al.* (2001). An Epstein–Barr-related herpesvirus from marmoset lymphomas. *Proc. Natl Acad. Sci. USA*, **98**, 1224–1229.

Clemens, M. J., Laing, K. G., Jeffrey, I. W. *et al.* (1994). Regulation of the interferon-inducible eIF-2a-protein kinase by small RNAs. *Biochimie*, **76**, 770–778.

Cohen, J. I. and Lekstrom, K. (1999). Epstein–Barr virus BARF1 protein is dispensable for B-cell transformation and inhibits α-interferon secretion from mononuclear cells. *J. Virol.*, **73**, 7627–7632.

Connolly, Y., Littler, E., Sun, N. *et al.* (2001). Antibodies to the Epstein–Barr virus thymidine kinase: a characteristic marker for the serological detection of nasopharyngeal carcinoma. *Int. J. Cancer*, **91**, 692–697.

Cook, I. D., Shanahan, F., and Farrell, P. J. (1994). Epstein–Barr virus SM protein. *Virology*, **205**, 217–227.

Countryman, J. and Miller, G. (1985). Activation of expression of latent Epstein–Barr herpesvirus after gene transfer with a small cloned subfragment of heterogeneous viral DNA. *Proc. Natl Acad. Sci. USA*, **82**.

Countryman, J., Jenson, H., Seibl, R., Wolf, H., and Miller, G. (1987). Polymorphic proteins encoded within BZLF1 of defective and standard Epstein–Barr viruses disrupt latency. *J. Virol.*, **61**, 3672–3679.

Cui, C., Griffiths, A., Li, G. *et al.* (2006). Prediction and identification of Herpes simplex virus 1-encoded microRNAs. *J. Virol.*, **80**, 5499–5508.

Cullen, B.R. (2006). Viruses and microRNAs. *Nature Genet. Suppl.*, **38**, S25–S30.

Dambaugh, T., Hennessy, K., Chamnankit, L., and Kieff, E. (1984). U2 region of Epstein–Barr virus DNA may encode Epstein–Barr nuclear antigen 2. *Proc. Natl. Acad. Sci. USA*, **81**, 7632–7636.

Dardari, R., Khyatti, M., Benider, A. *et al.* (2000). Antibodies to the Epstein–Barr virus transactivator protein (ZEBRA) as a valuable biomarker in young patients with nasopharyngeal carcinoma. *Int. J. Cancer*, **86**, 71–75.

Dawson, C. W., Eliopoulos, A. G., Dawson, J., and Young, L. S. (1995). BHRF1, a viral homologue of the Bcl-2 oncogene, disturbs epithelial cell differentiation. *Oncogene*, **9**, 69–77.

Dawson, C. W., Dawson, J., Jones, R., Ward, K., and Young, L. S. (1998). Functional differences between BHRF1, the EBV-encoded Bcl-2 homologue, and bcl-2 in human epithelial cells. *J. Virol.*, **72**, 9016–9024.

Dawson, C. W., Eliopoulos, A. G., Blake, S. M., Barker, R., and Young, L. S. (2000). Identification of functional differences between prototype Epstein–Barr virus-encoded LMP1 and a nasopharyngeal carcinoma-derived LMP1 in human epithelial cells. *Virology*, **272**, 204–217.

Dawson, C. W., Tramountanis, G., Eliopoulos, A. G., and Young, L. S. (2003). Epstein–Barr virus latent membrane protein 1 (LMP1) activates the PI3-K/Akt pathway to promote cell survival and induce actin filament remodelling. *J. Biol. Chem.*, **278**, 3694–3704.

de Jesus, O., Smith, P. R., Spender, L. C. *et al.* (2003). Updated Epstein–Barr virus (EBV) DNA sequence and analysis of a promoter for the BART (CST, BARF0) RNAs of EBV. *J. Gen. Virol.*, **84**, 1443–1450.

De Souza, Y. G., Greenspan, D., Felton, J. R., Hartzog, G. A., Hammer, M., and Greenspan, J. S. (1989). Localisation of Epstein–Barr virus DNA in the epithelial cells of oral hairy leukoplakia by *in situ* hybridisation of tissue sections. *N. Engl. J. Med.*, **320**, 1559–1560.

Deacon, E. M., Pallesen, G., Niedobitek, G. *et al.* (1993). Epstein–Barr virus and Hodgkin's disease: transcriptional analysis of virus latency in the malignant cells. *J. Exp. Med.*, **177**, 339–349.

Decaussin, G., Sbih-Lammali, F., de Turenne-Tessier, M., Bouguermouh, A., and Ooka, T. (2000). Expression of BARF1 gene encoded by Epstein–Barr virus in nasopharyngeal carcinoma biopsies. *Cancer Res.*, **60**, 5584–5588.

Deng, Z., Chen, C.-J., Chamberlin, M. *et al.* (2003). The CBP bromodomain and nucleosome targeting are required for Zta-directed nucleosome acetylation and transcription activation. *Mol. Cell Biol.*, **23**, 2633–2644.

Dolan, A., Addison, C., Gatherer, D., Davison, A.J., and McGeoch, D.J. (2006). The genome of Epstein-Barr virus type 2 strain AG876. *Virology*, **350**, 164–170.

Donaghy, G. and Jupp, R. (1995). Characterisation of the Epstein–Barr virus proteinase and comparison with the human cytomegalovirus proteinase. *J. Virol.*, **69**, 1265–1270.

Du, T. and Zamore, P.D. (2005). MicroPrimer: the biogenesis and function of microRNA. *Development*, **132**, 4645–4652.

Edson, C. M. and Thorley-Lawson, D. A. (1981). Epstein–Barr virus membrane antigens: characterisation, distribution, and strain differences. *J. Virol.*, **39**, 172–184.

Edwards, R. H., Seillier-Moiseiwitsch, F., and Raab-Traub, N. (1999). Signature amino acid changes in latent membrane protein 1 distinguish Epstein–Barr virus strains. *Virology*, **261**, 79–95.

Eliopoulos, A. G. and Young, L. S. (1998). Activation of the cJun N-terminal kinase (JNK) pathway by the Epstein-Barr virus-encoded latent membrane protein 1 (LMP1). *Oncogene*, **16**, 1731–1742.

Eliopoulos, A. G., Stack, M., Dawson, C. W. *et al.* (1997). Epstein–Barr virus-encoded LMP1 and CD40 mediate IL-6 production in epithelial cells via an NF-κB pathway involving TNF receptor-associated factors. *Oncogene*, **14**, 2899–2916.

Eliopoulos, A. G., Gallagher, N. J., Blake, S. M., Dawson, C. W., and Young, L. S. (1999). Activation of the p38 mitogen-activated protein kinase pathway by Epstein–Barr virus-encoded latent membrane protein 1 coregulates interleukin-6 and interleukin-8 production. *J. Biol. Chem.*, **274**, 16085–16096.

Eliopoulos, A. G., Davies, C., and Blake, S. M. (2002). The oncogenic protein kinase Tpl-2/Cot contributes to Epstein–Barr virus-encoded latent infection membrane protein 1-induced NF-κB signaling downstream of TRAF2. *J. Virol.*, **76**, 4567–4579.

Eliopoulos, A. G., Caamano, J. H., Flavell, J. R. *et al.* (2003). Epstein–Barr virus-encoded latent infection membrane protein 1 regulates the processing of p100 NFκB2 to p52 via an IKKγ/NEMO-independent signalling pathway. *Oncogene*, **22**, 7557–7569.

Ernberg, I. and Andersson, J. (1986). Acyclovir efficiently inhibits oropharyngeal excretion of Epstein–Barr virus in patients with acute infectious mononucleosis. *J. Gen. Virol.*, **67**, 2267–2272.

Ernberg, I. and Klein, G. (1979). EB virus-induced antigens. In Epstein, M. A. and Achong, B. G. (eds.), *The Epstein–Barr Virus*. Springer-Verlag, pp. 39–60.

Farina, A., Santarelli, R., Gonnella, R. *et al.* (2000). The BFRF1 gene of Epstein–Barr virus encodes a novel protein. *J. Virol.*, **74**, 3235–3244.

Faulkner, G. C., Burrows, S. R., Khanna, R., Moss, D. J., Bird, A. G., and Crawford, D. H. (1999). X-linked agammaglobulinemia patients are not infected with Epstein–Barr virus: implications for the biology of the virus. *J. Virol.*, **73**, 1555–1564.

Feederle, R., Kost, M., Baumann, M. *et al.* (2000). The Epstein–Barr virus lytic program is controlled by the co-operative functions of two transactivators. *EMBO J.*, **19**, 3080–3089.

Feng, P., Chan, S. H., Soo, M. Y. *et al.* (2001). Antibody response to Epstein–Barr virus Rta protein in patients with nasopharyngeal carcinoma: a new serologic parameter for diagnosis. *Cancer*, **92**, 1872–1880.

Fielding, C. A., Sandvej, K., Mehl, A. M., Brennan, P., Jones, M., and Rowe, M. (2001) Epstein–Barr virus LMP-1 natural sequence variants differ in their potential to activate cellular signaling pathways. *J. Virol.*, **75**, 9129–9141.

Fingeroth, J. D., Weis, J. J., Tedder, T. F., Strominger, J. L., Biro, P. A., and Fearon, D. T. (1984). Epstein–Barr virus receptor of human B lymphocytes is the C3d receptor CR2. *Proc. Natl Acad. Sci. USA*, **81**, 4510–4514.

Fixman, E. D., Hayward, G. S., and Hayward, S. D. (1992). Trans-acting requirements for replication of Epstein–Barr virus. *J. Virol.*, **66**, 5030–5039.

Flemington, E. K. (2001). Herpesvirus lytic replication and the cell cycle: arresting new developments. *J. Virol.*, **75**, 4475–4481.

Fones-Tan, A., Chan, S. H., Tsao, S. Y. *et al.* (1994). Enzyme-linked immunosorbent assay (ELISA) for IgA and IgG antibodies to Epstein–Barr-virus ribonucleotide reductase in patients with nasopharyngeal carcinoma. *Int. J. Cancer*, **59**, 739–742.

Fronko, G. E., Long, W. K., Wu, B., Papadopoulos, T., and Henderson, E. E. (1989). Relationship between methylation status and expression of an Epstein–Barr virus (EBV) capsid antigen gene. *Biochem. Biophys. Res. Commun.*, **159**, 263–270.

Fruehling, S. and Longnecker, R. (1997). The immunoreceptor tyrosine-based activation motif of Epstein–Barr virus LMPA2 is essential for blocking BCR-mediated signal transduction. *J. Virol.*, **235**, 241–251.

Fujii, K., Yokoyama, N., Kiyono, T. *et al.* (2000). The Epstein–Barr virus pol catalytic subunit physically interacts with the BBLF4-BSLF1-BBLF2/3 complex. *J. Virol.*, **74**, 2550–2557.

Furnari, F. B., Zacny, V., Quinlivan, E. B., Kenney, S. and Pagano, J. (1994). RAZ, an Epstein–Barr virus transdominant repressor that modulates the viral reactivation mechanism.

Gao, Z., Krithivas, A., Finan, J. E. *et al.* (1998). The Epstein–Barr virus lytic transactivator Zta interacts with the helicase–primase replication proteins. *J. Virol.*, **72**, 8559–8567.

Gires, O., Zimber-Strobl, U., Gonnella, R. *et al.* (1997). Latent membrane protein 1 of Epstein–Barr virus mimics a constitutively active receptor molecule. *EMBO J.*, **16**, 6131–6140.

Gires, O., Kohlhuber, F., Kilger, E. *et al.* (1999). Latent membrane protein 1 of Epstein–Barr virus interacts with JAK3 and activates STAT proteins. *EMBO J.*, **18**, 3064–3073.

Glaser, G., Vogel, M., Wolf, H., and Niller, H. H. (1998). Regulation of the Epstein–Barr viral immediate early BRLF1 promoter through a distal NF1 site. *Arch. Virol.*, **143**, 1967–1983.

Gong, M. and Kieff, E. (1990). Intracellular trafficking of two major Epstein–Barr virus glycoproteins, gp350/220 and gp110. *J. Virol.*, **64**, 1507–1516.

Gong, M., Ooka, T., Matsuo, T., and Kieff, E. (1987). Epstein–Barr virus glycoprotein homologous to herpes simplex virus gB. *J. Virol.*, **61**, 499–508.

Grundhoff, A., Sullivan, C. S., and Ganem, D. (2006). A combined computational and microarray-based approach identifies novel microRNAs encoded by human gamma-herpesviruses. *RNA*, **12**, 733–750.

Gratama, J. W., Oosterveer, M. A., Lepoutre, J. M. *et al.* (1990). Serological and molecular studies of Epstein–Barr virus infection in allogeneic marrow graft recipients. *Transplantation*, **49**, 725–730.

Gregory, C. D., Rowe, M., and Rickinson, A. B. (1990). Different Epstein–Barr virus-B cell interactions in phenotypically distinct clones of a Burkitt's lymphoma cell line. *J. Gen. Virol.*, **71**, 1481–1495.

Griffiths-Jones, S., Grocock, R. J., van Dongen, S., Bateman, A., and Enright, A. J. (2006). mirBase: microRNA sequences, targets and gene nomenclature. *Nucl. Acids Res.*, **34**, D140–D144.

Grossman, S. R., Johannsen, E., Tong, R., Yalamanchili, R., and Kieff, E. (1994). The Epstein–Barr virus nuclear antigen 2 transactivator is directed to response elements by the Jκ recombination signal binding protein. *Proc. Natl Acad. Sci. USA*, **91**, 7568–7572.

Gruffat, H., Batisse, J., Pich, D. *et al.* (2002a). Epstein–Barr virus mRNA export factor EB2 is essential for production of infectious virus. *J. Virol.*, **76**, 9635–9644.

Gruffat, H., Manet, E., and Sergeant, A. (2002b). MEF2-mediated recruitment of class II histone deacetylase at the EBV immediate early gene BZLF1 links latency and chromatin remodelling. *EMBO Rep.*, **3**, 141–146.

Gonnella, R., Farina, A., Santarelli, R. *et al.* (2005). Characterization and intracellular localization of the Epstein-Barr virus protein BFLF2: Interactions with BFRF1 and with the nuclear lamina. *J. Virol.*, **79**, 3713–3727.

Gu, S., Huang, T., Miaio, Y. *et al.* (1991). A preliminary study on the immunogenicity in rabbits and in human volunteers of a recombinant vaccinnia virus expressing Epstein–Barr virus membrane antigen. *Chin. Med. Sci. J.*, **6**, 241–243.

Gulley, M. L., Pulitzer, D. R., Eagan, P. A., and Schneider, B. G. (1996). Epstein–Barr virus infection is an early event in gastric carcinogenesis and is independent of bcl-2 expression and p53 accumulation. *Hum. Pathol.*, **27**, 20–27.

Gupta, A., Gartner, J. J., Sethupathy, P., Hatzigeorgiou, A. G., and Fraser, N. W. (2006). Anti-apoptotic function of a microRNA encoded by the HSV-1 latency-associated transcript. *Nature*, **442**, 82–85.

Haan, K. M., Lee, S. K., and Longnecker, R. (2001). Different functional domains in the cytoplasmic tail of glycoprotein B are involved in Epstein–Barr virus-induced membrane fusion. *Virology*, **290**, 106–114.

Hammerschmidt, W. and Sugden, B. (1988). Identification and characterisation of oriLyt, a lytic origin of DNA replication of Epstein–Barr virus. *Cell*, **55**, 427–433.

Hammerschmidt, W. and Sugden, B. (1989). Genetic analysis of immortalising functions of Epstein-Barr virus in human B lymphocytes. *Nature*, **340**, 393–397.

Harada, S. and Kieff, E. (1997). Epstein–Barr virus nuclear protein LP stimulates EBNA-2 acidic domain-mediated transcriptional activation. *J. Virol.*, **71**, 6611–6618.

Hardwick, J. M., Lieberman, P. M., and Hayward, S. D. (1988). A new Epstein–Barr virus transactivator, R, induces expression of a cytoplasmic early antigen. *J. Virol.*, **62**, 2274–2284.

Henderson, S., Rowe, M., Gregory, C. *et al.* (1991). Induction of bcl-2 expression by Epstein–Barr virus latent membrane protein 1 protects infected B cells from programmed cell death. *Cell*, **65**, 1107–1115.

Henderson, S., Huen, D. S., Rowe, M., Dawson, C. W., Johnson, G., and Rickinson, A. (1993). Epstein-Barr virus-coded BHRF1 protein, a viral homologue of Bcl-2, protects human B cells from programmed cell death. *Proc. Natl Acad. Sci. USA*, **90**, 8479–8483.

Henle, W., Henle, G., Ho, H.-C. *et al.* (1970). Antibodies to Epstein–Barr virus in nasopharyngeal carcinoma, other head and neck neoplasms and control groups. *J. Natl Cancer Inst.*, **44**, 225–231.

Herrold, R. E., Marchini, A., Fruehling, S., and Longnecker, R. (1996) Glycoprotein 110, the Epstein–Barr virus homolog of herpes simplex virus glycoprotein B, is essential for Epstein–Barr virus replication *in vivo*. *J. Virol.*, **70**, 2049–2054.

Higuchi, M., Kieff, E., and Izumi, K. M. (2002). The Epstein–Barr virus latent membrane protein 1 putative Janus Kinase 3 (JAK3) binding domain does not mediate JAK3 association or activation in B-lymphoma or lymphoblastoid cell lines. *J. Virol.*, **76**, 455–459.

Hinderer, W., Lang, D., Rothe, M., Vornhagen, R., Sonneborn, H. H., and Wolf, H. (1999). Serodiagnosis of Epstein–Barr virus infection by using recombinant viral capsid antigen fragments and autologous gene fusion. *J. Clin. Microbiol.*, **37**, 3239–3244.

Hitt, M. M., Allday, M. J., Hara, T. *et al.* (1989). EBV gene expression in an NPC-related tumour. *EMBO J.*, **8**, 2639–2651.

Hochberg, D., Middeldorp, J. M., Catalina, M., Sullivan, J. L., Luzuriaga, K., and Thorley-Lawson, D. A. (2004). Demonstration of the Burkitt's lymphoma Epstein–Barr virus phenotype in dividing latently infected memory cells *in vivo*. *Proc. Natl Acad. Sci. USA*, **101**, 239–244.

Hofelmayr, R., Strobl, L. J., Stein, C., Laux, G., Marschall, G., Bornkamm, G. W. and Zimber-Strobl, U. (1999). Activated mouse Notch1 transactivates Epstein–Barr virus nuclear antigen 2-regulated viral promoters. *J. Virol.*, **73**, 2770–2780.

Hofelmayr, H., Strobl, L. J., Marschall, G., Bornkamm, G. W., and Zimber-Strobl, U. (2001). Activated Notch1 can transiently substitute for EBNA2 in the maintenance of proliferation of LMP1-expressing immortalised B cells. *J. Virol.*, **75**, 2033–2040.

Hong, G. K., Delecluse, H-J., Gruffat, H. *et al.* (2004). The BRRF1 early gene of Epstein-Barr virus encodes a transcription factor that enhances induction of lytic infection by BRLF1. *J. Virol.* **78**, 4983–4992.

Huen, D. S., Henderson, S. A., Croom-Carter, D., and Rowe, M. (1995). The Epstein–Barr virus latent membrane protein-1 (LMP1) mediates activation of NF-κB and cell surface phenotype via two effector regions in its carboxy-terminal cytoplasmic domain. *Oncogene*, **10**, 549–560.

Humme, S., Reisbach, G., Feederle, R. *et al.* (2003). The EBV nuclear antigen enhances B cell immortalization several thousandfold. *Proc. Natl Acad. Sci. USA*, **100**, 10989–10994.

Hutt-Fletcher, L. M. and Lake, C. M. (2001). Two Epstein–Barr virus glycoprotein complexes. *Curr. Top. Microbiol. Immunol.*, **258**, 51–64.

Ikeda, M., Ikeda, A., Longan, L. C., and Longnecker, R. (2000). The Epstein–Barr virus latent membrane protein 2A PY motif recruits WW domain-containing ubiquitin-protein ligases. *Virology*, **268**, 178–191.

Izumi, K. M., Cahir McFarland, E. D., Riley, E. A., Rizzo, D., Chen, Y., and Kieff, E. (1999). The residues between the two transformation effector sites of Epstein–Barr virus latent membrane protein 1 are not critical for B-lymphocyte growth transformation. *J. Virol.*, **73**, 9908–9916.

Jackman, W. T., Mann, K. A., Hoffmann, H. J., and Spaete, R. R. (1999). Expression of Epstein-Barr virus gp350 as a single chain glycoprotein for an EBV subunit vaccine. *Vaccine*, **17**, 660–668.

Jansson, A., Masucci, M. G., and Rymo, L. (1992). Methylation of discrete sites within the enhancer region regulates the activity of the Epstein–Barr virus BamHI W promoter in Burkitt lymphoma lines. *J. Virol.*, **66**, 62–69.

Janz, A., Oezel, M., Kurzeder, C. *et al.* (2000). Infectious Epstein–Barr virus lacking major glycoprotein BLLF1 (gp350/220) demonstrates the existence of additional viral ligands. *J. Virol.*, **74**, 10142–10152.

Jenkins, P., Binne, U., and Farrell, P. J. (2000). Histone acetylation and reactivation of Epstein–Barr virus from latency. *J. Virol.*, **74**, 710–720.

Jiang, W. Q., Szekely, L., Wendel-Hansen, V., Ringertz, N., Klein, G., and Rosen, A. (1991). Colocalisation of the retinoblastoma protein and the Epstein–Barr virus-encoded nuclear antigen EBNA-5. *Exp. Cell Res.*, **197**, 314–318.

Johannsen, E., Luftig, M., Chase, M. R. *et al.* (2004). Proteins of purified Epstein–Barr virus. *Proc. Natl Acad. Sci. USA* **101**, 16286–16291.

Jones, R. J., Smith, L. J., Dawson, C. W., Haigh, T., Blake, N. W., and Young, L. S. (2003). Epstein–Barr virus nuclear antigen 1 (EBNA1) induced cytotoxicity in epithelial cells is associated with EBNA1 degradation and processing. *Virology*, **313**, 663–676.

Joseph, A.m., Babcock, G. J., and Thorley-Lawson, D. A. (2000). Cells expressing the Epstein–Barr virus growth program are present in and restricted to the naive B-cell subset of healthy tonsils. *J. Virol.*, **74**, 9964–9971.

Kaiser, C., Laux, G., Eick, D., Jochner, N., Bornkamm, G. W., and Kempkes, B. (1999). The proto-oncogene *c-myc* is a direct target gene of Epstein-Barr virus nuclear antigen 2. *Virology*, **73**, 4481–4484.

Karajannis, M. A., Hummel, M., Anagnostopoulos, I., and Stein, H. (1997). Strict lymphotropism of Epstein–Barr virus during acute infectious mononucleosis in non-immunocompromised individuals. *Blood*, **89**, 2856–2862.

Kato, K., Kawaguchi, Y., Tanaka, M. *et al.* (2001). Epstein–Barr virus-encoded protein kinase BGLF4 mediates hyperphosphorylation of cellular elongation factor 1delta (EF-1delta): EF-1delta is universally modified by conserved protein kinases of herpesviruses in mammalian cells. *J. Gen. Virol.*, **82**, 1467–1473.

Kawanishi, M. (1997). Epstein–Barr virus BHRF1 protein protects intestine 407 epithelial cells from apoptosis induced by tumour necrosis factor a and anti-Fas antibody. *J. Virol.*, **71**, 3319–3322.

Kelly, G., Bell, A., and Rickinson, A. B. (2002). Epstein–Barr virus-associated Burkitt lymphomagenesis selects for downregulation of the nuclear antigen EBNA1. *Nat. Med.*, **8**, 1098–1104.

Kennedy, G., Komano, J., and Sugden, B. (2003) Epstein–Barr virus provides a survival factor to Burkitt's lymphomas. *Proc. Natl Acad. Sci. USA*, **100**, 14269–14274.

Khanim, F., Yao, Q. Y., Niedobitek, G., Sihota, S., Rickinson, A. B., and Young, L. S. (1996). Analysis of Epstein–Barr virus gene polymorphisms in normal donors and in virus-associated tumours from different geographic locations. *Blood*, **88**, 3491–3501.

Khanim, F., Dawson, C. W., Meseda, C. A., Dawson, J., Mackett, M., and Young, L. S. (1997). BHRF1, a viral homologue of the Bcl-2 oncogene, is conserved at both the sequence and functional level in different Epstein–Barr virus isolates. *J. Gen. Virol.*, **78**, 2987–2999.

Kieff, E. and Rickinson, A. B. (2001). Epstein–Barr virus and its replication. In Knipe, D. M. and Howley, P. M. (eds.), *Fields Virology*. Philadelphia: Lippincott Williams & Wilkins, pp. 2511–2574.

Kieser, A., Kilger, E., Gires, O., Ueffing, M., Kolch, W., and Hammerschmidt, W. (1997). Epstein–Barr virus latent membrane protein-1 triggers AP-1 activity via the c-Jun N-terminal kinase cascade. *EMBO J.*, **16**, 6478–6485.

Kilger, E., Kieser, A., Baumann, M., and Hammerschmidt, W. (1998). Epstein-Barr virus-mediated B-cell proliferation is dependent upon latent membrane protein 1, which simulates an activated CD40 receptor. *EMBO J.*, **17**, 1700–1709.

Kim, V. N. and Nam, J-W. (2006). Genomics of microRNA. *Trends Genet.*, **22**, 165–173.

Kitagawa, N., Goto, M., Kurozumi, K. *et al.* (2000). Epstein-Barr virus-encoded poly(A)(-) RNA supports Burkitt's lymphoma growth through interleukin-10 induction. *EMBO J.*, **19**, 6742–6750.

Knox, P. G., Li, Q. X., Rickinson, A. B., and Young, L. S. (1996). In vitro production of stable Epstein–Barr virus-positive epithelial cell clones which resemble the virus: Cell interaction observed in nasopharyngeal carcinoma. *Virology*, **215**, 40–50.

Koffa, M. D., Clements, J. B., Izaurralde, E. *et al.* (2001). Herpes simplex virus ICP27 protein provides viral mRNAs with access to the cellular mRNA export pathway. *EMBO J.*, **20**, 5769–5778.

Komano, J., Maruo, S., Kurozumi, K., Oda, T., and Takada, K. (1999). Oncogenic role of Epstein–Barr virus-encoded RNAs in Burkitt's lymphoma cell line Akata. *J. Virol.*, **73**, 9827–9831.

Kraus, R. J., Perrigoue, J. G., and Mertz, J. E. (2003). ZEB negatively regulates the lytic switch BZLF1 gene promoter of Epstein–Barr virus. *J. Virol.*, **77**, 199–207.

Kudoh, A., Daikoku, T., and Sugaya, Y. (2004). Inhibition of S-phase cyclin-dependent kinase activity blocks expression of Epstein-Barr virus immediate–early and early genes, preventing viral lytic replication. *J. Virol.*, **78**, 104–115.

Kudoh, A., Fujita, M., Kiyono, T. *et al.* (2003). Reactivation of lytic replication from B cells latently infected with Epstein-Barr virus occurs with high S-phase cyclin-dependent kinase activity while inhibiting cellular DNA replication. *J. Virol.*, **77**, 851–861.

Laherty, C. D., Hu, H. M., Opipari, A. W., Wang, F., and Dixit, V. M. (1992). The Epstein–Barr virus LMP1 gene product induces A20 zinc finger protein expression by activating nuclear factor κB. *J. Biol. Chem.*, **267**, 24157–24160.

Laing, K. G., Elia, A., Jeffrey, I. W. *et al.* (2002). In vivo effects of the Epstein–Barr virus small RNA EBER-1 on protein synthesis and cell growth regulation. *Virology*, **297**, 253–269.

Lake, C. M. and Hutt-Fletcher, L. M. (2000). Epstein–Barr virus that lacks glycoprotein gN is impaired in assembly and infection. *J. Virol.*, **74**, 11162–11172.

Lake, C. M., Molesworth, S. J., and Hutt-Fletcher, L. M. (1998). The Epstein–Barr virus (EBV) gN homolog BLRF1 encodes a 15-kilodalton glycoprotein that cannot be authentically processed unless it is coexpressed with the EBV gM homolog BBRF3. *J. Virol.*, **72**, 5559–5564.

Lee, M. A. and Yates, J. L. (1992). BHRF1 of Epstein–Barr virus, which is homologous to human proto-oncogene bcl2, is not essential for transformation of B cells or for virus replication *in vitro*. *J. Virol.*, **66**, 1899–1906.

Lees, J. F., Arrand, J. R., Pepper, S. D., Stewart, J. P., Mackett, M., and Arrand, J. R. (1993). The Epstein–Barr Virus candidate vaccine antigen (gp340/220) is highly conserved between virus types A and B. *Virology*, **195**, 578–586.

Lerner, M. R., Andrews, N. C., Miller, G., and Steitz, J. A. (1981). Two small RNAs encoded by Epstein–Barr virus and complexed with protein are precipitated by antibodies from patients with systemic lupus erythematosus. *Proc. Natl Acad. Sci. USA*, **78**, 805–809.

Levitskaya, J., Coram, M., Levitsky, V., Imreh, S., Steigerwald-Mullen, P., and Masucci, M. G. (1995). Inhibition of antigen processing by the internal repeat region of the Epstein–Barr virus nuclear antigen-1. *Nature*, **375**, 685–688.

Li, S. N., Chang, Y. S., and Liu, S. T. (1996). Effect of a 10-amino acid deletion on the oncogenic activity of latent membrane protein 1 of Epstein–Barr virus. *Oncogene*, **12**, 2129–2135.

Liao, G., Wu, F. Y., and Hayward, S. D. (2001). Interaction with the Epstein–Barr virus helicase targets Zta to DNA replication compartments. *J. Virol.*, **75**, 8792–8802.

Lieberman, P. M., Hardwick, J. M., Sample, J., Hayward, G. S., and Hayward, S. D. (1990). The Zta transactivator involved in induction of lytic cycle gene expression in Epstein-Barr virus-infected lymphocytes binds to both AP-1 and ZRE sites in target promoter and enhancer regions. *J. Virol.*, **64**, 1143–1155.

Liu, M. Y., Wu, Y. L., Chen, L. S., Hsu, T. Y., Chen, J. Y., and Yang, C. S. (1994). Serological responses of patients with nasopharyngeal carcinoma to an N-terminal Epstein–Barr virus DNA polymerase protein expressed in prokaryotic cells. *J. Biomed. Sci.*, **1**, 119–124.

Liu, P. and Speck, S. H. (2003). Synergistic autoactivation of the Epstein-Barr virus immediate-early BRLF1 promoter by Rta and Zta. *Virology*, **10**, 199–206.

Liu, P., Liu, S., and Speck, S. H. (1998). Identification of a negative cis element within the ZII domain of the Epstein–Barr virus lytic switch BZLF1 gene promoter. *J. Virol.*, **72**, 8230–8239.

Lo, K.-W. and Huang, D. P. (2002). Genetic and epigenetic changes in nasopharyngeal carcinoma. *Semin. Cancer Biol.*, **12**, 451–462.

Longnecker, R. (2000). Epstein-Barr virus latency: LMP2, a regulator or means for Epstein–Barr virus persistence? *Adv. Cancer Res.*, **79**, 175–200.

Longnecker, R. and Kieff, E. (1990). A second Epstein–Barr virus membrane protein (LMP2) is expressed in latent infection and co-localises with LMP1. *J. Virol.*, **64**, 2319–2326.

Mackett, M., Conway, M. J., Arrand, J. R., Haddad, R. S., and Hutt-Fletcher, L. M. (1990). Characterisation and expression of a glycoprotein encoded by the Epstein–Barr virus BamHI I fragment. *J. Virol.*, **64**, 2545–2552.

Manet, E., Gruffat, H., Trscol-Biemont, M. C. *et al.* (1989). Epstein–Barr virus bicistronic mRNAs generated by facultative splicing code for two transcriptional transactivators. *EMBO J.*, **8**, 1819–1826.

Marchini, A., Tomkinson, B., Cohen, J. I., and Kieff, E. (1991). BHRF1, the Epstein–Barr virus gene with homology to Bc12, is dispensable for B-lymphocyte transformation and virus replication. *J. Virol.*, **65**, 5991–6000.

Miller, C. L., Burkhardt, A. L., Lee, J. H. *et al.* (1995). Integral membrane protein 2 of Epstein–Barr virus regulates reactivation from latency through dominant negative effects on protein-tyrosine kinases. *Immunity*, **2**, 155–166.

Miller, W. E., Cheshire, J. L., Baldwin, A. S. J., and Raab-Traub, N. (1998). The NPC derived C15 LMP1 protein confers enhanced activation of NKκB and induction of the EGFR in epithelial cells. *Oncogene*, **16**, 1869–1877.

Modrow, S., Hoflacher, B., and Wolf, H. (1992). Identification of a protein encoded in the EB-viral open reading frame BMRF2. *Arch. Virol.*, **127**, 379–386.

Moghaddam, A., Rosenzweig, M., Lee-Parritz, D., Annis, B., Johnson, R. P., and Wang, F. (1997). An animal model for acute and persistent Epstein–Barr virus infection. *Science*, **276**, 2030–2033.

Montalvo, E. A., Cottam, M., Hill, S., and Wang, Y.-C. (1995). YY1 binds to and regulates *cis*-acting negative elements in the Epstein–Barr virus BZLF1 promoter. *J. Virol.*, **69**, 4158–4165.

Moody, C. A., Scott, R. S., Tao, S., and Sixbey, J. W. (2003). Length of Epstein–Barr virus termini as a determinant of epithelial cell clonal emergence. *J. Virol.*, **77**, 8555–8561.

Moore, K. W., Vieira, P., Fiorentino, D. F., Trounstine, M. L., Khan, T. A., and Mosmann, T. R. (1990). Homology of cytokine synthesis inhibitory factor (IL-10) to the Epstein–Barr virus gene BCRFI. *Science*, **248**, 1230–1234.

Moore, K. W., de Waal Malefyt, T., Coffman, R. L., and O'Garra, A. (2001). Interleukin-10 and the interleukin-10 receptor. *Annu. Rev. Immunol.*, **19**, 683–765.

Murray, P. G., Lissauer, D., Junying, J. *et al.* (2003). Reactivity with a monoclonal antibody to Epstein–Barr virus (EBV) nuclear antigen 1 defines a subset of aggressive breast cancers in the absence of the EBV genome. *Cancer Res.*, **63**, 2338–2343.

Nanbo, A., Inoue, K., Adachi-Takasawa, K., and Takada, K. (2002). Epstein–Barr virus RNA confers resistance to interferon-a-induced apoptosis in Burkitt's lymphoma. *EMBO J.*, **21**, 954–965.

Nemerow, G. R., Houghten, R. A., Moore, M. D., and Cooper, N. R. (1989). Identification of an epitope in the major envelope protein of Epstein–Barr virus that mediates viral binding to the B lymphocyte EBV receptor (CR2). *Cell*, **56**, 369–377.

Neuhierl, B., Feederle, R., Hammerschmidt, W., and Delecluse, H. J. (2002). Glycoprotein gp110 of Epstein–Barr virus determines viral tropism and efficiency of infection. *Proc. Natl Acad. Sci. USA*, **99**, 15036–15041.

Niedobitek, G., Hamilton-Dutoit, S. J., Herbst, H. *et al.* (1989). Identification of Epstein–Barr virus-infected cells in tonsils of acuteinfectious mononucleosis by in situ hybridisation. *Hum. Pathol.*, **20**, 796–799.

Niedobitek, G., Young, L. S., Sam, C. K., Brooks, L., Prasad, U., and Rickinson, A. B. (1992). Expression of Epstein–Barr virus genes and of lymphocyte activation molecules in undifferentiated nasopharyngeal carcinomas. *Am. J. Pathol.*, **140**, 879–887.

Niedobitek, G., Agathanggelou, A., Rowe, M. *et al.* (1995). Heterogeneous expression of Epstein–Barr virus latent proteins in endemic Burkitt's lymphoma. *Blood*, **86**, 659–665.

Niedobitek, G., Baumann, I., Brabletz, T. *et al.* (2000). Hodgkin's disease and peripheral T-cell lymphoma: composite lymphoma with evidence of Epstein–Barr virus infection. *J. Pathol.*, **191**, 394.

Nitsche, F., Bell, A., and Rickinson, A. B. (1997). Epstein–Barr virus leader protein enhances EBNA-2-mediated transactivation of latent membrane protein 1 expression: A role for the W_1W_2 repeat domain. *J. Virol.*, **71**, 6619–6628.

Nonkwelo, C., Skinner, J., Bell, A., Rickinson, A. B., and Sample, J. (1996). Transcription start sites downstream of the Epstein–Barr virus (EBV) Fp promoter in early-passage Burkitt lymphoma cells define a fourth promoter for expression of the EBV EBNA-1 protein. *J. Virol.*, **70**, 623–627.

Nuebling, C. M. and Mueller-Lantzsch, N. (1989). Identification and characterisation of an Epstein–Barr virus early antigen that is encoded by the NotI repeats. *J. Virol.*, **63**, 4609–4615.

Olsen, L. C., Aasland, R., Wittwer, C. U., Krokan, H. E., and Helland, D. E. (1989). Molecular cloning of human uracil-DNA glycosylase, a highly conserved DNA repair enzyme. *EMBO J.*, **8**, 3121–3125.

Pallesen, G., Hamilton-Dutoit, S. J., Rowe, M., and Young, L. S. (1991). Expression of Epstein–Barr virus latent gene products in tumour cells of Hodgkin's disease. *Lancet*, **337**, 320–322.

Papworth, M. A., Van Dijk, A. A., Benyon, G. R., Allen, T. D., Arrand, J. R., and Mackett, M. (1997). The processing, transport and heterologous expression of Epstein–Barr virus gp110. *J. Gen. Virol.*, **78**, 2179–2189.

Parker, G. A., Crook, T., Bain, M., Sara, E. A., Farrell, P. J., and Allday, M. J. (1996). Epstein–Barr virus nuclear antigen (EBNA)3C is an immortalizing oncoprotein with similar properties to adenovirus E1A and papillomavirus E7. *Oncogene*, **13**, 2541–2549.

Parker, B. D., Bankier, A., Satchwell, S., Barrell, B., and Farrell, P. J. (1990). Sequence and transcription of Raji Epstein–Barr virus DNA spanning the B95-8 deletion region. *Virology*, **179**, 339–346.

Pellett, P. E., Jenkins, F. J., Ackermann, M., Sarmiento, M., and Roizman, B. (1986). Transcription initiation sites and nucleotide sequence of a herpes simplex virus 1 gene conserved in the Epstein–Barr virus genome and reported to affect the transport of viral glycoproteins. *J. Virol.*, **60**, 1134–1140.

Pertuiset, B., Boccara, M., Cebrian, J. *et al.* (1989). Physical mapping and nucleotide sequence of a herpes simplex virus type 1 gene required for capsid assembly. *J. Virol.*, **63**, 2169–2179.

Pfeffer, S., Zavolan, M., Grasser, F. A. *et al.* (2004). Identification of virus-encoded microRNAs. *Science*, **304**, 734–736.

Pizzo, P. A., Magrath, I. T., Chattopadhyay, S. K., Biggar, R. J., and Gerber, P. (1978). A new tumour-derived transforming strain of Epstein-Barr virus. *Nature*, **272**, 629–631.

Pudney, V. A., Leese, A. M., Rickinson, A. B., and Hislop, A.D. (2005). CD8+ immunodominance among Epstein-Barr virus lytic cycle antigens directly reflects the efficiency of antigen presentation in lytically infected cells. *J. Exp. Med.*, **201**, 349–360.

Raab-Traub, N. and Flynn, K. (1986). The structure of the termini of the Epstein–Barr virus as a marker of clonal cellular proliferation. *Cell*, **47**, 883–889.

Rabson, M., Gradoville, L., Heston, L., and Miller, G. (1982). Nonimmortalising P3J-HR-1 Epstein–Barr virus: a deletion mutant of its transforming parent, Jijoye. *J. Virol.*, **44**, 834–844.

Radkov, S. A., Bain, M., Farrell, P. J., West, M., Rowe, M., and Allday, M. J. (1997). Epstein–Barr virus EBNA3C represses Cp, the major promoter for EBNA expression, but has no effect on the promoter of the cell gene CD21. *J. Virol.*, **71**, 8552–8562.

Radkov, S. A., Touitou, R., Brehm, A., Rowe, M., West, M., Kouzarides, T. and Allday, M. J. (1999). Epstein–Barr virus nuclear antigen 3C interacts with histone deacetylase to repress transcription. *J. Virol.*, **73**, 5688–5697.

Ragoczy, T. and Miller, G. (1999). Role of the Epstein–Barr virus Rta protein in activation of distinct classes of viral lytic genes. *J. Virol.*, **73**, 9858–9866.

Ragoczy, T. and Miller, G. (2001). Autostimulation of the Epstein–Barr virus BRLF1 promoter is mediated through consensus Sp1 and Sp3 binding sites. *J. Virol.*, **75**, 5240–5251.

Reischl, U., Gerdes, C., Motz, M., and Wolf, H. (1996). Expression and purification of an Epstein–Barr virus encoded 23-kDa protein and charcterisation of its immunological properties. *J. Virol. Meth.*, **57**, 71–85.

Ressing, M. E., Keating, S. E., van Leeuwen, D. *et al.* (2005). Impaired transporter associated with antigen processing-dependent peptide transport during productive EBV infection. *J. Immunol.*, **174**, 6829–6838.

Rickinson, A. B. and Kieff, E. (2001). Epstein–Barr virus. In Knipe, D. M. and Howley, P. M. (eds.), *Fields Virology*. Lippincott Williams and Wilkins, Philadelphia, pp. 2575–2627.

Rickinson, A. B., Rowe, M., Hart, I. J. *et al.* (1984). T-cell-mediated regression of "spontaneous" and of Epstein–Barr virus-induced B-cell transformation *in vitro*: studies with cyclosporin A. *Cell. Immunol.*, **87**, 646–658.

Rivailler, P., Cho, Y., and Wang, F. (2002). Complete genomic sequence of an Epstein–Barr virus-related herpesvirus naturally infecting a new world primate: a defining point in the evolution of oncogenic lymphocryptoviruses. *J. Virol.*, **76**, 12055–12068.

Roberts, M. L. and Cooper, N. R. (1998). Activation of a ras-MAPK-dependent pathway by Epstein–Barr virus latent membrane protein 1 is essential for cellular transformation. *Virology*, **240**, 93–99.

Robertson, E. S. (1997). The Epstein–Barr virus EBNA3 protein family as regulators of transcription. *EBV Rep.*, **4**, 143–150.

Roizman, B. and Knipe, D. M. (2001). Herpes simplex viruses and their replication. In Knipe, D. M. and Howley, P. M. (eds.), *Fields Virology*. Lippincott Williams & Wilkins, Philadelphia, pp. 2399–2459.

Rooney, C. M., Rowe, D. T., Ragot, T., and Farrell, P. J. (1989). The spliced BZLF1 gene of Epstein–Barr virus (EBV) transactivates an early EBV promoter and induces the virus productive cycle. *J. Virol.*, **63**, 3109–3116.

Rowe, M., Rowe, D. T., Gregory, C. D. *et al.* (1987). Differences in B cell growth phenotype reflect novel patterns of Epstein–Barr virus latent gene expression in Burkitt's lymphoma cells. *EMBO J.*, **6**, 2743–2751.

Ruf, I. K., Rhyne, P. W., Yang, C., Cleveland, J. L., and Sample, J. T. (2000). Epstein–Barr virus small RNAs potentiate tumourigenicity of Burkitt lymphoma cells independently of an effect on apoptosis. *J. Virol.*, **74**, 10223–10228.

Sakai, T., Taniguchi, Y., Tamura, K. *et al.* (1998). Functional replacement of the intracellular region of the Notch1 receptor by Epstein–Barr virus nuclear antigen 2. *J. Virol.*, **72**, 6034–6039.

Salek-Ardakani, S., Stuart, A. D., Arrand, J. E., Lyons, S., Arrand, J. R., and Mackett, M. (2001). High level expression and purification of the Epstein–Barr virus encoded cytokine viral interleukin 10: efficient removal of endotoxin. *Cytokine*, **17**, 1–13.

Sam, C. K., Brooks, L. A., Niedobitek, G., Young, L. S., Prasad, U., and Rickinson, A. B. (1993). Analysis of Epstein–Barr virus infection in nasopharyngeal biospies from a group at high risk of nasopharyngeal carcinoma. *Int. J. Cancer*, **53**, 957–962.

Sample, J., Young, L., Martin, B. *et al.* (1990). Epstein–Barr virus types 1 and 2 differ in their EBNA-3A, EBNA-3B and EBNA-3C genes. *J. Virol.*, **64**, 4084–4092.

Sample, J. T., Henson, E., and Sample, C. (1992). The Epstein–Barr virus nuclear protein 1 promoter active in type 1 latency is autoregulated. *J. Virol.*, **66**, 4654–4661.

Saridakis, V., Sheng, Y., Sarkari, F. *et al.* (2005) Structure of the p53 binding domain of HAUSP/USP7 bound to Epstein-Barr nuclear antigen 1: implications for EBV-mediated immortalization. *Mol. Cell.*, **18,** 25–36.

Schepers, A., Pich, D., Manketz, J., and Hammerschmidt, W. (1993). *Cis*-acting elements in the lytic origin of replication of Epstein–Barr virus. *J. Virol.*, **67**, 4237–4245.

Schmaus, S., Wolf, H., and Schwarzmann, F. (2004). The reading frame BPLF1 of Epstein–Barr virus: a homologue of herpes simplex protein VP16. *Virus Genes*, **29**, 267–277.

Scholle, F., Bendt, K. M., and Raab-Traub, N. (2000). Epstein–Barr virus LMP2A transforms epithelial cells, inhibits cell differentiation, and activates Akt. *J. Virol.*, **74**, 10681–10689.

Segouffin, C., Gruffat, H., and Sergeant, A. (1996). Repression of RAZ of Epstein–Barr virus bZIP transcription factor EB1 is dimerization independent. *J. Gen. Virol.*, **77**, 1529–1536.

Semmes, O. J., Chen, L., Sarisky, R. T., Gao, Z., Zhong, L., and Hayward, S. D. (1998). Mta has properties of an RNA export protein and increases cytoplasmic accumulation of Epstein–Barr virus replication gene mRNA. *J. Virol.*, **72**, 9526–9534.

Serio, T. R., Kolman, J. L., and Miller, G. (1997). Late gene expression from the Epstein–Barr virus BcLF1 and BFRF3 promoters does not require DNA replication in cis. *J. Virol.*, **71**, 8726–8734.

Serio, T. R., Cahill, N., Prout, M. E., and Miller, G. (1998). A functionally distinct TATA box required for late progression through the Epstein–Barr virus life cycle. *J. Virol.*, **72**, 8338–8343.

Sheng, W., Decaussin, G., Sumner, S., and Ooka, T. (2001). N-terminal domain of BARF1 gene encoded by Epstein–Barr virus is essential for malignant transformation of rodent fibroblasts and activation of BCL-2. *Oncogene*, **20**, 1176–1185.

Sheng, W., Decaussin, G., Ligout, A., Takada, K., and Ooka, T. (2003). Malignant transformation of Epstein–Barr virus-negative Akata cells by introduction of the BARF1 gene carried by Epstein–Barr virus. *J. Virol.*, **77**, 3859–3865.

Silins, S. L. and Sculley, T. B. (1994). Modulation of vimentin, the CD40 activation antigen and Burkitt's lymphoma antigen (CD77) by the Epstein–Barr virus nuclear antigen EBNA-4. *Virology*, **202**, 16–24.

Sinclair, A. J. and Farrell, P. J. (1995). Host cell requirements for efficient infection of quiescent primary B lymphocytes by Epstein–Barr virus. *J. Virol.*, **69**, 5461–5468.

Sinclair, A. J., Brimmell, M., Shanahan, F., and Farrell, P. J. (1991). Pathways of activation of the Epstein–Barr virus productive cycle. *J. Virol.*, **65**, 2237–2244.

Sinclair, A. J., Palmero, I., Peters, G., and Farrell, P. J. (1994). EBNA-2 and EBNA-LP cooperate to cause G0 and G1 transition during immortalisation of resting human B lymphocytes by Epstein–Barr virus. *EMBO J.*, **13**, 3321–3328.

Sitki-Green, D., Covington, M., and Raab-Traub, N. (2003). Compartmentalization and transmission of multiple Epstein–Barr virus strains in asymptomatic carriers. *J. Virol.*, **77**, 1840–1847.

Smith, P. R., de Jesus, O., Turner, D. *et al.* (2000). Structure and coding content of CST (BART) family RNAs of Epstein–Barr virus. *J. Virol.*, **74**, 3082–3092.

Sommer, P., Kremmer, E., Bier, S. *et al.* (1996). Cloning and expression of the Epstein–Barr virus-encoded dUTPase: patients with acute, reactivated or chronic virus infection develop antibodies against the enzyme. *J. Gen. Virol.*, **77**, 2795–2805.

Speck, S., Chatila, T., and Flemington, E. K. (1997). Reactivation of Epstein–Barr virus: regulation and function of the BZLF1 gene. *Trends Microbiol.*, **5**, 399–405.

Speck, S. H. and Strominger, J. L. (1989). Transcription of Epstein–Barr virus in latently infected, growth-transformed lymphocytes. *Adv. Viral Oncol.*, **8**, 133–150.

Srivastava, G., Wong, K. Y., Chiang, A. K., Lam, K. Y., and Tao, Q. (2000). Coinfection of multiple strains of Epstein–Barr virus in immunocompetent normal individuals: reassessment of the viral carrier state. *Blood*, **95**, 2443–2445.

Stolzenberg, M. C., Debouze, S., Ng, M. *et al.* (1996). Purified recombinant EBV desoxyribonuclease in serological diagnosis of nasopharyngeal carcinoma. *Int. J. Cancer*, **66**, 337–341.

Strobl, L. J., Hofelmayr, H., Marschall, G., Brielmeier, M., Bornkamm, G. W., and Zimber-Strobl, U. (2000). Activated Notch1 modulates gene expression in B cells similarly to Epstein–Barr viral nuclear antigen 2. *J. Virol.*, **74**, 1727–1735.

Strockbine, L. D., Cohen, J. I., Farrah, T. *et al.* (1998). The Epstein–Barr virus BARF1 gene encodes a novel, soluble colony-stimulating factor-1 receptor. *J. Virol.*, **72**, 4014–4021.

Stuart, A. D., Stewart, J. P., Arrand, J. R., and Mackett, M. (1995). The Epstein–Barr virus encoded cytokine viral interleukin-10 enhances transformation of human B lymphocytes. *Oncogene*, **11**, 1711–1719.

Sugano, N., Chen, W., Roberts, M. L., and Cooper, N. R. (1997). Epstein–Barr virus binding to CD21 activates the initial viral promoter via NF-κB induction. *J. Exp. Med.*, **186**, 731–737.

Sugawara, Y., Mizugaki, Y., Uchida, T. *et al.* (1999). Detection of Epstein–Barr virus (EBV) in hepatocellular carcinoma tissue: a novel EBV latency characterised by the absence of EBV-encoded small RNA expression. *Virology*, **256**, 196–202.

Swaminathan, S., Tomkinson, B., and Kieff, E. (1991). Recombinant Epstein–Barr virus with small RNA (EBER) genes deleted transforms lymphocytes and replicates *in vivo*. *Proc. Natl Acad. Sci. USA*, **88**, 1546–1550.

Swaminathan, S., Hesselton, R., Sullivan, J., and Kieff, E. (1993). Epstein–Barr virus recombinants with specifically mutated BCRF1 genes. *J. Virol.*, **67**, 7406–7413.

Sylla, B. S., Hung, S. C., Davidson, D. M. *et al.* (1998). Epstein–Barr virus-transforming protein latent infection membrane protein 1 activates transcription factor NF-κB through a pathway that includes the NF-κB-inducing kinase and the IκB kinases IKKα and IKKβ. *Proc. Natl Acad. Sci. USA*, **95**, 10106–10111.

Szekely, L., Selivanova, G., Magnusson, K. P., Klein, G., and Wiman, K. G. (1993). EBNA-5, an Epstein–Barr virus-encoded nuclear antigen, binds to the retinoblastoma and p53 proteins. *Proc. Natl Acad. Sci. USA*, **90**, 5455–5459.

Szyf, M., Elasson, L., Mann, V., Klein, G., and Razin, A. (1985). Cellular and viral DNA hypomethylation associated with induction of Epstein–Barr virus lytic cycle. *Proc. Natl Acad. Sci. USA*, **82**, 8090–8094.

Tanner, J., Weis, J., Fearon, D. T., Whang, Y., and Kieff, E. (1987). Epstein–Barr virus gp350/220 binding to the B lymphocyte C3d receptor mediates adsorption, capping, and endocytosis. *Cell*, **50**, 203–213.

Tao, Q., Robertson, K. D., Manns, A., Hildesheim, A., and Ambinder, R. F. (1998). Epstein–Barr virus (EBV) in endemic Burkitt's lymphoma: Molecular analysis of primary tumour tissue. *Blood*, **91**, 1373–1381.

Tarodi, B., Subramanian, T., and Chinnadurai, G. (1994). Epstein–Barr virus BHRF1 protein protects against cell death induced by DNA-damaging agents and heterologous viral infection. *Virology*, **201**, 404–407.

Thomas, C., Dankesreiter, A., Wolf, H., and Schwarzmann, F. (2003). The BZLF1 promoter of Epstein–Barr virus is controlled by E box-/HI-motif-binding factors during virus latency. *J. Gen. Virol.*, **84**, 959–964.

Thorley-Lawson, D. A. (2001). Epstein–Barr virus: exploiting the immune system. *Nat. Rev. Immunol.*, **1**, 75–82.

Thorley-Lawson, D. A. and Poodry, C. A. (1982). Identification and isolation of the main component (gp350–gp220) of Epstein–Barr virus responsible for generating neutralising antibodies *in vivo*. *J. Virol.*, **43**, 730–736.

Toczyski, D. P., Matera, A. G., Ward, D. C., and Steitz, J. A. (1994). The Epstein–Barr virus (EBV) small RNA EBER1 binds and relocalises ribosomal protein L22 in EBV-infected human B lymphocytes. *Proc. Natl Acad. Sci. USA*, **91**, 3463–3467.

Tsurumi, T., Kobayashi, A., Tamai, K. *et al.* (1996). Epstein–Barr virus single-stranded DNA-binding protein: purification, characterisation, and action on DNA synthesis by the viral DNA polymerase. *Virology*, **222**, 352–364.

Tugizov, S. M., Berline, J. W., and Palefsky, J. M. (2003). Epstein–Barr virus infection of polarized tongue and nasopharyngeal epithelial cells. *Nat. Med.*, **9**, 307–314.

Uchida, J., Yasui, T., Takaoka-Shichijo, Y. *et al.* (1999). Mimicry of CD40 signals by Epstein–Barr virus LMP1 in B lymphocyte responses. *Science*, **286**, 300–303.

van Beek, J., Brink, A. A., Vervoort, M. B. *et al.* (2003). *In vivo* transcription of the Epstein–Barr virus (EBV) *Bam*HI-A region without associated *in vivo* BARF0 protein expression in multiple EBV-associated disorders. *J. Gen. Virol.*, **84**, 2647–2659.

van Grunsven, W. M., van Heerde, E. C., de Haard, H. J., Spaan, W. J., and Middeldorp, J. M. (1993). Gene mapping and expression of two immunodominant Epstein–Barr virus capsid proteins. *J. Virol.*, **67**, 3908–3916.

Walling, D. M. and Raab-Traub, N. (1994). Epstein–Barr virus intrastrain recombination in oral hairy leukoplakia. *J. Virol.*, **68**, 7909–7913.

Walling, D. M., Brown, A. L., Etienne, W., Keitel, W. A., and Ling, P. D. (2003). Multiple Epstein–Barr virus infections in healthy individuals. *J. Virol.*, **77**, 6546–6550.

Wang, F., Gregory, C., Sample, C. *et al.* (1990). Epstein–Barr virus latent membrane protein (LMP1) and nuclear proteins 2 and 3C are effectors of phenotypic changes in B lymphocytes: EBNA-2 and LMP1 cooperatively induce CD23. *J. Virol.*, **64**, 2309–2318.

Wei, M. X. and Ooka, T. (1989). A transforming function of the BARF1 gene encoded by Epstein–Barr virus. *EMBO J.*, **8**, 2897–2903.

Wei, M. X., Moulin, J. C., Decaussin, G., Berger, F., and Ooka, T. (1994). Expression and tumourigenicity of the Epstein–Barr virus BARF1 gene in human Louckes B-lymphocyte cell line. *Cancer Res.*, **54**, 1843–1848.

Wei, M. X., de Turenne-Tessier, M., Decaussin, G., Benet, G., and Ooka, T. (1997). Establishment of a monkey kidney epithelial cell line with the BARF1 open reading frame from Epstein–Barr virus. *Oncogene*, **14**, 3073–3081.

Wilson, J. B., Bell, J. L., and Levine, A. J. (1996). Expression of Epstein–Barr virus nuclear antigen1 induces B cell neoplasia in transgenic mice. *EMBO J.*, **15**, 3117–3126.

Wu, F. Y., Chen, H., Wang, S. E. *et al.* (2003). CCAAT/Enhancer binding protein a interacts with ZTA and mediates ZTA-induced p21CIP-1 accumulation and G1 cell cycle arrest during the Epstein–Barr virus lytic cycle. *J. Virol.*, **2003**, 1481–1500.

Yao, Q. Y., Ogan, P., Rowe, M., Wood, M., and Rickinson, A. B. (1989). Epstein–Barr virus infected B cells persist in the circulation of acyclovir-treated virus carriers. *Int. J. Cancer*, **43**, 67–71.

Yao, Q. Y., Rowe, M., Martin, B., Young, L. S., and Rickinson, A. B. (1991). The Epstein–Barr virus carrier state: dominance of a single growth transforming isolate in the blood and in the oropharynx of healthy virus carriers. *J. Gen. Virol.*, **72**, 1579–1590.

Yao, Q. Y., Tierney, R. J., Croom-Carter, D. *et al.* (1996a). Isolation of inter-typic recombinants of Epstein–Barr virus from T cell immunocompromised individuals. *J. Virol.*, **70**, 4895–4903.

Yao, Q. Y., Tierney, R. J., Croom-Carter, D. *et al.* (1996b). Frequency of multiple Epstein–Barr virus infections in T cell-immunocompromised individuals. *J. Virol.*, **70**, 4884–4894.

Yao, Q. Y., Croom-Carter, D., Tierney, R. J. *et al.* (1998). Epidemiology of infection with Epstein–Barr virus types 1 and 2: lessons from the study of a T-cell-immunocompromised haemophilic cohort. *J. Virol.*, **72**, 4352–4363.

Yokoyama, N., Fujii, K., Hirata, M. *et al.* (1999). Assembly of the Epstein–Barr virus BBLF4, BSLF1 and BBLF2/3 proteins and their interactive properties. *J. Gen. Virol.*, **80**, 2879–2887.

Young, L. S. and Murray, P. G. (2003). Epstein–Barr virus and oncogenesis: from latent genes to tumours. *Oncogene*, **22**, 5108–5121.

Young, L. S., Yao, Q. Y., Rooney, C. M. *et al.* (1987). New type B isolates of Epstien–Barr virus from Burkitt's lymphoma and from normal individuals in endemic areas. *J. Gen. Virol.*, **68**, 2853–2862.

Young, L. S., Dawson, C. W., Clark, D. *et al.* (1988). Epstein–Barr virus gene expression in nasopharyngeal carcinoma. *J. Gen. Virol.*, **69**, 1051–1065.

Zalani, S., Holley-Guthrie, E. and Kenney, S. (1995). The Zif268 cellular transcription factor activates expression of the Epstein–Barr virus immediate-early BRLF1 promoter. *J. Virol.*, **69**, 3816–3823.

Zalani, S., Coppage, A., Holley-Guthrie, E., and Kenney, S. (1997). The cellular YY1 transcription factor binds a *cis*-acting, negative regulating element in the Epstein–Barr virus BRLF1 promoter. *J. Virol.*, **71**, 3268–3274.

Zeng, Y., Gong, C. H., Jan, M. G., Fun, Z., Zhang, L. G., and Li, H. Y. (1983). Detection of Epstein–Barr virus IgA/EA antibody for diagnosis of nasopharyngeal carcinoma by immunoautoradiography. *Int. J. Cancer*, **31**, 599–601.

Zeng, Y., Middeldorp, J. M., Madjar, J. J., and Ooka, T. (1997). A major DNA binding protein encoded by BALF2 open reading frame of Epstein–Barr virus (EBV) forms a complex with other EBV DNA-binding proteins: DNAase, EA-D, and DNA polymerase. *Virology*, **239**, 285–295.

Zeng, M. S., Li, D. J., Liu, Q. L. *et al.* (2005). Genomic sequence analysis of Epstein–Barr virus strain GD1 from a nasopharyngeal carcinoma patient. *J. Virol.*, **79**, 15323–15330.

Zimmermann, J. and Hammerschmidt, W. (1995). Structure and role of the terminal repeats of Epstein–Barr virus in processing and packaging of virion DNA. *J. Virol.*, **69**, 3147–3155.

zur Hausen, H., Brink, A. A., Craanen, M. E., Middeldorp, J. M., Meijer, C. J., and van den Brule, A. J. (2000). Unique transcription pattern of Epstein–Barr virus (EBV) in EBV-carrying gastric adenocarcinomas: expression of the transforming BARF1 gene. *Cancer Res.*, **60**, 2745–2748.

28

KSHV gene expression and regulation

Thomas F. Schulz[1] and Yuan Chang[2]

[1]Department of Virology, Hannover Medical School, Germany
[2]Molecular Virology Program, University of Pittsburgh, PA, USA

Introduction

In this chapter, both in vivo and in vitro KSHV viral gene expression patterns are described. Observations in both systems have been critical for the identification of viral proteins contributing to the pathogenic properties of this virus and for our appreciation of how this virus persists and replicates in the course of naturally occurring infections, the vast majority of which are asymptomatic (see *Epidemiology*). In contrast to other human herpesviruses, cell-free infection with KSHV in vitro is still inefficient and only a few studies have investigated viral gene expression following *de novo* infection. However, informative studies using *in situ* hybridization (ISH), immunohistochemistry (IHC), and various methods of transcript analysis have been carried out with stably infected, primary effusion lymphoma (PEL)-derived cell lines and, to a lesser extent, biopsy samples. Gradually, a picture on viral gene expression patterns and their regulation in different cell types is beginning to emerge.

Viral gene expression patterns in culture

PEL derived cell lines

PEL cell lines remain the most tractable system for examining KSHV viral gene expression. The vast majority of cells are infected latently and express a restricted repertoire of genes, while a small percentage (this varies from cell line to cell line, usually in the order of 1%–5%) of cells spontaneously switch into the lytic replication cycle. Lytic reactivation can be enhanced (up to 20% in some cell lines) in this system by chemical treatment with butyrate or phorbol esters. Despite the convenience of working with PEL cell lines, limitations exist: (1) if a bulk analysis of all cells in such a culture is carried out using Northern blots or RT-PCR, both the group of genuinely latent genes and that of strongly expressed, albeit only in a few cells, lytic genes may be detected, (2) chemical manipulation may have extraneous and secondary effects on viral gene expression, and (3) expression patterns in PEL B cell lines may not extend to expression patterns in KSHV infected tissues, in particular, spindle cells. With these caveats in mind, Fig. 28.1 shows an overview of the KSHV viral genome and the position of individual viral genes. The color coding reflects their expression during the different stages of lytic replication or latency. The coding is the result of a comparison of three publications that used gene arrays covering the entire viral genome (Jenner *et al.*, 2001; Paulose-Murphy *et al.*, 2001; Nakamura *et al.*, 2003), and two earlier publications using Northern blots to investigate the basal expression and induction of KSHV genes in PEL cell lines following treatment with butyrate or phorbol esters (Sarid *et al.*, 1998; Sun *et al.*, 1999).

The first report to systematically analyze the expression pattern, by Northern blot, of the vast majority of KSHV genes in PEL cells before and after induction of the lytic cycle (Sarid *et al.*, 1998) distinguished three categories of viral genes: class I genes, expressed during latency and not upregulated by chemical induction; class II genes, characterized by a baseline expression of variable abundance (high, moderate, and low) before, and increased expression after, chemical induction; class III genes that are only expressed after chemical induction. Class I genes comprised those marked in red in Fig. 28.1, i.e. ORF73 (encoding LANA1), ORF72 (vCYC), and ORF71/K13 (vFLIP). Transcripts most likely related to ORFs K2 (vIL6), ORF70, K4 (vMIP-II), K5 (MIR1), K6 (vMIP-I), K7 (PAN/nut-1/T1.1 RNA), K8 (bZIP), ORF57, the vIRFs locus, and T0.7/Kaposin were classified as class II genes, as were at least another five transcripts that could not be unambiguously assigned to

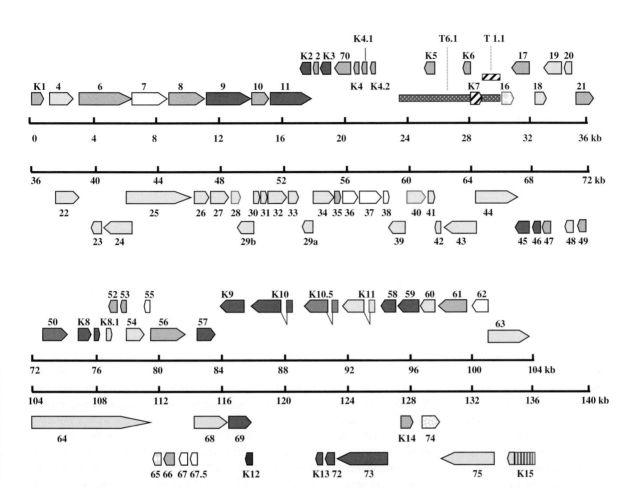

Fig. 28.1. KSHV gene expression in PEL cell lines and biopsy samples. This Figure summarizes the expression of individual KSHV genes in PEL cells during latency and following reactivation of the lytic cycle by treatment with TPA, Na-butyrate or heterologous expression of RTA by transfection or transduction. Also included are results from in situ hybridization or immunohistochemistry studies on biopsy samples of KS, MCD or PEL tumors. As discussed in the text, the color-coding is based on a comparison of several reports that studied KSHV genes by Northern blot, real time PCR or DNA array. (See color plate section.)

- ■ Latent gene
- ■ Latent gene in B cells only
- ■ Latent gene in KS spindle cells in vivo; early (in some studies delayed) expression kinetics in PEL cells in vitro
- ■ Immediate–early gene as judged by cycloheximide resistance
- ■ Very rapid onset of gene expression in at least 2 studies
- ▨ Early lytic transcript: TPA inducible, unaffected by PFA
- □ Delayed onset of gene expression
- □ Late gene expression profile
- □ Late gene expression profile confirmed by PAA sensitivity
- ▨ Discrepant results in different gene array studies

individual ORFs. The remainder were considered class III genes. The existence of Class II transcripts outside of the classical dichotomous lytic-latent classification may, in part, be explain by a recent publication from H. Chang and colleagues which showed that a subset of immunoregulatory and growth promoting KSHV genes can be activated by RTA-independent notch signaling. Further, detection of these transcripts was shown to be dissociated from the full repertoire of lytic viral gene expression (Chang et al. 2005).

A subsequent study (Sun et al., 1999) attempted to relate the pattern of viral gene expression seen following the induction of the lytic cycle by treatment with Na-butyrate or phorbol-12-myristate-13-acetate (TPA) to the conventional cascade of herpesviral gene expression

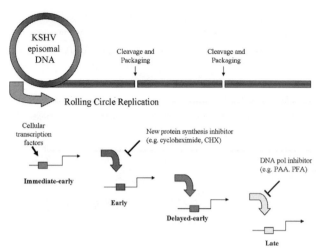

Fig. 28.2. KSHV lytic replication. Herpesvirus lytic replication is characterized by wide-spread gene activation, classically in an ordered cascade of sequential induction. The full expression of this cascade can be chemically manipulated to temporally distinguish immediate early, early and late lytic genes. Lytic activation is believed to result in a rapid increase in virion DNA as well as host cell death.

during lytic replication (Fig. 28.2). This conventional classification distinguishes immediate–early, early, and late genes: Immediate–early genes are expressed immediately following viral entry, do not require the *de novo* expression of viral proteins and are therefore resistant to treatment of the infected cell with cycloheximide. Early genes are sensitive to cycloheximide (i.e., require *de novo* protein synthesis in the infected cell) but are expressed prior to the replication of the viral genome and therefore are resistant to PAA or PFA.

Sun *et al.* (1999) classified ORF50 (RTA) as an immediate–early gene on the basis of its early onset of transcription (8 hours) following treatment with Na-butyrate and (only partial) resistance to cycloheximide. In spite of a similar rapid onset of expression seen with several other genes (e.g., h vIL6, vMIP-II, PAN/nut-1, vTS), none of these other genes examined by Sun *et al.* were resistant to cycloheximide and these therefore represent early genes. Since none of the gene array studies (see below) examined cycloheximide resistance, ORF50/RTA is therefore the only gene for which at least a partial resistance to cycloheximide has been demonstrated. It could be argued that the criterion of cycloheximide resistance should not be overinterpreted since reactivation rather than de novo infection (as in the classical experiments with alpha herpesviruses) was examined in all these studies, and that the designation of "immediate–early" for a KSHV gene on the basis of cycloheximide resistance is therefore problematic. However, ORF50/RTA stands out as the only KSHV gene with rapid expression kinetics for which this property has been demonstrated and is also the first viral gene to be expressed following *de novo* infection. Functional studies (see below and elsewhere in this book), as well as a systematic survey of viral genes whose expression is induced, directly or indirectly, by RTA (Nakamura *et al.*, 2003), have shown that RTA is the central regulator of the lytic replication cycle. It has therefore been labeled pink in Fig. 28.1.

In addition to ORF50/RTA, a few other viral genes have been shown to be resistant to cycloheximide in chemically induced PEL cell lines and thus to have immediate–early characteristics (Zhu *et al.*, 1999; Haque *et al.*, 2000; Rimessi *et al.*, 2001). In their study, Zhu *et al.* (1999) found the transcripts for ORFK8, ORF45 and ORFK4.2, in addition to that for ORF50/RTA, to have immediate-early characteristics. Haque *et al.* (2000) reported this for the ORFK5 transcript and Rimessi *et al.* (2001) for the ORFK3 mRNA.

Four groups (Jenner *et al.*, 2001; Paulose-Murphy *et al.*, 2001; Nakamura *et al.*, 2003; Fakhari & Dittmer, 2002; Dittmer, 2003) have recently examined KSHV gene expression patterns in PEL cells by DNA array or real time PCR methods. All studies attempted to group individual viral genes into categories reflecting their onset or rate of expression. The results correlate on the whole, except for a few genes classified differently by several studies. These are indicated by open boxes in Fig. 28.1. All studies group ORFs 73 (LANA1), 72 (vCYC), 71/K13 (vFLIP) together as expressed in PEL cell lines prior to, and increasing only moderately following, induction of the lytic cycle ("latent" or "constitutive" genes). Based on *in situ* hybridization or immunohistochemistry, these genes, or their proteins, are expressed in the majority of infected cells in vivo (see below). These are therefore, marked in red in Fig. 28.1. As outlined below, these three viral genes are expressed from two alternatively spliced mRNAs (Fig. 28.4), with vCYC and vFLIP expressed from the same bicistronic mRNA. In spite of the general consensus that these are latent transcripts, the study by Nakamura *et al.* observed an increased expression of these mRNAs early (ORF71/ORF72) or late (ORF73) after triggering the lytic cycle by RTA expression. Since this has not been seen when Na-butyrate or phorbol esters were used to induce the lytic cycle, it may reflect the more "physiological" induction of the lytic cycle by RTA in this experiment and indicate that this group of mRNAs, although expressed during latent persistence, may increase during lytic replication.

The non-coding nuclear RNA variously referred to as PAN, nut-1 or T1.1, and T0.7 or Kaposin, one of several transcripts derived from ORFK12, were the first abundant transcripts to be identified in KS biopsies (Zhong et al., 1996). On Northern blots from uninduced vs. induced PEL cell lines both mRNAs show basal expression that is increased upon induction of the lytic cycle (Sarid et al., 1998; Sun et al., 1999) and were designated as class II transcripts by Sarid et al. In a gene array study, Jenner et al. found that the expression kinetics of T0.7/Kaposin resembled that of ORFK10 (these were designated latent/lytic transcripts), while that of T1.1/PAN clustered with those of ORFK7, ORFK14 and other early genes, grouped together as "primary lytic" genes. However, in a similarly designed study by Paulose-Murphy et al. (2001) and in that by Nakamura et al. (2003) T0.7/Kaposin and K10 did not group together, with T0.7/Kaposin having later expression kinetics. Similarly, T1.1/PAN, ORFK7, ORFK14 did not group together in these two studies. We therefore chose a separate color coding in Fig. 28.1 for T0.7/Kaposin to reflect its probable latent nature in KS spindle cells in vivo. In spite of the controversial expression kinetics for T 1.1/PAN and K7, reflected in a hatched box in Fig. 28.1, it is clear that both are lytic genes.

Recently, in the region encompassing both T1.1/PAN and K7, Taylor et al. (2005) found a large transcript of approximately 6.1 kb by northern blot hybridization designated T6.1. This transcript is inducible with TPA, but is resistant to PFA. RACE identified the 5' end of the transcript at nucleotide 23,586, and 5 excised clones from a screening of a PEL cDNA lambda phage library identified the 3' end of the transcript at nucleotide 29,741 making the transcript co-terminal with T1.1/PAN (Fig. 28.1). This transcript encompasses K7 in the same orientation and ORFs K5 and K6 in the reverse orientation. Thus far, this 6.1 kb transcript is the largest found in the KSHV genome, but the presence of large lytic transcripts is not unique to KSHV and have been reported for other herpesviruses. Smuda et al. (1997) found high molecular mass overlapping early lytic transcripts of 6 kb, 8 kb, 10 kb, and 14 kb within the human cytomegalovirus genome. Wirth et al. (1989) identified a 6 kb immediate–early transcript and six late lytic transcripts ranging from 4.5 kb to >8 kb in bovine herpesvirus 1. It is unclear why these herpesviruses produce such large transcripts, although it has been postulated that their size may lead to RNA stability by the formation of pseudoknots. Regardless of function, the presence of this large transcript has implications in the examination of expression patterns for overlapping ORFs if DNA array and real time PCR methods are used.

The KSHV genome contains a region encoding a series of proteins with homologies to cellular interferon regulatory factors (IRFs). In this region one spliced gene, K10.5, shows latent gene expression in PEL cell lines in vitro (Rivas et al., 2001; Cunningham et al., 2003) and the corresponding protein, LANA2 or vIRF3, has been demonstrated by immunohistochemistry in all infected B cells in MCD and PEL in vivo, suggesting a B-lineage specific latent expression pattern (Rivas et al., 2001). However, the study by Nakamura et al. (2003) indicates that its expression is increased at a late stage following activation of the lytic cycle by RTA in a PEL cell line. Because of its B-cell specific expression pattern, K10.5/vIRF3 has been given its own (light brown) color coding in Fig. 28.1.

Three other genes in this locus, ORFs K9, K10, K11, are induced after activation of the lytic cycle (Cunningham et al., 2003; Nakamura et al., 2001; Paulose-Murphy et al., 2001; Jenner et al., 2001). Jenner et al. (2001) classified ORFK10, encoding vIRF4, as a "latent/lytic" gene, since its expression kinetics was similar to that of the T0.7/Kaposin transcript. The two other published gene array studies (Paulose-Murphy et al., 2001; Nakamura et al., 2003) concur to the extent that the ORFK10 transcript increases early after induction of the lytic cycle but group it with several other early transcripts. We have based our color coding of this gene on their results. In a similar manner, ORFK9 appears to be expressed relatively early, while in comparison ORFK11 expression appears to come on somewhat later. The upstream exon of K11, termed K11.1 in the study by Nakamura et al. (2003) and referred to as vIRF2 by Jenner et al. (2001), was classified in an earlier expression group than the second K11 exon by Nakamura et al. (2003), but in the same group as the second exon by Jenner et al. (2001).

Although the three gene array studies published so far do not always concur on the expression kinetics of individual viral genes, as illustrated by the above examples, there is broad agreement that viral proteins required for DNA replication or gene expression are produced earlier in the lytic cycle than viral structural proteins necessary for assembly of new virions. Likewise, lytic viral proteins known to be expressed in a slightly higher number of productively infected cells in vivo such as vIL6 or PF8 (see below) appear to be encoded by transcripts expressed in PEL cells early during the lytic cycle, whereas a structural glycoprotein encoded by ORFK8.1 and expressed only in few cells in vivo has been grouped with late transcripts. However, it needs to be emphasized that other factors than the stage of the lytic cycle may affect the expression of certain genes, e.g., vIL6, in vivo. However, in the case of vGPCR, the viral homologue of a G-coupled receptor that has been proposed to play an important role in KS pathogenesis by virtue of its ability to induce the secretion of VEGF and other paracrine factors from infected cells, the available data are controversial. While its expression kinetics in PEL cells resembled that of an early gene in the study by Jenner et al. and Nakamura et al., Paulose-Murphy et al. found a delayed onset and Sun et al. (1999) showed that its transcript was at least partially sensitive to PAA, suggesting late viral gene expression. However, using Northern blots Kirshner et al. (1999) did not see an inhibition of the vGPCR mRNA by PAA and classified it as an early lytic gene.

Viral gene expression in newly infected cultured endothelial, epithelial or fibroblast cultures

Experiments with KSHV released from PEL cell lines after chemical induction, or with recombinant KSHV preparations induced in Vero or 293 cells, have shown that KSHV can infect a wide variety of cultured cells belonging to several lineages (endothelial, epithelial, fibroblast) with the notable exception of lymphoid cell lines (Bechtel et al., 2003; Lagunoff et al., 2002; Moses et al., 1999; Vieira et al., 1997; Renne et al., 1998; Gao et al., 2003; Ciufo et al., 2001). It is not know at this time why B lymphocytes are resistant to de novo infection, however, Chen and Lagumoff have shown that naked DNA of a KSHV BAC, engineered with a selectable element, can be introduced into BJAB cells such that virus can be maintained in latency as well as undergo lytic reactivation (Chen and Lagunoff, 2005). In the majority of these reports, KSHV quickly established a latent infection, as defined by the expression of LANA1, in most infected cells. Only a small proportion of infected cells express viral transcripts or proteins characteristic of the lytic replication cycle such as ORF59/PFA, the K8.1 envelope glycoprotein, or the minor capsid protein mCP/SCIP encoded by ORF65 (Renne et al., 1998; Lagunoff et al., 2002; Ciufo et al., 2001; Vieira et al., 1997; Moses et al., 1999; Bechtel et al., 2003). In these latently KSHV-infected cells the lytic replication cycle can be reactivated using phorbol esters (as in PEL cell lines), or by superinfection with CMV (Vieira et al., 1997), and expression of RTA by transfection or transduction can do so in all cell types examined (Bechtel et al., 2003). A possible interpretation of these findings is that events upstream and controlling the expression of RTA are responsible for the blocked lytic replication and default latency in these cells. As discussed above, methylation of CpG residues in the ORF50/RTA promoter may represent such an event (Chen et al., 2001).

In one experimental system, which used a recombinant KSHV carrying a bacterial artificial chromosome and GFP cassette between ORFs 18 and 19, spontaneous transient lytic activation of KSHV in newly infected endothelial cells was observed during the first week of culture which subsided subsequently, giving way to long-term latent infection (Gao et al., 2003). Lytic reactivation in this experimental system was measured by the expression of the minor capsid protein SCIP, encoded by ORF65, and latent infection by expression of LANA1 (Gao et al., 2003).

Investigating early events following virus entry Dezube et al. (2002) found that rapid circularization of the viral genome occurred within 8 hours of infecting cultured endothelial cells with PEL-line derived KSHV. This was followed by the appearance of linear genomes, indicating lytic replication, approximately 72 hours after infection. Expression of the lytic transcripts T1.1/PAN and K8.1 could be detected by Northern blot at 3–6 days, and increased up to days 8–10, after infection. Latent transcripts for ORF72 (vCYC) and ORF73 (LANA1) were first detected on day 8. Interestingly, ORF74 (vGPCR) mRNA expression oscillated between days 1–8 (Dezube et al., 2002).

Viral gene expression early after *de novo* infection of endothelial cell and fibroblast cultures has also been investigated using a KSHV microarray (Krishnan et al., 2004). Following *de novo* infection, a limited number of KSHV genes are initially expressed (Fig. 28.3, Krishnan et al., 2004). However, with the exception of the latent transcripts for LANA1, vCYC and vFLIP, all mRNAs are down-regulated over the following 24 hours and KSHV therefore quickly adopts a transcriptional latency pattern. The first viral transcript to be expressed following *de novo* infection encodes ORF 50/RTA, the central regulator of the viral lytic replication cycle (Krishnan et al., 2004). However, only a limited number of RTA-activated viral genes (see below) show a transient expression. These include the genes for vIL6 (ORFK2), vMIP-II (ORFK4), MIR2 (ORFK5), vMIP-I (ORFK6), vIRF2 (ORF11) and the survivin homologue (ORFK7), which are all thought to play a role in modulating the response to interferon, cytotoxic T-lymphocytes, NK cells or apoptosis. In contrast, many KSHV genes involved in DNA synthesis or encoding structural proteins were not expressed. This pattern of viral gene expression suggests that, unlike α- or β-herpesviruses, KSHV quickly adopts a latent program of gene expression and only transiently expresses a set of genes that counteract the effects of the interferon system – which is induced in endothelial and fibroblast cells very early following KSHV infection (Naranatt et al., 2004) – or other components of the innate or adaptive immune system. Which viral or cellular factors determine this switch into latency and interfere with the completion of the full lytic transcription program is not understood at present and remains one of the most interesting aspects of the control of KSHV gene expression.

Viral gene expression in vivo

Despite the relative ease of working with KSHV infected PEL-derived cell lines, a major problem of studying viral gene expression in such a system is that expression patterns may not reflect that found in infected tissues.

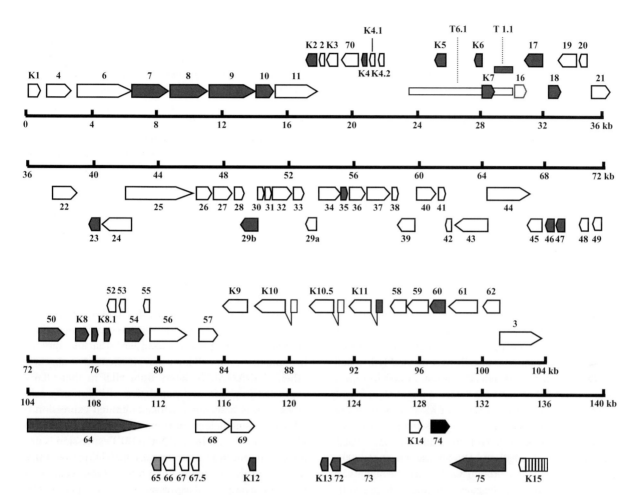

Fig. 28.3. KSHV gene expression pattern in endothelial and fibroblast cells following *de novo* infection. This figure summarizes the expression of individual KSHV genes following *de novo* infection of endothelial and fibroblast cultures reported in Ciufo *et al.*, 2001; Dezube *et al.*, 2002; Bechtel *et al.*, 2003; Gao *et al.*, 2003; Krishnan *et al.*, 2004.
■ Latent gene
■ Immediate-early gene in Krishnan *et al.* (2004)
■ Transient expression during the first days after de novo infection (Dezube *et al.*, 2002; Ciufo *et al.*, 2001; Bechtel *et al.*, 2003; Krishnan *et al.*, 2004)
□ Transient expression during first week of culture (Gao *et al.*, 2003)
▨ Cyclic expression pattern in the study by Dezube *et al.* (2002)

Initial results from immunohistochemistry suggest that some KSHV genes can become dysregulated in tissue culture and that tissue-specific patterns of expression exist. The lack of a KSHV-infected spindle cell line raises additional concerns regarding generalizing findings from infected B cell lines to endothelial-derived KS lesions.

KS lesions

The first studies on viral expression in KS lesions examined the abundance of the T1.1/PAN and T0.7/Kaposin transcripts by *in situ* hybridization. The vast majority of spindle cells comprising KS lesions expressed T0.7/Kaposin in a cytoplasmic distribution with a predicted membrane proclivity (Zhong *et al.*, 1996). By colocalization, a subpopulation (1%–10%) of T0.7/Kaposin positive cells also expressed T1.1/PAN transcripts and is thought to represent cells supporting lytic viral replication. The T1.1/PAN transcripts, although expressed in few cells, were present in high abundance ranging from an estimated 10 000 to 25 000 transcript copies per cell and were targeted to the nuclear compartment (Zhong *et al.*, 1996). Consistent with a transcript expressed in lytic replication, T1.1/PAN also co-localized to the same cell population with probes to the major capsid protein (ORF25) (Staskus et al., 1997) and to the viral GPCR (ORF74) (Kirschner et al., 1999). The transcripts of two other genes, K3, K8 were shown to have a similar distribution to T1.1/Kaposin in KS lesions (Rimessi et al., 2001).

By immunohistochemistry, LANA1 protein is expressed in almost all tumor spindle and endothelial cells (Rainbow et al., 1997; Dupin et al., 1999; Katano et al., 2000). This is consistent with in vivo hybridization studies using the T0.7/Kaposin riboprobe as a surrogate marker for viral latent replication. Although vCYC and vFLIP proteins have not been formally shown to be expressed in a similar manner as LANA1, *in situ* hybridization studies of their transcripts in KS lesions demonstrate their presence in the majority of spindle cells (Reed et al., 1998; Dittmer et al., 1998; Sturzl et al., 1999). Reed and colleagues additionally found vCYC transcripts in epithelial cells of eccrine ducts and scattered epidermal cells (Reed et al., 1998). In contrast to the expression of latent genes, only a few cells within KS tumors express proteins associated with lytic replication indicating a relatively tight regulation of lytic viral reactivation. The low number of cells hosting viral lytic reactivation in KS lesions is reflected in the numerous reports where lytic viral proteins are detected not at all or in only a few cells (<1%) when a series of KS lesions are examined. Viral proteins found to be expressing in rare cells of KS lesions include PF-8 (ORF59), (Katano et al., 1999a,b; Parravicini et al., 2000) and ORF50 (Katano et al., 2001). The expression of vIL6 protein was found to be highly variable. Parravicini and colleagues were unable to detect the protein in 15 KS lesions they examined, while Cannon and colleagues found its expression in one out of 13 KS cases in one series but 7 out of 7 KS cases in another series deliberately selected for the presence of lytic foci (Parravicini et al., 2000; Cannon et al., 1999). The vIRF1 protein has not been detected in KS lesions by immunohistocheminstry thus far (Parravicini et al., 2000). This is most likely due to antibody sensitivity, since cells hosting lytic replication would be expected to express the full spectrum of encoded proteins.

Primary effusion lymphomas

Due to the scarcity of these lymphomas, extensive sampling of *in vivo* viral gene expression has not been done in this disorder. In a pattern similar to that found in KS lesions, tumor cells in PEL all express LANA1 protein (Dupin et al., 1999; Katano et al., 1999a,b) and only rarely express ORF50 (Katano et al., 2001). The major difference detected between PEL and KS lesions at this point is the expression of LANA2 which appears to be lymphoid specific. In contrast to ORF50 protein which is rarely detected, vIL6 is present in up to 5% of the PEL tumor cells. This partial uncoupling of vIL6 gene expression from RTA activation has been confirmed by in vitro studies on PEL cell lines showing that the vIL6 gene has a promoter containing two interferon stimulated response elements (ISRE) with the ability to induce vIL6 expression in cells treated with IFN-α. Additional evidence that transcriptional regulation of vIL6 is unique comes from microarray studies showing that only vIL6 transcripts in PEL cell lines were upregulated in response to IFN-α in the presence of cycloheximide (Chatterjee et al., 2002). These results show that additional pathways, beyond the dichotomous latency-lytic pathways traditionally described for herpesviruses, regulate vIL6 transcription.

The LANA2/vIRF3 gene (K10.5) is one of the few KSHV proteins which has been found to be latently expressed in PEL and MCD cells in vivo; however, LANA2/vIRF3 is not expressed in the vast majority of KS spindle cells. This finding reinforces the concept that KSHV is capable of multiple latency expression programs, and genes that are expressed in some tissues or cell lines may be silenced or absent in others. LANA2/vIRF3 differs from vIL6 in that vIL6 is expressed in a minority population of PEL tumor cells. Since vIL6 is a secreted cytokine, limited expression of vIL6 may nonetheless contribute to the pathogenesis of PEL tumors. In contrast, LANA2/vIRF3 expression is uniformly present in PEL tumor cells, indicating that it may have a critical role in maintaining the PEL tumor cell phenotype. These patterns of expression could be expected if the vIL6 promoter is activated by cytokine signaling pathways that are dependent on the local cellular milieu, whereas the LANA2/vIRF3 promoter is activated by B-cell transcription factors. It bears repeating at this point that although PEL-derived cell lines also express LANA2/vIRF3 and vIL6 there is a greater percentage of cells positive for class II and class III proteins (see above) in vitro suggesting that regulation of KSHV protein expression may be different in culture (Parravicini et al., 2000).

Multicentric Castleman's disease

In MCD, the majority of cells in affected lymphoid tissues are not infected with KSHV: the LANA1 positive cells are largely confined to the mantle zone of lymphoid follicles. These KSHV-infected cells are negative for T-cell or monocytic markers and are felt to be B-cells, although only a minority express CD20 or CD79 B-cell markers. A subset of these LANA1 positive mantle zone cells also express vIL6, K8, K10, PF-8, and ORF65 proteins. However, in contrast to both PEL and KS lesions there are a higher percentage

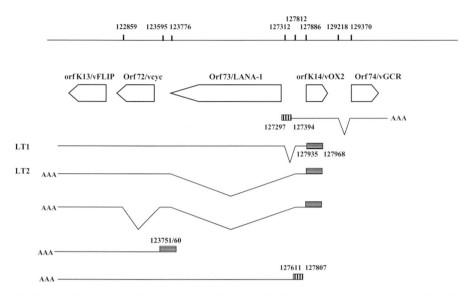

Fig. 28.4. Splicing pattern of latency-associated and neighboring transcripts. Two main transcripts, LT1 and LT2, and an additional minor transcript are directed by a latent promoter (horizontally striped box) and are translated to yield LANA1, vCYC and vFLIP. An additional latent promoter located in the 3′ end of the orf73/LANA1 gene (horizontally striped box) directs the expression of a bicistronic mRNA for vcyc and vFLIP. Both latent promoters also direct the expression of the kaposins and the viral miRNAs (see Fig. 29.8). In addition, expression of orf73/LANA1 can also be directed by a lytic promoter (vertically striped box). Overlapping with an intron spliced out of these transcripts is the promoter directing a bicistronic mRNA for ORFK14 and vGPCR. Numbering at the top refers to the position of splice donors and acceptors.

of LANA1 positive cells in MCD that express protein associated with lytic activation. Of these lytic cycle-associated genes, vIL6 appears to be expressed in a larger percentage of KSHV-infected cells. KSHV infected mantle zone cells therefore reproduce the pattern of viral gene expression observed in TPA-stimulated PEL-derived cell lines, in which a small, but significant subset of cells expresses class II and III genes (Parravicini et al., 2000; Katano et al., 2000).

Immunohistochemical techniques address critical aspects of virus behavior in infected tissue culture cells and pathological lesions that cannot be explored by mRNA studies. Although extensive mRNA mapping of viral gene expression has been performed in KSHV infected cell lines, tissue localization studies show that KS, PEL, and MCD are characterized by differing and unique patterns of KSHV protein expression.

Regulation of gene expression

Splicing

Genomic region containing KSHV latent genes and the viral chemokine receptor homologue

Gene expression in the locus encoding the major latent genes of KSHV, ORF73 (LANA1), ORF72 (vCYC), ORF71/K13 (vFLIP) is controlled by a constitutively active promoter located between nucleotides 127 935 and 129 370, with a minimal promoter region mapped to 127 935–127 968 of the prototypic KSHV sequence (Russo et al., 1996), as shown in Fig. 28.4. (Jeong et al., 2001). This promoter has the characteristics of a latent promoter, i.e. is not upregulated by treatment with phorbol esters or butyrate (Jeong et al., 2004) however, it may be regulated in a cell cycle specific manner (Sarid et al., 1999). It directs the expression of two more abundant and one rare mRNAs. The first transcript, latent transcript 1 (LT1; Fig. 28.4) encodes LANA1, while the second, LT2 represents a bicistronic mRNA from which both vCYC and vFLIP are translated. To enable efficient translation of the downstream reading frame for vFLIP, this mRNA contains an internal ribosomal entry site (IRES) located within ORF72 between nucleotides 122 973 and 123 206 (Bieleski & Talbot, 2001; Grundhoff & Ganem, 2001; Low et al., 2001). In addition, Grundhoff & Ganem (2001) reported the existence of a further spliced mRNA from which most of the ORF72 coding sequence was removed and only vFLIP could be translated (see Fig. 28.4). However, this doubly spliced mRNA was of low abundance and only detected by RT-PCR after induction of the lytic cycle suggesting a mechanism for increasing the expression of this normally latent (Low et al., 2001) anti-apoptotic protein during lytic replication. Low et al. (2001) have also suggested that the IRES dependent translation of vFLIP may allow its expression during apoptosis when normal cap-dependent translation is less efficient due to cleavage of eIF4G by caspase 3 (Low et al., 2001). A further bicistronic mRNA fo vcyc and vFLIP is directed by an additional latent promoter located in the 3′ end of the ORF73/LANA1 gene (Pearce et al., 2005; Cai et al., 2006). This promoter also directs the expression of a spliced mRNA, from which the Kaposin proteins are translated (see below and Fig. 28.8). In addition, un unspliced mRNA transcribed from his promoter serves as the precursor RNA for the viral miRNAs (see below and Fig 28.8).

Upregulation of LANA1 by the activator of the lytic cycle RTA shortly after infection of a cell by KSHV is directed by a lytic promoter (127,807–127,620) located downstream of the major constitutive (latent) LANA1 promoter. This lytic mRNA starts at position 127,611, i.e. within the intron in the LT1 latent mRNA (Matsumara et al., 2005).

A recent report (Canham and Talbot, 2004) suggests the existence of a further mRNA which is prematurely polyadenylated within ORF73 and would be predicted to encode a truncated variant of LANA1 lacking the 76 c-terminal amino acids. Based on a deletion analysis of the c-terminal end of LANA1 (Viejo-Borbolla et al., 2003) such a truncated version of LANA1 would be expected to be deficient in its interaction with the nuclear matrix and in its ability to activate heterologous promoters and to replicate viral episomal DNA (Canham and Talbot, 2004; Viejo-Borbolla et al., 2003).

The region upstream of ORF73 contains a second promoter that directs the expression of another bicistronic mRNA, expressed during the lytic replication cycle and oriented in the opposite direction (Fig. 28.4). This mRNA contains the reading frames K14 (vOX2) and 74 (vGPCR) (Talbot et al., 1999; Kirshner et al., 1999; Jeong et al., 2001; Nador et al., 2001; Chiou et al., 2002; see Fig. 28.4). This promoter is activated by RTA, the central regulator of the lytic cycle and the minimal region response to RTA has been mapped to nucleotides 127 297–127 394 (Jeong et al., 2004; Chiou et al., 2002). At this promoter, activation by RTA is mediated through its interaction with the cellular transcriptional repressor RBP-Jκ, rather than by direct DNA binding (Liang and Ganem 2004). The bicistronic ORFK14/ORF74 mRNA results from splicing out an intron located between these two viral genes (Kirshner et al., 1999; Talbot et al., 1999; Nador et al., 2001; Chiou et al., 2002; Fig. 28.4). Although there is clear evidence from immunohistochemical staining of KS, PEL and MCD samples, as well as of TPA-induced PEL cell lines in vitro, that the vGPCR protein is expressed in cells undergoing lytic replication (Chiou et al., 2002), it is not yet clear how this protein is translated from its downstream position in a bicistronic mRNA. Internal ribosomal entry, translational reinitiation, modified ribosomal scanning have been suggested as possible mechanisms (Kirshner et al., 1999). In addition, Nador et al. (2001) found an additional monocistronic mRNA encoding only ORF74/vGPCR which was however much less abundant than the bicistronic mRNA for ORFs K14 and 74. The significance of this monocistronic mRNA and its contribution to vGPCR translation is not clear at present.

Genomic region containing immediate–early genes

The immediate–early gene ORF50, encoding the activator of the lytic cycle RTA, is located next to the multiply spliced early gene ORFK8, which encodes another player in lytic cycle regulation, KbZIP or RAP (Fig. 28.5). RTA is translated from an mRNA which incorporates a small exon located upstream of ORF49 in addition to the originally predicted reading frame 50 (Russo et al., 1996; Lukac et al., 1999; Zhu et al., 1999; Saveliev et al., 2002). The immediate–early expression kinetics of ORF50 mRNA, which has been reported to be upregulated by some groups as early as 1 hour following TPA treatment of PEL cell lines, has been discussed above. Expression of this mRNA is directed from a promoter that is autonomous and dependent on cellular factors (Seaman et al., 1999; Deng et al., 2000). In transient transfection assays using constructs in which the RTA promoter was placed upstream of a reporter gene, its activity can be further upregulated by RTA itself, but also by Na-butyrate or phorbol ester treatment and by co-transfection of some other viral proteins, e.g., vGPCR (Deng et al., 2000; Chiou et al., 2002). The autoactivation of the RTA promoter by RTA itself was also seen in persistently infected PEL cell lines (Deng et al., 2000).

In latently infected cells the RTA promoter is partially silenced by methylation and it has been suggested that this provides a mechanism by which KSHV latency could be controlled (Chen et al., 2001). Methylation of CpG islands in the RTA promoter region is seen in persistently infected PEL cell lines in vitro, as well as in samples from KSHV-associated diseases (KS, PEL, MCD) or KSHV-infected cells in vivo (Chen et al., 2001). Treatment of PEL cell lines in vitro with 5-azacytidine, an inhibitor of methyltransferase, activates the lytic cycle (Chen et al., 2001). Activation of the lytic cycle in PEL cell lines by TPA involves demethylation of the ORF50 promoter (Chen et al., 2001). It has therefore been suggested that methylation of the ORF50 promoter is one of the mechanisms by which KSHV establishes latency in vivo (Chen et al., 2001).

KSHV gene expression and regulation 499

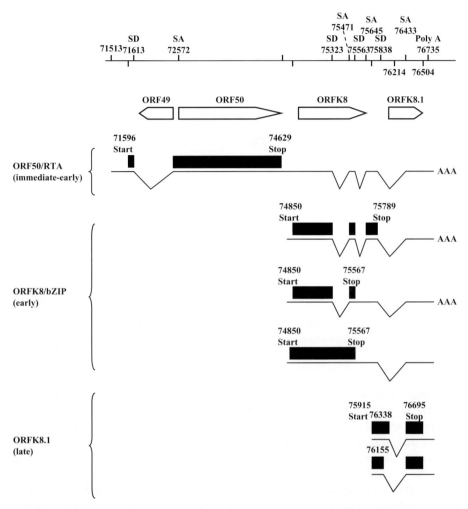

Fig. 28.5. Splicing pattern of transcripts originating in the immediate-early region of the KSHV genome. The region between ORFs 48 and 52 (see Fig. 28.1) encodes the immediate-early ORF50 transcript, as well as an early transcript for the ORFK8-derived proteins. The KbZIP protein involved in lytic replication consists of sequences included in 2 exons within the originally annotated ORFK8 in addition to a third, downstream exon encoding the leucine zipper region defining KbZIP. The mRNA for the ORFK8.1 glycoprotein also exists in two splice variants and has late expression kinetics (see Fig. 28.1).

The mRNA encoding ORF50 extends through two neighboring downstream genes, K8 and K8.1 (Fig. 28.5) but it is not clear whether there is any translation of these genes from this mRNA. However, a promoter located between ORF50 and K8 directs the expression of three alternatively spliced mRNAs, expressed at the ratio of 16:4:1 (Lin *et al.*, 1999; Fig. 28.5). One of these contains three splice events and consequently joins two exons from the originally predicted K8 reading frame to a downstream third exon which contains a leucine zipper region (Lin *et al.*, 1999; Gruffat *et al.*, 1999). Together with a basic region found in the second exon (Fig. 28.5) the resulting protein resembles members of the basic leucine-zipper transcription factors (bZIP) which includes jun, fos and the activator of the EBV lytic cycle, Zta or BZLF-1 (Sun *et al.*, 1998; Lin *et al.*, 1999; Gruffat *et al.*, 1999; Zhu *et al.*, 1999; Seaman *et al.*, 1999; further references in Sinclair, 2003). This protein, KbZIP or RAP is the predominant protein expressed in PEL cell lines after induction of the lytic cycle (Polson *et al.*, 2001). In contrast to Zta, KbZIP cannot on its own activate the lytic cycle (Lukac *et al.*, 1999; Polson *et al.*, 2001). On the contrary, it has been suggested that KbZIP, by binding to RTA, could repress the ability of RTA to activate some (e.g., ORF57), but not all (e.g., PAN/nut-1), lytic cycle genes (Izumiya *et al.*,

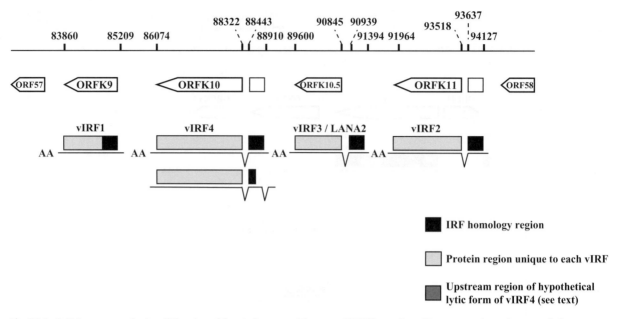

Fig. 28.6. Splicing patterns in the vIRF region of the viral genome. There are 4 KSHV proteins with sequence homology to cellular interferon regulatory factors (IRFs). The region of IRF homology is located at the amino terminal end of the viral proteins and encoded by a different exon in 3 out of 4 vIRFs.

2003a). The basic region of KbZIP is required for the interaction with RTA (Izumiya et al., 2003a), as well as for the more recently described binding to cyclin A/E-cdk2 and its consequent phosphorylation by cdks (Polson et al., 2001) and the resulting slowing of the cell cycle (Izuimya et al., 2003b). The expression kinetics of KbZIP indicates that it is an early gene, since the corresponding mRNAs are sensitive to treatment with cycloheximide, but not phosphonoacetic acid (Lin et al., 1999).

The fourth exon of the three K8/KbZIP mRNAs (Fig. 28.5) overlaps with another reading frame, ORFK8.1, encoding a structural glycoprotein incorporated into the KSHV virion and of importance for the binding of virions to glycosaminoglycans (Birkmann et al., 2001; Wang et al., 2001a, b). However, as shown in Fig. 28.5, this protein is translated from two alternatively spliced mRNAs, whose expression is controlled by a different promoter and which use the same splice acceptor at nt 76,433 as the K8/KbZIP mRNAs, but two different splice donors at nt 76,155 and nt 76,338 (Gruffat et al., 1999; Raab et al., 1998; Chandran et al., 1998). This results in two isoforms of the K8.1 glycoprotein which run at molecular weights of 35 and 38 kDa on SDS gels (Raab et al., 1998; Chandran et al., 1998; Birkmann et al., 2001; Wang et al., 2001). As befits a structural virion glycoprotein, the K8.1 mRNAs have late expression kinetics, with doubling of expression between 16 and 24 hrs after treatment of PEL cell lines with TPA or overexpression of RTA (Nakamura et al., 2003; Jenner et al., 2001; Gradoville et al., 2000) and sensitivity of the 0.9 kb K8.1 transcript to PAA (Gradoville et al., 2000).

vIRF Locus

A gene locus located between nt 83,500 and 94,200 of the KSHV genome contains several homologues of cellular interferon regulatory factors, termed vIRFs (Russo et al., 1996; Neipel et al., 1997). Although initially controversial, the gene expression and splicing patterns, as well as the proteins encoded by the different ORFs in this locus, have recently become clearer. A current consensus view is summarized in Fig. 28.6 (Cunningham et al., 2003). The first vIRF to be studied in detail, vIRF1 is encoded by an unspliced gene, ORFK9 (Gao et al., 1997; Chen et al., 2000; Wang et al., 2001a, b; Cunningham et al., 2003). ORFK9 shows expression kinetics compatible with its classification as an early gene: on Northern blots its expression is detected 8–12 hours after induction of PEL cell lines by TPA and is sensitive to treatment with cycloheximide but resistant to PAA (Wang et al., 2001a, b). In DNA array studies ORFK9 expression peaked at 24 hours (Paulose-Murphy et al., 2001; Nakamura et al., 2003) and was classified as a secondary lytic gene by Jenner et al. (2001). Immunofluorescence studies with an antibody to vIRF1 have also indicated a marked increase in vIRF1 expression following TPA stimulation of PEL cell lines (Parravicini et al., 2000).

In cells undergoing lytic viral replication a major transcriptional start site has been mapped to two adjacent nucleotides 74 and 77 bp upstream of the translational start codon by one group (Chen et al., 2001; Inagi et al., 1999) and to a neighboring nucleotide (–76 bp) by two other groups (Wang et al., 2001a, b; Cunningham et al., 2003). This start site is located 20–25 bp downstream of a TATA box. In addition, Chen et al. (2001) reported another transcriptional start site, found only in latently infected cells, approx. 84 bp upstream of the lytic start site. In contrast, in spite of finding 5' RACE products with varying start sites upstream of position – 77, Cunningham et al. (Cunningham et al., 2003) could not confirm the existence of a defined latent start site and the evidence for the existence of an additional latent promoter for vIRF1 must therefore be seen as inconclusive. In vivo, vIRF1 expression could only be seen by immunohistochemistry in MCD tissue, but not in KS or PEL tissues, in keeping with the notion, derived from the in vitro studies, that vIRF-1 is expressed early during the lytic cycle (Parravicini et al., 2000).

The neighboring viral gene, ORFK10, is also inducible in PEL cell lines (Jenner et al., 2001; Paulose-Murphy et al., 2001; Nakamura et al., 2003; Cunningham et al., 2003). Jenner et al. and Nakamura et al. noted the very rapid onset of expression following chemical induction of PEL cell lines and Jenner et al. classified ORFK10 as a "latent/lytic" gene because of the basal expression seen in uninduced PEL cell lines. The ORF K10 transcript is spliced (Fig. 28.6). The open reading frame originally designated as K10 (Russo et al., 1996) started at an ATG at position 88,164, i.e., within the larger downstream exon depicted in Fig. 28.6. For this reason, some authors refer to the smaller upstream exon as K10.1 (Jenner et al., 2001; Neipel et al., 1997). This upstream exon contains the protein regions with homology to the DNA binding domains of cellular IRFs (Jenner et al., 2001; Cunningham et al., 2003). However, analysis of the splicing patterns in the K10 region has shown that the original "K10" is expressed as part of a spliced mRNA that includes "K10.1" and consequently the inclusion of the IRF homology domains justifies the designation vIRF4 for the corresponding protein (Cunningham et al., 2003; Jenner et al., 2001; see Fig. 28.6). Cunningham et al. (2003) concluded that this spliced mRNA is inducible in PEL cells, while Jenner et al. (2001) considered this mRNA as "latent/lytic" but reported the existence of an additional alternatively spliced mRNA, found only in induced PEL cells, which eliminates the first 111 bp of the coding region in the upstream region. This would theoretically lead to a protein of 767 amino acids and a predicted molecular weight of 82 kDa, initiated at an internal ATG, which lacks the IRF homology region. However, Cunningham et al. (2003) found the alternative splice acceptor to be used by several mRNAs spliced to upstream viral regions as well as cellular sequences and queried whether this alternative transcript would be relevant physiologically. Using an antibody to K10, Katano et al. (2000) detected a dominant band of 100 kDa on Western Blots of induced but not uninduced PEL cell lines, in reasonable agreement with the predicted protein size of 98 kDa for the 905 aa translated from the singly spliced mRNA (Fig. 28.6). Although the existence of an additional minor protein cannot be completely ruled out, vIRF4, derived from the singly spliced mRNA, appears to be the dominant protein and expressed during the lytic cycle. By immunohistochemistry of pathology sections, vIRF4 was found to be expressed in 5% of KSHV-infected cells in MCD, but in less than 1% of cells in KS and PEL samples (Katano et al., 2000). This staining pattern is compatible with the expression of K10/vIRF4 during lytic viral replication.

ORFK10.5 is contained in a spliced mRNA (Lubyova and Pitha, 2000; Rivas et al., 2001; Jenner et al., 2001; Cunningham et al., 2003). In contrast to the original assignation of this ORF, the resulting protein (vIRF3, LANA2) contains sequences from both exons (Rivas et al., 2001; Cunningham et al., 2003; see Fig. 28.6). As in the case of the other vIRFs, a region with homology to cellular IRFs is located at the N-terminal end of vIRF3/LANA2 (Rivas et al., 2001; Cunningham et al., 2003; see Fig. 28.6) and derived from this first exon. While Lubyova and Pitha characterized this gene as inducible and Jenner et al. classified it as "secondary lytic" on their KSHV microarray using a probe for the upstream exon, Rivas et al. and Fakhari and Dittmer found it to be constitutively expressed in B-cells by northern blots or real time PCR. Using an antibody to vIRF3/LANA2, Rivas et al. could show its constitutive expression in latently infected PEL cell lines, as well as in PEL cell tumors and MCD specimens, but not in the endothelial and spindle cells of KS lesions. Cunningham et al. found several transcriptional start sites for the vIRF3/LANA2 transcript, none of which is in close proximity to a TATA box (Cunningham et al., 2003). The TATA box noted by Lubyova and Pitha is located approximately 500 bp further upstream and thus unlikely to direct the transcriptional start of the vIRF3/LANA2 mRNA. However, Cunningham et al. noted the sequence element AAGGTAATGAGGT approx. 250 bp upstream of most 5' RACE products in their study. This element is closely related to a motif AAGGTAAT-GAAAT in the latent LANA1 promoter (Talbot et al., 1999) and the Oct-1/TAATGARAT element of immediate–early promoters in other herpesviruses (O'Hare, 1993).

ORFK11, as originally assigned by Russo et al. (1996), is also part of a larger coding region generated by a splice event that joins it to an upstream exon. As in the case of vIRF3/LANA2 and vIRF4, this upstream exon contains the region showing homology with cellular IRFs (Cunningham et al., 2003). ORFK11/vIRF2 is an inducible gene in PEL cells (Sarid et al., 1998; Cunningham et al., 2003) which doubles

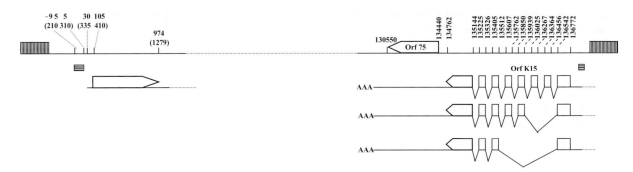

Fig. 28.7. Splicing pattern of transcripts and location of promoters at either end of the viral genome. The K1 gene at the "left" end of the viral genome is controlled by a promoter located next to the terminal repeat region. At the opposite end, the K15 gene is multiply and alternatively spliced to produce a group of proteins. A K15 promoter element is located adjacent to the terminal repeat region.

its basic expression level at about 20–24 hours after TPA treatment when measured on gene arrays (Jenner et al., 2001; Paulose-Murphy et al., 2001). In induced PEL cell lines, the vIRF2 mRNA has a single transcriptional start site located 23 nucleotides downstream from a TATA box (Cunningham et al., 2003). Using an antibody raised against ORFK11, Katano et al. (2000) could show that expression of the 110 kDa vIRF2 protein was only seen in TPA-induced PEL cells and that it is only rarely seen in KSHV-infected cells in KS, PEL or MCD, in keeping with its classification as a lytic gene product (Katano et al., 2000).

Terminal membrane proteins

Two viral genes, K1 and K15, located at either end of the virus genome, encode membrane-associated proteins, VIP and TMP, respectively, that can trigger several cellular signal transduction pathways (Lee et al., 1998a,b; Lee et al., 2000, 2002; Lagunoff et al., 1999, 2001; Glenn et al., 1999; Poole et al., 1999; Choi et al., 2000; Brinkmann et al., 2003). Both have no, or minimal, expression in uninduced PEL cells and mRNAs can be detected by northern blot, RT-PCR, RNAse protection or gene array following treatment with TPA or Na-butyrate (Lagunoff and Ganem, 1997; Sarid et al., 1998; Glenn et al., 1999; Choi et al., 2000; Jenner et al., 2001; Paulose-Murphy et al., 2001; Fakhari and Dittmer, 2002; Nakamura et al., 2003). ORFK1 encodes a type I transmembrane protein, containing two hypervariable extracellular domains and an ITAM (immunoreceptor tyrosine activation motif) in its cytoplasmic domain (Lagunoff and Ganem, 1997; Lee et al., 1998; Lagunoff et al., 1999; Poole et al., 1999; Cook et al., 1999). The K1 encoded protein has therefore been termed VIP for variable ITAM containing protein.

ORFK1 gene expression was reported to increase significantly 8–10 hrs following TPA addition and to peak after 24–72 hours. Lagunoff and Ganem (1997) found that the increase in its mRNA is not sensitive to PAA and therefore classified K1 as an early gene. The rate of increase of K1 gene expression led Jenner et al. (2001) to classify it as a 'tertiary lytic' gene, expressed with the same kinetics as many structural viral proteins. Similarly, Paulose-Murphy et al. (2001) placed it among the lytic genes with slightly delayed expression kinetics (peak expression after 36 hours). Nakamura et al. (2003) grouped K1 together with some structural proteins (ORF65/SCIP, a capsid protein; ORF47/gL, a virion glycoprotein; ORF62, a tegument gene), but also the ORF56 DNA replication protein and the ORF74/vGPCR chemokine receptor homologue.

The promoter for ORFK1 has been mapped to a region in the long unique region (LUR) of the viral genome immediately adjacent to the terminal repeats (Fig. 28.7). A 100 bp fragment corresponding to nucleotides 210–310 of the partial BCBL-1 sequence reported by Lagunoff and Ganem (1997), but located largely outside the prototypic KSHV genome sequence reported by Russo et al. (1996), can confer promoter activity to a heterologous indicator gene and has moderate but significant constitutive activity in B cells, epithelial cells and endothelial cells (Bowser et al., 2002). The ORFK1 promoter is activated directly by RTA and TPA in B cells and epithelial cells; however, in SLK endothelial cells this effect is only weak (Bowser et al., 2002). These results are in keeping with the reported lytic cycle expression kinetics of ORFK1. Lee et al. (2003) used monoclonal antibodies to the extracellular domain of K1 to demonstrate its expression early after induction of the lytic cycle in PEL cells and in a small proportion of KSHV-infected cells in MCD biopsies.

ORFK15, at the other end of the genome, consists of 8 exons, which are multiply and alternatively spliced (see Fig. 28.7) to give rise to a family of proteins that share a common c-terminal cytoplasmic domain encoded by exon 8 but vary in the number of membrane anchor domains encoded by exons 1–7 (Glenn *et al.*, 1999; Poole *et al.*, 1999; Choi *et al.*, 2000). The reading frame originally designated as ORFK15 by Russo *et al.* (1996) represents only a small part of this gene and overlaps with exon 2 (see Fig. 28.7). The designation of TMP (for terminal membrane protein) has recently been adopted for the K15 proteins. The largest of the K15/TMP proteins has an apparent molecular weight of 45 kDa on SDS-PAGE, is predicted to contain 12 such transmembrane segments in addition to the c-terminal cytoplasmic domain, and has recently been shown to be a potent activator of the Ras/ERK, JNK and NF-κB pathways (Brinkmann *et al.*, 2003).

Like K1, K15 is inducible in PEL cells and has been classified as a class III gene on the basis of its inducibility but lack of basal expression in PEL cells (Sarid *et al.*, 1998). One of the three published gene array studies classified K15 as "tertiary lytic" (Jenner *et al.*, 2001), another (Nakamura *et al.*, 2003) reported a relatively early (8 hours) onset of K15 transcription which continued to increase up to 48 hours, whereas a third (Paulose-Murphy *et al.*, 2001) observed peak expression at 24 hours with a subsequent decrease. In all three gene array studies (Nakamura *et al.* 2003; Jenner *et al.*, 2001; Paulose-Murphy *et al.*, 2001) K15 and K1 were grouped close to each other on cluster analysis. A promoter element directing the expression of the K15 gene has recently been identified in the long unique region between the first K15 exon and the terminal repeat region (Wong and Damania, 2006). A region derived from a terminal repeat subunit has promoter activity in vitro but is not responsive to RTA (Henke-Gendo, Rainbow & Schulz, unpublished data). In contrast to the similar expression kinetics of K1 and K15, regulation of K15 gene expression may therefore differ from that of K1.

At the protein level, different TMP isoforms have been demonstrated in transient transfection assays using expression constructs with differentially spliced mRNAs (Glenn *et al.*, 1999; Choi *et al.*, 2000; Sharp *et al.*, 2002; Brinkmann *et al.*, 2003). Recent findings suggest that the 45 kDa K15 protein is expressed in epithelial cell lines harboring a recombinant KSHV genome (M. M. Brinkmann *et al.*, unpublished data). A 21 kDa isoform, much smaller than the expected molecular weight of most TMPs, has been seen in some PEL cell lines and could represent a proteolytic cleavage fragment (Sharp *et al.*, 2002). Immunoreactive K15 protein has been detected in a small number of B cells in MCD biopsies using a monoclonal antibody to K15, in keeping with the predicted lytic expression pattern of K15 (Sharp *et al.*, 2002).

"Kaposin" locus

The region between nt 117,432 and nt 118,758 of the prototype KSHV sequence was originally predicted to contain an open reading frame, ORFK12, defined by a start ATG at position 117 919 and a stop codon at position 118 101 and expected to encode a small hydrophobic protein of 60 aa (Russo *et al.*, 1996; see Fig. 28.8). Independently, an 0.7 kb mRNA (T0.7) was cloned from a pulmonary KS sample and found to be latently expressed in KS biopsies and PEL cell lines by *in situ* hybridization (Zhong *et al.*, 1996; Staskus *et al.*, 1997; Stürzl *et al.*, 1997). By Northern blot, an mRNA originating in this region was also strongly expressed in uncultured PEL cells (Li *et al.*, 2002). K12/T0.7 has since been regarded as a marker of latently infected cells. However, in PEL cell lines, K12/T0.7 mRNA expression is induced by treatment with TPA or butyrate, with one group classifying it as a class II gene in view of its detectable basic expression in the BC-1 cell line in the absence of chemical treatment (Sarid *et al.*, 1998), while another classified it as an early gene because of the cycloheximide-sensitive induction of T0.7 mRNA 13 hours following Na-butyrate treatment of the same PEL cell line (Sun *et al.*, 1999). In more recent gene array experiments K12/T0.7 was classified as a latent/lytic gene (Jenner *et al.*, 2001) or as a lytic gene with relatively late doubling of expression (Paulose-Murphy *et al.*, 2001; Nakamura *et al.*, 2003). The contrast between the in vivo gene expression pattern (constitutive) and that in cultured PEL cell lines (inducible) suggests that the regulation of gene expression in PEL cells may have been affected by in vitro culture.

Although the term T0.7/Kaposin is now often used as a synonym for K12-derived transcripts, recent work has shown that in most PEL cell lines, in a primary PEL sample and in KS biopsies a larger transcript of varying size (approx. 1.4–2.4 kb, depending on the sample studied) predominates (Sadler *et al.*, 1999; Li *et al.*, 2002). The varying size of these transcripts is explained by the variable number of repeat units in two groups of repeats, DR1 and DR2 (Sadler *et al.*, 1999; Li *et al.*, 2002). This genomic arrangement has been seen in tumor samples or PEL lines of subtype A (see Fig. 28.8; Poole *et al.*, 1999). In addition to the variable length of the DR1 and DR2 repeats, additional repeat elements, I and IIa-c, have been described in a primary PEL sample of subtype B (Li *et al.*, 2002). However, the assignation of genomic subtypes in the K12 region is based on the sequence of the original K12 open reading frame (Fig. 28.8) and no extensive analysis of the genomic arrangement in the upstream repeat region in different KSHV subtypes has been carried out.

The larger mRNA encoded in this region originates at position 118,758 according to one report (Sadler *et al.*, 1999), or at position 123,842 between ORFs 72 (vCYC) and 73 (LANA1) and involving a splice event between nt 118,779 and 123,595 (Li *et al.*, 2002; see Fig. 28.8). The latter report found evidence for conservation of this splice

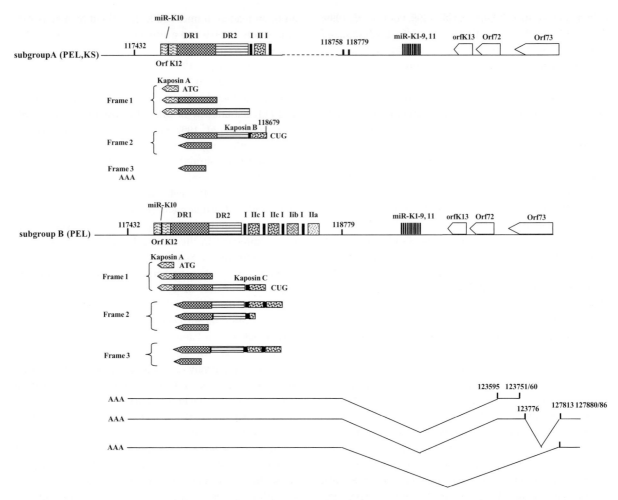

Fig. 28.8. Splicing patterns and translation products in the K12 region of the KSHV genome. Transcripts in the K12 region appear to originate upstream of K12. In the case of a primary PEL tumor, a promoter has been identified in the latent region of the genome, within ORF73. Translation appears to occur in different reading frames and from conventional (ATG) as well as unconventional (CTG) start codons.

event in all examined PEL cell lines and showed that the region between ORFs 72 and 73 contains a constitutive promoter element between nt 123,842 and 124,242, i.e., overlapping with ORF73 (LANA1) (Li *et al.*, 2002). The existence of this promoter has recently been confirmed by two other groups, although several start sites for the latent transcript originating at this promoter have been identified around 123751/60 (Pearce *et al.*, 2005; Cai *et al.*, 2006; see Fig. 28.8).

This latent mRNA uses alternative start codons (CUG, GUG) to translate several proteins in different frames whose sequence is derived from the repeats upstream of the original K12 (Sadler *et al.*, 1999; see Fig. 28.8). In frame 1 the original ORFK12 is also translated from a conventional ATG start codon, giving rise to the small (60 aa) hydropho-

bic membrane associated protein "kaposin A." Being thus located at the 3' end of a bicistronic mRNA it is not clear at present whether its translation involves an internal ribosomal entry site, the inefficient use of the upstream alternative CUG start codon, ribosomal scanning, or a separate smaller mRNA. However, evidence for its expression in PEL cell lines has been presented (Kliche *et al.*, 2001).

A CUG start codon (nt 118 679) in frame 2 directs the expression of "kaposin B", a 48 kDa protein; evidence for its expression comes from transfection studies with an expression vector that contained an epitope tag in frame with, and downstream of, the predicted "kaposin B" sequence (Sadler *et al.*, 1999). "kaposin B" was the predominant protein expressed from the repeat region upstream of K12

(Sadler et al., 1999) and also detected in a PEL cell line (Kliche et al., 2001). However, the CUG start codon used by "kaposin B" was absent from the subtype B PEL sample investigated by Li et al. (2002). Not all KSHV subtypes may therefore express "kaposin B." A further alternative start codon (CUG) in frame 1 could be used to translate a third protein, "kaposin C"; however, expression of this protein appeared inefficient in the studies by Sadler et al. (1999) and Kliche et al. (2001). It is conceivable that it predominates in other KSHV subtypes (Li et al., 2002), but no direct evidence for this currently exists.

As a consequence of the 23 bp repeat elements that constitute the DR1 and DR2 region the reading frame with regard to each individual element shifts in each consecutive element. The resulting proteins translated from the three different frames therefore share a repetitive 23 aa sequence motif (PGTWCPPPREPGALLPGNLVPSS for DR1; HPRNPARRTPGTRRGAPQEPGAA for DR2) and a monoclonal antibody to the DR1 motif will react with proteins translated in all three reading frames (Sadler et al., 1999). This antibody detects DR1 containing proteins in a subpopulation of latently infected KS spindle cells, underscoring the expression of at least some DR1-derived proteins in vivo (Sadler et al., 1999).

Viral microRNAs

In 2005, several groups independently identified a cluster of microRNAs (miRNAs) in the KSHV genome. Of 11 currently known miRNAs, 10 are encoded between the "Kaposin" locus and ORF71/K13 (miR K1-9,11), while a single miRNA has been identified in ORFK12 (Fig. 28.8). All KSHV miRNAs are derived from latent mRNAs directed by either the latency promoter in the 3' end of ORF73/LANA1 or the major latency promoter upstream of ORF73/LANA1 (position 127,935–127,968; see Figs. 28.4 and 28.8). While miR K10 is located in an exon present in all spliced forms of these latent mRNAs the miR K1-9, 11 cluster is located in an intron present in the corresponding pre-mRNAs (Fig. 28.8; Cai et al., 2005; Pfeffer et al., 2005; Samols et al., 2005; Grundhoff et al., 2006). This ensures the expression of these miRNAs during latency, suggesting a role in the regulation of latent persistence. Potential viral and cellular mRNAs that could be targeted by these viral miRNAs are currently being explored.

Other spliced genes in the KSHV genome
ORF4 (KSHV complement control protein-KCP)

ORF4 encompasses nucleotides 1,142 through 1,794 and shares homology with cellular genes encoding proteins referred to as regulators of complement activation. Northern blot analysis and RT-PCR studies in PEL-derived cell

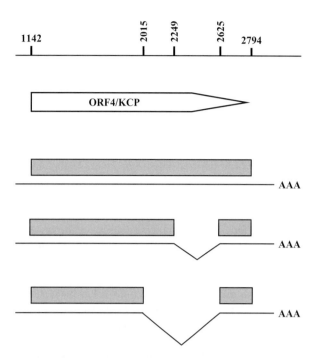

Fig. 28.9. Splicing patterns of ORF4 transcripts. Two of several alternatively spliced transcripts co-terminal with an unspliced full length transcript of ORF4, all inducible with TPA.

lines demonstrate at least two alternatively spliced co-terminal transcripts in addition to an unspliced, full length mRNA of 1,679 bp (Fig. 28.9) which are induced by TPA treatment (Spiller et al., 2003). These three transcripts encode proteins which retain C-terminal transmembrane domains and four N-terminal complement control protein (CCP) domains required for membrane attachment and complement regulation respectively. Analysis of complement regulation by soluble and membrane associated KCP demonstrated its ability to inhibit C3b deposition on cell surface and to act as a cofactor for factor I-mediated inactivation of complement proteins C3b and C4b, subunits of classical C3 convertase (Mullick et al., 2003; Spiller et al., 2003).

ORF40/41 (PAF)

ORF40 and ORF41 are both located on a spliced 2.2 kb mRNA that removes the region between these two ORFs and generates a long joint reading frame, ORF40/41, and has been shown to encode a protein of 75 kDa. Based on sequence homology, the 75 kDa protein is likely to be a primase-associated factor (PAF) (AuCoin and Pari, 2002; Wu et al., 2001). The joint ORF40/41 transcript starts at position 60, 226, eliminates the genomic region between nt 61,658 and 61,784 and uses a polyadenylation site at position 62,546 (AuCoin and Pari, 2002; Wu et al., 2001). A region

5′ to the start of this transcript has been found to contain a strong promoter activity when inserted into a luciferase vector (AuCoin and Pari, 2002). In addition, a second transcript of 0.7 kb initiates at nt 61,871 and thus only contains a part of ORF41; the corresponding protein is predicted to be translated from an ATG at position 61,908, within ORF41 (AuCoin and Pari, 2002). A 439 bp fragment upstream of the start site for this mRNA (nt 61,372–61,811) also has strong promoter activity (AuCoin and Pari, 2002). However, the existence of a protein translated from this mRNA has not yet been demonstrated. *ORF57*: The originally assigned ORF57 is located between nt 82,717 and 83,541 and was predicted to encode a homologue of an early herpesviral gene widely conserved among different herpesviruses, e.g., *herpesvirus saimiri* (HVS) ORF57, herpes simplex virus (HSV) ICP27 and Epstein–Barr Virus (EBV) BMLF1 (Russo *et al.*, 1996). For many of these homologues a role in RNA processing and nuclear export of unspliced mRNAs has been shown (detailed literature in Bello *et al.*, 1999). Subsequent RT-PCR studies, prompted by the smaller than expected size of KSHV ORF57, showed that the ORF57 mRNA is spliced and thus encodes a larger reading frame, of which the originally assigned ORF57 represents the c-terminal end. This splice removes an intron (nt 82,118–82,225) and with it an in frame stop codon upstream of the original ORF57. The spliced ORF57 mRNA initiates at nt 82,003, contains several in frame translational start codons in its first exon, uses the stop codon of the original ORF57 at 83,544 and a polyadenylation site at nt 83,608 (Bello *et al.*, 1999; Kirshner *et al.*, 2000). ORF57 is an early lytic gene whose expression becomes detectable on northern blots 2–4 hours after TPA induction of BCBL-1 cells, i.e., slightly later than ORF50/RTA and at about the same time as ORFK8/KbZIP, but before other early lytic genes (Lukac *et al.*, 1999). One of the more recent gene array studies classified it as a primary lytic gene (Jenner *et al.*, 2001), while another found a doubling of expression at 8h and a peak of expression at 72 h (Paulose-Murphy *et al.*, 2001). The ORF57 promoter is activated by RTA (Lukac *et al.*, 1999; Wang *et al.*, 2003a, b, c), placing ORF57 expression immediately downstream of the expression of RTA.

The ORF57 protein (SSM or MTA) enhances the expression of the bicistronic ORF59/ORF58 mRNA (as well as that of the ORF59/PFA protein), of the untranslated nuclear T1.1/PAN, RNA, and, in the presence of ORF50, RTA, of luciferase reporters driven by the nut-1 and kaposin promoters (Kirshner *et al.*, 1999). ORF57/MTA does not activate these promoters on its own, but enhances their ORF50/RTA-mediated activation. These findings suggest that ORF57 acts at a post-transcriptional level, but does so in a promoter-specific manner (Kirshner *et al.*, 2000).

ORFK3

The proteins encoded by ORFs K3 and K5 downmodulate major histocompatibility class I (MHC-I) proteins, NK receptors and coactivation molecules, thereby allowing KSHV-infected cells to escape both cytotoxic T-cell (CTL) and natural killer (NK) cell responses (Coscoy and Ganem, 2000; Haque *et al.*, 2000; Ishido *et al.*, 2000). Viral transcripts containing ORFK3 include three early (cycloheximide-sensitive) transcripts that also cover the neighboring ORF70 (TS). As shown in Fig. 28.10, one of these, an unspliced bicistronic mRNA, includes the entire ORF70 gene with the ORF70 translational start codon and presumably serves to translate the viral thymidylate synthase (Rimessi *et al.*, 2001). Another unspliced mRNA initiates downstream of the ORF70 start codon and could therefore translate a shortened ORF70 protein, or represent a monocistronic mRNA from which only the ORFK3 protein (MIR1, ZMP-B) could be translated. The third early mRNA splices out most of ORF70 and, although it does retain the ORF70 start codon and therefore represents a bicistronic transcript, could again serve to translate the ORFK3 protein. In addition to these early transcripts, an immediate-early, doubly spliced transcript that lacks most of the ORF70 coding region (but does retain the ORF70 ATG and is therefore bicistronic) could serve to translate the ORFK3 protein (Rimessi *et al.*, 2001).

Finally, a low abundance 2.5 kb latent transcript was recently identified by Taylor *et al.* (2005) which is coterminal with and encodes K3 in its entirety. When mapped, this transcript shows a complicated splicing pattern and encodes the entire K3 open reading frame (nt 18 585–19 671) along with 208 base pairs of the amino terminus of ORF70 (nt 20,096–20,304) and 70 base pairs of a region more than 3kb upstream (nt 23,770–23,840) (Fig. 28.10). Although low levels of ORFK3 protein expression has been documented in KS biopsies in vivo (Rimessi *et al.*, 2001), it is not yet clear which of these mRNAs is most efficiently translated to yield the ORFK3 protein and whether the novel 2.5kb latent transcript also plays a role in down-regulation of MHC class I during latent infection.

Events leading to the activation of immediate–early and early KSHV genes

In the experimental model commonly used to study the early stages of the lytic cycle, i.e., the induction of PEL cells by TPA or Na-butyrate, the immediate–early ORF50 gene, encoding RTA, is the earliest viral gene to be expressed. The ORF50/RTA promoter contains several transcription factor binding sites, including AP-1, Sp1, Oct 1, CEBP/alpha (Deng *et al.*, 2000; Sakakibara *et al.*, 2001; Wang *et al.*,

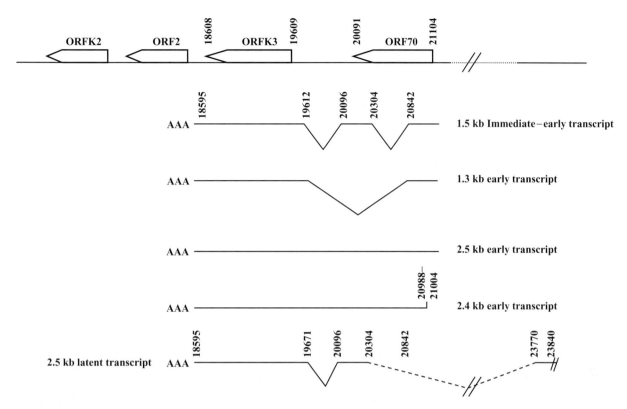

Fig. 28.10. Splicing patterns in the ORFK3-ORF70 region of the genome. Four transcripts are expressed during lytic induction of virus while a fifth transcript is detected at low levels during latent infection in PEL cell lines.

2003a,b,c). RTA activates its own promoter through two of three CEBP/alpha binding sites, most – likely by physically associating with CEBP/alpha (Wang et al., 2003a,b). RTA also increases the expression of CEBP/alpha, thereby generating an amplification loop that leads to the expression of not only the immediate–early ORF50/RTA gene, but also of other early genes (see below).

In persistently infected PEL cell lines the ORF50/RTA promoter appears to be methylated in a region (–315 to –255 of the transcriptional start site) located between the two CEBP/alpha sites that are important for RTA-mediated activation (Chen et al., 2001; Wang et al., 2003a,b). In KSHV-infected B-cells in vivo this regions also appears to be heavily methylated, whereas in PEL biopsies, MCD lesions and in KS tumors in vivo, the methylation pattern is lighter, with an inverse correlation between the expression of lytic viral proteins and the methylation status of the ORF50 promoter in individual samples (Chen et al., 2001). Treatment of persistently infected PEL cell lines with TPA or 5-azacytidine reduces the number of methylated CpG residues in the ORF50 promoter and activates the lytic cycle (Chen et al., 2001). It is therefore, conceivable that methylation of the ORF50 promoter during viral persistence regulates, at least in part, the spontaneous activation of the lytic cycle in persistently infected cells. However, given the presence of transcription factor sites that are targeted by components of signaling pathways known to be induced by TPA or Na-butyrate (e.g., AP-1) these could also contribute to the activation of the lytic cycle.

RTA also activates a number of viral early promoters, including those of ORF, K8 (KbZIP/RAP), nut-1 (T1.1/PAN), ORF57 (MTA), ORFK2 (vIL6), vMIP, ORFK12 (kaposin), ORF74 (vOX2/GPCR). In at least some target promoters, i.e., T1.1/PAN, ORFK12, vIL6, RTA binds to specific DNA sequence elements (type II RTA responsive elements; RRE) (Chang et al., 2002; Deng et al., 2002; Song et al., 2002; Wang et al., 2003a,b). In contrast, the promoters for ORF50 (RTA), ORFK8 (KbZIP/RAP), nut-1 (PAN), and ORF57 (MTA) contain CEBP/alpha binding sites and their activation by RTA involves an interaction of RTA with DNA-bound CEBP/alpha (Wang et al., 2003a,b).

In addition to the ability to directly bind DNA of target viral promoters, RTA can also target promoters lacking direct recognition elements by interaction with host DNA-binding factors such a RBP-Jκ. RBP-Jκ belongs to a family of sequence-specific transcriptional repressors which recruits other corepressors to silence gene activation. By binding to RBP-Jκ, it appears that RTA not only displaces associated corepressors, but also allows for ligand independent activation of target genes. Although specific genes including PAN, ORF57, and SSB have been individually shown to be regulated in this manner, the broader implication is that RTA-mediated redirection of RBP-Jκ activity from repression to activation is critical for lytic reactivation (Liang et al., 2002; Liang and Ganem, 2003).

The ORFK8 encoded protein, KbZIP or RAP, related to the EBV lytic-cycle Z transactivator (ZTA), as discussed above, contains a leucine zipper oligomerization domain and may interact with cellular transcription factors like CBP and CEBP/alpha (Wang et al., 2003b). Although it plays a role in the KSHV lytic replication cycle, as shown by its association with PML domains and recruitment into lytic replication compartments (Wu et al., 2001), it is, unlike EBV ZTA, not sufficient to trigger the activation of the lytic cycle and does not directly bind to viral DNA (Polson et al., 2001; Chiou et al., 2002). There is, however, evidence for its indirect association with the promoters for RTA, ORF57/MTA, as well as its own promoter, most likely as a consequence of its ability to associate with CEBP/alpha (Wang et al., 2003b).

Regulation of the lytic cycle by other viral proteins

In addition to the regulatory role of RTA, KbZIP/RAP and ORF57/MTA during the immediate–early and early phase of the lytic cycle several other KSHV proteins may have the role of modulating lytic replication. Thus the membrane-associated glycoprotein encoded by ORFK1 has been found to inhibit the TPA-induced activation of the lytic cycle in the BCBL-1 PEL cell line (Lee et al., 2002). A detailed analysis of the viral gene expression pattern in this cell line following the overexpression of K1 and treatment with TPA showed that the majority of viral genes appears to be downregulated as the result of K1 overexpression; however, a small number, including ORF72/vCYC, K15/TMP, ORF48 and K1 itself appeared to be upregulated. In contrast, K1 does not appear to affect the ORF50/RTA mediated activation of the lytic cycle, suggesting that TPA-induced events upstream of the ORF50/RTA promoter are modulated by K1. Among these the TPA-mediated activation of AP-1, NF-κB and Oct-1 in this PEL cell line appears to be inhibited by overexpression of K1 (Lee et al., 2002). Lagunoff et al. (2001) also reported that K1 may moderately augment the activation of the lytic replication cycle in a PEL cell line but did observe a dominant negative effect of K1 signaling defective mutants on the ORF50/RTA-mediated activation of the lytic replication cycle in the same PEL cell line (BCBL-1).

Other factors that increase lytic viral replication

Several clinical observations suggest that reactivation of KSHV could be mediated by environmental factors or injury. Thus the frequent localization of classic KS lesions on the feet has been linked to an exposure to volcanic soil (Ziegler, 1993) or to reduced blood flow and poor oxygenation of the lower extremities in elderly individuals. Experimentally, hypoxia has been shown to activate KSHV lytic replication in PEL cell lines (Davis et al., 2001). Haque et al. (2003) reported the presence of functional hypoxia response elements in the ORF50/RTA and ORF34 promoter. These elements are activated by either HIF-2 alpha (ORF50/RTA promoter) or by both HIF-1alpha and HIF-2alpha (ORF34 promoter) and hypoxia induces the transcription of ORF34 and ORF50/RTA mRNAs (Haque et al., 2001). Chang et al. (2000) and Zoeteweij et al. (2001) reported that calcium ionophores, such as ionomycin and thapsigargin, could activate KSHV lytic replication cycle in PEL cells and further synergized with the effects of phorbol esters (Chang et al., 2000). That KS lesions can arise in scar tissue or regions of traumatized skin (Köbner phenomenon) is another well-established clinical observation (Sachsenberg-Struder et al., 1999).

In addition, an extensive body of experimental work has suggested some inflammatory cytokines may accelerate the development of KS lesions in AIDS patients (for a review see Ensoli et al., 2001). Thus Monini et al. (1999) showed that inflammatory cytokines, and in particular interferon gamma, can increase the viral load in cultured PBMC of KSHV infected individuals. In a similar experiment Mercader et al. (2000) identified oncostatin M, hepatocyte growth factor/scatter factor and interferon gamma as cytokines that are released from HIV-1 infected T cells and can induce the expression of ORFK12 and ORF26 mRNA, as well as ORF59 and K8.1 proteins, in the BCBL-1 cell line. In vitro examination of KSHV infected cell lines demonstrates that inflammatory cytokines had diverse effects on KSHV induction. While interferon gamma consistently induced lytic activation, Chang et al. (2000) found other cytokines including tumor necrosis factor, IL-1, IL-2, IL-6, granulocyte-macrophage colony stimulating factor, and basic fibroblast growth factor did not. Further, interferon alpha inhibited KSHV induction (Monini et al., 1999; Chang et al., 2000).

Recently, it was shown that KSHV-infected keratinocytes could activate the lytic replication cycle upon epithelial differentiation in raft cultures (Johnson et al., 2005), suggesting that, similar to human papillomavirus, KSHV infected epithelial cells could be programmed to allow the production of new virions at the epithelial surface.

REFERENCES

AuCoin, D. P. and Pari, G. S. (2002). The human herpesvirus-8 (Kaposi's sarcoma-associated herpesvirus) ORF 40/41 region encodes two distinct transcripts. *J. Gen. Virol.*, **83**, 189–193.

Bechtel, J. T., Liang, Y., Hvidding, J., and Ganem, D. (2003). Host range of Kaposi's sarcoma-associated herpesvirus in cultured cells. *J. Virol.*, **77**, 6474–6481.

Bello, L. J., Davison, A. J., Glenn, M. A. *et al.* (1999). The human herpesvirus-8 ORF 57 gene and its properties. *J. Gen. Virol.*, **80** (12), 3207–3215.

Bieleski, L. and Talbot, S. J. (2001). Kaposi's sarcoma-associated herpesvirus vCYClin open reading frame contains an internal ribosome entry site. *J. Virol.*, **75**, 1864–1869.

Birkmann, A., Mahr, K., Ensser, A., Yaguboglu, S., Titgemeyer, F., Fleckenstein, B., and Neipel, F. (2001). Cell surface heparan sulfate is a receptor for human herpesvirus 8 and interacts with envelope glycoprotein K8.1. *J. Virol.*, **75**, 11583–11593.

Bowser, B. S., DeWire, S. M., and Damania, B. (2002). Transcriptional regulation of the K1 gene product of Kaposi's sarcoma-associated herpesvirus. *J. Virol.*, **76**, 12574–12583.

Brinkmann, M. M., Glenn, M., Rainbow, L., Kieser, A., Henke-Gendo, C., and Schulz, T. F. (2003). Activation of mitogen-activated protein kinase and NF-kappaB pathways by a Kaposi's sarcoma-associated herpesvirus K15 membrane protein. *J. Virol.*, **77**, 9346–9358.

Cai, S., Lu, S., Zhang, Z., Gonzalez, C. M., Damania, B., Cullen, B. R. (2005). Kaposi's sarcoma-associated herpesvirus expresses an array of viral micrRNAs in latently infected cells. *Proc. Natl. Acad. Sci. USA*, **102**, 5570–5575.

Cai, X. and Cullen, B. R. (2006). Transcriptional origin of Kaposi's sarcoma-associated herpesvirus micrRNAs. *J. Virol.*, **80**, 2234–2242.

Cai, X., Lu, S., Zhang, Z., Gonzalez, C. M., Damania, B., and Cullen, B. R. (2005). Kaposi's sarcoma-associated herpesvirus expresses an array of viral microRNAs in latently infected cells. *Proc. Natl Acad. Sci. USA*, **102**, 5570–5575.

Canham, M. and Talbot, S. J. (2004). A naturally occurring c-terminal truncated isoform of the latent nuclear antigen (LANA) of Kaposi's sarcoma-associated herpesvirus (KSHV) does not associate with viral episomal DNA. *J. Gen. Virol.*, **85**, in press.

Cannon, J. S., Nicholas, J., Orenstein, J. M. *et al.* (1999). Heterogeneity of viral IL-6 expression in HHV-8-associated diseases. *J. Infect. Dis.*, **180**, 824–828.

Chandran, B., Bloomer, C., Chan, S. R., Zhu, L., Goldstein, E., and Horvat, R. (1998). Human herpesvirus-8 ORF K8.1 gene encodes immunogenic glycoproteins generated by spliced transcripts. *Virology*, **249**, 140–149.

Chang, H., Dittmer, D. P., Chul, S-Y., Hong, Y., and Jung, J. U. (2006). Role of notch signal transduction in Kaposi's sarcoma-associated herpesvirus gene expression. *J. Virol.*, **79**, 14371–14382.

Chang, J., Renne, R., Dittmer, D. *et al.* (2000). Inflammatory cytokenes and the reactivation of Kaposi's sarcoma-associated herpesvirus lytic replication. *Virology*, **266**, 17–25.

Chang, P. J., Shedd, D., Gradoville, L. *et al.* (2002). Open reading frame 50 protein of Kaposi's sarcoma-associated herpesvirus directly activates the viral PAN and K12 genes by binding to related response elements. *J. Virol.*, **76**, 3168–3178.

Chatterjee, M., Osborne, J., Bestetti, G., Chang, Y., and Moore, P. S. (2002). Viral IL-6-induced cell proliferation and immune evasion of interferon activity. *Science*, **298**, 1432–1435.

Chen, L. and Lagunoff, M. (2005). Establishment and maintenance of Kaposi's sarcoma-associated herpesvirus latency in B cells. *J. Virol.*, **79**, 14383–14391.

Chen, J., Ueda, K., Sakakibara, S., Okuno, T., and Yamanishi, K. (2000). Transcriptional regulation of the Kaposi's sarcoma-associated herpesvirus viral interferon regulatory factor gene. *J. Virol.*, **74**, 8623–8634.

Chen, J., Ueda, K., Sakakibara, S. *et al.* (2001). Activation of latent Kaposi's sarcoma-associated herpesvirus by demethylation of the promoter of the lytic transactivator. *Proc. Natl Acad. Sci. USA*, **98**(7), 4119–4124.

Chiou, C. J., Poole, L. J., Kim, P. S. *et al.* (2002). Patterns of gene expression and a transactivation function exhibited by the vGCR (ORF 74) chemokine receptor protein of Kaposi's sarcoma-associated herpesvirus. *J. Virol.*, **76**, 3421–3439.

Choi, J. K., Lee, B. S., Shim, S. N. *et al.* (2000). Identifications of the novel K15 gene at the rightmost end of the Kaposi's sarcoma-associated herpesvirus genome. *J. Virol.*, **74**, 436–446.

Ciufo, D. M., Cannon, J. S., Poole, L. J. *et al.* (2001). Spindle cell conversion by Kaposi's sarcoma-associated herpesvirus: formation of colonies and plaques with mixed lytic and latent gene expression in infected primary dermal microvascular endothelial cell cultures. *J. Virol.*, **75**, 5614–5626.

Cook, P. M., Whitby, D., Calabro, M. L. *et al.* (1999). Variability and evolution of Kaposi's sarcoma-associated herpesvirus in Europe and Africa. International Collaborative Group. *AIDS*, **13**, 1165–1176.

Coscoy, L. and Ganem, D. (2000). Kaposi's sarcoma-associated herpesvirus encodes two proteins that block cell surface display of MHC class I chains by enhancing their endocytosis. *Proc. Natl Acad. Sci. USA*, **97**, 8051–8056.

Cunningham, C., Barnard, S., Blackbourn, D. J., and Davison, A. J. (2003). Transcription mapping of human herpesvirus 8 genes encoding viral interferon regulatory factors. *J. Gen. Virol.*, **84**, 1471–1483.

Davis, D. A., Rinderknecht, A. S., Zoeteweij, J. P. *et al.* (2001). Hypoxia induces lytic replication of Kaposi sarcoma-associated herpesvirus. *Blood*, **97**, 3244–3250.

Deng, H., Young, A., and Sun, R. (2000). Auto-activation of the rta gene of human herpesvirus-8/Kaposi's sarcoma-associated herpesvirus. *J. Gen. Virol.*, **81**, 3043–3048.

Deng, H., Chu, J. T., Rettig, M. B., Martinez-Maza, O., and Sun, R. (2002). Rta of the human herpesvirus 8/Kaposi sarcoma-associated herpesvirus up-regulates human interleukin-6 gene expression. *Blood*, **100**, 1919–1921.

Dezube, B. J., Zambela, M., Sage, D. R., Wang, J. F., and Fingeroth, J. D. (2002). Characterization of Kaposi sarcoma-associated herpesvirus/human herpesvirus-8 infection of human vascular endothelial cells: early events. *Blood*, **100**, 888–896.

Dittmer, D. P. (2003). Transcription profile of Kaposi's sarcoma-associated herpesvirus in primary Kaposi's sarcoma lesions as determined by real-time PCR arrays. *Cancer Res.*, **63**, 2010–2015.

Dittmer, D., Lagunoff, M., Renne, R. *et al.* (1998). A cluster of latently expressed genes in Kaposi's sarcoma-associated herpesvirus. *J. Virol.*, **72**, 8309–8315.

Dupin, N., Fisher, C., Kellam, P. *et al.* (1999). Distribution of human herpesvirus-8 latently infected cells in Kaposi's sarcoma, multicentric Castleman's disease, and primary effusion lymphoma. *Proc. Natl Acad. Sci. USA*, **96**, 4546–4551.

Ensoli, B., Sturzl, M., and Monini, P. (2001). Reactivation and role of HHV-8 in Kaposi's sarcoma initiation. *Adv. Cancer Res.*, **81**, 161–200.

Fakhari, F. D. and Dittmer, D. P. (2002). Charting latency transcripts in Kaposi's sarcoma-associated herpesvirus by whole-genome real-time quantitative PCR. *J. Virol.*, **76**, 6213–6223.

Gao, S. J., Boshoff, C., Jayachandra, S., Weiss, R. A., Chang, Y., and Moore, P. S. (1997). KSHV ORF K9 (vIRF) is an oncogene which inhibits the interferon signaling pathway. *Oncogene*, **15**, 1979–1985.

Gao, S. J., Deng, J. H., and Zhou, F. C. (2003). Productive lytic replication of a recombinant Kaposi's sarcoma-associated herpesvirus in efficient primary infection of primary human endothelial cells. *J. Virol.*, **77**, 9738–9749.

Glenn, M., Rainbow, L., Aurade, F., Davison, A., and Schulz, T. F. (1999). Identification of a spliced gene from Kaposi's sarcoma-associated herpesvirus encoding a protein with similarities to latent membrane proteins 1 and 2A of Epstein–Barr virus. *J. Virol.*, **73**, 6953–6963.

Gradoville, L., Geralach, J., Grogan, E. *et al.* (2000). Kaposi's sarcoma-associated herpesvirus (human herpesvirus-8) encodes a homologue of the Epstein–Barr virus bZip protein EB1. *J. Gen. Virol.*, **80**(3), 557–561.

Gruffat, H., Portes-Sentis, S., Sergeant, A., and Manet, E. (1999). Kaposi's sarcoma-associated herpesvirus (human herpesvirus-8) encodes a homologue of the Epstein–Barr virus bZip protein EB1. *J. Gen. Virol.*, **80**(3), 557–561.

Grundhoff, A. and Ganem, D. (2001). Mechanisms governing expression of the v-FLIP gene of Kaposi's sarcoma-associated herpesvirus. *J. Virol.*, **75**, 1857–1863.

Grundhoff, A., Sullivan, C. S., and Ganem, D. (2006). A combined computational and microarray-based approach identifies novel microRNAs encoded by human gamma-herpesviruses. *RNA*, **12**, 733–750.

Haque, M., Chen, J., Ueda, K. *et al.* (2000). Identification and analysis of the K5 gene of Kaposi's sarcoma associated herpesvirus. *J. Virol.*, **74**, 2867–2875.

Haque, M., Ueda, K., Nakano, K. *et al.* (2001). Major histocompatibility complex class I molecules are down-regulated at the cell surface by the K5 protein encoded by the Kaposi's sarcoma associated herpesvirus human herpesvirus-8. *J. Gen. Virol.*, **82**, 1175–1180.

Haque, M., Davis, D. A., Wang, V., Widmer, I., and Yarchoan, R. (2003). Kaposi's sarcoma-associated herpesvirus (human herpesvirus 8) contains hypoxia response elements: relevance to lytic induction by hypoxia. *J. Virol.*, **77**, 6761–6768.

Harrington, W., Jr., Sieczkowski, L., Sosa, C. *et al.* (1997). Activation of HHV-8 by HIV-1 tat. *Lancet*, **349**, 774–775.

Huang, L. M., Chao, M. F., Chen, M. Y. *et al.* (2001). Reciprocal regulatory interaction between human herpesvirus 8 and human immunodeficiency virus type 1. *J. Biol. Chem.*, **276**, 13427–13432.

Inagi, R., Okuno, T., Ito, M. *et al.* (1999). Identification and characterization of human herpesvirus 8 open reading frame K9 viral interferon regulatory factor by a monoclonal antibody. *J. Hum. Virol.*, **2**, 63–71.

Ishido, S., Choi, J. K., Lee, B. S. *et al.* (2000). Inhibition of natural killer cell-mediated cytotoxicity by Kaposi's sarcoma-associated herpesvirus K5 protein. *Immunity*, **13**, 365–374.

Izumiya, Y., Lin, S. F., Ellison, T. J. *et al.* (2003a). Cell cycle regulation by Kaposi's sarcoma-associated herpesvirus K-bZIP: direct interaction with cyclin-CDK2 and induction of G1 growth arrest. *J. Virol.*, **77**, 9652–9661.

Izumiya, Y., Lin, S. F., Ellison, T. *et al.* (2003b). Kaposi's sarcoma-associated herpesvirus K-bZIP is a coregulator of K-Rta: physical association and promoterdependent transcriptional repression. *J. Virol.*, **77**, 1441–1451.

Jenner, R. G., Alba, M. M., Boshoff, C., and Kellam, P. (2001). Kaposi's sarcoma-associated herpesvirus latent and lytic gene expression as revealed by DNA arrays. *J. Virol.*, **75**, 891–902.

Jeong, J., Papin, J., and Dittmer, D. (2001). Differential regulation of the overlapping Kaposi's sarcomaassociated herpesvirus vGPCR (ORF74) and LANA (ORF73) promoters. *J. Virol.*, **75**, 1798–1807.

Jeong, J. H., Orvis, J., Kim, J. W. *et al.* (2004). Regulation and autoregulation of the promoter for the latency-associated nuclear antigen of Kaposi's sarcoma-associated herpesvirus. *J. Biol. Chem.*, **279**, 16822–16831.

Johnson, A. S., Maronian, N., and Vieira, J. (2005). Activation of Kaposi's sarcoma-associated herpesvirus lytic gene expression during epithelial differentiation. *J. Virol.*, **79**, 13769–13777.

Katano, H., Sato, Y., Kurata, T., Mori, S., and Sata, T. (1999a). High expression of HHV-8-encoded ORF73 protein in spindle-shaped cells of Kaposi's sarcoma. *Am. J. Pathol.*, **155**, 47–52.

Katano, H., Sata, T., Suda, T. *et al.* (1999b). Expression and antigenicity of human herpesvirus 8 encoded ORF59 protein in AIDS-associated Kaposi's sarcoma. *J. Med. Virol.*, **59**, 346–355.

Katano, H., Sato, Y., Kurata, T., Mori, S., and Sata, T. (2000). Expression and localization of human herpesvirus 8-encoded proteins in primary effusion lymphoma, Kaposi's sarcoma, and multicentric Castleman's disease. *Virology*, **269**, 335–344.

Katano, H., Sato, Y., Itoh, H., and Sata, T. (2001). Expression of human herpesvirus 8 (HHV-8)-encoded immediate early protein, open reading frame 50, in HHV-8-associated diseases. *J. Hum. Virol.*, **4**, 96–102.

Kirshner, J. R., Staskus, K., Haase, A., Lagunoff, M., and Ganem, D. (1999). Expression of the open reading frame 74 (G-protein-coupled receptor) gene of Kaposi's sarcoma (KS)-associated herpesvirus: implications for KS pathogenesis. *J. Virol.*, **73**, 6006–6014.

Kirshner, J. R., Lukac, D. M., Chang, J., and Ganem, D. (2000). Kaposi's sarcoma-associated herpesvirus open reading frame 57 encodes a posttranscriptional regulator with multiple distinct activities. *J. Virol.*, **74**, 3586–3597.

Kliche, S., Nagel, W., Kremmer, E. *et al.* (2001). Signaling by human herpesvirus 8 kaposin A through direct membrane recruitment of cytohesin-1. *Mol. Cell*, **7**, 833–843.

Krishnan, H. H., Naranatt, P. P., Smith, M. S. *et al.* (2004). Concurrent expression of latent and a limited number of lytic genes with immune modulation and antiapoptotic function by Kaposi's sarcoma-associated herpesvirus early during infection of primary endothelial and fibroblast cells and subsequent decline of lytic gene expression. *J. Virol.*, **78**, 2601–2620.

Lagunoff, M. and Ganem, D. (1997). The structure and coding organization of the genomic termini of Kaposi's sarcoma-associated herpesvirus. *Virology*, **236**, 147–154.

Lagunoff, M., Majeti, R., Weiss, A. *et al.* (1999). Deregulated signal transduction by the K1 gene product of Kaposi's sarcoma-associated herpesvirus. *Proc. Natl Acad. Sci. USA*, **96**, 5704–5709.

Lagunoff, M., Lukac, D. M., and Ganem, D. (2001). Immunoreceptor tyrosine-based activation motifdependent signaling by Kaposi's sarcoma-associated herpesvirus K1 protein: effects on lytic viral replication. *J. Virol.*, **75**, 5891–5898.

Lagunoff, M., Bechtel, J., Venetsanakos, E. *et al.* (2002). De novo infection and serial transmission of Kaposi's sarcoma-associated herpesvirus in cultured endothelial cells. *J. Virol.*, **76**, 2440–2448.

Lee, B. S., Alvarez, X., Ishido, S., Lackner, A. A., and Jung, J. U. (2000). Inhibition of intracellular transport of B cell antigen receptor complexes by Kaposi's sarcoma-associated herpesvirus K1. *J. Exp. Med.*, **192**, 11–21.

Lee, B. S., Paulose-Murphy, M., Chung, Y. H., Connlole, M., Zeichner, S., and Jung, J. U. (2002). Suppression of tetradecanoyl phorbol acetate-induced lytic reactivation of Kaposi's sarcoma-associated herpesvirus by K1 signal transduction. *J. Virol.*, **76**, 12185–12199.

Lee, B. S., Connole, M., Tang, Z., Harris, N. L., and Jung, J. U. (2003). Structural analysis of the Kaposi's sarcoma-associated herpesvirus K1 protein. *J. Virol.*, **77**, 8072–8086.

Lee, H., Guo, J., Li, M. *et al.* (1998a). Identification of an immunoreceptor tyrosine-based activation motif of K1 transforming protein of Kaposi's sarcomaassociated herpesvirus. *Mol. Cell Biol.*, **18**, 5219–5228.

Lee, H., Veazey, R., Williams, K. *et al.* (1998b). Deregulation of cell growth by the K1 gene of Kaposi's sarcomaassociated herpesvirus. *Nat. Med.*, **4**, 435–440.

Li, H., Komatsu, T., Dezube, B. J., and Kaye, K. M. (2002). The Kaposi's sarcoma-associated herpesvirus K12 transcript from a primary effusion lymphoma contains complex repeat elements, is spliced, and initiates from a novel promoter. *J. Virol.*, **76**, 11880–11888.

Liang, Y. and Ganem, D. (2003). Lytic but not latent infection by Kaposi's sarcoma-associated herpesvirus requires host CSL protein, the mediator of Notch signaling. *Proc. Natl Acad. Sci. USA*, **100**, 8490–8495.

Liang, Y. and Ganem, D. (2004). RBP-J (CSL) is essential for activation of the K14/vGPCR promoter of Kaposi's sarcoma-associated herpesvirus by the lytic switch protein RTA. *J. Virol.*, **78**, 6818–6826.

Liang, Y., Chang, J., Lynch, S. J., Lukac, D. M., and Ganem, D. (2002). The lytic switch protein of KSHV activates gene expression via functional interaction with RBP-Jkappa (CSL), the target of the Notch signaling pathway. *Genes Dev.*, **16**, 1977–1989.

Lin, S. F., Robinson, D. R., Miller, G., and Kung, H. J. (1999). Kaposi's sarcoma-associated herpesvirus encodes a bZIP protein with homology to BZLF1 of Epstein–Barr virus. *J. Virol.*, **73**, 1909–1917.

Low, W., Harries, M., Ye, H., Du, M. Q., Boshoff, C., and Collins, M. (2001). Internal ribosome entry site regulates translation of Kaposi's sarcoma-associated herpesvirus FLICE inhibitory protein. *J. Virol.*, **75**, 2938–2945.

Lubyova, B. and Pitha, P. M. (2000). Characterization of a novel human herpesvirus 8-encoded protein, vIRF-3, that shows homology to viral and cellular interferon regulatory factors. *J. Virol.*, **74**, 8194–8201.

Lukac, D. M., Kirshner, J. R., and Ganem, D. (1999). Transcriptional activation by the product of open reading frame 50 of Kaposi's sarcoma-associated herpesvirus is required for lytic viral reactivation in B cells. *J. Virol.*, **73**, 9348–9361.

Matsumara, S., Fujita, Y., Gomez, E., Tanese, N., and Wilson, A. C. (2005). Activation of the Kaposi's sarcoma-associated herpesvirus major latency locus by the lytic switch protein RTA (ORF50). *J. Virol.*, **79**, 8493–8505.

Mercader, M., Taddeo, B., Panella, J. R., Chandran, B., Nickoloff, B. J., and Foreman, K. E. (2000). Induction of HHV-8 lytic cycle replication by inflammatory cytokines produced by HIV-1-infected T cells. *Am. J. Pathol.*, **156**, 1961–1971.

Monini, P., Colombini, S., Sturzl, M. *et al.* (1999). Reactivation and persistence of human herpesvirus-8 infection in B cells and monocytes by Th-1 cytokines increased in Kaposi's sarcoma. *Blood*, **93**, 4044–4058.

Moses, A. V., Fish, K. N., Ruhl, R. *et al.* (1999). Long-term infection and transformation of dermal microvascular endothelial cells by human herpesvirus 8. *J. Virol.*, **73**, 6892–6902.

Mullick, J., Bernet, J., Singh, A. K., Lambris, J. D., and Sahu, A. (2003). Kaposi's sarcoma-associated herpesvirus (human herpesvirus 8) open reading frame 4 protein (kaposica) is a functional homolog of complement control proteins. *J. Virol.*, **77**, 3878–3881.

Nador, R. G., Milligan, L. L., Flore, O. *et al.* (2001). Expression of Kaposi's sarcoma-associated herpesvirus G protein-coupled receptor monocistronic and bicistronic transcripts in primary effusion lymphomas. *Virology*, **287**, 62–70.

Nakamura, H., Muller, J. T., Chandrasekhar, S. et al. (2001). Multimodality therapy with a replication-conditional herpes simplex vius mutant that expresses yeast cytosine deaminase for intranumoral conversion of 5-fluorocytosine to 5-fluorouracil. *Cancer Res.*, **61**, 5447–5452.

Nakamura, H., Lu, M., Gwack, Y., Souvlis, J., Zeichner, S. L., and Jung, J. U. (2003). Global changes in Kaposi's sarcoma-associated virus gene expression patterns following expression of a tetracycline-inducible Rta transactivator. *J. Virol.*, **77**, 4205–4220.

Naranatt, P. P., Krishnan, H. H., Svojanovsky, S. R., Bloomer, C., Mathur, S., and Chandran, B. (2004). Host gene induction and transcriptional reprogramming in Kaposi's sarcoma-associated herpesvirus (KSHV/HHV-8)-infected endothelial, fibroblast, and B cells: insights into modulation events early during infection. *Cancer Res.*, **64**, 72–84.

Neipel, F., Albrecht, J. C., and Fleckenstein, B. (1997). Cell-homologous genes in the Kaposi's sarcomaassociated rhadinovirus human herpesvirus 8: determinants of its pathogenicity? *J. Virol.*, **71**, 4187–4192.

O'Hare, P. (1993). The virion transactivator of herpes simplex virus. *Semin. Virol.*, **4**, 145–155.

Parravicini, C., Chandran, B., Corbellino, M. et al. (2000). Differential viral protein expression in Kaposi's sarcoma-associated herpesvirus-infected diseases: Kaposi's sarcoma, primary effusion lymphoma, and multicentric Castleman's disease. *Am. J. Pathol.*, **156**, 743–749.

Paulose-Murphy, M., Ha, N. K., Xiang, C. et al. (2001). Transcription program of human herpesvirus 8 (kaposi's sarcoma-associated herpesvirus). *J. Virol.*, **75**, 4843–4853.

Pearce, M., Matsumara, S., and Wilson, A. C. (2005). Transcripts encoding K12, v-FLIP, v-cyclin, and the microRNA cluster of Kaposi's sarcoma-associated herpesvirus originate from a common promoter. *J. Virol.*, **79**, 14457–14464.

Pfeffer, S., Sewer, A., Lagos-Quintana, M. et al. (2005). Identification of microRNAs of the herpesvirus family. *Nature Methods*, **2**, 269–276.

Polson, A. G., Huang, L., Lukac, D. M. et al. (2001). Kaposi's sarcoma-associated herpesvirus K-bZIP protein is phosphorylated by cyclin dependent kinases. *J. Virol.*, **75**, 3175–3184.

Poole, L. J., Zong, J. C., Ciufo, D. M. et al. (1999). Comparison of genetic variability at multiple loci across the genomes of the major subtypes of Kaposi's sarcoma-associated herpesvirus reveals evidence for recombination and for two distinct types of open reading frame K15 alleles at the right-hand end. *J. Virol.*, **73**, 6646–6660.

Raab, M. S., Albrecht, J. C., Birkmann, A. et al. (1998). The immunogenic glycoprotein gp35–37 of human herpesvirus 8 is encoded by open reading frame K8.1. *J. Virol.*, **72**, 6725–6731.

Rainbow, L., Platt, G. M., and Simpson, G. R. (1997). The 222- to 234-kilodalton latent nuclear protein (LNA) of Kaposi's sarcoma-associated herpesvirus (human herpesvirus 8) is encoded by ORF73 and is a component of the latency-associated nuclear antigen. *J. Virol.*, **71**, 5915–5921.

Reed, J. A., Nador, R. G., Spaulding, D., Tani, Y., Cesarman, E., and Knowles, D. M. (1998). Demonstration of Kaposi's sarcoma-associated herpes virus cyclin D homolog in cutaneous Kaposi's sarcoma by colorimetric in situ hybridization using a catalyzed signal amplification system. *Blood*, **91**, 3825–3832.

Renne, R., Blackbourn, D., Whitby, D., Levy, J., and Ganem, D. (1998). Limited transmission of Kaposi's sarcoma-associated herpesvirus in cultured cells. *J. Virol.*, **72**, 5182–5188.

Rimessi, P., Bonaccorsi, A., Sturzl, M. et al. (2001). Transcription pattern of human herpesvirus 8 open reading frame K3 in primary effusion lymphoma and Kaposi's sarcoma. *J. Virol.*, **75**, 7161–7174.

Rivas, C., Thlick, A. E., Parravicini, C., Moore, P. S., and Chang, Y. (2001). Kaposi's sarcoma-associated herpesvirus LANA2 is a B-cell-specific latent viral protein that inhibits p53. *J. Virol.*, **75**, 429–438.

Roizman, B. and Knipe, D. M. (2001). Herpes Simplex viruses and their replication, p. 2399–2459. In D. M. Knipe and P. Howley, *Fields Virology*, ed. Lippincott Williams & Wilkins, Philadelphia.

Russo, J. J., Bohenzky, R. A., Chien, M. C. et al. (1996). Nucleotide sequence of the Kaposi sarcoma-associated herpesvirus (HHV8). *Proc. Natl Acad. Sci. USA*, **93**, 14862–14867.

Sachsenberg-Struder, E. M., Dobrynski, N., Sheldon, J. et al. (1999). Human herpesvirus S seropositive patient with skin and graft Kaposi's sarcoma after lung transplantation. *J. Am. Acad. Dermatol.*, **40**, 308–311.

Sadler, R., Wu, L., Forghani, B. et al. (1999). A complex translational program generates multiple novel proteins from the latently expressed kaposin (K12) locus of Kaposi's sarcoma-associated herpesvirus. *J. Virol.*, **73**, 5722–5730.

Sakakibara, S., Ueda, K., Chen, J., Okuno, T., and Yamanishi, K. (2001). Octamer-binding sequence is a key element for the autoregulation of Kaposi's sarcoma-associated herpesvirus ORF50/Lyta gene expression. *J. Virol.*, **75**, 6894–6900.

Samols, M. A., Hu, J., Skalsky, R. L., and Renne, R. (2005). Cloning and identification of a microRNA cluster within the latency-associated region of Kaposi's sarcoma-associated herpesvirus. *J. Virol.*, **79**, 9301–9305.

Sarid, R., Flore, O., Bohenzky, R. A., Chang, Y., and Moore, P. S. (1998). Transcription mapping of the Kaposi's sarcoma-associated herpesvirus (human herpesvirus 8) genome in a body cavity-based lymphoma cell line (BC-1). *J. Virol.*, **72**, 1005–1012.

Sarid, R., Wiezorek, J. S., Moore, P. S., and Chang, Y. (1999). Characterization and cell cycle regulation of the major Kaposi's sarcoma-associated herpesvirus (human herpesvirus 8) latent genes and their promoter. *J. Virol.*, **73**, 1438–1446.

Saveliev, A., Zhu, F., and Yuan, Y. (2002). Transcription mapping and expression patterns of genes in the major immediate-early region of Kaposi's sarcoma-associated herpesvirus. *Virology*, **299**, 301–314.

Seaman, W. T., Ye, D., Wang, R. X., Hale, E. E., Weisse, M., and Quinlivan, E. B. (1999). Gene expression from the ORF50/K8 region of Kaposi's sarcoma-associated herpesvirus. *Virology*, **263**, 436–449.

Sharp, T. V., Wang, H. W., Koumi, A. *et al.* (2002). K15 protein of Kaposi's sarcoma-associated herpesvirus. *Virology*, **263**, 436–449.

Sinclair, A. J. (2003). bZIP proteins of human gammaherpesviruses. *J. Gen. Virol.*, **84**, 1941–1949.

Song, M. J., Li, X., Brown, H. J., and Sun, R. (2002). Characterization of interactions between RTA and the promoter of polyadenylated nuclear RNA in Kaposi's sarcoma-associated herpesvirus/human herpesvirus 8. *J. Virol.*, **76**, 5000–5013.

Spiller, O. B., Blackbourn, D. J., Mark, L., Proctor, D. G., and Blom, A. M. (2003). Functional activity of the complement regulator encoded by Kaposi's sarcoma-associated herpesvirus. *J. Biol. Chem.*, **278**, 9283–9289.

Staskus, K. A., Zhong, W., Gebhard, K. *et al.* (1997). Kaposi's sarcoma-associated herpesvirus gene expression in endothelial (spindle) tumor cells. *J. Virol.*, **71**, 715–719.

Stürzl, M., Blasig, C., Schreier, A. *et al.* (1997). Expression of HHV-8 latency-associated T0.7 RNA in spindle cells and endothelial cells of AIDS-associated, classical and African Kaposi's sarcoma. *Int. J. Cancer*, **72**, 68–71.

Stürzl, M., Hohenadl, C., Zietz, C. *et al.* (1999). Expression of K13/v-FLIP gene of human herpesvirus 8 and apoptosis in Kaposi's sarcoma spindle cells. *J. Natl Cancer Inst.*, **91**, 1725–1733.

Smuda, C., Bogner, E., and Radsak, K. (1997). The human cytomegalovirus glycoprotein B gene (ORF UL55) is expressed early in the infectious cycle. *J. Gen. Virol.*, **78 (8)**, 1981–1992.

Sun, R., Lin, S. F., Gradoville, L., Yuan, Y., Zhu, F., and Miller, G. (1998). A viral gene that activates lytic cycle expression of Kaposi's sarcoma-associated herpesvirus. *Proc. Natl Acad. Sci. USA*, **95**, 10866–10871.

Sun, R., Lin, S. F., Staskus, K. *et al.* (1999). Kinetics of Kaposi's sarcoma-associated herpesvirus gene expression. *J. Virol.*, **73**, 2232–2242.

Talbot, S. J., Weiss, R. A., Kellam, P., and Boshoff, C. (1999). Transcriptional analysis of human herpesvirus-8 open reading frames 71, 72, 73, K14, and 74 in a primary effusion lymphoma cell line. *Virology*, **257**, 84–94.

Taylor, J. L. R., Bennett, H. N., Snyder, B. A., Moore, P. S., and Chang, Y. (2005). Identification of novel transcripts in Kaposi's sarcoma-associated herpesvirus (KSHV) genome. *J. Virol.*, **79**, 15099–15106.

Varthakavi, V., Smith, R. M., Deng, H., Sun, R., and Spearman, P. (2002). Human immunodeficiency virus type-1 activates lytic cycle replication of Kaposi's sarcoma-associated herpesvirus through induction of KSHV Rta. *Virology*, **297**, 270–280.

Vieira, J., Huang, M. L., Koelle, D. M., and Corey, L. (1997). Transmissible Kaposi's sarcoma-associated herpesvirus (human herpesvirus 8) in saliva of men with a history of Kaposi's sarcoma. *J. Virol.*, **71**, 7083–7087.

Vieira, J., O'Hearn, P., Kimball, L., Chandran, B., and Corey, L. (2001). Activation of Kaposi's sarcomaassociated herpesvirus (human herpesvirus 8) lytic replication by human cytomegalovirus. *J. Virol.*, **75**, 1378–1386.

Viejo-Borbolla, A., Kati, E., Shelodon, J. A. *et al.* (2003). A domain in the C-terminal region of latency-associated nuclear antigen 1 of Kaposi's sarcoma-associated herpesvirus affects transcriptional activation and binding to nuclear heterochromatin. *J. Virol.*, **77**, 7093–7100.

Wang, F. Z., Akula, S. M., Pramod, N. P., Zeng, L., and Chandran, B. (2001a). Human herpesvirus 8 envelope glycoprotein K8.1A interaction with the target cells involves heparan sulfate. *J. Virol.*, **75**, 7517–7527.

Wang, S. E., Wu, F. Y., Fujimuro, M., Zong, J., Hayward, S. D., and Hayward, G. S. (2003a). Role of CCAAT/enhancer-binding protein alpha (C/EBPalpha) in activation of the Kaposi's sarcoma-associated herpesvirus (KSHV) lytic-cycle replication-associated protein (RAP) promoter in cooperation with the KSHV replication and transcription activator (RTA) and RAP. *J. Virol.*, **77**, 600–623.

Wang, S. E., Wu, F. Y., Yu, Y., and Hayward, G. S. (2003b). CCAAT/enhancer-binding protein-alpha is induced during the early stages of Kaposi's sarcoma-associated herpesvirus (KSHV) lytic cycle reactivationand together with the KSHV replication and transcription activator (RTA) cooperatively stimulates the viral RTA, MTA, and PAN promoters. *J. Virol.*, **77**, 9590–9612.

Wang, X. P., Zhang, Y. J., Deng, J. H. *et al.* (2001b).Characterization of the promoter region of the viral interferon regulatory factor encoded by Kaposi's sarcoma-associated herpesvirus. *Oncogene*, **20**, 523–530.

Wang, Y. Li, H., Chan, M. Y. *et al.* (2003c). Kaposi's sarcoma-associated herpesvirus Ori-Lyt-dependent DNA replication: *cis*-acting requirements for replication and Ori-Lyt-associated RNA transcription. *J. Virol.*, **78**, 8615–8629.

Wirth, U. V., Gunkel, K., Engels, M., and Schwyzer, M. (1989). Spatial and temporal distribution of bovine herpesvirus 1 transcripts. *J. Virol.*, **63**, 4882–4889.

Wong, E. L. and Damania, B. (2006). Transcriptional regulation of the Kaposi sarcoma-associated herpesvirus K15 gene *J. Virol.*, **80**, 1385–1392.

Wu, F. Y., Ahn, J. H., Alcendor, D. J. *et al.* (2001). Origin-independent assembly of Kaposi's sarcoma-associated herpesvirus DNA replication compartments in transient cotransfection assays and association with the ORF-K8 protein and cellular PML. *J. Virol.*, **75**, 1487–1506.

Zhong, W., Wang, H., Herndier, B., and Ganem, D. (1996). Restricted expression of Kaposi sarcomaassociated herpesvirus (human herpesvirus 8) genes in Kaposi sarcoma. *Proc. Natl Acad. Sci. USA*, **93**, 6641–6646.

Zhu, F. X., Cusano, T., and Yuan, Y. (1999). Identification of the immediate-early transcripts of Kaposi's sarcoma-associated herpesvirus. *J. Virol.*, **73**, 5556–5567.

Ziegler, J. L. (1993). Endemic Kaposi's sarcoma in Africa and local volcanic soils. *Lancet*, **342**, 1348–1351.

Zoeteweij, J. P., Moses, A. V., and Rinderknecht, A. S. (2001). Targeted inhibition of calcineurin signaling blocks calcium-dependent reactivation of Kaposi sarcoma-associated herpesvirus. *Blood*, **97**, 2374–2380.

29

Effects on apoptosis, cell cycle and transformation, and comparative aspects of EBV with other known DNA tumor viruses

George Klein and Ingemar Ernberg

Microbiology and Tumor Biology Center, Karolinska Institutet, Stockholm, Sweden

The list of human viruses presently known to cause or to contribute to tumor development comprise four DNA viruses, Epstein–Barr virus, certain human papilloma virus subtypes, hepatitis B virus, and Kaposi sarcoma herpesvirus (HHV-8); and two RNA viruses, adult T-cell leukemia virus (HTLV-1) and hepatitis virus C. In addition, while HIV infection is not directly tumorigenic, it increases the incidence of certain tumors.

The purpose of this chapter is to consider EBV and HHV-8 in relation to the known DNA tumor viruses, with particular focus on tumorigenicity.

Viral strategy at the molecular level as a tumor risk factor

Altered genes or environmental factors are usually considered as major risk factors for tumor development. However, the strategy of certain viruses may constitute a risk factor in itself. Tumor-associated viruses in humans have a survival strategy, like other viruses, aiming to maintain, replicate and propagate their genomes, but some features of this strategy entail a risk to initiate or favor tumor development under certain circumstances. This implies that only a small minority of the infected cells enter the pathway towards a malignant tumor and even fewer succeed.

Three types of virus–host cell interactions may carry a risk

1. Blocking of late viral functions or blocking the replicative cycle, by mutation or deletion of genetic material, e.g., due to the integration of the viral genome, as exemplified by HPV or adenovirus transformation in vitro.

2. Infection of cells that are not fully permissive for viral replication, for species or tissue specific reasons. Permissiveness for the early but not the late functions of the viral cycle is particularly dangerous. The early viral proteins may exert continuous proliferation stimulating and/or apoptosis preventing effects. Infection of hamster or guinea pig cells with some of the human adenoviruses and SV40 infection of rodent cells may serve as examples.

3. Latent viral persistence may subvert normal controls. This can be illustrated by EBV infection of B-lymphocyes in immunodefective hosts.

Early history: up and down

Views on the role of viruses in the etiology of cancer have been polarized between two extreme positions during the major part of the last century. The belief that viruses have nothing to do with cancer was as widespread at certain times, as the suspicion that most and perhaps all tumors are caused by virus at other times. The field started with the discovery of Peyton Rous in 1911 that chicken sarcomas could be transmitted with cell-free filtrates (Rous, 1911). The tumors arose at the site of inoculation and were of the same histological type as the original sarcoma. This created great excitement: the cancer problem was solved! The enthusiasm subsided rapidly, however, when mouse and rat tumor filtrates failed to induce tumors. In retrospect we may see this as the consequence of exaggerated expectations, hasty experiments and increasing lack of confidence. It became the prevalent view that viruses may play a role for tumors in birds, but not in mammals.

Two decades later, Richard Shope (1933) found that benign warts could be transmitted from the wild cottontail to the domestic rabbit by cell-free filtrates. This did not change the climate of opinion. The rabbit was a mammalian but warts were benign tumors, not cancers. Several important points were overlooked by outside commentators, however. The initially benign rabbit papillomas turned occasionally into carcinomas. This could be accelerated by the topical application of chemical carcinogens. The term tumor progression was originally coined by Rous to designate this transition, or, in its generalized form, the process whereby "tumors go from bad to worse." Later, Leslie Foulds (1958) defined and extended the term. It refers to the development of tumors by multiple, stepwise changes in several "unit characteristics." Today we see them as distinct phenotypic traits. They are individually variable and reassort independently of each other. Tumor progression can therefore proceed along several alternative pathways and each tumor becomes individually unique from the biological point of view.

The early work on Shope papilloma was also interesting from the immunologist's point of view. The virally induced warts that did not progress to carcinoma were rejected simultaneously by a systemically acting host response, mediated by lymphocytes, rather than by antibodies. This was the first example of a tumor rejection response that targeted virally encoded proteins in DNA virus transformed cells.

In the 1930s, John Bittner (1936) discovered the milk factor, later called the mouse mammary tumor virus (MMTV). This discovery did not create any major change of opinion either. This may have been due, at least in part, to the way the findings were presented and discussed. The genetically oriented mouse mammary tumor biologists proceed by careful, gradual analysis that fitted the long duration of each experiment (2 years or more). It showed that MMTV could increase the frequency of mammary cancer, but it was neither necessary nor sufficient for tumor induction. Hormonal and genetic factors modified the risk considerably. The role of MMTV as a tumor-susceptibility factor in selectively inbred high cancer strains was readily accepted, but its role as a "tumor virus" remained questionable. It was appreciated, however, that the probability of tumor development could be influenced by multiple factors, including viruses.

Up again, and how!

A major paradigmatic shift occurred in the 1950s. It was triggered by the discovery of the murine leukemia virus by Ludwik Gross (1951) and the polyoma virus by Sarah Stewart and Bernice Eddy (Stewart *et al.*, 1958). Gross found that cell free filtrates prepared from the "spontaneous" leukemias of the high leukemic AKR strain could transmit the disease to a low leukemia strain, C3H. In contrast to many others who failed before him, Gross succeeded for three reasons: his serendipitous use of newborn, less than 24 hours old mice as recipients; his fortuitous choice of C3H, the only low leukemia strain available at the time that happened to be susceptible to the virus carried by the AKR strain, later called the Gross virus; and the dogged persistence of Ludvik Gross in an area where nobody expected positive results.

The scientific community received Gross's first report with surprise and disbelief. This attitude prevailed for 5 years, until the originator of the AKR strain, Jacob Furth, took pains to repeat Gross's experiments under the original conditions and with the same recipient C3H subline (Furth *et al.*, 1956). He succeeded, in contrast to others who were less meticulous in their choice of experimental conditions. Furth's confirmation has led to the immediate acceptance of Gross's findings. The discovery of the polyoma virus also stemmed from Gross's work, but in a more indirect fashion. Gross has observed occasional parotid tumors in C3H mice inoculated with AKR leukemia filtrates. He realized that they may have been induced by another virus, provisionally referred to as the parotid tumor agent.

Stewart and Eddy started out on the assumption that Gross's leukemia virus experiments were correct. Since the virus was apparently quite weak, however, they wished to amplify it by adding the leukemia filtrates to embryonic mouse fibroblast cultures. After a few days culturing, they inoculated the filtered supernatants into newborn mice. The mice developed a wide variety of sarcomas and carcinomas, but no leukemia. Due to its ability to induce many types of tumors, the virus was named polyoma.

Classes of experimental tumor viruses

The viruses so far mentioned fall into three major categories. Rous sarcoma virus belongs to the acute or class I RNA tumor viruses. The murine leukemia and the mammary tumor virus fall into the category of chronic or class II RNA tumor viruses. The Shope papilloma and the polyoma virus are DNA tumor viruses.

Some interesting generalizations can be made on the basis of this and later experimental work that has identified many additional viruses in all three categories.

All experimentally derived RNA tumor viruses belong to the retrovirus family. They carry their genetic information in RNA. Following their entry into a susceptible target cell, the virally encoded reverse transcriptase rewrites their RNA into proviral DNA that can insert into cellular

DNA at random. When virus production is activated again, the proviral DNA is transcribed into RNA. This is followed by viral RNA replication, the production of new viral proteins, the assembly of new viral particles, and their release by budding, but it is not accompanied by any cytopathic effect. Virus production is therefore compatible with cell proliferation.

Activation and transcription of the integrated provirus is an error-prone process. Adjacent cellular DNA may contribute to the RNA sequences carried by the viral particle. In the vast majority of the cases, this has no notable consequences, but occasionally the incorporated cellular sequence may originate from a gene whose activated product can stimulate the entry of the cell into the S-phase. Virus particles that carry such sequences may cause cell proliferation when they infect new recipient cells. The probability that this happens is very low, because every step in the process, from the integration of the virus into the "right place," through the production of the appropriately (in frame) fused viral–cellular messages, the release and the replication of competent virus and the subsequent new infection of a susceptible cell, are all low probability events. A tumorigenic virus variant is usually generated by the purposeful and often prolonged selection for tumorigenicity This requires great persistence on the part of the investigator. Following the early discovery of the Rous sarcoma virus, it took four decades before new acute or class I RNA tumor viruses were isolated that could induce tumors at the site of inoculation and to transform normal into tumor cells in vitro. Following the revival of viral oncology in the 1950s, some 40 such viral strains, carrying about 20 different cell derived oncogenes, as they were to be called, were isolated in rapid succession from fowl, rodent, feline and simian tumors.

Class I RNA tumor viruses are not known to play any tumorigenic role in nature. This is understandable, because most of them are defective, due to the replacement of essential viral genetic information, by the inserted cellular gene. With only some notable exceptions, they produce crippled virus particles that can only multiply in the presence of complete, but non-transforming "helper virus."

Chronic or class II RNA tumor viruses have no transforming activity in culture. They do not induce tumors at the site of inoculation and carry no cellular oncogenes. Insertion of the proviral DNA in the immediate neighborhood of a cellular oncogene is the most frequent mechanism whereby they contribute to the tumorigenic process. Since the proviral DNA integrates at random, the likelihood of such an insertion is low. Very high level of virus production, accompanied by viremia, is usually mandatory for tumorigenicity. This is the reason why only some mouse strains that can support virus replication and/or are deficient in their immunological responsiveness to the virus, are susceptible to the tumorigenic effect of murine leukemia virus or mammary tumor virus.

Insertion in the neighborhood of a cellular protooncogene is not the only mechanism whereby an RNA tumor virus can initiate tumor development, but other alternatives are less well documented. HTLV-1, or adult T cell leukemia (ATLV) virus, is an example of this. It is believed to stimulate the expansion of preneoplastic cell populations, paving the way to cellular changes that may be more directly involved in the tumorigenic process (Gallo *et al.*, 1983).

In conclusion, the RNA tumor viruses have provided a wealth of information about virus-cell interactions in relation to the tumorigenic process and have led, indirectly, to the discovery of numerous cell division regulating cellular genes. They can be regarded as a model of what can happen, but they give us very little information about what does actually happen in the genesis of human tumors.

The DNA tumor viruses provide a very different picture. They belong to several unrelated virus families. In contrast to the RNA tumor viruses that can replicate in growing cells without killing them, the DNA tumor viruses kill the cells in which they replicate. Their tumorigenic activity depends therefore on the blocking of the lytic viral cycle. This may occur in cells that are non-permissive for the lytic cycle due to their species and/or tissue derivation.

The transforming genes of all DNA tumor viruses are genuine constituents of the viral genome. The number of virally encoded transforming genes varies between one (SV40), two (adeno- and papillomaviruses) and six (EBV). The virally encoded transforming proteins are immunogenic, as a rule. The challenge of viral transformation is met by the immune surveillance of the host. Cells transformed by these viruses grow usually only in immunosuppressed hosts. They represent the major part of the "opportunistic tumors" that arise exclusively or predominantly in congenitally, iatrogenically (as after organ transplantation) or virally (e.g., by HIV) immunosuppressed persons.

Inactivation of Rb and p53 is an important prelude to viral replication, as discussed below. Early after primary infection, DNA tumor viruses induce a round of DNA replication in the recipient cells. This carries the risk of malignant proliferation. The host inhibits the progressive growth of the transformed cells by its immune response, however. While the immunocompetent host rejects virus driven, proliferating cells, the virus goes into hiding. It persists in non-proliferating cells where it is not "seen" by the immune response. The example of EBV provides a particularly interesting "success story" that favors the survival of both the virus and the host. A comparison with the smaller DNA tumor viruses, in the next section highlights both parallels and contrasts.

What does the type of virus-cell interaction tell us about tumorigenic risk?

There is a fundamental difference between the small DNA tumor viruses and the herpesviruses, with regard to potentially tumorigenic interactions with their host cell. Permissiveness for the early but not for the late (lytic) steps of the viral cycle constitute the main risk for the former group. Convergent evolution has provided SV40, the transforming adenoviruses and the tumor associated papillomaviruses with the ability to inactivate two of the main tumor suppressor pathways that involve p53 and Rb, respectively. Inactivation of the same two pathways appears to be mandatory for non-virally related tumor development. As discussed elsewhere in this chapter, this impairs two of the main controlling functions that prevent the replication of cells driven by illegitimately activated oncogenes.

Inactivation of both pathways by the small DNA tumor viruses is part of the viral strategy. Both the integrating and the episomal viruses need to induce an S-phase, as already mentioned, in order to integrate or to establish the appropriate chromosomal–episomal balance, respectively. They also need to protect the activated cell from apoptosis, in order to secure their persistence.

In the natural host cell, the growth stimulating and anti-apoptotic effects of these viruses have no lasting consequence, because virus production and cell lysis sets a natural endpoint.

In the case of the tumor associated herpesviruses and particularly of EBV, the possible tumorigenic contributions of the virus need to be considered in relation to the different forms of non-productive virus–cell interactions. EBV has evolved mechanisms to activate and expand its primary host cell population, the human B-lymphocyte. It is also capable of switching off its B-cell activating program and remain latent in long-lived resting memory B cells. The virus can thus use several non-lytic interaction programs, tailored to different B cell subclasses. They lead to different programs of viral expression that also differ in their ability to induce a CD8+ T-cell mediated immune response in the host that prevents the excessive proliferation of the virally transformed immunoblasts.

Unlike the small DNA tumor viruses, where tumorigenicity is favored by the structural or regulatory impairment of the lytic genes, the latent EBV-B cell interaction that occurs without any genetic defect in the virus, is a potential tumor risk in the immunodeficient host. This is due to the fact that, apart from the occasional activation of the viral cycle in EBV-carrying B cells, the interaction is largely non-lytic. In EBV-carrying immunoblastomas that arise in transplant recipients, or in certain congenitally T-cell defective patients (XLP in particular) as well as in part of the AIDS associated lymphomas (with immunoblastic morphology), the interaction of the virus with proliferating immunoblasts is comparable to or identical with the usual interaction of the virus with normal B-cells. The tumorigenic "accident" occurs at the level of the host and not at the level of the virus or the cell.

None of the other EBV-associated B-cell derived malignant lymphomas, such as BL, HL, or PEL or the unusual, EBV carrying T-cell lymphomas express the proliferation driving, blastogenic program of the virus. The virus expresses only minimalistic programs designated as latency I or II, in contrast to the full immunoblastic program (III). The tumor promoting contribution of the virus must therefore be sought in other, less direct effects.

In BL, one needs to depart from the fact that the lymphoma originates in the post-GC, centroblastic or centrocytic cell, that is either resting or is on its way to a long-lived resting memory cell, but cannot leave the cycling compartment because it is driven by an Ig/myc translocation. The translocation results from a faulty recombination that occurs in the course of physiological Ig gene rearrangement. Conceivably, EBV may contribute to the emergence of the virus carrying BL clone by expanding the original population or, alternatively, or in addition, by protecting the myc-driven, apoptosis prone cell from apoptosis. (See further in the section on EBV and BL below).

Human tumor viruses

Four of the six viruses known to be involved in the causation of human cancer in a direct or a contributory capacity are DNA viruses (EBV, HPV, HBV, HHV-8) while the remaining two are RNA viruses (HTLV-1 and HCV).

As discussed below, EBV is most directly involved in the causation of immunoblastomas that arise in immunodefective persons, such as transplant recipients, certain congenital immunodefectives, and HIV-infected persons. EBV may also play a role in Burkitt lymphoma (BL) and nasopharyngeal carcinoma (NPC), as indicated by the regularity of its association with these tumors, but the nature of the viral contribution is not fully understood.

Special subtypes of the human papilloma viruses are known to contribute to the genesis of cervical carcinomas and of skin tumors. Human herpesvirus no.8 (HHV8, also called KSHV) is associated with Kaposi sarcoma,

Castelman's disease and body cavity lymphoma. Hepatitis virus type B and C contribute to the genesis of primary liver cancer. The evidence for these virus-tumor associations is epidemiological and molecular, but the relative role of the virus and of cellular changes has not been properly established.

The following two sections deal with the two human tumor associated gamma herpesviruses, Epstein–Barr virus (EBV) and, to a minor extent, Kaposi sarcoma herpesvirus (KSHV or HHV-8).

Epstein-barr virus (EBV)

EBV is the causative agent of a self-limiting lymphoproliferative disease, infectious mononucleosis. In immunodefectives, the proliferation may proceed to progressively growing immunoblastomas. Multiple viral genomes, derived from a single infectious event, are regularly found in high endemic Burkitt lymphomas (BLs) and in low differentiated or anaplastic nasopharyngeal carcinomas (NPCs). EBV is also found, although less regularly, in Hodgkin's lymphomas, nasal T-cell lymphomas, gastric carcinomas, salivary gland tumors and leiomyosarcomas (Table 29.1).

EBV exploits B-cell specific regulatory mechanisms and signals

Normal B cell physiology is tightly regulated. The generation of B-cell receptor diversity by immunoglobulin gene rearrangements, activation of resting B cells by cognate antigen and associated molecules, expansion of the activated population, migration through germinal centers and concomitant hypermutation, generation of long-lived memory cells and differentiation into secretory subtypes, plasma cells in particular, is regulated both by internal programs and external signals, including antigens, ligands and cytokines that influence homing, proliferation, differentiation and death of the cells. EBV has a whole gamut of highly refined mechanisms that exploit normal B cell physiology. Unlike many other viruses, its strategy is not limited to the turning of its host cell into a viral protein factory with the single purpose of virus production and release to the environment, although it can switch on that mechanism when it enters the lytic cycle. Rather, the virus follows a "live and let live" principle. Its vast success in infecting all human populations and persisting in latent form over the lifetime of the host without causing disease, except by accident, testifies to the validity of this strategy, both for the virus and for the cells.

The exploitation of normal B-cell physiology by the virus manifests itself at many different points. Already the very

Table 29.1. EBV-associated tumors in man (the percentage figures indicate the frequency of EBV carrying tumors)

Lymphoid tissues		Epithelial tissues	
Burkitt's lymphoma, endemic	98%		
Burkitt's lymphoma, sporadic	25%	Gastric adenocarcinoma	5–10%
AIDS-immunoblastic lymphoma – in CNS	60% 100%	Nasopharyngeal carcinoma undifferentiated	100%
Post-transplant lymphoma	100%	Salivary gland carcinomas	<100%
Hodgkin's lymphoma	50%	Leiomyosarcoma in immunosuppressed	100%
T-cell lymphomas -lethal midline granuloma	10–30% >90%		

first step, viral attachment and penetration, is based on the use of a B-cell specific surface moiety, CD21 (also called the C3d receptor). This receptor is normally involved in B-cell activation by antigen, antibody and complement complexes. Activated B-blasts secrete cytokines and lymphokines that can stimulate B cell proliferation and express the corresponding receptors (e.g., CD 23), creating an autocrine loop. Moreover, the virus encodes three membrane proteins, LMP1, 2a and 2b, of which at least two control and modulate incoming signals, that participate in Ig-receptor activation, TNF-response and programmed cell death. As discussed in more detail below, the LMPs are constitutively active multifunctional membrane proteins. LMP1 interferes with TNF-α signaling. It can replace many CD40 induced functions and activates major signaling systems in B-lymphocytes and epithelial cells, such as NFkB, JNK-kinase and one JAK/STAT-pathway. Protection from apoptosis is one of its major downstream effects. LMP2a modulates kinase signaling from membrane receptors. Most notable are the eight N-terminal phosphotyrosine motifs that interact with the Ig-receptor induced kinases lyn and syk. LMP2a has an Immunoglobulin Transactivation Motif (ITAM) – with complete homology to the corresponding Ig-receptor ITAM-motif of its gamma-chain, that binds the syk kinase in its activated, phosphorylated state. Interspersed with these motifs are a PPPPY-motif that interacts with WW-domains of the Nedd-family of E3-ubiquitine ligases (Winberg et al., 2000). It is conceivable that LMP2a may attract the kinases and is involved in their fast destruction by guiding the complex to the ubiquitine –proteasome system. Characteristically, the expression of

Table 29.2. Overview of the EBNA proteins

Name	Sub-type	Viral functions	Interactive cellular proteins	Expression	Required for in vitro transformation
EBNA-1		Maintains viral episomes Regulates viral promoters	Karyopherins 2 α and β; TAP/p32; USP7 (HAUSP); RPA	All EBV-carrying cells	Yes
EBNA-2	A & B	Activates viral and cellular promoters	PU.1; hSNF5; Spi-B; RBP-J kappa; p300/CBP; DP103; p100; TFIIE;TFIIH; TFIIB; TAF40; myb; TBP	Latency III in B-cells	Yes
EBNA-3 (EBNA-3A)	A & B	Represses the RBP-J kappa dependent transcription	RBP-J kappa; RBP-2N; CtBP; epsilon-subunit of TCP-1; XAP-2; F538 (UK/UPRT); AhR	Latency III in B-cells	Yes
EBNA-4 (EBNA-3B)	A & B		RBP-J kappa; RBP-2N	Latency III in B-cells	No
EBNA-5 (EBNA-LP)		Enhances EBNA-2 dependent transcription	Hsp27; Hsp70 (Hsp72); Hsc70 (Hsp73); HAX-1; HA95; alpha & beta tubulins; prolyl-4-hydroxylase alpha-1 subunit; p14ARF; Fte-1/S3a	Latency III in B-cells	Yes
EBNA-6 (EBNA-3C)	A & B	Represses the RBP-J kappa dependent transcription	RBP-J kappa; RBP-2N; DP103; ProT-alpha; SMN; NM23-H1	Latency III in B-cells	Yes

these proteins still permits the corresponding physiological signaling pathways to operate.

For example, LMP1 can replace CD40 ligand-CD 40 signalling, but does not interfere with physiological CD40-reception. LMP2 does not completely abolish Ig-receptor signaling, although it is likely to increase the signal threshold. It may be noted that the HHV8 membrane proteins K 1 and K 15, in combination, carry many of the motifs that function in the LMPs, such as the NFkB activation site and ITAM-motifs. Their role in latency, lytic cycle and tumorigenesis remains to be elucidated.

The following section will deal with the EBV-encoded growth transformation associated proteins in some more detail.

Growth transformation associated EBV encoded proteins

Table 29.2 summarizes the information of the six nuclear proteins (EBNAs).

EBNA1 is encoded by the ORF/KBRF1. It is a DNA binding protein of highly variable size (60–100 kD) due to the presence of a glycine alanine repetitive sequence, inserted in the first molecule that is flanked by a highly basic domain. The C-terminal part of the protein contains a stretch of acidic amino acids. It is expressed in most EBV-carrying cells, with the possible exception of latently infected resting B-cells (Reedman & Klein, 1974; Lindahl et al., 1974; Andersson-Anvret et al., 1978; Hennessy & Kieff, 1983; Dillner et al., 1986a,b; Chen et al., 1995a,b). In all other cell types that have been studied, EBNA 1 is expressed irrespectively of the cell phenotype, level of differentiation or, in the case of lymphocytes, activation status (Niedobitek et al., 1989; Hamilton-Dutoit et al., 1991; Prevot et al., 1992; Zhou et al., 1994). It is the only latency associated EBV-encoded protein whose expression is not influenced by the cell phenotype. In somatic cell hybrids between EBV carrying immunoblasts that express the full type III program of six nuclear and three membrane proteins and EBV negative non-B cells where all B-cell specific markers are eclipsed, EBNA1 but not EBNA 2–6 remains expressed (Contreras-Salazar et al., 1989). EBNA1 is also the only member of the EBNA-family that remains associated with the chromosomes in metaphase (Ohno et al., 1977; Jiang et al., 1991). It is randomly distributed among the chromosomes, but binds specifically to the origin of latent viral DNA replication (OriP). This binding is necessary for the maintenance of the EBV episomes, by equal distribution to the daughter cells in mitosis (Jones et al., 1989). EBNA 1 has three specific binding regions in the viral DNA, each multiple. 20 binding sites are in the family of repeats (FR), four in the dyad symmetry, and two downstream of the Q promoter (Reisman & Sugden, 1986; Sugden & Warren, 1989; Ambinder et al., 1990; Rawlins et al., 1985).

The latent replication of the viral DNA starts from ori P. EBNA1 binds to ori P as a dimer. It is composed of a flanking domain and a core domain. The flanking domain includes a helix that projects into the major DNA grove and an extended chain that travels along the minor grove. This motif is responsible for all sequence determined contacts with DNA. The core domain makes no direct contact with DNA (Polvino-Bodnar et al., 1988). The binding to chromatin is mediated via chromatin protein (ref). EBNA1 binding to the chromosomes is essential for the precise division of the replicated DNA into the two daughter cells.

Through the multiple interactions with viral DNA, EBNA 1 causes DNA looping by multimerization. This increases the complexity of its promoter regulation. Dyad symmetry controls S-phase associated viral DNA replication. EBNA 1 regulates viral promoters via its multiple binding sites. FR acts as an enhancer for the C-promoter, directing all six EBNA transcripts and the Qp elements that are negative regulators of Qp-driven EBNA1 transcription through a negative feedback loop (Bodescot et al., 1987; Sample & Kieff, 1990).

EBNA1 contains a glycine–alanine repeat of variable length that inhibits its processing through the proetasomes and the subsequent MHC class 1 association of the derived peptides, a prerequisite for recognition by CD8 positive cytotoxic T-cells (Levitskaya et al., 1995). This results in a dramatically extended half life of EBNA 1 to more than 2 weeks, and may contribute to its presence in resting B-cells without *de novo* synthesis.

EBNA2

EBNA2 (ORF:BYRF1) is an 82 kD phosphoprotein. It contains a 14 AA long domain that is responsible for transactivation. In contrast to EBNA1, the expression of EBNA2 is restricted to immunoblasts (Dillner et al., 1985; Hennessy & Kieff, 1985; Ernberg et al., 1986). On primary infection of B-cells it acts as a transcriptional transactivator (Rickinson et al., 1987). It is essential for the transformation of B-cells into immunoblasts and the derivation of LCLs (Cohen et al., 1989). EBNA2 defective viral substrains cannot activate B-cells. EBNA2 is the EBV encoded oncoprotein that differs most extensively between EBV types 1 and 2 (Zimber et al., 1986). Type I EBV is a more efficient transformer of primary B lymphocytes than type 2 (Rowe et al., 1989). EBNA2 is associated with nucleoplasmic, chromatin and nuclear matrix fractions.

EBNA2 induces a variety of activation markers and other cellular proteins in B-cells, including CD23, CD21, c- fgr and c-myc. It is required for the expression of EBV encoded LMP1 and LMP2a in immunoblastic cells (Wang et al., 1987a,b, 1990; Aman et al., 1990).

The interaction of EBNA 2 with the cellular proteins p300 and CBP is critical for EBNA2 mediated transactivation, due to the intrinsic histone acetylase activities of the former and their interaction with transcription factors (Bornkamm & Hammerschmidt, 2001). CBP has been implicated in EBNA2 activation of c-myc promoter.

Even though EBNA2 is a potent activator of many cellular and viral genes, it does not bind directly to DNA. It influences the responding promoters through its interaction with RBP-Jk, PU1 and other cellular proteins. The complexes formed modify the affinity of histones for DNA. Further chromatin remodeling activity is achieved through an interaction between EBNA2 and hSFN5. Recruitment of EBNA2 to DNA is essential for the transforming activity of EBV and RBP-Jk is the most extensively studied partner. RBP-Jk functions as a downstream target of the cell surface receptor known as Notch. Notch genes encode cell surface receptors that regulate developmental processes in a wide variety of organisms. The cleaved product of Notch is targeted to the nucleus where it binds to RBP-Jk and can activate transcription, but with a lower efficiency than the intracellular part of Notch. The binding of ligand to the extracellular domain of Notch results in the cleavage of an intracellular domain. This intracellular fragment of Notch (Notch-IC) migrates to the nucleus, binds to DNA-bound RBP-Jk and converts thereby a repressor of transcription into an activator (Hsieh et al., 1996).

On the basis of these findings, EBNA2 is regarded as a constitutively active homologue of Notch. However, Notch can only partially substitute for EBNA2 in B-cell transformation experiments, probably because it does not upregulate the transcription of LMP1 or c-myc. The EBNA2 induced activation of the LMP1 promoter requires additional B lymphocyte specific factors, such as PU.1 (Johannsen et al., 1995) and RBPJK (Johannsen et al., 1996). Elements responsible for EBNA2 responsiveness have been characterized in EBV-Cp, LMP1 and LMP2 promoters and the cellular promoter for CD23. All have at least one RBP-Jk binding site.

As already mentioned, the interaction of EBNA2 with the cellular sequence specific DNA binding protein, RBP-Jk, is critical for transformation and LCL outgrowth. A sequence in EBNA2 closely mimics a corresponding sequence in the notch-receptor. Notch and EBNA2 may activate transcription from the RBP-Jk and PU.1 promoters by interacting with SKIP, a component of the HDAC2 corepressor complex. The EBNA2 domain that interacts with PU.1 includes the site that interacts with RBP-Jk. The targeting of PU.1 by the EBNA2 transactivator is an important aspect of EBV adaptation to lymphoid cells (Tamura et al., 1995).

The essential role of EBNA2 in the immortalization of B-cells is thus due to its transactivation of viral promoters

(Cp, LMP1 and 2) and a variety of cellular genes associated with B-cell activation and growth, among them c-myc. Myc activation in lymphocytes induces protein synthesis and increase in cell size, D-type cyclins, cyclin E. It downregulates the inhibitors p21 and p27. The induction of c-myc is regarded as a major link between EBNA2 and the cell cycle machinery (Kaiser et al., 1999).

EBNA2 is also required to maintain the EBV driven proliferation of B-cells, as shown in the conditional LCL designated as EREB2–5, that contains an EBNA2-estrogen receptor fusion protein. The removal of estrogen from the growth medium results in cell cycle arrest and apoptosis. Early reintroduction of estrogen stimulates renewed cell cycle entry and proliferation (Kempkes et al., 1995). EBNA2 can be replaced by the constitutive expression of exogenous c-myc. The switch from the EBNA2 driven to the myc-driven state is accompanied by a phenotypic change of the LCL-like cell to a more BL-like cell, resembling dividing germinal center B-cells (Polack et al., 1996).

Paradoxically, EBNA2 can also inhibit proliferation in established BL lines. EBNA2 is a transcriptional repressor of the immunoglobulin mu-gene. In BL lines where myc is controlled by the immunoglobulin mu enhancer, EBNA2 expression results in suppression of the myc transcription from the translocated myc gene, leading to growth arrest (Jochner et al., 1996).

EBNA5 (alternative name: **EBNA-LP**). **EBNA5** is a nuclear phosphoprotein that localizes to distinct subnuclear bodies. It is spliced from a variable number of W1-W2 exon pairs, 66 and 132 nucleotides long, respectively, forming 66 aminoacid long repeats and, from the Y1 and Y2 exons, a C-terminal 45 AA unique region. Its progenitor, the giant primary transcript originates from the W or C promoter in immunoblastic cells (and only there) (Dillner et al., 1986a,b; Wang et al., 1987a,b; Bodescot & Perricaudet, 1986). Together with EBNA2, EBNA5 is the earliest viral protein expressed in freshly infected B-cells. The two proteins can induce the entry of resting B-cells into the G1 phase. Coexpression of EBNA5 with EBNA2 enhances EBNA2 mediated transcriptional activation. EBNA5 is tightly associated with the nuclear matrix, and often accumulates in PML bodies (Pokrovskaja et al., 2001). It migrates together with various components of the proteasome dependent degradation machinery in heat shocked cells, and in cells treated with proteasome inhibitors, raising the possibility that EBNA5 participates in the regulation of specific protein degradation in the nucleus. Kashuba et al.'s experiments on EBNA5 also showed that it does not bind to Rb and p53 in the yeast two hybrid assay, but can exert an inhibitory effect on the p53-Rb axis by targeting the p53 regulator p14 ARF (Kashuba et al., 2003). The latter can bind MDM2, suppress its ability to mediate in the degradation of p53 and thereby increase the expression level of p53. It was suggested that EBNA5 participates in the elimination of the p14 ARF-HDM2- p53 complexes and thereby contributes to the downregulation of p14 ARF and p53 protein levels in EBV infected B-cells (see also Kanamori et al., 2004).

EBNA3 family

EBNA3 (ORF: BLRF3 + BERF1), **EBNA4** (ORF: BERF2a + BERF2b) and **EBNA6** (ORF: BERF3 + BERF4) are three large nuclear phosphoproteins in a size range of 140–180 kD. EBNA3 and EBNA6, but not EBNA4 is necessary for in vitro transformation. Individual sequences of these three EBNAs show little similarity, but they are all composed of a highly charged N-terminal half and a C-terminal half that contains numerous repeat elements. EBNA4 also contains an LxCxE motif. **EBNA6** is transactivator that induces CD21, 23 and LMP1 (alternative nomenclature: EBNA3a,b,c). All three proteins are encoded by tandemly arranged genes, localized in the middle of the viral genome (Hennessy et al., 1985; Dillner et al., 1986a,b; Shimizu et al., 1988). They are all highly hydrophilic. They are stable proteins that accumulate in intranuclear clumps, sparing the nucleolus. They are believed to act as transcriptional regulators and can interact with RBP-Jk (Radkov et al., 1997; Zhao et al., 2003; Hickabottom et al., 2002). The three proteins use unrelated peptide sequences for their interaction. EBNA3 and 6, but not EBNA4, are required for B-cell transformation (Parker et al., 1996). By and large, the EBNA 3 family member, have similar but more limited effects on cellular gene expression compared to EBNA 2. EBNA4, as also EBNA3 and 6, generate highly immunogenic peptides that can associate with MHC class I molecules. Some peptide-HLA class I combinations can induce CD8+ CTL mediated rejection in immunocompetent hosts.

The following further information on the two members of the EBNA 3 family involved in growth transformation, EBNA 3 and 6, are of interest.

EBNA 3 (alt: EBNA 3a)

Kashuba et al. (2000, 2002) have identified two EBNA3 interacting proteins, using a two-hybrid technique. TCP-1 is part of a chaperonine complex (Kashuba et al., 1999). EBNA3 binds to the epsilon subunit of TCP-1. Kashuba et al. proposed that nascent EBNA3 is folded by the TCP-1 containing chaperon complex through its binding to the apical region of the epsilon subunit. EBNA3 may thereby receive help for its proper folding.

Table 29.3. Overview of the EBV latent membrane proteins

Name	Variants	Functions	Major protein interactions	Expression	Necessary for in vitro transformation
LMP1	Latent form	Mimics CD 40 Activation of NFkB, JNK-kinase, JAK/ STAT, MAP kinase, Akt cell survival induction of adhesion and immune regulatory membrane proteins	TRAF 1, 2, 3 TRADD BRAM 1 LMP2A	B-cell latency II-III, BL, HL, DLBCL, T-cell lymphoma, NPC	Yes
	Lytic	Not known	Not known	Lytic cycle	No
LMP 2	LMP2A	Interacts with phosphotyrosine kinases incl Src-family and PI3-kinase Blocks lytic cycle Block BCR activation	Src, Lyn, Lck ZAP-70, Syk, AIP4/Nedd 4	B-cell latency I-III, HL, DLBCL, T-cell lymphoma, NPC	No
	LMP2B	Blockc LMP 2A?	Not known	B-cells latency III, DLBCL, NPC	No

Kashuba *et al.* (2000) also found that EBNA3 interacts with p38/XAP-2. In the presence of EBNA3, the cytoplasmic p38/XAP-2 translocates to the nucleus. XAP-2 also binds to the hepatitis B virus X antigen, believed to be involved in the oncogenic effect of hepatitis B virus. XAP-2 is known to be involved in the regulation of the aryl hydrocarbon receptor (AhR) pathway. AhR is a ligand activated transcription factor, a member of the HLH transcription family.

EBNA3 was also shown to interact with a new member of the UK/UPRT (uridine kinase/uridine phosphoribasyl transferase) family (Kashuba *et al.*, 1999). The predominantly cytoplasmic enzyme translocates to the nucleus in the presence of EBNA3. It was suggested that EBNA3 may influence the uridine salvage pathway by contributing to the increase of the nuclear UTP pool, required for active cell proliferation.

EBNA6 (alternative EBNA3c) is the only member of the EBNA3 family that has a leucine zipper (West *et al.*, 2004). EBNA6 associates with histone deacetylase and can repress transcription through the Notch signaling pathway. EBNA6 is unique among the EBNAs in its ability to coactivate the LMP1 promoter with EBNA2 (Lin *et al.*, 2002). EBNA6 has also a number of specific repressive effects (Touitou *et al.*, 2001; Radkov *et al.*, 1999). Moreover, EBNA6 associates with histone deacetylase and can repress transcription through the Notch signaling pathway (Radkov *et al.*, 1999).

EBNA6 can also cooperate with oncogenic mutant H-ras in the immortalization and transformation of REFs (Parker *et al.*, 2000). It can also override the suppression of this transformation by p16, by targeting the checkpoint at the G1/S transition, regulated by Rb. EBNA6 can induce aberrant nuclear division that results in multinucleated cells, polyploidy and eventually cell death (Allday review, sid.36). All this suggests that EBNA6 may disrupt multiple cell cycle checkpoints and produce a similar phenotype as the K cyclin of KSHV (Krauer *et al.*, 2004).

Table 29.3 summarizes some of the known interactions of the EBNAs with cellular proteins:

The latent membrane proteins (LMP) of EBV

In the course of infection, replication or persistence, viral gene products frequently interact with proteins that regulate signaling pathways in the host cell. This capacity to modify host cell signal transduction is particularly apparent in the control of EBV.

EBV can express three membrane proteins during latent infection, latent membrane protein (LMP) 1 and 2 A and B (LMP 2A and B) (Hennessy *et al.*, 1984; Laux *et al.*, 1988; Longnecker & Kieff, 1990). These proteins interfere with multiple cellular signal transduction pathways so as to modulate apoptosis and cell surface receptor signalling. They are both transmembrane proteins with six (LMP 1) or twelve (LMP 2) anchoring transmembrane domains, according to computer based structure predictions. No full crystal structures have been established. Neither one acts as a ligand-receptor, but through constitutive activation at cellular membranes (Gires *et al.*, 1997). If there are no ligands, why are they located as membrane proteins?

The main function of both membrane proteins appears to be directed towards interaction with signalling and adaptor molecules normally regulated by cell membrane receptors. They are highly multifunctional and interact with several cellular signalling pathways. Importantly both proteins are expressed at the cell surface membrane as well as in intracellular membranes of the Golgi and endoplasmic reticulum (Lynch *et al.*, 2002; Eliopoulos &

Young, 2001). The significance of this compartmentalization is not known, since the function of the intracellularly localized LMPs has not been the subject of focused studies. Both proteins can be expressed in two forms, one full length and one shorter variant where the first (LMP 1) or the last exon (LMP2B) is excluded by alternative promoter usage or alternative splicing. The shorter variants appear structurally competent to disrupt or block the constitutive activation of the full length protein, by interfering with activation mechanism. LMP 1 is activated by aggregation to trimeres or multimeres, mediated by the transmembrane domains. The truncated protein variant lacks the C-terminus and four of the transmembrane domains. LMP 2 depends on the N-terminal tail and its phosphorylation for activation, which cannot take place with LMP 2B. Both LMP1 and 2 are expressed in latency forms II and III immunoblasts and derived tumors and cell lines (Rea et al., 1994). LMP2A transcripts are also expressed in resting virus carrying B-lymphocytes in healthy individuals, the reservoir of persistently latent EBV (Chen et al., 1995a,b; Qu & Rowe, 1992; Tierney et al., 1994). Both proteins are also detected in epithelial tumors of the nasopharynx (NPC) and during the early stages of oral hairy leukoplakia (Pathmanathan et al., 1995; Webster-Cyriaque & Raab-Traub, 1998). In NPC between 35 and 65% of the tumors are LMP-positive. LMP1 and 2 are expressed in a coordinate fashion Their transcription is co-regulated via a 600 bp bi-directional promoter-enhancer control element designated as the LMP-regulatory sequence (LRS). LMP 2 can only be expressed from viral episomes, since the precursor transcript passes through the terminal repeats (Table 29.3).

The short variant of LMP1 has only been demonstrated during productive, lytic virus infection where it may block the constitutive action of full length LMP 1.

Latent membrane proteins 1 (LMP1)

LMP 1 is a 356 amino acid protein with a short intracellular N-terminus and 150 aa C-terminus.

LMP1 is essential for the transformation of B lymphocytes into lymphoblastoid cell lines (Dirmeier et al., 2003). It confers a survival advantage on EBV-infected B cells by protecting them from apoptosis. This is largely due to the LMP1-induced upregulation of the anti-apoptotic protein Bcl-2 and the block of p53 mediated apoptosis by the latter (Henderson et al., 1991).

EBV-encoded LMP1 can also transform established rodent fibroblasts in vitro (Baichwal et al., 1989; Fahraeus et al., 1990). Furthermore, expression of LMP1 is correlated with a more favorable influence of treatment (chemotherapy/irradiation) on patients with NPC (Kawanishi, 2000) or Hodgkin's lymphoma (Montalban et al., 2000). Clinical and follow-up data from 74 cases of NPC showed that LMP1 positive NPC grew faster and more expansively than LMP1 negative tumors.

LMP 1 almost completely mimicks the function of CD 40 mediated signalling and is thus functionally homologous to the TNF receptor (TNFR) family of proteins (Eliopoulos et al., 1996, 1997; Kilger et al., 1998; Zimber-Strobl et al., 1996; Lam & Sugden, 2003). LMP1 has been shown to interact with several proteins of the TNFR signaling pathway through its C-terminal activation region (CTAR) 1 and 2. Hence, LMP1 can bind TRAF (TNFR-associated factor) 1, 2 and 3, as well as TRADD (TNFR-associated death domain protein), an adaptor protein that serves to recruit caspases to the death-inducing signaling complex (DISC) of the TNFR (Mosialos et al., 1995; Devergne et al., 1996). These interactions result in the NFκB-dependent upregulation of a number of genes, including those encoding anti-apoptotic proteins such as A20 and Bcl-2 (Hatzivassiliou, 2002). Bone morphogenetic protein receptor IA-binding protein (BRAM1), a novel LMP1-interacting protein, interferes with LMP1-mediated NFκB activation and reverses the resistance of cells to TNFR-mediated apoptosis (Chung et al., 2002). Kawanishi (2000) has provided evidence that LMP1 domains CTAR1 and 2 are involved in the enhancement of TNF-induced apoptosis in epithelial cells.

It has been shown that EBV also modulates host apoptotic sensitivity by modifying the relative level of caspase-8, an initiator caspase and its competitor, FLIP (FLICE inhibitor protein (Tepper & Seldin, 1999). LMP1 may alter the ratio of caspase-8 and FLIP.

The findings of Zhang et al. (2002) suggest that the apoptotic modulation by LMP1 is stimulus dependent: tumor necrosis factor (TNF) induced apoptosis was inhibited while Fas ligation- and etoposide- induced apoptosis was potentiated. The attenuation of TNF induced apoptosis parallelled the induction of the anti-apoptotic zinc finger protein A20.

LMP 1 also induces IL 6 and IL 6-receptor expression via the JAK/STAT pathway and JNK-kinase and MAP-kinase (Eliopoulos et al., 1997; Gires et al., 1999; Kieser et al., 1997). Through its interference with a number of major signaling pathways in B-cells and epithelial cells, LMP 1 mediates deregulation of several hundred cellular proteins. LMP 1 also induces the expression of adhesion molecules such as ICAM-1 and LFA, and MHC Class I and II (Mehl et al., 2001; Rowe et al., 1995).

LMP2 modulation of signaling in B-cells and epithelial cells

LMP2A has an intracellular N-terminal cytoplasmic region of 119 residues, which is predicted to be followed by 12 membrane-spanning regions and a short C-terminal cytoplasmic tail, also intracellular. It has been reported to aggregate into "cap-like" structures at the plasma membrane and specifically associate with lipid rafts (Dykstra et al., 2001; Higuchi et al., 2001). The C-terminal tail of LMP2A has been reported to possess a clustering signal as well (Matskova et al., 2001).

LMP2, along with EBNA1 and LMP1, is consistently detected in some latently infected B cells and EBV-associated diseases in vivo, and plays presumably important roles in vivo, related to viral replication, persistence and EBV associated diseases (Qu & Rowe, 1992; Miyashita et al., 1997). A major role of LMP2A in relation to latent EBV infection may stem from its ability to inhibit the activation of lytic EBV replication by cell-surface-mediated signal transduction (Miller et al., 1994). This may prevent lytic replication in latently infected B-cells as they circulate in the blood, bone marrow or lymphatic tissues, where they might encounter antigens, superantigens or other ligands capable of engaging B-cell receptors and activating the viral cycle. In this context it may be relevant that LMP 2A also downregulates telomerase birth in B-cells and epithelial cells (Chen et al., 2004; Scholle et al., 2000).

LMP2A's ability to interfere with BCR signaling and to maintain viral latency may stem from protein–protein interaction motifs located within the amino-terminal tail (see Fig. 29.2). These include a YEEA (amino acid; single letter code) site that, when phosphorylated on the tyrosine residue (Y112), can serve as a binding site for the Src Homology 2 (SH2) domain of the Src family tyrosine kinase Lyn (Burkhardt et al., 1992; Miller et al., 1994; Frueling et al., 1998). In addition, LMP2A possesses an immunoreceptor tyrosine-based activation motif (ITAM) with the consensus sequence YXXI/V-X$_{(6-8)}$-YXXI/V which is found in a number of immunoreceptors including the BCR, the T-cell receptor (TCR), as well as the Fcε receptor that binds IgE. This motif in LMP2A, when phosphorylated on tyrosines 74 and 85, provides a binding site for the dual SH2 domains of the tyrosine kinase Syk (Fruehling & Longnecker, 1997). LMP2A also possesses 2 PPPPY (PY) motifs that can bind to the WW domains of the NEDD4 family of E3 ubiquitin ligases including AIP4, NEDD4-2, and WWP2 (Winberg et al., 2000; Ikeda et al., 2000). Binding to NEDD4 proteins is abrogated by mutation of both tyrosines in the PY motifs (Y60; Y101). NEDD4 family proteins contain HECT (homologous to E6-associated protein carboxy-terminus) domains that catalyze the ubiquitination of proteins such as those associated with the WW domains and target them for degradation via either the 26S proteasome or a lysosomal pathway. LMP2A and the LMP2A-associated kinases are substrates for the NEDD4 family of proteins, suggesting that LMP2A may not only sequester tyrosine kinases away from the BCR, but may also direct them to ubiquitin-mediated pathways including degradation.

Somewhat paradoxically, LMP2A has also been shown to mimic BCR signaling. When expressed as a B-lineage specific transgene in mice, it can both drive B-cell development and promote the survival of mature B cells in the absence of surface immunoglobulin (Ig) expression (Caldwell et al., 2000). Furthermore, this signal appears to be attenuated by the NEDD4 family protein, Itch, indicated by the finding that Itch −/− introduced into the LMP2A transgenic background enhanced LMP2A-mediated signaling (Ikeda et al., 2003). This suggests that LMP2A may act as a survival factor for EBV-positive B-cell tumors that have lost the expression of surface Ig, while also preventing virus reactivation, such as in HL.

LMP2A has also been shown to activate PI3 kinase and the downstream phosphorylation of Akt in epithelial cells and B cells. This may result influence cell growth and apoptosis (Swart et al., 2000).

EBV LMP2A and HHV8 K1 and K15 membrane proteins both target the BCR, but in different ways. While the LMP2A effects on cellular signal transduction have been widely studied, the functions of the HHV8 membrane proteins have been given equal attention (Choi et al., 2000; Lee et al., 2000).

The transforming HHV8 K1 transmembrane transforming protein associates spontaneously to form a trimer in the membrane, which, like LMP2A, carries ITAM motifs. K1 prevents cell surface expression of the BCR by the association of its N-terminal domain with the μ-chains of the BCR, thus preventing the CD79α and β chains from binding. The K1-BCR complex is retained in the ER. The ITAM-motif of K1 is thus available for interaction with cytoplasmic signaling proteins. It has been speculated that the ITAM motif is speculated to function by delivering growth and survival signals to the target cell (Lee et al., 2000). The K15 has a similar topology as LMP2A, with 12 transmembrane helices, but lacks the N-terminal signal transduction domain of LMP2A. It reportedly blocks BCR signaling but the mechanism is not known.

Thus, similar functional elements of function appear to have been conserved in the latent membrane protein of these two distantly related herpesviruses, although the protein structure differs.

In view of the puzzling fact that K1 appears to bind to the μ-chain of BCR in the ER, with intracellular retention of the complex as a result, it is important to determine whether its ITAM motifs bind the Syk tyrosine kinase or a different SH2-domain protein. This could answer the question how K15 can stimulate B-cell survival and proliferation.

The elucidation of the function of the gamma herpesvirus signal transduction mediators may thus allow a refined understanding of BCR signaling functions, by way of a perturbation analysis.

Immunoblastic lymphomas arise in bone marrow or organ transplant recipients (PTLD), congenital immunodeficiencies, particularly the X-linked lymphoproliferative syndrome (XLP) and in AIDS patients. In PTLD and XLP, EBV carrying immunoblasts proliferate, as in mononucleosis, but without being arrested by the immune response. Initially, the proliferation may be polyclonal but becomes eventually monoclonal. During the polyclonal phase, the progression of the disease can often be halted by viral DNA inhibitors such as acyclovir, indicating that virus release and recruitment of new virally transformed cells play a role in the initial development of the disease, but not after it has turned into a monoclonal lymphoma.

EBV carrying immunoblastomas express the full (type III) set of the virally encoded growth transformation associated antigens. They provide the virus carrying B-cells with proliferation drive and antiapoptotic protection. They include the highly immunogenic members of the EBNA3 triad (EBNA 3,4 and 6, also called EBNA 3a,b,c), explaining why passive immunotherapy with sensitized CD8+CTLs or with unsensitized but immunocompetent, histocompatible T-cells can bring about dramatic regression even of widely disseminated tumors.

The immunoblastomas and lymphomas that arise in AIDS patients show a broader picture. Only part of them resemble the post-transplant immunoblastomas. Others are more akin to EBV carrying Burkitt lymphomas, mainly because they carry BL-type Ig/myc translocations, as discussed in more detail below, but they have a more variable cellular and viral expression phenotype. In the strict (type I) phenotype, associated with high endemic BL (only EBNA1 and the EBERs are expressed), Ig/myc translocation carrying tumors with a more immunoblastic cellular and viral (typeIII) expression phenotype are also found. This may be related to the well established fact that EBV-carrying type I BL cells tend to drift towards a more immunoblastic phenotype and full (type III) antigen expression during in vitro culturing. The selective filter that normally removes the highly immunogenic immunoblasts is, not surprisingly, impaired in immunodefectives.

EBV and Burkitt lymphoma (BL)

EBV is associated with 98% of the high endemic BLs, but only with about 20% of sporadic BLs. Both types contain essentially similar Ig/myc translocations, with only minor differences (Magrath, 1990). Only EBNA1 and the EBERs but none of the growth transformation associated EBV proteins (EBNA 2–6, LMP1–2) are expressed in BLs. The virus can therefore not be held directly responsible for the proliferation of the tumor. The latter function is attributed to the constitutive activation of the c-myc protooncogene, resulting from its juxtaposition to one of the three Ig-loci by chromosomal translocation.

Phenotypically, BL cells differ from EBV transformed or mitogen activated immunoblasts. Their markers and their V-gene mutations identify them as post–germinal center memory cells. Even in the most highly BL prone areas of Africa where malaria is rampant and where the regularly high EBV antibody levels in most young children indicate early infection and a high viral load – proven risk factors for the development of BL (Geser et al., 1982) – only a very small fraction of normal B cells (<0.1%) carry the virus. The 98% EBV positivity of the BLs must therefore mean that the presence of the virus increases the probability of lymphoma development. This is the same as to say that the virus contributes to the development of the tumor.

Falling short of the activation of cell proliferation, EBV is likely to contribute to the genesis of BL in some other way. According to one theory, apoptosis protection by the EBERs may be responsible (Takada, 2001). Another indication of a possible apoptosis protecting role has been derived from experiments with EBV negative sublines of originally EBV positive BLs that have lost the virus accidentally, or after hydroxyurea treatment. Viral loss is accompanied by decreased clonability and tumorigenicity (Komano et al., 1998). Comparison of three independently established EBV carrying BLs and their EBV–loss variants showed a marked downregulation of the tcl-1 oncogene (Kiss et al., 2003). Tcl-1 is highly expressed on both T and B cell derived leukemias. EBV reinfection has upregulated tcl-1 again in the EBV-loss variants. Since originally EBV negative BLs express tcl-1 at a high level, we have suggested that the EBV negative BLs switch on tcl-1 constitutively during their neoplastic development. In the virus carriers, EBV is responsible for the upregulation. Tcl-1 activates the apoptosis protective AKT pathway and may thus further increase the apoptotic threshold in these myc-driven and thereby apoptosis prone cells. Conceivably, EBV may also act at the pretranslocation level, by contributing a strong B-cell proliferation, driving stimulus. This would be further enhanced by malaria associated immune dysregulation and opportunistic coinfections. This could expand the target population available for the critical myc-translocation.

The absence of the virus from the EBV negative BLs is consistent with the interpretation that the virus is a contributory, but not a mandatory factor for BL development. The Ig/myc translocation is, on the other hand, regularly found in all BLs and must therefore play a more central role in the origin of the tumor.

The Ig/myc translocation carrying murine tumor prototype, plasmacytoma (MPC) develops earlier and in a higher frequency when the precursors are infected with the pre-B-cell-immortalizing Abelson virus, that carries the v-abl oncogene that has a known antiapoptotic effect.

Since myc-driven cells are highly apoptosis prone, as already mentioned, it is hardly surprising that BL cells are protected against apoptosis at several different levels. Both the Rb and p53 pathways are crippled in BLs, as a rule. In most cases, the Rb pathway is impaired by p16 promoter hypermethylation. The p53 pathway can be inactivated in at least three alternative ways: p53 mutation, ARF mutation or deletion, and MDM2 amplification (Lindström & Wiman, 2002). In spite of this, the BL cell is still quite apoptosis prone, as indicated by its "starry sky" histology, where the "stars" are macrophages that have engulfed apoptotically generated nuclear fragments from the lymphoma cells, and also by the high chemotherapeutic sensitivity of the tumor.

The primary localization of African Burkitt lymphomas may be relevant in this context as well. It suggests that the cytokine environment associated with local tissue proliferation may favor the outgrowth of Ig/myc translocation carrying cells. Jaw tumors are frequent around the age of dentition, ovary and testis are frequent primary sites of BL in prepubertal and pubertal children. Lymphomas may arise in the long bones of teenagers, and BLs with a primary mammary localization have been seen in young lactating women. Some of them regressed when nursing was interrupted. Chronic inflammation may act in a similar way. EBV carrying body cavity lymphomas can be associated with pyothorax of 20 or more years' duration. They carry HHV-8 as well. They present as diffuse large cell lymphomas, sometimes with an immunoblastic appearance. This is in line with numerous examples in the experimental literature, showing that chronic inflammation may act as a tumor promotor.

Hodgkin's lymphoma (HL)

Almost half of the HL-cases in Western countries carry EBV-positive Hodgkin Reed-Sternberg (HRS) cells, that express EBERs, EBNA 1, LMP1 and presumably LMP2a, although this has been less extensively studied (Glaser et al., 1997; Levine et al., 1994; Ohshima et al., 1996; Lennette et al., 1995). The frequency of these presumably malignant cells is surprisingly low in the tumors (1–3%). Conceivably, the HRS cell orchestrates tissue derangement, by recruiting immune bystander cells such as non-neoplastic helper T lymphocytes, plasma cells, macrophages and eosinophilic granulocytes (Molin et al., 2001; Enblad et al., 1993; Weng et al., 2003). It is frequently surrounded by a rosette of CD4+ T-lymphocytes of both the Th1 and the Th2 type. EBV positive HLs show a shift towards Th1. The tumor is described as a "malignant inflammatory process." It produces a large variety of cytokines (Dukers et al., 2000). The HRS cells carry non-functionally rearranged immunoglobulin heavy chain genes and contain somatic mutations in a high frequency, indicating post-germinal center derivation (Kuppers et al., 2002; Muschen et al., 2000; Spieker et al., 2000). They may have been frozen in a non-physiological state that prevents further differentiation or apoptosis.

Several findings suggest that EBV positive HRS originate from latently EBV infected B cells. Like BL and NPC cells, HL cells carry complete viral genomes in the form of multiple covalently closed episomal DNA. TR analysis revealed that viral genomes were clonal, suggesting that they have originated in a common proliferating precursor (Langerak et al., 2002). This argues against any role of virus replication in the establishment of the tumor cell.

Enhanced permissiveness and virus replication may still have a role as a risk factor, HD patients frequently have elevated antibody titres to EBV early antigen (EA) already at the presentation of disease and often years before. Significantly increased EBV genome load has been detected in the blood several years before the disease (Drouet et al., 1999). This suggests that the disease may be preceded by increased EBV reactivation and deregulation of the virus-host balance. Moreover, it has been shown that patients with acute infectious mononucleosis run an increased risk of developing HD (Amini et al., 2000; Axdorph et al., 1999).

In contrast to BL-cells and LCLs, it is difficult to grow HRS-cells in vitro. Only a dozen HL-/HRS-dervied cell lines have been established in vitro. They are EBV-negative, with only one exception. EBV-positive and negative HLs show no convincing differences in phenotype or clinical behavior. But while HD is less common in developing countries, it is much more frequently EBV-positive, (up to 90%). This is reminiscent of the difference between African and sporadic BLs (98% vs. 20% EBV positives).

Two studies have shown no difference in the prognosis of EBV positive and negative cases of HD. Morente et al. (1997) found however, that EBV-positivity was associated with improved overall survival and resulted in a higher complete therapeutic response, together with a significantly longer disease free interval. According to a fourth study (Murray et al., 1999) EBV positive tumors are easier to treat and treatment leads to longer disease free intervals.

EBV and nasopharyngeal carcinoma

Low differentiated or anaplastic NPC is the most regularly EBV associated tumor. It is the commonest malignant tumor among men in Southern China, the Guangzhou region in particular. The carcinoma cells carry multiple viral episomes, like BL cells. Terminal repeat (TR) analysis revealed that they have been derived from a single infectious event like the EBV positive BLs.

Some apparent paradoxes need to be reconciled. Given that the virus replicates lytically in epithelial cells, as particularly well shown in oral hairy leukoplakia (OHL, see below), why does it remain latent in NPC where it expresses only EBNA1, the EBERs and the LMPs (latency II)? Is this due to the fact that NPC cells do not proceed to squamous differentiation? In OHL, the productive viral cycle is only switched on when the cells move upwards within the epithelium, to the level where they start engaging in squamous differentiation.

Early reports claiming that latent EBV could be detected in the basal layer of normal epithelia by in situ techniques have not been confirmed. Foci of lytic viral replication are only found in OHL, which is an EBV-induced lesion. It is found in immunodefectives and can be cursed by acylovir.

The robustly latent interaction between EBV and NPC is puzzling. It raises the question whether EBV inhibits the differentiation of NPC cells and, if so, whether this gives a clue to its role in the genesis of NPC.

It is not clear how and when the NPC-precursor cell becomes infected. In contrast to the EBV-infectability (and transformability) of B cells with EBV and the persistence of the virus in this compartment, epithelial cells are difficult to infect, unless a genetically engineered virus is used that carries a selectable marker like neomycin resistance.

Two experimental findings may offer possible clues. Comparing three different lines of EBV negative carcinoma cells with their EBV infected sublines, Nishikawa et al. (2003) found that the virus switched on the expression of a truncated basic hair keratin gene in all three lines. Conceivably, the truncated keratin may interfere with the production of full sized keratin and, thereby, differentiation.

But why would the keratin be truncated in the first place? This could stem from some of the multiple genetic changes found by PCR in NPC precursor lesions. Dolly Huang's group has shown that some of the changes, particularly the frequent deletions affecting chr.3p and 9p, occur prior to EBV infection (Lo & Huang, 2002). A possible scenario proceeds from an early genetic change that endows the precursor cell with the ability to produce a variant keratin, potentially capable of interfering with differentiation. This variant would be switched on by some viral product, expressed within the latency II program. From the viewpoint of viral strategy, such a scenario would protect the virus from self-elimination by lytic infection and secure its persistence in latently infected, dividing, and undifferentiated cells.

Viral expression in carcinoma cells, cell behavior and host relationships in NPC

About two thirds of NPC tumors express LMP1 in vivo. In the non-expressors, the promoter region of the gene is hypermethylated (Hu et al., 1991). A comparison between non expressed LMP1 genes taken from NPC biopsies and the corresponding genes from LMP1 expressing tumors, showed that the former but not the latter could confer immunogenicity (rejection inducing capacity) on a non-immunogenic mouse mammary carcinoma, transplanted to syngeneic hosts (Hu et al., 2000). This suggested that the LMP1 expressors may have been sculpted by immunoselection in vivo that favored cells with genetic or epigenetic LMP1 inactivation.

LMP1 has been shown to convey increased agarose clonability and tumorigenicity on immortalized epithelial cells in vitro (Hu et al., 1993). Moreover, LMP1 expressing NPCs grew more expansively in immunodefective mice than non-expressors (Hu et al., 1995). Nevertheless, patients with LMP1 positive tumors showed better survival in a retrospective study than patients with LMP1 negative tumors, suggesting that the immunoselective sculpting of the LMP1 positives may still have left the tumors with a certain residual immunogenicity.

In addition to NPC, EBV genomes were also found in other solid tumors, notably gastric carcinomas, salivary gland tumors and a case of thymic carcinoma. Since these associations are not equally regular, they will not be included in this comparative discussion.

Immune surveillance and the oncogenic herpesviruses – the role of immunological "anticipation"

Viewed as a group, four of the potentially oncogenic herpesviruses, Marek's disease herpesvirus (MDHV), H.

saimiri (HVS), *H. ateles* (HVA) and EBV provide us with some important lessons about surveillance mechanisms that can protect against viral tumorigenesis, without reducing the spread of the virus. This results in a largely non-pathogenic "live and let live" situation.

MDHV is the only known DNA tumor virus that can cause tumors by epizootic infection. Unlike the three other viruses, MDHV is not ubiquitous in its natural host, the chicken. Infection of immunologically naive birds can therefore cause horizontally spreading epizootics. The frequency of the lymphoproliferative tumors and the level of their malignancy is influenced both by genetic and evironmental (e.g., stress) factors. One of the genetic resistance factors is linked to MHC. This is in line with the known role of the locus as an immune response regulator. It is reasonable to assume that a more general spread of the agent in chickens would have selected the natural host species for a similarly solid resistance that has been achieved by the other three viruses.

HVS infection is ubiquitous in the natural New World primate host, the squirrel monkey, and the same applies for HVA and its natural host, the spider monkey. Neither of the two viruses are known to be associated with any disease. But the number of examined animals and the observation periods are not comparable to what is known about EBV and the human host. The effect of immune defects is not known for the two simian viruses either.

In distantly related but HVS and HVA naive New World primates, such as marmosets, both HVS and HVA cause rapidly proliferating T-cell malignancy. The tumorigenic potential of both viruses is also consistent with their ability to immortalize human T-lymphocytes.

What makes the natural host solidly resistant to the tumorigenic effect of transforming viruses that can cause rapidly growing malignancies in related but immunologically naive species? Some years ago we performed an experiment with Friedrich Deinhardt's group (Klein *et al.*, 1973) that may throw a certain light on this question. We compared the primary antibody response of squirrel monkeys and marmosets to HVS inoculation soon after birth. Since all previously tested squirrel monkeys were found to carry HVS, fully mature fetuses were removed by Cesarian section from their mothers and were kept virus free by isolation, surrogate mothers and bottle feeding. After a few weeks they were inoculated with live HVS, in parallel with young marmosets. Both species responded with antiviral antibody production but while the squirrel monkeys reached peak antibody titers already 10–12 days after inoculation, the marmosets started responding only after 3 weeks. By that time the lymphoproliferative disease was already in progress, however.

Even though this study was restricted to humoral antibodies and gave no information about the more important cell mediated arm of the immune response, the time difference in the onset of the reaction indicated that the natural host of the virus has been selected for some kind of "immunological anticipation" of the impact of HSV that succeeds in infecting most and perhaps all members of the species under natural conditions.

EBV is also ubiquitous in its natural human host and causes only a self-limiting proliferative disease, mononucleosis, and only in about half of the primarily infected adolescents and adults. The other half and most children under the age of ten respond with "silent," symptom-free seroconversion. Mononucleosis is characterized by the temporary proliferation of EBV transformed immunoblasts, followed by a rejection reaction, mediated by multiple immune effectors. In immunodefectives, whether of congenital (e.g., XLP) or iatrogenic (e.g., transplant recipient) or infectious (e.g., HIV) origin, immunoblastic proliferation may be fatal, as already discussed in the section on immunoblastomas. Moreover, and in further similarity to HVS and HVA, EBV can induce progressive lymphoproliferative malignancy in marmosets and owl monkeys, New World primates that do not have EBV-like viruses of their own. Old World primates that have their own EBV-like viruses carry cross reactive antibodies and are solidly resistant against EBV infection.

Neither BL nor NPC, nor any of the other malignancies where EBV is only found in a proportion of cases, are directly caused by EBV. Therefore, the relatively non-tumorigenic association of this ubiquitous virus with its natural human host is not very different from what HVS and HVA have achieved in their natural simian hosts. Our "immunological anticipation" of EBV is reflected by the surprisingly high frequencies of CD8+T-cells specific for latent and lytic EBV antigens in healthy virus carriers. As many as 5.5% circulating CD8+T cells in a virus carrier can be specific for a single EBV lytic protein epitope, as shown by tetramer staining (Tan *et al.*, 1999). Lymphocytes carrying TCRs specific for latent proteins were found at somewhat lower, but still considerable (0.4–3.8%) frequencies. The preparedness of the immune system for the encounter with EBV transformed B-cells is also reflected by the fact that autologous T cells, admixed to EBV infected B-cells, undergo blast transformation and generate cytotoxicity at equally high levels as allogeneic, MHC-incompatible mixed lymphocyte cultures.

Surveillance of the human host against the development of EBV carrying neoplasia is thus virtually watertight. Occasional tumor development is due to an immunological or cytogenetic accident. Directly EBV-driven immunoblastomas can only arise in immunodefective hosts. Burkitt lymphoma is driven by the unrelated accident of the Ig/myc translocation, probably assisted by an anti-apoptotic effect of the minimal, non proliferation driving type I viral expression program. In NPC, the role of EBV is even less clear. Our findings prompt the speculation that it may act by inhibiting squamous differentiation.

HHV-8 (KSHV)

This is the most puzzling virus of the DNA tumor virus family. It has hijacked more than a dozen cellular genes, many of which have potential tumor related functions. They include genes that influence the cell cycle, apoptosis, various other types of signaling and can create chromosomal imbalance. If a tumor biologist had been given the task of designing a tumor virus, he could not have done better. Surprisingly, however, the virus does not transform in vitro any target cell so far tested. The lack of an in vitro transformation system has hampered the functional analysis of tumorigenicity. Still, there are very good grounds to believe that the virus is responsible for three tumors, Kaposi sarcoma, multicentric Castleman's disease (CD, a polyclonal B cell hyperplasia) and PEL, monoclonal body cavity lymphoma of the B cell series. Each of the three major proliferative syndromes associated with HHV-8 has a partially different virus expression program.

Only the viral ORF73-coded nuclear antigen, LANA1, is regularly expressed in all three HHV-8 related neoplasms. LANA1 binds to the histone H-1 which tethers the viral DNA to the chromosomes during mitosis, securing the maintainance of HHV-8 episomal DNA in infected cells and the delivery of the viral progeny to the daughter cells. LANA1 is a highly immunogenic protein, expressed predominantly by latent virus in KS cells and in PEL lines. LANA1 represses p53 transcription in a highly specific fashion (Friborg et al., 1999).

The viral cyclin D homologue, K cyclin is expressed from the same polycistronic transcript as LANA1. It can promote apoptosis and growth arrest (Verschueren et al., 2002). DNA synthesis, but not mitosis, continues, leading to multinucleation and polyploidy. Centrosome amplification leads to aneuploidy. In the absence of functional p53, aneuploid cells survive and expand. K cyclin expression in p53−/− and also in wild-type mouse embryonic fibroblasts induces massive centrosome amplification with multiple spindles and fusion bridges. In p53 knockout mice, viral K cyclin induces lymphomas.

Similarly to the small DNA tumor viruses, HHV-8 impairs both the p53 and the Rb pathway. But, unlike the small DNA tumor viruses, HHV-8 has developed multiple tactics to corrupt Rb functions. The viral cyclin K which is, like LANA1, constitutively transcribed in HHV-8 carrying cell lines, inactivates Rb and activates EF2 related transcription (Radkov et al., 2000). LANA 1 and Rb coexist as a complex in vivo. Similarly to adenovirus E1A, papillomavirus E7 and SV-40LT, LANA 1 targets the hypophosphorylated, active form of Rb. Moreover, LANA 1 can overcome the flat cell phenotype, induced by the Rb protein in SAOS2 cells. In cooperation with ras, LANA 1 transforms primary REF cells and renders them tumorigenic. While LANA 1 thus resembles SV40LT in being able to interfere with both Rb and p53 function, its ability to inactivate the two main tumor suppressor pathways is not as complete as the action of LT, because LANA 1 cannot transform by itself.

Double HHV8/EBV carrying PEL cells

The majority of the body cavity (PEL) derived lymphoma lines carry both viruses while some carry only HHV-8. EBV expresses its minimal (type I) program, characteristic for BL. The growth transformation associated, proliferation driving genes, characteristic for the type III program of the LCLs, are not expressed, indicating that the double virus carrier lines are not driven by EBV. EBV may have a similar accessory function as it has in BL.

But are the PEL lines, whether single or double virus carriers, driven by HHV-8? This is a reasonable possibility, but it cannot be taken for granted. Body cavity lymphoma lines have numerous chromosomal changes. Some of them may be responsible for the proliferative activity. There is no single, common cytogenetic change like the Ig/myc translocations in BL. Multiple rearrangements may cover more specific changes, however, as in the cryptic Ig/myc translocations that often hide within the massively rearranged karyotypes of cell lines derived from human multiple myeloma, only detectable by the SKY technique (Gratama et al., 1988).

If HHV-8 occupies the driver's seat in the body cavity lymhomas, RNAi or antisense techniques directed against either LANA1 or viral cyclin K should cause growth arrest or apoptosis. This experiment could go a long way in clarifying the role of the virus in PEL. In the absence of direct transformation systems, such evidence may be quite crucial.

Other HHV-8 genes that may be directly relevant for tumorigenesis include the pirated MIR1 and 2 genes, encoded by K3 and K5. They inhibit MHC class I surface expression, through a unique mechanism not found in other viruses. They remove the MHC I proteins from the plasma membrane by enhanced endocytosis. V-FLIP, another pirated gene, is a powerful inhibitor of receptor mediated apoptosis. It is expressed constitutively on latent transcripts and it enhances the tumorigenicity of mouse lymphomas. In addition to the crippling of Rb and p53, and the virally encoded bcl-2, v-FLIP may provide additional protection against apoptosis.

Conclusions

EBV and HHV-8 associated malignancies show interesting parallels and contrasts. The main parallel is the universally occurring expression of the viral product required to maintain the viral episomes, EBNA1 in EBV, LANA1 in HHV-8. Both are nuclear proteins, but they act quite differently.

The most prominent and best known feature of EBV is its finely poised adaptation to the B cell compartment and its sophisticated exploitation of B cell biology – in different ways – for viral expansion, the control of that expansion, and for the latency of the persisting virus. It uses a B-cell surface receptor, CD21, as its receptor. It stimulates the infected B-cells to blast transformation, using or mimicking the normal immunoblastic transformation pathways, and it "immortalizes" its targets, driving them to continuous expansion in vivo and in vitro. The immune response of the host, directed against one of the immunogenic, growth transformation associated proteins (the choice depending on the MHC constitution of the host), rejects the expanded blasts, but not before they have substantially raised the viral load. Meanwhile, the virus secures its lifelong latency by downregulating its proliferation driving and its immunogenic proteins (the two categories overlap partly but not completely) and establishes permanent residence in long-lived, post-germinal center memory cells. Since successful bone marrow transplantation eradicates the resident virus population (Damania et al., 2000), all the persisting virus must reside in the hemopoetic compartment, and probably in B-cells.

We have no knowledge as yet of host cell gene expression pattern in latently HHV8 infected cells. It is therefore still an open issue whether the HHV8 tumorigenic process develops from a latent infection, from infection of "non-physiological" host cells or the abortion of a lytic infection. Several of the HHV8 proteins that have not yet been detected in tumors are interesting candidates in relation to tumor risks. Conceivably, the patterns of viral gene expression may differ in precursor cells of different phenotypes.

Interestingly, motifs of the two membrane proteins K1 and K15 mimic several features of LMP 2 a and LMP 1, which are frequently expressed in EBV-associated tumors. They contain potential NFkB- and ITAM-interacting motifs (Damania et al., 2000; Nicholas, 2003). In contrast to the smaller DNA tumor viruses, they may be less in need to control their long term persistence in the host cell and the fate of the host cell through long periods of time. On the other hand, that may be more dependent on modulators of the acute immune response and intracellular controls of proliferation and apoptosis, as part of their lytic virus replication.

Neither the proliferative, nor the resident phase of the viral life cycle requires crippling of the two main tumor suppressor pathways, Rb and p53. The situation is different in EBV carrying malignancies that are not driven to proliferate by EBV (like BL and NPC), but where the virus is present in an adjuvant capacity, probably as an accessory antiapoptotic device.

Most and perhaps all malignant tumors need to inactivate both the Rb and the p53 pathways. This can happen by a number of alternative mechanisms. In BL, the p53 pathway can be crippled by p53 mutation/deletion, ARF mutation or MDM2 amplification. The Rb pathway can be inactivated by Rb mutation/deletion, p16 inactivation or CDK4 amplification. There is no reason why the minimal (type I) EBV program expressed in BL cells should interfere with the Rb or the p53 pathway and there is no evidence that it does.

In HHV-8 associated tumors, the situation is quite different. In the absence of an in vitro transforming system, we cannot tell whether any of the viral genes (including the genes pirated from the host cell) can drive cell proliferation. We know, however, that two of the genes, LANA1, and viral cyclin K cripple the Rb and p53 pathways. This brings HHV-8 into the previously established DNA tumor virus fold.

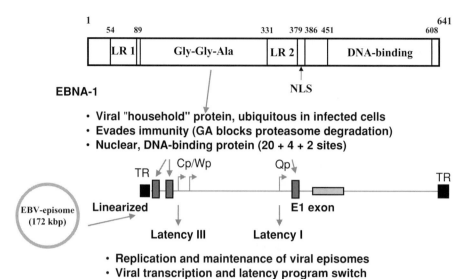

Fig. 29.1. Schematic representation of EBNA 1.

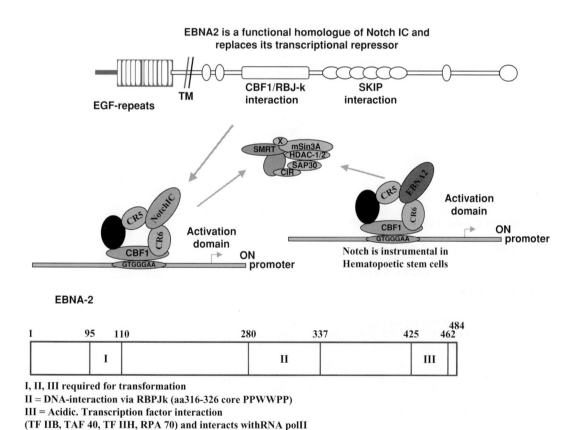

I, II, III required for transformation
II = DNA-interaction via RBPJk (aa316-326 core PPWWPP)
III = Acidic. Transcription factor interaction
(TF IIB, TAF 40, TF IIH, RPA 70) and interacts with RNA polII
machinery, p300, CBP, histone acetylases and bind Notch-
repressor hSNF5/Ini1
II can be replaced by HSV VP16

Fig. 29.2. Schematic representation of EBNA 2 and its major functions.

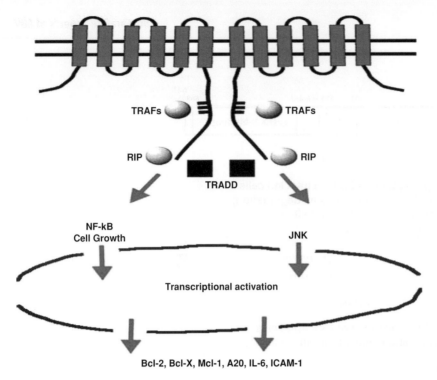

Fig. 29.3. Established major signaling pathways of LMP 1. Studies have revealed several functional domains of the cytoplasmic tail of LMP1 that are important for activation of transcription factor NF-kB, AP-1 and P38 through its interaction with TRAF and TRADD. These findings suggest that LMP1 mimics TNFR aggregation, which is essential for subsequent signal transduction.

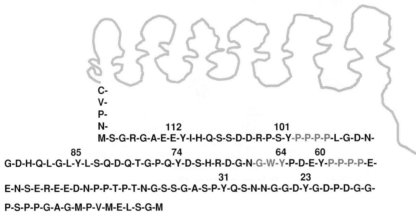

The N-terminus of EBV-LMP2a contains eight phosphotyrosine motifs and two PPPPY-motifs

```
C-
V-
P-
N-           112              101
   M-S-G-R-G-A-E-E-Y-I-H-Q-S-S-D-D-R-P-S-Y-P-P-P-P-L-G-D-N-
85                74              64      60
G-D-H-Q-L-G-L-Y-L-S-Q-D-Q-T-G-P-Q-Y-D-S-H-R-D-G-N-G-W-Y-P-D-E-Y-P-P-P-P-E-
                                  31          23
E-N-S-E-R-E-E-D-N-P-P-T-P-T-N-G-S-S-G-A-S-P-Y-Q-S-N-N-G-G-D-Y-G-D-P-D-G-G-
P-S-P-P-G-A-G-M-P-V-M-E-L-S-G-M
```

EBV-LMP2a eight phosphotyrosine motifs interact with SH2- and WW-domain kinases, adaptors and ubiquitin-pathway components

Aa pos	Motif	Associated proteins
112	A-E-E-Y	Lyn, Fyn, Lck, Src, Blk, Src family PTKs
101	R-P-S-Y-P-P-P-P	Csk, WW-domain (E3-ubiquitin)
85	L-G-L-Y	Syk (ITAM:YXXL)
74	L-P-Q-Y	Syk (ITAM:YXXL)
64	N-G-W-Y	None?
60	Y-P-D-E-Y-P-P-P-P	Abl, Crk, Nck, WW-domain (E3-ubiquitin)
31	A-S-P-Y	Shc, PI-3-kinase, PLCgamma2?
23	G-G-D-Y	None?

Fig. 29.4. N-terminal phosphotyrosine motifs of LMP 2 a.

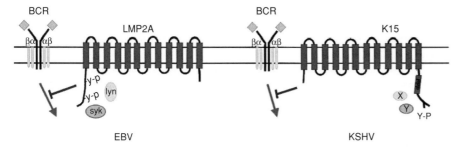

Fig. 29.5. Functional comparison between the Epstein–Barr virus LMP2a and the Kaposi Sarcoma virus (HHV8) K1 and K15 membrane proteins.

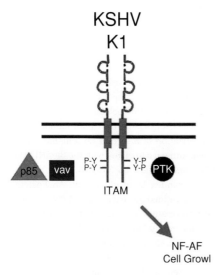

Fig. 29.6. HHV 8 K1 membrane protein.

REFERENCES

Ambinder, R. F., Shah, W. A., Rawlins, D. R., Hayward, G. S., and Hayward, S. D. (1990). Definition of the sequence requirements for binding of the EBNA-1 protein to its palindromic target sites in Epstein–Barr virus DNA. *J. Virol.*, **64**, 2369–2379.

Aman, P., Rowe, M., Kai, C. *et al.* (1990). Effect of the EBNA-2 gene on the surface antigen phenotype of transfected EBV-negative B-lymphoma lines. *Int. J. Cancer*, **45**, 77–82.

Andersson-Anvret, M., Klein, G., Forsby, N., and Henle, W. (1978). The association between undifferentiated nasopharyngeal carcinoma and Epstein–Barr virus shown by correlated nucleic acid hybridization and histopathological studies. *IARC Sci. Publ.*, **20**, 347–357.

Amini, R. M., Enblad, G., Gustavsson, A. *et al.* (2000). Treatment outcome in patients younger than 60 years with advanced stages (IIB-IV) of Hodgkin's disease: the Swedish National Health Care Programme experience. *Eur. J. Haematol.*, **65**, 379–389.

Axdorph, U., Porwit-MacDonald, A., Sjoberg, J. *et al.* (1999). Epstein–Barr virus expression in Hodgkin's disease in relation to patient characteristics, serum factors and blood lymphocyte function. *Br. J. Cancer*, **81**, 1182–1187.

Baichwal, V. R., Hammerschmidt, W., and Sugden, B. (1989). Characterization of the BNLF-1 oncogene of Epstein–Barr virus. *Curr. Top. Microbiol. Immunol.*, **144**, 233–239.

Bittner, J. J. (1936). Some possible effects of nursing on the mammary tumor incidence in mice. *Science*, **84**, 162–168.

Bodescot, M. and Perricaudet, M. (1986). Epstein–Barr virus mRNAs produced by alternative splicing. *Nucl. Acids Res.*, **14**, 7103–7114.

Bodescot, M., Perricaudet, M., and Farrell, P. J. (1987). A promoter for the highly spliced EBNA family of RNAs of Epstein–Barr virus. *J. Virol.*, **61**, 3424–3430.

Bornkamm, G. W. and Hammerschmidt, W. (2001). Molecular virology of Epstein–Barr virus. *Phil. Trans. R. Soc. Lond. B Biol. Sci.*, **356**, 437–459.

Burkhardt, A. L., Bolen, J. B., Kieff, E., and Longnecker, R. (1992). An Epstein–Barr virus transformation-associated membrane protein interacts with src family tyrosine kinases. *J. Virol.*, **66**, 5161–5167.

Caldwell, R. G., Brown, R. C., and Longnecker, R. (2000). Epstein–Barr virus LMP2A-induced B-cell survival in two unique classes of EmuLMP2A transgenic mice. *J. Virol.*, **74**, 1101–1113.

Chen, F., Hu, L. F., Ernberg, I., Klein, G., and Winberg, G. (1995a). A subpopulation of normal B cells latently infected with Epstein–Barr virus resembles Burkitt lymphoma cells in expressing EBNA-1 but not EBNA-2 or LMP1. *J. Virol.*, **69**, 3752–3758.

Chen, F., Zou, J. Z., di Renzo, L. *et al.* (1995b). A subpopulation of normal B cells latently infected with Epstein–Barr virus resembles Burkitt lymphoma cells in expressing EBNA-1 but not EBNA-2 or LMP1. *J. Virol.*, **69**, 3752–3758.

Chen, F., Chen, L., Lindvall, C., Xu, D., and Ernberg, I. (2004). Epstein–Barr virus latent membrane 2A (LMP2A) down-regulates telomerase reverse transcriptase (hTERT) in epithelial cell lines. *Int. J. Cancer*.

Choi, J. K., Lee, B. S., Shim, S. N., Li, M., and Jung, J. U. (2000). Identification of the novel K15 gene at the rightmost end of the Kaposi's sarcoma-associated herpesvirus genome. *J. Virol.*, **74**, 436–446.

Chung, P. J., Chang, Y. S., Liang, C. L., and Meng, C. L. (2002). Negative regulation of Epstein–Barr virus latent membrane protein 1-mediated functions by the bone morphogenetic protein receptor IA-binding protein, BRAM1. *J. Biol. Chem.*, **277**, 39850–39857.

Cohen, J. I., Wang, F., Mannick, J., and Kieff, E. (1989). Epstein–Barr virus nuclear protein 2 is a key determinant of lymphocyte transformation. *Proc. Natl Acad Sci. USA.*, **86**, 9558–9562.

Contreras-Salazar, B., Klein, G., and Masucci, M. G. (1989). Host cell-dependent regulation of growth transformation-associated Epstein–Barr virus antigens in somatic cell hybrids. *J. Virol.*, **63**, 2768–2772.

Damania, B., Choi, J. K., and Jung, J. U. (2000). Signaling activities of gammaherpesvirus membrane proteins. *J. Virol.*, **74**, 1593–1601.

Devergne, O., Hatzivassiliou, E., Izumi, K. M. *et al.* (1996). Association of TRAF1, TRAF2, and TRAF3 with an Epstein–Barr virus LMP1 domain important for B-lymphocyte transformation: role in NF-kappaB activation. *Mol. Cell Biol.*, **16**, 7098–7108.

Dillner, J., Kallin, B., Ehlin-Henriksson, B., Timar, L., and Klein, G. (1985). Characterization of a second Epstein–Barr virus-determined nuclear antigen associated with the BamHI WYH region of EBV DNA. *Int. J. Cancer*, **35**, 359–366.

Dillner, J., Kallin, B., Alexander, H. *et al.* (1986a). An Epstein–Barr virus (EBV) – determined nuclear antigen (EBNA5) partly encoded by the transformation-associated BamWYH region of EBV DNA: preferential expression in lymphoblastoid cell lines. *Proc. Natl Acad. Sci. USA*, **83**, 6641–6645.

Dillner, J., Kallin, B., Ehlin-Henriksson, B. *et al.* (1986b). The Epstein–Barr virus determined nuclear antigen is composed of at least three different antigens. *Int. J. Cancer*, **37**, 195–200.

Dirmeier, U., Neuhierl, B., Kilger, E., Reisbach, G., Sandberg, M. L., and Hammerschmidt, W. (2003). Latent membrane protein 1 is critical for efficient growth transformation of human B cells by Epstein–Barr virus. *Cancer Res.*, **63**, 2982–2989.

Drouet, E., Brousset, P., Fares, F. *et al.* (1999). High Epstein–Barr virus serum load and elevated titers of anti-ZEBRA antibodies in patients with EBV-harboring tumor cells of Hodgkin's disease. *J. Med. Virol.*, **57**, 383–389.

Dukers, D. F., Jaspars, L. H., Vos, W. *et al.* (2000). Quantitative immunohistochemical analysis of cytokine profiles in Epstein–Barr virus-positive and -negative cases of Hodgkin's disease. *J. Pathol.*, **190**, 143–149.

Dykstra, M. L., Longnecker, R., and Pierce, S. K. (2001). Epstein–Barr virus coopts lipid rafts to block the signaling and antigen transport functions of the BCR. *Immunity*, **14**, 57–67.

Eliopoulos, A. G. and Young, L. S. (2001). LMP1 structure and signal transduction. *Semin. Cancer Biol. Rev.*, **11**, 435–444.

Eliopoulos, A. G., Dawson, C. W., Mosialos, G. *et al.* (1996). CD40-induced growth inhibition in epithelial cells is mimicked by Epstein–Barr virus-encoded LMP1: involvement of TRAF3 as a common mediator. *Oncogene*, **13**, 2243–2254.

Eliopoulos, A. G., Stack, M., Dawson, C. W. *et al.* (1997). Epstein–Barr virus-encoded LMP1 and CD40 mediate IL-6 production in epithelial cells via an NF-kappaB pathway involving TNF receptor-associated factors. *Oncogene*, **14**, 2899–2916.

Ernberg, I., Kallin, B., Dillner, J. *et al.* (1986). Lymphoblastoid cell lines and Burkitt-lymphoma-derived cell lines differ in the expression of a second Epstein–Barr virus encoded nuclear antigen. *Int. J. Cancer*, **38**, 729–737.

Enblad, G., Sundstrom, C., and Glimelius, B. (1993). Infiltration of eosinophils in Hodgkin's disease involved lymph nodes predicts prognosis. *Hematol. Oncol.*, **11**, 187–193.

Fahraeus, R., Rymo, L., Rhim, J. S., and Klein, G. (1990). Morphological transformation of human keratinocytes expressing the LMP gene of Epstein–Barr virus. *Nature*, **345**, 447–449.

Foulds, L. (1958). The natural history of cancer. *J. Chronic Dis.*, **8**, 2–37.

Friborg, J., Kong, W., Hottiger, M., and Nabel, G. (1999). P53 inhibition by the LANA protein of KSHV protects against cell death. *Nature*, **402**, 889–894.

Fruehling, S. and Longnecker, R. (1997). The immunoreceptor tyrosine-based activation motif of Epstein–Barr virus LMP2A is essential for blocking BCR-mediated signal transduction. *Virology*, **235**, 241–251.

Fruehling, S., Swart, R., Dolwick, K. M., Kremmer, E., and Longnecker, R. (1998). Tyrosine 112 of latent membrane protein 2A is essential for protein tyrosine kinase loading and regulation of Epstein–Barr virus latency. *J. Virol.*, **72**, 7796–7806.

Furth, J., Buffett, R. F., Barasiewicz-Rodriguez, M., and Upton, A. C. (1956). Character of agent inducing leukemia in newborn mice. *Proc. Soc. Exp. Biol. Med.*, **93**, 165–172.

Gallo, R. C., Kalyanaraman, V. S., Sarngadharan, M. G. *et al.* (1983). Association of the human type-C retrovirus with a subset of adult T-cell cancers. *Cancer Res.*, **42**, 3892–3899.

Geser, A. D., De Thé, G., Lenoir, G. *et al.* (1982). Final case reporting from the Ugandan prospective study of the relationship between EBV and Burkitt's lymphoma. *Int. J. Cancer*, **29**, 397–400.

Gires, O., Zimber-Strobl, U., Gonnella, R. *et al.* (1997). Latent membrane protein 1 of Epstein–Barr virus mimics a constitutively active receptor molecule. *EMBO J.*, **16**, 6131–6140.

Gires, O., Kohlhuber, F., Kilger, E. *et al.* (1999). Latent membrane protein 1 of Epstein–Barr virus interacts with JAK3 and activates STAT proteins. *EMBO J.*, **18**, 3064–3073.

Glaser, S. L., Lin, R. J., Stewart, S. L. *et al.* (1997). Epstein–Barr virus-associated Hodgkin's disease: epidemiologic characteristics in international data. *Int. J. Cancer*, **70**, 375–382.

Gratama, J. W., Oosterveer, M. A. P., Zwaan, F. E., Lepoutre, J., Klein, G., and Ernberg, I. (1988). Eradication of Epstein–Barr virus by allogeneic bone marrow transplanation: implications for sites of viral latency. *Proc. Natl Acad. Sci. USA*, **85**, 8693–8696.

Gross, L. (1951). Spontaneous leukemia developing in C3H mice following inoculation in infancy with AK leukemic extracts of AK embryos. *Proc. Soc. Exp. Biol. Med.*, **76**, 27–32.

Hatzivassiliou, E. and Mosialos, G. (2002). Cellular signaling pathways engaged by the Epstein–Barr virus transforming protein LMP1. *Front Biosci.*, **7**, 319–329.

Hamilton-Dutoit, S. J., Pallesen, G., Karkov, J., Skinhoj, P., Franzmann, M. B., and Pedersen, C. (1989). Identification of EBV-DNA in tumour cells of AIDS-related lymphomas by in-situ hybridisation. *Lancet*, **1**, 554–562.

Hamilton-Dutoit, S. J., Pallesen, G., Franzmann, M. B. *et al.* (1991). Histopathology, immunophenotype, and association with Epstein–Barr virus as demonstrated by in situ nucleic acid hybridization. *Am. J. Pathol.*, **138**, 149–163.

Henderson, S., Rowe, M., Gregory, C. *et al.* (1991). Induction of bcl-2 expression by Epstein–Barr virus latent membrane protein 1 protects infected B cells from programmed cell death. *Cell*, **65**, 1107–1115.

Hennessy, K. and Kieff, E. (1983). One of two Epstein–Barr virus nuclear antigens contains a glycine–alanine copolymer domain. *Proc. Natl Acad. Sci. USA*, **80**, 5665–5669.

Hennessy, K. and Kieff, E. (1985). Second nuclear protein is encoded by Epstein–Barr virus in latent infection. *Science*, **227**, 1238–1240.

Hennessy, K., Heller, M., van Santen, V., and Kieff, E. (1983). Simple repeat array in Epstein–Barr virus DNA encodes part of the Epstein–Barr nuclear antigen. *Science*, **220**, 1396–1398.

Hennessy, K., Fennewald, S., Hummel, M., Cole, T., and Kieff, E. (1984). A membrane protein encoded by Epstein–Barr virus in latent growth-transforming infection. *Proc. Natl Acad. Sci. USA*, **81**, 7207–7211.

Hennessy, K., Fennewald, S., and Kieff, E. (1985). A third viral nuclear protein in lymphoblasts immortalized by Epstein–Barr virus. *Proc. Natl Acad. Sci. USA*, **82**, 5944–5948.

Hickabottom, M., Parker, G. A., Freemont, P., Crook, T., and Allday, M. J. (2002). Two nonconsensus sites in the Epstein–Barr virus oncoprotein EBNA3A cooperate to bind the co-repressor carboxyl-terminal-binding protein (CtBP). *J. Biol. Chem.*, **277**, 47197–47204.

Higuchi, M., Izumi, K. M., and Kieff, E. (2001). Epstein–Barr virus latent-infection membrane proteins are palmitoylated and raft-associated: protein 1 binds to the cytoskeleton through TNF receptor cytoplasmic factors. *Proc. Natl Acad. Sci. USA*, **98**, 4675–4680.

Hsieh, J. J., Henkel, T., Salmon, P., Robey, E., Peterson, M. G., and Hayward, S. D. (1996). Truncated mammalian Notch1 activates CBF1/RBPJk-repressed genes by a mechanism resembling that of Epstein–Barr virus EBNA2. *Mol. Cell Biol.*, **16**, 952–959.

Hu, L-F., Minarovits, J., Cao, S. L. *et al.* (1991). Variable expression of latent membrane protein in nasopharyngeal carcinoma can be related to methylation status of the Epstein–Barr virus BNLF-1 5′-flanking region. *J. Virol.*, **65**, 1558–1567.

Hu, L-F., Chen, F., Zheng, X. *et al.* (1993). Clonability and tumorigenicity of human epithelial cells expressing the EBV encoded membrane protein LMP1, *Oncogene*, **8**, 1575–1583.

Hu, L-F., Chen, F., Zhen, Q. *et al.* (1995). Differences in the growth pattern and clinical course of EBV-LMP1 expressing and non-expressing nasopharyngeal carcinomas. *Eur. J. Cancer*, **31**, 658–660.

Hu, L. F., Troyansky, B., Zhang, X. *et al.* (2000). Differences in the immunogenicity of latent membrane protein 1 (LMP1) encoded by Epstein–Barr virus genomes derived from LMP1-positive and – negative nasopharyngeal carcinoma. *Cancer Res.*, **60**, 5589–5593.

Ikeda, M., Ikeda, A., Longan, L. C., and Longnecker, R. (2000). The Epstein–Barr virus latent membrane protein 2A PY motif recruits WW domain-containing ubiquitin-protein ligases. *Virology*, **268**, 178–191.

Ikeda, M., Ikeda, A., Longnecker, R. (2002). Lysine-independent ubiquitination of Epstein–Barr virus LMP2A. *Virology*, **75**, 153–159.

Ikeda, A., Caldwell, R. G., Longnecker, R., and Ikeda, M. (2003). Itchy, a Nedd4 ubiquitin ligase, downregulates latent membrane protein 2A activity in B-cell signaling. *J. Virol.*, **77**, 5529–5534.

Jiang, W. Q., Wendel-Hansen, V., Lundkvist, A., Ringertz, N., Klein, G., and Rosen, A. (1991). Intranuclear distribution of Epstein–Barr virus-encoded nuclear antigens EBNA-1, -2, -3 and -5. *J. Cell Sci.*, **99**, 497–502.

Jochner, N., Eick, D., Zimber-Strobl, U., Pawlita, M., Bornkamm, G. W., and Kempkes, B. (1996). Epstein–Barr virus nuclear antigen 2 is a transcriptional suppressor of the immunoglobulin mu gene: implications for the expression of the translocated c-myc gene in Burkitt's lymphoma cells. *EMBO J.*, **15**, 375–382.

Johannsen, E., Koh, E., Mosialos, G., Tong, X., Kieff, E., and Grossman, S. R. (1995). Epstein–Barr virus nuclear protein 2 transactivation of the latent membrane protein 1 promoter is mediated by J kappa and PU. 1. *J. Virol.*, **69**, 253–262.

Johannsen, E., Miller, C. L., Grossman, S. R., and Kieff, E. (1996). EBNA-2 and EBNA-3C extensively and mutually exclusively associate with RBPJ kappa in Epstein–Barr virus-transformed B lymphocytes. *J. Virol.*, **70**, 4179–4183.

Jones, C. H., Hayward, S. D., and Rawlins, D. R. (1989). Interaction of the lymphocyte-derived Epstein–Barr virus nuclear antigen EBNA-1 with its DNA-binding sites. *J. Virol.*, **63**, 101–110.

Kaiser, C., Laux, G., Eick, D., Jochner, N., Bornkamm, G. W., and Kempkes, B. (1999). The proto-oncogene c-*myc* is a direct target gene of Epstein–Barr virus nuclear antigen 2. *J. Virol.*, **73**, 4481–4484.

Kanamori, M., Watanabe, S., Honma, R. *et al.* (2004). Epstein–Barr virus nuclear antigen leader protein induces expression of thymus – and activation-regulated chemokine in B cells. *J. Virol.*, **78**, 3984–3993.

Kashuba, E., Pokrovskaja, K., Klein, G., and Szekely, L. (1999). Epstein–Barr virus-encoded nuclear protein EBNA-3 interacts with the epsilon-subunit of the T-complex protein 1 chaperonin complex. *J. Hum. Virol.*, **2**, 33–37.

Kashuba, E., Kashuba, V., Pokrovskaja, K., Klein, G., and Szekely, L. (2000). Epstein–Barr virus encoded nuclear protein EBNA-3 binds XAP-2, a protein associated with Hepatitis B virus X antigen. *Oncogene*, **19**, 1801–1806.

Kashuba, E., Kashuba, V., Sandalova, T., Klein, G., and Szekely, L. (2002). Epstein–Barr virus encoded nuclear protein EBNA-3 binds a novel human uridine kinase/uracil phosphoribosyltransferase. *BMC Cell Biol.*, **3**, 23.

Kashuba, E., Mattsson, K., Pokrovskaja, K. *et al.* (2003). EBV-encoded EBNA-5 associates with P14ARF in extranucleolar inclusions and prolongs the survival of P14ARF-expressing cells. *Int. J. Cancer*, **105**, 644–653.

Kawanishi, M. (2000). The Epstein–Barr virus latent membrane protein 1 (LMP1) enhances TNF alpha-induced apoptosis of intestine 407 epithelial cells: the role of LMP1 C-terminal activation regions 1 and 2. *Virology*, **270**, 258–266.

Kaye, K. M., Izumi, K. M., Li, H. *et al.* (1999). An Epstein–Barr virus that expresses only the first 231 LMP1 amino acids efficiently initiates primary B-lymphocyte growth transformation. *J. Virol.*, **73**, 10525–10530.

Kempkes, B., Pawlita, M., Zimber-Strobl, U., Eissner, G., Laux, G., and Bornkamm, G. W. (1995). Epstein–Barr virus nuclear antigen 2-estrogen receptor fusion protein transactivate viral and cellular genes and interact with RBP-J kappa a conditional fashion. *Virology*, **214**, 675–679.

Kieser, A., Kilger, E., Gires, O., Ueffing, M., Kolch, W., and Hammerschmidt, W. (1997). Epstein–Barr virus latent membrane protein-1 triggers AP-1 activity via the c-Jun N-terminal kinase cascade. *EMBO J.*, **16**, 6478–6485.

Kilger, E., Kieser, A., Baumann, M., and Hammerschmidt, W. (1998). Epstein–Barr virus-mediated B-cell proliferation is dependent upon latent membrane protein 1, which simulates an activated CD40 receptor. *EMBO J.*, **17**, 1700–1709.

Kiss, C., Nishikawa, J., Takada, K., Trivedi, P., Klein, G., and Szekely, L. (2003). T cell leukemia 1 oncogene expression depends on the presence of Epstein–Barr virus in the virus-carrying Burkitt lymphoma lines. *Proc. Natl Acad. Sci. USA*, **100**, 4813–4818.

Klein, G., Pearson, G., Rabson, A. *et al.* (1973). Antibody reactions to herpesvirus Saimiri (HVS)-induced early and late antigens (EA and LA) in HVS-infected squirrel, marmoset and owl monkeys. *Int. J. Cancer*, **12**, 270–289.

Komano, J., Sugiura, M., and Takada, K. (1998). Epstein–Barr virus contributes to the malignant phenotype and to apoptosis resistance in Burkitt's lymphoma cell line AKATA. *J. Virol.*, **72**, 9150–9156.

Krauer, K. G., Burgess, A., Buck, M., Flanagan, J., Sculley, T. B., and Gabrielli, B. (2004). The EBNA-3 gene family proteins disrupt the G2/M checkpoint. *Oncogene*, **23**, 1342–1353.

Kuppers, R., Schwering, I., Brauninger, A., Rajewsky, K., and Hansmann, M. L. (2002). Biology of Hodgkin's lymphoma. *Ann. Oncol.*, **13** Suppl 1:11–18.

Lam, N., and Sugden, B. (2003). LMP1, a viral relative of the TNF receptor family, signals principally from intracellular compartments. *EMBO J.*, **22**, 3027–3038.

Langerak, A. W., Moreau, E., van Gastel-Mol, E. I., van der Burg, M., and van Dongen, J. J. (2002) Detection of clonal EBV episomes in lymphoproliferations as a diagnostic tool. *Leukemia*, **16**, 1572–1573.

Laux, G., Perricaudet, M., and Farrell, P. J. (1988). A spliced Epstein–Barr virus gene expressed in immortalized lymphocytes is created by circularization of the linear viral genome. *EMBO J.*, **7**, 769–774.

Lee, B. S., Alvarez, X., Ishido, S., Lackner, A. A., and Jung, J. U. (2000). Inhibition of intracellular transport of B cell antigen receptor complexes by Kaposi's sarcoma-associated herpesvirus K1. *J. Exp. Med.*, **192**, 11–21.

Lennette, E. T., Winberg, G., Yadav, M., Enblad, G., and Klein, G. (1995). Antibodies to LMP2A/2B in EBV-carrying malignancies. *Eur. J. Cancer*, **31A**, 1875–1878.

Levine, P. H., Pallesen, G., Ebbesen, P., Harris, N., Evans, A. S., and Mueller, N. (1994). Evaluation of Epstein–Barr virus antibody patterns and detection of viral markers in the biopsies of patients with Hodgkin's disease. *Int. J. Cancer*, 5948–5950.

Levitskaya, J., Coram, M., Levitsky, V. et al. (1995). Inhibition of antigen processing by the internal repeat region of the Epstein–Barr virus nuclear antigen-1. *Nature*, **375**, 685–688.

Lin, J., Johannsen, E., Robertson, E., and Kieff, E. (2002). Epstein–Barr virus nuclear antigen 3C putative repression domain mediates coactivation of the LMP1 promoter with EBNA-2. *J. Virol.*, **76**, 232–242.

Lindahl, T., Klein, G., Reedman, B. M., Johansson, B., and Singh, S. (1974). Relationship between Epstein–Barr virus (EBV) DNA and the EBV-determined nuclear antigen (EBNA) in Burkitt lymphoma biopsies and other lymphoproliferative malignancies. *Int. J. Cancer*, **13**, 764–772.

Lindström, M. and Wiman, K. G. (2002). Role of genetic and epigenetic changes in Burkitt lymphoma. *Semin. Cancer Biol.*, **12**, 381–387.

Lo, K. W. and Huang, D. P. (2002). Genetic and epigenetic changes in nasopharyngeal carcinoma. *Semin. Cancer Biol.*, **12**, 451–462.

Longnecker, R. and Kieff, E. (1990). A second Epstein–Barr virus membrane protein (LMP2) is expressed in latent infection and colocalizes with LMP1. *J. Virol.*, **64**, 2319–2326.

Lynch, D. T., Zimmerman, J. S., and Rowe, D. T. (2002). Epstein–Barr virus latent membrane protein 2B (LMP2B) co-localizes with LMP2A in perinuclear regions in transiently transfected cells. *J. Gen. Virol.*, **83**, 1025–1035.

Magrath, I. (1990). The pathogenesis of Burkitt's lymphoma, *Adv. Cancer Res.*, **55**, 133–269.

Matskova, L., Ernberg, I., Pawson, T., and Winberg, G. (2001). C-terminal domain of the Epstein–Barr virus LMP2a protein contains a clustering signal. *J. Virol.*, **75**, 10941–10949.

Mehl, A. M., Floettmann, J. E., Jones, M., Brennan, P., and Rowe, M. (2001). Characterization of intercellular adhesion molecule-1 regulation by Epstein–Barr virus-encoded latent membrane protein-1 identifies pathways that cooperate with nuclear factor kappa B to activate transcription. *J. Biol. Chem.*, **276**, 984–992.

Miller, C. L., Lee, J. H., Kieff, E., and Longnecker, R. (1994). An integral membrane protein (LMP2) blocks reactivation of Epstein–Barr virus from latency following surface immunoglobulin crosslinking. *Proc. Natl Acad. Sci. USA*, **91**, 772–776.

Miyashita, E. M., Yang, B., Babcock, G. J., and Thorley-Lawson, D. A. (1997). Identification of the site of Epstein–Barr virus persistence in vivo as a resting B cell. *J. Virol.*, **71**, 4882–4891.

Molin, D., Fischer, M., Xiang, Z. et al. (2001). Mast cells express functional CD30 ligand and are the predominant CD30L-positive cells in Hodgkin's disease. *Br. J. Haematol.*, **114**, 616–623.

Montalban, C., Abraira, V., Morente, M. et al. (2000). Epstein–Barr virus-latent membrane protein 1 expression has a favorable influence in the outcome of patients with Hodgkin's Disease treated with chemotherapy. *Leuk. Lymphoma*, **39**, 563–572.

Morente, M. M., Piris, M. A., Abraira, V. et al. (1997). Adverse clinical outcome in Hodgkin's disease is associated with loss of retinoblastoma protein expression, high Ki67 proliferation index, and absence of Epstein–Barr virus-latent membrane protein 1 expression. *Blood*, **90**, 2429–2436.

Mosialos, G., Birkenbach, M., Yalamanchili, R., VanArsdale, T., Ware, C., and Kieff, E. (1995). The Epstein–Barr virus transforming protein LMP1 engages signaling proteins for the tumor necrosis factor receptor family. *Cell.*, **80**, 389–399.

Murray, P. G., Billingham, L. J., Hassan, H. T., and Young, L. S. (1999). Epstein–Barr virus infection on response to chemotherapy and survival in Hodgkin's disease. *Blood*, **94**, 442–447.

Muschen, M., Re, D., Brauninger, A. et al. (2000). Somatic mutations of the CD95 gene in Hodgkin and Reed–Sternberg cells. *Cancer Res.*, **60**, 5640–5643.

Nicholas, J. (2003). Human herpesvirus-8-encoded signalling ligands and receptors. *J. Biomed. Sci.*, **10**, 475–489.

Niedobitek, G., Deacon, E. M., and Young, L. S. (1989). Epstein–Barr virus gene expression in Hodgkin's disease. *Blood*, **78**, 1628–1630.

Nishikawa, J., Kiss, C., Imai, S. et al. (2003). Upregulation or the truncated basic hair keratin 1(hHb1-ΔN) in carcinoma cells by Epstein–Barr virus (EBV). *Internat. J. Cancer*, **107**, 597–602.

Ohno, S., Luka, J., Lindahl, T., and Klein, G. (1977). Identification of a purified complement-fixing antigen as the Epstein–Barr-virus determined nuclear antigen (EBNA) by its binding to metaphase chromosomes. *Proc. Natl Acad. Sci. USA*, **74**, 1605–1609.

Ohshima, K., Suzumiya, J., Tasiro, K. et al. (1996). Epstein–Barr virus infection and associated products (LMP, EBNA2, vIL-10) in nodal non-Hodgkin's lymphoma of human immunodeficiency virus-negative Japanese. *Am. J. Hematol.*, **52**(1), 21–28.

Parker, G. A., Crook, T., Bain, M., Sara, E. A., Farrell, P. J., and Allday, M. J. (1996). Epstein–Barr virus nuclear antigen (EBNA)3C is an immortalizing oncoprotein with similar properties to adenovirus E1A and papillomavirus E7. *Oncogene*, **13**, 2541–2549.

Parker, G. A., Touitou, R., and Allday, M. J. (2000). Epstein–Barr virus EBNA3C can disrupt multiple cell cycle checkpoints and induce nuclear division divorced from cytokinesis. *Oncogene*, **19**, 700–709.

Pathmanathan, R., Prasad, U., Sadler, R., Flynn, K., and Raab-Traub, N. (1995). Clonal proliferations of cells infected with Epstein–Barr virus in preinvasive lesions related to nasopharyngeal carcinoma. *N. Engl. J. Med.*, **333**, 693–698.

Polack, A., Hortnagel, K., Pajic, A. et al. (1996). c-myc activation renders proliferation of Epstein–Barr virus (EBV)-transformed cells independent of EBV nuclear antigen 2 and latent membrane protein 1. *Proc. Natl Acad. Sci. USA*, **93**, 10411–10416.

Polvino-Bodnar, M., Kiso, J., and Schaffer, P. A. (1988). Mutational analysis of Epstein–Barr virus nuclear antigen 1 (EBNA1). *Nucl. Acids Res.*, **16**, 3415–3435.

Pokrovskaja, K., Mattsson, K., Kashuba, E., Klein, G., and Szekely, L. (2001). Inhibitor induces nucleolar translocation of Epstein–Barr virus-encoded EBNA-5. *J. Gen. Virol.*, **82**, 345–358.

Prevot, S., Hamilton-Dutoit, S., Audouin, J., Walter, P., Pallesen, G., and Diebold, J. (1992). Analysis of African Burkitt's and high-grade B cell non-Burkitt's lymphoma for Epstein–Barr virus genomes using in situ hybridization. *Br. J. Haematol*, **80**, 27–32.

Qu, L. and Rowe, D. T. (1992). Epstein–Barr virus latent gene expression in uncultured peripheral blood lymphocytes. *J. Virol.*, **66**, 3715–3724.

Radkov, S. A., Bain, M., Farrell, P. J., West, M., Rowe, M., and Allday, M. J. (1997). Epstein–Barr virus EBNA3C represses Cp, the major promoter for EBNA expression, but has no effect on the promoter of the cell gene CD21. *J. Virol.*, **71**, 8552–8562.

Radkov, S. A., Touitou, R., Brehm, A. *et al.* (1999). Epstein–Barr virus nuclear antigen 3C interacts with histone deacetylase to repress transcription. *J. Virol.*, **73**, 5688–5697.

Radkov, S., Kellam, P., and Boshoff, C. (2000). The latent nuclear antigen of Kaposi sarcoma-associated herpesvirus targets the retinoblastoma-E2F pathway and with the oncogene Hras transforms primary rat cells. *Nat. Med.*, **6**, 1121–1127.

Rawlins, D. R., Milman, G., Hayward, S. D., and Hayward, G. S. (1985). Sequence-specific DNA binding of the Epstein–Barr virus nuclear antigen (EBNA-1) to clustered sites in the plasmid maintenance region. *Cell*, **42**, 859–868.

Rea, D., Fourcade, C., Leblond, V. *et al.* (1994). Patterns of Epstein–Barr virus latent and replicative gene expression in Epstein–Barr virus B cell lymphoproliferative disorders after organ transplantation. *Transplantation*, **58**, 317–324.

Reedman, B. M. and Klein, G. (1973). Related Articles, Cellular localization of an Epstein–Barr virus (EBV)-associated complement-fixing antigen in producer and non-producer lymphoblastoid cell lines. *Int. J. Cancer*, **11**, 499–520.

Reisman, D. and Sugden, B. (1986). *Trans*-activation of an Epstein–Barr viral transcriptional enhancer by the Epstein–Barr viral nuclear antigen 1. *Mol. Cell Biol.*, **6**, 3838–3846.

Rickinson, A. B., Young, L. S., and Rowe, M. (1987). Influence of the Epstein–Barr virus nuclear antigen EBNA 2 on the growth phenotype of virus-transformed B cells. *J. Virol.*, **61**, 1310–1317.

Rous, P. (1911). A sarcoma of fowl transmissible by an agent from the tumor cells. *J. Exp. Med.*, **13**, 397–411.

Rowe, M., Young, L. S., Cadwallader, K., Petti, L., Kieff, E., and Rickinson, A. B. (1989). Distinction between Epstein–Barr virus type A (EBNA 2A) and type B (EBNA 2B) isolates extends to the EBNA 3 family of nuclear proteins. *J. Virol.*, **63**, 1031–1039.

Rowe, M., Khanna, R., Jacob, C. A. *et al.* (1995). Restoration of endogenous antigen processing in Burkitt's lymphoma cells by Epstein–Barr virus latent membrane protein-1: coordinate up-regulation of peptide transporters and HLA-class I antigen expression. *Eur. J. Immunol.*, **25**, 1374–1384.

Scholle, F., Bendt, K. M., and Raab-Traub, N. (2000). Epstein–Barr virus LMP2A transforms epithelial cells, inhibits cell differentiation, and activates Akt. *J. Virol.*, **74**, 10681–10689.

Sample, J. and Kieff, E. (1990). Transcription of the Epstein–Barr virus genome during latency in growth-transformed lymphocytes. *J. Virol.*, **64**, 1667–1674.

Shimizu, N., Yamaki, M., Sakuma, S., Ono, Y., and Takada, K. (1988). Three Epstein–Barr virus (EBV)-determined nuclear antigens induced by the BamHI E region of EBV DNA. *Int. J. Cancer*, **41**, 744–751.

Shope, R. E. (1933). Infectious papillomatosis of rabbits; with a note on the histopathology. *J. Exp. Med.*, **68**, 607–624.

Spieker, T., Kurth, J., Kuppers, R., Rajewsky, K., Brauninger, A., and Hansmann, M. L. (2000). Molecular single-cell analysis of the clonal relationship of small Epstein–Barr virus-infected cells and Epstein–Barr virus-harboring Hodgkin and Reed/Sternberg cells in Hodgkin disease. *Blood.*, **96**, 3133–3138.

Stewart, S-E., Eddy, B-E., and Borgear, N. (1958). Neoplasms in mice inoculated with a tumor agent carried in tissue culture. *J. Natl Cancer Inst.*, **20**, 1223–1243.

Sugden, B. and Warren, N. (1989). A promoter of Epstein–Barr virus that can function during latent infection can be transactivated by EBNA-1, a viral protein required for viral DNA replication during latent infection. *J. Virol.*, **63**, 2644–2649.

Swart, R., Ruf, I. K., Sample, J., and Longnecker, R. (2000). Latent membrane protein 2A-mediated effects on the phosphatidylinositol 3-kinase/Akt pathway. *J. Virol.*, **74**, 10838–10845.

Takada, K. (2001). Role of Epstein–Barr virus in Burkitt's lymphoma. *Curr. Top. Microbiol. Immunol.*, **258**, 141–161.

Tamura, K., Taniguchi, Y., Minoguchi, S. *et al.* (1995). Physical interaction between a novel domain of the receptor Notch and the transcription factor RBP-Jk. *Curr. Biol.*, **5**, 1416–1423.

Tan, L. C., Gudgeon, N., Annels, N. *et al.* (1999). Re-evaluation of the frequency of CD8+ T cells specific for EBV in healthy virus carriers. *J. Immunol.*, **162**, 1827–1835.

Tepper, C. and Seldin, M. (1999). Modulation of Casoase-8 and FLICE-inhibitory proytein expression as a potential mechanism of Epstein–Barr virus tumorigeneis in Burkitt's lymphoma. *Blood*, **94**, 1727–1737.

Tierney, R. J., Steven, N., Young, L. S., and Rickinson, A. B. (1994). Epstein–Barr virus latency in blood mononuclear cells: analysis of viral gene transcription during primary infection and in the carrier state. *J. Virol.*, **68**, 7374–7385.

Touitou, R., Hickabottom, M., Parker, G., Crook, T., and Allday, M. J. (2001). Physical and functional interactions between the corepressor CtBP and the Epstein–Barr virus nuclear antigen EBNA3C. *J. Virol.*, **75**, 7749–7755.

Verschueren, E. W., Klefstrom, J., Evan, G. I., and Jones, N. (2002). The oncogeneic potential of Kaposi's sarcoma-associated herpesvirus cyclin is exposed by p53 loss in vitro and in vivo. *Cancer Cell*, **2**, 229–241.

Wang, F., Gregory, C. D., Rowe, M. *et al.* (1987a). Epstein–Barr virus nuclear antigen 2 specifically induces expression of the B-cell activation antigen CD23. *Proc. Natl Acad. Sci. USA*, **84**, 3452–3456.

Wang, F., Petti, L., Braun, D., Seung, S., and Kieff, E. (1987b). Free in PMC A bicistronic Epstein–Barr virus mRNA encodes two nuclear proteins in latently infected, growth-transformed lymphocytes. *J. Virol.*, **61**, 945–954.

Wang, F., Gregory, C., Sample, C. *et al.* (1990). Epstein–Barr virus latent membrane protein (LMP1) and nuclear proteins 2 and 3C are effectors of phenotypic changes in B lymphocytes: EBNA-2 and LMP1 cooperatively induce CD23. *J. Virol.*, **64**, 2309–2318.

Webster-Cyriaque, J. and Raab-Traub, N. (1998). Transcription of Epstein–Barr virus latent cycle genes in oral hairy leukoplakia. *Virology*, **248**, 53–65.

Weng, A. P., Shahsafaei, A., and Dorfman, D. M. (2003). CXCR4/CD184 immunoreactivity in T-cell non-Hodgkin lymphomas with an overall Th1-Th2+ immunophenotype. *Am. J. Clin. Pathol.*, **119**, 424–430.

West, M. J., Webb, H. M., Sinclair, A. J., and Woolfson DN. (2004). Biophysical and mutational analysis of the putative bZIP domain of Epstein–Barr virus EBNA 3C. *J. Virol.*, **78**, 9431–9445.

Winberg, G., Matskova, L., Chen, F. *et al.* (2000). Latent membrane protein 2A of Epstein–Barr virus binds WW domain E3 protein-ubiquitin ligases that ubiquitinate B-cell tyrosine kinases. *Mol. Cell*, **20**, 8526–8535.

Zhang, X., Hu, L., Fadeel, B., and Ernberg, I. T. (2002). Apoptosis modulation of Epstein–Barr virus-encoded latent membrane protein 1 in the epithelial cell line HeLa is stimulus-dependent. *Virology*, **304**, 330–341.

Zhao, B., Dalbies-Tran, R., Jiang, H. *et al.* (2003). Transcriptional regulatory properties of Epstein–Barr virus nuclear antigen 3C are conserved in simian lymphocryptoviruses. *J. Virol.*, **77**, 5639–5648.

Zimber, U., Adldinger, H. K., Lenoir, G. M. *et al.* (1986). Geographical prevalence of two types of Epstein–Barr virus. *Virology*, **154**, 56–66.

Zimber-Strobl, U., Kempkes, B., Marschall, G. *et al.* (1996). Epstein–Barr virus latent membrane protein (LMP1) is not sufficient to maintain proliferation of B cells but both it and activated CD40 can prolong their survival. *EMBO J.*, **15**, 7070–7078.

Zhou, X. G., Hamilton-Dutoit, S. J., Yan, Q. H., and Pallesen, G. (1994). High frequency of Epstein–Barr virus in Chinese peripheral T-cell lymphoma. *Histopathology*, **24**, 115–122.

30

KSHV manipulation of the cell cycle and apoptosis

Patrick S. Moore

Molecular Virology Program, University of Pittsburgh Cancer Institute, Pittsburgh, PA USA

Disruptions of cell cycle and apoptotic regulatory control are primary hallmarks tumor cells. It is therefore not surprising that Kaposi's sarcoma-associated herpesvirus (KSHV/HHV8), a tumor virus, encodes viral proteins targeting these cell growth regulation mechanisms. The extent and range of KSHV genes devoted to manipulating these processes is, however, remarkable.

As described in previous chapters, herpesviral structural and replication-related genes are highly conserved among the herpesviruses, including KSHV. In contrast, regulatory genes generating proteins that modify the cellular environment – particularly during latency – are generally unique to each virus. As will become evident in this chapter, even though KSHV and EBV are closely related to each other, there are few sequence homologies among the oncogenes and non-structural regulatory genes found in the two viruses. Despite this, there is a striking functional similarity between the two viruses (Table 30.1). EBV encodes multiple highly evolved transcription factors and signaling proteins that induce many of the same cellular genes that KSHV has pirated into its genome. Further, once herpesvirus targeting of a cellular pathway has been found for one herpesvirus (e.g., HSV-1 downregulation of MHC I surface expression, Hill *et al.*, 1994), searching for functional similarities among other herpesviruses has been particularly rewarding (e.g., Coscoy *et al.*, 2000). It is therefore not surprising that KSHV and EBV share pathways for cell transformation although they achieve this through very different mechanisms.

Several general principles for KSHV regulatory gene functions that affect cell transformation and tumorigenesis can be made with the important caveat that exceptions exist to each rule.

1. Although there is little or no sequence homology among oncogenes encoded by different tumor viruses, the cellular targets for viral oncogenes are frequently conserved (Table 30.1). For example, direct inhibitors of p53 from KSHV, adenoviruses, polyomaviruses, and papillomaviruses have no apparent similarity to each other but all of these viral proteins target and inhibit p53 functions.

2. KSHV proteins encoded by viral genes pirated from the cellular genome have similar functions to their cellular counterparts. They generally differ in their regulation rather than their function. For example, the KSHV vCYC protein acts as D-type cyclin in cells but unlike cellular cyclins it is resistant to inhibition by cyclin-dependent kinase inhibitors but are modified to escape normal cellular regulation. The evolution of entirely new KSHV gene functions is uncommon and differences between cellular and KSHV homologues lie primarily in their expression and regulation (for an exception, however, see description of ORF36 mRNA shut-off functions in Chapter 56).

3. KSHV targeting of cellular tumor suppressor pathways also inhibits host defenses against viral infection which indeed may be the principle benefit to the virus for these proteins (Moore & Chang, 1996, see also Chapter 31). Signaling pathways controlling of tumor cell growth, such as Fas-FasL death receptor signaling, also critical for both innate and adaptive immune responses, and are targeted by putative KSHV oncoproteins.

This chapter describes the effects of individual KSHV proteins on cell cycle control, apoptosis, and cellular transformation. It is, by necessity, an artificial division of these functions, since cell growth control mechanisms are intimately tied into other aspects of the viral lifecycle such as maintenance of latency (Chapter 24) and immunoevasion (Chapter 31). Caution is warranted given the limitations to our ability to study how KSHV contributes to cancer. Our understanding of viral effects on cell growth are generally based on in vitro cell culture systems, e.g., PEL cell cultures, and on the study of individual genes in isolation. Much can be learned from this reductionist approach, but it is important to keep in mind that results from the bench-top do not always translate to the bedside, which is more fully addressed in Chapters 50 and 56).

Cell cycle and programmed cell death regulation

The normal cell cycle is actively regulated through specific protein-kinase regulatory subunits, cyclins (Murry, 2004), that are cyclicly expressed during the different phases of the cell cycle and degrade as the cell exits each phase (Fig. 30.1). Cyclins regulate the periodic oscillations of the cell cycle by coupling to cyclin-dependent kinases (which tend to be constitutively expressed) to phosphorylate specific cell cycle regulatory targets, for example, the retinoblastoma protein (pRB1) controlling expression of genes necessary for transit from G1 into S phase. The cyclin component of the dimeric complex generally serves as the targeting moiety directing CDK phosphorylation to specific substrates.

Some cyclins such as cyclin A and the D-type cyclins do not appear to be essential for intrinsic cell cycle periodicity but serve to regulate it (Kozar et al., 2004). pRB1 (a member of a family of related proteins that also includes p130) is a transcriptional repressor that binds and inactivates E2F family transcription factors involved in transcription of genes required for DNA synthesis prior to S phase. These enzymes include dihydrofolate reductase, thymidine kinase, and several other nucleotide synthesis enzymes expressed during the G1/S phase transition and have been pirated by KSHV (Russo et al., 1996). When pRB1 is hyperphosphorylated by cyclin D-CDK4 or CDK6, it is inactivated and releases E2F allowing expression of DNA synthesis enzymes. Thus pRB1 is a critical regulator for the transition between G1 and S phase and controls the cellular environment to prevent unscheduled DNA synthesis. Another substrate phosphorylated by cyclin-CDK complexes is the anaphase-promoting complex (APC), which controls chromosome separation during mitosis and acts as a checkpoint protein at the G2/M cell cycle transition.

Viral manipulation of cell cycle checkpoint proteins could be an obvious advantage to a virus, particularly during lytic viral replication when large amounts of viral DNA must be generated. But, interference with normal cell cycle regulatory circuits often activates cell cycle arrest or programmed cell death (apoptosis) signaling. Cell cycle and apoptotic pathways are characterized by extensive feedback interactions that not only serve to prevent tumor cell generation but also to inhibit viral replication within cells (Takaoka et al., 2003). Viral inhibition of pRB1, for example, results in p53 activation through p14ARF and MDM2 (Fig.

Table 30.1. Functional similarities between KSHV, EBV and other tumor viruses

	KSHV	EBV	Other viruses
pRB1 inactivation	vCYC	EBNA2/EBNA-LP	Ad, HPV, SV40
β-catenin stabilization	LANA1	LMP1	
p53 inhibition	LANA1, vIRF1, LANA2	LMP1	Ad, HPV, SV40
Anti-apoptotic, NF-κB activation	vBCL2, vIAP, vFLIP, LMP1	BHRF1, LMP1	Many viral proteins
BCR signaling	ORFK1, LAMP	LMP2	?
Death receptor inhibiton	vFLIP	LMP1	HVS, MCV
CBP/p300 inactivation,	vIRF1	EBNA2	Ad, CMV, HTLV I,
Interferon transcription factor inhibition	ORF45 protein		HPV, SV40
MHC down-regulation	MIR1/2	–	Ad, HSV, CMV
IL-6 signaling	vIL-6	LMP1	?
Telomerase activation	LANA1	?	HPV
Th2 Chemokines	vMIP 1-3	?	CMV

30.1). Thus, overexpression of individual cellular or viral oncoproteins may paradoxically result in cell cycle arrest or cell death rather than proliferation, as is the case for cellular cMYC, or adenoviral E1A (de Stanchina et al., 1998, Debbas and White, 1993; Zindy et al., 1998). Because of this feedback regulation, viral proteins that initiate dysregulated cell cycle entry can be mistaken to have the exact opposite effect, e.g., cell cycle arrest or apoptosis. Caution must be used to interpret the consequences of viral protein expression in the context of the actual viral lifecycle in which multiple KSHV proteins may be acting in concert.

Cell cycle dysregulation during viral latency

LANA-1

Although lytic KSHV replication may contribute to tumor formation in humans though paracrine mechanisms (see Chapter 56), most interest is focused on the latent viral genes constitutively expressed in tumor cells as oncogenes. Whereas latent virus replication is compatible with cell expansion, virion production generally leads to cell death. As described in Chapter 28, the division between "latent" genes and "lytic" genes, however, has become increasingly blurred. Intracellular notch (Chang et al., 2005) or interferon signalling (Chatterjee et al., 2002) can activate expression of genes such as K1 (KIS) and K2 (vIL-6) that are traditionally referred to as lytic genes without full lytic cascade

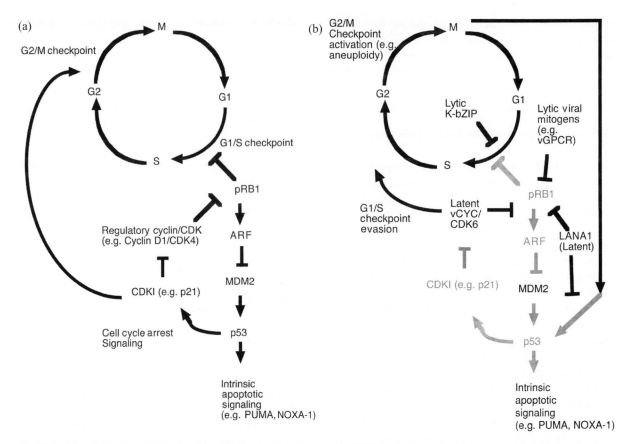

Fig. 30.1. A schematic diagram of cell cycle control interactions between the G1/S checkpoint retinoblastoma protein (pRB1) and p53. (a) Normal feedback control allows pRB1 to negatively regulate entry into the S phase by inhibition of E2F-regulated DNA synthesis genes and positively regulate p53 activity through ARF-dependent inhibition of the p53 E3-ligase, MDM2. Mitogenic cyclins such as cyclin D bind to cyclin-dependent kinases that than phosphorylate and inactivate pRB1, allowing S phase entry. Uncontrolled activation of this circuit will induce p53 activity to initiate cell cycle arrest or apoptosis. KSHV vCYC and LANA1 proteins act together during latent viral replication to inhibit both the pRB1 control functions and p53-dependent apoptosis. Inhibition of p53 may be particularly important since dysregulated entry into the cell cycle by vCYC can initiate aneuploidy and dysregulated cytokineses. During lytic replication a more complicated pattern arises since KSHV proteins can both block (K-bZIP) and enhance (vGPCR, vIL-6) G1/S cell cycle transit, to enhance virion production.

activation and cell death. Notch signaling in particular appears to be responsible for the Type II pattern of KSHV gene activation (Sarid et al., 1998), markedly increasing the number and range of KSHV genes having potential to play a role in KSHV-induced tumorigenesis. Intriguingly, the latent antigen LANA1 has been reported to activate notch signaling and intracellular notch activity is high in resting PEL cells (Lan et al., 2006).

LANA

The major latency locus on the right-hand end of the genome (Fig. 30.2) encodes three open reading frames (ORFs K13, 72 and 73) for the vFLIP, vCYC and LANA1 proteins. An additional long transcript expressed by polyadenylation site read-through from this promoter is processed into at a number of miRNAs that are also constitutively expressed (Pfeffer et al., 2005; Cai et al., 2005). While the viral or cellular targets for these miRNAs are unknown, they are of particular interest since cellular miRNAs have been closely associated with cancer cell regulation (Esquela-Kerscher and Slack, 2006). Recent studies also reveal the complexity of gene expression at this locus with some transcripts extending to the K12 region. Some overlapping transcripts for ORFs K12, K13, 72 and 73 have been shown to be induced during lytic replication demonstrating that the widely-held view that these genes are expressed in a static fashion is incomplete (Cai and Cullin, 2005; Pearce et al., 2005).

ORF73 encodes LANA1 (Latency-associated nuclear antigen)1, first discovered as a serologic antigen useful for

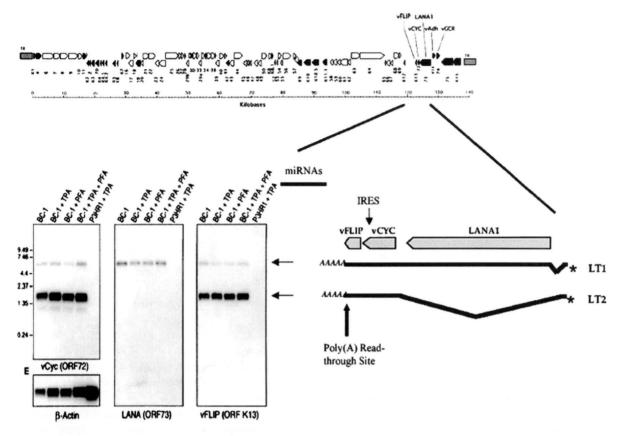

Fig. 30.2. Diagram of the KSHV major latency locus. Northern blots are shown for the major genes in this region under conditions of lytic induction (TPA) or viral DNA synthesis inhibition using the DNA polymerase inhibitor, phosphonoformic acid (PFA). The genes encoding LANA1, vCYC and vFLIP are expressed in the BC-1 cell line under all conditions, but they are also under cell cycle regulation. Less abundant transcripts, including transcripts expression KSHV miRNAs after read-through of the LT1/LT2 polyadenylation site, are not seen at this exposure. (From Sarid et al., 1999.)

Table 30.2. Major KSHV proteins affecting cell cycle control machinery

	Protein	Gene	Target(s)
Latency	LANA1	ORF73	pRB1
	vCYC	ORF72	pRB1, p27, ORC1, H1, Cdc25a
Lytic or Induced	vGPCR	ORF74	Akt, SAPK pathways
	KIS	ORF K1	ITAM signaling
	vIL-6	ORF K2	Interferon, IL-6 signaling
	vMIP 1–3	ORFs K4, 4.1 and 6	Angiogenesis
Lytic	K-bZIP (RAP1)	ORF K8	C/EBP-α, p21

detecting KSHV infection (Moore et al., 1996), that functions to maintain the viral episome by tethering it to cellular chromosomes during mitosis (Ballestas et al., 1999, see Chapter 24). LANA is mainly expressed from a polycistronic transcript (LT1) that includes vCYC and vFLIP (Figure 30.2). These two latter proteins are also expressed from a second transcript (LT2) that originates from the same promoter but splices out ORF73. The latency promoter is cell cycle-regulated with highest expression during late G1 (Sarid et al., 1998) and LANA1 positively autoregulates its own expression as well (Jeong, et al., 2004). Although LANA1 and vCYC proteins are translated from LT1 and LT2 respectively, vFLIP translation requires an internal ribosomal entry site (IRES) located at the 3' end of the vCYC message (Grundhoff and Ganem, 2001; Bieleski and Talbot, 2001; Low et al., 2001). Outside of the major latency locus, the ORF K10.5 gene product, vIRF3 or LANA2, is also constitutively expressed in KSHV-infected hematopoeitic cells but not KS tumor cells (Cunningham *et al.*, 2003). Other KSHV genes, including K12 (kaposin) are expressed during latency but are also induced during lytic replication and by other transcriptional activation, such as notch-signaling (Chang *et al.*, 2005).

LANA1 is a large protein (*ca.* 150 kDa) composed of basic, glutamine-rich amino- and carboxyl-terminal domains separated by a highly acidic, aspartic- and glutamic acid-rich repeat region that includes a leucine zipper domain (see Chapter 24). Because of its highly charged, amphipathic structure it runs as a 220–224 kDa doublet on denaturing gel electrophoresis. This multifunctional protein is reminiscent of the SV40 virus large T-antigen (LT ag), since it tethers the episome to cellular DNA during mitosis and also disrupts both cell cycle and p53-mediated apoptosis.

LANA1 abrogates cell cycle arrest through its binding to at least two of the many cellular interaction partners for LANA1 that have been described. Radkov and colleagues (Radkov *et al.*, 2000) found that LANA1 directly binds the hypophosphorylated (active) form of RB1, inhibiting RB1's ability to serve as a transcriptional repressor of the E2F family. LANA1 binds the pocket region of RB1, but not the related RB1-like protein p130, through interactions with a central region that includes the leucine zipper domain. This effectively sequesters RB1, allowing E2F transactivation (Figure 30.1). Dysregulation of the G1/S checkpoint by LANA1 can be functionally demonstrated rodent cell transformation assays. While LANA1 expression alone does not enhance cellular transformation, oncogenic cooperativity occurs when LANA1 is coexpressed with the activated H-Ras oncogene.

Aside from direct inhibition of RB1, LANA1 as a second pro-mitogenic activity through its ability to activate the Wnt signaling pathway. Hayward and colleagues identified glycogen synthase kinase – 3β (GSK-3β) as a protein interactor with LANA1 through yeast two-hybrid screening (Fujimuro and Hayward, 2003; Fujimuro *et al.*, 2003). GSK3-β normally phosphorylates β-catenin causing the cytoplasmic sequestration of this proto-oncoprotein. LANA1, however, inhibits GSK-3β regulation of β-catenin allowing it to accumulate in the nucleus and transactivate responsive promoters, including the cMYC promoter. cMYC has diverse mitogenic activity and activates the hTERT promoter, which may contribute to the ability LANA1 to activate telomerase activity in KSHV infected cell lines (Verma *et al.*, 2004; Wu *et al.*, 1999). GSK3-β inhibition could potentially also indirectly modulate cell cycle entry through its ability to phosphorylate D-type cyclins resulting in their cytoplasmic accumulation (Verschuren *et al.*, 2004b). These secondary consequences of LANA targeting of Wnt pathway signaling are speculative and remain to be examined but suggest novel and unexplored ways that LANA can contribute to cell transformation. As is the case for many KSHV signaling pathways, EBV has also been shown to stabilize β-catenin showing conservation of cell signaling pathway targeting by the two vriuses (Hayward *et al.*, 2006).

Viral Cyclin (vCYC)

While LANA1 has no homologue in the human genome, KSHV also uses its pirated cyclin to hijack cell cycle regulatory control mechanisms. The vCYC protein (ORF72) (Cesarman *et al.*, 1996; Chang *et al.*, 1996) is expressed together with LANA1 from the major latency locus. As previously described, cellular cyclins positively regulate various stages of the cell cycle by partnering with CDKs to phosphorylate specific cell cycle components. KSHV vCYC retains sequence similarity to the D-type cyclins (there are three cellular D cyclins-D1, D2, and D3 which have overlapping and apparently redundant activities), which target CDK4 and CDK6 to hyperphosphorylate RB1, thereby inhibiting this inhibitor of E2F-induced transcription. KSHV vCYC partners almost exclusively with CDK6 to achieve this effect (Chang *et al.*, 1996; Godden-Kent *et al.*, 1997; Li *et al.*, 1997), initiating illicit S phase entry and DNA replication (Laman *et al.*, 2001).

Although vCYC is structurally similar to D-type cyclins, several features of the protein are unique. Unlike D-type cyclins, vCYC (also referred to as K-cyclin) targets cell cycle control proteins that are more typical targets of other cyclins such as cyclins A and E which couple to the CDK2 kinase. These targets include histone H1, the CDKI p27, and Cdc25a, as well as ORC1 and Cdc6 (Ellis *et al.*, 1999; Laman *et al.*, 2001; Mann *et al.*, 1999) (for review see Verschuren *et al.*, 2004b). Unlike cellular cyclin D/CDK6 complex, which normally requires CDK6 phosphorylation through the action of a CDK-acitvating kinase (CAK), the vCYC/CDK6 is fully active in an unphosphorylated form (Child and Mann, 2001; Kaldis *et al.*, 2001).

The vCYC gene, ORF72, like the other genes encoded in the major latency locus, is expressed during late G1 in a cell cycle-dependent fashion (Sarid *et al.*, 1999). Although direct measurement of vCYC protein levels are difficult, vCYC lacks the cyclin destruction box motif that targets cyclins for rapid protein turnover (Klotzbucher *et al.*, 1996) suggesting that the viral protein may be long-lived and active at other portions of the cell cycle including the G2/M checkpoint (Van Dross *et al.*, 2005). Also absent from the viral protein are motifs required for docking to nuclear export proteins, which may indicate that vCYC abnormally accumulates in the nucleas and may escape regulations imposed on cellular cyclin proteins (Verschuren *et al.*,

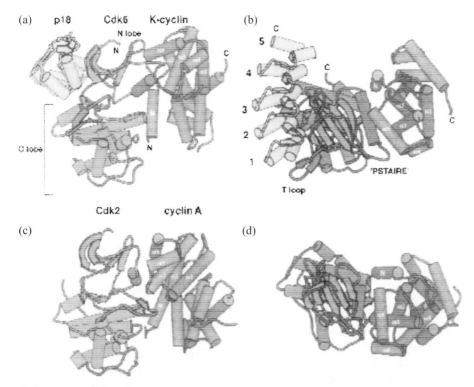

Fig. 30.3. The structure of the vCYC (purple), CDK6 (cyan), p18Inkb (yellow) complex from side (a) and top (b) views, compared to cellular cyclin A (purple), CDK2 (cyan) side (c) and top (d) views. Unlike cellular cyclins, the regulatory T-loop of CDK6 is excluded from interaction with vCYC but the PSTAIRE regulatory helix of CDK6 still forms an interface with vCYC. The PSTAIRE helix forms part of the ATP binding domain required for kinase activity while the T loop acts as a negative regulator of kinase activity and must be phosphorylated by cyclin-activating kinases (CAK) in cellular cyclin–CDK complexes. While CAK phosphorylation may enhance vCYC-CDK6 stability, displacement of the T loop by vCYC allows this complex to be active in the absence of CAK activity. The structure of vCYC-CDK6 also reveals loss of the binding pocket used by cyclin-dependent kinase inhibitors (CDKI) of the CIP1/KIP1 family. These and other features support experimental data showing the vCYC-CDK6 not only have a broader target range than cellular D-type cyclins but also escape many normal negative regulatory controls imposed on the cellular cyclin machinery. Reprinted with permission (Jeffrey et al., 2000). (See color plate section.)

2004b). This is supported by transgenic mouse experiments (see below) in which constitutive vCYC expression leads to defects in chromosome segregation, abnormal cytokinesis and polyploidy (Verschuren et al., 2002). Surprisingly, vCYC also phosphorylates and inactivates the antiapoptotic cellular protein BCL-2, but not the corresponding KSHV BCL-2 homologue, contributing to the pro-apoptotic properties of this protein when overexpressed in cells (Ojala et al., 2000).

Another critical difference between cellular cyclins and vCYC is that vCYC escapes from normal CDK inhibitor (CDKI) control. CDKIs, including p21 and p27 and members of the p16Ink4a family, act to inhibit cyclin-dependent phosphorylation and are a critical link for transmitting cell arrest signaling from p53 to the cell cycle machinery. vCYC/CDK6 is resistant to p21 and p27 CDKI inhibition (Swanton et al., 1997, 1999), but is still inhibited by Ink4 unless CDK6 is phosphorylated through the action of CAK (Jeffrey et al., 2000). This has allowed crystallographic analysis of the trimolecular vCYC/CDK6/p18Inkb structure (Fig. 30.3), which has been tremendously informative for understanding the structural basis for vCYC regulation as well as regulation of the cellular cyclins. vCYC phosphorylation of p27 also diminishes cellular levels of this inhibitor protein, contributing to positive cell cycle regulation. In summary, although vCYC has similar functionality to cellular cyclins, modifications to this protein allow the virus to escape normal cell cycle regulatory constraints and to couple CDK6 phosphorylation to RB1 and other cell cycle components (for review, see Mittnacht and Boshoff, 2000; Verschuren et al., 2004b).

A potential role for vCYC in cell tranformation and carcinogenesis has been uncovered using transgenic mice in which vCYC is expressed under an Eμ promoter (Verschuren et al., 2002, 2004a). Overexpression of vCYC both induces dysregulated DNA synthesis and leads to p53-dependent apoptosis. One mechanism by which this could occur is a circuit in which RB1 inactivation leads to E2F activation of p14ARF – a potent activator of p53 acting through MDM2. This, however, does not seem to be the case since p53-induced apoptosis is not reduced by mating the transgenic vCYC mice onto a p19ARF-null background. Instead, vCYC appears to dysregulate the G2/M checkpoint resulting in dysregulated cytokinesis and aneuploidy that in turn activates p53 through DNA-damage response pathways. When mice expressing vCYC are mated with p53-null mice, progeny develop lymphomas at an accelerated rate.

Other KSHV mitogenic signaling proteins

KSHV also possesses a number of proteins which act through mitogenic signaling pathways to achieve similar effects. Mitogenic signaling can occur through diverse signaling pathways which act on common regulatory points to induce cell cycle entry, such as activation of cyclin-dependent phosphorylation of RB1 (Sherr, 2004). While most of these molecules are thought to be expressed only during active lytic replication, evidence suggests that they have more complicated patterns of expression (see Chapter 28) in that at least several of them, such as the vIL-6 and the KSHV-encoded chemokines (Moore *et al.*, 1996; Parravicini *et al.*, 2000), are expressed at low levels during true viral latency (at least in tissue culture where the process can be readily examined) and are further activated during lytic viral replication or in response to specific signaling pathways. This is a similar pattern of expression to the EBV LMP1 protein. It is unclear what, if any, effects these mitogenic factors have during latency but these pathways have also received renewed interest related to the possibility that lytic virus replication contributes to the tumorigenesis, particularly in KS tumors (described more fully elsewhere in this volume).

Viral G-protein coupled receptor (vGPCR)

The best-studied example of a KSHV mitogenic signaling molecule is the vGPCR (ORF74), a seven-spanning G-protein coupled receptor that is expressed at early phases during lytic replication (Cesarman *et al.*, 1996). vGPCR is a constitutively active CXC receptor (Chiou *et al.*, 2002; Kirshner *et al.*, 1999), which activates MAPK, p38, Akt and NF-κB pathways resulting in expression of angiogenic factors, such as VEGF, and in cell transformation (Bais *et al.*, 1998; Cannon *et al.*, 2003; Masood *et al.*, 2002; Montaner *et al.*, 2001; Polson *et al.*, 2002). Although constitutively active, evidence suggests that its growth promoting activity is enhanced by host ligand binding (Holst *et al.*, 2001). The principal interest in this protein comes from the unique phenotype that it generates in transgenic mice which was first demonstrated by Lira and colleagues (Yang *et al.*, 2000) but has been confirmed using a variety of experimental systems by others (Guo *et al.*, 2003; Montaner *et al.*, 2003).

In these first experiments, vGPCR was expressed under control of the CD2 promoter, resulting in diffuse hematopoietic expression of the viral protein. Surprisingly, this resulted in endothelial tumors pathologically resembling Kaposi sarcoma tumors. These and similar results by Montaner and colleagues (Montaner *et al.*, 2003) suggest that KS tumors, unlike primary effusion lymphomas, may actually be dependent on active lytic viral replication and that KS tumor cell proliferation occurs in *trans* due to paracrine factors released by infected cells undergoing lytic replication. This is a unique pathogenic model in which paracrine factors, rather than endogenous genetic changes, are responsible for the neoplastic phenotype (Cesarman *et al.*, 2000).

Several findings, however, complicate this view. It is evident that virtually all tumor cells in KS tumors are infected with KSHV and so paracrine-effects of lytic replication appear to act in concert with endogenous viral gene expression to result in tumor cell outgrowth (Parravicini *et al.*, 2000, Katano *et al.*, 2000). KS development can be effectively prevented by antilytic DNA pol inhibitors, such as ganciclovir (Martin *et al.*, 1999), but there is no current evidence that these drugs have any effect on established KS tumors (Little *et al.*, 2003). Further, clinical studies suggest that some KS tumors arising during transplantation are donor derived (Barozzi *et al.*, 2003). Since these donors were ostensibly healthy, the prototumor was primarily latent, or at least subclinical, in the donor prior to the transplantation. Studies of cell and virus monoclonality do not clarify the origin of KS pathogenesis since both cellular monoclonality and multiclonality have been reported. KS tumors have KSHV terminal repeat patterns that are oligoclonal or monoclonal, with the possibility that tumors evolve into a monoclonal pattern over time (Judde *et al.*, 2000; Russo *et al.*, 1996). The role for paracrine-induced proliferation from vGCPR or other viral proteins may become clearer as KSHV gene regulation outside of the latent-lytic expression pattern is explored.

K1 Protein

On the opposite end of the KSHV genome (see Chapter 28), a second membrane signaling protein encoded by ORFK1, also called KIS (KSHV ITAM signaling protein), has strong mitogenic activity when expressed in cells. K1 protein is a type 1 transmembrane protein that aggregates through ectodomain disulfide bonds into a signaling complex (Lee *et al.*, 1998b). The cytoplasmic tail of the protein contains two immunoreceptor tyrosine signaling motifs (ITAMs) which recruit SH2-containing signaling kinases; NFAT, syk, vav and other downstream signaling effectors have been shown to be activated by K1, resulting in Akt signaling activation (Lagunoff et al., 1999, 2001; Lee et al., 1998a, 2003; Tomlinson and Damania, 2004, Wang et al., 2005). As a consequence of its mitogenic signaling activities, K1 transforms rodent fibroblasts and primary endothelial cells in vitro and when substituted into a herpesvirus saimiri backbone, induces lymphomas in rhesus macques (Lee et al., 1998b, Wang et al., 2005).

Clues to the functional advantage of this signaling protein for the virus, come from overlap between K1 signaling and signaling through the B cell receptor (BCR). The BCR is active as a non-specific innate immune signaling pathway. Intriguingly, K1 causes ER retention and degradation of the BCR, suggesting that K1 may serve as a decoy molecule after downregulation of this pathway (Lee et al., 2000). A consequence of K1 expression is induction of paracrine angiogenic factors including vascular endothelial growth factor (VEGF) and matrix metalloproteinase-9 (MMP-9), analogous to the paracrine mitogenic induction that can occur with vGPCR (Wang et al., 2004). The immunoevasion/mitogenic properties of K1 have analogy, together with the KSHV LAMP1 protein, to properties of EBV membrane proteins, LMP1 and LMP2 (Damania et al., 2000).

Virus-encoded chemokines and cytokines

In addition to both vGPCR and K1 protein, which induce secretion of proliferative cytokines, KSHV itself encodes three secreted chemokines, vCCL1 (*ORF K6*), vCCL2 (*ORF K4*) and vCCL3 (*ORF K4.1*), formerly known as vMIP-I/MIP-1a, vMIP-II/MIP-1b and vMIP-III/BCK, respectively and a functional, secreted vIL-6 (ORF K2) cytokine. The chemokines are believed to act to polarize local immune responses towards a Th2 phenotype. vCCL2 initiates a strong chemotactic response through CCR3 activation (Boshoff et al., 1997), while vCCL1 and vCCL3 activate CCR8 (Dairaghi et al., 1999, Endres et al., 1999) and CCR4 receptors (Stine et al., 2000). All three chemokines have angiogenic activity and stimulate endothelial and B-lymphocytic proliferation (Moore et al., 1996; Stine et al., 2000). While they are generally not expressed in PEL cells during latency, they may play a role in mitogenesis in KS tumors.

Like K1 protein, KSHV encoded vIL-6 has both immune evasion and cell cycle regulatory properties (Moore et al., 1996; Nicholas et al., 1997) (described in more detail in Chapter 31). vIL-6 is a secreted cytokine similar to the human cytokine (25% identity, 62% similarity) that activates IL-6 signaling pathways by binding directly to the gp130 signal transducer molecule without requiring interaction with the IL-6 specific recepor, gp80 (Burger et al., 1998; Chow et al., 2001; Molden et al., 1997; Mullberg et al., 2000; Osborne et al., 1999). Although this has not been directly examined, it is likely that the viral protein activates the same signaling pathways as hIL-6, resulting in RB1 hyperphosphorylation and mitogenesis (Urashima et al., 1996, 1997; Zhu et al., 1994). Studies of a non-adapted tissue culture PEL cell line, BCP-1, demonstrate that the cells are autocrine dependent on hIL-10 and vIL-6 (Jones et al., 1999), and can reinitiate DNA synthesis for serum-starved PEL cells (Chatterjee et al., 2002).

The role of vIL-6 in the lifecycle of KSHV reveals the intimate connection between cell cycle regulation and early innate immune responses (Chatterjee et al., 2002). Type I interferon signaling in PEL cells causes upregulation of p21 CDKI and initiates arrest. The vIL-6 promoter, however, has transcription elements responsive to interferon signaling and is simultaneously up-regulated. Evidence suggests that vIL-6 can block interferon signaling at the receptor resulting in a negative feedback loop that protects infected cells from cell-cycle arrest effects of interferon. Interferons are activated by viral infection and the autocrine loop formed by vIL-6 appears to block antiviral effects induced by KSHV infection itself. A consequence of vIL-6 hypersecretion may include neighboring cell proliferation as is seen in multicentric Castleman's disease (Parravicini et al., 1997). As an interesting aside, this demonstrates that a virus can sense and modify its environment, a property referred to as irritability, that is part of the fundamental definitions for living organisms.

Inhibition of cell cycle progression: K-BZIP/RAP

The proteins thus far described for KSHV act on cell cycle checkpoints to prevent cell cycle arrest. KSHV k-BZIP (also known as replication associated protein, RAP) encoded by ORF K8, paradoxically has opposing effects on cell cycle regulation. K-BZIP is an early spliced gene (corresponding by weak sequence homology to the EBV transactivator Zta or ZEBRA) possessing a basic-leucine zipper (bZIP) (Gruffat et al., 1999; Lin et al., 1999; Seaman et al., 1999). This protein interacts with p53 and may sequester p53 (together with the other major lytic transactivator RTA (Gwack et al., 2001b)) to promyelocytic leukemia (PML) bodies, presumably as a means of delaying p53-dependent apoptosis during the early phases of lytic reactivation (Park et al., 2000). Despite this, K-bZIP causes cell cycle arrest through induction of the CDKI p21, a downstream target of p53, and CCAAT/enhancer binding protein-α (C/EBP-α) resulting in G1 arrest during lytic replication (Wang et al., 2003a,b; Wu et al., 2003). K-bZIP is phosphorylated by CDKs (Polson et al., 2001) and also directly interacts with cyclin A/CDK2 complexes contributing to G1 arrest during early lytic replication (Izumiya et al., 2003).

The reasons for this effect remain speculative. Virus-induced cell cycle arrest may seem counterintuitive – particularly in view of the limited resource hypothesis for oncogene teleology developed from analyses of small DNA

Table 30.3. Major KSHV proteins targeting apoptotic control machinery

	Protein	Gene	Target(s)
Latency	LANA1	ORF73	p53
	LANA2 (vIRF-3)	ORF K10.5	p53
	vFLIP	ORF K13	Fas, NF-κB
Lytic or induced	RTA	ORF50	p53
	K-bZIP	ORF K8	p53/p300/CBP
	vIRF-1	ORF K9	p53/p300/CBP/ATM
	vBCL-2	ORF 16	BAX?
	VIAP	ORF K7	BAX, BH-3 proteins?

tumor viruses (Braithwaite and Russell, 2001; Russell et al., 2004), since S phase entry is thought to be required for viral DNA replication. Entry into a "senescent" phenotype, however, might have protective effects in preventing premature apoptosis during lytic replication. It is also unclear if expression of the lytic phase KSHV DNA synthesis enzymes whose cellular counterparts are under E2F-control (e.g., ribonucleotide reductase, thymidylate synthase, dihydrofolate reductase and thymidine kinase) can generate a quasi-S phase state in the face of K-BZIP induced cell cycle arrest. Conceivably, this may allow viral DNA replication during stasis in cellular DNA replication. K-BZIP acts during lytic replication whereas LANA1 and vCYC act during latency (possibly during lytic replication as well) indicating that the different phases of the viral life cycle require different cell cycle manipulations.

KSHV inhibition of apoptosis

Interference with cell cycle checkpoints activates cellular apoptotic pathways through p14ARF and other less well-defined mechanisms, presumably as a means to prevent tumor cell formation (Sherr, 1998, 2004). It is therefore not surprising that KSHV encodes antiapoptotic factors that mitigate this response. What is surprising, however, is the number, range and kind of anti-apoptotic factors encoded by KSHV (Table 30.3, for review see Lagunoff and Carroll, 2003). KSHV also activates survival factors, such as NF-κB, a trait shared with EBV and other B-lymphotrophic viruses.

Apoptotic signaling is divided into intrinsic and extrinsic pathways integrated with each other through the activity of the transcription factor p53 (Fig. 30.4). Extrinsic pathways are activated through apoptotic signaling receptors, such as Fas/CD95 and the tumor necrosis factor receptor (TNFR), whereas intrinsic pathways are activated in response to cellular stress and DNA damage (Danial and Korsmeyer, 2004).

Extrinsic apoptotic signaling is principally an immune response activated through death-inducing receptors by natural killer (NK) cells and cytotoxic lymphocytes (CTL). Receptors of the TNF-Fas receptor family can have either opposing proapoptotic or antiapoptotic signaling responses depending on the mechanism of activation and the cellular context of receptor activation. Extrinsic apoptotic signaling activates caspase cascade signaling which in turn results in mitochondrial release of apoptosis mediators including cytochrome C. p53 has been implicated in increasing apoptotic receptor transcription and priming other components of these pathways (Sheard et al., 2003).

Intrinsic apoptotic signaling directly activates p53 through a series of kinase cascades, ultimately resulting in mitochondrial apoptosis. Although this characterization of this response is rapidly evolving, current evidence suggest that sensors of DNA damage activate signaling cascades that ultimately result in cell cycle arrest and repair or, failing this, apoptosis. Responses may differ between types of DNA damage (e.g., mismatch damage vs. single and double-strand breaks) that activate different repair responses including nucleotide-excision repair, base-excision repair, or homologous and non-homologous recombination (for review see Wood et al., 2001).

One of the initial responses to DNA damage recognition is binding and activation of the MRE11- Rad51-NBS (MRN) complex, which sequentially activates Chk2 and ATM phosphorylation and subsequent phosphorylation of p53 (Banin et al., 1998; Lee and Paull, 2004). The importance of this pathway to viral replication is hinted at by viruses encoding proteins that target these early responses (Weitzman et al., 2004). KSHV vIRF1, for example, binds to and inactivates ATM downstream signaling to p53 (Shin et al., 2006). p53 phosphorylation causes conformational changes that promote p53 binding to specific DNA regulatory elements to initiate transcription of pro-apoptotic protein genes, such as PUMA and NOXA-1, BH3-only members (see below) of the BCL-2 factor family, which act at the mitochondria to initiate mitochondrial apoptotic responses (Oda et al., 2000; Yu et al., 2001). These BH3-only containing BCL-2 factors bind and sequester other anti-apoptotic BCL-2 members, including BCL-2 itself and BCL-x_L (Cheng et al., 2001; Schuler and Green, 2001).

Disarming the guardian: p53 inhibition

p53 has been called the "guardian of the genome" for its critical role in integrating apoptotic and cell cycle arrest signaling, most notably in response to DNA-damaging

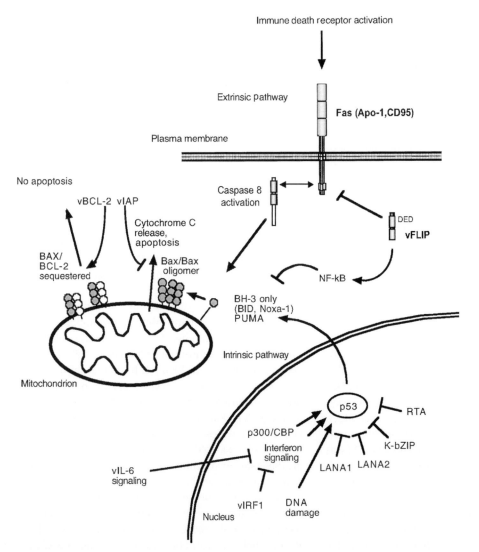

Fig. 30.4. KSHV inhibits both intrinsic and extrinsic apoptotic pathways at multiple points. Extrinsic signaling shown here is activated by cellular immune signaling (NK cell, cytotoxic lymphocyte responses) though activation of the Fas receptor. vFLIP directly inhibits this response through a dominant-negative binding to death effector domains (DED) in the death-inducing signaling complex (DISC) and also activate NF-kB through an alternative pathway which may inhibit B-cell apoptosis at the mitochondria and endoplasmic reticulum. Both vIAP and vBCL-2 act at the mitochondria to stabilize the mitochondrial membrane and inhibit the activating effects of BH3-only pro-apoptotic molecules. The central transcriptional integrator of apoptotic signaling, p53, plays a key role in mediating intrinsic apoptotic effects in response to DNA damage or interferon signaling. KSHV proteins including LANA1, LANA2, K-bZIP and RTA inhibit p53-induced apoptotic signaling either through direct binding or through inhibition of the p300/CBP coactivator used in p53 transcriptional signaling. Delaying apoptosis during lytic viral replication allows efficient production of infectious virions. Apoptotic signaling is also inhibited during latency. The reasons for viral targeting of the cell cycle and apoptotic pathways during latency remain poorly understood.

agents (Lane, 1992). p53 prevents germline transmission of mutations, since DNA damage will either cause p53-dependent arrest allowing repair prior to transmission to daughter cells or, if the damage is irreparable, commits the cell to p53-dependent apoptosis. The molecular decision-making process between apoptosis or cell cycle arrest remains unclear, although p21 has a key role in determining whether p53-activation results in arrest or cell death (Gorospe et al., 1997).

For somatic cells, the roles for p53 are less clear. As a tumor suppressor, p53 may prevent cell transformation resulting from DNA damage. More recently, evidence has accumulated that p53 also acts to prevent viral nucleic acid replication (Moore & Chang, 1998; Takaoka et al., 2003).

Replicating extrachromosomal DNA may activate ATM-p53 signaling, thus serving as an intracellular innate immune response. It is now widely accepted that cellular responses limiting viral replication include apoptosis (Benedict et al., 2002; Meinl et al., 1998), although programmed cell death is not universal for all viral infections and some viruses may actually capitalize on cell dissolution during apoptosis to enhance replication (Teodoro and Branton, 1997).

As a critical integrator of cell cycle regulation and apoptotic signaling, p53 is a common target for tumor viruses that have convergently evolved very different mechanisms to inhibit this major regulatory protein (for review, see Lagunoff and Carroll, 2003). KSHV is no exception to this, and it directly targets p53 during both latency and during lytic replication. Unlike many malignancies, apoptosis in not prominent in KSHV-related disorders, p53 is expressed in tumor cells and p53 mutations do not appear to be common in KSHV-induced tumors (Katano et al., 2001b).

LANA-1

To balance the cell cycle dysregulation effect of vCYC and LANA1 during latency, KSHV must also inhibit p53-mediated apoptotic signaling for infected cell survival. This is most clearly seen in unopposed vCYC transfection assays which induce apoptosis, and vCYC transgenic mice which have a dramatically increased rate of lymphomagenesis in a p53-null background. LANA1 encoded by ORF73 was the first p53 inhibitor discovered in KSHV (Friborg et al., 1999), in which the carboxyl terminus of the protein was shown to interact with p53 and inhibit its transcriptional activator function. This work has since been extended to other rhadinoviruses such as herpesvirus saimiri whose ORF73 protein – while structurally different from the KSHV LANA1 protein – also inhibits p53 activity (Borah et al., 2004).

LANA2/vIRF3

While LANA1 is expressed in all KSHV-infected cells, LANA2 (also known as vIRF3) encoded by the spliced gene ORF 10.5, is expressed exclusively in KSHV-infected hematopoeitic cells. LANA2 shares with LANA1 p53-inhibitory functions although evidence for direct interaction with p53 is less certain due to the inherent "stickiness" of the protein (Rivas et al., 2001). Transient expression of LANA2 abrogates apoptosis caused by activation of p53 signaling or by direct overexpression of p53 protein. Paradoxically, LANA2 simultaneously activates interferon transcription pathways (Lubyova et al., 2004)and inhibits NF-kB signaling pathways (Seo et al., 2004) – two signaling events that would be expected to induce lymphocyte apoptosis. The role, if any, of this molecule in PEL survival and transformation remains largely unknown.

RTA, K-bZIP and vIRF1

KSHV p53-inhibitory proteins active during lytic replication include the lytic transactivator proteins RTA (encoded ORF50) and K-bZIP (encoded by K8 and describe above), and the interferon regulatory factor homologue vIRF1 encoded by ORF K9. These three proteins appear to inhibit p53 transcriptional activity (Gwack et al., 2001b; Park et al., 2000; Nakamura et al., 2001) principally by binding to the p300/CBP family of histone acetyltransferases (HAT) that serve as transcriptional coadaptors for p53 (Gwack et al., 2001a; Hwang et al., 2001; Li et al., 2000; Lin et al., 2001). Direct binding by vIRF1 and K-bZIP to p53 may also occur. HAT activity is required to not only acetylate p53 itself, but also histones to prepare the operon for p53-directed transcription.

By sequestering HATs from the transcriptional complex, these KSHV proteins inhibit transcription not only at p53-regulated promoters but also (in the case of vIRF-1) interferon-regulated promoters (Gao et al., 1997; Lin et al., 2001; Zimring et al., 1998). K-bZIP may also directly sequester p53 to promyelocytic leukemia protein (PML) bodies rendering it inactive for participation in apoptotic signaling (Katano et al., 2001a). The use of CBP/p300 coadaptors is widespread in growth control transcriptional responses, and K-bZIP's ability to sequester CBP/p300 has also been shown to inhibit SMAD3 transcriptional response in the TGF-beta signaling cascade (Tomita et al., 2004).

Beyond p300/CBP sequestration, vIRF1 also activates p53 degradation, possibly by enhancing the E4 ubiquitin-ligase activity of p300/CBP (Shin et al., 2006). vIRF1 has the unusual property of binding to and inhibiting ATM, as well. Thus, vIRF1 has a multiple roles in inhibiting ATM-p53 activation during viral infection.

Induction of p53-mediated apoptosis during lytic viral replication is thus postponed by the activity of several proteins expressed during the earliest phases of viral replication. This presumably forestalls early cell death to optimize virion production. Since cells undergoing full viral replication eventually undergo apoptosis, it is clear that, in the struggle between the virus and the cell, the cell eventually wins–but presumably not before the virus is able to generate infectious progeny. The actual apoptotic triggers initiated by viral replication remain unknown. One possibility is that viral DNA breaks, as a consequence of massive but inefficient viral DNA replication, initiate ATM-p53 signaling. Other possibilities include endoplasmic reticulum stress due to hijacking of cellular protein synthesis machinery or the degradation of cellular mRNA with concomitant transcriptional inhibition by the KSHV ORF 37 protein (Glaunsinger and Ganem, 2004).

Inhibition of extrinsic apoptotic signaling

vFLIP

KSHV down-regulation of MHC I during both lytic (Coscoy and Ganem, 2000) and latent (Tomescu et al., 2003) viral replication leaves the infected cell open to NK cell attack (see Chapter 31). Intercellular killing is mediated by released membrane toxins (granzyme) and activation of Fas signaling. KSHV vFLIP encoded by ORF K13 potentially abrogates Fas-mediated apoptosis through two dominent-negative death-effector domains (DED) that block the formation of the death-induced signaling complex (DISC)(reviewed in Krueger et al., 2001).

vFLIP encoded by ORF K13 has generated considerable interest as an antiapoptic protein since it is expressed during latency through an IRES in the ORF 72 (vCYC) gene on LT1 and LT2 transcripts (Bieleski et al., 2004; Bieleski and Talbot, 2001; Grundhoff and Ganem, 2001; Low et al., 2001). While its caspase-inhibition functions have a clear benefit in preventing NK immune killing of an infected cell, the ability of this protein to activate NF-kB may have even greater importance in maintaining the infected tumor cell (Chaudhary et al., 1999). NF-kB is constitutively activated in PEL cells through IkB inhibitor phosphorylation due to vFLIP signaling (Field et al., 2003; Matta and Chaudhary, 2004) and this activity may inhibit BH3-only molecule-induced apoptosis (Fig. 30.4). Cesarman and colleagues have demonstrated the importance of this to PEL cell survival using specific NF-kB inhibitors which rapidly induce PEL cell apoptosis (Guasparri et al., 2004; Keller et al., 2000). Differentiating the effects of vFLIP on caspase inhibition from NF-kB activation suggests that the latter is critical for PEL cell survival in tissue culture. vFLIP activates NF-kB through direct interactions with the Ikappa B kinase (IKK) complex which targets inhibition of the NF-kB inhibitor, Ik-B (Liu et al., 2002). Evidence suggests this specifically activates an alternative NF-kB pathway that favors processing of the p52 subunit of NF-kB (Matta and Chaudhary, 2004). Latent expression of vFLIP makes this protein an attractive candidate for contributing to human tumors. Expression of vFLIP enhances tumorigenicity of mouse B lymphoma cells in immunocompetent mice strains (Djerbi et al., 1999), suggesting a role in human KSHV-induced tumors.

The mitochondrial anti-apoptotic proteins: vBCL-2, vIAP

Both intrinsic and extrinsic apoptotic signaling ultimately merge at mitochondria to initiate membrane depolarization, release of cytochrome c and formation of the apoptosomal proteins required for chromatin condensation and endonucleolytic cleavage, volume contraction and the breakdown and blebbing of membrane structures that result in apoptotic cell death (Danial and Korsmeyer, 2004).

As previously indicated, critical components of this process are the BCL-2 family of proteins (BCL-2 referring to the second B-cell lymphoma related rearrangement protein found (Bakhshi et al., 1985) with the cyclin D1 being "BCL-1"). BCL-2 members have up to four conserved BCL-2 homology (BH) domains and dimerize with each other in the mitochondrial membrane. BH1, BH2 and BH3 domains on antiapoptotic members form a hydrophobic pocket which sequesters proapoptotic BH3-only containing members, such as BID, of the BCL-2 family. Some proapoptotic BCL-2 family members, including BAX and BAK, possess all three BH domains but may have specific activation at the BH3 domain which initiates their proapoptotic activity (Danial and Korsmeyer, 2004).

KSHV and other DNA viruses (Cuconati and White, 2002) encode homologues to the cellular BCL-2 antiapoptic protein (Sarid et al., 1997). vBCL2 encoded by ORF16 was the first KSHV protein to be investigated for its apoptosis-inhibitory properties (Cheng et al., 1997; Sarid et al., 1997) and possesses BH1 and BH2 domains. Solution structure studies suggest structural similarities to BH3 and BH4 domains being present (Huang et al., 2002) allowing the KSHV protein to tightly bind pro-apoptotic Bak and Bax peptides, consistent with two-hybrid heterodimerization studies (Sarid et al., 1997). Whereas cellular BCL-2 can be cleaved by caspase proteolysis and converted to a proapoptotic version, KSHV vBCL-2 lacks this cleavage site and escapes cellular regulation (Bellows et al., 2000). Also, as previously indicated, vBCL-2 may serve a specific role in KSHV infected cells since it escapes inactivation by the KSHV vCYC protein which can occur for the cellular BCL-2 (Ojala et al., 2000).

Recent studies also suggest an novel role for viral BCL-2 members in preventing cell death. In addition to apoptosis, autophagy – programmed lysosomal degradation of cytosolic components – plays a critical role in inhibiting intracellular pathogens and initiating CD4+ antigen presentation (Schmid et al., 2006). Liang and colleagues demonstrated that the murine γHV-68 vBCL-2 binds to the autophagy signaling complex composed of UVRAG and Beclin-1 (Liang et al., 2006). vBCL-2 inhibition of autophagy is an attractive mechanism for gammaherpesviruses to escape this innate immune signaling pathway. Thus, vBCL-2 may help KSHV and related viruses escape both apoptotic and autophagic surveillance systems.

vBCL-2 is expressed as an early gene during lytic replication (Sarid et al., 1997; Sun et al., 1999), and presumably delays apoptosis to allow optimal virion production (Cuconati and White, 2002). Immunostaining of KS tissues shows vBCL-2 production in a minority of infected spindle cells of advanced nodular lesions also consistent with a role primarily in delaying lytic apoptosis in vivo (Widmer et al., 2002).

Another KSHV molecule acting as an antiapoptotic factor at the mitochondrial member is the recently investigated viral inhibitor of apoptosis protein (vIAP) encoded by ORF K7 (Feng et al., 2002; Wang et al., 2002). KSHV vIAP possesses a BH2 domain and localizes to mitochondrial membranes where it stabilizes mitochondrial membranes from apoptotic $Ca+2$ depolarization induced by a variety of agents (Feng et al., 2002). While a BCL-2-like interaction may account for some of the antiapoptotic properties of this protein, vIAP interacts with ubiquillin (also known as PLIC1) which regulates the proteosomal machinery. K7 binding to ubiquillin may enhance polyubiquitin-mediated proteolysis of key apoptotic signaling molecules including IK-B and p53 (Feng et al., 2004). vIAP is expressed during lytic replication, but also can be seen immediately after infection with KSHV suggesting a critical role for this protein in preparing the cell for successful viral invasion (Krishnan et al., 2004).

Conclusions

Further, recent studies suggest that many of these "lytic cycle" proteins are actually activated during latency by transcriptional signaling such as notch. Thus, there is a large array of KSHV nonstructural proteins that may contribute cell transformation, and by extension, to KSHV-related tumorigenesis.

In contrast to the small DNA tumor viruses that have only one, or a few, likely viral oncoproteins, KSHV possesses startlingly large number of nonstructural proteins targeting cellular control pathways that regulate cellular proliferation. Multiple KSHV proteins inhibit cellular controls of the cell cycle. Both LANA1 and vCYC directly target negative cell cycle regulators and bypass normal cellular feedback controls that limit cell proliferation. Similarly, KSHV inhibits intrinsic and extrinsic apoptotic signaling at multiple levels using many different proteins, that include direct targeting of p53 as well as targeting both upstream and downstream signaling pathways to p53.

While it is likely that only a few KSHV proteins principally contribute to oncogenesis, it remains to be determined which proteins this are. Latency-expressed proteins are the leading candidates but recent studies reveal that KSHV genes traditionally thought of as being lytic cycle genes can be induced during viral latency. In addition, paracrine contributions to neoplasia have long been thought to be important for KS tumors adding an additional layer of complexity to KSHV-induced cell transformation. One likely reason for the large number of KSHV proteins targeting cellular control machinery is that they act in different tissues that are infected with the virus. This is most obvious example for this is LANA2 which is not appreciably expressed in KS endothelial cells. Similarly, vIRF1 and K1 may have widespread expression in KS tumors that is not found in cultured PEL cells in the laboratory. Although KSHV appears to encode many more 'oncoproteins' than other viruses, this may be more apparent than real. KSHV molecular piracy makes identification of regulatory proteins relatively easy; it is possible that additional, functionally-similar proteins will be found in the other herpesviruses as well.

A more salient question is "Why does KSHV dysregulate the cell cycle and control apoptotic signaling?" One explanation is that during lytic replication, KSHV needs to generate a cell environment that can replicate thousands of copies of viral DNA. This view assumes a passive role for the cell during virus replication. It is becoming increasingly clear, however, that lytic virus replication activates host cell defenses that attempt to shutdown the cell cycle or to initiate apoptotic cell death. While the tumor suppressor feedback control machinery is traditionally thought to be a means of preventing spontaneous tumor cell generation, it works extremely well to also limit virus replication (Moore & Chang, 2003). Evidence for the interplay between innate immune signaling and tumor suppressor signaling (Takaoka et al., 2002) makes it increasingly likely that tumor suppressor pathways have evolved for the equally important role of controlling viral replication (Moore & Chang 1998). Seen from this light, KSHV 'oncoproteins' may actually be innate immunity evasion proteins that allow the virus to escape from hostile cellular responses to virus infection.

REFERENCES

Bais, C., Santomasso, B., Coso, O. et al. (1998). G-protein-coupled receptor of Kaposi's sarcoma-associated herpesvirus is a viral oncogene and angiogenesis activator. *Nature*, **391**(6662), 86–89.

Bakhshi, A., Jensen, J. P., Goldman, P. et al. (1985). Cloning the chromosomal breakpoint of t(14;18) human lymphomas: clustering around JH on chromosome 14 and near a transcriptional unit on 18. *Cell*, **41**(3), 899–906.

Banin, S., Moyal, L., Shieh, S. et al. (1998). Enhanced phosphorylation of p53 by ATM in response to DNA damage. *Science*, **281**(5383), 1674–1677.

Barozzi, P., Luppi, M., Facchetti, F. et al. (2003). Post-transplant Kaposi sarcoma originates from the seeding of donor-derived progenitors. *Nat. Med.*, **9**(5), 554–561.

Bellows, D. S., Chau, B. N., Lee, P., Lazebnik, Y., Burns, W. H., and Hardwick, J. M. (2000). Antiapoptotic herpesvirus bcl-2 homologs escape caspase-mediated conversion to proapoptotic proteins. *J. Virol.*, **74**(11), 5024–5031.

Benedict, C. A., Norris, P. S., and Ware, C. F. (2002). To kill or be killed: viral evasion of apoptosis. *Nat. Immunol.*, **3**(11), 1013–1018.

Bieleski, L., Hindley, C., and Talbot, S. J. (2004). A polypyrimidine tract facilitates the expression of Kaposi's sarcoma-associated herpesvirus vFLIP through an internal ribosome entry site. *J. Gen. Virol.*, **85**(3), 615–620.

Bieleski, L. and Talbot, S. J. (2001). Kaposi's sarcoma-associated herpesvirus vCyclin open reading frame contains an internal ribosome entry site. *J. Virol.*, **75**(4), 1864–1869.

Borah, S., Verma, S. C., and Robertson, E. S. (2004). ORF73 of Herpesvirus saimiri, a viral homolog of Kaposi's sarcoma-associated herpesvirus, modulates the two cellular tumor suppressor proteins p53 and pRb. *J. Virol.*, **78**(19), 10336–10347.

Boshoff, C., Endo, Y., Collins, P. D. et al. (1997). Angiogenic and HIV inhibitory functions of KSHV-encoded chemokines. *Science*, **278**, 290–294.

Braithwaite, A. W. and Russell, I. A. (2001). Induction of cell death by adenoviruses. *Apoptosis*, **6**(5), 359–370.

Burger, R., Neipel, F., Fleckenstein, B. et al. (1998). Human herpesvirus type 8 interleukin-6 homologue is functionally active on human myeloma cells. *Blood*, **91**(6), 1858–1863.

Cai, X. and Cullen, B. R. (2006). Transcriptional origin of Kaposi's sarcoma-associated herpesvirus microRNAs, *J. Virol.*, **80**(5), 2234–2242.

Cai, X., Lu, S., Zhang, Z., Gonzalez, C. M., Damania, B., and Cullen, B. R. (2005). Kaposi's sarcoma-associated herpesvirus expresses an array of viral microRNAs in latently infected cells, *Proc. Natl. Acad. Sci. USA*, **102**(15), 5570–5575.

Cannon, M., Philpott, N. J., and Cesarman, E. (2003). The Kaposi's sarcoma-associated herpesvirus G protein-coupled receptor has broad signaling effects in primary effusion lymphoma cells. *J. Virol.*, **77**(1), 57–67.

Cesarman, E., Nador, R. G., Bai, F. et al. (1996). Kaposi's sarcoma-associated herpesvirus contains G protein-coupled receptor and cyclin D homologs which are expressed in Kaposi's sarcoma and malignant lymphoma. *J. Virol.*, **70**(11), 8218–8223.

Cesarman, E., Mesri, E. A., and Gershengorn, M. C. (2000). Viral G protein-coupled receptor and Kaposi's sarcoma: a model of paracrine neoplasia? [comment]. *J. Exp. Med.*, **191**(3), 417–422.

Chang, Y., Moore, P. S., Talbot, S. J. et al. (1996). Cyclin encoded by KS herpesvirus. *Nature*, **382**, 410.

Chatterjee, M., Osborne, J., Bestetti, G., Chang, Y., and Moore, P. S. (2002). Viral IL-6-induced cell proliferation and immune evasion of interferon activity. *Science*, **298**(5597), 1432–1435.

Chaudhary, P. M., Jasmin, A., Eby, M. T., and Hood, L. (1999). Modulation of the NF-kappa B pathway by virally encoded death effector domains-containing proteins. *Oncogene*, **18**(42), 5738–5746.

Cheng, E. H., Nicholas, J., Bellows, D. S. et al. (1997). A Bcl-2 homolog encoded by Kaposi sarcoma-associated virus, human herpesvirus 8, inhibits apoptosis but does not heterodimerize with Bax or Bak. *Proc. Natl Acad. Sci. USA*, **94**(2), 690–694.

Cheng, E. H., Wei, M. C., Weiler, S. et al. (2001). BCL-2, BCL-X(L) sequester BH3 domain-only molecules preventing BAX- and BAK-mediated mitochondrial apoptosis. *Mol. Cell*, **8**(3), 705–711.

Child, E. S. and Mann, D. J. (2001). Novel properties of the cyclin encoded by Human Herpesvirus 8 that facilitate exit from quiescence, *Oncogene*, **20**(26), 3311–3322.

Chiou, C. J., Poole, L. J., Kim, P. S. et al. (2002). Patterns of gene expression and a transactivation function exhibited by the vGCR (ORF74) chemokine receptor protein of Kaposi's sarcoma-associated herpesvirus. *J. Virol.*, **76**(7), 3421–3439.

Chow, D.-C., He, X.-L., Snow, A. L., Rose-John, S., and Garcia, K. C. (2001). Structure of an extracellular gp130 cytokine receptor signaling complex. *Science*, **291**(5511), 2150–2155.

Coscoy, L. and Ganem, D. (2000). Kaposi's sarcoma-associated herpesvirus encodes two proteins that block cell surface display of MHC class I chains by enhancing their endocytosis. *Proc. Natl Acad. Sci. USA*, **97**(14), 8051–8056.

Cuconati, A. and White, E. (2002). Viral homologs of BCL-2: role of apoptosis in the regulation of virus infection. *Genes Dev.*, **16**(19), 2465–2478.

Dairaghi, D. J., Fan, R. A., McMaster, B. E., Hanley, M. R., and Schall, T. J. (1999). HHV8-encoded vMIP-I selectively engages chemokine receptor CCR8. Agonist and antagonist profiles of viral chemokines. *J. Biol. Chem.*, **274**(31), 21569–21574.

Damania, B., Choi, J. K., and Jung, J. U. (2000). Signaling activities of gammaherpesvirus membrane proteins. *J. Virol.*, **74**(4), 1593–1601.

Danial, N. N. and Korsmeyer, S. J. (2004). Cell death: critical control points, *Cell*, **116**(2), 205–219.

de Stanchina, E., McCurrach, M. E., Zindy, F. et al. (1998). E1A signaling to p53 involves the p19(ARF) tumor suppressor, *Genes Dev.*, **12**(15), 2434–2442.

Debbas, M. and White, E. (1993). Wild-type p53 mediates apoptosis by E1A, which is inhibited by E1B. *Genes Dev.*, **7**, 546–554.

Djerbi, M., Screpanti, V., Catrina, A. I., Bogen, B., Biberfeld, P., and Grandien, A. (1999). The inhibitor of death receptor signaling, FLICE-inhibitory protein defines a new class of tumor progression factors, *J. Exp. Med.*, **190**(7), 1025–1032.

Ellis, M., Chew, Y. P., Fallis, L. et al. (1999). Degradation of p27(Kip) cdk inhibitor triggered by Kaposi's sarcoma virus cyclin-cdk6 complex, *EMBO J.*, **18**(3), 644–653.

Endres, M. J., Garlisi, C. G., Xiao, H., Shan, L., and Hedrick, J. A. (1999). The Kaposi's sarcoma-related herpesvirus (KSHV)-encoded chemokine vMIP- I is a specific agonist for the CC chemokine receptor (CCR)8. *J. Exp. Med.*, **189**(12), 1993–1998.

Feng, P., Park, J., Lee, B. S., Lee, S. H., Bram, R. J., and Jung, J. U. (2002). Kaposi's sarcoma-associated herpesvirus mitochondrial K7 protein targets a cellular calcium-modulating cyclophilin ligand to modulate intracellular calcium concentration and inhibit apoptosis. *J. Virol.*, **76**(22), 11491–11504.

Feng, P., Scott, C. W., Cho, N. H. *et al.* (2004). Kaposi's sarcoma-associated herpesvirus K7 protein targets a ubiquitin-like/ubiquitin-associated domain-containing protein to promote protein degradation. *Mol. Cell. Biol.*, **24**(9), 3938–3948.

Field, N., Low, W., Daniels, M. *et al.* (2003). KSHV vFLIP binds to IKK-gamma to activate IKK, *J. Cell. Sci.*, **116**(18), 3721–3728.

Fraser, A. and James, C. (1998). Fermenting debate: do yeast undergo apoptosis? *Trends Cell. Biol.*, **8**(6), 219–221.

Friborg, J., Jr., Kong, W., Hottiger, M. O., and Nabel, G. J. (1999). p53 inhibition by the LANA protein of KSHV protects against cell death. *Nature*, **402**(6764), 889–894.

Fujimuro, M. and Hayward, S. D. (2003). The latency-associated nuclear antigen of Kaposi's sarcoma-associated herpesvirus manipulates the activity of glycogen synthase kinase-3beta. *J. Virol.*, **77**(14), 8019–8030.

Fujimuro, M., Wu, F. Y., ApRhys, C. *et al.* (2003). A novel viral mechanism for dysregulation of beta-catenin in Kaposi's sarcoma-associated herpesvirus latency. *Nat. Med.*, **9**(3), 300–306.

Gao, S.-J., Boshoff, C., Jayachandra, S., Weiss, R. A., Chang, Y., and Moore, P. S. (1997). KSHV ORF K9 (vIRF) is an oncogene that inhibits the interferon signaling pathway. *Oncogene*, **15**, 1979–1986.

Glaunsinger, B. and Ganem, D. (2004). Lytic KSHV infection inhibits host gene expression by accelerating global mRNA turnover. *Mol. Cell.*, **13**(5), 713–723.

Godden-Kent, D., Talbot, S. J., Boshoff, C. *et al.* (1997). The cyclin encoded by Kaposi's sarcoma-associated herpesvirus stimulates cdk6 to phosphorylate the retinoblastoma protein and histone H1. *J. Virol.*, **71**(6), 4193–4198.

Gorospe, M., Cirielli, C., Wang, X., Seth, P., Capogrossi, M. C., and Holbrook, N. J. (1997). p21(Waf1/Cip1) protects against p53-mediated apoptosis of human melanoma cells. *Oncogene*, **14**(8), 929–935.

Gruffat, H., Portes-Sentis, S., Sergeant, A., and Manet, E. (1999). Kaposi's sarcoma-associated herpesvirus (human herpesvirus-8) encodes a homologue of the Epstein–Barr virus bZip protein EB1. *J. Gen. Virol.*, **80**(3), 557–561.

Grundhoff, A. and Ganem, D. (2001). Mechanisms governing expression of the v-FLIP gene of Kaposi's sarcoma-associated herpesvirus. *J. Virol.*, **75**(4), 1857–1863.

Guasparri, I., Keller, S. A., and Cesarman, E. (2004). KSHV vFLIP is essential for the survival of infected lymphoma cells. *J. Exp. Med.*, **199**(7), 993–1003.

Guo, H. G., Sadowska, M., Reid, W., Tschachler, E., Hayward, G., and Reitz, M. (2003). Kaposi's sarcoma-like tumors in a human herpesvirus 8 ORF74 transgenic mouse. *J. Virol.*, **77**(4), 2631–2639.

Gwack, Y., Byun, H., Hwang, S., Lim, C., and Choe, J. (2001a). CREB-binding protein and histone deacetylase regulate the transcriptional activity of Kaposi's sarcoma-associated herpesvirus open reading frame 50. *J. Virol.*, **75**(4), 1909–1917.

Gwack, Y., Hwang, S., Byun, H. *et al.* (2001b). Kaposi's sarcoma-associated herpesvirus open reading frame 50 represses p53-induced transcriptional activity and apoptosis. *J. Virol.*, **75**(13), 6245–6248.

Hayward, S. D., Liu, J., and Fujimuro, M. (2006). Notch and Wnt signaling: mimicry and manipulation by gamma herpesviruses, *Sci. STKE*, **2006**(335), re4.

Hobeika, A. C., Subramaniam, P. S., and Johnson, H. M. (1997). IFNα induces the expression of the cyclin-dependent kinase inhibitor p21 in human prostate cancer cells. *Oncogene*, **14**(10), 1165–1170.

Holst, P. J., Rosenkilde, M. M., Manfra, D. *et al.* (2001). Tumorigenesis induced by the HHV8-encoded chemokine receptor requires ligand modulation of high constitutive activity. *J. Clin. Invest.*, **108**(12), 1789–1796.

Huang, Q., Petros, A. M., Virgin, H. W., Fesik, S. W., and Olejniczak, E. T. (2002). Solution structure of a Bcl-2 homolog from Kaposi sarcoma virus. *Proc. Natl Acad. Sci. USA*, **99**(6), 3428–3433.

Hwang, S., Gwack, Y., Byun, H., Lim, C., and Choe, J. (2001). The Kaposi's sarcoma-associated herpesvirus K8 protein interacts with CREB-binding protein (CBP) and represses CBP-mediated transcription. *J. Virol.*, **75**(19), 9509–9516.

Izumiya, Y., Lin, S. F., Ellison, T. J. *et al.* (2003). Cell cycle regulation by Kaposi's sarcoma-associated herpesvirus K-bZIP: direct interaction with cyclin-CDK2 and induction of G1 growth arrest. *J. Virol.*, **77**(17), 9652–9661.

Jeffrey, P. D., Tong, L., and Pavletich, N. P. (2000). Structural basis of inhibition of CDK–cyclin complexes by INK4 inhibitors. *Genes Dev.*, **14**(24), 3115–3125.

Jeong, J. H., Orvis, J., Kim, J. W., McMurtrey, C. P., Renne, R., and Dittmer, D. P. (2004). Regulation and autoregulation of the promoter for the latency-associated nuclear antigen of Kaposi's Sarcoma-associated herpesvirus. *J. Biol. chem.*, **279**, 16822–16831.

Jones, K. D., Aoki, Y., Chang, Y., Moore, P. S., Yarchoan, R., and Tosato, G. (1999). Involvement of interleukin-10 (IL-10) and viral IL-6 in the spontaneous growth of Kaposi's sarcoma herpesvirus-associated infected primary effusion lymphoma cells. *Blood*, **94**(8), 2871–2879.

Judde, J. G., Lacoste, V., Briere, J. *et al.* (2000). Monoclonality or oligoclonality of human herpesvirus 8 terminal repeat sequences in Kaposi's sarcoma and other diseases. *J. Natl Cancer Inst.*, **92**(9), 729–736.

Kaldis, P., Ojala, P. M., Tong, L., Makela, T. P., and Solomon, M. J. (2001). CAK-independent activation of CDK6 by a viral cyclin, *Mol. Biol. Cell*, **12**(12), 3987–3999.

Katano, H., Ogawa-Goto, K., Hasegawa, H., Kurata, T., and Sata, T. (2001a). Human-herpesvirus-8-encoded K8 protein colocalizes with the promyelocytic leukemia protein (PML) bodies and recruits p53 to the PML bodies. *Virology*, **286**(2), 446–455.

Katano, H., Sato, Y., and Sata, T. (2001b). Expression of p53 and human herpesvirus-8 (HHV-8)-encoded latency-associated nuclear antigen with inhibition of apoptosis in HHV-8-associated malignancies. *Cancer*, **92**(12), 3076–3084.

Keller, S. A., Schattner, E. J., and Cesarman, E. (2000). Inhibition of NF-kappa B induces apoptosis of KSHV-infected primary effusion lymphoma cells. *Blood*, **96**(7), 2537–2542.

Kirshner, J. R., Staskus, K., Haase, A., Lagunoff, M., and Ganem, D. (1999). Expression of the open reading frame 74 (G-protein-coupled receptor) gene of Kaposi's sarcoma (KS)-associated herpesvirus: implications for KS pathogenesis. *J. Virol.*, **73**(7), 6006–6014.

Klotzbucher, A., Stewart, E., Harrison, D., and Hunt, T. (1996). The 'destruction box' of cyclin A allows B-type cyclins to be ubiquitinated, but not efficiently destroyed. *EMBO J.*, **15**(12), 3053–3064.

Kozar, K., Ciemerych, M. A., Rebel, V. I. *et al.* (2004). Mouse development and cell proliferation in the absence of D-cyclins. *Cell*, **118**(4), 477–491.

Krishnan, H. H., Naranatt, P. P., Smith, M. S., Zeng, L., Bloomer, C., and Chandran, B. (2004). Concurrent expression of latent and a limited number of lytic genes with immune modulation and antiapoptotic function by Kaposi's sarcoma-associated herpesvirus early during infection of primary endothelial and fibroblast cells and subsequent decline of lytic gene expression. *J. Virol.*, **78**(7), 3601–3620.

Krueger, A., Baumann, S., Krammer, P. H., and Kirchhoff, S. (2001). FLICE-inhibitory proteins: Regulators of death receptor-mediated apoptosis. *Mol. Biol. Cell*, **21**(24), 8247–8254.

Lagunoff, M. and Carroll, P. A. (2003). Inhibition of apoptosis by the gamma-herpesviruses. *Int. Rev. Immunol.*, **22**(5–6), 373–399.

Lagunoff, M., Majeti, R., Weiss, A., and Ganem, D. (1999). Deregulated signal transduction by the K1 gene product of Kaposi's sarcoma-associated herpesvirus. *Proc. Natl Acad. Sci. USA*, **96**(10), 5704–5709.

Lagunoff, M., Lukac, D. M., and Ganem, D. (2001). Immunoreceptor tyrosine-based activation motif-dependent signaling by Kaposi's sarcoma-associated herpesvirus K1 protein: effects on lytic viral replication. *J. Virol.*, **75**(13), 5891–5898.

Laman, H., Coverley, D., Krude, T., Laskey, R., and Jones, N. (2001). Viral cyclin-cyclin-dependent kinase 6 complexes initiate nuclear DNA replication. *Mol. Cell Biol.*, **21**(2), 624–635.

Lan, K., Choudhuri, T., Murakami, M., Kuppers, D. A., and Robertson, E. S. (2006). Intracellular activated Notch1 is critical for proliferation of Kaposi's sarcoma-associated herpesvirus-associated B-lymphoma cell lines in vitro. *J. Virol.*, **80**(13), 6411–6419.

Lane, D. P. (1992). p53, guardian of the genome. *Nature*, **358**(6381), 15–16.

Lee, B. S., Alvarez, X., Ishido, S., Lackner, A. A., and Jung, J. U. (2000). Inhibition of intracellular transport of B cell antigen receptor complexes by Kaposi's sarcoma-associated herpesvirus K1. *J. Exp. Med.*, **192**(1), 11–21.

Lee, B. S., Connole, M., Tang, Z., Harris, N. L., and Jung, J. U. (2003). Structural analysis of the Kaposi's sarcoma-associated herpesvirus K1 protein. *J. Virol.*, **77**(14), 8072–8086.

Lee, H., Guo, J., Li, M. *et al.* (1998a). Identification of an immunoreceptor tyrosine-based activation motif of K1 transforming protein of Kaposi's sarcoma-associated herpesvirus. *Mol. Cell. Biol.*, **18**(9), 5219–5228.

Lee, H., Veazey, R., Williams, K. *et al.* (1998b). Deregulation of cell growth by the K1 gene of Kaposi's sarcoma-associated herpesvirus. *Nat. Med.*, **4**(4), 435–440.

Lee, J. H. and Paull, T. T. (2004). Direct activation of the ATM protein kinase by the Mre11/Rad50/Nbs1 complex. *Science*, **304**.(5667), 93–96.

Li, M., Lee, H., Yoon, D. W. *et al.* (1997). Kaposi's sarcoma-associated herpesvirus encodes a functional cyclin. *J. Virol.*, **71**(3), 1984–1991.

Li, M., Damania, B., Alvarez, X., Ogryzko, V., Ozato, K., and Jung, J. U. (2000). Inhibition of p300 histone acetyltransferase by viral interferon regulatory factor. *Mol. Cell. Biol.*, **20**(21), 8254–8263.

Liang, C., Feng, P., Ku, B., Dotan, I., Canaani, D., Oh, B. H., and Jung, J. U. (2006). Autophagic and tumour suppressor activity of a novel Beclin1-binding protein UVRAG, *Nat. Cell. Biol.*, **8**(7), 688–699.

Lin, S. F., Robinson, D. R., Miller, G., and Kung, H. J. (1999). Kaposi's sarcoma-associated herpesvirus encodes a bZIP protein with homology to BZLF1 of Epstein–Barr virus. *J. Virol.*, **73**(3), 1909–1917.

Lin, R., Genin, P., Mamane, Y. *et al.* (2001). HHV-8 encoded vIRF-1 represses the interferon antiviral response by blocking IRF-3 recruitment of the CBP/p300 coactivators. *Oncogene*, **20**(7), 800–811.

Liu, L., Eby, M. T., Rathore, N., Sinha, S. K., Kumar, A., and Chaudhary, P. M. (2002). The human herpes virus 8-encoded viral FLICE inhibitory protein physically associates with and persistently activates the Ikappa B kinase complex. *J. Biol. Chem.*, **277**(16), 13745–13751.

Low, W., Harries, M., Ye, H., Du, M. Q., Boshoff, C., and Collins, M. (2001). Internal ribosome entry site regulates translation of Kaposi's sarcoma-associated herpesvirus FLICE inhibitory protein. *J. Virol.*, **75**(6), 2938–2945.

Lubyova, B., Kellum, M. J., Frisancho, A. J., and Pitha, P. M. (2004). Kaposi's sarcoma-associated herpesvirus-encoded vIRF-3 stimulates the transcriptional activity of cellular IRF-3 and IRF-7, *J. Biol. Chem.*, **279**(9), pp. 7643–7654.

Mann, D. J., Child, E. S., Swanton, C., Laman, H., and Jones, N. (1999). Modulation of p27(Kip1) levels by the cyclin encoded by Kaposi's sarcoma-associated herpesvirus. *EMBO J.*, **18**(3), 654–663.

Martin, D. F., Kuppermann, B. D., Wolitz, R. A., Palestine, A. G., Li, H., and Robinson, C. A. (1999). Oral ganciclovir for patients with cytomegalovirus retinitis treated with a ganciclovir implant. *N. Engl. J. Med.*, **340**(14), 1063–1070.

Masood, R., Cesarman, E., Smith, D. L., Gill, P. S., and Flore, O. (2002). Human herpesvirus-8-transformed endothelial cells have functionally activated vascular endothelial growth factor/vascular endothelial growth factor receptor. *Am. J. Pathol.*, **160**(1), 23–29.

Matta, H. and Chaudhary, P. M. (2004). Activation of alternative NF-kappa B pathway by human herpes virus 8-encoded Fas-associated death domain-like IL-1 beta-converting enzyme inhibitory protein (vFLIP). *Proc. Natl Acad. Sci. USA*, **101**(25), 9399–9404.

Meinl, E., Fickenscher, H., Thome, M., Tschopp, J., and Fleckenstein, B. (1998). Anti-apoptotic strategies of lymphotropic viruses. *Immunol. Today*, **19**(10), 474–479.

Mittnacht, S. and Boshoff, C. (2000). Viral cyclins. *Rev. Med. Virol.*, **10**(3), 175–184.

Molden, J., Chang, Y., You, Y., Moore, P. S., and Goldsmith, M. A. (1997). A Kaposi's sarcoma-associated herpesvirus-encoded cytokine homolog (vIL-6) activates signaling through the shared gp130 receptor subunit, *J. Biol. Chem.*, **272**(31), 19625–19631.

Montaner, S., Sodhi, A., Pece, S., Mesri, E. A., and Gutkind, J. S. (2001). The Kaposi's sarcoma-associated herpesvirus G protein-coupled receptor promotes endothelial cell survival through the activation of Akt/protein kinase B. *Cancer Res.*, **61**(6), 2641–2648.

Montaner, S., Sodhi, A., Molinolo, A. *et al.* (2003). Endothelial infection with KSHV genes in vivo reveals that vGPCR initiates Kaposi's sarcomagenesis and can promote the tumorigenic potential of viral latent genes. *Cancer Cell*, **3**(1), 23–36.

Moore, P. S. (2003). Transplanting cancer: donor-cell transmission of Kaposi sarcoma. *Nat. Med.*, **9**(5), 506–508.

Moore, P. S. and Chang, Y. (1998). Antiviral activity of tumor-suppressor pathways: clues from molecular piracy by KSHV. *Trends Genet.*, **14**(4), 144–150.

Moore, P. S. and Chang, Y. (2001). Molecular virology of Kaposi's sarcoma-associated herpesvirus. *Phil. Trans. R. Soc. Lond. B Biol. Sci.*, **356**(1408), 499–516.

Moore, P. S. and Chang, Y. (2003). Kaposi's sarcoma-associated herpesvirus immunoevasion and tumorigenesis: two sides of the same coin? *Annu. Rev. Microbiol.*, **57**, 609–639.

Moore, P. S., Boshoff, C., Weiss, R. A., and Chang, Y. (1996). Molecular mimicry of human cytokine and cytokine response pathway genes by KSHV. *Science*, **274**(5293), 1739–1744.

Mullberg, J., Geib, T., Jostock, T. *et al.* (2000). IL-6 receptor independent stimulation of human gp130 by viral IL-6. *J. Immunol.*, **164**(9), 4672–4677.

Murray, A. W. (2004). Recycling the cell cycle: cyclins revisited, *Cell*, **116**(2), 221–234.

Nakamura, H., Li, M., Zarycki, J., and Jung, J. U. (2001). Inhibition of p53 tumor suppressor by viral interferon regulatory factor. *J. Virol.*, **75**(16), 7572–7582.

Nicholas, J., Ruvolo, V. R., Burns, W. H. *et al.* (1997). Kaposi's sarcoma-associated human herpesvirus-8 encodes homologues of macrophage inflammatory protein-1 and interleukin-6. *Nat. Med.*, **3**(3), 287–292.

Oda, E., Ohki, R., Murasawa, H. (2000). Noxa, a BH3-only member of the Bcl-2 family and candidate mediator of p53-induced apoptosis. *Science*, **288**(5468), 1053–1058.

Ojala, P. M., Yamamoto, K., Castanos-Velez, E., Biberfeld, P., Korsmeyer, S. J., and Makela, T. P. (2000). The apoptotic v-cyclin-CDK6 complex phosphorylates and inactivates Bcl-2. *Nat. Cell. Biol.*, **2**(11), 819–825.

Osborne, J., Moore, P. S., and Chang, Y. (1999). KSHV-encoded viral IL-6 activates multiple human IL-6 signaling pathways. *Hum. Immunol.*, **60**(10), 921–927.

Park, J., Seo, T., Hwang, S., Lee, D., Gwack, Y., and Choe, J. (2000). The K-bZIP protein from Kaposi's sarcoma-associated herpesvirus interacts with p53 and represses its transcriptional activity. *J. Virol.*, **74**(24), 11977–11982.

Parravicini, C., Corbellino, M. Paulli, M. *et al.* (1997). Expression of a virus-derived cytokine, KSHV vIL-6, in HIV-seronegative Castleman's disease. *Am. J. Pathol.*, **151**(6), 1517–1522.

Parravicini, C., Chandran, B., Corbellino, M. *et al.* (2000). Differential viral protein expression in Kaposi's sarcoma-associated herpesvirus-infected diseases: Kaposi's sarcoma, primary effusion lymphoma, and multicentric Castleman's disease. *Am. J. Pathol.*, **156**(3), 743–749.

Polson, A. G., Huang, L., Lukac, D. M. *et al.* (2001). Kaposi's sarcoma-associated herpesvirus K-bZIP protein is phosphorylated by cyclin-dependent kinases. *J. Virol.*, **75**(7), 3175–3140.

Polson, A. G., Wang, D., DeRisi, J., and Ganem, D. (2002). Modulation of host gene expression by the constitutively active G protein-coupled receptor of Kaposi's sarcoma-associated herpesvirus. *Cancer Res.*, **62**(15), 4525–4530.

Radkov, S. A., Kellam, P., and Boshoff, C. (2000). The latent nuclear antigen of Kaposi sarcoma-associated herpesvirus targets the retinoblastoma-E2F pathway and with the oncogene hras transforms primary rat cells. *Nat. Med.*, **6**(10), 1121–1127.

Rivas, C., Thlick, A. E., Parravicini, C., Moore, P. S., and Chang, Y. (2001). Kaposi's sarcoma-associated herpesvirus LANA2 is a B-cell-specific latent viral protein that inhibits p53. *J. Virol.*, **75**(1), 429–438.

Russell, I. A., Royds, J. A., and Braithwaite, A. W. (2004). Exploitation of cell cycle and cell death controls by adenoviruses: the road to a productive infection. *Prog. Mol. Subcell Biol.*, **36**, 207–243.

Russo, J. J., Bohenzky, R. A., Chien, M. C. *et al.* (1996). Nucleotide sequence of the Kaposi sarcoma-associated herpesvirus (HHV8). *Proc. Natl Acad. Sci. USA*, **93**(25), 14862–14867.

Sangfelt, O., Erickson, S., Einhorn, S., and Grander, D. (1997). Induction of Cip/Kip and Ink4 cyclin dependent kinase inhibitors by interferon-alpha in hematopoietic cell lines. *Oncogene*, **14**(4), 415–423.

Sarid, R., Sato, T., Bohenzky, R. A., Russo, J. J., and Chang, Y. (1997). Kaposi's sarcoma-associated herpesvirus encodes a functional bcl-2 homologue. *Nat. Med.*, **3**(3), 293–298.

Sarid, R., Wiezorek, J. S., Moore, P. S., and Chang, Y. (1999). Characterization and cell cycle regulation of the major Kaposi's sarcoma-associated herpesvirus (human herpesvirus 8) latent genes and their promoter. *J. Virol.*, **73**(2), 1438–1446.

Schuler, M. and Green, D. R. (2001). Mechanisms of p53-dependent apoptosis. *Biochem. Soc. Trans.*, **29**(6), 684–688.

Seaman, W. T., Ye, D., Wang, R. X., Hale, E. E., Weisse, M., and Quinlivan, E. B. (1999). Gene expression from the ORF50/K8 region of Kaposi's sarcoma-associated herpesvirus. *Virology*, **263**(2), 436–449.

Schmid, D., Dengjel, J., Schoor, O., Stevanovic, S., and Munz, C. (2006). Autophagy in innate and adaptive immunity against intracellular pathogens, *J. Mol. Med.*, **84**(3), 194–202.

Seo, T., Park, J., Lim, C., and Choe, J. (2004). Inhibition of nuclear factor kappa B activity by viral interferon regulatory factor 3 of Kaposi's sarcoma-associated herpesvirus, *Oncogene*, **23**(36), pp. 6146–6155.

Sheard, M. A., Uldrijan, S., and Vojtesek, B. (2003). Role of p53 in regulating constitutive and X-radiation-inducible CD95 expression and function in carcinoma cells. *Cancer Res.*, **63**(21), 7176–7184.

Sherr, C. J. (1998). Tumor surveillance via the ARF-p53 pathway. *Genes Dev.*, **12**(19), 2984–2991.

Sherr, C. J. (2004). Principles of tumor suppression. *Cell*, **116**(2), 235–246.

Shin, Y. C., Nakamura, H., Liang, X., Feng, P., Chang, H., Kowalik, T. F., and Jung, J. U. (2006). Inhibition of the ATM/p53 signal transduction pathway by Kaposi's sarcoma-associated herpesvirus interferon regulatory factor 1, *J. Virol.*, **80**(5), 2257–2266.

Stine, J. T., Wood, C., Hill, M. *et al.* (2000). KSHV-encoded CC chemokine vMIP-III is a CCR4 agonist, stimulates angiogenesis, and selectively chemoattracts TH2 cells. *Blood*, **95**(4), 1151–1157.

Sun, R., Lin, S. F., Staskus, K. *et al.* (1999). Kinetics of Kaposi's sarcoma-associated herpesvirus gene expression. *J. Virol.*, **73**(3), 2232–2242.

Swanton, C., Mann, D. J., Fleckenstein, B., Neipel, F., Peters, G., and Jones, N. (1997). Herpes viral cyclin/Cdk6 complexes evade inhibition by CDK inhibitor proteins. *Nature*, **390**(6656), 184–187.

Swanton, C., Card, G. L., Mann, D., McDonald, N., and Jones, N. (1999). Overcoming inhibitions: subversion of CKI function by viral cyclins. *Trends Biochem. Sci.*, **24**(3), 116–120.

Takaoka, A., Hayakawa, S., Yanai, H. *et al.* (2003). Integration of interferon-alpha/beta signalling to p53 responses in tumour suppression and antiviral defence. *Nature*, **424**(6948), 516–523.

Teodoro, J. G. and Branton, P. E. (1997). Regulation of apoptosis by viral gene products. *J. Virol.*, **71**, 1739–1746.

Tomescu, C., Law, W. K., and Kedes, D. H. (2003). Surface downregulation of major histocompatibility complex class I, PE-CAM, and ICAM-1 following de novo infection of endothelial cells with Kaposi's sarcoma-associated herpesvirus. *J. Virol.*, **77**(17), 9669–9684.

Tomita, M., Choe, J., Tsukazaki, T., and Mori, N. (2004). The Kaposi's Sarcoma-associated herpesvirus K-bZIP protein represses transforming growth factor beta signaling through interaction with CREB-binding protein. *Oncogene*, **23**, 8272-8281.

Tomlinson, C. C. and Damania, B. (2004). The K1 protein of Kaposi's sarcoma-associated herpesvirus activates the Akt signaling pathway. *J. Virol.*, **78**(4), 1918–1927.

Urashima, M., Ogata, A., Chauhan, D. *et al.* (1996). Interleukin-6 promotes multiple myeloma cell growth via phosphorylation of retinoblastoma protein. *Blood*, **88**(6), 2219–2227.

Urashima, M., Teoh, G., Chauhan, D. *et al.* (1997). Interleukin-6 overcomes p21WAF1 upregulation and G1 growth arrest induced by dexamethasone and interferon-gamma in multiple myeloma cells. *Blood*, **90**(1), 279–289.

Van Dross, R., Yao, S., Asad, S., Westlake, G., Mays, D. J., Barquero, L., Duell, S., Pietenpol, J. A., and Browning, P. J. (2005). Constitutively active K-cyclin/cdk6 kinase in Kaposi sarcoma-associated herpesvirus-infected cells, *J. Natl. Cancer Inst.*, **97**(9), 656–666.

Verma, S. C., Borah, S., and Robertson, E. S. (2004). Latency-associated nuclear antigen of kaposi's sarcoma-associated herpesvirus up-regulates transcription of human telomerase reverse transcriptase promoter through interaction with transcription factor Sp1. *J. Virol.*, **78**(19), 10348–10359.

Verschuren, E. W., Hodgson, J. G., Gray, J. W., Kogan, S., Jones, N., and Evan, G. I. (2004a). The role of p53 in suppression of KSHV cyclin-induced lymphomagenesis. *Cancer Res.*, **64**(2), 581–589.

Verschuren, E. W., Jones, N., and Evan, G. I. (2004b). The cell cycle and how it is steered by Kaposi's sarcoma-associated herpesvirus cyclin. *J. Gen. Virol.*, **85**(6), 1347–1361.

Verschuren, E. W., Klefstrom, J., Evan, G. I., and Jones, N. (2002). The oncogenic potential of Kaposi's sarcoma-associated herpesvirus cyclin is exposed by p53 loss in vitro and in vivo. *Cancer Cell*, **2**(3), 229–241.

Wang, L., Dittmer, D. P., Tomlinson, C. C., Fakhari, F. D., and Damania, B. (2006). Immortalization of primary endothelial cells by the K1 protein of Kaposi's sarcoma-associated herpesvirus, *Cancer Res.*, **66**(7), 3658–3666.

Wang, H. W., Sharp, T. V., Koumi, A., Koentges, G., and Boshoff, C. (2002). Characterization of an anti-apoptotic glycoprotein encoded by Kaposi's sarcoma-associated herpesvirus which resembles a spliced variant of human survivin. *EMBO J.*, **21**(11), 2602–2615.

Wang, L., Wakisaka, N., Tomlinson, C. C. *et al.* (2004). The Kaposi's sarcoma-associated herpesvirus (KSHV/HHV-8) K1 protein induces expression of angiogenic and invasion factors. *Cancer Res.*, **64**(8), 2774–2781.

Wang, S. E., Wu, F. Y., Fujimuro, M., Zong, J., Hayward, S. D., and Hayward, G. S. (2003a). Role of CCAAT/enhancer-binding protein alpha (C/EBPalpha) in activation of the Kaposi's sarcoma-associated herpesvirus (KSHV) lytic-cycle replication-associated protein (RAP) promoter in cooperation with the KSHV replication and transcription activator (RTA) and RAP. *J. Virol.*, **77**(1), 600–623.

Wang, S. E., Wu, F. Y., Yu, Y., and Hayward, G. S. (2003b). CCAAT/enhancer-binding protein-alpha is induced during the early stages of Kaposi's sarcoma-associated herpesvirus (KSHV) lytic cycle reactivation and together with the KSHV replication and transcription activator (RTA) cooperatively stimulates the viral RTA, MTA, and PAN promoters, *J. Virol.*, **77**(17), 9590–9612.

Weitzman, M. D., Carson, C. T., Schwartz, R. A., and Lilley, C. E. (2004). Interactions of viruses with the cellular DNA repair machinery, DNA *Repair (Amst)*, **3**(8–9), 1165–1173.

Widmer, I., Wernli, M., Bachmann, F., Gudat, F., Cathomas, G., and Erb, P. (2002). Differential expression of viral Bcl-2 encoded by Kaposi's sarcoma-associated herpesvirus and human Bcl-2 in primary effusion lymphoma cells and Kaposi's sarcoma lesions. *J. Virol.*, **76**(5), 2551–2556.

Wood, R. D., Mitchell, M., Sgouros, J., and Lindahl, T. (2001). Human DNA repair genes. *Science*, **291**(5507), 1284–1289.

Wu, K. J., Grandori, C., Amacker, M. *et al.* (1999). Direct activation of TERT transcription by c-MYC. *Nat. Genet.*, **21**(2), 220–224.

Wu, F. Y., Wang, S. E., Tang, Q. Q. *et al.* (2003). Cell cycle arrest by Kaposi's sarcoma-associated herpesvirus replication-associated protein is mediated at both the transcriptional and posttranslational levels by binding to CCAAT/enhancer-binding protein alpha and p21(CIP-1). *J. Virol.*, **77**(16), 8893–8914.

Yang, B. T., Chen, S. C., Leach, M. W. *et al.* (2000). Transgenic expression of the chemokine receptor encoded by human herpesvirus 8 induces an angioproliferative disease resembling Kaposi's sarcoma. *J. Exp. Med.*, **191**(3), 445–454.

Yu, J., Zhang, L., Hwang, P. M., Kinzler, K. W., and Vogelstein, B. (2001). PUMA induces the rapid apoptosis of colorectal cancer cells. *Mol. Cell*, **7**(3), 673–682.

Zhu, Y. M., Bradbury, D. A., Keith, F. J., and Russell, N. (1994). Absence of retinoblastoma protein expression results in autocrine production of interleukin-6 and promotes the autonomous growth of acute myeloid leukemia blast cells. *Leukemia*, **8**(11), 1982–1988.

Zimring, J. C., Goodbourn, S., and Offermann, M. K. (1998). Human herpesvirus 8 encodes an interferon regulatory factor (IRF) homolog that represses IRF-1-mediated transcription. *J. Virol.*, **72**(1), 701–707.

Zindy, F., Eischen, C. M., Randle, D. H. *et al.* (1998). Myc signaling via the ARF tumor suppressor regulates p53-dependent apoptosis and immortalization. *Genes Dev.*, **12**(15), 2424–2433.

Human gammaherpesvirus immune evasion strategies

Robert E. Means[1], Sabine M. Lang[1] and Jae U. Jung[2]

[1]Department of Pathology, Yale University School of Medicine, New Haven, CT, USA and
[2]Division of Tumor Virology, New England Primate Research Center, Harvard Medical School, Southborough, MA, USA

Introduction

The human γ-HVs are able to establish a lifelong, persistent infection that is largely clinically inapparent within the immunocompetent host. However, when these viruses are not kept in check, a variety of lymphoproliferative and neoplastic disorders result that will be detailed elsewhere within this volume. In brief, for HHV-8, also known as Kaposi's sarcoma-associated herpesvirus (KSHV), these neoplasias include Kaposi's sarcoma (KS), multicentric Castleman's disease (MCD) and primary effusion lymphoma (PEL). HHV-4, or Epstein–Barr virus (EBV), has been etiologically associated with infectious mononucleosis, Burkitt's lymphoma, nasopharyngeal carcinoma (NPC), Hodgkin's disease, hemophagocytic lymphohistiocytosis syndrome and some gastric cancers. Through coevolution with their hosts, these viruses have acquired a number of genes that act to set a fine balance between the uncontrolled, virally driven cellular proliferation seen in the immunocompromised host and complete elimination of infected cells by the immune responses. Several of these gene products cause selective suppression of normal immune system functioning and allow for an apathogenic, persistent infection.

Immune system overview

The immune system provides multiple mechanisms of protection from invading pathogens, whether viral, bacterial or parasitic. These immune responses include both broad spectrum, innate responses and highly specific, adaptive responses. Mechanisms of the innate response include the production of viral replication blocking interferons, opsonization and lysis by the complement cascade and natural antibodies, apoptosis, as well as clearance of infection by natural killer (NK) cells, macrophages, neutrophils and T-cells. The adaptive response mechanisms include the CD4$^+$ T-helper cell directed production of specific, high avidity neutralizing antibodies by the B-cells and elimination of infected cells by antigen-specific cytotoxic T-lymphocytes (CTL). A complex network of protein–protein interactions, providing numerous targets for viral intervention and deregulation, governs all of these processes.

Evasion of innate host immunity

By definition, the innate immune responses are the host's first line of defense against viral infection. These defenses can be roughly broken down into complement-mediated responses (both antibody-dependent and -independent), cytokine responses, apoptotic responses and cell-mediated responses. These responses are broad, able to target multiple pathogens, but by no means non-specific. The innate immune response utilizes a large number of germ line-encoded receptors capable of sensing moieties that are common to many pathogens. Other members of the innate immune system, such as the natural killer (NK) cells, have evolved mechanisms for determining the "health" of a cell by examining the cell for changes in the repertoire of surface molecules. This complexity built in to the innate immune responses excludes the possibility of non-specific targeting of host cells, but also provides a number of regulatory checkpoints which invading pathogens can usurp. Both of the known human γ-HVs have devised a number of strategies for thwarting the efforts of the innate immune system to clear them from the body and for deregulating the cross-talk between the innate and adaptive responses.

Complement deregulation

The complement response is mediated by a series of heat-labile plasma proteins, each given a number designation, whose cleavage and activation from an inactive circulating zymogen is controlled by a host of regulatory proteins. It is initiated through one of three pathways: the classical, alternative or mannan-binding-lectin-associated serine protease (MASP) pathways (for review see Medzhitov and Janeway, 2000). Triggering of the complement response results in activation and cleavage of the first zymogen to its active form, which then in turn cleaves and activates the next zymogen in the cascade. After cleavage, the resulting zymogen products are given lettered subscripts. For example, the cleavage of the C4 zymogen by active C1 results in production of C4a and C4b products (Fig. 31.1). The complement system protects against infection by both bacteria and viruses in three different ways. First, several of the complement proteins, when activated, can covalently bind to pathogens in a process called opsonization. Complement receptor-bearing phagocytes can then internalize and clear the infecting organism. This opsonization also contributes to the activation of the adaptive, humoral response. Second, multiple complement protein cleavage products act as anaphylotoxins, recruiting and activating circulating phagocytes. Third, several activated complement proteins can form a large multimeric structure called the membrane attack complex (MAC). This protein complex is capable of creating a pore in lipid membranes resulting in the lysis of cells, enveloped virus or bacteria onto which it has been deposited. While each pathway is initiated by a different triggering event, they converge at the production of the multi-component C3 convertase and ultimately, each result to different degrees in opsonization, anaphylotoxin production and MAC formation. Regulation of the complement cascade is complex, involving proteins that mediate the degradation of complement components into inactive fragments, as well as other inhibitory proteins capable of irreversible binding to and inactivation of complement proteins. The γ-HVs have taken advantage of this complexity by encoding viral genes that interfere with this regulation which are outlined in Table 31.1.

KSHV encodes a homologue of the human complement control protein CD46 (Neipel et al., 1997a,b). Like its human homologue, the ORF4 gene product, termed KCP or Kaposica, contains four short consensus (SCR) or sushi domains. These domains are characteristic of the cellular regulators of complement activation (RCA) (Klickstein et al., 1987; Law, 1988). The SCR are typically 60–70 amino acids in length and contain four conserved cysteine residues, which are disulfide-linked. KCP/Kaposica is encoded from a 1650 nucleotide long open reading frame and work by Spiller et al. (2003) has demonstrated that it is expressed as three alternatively spliced constructs, an unspliced 550 residue form and two singly spliced forms of 425 residues and 347 residues (depicted in Fig. 31.2). All three forms retain the putative membrane-spanning region. The unspliced product (ORF4-F) has 14 N-X-S/T, consensus N-linked glycosylation sites. However, the NetNGlyc neural network N-linked glycosylation prediction program (http://www.cbs.dtu.dk/services/NetNGlyc) (Gupta et al. 2002), indicates that only 10 of these have a significant probability of being glycosylated. The other two forms, designated ORF4-M and ORF4-S, have five and four probable sites, respectively. Additionally, ORF4-F has potential for modification by O-linked glycosylation in a serine/threonine-rich region just upstream of the predicted transmembrane domain, while the other forms lack this region. Examination of the lysates of TPA-treated PEL cells showed three anti-ORF4 antibody reactive bands at 175 kD, 82 kD and 62 kD (Spiller et al., 2003). Examination of culture supernatants demonstrated the presence of only the two more slowly migrating forms. At this time, the contribution of glycosylation or additional post-translational modifications to the higher than predicted molecular weights of these products or differences in the functioning of each product has not been clarified. Since all of the proposed products maintain a trans-membrane domain, the mechanism of secretion also needs further investigation.

KCP/Kaposica strongly enhances the decay of the classical C3 convertase (C4b2a) but poorly promotes decay of the alternative pathway C3 convertase (C3bBbP) compared with the host complement control proteins (Mullick et al., 2003; Spiller et al., 2003). It acts as a co-factor to aid Factor I (fI), a major cellular complement control protein, in its degradation of both C4b and C3b (Fig. 31.1). Unlike cellular fI co-factors, however, KCP/Kaposica is able to drive production of the C3d complement protein as a final product of fI-mediated cleavage of iC3b (Spiller et al., 2003). Production of this molecule is usually driven by a cellular protease in a non-fI-dependent manner. In addition to accelerating decay of the C3 convertase, thus preventing the action of complement, this production of C3d by KCP/Kaposica probably plays an additional role in KSHV biology. The C3d molecule is capable of binding to complement receptor 2 (CR2, CD21), which complexes with CD19 and CD81, resulting in a dramatic increase in B cell responsiveness to B cell receptor stimulation (Dempsey et al., 1996). So, the actions of KCP/Kaposica likely have some effects on B cell production of antibodies in response to viral antigens. Whether this directly alters anti-viral responses or aids the

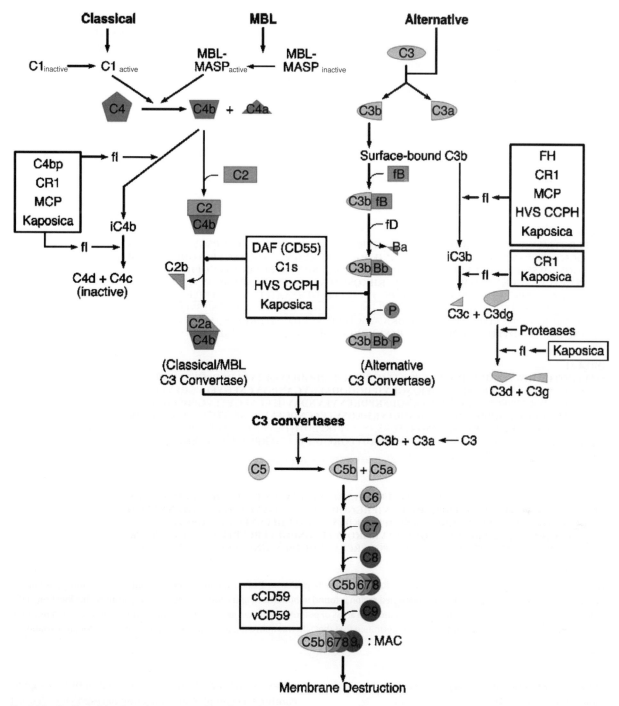

Fig. 31.1. Outline of the Complement cascade with interfering herpesvirus products noted. The complement cascade is a complex series of zymogens and regulating proteolytic enzymes. This high-level of complexity gives multiple opportunities for intervention by the herpesviruses. Additional details are given in the text.

Table 31.1. Viral complement regulators. Complement forms an important facet of the innate immune response. Not only does it play a role in direct defense, through lysis of infected cells or enveloped viruses, but it also helps to co-ordinate later adaptive responses. Both human γ-herpesviruses encode gene products with the potential to alter the complement response. The open reading frame, product and potential function are listed for each, with additional details in the text

	Gene	Product	Function
HHV-8	ORF4	KCP/Kaposica	Homologue of human CD46, accelerates the decay of the C3 convertases and drives production of C3d, which binds complement receptor 2 (CR2)
EBV	BLLF1a/b	gp350/220	Binds to CR2, might interfere with complement mediated B cell stimulation or aid in viral dissemination

ORF4-F
MAFLRQTLWILWTFTMVIGQDNEKCSQKTLIGYRLKMSRDGDIAVGETVELRCRSGYTTY ARNITA TCLQGGTWSEPTATCNKKSCPNPGEIQNGKVIFHGGQDALKYGANISYVCNEGYFLVGREYVRYCM IGASGQMAWSSSPPFCEKEKCHRPKIKNGDFKPDKDYYEYNDAVHFECNEGYTLVGPHSIACAVNNT WTSNMPTCELAGCKFPSVTHGYPIQGFSLTYKHKQSVTFACNDGFVLRGSPTITCNVTEWDPPLPKC VLEDIDDPNNSNPGRLHPTPNEKPNGNVFQRSNYTEPPTKPEDTHTAATCDTNCEQPPKILPTSEGFNETT TSNTITKQLEDEKTTSQPNTHITSALTSMKAKGNFTNKTNNSTDLHIASTPTSQDDATPSIPSVQTPNYNTNA PTRTLTSLHIEEGPSNSTTSEKATSSTLSHNSHKNDTGGIYTTLNKTTQLPSTNKPTNSQAKSSTKPRVETHN KTTSNPAISLTDSADVPQRPREPTLPPIFRPPASKNRYLEKQLVIGLLTAVALTCGLITLFHYLFFR

ORF4-M
MAFLRQTLWILWTFTMVIGQDNEKCSQKTLIGYRLKMSRDGDIAVGETVELRCRSGYTTYARNITA TCLQGGTWSEPTATCNKKSCPNPGEIQNGKVIFHGGQDALKYGANISYVCNEGYFLVGREYVRYCM IGASGQMAWSSSPPFCEKEKCHRPKVKNGDFKPDKDYYEYNDAVHFECNEGYTLVGPHSIACAVNN TWTSNMPTCELTGCKFPSVTHGYPIQGFSLTYKHKQSVTFACNDGFVLRGSPTITCNVTEWDPPLPK CVLEDIDDPNNSNPGRLHPTPNEKPNGNVFQRSNYTEPPTKPEDTHTAATCDTNCEQPPKILPTSEGFNET TTSNTITKQLEDEKTTSQPNTHITSALTSMKAKDSADVPQRPREPTLPPIFRPPASKNRYLEKQLVIGLLT AVALTCGLITLFHYLFFR

ORF4-S
MAFLRQTLWILWTFTMVIGQDNEKCSQKTLIGYRLKMSRDGDIAVGETVELRCRSGYTTYARNITA TCLQGGTWSEPTATCNKKSCPNPGEIQNGKVIFHGGQDALKYGANISYVCNEGYFLVGREYVRYCM IGASGQMAWSSSPPFCEKEKCHRPKVKNGDFKPDKDYYEYNDAVHFECNEGYTLVGPHSIACAVNN TWTSNMPTCELTGCKFPSVTHGYPIQGFSLTYKHKQSVTFACNDGFVLRGSPTITCNVTEWDPPLPK CVLEDIDDPNNSNPGRLHPTPNEKPNDSADVPQRPREPTLPPIFRPPASKNRYLEKQLVIGLLTAVALT CGLITLFHYLFFR

Fig. 31.2. Products of the Kaposica/KCP open reading frame. The Kaposica/KCP open reading frame has multiple splice forms. Regions in bold are shared by all three isoforms. The underlined region is found in both the M and F forms. Green residues indicate the location of the potential transmembrane domain. Blue residues indicate areas of potential N-linked glycosylation with the first residue colored red if the NetNGlyc neural network prediction program determined that that site was above the predicted probability threshold for glycosylation.

virus in recruiting additional target cells or possibly altering viral entry is still unclear.

While no EBV-encoded proteins to date have been shown to have a direct effect on complement regulation, EBV also targets CR2. The gp350/220 viral envelope protein is capable of binding to and mediating viral entry into CD21+ cells. The binding of gp350/220 to CR2, while not identical to C3d, probably overlaps the complement binding region (Moore *et al.*, 1991; Prota *et al.*, 2002). However, it is currently unclear if binding to this receptor by EBV significantly alters complement activation or responses. Again, it is possible that the virus utilizes this ability to aid in dissemination without effects on complement. It is clear, however, that binding of EBV or the gp350/220 glycoprotein to CR2 has effects on cytokine production and survival for several cell types and will be discussed in later sections.

A number of other viruses have been shown to incorporate host complement regulatory proteins into their envelopes including human cytomegalovirus and HIV (Saifuddin et al., 1994; Spiller et al., 1996). While no experimental evidence has yet been shown for a similar strategy employed by the human γ-HVs, this is a tantalizing possibility.

Cytokine responses

The cytokines are a large number of mostly soluble proteins, able to bind to a wide variety of cellular receptors expressed both on other immune effectors and non-immune related host cells. Through binding to their receptors they can induce proliferation, differentiation and activation both in the producer cell (autocrine effects) and in other targets (paracrine effects). Included in this large group of proteins are several super-families of proteins including the interleukins, interferons and chemokines. Generally, the interleukins (usually given an IL designation) are proteins that are produced by one leukocyte and act on another, however numerous examples exist that don't fall into this general definition. These proteins act to attract and activate a number of immune effector cells, activate the host acute-phase response and drive the differentiation of cells to result in a polarized immune response. The interferons (IFNs) are an evolutionarily conserved group of proteins that play a crucial role in the innate response to viruses. These proteins are able to mediate signaling through their receptors to induce the expression of a large number of cellular proteins that are able to alter cellular physiology to be less hospitable for viral replication. The chemokines interact with cellular 7-transmembrane, G-protein-coupled receptors (GPCRs) stimulating leukocyte trafficking and development, as well as regulating angiogenesis. Crucial to immune system functioning is their ability to recruit various effector cells to the site of inflammation. The spectrum of chemokines that are produced govern which cells respond to the site of inflammation and have a large influence in directing how the immune system reacts to invading pathogens. The signals that these cytokines transmit to the cells can stimulate the production of additional cytokines and chemokines, providing a complex cross-talk evolved to coordinate an effective immune response.

Two main subpopulations of CD4$^+$ T lymphocytes, termed T helper (Th)1 and Th2 cells, coordinate the type of immune response that is made to an infecting pathogen. Th1 cells predominantly secrete IFN-γ, GM-CSF and TNF-α, but also secrete TNF-β, IL-3 and IL-2. Additionally, they usually express CD40 ligand and/or CD95 ligand on their surface. These types of cells act to activate macrophages, direct B-cells to produce opsonizing antibodies and cause inflammatory cell infiltration of tissues. Thus, the Th1 cells select for cell-mediated immune responses against pathogens. Th2 cells secrete IL-4 and IL-5, but also IL-10, TGF-β, eotaxin and IL-3. They also express CD40 on their surface. These types of cells act to activate antigen-specific B-cells to produce neutralizing antibodies and thus direct the immune effectors toward a humoral response against the invading pathogen. Additionally, the cytokines released by Th2 cells tend to inhibit inflammation. These two populations of T-lymphocytes result from the differentiation of naïve CD4$^+$ T-cells in response to the cytokine milieu, cytokines which have been released from either infected cells or other immune effectors such as NK cells. Shifts in the dominance of Th1 or Th2 immune effectors can dramatically influence the type and importantly, the effectiveness of responses made against invading pathogens.

Interleukin and chemokine responses

KSHV expresses multiple chemokine homologues, homologues of the macrophage inflammatory proteins, vMIP-I, -II and –III, a homologue of the cellular IL-6 protein and a homologue of the cellular Ox2 protein, which is involved in the release of a number of different cytokines. A summary of these gene products is outlined in Table 31.2. The viral MIPs are able to bind to a variety of cellular chemokine receptors, acting as agonist and antagonists (Boshoff et al., 1997; Kledal et al., 1997; Sozzani et al., 1998; Dairaghi et al., 1999; Endres et al., 1999; Stine et al., 2000). The gene products of ORFs K6 and K4 of KSHV, vMIP-I (vCCL1) and v-MIP-II (vCCL2) respectively, share homology with the cellular CC chemokine macrophage inflammatory protein-1 alpha (MIP-1α) (Moore et al., 1996; Neipel et al., 1997a,b). The similar size of the K6 (95 residues) and K4 (94 residues) products and their high degree of sequence identity suggest that they arose through a gene duplication event. The third chemokine homologue, vMIP-III (vBCK, vCCL3) is 114 residues in length, encoded by the K4.1 ORF and has homology with MIP-1β as well as several other members of the cellular CC chemokine family (Neipel et al., 1997a,b; Stine et al., 2000). The target of the vMIPs seems to be the Th2 lineage CD4$^+$ T cells based on the fact that vMIP-I can act to induce chemotaxis of CCR8-bearing cells; vMIP-II, chemotaxis of CCR3-bearing cells; vMIP-III chemotaxis of CCR4-bearing cells, and all of these receptors are found on Th2 cells (Sallusto et al., 1998) (Fig. 31.3). Each of the vMIPs have been shown to induce the chemotaxis of Th2 cells (Stine et al., 2000). Further, Weber et al. demonstrated that vMIP-II is able to block the chemotactic effects of RANTES on Th1 cells and monocytes, thus inhibiting their recruitment to sites of vMIP production (Weber et al., 2001) (Fig. 31.3). Nakano et al. (2003), in contrast, demonstrated

Table 31.2. Viral chemokine regulators. Recruitment of immune effectors is critical to the generation of an effective immune response. The soluble chemokines play a large role in this recruitment. Both human γ-herpesviruses encode multiple gene products with the potential to alter the chemokine response. The open reading frame, product and potential function are listed for each, with additional details in the text

	Gene	Product	Function
HHV-8	K6	vMIP-I (vCCL1)	Alters chemotaxis, causes Th2 polarization, neo-angiogenesis, VEGF-A elicitation
	K4	vMIP-II (vCCL2)	Alters chemotaxis, causes Th2 polarization, neo-angiogenesis
	K4.1	vMIP-III (vCCL3, vBCK)	Alters chemotaxis, causes Th2 polarization
	K2	vIL-6	Acts as growth factor, stimulates elicitation of VEGF-B, causes Th2 polarization and Th1 inhibition, activates multiple signaling cascades
	Orf13	vFLIP	Binds TRAF2 causing the induction of cIL-6, causes Th2 polarization, acts as a growth factor
	K14	vOX2	Stimulates macrophage/monocytes to release IL-1β, IL-6, MCP, causes Th2 polarization, may have role in viral dissemination
EBV	LMP-1/EBI-3	cIL-12 subunit	Alters IL-12 signaling, Th2 polarization, might alter IL-4 and IFN-γ production, might effect NKT cells
	BCRF-1	vIL-10	Blocks IFN-γ and IL-2 production, inhibits dendritic cell maturation, Th2 polarization

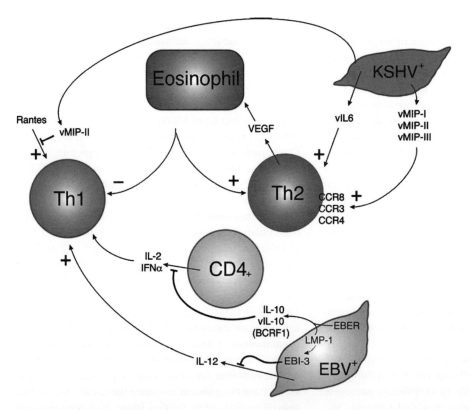

Fig. 31.3. Herpesvirus skewing of the Th1/Th2 balance by multiple gene products. Both KSHV and EBV express multiple gene products that mimic cellular cytokines. These proteins have multiple effects on a number of immune effectors including the CD4+ T helper cells, further detailed in the text. The web of viral and cellular cytokines have a net effect of favoring a Th2, humoral response.

that vMIP-I and –II induced chemotaxis of a monocyte cell line. However, these two groups used different experimental designs and much different target cells, a transformed monocyte cell line versus primary monocytes. The majority of the published data suggests that it is to the advantage of the virus to polarize the immune response to a Th2 pattern, suggesting that cellular adaptive immune responses are more likely to clear the virus from the body.

The vMIP proteins are also likely to have other effects in addition to their role in immune evasion. Both the vMIP-I and –II proteins are highly angiogenic in the chorioallantoic assay (Boshoff et al., 1997). Additionally, vMIP-1 can induce chemotaxis of endothelial cells through its interactions with the CCR8 receptor (Endres et al., 1999). Combined, this suggests that the vMIP proteins might be playing a large part in directing the development of the structure of the vascular KS lesions. Liu et al. (2001) have shown that addition of the vMIP-I protein to PEL cell lines resulted in the expression of vascular endothelial growth factor type A (VEGF-A). This VEGF-A can have both paracrine and autocrine effects, influencing PEL cell growth, extravasation and recruitment of other cells such as eosinophils, which can release Th2-type cytokines (Weber et al., 2001; Feistritzer et al., 2003) (Fig. 31.3). Again, pointing to a dual role for the vMIP proteins in directing KS lesion formation as well as altering anti-viral immune responses.

Further, supporting the thesis that KSHV better survives a Th2-biased immune response, the virus produces yet another soluble factor which favors the development of a Th2 response. Viral IL-6, encoded by KSHV ORF K2 is 204 residues in length and has approximately 25% homology with human IL-6 (Neipel et al., 1997a,b; Nicholas et al., 1997). Message for vIL-6 is very rapidly transcribed after infection (within 2 hours) and then is just as quickly downregulated, disappearing by 8 hours post-infection (Krishnan et al., 2004). Cellular IL-6 (cIL-6) performs multiple functions, including inducing the differentiation of B-cells into antibody-secreting plasma cells (Beagley et al., 1989). It promotes Th2 differentiation and simultaneously inhibits Th1 polarization through two independent molecular mechanisms. It also acts as both an autocrine and paracrine growth factor, delivering a signal through the IL-6 receptor, a heterodimer made up of gp80 and gp130 (Kawano et al., 1988; Klein et al., 1989; Kishimoto et al., 1995; Nakashima and Taga, 1998) (Fig. 31.3). This signal in many ways resembles the signal transmitted by INF-α/β interactions with its receptor, proceeding through members of the JAK kinase family to transmit a signal to the cellular STAT3, which can then stimulate transcription of a group of IL-6 responsive genes (Murakami et al., 1993; Narazaki et al., 1994; Stahl et al., 1994; Guschin et al., 1995). Additionally, STAT1 also becomes phosphorylated, dimerizing with STAT3 to bind and transactivate genes containing interferon-inducible GAS sequences (Feldman et al. 1994; Lutticken et al., 1994; Wegenka et al., 1994; Guschin et al., 1995). The stimulation of cells with cIL-6 also causes the phosphorylation of STAT5 and the induction of the MAP kinase pathway (Diehl and Rincon, 2002).

The KSHV vIL-6 protein, like cIL-6, has been shown to perform numerous functions. It is capable of activating STAT1, 3 and 5, as well as the MAP kinase signaling cascade (Molden et al., 1997; Osborne et al., 1999; Hideshima et al., 2000). However, unlike cIL-6, only the gp130 subunit of the IL-6 receptor is required, although the gp80 subunit can allow vIL-6 to signal more promiscuously (Molden et al., 1997; Aoki et al., 1999; Wan et al., 1999; Li et al., 2001; Klouche et al., 2002; Li and Nicholas, 2002). This ability to signal through the gp130 subunit alone probably allows vIL-6 to continue to transmit anti-apoptotic and growth stimulatory signals even after down regulation of the p80 protein, a normal cellular response to cIL-6 signaling. KSHV vIL-6 likely plays a critical role in the pathology of the virus. There are greater levels of expression in MCD and PEL samples than KS lesion samples, and one group has demonstrated high level vIL-6 production in KSHV-associated germinotropic lymphoproliferative disorder, a rare, newly described disease (Boshoff et al., 1996; Parravinci et al., 1997; Staskus et al., 1997; Du et al., 2002). Both cIL-6 and vIL-6 transmit a proliferative signal to PEL cell lines, both through induction of VEGF-B and induction of pro-survival pathways (Neipel et al., 1997a,b; Nicholas et al., 1997; Burger et al., 1998; Jones et al., 1999; Hideshima et al., 2000; Liu et al., 2001). Although there is great overlap in the functions of vIL-6, Foussat et al. demonstrated a clear need for cIL-6 in PEL cell tumor progression in mice (Foussat et al., 1999). Antibodies against cIL-6 slowed tumor growth even though vIL-6 was still being produced. In addition to a role of vIL-6 in delivering a positive growth signal and protecting from programmed cell death, it probably plays additional roles important to immune effector avoidance. As described above, cIL-6 is critical in driving immunoglobulin production from committed B-cells. The KSHV vIL-6 probably plays a similar role, further polarizing the immune responses, along with the other virally-encoded or –induced cytokines, toward a Th2 response. More recently, Klouche et al. demonstrated that unlike cIL-6, vIL-6 can induce the production of pentraxin-3 (PTX-3, TSG14) (Alles et al., 1994; Klouche et al., 2002). This acute-phase protein is capable of binding to apoptotic cells and preventing their recognition by dendritic cells, possibly preventing auto-immunity during the acute phase response in which there is a high amount of cell death (Rovere et al., 2000). Therefore, it is possible that the production of PTX-3 by vIL-6 helps to reduce recognition of virally-infected cells by APC. However, since PTX-3 only binds to C1q, the initiating protein of the classical complement pathway, or the surface of cells undergoing programmed cell death, the ability of vIL-6 to aid in immune avoidance through this mechanism requires additional experimental examination (Rovere et al., 2000; Mantovani et al., 2003; Nauta et al., 2003). Further underlining a potentially high importance of IL-6 to KSHV persistence or replication is the finding that the vFLIP protein, discussed later in detail, can induce the production of cIL-6 through interactions with TRAF2, which activates the JNK/AP1 pathway and induces IL-6 synthesis (An et al., 2003).

The cellular OX2 protein (CD200) plays a role in co-stimulation of activated T-cells and suppression of monocyte lineage cell responses (Borriello et al., 1997; Gorczynski et al., 1999). It has been shown to provide a co-stimulatory signal for activated T-cells, leading to an increase in IL-4 and TGF-β, but not IL-2 production (Borriello et al., 1997). In contrast OX2 delivers a negative signal to macrophage and monocytes, inhibiting their proliferation (Gorczynski et al., 1998; Gorczynski et al., 1999). Work by Foster-Cuevas et al. (2004) has shown that the interaction of OX2 with its receptor (CD200R) on activated macrophages results in a block to TNF-α production. In mice lacking OX2, dramatic increases in the macrophage and monocyte populations in the mesenteric lymph nodes supports the hypothesis that OX2 plays a role in negatively regulating these cell populations (Gorczynski et al., 1999).

KSHV encodes a gene product from ORF K14 with approximately 40% homology with human OX2. This viral protein is 271 residues in length, migrates with an apparent molecular weight of 55kDa and contains five putative N-linked glycosylation sites (Chung et al., 2002). The higher than predicted molecular weight and experiments with N-glycosidases suggest that all of the putative carbohydrate modification sites are used (Chung et al., 2002). The expression of vOX2 protein is increased after TPA-treatment of PEL cell lines. Although this homology is rather low it is still able to bind to CD200R with affinity and kinetics similar to OX2 (Foster-Cuevas et al., 2004). The biological activity of this viral OX2 is controversial. The experimental work of Chung et al. (2002) demonstrated that the viral protein, provided as a soluble GST-coupled protein, delivers a stimulatory signal to macrophage/monocyte and dendritic cells causing them to elicit several pro-inflamatory cytokines including interleukin-1β (IL-1β), IL-6, monocyte chemoattractant protein 1 (MCP-1), and TNF-alpha. Further, expression of vOX2 on the surface of a B-cell line could stimulate the production of TNF-α and IL-12 from U937 cells in the presence of IFN-γ. In contrast, Barclay's group found that when vOX2 expressed on the surface of Chinese hamster ovary (CHO) cells was presented to human peripheral monocyte-derived macrophages there was no increase in TNF-α production (Foster-Cuevas et al., 2004). To the contrary, there was an inhibition of TNF-α production, similar to what was seen when cOX2 was delivered in a similar manner. Reductions were also seen in the amounts of MCP-1 and G-CSF. However, the experimental methodologies of these two groups were radically different. It is a distinct possibility that the two groups were measuring the effects of vOX2 on different receptors. Further experimental verification is still required to determine the biological activity of this protein. The exact role of this protein and the advantage it conveys upon this virus also still requires further study. One possibility is that the virus is altering the cytokine response profile to control or misdirect anti-viral immune effector proliferation and recruitment. Increases in IL-6 production would be expected to bias $CD4^+$ Th2 cell generation. However, it is also possible that the virus is utilizing cellular cytokines to induce proliferation/recruitment of additional target cells as well as facilitating cytokine-mediated angiogenic proliferation to aid in viral dissemination. If vOX2 has a negative effect on monocyte stimulation it could be acting within KS lesions to block responses from the local infiltrating macrophages which could recruit other immune effectors.

EBV expresses a variety of genes that influence the cellular cytokine milieu. As mentioned previously, LMP-1 induces the expression of EBI-3 resulting in decrease in IL-12 production and increases in IL-27 secretion (Devergne et al., 1996, 1997). This has effects on IFN-γ and Th1 responses from both monocytes and $CD4^+$ T cells (Nieuwenhuis et al., 2002; Pflanz et al., 2002) (Fig. 31.3). Further, the BCRF1 gene, a homologue of IL-10, also modulates cytokine production. Its expression limits the production of both IL-1 and IL-2 from $CD4^+$ T-cells (de Waal Malefyt et al., 1991; Liu et al., 1997; Zeidler et al., 1997; Hayes et al., 1999). vIL-10 can also alter the responsiveness of dendritic cells to MIP-1α and MIP-1β. Although vIL-10 is expressed during the lytic program, LMP1 and the EBERs have been shown to induce production of cIL-10. Examination of immune responses against epitopes in LMP1 in EBV^+ and EBV^- individuals demonstrated that the majority of responding cells were Th1 cells, which secrete IL-10, suppressing T-cell proliferation and IFN-γ production (Marshall et al., 2003) (Fig. 31.3). In addition to these specific genes that have been mentioned, EBV likely possesses a number of additional mechanisms for altering the host chemokine and cytokine profile. These changes seem to play a large role in driving the pathophysiology of EBV infection.

As is seen for KSHV, EBV seems to alter the cytokine milieu to favor the development of a Th2 response. The IL-12 protein influences naïve CD4 T-cells to differentiate toward a Th1 profile. EBI-3 decreases IL-12 production, thus reducing one pro-Th1 factor. Further cellular IL-10 can inhibit Th1 cell generation. The BCRF1 viral protein likely plays a similar role and additionally, like cellular IL-10, inhibits the Th1 cytokines IL-2 and IFN-γ. Again, further in vivo investigation is required to better understand the correlates of an effective immune response against the γ-HVs.

Interferon responses
The interferons (IFN) are a family of critically important cytokines that act to modulate cell proliferation and play an important role in innate and adaptive immunity. The type I IFN-α/β and IFN-ω are produced by virally infected cells, whereas the type II IFN-γ is produced by innate immune system effectors cells, as well as adaptive response effectors such as Th1 cells and CD8$^+$ cells (Biron et al., 1999). These proteins act by binding a variety of cell surface receptors and transmitting a signal through the Janus protein kinases (JAKs) and signal transducers and activators of transcription (STATs) to induce expression of a variety of interferon response factors (IRFs) (reviewed in Leonard, 2001; Sato et al., 2001; Taniguchi et al., 2001). In turn, these IRFs regulate the transcription of a wide variety of genes containing either IFN-stimulated response elements (ISRE) or γ-interferon activation sequences (GAS) in their promoters. Regulated proteins include multiple protein kinases, the tumor necrosis factor receptor and MHC class I and class II proteins (Pober et al., 1983; Collins et al., 1984; Boehm et al., 1997; Stark et al., 1998). The interferon responsive proteins act to induce an anti-viral state in the expressing cells, targeting multiple steps in the life cycle of the virus. For example, through the action of the IFN-responsive oligoadenylate synthase, RNase L is activated. This endoribonuclease is active against double-stranded RNA (dsRNA), thus targeting those viruses with either dsRNA genomes, such as the *Reoviridae* (Miyamoto et al., 1983), or containing extensive dsRNA structure, such as the *Picornaviridae* (Robberson et al., 1982). Another major IFN-inducible gene is the protein kinase PKR, capable of phosphorylating the eIF-2α initiation factor, inhibiting mRNA translation and blocking the production of viral proteins (Thomis and Samuel, 1992). Yet a third major antiviral interferon response is the induction of the MxA protein. MxA is a dynamin-like GTPase that is able to bind to the nucleocapsids of some viruses altering their intracellular transport (Haller and Kochs, 2002; Kochs et al., 2002). Further, the IFNs are able to stimulate the production of a number of other chemokines and cytokines, influencing the immune response to invading pathogens.

Activation of the IFN response can occur in at least two ways. First, as described above, binding of interferon to its cognate receptor on the surface of the cell transmits a signal that modulates the IRFs. However, this mechanism requires that IFNs already have been synthesized, either by the responding cell or a surrounding cell. Activation can also occur by a much more direct method. The cellular IRF-3 is part of a complex of proteins called the double-stranded RNA-activated transcription factor complex (DRAF1), which also includes p300/CREB binding protein (CBP) (Weaver et al., 1998). DRAF1 is sensitive to the presence of dsRNA and becomes serine/threonine phosphorylated upon viral infection. This results in a nuclear accumulation of DRAF1, where it binds to and activates ISRE sequences (Kumar et al., 2000). This results in the up regulation of a number of "interferon-responsive" genes as well as production of IFN-α and -β, which can then act in both autocrine and paracrine activation of the interferon pathway (Weaver et al., 1998). A schematic of the multiple mechanisms that the herpesviruses use to interfere with the IFN response pathway is given in Fig. 31.4 and detailed in the text below.

KSHV was the first virus identified as carrying an IRF (Moore et al., 1996). The K9 protein, vIRF-1, is a 449 residue product with some limited homology to the cellular IRFs (Moore et al., 1996). It is capable of inhibiting both type I and II interferon signaling and additionally has transforming activity (Gao et al., 1997; Li et al., 1997; Inagi et al., 1999) (Table 31.3). Expression in NIH 3T3 cells allows growth in soft agar and at low serum concentration (Gao et al., 1997). Further, these vIRF-1-expressing NIH 3T3 cells lose contact inhibition and are tumorigenic in nude mice. These activities of vIRF-1 are the result of interactions with multiple cellular proteins including the cellular IRF-1 and IRF-3 transcription factors, however it does not effect IRF-7-mediated transactivation (Lin et al., 2001). Interactions with these cellular IRFs block production of IFN-β and the RANTES chemokine, important in directing the infiltration of a number of leukocytes including NK and effector T-cells (Lin et al., 2001). These interactions also block the ability of IRF-1 and IRF-3 to direct transcription from the ISG and IFNA4 promoters. However, at least for IRF-3, binding by vIRF-1 did not effect dimerization, nuclear translocation and DNA binding activity. Rather, vIRF-1 interacted with the p300/CBP and efficiently inhibited the formation of transcriptionally competent IRF-3-CBP/p300 complexes (Lin et al., 2001). The further implications of the ability of vIRF-1 to interact with p300/CBP will be discussed later. Additionally, the interaction of

Table 31.3. Viral interferon regulators. Both human γ-herpesviruses encode multiple gene products with the potential to alter the IFN response. The open reading frame, product and potential function are listed for each, with additional details in the text

	Gene	Product	Function
HHV-8	K9	vIRF-1	Blocks IFN-a, -β and -γ effects and production, anti-apoptotic, transforming
	K11.1	vIRF-2	Blocks IFN-α and -β effects, anti-apoptotic
	K11	?	?
	K10.5/10.6	vIRF-3/LNA-2	Inhibits IFN-α and -β production
	K2	vIL-6	Blocks IFN-α activation of p21CIP1/WAF1, allowing cell cycle progression
	ORF45	KIE-2	Reduces IFN-a production through inhibition of IRF-7 function
	ORF10	RIF	Blocks STAT1, STAT2 and Tyk2 phosphorylation, reducing ISG production
EBV	BCRF1	vIL-10	Blocks IFN-γ and IL-2 production, inhibits dendritic cell maturation, Th2 polarization
	BZLF1	ZTA	Blocks STAT1 activation, MHC class II up regulation and IFN-γ production, anti-apoptotic, disperses PML bodies
	BARF1	vCSF-1R	Blocks IFN-α production, inhibits macrophage proliferation, transforming
	LMP-1/EBI-3	cIL-12 subunit	Alters IL-12 signaling, Th2 polarization, might alter IL-4 and IFN-γ production, might effect NKT cells

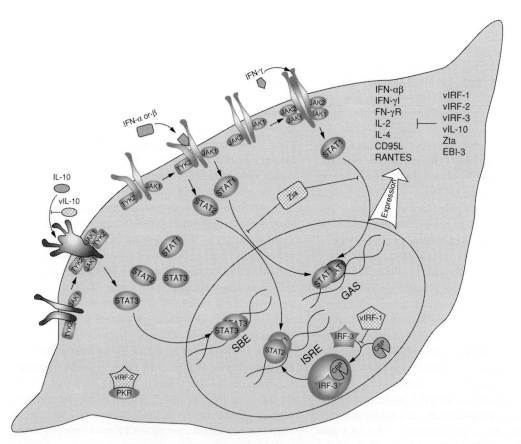

Fig. 31.4. Viral proteins involved in control of the anti-viral IFN responses. A number of γ-HV proteins, detailed in the text and shown in a checkered pattern, are capable of interfering with the IFN responses. Some prevent STAT assembly on GAS, ISRE or STAT binding element (SBE) DNA sequences in the nucleus. Others interfere with the down stream products of the IFN response, such as the binding of PKR by vIRF-2. Additional mechanisms of interference are discussed in the text.

vIRF-1 with the cellular IRF-1 is likely responsible for its ability to suppress CD95L up-regulation and FAS mediated cell death after TCR/CD3 stimulation (Kirchhoff *et al.*, 2002). However, this effect might also be a result of interactions with p300/CBP. More recently, the group of Seo *et al.* (2002) identified an additional binding partner of vIRF-1, retinoid-IFN-induced-mortality-19 (GRIM19). This gene enhances caspase-9 activity and induces apoptosis in response to signals from IFN and retinoic acid treatment of cells. vIRF-1 binding suppresses the ability of GRIM19 to induce apoptosis in HELA and MCF-7 cells. This inhibition of apoptosis through interactions with multiple transcription factors along with an ability to increase c-myc expression all contribute to the transformation ability of vIRF-1.

KSHV encodes three additional vIRFs, vIRF-2, a 489 bp ORF encoded by the ORFK11.1 gene and its close homologue encoded by the ORFK11 gene and vIRF–3, also termed LANA-2, encoded as a 1072 bp spliced product of the ORF K10.5 and 10.6 genes (Burysek *et al.*, 1999; Lubyova and Pitha, 2000). Over expression of these genes results in suppression of both IFN-α and -β signaling (Table 31.3). Unlike vIRF-1, the vIRF-2 protein does not seem to possess transforming activity (Burysek *et al.*, 1999). It is capable of binding to several cellular factors including IRF-1, IRF-2, interferon consensus sequence binding protein, RelA/p65 and CBP (Burysek *et al.*, 1999). vIRF-2 is capable of homodimerizing and binding to DNA encoding the NF-kB sequence (Burysek *et al.*, 1999). More recently it was shown that vIRF-2 is able to interact with the double-stranded RNA-activated protein kinase (PKR) and prevent its autophosphorylation (Burysek and Pitha, 2001). As detailed above, PKR targets the elongation initiation factor 2α (eIF-2α), critical to the initiation of protein synthesis, phosphorylating the GDP-bound inactive form. This phosphorylated form acts as a dominant negative, binding to the eIF-2β guanine nucleotide release factor, preventing the reloading of GTP onto other eIF-2α molecules, thus preventing the initiation of new rounds of protein synthesis (Thomis and Samuel, 1992). All of these abilities of vIRF-2 contribute to its ability to block the effects of the Type I interferons. Intriguingly, vIRF-2 transcripts are present at high levels within 2 hours of viral infection and then subside to undetectable levels by 8 hours post-infection (Krishnan *et al.*, 2004). Further, like vIRF-1, vIRF-2 is able to block FAS-mediated apoptosis through an ability to block up regulation of CD95L on the surface of expressing cells (Kirchhoff *et al.*, 2002).

The transcription pattern of vIRF-3 is more complicated than the other v-IRF genes. Its mRNA is a spliced product of two genomic regions previously thought to code for two separate proteins, ORF K10.6 and ORF K10.5 (Lubyova and Pitha, 2000). It has homology with the vIRF-2 and ORFK11 proteins as well as the cellular IRF-4 (Rivas *et al.*, 2001). It can block the activities of both IRF-3 and IRF-7 on the IFNA promoter, inhibiting the production of both α- and β-interferon (Lubyova and Pitha, 2000). More recent work from Rivas and colleagues has shown that vIRF-3 is able to block PKR-mediated apoptosis, but not oligoadenylate pathway-mediated apoptosis (Esteban *et al.*, 2003). In these studies the expression of vIRF-3 was able to prevent PKR mediated inhibition of protein synthesis, at least partially through a block to the phosphorylation of eIF-2α. Further, vIRF-3 was able to block the activation of caspase 3, a member of the FADD/caspase 8 pathway of apoptosis that is activated by PKR. However, no effects of vIRF-3 were observed on caspase 9, another PKR activated caspase. Since vIRF-2 also targets the PKR pathway, an exploration of the co-expression of these genes and their potentially additive effects on antiviral interferon responses would be interesting.

More recently, in a comprehensive screen of the KSHV lytic genes, Ganem's group identified a viral protein capable of blocking interferon signaling at a membrane proximal position, unlike the majority of KSHV gene products that block responses in the nucleus. ORF 10, now named RIF (regulator of Interferon Function), is able to block phosphorylation of STAT1, STAT2 and Tyk2 following IFN-α stimulation (A-L Page, SA Bisson and D Ganem, personal communication). Interestingly, this viral protein directly interacts with the STAT proteins, potentially blocking their multimerization. This mechanism seems distinct from that of the EBV BZLF1 gene product ZTA, which will be discussed in detail later in this section, as ZTA only blocks STAT1 phosphorylation following IFN-γ stimulation, not IFN-α (Morrison *et al.*, 2001).

The interferon responses typically take place very quickly after viral infection. Therefore, in order to persist within the host the virus must take immediate protective action. Zhu *et al.* have identified a KSHV protein encoded by ORF45 that is incorporated into the virus particle as a tegument protein (Zhu and Yuan, 2003). This protein, KIE-2, is able to bind to IRF-7, blocking its phosphorylation and accumulation in the nucleus (Zhu *et al.*, 2002). This results in a blockage of IFN-α and IFN-β transcription in response to viral infection. As its name suggests, KIE-2 is an immediate early protein of $\sim$78kDa and is found within the cytoplasm of expressing cells. Based on the presence of the protein in preparations of purified virus and its resistance to detergent treatment combined with sensitivity to detergent plus trypsin suggests that this protein is found in the tegument of the virus. This protein, therefore, would be available to block the interferon responses immediately following viral infection.

KSHV possess yet an additional way of mitigating the effects of interferon on viral replication and persistence. The viral IL6 homologue is able to block the induction of p21$^{\text{CIP1/WAF1}}$, a cyclin-dependant kinase inhibitor, by IFN-α (Table 31.3). Normally treatment of cells results in an up regulation of this protein, arresting the cells in G_1/S (Chatterjee et al., 2002). Further, treatment of cells with vIL-6 was shown to block the IFN-α stimulated binding of ISGF3 to ISRE probes. Interestingly, IFN-α downregulates the gp80 sub-unit of the IL-6 receptor blocking the ability of cIL-6 to transmit a signal. On the other hand, vIL-6 only requires the gp130 sub-unit to signal and thus, is not blocked by the down regulation of gp80. Additionally, vIL-6 expression is induced by IFN-α, providing a negative feedback loop to control this antiviral response in virally-infected cells.

One remaining question is why seven different gene products potentially involved in regulating the cellular IFN responses are encoded by the virus. Several non-exclusive answers exist. First, although each of the studied products possess similar functions, they are not identical. Given the importance of the IFN response in the control of other viruses, as well as a proven ability of interferon treatment to block KS progression in a large percentage of patients, this simplistic answer is probably also true (Von Roenn and Cianfrocca, 2001). Recent work by a number of groups using DNA array technology has pointed to another potential answer. When examining expression of each vIRF gene, it was found that the kinetics and tissue-expression of each differed (Jenner et al., 2001; Paulose-Murphy et al., 2001; Fakhari and Dittmer, 2002; Dittmer, 2003). Unlike vIRF-1, the vIRF-3/LANA-2 protein is detectable in primary effusion lymphoma (PEL) cell lines without TPA stimulation. The work of Fakhari and Dittmer demonstrated that the kinetics of vIRF-3/LANA-2 mRNA production mirrored that of LANA-1, v-FLIP and v-cyclin, all non-TPA induced, latency-associated genes in the BCBL-1 PEL cell line (Fakhari and Dittmer, 2002). In KS lesions, however, expression of vIRF-1 and not vIRF-3 clusters with LANA-1. So, a degree of tissue- or disease-specific expression might also contribute to the need for multiple genes to combat this facet of innate immunity. An understanding of the role of the vIRFs during infection is further complicated by the work of Pozharskaya et al. (2004). In experiments looking at vIRF-1 it was found that during latency in BCBL-1 PEL cells, only low levels of vIRF-1 are expressed and are not able to block the effects of IFN-α and while higher levels were initially expressed after TPA induction, these levels quickly fell off. Further, the vIL-6 gene is transcribed to high levels shortly after infection (Krishnan et al., 2004). In summary, KSHV expresses multiple genes capable of blunting the production and effects of the interferon genes. These genes are expressed during both the lytic and latent programs, underlining the importance of the interferon proteins in the control of viral infection.

Like KSHV, EBV encodes multiple genes that help it avoid the antiviral effects of interferon. Among these are BCRF1, BZLF1 and BARF1 (Table 31.3). Additionally, viral infection induces the expression of a cellular protein named EBI-3, also involved in regulating the effects of interferon. The mature BCRF1 gene product (vIL-10) possesses 84% identity with cellular interleukin-10 (Hsu et al., 1990). A 170 residue protein, it is expressed late in the lytic program, although one group reports expression of BCRF1 in a small number of patients with nasal type, extranodal natural killer (T(NK/T)-cell) lymphoma, which is usually associated with latent EBV infection (Swaminathan et al., 1993; Xu et al., 2001). This gene product indirectly effects the production of the type II IFN-γ by binding to the cellular IL-10 receptor. This results in a blockage of IL-2 and IFN-γ production (Liu et al., 1997; Takayama et al., 2001). Like cellular IL-10, vIL-10 can block the maturation of dendritic cells causing them to down regulate CCR7 and up regulate CCR5. This blunts their ability to stimulate T cell release of IFN-γ (Takayama et al., 2001). In addition to aiding the virus in escape from IFN responses this has profound effects on CTL induction, which will be discussed in a later section of this chapter. Viruses containing a truncated BCRF1 protein or completely deleted for the gene were functionally similar to wild-type virus (Swaminathan et al., 1993). Like the parental virus, BCRF1 deleted virus was able to transform B-lymphocytes into long-term lymphoblastoid cell lines (LCLs), and these LCLs were capable of inducing tumors in SCID mice to the same degree as wild-type derived LCLs (Swaminathan et al., 1993). This suggests that BCRF1 is playing a larger role in immune regulation than in viral pathogenesis.

The BZLF1 gene expresses an immediate early viral protein with a wide number of functions. Not only is it important in directing the lytic replication program through its binding to the lytic origin of replication and within several of the early lytic gene promoters, but it also blocks tyrosine phosphorylation and nuclear translocation of STAT1, an important molecule in IFN response signaling (Kenney et al., 1989; Rooney et al., 1989; Packham et al., 1990; Morrison et al., 2001). Additionally, this protein blocks IRF-1 activation and decreases the amount of IFN-γ α-chain receptor expression (Morrison et al., 2001). BZLF1 is able to decrease the ability of IFN-γ to activate a variety of important downstream target genes, such as IRF-1, p48, and CIITA, and prevents IFN-γ-induced class II MHC surface expression (Morrison et al., 2001). Like BCRF1, not only does BZLF1 affect interferon responses, but it also interferes with activation of helper T-cells and it possesses anti-apoptosis activity, both of which will be discussed in greater detail in later sections of this chapter. Interestingly, through competition for limiting amounts of the SUMO-1 protein, BZLF1 can also disperse nuclear PML bodies, which are induced by interferon and posited to have antiviral effects (Adamson and Kenney, 2001).

The BARF1 gene encodes a 31–33 kDa soluble receptor for colony stimulating factor 1 (CSF-1) that is expressed as an early lytic gene (Wei and Ooka, 1989; Strockbine et al., 1998). Its expression inhibits macrophage proliferation and blocks IFN-α production by monocytes (Cohen and Lekstrom, 1999). Additionally, BARF1 can act as an oncogene when expressed in fibroblasts, B-lymphoma cells and monkey kidney cells (Wei and Ooka, 1989; Wei et al., 1994, 1997). It increases c-myc, CD21 and CD23 expression and introduction into EBV$^-$ Akata cells resulted in increased Bcl-2 expression and tumor induction in SCID mice (Wei et al., 1994; Sheng et al., 2001, 2003). However, Cohen and Lekstrom (1992) demonstrated that a BARF1$^-$ virus was competent for B cell transformation. Groups have reported that in both gastric adenocarcinomas and NPC, BARF1 is strongly expressed along with a number of the other latent proteins (Hayes et al., 1999; Decaussin et al., 2000; zur Hausen et al., 2000). In the case of EBV positive gastric adenocarcinomas, this is in the absence of the LMP1 oncogene, giving greater weight to the ability of BARF1 to act as an oncogene, at least in certain tissues or cell-types. Fewer reports have been made concerning the potential immune evasion role of BARF1.

One final gene utilized by EBV to control the anti-viral interferon responses is encoded by the host and induced by the LMP1 protein (Devergne et al., 1996, 1998). EBV-induced gene-3 (EBI-3) is a 34 kDa glycoprotein which localizes primarily to the ER of expressing cells (Devergne et al., 1996). It is homologous to the IL-12 p40 subunit and can bind to IL-12 p35 (Devergne et al., 1996). IL-12 normally triggers Th1 polarization of naïve CD4$^+$ T-cells, which then secrete IFN-γ. Recently, Pflanz and coworkers (Pflanz et al., 2002) demonstrated that IL-27 is made up of a complex of EBI-3 and IL-12 p35. This interleukin is produced by activated antigen presenting cells and can drive expansion of naïve CD4$^+$ T cells, although the effects on EBV are not yet clear since IL-12 can synergize with IL-27 for IFN-γ production and effect both CTL and NK cell development (Pflanz et al., 2002). An EBI-3-knockout mouse has normal numbers of most immune effectors except invariant natural killer T cells. This results in decreased IL-4 production and some decreases in IFN-γ production. The cellular EBI-3 protein, therefore, is playing a critical role in the generation of Th2 immune responses and its induction by EBV infection probably drives polarization of the anti-viral immune response (Nieuwenhuis et al., 2002).

The LMP1 protein makes at least one potential additional contribution to viral avoidance of the interferon defenses. Quizzically, LMP1 induces the expression, activation and nuclear translocation of IRF-7, the same IRF that the KSHV ORF45 gene product inactivates (Zhang and Pagano, 2001; Zhang et al., 2001). It has been shown that expression of LMP-1 in cells induces a number of ISGs and can block the replication of vesicular stomatitis virus (Zhang et al., 2004). The paradoxical stimulation of what would seem to be an antiviral state within the cell most likely plays a role in controlling EBV latency and superinfection of EBV$^+$ cells by other viruses.

Thus, like KSHV, EBV encodes numerous proteins capable of altering the antiviral interferon responses. These proteins are expressed at multiple time points during the viral life cycle, highlighting how important the interferon responses are for the control of viral infections. Further examination of these groups of genes in an in vivo context should yield important information about how the interferon responses are modulated within the host.

Apoptosis responses

Apoptosis or programmed cell death plays a role both in innate immunity and normal cellular regulation. It is a mechanism by which intrinsic or extrinsic signals are capable of inducing cell death for the purposes of removing a diseased or unwanted cell from the body. Central to the intrinsic apoptotic responses are the members of the BCL-2 protein family. These proteins are capable of either inducing or suppressing apoptosis and possibly function through homo- or hetero-dimerizing with other family members, although this is controversial. The extrinsic responses, such as those triggered by CD8$^+$ CTL, largely depend on members of the tumor necrosis factor (TNF) receptor family. These receptors contain death response domains in their cytoplasmic tails and upon multimerization transmit a signal to the intracellular caspases that initiate the apoptosis response. It is critical that the γ-HV control apoptosis in order to insure that the infected cell is not eliminated prior to virion production.

Both EBV and KSHV encode homologues of the cellular Bcl-2 gene (Table 31.4). The KSHV Bcl-2 homologue (vBcl-2) is expressed from ORF16, but only possesses low homology with cellular Bcl-2 (Russo et al., 1996; Neipel et al., 1997a,b). Little is known of the mechanism of action of this protein. While it can inhibit Bax toxicity in yeast and fibroblasts, there is conflicting data concerning its ability to dimerize with the cellular Bcl-2 family members (Cheng

Table 31.4. Viral apoptosis regulators. Cellular suicide, whether self-induced or induced by other effectors, is an important immune response to control the replication and spread of viruses. Both human γ-herpesviruses encode multiple gene products with the potential to alter the cell suicide, apoptosis response. The open reading frame, product and potential function are listed for each, with additional details in the text

	Gene	Product	Function
HHV-8	Orf16	vBcl-2	blocks both Bax and vCyclin induced apoptosis
	Orf13	vFLIP	up regulates Bcl-x(L) through the NF-kB pathway blocking starvation-mediated apoptosis, up regulates IL-6 in a TRAF2/JNK/AP1 dependent fashion, blocks Fas-mediated apoptosis, interferes with caspase-3, -8 and -9, tumorigenic
	K9	vIRF-1	binds IRFs, GRIM19, p53 and p300/CBP, blocks p53 and IFN + retinoic acid induced apoptosis
	K7	K7/vIAP	binds CAML, cBcl-2 and caspase-3, preserves mitochondrial membrane potential, blocks TRAIL, staurosporin and thapsigargin-induced apoptosis
EBV	BHRF1	vBcl-2	preserves mitochondrial membrane potential, blocks TRAIL and Fas-mediated apoptosis
	BCRF1	vBcl-2	binds HAX-1 and Bcl-2 through EBNA-LP effecting apoptosis
	BALF1	vBcl-2	binds Bax and Bak, can modulate BHRF1 activity
	BNLF1	LMP-1	increases Bcl-2, A20 and Traf1 expression blocking TNF-mediated apoptosis, can induce bfl-1 blocking p53-mediated apoptosis

et al., 1997; Sarid et al., 1997). Additionally, vBcl-2 is capable of blocking the apoptosis induced by viral cyclin, so whether KSHV vBcl-2 is acting to protect virally infected cells against the extrinsic pro-apoptotic immune responses or intrinsic virally-mediated apoptotic responses is unclear (Ojala et al., 1999, 2000).

In addition to a Bcl-2 homologue, KSHV also encodes a homologue of the cellular FLICE inhibitory protein, termed vFLIP (Chang et al., 1994). It is expressed from ORF13 as a multi-cistronic transcript with ORF72 (vCyclin) and ORF73 (LANA) through either differential splicing or expression from an IRES element (Sarid et al., 1999; Grundhoff and Ganem, 2001; Low et al., 2001). FLICE, or caspase-8, is a member of the ICE family of cellular caspases, and is important in the apoptosis response (Muzio et al., 1996). Interestingly, all three of these genes are transcribed rapidly after infection, underscoring a potential need to combat the apoptotic response soon after viral entry into cells (Krishnan et al., 2004). The vFLIP protein has been shown to block pro-apoptotic signaling mediated by the Fas-receptor, resulting in decreases in caspase-8, -9 and -3 activity (Thome et al., 1997; Djerbi et al., 1999; Belanger et al., 2001). A recent study has shown that vFLIP can target the NF-kB pathway, up regulating Bcl-x(L) resulting in protection of cells from serum withdrawal (Sun et al., 2003). Additionally, vFLIP physically interacts with tumor necrosis factor receptor associated factor 2 (TRAF2) activating the JNK/AP1 pathway in a TRAF-dependent fashion (An et al., 2003). This modulation of the JNK/AP1 pathway results in the induction of IL-6, important in directing a Th2 polarization of the immune response and having proliferative effects as detailed earlier (An et al., 2003). Further, vFLIP expression promoted tumor formation after injection of syngeneic and semiallogeneic mouse strains with A20 cells expressing this protein (Djerbi et al., 1999).

The K9/vIRF-1 protein, able to block the anti-viral interferon responses as described above, also has a role in blocking programmed cell death. In addition to binding cellular IRF and GRIM19, vIRF-1 has been shown to bind both p53 and p300/CBP through tryptophan- and proline-rich sequences (Li et al., 2000; Seo et al., 2000; Nakamura et al., 2001; Seo et al., 2001). The irreversible cell cycle arrest and cell death induced by p53 are considered part of host surveillance mechanisms for detecting and preventing viral infection and tumor induction. The activity of p53 is regulated by a series of kinases, phosphatases and acetylases. Acetylation of the carboxyl-terminal region of p53 is mediated by p300 and p300/CBP-associated factor (PCAF) (Sakaguchi et al., 1998). This modification leads to increased DNA binding activity. Interactions of vIRF-1 with p53 and p300/CBP lead to decreased acetylation of p53 as well as decreased phosphorylation, resulting in a dramatic decrease in p53 activity (Nakamura et al., 2001). Blocking p53-dependent transcription suppresses Bax and p21 transcription, mediators of p53-mediated apoptosis, thus rescuing vIRF-1 expressing cells from programmed cell death (Nakamura et al., 2001; Seo et al., 2001). Additionally, interactions of vIRF-1 with CBP results in hypoacetylation of histones H3 and H4, reducing transcription from the early inflammatory gene promoter (Li et al., 1998).

KSHV encodes at least one additional protein that has anti-apoptotic activity. The K7 protein, also termed vIAP, localizes to the mitochondria of expressing cells where it can interact with the cellular calcium-modulating cyclophilin ligand (CAML) (Feng et al., 2002; Wang et al., 2002). This interaction helps to maintain the mitochondrial membrane potential after treatment with a variety of pro-apoptotic compounds including TRAIL, staurosporin and thapsigargin (Feng et al., 2002). Additionally, K7 has been shown to interact with the Protein-linking integrin-associated protein and cytoskeleton 1 (PLIC1) (Feng et al., 2004). PLIC1 is capable of dimerizing and binding to polyubiquitin containing proteins, as well as associating with the 19s unit of the proteasome (Feng et al., 2004). KSHV K7 is able to reduce the ability of PLIC1 to homodimerize and bind to ubiquitinylated proteins, with the end result that two of the targets of PLIC1 activity, Iκb and p53, are rapidly degraded in the presence of K7 (Feng et al., 2004). This reduction of p53 levels within the cell contributes to the anti-apoptotic action of K7. Finally, the K7 protein has also been shown to interact with cellular Bcl-2 and caspase-3, but not with Bax and these interactions are critical to its anti-apoptotic activity (Wang et al., 2002). Like the vFlip gene, K7 is transcribed rapidly after viral infection (Krishnan et al., 2004).

The EBV BHRF1 protein is an early lytic protein capable of blocking the pro-apoptotic actions of TNF-related apoptosis inducing ligand (TRAIL) and FAS (Cheng et al., 1997; Foghsgaard and Jaattela, 1997; Kawanishi, 1997; Kawanishi et al., 2002). TRAIL normally causes cleavage of Bid, a BCL-2 family member, via activation of caspase 8. BHRF1 doesn't block Bid cleavage, but it does block loss of mitochondrial membrane potential, an important downstream apoptotic effect (Kawanishi et al., 2002). Recently, the NMR structure of BHRF1 was solved, demonstrating some clear differences with the structure of its cellular counter-part (Huang et al., 2003). Unlike Bcl-2, it does not contain a hydrophobic groove important in homo- or hetero-dimerization with other apoptotic factors. Additionally, BHRF1 doesn't bind to peptides from Bak, Bax, Bik, and Bad, indicating it functions in a fundamentally different way than the cellular Bcl-x(L) or Bcl-2 (Kawanishi et al., 2002; Huang et al., 2003). BCRF1 protein is also able to complex with another EBV protein, EBV nuclear antigen leader protein (EBNA-LP) (Matsuda et al., 2003). Previously it was shown that EBNA-LP can bind to the HS1-associated protein X-1 (HAX-1), while more recently it was shown that this protein can bind to cellular Bcl-2 (Kawaguchi et al., 2000; Matsuda et al., 2003). The implications of this complex web of interactions to apoptosis is made more complicated by a third EBV protein, BALF1. BALF1 is also an early lytic, Bcl-2 homologue (Hatfull et al., 1988). It can interact with both the Bak and Bax BCL-2 family members and was originally demonstrated to have apoptotic effects (Marshall et al., 1999). More recent experiments have shown that BALF1 can block the action of BHRF1 through an unknown mechanism, but itself has no direct pro- or anti-apoptotic activity (Bellows et al., 2002).

The LMP-1 gene of EBV is expressed during latency and has been shown, in addition to its latency regulatory activity, to prevent apoptosis. It can increase the expression of cellular Bcl-2 as well as a number of other cellular proteins including A20 and TRAF1, important in the anti-apoptotic TNF receptor pathway, through its activation of NF-κB (Henderson et al., 1991; Devergne et al., 1998). LMP-1 is additionally able to induce the expression of bfl-1, a Bcl-2 homologue able to suppress p53 mediated apoptosis (D'Souza et al., 2000). Ectopic expression of bfl-1 in an EBV-positive cell line exhibiting a latency type I infection protects against apoptosis induced by growth factor deprivation, thereby providing a functional role for bfl-1 in this cellular context and adding bfl-1 to the list of anti-apoptotic proteins whose expression is modulated by EBV.

As outlined in this section, the γ-HVs encode a large number of proteins aimed at controlling the cellular apoptosis response. These proteins likely aid the virus in escape from immune effectors such as NK cells and CTL, as well as preventing viral replication from inducing cell death. Given the central importance of programmed cell death in immune function, additional viral mechanisms to avoid apoptosis are likely to be discovered.

Natural killer (NK) cell responses

The NK cells play a critical role in clearing virally-infected cells through direct lysis and the release of various cytokines, which coordinate other immune responses. Although the task that they perform is simple, their regulation is not. A complex set of cell:cell interactions determine whether the NK cell will release its deadly cargo of perforin and granzyme to induce programmed cell death in the target cell, secrete large amounts of IFN-γ to stimulate Th1 T cell production or release the target cell unharmed. The cell surface receptors that govern NK activity can be split into four classes (for review see Anderson et al., 2001; Boyington et al., 2001; LaBonte et al., 2001; Long et al., 2001; McVicar and Burshtyn, 2001; Volz et al., 2001). The killer cell immunoglobulin receptors (KIR) make up the first class. They are capable of binding to a variety of MHC class I haplotypes and generally transmit a negative signal. The second class is the C-type lectin receptor family composed of heterodimers of CD94 and one of several NKG2 proteins. Like the KIR, these receptors also bind MHC class I molecules, but only HLA-G and -E. The natural cytotoxicity receptors (NCR) compose the third class of receptors. The NCR don't interact with class I, but as of yet no cognate ligands have been identified. All identified NCR transmit

Table 31.5. Viral NK regulators. The immune system employs a number of specialized cellular effectors that perform general "house-keeping" function, including the elimination of diseased cells. The natural killer cells are a sub-set of these effectors that are capable of sensing the health of a cell through a number of cell surface receptors, including several which recognize MHC class I. Both human γ-herpesviruses encode gene products with the potential to alter the response of NK cells to infection. The open reading frame, product and potential function are listed for each, with additional details in the text

	Gene	Product	Function
HHV-8	K5	K5 (MIR-2)	Down regulates HLA-A and –B, B7.2 and ICAM-1, but leaves HLA-C on the surface of cells blocking NK cell lysis
EBV	LMP-1/EBI-3	cIL-12 subunit	Stabilizes HLA-G1 surface expression sending a negative signal to the NK cells

positive signals to their expressing NK cells, inducing killing and cytokine release in the absence of stronger negative signals. The fourth class, the leukocyte immunoglobulin-like receptor (LIR) family, similar to the class two receptors, can bind HLA-G to transmit a negative signal. The net overall strength of each positive and negative signal determine whether the NK cell will be turned on to make a response or induced to release the target cell.

Important to NK surveillance are multiple adhesion molecules on both the NK and target cell. These molecules include the integrins, intracellular adhesion molecule 1 (ICAM-1), CD2 and LFA3. Interactions between these molecules help to bring the NK cell into close conjugation with its target. This allows both for the NK cell to survey the target cell for the many positive and negative regulatory factors and to potentially deliver the perforin/granzyme payload specifically to the closely juxtaposed target. Antibodies that block the binding of the NK adhesion molecules to the target cell have been shown to block NK cell lysis (Papa *et al.*, 1994; Komatsu and Kajiwara, 1998). Experiments from Burshtyn *et al.* demonstrated that when the KIR interacts with MHC class I on the target cell and transmits a negative signal, there is a decrease in the ability of the NK cell to stay in conjugation with the target (Burshtyn *et al.*, 2000).

The KSHV K5 protein is capable of inducing the down regulation of several cell surface proteins through increasing their rate of endocytosis. This protein will be further discussed later, but as a brief introduction, K5 seems to act as an E3 ubiquitin ligase, targeting ICAM-1, B7.2 and some MHC class I haplotypes for destruction by the ubiquitin: proteasome system (Coscoy and Ganem, 2000; Ishido *et al.*, 2000a,b; Coscoy and Ganem, 2001; Coscoy *et al.*, 2001; Means *et al.*, 2002; Sanchez *et al.*, 2002). This destruction happens in a sequential manner with the targeted proteins first being endocytosed from the cell surface into the trans-Golgi network (Means *et al.*, 2002). Target proteins are then redirected into the lysosome, where they undergo destruction (Means *et al.*, 2002). While MHC I normally acts to transmit a negative signal to NK cells, the ICAM-1 and B7.2 molecules act as anchors to bring the NK cell into close conjugation with target cells. By removing these last two molecules from the surface of infected cells, K5 reduces the average time that the NK cell stays in contact with the K5-expressing target cell (Table 31.5). Thus, even without MHC class I present to transmit a negative signal through the KIR, the NK cell releases the K5-expressing cell unharmed, simply because it can't stay in contact long enough to get a strong positive signal and turn on granzyme/perforin or cytokine release (Ishido *et al.*, 2000a,b) (Fig 31.5).

Less information is available concerning the avoidance of NK cell responses by EBV. The work of Devergne *et al.* (2001) demonstrated that the EBV-induced EBI-3 protein is capable of stabilizing HLA-G presentation on the surface of cells (Table 31.5). HLA-G1 is capable of transmitting a negative signal to NK cells, preventing the activation of killing or cytokine elicitation (Adrian Cabestre *et al.*, 1999; Navarro *et al.*, 1999; Rajagopalan and Long, 1999). Further, HLA-G1 expression was shown to block the lysis of cells presenting HLA-A2-restricted influenza epitopes to specific CTL clones (Le Gal *et al.*, 1999). However, no experimental data has been presented to demonstrate that the LMP1-mediated up regulation of EBI-3 is able to convey these immune avoidance phenotypes in the context of EBV infection (Fig 31.5). One other mechanism that EBV may be using to avoid NK surveillance is through direct infection. While NK cells lack the CD21/CR2 EBV receptor, studies have shown that they become briefly CD21[+] after conjugation with CD21[+] B-cell targets (Tabiasco *et al.*, 2003). Acquisition of this molecule allows for EBV infection and likely underlies the genesis of EBV[+] NK cell lymphomas, while at the same time allowing for viral escape from NK surveillance.

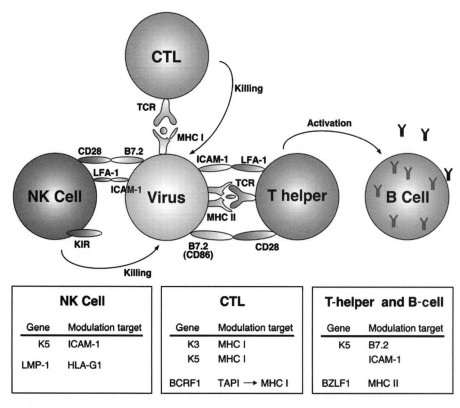

Fig. 31.5. Viral alteration of immunomodulatory proteins. Through the down regulation of multiple immunomodulatory proteins both KSHV and EBV are able to alter the ability of innate and adaptive immune effectors to recognize and mount responses against virally infected cells. Diagramed are some of the cellular proteins altered by viral gene products and their binding partners. The viral proteins and their targets are listed in the tables below the diagram. Details of the interactions are given in the text.

While it is clear that both of the human γ-HV interfere with NK cell surveillance the possibility of additional viral mechanisms for avoiding these effectors remains. For example, the human cytomegalovirus (HCMV), a β-herpesvirus, encodes the UL16 protein. This protein is able to bind and down regulate the cellular UL16-binding proteins (ULBP) 1 and 2, which are ligands for the c-type lectin NKG2D activating receptor on NK cells (Rolle *et al.*, 2003). This effectively protects HCMV-infected cells from NK cell lysis. To date, no human γ-HV protein has been shown to target an NK cell activating receptor.

Evasion of other innate cellular responses

The immune system employs a number of additional innate effectors which surveil the body, including the professional phagocytes, neutrophils and macrophage that internalize and destroy extracellular pathogens such as bacteria or virus, as well as eosinophils and basophils, both able to release a number of immunomodulatory proteins. Like NK cells, these cells represent the first line of defense against infecting pathogens and are able to modulate the later adaptive responses. It is therefore critical that the γ-HV deregulate or avoid recognition by these cells in order to establish a persistent infection.

EBV is able to infect both neutrophils and monocytes, macrophage-precursors. While EBV infection of neutrophils is abortive, multiple changes in cellular physiology important to the potential escape of the virus from immune avoidance occur (Larochelle *et al.*, 1998). First, viral infection causes the up regulation of Fas ligand. Neutrophils express CD95/Fas, which plays a role in immune privilege, and the increased expression of Fas ligand results in apoptosis (Griffith *et al.*, 1995; Larochelle *et al.*, 1998). This effectively eliminates responding neutrophils. However, EBV infection also triggers these cells to release a number of cytokines, including IL-8, MIP-1α, IL-1α, IL-1β and the IL-1R antagonist (Beaulieu *et al.*, 1995; McColl *et al.*, 1997; Roberge *et al.*, 1997). These chemokines, along with the highly-induced leukotrien B4, act to recruit additional leukocytes, potentially aiding in viral dissemination (Gosselin *et al.*, 2001).

Table 31.6. Viral CTL Regulators. CD8⁺ T-cell responses play a critical role in the elimination of virally-infected cells. Both human γ-herpesviruses encode multiple gene products with the potential to alter the ability of host CTLs to recognize and eliminate virally-infected cells. The open reading frame, product and potential function are listed for each, with additional details in the text

	Gene	Product	Function
HHV-8	K3	K3 (MIR-1)	Down-regulates MHC class I, blocking induction of CTL responses
	K5	K5 (MIR-2)	Down-regulates HLA-A and -B, B7.2 and ICAM-1 blocking CTL and T helper activation
	LANA	LANA	Block *in cis* CTL epitope presentation
EBV	BKRF1	EBNA-1	GAR region interferes with the proteasome and MHC class I presentation
	BCRF1	vIL-10	Down regulates TAP1 and cLMP2 interfering with MHC class I loading and presentation

In contrast, infection of monocytes, while highly inefficient, seems to be productive, resulting in transformed monocyte cell lines displaying type II latency (Masy *et al.*, 2002). The route of infection is unclear since monocytes do not express detectable levels of CD21, however, transient CD21 expression might result from the engulfment of CD21⁺ cells (Inghirami *et al.*, 1988). Addition of the gp350/220 glycoprotein of EBV to monocytes results in the elicitation of IL-1, IL-6 and TNF-α (D'Addario *et al.*, 1999; 2000). However, addition of the whole virus does not up regulate IL-1 expression and blocks TNF-α secretion (D'Addario, 1999; Gosselin *et al.*, 2001). Finally, EBV infection has been shown to decrease the production of prostaglandin E2 (Savard *et al.*, 2000). This would be expected to induce or favor a Th1 response, but in the face of other virally-elicited cytokines, it probably acts to elicit an inflammatory response, recruiting additional targets for viral infection.

These alterations in innate cellular responses along with the alterations in eosinophils function described earlier likely all contribute to long-term control of the anti-viral immune responses. By controlling the cells which initially determine the direction the immune response is to take, the γ-HV are able to insure that they are able to establish a persistent infection. Using these cells, the virus is able to skew responses made by the immune effectors such that the additional immunomodulatory genes are most effective.

Evasion of adaptive host immunity

The adaptive immune responses are mediated by the CD4⁺ and CD8⁺ T-cells and the antibody producing B-cells. Like the innate responses, there are multiple levels of regulation and therefore, multiple opportunities for viral intervention. The adaptive immune responses provide two critical "improvements" over the innate responses: the memory response, allowing the immune system to react more quickly and effectively to a previously seen pathogen, and response maturation, allowing for a more targeted, higher affinity response to a pathogen. These differences from the innate responses can also be taken advantage of by invading pathogens in the form of dominant epitopes or antigenic variation, both of which can mislead the immune system into making ineffective responses.

Evasion of CTL responses

The cytotoxic T-lymphocytes are CD8⁺ T cells that can directly lyse and induce apoptosis in infected cells, as well as releasing cytokines such as IFN-γ, TNF-α and TNF-β. Presentation of non-self antigens in complex with MHC class I on the surface of infected cells along with co-stimulatory molecules can activate this killing and the γ-HVs have devised several ways of preventing this from occurring as outlined in Table 31.6.

KSHV encodes two genes, K3 (MIR-1) and K5 (MIR-2), whose products are able to down regulate MHC class I from the surface. Respectively, they are the eleventh and fourteenth Orfs from the left end of the genome, encoding products with approximately 40% identity (Russo *et al.*, 1996). They are early lytic proteins and showed increased expression in TPA treated PEL cells (Sun *et al.*, 1999). Work from Krishnan *et al.*, (2004) demonstrated that the K5 gene product is also expressed very rapidly after infection with KSHV. The levels of this protein then slowly decline over the next several days. The K3 and K5 proteins are both type III integral membrane proteins containing a zinc-binding Really Interesting New Gene (RING-CH) sequence at the N-termini, two hydrophobic transmembrane regions and a series of protein motifs important in cellular trafficking in the C-terminus (Coscoy and Ganem, 2000; Ishido *et al.*, 2000; Means *et al.*, 2002; Sanchez *et al.*, 2002). Both have been shown to insert into the ER membrane such that the N- and C-termini are projecting into the cytosol (Sanchez *et al.*, 2002). The PHD domains of these proteins resemble those found in a number of E3 ubiquitin ligases and are capable of mediating self ubiquitinylation when fused to the GFP protein (Coscoy et al., 2001). While the exact mechanism of MHC class I molecule down regulation is still only partially understood, this ability of K3 and K5 to act as an E3 ligase seems critical. The transmembrane regions of these two proteins probably play at least two roles. First, they define the target specificity. K3 is able to down regulate multiple HLA haplotypes, whereas K5 down-regulates a much more restricted set. However, K5 is additionally able to target the cellular B7.2 costimulatory molecule and ICAM-1 adhesion molecule for down-regulation (Coscoy and Ganem, 2000; Ishido et al., 2000; Means et al., 2002; Sanchez et al., 2002). The selection of targets is regulated by the transmembrane domains (Sanchez et al., 2002). Second, these sequences probably allow K3 and K5 multimerization, although it isn't clear what role this plays in their function (Sanchez et al., 2002). Downstream of the transmembrane regions, both contain a conserved series of residues identified as being important in protein:protein interactions and cellular trafficking (Means et al., 2002; Sanchez et al., 2002). Several of these motifs, including a Y–X–X–ϕ endocytosis sequence, direct internalization of the target proteins from the cell surface into the trans-Golgi network (TGN) (Means et al., 2002). From there other motifs, primarily two stretches of acidic amino acids, redirect the target proteins to the endosomal/lysosomal compartment where they undergo destruction by the ubiquitin:proteasome system (Lorenzo et al., 2002; Means et al., 2002). Without MHC class I on the cell surface, no peptides are presented to induce CL activation and K3/K5 expressing cells are able to escape killing (Ishido et al., 2000) (Fig. 31.5). Down regulation of ICAM-1 likely also reduces the non-specific surveillance of cells by $CD8^+$ effectors.

EBV also regulates MHC class I presentation of viral peptides. EBV nuclear antigen (EBNA)-1 is a latent viral protein and contains a glycine, alanine repeat (GAR) region and plays a critical role in maintenance and segregation of the viral episome (Hennessy and Kieff, 1983; Yates et al., 1984). The GAR region inhibits proteasome functioning, greatly decreasing presentation of EBNA-1 peptides derived from full-length protein, as well as limiting EBNA-1 mRNA translation (Levitskaya et al., 1997; Yin et al., 2003; Blake et al., 1997). This has the effect of keeping the levels of EBNA-1 low, but stable, in latently infected cells. In addition to proteasome-independent presentation of EBNA-1 peptides, most likely by professional APCs that take up dead or dying EBV-infected cells, EBNA-1 peptides are probably also generated by degradation of aberrant translation products in a proteasome-dependant manner (Khanna et al., 1996; Lee et al., 1996; Lautscham et al., 2003).

Several papers have now shown that the anti-EBNA-1 $CD8^+$ T-cells are present in most EBV-infected healthy individuals, however, only with more sensitive IFN-γ detection are these CTL detected and not with less sensitive killing assays (Meij et al., 2002; Lee et al., 2004; Tellam et al., 2004; Voo et al., 2004). Given this new information the overall role of EBNA-1 in protection from $CD8^+$ T-cell responses needs to be evaluated. There is a possibility that EBV has evolved a mechanism for allowing limited CTL recognition of infected cells in order to maintain its latency program.

KSHV, like EBV, seems to have evolved a similar mechanism for blocking CTL recognition of its major latency-associated protein, LANA. Like EBNA-1 for EBV, LANA acts in maintenance of the KSHV episome by tethering it to the cellular chromosome (Barbera et al., 2006). Also like EBNA-1, LANA contains long repetitive sequences, that can be broken up into three sections composed of repeats of aspartic acid and glutamic acid, glutamine and glutamic acid, or aspartic acid and glutamine, respectively. These repeat sequences are capable of blocking the processing of CTL epitopes in cis, but not in trans (Zaldumbide et al., 2006). Further exploration of this function by the Moore group has demonstrated that the block occurs both through synthesis retardation and reduced defective ribosomal product (DRiP) formation and processing (P Moore, personal communication). The overall contribution of this viral impediment to MHC class I antigen presentation on viral immune escape still requires further investigation.

The BCRF1 protein, described earlier in this chapter as a deregulator of the interferon responses, is also able to block MHC class I-dependent CTL responses against viral antigens (Fig. 31.5). This protein, like cellular IL-10, is able to down regulate the transporter associated with antigen processing subunit 1 (TAP1) and a proteasome subunit, low molecular weight protein 2 (LMP2), but not the TAP2 protein (Zeidler et al., 1997). The TAP proteins act to transport peptides from the cytosol into the ER, where they can be loaded onto MHC class I, while LMP2 is a constituent of the proteasome, which degrades antigenic proteins into peptides. After treatment of primary tonsillar B cells with human or viral IL-10 both TAP1 and LMP2 mRNA levels were seen to decrease dramatically (Zeidler et al., 1997). So, EBV has hijacked an immunoregulatory cytokine, which likely plays a role in preventing autoimmune responses, to dramatically decreases the $CD8^+$ CTL antiviral responses (Fig. 31.5).

Evasion of $CD4^+$ T helper cell and B cell responses

The $CD4^+$ T helper (Th) cells are able aid in the recognition and elimination of pathogens in multiple ways. The

Table 31.7. Viral B-cell regulators. The B-cell response is controlled both by signals given directly to the antibody-producing B-cell and signals transmitted to T-helper cells, which in turn aid the B-cell response. Both human γ-herpesviruses encode multiple gene products with the potential to alter the host's humoral response through interfering with both of these aspects of B-cell stimulation. The open reading frame, product and potential function are listed for each, with additional details in the text

	Gene	Product	Function
HHV-8	ORF4	KCP/Kaposica	Accelerates the decay of the C3 convertases and drives production of C3d, which binds complement receptor 2 (CR2) found on B cells
	K5	K5 (MIR-2)	Down regulates ICAM-1 and B7.2 reducing T helper cell activation and reducing the B cell response
EBV	BLLF1a/b	gp350/220	Binds to CR2, might interfere with complement mediated B cell stimulation or aid in viral dissemination
	BZLF1	Zta	Down-regulates MHC class II through CIITA inhibition blocking T helper cell activation

Th1 cells, after recognition of foreign peptides complexed with MHC class II, are able to activate macrophages, as well as activating B cells to produce certain subclasses of antibodies. The CD Th2 cells, in an analogous way, are able to drive the activation and differentiation of B-cells such that they produce a wide variety of immunoglobulins. The B-cell responses are closely tied to this activation of the $CD4^+$ T helper cells and binding of non-self peptides by MHC class II. On the surface of B cells, the B cell antigen receptor (BCR) can bind to antigens, which are then internalized and degraded into peptides that are loaded onto MHC class II. These complexes are transported to the cell surface, where they can be recognized by antigen-specific Th2 cells causing the T-cell to produce both cell surface and secreted proteins. This T-cell help causes the B cell to proliferate and its progeny to differentiate into antibody-secreting cells. The threshold of this proliferation and antibody production can be significantly lowered if the B cell is additionally stimulated through the B-cell coreceptor made up of CD19, CD21 and CD18. Antibodies produced by the activated, differentiated B-cells can then act to neutralize and clear free virus, as well as drive antibody-dependent cell-mediated cytotoxicity (ADCC) reactions where NK cells can target infected cells through Fc receptors on their surface.

Both KSHV and EBV have mechanisms by which they can possibly block B-cell responses as outlined in Table 31.7 and in Fig. 31.5. One component of the B-cell coreceptor, CD21, is capable of binding to C3d. The KSHV KCP/Kaposica protein drives inactivation of the complement C3 convertase and production of C3d, detailed more fully earlier in this chapter (Spiller et al., 2003). It is unclear whether this aberrant production of C3d is capable of altering B-cell responses. It is also possible that C3d is produced in order to attract $CD21^+$ B-cells, which KSHV can then target for infection. EBV also targets CD21 through its gp350/220 envelope protein. This protein is a constituent of the viral envelope and is capable of binding to CD21 to aid in viral entry. Again, it is unclear what implications this has for anti-viral B cell responses.

Much in the same way that the KSHV K5 (MIR-2) protein was able to block the anti-viral activities of the NK cells, it is also able to inhibit T-helper cell activation (Coscoy and Ganem, 2001). Both ICAM-1 and B7.2 play crucial roles in inducing T-help. The down regulation and destruction of these molecules, therefore, prevents the induction of a vigorous B cell response (Coscoy and Ganem, 2001). The presence of multiple cytokines that enhance the Th2 response, however, might diminish the immune evasion potential of this mechanism.

The EBV BZLF1 protein, earlier introduced as having a role in altering interferon responses, is able to block IFN-γ-induced MHC class II surface expression by inhibiting the CIITA transcription factor (Morrison et al., 2001). This has the effect of shutting down T-helper cell activation, limiting the humoral response. While a similar mechanism has not been described for KSHV, the presence of multiple genes capable of interfering with the actions of IFN-γ leave open the possibility that MHC class II induction and stimulation of T-help is being blocked in a similar manner.

Finally, the GAR region of the EBNA-1 protein of EBV was originally thought to limit the $CD4^+$ T-cell responses. This doesn't, however, seem to be true. Several groups have demonstrated an ability to detect strong EBNA-1 $CD4^+$ Th1 responses in healthy individuals (Munz et al., 2000; Bickham et al., 2001; Leen et al., 2001; Paludan et al., 2002; Voo et al., 2002). These cells are capable of recognizing LCLs, EBV transformed cells and Burkitt's lymphoma cell lines (Munz et al., 2000; Bickham et al., 2001; Paludan et al., 2002; Voo et al., 2002). Thus, the role of EBNA-1 in escape from Th and B-cell responses needs further evaluation.

Conclusions

An understanding of the mechanisms by which these viruses evade the antiviral immune responses is informative on several levels. First, by examining viral inhibition of specific immune responses much can be learned about regulation and functioning of the immune system. Second, virally-associated neoplasms can be viewed as aberrations where the normal balance between control of the virus by the host immune responses and avoidance of those same responses by the virus has been corrupted. By understanding what responses are capable of controlling viral proliferation in the case of the immunocompetent host then more effort can be directed at vaccinating to induce protective responses.

REFERENCES

Adamson, A. L. and Kenney, S. (2001). Epstein–Barr virus immediate-early protein BZLF1 is SUMO-1 modified and disrupts promyelocytic leukemia bodies. *J. Virol.*, **75**(5), 2388–2399.

Adrian Cabestre, F., Moreau, P., Riteau, B. *et al.* (1999). HLA-G expression in human melanoma cells: protection from NK cytolysis. *J. Reprod. Immunol.*, **43**(2), 183–193.

Alles, V. V., Bottazzi, B., Peri, G. *et al.* (1994). Inducible expression of PTX3, a new member of the pentraxin family, in human mononuclear phagocytes. *Blood*, **84**(10), 3483–3493.

An, J., Sun, Y., Sun, R., and Rettig, M. B. (2003). Kaposi's sarcoma-associated herpesvirus encoded vFLIP induces cellular IL-6 expression: the role of the NF-kappaB and JNK/AP1 pathways. *Oncogene*, **22**(22), 3371–3385.

Anderson, S. K., Ortaldo, J. R., and McVicar, D. W. (2001). The ever-expanding Ly49 gene family: repertoire and signaling. *Immunol. Rev.*, **181**, 79–89.

Aoki, Y., Jaffe, E. S., Chang, Y. *et al.* (1999). Angiogenesis and hematopoiesis induced by Kaposi's sarcoma-associated herpesvirus-encoded interleukin-6. *Blood*, **93**(12), 4034–4043.

Barbera, A. J., Chodaparambil, J. V., Kelley-Clarke, B. *et al.* (2006). Kaposi's sarcoma-associated herpesvirus LANA hitches a ride on the chromosome. *Cell Cycle*, **5**(10), 1048–1052.

Beagley, K. W., Eldridge, J. H., Lee, F., *et al.* (1989). Interleukins and IgA synthesis. Human and murine interleukin 6 induce high rate IgA secretion in IgA-committed B cells. *J. Exp. Med.*, **169**(6), 2133–2148.

Beaulieu, A. D., Paquin, R., and Gosselin, J. (1995). Epstein–Barr virus modulates de novo protein synthesis in human neutrophils. *Blood*, **86**(7), 2789–2798.

Belanger, C., Gravel, A., Tomoiu, A. *et al.* (2001). Human herpesvirus 8 viral FLICE-inhibitory protein inhibits Fas- mediated apoptosis through binding and prevention of procaspase-8 maturation. *J. Hum. Virol.*, **4**(2), 62–73.

Bellows, D. S., Howell, M., Pearson, C., Hazlewood, S. A., and Hardwick, J. M. (2002). Epstein–Barr virus BALF1 is a BCL-2-like antagonist of the herpesvirus antiapoptotic BCL-2 proteins. *J. Virol.*, **76**(5), 2469–2479.

Bickham, K., Munz, C., Tsang, M. L. *et al.* (2001). EBNA1-specific CD4+ T cells in healthy carriers of Epstein-Barr virus are primarily Th1 in function. *J. Clin. Invest.*, **107**(1), 121–130.

Biron, C. A., Nguyen, K. B., Pien, G. C., Cousens, L. P., and Salazar-Mather, T. P. (1999). Natural killer cells in antiviral defense: function and regulation by innate cytokines. *Annu. Rev. Immunol.*, **17**, 189–220.

Blake, N., Lee, S., Redchenko, I. *et al.* (1997). Human CD8+ T cell responses to EBV EBNA1: HLA class I presentation of the (Gly–Ala)-containing protein requires exogenous processing. *Immunity*, **7**(6), 791–802.

Boehm, U., Klamp, T., Groot, M., and Howard, J. C. (1997). Cellular responses to interferon-gamma. *Annu. Rev. Immunol.*, **15**, 749–795.

Borriello, F., Lederer, J., Scott, S., and Sharpe, A. H. (1997). MRC OX-2 defines a novel T cell costimulatory pathway. *J. Immunol.*, **158**(10), 4548–4554.

Boshoff, C., Endo, Y., Collins, P. D. *et al.* (1997). Angiogenic and HIV-inhibitory functions of KSHV-encoded chemokines. *Science*, **278**(5336), 290–294.

Boyington, J. C., Brooks, A. G., and Sun, P. D. (2001). Structure of killer cell immunoglobulin-like receptors and their recognition of the class I MHC molecules. *Immunol. Rev.*, **181**; 66–78.

Burger, R., Neipel, F., Fleckenstein, B. *et al.* (1998). Human herpesvirus type 8 interleukin-6 homologue is functionally active on human myeloma cells. *Blood*, **91**(6), 1858–1863.

Burshtyn, D. N., Shin, J., Stebbins, C., and Long, E. O. (2000). Adhesion to target cells is disrupted by the killer cell inhibitory receptor. *Curr. Biol.*, **10**(13), 777–780.

Burysek, L. and Pitha, P. M. (2001). Latently expressed human herpesvirus 8-encoded interferon regulatory factor 2 inhibits double-stranded RNA-activated protein kinase. *J. Virol.*, **75**(5), 2345–2352.

Burysek, L., Yeow, W. S., and Pitha, P. M. (1999). Unique properties of a second human herpesvirus 8-encoded interferon regulatory factor (vIRF-2). *J. Hum. Virol.*, **2**(1), 19–32.

Chang, Y., Cesarman, E., Pessin, M. S. *et al.* (1994). Identification of herpesvirus-like DNA sequences in AIDS-associated Kaposi's sarcoma. *Science*, **266**(5192), 1865–1869.

Chatterjee, M., Osborne, J., Bestetti, G., Chang, Y., and Moore, P. S. (2002). Viral IL-6-induced cell proliferation and immune evasion of interferon activity. *Science*, **298**(5597), 1432–1435.

Cheng, E. H., Nicholas, J., Bellows, D. S. *et al.* (1997). A Bcl-2 homolog encoded by Kaposi sarcoma-associated virus, human herpesvirus 8, inhibits apoptosis but does not heterodimerize with Bax or Bak. *Proc. Natl Acad. Sci. USA*, **94**(2), 690–694.

Chung, Y. H., Means, R. E., Choi, J. K., Lee, B. S., and Jung, J. U. (2002). Kaposi's sarcoma-associated herpesvirus OX2 glycoprotein activates myeloid-lineage cells to induce inflammatory cytokine production. *J. Virol.*, **76**(10), 4688–4698.

Cohen, J. I. and Lekstrom, K. (1999). Epstein–Barr virus BARF1 protein is dispensable for B-cell transformation and inhibits alpha interferon secretion from mononuclear cells. *J. Virol.*, **73**(9), 7627–7632.

Collins, T., Korman, A. J., Wake, C. T. *et al.* (1984). Immune interferon activates multiple class II major histocompatibility complex genes and the associated invariant chain gene in human endothelial cells and dermal fibroblasts. *Proc. Natl Acad. Sci. USA*, **81**(15), 4917–4921.

Coscoy, L. and Ganem, D. (2000). Kaposi's sarcoma-associated herpesvirus encodes two proteins that block cell surface display of MHC class I chains by enhancing their endocytosis. *Proc. Natl Acad. Sci. USA*, **97**(14), 8051–8056.

Coscoy, L. and Ganem, D. (2001). A viral protein that selectively downregulates ICAM-1 and B7-2 and modulates T cell costimulation. *J. Clin. Invest.*, **107**(12), 1599–1606.

Coscoy, L., Sanchez, D. J., and Ganem, D. (2001). A novel class of herpesvirus-encoded membrane-bound E3 ubiquitin ligases regulates endocytosis of proteins involved in immune recognition. *J. Cell. Biol.*, **155**(7), 1265–1273.

D'Addario, M., Ahmad, A., Xu, J. W., and Menezes, J. (1999). Epstein-Barr virus envelope glycoprotein gp350 induces NF-kappaB activation and IL-1beta synthesis in human monocytes-macrophages involving PKC and PI3-K. *FASEB J.*, **13**(15), 2203–2213.

D'Addario, M., Ahmad, A., Morgan, A., and Menezes, J. (2000). Binding of the Epstein-Barr virus major envelope glycoprotein gp350 results in the upregulation of the TNF-alpha gene expression in monocytic cells via NF-kappaB involving PKC, PI3-K and tyrosine kinases. *J. Mol. Biol.*, **298**(5), 765–778.

D'Souza, B., Rowe, M., and Walls, D. (2000). The bfl-1 gene is transcriptionally upregulated by the Epstein–Barr virus LMP1, and its expression promotes the survival of a Burkitt's lymphoma cell line. *J. Virol.*, **74**(14), 6652–6658.

Dairaghi, D. J., Fan, R. A., McMaster, B. E., Hanley, M. R., and Schall, T. J. (1999). HHV8-encoded vMIP-I selectively engages chemokine receptor CCR8. Agonist and antagonist profiles of viral chemokines. *J. Biol. Chem.*, **274**(31), 21569–21574.

de Waal Malefyt, R., Haanen, J., Spits, H. *et al.* (1991). Interleukin 10 (IL-10) and viral IL-10 strongly reduce antigen-specific human T cell proliferation by diminishing the antigen-presenting capacity of monocytes via downregulation of class II major histocompatibility complex expression. *J. Exp. Med.*, **174**(4), 915–924.

Decaussin, G., Sbih-Lammali, F., de Turenne-Tessier, M., Bouguermouh, A., and Ooka, T. (2000). Expression of BARF1 gene encoded by Epstein-Barr virus in nasopharyngeal carcinoma biopsies. *Cancer Res.*, **60**(19), 5584–5588.

Dempsey, P. W., Allison, M. E., Akkaraju, S., Goodnow, C. C., and Fearon, D. T. (1996). C3d of complement as a molecular adjuvant: bridging innate and acquired immunity. *Science*, **271**(5247), 348–350.

Devergne, O., Hummel, M., Koeppen, H. *et al.* (1996). A novel interleukin-12 p40-related protein induced by latent Epstein–Barr virus infection in B lymphocytes. *J. Virol.*, **70**(2), 1143–1153.

Devergne, O., Birkenbach, M., and Kieff, E. (1997). Epstein–Barr virus-induced gene 3 and the p35 subunit of interleukin 12 form a novel heterodimeric hematopoietin. *Proc. Natl Acad. Sci USA*, **94**(22), 12041–12046.

Devergne, O., Cahir McFarland, E. D., Mosialos, G. *et al.* (1998). Role of the TRAF binding site and NF-kappaB activation in Epstein–Barr virus latent membrane protein 1-induced cell gene expression. *J. Virol.*, **72**(10), 7900–7908.

Devergne, O., Coulomb-L'Hermine, A., Capel, F., Moussa, M., and Capron, F. (2001). Expression of Epstein-Barr virus-induced gene 3, an interleukin-12 p40-related molecule, throughout human pregnancy: involvement of syncytiotrophoblasts and extravillous trophoblasts. *Am. J. Pathol.*, **159**(5), 1763–1776.

Diehl, S. and Rincon, M. (2002). The two faces of IL-6 on Th1/Th2 differentiation. *Mol. Immunol.*, **39**(9), 531–536.

Dittmer, D. P. (2003). Transcription profile of Kaposi's sarcoma-associated herpesvirus in primary Kaposi's sarcoma lesions as determined by real-time PCR arrays. *Cancer Res.*, **63**(9), 2010–2015.

Djerbi, M., Screpanti, V., Catrina, A. I. *et al.* (1999). The inhibitor of death receptor signaling, FLICE-inhibitory protein defines a new class of tumor progression factors. *J. Exp. Med.*, **190**(7), 1025–1032.

Du, M. Q., Diss, T. C., Liu, H. *et al.* (2002). KSHV- and EBV-associated germinotropic lymphoproliferative disorder. *Blood*, **100**(9), 3415–3418.

Endres, M. J., Garlisi, C. G., Xiao, H., Shan, L., and Hedrick, J. A. (1999). The Kaposi's sarcoma-related herpesvirus (KSHV)-encoded chemokine vMIP-I is a specific agonist for the CC chemokine receptor (CCR)8. *J. Exp. Med.*, **189**(12), 1993–1998.

Esteban, M., Garcia, M. A., Domingo-Gil, E. *et al.* (2003). The latency protein LANA2 from Kaposi's sarcoma-associated herpesvirus inhibits apoptosis induced by dsRNA-activated protein kinase but not RNase L activation. *J. Gen. Virol.*, **84**(6), 1463–1470.

Fakhari, F. D. and Dittmer, D. P. (2002). Charting latency transcripts in Kaposi's sarcoma-associated herpesvirus by whole-genome real-time quantitative PCR. *J. Virol.*, **76**(12), 6213–6223.

Feistritzer, C., Kaneider, N. C., Sturn, D. H. *et al.* (2003). Expression and function of the vascular endothelial growth factor receptor FLT1 in human eosinophils. *Am. J. Respir. Cell. Mol. Biol.*,

Feldman, G. M., Petricoin, E. F., 3rd, David, M., Larner, A. C., and Finbloom, D. S. (1994). Cytokines that associate with the signal transducer gp130 activate the interferon-induced transcription factor p91 by tyrosine phosphorylation. *J. Biol. Chem.*, **269**(14), 10747–10752.

Feng, P., Park, J., Lee, B. S. *et al.* (2002). Kaposi's sarcoma-associated herpesvirus mitochondrial K7 protein targets a cellular calcium-modulating cyclophilin ligand to modulate intracellular calcium concentration and inhibit apoptosis. *J. Virol.*, **76**(22), 11491–11504.

Feng, P., Scott, C. W., Cho, N. H. *et al.* (2004). Kaposi's sarcoma-associated herpesvirus K7 protein targets a ubiquitin-like/ubiquitin-associated domain-containing protein to promote protein degradation. *Mol. Cell. Biol.*, **24**(9), 3938–3948.

Foghsgaard, L. and Jaattela, M. (1997). The ability of BHRF1 to inhibit apoptosis is dependent on stimulus and cell type. *J. Virol.*, **71**(10), 7509–7517.

Foster-Cuevas, M., Wright, G. J., Puklavec, M. J., Brown, M. H., and Barclay, A. N. (2004). Human herpesvirus 8 K14 protein mimics CD200 in down-regulating macrophage activation through CD200 receptor. *J. Virol.*, **78**(14), 7667–7676.

Foussat, A., Wijdenes, J., Bouchet, L. *et al.* (1999). Human interleukin-6 is in vivo an autocrine growth factor for human herpesvirus-8-infected malignant B lymphocytes. *Eur. Cytokine Netw.*, **10**(4), 501–508.

Gao, S. J., Boshoff, C., Jayachandra, S. *et al.* (1997). KSHV ORF K9 (vIRF) is an oncogene which inhibits the interferon signaling pathway. *Oncogene*, **15**(16), 1979–1985.

Gorczynski, R. M., Chen, Z., Fu, X. M., and Zeng, H. (1998). Increased expression of the novel molecule OX-2 is involved in prolongation of murine renal allograft survival. *Transplantation*, **65**(8), 1106–1114.

Gorczynski, R. M., Cattral, M. S., Chen, Z. *et al.* (1999). An immunoadhesin incorporating the molecule OX-2 is a potent immunosuppressant that prolongs allo- and xenograft survival. *J. Immunol.*, **163**(3), 1654–1660.

Gosselin, J., Savard, M., Tardif, M., Flamand, L., and Borgeat, P. (2001). Epstein–Barr virus primes human polymorphonuclear leucocytes for the biosynthesis of leukotriene B4. *Clin. Exp. Immunol.*, **126**(3), 494–502.

Griffith, T. S., Brunner, T., Fletcher, S. M., Green, D. R., and Ferguson, T. A. (1995). Fas ligand-induced apoptosis as a mechanism of immune privilege. *Science*, **270**(5239), 1189–1192.

Grundhoff, A. and Ganem, D. (2001). Mechanisms governing expression of the v-FLIP gene of Kaposi's sarcoma- associated herpesvirus. *J. Virol.*, **75**(4), 1857–1863.

Gupta, R., Jung, E., and Brunak, S. (2002). Prediction of N-glycosylation sites in human proteins. *In preparation.*

Guschin, D., Rogers, N., Briscoe, J. *et al.* (1995). A major role for the protein tyrosine kinase JAK1 in the JAK/STAT signal transduction pathway in response to interleukin-6. *EMBO J.*, **14**(7), 1421–1429.

Haller, O. and Kochs, G. (2002). Interferon-induced mx proteins: dynamin-like GTPases with antiviral activity. *Traffic*, **3**(10), 710–717.

Hatfull, G., Bankier, A. T., Barrell, B. G., and Farrell, P. J. (1988). Sequence analysis of Raji Epstein–Barr virus DNA. *Virology*, **164**(2), 334–340.

Hayes, D. P., Brink, A. A., Vervoort, M. B. *et al.* (1999). Expression of Epstein-Barr virus (EBV) transcripts encoding homologues to important human proteins in diverse EBV associated diseases. *Mol. Pathol.*, **52**(2), 97–103.

Henderson, S., Rowe, M., Gregory, C. *et al.* (1991). Induction of bcl-2 expression by Epstein-Barr virus latent membrane protein 1 protects infected B cells from programmed cell death. *Cell*, **65**(7), 1107–1115.

Hennessy, K. and Kieff, E. (1983). One of two Epstein–Barr virus nuclear antigens contains a glycine-alanine copolymer domain. *Proc. Natl Acad. Sci. USA*, **80**(18), 5665–5669.

Hideshima, T., Chauhan, D., Teoh, G. *et al.* (2000). Characterization of signaling cascades triggered by human interleukin-6 versus Kaposi's sarcoma-associated herpes virus-encoded viral interleukin 6. *Clin. Cancer Res.*, **6**(3), 1180–1189.

Hsu, D. H., de Waal Malefyt, R., Fiorentino, D. F. *et al.* (1990). Expression of interleukin-10 activity by Epstein–Barr virus protein BCRF1. *Science*, **250**(4982), 830–832.

Huang, Q., Petros, A. M., Virgin, H. W., Fesik, S. W., and Olejniczak, E. T. (2003). Solution structure of the BHRF1 protein from Epstein–Barr virus, a homolog of human Bcl-2. *J. Mol. Biol.*, **332**(5), 1123–1130.

Inagi, R., Okuno, T., Ito, M. *et al.* (1999). Identification and characterization of human herpesvirus 8 open reading frame K9 viral interferon regulatory factor by a monoclonal antibody. *J. Hum. Virol.*, **2**(2), 63–71.

Inghirami, G., Nakamura, M., Balow, J. E., Notkins, A. L., and Casali, P., (1988). Model for studying virus attachment: identification and quantitation of Epstein–Barr virus-binding cells by using biotinylated virus in flow cytometry. *J. Virol.*, **62**(7), 2453–2463.

Ishido, S., Choi, J. K., Lee, B. S. *et al.* (2000a). Inhibition of natural killer cell-mediated cytotoxicity by Kaposi's sarcoma-associated herpesvirus K5 protein. *Immunity*, **13**(3), 365–374.

Ishido, S., Wang, C., Lee, B. S., Cohen, G. B., and Jung, J. U. (2000b). Downregulation of major histocompatibility complex class I molecules by Kaposi's sarcoma-associated herpesvirus K3 and K5 proteins. *J. Virol.*, **74**(11), 5300–5309.

Jenner, R. G., Alba, M. M., Boshoff, C., and Kellam, P. (2001). Kaposi's sarcoma-associated herpesvirus latent and lytic gene expression as revealed by DNA arrays. *J. Virol.*, **75**(2), 891–902.

Jones, K. D., Aoki, Y., Chang, Y. *et al.* (1999). Involvement of interleukin-10 (IL-10) and viral IL-6 in the spontaneous growth of Kaposi's sarcoma herpesvirus-associated infected primary effusion lymphoma cells. *Blood*, **94**(8), 2871–2879.

Kawaguchi, Y., Nakajima, K., Igarashi, M. *et al.* (2000). Interaction of Epstein–Barr virus nuclear antigen leader protein (EBNA-LP) with HS1-associated protein X-1: implication of cytoplasmic function of EBNA-LP. *J. Virol.*, **74**(21), 10104–10111.

Kawanishi, M. (1997). Epstein–Barr virus BHRF1 protein protects intestine 407 epithelial cells from apoptosis induced by tumor necrosis factor alpha and anti-Fas antibody. *J. Virol.*, **71**(4), 3319–3322.

Kawanishi, M., Tada-Oikawa, S., and Kawanishi, S. (2002). Epstein–Barr virus BHRF1 functions downstream of Bid cleavage and upstream of mitochondrial dysfunction to inhibit TRAIL-induced apoptosis in BJAB cells. *Biochem. Biophys. Res. Commun.*, **297**(3), 682–687.

Kawano, M., Hirano, T., Matsuda, T. *et al.* (1988). Autocrine generation and requirement of BSF-2/IL-6 for human multiple myelomas. *Nature*, **332**(6159), 83–85.

Kenney, S., Holley-Guthrie, E., Mar, E. C., and Smith, M. (1989). The EpsteinBarr virus BMLF1 promoter contains an enhancer element that is responsive to the BZLF1 and BRLF1 transactivators. *J. Virol.*, **63**(9), 3878–3883.

Khanna, R., Burrows, S. R., Moss, D. J., and Silins, S. L. (1996). Peptide transporter (TAP-1 and TAP-2)-independent endogenous processing of EpsteinBarr virus (EBV) latent membrane protein

2A: implications for cytotoxic T-lymphocyte control of EBV-associated malignancies. *J. Virol.*, **70**(8), 5357–5362.

Kirchhoff, S., Sebens, T., Baumann, S. *et al*. (2002). Viral IFN-regulatory factors inhibit activation-induced cell death via two positive regulatory IFN-regulatory factor 1-dependent domains in the CD95 ligand promoter. *J. Immunol.*, **168**(3), 1226–1234.

Kishimoto, T., Tanaka, T., Yoshida, K., Akira, S., and Taga, T. (1995). Cytokine signal transduction through a homo- or heterodimer of gp130. *Ann. NY Acad. Sci.*, **766**: 224–234.

Kledal, T. N., Rosenkilde, M. M., Coulin, F. *et al*. (1997). A broad-spectrum chemokine antagonist encoded by Kaposi's sarcoma-associated herpesvirus. *Science*, **277**(5332), 1656–1659.

Klein, B., Zhang, X. G., Jourdan, M. *et al*. (1989). Paracrine rather than autocrine regulation of myeloma-cell growth and differentiation by interleukin-6. *Blood*, **73**(2), 517–526.

Klickstein, L. B., Wong, W. W., Smith, J. A. *et al*. (1987). Human C3b/C4b receptor (CR1). Demonstration of long homologous repeating domains that are composed of the short consensus repeats characteristics of C3/C4 binding proteins. *J. Exp. Med.*, **165**(4), 1095–1112.

Klouche, M., Brockmeyer, N., Knabbe, C., and Rose-John, S. (2002). Human herpesvirus 8-derived viral IL-6 induces PTX3 expression in Kaposi's sarcoma cells. *Aids*, **16**(8), F9–F18.

Kochs, G., Janzen, C., Hohenberg, H., and Haller, O. (2002). Antivirally active MxA protein sequesters La Crosse virus nucleocapsid protein into perinuclear complexes. *Proc. Natl Acad. Sci. USA*, **99**(5), 3153–3158.

Komatsu, F. and Kajiwara, M. (1998). Relation of natural killer cell line NK-92-mediated cytolysis (NK-92- lysis) with the surface markers of major histocompatibility complex class I antigens, adhesion molecules, and Fas of target cells. *Oncol. Res.*, **10**(10), 483–489.

Krishnan, H. H., Naranatt, P. P., Smith, M. S. *et al*. (2004). Concurrent expression of latent and a limited number of lytic genes with immune modulation and antiapoptotic function by Kaposi's sarcoma-associated herpesvirus early during infection of primary endothelial and fibroblast cells and subsequent decline of lytic gene expression. *J. Virol.*, **78**(7), 3601–3620.

Kumar, K. P., McBride, K. M., Weaver, B. K., Dingwall, C., and Reich, N. C. (2000). Regulated nuclear-cytoplasmic localization of interferon regulatory factor 3, a subunit of double-stranded RNA-activated factor 1. *Mol. Cell. Biol.*, **20**(11), 4159–4168.

LaBonte, M. L., Hershberger, K. L., Korber, B., and Letvin, N. L. (2001). The KIR and CD94/NKG2 families of molecules in the rhesus monkey. *Immunol. Rev.*, **183**: 25–40.

Larochelle, B., Flamand, L., Gourde, P., Beauchamp, D., and Gosselin, J. (1998). Epstein–Barr virus infects and induces apoptosis in human neutrophils. *Blood*, **92**(1), 291–299.

Lautscham, G., Rickinson, A., and Blake, N. (2003). TAP-independent antigen presentation on MHC class I molecules: lessons from Epstein–Barr virus. *Microbes Infect.*, **5**(4), 291–299.

Law, S. K. (1988). C3 receptors on macrophages. *J. Cell. Sci. Suppl.*, **9**, 67–97.

Le Gal, F. A., Riteau, B., Sedlik, C. *et al*. (1999). HLA-G-mediated inhibition of antigen-specific cytotoxic T lymphocytes. *Int. Immunol.*, **11**(8), 1351–1356.

Lee, S. P., Thomas, W. A., Blake, N. W., and Rickinson, A. B. (1996). Transporter (TAP)-independent processing of a multiple membrane-spanning protein, the Epstein–Barr virus latent membrane protein 2. *Eur. J. Immunol.*, **26**(8), 1875–1883.

Lee, S. P., Brooks, J. M., Al-Jarrah, H. *et al*. (2004). CD8 T cell recognition of endogenously expressed epstein-barr virus nuclear antigen 1. *J. Exp. Med.*, **199**(10), 1409–1420.

Leen, A., Meij, P., Redchenko, I. *et al*. (2001). Differential immunogenicity of Epstein–Barr virus latent-cycle proteins for human CD4(+) T-helper 1 responses. *J. Virol.*, **75**(18), 8649–8659.

Leonard, W. J. (2001). Role of Jak kinases and STATs in cytokine signal transduction. *Int. J. Hematol.*, **73**(3), 271–277.

Levitskaya, J., Sharipo, A., Leonchiks, A., Ciechanover, A., and Masucci, M. G. (1997). Inhibition of ubiquitin/proteasome-dependent protein degradation by the Gly-Ala repeat domain of the Epstein–Barr virus nuclear antigen 1. *Proc. Natl Acad. Sci. USA*, **94**(23), 12616–12621.

Li, H. and Nicholas, J. (2002). Identification of amino acid residues of gp130 signal transducer and gp80 alpha receptor subunit that are involved in ligand binding and signaling by human herpesvirus 8-encoded interleukin-6. *J. Virol.*, **76**(11), 5627–5636.

Li, H., Wang, H., and Nicholas, J. (2001). Detection of direct binding of human herpesvirus 8-encoded interleukin- 6 (vIL-6) to both gp130 and IL-6 receptor (IL-6R) and identification of amino acid residues of vIL-6 important for IL-6R-dependent and -independent signaling. *J. Virol.*, **75**(7), 3325–3334.

Li, M., Lee, H., Yoon, D. W. *et al*. (1997). Kaposi's sarcoma-associated herpesvirus encodes a functional cyclin. *J. Virol.*, **71**(3), 1984–1991.

Li, M., Lee, H., Guo, J. *et al*. (1998). Kaposi's sarcoma-associated herpesvirus viral interferon regulatory factor. *J. Virol.*, **72**(7), 5433–5440.

Li, M., Damania, B., Alvarez, X. *et al*. (2000). Inhibition of p300 histone acetyltransferase by viral interferon regulatory factor. *Mol. Cell. Biol.*, **20**(21), 8254–8263.

Lin, R., Genin, P., Mamane, Y. *et al*. (2001). HHV-8 encoded vIRF-1 represses the interferon antiviral response by blocking IRF-3 recruitment of the CBP/p300 coactivators. *Oncogene*, **20**(7), 800–811.

Liu, C., Okruzhnov, Y., Li, H., and Nicholas, J. (2001). Human herpesvirus 8 (HHV-8)-encoded cytokines induce expression of and autocrine signaling by vascular endothelial growth factor (VEGF) in HHV-8-infected primary-effusion lymphoma cell lines and mediate VEGF-independent antiapoptotic effects. *J. Virol.*, **75**(22), 10933–10940.

Liu, Y., de Waal Malefyt, R., Briere, F. *et al*. (1997). The EBV IL-10 homologue is a selective agonist with impaired binding to the IL-10 receptor. *J. Immunol.*, **158**(2), 604–613.

Long, E. O., Barber, D. F., Burshtyn, D. N. *et al.* (2001). Inhibition of natural killer cell activation signals by killer cell immunoglobulin-like receptors (CD158). *Immunol. Rev.*, **181**: 223–233.

Lorenzo, M. E., Jung, J. U., and Ploegh, H. L. (2002). Kaposi's sarcoma-associated herpesvirus K3 utilizes the ubiquitin-proteasome system in routing class major histocompatibility complexes to late endocytic compartments. *J. Virol.*, **76**(11), 5522–5531.

Low, W., Harries, M., Ye, H. *et al.* (2001). Internal ribosome entry site regulates translation of Kaposi's sarcoma-associated herpesvirus FLICE inhibitory protein. *J. Virol.*, **75**(6), 2938–2945.

Lubyova, B. and Pitha, P. M. (2000). Characterization of a novel human herpesvirus 8-encoded protein, vIRF-3, that shows homology to viral and cellular interferon regulatory factors. *J. Virol.*, **74**(17), 8194–8201.

Lutticken, C., Wegenka, U. M., Yuan, J. *et al.* (1994). Association of transcription factor APRF and protein kinase Jak1 with the interleukin-6 signal transducer gp130. *Science*, **263**(5143), 89–92.

Mantovani, A., Garlanda, C., and Bottazzi, B. (2003). Pentraxin 3, a non-redundant soluble pattern recognition receptor involved in innate immunity. *Vaccine*, **21** (Suppl. 2), S43–S47.

Marshall, N. A., Vickers, M. A., and Barker, R. N. (2003). Regulatory T cells secreting IL-10 dominate the immune response to EBV latent membrane protein 1. *J. Immunol.*, **170**(12), 6183–6189.

Marshall, W. L., Yim, C., Gustafson, E. *et al.* (1999). Epstein–Barr virus encodes a novel homolog of the bcl-2 oncogene that inhibits apoptosis and associates with Bax and Bak. *J. Virol.*, **73**(6), 5181–5185.

Masy, E., Adriaenssens, E., Montpellier, C. *et al.* (2002). Human monocytic cell lines transformed in vitro by Epstein–Barr virus display a type II latency and LMP-1-dependent proliferation. *J. Virol.*, **76**(13), 6460–6472.

Matsuda, G., Nakajima, K., Kawaguchi, Y., Yamanashi, Y., and Hirai, K. (2003). Epstein–Barr virus (EBV) nuclear antigen leader protein (EBNA-LP) forms complexes with a cellular anti-apoptosis protein Bcl-2 or its EBV counterpart BHRF1 through HS1-associated protein X-1. *Microbiol. Immunol.*, **47**(1), 91–99.

McColl, S. R., Roberge, C. J., Larochelle, B., and Gosselin, J. (1997). EBV induces the production and release of IL-8 and macrophage inflammatory protein-1 alpha in human neutrophils. *J. Immunol.*, **159**(12), 6164–6168.

McVicar, D. W. and Burshtyn, D. N. (2001). Intracellular signaling by the killer immunoglobulin-like receptors and Ly49. *Sci. STKE*, 2001(**75**), RE1.

Means, R. E., Ishido, S., Alvarez, X., and Jung, J. U. (2002). Multiple endocytic trafficking pathways of MHC class I molecules induced by a Herpesvirus protein. *EMBO J.*, **21**(7), 1–12.

Medzhitov, R. and Janeway, C., Jr. (2000). Innate immunity. *N. Engl. J. Med.*, **343**(5), 338–344.

Meij, P., Leen, A., Rickinson, A. B. *et al.* (2002). Identification and prevalence of CD8(+) T-cell responses directed against Epstein–Barr virus-encoded latent membrane protein 1 and latent membrane protein 2. *Int. J. Cancer*, **99**(1), 93–99.

Miyamoto, N. G., Jacobs, B. L., and Samuel, C. E. (1983). Mechanism of interferon action. Effect of double-stranded RNA and the 5′-O-monophosphate form of 2′,5′-oligoadenylate on the inhibition of reovirus mRNA translation in vitro. *J. Biol. Chem.*, **258**(24), 15232–15237.

Molden, J., Chang, Y., You, Y., Moore, P. S., and Goldsmith, M. A. (1997). A Kaposi's sarcoma-associated herpesvirus-encoded cytokine homolog (vIL-6) activates signaling through the shared gp130 receptor subunit. *J. Biol. Chem.*, **272**(31), 19625–19631.

Moore, M. D., Cannon, M. J., Sewall, A. *et al.* (1991). Inhibition of Epstein–Barr virus infection in vitro and in vivo by soluble CR2 (CD21) containing two short consensus repeats. *J. Virol.*, **65**(7), 3559–3565.

Moore, P. S., Boshoff, C., Weiss, R. A., and Chang, Y. (1996). Molecular mimicry of human cytokine and cytokine response pathway genes by KSHV. *Science*, **274**(5293), 1739–1744.

Morrison, T. E., Mauser, A., Wong, A., Ting, J. P., and Kenney, S. C. (2001). Inhibition of IFN-gamma signaling by an Epstein–Barr virus immediate-early protein. *Immunity*, **15**(5), 787–799.

Mullick, J., Bernet, J., Singh, A. K., Lambris, J. D., and Sahu, A. (2003). Kaposi's sarcoma-associated herpesvirus (human herpesvirus 8) open reading frame 4 protein (kaposica) is a functional homolog of complement control proteins. *J. Virol.*, **77**(6), 3878–3881.

Munz, C., Bickham, K. L., Subklewe, M. *et al.* (2000). Human CD4(+) T lymphocytes consistently respond to the latent Epstein–Barr virus nuclear antigen EBNA1. *J. Exp. Med.*, **191**(10): 1649–1660.

Murakami, M., Hibi, M., Nakagawa, N. *et al.* (1993). IL-6-induced homodimerization of gp130 and associated activation of a tyrosine kinase. *Science*, **260**(5115), 1808–1810.

Muzio, M., Chinnaiyan, A. M., Kischkel, F. C. *et al.* (1996). FLICE, a novel FADD-homologous ICE/CED-3-like protease, is recruited to the CD95 (Fas/APO-1) death–inducing signaling complex. *Cell*, **85**(6), 817–827.

Nakamura, H., Li, M., Zarycki, J., and Jung, J. U. (2001). Inhibition of p53 tumor suppressor by viral interferon regulatory factor. *J. Virol.*, **75**(16), 7572–7582.

Nakano, K., Isegawa, Y., Zou, P. *et al.* (2003). Kaposi's sarcoma-associated herpesvirus (KSHV)-encoded vMIP-I and vMIP-II induce signal transduction and chemotaxis in monocytic cells. *Arch. Virol.*, **148**(5), 871–890.

Nakashima, K. and Taga, T. (1998). gp130 and the IL-6 family of cytokines: signaling mechanisms and thrombopoietic activities. *Semin. Hematol.*, **35**(3), 210–221.

Narazaki, M., Witthuhn, B. A., Yoshida, K. *et al.* (1994). Activation of JAK2 kinase mediated by the interleukin 6 signal transducer gp130. *Proc. Natl Acad. Sci. USA*, **91**(6), 2285–2289.

Nauta, A. J., Bottazzi, B., Mantovani, A. *et al.* (2003). Biochemical and functional characterization of the interaction between pentraxin 3 and C1q. *Eur. J. Immunol.*, **33**(2), 465–473.

Navarro, F., Llano, M., Bellon, T. *et al.* (1999). The ILT2(LIR1) and CD94/NKG2A NK cell receptors respectively recognize HLA-G1 and HLA-E molecules co-expressed on target cells. *Eur. J. Immunol.*, **29**(1), 277–283.

Neipel, F., Albrecht, J. C., Ensser, A. *et al.* (1997a). Human herpesvirus 8 encodes a homolog of interleukin-6. *J. Virol.*, **71**(1), 839–842.

Neipel, F., Albrecht, J. C., and Fleckenstein, B. (1997b). Cell-homologous genes in the Kaposi's sarcoma-associated rhadinovirus human herpesvirus 8: determinants of its pathogenicity? *J. Virol.*, **71**(6), 4182–4187.

Nicholas, J., Ruvolo, V., Zong, J. *et al.* (1997a). A single 13-kilobase divergent locus in the Kaposi sarcoma-associated herpesvirus (human herpesvirus 8) genome contains nine open reading frames that are homologous to or related to cellular proteins. *J. Virol.*, **71**(3), 1963–1974.

Nicholas, J., Ruvolo, V. R., Burns, W. H. *et al.* (1997b). Kaposi's sarcoma-associated human herpesvirus-8 encodes homologues of macrophage inflammatory protein-1 and interleukin-6. *Nat. Med.*, **3**(3), 287–292.

Nieuwenhuis, E. E., Neurath, M. F., Corazza, N. *et al.* (2002). Disruption of T helper 2-immune responses in Epstein-Barr virus-induced gene 3-deficient mice. *Proc. Natl Acad. Sci. USA*, **99**(26), 16951–19956.

Ojala, P. M., Tiainen, M., Salven, P. *et al.* (1999). Kaposi's sarcoma-associated herpesvirus-encoded v-cyclin triggers apoptosis in cells with high levels of cyclin-dependent kinase 6. *Cancer Res.*, **59**(19), 4984–4989.

Ojala, P. M., Yamamoto, K., Castanos-Velez, E. *et al.* (2000). The apoptotic v-cyclin-CDK6 complex phosphorylates and inactivates Bcl-2. *Natl Cell. Biol.*, **2**(11), 819–825.

Osborne, J., Moore, P. S., and Chang, Y. (1999). KSHV-encoded viral IL-6 activates multiple human IL-6 signaling pathways. *Hum. Immunol.*, **60**(10), 921–927.

Packham, G., Economou, A., Rooney, C. M., Rowe, D. T., and Farrell, P. J. (1990). Structure and function of the Epstein-Barr virus BZLF1 protein. *J. Virol.*, **64**(5), 2110–2116.

Paludan, C., Bickham, K., Nikiforow, S. *et al.* (2002). Epstein–Barr nuclear antigen 1-specific CD4(+) Th1 cells kill Burkitt's lymphoma cells. *J. Immunol.*, **169**(3), 1593–1603.

Papa, S., Gregorini, A., Pascucci, E. *et al.* (1994). Inhibition of NK binding to K562 cells induced by MAb saturation of adhesion molecules on target membrane. *Eur. J. Histochem.*, **38** (Suppl 1), 83–90.

Parravinci, C., Corbellino, M., Paulli, M. *et al.* (1997). Expression of a virus-derived cytokine, KSHV vIL-6, in HIV-seronegative Castleman's disease. *Am. J. Pathol.*, **151**(6), 1517–1522.

Paulose-Murphy, M., Ha, N. K., Xiang, C. *et al.* (2001). Transcription program of human herpesvirus 8 (kaposi's sarcoma-associated herpesvirus). *J. Virol.*, **75**(10), 4843–4853.

Pflanz, S., Timans, J. C., Cheung, J. *et al.* (2002). IL-27, a heterodimeric cytokine composed of EBI3 and p28 protein, induces proliferation of naive CD4(+) T cells. *Immunity*, **16**(6), 779–790.

Pober, J. S., Gimbrone, M. A., Jr., Cotran, R. S. *et al.* (1983). Ia expression by vascular endothelium is inducible by activated T cells and by human gamma interferon. *J. Exp. Med.*, **157**(4), 1339–1353.

Pozharskaya, V. P., Weakland, L. L., Zimring, J. C. *et al.* (2004). Short duration of elevated vIRF-1 expression during lytic replication of human herpesvirus 8 limits its ability to block antiviral responses induced by alpha interferon in BCBL-1 cells. *J. Virol.*, **78**(12), 6621–6635.

Prota, A. E., Sage, D. R., Stehle, T., and Fingeroth, J. D. (2002). The crystal structure of human CD21: Implications for Epstein-Barr virus and C3d binding. *Proc. Natl Acad. Sci. USA*, **99**(16), 10641–10646.

Rajagopalan, S. and Long, E. O. (1999). A human histocompatibility leukocyte antigen (HLA)-G-specific receptor expressed on all natural killer cells. *J. Exp. Med.*, **189**(7), 1093–1100.

Rivas, C., Thlick, A. E., Parravicini, C., Moore, P. S., and Chang, Y. (2001). Kaposi's sarcoma-associated herpesvirus LANA2 is a B-cell-specific latent viral protein that inhibits p53. *J. Virol.*, **75**(1), 429–498.

Robberson, D. L., Thornton, G. B., Marshall, M. V., and Arlinghaus, R. B. (1982). Novel circular forms of mengovirus-specific double-stranded RNA detected by electron microscopy. *Virology*, **116**(2), 454–467.

Roberge, C. J., Larochelle, B., Rola-Pleszczynski, M., and Gosselin, J. (1997). Epstein–Barr virus induces GM-CSF synthesis by monocytes: effect on EBV-induced IL-1 and IL-1 receptor antagonist production in neutrophils. *Virology*, **238**(2), 344–352.

Rolle, A., Mousavi-Jazi, M., Eriksson, M. *et al.* (2003). Effects of human cytomegalovirus infection on ligands for the activating NKG2D receptor of NK cells: up-regulation of UL16-binding protein (ULBP)1 and ULBP2 is counteracted by the viral UL16 protein. *J. Immunol.*, **171**(2), 902–9028.

Rooney, C. M., Rowe, D. T., Ragot, T., and Farrell, P. J. (1989). The spliced BZLF1 gene of Epstein-Barr virus (EBV) transactivates an early EBV promoter and induces the virus productive cycle. *J. Virol.*, **63**(7), 3109–3116.

Rovere, P., Peri, G., Fazzini, F. *et al.* (2000). The long pentraxin PTX3 binds to apoptotic cells and regulates their clearance by antigen-presenting dendritic cells. *Blood*, **96**(13), 4300–4306.

Russo, J. J., Bohenzky, R. A., Chien, M. C. *et al.* (1996). Nucleotide sequence of the Kaposi sarcoma-associated herpesvirus (HHV8). *Proc. Natl Acad. Sci. USA*, **93**(25), 14862–14867.

Saifuddin, M., Ghassemi, M., Patki, C., Parker, C. J., and Spear, G. T. (1994). Host cell components affect the sensitivity of HIV type 1 to complement-mediated virolysis. *AIDS Res Hum Retroviruses*, **10**(7), 829–837.

Sakaguchi, K., Herrera, J. E., Saito, S. *et al.* (1998). DNA damage activates p53 through a phosphorylation-acetylation cascade. *Genes Dev.*, **12**(18), 2831–2841.

Sallusto, F., Lenig, D., Mackay, C. R., and Lanzavecchia, A. (1998). Flexible programs of chemokine receptor expression on human polarized T helper 1 and 2 lymphocytes. *J. Exp. Med.*, **187**(6), 875–883.

Sanchez, D. J., Coscoy, L., and Ganem, D. (2002). Functional Organization of MIR2, a Novel Viral Regulator of Selective Endocytosis. *J. Biol. Chem.*, **277**(8), 6124–6130.

Sarid, R., Sato, T., Bohenzky, R. A., Russo, J. J., and Chang, Y. (1997). Kaposi's sarcoma-associated herpesvirus encodes a functional bcl-2 homologue. *Natl Med.*, **3**(3), 293–298.

Sarid, R., Wiezorek, J. S., Moore, P. S., and Chang, Y. (1999). Characterization and cell cycle regulation of the major Kaposi's sarcoma-associated herpesvirus (human herpesvirus 8) latent genes and their promoter. *J. Virol.*, **73**(2), 1438–1446.

Sato, M., Taniguchi, T., and Tanaka, N. (2001). The interferon system and interferon regulatory factor transcription factors – studies from gene knockout mice. *Cytokine Growth Factor Rev.*, **12**(2–3), 133–142.

Savard, M., Belanger, C., Tremblay, M. J. *et al.* (2000). EBV suppresses prostaglandin E2 biosynthesis in human monocytes. *J. Immunol.*, **164**(12), 6467–6473.

Seo, T., Lee, D., Lee, B., Chung, J. H., and Choe, J. (2000). Viral interferon regulatory factor 1 of Kaposi's sarcoma-associated herpesvirus (human herpesvirus 8) binds to, and inhibits transactivation of, CREB-binding protein. *Biochem. Biophys. Res. Commun.*, **270**(1), 23–27.

Seo, T., Park, J., Lee, D., Hwang, S. G., and Choe, J. (2001). Viral interferon regulatory factor 1 of Kaposi's sarcoma-associated herpesvirus binds to p53 and represses p53-dependent transcription and apoptosis. *J. Virol.*, **75**(13), 6193–6198.

Seo, T., Lee, D., Shim, Y. S. *et al.* (2002). Viral interferon regulatory factor 1 of Kaposi's sarcoma-associated herpesvirus interacts with a cell death regulator, GRIM19, and inhibits interferon/retinoic acid-induced cell death. *J. Virol.*, **76**(17), 8797–8807.

Sheng, W., Decaussin, G., Sumner, S., and Ooka, T. (2001). N-terminal domain of BARF1 gene encoded by Epstein–Barr virus is essential for malignant transformation of rodent fibroblasts and activation of BCL-2. *Oncogene*, **20**(10), 1176–1178.

Sheng, W., Decaussin, G., Ligout, A., Takada, K., and Ooka, T. (2003). Malignant transformation of Epstein-Barr virus-negative Akata cells by introduction of the BARF1 gene carried by Epstein-Barr virus. *J. Virol.*, **77**(6), 3859–3865.

Sozzani, S., Luini, W., Bianchi, G. *et al.* (1998). The viral chemokine macrophage inflammatory protein-II is a selective Th2 chemoattractant. *Blood*, **92**(11), 4036–4039.

Spiller, O. B., Blackbourn, D. J., Mark, L., Proctor, D. G., and Blom, A. M. (2003). Functional activity of the complement regulator encoded by Kaposi's sarcoma-associated herpesvirus. *J. Biol. Chem.*, **278**(11), 9283–9289.

Spiller, O. B., Morgan, B. P., Tufaro, F., and Devine, D. V. (1996). Altered expression of host-encoded complement regulators on human cytomegalovirus-infected cells. *Eur. J. Immunol.*, **26**(7), 1532–1538.

Spiller, O. B., Robinson, M., O'Donnell, E. *et al.* (2003b). Complement regulation by Kaposi's sarcoma-associated herpesvirus ORF4 protein. *J. Virol.*, **77**(1), 592–599.

Stahl, N., Boulton, T. G., Farruggella, T. *et al.* (1994). Association and activation of Jak-Tyk kinases by CNTF-LIF-OSM-IL-6 beta receptor components. *Science*, **263**(5143), 92–95.

Stark, G. R., Kerr, I. M., Williams, B. R., Silverman, R. H., and Schreiber, R. D. (1998). How cells respond to interferons. *Annu. Rev. Biochem.*, **67**, 227–264.

Staskus, K. A., Zhong, W., Gebhard, K. *et al.* (1997). Kaposi's sarcoma-associated herpesvirus gene expression in endothelial (spindle) tumor cells. *J. Virol.*, **71**(1), 715–719.

Stine, J. T., Wood, C., Hill, M. *et al.* (2000). KSHV-encoded CC chemokine vMIP-III is a CCR4 agonist, stimulates angiogenesis, and selectively chemoattracts TH2 cells. *Blood*, **95**(4), 1151–1157.

Strockbine, L. D., Cohen, J. I., Farrah, T. *et al.* (1998). The Epstein–Barr virus BARF1 gene encodes a novel, soluble colony-stimulating factor-1 receptor. *J. Virol.*, **72**(5), 4015–4021.

Sun, Q., Matta, H., and Chaudhary, P. M. (2003). The human herpes virus 8-encoded viral FLICE inhibitory protein protects against growth factor withdrawal-induced apoptosis via NF-kappa B activation. *Blood*, **101**(5), 1956–1961.

Sun, R., Lin, S. F., Staskus, K. *et al.* (1999). Kinetics of Kaposi's sarcoma-associated herpesvirus gene expression. *J. Virol.*, **73**(3), 2232–2242.

Swaminathan, S., Hesselton, R., Sullivan, J., and Kieff, E. (1993). Epstein–Barr virus recombinants with specifically mutated BCRF1 genes. *J. Virol.*, **67**(12), 7406–7413.

Tabiasco, J., Vercellone, A., Meggetto, F. *et al.* (2003). Acquisition of viral receptor by NK cells through immunological synapse. *J. Immunol.*, **170**(12), 5993–5998.

Takayama, T., Morelli, A. E., Onai, N. *et al.* (2001). Mammalian and viral IL-10 enhance C-C chemokine receptor 5 but down-regulate C-C chemokine receptor 7 expression by myeloid dendritic cells: impact on chemotactic responses and in vivo homing ability. *J. Immunol.*, **166**(12), 7136–71643.

Taniguchi, T., Ogasawara, K., Takaoka, A., and Tanaka, N. (2001). IRF family of transcription factors as regulators of host defense. *Annu. Rev. Immunol.*, **19**: 623–655.

Tellam, J., Connolly, G., Green, K. J. *et al.* (2004). Endogenous presentation of CD8+ T cell epitopes from Epstein–Barr virus-encoded nuclear antigen 1. *J. Exp. Med.*, **199**(10), 1421–1431.

Thome, M., Schneider, P., Hofmann, K. *et al.* (1997). Viral FLICE-inhibitory proteins (FLIPs) prevent apoptosis induced by death receptors. *Nature*, **386**(6624), 517–521.

Thomis, D. C. and Samuel, C. E. (1992). Mechanism of interferon action: autoregulation of RNA-dependent P1/eIF-2 alpha protein kinase (PKR) expression in transfected mammalian cells. *Proc. Natl Acad. Sci. USA*, **89**(22), 10837–10841.

Volz, A., Wende, H., Laun, K., and Ziegler, A. (2001). Genesis of the ILT/LIR/MIR clusters within the human leukocyte receptor complex. *Immunol. Rev.*, **181**, 39–51.

Von Roenn, J. H. and Cianfrocca, M. (2001). Treatment of Kaposi's sarcoma. *Cancer Treat. Res.*, **104**, 127–148.

Voo, K. S., Fu, T., Heslop, H. E. *et al.* (2002). Identification of HLA-DP3-restricted peptides from EBNA1 recognized by CD4(+) T cells. *Cancer Res.*, **62**(24), 7195–7199.

Voo, K. S., Fu, T., Wang, H. Y. *et al.* (2004). Evidence for the presentation of major histocompatibility complex class I-restricted Epstein-Barr virus nuclear antigen 1 peptides to CD8+ T lymphocytes. *J. Exp. Med.*, **199**(4), 459–470.

Wan, X., Wang, H., and Nicholas, J. (1999). Human herpesvirus 8 interleukin-6 (vIL-6) signals through gp130 but has structural and receptor-binding properties distinct from those of human IL-6. *J. Virol.*, **73**(10), 8268–8278.

Wang, H. W., Sharp, T. V., Koumi, A., Koentges, G., and Boshoff, C. (2002). Characterization of an anti-apoptotic glycoprotein encoded by Kaposi's sarcoma-associated herpesvirus which resembles a spliced variant of human survivin. *EMBO J.*, **21**(11), 2602–2615.

Weaver, B. K., Kumar, K. P., and Reich, N. C. (1998). Interferon regulatory factor 3 and CREB-binding protein/p300 are subunits of double-stranded RNA-activated transcription factor. *Mol. Cell. Biol.*, **18**(3), 1359–1368.

Weber, K. S., Grone, H. J., Rocken, M. *et al.* (2001). Selective recruitment of Th2-type cells and evasion from a cytotoxic immune response mediated by viral macrophage inhibitory protein-II. *Eur. J. Immunol.*, **31**(8), 2458–2466.

Wegenka, U. M., Lutticken, C., Buschmann, J. *et al.* (1994). The interleukin-6-activated acute-phase response factor is antigenically and functionally related to members of the signal transducer and activator of transcription (STAT) family. *Mol. Cell. Biol.*, **14**(5), 3186–3196.

Wei, M. X. and Ooka, T. (1989). A transforming function of the BARF1 gene encoded by Epstein-Barr virus. *EMBO J.*, **8**(10), 2897–2903.

Wei, M. X., Moulin, J. C., Decaussin, G., Berger, F., and Ooka, T. (1994). Expression and tumorigenicity of the Epstein–Barr virus BARF1 gene in human Louckes B-lymphocyte cell line. *Cancer Res.*, **54**(7), 1843–1848.

Wei, M. X., de Turenne-Tessier, M., Decaussin, G., Benet, G., and Ooka, T. (1997). Establishment of a monkey kidney epithelial cell line with the BARF1 open reading frame from Epstein–Barr virus. *Oncogene*, **14**(25), 3073–3081.

Xu, Z. G., Iwatsuki, K., Oyama, N. *et al.* (2001). The latency pattern of Epstein–Barr virus infection and viral IL-10 expression in cutaneous natural killer/T-cell lymphomas. *Br. J. Cancer.*, **84**(7), 920–925.

Yates, J., Warren, N., Reisman, D., and Sugden, B. (1984). A cis-acting element from the Epstein-Barr viral genome that permits stable replication of recombinant plasmids in latently infected cells. *Proc. Natl Acad. Sci. USA*, **81**(12), 3806–3810.

Yin, Y., Manoury, B., and Fahraeus, R. (2003). Self-inhibition of synthesis and antigen presentation by Epstein-Barr virus-encoded EBNA1. *Science*, **301**(5638), 1371–1374.

Zaldumbide, A., Ossevoort, M., Wiertz, E. J. H. J., and Hoeben, R. C. (2006). *In cis* inhibition of antigen processing by the latency-associated nuclear antigen I of Kaposi sarcoma Herpes virus. *Mol. Immunol.*, e-pub.

Zeidler, R., Eissner, G., Meissner, P. *et al.* (1997). Downregulation of TAP1 in B lymphocytes by cellular and Epstein–Barr virus-encoded interleukin-10. *Blood*, **90**(6), 2390–2397.

Zhang, J., Das, S. C., Kotalik, C., Pattnaik, A. K., and Zhang, L. (2004). The latent membrane protein 1 of Epstein–Barr virus establishes an antiviral state via induction of interferon-stimulated genes. *J. Biol. Chem.*

Zhang, L. and Pagano, J. S. (2001). Interferon regulatory factor 7 mediates activation of Tap-2 by Epstein-Barr virus latent membrane protein 1. *J. Virol.*, **75**(1), 341–350.

Zhang, L., Wu, L., Hong, K., and Pagano, J. S. (2001). Intracellular signaling molecules activated by Epstein-Barr virus for induction of interferon regulatory factor 7. *J. Virol.*, **75**(24), 12393–12401.

Zhu, F. X. and Yuan, Y. (2003). The ORF45 protein of Kaposi's sarcoma-associated herpesvirus is associated with purified virions. *J. Virol.*, **77**(7), 4221–4230.

Zhu, F. X., King, S. M., Smith, E. J., Levy, D. E., and Yuan, Y. (2002). A Kaposi's sarcoma-associated herpesviral protein inhibits virus-mediated induction of type I interferon by blocking IRF-7 phosphorylation and nuclear accumulation. *Proc. Natl Acad. Sci. USA*, **99**(8), 5573–5578.

zur Hausen, A., Brink, A. A., Craanen, M. E. *et al.* (2000). Unique transcription pattern of Epstein-Barr virus (EBV) in EBV-carrying gastric adenocarcinomas: expression of the transforming BARF1 gene. *Cancer Res.*, **60**(10), 2745–2748.

Part III

Pathogenesis, clinical disease, host response, and epidemiology: alphaherpes viruses

Edited by Ann Arvin and Richard Whitley

part III

Pathogenesis, clinical disease, host response,
and epidemiology: alphaherpes viruses

Edited by Ann Arvin and Richard Whitley

Pathogenesis and disease

Richard Whitley[1], David W. Kimberlin[2], and Charles G. Prober[3]

[1]Department of Pediatrics, Microbiology, Medicine and Neurosurgery, University of Alabama at Birmingham, Birmingham, AL, USA
[2]Department of Pediatrics University of Alabama at Birmingham, Birmingham, AL, USA
[3]Department of Pediatrics, Stanford University School of Medicine, Scientific Director, Glaser Pediatric Research Network, Stanford University Medical Center, Stanford, CA, USA

Pathogenesis

The transmission of herpes simplex virus (HSV) infection is dependent upon intimate, personal contact of a susceptible seronegative individual with someone excreting HSV. Virus must come in contact with mucosal surfaces or abraded skin for infection to be initiated. With viral replication at the site of primary infection, either an intact virion or, more simply, the capsid is transported retrograde by neurons to the dorsal root ganglia where, after another round of viral replication, latency is established (Fig. 32.1(a), left panel). The more severe the primary infection, as reflected by the size, number, and extent of lesions, the more likely it is that recurrences will ensue. Although replication sometimes leads to disease and, infrequently, results in life-threatening infection (e.g., encephalitis), the host-virus interaction leading to latency predominates. After latency is established, a proper stimulus causes reactivation; virus becomes evident at mucocutaneous sites, appearing as skin vesicles or mucosal ulcers (Fig. 32.1(b), right panel).

Infection with HSV-1 generally occurs in the oropharyngeal mucosa. The trigeminal ganglion becomes colonized and harbors latent virus. However, it has been increasingly common to detect evidence of HSV-1 in the genital tract, usually the consequence of oral-genital sex. When such occurs, recurrences of HSV-1 in the genital tract are uncommon. Acquisition of HSV-2 infection is usually the consequence of transmission by genital contact. Virus replicates in the genital, perigenital or anal skin sites with seeding of the sacral ganglia (Fig. 32.2). As is the case of HSV-1's ability to infect the genital tract, HSV-2 can infect the mouth. Recurrences at this site are uncommon.

Operative definitions of the nature of the infection are of pathogenic relevance. Susceptible individuals (namely, those without pre-existing HSV antibodies) develop primary infection after the first exposure to either HSV-1 or HSV-2. A recurrence of HSV is known as "recurrent infection." Initial infection is when an individual with pre-existing antibodies to one type of HSV (namely, HSV-1 or HSV-2) can experience a first infection with the opposite virus type (namely, HSV-2 or HSV-1, respectively). Primary infection has, more recently, been labeled first-episode disease because some individuals present with what appears to be a clinically severe primary infection but have pre-existing antibodies to the causative type. This observation indicates that individuals may have a well-established latent infection before the first episode of clinically evident disease occurs.

Reinfection with a different strain of HSV can occur, albeit extremely uncommon in the normal host and is called exogenous reinfection. Cleavage of DNA from an HSV isolate by restriction endonuclease enzymes yields a characteristic pattern of subgenomic products. Analyses of numerous HSV-1 and HSV-2 isolates from a variety of clinical situations and widely divergent geographic area demonstrates that epidemiologically unrelated strains yield distinct HSV DNA fragment patterns. In contrast, fragments of HSV DNA derived from the same individual obtained years apart, from monogamous sexual partners, or following short and long passages *in vitro*, have identical fragments after restriction endonuclease cleavage (Buchman *et al.*, 1978). Utilizing endonuclease technology, exogenous reinfection is exceedingly low in the immune competent host.

Unique biologic properties of HSV that influence pathogenesis

HSV-1 and HSV-2 exhibit two unique biologic properties that influence pathogenesis and subsequent human disease. Both viruses have the capacity to invade and replicate

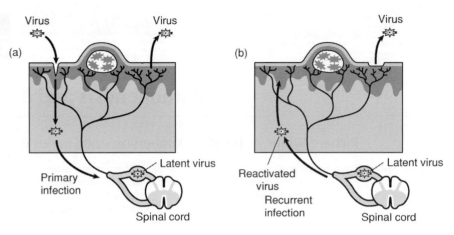

Fig. 32.1. (a) Primary infection. (b) Recurrent infection.

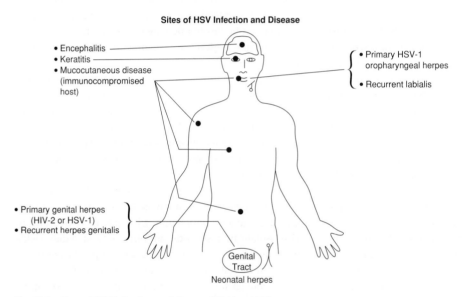

Fig. 32.2. Sites of HSV infection and disease (Whitley, 2001).

in the CNS and the capacity to establish a latent infection in dorsal root ganglia (Roizman and Pellett, 2001).

The term, neurovirulence, encompasses both neuroinvasiveness from peripheral sites and replication in neuronal cells. When paired isolates (brain and lip) from patients with HSV encephalitis are evaluated by PFU/LD_{50} ratios following direct intracerebral inoculation in mice, the encephalitis isolates have lower PFU/LD_{50} ratios than isolates from lip lesions. Neurovirulence appears to be the function of numerous genes (Roizman and Knipe, 2001). In fact, deletion of virtually any of the genes dispensable for viral replication in cell culture reduces the capacity of the virus to invade and replicate in CNS. Mutations affecting neuroinvasiveness have also been mapped in genes encoding glycoproteins. Access to neuronal cells from usual portals of entry into the body requires postsynaptic transmission of virus and, therefore, a particularly vigorous capacity to multiply and to direct the virions to appropriate membranes. In addition, since neuronal cells are terminally differentiated and do not make cellular DNA, they lack the precursors for viral DNA synthesis that are also encoded by the viral genes dispensable for growth in cell culture. Of particular interest, however, is the role of $\gamma_1 34.5$ gene in neurovirulence (Chou et al., 1990; Chou and Roizman, 1986; Hesselgesser and Horuk, 1999; Whitley et al., 1993). Although $\gamma_1 34.5$ deletion mutants multiply well in a variety of cells in culture, they are among the most avirulent mutants identified to date in vivo.

Latency has been recognized biologically since the beginning of the century (Baringer and Swoveland, 1973; Bastian et al., 1972; Stevens and Cook, 1971) and has been extensively reviewed (Roizman and Knipe, 2001; Nahmias and Roizman, 1973; Roizman and Sears, 1987). The molecular basis for latency is addressed in Chapter 33. Following entry, both HSV-1 and HSV-2 infect nerve endings and translocate by retrograde transport to the nuclei of sensory ganglia. The virus multiplies in a small number of sensory neurons, which are ultimately destroyed. In the vast majority of the infected neurons, the viral genome remains for the entire life of the individual in an episomal state. In a fraction of individuals, the virus reactivates and is moved by anterograde transport to a site at or near the portal of entry. Reactivations occur following a variety of local or systemic stimuli.

Patients treated for trigeminal neuralgia by sectioning a branch of the trigeminal nerve develop herpetic lesions along the innervated areas of the sectioned branch (Carton and Kilbourne, 1952; Cushing, 1905; Goodpasture, 1929; Pazin et al., 1978). Reactivation of latent virus appears dependent upon an intact anterior nerve route and peripheral nerve pathways. Latent virus can be retrieved from the trigeminal, sacral, and vagal ganglia of humans either unilaterally or bilaterally (Bastian et al., 1972). The recovery of virus by in vitro cultivation of trigeminal ganglia helps explain the observation of vesicles that recur at the same site in humans, usually the vermilion border of the lip. Recurrences occur in the presence of both cell-mediated and humoral immunity. Recurrences are spontaneous, but there is an association with physical or emotional stress, fever, and exposure to ultraviolet light, tissue damage, and immune suppression. Recurrent herpes labialis is three times more frequent in febrile patients than in non-febrile controls (Baringer and Swoveland, 1973; Roizman and Sears, 1987; Selling and Kibrick, 1964).

Little is known regarding the mechanisms by which the virus establishes and maintains a latent state or is reactivated. There are in fact disagreements on the fate of neurons in which latent virus became reactivated. The relevant issues may be summarized as follows.

1. Sensory neurons harboring virus contain nuclear transcripts arising from approximately 8.5 kbp of the sequences flanking the U_L sequence. These transcripts are known as the latency associated transcripts or LATs. A shorter region is more abundantly represented in the nuclei. The RNA transcribed from this region forms two populations 2 kbp and 1.5 kbp, respectively, and represents stable introns of an unknown, and relatively unstable transcript. The abundant 2.5 and 1.5 kbp RNA play no role in the establishment or maintenance of the latent state although they may play a role in reactivation. These LATs may have an apoptotic function, which might explain the higher efficiency of reactivation of viruses expressing LATs.

   The source of genetic functions required for the establishment or maintenance of the latent state remains unknown. All of the deletion mutants tested to date establish latency but not all reactivate. Whereas establishment or maintenance of latency are functions expressed by dorsal root neurons, the activation of viral gene expression that leads to viral replication does require a full complement of viral gene.
2. Usually, replication of HSV-1 and HSV-2 destroys the infected cell, but reactivation of latent virus may not destroy neurons harboring the virus. This suggestion is based on the observation that patients do not suffer from local anesthesia at the site of frequent, multiple recurrences. An alternative explanation is that nerve endings from adjacent tissues innervated by other neurons extend into the site of the healed lesion (Roizman and Knipe, 2001; Roizman and Sears, 1987).

Pathology

The histopathologic characteristics of a primary or recurrent HSV (Fig. 32.3) reflect viral-mediated cellular death and associated inflammatory response. Viral infection induces ballooning of cells with condensed chromatic within the nuclei of cells, followed by nuclear degeneration, generally within parabasal and intermediate cells of the epithelium. Cells lose intact plasma membranes and form multinucleated giant cells. With cell lysis, a clear (referred to as vesicular) fluid containing large quantities of virus appears between the epidermis and dermal layer. The vesicular fluid contains cell debris, inflammatory cells, and often multinucleated giant cells. In dermal substructures there is an intense inflammatory response, usually in the corium of the skin, more so with primary infection than with recurrent infection. With healing, the vesicular fluid becomes pustular with the recruitment of inflammatory cells and scabs. Scarring is uncommon. When mucous membranes are involved, vesicles are replaced by shallow ulcers.

Pathology of central nervous system disease

HSE results in acute inflammation, congestion and/or hemorrhage, most prominently in the temporal lobes and usually asymmetrically in adult (Boos and Esiri, 1986) and

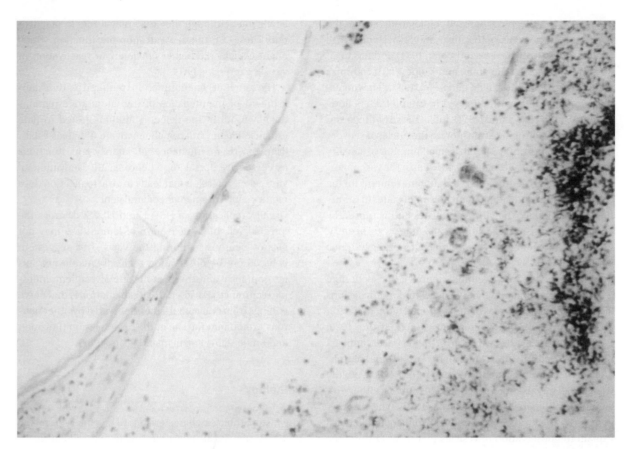

Fig. 32.3. Histopathology of herpes simplex virus infection (Whitley, 2001).

more diffusely in the newborn. Adjacent limbic areas show involvement as well. The meninges overlying the temporal lobes may appear clouded or congested. After approximately 2 weeks, these changes proceed to frank necrosis and liquefication, as shown in Fig. 30.4. Microscopically, involvement extends beyond areas that appear grossly abnormal. At the earliest stage, the histologic changes are not dramatic and may be non-specific. Congestion of capillaries and other small vessels in the cortex and subcortical white matter is evident; other changes are also evident, including petechiae. Vascular changes that have been reported in the area of infection include areas of hemorrhagic necrosis and perivascular cuffing (Fig. 32.5(a), (b)). The perivascular cuffing becomes prominent in the second and third weeks of infection. Glial nodules are common after the second week (Boos and Kim, 1984; Kapur *et al.*, 1994). The microscopic appearance becomes dominated by evidence of necrosis and, eventually, inflammation; the latter is characterized by a diffuse perivascular subarachnoid mononuclear cell infiltrate, gliosis, and satellitosis-neuronophagia (Boos and Esiri, 1986; Garcia *et al.*, 1984).

In such cases, widespread aras of hemorrhagic necrosis, mirroring the area of infection, become most prominent. Oligodendrycytic involvement and bliosis (as well as astrocytosis) are common, but these changes develop very late in the disease. Although found in only approximately 50% of patients, the presence of intranuclear inclusions supports the diagnosis of viral infection, and these inclusions are most often visible in the first week of infection. Intranuclear inclusions (Cowdry type A inclusions) are characterized by an eosinophilic homogeneous appearance and are often surrounded by a clear, unstained zone beyond which lies a rim of marginated chromatin, as shown in Fig. 32.6.

Impact of host response to infection on disease

The pathogenesis of HSV infections is influenced by both specific and non-specific host defense mechanisms (Lopez *et al.*, 1993). With the appearance of non-specific inflammatory changes, paralleling a peak in viral replication, specific host responses can be quantitated but vary from one

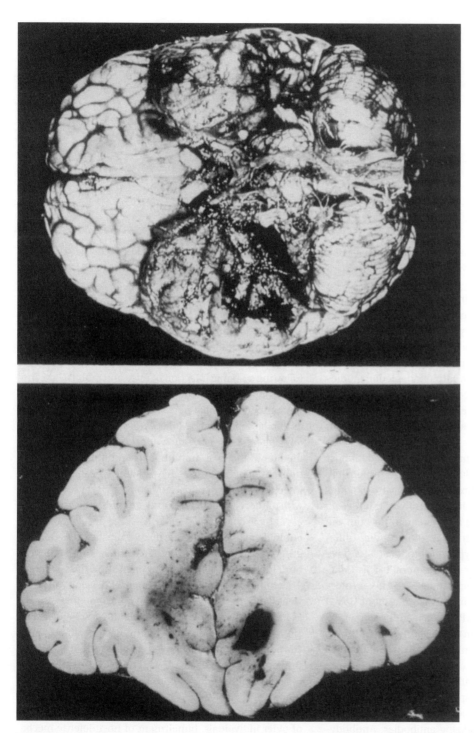

Fig. 32.4. Gross pathologic findings in HSE, illustrating hemorrhagic necrosis of the inferior medial portion of the temporal lobe (Whitley, 2001).

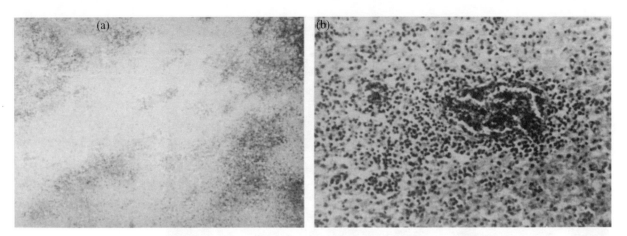

Fig. 32.5. (a) Hemorrhagic necrosis on microscopic examination (Whitley, 2001). (b) Perivascular cuffing on histopathologic examination of a patient with HSE (Whitley, 2004).

animal system to the next. In the mouse, delayed-type hypersensitivity responses are identified within 4–6 days after disease onset, followed by a cytotoxic T-cell response and by the appearance of both IgM- and IgG-specific antibodies. Host responses in humans are delayed, developing approximately 7–10 days later. Immunodepletion studies have identified the importance of cytotoxic T-cells (CTLs) in resolving cutaneous disease. Adoptive transfer of CD8+ or HSV-immune CD4+ T cells also reduces viral replication or protection from challenge.

T-cell lymphocyte subsets have been examined for host susceptibility to infection, including those cells responsible either for H2-restricted cytotoxicity or for in vitro or adoptive transfer of delayed-type hypersensitivity (Kohl et al., 1989). These latter cells have a requirement for both the IA and H2 K/D regions (Nash et al., 1981). Studies utilizing a specific infected cell polypeptide product (ICP4) have identified its requirement for mediation of T-cells (Martin et al., 1988). Prior immune responses to HSV-1 infection have a protective effect on the acquisition of HSV-2 infection (Mertz et al., 1992). Polyclonal antibody therapy will decrease mortality rates in the newborn mouse (Brown et al., 1991). In addition, administration of these antibodies can limit progression of both neurologic and ocular disease. Protection can be achieved with monoclonal antibodies to specific viral polypeptides, especially the envelope glycoproteins. Such results have been accomplished with both neutralizing and non-neutralizing antibodies. Antibody-dependent cell-mediated cellular cytoxic host responses also correlate with improved clinical outcome, as will be noted below for neonatal HSV infections.

Numerous reports have incriminated or refuted HLA associations with human HSV infections. For recurrent fever blisters, these studies have included HLA-A1, HLA-A2, HLA-A9, HLA-BW16, and HLA-CW2. Recurrent ocular HSV infections have been associated with HLA-A1, HLA-A2, HLA-A9, and HLA-DR3. These conflicting associations can be faulted by population selection bias.

Humoral immune responses of humans parallel those following systemic infection of mice and rabbits. IgM antibodies appear transiently and are followed by IgG and IgA antibodies, which persist over time. Neutralizing and antibody-dependent cellular cytotoxic antibodies generally appear 2–6 weeks after infection and persist for the lifetime of the host. Immunoblot and immunoprecipitation antibody responses have defined host response to infected cell polypeptides and correlated these responses with the development of neutralizing antibodies (Bernstein et al., 1985; Eberle et al., 1981). After the onset of infection, antibodies appear which are directed against gD, gB, ICP-4, gE, gG-1 or gG-2, and gC. Both IgM and IgG antibodies can be demonstrated, depending upon the time of assessment.

Lymphocyte blastogenesis responses develop within 4–6 weeks after the onset of infection and sometimes as early as 2 weeks (Corey et al., 1978; Russell, 1974; Sullender et al., 1987). With recurrences, boosts in blastogenic responses can be defined promptly; however, these responses, as after primary infection, decrease with time. Non-specific blastogenic responses do not correlate with a history of recurrences.

Host response of the newborn to HSV differs from that of older individuals. Impairment of host defense mechanisms contributes to the increased severity of some infectious agents in the fetus and the newborn. Factors which must be considered in defining host response of the newborn include the mode of transmission of the agent (viremia vs mucocutaneous infection without blood-borne spread), and time of acquisition of infection.

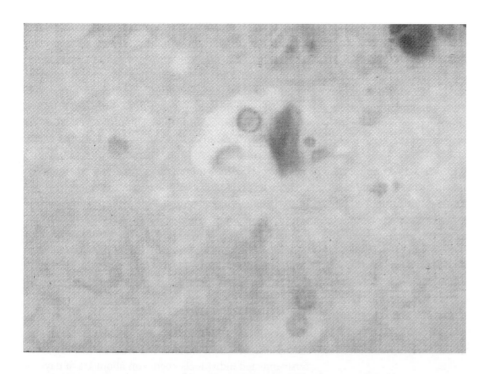

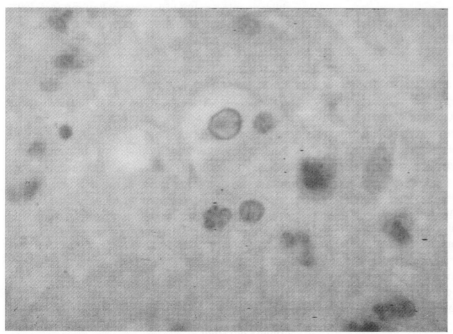

Fig. 32.6. Intranuclear inclusions (Whitley, 2004).

Humoral immunity does not prevent either recurrences or exogenous reinfection. Thus, it is not surprising that transplacentally acquired antibodies from the mother are not totally protective against newborn infection (Kohl *et al.*, 1989; Sullender *et al.*, 1987). The quantity of neutralizing antibodies is higher in those newborns who do not develop infection when exposed to HSV at delivery (Prober *et al.*, 1987). Transplacentally acquired neutralizing antibodies either prevent or ameliorate infection in exposed newborns, as do antibody-dependent cell-mediated cytotoxic antibodies (Prober *et al.*, 1987). Nevertheless, the presence of antibodies at the time of disease presentation does not necessarily influence the subsequent outcome (Whitley et al., 1988; Whitley et al., 1980).

Infected newborns produce IgM antibodies (as detected by immunofluorescence) specific for HSV within the first 3 weeks of infection and increase rapidly during the first 2–3 months, being detectable for as long as 1 year after infection. The most reactive immunodeterminants are the surface viral glycoproteins, particularly gB and gD (Sullender et al., 1987).

Newborns infected by HSV have a delayed T-lymphocyte proliferative response as compared to that of older individuals (Sullender et al., 1987). Most infants have no detectable T-lymphocyte responses to HSV 2–4 weeks after the onset of clinical symptoms (Sullender et al., 1987; Rasmussen and Merigan, 1978). These delayed responses may be associated with disease progression (Sullender et al., 1987).

Infected newborns have decreased α-interferon production in response to HSV antigen as compared to adults with primary HSV infection (Sullender et al., 1987). Lymphocytes from infected babies also have decreased responses to α-interferon generation (Sullender et al., 1987).

Disease consequences

Most individuals who have prior serologic evidence of infection with HSV-1 and/or HSV-2 do not recognize that they have been infected (Whitley and Roizman, 2001). Therefore, most infections are asymptomatic or associated with non-specific signs and symptoms. However, when symptoms do occur, they tend to be more severe with primary compared with recurrent infections. Also, whether accompanied by symptoms or not, viral excretion during primary infection is more prolonged than shedding during recurrent infection.

The most common sites of HSV infection include the skin and mucosal surfaces. HSV-1 and HSV-2 infections tend to be transmitted by different routes and infect different areas of the body but signs and symptoms of infection with either virus are similar (Whitley and Roizman, 2001). In general, infections caused by HSV-1 occur above the waist and those caused by HSV-2 occur below the waist. However, over the last several decades considerable overlap in site of infection has evolved.

Orolabial infection

Primary infection

The oropharynx is the most common site of infection caused by HSV-1. Although most primary orolabial infections appear to be mild or asymptomatic, some young children develop extensive orolabial lesions accompanied by systemic symptoms. A typical course of severe infection includes, high fever, irritability, tender submandibular lymphadenopathy, and a widespread mucocutaneous eruption. Vesiculo-ulcerative lesions involve the palate, gingiva, tongue, lip, and perioral area (Kuzushima et al., 1991). Dehydration, due to impaired eating and drinking, is the most common reason for hospital admission (Cesario et al., 1969). Symptomatic primary infection may evolve over 2 to 3 weeks.

Primary HSV infection in older children and adults can present as pharyngitis. HSV has been isolated from the posterior pharynx of up to 24% of college students with symptoms of pharyngitis, including pharyngeal erythema, exudative or ulcerative lesions on the posterior pharynx and tonsils, enlarged cervical lymph nodes, and fever (McMillan et al., 1993).

Reactivation

Reactivation of HSV from the trigeminal ganglia often is asymptomatic; silent excretion of virus by healthy previously infected individuals occurs on about 1% of days for children and 5% to 10% of days for adults (Scott et al., 1997). In some individuals, viral reactivation, with or without associated symptoms occurs in association with fever, exposure to ultraviolet radiation or wind, non-specific stresses, manipulation of the trigeminal nerve root, or dental extraction (Openshaw and Bennett, 1982). It is estimated that 20 to 40% of adults experience recurrent herpes labialis (Bader et al., 1978; Lowhagen et al., 2002).

The outer edge of the vermilion border is the most common site of reactivation; on average three to five lesions are present. The lesions usually begin as vesicles, evolve into pustules or ulcers after 1 to 2 days, and heal within 8 to 10 days. Prodromal symptoms including burning, itching, or tingling may precede the outbreak by several hours and pain, when evident, is maximum at the onset of eruption, resolving after 4 to 5 days (Spruance et al., 1977).

Genital infection

Primary infection

The majority of primary genital herpes infections occur in the absence of symptoms. When symptoms do occur, they tend to be more severe when infection is caused by HSV-2 than HSV-1 (Whitley, 2001). Systemic symptoms, including headache, fever, myalgia, and backache occur in about 70% of women and 40% of men seeking medical care for primary genital herpes (Corey et al., 1983). These symptoms peak during the first 4 days of infection and abate over the subsequent 7 to 10 days. Itching and local pain often precede visible lesions by 1 to 2 days. Lesions erupt over 7 to 8 days and evolve from vesicles and pustules to wet ulcers over approximately 10 days; crusting and healing follows over the ensuing 10 days. Common sites for lesions in women are the labia majora, labia minora, mons pubis, vaginal mucosa, and cervix. Lesions in men typically are found on the shaft of the penis. More than 80% of women and 40% of men have dysuria for 7 to 10 days. Tender inguinal adenopathy appears during the second to third week of illness and is generally the last sign to resolve. Complications are more common in women than men and include aseptic meningitis, paraesthesias and dysaesthesias of the legs and perineum, mucocutaneous lesions beyond the genital area, pharyngitis, and visceral dissemination. Perianal infection and proctitis are common in men who have sex with men.

Reactivation

Most recurrences of genital herpes are asymptomatic and, on any given day, symptomless shedding occurs in approximately 3 to 5% of women previously infected with HSV-2 (Wald *et al.*, 1997). Importantly, when PCR is used to detect evidence of HSV excretion in the genital tract of women known to have genital herpes, infectivity increases by at least fourfold. Thus, these women can be infectious as often as one out of four days. When symptoms do occur, they tend to be mild; constitutional complaints are present in less than 10% of patients and local prodromal symptoms are apparent in less than 50% (Corey *et al.*, 1983). Genital lesions are few in number and localized; they typically evolve from vesicle to healing in 8 to 10 days. The buttock, thighs and perianal mucosa may be unrecognized sites of recurrent infection. It has been suggested that herpes infection be considered in the differential diagnosis of unexplained recurrent itching, burning, blistering, or erythema at any site below the waist (Simmons, 2002). Approximately one-third of patients will not have recurrent infections, one-third will have two recurrences per year, and one third will have more than six recurrences per year (Whitley, 2001). Emotional stress, menses, and sexual intercourse have been some of the factors implicated in precipitating recurrences.

Keratoconjunctivitis

Herpes simplex virus is a major cause of ocular scarring and visual loss (Simmons, 2002). It is estimated that in excess of 300 000 cases of HSV eye infections are diagnosed each year in the United States (Whitley *et al.*, 1998). Beyond the neonatal period, the majority of these infections are caused by HSV-1. Infection may be unilateral or bilateral, beginning with follicular conjunctivitis associated with pain, photophobia, and tearing and followed by chemosis, periorbital edema, and preauricular lymphadenopathy (Pavan-Langston, 1990). Progressive infection may result in sight-threatening corneal ulcers, characterized by pathognomonic branching dendritic lesions. Healing may be slow, requiring more than 1 month. About one-third of individuals develop recurrences during the ensuing 5 years.

Cutaneous infections

HSV can infect virtually any part of the skin or mucosa. One of the most common cutaneous sites for HSV-1 or HSV-2 infection is the pulp or nail bed of the finger. This is referred to as herpetic whitlow and most commonly occurs in medical and dental professionals, in whom it results from digital contamination with genital or oral secretions (Feder and Long, 1983). When a young child develops herpetic whitlow, it may result from autoinoculation during primary oral herpes infection or when an infected adult trims the child's nails by biting (Feder and Long, 1983). The typical clinical course of whitlow involves the initial appearance of discrete vesicular or pustular lesions over the distal phalynx which subsequently coalesce over several days. Pain often is associated with a tingling or burning sensation. Fever, lymphangitis, and tender swelling of local lymph nodes may be present. The diagnosis of herpetic whitlow is most often confused with bacterial cellulitis.

Close contact between abraded skin and oral secretions results in cutaneous infections caused by HSV-1 among participants in certain contact sports including wrestlers (herpes gladiatorum) and rugby players (scrumpox) (Becker *et al.*, 1988; Stacey and Atkins, 2000). In descending order, the most common sites of infection among wrestlers are the head, extremities, and trunk (Belongia *et al.*, 1991). About 40% of infected athletes have associated sore throat and 25% have fever, chills, and headache (Belongia *et al.*, 1991). Herpes infections also can result in severe cutaneous infection when they occur on skin damaged by diaper dermatitis, burns, or atopic dermatitis (Jenson and Shapiro, 1987; Wheeler and Abele, 1966; McMill and Cartotto, 2000). Finally, HSV is the most common precipitating factor for recurrent erythema multiforme (Orton *et al.*, 1984).

Central nervous system infections

Herpes simplex viruses cause a variety of peripheral and CNS illnesses of infectious and post-infectious nature

(Simmons, 2002; Schmutzhard, 2001). HSV-1 is the most common cause of sporadic severe encephalitis in the United States, accounting for an estimated 10 to 20% of all cases (Lakeman et al., 1995). Without treatment, more than 70% of infected patients die and virtually all survivors have severe sequelae (Whitley, 2001). Encephalitis can result from a primary or, more commonly, a reactivated HSV infection.

Patients typically present with altered state of consciousness, bizarre behavior, and focal neurologic findings, referable to the temporal lobe. Typical abnormalities in the cerebrospinal fluid (CSF) of patients with HSV encephalitis include a few hundred white blood cells/mm^3, with a predominance of lymphoid cells (75% to 100%) and an increased number of red blood cells (Koskiniemi et al., 1984). Protein concentration is normal in about one-half of CSF specimens obtained during the first week of illness, but thereafter concentrations as high as 500 to 1200 mg/dl are common (Koskiniemi et al., 1984). Virus rarely is isolated from CSF but the presence of HSV DNA, identified by polymerase chain reaction (PCR), is sensitive and specific for the diagnosis of HSV encephalitis (Lakeman et al., 1995; Tang et al., 1999).

Typical findings on electroencephalography include focal spike and slow-wave abnormalities, with characteristic paroxysmal lateralizing epileptiform discharges. Focal edema associated with hemorrhagic necrosis may be present on neurodiagnostic images; abnormalities tend to be evident earlier on magnetic resonance imaging than computed tomography.

Other neurologic syndromes associated with HSV infection include recurrent aseptic meningitis (Mollaret's meningitis), brainstem encephalitis, ascending myelitis, post infectious encephalomyelitis, a variety of movement disorders and atypical pain syndromes, and temporal lobe epilepsy (Simmons, 2002; Schmutzhard, 2001).

Neonatal infection

Over 90% of neonatal infections caused by HSV are contracted at the time of delivery (intrapartum infection) but about 5% are contracted in utero (congenital infection). Manifestations of congenital infection include skin lesions and scars, chorioretinitis, microcephaly, hydranencephaly, and microphthalmia (Hutto et al., 1987).

Neonates infected perinatally present with a range of manifestations, categorized as localized to the skin eye and mouth (SEM) or the CNS, or as disseminated infection. In a recent cohort of 79 neonates with HSV infection who were enrolled into a clinical study between 1989 and 1997, 13% had SEM, 35% had CNS, and 52% had disseminated infection (Kimberlin et al., 2001).

Neonates with SEM disease usually present during the first 2 weeks of life; occasionally skin lesions are evident in the delivery room. The cutaneous lesions first appear where there has been trauma, such as the site of attachment of fetal scalp electrodes, the margin of the eyes, or over the presenting body part. Initially the lesions appear as macules but they rapidly evolve to vesicles. Outcome of SEM disease is excellent if diagnosis is considered, and antiviral therapy administered, in a timely fashion (Kimberlin et al., 2001).

Neonatal HSV infection involving the CNS usually results in fever and lethargy, first appearing between the second and third weeks of life. The sign most specific for HSV infection is the presence of skin lesions. However, approximately one-third infants with CNS disease due to HSV infection do not have skin lesions at the time of clinical presentation (Kimberlin et al., 2001). A common but not as specific sign of neonatal HSV infection of the CNS is the sudden onset of seizures that tend to be focal and difficult to control. Usual CSF abnormalities include a mononuclear pleocytosis (<100 white blood cells/mm^3), slightly reduced glucose, and modestly to markedly elevated protein concentration. The electroencephalogram typically is diffusely abnormal and magnetic resonance imaging reveals either temporal or diffuse cerebral disease. If untreated, most neonates with CNS infection caused by HSV die and almost all survivors are left severely neurologically impaired.

Signs of disseminated infection caused by HSV may mimic severe bacterial infection with onset during the first week of life. Common clinical manifestations include vascular instability, hepatomegaly, jaundice, bleeding, and respiratory dysfunction. Approximately 60% of patients develop skin lesions during their illness, but lesions may be absent at the onset of symptoms (Kimberlin et al., 2001). Progression of infection is rapid, with death resulting from shock, liver failure with bleeding, respiratory failure, or neurologic compromise.

Infection in compromised hosts

The likelihood of complicated HSV, with attendant substantial morbidity, parallels the degree of compromise of cellular immune function (Rand et al., 1977). The most frequent complication of HSV infections among immunocompromised patients is slowly progressive and chronic mucocutaneous infections, accompanied by extensive tissue damage and necrosis (Whitley et al., 1984; Whitley, 2004). Contiguous mucosal spread resulting in esophageal, tracheal, pulmonary involvement or visceral dissemination also can occur but fatal infections are not common. Organ transplant recipients, particularly human stem cell transplant recipients, and individuals with HIV/AIDS are at particular risk for both severe and frequently recurrent infections.

Acknowledgment

This project has been funded in whole or in part with Federal funds from the National Institute of Allergy and Infectious Diseases, National Institutes of Health, Department of Health and Human Services, under Contract (NO1-AI -65306, NO1-AI-15113, NO1-AI-62554, NO1-AI-30025), the General Clinical Research Unit (RR-032), and the State of Alabama.

REFERENCES

Bader, C., Crumpacker, C. S., Schnipper, L. E. *et al.* (1978). The natural history of recurrent facial–oral infection with herpes simplex virus. *J. Infect. Dis.*, **138**, 897–905.

Baringer, J. R. and Swoveland, P. (1973). Recovery of herpes simplex virus from human trigeminal ganglions. *N. Engl. J. Med.*, **288**, 648–650.

Bastian, F. O., Rabson, A. S., and Yee, C. L. (1972). Herpesvirus hominis: Isolation from human trigeminal ganglion. *Science*, **178**, 306.

Becker, T. M., Kodsi, R., Bailey, P., Lee, F., Levandowski, R., and Nahmias, A. J. (1988). Grappling with herpes: herpes gladiatorum. *Am. J. Sports Med.*, **16**, 665–669.

Bernstein, D. I., Garratty, E., Lovett, M. A., and Bryson, Y. J. (1985). Comparison of Western Blot analysis to microneutralization for the protection of type-specific herpes simplex virus antibodies. *J. Med. Virol.*, **15**, 223–230.

Belongia, E. A., Goodman, J. L., Holand, E. J. *et al.* (1991). An outbreak of herpes gladiatorum at a high school wrestling camp. *N. Engl. J. Med.*, **325**, 906–910.

Boos, J. and Esiri, M. M. (1986). Sporadic encephalitis I. *Viral Encephalitis: Pathology, Diagnosis and Management*. Oxford, UK: Blackwell Scientific Publishers, 55–93.

Boos, J. and Kim, J. H. (1984). Biopsy histopathology in herpes simplex encephalitis and in encephalitis of undefined etiology. *Yale J. Biol. Med.*, **57**, 751–755.

Brown, Z. A., Benedetti, J., Ashley, R. *et al.* (1991). Neonatal herpes simplex virus infection in relation to asymptomatic maternal infection at the time of labor. *N. Engl. J. Med.*, **324**, 1247–1252.

Buchman, T. G., Roizman, B., Adams, G., and Stover, B. H. (1978). Restriction endonuclease fingerprinting of herpes simplex DNA: a novel epidemiological tool applied to a nosocomial outbreak. *J. Infect. Dis.*, **138**, 488–498.

Carton, C. A. and Kilbourne, E. D. (1952). Activation of latent herpes simplex by trigeminal sensory-root section. *N. Engl. J. Med.*, **246**, 172–176.

Cesario, T. C., Poland, J. D., Wulff, H., Chin, T. D., and Wenner, H. A. (1969). Six years experiences with herpes simplex virus in a children's home. *Am. J. Epidemiol.*, **90**, 416–422.

Chou, J. and Roizman, B. (1986). The terminal sequence of the herpes simplex virus genome contains the promoter of a gene located in the repeat sequences of the L component. *J. Virol.*, **57**, 629–637.

Chou, J., Kern, E. R., Whitley, R. J., and Roizman, B. (1990). Mapping of herpes simplex virus-1 neurovirulence to gamma$_1$34.5, a gene nonessential for growth in culture. *Science*, **250**, 1262–1266.

Corey, L., Reeves, W. C., and Holmes, K. K. (1978). Cellular immune response in genital herpes simplex virus infection. *N. Engl. J. Med.*, **299**, 986–991.

Corey, L., Adams, H. G., Brown, Z. A., and Holmes, K. K. (1983). Genital herpes simplex virus infections: clinical manifestations, course and complications. *Ann. Intern. Med.*, **98**, 958–972.

Cushing, H. (1905). Surgical aspects of major neuralgia of trigeminal nerve: report of 20 cases of operation upon the Gasserian ganglion with anatomic and physiologic notes on the consequences of its removal. *J. Am. Med. Assoc.*, **44**, 3773–3379, 860–865, 920–929, 1002–1008.

Eberle, R., Russell, R. G., and Rouse, B. T. (1981). Cell-mediated immunity to herpes simplex virus: recognition of type-specific and type-common surface antigens by cytotoxic T cell populations. *Infect. Immun.*, **34**, 795–803.

Feder, H. M., Jr. and Long, S. S. (1983). Herpetic whitlow. Epidemiology, clinical characteristics, diagnosis, and treatment. *Am. J. Dis. Child.*, **137**, 861–863.

Garcia, J. H., Colon, L. E., Whitley, R. J., Kichara, J., and Holmes, F. J. (1984). Diagnosis of viral encephalitis by brain biopsy. *Semin. Diagn. Pathol.*, **1**, 71–80.

Goodpasture, E. W. (1929). Herpetic infections with special reference to involvement of the nervous system. *Medicine*, **8**, 223–243.

Hesselgesser, J. and Horuk, R. (1999). Chemokine and chemokine receptor expression in the central nervous system. *J. Neurovirol.*, **5**, 13–26.

Hutto, C., Arvin, A., Jacobs, R. *et al.* (1987). Intrauterine herpes simplex virus infections. *J. Pediatr.*, **110**, 97–101.

Jenson, H. B. and Shapiro, E. D. (1987). Primary herpes simplex virus infection of a diaper rash. *Pediatr. Infect. Dis. J.*, **6**, 1136–1138.

Kapur, N., Barker, S., Burrows, E. H. *et al.* (1994) Herpes simplex encephalitis: long term magnetic resonance imaging and neuropsychological profile. *J. Neurol. Neurosurg. Psychiatry*, **57**, 1334–1342.

Kimberlin, D. W., Lin, C.-Y., Jacobs, R. F. *et al.* (2001). Natural history of neonatal herpes simplex virus infections in the acyclovir era. *Pediatrics*, **108**, 223–229.

Kohl, S., West, M. S., Prober, C. G., Sullender, W. M., Loo, L. S., and Arvin, A. M. (1989). Neonatal antibody-dependent cellular cytoxic antibody levels are associated with the clinical presentation of neonatal herpes simplex virus infection. *J. Infect. Dis.*, **160**, 770–776.

Koskiniemi, M., Vaheri, A., and Taskinen, E. (1984). Cerebrospinal fluid alterations in herpes simplex virus encephalitis. *Rev. Infect. Dis.*, **6**, 608–618.

Kuzushima, K., Kimura, H., Kino, Y. *et al.* (1991). Clinical manifestations of primary herpes simplex virus type 1 infection in a closed community. *Pediatrics*, **87**, 152–158.

Lakeman, F. D., Whitley, R. J., and the National Institute of Allergy and Infectious Diseases Collaborative Antiviral Study Group. (1995). Diagnosis of herpes simplex encephalitis: Application of polymerase chain reaction to cerebrospinal fluid from brain biopsied patients and correlation with disease. *J. Infect. Dis.*, **172**, 857–863.

Lopez, C., Arvin, A. M., and Ashley, R. (1993). Immunity to herpesvirus infections in humans. In *The Human Herpesviruses*, ed. B. Roizman, R. J. Whitley, and C. Lopez. New York: Raven Press, 397–425.

Lowhagen, G. B., Bonde, E., Eriksson, B., Nordin, L., Tunback, P., and Krantz, I. (2002). Self-reported herpes labialis in a Swedish population. *Scand. J. Infect. Dis.*, **34**, 664–667.

McMill, S. N. and Cartotto, R. C. (2000). Herpes simplex virus infection in a pediatric burn patient: case report and review. *Burns*, **26**, 194–199.

McMillan, J. A., Weiner, L. B., Higgins, A. M., and Lamparella, V. J. (1993). Pharyngitis associated with herpes simplex virus in college students. *Pediatr. Infect. Dis.*, **12**, 280–284.

Martin, S., Courtney, R., Fowler, G., and Rouse, B. T. (1988). Herpes simplex virus type 1 specific cytotoxic T lymphocytes recognize virus structure proteins. *J. Virol.*, **62**, 2265–2273.

Mertz, G. J., Benedetti, J., Ashley, R., Selke, S., and Corey, L. (1992). Risk factors for the sexual transmission of genital herpes. *Ann. Intern. Med.*, **116**, 197–202.

Nahmias, A. J. and Roizman, B. (1973). Infection with herpes simplex viruses 1 and 2. *N. Engl. J. Med.*, **289**, 667–674;719–725;781–789.

Nash, A. A., Phelan, J., and Wildy, P. (1981). Cell-mediated immunity to herpes simplex virus-infected mice: H-2 mapping of the delayed-type hypersensitivity response and the antiviral T-cell response. *J. Immunol.*, **126**, 1260–1262.

Openshaw, H. and Bennett, H. E. (1982). Recurrence of herpes simplex virus after dental extraction. *J. Infect. Dis.*, **146**, 707.

Orton, P., Huff, J. C., Tonnesen, M. G., and Weston, W. L. (1984). Detection of herpes simplex viral antigen in skin lesions of erythema multiforme. *Ann. Intern. Med.*, **101**, 48–50.

Pavan-Langston, D. R. (1990). Major ocular viral diseases. In *Antiviral Agents and Viral Diseases of Man*. 3rd edn, ed. G. Galasso, R. J. Whitley, and T. Merigan. New York: Raven Press, 183–233.

Pazin, G. J., Ho, M., and Jannetta, P. J. (1978). Reactivation of herpes simplex virus after decompression of the trigeminal nerve root. *J. Infect. Dis.*, **138**, 405–409.

Prober, C. G., Sullender, W. M., Yasukawa, L. L., Au, D. S., Yeager, A. S., and Arvin, A. M. (1987). Low risk of herpes simplex virus infections in neonates exposed to the virus at the time of vaginal delivery to mothers with recurrent genital herpes simplex virus infections. *N. Engl. J. Med.*, **316**, 240–244.

Rand, K. H., Rasmussen, L. E., Pollard, R. B., Arvin, A. M., and Merigan, T. C. (1977). Cellular immunity and herpes virus infections in cardiac transplant patients. *N. Engl. J. Med.*, **296**, 1372–1377.

Rasmussen, L. and Merigan, T. C. (1978). Role of T-lymphocytes in cellular immune responses during herpes simplex virus infection in humans. *Proc. Natl Acad. Sci. USA*, **75**, 3957–3961.

Roizman, B. and Knipe, D. M. (2001). Herpes simplex viruses and their replication. In *Fields' Virology*. 4th edn, ed. D. M. Knipe, and R. M. Howley. Philadelphia: Lippincott Williams & Wilkins, 2399–2459.

Roizman, B. and Pellett, P. E. (2001). Herpesviridae. In *Fields' Virology*. 4th edn. ed. D. M. Knipe and R. M. Howley. Philadelphia: Lippincott Williams & Wilkins, 2381–2397.

Roizman, B. and Sears, A. (1987). An Inquiry into the mechanisms of herpes simplex virus latency. *Annu. Rev. Microbiol.*, **41**, 543–571.

Russell, A. S. (1974). Cell-mediated immunity to herpes simplex virus in man. *J. Infect. Dis.*, **129**, 142–146.

Schmutzhard, E. S. (2001). Viral infections of the CNS with special emphasis on herpes simplex infections. *J. Neurol.*, **248**, 469–477.

Scott, D. A., Coulter, W. A., and Lamey, P. J. (1997). Oral shedding of herpes simplex virus type 1: a review. *J. Oral Pathol. Med.*, **26**, 441–447.

Selling, B. and Kibrick, S. (1964) An outbreak of herpes simplex among wrestlers (herpes gladiatorum). *N. Engl. J. Med.*, **270**, 979–982.

Simmons, A. (2002). Clinical manifestations and treatment considerations of herpes simplex virus infections. *J. Infect. Dis.*, **186** (Suppl. 1):S71–S77.

Spruance, S. L., Overall, J. C., Jr., Kern, E. R., Krueger, G. G., Pliam, V., and Miller, W. (1977). The natural history of recurrent herpes simplex labialis – implications for antiviral therapy. *N. Engl. J. Med.*, **297**, 69–75.

Stacey, A. and Atkins, B. (2000). Infectious diseases in rugby players: incidence, treatment and prevention. *Sports Med.*, **29**, 211–220.

Stevens, J. G. and Cook, M. L. (1971). Latent herpes simplex virus in spinal ganglia. *Science*, **173**, 843–845.

Sullender, W. M., Miller, J. L., Yasukawa, L. L. *et al.* (1987). Humoral and cell-mediated immunity in neonates with herpes simplex virus infection. *J. Infect. Dis.*, **155**, 28–37.

Tang, Y.-W., Mitchell, P. S., Espy, M. J., Smith, T. F., and Persing, D. H. (1999). Molecular diagnosis of herpes simplex virus infections in the central nervous system. *J. Clin. Microbiol.*, **37**, 2127–2136.

Wald, A., Corey, L., Cone, R., Hobson, A., Davis, G., and Zeh, J. (1997). Frequent genital herpes simplex virus 2 shedding in immunocompetent women: effect of acyclovir treatment. *J. Clin. Investig.*, **99**, 1092–1097.

Wheeler, C. E., Jr. and Abele, D. C. (1966). Eczema herpeticum, primary and recurrent. *Arch. Dermatol.*, **93**, 162–173.

Whitley, R. J. (2001). Herpes simplex virus. In *Fields' Virology*, 4th edn, ed. D. M. Knipe, R. M. Howley, D. Griffin, R. Lamb,

M. Martin and S. E. Straus. New York: Lippincott Williams & Wilkins, 2461–2509.

Whitley, R. J. (2004). Herpes simplex virus. In *Infections of the Central Nervous System*, 3rd edn, ed. W. M. Scheld, R. J. Whitley, and C. M. Marra. New York: Lippincott Williams & Wilkins, 123–144.

Whitley, R. J. and Roizman, B. (2001). Herpes simplex viruses. *Lancet*, **357**, 1513–1518.

Whitley, R. J., Nahmias, A. J., Visitine, A. M., Fleming, C. L., Alford, C. A., Jr., and the National Institute of Allergy and Infectious Diseases Collaborative Antiviral Study Group. (1980). The natural history of herpes simplex virus infection of mother and newborn. *Pediatrics*, **66**, 489–494.

Whitley, R. J., Levin, M., Barton, N. *et al.* (1984). Infections caused by herpes simplex virus in the immunocompromised host: natural history and topical acyclovir therapy. *J. Infect. Dis.*, **150**, 323–329.

Whitley, R. J., Corey, L., Arvin, A. *et al.* (1988). Changing presentation of herpes simplex virus infection in neonates. *J. Infect. Dis.*, **158**, 109–116.

Whitley, R. J., Kern, E. R., Chatterjee, S., Chou, J., and Roizman, B. (1993). Replication, establishment of latency, and induced reactivation of herpes simplex virus $\gamma_1 34.5$ deletion mutants in rodent models. *J. Clin. Invest.*, **91**, 2837–2843.

Whitley, R. J., Kimberlin, D. W., and Roizman, B. (1998). Herpes simplex virus. *Clin. Infect. Dis.*, **26**, 541–555.

Molecular basis of HSV latency and reactivation

Chris M. Preston[1] and Stacey Efstathiou[2]

[1] Medical Research Council Virology Unit, Scotland, UK
[2] Division of Virology, Department of Pathology, University of Cambridge, UK

Introduction

Primary infection with HSV-1 or HSV-2 results in productive replication of the virus at the site of infection, following the pattern of gene expression described elsewhere in this volume. During this initial phase, virus enters sensory neurons via their termini and retrograde transport takes the genome to the neuronal nuclei in the sensory ganglia that innervate the infected dermatome. At early times after infection, virus replication occurs in ganglionic neurons but within a few days no virus can be detected. The genome, however, persists in neurons in a latent state from which it reactivates periodically to resume replication and produce infectious virus. This reactivation event may be "spontaneous" but is generally thought to be provoked by stress stimuli that act on the neuron, or at a peripheral site innervated by the infected ganglion, or systemically. Three phases of latency are recognized. Establishment occurs during the period following primary infection, and although virus replication can be detected in a proportion of neurons during this phase, the initiation and normal progression of productive infection and cell death is arrested in those neurons destined to become latently infected. Unravelling the way in which the seemingly inexorable progression of the gene expression program is blocked constitutes a major challenge for the molecular virologist. The maintenance phase of latency is characterized by the lifelong retention of the HSV genome in a silent state, characterized by repression of all viral lytic genes. One region, encoding the latency-associated transcripts (LATs), remains active during latency. Questions relating to the maintenance of the latent state focus on the structure of the genome, the mechanisms that silence it, and the specific properties of the LAT transcription unit that enable it to remain active. During the reactivation phase the silent genome responds to cellular signals that provoke the resumption of viral gene expression. The molecular basis for this dramatic functional reversal is poorly understood and is the subject of considerable research effort. In view of the specific association of LAT with the latent state, questions concerning the role of this transcript pervade all aspects of latency.

Model systems to study latency

Animal systems provide the most relevant means of studying HSV latency. In mice, latency can be established efficiently and relatively reproducibly after inoculation with HSV-1 in the cornea, ear, footpad, or at other peripheral sites. The virus replicates at the site of inoculation, and as a consequence the exact dose applied to nerve termini is undefined and changing over the first few days. These factors complicate quantitative aspects of latency studies. Reactivation is difficult to achieve in mice and most investigations have relied on explantation of ganglia, with subsequent culture in the laboratory, to recover virus (Stevens and Cook, 1971). An in vivo protocol has been developed in which reactivation is achieved by exposure of mice to transient hyperthermia (Sawtell and Thompson, 1992b). While this method is inefficient in terms of the number of reactivation events per animal, it represents the most relevant mouse model currently available for paralleling latency in humans. In the rabbit, inoculation of the cornea results in latency that, for certain strains of HSV-1 such as McKrea, is characterized by long-term periodic virus shedding, described as spontaneous reactivation. Production of virus can be enhanced by procedures such as iontophoresis of epinephrine into the eye. For HSV-2, inoculation into the guinea pig vagina results in latency in which virus is periodically shed to form lesions that can be scored. Therefore, the rabbit and guinea pig provide reasonable models for

HSV-1 and HSV-2, respectively, in humans but they are more difficult and expensive to use than the mouse. All animal systems entail inoculation with relatively high virus doses, often just short of fatal, and it is by no means clear how this relates to natural infection. A further problem is the considerable variation in the efficiency of establishment of latency and reactivation between strains of HSV, a factor that frequently causes confusion when comparisons are made between the results from different laboratories.

As a more tractable system, infection of cultured neurons has been investigated (Wilcox and Johnson, 1988; Arthur et al., 2001). These cells are susceptible to lytic infection with HSV, but if measures are taken to prevent virus replication, long-term retention of the viral genome can be achieved. LAT can be detected in a proportion of neurons, but all other viral genes are repressed. Production of virus can be induced by removal of nerve growth factor (NGF), inhibition of histone deacetylases, or various treatments that activate signal transduction pathways (Smith et al., 1992). Alternatively, cultures may be made from ganglia dissected from mice harboring latent HSV; in this case, heat shock or treatment with dexamethasone are the most effective reactivation stimuli (Halford et al., 1996).

The final type of model involves the infection of standard tissue culture cells, usually human fibroblasts, with HSV-1 mutants that are impaired for immediate early (IE) gene expression and thus do not kill cells (Preston and Nicholl, 1997; Samaniego et al., 1998). The viral genome is retained in a quiescent state in which all gene expression, including that of LAT, is repressed. The only known way of reactivating quiescent virus is to provide the HSV IE protein ICP0 by superinfection of cultures. Fibroblast systems may mimic some, but certainly not all, aspects of latency.

The latent genome

Latent HSV DNA does not contain detectable termini and almost certainly exists as a circular episome, in contrast to the linear state in the virus particle (Rock and Fraser, 1983; Efstathiou et al., 1986). Quiescent genomes stably retained in fibroblasts are also circular (Jamieson et al., 1995; Jackson and DeLuca, 2003). Various methods of quantifying viral DNA load revealed that latently infected neurons must contain, on average, many more than one HSV genome copy per infected cell. This conclusion has been verified by the use of "contextual analysis" (CXA), in which individual neurons or small groups of cells are separated and analyzed by polymerase chain reaction (PCR) (Sawtell, 1997). The latent viral genome copy number varied generally between 1 and 100, but a small proportion of neurons contained more than 1000 viral DNA molecules per cell. Likely, the retention of such high copy numbers has an influence on neuronal physiology, and recent studies have shown that latently infected ganglia contain increased levels of certain cellular gene products (Kramer et al., 2003). Furthermore, analysis of latent DNA at a gross level is skewed towards the few neurons containing thousands of viral genomes. Surprisingly, for reasons that are not understood, latent viral DNA cannot be detected by *in situ* hybridization (ISH), therefore *in situ* PCR has been applied to investigate the number of neurons that harbor HSV genomes. This approach shows that many more cells contain DNA than are detected by ISH for LAT; thus, LAT is not an unambiguous marker for latent HSV. Laser capture microdissection, in which individual neurons are excised and analyzed by PCR, confirmed that viral genomes can be isolated from LAT-negative (LAT-) neurons and essentially agreed with the quantification from CXA (Chen et al., 2002). The conclusion that there is a population of latently infected neurons that does not express LAT may depend on the sensitivity of ISH, since a study using *in situ* RT-PCR suggested that LAT was present in all HSV DNA-containing neurons, albeit at low concentration in many (Ramakrishnan et al., 1996).

In cells, silencing of large gene blocks occurs at the level of chromatin structure, and it is therefore suspected that an organization of this type applies to the latent viral genome. One study has addressed this issue and found that all regions of HSV DNA examined, including the LAT region, exhibit a regular nucleosomal pattern in mouse brain stem (Deshmane and Fraser, 1989). Interpretation of this result is complicated by the fact that reactivation from brain stem is inefficient and, unfortunately, it was not possible to obtain sufficient material from trigeminal ganglia for similar analyses. More recently, the application of chromatin immunoprecipitation (ChiP) assays has demonstrated the importance of histone modifications in the maintenance of latency. It is well established that post-translational modification of the amino terminal tails of histones is involved in the regulation of transcription. Thus hyperacetylation of histones is generally associated with an "open chromatin" conformation and transcriptional activity, whilst histone hypoacetylation is associated with condensed chromatin and gene silencing. Recent work on HSV-1 suggests that chromatinization of the viral genome and certain accompanying histone modifications offer a means to regulate virus gene expression during lytic infection (Herrera and Triezenberg, 2004; Kent et al., 2004). In the context of latency it is of particular significance that ChiP assays have shown the LAT promoter to be enriched with acetylated histone H3 whilst representative lytic cycle promoters exhibit a decreased association with acetylated histones (Kubat et al., 2004a,b). The demonstration that enrichment of acetylated histones on the ICP0 promoter following the application of a reactivation stimulus by ganglionic explantation strongly supports the view that genome derepression is linked to the acetylation status of histones positioned on lytic cycle promoters (Amelio et al., 2006). Furthermore, it has been shown that a LAT- mutant exhibits enrichment of histone modifications associated with transcriptional activation during latency, suggesting that LAT-encoded functions facilitate maintenance of a repressed chromatinized genome (Wang et al., 2005). Since HSV replication in ganglia precedes latency, it has long been suspected that some viral genomes are derived from residual replication intermediates rather than from virions delivered from the periphery. During infection with TK-mutants, which replicate at the site of inoculation but not in neurons, high copy number retention of TK-virus genomes is possible and therefore some neurons can receive hundreds of viruses from the periphery (Thompson and Sawtell, 2000). In general, however, TK-mutants deposit less latent DNA than wild type virus. However, depending on the site of inoculation, TK-mutants replicate less efficiently peripherally. Thus, apparently normal latency can be established without viral replication in neurons.

The latency-associated transcripts

The only transcripts detectable during latency are the LATs, which map to the viral repeats flanking U_L (Fig. 33.1). These have been detected in latently infected neuronal tissues from experimentally infected animals and following natural infection in humans (Stevens et al., 1987). Similar transcripts are synthesized during latent infection by HSV-2 and other alphaherpesviruses such as bovine herpesvirus-1 (BHV-1) and pseudorabies virus.

Structure of LATs

In HSV-1, the LATs comprise a series of colinear predominantly nuclear transcripts. They consist of a highly abundant non-polyadenylated major species of 2.0 kb that is derived by splicing from a less abundant precursor RNA termed minor (m) LAT. The mLAT is transcribed antisense to the ICP0 gene and extends to a polyadenylation signal in the short repeat region. Based on the sequence analysis of HSV-1 strain 17, in LAT spans nucleotides 118 801 to 127 143 and consists of a primary transcript of 8.3 kb. Current evidence supports the view that the 2.0 kb major LAT is an unusually stable intron which is present to at least 40 000 copies per cell. The stability of this RNA is a consequence of inefficient debranching of the intron, due to the presence of a unique non-consensus guanosine branchpoint resulting in persistence of major LAT as a lariat. Further splicing of the 2.0 kb major LAT RNA occurs within neurons to produce an additional stable RNA species of 1.5 kb, which is also considered to accumulate as a stable lariat (Zabolotny et al., 1997). A less complex pattern of transcription is observed during lytic infection of cells in culture. In this setting, synthesis of the 2.0 kb LAT can be detected late in infection but there is a notable absence of the 1.5 kb major LAT species. Furthermore, a fully processed transcript composed of the spliced exons of the primary transcript has not been detected during productive or latent infection, presumably reflecting the rapid degradation of this RNA species. ISH studies of latently infected sensory neurons have shown that major LATs have a diffuse nuclear localization pattern whereas mLATs are localized within discrete nuclear foci that may represent sites of accumulation or synthesis (Arthur et al., 1993). In contrast, during productive infection of cells in culture the 2 kb LAT intron is also found in the cytoplasm and associates with both ribosomal and splicing complexes in infected cells (Ahmed and Fraser, 2001). More recently it has been shown that herpesviruses, including HSV-1, encode micro (mi) RNAs (Pfeffer et al., 2005; Cui et al., 2006). Interestingly, a single miRNA generated from the exon 1 region of LATs has been shown to exert an anti-apoptotic effect by targeting transforming growth factor (TGF) beta and SMAD3 expression (Gupta et al., 2006).

The LAT promoter

Analyses of the HSV-1 DNA sequence upstream from the minor LAT transcription start site identified a TATA box (nt 118 647), a CAAT box (nt 118 647), two CREB binding sites, and SP1 binding sites, making this a candidate LAT promoter element (LAP1). To define the role played by LAP1 in LAT synthesis, a small fragment including the TATA box was deleted (Dobson et al., 1989). Although such a virus could establish latency, no LATs were produced. In addition when the rabbit beta-globin gene was inserted downstream of the TATA box, beta-globin specific RNA, but no major LATs, were transcribed in latently infected neurons. These data are consistent with latent phase transcription initiating from LAP1 to produce the large mLAT species, which is subsequently processed to generate the stable major LAT species. Considerable effort has gone into studying the activity of LAP1 in transient assays. These studies have revealed that this promoter has a high basal activity in

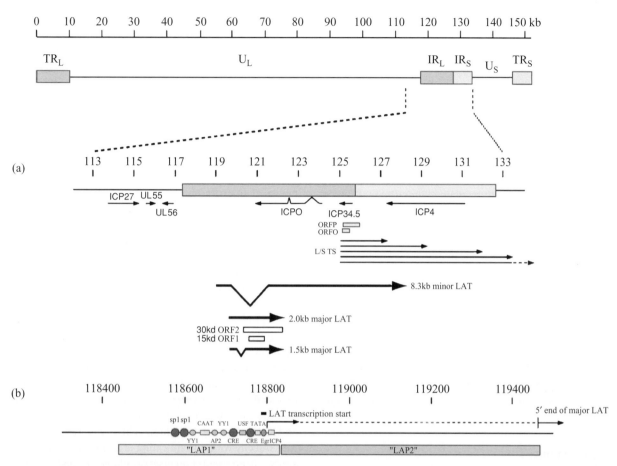

Fig. 33.1. Location and organization of HSV-1 LATs. The IR_L/IR_S region of the genome is expanded in part (a). In addition to the LATs, the positions of lytic cycle genes and a set of transcripts known as L/STs, which specify ORFs O and P, are shown. The functions of L/STs are unclear. The LAP1 and LAP2 promoters are depicted in (b).

a variety of non-neuronal cell types and shows enhanced activity in cells of neuronal origin, an observation consistent with the identification of neuron specific transcription factors which bind to upstream regions of the promoter. Since LATs are expressed to high levels in only a small proportion of latently infected neurons it is likely that their expression is tightly regulated during the various stages of latency. In support of this view, transient promoter assays in PC12 cells have identified *cis*-acting sequences which are required for activation by NGF and sodium butyrate, which mediate their affects via the Ras and Raf signalling pathways (Frazier *et al.*, 1996). The in vivo significance of these observations is unclear, although it has been suggested that the upregulation of LATs *via* expression of neurotrophins could function to block reactivation.

LAP1 contains two cAMP response elements (CREs), located at −38 bp (CRE1) and −77 bp (CRE2) relative to the LAT transcription start site, which appear to play an important role in virus reactivation. The CRE1 element has been shown to facilitate both epinephrine-induced reactivation in rabbits and reactivation in mice induced by hyperthermic stress or explantation of ganglia (Bloom *et al.*, 1996, 1997; Marquart *et al.*, 2001). Although these studies suggested that cAMP mediated up-regulation of LATs may be associated with reactivation, it is of interest to note that an *in vitro* neuronal latency model has linked expression of inducible cAMP repressors (ICERs) with downregulation of LATs and subsequent virus reactivation (Colgin *et al.*, 2001). Located adjacent to the LAP1 transcription start site is a binding site for ICP4 which functions to repress expression of LATs during lytic cycle replication. The mechanism by which the LAT promoter remains active during latency and escapes the otherwise global repression which is so efficiently imposed on the latent genome has been subject to much investigation. The observation that LAP1 deleted viruses are able to express 2 kb major LAT during lytic infection in culture but not during latency in vivo implied the existence of a second promoter between LAP1 and the start of the major LAT intron (Nicosia et al., 1993). A 600 bp fragment within this region was subsequently shown to exhibit promoter activity and was designated LAP2. This second latency associated promoter drives low level reporter gene expression when inserted at an ectopic site in the virus genome. However, despite its designation it would appear that LAP2 functions principally during lytic infection and appears to make a minimal contribution to LATs expression during latency (Chen et al., 1995).

LAP1 is insufficient to mediate long-term latent phase expression, because insertion of reporter genes downstream of LAP1 results in only transient latent phase gene expression. Such studies indicate that although LAP1 contains elements necessary for neuronal expression, additional regulatory sequences are necessary for long-term promoter activity. A long-term expression element (LTE) has been shown to reside downstream of the LAP transcription start site and corresponds to a 1.5 kb fragment which contains an enhancer element and LAP2. Despite extensive efforts it has proven difficult to genetically dissect the downstream LTE sequence. This raises the possibility that the LTE cooperates with LAP1 to direct latent phase transcription (Lachmann and Efstathiou, 1997; Berthomme et al., 2001).

Major LAT ORFs

Major LAT contains two prominent ORFs with the potential to encode proteins of 30 and 15 kd (Fig. 33.1). The lack of conservation of these ORFs between HSV-1 and HSV-2 and the lack of any detectable in vivo latency phenotypes of mutants in which these ORFs are disrupted has suggested that they are unlikely to be of functional significance. Nonetheless, cell lines expressing the 30 kd ORF2 can support the replication of virus mutants defective for IE gene expression and therefore that the ORF can overcome the repression characteristic of quiescent HSV (Thomas et al., 2002). This raises the possibility that this ORF could play a role in reactivation. The significance of these observations remains unclear since there is currently no evidence for the expression of this ORF during infection or following the induction of reactivation from latency; further research in this area is clearly warranted.

Establishment of latency

Specific features of the neuron must be crucial for the interruption of the normal gene expression program during the establishment of latency. The point of arrest in neurons is not known at present, but a number of possibilities, not necessarily mutually exclusive, have been proposed. A description that includes all of the current data and hypotheses in a consistent manner cannot be presented, thus the concepts that are currently favored will be considered separately.

A block to HSV IE transcription

The hypothesis that viral IE transcription fails in neurons has its origins in the observation from tissue culture studies that synthesis of IE proteins is essential for virus replication. HSV mutants with mutations that prevent IE gene expression are not cytotoxic but instead are retained in a quiescent state; therefore, artificial measures to block IE protein production lead to a latency-like interaction in fibroblasts. In mouse ganglia, neurons express either viral antigens or LAT but rarely both during the first few days after infection, suggesting that early events determine the outcome of infection and that latency is incompatible with productive replication (Margolis et al., 1992). Virus mutants that are unable to replicate in neurons still can establish latency. In particular, long term latent promoter activity was observed after inoculation of mice with high doses of HSV-1 mutants that lack the three major transcription activators VP16, ICP0 and ICP4 (Marshall et al., 2000). These mutants enter neurons directly without replicating at a peripheral site. This approach represents the closest available to direct infection of the target cell. The results show that latency can be established in the absence of IE proteins; thus, a natural block to IE transcription in neurons is compatible with the latent state. Ideas on the mechanism by which gene expression in neurons may fail at this stage focus on the requirement for the formation of a TAATGARAT-binding multiprotein complex between VP16, Oct-1 and HCF to initiate IE transcription.

The infecting virion must travel long distances to reach the ganglion, and the structure of the subviral particle that is ultimately delivered to the neuronal nucleus is not known. One idea is that VP16, a tegument protein, fails to be transported to the ganglion with the viral genome, due either to physical loss during retrograde transport or to different uncoating mechanisms in the neuron (Kristie and Roizman, 1988). Alternatively, correct phosphorylation of VP16, especially at serine residue 375 within the Oct-1/HCF recognition domain, is required for its transcriptional activity, and this modification may be affected in neurons (O'Reilly et al., 1997). Absence of functional VP16, even if Oct-1 and HCF are present, would be expected to reduce IE transcription and might, by analogy with observations in cell cultures, predispose the genome to latency.

Oct-1 is a ubiquitous cellular protein initially defined by its ability to bind to the 'octamer' element ATGCAAAT. The protein participates in a variety of important cellular processes including transcription, and is utilized by many viruses for gene expression or replication. Oct-1 contains a 'POU' domain, which contains the DNA-binding elements and the sites for interaction with many different proteins including VP16. Sensory neurons contain Oct-1 in a form that is functional *in vitro;* thus it is unlikely that absence of this factor underlies a failure of IE transcription (Hagmann et al., 1995). It is possible, however, that neuron-specific members of the POU-containing family interfere with the binding of Oct-1 to viral target sequences. Many POU-containing proteins bind to TAATGARAT elements in IE promoters but do not interact with VP16, and it would be expected that such proteins could compete with Oct-1 and thereby block gene activation (Latchman, 1999). Rodent Oct-1 varies from the human protein specifically at a few residues that are important for binding of human Oct-1 to VP16 and HCF (Cleary et al., 1993). Thus, VP16 forms the multiprotein complex less efficiently with murine Oct-1, raising concerns about the relevance of the mouse models of latency. Possibly, latency is relatively favored over lytic replication in mice compared with humans. Murine Oct-1 must function to some extent in vivo, however, because HSV-1 VP16 mutants are severely attenuated for replication in mice; if Oct-1 were inactive, the absence of VP16 function would probably be inconsequential.

HCF is a large cellular protein of 2035 amino acids that undergoes internal proteolytic cleavage but nonetheless can participate in activation of transcription with only a heterodimer of the critical N- and C- terminal fragments. The N-terminal portion contains six repeats with homology to the *Drosophila* protein Kelch, that are predicted to form a propeller-like structure which binds VP16 (Wilson et al., 1993). One major function of HCF appears to be stabilization of the Oct-1/VP16/HCF complex, but more recent studies suggest that HCF itself contains activating regions that may contribute to stimulation of gene expression (Lociano and Wilson, 2002). In proliferating cells HCF is associated with chromatin and is important for cell division, since a cell line harboring a temperature sensitive mutation in HCF arrests predominantly at G0/G1 upon shift to the non-permissive temperature. In sensory neurons in vivo, HCF appears to be cytoplasmic, possibly reflecting the non-dividing state of the cells (Kristie et al., 1999). This localization, if maintained after infection, would prevent activation of IE transcription through the VP16-mediated pathway. Cellular proteins have been identified that, like VP16, contain the short motif $^D/_E$HXY which interacts with the Kelch domain of HCF. One of these, named LZIP or Luman, is cytoplasmic in tissue culture cells and, when over-expressed, redistributes HCF from the nucleus to the endoplasmic reticulum (ER) (Freiman and Herr, 1997; Lu and Misra, 2000). Transfected tissue culture cells expressing Luman are impaired for productive HSV-1 replication, presumably because HCF is sequestered at the ER. Another HCF-binding protein, Zhangfei, is selectively expressed in human neurons and also blocks HSV-1 replication when ectopically expressed in tissue culture cells, possibly by counteracting VP16 (Akhova et al., 2005). Clearly, if Luman, Zhangfei or other HCF-binding proteins are present in neurons, activation of IE transcription may be impaired, due to relocation of HCF to the ER, to competition for VP16-binding sites, or to interaction with VP16.

Role of LAT in the establishment of latency

Expression of LAT is not essential for any phase of latency, but there is considerable evidence that it plays a modulatory role. When LAT+ and LAT− viruses are compared virus production at the periphery and in the ganglion is generally equivalent, although early studies suggested that LAT− mutants produce greater quantities of lytic transcripts and proteins in neurons (Garber et al., 1997). In general, however, LAT− mutants reactivate inefficiently and much experimentation has centered on whether this reflects a defect in reactivation *per se* or is a consequence of reduced ability to establish latency. Analysis of ganglionic viral DNA contents by direct PCR yields equivocal results, with some investigators reporting a deficit of around threefold and others detecting no significant difference. Errors in these estimations are inherently large, thus relevant differences might not score as statistically significant. The application of CXA revealed that corneal infection with LAT− mutants results in approximately threefold fewer latently infected neurons in trigeminal ganglia, although the HSV-1 genome content distribution within cells was indistinguishable from that of mice infected with a LAT+ virus (Thompson and Sawtell, 1997). These results suggest that LAT affects the number of neurons that ultimately harbor the latent genome rather than copy number within individual cells, and this conclusion is supported by investigation of the effect of LAT on neuronal survival (Perng et al., 2000). Infected rabbit ganglia exhibited greater neuronal apoptosis after infection with a LAT− virus than with a LAT+ counterpart. This effect was maximal at 7 days post-infection, and, surprisingly, few apoptotic neurons were detected at 3 days post-infection, when virus replication was at its peak. It is proposed that LAT has an anti-apoptotic activity that could result in a greater number of neurons surviving in animals infected with the LAT+ virus, thereby increasing establishment of latency. In mice, the basic observation that LAT improves neuronal survival also holds, although there is currently debate concerning whether death is through apoptosis or an alternative route (Thompson and Sawtell, 2001; Ahmed et al., 2002). In tissue culture cells, expression of LAT from transfected plasmids or viruses inhibits apoptosis induced by toxic agents or by virus infection itself, supporting the idea of an anti-apoptotic role (Inman et al., 2001). Furthermore, recent data showing that a miRNA encoded by the HSV-1 LAT gene regulates apoptosis induction by modulating TGF-beta signalling adds considerable support to the view that an important biological function of LATs is to prevent neuronal apoptosis during latency establishment and/or reactivation (Gupta et al., 2006).

LAT has been proposed to block IE gene expression, possibly by antisense inhibition of ICP0 synthesis, an hypothesis that could explain the greater toxicity of LAT-mutants for neurons. Cultured neuroblastoma cells transformed stably to express the 2 kb LAT exhibited reduced permissiveness to HSV-1 infection and a reduction in the levels of all IE-specific mRNAs, suggesting an inhibitory effect of LAT on IE RNA production through a *trans*-acting mechanism (Mador et al., 1998). However, no reduction in ICP0-specific transcript or protein levels was found in human 293T cells engineered to express 2 kb LAT (Burton et al., 2003).

Alternative models for establishment of latency

In studies with cultured neurons ICP0 was not detected in the nucleus, even though ICP0-specific RNA was expressed (Chen et al., 2000). The reasons for the failure to detect the protein are not clear, although post-transcriptional mechanisms are implicated. The absence of ICP0 might predispose the virus to latency.

All models for the establishment of latency are complicated by the fact that neurons are not inherently resistant to HSV infection because a proportion is able to support productive replication during the first few days after inoculation of animals. There is some evidence that specific neuronal subtypes may differ in susceptibility, but an absolute distinction between permissive and non-permissive cells has not been made to date. Most of the viral DNA produced during the acute phase is eliminated by a rapidly evolving immune response; however, there remains the possibility that some of the latent genomes are derived from replicated molecules rather than transport from peripheral sites. Studies with TK-mutants argue against this hypothesis for snout and corneal inoculation of mice, but in a flank inoculation model evidence was obtained for retention of replicated DNA in neurons that directly innervate the site of infection (Simmons et al., 1992).

An all-encompassing model does not exist to describe the molecular basis for the establishment of latency. If the idea of an early decision between lytic infection and latency, with a primary block at the level of IE gene expression, is accepted, then there would be no apoptotic stimulus (in the form of *de novo* synthesized viral proteins) to the neuron. This is difficult to reconcile with the hypothesis that LAT antagonizes a response to the presence of viral proteins, which presupposes that the gene expression program proceeds past the IE stage. Possibly, there is heterogeneity in the responses of individual infected neurons, such that some escape an IE block but are arrested at a later stage by LAT. Understanding the cause of neuronal death in infected ganglia is critical to a resolution of these issues. The effect of LAT on the establishment of latency is anatomical site-specific, since LAT− mutants apparently show no difference from LAT+ HSV-1 when latency in dorsal root ganglia is examined after inoculation of the footpad (Sawtell and Thompson, 1992a).

Maintenance of latency

The stability of the latent state, together with the failure to detect viral gene expression apart from that of LAT, supports the concept that the majority of the genome is in a silent state that can be reversed only by specific triggers. Studies in the mouse using sensitive RT-PCR, however, demonstrated that transcripts from the ICP4 and TK regions of the genome could be detected in ganglia during latency (Kramer et al., 1998). This observation is supported by experiments in which sections from many mouse ganglia were analyzed by ISH (Feldman et al., 2002). Approximately one neuron per 10 sections was found to be positive for transcripts representing the lytic genes ICP4, TK and glycoprotein C. In addition, antigen positive neurons were detected at approximately the same frequency, and these cells were surrounded by an immune infiltrate. The most reasonable explanation for the results is that a few neurons support viral gene expression in the mouse, a view that is supported by the finding that interferon gamma and CD8+ T cells are present in murine ganglia at latent times, suggesting that active immune surveillance may operate to maintain latency (Cantin et al., 1995; Khanna et al., 2003). Further discussion of these results is given elsewhere in this volume. Therefore, although the majority of latent genomes are retained in an untranscribed state, the possibility exists that some neurons express HSV-specific proteins and are prevented from producing virus by host immune responses.

Reactivation

Since viral gene products characteristic of the lytic cycle cannot, in general, be detected in latently infected neurons, cellular mechanisms must be important for reactivation. The crucial cellular events are not understood at the molecular level and are still vaguely described as applying 'stress' to the neuron. Furthermore, the models for reactivation may rely on very different cellular stimuli and hence the mechanisms involved may vary between both animals and systems. For instance, explantation is probably a more severe stress than in vivo treatments. A further serious complication arises from the fact that reactivation is an inefficient process with only a small proportion of the neurons that harbor viral genomes responding by production of virus. This means that the genomes detected at a gross level during latency may not represent those able to reactivate, with the latter possibly forming a small subset of the total. In addition, in a comparison between HSV-1 strains that differ in their abilities to respond to hyperthermia in vivo, the efficiency of reactivation correlated with the genome copy number distribution but not the number of neurons harboring latent virus (Sawtell, 1998). Therefore, the neurons containing large amounts of HSV DNA may be more susceptible to reactivation stimuli in vivo.

Models for reactivation depend critically on understanding the mechanism of establishment of latency. Thus, if the view is taken that a block in IE transcription leads to establishment, the route to reactivation can be subdivided into two basic concepts, depending on the consequences of the IE block. If, as in fibroblast models, failure of IE gene expression results in conversion of the genome into a quiescent state that is disrupted by ICP0 but is unresponsive to changes in cell physiology such as activation of signal transduction pathways, it follows that reactivation must be provoked either by the action of cellular proteins that mimic the activity of ICP0 or by induction of ICP0 synthesis. An alternative, more popular, view is that viral promoters are not repressed thoroughly, as in fibroblasts, but are inactive and potentially responsive to cellular signals provided by reactivation stimuli. The two models overlap if the genome is generally repressed but the ICP0 promoter specifically escapes repression. In this case, reactivation stimuli would initially be targeted to the ICP0 promoter, with the subsequent reversal of genome repression by the ICP0 protein. A role for LAT in reactivation is suggested by a number of experimental observations, although the interpretation of the data again depends on the events leading to establishment.

The role of ICP0 in reactivation

ICP0 was first characterized as a transcription activator that is not sequence-specific, but recent studies have shown that its primary mode of action is as an ubiquitin E3 ligase that mediates the targeted proteolysis of cellular proteins, particularly those of the nuclear structures known as ND10 (Everett, 2000; Van Sant et al., 2001; Boutell et al., 2002). Indeed, ICP0 rapidly and effectively mediates the disruption of all ND10 in the cell, with accompanying degradation of many of the component proteins. Since transcriptionally active input HSV genomes initially associate with ND10, it is thought that ICP0 creates an environment that is conducive to transcription, probably by directing the destruction of cellular repressors. Histone deacetylases (HDACs) promote the formation of inactive chromatin, thus it is interesting that ICP0 interacts with HDACs 4, 5 and 7 (Lomonte et al., 2004). ICP0 also dissociates HDAC 1 and 2 from CoREST/REST, a protein complex that represses transcription, thereby possibly relieving repression (Gu et al., 2005). These data suggest an important role for ICP0 in antagonizing histone-mediated gene silencing. The dramatic reversal of the quiescent state by ICP0 in cell culture suggests that this protein may be important for reactivation of latent HSV. Early in vivo studies showed that ICP0-deficient mutants were impaired for latency, as measured by reactivation efficiency after explantation, but it was not possible to distinguish between a true effect on reactivation and inefficient establishment due to the known reduction in replication at the periphery and in the ganglion. Immunosuppression of mice enables ICP0 null mutants to establish latency as efficiently as wild-type virus as judged by latent genome copy number, and ICP0 null mutants exhibit reduced reactivation efficiency in the explant model even when viral DNA loads in the ganglia are equivalent (Halford and Schaffer, 2001). ICP0 is therefore important for explant reactivation, but the exact stage at which it functions is unclear. Explantation might specifically induce the synthesis of ICP0, but an alternative interpretation is that ICP0 merely improves the replication, and hence detection, of HSV-1 once the reactivation stimulus has acted. The former hypothesis predicts that the promoter, or other important sequences controlling ICP0, contains elements that respond to reactivation stimuli.

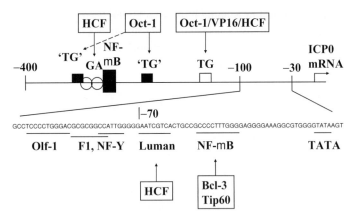

Fig. 33.2. Binding sites for transcription factors in the ICP0 promoter. The region to nucleotide −400 is shown, with the −100 to −30 sequences expanded. The major TAATGARAT element (TG), and two TAATGARAT homologies that have not been demonstrated to bind VP16 and HCF ('TG') are shown. Other sites in the −400 to −100 region predicted to bind GABP (GA; two sites) and NF-κB are also shown. There are functional data to support the binding of Olf-1, F1 plus NF-Y, and Luman to the indicated sites. The CCCCTTTGGGG motif at −57 is predicted to bind NF-κB on the basis of sequence homology.

The ICP0 promoter as a possible target for reactivation signals

The ICP0 promoter has many motifs, in addition to the TAATGARATs, that bind transcription factors, and these sites might be targets for reactivation stimuli (Fig. 33.2). Nucleotides −79 to −97 bind Olf-1, a neuron-specific factor that activates transcription (Devireddy and Jones, 2000), and sequences between −74 and −89 are recognized by two proteins, NF-Y and one of unknown identity (named F1), in the human neuroblastoma line IMR-32 (O'Rourke and O'Hare, 1993). Gene array analysis demonstrated that explantation of ganglia induces the synthesis of Bcl-3 (as well as other gene products) in neurons (Tsavachidou et al., 2001). This is interesting because Bcl-3 associates with a dimer of the p50 subunit of NF-κB, and the ICP0 promoter contains NF-κB consensus binding sites at −51 and −273. Phosphorylation influences the binding of Bcl-3 to p50, thus explantation may activate kinases that promote the interaction of these proteins. Bcl-3 also interacts with Tip60, a histone acetylase, and therefore may mediate its effects by recruiting this protein and modifying chromatin structure at the ICP0 promoter. In ganglia, HCF is found in the cytoplasm of neurons but is transported to the nucleus within 20 minutes of explantation (Kristie et al., 1999). If the HSV genome, or strategic regions such as the ICP0 promoter, is available for transcription then HCF, by virtue of its intrinsic activation domain, could trigger the viral gene expression program. This hypothesis requires that a mechanism exists for localizing HCF to the promoter, and binding to Oct-1 is the obvious candidate. However, HCF interacts with the ETS family member GABP, which binds to motifs of consensus CGGAAR (Vogel and Kristie, 2000). There are GABP recognition sites in the ICP0 promoter, and these might direct activation of transcription through a GABP/HCF complex. Another HCF-binding protein, Luman, is cytoplasmic in tissue culture cells but is, in essence, a basic leucine zipper transcription factor of the ATF/CREB family that can bind to CREs and activate transcription in an HCF-dependent manner (Lu and Misra, 2000). In tissue culture cells, Luman is released from the ER by the action of the site 1 protease, an enzyme that catalyzes the regulated intramembrane proteolysis (RIP) of membrane-bound transcription factors, releasing them for transport to the nucleus and activation of transcription (Raggo et al., 2002). Various stress stimuli trigger RIP, thus reactivation signals may result in the release of Luman from the ER of neurons, thereby relocating a complex of this protein plus HCF to the nucleus. The proposed site of action is a CRE at position −67 in the ICP0 promoter.

Hypotheses on the significance of transcription factor binding to the ICP0 promoter must include the possibility that such binding may be relevant to replication in neurons at the early stages of infection rather than to reactivation. In addition, all of the above ideas must take account of studies on an HSV-1 mutant deleted for nucleotides −70 to −420 in the ICP0 promoter, thus lacking most of the factor-binding sequences mentioned above (Davido and Leib, 1996). This mutant established latency and displayed normal reactivation efficiency in the explantation system even though replication in cell culture was impaired, suggesting that the region between −70 and −420 in the ICP0 promoter, which includes most of the important known elements controlling expression in cell culture systems, does not contain critical target sequences for explant reactivation of latent virus. Notably, the NF-κB binding site at −51 and the CRE at −67 lie outwith the dispensable region.

Cellular reactivation signals

Among the many changes that occur in neurons following explantation of ganglia, the cyclin-dependent kinases cdk2, cdk4 and cdk7 exhibit alterations in abundance and location (Davido et al., 2002). Increases in the level of cdk2 were observed, and this enzyme was found predominantly in the nucleus. In the case of cdk4, the protein was found mainly in the cytoplasm immediately after plating of explanted ganglia, but became nuclear during culture. A dramatic drop in cdk7 levels occurred within the first day of explant. HSV-1-specific antigens were found exclusively in those neurons containing nuclear cdk2 and cdk4, suggesting that changes in the kinases might be required for reactivation. Roscovitine, an inhibitor of cdk2 that blocks HSV-1 replication in tissue culture, also prevented virus reactivation. Furthermore, no HSV-1 antigen reactivity could be detected in the presence of roscovitine, suggesting that the inhibitor blocks reactivation at an early stage rather than during spread of virus in the explanted ganglion. In tissue culture systems, roscovitine affects many aspects of HSV-1 replication, but it is noteworthy that the compound blocks the function of ICP0 due to alteration of post-translational modification. Therefore, cdk2 and cdk4 may be important for reactivation due to their roles in ensuring the activity of ICP0. In cultured primary rat neurons, withdrawal of NGF results in the rapid resumption of virus replication, to an extent mimicking one of the effects of explantation, in which the in vivo supply of NGF is disrupted (Wilcox and Johnson, 1988). Inhibition of deacetylases also reactivates latent virus in cultured neurons, suggesting a requirement for modification of chromatin structure (Arthur et al., 2001). Treatment of cells with agents that activate signal transduction pathways through cAMP-mediated mechanisms is effective, and recent studies have indicated an involvement of inducible cAMP early repressors (ICER) in this process (Colgin et al., 2001). ICER can heterodimerize with CREB/ATF transcription family members that mediate the transcriptional changes induced by cAMP, but since ICER lacks an activation domain the complexes act as repressors when bound to CREs. Expression of ICER itself is activated by cAMP and, intriguingly, by heat stress of neurons. Crucially, reactivation of latent HSV-1 was induced by infection of neuronal cultures with an adenovirus recombinant expressing ICER. In concert with reactivation, the levels of LAT decreased, leading to the suggestion that the known CREs in the LAT promoter mediate repression by ICER. This observation is difficult to reconcile with suggestions of a positive role for LAT in reactivation, as discussed below. However, in a model that uses cultured cells from dissociated ganglia of latently infected mice, transient heat shock or addition of dexamethasone induced reactivation but elevation of cAMP levels did not (Halford et al., 1996). The nature of the reactivating stimuli therefore differs in the various cell culture systems currently available.

The role of LAT in reactivation

Early work ascertained that, in most cases, LAT− virus mutants reactivate less efficiently than their LAT+ counterparts. This observation was made in mice, for both explant and in vivo reactivation, in rabbits, and in guinea pigs infected with HSV-2. The conclusion that LAT has a role in reactivation is therefore widely accepted. This assumption is complicated by the findings, discussed above, that LAT− mutants establish latency less efficiently in some systems; clearly if fewer neurons harbor HSV genomes, a lower reactivation potential would be expected. Studies in mice, analyzing neuronal DNA contents by CXA, concluded that the impaired reactivation of LAT− mutants in trigeminal ganglia can be entirely accounted for by reduced establishment of latency (Thompson and Sawtell, 1997). Tellingly, it was possible to increase the efficiency of establishment by LAT− mutants to that of wild-type HSV-1 if hyperthermic treatment was applied during the first three days after infection. An equivalent rise in in vivo reactivation frequency to wild-type levels accompanied the increased establishment, strongly suggesting that the primary role of LAT in the mouse trigeminal ganglion is at the level of establishment of latency. In the rabbit eye model, LAT− mutants exhibit reduced efficiency of both spontaneous and induced reactivation. Analysis of latent DNA levels is difficult in this model, however, and although most studies conclude that LAT− and LAT+ mutants establish latency with equivalent efficiencies, variation in the data could obscure a three-fold difference. The question of whether LAT affects establishment or reactivation, or both, in the rabbit remains open. Intriguingly, replacement of the LAT region of HSV-2 with the equivalent region from HSV-1 revealed a role of LAT in anatomical-site specificity of reactivation (Yoshikawa et al., 1996). The recombinant acquired HSV-1-like characteristics, displaying an increased response to iontophoresis of epinephrine in the rabbit but a reduced reactivation frequency in the guinea pig. Only the first 1.5 kb of the mLAT transcript, representing the LAP2 region and part of the stable LAT, is required for efficient spontaneous reactivation in the rabbit (Perng et al., 1996). Re-introduction of sequences encoding this region, plus 1.8 kbp of the LAT promoter, between the UL37 and UL38 coding sequences of a LAT− mutant restored the defect and resulted in a virus exhibiting normal reactivation phenotype. Comparison between strains suggested that none of the ORFs that can be detected in the 1.5 kbp fragment is functionally important for reactivation (Drolet et al., 1998). In addition, inhibition of apoptosis by HSV-1 LAT in tissue culture cells also maps to the 1.5 kbp region (Inman et al., 2001). Thus, in the rabbit, the 1.5 kbp region is thought to mediate increased spontaneous reactivation by virtue of its anti-apoptotic activity. This view is strengthened by the finding that the reduced reactivation efficiency of LAT-viruses can be reversed by insertion of sequences that encode a baculovirus anti-apoptotic protein (Jin et al., 2005). Therefore, the anti-apoptotic function of the LAT region may be important for prolonging survival of the reactivating cells and increasing the production of infectious virus. Deletion of a subfragment of the 1.5 kbp region, consisting of a part of LAP2, dramatically reduced the efficiency of epinephrine-induced reactivation in the rabbit (Bloom et al., 1996). This deleted region lies within the mLAT region and does not affect the accumulation of major LAT; thus, presumably either the expression of a transcript or a *cis* effect accounts for the activity of the LAP2-derived element and probably the entire 1.5 kbp region.

All of the ideas described above on the mechanism of reactivation assume that latency is essentially "static," with a switch required to reverse the silencing of the genome. The alternative "dynamic" model, in which continual low level production of virus occurs with lesions only occurring sporadically, does not readily fit with known ideas of viral gene expression but may be consistent with the detection of CD8+ T cells in ganglia (Khanna et al., 2003). The use of PCR has demonstrated that ayrnptomatic shedding of HSV-1 and HSV-2 occurs with surprisingly high frequency in humans (Wald et al., 1997), suggesting that the dynamic model, an interaction which could be envisaged as a slow persistent infection, deserves consideration.

Concluding remarks

Latency is clearly very complex at the molecular level, and the difficulties inherent in the model systems ensure that it will not be unraveled easily. The non-uniformity of latency, in terms of viral genome copy number, LAT expression and nature of reactivation stimulus, may be of fundamental benefit to the virus. If latency was uniform, a single stimulus might induce reactivation in the entire latent reservoir and result in clearance of the virus from the host. Perhaps the different virus/cell interactions respond to different host signals, explaining why it has been so difficult to arrive at a simple model for the molecular basis of latency.

Acknowledgments

We thank Valerie Preston for constructive comments on the manuscript, and Robin Lachmann for help with Figure 33.1.

REFERENCES

Ahmed, M. and Fraser, N. W. (2001). Herpes simplex virus type 1 2-kilobase latency-associated transcript intron associates with ribosomal proteins and splicing factors. *J. Virol.*, **75**, 12070–12080.

Ahmed, M., Lock, M., Miller, C. G., and Fraser, N. W. (2002). Regions of the herpes simplex virus type 1 latency-associated transcript that protect cells from apoptosis in vitro and protect neuronal cells in vivo. *J. Virol.*, **76**, 717–729.

Akhova, O., Bainbridge, M. and Misra, V. (2005). The neuronal host cell factor-binding protein Zhangfei inhibits herpes simplex virus replication. *J. Virol.* **79**, 14708–14718.

Amelio, A. L., Giordani, N. V., Kubat, N. J., O'Neil, J. E. and Bloom, D. C. (2006). Deacetylation of the herpes simplex virus type 1 latency-associated transcript (LAT) enhancer and a decrease in LAT abundance precede an increase in ICP0 transcriptional permissiveness at early times postexplant. *J. Virol.* **80**, 2063–2068.

Arthur, J., Efstathiou, S., and Simmons, A. (1993). Intranuclear foci containing low abundance herpes simplex virus latency-associated transcripts visualized by non-isotopic *in situ* hybridization. *J. Gen. Virol.*, **74**, 1363–1370.

Arthur, J. L., Scarpini, C. G., Connor, V., Lachmann, R. H., Tolkovsky, A. M., and Efstathiou, S. (2001). Herpes simplex virus type 1 promoter activity during latency establishment, maintenance, and reactivation in primary dorsal root neurons in vitro. *J. Virol.*, **75**, 3885–3895.

Berthomme, H., Thomas, J., Texier, P., Epstein A., and Feldman, L. T. (2001). Enhancer and long-term expression functions of herpes simplex virus type 1 latency-associated promoter are both located in the same region. *J. Virol.*, **75**, 4386–4393.

Bloom, D. C., Hill, J. M., Devi-Rao, G. B., Wagner, E. K., Feldman, L. T., and Stevens, J. G. (1996). A 348-base-pair region in the latency-associated transcript facilitates herpes simplex virus type 1 reactivation. *J. Virol.*, **70**, 2449–2459.

Bloom, D. C., Stevens, J. G., Hill, J. M., and Tran, R. K. (1997). Mutagenesis of a cAMP response element within the latency-associated transcript promoter of HSV-1 reduces adrenergic reactivation. *Virology*, **236**, 202–207.

Boutell, C., Sadis, S., and Everett, R. D. (2002). Herpes simplex virus type 1 immediate-early protein ICP0 and its isolated RING finger domain act as ubiquitin E3 ligases in vitro. *J. Virol.*, **76**, 841–850.

Burton, E. A., Hong, C. S., and Glorioso, J. C. (2003). The stable 2.0-kilobase intron of the herpes simplex virus type 1 latency-associated transcript does not function as an antisense repressor of ICP0 in nonneuronal cells. *J. Virol.*, **77**, 3516–3530.

Cantin, E. M., Hinton, D. R., Chen, J. D. and Openshaw, H. (1995). Gamma interferon expression during acute and latent nervous system infection by herpes simplex virus type 1. *J. Virol.* **69**, 4898–4905.

Chen, X., Schmidt, M. C., Goins, W. F., and Glorioso, J. C. (1995). Two herpes simplex virus type 1 latency-active promoters differ in their contributions to latency-associated transcript expression during lytic and latent infections. *J. Virol.*, **69**, 7899–7908.

Chen, X.-P., Li, J. Mata, M. Goss, J. Wolfe, D. Glorioso, J. C. and Fink, D. J. (2000). Herpes simplex virus type 1 ICP0 protein does not accumulate in the nucleus of primary neurons in culture. *J. Virol.*, **74**, 10132–10141.

Chen, X.-P., Mata, M., Kelley, M., Glorioso, J. C., and Fink, D. J. (2002). The relationship of herpes simplex virus latency associated transcript expression to genome copy number: a quantitative study using laser capture microdissection. *Journal of Neurovirology*, **8**, 204–210.

Cleary, M. A., Stern, S., Tanaka, M., and Herr, W. (1993). Differential positive control by Oct-1 and Oct-2 – activation of a transcriptionally silent motif through Oct-1 and VP16 recruitment. *Genes Dev.*, **7**, 72–83.

Cui, C., Griffiths, A., Li, G. L., Silva, L. M., Kramer, M. F., Gaasterland, T., Wang, X. J. and Coen, D. M. (2006). Prediction and identification of herpes simplex virus 1-encoded microRNAs. *J. Virol.* **80**, 5499–5508.

Colgin, M. A., Smith, R. L., and Wilcox, C. L. (2001). Inducible cyclic AMP early repressor produces reactivation of latent herpes simplex virus type 1 in neurons in vitro. *J. Virol.*, **75**, 2912–2920.

Davido, D. J. and Leib, D. A. (1996). Role of *cis*-acting sequences of the ICP0 promoter of herpes simplex virus type 1 in viral pathogenesis, latency and reactivation. *J. Gen. Virol.*, **77**, 1853–1863.

Davido, D. J., Leib, D. A., and Schaffer, P. A. (2002). The cyclin-dependent kinase inhibitor roscovitine inhibits the transactivating activity and alters the posttranslational modification of herpes simplex virus type 1 ICP0. *J. Virol.*, **76**, 1077–1088.

Deshmane, S. L. and Fraser, N. W. (1989). During latency, herpes simplex virus type 1 DNA is associated with nucleosomes in a chromatin structure. *J. Virol.*, **63**, 943–947.

Devireddy, L. R. and Jones, C. J. (2000). Olf-1, a neuron-specific transcription factor, can activate the herpes simplex virus type 1-infected cell protein 0 promoter. *J. Biol. Chem.*, **275**, 77–81.

Dobson, A., Sederati, F., Devi-Rao, G., Flanagan, W. M., Farrell, M., Stevens, J., Wagner, E., and Feldman, L. T. (1989). Identification of the latency-associated transcript promoter by expression of rabbit beta-globin mRNA in sensory nerve ganglia latently infected with a recombinant herpes simplex virus. *J. Virol.*, **63**: 3844–3851.

Drolet, B. S., Perng, G. C., Cohen, J. *et al.* (1998). The region of herpes simplex virus type 1 LAT gene involved in spontaneous reactivation does not encode a functional protein. *Virology*, **242**, 221–232.

Efstathiou, S., Minson, A. C., Field, H. J., Anderson, J. R. and Wildy, P. (1986). Detection of herpes simplex virus-specific DNA sequences in latently infected mice and in humans. *J. Virol.* **57**, 446–455.

Everett, R. D. (2000). ICP0, a regulator of herpes simplex virus during lytic and latent infection. *Bioessays*, **22**, 761–770.

Feldman, L. T., Ellison, A. R., Voytek, C. C., Yang, L., Krause, P., and Margolis, T. (2002). Spontaneous molecular reactivation of herpes simplex virus type 1 latency in mice. *Proc. Natl Acad. Sci. USA*, **99**, 978–983.

Frazier, D. P., Cox, D., Godshalk, E. M., and Schaffer, P. A. (1996). Identification of cis-acting sequences in the promoter of the herpes simplex virus type 1 latency-associated transcripts required for activation by nerve growth factor and sodium butyrate in PC12 cells. *J Virol.*, **70**, 7433–7444.

Freiman, R. N. and Herr, W. (1997). Viral mimicry: common mode of association with HCF by VP16 and the cellular protein LZIP. *Genes Dev.*, **11**, 3122–3127.

Garber, D. A., Schaffer, P. A., and Knipe, D. M. (1997). A LAT-associated function reduces productive-cycle gene expression during acute infection of murine sensory neurons with herpes simplex virus type 1. *J. Virol.*, **71**, 5885–5893.

Gu, H., Liang, Y., Mandel, G. and Roizman, B. (2005). Components of the REST/CoREST/histone deacetylase repressor complex arre disrupted, modified, and translocated in HSV-1-infected cells. *Proc Natl Acad Sci U S A* **102**, 7571–7576.

Gupta, A., Gartner, J. J., Sethupathy, p., Hatzigeorgiou, A. G. and Fraser, N. W. (2006). Anti-apoptotic function of a microRNA encoded by the HSV-1 latency-associated transcript. *Nature* **442**, 82–85.

Hagmann, M., Georgiev, O., Schaffner, W., and Douville, P. (1995). Transcription factors interacting with herpes simplex virus α gene promoters in sensory neurons. *Nucl. Acids Res.*, **23**, 4978–4985.

Halford, W. P. and Schaffer, P. A. (2001). ICP0 is required for efficient reactivation of herpes simplex virus type 1 from neuronal latency. *J. Virol.*, **75**, 3240–3249.

Halford, W. P., Gebhardt, B. M., and Carr, D. J. (1996). Mechanisms of herpes simplex virus type 1 reactivation. *J. Virol.*, **70**, 5051–5060.

Herrera, F. J. and Triezenberg, S. J. (2004). VP16-dependent association of chromatin-modifying coactivators and underrepresentation of histones at immediate-early gene promoters during herpes simplex virus infection. *J. Virol.* **78**, 9689–9696.

Inman, M., Perng, G.-C., Henderson, G., Ghiasi, H., Nesburn, A. B., Wechsler, S. L., and Jones, C. (2001). Region of herpes simplex virus type 1 latency-associated transcript sufficient for wild-type spontaneous reactivation promotes cell survival in tissue culture. *J. Virol.*, **75**, 3636–3646.

Jackson, S. A. and DeLuca, N. A. (2003). Relationship of herpes simplex virus genome configuration to productive and persistent infections. *Proc. Natl Acad. Sci. USA*, **100**, 7871–7876.

Jamieson, D. R. S., Robinson, L. H., Daksis, J. I., Nicholl, M. J., and Preston, C. M. (1995). Quiescent viral genomes in human fibroblasts after infection with herpes simplex virus Vmw65 mutants. *J. Gen. Virol.*, **76**, 1417–1431.

Jin, L., Perng, G. C., Mott, K. R. *et al.* (2005). A herpes simplex virus type 1 mutant expressing a baculovirus inhibitor of apoptosis gene in place of latency-associated transcript has a wild-type reactivation phenotype in the mouse. *J. Virol.* **79**, 12286–12295.

Kent, J. R., Zeng, P.-Y., Atanasiu, D., Gardner, J., Fraser, N. W. and Berger, S. L. (2004). During lytic infection herpes simplex virus type 1 is associated with histones bearing modifications that correlate with active transcription. *J. Virol.* **78**, 10178–10186.

Khanna, K. M., Bonneau, R. H., Kinchington, P. R., and Hendricks, R. L. (2003). Herpes simplex virus -specific memory CD8+ T cells are selectively activated and retained in latently infected sensory ganglia. *Immunity*, **18**, 593–603.

Kramer, M. F., Chen, S. -H., Knipe, D. M., and Coen, D. M. (1998). Accumulation of viral transcripts and DNA during establishment of latency by herpes simplex virus. *J. Virol.*, **72**, 1177–1185.

Kramer, M. F., Cook, W. J., Roth, F. P. *et al.* (2003). Latent herpes simplex virus infection of sensory neurons alters neuronal gene expression. *J. Virol.*, **77**, 9533–9541.

Kristie, T. M. and Roizman, B. (1988). Differentiation and DNA contact points of the host proteins binding at the *cis* site for virion-mediated induction of herpes simplex virus 1 α genes. *J. Virol.*, **62**, 1145–1157.

Kristie, T. M., Vogel, J. L., and Sears, A. E. (1999). Nuclear localization of the C1 factor (host cell factor) in sensory neurons correlates with reactivation of herpes simplex virus from latency. *Proc. Natl Acad. Sci. USA*, **96**, 1229–1233.

Kubat, N. J., Amelio, A. L., Giordani, N. V. and Bloom, D. C. (2004a). The herpes simplex virus type 1 latency-associated transcript (LAT) enhancer/rcr is hyperacetylated during latency independently of LAT transcription. *J. Virol.* **78**, 12508–12518.

Kubat, N. J., Tran, R. K., McAnany, P. K. and Bloom, D. C. (2004b). Specific histone tail modification and not DNA methylation is a determinant of herpes simplex virus type 1 latent gene expression. *J. Virol.* **78**, 1139–1149.

Lachmann, R. H. and Efstathiou, S. (1997). Utilization of the herpes simplex virus type 1 latency-associated regulatory region to drive stable reporter gene expression in the nervous system. *J. Virol.*, **71**, 3197–3207.

Latchman, D. S. (1999). POU family transcription factors in the nervous system. *J. Cell. Physiol.*, **80**, 1271–1282.

Lociano, R. L. and Wilson, A. C. (2002). An activation domain in the C-terminal subunit of HCF-1 is important for transactivation by VP16 and LZIP. *Proc. Natl Acad. Sci. USA*, **99**, 13403–13408.

Lu, R. and Misra, V. (2000). Potential role for luman, the cellular homologue of herpes simplex virus VP16 (alpha gene trans-inducing factor), in herpesvirus latency. *J. Virol.*, **74**, 934–943.

Lomonte, P., Thomas, J., Texier, P., Caron, C., Khochbin, S. and Epstein, A. L. (2004). Functional interaction between class II histone deacetylases and ICP0 of herpes simplex type 1. *J. Virol.* **78**, 6744–6757.

Mador, N., Goldenberg, D., Cohen, O., Panet, A., and Steiner I. (1998). Herpes simplex virus type 1 latency-associated transcripts suppress viral replication and reduce immediate-early gene mRNA levels in a neuronal cell line. *J. Virol.*, **72**, 5067–5075.

Margolis, T., Sederati, F., Dobson, A. T., Feldman, L. T., and Stevens, J. G. (1992). Pathways of viral gene expression during acute neuronal infection with HSV-1. *Virology*, **189**, 150–160.

Marquart, M. E., Zheng, X., Tran, R. K., Thompson, H. W., Bloom, D. C., and Hill, J. M. (2001). A cAMP response element within the latency-associated transcript promoter of HSV-1 facilitates induced ocular reactivation in a mouse hyperthermia model. *Virology*, **284**, 62–69.

Marshall, K. R., Lachmann, R. H., Efstathiou, S., Rinaldi, A., and Preston, C. M. (2000). Long-term transgene expression in mice infected with a herpes simplex virus type 1 mutant severely impaired for immediate-early gene expression. *J. Virol.*, **74**, 956–964.

Nicosia, M., Deshmane, S. L., Zabolotny, J. M., Valyi-Nagy, T., and Fraser, N. W. (1993). Herpes simplex virus type 1 latency-associated transcript (LAT) promoter deletion mutants can express a 2-kilobase transcript mapping to the LAT region. *J. Virol.*, **67**, 7276–7283.

O'Reilly, D., Hanscombe, O., and O'Hare, P. (1997). A single serine residue at position 375 of VP16 is critical for complex assembly with Oct-1 and HCF and is a target of phosphorylation by casein kinase II. *EMBO J.*, **16**, 2420–2430.

O'Rourke, D. and O'Hare, P. (1993). Mutually exclusive binding of two cellular factors within a critical promoter region of the gene for the IE110k protein of herpes simplex virus. *J. Virol.*, **67**, 7201–7214.

Perng, G., Ghiasi, H., Slanina, S., Nesburn, A., and Wechsler, S. (1996). The spontaneous reactivation function of the herpes simplex virus type 1 LAT gene resides completely within the first 1.5 kilobases of the 8.3- kilobase primary transcript. *J. Virol.*, **70**, 976–984.

Perng, G., Jones, C., Ciacci-Zanella, J. *et al.* (2000). Virus-induced neuronal apoptosis blocked by the herpes simplex virus latency-associated transcript. *Science*, **287**, 1500–1503.

Pfeffer, S., Sewer, A., Lagos-Quintana, M., Sheridan, R., Sander, C., Grasser, F. A., van Dyk, L. F., Ho, C. K., Shuman, S., Chien, M., Fusso, J. J., Ju, J., Randall, G., Lindenbach, B. D., Rice, C. M., Simon, V., Ho, D. D., Zavolan, M. and Tuschl, T. (2005). Identification of microRNAs of the herpesvirus family. *Nature Methods* **2**, 269–276.

Preston, C. M. and Nicholl, M. J. (1997). Repression of gene expression upon infection of cells with herpes simplex virus type 1 mutants impaired for immediate-early protein synthesis. *J. Virol.*, **71**, 7807–7813.

Raggo, C., Rapin, N., Stirling, J. *et al.* (2002). Luman, the cellular counterpart of herpes simplex virus VP16, is processed by regulated intramembrane proteolysis. *Mol. Cell. Biol.*, **22**, 5639–5649.

Ramakrishnan, R., Poliani, P. L., Levine, M., Glorioso, J. C., and Fink, D. J. (1996). Detection of herpes simplex virus type 1 latency-associated transcript expression in trigeminal ganglia by in situ reverse transcriptase PCR. *J. Virol.*, **70**, 6519–6523.

Rock, D. L. and Fraser, N. W. (1983). Detection of HSV-1 genome in central nervous system of latently infected mice. *Nature*, **302**, 523–525.

Samaniego, L. A., Neiderhiser, L., and DeLuca, N. A. (1998). Persistence and expression of the herpes simplex virus genome in the absence of immediate-early proteins. *J. Virol.*, **72**, 3307–3320.

Sawtell, N. M. (1997). Comprehensive quantification of herpes simplex virus latency at the single-cell level. *J. Virol.*, **71**, 5423–5431.

Sawtell, N. M. (1998). The probability of in vivo reactivation of herpes simplex virus type 1 increases with the number of latently infected neurons in the ganglia. *J. Virol.*, **72**, 6888–6892.

Sawtell, N. M. and Thompson, R. L. (1992a). Herpes simplex virus type 1 latency-associated transcription unit promotes anatomical site-dependent establishment and reactivation from latency. *J. Virol.*, **66**, 2157–2169.

Sawtell, N. M. and Thompson, R. L. (1992b). Rapid in vivo reactivation of herpes simplex virus in latently infected murine ganglionic neurons after transient hyperthermia. *J. Virol.*, **66**, 2150–2156.

Simmons, A., Slobedman, B., Speck, P., Arthur, J., and Efstathiou, S. (1992). Two patterns of persistence of herpes simplex virus DNA sequences in the nervous system of latently infected mice. *J. Gen. Virol.*, **73**: 1287–1291.

Smith, R. L., Escudero, J. M., and Wilcox, C. L. (1992). Activation of second messenger pathways activates latent herpes simplex virus in neuronal cultures. *Virology*, **188**, 311–318.

Stevens, J., Wagner, E., Devi-Rao, G. B., Cook, M. L., and Feldman, L. T. (1987). RNA complementary to a herpesvirus alpha gene mRNA is predominant in latently infected neurons. *Science*, **235**, 1056–1059.

Stevens, J. G. and Cook, M. L. (1971). Latent herpes simplex virus in spinal ganglia of mice. *Science*, **173**, 843–845.

Thomas, S. K., Lilley, C. E., Latchman, D. S., and Coffin, R. S. (2002). A protein encoded by the herpes simplex virus (HSV) type 1 2-kilobase latency-associated transcript is phosphorylated, localized to the nucleus, and overcomes the repression of expression from exogenous promoters when inserted into the quiescent HSV genome. *J. Virol.*, **76**, 4056–4067.

Thompson, R. L. and Sawtell, N. M. (1997). The herpes simplex virus type 1 latency-associated transcript gene regulates the establishment of latency. *J. Virol.*, **71**, 5432–5440.

Thompson, R. L. and Sawtell, N. M. (2000). Replication of herpes simplex virus type 1 within trigeminal ganglia is required for high frequency but not high viral genome copy number latency. *J. Virol.*, **74**, 965–974.

Thompson, R. L. and Sawtell, N. M. (2001). Herpes simplex virus type 1 latency-associated transcript gene promotes neuronal survival. *J. Virol.*, **75**, 6660–6675.

Tsavachidou, D., Podrzucki, W., Seykora J., and Berger, S. L. (2001). Gene array analysis reveals changes in peripheral nervous system gene expression following stimuli that result in reactivation of latent herpes simplex virus type 1: induction of transcription factor Bcl-3. *J. Virol.*, **75**, 9909–9917.

Van Sant, C., Hagglund, R., Lopez, P., and Roizman, B. (2001). The infected cell protein 0 of herpes simplex virus 1 dynamically interacts with proteasomes, binds and activates the cdc34 E2 ubiquitin-conjugating enzyme, and possesses in vitro E3 ubiquitin ligase activity. *Proc. Natl Acad. Sci. USA*, **98**, 8815–8820.

Vogel, J. L. and Kristie, T. M. (2000). The novel coactivator C1 (HCF) coordinates multiprotein enhancer formation and mediates transcription activation by GABP. *EMBO J.*, **19**, 683–690.

Wald, A., Corey, L., Cone, R., Hobson, A., Davis, G., and Zeh, J. (1997). Frequent genital herpes simplex virus 2 shedding in immunocompetent women. Effect of acyclovir treatment. *J. Clin. Investig.*, **99**, 1092–1097.

Wang, Q. Y., Zhou, C. H., Johnson, K. E., Colgrove, R. C., Coen, D. M. and Knipe, D. M. (2005). Herpesviral latency-associated transcript gene promotes assembly of heterochromatin on viral lytic-gene promoters in latent infection. *Proc. Natl. Acad. Sci. USA* **102**, 16055–16059.

Wilcox, C. L. and Johnson, E. (1988). Characterization of nerve growth factor-dependent herpes simplex virus latency in neurons in vitro. *J. Virol.*, **62**, 393–399.

Wilson, A. C., LaMarco, K., Peterson, M. G., and Herr, W. (1993). The VP16 accessory protein HCF-1 is a family of polypeptides processed from a large precursor protein. *Cell*, **74**, 115–125.

Yoshikawa, T., Hill, J. M., Stanberry, L. R., Bourne, N., Kurawadwala, J. F., and Krause, P. R. (1996). The characteristic site-specific reactivation phenotypes of HSV-1 and HSV-2 depend upon the latency-associated transcript region. *J. Exp.* Med., **184**, 659–664.

Zabolotny, J. M., Krummenacher, C., and Fraser, N. W. (1997). The herpes simplex virus type 1 2.0-kilobase latency-associated transcript is a stable intron which branches at a guanosine. *J. Virol.*, **71**, 4199–4208.

34

Immunobiology and host response

David M. Koelle

Department of Medicine, University of Washington School of Medicine, Seattle, WA, USA

Introduction

Herpesviruses began to evolve prior to the development of acquired immunity (Arzul *et al.*, 2002). It is therefore likely that evasion of innate immunity is an ancient function of alphaherpesviruses. Additional immune evasion functions have developed to adapt to the diverse repertoires of B- and T-cell immune receptors that characterize acquired immunity (Roizman and Pellet, 2001; Littman *et al.*, 1999). Immune evasion is covered in detail elsewhere in this volume. The innate and acquired immune responses to HSV are relevant to preventative and therapeutic vaccines for HSV, HSV-induced immunopathology, and the use of modified HSV for gene or cancer therapy. While human studies are, of necessity, observational or ex vivo in nature and seldom access sites of neuronal latency, we review them in detail because of their medical relevance. The excellent tools available for murine studies, including exquisite control of the DNA sequence of HSV challenge strains, and of the phenotype and genotype of recipient animals, are yielding dramatic new insights as well. Reactivation of HSV from neuronal latency is less frequent in mice than in humans, limiting immunologic studies of this challenging phenomenon. Readers are referred to excellent reviews (Schmid and Rouse, 1992; Nash, 2000; Lopez *et al.*, 1993, Simmons *et al.*, 1992; Kohl,1992) for models and materials that cannot be covered in detail.

HSV interactions with dendritic cells

Dendritic cells (DC) are a major link between innate and acquired immunity. DC are mobile cells that can potently initiate acquired immunity. Priming of the HSV-specific CD8 response occurs promptly and vigorously, suggesting the involvement of DC. After HSV-1 footpad inoculation, draining lymph nodes (DLN) of C57BL/6 mice are infiltrated by large, activated (CD44+), CD8+, CD62L− cells that express Vβ10. In these mice, the CD8 T-cell response to HSV-1 is dominated by Vβ10+, K^b-restricted, HSV-1 gB$_{498-505}$-specific cells (Cose *et al.*, 1995; Wallace *et al.*, 1999). HSV-specific cells are detectable in DLN by tetramer staining by day 2 (Coles *et al.*, 2002), and peak at day 5 at about 5% of the total DLN CD8+ cells (Cose *et al.*, 1997; Jones *et al.*, 2000; Coles *et al.*, 2002). The low direct ex vivo HSV-specific cytotoxic T-lymphocyte CTL activity of DLN cells increases about 40-fold during simple "holding" of the cells in vitro for a few days. This functional maturation correlates with a 35-fold increase in the number of HSV-specific CD8+ cells during culture. These results imply profound in vivo stimulation of naive HSV-specific cells in vivo, which continues in vitro.

Infectious virus was not detected in the DLN (Jones *et al.*, 2000), suggesting that mobile antigen presenting cells (APC) acquire HSV antigen in the periphery and cross-present antigen to naïve CD8 T-cells in DLN. While cross-priming of HSV to naïve CD8 T-cells has not been reconstituted in vitro, fibroblastoid cells, as expected, were not competent for this function (Mueller *et al.*, 2003). The quickness of CD8 T-cell priming after HSV infection is impressive. Naïve wild-type mice were adoptively treated with syngeneic, naïve HSV-specific CD8 cells (from transgenic mice) and then infected. The HSV antigen is presented in the DLN by 6 hours after footpad infection, as detected by CD69 expression or a reporter gene, with the first cell division occurring within 24 hours. The HSV-specific cells gained effector CTL function simultaneously with replication. De novo HSV protein synthesis, rather than delivery of protein in the inoculum, was required for naïve T-cell stimulation, as demonstrated with mutant viruses incapable of encoding the dominant epitope. Detection of viral DNA in the DLN again did not correlate with the priming of HSV-TCR (T-cell receptor) cells (Coles et al., 2002).

DC subsets can be defined by tissue distribution, morphology, surface markers (which can differ between species), and responses to pathogens or other stimuli. To study which were DC involved in priming for HSV, DLN cells from two days after footpad infection were fractionated and admixed with naïve HSV-TCR cells (Smith et al., 2003). B-cells, T-cells, CD11b+ macrophages, and Langerhans cells were not active APC. Depletion of cells expressing CD11c, CD8α, or DEC205 abrogated antigen presentation. The biologically active cells were CD8α+ CD45− cells, distinct from CD45+ plasmacytoid DC (O'Keeffe et al., 2002). These "conventional" DC (CD8α+ in mice) are efficient cross-presenters (Iyoda et al., 2002; den Haan et al., 2000). While the DLN cells contained HSV DNA (Jones et al., 2000; Smith et al., 2003), other studies in this system (Jones et al., 2000) showed no infectious virus. Similar studies were performed after flank skin inoculation with HSV, which results in a strictly epidermal infection. DC again accumulated in DLN that can prime naïve HSV-specific cells. No HSV DNA signal was detected in the active DLN cells (Mueller et al., 2002). Fractionation studies (Allan et al., 2003) revealed that the active APC were "conventional" CD11c+, CD8αhigh, CD205+, CD45RA− DC. Langerhans cells and plasmacytoid DC were detected in DLN, but did not have direct APC activity. Recently, the Carbone and Heath group determined that migratory DC do not directly present HSV antigen to naïve T-cells. Rather, DLN-resident CD8α+ DC appear to acquire antigen from migratory DC (Allan et al., 2006). Local plasmacytoid DC-like cells and interferon-alpha may also play an important role in assisting priming of HSV-specific CD8 CTL responses (Yoneyama et al., 2005). Taken together, multiple DC subsets appear to work together to prime cellular immunity after cutaneous HSV infection (Randolph, 2006).

The DC implicated in the priming of murine CD4 responses after HSV-2 vaginal inoculation may have a slightly different phenotype. Infection of steroid-treated mice with a tk- HSV-2 strain is confined to the epithelium. Zhao et al. found that CD11b+, CD11c+ cells migrated to the submucosa in areas subjacent to HSV-2 infection. DLN CD11c+ cells displayed up-regulation of costimulatory molecules for several days after inoculation. By day 2, DLN CD11c+ cells specifically stimulated HSV-specific CD4 T-cells, presumably due to presentation of HSV-2 antigen acquired in vivo. Fractionation showed that CD11c+, CD11b+ cells, but not B cells, were active APC. In contrast to the CD8 T-cell priming studies, the APC were CD8α−.

Again, the active cells did not have features of Langerhans or plasmacytoid DC. No HSV DNA was detected in the DLN cells (Zhao et al., 2003). Combined, these recent studies of priming after HSV infection demonstrate that specific DC subsets prime HSV-specific CD4 and CD8 T-cells in the apparent absence of their direct infection by HSV.

The APC involved in T-cell priming during primary HSV infections of humans are unknown. Langerhans cell numbers are decreased in HSV-infected skin, possibly consistent with their emigration and a role in antigen presentation (Memar et al., 1995). Skin-derived Langerhans cells have APC function for HSV-specific memory HLA class II-restricted (CD4) responses in vitro (Vestey et al., 1990). The ability of other cell types to present HSV antigen in the recall context is reviewed below.

In some viral infections, specific interactions with dendritic cells, such as direct infection, have roles in pathogenesis (Servet-Delprat et al., 2003). Several groups have examined HSV infection of DC and the activity of immune evasion functions in these cells (Becker, 2003.) Human in vitro-generated myeloid DC express HSV entry receptors (Salio et al., 1999) and can be productively infected by a clinical HSV-1 strain (Mikloska et al., 2001). Efficient entry, but restricted immediate early gene expression, and little or no production of daughter virus was observed with various lab strains of HSV-1 (Rong et al., 2003; Kruse et al., 2000; Pollara et al., 2003; Samady et al., 2003). HSV is pathogenic in both murine and human DC even in the absence of productive infection (Jones et al., 2003; Samady et al., 2003; Pollara et al., 2003). There is more agreement that HSV infection generally inhibits DC maturation and function. Addition of infectious HSV generally blocks LPS-mediated maturation of myeloid DC, as measured by up-regulation of T-cell co-stimulatory molecules, with some evidence that "bystander" uninfected DC may be activated to mature by factors released from infected DC (Salio et al., 1999; Samady et al., 2003; Pollara et al., 2003). Bystander DC were not adversely affected in terms of cytokine secretion and T-cell stimulatory capacity for third-party responses, while infected cells were markedly functionally impaired (Salio et al., 1999; Pollara et al., 2003). Infection of mature myeloid DC can specifically down-regulate CD83 (Kruse et al., 2000). Some genes responsible for this inhibition have been identified. In HSV-1, vhs (unique long gene 41, *UL41*) may be involved (Samady et al., 2003). For HSV-1, deletion of vhs and US12 (encoding unique short gene 12, infected cell protein 47, ICP47) has been reported to improve DC antigen presentation (Sun et al., 2003). The complex, mainly inhibitory effects of HSV on DC function were examined in the context of stimulating recall T-cell responses to HSV itself. Lower MOIs permitted detection of memory responses, which were abrogated by high-dose infection of human myeloid DC (Pollara et al., 2003).

CD8 T-cell responses to HSV

The long-term consequences of primary infection include immunologic priming and latent infection of ganglia. Events of immunologic interest in the ganglia are reviewed first, followed by a discussion of memory CD8 responses in the blood and peripheral tissues. While mice do not have spontaneous HSV recurrences, virologic and immunologic data are consistent with chronic, low level HSV gene expression and immune recognition in dorsal root ganglia (DRG). High subclinical HSV shedding rates in humans are consistent with chronic or very frequent, intermittent reactivation (4). HSV may be fundamentally less tightly controlled in human than in murine ganglia.

After recovery from HSV-1 infection, latently infected murine ganglia show persistent evidence of inflammation. Feldman et al. 2002) studied trigeminal ganglia (TG) of mice 5 to 7 weeks after recovery from ocular inoculation with HSV-1. mRNA for lytic HSV genes were localized to rare neuron-like cells surrounded by mononuclear leukocytes, while LAT (+) neurons lacked this infiltrate. The ratio of LAT RNA (+) to lytic RNA (+) cells was about 5000. Late protein (gC) was detected by immunohistochemistry in rare neuron-like cells. These data extend RT-PCR analyses of latently infected ganglia that detect lytic HSV-1 mRNA (Kramer and Coen, 1995). Latently infected ganglia are also enriched for mRNA encoding pro-inflammatory and lymphocyte-specific proteins such as IFN-γ. The cellular source of this IFN-γ mRNA is somewhat obscure (Tscharke and Simmons, 1999) despite the detection of HSV-specific, IFN-γ-producing cells in infected ganglia (below). Levels of these host response transcripts do not strictly correlate with the ability to reactivate: mutant *tk*- strains, which cannot reactivate to make infectious virus, still lead to persistent inflammation (Chen et al., 2000). Possibly, specific viral proteins, or HSV DNA, which is rich in potentially immunostimulatory CpG sequences (McGeoch et al., 1988), stimulate inflammation in the absence of complete reactivation. Therapy that interrupts HSV DNA replication reduces (but does not eliminate) inflammation in murine TG latently infected with a different HSV-1 strain (Halford et al., 1997).

The CD8 response in murine ganglia can be separated into acute and latent phases. In A/J mice, the earliest cells infiltrating the TG after corneal HSV-1 strain RE infection are NK-like cells and macrophages (Liu et al., 1996). Virus is cleared by day 7; TCR $\gamma\delta$ cells start to appear at this time.

The CD8 infiltrate peaks on day 12, most after viral antigen becomes undetectable. In this model, a significant number of CD4, CD8, TCR $\gamma\delta$, macrophage-like, and NK-like cells, and cells positive for TNF, persist in the ganglia for up to 90 days. After flank scarification of mice, CD8+ cells are involved in control of HSV-1 replication in the draining ganglia (Simmons and Tscharke, 1992). Temporally, there is a good correlation between CD8 cell infiltration and viral control (Speck and Simmons, 1998). MHC class I molecules are observed to be up-regulated on ganglionic cells during this phase, and neuronal cell death is not observed (Pereira and Simmons, 1999; Speck and Simmons, 1998; Pereira et al., 1994).

CD8+ cells may "monitor" the HSV-1-infected murine ganglia and contribute to the maintenance of clinical latency. Explanted, HSV-1 latently-infected TG contain endogenous CD8+ cells that suppress reactivation. Exogenous, immune CD8+ T-cells can serve the same function in an MHC-restricted fashion (Liu et al., 2000; Khanna et al., 2003). A non-lytic mechanism is suggested by the continuing presence of HSV genomes (presumably in latently infected neurons) in "suppressed" cultures. IFN-γ may exert an antiviral effect. The release of IFN-γ from TG in culture is inhibited by acyclovir, implying that lymphocyte recognition of viral protein is a step in lymphokine secretion. In addition, exogenous IFN-γ protects against reactivation from latency in ganglionic explants in a model which includes initial acyclovir blockade (Liu et al., 2001). Direct effects of IFN-γ on neurons, and indirect effects mediated by CD8+ cells, were both detected. Another possible effector molecule is granzyme A, a constituent of CD8 T-cell and NK cell granules (Lieberman and Fan, 2003). Animals deficient in granzyme A show decreased viral clearance from draining DRG after peripheral HSV-1 inoculation (Pereira et al., 2000).

Direct evidence for involvement of HSV-1-specific "classic" CD8 T-cells in viral control in TG has been obtained in C57BL/6 mice. Cells recognizing the dominant K^b-restricted, HSV-1 $gB_{498-505}$ epitope infiltrate TG 2 to 5 weeks after ocular HSV-1 infection, as shown by tetramer staining (in situ and after dissociation of TG) and IFN-γ responses (Khanna et al., 2003). Interestingly, these cells appear to become increasing activated from day 14 to day 34. The functional antiviral activity of the ganglionic CD8 cells appeared to wane somewhat by day 34 (Liu et al., 2000). The duration of ganglionic localization is of interest, given the chronicity of HSV infections in humans. It is not known whether the HSV-specific CD8 cells are reacting to low levels of lytic protein expression, and/or somehow sense, or assist with the maintenance of, latent gene transcription. The factors involved in T-cell trafficking to ganglia are unknown. Taken together, these data are consistent with a model in which HSV-specific CD8+ T-cells are persistently localized to HSV-infected ganglia. Recently, the group of Verjans and Osterhaus (Osterhaus et al., 2006) has demonstrated that human trigeminal ganglia latently infected by HSV-1, contain HSV-specific CD8 T-cells capable of producing IFN-γ. It will be of great interest to determine the effector functions, phenotype, and fine specificity of these T-cells. In contrast to ganglia, DLN HSV-specific murine CD4 (Zhao et al., 2003) and CD8 (Andersen et al., 2000) T-cells decline dramatically in after recovery from peripheral HSV inoculation, as expected for classic cellular immune responses.

The functional importance of CD8 T-cells in mice is somewhat dependent on the details of the experimental model. Mice deficient in β2-microglobulin, and therefore in CD8 T-cells, have decreased containment of HSV infection in some models (Holterman et al., 1999; Manickan and Rouse, 1995). However, these mice also lack CD1d-restricted NKT cells. Deletion of ICP47 from HSV-1 can decrease neurovirulence, consistent with an effect due to increased recognition of infected cells by CD8 T-cells (Goldsmith et al., 1998). CD8 T-cells alone can provide protection against HSV-1. This was established by immunizing MHC-suitable mice with the $gB1_{498-505}$ epitope, albeit in a specialized vaccinia format (Blaney et al., 1998). The immunodominance of $gB1_{498-505}$ in $H-2^b$ mice was recently exploited to study the relationship between T-cell avidity and diversity and functional protection (Messaoudi et al., 2002). Mice with an allelic variant of $H-2^b$ were found to be relatively resistant to acute HSV-1 lethal infection compared to wild-type $H-2^b$ congenics. The resistant mice had a higher diversity of $gB1_{498-505}$-specific CD8 T-cells in their repertoire, which included cells with very high avidity for peptide-MHC, compared to the wild-type $H-2^b$ mice. The cause of this diversity was hypothesized to be differences in thymic T-cell positive selection, prior to viral infection. Diversity in HLA class I alleles, and hence of the T-cell repertoire, gives a selective advantage in human HIV-1 infection (Trachtenberg et al., 2003) but has not yet been studied for HSV. Contributions to TCR repertoire variability from previous viral infections (Brehm et al., 2002), allelic variations at non-restricting self MHC (Burrows et al., 1995), and minor histocompatibility (Roopenian et al., 2002) loci are well documented and are likely applicable to HSV immunology.

Human CD8 and other immune responses may be expected to differ from murine responses. Lytic replication occurs intermittently in essentially all infected people (Wald et al., 2000), perhaps maintaining or "maturing" responses. Some immune evasion mechanisms, such as transporter of antigen processing (TAP) inhibition by ICP47, are much stronger in humans (Tomazin et al., 1998), potentially influencing CD8 responses. On the balance, HSV stimulates readily detectable CD8 responses in humans. Based on limited tetramer analyses of chronically infected persons, responses are lower than those seen for CMV and EBV (Koelle et al., 2002b; Barouch and Letvin, 2001). HSV infects mainly non-professional APC in a relatively small tissue volume. Some other chronic viral infections such as HPV, HCV, and HBV stimulate even lower-abundance CD8 responses as assessed in the blood. The reasons for this variability remain unknown.

Data concerning the importance of CD8 responses in humans is indirect. The frequency ("pCTL") of circulating CD8+ cells which, in response to HSV-2 antigen, give rise to progeny which kill autologous infected cells in classical limiting dilution assays, is on the order of 1 in 6000 peripheral blood mononuclear cells (PBMC) (perhaps 1 in 1500 or so CD8 T-cells) (Posavad et al., 1996). Among HIV and HSV-2 co-infected persons, the pCTL was inversely correlated with HSV-2 disease severity (Posavad et al., 1997). HLA correlation studies support a functional role for CD8 T-cells as some have shown associations between HLA class I alleles and HSV-2 infection or severity (Lekstrom-Himes et al., 1999). CD8 T-cells with HSV-specific CTL and IFN-γ secretion localize to recurrent genital HSV-2 lesions, and the infiltration of CTL is temporally correlated with clearance of culturable virus (Koelle et al., 1998b). It is not clear if this is simply a reactive "mop-up brigade," or if similar cells are capable of holding HSV replication below clinical threshold or even below the threshold of subclinical shedding (Wald et al., 2000).

HSV-specific CD8 T-cells likely interact with many APC in vivo, including DC, ganglionic cells, and infected cells in the periphery, with different outcomes. The type and condition of APC used in vitro to characterize CD8 responses is also critically important. Fibroblasts are more susceptible than B cells to HSV-mediated down-regulation of HLA class I (Koelle et al., 1993) and poorly re-stimulate memory CD8 responses (Yasukawa et al., 1989; Tigges et al., 1992). Recognition of fibroblasts can be obtained, but knock-out of one or both the immune evasion-related genes, US12 and vhs, or pre-treatment with IFN-γ, is required (Koelle et al., 2001; Tigges et al., 1996). Similarly, recognition of keratinocytes, representative of the likely in vivo target cell in the periphery, requires IFN-γ and specific infection conditions (Mikloska et al., 1996, 2001; Koelle et al., 2001). In vivo, HSV lesions are rich in IFN-γ and display signs of local IFN-γ effects (up-regulation of keratinocyte HLA class II) quite early on (Cunningham et al., 1985; Koelle and Corey, 1995), so these systems may be somewhat physiological. EBV-transformed B cells are more frequently used as APC in the readout phase of cytotoxicity assays, but their in vivo relevance is questionable. Human HSV-specific CD8 CTL can recognize and kill bystander CD8 T-cells (Raftery et al., 1999), but it is not clear if T-cells are a physiologically important target in vivo.

The number and functional characteristics of human HSV-specific CD8 cells are of interest given their potential varied roles in the nervous system and periphery. Assays of IFN-γ secretion by circulating CD8+ cells in response to HSV-2-infected DC reveals responses (median 0.64%) higher than pCTL estimates (Posavad et al., 2003). While tetramer staining can reveal populations of up to 0.6% of circulating CD8+ cells to be HSV-2-specific (Koelle et al., 2002b), it is not known how many of these cells have CTL, IFN-γ, or both activities. CD8 clones with CTL activity have each displayed specific IFN-γ secretion (Koelle et al., 2001, 2002b). The cytolytic pathways used by HSV-specific CD8 cells are unknown, and are relevant given HSV inhibition of CTL-induced apoptosis (Cartier et al., 2003). Reductions in viral output after interaction with infected target cells, noted for HSV-specific CD4 and NK cells (Yasukawa and Kobayashi, 1985), and for virus-specific CD8 cells in other systems (Yang et al., 2003), are little studied for HSV and CD8 cells. Circulating HSV-2-specific CD8 cells specific for one epitope in virion protein 22 (VP22) are largely CD28+, consistent with a capacity for self-renewal through co-stimulation (Hamann et al., 1997). In other human viral infections, CD28 can vary from epitope to epitope (Koelle et al., 2001). Comparisons by epitope are not yet available for HSV, but we were able to recover HSV-2-specific CD8 CTL of diverse fine specificity using expression of CD28 as a selection criteria (Koelle and Corey, 2003). HSV-specific CD8 cells detected during chronic infection also express CD62L and CCR7 (+), molecules thought to assist in homing to lymph nodes (Sallusto et al., 1999).

The first human CD8 epitopes in HSV were found several years ago, in gB2 and gD2, using a small panel of recombinant vaccinia viruses (Tigges et al., 1992, 1996). Additional HSV antigens recognized by human CD8 T-cells have recently been described with methods such as ORF-spanning peptide pools (Hosken et al., 2006) and expression cloning using whole HSV genome libraries (Koelle et al., 2001, 2002a, 2003). HSV-2 proteins from diverse structural and kinetic classes are now known to be CD8 targets. Known human HSV-1 epitopes are limited to two cross-reactive epitopes in gB and VP13/14 (Tigges et al., 1996; Koelle, 2003). CD8 antigens include, for HSV-2, glycoproteins gB, gD, and gE, the capsid or scaffold protein products of the *UL26* (or in-frame overlapping *UL26.5*) and *UL25* genes, and the tegument proteins VP16 (*UL48*), VP22 (*UL49*), VP13/14 (*UL47*), and the *UL7* gene product. The immediate early non-structural proteins ICP0, ICP4, and ICP27 are also recognized (Mikloska et al., 2001; Koelle, 2003; Koelle et al., 2001, 2002b, 1992; Tigges et al., 1996). IFN-γ ELISPOT surveys have revealed stimulatory peptides in many other ORFS (Hosken et al., 2006) and await complementary studies such as CTL assays and effector cell enrichment from PBMC.

Functional data from longitudinal biopsy studies of genital HSV-2 lesions in humans, in which serial specimens are used for culture of skin-infiltrating lymphocytes, have also been used to probe the CD8 response. HSV-2-specific CD8 T-cells were shown to be dramatically locally enriched, compared to the blood (Koelle et al., 1998b). The mechanism of homing to skin was investigated with HSV-specific tetramers and antibodies to a skin homing-associated molecule, CLA (cutaneous lymphocyte-associated antigen) (Fig. 34.1). Pronounced expression of CLA was detected on HSV-specific cells; expression by control CD8 cells specific for the non skin-associated pathogens EBV and CMV was low (Koelle et al., 2002b). CLA expression enables one-step enrichment of HSV-2-reactive CD8 CTL from blood (Koelle, 2003). Both CLA-positive cells and E-selectin up-regulation are present in human genital HSV-2 lesions (Koelle et al., 2002b). The pathway by which naïve HSV-specific CD8 cells become "programmed" to express CLA is unknown. The cytokines IL-12, TGF-β, and class I IFN are present in HSV lesions (Van Voorhis et al., 1996; Kokuba et al., 1999; Overall et al., 1981), and can synergize with T-cell stimulation through TCR to enhance CLA expression. Plasmacytoid DC can prime CLA on human CD8 T-cells (Salio et al., 2003) and react with HSV as discussed below, but have yet to be documented in HSV lesions.

A CLA-associated determinant binds to E-selectin, a lumenal venular endothelial adhesion molecule up-regulated in the inflamed skin and genital tract (Johansson et al., 1999). Known up-regulators of E-selectin, IL-1, IFN-γ and TNF-α, are enriched in HSV lesions (Doukas and Pober, 1990; Xia et al., 1998; Cunningham et al., 1985; Keadle et al., 2000). In immune mice, treatment with anti-IFN-γ decreases recruitment of lymphocytes adherence to endothelium after vaginal HSV challenge (Parr and Parr, 2003), possibly via decreases in adhesion molecule expression. Parr and Parr documented up-regulation of ICAM-1 and VCAM-1, but not E-selectin or MadCAM-1 ($A_E B_7$ integrin ligand) in the HSV-2 infected mouse vagina (Parr and Parr, 2000).

Note was made above of the immunodominance of CD8 responses to a specific peptide in $H-2^b$ haplotype mice. There is little information concerning diversity and dominance within the CD8 response in individual HSV-infected

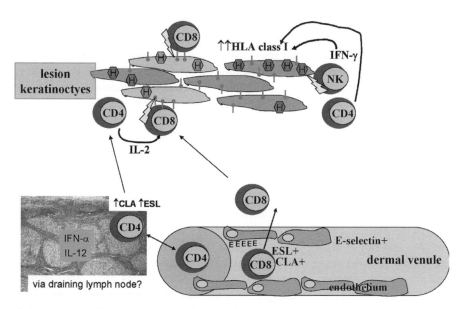

Fig. 34.1. Model of human recurrent genital HSV-2 lesion.

persons. Recently, CLA expression was used to derive panels of HSV-2-specific CD8 CTL clones from blood samples, without secondary in vitro re-stimulation with antigen. The fine specificity of each resultant clone was determined. For most subjects, clonal enumeration detected responses that were focused on one to three HSV-2 peptides per person (Koelle, 2003). Likely, subdominant responses were missed. Similar to other viral systems in humans (Betts et al., 2000), the presence of a specific HLA class I allele did not exert a dominant effect over the selection of viral epitopes for recognition. In some individuals with prevalent alleles such as HLA A*0201 or B*0702, clones restricted by these alleles predominated, while the major response "ignored" these alleles in other persons. Tegument-derived peptides were recognized the most frequently when clonal specificities were categorized by viral structural and kinetic class. Virion input tegument proteins to be recognized in infected APC without a requirement for de novo protein synthesis (Koelle et al., 2001), but it is not known if this contributes to the relatively frequent recovery of clones specific for tegument proteins.

Higher estimates of the diversity of the human CD8 response to HSV-2 have recently been obtained using overlapping peptide sets covering about half of the proteome and IFN-γ secretion as the readout. The median number of ORFs recognized per person was 11. Tegument and immediate early targets of the CD8 response were particularly well represented. The cumulative frequency of IFN-γ producing cells was generally well under 1% of CD8 cells (Hosken et al., 2006). As with the tetramer readouts mentioned above, peptide interrogation of IFN-γ secreting cells show that the integrated CD8 response to HSV-2 in the PBMC compartment is likely much smaller than the response to CMV (Sylwester et al., 2005).

CD4 T-cell responses to HSV

CD4 T-cells have several potential antiviral functions including B-cell help (Yasukawa et al., 1988), CD8 help (Lu et al., 2000), secretion of antiviral (Wong and Goeddel, 1986) and immune-enhancing cytokines such as IFN-γ and TNF-α, and direct cytotoxicity (Yasukawa and Zarling, 1984). These cells localize by day two to recurrent human genital HSV-2 lesions (Koelle et al., 1998b), and also to the uterine cervix (Koelle et al., 2000b) and to the cornea and retina in human ocular HSV infections (Verjans et al., 1996, 1998; Koelle et al., 2000a). Brisk lymphoproliferative responses by PBMC to killed whole HSV reflect a fairly high frequency of HSV-specific CD4 cells in seropositive persons. Quantitative estimates range from about 0.1% of PBMC by limiting dilution proliferation assays (Posavad et al., 1997) to 0.2%–0.4% of circulating CD4+ lymphocytes by IFN-γ intracellular cytokine cytometry (ICC) (Asanuma et al., 2000), and TNFβ ELISPOT (Schmid et al., 1997). CD40L up-regulation, a vital step in B-cell and CD8 T-cell help via DC conditioning, is also detectable on about 0.5% of peripheral blood CD4 cells in response to HSV-2 antigen (Gonzalez et al., 2005). The responder estimates for a specific peptide epitope are quite low (0.002% of CD4 cells) (Kwok et al., 2000). Data are limited, but the response appears to be diverse within infected persons: a median of four HSV-2 ORFs were recognized among seven ORFs tested (Koelle et al., 2000c). The CD4 response coexists with CD4-directed immune evasion strategies (Lewandowski et al., 1993; Barcy and Corey, 2001; Neumann et al., 2003; Trgovcich et al., 2002), covered in detail elsewhere in this volume.

CD4+ cells contribute to protection against HSV in mice. In a zosteriform model, passive transfer of immune CD4+ cells was sufficient to confer protection, and ablation of CD4 cells increased susceptibility in naïve animals (Manickan and Rouse, 1995; Manickan et al., 1995a, b). The CD4 effect was mouse strain-dependent. In the murine vaginal HSV-2 model, recently reviewed (Parr and Parr, 2003), progestin treatment thins the epithelium, increases the susceptibility of naïve animals, and alters local immune responses to HSV-2 (Kaushic et al., 2003). Attenuated (tk mutant) intravaginal inoculation is non-fatal, and results in high-level, sterilizing, protective immunity against challenge with wild-type virus. In this model, depletion of CD4 T-cells delayed viral clearance after challenge (Milligan et al., 1998). Qualitative parameters in the murine CD4 response generally support the importance of Th1-like IFN-γ responses. A survey of "long" gD1 peptides predicted to be antigenic by a computer algorithm revealed distinct elicitation of Th1 (IFN-γ-high IL-4 low) and Th2 (IFN-γ-low IL-4 high) responses by individual peptides given with an oil-in-water adjuvant. The Th1 peptides were more protective against an ocular HSV-1 challenge than were the Th2 peptides, and protection was mediated by CD4+ cells (BenMohamed et al., 2003).

Recently, a subset of CD4+ T-cells with constituitive expression of CD25 (T_{reg}) have been described that have suppressor or regulatory activity (Chatenoud et al., 2001). Depletion of T_{reg} in mice led to increased CD8 CTL responses against the HSV $gB1_{498-505}$ epitope, which persisted into the memory phase after T_{reg} recovery (Suvas et al., 2003). CD25 depletion lead to a short window period of faster viral clearance from the inoculation site, while adoptive transfer of CD4+CD25+ cells (from naïve mice) led to delayed clearance. HSV-1 infection of mice increased the in vitro, per-cell suppressor activity of their CD4+CD25+ splenocytes. Interestingly, CD25+ cell depletion worsened CD4 T-cell mediated corneal immunopathology in a mouse model of HSV keratitis, even though it sped viral clearance (Suvas et al., 2004). Recently, blood CD4+ CD25^{high} cells have been shown to suppress recall lymphoproliferative responses to HSV-2 antigen in humans (Diaz and Koelle, 2006). While T_{reg} have functional TCR, they often act in an antigen non-specific manner and it is not known if HSV-specific T_{reg} occur in mice or humans.

It is not yet clear if CD4 responder cell numbers or function correlate with disease severity in humans. A general relationship is present between lower overall CD4 cell numbers and HSV shedding among HIV-infected men (Schacker et al., 1998). However, in a cross-sectional study of HSV-2/HIV-1 co-infected men, HSV-2 severity did not correlate with HSV-2-specific CD4 cell numbers (Posavad et al., 1997). Data from small numbers of subjects indicate that proliferative responses to specific viral proteins may be higher in symptomatic than asymptomatic persons (Spatz et al., 2000). Responses to whole virus may be lower in symptomatic than in asymptomatic persons (reaching significance on one study (Frenkel et al., 1989) and trending to significance in a small study (Singh, 2003a). Studies of HSV-1 disease severity and IFN-γ responses (likely, but not proven, to be CD4 mediated) were close to (Spruance et al., 1995) or achieved (McKenna et al., 2001) statistical significance for association between higher responses and milder disease. In a small study of HSV-2 infected persons with proliferative responses to HSV antigen were measured, asymptomatic seropositives had higher IFN-γ and lower IL-10 responses to HSV than did persons with symptomatic disease (Singh, 2003a). Longitudinal studies revealed a trend to decreased PBMC IFN-γ responses to HSV antigen over time after episodic acyclovir therapy of a genital herpes outbreak (Singh, 2003a). Two recent vaccine trials (Corey et al., 1999; Stanberry et al., 2002), used similar purified recombinant HSV-2 protein antigens, but different adjuvants. Partial clinical efficacy was reported only for the vaccine that included an adjuvant (alum and 3d-MPL) that elicits Th1-like CD4 responses, although head-to-head comparisons are not possible. In the recent human vaccine experience, elicitation of CD4 (and antibody) responses has not provided high-level protection from genital HSV-2 infection or disease (Koelle and Corey, 2003).

HSV-specific CD4 clones have diverse functional activities in vitro. They are heterogeneous with regards to cytotoxicity towards HSV-2-infected B-cells. All blood and genital lesion-derived CD4 clones have cytolytic potential, as all display cytotoxicity when maximally stimulated by peptide-pulsed B cells (Koelle et al., 1998a; 2000a). We can speculate that CD4 immune evasion mechanisms differentially modulate the killing of infected cells by HSV-specific CD4 clones; differential resistance to CD4 CTL-induced apoptosis has been demonstrated (Jerome et al., 1998). Cornea-derived HSV-1-reactive CD4 clones, in contrast, have not had CTL activity even when maximally stimulated (Koelle et al., 2000a). Killing of infected keratinocytes is detectable if they are pre-treated with IFN-γ (Mikloska et al., 1996). For blood-derived CD4 clones, the cytolytic mechanism for B cell targets appears to involve granules and not the Fas/FasL pathway (Yasukawa et al., 1999).

The CD4 response to HSV is broadly directed. Published targets are non-structural proteins ICP8 and the *UL50* product dUTPase, glycoproteins gB, gC, gD, gE, and gH, tegument proteins VP11/12, VP13/14, VP16, VP22, and the *UL21* gene product, and the capsid protein VP5 (Koelle and Corey, 2003). Responses to the *UL29* gene product, a DNA binding protein, were detected in the blood of an HSV-2-exposed, but HSV-1/HSV-2 seronegative person and possibly represent sensitization without seroconversion (Posavad *et al.*, 2003). The HLA DR, DP and DQ loci are each well represented among alleles restricting peptide-specific responses. The population prevalence of responses to the candidate vaccine compounds gB2 and gD2 is quite high, over 80%, among HSV-2 seropositives. Responses to some of the tegument proteins can match these levels (Koelle *et al.*, 2000c).

T-cells are required in the immunopathogensis of experimental herpes simplex interstitial keratitis (HSK) in mice (Metcalf *et al.*, 1979). Controversy surrounds the requirement for HSV-specific CD4 T-cells in the pathogenesis of this disease. In humans, tissue from end-stage lesions, namely, corneas removed for blinding HSK have been examined for the presence of HSV-specific T-cells. Two research groups are in agreement (Verjans *et al.*, 1998; Koelle *et al.*, 2000a) that HSV-specific, HLA class II-restricted, CD4+ T-cell clones are readily established from these specimens. These cells recognize HSV-1/HSV-2 cross-reactive tegument protein epitopes in some instances, and generally have a Th1-like cytokine profile. A minority of patients with more superficial corneal HSV infections progress to HSK. The effects of potent immunotherapy directed at genital herpes on the natural history of ocular HSV infections deserve close medical attention.

T-cell costimulation and HSV

Both CD4 and CD8 T-cells require costimulation during primary, and to a lesser extent, recall, responses. The two-signal model of T-cell activation holds that in addition to an agonistic ligand of the T-cell receptor, usually MHC plus peptide, one or more additional signals instruct a T-cell to become activated. Major co-stimulatory pathways include CD80 and CD86 on APC interacting with CD28 on T-cells, and CD40 on APC interacting with CD154 on T-cells. In vivo, a complex mixture of activatory and inhibitory stimuli are integrated by signal transduction pathways.

The CD40-CD40L system is required for immunoglobulin class switching and the development of Th1 CD4 responses. One human with a mutation in CD40 has been found to be hypersusceptible to HSV disease (Fuleihan, 2001; Garcia-Perez, 2003). Increased monocyte CD80 and CD86 expression after incubation of immune human PBMC with HSV is not inhibited by anti-IFN-γ, and may be due to CD40L conditioning of monocytes (Singh, 2003b). Deletion of CD40L or administration of anti-CD40L antibody decreased survival after HSV-1 footpad or vaginal inoculation, and delayed DLN CD4 responses to HSV antigen (Edelmann and Wilson, 2001; Inagaki-Ohara *et al.*, 2002). Enhancement of CD40L expression via an exogenous plasmid co-administered with a gD2 plasmid vaccine increased splenocyte memory Th1 responses to gD2 protein, and also increased survival in a murine HSV-2 challenge model (Sin *et al.*, 2001). As CD40L induces B cell maturation, the increased survival after HSV-1 challenge of mice with GVHD associated with CD40L protein administration was ascribed to enhanced anti-HSV antibodies (Beland *et al.*, 1998).

CD40 and CD40L are each members of the large TNF receptor and TNF families, respectively (Croft, 2003). Other members of these families have also been implicated in HSV pathogenesis. Lopez observed in 1975 that Balb/c mice were more susceptible than C57BL/6 mice to mortality after intraperitoneal infection with HSV-1 (Lopez, 1975). The exact genetic basis of this difference remains unknown, but at least one prominent locus has been mapped to a region of murine chromosome 6 which contains TNF receptor genes (Lundberg *et al.*, 2003). CD137 (4–1BB) is a TNF family member expressed by T-cells. CD137 provides a positive co-stimulatory signal which can augment anti-viral immunity (Halstead *et al.*, 2002). Mice deficient in CD137 or treated with anti-CD137L mAb show less corneal pathology in a HSV keratitis model (Seo *et al.*, 2003). HVEM, a member of the TNFR family, is best known as a receptor for HSV entry. Less is known concerning the potential for immune modulation by gD ligation of HVEM, which is expressed by many APC and lymphocytes (La *et al.*, 2002).

An expanding family of membrane proteins in the B7 family (Prasad *et al.*, 2003) expressed by APC and stromal cells have complex positive and negative effects on members of the CD28 family (Rudd and Schneider, 2003) expressed on T-cells. CD80 or CD86, when separately coadministered with gD2 as plasmids in mice, had adjuvant and suppressive effects, respectively, using immunologic and clinical end-points (Flo *et al.*, 2000, 2001). In a vaginal model of HSV-2 infection, mice deficient in both CD80 and CD86 failed to control the infection (Thebeau and Morrison, 2002). Immune correlates included decreases in CTL responses, local IFN-γ secreting T-cells, and CD40L up-regulation by CD4 T-cells in response to antigen, and alterations in HSV-specific immunoglobulin isotypes (Thebeau and Morrison, 2003). Systemic interruption of

B7 family/CD28 family interactions with CTLA4-Ig fusion ameliorates the course of HSK in mice, correlating with decreased memory CD4 responses to HSV (Gangappa et al., 1998). Local blockade of B7–1 and B7–2 (CD80 and CD86), which are present on corneal LC, also prevents HSK in mice (Chen and Hendricks, 1998). Thus far, few data link the B7 pathway and HSV in humans. A small study found that monocytes from HSV-infected persons displayed impaired CD80 and CD86 up-regulation in response to exogenous IFN-γ (Singh, 2003a).

Antibody responses to HSV

Antibody responses to HSV are known to be functionally important in the context of neonatal infection. The risk of clinically significant infection after delivery through a HSV culture-positive cervicovaginal tract is much higher during primary than during recurrent maternal infection (Brown et al., 2003). In the latter instance, maternal IgG antibodies are transferred to the neonate across the placenta. Antibodies cooperate with neutrophils, monocytes, and NK-like cells in mediating antibody-dependent cell-mediated cytotoxicity (ADCC) (Kohl, 1991). Of interest, recent candidate vaccines with limited efficacy stimulated low ADCC titers, despite eliciting high levels of binding and neutralizing antibody (Kohl et al., 2000).

Local antibody responses are of interest in the female genital tract. In the murine vaginal HSV-2 model, mice are protected by non-lethal vaginal infection with a tk- HSV-2 strain (Parr and Parr, 2003). Antibody plays a significant role in early virus containment after vaginal challenge, as shown with B-cell knock-out mice (Parr and Parr, 2003). Little evidence for local secretory IgA as an effector molecule was found, similar to findings in human genital secretions (Boggess et al., 1997). In contrast, local IgG with neutralizing activity was readily detected. Attempts to induce vaginal immunity in mice through a "common mucosal immune system" pathway, via intranasal or oral immunization, have been successful in some models, but protection has not been mechanistically linked with local IgA. Human IgG immunoblot kinetic patterns differ between serum and cervical samples, suggesting that genital tract IgG may reflect local synthesis in addition to diffusion of plasma protein (Ashley et al., 1994). Similar data has been presented for local antibody synthesis in HSV infections of the eye (Peek et al., 2002) and CNS, especially late into HSV encephalitis (Sauerbrei et al., 2000). Vaginal tissues from vaginally immunized mice contain many fairly persistent IgG-producing plasma cells, while similar vaccinations at other sites do not lead to this cell localization (Parr and Parr, 2003). Recently, specific expression of the mucosal homing molecule A_4B_7 integrin (MLA, CD103) has been demonstrated for B-cells specific for a gastrointestinal pathogen (Gonzalez et al., 2003). Similar B-cell homing to the genital tract is rational but has not yet been demonstrated.

The development of a specific immune evasion function for antibodies is additional evidence of the functional importance of the antibody response (Nagashunmugam et al., 1998). The HSV-encoded gE-gI high-affinity FcγR receptor is expressed on infected cells. gE-gI binds human, but not mouse, Fcγ, so a murine zosteriform spread model combines injection of human immune serum and challenge with wild-type or gE knockout HSV-1. The gE knockout has decreased virulence in the context of immune but not pre-immune human serum treatment (Lubinski et al., 2002), consistent with an effect on pathogenesis mediated through immune escape. Recently, a region of gE1 capable of eliciting blocking antibodies that reduce Fcγ binding was identified (Lin et al., 2003), and it has been proposed that inclusion of such an immunogen could assist vaccination against HSV (Lin et al., 2004).

Neutralization of clinical HSV isolates by rabbit antisera to HSV-1 vs. HSV-2 formed the basis for early HSV typing methods. Antibodies that inhibit the absorption, or neutralize, HSV in vitro are specific for gB, gC, gD, or gH/gL (Fuller et al., 1989; Fuller and Spear, 1987, 1985; Sanchez-Pescador et al., 1992). Antibodies to gB or gD inhibit neuron to keratinocyte spread in a two-cell model (Mikloska et al., 1999). Passive transfer of antibodies specific for several of these glycoproteins is protective in animals (Su et al., 1996; Balachandran et al., 1982); in some cases, ADCC may be involved rather than classic neutralization (Kohl et al., 1986). Recent advances in the study of HSV receptors, particularly for gD, have provided a structural basis for the differential neutralization of various gD-specific mAb (Whitbeck et al., 1999). Local application of neutralizing mAb can prevent disease after vaginal inoculation (Whaley et al., 1994). As reviewed elsewhere (Koelle and Corey, 2003), vaccines eliciting neutralizing titers above those seen in natural infection have not been clinically effective.

Innate immunity

The importance of innate immunity is readily demonstrable in primary infection and in acute lethality models. HSV immune escape mechanisms that target innate complement and class I interferon responses are reviewed elsewhere in this volume. Mobile leukocytes and tissue stromal cells collaborate in innate immunity. As reviewed at the outset of this chapter, dendritic cells form a crucial bridge between innate and adaptive immunity. Distinctions between innate and acquired are becoming increasingly arbitrary, as specialized pattern recognition receptors such as toll-like receptors (TLR) and NK-cell activatory receptors that recognize viral proteins in highly specific fashions (Arase et al., 2002) are being described.

Complement is another major bridge between innate and acquired immunity (Mullick et al., 2003). As discussed elsewhere in this volume, HSV gC specifically binds to and inactivates certain complement components (Lubinski et al., 2002). Elegant studies in complement-deficient mice have shown through genetic "complementation" that gC is a virulence factor in intact animals (Lubinski et al., 1999). Clinically, persons with complement deficiencies are not generally felt to have more serious HSV infections than the general population (Walport, 2001). This can be interpreted in two ways: either complement is already maximally disabled, or complement-dependent mechanisms, while active, are redundant in the otherwise normal host.

Neutrophils are not typically considered major antiviral effector cells. Neutropenic patients can have severe HSV infections, but usually in settings in which lymphocyte number or function are also impaired. Isolated neutropenia, or disorders of phagocyte effector functions such as chronic granulomatous disease (CGD), are not generally clinically associated with severe HSV infections (Andrews and Sullivan, 2003). Neutrophils do strongly infiltrate genital HSV lesions in humans at the pustule stage. Giemsa stains of cytospin preps of pustule cells from day 2–3 HSV-2 buttock or thigh lesions show >95% neutrophils (D. M. Koelle et al., unpublished data). HSV vesicle fluid is rich in chemokines that can attract neutrophils (Mikloska et al., 1998), and mice with genetic knock-out of chemokines which attract neutrophils have alterations in HSV pathogenesis (Tumpey et al., 1998). IL-17 can assist in chemokine synthesis, is up-regulated in infected human corneas, and made by keratocytes in response to HSV infection (Maertzdorf et al., 2002). Neutrophils localize to the HSV-2-infected vagina in mice. Depletion of neutrophils has measurable effects on viral clearance in both primary and vaccination/challenge models, especially at early time points and locally in the vagina (Milligan, 1999; Milligan et al., 2001). Neutrophil antiviral effector functions are not well characterized. CGD neutrophils, which have defects in the formation of reactive oxygen species, digest HSV normally (Van Strijp et al., 1990). Neutrophils have ADCC activity against infected cells (Siebens et al., 1979). Some defensins that are expressed by neutrophils have potent anti-HSV activity (Sinha et al., 2003). Neutrophils matrix metalloproteinases have been implicated in tissue damage related to HSV infection (Lee et al., 2002b).

Many cells respond to viral infection by the production of class I interferons. Protein products of this multigene family (interferon alphas and beta) have autocrine and paracrine activity and trigger the expression of a characteristic pattern of genes (interferon-stimulated genes, ISG). Class I interferons have pronounced anti-HSV activity in vitro and in animals (Connell et al., 1985) and appear to also be active in humans (Lebwohl et al., 1992). Limitin is a class I interferon-related protein with anti-HSV activity in an acute murine HSV-1 lethality model (Kawamoto et al., 2003) and potentially less toxicity.

The ISG pattern has been detected with expression arrays after infection of several cell types with HSV. Deletion of immediate early genes has been helpful to unmask this response (Nicholl et al., 2000). The canonical class I interferon signaling pathway through TyK2, JAK1, and STAT1 is not required for ISG up-regulation. Therefore, an autocrine class I interferon effect is unlikely be responsible for ISG activation. HSV virions, or VP16-mutated HSV which cannot replicate in fibroblasts, also elicits ISG expression without eliciting an interferon biological activity. Cells may have an alternative sensor mechanism to trigger the ISG pathway (Mossman et al., 2001). If VP16 is restored, ISG up-regulation is not detected, while cycloheximide restores ISG mRNA up-regulation during infection with wild-type HSV. HSV may therefore direct the synthesis of protein(s) that block ISG transcription, with some data suggesting ICP0 can mediate this function (Eidson et al., 2002; Harle et al., 2002). HSV evasion of class I interferon through $\gamma 34.5$ is discussed elsewhere in this volume and was recently reviewed (Leib, 2002). In brief, $\gamma 34.5$ antagonizes the protein kinase R (PKR) effector pathway for class I interferons. While PKR phosphorylates, and inactivates, EIF2α, thus reducing viral protein synthesis, $\gamma 34.5$ has or induces a phosphatase activity which removes this block. Deletion of $\gamma 34.5$ reduces the virulence of HSV by several orders of magnitude (Chou et al., 1990), an effect that disappears in IFN-α receptor or PKR knock-out, but not RNAse-L knock-out, mice (Leib et al., 1999; 2000).

Interferon-alpha is confusingly known as leukocyte interferon, in contrast to interferon-gamma, which is made more or less exclusively by lymphocytes (which are leukocytes). It was recognized very early that PBMC exposed to HSV make large amounts of interferon-alpha, regardless of donor HSV serostatus (Haahr et al., 1976). Rare leukocytes in PBMC that respond to HSV by producing IFN-α have been termed natural interferon producing cells (NIPC). A prominent NIPC was recently identified as dendritic cell subtype termed plasmacytoid dendritic cells or pDC (Siegal et al., 1999; Colonna et al., 2002; Fitzgerald-Bocarsly, 2002). These rare (<1% of PBMC) cells produce enormous amounts of IFN-α on a per-cell basis by up-regulating IFN mRNA after stimulation. The phenotype of pDC varies slightly from humans (CD4+ CD11c−) to mice (CD11c+CD11b-Gr-1+B220+). pDC recognize many DNA and RNA viruses, produce several different IFN-α gene products and IFN-β, and are decreased in advanced HIV infection (Chehimi et al., 2002), a condition characterized by susceptibility to viral infections. Their selective expression of TLR7 (Hornung et al., 2002) makes them a logical target for imidazoquinolines, TLR7 agonists (Hemmi et al., 2002) with anti-HSV activity (Spruance et al., 2001). It is not yet known if pDC localize to HSV-2 lesions, but pDC-like cells express CLA, a skin-homing molecule (Schmitt et al., 2000), and localize to melanoma lesions (Salio et al., 2003) and some inflammatory skin conditions (Wollenberg et al., 2002).

Clearly, several cell types in PBMC are capable of innate responses to viral stimuli. For example, monocytes, while secreting less IFN-α than pDC on a per-cell basis (Fitzgerald-Bocarsly, 2002), are more abundant in the blood and are the main NIPC for Sendai virus (Feldman et al., 1994). Dendritic cell plasticity allows non-pDC to make large amounts of IFN-α in response to some viruses (Diebold et al., 2003). Monocyte-lineage dendritic cells (derived in vitro with GM-CSF and maturation stimuli) also produce IFN-α in response to HSV (Rong et al., 2003). Other monocyte pro-inflammatory responses to HSV are discussed below.

The viral factor(s) involved in the detection of HSV by the innate immune system have been incompletely defined and may vary between different host responses and responder cell types. UV-inactivated virus or aldehyde-fixed, HSV-infected cells can stimulate PBMC IFN-α responses, indicating that viral replication may not be required (Rong et al., 2003; Lebon, 1985). Ankel et al. (1998) have presented data that glycoprotein D of HSV-1 or HSV-2 is a potent trigger of IFN-α production by human PBMC. Insect cells expressing plasma membrane gD (Sf9-gD1), but not other HSV-1 glycoproteins, or soluble truncated gD1, but not soluble gH/gL complexes, stimulate PBMC IFN-α secretion. Responses to HSV-1 or Sf9-gD1 were inhibited by HSV immune human sera and also monoclonal anti-gD (Fitzgerald-Bocarsly et al., 1991; Ankel et al., 1998). Inter-strain differences in the ability of HSV-1 strains to stimulate various NIPC have been detected (Rong et al., 2003), but their structural or genetic basis is unknown.

The host factors by which cells detect HSV and other viruses are under intense study (Vaidya and Cheng, 2003). TLR2, but not TLR4, has been implicated in sensing HSV-1 in a mouse intraperitoneal challenge model (Wakimoto et al., 2003; Finberg et al., 2003). A study of pDC isolated from bone marrow of gene knock-out mice, using IFN-α production as the readout, suggests a role for TLR9, but not TLR4, for responses to HSV-2 (Lund et al., 2003). Both human and mouse pDC express TLR9 (Kadowaki et al., 2001; Boonstra et al., 2003).

MyD88 knock-out also reduced IFN-α production, but this adaptor molecule is downstream of many receptors (Takeuchi and Akira, 2002). Confirmatory evidence of the TLR9 and MyD88-dependence of pDC IFN-α responses to HSV-1 was obtained using pDC sorted from splenocytes (Krug et al., 2003). HSV replication was not required, as UV-inactivated HSV-1 was able to stimulate IFN-α. In vivo, neither TLR9 knock out (in the Balb/c background) nor MyD88 knock out (in the C57BL/6 background) had any deleterious effect on the local control of HSV-1 infection. Because mice with deficiency of either the class I IFN receptor or PKR fail to contain HSV-1 infection (Luker et al., 2003; Leib et al., 2000), these data suggest that MyD88- and TLR-independent activation of the class I IFN pathway is possible.

Certain unmethylated CpG oligodeoxynucleotide sequences are the primary known ligands for TLR9. The IFN-α response of PBMC is inhibited by the lysosomotropic agent chloroquine, consistent with a requirement for the acidification of endosomes containing the triggering signal (Feldman et al., 1994). Of note, TLR9 has been reported to be primarily expressed intracellularly (Ahmad-Nejad et al., 2002). A possible link between endocytosis and TLR9 comes from the demonstration that mannose receptors (MR) on DC are involved in NIPC responses (Milone and Fitzgerald-Bocarsly, 1998). Anti-MR sera block NIPC responses, and NIPC with characteristics of human pDC (CD4+) express MR. MR is involved in internalizing ligands via endocytosis. If gD is a primary trigger for IFN-α, HSV receptors (Spear et al., 2000), including an MR (Brunetti et al., 1995), that recognize gD are logical candidates. Monoclonal antibodies to galactosyl cerebroside/sulfatide can block IFN-α production by PBMC in response to HSV-1 or gD (Ankel et al., 1998); related structures are present on some HSV receptors (Shukla and Spear, 2001).

The consequences of NIPC interactions with HSV have only begun to be described. In addition to secreting IFN-α, pDC can secrete other cytokines that influence priming such as IL-10 or IL-12 (Krug et al., 2003), prime T-cells (Fonteneau et al., 2003), increase T_{reg} activity ((Gilliet and Liu, 2002), or be tolerogenic (Kuwana et al., 2001). PDC priming of pseudo-naïve CD8 cells specific for a melanoma antigen reportedly up-regulated CLA expression (Salio et al., 2003); as noted above, HSV-2-specific CD8 cells express CLA, but thus far animal models have not indicated that pDC are functional APC for HSV-1 (Allan et al.,

2003). HSV-2 interaction with pDC leads to secretion of IFN-α and IL-12, which promote the expression of CLA on human memory HSV-2-specific CD4 T-cells in an ex vivo reconstitution system (Koelle et al., 2006). IFN-α biases Th responses to the Th1 phenotype in humans (Rogge et al., 1998). Murine NIPC (Asselin-Paturel et al., 2001) secrete IFN-α in response to HSV, but IFN-α biasing towards Th1 responses is altered in mice (Rogge et al., 1998), limiting the application of murine studies to humans. Other host cytokines can have modulatory effects on NIPC responses to HSV in vitro (Gary-Gouy et al., 2002; Payvandi et al., 1998) and may also influence pDC in vivo.

In addition to IFN-α, monocytes and macrophages secrete other immunomodulatory cytokines after exposure to HSV. TNF-α has anti-HSV activity by synergizing with IFN-γ (Wong and Goeddel, 1986) and up-regulating nitric oxide (Kodukula et al., 1999) and has both protective and immunopathologic roles in various HSV models (Kodukula et al., 1999; Keadle et al., 2000; Croen, 1993; Adler et al., 1997). Murine IFN-γ-primed macrophage-like cells produce TNF-α in response to HSV. UV- or formaldehyde-killed virus, a gL-deficient mutant (unable to enter cells), and a VP16 mutant unable to initiate transcription elicit TNF-α elicit partial TNF-α responses, while purified gD1 is a potent stimulator in this system. Responses to HSV-2 involved transcriptional (NF-κB, ATF/Jun) and translational control (Paludan et al., 2001). The use of gD vaccines (Stanberry et al., 2002) and anti-TNF therapies (Bresnihan and Cunnane, 2003) in humans raises interest in studying HSV-TNF-α biology in the natural host.

IL-12 is a cytokine with prominent effects on T-helper polarization. IL-12 p40 mRNA is increased in human genital HSV-2 lesions (Van Voorhis et al., 1996) and after infection of mice with HSV-1 (Kanangat et al., 1996). In contrast to TNF-α, murine macrophage-like cells had poor IL-12 p40 production in response to UV- or heat-killed HSV-1. Corneal epithelial cells are poor sources of IL-12 in response to HSV when compared to macrophage-lineage cells, but produce an uncharacterized activity that induces IL-12 in macrophages. Infected macrophages are also low producers of IL-12, based on two-color confocal microscopy, indicating that paracrine induction may also take place when macrophages are infected with HSV-1. In contrast to some monokines, viral protein synthesis appears to be required for macrophage IL-12 responses to HSV (Kumaraguru and Rouse, 2002). Detectable IL-12 is present in human HSV-1 vesicle fluid, and fetal and adult keratinocytes synthesize IL-12 in response to live HSV-1 infection (Mikloska et al., 1998).

IL-12 is one of several cytokines with adjuvant activity for HSV vaccines (Lee et al., 2003). In a murine intravaginal HSV-2 model, IL-12 knock-out mice had faster mortality than wild-type controls (Harandi et al., 2001a). IL-12 has anti-angiogenic activity in the cornea, mediated through IFN-γ and IFN-γ up-regulated chemokines, which may be relevant in herpes keratitis (reviewed by Dr. Rouse elsewhere in this volume) (Lee et al., 2002a). IL-18 is an IL-1 family cytokine which synergizes with IL-12 in inducing IFN-γ secretion by T cells. When leukocytes from HSV-naïve mice are stimulated with live HSV-2, roles for IL-12, IL-18, and also IFN-αβ can be demonstrated for IFN-γ secretion (Malmgaard and Paludan, 2003). Exogenous IL-18 improves survival in an acute HSV-1 lethality model, an effect that depended on IFN-γ but not NK cells (Fujioka et al., 1999). Knock-out of IL-18 alone accelerated death in a murine HSV-2 intravaginal acute lethality model. Depletion of IL-18 on an IL-12 deficient background further compromised survival. In the setting of sublethal attenuated HSV-2 vaccination, followed by a vaginal HSV-2 challenge, knock-out of either IL-12, IL-18, or both had no effect on survival, despite alterations in lymphoproliferation and immunoglobulin isotype switching (Harandi et al., 2001a).

IL-15 is an IL-2-related cytokine with profound effects on NK cells. HSV increases IL-15 in vivo in mice (Tsunobuchi et al., 2000) and in human PBMC; HSV-mediated increases in NK activity in these cultures are dependent on IL-15, and IL-15 neutralization increases productive HSV infection (Ahmad et al., 2000). Exogenous IL-15 can be protective in a murine HSV challenge model (Tsunobuchi et al., 2000). IL-15-deficient mice are about 100-fold more susceptible to acute lethality after vaginal HSV-2 inoculation (in the setting of progesterone treatment) than are wild-type congenics (Ashkar and Rosenthal, 2003). IL-15 can also increase acquired responses to HSV in the context of HSV DNA/cytokine cDNA co-vaccination (Sin et al., 1999).

Experimental HSV studies in mice typically use gene disruptions, antibody blockade, or cell depletion to study innate immunity. Fewer studies have addressed the human host and natural infection. CD40 assists priming at an intersection between innate and acquired responses, and as mentioned above, a person with a CD40 mutation and severe HSV has been described. Mutations affecting IFN-γ receptors or IL-12/IL-12R are not uncommon, but no instances of severe viral infection have been reported (Fieschi et al., 2003; Fieschi and Casanova, 2003). Homozygous mutations in the C-terminal phosphorylation domain of STAT1 reduce both IFN-α/β and IFN-γ signal transduction (Dupuis et al., 2003). As in *IFNGR1* (IFN-γ receptor ligand-binding chain), *IFNGR2* (IFN-γ receptor signaling chain), *IL12B* (IL-12 p40 protein), and *IL12RB1* (IL-12 receptor β1 chain) mutations, disseminated bacillus Calmette-Guerin (BCG) infections occur. Disseminated, fatal childhood infection with HSV-1 is also observed. Cell lines from these subjects are resistant to the anti-HSV effects of IFN-α in vitro (Dupuis et al., 2003). NK cell deficiencies are discussed below. Mutations in UNC-93B, an endoplasmic reticulum protein of unknown function, have recently been associated with lethal HSV infections and impairment of the PBMC IFN-α response to HSV virions (Casrouge et al., 2006).

IL-10 is another monocyte product with pleotropic anti-inflammatory and immune modulatory activities. In models of HSV keratitis, IL-10 administered in a variety of formats decreases interstitial keratitis without increasing viral replication (Daheshia et al., 1997). IL-10 mRNA is locally enriched in genital HSV-2 in humans (Van Voorhis et al., 1996) and protein is detected in areas of murine (Stumpf et al., 2002) and human (Mikloska et al., 1998; Ongkosuwito et al., 1998) HSV-1 infection. The sources of IL-10 in herpes infection in vivo are not known, and could include parenchymal cells (Zak-Prelich et al., 2001) and responding lymphocytes (Koelle et al., 2000a). An association between a homozygous polymorphism in the IL-10 promoter and HSV serostatus (Hurme et al., 2003) awaits confirmation.

Immunomodulators and HSV

Several groups have attempted to modulate HSV infection by altering innate or HSV-specific immune responses. CpG ODN co-administration potentiates the immunogenicity and efficacy (against subsequent vaginal HSV-1 challenge) of vaccination with an immunodominant HSV CD8 peptide (Gierynska et al., 2002). CpG also had an adjuvant effect when given prior to vaccination with an intravaginal sublethal dose of live HSV-2 (Harandi et al., 2003). CpG ODN given intravaginally without an HSV constituent protects against subsequent intravaginal HSV-2 challenge and can also be therapeutic (Harandi et al., 2003; Ashkar et al., 2003; Pyles et al., 2002). IFN-γ and the IFN-γ inducers IL-12 and IL-18 were induced locally by CpG ODN. Knock-out of IL-12 and IL-18 reduced protection in one model, while the effect of IFN-γ knock-out on CpG ODN protection may depend on CpG and virus dosing. Infiltration of NK1.1 (+) NK or NKT cells and CD11b+ cells (likely DC) and proliferative changes in the genital mucosa were associated with CpG ODN but not control ODN administration. The imidazoquinoline resiquimod is a TLR7 agonist that increases local IFN-α levels after topical application (Hemmi et al., 2002; Arany et al., 1999). Unfortunately, a phase III clinical trial of topical resiquimod for recurrent genital HSV-2 in humans was stopped without evidence of clinical activity (February 2003).

Chemokines

Chemokines are a large family of small, basic proteins with diverse cellular sources and biological activities (Bacon et al., 2002). HSV-1 is not known to encode chemokine or chemokine receptor homologues. HSV-1 vesicle fluid from humans contains high levels of CCL5 (RANTES), CCL3 (MIP-1α), and CCL4 (MIP-1β) (Mikloska et al., 1998). Cultured human keratinocytes synthesize these chemokines in response to live HSV-1 infection, despite cytopathic effect. The chemokines CCL2 (MCP-1), CCL3, CCL5, and CXCL8 (IL-8) are significantly increased the cerebrospinal fluid in HSV encephalitis in humans (Rosler et al., 1998).

Chemokines have been hypothesized to assist with recruitment of lymphocytes and monocytes to areas of infection (Mikloska et al., 1998). Studies of HSV infection and vaccination in wild-type and knock-out animals, and in vitro studies, have implicated chemokines and their receptors in adaptive, and pathogenic, host responses. Local CCL5 (RANTES) and CCL2 (MCP-1) levels are increased in the vagina after HSV-2 infection. Innate and acquired immunity both contribution to CCL5 accumulation as accelerated, heightened responses are observed in previously vaccinated animals. For CCL2, in contrast, vaginal levels were decreased after challenge of vaccinated vs. non-vaccinated animals, and local CCL2 was correlated with tissue inflammation and damage. Vaginal CCL5 protein levels were partially dependent on IFN-γ after challenge of vaccinated wild-type vs. IFNγ -/- mice (Harandi et al., 2001b). CCL5 is persistently expressed in latently infected murine ganglia (Halford et al., 1996). Knockout of CCL3 (MIP-1α) (Menten et al., 2002) lessens histologic HSK in mice, correlating with decreased ingress of CD4+ cells and decreased IFN-γ and IL-2 mRNA levels, without effecting HSV-1 clearance (Tumpey et al., 1998). Neutralization of CXCL10 (IP-10) also lessened leukocyte infiltration and pathology while transiently increasing corneal HSV-1 replication after scarification (Carr et al., 2003). As with T$_{reg}$ cells, chemokines can have complex influences on HSV pathogenesis. CXCR3-deficient mice have decreased clearance of HSV-1 in a CNS infection model, but also show increased survival (Wickham et al., 2005).

NK cells

Human NK cells with activity against non HLA-restricted cytotoxicity against HSV-infected fibroblasts have long been described (Lopez et al., 1982). NK activity against HSV-infected fibroblasts was always observed to take many hours, in contrast to the killing of tumor cells such as K562, and some distinctions were found between the two effector functions. The recognition that IL-12, IL-15, and IFN-α are induced upon exposure of mixed PBMC to HSV, and are profound inducers of NK cell activity (reviewed above), may explain the time course of NK action against HSV-infected target cells.

NK recognition of HSV-infected cells is not unexpected, as HSV down-regulates HLA class I (Hill et al., 1995), and this precise absence is detected by NK cells through loss of inhibitory ligand recognition (Moser et al., 2002). Introduction of HSV-1 ICP47 into target cells can increase their susceptibility to NK cell lysis, as expected from decreased surface HLA class I (Huard and Fruh, 2000). However, it is increasingly recognized that NK cell activation can include ligation of specific activatory receptors in addition to loss of inhibition, and several examples of interactions between virally-encoded proteins and NK receptors have been discovered (Arase et al., 2002; Mandelboim et al., 2001). We believe it is likely that NK cells are involved in controlling virus in recurrent genital HSV-2 lesions that reach clinical threshold, as both NK cell numbers and NK activity were dramatically increased in cells expanded from lesional biopsies compared to normal skin (Koelle et al., 1998b). No activatory interactions between HSV proteins and NK cells are known, but little work was been done in this area. Some early work suggested specific recognition of HSV-1 glycoproteins (Bishop et al., 1984, 1986). In contrast, other work with replication inhibitors and mutant viruses suggest that immediate early gene expression may be sufficient to sensitize HSV-infected targets to NK lysis (Fitzgerald-Bocarsly et al., 1991). With hindsight, it is possible to hypothesize that these HSV glycoproteins were triggering innate immune responses which facilitate NK cell cytotoxicity, or alternatively that direct interactions between NK surface activatory molecules and HSV glycoproteins are occurring ... we have little real data. NK clones with cytolytic and anti-viral activities against HSV-infected cells from human blood (Yasukawa and Zarling, 1983; Yasukawa and Kobayashi, 1985), expressing clonally distributed NK receptors (Pietra et al., 2000), may assist in determining the molecular basis of NK cell recognition of HSV.

Clinically, low NK cell activity has been linked with severe, usually primary, HSV infections (Biron et al., 1989; Lopez et al., 1983). A homozygous mutation was detected in the FcγRIIIa gene of a child with severe HSV infection, and low NK cell number and function, although ADCC function was not abnormal (Jawahar et al., 1996). Tantalizing older literature has linked high HSV disease severity with low PBMC NK activity (Sirianni et al., 1986). As with many immune assays, re-evaluation may be in order using objective measures of HSV severity such as viral shedding rates (Wald et al., 2000), which can differ greatly between immunocompetent persons. Some functional data indicate that NK cells are active in acute HSV lethality models in mice (Rager-Zisman et al., 1987; Bukowski and Welsh, 1986). The difference in lethal dose for 50% of animals (LD_{50}) for acute HSV-1 infection between C57BL/6 and Balb/c mice (Lopez, 1975), discussed above in the context of a TNF-receptor locus, has also been genetically mapped by a second research group to a region containing many NK-cell receptors (Pereira et al., 2001). However, it is not yet known precisely what gene (or genes) is involved.

NKT cells

Several populations of NKT cells, broadly defined as expressing both TCR $\alpha\beta$ heterodimers and NK markers such as NK1.1 or CD161, are now recognized (Kronenberg and Gapin, 2002). NKT cells can make large amounts of cytokines such as IL-4 or IFN-γ after activation (Benlagha et al., 2002). In mice, many NKT cells expressing the semi-variant Vα14-Jα281 TCR. Deletion of either CD1d or Jα281 from the germline increases the early pathogenicity of HSV for zosteriform spread in the normally resistant C57BL6 background (Grubor-Bauk et al., 2003). While a subset of NKT cells recognize antigens presented by CD1, the viral or host molecules involved in possible activation of NKT cells by HSV have not been defined. An NKT-like infiltrate in a region of HSV infection has been reported in a human (Taddesse-Heath et al., 2003), but in vitro studies have not documented interactions between murine or human NKT cells and HSV.

TCR$\gamma\delta$ cells

T-cell expressing the gamma and delta T-cell receptor molecules (TCR$\gamma\delta$ cells) can recognize HSV-infected cells. Non-MHC-restricted recognition of a peptide from HSV-1 gI has been documented (Sciammas and Bluestone, 1998). TCR$\gamma\delta$ cells contribute to HSV-1 clearance in an acute cerebral infection model in mice (Sciammas et al., 1997) and localize to some sites of infection (Liu et al., 1996), but other models have not shown an effect when TCR$\gamma\delta$ cells are missing (Nass et al., 2001). Human TCR$\gamma\delta$ clones can recognize HSV-1-infected cells in a non HLA-restricted manner (Maccario et al., 1995). These cells can be expanded from the blood by incubation with HSV (Maccario et al., 1993). The jury is still out on the importance of rare

T-cell subsets such as NKT and TCRγδ cells in human HSV infection.

Additional interactions between HSV and the immune system

Chronic stress has been linked to recurrences of symptomatic HSV disease (Cohen *et al.*, 1999) although not, as yet, to quantitatively measured HSV shedding. Broadly, stressors could affect neuronal events and/or immunologic responsiveness. For example, ciliary neurotrophic growth factor and IL-6 share a receptor subunit, and have been reported to worsen clinical HSV infections in humans or promote reactivation from ganglia in culture (Kriesel *et al.*, 1994, 1997a,b). Manipulations of sympathetic enervation can reduce primary and memory HSV-specific CTL responses in mice and worsen HSV pathogenesis (Leo and Bonneau, 2000). Some data link stress and immune suppression in humans, including relevant effector functions such as NK cell number and activity and lymphocyte proliferation (Zorrilla *et al.*, 2001). Bonneau *et al.* have been studying the relationship between the nervous system, stressors and HSV-specific CD8 CTL activity in C57BL/6 mice. Stress increases the pathogenesis of HSV infection in several models (Bonneau *et al.*, 1991, 1997). Using mice previously immunized with the immunodominant gB1 epitope in a recombinant vaccinia format, the effects of restraint stress and mAb-mediated CD8 depletion were compared for intravaginal or intranasal HSV challenges (Wonnacott and Bonneau, 2002). Both stress and CD8 depletion caused similar, significant increases in acute mortality and increases in vaginal HSV replication.

Very recently, a possible mechanistic link has been suggested by the finding that structured stress decreased the number of HSV-specific CD8 T-cells in the ganglia of HSV-infected mice (Hendricks, 2006). Ongoing work will hopefully elucidate mechanisms that connect stress and the nervous and immune systems.

Summary

The broad host range of HSV and the prevalence of HSV infections in humans have enabled several decades of excellent studies, well beyond the capacity of this review or this reviewer. Despite this, it is fair to say that our understanding of the immune response to HSV is still primitive, and inadequate to address clinical and basic science issues. For example, we do not know if "immunology" can explain the variation in disease severity, how to make an effective vaccine or immunotherapy, or what goes wrong in HSK. HSV research has benefited tremendously from advances in basic immunology, such as the definition of leukocyte subsets, leukocyte-specific proteins, cytokines, and chemokines. The huge effort that has gone into human retrovirus and cancer immunology has led to the development of technique and reagents that have been very useful in the study of acquired responses to HSV in humans. Research accompanying the resurgence of interest in innate immunity over the last decade has revealed that HSV is a strong initiator of innate responses, and that HSV infection can be powerfully modified by innate immunity. Laboratory studies with materials from "outlier" patients with severe HSV, and well-characterized subjects with more routine HSV infections, together with the continuing application of animal models as new key host and viral molecules and pathways are defined, will continue to be rational lines of inquiry. Insights into basic immunology, such as the NIPC and APC identification studies discussed above, are likely to continue to result from HSV research. The challenging synthesis of HSV-specific and broader studies may hopefully lead to clinical advances in the not-too-distant future.

REFERENCES

Adler, H., Beland, J. L., Del-Pan, N. C. *et al.* (1997). Suppression of herpes simplex virus type 1 (HSV-1)-induced pneumonia in mice by inhibition of inducible nitric oxide synthase (iNOS, NOS2). *J. Exp. Med.*, **185**, 1533–1540.

Ahmad, A., Sharif-Askari, E., Fawaz, L., and Menezes, J. (2000). Innate immune response of the human host to exposure with herpes simplex virus type 1: in vitro control of the virus infection by enhanced natural killer activity via interleukin-15 induction. *J. Virol.*, **74**, 7196–7203.

Ahmad-Nejad, P., Hacker, H., Rutz, M., Bauer, S., Vabulas, R. M., and Wagner, H. (2002). Bacterial CpG-DNA and lipopolysaccharides activate Toll-like receptors at distinct cellular compartments. *Eur. J. Immunol.*, **32**, 1958–1968.

Allan, R. S., Smith, C. M., Belz, G. T. *et al.* (2003). Epidermal viral immunity induced by CD8alpha+ dendritic cells but not by Langerhans cells. *Science*, **301**, 1925–1928.

Allan, R. S., Waithman, J., Bedoui, S. *et al.* (2006). Migratory dendritic cells transfer antigen to a lymph node-resident dendritic cell population for efficient CTL priming. *Immunity* **25**, 153.

Andersen, H., Dempsey, D., Chervenak, R., and Jennings, S. R. (2000). Expression of intracellular IFN-gamma in HSV-1-specific CD8+ T cells identifies distinct responding subpopulations during the primary response to infection. *J. Immunol.*, **165**, 2101–2107.

Andrews, T., and Sullivan, K. E. (2003). Infections in patients with inherited defects in phagocytic functions. *Clin. Microbiol. Rev.*, **16**, 597–621.

Ankel, H., Westra, D. F., Welling-Wester, S., and Lebon, P. (1998). Induction of interferonalpha by glycoprotein D of herpes simplex virus: a possible role of chemokine receptors. *Virology*, **251**, 317–326.

Arany, I., Tyring, S. K., Stanley, M. A. *et al.* (1999). Enhancement of the innate and cellular immune response in patients with genital warts treated with topical imiquimod cream 5%. *Antiviral Res.*, **43**, 55–63.

Arase, H., Mocarski, E. S., Campbell, A. E., Hill, A. B., and Lanier, L. L. (2002). Direct recognition of cytomegalovirus by activating and inhibitory NK cell receptors. *Science*, **296**, 1323–1326.

Arzul, I., Renault, T., Thebault, A., and Gerard, A. (2002). Detection of oyster herpesvirus DNA and proteins in asymptomatic *Crassostrea gigas* adults. *Virus Res.*, **84**, 151–160.

Asanuma, H., Sharp, M., Maecker, H. T., Maino, V. C., and Arvin, A. M. (2000). Frequencies of memory T cells specific for varicella-zoster virus, herpes simplex virus and cytomegalovirus determined by intracellular detection of cytokine expression. *J. Infect. Dis.*, **181**, 859–866.

Ashkar, A. A., and Rosenthal, K. L. (2003). Interleukin-15 and natural killer and NKT cells play a critical role in innate protection against genital herpes simplex virus type 2 infection. *J. Virol.*, **77**, 10168–10171.

Ashkar, A. A., Bauer, S., Mitchell, W. J., Vieira, J., and Rosenthal, K. L. (2003). Local delivery of CpG oligodeoxynucleotides induces rapid changes in the genital mucosa and inhibits replication, but not entry, of herpes simplex virus type 2. *J. Virol.*, **77**, 8948–8956.

Ashley, R. L., Corey, L., Dalessio, J. *et al.* (1994). Protein-specific cervical antibody responses to primary genital herpes simplex virus type 2 infections. *J. Infect. Dis.*, **170**, 20–26.

Asselin-Paturel, C., Boonstra, A., Dalod, M. *et al.* (2001). Mouse type I IFN-producing cells are immature APCs with plasmacytoid morphology. *Nat. Immunol.*, **2**, 1144–1150.

Bacon, K., Baggiolini, M., Broxmeyer, H. *et al.* (2002). Chemokine/chemokine receptor nomenclature. *J. Interferon Cytokine Res.*, **22**, 1067–1068.

Balachandran, N., Bacchetti, S., and Rawls, W. E. (1982). Protection against lethal challenge of Balb/c mice by passive transfer of monoclonal antibodies to five glycoproteins of herpes simplex virus type 2. *Infect. Immun.*, **37**, 1132–1137.

Barcy, S. and Corey, L. (2001). Herpes simplex inhibits the capacity of lymphoblastoid B cell lines to stimulate CD4+ T cells. *J. Immunology*, **166**, 6242–6249.

Barouch, D. H. and Letvin, N. L. (2001). CD8+ cytotoxic T lymphocyte responses to lentiviruses and herpesviruses. *Curr. Opin. Immunol.*, **13**, 479–482.

Becker, Y. (2003). Immunological and regulatory functions of uninfected and virus infected immature and mature subtypes of dendritic cells – a review. *Virus Genes*, **26**, 119–130.

Beland, J. L., Alder, H., Del-Pan, N. C. *et al.* (1998). Recombinant CD40L treatment protects allogeneic murine bone marrow transplant recipients from death caused by herpes simplex virus-1 infection. *Blood*, **92**, 4472–4478.

Benlagha, K., Kyin, T., Beavis, A., Teyton, L., and Bendelac, A. (2002). A thymic precursor to the NK T cell lineage. *Science*, **296**, 553–555.

BenMohamed, L., Bertrand, G., McNamara, C. D. *et al.* (2003). Identification of novel immunodominant CD4+ Th1-type T-cell peptide epitopes from herpes simplex virus glycoprotein D that confer protective immunity. *J. Virol.*, **77**, 9463–9473.

Betts, M. R., Casazza, J. P., Patterson, B. A. *et al.* (2000). Putative immunodominant human immunodeficiency virus-specific CD8+ T-cell responses cannot be predicted by major histocompatibility complex class I haplotype. *J. Virol.*, **74**, 9144–9151.

Biron, C. A., Byron, K. S., and Sullivan, J. L. (1989). Severe herpesvirus infections in an adolescent without natural killer cells. *N. Engl. J. Med.*, **320**, 1731–1735.

Bishop, G. A., Marlin, S. D., Schwartz, S. A., and Glorioso, J. C. (1984). Human natural killer cell recognition of herpes simplex virus type 1 glycoproteins: specificity analysis with the use of monoclonal antibodies and antigenic variants. *J. Immunol.*, **133**, 2206–2214.

Bishop, G. A., Kumel, G., Schwartz, S. A., and Glorioso, J. C. (1986). Specificity of human natural killer cells in limiting dilution culture for determinants of herpes simplex virus type 1 glycoproteins. *J. Virol.*, **57**, 294–300.

Blaney, J. E., Nobusawa, E., Brehm, M. A. *et al.* (1998). Immunization with a single major histocompatibility class I-restricted cytotoxic T-lymphocyte recognition epitope of herpes simplex virus type 2 confers protective immunity. *J. Virol.*, **72**, 9567–9574.

Boggess, K. A., Watts, D. H., Hobson, A. C., Ashely, R. L., Brown, Z. A., and Corey, L. (1997). Herpes simplex virus type 2 detection by culture and polymerase chain reaction and relationship to genital symptoms and cervical antibody status during the third trimester of pregnancy. *Am. J. Obstet. Gynecol.*, **176**, 443–451.

Bonneau, R. H., Sheridan, J. F., Feng, N. G., and Glaser, R. (1991). Stress-induced suppression of herpes simplex virus (HSV)-specific cytotoxic T lymphocyte and natural killer cell activity and enhancement of acute pathogenesis following local HSV infection. *Brain Behav. Immun.*, **5**, 170–192.

Bonneau, R. H., Brehm, M. A., and Kern, A. M. (1997). The impact of psychological stress on the efficacy of anti-viral adoptive immunotherapy in an immunocompromised host. *J. Neuroimmunol.*, **78**, 19–33.

Boonstra, A., Asselin-Paturel, C., Gilliet, M. *et al.* (2003). Flexibility of mouse classical and plasmacytoid-derived dendritic cells in directing T helper type 1 and 2 cell development: dependency on antigen dose and differential toll-like receptor ligation. *J. Exp. Med.*, **197**, 101–109.

Brehm, M. A., Pinto, A. K., Daniels, K. A., Schneck, J. P., Welsh, R. M., and Selin, L. K. (2002). T cell immunodominance and maintenance of memory regulated by unexpectedly cross-reactive pathogens. *Nat. Immunol.*, **3**, 627–634.

Bresnihan, B. and Cunnane, G. (2003). Infection complications associated with the use of biologic agents. *Rheum. Dis. Clin. North Am.*, **29**, 185–202.

Brown, Z. A., Wald, A., Morrow, R. A., Selke, S., Zeh, J., and Corey L. (2003). Effect of serologic status and cesarean delivery on transmission rates of herpes simplex virus from mother to infant. *J. Am. Med. Assoc.*, **289**, 203–209.

Brunetti, C. R., Burke, R. L., Hoflack, B., Ludwig, T., Dingwell, K. S., and Johnson, D. C. (1995). Role of mannose-6-phosphate receptors in herpes simplex virus entry into cells and cell-to-cell transmission. *J. Virol.*, **69**, 3517–3528.

Bukowski, J. F. and Welsh, R. M. (1986). The role of natural killer cells and interferon in resistance to acute infection of mice with herpes simplex virus type 1. *J. Immunol.*, **136**, 3481–3485.

Burrows, S. R., Silins, S. L., Moss, D. J., Khanna, R., Misko, I. S., and Argaet, V. P. (1995). T cell receptor repertoire for a viral epitope in humans is diversified by tolerance to a background major histocompatibility complex antigen. *J. Exp. Med.*, **182**, 1703–1715.

Carr, D. J., Chodosh, J., Ash, J., and Lane, T. E. (2003). Effect of anti-CXCL10 monoclonal antibody on herpes simplex virus type 1 keratitis and retinal infection. *J. Virol.*, **77**, 10037–10046.

Cartier, A., Broberg, E., Komai, T., Henriksson, M., and Masucci, M. G. (2003). The herpes simplex virus-1 Us3 protein kinase blocks CD8T cell lysis by preventing the cleavage of Bid by granzyme B. *Cell Death Differ.*

Casrouge, A., Zhang, S. Y., Eidenschenk, C. Herpes simplex virus encephalitis in human UNC-93B deficiency. *Science*, **314**, 308–312.

Chatenoud, L., Salomon, B., and Bluestone, J. A. (2001). Suppressor T cells-they're back and critical for regulation of autoimmunity! *Immunol. Rev.*, **182**, 149–163.

Chehimi, J., Campbell, D. E., Azzoni, L. *et al.* (2002). Persistent decreases in blood plasmacytoid dendritic cell number and function despite effective highly active antiretroviral therapy and increased blood myeloid dendritic cells in HIV-infected individuals. *J. Immunol.*, **168**, 4796–4801.

Chen, H. and Hendricks, R. L. (1998). B7 costimulatory requirements of T cells at an inflammatory site. *J. Immunol.*, **160**, 5045–5052.

Chen, S. H., Garber, D. A., Schaffer, P. A., Knipe, D. M., and Coen, D. M. (2000). Persistent elevated expression of cytokine transcripts in ganglia latently infected with herpes simplex virus in the absence of ganglionic replication or reactivation. *Virology*, **278**, 207–216.

Chou, J., Kern, E. R., Whitley, R. J., and Roizman, B. (1990). Mapping of herpes simplex virus 1 neurovirulence to gamma 1 34.5, a gene nonessential for growth in cell culture. *Science*, **252**, 1262–1266.

Cohen, F., Kemeny, M. E., Zegans, L. S., Neuhaus, J. M., and Conant, M. A. (1999). Persistent stress as a predictor of genital herpes recurrence. *Arch. Intern. Med.*, **159**, 2330–2336.

Coles, R. M., Mueller, S. N., Heath, W. R., Carbone, F. R., and Brooks, A. G. (2002). Progression of armed CTL from draining lymph node to spleen shortly after localized infection with herpes simplex virus 1. *J. Immunol.*, **168**, 834–838.

Colonna, M., Krug, A., and Cella, M. (2002). Interferon-producing cells: on the front line in immune responses against pathogens. *Curr. Opin. Immunol.*, **14**, 373–379.

Connell, E. V., Cerruti, R. L., and Trown, P. W. (1985). Synergistic activity of combinations of recombinant human alpha interferon and acyclovir, administered concomitantly and in sequence, against a lethal herpes simplex type 1 infection in mice. *Antimicrob. Agents Chemother.*, **28**, 1–4.

Corey, L., Langenberg, A. G. M., Ashley, R. *et al.* (1999). Two double-blind, placebo-controlled trials of a vaccine containing recombinant gD2 and gB2 antigens in MF59 adjuvant for the prevention of genital HSV-2 acquisition. *J. Am. Med. Assoc.*, **282**, 331–340.

Cose, S. C., Kelly, J. M., and Carbone, F. R. (1995). Characterization of a diverse primary herpes simplex virus type 1 gB-specific cytotoxic T-cell response showing a preferential V beta bias. *J. Virol.*, **69**, 5849–5852.

Cose, S. C., Jones, C. M., Wallace, M. E., Heath, W. R., and Carbone, F. R. (1997). Antigen-specific CD8+ T cell subset distribution in lymph nodes draining the site of herpes simplex virus infection. *Eur. J. Immunol.*, **27**, 2310–2316.

Croen, K. D. (1993). Evidence for antiviral effect of nitric oxide. Inhibition of herpes simplex virus type 1 replication. *J. Clin. Invest.*, **91**, 2446–2452.

Croft, M. (2003). Co-stimulatory members of the TNFR family: keys to effective T-cell immunity? *Nat. Rev. Immunol.*, **3**, 609–620.

Cunningham, A. L., Turner, R. R., Miller, A. C., Para, M. F., and Merigan, T. C. (1985). Evolution of recurrent herpes simplex lesions: an immunohistologic study. *J. Clin. Invest.*, **75**, 226–233.

Daheshia, M., Kuklin, N., Kanangat, S., Manickan, E., and Rouse, B. T. (1997). Suppression of ongoing ocular inflammatory disease by topical administration of plasmid encoding IL-10. *J. Immunol.*, **159**, 1945–1952.

den Haan, J. M., Lehar, S. M., and Bevan, M. J. (2000). CD8(+) but not CD8(–) dendritic cells cross-prime cytotoxic T cells in vivo. *J. Exp. Med.*, **192**, 1685–1696.

Diaz, G. A. and Koelle, D. M., (2006). Human CD4+ CD25high cells suppress proliferative memory lymphocyte responses to herpes simplex virus type 2. *J. Virol.* **80**, 8271.

Diebold, S. S., Montoya, M., Unger, H. *et al.* (2003). Viral infection switches non-plasmacytoid dendritic cells into high interferon producers. *Nature*, **424**, 324–328.

Doukas, J. and Pober, J. S. (1990). IFN-gamma enhances endothelial activation induced by tumor necrosis factor but not IL-1. *J. Immunol.*, **145**, 1727–1733.

Dupuis, S., Jouanguy, E., Al-Hajjar, S. *et al.* (2003). Impaired response to interferon-alpha/beta and lethal viral disease in human STAT1 deficiency. *Nat. Genet.*, **33**, 388–391.

Edelmann, K. H. and Wilson, C. B. (2001). Role of CD28/CD80–86 and CD40/CD154 costimulatory interactions in host defense to primary herpes simplex virus infection. *J. Virol.*, **75**, 612–621.

Eidson, K. M., Hobbs, W. E., Manning, B. J., Carlson, P., and DeLuca, N. A. (2002). Expression of herpes simplex virus ICP0 inhibits the induction of interferon-stimulated genes by viral infection. *J. Virol.*, **76**, 2180–2191.

Feldman, L. T., Ellison, A. R., Voytek, C. C., Yang, L., Krause, P., and Margolis, T. P. (2002). Spontaneous molecular reactivation of herpes simplex virus type 1 latency in mice. *Proc. Natl Acad. Sci. USA*, **99**, 978–983.

Feldman, S. B., Ferraro, M., Zheng, H.-M., Patel, N., Gould-Fogerite, S. and Fitzgerald, Bocarsly, P. (1994). Viral induction of low frequency interferon-à producing cells. *Virology*, **204**, 1–7.

Fieschi, C. and Casanova, J. L. (2003). The role of interleukin-12 in human infectious diseases: only a faint signature. *Eur. J. Immunol.*, **33**, 1461–1464.

Fieschi, C., Dupuis, S., Catherinot, E. *et al.* (2003). Low penetrance, broad resistance, and favorable outcome of interleukin 12 receptor beta 1 deficiency: medical and immunological implications. *J. Exp. Med.*, **197**, 527–535.

Finberg, R. W., Kurt-Jones, E. A., Zhu, J., Arnold, M., and Knipe, D. (2003). Presented at the 28th International Herpesvirus Workshop, July 2003.

Fitzgerald-Bocarsly, P. (2002). Natural interferon-alpha producing cells: the plasmacytoid dendritic cells. *Biotechniques* Suppl, 16–20, 22, 24–29.

Fitzgerald-Bocarsly, P., Howell, D. M., Pettera, L., Tehrani, S., and Lopez, C. (1991). Immediate-early gene expression is sufficient for induction of natural killer cell-mediated lysis of herpes simplex virus type 1-infected fibroblasts. *J. Virol.*, **65**, 3151–3160.

Flo, J., Tismintezky, S., and Baralle, F. (2000). Modulation of the immune response to DNA vaccina by co-delivery of costimulatory molecules. *Immunology*, **100**, 259–267.

Flo, J., Tismintezky, S., and Baralle, F. (2001). Codelivery of DNA coding for the soluble form of CD86 results in the down-regulation of the immune response to DNA vaccines. *Cell. Immunol.*, **209**, 120–131.

Fonteneau, J. F., Gilliet, M., Larsson, M. *et al.* (2003). Activation of influenza virus-specific CD4+ and CD8+ T cells: a new role for plasmacytoid dendritic cells in adaptive immunity. *Blood*, **101**, 3520–3526.

Frenkel, L., Pineda, E., Hall, H., Dillon, M., and Bryson, Y. (1989). A prospective study of the effects of acyclovir treatment on the HSV-2 lymphoproliferative response of persons with frequently recurring HSV-2 genital infections. *J. Infect. Dis.*, **159**, 845–850.

Friedman, H. M. (2000). (letter) Immunologic strategies for herpes vaccination. *J. Am. Med. Assoc.*, **283**, 746.

Fujioka, N., Akazawa, R., Ohashi, K., Fujii, M., Ikeda, M., and Kurimoto, M. (1999). Interleukin-18 protects mice against acute herpes simplex virus type 1 infection. *J. Virol.*, **73**, 2401–2409.

Fuleihan, R. L. (2001). Hyper IgM syndrome: the other side of the coin. *Curr. Opin. Pediatr.*, **13**, 528–532.

Fuller, A. O. and Spear, P. G. (1985). Specificities of monoclonal and polyclonal antibodies that inhibit adsorption of herpes simplex virus to cells and lack of inhibition by potent neutralizing antibodies. *J. Virol.*, **55**, 475–482.

Fuller, A. O. and Spear, P. G. (1987), Anti-glycoprotein D antibodies that permit adsorption but block infection by herpes simplex virus 1 prevent virion-cell fusion at the cell surface. *Proc. Natl Acad. Sci. USA*, **84**, 5454–5458.

Fuller, A. O., Santos, R. E., and Spear, P. G. (1989). Neutralizing antibodies specific for glycoprotein H of herpes simplex virus permit viral attachment to cells but prevent penetration. *J. Virol.*, **63**, 3435–3443.

Gangappa, S., Manickan, E., and Rouse, B. T. (1998). Control of herpetic stromal keratitis using CTLA 4Ig fusion protein. *Clin. Immunol. Immunopathol.*, **86**, 88–94.

Garcia-Perez, M. A., Paz-Artal, E., Correll, A. *et al.* (2003). Mutations of CD40L ligand in two patients with hyper-IgM syndrome. *Immunobiology*, **207**, 285–294.

Gary-Gouy, H., Lebon, P., and Dalloul, A. H. (2002). Type I interferon production by plasmacytoid dendritic cells and monocytes is triggered by viruses, but the level of production is controlled by distinct cytokines. *J. Interferon Cytokine Res.*, **22**, 653–659.

Gierynska, M., Kumaraguru, U., Eo, S. K. (2002). Induction of CD8 T-cell-specific systemic and mucosal immunity against herpes simplex virus with CpG-peptide complexes. *J. Virol.*, **76**, 6568–6576.

Gilliet, M. and Liu, Y. J. (2002). Generation of human CD8 T regulatory cells by CD40 ligand-activated plasmacytoid dendritic cells. *J. Exp. Med.*, **195**, 695–704.

Goldsmith, K., Chen, W., Johnson, D. C., and Hendricks, R. L. (1998). Infected cell protein (ICP)47 enhances herpes simplex virus neurovirulence by blocking the CD8 T cell response. *J. Exp. Med.*, **187**, 341–348.

Gonzalez, A. M., Jaimes, M. C., Cajiao, I. *et al.* (2003). Rotavirus-specific B cells induced by recent infection in adults and children predominantly express the intestinal homing receptor alpha4beta7. *Virology*, **305**, 93–105.

Gonzalez, J. C., Kwok, W. W., Wald, A., McClurkan, C. L., and Koelle, D. M. (2005). Programmed expression of cutaneous lymphocyte-associated antigen amongst circulating memory T-cells specific for HSV-2. *J. Infect. Dis.*, **191**, 243–254.

Grubor-Bauk, B., Simmons, A., Mayrhofer, G., and Speck, P. G. (2003). Impaired clearance of herpes simplex virus type 1 from mice lacking CD 1d or NKT cells expressing the semi-variant V alpha 14-J alpha 281 TCR. *J. Immunol.*, **170**, 1430–1434.

Haahr, S., Rasmussen, L., and Merigan, T. C. (1976). Lymphocyte transformation and inter interferon production in human mononuclear cell microcultures for assay of cellular immunity to herpes simplex virus. *Infect. Immunol.*, **14**, 47–54.

Halford, W. P., Gebhardt, B. M., and Carr, D. J. (1996). Persistent cytokine expression in trigeminal ganglion latently infected with herpes simplex virus type 1. *J. Immunol.*, **157**, 3542–3549.

Halford, W. P., Gebhardt, B. M., and Carr, D. J. J. (1997). Acyclovir blocks cytokine gene expression in trigeminal ganglia latently infected with herpes simplex virus type 1. *Virology*, **238**, 53–63.

Halstead, E. S., Mueller, Y. M., Altman, J. D., and Katsikis, P. D. (2002). In vivo stimulation of CD 137 broadens primary antiviral CD8+ T cell responses. *Nat. Immunol.*, **3**, 536–541.

Hamann, D., Baars, P. A., Rep, M. H. *et al.* (1997). Phenotypic and functional separation of memory and effector human CD8+ T cells. *J. Exp. Med.*, **186**, 1407–1418.

Harandi, A. M., Svennerholm, B., Holmgren, J., and Eriksson, K. (2001a). Interleukin-12 (IL-12) and IL-18 are important in innate defense against genital herpes simplex virus type 2 infection in mice but are not required for the development of acquired gamma interferonmediated protective immunity. *J. Virol.*, **75**, 6705–6709.

Harandi, A. M., Svennerholm, B., Holmgren, J., and Eriksson, K. (2001b). Protective vaccination against genital herpes simplex virus type 2 (HSV-2) infection in mice is associated with a rapid induction of local IFN-gamma-dependent RANTES production following a vaginal viral challenge. *Am. J. Reprod. Immunol.*, **46**, 420–424.

Harandi, A., M., Eriksson, K., and Holmgren, J. (2003). A protective role of locally administered immunostimulatory CpG oligodeoxynucleotide in a mouse model of genital herpes infection. *J. Virol.*, **77**, 953–962.

Harle, P., Sainz, B. Jr., Carr, D. J. and Halford, W. P. (2002). The immediate-early protein, ICP0 is essential for the resistance of herpes simplex virus to interferon-alpha/beta. *Virology*, **293**, 295–304.

Hemmi, H., Kaisho, T., Takeuchi, O. *et al.* (2002). Small antiviral compounds activate immune cells via the TLR7 MyD88-dependent signaling pathway. *Nat. Immunol.*, **3**, 196–200.

Hendricks, R. L. (2006). Stress-induced dysregulation of HSV-specific immunity in latently-infected sensory ganglia. In *31st International Herpesvirus Workshop*, Seattle, Washington, USA, p. Abstract 9.57.

Hill, A., Jugovic, P., York, I. *et al.* (1995). Herpes simplex virus turns off the TAP to evade host immunity. *Nature*, **375**, 411–415.

Holterman, A.-X., Rogers, K., Edelmann, K., Koelle, D. M., Corey, L., and Wilson, C. B. (1999). An important role for MHC class I restricted T cells, and limited role for IFN-gamma, in protection against herpes simplex virus infection in C57BL/6 mice. *J. Virol.*, **73**, 2058–2063.

Hornung, V., Rothenfusser, S., Britsch, S. *et al.* (2002). Quantitative expression of toll-like receptor 1–10 mRNA in cellular subsets of human peripheral blood mononuclear cells and sensitivity to CpG oligodeoxynucleotides. *J. Immunol.*, **168**, 4531–4537.

Hosken, N., McGowan P., Meier A. *et al.* (2006). Diversity of the CD8+ T cell response to herpes simpolex virus type 2 proteins among persons with genital herpes. *J. Virol.* **80**, 5509.

Huard, B. and Fruh, K. (2000). A role for MHC class I down-regulation in NK cell lysis of herpes virus-infected cells. *Eur. J. Immunol.*, **30**, 509–515.

Hurme, M., Haanpaa, M., Nurmikko, T. *et al.* (2003). IL-10 gene polymorphism and herpesvirus infections. *J. Med. Virol.*, **70 Suppl 1**, S48–S50.

Inagaki-Ohara, K., Kawabe, T., Hasegawa, Y., Hashimoto, N., and Nishiyama, Y. (2002). Critical involvement of CD40 in protection against herpes simplex virus infection in a murine model of genital herpes. *Arch. Virol.*, **147**, 187–194.

Iyoda, T., Shimoyama, S., Liu, K. *et al.* (2002). The CD8+ dendritic cell subset selectively endocytoses dying cells in culture and in vivo. *J. Exp. Med.*, **195**, 1289–1302.

Jawahar, S., Moody, C., Chan, M., Finberg, R., Geha, R., and Chatila, T. (1996). Natural Killer (NK) cell deficiency associated with an epitope-deficient Fc receptor type IIA (CD16-II). *Clin. Exp. Immunol.*, **103**, 408–413.

Jerome, K. R., Tait, J. F., Koelle, D. M., and Corey, L. (1998). Herpes simplex virus type 1 renders infected cells resistant to cytotoxic T-lymphocyte-induced apoptosis. *J. Virol.*, **72**, 436–441.

Johansson, E. L., Rudin, A., Wassen, L., and Holmgren, J. (1999). Distribution of lymphocytes and adhesion molecules in human cervix and vagina. *Immunology*, **96**, 272–277.

Jones, C. A., Fernandez, M., Herc, K. *et al.* (2003). Herpes simplex virus type 2 induces rapid cell death and functional impairment of murine dendritic cells in vitro. *J. Virol.*, **77**, 11139–11149.

Jones, S. M., Cose, S. C., Coles, R. M. *et al.* (2000). Herpes simplex virus type 1-specific cytotoxic T-lymphocyte arming occurs within lymph nodes draining the site of cutaneous infection. *J. Virol.*, **74**, 2414–2419.

Kadowaki, N., Ho, S., Antonenko, S. *et al.* (2001). Subsets of human dendritic cell precursors express different toll-like receptors and respond to different microbial antigens. *J. Exp. Med.*, **194**, 863–869.

Kanangat, S., Thomas, J., Gangappa, S., Babu, J. S., and Rouse, B. T. (1996). Herpes simplex virus type 1-mediated up-regulation of IL-12 (p40) mRNA expression. Implications in immunopathogenesis and protection. *J. Immunol.*, **156**, 1110–1116.

Kaushic, C., Ashkar, A. A., Reid, L. A., and Rosenthal, K. L. (2003). Progesterone increases susceptibility and decreases immune responses to genital herpes infection. *J. Virol.*, **77**, 4558–4565.

Kawamoto, S., Oritani, K., Asada, H. *et al.* (2003). Antiviral activity of limitin against encephalomyocarditis virus, herpes simplex virus, and mouse hepatitis virus: diverse requirements by limitin and alpha interferon for interferon regulatory factor 1. *J. Virol.*, **77**, 9622–9631.

Keadle, T. L., Usui, N., Laycock, K. A., Miller, J. K., Pepose, J. S., and Stuart, P. M. (2000). IL-1 and TNF-alpha are important factors in the pathogenesis of murine recurrent herpetic stromal keratitis. *Invest. Ophthalmol. Visual. Sci.*, **41**, 96–102.

Khanna, K. M., Bonneau, R. H., Kinchington, P. R., and Hendricks, R. L. (2003). Herpes simplex virus-specific memory CD8(+) T cells are selectively activated and retained in latently infected sensory Ganglia. *Immunity*, **18**, 593–603.

Kodukula, P., Liu, T., Rooijen, N. V., Jager, M. J., and Hendricks, R. L. (1999). Macrophage control of herpes simplex virus type

1 replication in the peripheral nervous system. *J. Immunol.*, **162**, 2895–2905.

Koelle, D. M. and Corey, L. (1995). Role of cellular immune response to human genital herpes. *Herpes*, **2**, 83–88.

Koelle, D. M. and Corey, L. (2003). Recent progress in herpes simplex virus immunobiology and vaccine research. *Clin. Microbiol. Rev.*, **16**, 96–113.

Koelle, D. M., Tigges, M. A., Burke, R. L. *et al.* (1993). Herpes simplex virus infection of human fibroblasts and keratinocytes inhibits recognition by cloned CD8+ cytotoxic T lymphocytes. *J. Clin. Invest.*, **91**, 961–968.

Koelle, D. M., Frank, J. M., Johnson, M. L., and Kwok, W. W. (1998a). Recognition of herpes simplex virus type 2 tegument proteins by CD4 T cells infiltrating human genital herpes lesions. *J. Virol.*, **72**, 7476–7483.

Koelle, D. M., Posavad, C. M., Barnum, G. R., Johnson, M. L., Frank, J. M., and Corey, L. (1998). Clearance of HSV-2 from recurrent genital lesions correlates with infiltration of HSV-specific cytotoxic T lymphocytes. *J. Clin. Invest.*, **101**, 1500–1508.

Koelle, D. M., Reymond, S. N., Chen, H. *et al.* (2000a). Tegument-specific, virus-reactive CD4 T-cells localize to the cornea in herpes simplex virus interstitial keratitis in humans. *J. Virol.*, **74**, 10930–10938.

Koelle, D. M., Schomogyi, M., and Corey, L. (2000b). Recovery of antigen-specific T-cells from the uterine cervix of women with genital herpes simplex virus type 2 virus infection. *J. Infect. Dis.*, **182**, 662–670.

Koelle, D. M., Schomogyi, M., McClurkan, C., Reymond, S. N., and Chen, H. B. (2000c). CD4 T-cell responses to herpes simplex virus type 2 major capsid protein VP5: comparison with responses to tegument and envelope glycoproteins. *J. Virol.*, **74**, 11422–11425.

Koelle, D. M., Chen, H., Gavin, M. A., Wald, A., Kwok, W. W., and Corey, L. (2001). CD8 CTL from genital herpes simplex lesions: recognition of viral tegument and immediate early proteins and lysis of infected cutaneous cells. *J. Immunol.*, **166**, 4049–4058.

Koelle, D. M., Chen, H. B., McClurkan, C. M., and Petersdorf, E. W. (2002a). Herpes simplex virus type 2-specific CD8 cytotoxic T lymphocyte cross-reactivity against prevalent HLA class I alleles. *Blood*, **99**, 3844–3847.

Koelle, D. M., Liu, Z., McClurkan, C. M. *et al.* (2002b). Expression of cutaneous lymphocyte-associated antigen by CD8+ T-cells specific for a skin-tropic virus. *J. Clin. Invest.*, **110**, 537–548.

Koelle, D. M., Liu, Z., McClurkan, C. L. *et al.* (2003). Immunodominance among herpes simplex virus-specific CD8 T-cells expressing a tissue-specific homing receptor. *Proc. Natl Acad. Sci. USA*, **100**, 12899–12904.

Koelle, D. M., Huang, J., Hensel, M. T., and McClurkan, C. L. (2006). Innate immune responses to herpes simplex virus type 2 influence skin homing molecule expression by memory CD4+ lymphocytes. *J. Virol.* **80**, 2863.

Kohl, S. (1991). Role of antibody-dependent cellular cytotoxiciy in defense against herpes simplex virus infections. *Rev. Infect. Dis.*, **13**, 108–114.

Kohl, S. (1992). The role of antibody in herpes simplex virus infection in humans. *Curr. Top. Microbiol. Immunol.*, **179**, 75–88.

Kohl, S., Loo, L. S., Schmalstieg, F. S., and Anderson, D. C. (1986). The genetic deficiency of leukocyte surface glyoprotein Mac-1, LFA-1, p150,95 in humans is associated with defective antibody-dependent cellular cytotoxicity in vitro and defective protection against herpes simplex infection in vivo. *J. Immunol.*, **137**, 1688–1694.

Kohl, S., Charlebois, E. D., Sigouroudinia, M. *et al.* (2000). Limited antibody-dependent cellular cytotoxicity antibody response induced by a herpes simplex virus type 2 subunit vaccine. *J. Infect. Dis.*, **181**, 335–339.

Kokuba, H., Aurelian, L., and Burnett, J. (1999). Herpes simplex virus associated erythema multiforme (HAEM) is mechanistically distinct from drug-induced erythema multiforme: interferon-gamma is expressed in HAEM lesions and tumor necrosis factor-alpha in druginduced erythema multiforme lesions. *J. Invest. Dermatol.*, **113**, 808–815.

Kramer, M. F. and Coen, D. M. (1995). Quantification of transcripts from the ICP4 and thymidine kinase genes in mouse ganglia latently infected with herpes simplex virus. *J. Virol.*, **69**, 1389–1399.

Kriesel, J. D., Araneo, B., Petajan, J. P., Spruance, S. L., and Stromatt, S. (1994). Herpes labialis associated with recombinant human ciliary neurotrophic factor. *J. Infect. Dis.*, **170**, 1046.

Kriesel, J. D., Gebhardt, B. M., Hill, J. M. *et al.* (1997a). Anti-interleukin-6 antibodies inhibit herpes simplex virus reactivation. *J. Infect. Dis.*, **175**, 821–827.

Kriesel, J. D., Ricigliano, J., Spruance, S. L., Garza, H. H. Jr., and Hill, J. M. (1997b). Neuronal reactivation of herpes simplex virus may involve interleukin-6. *J Neurovirol*, **3**, 441–448.

Kronenberg, M. and Gapin, L. (2002). The unconventional lifestyle of NKT cells. *Nat. Rev. Immunol.*, **2**, 557–568.

Krug, A., Luker, G. D., Barchet, W., Leib, D. A., Akira, S., and Colonna, M. (2003). Herpes simplex virus type 1 (HSV-1) activates murine natural interferon-producing cells through toll-like receptor 9. *Blood*, In Press.

Kruse, M., Rosorius, O., Kratzer, F. *et al.* (2000). Mature dendritic cells infected with herpes simplex virus type 1 exhibit inhibited T-cell stimulatory capacity. *J. Virol.*, **74**, 7127–7136.

Kumaraguru, U. and Rouse, B. T. (2002). The IL-12 response to herpes simplex virus is mainly a paracrine response of reactive inflammatory cells. *J. Leukoc. Biol.*, **72**, 564–570.

Kuwana, M., Kaburaki, J., Wright, T. M., Kawakami, Y., and Ikeda, Y. (2001). Induction of antigen-specific human CD4(+) T cell anergy by peripheral blood DC2 precursors. *Eur. J. Immunol.*, **31**, 2547–2557.

Kwok, W. W., Liu, A. W., Novak, E. J. *et al.* (2000). HLA-DQ tetramers identify epitope-specific T-cells in peripheral blood of herpes simplex virus-2-infected individuals: direct detection of immunodominant antigen responsive cells. *J. Immunol.*, **164**, 4244–4249.

La, S., Kim, J., and Kwon, B. S., Kwon, B. (2002). Herpes simplex virus type 1 glycoprotein D inhibits T-cell proliferation. *Mol. Cells*, **14**, 398–403.

Lebon, P. (1985). Inhibition of herpes simplex virus type 1-induced interferon synthesis by monoclonal antibodies against viral glycoprotein D and by lysosomotropic drugs. *J. Gen. Virol.*, **66**, (Pt 12):2781–2786.

Lebwohl, M., Sacks, S., Conant, M. *et al.* (1992). Recombinant alpha-2 interferon gel treatment of recurrent herpes genitalis. *Antiviral. Res.*, **17**, 235–243.

Lee, S., Zheng, M., Deshpande, S., Eo, S. K., Hamilton, T. A., and Rouse, B. T. (2002a). IL-12 suppresses the expression of ocular immunoinflammatory lesions by effects on angiogenesis. *J. Leukoc. Biol.*, **71**, 469–476.

Lee, S., Zheng, M., Kim, B., and Rouse, B. T. (2002b). Role of matrix metalloproteinase-9 in angiogenesis caused by ocular infection with herpes simplex virus. *J. Clin. Invest.*, **110**, 1105–1111.

Lee, S., Gierynska, M., Eo, S. K., Kuklin, N., and Rouse, B. T. (2003). Influence of DNA encoding cytokines on systemic and mucosal immunity following genetic vaccination against herpes simplex virus. *Microbes Infect.*, **5**, 571–578.

Leib, D. A. (2002). Counteraction of interferon-induced antiviral responses by herpes simplex viruses. *Curr. Top. Microbiol. Immunol.*, **269**, 171–185.

Leib, D. A., Harrison, T. E., Laslo, K. M., Machalek, M. A., Moorman, N. J., and Virgin, H. W. (1999). Interferons regulate the phenotype of wild-type and mutant herpes simplex viruses in vivo. *J. Exp. Med.*, **189**, 663–672.

Leib, D. A., Machalek, M. A., Williams, B. R., Silverman, R. H., and Virgin, H. W. (2000). Specific phenotypic restoration of an attenuated virus by knockout of a host resistance gene. *Proc. Natl Acad. Sci.*, **97**, 6097–6101.

Lekstrom-Himes, J. A., Hohman, P., Warren, T. *et al.* (1999). Association of major histocompatibility complex determinants with the development of symptomatic and asymptomatic genital herpes simplex virus type 2 infections. *J. Infect. Dis.*, **179**, 1077–1085.

Leo, N. A. and Bonneau, R. H. (2000). Chemical sympathectomy alters cytotoxic T lymphocyte responses to herpes simplex virus infection. *Ann. NY Acad. Sci.*, **917**, 923–934.

Lewandowski, G. A., Lo, D., and Bloom, F. E. (1993). Interference with major histocompatibility complex class II-restricted antigen presentation in the brain by herpes simplex virus type 1; a possible mechanism of evasion of the immune system. *Proc. Natl Acad. Sci. USA.*, **90**, 2005–2009.

Lieberman, J. and Fan, Z. (2003). Nuclear war: the granzyme A-bomb. *Curr. Opin. Immunol.*, **15**, 553–559.

Lin, X., Lubinksi, J. M., and Friedman, H. M. (2003). Presented at the 28th International Herpesvirus Workshop.

Lin, X., Lubinski, J. M., and Friedman, H. M. (2004). Immunization strategies to block the herpes simplex virus type 1 immunoglobulin G Fc receptor. *J. Virol.* **78**, 2562.

Litman, G. W., Anderson, M. K., and Rast, J. P. (1999). Evolution of antigen binding receptors. *Annu. Rev. Immunol.*, **17**, 109–147.

Liu, T., Tang, Q., and Hendricks, R. L. (1996). Inflammatory infiltration of the trigeminal ganglion after herpes simplex virus type 1 corneal infection. *J. Virol.*, **70**, 264–271.

Liu, T., Khanna, K. M., Chen, X., Fink, D. J., and Hendricks, R. L. (2000). CD8(+) T cells can block herpes simplex virus type 1 (HSV-1) reactivaton from latency in sensory neurons. *J. Exp. Med.*, **191**, 1459–1466.

Liu, T., Khanna, K. M., Carriere, B. N., and Hendricks, R. L. (2001). Gamma interferon can prevent herpes simplex virus type 1 reactivation from latency in sensory neurons. *J. Virol.*, **75**, 11178–11184.

Lopez, C. (1975). Genetics of natural resistance to herpes virus infections in mice. *Nature*, **258**, 1352–1353.

Lopez, C., Kirkpatrick, D., Fitzgerald, P. A. *et al.* (1982). Studies of the cell lineage of the effector cells that spontaneously lyse HSV-1 infected fibroblasts (NK(HSV-1)). *J. Immunol.*, **129**, 824–828.

Lopez, C., Kirkpatrick, D., Read, S. E. *et al.* (1983). Correlation between low natural killing of fibroblasts infected with herpes simplex virus type 1 and susceptibility to herpesvirus infections. *J. Infect. Dis.*, **147**, 1030–1035.

Lopez, C., Arvin, A. M., and Ashley, R. (1993). Immunity to herpesvirus infections in humans, p. 397–425. In Roizman, B., Whitley, R. J., and Lopez, C., (ed.). The Human Herpesviruses. New York: Raven Press.

Lu, Z., Yuan, L., Zhou, X., Sotomayor, E., Levitsky, H. I., and Pardoll, D. M. (2000). CD40-independent pathways of T cell help for priming of CD8(+) cytotoxic T lymphocytes. *J. Exp. Med.*, **191**, 541–550.

Lubinski, J., Wang, L., Mastellos, D., Sahu, A., Lambris, J. H., and Friedman, H. M. (1999). In vivo role of complement-interacting domains of herpes simplex virus type 1 glycoprotein gC. *J. Exp. Med.*, **190**, 1637–1646.

Lubinski, J. M., Jiang, M., Hook, L. *et al.* (2002). Herpes simplex virus type 1 evades the effects of antibody and complement in vivo. *J. Virol.*, **76**, 9232–9241.

Luker, G. D., Prior, J. L., Song, J., Pica, C. M., and Leib, D. A. (2003). Bioluminescence imaging reveals systemic dissemination of herpes simplex virus type 1 in the absence of interferon receptors. *J. Virol.*, **77**, 11082–11093.

Lund, J., Sato, A., Akira, S., Medzhitov, R., and Iwasaki, H. (2003). Toll-like receptor 9-mediated recognition of herpes simplex virus-2 by plasmacytoid dendritic cells. *J. Exp. Med.*, **198**, 513–520.

Lundberg, P., Welander, P., Openshaw, H. *et al.* (2003). A locus on mouse chromosome 6 that determines resistance to herpes simplex virus also influences reactivation, while an unlinked locus augments resistance of female mice. *J. Virol.*, **77**, 11661–11673.

Maccario, R., Revello, M. G., Comoli, P., Montagna, D., Locatelli, F., and Gerna, G. (1993). HLA-unrestricted killing of HSV-1-infected mononuclear cells. *J. Immunol.*, **150**, 1437–1445.

Maccario, R., Comoli, P., Percivalle, E., Montagna, D., Locatelli, F., and Gerna, G. (1995). Herpes simplex virus-specific human cytotoxic T-cell colonies expressing either gamma-delta or alpha-beta T-cell receptor: role of accessory molecules on HLA-unrestricted killing of virus-infected targets. *Immunology*, **85**, 49–56.

Maertzdorf, J., Osterhaus, A. D., and Verjans, G. M. (2002). IL-17 expression in human herpetic stromal keratitis: modulatory effects on chemokine production by corneal fibroblasts. *J. Immunol.*, **169**, 5897–5903.

Malmgaard, L. and Paludan, S. R. (2003). Interferon (IFN)-alpha/beta, interleukin (IL)-12 and IL-18 coordinately induce production of IFN-gamma during infection with herpes simplex virus type 2. *J. Gen. Virol.*, **84**, 2497–2500.

Mandelboim, O., Lieberman, N., Lev, M. et al. (2001). Recognition of haemagglutinins on virus-infected cells by NK p46 activates lysis by human NK cells. *Nature*, **409**:1055–1060.

Manickan, E. and Rouse, B. T. (1995). Roles of different T-cell subsets in control of herpes simplex virus infection determined by using T-cell-deficient mouse models. *J. Virol.*, **69**, 8178–8179.

Manickan, E., Francotte, M., Kuklin, N. et al. (1995a). Vaccination with recombinant vaccinia viruses expressing ICP27 induces protecting immunity against herpes simplex virus through CD4+ Th1+ T cells. *J. Virol.*, **69**, 4711–4716.

Manickan, E., Rouse, R. J., Yu, Z., Wire, W. S., and Rouse, B. T. (1995b). Genetic immunization against herpes simplex virus. Protection is mediated by CD4+ T lymphocytes. *J. Immunol.*, **155**, 259–265.

McGeoch, D. J., Dalrymple, M. A., Davison, A. J. et al. (1988). The complete DNA sequence of the long unique region of herpes simplex virus type 1. *J. Gen. Virol.*, **69**, 1531–1574.

McGowan, P., Wagener, F., Posavad, C. et al. (2003). Presented at the 28th International Herpesvirus Workshop, Madison, WI.

McKenna, D. B., Neill, W. A., and Norval, M. (2001). Herpes simplex virus-specific immune responses in subjects with frequent and infrequent orofacial recurrences. *Br. J. Dermatol.*, **144**, 459–464.

Memar, O. M., Arany, I., and Tyring, S. K. (1995). Skin-associated lymphoid tissue in human immunodeficiency virus-1, human papillomavirus, and herpes simplex virus infections. *J. Invest. Dermatol.*, **105**, 99S-104S.

Menten, P., Wuyts, A., and Van Damme, J. (2002). Macrophage inflammatory protein-1. *Cytokine Growth Factor Rev.*, **13**, 455–481.

Messaoudi, I., Guevara Patino, J. A., Dyall, R., LeMaoult, J., and Nikolich-Zugich, J. (2002). Direct link between mhc polymorphism, T cell avidity, and diversity in immune defense. *Science*, **298**, 1797–1800.

Metcalf, J. F., Hamilton, D. S., and Reichert, R. W. (1979). Herpetic keratitis in athymic (nude) mice. *Infect. Immun.*, **26**, 1164–1171.

Mikloska, A., Kesson, A. M., Penfold, M. E. T., and Cunningham, A. L. (1996). Herpes simplex virus protein targets for CD4 and CD8 lymphocyte cytotoxicity in cultured epidermal keratinocytes treated with interferon-gamma. *J. Infect. Dis.*, **173**, 7–17.

Mikloska, Z., Danis, V. A., Adams, S., Lloyd, A. R., Adrian, D. L., and Cunningham, A. L. (1998). In vivo production of cytokines and beta (C-C) chemokines in human recurrent herpes simplex lesions-do herpes simplex virus-infected keratinocytes contribute to their production? *J. Infect. Dis.*, **177**, 827–838.

Mikloska, Z., Sanna, P. P., and Cunningham, A. L. (1999). Neutralizing antibodies inhibit axonal spread of herpes simplex virus type 1 to epidermal cells in vitro. *J. Virol.*, **73**, 5934–5944.

Mikloska, Z., Ruckholdt, M., Ghadiminejad, I, Dunckley, H. Denis, M., and Cunningham, A. L. (2001). Monophosphoryl lipid A and QS21 increase CD8 T lymphocyte cytotoxicity to herpes simplex virus-2 infected cell proteins 4 and 27 through IFN-gamma and IL-12 production. *J. Immunol.*, **164**, 5167–5176.

Mikloska, Z., Bosnjak, L., and Cunningham, A. L. (2001). Immature monocyte-derived dendritic cells are productively infected with herpes simplex virus type 1. *J. Virol.*, **75**, 5958–5964.

Milligan, G. N. (1999). Neutrophils aid in protection of the vaginal mucosae of immune mice against challenge with herpes simplex virus type 2. *J. Virol.*, **73**, 6380–6386.

Milligan, G. N., Bernstein, D. I., and Bourne, N. (1998). T lymphocytes are required for protection of the vaginal mucosae and sensory ganglia of immune mice against reinfection with herpes simplex virus type 2. *J. Immunol.*, **160**, 6093–6100.

Milligan, G. N., Bourne, N., and Dudley, K. L. (2001). Role of polymorphonuclear leukocytes in resolution of HSV-2 infection of the mouse vagina. *J. Reprod. Immunol.*, **49**, 49–65.

Milone, M. C. and Fitzgerald-Bocarsly, P. (1998). The mannose receptor mediates induction of IFN-alpha in peripheral blood dendritic cells by enveloped RNA and DNA viruses. *J. Immunol.*, **161**, 2391–2399.

Moser, J. M., Byers, A. M. and Lukacher, A. E. (2002). NK cell receptors in antiviral immunity. *Curr. Opin. Immunol.* **14**, 509–516.

Mossman, K. L., Macgregor, P. F., Rozmus, J. J., Goryachev, A. B., Edwards, A. M., and Smiley, J. R. (2001). Herpes simplex virus triggers and then disarms a host antiviral response. *J. Virol.*, **75**, 750–758.

Mueller, S. N., Jones, C. M., Smith, C. M., Health, W. R., and Carbone, F. R. (2002). Rapid cytotoxic T lymphocyte activation occurs in the draining lymph nodes after cutaneous herpes simplex virus infection as a result of early antigen presentation and not the presence of virus. *J. Exp. Med.*, **195**, 651–656.

Mueller, S. N., Jones, C. M., Chen, W. (2003). The early expression of glycoprotein B from herpes simplex virus can be detected by antigen-specific CD8+ T cells. *J. Virol.*, **77**, 2445–2451.

Mullick, J., Kadam, A., and Sahu, A. (2003). Herpes and pox viral complement control proteins: 'the mask of self'. *Trends Immunol.*, **24**, 500–507.

Nagashunmugam, T., Lubinski, J., Wang, L. et al. (1998). In vivo immune evasion mediated by the herpes simplex virus type 1 immunoglobulin G Fc receptor. *J. Virol.*, **72**, 5351–5359.

Nash, A. A. (2000). T cells and the regulation of herpes simplex virus latency and reactivation. *J. Exp. Med.*, **191**, 1455–1458.

Nass, P. H., Elkins, K. L., and Weir, J. P. (2001). Protective immunity against herpes simplex virus generated by DNA vaccination compared to natural infection. *Vaccine*, **19**, 1538–1546.

Neumann, J., Eis-Hubinger, A. M., and Kock, N. (2003). Herpes simplex virus type 1 targets the MHC class II processing pathway for immune evasion. *J. Immunol.*, **171**, 3075–3083.

Nicholl, M. J., Robinson, L. H., and Preston, C. M. (2000). Activation of cellular interferon-responsive genes after infection of human cells with herpes simplex virus type 1. *J. Gen. Virol.*, **81**, 2215–2218.

O'Keeffe, M., Hochrein, H., Vremec, D. *et al.* (2002). Mouse plasmacytoid cells: long-lived cells, heterogeneous in surface phenotype and function, that differentiate into CD8(+) dendritic cells only after microbial stimulus. *J. Exp. Med.*, **196**, 1307–1319.

Ongkosuwito, J. V., Feron, E. J., van Doornik, C. E. *et al.* (1998) Analysis of immunoregulatory cytokines in ocular fluid samples from patients with uveitis. *Invest. Ophthalmol. Vis. Sci.*, **39**, 2659–2665.

Osterhaus, A. D., Hintzen, R. Q., van Dun, J. M., Poot, A, Verjans, G. M. (2006). Selective accumulation of differentiated HSV serotype-specific CD8+ T cells within human HSV-1 latently infected trigeminal ganglia. In *31st International Herpesvirus Workshop*, Seattle, Washington, USA, p. Abstract 9.02.

Overall, J. C., Spruance, S. L., and Green, J. A. (1981). Viral-induced leukocyte interferon in vesicle fluid from lesions of recurrent herpes labialis. *J. Infect. Dis.*, **143**, 543–547.

Paludan, S. R., Ellerman-Eriksen, S., Kruys, V., and Mogensen, S. C. (2001). Expression of TNF-alpha by herpes simplex virus-infected macrophages is regulated by a dual mechanism: transcriptional regulation by NF-kappa-B and activating transcription factor 2/jun and translational regulation through the AU-rich region of the 3' untranslated region. *J. Immunol.*, **167**, 2202–2208.

Parr, M. B. and Parr, E. L. (2000). Interferon-gamma up-regulates intercellular adhesion molecule-1 and vascular cell adhesion molecule-1 and recruits lymphocytes into the vagina of immune mice challenged with herpes simplex virus-2. *Immunology*, **99**, 540–545.

Parr, M. B. and Parr, E. L. (2003). Vaginal immunity in the HSV-2 mouse model. *Int. Rev. Immunol.*, **22**, 43–63.

Payvandi, F., Amrute, S., and Fitzgerald-Bocarsly, P. (1998). Exogenous and endogenous IL-10 regulate IFN-alpha production by peripheral blood mononuclear cells in response to viral stimulation. *J. Immunol.*, **160**, 5861–5868.

Peek, R., Verjans, G. M., and Meek, B. (2002). Herpes simples virus infection of the human eye induces a compartmentalized virus-specific B cell response. *J. Infect. Dis.*, **186**, 1539–1546.

Pereira, R. A. and Simmons, A. (1999). Cell surface expression of H2 antigens on primary sensory neurons in response to acute but not latent herpes simplex virus infection in vivo. *J. Virol.*, **73**, 6484–6489.

Pereira, R. A., Tscharke, D. C., and Simmons, A. (1994). Upregulation of class I major histocompatibility complex gene expression in primary sensory neurons, satellite cells, and Schwann cells in mice in response to acute but not latent herpes simplex virus infection in vivo. *J. Exp. Med.*, **180**, 841–850.

Pereira, R. A., Simon, M. M., and Simmons, A. (2000). Granzyme A, anoncytolytic component of CD8(+) cell granules, restricts the spread of herpes simples virus in the peripheral nervous systems of experimentally infected mice. *J. Virol.*, **74**, 1029–1032.

Pereira, R. A., Scalzo, A., and Simmons, A. (2001). Cutting edge: a NK complex-linked locus governs acute versus latent herpes simplex virus infection of neurons. *J. Immunol.*, **166**, 5869–5873.

Pietra, G., Semino, C., Cagnoni, F. *et al.* (2000). Natural killer cells lyse autologous herpes simplex virus infected targets using cytolytic mechanisms distributed clonotypically. *J. Med. Virol.*, **62**, 354–363.

Pollara, G., Speidel, K., Samady, L. *et al.* (2003). Herpes simplex virus infection of dendritic cells: balance among activation, inhibition, and immunity. *J. Infect. Dis.* **187**, 165–178.

Posavad, C. M., Koelle, D. M., and Corey, L. C. (1996). High frequency of CD8+ cytotoxic Tlymphocyte precursors specific for herpes simplex viruses in persons with genital herpes. *J. Virol.*, **70**, 8165–8168.

Posavad, C. M., Koelle, D. M., Shaughnessy, M. F., and Corey, L. (1997). Severe genital herpes infections in HIV-infected individuals with impaired HSV-specific CD8+ cytotoxic T lymphocyte responses. *Proc. Nat. Acad. Sci.*, **94**, 10289–10294.

Posavad, C. M., Wald, A., Hosken, N., Huang, M.-L., Koelle, D. M., and Corey, L. (2003). T cell immunity to herpes simplex virus in seronegative persons: silent infection or acquired immunity. *J. Immunol.*, **170**, 4380–4388.

Prasad, D. V., Richards, S., Mai, X. M., and Dong, C. (2003). B7S1, a novel B7 family member that negatively regulates T cell function. *Immunity*, **18**, 863–873.

Pyles, R. B., Higgins, D., Chalk, C. *et al.* (2002). Use of immunostimulatory sequence-containing oligonucleotides as topical therapy for genital herpes simplex virus type 2 infection. *J. Virol.*, **76**, 11387–11396.

Raftery, M. J., Behrens, C. K., Muller, A., Krammer, A., Walczak, H., and Schonrich, G. (1999). Herpes simplex virus type 1 infection of activated cytotoxic T cells: induction of fratricide as a mechanism of viral immune evasion. *J. Exp. Med.*, **190**, 1103–1114.

Rager-Zisman, B., Quan, P. C., Rosner, M., Moller, J. R., and Bloom, B. R. (1987). Role of NK cells in protection of mice against herpes simplex virus-1 infection. *J. Immunol.*, **138**, 884–888.

Randolph, G. J. (2006). Migratory dendritic cells: sometimes simply ferries? *Immunity* **25**, 15.

Rogge, L., D'Ambrosio, D., Biffi, M., Penna, G., Minetti, L. J., Presky, D. H., Adorini, L., and Sinigaglia, F. (1998). The role of Stat4 in species-specific regulation of Th cell development by type I IFNs. *J. Immunol.*, **161**, 6567–6574.

Roizman, B. and Pellett, P. E. (2001). The family herpesviridae: a brief introduction, p. 2381–2397. *In* P. M. Howley, (ed.), Fields Virology, Fourth ed, vol. 2. Lippincott, Philadelphia.

Rong, Q., Alexander, T. S., Koski, G. K., and Rosenthal, K. S. (2003). Multiple mechanisms for HSV-1 induction of interferon alpha production by peripheral blood mononuclear cells. *Arch. Virol.*, **148**, 329–344.

Roopenian, D., Chio, E. Y., and Brown, A. (2002). The immunogenomics of minor histocompatibility antigens. *Immunol. Rev.*, **190**, 86–94.

Rosler, A., Pohl, M., Braune, H. J., Oertel, W. H., Gemsa, D., and Sprenger, H. (1998). Time course of chemokines in the cerebrospinal fluid and serum during herpes simplex type 1 encephalitis. *J. Neurol. Sci.*, **157**, 82–89.

Rudd, C. E. and Schneider, H. (2003). Unifying concepts in CD28, ICOS and CTLA4 co-receptor signalling. Nature Reviews *Immunology*, **3**, 544–556.

Salio, M., Cella, M., Suter, M., and Lanzavecchia, A. (1999). Inhibition of dendritic cell maturation by herpes simplex virus. *Eur. J. Immunol.*, **29**, 3245–3253.

Salio, M., Cella, M., Vermi, W. *et al.* (2003). Plasmacytoic dendritic cells prime IFN-gammasecreting melanoma-specific CD8 lymphocytes and are found in primary melanoma lesions. *Eur. J. Immunol.*, **33**, 1052–1062.

Sallusto, F., Lenig, D., Forster, R., Lipp, M., and Lanzavecchia, A. (1999). Two subsets of memory T lymphocytes with distinct homing potentials and effector functions. *Nature*, **401**, 708–712.

Samady, L., Costigliola, E., MacCormac, L. *et al.* (2003). Deletion of the virion host shutoff protein (vhs) from herpes simplex virus (HSV) relieves the viral block to dendritic cell activation: potential of vhs- HSV vectors for dendritic cell-mediated immunotherapy. *J. Virol.*, **77**, 3768–3776.

Sanchez-Pescador, L., Paz, P., Navarro, D., Pereira, L., and Kohl, S. (1992). Epitopes of herpes simplex virus type 1 glycoprotein B that bind type-common neutralizing antibodies elicit type-specific antibody-dependent cellular cytotoxicity. *J. Infect. Dis.*, **166**, 623–627.

Sauerbrei, A., Eichhorn, U., Hottenrott, G., and Wutzler, P. (2000). Virological diagnosis of herpes simplex encephalitis. *J. Clin. Virol.*, **17**, 31–63.

Schacker, T., Zeh, J., Hu, H.-L., Hill, E., and Corey, L. (1998). Frequency of symptomatic and asymptomatic herpes simplex virus type 2 reactivations among human immunodeficiency virus-infected men, *J. Infect. Dis.*, **178**, 1616–1622.

Schmid, D. S. and Rouse, B. T. (1992). The role of T cell immunity in control of herpes simplex virus. *Curr. Top. Microbiol. Immuno.*, **179**, 57–74.

Schmid, D. S., Thieme, M. L., Gary, H. E., and Reeves, W. C. (1997). Characterization of T cell responses to herpes simplex virus type 1 (HSV-1) and herpes simplex virus type 2 (HSV-2) using a TNF-beta ELISpot cytokine assay. *Arch. Virol.*, **142**, 1659–1671.

Schmitt, C., Fohrer, H., Beaudet, S. *et al.* (2000). Identification of mature and immature human thymic dendritic cells that differentially express HLA-DR and interleukin-3 receptor in vivo. *J. Leukoc. Biol.*, **68**, 836–844.

Sciammas, R. and Bluestone, J. A. (1998). HSV-1 glycoprotein I-reactive TCR gamma delta cells directly recognize the peptide backbone in a conformationally dependent manner. *J. Immunology*, **161**, 5187–5192.

Sciammas, R., Kodukula, P., Tang, Q., Hendricks, R. L., and Bluestone, J. A. (1997). T cell receptor-gamma-delta cells protect mice from herpes simplex virus type 1-induced lethal encephalitis. *J. Exp. Med.*, **185**, 1969–1975.

Seo, S. K., Park, H. Y., Choi, J. H. *et al.* (2003). Blocking 4–1 BB/4–1BB ligand interactions prevents herpetic stromal keratitis. *J. Immunol.*, **171**, 576–583.

Servet-Delprat, C., Vidalain, P. O., Valentin, H., and Rabourdin-Combe, C. (2003). Measles virus and dendritic cell functions: how specific response cohabits with immunosuppression. *Curr. Top. Microbiol. Immuno.*, **276**, 103–123.

Shukla, D. and Spear, P. G. (2001). Herpesviruses and heparan sulfate: an intimate relationship in aid of viral entry. *J. Clin. Invest.*, **108**, 503–510.

Siebens, H., Tevethia, S. S., and Babior, B. M. (1979). Neutrophil-mediated antibody-dependent killing of herpes-simplex-virus-infected cells. *Blood*, **54**, 88–94.

Siegal, F. P., Kadowaki, N., Shodell, M. *et al.* (1999). The nature of the principle type 1 interferon-producing cells in human blood. *Science*, **284**, 1835–1837.

Simmons, A. and Tscharke, D. C. (1992). Anti-CD8 impairs clearance of herpes simplex virus from the nervous system: implications for the fate of virally infected neurons. *J. Exp. Med.*, **175**, 1337–1344.

Simmons, A., Tscharke, D., and Speck, P. (1992). The role of immune mechanisms in control of herpes simplex virus infection of the peripheral nervous system. *Curr. Top. Microbiol. Immunol.*, **179**, 31–56.

Sin, J. I., Kim, J. J., Boyer, J. D., Ciccarelli, R. B., Higgins, T. J., and Weiner, D. B. (1999). In vivo modulation of vaccine-induced immune responses toward a Th1 phenotype increases potency and vaccine effectiveness in a herpes simplex type 2 mouse model. *J. Virol.*, **73**, 501–509.

Sin, J. I., Kim, J. J., Zhang, D., and Weiner, D. B. (2001). Modulation of cellular responses by plasmid CD40L: CD40L plasmid vectors enhance antigen-specific helper T cell type 1 CD4+ T cell-mediated protective immunity against herpes simplex virus type 2 in vivo. *Hum. Gene Ther.*, **12**, 1091–1102.

Singh, R., Kumar, A., Creery, W. D., Ruben, M., Guiluvi, A., and Diaz-Mitoma, F. (2003a). Dysregulated expression of IFN-gamma and IL-10 and imparied IFN-gamma-mediated responses at different disease stages in patients with genital herpes simplex virus-2 infection. *Clin. Exp. Immunol*, **133**, 97–107.

Singh, R., Kumar, A., and Diaz-Mitoma, F. (2003b). Augmentation of B7 expression by herpes simplex virus antigen. *Hum. Immunol.*, **64**, 780–786.

Sinha, S., Cheshenko, N., Lehrer, R. I., and Herold, B. C. (2003). NP-1, a rabbit alphadefensin, prevents the entry and intercellular spread of herpes simplex virus type 2. *Antimicrob. Agents Chemother.*, **47**, 494–500.

Sirianni, M. C., Bonomo, R., Scarpati, B. *et al.* (1986). Immunological responses of patients with recurrent herpes genitalis. *Diagn. Immunol.*, **4**, 294–298.

Smith, C. M., Belz, G. T., Wilson, N. S. *et al.* (2003). Cutting edge: conventional CD8alpha(+) dendritic cells are preferentially involved in CTL priming after footpad infection with herpes simplex virus-1. *J. Immunol.*, **170**, 4437–4440.

Spatz, M., Wolf, H. M., Thon, V., Gampfer, J. M., and Eibl, M. M. (2000). Immune response to the herpes simplex type 1 regulatory proteins ICP8 and VP16 in infected persons. *J. Med. Virol.*, **62**, 29–36.

Spear, P. G., Eisenberg, R. J., and Cohen, G. H. (2000). Three classes of surface receptors for alphaherpesvirus entry. *Virol.*, **275**, 1–8.

Speck, P. and Simmons, A. (1998). Precipitous clearance of herpes simplex virus antigens from the peripheral nervous systems of experimentally infected C57BL/10 mice. *J. Gen. Virol.*, **79**, 561–564.

Spruance, S. L., Evans, T. G., McKeough, M. B. *et al.* (1995). Th1/Th2-like immunity and resistance to herpes simplex labialis. *Antiviral Res.*, **28**, 39–55.

Spruance, S. L., Tyring, S. K., Smith, M. H., and Meng, T. C. (2001). Application of a topical immune response modifier, resiquimod gel, to modify the recurrence rate of recurrent genital herpes: a pilot study. *J. Infect. Dis.*, **184**, 196–200.

Stanberry, L. R., Spruance, S., Cunningham, A. L. *et al.* (2002). Prophylactic vaccination against genital herpes with adjuvanted recombinant glycoprotein D vaccine: two randomized contolled trials. *N. Engl. J. Med.*, **347**, 1652–1661.

Stumpf, T. H., Case, R., Shimeld, C., Easty, D. L., and Hill, T. J. (2002). Primary herpes simplex virus type 1 infection of the eye triggers similar immune responses in the cornea and the skin of the eyelids. *J. Gen. Virol.*, **83**, 1579–1590.

Su, Y. H., Yan, X. T., Oakes, J. E., and Lausch, R. N. (1996). Protective antibody therapy is associated with reduced chemokine transcripts in herpes simplex virus type 1 corneal infection. *J. Virol.*, **70**, 1277–1281.

Sun, M.-Y., Brown, J., Liu, B. *et al.* (2003). Presented at the AIDS Vaccine 2003, New York, New York.

Suvas, S., Kumaraguru, U., Pack, C. D., Lee, S., and Rouse, B. T. (2003). CD4+ CD25+ T cells regulate virus-specific primary and memory CD8+ T cell responses. *J. Exp. Med.*, **198**, 889–901.

Suvas, S., Azkur, A. K., Kim, B. S., Kumaraguru, U., and Rouse, B. T. (2004). CD4(+)CD25(+) regulatory T cells control the severity of viral immunoinflammatory lesions. *J. Immunol.* **172**; 4123.

Sylwester, A. W., Mitchell, B. L., Edgar *et al.* (2005). Broadly targeted human cytomegalovirus-specific CD4+ and CD8+ T cells dominate the memory compartments of exposed subjects. *J. Exp. Med.* **202**, 673.

Taddesse-Heath, L., Feldman, J. I., Fahle, G. A. *et al.* (2003). Florid CD4+, CD56+ T-cell infiltrate associated with herpes simplex infection simulating nasal NK-/T-cell lymphoma. *Mod. Pathol.*, **16**, 166–172.

Takeuchi, O. and Akira, S. (2002). MyD88 as a bottleneck in Toll/IL-1 signaling. *Curr. Top. Microbiol. Immunol.*, **270**, 155–167.

Thebeau, L. G. and Morrison, L. A. (2002). B7 costimulation plays an important role in protection from herpes simplex type 2-mediated pathology. *J. Virol.*, **76**, 2563–2566.

Thebeau, L. G. and Morrison, L. A. (2003). Mechanism of reduced T-cell effector functions and class-switched antibody responses to herpes simplex virus type 2 in the absence of B7 costimulation. *J. Virol.*, **77**, 2426–2435.

Tigges, M. A., Koelle, D. M., Hartog, K., Sekulovich, R. E., Corey, L., and Burke, R. L. (1992). Human CD8+ herpes simplex virus-specific cytotoxic T lymphocyte clones recognize diverse virion protein antigens. *J. Virol.*, **66**, 1622–1634.

Tigges, M. A., Leng, S., Johnson, D. C., and Burke, R. L. (1996). Human herpes simplex (HSV)-specific CD8+ CTL clones recognize HSV-2-infected fibroblasts after treatment with IFN-gamma or when virion host shutoff functions are disabled. *J. Immunol.*, **156**, 3901–3910.

Tomazin, R., van Schoot, N. E., Goldsmith, K. *et al.* (1998). Herpes simplex virus type 2 ICP47 inhibits human TAP but not mouse TAP. *J. Virol.*, **72**, 2560–2563.

Trachtenberg, E., Korber, B., Sollars, C. *et al.* (2003). Advantage of rare HLA supertype in HIV disease progression. *Nat. Med.*, **9**, 928–935.

Trgovcich, J., Johnson, D., and Roizman, B. (2002). Cell surface major histocompatibility complex class II proteins are regulated by the products of the gamma(1)34.5 and U(L)41 genes of herpex simplex virus 1. *J. Virol.*, **76**, 6974–6986.

Tscharke, D. C. and Simmons, A. (1999). Anti-CD8 treatment alters interleukin-4 but not interferon-gamma mRNA levels in murine sensory ganglia during herpes simplex virus infection. Brief report. *Arch. Virol.*, **144**, 2229–2238.

Tsunobuchi, H., Nishimura, H., Goshima, F. *et al.* (2000). A protective role of interleukin-15 in a mouse model for systemic infection with herpes simplex virus. *Virology*, **275**, 57–66.

Tumpey, T. M., Cheng, H., Cook, D. N., Smithies, O., Oakes, J. E., and Lausch, R. N. (1998). Absence of macrophage inflammatory protein-1 alpha prevents the development of blinding herpes stromal keratitis. *J. Virol.*, **72**, 3705–3710.

Vaidya, S. A. and Cheng, G. (2003). Toll-like receptors and innate antiviral responses. *Curr. Opin. Immunol.*, **15**, 402–407.

Van Strijp, J. A., Miltenburg, L. A., van der Rol, M. E., Van Kessel, K. P., Fluit, A. C., and Verhoef, J. (1990). Degradation of herpes simplex virions by human polymorphonuclear leukocytes and monocytes. *J. Gen. Virol.*, **71**, 1205–1209.

Van Voorhis, W. C., Barrett, L. K., Koelle, D. M., Nasio, J. M., Plummer, F. A., and Lukehart, S. A. (1996). Primary and secondary syphilis lesions contain mRNA for Th1 cytokines and activated cytolytic T cells. *J. Infect. Dis.*, **173**:491–495.

Verjans, G. M., Baarmsa, G. S., Van der Lelij, A., Kijaltra, A., and Osterhaus, A. D. M. E. (1996). Characterization of herpes simplex virus (HSV) specific T cell clones from vitreous fluid of a patient with HSV mediated acute retinal necrosis. *Invest. Ophthalmol. Vis. Sci.*, **37**, S45.

Verjans, G. M. G. M., Remeijer, L., and van Binnendijk, R. S. (1998). Identification and characterization of herpes simplex virus-specific CD4+ T cells in corneas of herpetic stromal keratitis patients. *J. Infect. Dis.*, **177**, 484–488.

Vestey, J. P., Norval, M., Howie, S. E. M., Manigay, J. P., and Neill, W. (1990). Antigen presentation in patients with recrudescent orofacial herpes simplex virus infections. *Br. J. Dermatol.*, **122**, 33–42.

Wakimoto, H., Johnson, P. R., Knipe, D. M., and Chiocca, E. A. (2003). Effects of innate immunity on herpes simplex virus and its ability to kill tumor cells. *Gene Ther.*, **10**, 983–990.

Wald, A., Zeh, J., Selke, S. *et al.* (2000). Reactivation of genital herpes type 2 infection in asymptomatic seropositive persons. *N. Engl. J. Med.*, **342**, 844–850.

Wallace, M. E., Keating, R., Heath, W. R., and Carbone, F. R. (1999). The cytotoxic T-cell response to herpes simplex virus type 1 infection of C57BL/6 mice is almost entirely directed against a single immunodominant determinant. *J. Virol.*, **73**, 7619–7626.

Walport, M. J. (2001). Complement. First of two parts. *N. Engl. J. Med.*, **344**, 1058–1066.

Whaley, K. J., Zeitlin, L., Barratt, R. A., Hoen, T. E., and Cone, R. A. (1994). Passive transfer of the vagina protects mice against vaginal transfer of genital herpes infections. *J. Infect. Dis.*, **144**, 142–146.

Whitbeck, J. C., Muggeridge, M. I., Rux, A. H. *et al.* (1999). The major neutralizing antigenic site on herpes simplex virus glycoprotein D overlaps a receptor-binding domain. *J. Virol.*, **73**, 9879–9890.

Wickham, S., Lu, B., Ash, J. and Carr, D. J. (2005). Chemokine receptor deficiency is associated with increased chemokine expression in the peripheral and central nervous systems and increased resistance to herpetic encephalitis. *J. Neuroimmunol.* **162**, 51.

Wollenberg, A., Wagner,. M., Gunther, S. *et al.* (2002). Plamacytoid dendritic cells: a new cutaneous dendritic cell subset with distinct role in inflammatory skin diseases. *J. Invest. Dermatol.*, **119**, 1096–1102.

Wong, G. H. and Goeddel, D. V. (1986). Tumour necrosis factors alpha and beta inhibit virus replication and synergize with interferons. *Nature*, **323**, 819–822.

Wonnacott, K. M. and Bonneau, R. H. (2002). The effects of stress on memory cytotoxic T lymphocyte-medicated protection against herpes simplex virus infection at mucosal sites. *Brain Behav. Immunol.*, **116**, 104–117.

Xia, P., Gamble, J. R., Rye, K. A. *et al.* (1998). Tumor necrosis factor-alpha induces adhesion molecule expression through the sphingosine kinase pathway. *Proc. Natl Acad. Sci. USA*, **95**, 14196–14201.

Yang, O. O., Sarkis, P. T., Trocha, A., Kalams, S. A., Johnson, R. P., and Walker, B. D. (2003). Impacts of avidity and specificity on the antiviral efficiency of HIV-1-specific CTL. *J. Immunol.*, **171**, 3718–3724.

Yasukawa, M. and Kobayashi, Y. (1985). Inhibition of herpes simplex virus replication in vitro by human cytotoxic T cell clones and natural killer cell clones. *J. Gen. Virol.*, **66**, 2225–2229.

Yasukawa, M. and Zarling, J. M. (1983). Autologous herpes simplex virus-infected cells are lysed by human natural killer cells. *J. Immunol.*, **131**, 2011–2016.

Yasukawa, M. and Zarling, J. M. (1984). Human cytotoxic T cell clones directed against herpes simplex virus-infected cells. I. Lysis restricted by HLA Class II MB and DR antigens. *J. Immunol.*, **133**, 422–427.

Yasukawa, M., Inatsuki, A., and Kobayashi, Y. (1988). Helper activity in antigen-specific antibody production mediated by CD4+ human cytotoxic T cell clones directed against herpes simplex virus. *J. Immunol.*, **140**, 3419–3425.

Yasukawa, M., Inatsuki, A., and Kobayashi, Y. (1989). Differential in vitro activation of CD4+CD8- and CD8+CD4- herpes simplex virus-specific human cytotoxic T cells. *J. Immunol.*, **143**, 2051–2057.

Yasukawa, M., Ohminami, H., Yakushijin, Y. *et al.* (1999). Fas-independent cytotoxicity mediated by CD4+ CTL directed against herpes simplex virus-infected cells. *J. Immunol.*, **162**, 6100–6106.

Yoneyama, H., Matsuno, K., Toda, E. *et al.* (2005). Plasmacytoid DCs help lymph node DCs to induce anti-HSV CTLs. *J. Exp. Med.* **202**, 425.

Zak-Prelich, M., Halliday, K. E., Walker, C., Yates, C. M., Norval, M., and McKenzie, R. C. (2001). Infection of murine keratinocytes with herpes simplex virus type 1 induces the expression of interleukin-10, but not interleukin-1 alpha or tumour necrosis factor-alpha. *Immunology*, **104**, 468–475.

Zhao, X., Deak, E., Soderberg, K. *et al.* (2003). Vaginal submucosal dendritic cells, but not Langerhans cells, induce protective Th1 responses to herpes simplex virus-2. *J. Exp. Med.*, **197**, 153–162.

Zorrilla, E. P., Luborsky, L., McKay, J. R. *et al.* (2001). The relationship of depression and stressors to immunological assay: a meta-analytic review. *Brain Behav. Immun.*, **15**, 199–226.

35

Immunopathological aspects of HSV infection

Kaustuv Banerjee and Barry T. Rouse

Department of Microbiology, College of Veterinary Medicine, University of Tennessee, Knoxville, TN, USA

Introduction

"What is food to one man is bitter poison to others" Lucretius *De Rerum Natura* (50BCE)

Foreign material entering multicellular organisms triggers a range of defense reactions which, when successful, subjugates and removes the invaders. Invertebrates and plants have natural defense systems, which recognize commonly shared patterns and usually react in a stereotypical manner. Long-lived animals such as vertebrates add to these natural defenses with adaptive systems that show discriminating recognition machinery, complex and varying effector mechanisms and development of persistent or "memory" responses. Under ideal circumstances, immune defense proceeds with minimal or inapparent damage to the host. In other situations, the defense system is less successful and the host tissues become damaged by the reaction. We usually consider the former situation as immunity and the latter as immunopathology. However, in both instances, mechanisms at play may be similar and deciding if the process is one or the other may require Lucretian logic.

With microorganisms, the commonest circumstance that results in immunopathology is where the microbe persists and continues to cause an innate and adaptive response. These, however, prove ineffective to remove or neutralize the agent. Thus the reaction becomes chronic and host tissues become damaged as a consequence. This situation occurs in tuberculosis as well as hepatitis B and C virus infections. Over time, many microbes with a long association with a host species find ways of persisting by evading responses that would either eliminate them or cause too much tissue damage. Human CMV infection in immunocompetent adults provides an example of this scenario (Reddehase, 2002). Other circumstances that result in immunopathology involve settings where one or more components of normal immune defense are compromised for genetic or other reasons. Prolonged severe genital herpes simplex virus (HSV) lesions in AIDS patients with very low CD4+ T-cells represent such an example (Koelle and Corey, 2003). Atopics too often have problems clearing HSV and hence often develop skin and eye lesions (Pepose, 1991a). In addition, some microbes are considered as able to trigger immune reactions that target host components themselves (autoimmune disease) or cause infected cells to undergo neoplastic transformation. The herpesvirus EBV provides an example of the latter in genetically susceptible individuals (Kieff and Rickinson, 2001). There are no undisputed examples wherein herpesviruses cause autoimmune diseases. However, HHV-6 has been proposed to cause multiple sclerosis (Swanborg *et al.*, 2003) and HSV infection may cause an autoimmune corneal inflammatory lesion (Streilein *et al.*, 1997).

Herpes simplex virus is a pathogen that only rarely appears to be involved in immune mediated tissue damage. Characteristically, primary or recurrent infections at superficial mucosal or dermal sites result in viral replication and destruction of most cells that support infection. This process induces an innate inflammatory reaction that contributes to infection control. Some cells, likely Langerhans dendritic cells, leave the site and carry viral antigens to draining lymph nodes where an adaptive response is induced or recalled. After a few days, effectors of adaptive immunity are recruited to the site, initially CD4+ T-cells followed by CD8+ cells, and these T-cells, probably assisted by antibody, complete the task of recovery (Koelle and Corey, 2003). Virus is removed and the inflammatory reaction subsides usually without trace. These events can be judged to represent immunity. When T cell function is impaired, as can happen in AIDS patients, HSV removal is impaired and the inflammatory reaction becomes unusually severe and prolonged. This situation can be taken to represent immunopathology.

Certain tissue sites are particularly vulnerable to damage by an inflammatory response. These are sites where virus is difficult to dislodge, so the inflammatory reaction becomes prolonged and destructive, or where tissue repair leaves a functionally damaged organ. The eye is the site which best exemplifies such circumstances. In this organ, where inflammation or scar tissue along the visual axis impairs function, HSV infection may permanently impair vision. The most frequent example is herpetic stromal keratitis (SK). This chronic inflammatory reaction damages the stroma and can become sufficiently severe to merit corneal transplantation. About 20% of ocular HSV infections in humans result in stromal keratitis (Pepose et al., 1996). In most instances, these are caused by HSV-1 and result from reactivation from latent infection in the trigeminal ganglion (Pepose et al., 1996). Most of our understanding of the immunopathogenesis of SK comes from studies in animal models, in former times mostly the rabbit and now most usually the mouse.

Human HSV infections may also cause anterior as well as posterior uveitis (retinitis). These are rarer manifestations of HSV infection and much of the damage may result from direct viral damage more than from immunopathology. However, uveitis lesions in the rabbit and mouse models have a definite immunopathological component. Finally, HSV is the cause of a vision destroying reaction in the retina termed acute retinal necrosis (ARN). This lesion occurs both in children infected neonatally or later with HSV-2 as well as in adults where HSV-1 is usually involved (Margolis and Atherton, 1996). Acute retinal necrosis has also been studied in animal models, where lesions were shown to be immunopathological in part (Atherton, 2001).

Inflammatory reactions associated with HSV infection in the peripheral and central nervous systems may also be judged as immune mediated. The best studied example is ganglionitis, an HSV induced lesion that occurs in heterologous hosts but may not be a feature of the natural human disease. Lesions caused by HSV in the CNS are the most dramatic and devastating manifestations of HSV infection of humans. This rare disease is usually caused by HSV-1 infection in adults and is mostly a direct virologic lesion. However, immunopathological events such as demyelination may also occur in a few cases. In infants and children, encephalitis is more commonly associated with neonatal infection with HSV-2 and this lesion appears to be the direct result of a lytic virus infection.

Finally, there are some chronic inflammatory reactions that have been associated with HSV infection especially with the widespread use of modern technology to detect viral DNA. Some reports suggest that the virus or an immune response against it accounts for such HSV associated diseases as erythema multiforme, arteritis, Alzheimer's disease, Bell's palsy and Behcet's disease.

Herpes infections and ocular disease

At least four human herpesviruses have been implicated as causes of ocular disease. Two alphaherpesviruses, HSV and varicella zoster virus (VZV), the betaherpes virus CMV and the gammaherpesvirus EBV. CMV is a cause of retinitis, a lesion found only in immunosuppressed individuals, the majority of which were formerly AIDS patients, but now transplant recipients, especially recipients of bone marrow (Holland et al., 1996). With the widespread use of protease inhibitors to control HIV, CMV retinitis is now mainly a disease of transplant recipients. The lesion itself is likely a direct consequence of viral replication in retinal cells. EBV is an occasional cause of SK lesions. These are characterized by an abundance of lymphoma like cells, in the stroma that are presumed to be mainly B cells (Matoba, 1990).

More commonly both HSV and VZV cause lesions in the anterior segment, principally the cornea. Both HSV and VZV can also cause uveitis and acute retinal necrosis (ARN).

Keratitis in humans

Both HSV and VZV can infect multiple structures in the eye. Lesions caused by HSV are much more common. The incidence of HSV ocular disease ranges from 4.1–20.7 cases/100 000 patient years representing the commonest single infectious cause of vision impairment in the western world (Pepose et al., 1996). Of the three general types of HSV corneal disease, Infectious Epithelial Keratitis (IEK) is the most common lesion and appears to be a result of the direct effect of viral infection. Both disciform keratitis (HSV endotheliitis) and SK are thought to be mainly the consequence of immune mediated mechanisms rather than direct viral damage. IEK lesions are a result of viral replication and spread in the superficial epithelial layer of the cornea. This condition is usually self-limiting and no permanent corneal damage results. The quick remission seen with timely antiviral therapy suggests a simple viral cytolytic mechanism. However, virus invariably infects nervous ramifications in the cornea that have free ends within the epithelial layer, thus allowing retrograde transport and establishment of latency (Shimeld et al., 2001). In addition, as a consequence of epithelial damage, virus can spread to the underlying stromal keratocytes and cause what is usually termed a necrotizing form of stromal keratitis (Liesegang, 1999). This terminology is not used by many ophthalmologists since necrosis also occurs in immune mediated SK (T. P. Margolis, personal communication, 2003).

Disciform keratitis (DK) is a lesion in which the corneal endothelium is the primary site of damage. This form of ocular disease appears immunopathological based upon the fact that early intervention with corticosteroids leads to complete resolution (Liesegang, 1999). In DK, the inflammatory reaction of the endothelium sometimes results in secondary stromal and epithelial edema but there is usually no stromal infiltrate or neovascularization. One of the characteristic findings is the demonstration of keratic precipitates or KP (Liesegang, 1999). The exact nature of the KP is unknown but they could be aggregates of macrophages or NK cells attracted by the immunoglobulins on the surfaces of infected cells (Liesegang, 1999). An alternative idea is that KP represent cytotoxic T-cells recognizing viral epitopes on the endothelial cells (Liesegang, 1999). The role of live virus in disease development is supported by finding antigens, live virus and DNA in the anterior chamber and perhaps also corneal endothelial cells (Kaufman et al., 1971; Sundmacher and Neumann-Haefelin, 1979a). It has been postulated that productive infection of the endothelial cell elicits a cellular and humoral immune response (Sundmacher and Neumann-Haefelin, 1979b), but this evidence is only circumstantial. Alternative suggestions include a possible delayed type hypersensitivity reaction to persisting HSV antigens within the stroma or the endothelium (Pepose, 1991b). It is difficult to resolve the nature of DK pathogenesis since animal models to study it are less than ideal. Disciform disease is seen in rabbits with an intracorneal injection of soluble viral antigen (Williams et al., 1965). Using the rabbit model for DK, some have suggested that the lesions involve immune complex formation and antibody dependent cell mediated cytotoxicity (Meyers and Chitjian, 1976).

Inflammation of the corneal stroma (SK) as a result of HSV-1 (rarely HSV-2) infection can lead to a blinding immuno-inflammatory lesion of the stroma. This only accounts for approximately 2% of initial episodes of ocular disease but approximately 50% of recurrent ocular HSV disease (Norn, 1970). A similar, but even more devastating lesion can be caused by VZV infection. Fortunately, this is quite rare and also usually occurs as a consequence of reactivation (zoster). The infections usually heal quickly unless the patient is immuno-suppressed (Pepose et al., 2003). Recurrent lesions can be very severe and most difficult to treat and control. Frequently, corneal lesions are accompanied by conjunctivitis, anterior uveitis and lipid keratopathy (Pepose et al., 2003). If the virus is not controlled, it spreads to involve the iris and the corneal stroma. Stromal lesions can become sclerotic and very persistent and is believed to be immune mediated, however, the mechanism is not known and is difficult to study. Patients often lose sensitivity of the cornea and involuntary physical damage can result in secondary bacterial infection.

Table 35.1. Immunopathological basis for SK in humans

Lesions in the absence of virus or viral antigens
Indefinite corticosteroid therapy
Uncommon in immunosuppressed individuals
T-lymphocytes with reactivity to viral epitopes detectable in corneas with chronic lesions

Several observations suggest the operation of an immune etiology behind HSV induced SK (see Table 35.1). These include the fact that the lesions are persistent and are manifest well beyond the time that virus or viral antigens can be demonstrated. Lesions often need to be managed with indefinite corticosteroid treatment and reactivation lesions, except initially, do not benefit from acyclovir antiviral treatment. Also making a case for the pathogenesis of SK involving immunopathology is the fact that the lesion is very uncommon in immunosuppressed patients. Finally, clones of T-lymphocytes reactive to viral epitopes and possessing cytotoxic activity can be cultured from corneas showing chronic SK lesions (Verjans et al., 1998; Koelle et al., 2000).

Approximately 90% of patients maintain good visual acuity despite prolonged disease. However, in many cases resolution of inflammation is associated with a permanent loss of vision resulting from corneal scarring and ulceration. This necessitates treatment by corneal transplantation, which in itself can sometimes be a high risk factor for recrudescent herpetic keratitis (also called newly acquired herpetic keratitis) (Remeijer et al., 1997) and super-infection with a different strain (Remeijer et al., 2002)

The corneal stroma may be affected by several mechanisms; this may be secondary to disease of the epithelium (IEK) or endothelium (DK) or as a stromal edema resulting from a damaged endothelium. In humans, SK manifests itself in two primary forms that are perhaps mis-termed necrotizing SK and immune SK (Liesegang, 1999). While the former is thought to result from direct viral invasion of the stroma, chronic immune mechanisms, possibly of an autoimmune nature (yet unproven), are suspected in pathogenesis of the latter (Pepose et al., 1996). These divisions are not mutually exclusive and necrosis can definitely occur in the immune form of disease. Intact virions and antigens can be detected in corneal keratocytes, endothelial cells and foci of epithelial cells in specimens from patients with acute (necrotizing) stromal keratitis (Kobayashi et al., 1972; Metcalf and Kaufman, 1976). This suggests that replicating virus and the resulting host inflammatory response leads to stromal cell destruction. This acute necrotizing form of SK eventually may become chronic, then considered to be the immune form of SK, when viral antigens are no longer present. The signs of SK are generally quite variable but they include the influx of a large number of different kinds of cells including polymorphonuclear leukocytes (PMN), macrophages, Langerhans' cells, natural killer (NK) cells, plasma cells and T-lymphocytes (Pepose et al., 1985a; Youinou et al., 1985, 1986; Miller et al., 1993). In chronic herpetic SK in humans, the predominant population are macrophages and T-lymphocytes (Youinou et al., 1985). Excess neovascularization also occurs in some patients.

The original mechanism proposed for the pathogenesis of the immune form of SK focused on the role of anti-HSV antibodies. This was based on the finding that rings (Wessely rings) seen in the mid-stroma of the cornea in immune stromal keratitis were positive for IgM, IgG and IgA (Meyers-Elliot et al., 1980). Herpes virus particles have been demonstrated in these rings, many of them defective or incomplete (Meyers-Elliot et al., 1980). In addition, viral antigens have been found localized in the keratocytes of the corneal stroma in transplanted corneas (Youinou et al., 1986; Easty et al., 1987). Hence it has been speculated that viral antigens trapped in the stroma acted as a nidus for deposition of anti-HSV antibodies that fix complement and leads to cellular damage (Pepose et al., 1996). Viral antigens can also be presented to the infiltrating T-lymphocytes. In clinical specimens, increased levels of class I and II HLA antigens have been noted in areas of the greatest infiltrate, suggesting active presentation of antigens (Pepose et al., 1985b). Both CD4+ and CD8+ T-cells occur in chronic herpetic SK with the former dominating the total T-cell numbers (Youinou et al., 1986). Most of these cells are reactive against HSV antigens with the CD4+ subset reactive to peptide epitopes from UL21 and UL49 tegument proteins of HSV (Verjans et al., 1998; Koelle et al., 2000). They do not apparently recognize antigens derived from corneal tissues which would provide evidence for an auto-immune mechanism (Verjans et al., 1998). Corneal derived CD4+ cells have been shown to possess cytotoxic activity suggesting the possible operation of this mechanism in stromal cell injury (Verjans et al., 1998; Koelle et al., 2000).

Animal models for SK

Understanding the pathogenesis of human SK from clinical observations, transplant material and the occasional samples obtained at biopsy is difficult. Fortunately, convenient animal models exist wherein HSV infection of the eye reproducibly generates a stromal inflammatory response. Moreover, this appears to reflect human immune SK at least before it is treated. The usual animal models are the mouse and rabbit with the latter now rarely used except for studies on therapy. Events in SK pathogenesis are mainly studied in primary infection of various mouse strains. Since human SK is most commonly a sequel to reactivated HSV, a better animal model should be one where lesions follow reactivation. Such models have in fact, been described for both mice and rabbit (Myers-Elliot and Chitjian, 1983; Shimeld et al., 1989) but these are expensive and inconvenient and have contributed minimally to the understanding of pathogenesis. Rabbit reactivation can be achieved by ocular iontophoresis but this seldom gives rise to SK lesions (Myers-Elliot and Chitjian, 1983). The mouse reactivation model can be achieved by infecting mice under a cover of neutralizing antibody, then after some weeks asymptomatic animals are exposed to UV light. In usually a minority of animals, virus reactivates and generates an inflammatory reaction in the stroma (Shimeld et al., 1989). Few papers have employed the model, and the results of these usually support the basic findings of the primary infection model; namely that SK is an immuno-inflammatory lesion mainly orchestrated by CD4+ T cells (Shimeld et al., 1996).

The primary infection model usually uses strain HSV-1 RE and involves virus application to a lightly scratched cornea. Replication begins in epithelial cells of the cornea and usually the conjunctiva, but in immuno-competent mice rarely spreads to involve stromal cells or cells in uveal tissue. Characteristically, the viral replication events are over by 5–6 days and viral gene expression, as judged by protein detection or viral mRNA, are undetectable beyond a further 2–3 days (Babu et al., 1996). Viral DNA, however, can be detected for prolonged periods although copy numbers, detectable by real-time PCR, do not exceed 2000–5000 copies per cornea by 14 days p.i. (our unpublished results). When looked at with an ophthalmoscope, the initial viral replication events are accompanied by a barely detectable inflammatory reaction with new blood vessel growth from the limbus (the location of blood vessels at the edge of the vessel free normal cornea) the most obvious feature. This is often referred to as the preclinical phase, although in fact with appropriate tests is readily observable.

Innate reactions to infection in the mouse model

HSV infection of the corneal epithelium sets off a range of humoral and cellular events that taken together help contain infection. Unfortunately, some of these also set the stage for subsequent immunopathology. A prominent early cellular event is the influx of polymorphonuclear neutrophils (PMN). This occurs mainly into stromal tissues subjacent to the infected epithelium. Such PMN escape from blood vessels at the limbus presumably in response to signaling molecules generated from virus infected cells. The nature of such signaling molecules is unclear but several chemokines, including those known to be chemotactic to PMN, can be demonstrated within 12 hr p.i. (Su et al., 1996; Thomas et al., 1998)

The PMN response is at its peak around 48 hrs and it seems that this response helps control viral replication. Thus depleting PMN with specific monoclonal antibodies results in more intense and prolonged virus infection in the cornea (Tumpey et al., 1996; Thomas et al., 1997). Moreover, PMN suppressed animals may succumb to encephalitis since virus now spreads to the brain. Such observations indicate that PMN are part of the antiviral defense system although it is unclear how this function is performed. Accordingly, virus infected cells and PMN are usually not in direct contact implying that the protective function is indirect. Ideas for the mediation of such defenses include IFNγ and TNFα production as well as nitric oxide production by PMN (Daheshia et al., 1998a). This topic has not been fully explored using, for example, knockout mice and other means of implicating potential antiviral mechanisms.

The PMN response to virus is not only a defense reaction. Indeed products released from PMN have been proposed to contribute to corneal damage possibly unmasking autoantigens subsequently involved in the immunopathology (Thomas et al., 1997). In addition, PMN contribute to the process of neovascularization, a prominent feature of SK and a necessary step in its pathogenesis (Zheng et al., 2001a; Lee et al., 2002a). It appears that PMN may be a source of angiogenesis factors such as VEGF as well as tissue degrading enzymes which breakdown the stromal matrix and facilitates the growth of new blood vessels. One such enzyme released by the granules of activated PMN is MMP9 (Lee et al., 2002a). Since infected mice given the MMP-9 inhibitor TIMP-1 as well as MMP9-/- mice have reduced angiogenic and SK responses, MMP9 appears to be intricately involved in SK pathogenesis (Lee et al., 2002a).

Although PMN dominate the early inflammatory reaction to ocular HSV infection, other cell types can also be demonstrated. These include macrophages, dendritic cells (DC), NK cells but not B or αβ TCR T cells. The roles for these other cell types have received minimal investigation. It is likely, however that the macrophage is a source of angiogenic factors such as VEGF and FGF as well as the angiogenic CXC chemokines. For example MIP-2 (CXCL8) appears important since infected mice lacking the receptor for MIP-2 have an impaired PMN response (Banerjee et al., 2004a). In addition, in vivo neutralization of MIP-2 in HSV infected mice reduces PMN migration (Yan et al., 1998). Macrophages, along with DC, also act as a source of cytokines demonstrable early after infection. Most prominent of these are IL-1 and IL-6, both of which can also be produced by virus infected epithelial cells themselves (Tran et al., 1998; Kanangat et al., 1996). Indeed, it could be that these two cytokines are critical signaling molecules responsible for the many paracrine events set off by virus infected epithelial cells. The other early events described include the production of IL-12, VEGF and TNFα, but none of these are thought to be products of virus-infected cells themselves (Zheng et al., 2001b; Kumaraguru and Rouse, 2002). We have demonstrated that IL-6, for example, can cause macrophages in vitro to generate VEGF (Banerjee et al., 2004a), and IL-1 is well known to cause mononuclear cells to produce TNFα and other cytokines (Neta et al., 1992). Our recent findings also indicate that within HSV infected corneas, IL-1 maybe responsible for IL-6 expression, which in turn upregulates VEGF production (Biswas et al., 2004).

The cytokine IL-12 appears as a pivotal molecule in SK pathogenesis. Knockout mice, for example, unable to produce IL-12 have only mild SK lesions (Osorio et al., 2002). The source of IL-12 following HSV infection remains to be clarified, since as mentioned it does not appear to be HSV-infected cells themselves (Kumaraguru and Rouse, 2002) However conceivably viral DNA that has pathogen associated molecular pattern (PAMP) activity could represent such a stimulus (Zheng et al., 2002). The most likely producer cell types are DC and macrophages. The DC initially involved would seem to be the resident cells only recently demonstrated as present in normal non-inflamed corneas (Hamrah et al., 2003). A prominent feature of the injured cornea, including that caused by HSV, is the invasion of Langerhans DC, likely from the conjunctiva, into the cornea (Jager et al., 1991). However, this event takes several days to occur. Likely such cells also act as a source of cytokines and chemokines but their major function in SK pathogenesis is transport of viral antigens to lymphoid tissue where the adaptive immune response is initiated (discussed later).

The cytokine IL-12 has several downstream effects that impact on SK pathogenesis. The primary effect is induction of IFNγ production by cells with IL-12 receptors. Although not proven in the eye, the most likely cells that respond and produce IFNγ are natural killer (NK) cells. Such cells in non-ocular systems have been shown to be important for resistance to HSV. In fact, removing them results in heightened susceptibility (Rager-Zisman et al., 1987). An early study of SK indicated that NK removal ameliorated SK (Tamesis et al., 1994; Bouley et al., 1996), although this issue warrants further investigation. Whatever the source of IFNγ, this molecule appears to be intricately involved in antigen processing as well as other events critical for

SK pathogenesis. These include up-regulation of the cell adhesion molecule PECAM-1 on vascular endothelial cells, at the limbus (Tang and Hendricks, 1996). This is a necessary step for normal PMN invasion as evidenced by the fact that neutralization of IFNγ or PECAM-1 results in diminished PMN ingress (Tang and Hendricks, 1996).

The importance of IFNγ in facilitating cell migration is further underscored by studies with human corneas. Stimulation of human corneal cells in vitro with IFNγ, and also IL-1 and TNFα, rapidly up-regulates ICAM-1 expression (another cell adhesion molecule that participates in the adhesion and extravasation of cells) (Pavilack et al., 1992). IFNγ also upregulates MHC Class II expression on the antigen presenting cells involved in the induction of the initial antigen specific CD4+ T-cell response in local draining lymph nodes (Dreizen et al., 1988; Foets et al., 1991). On the other hand, IFNγ could help modulate lesion development since it also induces angiostatic chemokines such as IP-10 and MIG (Lee et al., 2002b). Accordingly the IL-12 response to HSV infection indirectly impacts on both inflammatory and regulatory effects on SK.

In Fig. 35.1 several critical events are shown that are set into play by HSV during the first 6–7 days postinfection. By the end of this often-called preclinical phase, the corneal tissues show little or no damage. The epithelium is fully intact, the stroma has few if any inflammatory cells and cytokine/chemokine levels have fallen significantly. The most obvious sign of change is a neovascular bed that continues to expand slowly beyond the limbal region. Nevertheless, in spite of the quiet appearance, notable changes begin to occur which constitute the true immunopathological events of SK. Accordingly, the T-cell orchestrators begin to invade via the new blood vessels and an intense inflammatory response ensues. This becomes obvious upon ophthalmoscopic examination and is frequently referred to as the clinical phase.

Adaptive immunity in SK

Migration of T-cells that express appropriate homing molecules escaping from the newly established blood vessels represents a crucial step in SK pathogenesis. Mice without T-cells never develop typical SK lesions (Metcalf et al., 1979; Mercadal et al., 1993), but do if given T-cell transfers (Russell et al., 1984; Mercadal et al., 1993). Although debated early on, most investigators now agree that CD4+ T-cells, with the type 1 producing cytokine phenotype, are the main aggressors in HSK (Niemialtowski and Rouse, 1992; Mercadal et al., 1993). Such cells trigger the invasion of non-specific inflammatory cells, surprisingly once again dominated by PMN, giving rise to a peak response around 15 days after initial infection. The inflammatory response considerably thickens the stroma and neovascularization

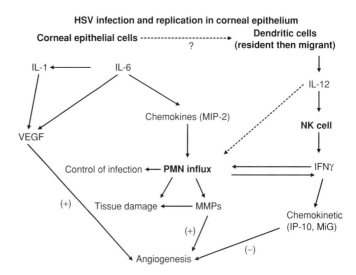

Fig. 35.1. Some early critical events occurring after HSV-1 ocular infection.

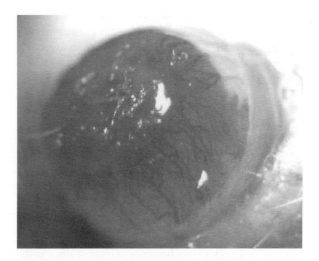

Fig. 35.2. Corneal blood vessels at the peak of HSK lesions in the mouse (day 15) with evidence of corneal opacity, necrosis and epithelial ulcers.

continues almost reaching the central cornea (see Fig. 35.2). Severe lesions have areas of necrosis and epithelial ulcers and uveal tissues may also be involved. The lesional T-cells, which account for only a minority of the inflammatory cells present, are mainly CD4+ T-cells. Judging from a variety of approaches, the principal cytokine necessary for the lesion expression is IFNγ (Tang and Hendricks, 1996; Deshpande et al., 2002). However, SK can still be induced in animals lacking this cytokine (Bouley et al., 1995). In cases where lesions do diminish in severity, the cytokine IL-10 is upregulated (Babu et al., 1995). Furthermore, the artificial expression of IL-10 or IL-4 early in the syndrome can markedly diminish lesions (Daheshia et al., 1998b).

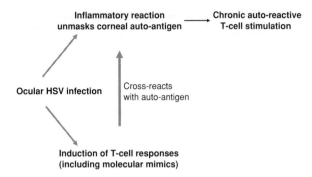

Fig. 35.3. The autoimmunity model of SK pathogenesis.

Such observations indicate that CD4+ Th1 are the principal aggressors but if a type 2 response can be induced, lesions will resolve. Whether such ideas can be applied usefully to the human system warrants investigation.

Very recently the severity of SK lesions was shown to be modulated by a second species of CD4+ T-cells (Suvas et al., 2004). These were CD4+CD25+ T-regulatory cells (T_{reg}) found operative in autoimmune inflammatory lesions (Shevach, 2000). Accordingly, in animals unable to generate T_{reg} responses, SK lesions were more severe and animals more susceptible to a low dose of infection (Suvas et al., 2004). In addition, there is evidence that the CD8 T cell response to HSV provides a protective function against SK (Mercadal et al., 1993; Gangappa et al., 1999; Banerjee et al., 2004b, 2005). The mechanisms by which T_{reg} or CD8+ T-cells exert controlling effects on SK expression are not currently understood but are being actively explored.

A central issue in SK pathogenesis is the nature of antigens recognized by the CD4+ T-cell orchestrators and if such recognition occurs in the extra-lymphoid or lymphoid sites (or both). This issue becomes of interest since at the time when T-cells invade the cornea, replicating virus has usually disappeared (Babu et al., 1996). Moreover, certainly at the time of peak lesions (15 days), the presence of viral antigens in stromal tissues cannot be demonstrated (Babu et al., 1996). Conceivably, viral peptides expressed by DC could still be present in the cornea and draining lymph nodes, although usually T-cell target peptides turn over within 2–3 days after protein processing. Since new protein formation appears to have ceased by 6 days p.i., it is difficult to support the logical notion that peptides derived from viral proteins are the target antigens recognized by the $T_{aggressors}$.

An alternative concept is that viral specific T-cells are initially responsible for the immunopathology but subsequently the chronic phase is maintained by an autoreactive response (Deshpande et al., 2002). Here the

Table 35.2. Lack of evidence for molecular mimicry between HSV UL6 peptide and corneal antigen

1. Failure to demonstrate an immune response directed to UL6 peptide after HSV ocular infection	Deshpande et al., 2001a
2. Ocular infection with vaccinia virus expressing UL6 fails to induce HSK	Deshpande et al., 2001a
3. CD4+ T-cells that are apparently tolerized to molecular mimics are able to induce SK lesions upon adoptive transfer to SCID mice	Thomas and Rouse, 1998
4. T-cells extracted from human corneas show no reactivity to HSV UL6	Verjans et al., 1998; Koelle et al., 2000
5. T-cells extracted from human corneas are not reactive to corneal antigens	Verjans et al., 1998
6. Variation in clinical presentation of SK is not due to genetic variation in the UL6 epitope	Ellison et al., 2003

idea is that the virus infection results in unmasking of the some corneal autoantigen (see Fig. 35.3), tolerance is broken and the autoreactive T-cells induced are responsible for orchestrating lesions. A modification of this idea favored by the Cantor group is that the autoimmune process is set off by some viral peptide sharing reactivity to the unmasked corneal autoantigen (Zhao et al., 1998). Thus the initial antiviral response subsequently becomes sustained by autoreactive $T_{aggressor}$ cells. This concept of molecular mimicry has aroused much interest and discussion (Deshpande et al., 2002). Its best support comes from studies on closely related inbred mice. Here it would seem that the UL6 protein of HSV possesses molecular mimicry with an autopeptide that in fact represents a sequence also found on an immunoglobulin isotype (Zhao et al., 1998). The molecular mimicry idea is not accepted by other groups for a number of reasons (See Table 35.2). Most, especially the UL6 proteins of HSV appear not to induce T cell responses in animals following infection with HSV (Deshpande et al., 2001a). In humans also the UL6 protein appears not to be recognized (Verjans et al., 1998; Koelle et al., 2000; Ellison et al., 2003).

An alternative idea to explain how CD4+ T-cells become activated is that the inflammatory process could be initiated by viral antigen recognizing T-cells, but subsequently is maintained by cells of the effector memory phenotype that escape into the cornea because of the highly permeable neovascular bed. Such cells, in turn, become activated by inflammatory molecules initially released by viral antigen reactive cells. The responding cells, release inflammatory cytokines and so the process continues (see Fig. 35.4). This idea is supported by the observation that abundant non-antigen T-cells can be demonstrated and that it is possible to develop lesions identical to SK in animals whose T-cells are genetically incapable of recognizing viral antigens (Gangappa et al., 1998; Deshpande et al., 2001b; Banerjee et al., 2002). Such was shown in several T-cell transgenic mice on SCID or RAG–/– backgrounds whose recognition repertoire did not include HSV antigen recognition (Gangappa et al., 1998; Deshpande et al., 2001b; Banerjee et al., 2002). In these models, the chronic source of activating cytokines were cells dying of HSV infection since in this instance virus persisted and spread to the stromal site of inflammation (Gangappa et al., 1998; Deshpande et al., 2001b; Banerjee et al., 2002).

Other ideas have also been advocated to explain which agonists drive SK, especially in the chronic phase, but the issue remains unresolved. The candidate agonists include PAMP expressed by virus, superantigen expression and inflammatory reactions driven by stress proteins (Deshpande et al., 2002). Currently, a favored idea is that the HSV DNA could itself be pro-inflammatory because of its high content of bioactive CpG containing deoxynucleotide motifs (Zheng et al., 2002). Such ideas await verification.

Human Uveitis

Herpes simplex virus infection of the iris, ciliary body and the choroid results in an inflammatory condition known as HSV uveitis. This lesion usually accompanies SK or DK but occasionally it can stand alone. In many cases, it can occur in the absence of a previous history of HSV infection. Ophthalmoscopic examination reveals the presence of fine keratic precipitates (KP) and anterior chamber inflammation that ranges from mild to severe (Liesegang, 1999). The virus can be detected in the inflamed iris by electron microscopy. There seems to be a lack of consensus about the isolation of infectious virus from the anterior chamber of patients with HSV uveitis (Kimura, 1962; Sundmacher and Neumann-Haefelin, 1979b). This disparity may, however, result from differences among patients in the relative concentrations of anti-HSV antibodies to the virus in the anterior chamber that is needed to clear virus. Interestingly, intra-ocular antibodies recognize different viral antigens than those recognized by antibodies in the systemic immune response (Peek et al., 2002). The implications of this finding are unclear but possibly persisting intraocular antibodies could be involved in the development of secondary uveitis by the formation of toxic immune complexes. Currently, the only evidence supporting an immunopathological basis for HSV uveitis in humans is the benefit of treatment achieved

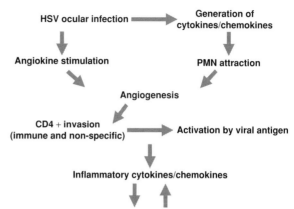

Fig. 35.4. Bystander activation model for SK pathogenesis.

with administration of topical corticosteroids along with systemic acyclovir (Liesegang, 1999). Anterior chamber uveitis can precede ARN, the latter lesion initially virologic, but later on includes immune mediated events (discussed later).

The rabbit model for HSV uveitis

The possible immunopathological nature of HSV uveitis has been revealed in studies with the rabbit model (Oh, 1976). Injection of live virus directly into the vitreous humor (intravitreal injections) of the rabbit eye results in a slowly progressing inflammation of the uveal tract. Eventually an HSV neutralizing antibody response in the infected eyes, clears the virus. Only live virus is capable of producing primary uveitis. However in eyes that have recovered, secondary uveitis can be induced by injection of inactivated virus (Oh, 1976). The disease kinetics of this secondary disease is faster than that seen with the primary infection. Such results indicate that in cases of secondary uveitis the pathogenic mechanism is likely to be immune mediated.

Acute retinal necrosis (ARN) in humans

This dramatic and devastating lesion can be caused by VZV or more commonly by HSV. Lesions can result from primary or recurrent infection and in the case of VZV can stand alone or accompany chicken pox or zoster (Ganatra et al., 2000). Without treatment the virus destroys the retina in 7–14 days. The initial stages of acute retinal necrosis (ARN) appear to be the direct result of viral damage but later stages involve immune mediated events.

Either HSV-1 or 2 can be involved. HSV-2 is usually the cause in infants, children and young adults (average age 27). In adults HSV-1 is usually the culprit (average age 50). With

HSV-2 induced ARN there is often a history of encephalitis and meningitis. It is thought that virus remains in the brain after such lesions, but then passes from that site to affect the retina (Margolis and Atherton, 1996). Typically, ARN starts off as a virologic lesion, but subsequently becomes immune mediated. The vitreous fills up with inflammatory cells and occlusive vasculitis can occur which deprives the retina of its blood supply (Margolis and Atherton, 1996). In addition, both CD4+ and CD8+ T-cells, possessing cytolytic and cytokine secreting functions, have been isolated from intraocular fluids of patients. These cells have been found to be reactive with HSV UL46 and UL47 encoded tegument proteins VP11/12 and VP13/14 (Verjans et al., 2000).

In adults where HSV-1 is the usual cause, ARN is most commonly unilateral and usually associated with encephalitis. However there are two cases of retinitis that have occurred years after recovery from encephalitis (Margolis and Atherton, 1996).

The mouse model of ARN

Both the mouse and the rabbit model have been employed to study the pathogenesis of ARN and have yielded interesting clues for pathogenesis. If injected intra-cerebrally, virus spreads to the retina via the optic nerve (Atherton, 2001), providing evidence that a similar effect could occur in humans accounting for ARN long after an episode of encephalitis (Margolis and Atherton, 1996). ARN can also be induced by injecting HSV into the anterior chamber. Such infection usually fails to cause lesions in the injected eye, that is presumed to be protected by an IFNα response (Atherton, 2001). However, after a few days the contralateral eye develops a severe retinitis. This response is assumed to be immune mediated since it is of much milder extent in T-deficient mice. Moreover, reconstituting such mice with CD4+ immune T-cells, but not CD8+, restores lesion expression (Atherton, 2001).

Taken together, results from the mouse and human studies support the idea that a combination of viral infection of the retina and virus specific T-lymphocytes is likely involved in the pathogenesis of ARN.

Herpes simplex virus in the nervous system

In humans the most dramatic and devastating disease associated with HSV infection is herpes simplex encephalitis (HSE). Fortunately this is a rare syndrome for it is usually lethal or leaves patients with serious neurological damage. In adults, HSE is usually caused by HSV-1 and can occur following primary or more commonly recurrent infection (Whitley, 2001). Lesions are mainly considered to be the direct cytolytic effect of the virus. However, inflammatory reactions occur that include both CD4+ and CD8+ T-cells. In about 3% of adult cases demyelination has been noted likely a consequence of a T cell mediated immunopathological reaction (R. J. Whitley, 2003, personal communication). HSE in infants is occasionally associated with involvement of the retina (ARN).

Whereas HSE is a very rare disease in humans, heterologous hosts infected with this alphaherpesvirus are far more likely to suffer from HSE. Thus primary infection of susceptible mouse strains, especially with HSV-2, results in spread to the CNS and death from encephalitis (Hudson et al., 1991; Whitley, 2001). Whereas in humans there is no evidence of neurotropic strains of HSV, in mice some viral strains are far more neurotropic than others (LaVail et al., 1997). In some cases, the neurotropism has been associated with known amino acids in a single protein (Diefenbach et al., 2002). The rodent form of HSE largely represents a direct effect of viral destruction, but immunopathology can play a role (Kastrukoff et al., 1993; Hudson and Strelein, 1994). Multifocal brain demyelination (MBD) has been reported in susceptible mouse strains upon lip inoculation with HSV-1 and immunosuppression prevents the development of such lesions (Kastrukoff et al., 1987; Kastrukoff et al., 1993). Of the two major T-subsets, CD8+ T-cells appear to be involved in the focal lesions of the brain and depleting such cells prevents lesion development (Hudson and Streilein, 1994). Other studies indicate that CD8+ T-cells play both a protective and pathogenic role in encephalitis (Anglen et al., 2003). These studies evaluated the role of such cells in stress induced HSE. If present prior to an infection, protection ensues, possibly by limiting the HSV replication and spread within the CNS; the delayed entrance of CD8+ T-cells could result in pathology, based on limited evidence (Anglen et al., 2003).

Ganglionitis

A characteristic feature of all alphaherpesviruses is that they succeed in gaining access to sensory nerve fibers during primary infection and pass by retrograde axonal transport to the nerve cell bodies in the appropriate ganglion. At that site, whereas some neurons appear to support a productive infection, in others an alternative replication cycle is initiated that results in latency (Roizman and Knipe, 2001). With HSV, at least, latency is thought to be an immunologically cryptic situation, since the viral transcripts expressed have no protein product (Roizman and Knipe, 2001). Latency in a particular neuron can be maintained indefinitely, but some infected neurons restart the productive cycle and progeny virus spreads by anterograde transport to peripheral sites, such as the cornea. In their homologous hosts, alphaherpesviruses rarely spread to the CNS after primary infection. Such events are quite common in heterologous hosts such as HSV in the mouse. Moreover, reactivation in homologous hosts often results in recrudescent lesions, but such are rare in heterologous situations. In the mouse latently infected with HSV, occasional neurons undergo reactivation (about 1 neuron in 5 days) and this induces a notable local inflammatory reaction (Feldman et al., 2002). This likely prevents widespread dissemination in the ganglion.

Another event that characterizes HSV infection in heterologous hosts is a marked and prolonged ganglionitis that occurs after primary infection (Shimeld et al., 1995; Liu et al., 1996). This represents an immune mediated event that mainly involves CD8 + T-cells (Liu et al., 1996; Liu et al., 2000; Khanna et al., 2003). The CD8 + T-cells seemingly function to purge productively infected neurons of virus, rather than killing them by a cytotoxic mechanism (Liu et al., 2000; Khanna et al., 2003). Hence there is no tissue damage and strictly speaking no pathology. Currently, the relevance of heterologous ganglionitis is not understood nor is it known if a similar phenomenon occurs in infected human ganglia. Ganglionitis, may be another example of events that occur only in heterologous hosts infected with alphaherpesviruses.

The course of events in the mouse ganglion has been carefully studied and they tell an intriguing story (Liu et al., 1996; Liu et al., 2000; Khanna et al., 2003). The initial events involve viral replication and an inflammatory cascade that resembles that described for SK. However, after 7–10 days, CD4+ cells appear to enter and orchestrate subsequent events in SK whereas a remarkably high percentage of the inflammatory cells in the ganglia are CD8+ T-cells. Moreover, most of these are viral antigen specific and maintain this phenotype for months, which would indicate their continuous activation by antigen. However, demonstrating such antigen has proven impossible and most would agree that, after 10 days or so, virus is latent in neurons. The ganglionitis studies, however, imply that some antigen might be expressed by neurons but these are not sacrificed (Liu et al., 2000; Khanna et al., 2003); instead they are spared by the ability of the CD8+ T-cells to purge them of their offending virus (Liu et al., 2000; Khanna et al., 2003). These ideas remain to be proven and shown to be not purely a murine idiosyncrasy.

Other possible HSV induced immune mediated conditions

Herpes simplex virus affects the majority of mankind and it usually persists in some form in all it infects. Indeed, the latest sensitive molecular approaches have revealed that HSV DNA can be found in many tissues previously not recognized as an infection site. Such observations have led to the speculation that HSV could contribute to the cause of several chronic inflammatory diseases. For example, some have associated HSV with Alzheimer's disease based on the high correlation between HSV-1 in the brain and Alzheimer's disease (Pyles, 2001). On the same grounds, HSV-1 has been suggested to be a risk factor in other conditions like in Behcet's disease, Bell's palsy and Parkinson's disease (Hegab and Al-Mutawa, 2000; Simmons, 2002; Hemling et al., 2003). Furthermore, HSV could also be a contributory cause of arteritis leading to atherosclerosis, an idea supported by some animal studies (Leinonen and Saikku, 2002).

In all cases where HSV is associated with chronic inflammatory lesions, experimental verification of a causative role is lacking.

REFERENCES

Anglen, C. S., Truckenmiller, M. E., Schell, T. D., and Bonneau, R. H. (2003). The dual role of CD8+ T lymphocytes in the development of stress-induced herpes simplex encephalitis. J. Neuroimmunol., 140(1–2), 13–27.

Atherton, S. S. (2001). Acute retinal necrosis: insights into pathogenesis from the mouse model. Herpes, 8(3), 69–73.

Babu, J. S., Kanangat, S., and Rouse, B. T. (1995). T cell cytokine mRNA expression during the course of the immunopathologic ocular disease herpetic stromal keratitis. J. Immunol., 154(9), 4822–4829.

Babu, J. S., Thomas, J., Kanangat, S., Morrison, L. A., Knipe, D. M., and Rouse, B. T. (1996). Viral replication is required for induction of ocular immunopathology by herpes simplex virus. J. Virol., 70(1), 101–107.

Banerjee, K., Deshpande, S., Zheng, M., Kumaraguru, U., Schoenberger, S. P., and Rouse, B. T. (2002). Herpetic stromal keratitis in the absence of viral antigen recognition. Cell Immunol., 219(2), 108–118.

Banerjee, K, Biswas, P. S, Kim, B, Lee, S., and Rouse, B. T. (2004a). CXCR2-/- mice show enhanced susceptibility to herpetic stromal keratitis: a role for IL-6-induced neovascularization. J. Immunol., 172(2), 1237–1245.

Banerjee, K., Biswas, P. S., Kumaraguru, U., Schoenberger, S. P., and Rouse, B. T. (2004b). Protective and pathological roles of virus-specific and bystander CD8+ T cells in herpetic stromal keratitis. J. Immunol., 173(12), 7575–7583.

Banerjee, K., Biswas, P. S., and Rouse B, T. (2005). Elucidating the protective and pathologic T cell species in the virus-induced corneal immunoinflammatory condition herpetic stromal keratitis. J. Leukoc. Biol., 77(1), 24–32.

Biswas, P. S, Banerjee, K, Kim, B., and Rouse, B. T. (2004). Mice transgenic for IL-1 receptor antagonist protein are resistant to herpetic stromal keratitis: possible role for IL-1 in herpetic stromal keratitis pathogenesis. J. Immunol., 172(6): 3736–3744.

Bouley, D. M., Kanangat, S., Wire, W., and Rouse, B. T. (1995). Characterization of herpes simplex virus type-1 infection and herpetic stromal keratitis development in IFN-gamma knockout mice. *J. Immunol.*, **155**(8), 3964–3971.

Bouley, D. M., Kanangat, S., and Rouse, B. T. (1996). The role of the innate immune system in the reconstituted SCID mouse model of herpetic stromal keratitis. *Clin. Immunol. Immunopathol.*, **80**(1), 23–30.

Daheshia, M., Kanangat, S., and Rouse, B. T. (1998a). Production of key molecules by ocular neutrophils early after herpetic infection of the cornea. *Exp. Eye Res.*, **67**(6), 619–624.

Daheshia, M., Kuklin, N., Manickan, E., Chun, S., and Rouse, B. T. (1998b). Immune induction and modulation by topical ocular administration of plasmid DNA encoding antigens and cytokines. *Vaccine*, **16**(11–12), 1103–1110.

Deshpande, S. P., Lee, S., Zheng, M. et al. (2001a). Herpes simplex virus-induced keratitis: evaluation of the role of molecular mimicry in lesion pathogenesis. *J. Virol.*, **75**(7), 3077–3088.

Deshpande, S., Zheng, M., Lee, S. et al. (2001b). Bystander activation involving T lymphocytes in herpetic stromal keratitis. *J. Immunol.*, **167**(5), 2902–2910.

Deshpande, S. P., Zheng, M, Lee, S., and Rouse, B. T. (2002). Mechanisms of pathogenesis in herpetic immunoinflammatory ocular lesions. *Vet. Microbiol.*, **86**(1–2), 17–26.

Diefenbach, R. J., Miranda-Saksena, M., Diefenbach, E. et al. (2002). Herpes simplex virus tegument protein US11 interacts with conventional kinesin heavy chain. *J. Virol.*, **76**(7), 3282–3291.

Dreizen, N. G., Whitsett, C. F., and Stulting, R. D. (1988). Modulation of HLA antigen expression on corneal epithelial and stromal cells. *Invest. Ophthalmol. Vis. Sci.*, **29**(6), 933–939.

Easty, D. L., Shimeld, C., Claoue, C. M., and Menage, M. (1987). Herpes simplex virus isolation in chronic stromal keratitis: human and laboratory studies. *Curr. Eye Res.*, **6**(1), 69–74.

Ellison, A. R., Yang, L., Cevallos, A. V., and Margolis, T. P. (2003). Analysis of the herpes simplex virus type 1 UL6 gene in patients with stromal keratitis. *Virology*, **310**(1), 24–28.

Feldman, L. T., Ellison, A. R., Voytek, C. C., Yang, L., Krause, P., and Margolis, T. P. (2002). Spontaneous molecular reactivation of herpes simplex virus type 1 latency in mice. *Proc. Natl Acad. Sci. USA*, **99**(2), 978–983.

Foets, B. J., van den Oord, J. J., Billiau, A., Van Damme, J., and Missotten, L. (1991). Heterogeneous induction of major histocompatibility complex class II antigens on corneal endothelium by interferon-gamma. *Invest. Ophthalmol. Vis. Sci.*, **32**(2), 341–345.

Ganatra, J. B., Chandler, D., Santos, C., Kuppermann, B., and Margolis, T. P. (2000). Viral causes of the acute retinal necrosis syndrome. *Am. J. Ophthalmol.*, **129**(2), 166–172.

Gangappa, S., Babu, J. S., Thomas, J., Daheshia, M., and Rouse, B. T. (1998). Virus-induced immunoinflammatory lesions in the absence of viral antigen recognition. *J. Immunol.*, **161**(8), 4289–4300.

Gangappa, S, Deshpande, S. P., and Rouse, B. T. (1999). Bystander activation of CD4(+) T cells can represent an exclusive means of immunopathology in a virus infection. *Eur. J. Immunol.*, **29**(11), 3674–3682.

Hamrah, P., Liu, Y., Zhang, Q., and Dana, M. R. (2003). The corneal stroma is endowed with a significant number of resident dendritic cells. *Invest. Ophthalmol. Vis. Sci.*, **44**(2), 581–589.

Hegab, S. and Al-Mutawa, S. (2000). Immunopathogenesis of Behcet's disease. *Clin. Immunol.*, **96**(3), 174–186.

Hemling, N., Roytta, M., Rinne, J. et al. (2003). Herpesviruses in brains in Alzheimer's and Parkinson's diseases. *Ann. Neurol.*, **54**(2), 267–271.

Holland, G. N., Tufail, A., and Jordan, C. N. (1996). Cytomegalovirus diseases. In *Ocular Infection and Immunity*, ed. J. S., Pepose, G. N., Holland, and K. R. Wilhelmus, pp. 1088–1130. St. Louis: Mosby.

Hudson, S. J. and Streilein, J. W. (1994). Functional cytotoxic T cells are associated with focal lesions in the brains of SJL mice with experimental herpes simplex encephalitis. *J. Immunol.*, **152**(11), 5540–5547.

Hudson, S. J., Dix, R. D., and Streilein, J. W. (1991). Induction of encephalitis in SJL mice by intranasal infection with herpes simplex virus type 1: a possible model of herpes simplex encephalitis in humans. *J. Infect. Dis.*, **163**(4), 720–727.

Jager, M. J., Atherton, S., Bradley, D., and Streilein, J. W. (1991). Herpetic stromal keratitis in mice: less reversibility in the presence of Langerhans cells in the central cornea. *Curr. Eye Res.*, **10** Suppl, 69–73.

Kanangat, S., Babu, J. S., Knipe, D. M., and Rouse, B. T. (1996). HSV-1-mediated modulation of cytokine gene expression in a permissive cell line: selective upregulation of IL-6 gene expression. *Virology*, **219**(1), 295–300.

Kastrukoff, L. F., Lau, A. S., and Kim, S. U. (1987). Multifocal CNS demyelination following peripheral inoculation with herpes simplex virus type 1. *Ann. Neurol.*, **22**(1), 52–59.

Kastrukoff, L. F., Lau, A. S., Leung, G. Y., and Thomas, E. E. (1993). Contrasting effects of immunosuppression on herpes simplex virus type I (HSV I) induced central nervous system (CNS) demyelination in mice. *J. Neurol. Sci.*, **117**(1–2), 148–158.

Kaufman, H. E., Kanai, A., and Ellison, E. D. (1971). Herpetic iritis: demonstration of virus in the anterior chamber by fluorescent antibody techniques and electron microscopy. *Am. J. Ophthalmol.*, **71**(2), 465–469.

Khanna, K. M., Bonneau, R. H., Kinchington, P. R., and Hendricks, R. L. (2003). Herpes simplex virus-specific memory CD8+ T cells are selectively activated and retained in latently infected sensory ganglia. *Immunity*, **18**(5), 593–603.

Kieff, E. and Rickinson, A. B. (2001). Epstein–Barr virus and its replication. In *Fields Virology*, ed. D. M. Knipe and P. M. Howley, pp. 2511–2574. Philadelphia: Lipincott Williams and Wilkins.

Kimura, S. J. (1962). Herpes Simplex Uveitis: A clinical and experimental study. *Trans. Am. Ophthalmol. Soc.*, **60**, 440–470.

Kobayashi, S., Shogi, S., and Ishizu, M. (1972). Electron microscopic demonstration of virus particles in keratitis. *Jpn J. Ophthalmol.*, **16**, 247–250.

Koelle, D. M. and Corey, L. (2003). Recent progress in herpes simplex virus immunobiology and vaccine research. *Clin. Microbiol. Rev.*, **16**(1), 96–113.

Koelle, D. M., Reymond, S. N., Chen, H. *et al.* (2000). Tegument-specific, virus-reactive CD4 T cells localize to the cornea in herpes simplex virus interstitial keratitis in humans. *J. Virol.*, **74**(23), 10930–10938.

Kumaraguru, U. and Rouse, B. T. (2002). The IL-12 response to herpes simplex virus is mainly a paracrine response of reactive inflammatory cells. *J. Leukoc. Biol.*, **72**(3), 564–570.

LaVail, J. H., Topp, K. S., Giblin, P. A., and Garner, J. A. (1997). Factors that contribute to the transneuronal spread of herpes simplex virus. *J. Neurosci. Res.*, **49**(4), 485–496.

Lee, S., Zheng, M., Kim, B., and Rouse, B. T. (2002a). Role of matrix metalloproteinase-9 in angiogenesis caused by ocular infection with herpes simplex virus. *J. Clin. Invest.*, **110**(8), 1105–1111.

Lee, S., Zheng, M., Deshpande, S., Eo, S. K., Hamilton, T. A., and Rouse, B. T. (2002b). IL-12 suppresses the expression of ocular immunoinflammatory lesions by effects on angiogenesis. *J. Leukoc. Biol.*, **71**(3), 469–476.

Leinonen, M. and Saikku, P. (2002). Evidence for infectious agents in cardiovascular disease and atherosclerosis. *Lancet Infect. Dis.*, **2**(1), 11–17.

Liesegang, T. J. (1999). Classification of herpes simplex virus keratitis and anterior uveitis. *Cornea.*, **18**(2), 127–143.

Liu, T., Tang, Q., and Hendricks, R. L. (1996). Inflammatory infiltration of the trigeminal ganglion after herpes simplex virus type 1 corneal infection. *J. Virol.*, **70**(1), 264–271.

Liu, T., Khanna, K. M., Chen, X., Fink, D. J., and Hendricks, R. L. (2000). CD8(+) T cells can block herpes simplex virus type 1 (HSV-1) reactivation from latency in sensory neurons. *J. Exp. Med.*, **191**(9), 1459–1466.

Margolis, T. P. and Atherton, S, S. (1996). Herpes simplex virus diseases: Posterior segment of the eye. In *Ocular Infection and Immunity*. Pepose, J. S., Holland, G. N., and Wilhelmus, K. R. eds, pp. 1155–1168. St. Loius: Mosby.

Matoba, A. Y. (1990). Ocular disease associated with Epstein–Barr virus infection. *Surv. Ophthalmol.*, **35**(2), 145–150.

Mercadal, C. M., Bouley, D. M., DeStephano, D., and Rouse, B. T. (1993). Herpetic stromal keratitis in the reconstituted scid mouse model. *J. Virol.*, **67**(6), 3404–3408.

Metcalf, J. F. and Kaufman, H. E. (1976). Herpetic stromal keratitis-evidence for cell-mediated immunopathogenesis. *Am. J. Ophthalmol.*, **82**(6), 827–834.

Metcalf, J. F., Hamilton, D. S., and Reichert, R. W. (1979). Herpetic keratitis in athymic (nude) mice. *Infect. Immun.*, **26**(3), 1164–1171.

Meyers, R. L. and Chitjian, P. A. (1976). Immunology of herpesvirus infection: immunity to herpes simplex virus in eye infections. *Surv. Ophthalmol.*, **21**(2), 194–204.

Meyers-Elliott, R. H., Pettit, T. H., and Maxwell, W. A. (1980). Viral antigens in the immune ring of Herpes simplex stromal keratitis. *Arch. Ophthalmol.*, **98**(5), 897–904.

Meyers-Elliot, R. H., Chitjian, P. A., and Dethiefs, B. A (1983). Experimental herpesvirus keratitis in the rabbit: topical versus intrastromal infection routes. *Ophthalmic Res.*, **15**, 240–256.

Miller, J. K., Laycock, K. A., Nash, M. M., and Pepose, J. S. (1993). Corneal Langerhans cell dynamics after herpes simplex virus reactivation. *Invest. Ophthalmol. Vis. Sci.*, **34**(7), 2282–2290.

Neta, R., Sayers, T. J., and Oppenheim, J. J. (1992). Relationship of TNF to interleukins. *Immunol. Ser.*, **56**, 499–566.

Niemialtowski, M. G. and Rouse, B. T. (1992). Predominance of Th1 cells in ocular tissues during herpetic stromal keratitis. *J. Immunol.*, **149**(9), 3035–3039.

Norn, M. S. (1970). Dendritic (herpetic) keratitis. I. Incidence-seasonal variations – recurrence rate–visual impairment–therapy. *Acta Ophthalmol.*, **48**(1), 91–107.

Oh, J. O. (1976). Primary and secondary herpes simplex uveitis in rabbits. *Surv. Ophthalmol.*, **21**(2), 178–184.

Osorio, Y., Wechsler, S. L., Nesburn, A. B., and Ghiasi, H. (2002). Reduced severity of HSV-1-induced corneal scarring in IL-12-deficient mice. *Virus Res.*, **90**(1–2), 317–326.

Pavilack, M. A., Elner, V. M., Elner, S. G., Todd, R. F 3rd., and Huber, A. R. (1992). Differential expression of human corneal and perilimbal ICAM-1 by inflammatory cytokines. *Invest. Ophthalmol. Vis. Sci.*, **33**(3), 564–573.

Peek, R., Verjans, G. M., and Meek, B. (2002). Herpes simplex virus infection of the human eye induces a compartmentalized virus-specific B cell response. *J. Infect. Dis.*, **186**(11), 1539–1546.

Pepose, J. S. (1991a). External ocular herpesvirus infections in immunodeficiency. *Curr. Eye Res.*, **10** Suppl, 87–95.

Pepose, J. S. (1991b). Herpes simplex keratitis: role of viral infection versus immune response. *Surv. Ophthalmol.*, **35**(5), 345–352.

Pepose, J. S., Nestor, M. S., Gardner, K. M., Foos, R. Y., and Pettit, T. H. (1985a). Composition of cellular infiltrates in rejected human corneal allografts. *Graefes Arch. Clin. Exp. Ophthalmol.*, **222**(3), 128–133.

Pepose, J. S., Gardner, K. M., Nestor, M. S., Foos, R. Y., and Pettit, T. H. (1985b). Detection of HLA class I and II antigens in rejected human corneal allografts. *Ophthalmology*, **92**(11), 1480–1484.

Pepose, J. S., Leib, D. A., Stuart, M., and Easty, D. (1996). Herpes simplex virus diseases: anterior segment of the eye. In *Ocular Infection and Immunity*, ed. J. S., Pepose, G. N., Holland, and K. R. Wilhelmus, pp. 905–932. St. Louis: Mosby.

Pepose, J. S., Margolis, T. P., LaRussa, P., and Pavan-Langston, D. (2003). Ocular complications of smallpox vaccination. *Am. J. Ophthalmol.*, **136**(2), 343–352.

Pyles, R. B. (2001). The association of herpes simplex virus and Alzheimer's disease: a potential synthesis of genetic and environmental factors. *Herpes*, **8**(3), 64–68.

Rager-Zisman, B., Quan, P. C., Rosner, M., Moller, J. R., and Bloom, B. R. (1987). Role of NK cells in protection of mice against herpes simplex virus-1 infection. *J. Immunol.*, **138**(3), 884–888.

Reddehase, M. J. (2002). Antigens and immunoevasins: opponents in cytomegalovirus immune surveillance. *Nat. Rev. Immunol.*, **2**, 831–844.

Remeijer, L., Doornenbal, P., Geerards, A. J., Rijneveld, W. A., and Beekhuis, W. H. (1997). Newly acquired herpes simplex virus keratitis after penetrating keratoplasty. *Ophthalmology.*, **104**(4) 648–652.

Remeijer, L., Maertzdorf, J., Buitenwerf, J., Osterhaus, A. D., and Verjans, G. M. (2002). Corneal herpes simplex virus type 1 superinfection in patients with recrudescent herpetic keratitis. *Invest. Ophthalmol. Vis. Sci.*, **43**(2), 358–363.

Roizman, B. and Knipe, D. M. (2001). Herpes simplex viruses and their replication. In *Fields Virology*, ed. D. M. Knipe, and P. M. Howley, pp. 2399–2460. Philadelphia: Lipincott Williams and Wilkins.

Russell, R. G., Nasisse, M. P., Larsen, H. S., and Rouse, B. T. (1984). Role of T-lymphocytes in the pathogenesis of herpetic stromal keratitis. *Invest. Ophthalmol. Vis. Sci.*, **25**(8), 938–944.

Shevach, E. M. (2000). Regulatory T cells in autoimmmunity. *Annu. Rev. Immunol.*, **18**, 423–449.

Shimeld, C., Hill, T., Blyth, B., and Easty, D. (1989). An improved model of recurrent herpetic eye disease in mice. *Curr. Eye Res.*, **8**(11), 1193–1205.

Shimeld, C., Whiteland, J. L., Nicholls, S. M., *et al.* (1995). Immune cell infiltration and persistence in the mouse trigeminal ganglion after infection of the cornea with herpes simplex virus type 1. *J. Neuroimmunol.*, **61**(1), 7–16.

Shimeld, C., Whiteland, J. L., Nicholls, S. M., Easty, D. L., and Hill, T. J. (1996). Immune cell infiltration in corneas of mice with recurrent herpes simplex virus disease. *J. Gen. Virol.*, **77** (5), 977–985.

Shimeld, C., Efstathiou, S., and Hill T. (2001). Tracking the spread of a lacZ-tagged herpes simplex virus type 1 between the eye and the nervous system of the mouse: comparison of primary and recurrent infection. *J. Virol.*, **75**(11), 5252–5262.

Simmons, A. (2002). Clinical manifestations and treatment considerations of herpes simplex virus infection. *J. Infect Dis.*, **186** Suppl 1: S71–577.

Streilein, J. W., Dana, M. R., and Ksander, B. R., (1997). Immunity causing blindness: five different paths to herpes stromal keratitis. *Immunol. Today*, **18**(9), 443–449.

Su, Y. H., Yan, X. T., Oakes, J. E., and Lausch, R. N. (1996). Protective antibody therapy is associated with reduced chemokine transcripts in herpes simplex virus type 1 corneal infection. *J. Virol.*, **70**(2), 1277–1281.

Sundmacher, R. and Neumann-Haefelin, D. (1979a). Herpes simplex virus isolations from the aqueous humor of patients suffering from focal iritis, endotheliitis, and prolonged disciform keratitis with glaucoma. *Klin. Monatsbl. Augenheilkd.*, **175**(4), 488–501.

Sundmacher, R. and Neumann-Haefelin, D. (1979b). Herpes simplex virus-positive and negative keratouveitis. In *Immunology and Immunopathology of the Eye*. ed. A, M. Silverstein, and G. R. O'Connor, pp. 225–229. New York: Masson Publishing.

Suvas, S, Azkur, A. K, Kim, B. S, Kumaraguru, U., and Rouse, B. T. (2004). CD4+CD25+ regulatory T cells control the severity of viral immunoinflammatory lesions. *J. Immunol.*, **172**(7), 4123–4132.

Swanborg, R. H., Whittum-Hudson, J. A., and Hudson, A. P. (2003). Infectious agents and multiple sclerosis – are *Chlamydia pneumoniae* and human herpes virus 6 involved? *J. Neuroimmunol.*, **136**(1–2), 1–8.

Tamesis, R. R., Messmer, E. M., Rice, B. A., Dutt, J. E., and Foster, C. S. (1994). The role of natural killer cells in the development of herpes simplex virus type 1 induced stromal keratitis in mice. *Eye*, **8**(Pt 3), 298–306.

Tang, Q. and Hendricks, R. L. (1996). Interferon gamma regulates platelet endothelial cell adhesion molecule 1 expression and neutrophil infiltration into herpes simplex virus-infected mouse corneas. *J. Exp. Med.*, **184**(4), 1435–1447.

Thomas, J. and Rouse, B. T. (1998). Immunopathology of herpetic stromal keratitis: discordance in CD4+ T cell function between euthymic host and reconstituted SCID recipients. *J. Immunol.*, **160**, 3965–3970.

Thomas, J., Gangappa, S., Kanangat, S., and Rouse, BT. (1997). On the essential involvement of neutrophils in the immunopathologic disease: herpetic stromal keratitis. *J. Immunol.*, **158**(3), 1383–1391.

Thomas, J, Kanangat, S., and Rouse, B. T. (1998). Herpes simplex virus replication-induced expression of chemokines and proinflammatory cytokines in the eye: implications in herpetic stromal keratitis. *J. Interferon Cytokine Res.*, **18**(9), 681–690.

Tran, M. T., Dean, D. A., Lausch, R. N., and Oakes, J. E. (1998). Membranes of herpes simplex virus type-1-infected human corneal epithelial cells are not permeabilized to macromolecules and therefore do not release IL-1alpha. *Virology*, **244**(1), 74–48.

Tumpey, T. M., Chen, S. H., Oakes, J. E., and Lausch, R. N. (1996). Neutrophil-mediated suppression of virus replication after herpes simplex virus type 1 infection of the murine cornea. *J. Virol.*, **70**(2), 898–904.

Verjans, G. M., Remeijer, L., van Binnendijk, R. S. *et al.* (1998). Identification and characterization of herpes simplex virus-specific CD4+ T cells in corneas of herpetic stromal keratitis patients. *J. Infect. Dis.*, **177**(2), 484–488.

Verjans, G. M., Dings, M. E., McLauchlan, J *et al.* (2000). Intraocular T cells of patients with herpes simplex virus (HSV)-induced acute retinal necrosis recognize HSV tegument proteins VP11/12 and VP13/14. *J. Infect. Dis.*, **182**(3), 923–927.

Whitley, R. J. (2001). Herpes simplex viruses. In *Fields Virology.*, ed. D. M. Knipe, and P. M. Howley, pp. 2461–2510. Philadelphia: Lippincott Williams and Wilkins.

Williams, L. E., Nesburn, A. B., and Kaufman, H. E. (1965). Experimental induction of disciform keratitis. *Arch. Ophthalmol.*, **73**, 112–118.

Yan, X. T., Tumpey, T. M., Kunkel, S. L., Oakes, J. E., and Lausch, R. N. (1998). Role of MIP-2 in neutrophil migration and tissue injury in the herpes simplex virus-1-infected cornea. *Invest. Ophthalmol. Vis. Sci.*, **139**(10), 1854–1862.

Youinou, P., Colin, J., and Mottier, D. (1985). Immunological analysis of the cornea in herpetic stromal keratitis. *J. Clin. Lab. Immunol.*, **17**(2), 105–106.

Youinou, P., Colin, J., and Ferec, C. (1986). Monoclonal antibody analysis of blood and cornea T lymphocyte subpopulations in herpes simplex keratitis. *Graefes Arch. Clin. Exp. Ophthalmol.*, **224**(2), 131–133.

Zhao, Z. S., Granucci, F., Yeh, L., Schaffer, P. A., and Cantor, H. (1998). Molecular mimicry by herpes simplex virus-type 1: autoimmune disease after viral infection. *Science.*, **279**(5355), 1344–137.

Zheng, M., Schwarz, M. A., Lee, S., Kumaraguru, U., and Rouse, B. T. (2001a). Control of stromal keratitis by inhibition of neovascularization. *Am. J. Pathol.*, **159**(3), 1021–1029.

Zheng, M., Deshpande, S., Lee, S., Ferrara, N., and Rouse, B. T. (2001b). Contribution of vascular endothelial growth factor in the neovascularization process during the pathogenesis of herpetic stromal keratitis. *J. Virol.*, **75**(20), 9828–9835.

Zheng, M., Klinman, D. M., Gierynska, M., and Rouse, B. T. (2002). DNA containing CpG motifs induces angiogenesis. *Proc. Natl Acad. Sci. USA*, **99**(13), 8944–8949.

36

Persistence in the population: epidemiology, transmission

Anna Wald[1] and Lawrence Corey[2]

[1] University of Washington, USA
[2] University of Washington, Fred Hutchinson Cancer Research Center, WA, USA

Epidemiology of HSV-1 and HSV-2

Herpes simplex viruses are among the most ubiquitous of human infections. The frequency of HSV infection has been measured by testing various populations for the presence of antibody, as both virus and the immune response are thought to persist after infection for the life of the host. Worldwide, ~90% of people have one or both viruses. HSV-1 is the more prevalent virus, with 65% of persons in the United States having antibodies to HSV-1 (Xu et al., 2002). The epidemiology in Europe is similar, with at least half of the population seropositive for HSV-1. In the developing world, HSV-1 is almost universal, and usually acquired from intimate contact with family in early childhood (Whitley et al., 1998). After childhood, the HSV-1 prevalence rates increase minimally with age. Rates of HSV-1 infection are similar for men and women. In the United States, African-Americans and Asians have higher rates of HSV-1 infection than whites. The majority of infections are oral, although most are asymptomatic. Some data suggest that in developed countries, acquisition of HSV-1 is delayed from early childhood to adolescence or young adulthood (Hashido et al., 1999; Mertz et al., 2003).

HSV-2 infections are markedly less frequent than HSV-1 infections, with 15%–80% of people in various populations infected (Corey and Wald, 1999). The rates of infection vary with country as well as levels of sexual activity. In some countries, such as Spain and the Philippines, the HSV-2 prevalence hovers around 10%, increasing to 20%–30% range for most European countries and the United States (Varela et al., 2001; Smith et al., 2001; Enders et al., 1998; Malkin et al., 2002). Developing countries bear a much higher burden of HSV-2 infection, with many populations in Africa having >50% prevalence in the general population (Weiss et al., 2001). Because HSV-2 infections are transmitted almost exclusively during sexual activity, the risk of HSV-2 reflects a person's level of sexual activity and the number of partners, and background prevalence of infection in the community. In communities with relatively low rates of infection, the risk of HSV-2 infection reflects more closely sexual activity of the person. However, in communities with high prevalence of infection, demographic rather than behavioral factors reflect HSV-2 risk more accurately (Sucato et al., 2001; Rosenthal et al., 1997; Austin et al., 1999). Women have a greater risk of HSV-2 acquisition, reflecting both increased biologic susceptibility and pattern of relationships with older men, who are more likely to be HSV-2 seropositive. HSV-2 prevalence in the United States is higher among African-Americans than among whites and Asians (Fleming et al., 1997). As a result, there is great disparity in infection rates according to both gender and race. For example, for white women, the risk of HSV-2 increases from about 18% among those with 2–4 lifetime partners to 35% for those with 10 to 49 lifetime partners (Fleming et al., 1997). In contrast, for African-American women the risk increases steeply even with fewer partners, and exceeds 60% for women with more than 4 lifetime partners. For white men, the risk is ~10% among those who report 2 to 9 lifetime partners, and reaches 40% in those with >50 lifetime partners. Among African-American men, the risk rises from 35% in those with 2–4 lifetime partners to ~ 50% in those reporting >50 lifetime partners. The increase in the frequency of HSV-2 antibodies starts in adolescence, reflecting the initiation of sexual activity, and levels off in the 40s, probably reflecting cessation of new partner acquisition (Blower and Boe, 1993). In the United States, most people acquire HSV-2 in their 20s with a mean age at presentation of 24 years. In contrast, in South Africa, girls acquire HSV-2 infection in adolescence and >60% are infected by the age of 21 (Chen et al., 2000).

The advent of the HIV epidemic initially eclipsed HSV-2 as a viral sexually transmitted disease of importance, but recent data have increasingly showed multiple interactions between the two viral infections (Corey *et al.*, 2004a). The development of molecular diagnostics has revealed that HSV-2 is the most common etiologic agent of genital ulcers in the developed and developing world (Chen *et al.*, 2000; Serwadda *et al.*, 2003). Even in regions in which syphilis and chancroid have been historically considered responsible for most genital ulcerations, the use of PCR-based techniques has clearly shown a predominance of HSV (Beyrer *et al.*, 1998; Morse *et al.*, 1997). In almost all studies, and in all populations, having HSV-2 infection increases the risk of HIV acquisition (Wald and Link 2002; Freeman *et al.*, 2006). The mechanism probably involves both HSV-2 induced skin or mucosal ulcerations, as well as influx of CD4+ cells into the herpetic lesions, cells that provide receptor for entry of HIV (Koelle *et al.*,1994). As transmission is more difficult to study than acquisition, the role of HSV-2 in the transmission of HIV is less well defined (Cameron *et al.*, 1989). However, the biology also suggests that HSV-2 infection may amplify HIV transmission, as HIV virions have been demonstrated in herpes ulcers (Schacker *et al.*, 1998c; Ballard, 2001). This topic of HSV and HIV interactions has been recently reviewed (Corey *et al.*, 2004a).

Spectrum of clinical disease

HSV can cause both mucocutaneous and systemic disease, and both HSV-1 and HSV-2 can cause the same syndromes, although the viruses are preferentially more likely to be associated with some syndromes than others. The variability in clinical expression is poorly understood, but the host immune system appears to be the main determinant of the clinical manifestations of HSV infections. The most severely affected are neonates, who usually acquire the disease during birth through exposure to infected genital secretions (Whitley *et al.*,1980). Rarely, adults can develop severe or fatal HSV infection during acquisition, and pregnant women appear to have a higher risk for this syndrome (Kobberman *et al.*, 1980; Sutton *et al.*, 1974). In most persons, HSV infections are confined to skin and mucosa. However, these can be severe, especially in persons immunocompromised either by other diseases (HIV, lupus), or iatrogenic immunosuppression or transplant, or extensive skin disease, such as eczema (Luchi *et al.*, 1995; Wheeler, Jr and Abele, 1966). Certain HSV-associated syndromes, such as HSV uveitis, have a strong immunopathogenic component and respond to immunosuppressive therapy (Balfour, 1994; Lairson *et al.*, 2003).

Immunocompetent host

Oral herpes

HSV-1 causes oral and labial, and occasionally facial, lesions. Initial infection is the most severe with ulcerative, painful stomatitis that usually occurs in children and is often associated with fever, anorexia and local edema of oral mucosa interfering with swallowing (Amir *et al.*, 1999). The lesions last a mean of 12 days and HSV-1 can be isolated in culture for the initial 7 days. The most common complication is dehydration requiring intravenous fluids, although secondary bacterial infection can also occur. In young adults, the presentation of initial oral HSV-1 infection can include pharyngitis, and tonsillectomy is occasionally (and erroneously) performed (Evans and Dick, 1964; Langenberg *et al.*, 1999).

Reactivation of HSV-1 in the mouth usually causes lesions on the lip ("fever blisters" or "cold sores"). The initial symptoms of pain, tingling, and itching occur prior to lesion appearance and are termed "prodrome" (Spruance, 1984). Initial lesion is an erythematous papule that evolves into a fluid-filled blister (Spruance *et al.*, 1997). Often there is a cluster of blisters, usually on a localized part of the lip, most often at the vermillion border. The lesions can also extend to skin on the face, and sometimes occur only on the face. The vesicles dry into a crust, and eventually re-epithelialize without scarring. The episodes last an average of 5 to 7 days. Only about 30% of persons with serologic evidence of HSV-1 have recurrent oro-labial herpes. Among those, 40% will have more than one recurrence per year. Known triggers of HSV-1 reactivation include facial trauma, surgery, fever and exposure to UV light (Spruance *et al.*, 1991). Oral labial HSV lesions were often associated with pneumococcal pneumonia and thought to be stimulated by the rapid rise in body temperature. Reactivation by UV light, such as occurs in skiers, can be abrogated by preventative use of sunscreen or antivirals (Spruance *et al.*, 1988). Recent popularity of laser skin resurfacing has been associated with severe HSV outbreaks resulting in recommendations that these procedures should be prophylaxed by antiviral therapy (Alster and Nanni, 1999; Beeson and Rachel, 2002). These triggers suggest that both systemic and skin factors can result in HSV reactivation (Hill *et al.*, 1978).

Genital herpes

HSV also causes ulcerations of genital mucosa and skin. The more common cause of genital herpes is HSV-2. However, recent studies suggest that 20%-50% of incident episodes of genital herpes are caused by HSV-1 and the proportion of such incident cases due to HSV-1 may be increasing (Lafferty et al., 2000; Lowhagen et al., 2000; Vyse et al.,2000; Mertz et al., 2003; Ross et al., 1993). The reasons for this are not entirely clear but decreased HSV-1 acquisition in childhood and preferential practice of oral–genital sex during adolescence may be partly responsible. The clinical course of the initial and subsequent episodes is the same for both viruses; however, the frequency of recurrences and shedding is quite different, with HSV-1 reactivating infrequently in comparison to HSV-2 (Lafferty et al., 1987; Benedetti et al., 1994; Engelberg et al., 2003). As such, it is important to identify the type of virus that causes the infection.

The severity of infection with HSV depends on previous immunity to HSV. Primary infection, defined as the first encounter with HSV-1 or HSV-2, is clinically most severe, and most likely to be symptomatic (Corey and Spear, 1986; Corey et al., 1983). Non-primary infection is a new HSV-2 infection in a person with prior HSV-1 infection. New infections are diagnosed by detecting the virus on the mucosa in a person without concomitant antibody to the same type of virus. Recurrent infections occur as a result of reactivation of a previous, latent infection, and are identified by the presence of antibody at the time of initial presentation. It is important to note that accurate classification of an episode must include both virologic information as well as determination of antibody status because there is a wide overlap in clinical manifestations of the infection. Although primary infection is more likely to be symptomatic than an episode of reactivation, only up to 39% of people who acquire primary HSV will be diagnosed with the infection at that time (Langenberg et al., 1999). A substantial proportion will become symptomatic at some point during the disease and present with a first clinical episode of genital herpes (Bernstein et al., 1984; Diamond et al., 1999). In a recent study of 401 persons presenting with a first episode of genital herpes, 91 (23%) had primary infection with HSV-1, 139 (35%) had primary infection with HSV-2, 36 (9%) had non-primary initial HSV-2 and 135 (37%) had a first recognized recurrence of HSV-2.

The painful genital vesicles and ulcers accompanied by inguinal adenopathy and systemic flu-like illness are part of the classic presentation of first episode of genital herpes (Corey et al., 1983). The evolution of lesions is similar to those of oral herpes, usually with more rapid progression to ulcers in women, and often a prolonged vesicular phase in men. The lesions are widely distributed in the genital area, and multiple (up to 100 lesions) can be seen. During an initial episode, lesions last up to 3 weeks, and new lesion formation continues for 10–14 days. Itching, tingling and pain can be severe. Neurologic complications, such as meningitis and bladder paresis, usually transient, occur in ∼10% and are more common among women. External dysuria is also common among women. Proctitis is common among MSM and can be associated with transient bowel dysfunction (Quinn et al., 1981).

Recurrent episodes of genital HSV-2 occur a median of 4 (women) to 5 (men) times during the first year (Benedetti et al., 1994). However, there is great variability in the frequency of recurrences, even during the first year. In a study of 457 persons with newly acquired HSV-2 infection, 38% had 6 or more recurrences and 20% had more than 10 recurrences during the first year. 14% of women and 26% of men had more than 10 recurrences and only 26% of women and 8% of men had no or 1 recurrence in the first year of infection (Benedetti et al., 1994). Subsequently, the frequency of episodes slowly decreases, with an average decrease of 2 recurrences between years 1 and 5 of infection. As such, most patients will not perceive the decrease in severity until several years have elapsed. This improvement is not universal, and some people will continue to have very frequent or even more frequent recurrent episodes many years into the infection. In contrast, HSV-1 infection recurs infrequently, with a median of 195 days to first recurrence among women and 567 days among men after documented new genital HSV-1. Subsequently, the rate of recurrences falls even further with only 19% having 1 recurrence, and 15% having two or more recurrences during the second year after genital HSV-1 infection (Engelberg et al., 2003).

Genital herpes is often associated with psychosocial distress, caused by having an incurable STD, stigma of having such disease, and anxiety about resuming normal sexual life after acquisition (Catotti et al., 1993; Carney et al., 1994; Swanson and Chenitz, 1990). The distress is usually greater among women than men and in many persons it surpasses the physical discomfort caused by the infection. Over time, most people adjust to living with herpes, although recurrences of depression and feelings of worthlessness tend to return during recurrences. Oral herpes can also be associated with feelings of being damaged, as it is cosmetically more obvious; however, it is clearly associated with less social stigma.

Other mucocutaneous infections

Despite the common involvement of oral or genital mucosa in the acquisition of HSV, cutaneous infections at other body sites are also well recognized. Eczema herpeticum occurs occasionally in persons with atopic dermatitis, regardless of whether they are receiving topical steroids (Wollenberg et al., 2003; Yoshida and Amatsu,

2000). Outbreaks of herpes gladiatorum occur among young athletes involved in contact sports, often high-school wrestlers (Anderson, 2003; Becker,1992; Belongia et al., 1991). Both infections are usually caused by HSV-1, and respond to therapy with antiviral medication (Niimura and Nishikawa,1988; Anderson, 1999).

Herpetic whitlow results from infection of the distal finger with HSV. Historically, this disease was caused by HSV-1 and was acquired among dental or nursing professionals (Stern et al., 1959; Manzella et al., 1984). More recently, with the adoption of universal precautions, the incidence of HSV-1 whitlow has decreased, and most distal finger infections arise in the setting of primary genital HSV-2 infections.

Recent studies have shown a link between erythema multiforme and recurrent HSV infections (Huff et al., 1983). While the pathogenesis is not completely understood, strong association of erythema multiforme with particular HLA-DQ alleles is consistent with an immunopathologic basis (Malo et al., 1998; Kampgen et al., 1988). Molecular studies of the involved skin have demonstrated HSV DNA in the erythema multiforme lesions, and reports of prevention of attacks with oral acyclovir support HSV as an etiologic factor in this disease (Brice et al., 1989; Miura et al., 1992; Ng et al., 2003; Lemak et al., 1986).

HSV infection in CNS

Reactivation of HSV in the CNS is associated with 2 distinct syndromes with vastly different prognoses. Recent studies have shown that recurrent benign meningitis, or Mollaret's meningitis, results from HSV infection (Cohen et al., 1994; Picard et al., 1993). Most often HSV-2 is implicated, although HSV-1 has also been reported (Yamamoto et al., 1991). Women are at higher risk for this complication than men, and often develop the initial episode during acquisition of genital HSV-2, with subsequent recurrent episodes. Thus, the epidemiology of Mollaret's meningitis parallels that of genital herpes. However, not infrequently the meningitis is the presenting complaint, and the association with HSV-2 is not always recognized. Spinal fluid findings are consistent with "aseptic meningitis" with a lymphocyte predominance, fairly normal protein and glucose, and sterile fluid. HSV DNA can be detected by PCR (Yamamoto et al., 1991; Cohen et al., 1994). While unpleasant, this condition is benign, and anecdotal data suggest that individual episodes respond well to antiviral therapy and further episodes can be abrogated in large part by suppressive antiviral therapy. In contrast, HSV encephalitis is a disease of severe morbidity (Whitley and Lakeman 1995). The usual agent is HSV-1, although HSV-2 meningoencephalitis has also been described in immunosuppressed patients (Gateley et al., 1990; Linnemann et al., 1976). HSV encephalitis is the most common cause of sporadic encephalitis in adults, with an estimated frequency of 1 in 200,000 to million persons. There is no gender predilection, and the age distribution appears bimodal, with a smaller peak among youth and a larger peak among the elderly. Encephalitis can develop both during primary infection (usually among younger people) and during reactivation (usually among older people) of HSV. Classically, the patient presents with fever and signs of focal encephalitis, such as seizures, headache and focal neurologic deficits. However, the initial symptoms can be insidious and include personality and cognitive disturbances. Fever is common. Spinal fluid shows increased white count, usually but not always with lymphocyte predominance, and can be bloody with abnormal chemistry. Imaging studies are not pathognomic, although temporal lobe disease is typical. The diagnosis should always be confirmed virologically. Most cases are diagnosed with the use of PCR that has surpassed the "gold standard" of brain biopsy because of similar sensitivity but virtually no risk (Lakeman and Whitley, 1995; Puchhammer-Stockl et al., 1993). However, lack of positive PCR in the spinal fluid does not rule out the diagnosis of HSV, especially early in the disease, and intravenous acyclovir should be initiated if the clinical picture is compatible, no alternative diagnosis is made, and the PCR is negative (Whitley et al., 1986). The lumbar puncture should be repeated in 24–48 hours and CSF submitted for PCR testing again. Untreated HSV encephalitis has >70% fatality rate. Even with therapy, HSV encephalitis results in death in a substantial proportion of patients and only a few percent return to normal function.

Eye disease

Occasionally, oral HSV-1 infection is associated with blepheritis or conjunctivitis (Souza et al., 2003). While these are benign manifestations of herpetic eye infection, herpetic keratitis causes significant morbidity (Liesegang, 2001). Clinically, the disease is manifested by pain, photophobia and visual impairment. Dendritic ulcers can be visualized on examination with fluorescein staining. Recurrent episodes of reactivation are associated with stromal involvement and lead to progressive loss of vision and scarring, requiring penetrating keratoplasty or corneal transplants. Since the onset of keratitis is rarely coincidental with initial acquisition of HSV infection, the corneal infection may either result from direct inoculation of the virus into the eye, or more likely, from reactivation of HSV in the distribution that enervates the eye. The predisposition to herpes keratitis is not well understood but the infiltrate of HSV-specific T lymphocytes supports the immunopathologic basis for this disease (Deshpande et al., 2001; Koelle et al., 2000; Thomas et al., 1997; Thomas and Rouse, 1998; Verjans et al., 2000). The complications of HSV-1 keratitis are the leading cause of infectious blindness in the United States (Lairson et al., 2003). Clinical trials have demonstrated the benefit of suppressive acyclovir in the prevention of herpetic keratitis recurrences (Herpetic Eye Disease Study Group 1997, Wilhelmus et al., 1998).

Acute retinal necrosis is another HSV-related syndrome that often results in blindness. The pathogenesis is poorly understood, and HSV-2 is detected more often than HSV-1 in this disease (Itoh et al., 2000; Thompson et al., 1994; Tran et al., 2004). Immunosuppression appears to be a risk factor, as the acute retinal necrosis appears to be more common among patients with AIDS, although this syndrome has also been observed in persons with iatrogenic immunosuppression (Guex-Crosier et al., 1997). The presentation is often rapid, and loss of sight is frequent. Antiviral therapy may prevent involvement of the contralateral eye, even if it does not restore vision in the affected eye (Tran et al., 2004).

Other syndromes

Other, infrequent manifestations of HSV have also been reported. Of note is disseminated HSV, which occurs occasionally in persons who appear immunocompetent and has a high fatality rate (Goyette and Donowho, 1974; Flewett et al., 1969; Keane et al., 1976; Frederick et al., 2002; Chase et al., 1987). While the infection most likely begins as oral or genital herpes, these localized symptoms are often not recognized, and patients present with fulminant hepatitis with transaminases in the thousands, diffuse rash, or other systemic manifestations. Death results from sepsis with DIC, ARDS, or progressive hepatic failure. This syndrome occurs more frequently among women in the second half of pregnancy although occasional cases are reported among non-pregnant women and men. Factors predisposing to this have not been described. Early administration of acyclovir is often effective, but the disease is often not diagnosed premortem.

Neonatal herpes

The frequency of neonatal herpes varies by region and is estimated to occur from 1 in 3200 to 1 in 15 000 pregnancies (Sullivan-Bolyai et al., 1983a; Tookey and Peckham, 1996; Mindel et al., 2000; Brown et al., 2003; Gutierrez et al., 1999). Reasons for the variant frequency are poorly understood but are likely to result from interplay between sexual behavior in the population and the baseline prevalence and incidence of HSV-1 and HSV-2. Over 85% of neonatal herpes is acquired from intrapartum exposure of the newborn to infected maternal secretions. In 5% of cases, congenital infection of the fetus in the setting of new acquisition of HSV during pregnancy has been reported (Florman, 1973; Sullivan-Bolyai et al., 1983a). These infants are born with clinical evidence of disseminated disease, often including skin lesions, may be premature and have a poor prognosis. Post-natal acquisition of HSV, often from non-maternal sources, has also been reported in about 10% of cases, and is associated with HSV-1 infection.

Recent prospective studies have clarified risk factors for HSV transmission during delivery (Brown et al., 1997; Arvin et al., 1986; Prober et al., 1992). The greatest risk of neonatal herpes is conferred by viral shedding, defined as HSV isolation in maternal genital secretions at the time of parturition, with a relative risk of neonatal HSV of >300 compared with women who do not have HSV isolated during labor (Brown et al., 2003). However, some infants acquire neonatal herpes despite lack of culturable virus at the time of delivery. In some of these cases, HSV DNA can be detected by PCR despite negative viral culture, suggesting that culture can be falsely negative. Of greater concern is the observation that only 5% of women who have HSV isolated from the genital tract at the time of delivery transmit HSV to the infant. As such, these women are at potential risk of unnecessary interventions.

Among women who are shedding HSV in genital secretions at labor, risk factors for neonatal herpes include newly acquired HSV infection (RR = 59), cervical vs. vulvar viral isolation (RR = 15), young mother (RR = 2.7 for women aged <21), and HSV-1 vs. HSV-2 isolation (RR = 35). Cesarean deliveries appear protective as women who are delivered abdominally had a significantly lower risk of HSV transmission compared with women who had vaginal delivery (RR = 0.14). Because even the largest series of neonatal herpes contain only a handful of cases, the exact contribution of each risk factor is difficult to measure. However, overall, most cases of neonatal herpes appear to occur among women who acquire subclinically new genital HSV-1 or HSV-2 and who deliver vaginally (Arvin et al., 1982, Whitley et al., 1991b). In one study, 4 of 9 women who acquired HSV so late in pregnancy that they did not seroconvert by the time of delivery transmitted the virus to their infant (Brown et al., 1997). Management of recognized newly acquired genital herpes at the end of pregnancy needs to be individualized and should include consideration of administration of acyclovir to women toward the end of pregnancy, scheduled abdominal delivery prior to rupture of membranes, and prophylactic antiviral therapy of the newborn (Prober et al., 1992; Sheffield et al., 2003).

Infants with neonatal herpes often present with non-specific complaints such as fever, fussiness, sepsis, or seizures (Whitley et al., 1998). Typical skin lesions are not noted universally, and depending on the disease classification, may develop only in up to 80% of patients. Clinically, neonatal herpes has been divided into 3 syndromes. In recent studies, skin, eye and mouth disease accounted for 42% of cases, and is defined by disease that is present only on skin or mucosa (Whitley et al., 1998, Kimberlin et al., 2001a). This form of infection has the best prognosis with negligible mortality and up to 70% of treated infants having normal development. Of interest, even those infants who did not have any evidence of CNS involvement may subsequently present with neurologic deficits, suggesting that subclinical and/or delayed involvement of the brain is not uncommon. Disseminated disease accounts for 23% of cases and has the highest mortality (60% with therapy). Among the survivors, normal development is noted in about 60%. CNS disease comprises the remaining 35% of newborns with neonatal herpes. Mortality is low, but this form of disease is associated with highest morbidity as less than 50% will have normal development. Comparison of secular trends suggests that a greater proportion of cases are diagnosed with SEM disease in recent years compared with an earlier cohort (Whitley et al., 1988, 1991a, b). A potential explanation is that the diagnosis is made earlier, prior to dissemination or CNS invasion. Many cases are still diagnosed late, or post-mortem, and administration of acyclovir to infants with sepsis-like syndrome is not universally done. Prompt antiviral therapy is associated with decreased morbidity and mortality, but the prognosis remains grave for most children. HSV-2 appears more neuroinvasive in newborns than HSV-1, and as such, has a worse prognosis (Corey et al., 1988).

The observations about risk factors for neonatal herpes suggest that prevention of neonatal herpes relies on prevention of HSV acquisition in late pregnancy. This strategy, in turn, relies on identification of women at risk for HSV infection with the use of type-specific serology, and, potentially, the serologic testing of their sex partners. This approach has not been widely accepted (Wilkinson et al., 2000; Brown, 2000). Reasons for resistance are numerous, including lack of confidence in the performance of commercial type-specific serologies, perception that counseling about results of HSV serologies is burdensome to both providers and patients, lack of simple interventions, and the relative rarity of neonatal HSV. Of note, after institution of universal testing for Group B streptococcus (GBS) during the last trimester, the frequency of neonatal GBS sepsis now approaches that of neonatal HSV (Gibbs et al., 1994; Chuang et al., 2002; Schrag and Schuchat, 2004).

Immunocompromised persons

Immunosuppression, regardless of etiology, is associated with greater risk of HSV reactivation, prolonged viral shedding and more severe clinical recurrences (Meyers et al., 1980; Siegal et al., 1981). While even in severely immunocompromised patients most disease is mucocutaneous, extension to internal organs, such as esophagus, or dissemination, can also occur. Other syndromes include hepatitis and pneumonia (Ramsey et al., 1982). Patients receiving cancer chemotherapy are at risk for HSV recurrences during periods of neutropenia; the risk in organ or marrow transplant patients is prolonged and parallels the duration of immunosuppression (Wade et al., 1984a). However, the greatest risk of HSV reactivation after bone marrow transplant occurs early during the initial neutropenia associated with myeloablation. This is in contrast to other herpesvirus infections, such as VZV and CMV, which tend to occur later during the post-transplant period during maximal suppression of cell-mediated immunity. Because HSV has a significant impact on post-chemotherapy and post-transplant morbidity, acyclovir prophylaxis is administered routinely in this population (Wade et al., 1984b).

In the last two decades, HIV has emerged as the most common cause of immunosuppression worldwide. Not surprisingly, early clinical reports of patients with HIV document extensive clinical HSV recurrences (Siegel et al., 1988). The disease burden is especially great, as persons at risk for sexually transmitted HIV are more likely to have HSV-2 infection than the general population. Prior to the introduction of effective antiretroviral therapy, chronic HSV ulcers accounted for a small proportion of newly diagnosed persons with AIDS, and developed in many other persons as immunosuppression progressed. Despite the frequent presence of HSV-1 and HSV-2 infection (90% overall) in patients with HIV, extensive clinical disease develops only in a minority of patients (Bagdades et al., 1992). The immunologic and virologic risk factors for developing severe disease are not understood. Systematic study of clinical and virologic aspects of genital HSV-2 shows that even in the absence of overt clinical disease, HIV infected persons have high rates of viral shedding. Among a group of 68 men who have sex with men with HIV infection and a

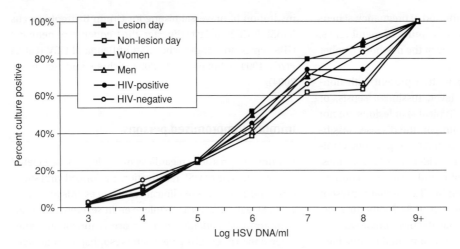

Fig. 36.1. The relationship between the probability of HSV isolation in viral culture and the number of copies of HSV DNA as detected by PCR (adapted from Wald (Wald *et al.*, 2003)).

mean CD4 count of 351, the rate of genital HSV isolation was 9.7% of days, and the perianal area accounted for 79% of isolates (Schacker *et al.*, 1998b). The relative risk of total viral shedding was elevated at 3.3 compared with men who are HIV negative, but an even greater relative risk of 6.9 was shown for subclinical shedding. These observations show that HIV has a greater effect on the virologic than clinical aspects of the natural history of HIV and may provide an explanation for a burgeoning epidemic of HSV-2 in parallel with HIV in sub-Saharan Africa.

Immune reconstitution with antiretroviral therapy (ART) has resulted in a decrease in risk of several opportunistic infections, and has allowed for stopping of prophylaxis in those patients with vigorous CD4 response. Unfortunately, the data suggest that the increase in CD4 cells associated with ART prevents lesions, with significantly lower risk of mucocutaneous lesions among patients treated with ART compared with patients who are untreated, but has a negligible effect on viral shedding (Posavad *et al.*, 2001). As such, HSV-2 & HIV seropositive patients are likely to continue to be infectious for HIV and HSV-2 and suppressive HSV therapy should be considered in that setting.

Viral shedding

HSV is present intermittently on skin or mucosa in between symptomatic recurrences. This phenomenon, defined as asymptomatic or subclinical shedding, has been described since the early clinical descriptions of genital herpes. However, the frequency, pattern, and the importance of subclinical shedding for transmission of HSV have only recently been elucidated.

The frequency of viral shedding has been measured both by culture and by PCR. Studies using amplification techniques show that HSV DNA PCR is up to 400% more sensitive for detection of HSV on mucosal surfaces than viral isolation (Wald *et al.*, 2003) (Fig. 36.1). The frequency of viral shedding varies with type of HSV, duration of infection, gender, and immune status. Most variability observed in the frequency of viral reactivation is not explained by these risk factors, suggesting that there is a strong host immunogenetic (or viral strain) factor in determining the severity of disease.

The initial study examining prospectively viral shedding among women with recent genital HSV-2 infection showed that HSV was detected by PCR on 28% of days sampled (Wald *et al.*, 1997). However, as shown in Fig. 36.2, the variability in the frequency of reactivation is great, even among this homogeneous group of women. Subsequent studies have also examined viral shedding among men. In a group of men with either recent acquisition of genital HSV-2 or a history of frequent recurrences, the overall rate of HSV detection from the genital area by PCR was 32% (median 30%; range 0 to 92%) (Wald *et al.*, 2002b). Despite the rough parallel between the frequency of viral shedding and the frequency of recurrent lesions, these two processes are somewhat independent, with some persons having frequent days with lesions, or prolonged lesions, and others having frequent viral shedding but without many recurrences. These observations suggest that the immunologic mechanisms that control viral shedding may differ from those that control lesion formation and resolution. Animal experiments, and findings in persons with immune compromise, indicate that the CD4 response predominates in control of lesions, while CD8 response is more important for control of viral reactivation (see Chapter 34).

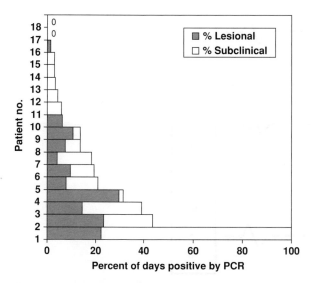

Fig. 36.2. Variability in symptomatic and subclinical shedding among 26 women with genital HSV-2 infection for less than 2 years.

Transmission dynamics

Figure 36.3 illustrates the pattern of viral shedding during inadvertent sexual transmission of HSV-2 infection. The woman participating in a daily home sampling study had symptomatic genital HSV-2 infection for 3.5 years, and had initiated a new relationship with a partner who was HSV seronegative. Despite having occasional non-specific symptoms, she did not notice a recurrence during the episode of subclinical viral shedding that resulted in transmission of HSV-2. Studies consistently indicate that transmission to sex partners, or to neonates, usually occurs during such episodes of subclinical shedding (Barton et al., 1987; Mertz et al., 1992).

Prospective studies of HSV-2 discordant couples have been used to estimate rate of transmission and ascertain risk factors for transmission. Unfortunately, only a few such studies have been done that included a sufficiently large number of persons to obtain reliable estimates of rates of transmission and risk factors (Mertz et al., 1988, 1992; Stanberry et al., 2002; Bryson et al., 1993; Wald et al., 2001; Corey et al., 2004b). The rate of HSV-2 acquisition among persons at risk varies from a high of 8.6 per 100 person-years for women, to a low of 2.7 per 100 person-years among men. These studies have also shown that (1) women are at 2-to-6 fold higher risk for HSV-2 acquisition than men; (2) prior infection with HSV-1 does not protect against HSV-2 acquisition; (3) symptoms of first episode HSV-2 infection are less prominent among those with previous HSV-1 infection; (4) frequent sexual activity is a risk factor for HSV-2 transmission, and (5) HSV-2 is transmitted more easily than HSV-1 infection. Other characteristics that have been associated with increased risk of HSV-2 transmission, but inconsistently, or without reaching statistical significance, include short duration of relationship and short duration of genital herpes in the source partner prior to study participation, and sex during recurrences (Corey et al., 2004b). Condoms appear to be protective, but the degree of protection afforded by consistent use, and effect of condom use on female-to-male vs. male-to-female transmission varies among the studies (Wald et al., 2001). In addition, the use of condoms in monogamous, long-term relationships is rare, even in the settings of known HSV-2 discordance and extensive counseling in the context of a clinical trial. Available data indicate that consistent condom use offers partial protection (∼ 50%) against HSV-2 acquisition at best. A recent study of daily suppressive valacyclovir has shown that transmission is decreased by 48% among those couples who were randomized to receive antiviral therapy (Corey et al., 2004b). These results offer couples another option to use to decrease the risk of HSV-2 transmission, and are an added benefit to the use of daily antiviral therapy (see below).

Management and Prevention

Treatment

The advent of antiviral drugs for HSV-1 and HSV-2 infections has made clinical management of these infections a part of standard clinical practice (Table 36.1). For mucocutaneous and visceral HSV infections, acyclovir and its related compounds famciclovir and valacyclovir have been the mainstay of therapy (Whitley and Gnann Jr, 1992). Several antiviral agents are available for topical use in HSV eye infections: idoxuridine, trifluorothymidine and topical vidarabine. For HSV encephalitis and neonatal herpes, intravenous acyclovir is the treatment of choice. Acyclovir resistant virus can be encountered in immunocompromised hosts (Erlich et al., 1989; Reyes et al., 2003).

Acyclovir was the first antiviral clearly demonstrated to be effective against HSV infections (Elion et al., 1977). It is an acyclic nucleoside analogue that is a substrate for HSV-specific thymidine kinase. Acyclovir is selectively phosphorylated by HSV-infected cells to acyclovir-monophosphate. Cellular enzymes then phosphorylate acyclovir-monophosphate to acyclovir-triphosphate, a competitive inhibitor of viral DNA polymerase. Acyclovir-triphosphate is incorporated into the growing DNA chain of the virus and causes chain termination. Acyclovir has potent in vitro activity against both HSV-1 and HSV-2.

Valacyclovir is the valyl ester of acyclovir and is metabolized in the gut, liver and epithelium to acyclovir and

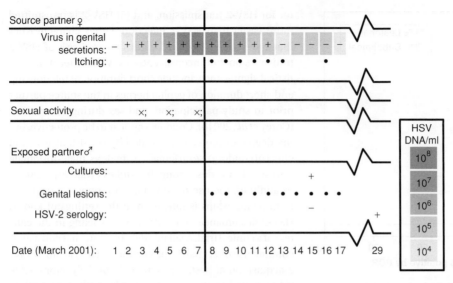

Fig. 36.3. Sexual transmission of HSV-2 during subclinical shedding.

produces much higher levels of drug leading to more convenient therapy (Soul-Lawton et al., 1995). Famciclovir, the oral formulation of penciclovir, is also clinically effective in the treatment of a variety of HSV-1 and HSV-2 infections (Pue and Benet, 1993). Ganciclovir has activity against both HSV-1 and HSV-2, but because it is more toxic than acyclovir, valacyclovir, and famciclovir, it is generally not recommended for treatment of HSV infections. Numerous trials of acyclovir in mucocutaneous HSV infections of immunocompetent and immunosuppressed host have been conducted. General recommendations are outlined below (Centers for Disease Control and Prevention 2002). Increasingly, shorter courses of therapy are being utilized for treatment of recurrent mucocutaneous HSV-1 or HSV-2 in immunocompetent patients.

Treatment of recurrent mucocutaneous herpes

Among immunocompetent patients, recent studies have shown the effectiveness of short course therapy to reduce the signs and symptoms of oral and genital HSV infection. These include 2 g twice daily for one day of valacyclovir for oral-labial HSV and 2 and 3 day courses of acyclovir or valacyclovir for recurrent episode genital herpes (Spruance et al., 2003; Leone et al., 2002; Wald et al., 2002a). One-day therapy with famciclovir for genital herpes also appears to increase the probability of an aborted recurrence and to shorten the duration of lesions and symptoms, compared with placebo (Aoki et al., 2006).

Suppression of mucocutaneous herpes

Recognition of the high frequency of subclinical reactivation has provided increasing rationale for the use of daily antiviral therapy to suppress reactivations of HSV. This is especially useful for persons with frequent clinical reactivations such as those with recently acquired genital HSV infection. Immunosuppressed persons, including those with HIV infection, may also benefit from daily antiviral therapy. A variety of dosages have been utilized.

Reduction in transmission to sexual partners

Once daily valacyclovir (500mg) has been shown to reduce transmission of HSV in partnerships in which one partner has symptomatic genital HSV-2 and the other partner is susceptible (Corey et al., 2004b). Serologic screening can be used to identify at risk couples, as many couples identified as discordant by history are concordant on serologic evaluation.

Severe HSV infection

Intravenous acyclovir (30 mg/kg/day, given as a 10 mg/kg infusion over 1 hour at 8-hour intervals) is effective in reducing the morbidity and mortality from HSV encephalitis (Whitley, 1988; Whitley and Lakeman, 1995). Early initiation of therapy is a critical factor in outcome. The major side effect associated with intravenous acyclovir is transient renal insufficiency, usually caused by crystallization of the compound in the renal parenchyma. This adverse reaction can be avoided if the medication is given slowly over 1 hour and the patient is well hydrated. Because CSF levels of acyclovir average only 30% to 50% of plasma levels, the dosage of acyclovir used for treatments of CNS infection (30 mg/kg per day) is double that used for the treatment of mucocutaneous or visceral disease (15 mg/kg per day). For neonatal HSV, high-dose intravenous therapy is

Table 36.1. Treatment of HSV infections

Infections in immunosuppressed patients
   Acute symptomatic first or recurrent episodes: IV acyclovir (5 mg/kg q 8 h), or oral acyclovir (400 mg qid), famciclovir (500 mg po tid) or valacyclovir (500 mg po bid). Treatment duration may vary from 7 to 14 days.
   Suppression of reactivation disease: IV acyclovir (5 mg/kg q 8 h), valacyclovir (500 mg po bid) or oral acyclovir (400–800 mg 3–5 times per day) prevent recurrences during the immediate 30 day post transplantation period. Longer term suppression is often used for persons with continued immunosuppression. In bone marrow and renal transplant patients, valacyclovir 2 grams 4 times daily is also effective in preventing CMV infection (Dignani *et al.*, 2002, Lowance *et al.*, 1999). Valacyclovir 8 gm daily has been associated with thrombotic microangiopathy after extended use in HIV positive persons (Bell *et al.*, 1997). In HIV-infected persons, oral famciclovir (500 mg bid) is effective in reducing clinical and subclinical reactivations of HSV-1 and 2, and valacyclovir 500mg bid decreases the frequency of genital HSV-2 recurrences (Schacker *et al.*, 1998a, Romanowski *et al.*, 2000, DeJesus *et al.*, 2003).

Genital herpes
   First episodes: Oral acyclovir (200 mg 5 times per day or 400 mg tid), oral valacyclovir (1000 mg bid) or famciclovir (250 mg bid) for 10–14 days are effective. IV acyclovir (5 mg/kg q 8 h for 5 days) is given for severe disease or neurologic complications such as aseptic meningitis.
   Symptomatic recurrent genital herpes: Oral acyclovir (200 mg 5 times per day for 5 days, 800 mg po tid for 2 days), valacyclovir (500 mg bid for 3 or 5 days) or famciclovir (125 mg bid for 5 days). All these therapies are effective in shortening duration of lesions, viral shedding and symptoms.
   Suppression of recurrent genital herpes: Oral acyclovir (200-mg capsules bid or tid, 400 mg bid, or 800 mg qd), famciclovir (250 mg bid), or valacyclovir (500 mg or 1000 mg qd or 500 mg bid) prevents symptomatic reactivation. Persons with frequent reactivation (<9 episodes) can take 500 mg daily; those with >9 should take 1000 mg/daily or 500 mg bid (Reitano *et al.*, 1998).

Oral-labial HSV infections:
   First episode: Oral acyclovir (200 mg) is given 4 or 5 times per day. Famciclovir (250 mg bid) or valacyclovir (1000 mg bid) has been used clinically.
   Recurrent episodes: Valacyclovir 1000 mg bid for 1 day or 500 mg bid for 3 days is effective in reducing pain and speeding healing. Self-initiated therapy with 6 times daily topical penciclovir cream is effective in speeding the healing of oral-labial HSV, topical acyclovir cream has also been shown to speed healing (Spruance *et al.*, 1997).
   Suppression of reactivation of oral-labial HSV: Oral acyclovir (400 mg bid), if started before exposure and continued for the duration of exposure (usually 5–10 days), will prevent reactivation of recurrent oral-labial HSV infection associated with severe sun exposure (Spruance *et al.*, 1988).
   Herpetic whitlow: Regimens used for treating genital herpes can be utilized but clinical trial data are lacking.
   HSV proctitis: Oral acyclovir (400 mg 5 times per day) is useful in shortening the course of infection (Rompalo *et al.*, 1988); less frequent dosing is also likely to be effective. In immunosuppressed patients or in patients with severe infection, IV acyclovir (5 mg/kg q 8 h) may be useful.
   Herpetic eye infections: In acute keratitis, topical trifluorothymidine, vidarabine, idoxuridine, acyclovir, penciclovir, and interferon are all beneficial. Debridement may be required; topical steroids may worsen disease.

CNS HSV infections
   HSV encephalitis: Intravenous acyclovir (10 mg/kg q 8 h; 30 mg/kg per day) for 10 days is preferred.
   HSV aseptic meningitis: No studies of systemic antiviral chemotherapy exist. If therapy is to be given, IV acyclovir (15–30 mg/kg per day) should be used in severely affected patients, followed by oral course of valacyclovir.
   Autonomic radiculopathy: No studies are available.

Neonatal HSV infections: Acyclovir (60 mg/kg per day, divided into 3 doses) is given. The recommended duration of treatment is 21 days. Monitoring for relapse should be undertaken and some authorities recommend continued suppression with oral acyclovir suspension for 3 to 4 months (Kimberlin *et al.*, 1996).

Visceral HSV infections
   HSV esophagitis: IV acyclovir (15 mg/kg per day). In some patients with a milder degree of immunosuppression, oral therapy with valacyclovir or famciclovir is effective.
   HSV pneumonitis: No controlled studies exist. IV acyclovir (15 mg/kg per day) should be considered.

Disseminated HSV infections: No controlled studies exist. Intravenous acyclovir nevertheless should be tried, and in some cases has been reported to result in survival.

recommended (60 mg/kg per day in three divided doses) (Kimberlin et al., 2001b). Intravenous therapy for neonatal herpes should be given for 21 days. Increasingly, serial testing of CSF HSV DNA has been utilized to guide the duration of therapy, and most experts advocate treating until HSV DNA is no longer detected. In immunosuppressed patients, IV acyclovir or oral valacyclovir are utilized to prevent HSV reactivations during transplantation or chemotherapy, and high doses of oral valacyclovir also prevent CMV reactivation (Dignani et al., 2002; Lowance et al., 1999).

Acyclovir-resistant strains of HSV have been identified, especially in HIV-infected persons. Almost all clinically significant acyclovir resistance has been seen in immunocompromised patients. Most acyclovir-resistant strains of HSV have a deficiency in thymidine kinase, the enzyme that phosphorylates acyclovir (Darby et al., 1981). Thus, cross-resistance to famciclovir is usually found. Occasionally, an isolate with altered thymidine kinase specificity will arise and will be sensitive to famciclovir but not to acyclovir. In some patients infected with thymidine kinase–deficient virus, higher doses of acyclovir are associated with clearing of lesions. In others, clinical disease progresses despite high-dose therapy. Isolation of HSV from persisting lesions despite adequate dosages and blood levels of acyclovir should raise the suspicion of acyclovir resistance (Safrin et al., 1992, 1994). In such cases therapy with the antiviral drug foscarnet is useful (Safrin et al., 1991). Because of its toxicity and cost, this drug is usually reserved for patients with extensive mucocutaneous infections. Cidofovir is a nucleotide analogue (Snoeck et al., 1994). Most thymidine kinase–deficient strains of HSV are sensitive to cidofovir. Cidofovir ointment has been shown to speed healing of acyclovir-resistant lesions (Lalezari et al., 1997). Similarly, trifluorothymidine ointment has also been reported to be of utility (Birch et al., 1992).

REFERENCES

Alster, T. S. and Nanni, C. A. (1999). Famciclovir prophylaxis of herpes simplex virus reactivation after laser skin resurfacing. *Dermatol. Surg*, **25**, 242–246.

Amir, J., Harel, L., Smetana, Z., and Varsano, I. (1999). The natural history of primary herpes simplex type 1 gingivostomatitis in children. *Pediatr. Dermatol.*, **16**, 259–263.

Anderson, B. J. (1999). The effectiveness of valacyclovir in preventing reactivation of herpes gladiatorum in wrestlers. *Clin. J. Sport Med.*, **9**, 86–90.

Anderson, B. J. (2003). The epidemiology and clinical analysis of several outbreaks of herpes gladiatorum. *Med. Sci. Sports Exerc.*, **35**, 1809–1814.

Aoki, F. Y., Tyring, S., Diaz-Mitoma, F., Gross, G., Gao, J. and Hamed, K. (2006). Single-day, patient-initiated famciclovir therapy for recurrent genital herpes: a randomized, double-blind, placebo-controlled trial. *Clin. Infect. Dis.*, **42**(1), 8–13.

Arvin, A., Yeager, A., Bruhn, F., and Grossman, M. (1982). Neonatal herpes simplex infection in the absence of mucocutaneous lesions. *J. Pediatrics*, **100**, 715–721.

Arvin, A., Hensleigh, P., Prober, C. et al. (1986). Failure of antepartum maternal cultures to predict the infant's risk of exposure to herpes simplex virus at delivery. *N. Engl. J. Med.*, **315**, 796–800.

Austin, H., Macaluso, M., Nahmias, A. et al. (1999). Correlates of herpes simplex virus seroprevalence among women attending a sexually transmitted disease clinic. *Sex Transm. Dis.*, **26**, 329–334.

Bagdades, E., Pillay, D., Squire, S., O'Neil, C., Johnson, M., and Griffiths, P. (1992). Relationship between herpes simplex virus ulceration and CD4+ cell counts in patients with HIV infection. *AIDS*, **6**, 1317–1320.

Balfour H. (1994). Recurrent ocular herpes simplex infection. *Pediatr. Infect. Dis. J.*, **13**, 170.

Ballard R. (2001). In *ASHA Summit on HSV Diagnostics* Seattle.

Barton, S. E., Davis, J. M., Moss, V. W., Tyms, A. S., and Munday, P. E. (1987). Asymptomatic shedding and subsequent transmission of genital herpes simplex virus. *Genitourin. Med.*, **63**, 102–105.

Becker, T. M. (1992). Herpes gladiatorum: a growing problem in sports medicine. *Cutis*, **50**, 150–152.

Beeson, W. H. and Rachel, J. D. (2002). Valacyclovir prophylaxis for herpes simplex virus infection or infection recurrence following laser skin resurfacing. *Dermatol Surg.*, **28**, 331–336.

Bell, W., Chulay, J., and Feinberg, J. (1997). Manifestations resembling thrombotic microangiopathy in patients with advanced HIV disease in a cytomegalovirus prophylaxis trial (ACTG 204). *Medicine*, **76**, 369–380.

Belongia, E., Goodman, J., Holland, E. et al. (1991). An outbreak of herpes gladiatorum at a high school wrestling camp. *N. Engl. J. Med.*, **325**, 906–910.

Benedetti, J. K., Corey, L., and Ashley, R. (1994). Recurrence rates in genital herpes after symptomatic first-episode infection. *Ann. Intern. Med.*, **121**, 847–854.

Bernstein, D. I., Lovett, M. A., and Bryson, Y. J. (1984). Serologic analysis of first-episode nonprimary genital herpes simplex virus infection. Presence of type 2 antibody in acute serum samples. *Am. J. Med.*, **77**, 1055–1060.

Beyrer, C., Jitwatcharanan, K., Natpratan, C. et al. (1998). Molecular methods for the diagnosis of genital ulcer disease in a sexually transmitted disease clinic population in northern Thailand: predominance of herpes simplex virus infection. *J. Infect. Dis.*, **178**, 243–246.

Birch, C., Tyssen, D., Tachedjian, G. et al. (1992). Clinical effects and in vitro studies of trifluorothymidine combined with interferon-alpha for treatment of drug-resistant and -sensitive herpes simplex virus infections. *J. Infect. Dis.*, **166**, 108–112.

Blower, S. and Boe, C. (1993). Sex acts, sex partners, and sex budgets: implications for risk factor analysis and estimation of HIV transmission probabilitites. *J. Acq. Immun. Def. Syndn.*, **6**, 1347–1352.

Brice, S., Krzemien, D., Weston, W., and Huff, J. (1989). Detection of herpes simplex virus DNA in cutaneous lesions of erythema multiforme. *J. Invest. Dermatol.*, **93**, 183–187.

Brown, Z. A. (2000). HSV-2 specific serology should be offered routinely to antenatal patients [In Process Citation]. *Rev. Med. Virol.*, **10**, 141–144.

Brown, Z. A., Selke, S. A., Zeh, J. *et al.* (1997). Acquisition of herpes simplex virus during pregnancy. *N. Engl. J. Med.*, **337**, 509–515.

Brown, Z. A., Wald, A., Morrow, R. A., Selke, S., Zeh, J., and Corey, L. (2003). Effect of serologic status and cesarean delivery on transmission rates of herpes simplex virus from mother to infant. *J. Am. Med. Assoc.*, **289**, 203–209.

Bryson, Y. J., Dillon, M., Bernstein, D. I., Radolf, J., Zakowski, P., and Garratty, E. (1993). Risk of acquisition of genital herpes simplex virus type 2 in sex partners of persons with genital herpes: a prospective couple study. *J. Infect. Dis.*, **167**, 942–946.

Cameron, D. W., Simonsen, J. N., D'Costa, L. J. *et al.* (1989). Female to male transmission of human immunodeficiency virus type 1: risk factors for seroconversion in men. *Lancet*, 403–407.

Carney, O., Ross, E., Bunker, C., Ikkos, G., and Mindel, A. (1994). A prospective study of the psychological impact on patients with a first episode of genital herpes. *Genitourin. Med.*, **70**, 40–45.

Catotti, D. N., Clarke, P., and Catoe, K. E. (1993). Herpes revisited: still a cause of concern. *Sex Transm. Dis.*, **20**, 77–80.

Centers for Disease Control and Prevention (2002). Sexually transmitted diseases treatment guidelines 2002. *MMWR Recomm. Rep.*, **51**, 1–82.

Chase, R. A., Pottage, J. C., Jr., Haber, M. H., Kistler, G., Jensen, D., and Levin, S. (1987). Herpes simplex viral hepatitis in adults: two case reports and review of the literature. *Rev. Infect. Dis.*, **9**, 329–333.

Chen, C. Y., Ballard, R. C., Beck-Sague, C. M. *et al.* (2000). Human immunodeficiency virus infection and genital ulcer disease in South Africa: the herpetic connection [see comments]. *Sex Transm. Dis.*, **27**, 21–29.

Chuang, I., Van Beneden, C., Beall, B., and Schuchat, A. (2002). Population-based surveillance for postpartum invasive group A streptococcus infections, 1995–2000. *Clin. Infect. Dis.*, **35**, 665–670.

Cohen, B., Rowley, A., and Long, C. (1994). Herpes simplex type 2 in a patient with Mollaret's meningitis: demonstration by polymerase chain reaction. *Ann. Neurol.*, **35**, 112–116.

Corey, L. and Spear, P. G. (1986). Infections with herpes simplex viruses (part 1). *N. Engl. J. Med.*, **314**, 686–691.

Corey, L., and Wald, A. (1999). *In Sexually Transmitted Diseases*, ed. Holmes, K., Sparling, P., PA, M., Lemon, S., Stamm, W., Piot, P., Wasserheit, J. New York: McGraw-Hill.

Corey, L., Adams, H. G., Brown, Z. A., and Holmes, K. K. (1983). Clinical course of genital herpes simplex virus infections in men and women. *Ann. Intern. Med.*, **48**, 973.

Corey, L., Whitley, R. J., Stone, E. F., and Mohan, K. (1988). Difference between herpes simplex virus type 1 and type 2 neonatal encephalitis in neurological outcome. *Lancet*, **1**, 1–4.

Corey, L., Wald, A., Celum, C. L., and Quinn, T. C. (2004a). The effects of herpes simplex virus-2 on HIV-1 acquisition and transmission: a review of two overlapping epidemics. *J. Acquir. Immune Defic. Syndr.*, **35**, 435–445.

Corey, L., Wald, A., Patel, R. *et al.* (2004b). Once-daily valacyclovir to reduce the risk of transmission of genital herpes. *N. Engl. J. Med.*, **350**, 11–20.

Darby, G., Field, H., and Salisbury, S. (1981). Altered substrate specificity of herpes simplex virus thymidine kinase confers acyclovir-resistance. *Nature*, **289**, 81–83.

DeJesus, E., Wald, A., Warren, T. *et al.* (2003). Valacyclovir for the suppression of recurrent genital herpes in human immunodeficiency virus-infected subjects. *J. Infect Dis*, **188**, 1009–1016.

Deshpande, S. P., Lee, S., Zheng, M. *et al.* (2001). Herpes simplex virus-induced keratitis: evaluation of the role of molecular mimicry in lesion pathogenesis. *J. Virol*, **75**, 3077–3088.

Diamond, C., Selke, S., Ashley, R., Benedetti, J., and Corey, L. (1999). Clinical course of patients with serologic evidence of recurrent genital herpes presenting with signs and symptoms of first episode disease. *Sex. Transm. Dis.*, **26**, 221–225.

Dignani, M. C., Mykietiuk, A., Michelet, M. *et al.* (2002). Valacyclovir prophylaxis for the prevention of Herpes simplex virus reactivation in recipients of progenitor cells transplantation. *Bone Marrow Transpl.*, **29**, 263–267.

Elion, G., Furman, P., Fyfe, J., deMiranda, P., Beauchamp, L., and Schaeffer, H. (1977). The selectivity of action of an antiherpetic agent, 9-(2-hydroxyethoxymethyl) guanine. *Proc. Natl Acad. Sci. USA*, **74**, 5716–5720.

Enders, G., Risse, B., Zauke, M., Bolley, I., and Knotek, F. (1998). Seroprevalence study of herpes simplex virus type 2 among pregnant women in Germany using a type-specific enzyme immunoassay [In Process Citation]. *Eur. J. Clin. Microbiol. Infect. Dis.*, **17**, 870–872.

Engelberg, R., Carrell, D., Krantz, E., Corey, L., and Wald, A. (2003). Natural history of genital herpes simplex virus type 1 infection. *Sex. Transm. Dis.*, **30**, 174–177.

Erlich, K., Mills, J., Chatis, P. *et al.* (1989). Acyclovir-resistant herpes simplex virus infections in patients with the acquired immunodeficiency syndrome. *N. Engl. J. Med.*, **320**, 293–296.

Evans, A. and Dick, E. (1964). Acute pharyngitis and tonsilitis in University of Wisconsin students. *J. Am. Med. Assoc.*, **190**, 699.

Fleming, D., McQuillan, G., Johnson, R. *et al.* (1997). Herpes simplex virus type 2 in the United States, 1976 to 1994. *N. Engl. J. Med.*, **337**, 1105–1111.

Flewett, T., Parker, R., and Philip, W. (1969). Acute hepatitis due to herpes simplex in an adult. *J. Clin. Pathol.*, **22**, 60–66.

Florman, A. (1973). Intrauterine infection with herpes simplex virus: resultant congenital malformations. *J. Am. Med. Assoc.*, **225**, 129.

Frederick, D. M., Bland, D., and Gollin Y. (2002). Fatal disseminated herpes simplex virus infection in a previously healthy pregnant woman. A case report. *J Reprod Med.*, **47**, 591–596.

Freeman, E. E., Weiss, H. A., Glynn, J. R., Cross, P. L., Whitworth, J. A., and Hayes, R. J. (2006). Herpes simplex virus 2 infection increases HIV acquisition in men and women: systematic review and meta-analysis of longitudinal studies. *AIDS*, **20**(1), 73–83.

Gateley, A., Gander, R., Johnson, P., Kit, S., Otsuka, H., and Kohl, S. (1990). Herpes simplex virus 2 meningoencephalitis resistant to acyclovir in a patient with AIDS. *J. Infect. Dis.*, **161**, 711–715.

Gibbs, R. S., McDuffie, R. S., Jr., McNabb, F., Fryer, G. E., Miyoshi, T., and Merenstein, G. (1994). Neonatal group B streptococcal sepsis during 2 years of a universal screening program. *Obstet. Gynecol.*, **84**, 496–500.

Goyette, R., and Donowho E. (1974). Fulminant hepatitis during pregnancy. *Obstet. Gynecol.*, **43**, 191–195.

Guex-Crosier, Y., Rochat, C., and Herbort, C. P. (1997). Necrotizing herpetic retinopathies. A spectrum of herpes virus-induced diseases determined by the immune state of the host. *Ocul. Immunol. Inflamm.*, **5**, 259–265.

Gutierrez, K. M., Halpern MSF, Maldonado, Y., and Arvin, A. M. (1999). The epidemiology of neonatal herpes simplex virus infections in California from 1985 to 1995. *J. Infect. Dis.*, **180**, 199–202.

Hashido, M., Kawana, T., Matsunaga, Y., and Inouye S. (1999). Changes in prevalence of herpes simplex virus type 1 and 2 antibodies from 1973 to 1993 in the rural districts of Japan. *Microbiol. Immunol.*, **43**, 177–180.

Herpetic Eye Disease Study Group (1997). A controlled trial of oral acyclovir for the prevention of stromal keratitis or iritis in patients with herpes simplex virus epithelial keratitis. The Epithelial Keratitis Trial. *Arch. Ophthalmol.*, **115**, 703–712.

Hill, T., Blyth, W., and Harbour, D. (1978). Trauma to the skin causes recurrence of herpes simplex in the mouse. *J. Gen. Virol.*, **39**, 21–28.

Huff, J., Weston, W., and Tonnesen M. (1983). Erythema multiforme: A critical review of characteristics, diagnostic criteria, and causes. *J. Am. Acad. Dermatol.*, **6**, 763–775.

Itoh, N., Matsumura, N., Ogi, A. *et al.* (2000). High prevalence of herpes simplex virus type 2 in acute retinal necrosis syndrome associated with herpes simplex virus in Japan. *Am. J. Ophthalmol.*, **129**, 404–405.

Kampgen, E., Burg, G., and Wank, R. (1988). Association of herpes simplex virus-induced erythema multiforme with the human leukocyte antigen DQw3. *Arch. Dermatol.*, **124**, 1372–1375.

Keane, J., Malkinson, F., Bryant, J., and Levin, S. (1976). Herpesvirus hominis hepatitis and disseminated intravascular coagulation: occurrence in an adult with pemphigus vulgaris. *Arch. Dermatol.*, **93**, 1312–1317.

Kimberlin, D., Lin C-Y., Jacobs, R. *et al.* (2001a). Natural history of neonatal herpes simplex virus infections in the acyclovir era. *Pediatrics*, **108**, 223–229.

Kimberlin, D., Lin, C.-Y., Jacobs, R. *et al.* (2001b). The safety and efficacy of high-dose acyclovir in the management of neonatal herpes simplex virus infections. *Pediatrics*, **108**, 230–238.

Kimberlin, D., Powell, D., Gruber, W., *et al.* (1996). Administration of oral acyclovir suppressive therapy after neonatal herpes simplex virus disease limited to the skin, eyes and mouth: results of a phase I/II trial. *Pediatr. Infect. Dis. J.*, **15**, 247–254.

Kobberman, T., Clark, L., and Griffin, W. (1980). Maternal death secondary to disseminated herpesvirus hominis. *Am. J. Obstet. Gyn.*, **137**, 742–743.

Koelle, D. M., Abbo, H., Peck, A., Ziegweld, K., and Corey, L. (1994). Direct recovery of herpes simplex virus (HSV) – specific T lymphocyte clones from recurrent genital HSV-2 lesions. *J. Infect. Dis.*, **169**, 956–961.

Koelle, D. M., Reymond, S. N., Chen, H. *et al.* (2000). Tegument-specific, virus-reactive CD4 T cells localize to the cornea in herpes simplex virus interstitial keratitis in humans. *J. Virol.*, **74**, 10930–10938.

Lafferty, W. E., Coombs, R. W., Benedetti, J., Critchlow, C., and Corey, L. (1987). Recurrences after oral and genital herpes simplex virus infection: influence of anatomic site and viral type. *N. Engl. J. Med.*, **316**, 1444–1449.

Lafferty, W. E., Downey, L., Celum, C., and Wald, A. (2000). Herpes simplex virus type 1 as a cause of genital herpes: impact on surveillance and prevention. *J. Infect. Dis.*, **181**, 1454–1457.

Lairson, D. R., Begley, C. E., Reynolds, T. F., and Wilhelmus, K. R. (2003). Prevention of herpes simplex virus eye disease: a cost-effectiveness analysis. *Arch. Ophthalmol.*, **121**, 108–112.

Lakeman, F. and Whitley, R. (1995). Diagnosis of herpes simplex encephalitis: application of polymerase chain reaction to cerebrospinal fluid from brain-biopsied patients and correlation with disease. *J. Infect. Dis.*, **171**, 857–863.

Lalezari, J., Schacker, T., Feinberg, J. *et al.* (1997). A randomized, double-blind, placebo-controlled trial of cidofovir topical gel for the treatment of acyclovir-unresponsive mucocutaneous herpes simplex infection in patients with AIDS. *J. Infect. Dis.*, **176**, 892–898.

Langenberg, A., Corey, L., Ashley, R., Leong, W., and Straus, S. (1999). A prospective study of new infections with herpes simplex virus type 1 and type 2. *N. Engl. J. Med.*, **341**, 1432–1438.

Lemak, M., Duvic, M., Bean, S. (1986). Oral acyclovir for the prevention of herpes-associated erythema multiforme. *J. Am. Acad. Dermatol.*, **15**, 50–54.

Leone, P. A., Trottier, S., and Miller, J. M. (2002). Valacyclovir for episodic treatment of genital herpes: a shorter 3-day treatment course compared with 5-day treatment. *Clin. Infect. Dis.*, **34**, 958–962.

Liesegang, T. J. (2001). Herpes simplex virus epidemiology and ocular importance. *Cornea*, **20**, 1–13.

Linnemann, C., First, M., Alvira, M., Alexander, J., and Schiff, G. (1976). Herpesvirus hominis type 2 meningoencephalitis following renal transplantation. *Am. J. Med.*, **61**, 703–708.

Lowance, D., Neumayer, H. H., Legendre, C. M. *et al.* (1999). Valacyclovir for the prevention of cytomegalovirus disease after renal transplantation. International Valacyclovir Cytomegalovirus Prophylaxis Transplantation Study Group. *N. Engl. J. Med.*, **340**, 1462–1470.

Lowhagen, G. B., Tunback, P., Andersson, K., Bergstrom, T., and Johannisson, G. (2000). First episodes of genital herpes in a Swedish STD population: a study of epidemiology and transmission by the use of herpes simplex virus (HSV) typing and specific serology. *Sex. Transm. Infect.*, **76**, 179–182.

Luchi, M., Feldman, M., and Williams, W. (1995). Fatal disseminated herpes simplex II infection in a patient with systemic lupus erythematosus. *J. Rheumatol.* (*letter to editors*), **22**, 799–801.

Malkin, J. E., Morand, P., Malvy, D. *et al.* (2002). Seroprevalence of HSV-1 and HSV-2 infection in the general French population. *Sex. Transm. Infect.*, **78**, 201–203.

Malo, A., Kampgen, E., and Wank, R. (1998). Recurrent herpes simplex virus-induced erythema multiforme: different HLA-DQB1 alleles associate with severe mucous membrane versus skin attacks. *Scand. J. Immunol.*, **47**, 408–411.

Manzella, J. P., McConville, J. H., Valenti, W., Menegus, M. A., Swierkosz, E. M., and Arens, M. (1984). An outbreak of herpes simplex virus type I gingivostomatitis in a dental hygiene practice. *J. Am. Med. Assoc.*, **252**, 2019–2022.

Mertz, G. J., Coombs, R. W., Ashley, R. *et al.* (1988). Transmission of genital herpes in couples with one symptomatic and one asymptomatic partner: a prospective study. *J. Infect. Dis.*, **157**, 1169–1177.

Mertz, G. J., Benedetti, J., Ashley, R., Selke, S. A., and Corey, L. (1992). Risk factors for the sexual transmission of genital herpes. *Ann. Intern. Med.*, **116**, 197–202.

Mertz, G. J., Rosenthal, S. L., and Stanberry, L. R. (2003). Is herpes simplex virus type 1 (HSV-1) now more common than HSV-2 in first episodes of genital herpes? *Sex. Transm. Dis.*, **30**, 801–802.

Meyers, J., Flournoy, N., and Thomas, E. (1980). Infection with herpes simplex virus and cell-mediated immunity after marrow transplant. *J. Infect. Dis.*, **142**, 338–346.

Mindel, A., Taylor, J., Tideman, R. L. *et al.* (2000). Neonatal herpes prevention: a minor public health problem in some communities. *Sex. Transm. Infect.*, **76**, 287–291.

Miura, S., Smith, C., Burnett, J., and Aurelian, L. (1992). Detection of viral DNA within skin of healed recurrent herpes simplex infection and erythema multiforme lesions. *J. Invest. Dermatol.*, **98**, 68–72.

Morse, S. A., Trees, D. L., Htun, Y. *et al.* (1997). Comparison of clinical diagnosis and standard laboratory and molecular methods for the diagnosis of genital ulcer disease in Lesotho: association with human immunodeficiency virus infection. *J. Infect. Dis.*, **175**, 001–007.

Ng, P. P., Sun, Y. J., Tan, H. H., and Tan, S. H. (2003). Detection of herpes simplex virus genomic DNA in various subsets of *Erythema multiforme* by polymerase chain reaction. *Dermatology*, **207**, 349–353.

Niimura, M., and Nishikawa, T. (1988). Treatment of eczema herpeticum with oral acyclovir. *Am. J. Med.*, **85**, 49–52.

Picard, F., Dekaban, G., Silva, J., and Rice, G. (1993). Mollaret's meningitis associated with herpes simplex type 2 infection. *Neurology*, **43**, 1722–1727.

Posavad, C. M., Wald, A., Kuntz, S. *et al.* (2001). In *Conf. Retroviruses Opportunistic Infect.*, Chicago, IL pp. 211.

Prober, C. G., Corey, L., Brown, Z. A. *et al.* (1992). The management of pregnancies complicated by genital infections with herpes simplex virus. *Clin. Infect. Dis.*, **15**, 1031–1038.

Puchhammer-Stockl, E., Heinz, F., Kundi, M. *et al.* (1993). Evaluation of the polymerase chain reaction for diagnosis of herpes simplex virus encephalitis. *J. Clin. Microbiol.*, **31**, 146–148.

Pue, M. A. and Benet, L. Z. (1993). Pharmacokinetics of famciclovir in man. *Antiviral Chem. Chemother*, **4**(S1), 47–55.

Quinn, T. C., Corey, L., Chaffee, R. G., Schuffler, M. D., Brancato, F. P., and Holmes, K. K. (1981). The etiology of anorectal infection in homosexual men. *Am. J. Med.*, **71**, 395–406.

Ramsey, P., Fife, K., Hackman, R., Meyers, J., and Corey, L. (1982). Herpes simplex virus pneumonia: clinical, virologic, and pathologic features in 20 patients. *Ann. Intern. Med.*, **97**, 813–820.

Reitano, M., Tyring, S., Lang, W. *et al.* (1998). Valaciclovir for the suppression of recurrent genital herpes simplex virus infection: a large-scale dose range-finding study. *J. Infect. Dis.*, **178**, 603–610.

Reyes, M., Shaik, N. S., Graber, J. M. *et al.* (2003). Acyclovir-resistant genital herpes among persons attending sexually transmitted disease and human immunodeficiency virus clinics. *Arch. Intern. Med.*, **163**, 76–80.

Romanowski, B., Aoki, F. Y., Martel, A. Y., Lavender, E. A., Parsons, J. E., and Saltzman, R. L. (2000). Efficacy and safety of famciclovir for treating mucocutaneous herpes simplex infection in HIV-infected individuals. Collaborative Famciclovir HIV Study Group [In Process Citation]. *AIDS*, **14**, 1211–1217.

Rompalo, A., Mertz, G., Davis, L., *et al.* (1988). Oral acyclovir for treatment of first-episode herpes simplex virus proctitis. *J. Am. Med. Assoc.*, **259**, 2879–2881.

Rosenthal, S. L., Stanberry, L. R., Biro, F. M., *et al.* (1997). Seroprevalence of herpes simplex virus types 1 and 2 and cytomegalovirus in adolescents. *Clin. Infect. Dis.*, **24**, 135–139.

Ross, J. D. C., Smith, I. W., and Elton, R. A. (1993). The epidemiology of herpes simplex types 1 and 2 infection of the genital tract in Edinburgh 1978–1991. *Genitourin. Med.*, **69**, 381–383.

Safrin, S., Crumpacker, C., Chatis, P., *et al.* (1991). A controlled trial comparing foscarnet with vidarabine for acyclovir-resistant mucocutaneous herpes simplex in the acquired immunodeficiency syndrome. *N. Engl. J. Med.*, **325**, 551–555.

Safrin, S., Elbaggari, A., and Elbeik, T. (1992). Risk factors for the development of acyclovir-resistant herpes simplex virus infection. *VII International AIDS Conference 1992; Abstract B. 1548.*

Safrin, S., Elbeik, T., Phan, L., *et al.* (1994). Correlation between response to acyclovir and foscarnet therapy and in vitro susceptibility result for isolates of herpes simplex virus from human immunodeficiency virus-infected patients. *Antimicrob. Agents Chemother*, **38**, 1246–1250.

Schacker, T., Hu, H. L., Koelle, D. M. *et al.* (1998a). Famciclovir for the suppression of symptomatic and asymptomatic herpes simplex virus reactivation in HIV-infected persons. A double-blind, placebo-controlled trial. *Ann. Intern. Med.*, **128**, 21–28.

Schacker, T., Zeh, J., Hu, H. L., Hill, J., and Corey, L. (1998b). Frequency of symptomatic and asymptomatic HSV-2 reactivations among HIV-infected men. *J. Infect. Dis.*, **178**, 1616–1622.

Schacker, T. W., Ryncarz, A. J., Goddard, J., Diem, K., Shaughnessy, M., and Corey, L. (1998c). Frequent recovery of HIV-1 from genital herpes simplex virus lesions in HIV-1–infected men. *J. Am. Med. Assoc.*, **280**, 61–66.

Schrag, S. J., and Schuchat, A. (2004). Easing the burden: characterizing the disease burden of neonatal group B streptococcal disease to motivate prevention. *Clin. Infect. Dis.*, **38**, 1209–1211.

Serwadda, D., Gray, R. H., Sewankambo, N. K., *et al.* (2003). Human immunodeficiency virus acquisition associated with genital ulcer disease and herpes simplex virus type 2 infection: a nested case-control study in Rakai, Uganda. *J. Infect. Dis.*, **188**, 1492–1497.

Sheffield, J. S., Hollier, L. M., Hill, J. B., Stuart, G. S., and Wendel, G. D. (2003). Acyclovir prophylaxis to prevent herpes simplex virus recurrence at delivery: a systematic review. *Obstet. Gynecol.*, **102**, 1396–1403.

Siegal, F., Lopez, C., Hammer, G. *et al.* (1981). Severe acquired immunodeficiency in male homosexuals, manifested by chronic perianal ulcerative herpes simplex lesions. *N. Engl. J. Med.*, **305**, 1439–1444.

Smith, J. S., Herrero, R., Munoz, N. *et al.* (2001). Prevalence and risk factors for herpes simplex virus type 2 infection among middle-age women in Brazil and the Philippines. *Sex. Transm. Dis.*, **28**, 187–194.

Snoeck, R., Andrei, G., Gerard, M. *et al.* (1994). Successful treatment of progressive mucocutaneous infection due to acyclovir- and foscarnet-resistant herpes simplex virus with (S)-1(3–hydroxy-2-phosphonylmethoxypropyl) cytosine (HPMPC). *Clin. Infect. Dis.*, **18**, 570–578.

Soul-Lawton, J., Seaber, E., On, N., Wootton, R., Rolan, P., and Posner, J. (1995). Absolute bioavailability and metabolic disposition of valaciclovir, the L-Val ester of acyclovir, following oral administration to humans. *Antimicrob Agents Chem.*, **36**, 2759–2764.

Souza, P. M., Holland, E. J., and Huang, A. J. (2003). Bilateral herpetic keratoconjunctivitis. *Ophthalmology*, **110**, 493–496.

Spruance, S. (1984). Pathogenesis of herpes simplex labialis: excretion of virus in the oral cavity. *J. Clin. Microbiol.*, **19**, 675–679.

Spruance, S., Overall, J., Kern, E., Krueger, G., Pliam, V., and Miller, W. (1977). The natural history of recurrent herpes simplex labialis: implications for antiviral therapy. *N. Engl. J. Med.*, **297**, 69–75.

Spruance, S., Hamill, M., Hoge, W., Davis, L., and Mills, J. (1988). Acyclovir prevents reactivation of herpes simplex labialis in skiers. *J. Am. Med. Assoc.*, **260**, 1597–1599.

Spruance, S., Freeman, D., Stewart, J. *et al.* (1991). The natural history of ultraviolet radiation-induced herpes simplex labialis and response to therapy with peroral and topical formulations of acyclovir. *J. Infect. Dis.*, **163**, 728–734.

Spruance, S., Rea, T., Thoming, C., Tucker, R., Saltzman, R., and Boon, R. (1997). Penciclovir cream for the treatment of herpes simplex labialis: a randomized, multicenter, double-blind, placebo-controlled trial. *J. Am. Med. Assoc.*, **277**, 1374–1379.

Spruance, S. L., Jones, T. M., Blatter, M. M. *et al.* (2003). High-dose, short-duration, early valacyclovir therapy for episodic treatment of cold sores: results of two randomized, placebo-controlled, multicenter studies. *Antimicrob. Agents Chemother.*, **47**, 1072–1080.

Stanberry, L. R., Spruance, S. L., Cunningham, A. L. *et al.* (2002). Glycoprotein-D-adjuvant vaccine to prevent genital herpes. *N. Engl. J. Med.*, **347**, 1652–1661.

Stern, H., Elek, S., Millar, D., and Anderson, H. (1959). Herpetic whitlow, a form of cross-infection in hospitals. *Lancet*, **2**, 871–874.

Sucato, G., Celum, C., Dithmer, D., Ashley, R., and Wald, A. (2001). Demographic rather than behavioral risk factors predict herpes simplex virus type 2 infection in sexually active adolescents. *Pediatr. Infect. Dis. J.*, **20**, 422–426.

Sullivan-Bolyai, J., Hull, H. F., Wilson, C., and Corey, L. (1983). Neonatal herpes simplex virus infection in King County, Washington: increasing incidence and epidemiological correlates. *J. Am. Med. Assoc.*, **250**, 3059–3062.

Sutton, A., Smithwick, E., Seligman, S., and Kim, D. (1974). Fatal disseminated herpesvirus hominis type 2 infection in an adult with associated thymic dysplasia. *Am. J. Med.*, **56**, 545–553.

Swanson, J. and Chenitz, W. (1990). Psychosocial aspects of genital herpes: a review of the literature. *Pub. Health Nurs.*, **7**, 96–104.

Thomas, J., and Rouse, B. T. (1998). Immunopathology of herpetic stromal keratitis: discordance in CD4+ T cell function between euthymic host and reconstituted SCID recipients. *J. Immunol.*, **160**, 3965–3970.

Thomas, J., Gangappa, S., Kanangat, S., and Rouse, B. T. (1997). On the essential involvement of neutrophils in the immunopathologic disease: herpetic stromal keratitis. *J. Immunol*, **158**, 1383–1391.

Thompson, W., Culbertson, W., Smiddy, W., Robertson, J., and Rosenbaum, J. (1994). Acute retinal necrosis caused by reactivation of herpes simplex virus type 2. *Am. J. Opthalmol.*, **118**, 205–211.

Tookey, P. and Peckham, C. S. (1996). Neonatal herpes simplex virus infection in the British Isles. *Paediatr. Perinat. Epidemiol.*, **10**, 432–442.

Tran, T. H., Stanescu, D., Caspers-Velu, L. *et al.* (2004). Clinical characteristics of acute HSV-2 retinal necrosis. *Am. J. Ophthalmol.*, **137**, 872–879.

Varela, J. A., Garcia-Corbeira, P., Aguanell, M. V. *et al.* (2001). Herpes simplex virus type 2 seroepidemiology in Spain: prevalence and seroconversion rate among sexually transmitted disease clinic attendees. *Sex. Transm. Dis.*, **28**, 47–50.

Verjans, G. M., Remeijer, L., Mooy, C. M., and Osterhaus, A. D. (2000). Herpes simplex virus-specific T cells infiltrate the cornea of patients with herpetic stromal keratitis: no evidence for autoreactive T cells. *Invest. Ophthalmol. Vis. Sci.*, **41**, 2607–2612.

Vyse, A. J., Gay, N. J., Slomka, M. J. *et al.* (2000). The burden of infection with HSV-1 and HSV-2 in England and Wales: implications for the changing epidemiology of genital herpes. *Sex. Transm. Infect.*, **76**, 183–187.

Wade, J., Day, L., Crowley, J., and Meyers, J. (1984a). Recurrent infection with herpes simplex virus after marrow transplantation: role of the specific immune response and acyclovir treatment. *J. Infect. Dis.*, **149**, 750–756.

Wade, J., Newton, B., Flournoy, N., and Meyers, J. (1984b). Oral acyclovir for prevention of herpes simplex virus reactivation after marrow transplantation. *Ann. Int. Med.*, **100**, 823–828.

Wald, A. and Link, K. (2002). Risk of human immunodeficiency virus (HIV) infection in herpes simplex virus type-2 (HSV-2) seropositive persons: a meta-analysis. *J. Infect. Dis.*, **185**, 45–52.

Wald, A., Corey, L., Cone, R., Hobson, A., Davis, G., and Zeh, J. (1997). Frequent genital HSV-2 shedding in immunocompetent women. *J. Clin. Invest.*, **99**, 1092–1097.

Wald, A., Langenberg, A., Link, K. *et al.* (2001). Effect of condoms on reducing the transmission of herpes simplex virus type 2 from men to women. *J. Am. Med. Assoc.*, **285**, 3100–3106.

Wald, A., Carrell, D., Remington, M., Kexel, E., Zeh, J., and Corey, L. (2002a). Two-day regimen of acyclovir for treatment of recurrent genital herpes simplex virus type 2 infection. *Clin. Infect. Dis.*, **34**, 944–948.

Wald, A., Zeh, J. E., Selke, S. A., Warren, T., Ashley, R. L., and Corey, L. (2002b). Genital shedding of herpes simplex virus among men. *J. Infect. Dis.*, **186 Suppl 1**, S34–S39.

Wald, A., Huang, M. L., Carrell, D., Selke, S., and Corey, L. (2003). Polymerase chain reaction for detection of herpes simplex virus (HSV) DNA on mucosal surfaces: comparison with HSV isolation in cell culture. *J. Infect. Dis.*, **188**, 1345–1351.

Weiss, H., Buve, A., Robinson, N. *et al.* (2001). The epidemiology of HSV-2 infection and its association with HIV infection in four urban African populations. *AIDS*, **15 (suppl 4)**, S97–S108.

Wheeler, Jr. C. and Abele, D. (1966). Eczema herpeticum, primary and recurrent. *Arch. Dermatol.*, **93**, 162.

Whitley, R. (1988). The frustrations of treating herpes simplex virus infections of the central nervous system. *J. Am. Med. Assoc.*, **259**, 1067.

Whitley, R. J. and Gnann Jr, J. W. (1992). Acyclovir: a decade later. *N. Engl. J. Med.*, **327**, 782–789.

Whitley, R. and Lakeman, F. (1995). Herpes simplex virus infections of the central nervous system: therapeutic and diagnostic considerations. *Clin. Infect. Dis.*, **20**, 414–420.

Whitley, R., Nahmias, A., Visintine, A., Fleming, C., and Alford, C. (1980). The natural history of genital herpes simplex virus infection of mother and newborn. *Pediatrics*, **66**, 489.

Whitley, R. J., Alford, C. A., Hirsch, M. S. *et al.* (1986). Vidarabine versus acyclovir therapy in herpes simplex encephalitis. *N. Engl. J. Med.*, **314**, 144–149.

Whitley, R., Corey, L., Arvin, A. *et al.* (1998). Changing presentation of herpes simplex virus infection in neonates. *J. Infect. Dis.*, **158**, 109–116.

Whitley, R., Arvin, A., Prober, C. *et al.* (1991b). A controlled trial comparing vidarabine with acyclovir in neonatal herpes simplex virus infection. *N. Engl. J. Med.*, **324**, 444–449.

Whitley, R., Arvin, A., Prober, C. *et al.* (1991b). Predictors of morbidity and mortality in neonates with herpes simplex infections. *N. Engl. J. Med.*, **324**, 450–454.

Whitley, R. J., Kimberlin, D. W., and Roizman, B. (1998). Herpes simplex viruses. *Clin. Infect. Dis.*, **26**, 541–553; quiz 554–555.

Wilhelmus, K., Beck, R., Moke, P. *et al.* (1998). Acyclovir for the prevention of recurrent herpes simplex virus eye disease. Herpetic Eye Disease Study Group. *N. Engl. J. Med.*, **339**, 300–306.

Wilkinson, D., Barton, S., and Cowan, F. (2000). HSV-2 specific serology should not be offered routinely to antenatal patients [In Process Citation]. *Rev. Med. Virol.*, **10**, 145–153.

Wollenberg, A., Zoch, C., Wetzel, S., Plewig, G., and Przybilla, B. (2003). Predisposing factors and clinical features of eczema herpeticum: a retrospective analysis of 100 cases. *J. Am. Acad. Dermatol.*, **49**, 198–205.

Xu, F., Schillinger, J. A., Sternberg, M. R. *et al.* (2002). Seroprevalence and coinfection with herpes simplex virus type 1 and type 2 in the United States, 1988–1994. *J. Infect. Dis.*, **185**, 1019–1024.

Yamamoto, L., Tedder, D., Ashley, R., and Levin, M. (1991). Herpes simplex virus type 1 DNA in cerebrospinal fluid of a patient with Mollaret's meningitis. *N. Engl. J. Med.*, **325**, 1082–1085.

Yoshida, M. and Amatsu, A. (2000). Asymptomatic shedding of herpes simplex virus into the oral cavity of patients with atopic dermatitis. *J. Clin. Virol.*, **16**, 65–69.

Part III

Pathogenesis, clinical disease, host response, and epidemiology: alphaherpes viruses VZV

Ann Arvin and Richard Whitley

Part III

Pathogenesis, clinical disease, host response, and epidemiology: alphaherpes viruses VZV

Ann Arvin and Richard Whitley

VZV: pathogenesis and the disease consequences of primary infection

Jennifer Moffat[1], Chia-Chi Ku[2], Leigh Zerboni[2], Marvin Sommer[2] and Ann Arvin[2]

[1] Suny Upstate Medical University, Syracuse, NY, USA
[2] Stanford University, CA, USA

Introduction

VZV is a human alphaherpesvirus that causes varicella (chickenpox) as the primary infection and establishes latency in sensory ganglia. VZV reactivation results in herpes zoster (shingles). During the course of varicella and zoster, VZV infects differentiated human cells that exist within unique tissue microenvironments in humans. The tropism of VZV for skin is the most obvious clinical manifestation of VZV infection, producing the vesicular cutaneous lesions that are associated with varicella and zoster. The site of initial VZV infection in naïve hosts is thought to be mucosal epithelial cells of the upper respiratory tract. Entry is presumed to follow inoculation of the respiratory epithelium with infectious virus transmitted by aerosolized respiratory droplets or by contact with virus in varicella or zoster skin lesions (Arvin, 2001a; Grose, 1981). VZV in respiratory or conjunctival mucosal cells has the opportunity to interact with and infect local immune system cells and those in adjacent lymphoid tissues. Trafficking of infected peripheral blood mononuclear cells (PBMC), which appear to be predominantly T-cells, to the skin is thought to give rise to crops of cutaneous vesicles. Skin lesions contain VZV material associated with necrotic debris and, unlike virus grown in vitro, cell-free, infectious particles are detected in vesicular fluid (Williams et al., 1962). The life cycle of VZV is completed upon its transmission to a susceptible host from an individual with varicella, or it can be postponed for decades by establishing latency in neurons and transmitting to future generations during episodes of zoster.

VZV shares its tropism for epithelial tissues with its relatives, HSV-1 and HSV-2, as well as with the non-human alphaherpesviruses. VZV also shares the neurotropism of these viruses, as discussed elsewhere in this volume. However, VZV seems to be more akin to the betaherpesviruses, HHV6 and HHV7, in its apparent tropism for T-cells (Ku et al., 2002, 2004; Takahashi et al., 1989). VZV infection of T-cells appears to represent a critical phase of its life cycle, providing a mechanism for viral transport from sites of initial infection to the skin. Sensory nerve axons terminate in the dermis and may be infected with VZV, allowing for retrograde transport to sensory ganglia, as it spreads through the skin layers (Annunziato et al., 2000). VZV may also reach neurons by hematogenous spread. The outcome of VZV infection in these various cell types, which are differentiated and non-dividing, depends on interactions between virus proteins and host factors at the cellular level and is modulated by the innate and adaptive immune responses of the infected host (Chapter 39). VZV infection of dendritic cells is described in Chapter 39, and investigations of latency and reactivation in the human host and in rodent models are reviewed in Chapter 38. The goals of this chapter are to discuss VZV infection of T-cells and skin, which are essential target cells of the virus during primary infection, and the disease consequences of varicella in healthy and immunocompromised individuals.

Systems for evaluating determinants of VZV pathogenesis in human skin and T-cells

Immunodeficient (*scid/scid*) mice with thymus/liver (T-cell) or skin xenografts have provided a useful experimental model for examining VZV pathogenesis in vivo, known as the SCID-hu model of VZV infection (Moffat et al., 1995). In this model, VZV-infected fibroblasts are injected into human tissue xenografts, which are then removed at intervals up to 21–28 days after infection. Initial experiments with T-cell xenografts showed that VZV proteins were expressed in CD4+, CD8+ and CD4/CD8+ T-cells and VZV was cultured from each T-cell subpopulation. T-cells released infectious VZV, which was an important

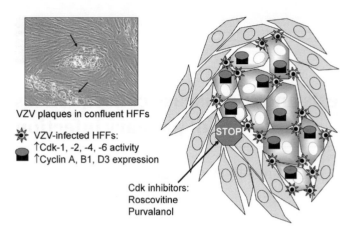

Fig. 37.1. Activation of host cyclin-dependent kinases in VZV-infected fibroblasts. VZV infects quiescent cells such as dermal fibroblasts (HFFs) to cause skin lesions. The photo of VZV plaques in HFFs (arrows) shows that the infected cells are rounded and have not fused into syncytia, though they are adherent (magnification, 10X). The uninfected cells are confluent and contact inhibited. Since they are not dividing, HFFs express basal levels of cyclin D3, and the cyclin-dependent kinases (Cdks) are inactive. Upon infection with VZV, unscheduled cyclin expression results in high levels of cyclins A, B1, and D3, which does not reflect a normal phase of the cell cycle. In association with these cyclins, several cdks are activated in VZV-infected HFFs: Cdk-1, −2, −4, and −6 (depicted as oval/rectangle heterodimers). It is not known how VZV infection dysregulates cdks or how this favors virus replication. However, when cdk activity is inhibited with roscovitine or purvalanol, VZV spread is reversibly blocked, and viral DNA synthesis is shut off. (Adapted from (Moffat et al., 2004b), photo provided by Stacey Leisenfelder.)

observation because VZV replication in vitro is highly cell-associated. VZV-infected skin implants exhibited epidermal lesions that were indistinguishable from the characteristic lesions of varicella. Experiments with VZV mutants in the SCIDhu model indicate that VZV is challenged to employ more gene functions to replicate successfully in skin and T-cells in vivo, because the cellular environment in intact tissues is fundamentally different from that in cultured cells. Host cell factors such as innate immunity, cellular kinase activation, cellular transactivating proteins and protein trafficking pathways, are likely to affect virulence such that the full range of VZV gene products is needed to modify the tissue environment for effective viral pathogenesis.

Information about the molecular pathogenesis of VZV has been obtained by generating VZV recombinants with selected mutations in the viral genome using cosmid systems. Sets of four or five cosmids have been derived using genomic DNA from the parent Oka strain, pOka, a clinical isolate from Japan from which the live, attenuated varicella vaccine virus, vOka, was made (Niizuma et al., 2003) and from the vOka strains used by Merck & Co., Inc. (Kemble et al., 2000) and the strain deposited at the American Type Culture Collection (Cohen and Seidel, 1993). To obtain mutant viruses, alterations are made in selected VZV open reading frames (ORFs) and introduced into the cosmid that carries the gene of interest. The altered cosmid and the three or four other cosmids are transfected or transduced together into human melanoma cells. Homologous recombination between overlapping sequences generates an intact VZV genome, and if the mutation is not lethal, the virus propagates by cell-cell spread and plaques appear in the transfected cells. To discern phenotypes beyond lethality, mutant viruses are compared to isogenic parent viruses and a repaired strain, also made from cosmids. These "matched sets" of mutant, parent, and repaired viruses are evaluated in vitro using primary cell cultures and in the SCIDhu model in vivo.

Effects of VZV replication on cellular cyclin-dependent kinases and cyclins

The primary reason why VZV pathogenesis must be studied in vivo using the SCIDhu model is that the intracellular environment in human skin and thymus tissues differs greatly from the conditions in cultured cells. VZV is commonly cultivated in human melanoma cells (MeWo) or in subconfluent human fibroblasts (HFF, HELF, MRC-5, WI-38) that contain abundant metabolic precursors and enzymes involved in cell growth and division. In contrast, dermal fibroblasts, differentiated keratinocytes, and single-positive CD4+ or CD8+ T cells in xenografts in SCIDhu mice are not dividing. In these quiescent cells, regulatory proteins such as Rb and p27 suppress biosynthetic pathways for DNA replication and cell division by inhibiting transcription of cyclins and the activity of cyclin-dependent kinases (CDKs) (Olashaw and Pledger, 2002). VZV infection subverts these suppression mechanisms in an unknown manner and causes unscheduled cyclin expression and dysregulation of cyclin-dependent kinases (Fig. 37.1). In VZV-infected, confluent HFFs, high levels of CDK activity are associated with simultaneous expression of cyclins A, B1, and D3 (Leisenfelder and Moffat, 2006). This unusual protein profile is likely induced by VZV since it does not correspond with CDK and cyclin expression patterns found in cellular G0/1, S, G2, or M phases.

VZV alters the intracellular environment of resting cells by inducing kinase activity, an effect that appears to be an essential step in virus replication because compounds that inhibit CDK activity prevent VZV spread. Roscovitine and purvalanol A are specific inhibitors of CDKs 1, 2, 5, 7, and 9 that have potent antiviral effects on VZV and other viruses (Moffat et al., 2004b; Taylor et al., 2004). Interestingly, as little as 5μM roscovitine or 2μM purvalanol is needed to prevent VZV replication and yet 10-fold more is needed to cause cell cycle arrest in MeWo cells. Thus VZV is acutely sensitive to levels of CDK activity, which the virus may utilize for initiation of transcription from viral promoters (CDK7 and CDK9), phosphorylation of the C-terminus of glycoprotein I (CDK1) (Ye et al., 1999), and for numerous potential viral and cellular protein targets. An important role for kinase activity associated with cyclin B, presumably CDK1, is phosphorylation of IE62 since these proteins interact in the cytoplasm. Recognition sites for CDK1 are plentiful in IE62, and point mutagenesis confirmed that several are targeted by the kinase in vitro (Leisenfelder and Moffat, unpublished observations).

Investigation of events in the pathogenesis of primary VZV infection in the SCIDhu model

The clinical experience documents that primary VZV infection is initiated by inoculation of the respiratory mucosal epithelium and that the varicella rash appears after a 10–21 day incubation period (Arvin, 2001a; Cohen and Straus, 2001). Given the extreme host-range restriction of VZV, concepts about the pathogenesis of primary VZV infection have been derived from the sequence of events during primary mousepox infection (Grose, 1981). Based on this model, VZV has been thought to reach mononuclear cells in regional lymph nodes, causing a primary viremia that transports the virus to reticuloendothelial organs, such as the liver, for a phase of viral amplification. The theory has been that this amplification stage is followed by a secondary viremia in the late incubation period that carries VZV to skin sites. Recently, work using the SCIDhu model has provided experimental evidence to refine hypotheses about primary VZV pathogenesis (Ku et al., 2004). According to our new model of VZV pathogenesis, VZV tropism for T-cells may facilitate viral transfer to skin (Fig. 37.2). Previous investigations in cultured cells demonstrated that T cells could be infected with VZV (Koropchak et al., 1989; Soong et al., 2000) and that tonsil T-cells, especially activated, memory subpopulations, are highly permissive for VZV infection (Ku et al., 2002). In addition, VZV preferentially infected the activated, memory CD4+ T-cells that constitute >20% of tonsil T-cells. T-cell sub-populations that expressed the skin homing markers, cutaneous leukocyte antigen (CLA), and chemokine receptor CCR4, were also more likely to be infected and VZV did not disrupt the important chemotaxis functions of these cells. In order to investigate the hypothesis that VZV could be transferred to skin by tonsil T-cells, VZV-infected human tonsil T-cells were adoptively transferred to SCIDhu mice via intravenous injection (Ku et al., 2004). The microcirculation within these skin xenografts is formed by human CD31+ endothelial cells, which permits interaction with human T-cells. CD3+ T cells were detected within the epidermis, dermis and around the hair follicles in skin tissues within 24 h after injection into the mouse circulation. T-cells expressing the memory marker, CD45RO, were the predominant population. When skin xenografts were harvested at intervals after inoculation of infected T-cells, characteristic cutaneous VZV lesions were formed and progressed in size and production of infectious virus over 10–21 days. Intravenous injection of VZV-infected fibroblasts did not result in VZV transfer into skin xenografts. T-cell transfer of the virus resulted in lesions expressing the VZV proteins needed for lytic infection, such as the major immediate early ORF62 (IE62) transactivator, the ORF47 kinase and glycoprotein E (gE). VZV infection of skin resulted in extensive formation of multi-nucleated polykaryocytes, a gradual thickening of the epidermis, epidermal cell proliferation, destruction of basement membranes, and cellular degeneration. Foci of VZV-infected cells eventually extended up to surface keratinocytes but only after 14–21 days. Infectious VZV was produced throughout this period of progressive cutaneous lesion formation. Thus, the time required for VZV lesions to penetrate through the keratinocyte layer at the skin surface implies that VZV must reach cutaneous sites of replication at an early, rather than a late stage of the incubation period.

VZV alters the intracellular environment and produces lytic infection within 2 days in cultured cells in vitro. In contrast, VZV infection in skin xenografts evolved much more slowly. These observations suggested that innate immune mechanisms within the intact cutaneous tissue microenvironment in vivo might modulate VZV replication. Analyses of skin xenografts showed that interferon-α (IFN-α) and interleukin 1-α (IL-1α) were expressed constitutively in the cytoplasm of epidermal cells in uninfected skin (Ku et al., 2002). After VZV infection, IL-1α was translocated to the nuclei of cells expressing VZV proteins, but remained in the cytoplasm of adjacent, uninfected cells. TNF-α expression was not present in uninfected skin and was not induced by VZV infection. Importantly, interferon-α (IFN-α) was not expressed in VZV-infected cells but was up-regulated in neighboring uninfected epidermal cells within the skin

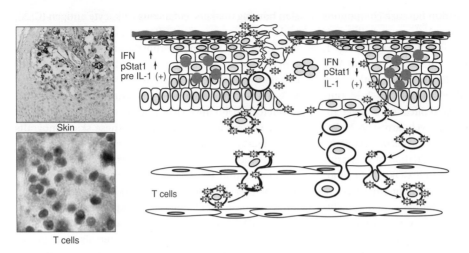

Fig. 37.2. A model of the pathogenesis of primary VZV infection. This figure illustrates new concepts about VZV pathogenesis and immunobiology that have emerged from experiments in the SCIDhu mouse model. The upper left panel shows the appearance of a mature VZV lesion in a SCIDhu skin xenograft, stained for VZV protein expression with a polyclonal human anti-VZV IgG antiserum. The lower left panel shows VZV infection of T-cells in a SCIDhu T-cell xenograft, detected by *in situ* hybridization with a VZV DNA probe. The right panel is a diagram depicting proposed events in the pathogenesis of VZV infection of skin. According to this model, T-cells within the tonsil lymphoid tissues become infected by VZV transfer into these migratory cells of the immune system following the initial inoculation of respiratory epithelial cells with the virus. Infected T-cells enter the circulation and transport the virus to the skin shortly thereafter, exiting through capillary endothelium by the usual mechanisms for trafficking of migratory T-cells. The infected T-cells then release infectious VZV at skin sites of replication. The remainder of the 10–21-day incubation period is the interval required for VZV to overcome the innate IFN-α response in enough epidermal cells to create the typical vesicular lesions containing VZV at the skin surface, as shown in the upper left panel. Signaling of enhanced IFN-α production in adjacent skin cells prevents a rapid, uncontrolled cell-cell spread of VZV. Additional crops of varicella lesions may result when T-cells traffic through early stage cutaneous lesions, become infected and produce a secondary viremia. This process continues until host immune responses trigger the up-regulation of adhesion molecules and mediates the clearance of the virus by VZV-specific antiviral T-cells. (Adapted from Ku *et al.*, 2004.)

xenograft. The phosphorylation state of Stat1 protein is a marker for activation or suppression of the IFN-α pathway because IFN-α binding to its receptors induces Stat1 phosphorylation by JAK kinases. Without phosphorylation, Stat1 is not translocated to cell nuclei and production of IFN-α does not occur. In VZV-infected skin, phosphorylated Stat1 was localized to nuclei in neighboring uninfected epidermal cells, but it was not detected in cells expressing VZV proteins. In uninfected skin, Stat1 was not phosphorylated and Stat1 and IFN-α remained cytoplasmic. Another mediator of the innate immune response, the transcription factor NF-κB, also remained in the cytoplasm of VZV-infected skin cells in SCIDhu implants (Jones and Arvin, 2006). These experiments indicated that VZV replication was associated with expression of a gene product(s) that inhibited antiviral IFN-α production in foci of infected skin cells in vivo by interference with Stat1 activation. To further document the role of the IFN-α response in regulating VZV infection and cell-cell spread between epidermal cells within intact skin tissue in vivo, skin xenografts were inoculated with VZV and SCIDhu mice were given neutralizing antibody against the human IFN-α/β receptor, in order to block type I IFN activity. In these experiments, infectious VZV titers were ten-fold higher in skin specimens when IFN signaling was inhibited by receptor blocking and the cutaneous lesions were substantially larger.

Because SCID mice lack the capacity to develop an adaptive, antigen-specific immune response, the progression of VZV infection in skin xenografts is controlled only by innate immunity. In the intact human host, biopsies of varicella skin lesions show a local inflammatory response surrounding the infected cells. The migration of immune cells into damaged tissues is signaled by the up-regulation of adhesion molecules on the vascular endothelial cells. Comparative analyses of infected skin xenografts and human VZV lesion biopsies permitted an examination of whether these changes could be induced by viral replication *per se*. Cutaneous lesions in patients biopsied at the onset of the varicella rash showed extensive expression of E-selectin, ICAM-1, and VCAM-1, whereas these proteins were not detected in capillaries of infected skin xenografts. Many infiltrating mononuclear cells were detected, most of which expressed CD4 or CD8, and included predominantly CD45RO+ memory T-cells and skin homing CLA+ and CCR4+ T-cells. In contrast, adoptive transfer of PBMC to SCIDhu mice showed no enrichment for these effector T-cell populations in VZV infected skin. These differences in adhesion molecule expression and in mononuclear cell profiles in VZV lesion biopsies and in VZV-infected skin xenografts suggested that recruitment and/or retention of inflammatory T-cells required signals provided by host cellular immunity.

Considered together, data showing VZV infection of T cells in vitro (Ku et al., 2002; Soong et al., 2000) and these experiments in the SCIDhu model suggest that T-cell tropism plays an essential role in VZV pathogenesis. The prolonged varicella incubation period appears to represent the time required for VZV to overcome previously unrecognized, but potent innate antiviral responses, especially IFN-α production, mediated directly by epidermal cells in vivo. The initial phase of VZV pathogenesis is also likely to be facilitated by the failure of VZV to trigger up-regulation of inflammatory adhesion molecules on capillary endothelial cells in skin and virus-mediated modulation of MHC I and MHC II expression (see elsewhere in this volume).

The role of VZV glycoproteins in T-cell and skin tropism

As is true of all herpesviruses, VZV glycoproteins have multiple functions that affect tissue tropism both within cells during virus assembly, and outside cells when they are expressed on plasma membranes and virion envelopes. VZV encodes glycoproteins designated gB, gC, gE, gH, gI, gK, gL, gM and gN. However, characterization of the functions of most of these proteins is limited. VZV is unique among the alphaherpesviruses in having no gD homologue. In transfected and VZV-infected cells, glycoproteins form gE/gI and gH/gL heterodimers and gE homodimers; noncovalent interactions between gB/gE and gH/gE have also been identified (Cole and Grose, 2003). Recycling of glycoproteins from the cell surface to the trans-Golgi network (TGN) is regulated to balance envelopment in the TGN, where infectious virions are formed, with the cell fusion that spreads VZV genomes to neighboring cells even when formation of intact virion particles is limited. The VZV glycoproteins, gB, gC, gE, gH, gI, gK, and gL have been shown to be or are likely to be structural components of the virus (Cohen and Straus, 2001; Mo et al., 1999, 2002). In addition to studies of the glycoproteins using expression systems, deletions or targeted mutations of these genes that are not lethal have yielded recombinant VZV mutants for investigation of glycoprotein function in cultured cells and in SCIDhu T cell and skin xenografts in vivo. VZV gB, gE and gK have been demonstrated to be essential for VZV replication in cultured cells, based on failure to generate infectious virus from cosmids with deletions of these genes, and the rescue of infectivity when the deletion is complemented by insertion of the gene into a non-native site and in cell lines. In the SCIDhu model, interactions between VZV glycoproteins at internal sites of virion assembly and surface membranes determine the ability of VZV to replicate in differentiated human T-cells and skin. This summary focuses particularly on evaluations of the contributions of VZV glycoproteins to viral pathogenesis in T-cell and skin xenografts in vivo.

Glycoprotein C

VZV gC is the product of ORF14 (Davison and Scott, 1986). The role of gC in infectivity for human skin was assessed using gC negative mutants of vOka and VZV-Ellen (Moffat et al., 1998). Whereas all of these VZV strains replicated well in tissue culture, only low passage clinical isolates were fully virulent in skin, as shown by infectious virus yields and analysis of xenografts for VZV DNA and viral protein synthesis. All strains except the gC-null Ellen strain retained some capacity to replicate in human skin, but cell-free virus was recovered only from xenografts infected with pOka or VZV-S. An HSV-1 mutant lacking gC expression was also deficient in skin infectivity. These SCID-hu mouse experiments show that gC, which is dispensable for replication in tissue culture, plays a critical role in the virulence of the human alphaherpesviruses, VZV and HSV-1, for human skin.

Glycoprotein E

Whereas the homologous protein in the other alphaherpesviruses is dispensable in cultured cells, VZV gE, encoded by ORF68, is essential for replication (Ku et al., 2002). The functions of gE were analyzed further by creating point mutations or deleting the short 62 amino acid C-terminal domain (Moffat et al., 2004a). These mutants were designed based on observations about functional motifs made using gE expression systems (Cole and Grose, 2003). Mutations were introduced in YAGL (aa582–585), which mediates gE endocytosis, AYRV (aa568–571), the motif that targets gE to the trans-Golgi network (TGN), and SSTT, which is an "acid cluster" comprising a phosphorylation motif (aa588–601). A substitution Y582G in YAGL prevented gE endocytosis, and the Y569A mutation interfered with gE shuttling from the Golgi to the TGN in reports using transient expression methods. These changes were introduced into the viral genome using VZV cosmids and residues S593, S595, T596, and T598 were changed to alanines to alter phosphorylation. These experiments demonstrated a hierarchy in the contributions of gE C-terminal motifs to VZV replication in vitro and to virulence in the SCIDhu model. Deleting the gE C-terminus or mutating the YAGL motif were lethal for VZV replication in vitro. Mutations of AYRV and SSTT were compatible with recovery of VZV, but the AYRV mutation resulted in decreased plaque size and virus production in vitro. When the rOka-gE-AYRV and rOka-gE-SSTT mutants were evaluated in skin and T cell xenografts in SCIDhu mice, interference with TGN targeting was associated with substantial attenuation, especially in skin, whereas the SSTT mutation did not alter VZV infectivity in vivo. Thus, the gE C-terminus contains domains that are essential for VZV replication or are determinants of VZV virulence in differentiated dermal and epidermal cells and T-cells within intact tissue microenvironments in vivo. In addition to C-terminal functions, VZV gE has a unique N-terminal region from amino acids 1–188 (Berarducci et al., 2006). Mutagenesis of this gE ectodomain region identified subdomains essential for replication, cell-cell spread and secondary envelopment and for VZV skin tropism.

Whereas VZV has been considered to be highly antigenically stable, VZV-MSP is a recently discovered wild type virus that has lost an immunodominant B-cell epitope in the gE ectodomain (Mo et al., 2002). This gE "escape mutant" virus exhibited an unusual pattern of egress. When VZV-MSP was evaluated in SCIDhu skin xenografts, the spread of the VZV-MSP variant was accelerated significantly. The cytopathologic changes produced after 21 days by isolates that had the prototypical gE sequence were demonstrated at 14 days in skin xenografts infected with VZV-MSP. Thus, VZV-MSP is a naturally occurring variant with a gE mutation that is associated with a phenotype of enhanced cell–cell spread in vitro and in vivo.

Glycoprotein I

VZV mutants with deletions of gI, encoded by ORF67, can replicate in melanoma cells and fibroblasts, although not in Vero cells (Cohen and Nguyen, 1997; Mallory et al., 1997). Since gI was dispensable in cell culture, gI deletion mutants were evaluated for their capacity to infect human cells in SCIDhu xenografts. Deleting gI was lethal for VZV replication in differentiated skin and T cells in vivo (Moffat et al., 2002). Restoring gI into the mutated VZV genome was associated with the recovery of VZV virulence. Thus, gI is essential for VZV pathogenesis.

Analyses of the gI promoter in expression systems has demonstrated that it contains an activating upstream sequence (AUS) that binds cellular transcription factors Sp1 and USF (Specificity factor 1, Upstream Stimulatory Factor), and the viral transactivator ORF29 DNA binding protein which mediates enhancement of immediate early 62 (IE62)-induced transcription (He et al., 2001). This information was used to design mutants from VZV cosmids in order to evaluate the contributions of these motifs to VZV replication in vitro and in vivo (Ito et al., 2003). Recombinants rOkagI-Sp1 and rOkagI-USF, with two substitutions in Sp1 or USF sites, replicated like rOka in vitro, but infectivity of rOkagI-Sp1 was significantly impaired in skin and T cells in vivo. A double mutant, rOKAgI-Sp1/USF, did not replicate in skin, but yielded low titers of infectious virus in T-cells. The repair, rOkagI:rep-Sp1/USF, was as infectious as rOka. Thus, disrupting gI promoter sites for cellular transactivators altered VZV virulence in vivo, with variable consequences related to the cellular factor and the host cell type. Mutations in the ORF29 responsive element of the gI promoter were made by substituting each of four 10 base pair blocks in this region with a 10 base pair sequence, GATAACTACA, that was predicted to interfere with enhancer effects of the ORF29 protein. One of these mutants, designated rOKAgI-29RE-3, had diminished replication in skin and T-cells, indicating that ORF29 protein-mediated enhancement of gI expression contributes to VZV virulence. These experiments demonstrated that VZV pathogenesis is influenced by interactions of cellular transactivators with the gI promoter. Significantly, comparisons of the effects of the gI promoter mutants on growth in skin and T-cells indicated that cellular transactivators can have consequences for virulence that are cell-type specific. Mutations within promoters of viral genes that are non-essential in vitro should allow construction of recombinant herpesviruses that have altered virulence in specific host cells in vivo, and may be useful for designing herpesvirus gene therapy vectors and attenuated vaccines.

The role of regulatory proteins and viral kinases in T-cell and skin tropism

Although the difficulty of generating sufficient quantities of infectious cell-free virus has prevented experimental analysis, VZV replication is presumed to occur through a sequential expression of immediate early, early and late genes (Chapter 10). VZV regulatory proteins include viral transactivating proteins and viral kinases, which may also be structural components of the virion tegument. While the task is far from complete, some of these genes have been analyzed for their contributions to VZV replication in cultured cells and in the SCIDhu model of VZV pathogenesis in vivo.

IE62 protein

The IE62 protein is the major VZV transactivating protein, required for expression of all viral genes tested to date (Kinchington et al., 1992, 1994). It is encoded by the duplicated genes, ORF62 and ORF71. Experiments in which pOka cosmids were mutated to delete ORF62, ORF71, or the ORF62/71 gene pair demonstrated that at least one copy of ORF62 was required for VZV replication, as expected (Sato et al., 2003a). Restoring a single copy of ORF62 into a non-native site in the U_S region of the VZV genome resulted in some, albeit reduced, VZV replication in vitro. VZV replication persisted despite introducing targeted mutations in IE62 binding sites that mediate interaction with the IE4 protein. Related experiments demonstrated that the ORF4 gene is essential in VZV (Sato et al., 2003b). Interestingly, when a single copy of ORF62 or ORF71 was deleted, recombination events during cosmid transfection repaired the defective repeat region in some progeny viruses. Mixtures of single copy rOkaΔ62 or rOkaΔ71 and repaired rOka generated by recombination of the single copy deletion mutants was detected in some skin xenografts infected with these recombinants. The diminished replication of the pOka mutants with a single copy of ORF62 at the non-native site was associated with a complete block in VZV infection of skin xenografts in vivo. Although insertion of ORF62 into the non-native site permitted replication in cell culture, ORF62 expression from its native site was necessary for cell-cell spread in differentiated human skin tissues in vivo.

IE63 protein

The IE63 protein is encoded by ORF63 and is duplicated in the VZV genome as ORF70. IE63 protein is a nuclear phosphoprotein with some homology to HSV-1 ICP22. Sequence analysis indicates that IE63 is related to HSV-1 $U_S1.5$ protein, which is expressed colinearly with ICP22 (U_S1) (Baiker et al., 2004). Removing one copy of the duplicated gene, either ORF63 or ORF70, was compatible with VZV replication in vitro (Sommer et al., 2001). VZV was not recovered from transfections done with a dual deletion cosmid, but infectious virus was generated when ORF63 was cloned into the non-native site in the Us region. IE63 protein interacts directly with ORF62, the major immediate early transactivating protein of VZV. The importance of IE62 protein for VZV replication is suggested by the observation that ORF63/ORF70 could be removed and yield infectious virus in vitro if deleted cosmids were transfected along with a plasmid expressing IE62 (Cohen et al., 2004).

The potential functional domains of IE63 protein were analyzed by creating 22 ORF63 mutations in expression plasmids and in the VZV genome. The effects of IE63 phosphorylation and nuclear localization, and IE63 binding to IE62, were evaluated by transient transfection and by replication of the mutant viruses. Briefly, IE63 aa55–67 constituted the IE62 binding site, with R59/L60 being critical residues; S165, S173 and S185 in the IE63 center region were phosphorylated by cellular kinases; and mutations in two putative nuclear localization signal (NLS) sequences changed intracellular IE63 distribution from a nuclear to a cytoplasmic/nuclear pattern. Infectious VZV was recovered with three of the 22 mutations in ORF63. Each of these three IE63 mutants had a single alanine substitution (T171A, S181A or S185A). The IE63 mutants, rOka/ORF63rev[T171], rOka/ORF63rev[S181] and rOka/ORF63rev[S185], replicated less efficiently, had a small plaque phenotype in vitro and had less production of gE and ORF47, indicating that IE63 was involved in expression of these early and late gene products. Virulence of the three IE63 mutants was reduced markedly in skin xenografts, but infection of T-cell xenografts was not affected. The fact that these IE63 mutants were attenuated in skin but not T-cells, suggests that the contribution of the IE63 tegument/regulatory protein to VZV pathogenesis differs depending on the human cell types and tissues that are targeted for infection.

ORF64 protein

ORF64 is duplicated as ORF69 and it has some sequence homology to the HSV-1 Us10 gene, which exists as a single copy. When ORF64 and ORF69 were deleted, either separately or together, one copy at either location in the genome was sufficient to yield infectious virus with growth kinetics and plaque morphology indistinguishable from the parent virus (Sommer et al., 2001). Removing both ORF64 and ORF69 caused an abnormal plaque phenotype made up of very large multinucleated syncytia. Single and dual ORF64/ORF69 mutants were as infectious as the parent and repaired viruses when evaluated in human T-cells in vitro and in human skin xenografts in the SCIDhu mouse model of VZV pathogenesis.

ORF10 Protein

ORF10 encodes a tegument protein that enhances transactivation of VZV genes. Analysis of pOkaΔ10 and ORF10 point mutants with disruption of the acidic activation domain and the putative motif for binding human cellular factor-1 (HCF-1) showed no effects on replication, IE gene transcription or virion assembly in vitro (Che et al., 2006). However, epidermal cells in SCIDhu skin xenografts infected with pOkaΔ10 had significantly fewer DNA-containing nucleocapsids and complete virions; extensive aggregates of intracytoplasmic viral particles were also observed. Altering the activation or the putative HCF-1 domains of ORF10 protein had no consequences for VZV skin infection. Deleting ORF10 did not impair VZV T-cell tropism in vivo. Thus, ORF10 protein is necessary for efficient VZ virion assembly and is a VZV virulence determinant in epidermal and dermal cells in vivo.

ORF47 protein

ORF47 encodes a serine/threonine protein kinase that is in a class of conserved herpesvirus proteins that are homologous to HSV-1 $U_L 13$. ORF47 protein also has similarities to the casein kinase II family of cellular proteins (Cole and Grose, 2003). ORF47 appears to be a component of the virion tegument. VZV mutants that did not express ORF47 protein were made by inserting stop codons into the gene, producing ROka47S, which was shown to replicate as well as intact ROka in an infectious focus assay (Heineman et al., 1996). However, these findings were not predictive of the consequences of blocking ORF47 protein synthesis in vivo, since ORF47 protein was essential for VZV infection of human T cells and skin (Moffat et al., 1998). Restoring ORF47 into the genome of the ROKA47S mutant reconstituted the T cell and skin tropism of the virus. Thus, ORF47 protein functions are necessary in differentiated cells that are involved in VZV pathogenesis in vivo.

In order to further investigate the role of the ORF47 protein, VZV mutants were made that expressed a truncated ORF47 protein, by deleting the C-terminus, and that had mutations that disrupted conserved putative kinase motifs in ORF47 protein (Besser et al., 2003). The mutants were tested for replication, phosphorylation and protein-protein interactions in vitro and allowed an assessment of the effects of specifically eliminating the kinase activity of ORF47 protein on VZV replication in vivo. The ORF47 C-terminal truncation mutants (rOka47ΔC) and those that disrupted the DYS kinase motif (rOka47D-N) had no ORF47 kinase activity. However, binding to IE62 protein was mapped to the N-terminal domain and was preserved. Cells infected with these ORF47 kinase defective mutants exhibited marked nuclear retention of ORF47 and IE62 proteins in vitro. Even though virus titers were not altered based on an infectious focus assay, the electron microscopy analysis of cultured cells infected with the kinase defective mutants showed severely impaired virion assembly and transport of virions to cell surfaces. Normal VZV virion assembly appears to require ORF47 kinase function. Nevertheless, rOka47ΔC or rOka47D-N-infected cells showed VZV-induced cell fusion and syncytia formation.

With regard to pathogenesis, ORF47 protein mutations that eliminated the ORF47 kinase function caused substantial reductions in the capacity to replicate and produce cutaneous lesions in skin xenografts in the SCIDhu model. However, in contrast to the complete ORF47 null mutant, rOKA47S, some replication occurred in skin in vivo if the capacity of ORF47 protein to bind IE62 protein was intact, as shown in experiments with rOka47ΔC and rOka47D-N. ORF47 kinase activity was important for VZV infection and cell-cell spread in human skin in vivo, but preserving the capacity of ORF47 protein to form complexes with IE62 protein, both of which are VZV tegument components, appeared to be the *sine qua non* for VZV infection of skin in vivo. In contrast to the skin experiments, when the kinase defective rOka47ΔC and rOka47D-N mutants were evaluated in T-cell xenografts, no infectious virus was made in vivo (Besser et al., 2004). These observations were similar to the data obtained in T-cell xenografts infected with ROka47S, when no ORF47 protein was made. The comparison of the growth of kinase-defective ORF47 mutants in skin vs. T-cells suggested the hypothesis that fundamental requirements for VZV pathogenesis in skin and T-cells differ in vivo. Even though virion assembly was much diminished and intracellular trafficking of ORF47 and IE62 proteins, both components of the tegument, and of gE, was aberrant in skin in the absence of ORF47 kinase activity, VZV polykaryocytes were generated by rOka47ΔC and rOka47D-N. Thus, some cell fusion was induced by ORF47 mutants in skin and cell–cell spread occurred even though virion formation was deficient. In contrast, impaired virion assembly by ORF47 mutants was associated with a complete elimination of the capacity to infect T-cells in vivo. Since VZV-infected T-cells do not undergo cell fusion even when most cells in the T cell xenograft have been infected, transfer of incomplete virions by cell–cell fusion does not occur. Instead, virus appears to be released from T-cells for entry into uninfected T-cells in other regions of the xenograft. Considered together, these observations make it plausible to suggest that formation of complete virions and their release is essential for VZV T-cell tropism, creating a differential requirement for virion assembly during the pathogenesis of VZV infection of T-cells and skin.

ORF66 protein

ORF66 encodes a second serine/threonine protein kinase homologous to HSV U_S 3. Like the ORF47 protein kinase, ORF66 protein was shown to be dispensable for VZV replication in cultured cells by creating ROka66S stop codon mutants. Again, ROka66 mutants replicated as well as intact ROka in cultured cells. Eliminating ORF66 expression did not impair replication in SCIDhu skin xenografts, as compared to the vaccine-derived ROka parent (Moffat et al., 1998). In contrast, ORF66 defective VZV mutants had a significant decrease in their capacity to replicate in T-cell xenografts in vivo. Thus, ORF66 protein appears to be a viral kinase that is necessary to VZV T-cell tropism. When ORF66 expression was blocked in pOka, growth and VZ virion formation was reduced in T-cells in vivo, infected T-cells were more susceptible to apoptosis and pOka66S mutants had less capacity to interfere with induction of the interferon (IFN) signaling pathway (Schaap et al., 2005). Thus, ORF66 kinase appears to have a unique role during T-cell infection and supports VZV T cell tropism by contributing to immune evasion and enhancing survival of infected T-cells.

Disease consequences of primary VZV infection in healthy and immunocompromised hosts

The clinical pattern of primary VZV infection is highly predictable, beginning with an incubation period of 10–21 days following a close exposure of a susceptible individual to another person with varicella or in some cases, herpes zoster (Arvin, 2001b). In contrast to other herpesviruses, primary VZV infection almost always causes symptoms although the diagnosis is missed when the child has only a few lesions and no identified exposure. Varicella often begins with a prodrome of fever, malaise, headache and abdominal pain. These initial symptoms last about 24–48 hours before skin vesicles are noted and are more common in older children and adults. The occurrence of a cell-associated VZV viremia has been well documented during the last few days of the incubation period and for a few days after the cutaneous rash appears, when specimens are tested by tissue culture or for VZV DNA (Asano et al., 1990; Gershon et al., 1978; Koropchak et al., 1989, 1991; Ozaki et al., 1986). Viral cultures of PBMC demonstrate that infectious virus can be recovered from PBMC; VZV was isolated from 11%–24% of PBMC samples taken from healthy individuals with varicella less than 24 h after the rash had appeared. DNA methods are more sensitive, with VZV being detected in 67%–74% of samples tested by in situ hybridization or PCR. Although viral cultures do not yield infectious virus, PCR methods indicate that VZV is present in oropharyngeal specimens just before and after the appearance of skin lesions. The estimated frequency of VZV infection of PBMC from healthy individuals with varicella was approximately 0.01%–0.001%, as detected by in situ hybridization (Koropchak et al., 1989). According to our proposed model of the pathogenesis of primary VZV, this viremic phase may represent the infection of T cells migrating through infected skin sites and re-entering the circulation (Fig. 37.1). This early phase of the illness is usually associated with systemic symptoms, including fever and fatigue, presumably related to cytokine responses; varicella-related fever is usually mild (less than 101.5 °F). The cell-associated VZV viremia is transient, usually resolving within 24–72 hours after the onset of the rash in healthy children and adults. Primary VZV infection is often accompanied by a reduction in the numbers of circulating lymphocytes but this finding is probably secondary, rather than being due to cell destruction by the virus. Mild upper respiratory symptoms and diarrhea may occur but severe respiratory or gastrointestinal illness is rare.

The lesions caused by VZV replication in the skin appear first as small erythematous papules, each of which then evolves within about 12–24 hours to surface vesicles that are filled with clear fluid and surrounded by erythema – the so-called "dew drop on a rose petal." The first skin lesions in patients with varicella often appear on the face and scalp, or on the chest or back and are pruritic. Formation of multinucleated epithelial cells with intranuclear eosinophilic inclusions and vasculitis involving small blood vessels occurs during the early maculopapular stage. VZV virions are detected in keratinocytes and also in capillary endothelial cells by electron microscopy. VZV is delivered to mucous membrane sites as well as to skin, where it produces ulcers in the oropharynx, conjunctivae and vagina. Vesicles result from a progressive ballooning degeneration of epithelial cells and coalescence of fluid-filled vacuoles between cells. The numbers of VZV-infected cells at the base of the lesion increases during this phase and cell-free virus is released into vesicular fluid. Each lesion begins to become cloudy and crusted within about 48 hours and infectious virus is usually no longer detected after about 72–96 hours. Healing reflects the replacement of epithelial cells at the base of the lesion by cellular proliferation. New skin and mucous membrane lesions continue to develop for a period of 3–5 days in most children, with a range of 1–7 days. Over the 1–7 day course of primary VZV infection, as few as 10 to more than 1500 lesions may appear; on average, healthy children have about 100–300 lesions. Older children and adults, those who are secondary household cases and patients with skin trauma, such as sunburn or eczema are more likely to have more cutaneous and mucous membrane lesions. The crops of lesions that appear later in the clinical course of varicella are usually on the arms and legs. Vesicle formation may be abortive, with little or no infectious virus being detected, presumably due to the induction of antigen-specific T cells by this point in the infection (Chapter 39). VZV lesions are usually superficial and do not leave scars except at the sites of the earliest skin replication; residual scars can often be seen along the hairline or eyebrows.

Secondary bacterial infection of skin lesions is the most common complication of primary VZV infection in healthy children. These infections are most often due to *Staphylococcus aureus* or *Streptococcus pyogenes* (group A beta-hemolytic streptococcus) (Dunkle *et al.*, 1991; Jackson *et al.*, 1992). Skin and mucosal damage may provide a portal of entry for these organisms such that bacteremia occurs and the organisms reach deep tissue sites. Thus, varicella may be associated with staphylococcal or streptococcal pneumonia, arthritis or osteomyelitis. Varicella lesions often involve the eyelids and ocular conjunctivae but serious eye complications are rare; unilateral anterior uveitis or corneal lesions may develop but long-term damage is unusual (Liesegang, 1991).

VZV has the capacity to infect the epithelial cells that line the pulmonary alveoli, and to induce edema and an extensive infiltration of mononuclear cells into the alveolar septae. The result of this process can be a severe viral pneumonia. Active VZV replication in the lungs is very unusual in healthy children with varicella. However, the increased morbidity and mortality caused by primary VZV infection in adults is accounted for by their much greater susceptibility to varicella pneumonia (Krugman *et al.*, 1957). Interstitial inflammation and the desquamation of alveolar lining cells into the alveoli has the potential to block the effective transfer of oxygen from the alveolar spaces into the pulmonary capillaries. The consequence is severe hypoxemia and respiratory failure. Most patients with varicella pneumonia develop cough and dyspnea several days after the onset of the cutaneous rash, which suggests that the virus reaches pulmonary epithelial sites during the later viremic phase. Physical abnormalities associated with varicella pneumonia may be difficult to detect because early signs are often limited to fever and tachypnea. The chest radiograph usually shows interstitial pneumonitis with diffuse bilateral infiltrates and perihilar nodular densities but may appear relatively benign even when patients have severe hypoxia. Severe varicella pneumonia may be fatal even with antiviral therapy (Chapter 65) and assisted ventilation.

Healthy children with varicella often have mild, sub clinical hepatitis, detected by minor abnormalities of liver function tests. These abnormalities may reflect an inflammatory response or some limited viral replication in the liver during primary VZV infection. Liver involvement is usually asymptomatic but children with the highest elevation of liver function tests may have severe vomiting. Extensive VZV infection of hepatocytes, with widespread hepatocellular destruction due to virus-induced cell lysis is a rare occurrence but is associated with fulminant hepatic failure.

In addition to its neurotropism for cells in the sensory ganglia, VZV can cause encephalitis and cerebellar ataxia. Meningoencephalitis and cerebellar ataxia are the major clinical signs of VZV-related damage to the central nervous system; some patients have signs of both cerebral and cerebellar disease (Johnson and Milbourn, 1970; Peters *et al.*, 1978). VZV was the cause of encephalitis in 13% of cases of defined etiology in CDC surveillance studies from 1972 and 1977. Although these syndromes are the most common neurologic complications of varicella, information about the pathogenesis of these disorders is limited because most children recover. How primary VZV infection might produce cerebellar ataxia is of interest because VZV is the most common cause of this syndrome in healthy children. VZV has been recovered from the brain tissue of immunocompromised children with fatal varicella encephalitis, suggesting that this syndrome might be caused by direct infection. However, it is speculated that these neurologic manifestations of primary VZV infection may be immune-mediated, for the most part. The symptoms are typically transient but neurologic complications are the second most frequent indication for hospitalization of otherwise healthy children with varicella. The onset of neurologic complications follows the appearance of the rash by several days but a few case reports describe encephalitis and ataxia beginning before skin lesions have appeared. The symptoms of encephalitis are sudden changes in the level of consciousness and generalized seizures; the signs may be meningeal, e.g., nucal rigidity, rather than encephalitic in some cases. The cerebellar syndrome is characterized by a gradual onset of irritability, ataxia, nystagmus and speech disturbances. The cerebrospinal fluid usually shows a mild mononuclear cell inflammatory pattern, with a predominance of lymphocytes, a somewhat elevated protein (<200 mg) and normal glucose, or in some cases, the cerebrospinal fluid may be normal (Gershon *et al.*, 1980).

Children under 5 and adults appear to be the most susceptible to central nervous system complications. Not surprisingly, the highest risk of fatal complications appears to be associated with encephalitis rather than cerebellar ataxia. Varicella encephalitis usually resolves within 24–72 hours, even without antiviral therapy. Information about the risk of long-term sequelae after varicella encephalitis is limited; whereas most recover fully, some patients have recurrent seizures and permanent neurologic deficits (Johnson and Milbourn, 1970). The signs of cerebellar ataxia can persist for days or weeks. Among the rare neurologic complications of varicella are transverse myelitis, optic neuritis and very rarely, Guillain-Barre syndrome.

Primary VZV infection can be associated with thrombocytopenia and coagulopathy, although these manifestations are unusual in healthy individuals. The signs of these complications include hemorrhage into the skin vesicles, petechiae, purpura, epistaxis, hematuria and gastrointestinal bleeding. The mechanisms by which thrombocytopenia may be induced include reduced production of platelets and decreased platelet survival; vasculitis, transient hypersplenism or intravascular coagulopathy may be involved. As described for varicella pneumonia, adults are at higher risk for acute hemorrhagic complications of varicella than children. Purpura fulminans, due to arterial thrombosis, is a very rare but life-threatening complication of varicella. Immune-mediated thrombocytopenia may also occur, with symptoms developing from 1 to 2 weeks or longer after varicella. Whether acute or later in their onset, bleeding complications may last for several weeks, but the thrombocytopenia usually resolves completely. Inflammatory damage to the kidneys, presenting as nephritis, is an unusual, late complication in children and adults with varicella; it is possible that this syndrome is due to secondary group A streptococcal infection. A few cases of nephritic syndrome and hemolytic uremic syndrome have been described in children with primary VZV infection. Viral arthritis, diagnosed by the isolation of VZV from joint fluid, is unusual and resolves spontaneously within 3–5 days and has not been associated with residual damage. Myocarditis, pericarditis, pancreatitis and orchitis are other very rare complications of primary VZV infection. The risks of varicella in healthy children and adults have been reduced substantially by the introduction of live attenuated varicella vaccines (Chapter 70).

Varicella in the immunocompromised host

Primary VZV infection was often a life-threatening illness in immunocompromised children before the introduction of acyclovir (Chapter 65) and can be attributed to the delayed or failed induction of VZV-specific cellular immunity (Chapter 39). Most information about the clinical course of varicella in high-risk patients is based on observations in children with leukemia and other childhood malignancies. These children often have prolonged fever and a much more extensive rash and continued formation of new lesions. Serious complications result from unchecked viral dissemination by cell-associated viremia to the lungs, liver and in some cases to the central nervous system. Immunocompromised children develop varicella pneumonia, hepatitis, coagulopathy and meningoencephalitis (Feldman and Lott, 1987; Myers, 1979). Whereas new varicella lesions are unusual after 3–5 days in most healthy children, new lesions may appear for >7 days and resolution of the lesions may take 14 days. Susceptibility to secondary bacterial infections is typically enhanced in children receiving chemotherapy or radiation because of the granulocytopenia induced by treatment of the malignancy. As is the case in healthy adults, most varicella-related deaths result from pneumonia that develops shortly after the appearance of the rash. Before antiviral drugs were available, varicella pneumonia progressed rapidly with most deaths occurring within a few days due to untreatable hypoxemia. Varicella pneumonia is often associated with hepatitis, which can progress to liver failure. Again, as is true in healthy adults, hemorrhage into varicella lesions is a clinical sign of life-threatening coagulopathy, due to thrombocytopenia and altered production of clotting factors. VZV dissemination can also cause meningoencephalitis. Severe abdominal or back pain is a clinical sign of serious primary VZV infection in high-risk patients but the etiology of the symptoms is unknown; it is possible that it is related to early infection of sensory ganglia by hematogenous spread of the virus. Other complications of disseminated varicella in children with malignancy include myocarditis, nephritis, pancreatitis, necrotizing splenitis, esophagitis, and enterocolitis.

Children who receive kidney, liver or other solid organ transplants may also develop progressive varicella as a result of the immunosuppressive drugs given to prevent rejection of the transplanted organ (Feldhoff *et al.*, 1981). Varicella pneumonia appears to be a less frequent complication than hepatitis and coagulopathy in kidney transplant patients. Steroid therapy for chronic diseases, including rheumatoid arthritis, nephrotic syndrome and ulcerative colitis, may lead to severe varicella. Asthma patients given high doses of prednisone, especially during the incubation period, are also at risk, but chronic low-dose steroid therapy does not usually result in varicella complications. The immunologic deficits caused by human immunodeficiency virus (HIV) infection are associated with prolonged, recurrent varicella and with chronic, hyperkaratotic skin lesions but varicella pneumonia, hepatitis and other manifestations of dissemination are unusual compared to children with malignancies or organ transplants (Jura *et al.*, 1989; Kelley *et al.*, 1994). Any of the rare genetic disorders that interfere with the acquisition of antigen-specific T cell immunity results in very high risk of fatal varicella. These diseases include severe combined immunodeficiency disorder, adenosine deaminase deficiency, nucleoside phosphorylase deficiency and cartilage hair hypoplasia/short-limbed dwarfism; serious varicella also occurs in some children with Wiskott–Aldrich syndrome and ataxia telangiectasia.

Varicella in pregnancy and the newborn

Most adults are immune, but susceptible pregnant women appear to be predisposed to severe varicella at rates higher than the enhanced risk associated with primary VZV infection in all healthy adults. Varicella pneumonia is the predominant complication and appears to be more common with varicella acquired in late gestation (Pastuszak *et al.*, 1994). From the limited information available, the risk of fatal varicella, due to pneumonia, appears to be ∼1%–2% (Enders *et al.*, 1994). When primary VZV infection occurs in early pregnancy, the virus can be transferred across the placenta to the developing fetus. The frequency of viral transfer is higher than the risk of fetal damage, as shown by postnatal testing of infants for VZV-specific immunity and the occurrence of zoster in early childhood among infants with no symptoms of intrauterine VZV infection (Dworsky *et al.*, 1980). The estimated incidence of varicella embryopathy is <1%, with most damage due to maternal infection acquired in the first 20 weeks of gestation. The congenital varicella syndrome is most often recognized by unusual cutaneous defects and atrophy of an extremity. Infants often have microcephaly, cortical atrophy and intracranial calcifications secondary to intrauterine VZV encephalitis, with seizures and mental retardation. Damage to the autonomic nervous system is common and produces severe gastroesophogeal reflux and neurogenic bladder, hydroureter and hydronephrosis. Eye damage, manifesting as chorioretinitis, microophthalmia, and cataracts, is typical. Although intrauterine damage is not observed, infants whose mothers develop primary VZV infection just before delivery often develop varicella during the newborn period (Preblud *et al.*, 1985). The risk of transfer of virus to the infant is highest when maternal infection begins 4 days before to 2 days after delivery, suggesting that the virus crosses the placenta during the viremia associated with lesion formation. Because of the early stage of the maternal infection, viral transfer is not associated with transplacental transport of maternal VZV IgG antibodies. Neonatal varicella can be progressive, presumably due to deficiencies in the capacity of the infant to develop VZV-specific T cell responses. Dissemination causes pneumonia and hepatitis, with a risk of meningoencephalitis. These infants require antiviral therapy to prevent such complications. Infants exposed to late gestation maternal varicella can be protected to some extent by administration of passive antibodies, given as varicella immune globulin. Some infants whose mothers have varicella more than 4–5 days before delivery are born with varicella lesions or develop lesions within a few days after birth; these infants appear to be at low risk for complications. Herpes zoster in pregnant women has not been associated with varicella embryopathy.

Summary

The principal host cell targets during the life cycle of VZV include the respiratory mucosal epithelium as a portal of entry, immune system cells, especially T-cells, for delivery of the virus to skin sites of replication, and sensory ganglia, where latency is established. VZV transmission to susceptible hosts is ensured by the release of cell-free virus into mucocutaneous lesions during varicella or herpes zoster. Like HSV-1 and HSV-2, VZV is an alphaherpesvirus that has achieved an equilibrium with the human host that has ensured its persistence in the species for millions of years.

REFERENCES

Annunziato, P. W., Lungu, O., Panagiotidis, C. *et al.* (2000). Varicella-zoster virus proteins in skin lesions: implications for a novel role of ORF29p in chickenpox. *J. Virol.*, **74**(4), 2005–2010.

Arvin, A. M. (2001a). Varicella-zoster virus. 4th edn. In *Fields Virology*, D. M. Knipe, and P. M. Howley, eds., Vol. 2, pp. 2731–2768. Philadelphia: Lippincott-Raven.

Arvin, A. M. (2001b). Varicella-zoster virus: molecular virology and virus–host interactions. *Curr. Opin. Microbiol.*, **4**(4), 442–449.

Asano, Y., Itakura, N., Kajita, Y. *et al.* (1990). Severity of viremia and clinical findings in children with varicella. *J. Infect. Dis.*, **161**(6), 1095–1098.

Baiker, A., Bagowski, C., Ito, H. *et al.* (2004). The immediate-early 63 protein of Varicella-Zoster virus: analysis of functional domains required for replication in vitro and for T-cell and skin tropism in the SCIDhu model in vivo. *J. Virol.*, **78**(3), 1181–1194.

Berarducci, B., Ikoma, M., Stamatis, S., Sommer, M., Grose, C. and Arvin, A. M. (2006). Essential functions of the unique

N-terminal region of the Varicella-zoster virus glycoprotein E ectodomain in viral replication and in the pathogenesis of skin infection, *J. Virol.*, in press.

Besser, J., Ikoma, M., Fabel, K. *et al.* (2004). Differential requirement for cell fusion and virion formation in the pathogenesis of varicella-zoster virus infection in skin and T cells. *J. Virol.*, **78**(23), 13293–13305.

Besser, J., Sommer, M. H., Zerboni, L. *et al.* (2003). Differentiation of varicella-zoster virus ORF47 protein kinase and IE62 protein binding domains and their contributions to replication in human skin xenografts in the SCID-hu mouse. *J. Virol.*, **77**(10), 5964–5974.

Che, X., Zerboni, L., Sommer, M. H., and Arvin, A. M. (2006). Varicella-zoster virus open reading frame 10 is a virulence determinant in skin cells but not in T-cells *in vivo*. *J. Virol.*, **7**, 3238–3248.

Cohen, J. I. and Nguyen, H. (1997). Varicella-zoster virus glycoprotein I is essential for growth of virus in Vero cells. *J. Virol.*, **71**(9), 6913–6920.

Cohen, J. I. and Seidel, K. E. (1993). Generation of varicella-zoster virus (VZV) and viral mutants from cosmid DNAs: VZV thymidylate synthetase is not essential for replication in vitro. *Proc. Natl Acad. Sci. USA*, **90**, 7376–7380.

Cohen, J. I. and Straus, S. E. (2001). Varicella-zoster virus and its replication. 4th edn. In *Fields Virology*, D. M. Knipe, and P. M. Howley, eds., Vol. 2, pp. 2707–2730. Philadelphia: Lippincott-Raven.

Cohen, J. I., Cox, E., Pesnicak, L., Srinivas, S., and Krogmann, T. (2004). The varicella-zoster virus open reading frame 63 latency-associated protein is critical for establishment of latency. *J. Virol.*, **78**(21), 11833–11840.

Cole, N. L. and Grose, C. (2003). Membrane fusion mediated by herpesvirus glycoproteins: the paradigm of varicella-zoster virus. *Rev. Med. Virol.*, **13**(4), 207–222.

Davison, A. J. and Scott, J. E. (1986). The complete DNA sequence of varicella-zoster virus. *J. Gen. Virol.*, **67**, 1759–1816.

Dunkle, L. M., Arvin, A. M., Whitley, R. J. *et al.* (1991). A controlled trial of acyclovir for chickenpox in normal children. *N. Engl. J. Med.*, **325**(22), 1539–1544.

Dworsky, M., Whitley, R., and Alford, C. (1980). Herpes zoster in early infancy. *Am. J. Dis. Child.*, **134**(6), 618–619.

Enders, G., Miller, E., Cradock-Watson, J., Bolley, I., and Ridehalgh, M. (1994). Consequences of varicella and herpes zoster in pregnancy: prospective study of 1739 cases. *Lancet*, **343**(8912), 1548–1551.

Feldhoff, C. M., Balfour, H. H., Jr., Simmons, R. L., Najarian, J. S., and Mauer, S. M. (1981). Varicella in children with renal transplants. *J. Pediatr.*, **98**(1), 25–31.

Feldman, S. and Lott, L. (1987). Varicella in children with cancer: impact of antiviral therapy and prophylaxis. *Pediatrics*, **80**(4), 465–472.

Gershon, A. A., Steinberg, S., and Silber, R. (1978). Varicella-zoster viremia. *J. Pediatr.*, **92**(6), 1033–1034.

Gershon, A., Steinberg, S., Greenberg, S., and Taber, L. (1980). Varicella-zoster-associated encephalitis: detection of specific antibody in cerebrospinal fluid. *J. Clin. Microbiol.*, **12**(6), 764–767.

Grose, C. (1981). Variation on a theme by Fenner: the pathogenesis of chicken pox. *Pediatrics*, **68**, 735–737.

He, H., Boucaud, D., Hay, J., and Ruyechan, W. T. (2001). Cis and trans elements regulating expression of the varicella zoster virus gI gene. *Arch. Virol. Suppl.*(17), 57–70.

Heineman, T. C., Seidel, K., and Cohen, J. I. (1996). The varicella-zoster virus ORF66 protein induces kinase activity and is dispensable for viral replication. *J. Virol.*, **70**(10), 7312–7317.

Ito, H., Sommer, M. H., Zerboni, L. *et al.* (2003). Promoter sequences of varicella-zoster virus glycoprotein I targeted by cellular transactivating factors Sp1 and USF determine virulence in skin and T cells in SCIDhu mice in vivo. *J. Virol.*, **77**(1), 489–498.

Jackson, M. A., Burry, V. F., and Olson, L. C. (1992). Complications of varicella requiring hospitalization in previously healthy children. *Pediatr. Infect. Dis. J.*, **11**(6), 441–445.

Johnson, R. and Milbourn, P. E. (1970). Central nervous system manifestations of chickenpox. *Can. Med. Assoc. J.*, **102**(8), 831–834.

Jones, J. O. and Arvin, A. M. (2006). Inhibition of the NF-κB pathway by varicella-zoster virus in vitro and in human epidermal cells in vivo. *J. Virol.*, **80**(11), 5113–5124.

Jura, E., Chadwick, E. G., Josephs, S. H. *et al.* (1989). Varicella-zoster virus infections in children infected with human immunodeficiency virus. *Pediatr. Infect. Dis. J.*, **8**(9), 586–590.

Kelley, R., Mancao, M., Lee, F., Sawyer, M., Nahmias, A., and Nesheim, S. (1994). Varicella in children with perinatally acquired human immunodeficiency virus infection. *J. Pediatr.*, **124**(2), 271–273.

Kemble, G. W., Annunziato, P., Lungu, O. *et al.* (2000). Open reading frame S/L of varicella-zoster virus encodes a cytoplasmic protein expressed in infected cells. *J. Virol.*, **74**(23), 11311–11321.

Kinchington, P. R., Hougland, J. K., Arvin, A. M., Ruyechan, W. T., and Hay, J. (1992). The varicella-zoster virus immediate-early protein IE62 is a major component of virus particles. *J. Virol.*, **66**(1), 359–366.

Kinchington, P. R., Vergnes, J. P., Defechereux, P., Piette, J., and Turse, S. E. (1994). Transcriptional mapping of the varicella-zoster virus regulatory genes encoding open reading frames 4 and 63. *J. Virol.*, **68**(6), 3570–3581.

Koropchak, C. M., Diaz, P. S., and Arvin, A. M. (1989). Investigation of varicella-zoster virus infection of lymphocytes by in situ hybridization. *J. Virol.*, **63**, 2392–2395.

Koropchak, C. M., Graham, G., Palmer, J. *et al.* (1991). Investigation of varicella-zoster virus infection by polymerase chain reaction in the immunocompetent host with acute varicella. *J. Infect. Dis.*, **163**, 1016–1022.

Krugman, S., Goodrich, C. H., and Ward, R. (1957). Primary varicella pneumonia. *N. Engl. J. Med.*, **257**(18), 843–848.

Ku, C. C., Padilla, J. A., Grose, C., Butcher, E. C., and Arvin, A. M. (2002). Tropism of varicella-zoster virus for human tonsillar CD4(+) T lymphocytes that express activation, memory, and skin homing markers. *J. Virol.*, **76**(22), 11425–11433.

Ku, C. C., Zerboni, L., Ito, H., Graham, B. S., Wallace, M., and Arvin, A. M. (2004). Varicella-zoster virus transfer to skin by T Cells and modulation of viral replication by epidermal cell interferon-alpha. *J. Exp. Med.*, **200**(7), 917–925.

Leisenfelder, S. A. and Moffat, J. F. (2006). Varicella-zoster virus infection of human foreskin fibroblast cells results in atypical cyclin expression and cyclin-dependent kinase activity. *J. Virol.* **80**(11), 5577–5587.

Liesegang, T. J. (1991). Diagnosis and therapy of herpes zoster ophthalmicus. *Ophthalmology*, **98**(8), 1216–1229.

Mallory, S., Sommer, M., and Arvin, A. M. (1997). Mutational analysis of the role of glycoprotein I in varicella-zoster virus replication and its effects on glycoprotein E conformation and trafficking. *J. Virol.*, **71**(11), 8279–8288.

Mo, C., Suen, J., Sommer, M., and Arvin, A. (1999). Characterization of Varicella-Zoster virus glycoprotein K (open reading frame 5) and its role in virus growth. *J. Virol.*, **73**(5), 4197–4207.

Mo, C., Lee, J., Sommer, M., Grose, C., and Arvin, A. M. (2002). The requirement of varicella zoster virus glycoprotein E (gE) for viral replication and effects of glycoprotein I on gE in melanoma cells. *Virology*, **304**(2), 176–186.

Moffat, J., Ito, H., Sommer, M., Taylor, S., and Arvin, A. M. (2002). Glycoprotein I of varicella-zoster virus is required for viral replication in skin and T cells. *J. Virol.*, **76**(16), 8468–8471.

Moffat, J., Mo, C., Cheng, J. J. *et al.* (2004a). Functions of the C-terminal domain of varicella-zoster virus glycoprotein E in viral replication in vitro and skin and T-cell tropism in vivo. *J. Virol.*, **78**(22), 12406–12415.

Moffat, J. F., McMichael, M. A., Leisenfelder, S. A., and Taylor, S. L. (2004b). Viral and cellular kinases are potential antiviral targets and have a central role in varicella zoster virus pathogenesis. *Biochim. Biophys. Acta.*, **1697**(1–2), 225–231.

Moffat, J. F., Stein, M. D., Kaneshima, H., and Arvin, A. M. (1995). Tropism of varicella-zoster virus for human CD4+ and CD8+ T lymphocytes and epidermal cells in SCID-hu mice. *J. Virol.*, **69**(9), 5236–5242.

Moffat, J. F., Zerboni, L., Sommer, M. H. *et al.* (1998). The ORF47 and ORF66 putative protein kinases of varicella-zoster virus determine tropism for human T cells and skin in the SCID-hu mouse. *Proc. Natl Acad. Sci. USA*, **95**(20), 11969–11974.

Myers, M. G. (1979). Viremia caused by varicella-zoster virus: association with malignant progressive varicella. *J. Infect. Dis.*, **140**, 229–233.

Niizuma, T., Zerboni, L., Sommer, M. H., Ito, H., Hinchliffe, S., and Arvin, A. M. (2003). Construction of varicella-zoster virus recombinants from parent oka cosmids and demonstration that ORF65 protein is dispensable for infection of human skin and T cells in the SCID-hu mouse model. *J. Virol.*, **77**(10), 6062–6065.

Olashaw, N. and Pledger, W. J. (2002). Paradigms of growth control: relation to Cdk activation. *Sci. STKE*, **2002**(134), RE7.

Ozaki, T., Ichikawa, T., Matsui, Y. *et al.* (1986). Lymphocyte-associated viremia in varicella. *J. Med. Virol.*, **19**, 249–253.

Pastuszak, A. L., Levy, M., Schick, B. *et al.* (1994). Outcome after maternal varicella infection in the first 20 weeks of pregnancy. *N. Engl. J. Med.*, **330**(13), 901–905.

Peters, A. C., Versteeg, J., Lindeman, J., and Bots, G. T. (1978). Varicella and acute cerebellar ataxia. *Arch. Neurol.*, **35**(11), 769–771.

Preblud, S. R., Bregman, D. J., and Vernon, L. L. (1985). Deaths from varicella in infants. *Pediatr. Infect. Dis.*, **4**(5), 503–507.

Sato, B., Ito, H., Hinchliffe, S., Sommer, M. H., Zerboni, L., and Arvin, A. M. (2003a). Mutational analysis of open reading frames 62 and 71, encoding the varicella-zoster virus immediate-early transactivating protein, IE62, and effects on replication in vitro and in skin xenografts in the SCID-hu mouse in vivo. *J. Virol.*, **77**(10), 5607–5620.

Sato, B., Sommer, M., Ito, H., and Arvin, A. M. (2003b). Requirement of varicella-zoster virus immediate-early 4 protein for viral replication. *J. Virol.*, **77**(22), 12369–12372.

Schaap, A., Fortin, J. F., Sommer, M. *et al.* (2005). T-cell tropism and the role of ORF66 protein in the pathogenesis of varicella-zoster virus infection. *J. Virol.*, **79**, 12921–33.

Sommer, M. H., Zagha, E., Serrano, O. K. *et al.* (2001). Mutational analysis of the repeated open reading frames, ORFs 63 and 70 and ORFs 64 and 69, of varicella-zoster virus. *J. Virol.*, **75**(17), 8224–8239.

Soong, W., Schultz, J. C., Patera, A. C., Sommer, M. H., and Cohen, J. I. (2000). Infection of human T lymphocytes with varicella-zoster virus: an analysis with viral mutants and clinical isolates. *J. Virol.*, **74**(4), 1864–1870.

Takahashi, K., Sonoda, S., Higashi, K. *et al.* (1989). Predominant CD4 T-lymphocyte tropism of human herpesvirus 6-related virus. *J. Virol.*, **63**(7), 3161–3163.

Taylor, S. L., Kinchington, P. R., Brooks, A., and Moffat, J. F. (2004). Roscovitine, a cyclin dependent kinase inhibitor, prevents replication of varicella-zoster virus. *J. Virol.*, **78**(6), 2853–2862.

Williams, M. G., Almeida, J. D., and Howatson, A. F. (1962). Electron microscope studies on viral skin lesions. *Arch. Dermatol.*, **86**, 290–297.

Ye, M., Duus, K. M., Peng, J., Price, D. H., and Grose, C. (1999). Varicella-zoster virus Fc receptor component gI is phosphorylated on its endodomain by a cyclin-dependent kinase. *J. Virol.*, **73**(2), 1320–1330.

VZV: molecular basis of persistence (latency and reactivation)

Jeffrey I. Cohen

Laboratory of Clinical Infectious Diseases, National Institutes of Health, Bethesda, MD, USA

Primary infection with varicella-zoster virus (VZV) causes varicella manifested by fever and a vesicular rash. During primary infection the virus disseminates in lymphocytes to the skin and other organs, and replicates in and establishes a latent infection in the nervous system (Croen *et al.*, 1988). Early studies demonstrated viral DNA in human trigeminal and dorsal root ganglia by in situ hybridization and Southern blotting (Gilden *et al.*, 1983, 1987; Hyman *et al.*, 1983). More recent studies, using PCR, have demonstrated latent VZV in multiple cranial nerve, dorsal root, and autonomic ganglia (Furuta *et al.*, 1992, 1997; Gilden *et al.*, 2001; Mahalingham *et al.*, 1990). The virus can reactivate from these sites to cause herpes zoster.

The structure of the VZV genome during latency is not certain. Clarke *et al.* (1995) performed PCR on human ganglia DNA using pairs of primers specific for the unique long internal and terminal regions of the genome. Analysis of the ratio of the signals of the PCR products indicated that the termini of the genome are adjacent during latency, suggesting that the VZV genome is probably episomal.

Site of VZV latency

A number of studies have attempted to identify the cell type in which VZV is latent in human ganglia (Table 38.1). While early studies using in situ hybridization suggested that the virus was present in neurons (Hyman *et al.*, 1983; Gilden *et al.*, 1987), other studies suggested that viral RNA was latent exclusively in satellite cells that surround the neurons (Croen *et al.*, 1988). Lungu and colleagues (1995) found VZV nucleic acid in both satellite cells and neurons.

Further studies by Dueland *et al.* (1995) and Kennedy *et al.* (1998, 1999) using in situ PCR showed that VZV is latent predominantly in neurons. LaGuardia *et al.* (1999) isolated human trigeminal ganglia, fixed the tissue, minced it, treated it with collagenase, and filtered the cells through various pore sizes of nylon mesh to separate neurons from non-noneuronal cells. PCR analysis of the neurons and non-neuronal cells showed that VZV DNA was present only in neurons. Levin and colleagues (2003) purified neurons and satellite cells and found VZV in 1.5% of neurons and in none of over 20 000 satellite cells tested. Additional studies using antibodies to VZV proteins expressed during latency detected viral proteins in neurons, but not in satellite cells (Mahalingam *et al.*, 1996; Lungu *et al.*, 1998). Wang *et al.* (2005) performed laser capture microdissection isolating single neurons or non-neuronal cells from human trigeminal ganglia. VZV DNA was present in neurons, but rarely if ever in non-neuronal cells. Theil *et al.* (2003) used double fluorescence in situ hybridization to detect VZV neurons from human trigeminal ganglia; rare satellite cells were positive for VZV. A few neurons were infected with both VZV and HSV.

In summary, while a number of studies have detected VZV RNA in both neurons and satellite cells, most recent studies indicate that neurons are the principal site of latency.

Quantification of VZV DNA load during latency

Initial studies to quantify the latent viral load used competitive PCR in which an internal mutant template is added to the unknown sample in the PCR mixture to determine the copy number of VZV genomes in human ganglia (Mahalingam *et al.*, 1993). Using this method Mahalingam and colleagues estimated that there were 9 to 53 copies of VZV DNA per ug of ganglion DNA which corresponds to 6 to 31 copies of VZV DNA per 10^5 ganglionic cells (Table 38.2). This number is considerably lower than the 1 000 to 10 000

Table 38.1. Site of VZV latency in human ganglia

Site	% neurons with VZV	%non-neuronal cells with VZV	Technique	Reference
Neuron	0.1–0.3	0	ISH	Hyman et al., 1983
Neuron	"most"	0	ISH	Gilden et al., 1987
Satellite	0	0.01–0.15	ISH	Croen et al., 1988
Neuron = Satellite	5–30%	5–30%	ISH	Lungu et al., 1995
Neuron > Satellite	2–5%	<0.1%	ISH	Kennedy et al., 1998
Neuron > Satellite	2–5%	rare	IS-PCR	Kennedy et al., 1999
Neuron	"many"	0	IS-PCR	Dueland et al., 1995
Neuron	ND	0	Diss-PCR	LaGuardia et al., 1999
Neuron	1.5%	0	Diss-PCR	Levin et al., 2003
Neuron	4.1%	0.06	LCM	Wang et al., 2005

ISH = in situ hybridization; IS PCR = in situ PCR; Diss-PCR = dissociated trigeminal cells and PCR; LCM = laser capture microdissection.

Table 38.2. Latent VZV DNA load

Copies per 10^5 cells		Ratio		
VZV DNA	HSV-1 DNA	VZV/HSV	Method	Reference
6–31		(0.003)	cPCR	Mahalingham et al., 1993
	10^3 to 10^4			Efstathiou et al., 1986
20–50		(0.005)	cPCR	LaGuardia et al., 1999
258	2902	0.1	rPCR	Pevenstein et al., 1999
9046	3042	3	rPCR	Cohrs et al., 2000
38–179			cPCR	Levin et al., 2003
283	711	0.4	LCM	Wang et al., 2005

cPCR = quantitative DNA PCR; rPCR = real time PCR; LCM = laser capture microdissection.

copies of HSV DNA per 10^5 ganglionic cells (Efstathiou et al., 1986).

LaGuardia and colleagues (1999) performed PCR on sets of 100 neurons obtained from human trigeminal ganglia; of PCR-positive sets of neurons, there were two to five copies of VZV DNA per 100 neurons. Assuming that there are 100 cells per neuron in human ganglia (Mahalingam et al., 1993), these results correspond to 20–50 copies of VZV DNA per 10^5 ganglionic cells. Levin et al. (2003) performed PCR on purified neurons and detected an average of 4.7 copies of VZV per latently infected neuron. Since they found that 0.8%–3.8% of neurons were latently infected, this corresponds to 3.8–17.9 copies per 100 neurons or 38–179 copies per 10^5 ganglionic cells.

Pevenstein et al. (1999) used real time PCR to determine the number of copies of VZV and HSV-1 DNA in human trigeminal ganglia. They estimated that the copy number of VZV DNA was 177 to 299 per 10^5 ganglion cells, while the copy number of HSV-1 DNA was 2902 per 10^5 ganglia cells. This suggests that there is about tenfold more HSV-1 DNA than VZV DNA in latently infected ganglia.

Cohrs et al. (2000) also used real time PCR to estimate copy numbers in human trigeminal ganglia. The mean VZV DNA copy number was 580 copies per 100 ng of ganglia DNA (corresponding to 9,046 copies per 10^5 cells) and the mean HSV-1 DNA copy number was 195 per 100 ng of DNA (corresponding to 3,042 copies per 10^5 cells). This suggests that there is about a 3-fold lower amount of HSV-1 than VZV DNA in latently infected human ganglia.

Wang et al. (2005), using laser capture microdissection to measure VZV DNA in trigeminal ganglia from 10 subjects, found a median of 6.9 copies of VZV per positive neuron. Since 4.1% of neurons were VZV positive, and there are about 100 cells per neuron in human ganglia, this corresponds to a median of 283 VZV DNA copies per 10^5 ganglionic cells. The same authors measured HSV DNA in ganglia from 6 subjects and found a median of 11.3 copies of HSV per positive neuron and 6.3% of neurons were positive of HSV. This corresponds to a median of 711 HSV copies per 10^5 cells.

The difference between the three studies (Cohrs et al., 2000; Pevenstein et al., 1999; Wang et al., 2005) may be due to the difference in age of the subjects; those in the study by Cohrs et al. were older and may have had more episodes of asymptomatic reactivation with increased seeding of ganglia with VZV DNA. Alternatively, the differences may be due to the relatively small number of subjects tested (<20) in each study and the wide range in the amount of VZV DNA detected in ganglia from different subjects.

Animal models for VZV latency

Inoculation of several rodent species with VZV results in a latent infection of the nervous system. VZV was detected in trigeminal and thoracic ganglia from hairless guinea pigs by PCR after inoculation with a guinea pig adapted strain of virus (Lowry et al., 1993). VZV DNA was present in mouse trigeminal ganglia 1 month after corneal inoculation with the virus (Wroblewska et al., 1993). Inoculation of adult rats with VZV in the footpad or by paraspinal intramuscular injection results in latent virus infection in the dorsal root ganglia (Debrus et al., 1995; Sadzot-Delvaux et al., 1990; Annunziato et al., 1998). Using this system, Sadzot-Delvaux and colleagues (1995) found that viral DNA was present as early as 2 days after infection and up to 9 months later. In most animals, only the ganglia innervating the inoculation site were latently infected, indicating that ganglia were infected by retrograde transport of virus up the axon, rather than by viremia. Up to 80% of neurons were infected; some non-neuronal cells were also infected. The pattern of latent viral transcription and protein expression was similar in rats to that seen in humans. Kennedy and colleagues (2001) were able to detect latent transcripts in rat ganglia up to 18 months after inoculation. Sato et al. (2002b) inoculated cotton rats with VZV and obtained latent infection, based on DNA and RNA transcripts, in dorsal root ganglia of 50% to 70% of animals. Inoculation of animals with heat-inactivated virus-infected cells failed to result in latency. VZV was not detected in the lungs and usually not in the brain of animals (Sato et al., 2003b). Brunell and colleagues (1999) inoculated neonatal rats with an early passage isolate of VZV intraperitoneally, and detected a latent viral transcript in trigeminal ganglia.

Baiker et al. (2004) transplanted fetal human brain stem cells into NOD-SCID mice and then inoculated the animals with VZV-infected melanoma cells. VZV infected both neural and glial cells. While latency-associated proteins (ORF62, ORF63, ORF47 proteins) were detected and a late protein not associated with latency (gE) was rarely detected in the animals, the localization of the latency-associated proteins was either in the nucleus or in the nucleus and the cytoplasm, unlike that seen in latently infected human neurons (see below). Zerboni et al. (2005) implanted human fetal dorsal root ganglia under the capsule of the kidney of SCID mice and then either injected the implants with VZV-infected fibroblasts or injected the animals intravenously with VZV-infected tonsil T cells. Direct injection of the ganglia resulted in a lytic infection followed by latency with expression of the ORF63 latency gene, but not the ORF62 latency gene or gB 8 weeks after infection. Intravenous injection of T cells resulted in a lytic infection in the ganglia 2 weeks after injection.

Simian varicella virus (SVV) is the simian counterpart of VZV, and the two viruses share nearly all the same open reading frames (Gray et al., 2001; Gray, 2004). Intratracheal inoculation of SVV into African green monkeys results in infection of the trigeminal and dorsal root ganglia (Mahalingam et al., 1991); however, other sites including peripheral blood mononuclear cells and lungs show persistent infection (White et al., 2002). Naturally acquired SVV infection, transmitted from one African green monkey to another, results in a mild rash followed by latent infection of multiple ganglia, but not infection of other tissues (Mahalingam et al., 2002). SVV DNA is present only in neu-

Table 38.3. VZV transcripts consistently expressed during latency[a]

Transcript	Species	Method	Reference
4 (IE)[b]	human	ISH	Kennedy et al., 1999; Kennedy et al., 2000
	rat	Northern & PCR	Sadzot-Delvaux et al., 1995
21 (E)	human	cDNA library	Cohrs et al., 1996
	human	real time PCR	Cohrs et al., 2000
	human	ISH	Kennedy et al., 1999; Kennedy et al., 2000
	neonatal rat	RT-PCR	Brunell et al., 1996
	rat	ISH	Kennedy et al., 2001
29 (E)	human	Northern	Meier et al., 1993
	human	cDNA library	Cohrs et al., 1996
	human	real time PCR	Cohrs et al., 2000
	human	ISH	Kennedy et al., 1999; Kennedy et al., 2000
	rat	Northern & PCR	Sadzot-Delvaux et al., 1995
	rat	ISH	Kennedy et al., 2001
62 (IE)	human	Northern	Meier et al., 1993
	human	cDNA library	Cohrs et al., 1996
	human	ISH	Kennedy et al., 2000
	rat	Northern & PCR	Sadzot-Delvaux et al., 1995
	rat	ISH	Kennedy et al., 2001
	human	FISH	Thiel et al., 2003
63 (IE)	human	cDNA library	Cohrs et al., 1996
	human	real time PCR	Cohrs et al., 2000
	human	ISH	Kennedy et al., 1999; Kennedy et al., 2000
	rat	Northern & PCR	Sadzot-Delvaux et al., 1995
	rat	ISH	Kennedy et al., 2001
	cotton rat	RT-PCR	Sato et al., 2002b
66 (E)	human	ISH, RT-PCR	Cohrs et al., 2003

[a]Generally not expressed during latency: 10 (L), 14 (L), 28 (E), 36 (E), 40 (L), 61, 67 (L), 68 (L).
[b]Predicted temporal class of transcription: immediate-early (IE), early (E), late (L).

rons of latently infected monkeys (Kennedy et al., 2004) At least one VZV gene shown to be expressed during latency, ORF21, is expressed in ganglia from monkeys infected with SVV (Clarke et al., 1996). The SVV model is the only animal model for VZV that recapitulates the features of varicella, latency, and reactivation.

VZV transcripts expressed during latency

A number of laboratories have detected transcripts corresponding to various VZV genes in human ganglia and from experimentally infected rodents (Table 38.3). Meier et al. (1993) detected transcripts for VZV ORF 29 and ORF62, but

Table 38.4. Latent VZV and HSV-1 RNA loads in human trigeminal ganglia[a]

VZV RNA Transcript	Median Copy Number[b] (range)	% Positive Ganglia	Median VZV DNA Copy Number[c] (range)	% Positive Ganglia
21	6.2 (0.6–85.5)	23%	223 (24.9–4027)	100%
29	427 (56–1,154)	13%		
63	121 (17–2,786)	86%		
HSV RNA Transcript	Median Copy Number (range)	% Positive ganglia	Median HSV-1 DNA copy number (range)	% Positive ganglia
LAT	1188 (44–23,070)	68%	162 (22.5–289)	68%

[a]Data from Cohrs et al., 2000.
[b]Expressed as number of virus gene transcripts/number of GADPH transcripts × 10^4.
[c]Expressed per 100 ng of DNA.

Table 38.5. VZV Proteins expressed during latency[a]

Protein	Species	Method	Reference
4 (IE)[b]	human	IH	Lungu et al., 1998
62 (IE)	human	IH	Lungu et al., 1998; Kennedy et al., 2004
63 (IE)	rat	IH	Debrus et al., 1995; Kennedy et al., 2001
	human	IH	Mahalingham et al., 1996; Lungu et al., 1998; Kennedy et al., 2000; Kennedy et al., 2004
21 (E)	human	IH	Lungu et al., 1998; Kennedy et al., 2004
29 (E)	human	IH	Lungu et al., 1998; Kennedy et al., 2004
66 (E)	human	IH	Cohrs et al., 2003

[a]VZV proteins ORF 10 (L), 14 (L), 67 (L) not detected.
[b]Predicted temporal class of transcription: immediate-early (IE), early (E), late (L).

not ORF28 by Northern blot analysis of RNA extracted from pooled human trigeminal ganglia.

Cohrs et al. (1996) detected VZV ORFs 21, 29, 62, and 63 from cDNA obtained by isolating RNA from pooled human trigeminal ganglia. They were unable to detect transcripts for ORFs 4, 10, 40, 51, and 61 in the library. ORF66 was also detected in latently infected human ganglia (Cohrs et al., 2003).

Kennedy et al. (1999, 2000) used in situ hybridization and detected VZV transcripts for ORFs 21, 29, 62, and 63 during latency. ORF21 transcripts were detected in 64% of ganglia from HIV-negative subjects and in 60% from those with HIV; ORF29 transcripts were found in 38% of ganglia from HIV-negative persons and in 100% from those with HIV; ORF62 transcripts were noted in 40% of ganglia from HIV-negative subjects and in 67% from those with HIV; ORF63 transcripts were detected in 47% of transcripts from HIV-negative persons and in 80% from those with HIV. Transcripts for VZV ORFs 4 and 18 were infrequently expressed, while those for VZV ORFs 28, 40, and 61 were rarely expressed.

Cohrs et al. (2000) used real time PCR to detect transcripts for VZV ORF 63 from 86% of human trigeminal ganglia assayed. Transcripts for ORFs 21 and 29 were detected less frequently in 23% and 13% of ganglia, respectively. While the copy numbers for ORF63 transcripts varied over a wide range, they were consistently lower than the copy numbers for HSV-1 LAT transcripts from the same ganglia (Table 38.4).

Several studies have looked at rodents (adult rats, neonatal rats, and adult cotton rats) latently infected with VZV (Table 38.3). Transcripts for ORFs 4, 21, 29, 62 and 63 have been detected in these animals (Kennedy et al., 2001; Sadzot-Delvaux et al., 1990; Brunell et al., 1999; Sato et al., 2002b). Transcripts for ORFs 4, 28, 36, 40, and 68 were not detected. VZV gene expression during latency may be regulated by epigenetic mechanisms. Gary et al. (2006) showed that the VZV ORF62 and 63 promoters are associated with a histone protein (acetylated H3K9) and thereby maintained in a euchromatic state during latency and thus can be transcribed. In contrast, the ORF14 and 36 promoters whose genes are not expressed during latency are not associated with the histone protein and instead are maintained in a heterochromatic state.

In summary, a number of studies from several different laboratories have detected 6 different viral transcripts during latency in humans and in rodents. These are predicted to encode immediate-early and early proteins. In contrast, other putative early (ORFs 28, 36, 51) and late (ORFs 10, 40, 68) transcripts have not been found in latently infected human or rodent ganglia.

VZV proteins expressed during latency

Six VZV proteins have also been detected during latency (Table 38.5). Three laboratories (Mahalingham et al., 1996; Kennedy et al., 2000, 2004; Lungu et al., 1998) have detected ORF63 protein in human ganglia using antibody to the protein. In all four studies, ORF63 protein was found either predominantly or exclusively in the cytoplasm of neurons. This is in contrast to its usual localization in both the nucleus and cytoplasm early during lytic infection, and in the nucleus late in lytic infection in vitro (Debrus et al., 1995).

Debrus et al. (1995) and Kennedy et al. (2001) inoculated rats in the footpad with VZV and detected ORF63 protein in lumbar ganglia. ORF63 protein was present in both the cytoplasm and nucleus of neurons using either a polyclonal (Debrus et al., 1995) or monoclonal (Kennedy et al., 2001) antibody to the protein.

In addition to ORF63 protein, ORFs 4, 21, 29, and 62 proteins were detected exclusively in the cytoplasm of neurons of latently infected human ganglia using polyclonal antibodies in one study (Lungu et al., 1998) and ORFs 21, 29, and 62 proteins were detected predominantly in the cytoplasm of neurons in another study (Kennedy et al., 2004). During lytic infection in vitro, ORF21, 29, and 62 proteins are present predominantly in the nucleus, while ORF4 protein is present mostly in the cytoplasm. Lungu et al. (1998) postulated that these proteins are sequestered from the nucleus during latency and cannot function to transactivate genes or replicate viral DNA. VZV ORF 10, 14, and 67 proteins were not detected by the authors in human ganglia. Cohrs et al. (2003) detected ORF66 protein exclusively in the cytoplasm of neurons.

Function of VZV latency-associated proteins

Three of the VZV genes expressed during latency (ORFs 4, 62, 63) have been identified as immediate-early proteins. ORF62 protein is the major viral transactivator and up-regulates expression of all VZV genes that have been tested in transient expression assays (reviewed in Cohen and Straus, 2001). ORF4 protein transactivates expression of certain VZV genes and enhances the ability of ORF62 to transactivate VZV gene expression. VZV ORF63 down-regulates expression of ORF62 transcripts and protein (Hoover et al., 2006). Cells infected with VZV ORF63 deletion mutants that are impaired for latency show an increase in ORF62 transcription relative to those infected with parental virus, while cells infected with ORF63 mutants not impaired for latency show levels of ORF62 transcription similar to parental virus. Thus, expression of ORF63 during latency may allow the cell to down-regulate ORF62 transcription and limit lytic gene expression. ORF63 protein may have a role in inhibiting apoptosis. Expression of ORF63 protein in rat neurons inhibited apoptosis induced by withdrawal of nerve growth factor (Hood et al., 2006); however, ganglia from cotton rats acutely infected with an ORF63 deletion mutant did not show an increase in apoptosis (Cohen et al., 2004). ORF4, ORF62, and ORF63 proteins are all present in the viral tegument.

VZV ORF29 is predicted to encode an early protein, while ORFs 21 and 66 are predicted to encode late proteins, based on their homology with HSV genes. VZV ORF21 protein is present in the viral nucleocapsid and ORF29 protein is a single-stranded DNA binding protein that regulates gene expression from the gI promoter. ORF66 encodes a serine-threonine protein kinase that phosphorylates the ORF62 protein. The actual function of these six VZV genes during latent infection is unknown.

VZV genes required for establishment of latent infection

The cotton rat model has been used to test the ability of several VZV mutants to establish a latent infection. VZV ORFs 1, 2, 13, 32, and 57 encode proteins that do not have HSV homologues. Inoculation of cotton rats with VZV mutants unable to express each of these proteins showed that each is dispensable for establishment of latency (Sato et al., 2002b, 2003b). VZV ORF10, ORF14, ORF17, ORF61, and ORF67 encode the homologues of the HSV VP16 transactivator, glycoprotein C, viral host shut off protein, ICP0 immediate-early protein, and glycoprotein I, respectively. All five of these VZV proteins are dispensable for latency in the cotton rat (Kennedy et al., 2004; Sato et al., 2002a, 2003a, b). ORF21 and ORF66 proteins, which are expressed during VZV latency, are also dispensable for establishment of latent infection (Sato et al., 2003b; Xia et al., 2002). VZV ORF47 protein, which is required for infection of human T cells and skin is dispensable for latency. In contrast, deletion of ORF4 or ORF63 results in a virus that is impaired for establishment of latency (Cohen et al., 2004, 2005b).

In vitro models for VZV latency

Several investigators have infected human neurons with VZV in vitro in attempts to produce models for latency. Infection of human fetal dorsal root ganglia neurons with cell associated or cell-free VZV resulted in a productive infection, but neurons were less susceptible to infection or had a slower rate of infection than non-neuronal cells (Wigdahl et al., 1986; Assouline et al., 1990). Somekh and colleagues (1992) prepared human fetal neuron, satellite cell, or mixed neuron and satellite cell cultures from dorsal root ganglia and infected the cells with cell-free VZV in the presence of BVaraU. After 1 week BVaraU was removed, and 1 to 3 weeks later the cells were plated onto human fibroblasts. VZV "reactivated" from 56% of mixed cultures (neurons and satellite cells), but not from pure neuron or satellite cell cultures.

Merville-Louis et al. (1989) infected adult rat dorsal root ganglia neurons with cell associated or cell-free VZV and observed all three kinetic classes of VZV transcripts in the cells; CPE was not observed and virus was not produced. This suggests that the cells underwent an abortive, but not latent infection. In contrast, Kress et al. (2001) infected adult rat dorsal root ganglia with cell-associated virus and noted productive infection with death of the cells. Hood et al. (2003) infected human dorsal root ganglion neurons with cell-associated VZV and observed expression of all three kinetic classes of VZV proteins, but apoptosis did not occur, in contrast to the marked apoptosis observed in virus-infected fibroblasts.

Chen et al. (2003) infected guinea pig enteric neurons with cell-free or cell-associated virus. Infection with cell-associated virus resulted in a productive infection of the neurons, while infection with cell-free virus resulted in a latent pattern of infection. The latently infected neurons expressed VZV ORF4, 21, 29, 62, and 63 proteins in the cytoplasm of the cells; however, glycoproteins were not expressed. The authors postulated that cell-free VZV, unlike cell-associated virus, lacks some of the proteins that are present in virus-infected cells at the onset of infection and therefore is not able to initiate virus replication in neurons. Stallings et al. (2006) showed that while ORF29 and ORF62 proteins are excluded from the nucleus of cultured guinea pig enteric neurons infected with VZV, expression of VZV ORF61 protein in these cells resulted in translocation of ORF29 and ORF62 proteins to the nucleus. These studies suggest that VZV ORF61 protein may contribute to reactivation of virus from latency.

While these in vitro models recapitulate some of the features of latent VZV infection, it is not clear how well they emulate latency in vivo. The limitations of cell culture based models of HSV latency to simulate latency in vivo, and the lack of understanding of what actually constitutes latency in vivo, suggests that in vitro models for VZV may also have limitations.

Reactivation of VZV

VZV reactivation, which presents as zoster, occurs more frequently in immuncompromised persons and in the elderly. A decline in the frequency of VZV-specific T-cells is thought to allow the virus to clinically reactivate. VZV-specific cytotoxic T-lymphocytes (CTLs) have been detected that recognize the ORF4, 29, 62, and 63 latency proteins (Sadzot-Delvaux et al., 1997; Arvin et al., 2002). These CTLs may help to prevent reactivation of VZV from latency. The demonstration that vaccination of adults with varicella-zoster virus vaccine can reduce the incidence of zoster and postherpetic neuralgia, suggests that augmentation of the cellular immune response to VZV can reduce reactivation (Oxman et al., 2005).

The molecular basis of reactivation is not known. While HSV can be cocultivated from human ganglia, infectious VZV has never been recovered from human ganglia. Vafai et al. (1988) cultured human ganglia in tissue culture media for 11 to17 days and detected 7 major VZV-specific proteins of 35 to 200 kDa. While these proteins were not identified, lysates from the cultivated ganglia did not react with monoclonal antibodies to VZV proteins expressed during the late phase of the replicative cycle, indicating that viral replication did not occur in vitro. Kennedy et al. (2000) studied human trigeminal and dorsal root ganglia that were cocultivated with monkey kidney cells for 3 to 11 days. Transcripts associated (ORFs 29 and 63) and not associated (ORFs 18, 28, and 40) with latency were detected in most of the ganglia. This pattern was very different from that observed in ganglia that were not cocultivated, suggesting that reactivation had occurred. No evidence of infectious VZV was detected after cocultivation. In one report, VZV was said to have reactivated, as detected by cytopathic effects and in situ hybridization, from VZV-infected rats after cocultivation of dissociated ganglia with human fibroblasts and repeated treatment of the cells with trypsin (Sadzot-Delvaux et al., 1990). This finding has not yet been confirmed by others.

Analysis of VZV DNA in dorsal root ganglia from a person with zoster showed that viral DNA was present both in neurons and satellite cells of ganglia innervating the sites of reactivation (Lungu et al., 1995). VZV DNA was present in both the nucleus and the cytoplasm of reactivating ganglia, and a late viral protein, gI, was present in the cytoplasm of these ganglia. A subsequent study showed that while latency associated proteins were present in only the cytoplasm during latency, these proteins translocated to both the cytoplasm and nucleus of neurons in ganglia undergoing reactivation (Lungu et al., 1998). Latency associated proteins were not detected in the satellite cells of the ganglia.

Comparison of VZV latency with that of other alphaherpesviruses

VZV latency has a number of different features than that seen in HSV (Table 38.6). During latency of other alphaherpesvirus, such as HSV, bovine herpesvirus (BHV), or pseudorabies virus (PRV), only the latency associated transcripts (LAT) are expressed. The BHV LAT encodes a protein, while no HSV LAT protein has been detected in latently infected humans or animals. PRV, like VZV, is a member of the varicellovirus family, however, only the PRV LAT transcript has been detected during latency. At present it is unclear why latent gene expression in VZV is different from that of the other alphaherpesviruses.

Is the large number of transcripts in VZV latency due to reactivation?

A number of observations suggest that the large number of VZV transcripts that are detected during latency in humans is not an artifact due to reactivation. First, comparison of transcripts detected from human ganglia shortly after death, with those obtained after ganglia are explanted show different patterns of gene expression (Kennedy *et al.*, 2000). Second, similar studies in which human ganglia are obtained after death detect only a single latency-associated transcript for HSV-1 (Croen *et al.*, 1988). Since HSV can undergo reactivation with productive infection in cell culture, apparently the brief period of time between death and processing the ganglia to detect latent transcripts is insufficient to induce reactivation and may also hold true for VZV. Third, the time between death and obtaining tissue at autopsy did not correlate with the number of VZV genome copies (Cohrs *et al.*, 2000). Fourth, only certain immediate-early and early VZV genes are expressed during latency. Finally, animal models of VZV, in which ganglia are processed immediately after death, show a similar pattern of VZV transcription and protein expression during latency as occurs in human ganglia (Sadzot-Delvaux *et al.*, 1995).

Models for VZV latency

The relatively large number of transcripts that are expressed during latency along with the presence of viral proteins, in latently infected neurons indicates that the mechanism of latency for VZV differs from that of herpes simplex virus. Two models may be proposed to explain the ability of the virus to remain latent, despite expression of several gene products.

VZV proteins localize to the cytoplasm, instead of the nucleus of neurons and thus are unable to carry out their activities

VZV ORF21, 29, 62, and 63 proteins, are usually present in the nucleus of cells during lytic replication. Four

Table 38.6. Differences between VZV and HSV-1 infection, latency, and reactivation

Property	VZV	HSV-1
Primary infection	Disseminated	Localized
Entry into ganglia	Viremia, neural	Neural
Frequency of reactivation	Usually once	Multiple
Likelihood of reactivation	Increases with age	Decreases with age
Asymptomatic reactivation with virus shedding	No	Frequent
Distribution	Dermatome (ganglia)	Focal (sensory nerve)
Reactivation stimuli	None	UV, fever
Reactivation symptoms	Severe pain	Mild or none
Time to recurrence after immunosuppression	2–6 months	1–4 weeks
Latency associated RNAs and proteins	ORFs4, 21, 29, 62, 63, 66 RNA and protein	LAT RNA only

studies (Mahalingam *et al.*, 1996; Grinfeld and Kennedy, 2004; Kennedy *et al.*, 2000; Lungu *et al.*, 1998) have shown that ORF63 is located in the cytoplasm of latently infected neurons. Furthermore, Lungu and colleagues (1998) detected ORF21, 29, and 62 proteins exclusively in the cytoplasm of latently infected neurons. Segregated to the cytoplasm, ORF62 protein would not be able to transactivate VZV promoters, and ORF29 protein would not be able to bind to single-stranded DNA to perform its regulatory activities during DNA replication. While the functions of ORF21 and ORF63 are not known, their sequestration in the cytoplasm during latency, away from the nucleus, suggests that they might be unable to carry out their activities during latency.

How might these latency-associated proteins be sequestered in the cytoplasm during latency? Bontems *et al.* (2002) showed that the phosphorylation status of IE63 protein determines its localization in either the cytoplasm or nucleus. Transient expression of wild-type ORF63 protein resulted in a predominantly nuclear localization in Vero cells, while mutation of several serine or threonine residues that are sites of phosphorylation resulted in a predominantly cytoplasmic localization. While the phosphorylation pattern of ORF63 protein may appear to regulate its localization, the same authors showed that ORF63 protein localized to the nucleus of a neural cell line regardless of its phosphorylation status. In addition, localization of different phosphorylated forms of ORF63 is apparently dependent on whether the protein is expressed alone (Bontems *et al.*, 2002) or in the context of the rest of the genome (Cohen *et al.*, 2005a).

The phosphorylation status of ORF62 protein also regulates its localization (Kinchington et al., 2000). ORF66 protein phosphorylates ORF62 protein and keeps it sequestered to the cytoplasm. Since ORF66 is expressed during latency, this might be a mechanism to keep ORF62 protein from activating transcription during latency. However, a VZV mutant that is unable to express ORF66 still maintains latent infection in an animal model (Sato et al., 2003b). Thus, there are likely to be factors in addition to phosphorylation that are important for inhibiting the lytic functions of ORF63 and ORF62 protein during latency.

This model still leaves a number of questions unanswered. It is unclear from this model how ORF 21 and ORF29 are expressed if ORF62 is sequestered in the cytoplasm. Furthermore it is unclear why gene expression is limited to selected immediate-early and early genes and not other early or late genes.

VZV proteins have different activities in neurons than in permissive cells due to differences in cellular proteins

Differences in cellular proteins, such as transcription factors, may be responsible for the different activity of VZV in latently infected neurons compared to permissive cells. ORF29 protein augments the ability of ORF62 protein to transactivate the gI promoter in fibroblasts and T-cells; however, ORF29 inhibits the ability of ORF62 protein to activate the gI promoter in neuronal (PC-12) cells (Boucaud et al., 1998). Similarly, ORF63 protein activates the EF-1α promoter in melanoma cells, but not in neuroblastoma cells (Zuranski et al., 2005). This suggests that either neuronal cells lack an activator or that these cells express a repressor that is lacking in fibroblasts and T cells.

Neuronal cells may lack transcription factors, or may have transcription factors that are in an inactive form. VZV ORF10 forms a complex with TAATGARAT-like elements, Oct1 and host cell factor (HCF) to transactivate the ORF62 promoter (Moriuchi et al., 1995). HCF is sequestered in the cytoplasm in sensory neurons, but translocates to nucleus during stimuli that induce reactivation of HSV (Kristie et al., 1999). If HCF is important for reactivation of VZV, its normal sequestration in the cytoplasm may help VZV to maintain a latent infection.

Alternatively, transcription factors may act as repressors in neurons, but not in permissive cells. Transient expression Oct 2 in hamster kidney cells (in which the protein is normally not expressed) increases the basal activity of the ORF62 promoter (Patel et al., 1998). In contrast, expression of Oct2 in a neuronal cell line represses the activity of the ORF62 promoter. Since Oct2 is normally expressed only in neuronal and B-cells, Oct2 may repress the ORF62 promoter in these cells and help to maintain latency.

Oct 2 can also inhibit transactivation of the ORF62 promoter by the ORF10 protein. Transient expression of Oct2 with the ORF10 transactivator and an ORF62 promoter driving CAT as a reporter construct inhibited the ability of ORF10 protein to transactivate the ORF62 promoter. Thus, expression of Oct2 in neurons may inhibit the transactivating activity of ORF10, which might otherwise stimulate reactivation of VZV in neurons.

Future directions

While the last several years have resulted in much new information about VZV latency, many issues still remain. Further studies are needed from other laboratories to confirm the pattern of VZV protein expression during latency, preferably using monoclonal antibodies.

Additional studies using animal models will be critical in studies of VZV latency. Since animals can be sacrificed and ganglia removed quickly, reactivation is less of an issue. The simian varicella virus is a particularly attractive model since one can study acute and latent disease in the natural animal model. While the simian virus is the closest homologue to VZV, there are some differences in the genomes of the two viruses, and it is uncertain if these differences would result in different mechanisms of latency.

A number of questions regarding latency remain unanswered. At present it is unclear why VZV, unlike the other alphaherpesvirus, expresses so many viral genes during latency. Why are many of the immediate-early genes, which normally initiate VZV infection, expressed during latency? What are the molecular mechanisms involved in maintaining latency and in inducing reactivation?

REFERENCES

Annunziato, P., LaRussa, P., Lee, P. et al. (1998). Evidence of latent varicella-zoster virus in rat dorsal root ganglia J. Infect. Dis., **178** (Suppl 1), S48–S51.

Arvin, A. M., Sharp, M., Moir, M. et al. (2002). Memory cytotoxic T cell responses to viral tegument and regulatory proteins encoded by open reading frames 4, 10, 29, and 62 of varicella-zoster virus. Viral Immunol., **15**, 507–516.

Assouline J. G., Levin, M. J., Major, E. O., Forghani, B., Straus, S. E., and Ostrove, J. M. (1990). Varicella-zoster virus infection of human astrocytes, Schwann cells, and neurons. Virology, **179**, 834–844.

Baiker, A., Fabel, K., Cozzio, A. et al. (2004). Varicella-zoster virus infection of human neural cells in vivo. *Proc. Natl Acad. Sci. USA*, **101**, 10792–10797

Bontems, S., Di Valentin, E., Baudoux, L., Rentier, B., Sadzot-Delvaux, C., and Piette, J. (2002). Phosphorylation of varicella-zoster virus IE63 protein by casein kinases influences its cellular localization and gene regulation activity. *J. Biol. Chem.*, **277**, 21050–21060.

Boucaud, D., Yoshitake, H., Hay, J., and Ruyechan, W. (1998). The varicella-zoster virus (VZV) open-reading frame 29 protein acts as a modulator of a late VZV gene promoter. *J. Infect. Dis.*, **178** (Suppl. 1), S34–S38.

Brunell, P. A., Ren, L. C., Cohen, J. I., and Straus, S. E. (1999). Viral gene expression in rat trigeminal ganglia following neonatal infection with varicella-zoster virus. *J. Med. Virol.*, **58**, 286–290.

Chen J. J., Gershon, A. A., Li, Z. S., Lungu, O., and Gershon, M. D. (2003). Latent and lytic infection of isolated guinea pig enteric ganglia by varicella zoster virus. *J. Med. Virol.*, **70** (Suppl. 1), S71–S78

Clarke, P., Beer, T., Cohrs, R., and Gilden, D. H. (1995). Configuration of latent varicella-zoster virus DNA. *J. Virol.*, **69**, 8151–8154.

Clarke, P., Matlock, W. L., Beer, T. and Gilden, D. H. (1996). A simian varicella virus (SVV) homolog to varicella-zoster virus gene 21 is expressed in monkey ganglia latently infected with SVV. *J. Virol.*, **70**, 5711–5715.

Cohen, J. I., Cox, E., Pesnicak, L., Srinivas, S., and Krogmann T. (2004). The varicellazoster virus ORF63 latency-associated protein is critical for establishment of latency. *J. Virol.*, **78**, 11833–11840.

Cohen, J. I., Krogmann, T., Bontems, S., Sadzot-Delvaux, C., and Pesnicak, L. (2005a). Regions of the varicella-zoster virus open reading from 63 latency-associated protein important for replication in vitro are also critical for efficient establishment of latency. *J. Virol.*, **79**, 5069–5077.

Cohen, J. I. and Straus, S. E. (2001). Varicella-zoster virus and its replication. In *Fields Virology*, ed. D. M. Knipe, P. M. Howley et al. pp. 2707–2730. Philadelphia, PA: Lippincott-Williams & Wilkins.

Cohen J. I., Krogmann, T., Ross, J. P. et al. (2005b). Varicella-zoster virus ORF4 latency-associated protein is important for establishment of latency. *J. Virol.*, **79**, 6969–6975.

Cohrs R. J., Barbour, M. B., and Gilden, D. H. (1996). Varicella-zoster virus (VZV) transcription during latency in human ganglia: detection of transcripts mapping to genes 21, 29, 62, and 63 in a cDNA library enriched for VZV RNA. *J. Virol.*, **70**, 2789–2796

Cohrs, R. J., Randall, J., Smith, J. et al. (2000). Analysis of individual human trigeminal ganglia for latent herpes simplex virus type 1 and varicella-zoster virus nucleic acids using real-time PCR. *J. Virol.*, **74**, 11464–11471.

Cohrs R. J., Gilden, D. H., Kinchington, P. R., Grinfeld, E., and Kennedy, P. G. E. (2003). Varicella-zoster virus gene 66 transcription and translation in latently infected human ganglia. *J. Virol.*, **77**, 6660–6665.

Croen, K. D., Ostrove, J. M., Dragovic, L. J., and Straus, S. E. (1988). Patterns of gene expression and sites of latency in human nerve ganglia are different for varicella-zoster and herpes simplex viruses. *Proc. Natl Acad. Sci. USA*, **85**, 9773–9777.

Debrus, S., Sadzot-Delvaux, C., Nikkels, A. F., Piette, J., and Rentier, B. (1995). Varicella-zoster virus gene 63 encodes an immediate-early protein that is abundantly expressed during latency. *J. Virol.*, **69**, 3240–3245.

Dueland, A. N., Rannenbery-Nilsen, T., and Degre, M. (1995). Detection of latent varicella-zoster virus DNA and human gene sequences in human trigeminal ganglia by in situ amplification combined with in situ hybridization. *Arch. Virol.*, **140**, 2055–2066.

Efstathiou, S. E., Minson, A. C., Field, H. J., Anderson, J. R., and Wildy, P. (1986). Detection of herpes simplex virus-specific DNA sequences in latently infected mice and humans. *J. Virol.*, **57**, 446–455.

Furuta, Y., Takasu, T., Fukuda, S. et al. (1992). Detection of varicella-zoster virus DNA in human geniculate ganglia by polymerase chain reaction. *J. Infect. Dis.*, **166**, 1157–1159.

Furuta, Y., Takasu, T., Suzuki, S., Fukuda, S., Inuyama, Y., and Nagashima, K. (1997). Detection of latent varicella-zoster virus infection in human vestibular and spiral ganglia. *J. Med. Virol.*, **51**, 214–216.

Gary, L., Gilden, D. H., and Cohrs, R. J. (2006). Epigenetic regulation of varicella-zoster virus open reading frame 62 and 63 in latently infected human trigeminal ganglia. *J. Virol.*, **80**, 4921–4926.

Gilden, D. H., Vafai, A., Shtram, Y., Becker, Y., Devlin, M., and Wellish, M. (1983). Varicella-zoster virus DNA in human sensory ganglia. *Nature*, **306**, 478–480.

Gilden, D. H., Rosenman, Y., Murray, R., Devlin, A., and Vafai, A. (1987). Detection of varicella-zoster virus nucleic acid in neurons of normal human thoracic ganglia. *Ann. Neural.*, **22**, 377–380.

Gilden, D. H., Gesser, R., Smith, J. et al. (2001). Presence of VZV and HSV-1 DNA in human nodose and celiac ganglia. *Virus Genes*, **23**, 145–147.

Gray, W. L. (2004). Simian varicella: a model for human varicella-zoster virus infection. *Rev. Med. Virol.*, **14**, 363–381.

Gray, W. L., Starnes, B., White, M. W., and Mahalingam, R. (2001). The DNA sequence of the simian varicella virus genome. *Virology*, **284**, 123–130.

Grinfeld, E. and Kennedy, P. G. E. (2004). Translation of varicella-zoster virus genes during human ganglionic latency. *Virus Genes*, **29**, 317–319.

Grinfeld, E., Sadzot-Delvaux, C., and Kennedy, P. G. E. (2004). Varicella-zoster virus proteins encoded by open reading frames 14 and 67 are both dispensable for the establishment of latency in a rat model. *Virology*, **323**, 85–90.

Hood, C. Cunningham, A. L., Slobedman, B., Boadle, R. A., and Abendroth, A. (2003). Varicella-zoster virus-infected human sensory neurons are resistant to apoptosis, yet human foreskin fibroblasts are susceptible: evidence for a cell-type-specific apoptotic response. *J. Virol.*, **77**, 12852–12864.

Hood, C., Cunningham, A. L., Slobedman, B., et al. (2006). Varicella-zoster virus ORF63 inhibits apoptosis of primary human neurons. *J. Virol.* **80**, 1025–1031.

Hoover, S. E., Cohrs, R. J., Rangel, Z. G., Gilden, D. H., Munson, P., and Cohen, J. I. (2006). Downregulation of varicella-zoster virus (VZV) immediate-early ORF62 transcription by VZV ORF63 correlates with virus replication in vitro and with latency. *J. Virol.* **80**, 3459–3468

Hyman, R. W., Ecker, J. R., and Tenser, R. B. (1983). Varicella-zoster virus RNA in human trigeminal ganglia. *Lancet*, **ii**, 814–816.

Kennedy, P. G., Grinfeld, E., Bontems, S., and Sadzot-Delvaux, C. (2001). Varicella-zoster virus gene expression in latently infected rat dorsal root ganglia. *Virology*, **289**, 218–223.

Kennedy, P. G., Grinfeld, E., Traina-Dorge, V., Gilden, D. H., and Mahalingam, R. (2004). Neuronal localization of simian varicella virus DNA in ganglia of naturally infected African green monkeys. *Virus Genes*, **28**, 273–276.

Kennedy, P. G. E., Grinfield, E., and Gow, J. W. (1998). Latent varicella-zoster virus is located predominantly in neurons in human trigeminal ganglia. *Proc. Natl Acad. Sci. USA*, **95**, 4658–4662.

Kennedy. P. G. E., Grinfeld, E., and Gow, J. W. (1999). Latent varicella-zoster virus in human dorsal root ganglia. *Virology*, **258**, 451–454.

Kennedy, P. G. E., Grinfeld, E., and Bell, J. E. (2000). Varicella-zoster virus gene expression in latently infected and explanted human ganglia. *J. Virol.*, **74**, 11893–11898.

Kinchington, P. R., Fite, K, and Turse, S. E. (2000). Nuclear accumulation of IE62, the varicella-zoster virus (VZV) major transcriptional regulatory protein, is inhibited by phosphorylation mediated by the VZV open reading frame 66 protein kinase. *J. Virol.*, **74**, 2265–2277.

Kress, M. and Fickenscher, H. (2001). Infection by human varicella-zoster virus confers norepinephrine sensitivity to sensory neurons from rat dorsal root ganglia. *FASEB J.*, **15**, 1037–1043.

Kristie, T. M., Vogel, J. L., and Sears, A. E. (1999). Nuclear localization of the C1 factor (host cell factor) in sensory neurons correlates with reactivation of herpes simplex from latency. *Proc. Natl Acad. Sci.*, **96**, 1229–1233.

LaGuardia, J. J., Cohrs, R. J., and Gilden, D. H. (1999). Prevalence of varicella-zoster virus DNA in dissociated human trigeminal ganglion neurons and nonneuronal cells. *J. Virol.*, **73**, 8571–8577.

Levin, M. J., Cai, G. Y., Manchak, M. D., and Pizer, L. I. (2003). Varicella-zoster virus DNA in cells isolated from human trigeminal ganglia. *J. Virol.*, **77**, 6979–6987.

Lowry, P. W., Sabella, C., Koropchak, C. M. et al. (1993). Investigation of the pathogenesis of varicella-zoster virus infection in guinea pigs by using polymerase chain reaction *J. Infect. Dis.*, **167**, 78–83.

Lungu, O., Annunziato, P. W., Gershon, A. et al. (1995). Reactivated and latent varicella-zoster virus in human dorsal root ganglia. *Proc. Natl Acad. Sci. USA*, **92**, 10980–10984.

Lungu, O., Panagiotidis, C. A., Annunziato, P. W., Gershon, A. A., and Silverstein, S. J. (1998). Aberrant intracellular localization of varicella-zoster virus regulatory proteins during latency. *Proc. Natl Acad. Sci. USA*, **95**, 7080–7085.

Mahalingam, R., Wellish, M., Wolf, Q. et al. (1990). Latent varicella-zoster virus DNA in human trigeminal and thoracic ganglia. *N. Engl. J. Med.*, **323**, 627–631.

Mahalingam, R., Smith, D., Wellish, M. et al. (1991). Simian varicella virus DNA in dorsal root ganglia. *Proc. Natl Acad. Sci. USA*, **88**, 2750–2752.

Mahalingam, R., Wellish, M., Lederer, D., Forghani, B., Cohrs, R., and Gilden, D. (1993). Quantitation of latent varicella-zoster virus DNA in human trigeminal ganglia by polymerase chain reaction. *J. Virol.*, **67**, 2381–2384.

Mahalingam, R., Wellish, M., Cohrs, R. et al. (1996). Expression of protein encoded by varicella-zoster virus open reading frame 63 in latently infected human ganglionic neurons. *Proc. Natl Acad. Sci. USA*, **93**, 2122–2124.

Mahalingam, R., Traina-Dorge, V., Wellish, M., Smith, J., and Gilden, D. (2002). Naturally acquired simian varicella virus infection in African green monkeys. *J. Virol.*, **76**, 8548–8550.

Meier, J. L., Holman, R. P., Croen, K. D., Smialek, J. E., and Straus, S. E. (1993). Varicella-zoster virus transcription in human trigeminal ganglia. *Virology*, **193**, 193–200.

Merville-Louis, M. P., Sadzot-Delvaux, S. Delree, P., Piette, J., Moonen, G., and Rentier, B. (1989). Varicella-zoster virus infection of adult rat sensory neurons in vitro. *J. Virol.*, **63** 3155–3160.

Moriuchi, H., Moriuchi, M., and Cohen, J. I. (1995). Proteins and *cis*-acting elements associated with transactivation of the varicella-zoster virus (VZV) immediate-early gene 62 promoter by VZV open reading frame 10 protein. *J. Virol.*, **69**, 4693–4701.

Oxman, M. N., Levin, M. J., Johnson, G. R. et al. (2005). A vaccine to prevent herpes zoster and postherpetic neuralgia. *N. Eng. J. Med.*, **352**, 2271–2284.

Patel, Y., Gough, G., Coffin, R. S., Thomas, S., Cohen, J. I., and Latchman, D. S. (1998). Cell type specific repression of the varicella-zoster virus immediate-early gene 62 promoter by the cellular Oct-2 transcription factor. *Biochim. Biophys. Acta*, **1397**, 268–274.

Pevenstein, S. R., Williams, R. K., McChesney, D., Mont, E. K., Smialek, J. E., and Straus, S. E. (1999). Quantitation of latent varicella-zoster virus and herpes simplex virus genomes in human trigeminal ganglia. *J. Virol.*, **73**, 10514–10518.

Sadzot-Delvaux, C., Merville-Louis, S., and Delree, M. P. (1990). An in vivo model of varicella-zoster virus latent infection of dorsal root ganglia. *J. Neurosci. Res.*, **26**, 83–89.

Sadzot-Delvaux, C., Debrus, S., Nikkels, A., Piette, J., and Rentier, B. (1995). Varicella-zoster virus latency in the adult rat is a useful model for human latent infection. *Neurology*, **45** (Suppl. 8), S18–S20.

Sadzot-Delvaux, C., Kinchington, P. R., Debrus, S., Rentier, B., and Arvin, A. M. (1997). Recognition of the latency-associated immediate early protein IE63 of varicella-zoster virus by human memory T lymphocytes. *J. Immunol.*, **159**, 2802–2806.

Sato, H., Callanan, L. D., Pesnicak, L., Krogmann, T., and Cohen, J. I. (2002a). Varicella-zoster virus (VZV) ORF17 protein induces RNA cleavage and is critical for replication of VZV at 37 °C, but not 33 °C. *J. Virol.*, **76**, 11012–11023.

Sato, H., Pesnicak, L., and Cohen, J. I. (2002b). Varicella-zoster virus open reading frame 2 encodes a membrane phosphoprotein that is dispensable for viral replication and for establishment of latency. *J. Virol.*, **76**, 3575–3578.

Sato, H., Pesnicak, L., and Cohen, J. I. (2003a). Use of a rodent model to show that varicella-zoster virus ORF61 is dispensable for establishment of latency. *J. Med. Virol.*, **70** (Suppl 1), S79–S81.

Sato, H., Pesnicak, L., and Cohen, J. I. (2003b). Varicella-zoster virus ORF47 protein kinase which is required for replication in human T cells, and ORF66 protein kinase which is expressed during latency, are dispensable for establishment of latency. *J. Virol.*, **77**, 11180–11185.

Somekh, E., Tedder, D. G., Vafai, A. *et al.* (1992). Latency in vitro of varicella-zoster virus in cells derived from human fetal dorsal root ganglia. *Pediatr. Res.*, **32**, 699–703.

Stallings, C. L., Duigou, G. J., Gershon, A. A., Gershon, M. D., and Silverstein, S. J. (2006). The cellular localization pattern of varicella-zoster virus ORF29p is influenced by proteosome-mediated degradation. *J. Virol.*, **80**, 1497–1512.

Theil, D., Paripovic, I., Derfuss, T. *et al.* (2003). Dually infected (HSV-1/VZV) single neruons in human trigeminal ganglia. *Ann. Neurol.*, **54**, 678–681.

Vafai, A., Murray, R. S., Wellish, M., Devlin, M., and Gilden, D. H. (1988). Expression of varicella-zoster virus and herpes simplex virus in normal human trigeminal ganglia. *Proc. Natl Acad. Sci. USA*, **85**, 2362–2366.

Wang, K., Lau, T. Y., Morales, M., Mont, E. K., and Straus, S. E. (2005). Laser-capture microdissection: refining estimates of the quantity and distribution of latent herpes simplex virus 1 and varicella-zoster virus DNA in human trigeminal ganglia at the single-cell level. *J. Virol.* **79**, 14079–14087.

White, T. M., Mahalingam, R., Traina-Dorge, V., and Gilden, D. H. (2002). Simian varicella virus DNA is present and transcribed months after experimental infection of adult African green monkeys. *J. Neurovirol.*, **8**, 191–205.

Wigdahl, B., Rong, B. L., and Kinney-Thomas, E. (1986). Varicella-zoster virus infection of human sensory neurons. *Virology*, **152**, 384–399.

Wroblewska, Z., Valyi-Nagy, T., Otte, J. *et al.* (1993). A mouse model for varicella-zoster virus latency. *Microbiol. Pathogen.*, **15**, 141–151.

Xia, D. M., Srinivas, S., Sato, H., Pesnicak, L., Straus, S. E., and Cohen, J. I. (2002). Varicella-zoster virus ORF21, which is expressed during latency, is essential for virus replication but dispensable for establishment of latency. *J. Virol.*, **77**, 1211–1218.

Zerboni, L., Ku, C.-C., Jones, C. D., Zehnder, J. L., and Arvin, A. M. (2005). Varicella-zoster virus infection of human dorsal root ganglia in vivo. *Proc. Natl Acad. Sci. USA*, **102**, 6490–6495.

Zuranski, T., Nawar, H., Czechowski, D. *et al.* (2005). Cell-type-dependent activation of the cellular EF-1α promoter by the varicella-zoster virus IE63 protein. *Virology*, **338**, 35–42.

39

VZV immunobiology and host response

Ann Arvin[1] and Allison Abendroth[2]

[1]Departments of Pediatrics and Microbiology & Immunology, Stanford University School of Medicine, Stanford, CA, USA
[2]Centre for Virus Research, Westmead Millennium Institute and University of Sydney, Westmead, NSW, Australia

Immunobiology

Introduction

Varicella zoster virus (VZV) like the other herpesvirus family members is a highly successful and ubiquitous human pathogen. In order for VZV to persist in the human population, the virus has evolved strategies to avoid immune detection and potentially promote viral pathogenesis. We have demonstrated that VZV encodes two separate immune evasion strategies by specifically down-regulating cell-surface MHC class I (Abendroth et al., 2001a) and inhibiting the up-regulation of interferon-γ-induced MHC class II expression (Abendroth et al., 2000) during productive infection of primary human foreskin fibroblasts (HFFs). Given that VZV appears to evade host recognition by T-cells during the prolonged, 10–21 day incubation period, viral genes encoding immunomodulatory proteins are likely to delay the initial clonal amplification of VZV specific $CD4^+$ and $CD8^+$ T-lymphocytes and at least transiently enhance the ability of VZV to replicate at cutaneous sites. Recently we have studied the interaction of VZV with human dendritic cells (DCs) and T-lymphocytes. VZV has the ability to infect immature DCs and transfer virus to T-lymphocytes (Abendroth et al., 2001b). VZV also readily infects tonsil T-cells (Ku et al., 2002). The analysis of VZV interactions with T-cells during viral pathogenesis is described in Chapter 37. These capacities of VZV to infect DC and T-cells provide new models of viral dissemination during primary and recurrent VZV infections. Further studies assessing mature DCs have revealed a third immune evasion mechanism for VZV whereby the virus is able to productively infect a specialized immune cell (representing the most potent antigen presenting cell type), and in doing so impairs its ability to function properly.

More recently we have revealed that VZV has evolved a mechanism to limit host cell anti-viral defenses by impairing NF_{KB} activation in cultured fibroblasts and in differentiated epidermal cells in Skin xenografts in SCID by mice infected in vivo (Jones and Arvind, 2006).

VZV encoded downmodulation of cell-surface MHC class I expression

Our initial studies on VZV encoded immunomodulation began with the observation that VZV could downregulate cell-surface MHC class I expression in HFFs, which are the optimal cell-type for VZV infection and replication in vitro (Arvin, 2001). Cell-surface MHC class I and VZV antigen expression was examined by flow cytometry on HFFs infected with a low passage clinical VZV isolate (strain S) (Abendroth et al., 2001a). In cells where no viral antigen was observed, approximately 70%–80% of cells had detectable MHC class I expression, whereas only about 20%–30% of the cells that had detectable VZV antigen synthesis also expressed cell-surface MHC class I. VZV selectively down-regulated cell-surface MHC class I expression on HFFs as flow cytometry of these cells for transferrin receptor (CD71) expression, revealed that VZV infection did not alter cell-surface CD71 expression (Fig. 39.1). Cohen and co-workers have also found that infection of human fibroblasts with VZV results in the specific downregulation of cell-surface MHC class I expression (Cohen, 1998). We have further demonstrated that VZV isolates, whether fresh clinical isolates or tissue-culture passaged virus, specifically down-regulate MHC class I expression in primary and transformed human cells.

Given this evidence for MHC class I down-regulation following VZV infection of tissue culture cells, we sought to determine the potential biological significance of this effect in facilitating VZV pathogenesis. Based on our previous

(a)
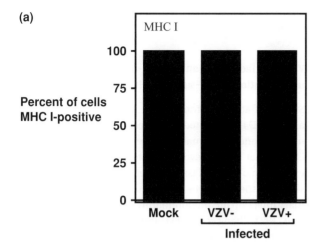

(b)
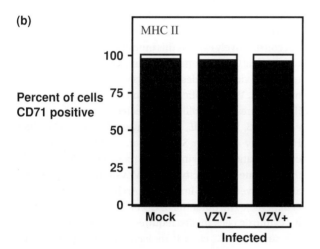

Fig. 39.1. FACS analysis of MHC class I, transferrin receptor (CD71) and VZV proteins on VZV infected cells. HFF were either infected with VZV for 24 hr or mock infected, cell preparations were stained with antibodies and fluorescent conjugates to MHC I and VZV proteins or to transferrin receptor (CD71) and VZV proteins. The percentage of VZV+ and VZV− cell populations expressing cell surface MHC I and transferrin receptor is shown using analysis by flow cytometry.

studies showing that VZV causes cell-associated viremia during the incubation period of primary infection without inducing a detectable immune response, we evaluated whether VZV infection altered MHC class I expression on human T-cells in vivo using the SCID-hu mouse model. We have previously demonstrated that VZV infects human CD4+ and CD8+ T-cells as well as immature CD4+CD8+ in SCID-hu thymus/liver implants *in vivo* (Moffat et al., 1995). To determine whether VZV infection alters MHC class I expression on human T-cells, human fetal thymus/liver implants placed under the kidney capsule of SCID-hu mice were inoculated with VZV according to our standard protocol (Moffat et al., 1995). Cells from the infected and uninfected implants were immunostained with antibodies to the CD3 T-cell marker, MHC class I and VZV proteins and analysed by flow cytometry. In all mice inoculated with VZV, CD3 positive T-cells expressing viral antigens were readily detectable (range of 11%–20%). The percentage of T-cells that expressed MHC class I within the population of cells that was positive for both CD3 and VZV proteins was significantly decreased when compared to the population that was positive for CD3 but had no detectable VZV proteins. Thus, VZV replication has the capacity to cause MHC class I down-regulation on human CD3 T cells a cell-type critical for the viremic phase of VZV pathogenesis. This observation is consistent with the concept that this immunomodulatory mechanism may provide the virus with a transient advantage, allowing viral dissemination to skin sites of replication that are required to achieve transmission.

Recently, we identified the first VZV immunomodulatory gene product and described the mechanism by which VZV alters cell-surface MHC class I expression (Abendroth et al., 2001a). To identify the compartment of MHC class I retention within the cell, we assessed the localization of MHC class I complexes with organelle specific markers in uninfected and VZV infected cells by confocal microscopy. Uninfected HFFs showed a uniform distribution of MHC class I throughout the cell cytoplasm and surface. In contrast, VZV infected HFs showed a strong perinuclear staining pattern for MHC class I molecules that colocalized with ceramide which labelled the membranes of the Golgi complex. The intracellular localization of MHC class I molecules to the Golgi in VZV infected cells suggests that a viral protein may interact specifically with a component of the MHC class I complex, thereby preventing efficient MHC class I transport to the cell-surface. In this respect, other herpesviruses, including HSV and human and murine CMV, have been shown to encode immunomodulatory proteins that directly associate with components of the MHC class I biosynthesis pathway (York et al., 1994; Fruh et al., 1995; Hill et al., 1995; Ahn et al., 1996; Jones et al., 1996; Tomazin et al., 1996; Wiertz et al., 1996; Galocha et al., 1997; Jones and Sun, 1997; Kleijnen et al., 1997; Machold et al., 1997; Reusch et al., 1999). Immunoprecipitation of radiolabelled MHC class I molecules in VZV and mock infected cells did not reveal binding of a viral protein but a modified, ~40 KDa MHC class I was detected consistently in VZV infected cells, which may reflect accelerated degradation of MHC class I molecules retained in the Golgi.

Despite the sequence similarities between the VZV and HSV genomes, VZV does not encode an ICP47 homologue.

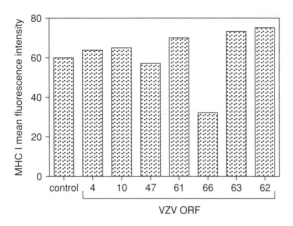

Fig. 39.2. Analysis of MHC I downregulation in cells transfected with plasmids expressing VZV proteins. HFF were transiently transfected with plasmids expressing VZV ORF4, ORF10, ORF47, ORF61, ORF62, ORF63, ORF66, or a parental control plasmid (control). 48 hr post-transfection cell preparations were stained for MHC I. Data is shown as the mean fluorescence intensity of specific cell surface MHC I staining.

In addition, VZV does not contain any identifiable homologues to the gene products of the other herpesviruses known to alter cell-surface MHC class I expression. Nonetheless, experiments using PAA to inhibit viral DNA replication suggest that an immediate-early or early VZV gene product(s) is involved in the down-modulation of cell-surface MHC class I molecules, whereas late genes were not required. VZV encodes several genes which have been reported to be expressed under immediate-early conditions (Kinchington and Cohen, 2000). To test whether these immediate-early proteins might play a role in MHC class I downregulation, HFs were transfected with the plasmids expressing ORF62, ORF63, ORF4 and ORF61. In addition, plasmids encoding the early gene products ORF10, ORF47 and ORF66 were also tested. After 48 hours, transfected cells were stained for cell-surface MHC class I expression and the mean fluorescence intensity of cell-surface MHC class I staining was determined for each transfected population of HFs by flow cytometry. Compared to the parental control plasmid, those expressing ORFs 4, 10, 47, 61, 62 and 63 did not significantly alter cell-surface MHC class I expression. In contrast, the mean fluorescence intensity of cell-surface MHC class I staining was significantly decreased on cultures transfected with the ORF66 expressing plasmid (Fig. 39.2). This is the first identification of a VZV immunomodulatory gene product that alters cell-surface MHC class I expression. Other VZV genes are also likely to encode the ability to downregulate MHC class I as another herpesvirus, HCMV, encodes no fewer than four viral genes which function to down-regulate MHC class I (Fruh et al., 1999).

VZV encoded inhibition of IFN γ-mediated up-regulation of cell-surface MHC class II

Studies of adaptive immunity to VZV reveal the importance of CD4+ restricted T-cell responses during primary infection and in the maintenance of latency. Therefore, it is likely that VZV has evolved strategies for modulating the expression of MHC class II, as well as MHC class I expression. VZV specific CD4+ T-cells that are elicited during primary infection are predominantly of the Th1 type (Bergen et al., 1991; Zhang et al., 1994) and function to produce high levels of IFN-γ which potentiates the clonal expansion of VZV specific T-cells (Arvin et al., 1986a,b; Jenkins et al., 1998; Wallace, et al., 1994). This cytokine is also essential for the up-regulation of MHC class II on cell types that usually do not constitutively express this immune molecule. Although the classical CTL response is mediated by CD8+ T-cells that recognize viral peptides in association with MHC class I molecules, VZV specific CTLs can also exhibit MHC class II (CD4+) restricted killing of infected target cells (Cooper et al., 1988; Diaz et al., 1989; Hayward et al., 1986, 1989; Hickling et al., 1987; Sharp et al., 1992). Peripheral T-cell populations contain high frequencies of CD4+ T-cells that mediate cytotoxicity against VZV-infected targets, as is also observed in HSV immunity (Arvin et al., 1991; Zarling et al., 1986). The potential of CD4+ T-cells to act as effective cytotoxic cells in vivo requires that target cells express cell-surface MHC class II molecules. These proteins are induced at sites of local inflammation, as in the case of cutaneous VZV lesions. Other herpesviruses such as human and mouse CMV have been shown to inhibit the upregulation of MHC class II expression induced by IFN-γ (Heise et al., 1998; Miller et al., 1998). Escape from CD4+ T-cell recognition by disrupting MHC class II expression is likely to be another VZV immune evasion strategy that has clinical significance. The block of IFNγ effects on MHC class II regulation could limit primary sensitization of T-cells to VZV peptides and delay the early amplification of VZV-specific CD4+ helper T-cells and release of cytokines at cutaneous sites of VZV replication. In vivo fibroblasts are infected by VZV and require IFNγ stimulation to up-regulate cell-surface MHC class II expression (Abendroth et al., 2000). Therefore, we assessed the impact of VZV infection on IFN γ-stimulated expression of MHC class II on HFFs and the induction of genes associated with surface MHC class II expression. In these experiments, HFFs were infected with VZV and treated with 100 U/ml of IFNγ for 48 hours, beginning 12 hours post-infection.

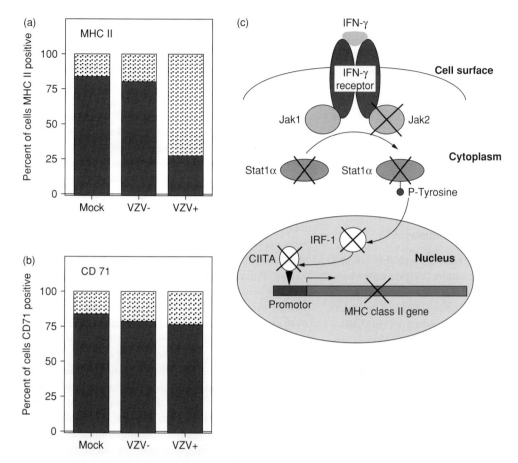

Fig. 39.3. FACS analysis of MHC class II, transferrin receptor (CD 71) and VZV proteins on VZV-infected cells treated with IFN-γ. Right panel: At 12 hours after VZV infection, HFF were treated with IFN-γ for 36 hours; cell preparations were stained with antibodies and fluorescent conjugates to MHC class II and VZV proteins or to transferrin receptor (CD71) and VZV proteins. The percentage of VZV$^+$ and VZV$^-$ cell populations expressing cell surface MHC class II or CD71 is shown. Left panel: Jak/Stat signal transduction pathway, showing cellular proteins affected by VZV.

Flow cytometry analysis of VZV and cell-surface MHC class II (HLA-DR) protein expression demonstrates that IFNγ treatment induced MHC class II expression in the majority of uninfected HFs but rarely in VZV infected HFFs (Fig. 39.3). With regard to the mechanism of inhibition of IFNγ induced MHC class II gene expression, we found that MHC Class II DRα, CIITA and IRF-1 transcripts did not accumulate in VZV infected cells after treatment with IFN-γ. Stat1α and Jak2 protein synthesis was reduced compared with Jak1 and CD71, which remained unchanged (Fig. 39.3). These observations indicate that the pathway by which VZV infection alters induction of MHC class II by IFN-γ differs from the effects of HCMV and MCMV. HCMV inhibits MHC class II expression in HFFs by blocking Jak/Stat signal transduction through a specific decrease in Jak1 expression. In contrast, MCMV inhibits IFN-γ stimulated MHC class II expression in murine macrophages by a mechanism that does not involve Jak/Stat signal transduction (Heise *et al.*, 1998). Thus, among the herpesviruses, VZV, HCMV and MCMV employ different strategies to reduce MHC class II antigen presentation pathways.

The significance of the in vitro studies is substantiated by examination of skin biopsies of human varicella and herpes zoster lesions for MHC class II and VZV RNA synthesis by non-isotopic *in situ* hybridization. Cutaneous VZV lesions showed a distinct separation of VZV infected cells and cells positive for MHC class II transcripts. These experiments demonstrated that dermal and epidermal cells infected with VZV were not expressing MHC class II transcripts in vivo at early stages of lesion formation.

The persistence of VZV as a human pathogen depends upon its transmission from the cutaneous lesions that are associated with varicella, caused by primary VZV infection, and herpes zoster, which results from reactivation of the virus from neuronal sites of latency. The ability of VZV to inhibit MHC class II expression in most infected human fibroblasts, despite exposure to high concentrations of IFNγ, provides a mechanism by which the virus can limit the consequences of immune surveillance by CD4+ T-cells. Impaired recognition of VZV-infected cells by CD4+ T-cells, which requires interaction of the T-cell receptor and viral peptides complexed with MHC class II molecules, can be predicted to allow transient viral replication in dermal and epidermal cells that is necessary for VZV transmission to susceptible individuals.

VZV interference with the NF-kB pathway

Since activation of the NF-kB pathway elicits IFN-a/b and other antiviral cytokines and proteins, herpesviruses have acquired mechanisms that inhibit this pathway. VZV interferes with NF-kB activation in cultured fibroblasts and in differentiated epidermal cells in skin xenografts in SCIDhu mice infected in vivo (Jones and Arvin, 2005). After a transient nuclear localization of the cononical NF-kB family members, p50 and p65 (Rel-A), these proteins become sequestered in the cytoplasm of VZV-infected fibroblasts. Nuclear exclusion of NF-kB proteins occurs because IkBa, which binds p50 and p65, is not degraded in VZV infected cells even though it is phosphorylated and ubiquitinated, and the 26S proteasome remains functional. VZV infection also inhibited the characteristic degradation of IkBa that is induced by exposure of fibroblasts to tumor necrosis factor alpha (TNF-α). The cytoplasmic retention of NF-kB proteins depended upon VZV replication and was in contrast to HSV-1, which induces persistent nuclear localization of p50 and p65, in a process that is required for normal HSV-1 replication. Thus, VZV has evolved a mechanism to limit host cell antiviral defenses by sequestering NF-kB proteins in the cytoplasm, a strategy that appears to be unique among the herpesviruses.

VZV infection of human dendritic cells and transmission to T-cells

The initial stage of primary VZV infection, involves the inoculation of mucosal sites with virus from respiratory droplets or cutaneous vesicle fluid from an infected individual. After inoculation, the virus remains undetected by the host immune system. (Arvin *et al., 1996*; Grose, 1981). The lymphotropism of VZV is critical for the dissemination of virus from peripheral blood mononuclear cells (PBMC) to epithelial cells, resulting in infection of the skin and the characteristic varicella rash (Arvin *et al.*, 1996). It remains unclear how VZV is transmitted from mucosal sites of inoculation to T-cells. Some T-cells may become infected in tonsillar tissues by direct transfer from infected mucosal epithelial cells (Ku *et al.*, 2004). At the same time, dendritic cells (DCs) of the respiratory mucosa may be among the first target cells to encounter VZV during primary infection and subsequently transport virus to the draining lymph nodes to enable T-cell infection as well as initiating a virus specific immune response (Jenkins *et al.*, 1999).

DCs are bone marrow-derived potent antigen presenting cells that are located in most tissues including the skin, blood, lymph and mucosal surfaces (Klagge and Schneider-Schaulies, 1999). Dendritic cells play a major role in initiating and maintaining the adaptive immune responses to pathogens such as viruses (Banchereau and Steinman, 1998; Banchereau *et al.*, 2000). Several human viruses including human immunodeficiency virus (HIV), measles virus, influenza virus, human herpes virus 6, human cytomegalovirus and herpes simplex virus have been shown to infect human DCs (Asada *et al.*, 1999; Bender *et al.*, 1998; Fugier-Vivier *et al.*, 1997; Grosjean *et al.*, 1997; Riegler *et al.*, 2000; Salio *et al.*, 1999; Schnorr *et al.*, 1997; Warren *et al.*, 1997). There is evidence that viruses exploit DCs as transport vehicles into lymphoid tissue and ultimately contribute to the transmission of the virus in the host. Viruses are also capable of modulating or interfering with the maturation, migration and function of DCs, thereby enabling potential evasion of the immune response.

Our initial interest in DCs began with determining whether VZV could infect human dendritic cells and subsequently transfer virus to T-cells. In this study, human monocyte derived dendritic cells were inoculated with VZV strain-S and assessed by flow cytometry for VZV and dendritic cell (CD1a) antigen expression (Abendroth *et al.*, 2001b). In all human DCs inoculated with VZV, CD1a positive DCs expressing viral antigens were readily detectable (range of 15%–40%). Dendritic cells were also shown to be susceptible to VZV infection by the immunoflourescence and confocal microscopy detection of immediate-early (IE62), early (ORF29) and late (gC) gene products in CD1a+ DCs. Infectious virus was recovered from infected DCs and cell-to-cell contact was required for virus transmission to permissive fibroblasts. Significantly, VZV-infected dendritic cells were capable of transferring virus to autologous human T lymphocytes, causing productive infection of these cells. This study provides the first evidence that DC are permissive to VZV infection and that infected DCs can transfer infectious virus to T-lymphocytes.

Two possible outcomes resulting from the interaction of VZV with DCs could account for transfer of infectious

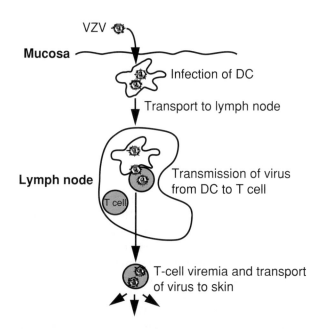

Fig. 39.4. Model of the potential role of VZV infection of dendritic cells.

virus to other cell types. Firstly, VZV may productively infect DCs and transfer new progeny virus to other cells (e.g., T-cells). Alternatively, because VZV envelope glycoproteins are known to bind mannose receptors which are found on immature DCs, the virus may be captured by DCs and internalised into trypsin resistant compartments and subsequently transmitted to other cells. Our current data clearly support the former as we were able to readily detect (by IFA and confocal microscopy) viral antigen expression from all three kinetic gene classes in sub-cellular locations consistent with those reported during productive infection of fully permissive fibroblasts (Kinchington and Cohen, 2000). This study proposed a model of VZV dissemination following primary inoculation (Fig. 39.4). In this model, upon entering the host at respiratory mucosa VZV infects DCs (Langerhans cells), which are then triggered to mobilize and migrate to the T-cell rich areas of regional lymph nodes. At this site the direct interaction of productively infected DCs with T-cells would then result in virus transmission and the productive infection of T-cells. This model, together with the potential for direct infection of T-cells by virus from VZV-infected respiratory epithelial cells are mutually compatible and consistent with a redundancy in the mechanisms by which VZV reaches T-cells. VZV pathogenesis should be facilitated by dual strategies for transfer of infectious virus into migratory T-cells. Once infection of T-cells occurs the virus should be disseminated to other sites of the body, infecting cutaneous epithelial cells with the formation of the characteristic vesicular rash of varicella. It is also possible that VZV is only captured by DCs and studies are underway to determine the mechanism of VZV entry into human DCs. Interestingly, it has been reported that HIV can either productively infect or be captured by DCs and that these two outcomes are mediated by separate pathways (Blauvelt et al., 1997). Further analysis of VZV-DC interactions, including the potential to isolate infected DCs from patients undergoing primary (varicella) or recurrent (herpes zoster) infection are likely to provide additional information on these outcomes.

DCs function to present antigenic peptides on the cell surface and to stimulate T-cells. Jenkins et al. demonstrated that a naïve T-cell response can be induced in vitro by VZV antigenic peptides, suggesting that DCs may be involved in the initiation of the primary immune response in vivo (Jenkins et al., 1999). The induction of the primary T-cell response involves not only the recognition of antigenic peptides in association with cell-surface MHC molecules, but also the interaction of co-stimulatory molecules (Marland et al., 1996). Several molecules are involved in this process include CD86, CD80, CD40, CD54 and CD83 and the absence or decreased expression of these immune molecules can render a DC less capable of inducing a T-cell response (Klagge and Schneider-Schaulies, 1999). It has been postulated that interference with DC function following virus infection may enable viruses to avoid immune recognition. In this respect, measles virus and HSV have been shown to interfere with the antigen presenting capability of infected DCs by a variety of mechanisms. Measles virus can productively infect DCs and interfere with the cells ability to induce the proliferation of CD4+ naïve T-cells (Grosjean et al., 1997). HSV infection of mature DCs results in a decreased T-cell stimulatory capacity and the specific degradation of the CD83 cell-surface molecule (Salio et al., 1999). However, not all viruses which infect DCs interfere with DC antigen presenting function. For example, HHV-6 productively infects DCs but these cells can still function as antigen presenting cells (Asada et al., 1999). As outlined above VZV has been shown to encode the ability to specifically down-modulate cell-surface MHC class I and IFNγ-induced MHC class II expression during productive infection of primary human fibroblasts (Abendroth et al., 2001a, 2000). VZV-infected immature DCs showed little or no change in the level of cell-surface expression of MHC class I, MHC class II, CD40 and CD86. Current studies are in progress to determine whether VZV infection of immature DCs inhibits DC maturation given that the transition from an immature to a mature state is essential for DCs to migrate and perform their antigen presentation function. To date, several other herpesviruses including HSV, HCMV and MCMV have been shown to inhibit the maturation of immature DCs by preventing up-regulation and expression of selective cell-surface immune molecules (Kruse *et al.*, 2000).

VZV encodes an immune evasion strategy during the productive infection of mature dendritic cells

DCs located in the periphery exist as immature cells, expressing low levels of MHC class I and MHC class II molecules and costimulatory molecules such as CD80 and CD86. Immature DCs readily take up antigen and are induced to migrate to the secondary lymphoid organs where they undergo maturation and present processed antigens to antigen specific T-lymphocytes (Steinman, 1991; Steinman *et al.*, 1997; Banchereau and Steinman, 1998). Maturation of DCs results in the down-regulation of antigen uptake and processing properties and the upregulation of MHC class I and MHC class II molecules, increased surface expression of costimulatory molecules CD80, CD86, CD40 and the maturation molecule CD83 and upregulation of adhesion molecules such as ICAM-1 (CD54) (Young and Steinman,1990; Young *et al.*, 1992; Zhou *et al.*, 1992; Zhou and Tedder, 1995; Cella *et al.*, 1997; Banchereau and Steinman, 1998; Steinman, 1999; Lechmann *et al.*, 2002). The ability of mature DCs to efficiently activate naïve T-lymphocytes which subsequently eliminate virus-infected cells has been attributed to their expression of these specific cell-surface immune molecules (Bhardwaj, 1997).

DCs should be an ideal target for viruses seeking to evade or delay the immune response by disrupting their function (Bhardwaj, 1997). In this respect, viruses including HSV-1 (Klagge and Schneider-Schaulies, 1999), HCMV (Raftery *et al.*, 2001), human herpesvirus 6 (HHV-6) (Kakimoto *et al.*, 2002), measles virus (Fugier-Vivier *et al.*, 1997; Grosjean *et al.*, 1997; Schnorr *et al.*, 1997), HIV (Blauvelt *et al.*, 1997) and lymphocytic choriomeningitis virus (LCMV) (Sevilla *et al.*, 2000) have been shown to interfere with the immune function of infected DCs by a variety of mechanisms. However, not all viruses which infect DCs interfere with DC antigen-presenting function. For example, influenza virus productively infects DCs, but these cells can still function as antigen-presenting cells (Bhardwaj *et al.*, 1994).

Given the pivotal role mature DCs play in the induction of successful anti-viral immune responses, we investigated whether VZV could infect mature DCs and interfere with their immune function. In this study, we demonstrated by flow cytometry, immunofluorescence and infectious center assays that VZV can productively infect human mature DCs and produce infectious virus (Morrow *et al.*, 2003). Following the assessment of the cell-surface expression of MHC class I, MHC class II, CD80, CD83 and CD86 by flow cytometry we found that with the exception of MHC class II, all of these molecules were down-regulated on VZV infected mature Dcs. These observations indicate that the mechanism by which VZV alters immune molecule expression on mature DCs appears novel, since the pattern of immune molecule alteration differs from that of other viruses which infect and alter mature DCs. In comparison, HSV-1 infection of mature DCs results in the down-regulation only of CD83 (Kruse *et al.*, 2000) and HSV-2 infection causes down-regulation of MHC class I, MHC class II, CD40, CD80 and CD86 on murine DCs (Jones *et al.*, 2003). It should be noted, however, that the source of cells and/or the DC maturation stimuli may have a significant bearing on the expression of immune molecules and subsequent DC function following virus infection. In this respect, HCMV has been shown to down-regulate MHC class I and MHC class II on monocyte derived DCs induced to mature with LPS or TNF-α, yet CD34$^+$ bone marrow-derived DCs induced to mature with CD40 display a down-regulation of MHC class I, MHC (Hertel *et al.*, 2003) class II, CD80, CD83, CD86 and CCR7 (E.S. Mocarski, personal communication, July 2002). Thus, among the human herpesviruses studied to date, there appear to be multiple strategies to interfere with DC immune molecule expression and the present study provides evidence that VZV has done likewise.

The most distinctive functional characteristic of mature DCs is their ability to stimulate T-cells (Banchereau and Steinman, 1998; Cella *et al.*, 1997; Steinman, 1999). Therefore, we assessed the functional consequences of the selective immune molecule alteration observed on VZV infected mature DCs. We found that VZV infection of mature DCs significantly reduced their ability to stimulate the proliferation of allogeneic T-lymphocytes. The identity of the VZV gene or genes involved in the downregulation of immune molecules and reduced T cell stimulation capacity during productive infection of mature DCs is yet to be determined. To date, ORF66 is the only identified VZV immunomodulatory gene product (Abendroth *et al.*, 2001b). Additional studies assessing ORF66 together with other viral ORFs are a focus of current experiments aimed at identifying the VZV genes responsible for the inhibition of mature DC function.

Thus, current evidence indicates that VZV is DC-tropic, and can target two distinct aspects of DC function represented by immature and mature DCs. This ability to infect both DC types confers upon the virus the potential to both increase virus dissemination in the host as well as evade the immune response.

The host immune response

Immunity during primary VZV infection

Innate immune responses are presumed to mediate the initial control of primary VZV infection. Interferon-α (IFN-α) inhibits VZV replication and is released by PBMC from naive donors exposed to VZV antigens in vitro. Early clinical trials demonstrated that the severity of varicella was reduced when immunocompromised children with varicella were given exogenous IFN-α. Our recent analysis of VZV infection of human skin xenografts in the SCIDhu mouse model of VZV pathogenesis demonstrated a dramatic increase in IFN-α production, accompanied by nuclear translocation of pStat protein within uninfected epidermal cells that surrounded skin cells actively infected with VZV (Ku et al., 2004). When animals were given antibody to IFN-α/β receptor, VZV titers increased tenfold and cytopathic changes in the skin were much more extensive. Innate antiviral immunity is also mediated by natural killer (NK) cells. NK cells from naive individuals have the capacity to lyze VZV-infected targets in vitro; non-specific cytotoxicity is mediated by CD16+ T-cells and is enhanced by IL-2.

Adaptive T-cell responses, manifest as an initial burst in VZV-specific T cells, appear to be critical for resolving primary VZV infection (Fig. 39.5). Primary VZV infection is associated with an incubation period of 10–21 days before skin lesions appear. T-cell recognition of VZV is not detected in individuals tested during the incubation period, suggesting that viral mechanisms for evading immune surveillance are very effective during the initial phase of primary VZV infection (Arvin, 1999). When acquisition of VZV-specific T-cell immunity is delayed, life-threatening dissemination of the virus occurs, as described in patients with congenital T-cell immunodeficiency diseases, malignancy or immunosuppression and in newborn infants. In our early studies of antiviral immunity in immunocompromised children with varicella and malignancy, only one (7.7%) of 13 immunocompromised patients had a detectable VZV-specific T-cell proliferation response within three days after the onset of varicella compared with 19 (42%) of 45 healthy subjects ($P<0.05$) (Arvin et al., 1986a). Diminished VZV-specific cellular immunity was associated with persistent VZV viremia, continued formation of new skin lesions and viral dissemination to lungs, liver and other organs. Children with HIV may develop chronic varicella, which also suggests the significance of antiviral T cell-mediated immunity in the host response to VZV. In contrast, VZV IgG and IgM antibody titers measured within the first three days, did not correlate with the severity of varicella in healthy or immunodeficient children (Arvin

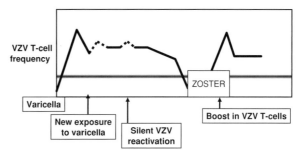

Fig. 39.5. Schema of the T-cell response to VZV.

et al., 1986a,b) and varicella appears to be uncomplicated in patients with agammaglobulinemia.

In the healthy host with acute varicella, VZV-specific T-cell proliferation responses were detected in 12%, 31% and 47% of subjects tested at one, two and three days after the onset of rash, respectively (Arvin et al., 1986a). A higher VZV-specific T-cell proliferation response, measured as the mean stimulation index (SI) at three days, was associated with fewer varicella lesions (Arvin et al., 1986a). The mean VZV SI was 7.5±10.43 SD in those who had fewer than 100 lesions/m^2 when new lesion formation had stopped, compared with 1.4 ± 1.85 SD for those with >400 lesions/m^2 ($P < 0.05$). In these early experiments, activated CD4+ and CD8+ T-cells were present in peripheral blood by flow cytometry before T-cell proliferation to VZV was detected. Primary VZV infection also elicits virus-specific CD4+ T-cells that produce IL-2 and IFN-γ, which are considered Th1 cytokines. In contrast, very few VZV specific CD4+ T-cells release IL-4, a cytokine made by the Th2 subset of CD4+ T-cells (Zhang et al., 1994). As expected, based on the CD4+ T cell cytokine profiles, IL-2 and IFN-γ, as well as IFN-α concentrations are increased in sera from healthy individuals with varicella (Wallace et al., 1994; Arvin et al., 1986a,b). Like IFN-α, IFN-γ has antiviral activity against VZV. IFN-γ, which enhances clonal expansion of antiviral T-cells, was diminished in adults with primary VZV infection compared to children. This difference may help to explain the severe cases of varicella observed in healthy adults.

Information about the VZV proteins that are recognized during the initial T cell response to primary infection is limited. Clonal expansion of T cells that recognize glycoproteins, gE and gH, and the IE62 major tegument/regulatory protein has been documented (Arvin et al., 1986b). The pattern of VZV proteins that were recognized by early virus-specific CD4+ T-cells from individuals with primary VZV was variable; gE was the predominant target in 67% of healthy individuals, gH in 71% and IE62 protein in 57% of subjects. Regardless of the predominant protein target, varicella was uncomplicated in all cases. As noted, up-regulation of class II expression permits lysis of infected cells by CD4+ cytotoxic T-cells and IFN-γ also enhances class I restricted cytotoxicity mediated by CD8+ T-cells. Although sub-populations of effector cells were not identified, high frequencies of CTL that lyze targets expressing VZV gE and IE62 protein were documented in healthy individuals with acute varicella (Diaz et al., 1989).

VZV immunity during latency

VZV-specific IgG antibodies and CD4+ and CD8+ T-cells persist for decades after primary VZV infection (Arvin, 2001). VZV-specific IgG antibodies are directed against many VZV polypeptides and have functional capacities that include viral neutralization and antibody-dependent cytotoxicity (ADCC) against VZV infected targets. Most healty immune individuals also have serum antibodies to VZV.

Immune adults have VZV-specific memory T cells in peripheral blood with frequencies of approximately 1:40 000 PBMC. Glycoproteins, gE, gB, gC and gH, and the IE62 protein were recognized by T-cells in proliferation and cytokine release assays (Arvin et al., 1986a). CD4+ T-cell clones specific for epitopes of gE, gB, gH or gI were derived from VZV immune donors and some clones specific for gB or gI had dual helper and cyotutoxic functions. Using synthetic peptides to stimulate T-cells confirmed that regions of IE62, gB, gE and gI functioned as T-cell epitopes. In addition, VZV specific memory T-cells have been recovered from lymphoid tissue. As was reported during primary VZV infection, cytokine profiles of memory CD4+ T-cells showed that up to 85% of proliferating cells produced IFN-γ whereas only 10% released IL-4 (Hayward et al., 1989). Intradermal inoculation of inactivated VZV antigens elicits delayed hypersensitivity reactions in immune children and adults (Kamiya et al., 1977).

MHC class I or class II restricted cytotoxic T-cells that recognize VZV proteins persist for many years after primary VZV infection (Diaz et al., 1989; Hayward et al., 1986; Sharp et al., 1992). Memory CD4+ CTL are detected with secondary VZV stimulation and using autologous lymphoblastoid cells infected with VZV or vaccinia recombinants that express VZV proteins as targets, and CD8+ CTL can be detected with VZV-infected fibroblast targets, that express only MHC class I antigen, or with highly purified preparations of CD8+ T-cells tested against lymphoblastoid cells expressing VZV proteins. Viral protein targets that have been documented include gC, gE, gI and IE62 and IE63 proteins (Sharp et al., 1992). Memory CTL specific for the IE62 protein were found at frequencies of 1:105 000 ± 85 000

SD in VZV immune subjects tested > 20 years after varicella. Mean frequencies of anti-VZV gE CTL were 1:121 000 ± 86 000 SD. Using these methods, mean frequencies of CD4+ CTLs that recognized IE62 protein were 1:108 000 and 1:74 000 in the CD8+ population, which was not significantly different. VZV gE specific CD4+ CTL frequencies were 1:119 000 compared to 1:31 000 in the CD8+ population (NS).

Persistence of VZV-specific memory

The host response to VZV must protect against new exposures to varicella and against VZV reactivation from latently infected cells in the sensory ganglia (Fig. 39.5). At the same time, these exogenous and endogenous exposures to infectious VZV, constitute mechanisms by which VZV immunity may be boosted. VZV immune adults and children tested after household exposures to varicella have been found to develop increases in VZV IgG, IgM and IgA antibodies and in VZV-specific T-cell proliferation as well as enhanced delayed hypersensitivity to VZV skin test antigens (Gershon et al., 1984).

Preserving VZV immunity is also important for maintaining VZV latency. VZV may undergo periodic reactivations that are asymptomatic or result in mild, undiagnosed episodes of zoster. Endogenous reactivation of VZV provides a second potential mechanism for sustaining VZV immunity over all or most of the lifetime of the host. Whereas other herpesviruses are readilty shown to reactivate at mucosal surfaces asymptomatically, VZV shedding at mucosal sites has not been documented. Evidence that subclinical VZV reactivation occurs has been suggested in studies monitoring VZV immune markers over time in healthy adults with no recent exposure to varicella. Intermittent increases in these responses may represent responses to asymptomatic VZV. The re-appearance of VZV IgM antibodies has been considered such a marker (Gershon et al. 1984). More directly, we found that 19% of bone marrow transplant patients tested during the period of highest risk for herpes zoster in these patients had subclinical cell-associated VZV viremia as detected by PCR. VZV DNA has also been detected in PBMC from some elderly individuals (Devlin et al. 1992). A relationship between VZV reactivation and preservation of cell-mediated immunity was suggested by the fact that many bone marrow transplant recipients had reconstitution of VZV-specific T-cell responses during the first year after transplantation, without having had any exposures to varicella or clinical signs of zoster. Recovery of VZV-specific CTL function was also observed in 50% of BMT patients who had remained asymptomatic.

Immunity during VZV reactivation

The clinical experience demonstrates a direct correlation between the increased risk of zoster and diseases or treatments that interfere with T cell function. Patients with HIV infection who have progressive depletion of CD4+ T-cells also have a high incidence of zoster. The age-related increase in the risk of zoster in healthy elderly people is also well documented and several studies have shown that VZV-specific T cell responses decline with age. In contrast, VZV IgG antibodies do not decline in high risk populations and lower titers do not predict a higher risk of VZV reactivation, causing zoster (Webster et al., 1989). Elderly peole have decreases in frequencies of memory T-cells that recognize VZV in proliferation and CTL assays and delayed hypersensitivity responses to VZV skin testing are absent or diminished. In limiting dilution proliferation assays, older individuals showed reduced frequencies of CD4+ T-cells, primarily within the IFN-γ producing Th1 subset, as compared to IL-4 positive CD4+ T-cells.

In the healthy individual with zoster, the equilibrium between the virus and the host is re-established rapidly. Viral replication at skin sites is usually controlled within 1 or 2 weeks. Transfer of infectious virus into T-cells from sites of virus replication in dorsal root ganglia or skin appears to be unusual, since skin lesions are rarely found beyond the affected dermatome. In immunocompromised patients, severe, prolonged suppression of cellular immunity is associated with the highest risk of herpes zoster and of life-threatening dissemination of the virus, resulting from cell-associated VZV viremia (Arvin, 1999). Among bone marrow transplant recipients, memory CD8+ T-cells are generated after in vitro stimulation with VZV antigen in numbers comparable to those of healthy immune individuals whereas CD4+ CTL function is difficult to detect during the period after transplantation when these patients are at high risk for VZV recurrences. The observation that the risk of herpes zoster increases when patients with HIV infection have low CD4+ T-cell numbers is consistent with a role for CD4+ as well as CD8+ T-cells in the restriction of viral replication in vivo. Immunocompromised patients often have scattered cutaneous lesions indicating the occurrence of viremia during zoster. Under these circumstances, VZV may enter DC in the involved skin area and reach T-cells in regional lymph nodes, or it may be transferred into migratory T-cells, causing viremia as a result of the limitations of the host response.

Herpes zoster is followed by increased VZV IgG, IgM and IgA antibodies in healthy and immunocompromised patients. The humoral immune response is directed against a broad range of VZV proteins, including early, structural/regulatory proteins, viral enzymes and glycoproteins. Nevertheless, the contribution of humoral immunity to resolving VZV reactivation is not certain. Some individuals who have early responses with high titers of VZV IgG and IgM antibodies have severe herpes zoster whereas those with mild clinical disease may have limited increases in VZV antibody titers. Viral replication at local cutaneous sites was not inhibited when VZV immune globulin was given to immunocompromised individuals with herpes zoster before treatment with antiviral drugs was possible. However, there was some evidence that a diminished humoral immune response early in the clinical course was associated with a higher risk of viremia and viral dissemination in immunocompromised patients.

Healthy adults with herpes zoster develop a marked increase in VZV-specific T-cell responses, as shown by comparing VZV T-cell proliferation within one week after onset with responses tested from two to four weeks later. IFN-α is detected in vesicle fluid from the cutaneous zoster lesions, increasing as the lesions resolve in healthy subjects (Stevens et al., 1975). Herpes zoster in immunocompromised patients is associated with delayed boosting of VZV T-cell responses. In one study of patients with malignancy and zoster, the mean SI was 1.8 ± 0.85 SD during the first week and had increased only to 5.7 ± 3.03 SD by 2 to 4 weeks. IFN-α concentrations were also low in zoster lesions in these high-risk patients and IFN-α treatment accelerated the resolution of zoster in such patients (Merigan et al., 1978).

The introduction of the live attenuated varicella vaccine has introduced new considerations about the persistence of memory immunity to VZV, which are discussed in Chapter 37. Such vaccines may prove to be useful clinically as a strategy for reversing the waning VZV T cell immunity that occurs with age. In a recent study, we provided a "proof of concept" for this approach by demonstrating that inactivated varicella vaccine given to hematopoeitic cell transplant recipients resulted in early reconstitution of VZV-specific CD4 T cell proliferation and a reduced risk of symptomatic episodes of zoster (Hata et al., 2002). Since the live attenuated varicella vaccine can boost VZV T cell immunity in healthy elderly adults, the successful outcome of studies to examine its effectiveness for preventing or modifying the severity of zoster suggests that VZV-specific T cells help to block the progression of VZV reactivation from latency to clinically symptomatic infection (Oxman et al., 2005).

REFERENCES

Abendroth, A., Slobedman, B., Eunice, L., Mellins, E., Wallace, M., and Arvin, A. M. (2000). Modulation of MHC class II protein expression by varicella zoster virus. J. Virol., **74**, 1900–1907.

Abendroth, A., Lin, I., Slobedman, B., Ploegh, H., and Arvin, A. M. (2001a). Varicella-zoster virus retains major histocompatibility complex class I proteins in the Golgi compartment of infected cells. *J. Virol.*, **75**, 4878–4888.

Abendroth, A., Morrow, G., Cunningham, A. L. and Slobedman, B. (2001b). Varicella-zoster virus infection of human dendritic cells and transmission to T cells: Implications for virus dissemination in the host. *J. Virol.*, **75**, 6183–6192.

Ahn, K., Meyer, T. H., Uebel, S. *et al.* (1996). Molecular mechanism and species specificity of TAP inhibition by herpes simplex virus ICP47. *EMBO. J.*, **15**, 3247–3255.

Arvin, A. M. (1999). Varicella-zoster virus. In *Persistent Viral Infections of Humans*. eds. Ahmed, R. and Chen, I. S. Y., pp. 183–208. Chicheaces, UK: John Wiley.

Arvin, A. M. (2001). Varicella-zoster virus. In *Fields' Virology*, ed. Howley, P. and Knipe, D. M. 4th edn, pp. 2731–2768. Philadelphia: Lippincott-Williams & Wilkins.

Arvin, A. M., Koropchak, C. M., Williams, B. R., Grumet, F. C., and Foung, S. K. (1986a). Early immune response in healthy and immunocompromised subjects with primary varicella-zoster virus infection. *J. Infect. Dis.*, **154**, 422–429.

Arvin, A. M., Kinney-Thomas, E., Shriver, K. *et al.* (1986b). Immunity to varicella-zoster viral glycoproteins, gp I (90/58) and gp III (gp 118) and to a nonglycosylated protein, p170. *J. Immunol.*, **137**, 1346.

Arvin, A. M., Sharp, M., Smith, S. *et al.* (1991). Equivalent recognition of a varicella-zoster virus immediate early protein (IE62) and glycoprotein I by cytotoxic T lymphocytes of either CD4+ or CD8+ phenotype. *J. Immunol.*, **146**, 257–264.

Arvin, A. M., Moffat, J. F., and Redman, R. (1996). Varicella-zoster virus: aspects of pathogenesis and host response to natural infection and varicella vaccine. *Adv. Virus Res.*, **46**, 263–309.

Asada, H., Klaus-Kovtun, V., Golding, H., Katz, S. I. and Blauvelt., A. (1999). Human herpesvirus-6 infects dendritic cells and suppresses human immunodeficiency virus type-1 replication in coinfected cultures. *J. Virol.*, **73**, 4019–4028.

Auwaerter, P. G., Kaneshima, H., McCune, J. M., Wiegand, G. and Griffin, D. E. (1996). Measles virus infection of thymic epithelium in the SCID-hu mouse leads to thymocyte apoptosis. *J. Virol.*, **70**, 3734–3740.

Bancherau, J. and Steinman, R. M. (1998). Dendritic cells and the control of immunity. *Nature*, **392**, 245–252.

Bancherau, J., Briere, F., Caux, C. *et al.* (2000). Immunobiology of dendritic cells. *Annu. Rev. Immunol.*, **18**, 767–811.

Bender, A., Albert, M., Reddy, A. *et al.* (1998). The distinctive features of influenza virus infection of dendritic cells. *Immunobiology*, **198**, 552–567.

Bergen, R. E., Sharp, M., Sanchez, A., Judd, A. K., and Arvin, A. M. (1991). Human T cells recognize multiple epitopes of an immediate early/tegument protein (IE62) and glycoprotein I of varicella zoster virus. *Viral Immunol.*, **4**, 151–166.

Bhardwaj, N. (1997). Interactions of Viruses with dendritic cells: a double-edged sword. *J. Exp. Med.*, **186**, 795–799.

Bhardwaj, N., Bender, A., Gonzalez, N. *et al.* (1994). Influenza virus-infected dendritic cells stimulate strong proliferative and cytolytic responses from human CD8+ T cells. *J. Clin. Invest.*, **94**, 797–807.

Blauvelt, A., Asada, H., Saville, W. M. *et al.* (1997). Productive infection of dendritic cells by HIV-1 and their ability to capture virus are mediated through separate pathways. *J. Clin. Invest.*, **100**, 2043–2053.

Cella, M., Engering, A., Pinet, V., Pieters, J. and Lanzavecchia, A. (1997). Inflammatory stimuli induce accumulation of MHC class II complexes on dendritic cells. *Nature*, **388**, 782–787.

Cohen, J. I. (1998). Infection of cells with varicella-zoster virus down-regulates surface expression of class I major histocompatibility complex antigens. *J. Infect. Dis.*, **177**, 1390–1393.

Cohen, O. J. and Fauci, A. S. (2001). Pathogenesis and medical aspects of HIV-1 infection In *Fields' Virology* 4th edn, Knipe, D. M. and Howley, P. M. eds, pp. 2043–2094. Philadelphia: Lippincott Williams & Wilkins

Cooper, E. C., Vujcic, L. K., and Quinnan, G. V. Jr. 1988. Varicella-zoster virus-specific HLA-restricted cytotoxicity of normal immune adult lymphocytes after in vitro stimulation. *J. Infect. Dis.*, **158**, 780–788.

Devlin, M. E., Gilden, D. H., Mahalingam, R. *et al.* (1992). Peripheral blood mononuclear cells of the elderly contain varicella-zoster virus DNA. *J. Infect. Dis.*, **165**, 619.

Diaz, P. S., Smith, S., Hunter, E., and Arvin, A. M. (1989). T lymphocyte cytotoxicity with natural varicella-zoster virus infection and after immunization with live attenuated varicella vaccine. *J. Immun.*, **142**, 636–641.

Esolen, L. M., Park, S. W., Hardwick, J. M., and Griffin. D. E. (1995). Apoptosis as a cause of death in measles virus-infected cells. *J. Virol.*, **69**, 3955–3958.

Frey, C. R., Sharp, M. A., Min, A. S., Schmid, D. S., Loparev, V., and Arvin, A. M. (2003). Identification of CD8+ T cell epitopes in the immediate early protein 62 of varicella-zoster virus and evaluation of CD8+ T cell responder frequencies to the immediate early protein 62 using IE62 peptides after varicella vaccination. *J. Infect. Dis.*, **188**, 40–52.

Fruh, K., Ahn, K., Djaballah, H. *et al.* (1995). A viral inhibitor of peptide transporters for antigen presentation. *Nature*, **375**, 415–418.

Fruh, K., Gruhler, A., Krishna, R., and Schoenhals, G. (1999). A comparison of viral immune escape strategies targeting the MHC class I assembly pathway. *Immunol. Revs.*, **168**, 157–166.

Fugier-Vivier, I., Servat-Delprat, C., Rivailler, P., Rissoan, M. C., Liu, Y. J. and Rabourdin-Combr, C. (1997). Measles virus suppresses cell mediated immunity by interfering with the survival and function of dendritic and T-cells. *J. Exp. Med.*, **186**, 813–823.

Galocha, B., Hill, A., Barnett, B. *et al.* (1997). The active site of ICP47, a herpes simplex virus-encoded inhibitor of major histocompatibility complex (MHC)-encoded peptide transport associated with antigen processing (TAP), maps to the NH2-terminal 35 residues. *J. Exp. Med.*, **185**, 1565–1572.

Gershon, A. A., Steinberg, S. P., and Gelb, L. (1984). Clinical reinfection with varicella-zoster virus. *J. Infect. Dis.*, **149**, 137.

Grose, C. (1981). Variation on a theme by Fenner: the pathogenesis of chicken pox. *Pediatrics*, **68**, 735–737.

Grosjean, I., Caux, C., Bella, C. et al. (1997). Measles virus infects human dendritic cells and blocks their allostimulatory properties for CD4+ T-cells. *J. Exp. Med.*, **186**, 801–812.

Hata, A., Asanuma, H., Rinki, M. et al. (2002). Protection of hematopoietic cell transplant recipients from herpes zoster by an inactivated varicella vaccine. *N. Engl. J. Med.*, **347**, 26–34.

Hayward, A. R., Pontesilli, O., Herberger, M., Laszlo, M., and Levin. M. (1986). Specific lysis of varicella zoster virus-infected B lymphoblasts by human T cells. *J. Virol.*, **58**, 179–184.

Hayward, A., Giller, R., and Levin, M. (1989). Phenotype, cytotoxic, and helper functions of T cells from varicella zoster virus stimulated cultures of human lymphocytes. *Viral Immun.*, **2**, 175–184.

Heise, M. T., Connick, M., and Virgin, H. W. T. (1998). Murine cytomegalovirus inhibits interferon gamma-induced antigen presentation to CD4 T cells by macrophages via regulation of expression of major histocompatibility complex class II-associated genes. *J. Exp. Med.*, **187**, 1037–1046.

Hertel, L., Lacaille, V. G., Strobl, H., Mellins, E. D., and Mocarski, E. S. (2003). Susceptibility of immature and mature Langerhans cell-type dendritic cells to infection and immunomodulation by human cytomegalovirus. *J. Virol.* **77**(13), 7563–7574.

Hickling, J. K., Borysiewicz, L. K., and Sissons, J. G. (1987). Varicella-zoster virus-specific cytotoxic T lymphocytes (Tc): detection and frequency analysis of HLA class I-restricted Tc in human peripheral blood. *J. Virol.*, **61**, 3463–3469.

Hill, A., Jugovic, P., York, I. et al. (1995). Herpes simplex virus turns off the TAP to evade host immunity. *Nature.*, **375**, 411–415.

Ihara, T., Kato, T., Torigoe, S. et al. (1991). Antibody response determined with antibody-dependent cell-mediated cytotoxicity (ADCC), neutralizing antibody, and varicella skin test in children with natural varicella and after varicella immunization. *Acta Paediatr. Jap.* **33**, 43.

Jenkins, D. E., Redman, R. L., Lam, E. M., Liu, C., Lin, I., and Arvin, A. M. (1998). Interleukin (IL)-10, IL-12, and interferon-gamma production in primary and memory immune responses to varicella-zoster virus. *J. Infect. Dis.*, **178**, 940–948.

Jenkins, D. E., Yasukawa, L. L., Bergen, R., Benike, C., Engleman, E. G., and Arvin. A. M. (1999). Comparison of primary sensitization of naive human T cells to varicella zoster virus peptides by dendritic cells in vitro with responses elicited in vivo by varicella vaccination. *J. Immunol.*, **162**, 550–567.

Jones, J. O. and Arvin A. M. (2006). Inhibition of the NF-kB pathway by varicella-zoster virus in vitro and in human epidermal cells in vivo. *J. Virol.*, **80**, 5113–5124.

Jones, T. and Sun, L. (1997). Human cytomegalovirus US2 destabilizes major histocompatibility complex class I heavy chains. *J. Virol.*, **71**, 2970–2979.

Jones, T. R., Wiertz, E. J., Sun, L., Fish, K. N., Nelson, J. A., and Ploegh, H. L. (1996). Human cytomegalovirus US3 impairs transport and maturation of major histocompatibility complex class I heavy chains. *Proc. Natl Acad. Sci. USA*, **93**, 11327–11330.

Jones, C. A., Fernandez, M., Herc, K. et al. (2003). Herpes simplex virus type 2 induces rapid cell death and functional impairment of murine dendritic cells in vitro. *J. Virol.*, **77**(20), 11139–11149.

Kakimoto, M., Hasegawa, A., Fujita, S., and Yasukawa, M. (2002). Phenotypic and functional alterations of dendritic cells induced by human herpesvirus 6 infection. *J. Virol.*, **76**, 10338–10345.

Kinchington, P. R. and Cohen, J. I. (2000). Varicella zoster virus proteins In *Varicella Zoster Virus. Virology and Clinical Management*. Arvin, A. M. and Gershon, A. A., eds., pp. 74–104. Cambridge, UK: Cambridge University Press.

Klagge, I. M. and Schneider-Schaulies, S. (1999). Virus interactions with dendritic cells. *J. Gen. Virol.*, **80**, 823–833.

Kleijnen, M., Huppa, J., Lucin, P. et al. (1997). A mouse cytomegalovirus glycoprotein, gp34, forms a complex with folded class I MHC molecules in the ER which is not retained but is transported to the cell surface. *EMBO J.*, **16**, 685–694.

Ku, C. C., Padilla, J., Grose, C., Butcher, E. C., and Arvin, A. M. (2002). Tropism of varicella-zoster virus for human tonsillar CD4+ T lymphocytes that express activation, memory and skin homing markers. *J. Virol.*, **76**, 11425–11433.

Kruse, M., Rosorius, O., Kratzer, F. et al. (2000). Mature dendritic cells infected with herpes simplex virus type 1 exhibit inhibited T-cell stimulatory capacity. *J. Virol.*, **74**, 7127–7136.

Ku, C.-C., Zerboni, L., Besser, J., Ito, H., and Arvin, A. M. (2004) (Transport) of varicella-zoster virus to skin by infected CD4 T cells and modulation of skin infection by innate immunity in vivo. *J. Exp. Med.*, **200**, 917–925.

Lechmann, M., Berchtold, S., Hauber, J., and Steinkasserer, A. (2002). CD83 on dendritic cells: more than just a marker for maturation. *Trends Immunol.*, **23**, 273–275.

Macatonia, S. E., Gompels, M., Pinching, A. J., Patterson, S., and Knight, S. C., (1992). Antigen-presentation by macrophages but not by dendritic cells in human immunodeficiency virus (HIV) infection. *Immunology*, **75**, 576–581.

Machold, R., Wiertz, E., Jones, T., and Ploegh, H. (1997). The HCMV gene products US11 and US2 differ in their ability to attack allelic forms of murine major histocompatibility complex (MHC) class I heavy chains. *J. Exp. Med.*, **185**, 363–366.

Marland, G., Bakker, B., Adema, G. J., and Figdor, C. G. (1996). Dendritic cells in immune response induction. *Stem Cells*, **14**, 501.

Merigan, T. C., Rand, K. H., Pollard, R. B. et al. (1978). Human leukocyte interferon for the treatment of herpes zoster in patients with cancer. *N. Engl. J. Med.*, **298**, 981.

Miller, D. M., Rahill, B. M., Boss, J. M. et al. (1998). Human cytomegalovirus inhibits major histocompatibility complex class II expression by disruption of the Jak/Stat pathway. *J. Exp. Med.*, **187**, 675–683.

Moffat, J. F., Stein, M. D., Kaneshima, H., and Arvin, A. M. (1995). Tropism of varicella zoster virus for human CD4+ and CD8+ T-lymphocytes and epidermal cells in SCID-hu mice. *J. Virol.*, **69**, 5236–5242.

Morrow, G., Slobedman, B., Cunningham, A. L., and Abendroth, A. (2003). Varicella zoster virus productively infects mature dendritic cells and alters their immune function. *J. Virol.*, **77**(8), 4950–4959.

Oxman, M. N., Levin, M. J., Johnson, G. R. et al. (2005). A vaccine to prevent herpes zoster and postherpetic neuralgia in order adults. *N. Eng. J. Med.*, **352**(22), 2271–2284.

Raftery, M. J., Schwab, M., Eibert, S. M., Samstag, Y., Walczak, H., and Schonrich, G. (2001). Targeting the function of mature dendritic cells by human cytomegalovirus: a multilayered viral defense strategy. *Immunity*, **15**, 997–1009.

Reusch, U., Muranyi, W., Lucin, P., Burgert, H., Hengel, H., and Koszinowski, U. (1999). A cytomegalovirus glycoprotein reroutes MHC class I complexes to lysosomes for degradation. *EMBO J.*, **18**, 1081–1091.

Riegler, S., Hebart, H., Einsele., Brossart, P., Jahn, G., and Sinzger, C. (2000). Monocyte derived dendritic cells are permissive to the complete replicative cycle of human cytomegalovirus. *J. Gen. Virol.*, **81**, 393–399.

Salio, M., Cella, M., Suter, M., and Lanzavecchia, A. (1999). Inhibition of dendritic cell maturation by herpes simplex virus. *Eur. J. Immunol.*, **29**, 3245–3253.

Schnorr, J. J., Xanthakos, S., Keikavoussi, P., Kampgen, E., ter Meulen, V., and Schneider-Schaulies, S. (1997). Induction of maturation of human blood dendritic cell precursors by measles virus in association with immunosuppression. *Proc. Natl Acad. Sci. USA*, **92**, 5326–5331.

Sevilla, N., Kunz, S., Holz, A. et al. (2000). Immunosuppression and resultant viral persistence by specific viral targeting of dendritic cells. *J. Exp. Med.*, **192**, 1249–1260.

Sharp, M., Terada, K., Wilson, A. et al. (1992). Kinetics and viral protein specificity of the cytotoxic T lymphocyte response in healthy adults immunized with live attenuated varicella vaccine. *J. Infect. Dis.*, **165**, 852–858.

Steinman, R. M. (1991). The dendritic cell system and its role in immunogenicity. *Annu. Rev. Immunol.*, **9**, 271–296.

Steinman, R. M. (1999). Dendritic cells. In *Fundamental Immunology*, 4th edn. Paul, W. E., ed., pp. 547–573. Philadelphia: Lippincott Raven Publishers.

Steinman, R. M., Pack, M., and Inaba, K. (1997). Dendritic cell development and maturation. *Adv. Exp. Med. Biol.*, **417**, 1.

Stevens, D. A., Ferrington, R. A., Jordan, G. W., et al. (1975) Cellular events in zoster vesicles: relation to clinical course and immune parameters. *J. Infect. Dis.*, **131**, 509.

Tomazin, R., Hill, A. B., Jugovic, P. et al. (1996). Stable binding of the herpes simplex virus ICP47 protein to the peptide binding site of TAP. *EMBO J.*, **15**, 3256–3266.

Wallace, M. R., Woelfl, I., Bowler, W. A. et al. (1994). Tumor necrosis factor, interleukin-2, and interferon-gamma in adult varicella. *J. Med. Virol.*, **43**, 69–71.

Warren, M. K., Rose, W. L., Cone, J. L., Rice, W. G., and Turpin, J. A. (1997). Differential infection of CD34+ cell derived dendritic cells and monocytes with lymphocyte tropic and monocyte tropic HIV strains. *J. Immunol.*, **158**, 5035–5042.

Webster, A., Grint, P., Brenner, M.K. et al. (1989). Titration of IgG antibodies against varicella zoster virus before bone marrow transplantation is not predictive of future zoster. *J. Med. Virol.*, **27** 117.

Wiertz, E. J., Jones, T. R., Sun, L., Bogyo, M., Geuze, H. J., and Ploegh, H. L. (1996). The human cytomegalovirus US11 gene product dislocates MHC class I heavy chains from the endoplasmic reticulum to the cytosol. *Cell*, **84**, 769–779.

York, I. A., Roop, C., Andrews, D. W., Riddell, S. R., Graham, F. L., and Johnson, D. C. (1994). A cytosolic herpes simplex virus protein inhibits antigen presentation to CD8+ T lymphocytes. *Cell*, **77**, 525–535.

Young, J. W. and Steinman, R. M. (1990). Dendritic cells stimulate primary human cytolytic lymphocyte responses in the absence of CD4+ helper T cells. *J. Exp. Med.*, **171**, 1315–1332.

Young, J. W., Koulova, L., Soergel, S. A., Clark, E. A., Steinman, R. M., and Dupont, B. (1992). The B7/BB1 antigen provides one of several costimulatory signals for the activation of CD4+ T lymphocytes by human blood dendritic cells in vitro. *J. Clin. Invest.*, **90**, 229–237.

Zarling, J. M., Moran, P. A., Burke, R. L., Pachl, C., Berman, P. W., and Lasky, L. A. (1986). Human cytotoxic T cell clones directed against herpes simplex virus-infected cells. IV. Recognition and activation by cloned glycoproteins gB and gD. *J. Immunol.*, **136**, 4669–4673.

Zhang, Y., Cosyns, M., Levin, M. J., and Hayward, A. R. (1994). Cytokine production in varicella zoster virus-stimulated limiting dilution lymphocyte cultures. *Clin. Exp. Immunol.*, **98**, 128–133.

Zhou, L. J., Schwarting, R., Smith, H. M., and Tedder, T. F. (1992). A novel cell-surface molecule expressed by human interdigitating reticulum cells, Langerhans cells, and activated lymphocytes is a new member of the Ig superfamily. *J. Immunol.*, **149**, 735–742.

Zhou, L. J. and Tedder, T. F. (1995). Human blood dendritic cells selectively express CD83, a member of the immunoglobulin superfamily. *J. Immunol.*, **154**, 3821–3835.

VSV: persistence in the population

Jane Seward and Aisha Jumaan

National Immunization Program Centers for Disease Control and Prevention, Atlanta, GA, USA

Like other herpes viruses, varicella zoster virus (VZV) causes disease due to the primary infection (varicella) and due to reactivation (herpes zoster). However, VZV differs from other herpes viruses in causing primary and reactivation infections that are easily recognized clinical diseases, even by the lay public. Because of this, the epidemiology of varicella and herpes zoster has been well described from clinically recognized disease (incidence, severe disease outcomes and deaths) with seroprevalence data providing additional information on the epidemiology of varicella especially in populations where varicella disease history may not be available.

Varicella occurs worldwide with ongoing endemic transmission in areas where populations are sufficiently large to support such transmission. However the epidemiology of varicella varies between temperate and tropical climates (Lee, 1998). Universal childhood vaccination programs have changed the epidemiology of varicella in countries implementing such programs with significant declines in disease. Most experience has been gained in the United States where a varicella vaccination program was initiated in 1995. Herpes zoster infections also occur throughout the world although the epidemiology of herpes zoster is less well described globally. Because the incidence of herpes zoster increases dramatically with age, countries with lower life expectancies may have lower health burdens due to this disease. A vaccine for prevention of herpes zoster and post-herpetic neuralgia was licensed in the USA in May, 2006 (Oxman et al., 2005). This chapter reviews pre- and post-vaccine epidemiology of varicella and herpes zoster.

Varicella: prevaccine epidemiology

Transmission

Varicella is a highly infectious viral disease caused by the varicella zoster virus (VZV) that results from exposure to cases of varicella or herpes zoster. Herpes zoster cases represent a method for regular exposure and reintroduction of VZV into communities that otherwise may not be large enough to sustain endemic transmission of the virus. Herpes zoster is less transmissible than varicella. This may relate both to the limited number of lesions and to modes of transmission; the infection is most commonly localized and is not thought to involve the respiratory tract. Varicella can be transmitted by respiratory droplets, from skin lesions, by direct contact or possibly by aerosolization of virus from skin lesions and also, presumably from lesions in the mouth (enanthem). Studying transmission of varicella has been challenging due to the strong cell association of the virus. VZV has been consistently difficult to culture from the throat but easy to culture from skin lesions. Finally, infection of a pregnant woman in the first 2 trimesters of pregnancy may result in transplacental transmission of VZV resulting in a severe congenital infection in the fetus or newborn known as congenital (fetal) varicella syndrome (Enders et al., 1994).

Varicella transmission has been described from household studies where secondary attack rates among susceptible children following household exposure has ranged from 61% to 100% (Asano et al., 1977; Hope-Simpson, 1952; Ross, 1962). The highest estimates come from small groups of seronegative children involved in postexposure vaccine effectiveness studies in household settings. The lowest estimate is from observations in a general practice in England where children <15 years with a negative disease history were followed after exposure to a primary household case (Hope-Simpson, 1952). Hope-Simpson described transmissibility of varicella to be lower than measles (76%) but higher than mumps (32%). In a large study in the United States of the effect of gamma globulin on modifying varicella infections, Ross described a secondary attack rate of 87% among untreated children aged 6 months to 12 years with a negative disease history (Ross, 1962).

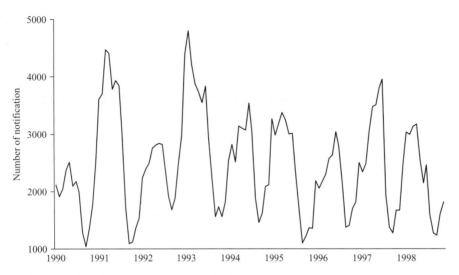

Fig. 40.1. Notification of varicella in Scotland, 4-week periods, 1990–1998.

Compared with households, transmission is lower in community settings; the relatively few published estimates available come from varicella outbreak investigations that have included vaccinated as well as unvaccinated children. In these situations, due to continuing exposure, outbreaks in child care centers may ultimately achieve a cumulative attack rate among history and vaccine negative children as high as 80%–88% (Galil *et al.*, 2002b; Izurieta *et al.*, 1997) though, depending on the size of the child care center, this may take weeks or months of transmission. In elementary schools, cumulative attack rates among susceptible children tend to be lower (30%–54%) perhaps due to different mixing patterns resulting in lower risk of exposure (Dworkin *et al.*, 2002). Yorke and London, in analyses of 30 to 35 years of monthly reported measles and varicella cases from New York City and Baltimore, suggested that varicella is only 35%–65% as infectious as measles in the community (Yorke and London, 1973).

Herpes zoster represents a method for reintroduction of VZV into the community in the absence of epidemic varicella. Patients with herpes zoster are less contagious than cases of varicella because their infection is localized and it is not thought to involve the respiratory tract. However, some studies have identified VZV antigen (by PCR) in throat samples of healthy persons with localized herpes zoster. There are few published studies on the transmissibility of herpes zoster probably because of the limited opportunities for exposure of susceptible persons to herpes zoster cases which occur predominantly, among older adults. However, Seiler reported that 11 (15.5%) of 71 susceptible children <15 years of age exposed to herpes zoster in household settings developed varicella (Seiler, 1949). This proportion increased to 17% if infants <1 year of age, who may be protected by maternally acquired antibodies, were excluded from the calculation. Young children with herpes zoster may be more contagious. In a daycare setting, a 3-year-old boy with herpes zoster transmitted in the secondary generation to ∼30% of susceptible children in the day care he attended and to both his susceptible siblings (Reigle and Cooperstock, 1985). The child was reported to "lift his shirt repeatedly to scratch or to show everyone his lesions." As varicella disease declines in countries implementing universal childhood vaccination programs, transmission from herpes zoster may become more apparent.

Periodicity and seasonality

Worldwide, varicella is an endemic disease that exhibits a marked seasonal pattern in temperate climates and most temperate climates where this has been studied (Bramley and Jones 2000; Degeun *et al.*, 1998; Lee, 1998; Seward *et al.*, 2002; Tobias *et al.*, 1998) (Fig. 40.1). The exception is Singapore where seasonality has not been described from surveillance data (Ooi *et al.*, 1992). In temperate and tropical climates, the peak disease incidence is most commonly reported in the cooler, drier months during winter or spring. Periodicity with interepidemic cycles of 2–5 years is described from many countries (Bramley and Jones, 2000; Degeun *et al.*, 1998; Seward *et al.*, 2000; Tobias *et al.*, 1998) while a time period as long as 15 years between major epidemics has been described from Singapore (Ooi *et al.*, 1992).

Congenital (fetal) varicella syndrome

This condition was first described in 1947 (Laforet and Lynch, 1947). It is characterized by cicatricial skin lesions and neurologic, eye and skeletal anomalies which may include limb paresis, hypoplasia of upper or lower extremities, chorioretinitis, cataracts and cortical atrophy. Based on a large, multicenter study where 1373 women with varicella and 366 with herpes zoster during pregnancy were prospectively studied, the risk of congenital (fetal) varicella syndrome was found to be approximately 0.4% if varicella infection was acquired in the first 12 weeks of pregnancy and 2.0% from 13–20 weeks (Enders et al., 1994). Maternal zoster was not associated with fetal abnormalities. Based on this study, Enders estimated that the rate of fetal varicella syndrome may be 1.6 per 100 000 births. Enders and Miller used these findings to estimate the number of cases of congenital varicella syndrome that may occur every year by applying a varicella age-specific incidence of 2/1000 population among women of child-bearing age to the number of births per year, taking into account the risk of infection occurring in the first 20 weeks of pregnancy. They calculated that, in the prevaccine era, there may have been 44 cases of congenital varicella syndrome every year in the United States, 8 in England and Wales and 9 in Germany (Enders and Miller, 2000). Incidence is likely to be higher in countries where VZV susceptibility is higher among adults though data are lacking.

Incidence and seroprevalence

Age and climate

Varicella is a highly contagious disease that occurs worldwide. The epidemiology of varicella varies between temperate and tropical climates. Though incompletely understood, these differences may relate to agent, host, environmental or a combination of these factors (Garnett et al., 1993; Lolekha et al., 2001; Mandal et al., 1998; Seward et al., 2000). Because climatic differences (as distinguished from an "island" effect reflecting reduced risk of exposure) are not observed for other highly contagious diseases such as measles, and VZV is known to be heat labile, a partial explanation may be that heat diminishes the ability of the virus to survive in the environment and thereby decreases transmission. In most temperate climates, >90% of persons are infected by 15 years of age with the highest incidence of disease occurring among children <10 years of age (Seward et al., 2000; Wharton, 1996). In tropical climates, cases are acquired at older ages with a higher proportion of cases and higher susceptibility among adults (Lee, 1998).

Varicella incidence data has been described mainly from developed countries where data are collected from notifiable disease reporting, surveys or studies based on medical record encounters. Prior to the national varicella vaccination program in the United States, total annual varicella incidence measured from national household survey data, averaged over a decade, was 15.0–16.0 cases per 1000 population (Guess et al., 1986; Seward et al., 1998). In other temperate climates, reported incidence using different methods of data collection have been generally lower than US rates varying from <5 to ~13.0 cases per 1000 total population (Boelle and Hanslik, 2002; Bramley and Jones, 2000; Choo et al., 1995; Fairley and Miller, 1996). Higher rates, especially from a single year of data collection, may reflect an epidemic disease year (Chant et al., 1998) (Table 40.1).

Infectiousness of diseases is reflected in age-specific incidence. As stated by Hope-Simpson following studies of the infectiousness of measles, varicella and mumps in the household "the more infectious the disease, the younger is the age at which an attack is likely to be received" (Hope-Simpson, 1952). Studies from earlier in the twentieth century in the US showed the highest varicella age-specific incidence was among children aged 6–7 years, in the first 2 years of school (Fales, 1928). To understand age-specific disease patterns, single years of age or small age groups should be studied; grouping ages 5–14 years, for example, may mask considerable variations in incidence within this broad age span. Age-specific incidence among children 5–9 years from US national data in the 1970s and 1980s was ~90/1000 children (Guess et al., 1986; Wharton, 1996). However, by the 1990s, varicella was being acquired at earlier ages. Before introduction of varicella vaccine in the United States in 1995, varicella age-specific incidence had shifted to earlier ages with preschool aged children (1–4 years) having higher age specific incidence than the 5–9-year-old age group (Seward, 1998) (Table 40.1). These data are consistent with findings in many countries including France, Italy, England and Wales, Scotland and Slovenia where the highest age-specific incidence in the 1990s has been reported among preschool-aged children <5 years (Bramley and Jones, 2000; Degeun et al., 1998; Fornaro et al., 1999; Ross and Fleming, 2000) with peak incidence in some studies as young as 1 or 2 years (Socan et al., 2001, Yawn et al., 1997). These changes in epidemiology are thought to reflect earlier exposure through attendance in child care (Wharton 1996; Yawn et al. 1997; Ross and Fleming, 2000)

Varicella seroprevalence data reflect age-specific disease incidence and in countries where incidence data are not available, VZV age-specific seroprevalence provide an excellent method for understanding the epidemiology of

Table 40.1. Varicella age-specific and total incidence, selected studies

Country, author, publication year	Study method	Years data collection	Age (years)						Annual total varicella incidence/1000 population
			<1	1–4	5–9	10–14	15–19	20+	
United States (Guess et al., 1986)	National survey	1970–1978	33.8	82.1	90.3	17.5	2.9	0.3	16.0
United States (Seward et al., 1998)	National survey	1990–1994	56.7	100.4	91.0	19.5	4.9	1.5	15.0
France (Boelle et al., 2002)	Sentinel physician reporting	1990–1999	49.8	121.2		36.0		3.4	12.6
United States (Choo et al., 1995)	Health maintenance organization records	July 1990–June 1991 July 1991–June 1992		52.3	41.3	14.0	6.1	1.8	7.6, 12.0
England and Wales (Fairley and Miller, 1996)	Sentinel physician reporting	1989–1990		40.0		17.3	3.1 (15–44 years)		6.3
Scotland (Bramley and Jones, 2000)	Sentinel physician reporting	1989–1990	14.5–35.0	31.4–63.4	16.4–27.8		2.3–6.1 (15–24 years)		5.4–8.9 (European standardized rate)
Australia (Chant et al., 1998)	Local survey	1995		110	130	60	40		33.9

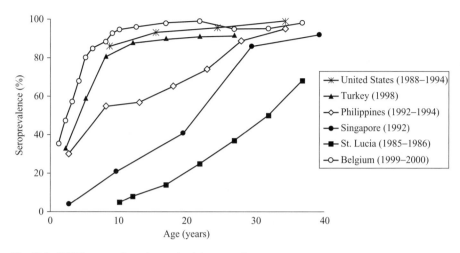

Fig. 40.2. VZV Seroprevalence by age in eight countries.

the disease. Comparing results from serosurveys should take into account improvements in sensitivity and specificity of laboratory methods over time. In addition, these studies represent a snapshot of the seroprevalence status in a community; seroprevalence will be higher if samples are obtained after a varicella epidemic. In temperate climates, >90% of adolescents or young adults are VZV seropositive (Fig. 40.2) (Kanra et al., 2002; Kilgore et al., 2003; Seward et al., 2000; Thiry et al., 2002). Slightly lower seroprevalence rates in adolescents (10–15 years) (82%) are reported from Italy whereas a study in South Africa reported a seroprevalence of 81% among adults 20–29 years (Gabutti et al., 2001; Schoub et al., 1985). In tropical climates, serological studies show higher susceptibility among adults reflecting a higher mean age of infection than in temperate climates (Fig. 40.2). In such countries, seroprevalence among adolescents or young adults has varied widely from less than 20% in St. Lucia (an island community in the West Indies) to >90% in tropical areas in Brazil and urban Calcutta, India (Barzaga et al., 1994; Garnett et al., 1993; Lee, 1998; Mandal et al., 1998; Ooi et al., 1992; Reis et al., 2003).

Urban/rural (risk of exposure)

Urban/rural differences in varicella epidemiology are likely to be due to varying risks of exposure due to differences in population density. Analysis of surveillance data collected in the 1920s in Maryland, US, between 1913 and 1917, showed an earlier mean age of varicella infection among urban (6.7 years) compared with rural children (8.6 years) (Fales, 1928). Studies exploring reasons why the epidemiology of varicella differs between temperate and tropical climates have examined the effect of climate and population density on VZV seroprevalence. In Thailand, significantly lower age-adjusted VZV seroprevalence was found in the warmer than in the cooler regions and in the warmer regions only, the age-specific seroprevalence was significantly higher in the urban population than the rural population (Lolekha et al., 2001). Urban/rural differences have also been described in Calcutta and neighboring rural areas in India. Mandel found that 96% of urban young adults aged 17–25 years were immune compared with 42% of similarly aged rural adults (Mandal et al., 1998). In Eritrea, VZV seroprevalence among an isolated adult population was 44% compared with other adult groups in the same areas where immunity ranged from 91%–96% (Ghebrekidan et al., 1999). Although these data suggest that the higher susceptibility in the tropics may reflect reduced exposure, this is not the only explanation for the differences described. In St. Lucia, seroprevalence for VZV was lower than for mumps, a far less infectious disease and in Singapore, which is densely populated, VZV seroprevalence among young adults has consistently been lower than in countries with temperate climates (Garnett et al., 1993; Ooi et al., 1992).

Other factors: sex, race, number of siblings in the household and child care

Most studies show no differences in seroprevalence by sex. In the United States, national data and studies conducted among military recruits have described differences in varicella susceptibility by race with higher susceptibility among African Americans compared with whites (Jerant et al., 1998; Kilgore et al., 2003). In the national data, these differences narrow with increasing age and are not apparent after approximately age 40. Some studies have shown differences in seroprevalence according to number of siblings in the household during childhood (Jerant et al., 1998; Ryan et al., 2003). Because of its high incidence in young children, varicella is one of the most common communicable diseases in child care centers and attendance in child care or preschools provides the opportunity for exposure to the varicella zoster virus (VZV) at younger ages. Children attending day care have higher incidence or prevalence of varicella and an increased risk of exposure to varicella with increasing size of the center (Hurwitz et al., 1991; Seward et al., 2000).

Hospitalization and deaths

Though often considered a benign childhood disease, varicella may result in serious complications and death. This health burden assumes greater importance as other infectious causes of morbidity and mortality such as polio, measles and *H. influenzae* are controlled through vaccination (Rawson et al., 2001). Assessing the severe health burden due to varicella in terms of economic and societal costs is important for vaccine policy decision making and to monitor the impact of vaccination programs. Data on population-based varicella mortality, case fatality and hospitalizations are rarely available from developing countries or countries with tropical climates where a higher proportion of cases occur among adults. Additionally, methodological differences in data collection as well as issues such as access to health care should be considered when comparing studies, especially across countries. Finally, calculating case fatality rates and risks of hospitalization for varicella cases is dependent on having accurate incidence data available.

In the United States, in the 5–8 years before licensure of varicella vaccine, varicella resulted in an average of 10 632 hospitalizations and 100 deaths per year (Galil et al., 2002a; Meyer et al., 2000); two-thirds of the hospitalizations and about half the deaths occurred in children. Although varicella is a more severe infection in immunocompromised persons, the majority of severe morbidity and mortality in developed countries occurs among healthy persons. In France (1990–1997), 70% of all varicella deaths and in the United States (1990–1994), 89% of varicella deaths among children and 75% of varicella deaths among adults occurred in persons without underlying high risk medical conditions (including HIV/AIDS, leukemia and other malignancies, other forms of blood dyscrasia and immune deficiencies) (Boelle and Hanslik, 2002; Meyer et al., 2000).

In the US, between 1970 and 1994, before the use of varicella vaccine, crude varicella mortality rates (examining varicella as the underlying cause of death) declined from 0.7 per million population in 1973 to 0.2 in 1986 and then increased to average 0.4 per million population from 1990–1994 (Meyer et al., 2000). Similar crude mortality rates are reported from Australia (0.3/million), France (0.35/million), England and Wales (0.5/million), Scotland (0.5/million) and Singapore (0–0.8/million) (Boelle and Hanslik, 2002; Bramley and Jones, 2000; Chant et al., 1998; Fairley and Miller, 1996; Lam et al., 1993; Rawson et al., 2001). Reflecting the high incidence of varicella in children, varicella mortality rates are highest among children especially those <1 year of age (1.1–3.6 deaths per million population) and lowest among adults (0.2–0.3 deaths per million population).

The risk of dying from varicella is measured by the case fatality rate (CFR). In the US, data from 1970–1994 show higher case fatality rates in infants <1 year and adults ≥20 years of age compared with children 1–9 years (Meyer et al., 2000). Even though CFRs among adults declined substantially from the 1970s to the 1990s, during 1990–1994, adults still had a 27 times higher risk of dying from varicella (CFR 21.3 per 100 000 cases) than children 1–4 years (0.8/100 000 cases). Similar CFRs are reported from France from 1990–97 (CFR 1.0/100 000 for children <15 years and 22.8 for persons ≥15 years) and England and Wales from 1988–1992 for persons <45 years (0.7 for 0–4 years, 1.4 for 5–14 years and 20 for persons 15–44 years of age) (Boelle and Hanslik, 2002; Fairley and Miller, 1996). Though extremely high CFRs (471 and 535) are reported for adults ≥65 years in England and Wales, and France respectively, in this age group, misclassification of varicella with herpes zoster is more likely to occur, as documented in US hospitalization and mortality data (Choo et al., 1995; Galil et al., 2002c).

Population-based mortality data are lacking from developing countries and from countries with tropical climates. Because of the older age of infection and case severity among adults, tropical countries may experience greater morbidity and mortality from varicella and its complications, including congenital varicella syndrome. The eradication of smallpox afforded an opportunity to study varicella in developing countries in the 1970s in more detail than has been possible since. When smallpox was still endemic, varicella was the rash illness most commonly confused with smallpox (Jezek et al., 1978a). For several years after smallpox eradication, heightened surveillance for febrile rash illnesses was conducted. In India, 862 155 varicella cases and 433 varicella deaths were reported from January to December 1976 for a CFR of 5.2 per 10 000 reported cases, 50 times higher than in developed countries (Jezek et al., 1978b). Reasons for the higher case fatality may include incomplete ascertainment of cases (reporting bias for more severe cases) compared with deaths, varicella epidemiology in India, and access to, and quality of, medical care. For 400 deaths where both age and sex were recorded, 80% occurred among adults >15 years and 71%

were male, reflecting varicella epidemiology in tropical climates and perhaps a reporting bias and/or medical access differences for adults and for males compared with females (Jezek et al., 1978a).

Varicella hospitalizations represent severe morbidity or health burden due to varicella and its consequences, and the infection control burden due to varicella infections in hospitals. As pointed out by Wharton, "ascertaining the reason for hospitalization from hospital discharge diagnoses, in the absence of additional information from the clinical record, is difficult due to lack of standard procedures for ordering hospital discharge diagnoses" (Wharton, 1996). Some studies have validated hospital discharge codes (Choo et al., 1995). Thus, when comparing studies of hospitalizations, especially across countries, it is important to consider differences in methods that may result in higher or lower estimates including how hospitalizations were identified (from discharge codes or from reviewing medical records), whether the primary discharge or all discharge codes were searched for varicella, the validity of discharge codes and how hospital admission practices, billing and coding may change over time.

Estimates of annual hospitalizations for varicella in the US during the 1970s and 1980s ranged from approximately 4000 to 9000 depending on the dates of the study, the population studied, and study methods (Guess et al., 1986; Wharton, 1996). More recent estimates indicate annual hospitalizations attributable to varicella of 10 632 per year (Galil et al., 2002a) and almost 15 000 per year if all varicella hospitalizations are included (Ratner, 2002). Reflecting the range of these estimates, crude varicella hospitalization rates from the US, France, Australia, Scotland, and England and Wales have varied from approximately 2–6 per 100 000 population with more recent estimates attempting to describe attributable hospitalizations in the US varying from 3.1–4.1 per 100 000 population (Boelle and Hanslik, 2002; Bramley and Jones, 2000; Chant et al., 1998, Fairley and Miller, 1996; Galil et al., 2002a, Ratner, 2002). The majority of varicella hospitalizations occur among children (56%–67%) reflecting the fact that 90% of varicella cases occur among this age group.

For all ages combined, overall rates of hospital admission per 1000 varicella cases have ranged from 2.2 to 4.7 in national studies in the US and France (Boelle and Hanslik, 2002; Galil et al., 2002a; Ratner, 2002). The highest rate from France included principal and associated varicella hospitalizations. In the 1990s, among children <13 with varicella, a hospitalization rate of 5.5 per 1000 cases was reported from Minnesota (Yawn et al., 1997). The risk of hospitalization varies by age. The pattern of age-specific risks for hospitalizations is similar to that of age-specific case fatality rates with infants and adults having higher risks of hospitalization than young children. Except in France where the risk for hospitalization is higher in infants than in adults, studies consistently report the highest risk of hospitalization in adults, an increased risk in infants and the lowest risk in children 1–4 years or 5–9 years of age (Boelle and Hanslik, 2002; Fairley and Miller, 1996; Galil et al., 2002a; Guess et al., 1986; Wharton, 1996).

Studies of varicella hospitalizations in developing countries are sparse and population-based hospitalization rates are commonly not available for comparison with data from developed countries. However, similar to reported varicella mortality described above (Jezek et al., 1978a), studies of varicella hospitalizations in tropical climates also describe a high proportion of hospitalized cases among adults and also males, which may, in part, reflect hospital admission practices (Seward et al., 2000).

The HIV epidemic may also be expected to influence the epidemiology of varicella. In countries with high HIV prevalence, varicella may cause more severe morbidity and mortality however there are few population-based data examining these issues. A retrospective review of all children admitted to the only isolation facility in Durban, South Africa from 1986–1996, showed a decline in all disease mortality of 86% over the study period mainly attributed to a decline in measles deaths. However, between 1994 and 1996, 15% of varicella admissions and 75% of varicella deaths occurred in HIV co-infected children (Jeena et al., 1998).

Varicella epidemiology: post-vaccine era

A vaccination program is implemented in order to reduce, eliminate or eradicate disease. Because current strains of live attenuated varicella vaccine are neurotropic and are capable of reactivating to cause herpes zoster, albeit at lower rates than wild virus, eradication of VZV infections is not possible with currently licensed vaccines. The goal of a universal varicella vaccination program is to greatly reduce or eliminate varicella disease, especially severe disease.

The United States was the first country to implement a national varicella vaccination program in 1995 and active surveillance for varicella was established in sentinel sites to monitor impact of the vaccination program. By 2000, in these communities, vaccine coverage among children 19–35 months had reached 74%–84% and reported total varicella cases and hospitalizations had declined 71%–84% (Seward et al., 2002) (Fig. 40.3, Table 40.2). Although incidence declined to the greatest extent (83%–90%) among children 1 to 4 years, incidence declined in all age groups including infants and adults indicating herd immunity effects. In the combined surveillance

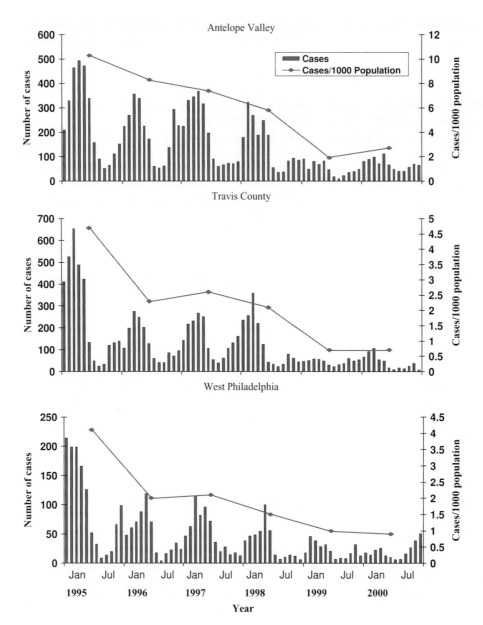

Fig. 40.3. Reported varicella cases by month and annual rates of reported cases per 1000 population in three surveillance areas, 1995–2000.

areas, varicella-related hospitalizations declined from a range of 2.7–4.2 per 100 000 population from 1995 to 1998 to 0.6 and 1.5 per 100 000 population in 1999 and 2000, respectively.

In the USA, a decline in varicella incidence has also been documented from passive surveillance systems. In four states with adequate ($\geq$5% of expected cases) and consistent rates of reporting to the national notifiable disease surveillance system, compared with the average incidence for 1990–1994, reductions in varicella incidence in 2001 ranged from 67% to 82% with vaccine coverage among children 19–35 months ranging from 57%-84% (Centers for Disease Control & Prevention, 2003). Additionally, implementation of a varicella serological screening and vaccination program in Navy military recruits has been followed by an 80% decline in cases in this population (Ryan *et al.*, 2003). At the national level, significant declines in varicella mortality, and in varicella-related

Table 40.2. Percent reduction of reported varicella cases in 2000 compared to 1995, three surveillance areas, United States

Age	Antelope Valley, California	Travis County, Texas	West Philadelphia, Pennsylvania
	%	%	%
<1	69	81	68
1–4	83	90	83
5–9	63	77	77
10–14	65	75	80
15–19	85	83	81
≥20	66	64	68
Total	71	84	79

Note: From Seward, J. F, Watson, B. M., Peterson, C. L. et al. (2002).

hospitalizations and their attendant costs have been also been documented in the United States (Nguyen et al., 2005; Zhou et al., 2005; Davis et al., 2004). Among persons less than 50 years of age, varicella deaths declined 74% or more from the immediate pre-vaccine era (1990–1994) to 1999 to 2001 and deaths in children 1 to 9 years of age declined approximately 90% (Nguyen et al., 2005). For hospitalizations, from the prevaccination period to 2002, hospitalizations due to varicella declined by 88% and ambulatory visits declined 59% (Zhou, 2005).

Routine childhood vaccination programs are the most effective strategy for interrupting disease transmission and reducing varicella mortality and morbidity in both temperate and tropical climates. Achieving high vaccination coverage among children will provide the additional benefits of herd immunity with protection of susceptible adults, infants and other persons at high risk for severe varicella disease who are not eligible for vaccination. For programs that achieve high vaccination coverage, the most dramatic effect will be a marked reduction in varicella cases, severe complications and deaths in the population as is now occurring in the United States (Seward et al., 2002; CDC unpublished data, 2003). Among the remaining greatly reduced number of varicella cases, a higher proportion is expected to occur among older persons, as was seen following the introduction of vaccines against measles, mumps and rubella. The shift in the proportion of cases to older persons will be minimized by catch-up vaccination of older children and adolescents. In contrast, vaccination programs targeting only adolescents and adults will have little impact on the epidemiology of varicella in temperate climates. In the US such a targeted program, assuming that all susceptible adults could be vaccinated, would be expected to result in only a 5%–10% decline in cases, a 33% decline in hospitalizations and a 50% decline in deaths. In tropical countries, providing vaccine for susceptible adolescents and adults in addition to infants and children may be more important because a higher proportion of adults are likely to be susceptible.

Although some other countries, including Uruguay, Qatar, Australia, Canada, and Germany (2005) have implemented universal childhood varicella vaccination programs, no data are yet available on the impact of these programs. Some countries are waiting for the availability of a combination MMRV vaccine (licenced in the USA in 2005) before implementing a universal vaccination program and others are considering adolescent vaccination programs. Varicella vaccines are now widely available through the private sector throughout the world. If partial and sustained vaccine uptake occurs through the private sector reaching coverage levels in the range of 30%–60%, adverse epidemiological effects may occur resulting in an increase in incidence or severe morbidity in adolescents and adults similar to those predicted for selective rubella vaccine use (Vynnycky et al., 2003).

A varicella vaccination program has the potential to change the epidemiology of herpes zoster as well as varicella. Therefore, surveillance for herpes zoster as well as varicella is important for monitoring the vaccination program.

Herpes zoster epidemiology

Methodological issues

Studies of herpes zoster (HZ) incidence, morbidity and mortality have used various methodologies; the most reliable data come from prospective cohort studies. Herpes zoster incidence has been described from surveillance data where there is likely to be significant under-reporting of cases, retrospective cohort studies that use medical records thus missing cases that do not seek medical attention, and surveys that may encounter non responders. Thus, differences in the method of data collection must be taken into account when comparing HZ incidence data. In addition, because HZ incidence increases dramatically with age, comparing HZ incidence rates across studies needs to take this into account by standardizing rates to a reference population. Other methodological issues arise, especially when assessing disease burden due to HZ. Herpes zoster is more common among elderly adults, an age group that is likely to have chronic medical conditions that may cause lengthy hospitalizations or death; therefore, it is important to describe the attributable health burden or mortality from HZ. Otherwise, coincidental HZ infections that occur during hospitalization and that may be listed in hospital discharge codes and on death certificates may inflate health burden and mortality due to HZ. MacIntyre *et al.* (2003) reported that only 40% of 4718 hospitalizations that listed HZ in discharge codes had HZ as the primary diagnosis, and that these cases had significantly shorter hospitalization stay and were less likely to die (1%) than those with a secondary HZ diagnosis (6%).

Seasonality and clustering

Because HZ results from reactivation of latent VZV, the disease does not occur in epidemics and periodicity is not described. Most studies report no seasonal variations in the incidence of HZ (Brisson *et al.*, 2001; Hope-Simpson, 1965; McGregor, 1957; Ragozzino *et al.*, 1982); however several studies report seasonality with peak incidence in the summer and some authors speculate that this may be associated with ultraviolet radiation that peaks in the summer months (Glynn *et al.*, 1990; Wilson, 1986; Zak-Prelich *et al.*, 2000).

Although small clusters of HZ cases have been reported (Hope Simpson, 1965; Palmer *et al.*, 1985; Schimpff *et al.*, 1972), most authors report no clustering, or if clustering occurred they were considered to represent coincidental episodes of disease (Brisson *et al.*, 2001; Donahue *et al.*, 1995; Glynn *et al.*, 1990; Hope-Simpson, 1965; Wilson, 1986). A few authors suggest that clusters may represent a clinical manifestation of exogenous reinfection, or stimulation of endogenous VZV reactivation, (Palmer *et al.*, 1985; Schimpff *et al.*, 1972).

Secular trends

Several studies have suggested that HZ rates are increasing. In a study in the United States spanning 15 years from 1945–1959, Ragozzino *et al.* (1982) reported an increase in the annual age standardized (1970 US white population) incidence from 1.1 to 1.5 per 1000 person years. In his study in the 1990s, Donahue *et al.* (1995) reported that once the HZ incidence rates he observed were standardized to the 1970 US white population, they increased to 2.9 per 1000 person–years, more than double that reported by Ragazzino. The increase was not associated with aging of the population or with an increase in immunosuppressed individuals. In addition, from 1979 to 1997, increases in HZ incidence of 35% and 21% have been described in Canada and England, respectively (Brisson *et al.*, 2001).

Dermatomal distribution

Most studies report no laterality to the HZ rash with both the right and left sides affected equally. The rash affects mainly one dermatome with the thoracic, cervical, lumbar, and cranial dermatomes accounting for over 90% of the dermatomes affected (di Luzio Paparatti *et al.*, 1999; Guess *et al.*, 1985; Hope-Simpson, 1965; McGregor, 1957; Petursson *et al.*, 1998; Ragozzino *et al.*, 1982). Hope-Simpson noted that the HZ rash distribution correlates with the distribution of the varicella rash that follows a centripetal distribution. The rash affects mostly the trunk (thoracic 50%), and face (cranial 13%) with similar percentages for the cervical (14%) and lumbar (13%) regions, and spares the limbs. Similar findings were reported for HZ rashes in children (Guess *et al.*, 1985; Takayama *et al.*, 2000).

Incidence

Age

It is estimated that about 10%–30% of people will get HZ during their lifetime, resulting in about 300 000–900 000 cases of HZ in the US, and 260 000 cases in the UK each year (Brisson *et al.*, 2001; Schmader, 2001). The incidence of HZ varies markedly in published studies. The total population incidence of HZ, unadjusted for age differences between populations, ranges from 1.3 to 4.8 per 1000 person–years (Table 40.3) (Chidiac *et al.*, 2001; McGregor, 1957; Ragozzino *et al.*, 1982). The differences in the rates observed across studies may be due to differences in the methods used for ascertainment of cases, case definitions, determination of population at risk, health systems capturing cases, and age distribution of population studied (that may be skewed or not reflective of the overall population) rather than to true population differences. In a prospective cohort study of all patients in his general practice in Cirencester, UK from 1947–1962, Hope-Simpson reported an annual incidence rate of 3.4 per 1000 person–years (Hope-Simpson, 1965). Much lower incidence rates were found in a community-based study in the US in which cases were identified retrospectively from medical records in a central diagnosis system that included all providers in the community (Ragozzino *et al.*, 1982). The denominator included the population of Rochester, Minnesota, obtained from census data. Other studies used well defined populations for denominators such as enrollees in a health plan in Massachusetts (Donahue *et al.*, 1995), attendants at general practices in Scotland (McGregor, 1957), England, (Hope-Simpson, 1965), and Italy (di Luzio Paparatti *et al.*, 1999). The study in France (Chidiac *et al.*, 2001) was a prospective study that did not include cases from pediatricians or from residents in institutions, and used the population from the census for the denominator. Therefore, it is important to adjust rates of studies that report age-specific incidence to a standard population for comparison purposes. The

Table 40.3. Herpes zoster age-specific and total incidence, selected studies

Country, author, publication year	Study method and population	Number of cases	Years data collection	Age (years)									Annual total zoster incidence/ 1000 population
				0–9	10–19	20–39	40–49	50–59	60–69	70–79	80+		
United Kingdom (Hope-Simpson, 1965)	Prospective General practices	192	1947–1962	0.7	1.4	2.4	2.9	5.1	6.8	6.4	9.4		3.4
France (Chidiac et al., 2001)	Prospective General practices and dermatologists	8103	1997–1998	2.2		2.4		5.4	9.9 (60–74 yrs)	12.8 (75+yrs)			4.8
				0–4 yrs	5–9 yrs	10–14 yrs	15–19 yrs					0–19 yrs	
United States (Guess et al., 1985)	Retrospective Medical records for Population	173	1960–1981	0.20	0.30	0.59	0.63		NA			0.42	
Iceland (Petursson et al., 1998)	Prospective General practices	121	1990–1995	0.8	1.5	2.3	1.8		NA			1.6	

Country, author, publication year	Study method and population	Number of cases	Years data collection	Age (years)								Annual total zoster incidence/ 1000 population
				0–14	15–24	25–44	45–54	55–64	65–74	75+		
United States (Ragozzino et al., 1982)	Retrospective Medical Records of the Population	590	1945–1959	0.30	0.8	1.0	1.5	2.4	3.4	4.4		1.3
United States (Donahue et al., 1995)	Retrospective Health maintenance organization records	1075	1990–1992	0.46	1.03	2.10	3.13	5.71	9.99	14.24		2.15
Netherlands (Opstelten et al., 2002)	Retrospective Medical records in General Practices	837	1990–1995		2.1 (0–44 yrs)		3.6	5.8	6.5	9.1		3.4
England (Brisson and Edmunds, 2003)	Surveillance of General Practices	Not available	1991–2003	0.92 (0–4 yrs)	2.19 (5–14 yrs)	2.12 (15–44 yrs)	7.12 (45–64 yrs)		9.32 (65+ yrs)			3.73
Scotland (McGregor, 1957)	Prospective General Practice	81	1948–1955	1.2 (0–5 yrs)		2.2 (15–44 yrs)	8.1 (45–64 yrs)		10.4 (65+ yrs)			4.8

differences in incidence rates for two studies (Donahue *et al.*, 1995; Hope-Simpson, 1965) narrowed from 2.1 and 3.4 per 1000 person–years respectively to 3.2 and 3.3 per 1000 person–years as a result of adjusting the crude rated to the 2000 US population, highlighting the need for such adjustments before comparing rates between studies.

The majority of studies report that a small proportion of persons infected with HZ may experience a second or a third episode. Hope-Simpson (1965) reported that the rate of second or more infections in persons previously infected is similar to that of first infection in the general population with 8 (4.1%) of 192 cases reporting a second episode, and one person a third episode, resulting in a rate of 3.1 per 1000 person–years. These findings were supported by other studies with recurrence ranging from 1.7%–5.2% (Donahue *et al.*, 1995; Ragozzino *et al.*, 1982; Wilson, 1982). A much higher recurrence rate of 45% was reported in one English study in persons with a first infection occurring over the age of 45 years (Edmunds *et al.*, 2001).

All published studies report that the incidence of HZ increases with increasing age (Brisson *et al.*, 2001; Chidiac *et al.*, 2001; Donahue *et al.*, 1995; McGregor, 1957; Hope-Simpson, 1965; Ragozzino *et al.*, 1982; Opstelten *et al.*, 2002) (Table 40.3). Most studies report an approximately 10 fold increase in risk with increasing age; Hope-Simpson reported incidence increasing from 0.74 among children less than 10 years of age to 10.1 per 1000 person–years among individuals aged 80–89 years. This marked increase in incidence with age results in up to 50% of people who live to 85 years acquiring HZ (Brisson *et al.*, 2001; Schmader, 2001).

Because children may not have acquired varicella and therefore may not yet be at risk for reactivation of VZV, the incidence of HZ also depends on varicella epidemiology. Therefore, comparison of HZ incidence rates in children need to take into account both the age distribution of children in the studies and the age-specific incidence of varicella which may vary across populations. Hope-Simpson, 40 years ago, speculated that the increase in HZ incidence in persons 0–20 years reflected the increase in the number of children infected with VZV, placing them at risk for HZ. He suggested that the incidence observed in the third decade, by which time almost everyone in temperate climates is latently infected with VZV, reflects the incidence in a maximally infected population. Studies of HZ in children report annual incidence rates ranging from 0.25 to 1.15 per 1000 population for children <10 years and from 0.43 to 1.60 for those <20 years (Chidiac *et al.*, 2001; Guess *et al.*, 1985; Hope-Simpson, 1965; Petursson *et al.*, 1998) (Table 40.3). Other studies used different age groups such as <5, and 5–14 years, or <14 years making comparison between studies difficult (Brisson *et al.*, 2001; Donahue *et al.*, 1995; McGregor, 1957; Ragozzino *et al.*, 1982). Guess *et al.* (1985) in Rochester, Minnesota, during the period 1960–1981, reported that the incidence of HZ increased with age from 0.20 cases per 1000 person–years in children less than 5 years of age to 0.63 cases per 1000 person–years in those 15 to 19 years of age. In contrast, Petursson *et al.* (1998) in Iceland, during 1990–1996, reported rates that ranged from 0.80 per 1000 person-years in children less than 5 years to 1.80 in those 15–19 years of age (Table 40.3). These four fold differences in rates of HZ in children in narrow (5 year) age groupings are more likely to signify differences in study methods including completeness of ascertainment than differences between populations (Guess *et al.*, 1985; Petursson *et al.*, 1998). Further studies to understand such differences are needed. Maternal varicella during pregnancy and varicella or variable exposure during the first few months of life are associated with HZ in childhood.

Sex

The majority of studies among all ages or among the elderly find no significant differences between males and females in crude or age-adjusted HZ incidence (Brisson *et al.*, 2001; Donahue *et al.*, 1995; Guess *et al.*, 1985; MacIntyre *et al.*, 2003; Wilson, 1986; Petursson *et al.*, 1998; Ragozzino *et al.*, 1982; Schmader *et al.*, 1995), while some studies report slight differences in rates between males and females (di Luzio Paparatti *et al.*, 1999; Hope-Simpson, 1965; McGregor, 1957), and others report higher rates among females (Chant *et al.*, 1998; Chidiac *et al.*, 2001; Cooper, 1987; Thomas and Hall, 2004). Wilson (1986) found that younger males 0–20 years had a higher incidence when compared to females of the same age. One study in the US found that females had a higher crude hospitalization rate of 18.5 compared to 13.4 among males; however, once age adjusted, the differences disappeared (Lin and Hadler, 2000). Although a study from Australia reported a 2.2 times higher HZ mortality rate among females (0.092 per 100 000) compared to males (0.043); these rates were not age adjusted and may be affected by the longer life expectancy in females (Chant *et al.*, 1998).

Race

The effect of race on incidence of HZ has been studied mainly by Schmader in the United States. In several studies among elderly racially diverse populations in North Carolina, blacks had a significantly lower lifetime occurrence and annual incidence of HZ than whites. In a community-based study among persons >64 years old in North Carolina, Schmader *et al.* (1995) reported that 16.1% of elderly white persons reported HZ compared with only 4.5% of elderly blacks ($P < 0.0001$). Even after controlling for age, cancer, and demographic factors, blacks were 4 times less likely than whites to have experienced HZ (adjusted odds ratio (aOR), 0.25, 95% Confidence Interval (CI), 0.18–0.35). In a follow-up prospective study in the same community between 1989 and 1994, Schmader et al. (1998) reported that after controlling for age, sex, education, cancer, other chronic diseases, hospitalization, activities of daily living, self-rated health, depression, and cigarette smoking, black individuals were a little over a third as likely to develop HZ than were white individuals (aOR, 0.37; 95% CI, 0.26, 0.53; $P = 0.0001$). Hypothesized reasons for the lower risk of HZ among elderly blacks include age at onset of varicella, racial differences in VZV immunity, and lifetime exposures to varicella (Schmader, 2000). Thomas and Hall (2004), in a recent analysis of Morbidity Statistics from General Practice (MSGP) studies in the UK, have corroborated these findings with black adults having less than half the risk of HZ after adjusting for age, sex and country of birth (risk ratio (RR), 0.46, 95% CI, 0.21–0.97). However, in this analysis, the protective effect for blacks was not associated with household exposure to children.

Stress

Few studies have examined the effect of psychological stress on risk of HZ although there are case reports of HZ occurring after a stressful event. Schmader has studied psychological stress as a risk factor for HZ (Schmader et al. (1990). In a community-based case control study where HZ cases were matched for age, sex, and race, he reported that psychologically stressful life events were risk factors for HZ. Cases experienced negative life events significantly more often than controls 2 months before (OR, 2.60, 95% CI, 1.13, 6.27), 3 months before (OR, 2.64, 95% CI, 1.20, 6.04), or 6 months before HZ onset (OR, 2.00, 95% CI, 1.04, 3.93). Cases were more likely to perceive recent events as stressful compared to controls. In a prospective study where recall bias was not an issue, stressful life events increased the risk of HZ but the result was borderline for statistical significance (aOR, 1.38; 95% CI, 0.96–1.97) (Schmader et al., 1998).

Age of varicella infection

Some researchers have speculated that the lower risk of HZ among elderly black adults may be due to later age of acquisition of varicella. Thomas and Hall (2004) attempted to address this question for adults born in tropical climates where age of varicella infections are later than in temperate climates. Persons born in countries described as having stronger evidence of late-onset varicella (the Caribbean, Central America, India, Pakistan, Sri Lanka, Bangladesh, Singapore and Malaysia), had a lower risk of HZ compared with adults born in the UK after adjusting for age and sex (RR, 0.56, 95% CI 0.28–1.12, $P = 0.072$) although these differences were not statistically significant (Thomas and Hall, 2004). Additional studies are needed to verify that this is due to age at varicella infection and not other factors related to country of birth or migration.

Exposure to varicella

Hope-Simpson first speculated that immunity to VZV may be maintained by periodic internal reactivation of VZV, external boosting of immunity through exposures to varicella or HZ or both. A number of studies have either directly or indirectly examined the role of contacts with varicella in both immunocompromised and healthy populations. Garnett and Grenfell (1992) examined weekly reported data in a time series analysis and reported no association between varicella and HZ although they reported some correlation with the annual data for some age groups. Three other studies suggest that contact with varicella cases appear to lower the risk of HZ in adults (Solomon et al., 1998; Terada et al., 1995; Thomas et al., 2002). However, the level of exposure reported to affect herpes zoster in the above studies is unlikely to occur for most of the population. Two analyses reported that exposure to children was associated with a lower HZ risk (Brisson et al., 2001; Thomas and Hall, 2004). A detailed discussion of this topic is presented in the "Impact of vaccination" section below.

Immunocompromising states

Herpes zoster is more common among individuals with depressed cell-mediated immunity from immunosuppressive disorders including cancer, especially hematological cancers (certain leukemias and lymphomas), HIV infection and transplants, and from immunosuppressive medications. A higher proportion of persons with HZ are immunosuppressed compared to the general population (Ragozzino et al., 1982; Guess et al., 1985; Rusthoven, 1994; Donahue et al., 1995; Lin and Hadler, 2001). Guinee et al. (1985) conducted a retrospective cohort study of HZ from six cancer centers over a 3-year period. The cumulative incidence of HZ in the 717 patients identified with Hodgkin's disease was 9.5% after 1 year, 16.6% after 2 years and 20.6% after 3 years. To further study this issue, in a large prospective study in Canada of HZ in cancer patients >15 years of age with a minimum of 5 years of follow-up, Rusthoven et al. (1988) found that the cumulative incidence rate of HZ 5 years after diagnosis was highest in hematological malignancies (14% in Hodgkin's disease, 10% in leukemia and 5% in non-Hodgkin's lymphoma) compared with solid tumors (breast 2%, lung 2%, and gynecological malignancies 1%). These differences were not due to age; in fact the median age of HZ patients with hematological malignancies was younger (51 years) than patients with solid tumors (59 years, $P < 0.005$). The finding of the highest risk of HZ in patients with Hodgkin's disease has been reported by other investigators in both pediatric and adult populations (Rusthoven, 1994; Schmader, 2000). Persons with cancers of any kind have an increased HZ risk with the administration of chemotherapy and radiation (Rusthoven, 1994). Feld et al. (1980) reported that 13 (8.1%) of patients with small-cell anaplastic carcinoma of the lung treated with chemotherapy and radiation developed HZ.

Persons with HIV infection also have a higher risk of incident and recurrent HZ although the risks are more comparable to solid tumors than hematological malignancies. Studies from the US, the Netherlands, Australia and Uganda that have compared rates of HZ in HIV-positive and HIV-negative persons have described 12–17 times higher risk among HIV-positive persons (Buchbinder et al., 1992; McNulty et al., 1997; Morgan et al., 2001; Veenstra et al., 1996). Incidence rates among HIV-positive persons varied in the above studies from 29.4 cases to 51.5 per 1000 person–years. Recurrence rates also varied according to the length of follow up, ranging from 10% to 25.6% (Morgan et al., 2001; Veenstra et al., 1996). In the Ugandan study, the incidence of HZ increased with increasing time since seroconversion to HIV + status from 7.6% at 2 years to 24.0% at 6 years. Differences in rates across studies in HIV+ populations may relate to differences in immune status and viral load because of differences in availability of effective treatment.

Persons who undergo allogeneic or autologous bone marrow transplant (BMT) experience a high risk of HZ, soon after the procedure. A variety of studies in different countries have reported this risk to range from 17%–52% (Locksley et al., 1985; Nader et al., 1995; Rusthoven, 1994; Schuchter et al., 1989; Tzeng et al., 1995). The risk is highest in the months immediately following the procedure; the majority of HZ cases occur within a year of transplantation. Schuchter reported that 28% of 151 autologus BMT patients developed HZ after the procedure, and that 91% of the cases occurred within the first year; these findings were supported by another study in which 82% of the HZ cases occurred within the first year following BMT (Tzeng et al., 1995).

Complications

Herpes zoster may lead to complications such as persistent pain (postherpetic neuralgia), bacterial infection of the lesions, pneumonia, encephalitis, and hemorrhagic complications. A number of risk factors have been found to be associated with complications, the most important of which are older age and immunosuppression. Persons >64 years have about eight times the risk of complications compared to those <25 years (Galil et al., 1997). Other factors include trigeminal distribution of the HZ rash, involvement of more than one dermatome (di Luzio Paparatti et al., 1999; Galil et al., 1997), severe pain, rash or prodromal symptoms at HZ presentation (Choo et al., 1997; Dworkin et al., 2001; Nagasako et al., 2002; Whitley et al., 1998), persisting abnormal sensations in the affected dermatome (Decroix et al., 2000) and scarring, presumed to be a consequence of rash severity (Battcock et al., 1990; Bowsher, 1999). Patients who presented with severe or incapacitating pain and a large number of lesions were 18 times less likely to achieve resolution of both acute neuritis and HZ-associated pain (Whitley et al., 1999).

Postherpetic neuralgia (PHN), a chronic pain syndrome, is the most common complication of HZ (Johnson, 2002; Lojeski and Stevens, 2000; Ragozzino et al., 1982; Stankus et al., 2000). The variability in the intensity and duration of the pain has made it complicated for researchers to agree on a standard definition making it difficult to compare results across studies. Studies have variously defined onset of PHN at rash onset or rash resolution. Study end points vary from 1, 3, 6 and 12 months after rash onset or resolution. At one month past rash onset, reported proportions of persons with PHN range from 6.5% to 45% (Haanpaa et al., 2000; Opstelten et al., 2002), at 3 months, the range is from 7.2% to 25% (Haanpaa et al., 2000; Helgason et al., 2000), and at 12 months, 3.4% to 10% (Bowsher, 1999; Helgason et al., 2000). The varying proportions in PHN at the different time periods may be affected by several factors including age and percent of immunosuppressed in the population under study.

The risk of PHN increases with increasing age although the magnitude of the effect varies across studies. PHN is more common among adults older than 50 years (Bowsher, 1999; Decroix et al., 2000; di Luzio Paparatti et al., 1999; Dworkin et al., 2001). It is estimated that about 27–68% of HZ cases over 60 years of age experience PHN (Dworkin et al., 2001; Kurokawa et al., 2002). In an Iceland study, older age was a significant and independent predictor of PHN; persons 55–74 years were 4.2 times more likely to develop PHN one month after rash onset compared to those younger than 55 years; while those over 75 years of age were 10.7 more likely to develop PHN (Opstelten et al., 2002). An even stronger association with older age was reported in a U.S. study where age ≥50 years compared to age <50 years was associated with a 14.7-fold higher prevalence of PHN at 1 month and a 27.4-fold higher prevalence at 2 months after developing HZ (Choo et al., 1997). Finally, in Singapore, Goh and Khoo (1997) reported that 20% of patients older than 50 years suffered from PHN compared to 7% of persons less than 30 years of age. Some of the difference in magnitude of the effect of older age on PHN may be due to the fact that baseline comparison groups used in the above studies differed. Furthermore, some studies controlled for other risk factors (Choo et al., 1997; Opstelten et al., 2002) while others did not (Goh and Khoo, 1997).

Herpes zoster hospitalizations and complications in healthy children are rare. Guess et al. (1985) found low morbidity among children compared to adults. Among 173 HZ cases in person <20 years of age, there were no occurrences of post-herpetic neuralgia or other late complications and only 2 (1%) were hospitalized. Furthermore, in Iceland, none of the 112 (118 episodes) cases <20 years of age developed moderate or severe pain during the acute illness or postherpetic neuralgia (95% CI, 0 to 0.03) (Petursson et al., 1998).

Hospitalizations

Fewer population-based data are available on HZ hospitalizations and no studies report hospitalization rates that are adjusted for age and high risk conditions. As with HZ incidence, the hospitalization rates increase with increasing age and high rates are seen in persons with suppressed immune systems. In the US, statewide hospital discharge data from Connecticut from 1986–1995 showed an annual crude HZ hospitalization rate of 16.1 per 100 000 person years (Lin and Hadler, 2000). A much lower crude incidence rate was observed in Northern California (2.1 per 100 000 health maintenance organization members) (Coplan et al., 2001), and an intermediate rate of 4.4 per 100 000 was reported in England for 1995 to 1996 (Brisson and Edmunds, 2003). However, because the Connecticut study included all HZ diagnoses rather than HZ as the primary discharge diagnosis, hospitalization rates may have been over-estimated by including individuals with coincidental HZ (Lin and Hadler, 2000). In this study, 31.4% of all hospitalized HZ cases and the majority of HZ hospitalizations among person <50 years of age (61%) had at least one underlying condition that increased the risk or severity of HZ; the majority of these were immunocompromising conditions (82% malignancies, and 8% HIV infection). In contrast, only 8% of the HZ hospitalized cases in England had at least one underlying condition; malignancies accounted for 87% and HIV infection for 6% of the conditions listed (Brisson and Edmunds, 2003). Finally, 67% of the hospitalized cases in the Connecticut study were 64 years or older, while only 55% of those in the California study were 60 years or older emphasizing the importance of age adjustment when comparing studies.

The rates of HZ hospitalizations increase sharply among the elderly (Chant et al., 1998; Coplan et al., 2001; Lin and Hadler, 2000). In one US study, HZ hospitalization rates increased from 21.3 per 100 000 populations among individuals <30 years of age to 1604.5 per 100 000 among those 85 years of age or older. The steepest increase in rates occurred among those over 64 years of age (Lin and Hadler, 2000). Similar patterns are seen in other studies and other countries with hospitalization rates increasing after age 50 or 60 years though rates vary across studies (Brisson et al., 2001; Brisson and Edmunds, 2003; MacIntyre et al., 2003). In Australia, HZ hospitalization remained stable at about 25 per 100 000 populations among persons <60 years of age, then increased from about 50 per 100 000 for the 60–64 age groups to over 300 for the persons 85 years and older (MacIntyre et al., 2003). In England and Canada, HZ hospitalization rates increased from 2 and 1 per 100 000 population in children aged <5 years to 148 and 86 in adults older than 64 years of age, respectively (Brisson et al., 2001).

Some studies of HZ hospitalization did not report rates. In Singapore, between 1993 and 1994, HZ accounted for 3% of total hospitalizations with a mean age of 50 years (range 23 months to 88 years); 58% of HZ hospitalizations were older than 50 years of age (Oh et al. 1997). In contrast, HZ hospitalization in Australia accounted for 0.08% of all hospitalizations between 1998 and 1999 with a mean age of 69 years and 53% were older than 50 years (MacIntyre et al., 2003). Chant et al. (1998) reported that more women in Australia than men were hospitalized for HZ (ratio of women to men was 1.4:–1.6:1), while Oh et al. (1997) reported no sex differences in hospitalization in Singapore.

Deaths

Studies on HZ mortality are few and study methods may not be comparable. As with incidence, hospitalizations, and complications, HZ mortality is more common among the elderly and those with suppressed immune systems. Schmader (2000) surmized based on clinical experience and the absence of HZ-related deaths in cohort studies, that HZ mortality appears to be an infrequent event at least among healthy persons. In Australia during 1971–1993, Chant et al. (1998) reported that 92% of HZ deaths per year occurred among persons older than 65 years. The average crude death rate for the study period was 0.068 per 100 000 population and was 10 times higher for the elderly >65 years (mortality rate 0.60). Females had more than double the rate of death compared to males however these crude mortality rates are not age adjusted (Chant et al., 1998). In Lin's study in the US, 5.3% of all HZ-related hospitalizations resulted in death and about 52% of those who died had at least one underlying high risk condition, including malignancies; leukemia, and HIV. The risk of death was higher for those with underlying high risk conditions (8.7%) than for those without any high risk conditions (3.7%). In a more recent study in Australia, 4% of 4718 hospitalized for HZ died; however, death was much less common in the group with primary HZ hospitalization (1%) compared to the group with HZ as the secondary diagnosis for hospitalization (6%) (MacIntyre et al., 2003). Finally, in a study in England and Wales from 1993 to 2000, the overall HZ mortality rate was 0.094 per 100 000 person–years however, the number of HZ deaths decreased from 64 in 1993–1994 to 40 in 1999–2000 (Brisson and Edmunds, 2003). The risk of death was <0.014 per 100 000 person–years in persons aged <64 years then increased sharply to 0.566 for persons older than 64 years. Finally, similar results were observed for case fatality ranging from <2 per 100 000 HZ cases in persons <65 years of age to 61 per 100 000 HZ cases in persons older than 64 years of age (Brisson and Edmunds, 2003).

Impact of vaccination

The impact of child and adult vaccination against VZV on the incidence of HZ and PHN remains to be determined. In the US, where there are 9 years of experience with a universal varicella vaccination program, varicella incidence, hospitalizations, and mortality have declined dramatically (Seward et al., 2002; Nguyen et al., 2005; Zhou, 2005). In a study using data from a large Health Maintenance Organization, there was no change in the overall or age-specific incidence of HZ between 1992 and 2002 in an area with about 70% varicella vaccination coverage and a decline in varicella disease that started in 1999 (Jumaan et al., 2005). Survey data from 2000 onwards from Massachusetts show an increase in herpes zoster (Yih et al., 2005).

In 1965, Hope-Simpson hypothesized that the long interval observed between the infection with varicella disease, resulting in the establishment of the latent virus, and the reactivation to cause HZ may be due to internal and external boosting. The external boosting hypothesis, suggesting the need for frequent exposures to VZV to maintain immunity against reactivation of the latent virus has attracted attention, especially with the licensure of the varicella vaccine. Some researchers have speculated that a universal varicella vaccination program, with its associated decline in varicella disease, may have the unintended effect of increasing the incidence of HZ. They note that the decline in varicella disease due to the vaccination program leads to fewer opportunities for persons with a latent virus to boost their immunity through exposure to children with wild-type VZV infection.

Modeling the impact of universal varicella vaccination predicts an initial increase in the incidence of HZ that will occur within 50 years until HZ declines as vaccinated cohorts replace those with a history of varicella disease (Brisson et al., 2002; Garnett and Ferguson, 1996). Although the incidence of HZ is much lower than that of varicella, some studies suggest that the health burden due to HZ is greater than that due to varicella because of the higher rates of complications, hospitalizations and deaths (Lin and Hadler, 2000; Brisson and Edmunds, 2003; Chant et al., 1998; MacIntyre et al., 2003). This has been raised as a serious potential concern in other developed countries considering a varicella vaccination program. However, the health burden on HZ may be overestimated. In a study in England, varicella and HZ hospitalization rates were similar at 4.5 and 4.4 per 100 000 population, respectively (Brisson and Edmunds, 2003). Furthermore, in another study in England and Canada, the reported age specific proportion of cases hospitalized and in-patient days hospitalized were only slightly higher for HZ compared to varicella (Brisson et al., 2001). However, because HZ occurs mainly in the elderly compared to varicella, the overall burden on in-patient hospitalization for HZ is reported to be considerably higher (Brisson et al., 2001; Brisson and Edmunds, 2003; MacIntyre, 2003). In a US study of HZ hospitalizations, the authors did not differentiate between primary vs coincidental cause of HZ hospitalization or death (Lin and Hadler, 2000). Coincidental cases of HZ may be quite common especially among elderly hospitalized adults with long hospital stays, some of whom will die from other causes (MacIntyre et al., 2003). This may contribute to overestimation of the health burden due to HZ.

Several studies reported lower HZ rates among persons exposed to varicella cases (Solomon et al., 1998; Terada et al., 1995; Thomas et al., 2002), compared to those without any exposure. Thomas showed that contacts with ≥ 5 varicella cases were associated with a strong protective effect against HZ after controlling for occupational and social (OR = 0.29, 95% CI 0.10–0.8) compared to those with no contacts. The two other smaller studies with methodological limitations reported that pediatricians had lower HZ incidence than the general population (Terada et al., 1995), and dermatologists or psychiatrists (Solomon et al., 1998). Terada based his findings on small numbers of cases; while Solomon's findings were based on low response rates (31% paediatricians) and found no differences between dermatologists and psychiatrists, groups considered to have different rates of exposure to varicella cases. Finally, in all three studies, protection was observed for groups with more exposure to varicella than is generally experienced by the general population.

Other studies have used exposure to children as a proxy for exposure to varicella. Two observational studies in England reported that household or occupational exposure to children was associated with a lower HZ incidence (Brisson et al., 2002; Thomas and Hall, 2004). Brisson reported that people living with children had a significantly lower rate of developing HZ (RR, 0.75 95% CI 0.63–0.89). In a subsequent analysis of the same data, Thomas reported that individuals who reported working with young children (primary school teachers, nursery nurses, playgroup leaders and other child care providers) were significantly less likely to develop HZ after adjusting for age, sex, ethnicity and a child living in the household (RR, 0.70, 95% CI 0.58–0.85). However, it is not clear how other factors that could have contributed to such findings were adjusted for in the analysis including the fact that people with other medical health problems, who are at a higher risk for HZ, are less likely to live with children. Furthermore, Thomas and Hall (2004) in their review of risk factors for HZ report that women in general have higher incidence rates of HZ compared to males; they comment that these findings conflict with the suggested reduced HZ risk associated with exposure to varicella cases or children.

The protection against HZ due to varicella exposure is plausible and is supported by immunologic studies. One reported that 71% of adults who had household exposure to varicella experienced a boost in cellular immune responses (Arvin et al., 1983), and the other found that vaccinated leukemic children with household exposure to varicella were less likely to develop HZ than vaccinated leukemic children without such an exposure (Gershon et al., 1996; Hardy et al., 1991). Yet, other issues still remain unknown, including factors that contribute to immune boosting, the duration of protection from such exposures, and other factors that influence VZV reactivation. Herpes zoster affects mainly the elderly, and if there is a protection from exposure to varicella, the duration of this protection is not known. However, modeling, based on the assumption that the boosting effect lasts for 20 years, suggests that an increase in HZ incidence will occur as early as five (Garnett and Ferguson, 1996) to seven (Brisson et al., 2002) years following the implementation of a mass vaccination program.

Herpes zoster in vaccinated children

Current data suggest that vaccinated children experience a lower HZ incidence rate than those who have had wild varicella. Herpes zoster incidence among healthy children who received varicella vaccine is reported to be rare; the incidence of HZ among these children was reported to be approximately 13 cases per 100 000 person–years (Gershon et al., 2004) however, longer follow-up is needed. Furthermore, studies in leukemic children have found a much lower incidence of HZ among vaccinated (2%) than among age matched children with a history of varicella (15%) (Hardy et al.,1991). Therefore, it is expected that HZ incidence will decline over the long term, as vaccinated cohorts replace those in the community with naturally acquired varicella.

Vaccination for prevention of herpes zoster

As populations age and the survival of people with chronic and immunocompromised conditions improves, the incidence of HZ and PHN is expected to increase. Several studies have suggested that declines in VZV-specific CMI increase the risk and severity of HZ (Arvin 1996; Miller, 1980; Oxman, 1995). Early studies on administration of a higher titer varicella vaccine to older adults 55+ have shown that vaccinated persons experience an increased VZV-specific CMI responses to levels typical of those observed in younger persons, in whom the incidence and severity of HZ are lower (Levin et al., 1998; Levin, 2001). A recent study reported on the boosting in VZV-specific cell-mediated immunity from a booster dose of VZV vaccine administered ≥ 5 years after the first dose (Levin et al., 2003). In 2005, the results of a large placebo-controlled clinical trial to test whether a shingles vaccine in persons 60 years and older would prevent or reduce the risk or severity of HZ and its complications became available. The vaccine was 51.3% efficacious in reducing herpes zoster incidence, 66.6% efficacious in reducing the incidence of postherpetix neuralgia (largely through preventing herpes zoster) and 61.1% efficacious in reducing the burden of illness due to herpes zoster (Oxman et al., 2005). This vaccine, now licensed in the USA with expected licensure in other countries, has the potential to reduce the incidence of HZ or reduce/attenuate the severity of PHN, and complications of HZ. (Johnson et al., 2002; Schmader, 2001; Gilden, 2005). In the U.S. Zoster vaccine was recommended for use in all adults ≥ 60 years without a contraindication in October 2006 (CDC, 2006).

Acknowledgements

The authors thank Melinda Wharton, MD, MPH, CDC for comments? Dr. Claire Cameron (Health Protection Scotland) for providing data for Fig. 40.1 and staff in the varicella Active Surveillance Project sites for providing data on varicella in the post-vaccine era in the United States.

REFERENCES

Arvin, A. M. (1996). Varicella-zoster virus: overview and clinical manifestations. *Semin. Dermatol.*, **15**(2 Suppl. 1), 4–7. Review.

Arvin, A. M., Koropchak, C. M., and Wittek, A. E., (1983). Immunological evidence of re-infection with varicella zoster virus. *J. Infect. Dis.*, **148**, 200–205.

Asano, Y., Nakayama, H., Yazaki, T. *et al.* (1977). Protection against varicella in family contacts by immediate inoculation with live varicella vaccine. *Pediatrics*, **59**, 3–7.

Barzaga, N. G., Roxas, J. R., and Florese, R. H. (1994). Varicella zoster virus prevalence in metro Manila, Philippines. *J. Am. Med. Assoc.* (SE Asia), **274**, S633–S635.

Battcock, T. M., Finn, R., Barnes, R. M. *et al.* (1990). Observations on herpes zoster: 1. Residual scarring and post-herpetic neuralgia; 2. Handedness and the risk of infection. *Br. J. Clin. Pract.*, **44**(12), 596–598.

Boelle, P. Y. and Hanslik, T. (2002). Varicella in non-immune persons: incidence, hospitalization and mortality rates. *Epidemiol. Infect.*, **129**, 599–606.

Bowsher, D.(1999). The lifetime occurrence of herpes zoster and prevalence of postherpetic neuralgia: a retrospective survey in an elderly population. *Eur. J. Pain*, **3**, 335–342.

Bramley, J. C. and Jones, I. G. (2000). Epidemiology of chickenpox in Scotland: 1981 to 1998. *Commun. Dis. Public Health*, **3**, 82–87.

Brisson, M. and Edmunds, J. W. (2003). Epidemiology of Varicella-Zoster Virus in England and Wales. *J. Med. Virol.*, **70**(Suppl 1), S9–S14.

Brisson, M., Edmunds, W. J., Law, B. *et al.* (2001). Epidemiology of varicella zoster virus infection in Canada and the United Kingdom. *Epidemiol. Infect.* **127**(2), 305–314.

Brisson, M., Gay, N. J., Edmunds, W. J. *et al.* (2002). Exposure to varicella boosts immunity to herpes-zoster: implications for mass vaccination against chickenpox. *Vaccine*, **20**(19–20), 2500–2507.

Buchbinder, S. P., Katz, M. H., Hessol, N. A. *et al.* (1992). Herpes zoster and human immunodeficiency virus infection. *J. Infect. Dis.*, **166**(5), 1153–1156.

Centers for Disease Control and Prevention. (2003). Decline in annual incidence of varicella – selected states, 1990–2001. *Morb. Mortal. Wkly Rep.*, **52**(37), 884–885.

Chant, K. G., Sullivan, E. A., Burgess, M. A. *et al.* (1998). Varicella-zoster virus infection in Australia. *Aust. N Z J. Public Health*, **22**, 413–418.

Chidiac, C., Bruxelle, J., Daures, J. P. *et al.* (2001). Characteristics of patients with herpes zoster on presentation to practitioners in France. *Clin. Infect. Dis*, **33**, 62–69.

Choo, P. W., Donahue, J. G., Manson, J. E., and Platt, R. (1995). The epidemiology of varicella and its complications. *J. Infect. Dis.*, **172**, 706–712.

Choo, P. W., Galil, K., Donahue J. G. *et al.* (1997). Risk factors for postherpetic neuralgia. *Arch. Intern. Med.*, **157**(11), 1217–1224.

Cooper, M. (1987). The epidemiology of herpes zoster. *Eye*, **1**(Pt 3), 413–421.

Coplan, P., Black, S., Rojas, C. *et al.* (2001). Incidence and hospitalization rates of varicella and herpes zoster before varicella vaccine introduction: a baseline assessment of the shifting epidemiology of varicella disease. *Pediatr. Infect. Dis.*, **20**(7), 641–645.

Davis, M. M., Patel, M. S., Chen, B. S. *et al.* (2004). Decline in varicella-related hospitalization and expenditures for children and adults after introduction of varicella vaccine in the United States. *Pediatrics*, **114**(3), 786–792.

Decroix, J., Partsch, H., Gonzalez, R. *et al.* (2000). Factors influencing pain outcome in herpes zoster: an observational study with valaciclovir. Valaciclovir International Zoster Assessment Group (VIZA). *J. Eur. Acad. Dermatol. Venereol.*, **14**(1), 23–33.

Degeun, S., Chau, N. P., and Flahault, A. (1998). Epidemiology of chickenpox in France (1991–1995). *J. Epidemiol. Commun. Health*, **52**, 46S–98S.

di Luzio Paparatti, U., Arpinelli, F., and Visona, G. (1999). Herpes zoster and its complications in Italy: an observational survey. *J. Infect.*, **38**(2), 116–120.

Donahue, J. G., Choo, P. W., and Manson, J. E. (1995). The incidence of herpes zoster. *Arch. Intern. Med.*, **155**, 1605–1609.

Dworkin, R. H., Nagasako, E. M., Johnson, R. W., and Griffin, D. R. (2001). Acute pain in herpes zoster: the famciclovir database project. *Pain*, **94**(1), 113–119.

Dworkin, M. S., Jennings, C. E., Roth-Thomas, J. *et al.* (2002). An Outbreak of Varicella among children attending preschool and elementary school in Illinois. *Clin. Infect. Dis.*, **35**(1), 102–104. Epub 2002 Jun 05.

Edmunds, W. J., Brisson, M., and Rose, J. D. (2001). The epidemiology of herpes zoster and potential cost-effectiveness of vaccination in England and Wales. *Vaccine*, **19**(23–24), 3076–3090.

Enders, G. and Miller, E. (2000). Varciella and herpes zoster in pregnancy and the newborn. In Arvin, A. and Gershon, A, eds. *Varicella-Zoster Virus*, pp. 317–347. Cambridge: Cambridge University Press.

Enders, G., Miller, E., Cradock-Watson, J. *et al.* (1994). Consequences of varicella and herpes zoster in pregnancy: prospective study of 1739 cases. *Lancet*, **343**(8912), 1548–1551.

Fairley, C. K. and Miller, E. (1996). Varicella-zoster virus epidemiology – a changing scene? *J. Infect. Dis.*, **174**(suppl 3), S314–S319.

Fales, W. T. (1928). The age distribution of whooping cough, measles, chickenpox, scarlet fever and diphtheria in various areas in the United States. *Am. J. Hyg.*, **8**, 759–799.

Feld, R., Evans, W. K., and DeBoer, G. (1980). Herpes zoster in patients with small-cell carcinoma of the lung receiving combined modality treatment. *Ann. Intern. Med.*, **93**(2), 282–283.

Fornaro, P., Gandini, F., Marin, M. *et al.* (1999). Epidemiology and cost analysis of varicella in Italy: results of a sentinel study in the pediatric practice. *Pediatr. Infect. Dis. J.*, **18**, 414–419.

Gabutti, G., Penna, C., Rossi, M. *et al.* (2001). The seroepidemiology of varicella in Italy. *Epidemiol. Infect.*, **126**, 433–440.

Galil, K., Choo, P. W., Donahue, J. G., and Platt, R. (1997). The sequelae of herpes zoster. *Arch. Intern. Med.*, **157**(11), 1209–1213.

Galil, G., Brown, C., Lin, F., and Seward, J. (2002a). Hospitalizations for varicella in the United States, 1988–1999. *Pediatr. Infect. Dis. J.*, **21**, 931–934.

Galil, K., Lee, B., Strine, T. *et al.* (2002b). Outbreak of varicella at a day-care center despite vaccination. *N. Engl. J. Med.*, **347**(24), 1909–1915.

Galil, K., Pletcher, M. J., Wallace, B. J. *et al.* (2002c). Tracking varicella deaths: accuracy and completeness of death certificates and hospital discharge records, New York State, 1989–1995. *Am. J. Public Health*, **92**, 1248–1250.

Garnett, G. P. and Ferguson, N. M. (1996). Predicting the Effect of Varicella Vaccine on Subsequent Cases of Zoster and Varicella. *Rev. Med. Virol.*, **6**(3), 151–161.

Garnett, G. P. and Grenfell, B. T. (1992). The epidemiology of varicella-zoster virus infections: the influence of varicella on the prevalence of herpes zoster. *Epidemiol. Infect.*, **108**(3), 513–528.

Garnett, G. P., Cox, M. J., Bundy, D. A. P. *et al.* (1993). The age of infection with varicella-zoster virus in St, Lucia, West Indies. *Epidemiol. Infect.*, **110**, 361–372.

Gershon, A. A., LaRussa, P., Steinberg, S. *et al.* (1996). The protective effect of immunologic boosting against zoster: an analysis in leukemic children who were vaccinated against chickenpox. *J. Infect. Dis.*, **173**(2), 450–453.

Gershon, A., Takahashi, M., and Seward, J. (2004). Varicella vaccine. In *Vaccines*, 4th edn, pp. 783–823, New York: W. B. Saunders.

Ghebrekidan, H. Ruden, U., Cox, S. *et al.* (1999). Prevalence of herpes simplex virus types 1 and 2, cytomegalovirus, and varicella-zoster virus infections in Eritrea. *J. Clin. Virol.*, **12**, 53–64.

Gilden, D. H. (2005). Varicella-zoster virus vaccine – grown-ups need it too. *N. Engl. J. Med.*, **352**(22), 2344–2345.

Glynn, C., Crockford, G., Gavaghan, D. *et al.* (1990). Epidemiology of shingles. *J. Roy. Soc. Med.*, **83**(10), 617–619.

Goh, C. L. and Khoo, L. (1997). A retrospective study of the clinical presentation and outcome of herpes zoster in a tertiary dermatology outpatient referral clinic. *Int. J. Dermatol.*, **36**(9), 667–672.

Guess, H. A., Broughton, D. D., Melton, L. J., III, and Kurland, L. T. (1985). Epidemiology of herpes zoster in children and adolescents: a population-based study. *Pediatrics*, **76**, 512–517.

Guess, H. A., Broughton, D. D., Melton, L. J. III. *et al.* (1986). Population-based studies of varicella complications. *Pediatrics*, **78**, S723–S727.

Guinee, V. F., Guido, J. J., Pfalzgraf, K. A. *et al.* (1985). The incidence of herpes zoster in patients with Hodgkin's disease. An analysis of prognostic factors. *Cancer*, **56**(3), 642–648.

Haanpaa, M., Laippala, P., and Nurmikko, T. (2000). Allodynia and pinprick hypesthesia in acute herpes zoster, and the development of postherpetic neuralgia. *J. Pain Symptom Manage.*, **20**(1), 50–58.

Hardy, I., Gershon, A. A., Steinberg, S. P., and LaRussa P. (1991). The incidence of zoster after immunization with live attenuated varicella vaccine. A study in children with leukemia. *N. Engl. J. Med.*, **325**(22), 1545–1550.

Helgason, S., Petursson, G., Gudmundsson, S., and Sigurdsson, J. A. (2000). Prevalence of postherpetic neuralgia after a first episode of herpes zoster: prospective study with long term follow up. *Br. Med. J.*, **321**, 794–796.

Hope-Simpson, R. E. (1952). Infectiousness of communicable diseases in the household (measles, chickenpox and mumps). *Lancet*, **ii**, 549–554.

Hope-Simpson, R. E. (1965). The nature of herpes zoster: a long-term study and a new hypothesis. *Proc. Roy. Soc. Med.*, **58**, 2–20.

Hurwitz, E. S., Gunn, W. J., Pinsky, P. F. *et al.* (1991). Risk of respiratory illness associated with day-care attendance: a nationwide study. *Pediatrics*, **87**, 62–69.

Izurieta, H. S., Strebel, P. M., and Blake, P. A. (1997). Postlicensure effectiveness of varicella vaccine during an outbreak in a child care center. *J. Am. Med. Assoc.*, **278**, 1495–1499.

Jeena, P. M., Wesley, A. G., and Coovadia, H. M. (1998). Infectious diseases at the paediatric isolation units of Clairwood and King Edward VII hospitals, Durben. Trends in admission and mortality rates (1985–1996) and the early impact of HIV (1994–1996). *S. Afr. Med. J.*, **88**(7), 867–872.

Jerant, A. F., DeGaetano, J. S., Epperly, T. D. *et al.* (1998). Varicella susceptibility and vaccination strategies in young adults. *J. Am. Board Fam. Pract.*, **11**, 296–306.

Jezek, Z., Basu, R. N., and Arya, Z. S. (1978a). Investigation of smallpox suspected cases in the final stage of Indian smallpox eradication programme. *Ind. J. Public Health*, **22**(1), 107–112.

Jezek, Z., Basu, R. N., Arya, Z. S. *et al.* (1978b). Fever with rash surveillance in India. *Ind. J. Public Health*, **22**(1), 120–126.

Johnson, R. W. Consequences and management of pain in herpes zoster. (2002). *J. Infect. Dis.*, **15**, 186(Suppl 1), S83–90. Review.

Jumaan, A. O., Yu, O., Jackson, L. A., Bohlke, K., Galil, K., and Seward, J. F. (2005). Incidence of herpes zoster, before and after varicella-vaccination-associated decreases in the incidence of varicella, 1992–2002. *J. Infect. Dis.*, **191**(12), 2002–2007.

Kanra, G., Tezcan, S., Badur, S. and the Turkish National Study Team. (2002). Varicella seroprevalence in a random sample of the Turkish population. *Vaccine*, **20**(9–10), 1425–1428.

Kilgore, P. E, Kruszon-Moran, D., Seward, J. F. *et al.* (2003). Varicella in Americans from NHANES III: implications for control through routine immunization. *J. Med. Virol.*, **70**(Suppl 1), S111–S118.

Kurokawa, I., Kumano, K., Murakawa, K. *et al.* (2002). Clinical correlates of prolonged pain in Japanese patients with acute herpes zoster. *J. Int. Med. Res.*, **30**(1), 56–65.

Laforet, E. G. and Lynch, C. L. (1947). Multiple congenital defects following maternal varicella. *N. Engl. J. Med.*, **236**(15), 534–537.

Lam, M. S., Chew, S. K., Allen, D. M., and Monteiro, E. H. (1993). Fatal varicella infections in Singapore. *Singapore Med. J.*, **34**, 213–215.

Lee, B. W. (1998). Review of varicella zoster seroepidemiology in India and Southeast Asia. *Trop. Med. Int. Health*, **3**(11), 886–890. Review.

Levin, M. J. (2001). Use of varicella vaccines to prevent herpes zoster in older individuals. *Arch. Virol. Suppl*, **17**, 151–160. Review.

Levin, M. J., Barber, D., Goldblatt, E. *et al.* (1998). Use of a live attenuated varicella vaccine to boost varicella-specific immune responses in seropositive people 55 years of age and older: duration of booster effect. *J. Infect. Dis.*, **178**(Suppl 1), S109–S112.

Levin, M. J., Smith, J. G., Kaufhold, R. M. *et al.*(2003). Decline in varicella-zoster virus (VZV)-specific cell-mediated immunity with increasing age and boosting with a high-hose VZV vaccine. *J. Infect. Dis.*, **188**(9), 1336–1344.

Lin, F. and Hadler, J. L. (2000). Epidemiology of primary varicella and herpes zoster hospitalizations: the pre-varicella vaccine era. *J. Infect. Dis.*, **181**(6), 1897–1905.

Locksley, R. M., Flournoy, N., Sullivan, K. M. *et al.* (1985). Infection with varicella-zoster virus after marrow transplantation. *J. Infect. Dis.*, **152**(6), 1172–1181.

Lojeski, E. and Stevens, R. A. (2000). Postherpetic neuralgia in the cancer patient. *Curr. Rev. Pain*, **4**(3), 219–226.

Lolekha, S., Tanthiphabha, W., Sornchai, P. *et al.* (2001). Effect of climatic factors and population density on varicella zoster virus epidemiology within a tropical country. *Am. J. Trop. Med. Hyg.*, **64**, 131–136.

MacIntyre, C. R., Chu, C. P., and Burgess, M. A. (2003). Use of hospitalization and pharmaceutical prescribing data to compare the prevaccination burden of varicella and herpes zoster in Australia. *Epidemiol. Infect.*, **131**(1), 675–682.

Mandal, B. K., Mukherjee, P. P., Murphy, C. *et al.* (1998). Adult susceptibility to varicella in the tropics is a rural phenomenon due to lack of previous exposure. *J. Infect. Dis.*, **178**(Suppl.), S52–S54.

McGregor, R. M. (1957). Herpes zoster, chicken pox and cancer in general practice. *Br. Med. J.*, **1**, 84–87.

McNulty, A., Li, Y., Radtke, U. *et al.* (1997). Herpes zoster and the stage and prognosis of HIV-1 infection. *Genitourin. Med.*, **73**(6), 467–470.

Meyer, A., Seward, J. F., Jumaan, A. O., and Wharton, M. (2000). Varicella mortality: trends before vaccine licensure in the United States, 1970–94. *J. Infect. Dis.*, **182**, 383–390.

Miller, A. E. (1980). Selective decline in cellular immune response to varicella-zoster in the elderly. *Neurology*, **30**(6), 582–587.

Morgan, D., Mahe, C., Malamba, S. *et al.* (2001). Herpes zoster and HIV-1 infection in a rural Ugandan cohort. *AIDS*, **15**(2), 223–229.

Nader, S., Bergen, R., Sharp, M., and Arvin, A. M. (1995). Age-related differences in cell-mediated immunity to varicella-zoster virus among children and adults immunized with live attenuated varicella vaccine. *J. Infect. Dis.*, **171**(1), 13–17.

Nagasako, E. M., Johnson, R. W., Griffin, D. R. *et al.* (2002). Rash severity in herpes zoster: correlates and relationship to postherpetic neuralgia. *J. Am. Acad. Dermatol.*, **46**(6), 834–839.

Nguyen, H., Jumaan, A. O., and Seward, J. F. (2005). Decline in mortality due to varicella after implementation of varicella vaccination in the United States. *N. Engl. J. Med.*, **352**, 450–458.

Oh, H. M., Ho, A. Y., Chew, S. K. *et al.* (1997). Clinical presentation of herpes zoster in a Singapore hospital. *Singapore Med. J.*, **38**(11), 471–474.

Ooi, P. L., Goh, K. T., Doraisingham, S., and Ling, A. E. (1992). Prevalence of varicella-zoster virus infection in Singapore. *Southeast Asian J. Trop. Med. Public Health*, **23**, 22–25.

Opstelten, W., Mauritz, J. W., de Wit, N. J. *et al.* (2002). Herpes zoster and postherpetic neuralgia: incidence and risk indicators using a general practice research database. *Fam. Pract.*, **19**(5), 471–475.

Oxman, M. N. (1995). Immunization to reduce the frequency and severity of herpes zoster and its complications. *Neurology*, **45**(Suppl. 8), S41–S46.

Oxman, M. N., Levin, M. J., Johnson, G. R. *et al.* (2005). A vaccine to prevent herpes zoster and postherpetic neuralgia in order adults. *N. Engl. J. Med.*, **352**(22), 2271–2284.

Palmer, S. R., Caul, E. O., Donald, D. E., Kwantes, W., and Tillett, H. (1985). An outbreak of shingles? *Lancet*, **2**(8464), 1108–1111.

Petursson, G., Helgason, S., Gudmundsson, S. *et al.* (1998). Herpes zoster in children and adolescents. *Pediatr. Infect. Dis. J.*, **17**(10), 905–908.

Ragozzino, M. W., Melton, L. J. 3rd, Kurland, L. T. *et al.* (1982). Population-based study of herpes zoster and its sequelae. *Medicine (Baltimore)*, **61**(5), 310–316.

Ratner, A. J. (2002). Varicella-related hospitalizations in the vaccine era. *Pediatr. Infect. Dis. J.*, **21**, 927–930.

Rawson, H., Crampin, A., and Noah, N. (2001). Deaths from chickenpox in England and Wales 1995–97: analysis of routine mortality date. *Br. Med. J.*, **323**, 1091–1093.

Reigle, L. and Cooperstock, M. (1985). Contagiousness of zoster in a day care setting. *Pediatr. Infect. Dis.*, **4**(4), 413.

Reis, A. D., Pannuti, C. S., and de Souza, V. A. (2003). Prevalence of varicella-zoster virus antibodies in young adults from different Brazilian climatic regions. *Rev. Soc. Bras. Med. Trop.*, **36**(3), 317–320. Epub 2003 Jul 31.

Ross, A. H. (1962). Modification of chickenpox in family contacts by administration of gamma globulin. *N. Engl. J. Med.*, **267**, 369–376.

Ross, A. M. and Fleming, D. M. (2000). Chickenpox increasingly affects preschool children. *Commun. Dis. Public Health*, **3**, 213–215.

Rusthoven, J. J. (1994). The risk of varicella-zoster infections in different patient populations: a critical. *Transfus. Med. Rev.*, **8**(2), 96–116.

Rusthoven, J. J., Ahlgren, P., Elhakim, T. *et al.* (1988). Risk factors for varicella zoster disseminated infection among adult cancer patients with localized zoster. *Cancer*, **62**(8), 1641–1646.

Rusthoven, J. J., Ahlgren, P., Elhakim, T. *et al.* (1988). Varicella-zoster infection in adult cancer patients. A population study. *Arch. Intern. Med.*, **148**(7), 1561–1566.

Ryan, M. A., Smith, T. C., Honner, W. K. *et al.* (2003). Varicella susceptibility and vaccine use among young adults enlisting in the United States Navy. *J. Med. Virol.*, **70**(Suppl 1), S15–S19.

Schimpff, S., Serpick, A., Stoler. B. *et al.* (1972). Varicella-Zoster infection in patients with cancer. *Ann. Intern. Med.*, **76**(2), 241–254.

Schmader, K. (2000). Epidemiology of herpes zoster. In Arvin, A. and Gershon, A., eds. *Varicella-Zoster Virus*, pp. 220–245, Cambridge: Cambridge University Press.

Schmader, K. (2001). Herpes zoster in older adults. *Clin. Infect. Dis.*, **32**(10), 1481–1486.

Schmader, K., Studenski, S., MacMillan, J. *et al.* (1990). Are stressful life events risk factors for herpes zoster? *J. Am. Geriatr. Soc.*, **38**(11), 1188–1194.

Schmader, K., George, L. K., Burchett, B. M. *et al.* (1995). Racial differences in the occurrence of herpes zoster. *J. Infect. Dis.*, **171**(3), 701–704.

Schmader, K., George. L. K., Burchett, B. M. *et al.* (1998). Race and stress in the incidence of herpes zoster in older adults. *J. Am. Geriatr. Soc.*, **46**(8), 973–977.

Schoub, B. D., Johnson. S., McAnerney, J. M. *et al.* (1985). Prevalence of antibodies to varicella zoster virus in healthy adults. *S. Afr. Med. J.*, **8, 67**(23), 929–931.

Schuchter, L. M., Wingard, J. R., Piantadosi, S. *et al.* (1989). Herpes zoster infection after autologous bone marrow transplantation. *Blood*, **74**(4), 1424–1427.

Seiler, H. E. (1949). A study of herpes zoster particularly in relation to chickenpox. *J. Hyg. (Lond.)*, **47**, 253–262.

Seward, J. Meyer, P., Singleton, J. *et al.* (1998). Varicella incidence and mortality, USA 1970–1994. *Infectious Disease Society of America*. 36th Annual Meeting, Denver, CO.

Seward, J., Galil, K., and Wharton, M. (2000). Epidemiology of varicella. In Arvin, A. and Gershon, A., eds. *Varicella-Zoster Virus*, pp. 187–205. Cambridge University Press.

Seward, J. F., Watson, B. M., Peterson, C. L. *et al.* (2002). Varicella disease after introduction of varicella vaccine in the United States, 1995–2000. *J. Am. Med. Assoc.*, **287**, 606–611.

Socan, M., Kraigher, A., and Pahor, L. (2001). Epidemiology of varicella in Slovenia over a 20-year period (1979–1998). *Epidemiol. Infect.*, **126**, 279–283.

Solomon, B.A., Kaporis, A.G., Glass, A.T. *et al.* (1998). Lasting immunity to varicella in doctors study (L.I.V.I.D. study). *Am. Acad. Dermatol.*, **38**, 763–765.

Stankus, S. J., Dlugopolski, M., Packer, D. *et al.* (2000). Management of herpes zoster (shingles) and postherpetic neuralgia. *Am. Fam. Physician*, **61**(8), 2437–2444, 2447–2448. Review.

Takayama, N., Yamada, H., Kaku, H. *et al.* (2000). Herpes zoster in immunocompetent and immunocompromised Japanese. *Pediatr. Int.*, **42**(3), 275–279.

Terada, K., Hirago, U., Kawano, S. *et al.* (1995). Incidence of herpes zoster in pediatricians and history of reexposure to varicella-zoster virus in patients with herpes zoster. *Kansenshogaku Zasshi*, **69**(8), 908–912.

Thiry, N., Beutels, P., Shkedy, Z. *et al.* (2002). The seroepidemiology of primary varicella-zoster virus infection in Flanders (Belgium). *Eur. J. Pediatr.*, **161**, 588–593.

Thomas, S.L. and Hall, A.J. (2004). What does epidemiology tell us about risk factors for herpes zoster? *Lancet Infect. Dis.*, **4**(1), 26–33. Review.

Thomas, S. L., Wheeler, J. G., Hall, A. J. *et al.* (2002). Contacts with varicella or with children and protection against herpes zoster in adults: a case-control study. *Lancet*, **31**, 360 (9334), 678–682.

Tobias, M., Reid, S., Lennon, D. *et al.* (1998). Chickenpox immunization in New Zealand. *N Z Med. J.*, **111**, 274–281.

Tzeng, C. H., Liu, J. H., Fan, S. *et al.* (1995). Varicella zoster virus infection after allogeneic or autologous hemopoietic stem cell transplantation. Factors contributing to severity of herpes zoster in children. *Pediatrics*, **67**(5), 763–771.

Veenstra, J., van Praag, R.M., Krol, A. *et al.* (1996) Complications of varicella zoster virus reactivation in HIV-infected homosexual men. *AIDS*, **10**(4), 393–399.

Vynnycky, E. Gay, N. J., and Cutts, F. T. (2003). The predicted impact of private sector MMR vaccination on the burden of Congenital Rubella Syndrome. *Vaccine*, **21**(21–22), 2708–2719.

Wharton, M. (1996). The epidemiology of varicella-zoster virus infections. *Infect. Dis. Clin. North. Am.*, **10**(3), 571–581.

Whitley, R. J., Shukla, S., Crooks, R. J. *et al.* (1998). The identification of risk factors associated with persistent pain following herpes zoster. *J. Infect. Dis.*, **178**(Suppl 1), S710–S715.

Whitley, R. J., Weiss H. L., Soong, S. J. *et al.* (1999). Herpes zoster: risk categories for persistent pain. *J. Infect. Dis.*, **179**, 9–15.

Wilson, J. B. (1986) Thirty one years of herpes zoster in a rural practice. Br. Med. J. (Clin. Res. edn), **293**, 1349–1351.

Yawn, B. P., Yawn, R. A., and Lydick, E. (1997). Community impact of childhood varicella infections. *J. Pediatr.*, **130**, 759–765.

Yih, W. K., Brooks, D. R., Lett, S. M. *et al.* (2005). The incidence of varicella and herpes zoster in Massachusetts as measured by the Behavioral Risk Factor Surveillance System (BRFSS) during a period of increasing varicella vaccine coverage, 1998–2003. *BMC Public Health*, **5**(1), 68.

Yorke, J. A. and London, W. P. (1973). Recurrent outbreaks of measles, chickenpox and mumps. II. Systematic differences in contact rates and stochastic effects. *Am. J. Epidemiol.*, **98**(6), 469–482.

Zak-Prelich, M., Borkowski, J. L., Alexander, F. *et al.* (2000). The role of solar ultraviolet irradiation in zoster. *Epidemiol. Infect*, **129**(3), 593–597.

Zhou, F., Harpaz, R., Jumaan, A. O., Winston, C. A., and Shefer, A. (2005). Impact of varicella vaccination on health care utilization. *J. Am. Med. Assoc.*, **294**(7), 797–802.

Part III

Pathogenesis, clinical disease, host response, and epidemiology: betaherpesviruses

Edited by Ann Arvin and Richard Whitley

Part III

Pathogenesis, clinical disease, host response, and epidemiology: betaherpesviruses

Edited by Ann Arvin and Richard Whitley

41

Virus entry into host, establishment of infection, spread in host, mechanisms of tissue damage

William Britt

Department of Pediatrics, University of Alabama at Birmingham, AL, USA

Introduction

Cytomegaloviruses (CMV) were initially identified by distinct histopathological findings that were observed in tissue from a variety of infected mammals, including humans. Perhaps the most well-recognized finding were inclusion bearing cells in the salivary glands of infected animals (Jesionek and Kiolemenoglou, 1904; Ribbert, 1904; Goodpasture and Talbot, 1921; Cole and Kuttner, 1926). Similar histopathologic findings of intracellular inclusions were noted in tissues from infants dying as a result of severe congenital (present at birth) cytomegalovirus infection leading to the designation of this clinical syndrome as cytomegalic inclusion disease (Farber and Wolbach, 1932). Studies by several groups of investigators provided compelling evidence from natural history studies that HCMV was a relatively frequent cause of disease in infants infected in utero and, that this viral infection could result in neurologic impairment in infected infants (Hanshaw, 1971; Stagno et al., 1977; Pass et al., 1980; Williamson et al., 1982; Bale, 1984; Fowler et al., 1992). Importantly, these early studies demonstrated that even infants with subclinical or silent infections could develop neurological sequelae (Stagno et al., 1982, 1983; Williamson et al., 1992). In the late 1960s, HCMV was recognized as a significant cause of disease in allograft recipients and in the case of hematopoietic allograft recipients, HCMV infection became recognized as one of the most frequent causes of death in the post-transplant period (Rifkind, 1965; Myers et al., 1975; Ho, 1977; Rubin et al., 1979; Winston et al., 1979; Rubin et al., 1981; Rubin and Colvin, 1986; Rubin, 1990). Significant morbidity and mortality rates were reported in allograft recipients infected with HCMV until efficacious antiviral chemotherapy was developed for this agent (Emanuel et al., 1988; Schmidt et al., 1991; Goodrich et al., 1993; Winston et al., 1993). Similarly, HCMV rapidly emerged as a major opportunistic pathogen in patients with HIV infection, particularly those in the late stages of the retroviral infection (Klatt and Shibata, 1988; Gallant et al., 1992; Bowen et al., 1995; Selik et al., 1996; Spector et al., 1999). The spectrum of diseases associated with infection with HCMV has been well described in immunocompromised patients with acute infectious syndromes in which virus replication can be correlated with end-organ disease. Because immunocompromised patients often present with multiorgan dysfunction secondary to chronic underlying disease and in some cases the pharmacologic agents utilized to treat allograft rejection, it has been difficult to completely define the spectrum of clinical disease associated with HCMV infection. In contrast to findings in allograft recipients, the disease manifestations of congenitally (present at birth) infected infants can be related directly to HCMV infection. Yet even in this group of patients the contribution of organogenesis particularly that of the developing central nervous system, to the pathogenesis of disease in HCMV infected infants is not completely understood. As a result, it is sometimes difficult to directly translate the clinical features of congenital HCMV infections and end-organ disease to clinical syndromes observed in other patient populations such as allograft recipients. Lastly, it should be stressed that, in nearly all cases, symptomatic disease following acute HCMV infection is limited to patients with deficits in their immune system and clinical evidence of acute HCMV infection is rarely seen in normal hosts.

In contrast to the obvious role of HCMV in acute infectious syndromes in immunocompromised hosts, the role of this agent in chronic disease syndromes remains controversial even after decades of study. Early studies suggested a role of HCMV in several chronic diseases that are more prevalent in middle-aged and older individuals such as coronary atherosclerosis (Petrie et al., 1988). In addition, epidemiological studies have suggested a link between infection with HCMV and human cancers (Rapp and Robbins, 1984; Shen et al., 1993; Hsieh et al., 1999). More recent studies have provided convincing evidence for a role of HCMV in the accelerated vascular disease that is observed in solid organ allograft recipients, a disease process that may represent the extreme of the spectrum of HCMV-induced vascular disease (Grattan et al., 1989; Melnick et al., 1993; Epstein et al., 1996; Zhu et al., 1999). Recent studies have also demonstrated HCMV nucleic acids and viral proteins in human cancers, providing provocative evidence for a potential role of this virus in malignant behavior of at least some human tumors (Geder et al., 1977; Shen et al., 1993; Cobbs et al., 2002; Harkins et al., 2002). The life-long persistence of the virus in the infected host, the ubiquitous nature of the infection in the population, and the recently recognized disruption of normal host cellular functions suggests that careful investigations into the role of this virus in chronic diseases should remain a major focus of research in diseases associated with HCMV infection.

Acquisition of HCMV: Sources of virus and transmission within populations

Human CMV infection, as defined by serological evidence of previous infection, is ubiquitous in most populations with HCMV seroprevalence ranging from 20%–100% in different regions of the world (Alford et al., 1981; Krech and Tobin, 1981; Gold and Nankervis, 1982). In general, individuals from resource constrained countries have an increased HCMV seroprevalence and studies from sub-Saharan Africa, South America, and India have suggested that by early adulthood nearly 100% of individuals have been infected with HCMV (Alford et al., 1981). In contrast, in well-developed countries in Northern Europe and North America, the seroprevalence can range from 20%–100% in adults. Seroprevalence studies in the United States, Great Britain, Italy, and Scandinavia have provided clues as to routes of virus acquisition and sources of exposure in the community (Weller, 1971). Similarly, careful epidemiological studies aided by genetic analysis of virus isolates have helped define sources of virus infection in young children attending child-care centers, hospitalized patients and hospital staff.

Sources of HCMV in the community

Infectious virus has been recovered from saliva, tears, breast milk, semen, blood products, urine, and cervical secretions. With the exception of blood products, persistent virus infection of epithelial cells in secretory glands remains a constant theme for HCMV infection. Although the phenomena of virus persistence in the salivary glands of small animal models of the HCMV infection have been intensively studied, mechanisms leading persistence of the virus in epithelial cells of apacrine glandular tissue remain incompletely described. Similarly, the question of latency with abortive virus replication vs. a chronic persistent productive infection in these tissues has not been resolved. Studies in animal models and in vitro cell culture system indicate that latent infection can occur, yet these findings have been validated in only limited types of human cells (Jordan and Mar, 1982; Jordan et al., 1982; Kondo et al., 1996; Sinclair and Sissons, 1996; Kurz et al., 1997; Soderberg-Naucler et al., 1997; Hahn et al., 1998; Kurz et al., 1999; Goodrum et al., 2002). Regardless of whether the virus is maintained as a latent infection with periodic reactivation or as a chronic persistent infection yielding low titers of infectivity, the virus readily spreads within a population. Characteristics of HCMV infection such as prolonged virus shedding that may last for over 6 months in some individuals with acute HCMV infection favor spread within susceptible populations. In young infants, HCMV infection acquired in the perinatal period or even during infancy can result in the virus excretion lasting several years (Stagno et al., 1975a,b). Thus, in contrast to periods of communicability for respiratory viruses that are often measured in weeks, acutely infected hosts can remain contagious for months to years after HCMV infection. Although the mechanisms underlying its persistence are far from understood, during its evolution with its human host the virus has developed multiple strategies for persistence in the host and in populations. Persistence in the population has been accomplished without the necessity for a secondary animal reservoir or non-human vectors for transmission.

Although infection with HCMV has been shown to be endemic in all populations studied in the world, transmissibility of the virus has been suggested to be limited based on observations that close contact is required for infection within a population. Even though the efficiency of transmission may be limited either secondary to the liability of the virus or low levels of infectious virus excretion, its persistence favors repeated exposures of susceptible hosts to infectious virus. This is perhaps best illustrated by the finding that in almost all reported studies, acquisition of HCMV serological reactivity increases with age (Alford et al., 1981). In developed countries, primarily Northern Europe and North America, numerous serological studies have been carried out and together with more limited findings in populations from the developing world, have provided some understanding of the sources of HCMV in the community and modes of virus infection. In the developed

Table 41.1. Sources of community-acquired HCMV infections

Source	Infectious fluid	Mode of transmission
Pregnant women	Blood; genital secretions	Blood-borne transmission to Fetus; intrapartum ingestion of infected genital secretions
Lactating women	Breast milk	Ingestion of cell free virus by breast feeding infants
Young children	Saliva; urine	Ingestion
Adolescents/adults	Saliva; genital secretions	Ingestion; sexual contact

Table 41.2. Relationship between age and acquisition of HCMV. Estimated age for >50% seropositivity of population based on published seroprevalence and age

Location	Age at which 50% seropositive
Chile	6 mo–1 yr
Ivory Coast	< 1 yr
Birmingham, Al (low SES)	4–9 yrs
Rochester, NY (high SES)	>28–35 yrs
Tanzania	< 1 yr
India	1 yr
London	> 28–35

From Alford et al., 1981.

world, the variation in the prevalence of HCMV infection has been related to age, child-care practices, sexual activity, and socioeconomic status. These epidemiological associations are consistent with the finding of infectious virus in saliva, tears, breast milk, semen, urine, and cervical secretions (Table 41.1).

Serological evidence of HCMV infection has been used as a measure of exposure to HCMV in different population. Because no specific genetic linkage has been associated with susceptibility or resistance to HCMV infection, it follows that increasing rates of serologic reactivity reflect the relative risk of HCMV exposure of individuals in that population. When HCMV sero-prevalence is compared to age in different populations, it is apparent that near universal seroreactivity in young adults from less developed regions of the world are also associated with early acquisition of HCMV (Table 41.2).

In some parts of the world such as sub-Saharan Africa and southern Asia, nearly 100% of young children are seropositive for HCMV suggesting that exposure to HCMV is universal in these populations (Alford et al., 1981). In contrast, early studies in North America and Northern Europe suggested that between 10–50% of young children were seropositive for HCMV (Alford et al., 1981). Increased rates of serologic evidence of HCMV infection have been noted in children from lower socioeconomic groups in the USA, although these rates do not approach those observed in similarly aged children in the developing world. In addition, increased rates of seropositivity were noted in children from populations in which breast feeding was common and in populations in which group child care was commonly utilized (Weller, 1971). There is no single explanation that accounts for the differences in the age of HCMV acquisition that has been observed in children from Northern Europe and North America and young children from the southern hemisphere. The most frequently offered explanation is that increased rates of infection in Africa and Asia are secondary to near universal breast feeding and possibly to overcrowding in homes with young children (Stagno, 1995a,b). These explanations are consistent at least with observations from child care centers in the USA which have demonstrated an increased rate of virus transmission between children attending child care centers (Pass et al., 1984; CDC, 1985; Hutto et al., 1985; Murph et al., 1986; Adler, 1988; Dobbins et al., 1993). The other component of this explanation is the observed efficient spread of HCMV through breast milk to nursing infants (Stagno et al., 1980; Dworsky et al., 1983a,b; Ahlfors and Ivarsson, 1985; Minamishima et al., 1994; Vochem et al., 1998). Breast milk has been shown to contain significant amounts of infectious virus, much of which is cell free and readily transmitted (Asanuma et al., 1996; Vochem et al., 1998). Studies have documented that over 60% of breast fed infants born to a HCMV infected mother will become infected with HCMV (Stagno et al., 1980; Dworsky et al., 1983). This rate likely underestimates the efficiency of breast milk transmission, particularly in populations in which infants are exclusively breast fed. Because young infants infected following ingestion of infected breast milk excrete significant amounts of virus for extended periods of time, infected infants readily transmit virus to household and community contacts. The rate of breast feeding in countries from the developing world far exceed those in many populations in North America and Northern Europe, particularly when compared to the decreased rates of breast feeding in women from lower socioeconomic groups in the USA. Thus, it is likely that early childhood acquisition of HCMV in populations with high rates of HCMV infection in women of childbearing age can be explained by exposure to virus containing breast milk coupled with crowded living conditions that favor spread of HCMV among young children and other members of the household.

Young children as a source of HCMV

Young children have also been documented to be an important reservoir of infectious virus in the community. Transmission of HCMV between young children appears to be very efficient, presumably because of frequent physical contact, repeated hand-to-mouth contact, and the limited personal hygiene practices of infants and toddlers (Hutto et al., 1986). The initial speculation by Weller that high rates of infection in Swedish children as compared to infants in New York was secondary to the increased use of group child-care centers in Sweden was subsequently confirmed by a number of studies (Weller, 1971). Studies carried out in child-care facilities in the United States have consistently documented increased rates of HCMV infection in young children, particularly those less than 18 months of age (Table 41.2) (Pass et al., 1984; CDC, 1985; Murph et al., 1986; Pass et al., 1987; Adler, 1991a,b). In a study of a group care center that enrolled infants of middle and upper-middle class parents, the seroprevalence in the infants increased from about 10% in the first year of life to over 80% in the second year of life (Pass et al., 1982a,b). Similar results were reported by Adler et al. who also noted that over 50% of initially seronegative infants acquired a day-care related strain of HCMV over a 26-month period as determined by restriction fragment length polymorphism (RFLP) of viral DNA (Adler, 1985). In addition, this study as well as other studies has documented HCMV shedding in 20%–40% young children attending day-care centers (Pass et al., 1987). The ease with which HCMV can be transmitted between young children together with the prolonged duration of virus excretion in infants with congenital and perinatal infections attending child-care centers provides an ideal setting for spread of this virus to young children in group care facilities. Furthermore, infants infected following exposure in child-care centers also excrete significant amounts of virus for extended periods of time, increasing the reservoir of transmissible virus in a group-care setting. Thus, group child-care settings could mimic the exposure of young infants in developing countries in which child-care is often shared among members of the community. The routes of HCMV transmission between children has not been defined but is thought to be primarily through hand-to-mouth contact.

Young children not only readily transmit HCMV to other children but also serve as an important source of HCMV infection of adults (Taber et al., 1985; Pass et al., 1986; Adler, 1988, 1989, 1991; Murph et al., 1991). Early studies utilizing RFLP clearly demonstrated that HCMV could be transmitted from young children to adults (Spector and Spector, 1982; Dworsky et al., 1984). Similarly, several epidemiologic studies related exposure to young children with acquisition of HCMV (Yeager, 1983). These studies have documented increased annualized seroconversion rates in women exposed to young children as compared to women in homes without young children. Later studies included the parents of children attending child-care centers and at least two groups of investigators documented infections in 33%–45% for women whose children were shedding HCMV (Pass et al., 1986; Adler, 1988). Interestingly, the increased rates of virus infection were not limited to the parents of children attending child-care centers but were also noted in workers in child-care centers (Adler, 1989; Pass et al., 1990; Dobbins et al., 1993). An approximate five fold increase in the rate of HCMV infection as measured by seroconversion was noted in one group of women employees at child care centers (Adler, 1989). Analysis by RFLP of DNA from viruses isolated from children in the childcare centers and infected workers revealed similar patterns, suggesting a common source of infection (Adler, 1989). Although it is clear that child-care workers are at risk for acquisition of HCMV secondary to their exposure to young children, an increased risk of HCMV infection has not been demonstrated in hospital workers, including nurses caring for infants with perinatal HCMV infections (Yeager, 1975; Dworsky et al., 1983a,b; Adler et al., 1986; Balfour and Balfour, 1986). These findings argued that with adequate attention to routine hygienic practices, the risk for acquisition of HCMV is no greater for individuals caring for children than that of the general population. Finally, in several prospective natural history studies, maternal HCMV infection and the delivery of a congenitally infected baby have been linked to exposure to young children (Pass et al., 1987; Fowler et al., 1997). Thus, HCMV-infected children are efficient vectors for transmission of the virus to other children and their caretakers because they serve as a reservoir of virus by shedding virus for a prolonged period and because their behavior facilitates virus spread to susceptible contacts.

Acquisition of HCMV by sexual contact

As described above, HCMV infection occurs at an early age in populations in the developing world and virus acquisition through sexual contact is likely of limited importance in primary infection of HCMV in these populations. In contrast, in some populations in North America and northern Europe, a second rapid increase in HCMV seroprevalence has been observed during adolescence, suggesting that virus is acquired through sexual contact. A large number of epidemiological studies have supported the classification of HCMV as a sexually transmitted infection (STI). The associations between sexual activity and HCMV infection are listed in Table 41.3.

Studies of women attending sexually transmitted disease clinics have noted an increase in both HCMV seroprevalence and definitive evidence of HCMV transmission between sexual partners (Jordan *et al.*, 1973; Chandler *et al.*, 1985, 1987; Handsfield *et al.*, 1985; Collier *et al.*, 1990; Coonrod *et al.*, 1998). In addition, it appeared that previously infected individuals could be re-infected by a second strain of virus (see following section) (Handsfield *et al.*, 1985). Other associations between sexual activity and HCMV infection have included: (1) number of sexual partners, (2) number of lifetime sexual partners, and (3) co-infection with other sexually transmitted infections such as trichomonas, gonorrhea, and bacterial vaginosis (Chandler *et al.*, 1985, 1987; Handsfield *et al.*, 1985; Collier *et al.*, 1990; Fowler and Pass, 1991; Sohn *et al.*, 1991; Coonrod *et al.*, 1998). Similarly, in a sexually active male homosexual population it has been reported that over 90% of these men were infected with HCMV (Drew *et al.*, 1981; Drew and Mintz, 1984).

The association between HCMV infection and sexual activity is consistent with the shedding of this virus in the genitourinary tract. Both cervical secretions and vaginal fluid are frequent sites of virus recovery in populations of younger women (Reynolds *et al.*, 1973; Stagno *et al.*, 1975a,b; Waner *et al.*, 1977; Collier *et al.*, 1995; Coonrod *et al.*, 1998). Semen has been reported to be a rich source of virus and quantitation of viral DNA in semen has been used to monitor the in vivo response to antiviral drugs in clinical studies (Lang and Kummer, 1975; Drew and Mintz, 1984 ; Rinaldo *et al.*, 1992; Yang *et al.*, 1995; Liesnard *et al.*, 1998; Diamond *et al.*, 2000). The frequency with which HCMV can be isolated from the female genital tract varies between populations and interestingly, with the age of the woman (Collier *et al.*, 1995; Coonrod *et al.*, 1998). In some studies virus could be recovered from the genital tract of over 50% of women attending a STD clinic, whereas the rate of recovery from HCMV infected women in the post partum period were significantly lower (Pass *et al.*, 1982a,b). Thus, it is unclear if the increased rates of recovery of HCMV from women attending an STD clinic reflect increased shedding from a previous chronic infection or repeated re-infections. A second interesting observation is that age appears to influence the frequency of HCMV shedding in the genital tract of women such that young women infected with HCMV are more likely to shed virus from the genital tract as compared to older women (Fowler *et al.*, 1993; Collier *et al.*, 1995; Coonrod *et al.*, 1998). However, the relationship between risk of re-exposure to HCMV through sexual contact in these two populations and rates of genital shedding

Table 41.3. Representative studies that have associated HCMV infection with sexually transmitted infections

Population	Evidence of sexual transmission
Sexually active male homosexuals	Increased seroprevalence (> 90% +) as compared to general population (Drew *et al.*, 1981).
Women attending STD clinic	Increased seroprevalence; increased rate of cervical shedding; increased rates of seroconversion (Chandler *et al.*, 1985; Handsfield *et al.*, 1985; Collier *et al.*, 1990; Coonrod *et al.*, 1998).
Young women	HCMV infection associated with STIs including bacterial vaginosis, trichomonas and gonorrhea (Chandler *et al.*, 1985; Fowler and Pass, 1991; Sohn *et al.*, 1991)
Young women	Increased rates of HCMV seroconversion correlated with increased number of sexual partners (Collier *et al.*, 1990; Fowler and Pass, 1991)

of virus remains inadequately defined. Alternatively, it has been argued that primary HCMV infection leads to more prolonged shedding of virus and the more frequent recovery of virus from the genital tract of younger women could reflect the natural history of a resolving primary infection. These two possible explanations have not been reconciled.

Sources of HCMV in hospitalized patients and health-care workers

Some of the earliest reports of the clinical syndromes associated with HCMV infection described patients infected with HCMV by nosocomial routes. Several routes of nosocomial transmission have been described but the three most frequently routes of transmission include: (1) allograft transplantation, (2) blood products, and (3) breast milk. Transfusion associated HCMV infection was recognized in cardiac surgery patients who in the past often required significant quantities of blood as a result of cardiac bypass procedures. A syndrome of fever, atypical lymphocytosis, elevated liver transaminases, and splenomegaly was associated with these procedures and the phrase post-perfusion syndrome or post-perfusion mononucleosis was coined (Holsward *et al.*, 1963; Reyman, 1966; Paloheimo *et al.*, 1968). Subsequent studies revealed that HCMV infection could be related to up 50% of these cases and it was argued that HCMV was transmitted by blood products utilized in these procedures (Prince *et al.*, 1971). From a series of studies in seronegative patients receiving blood products it was estimated that risk of acquiring HCMV infection was about 2.5% per unit of blood transfusion (Stevens *et al.*, 1970; Armstrong *et al.*, 1976; Bowden, 1995). Because the total amount of blood products also correlated with the risk of acquiring HCMV, patient populations requiring large amounts of blood and blood products secondary to their underlying disease or complications of therapy were at increased risk for HCMV infection. In addition, the type of blood product transfused also influenced risk for transmission of HCMV. Studies in allograft recipients revealed that blood products that contain white blood cells or platelets were more likely to transmit HCMV to the recipient. As a result, several modifications were introduced to limit white blood cell contamination of blood, including the use of filters that can remove white blood cells from red blood cell transfusions and the use of frozen red blood cell preparations (Brady et al., 1984; Bowden et al., 1991; Ljungman et al., 2002a,b). Both approaches have been shown to reduce the incidence of transfusion acquired HCMV infection. The second approach involved screening blood donors and selecting those without serological evidence of past HCMV infection. This approach has proven successful in reducing the incidence of HCMV infection in transfusion recipients, particularly in bone marrow allograft recipients (Bowden et al., 1991; Bowden, 1995). However, two limitations have become apparent. The first is that in some donor populations over 50% of patients have serological evidence of HCMV infection, thus restricting the donor population and limiting the availability of blood products. The second more recent observation is that perhaps up to 15% of donors without serological evidence of HCMV infection can be shown to have evidence of previous HCMV infection when analyzed by more sensitive techniques such as PCR (Roback et al., 2001; Drew et al., 2003). The interpretation of this interesting finding is not straightforward as it is unclear what proportion of blood products from these serologically negative, PCR positive donors transmitted HCMV to recipients.

HCMV infections resulting from transfusions of blood products have also been shown to cause significant disease in newborn infants, particularly premature infants and infants born to women without serological immunity to HCMV (Yeager et al., 1981; Adler, 1983; Adler et al., 1983). Because extremely premature infants, regardless of their mothers' HCMV serologic status, are delivered prior to significant transplacental transfer of maternal antibodies, they often lack passively acquired antibody immunity to HCMV. Thus, these infants are at risk for severe HCMV infections. Perhaps one of the more interesting findings from these studies of nosocomial infections in premature infants was that passively acquired anti-HCMV antibodies provided some protective immunity. In a prospective study, infected infants with antiviral antibodies exhibited a milder disease than infected infants without passively acquired anti-HCMV antibodies and appeared to be protected from severe HCMV infections and in some cases, death (Yeager et al., 1981). This observation also provided one of the most compelling arguments for a role of antiviral antibodies in host protective responses to HCMV that limit disease.

Breast milk transmission of HCMV is well described (see above) and infection of extremely premature infants as a result of ingestion of infected breast milk can be associated with severe disease (Vochem et al., 1998). The finding that breast milk transmitted HCMV could result in significant disease in young infants defined an additional risk in the use of banked breast milk as nutritional support for premature infants. The lack of antiviral antibodies in premature infants was associated with symptomatic infection following breast milk acquisition of HCMV similar to infections associated with transfusions. Even though breast milk from HCMV seropositive women contains virus neutralizing antibodies of both the IgG and IgA isotypes, virus can be readily transmitted to infants. This finding suggests that antiviral antibodies cannot prevent virus transmission even if present in the inoculum.

Transmission of HCMV by transplantation of an allograft from donor previously infected with HCMV represents a major clinical problem in allograft transplantation. Human cytomegalovirus is the most common cause of infection in the post transplant period and the transplanted allograft represents the most important source of HCMV infection in allograft recipients (Peterson et al., 1980; Rubin 1990; Rubin and Colvin, 1986, Griffiths et al., 2000; Ljungman, 2002; Ljungman et al., 2002a,b). It is estimated up to 90% of allograft recipients who have received an allograft from a HCMV infected donor will become infected with HCMV; however, it is likely that all recipients of allografts from HCMV infected donors will become infected with HCMV present in the donor allograft, regardless of their serological status prior to transplantation. Although prior experience with HCMV either as the result of natural infection or live virus vaccines has been shown to provide some protection from severe infection and end-organ disease, pre-existing immunity does not prevent infection (Plotkin et al., 1991). Viral nucleic acids have been detected in the kidneys from HCMV infected donors indicating that the transplanted organ can serve as a source of virus in transplanted allografts (Gnann et al., 1988). In addition, bone marrow allografts from HCMV seropositive donors readily transmit HCMV to recipients, a finding consistent with the demonstration that the cells of macrophage/monocyte lineage can harbor latent HCMV (Soderberg-Naucler et al., 1997). Reactivation of latent HCMV from macrophages derived from HCMV seropositive donors has been demonstrated in-vitro, providing an explanation for the transmission of HCMV from both hematopoietic allografts as well as solid organs that almost certainly contain contaminating macrophages (Soderberg-Naucler et al., 1997). Together with transfusion acquired

HCMV infection, infection in allograft recipients from the virus in allograft represent the most common mode of nosocomial transmission of HCMV.

Transmission of HCMV from patients shedding HCMV to health-care workers is exceedingly rare. Shedding of significant titers of infectious virus is usually limited to hospitalized infants and young children and studies have shown that nurses exposed to these infected infans are no more likely to become infected with HCMV than control populations in the community (Dworsky *et al.*, 1983; Adler *et al.*, 1986; Demmler *et al.*, 1987). In the case of adults, HCMV shedding in hospitalized patients is usually only observed in severely immunocompromised patients such as allograft recipients and patients with AIDS. With the implementation of universal precautions in the care of hospitalized patients, the risk of nosocomial transmission of HCMV to a healthcare worker is almost certainly lower than the risk of community acquisition of this virus.

Reinfection: acquisition of HCMV by a previously infected host

Superinfection or reinfection of previously infected immunocompromised allograft recipients has been well described (Chou, 1986, 1987; Grundy *et al.*, 1988). In addition, numerous studies in patients infected with HIV demonstrated multiple infections with HCMV and in some patients, several genetically distinct strains of HCMV could be detected simultaneously (Drew *et al.*, 1984; Spector *et al.*, 1984; Chern *et al.*, 1998). These studies provided evidence that pre-existing immunity to HCMV, both antiviral antibodies and HCMV-specific cellular immune responses, failed to prevent infection with an unrelated strain of HCMV. Anecdotal reports have suggested that normal seropositive individuals could be superinfected with new strains of HCMV; however, it was argued that reinfections were only common in immunocompromised hosts. A study of vaccine immunity following inoculation with a candidate replicating virus vaccine demonstrated that individuals infected with the vaccine strain of HCMV could be reinfected with a challenge strain of HCMV (Plotkin *et al.*, 1989). A more recent study also demonstrated that normal women infected with a vaccine strain of HCMV could be reinfected following natural exposure to young children shedding HCMV (Adler *et al.*, 1995). These studies provided definitive evidence that prior infection in a normal host could not prevent a second infection (Table 41.4). In this latter report, the authors speculated that reinfection resulted from a failure of the vaccine to induce immunity that was similar to that following natural infection with a wild type strain of HCMV (Adler *et al.*, 1995).

Table 41.4. Infection in normal hosts with preexisting immunity to HCMV. Studies demonstrating the acquisition of a second strain of HCMV in a previously infected host

Population	Evidence of reinfection
Vaccine recipients	Clinical symptoms with virus challenge; virus excretion with virus challenge (Plotkin *et al.*, 1989).
Vaccine recipients	serologic boost in previously infected host following community acquired infection; recovery of non-vaccine strain of virus in recipients of live virus vaccine (Adler *et al.*, 1995)
Infants in day care	recovery of genetically distinct viruses over time from infants in day care center (Bale *et al.*, 1996)
Women with congenitally infected infants	serological evidence of acquisition of new gentoype in women with prior HCMV infection; delivery of infected infant following reinfection (Boppana *et al.*, 2001a,b)
experimental animals	serologic and virologic evidence of reinfection in both wild and captive mouse populations; reinfection in captive non-human primates (Moro *et al.*, 1999)

More recent findings in adults as well studies in young children have demonstrated that individuals with prior HCMV immunity can be readily reinfected with a second (or possibly third, fourth, etc.) strain of HCMV as a result of natural exposure. The spread of HCMV in young children attending a child care facility clearly demonstrated that previously infected young children could be reinfected with a second strain of HCMV (Bale *et al.*, 1996). More recently, reinfection of normal women by a genetically unrelated strain of HCMV was studied utilizing an antigenic polymorphism in glycoprotein H that allowed the detection of reinfection by serologic reactivity (Boppana *et al.*, 2001a,b). In this study, reinfection of women previously infected with HCMV with a new viral strain that encoded a unique serologic determinant was shown to occur in nearly 30% of women enrolled in the study (Boppana *et al.*, 2001a,b). Interestingly, reinfection in this population was associated with intrauterine transmission of HCMV during subsequent pregnancies and damaging congenital infection was observed in three infants infected in utero as a result of maternal reinfection (Boppana *et al.*, 2001a,b). Subsequent studies in this same population have indicated that approximately 12% of women are reinfected with a second virus strain each year. It is important to note that the serologic methods utilized in this study likely underestimates the frequency of reinfection because only two antigenic variants could be detected (Boppana *et al.*, 2001a,b). Because of this limitation, it is highly likely that women in this population are frequently reinfected with genetically different strains of HCMV. In view of the reported case of recombination between strains of HCMV, some individuals may harbor HCMV of significant genetic diversity, perhaps approaching a so-called swarm of viruses.

The importance of reinfection as a source of HCMV in a population is unclear but the ease with which HCMV can spread within populations and the apparent lack of protective immunity suggests that reinfection with new strains of HCMV are common in all populations and dependent only on the risk of exposure to infectious virus. In experimental animal model systems reinfection has been documented, including in the rhesus macaques (personal communication, J. Nelson, Oregon Health Sciences University, Portland, Or.) and mice. The spread of murine CMV in wild mice has been documented and multiple genetically unique strains of viruses have been found in a single mouse, indicating that multiple infections also occur in normal mice (Moro et al., 1999). Thus, when the spread of HCMV in populations is defined it is critical to include not only seronegative individuals, a group previously viewed to be the sentinel for HCMV spread in a population, but also seropositive individuals as both populations can be readily infected with HCMV. The design and strategy for vaccine control of HCMV must keep these possibilities in mind.

Entry and spread within susceptible hosts

Infection following community exposure

Infection with HCMV following community exposure presumably occurs as a result of exposure of mucosal surfaces of the upper respiratory tract or the genital tract to infectious HCMV. Although the cellular target of HCMV infection remains incompletely defined, the widespread expression of putative cell surface receptors including, proteoglycans, integrins, and epidermal growth factor receptor, suggest that the tropism of virus is not limited to specific cell types on the mucosal surface. Presumably virus attaches and enters susceptible epithelial cells and undergoes lytic replication. Following the release of progeny virions, adjacent cells including non-epithelial cells of the underlying submucosa are infected. This earliest phase of cytomegalovirus infection has not been well studied in humans or experimental animal models and the pathway of infection and local amplification that is postulated is based on modes of virus exposure that lead to infection. The steps following local amplification leading to disseminated spread of virus to the liver and spleen and eventually to sites of persistence are essentially unknown in humans. Studies in experimental animals including mice and primates have demonstrated that infection of the oral mucosa leads to dissemination and widespread infection of organs such as the liver and spleen (Kern, 1999; Lockridge et al., 1999). In a primate model of HCMV infection, Lockridge et al. observed that both intravenous and oral inoculation of rhesus macaques with rhesus CMV led to dissemination and widespread viral infection in a variety of organs (Lockridge et al., 1999). Perhaps the most surprising observation made in this study was that oral inoculation lead to virus dissemination and infection of liver and spleen as efficiently as intravenous inoculation of equivalent amounts of infectious virus (Lockridge et al., 1999). However, the kinetics of virus spread for the intravenously inoculated animals was accelerated as compared to the orally infected animals (Lockridge et al., 1999). Because peak of viremia was not detected until approximately 1 week later in the animal inoculated by mucosal exposure as compared to those given virus intravenously, it could be argued that following mucosal exposure, the virus undergoes a local amplification and then spread to secondary sites of infection such as the liver and spleen and regional lymph nodes (Lockridge et al., 1999). Studies in other experimental models such as mice and guinea pigs are consistent with this mode of spread in the host (Bernstein and Bourne, 1999; Kern, 1999). Thus, it appears that HCMV infection could follow a similar pathway of infection and spread as has been described for varicella-zoster virus (Grose, 1994). After mucosal infection with HCMV there is local amplification, an initial viremia that leads to infection of visceral structures such as the liver and spleen. Infection of these organs is then followed by a secondary viremia that leads to a more generalized infection. From studies in experimental animals and transfusion acquired HCMV infections, it is clear that the magnitude of the inoculum, the kinetics of virus replication at the primary site, and the host derived innate responses can influence the kinetics, duration, and magnitude of the virus replication/spread. Although the oral exposure of animals leads to widespread virus dissemination and infection of a similar spectrum of tissues, animals remained asymptomatic following oral inoculation and also did not demonstrate abnormalities in hematologic parameters that have been associated with HCMV infection (Lockridge et al., 1999). In contrast, animals inoculated intravenously developed a mononucleosis syndrome that was associated with monocytosis, thrombocytopenia, and leukocytosis (Lockridge et al., 1999). These observations parallel clinical observations in human subjects infected inadvertently by blood transfusion or transplantation of an infected allograft. Because intravenous (or by an allograft) inoculation allows direct access to the circulatory system, there is likely no requirement for virus amplification in local tissue prior to spread to visceral organs and regional lymphoid tissue. Thus, the virus can replicate to higher titers earlier in the course of the infection and presumably overwhelm the host innate immune responses. Clinical disease following acute CMV infection has been correlated with increased levels of replicating virus in humans as well as in experimental animal models of HCMV disease (Cope *et al.*, 1997; Spector *et al.*, 1998; Bernstein and Bourne, 1999; Kern, 1999; Emery *et al.*, 2000; Sequar *et al.*, 2002).

Following amplification in regional lymphoid tissue and the spleen and liver, dissemination of infectious virus results in the infection of sites that have been postulated to support persistent infection *in-vivo* and include salivary gland and breast secretory epithelium, prostatic epithelium, endometrium, and renal tubule epithelium (Becroft, 1981; Borisch *et al.*, 1988; Bale *et al.*, 1989; Sinzger *et al.*, 1995). Based on studies in experimental animal models and the findings that bone marrow and lung allografts can transmit infection, other sites such as the bone marrow and lung are also infected (Myerson *et al.*, 1984; Balthesen *et al.*, 1993; Kurz *et al.*, 1997; Salzberger *et al.*, 1997). The sites of long-term persistence, be it chronic productive infection or true latency, in humans are thought to include epithelium within exocrine glands, macrophage/monocytic cells, and hematopoietic stem cells. Pivotal aspects of the earliest phases of acute HCMV infection and dissemination remain inadequately studied. As an example, local amplification of virus following mucosal exposure has been postulated based on the kinetics of virus replication in the liver and spleen, yet there is little experimental evidence supporting this proposed mechanism. Alternatively, the virus could be transported to the regional lymph nodes, liver and spleen by circulating leucocytes prior to significant amplification in local tissue. The cell types that support local amplification are unknown and interactions between these cells and the innate immune system are not well described. The local host innate immune responses to naturally acquired HCMV infection could play a key role in the ultimate outcome of the infection, *i.e.* the level of virus replication and subsequent spread to the distant sites of infection. In contrast to the well documented role of the adaptive immune responses such as cytotoxic T lymphocytes and antiviral antibodies in the control and resolution of CMV infections, the importance of early innate responses at the site of inoculation to the course of infection with this virus remain poorly understood.

Transfusion and allograft-acquired infection

Infection with HCMV that follows exposure to blood products or an allograft more often resembles the symptomatic mononucleosis like syndrome that occurs in a minority of individuals who acquire HCMV by community exposure (Foster and Jack, 1969; Bowden, 1995). Presumably, development of symptomatic infection results from either the exposure to a large inoculum, delivery of infectious virus directly into the circulatory system, or by a combination of the two. In addition, allograft recipients as well as some recipients of blood products are often immunocompromised. Thus, the increase in HCMV burden is generally accelerated and the duration of active viral replication is increased secondary to the lack of normal immune responses to this virus. Clinical characteristics of this syndrome include fever, hematological abnormalities including leukocytosis often with monocytosis, and evidence of hepatocellular damage. Some patients will develop splenic enlargement and lymphadenopathy. Similar findings have been noted in animal models of acute HCMV infection (Bernstein and Bourne, 1999; Kern, 1999; Lockridge *et al.*, 1999). During peak virus replication, HCMV disseminates to end organs and sites of persistence as described above. Resolution of active virus replication is associated with control of clinical disease but virus excretion can continue for extended periods of time.

A consistent feature of HCMV infection in allograft recipients is the temporal sequence associated with virus replication and disease. In solid organ allograft recipients such as renal transplant recipients, virus replication and clinical symptoms are commonly observed several weeks following transplantation (Rubin and Colvin, 1986; Singh *et al.*, 1988; Rubin, 2002). The seemingly prolonged interval between transplantation and expression of an acute disease syndrome remains unexplained based on an expectation that virus reactivation/replication begins shortly after transplantation. It is possible that only vanishing amounts of virus are present in the allograft and replication of sufficient amounts of virus to induce disease requires this time interval. Consistent with this speculation is the finding that the virus burden in the blood closely parallels the development of disease in these patients and has been shown to increase exponentially in the time period preceding the development of disease (Cope *et al.*, 1997; Mendez *et al.*, 1998; Emery *et al.*, 2000; Nichols *et al.*, 2001). In contrast, disease in bone marrow allograft patients characteristically developed around 60 days post-transplantation and, based on these early studies in bone marrow allograft recipients, it was subsequently shown that detection of HCMV around day 35 post transplant in patients without clinical symptoms could be successfully treated with antiviral agents (Myers *et al.*, 1975; Schmidt *et al.*, 1991; Boeckh and Bowden, 1995; Boeckh *et al.*, 1997; Boeckh and Boivin, 1998; Nichols *et al.*, 2001). This finding is in agreement with the general time frame of HCMV replication in solid organ transplant recipients and again suggests that HCMV must first establish a productive infection and amplify its genome copy number prior to dissemination to distant sites. Studies with murine CMV and immunocompromised mice have documented the importance of virus dissemination in the development of disease following reactivation of virus (Jonjic et al., 1994; Reddehase et al., 1994).

Spread within the host

Cell-associated spread within the host

Although it is has been suggested that cell free virus is responsible for community acquired HCMV infection, only limited data supports this claim. Perhaps the most convincing evidence comes from studies in breast feeding women that have demonstrated that infectious virus is present in the cell-free fraction of breast milk (Hamprecht et al., 1998). This finding suggests that cell free virus can infect a mucosal surface. Animal models of CMV infection have utilized either intraperitoneal or subcutaneous inoculations almost exclusively; however oral inoculation with cell free murine CMV has been accomplished (personal communication, S. Jonjic, University of Rijeka, Rijeka, Croatia). In contrast to initial infection, the spread of HCMV within an infected host is likely to be cell associated based on findings from immuncompromised patients and studies in experimental animal models. In all but the most severely immunocompromised patients, infectivity that can be demonstrated in the blood compartment is most frequently associated with peripheral blood leukocytes and endothelial cells (Percivalle et al., 1993; Waldman et al., 1995; Salzberger et al., 1997; Gerna et al., 1998; Pooley et al., 1999; Maidji et al., 2002). The highest titers of infectious virus have been found associated with polymorphonuclear leukocytes from the buffy coat fraction of peripheral blood (Gerna et al., 1992; Schafer et al., 2000; Liapis et al., 2003). Polymorphonuclear leukocytes cannot support virus replication but have been shown to carry infectious virus and viral gene products (Gerna et al., 2000; Kas-Deelen et al., 2001). In a series of in vitro experiments, Gerna and colleagues have demonstrated that HCMV infected endothelial cells or fibroblasts can transfer infectious virus to PMNs and in turn, these cells can transmit virus to susceptible fibroblasts (Gerna et al., 2000). These studies have argued that microfusion events between virus containing vesicles and PMN are responsible for transmission of virus between cells (Gerna et al., 2000). Although such a mechanism has not been experimentally verified in animal models of HCMV infection, the role of PMN in transmission of infectious HCMV in vivo is well accepted and the correlation between HCMV antigen positive PMN (antigenemia assay) and disseminated infection has been repeatedly shown to be a reliable diagnostic tool for the identification of patients at risk for invasive infection with HCMV (van der Bij et al., 1988; The et al., 1990; Gerna et al., 1991; Erice et al., 1992; Landry and Ferguson, 1993; Boeckh et al., 1996; Nichols and Boeckh, 2000; Singh et al., 2000). Interestingly, antigen positive PMN can be detected in normal hosts infected with HCMV but with a drastically reduced frequency as compared to immunocompromised patients, suggesting that even in normal hosts that PMN may be a common mode of virus dissemination. Other cells within the leukocyte fraction of peripheral blood cells support HCMV persistence and also transmit infectious virus. These include monocyte and macrophages derived by differentiation of blood monocytes (Rice et al., 1984; Taylor-Wiedeman et al., 1991; Fish et al., 1995; Waldman et al., 1995; Sinclair and Sissons, 1996; Guetta et al., 1997; Soderberg-Naucler et al., 1998; Hanson et al., 1999; Jahn et al., 1999; Riegler et al., 2000). Cells derived from granulocyte/monocyte progenitor cells have been proposed as sites of latency based on in-vitro infections and can be detected as antigen containing cells in immunocompromised patients with disseminated HCMV infection (Taylor-Wiedeman et al., 1991; Fish et al., 1995; Kondo et al., 1996; Sinclair and Sissons, 1996; Soderberg-Naucler et al., 1997; Hahn et al., 1998). In contrast, macrophages derived from peripheral blood of monocytes have been shown to harbor infectious HCMV upon stimulation with specific cytokines, including TNF-α (Taylor-Wiedeman et al., 1994; Hummel et al., 2001; Soderberg-Naucler et al., 2001). Viral replication and expression of a variety of early and late proteins can be demonstrated in macrophages following infection with HCMV, although only recently derived clinical viral isolates efficiently infect these cells. This latter observation has been made independently by numerous laboratories and will be discussed in more detail in subsequent sections of this volume. The findings that individual strains of virus exhibited different biological behaviors in tissue culture have confirmed several observations that were first noted in the earliest in vitro studies of HCMV. Current studies are directed at deciphering the viral genes that account for these in-vitro phenotypes and may yield important new findings to help define the pathogenesis of HCMV infections.

A second cell lineage that is critical to the in-vivo spread of HCMV is the endothelial cell in a variety of microvascular beds in the human host. Endothelial cells have long been known to be a target for HCMV replication in vitro and infection of these cells results in a variety of cellular responses, including the release of cytokines and chemokines (Waldman et al., 1991; Sinzger et al., 1995,

1997; Waldman et al., 1995; Plachter et al., 1996; Fish et al., 1998; Gerna et al., 1998; Evans et al., 1999; Kas-Deelen et al., 2000; Brune et al., 2001a,b; Maidji et al., 2002; Odeberg et al., 2002). Both lytic and non-lytic productive infections have been described in endothelial cells suggesting that depending on the source of cells and the infecting virus, endothelial cells can respond very differently to infection (Sinzger et al., 1997, 2000; Fish et al., 1998; Kahl et al., 2000). Virus infection of endothelial cells is thought to be critical for infection of various tissues during HCMV dissemination and likewise, endothelial cell infection and virus release appears to be critical for the hematogenous spread from infected tissue (Waldman et al., 1995; Gerna et al., 2000; Maidji et al., 2002). Early studies in transplant populations described viral antigen containing cells circulating in the blood of viremic transplant patients that subsequently were shown to be infected endothelial cells (Grefte et al., 1993; Percivalle et al., 1993; Gerna et al., 1998). These cells contain infectious virus and are thought to represent infected endothelium that sloughs into the circulation, presumably secondary to local infection and/or inflammation. These cells are usually detected only in the most immunocompromised patients but these observations serve to illustrate that HCMV infection in these patients can be associated with an endothelitis that likely seeds the blood compartment with infectious virus containing cells. A similar role for endothelial cells in spread of CMV in both the murine model and guinea pig CMV model is assumed but has not been adequately explored (Brune et al., 2001a,b).

Viral genes associated with virulence: viral dissemination and in vivo tropism

The large coding capacity of the HCMV genome in comparison to other herpes viruses has raised the possibility that a sizable number of these genes may encode functions that facilitate efficient in vivo replication, spread and persistence. This indeed appears to be the case as genetic comparisons between commonly used laboratory viruses and recent clinical isolates have demonstrated that laboratory isolates have large scale deletions yet replicate in vitro to levels that often exceed those of clinical isolates (Cha et al., 1996). Studies utilizing laboratory isolates and recent clinical isolates have dramatic differences in tropism when cell types other than permissive human fibroblasts are used for in vitro propagation (Waldman et al., 1991; Fish et al., 1998; Soderberg-Naucler et al., 1998; Jarvis et al., 1999; Sinzger et al., 1999, 2000; Bolovan-Fritts and Wiedeman, 2001; Brune et al., 2001a,b; Gerna et al., 2002). It is also almost certain that the phenotype of some viral genes that contribute to growth and persistence can only be defined in vivo and therefore will be extremely difficult to dissect in vitro. Studies in experimental animals, particularly the mouse have been quite revealing and point to the importance of viral genes in the initial replication and spread of CMVs. In studies investigating the spread of murine CMV from the site of inoculation to distant sites, infection has been was shown to be primarily associated with peripheral blood mononuclear cells. In these models the importance of an initial viremic spread to the liver and spleen was demonstrated and the role of peripheral blood mononuclear cell spread of virus to sites of persistence such as salivary glands was carefully documented (Bale and O'Neil, 1989; Collins et al., 1994; Stoddart et al., 1994; Mitchell et al., 1996; Hanson et al., 1999; Kern, 1999; Reddehase et al., 2002). More recently, several reports have demonstrated the importance of individual viral genes in a murine model of CMV pathogenesis. At least three viral genes encoded by m139, 140, 141 orfs of MCMV have been shown to play a critical role in viral replication in monocyte/macrophages but have little to no effects on the replication of the virus in mouse fibroblasts (Saederup et al., 1999; Hanson et al., 2001; Saederup et al., 2001; Menard et al., 2003). The finding that viruses in which these genes have been deleted exhibit limited spread in vivo following intraperitoneal inoculation illustrates a potential role for these orfs in the in vivo pathogenesis of murine CMV (Saederup et al., 2001; Mocarski, 2002). To date, the mechanism that accounts for restricted replication in monocytes of MCMV with deletions in these orf is unknown. The HCMV gene(s) that permit replication in monocyte/macrophages has not been definitively identified. Although it is far from clear if the observed expanded tropism of some strains of HCMV is required for the spread of HCMV in the infected host, the conservation of this phenotype amongst low passage clinical isolates and the subsequent loss of this phenotype upon passage in tissue culture would argue that monocyte/macrophage tropism contributes to the spread of the virus in the infected host. Genetic analysis of murine CMV indicated that endothelial cell tropism can be linked to a single viral gene, M45, the viral encoded ribonucleotide reductase and may be associated with resistance of endothelial cells to murine CMV induced apoptosis (Brune et al., 2001a,b). The deletion of the homologous reading frame in HCMV was not associated with the loss of endothelial tropism (Hahn et al., 2002). More recently, the importance of the VL129–131 of HCMV in endothelial tropism and presumably replication in vivo has been demonstrated by several laboratories (Hahn et al., 2004; Wang and Shenk, 2005a,b). Thus, the viral genes and the mechanism by which products of the viral genes contribute to the expanded tropism of some clinical viral isolates of HCMV remain poorly understood.

Human cytomegalovirus encodes three G coupled protein receptor (GPCR) like molecules in orfs UL33, UL78,

US 27 and US28 (Margulies et al., 1996; Streblow et al., 1999; Rosenkilde et al., 2001; Beisser et al., 2002). The most extensively studied is US28, a GPCR that is constitutively activated and more importantly, can also signal after interaction with chemokines including RANTES, MCP-1, and fractalkine (Bodaghi et al., 1998; Streblow et al., 1999; Billstrom Schroeder and Worthen, 2001). Several laboratories have reported possible roles for this molecule in the spread of HCMV in vivo including, (i) acting as a chemokine sink to limit host cell chemotaxis to HCMV infected cells, (ii) providing an anti-apoptotic function, (iii) the recruitment of infected mononuclear cells to the sites of inflammation leading to dissemination of virus and (iv) perhaps even by binding of virus or virus infected cells to chemokine expressing endothelial cells based on observations of US28 binding membrane bound fractalkine (Bodaghi et al., 1998; Kledal et al., 1998; Billstrom Schroeder and Worthen, 2001; Beisser et al., 2002; Billstrom Schroeder et al., 2002; Randolph-Habecker et al., 2002). In addition, infected smooth muscle cells expression US28 have been shown to migrate down chemokine gradients, thus providing an additional mechanism for the localization of HCMV infected cells to sites containing inflammatory cellular infiltrates (Streblow et al., 1999). Although the role of US28 in HCMV induced vascular disease has been well studied and supported by in vitro models of smooth muscle cell migration, the importance of US28 in virus dissemination from local site of infection remains unclear. In murine CMV, two GPCR like gene products have been identified, M33 and M78 (Davis-Poynter et al., 1997; Oliveira and Shenk, 2001; Waldhoer et al., 2002). Studies have suggested that M33 is required for efficient virus dissemination to the salivary glands, a finding consistent with a potential role of US28 in the spread of HCMV (Davis-Poynter et al., 1997). Recently, the US28 homologue of rhesus CMV has been identified (Penfold et al., 2003). The phenotype of the M78 deletion virus suggests that the gene product of this orf is important in the replication of murine CMV in both monocytes/macrophages in vitro and in vivo (Oliveira and Shenk, 2001).

Another viral gene that appears to influence the spread of HCMV in vivo is UL146 (Penfold et al., 1999). The protein encoded by this orf is a secreted protein that appears to function as a CXCL chemokine (v-CXCL1) that can induce chemotaxis and degranulation of PMNs (Penfold et al., 1999). Interestingly this orf exhibits considerable sequence variability but maintains an amino terminal motif defining it as a CXCL chemokine (Penfold et al., 1999). It is thought that this viral chemokine can recruit PMNs in vivo and thus could serve to disseminate HCMV from sites of infection. In severely immunocompromised hosts such as AIDs patients with gastrointestinal and retinal disease secondary to disseminated HCMV infection, neutrophil infiltration can be observed in the lamina propria as well as in the retina (Pepose et al., 1985; Jacobson et al., 1988; Francis et al., 1989; Wilcox et al., 1998). Infection of lamina propria macrophages with HCMV in vitro results in the induction of IL-8 release from these cells, suggesting that HCMV can both induce IL-8 release and encode a viral IL-8 like molecule (Redman et al., 2002). Such findings are consistent with the proposed mechanism of chemokine expression and HCMV dissemination from sites of virus replication. Although this mechanism of dissemination is consistent with the histopathologic findings noted in severely immunocompromised patients, a neutrophil infiltrate is not an invariant feature of the histopathology of naturally acquired HCMV infections suggesting that interactions between this viral chemokine and other peripheral blood leukocytes that express its cognate cell surface receptor, CXCR2, also is required for virus dissemination. Alternatively, the recent findings that HCMV engages Toll-like receptors with resultant induction of pro-inflammatory cytokines and chemokines cascades suggests that the virus infection alone can recruit cells such as monocytes and PMN to sites of infection without the requirement of a specific viral chemokine (Compton et al., 2003). Regardless of the specific mechanism and the role of a viral chemokine such as that encoded by orf 146, the intimate relationship between HCMV and components of the host inflammatory response likely represents a key step in the dissemination of HCMV.

As noted previously, studies in the murine model of CMV infection have provided data consistent with cell-associated virus spread (Bale and O'Neil, 1989; Collins et al., 1994; Stoddart et al., 1994; Mitchell et al., 1996). Murine CMV encodes a related chemokine (orf m131), MCK-1, that initially was reported to function as a chemoattractant for monocyte/macrophages (Fleming et al., 1999; Saederup et al., 2001; Saederup and Mocarski, 2002). MCK-1 has been shown to induce calcium signaling and adherence of macrophages suggesting that it was a functional chemokine (Saederup et al., 1999). In addition, these investigators suggested that its cellular receptor was the chemokine receptor, CCR3 (Saederup et al., 1999). Later studies demonstrated that the major transcript and virus-expressed product of orf 131 was actually a spliced product in which the 5' end of the 131 ORF was fused with the entire 129 orf to generate a spliced gene termed MCK-2 (MacDonald et al., 1999). The protein product of MCK-2 shares a common chemokine domain encoded by m131 and thus is assumed to have similar activity as a chemokine (Mocarski, 2002). Perhaps the most interesting findings from this series of studies was that expression of the MCK-2 protein is non-essential for growth in fibroblasts in vitro, but virus with deletions in this viral gene have a remarkable phenotype in vivo. The deletion of MCK-2 results in virus that cannot disseminate from local sites of infection and fails to disseminate in blood monocytes (Saederup et al., 2001; Noda et al., 2006). Histopathological studies demonstrated that the MCK-2 deletion virus did not induce the same degree of tissue inflammation and cellular (PMN) infiltrate as the wild type virus suggesting that this virus encoded chemokine facilitated spread from local sites of infection to distant sites of virus replication, presumably by recruiting monocytes and PMN to the initial sites of virus replication (Saederup et al., 2001). Infection of these cells would then allow blood-borne dissemination of virus as infected leukocytes. This mechanism together with recent findings that envelope glycoproteins of HCMV can engage cellular Toll-like receptors (see above) and induce patterned responses of the innate immune system suggest that CMVs have subverted responses of the innate immune system to enhance their spread in vivo. Undoubtedly, additional mechanisms of virus dissemination will be uncovered as future studies unravel the function of the myriad on viral genes that are non-essential for in vitro virus replication in permissive cells. In addition, the development of more representative models of HCMV infection such as the rhesus macaque will also likely lead to a greater understanding of the role of various viral genes in the spread of HCMV in the infected host.

Disease and HCMV infection: pathogenesis of end-organ disease in acute infection

Disease associated with HCMV infection can be arbitrarily divided into manifestations that follow acute infection and diseases that appear to be associated with chronic infections. Considerably more is known about disease syndromes that follow acute infection because readily definable clinical abnormalities can be related to HCMV infection. In addition, disease can be temporally related to acquisition of the virus and often to levels of virus replication. Clinical disease has been most often related to the level of virus replication which in turn is dependent on characteristics of the host response, perhaps most importantly the host immune response. In severe infections, multiorgan involvement is often present and symptomatic disease is most commonly associated with some degree of organ system dysfunction or failure. The degree of organ dysfunction and overall disease has been most closely correlated with virus replication such that higher levels of virus replication are associated with more severe disease (Bowen et al., 1996; Cope et al., 1997; Baldanti et al., 1998; Spector et al., 1999; Emery et al., 2000; Boppana et al., 2001a,b; Nichols et al., 2001; Boeckh et al., 2003). In the absence of antiviral chemotherapy or the reconstitution of HCMV specific immune responsiveness, these patients often succumb to multiorgan failure. Studies in experimental animal models of HCMV disease, particularly those utilizing immunocompromised animals are consistent with many aspects of human disease, including the relationship between virus replication and disease (Kern, 1999; Lockridge et al., 1999; Brune et al., 2001a,b; Sequar et al., 2002). When the data from numerous studies of HCMV infection in immunocompromised populations are examined, there appears to be no absolute level of viral burden that has been associated with disease. In fact, in these patients the relative increase in virus burden appears more predictive of disease. These findings would argue that the absolute level of virus replication as measured in body compartments such as the blood or urine merely indicates virus dissemination, whereas the rate of increase in virus replication (viral burden) could more accurately reflect the loss of immunological control of virus replication in infected organs and represents a harbinger of invasive disease and end-organ dysfunction. Results from studies in an experimental murine model of HCMV infections have indicated that monitoring the viral burden in the blood compartment only indirectly correlates with viral replication in infected organs and then only in immunocompromised animals (Brune et al., 2001a,b). This experimental finding provides a possible explanation for the lack of a linear correlation between viral burden and disease and suggests that increasing viral burdens are of more diagnostic value in immunocompromised hosts and should be taken as evidence of continued virus replication and dissemination.

The histopathology of tissue from patients with acute HCMV syndromes suggests that organ dysfunction and disease is secondary to both direct viral cytopathogenic effects and indirectly through bystander damage secondary effector functions of the host as evidenced by the presence of inflammatory cells in histological tissue sections. The pathognomonic finding of HCMV infection in biopsy and autopsy specimens is the finding of so called owl-eye inclusions in large cells. These cells have been shown to be HCMV infected and their presence correlates with substantial HCMV replication (Mattes et al., 2000). In experimental animal models of HCMV infection, increased viral copy number in target organs such as the liver, adrenal gland, and lung are associated with the level of tissue damage and the severity of disease (Brody and Craighead, 1974; Kern, 1999; Lockridge et al., 1999). Similarly in humans with disseminated HCMV infections, virus-induced damage associated with histological evidence of HCMV infection can be demonstrated in the liver, adrenal glands, lung, pancreas, colon, esophagus, eyes and CNS (Bale et al., 1989; Sinzger and Jahn, 1996). Although virus-induced cytolysis and cellular necrosis could explain the disease manifestations of acute HCMV infection, additional mechanisms of cellular damage, including apoptosis have been suggested based on in vitro studies and in limited studies in experimental animal models (Kosugi et al., 1998; Goldmacher et al., 1999; Brune et al., 2001a,b).

Early observations in bone marrow allograft recipients raised the possibility that HCMV pneumonitis in the post-transplant period was secondary to both the host immune response to HCMV and direct viral cytopathic effects (Grundy et al., 1987; Barry et al., 2000). Several lines of evidence are consistent with the hypothesis that the immune response to HCMV contribute to the pathogenesis of disease including; (i) the initial development of disease in the transplanted allograft, particularly in solid organ allograft recipients, (ii) the disparity between the limited distribution of virus infection in affected organs such as the lungs and the severity of clinical disease in patients with HCMV infection, (iii) the presence of inflammatory cellular infiltration and progressive disease in AIDs patients with invasive HCMV infections, (iv) the development of accelerated disease (immune vitritis) in AIDS patients with HCMV retinitis following reconstitution of antiviral adaptive immune responses (Karavellas et al., 1998; Holland, 1999; Mutimer et al., 2002). Together these data have argued that the host immune response represents at least one component of the pathogenesis of diseases associated with invasive HCMV infections. In contrast to the observations in AIDs patient following reconstitution of cellular immune responses, the control of virus replication by adaptive immunotherapy with HCMV specific CTL has been shown to decrease disease in allograft recipients (Walter et al., 1995). This finding suggests that HCMV specific adaptive immune responses do not directly contribute to disease in the post-transplant period if present prior to widespread viral dissemination. Thus, it could be argued that the failure to restrict virus replication by more efficient host responses such as adaptive immunity could lead to end-organ damage secondary to the non-specific activities of cells of the innate immune system. In addition, the functional activity of virus-encoded cytokines, chemokine and chemokine receptors in HCMV disease in allograft rejection could also promote HCMV associated disease in allograft recipients by the recruitment of inflammatory myeloid cells into virus infected tissue Thus, the pathogenesis of disease observed during acute HCMV infection undoubtedly requires virus replication and expression of viral gene products, but also a significant but as yet unquantifiable contribution from the host immune response.

Although it can be argued that disease in immunocompromised hosts following acute infection with HCMV can be related to the level of virus replication, the variability of disease manifestations in different patient populations indicates that additional host factors contribute to the pathogenesis of this infection. As examples, the most common disease presentations in long-lived AIDs patients are retinitis and colitis (Blaser and Cohn, 1986; Pepose et al., 1987; Francis et al., 1989; Dieterich and Rahmin, 1991; Drew, 1992; Gallant et al., 1992; Wilcox et al., 1998; Pecorella et al., 2000). Although HCMV colitis occurs in severely immunocompromised transplant patients, eye involvement is rare (Aldrete et al., 1975; Kaplan et al., 1989; Reed et al., 1990). Similarly, in congenitally infected infants colitis is not a well described component of disseminated HCMV infection. Central nervous system involvement is a hallmark of congenital HCMV infections whereas it is rarely reported in transplant recipients and when present in AIDS patients, appears to be associated with similar CNS pathology and clinical features (Becroft, 1981; Morgello et al., 1987; Wiley and Nelson, 1988; Schmidbauer et al., 1989; Vinters et al., 1989; Gallant et al., 1992; Perlman and Argyle, 1992; Achim et al., 1994; Arribas et al., 1996). More recent studies of allograft recipients suggest that focal HCMU encephalitis may be more frequent that previously appreciated (Ribalta et al., 2002). A variety of hypotheses have been put forth to account for the variability in disease between these groups of immunocompromised patients, yet none has adequately explained the differences in the manifestations of clinical disease. However, it is evident that virus dissemination and increased virus replication alone cannot account for the pathogenesis of acute HCMV infections. The balance between host innate and adaptive immune responses and the modulation of these responses by viral gene products is almost certainly central to our understanding of the pathogenesis of acute HCMV infection; however, it is also likely that other host responses unrelated to host immunity also play a significant role in the outcome of HCMV infection.

Disease and HCMV infection: pathogenesis of end-organ disease related to chronic infections

Although clinical syndromes associated with acute HCMV infections have received the bulk of experimental and clinical study, the role of the virus in chronic human disease has only recently become the subject of more intense study. As discussed previously, several laboratories have raised the possibility that HCMV infection was associated with a variety of human diseases including coronary atherosclerotic heart disease, gastric ulcer disease, rheumatologic disorders, and some human cancers. Note that each of these chronic diseases is also associated with inflammation, a host response that is also linked to HCMV replication and gene expression (Zhu et al., 2002). Definitive evidence demonstrating a role for HCMV in any of these diseases has not been reported, yet in the last decade a significant volume of observational data has linked HCMV infection with several of these diseases, including atherosclerotic vascular disease. In addition, studies in cardiac allograft recipients have reported the relationship between the development of transplant associated vascular sclerosis and HCMV infection (Grattan et al., 1989; McDonald et al., 1989; Loebe et al., 1990; Everett et al., 1992; Koskinen et al., 1993; Hosenpud, 1999; Koskinen et al., 1999; Streblow et al., 2001). Aspects of many of these studies remain controversial but when viewed as a group, the data appear to support a role of HCMV in vascular disease (Table 41.5).

Perhaps more convincing support can be found in studies carried out in experimental animal models of allograft rejection and transplant associated vascular sclerosis. These studies have provided compelling evidence for the role of rodent CMVs in the development of post-transplant vasculopathy and coronary arteriosclerosis (Lemstrom et al., 1995; Lemstrom et al., 1997; De La Melena et al., 2001). The relationship of HCMV infection to other chronic human diseases such as cancer is provocative yet far from conclusive (Huang and Pagano, 1978; Rapp and Robbins, 1984; Shen et al., 1993; Cinatl et al., 1996; Cobbs et al., 2002; Harkins et al., 2002). The impact of HCMV on the cell cycle during permissive infection and the less well understood relationship between viral gene expression during abortive infections and cell proliferation suggests that HCMV could at least facilitate the development of the malignant phenotype in some human cancers (Zhu et al., 1995; Shen et al., 1997; Fortunato et al., 2000; Browne et al., 2001a,b; Kalejta and Shenk, 2002; Kalejta et al., 2003; Kalejta and Shenk, 2003). To unravel the possible roles of HCMV in human cancer, more comprehensive epidemiologic studies designed to determine possible relationships between infection with this ubiquitous virus and human cancer must be accomplished. In addition, it will be necessary to develop more informative in vitro model systems of cellular transformation following infection with HCMV.

In contrast to the relationship between the levels of virus replication and disease syndromes associated with acute HCMV infections, a similar relationship between HCMV virus replication and chronic diseases such as atherosclerosis in both normal and immunocompromised hosts has not been reported. To further complicate the study of HCMV infection and diseases such as coronary artery disease, it has been proposed that productive HCMV replication is not required for disease and that HCMV gene expression at a distant site could trigger disease in a target organ such as the heart (Zhou et al., 1999). Finally, in vitro studies have also demonstrated that HCMV infection could be responsible for hit and run transformation event

Table 41.5. Evidence linking HCMV infection and vasculature disease. Studies that have demonstrated a link between HCMV infection and vascular disease

Study	Findings and interpretation
HCMV infection and coronary restenosis (Zhou et al., 1996)	Increased rate of restenosis following coronary artery atherectomy in HCMV infected patients
HCMV antibody levels and carotid atherosclerosis (Nieto et al., 1996)	Increased antibody titers correlated with more rapid onset of carotid vasculature disease
HCMV nucleic acids and antigen in coronary artery plaques (Wu et al., 1992; Speir et al., 1994)	HCMV directly associated with diseased vasculature
HCMV seropositivity and coronary artery disease (Melnick et al., 1993; Epstein et al., 1996; O'Connor et al., 2001)	HCMV infection risk factor for development of coronary artery disease
HCMV infection and coronary vasculature disease in cardiac allograft recipients (Grattan et al., 1989; Everett et al., 1992; Hosenpud, 1999; Koskinen et al., 1999; Valantine et al., 2001)	Increased rate of vascular disease and graft loss in patients with HCMV infection

(Shen et al., 1997). Thus, it is a daunting task to design a natural history study with sufficient power to identify a relationship between the development of a common disease such as coronary atherosclerotic heart disease or cancer and HCMV infection in populations in which the seroprevalence rates exceeds 60%–80%. Yet when the incredibly complex relationship between HCMV and the host cell and the life-long persistence of this virus in the host are considered together, it readily follows that HCMV could contribute to the pathogenesis of many of the diseases that have been only loosely associated with HCMV infection.

The inflammatory nature of many chronic diseases and the relationship between HCMV and inflammation has raised the possibility that HCMV is merely a passenger or bystander in these disease states and not causal. However, studies in transplant patients with accelerated vascular disease have provided strong support for a role of HCMV in chronic vascular disease observed in the normal host. The mechanisms by which HCMV promotes disease such as atherosclerosis or transplant vasculopathies are not completely understood but likely result from bi-directional interactions between HCMV and the host immune system. Studies from a number of laboratories have demonstrated that HCMV infection of host cells, including monocytes and endothelial cells, can induce expression of a variety of key mediators of the inflammatory response including adhesion molecules, chemokines, cytokines, and

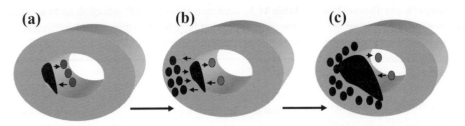

Vessel with developing plaque and/or focal area of damaged endothelium. (A) Inflammatory cellular infiltrate (●) into area increasing local inflammation with additional damage to endothelium. (B) Release of chemokines and other attractants by mononuclear cells promotes migration of virus-infected smooth muscle cells (●) into area. (C) Continued migration of smooth muscle cells into area leads to intimal thickening and narrowing of artery.

Fig. 41.1. Possible pathway of vasculopathy associated with HCMV infection of vessels.

pro-inflammatory host enzymes such as COX-2 (Van Dam-Mieras et al., 1987; Taylor et al., 1992; Koskinen, 1993; Sedmak et al., 1994; Waldman and Knight, 1996; Yilmaz et al., 1996; Craigen et al., 1997; Grundy et al., 1998; Speir et al., 1998; Burns et al., 1999; Redman et al., 2002; Zhu et al., 2002). In addition, HCMV encodes a number of immunomodulatory functions including chemokine receptors, chemokines (UL146), and cytokines (IL-10) as well as a plethora of viral evasion functions that favor viral persistence (Penfold et al., 1999; Kotenko et al., 2000; Spencer et al., 2002). Together, interactions between virus infected cells and inflammatory cells could foster virus persistence while at the same time fueling chronic inflammation.

The proposed pathogenesis of HCMV associated vasculopathies in transplant patients is particularly revealing. Studies have reported that HCMV infection in the post-transplant period is a risk factor for graft dysfunction, including the development of vascular sclerosis in the transplant organ (Richardson et al., 1981; Koskinen et al., 1999; Browne et al., 2001a,b; Soderberg-Naucler and Emery, 2001; Tolkoff-Rubin et al., 2001). In cardiac allograft recipients, HCMV infection has been shown to be a risk factors for the development of a distinctive form of coronary arteriosclerosis in the transplanted heart (Grattan et al., 1989; Koskinen et al., 1994; Hosenpud, 1999; Koskinen et al., 1999; Streblow et al., 2003). A less than definitive clinical trial in cardiac allograft recipients with the antiviral agent ganciclovir suggested that inhibition of HCMV replication could limit the rate of development of vascular disease (Valantine et al., 1999). Animal models of this disease process have been developed and data consistent with the observations in human disease have also been obtained (Lemstrom et al., 1995; De La Melena et al., 2001). In the rat model, rat CMV infection of animals with damaged endothelium is associated with infiltration of the intima with smooth muscle cells and narrowing of the lumen of coronary vessels of the transplanted heart (Lemstrom et al., 1995; Vossen et al., 1996; Li et al., 1998; Zhou et al., 1999; Streblow et al., 2001). Early, but not late treatment of infected animals with antivirals can dramatically slow the development of these arterial lesions (Lemstrom et al., 1997). From these experiments it appears that endothelial damage, inflammation and virus infection are required for the development of disease (Lemstrom et al., 1995; Li et al., 1998; Zhou et al., 1999; Streblow et al., 2003). Several models of the pathogenesis of this disease that combine these observations have been proposed. Some investigators have argued that CMV infection promotes systemic inflammation leading to an enhanced host inflammatory response that accelerates the development of vascular sclerosis in the transplanted organ. Other groups have argued that local expression of specific viral gene products in the target organ lead to disease in these animals. An example of such a viral gene product is the functional chemokine receptor HCMV US28. It has been shown that smooth muscle cells expressing the US28 viral gene product migrate down chemokine gradients (Streblow et al., 1999; Streblow et al., 2003). As illustrated in Fig. 41.1, damage to the endothelium either from virus infection, plaque deposition, or following allograft rejection in the case of cardiac allograft recipients, can lead to migration of infected smooth muscle cells expressing the viral chemokine receptor down a gradient of chemokines established by the infiltrating mononuclear cells or endothelial cells. The continued migration of these cells towards the gradient established by persistent local inflammation could account for the accumulation of these cell types in the intima of arteriosclerotic vessels. Because these virus infected smooth muscle cells also release inflammatory mediators, persistent HCMV infection could effectively recruit additional mononuclear cells into the focus of infection. Infected cells, including activated mononuclear cells, can release inflammatory mediators that can further activate HCMV gene expression. Thus, infection with the virus establishes a paracrine loop that can utilize the products of host inflammation to drive viral gene expression and recruit uninfected and infected cells into an area of virus infection. Once a balance between virus replication and the elimination of virus infected cells is reached, HCMV can persist in the face of chronic host inflammation. Diseases such as coronary arteriosclerosis or transplant vasculopathy could then develop from a combination of HCMV infection and ongoing host inflammation. Although this pathway is consistent with observations made in experimental models of HCMV associated vascular disease, particularly in models of transplant vascular sclerosis, it remains to be shown if a similar pathway can be related to disease in humans. However, it is well accepted that chronic human diseases such as coronary artery disease have inflammation as a major component in their pathogenesis (Zhu et al., 1999; Libby, 2002, 2003). Whether CMV plays a key role in chronic diseases such as coronary atherosclerosis remains unclear, yet this virus can be easily linked to chronic host inflammation and therefore remains a leading candidate as an infectious etiology of several chronic human diseases.

REFERENCES

Achim, C. L., Nagra, R. M. Wang, R., Nelson, J. A., and Wiley, C. A. (1994). Detection of cytomegalovirus in cerebrospinal fluid autopsy specimens from AIDS patients. *J. Infect. Dis.*, **169**, 623–627.

Adler, S. P. (1983). Transfusion-associated cytomegalovirus infections. *Rev. Infect. Dis.*, **5**, 977–993.

Adler, S. P. (1985). The molecular epidemiology of cytomegalovirus transmission among children attending a day care center. *J. Infect. Dis.*, **152**, 760–768.

Adler, S. P. (1988a). Cytomegalovirus transmission among children in day care, their mothers and caretakers. *Pediatr. Infect. Dis. J.*, **7**, 279–285.

Adler, S. P. (1988b). Molecular epidemiology of cytomegalovirus: viral transmission among children attending a day care center, their parents, and caretakers. *J. Pediatr.*, **112**, 366–372.

Adler, S. P. (1989). Cytomegalovirus and child day care. Evidence for an increased infection rate among day-care workers. *N. Engl. J. Med.*, **321**, 1290–1296.

Adler, S. P. (1991a). Cytomegalovirus and child day care: risk factors for maternal infection. *Pediatr. Infect. Dis. J.*, **10**, 590.

Adler, S. P. (1991b). Molecular epidemiology of cytomegalovirus: a study of factors affecting transmission among children at three day-care centers. *Pediatr. Infect. Dis. J.*, **10**, 584–590.

Adler, S. P., Chandrika, T., Lawrence, L., and Baggett, J. (1983). Cytomegalovirus infections in neonates due to blood transfusions. *Pediatr. Infect. Dis.*, **2**, 114–118.

Adler, S. P., Baggett, J., Wilson, M., Lawrence L., and McVoy, M. (1986). Molecular epidemiology of cytomegalovirus in a nursery: lack of evidence for nosocomial transmission. *J. Pediatr.*, **108**, 117–123.

Adler, S. P., Starr, S. E., Plotkin, S. A. *et al.* (1995). Immunity induced by primary human cytomegalovirus infection protects against secondary infection among women of childbearing age. *J. Infect. Dis.*, **171**, 26–32.

Ahlfors, K. and Ivarsson, S. A. (1985). Cytomegalovirus in breast milk of Swedish milk donors. *Scand. J. Infect. Dis.*, **17**, 11.

Aldrete, J. S., Sterlin, W. A., Hathway, B. M., Morgan, J. M., and Diethelm. A. G. (1975). Gastrointestinal and hepatic complications affecting patients with renal allografts. *Am. J. Surg.*, **129**, 115–124.

Alford, C. A., Stagno, S., Pass, R. F., and Huang, E. S. (1981). Epidemiology of cytomegalovirus. In *The Human Herpesviruses: An Interdisciplinary Perspective*, ed A. Nahmais, W. Dowdle, and R. Schinazi, pp. 159–171. New York: Elsevier.

Arribas, J. R., Storch, G. A., Clifford, D. B., and Tselis, A. C., (1996). Cytomegalovirus encephalitis. *Ann. Int. Med.*, **125**, 577–587.

Armstrong, J. A., Tarr, G. C., Youngblood, L. A. *et al.* (1976). Cytomegalovirus infection in children undergoing open heart surgery. *Yale. J. Biol. Med.*, **49**, 83–91.

Asanuma, H., Numazaki, K., Nagata, N., Hotsubo, T., Horino, K., and Chiba, S. (1996). Role of milk whey in the transmission of human cytomegalovirus infection by breast milk. *Microbiol. Immunol.*, **40**, 201–204.

Baldanti, F., Revello, M. G., Percivalle, E., and Gerna, G. (1998). Use of the human cytomegalovirus (HCMV) antigenemia assay for diagnosis and monitoring of HCMV infections and detection of antiviral drug resistance in the immunocompromised. *J. Clin. Virol.*, **11**, 51–60.

Bale, J. F. (1984). Human cytomegalovirus infection and disorders of the nervous system. *Arch. Neurol.*, **41**, 310–320.

Bale, J. F., Jr. and O'Neil, M. E. (1989). Detection of murine cytomegalovirus DNA in circulating leukocytes harvested during acute infection of mice.[erratum appears in *J. Virol.* 1989 Sep;**63**(9):4120]. *J. Virol.*, **63**, 2667–2673.

Bale, J. F., Jr., O'Neil, M. E., Hart, M. N., Harris, J. D., and Stinski M.F. (1989). Human cytomegalovirus nucleic acids in tissues from congenitally infected infants. *Pediatr. Neurol.* **5**, 216–220.

Bale, J. F., Jr., Petheram, S. J., Souza, I. E., and Murph, J. R. (1996). Cytomegalovirus reinfection in young children. *J. Pediatr.* **128**, 347–352.

Balfour, C. L. and Balfour, H. H. (1986). Cytomegalovirus is not an occupational risk for nurses in renal transplant and neonatal units. *J.Am.Med. Assoc.*, **256**, 1909–1914.

Balthesen, M., Messerle, M., and Reddehase, M. J. (1993). Lungs are a major organ site of cytomegalovirus latency and recurrence. *J. Virol.*, **67**, 5360–5366.

Barry, S. M., Johnson, M. A., and Janossy, G. (2000). Cytopathology or immunopathology? The puzzle of cytomegalovirus pneumonitis revisited. *Bone Marrow Transpl.* **26**, 591–597.

Becroft, D. M. O. (1981). Prenatal cytomegalovirus infection: epidemiology, pathology, and pathogenesis. In *Perspective in*

Pediatric Pathology, vol. 6, ed. H. S. Rosenberg and J. Bernstein, pp. 203–241. New York; Masson Press.

Beisser, P. S., Goh, C. S., Cohen, F. E., and Michelson, S.(2002). Viral chemokine receptors and chemokines in human cytomegalovirus trafficking and interaction with the immune system. CMV chemokine receptors. *Curr Top. Microbiol. Immunol.*, **269**, 203–234.

Bernstein, D. I. and Bourne, N. (1999). Animal models for cytomegalovirus infection: guinea-pig CMV. In *Handbook of Animal Models of Infection*, ed. M. S. O. Zak. London: Academic Press.

Billstrom Schroeder, M. and Worthen, G. S. (2001). Viral regulation of RANTES expression during human cytomegalovirus infection of endothelial cells. *J. Virol.*, **75**, 3383–3390.

Billstrom Schroeder, M., Christensen, R., and Worthen, G. S. (2002). Human cytomegalovirus protects endothelial cells from apoptosis induced by growth factor withdrawal. *J. Clini. Virol.*, **25**, S149–S157.

Blaser, M. J. and Cohn D. L. (1986). Opportunistic infections in patients with AIDS: clues to the epidemiology of AIDS and the relative virulence of pathogens. *Rev. Infect. Dis.*, **8**, 21–30.

Bodaghi, B., Jones, T. R., Zipeto, D. *et al.* (1998). Chemokine sequestration by viral chemoreceptors as a novel viral escape strategy: withdrawal of chemokines from the environment of cytomegalovirus-infected cells. *J. Exp. Medi.* **188**, 855–866.

Boeckh, M. and Boivin, G. (1998). Quantitation of cytomegalovirus: methodologic aspects and clinical applications. *Clin. Microbiol. Rev.* **11**, 533–554.

Boeckh, M. and Bowden, R. (1995). Cytomegalovirus infection in marrow transplantation. In C. D. Buckner (ed.), *Technical and Biological Components of Marrow Transplantation*, ed. C. D. Buckner, pp. 97–136. Boston: Kluwer Academic Publishers.

Boeckh, M., Gooley, T. A., Myerson, D., Cunningham, T., Schoch, G., and Bowden, R. A., (1996). Cytomegalovirus pp65 antigenemia-guided early treatment with ganciclovir versus ganciclovir at engraftment after allogeneic marrow transplantation: a randomized double-blind study. *Blood*, **88**, 4063–4071.

Boeckh, M., Gallez-Hawkins, G. M., Myerson, D., Zaia, J. A., and Bowden R. A. (1997). Plasma polymerase chain reaction for cytomegalovirus DNA after allogeneic marrow transplantation: comparison with polymerase chain reaction using peripheral blood leukocytes, pp65 antigenemia, and viral culture. *Transplantation*, **64**, 108–113.

Boeckh, M., Leisenring, W., Riddell, S. R. *et al.* (2003). Late cytomegalovirus disease and mortality in recipients of allogeneic hematopoietic stem cell transplants: importance of viral load and T–cell immunity. *Blood*, **101**, 407–414.

Bolovan-Fritts, C. and Wiedeman, J. A. (2001). Human cytomegalovirus strain Toledo lacks a virus-encoded tropism factor required for infection of aortic endothelial cells. *J. Infect. Dis.*, **184**, 1252–1261.

Boppana, S. B., Rivera, L. B., Fowler, K. B., Mach, M., and Britt W. J. (2001a). Intrauterine transmission of cytomegalovirus to infants of women with preconceptional immunity. *N. Engl. J. Medi.*, **344**, 1366–1371.

Boppana, S. B., Rivera, L. B., Fowler, K. B., Yang, J., and Britt, W. J. (2001b). Presented at the 41st Interscience Conference on Antimicrobial Agents and Chemotherapy, Chicago, IL, December 16–19.

Borisch, B., Jahn, G., Scholl, B. C. *et al.* (1988). Detection of human cytomegalovirus DNA and viral antigens in tissues of different manifestations of CMV infections. *Virch. Arch.[B]*, **55**, 93–99.

Bowden, R. A. (1995). Transfusion-transmitted cytomegalovirus infection. *Hematol. – Oncol. Clini. N. Am.* **9**, 155–166.

Bowden, R. A., Slichter, S. J., Sayers, M. H., Mori, M., Cays, M. J., and Meyers, J. D. (1991). Use of leukocyte-depleted platelets and cytomegalovirus-seronegative red blood cells for prevention of primary cytomegalovirus infection after marrow transplant. *Blood*, **78**, 246–250.

Bowen, E. F., Wilson, P., Atkins, M., *et al.* (1995). Natural history of untreated cytomegalovirus retinitis. *Lancet*, **346**, 1671–1673.

Bowen, E. F., Wilson, P., Cope, A. *et al.* (1996). Cytomegalovirus retinitis in AIDS patients: influence of cytomegaloviral load on response to ganciclovir, time to recurrence and survival. *AIDS* **10**, 1515–1520.

Brady, M. T., Milam, J. D. Anderson, D.C. *et al.* (1984). Use of deglycerolized red blood cells to prevent posttransfusion infection with cytomegalovirus in neonates. *J. Infect. Dis.*, **150**, 334–339.

Brody, A. R. and Craighead, J. E. (1974). Pathogenesis of pulmonary cytomegalovirus infection in immunosuppressed mice. *J. Infect. Dis.*, **129**, 677.

Browne, E. P., Wing, B., Coleman, D., and Shenk, T., (2001a). Altered cellular mRNA levels in human cytomegalovirus-infected fibroblasts: viral block to the accumulation of antiviral mRNAs. *J. Virol.*, **75**, 12319–12330.

Browne, G., Whitworth, C., Bellamy, C., and Ogilvie, M.M. (2001b). Acute allograft glomerulopathy associated with CMV viraemia. *Nephrol. Dial. Transpl.*, **16**, 861–862.

Brune, W., Hasan, M., Krych, M., Bubic, I., Jonjic, S., and Koszinowski U. H. (2001a). Secreted virus-encoded proteins reflect murine cytomegalovirus productivity in organs. *J. Infect. Dis.* **184**, 1320–1324.

Brune, W., Menard, C. Heesemann, J., and Koszinowski, U. H. (2001b). A ribonucleotide reductase homolog of cytomegalovirus and endothelial cell tropism. *Science*, **291**, 303–305.

Burns, L. J., Pooley, J. C., Walsh D. J., Vercellotti, G. M., Weber, M. L., and Kovacs A. (1999). Intercellular adhesion molecule–1 expression in endothelial cells is activated by cytomegalovirus immediate early proteins. *Transplantation*, **67**, 137–144.

CDC (1985). Prevalence of cytomegalovirus excretion from children in five day care centers – Alabama. *Morb. Mortal. Wkly Rep.*, **34**, 49–51.

Cha, T., Tom, E. Kembel, G. W., Duke, G. M., Mocarski, E. S., and Spaete, R. R. (1996). Human cytomegalovirus clinical isolates carry at least 19 genes not found in laboratory strains. *J. Virol.* **70**, 78–83.

Chandler, S. H., Holmes, K. K., Wentworth, B. B. *et al.* (1985). The epidemiology of cytomegaloviral infection in women attending a sexually transmitted disease clinic. *J. Infect. Dis.*, **152**, 597–605.

Chandler, S. H., Handsfield, H. H., and McDougally, J. K. (1987). Isolation of multiple strains of cytomegalovirus from women attending a clinic for sexually transmitted disease. *J. Infect. Dis.* **155**, 655–660.

Chern, K. C., Chandler, D. B., Martin, D. F., Kuppermann, B. D., Wolitz, R. A., and Margolis, T. P. (1998). Glycoprotein B subtyping of cytomegalovirus (CMV) in the vitreous of patients with AIDS and CMV retinitis. *J. Infect. Dis.*, **178**, 1149–1153.

Chou, S. W. (1986). Acquisition of donor strains of cytomegalovirus by renal-transplant recipients. *N. Engl. J. Med.*, **314**, 1418–1423.

Chou, S. W. (1987). Cytomegalovirus infection and reinfection transmitted by heart transplantation. *J. Infect. Dis.*, **155**, 1054–1056.

Cinatl, J., Jr., Cinatl, J., Vogel, J. U., Rabenau, H., Kornhuber, B., and Doerr, H. W. (1996). Modulatory effects of human cytomegalovirus infection on malignant properties of cancer cells. *Intervirology*, **39**, 259–269.

Cobbs, C. S., Harkins, L., Samanta, M. *et al.* (2002). Human cytomegalovirus infection and expression in human malignant glioma. *Cancer Res.*, **62**, 3347–3350.

Cole, R. and Kuttner, A. G. (1926). A filtrable virus present in the submaxillary glands of guinea pigs. *J. Exp. Med.* **44**, 855–873.

Collier, A. C., Handsfield, H. H., Roberts, P. L. *et al.* (1990). Cytomegalovirus infection in women attending a sexually transmitted disease clinic. *J. Infect. Dis.*, **162**, 46–51.

Collier, A. C., Handsfield, H. H., Ashley R. *et al.* (1995). Cervical but not urinary excretion of cytomegalovirus is related to sexual activity and contraceptive practices in sexually active women. *J. Infect. Dis.*, **171**, 33–38.

Collins, T. M., Quirk, M. R., and Jordan, M. C. (1994). Biphasic viremia and viral gene expression in leukocytes during acute cytomegalovirus infection of mice. *J. Virol.*, **68**, 6305–6311.

Compton, T., Kurt-Jones, E. A. Bochme, K. W. *et al.* (2003). Human cytomegalovirus activates inflammatory cytokine responses via CD14 and Toll-like receptor 2. *J. Virol.*, **77**, 4588–4596.

Coonrod, D., Collier, A. C., Ashley, R., DeRouen, T., and Corey, L. (1998). Association between cytomegalovirus seroconversion and upper genital tract infection among women attending a sexually transmitted disease clinic: a prospective study. *J. Infect. Dis.* **177**, 1188–1193.

Cope, A. V., Sabin, C., Burroughs, A., Rolles, K., Griffiths, P. D., and Emery V. C. (1997). Interrelationships among quantity of human cytomegalovirus (HCMV) DNA in blood, donor-recipient serostatus, and administration of methylprednisolone as risk factors for HCMV disease following liver transplantation. *J. Infect. Dis.*, **176**, 1484–1490.

Craigen, J. L., Yong, K. L., Jordan, N. J. *et al.* (1997). Human cytomegalovirus infection up-regulates interleukin–8 gene expression and stimulates neutrophil transendothelial migration. *Immunology*, **92**, 138–145.

Davis-Poynter, N. J., Lynch, D. M., Vally, H. *et al.* (1997). Identification and characterization of a G protein-coupled receptor homolog encoded by murine cytomegalovirus. *J. Virol.*, **71**, 1521–1529.

De La Melena, V. T., Kreklywich, C. N., Streblow, D. N. *et al.* (2001). Kinetics and development of CMV–accelerated transplant vascular sclerosis in rat cardiac allografts is linked to early increase in chemokine expression and presence of virus. *Transpl. Proc* **33**, 1822–1823.

Demmler, G. J., Yow, M. D., Spector, S. A. *et al.* (1987). Nosocomial cytomegalovirus infections within two hospitals caring for infants and children. *J. Infect. Dis.*, **156**, 9–16.

Diamond, C., Speck, C., Huang, M. L., Corey, L., Coombs, R. W., and Krieger, J. N. (2000). Comparison of assays to detect cytomegalovirus shedding in the semen of HIV–infected men. *J. Virol. Methods*, **90**, 185–191.

Dieterich, D. T. and Rahmin, M. (1991). Cytomegalovirus colitis in AIDS: presentation in 44 patients and a review of the literature. *J. AIDS*, **4**, S29–S35.

Dobbins, J. G., Adler, S. P., Pass, R. F., Bale, J. F., Grillner, L., and Stewart, J. A. (1993). The risks and benefits of cytomegalovirus transmission in child day care. *Am. J. Publ. Hlth* **in press**.

Drew, W. L. (1992). Cytomegalovirus infection in patients with AIDS. *Clin. Infect. Dis.*, **14**, 608–615.

Drew, W. L. and Mintz, L. (1984). Cytomegalovirus infection in healthy and immune-deficient homosexual men. In *The Acquired Immune Deficiency Syndrome and Infections of Homosexual Men*, ed. P. Ma and D. Armstrong, pp. 117–123. New York: Yorke Medical Books.

Drew, W. L., Mintz, L., Miner, R. C., Sands, M., and Ketterer, B. (1981). Prevalence of cytomegalovirus infection in homosexual men. *J. Infect. Dis.*, **143**, 188–192.

Drew, W. L., Sweet, E. S., Miner, R. C., and Mocarski, E. S. (1984). Multiple infections by cytomegalovirus in patients with acquired immunodeficiency syndrome: documentation by Southern blot hybridization. *J. Infect. Dis.*, **150**, 952–953.

Drew, W. L., Tegtmeier, G., Alter, H. J., Laycock, M. E., Miner, R. C., and Busch, M. P. (2003). Frequency and duration of plasma CMV viremia in seroconverting blood donors and recipients.[comment]. *Transfusion*, **43**, 309–313.

Dworsky, M., Welch, K., Cassady, G., and Stagno, S. (1983a). Occupational risk for primary cytomegalovirus infection among pediatric health care workers. *N. Engl. J. Med.*, **309**, 950–953.

Dworsky, M., Yow, M., Stagno, S., Pass, R. F., and Alford, C. (1983b). Cytomegalovirus infection of breast milk and transmission in infancy. *Pediatrics*, **72**, 295–299.

Dworsky, M., Lakeman, A., and Stagno, S. (1984). Cytomegalovirus transmission within a family. *Pediatr. Infect. Dis.* **3**, 236–238.

Emanuel, D., Cunningham, I., Jules-Elysee, K. *et al.* (1988). Cytomegalovirus pneumonia after bone marrow transplantation successfully treated with the combination of ganciclovir and high-dose intravenous immune globulin. *Ann. Intern. Med.*, **109**, 777–782.

Emery, V. C., Sabin, C. A., Cope, A. V., Gor, D., Hassan-Walker, A. F., and Griffiths, P. D. (2000). Application of viral-load kinetics to identify patients who develop cytomegalovirus disease after transplantation.[comment]. *Lancet*, **355**, 2032–2036.

Epstein, S. E., Speir, E., Zhou, Y. F., Guetta, E., Leon, M., and Finkel, T. (1996). The role of infection in restenosis and atherosclerosis: focus on cytomegalovirus. *Lancet*, **348**, s13–s17.

Erice, A., Holm, M. A., Gill, P. C. *et al.* (1992). Cytomegalovirus (CMV) antigenemia assay is more sensitive than shell vial cultures for rapid detection of CMV in polymorphonuclear blood leukocytes. *J. Clin. Microbiol.*, **30**, 2822–2825.

Evans, P. C., Coleman, N., Wreghitt, T. G., Wight, D. G., and Alexander, G. J. (1999). Cytomegalovirus infection of bile duct epithelial cells, hepatic artery and portal venous endothelium in relation to chronic rejection of liver grafts. *J. Hepatol.*, **31**, 913–920.

Everett, J. P., Hershberger, R. E., Norman, D. J. et al. (1992). Prolonged cytomegalovirus infection with viremia is associated with development of cardiac allograft vasculopathy. *J. Heart Lung Transpl.*.

Farber, S. and Wolbach, S. B. (1932). Intranuclear and cytoplasmic inclusions ("protozoan-like bodies") in the salivary glands and other organs of infants. *Am. J. Pathol. Child.*, **8**, 123–126.

Fish, K. N., Stenglein, S. G., Ibanez, C., and Nelson, J. A. (1995). Cytomegalovirus persistence in macrophages and endothelial cells. *Scand. J. Infect. Dis.* – Sppl. **99**, 34–40.

Fish, K. N., Soderberg-Naucler, C., Mills, L. K., Stenglein, S., and Nelson, J. A. (1998). Human cytomegalovirus persistently infects aortic endothelial cells. *J. Virol.*, **72**, 5661–5668.

Fleming, P., Davis-Poynter, N., Degli-Eposti, M. et al. (1999). The murine cytomegalovirus chemokine homolog, m131/129, is a determinant of viral pathogenicity. *J. Virol.*, **73**, 6800–6809.

Fortunato, E. A., McElroy, A. K., Sanchez, I., and Spector, D. H. (2000). Exploitation of cellular signaling and regulatory pathways by human cytomegalovirus. *Trends Microbiol.*, **8**, 111–119.

Foster, K. M. and Jack, I. (1969). A prospective study of the role of cytomegalovirus in post-transfusion mononucleosis. *N. Engl. J. Med.*, **280**, 1311–1315.

Fowler, K. B. and Pass, R. F. (1991). Sexually transmitted diseases in mothers of neonates with congenital cytomegalovirus infection. *J. Infect. Dis.*, **164**, 259–264.

Fowler, K. B., Stagno, S., Pass, R. F., Britt, W. J., Boll, T. J., and Alford, C. A. (1992). The outcome of congenital cytomegalovirus infection in relation to maternal antibody status. *N. Engl. J. Med.*, **326**, 663–667.

Fowler, K. B., Stagno, S., and Pass, R. F. (1993). Maternal age and congenital cytomegalovirus infection: screening of two diverse newborn populations, 1980–1990. *J. Infect. Dis.*, **168**, 552–556.

Fowler, K. B., Pass, R. F., and Stagno, S. (1997). Presented at the Society for Pediatric Epidemiological Research 10th Annual Meeting, Edmonton, Alberta, Canada, June 10–11.

Francis, N. D., Boylston, A. W., Roberts, A. H., Parkin, J. M., and Pinching, A. J. (1989). Cytomegalovirus infection in gastrointestinal tracts of patients infected with HIV-1 or AIDS. *J. Clin. Pathol.*, **42**, 1055–1064.

Gallant, J. E., Moore, R. D., Richman, D. D., Keruly, J., and Chaisson, R. E. (1992). Incidence and natural history of cytomegalovirus disease in patients with advanced human immunodeficiency virus disease treated with zidovudine. The Zidovudine Epidemiology Study Group. *J. Infect. Dis.*, **166**, 1223–1227.

Geder, L., Sanford, E. J., Rohner, T. J., and Rapp, F. (1977). Cytomegalovirus and cancer of the prostate: in vitro transformation of human cells. *Cancer Treat. Rep.*, **61**, 139–146.

Gerna, G., Zipeto, D., Parea, M. et al. (1991). Monitoring of human cytomegalovirus infections and ganciclovir treatment in heart transplant recipients by determination of viremia, antigenemia, and DNAemia. *J. Infect. Dis.*, **164**, 488–498.

Gerna, G., Zipeto, D., Percivalle, E. et al. (1992). Human cytomegalovirus infection of the major leukocyte subpopulations and evidence for initial viral replication in polymorphonuclear leukocytes from viremic patients. *J. Infect. Dis.*, **166**, 1236–1244.

Gerna, G., Zavattoni, M., Baldanti, F. et al. (1998). Circulating cytomegalic endothelial cells are associated with high human cytomegalovirus (HCMV) load in AIDS patients with late-stage disseminated HCMV disease. *J. Med. Virol.*, **55**, 64–74.

Gerna, G., Percivalle, E., Baldanti, F. et al. (2000). Human cytomegalovirus replicates abortively in polymorphonuclear leukocytes after transfer from infected endothelial cells via transient microfusion events. *J. Virol.*, **74**, 5629–5638.

Gerna, G., Percivalle, E., Baldanti, F., and Revello, M. G. (2002). Lack of transmission to polymorphonuclear leukocytes and human umbilical vein endothelial cells as a marker of attenuation of human cytomegalovirus. *J. Med. Virol.*, **66**, 335–339.

Gnann, J. W., Jr., Ahlmen, J., Svalander, C., Olding, L., Oldstone, M. B., and Nelson, J. A. (1988). Inflammatory cells in transplanted kidneys are infected by human cytomegalovirus. *Am. J. Pathol.*, **132**, 239–248.

Gold, E. and Nankervis, G. A. (1982). Cytomegalovirus. In *Viral Infections of Humans: Epidemiology and Control*, 2nd ed, ed. A. S. Evans, pp.167–186. New York: Plenum Press.

Goldmacher, V. S., Bartle, L. M., Skaletskaya, A. et al. (1999). A cytomegalovirus-encoded mitochondria-localized inhibitor of apoptosis structurally unrelated to Bcl-2. *Proc. Natl Acad. Sci. USA*, **96**, 12536–12541.

Goodpasture, E. W. and Talbot, F. B. (1921). Concerning the nature of "proteozoan-like" cells in certain lesions of infancy. *Am. J. Dis. Child.*, **21**, 415–421.

Goodrich, J. M., Bowden, R. A., Fisher, L. et al. (1993). Ganciclovir prophylaxis to prevent cytomegalovirus disease after allogeneic marrow transplant. *Ann. Intern. Med.*, **118**, 173–178.

Goodrum, F. D., Jordan, C. T., High, K., and Shenk, T. (2002). Human cytomegalovirus gene expression during infection of primary hematopoietic progenitor cells: a model for latency. *Proc. Natl Acad. Sci. USA*, **99**, 16255–16260.

Grattan, M. T., Moreno-Cabral, C. E., Starnes, V. A., Oyer, P. E., Stinson, E. B., and Shumway. N. E. (1989). Cytomegalovirus infection is associated with cardiac allograft rejection and atherosclerosis. *J. Am. Med. Assoc.*, **261**, 3561–3566.

Grefte, A., van der Giessen, M., van Son, W., and The, T. H. (1993). Circulating cytomegalovirus (CMV)-infected endoethelial cells in patients with an active CMV infection. *J. Infect. Dis.*, **167**, 270–277.

Griffiths, P. D., Clark, D. A., and Emery, V. C. (2000). Betaherpesviruses in transplant recipients. *J. Antimicrob. Chemother.*, **45**, 29–34.

Grose, C. (1994). Varicella zoster virus infections: chickenpox, shingles, and varicella vaccine. In *Herpesvirus Infections*, ed. R. Glaser and J. F. Jones, pp. 117–185. New York: Marcel Dekker, Inc.

Grundy, J. E., Shanley, J. D., and Griffiths, P. D. (1987). Is cytomegalovirus interstitial pneumonitis in transplant recipients an immunopathological condition? *Lancet*, **2**, 996–999.

Grundy, J. E., Lui, S. F., Super, M. *et al.* (1988). Symptomatic cytomegalovirus infection in seropositive kidney recipients: reinfection with donor virus rather than reactivation of recipient virus. *Lancet*, **2**, 132–135.

Grundy, J. E., Lawson, K. M., MacCormac, L. P., Fletcher, J. M., and Yong, K. L. (1998). Cytomegalovirus-infected endothelial cells recruit neutrophils by the secretion of C–X–C chemokines and transmit virus by direct neutrophil-endothelial cell contact and during neutrophil transendothelial migration. *J. Infect. Dis.*, **177**, 1465–1474.

Guetta, E., Guetta, V., Shibutani, T., and Epstein, S. E. (1997). Monocytes harboring cytomegalovirus: interactions with endothelial cells, smooth muscle cells, and oxidized low-density lipoprotein. Possible mechanisms for activating virus delivered by monocytes to sites of vascular injury. *Circ. Res.*, **81**, 8–16.

Hahn, G., Jores, R., and Mocarski, E. S. (1998). Cytomegalovirus remains latent in a common precursor of dendritic and myeloid cells. *Proc. Natl Acad. Sci. USA*, **95**, 3937–3942.

Hahn, G., Khan, H., Baldanti, F., Koszinowski, U. H., Revello, M. G., and Gerna, G. (2002). The human cytomegalovirus ribonucleotide reductase homolog UL45 is dispensable for growth in endothelial cells, as determined by a BAC-cloned clinical isolate of human cytomegalovirus with preserved wild-type characteristics. *J. Virol.*, **76**, 9551–9555.

Hahn, G., Revello, M. G., Patrone, M., *et al.* (2004). Human cytomegalovirus UL131–128 genes are indispensable for virus growth in endothelial cells and virus transfer to leukocytes. *J. Virol.*, **78**, 10023–10033.

Hamprecht, K., Vochem, M., Baumeister, A., Boniek, M., Speer, C. P., and Jahn, G. (1998). Detection of cytomegaloviral DNA in human milk cells and cell free milk whey by nested PCR. *J. Virol. Method*, **70**, 167–176.

Handsfield, H. H., Chandler, S. H., Caine, V. A. *et al.* (1985). Cytomegalovirus infection in sex partners: evidence for sexual transmission. *J. Infect. Dis.*, **151**, 344–348.

Hanshaw, J. B. (1971). Congenital cytomegalovirus infection: a fifteen year perspective. *J. Infect. Dis.*, **123**, 555–561.

Hanson, L. K., Slater, J. S., Karabekian, Z. *et al.* (1999). Replication of murine cytomegalovirus in differentiated macrophages as a determinant of viral pathogenesis. *J. Virol.*, **73**, 5970–5980.

Hanson, L. K., Slater, J. S., Karabekian, Z., Ciocco-Schmitt, G., and Campbell, A. E. (2001). Products of US22 genes M140 and M141 confer efficient replication of murine cytomegalovirus in macrophages and spleen. *J. Virol.*, **75**, 6292–6302.

Harkins, L., Volk, A. L., Samanta, M. *et al.* (2002). Specific localisation of human cytomegalovirus nucleic acids and proteins in human colorectal cancer. *Lancet*, **360**, 1557–1563.

Ho, M. (1977). Virus infections after transplantation in man. *Arch. Virol.*, **55**, 1–24.

Holland, G. N. (1999). Immune recovery uveitis. *Ocular Immunol. Inflammation*, **7**, 215–221.

Holsward, T. R., Engle, M. A. Redo, S. F. Goldsmith, E. I., and Barondess, J. A. (1963). Development of viral diseases and a viral disease-like syndrome after extracorporeal circulation. *Circulation*, **27**, 812–815.

Hosenpud, J. D. (1999). Coronary artery disease after heart transplantation and its relation to cytomegalovirus. *Am. Heart J.*, **138**, S469–S472.

Hsieh, C. Y., You, S. L., Kao, C. L., and Chen, C. J. (1999). Reproductive and infectious risk factors for invasive cervical cancer in Taiwan. *Anticancer Res.*, **19**, 4495–4500.

Huang, E. S. and Pagano. J. S. (1978). Cytomegalovirus DNA and adenocarcinoma of the colon: evidence for latent infection. *Lancet*, **1**, 957–960.

Hummel, M., Zhang, Z., Yan, S. *et al.* (2001). Allogeneic transplantation induces expression of cytomegalovirus immediate-early genes in vivo: a model for reactivation from latency. *J. Virol.*, **75**, 4814–4822.

Hutto, S. C., Ricks, R. E., Garvie, M., and Pass, R. F. (1985). Epidemiology of cytomegalovirus infections in young children: day care vs home care. *Pediatr. Infect. Dis.*, **4**, 149–152.

Hutto, C., Little, E. A., Ricks, R., Lee, J. D., and Pass, R. F. (1986). Isolation of cytomegalovirus from toys and hands in a day care center. *J. Infect. Dis.*, **154**, 527–530.

Jacobson, M. A., O'Donnell, J. J., Porteus, D., Brodie, H. R., Feigal, D., and Mills, J. (1988). Retinal and gastrointestinal disease due to cytomegalovirus in patients with the acquired immune deficiency syndrome: prevalence, natural history and response to ganciclovir therapy. *Quart. J. Med.*, **67**, 473.

Jahn, G., Stenglein, S., Riegler, S., Einsele, H., and Sinzger, C. (1999). Human cytomegalovirus infection of immature dendritic cells and macrophages. *Intervirology*, **42**, 365–372.

Jarvis, M. A., Wang, C. E., Meyers, H. L. *et al.* (1999). Human cytomegalovirus infection of Caco-2 cells occurs at the basolateral membrane and is differentiation state dependent. *J. Virol.*, **73**, 4552–4560.

Jesionek, A. and Kiolemenoglou, B. (1904). Uber einen befund von protozoenartigen gebilden in den organen eines heriditarluetischen fotus. *Munch. Med. Wochenschr.*, **51**, 1905–1907.

Jonjic, S., Pavic, I., Polic, B., Crnkovic, I., Lucin, P., and Koszinowski, U. H. (1994). Antibodies are not essential for the resolution of primary cytomegalovirus infection but limit dissemination of recurrent virus. *J. Exp. Med.*, **179**, 1713–1717.

Jordan, M. C. and Mar, V. L. (1982). Spontaneous activation of latent cytomegalovirus from murine spleen explants. Role of lymphocytes and macrophages in release and replication of virus. *J. Clin. Invest.*, **70**, 762–768.

Jordan, M. C., Rousseau, W. E., Noble, G. R., Stewart, J. A., and Chin, T. D. Y. (1973). Association of cervical cytomegaloviruses with venereal disease. *N. Engl. J. Med.*, **288**, 932–934.

Jordan, M. C., Takagi, J. L., and Stevens, J. G. (1982). Activation of latent murine cytomegalovirus in vivo and in vitro: a pathogenetic role for acute infection. *J. Infect. Dis.*, **145**, 699–705.

Kahl, M., Siegel-Axel, D., Stenglein, S., Jahn, G., and Sinzger, C. (2000). Efficient lytic infection of human arterial endothelial cells by human cytomegalovirus strains. *J. Virol.*, **74**, 7628–7635.

Kalejta, R. F. and Shenk, T. (2002). Manipulation of the cell cycle by human cytomegalovirus. *Frontiers Biosci.*, **7**, d295–d306.

Kalejta, R. F. and Shenk, T. (2003). The human cytomegalovirus UL82 gene product (pp71) accelerates progression through the G1 phase of the cell cycle. *J. Virol.*, **77**, 3451–3459.

Kalejta, R. F., Bechtel, J. T., and Shenk, T. (2003). Human cytomegalovirus pp71 stimulates cell cycle progression by inducing the proteasome-dependent degradation of the retinoblastoma family of tumor suppressors. *Mol. Cell. Biol.*, **23**, 1885–1895.

Kaplan, C. S., Petersen, E. A., Icenogle, T. B. *et al.* (1989). Gastrointestinal cytomegalovirus infection in heart and heart-lung transplant recipients. *Arch. Intern. Med.*, **149**, 2095–2100.

Karavellas, M. P., Lowder, C. Y., Macdonald, C., Avila, C. P., Jr., and Freeman, W. R. (1998). Immune recovery vitritis associated with inactive cytomegalovirus retinitis: a new syndrome. *Arch. Ophthalmol.*, **116**, 169–175.

Kas-Deelen, A. M., de Maar, E. F., Harmsen, M. C., Driessen, C., van Son, W. J., and The, T. H. (2000). Uninfected and cytomegalic endothelial cells in blood during cytomegalovirus infection: effect of acute rejection. *J. Infect. Dis.*, **181**, 721–724.

Kas-Deelen, A. M., The, T. H., Blom, N. *et al.* (2001). Uptake of pp65 in in vitro generated pp65-positive polymorphonuclear cells mediated by phagocytosis and cell fusion? *Intervirology*, **44**, 8–13.

Kern, E. R. (1999). Animal models for cytomegalovirus infection: murine CMV. In *Handbook of Animal Models of Infection*, ed. O. Zak and M. Sande, pp. 927–934. London: Academic Press.

Klatt, E. C. and Shibata, D. (1988). Cytomegalovirus infection in the acquired immunodeficiency syndrome. Clinical and autopsy findings. *Arch. Pathol. Lab. Med.*, **112**, 540–544.

Kledal, T. N., Rosenkilde, M. M., and Schwartz, T. W. (1998). Selective recognition of the membrane-bound CX3C chemokine, fractalkine, by the human cytomegalovirus-encoded broad-spectrum receptor US28. *FEBS Lett.*, **441**, 209–214.

Kondo, K., Xu, J., and Mocarski, E. S. (1996). Human cytomegalovirus latent gene expression in granulocyte-macrophage progenitors in culture and in seropositive individuals. *Proc. Natl. Acad. Sci. USA*, **93**, 11137–11142.

Koskinen, P. K. (1993). The association of the induction of vascular cell adhesion molecule-1 with cytomegalovirus antigenemia in human heart allografts. *Transplantation*, **56**, 1103–1108.

Koskinen, P. K., Nieminen, M. S., Krogerus, L. A. *et al.* (1993). Cytomegalovirus infection and accelerated cardiac allograft vasculopathy in human cardiac allografts. *J. Heart Lung Transpl.*, **12**, 724–729.

Koskinen, P., Lemstrom, K., Bruggeman, C., Lautenschlager, I., and Hayry, P. (1994). Acute cytomegalovirus infection induces a subendothelial inflammation (endothelialitis) in the allograft vascular wall. A possible linkage with enhanced allograft arteriosclerosis. *Am. J. Pathol.*, **144**, 41–50.

Koskinen, P. K., Kallio, E. A., Tikkanen, J. M., Sihvola, R. K., Hayry, P. J., and Lemstrom, K. B. (1999). Cytomegalovirus infection and cardiac allograft vasculopathy. *Transpl. Infect. Dis.*, **1**, 115–126.

Kosugi, I., Shinmura, Y., Li, R. Y. *et al.* (1998). Murine cytomegalovirus induces apoptosis in non-infected cells of the developing mouse brain and blocks apoptosis in primary neuronal culture. *Acta Neuropath.*, **96**, 239–247.

Kotenko, S. V., Saccani, S., Izotova, L. S., Mirochnitchenko, O. V., and Pestka, S. (2000). Human cytomegalovirus harbors its own unique IL-10 homolog (cmvIL-10). *Proc. Natl Acad. Sci. USA*, **97**, 1695–1700.

Krech, U. and Tobin, J. (1981). A collaborative study of cytomegalovirus antibodies in mothers and young children in 19 countries. *Bull. WHO*, **59**, 605–610.

Kurz, S., Steffens, H. P., Mayer, A., Harris, J. R., and Reddehase, M. J. (1997). Latency versus persistence or intermittent recurrences: evidence for a latent state of murine cytomegalovirus in the lungs. *J. Virol.*, **71**, 2980–2987.

Kurz, S. K., Rapp, M., Steffens, H. P., Grzimek, N. K., Schmalz, S., and Reddehase, M. J. (1999). Focal transcriptional activity of murine cytomegalovirus during latency in the lungs. *J. Virol.*, **73**, 482–494.

Landry, M. L. and Ferguson, D. (1993). Comparison of quantitative cytomegalovirus antigenemia assay with culture methods and correlation with clinical disease. *J. Clin. Microbiol.*, **31**, 2851–2856.

Lang, D. J. and Kummer, J. F. (1975). Cytomegalovirus in semen: observations in selected populations. *J. Infect. Dis.*, **132**, 472–473.

Lemstrom, K., Koskinen, P., Krogerus, L., Daemen, M., Bruggeman, C., and Hayry, P. (1995). Cytomegalovirus antigen expression, endothelial cell proliferation, and intimal thickening in rat cardiac allografts after cytomegalovirus infection. *Circulation*, **92**, 2594–2604.

Lemstrom, K., Sihvola, R., Bruggeman, C., Hayry, P., and Koskinen, P. (1997). Cytomegalovirus infection-enhanced cardiac allograft vasculopathy is abolished by DHPG prophylaxis in the rat. *Circulation*, **95**, 2614–2616.

Li, F., Yin, M., Van Dam, J. G., Grauls, G., Rozing, J., and Bruggeman, C. A. (1998). Cytomegalovirus infection enhances the neointima formation in rat aortic allografts: effect of major histocompatibility complex class I and class II antigen differences. *Transplantation*, **65**, 1298–1304.

Liapis, H., Storch, G. A., Hill, D. A., Rueda, J., and Brennan, D. C. (2003). CMV infection of the renal allograft is much more common than the pathology indicates: a retrospective analysis of qualitative and quantitative buffy coat CMV-PCR, renal biopsy pathology and tissue CMV-PCR. *Nephrol. Dial. Transpl.*, **18**, 397–402.

Libby, P. (2002). Inflammation in atherosclerosis. *Nature*, **420**, 868–874.

Libby, P. (2003). Vascular biology of atherosclerosis: overview and state of the art. *Am. J. Cardiol.*, **91**, 3A–6A.

Liesnard, C. A., Revelard, P., and Englert, Y. (1998). Is matching between women and donors feasible to avoid cytomegalovirus infection in artificial insemination with donor semen? [comment]. *Hum. Reprod.*, **13**, 25–31; discussion 32–34.

Ljungman, P. (2002). Beta-herpesvirus challenges in the transplant recipient. *J. Infect. Dis.*, **186**, S99–S109.

Ljungman, P., Griffiths, P., and Paya, C. (2002a). Definitions of cytomegalovirus infection and disease in transplant recipients. *Clin. Infect. Dis.*, **34**, 1094–1097.

Ljungman, P., Larsson, K. Kumlien, G. et al. (2002b). Leukocyte depleted, unscreened blood products give a low risk for CMV infection and disease in CMV seronegative allogeneic stem cell transplant recipients with seronegative stem cell donors. *Scand. J. Infect. Dis.*, **34**, 347–350.

Lockridge, K. M., Sequar, G., Zhou, S. S., Yue, Y., Mandell, C. P., and Barry, P. A. (1999). Pathogenesis of experimental rhesus cytomegalovirus infection. *J. Virol.*, **73**, 9576–9583.

Loebe, M., Schuler, S., Zais, O., Warnecke, H., Fleck, E., and Hetzer, R. (1990). Role of cytomegalovirus infection in the development of coronary artery disease in the transplanted heart. *J. Heart Transpl.*, **9**, 707–711.

MacDonald, M. R., Burney, M. W., Resnick, S. B., and Virgin, H. I. (1999). Spliced mRNA encoding the murine cytomegalovirus chemokine homolog predicts a beta chemokine of novel structure. *J. Virol.*, **73**, 3682–3691.

Maidji, E., Percivalle, E., Gerna, G., Fisher, S., and Pereira, L. (2002). Transmission of human cytomegalovirus from infected uterine microvascular endothelial cells to differentiating/invasive placental cytotrophoblasts. *Virology*, **304**, 53–69.

Margulies, B. J., Browne, H., and Gibson, W. (1996). Identification of the human cytomegalovirus G protein-coupled receptor homologue encoded by UL33 in infected cells and enveloped virus particles. *Virology*, **225**, 111–125.

Mattes, F. M., McLaughlin, J. E., Emery, V. C., Clark, D. A., and Griffiths, P. D. (2000). Histopathological detection of owl's eye inclusions is still specific for cytomegalovirus in the era of human herpesviruses 6 and 7. *J. Clin. Pathol.*, **53**, 612–614.

McDonald, K., Rector, T. S., Braulin, E. A., Kubo, S. H., and Olivari, M. T. (1989). Association of coronary artery disease in cardiac transplant recipients with cytomegalovirus infection. *Am. J. Cardiol.*, **64**, 359–362.

Melnick, J. L., Adam, E., and Debakey, M. E. (1993). Cytomegalovirus and atherosclerosis. *Eur. Heart. J.*, **14**, 30–38.

Menard, C., Wagner, M., Ruzsics, Z. et al. (2003). Role of murine cytomegalovirus US22 gene family members in replication in macrophages. *J. Virol.*, **77**, 5557–5570.

Mendez, J., Espy, M., Smith, T. F., Wilson, J., Wiesner, R., and Paya, C. V. (1998). Clinical significance of viral load in the diagnosis of cytomegalovirus disease after liver transplantation. *Transplantation*, **65**, 1477–1481.

Minamishima, I., Ueda, K., Minematsu, T. et al. (1994). Role of breast milk in acquisition of cytomegalovirus infection. *Microbiol. Immunol.*, **38**, 549–552.

Mitchell, B. M., Leung, A., and Stevens, J. G. (1996). Murine cytomegalovirus DNA in peripheral blood of latently infected mice is detectable only in monocytes and polymorphonuclear leukocytes. *Virology*, **223**, 198–207.

Mocarski, E. S., Jr. (2002). Immunomodulation by cytomegaloviruses: manipulative strategies beyond evasion. *Trends Microbiol.*, **10**, 332–339.

Morgello, S., Cho, E. S., Nielson, S., Devinsky, O., and Petito, C. K. (1987). Cytomegalovirus encephalitis in patients with acquired immunodeficiency syndrome: an autopsy study of 30 cases and a review of the literature. *Hum. Pathol.*, **18**, 289–297.

Moro, D., Lloyd, M. L., Smith, A. L., Shellam, G. R., and Lawson, M. A. (1999). Murine viruses in an island population of introduced house mice and endemic short-tailed mice in Western Australia. *J. Wildlife Dis.*, **35**, 301–310.

Murph, J. R., Bale, J. F., Murray, J. C., Stinski, M. F., and Perlman, S. (1986). Cytomegalovirus transmission in a Midwest day care center: possible relationship to child care practices. *J. Pediatr.*, **109**, 35–39.

Murph, J. R., Baron, J. C., Brown, K., Ebelhack, C. L., and Bale, J. F. (1991). The occupational risk of cytomegalovirus infection among day care providers. *J. Am. Med. Assoc.*, **265**, 603–608.

Mutimer, H. P., Akatsuka, Y., Manley, T. et al. (2002). Association between immune recovery uveitis and a diverse intraocular cytomegalovirus-specific cytotoxic T cell response. *J. Infect. Dis.*, **186**, 701–705.

Myers, J. D., Spencer, H. C., Jr., Watts, J. C. et al. (1975). Cytomegalovirus pneumonia after human marrow transplantation. *Ann. Int. Med.*, **82**, 181–188.

Myerson, D., Hackman, R. C., Nelson, J. A. et al. (1984). Widespread presence of histologically occult cytomegalovirus. *Hum. Pathol.*, **15**, 430–439.

Nichols, W. G. and Boeckh, M. (2000). Recent advances in the therapy and prevention of CMV infections. *J. Clini. Virol.*, **16**, 25–40.

Nichols, W. G., Corey, L., Gooley, T. et al. (2001). Rising pp65 antigenemia during preemptive anticytomegalovirus therapy after allogeneic hematopoietic stem cell transplantation: risk factors, correlation with DNA load, and outcomes. *Blood*, **97**, 867–874.

Nieto, F. J., Adam, E., Sorlie, P. et al. (1996). Cohort study of cytomegalovirus infection as a risk factor for carotid intimalmedial thickening, a measure of subclinical atherosclerosis. *Circulation*, **94**, 922–927.

Noda, S., Aguirre, S. A., Bitmansour, A. et al. (2006) Cytomegalovirus MCK-2 controls mobilization and recruitment of myeloid progenitor cells to facilitate dissemination. *Blood*, **107**, 30–38.

O'Connor, S., Taylor, C., Campbell, L. A., Epstein, S., and Libby, P. (2001). Potential infectious etiologies of atherosclerosis: a multifactorial perspective. *Emerg. Infect. Dis.*, **7**, 780–788.

Odeberg, J., Cerboni, C., Browne, H. et al. (2002). Human cytomegalovirus (HCMV)-infected endothelial cells and macrophages are less susceptible to natural killer lysis independent of the downregulation of classical HLA class I molecules or expression of the HCMV class I homologue, UL18. *Scand. J. Immunol.*, **55**, 149–161.

Oliveira, S. A. and Shenk, T. E. (2001). Murine cytomegalovirus M78 protein, a G protein-coupled receptor homologue, is a constituent of the virion and facilitates accumulation of immediate-early viral mRNA. *Proc. Natl Acad. Sci. USA*, **98**, 3237–3242.

Paloheimo, J. A., von Essen, R., Klemola, E., Kaariainen, L., and Siltanen, P. (1968). Subclinical cytomegalovirus infections and cytomegalovirus mononucleosis after open heart surgery. *Am. J. Cardiol.*, **22**, 624–630.

Pass, R. F., Stagno, S., Myers, G. J., and Alford, C. A. (1980). Outcome of symptomatic congenital CMV infection: results of long-term longitudinal follow-up. *Pediatrics*, **66**, 758–762.

Pass, R. F., August, A. M., Dworsky, M. E., and Reynolds, D. W. (1982a). Cytomegalovirus infection in a day care center. *N. Engl. J. Med.*, **307**, 477–479.

Pass, R. F., Stagno, S., Dworsky, M. E., Smith, R. J., and Alford, C. A. (1982b). Excretion of cytomegalovirus in mothers: observation after delivery of congenitally infected and normal infants. *J. Infect. Dis.*, **146**, 1–6.

Pass, R. F., Hutto, C., Reynolds, D. W., and Polhill, R. B. (1984). Increased frequency of cytomegalovirus in children in group day care. *Pediatrics*, **74**, 121–126.

Pass, R. F., Hutto, S. C., Ricks, R., and Cloud, G. A. (1986). Increased rate of cytomegalovirus infection among parents of children attending day care centers. *N. Engl. J. Med.*, **314**, 1414–1418.

Pass, R. F., Little, E. A., Stagno, S., Britt, W. J., and Alford, C. A. (1987). Young children as a probable source of maternal and congenital cytomegalovirus infection. *N. Engl. J. Med.*, **316**, 1366–1370.

Pass, R. F., Hutto, C., Lyon, M. D., and Cloud, G. (1990). Increased rate of cytomegalovirus infection among day care center workers. *Pediatr. Infect. Dis. J.*, **9**, 465–470.

Pecorella, I., Ciardi, A., Garner, A., McCartney, A. C., and Lucas, S. (2000). Postmortem histological survey of the ocular lesions in a British population of AIDS patients. *Br. J. Ophthalmol.*, **84**, 1275–1281.

Penfold, M. E., Dairaghi, D. J., Duke, G. M. *et al.* (1999). Cytomegalovirus encodes a potent alpha chemokine. *Proc. Natl Acad. Sci. USA*, **96**, 9839–9844.

Penfold, M. E., Schmidt, T. L., Dairaghi, D. J., Barry, P. A., and Schall, T. J. (2003). Characterization of the rhesus cytomegalovirus US28 locus. *J. Virol.*, **77**, 10404–10413.

Pepose, J. S., Holland, G. N., Nestor, M. S., Cochran, A. J., and Foos, R. Y. (1985). Acquired immune deficiency syndrome. Pathogenic mechanisms of ocular disease. *Ophthalmology*, **92**, 472–484.

Pepose, J. S., Newman, C., Bach, M. C. *et al.* (1987). Pathologic features of cytomegalovirus retinopathy after treatment with the antiviral agent ganciclovir. *Ophthalmology*, **94**, 414–424.

Percivalle, E., Revello, M. G., Vago, L., Morini, F., and Gerna, G. (1993). Circulating endothelial giant cells permissive for human cytomegalovirus (HCMV) are detected in disseminated HCMV infections with organ involvement. *J. Clin. Invest.*, **92**, 663–670.

Perlman, J. M. and Argyle, C. (1992). Lethal cytomegalovirus infection in preterm infants: clinical, radiological, and neuropathological findings. *Ann. Neurol.*, **31**, 64–68.

Peterson, P. K., Balfour, H. H., Marker, S. C. *et al.* (1980). Cytomegalovirus disease in renal allograft recipients: a prospective study of the clinical features, risk factors and impact on renal transplantation. *Medicine*, **59**, 283–300.

Petrie, B. L., Adam, E., and Melnick, J. L. (1988). Association of herpesvirus/cytomegalovirus infections with human atherosclerosis. *Progr. Med. Virol.*, **35**, 21–42.

Plachter, B., Sinzger, C., and Jahn, G. (1996). Cell types involved in replication and distribution of human cytomegalovirus. *Adv. Virus Res.*, **46**, 195–261.

Plotkin, S. A., Starr, S. E., Friedman, H. M. *et al.* (1989). Protective effects of Towne cytomegalovirus vaccine against low-passage cytomegalovirus administered as a challenge. *J. Infect. Dis.*, **159**, 860–865.

Plotkin, S. A., Starr, S. E., Friedman, H. M. *et al.* (1991). Effect of Towne live virus vaccine on cytomegalovirus disease after renal transplant. A controlled trial. *Ann. Intern. Med.*, **114**, 525–531.

Pooley, R. J., Jr., Peterson, L., Finn, W. G., and Kroft, S. H. (1999). Cytomegalovirus-infected cells in routinely prepared peripheral blood films of immunosuppressed patients. *Am. J. Clin. Pathol.*, **112**, 108–112.

Prince, A. M., Szumuness, W., Millian, S. J., and David, D. S. (1971). A serologic study of cytomegalovirus infections associated with blood transfusions. *N. Engl. J. Med.*, **284**, 1125–1131.

Randolph-Habecker, J. R., Rahill, B., Torok-Storb, B. *et al.* (2002). The expression of the cytomegalovirus chemokine receptor homolog US28 sequesters biologically active CC chemokines and alters IL-8 production. *Cytokine*, **19**, 37–46.

Rapp, F. and Robbins, D. (1984). Cytomegalovirus and human cancer. *Birth Defects: Original Article Series*, **20**, 175–192.

Reddehase, M. J., Balthesen, M., Rapp, M., Jonjic, S., Pavic, I., and Koszinowski, U. H. (1994). The conditions of primary infection define the load of latent viral genome in organs and the risk of recurrent cytomegalovirus disease. *J. Exp. Med.*, **179**, 185–193.

Reddehase, M. J., Podlech, J., and Grzimek, N. K. (2002). Mouse models of cytomegalovirus latency: overview. *J. Clin. Virol.*, **25**, S23–S36.

Redman, T. K., Britt, W. J., Wilcox, C. M., Graham, M. F., and Smith, P. D. (2002). Human cytomegalovirus enhances chemokine production by lipopolysaccharide-stimulated lamina propria macrophages. *J. Infect. Dis.*, **185**, 584–590.

Reed, E. C., Wolford, J. L., Kopecky, K. J., Lilleby, K. E., Dandliker, P. S., and Todaro, J. L. (1990). Ganciclovir for the treatment of cytomegalovirus gastroenteritis in bone marrow transplant patients. A randomized, placebo-controlled trial. *Ann. Intern. Med.*, **112**, 505–510.

Reyman, T. A. (1966). Postperfusion syndrome: a review and report of 21 cases. *Am. Heart J.*, **72**, 116–123.

Reynolds, D. W., Stagno, S., Hosty, T. S., Tiller, M., and Alford, C. A. (1973). Maternal cytomegalovirus excretion and perinatal infection. *N. Engl. J. Med.*, **289**, 1–5.

Ribalta, T., Martinez, A. J., Jares, P. *et al.* (2002). Presence of occult cytomegalovirus infection in the brain after orthotopic liver transplantation. An autopsy study of 83 cases. [see comment]. *Virchows Arch.*, **440**, 166–171.

Ribbert, D. (1904). Uber protozoenartige zellen in der niere eines syphilitischen neugoborenen und in der parotis von kindern. *Zentralbl. Allg. Pathol.*, **15**, 945–948.

Rice, G. P. A., Schrier, R. D., and Oldstone, M. B. A. (1984). Cytomegalovirus infects human lymphocytes and monocytes: virus expression is restricted to immediate-early gene products. *Proc. Natl. Acad. Sci. USA*, **81**, 6134.

Richardson, W. P., Colvin, R. B., Cheeseman, S. H. *et al.* (1981). Glomerulopathy associated with cytomegalovirus viremia in renal allografts. *N. Engl. J. Med.*, **305**, 57–63.

Riegler, S., Hebart, H., Einsele, H., Brossart, P., Jahn, G., and Sinzger, C. (2000). Monocyte-derived dendritic cells are permissive to the complete replicative cycle of human cytomegalovirus. *J. Gen. Virol.*, **81**, 393–399.

Rifkind, D. (1965). Cytomegalovirus infection after renal transplantation. *Arch. Intern. Med.*, **116**, 554–558.

Rinaldo, C. R., Jr., Kingsley, L. A., Ho, M., Armstrong, J. A., and Zhou, S. Y. (1992). Enhanced shedding of cytomegalovirus in semen of human immunodeficiency virus-seropositive homosexual men. *J. Clin. Microbiol.*, **30**, 1148–1155.

Roback, J. D., Hillyer, C. D., Drew, W. L. *et al.* (2001). Multicenter evaluation of PCR methods for detecting CMV DNA in blood donors. *Transfusion.*, **41**, 1249–1257.

Rosenkilde, M. M., Waldhoer, M., Luttichau, H. R., and Schwartz, T. W. (2001). Virally encoded 7TM receptors. *Oncogene*, **20**, 1582–1593.

Rubin, R. H. (1990). Impact of cytomegalovirus infection on organ transplant recipients. *Rev. Infect. Dis.*, **12**, S754–S766.

Rubin, R. (2002). Clinical approach to infection in the compromised host, In *Infection in the Organ Transplant Recipient*, ed. R. Rubin, pp. 573–679 New York: Kluwer Academic Press.

Rubin, R. H. and Colvin, R. B. (1986). Cytomegalovirus infection in renal transplantation: clinical importance and control. In *Kidney Transplant Rejection: Diagnosis and Treatment*, ed. G. M. Williams, J. F. Burdick, and K. Solez, pp. 283–304. New York: Dekker.

Rubin, R. H., Russell, P. S., Levin, M., and Cohen, C. (1979). From the National Institutes of Health. Summary of a workshop on cytomegalovirus infections during organ transplantation. *J. Infect. Dis.*, **139**, 728–734.

Rubin, R. H., Wolfson, J. S., Cosimi, A. B. *et al.* (1981). Infection in the renal transplant recipient. *Am. J. Med.*, **70**, 405–411.

Saederup, N., Lin, Y. C., Dairaghi, D. J., Schall, T. J., and Mocarski, E. S. (1999). Cytomegalovirus-encoded beta chemokine promotes monocyte-associated viremia in the host. *Proc. Natl Acad. Sci. USA*, **96**, 10881–10886.

Saederup, N., Aguirre, S. A., Sparer, T. E., Bouley, D. M., and Mocarski, E. S. (2001). Murine cytomegalovirus CC chemokine homolog MCK-2 (m131–129) is a determinant of dissemination that increases inflammation at initial sites of infection. *J. Virol.*, **75**, 9966–9976.

Saederup, N. and Mocarski, E. S. Jr, (2002). Fatal attraction: cytomegalovirus-encoded chemokine homologs. *Curr. Top. Microbiol. Immunol.*, **269**, 235–256.

Salzberger, B., Myerson, D., and Boeckh, M. (1997). Circulating cytomegalovirus (CMV)-infected endothelial cells in marrow transplant patients with CMV disease and CMV infection. *J. Infect. Dis.*, **176**, 778–781.

Schafer, P., Tenschert, W., Cremaschi, L., Schroter, M., Gutensohn, K., and Laufs, R. (2000). Cytomegalovirus cultured from different major leukocyte subpopulations: association with clinical features in CMV immunoglobulin G-positive renal allograft recipients. *J. Med. Virol.*, **61**, 488–496.

Schmidbauer, M., Budka, H., Ulrich, W., and Ambros, P. (1989). Cytomegalovirus (CMV) disease of the brain in AIDS and connatal infection: a comparative study by histology, immunocytochemistry and in situ DNA hybridization. *Acta Neuropathol. (Berl.)*, **79**, 286–293.

Schmidt, G. M., Horak, D. A., Niland, J. C., Duncan, S. R., Forman, S. J., and Zaia, J. A. (1991). A randomized, controlled trial of prophylactic ganciclovir for cytomegalovirus pulmonary infection in recipients of allogeneic bone marrow transplants; The City of Hope-Stanford-Syntex CMV Study Group. *N. Engl. J. Med.*, **324**, 1005–1011.

Sedmak, D. D., Knight, D. A., Vook, N. C., and Waldman, J. W. (1994). Divergent patterns of ELAM-1, ICAM-1, and VCAM-1 expression on cytomegalovirus-infected endothelial cells. *Transplantation*, **58**, 1379–1385.

Selik, R. M., Chu, S. Y., and Ward, J. W. (1996). Trends in infectious diseases and cancers among persons dying of HIV infection in the United States from 1987 to 1992. *Ann. Intern. Med.*, **123**, 933–936.

Sequar, G., Britt, W. J., Lakeman, F. D. *et al.* (2002). Experimental coinfection of rhesus macaques with rhesus cytomegalovirus and simian immunodeficiency virus: pathogenesis. *J. Virol.*, **76**, 7661–7671.

Shen, C. Y., Ho, M. S., Chang, S. F. *et al.* (1993). High rate of concurrent genital infections with human cytomegalovirus and human papillomaviruses in cervical cancer patients. *J. Infect. Dis.*, **168**, 449–452.

Shen, Y., Zhu, H., and Shenk, T. (1997). Human cytomagalovirus IE1 and IE2 proteins are mutagenic and mediate "hit-and-run" oncogenic transformation in cooperation with the adenovirus E1A proteins. *Proc. Natl Acad. Sci. USA*, **94**, 3341–3345.

Sinclair, J. and Sissons, P. (1996). Latent and persistent infections of monocytes and macrophages. *Intervirology*, **39**, 293–301.

Singh, N., Dummer, J. S., Kusne, S. *et al.* (1988). Infections with cytomegalovirus and other herpesviruses in 121 liver transplant recipients: transmission by donated organ and the effect of OKT3 antibodies. *J. Infect. Dis.*, **158**, 124–131.

Singh, N., Paterson, D. L., Gayowski, T., Wagener, M. M., and Marino, I. R. (2000). Cytomegalovirus antigenemia directed pre-emptive prophylaxis with oral versus I.V. ganciclovir for the prevention of cytomegalovirus disease in liver transplant recipients: a randomized, controlled trial. *Transplantation*, **70**, 717–722.

Sinzger, C. and Jahn, G. (1996). Human cytomegalovirus cell tropism and pathogenesis. *Intervirology*, **39**, 302–319.

Sinzger, C., Grefte, A., Plachter, B., Gouw, A. S., The, T. H., and Jahn, G. (1995). Fibroblasts, epithelial cells, endothelial cells and smooth muscle cells are major targets of human cytomegalovirus infection in lung and gastrointestinal tissues. *J. Gen. Virol.*, **76**, 741–750.

Sinzger, C., Knapp, J., Plachter, B., Schmidt, K., and Jahn, G. (1997). Quantification of replication of clinical cytomegalovirus isolates in cultured endothelial cells and fibroblasts by a focus expansion assay. *J. Virol. Methods*, **63**, 103–112.

Sinzger, C., Schmidt, K., Knapp, J. *et al.* (1999). Modification of human cytomegalovirus tropism through propagation in vitro is associated with changes in the viral genome. *J. Gen. Virol.*, **80**, 2867–2877.

Sinzger, C., Kahl, M., Laib, K. *et al.* (2000). Tropism of human cytomegalovirus for endothelial cells is determined by a post-entry step dependent on efficient translocation to the nucleus. *J. Gen. Virol.*, **81**, 3021–3035.

Soderberg-Naucler, C. and Emery, V. C. (2001). Viral infections and their impact on chronic renal allograft dysfunction. *Transplantation.*, **71**, SS224–SS230.

Soderberg-Naucler, C., Fish, K. N., and Nelson, J. A. (1997). Reactivation of latent human cytomegalovirus by allogeneic stimulation of blood cells from healthy donors. *Cell*, **91**, 119–126.

Soderberg-Naucler, C., Fish, K. N., and Nelson, J. A. (1998). Growth of human cytomegalovirus in primary macrophages. *Methods (Duluth)*, **16**, 126–138.

Soderberg-Naucler, C., Streblow, D. N., Fish, K. N., Allan-Yorke, J., Smith, P. P., and Nelson, J. A. (2001). Reactivation of latent human cytomegalovirus in CD14(+) monocytes is differentiation dependent. *J. Virol.*, **75**, 7543–7554.

Sohn, Y. M., Oh, M. K., Balcarek, K. B., Cloud, G. A., and Pass, R. F. (1991). Cytomegalovirus infection in sexually active adolescents. *J. Infect. Dis.*, **163**, 460–463.

Spector, S. A. and Spector, D. H. (1982). Molecular epidemiology of cytomegalovirus infections in premature twin infants and their mother. *Pediatr. Infect. Dis. J.*, **1**, 405–409.

Spector, S. A., Hirata, K. K., and Newman, T. R. (1984). Identification of multiple cytomegalovirus strains in homosexual men with acquired immunodeficiency syndrome. *J. Infect. Dis.*, **150**, 953–956.

Spector, S. A., Wong, R., Hsia, K., Pilcher, M., and Stempien, M. J. (1998). Plasma cytomegalovirus (CMV) DNA load predicts CMV disease and survival in AIDS patients. *J. Clin. Invest.*, **101**, 497–502.

Spector, S. A., Hsia, K., Crager, M., Pilcher, M., Cabral, S., and Stempien, M. J. (1999). Cytomegalovirus (CMV) DNA load is an independent predictor of CMV disease and survival in advanced AIDS. *J. Virol.*, **73**, 7027–7030.

Speir, E., Modali, R., Huang, E. S. *et al.* (1994). Potential role of human cytomegalovirus and p53 interaction in coronary restenosis. *Science*, **265**, 391–394.

Speir, E., Yu, Z. X., Ferrans, V. J., Huang, E. S., and Epstein, S. E. (1998). Aspirin attenuates cytomegalovirus infectivity and gene expression mediated by cyclooxygenase-2 in coronary artery smooth muscle cells. *Circ. Res.*, **83**, 210–216.

Spencer, J. V., Lockridge, K. M., Barry, P. A. *et al.* (2002). Potent immunosuppressive activities of cytomegalovirus-encoded interleukin-10. *J. Virol.*, **76**, 1285–1292.

Stagno, S. (1995). Cytomegalovirus, In *Infectious Diseases of the Fetus and Newborn Infant*, 4th ed, ed. J. S. Remington and J. O. Klein, pp. 312–353. Philadelphia: W.B. Saunders.

Stagno, S., Reynolds, D. W., Tsiantos, A. *et al.* (1975a). Cervical cytomegalovirus excretion in pregnant and nonpregnant women: suppression in early gestation. *J. Infect. Dis.*, **131**, 522–527.

Stagno, S., Reynolds, D. W., Tsiantos, A., Fucillo, D. A., Long, W., and Alford, C. A. (1975b). Comparative, serial virologic and serologic studies of symptomatic and subclinical congenital and natally acquired cytomegalovirus infection. *J. Infect. Dis.*, **132**, 568–577.

Stagno, S., Reynolds, D. W., Amos, C. S. *et al.* (1977). Auditory and visual defects resulting from symptomatic and subclinical congenital cytomegaloviral and toxoplasma infections. *Pediatrics*, **59**, 669–678.

Stagno, S., Reynolds, D. W., Pass, R. F., and Alford, C. A. (1980). Breast milk and the risk of cytomegalovirus infection. *N. Engl. J. Med.*, **302**, 1073–1076.

Stagno, S., Pass, R. F., Dworsky, M. E. *et al.* (1982). Congenital cytomegalovirus infection: the relative importance of primary and recurrent maternal infection. *N. Engl. J. Med.*, **306**, 945–949.

Stagno, S., Pass, R. F., Dworsky, M. E., and Alford, C. A. (1983). Congenital and perinatal cytomegaloviral infections. *Semin. Perinatol.*, **7**, 31–42.

Stevens, D. P., Barker, L. F., Ketcham, A. S., and Meyer, H. M. (1970). Asymptomatic cytomegalovirus infection following blood transfusion in tumor surgery. *J. Am. Med. Assoc.*, **211**, 1341–1344.

Stoddart, C. A., Cardin, R. D., Boname, J. M., Manning, W. C., Abenes, G. B., and Mocarski, E. S. (1994). Peripheral blood mononuclear phagocytes mediate dissemination of murine cytomegalovirus. *J. Virol.*, **68**, 6243–6253.

Streblow, D. N., Soderberg-Naucler, C., Vieira, J. *et al.* (1999). The human cytomegalovirus chemokine receptor US28 mediates vascular smooth muscle cell migration. *Cell.*, **99**, 511–520.

Streblow, D. N., Orloff, S. L., and Nelson, J. A. (2001). Do pathogens accelerate atherosclerosis? *J. Nutrit.*, **131**, 2798S–2804S.

Streblow, D. N., Kreklywich, C., Yin, Q. *et al.* (2003). Cytomegalovirus-mediated upregulation of chemokine expression correlates with the acceleration of chronic rejection in rat heart transplants. *J. Virol.*, **77**, 2182–2194.

Taber, L. H., Frank, A. L., Yow, M. D., and Bagley, A. (1985). Acquisition of cytomegaloviral infections in families with young children: a serological study. *J. Infect. Dis.*, **151**, 948–952.

Taylor, P. M., Rose, M. L., Yacoub, M. H., and Pigott, R. (1992). Induction of vascular adhesion molecules during rejection of human cardiac allografts. *Transplantation*, **54**, 451–457.

Taylor-Wiedeman, J., Sissons, J. G., Borysiewicz, L. K., and Sinclair, J. H. (1991). Monocytes are a major site of persistence of human cytomegalovirus in peripheral blood mononuclear cells. *J. Gen. Virol.*

Taylor-Wiedeman, J., Sissons, P., and Sinclair, J. (1994). Induction of endogenous human cytomegalovirus gene expression after differentiation of monocytes from healthy carriers. *J. Virol.*, **68**, 1597–1604.

The, T. H., van der Bij, W., van den Berg, A. P. *et al.* (1990). Cytomegalovirus antigenemia. *Rev. Infect. Dis.*, **12(S)**, 734–744.

Tolkoff-Rubin, N. E., Fishman, J. A., and Rubin, R. H. (2001). The bidirectional relationship between cytomegalovirus and allograft injury. *Transpl. Proc.*, **33**, 1773–1775.

Valantine, H. A., Gao, S. Z., Menon, S. G. *et al.* (1999). Impact of prophylactic immediate posttransplant ganciclovir on development of transplant atherosclerosis: a post hoc analysis of a randomized, placebo-controlled study. *Circulation*, **100**, 61–66.

Valantine, H. A., Luikart, H., Doyle, R. *et al.* (2001). Impact of Cytomegalovirus hyperimmune globulin on outcome after cardiothoracic transplantation: a comparative study of combined prophylaxis with CMV hyperimmune globulin plus ganciclovir versus ganciclovir alone. *Transplantation*, **72**, 1647–1852.

Van Dam-Mieras, M. C., Bruggeman, C. A., Muller, A. D., Debie, W. H., and Zwaal, R. F. (1987). Induction of endothelial cell procoagulant activity by cytomegalovirus infection. *Thromb. Res.*, **47**, 69–75.

van der Bij, W., Schirm, J., Torensma, R., van Son, W. J., Tegzess, A. M., and The, T. H. (1988). Comparison between viremia and antigenemia for detection of cytomegalovirus in blood. *J. Clin. Microbiol.*, **26**, 2531–2535.

Vinters, H. V., Kwok, M. K., Ho, H. W. *et al.* (1989). Cytomegalovirus in the nervous system of patients with the acquired immune deficiency syndrome. *Brain*,

Vochem, M., Hamprecht, K., Jahn, G., and Speer, C. P. (1998). Transmission of cytomegalovirus to preterm infants through breast milk. *Pediatr. Infect. Dis. J.*, **17**, 53–58.

Vossen, R. C., van Dam-Mieras, M. C., and Bruggeman, C. A. (1996). Cytomegalovirus infection and vessel wall pathology. *Intervirology*, **39**, 213–221.

Waldhoer, M., Kledal, T. N., Farrell, H., and Schwartz, T. W. (2002). Murine cytomegalovirus (CMV) M33 and human CMV US28 receptors exhibit similar constitutive signaling activities. *J. Virol.*, **76**, 8161–8168.

Waldman, W. J. and Knight, D. A. (1996). Cytokine-mediated induction of endothelial adhesion molecule and histocompatibility leukocyte antigen expression by cytomegalovirus-activated T cells. *Am. J. Pathol.*, **148**, 105–119.

Waldman, W. J., Roberts, W. H., Davis, D. H., Williams, M. V. Sedmak, D. D., and Stephens, R. E. (1991). Preservation of natural endothelial cytopathogenicity of cytomegalovirus by propagation in endothelial cells. *Arch. Virol.*, **117**, 143–164.

Waldman, W. J., Knight, D. A., Huang, E. H., and Sedmak, D. D. (1995). Bidirectional transmission of infectious cytomegalovirus between monocytes and vascular endothelial cells: an in vitro model. *J. Infect. Dis.*, **171**, 263–272.

Walter, E. A., Greenberg, P. D., Gilbert, M. J. *et al.* (1995). Reconstitution of cellular immunity against cytomegalovirus in recipients of allogeneic bone marrow by transfer of T-cell clones from the donor. *N. Engl. J. Med.*, **333**, 1038–1044.

Waner, J. L., Hopkins, D. R., Weller, T. H., and Allard, E. N. (1977). Cervical excretion of cytomegalovirus: correlation with secretory and humoral antibody. *J. Infect. Dis.*, **136**, 805–809.

Wang, D. and Shenk, T. (2005a). Human cytomegaloviruses virion protein complex required for epithelial and edothelial cell tropism. *Proc. Nat. Acad. Sci. USA*, **102**, 18153–18158.

Wang, D. and Shenk T. (2005b). Human cytomegaloviruses UL131 open reading frame is required of epithelial cell tropism. *J. Virol.*, **79**, 10330–10338.

Weller, T. H. (1971). The cytomegaloviruses: ubiquitous agents with protean clinical manifestations. *N. Engl. J. Med.*, **285**, 203–214.

Wilcox, C. M., Chalasani, N., Lazenby, A., and Schwartz, D. A. (1998). Cytomegalovirus colitis in acquired immunodeficiency syndrome: a clinical and endoscopic study. *Gastrointest. Endosc.*, **48**, 39–43.

Wiley, C. A. and Nelson, J. A. (1988). Role of human immunodeficiency virus and cytomegalovirus in AIDS encephalitis. *Am. J. Pathol.*, **133**, 73–81.

Williamson, W. D., Desmond, M. M., LaFevers, N., Taber, L. H., Catlin, F. I., and Weaver, T. G. (1982). Symptomatic congenital cytomegalovirus: disorders of language, learning and hearing. *Am. J. Dis. Child.*, **136**, 902–905.

Williamson, W. D., Demmler, G. J., Percy, A. K., and Catlin, F. I. (1992). Progressive hearing loss in infants with asymptomatic congenital cytomegalovirus infection. *Pediatrics*, **90**, 862–866.

Winston, D. J., Gale, R. P., Meyers, D. V. *et al.* (1979). Infectious complications of human bone marrow transplantation. *Medicine*, **58**, 1–31.

Winston, D. J., Ho, W. G., Bartoni, K. *et al.* (1993). Ganciclovir prophylaxis of cytomegalovirus infection and disease in allogeneic bone marrow transplant recipients. Results of a placebo-controlled, double-blind trial. *Ann. Intern. Med.*, **118**, 179–184.

Wu, T. C., Hruban, R. H., Ambinder, R. F. *et al.* (1992). Demonstration of cytomegalovirus nucleic acids in the coronary arteries of transplanted hearts. *Am. J. Pathol.*, **140**, 739–747.

Yang, Y. S., Ho, H. N., Chen, H. F. *et al.* (1995). Cytomegalovirus infection and viral shedding in the genital tract of infertile couples. *J. Med. Virol.*, **45**, 179–182.

Yeager, A. S. (1975). Longitudinal, serological study of cytomegalovirus infections in nurses and in personnel without patient contact. *J. Clin. Microbiol.*, **2**, 448–450.

Yeager, A. S. (1983). Transmission of cytomegalovirus to mothers by infected infants: another reason to prevent transfusion-acquired infections. *Pediatr. Infect. Dis.*, **2**, 295.

Yeager, A. S., Grumet, F. C., Hafleigh, E. B., Arvin, A. M., Bradley, J. S., and Prober, C. G. (1981). Prevention of transfusion-acquired cytomegalovirus infections in newborn infants. *J. Pediatr.*, **98**, 281–287.

Yilmaz, S., Koskinen, P. K., Kallio, E., Bruggeman, C. A., Hayry, P. J., and Lemstrom, K. B. (1996). Cytomegalovirus infection-enhanced chronic kidney allograft rejection is linked with intercellular adhesion molecule-1 expression. *Kidney Int.*, **50**, 526–537.

Zhou, Y. F., Leon, M. B., Waclawiw, M. A. *et al.* (1996). Association between prior cytomegalovirus infection and the risk of restenosis after coronary atherectomy. *N. Engl. J. Med.*, **335**, 624–630.

Zhou, Y. F., Shou, M., Guetta, E. *et al.* (1999). Cytomegalovirus infection of rats increases the neointimal response to vascular injury without consistent evidence of direct infection of the vascular wall. *Circulation*, **100**, 1569–1575.

Zhu, H., Shen, Y., and Shenk, T. (1995). Human cytomegalovirus IE1 and IE2 proteins block apoptosis. *J. Virol.*, **69**, 7960–7970.

Zhu, H., Cong, J. P., Bresnahan, W. A., and Shenk, T. E, (2002). Inhibition of cyclooxygenase 2 blocks human cytomegalovirus replication. *Proc. Natl Acad. Sci. USA*, **99**, 3932–3937.

Zhu, J., Quyyumi, A. A., Norman, J. E., Csako, G., and Epstein, S. E. (1999). Cytomegalovirus in the pathogenesis of atherosclerosis: the role of inflammation as reflected by elevated C-reactive protein levels. *J. Am. Coll. Cardiol.*, **34**, 1738–1743.

Molecular basis of persistence and latency

Michael A. Jarvis[1] and Jay A. Nelson[1,2]

[1]Vaccine and Gene Therapy Institute, Oregon Health Science University, Portland, OR, USA
[2]Department of Molecular Microbiology and Immunology, Oregon Health Sciences University, Portland, OR, USA

Introduction

Human cytomegalovirus (HCMV) is an ubiquitous β-herpesvirus that establishes a lifelong infection within the host. Although HCMV is generally asymptomatic within the normal individual, the virus causes severe and incapacitating disease in immune compromised patients (Pass, 2001). A critical component for HCMV persistence in the non-immune compromised host is the ability of the virus to establish cellular sites of latency as well as persistent infection. During latency, the HCMV genome is maintained within the cell with limited viral gene expression reactivating virus upon cellular stimulation. In HCMV persistent infection, infectious virus is continually produced in the cell with minimal cytopathic effect thereby enabling long-term infection. Endothelial cells (ECs) and specific subpopulations of the myeloid lineage are believed to represent important sites of persistent HCMV replication and latency, respectively. Recent studies of HCMV and the closely related murine cytomegalovirus (MCMV) are beginning to identify the virally encoded genetic determinants required for replication in these cell types. The establishment of latent infection in myeloid cells that are critical cellular components of the host immune system, also closely interconnects HCMV and the host immune response. This chapter will focus on the role of ECs and myeloid cells as sites of CMV persistent replication and latency, and the viral mechanisms that modulate cellular functions to ensure survival and reactivation within the host.

Sites of HCMV persistence and latency

HCMV infects many different cell types within the host, including: ECs, monocyte-derived macrophages (MDM), smooth muscle cells (SMCs), epithelial cells, fibroblasts, T-lymphocytes, granulocytes, stromal cells, neuronal cells and hepatocytes (Dankner *et al.*, 1990; Einhorn & Ost, 1984; Gnann *et al.*, 1985; Howell *et al.*, 1979; Myerson *et al.*, 1984; Schreier *et al.*, 1985; Sinzger *et al.*, 1995; Soderberg *et al.*, 1993; Wiley and Nelson, 1988). Recent studies have implicated ECs and specific cell types of the myeloid lineage [CD34+ hematopoietic progenitors, CD33+ granulocyte-macrophage progenitors (GM-Ps) and MDM] as critical sites of HCMV persistence and latency. The utilization of these sites as viral reservoirs appears to play an important role in enabling the virus to establish lifelong infection within the host. However, identification of these cell types as viral reservoirs does not preclude the existence of other sites of virus persistence within the host. For example, HCMV DNA has been identified in SMCs from the large arteries of healthy seropositive individuals (Gyorkey *et al.*, 1984; Hendrix *et al.*, 1989, 1990; Petrie *et al.*, 1987; Yamashiroya *et al.*, 1988). The absence of detectable viral gene expression in these HCMV DNA positive cells suggests that SMCs may represent a site of HCMV latency. The high incidence of HCMV transmission following bone marrow transplantation (BMT) (Ho, 1990) indicates that bone marrow stromal cells may also be a site of latency or persistent HCMV replication (Mayerson *et al.*, 1984). This observation is further supported by the ability to isolate infectious virus from the stroma of patients with HCMV disease, as well as the capacity to productively infect stromal cells with HCMV in vitro (Simmons *et al.*, 1990; Torok-Storb *et al.*, 1992). However, bone marrow stroma is composed of many different cell types, and ECs and myeloid progenitor cells within this heterogeneous population may actually represent the sites of virus persistence.

ECs are a site of persistent HCMV replication

ECs form the inner lining of blood vessels and are involved in a variety of processes regulating tissue homeostasis and

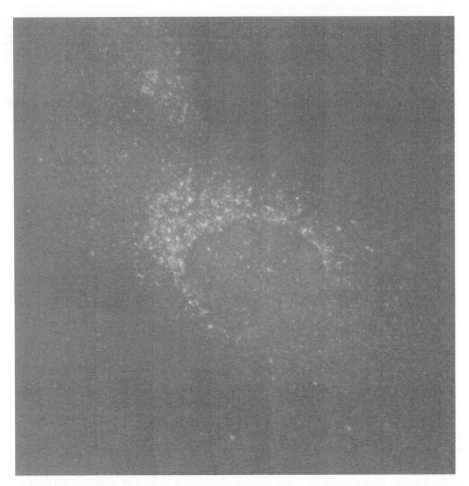

Fig. 42.1. Immunofluorescent micrograph of HCMV-infected AEC. Telomerase life-extended human AEC were infected with HCMV. Cells were fixed and stained for the presence of HCMV protein, glycoprotein B (a late product; green) and a cellular marker of the *trans*-Golgi network (TGN46; red). (See color plate section.)

inflammation. Results from a number of studies investigating the growth of HCMV in ECs have suggested a role for this cell type as an important reservoir of HCMV in the host (Fig. 42.1). The ability to infect cells with induction of minimal cytopathology is a critical requirement for a site of viral persistence. This virus-host cell interaction enables a persistent productive infection to be established for extended periods without cell death. Consistent with this requirement, early histological studies of BMT patients with acute HCMV disease showed that, in many cases, HCMV infection produced only minimal cytopathology in ECs (Friedman *et al.*, 1981). Subsequent studies identifying HCMV in the vessel walls of healthy individuals indicated that ECs also represented a site of persistent infection in individuals with normal immune function (Hendrix *et al.*, 1989; Pampou *et al.*, 2000; Smiley *et al.*, 1988; Speir *et al.*, 1994).

Recent studies have added considerably to our understanding of HCMV growth in ECs. ECs exhibit phenotypic differences that are dependent on the source (adult vs. fetal), vessel size (micro- vs. macrovascular) and anatomical location of the ECs (Page *et al.*, 1992; Turner *et al.*, 1987). Recent phage display-based assays using phage libraries expressing random peptides further emphasize the remarkable level of EC diversity, with ECs from different vascular beds expressing unique tissue-specific molecules (Rajotte *et al.*, 1998). EC origin also has a major influence on characteristics of HCMV replication. Studies comparing HCMV infection in human brain microvascular ECs (BMVEC) and macrovascular aortic ECs (AEC) have shown that HCMV replication differs significantly in these two cell types (Fish *et al.*, 1998). BMVEC, which together with astrocytes compose the blood brain barrier, possess specific transporter systems to allow the transfer of specific metabolites from the blood to the brain parenchyma. Due to these specialized functional requirements, BMVEC are functionally and biochemically distinct from AEC (Joo, 1992; Moses & Nelson, 1994; Page *et al.*, 1992; Turner *et al.*, 1987). Although both BMVEC and AEC express viral proteins and support HCMV replication, virus fails to accumulate intracellularly in AEC resulting in a reduced level of cell-associated compared to supernatant virus (Fish *et al.*, 1998). In contrast, virus accumulates intracellularly in BMVEC resulting in comparable levels of cell-associated and supernatant virus. This difference in the distribution of virus corresponds to HCMV infection resulting in a lytic infection in BMVEC, but not AEC, suggesting that efficient removal of mature intracellular virions (by either export or degradation) may enable prolonged cell survival. Importantly, this ability of HCMV to produce a persistent long-term productive infection in AEC suggests that AEC may represent a site of persistence within the host.

Differences between individual HCMV strains also have a profound influence on HCMV growth in ECs. Results from a number of laboratories suggest that EC and non-EC tropic HCMV strains are comparable in their ability to enter ECs. However, non-EC strains appear to be deficient in the ability to translocate the viral genome to the nucleus (Bolovan-Fritts and Wiedeman, 2001; Sinzger *et al.*, 2000; Slobbe-van Drunen *et al.*, 1998). Interpretation of results from these studies has been complicated by observed differences in the capacity of even identical strains of HCMV to replicate in ECs (Bolovan-Fritts and Wiedeman, 2001; Kahl *et al.*, 2000). These discrepancies may result from differences in virus preparation and EC culture or HCMV strain derivation. For example, when compared to the United Kingdom (UK) strain, the same HCMV laboratory strain from the American Tissue Culture Collection (ATCC) was shown to differ by the presence of a 929-bp genomic region (Dargan *et al.*, 1997; Mocarski *et al.*, 1997). The cloning of an increasing number of HCMV strains as genetically stable bacterial artificial chromosomes (BACs) is overcoming many of these technical problems and is beginning to facilitate the identification of genetic determinants of HCMV EC tropism (Borst *et al.*, 1999; Hahn *et al.*, 2002, 2003; Marchini *et al.*, 2001; Yu *et al.*, 2002).

The endothelium represents the cellular interface between the blood and underlying tissues. A number of studies indicate that HCMV may facilitate hematogenous spread of virus by modulating interactions between ECs and monocytes (an important site of latent HCMV infection; see below) (Cebulla *et al.*, 2000; Knight *et al.*, 1999; Waldman *et al.*, 1995). HCMV infection of ECs increases expression of cell adhesion molecules such as ICAM-1, which corresponds to an increased interaction between ECs and monocytes resulting in monocyte infection (Knight *et al.*, 1999). Monocytes infected in this manner were capable of transmitting virus to uninfected ECs suggesting a possible mechanism for HCMV dissemination in vivo (Waldman *et al.*, 1995). ICAM-1 was shown to be upregulated at the transcriptional level by the interaction of two HCMV transcriptional activators (IE1 and IE2) with the ICAM-1 promoter (Burns *et al.*, 1999). HCMV infection also upregulates adhesion molecules indirectly by the induction of proinflammatory cytokines. HCMV-infected ECs have been shown to induce vigorous lymphocyte proliferative responses in allogeneic HCMV seropositive-derived T cells resulting in the release of IFN-γ and TNF-α (Waldman and Knight, 1996). The ability of HCMV to induce TNF-α expression in monocytes may play a critical role in disease progression due to the role of this cytokine in HCMV reactivation from this cell type (see below). These proinflammatory cytokines were also shown to induce expression of immune response molecules (ICAM-1, VCAM-1, MHC-I and MHC-II) in neighboring uninfected EC (Waldman and Knight, 1996). Clinically, CMV-mediated upregulation of adhesion and immune response molecules within transplants of solid organ transplant (SOT) and BMT patients may also increase the immunogenicity of the graft resulting in increased incidence of graft rejection (a serious complication of transplantation closely associated with HCMV infection) (Girgis *et al.*, 1996; Grattan *et al.*, 1989; Humar *et al.*, 1999a; Keenan *et al.*, 1991; Koskinen *et al.*, 1996; Smith *et al.*, 1998).

Determinants of EC tropism

The dependence of HCMV replication in ECs on the virus strain suggests that specific viral genes are required for efficient replication in this cell type (Kahl *et al.*, 2000; MacCormac and Grundy, 1999; Sinzger *et al.*, 1999). However, until the recent ability to clone CMV genomes as BACs (for review see: (Wagner *et al.*, 2002)), the instability of EC tropism during in vitro culture of HCMV posed a major problem to the identification of EC tropism determinants. Although, most low passage clinical isolates can initially replicate in both ECs and fibroblasts, these isolates consistently lose their ability to replicate in ECs following repeated passage in fibroblasts (MacCormac and Grundy, 1999; Sinzger *et al.*, 1999). However, initial plaque purification of EC tropic strains and isolation of single clones results in stable maintenance of EC tropism (even after long-term passage in fibroblasts). This result suggests that loss of EC tropism results from selection of viral variants within the initial clinical isolate rather than from viral mutants derived by *de novo* mutation or from non-genetic alterations of the virus (Sinzger *et al.*, 1999). The presence of multiple genetic determinants directing EC tropism is suggested by the observation that recent clinical isolates exhibit a gradation in their ability to replicate in ECs (Sinzger et al., 1999). Alternatively, this observation could be explained by differences in expression level of a single gene or the existence of polymorphic forms of a single genetic determinant. However, the existence of multiple genes for EC tropism is further supported by the observation that co-infection with two distinct non-EC tropic strains resulted in production of a genetically stable EC-tropic recombinant virus (Sinzger et al., 1999). This result could be explained by two mutations present in the same gene having been repaired by a recombination event. Alternatively, a more likely explanation is one of recombination relocating two distinct genetic loci required for EC tropism within the same recombinant genome.

More recently, BAC-based deletional mutagenesis studies have identified a "genomic tropism island" composed of three HCMV ORFs: UL128, UL130 and UL131A that is required for replication in ECs (Hahn et al., 2004). Deletional mutagenesis identified UL128, UL130 and UL131A as each individually required for replication in human umbilical vein ECs (HUVECs). The inability of a number of laboratory strains to replicate in ECs was also consistent with these viruses encoding inactivated forms of UL128, UL130 and UL131A. Heterologous expression of products of each these ORFs recovered EC tropism of viruses that expressed inactivated versions of the respective ORF, identifying the product of each ORF as individually required for EC tropism. The pUL130 and pUL128 proteins are components of the virion envelope (Patrone et al., 2005; Wang and Shenk, 2005b) that form a complex with two essential envelope glycoproteins (gH and gL) (Wang and Shenk, 2005b). The gH and gL glycoproteins had previously been known to complex with a third glycoprotein, gO, and to be required for replication in fibroblasts (Hobom et al., 2000). Two distinct complexes have been identified in EC-tropic virions comprised of gH/gL complexed with either pUL128/pUL130 or gO (Wang and Shenk, 2005b). Antibodies directed against either pUL130 and pUL128 inhibit infection of ECs (HUVECs), but not fibroblasts. Together, these results support a model wherein the pUL128/pUL130 and the gO containing gH/gl complex are required for infection of ECs and fibroblasts, respectively. The pUL131A has not been detected in the gH/gl complex with pUL128 and pUL130. However, a functional UL131A ORF is required for incorporation of pUL128 and pUL130 into the gH/gl virion associated complex (Wang and Shenk, 2005b), and UL131A is required for an early stage of the virus replication cycle in ECs (Wang and Shenk, 2005a). These observations suggest that UL131A is also probably involved in mediating virus entry into ECs, but may be required at submolar levels, or perhaps is more weakly associated with the complex. UL131A is also required for HCMV replication in lung microvascular ECs and a variety of epithelial cell types (Wang and Shenk, 2005a), as well as monocyte-derived dendritic cells (GM-CSF and IL-4 derived) (Gerna et al., 2005). The requirement of these ORFs for replication in other biologically relevant types of ECs as well as MDM is unknown.

Studies in the closely related MCMV model have also identified a number of viral genes required for growth in ECs as well as macrophages (see below). These studies have similarly relied heavily on BAC-based technology and further emphasize the strength of bacterial-based genetic approaches to address these questions. A recent forward genetic approach identified the MCMV encoded ribonucleotide reductase R1 subunit homologue, M45, as necessary for MCMV growth in murine ECs in vitro (Brune et al., 2001). M45 was also required for normal in vitro replication in macrophages, but not fibroblasts, bone marrow stromal cells or hepatocytes. ECs infected with M45 deletion mutants died rapidly from apoptosis indicating that this gene enabled MCMV replication in ECs by preventing apoptosis of the infected cell. Since ECs represent a site of persistent virus infection, the ability to prevent the normal apoptotic death response of these cells to viral infection may be crucial for CMV replication in this cell type. However, a subsequent study showed that the HCMV M45 homologue (UL45) is not required for growth of a BAC cloned recent clinical isolate (RVFIX) in ECs (HUVEC) indicating that homologous genes in HCMV and MCMV may not always be functionally interchangeable (Hahn et al., 2002). Alternatively, given the heterogeneity of ECs, the function of UL45 during infection of HUVEC may not accurately reflect the role of this gene during HCMV replication in EC types normally infected in vivo. The specific level within the apoptotic pathway that the M45 product functions is unknown. A study from our laboratory investigating determinants of rhesus cytomegalovirus (RhCMV) cellular tropism has identified a virally encoded cyclooxygenase 2 (vCOX-2; Rh10) as a critical determinant of RhCMV EC tropism (Rue et al., 2004). The vCOX-2 appears to mediate EC tropism by inhibiting production of the cellular antiviral molecule, nitric oxide (NO). Although HCMV does not encode a COX-2 homologue, the virus is known to induce cellular COX-2 expression, suggesting that COX-2-mediated inhibition of NO synthesis may be an important determinant for EC tropism.

Myeloid lineage cells are a site of HCMV latency

In addition to ECs as a site of HCMV persistent infection, specific subpopulations of cells of the myeloid lineage have been identified as potential sites of HCMV latency. Within the periphery, CD14+ monocytes are a known site of latent HCMV infection. The ability to reactivate virus from naturally infected CD14+ monocytes by differentiation into MDM in vitro definitively identifies these cells as a site of latent HCMV infection. Within the bone marrow, CD34+ hematopoietic progenitors and GM-Ps have also been identified as potential sites of HCMV latency. However, reactivation of HCMV from these cell types has been observed only following *in vitro* infection. Consequently, the role of these cell types as sites of HCMV latency in vivo remains unclear.

CD14+ monocytes and MDM

The high level of HCMV transmission associated with the transfusion of blood products (Bowden, 1995; Bowden et al., 1995; Hersman et al., 1982; Tegtmeier, 1989), and specifically with cells of the leukocyte fraction, was the initial indication that leukocytes represented a significant source of latent or persistent virus (Adler et al., 1983, 1983; Tegtmeier, 1986). Subsequently, PCR analysis for HCMV DNA identified CD14+ monocytes as the predominant HCMV-infected cell type in the blood of normal immune competent HCMV seropositive individuals (Taylor-Wiedeman et al., 1991, 1993). PCR analysis showed that only a small number of monocytes in the peripheral blood contained HCMV DNA (<1 in 10^4) (Slobedman and Mocarski, 1999), and viral gene expression in these cells was shown either to be undetectable or restricted to immediate-early gene expression (Dankner et al., 1990; Taylor-Wiedeman, et al., 1991, 1993). These in vivo infection results were consistent with findings from in vitro studies, wherein HCMV infection of monocytes was inefficient, with viral replication being absent or restricted to early events of gene expression (Einhorn and Ost, 1984; Rice et al., 1984; Söderberg et al., 1993). Importantly, the ability of the leukocyte fraction to transmit infection, combined with the absence of viral gene expression in the major infected cell type within this population (CD14+ monocytes), identified CD14+ monocytes as a potential site of viral latency. Consistent with monocytes representing a site of HCMV latency, the HCMV genome in these cells was shown to be maintained at a relatively low copy number (6–13 copies/cell) (Slobedman and Mocarski, 1999) and in an episomal circular form (Bolovan-Fritts et al., 1999) comparable to the latent genome structure of other herpesviruses.

Definitive evidence identifying CD14+ monocytes as a site of HCMV latency requires demonstration of an ability to reactivate virus from naturally infected cells. However, initial attempts to reactivate virus from naturally infected monocytes (Ibanez et al., 1991; Taylor-Wiedeman et al., 1994), or even to establish productive replication following in vitro infection were unsuccessful (Einhorn and Ost, 1984; Rice et al., 1984; Söderberg et al., 1993). In one study, productive HCMV replication following in vitro infection was detected, but infection was extremely inefficient with levels of virus progeny at 0.1% of the level observed in fibroblasts (Maciejewski et al., 1993). A major break-through came with a series of experiments that revealed the importance of monocyte/MDM differentiation-state for HCMV replication (Fig. 42.2) (Ibanez et al., 1991). Specifically, differentiation of monocytes into MDM by co-culture with concanavalin A (Con A)-stimulated non-adherent cells dramatically increased the ability of HCMV to replicate in these cells with approximately 40% of MDM (designated Con A-MDM) supporting productive HCMV replication following in vitro infection (Ibanez et al., 1991). Subsequent studies demonstrated that differentiation of naturally infected peripheral CD14+ monocytes into MDM (designated Allo-MDM) by allogeneic stimulation with non-adherent peripheral blood mononuclear cells (PBMC) was able to reactivate virus from these cells (Söderberg-Naucler et al., 1997b). This report was the first study to conclusively identify myeloid lineage cells as a reservoir for HCMV latency, and has enabled the study of mechanisms of reactivation of latent virus from naturally infected cells.

Growth of HCMV in Con A-MDM

The initial studies using cocultivation with Con A-stimulated autologous non-adherent PBMCs to induce monocyte differentiation resulted in production of the Con A-MDM phenotype that was permissive to HCMV, and resulted in a nonlytic infection that produced exclusively cell-associated virus (Ibanez et al., 1991; Söderberg-Naucler et al., 1997a). Generation of this Con A-MDM phenotype was shown to require CD8+ T-lymphocytes and the proinflammatory cytokines IFN-γ and TNF-α (but not IL-1, IL-2, TGF-β or GM-CSF) (Söderberg-Naucler et al., 1997a). Addition of recombinant IFN-γ or TNF-α alone to monocyte cultures was sufficient to produce MDM that were comparable to Con A-MDM in their level of virus production (Söderberg-Naucler et al., 1997a). These observations suggest a model wherein production of IFN-γ and TNF-α by Con A-activated CD8+ T-lymphocytes induces monocyte differentiation into HCMV permissive Con A-MDM (Fig. 42.3), and indicate a critical role for immune stimulation in the production of HCMV-permissive MDM. Interestingly, IFN-γ and TNF-α were also shown to reactivate HCMV from latently in vitro infected GM-Ps (Hahn et al., 1998) identifying a common requirement for these cytokines in the production of an HCMV-permissive cellular phenotype. A more direct role of TNF-α in HCMV

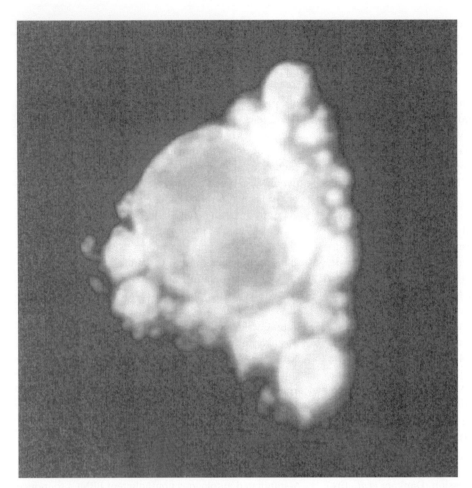

Fig. 42.2. Immunofluorescent micrograph of HCMV-infected MDM. MDM were infected with HCMV. Cells were fixed and stained for the presence of HCMV proteins, pp65 (an early late product; green) and IE-2 (an immediate-early product; red). (See color plate section.)

reactivation is also suggested by the ability of this cytokine to stimulate the IE promoter in myeloid cells by activation of NFκB. Activated NFκB translocates to the nucleus and binds directly to NFκB binding motifs in the IE enhancer thereby activating expression of the two main transcriptional activators of the virus (Prösch et al., 1995, 2001; Ritter et al., 2000; Stein et al., 1993; Zhang et al., 2001). The Con A-MDM model was a major advance in understanding mechanisms of HCMV reactivation. However, the inability to reactivate HCMV from naturally infected Con A-MDM prevented the definitive identification of CD14+ monocytes as a site of HCMV latency in vivo.

Growth of HCMV in Allo-MDM

Allogeneically stimulated PBMC have recently been used to induce MDM differentiation in a cellular microenvironment more closely resembling the milieu believed to exist during in vivo reactivation of HCMV from monocytes. In this system, coculture of HLA-mismatched donor PBMC populations resulted in the production of MDM (designated Allo-MDM) that were permissive to HCMV infection and enabled reactivation of latent virus from CD14+ monocytes naturally infected in vivo (Söderberg-Naucler et al., 1997b). Allo-MDM express both macrophage (CD14/CD64) and dendritic (CD1a/CD83) cell markers. In contrast to Con A-MDM, in vitro infection of Allo-MDM is characterized by vigorous lytic replication in a large number of cells (>50%) and results in accumulation of extracellular virus (Söderberg-Naucler et al., 2001). Importantly, latent HCMV can be reactivated from naturally infected Allo-MDM, which is not possible using other MDM culture systems (Söderberg-Naucler et al., 1997a, b, 2001) and emphasizes the importance of the specific MDM differentiation pathway for HCMV reactivation.

In the Allo-MDM system, cellular depletion and cytokine neutralization experiments showed that both CD4+ and

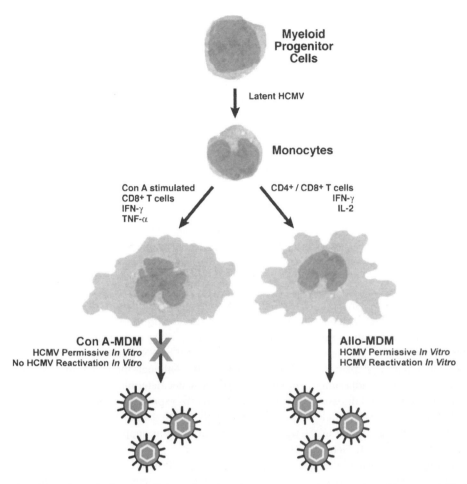

Fig. 42.3. Schematic showing cellular and cytokine factors necessary for generation of Con A- and Allo-MDM.

CD8+ T lymphocytes and the cytokines IFN-γ and IL-2 (but not IL-1, TNF-α or TGF-β) were required for generation of the HCMV-permissive phenotype (Fig. 42.3) (Söderberg-Naucler et al., 2001). These cytokines were required for induction of an Allo-MDM phenotype able to support HCMV replication following in vitro infection. However, reactivation of latent virus from naturally infected cells required additional factors. Conditioned media from Allo-MDM cultures stimulated reactivation of HCMV in the absence of allogeneic stimulation. Thus, soluble factors released during allogeneic stimulation are sufficient to produce a MDM phenotype capable of HCMV reactivation. The presence of IFN-γ (but not IL-1, IL-2, TNF-α, TGF-β or GM-CSF) within the first 48 hours of allogeneic stimulation was necessary for efficient reactivation of latent HCMV. However, IFN-γ alone was not sufficient for the induction of a MDM phenotype capable of reactivating virus. Analysis of the cytokines released during Allo- compared to Con A-MDM differentiation has revealed considerable differences in the kinetics as well as in the type of cytokines released by the two differentiation pathways. IL-13 was observed only in Allo-MDM cultures. IL-13 has previously been shown to increase, albeit at low levels, HCMV gene expression and replication in in vitro infected alveolar macrophages and may be important in the reactivation of HCMV from latency (Hatch et al., 1997). These studies suggest a model (Fig. 42.4) wherein latently infected CD14+ monocytes in the peripheral blood are activated by an immune response (ie., allogeneic organ transplantation or blood transfusion). During this activation, CD4+ and CD8+ lymphocytes play a critical role, with IL-2 released from CD4+ lymphocytes inducing the release of soluble factors from CD8+ lymphocytes. These soluble factors, which include IFN-γ, induce differentiation of CD14+ monocytes into the Allo-MDM phenotype required for reactivation of latent virus.

Consistent with the Allo-MDM in vitro model, a number of studies support a role for immune activation accompanied by release of proinflammatory cytokines

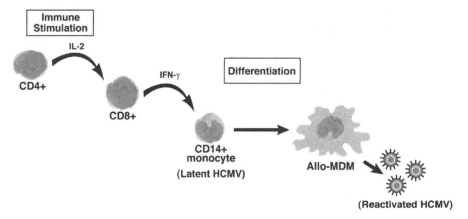

Fig. 42.4. Model for reactivation of latent HCMV in vivo. Allogeneic reaction during transplantation or blood transfusion results in IL-2 production by CD4+ T cells with subsequent stimulation of IFN-γ secretion by CD8+ T cells. In concert with other factors, IFN-γ induces CD14+ monocyte differentiation into Allo-MDM, reactivating latent virus and resulting in the production of infectious virus.

in HCMV reactivation and replication in vivo. In SOT patients, the recipient immune system launches a vigorous allogeneic immune response within the graft in an attempt to remove the transplanted tissue. This response is associated with the release of proinflammatory cytokines, chemokines and an increased expression of adhesion molecules. High levels of HCMV reactivation and disease are consistently observed in allogeneic graft tissue, and elevated plasma levels of IFN-γ and TNF-α are found in patients with HCMV disease (Docke *et al.*, 1994; Fietze *et al.*, 1994; Humar *et al.*, 1999a,b). This association of HCMV disease with proinflammatory cytokine levels is also observed in SOT patients receiving anti-lymphocyte γ globulin (ALG). In these cases, increased TNF-α levels associated with ALG treatment correspond to an increase in severity of HCMV disease (Tolkoff-Rubin and Rubin, 1994). The clinical significance of this extensive reactivation and induction of viral replication within the graft is illustrated by the high incidence of HCMV cytopathology and disease within the transplanted organ (Ho, 1990). For example, HCMV hepatitis is normally asymptomatic in non-hepatic SOT patients; however, in liver transplant recipients, HCMV hepatitis is frequently observed. Similarly, in heart–lung transplant recipients the incidence of HCMV pneumonia is significantly elevated as compared to other SOT patients (Ho, 1990). Since blood transfusion is commonly performed over histocompatibility barriers, reactivation of HCMV through allogeneic stimulation of PBMC would also be expected to play a role in HCMV transmission following transfusion. The high levels of HCMV antigenemia observed in patients with chronic plaque psoriasis are also consistent with the increased TNF-α expression observed in these patients (Asadullah *et al.*, 1999). In experimental studies of MCMV, allogeneic transplantation induces expression of CMV IE genes in vivo, which is accompanied by an increased expression of transcripts for IL-2, TNF-α, IFN-γ and activation of NFκB (Hummel *et al.*, 2001). Although the ability to reactivate productive virus was not determined, a separate study showed that MCMV IE expression could be induced in the lung of latently infected mice in vivo by treatment with TNF-α without immune suppression (Koffron *et al.*, 1999).

Other inflammatory cytokines and chemokines have also been associated with increased HCMV replication and disease following transplantation (Nordoy *et al.*, 1999; 2000a, b). IL-8 was shown to increase HCMV replication in MRC-5 fibroblasts (Murayama *et al.*, 1998), and may be of particular importance due to the high levels of IL-8 that are secreted from a variety of cells in response to proinflammatory cytokines released from allogeneically activated MDM within the graft (Harada *et al.*, 1994). HCMV has also been shown to induce IL-8 expression (Murayama *et al.*, 1998), and studies suggest that IL-8 may function by inhibition of the antiviral IFN-γ response pathway or by increasing neutrophil-mediated HCMV dissemination by attracting neutrophils to sites of HCMV replication (Grundy *et al.*, 1998). High levels of the anti-inflammatory cytokine IL-10 have been shown to be associated with HCMV disease in renal SOT recipients (Nordoy *et al.*, 2000b). An HCMV encoded IL-10 homologue (cmvIL-10) encoded by ORF UL111a was recently identified (Kotenko *et al.*, 2000). The cmvIL-10 shares low sequence homology (27%) with cellular IL-10; however, cmvIL-10 binds to the cellular IL-10 receptor and competes with cellular IL-10 for binding to this receptor. The biological activity of cmvIL-10 and cellular IL10 also appear comparable (Spencer et al., 2002). Paradoxically, IL-10 has been shown to inhibit monocyte and macrophage function, including inhibiting the release of TNF-α from activated MDM (Oswald et al., 1992). However, recent studies indicate that IL-10 is involved in macrophage differentiation (Allavena et al., 1998), and therefore high IL-10 levels may induce differentiation of MDM into a phenotype that is permissive for HCMV. Together, results from these studies suggest that immune activation with concomitant production of proinflammatory cytokines plays a critical role in virus reactivation and replication in vivo in naturally infected patients, which is recapitulated in vitro in the Allo-MDM system.

CD34+ hematopoietic and CD33+ GM-Ps

Peripheral blood monocytes are clearly an important site of HCMV latency. However, these cells are short-lived, non-replicating and are present in the circulation for only a brief period of time before entering the tissue and differentiating into MDM. These characteristics suggest another site of HCMV latency existing in a myeloid progenitor population that gives rise to latently infected CD14+ monocytes in the peripheral blood. HCMV has previously been reported to infect CD34+ pluripotent stem cells both in vitro (Goodrum et al., 2002; Maciejewski et al., 1992; Minton et al., 1994; Movassagh et al., 1996; Sindre et al., 1996) and in vivo (Mendelson et al., 1996; Torok-Storb et al., 1992; von Laer et al., 1995a,b). However, since CD34+ stem cells are a common precursor for all peripheral blood cell types, the absence of virus from many peripheral blood cell lineages suggests that CD34+ stem cells may not represent a major site for HCMV latency (Brytting et al., 1995; Schrier et al., 1995; Söderberg et al., 1993; Taylor-Wiedeman et al., 1993; von Laer et al., 1995a,b). This observation would predict that a precursor population further differentiated along the myeloid pathway would be a more biologically significant site of HCMV latency in vivo. Alternatively, HCMV may alter CD34+ cell differentiation, leading to differentiation of only specific cell lineages, or the HCMV genome may be maintained only within specific cell lineages during differentiation.

CD33+ GM-Ps have been identified as one possible precursor population representing a more differentiated site of HCMV latency. Following in vitro infection, HCMV has been shown to infect and establish a latent infection in fetal liver-derived CD33+ GM-Ps (Kondo et al., 1994; 1996; Hahn et al., 1998). Virus was reactivated from CD33+ cells co-expressing either CD15 (granulocyte marker), CD14 (monocyte marker) or CD15 and CD1a (dendritic lineage marker) (Kondo et al., 1994; Hahn et al., 1998). IFN-γ and TNF-α reactivated HCMV from latently in vitro infected GM-Ps (Hahn et al., 1998), closely linking reactivation with immune activation and cellular differentiation state as had been observed with Allo-MDM (Söderberg-Naucler et al., 1997b). However, for both CD34+ precursors and CD33+ GM-Ps, conclusive evidence that these populations represent a site of HCMV latency in vivo awaits demonstration of HCMV reactivation from these cells in vitro following their natural infection in healthy individuals.

The mechanisms controlling HCMV latency and reactivation in these cell types are currently unknown. CMV latency-associated transcripts (CLTs) have been detected in latently infected GM-Ps suggesting a possible role of CLTs in the control of latency. CLTs are represented by sense (ORF94) and antisense transcripts (ORF152 and 154), expressed from the UL122/UL123 region of the genome. This region is normally involved in the expression of transcriptional activators (IE1 and IE2) that are required for lytic replication (Kondo et al., 1996). The presence of CLTs in bone marrow aspirates from healthy HCMV seropositive individuals, as well as the presence of antibodies directed against proteins encoded by ORF94 and ORF152 in the serum of healthy HCMV seropositive individuals (Kondo et al., 1996), have implicated CLTs in the control of HCMV latency in vivo. However, in the in vitro GM-P latency model, only a small proportion of latently infected GM-Ps have been shown to contain detectable CLTs (1.8%–3.6%) even though greater than 90% of GM-Ps are latently infected (Slobedman and Mocarski, 1999). Furthermore, inactivation of ORF94 does not affect the ability of latent HCMV to reactivate in this latency model (White et al., 2000) and CLTs have never been observed in the Allo-MDM model. Together, these observations suggest that CLTs play a minimal role in the regulation of HCMV latency and reactivation. Recently, DNA array analysis using an *in vitro* CD34+ latency model has revealed an expression profile of HCMV genes that is unique to the latent, compared to lytic, state of infection (Goodrum et al., 2002). The role of this latency-associated gene expression profile for the maintenance of latency in these cells is currently unknown. Further investigation may lead to the identification of HCMV ORFs involved in regulating virus reactivation.

Determinants of myeloid lineage cell tropism

Early studies identified differences in the ability of individual HCMV strains to infect monocytes and macrophages indicating that HCMV tropism for monocyte/MDM is genetically determined (Einhorn and Ost, 1984; Rice et al., 1984). Although the genetic determinants for HCMV growth in MDM have not been identified, the MCMV model has provided considerable insight into the role of specific genes in CMV replication in MDM. In the murine model, initial studies identified M45, M140 and M141 as virally encoded genetic determinants necessary for normal MCMV replication in macrophages in vitro (Brune *et al.*, 2001; Hanson *et al.*, 1999a,b 2001). In animal studies, M140 and M141 were shown to be essential for normal virus replication in the MDM-rich spleen, but not liver, indicating a role of these genes for determination of tropism in vivo (Hanson *et al.*, 2001). Importantly, viruses deleted of M140 and M141 had reduced pathogenicity indicating a role of MDM tropism in virus pathogenicity. Individual deletion of M140 and M141 resulted in decreased viral replication in macrophages; however, a low level of replication remained suggesting a redundancy of function or the existence of additional genes mediating virus replication in MDM. The M140 and M141 gene products are homologues of the HCMV US22 gene family. A study utilizing BAC-based technology has analyzed the function of the 12 US22 MCMV homologues in mediating macrophage tropism (Menard *et al.*, 2003). Results from this study confirmed the role of M140 and M141 as determinants of macrophage tropism, and identified two additional MCMV genes necessary for MCMV growth in macrophages (M36 and m139) (Menard *et al.*, 2003). However, M36 alone was required for growth in primary macrophages as well as macrophage cell lines. The identification of m139 as necessary for growth in macrophages contrasts with results from the earlier studies. This may be a consequence of sequence differences between viruses used by the different laboratories. The function of the HCMV US22 gene family members in mediating HCMV macrophage tropism has not been determined.

Role of apoptotic inhibitors in EC and MDM tropism

Similar to M45 (see above), the M36 product exhibits an anti-apoptotic function suggesting that an ability to inhibit apoptosis may be a common requirement for growth of cytomegalovirus in ECs and macrophages. Studies using a BAC-cloned recent clinical isolate (RVFIX) have shown that the HCMV M45 homologue (UL45) is not involved in the modulation of apoptosis and is dispensable for replication in HUVECs (Hahn *et al.*, 2002) (see above). However, the function of UL45 for replication in macrophages remains to be determined. Four additional HCMV genes, IE1, IE2, UL36/viral inhibitor of caspase-8-induced apoptosis (vICA) and UL37x1/viral mitochondria-localized inhibitor of apoptosis (vMIA) have also been shown to inhibit apoptosis following over-expression of recombinant protein (Goldmacher *et al.*, 1999; Skaletskaya *et al.*, 2001; Zhu *et al.*, 1995). All of these genes except UL36/vICA are essential for virus replication in fibroblasts (Goldmacher, 2002; Marchini *et al.*, 2001; Patterson, and Shenk, 1999) (observed at only low multiplicities of infection for IE1) (Greaves and Mocarski, 1998). The requirement of the HCMV M36 homologue (UL36/vICA) for replication in macrophages or ECs is unknown. However, the M36 and UL36/vICA products appear to share a similar function, with the products of both genes (pM36 and pUL36/vICA, respectively) inhibiting apoptosis at a comparable level within the apoptotic pathway (Menard *et al.*, 2003).

Results from a number of studies have given considerable insight into the mechanisms by which pUL36/vICA and the product of UL37×1/vMIA (pUL37×1/vMIA) inhibit the apoptotic pathway (Goldmacher, 2000; Skaletskaya *et al.*, 2001). The pUL36/vICA and pUL37×1/vMIA appear to function at distinct steps in the apoptotic pathway. During apoptosis, death stimuli (e.g., Fas-ligation) activate caspase 8 resulting in permeabilization of the mitochondrial membrane leading to the release of mitochondrial proteins into the cytoplasm. These mitochondrial proteins activate downstream caspases and nucleases leading to the apoptotic death of the cell. The pUL36/vICA appears to function early in the apoptotic pathway by binding to the prodomain of caspase 8 and inhibiting activation. In contrast, pUL37×1/vMIA is localized to mitochondria (Colberg-Poley *et al.*, 2000; Goldmacher *et al.*, 1999), and has been shown to prevent apoptosis by inhibition of BID-mediated permeabilization of the mitochondrial membrane (Goldmacher, 2002). The function of pUL36/vICA and pUL37×1/vMIA at separate steps in the apoptotic pathway is further supported by the ability of pUL36/vICA, but not pUL37×1/vMIA, to inhibit Fas-mediated apoptosis in type I cells where caspase 8 can directly activate caspase 3 and thereby bypass the mitochondria (Skaletskaya *et al.*, 2001). As indicated above, deletional analysis has shown that UL37×1/vMIA, but not UL36/vICA, is essential for HCMV replication in fibroblasts (Borst *et al.*, 1999; Goldmacher, 2002). Although UL37×1/vMIA is required for oriLyt-dependent viral DNA synthesis (Smith and Pari, 1995), the anti-apoptotic function of pUL37×1/vMIA appears to be critical for replication in fibroblasts, since pUL37×1/vMIA-deficient HCMV replication was rescued by co-expression of other apoptosis inhibitors (Goldmacher, 2002; Reboredo *et al.* 2004). Although the requirement of IE1, IE2, pUL36/vICA and pUL37×1/vMIA for HCMV replication has been determined in fibroblasts, the role of these proteins as determinants of HCMV tropism in other permissive cell types has not been investigated.

Summary

ECs and myeloid lineage cell populations are important sites of HCMV persistence and latency within the host.

The use of cells of the myeloid lineage as a virus reservoir closely links HCMV replication to the immune system, and the virus has exploited immune activation to provide the necessary signals for reactivation of latent virus. The utilization of in vitro culture systems is beginning to increase our understanding of reactivation, persistence and replication of HCMV within EC and myeloid cell populations. The ability of CMV to replicate in EC and MDM is determined by genetic determinants of the virus. The MCMV model has enabled identification of a number of genes that are critical for virus replication in these cells. Ongoing studies in a number of laboratories, in large part using BAC-cloned CMV, are further defining viral determinants of CMV tropism. Recently, a tropism island comprising UL128, Ul130, and UL131A has been identified as necessary for HCMV replication in ECs. These studies are expected to yield exciting insights into the necessary requirements for virus replication in these cells.

Acknowledgments

We thank Drs. Markus Wagner and Hanna Välimaa, and Patsy Smith for their constructive comments during the preparation of the manuscript. We also thank Andrew Townsend for his help with the graphics.

REFERENCES

Adler, S. P., Chandrika, T., Lawrence, L., and Baggett, J. (1983). Cytomegalovirus infections in neonates acquired by blood transfusions. *Pediatr. Infect. Dis.*, **2**, 114–118.

Adler, S. P., Baggett, J., and McVoy M. (1985). Transfusion-associated cytomegalovirus infections in seropositive cardiac surgery patients. *Lancet*, **2**, 743–747.

Allavena, P., Piemonti, L., Longoni, D., Bernasconi, S., Stoppacciaro, A., Ruco, L., and Mantovani, A. (1998). IL-10 prevents the differentiation of monocytes to dendritic cells but promotes their maturation to macrophages. *Eur. J. Immunol.*, **28**, 359–369.

Asadullah, K., Prosch, S., Audring, H. *et al.* (1999). A high prevalence of cytomegalovirus antigenaemia in patients with moderate to severe chronic plaque psoriasis: an association with systemic tumour necrosis factor alpha overexpression. *Br. J. Dermatol.*, **141**, 94–102.

Bolovan-Fritts, C. and Wiedeman J. A. (2001). Human cytomegalovirus strain Toledo lacks a virus-encoded tropism factor required for infection of aortic endothelial cells. *J. Infect. Dis.*, **184**, 1252–1261.

Bolovan-Fritts, C. A., Mocarski, E. S., and Wiedeman J. A. (1999). Peripheral blood CD14(+) cells from healthy subjects carry a circular conformation of latent cytomegalovirus genome. *Blood*, **93**, 394–398.

Borst, E. M., Hahn, G., Koszinowski, U. H., and Messerle, M. (1999). Cloning of the human cytomegalovirus (HCMV) genome as an infectious bacterial artificial chromosome in *Escherichia coli*: a new approach for construction of HCMV mutants. *J. Virol.*, **73**, 8320–8329.

Bowden, R. A. (1995). Transfusion-transmitted cytomegalovirus infection. *Hematol. Oncol. Clin. North Am.*, **9**, 155–166.

Bowden, R. A., Slichter, S. J., Sayers, M. *et al.* (1995). A comparison of filtered leukocyte-reduced and cytomegalovirus (CMV) seronegative blood products for the prevention of transfusion-associated CMV infection after marrow transplant. *Blood*, **86**, 3598–3603.

Brune, W., Menard, C., Heesemann, J., and Koszinowski, U. H. (2001). A ribonucleotide reductase homolog of cytomegalovirus and endothelial cell tropism. *Science*, **291**, 303–305.

Brytting, M., Mousavi-Jazi, M., Bostrom, L. *et al.* (1995). Cytomegalovirus DNA in peripheral blood leukocytes and plasma from bone marrow transplant recipients. *Transplantation*, **60**, 961–965.

Burns, L. J., Pooley, J. C., Walsh, D. J., Vercellotti, G. M., Weber, M. L. and Kovacs, A. (1999). Intercellular adhesion molecule-1 expression in endothelial cells is activated by cytomegalovirus immediate early proteins. Transplantation, **67**, 137–44.

Cebulla, C. M., Miller, D. M., Knight, D. A., Briggs, B. R., McGaughy, V. and Sedmak, D. D. (2000). Cytomegalovirus induces sialyl Lewis(x) and Lewis(x) on human endothelial cells. *Transplantation*, **69**, 1202–1209.

Colberg-Poley, A. M., Patel, M. B., Erezo, D. P., and Slater, J. E. (2000). Human cytomegalovirus UL37 immediate-early regulatory proteins traffic through the secretory apparatus and to mitochondria. *J. Gen. Virol.*, **81**, 1779–1789.

Dankner, W. M., McCutchan, J. A., Richman, D. D., Hirata, K., and Spector, S. A. (1990). Localization of human cytomegalovirus in peripheral blood leukocytes by in situ hybridization. *J. Infect. Dis.*, **161**, 31–36.

Dargan, D. J., Jamieson, F. E., MacLean, J., Dolan, A., Addison, C., and McGeoch, D. J. (1997). The published DNA sequence of human cytomegalovirus strain AD169 lacks 929 base pairs affecting genes UL42 and UL43. *J. Virol.*, **71**, 9833–9836.

Docke, W. D., Prosch, S., Fietze, E. *et al.* (1994). Cytomegalovirus reactivation and tumour necrosis factor. *Lancet*, **343**, 268–269.

Einhorn, L. and Ost, A. (1984). Cytomegalovirus infection of human blood cells. *J. Infect. Dis.*, **149**, 207–214.

Fietze, E., Prosch, S., Reinke, P. (1994). Cytomegalovirus infection in transplant recipients. The role of tumor necrosis factor. *Transplantation*, **58**, 675–680.

Fish, K. N., Söderberg-Naucler, C., Mills, L. K., Stenglein, S., and Nelson, J. A. (1998). Human cytomegalovirus persistently infects aortic endothelial cells. *J. Virol.*, **72**, 5661–5668.

Friedman, H. M., Macarak, E. J., MacGregor, R. R., Wolfe, J., and Kefalides, N. A. (1981). Virus infection of endothelial cells. *J. Infect. Dis.*, **143**, 266–273.

Gerna, G., Percivalle, E., Lilleri, D. *et al.* (2005). Dendritic-cell infection by human cytomegalovirus is restricted to strains carrying functional UL131–128 genes and mediates efficient viral antigen presentation to CD8+ T cells. *J. Gen. Virol.*, **86**, 275–84.

Girgis, R. E., Tu, I., Berry, G. J. *et al.* (1996). Risk factors for the development of obliterative bronchiolitis after lung transplantation. *J. Heart Lung Transpl.*, **15**, 1200–1208.

Gnann, J. W., Jr., Ahlmen, J., Svalander, C., Olding, L., Oldstone, M. B., and Nelson, J. A. (1988). Inflammatory cells in transplanted kidneys are infected by human cytomegalovirus. *Am. J. Pathol.*, **132**, 239–248.

Goldmacher, V. S. (2002). vMIA, a viral inhibitor of apoptosis targeting mitochondria. *Biochimie*, **84**, 177–185.

Goldmacher, V. S., Bartle, L. M., Skaletskaya, A. *et al.* (1999). A cytomegalovirus-encoded mitochondria-localized inhibitor of apoptosis structurally unrelated to Bcl-2. *Proc. Natl Acad. Sci. USA*, **96**, 12536–12541.

Goodrum, F. D., Jordan, C. T., High, K., and Shenk, T. (2002). Human cytomegalovirus gene expression during infection of primary hematopoietic progenitor cells: a model for latency. *Proc. Natl. Acad. Sci. USA*, **99**, 16255–16260.

Grattan, M. T., Moreno-Cabral, C. E., Starnes, V. A., Oyer, P. E. Stinson, E. B., and Shumway, N. E. (1989). Cytomegalovirus infection is associated with cardiac allograft rejection and atherosclerosis. *J. Am. Med. Assoc.*, **261**, 3561–3566.

Greaves, R. F. and Mocarski, E. S. (1998). Defective growth correlates with reduced accumulation of a viral DNA replication protein after low-multiplicity infection by a human cytomegalovirus ie1 mutant. *J. Virol.*, **72**, 366–379.

Grundy, J. E., Lawson, K. M., MacCormac, L. P., Fletcher, J. M., and Yong, K. L. (1998). Cytomegalovirus-infected endothelial cells recruit neutrophils by the secretion of C–X–C chemokines and transmit virus by direct neutrophil– endothelial cell contact and during neutrophil transendothelial migration. J. Infect. Dis., 177, 1465–1474.

Gyorkey, F., Melnick, J. L., Guinn, G. A., Gyorkey, P., and DeBakey, M. E. (1984). Herpesviridae in the endothelial and smooth muscle cells of the proximal aorta in arteriosclerotic patients. *Exp. Mol. Pathol.*, **40**, 328–339.

Hahn, G., Jores, R., and Mocarski, E. S. (1998). Cytomegalovirus remains latent in a common precursor of dendritic and myeloid cells. *Proc. Natl Acad. Sci. USA*, **95**, 3937–3942.

Hahn, G., Khan, H., Baldanti, F., Koszinowski, U. H., Revello, M. G. and Gerna, G. (2002). The human cytomegalovirus ribonucleotide reductase homolog UL45 is dispensable for growth in endothelial cells, as determined by a BAC-cloned clinical isolate of human cytomegalovirus with preserved wild-type characteristics. *J. Virol.*, **76**, 9551–9555.

Hahn, G., Rose, D., Wagner, M., Rhiel, S., and McVoy, M. A. (2003). Cloning of the genomes of human cytomegalovirus strains Toledo, TownevarRIT3, and Towne long as BACs and site-directed mutagenesis using a PCR-based technique. *Virology*, **307**, 164–177.

Hahn, G., Revello, M. G., Patrone, M. *et al.* (2004). Human cytomegalovirus UL131-128 genes are indispensable for virus growth in endothelial cells and virus transfer to leukocytes. *J. Virol.* **78**, 10023–10033.

Hanson, L. K., Dalton, B. L., and Karabekian, Z. (1999a). Transcriptional analysis of the murine cytomegalovirus HindIII-I region: identification of a novel immediate-early gene region. *Virology*, **260**, 156–164.

Hanson, L. K., Slater, J. S., Karabekian, Z. *et al.* (1999b). Replication of murine cytomegalovirus in differentiated macrophages as a determinant of viral pathogenesis. *J. Virol.*, **73**, 5970–5980.

Hanson, L. K., Slater, J. S., Karabekian, Z. Ciocco-Schmitt, G. and Campbell, A. E. (2001). Products of US22 genes M140 and M141 confer efficient replication of murine cytomegalovirus in macrophages and spleen. *J. Virol.*, **75**, 6292–6302.

Harada, A., Sekido, N., Akahoshi, T., Wada, T., Mukaida, N., and Matsushima, K. (1994). Essential involvement of interleukin-8 (IL-8) in acute inflammation. *J. Leukoc. Biol.*, **56**, 559–564.

Hatch, W. C., Freedman, A. R., Boldthoule, D. M., Groopman, J. E., and Terwilliger, E. F. (1997). Differential effects of interleukin-13 on cytomegalovirus and human immunodeficiency virus infection in human alveolar macrophages. *Blood*, **89**, 3443–3450.

Hendrix, M., Dormans, P. H. J., Kitseelar, P., Bosman, F., and Bruggeman, C. A. (1989). The presence of CMV nucleic acids arterial walls of atherosclerotic and non-atherosclerotic patients. *Am. J. Path.*, **134**, 1151–1157.

Hendrix, M. G., Salimans, M. M. van Boven, C. P., and Bruggeman, C. A. (1990). High prevalence of latently present cytomegalovirus in arterial walls of patients suffering from grade III atherosclerosis. *Am. J. Pathol.*, **136**, 23–28.

Hersman, J., Meyers, J. D., Thomas, E. D., Buckner, C. D., and Clift, R. (1982). The effect of granulocyte transfusions on the incidence of cytomegalovirus infection after allogeneic marrow transplantation. *Ann. Intern. Med.*, **96**, 149–152.

Ho, M. (1990). Epidemiology of cytomegalovirus infections. *Rev. Infect. Dis.*, **12** (Suppl. 7), S701–S710.

Hobom, U., Brune, W., Messerle, M., Hahn, G., and Koszinowski, U. H. (2000). Fast screening procedures for random transposon libraries of cloned herpesvirus genomes: mutational analysis of human cytomegalovirus envelope glycoprotein genes. *J. Virol.*, **74**, 7720–7729.

Howell, C. L., Miller, M. J., and Martin, W. J. (1979). Comparison of rates of virus isolation from leukocyte populations separated from blood by conventional and Ficoll-Paque/Macrodex methods. *J. Clin. Microbiol.*, **10**, 533–537.

Humar, A., Gillingham, K. J., Payne, W. D., Dunn, D. L., Sutherland, D. E., and Matas, A. J. (1999a). Association between cytomegalovirus disease and chronic rejection in kidney transplant recipients. *Transplantation*, **68**, 1879–1883.

Humar, A., St Louis, P., Mazzulli, T. *et al.* (1999b). Elevated serum cytokines are associated with cytomegalovirus infection and disease in bone marrow transplant recipients. *J. Infect. Dis.*, **179**, 484–488.

Hummel, M., Zhang, Z., Yan, S. (2001). Allogeneic transplantation induces expression of cytomegalovirus immediate-early genes in vivo: a model for reactivation from latency. *J. Virol.*, **75**, 4814–4822.

Ibanez, C. E., Schrier, R., Ghazal, P., Wiley, C., and Nelson, J. A. (1991). Human cytomegalovirus productively infects primary differentiated macrophages. *J. Virol.*, **65**, 6581–6588.

Joo, F. (1992). The cerebral microvessels in culture, an update. *J. Neurochem.*, **58**, 1–17.

Kahl, M., Siegel-Axel D., Stenglein S., Jahn, G., and Sinzger, C. (2000). Efficient lytic infection of human arterial endothelial cells by human cytomegalovirus strains. *J. Virol.*, **74**, 7628–7635.

Keenan, R. J., Lega, M. E., Dummer, J. S. *et al.* (1991). Cytomegalovirus serologic status and postoperative infection correlated with risk of developing chronic rejection after pulmonary transplantation. *Transplantation*, **51**, 433–438.

Knight, D. A., Waldman, W. J., and Sedmak, D. D. (1999). Cytomegalovirus-mediated modulation of adhesion molecule expression by human arterial and microvascular endothelial cells. *Transplantation*, **68**, 1814–1818.

Koffron, A., Varghese, T., and Hummel, M. (1999). Immunosuppression is not required for reactivation of latent murine cytomegalovirus. *Transpl. Proc.*, **31**, 1395–1396.

Kondo, K., Kaneshima, H., and Mocarski, E. S. (1994). Human cytomegalovirus latent infection of granulocyte-macrophage progenitors. *Proc. Natl Acad. Sci. U S A*, **91**, 11879–11883.

Kondo, K., Xu, J., and Mocarski, E. S. (1996). Human cytomegalovirus latent gene expression in granulocyte-macrophage progenitors in culture and in seropositive individuals. *Proc. Natl Acad. Sci. USA*, **93**, 11137–11142.

Koskinen, P., Lemstrom, K., Mattila, S., Hayry, P., and Nieminen, M. S. (1996). Cytomegalovirus infection associated accelerated heart allograft arteriosclerosis may impair the late function of the graft. *Clin. Transpl.*, **10**, 487–493.

Kotenko, S. V., Saccani, S., Izotova, L. S., Mirochnitchenko, O. V., and Pestka, S. (2000). Human cytomegalovirus harbors its own unique IL-10 homolog (cmvIL-10). *Proc. Natl Acad. Sci. USA*, **97**, 1695–1700.

MacCormac, L. P. and Grundy, J. E. (1999). Two clinical isolates and the Toledo strain of cytomegalovirus contain endothelial cell tropic variants that are not present in the AD169, Towne, or Davis strains. *J. Med. Virol.*, **57**, 298–307.

Maciejewski, J. P., Bruening, E. E., Donahue, R. E., Mocarski, E. S., Young, N. S., and St Jeor, S. C. (1992). Infection of hematopoietic progenitor cells by human cytomegalovirus. *Blood*, **80**, 170–178.

Maciejewski, J. P., Bruening, E. E., Donahue, R. E. *et al.* (1993). Infection of mononucleated phagocytes with human cytomegalovirus. *Virology*, **195**, 327–336.

Marchini, A., Liu, H., and Zhu, H. (2001). Human cytomegalovirus with IE-2 (UL122) deleted fails to express early lytic genes. *J. Virol.*, **75**, 1870–1878.

Menard, C., Wagner, M., and Ruzsics, Z. (2003). Role of murine cytomegalovirus US22 gene family members in replication in macrophages. *J. Virol.*, **77**, 5557–5570.

Mendelson, M., Monard, S., Sissons, P., and Sinclair, J. (1996). Detection of endogenous human cytomegalovirus in CD34+ bone marrow progenitors. *J. Gen. Virol.*, **77**, 3099–3102.

Minton, E. J., Tysoe, C., Sinclair, J. H., and Sissons, J. G. (1994). Human cytomegalovirus infection of the monocyte/macrophage lineage in bone marrow. *J. Virol.*, **68**, 4017–4021.

Mocarski, E. S., Prichard, M. N., Tan, C. S., and Brown, J. M. (1997). Reassessing the organization of the UL42–UL43 region of the human cytomegalovirus strain AD169 genome. *Virology*, **239**, 169–175.

Moses, A. V. and Nelson, J. A. (1994). HIV infection of human brain capillary endothelial cells – implications for AIDS dementia. *Adv. Neuroimmunol.*, **4**, 239–247.

Movassagh, M., Gozlan, J., Senechal, B., Baillou, C., Petit, J. C., and Lemoine, F. M. (1996). Direct infection of CD34+ progenitor cells by human cytomegalovirus: evidence for inhibition of hematopoiesis and viral replication. *Blood*, **88**, 1277–1283.

Murayama, T., Mukaida, N., Khabar, K. S., and Matsushima, K. (1998). Potential involvement of IL-8 in the pathogenesis of human cytomegalovirus infection. *J. Leukoc. Biol.*, **64**, 62–67.

Myerson, D., Hackman, R. C., Nelson, J. A., Ward, D. C., and McDougall, J. K. (1984). Widespread presence of histologically occult cytomegalovirus. *Hum. Pathol.*, **15**, 430–439.

Nordoy, I., Muller, F., Nordal, K. P. *et al.* (1999). Immunologic parameters as predictive factors of cytomegalovirus disease in renal allograft recipients. *J. Infect. Dis.*, **180**, 195–198.

Nordoy, I., Muller, F., Nordal, K. P., Rollag, H., Aukrust, P., and Froland, S. S. (2000a). Chemokines and soluble adhesion molecules in renal transplant recipients with cytomegalovirus infection. *Clin. Exp. Immunol.*, **120**, 333–337.

Nordoy, I., Muller, F., Nordal, K. P. *et al.* (2000b). The role of the tumor necrosis factor system and interleukin-10 during cytomegalovirus infection in renal transplant recipients. *J. Infect. Dis.*, **181**, 51–57.

Oswald, I. P., Wynn, T. A., Sher, A., and James, S. L. (1992). Interleukin 10 inhibits macrophage microbicidal activity by blocking the endogenous production of tumor necrosis factor alpha required as a costimulatory factor for interferon gamma-induced activation. *Proc. Natl Acad. Sci. USA*, **89**, 8676–8680.

Page, C., Rose, M., Yacoub, M., and Pigott, R. (1992). Antigenic heterogeneity of vascular endothelium. *Am. J. Pathol.*, **141**, 673–683.

Pampou, S., Gnedoy, S. N., Bystrevskaya, V. B. *et al.* (2000). Cytomegalovirus genome and the immediate-early antigen in cells of different layers of human aorta. *Virchows Arch.*, **436**, 539–552.

Pass, R. F. (2001). Cytomegalovirus. In Knipe, D. M., Griffin, D. E., Lamb, R. A., Martin, M. A., Roizman, B., and Straus, S. E. (eds.), *Fields Virology*, 4th edn. pp. 2675–2705 Philadelphia: Lippincott Williams & Wilkins.

Patrone, M., Secchi, M., Fiorina, L., Ierardi, M., Milanesi, G., and Gallina, A. (2005). Human cytomegalovirus UL130 protein promotes endothelial cell infection through a producer cell modification of the virion. *J. Virol.*, **79**, 8361–8373.

Patterson, C. E. and Shenk, T. (1999). Human cytomegalovirus UL36 protein is dispensable for viral replication in cultured cells. *J. Virol.*, **73**, 7126–7131.

Petrie, B. L., Melnick, J. L., Adam, E., Burek, J., McCollum, C. H., and DeBakey, M. E. (1987). Nucleic acid sequences of human cytomegalovirus in cells cultured from human arterial tissue. *J. Infect. Dis.*, **155**, 158–159.

Prösch, S., Staak, K., Stein, J. et al. (1995). Stimulation of the human cytomegalovirus IE enhancer/promoter in HL-60 cells by TNFalpha is mediated via induction of NF-kappaB. *Virology*, **208**, 197–206.

Prösch, S., Heine, A. K., Volk, H. D., and Kruger, D. H. (2001). CCAAT/enhancer-binding proteins alpha and beta negatively influence the capacity of tumor necrosis factor alpha to up-regulate the human cytomegalovirus IE1/2 enhancer/promoter by nuclear factor kappa B during monocyte differentiation. *J. Biol. Chem.*, **276**, 40712–40720.

Rajotte, D., Arap, W., Hagedorn, M., Koivunen, E., Pasqualini, R., and Ruoslahti, E. (1998). Molecular heterogeneity of the vascular endothelium revealed by in vivo phage display. *J. Clin. Invest.*, **102**, 430–437.

Reboredo, M., Greaves, R. F., and Hahn, G. (2004). Human cytomegalovirus proteins encoded by UL37 exon 1 protect infected fibroblasts against virus-induced apoptosis and are required for efficient virus replication. *J. Gen. Virol.*, **85**, 3555–35567.

Rice, G. P., Schrier, R. D., and Oldstone, M. B. (1984). Cytomegalovirus infects human lymphocytes and monocytes: virus expression is restricted to immediate-early gene products. *Proc. Natl Acad. Sci. USA*, **81**, 6134–6138.

Ritter, T., Brandt, C., Prosch, S. et al. (2000). Stimulatory and inhibitory action of cytokines on the regulation of hCMV-IE promoter activity in human endothelial cells. *Cytokine*, **12**, 1163–1170.

Rue, C. A., Jarvis, M. A., Knoche, A. J. et al. (2004). A cyclooxygenase-2 homologue encoded by rhesus cytomegalovirus is a determinant for endothelial cell tropism. *J. Virol.*, **78**, 12529–12536.

Schrier, R. D., Nelson, J. A., and Oldstone, M. B. (1985). Detection of human cytomegalovirus in peripheral blood lymphocytes in a natural infection. *Science*, **230**, 1048–1051.

Simmons, P., Kaushansky, K., and Torok-Storb, B. (1990). Mechanisms of cytomegalovirus-mediated myelosuppression: perturbation of stromal cell function versus direct infection of myeloid cells. *Proc. Natl Acad. Sci. USA*, **87**, 1386–1390.

Sindre, H., Tjonnfjord, G. E., Rollag, H. et al. (1996). Human cytomegalovirus suppression of and latency in early hematopoietic progenitor cells. *Blood*, **88**, 4526–4533.

Sinzger, C., Grefte, A., Plachter, B., Gouw, A. S., The, T. H., and Jahn, G. (1995). Fibroblasts, epithelial cells, endothelial cells and smooth muscle cells are major targets of human cytomegalovirus infection in lung and gastrointestinal tissues. *J. Gen. Virol.*, **76**, 741–750.

Sinzger, C., Schmidt, K., Knapp, J. et al. (1999). Modification of human cytomegalovirus tropism through propagation in vitro is associated with changes in the viral genome. *J. Gen. Virol.*, **80**, 2867–2877.

Sinzger, C., Kahl, M., Laib, K. et al. (2000). Tropism of human cytomegalovirus for endothelial cells is determined by a post-entry step dependent on efficient translocation to the nucleus. *J. Gen. Virol.*, **81** (Pt 12), 3021–3035.

Skaletskaya, A., Bartle, L. M., Chittenden, T., McCormick, A. L., Mocarski, E. S., and Goldmacher, V. S. (2001). A cytomegalovirus-encoded inhibitor of apoptosis that suppresses caspase-8 activation. *Proc. Natl Acad. Sci. USA*, **98**, 7829–7834.

Slobbe-van Drunen, M. E., Hendrickx, A. T., Vossen, R. C., Speel, E. J., van Dam-Mieras, M. C., and Bruggeman, C. A. (1998). Nuclear import as a barrier to infection of human umbilical vein endothelial cells by human cytomegalovirus strain AD169. *Virus Res.*, **56**, 149–156.

Slobedman, B. and Mocarski, E. S. (1999). Quantitative analysis of latent human cytomegalovirus. *J. Virol.*, **73**, 4806–4812.

Smiley, M. L., Mar, E. C., and Huang, E. S. (1988). Cytomegalovirus infection and viral-induced transformation of human endothelial cells. *J. Med. Virol.*, **25**, 213–226.

Smith, J. A. and Pari, G. S. (1995). Expression of human cytomegalovirus UL36 and UL37 genes is required for viral DNA replication. *J. Virol.*, **69**, 1925–1931.

Smith, M. A., Sundaresan, S., Mohanakumar, T. et al. (1998). Effect of development of antibodies to HLA and cytomegalovirus mismatch on lung transplantation survival and development of bronchiolitis obliterans syndrome. *J. Thorac. Cardiovasc. Surg.*, **116**, 812–820.

Söderberg, C., Larsson, S., Bergstedt-Lindqvist, S., and Moller, E. (1993). Definition of a subset of human peripheral blood mononuclear cells that are permissive to human cytomegalovirus infection. *J. Virol.*, **67**, 3166–3175.

Söderberg-Naucler, C., Fish, K. N., and Nelson, J. A. (1997a). Interferon-gamma and tumor necrosis factor-alpha specifically induce formation of cytomegalovirus-permissive monocyte-derived macrophages that are refractory to the antiviral activity of these cytokines. *J. Clin. Invest.*, **100**, 3154–3163.

Söderberg-Naucler, C., Fish, K. N., and Nelson, J. A. (1997b). Reactivation of latent human cytomegalovirus by allogeneic stimulation of blood cells from healthy donors. *Cell*, **91**, 119–126.

Söderberg-Naucler, C., Streblow, D. N., Fish, K. N., Allan-Yorke, J., Smith, P. P., and Nelson, J. A. (2001). Reactivation of latent human cytomegalovirus in CD14(+) monocytes is differentiation dependent. *J. Virol.*, **75**, 7543–7554.

Speir, E., Modali, R., Huang, E. S., Leon, M. B., Shawl, F., Finkel, T., and Epstein, S. E. (1994). Potential role of human cytomegalovirus and p53 interaction in coronary restenosis. *Science*, **265**, 391–394.

Spencer, J. V., Lockridge, K. M., Barry, P. A. et al. (2002). Potent immunosuppressive activities of cytomegalovirus-encoded interleukin-10. *J. Virol.*, **76**, 1285–1292.

Stein, J., Volk, H. D., Liebenthal, C., Kruger, D. H., and Prosch, S. (1993). Tumour necrosis factor alpha stimulates the activity of the human cytomegalovirus major immediate early enhancer/promoter in immature monocytic cells. *J. Gen. Virol.*, **74**, 2333–2338.

Taylor-Wiedeman, J., Sissons, J. G., Borysiewicz, L. K., and Sinclair, J. H. (1991). Monocytes are a major site of persistence of human cytomegalovirus in peripheral blood mononuclear cells. *J. Gen. Virol.*, **72**, 2059–2064.

Taylor-Wiedeman, J., Hayhurst, G. P., Sissons, J. G., and Sinclair, J. H. (1993). Polymorphonuclear cells are not sites of persistence of human cytomegalovirus in healthy individuals. *J. Gen. Virol.*, **74**, 265–268.

Taylor-Wiedeman, J., Sissons, P., and Sinclair, J. (1994). Induction of endogenous human cytomegalovirus gene expression after differentiation of monocytes from healthy carriers. *J. Virol.*, **68**, 1597–1604.

Tegtmeier, G. E. (1989). Posttransfusion cytomegalovirus infections. *Arch. Pathol. Lab. Med.*, **113**, 236–245.

Tegtmeier, G. E. (1986). Transfusion-transmitted cytomegalovirus infections: significance and control. *Vox Sang.*, **51**(Suppl 1), 22–30.

Tolkoff-Rubin, N. E. and Rubin, R. H. (1994). The interaction of immunosuppression with infection in the organ transplant recipient. *Transpl. Proc.*, **26**, 16–19.

Torok-Storb, B., Simmons, P., Khaira, D., Stachel, D., and Myerson, D. (1992). Cytomegalovirus and marrow function. *Ann. Hematol.*, **64**(Suppl), A128–A131.

Turner, R. R., Beckstead, J. H., Warnke, R. A., and Wood, G. S. (1987). Endothelial cell phenotypic diversity. In situ demonstration of immunologic and enzymatic heterogeneity that correlates with specific morphologic subtypes. *Am. J. Clin. Pathol.*, **87**, 569–575.

von Laer, D., Meyer-Koenig, U., Serr, A. *et al.* (1995a). Detection of cytomegalovirus DNA in CD34+ cells from blood and bone marrow. *Blood*, **86**, 4086–4090.

von Laer, D., Serr, A., Meyer-Konig, U., Kirste, G., Hufert, F. T., and Haller, O. (1995b). Human cytomegalovirus immediate early and late transcripts are expressed in all major leukocyte populations in vivo [see comments]. *J. Infect. Dis.*, **172**, 365–370.

Wagner, M., Ruzsics, Z., and Koszinowski, U. H. (2002). Herpesvirus genetics has come of age. *Trends Microbiol.*, **10**, 318–324.

Waldman, W. J. and Knight, D. A. (1996). Cytokine-mediated induction of endothelial adhesion molecule and histocompatibility leukocyte antigen expression by cytomegalovirus-activated T cells. *Am. J. Pathol.*, **148**, 105–119.

Waldman, W. J., Knight, D. A., Huang, E. H., and Sedmak, D. D. (1995). Bidirectional transmission of infectious cytomegalovirus between monocytes and vascular endothelial cells: an in vitro model. *J. Infect. Dis.*, **171**, 263–272.

Wang, D. and Shenk, T. (2005a). Human cytomegalovirus UL131 open reading frame is required for epithelial cell tropism. *J. Virol.*, **79**, 10330–10338.

Wang, D. and Shenk, T. (2005b). Human cytomegalovirus virion protein complex required for epithelial and endothelial cell tropism. *Proc. Natl. Acad. Sci. USA*, **102**, 18153–18158.

White, K. L., Slobedman, B., and Mocarski, E. S. (2000). Human cytomegalovirus latency-associated protein pORF94 is dispensable for productive and latent infection. *J. Virol.*, **74**, 9333–9337.

Wiley, C. A. and Nelson, J. A. (1988). Role of human immunodeficiency virus and cytomegalovirus in AIDS encephalitis. *Am. J. Pathol.*, **133**, 73–81.

Yamashiroya, H. M., Ghosh, L., Yang, R., and Robertson, A. L. (1988). Herpesviridae in the coronary arteries and aorta of young trauma victims. *Am. J. Path.*, **130**, 71–79.

Yu, D., Smith, G. A., Enquist, L. W., and Shenk, T. (2002). Construction of a self-excisable bacterial artificial chromosome containing the human cytomegalovirus genome and mutagenesis of the diploid TRL/IRL13 gene. *J. Virol.*, **76**, 2316–2328.

Zhang, H., Fu, S., Busch, A., Chen, F., Qin, L., and Bromberg, J. S. (2001). Identification of TNF-alpha-sensitive sites in HCMVie1 promoter. *Exp. Mol. Pathol.*, **71**, 106–114.

Zhu, H., Shen Y., and Shenk T. (1995). Human cytomegalovirus IE1 and IE2 proteins block apoptosis. *J. Virol.*, **69**, 7960–7970.

43

Immunobiology and host response

Mark R. Wills, Andrew J. Carmichael, J. H. Sinclair, and J. G. Patrick Sissons

Department of Medicine, School of Clinical Medicine, University of Cambridge, UK

Introduction

HCMV, as all persistent viruses, has to survive in the host in the face of an immune response. Antibody, and probably T-cells in particular, contain the infection in the normal host but impaired T-cell immunity is associated with HCMV disease. The virus encodes functions which can counter this immune response and may also use immune cells as sites of latency. Although our knowledge of many aspects of the virus/host relationship is still incomplete, studies on HCMV over the past 20 years have given insight into how a large DNA virus achieves this coexistence with the normal immune response. Other chapters also contain relevant material.

Cells of the immune system as sites of latency and reactivation for HCMV

Consideration of the immune response to HCMV has to take account of the fact that some cells of the immune system are strong candidates for being sites of latency (see elsewhere in this volume). It is a longstanding clinical observation that HCMV can be transmitted by blood transfusion, but the most sensitive PCR based techniques do not detect HCMV DNA in plasma or serum of healthy virus carriers (although they do in patients with active HCMV disease), implying HCMV is most likely transmitted by cells in peripheral blood. Evidence from several laboratories suggests that HCMV is latent in myeloid lineage cells (Sinclair and Sissons, 2006). Using highly sensitive PCRs (of considerably greater sensitivity than those used for diagnostic assays) HCMV DNA can be detected in CD14+ peripheral blood mononuclear cells and in CD34+ cells in bone marrow (Mendelson et al., 1996; Taylor-Wiedeman et al., 1991). HCMV DNA is also reported in CD33+ cells in bone marrow (Hahn et al., 1998; Kondo et al., 1994). No infectious virus can normally be detected in freshly isolated peripheral blood monocytes or myeloid lineage progenitors, although the induction of HCMV immediate early gene expression can be detected by highly sensitive RT PCR when peripheral blood monocytes are differentiated with interferon-γ (IFN-γ) and GM CSF (Taylor-Wiedeman et al., 1994). In order to demonstrate that a particular cell type is really harboring latent virus capable of reactivation, it is necessary to show that infectious virus can be rescued from such putatively latently infected cells. One group has reported that differentiation of peripheral blood monocytes from seropositive subjects to monocyte-derived macrophages in vitro in the presence of allogeneic T cells results in detection of infectious HCMV by co-cultivation of the cells with fibroblasts (Soderberg-Naucler et al., 1997, 2001). There is also evidence that dendritic cells (DC) may be a specific site of latency and that their differentiation to mature DC in vitro may be associated with reactivation (Reeves et al., 2005).

These observations all relate to the detection of endogenous HCMV DNA in cells of normal seropositive subjects, rather than the detection of HCMV which has been exogenously added to such cells during in vitro culture. Although the latter type of experiment with exogenous HCMV in general supports the evidence from detecting endogenous HCMV DNA that myeloid lineage cells are a site of persistence, it is always difficult to exclude the possibility that low level virus replication (rather than true latency) is maintaining HCMV DNA in such experimental in vitro systems.

Considering all of the current evidence from the literature, the most plausible picture of HCMV latency and reactivation in cells of the bone marrow and blood is that HCMV is carried in myeloid lineage progenitor cells in the bone marrow and is maintained in the cells as they divide down the myeloid lineage into peripheral blood monocytes and dendritic cells, albeit at a very low frequency – perhaps 0.01% of mononuclear cells – and virus then reactivates when latently infected monocytes differentiate into macrophages (probably after exiting the circulation into tissues) under the influence of cytokines. However, unanswered questions include the following. (i) Is there a reservoir of HCMV in bone marrow which maintains virus in some stem cell population ? (ii) What is the mechanism by which viral DNA is maintained in myeloid lineage cells as they divide ? (iii) Is there a subpopulation of mononuclear cells, particularly DC, which is critical for maintenance of HCMV latency? (iv) What are the precise cytokines and pathways which differentiate peripheral blood mononuclear cells into the cell phenotype needed to permit reactivation of latent virus ? (v) Are there a limited set of HCMV RNA transcripts that are necessary for the maintenance of HCMV latent DNA (analogous to the LATs of HSV)?. There are reports of HCMV latency-associated transcripts in myeloid lineage cells in both natural and experimental infection, but it is unclear whether they are truly specific for latency and what their function might be (White et al., 2000; Bego et al., 2005). The subject is further discussed in the chapter by Nelson and colleagues.

The balance of evidence suggests that HCMV is not latent in other cell types in peripheral blood (Taylor-Wiedeman et al., 1993). In healthy carriers, lymphocytes and peripheral blood neutrophils appear not to carry virus – although neutrophils may contain CMV antigens during active HCMV disease, there is no evidence they do this in normal seropositive subjects and the evidence is against their being a site of replication for the virus (Sinzger et al., 1996).

The immune response to HCMV in the human host

Lessons from animal models of CMV disease

Murine cytomegalovirus (MCMV) infection of inbred mice has been extensively utilized as a model system to help to further understand HCMV infections, including aspects of immune responses, latency and immunopathology. This work has generated a substantial literature and made an important contribution to our understanding of the immunobiology of HCMV. The work cannot be reviewed here but is well summarized in several excellent recent reviews on the immune response to (Polic et al., 1998; Reddehase, 2002), and latency of (Reddehase et al., 2002), MCMV.

Antibody and complement

Following primary infection, antibodies specific to numerous HCMV encoded proteins are readily detectable in serum (for review see Britt, 1991; Landini and Michelson, 1988). These include structural tegument proteins (such as pp65 and pp150), envelope glycoproteins (predominantly gB and gH) as well as non-structural proteins such as the Immediate Early 1 protein (IE1, UL123) and a DNA binding protein (UL44). Viral neutralizing activity in vitro is predominantly mediated by antibodies specific for gB and gH (Britt et al., 1988; Urban et al., 1996). Both mouse and guinea pig animal models suggest that antibody is important in protection from a lethal infective dose and in reducing fetal infection (Rapp et al., 1992; Harrison et al., 1995). In humans, pre-existing humoral immunity to cytomegalovirus also plays an important role in preventing congenital infection of the fetus during pregnancy (Fowler et al., 1992) and in preventing transfusion-associated infection in premature infants (Yeager et al., 1981). The role of humoral immunity in the pathogenesis of HCMV disease in immunosuppressed patients is uncertain. Prior infection and thus the existence of preformed antibody to HCMV may be an important factor in limiting reactivation and protecting from re-exposure: however there is very limited evidence for the benefits of administration of HCMV-specific antibody to immunosuppressed transplant patients who are undergoing a primary infection or reactivation, with some studies reporting beneficial results and others suggesting no benefit (Guglielmo et al., 1994; Munoz et al., 2001).

gB in its mature form is composed of two disulfide bonded subunits gp116 and gp58 derived by the proteolytic cleavage of a glycosylated precursor molecule (Britt and Mach, 1996). The vast majority of HCMV-infected individuals mount an antibody response directed against gB, and a large proportion of neutralizing antibodies produced in response to viral infection are gB-specific (Britt et al., 1990; Gonczol et al., 1991; Marshall et al., 1992; Schoppel et al., 1997). The antibody response to gB has consequently been extensively studied, and three antigenic domains have been identified AD-1 (aa 552–635), AD-2 (aa50–77) and AD-3 (aa783–906). AD-2 has been further defined and is composed of two antibody binding sites, Site I (aa68–77) and Site II (aa50 to 54). Antibodies which bind AD-1 and AD-2 site II mediate viral neutralization (Kniess et al., 1991; Meyer et al., 1992; Wagner et al., 1992). The AD-1 site is large, consisting of a run of 75 amino acids: within this run, cysteine residues at positions 573 and 610 form a disulfide bond which is required for binding of antibodies directed at AD-1 (Speckner et al., 1999).

Of possible relevance to humoral immunity to HCMV is the existence of virus-associated Fc receptors. It has been recognized for some time that HCMV-infected cells are able to bind IgG isotype from human and other species, independent of any specific antibody activity to HCMV (Furukawa et al., 1975; Keller et al., 1976; Mackowiak and

Marling-Cason, 1987). However only recently has this IgG Fc binding activity been ascribed to viral encoded gene products rather than virus-induced cellular Fc binding proteins. Two proteins have been described to date. The first is a 34 KDa Fc binding protein (Fc-BP) encoded by the TRL11 and IRL11 ORFs and predicted to be a type I membrane glycoprotein with no homology to other herpesvirus encoded viral Fc binding proteins (Lilley et al., 2000). The second protein is 68KDa and also a type I membrane glycoprotein encoded by the UL119-UL118 genes involving mRNA splicing (Atalay et al., 2002). These may represent one of the many levels at which HCMV is modulating the host immune response – it has been suggested that binding of IgG could reduce the levels of neutralizing antibody directed at the virus. These Fc-BPs proteins have a rapid rate of endocytosis and endolysosomal degradation providing for an efficient antibody capture and disposal system. Binding of HCMV-specific IgG via the Fc region might also interfere with complement activation and antibody-dependent cellular cytotoxicity (Atalay et al., 2002).

The HCMV specific CD8+ T-cell response

Given the inferential evidence for the importance of T cell immunity in controlling HCMV infection, and the evidence for the importance of the CD8+ T-cell response to MCMV, more attention has focussed on the CD8+ T-cell response to HCMV than on any other aspect of the immune response. HCMV specific CD8+ cytotoxic T-lymphocytes (CTL) were first detected in the peripheral blood lymphocytes (PBL) of patients with overt HCMV infection in the early 1980s and a short time later MHC restricted HCMV specific CTL precursors (CTLp) were stimulated to grow and mediate cytotoxicity from the PBL of normal healthy HCMV carriers (Borysiewicz et al., 1983). Since then a large body of work has identified individual viral encoded proteins which are recognized by T-cells, defined minimal antigenic peptides within these proteins together with their MHC Class I restrictions, enumerated the frequency of HCMV-specific CD8+ T-cells in normal healthy carriers as well as immunosuppressed transplant patients, and analyzed in detail the clonal composition of HCMV specific CD8+ T-cells and the phenotypic characteristics of these long-term memory T-cells.

The cytomegalovirus gene products that are targets for the human CD8+ T cell response have been studied for over 20 years. Most recently a study produced overlapping peptides to the whole HCMV proteome (213 open reading frames) in order to comprehensively map all CD8 and CD4 epitopes. Previous to this work.

CD8+ T-cells specific for IE1 (UL123), the viral matrix proteins (pp65 (UL83), pp150 (UL32), pp28 (UL98), pp50 (UL44)), the surface viral glycoproteins (gB (UL55), gH (UL75)) and a number of other viral proteins (US2, US3, US6, US11, UL16 and UL18) have been detected using either interferon-γ secretion (ELISPOT or intracellular flow cytometry), or cytotoxicity using either bulk polyclonal T cell populations or T-cell clones as effector cells in radioactive Chromium release cytotoxicity assays (Borysiewicz et al., 1983; Wills et al., 1996; McLaughlin-Taylor et al., 1994; Elkington et al., 2003; Kern et al., 2002; Longmate et al., 2001).

The work of Riddell and colleagues first suggested a large proportion of the CD8+ T-cell response to HCMV was directed at the lower matrix protein pp65: these workers generated CD8+ T-cell clones for infusion into bone marrow transplant recipients by secondary in vitro restimulation of PBMC from their HCMV seropositive donors, and found the majority of clones were specific for this protein (Walter et al., 1995). A number of subsequent studies concluded that the majority of the CD8+ T-cell response to HCMV in a given virus carrier is directed at pp65 (Wills et al., 1996; Boppana and Britt, 1996). By comparing the killing of target cells infected with AD169 strain HCMV or a pp65 gene deletion mutant (RVAd65) in limiting dilution assays, the contribution of pp65-specific CTLp to the total HCMV-specific CTLp frequency was quantified in healthy seropositive virus carriers at between 70 and 90%, suggesting that pp65 is an immunodominant viral antigen. CD8+ T-cells specific for IE1 have also been isolated from seropositive carriers, although the frequencies of IE1-specific CTLp have been estimated as being on average ten fold lower than those for pp65-specific CTLp (Wills et al., 1996). pp150-specific CTL have also been isolated from some donors at about a four fold lower frequency as compared to pp65. The frequency of CTLp specific for gB, gH, pp50 or pp28 has been reported as < 10 CTLp/million CD8+ T cells which is at the limit of detection of this assay (Boppana and Britt, 1996).

Estimations of the frequency of virus-specific CTLp in assays based on in vitro restimulation with antigen depend on the CTL precursors being exposed to all the appropriate CTL epitopes. When autologous HCMV-infected fibroblasts are used for restimulation in vitro, viral encoded proteins (US2, US3, US6 and US11) which interfere with antigen processing and presentation (Reddehase, 2002) may lead to selective presentation of particular virus peptides by surface MHC Class I, with a consequent underestimation of CTLp frequencies against certain antigens. The view that pp65 is immunodominant has been refined in the light of further data over the past few years. Panels of synthetic peptides spanning complete proteins combined with rapid epitope screening assays (based on intracellular

IFN-γ production detected by flow cytometry) have been used to reassess the frequency of IE1-specific CD8+ T-cells (Kern et al., 2002). Previous observations that only a proportion of virus carriers have CD8+ T-cell responses to IE1 were confirmed, but this work also found much higher frequencies of IE1-specific T-cells similarly high to those specific for pp65 (Kern et al., 2002). It has been shown that de novo protein synthesis is not required to sensitize target cells to killing by pp65-specific CTL (McLaughlin-Taylor et al., 1994): pp65 is present in virions as a preformed structural protein which is delivered to the cytosol during virus infection, from which pp65 can enter the MHC Class I antigen processing pathway. In contrast IE1 has to be synthesized de novo after virus infection at a time in the virus replication cycle when the ability of the infected cell to present new MHC Class I-peptide complexes is impaired. Direct stimulation of CD8+ T-cells using synthetic peptides in the absence of any influence of other viral proteins, has demonstrated much higher frequencies of IE1-specific CD8+ T-cells than previously reported and this may hold true for other HCMV antigens. A recent investigation utilizing a bioinformatics approach to predict CD8+ T-cell epitopes has described dozens of new HCMV T-cell epitopes within 14 HCMV encoded proteins. The new epitopes were verified using an ELISPOT assay measuring IFN-γ production, and some of the epitopes were also used to generate functional CTL (Elkington et al., 2003). Although this approach clearly indicates that many other HCMV-encoded proteins can act as CD8+ T cell antigens, this work also confirms the previous findings that pp65-specific and IE-specific T-cells dominate the CD8+ T-cell response in most individuals.

In a recent and comprehensive study 13 687 consecutive 15-mer peptides overlapping each other by 10 amino acids and comprising 213 potential ORFs were synthesized and used in intracellular IFN gamma assays in order to identify all ORFs from HCMV that could be recognized by either CD4+ or CD8+ T cells derived from a cohort of 33 HCMV positive donors of diverse HLA haplotypes. The results showed that 47% of HCMV ORFs were recognized by CD8 T cells from at least one of the 33 donors, and on average, each donor exhibited CD8+ T cell responses to 7 different ORFs. Traditionally studied ORFs like pp65 (UL83) and IE1 (UL123) were among the most common, being recognized by more than half the subjects: however this study showed that many other ORFs are also commonly recognized and pp65 and IE1 are by no means universally immunodominant in such a diverse cohort (Sylwester et al., 2005).

The production of soluble tetrameric MHC class I molecules loaded with specific viral peptide, then biotinylated and labeled with a fluorescent tag, provides a reagent which binds directly to the T-cell receptor (TCR) of peptide-specific CD8+ T-cells. These labelled Class I tetramers allow the visualization of antigen-specific T-cells by flow cytometry and have made an important contribution to the analysis of virus-specific T-cell responses to many human virus infections including HCMV. Tetramers have been constructed to pp65 peptides presented by HLA-A0201, A2402, B0702 B0801 and B3501 (Gillespie et al., 2000; Hassan-Walker et al, 2001; Kuzushima et al., 2001), and IE1 peptides presented by HLA-A0201 and B0801 (Khan et al., 2002a,b; Wills et al., 2002), and used to determine the frequencies of virus-specific CD8+ T-cell frequencies in a large number of HCMV seropositive subjects. The results confirm the very high frequency response to pp65 and IE1 in most HCMV seropositive subjects and also demonstrate that functional assays such as LDA tend to underestimate the HCMV-specific frequency (as has been noted in other virus sytems).

It is clear that primary HCMV infection elicits strong virus-specific CD8+ responses to numerous viral proteins: evidence suggesting that these specific CD8+ responses are protective is provided both by murine models of CMV, and by data obtained from patients undergoing reconstitution of their immune systems following bone marrow transplantation (BMT) or stem cell transplantation. Mice are protected from lethal MCMV challenge by CD8+ cells specific for immediate early antigens (Reddehase et al., 1987). In a murine model of CMV reactivation (deficient in B-cell responses) it has been demonstrated that CD4+ and NK cells can substitute for CD8+ T-cells. However in murine models of BMT, removal of reconstituted CD8+ cells leads to lethal disease and reconstituted CD8+ cells transferred to immunocompromised mice could prevent disease (Polic et al., 1998). Following BMT in humans there was a strong correlation between the recovery of cytolytic T-cell activity and recovery from HCMV infection. Subsequent studies quantifying T-cell recovery using virus-specific tetramers estimate that a recovery of virus-specific cells of >10 per μl of blood was protective against serious HCMV disease (Cwynarski et al., 2001).

The availability of HCMV-specific MHC Class I tetramers, monoclonal antibodies against cell surface molecules and multi-parameter flow cytometry, and techniques for T-cell receptor analysis have made possible the detailed characterization of antigen-experienced HCMV-specific CD8+ T-cells.

Analysis of the clonal composition of the memory CD8+ T-cells specific for defined pp65 epitopes by sequencing of the TCRs of multiple independently derived epitope-specific CTL clones, reveals a high degree of clonal focusing: in a given virus carrier, the majority of CTL clones specific to a defined pp65 peptide use only one or two different TCRs at the level of the nucleotide sequence. Thus in a given carrier the large population of circulating HCMV peptide-specific CD8+ T cells is in fact composed of only a few individual CD8+ clones that have undergone extensive clonal expansion in vivo (Weekes et al., 1999). It is also clear that cells of an individual antigen-experienced pp65-specific clone persists in the virus carrier for years, because the same clones can be repeatedly isolated over time. CD8+ T-cells obtained from unrelated subjects that recognize the same defined peptide–MHC complex often use the same TCR Vβ segment, and have similar amino acid sequences within the hypervariable VDJ region of the TCR that binds to the viral peptide. Similar observations of clonal T cell focusing have also been made for CTL specific for a number of IE1 peptides (Khan et al., 2002a,b). Other persistent virus infections (EBV and HIV) are also associated with this tendency to develop large oligoclonal T-cell populations. The focused pp65-specific and IE-specific CD8+ T-cell response observed in HCMV carriers may be the result of repeated exposure to viral antigen upon periodic reactivation of HCMV, with selection of CD8+ T-cells that express certain high affinity TCRs, and persistence of these clones in long-term memory. It is interesting to note that a study of HCMV-specific T-cell responses in elderly subjects showed that the frequency can increase over time to very large numbers (up to 25% of all CD8+ cells in an individual) and that the T-cell repertoires become more oligoclonal (Khan et al., 2002a,b). It remains unclear how soon after primary HCMV infection the pattern of CD8+ T cell clonal focussing develops and to what extent the relative clonal dominance changes in long-term virus carriers. Following allogeneic BMT from HCMV-seropositive donors to HCMV-seropositive recipients, individual dominant HCMV-specific CD8+ clones present in the donor are typically transferred in the allograft, undergo expansion and are maintained long-term in the recipient; in addition, delayed emergence of different donor-derived clonotypes can be observed more than 6 months after transplantation (Gandhi et al., 2003).

Detailed analysis of the phenotype of peptide-specific CD8+ T-cells has been undertaken using oligonucleotide clonotype probing (which can quantify a virus-specific T-cell receptor rearrangement directly from peripheral blood) or HCMV-specific tetramers, in combination with monoclonal antibodies to cell surface markers. The expression of the CD45RA and CD45RO isoforms of CD45 was previously thought to distinguish naïve (CD45RAhigh) from memory T-cells (CD45ROhigh). However in healthy carriers, cells of a single antigen-experienced HCMV-specific CD8+ T-cell clone are present in both the CD45RO(high) and CD45RA(high) T-cell subpopulations. During primary HCMV infection, all the highly activated effector HCMV-specific T-cells express CD45RO, but during convalescence they accumulate in the CD45RA(high) subpopulation consistent with reversion from CD45RO(high) cells (revertant memory) (Wills et al., 1999). The same phenomenon has also been described following primary EBV infection (Faint et al., 2001). Further analysis of the CD45RA(high) HCMV-specific T-cells using markers to cell surface adhesion, costimulation and chemokine receptor molecules has shown that they lack the costimulatory molecule CD28 and the chemokine receptor CCR7. However, in contrast to previous suggested models of CD8+ T-cell memory, these CD28(−) CD45RA(high) CCR7(−) cells are not terminally differentiated, because following stimulation in vitro with specific HCMV peptide these cells undergo sustained clonal proliferation, up-regulate CD45RO and CCR5, and show strong peptide-specific cytotoxic activity. In an individual with acute primary HCMV infection, HCMV pp65-specific CD8+ T-cells are predominantly CD28(−) CD45RO(high) CCR7(−). During convalescence, an increasing proportion of pp65-specific CD8+ T-cells were CD28(−) CD45RA(high) CCR7(−). Thus CD8+ T-cell memory to HCMV is maintained by cells of expanded HCMV-specific clones that show heterogeneity of activation state and costimulation molecule expression within both CD45RO(high) and CD28(−)CD45RA(high) T-cell pool (Wills et al., 2002). Similar techniques have been used by a number of groups to examine the memory T-cells generated in response to EBV: it is interesting to note that T-cells specific for lytic EBV antigens display very similar phenotypic profiles to HCMV pp65-specific T-cells. It is also of interest that this does not hold for all persistent virus infections (Faint et al., 2001; Appay et al., 2002).

The capacity of viruses to encode functions which may enable them to evade the effector function of cytotoxic T-cells has generated enormous interest over the last 5 years. Investigation of the ways in which HCMV can disrupt the normal MHC Class I antigen processing pathways has revealed a surprising number of mechanisms: these include the degradation of newly synthesised MHC Class I heavy chains (mediated by US2 (Wiertz et al., 1996b) and US11 (Wiertz et al., 1996a; Jones et al., 1995), retention of MHC Class I peptide complexes in the endoplasmic reticulum (ER) (mediated by US3 (Jones et al., 1996) and blockade of peptide translocation into the ER (mediated by US6 (Ahn et al., 1997). Further details are available elsewhere in this volume and in a recent review by Reddehase et al. (2002). The sequential expression of the US3 and US11 gene products which would lead to MHC Class I-peptide complex retention in the ER (US3) followed by degradation of de novo MHC Class I heavy chains (US11) may be very efficient. The combination of US2 and US11 may allow many different MHC Class I heavy chains (as would be found in an outbred population) to be redirected to the cytosol for degradation. HCMV infects and becomes latent in a number of different cell types in vivo and it is conceivable that some of these viral gene products are more efficient in some cell types as compared to others. The human immune system and HCMV have co-evolved to a considerable extent, and it is possible that the diversity of immune evasion mechanisms reflects this co-evolution of the virus and the immune system, and that some of the immune evasion mechanisms are vestigial.

It is clear that in spite of viral immune evasion genes, upon primary HCMV infection the host mounts a strong T-cell response composed of both CD8+ CTL and CD4+ helper T-cells which produce antiviral cytokines: the outcome is that acute primary infection is resolved, although HCMV is not cleared from the host but becomes latent with periodic reactivation and production of new virions. It is also clear that during long term carriage of the virus there is a balance between the cell-mediated immune response and viral activity. This balance is lost in the immunocompromised host where reactivation of latent virus or primary infection can lead to uncontrolled viral replication which may cause serious disease and death. Although the functional significance of the immune evasion genes in vivo remains to be determined, a plausible hypothesis is that the immune evasion mechanisms give the virus a "window of protection" during reactivation from latency in the face of an expanded population of antigen-experienced T-cells, enabling the virus to complete its life cycle to produce new virions. During reactivation the IE proteins are abundant at a time when the virus is retaining MHC Class I complexes in the ER, blocking antigen presentation and preventing T-cell surveillance. The virus may thus be able to replicate and release progeny virus from the cell: however, subsequent infection of neighboring cells will deliver preformed viral structural proteins to the cytosol which can enter the antigen processing pathway and be presented at the infected cell surface for T-cell recognition, resulting in local containment of the reactivation episode.

The HCMV-specific CD4+ T-cell response

CD4+ T-cells play a key role in the control of virus infections, by the activation of dendritic cells (by ligation of CD40 on the dendritic cell by CD154 on the T-cell), by providing help for virus-specific B-cells (ligation of CD40 on the B-cell induces immunoglobulin gene somatic hypermutation and class switching), and by secreting cytokines that facilitate the proliferation and differentiation of virus-specific CD8+ T-cells. In murine CMV infection, long-term selective depletion of CD4+ T-cells in vivo is associated with persistent virus replication at specific sites (Jonjic et al., 1989). Analysis of the HCMV-specific CD4+ T-cell response in humans has been greatly enhanced by the development of flow cytometry methods to detect intracellular cytokine expression by antigen-specific T cells (Waldrop et al., 1997, 1998). At present the production of peptide-MHC Class II tetramers to identify HCMV-specific CD4+ T-cells is technically demanding; when such tetramers become widely available, not only the analysis but also the therapeutic manipulation of HCMV-specific CD4+ T-cells may become possible in the future.

Using in vitro restimulation of PBMC with whole HCMV antigen and detection of intracellular cytokine expression by flow cytometry, in healthy HCMV carriers typically 1%–2% of all circulating CD4+ T-cells are specific for HCMV (Waldrop et al., 1998; Rentenaar et al., 2000) with one report of much higher frequencies (Sester et al., 2002). In approximately 60% of HCMV carriers, virus-specific CD4+ T-cells recognize the lower matrix protein pp65, and in a given carrier, CD4+ T-cells typically focus on one or a few peptide epitopes within pp65 (Beninga et al., 1995; Kern et al., 2002). The recent examination of the whole HCMV proteome for CD8 T cell specific responses also included CD4+ T cell responses: the results show that 44 unique ORFs are antigens for CD4+ T cells and that 81 ORFs are targets for both CD4 and CD8 responses (Sylwester et al., 2005). In part because fewer peptide binding motifs are known for MHC Class II alleles than for MHC Class I alleles, relatively few MHC Class II restricted epitopes within pp65 have been identified (Kern et al., 2002; Khattab et al., 1997; Le Pira et al., 2004; Weekes et al., 2004).

In healthy virus carriers, the surface phenotype of HCMV-specific CD4+ T-cells has been analyzed by staining of HCMV-stimulated PBMC with two or three different fluorochrome-linked monoclonal antibodies. CD4+ T-cells responding to stimulation by whole HCMV are enriched within CD45RO+, CD27−, CD62L−, CD11a^{high} and CCR7− subpopulations (Rentenaar et al., 2000; Sester et al., 2002; Bitmansour et al., 2002). Most peripheral blood HCMV-specific CD4+ T-cells secrete IFN-γ, a proportion of which also secrete TNFα and IL-2; very few HCMV-specific CD4+ T-cells secrete IL-4 (Rentenaar et al., 2000; Bitmansour et al., 2002). Many HCMV specific CD4+ cells are also cytotoxic and MHC Class II restricted (van Leeuwen et al., 2006; Weekes et al., 2004).

In healthy HCMV carriers, the circulating population of HCMV-specific CD4+ T-cells is oligoclonal. Following in vitro stimulation with whole HCMV antigen, responding HCMV-specific CD4+ T-cells showed striking focussing of TCR Vβ segment usage by monoclonal antibody staining. When HCMV-specific CD4+ T-cells were sorted and analyzed by RT-PCR, the TCR Vβ expansions were composed of a limited number of clonotypes in which 1–3 clones dominated the response together with a cohort of subdominant clones and numerous minor clones. The same dominant clonotypes were identified when CD4+ T-cells were stimulated with individual pp65 peptides (Bitmansour et al., 2002). Cells of an individual expanded clone showed a spectrum of triggering thresholds consistent with TCR-independent threshold regulation, including different thresholds for secretion of IFN-γ and IL-2, but the triggering thesholds did not differ between CD27+ and CD27− cells of the given clonotype. These results indicate that a given antigen-experienced CD4+ clonotype can give rise to qualitatively distinct functional responses depending upon epitope dose and availability of costimulation (Bitmansour et al., 2002).

To study the CD4+ T-cell response during natural primary HCMV infection in immunocompetent subjects is difficult; usually the time at which infection began is uncertain, and subjects have often had symptoms for a number of days before primary HCMV infection is confirmed by detection of anti-HCMV IgM. Longitudinal studies of primary HCMV infection have been performed in the setting of HCMV-seronegative individuals who received a renal transplant from a HCMV-seropositive donor (D+/R−) without prophylactic Ganciclovir treatment, although the introduction of HCMV via a solid organ that lacks lymphatic drainage and the concurrent use of immunosuppressant therapy (to prevent graft rejection) may modify the kinetics of infection and of the host T cell response (Rentenaar et al., 2000; Gamadia et al., 2003). HCMV DNAemia was first detected at a median of 25 days (range 18–29 days) after transplantation, and HCMV-specific IFN-γ-producing CD4+ T-cells were first detected (by intracellular cytokine staining following in vitro restimulation with whole HCMV antigen) at a median of 7 days (range 4–14 days) after first detection of HCMV DNAemia. In four of five subjects, HCMV-specific CD4+ T-cells were detected 3–10 days before anti-HCMV IgM. The HCMV-specific CD4+ T cell response developed rapidly, reached peak frequencies of 0.46% to 2.5% of peripheral blood CD4+ T-cells, and decreased rapidly to a low level over at least the next 10 weeks. In contrast to the phenotype observed in long-term virus carriers, during primary infection HCMV-specific CD4+ T-cells were predominantly CD38+, many were CD27+, and most showed co-expression of CD45RO and CD45RA. During primary infection a proportion of HCMV-specific CD4+ T cells were in cell cycle, as indicated by Ki67 expression (Rentenaar et al., 2000). In a second study, compared to asymptomatic primary infection, symptomatic primary HCMV infection was associated with delayed appearance of HCMV-specific CD4+ T-cells in peripheral blood. Among nine subjects who developed primary HCMV infection following D+/R− renal transplantation, four subjects had symptomatic infection that required Ganciclovir treatment, while the other five subjects had asymptomatic infection. In the symptomatic subjects the time at which HCMV DNAemia was first detected after transplantation (median 27 days) was similar to that in asymptomatic subjects, but the peak viral load and duration of HCMV DNAemia was greater in the symptomatic subjects. The time from first detection of HCMV DNAemia to first detection of HCMV-specific CD4+ T-cells by intracellular cytokine staining was significantly longer in symptomatic infection (median 39 days, range 28–53) compared to asymptomatic infection (median 10 days, range 0–17). In symptomatic subjects, HCMV-specific CD4+ T-cells only became detectable after starting Ganciclovir therapy, and reached peak frequencies of 0.36% to 1.42% of peripheral blood CD4+ T-cells. There were no differences in the kinetics of antibody or CD8+ T-cell responses between symptomatic and asymptomatic subjects; the time from first detection of HCMV DNAemia to first detection of either anti-HCMV antibody (15 days vs. 17 days) or HCMV-specific CD8+ T-cells by peptide MHC Class I tetramer staining (21 days vs. 24 days) was similar in symptomatic and asymptomatic subjects (Gamadia et al., 2003).

HCMV, innate immunity and natural killer (NK) cells

NK cells were originally described for their ability to mediate cytotoxicity against certain tumors without prior activation; they are characterized by the lack of both T- and B-cell markers, and are a component of the innate immune system. An important role for NK cells in the early control of viral infections is emerging (Tay et al., 1998; Biron et al., 1999). There is only limited evidence for the role of NK cells in the control of HCMV infection (Biron et al., 1989, 1999). However the virus encodes a variety of NK cell evasion mechanisms which are discussed in this section, which provides indirect evidence for the importance of these cells in the innate response to HCMV. In the MCMV murine model system the evidence for their protective role is much stronger. Newborn mice are highly susceptible to lethal MCMV infection until NK responses become apparent at 3 weeks. Adoptive transfer of NK cells into these mice or adult SCID mice can confer protection reviewed in (Tay et al., 1998). Inbred mouse strains have differing resistance to MCMV (Scalzo *et al.*, 1992), and the dominant Cmv1 resistance locus has been mapped to the NK cell gene complex on chromosome 6. The Cmv1 resistance gene has now been shown to encode an activating NK cell receptor Ly49H (Brown *et al.*, 2001; Lee *et al.*, 2001; Daniels *et al.*, 2001).

Activation of NK cells is promoted by signals from activating NK receptors, but inhibited by signals received through the inhibitory NK receptors which interact with specific MHC class I molecules on the surface of the target cell. Individual NK cell clones express distinct patterns of inhibitory NK receptors, which include immunoglobulin supergene family members and C-type lectin family members (for review see Lanier, 2005). The C-type lectin heterodimer CD94/NKG2A is present on the surface of the NK cell and ligates HLA-E on a normal cell surface (Braud *et al.*, 1998). HLA-E is stabilized and translocated to the cell surface when it binds certain signal sequence peptides derived from the normal turnover of HLA-A, HLA-B and HLA-C molecules (Braud *et al.*, 1997).

As discussed earlier, HCMV encodes a number of genes responsible for the retention and destruction of MHC Class I molecules. Upon HCMV reactivation (Sissons *et al.*, 2002), the early interference with the MHC Class I pathway may impede the presentation of viral derived peptides to the host CD8+ T cells and hence avoid recognition. However, the reduced levels of surface Class I MHC on HCMV-infected cells might be expected to favor activation of host NK cells (Karre *et al.*, 1986). This has led to the suggestion that HCMV would also have to evade NK cell recognition in order to safeguard this window in which a latent genome within a cell can reactivate, and have enough time to assemble and release infectious virus. The observation in a number of experimental systems that HCMV-infected cells are relatively resistant to NK-mediated lysis suggests that HCMV has evolved viral encoded functions to evade NK surveillance (Reyburn *et al.*, 1997; Vales-Gomez *et al.*, 2003; Wang *et al.*, 2002; Cerboni *et al.*, 2000; Fletcher *et al.*, 1998; Arnon *et al.*, 2005; Tomasec *et al.*, 2005; Wills *et al.*, 2005). Six distinct virus encoded proteins and mechanisms have been proposed to prevent NK activation and lysis of HCMV-infected cells.

HCMV expresses a viral MHC Class I homologue gpUL18 which was reported to inhibit NK lysis (Reyburn *et al.*, 1997), although this report has been contradicted by a subsequent investigation which suggested that UL18 may activate NK cells (Leong *et al.*, 1998). These data might now be explicable in the light of the recent identification in MCMV of a new MHC Class I-like molecule (m157) which can engage an inhibitory NK receptor in one strain of mouse and an activating receptor in others (Arase *et al.*, 2002). It has subsequently been shown that HCMV UL18 binds LIR-1/ILT2 which is present on only a subset of NK cells (Cosman *et al.*, 1997). At present it remains unclear whether UL18 expression on HCMV-infected cells activates or inhibits specific populations of NK cells.

The viral protein encoded by HCMV UL40 also includes a signal sequence peptide similar to those of Class I molecules, and expression of UL40 has been reported to stabilize HLA-E (Tomasec *et al.*, 2000). HLA-E expression is not affected by the US2-11 gene products, and the maintenance of surface HLA-E expression by providing an appropriate signal peptide from UL40 has been proposed as another novel NK cell evasion strategy for HCMV (Wang *et al.*, 2002). However other groups have not observed this effect of UL40 in their systems (Falk *et al.*, 2002).

Some activating NK receptors recognize host cell proteins which are upregulated on the surface of stressed cells, for example, the activating receptor NKG2D recognizes MICA and MICB. A third mechanism of NK cell evasion is mediated by the viral membrane glycoprotein UL16 which is able to bind to MICB, ULBP-1 and ULBP-2 and sequester them in the endoplasmic reticulum/cis-Golgi, thereby preventing them interacting with NK cells bearing NKG2D and delivering an activating signal to the NK cell (Dunn *et al.*, 2003; Cosman *et al.*, 2001; Sutherland *et al.*, 2001).

A structural protein (pp65) from the virus tegument has been shown to interact with an activating NK receptor NKp30 leading to dissociation of the linked CD3zeta from NKp30 and thus reducing NK cell mediated killing (Arnon *et al.*, 2005).

In addition to these data, a comparison of the ability of different stains of HCMV to resist NK mediated lysis of infected fibroblasts has demonstrated a striking difference between the laboratory adapted strain AD169, and strains of the virus (including Toledo) that are more closely related to clinical isolates (Cerboni *et al.*, 2000; Fletcher *et al.*, 1998). As both laboratory adapted and clinical strains of the virus possess the UL16, UL18 and UL40 open reading frames these observations imply that other viral genes are responsible for this phenotype. Fletcher *et al.* (1998) reported that clinical strains of the virus downregulated lymphocyte function-associated antigen-3 (LFA-3) whereas AD169 did not, and speculated that this may be responsible for the difference in phenotype: however, Cerboni *et al.* (2000), while also observing the difference between clinical and laboratory strains, were not able to show any correlation with LFA-3 downregulation. It has been recognized since 1996 that clinical isolates of the virus have a larger genome, and comparison of AD169 with Toledo virus shows that Toledo has a 13.5 kb insert which encodes 20 predicted ORFs (Davison *et al.*, 2003) that are absent from AD169. It seems likely that some of the genes encoded in the UL b' region are responsible for rendering infected fibroblasts resistant to NK lysis Two genes encoded in the Ulb' region have now been shown to mediate inhibition of NK cell lysis. ORF UL141 is able to inhibit NK cell mediated lysis in a clonally dependent manner, by sequestering CD155 in the ER and thus preventing it engaging an NK activating receptor DNAM-1 (Tomasec et al., 2005). ORF UL142 is a novel HCMV encoded MHC class I related molecule which also inhibits NK cell killing in a clonally dependent manner. UL142 is also localized to the ER and it is likely that it sequesters virus induced stress molecules that would otherwise traffic to the cell surface to be recognized by activating NK cell receptors (Wills et al., 2005).

The immune response and pathology in immunocompromised subjects

Immunosuppression by CMV

It is frequently stated that HCMV is "immunosuppressive." At a clinical level, the association is somewhat anecdotal: obviously CMV disease frequently arises in the context of immunosuppression, iatrogenic or otherwise, and it is difficult conclusively to implicate HCMV in the causation of immunosuppression. The disease associated with primary HCMV infection in the normal immunocompetent host is characterized by marked T cell proliferation, but not obviously associated with immunosuppression.

The possession of a large number of gene functions which modulate the expression of MHC molecules, cytokines and NK cell interactions, is really the most specific evidence that HCMV exerts "immunosuppressive" effects, although it is obvious these effects do not prevent the normal host from mounting a sustained and effective immune response against the virus. In the whole organism the effect of HCMV- induced downregulation of MHC molecules may be counteracted by other influences – for instance, it has been shown that IFN-γ and TNFγ can upregulate MHC Class I molecules and counteract the downregulating effect of the HCMV genes referred to above (Hengel et al., 1995).

Much of the in vitro evidence for "immunosuppression" comes from experiments in which investigators have added HCMV to cultures of peripheral blood mononuclear cells and then used a readout such as T cell proliferation in response to exogenous mitogens or a similar assay. Given that HCMV, particularly recent clinical isolates, can infect differentiated macrophages, it can be envisaged that infection in this sort of in vitro system at high multiplicities may well cause impairment of such assays. More recently, it has been shown that HCMV can exogenously infect dendritic cells (DC) in vitro (Raftery et al., 2001), with enhanced expression of their costimulatory molecules and partial downregulation of MHC molecules, with upregulation of apoptosis-inducing ligands CD95L (FasL) and tumor necrosis factor related apoptosis-inducing ligand (TRAIL). This would result in HCMV-infected DC potentially being able to delete activated T-cells. There is emerging evidence that dendritic cells may well be a site of HCMV latency and, although it can be envisaged this sort of mechanism might operate in vivo, it is difficult to know how valid it is to extrapolate from in vitro experiments in which large numbers of DC are infected to the situation likely to obtain in vivo, where HCMV infection of DC would seem likely to be a low frequency event. Murine DC have also been shown to be permissive for murine CMV infection in vitro: again, MCMV infected DC were unable to deliver the signals necessary for T-cell activation and it has consequently been suggested they may be involved in CMV-induced immunosuppression in the mouse (Andrews et al., 2001).

In summary, the issue of whether HCMV can exert generalized immunosuppressive effects in vivo is unresolved. The clinical settings in which disseminated HCMV disease occurs are usually characterized by multiple variables operating simultaneously – such as pre-existing immunosuppression due to other disease or the administration of immunosuppressive drugs, the simultaneous administration of anti-rejection therapy, and other opportunistic infections. Given the in vitro evidence, it is plausible to suggest that CMV disease may be causally associated with immunosuppression but the case has to be regarded as not proven.

Immunopathology in human CMV disease
CMV pneumonitis

Pneumonitis is the most serious manifestation of HCMV infection after bone marrow transplantation (BMT), occurring in 10–15% of allogeneic BMT recipients, with a mortality of 80% prior to antiviral therapy. There is interstitial pneumonitis in the absence of any other identifiable pathogen, with increasing arterial hypoxemia, and progression to respiratory failure. It is suggested that graft versus host disease (GVHD) may contribute to the lung injury in HCMV pneumonitis in BMT recipients. The relationship between HCMV and GVHD is controversial, with proposals both that HCMV may predispose to GVHD, and vice versa. The striking rarity of pneumonitis attributable to HCMV in patients with AIDS, implies that factors other than immunosuppression alone contribute to its occurrence in BMT recipients. It has been hypothesized that CMV pneumonitis is mediated by an immunopathological mechanism, consequent on the regenerating immune system following bone marrow transplantation reacting against CMV infected cells in the lung. It has been suggested that CD4+ T cells might be particularly involved and that the absence of CD4+ cells in HIV infection might explain the rarity of CMV pneumonitis in that setting: however, in fact cells recovered from bronchoalveolar lavage during CMV pneumonitis in bone marrow transplant patients are mainly NK cells and CD8+ cells. An alternative suggestion has been that uncontrolled virus replication might trigger a dramatic release of cytokines such as TNFγ and this might mediate the pneumonitis – although any direct evidence for this is lacking (Barry et al., 2000).

Reddehase and colleagues (Podlech et al., 2000) have used the model of syngeneic bone marrow transplantation and simultaneous infection of BALB/c mice with MCMV to study the mechanisms of CMV interstitial pneumonitis in a longitudinal fashion. These authors have taken care to adapt the mouse model to mimic as closely as possible the events surrounding allogeneic bone marrow transplantation in humans. When reconstituting CD8+T-cells were depleted, there was a disseminated cytopathic MCMV infection of the lungs with high mortality. When hematopoietic reconstitution with both CD8+ and CD4+ T-cells occurred, viral replication in the lungs was much less and restricted to focal areas – after clearance of the infection, memory CD8+ T-cells persisted in the lung tissue with little MCMV present. These authors concluded there is no evidence for CD8+ T-cells exerting an immunopathological effect, but rather of their protecting against MCMV infection in the lungs. They make the point that the late phase appearances with persisting memory cells in the lung could be misinterpreted as CMV-induced immunopathology and conclude that this mouse model provides no evidence for immunopathologically mediated interstitial pneumonitis in human BMT recipients.

CMV retinitis and immune recovery vitritis

HCMV disease is one of the most frequent opportunistic infections in patients with advanced HIV infection, of whom 40% develop sight or life threatening HCMV disease. A CD4+ T-cell count of < 50/µl carries a particular risk of disease, although the widespread use of highly active antiretroviral therapy (HAART) in developed countries means that relatively few patients now have such low CD4+ T-cell counts, and the incidence of HCMV disease in patients with AIDS has consequently declined significantly. The commonest manifestation is HCMV retinitis which was seen in up to 25% of patients with AIDS prior to effective antiretroviral therapy. It is characterized by hemorrhagic retinal necrosis, spreading along retinal vessels, and threatening sight when disease encroaches on the macula (Whitcup, 2000).

However a newly recognized syndrome consequent on the use of HAART is "immune recovery vitritis." This is characterized by posterior segment inflammation and occurs in patients with inactive previously treated CMV retinitis, as the CD4+ T-cell count reconstitutes on antiretroviral therapy. In one series 60% of patients with prior HCMV retinitis who responded to HAART developed the syndrome (Karavellas et al., 1999). Although attributed to infiltrating T-cells reacting to HCMV antigens in the eye, this mechanism (whilst plausible) is not yet proven, although T cells are present in histopathological specimens of epiretinal membrane in the disease. The inflammation responds to steroids alone.

CMV and inflammatory demyelinating neuropathy

The pathogen most frequently associated with acute inflammatory demyelinating neuropathy, also known as Guillain–Barré syndrome (GBS), is *Campylobacter jejuni*. However a proportion (5%–10%) of patients with GBS show serological evidence of primary HCMV infection, and are more likely to have IgM antibodies to the GM2 ganglioside than other patients with GBS (Khalili-Shirazi et al., 1999): a causal relationship is postulated. CMV-infected fibroblasts have been shown to express the GM2 epitope (Ang et al., 2000) and "molecular mimicry" has been postulated as a possible cause of the association (Yuki, 2001).

CMV and organ transplant rejection

The risk of HCMV disease is 3–5 times greater in a seronegative than a seropositive recipient receiving an organ allograft from a seropositive donor, and disease is much more severe. Many centers "match" seronegative donors to seronegative recipients, although this is often thwarted by organ shortage. Disease often presents with specific organ involvement not seen in the normal subject. Interstitial pneumonitis due to HCMV carries a poor prognosis; disease in the gastrointestinal tract includes oesophagitis, gastritis and gastric ulceration, and colitis; HCMV retinitis may occur in severely immunosuppressed patients (Rubin, 2001; van der Bij and Speich, 2001).

There has been much circumstantial suggestion in the literature that CMV, even more so than other virus infections, may be somehow involved in the pathogenesis of rejection of solid organ allografts. There is suggestive epidemiological evidence that clinically significant HCMV infection is commoner in subjects who develop graft rejection, although it can be difficult to dissect out whether HCMV infection is a consequence of the immunosuppressive therapy in use, or preceded the treatment of rejection episodes – the latter would make a causal association more plausible (Kashyap et al., 1999; Borchers et al., 1999). Possible mechanisms which have been invoked to explain how CMV might be causally associated with rejection have focussed mainly on changes which the virus might induce in endothelial cells and in the expression of Class II MHC molecules. It is postulated that CMV-induced upregulation of adhesion molecules on endothelial cells might promote the infiltration of allospecific T-cells (Borchers et al., 1999; Craigen and Grundy, 1996). There is some evidence for increased expression of Class II MHC molecules on cells in solid organs in association with CMV infection – given the evidence that, if anything, CMV may downregulate class II MHC molecules in isolated cell types in vitro, such upregulation seems more likely to be mediated by cytokine release related to virus infection, such as IFN-γ or others. There is some evidence from the model of rat CMV infection that rat CMV can enhance chronic kidney allograft rejection in a transplant model (Lautenschlager et al., 1997) and that this is associated with increased vascular endothelial and tubular epithelial expression of ICAM-1 and increased interstitial inflammation (Yilmaz et al., 1996).

One group has reported that CD13 (Aminopeptidase N, a cell surface zinc metalloproteinase) is incorporated into virions, and that this may be associated with the development of autoantibodies to CD13. In the allogeneic bone marrow transplant setting, the presence of antibodies to CD13 correlated with the development of GVHD, and it was suggested CMV induced CD13 specific autoimmunity was contributing to the mediation of the GVHD (Moller et al., 1999).

The other aspect of solid organ allograft rejection in which CMV has been implicated is the chronic vasculopathy which may be a feature of chronic rejection. In cardiac transplantation, the most common cause of death following transplantation is cardiac allograft vasculopathy, an obliterative progressive vascular disease of the coronary arteries which is believed to be a form of chronic rejection (Orbaek Anderson, 1999). A number of studies have indicated an association between CMV and cardiac allograft vasculopathy (Weill, 2001), and it has been postulated that CMV may promote vasculopathy by the sort of mechanisms discussed above. Again, these suggestions are largely based on circumstantial evidence, although the virus may enhance the development of allograft vasculopathy in the rat CMV model of heterotopic heart or aortic transplantation, (Hosenpud, 1999; Koskinen et al., 1999).

REFERENCES

Ahn, K., Gruhler, A., Galocha, B. et al. (1997). The ER-luminal domain of the HCMV glycoprotein US6 inhibits peptide translocation by TAP. *Immunity*, **6**, 613–621.

Andrews, D. M., Andoniou, C. E., Granucci, F., Ricciardi-Castagnoli, P., and Degli-Esposti M. A. (2001). Infection of dendritic cells by murine cytomegalovirus induces functional paralysis. *Nat. Immunol.*, **2**, 1077–1084.

Ang, C. W., Jacobs, B. C., Brandenburg, A. H. et al. (2000). Cross-reactive antibodies against GM2 and CMV-infected fibroblasts in Guillain–Barre syndrome. *Neurology*, **54**, 1453–1458.

Appay, V., Dunbar, P. R., Callan, M. et al. (2002). Memory CD8+ T cells vary in differentiation phenotype in different persistent virus infections. *Nat. Med.*, **8**, 379–385.

Arase, H., Mocarski, E. S., Campbell, A. E., Hill, A. B., and Lanier L. L. (2002). Direct recognition of cytomegalovirus by activating and inhibitory NK cell receptors. *Science*, **296**, 1323.

Arnon, T. I., Achdout, H., Levi, O. et al. (2005). Inhibition of the NKp30 activating receptor by pp65 of human cytomegalovirus. *Nat. Immunol.*, **6**, 515–523.

Atalay, R., Zimmermann, A., Wagner, M. et al. (2002). Identification and expression of human cytomegalovirus transcription units coding for two distinct Fcgamma receptor homologs. *J. Virol.*, **76**, 8596–8608.

Barry, S. M., Johnson, M. A., and Janossy, G. (2000). Cytopathology or immunopathology? The puzzle of cytomegalovirus pneumonitis revisited. *Bone Marrow Transpl.*, **26**, 591–597.

Bego, M., Maciejewski, J., Khaiboullina, S., Pari, G., and St Jeor, S. (2005). Characterization of an antisense transcript spanning the UL81-82 locus of human cytomegalovirus. *J. Virol.*, **79**, 11022–11034.

Beninga, J., Kropff, B., and Mach, M. (1995). Comparative analysis of fourteen individual human cytomegalovirus proteins for helper T cell response. *J. Gen. Virol.*, **76**(Pt 1), 153–160.

Biron, C. A., Byron, K. S., and Sullivan, J. L. (1989). Severe herpesvirus infections in an adolescent without natural killer cells. *N. Engl. J. Med.*, **320**, 1731–1735.

Biron, C. A., Nguyen, K. B., Pien, G. C., Cousens, L. P., and Salazar-Mather, T. P. (1999). Natural killer cells in antiviral defense: function and regulation by innate cytokines. *Annu. Rev. Immunol.*, **17**, 189–220.

Bitmansour, A. D., Douek, D. C., Maino, V. C., and Picker, L. J. (2002). Direct ex vivo analysis of human CD4(+) memory T cell activation requirements at the single clonotype level. *J. Immunol.*, **169**, 1207–1218.

Boppana, S. B. and Britt, W. J. (1996). Recognition of human cytomegalovirus gene products by HCMV-specific cytotoxic T cells [Full text delivery]. *Virology*, **222**, 293–296.

Borchers, A. T., Perez, R., Kaysen, G., Ansari, A. A., and Gershwin, M. E. (1999). Role of cytomegalovirus infection in allograft rejection: a review of possible mechanisms. *Transpl. Immunol.*, **7**, 75–82.

Borysiewicz, L. K., Morris, S., Page, J. D., and Sissons, J. G. (1983). Human cytomegalovirus-specific cytotoxic T lymphocytes: requirements for in vitro generation and specificity. *Eur. J. Immunol.*, **13**, 804–809.

Braud, V., Jones, E. Y., and McMichael, A. (1997). The human major histocompatibility complex class Ib molecule HLA-E binds signal sequence-derived peptides with primary anchor residues at positions 2 and 9. *Eur. J. Immunol.*, **27**, 1164–1169.

Braud, V. M., Allan, D. S., O' Callaghan, C. A. *et al.* (1998). HLA-E binds to natural killer cell receptors CD94/NKG2A, B and C. *Nature*, **391**, 795–799.

Britt, W. J. (1991). Recent advances in the identification of significant human cytomegalovirus-encoded proteins. *Transpl. Proc.*, **23**, 64–69.

Britt, W. J. and Mach, M. (1996). Human cytomegalovirus glycoproteins. *Intervirology*, **39**, 401–412.

Birtt, W. J., Vugler, L., and Stephens, E. B. (1988). Induction of complement-dependent and -independent neutralizing antibodies by recombinant-derived human cytomegalovirus gp55–116 (gB). *J. Virol.*, **62**, 3309–3318.

Britt, W. J., Vugler, L., Butfiloski, E. J., and Stephens, E. B. (1990). Cell surface expression of human cytomegalovirus (HCMV) gp55–116 (gB): use of HCMV-recombinant vaccinia virus-infected cells in analysis of the human neutralizing antibody response. *J. Virol.*, **64**, 1079–1085.

Brown, M. G., Dokun, A. O., Heusel, J. W. *et al.* (2001). Vital involvement of a natural killer cell activation receptor in resistance to viral infection. *Science*, **292**, 934–937.

Cerboni, C., Mousavi-Jazi, M., Linde, A. *et al.* (2000). Human cytomegalovirus strain-dependent changes in NK cell recognition of infected fibroblasts. *J. Immunol.*, **164**, 4775–4782.

Cosman, D., Fanger, N., Borges L. *et al.* (1997). A novel immunoglobulin superfamily receptor for cellular and viral MHC class I molecules. *Immunity*, **7**, 273–282.

Cosman, D., Mullberg, J., Sutherland, C. L. *et al.* (2001). ULBPs, novel MHC class I-related molecules, bind to CMV glycoprotein UL16 and stimulate NK cytotoxicity through the NKG2D receptor. *Immunity*, **14**, 123–133.

Craigen, J. L. and Grundy, J. E. (1996). Cytomegalovirus induced up-regulation of LFA-3 (CD58) and ICAM-1 (CD54) is a direct viral effect that is not prevented by ganciclovir or foscarnet treatment. *Transplantation*, **62**, 1102–1108.

Cwynarski, K., Ainsworth, J., Cobbold, M. *et al.* (2001). Direct visualization of cytomegalovirus-specific T-cell reconstitution after allogeneic stem cell transplantation. *Blood*, **97**, 1232–1240.

Daniels, K. A., Devora, G., Lai, W. C., O'Donnell, C. L., Bennett, M., and Welsh, R. M. (2001). Murine cytomegalovirus is regulated by a discrete subset of natural killer cells reactive with monoclonal antibody to Ly49H. *J. Exp. Med.*, **194**, 29–44.

Davison, A. J., Dolan, A., Akter, P. *et al.* (2003). The human cytomegalovirus genome revisited: comparison with the chimpanzee cytomegalovirus genome. *J. Gen. Virol.*, **84**, 17–28.

Dunn, C., Chalupny, N. J., Sutherland, C. L. *et al.* (2003). Human cytomegalovirus glycoprotein UL16 causes intracellular sequestration of NKG2D ligands, protecting against natural killer cell cytotoxicity. *J. Exp. Med.*, **197**, 1427–1439.

Elkington, R., Walker, S., Crough, T. *et al.* (2003). Ex vivo profiling of CD8+-T-cell responses to human cytomegalovirus reveals broad and multispecific reactivities in healthy virus carriers. *J. Virol.*, **77**, 5226–5240.

Faint, J. M., Annels, N. E., Curnow, S. J. *et al.* (2001). Memory T cells constitute a subset of the human CD8(+)CD45RA(+) pool with distinct phenotypic and migratory characteristics. *J. Immunol.*, **167**, 212–220.

Falk, C. S., Mach, M., Schendel, D. J., Weiss, E. H., Hilgert, I., and Hahn, G. (2002). NK cell activity during human cytomegalovirus infection is dominated by US2–11-mediated HLA class I down-regulation. *J. Immunol.*, **169**, 3257–3266.

Fletcher, J. M., Prentice, H. G., and Grundy, J. E. (1998). Natural killer cell lysis of cytomegalovirus (CMV)-infected cells correlates with virally induced changes in cell surface lymphocyte function-associated antigen-3 (LFA-3) expression and not with the CMV-induced down-regulation of cell surface class I HLA. *J. Immunol.*, **161**, 2365–2374.

Fowler, K. B., Stagno, S., Pass, R. F., Britt, W. J., Boll, T. J., and Alford, C. A. (1992). The outcome of congenital cytomegalovirus infection in relation to maternal antibody status. *N. Engl. J. Med.*, **326**, 663–667.

Furukawa, T., Hornberger, E., Sakuma, S., and Plotkin, S. A. (1975). Demonstration of immunoglobulin G receptors induced by human cytomegalovirus. *J. Clin. Microbiol.*, **2**, 332–336.

Gamadia, L. E., Remmerswaal, E. B., Weel, J. F., Bemelman, F., van Lier, R. A., and Ten Berge, I. J. (2003). Primary immune responses to human CMV: a critical role for IFN-gamma-producing CD4+ T cells in protection against CMV disease. *Blood*, **101**, 2686–2692.

Gandhi, M. K., Wills, M. R., Okecha, G. *et al.* (2003). Late diversification in the clonal composition of human cytomegalovirus-specific CD8+ T cells following allogeneic hemopoietic stem cell transplantation. *Blood*, **102**, 3427–3438.

Gillespie, G. M., Wills, M. R., Appay, V. *et al.* (2000). Functional heterogeneity and high frequencies of cytomegalovirus-specific CD8(+) T lymphocytes in healthy seropositive donors. *J. Virol.*, **74**, 8140–8150.

Gonczol., E., de Taisne, C., Hirka, G. *et al.* (1991). High expression of human cytomegalovirus (HCMV)-gB protein in cells infected with a vaccinia-gB recombinant: the importance of the gB protein in HCMV immunity. *Vaccine*, **9**, 631–637.

Guglielmo, B. J., Wong-Beringer, A., and Linker, C. A. (1994). Immune globulin therapy in allogeneic bone marrow transplant: a critical review. *Bone Marrow Transpl.*, **13**, 499–510.

Hahn, G., Jores, R., and Mocarski, E. S. (1998). Cytomegalovirus remains latent in a common precursor of dendritic and myeloid cells. *Proc. Natl Acad. Sci. USA*, **95**, 3937–3942.

Harrison, C. J., Britt, W. J., Chapman, N. M., Mullican, J., and Tracy, S. (1995). Reduced congenital cytomegalovirus (CMV) infection after maternal immunization with a guinea pig CMV glycoprotein before gestational primary CMV infection in the guinea pig model. *J. Infect. Dis.*, **172**, 1212–1220.

Hassan-Walker, A. F., Vargas Cuero, A. L., Mattes, F. M. *et al.* (2001). CD8+ cytotoxic lymphocyte responses against cytomegalovirus after liver transplantation: correlation with time from transplant to receipt of tacrolimus. *J. Infect. Dis.*, **183**, 835–843.

Hengel, H., Esslinger, C., Pool, J., Goulmy, E., and Koszinowski, U. H. (1995). Cytokines restore MhC Class-I complex-formation and control antigen presentation in human cytomegalovirus infected cells. *J. Gen. Virol.*, **76**, 2987–2997.

Hosenpud, J. D. (1999). Coronary artery disease after heart transplantation and its relation to cytomegalovirus. *Am. Heart J.*, **138**, S469–S472.

Jones, T. R., Hanson, L. K., Sun, L., Slater, J. S., Stenberg, R. M., and Campbell. A. E. (1995). Multiple independent loci within the human cytomegalovirus unique short region down-regulate expression of major histocompatibility complex class I heavy chains. *J. Virol.*, **69**, 4830–4841.

Jones, T. R., Wiertz, E., Sun, L., Fish, K. N., Nelson, J. A., and Ploegh, H. L. (1996). Human cytomegalovirus US3 impairs transport and maturation of major histocompatability complex class I heavy chains. *Proc. Natl Acad. Sci. USA*, **93**, 11327–11333.

Jonjic, S., Mutter, W., Weiland, F., Reddehase, M. J., and Koszinowski, U. H. (1989). Site-restricted persistent cytomegalovirus infection after selective long-term depletion of CD4+ T lymphocytes. *J. Exp. Med.*, **169**, 1199–1212.

Kern, F., Bunde, T., Faulhaber, N. *et al.* (2002). Cytomegalovirus (CMV) phosphoprotein 65 makes a large contribution to shaping the T cell repertoire in CMV-exposed individuals. *J. Infect. Dis.*, **185**, 1709–1716.

Khalili-Shirazi, A., Gregson, N., Gray, I., Rees, J., Winer, J., and Hughes, R. (1999). Antiganglioside antibodies in Guillain-Barre syndrome after a recent cytomegalovirus infection. *J. Neurol. Neurosurg. Psychiatry*, **66**, 376–379.

Khan, N., Cobbold, M., Keenan, R., and Moss, P. A. (2002a). Comparative analysis of CD8+ T cell responses against human cytomegalovirus proteins pp65 and immediate early 1 shows similarities in precursor frequency, oligoclonality, and phenotype. *J. Infect. Dis.*, **185**, 1025–1034.

Khan, N., Shariff, N., Cobbold, M. *et al.* (2002b). Cytomegalovirus seropositivity drives the CD8 T cell repertoire toward greater clonality in healthy elderly individuals. *J. Immunol.*, **169**, 1984–1992.

Khattab, B. A., Lindenmaier, W., Frank, R., and Link, H. (1997). Three T-cell epitopes within the C-terminal 265 amino acids of the matrix protein pp65 of human cytomegalovirus recognized by human lymphocytes. *J. Med. Virol.*, **52**, 68–76.

Kondo, K., Kaneshima, H., and Mocarski, E. S. (1994). Human cytomegalovirus latent infection of granulocyte-macrophage progenitors. *Proc. Nat. Acad. Sci. USA*, **9**, 11879–11883.

Kniess, N., Mach, M., Fay, J., and Britt, W. J. (1991). Distribution of linear antigenic sites on glycoprotein gp55 of human cytomegalovirus. *J. Virol.*, **65**, 138–146.

Koskinen, P. K., Kallio, E. A., Tikkanen, J. M., Sihvola, R. K., Hayry, P. J., and Lemstrom, K. B. (1999). Cytomegalovirus infection and cardiac allograft vasculopathy. *Transpl. Infect. Dis.*, **1**, 115–126.

Kuzushima, K., Hayashi, N., Kimura, H., and Tsurumi, T. (2001). Efficient identification of HLA-A*2402-restricted cytomegalovirus-specific CD8(+) T-cell epitopes by a computer algorithm and an enzyme-linked immunospot assay. *Blood*, **98**, 1872–1881.

Landini, M. P. and Michelson, S. (1988). Human cytomegalovirus proteins. *Prog. Med. Virol.*, **35**, 152–185.

Lanier, L. L. (2005). NK cell recognition. *Annu. Rev. Immunol.*, **23**, 225–274.

Lautenschlager, I., Soots, A., Krogerus, L. *et al.* (1997). Effect of cytomegalovirus on an experimental model of chronic renal allograft rejection under triple-drug treatment in the rat. *Transplantation*, **64**, 391–398.

Lee, S. H., Girard S., Macina, D. *et al.* (2001). Susceptibility to mouse cytomegalovirus is associated with deletion of an activating natural killer cell receptor of the C-type lectin superfamily. *Nat. Genet.*, **28**, 42–45.

Leong, C. C., Chapman, T. L., Bjorkman, P. J. *et al.* (1998). Modulation of natural killer cell cytotoxicity in human cytomegalovirus infection: the role of endogenous class I major histocompatibility complex and a viral class I homolog. *J. Exp. Med.*, **187**, 1681–1687.

Lilley, B. N., Ploegh, H. L., and Tirabassi, R. S. (2000). Human cytomegalovirus open reading frame TRL11/IRL11 encodes an immunoglobulin G Fc-binding protein. *J. Virol.*, **75**, 11218–11221.

Li Pira, G., Bottone, L., Ivaldi, F. *et al.* (2004). Identification of new Th peptides from the cytomegalovirus protein pp65 to design a peptide library for generation of CD4 T cell lines for cellular immunoreconstitution. *Int. Immunol.*, **16**, 635–642.

Longmate, J., York, J., La Rosa, C. *et al.* (2001). Population coverage by HLA class-I restricted cytotoxic T-lymphocyte epitopes. *Immunogenetics*, **52**, 165–173.

Mackowiak, P. A. and Marling-Cason, M. (1987). Immunoreactivity of cytomegalovirus-induced Fc receptors. *Microbiol. Immunol.*, **31**, 427–434.

Marshall, G. S., Rabalais, G. P., Stout, G. G., and Waldeyer, S. L. (1992). Antibodies to recombinant-derived glycoprotein B after natureal human cytomegalovirus infection correlate with neutralizing activity. *J. Infect. Dis.*, **165**, 381–384.

McLaughlin-Taylor, E., Pande, H., Forman, S. J. *et al.* (1994). Identification of the major late human cytomegalovirus matrix protein pp65 as a gen for CD8+ virus-specific cytotoxic T lymphocytes. *J. Med. Virol.*, **43**, 103–110.

Mendelson, M., Monard, S., Sissions, P., and Sinclair, J. (1996). Detection of endogenous human cytomegalovirus in CD34+ bone marrow progenitors. *J. Gen. Virol.*, **77**, 3099–3102.

Meyer, H., Sundqvist, V. A., Pereira, L., and Mach, M. (1992). Glycoprotein gp 116 of human cytomegalovirus contains epitopes for strain-common and strain-specific antibodies. *J. Gen. Virol.*, **73**(Pt 9), 2375–2388.

Moller, E., Soderberg-Naucler, C., and Sumitran-Karuppan, S. (1999). Role of alloimmunity in clinical transplantation. *Rev. Immunogenet.*, **1**, 309–322.

Munoz, I., Gutierrez, A., Gimeno, C. *et al.* (2001). Lack of association between the kinetics of human cytomegalovirus (HCMV) glycoprotein B (gB)-specific and neutralizing serum antibodies and development or recovery from HCMV active infection in patients undergoing allogeneic stem cell transplant. *J. Med. Virol.*, **65**, 77–84.

Orback Andersen, H. (1999). Heart allograft vascular disease: an obliterative vascular in transplanted hearts. *Atherosclerosis*, **142**, 243–263.

Podlech, J., Holtappels, R., Pahl-Seibert, M. F., Steffens, H. P., and Reddehase, M. J. (2000). Murine model of interstitial cytomegalovirus pneumonia in syngeneic bone marrow transplantation: persistence of protective pulmonary CD8-T-cell infiltrates after clearance of acute infection. *J. Virol.*, **74**, 7496–7507.

Polic, B., Hengel, H., Krmpotic, A. et al. (1998). Hierarchical and redundant lymphocyte subset control precludes cytomegalovirus replication during latent infection. *J. Exp. Med.*, **188**, 1047–1054.

Quinnan, G. V., Jr., Kirmani, N., Rook, A. H. et al. (1982). Cytotoxic t cells in cytomegalovirus infection: HLA-restricted T-lymphocyte and non-T-lymphocyte cytotoxic responses correlate with recovery from cytomegalovirus infection in bone-marrow-transplant recipients. *N. Engl. J. Med.*, **307**, 7–13.

Raftery, M. J., Schwab, M., Eibert, S. M., Samstag, Y., Walczak, H., and Schonrich, G. (2001). Targeting the function of mature dendritic cells by human cytomegalovirus: a multilayered viral defense strategy. *Immunity*, **15**, 997–1009.

Rapp, M., Messerle, M., Buhler, B., Tannheimer, M., Keil, G. M., and Koszinowski, U. H. (1992). Identification of the murine cytomegalovirus glycoprotein B gene and its expression by recombinant vaccinia virus. *J. Virol.*, **66**, 4399–4406.

Reeves, M. B., MacAry, P. A., Lehner, P. J., Sissons, J. G., and Sinclair, J. H. (2005). Latency, chromatin remodeling, and reactivation of human cytomegalovirus in the dendritic cells of healthy carriers. *Proc. Natl. Acad. Sci. USA*, **102**, 4140–4145.

Reddehase, M. J. (2002). Antigens and immunoevasins: opponents in cytomegalovirus immune surveillance. *Nat. Rev. Immunol.*, **2**, 831–844.

Reddehase, M. J., Mutter, W., Munch, K., Buhring, H. J., and Koszinowski, U. H. (1987). CD8-positive T lymphocytes specific for murine cytomegalovirus immediate-early antigens mediate protective immunity. *J. Virol.*, **61**, 3102–3108.

Reddehase, M. J., Podlech, J., and Grzimek, N. K. (2002). Mouse models of cytomegalovirus latency: overview. *J. Clin. Virol.*, **25**, Suppl. 2, S23–S36.

Rentenaar, R. J., Gamadia, L. E., van DerHoek, N. et al. (2000). Development of virus-specific CD4(+) T cells during primary cytomegalovirus infection. *J. Clin. Invest.*, **105**, 541–548.

Reyburn, H. T., Mandelboim, O., Vales-Gomez, M., Davis, D. M., Pazmany, L., and Strominger, J. L. (1997). The class I MHC homologue of human cytomegalovirus inhibits attack by natural killer cells. *Nature*, **386**, 514–517.

Rubin, R. H. (2001). Cytomegalovirus in solid organ transplantation. *Transpl. Infect. Dis.*, **3** Suppl. 2, 1–5.

Scalzo, A. A., Fitzgerald, N. A., Wallace, C. R. et al. (1992). The effect of the Cmv-1 resistance gene, which is linked to the natural killer cell gene complex, is mediated by natural killer cells. *J. Immunol.*, **149**, 581–589.

Schoppel, K., Kropff, B., Schmidt, C., Vornhagen, R., and Mach, M. (1997). The humoral immune response against human cytomegalovirus is characterized by a delayed synthesis of glycoprotein-specific antibodies. *J. Infect. Dis.*, **175**, 533–544.

Sester, M., Sester, U., Gartner, B. et al. (2002). Sustained high frequencies of specific CD4 T cells restricted to a single persistent virus. *J. Virol.*, **76**, 3748–3755.

Sinclair, J. and Sissons, J. G. P. (2006). Latency and reactivation of human cytomegalovirus. *J. Gen. Virol.*, **87**, 1763–1779.

Sinzger, C., Plachter, B., Grefte, A., The, T. H., and Jahn, G. (1996). Tissue macrophages are infected by human cytomegalovirus in vivo. *J. Infect. Dis.*, **173**, 240–245.

Sissons, J. G., Bain, M., and Wills, M. R. (2002). Latency and reactivation of human cytomegalovirus. *J. Infect.*, **44**, 73–77.

Soderberg Naucler, C., Fish, K. N., and Nelson, J. A. (1997). Reactivation of latent human cytomegalovirus by allogeneic stimulation of blood cells from healthy donors. *Cell*, **91**, 119–126.

Speckner, A., Glykofrydes, D., Ohlin, M., and Mach, M. (1999). Antigenic domain 1 of human cytomegalovirus glycoprotein B induces a multitude of different antibodies which, when combined, results in incomplete virus neutralization. *J. Gen. Virol.*, **80** (Pt8), 2183–2191.

Soderberg-Naucler, C., Streblow, D. N., Fish, K. N., Allan-Yorke, J., Smith, P. P., and Nelson, J. A. (2001). Reactivation of latent human cytomegalovirus in CD14(+) monocytes is differentiation dependent. *J. Virol.*, **75**, 7543–7554.

Sutherland, C. L., Chalupny, N. J., and Cosman, D. (2001). The UL16-binding proteins, a novel family of MHC class I-related ligands for NKG2D, activate natural killer cell functions. *Immunol. Rev.*, **181**, 185–192.

Sylwester, A. W., Mitchell, B. L., Edgar, J. B. et al. (2005). Broadly targeted human cytomegalovirus-specific CD4+ and CD8+ T cells dominate the memory compartments of exposed subjects. *J. Exp. Med.*, **202**, 673–685.

Tay, C. H., Szomolanyi-Tsuda, E., and Welsh, R. M. (1998). Control of infections by NK cells. *Curr. Top. Microbiol. Immunol.*, **230**, 193–220.

Taylor-Wiedeman, J., Sissons, J. G. P., Borysiewicz, L. K., and Sinclair, J. H. (1991). Monocytes are a major site of persistence of human cytomegalovirus in peripheral-blood mononuclear-cells. *J. Gen. Virol.*, **72**, 2059–2064.

Taylor-Wiedeman, J., Hayhurst, G. P., Sissons, J. G., and Sinclair, J. H. (1993). Polymorphonuclear cells are not sites of persistence of human cytomegalovirus in healthy individuals. *J. Gen. Virol.*, **74** (Pt2), 265–268.

Taylor-Wiedeman, J., Sissons, J. G. P., and Sinclair, J. (1994). Induction of endogenous human cytomegalovirus gene expression after differentiation of monocytes from healthy carriers. *J. Virol.*, **68**, 1597–1604.

Tomasec, P., Braud V. M., Rickards, C. et al. (2000). Surface expression of HLA-E, an inhibitor of natural killer cells, enhanced by human cytomegalovirus gpUL40. *Science*, **287**, 1031–1035.

Tomasec, P., Wang, E. C., Davison, A. J. *et al.* (2005). Downregulation of natural killer cell-activating ligand CD155 by human cytomegalovirus UL141. *Nat. Immunol.*, **6**, 181–188.

Urban, M., Klein, M., Britt, W. J., Hassfurther, E., and Mach, M. (1996). Glycoprotein H of human cytomegalovirus is a major antigen for the neutralizing humoral immune response. *J. Gen. Virol.*, (Pt 7), 1537–1547.

Vales-Gomez, M., Browne, H., and Reyburn, H. T. (2003). Expression of the UL16 glycoprotein of Human Cytomegalovirus protects the virus-infected cell from attack by natural killer cells. *BMC Immunol.*, **4**, 4–8.

van der Bij, W. and Speich, R. (2001). Management of cytomegalovirus infection and disease after solid-organ transplantation. *Clin. Infect. Dis.*, **33** (*Suppl. 1*), S32–S37.

van Leeuwen, E. M., Remmerswaal, E. B., Heemskerk, M. H., Ten Berge, I. J., and van Lier, R. A. (2006). Strong selection of virus-specific cytotoxic CD4+ T cell clones during primary human cytomegalovirus infection. *Blood*, in press.

Wagner, B., Kropff, B., Kalbacher, H. *et al.* (1992). A continuous sequence of more than 70 amino acids is essential for antibody binding to the dominant antigenic site of glycoprotein gp58 of human cytomegalovirus. *J. Virol.*, **66**, 5290–5297.

Waldrop, S. L., Pitcher, C. J., Peterson, D. M., Maino, V. C., and Picker, L. J. (1997). Determination of antigen-specific memory/effector CD4+T cell frequencies by flow cytometry: evidence for a novel, antigen-specific homeostatic mechanism in HIV-associated immunodeficiency. *J. Clin. Invest.*, **99**, 1739–1750.

Waldrop, S. L., Davis, K. A., Maino, V. C., and Picker, L. J. (1998). Normal human CD4+ memory T cells display broad heterogeneity in their activation threshold for cytokine synthesis. *J. Immunol.*, **161**, 5284–5295.

Walter, E. A., Greenberg, P. D., Gilbert, M. J. (1995). Reconstitution of cellular immunity against cytomegalovirus in recipients of allogeneic bone marrow by transfer of T-cell clones from the donor [see comments]. *N. Engl. J. Med.*, **333**, 1038–1044.

Wang, E. C., McSharry, B., Retiere, C. *et al.* (2002). UL40-mediated NK evasion during productive infection with human cytomegalovirus. *Proc. Natl Acad. Sci. USA*, **99**, 7570–7575.

Weekes, M. P., Wills, M. R., Mynard, K., Carmichael, A. J., and Sissons. J. G. (1999). The memory cytotoxic T-lymphocyte (CTL) response to human cytomegalovirus infection contains individual peptide-specific CTL clones that have undergone extensive expansion in vivo. *J. Virol.*, **73**, 2099–2108.

Weekes, M. P., Wills, M. R., Sissons, J. G., and Carmichael, A. J. (2004). Long-term stable expanded human CD4+ T cell clones specific for human cytomegalovirus are distributed in both CD45RAhigh and CD45ROhigh populations. *J. Immunol.*, **173**, 5843–5851.

Weill, D. (2001). Role of cytomegalovirus in cardiac allograft vasculopathy. *Transpl. Infect. Dis.*, **3**, (*Suppl.* 2), 44–48.

Whitcup, S. M. (2000). Cytomegalovirus retinitis in the era of highly active antiretroviral therapy. *J. Am. Med. Assoc.*, **283**, 653–657.

White, K. L., Slobedman, B., and Mocarski, E. S. (2000). Human cytomegalovirus latency-associated protein pORF94 is dispensable for productive and latent infection. *J. Virol.*, **74**, 9333–9337.

Wiertz, E. J., Jones, T. R., Sun, L., Bogyo, M., Geuze, H. J., and Ploegh, H. L. (1996a). The human cytomegalovirus US11 gene product dislocates MHC class I heavy chains from the endoplasmic reticulum to the cytosol. *Cell*, **84**, 769–779

Wiertz, E. J., Tortorella, D., Bogyo, M. *et al.* (1996b). Sec61-mediated transfer of a membrane protein from the endoplasmic reticulum to the proteasome for destruction [see comments]. *Nature*, **384**, 432–438.

Wills, M. R., Carmichael, A. J., Mynard, K. *et al.* (1996). The human cytotoxic T-lymphocyte (CTL) response to cytomegalovirus is dominated by structural protein pp65: frequency, specificity, and T-cell receptor usage of pp65-specific CTL. *J. Virol.*, **70**, 7569–7579.

Wills, M. R., Carmichael, A. J., Weekes, M. P. *et al.* (1999). Human virus-specific CD8+ CTL clones revert from CD45ROhigh to CD45RAhigh in vivo: CD45RAhighCD8+ T cells comprise both naive and memory cells. *J. Immunol.*, **162**, 7080–7087.

Wills, M. R., Okecha, G., Weekes, M. P., Gandhi, M. K., Sissons, P. J., and Carmichael, A. J. (2002). Identification of naive or antigen-experienced human CD8(+) T cells by expression of costimulation and chemokine receptors: analysis of the human cytomegalovirus-specific CD8(+) T cell response. *J. Immunol.*, **168**, 5455–5464.

Wills, M. R., Ashiru, O., Reeves, M. B. *et al.* (2005). Human cytomegalovirus encodes an MHC class I-like molecule (UL142) that functions to inhibit NK cell lysis. *J. Immunol.*, **175**, 7457–7465.

Yeager, A. S., Grumet, F. C., Hafleigh, E. B., Arvin, A. M., Bradley, J. S., and Prober, C. G. (1981). Prevention of transfusion-acquired cytomegalovirus infections in newborn infants. *J. Pediatr.*, **98**, 281–287.

Yilmaz, S., Koskinen, P., K. Kallio, E., Bruggeman, C. A., Hayry, P. J., and Lemstrom, K. B. (1996). Cytomegalovirus infection-enhanced chronic kidney allograft rejection is linked with intercellular adhesion molecule-1 expression. *Kidney Int.*, **50**, 526–537.

Yuki, N. (2001). Infectious origins of, and molecular mimicry in, Guillain–Barré and Fisher syndromes. *Lancet Infect. Dis.*, **1**, 29–37.

44

Persistence in the population: epidemiology and transmisson

Suresh B. Boppana[1] and Karen B. Fowler[2]

[1]Departments of Pediatrics and Microbiology, University of Alabama School of Medicine, AL, USA
[2]Departments of Pediatrics, Epidemiology and Maternal & Child Health, University of Alabama School of Medicine, AL, USA

Introduction

Cytomegaloviruses (CMVs) are ubiquitous but highly species specific agents and are a common cause of infections in many animal species including humans (Weller, 1971). The characteristic cellular changes caused by CMV including cell enlargement with intranuclear inclusions were first reported in 1881 by Ribbert in the kidneys of a stillborn infant with congenital syphilis (Ribbert, 1904). Subsequent reports have described similar findings in the parotid glands of children and in the salivary glands from guinea pigs. It was initially thought that cytomegalic inclusion disease (CID) of the newborn was the sole manifestation of human CMV (HCMV) infection (Goodpasture and Talbot, 1921; Lipschutz, 1921; Cole and Kuttner, 1926; Lowenstein, 1907). Several groups of investigators have simultaneously isolated and propagated HCMV from infants and children with CID and from adenoidal tissue of children undergoing adenoidectomy (Rowe et al., 1956; Smith, 1956; Weller et al., 1957). As tissue culture isolation and serological assays became more widely available, HCMV was linked to a variety of illnesses, many of which have subsequently been shown to be unrelated to HCMV. A common characteristic of patients at risk for invasive HCMV infections is the suppression of host immune responsiveness. The onset of AIDS epidemic in the early 1980s has led to a dramatic expansion of the spectrum of HCMV disease. HCMV was the most common opportunistic infection in patients with AIDS and a major cause of morbidity and mortality in these patients until the introduction of highly active antiretroviral therapy (Jacobson et al., 1988; Gallant et al., 1992; Munoz et al., 1993; Spector et al., 1999). Currently, HCMV continues to cause disease in patients with AIDS, but similar to other opportunistic infections in AIDS patients responding to antiretroviral therapy, the incidence of invasive HCMV disease is extremely low even in those with minimally reconstituted immune systems (Jacobson et al., 2001). Currently, HCMV is a cause of significant morbidity and mortality in newborn infants who acquire HCMV prenatally and in allograft recipients.

Epidemiology of HCMV infection

Human cytomegalovirus infections have been recognized in every human population that has been studied (Krech et al., 1971; Gold and Nankervis, 1976). HCMV infection is endemic without seasonal variation (Gold and Nankervis, 1976). HCMV is acquired early in life in most populations with the exception of people in economically well developed countries of northern Europe and North America. The patterns of HCMV acquisition vary greatly based on geographic and socioeconomic backgrounds of the population and the seroprevalence increases generally with age (Alford et al., 1981). In the developing world, acquisition of HCMV is nearly universal in early childhood. Studies have shown that most preschool children (>90%) in South America, Sub-Saharan Africa, East Asia, and India are HCMV antibody positive (Gold and Nankervis, 1982; Stagno, 2001). In contrast, seroepidemiologic surveys in Great Britain and in certain populations in the United States have found that less than 20% of children of similar age are seropositive (Huang et al., 1980; Gold and Nankervis, 1982).

In Chengdu, China a population survey observed 60% of children 4 to 7 years of age were HCMV seropositive (Liu et al., 1990). Similiarly, 58% of children 4 to 12 years of age in Taipei, Taiwan, 61% of hospitalized pediatric patients from a low income population in Rio de Janeiro, Brazil and 56% of children aged 1 to 4 years in Jamaica were HCMV antibody positive (Prabhakar et al., 1992; Shen et al., 1992; Suassuna et al., 1995). In Finland the HCMV seroprevalence rate increased from 27% in children 7 months of age to 41% in children 8 years of age in a cohort of children followed for 8 years (Aarnisalo et al., 2003). In a population survey in Parma, Italy, age-specific HCMV seroprevalence increased from 28% in two year olds to 96% in 45–54-year-old residents (Natali et al., 1997). Similiarly, in Spain, the CMV seroprevalence rate in children 2 to 5 years of age was 42% increasing to 79% in adults 31 to 40 years of age (de Ory et al., 2004). Recent studies in blood donors have demonstrated that populations in Asia and Africa continue to have CMV seropositivity rates of 95%–100% (Urwijitaroon et al., 1993; Lu et al., 1999; Pultoo et al., 2001; Kothari et al., 2002) whereas in Germany the HCMV seropositivity rates in blood donors are lower ranging from 30% in 18 to 20 year olds to >70% in adults >65 years of age (Hecker et al., 2004).

Although the exact mode of HCMV acquisition is unknown, it is assumed to be through direct contact with body fluids from an infected person. The differences in age-related prevalence probably reflect differences in child rearing practices, sexual behaviors, and possibly, living conditions. Breastfeeding, group care of children, crowded living conditions, and sexual activity have all been associated with high rates of HCMV infections. Sources of virus include oropharyngeal secretions, urine, cervical and vaginal secretions, semen, breast milk, blood products, and allografts (Hayes et al., 1972; Reynolds et al., 1973; Lang, 1975; Alford et al., 1980). Presumably, exposure to saliva and other body fluids containing infectious virus is a primary mode of spread and because infected infants typically excrete significant amounts of HCMV for months to years following infection. Even older children and adults shed virus for prolonged periods (>6 months) following a primary HCMV infection. In addition, a significant proportion of seropositive individuals continue to shed virus intermittently.

An important determinant of the frequency of congenital and perinatal HCMV infections is the seroprevalence rate in women of child-bearing age. The incidence of congenital HCMV infection is directly related to the seroprevalence rates. Studies from United States and Europe have shown that the seropositivity rates in young women range from less than 50% to 85% (Krech et al., 1971; Gold and Nankervis, 1982). In contrast, most women of child bearing age in less well developed regions are HCMV antibody positive (Schopfer et al., 1978; Stagno et al., 1982; Vial et al., 1985). Prospective studies of pregnant women in the United States have shown that the rate of HCMV acquisition in young women of lower income is about 6% per year compared with about 2% in women of middle to upper income background (Stagno et al., 1986).

Perinatal HCMV acquisition, including congenital infection contributes significantly to the spread of HCMV in the population because infected infants excrete large amounts of virus for prolonged periods of time. An additional and less well appreciated mode of virus spread is through breast milk. It is estimated that over 80% of breast-fed infants of persistently infected mothers will be exposed to HCMV as a result of breast feeding (Hayes et al., 1972; Stagno et al., 1980). Similar to congenital infections, infants infected through breast feeding will excrete virus for prolonged periods of time, making them ideal vectors for the spread of virus. Children continue to acquire HCMV infection throughout childhood and the rate of infection continues to increase during adolescence and early adulthood secondary to sexual exposure. Significant titers of infectious HCMV can be found in semen and cervical secretions, suggesting that exposure to the body fluids could result in the transmission of HCMV (Jordan et al., 1973; Willmott, 1975; Drew et al., 1981; Chandler et al., 1985a,b). The natural history of HCMV infection in adolescents and adults has been shown to parallel sexually transmitted diseases (STDs) (Knox et al., 1979; Sohn et al., 1991). Homosexual men and women attending STD clinics have an increased incidence of HCMV infection (Drew et al., 1981). Thus, HCMV should be considered an STD in adults that can effectively spread through a sexually active population (Table 44.1).

Transmission of HCMV by mothers to infants: perinatal infections

Studies of mothers and infants from various countries in previous decades suggest that HCMV infections in young infants are acquired from their mothers (Numazaki et al., 1970; Hayes et al., 1972; Reynolds et al., 1973; Granstrom and Leinikki, 1978; Alford et al., 1980; Stagno et al., 1980; Dworsky et al., 1983a,b). HCMV may be transmitted from the mother to the infant either through the genital tract at delivery or through breast milk (Hayes et al., 1972; Reynolds et al., 1973; Stagno et al., 1975; Alford et al., 1980; Stagno et al., 1980; Dworsky et al., 1983a,b). As seen in Table 44.2, the rates of HCMV excretion in infants differ by country (Stagno et al., 1980). Children from countries such as Japan, Thailand, and Guatemala, where the practice of breast-feeding is almost universal and the majority of women of childbearing age are seroimmune to HCMV, have higher rates of HCMV excretion during the first year of life than infants from other countries where breast-feeding is less common (Stagno et al., 1980; Stagno and Cloud, 1990). (Table 44.2)

Table 44.1. Sources and routes of transmission of HCMV infection

	Mode of exposure and transmission
Community acquired, age	
Perinatal	Intrauterine fetal infection (congenital); intrapartum exposure to virus; breast milk acquired; mother-to-infant transmission
Infancy and childhood	Exposure to saliva and other body fluids; child-to-child transmission
Adolescence and adulthood	Exposure to young children; sexual transmission; possible occupational exposures
Hospital acquired, source	
Blood products	Blood products from seropositive donors; multiple transfusions; white blood cell containing blood products
Allografts	Allograft from seropositive donors
Donor semen	Artificial insemination using semen from seropositive donors

Breastfeeding practices have a major influence on the epidemiology of postnatal HCMV infections (Stagno and Cloud, 1994; Bryant et al., 2002). HCMV isolation from breast milk was first described over 35 years ago by Diosi et al., (1967). The importance of breast milk as a source of HCMV was first recognized by Hayes et al. (1972). HCMV has been detected in breast milk in 13% to 50% of lactating women using conventional virus isolation techniques (Yeager, 1975; Stagno et al., 1980; Dworsky et al., 1983). More recent studies utilizing the more sensitive PCR technology demonstrated the presence of HCMV DNA in breast milk from >90% of seropositive women (Hamprecht et al., 1998, 2001; Maschmann et al., 2001). The mechanisms of HCMV reactivation and excretion of HCMV in breast milk have not been defined. The early appearance of viral DNA in milk whey, the presence of infectious virus in milk whey, and higher viral load in breast milk have been shown to be risk factors for transmission of HCMV infection (Hamprecht et al., 1998, 2001; van der Strate et al., 2001).

In term infants, the consequences of HCMV infection acquired via breast milk has been reported to be negligible (Hayes et al., 1972; Stagno et al., 1980; Dworsky et al., 1983). In contrast, postnatal HCMV infection can lead to symptomatic infection in about 10% to 50% of preterm infants leading to significant morbidity (Alford et al., 1980; Dworsky et al., 1983; Yeager, 1983; Paryani et al., 1985; Hamprecht et al., 1998, 2001). A prospective study of 41 seropositive mothers and their infants revealed that 12/31 infants who were breastfed for >1 month acquired HCMV infection compared with none of the 10 infants who were breastfed for <1 month (Dworsky et al., 1983). Although it is clear that postnatal HCMV infection acquired through breast milk causes symptomatic infection such as sepsis-like syndrome in preterm infants, there is conflicting data on the occurrence of long-term sequelae. The association between postnatal HCMV infection and adverse neurodevelopmental outcome in preterm infants was reported in an earlier study

Table 44.2. Urinary HCMV excretion rates during the first two years of life[a]

Country	Total number of infants	% excreting HCMV by age							
		At birth	1 m	2 m	3 m	6 m	9 m	12 m	24 m
Japan	257	–	6	10	20	56	44	22	7
Thailand	140	–	–	–	38	55	18	15	–
Guatemala	109	–	–	–	23	42	40	35	–
Finland	105	2.3	–	12	23	35	25	33	41
Finland	148	2	–	16	32	36	–	39	–
Sweden	326	1	12	–	–	–	–	23	–
US, Seattle	92	1	3	–	11	13	–	11	–
UK	118	2.5	–	–	–	9	–	–	–
UK	1395	0.4	–	1.8	3.2	–	5.8	–	4
US, Birmingham	154	1.3	2	4	7	8	8	8	9

[a]Table used by permission (Stagno et al., 1980).

by Paryani et al., (1985). However, a more recent prospective study demonstrated that none of the 22 preterm infants with early postnatally acquired HCMV infection developed hearing loss or other neurologic sequelae (Vollmer et al., 2004).

Children-to-children transmission of HCMV

Young children are a known source of HCMV infection in the population. After early infancy where mother-to-child transmission occurs, young children likely acquire HCMV through horizontal transmission from other children or possibly indirectly through environmental contamination. Children who do not attend day-care centers have rates of HCMV seropositivity that remain generally stable until school age (Alford et al., 1980; Yow et al., 1987; Stagno and Cloud, 1994). However, studies in day-care centers

Table 44.3. HCMV excretion among children in day-care centers

Author	Year	Study location	% (number excreting virus/number of children)[a]
Strangert	1976	Sweden	35 (7/20)
Strom	1979	Sweden	72 (13/18)
Pass	1984	US, Birmingham	57 (59/103)
Adler	1985	US, Richmond	24 (16/66)
Hutto	1985	US, Birmingham	41 (77/188)
Jones	1985	US, San Francisco	22 (31/140)
Murph	1986	US, Iowa City	21 (17/80)
Grillner	1986	Sweden	27 (16/60)
Nelson	1987	UK	27 (32/117)
Adler	1988	US, Richmond	53 (55/104)
Volpi	1988	Italy	13 (33/253)
de Mello	1996	Brazil	52 (31/60)
Ford-Jones	1996	Canada	17 (79/471)
Kashiwagi	1999	Japan	22 (12/54)

[a]Virus excretion either from saliva or urine or both.

throughout the world have demonstrated that young children shed virus in saliva and urine creating exposure opportunities for virus transmission to other children in the day-care setting, to their parents and to the day-care or nursery workers. As illustrated in Table 44.3, HCMV excretion is common in children who attend day-care centers, although the percentage of children excreting virus varies by location (Strangert et al., 1976; Strom, 1979; Pass et al., Adler, Hutto et al., 1985; Jones et al., 1985; Grillner and Strangert, 1986; Murph et al., 1986; Nelson et al., 1987; Adler, 1988a,b; Volpi et al., 1988; de Mello et al., 1996; Ford-Jones et al., 1996; Kashiwagi et al., 2001) (Table 44.3).

Prospective studies in day-care centers have provided evidence of child-to-child transmission by documenting acquisition of HCMV in children previously known to be uninfected upon enrollment in the day care centers (Pass et al., 1984; Adler, 1988a,b; de Mello et al., 1996). Pass et al. followed a cohort of children <12 months of age in a day care center and found that <10% were shedding virus at enrollment but 6 to 12 months later 78% of the children in the cohort were shedding virus (Pass et al., 1984). Similarly, Adler followed a group of children for 26 months in a day-care center in Richmond, Virginia and found that virus excretion increased from 25 to 61% in children <3 years of age (Adler, 1988a,b). A study in a day-care center in Sao Paulo, Brasil identified 37 children who were initially HCMV seronegative upon enrollment into the study and demonstrated that 6 to 12 months later, 50% of these children excreted HCMV in either their saliva or urine (de Mello et al., 1996).

Studies that have provided appropriate control groups for comparing the day-care center populations have found that the prevalence of HCMV excretion is significantly higher in the children who attend a day-care center than in the control children who did not attend a day-care center (Hutto et al., 1985; Adler, 1988a,b). In both Richmond, Virginia (odds ratio (OR) = 4.3, 95% confidence interval (CI), 2.2–8.1) and Birmingham, Alabama (OR = 3.9, 95% CI, 1.8–9.0), children attending day-care centers were approximately four times more likely to shed HCMV than children who were not enrolled in day-care centers (Adler, 1985; Hutto et al., 1985).

Besides child-to-child transmission, HCMV is also found on toys and other environmental surfaces in day-cares providing another viral source for HCMV infection (Faix, 1985; Hutto et al., 1986; Schopfer et al., 1986). Although HCMV is usually considered labile under most environmental conditions, a study led by Hutto, found that HCMV survived on toys for up to 30 minutes in a day-care where children aged six to 30 months of age were placing a hand or toy in their mouths every one to two minutes (Hutto et al., 1986). Likely horizontal transmission of HCMV from child to child occurs through saliva on hands and toys. As seen in Fig. 44.1, the highest rates of HCMV excretion in day-care settings are usually seen among toddlers and young children (ages 12–24 months and 25–36 months) supporting the theory that HCMV transmission occurs through saliva on hands and toys as children play together (Strangert et al., 1976; Strom, 1979; Pass et al., 1984; Adler et al., 1985; Jones et al., 1985; Murph et al., 1986; Ford-Jones et al., 1996; Kashiwagi et al., 2001). (Fig. 44.1)

The strongest evidence to support child-to-child transmission of HCMV has been obtained by the analysis of the restriction endonuclease digestion patterns of HCMV DNA of isolates obtained from HCMV infected children attending day-care centers. Adler examined the restriction endonuclease patterns of HCMV isolates obtained from 16 children at a single day-care center and found that one group of seven children and another group of four children were excreting identical strains (Adler, 1988a,b). The seven children in one group were all <29 months of age and all but one of these children shared the same classroom. The four children in the second group were >36 months of age and three of the children were in the same room. In another prospective study by Adler, 104 children from a day-care center were followed and 14 different strains of HCMV were identified by restriction endonuclease analysis (Adler, 1988). Three of the 14 strains infected 44 of the children attending the day-care center. All children infected with one of the three strains of HCMV were younger than 3 years of age indicating frequent child-to-child transmission of

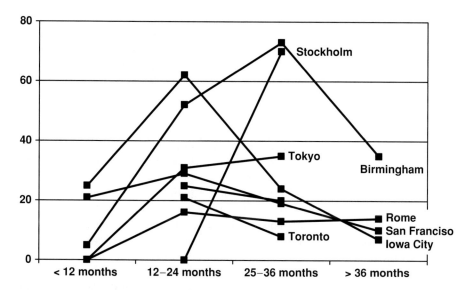

Fig. 44.1. Age-related HCMV excretion in various day-care center populations.

HCMV in these young children within the day-care setting. Other studies using restriction endonuclease analysis of HCMV DNA in different populations have also found identical HCMV strains are shared among children in group day-care confirming that HCMV is efficiently transmitted from child to child in day-care settings (Grillner and Strangert 1986; Murph et al., 1991).

The higher HCMV excretion rates in young children attending day-care centers ranging from 13% to 72% compared to children who do not attend day care; the highest rates of HCMV excretion observed in toddlers and young children; the documentation of HCMV shedding in children previously known to be uninfected after day-care center attendance in prospective studies; the isolation of HCMV from toys and other objects in day-care settings; and the identification of similar strains of HCMV within day-care centers provides compelling evidence for child-to-child transmission among young children in day-care settings.

Transmission of HCMV by children to parents

Children excreting virus often become the source of HCMV infection for susceptible parents and others in the household. Studies by Spector et al., and Dworsky et al., using restriction endonuclease analysis, have demonstrated that infants with perinatal HCMV infections may transmit HCMV to an uninfected parent or other adult family member (Spector and Spector, 1982; Dworsky et al., 1984). Seroconversion rates for parents when children reside in the household are higher than the rates reported for households with only adults in residence. In a study by Yeager et al., infants who were nosocomially infected with HCMV by transfusion transmitted HCMV infection to their seronegative mothers (Yeager, 1975). Of the mothers who were seronegative and exposed to infected infants, 47% (7/15) seroconverted within a year after the child was discharged from the hospital compared to 4% of the mothers whose infants were uninfected at the time of discharge. Dworsky et al. studied 372 women between pregnancies and observed these women had an annual seroconversion rate of 5.5% compared to 2.2% for women who were pregnant for the first time (Dworsky et al., 1983). Taber et al., in a family HCMV study, demonstrated an increased seroconversion rate within the family setting (Taber et al., 1985). The annual seroconversion rate for parents with young children in the household was 10.6% for mothers and 10% for fathers in this study. In 10 of 14 families where the initial family member who seroconverted could be identified, the index case was a child. In another study by Pass et al., virus isolates were collected from the members of five families where the mother had evidence of a primary maternal infection during her most recent pregnancy and a child less than three years of age who was excreting HCMV residing in the home (Pass et al., 1987). In each of the five families, the HCMV strains were identical by restriction endonuclease analysis. In two families, acquisition of HCMV by the child in a day-care center was followed by both maternal seroconversion and maternal excretion of the same identical strain of HCMV as shed by her child. This study provides further evidence that children in the household, especially

Table 44.4. Risk factors for primary HCMV infection in women attending an STD clinic (Chandler. et al., 1985a,b)

Factor	Seroconversion (11/84, 13%)	Remained seronegative (15/84, 18%)	P value
Age (years)	20.4 ± 0.9	22.3 ± 0.5	NS
>two recent sexual partners	67%	14%	0.01
History of STDs	73%	32%	0.02
STDs during study	73%	63%	NS

those attending group day-care may transmit HCMV to other family members.

Other studies in day-care centers have provided compelling evidence of the acquisition of HCMV by children in day care with the subsequent seroconversion of their parents (Adler, 1985; Pass et al., 1986; Adler, 1991). In a longitudinal follow-up study of seronegative parents with children in day-care centers and a control group of parents whose children were not in day-care centers, 21% (14/67) of the parents whose children were in the day-care centers seroconverted whereas none (0/31) of the controls seroconverted (Pass et al., 1986). All of the parents who seroconverted had a child who was shedding HCMV either in saliva or urine. Parents at greatest risk of HCMV infection were the parents of children who were found to be shedding HCMV (45%, 9/20) and were <18 months of age at enrollment. In a similar study, Adler observed that 39% (7/18) of mothers seroconverted within 3 to 7 months after their children became infected at the day-care center (Adler, 1988a,b). The HCMV strains isolated were identical in both the mothers and their children, and in six of the mothers the HCMV strain was associated with the day-care center. An additional study from Adler prospectively followed 96 seronegative mothers of children attending three day-care centers (Adler, 1991). Among the 50 mothers with HCMV infected children, 19 seroconverted (38%) whereas, only 2 of the 46 seronegative mothers of uninfected children seroconverted (4%). Of the 19 mothers who seroconverted, 9 shed HCMV and the virus was an identical isolate as was shed by their child. All of these studies provide evidence that young children contribute to parental HCMV infections and mothers of these young children are at an increased risk of HCMV infection that might result in congenital infections for their future offspring (Pass et al., 1987).

HCMV transmission through sexual activity

An important source of HCMV infection is through the intimate contact with oral and genital secretions (Britt and Alford, 1996). Salivary glands are a site of virus persistence in humans and it is likely that reactivations leads to the presence of infectious virus in oral secretions. Infectious virus can often be cultured from cervical secretions and semen has been shown to be a rich source of virus in seropositive men (Lang, 1975; Knox et al., 1979; Stagno et al., 1975). High rates of HCMV seropositivity have been reported in women attending STD clinics and couples discordant for HCMV have been shown to readily transmit virus and in some cases, reinfect previously infected partners (Handsfield et al., 1985; Chandler et al., 1985a,b, 1987).

Chandler et al., examined the association between HCMV infection and indices of sexual activity in 347 women attending an STD clinic (Chandler et al., 1985a,b). To determine the annual incidence of primary HCMV infection, 84 seronegative women were followed for a mean duration of 18.4 weeks with documented seroconversion in 11 (13%). Based on this study, the annualized incidence of primary HCMV infection was estimated to be 37% (Table 44.4). As can be seen in Table 44.4, the risk factors acquisition of HCMV infection in seronegative women in this population include the history of STDs and >2 sexual partners in the month preceding seroconversion. However, the majority of subjects included in the study were selected based on the presence of mucopurulent cervical discharge or cervical ectopy which may have resulted in the inclusion of more women with STDs in the study. In a more recent study from Seattle by Coonrod et al., 245 HCMV seronegative women attending an STD clinic were followed for a median duration of 23 months. During the study, seroconversion was documented in 36 (15%) women, an annualized rate of 10%–12% (Coonrod et al., 1998). The risk factors that were associated with seroconversion in that study include young age, younger age at sexual debut, greater number of sexual partners, and more recent sexual partners. In addition, seroconverters were more likely to have gonorrhea, chlamydia or pelvic inflammatory disease. (Table 44.4)

The shedding of HCMV in genital tract secretions was examined in studies of selected populations (Pereira et al., 1990; Fairfax et al., 1994; Shen et al., 1994; Clarke et al., 1996). Collier et al., studied the association between HCMV shedding and sexual activity in 1481 women attending an STD clinic (Collier et al., 1995). HCMV was isolated in cervical secretions from 9.4% of the 951 seropositive women. Cervical HCMV excretion was associated with concomitant gonococcal infection and was less frequent in women using barrier contraception. Higher frequency of HCMV-IgM antibodies were observed in seroconverters, suggesting recent HCMV infection and possible exogenous reinfection. The frequency and the factors associated with cervical shedding of HCMV were compared between a group of 195 licensed prostitutes and 187 women attending an

STD clinic in Taiwan (Shen et al., 1994). About a third of the women in both groups shed HCMV in cervical secretions. The factors that were associated with cervical HCMV shedding are multiple sexual partners, and history of STDs. In another study of STD clinic attendees by Pereira et al., age less than 23 years and concomitant gonococcal infection were independently associated with cervical HCMV excretion (Pereira et al., 1990). Women with another genital tract infection were 6.5 times more likely to have HCMV than those without other genital infections. In a more recent study by Clarke et al., HCMV shedding in HIV seronegative and HIV seropositive women from an urban minority community was examined (Clarke et al., 1996). HCMV seropositivity was >90% in both groups. Cervicovaginal shedding was detected in 4.4% of HIV-negative women and 19.6% of HIV-positive subjects (odds ratio, 5.28; $P < 0.001$). Multiple logistic regression analysis revealed that HCMV shedding was associated with younger age (OR = 0.90; $P < 0.001$), and concurrent chlamydial or gonococcal infection (OR = 3.60; $P < 0.08$). Among HIV-positive subjects, CMV shedding was significantly higher in women with CD4 cell counts $<500 \times 10^6$/L. The data from the studies described above provides evidence that cervicovaginal HCMV infection is related to sexual activity, and the presence of other genital tract infections.

Several studies have identified the risk factors for seropositivity to HCMV in women attending STD clinics, in pregnant women, sexually active adolescent girls, and HIV infected women (Chandler et al., 1985a, b; Collier et al., 1990; Sohn et al., 1991; Shen et al., 1994; Clarke et al., 1996; Coonrod et al., 1998). The results from these studies have been summarized in Table 44.5. In a study of 347 women attending an STD clinic, a stepwise logistic regression analysis showed that HCMV seropositivity was associated with non-white race, number of lifetime sexual partners, and young age at sexual debut (Chandler et al., 1985a,b). However, the majority of women included in the study had cervical abnormalities. A latter study from the same STD clinic including unselected study subjects and larger sample size has attempted to define the relationship between sexual practices and HCMV seropositivity in African American and Caucasian women (Collier et al., 1990). The risk factors associated with HCMV seroprevalence are similar in both African American and Caucasian women and these include more recent new sexual partners, more lifetime sexual partners, and the presence of chlamydial infection. Additional risk factors in Caucasian women included young age at sexual debut and not using barrier contraception. In another study from Seattle, the risk factors for the presence of HCMV antibodies were determined in 1129 pregnant women (Chandler et al., 1985a,b). Fifty seven percent of women were HCMV seropositive. Logistic regression

Table 44.5. Risk factors for CMV seropositivity in adolescents, contraceptive and STD clinics

Author and Year published, location	Study population	Risk factors for CMV seropositivity
Chandler, 1985 Seattle, US	347 STD clinic clients (219 with cervical abnormalities	Young age sexual debut More lifetime sexual partners More recent sexual partners
Collier, 1990 Seattle. US	1481 STD clinic clients	*African Americans*: Recent sexual partners New sexual partners Cervical chlamydial infection *Caucasians*: Young sexual debut Recent new sexual partners More lifetime sexual partners Lack of barrier contraception
Sohn, 1991 Birmingham, US	254 adolescent girls (12–18 years)	African American race STDs >2 sexual partners >3 years of sexual activity
Hyams, 1993 Philippines	470 male military personnel presenting at a STD clinic	History of STDs
Shen, 1994 Taiwan	195 licensed prostitutes 187 STD clinic clients 70 women attending a gynecologic clinic	Presence of cervical CMV shedding
Ray, 1997 India	368 in STD and antenatal clinics	Chlamydial endocervicitis
Rosenthal, 1997 Cincinnati, US	399 adolescents	African American race Female sex
Coonrod, 1998 Seattle, US	245 STD clinic clients	More sexual partners New sexual partners Gonorrhea Chlamydia Pelvic inflammatory disease

analysis showed the seropositivity correlated with lower socioeconomic status, older age, history of abnormal cervical cytology, infection with *Trichomonas vaginalis*, and greater number of sexual partners.

In a study of 254 adolescent girls attending a contraceptive counseling clinic, Sohn et al., demonstrated a strong association between indicators of sexual activity and the presence of CMV-IgG antibodies (Sohn et al., 1991). Using logistic regression analysis, the presence of two more sexual activity risk factors (young age at sexual debut, years of sexual activity, number of lifetime partners) was the most important predictor of HCMV infection. After controlling for confounders, African-American race was associated with an increased risk of infection (OR = 3.4) whereas oral contraceptive use was protective (OR = 0.6) for HCMV infection. The association between sexual activity and the HCMV seropositivity has also been documented in other studies from different geographic regions (Table 44.5) (Berry et al., 1988; Pereira et al., 1990; Hyams et al., 1993; Shen et al., 1994; Coonrod et al., 1998). (Table 44.5)

Further support for the sexual transmission of HCMV was provided by a study of HCMV infection in sexual partners by Handsfield et al. (1985). This study demonstrated that 74% of men whose female partners were seropositive were antibody positive compared to 34% of those whose partners were seronegative ($P = 0.008$). Restriction endonuclease analysis of HCMV isolates from three pairs of sexual partners identified that two of the couples were infected with common strains. To determine the frequency of HCMV reinfection, Chandler et al. examined serial isolates from eight women attending an STD clinic and seven women receiving routine prenatal care (Chandler et al., 1987). Using restriction digestion analysis, the authors demonstrated that four of the eight women from the STD clinic were infected with more than one virus strain. Two women shed different strains in serial samples, and two women shed different strains simultaneously from different body sites. These findings provide evidence that reinfection with different virus strains is not uncommon in women with increased exposure to HCMV.

The association between sexual activity and HCMV transmission can be summarized as follows: (a) the prevalence of HCMV antibody more than doubles during the years beginning sexual activity (15–30 yrs) (Wentworth and Alexander, 1971), (b) higher rates of seropositivity in male partners of seropositive women as compared to seronegative women (Numazaki et al., 1970; Handsfield et al., 1985), (c) HCMV has been isolated from cervix of 13% to 35% of women with suspected STDs (Knox et al., 1979; Shen et al., 1994), (d) seropositivity correlated with the presence of other STDs (Chandler et al., 1985a,b; Collier et al., 1995; Coonrod et al., 1998), (e) among seronegative women attending an STD clinic, the annual HCMV seroconversion rate was noted to be 37% vs. 1% to 2% per year in the general population (Table 44.5) (Chandler et al., 1985a,b), (f) seropositivity correlated with number of lifetime sexual partners and young age at onset of sexual activity (Collier et al., 1990; Pereira et al., 1990; Shen et al., 1992) and, (g) a negative correlation between the use of barrier contraception and seropositivity (Collier et al., 1990, 1995).

Thus, there is strong epidemiological evidence that acquisition and transmission of HCMV infection is associated with sexual activity and STDs. However, the mechanisms and pathogenesis of this association have not been defined. Although frequent and repeated exposure is an important determinant for HCMV infection in individuals with STDs, it is also possible that the presence of genital tract inflammation plays an important role by providing a local milieu that is conducive to HCMV replication and transmission. However, the relationship between genital tract inflammation and the local HCMV replication has not been studied.

Transmission of HCMV to child-care providers

Children in day-care settings may be an important source of HCMV infection for child-care personnel. Numerous studies in the past decades have described the risk of HCMV infection for women who provide care for children in an occupational setting, as seen in Table 44.6 (Jones et al. 1985; Blackman et al., 1987; Nelson et al., 1987; Adler, 1989; Pass et al., 1990; Murph et al., 1991; Ford-Jones et al., 1996; Bale et al., 1999; De Schryver et al., 1999). Overall, the annual seroconversion rates in day-care workers who care for young children range from 0% to 20%. Variations in seroconversion rates within differing populations may reflect underlying factors such as socioeconomic status and race and their impact on HCMV infection. The populations with the highest seroconversion rates were those that studied day-care providers in various regions of the US and Canada (Adler, 1989; Pass et al., 1990; Murph et al., 1991; Ford-Jones et al., 1996; Bale et al., 1999). Studies in England and Belgium found lower seroconversion rates among individuals who were exposed to children in occupational settings (Nelson et al., 1987; De Schryver et al., 1999). This lower transmission rate may be due to the smaller sample sizes and the shorter follow up periods for the detection of seroconversion. It is also possible that lower levels of virus shedding or the virologic characteristics including the infectivity of the circulating HCMV strains might account for the lower rates of transmission. Another explanation could be that child care personnel in these countries are better educated and adhere to standard hygiene practices when caring for young children thereby interrupting the transmission of the virus. Although HCMV seroconversion rates in child care providers vary in different populations and studies, the higher seroconversion rates observed in the larger cohort studies provide evidence that in some populations, young children play an important role in transmitting HCMV to their care providers (Adler, 1989; Pass et al., 1990; Murph et al., 1991; Ford-Jones et al., 1996; Bale et al., 1999). (Table 44.6).

Table 44.6. Annual HCMV seroconversion rates among child care personnel

Author, year, and location	Population	HCMV seropositivity, %	Annual seroconversion rate, %
Jones, 1985 US, San Francisco	130 infant development center workers	50	0
Blackman, 1987 US, Iowa City	57 preschool workers for physical and mentally impaired children program	35	0
	53 home-based early intervention program workers	40	7.7
	66 hospital clinic staff	38	0
Nelson, 1987 England	41 day-care teachers	66	0
	500 matched controls in their first pregnancy	53	NR[a]
Adler, 1989 US, Richmond	610 day-care workers	41	11
	565 hospital workers	47	2.2
Pass, 1990 US, Birmingham	509 day-care workers	62	20
Murph, 1991 US, Iowa City	252 day-care workers	38	7.9
Ford-Jones, 1996 Canada	206 day-care worlers	67	12.5
Bale, 1999 US, Iowa City	132 women providing child care in their homes	58	6.8
de Schryver, 1999 Belgium	283 educators for mentally disabled children	15.9	1.03
	294 nurses for the elderly	18.4	1.42

[a]NR = Not reported.

Risk factors for HCMV serconversion of child care providers have included workers <30 years of age, not wearing gloves when changing diapers, and caring for children ≤3 years of age for 20 hours a week (Pass *et al.*, 1990; Ford-Jones *et al.*, 1996). However, other studies did not find that seroconversion of day care providers was related to caring for children ≤3 years age (Adler, 1989; Murph *et al.*, 1991; Ford-Jones *et al.*, 1996). None of the studies found that race or the presence of other children in the home were associated with seroconversion in an occupational setting (Adler *et al.*, 1990; Murph *et al.*, 1991; Ford-Jones *et al.*, 1996). In several studies where day care children were evaluated for virus shedding, similar viral isolates were found in both the children and in the day-care providers who seroconverted suggesting that HCMV infection in the workers were acquired from the children in their care (Adler, 1989; Murph *et al.*, 1991; Bale *et al.*, 1999).

Seroprevalence studies of child care personnel have identified factors associated with HCMV seropositivity in these workers as illustrated in Table 44.7 (Blackman *et al.*, 1987; Volpi *et al.*, 1988; Adler, 1989; Pass *et al.*, 1990; Murph *et al.*, 1991; Ford-Jones *et al.*, 1996; Jackson *et al.*, 1996; Bale *et al.*, 1999; De Schryver *et al.*, 1999; Kiss *et al.*, 2002). The risk factors observed for HCMV seropositivity include factors that are associated with HCMV in the general population such as parity, age and race (Chandler *et al.*, 1985a,b; Collier *et al.*, 1990; Sohn *et al.*, 1991) and also additional risk factors related to occupation as a child-care provider. These occupational risk factors suggest that HCMV infection in occupational settings may result from the exposure to young children who are shedding virus. However, none of these studies can provide with certainty that all HCMV infections observed in the day-care personnel are due to child-to-worker transmission since other HCMV exposure opportunities may exist in the environment and the population from other sources. (Table 44.7)

Transmission of CMV in health-care settings

The possibility that CMV may be transmitted in health care settings has been explored over the last three decades. In 1969, Haldane *et al.*, reported a significantly higher incidence of birth defects among the offspring of nurses caring for children with CMV infection (Haldane *et al.*, 1969). Following this report, many studies (Table 44.8) have evaluated the risk of CMV infection in nurses who cared for young infants and children in the newborn nurseries or pediatric wards of hospitals and provided conflicting results (Yeager, 1975; Haneberg *et al.*, 1980; Ahlfors *et al.*, 1981; Dworsky *et al.*, 1983a,b; Friedman *et al.*, 1984; Hatherley, 1985; Adler *et al.*, 1986; Balfour and Balfour, 1986; Hatherley, 1986; Demmler *et al.*, 1987). Overall, the studies with appropriate control groups found the combined risk of CMV infection in nurses who cared for children to be almost three times (risk ratio (RR) 2.7, 95% CI, 1.3 – 5.5) greater than the controls (Yeager, 1975; Ahlfors *et al.*, 1981; Dworsky *et al.*, 1983; Friedman *et al.*, 1984; Balfour and Balfour, 1986; Hatherley,

Table 44.7. Risk factors for HCMV seropositivity among child care personnel

Author, year, and location	Population	HCMV seropositivity, %	Risk factors
Blackman, 1987 Iowa City, US	57 preschool workers for physical and mentally impaired children program	35	Older age
	53 home-based early intervention program workers	40	
	66 hospital clinic staff	38	
Volpi, 1988 Italy	82 day-care workers	96	Multiparous[a]
	82 housewife controls	84	
	229 female day-care students in training	85	
Adler, 1989 Richmond, US	610 day-care workers	41	Cared for children <2 years of age
	565 hospital workers	47	
Pass, 1990 Birmingham, US	509 day-care workers	62	Older age
			Non-white race Working with children <2 years of age for 8 hours/week
Murph, 1991 Iowa City, US	252 day-care workers	38	Older age
			Non-white race Children residing in home
Ford-Jones, 1996 Canada	206 day-care worlers	67	Born outside of Canada
			Children <5 residing in house Household size >3 people
Jackson, 1996 Seattle, US	360 child care workers	62	Non-white race
			Changing diapers ≥3 days/week at work
			Children residing in house
Bale, 1999 Iowa City, US	132 women providing child care in their homes	58	Caring for toddlers (1–2 yrs)
			Longer time as a child care provider
de Schryver, 1999 Belgium	283 educators for mentally disabled children	16	Muliparous
	294 nurses for the elderly	18	
Kiss, 2002 Belgium	211 kindergarten teachers	29%[b]	Children residing in house
	283 administrative workers		Kindergarten teaching

[a]Borderline significance.
[b]Reported for the combined groups.

1986; Flowers et al., 1988). However, when person–year analysis was performed to take into account the follow-up period, a trend toward an increased risk in nurses remained but failed to reach statistical significance (RR 1.8, 95% CI, 0.9 – 3.6) (Flowers et al., 1988).

Studies of health-care personnel including staff in children's hospitals have shown that CMV seroconversion rates do not differ between the employees, and the general population (Tolkoff-Rubin et al., 1978; Dworsky et al., 1983; Balfour and Balfour 1986; Demmler et al., 1987; Balcarek et al., 1990; Gerberding, 1994). However, all of the studies of health care personnel have low sample sizes, inadequate statistical power and have not provided information on potential confounding factors such as CMV sexual exposure or exposure to children outside of the workplace that could impact their risk for HCMV infection (Flowers et al., 1988; Farr and Torner, 1990). These limitations and also the widespread adoption of universal precautions (CDC, 1987, 1988) in health-care settings in the late 1980s have made it difficult to estimate whether an increased risk of CMV infection exists within occupational settings. As illustrated in Table 44.9, several studies have evaluated risk factors for CMV seropositivity in health-care providers although these studies did not account for other possible non-occupational CMV exposures (Gerberding, 1994; Herbert et al., 1995; Sobaszek et al., 2000). Studies using molecular epidemiologic techniques demonstrated that health care workers are at low risk for occupational CMV transmission (Dworsky et al., 1983; Adler, 1986; Peckham et al., 1986; Demmler et al., 1987). In these studies, molecular analysis of CMV isolates demonstrated that some of the CMV infections identified in the workers were similar to CMV isolates from other family members and were not occupationally acquired (Dworsky et al., 1983; Demmler et al., 1987). Without a large collaborative study or the pooling of results of multiple well-designed studies, the question about the relative contribution of CMV infection in health-care settings cannot be fully elucidated at this time. However,

Table 44.8. Seroconversion rates for personnel in health care settings

Study, year published, and location	Study groups	CMV seroconversion rates % (number/total)
Yeager 1975	Pediatric ward nurses	9.7 (3/31)
Denver, US	Nursery nurses	5.9 (2/34)
	Controls	0 (0/27)
Tolkoff-Rubin, 1978	Hemodialysis staff	0 (0/26)
Boston, US	Hemodialysis patients	13 (10/80)
Haneberg, 1980 Norway	Pediatric student nurses	9.4 (6/64)
Ahlfors, 1981	Pediatric ward nurses	6.9 (2/29)
Sweden	Pediatric nurses	0 (0/31)
	Controls	1.9 (1/52)
Dworsky, 1983	Nursery nurses	3.3 (4/61)
Birmingham, US	Controls (pregnant women)	1.5 (23/1549)
	Medical students	0.6 (1/89)
	Medical house staff	2.7 (1/25)
Friedman, 1984	Pediatric intensive care nurses	8.7 (2/23)
Philadelphia, US	Nursery nurses	7.7 (3/39)
	Pediatric ward nurses	4.6 (3/65)
	Controls	2.9 (1/35)
Hatherley, 1985 Australia	Nursery nurses	4.4 (2/45)
Hatherley, 1986	Nursery nurses	1.9 (3/154)
Australia	Controls	0 (0/12)
Adler, 1986	Pediatric ward nurses	6.5 (2/31)
Richmond, US	Nursery nurses	2.5 (1/40)
Balfour, 1986	Neonatal intensive care nurses	4.2 (4/96)
Minneapolis, US	Student nurses	5.0 (7/139)
	Renal transplant/hemodialysis nurses	1.7 (2/117)
	Controls	1.8 (3/167)
Brady, 1985	Nursery nurses	6.0 (4/67)
Houston, US	Medical house staff	9.5 (2/21)
Demmler, 1987	Nursery nurses	5.4 (2/37)
Houston, US	Pediatric chronic care ward nurses	0 (0/21)
	Pediatric chronic care ward therapists	0 (0/37)
Balcarek, 1990	Children hospital employees, patient care	4.4 (8/183)
Birmingham, US	Children hospital employees, administrative	3.6 (2/56)
	Children hospital employees, support	4.1 (2/49)
	Children hospital employees, laboratory	8.3 (1/12)
Gerberding, 1994	Health care providers at one hospital	6.6 (25/378)
San Francisco, US		

the existing data suggest that the risk of CMV infection in a health-care setting is low and likely does not differ from the risk of CMV infection in the general population. (Tables 44.8 and 44.9).

Transfusion acquired HCMV infection

Transfusion associated HCMV infection was first described in 1966 and since that time, has been demonstrated to be a cause of significant morbidity and mortality in a wide variety of clinical circumstances (Kaariainen et al., 1966; Hillyer et al., 1990; Meyers, 1991). HCMV infection following transfusion has been associated with transfused red cell, platelet concentrates, and granulocyte concentrates whereas, fresh-frozen plasma and cryoprecipitates have not been reported to cause HCMV transmission (Bowden and Sayers, 1990). HCMV is believed to establish latency in the cells of myeloid lineage and the virus can be reactivated and cause disease in seropositive immunocompromized hosts. Transfusion of unscreened cellular components results in HCMV transmission in approximately 30%

Table 44.9. Risk factors for CMV seropositivity in health care workers

Study, year published, and location	Study groups	Risk factors for CMV seropositivity evaluated	Odds ratio (95% confidence interval)
Gerberding, 1994 San Francisco, US	976 health care providers at San Francisco General Hospital	Older age	1.4 (1.2–1.7)[a]
		Female	1.8 (1.3–2.5)
		Being a physician	0.4 (0.3–0.6)
		Working on an AIDS clinical unit	NS[b]
Herbert, 1995 England	81 preclinical dental students and 81 matched controls 53 clinical dental students and 53 matched controls 103 dental surgeons and 103 matched controls	Protective workwear	NS[b]
Sobaszek, 2000 France	400 female health care workers who had contact with children or immunosuppressed patients	Number of children ≥1	1.9 (1.2–3.0)
		Close contact nursing tasks	2.2 (1.4–3.3)
		Older age	1.7 (1.0–3.0)

[a] For an increase of one decade.
[b] NS, Not significant.

(range 10%–70%) in seronegative recipients, as determined by seroconversion and/or virus isolation (Wilhelm et al., 1986; Preiksaitis et al., 1988). The risk of transfusion associated HCMV infection is directly related the number of components transfused and the quantity of leukocytes transfused. HCMV can also be transmitted via organ or marrow grafts (Wreghitt et al., 1988; Reusser et al., 1991). The use of blood products from seronegative donors and using procedures which limit the quantity of leukocytes in the transfused blood have considerably reduced the risk of transfusion associated HCMV infection (Lang et al., 1977; Brady et al., 1984; Preiksaitis et al., 1988; Miller et al., 1991). These findings suggest that leukocytes are the cellular components of blood products responsible for most transfusion-associated HCMV infection.

Transfusion-associated HCMV infection can result in significant morbidity and mortality in preterm infants, allograft recipients, following cardiac surgery and other immunocompromised hosts (Yeager et al., 1981; Brady et al., 1984; Adler, 1985; Bowden, 1991). The rate of HCMV acquisition in preterm infants of seronegative mothers who received multiple transfusion has been shown be between 9% and 13.5% (Yeager et al., 1981; Adler, 1983). The percentage of units of blood capable of transmitting HCMV has been estimated to be between 2.5% and 12.5%. A controlled trial in low birth weight HCMV seronegative infants born to HCMV-seronegative mothers compared the use of filtered and unfiltered red cell components for the prevention of transfusion associated HCMV infection (Gilbert et al., 1989). Twenty-one percent (9/42) of the recipients of unscreened, unfiltered blood acquired HCMV infection compared with none of 59 infants who received unscreened, filtered components. Additional studies have confirmed the effectiveness of the leukofiltration in reducing the transmission of HCMV in other population groups including immunocompromised hosts (Eisenfeld et al., 1992).

Transplantation and HCMV infection

Allografts from donors previously infected with HCMV represent a major risk factor for HCMV transmission. In all but the bone marrow allograft recipients, the transplantation of an organ from a donor previously infected with HCMV into a seronegative recipient has been shown to be the single most important risk factor for primary HCMV infection (Rubin et al., 1985; Ho, 1991). In solid organ transplantation, primary infections that develop from the allograft have a more profound impact on the outcomes than infections acquired via transfusions (Falagas et al., 1996). The natural history of HCMV infection in transplant recipients suggests that infection is nearly universal in those exposed, but the clinical disease is dependent on specific risk factors, in particular, the immunosuppressive regimen. As the severity of immunosuppression increases, so does the severity of HCMV disease, as evidenced by the often fatal HCMV infections that occur in bone marrow allograft recipients

(Meyers et al., 1982; Winston et al., 1990; Schmidt et al., 1991). In renal allograft recipients following HCMV mismatched donor-recipient transplantation, disease rates as high as 70% have been described (Rubin and Colvin, 1986). Mortality rates in excess of 50% in heart/lung transplantation have limited the mismatched donor-recipient transplantation in some centers (Smyth et al., 1991).

Historically, HCMV interstitial pneumonitis occurred in 10% to 30% of bone marrow transplant recipients, with mortality rates of over 80% in some studies, even after the introduction of ganciclvir (Wingard et al., 1988; Winston et al., 1988). However, the incidence of HCMV infection and disease in hematopoietic stem cell transplant recipients has decreased somewhat over the past 15 years due to changes in patient management. These changes include the avoidance of HCMV positive cellular blood products in susceptible, HCMV-negative recipients, and the use of prophylactic and/or pre-emptive antiviral therapy to limit HCMV reactivation and disease. Since, the advent of prophylactic and pre-emptive antiviral therapy, the onset time of HCMV pneumonia has been delayed from a median time of 44 days after transplant to between 92 and 188 days (Goodrich et al., 1993; Nguyen et al., 1999; de Medeiros et al., 2000; Machado et al., 2000; Ljungman, 2001). In a study of liver transplant recipients, despite the significant increase in the proportion of high risk patients (HCMV recipient-/donor+) and the increase in the rate of HCMV infection, the incidence of HCMV disease has decreased significantly (Singh et al., 2004). The authors of that study noted that the HCMV infection rate neither confounded the use of antiviral prophylaxis nor selective testing for HCMV. In addition to the morbidity and mortality associated with HCMV disease, the survival of the allografts has been adversely affected by HCMV.

HCMV transmission from artificial insemination by donor semen

The advent of artificial insemination with donor semen suggests another possible transmission route for HCMV in the population. HCMV has been cultured from semen even in cases in which urine, saliva or blood specimens have been negative for infectious virus (Lang and Kummer, 1975; Biggar et al., 1983; Mascola and Guinan, 1986; Tjiam et al., 1987). It has been demonstrated that HCMV transmission can occur through therapeutic donor insemination (Prior et al., 1994). However, most of the studies examining the presence of HCMV in semen have included individuals attending STD clinics. In a more recent study from France, Masat et al. examined the presence of HCMV in cryopreserved semen samples collected for therapeutic donor insemination (Mansat et al., 1997). Using cell culture and PCR, HCMV was detected in 5.1% of the semen specimens suggesting that cryopreserved semen from healthy donors may represent a potential source of HCMV infection. The American Fertility Society recommended that all semen donors be screened for the presence of HCMV antibodies and that semen from seropositive donors may only be used to inseminate seropositive recipients. Although the risk to offspring via donor insemination has not been defined, the British Andrology Society recommends that only semen from seronegative donors be stored for clinical use (British Andrology Society, 1999).

Summary

HCMV remains a ubiquitous infectious agent and a cause of significant disease in individuals with immature or suppressed immune responses. In most human populations examined, HCMV is acquired predominantly through exposure to young children, breast feeding and sexual activity. Although a strong epidemiologic association between these risk factor and acquisition of HCMV has been demonstrated, the exact mechanism and pathogenesis of HCMV transmission have not been defined. Furthermore, the roles of virologic characteristics including strain variation and reinfections in the transmission of HCMV have not been delineated. Today, HCMV is primarily a cause of disease in newborn infants and in allograft recipients. Perhaps of even greater potential medical importance is the proposed role of chronic HCMV infections in diseases such as coronary atherosclerosis and human cancers, two areas of active research (Everett et al., 1992; Zhou et al., 1996; Hosenpud, 1999; Zhu et al., 1999; Streblow et al., 2000).

REFERENCES

Aarnisalo, J., Ilonen, J., Vainionpaa, R., Volanen, I., Kaitosaari, T., and Simell, O. (2003). Development of antibodies against cytomegalovirus, varicella-zoster virus and herpes simplex virus in Finland during the first eight years of life: a prospective study. *Scand. J. Infect. Dis.*, **35**(10), 750–753.

Adler, S. P. (1983). Transfusion-associated cytomegalovirus infections.' *Rev. Infect. Dis.*, **5**, 977–993.

Adler, S. P. (1985). The molecular epidemiology of cytomegalovirus transmission among children attending a day care center. *J. Infect. Dis.*, **152**, 760–768.

Adler, S. P. (1986). Cytomegalovirus infection in parents of children at day-care centers (Letter). *N. Engl. J. Med.*, **315**(18), 1164–1165.

Adler, S. P. (1988a). Cytomegalovirus transmission among children in day care, their mothers and caretakers. *Pediatr. Infect. Dis. J.*, **7**, 279–285.

Adler, S. P. (1988b). Molecular epidemiology of cytomegalovirus: viral transmission among children attending a day care center, their parents, and caretakers. *J. Pediatr.*, **112**, 366–372.

Adler, S. P. (1989). Cytomegalovirus and child day care. Evidence for an increased infection rate among day-care workers. *N. Engl. J. Med.*, **321**, 1290–1296.

Adler, S. P. (1991). Cytomegalovirus and child day care: risk factors for maternal infection. *Pediatr. Infect. Dis. J.*, **10**, 590.

Adler, S. P., Wilson, M. S., and Lawrence, L. T. (1985). Cytomegalovirus transmission among children attending a day care center. *Pediatr. Res.*, **19**, 285A.

Adler, S. P., Baggett, J., Wilson, M., Lawrence, L., and McVoy, M. (1986). Molecular epidemiology of cytomegalovirus in a nursery: lack of evidence for nosocomial transmission. *J. Pediatr.*, **108**, 117–123.

Ahlfors, K., Ivarsson, S., Johnsson, T., and Renmarker, K. (1981). Risk of cytomegalovirus infection in nurses and congenital infection in their offspring. *Acta. Paediatr. Scand.*, **70**, 819–823.

Alford, C. A., Stagno, S., and Pass, R. F. (1980). Natural history of perinatal cytomegalovirus infection. In *Perinatal Infections*. pp. 125–147. Amsterdam: Excerpta Medica.

Alford, C. A., Stagno, S., Pass, R. F., and Huang, E. S. (1981). Epidemiology of cytomegalovirus. *The Human Herpesviruses: An Interdisciplinary Perspective*. A. Nahmais, W. Dowdle and R. Schinazi. eds. pp. 159–171. New York: Elsevier.

Balcarek, K. B., Bagley, R., Cloud, G. A., and Pass, R. F. (1990). Cytomegalovirus infection among employees of a childrens' hospital: no evidence for increased risk associated with patient care. *J. Am. Med. Assoc.*, **263**, 840–844.

Bale, J. F., Zimmerman, B., Dawson, J. D., Souza, I. E., Petheram, S. J., and Murph, J. R. (1999). Cytomegalovirus transmission in child care homes. *Arch. Pediatr. Adolesc. Med.*, **153** (75–79).

Balfour, C. L. and Balfour, H., H. (1986). Cytomegalovirus is not an occupational risk for nurses in renal transplant and neonatal units. *J. Am. Med. Assoc.*, **256**, 1909–1914.

Berry, N. J., Burns, D. M., Wannamethee, G. *et al.* (1988). Seroepidemiologic studies on the acquisition of antibodies to cytomegalovirus, herpes simplex virus, and human immunodeficiency virus among general hospital patients and those attending a clinic for sexually transmitted diseases. *J. Med. Virol.*, **24**, 385–393.

Biggar, R. J., Anderson, H. K., Ebbeson, P. *et al.* (1983). Seminal fluiid excretion of cytomegalovirus related to immunosuppression in homosexual men. *Br. Med. J.*, **286**, 2010–2012.

Blackman, J., Murph, J., and Bade, J. F., Jr. (1987). Risk of cytomegalovirus infection among educators and health care professionals serving disabled children. *Pediatr. Infect. Dis. J.*, **6**(8), 725–729.

Bowden, R. and Sayers, M. (1990). The risk of transmitting cytomegalovirus infection by fresh frozen plasma. *Transfusion*, **30**, 762–763.

Bowden, R. A. (1991). Cytomegalovirus infections in transplant patients: methods of prevention of primary cytomegalovirus. *Transpl. Proc.*, **23**, 136–138.

Brady, M. T., Milam, J. D., Anderson, D. C. *et al.* (1984). Use of deglycerolized red blood cells to prevent posttransfusion infection with cytomegalovirus in neonates. *J. Infect. Dis.*, **150**, 334–339.

British Andrology Society (1999). British Andrology Society guidelines for the screening of semen donors for donor insemination (1999). *Hum. Reprod.*, **14**, 1823–1826.

Britt, W. J. and Alford, C. A. (1996). Cytomegalovirus. In *Fields Virology*, Fields, B. N., Knipe, D. M., Howley, P. M. *et al.*, eds, Philadelphia: Lippincott-Raven Publishers 2493–2593.

Bryant, P., Morley, C., Garland, S., and Curtis, N. (2002). Cytomegalovirus transmission from breast milk in premature babies: does it matter? *Arch. Dis. Child Fetal Neonatal Ed.*, **87**, F75-F77.

CDC (1987). Recommendations for prevention of HIV transmission in health-care settings. *Morb. Mortal. Wkly Rep.*, **36**(2S).

CDC (1988). Perspectives in diseases prevention and health promotion update: universal precautions for prevention of transmission of human immunodeficiency virus, hepatitis B virus, and other bloodborne pathogens in health-care settings. *Morb. Mortal. Wkly Rep.*, **37**(24), 377–388.

Chandler, S. H., Alexander, E. R., and Holmes, K. K. (1985a). Epidemiology of cytomegaloviral infection in a heterogeneous population of pregnant women. *J. Infect. Dis.*, **152**, 249–256.

Chandler, S. H., Holmes, K. K., Wentworth, B. B. *et al.* (1985b). The epidemiology of cytomegaloviral infection in women attending a sexually transmitted disease clinic. *J. Infect. Dis.*, **152**, 597–605.

Chandler, S. H., Handsfield, H. H., and McDongall, J. K. (1987). Isolation of multiple strains of cytomegalovirus from women attending a clinic for sexually transmitted diseases. *J. Infect. Dis.*, **155**, 655–660.

Clarke, L. M., Duerr, A., Feldman, J., Sierra, M. F., Daidone, B. J., and Landesman, S. H. (1996). Factors associated with cytomegalovirus infection among human immunodeficiency virus type 1-seronegative and -seropositive women from an urban minority community. *J. Infect. Dis.*, **173**, 77–82.

Cole, R. and Kuttner, A. G. (1926). A filtrable virus present in the submaxillary glands of guinea pigs. *J. Exp. Med.*, **44**, 855–873.

Collier, A. C., Handsfield, H. H., Roberts, P. L. *et al.* (1990). Cytomegalovirus infection in women attending a sexually transmitted disease clinic. *J. Infect. Dis.*, **162**, 46–51.

Collier, A. C., Handsfield, H. H., Ashley, R. *et al.* (1995). Cervical but not urinary excretion of cytomegalovirus is related to sexual activity and contraceptive practices in sexually active women. *J. Infect. Dis.*, **171**, 33–38.

Coonrod, D., Collier, A. C., Ashley, R., De Rouen, T., and Corey, L. (1998). "Association between cytomegalovirus seroconversion and upper genital tract infection among women attending a sexually transmitted diseases clinic: a prospective study. *J. Infect. Dis.*, **177**, 1188–1193.

Craig, J. M., Macauley, J. C., Weller, T. H., and Wirth, P. (1957). Isolation of intranuclear inclusion producing agents from infants with illnesses resembling cytomegalic inclusion disease. *Proc. Soc. Exp. Biol. Med.*, **94**, 4–12.

de Medeiros, C. R., Moreira, V. A., and Pasquini R. (2000). Cytomegalovirus as a cause of late interstitial pneumonia after bone marrow transplantation. *Bone Marrow Transpl.*, **26**(4), 443–444.

de Mello, A., Ferreira, E. C., Vilas Boas, L. S., and Pannuti, C. S. (1996). Cytomegalovirus infection in a day-care center in the municipality of Sao Paulo. *Rev. Inst. Med. Trop. Sao Paulo*, **38**(3), 165–169.

de Ory, F., Ramirez, R., Garcia Comas L. et al. (2004). Is there a change in cytomegalovirus seroepidemiology in Spain? *Eur. J. Epidemiol.*, **19**(1), 85–89.

De Schryver, A., Glazemakers, J., De Bacquer, D., DeBacker, G., and Lust, E. (1999). Risk of cytomegalovirus infection among educators and health care personnel serving mentally disabled children. *J. Infect.*, **38**(1), 36–40.

Demmler, G. J., Yow, M. D., Spector, S. A. et al. (1987). Nosocomial cytomegalovirus infections within two hospitals caring for infants and children. *J. Infect. Dis.*, **156**, 9–16.

Diosi, P., Babusceac, L., Nevinglovschi, O., and Kun-Stoicu, G. (1967). Cytomegalovirus infection associated with pregnancy. *Lancet*, **1**, 1063–1066.

Drew, W. L., Mintz, L., Miner, R. C., Sands, M., and Ketterer, B. (1981). Prevalence of cytomegalovirus infection in homosexual men. *J. Infect. Dis.*, **143**, 188–192.

Dworsky, M., Welch, K., Cassady, G., and Stagno, S. (1983a). Occupational risk for primary cytomegalovirus infection among pediatric health care workers. *N. Engl. J. Med.*, **309**, 950–953.

Dworsky, M., Yow, M., Stagno, S., Pass, R. F., and Alford, C. (1983b). Cytomegalovirus infection of breast milk and transmission in infancy. *Pediatrics*, **72**, 295–299.

Dworsky, M., Lakeman, A., and Stagno, S. (1984). Cytomegalovirus transmission within a family. *Pediatr. Infect. Dis.*, **3**(3), 236–238.

Eisenfeld, L., Silver, H., McLaughlin, J. et al. (1992). Prevention of transfusion-associated cytomegalovirus infection in neonatal patients by removal of white cell from blood. *Transfusion*, **32**(3), 505–509.

Everett, J. P., Hershberger, R. E., Norman, D. J. et al. (1992). Prolonged cytomegalovirus infection with viremia is associated with development of cardiac allograft vasculopathy. *J. Heart. Lung. Transpl.*, **11**, 133–137.

Fairfax, M. R., Schacker, T., and Cone, R. W. (1994). Human herpesvirus 6 DNA in blood cells of human immunodeficiency virus-infected men: correlation of high levels with high CD4 cell counts. *J. Infect. Dis.*, **169**, 1342–1345.

Faix, R. G. (1985). Survival of cytomegalovirus on environmental surfaces. *J. Pediatr.*, **106**, 649–652.

Falagas, M. E., Snydman, D. R., Ruthazer, R., Griffin, J., and Werner, B. G. (1996). Primary cytomegalovirus infection in liver transplant recipients: comparison of infectios transmitted via donor organ and via transfusion. *Clin. Infect. Dis.*, **23**, 292–297.

Farr, B. and Torner, J. (1990). Cytomegalovirus infection among employees of a childrens hospital (Letter). *J. Am. Med. Assoc.*, **264**(2), 185.

Flowers, R., Torner, J., and Farr, B. M. (1988). Primary cytomegalovirus infection in pediatric nurses: a meta-analysis. *Infect. Control Hosp. Epidemiol.*, **9**(10), 491–496.

Ford-Jones, E., Kitai, I., Davis, L. et al. (1996). Cytomegalovirus infections in Toronto child-care centers: a prospective study of viral excretion in children and seroconversion among day-care providers. *Pediatr. Infect. Dis. J.*, **15**(6), 507–514.

Friedman, H. M., Lewis, M. R., Nemerofsky, D. M., and Plotkin, S. A. (1984). Acquisition of cytomegalovirus infection among female employees at a pediatric hospital. *Pediatr. Infect. Dis. J.*, **3**, 233–235.

Gallant, J. E., Moore, R. D., Richman, D. D., Keruly, J., and Chaisson, R. E. (1992). Incidence and natural history of cytomegalovirus disease in patients with advanced human immunodeficiency virus disease treated with zidovudine. *J. Infect. Dis.*, **166**, 1223–1227.

Gerberding, J. (1994). Incidence and prevalence of human immunodeficiency virus, hepatitis B virus, hepititis C virus, and cytomegalovirus among health care personnel at risk for blood exposure: final report from a longitudinal study. *J. Infect. Dis.*, **170**, 1410–1417.

Gilbert, G. L., Hayes, K., Hudson, I., and James, J. (1989). Prevention of transfusion-acquired cytomegalovirus infection in infants by blood filtration to remove leucocytes. *Lancet*, **1**, 1228–1231.

Gold, E. and Nankervis, G. A. (1976). Cytomegalovirus. In *Viral Infections of Humans: Epidemiology and Control*. A. S. Evans, ed., pp. 143–161. New York: Plenum Press.

Gold, E. and Nankervis, G. A. (1982). Cytomegalovirus. In *Viral Infections of Humans: Epidemiology and Control, 2nd edn*. A. S. Evans, ed., pp. 167–186. New York: Plenum Press.

Goodpasture, E. W. and Talbot, F. B. (1921). Concerning the nature of "proteozoan-like" cells in certain lesions of infancy. *Am. J. Dis. Child.*, **21**, 415–421.

Goodrich, J. M., Bowden, R. A., Fisher, L., Keller, C., Schoch, G., and Meyers, J. D. (1993). Ganciclovir prophylaxis to prevent cytomegalovirus disease after allogeneic marrow transplant. *Ann. Intern. Med.*, **118**, 173–178.

Granstrom, M. L. and Leinikki, P. (1978). Illnesses during the first two years of life and their association with perinatal CMV infection. *Scand. J. Infect. Dis.*, **10**, 257–264.

Grillner, L. and Strangert, K. (1986). Restriction endonulcease analysis of cytomegalovirus DNA from strains isolated in day care centers. *Pediatr. Infect. Dis.*, **5**(2), 184–187.

Haldane, E. V., Embil, J. A., and Wall, A. D. (1969). A serological study of cytomegalovirus infection in the population of Easter Island. *Bull. WHO*, **40**, 969–973.

Hamprecht, K., Vochem, M., Baumeister, A., Boniek, M., Speer, C. P., and Jahn, G. (1998). Detection of cytomegaloviral DNA in human milk cells and cell free milk whey by nested PCR. *J. Virol. Method*, **70**, 167–176.

Hamprecht, K., Maschmann, J., Vochem, M., Dietz, K., Speer, C. P., and Jahn, G. (2001). Epidemiology of transmission of cytomegalovirus from mother to preterm infants by breast-feeding. *Lancet*, **357**, 513–518.

Handsfield, H. H., Chandler, S. H., Caine, V. A. *et al.* (1985). Cytomegalovirus infection in sex partners: evidence for sexual transmission. *J. Infect. Dis.*, **151**, 344–348.

Haneberg, B., Bertnes, E., and Haukenes, G. (1980). Antibodies to cytomegalovirus among personnel at a childrens hospital. *Acta. Paediatr. Scand.*, **69**, 407–409.

Hatherley, L. (1985). Prevalence of cytomegalovirus antibodies in obstetric nurses. A study in a specialist metropolitan teaching hospital. *Med. J. Aust.*, **142**, 186–189.

Hatherley, L. (1986). Is primary cytomegalovirus infection an occupational hazard for obstetric nurses? A serological study. *Infect. Control.*, **7**(9), 452–455.

Hayes, D., Danks, M., Gibas, H., and Jack, I. (1972). Cytomegalovirus in human milk. *N. Engl. J. Med.*, **287**, 177.

Hecker, M., Qiu, D., Marquardt, K., Bein, G., and Hackstein, H. (2004). Continuous cytomegalovirus seroconversion in a large group of healthy blood donors. *Vox Sang.*, **86**(1), 41–44.

Herbert, A.-M., Bagg, J., Walker, D. M., Davies, K. J., and Westmoreland, D. (1995). Seroepidemiology of herpes virus infections among dental personnel. *J. Dentistry*, **23**(6), 339–342.

Hillyer, C. D., Syndman, D. R., and Berkman, F. M. (1990). The risk of cytomegalovirus infection in solid organ and bone marrow transplant recipients; transfusion of blood products. *Transfusion*, **30**, 659–666.

Ho, M. (1991). Observations from transplantation contributing to the understanding of pathogenesis of CMV infection. *Transpl. Proc.*, **23**, 104–109.

Hosenpud, J. D. (1999). Coronary artery disease after heart transplantation and its relation to cytomegalovirus. *Am. Heart. J.*, **138**(5), S469–S472.

Huang, E. S., Alford, C. A., Reynolds, D. W., Stagno, S., and Pass, R. F. (1980). Molecular epidemiology of cytomegalovirus infections in women and their infants. *N. Engl. J. Med.*, **303**, 958–962.

Hutto, C., Ricks, R., Garvie, M., and Pass, R. F. (1985). Epidemiology of cytomegalovirus infections in young children: day care vs. home care. *Pediatr. Infect. Dis.*, **4**(2), 149–152.

Hutto, C., Little, A., Ricks, R., Lee, J. D., and Pass, R. F. (1986). Isolation of cytomegalovirus from toys and hands in a day care center. *J. Infect. Dis.*, **154**(3), 527–530.

Hyams, K. C., Krogwald, R. A., Brock, S., Wignall, F. S., Cross, E., and Hayes, C. (1993). Heterosexual transmission of viral hepatitis and cytomegalovirus infection among United States military personnel in western Pacific. *Sex. Trans. Dis.*, **20**(1), 36–41.

Jackson, L., Stewart, L., Solomon, S. L. *et al.* (1996). Risk of infection with hepatitis A, B or C, cytomegalovirus, varicella or measles among child care providers. *Pediatr. Infect. Dis. J.*, **15**(7), 584–589.

Jacobson, M. A., Crowe, S., Levy, J. *et al.* (1988). Effect of foscarnet therapy on infection with human immunodeficiency virus in patients with AIDS. *J. Infect. Dis.*, **158**, 862–865.

Jacobson, M. A., Schrier, R., McCune, J. M. *et al.* (2001). Cytomegalovurs (CMV)-specific CD4+ T-lymphocyte function in long-term survivors of AIDS-related end organ disease who are receiving potent antiretoviral therapy. *J. Infect. Dis.*, **183**(9), 1399–1404.

Jones, L. A., Duke-Duncan, P. M., Yeager, A. S. *et al.* (1985). Cytomegaloviral infections in infant-toddler centers: centers for the developmentally delayed versus regular day care. *J. Infect. Dis.*, **151**, 953–955.

Jordan, M. C., Rousseau, W. E., Noble, G. R., Steward, J. A., and Chin, T. D. (1973). Association of cervical cytomegaloviruses with venereal disease. *N. Engl. J. Med.*, **288**, 932–934.

Kaariainen, L., Klemola, E., and Paloheimo, J. (1966). Rise of cytomegalovirus antibodies in an infectious mononucleosis-like syndrome after transfusion. *Br. Med. J.*, **1**, 1270–1272.

Kashiwagi, Y., Nemoto, S., Kawashima, H. *et al.* (2001). Cytomegalovirus DNA among children attending two day-care centers in Tokyo. *Pediatr. Int.*, **43**, 493–495.

Kiss, P., De Bacquer, D., Sergooris, L., De Meester, M., and Van Hoorne, M. (2002). Cytomegalovirus infection: an occupational hazard to kindergarten teachers working with children aged 2.5–6 years. *Int. J. Occup. Environ. Health*, **8**, 79–86.

Knox, G. E., Pass, R. F., Reynolds, D. W., Stagno, S., and Alferd, C. A. (1979). Comparative prevalence of subclinical cytomegalovirus and herpes simplex virus infections in the genital and urinary tracts of low income, urban females. *J. Infect. Dis.*, **140**, 419–422.

Kothari, A., Ramachandran, V. G., Gupta, B., and Talwar, V. (2002). Seroprevalence of cytomegalovirus among voluntary blood donors in Delhi, India. *J. Health Popul. Nutr.*, **20**(4), 348–351.

Krech, U., Konjajev, Z., and Jung, M. (1971). Congenital cytomegalovirus infection in siblings from consecutive pregnancies. *Helv. Paediatr. Acta.*, **26**, 355–362.

Lang, D. J. (1975). The epidemiology of cytomegalovirus infections: interpretation of recent observations. In *Infections of the Fetus and Newborn Infant.* S. Krugman and A. A. Gershon, eds., vol. 3, pp. 35–45. New York: Alan R. Liss.

Lang, D. J. and Kummer, J. F. (1975). Cytomegalovirus in semen: observations in selected populations. *J. Infect. Dis.*, **132**, 472–473.

Lang, D. J., Ebert, P. A., Rodgers, B. M., Boggess, H. P., and Rixse, R. S. (1977). Reductions of post-perfusion cytomegalovirus infections following the use of leucocyte depleted blood. *Transfusion*, **17**, 391–395.

Lipschutz, B. (1921). Untersuchungen uber die atiologie der krankheiten der herpesgruppe (herpes zoster, herpes genitalis, herpes febrilis). *Arch. Derm. Syph. (Berl.)*, **136**, 428–482.

Liu, Z., Wang, E., Taylor, W. *et al.* (1990). Prevalence survey of cytomegalovirus infection in children in Chengdu. *Am. J. Epidemiol.*, **131**(1), 143–150.

Ljungman, P. (2001). Prophylaxis against herpesvirus infections in transplant recipients. *Drugs*, **61**, 187–196.

Lowenstein, C. (1907). Uber protozoenartigen gebilden in den organen von dindern. *Žentralbl. Allg. Pathol.*, **18**, 513–518.

Lu, S. C., Chin, L. T., Wu, F. M. *et al.* (1999). Seroprevalence of CMV antibodies in a blood donor population and premature neonates in the south-central Taiwan. *Kaohsiung J. Med. Sci.*, **15**(10), 603–610.

Machado, C. M., Dulley, F. L., Boas, L. S. et al. (2000). CMV pneumonia in adult allogeneic blood and bone marrow transplant recipients. *Bone Marrow Transpl.*, **26**, 413–417.

Mansat, A., Mengelle, C., Chalet, M. et al. (1997). Cytomegalovirus detection in cryopreserved semen samples collected for therapeutic donor insemination. *Hum. Reprod.*, **12**(8), 1663–1666.

Maschmann, J., Hamprecht, K., Dietz, K. H., Jahn, G., and Speer, C. P. (2001). Cytomegalovirus infection of extremely low-birth weight infants via breast milk. *Clin. Infect. Dis.*, **33**, 1998–2003.

Mascola, L. and Guinan, M. E. (1986). Screening to reduce transmission of sexually transmitted diseases in semen used for artificial insemination. *N. Engl. J. Med.*, **314**, 354–359.

Meyers, J. D. (1991). Prevention and treatment of cytomegalovirus infection. *Ann. Rev. Med.*, **42**, 179–187.

Meyers, J. D., McGuffin, R. W., Bryson, Y. J., Cantell, K., and Thomas, E. D. (1982). Treatment of cytomegalovirus pneumonia after marrow transplant with combined vidarabine and human leukocyte interferon. *J. Infect. Dis.*, **146**, 80–84.

Miller, W. J., McCullough, J., Balfour, H. H. Jr. et al. (1991). Prevention of cytomegalovirus infection following bone marrow transplantation: a randomized trial of blood product screening. *Bone Marrow Transpl.*, **7**(3), 227–234.

Munoz, A., Schrager, L. K., Bacellar, H. et al. (1993). Trends in the incidence of outcomes defining acquired immunodeficiency syndrome (AIDS) in the Multicenter AIDS Cohort Study: 1985–1991. *Am. J. Epidemiol.*, **137**(4), 423–438.

Murph, J. R., Bale, J. F., Jr., Murray, J. C., Stinski, M. F., and Perlman, S. (1986). Cytomegalovirus transmission in a Midwest day care center: possible relationship to child care practices. *J. Pediatr.*, **109**, 35–39.

Murph, J. R., Baron, J. C., Brown, C. K., Ebelhack, C. L., and Bale, J. F., Jr. (1991). The occupational risk of cytomegalovirus infection among day care providers. *J. Am. Med. Assoc.*, **265**, 603–608.

Natali, A., Valcavi, P., Medici, M. C., Dieci, E., Montali, S., and Chezzi, C. (1997). Cytomegalovirus infection in an Italian population: antibody prevalence, virus excretion and maternal transmission. *New Microbiol.*, **20**(2), 123–133.

Nelson, D., Peckham, C., Pearl, K. N., Chin, K. S., Garrett, A. J., and Warren, D. E. (1987). Cytomegalovirus infection in day nurseries. *Arch. Dis. Child.*, **62**, 329–332.

Nguyen, Q., Champlin, R., Giralt, S. et al. (1999). Late cytomegalovirus pneumonia in adult allogeneic blood and marrow transplant recipients. *Clin. Infect. Dis.*, **28**(3), 618–623.

Numazaki, Y., Yano, N., Morizuka, T., Takai, S., and Ishida, N. et al. (1970). Primary infection with human cytomegalovirus: virus isolation from healthy infants and pregnant women. *Am. J. Epidemiol.*, **91**, 410–417.

Paryani, S. G., Yeager, A. S., Hosford-Dunn, H. et al. (1985). Sequelae of acquired cytomegalovirus infection in premature and sick term infants. *J. Pediatr.*, **107** 451–456.

Pass, R. F., Hutto, C., Reynolds, D. W., and Polhill, R. B. (1984). Increased frequency of cytomegalovirus in children in group day care. *Pediatrics*, **74**, 121–126.

Pass, R. F., Hutto, C., Ricks, R., and Cloud, G. A. (1986). Increased rate of cytomegalovirus infection among parents of children attending day care centers. *N. Engl. J. Med.*, **314**, 1414–1418.

Pass, R. F., Little, E. A., Stagno, S., Britt, W. J., and Alferd, C. A. (1987). Young children as a probable source of maternal and congenital cytomegalovirus infection. *N. Engl. J. Med.*, **316**, 1366–1370.

Pass, R. F., Hutto, C., Lyon, M. D., and Cloud, G. (1990). Increased rate of cytomegalovirus infection among day care center workers. *Pediatr. Infect. Dis. J.*, **9**, 465–470.

Peckham, C., Garrett, A., Chin, K. S., Preece, P. M., Nelson, D. B., and Warren, D. E. (1986). Restriction enzyme analysis of cytomegalovirus DNA to study transmission of infection. *J. Clin. Pathol.*, **39**(3), 318–324.

Pereira, L. H., Embil, J. A., Hasse, D. A., and Marley, K. M. (1990). Cytomegalovirus infection among women attending a sexually transmitted disease clinic: association with clinical symptoms and other sexually transmitted diseases. *Am. J. Epidemiol.*, **131**, 683–692.

Prabhakar, P., Bailey, A., Smikle, M. F., and Ashley, D. (1992). Seroprevalence of cytomegalovirus infection in a selected population in Jamaica. *West Indian Med. J.*, **41**(4), 133–135.

Preiksaitis, J. K., Brown, L., and McKenzie, M. (1988). Transfusion-acquired cytomegalovirus infection in neonates. *Transfusion*, **28**, 205–209.

Prior, J. R., Morrol, D. R., Birks, A. G., Matson, P. L., and Lieberman, B. A. (1994). The screening for cytomegalovirus antibody in semen donors and recipients within a donor insemination program. *Hum. Reprod.*, **9**, 2076–2078.

Pultoo, A., Meetoo, G., Pyndiah, M. N., and Khittoo, G. (2001). Seroprevalence of cytomegalovirus infection in Mauritian volunteer blood donors. *Indian J. Med. Sci.*, **55**(2), 73–78.

Reusser, P., Riddell, S. R., Meyers, J. D., and Greenberg, P. D. (1991). Cytotoxic T-lymphocyte response to cytomegalovirus after human allogeneic bone marrow transplantation: pattern of recovery and correlation with cytomegalovirus infection and disease. *Blood*, **78**, 1373–1380.

Reynolds, D. W., Stagno, S., Hosty, T. S., Tiller, M., and Alford, C. A., Jr. (1973). Maternal cytomegalovirus excretion and perinatal infection. *N. Engl. J. Med.*, **289**, 1–5.

Ribbert, D. (1904). Uber protozoenartige zellen in der niere eines syphilitischen neugoborenen und in der parotis von kindern. *Zentralbl. Allg. Pathol.*, **15**, 945–948.

Rowe, W. P., Hartley, J. W., Waterman, S., Turner, H. C., and Huebner, R. J. (1956). Cytopathogenic agents resembling human salivary gland virus recovered from tissue cultures of human adenoids. *Proc. Soc. Exp. Biol. (NY)*, **92**, 418–424.

Rubin, R. H. and Colvin, R. B. (1986). Cytomegalovirus infection in renal transplantation: clinical importance and control. *Kidney Transplant Rejection: Diagnosis and Treatment*. ed. G. M. Williams, J. F. Burdick, and K. Solez, eds., pp. 283–304. New York: Dekker: 283–304.

Rubin, R. H., Tolkoff-Rubin, N. E., Oliver, D. et al. (1985). Multicenter seroepidemiologic study of the impact of cytomegalovirus infection on renal transplantation. *Transplantation*, **40**, 243–249.

Schmidt, G. M., Horak, D. A., Niland, J. C., Duncan, S. R., Forman, S. J., and Zaia J. A. (1991). A randomized, controlled trial of prophylactic ganciclovir for cytomegalovirus pulmonary infection in recipients of allogeneic bone marrow transplants. *N. Engl. J. Med.*, **324**, 1005–1011.

Schopfer, K., Lauber, E., and Krech, U. (1978). Congenital cytomegalovirus infection in newborn infants of mothers infected before pregnancy. *Arch. Dis. Child.*, **53**, 536–539.

Schupfer, P., Murph, J. R., and Bale, J. F., Jr. (1986). Survival of cytomegalovirus in paper diapers and saliva. *Pediatr. Infect. Dis.*, **5**(6), 677–679.

Shen, C. Y., Chang, W. W., Chao, M. F., Huang, E. S., and Wu, C. W. (1992). Seroepidemiology of cytomegalovirus infection among children between the ages of 4 and 12 years in Taiwan. *J. Med. Virol.*, **37**(1), 72–75.

Shen, C. Y., Chang, S. F., Lin, H. J. et al. (1994). Cervical cytomegalovirus infection in prostitutes and in women attending a sexually transmitted diseases clinic. *J. Med. Virol.*, **43**, 362–366.

Singh, N., Wannstedt, C., Keyes, L. et al. (2004). Impact of evolving trends in recipient and donor characteristics on cytomegalovirus infection in liver transplant recipients. *Transplantation*, **77**(1), 106–110.

Smith, M. G. (1956). Propagation in tissue cultures of a cytopathogenic virus from human salivary gland virus disease. *Proc. Soc. Exp. Biol. (NY)*, **92**, 424–430.

Smyth, R. L., Scott, J. P., Borysiewicz, L. K. et al. (1991). Cytomegalovirus infection in heart-lung transplant recipients: risk factors, clinical associations, and response to treatment. *J. Infect. Dis.*, **164**, 1045–1050.

Sobaszek, A., Fantoni-Quinton, S., Frimat, P., Leroyer, A., Iaynat, A., and Edme, J. L. (2000). Prevalence of cytomegalovirus infection among health care workers in pediatric and immunosuppressed adult units. *J. Occup. Environ. Med.*, **42**(11), 1109–1114.

Sohn, Y. M., Oh, M. K., Balcarek, K. B., Cloud, G. A., and Pass, R. F. (1991). Cytomegalovirus infection in sexually active adolescents. *J. Infect. Dis.*, **163**, 460–463.

Spector, S. A. and Spector, D. H. (1982). Molecular epidemiology of cytomegalovirus infections in premature twin infants and their mother. *Pediatr. Infect. Dis. J.*, **1**, 405–409.

Spector, S. A., Hsia, K., Crager, M., Pilcher, M., Cabral, S., and Stempien, M. J. (1999). Cytomegalovirus (CMV) DNA load is an independent predictor of CMV disease and survival in advanced AIDS. *J. Virol.*, **73**(8), 7027–7030.

Stagno, S. (2001). Cytomegalovirus. In *Infectious Diseases of the Fetus and Newborn Infant*, 5th edn. J. S. Remington and J. O. Klein, eds., pp. 389–424. Philadelphia: W.B. Saunders.

Stagno, S. and Cloud, G. A. (1990). Changes in the epidemiology of cytomegalovirus. In *Immunology and Prophylaxis of Human Herpesvirus Infections*. C. Lopez, ed., pp. 93–104, New York: Plenum Press.

Stagno, S. and Cloud G. (1994). Working parents: the impact of day care and breast-feeding on cytomegalovirus infections in offspring. *Proc. Natl. Acad. Sci. USA*, **91** 2384–2389.

Stagno, S., Reynolds, D. W., Tsiantos, A. et al. (1975). Comparative, serial virologic and serologic studies of symptomatic and subclinical congenital and natally acquired cytomegalovirus infection. *J. Infect. Dis.*, **132**, 568–577.

Stagno, S., Reynolds, D. W., Pass, R. F., and Alford, C. A. (1980). Breast milk and the risk of cytomegalovirus infection. *N. Engl. J. Med.*, **302**, 1073–1076.

Stagno, S., Pass, R. F., Dworsky, M. E., and Alford, C. A., Jr. (1982). Maternal cytomegalovirus infection and perinatal transmission. *Clin. Obstet. Gynecol.*, **25**, 563–576.

Stagno, S., Pass, R. F., Cloud, G. et al. (1986). Primary cytomegalovirus infection in pregnancy. Incidence, transmission to fetus, and clinical outcome. *J.Am. Med. Assoc.*, **256**, 1904–1908.

Strangert, K., Carlstrom, G., Jeansson, S., and Nord, C. E. (1976). Infections in preschool children in group day care. *Acta. Paediatr. Scand.*, **65**, 455–463.

Streblow, D. N., Soderberg-Naucler, C., Vieira, J. et al. (2000). The human cytomegalovirus chemokine receptor US28 mediates vascular smooth muscle cell migration. *Cell* in press.

Strom, J. (1979). A study of infections and illnesses in a day nursery based on inclusion-bearing cells in the urine and infectious agent in faeces, urine and nasal secretion. *Scand. J. Infect. Dis.*, **11**(4), 265–269.

Suassuna, J. H., Leite, L. L., and Villela, L. H. (1995). Prevalence of cytomegalovirus infection in different patient groups of an urban university in Brazil. *Rev. Soc. Bras. Med. Trop.*, **28**(2), 105–108.

Taber, L. H., Frank, A., Yow, M. D., and Bagley, A. (1985). Acquisition of cytomegaloviral infections in families with young children: a serological study. *J. Infect. Dis.*, **151**(5), 948–952.

Tjiam, K. H., van Heijst, B. Y., Polak-Vogelzang, A. A. et al. (1987). Sexually communicable micro-organisms in human semen samples to be used for artificial insemination by donor. *Genitourin. Med.*, **63**, 116–118.

Tolkoff-Rubin, N., Rubin, R., Keller, E. E., Baker, G. P., Stewart, J. A., and Hirsch, M. S. (1978). Cytomegalovirus infection in dialysis patients and personnel. *Ann. Intern. Med.*, **89**, 625–628.

Urwijitaroon, Y., Teawpatanataworn, S., and Kitjareontarm, A. (1993). Prevalence of cytomegalovirus antibody in Thai-northeastern blood donors. *Southeast Asian J. Trop. Med. Public Health*, **24**(S1), 180–182.

van der Strate, B. W., Harmsen, M. C., Schafer, P. et al. (2001). Viral load in breast milk correlates with transmission of human cytomegalovirus to preterm neonates, but lactoferrin concentrations do not. *Clin. Diag. Lab. Immunol.*, **8**, 818–821.

Vial, P., Torres-Pereyra, J., Stagno, S. et al. (1985). Serological screening for cytomegalovirus, rubella virus, herpes simplex virus, hepatitis B virus and *Toxoplasma gondii* in two populations of pregnant women in Chile. *Bol. Sanit. Panam.*, **99**, 528–538.

Vollmer, B., Seibod-Weiger, K., Schmitz-Salue, C. et al. (2004). Postnatally acquired cytomegalovirus infection via breast milk: effects on hearing and development in preterm infants. *Pediatr. Infect. Dis. J.*, **23**(4), 322–327.

Volpi, A., Pica, F., Caoletti, M., Pana, A., and Rocchi, G. (1988). Cytomegalovirus infection in day care centers in Rome, Italy: viral excretion in children and occupational risk among workers. *J. Med. Virol.*, **26**, 119–125.

Weller, T. H. (1971). The cytomegaloviruses: ubiquitous agents with protean clinical manifestations. *N. Engl. J. Med.*, **285**, 203–214.

Wentworth, B. B. and Alexander, E. R. (1971). Seroepidemiology of infections due to members of herpesvirus group. *Am. J. Epidemiol.*, **94**, 496–507.

Wilhelm, J. A., Matter, L., and Schopfer, K. (1986). The risk of transmitting cytomegalovirus to patients receiving blood trasnsfusion. *J. Infect. Dis.*, **154**, 169–171.

Willmott, F. E. (1975). Cytomegalovirus in female patients attending a VD clinic. *Br. J. Vener. Dis.*, **51**, 278–280.

Wingard, J. R., Mellits, E. D., Sostrin, M. B. *et al.* (1988). Interstitial pneumonitis after allogeneic bone marrow transplantation. *Medicine*, **67**, 175–186.

Winston, D. J., Ho, W. G., Bartoni, K. *et al.* (1988). Ganciclovir therapy for cytomegalovirus infections in recipients of bone marrow transplants and other immunosuppressed patients. *Rev. Infect. Dis.*, **10**, S547-S553.

Winston, D. J., Ho, W. G., and Champlin, R. E. (1990). Cytomegalovirus infections after bone marrow transplantation. *Rev. Infect. Dis.*, **12**, S776-S792.

Wreghitt, T. G., Hakim, M., Gray, J. J., Kucia, S., Wallwork, J., and English, T. A. (1988). Cytomegalovirus infections in heart and heart and lung transplant recipients. *J. Clin. Pathol.*, **41**, 660–667.

Yeager, A. S. (1975). Longitudinal, serological study of cytomegalovirus infections in nurses and in personnel without patient contact. *J. Clin. Microbiol.*, **2**, 448–450.

Yeager, A. S. (1983). Transmission of cytomegalovirus to mothers by infected infants: another reason to prevent transfusion-acquired infections. *Pediatr. Infect. Dis.*, **2**, 295.

Yeager, A. S., Grumet, F. C., Hafleigh, E. B., Arvin, A. M., Bradley, J. S., and Prober, C. (1981). Prevention of transfusion-acquired cytomegalovirus infections in newborn infants. *J. Pediatr.*, **98**, 281–287.

Yow, M. D., White, N., Taber, L. H. *et al.*, (1987). Acquisition of cytomegalovirus infection from birth to 10 years: a longitudinal serologic study. *J. Pediatr.*, **110**, 37–42.

Zhou, X. J., Gruber, W., Demmler, G. *et al.* (1996). Population pharmacokinetics of ganciclovir in newborns with congenital cytomegalovirus infections. *Antimicrob. Agent Chemother.*, **40**, 2202–2205.

Zhu, J., Quyyumi, A. A., Csako, G., and Epstein, S. E. (1999). Cytomegalovirus in the pathogenesis of atherosclerosis: the role of inflammation as reflected by elevated C-reactive protein levels. *J. Am. Coll. Cardiol.* **34**(6), 1738–1743.

45

HCMV persistence in the population: potential transplacental transmission

Lenore Pereira, Ekaterina Maidji, Susan J. Fisher, Susan McDonagh, and Takako Tabata

Departments of Cell and Tissue Biology, Anatomy, Pharmaceutical Chemistry, and the Biomedical Sciences Graduate Program, and the Oral Biology Graduate Program, University of California San Francisco, CA, USA

Congenital cytomegalovirus infection and the placenta

Congenital CMV infection

Human cytomegalovirus (CMV) is a ubiquitous virus that causes asymptomatic infections in healthy individuals (for review see Pass, 2001). Because breast feeding (Stagno et al., 1980), exposure to young children (Pass et al., 1987) and sexual contact (Fowler and Pass, 1991) are major risk factors for infection, most adults are seropositive. Diverse organs and specialized cells, including polarized epithelial cells (Tugizov et al., 1996) and endothelial cells (Fish et al., 1998; Maidji et al., 2002), are susceptible to CMV infection. CMV establishes latent infection in granulocyte-macrophage progenitors (Kondo et al., 1996) and reactivates upon cellular differentiation (Hahn et al., 1998; Soderberg-Naucler et al., 1997). Congenital CMV infection is estimated to affect 1 to 3% of infants in the United States annually and remains an important public health problem causing significant morbidity and mortality (for review see Britt, 1999).

It has long been appreciated that maternal neutralizing antibodies reduce the risk of symptomatic congenital disease in the fetus (Ahlfors et al., 1984; Boppana and Britt, 1995; Fowler et al., 2003; Stagno et al., 1982). The importance of adaptive immunity to CMV is apparent in women with primary infection, often with low-avidity neutralizing antibodies (Boppana and Britt, 1995; Lazzarotto et al., 1998; Revello et al., 2002). Approximately 15% of these women spontaneously abort in early gestation (Griffiths and Baboonian, 1984). Examination of placentas infected with CMV in vitro and in utero has suggested potential routes of virus transmission from the uterus to the placenta (Fisher et al., 2000; Pereira et al., 2003). Importantly, these studies suggest that placental involvement precedes virus transmission and infection of the embryo/fetus. Progression of infection hinges on maternal immunity to CMV, the mechanics of cytotrophoblast development and the presence of other pathogens at the maternal–fetal interface. In this chapter, we describe patterns of CMV infection in early gestation, routes of viral transmission at the maternal-fetal interface and dysregulation of cytotrophoblast differentiation and function secondary to CMV infection in vitro.

CMV infects specialized cells in the placenta

Numerous reports indicate that placentas from pregnancies complicated by congenital CMV infection contain viral DNA and proteins (Benirschke and Kaufmann, 2000; Muhlemann et al., 1992; Nakamura et al., 1994; Sinzger et al., 1993). Later in pregnancy, CMV infection is associated with premature delivery and, in 25% of affected infants, intrauterine growth retardation (Istas et al., 1995), outcomes that are often associated with placental pathologies. CMV replicates in cytotrophoblasts isolated from early and late gestation placentas in vitro (Fisher et al., 2000; Halwachs-Baumann et al., 1998; Hemmings et al., 1998). The routes of virus transmission and the types of immune responses elicited are likely linked to the unusual nature of cytotrophoblast interactions with maternal cells at the uterine-placental interface. A diagram of the maternal-fetal interface midway through gestation with potential sites of CMV infection is shown in Fig. 45.1.

Placental development in early gestation

Diverse cell types in the uterus

Immunologically competent cells are detected in the uterine endometrium and decidua (Kamat and Isaacson,

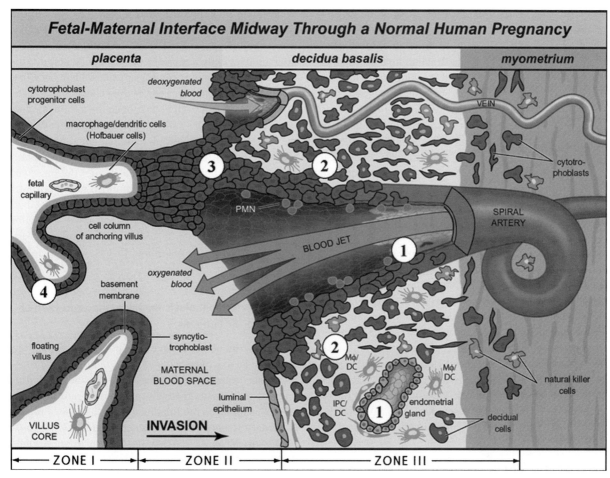

Fig. 45.1. Diagram of the histologic organization of the human maternal-fetal interface at midgestation. In this location, cytotrophoblasts, which are specialized (fetal) epithelial cells of the placenta, differentiate and invade the uterine wall, where they also breach maternal blood vessels. The basic structural unit of the placenta is the chorionic villus, composed of a stromal core with blood vessels, surrounded by a basement membrane and overlain by cytotrophoblast progenitor cells. As part of their differentiation program, these cells detach from the basement membrane and adopt one of two lineage fates. They either fuse to form the syncytiotrophoblasts that cover floating villi or join a column of extravillous cytotrophoblasts at the tips of anchoring villi. The syncytial covering of floating villi mediates nutrient, gas, and waste exchange and transfer of IgG from maternal blood to the fetus (Zone 1). The anchoring villi, through the attachment of cytotrophoblast columns, establish physical connections between the fetus and the mother (Zone II). Invasive cytotrophoblasts penetrate the uterine wall up to the first third of the myometrium (Zone III). A portion of the extravillous cytotrophoblasts home to uterine spiral arterioles and remodel these vessels by destroying their muscular walls and replacing their endothelial linings. To a lesser extent they also remodel uterine veins. At term, few cytotrophoblast progenitor cells remain, the syncytiotrophoblast layer thins, and the volume of the stromal cores expand. Sites proposed as routes of CMV infection in utero are numbered 1 to 4. Diagram modified from (Hoang et al., 2001).

1987). Early studies of leukocyte antigens by using immunohistologic approaches suggested that cells in the endometrium of cycling women in the mid-secretory phase (7–10 days after ovulation) resemble leukocytes in early gestation decidua (King et al., 1989). Granulated lymphocytes with an unusual antigenic phenotype (CD56+ high, CD16−), known as natural killer (NK) cells, constitute a substantial proportion of these cells (Bulmer et al., 1991; Starkey et al., 1988), increasing from the proliferative endometrium to the late secretory endometrium. Macrophages increase prior to menstruation (Kamat and Isaacson, 1987). CD83+ dendritic cells in the uterine stratum basale are present in the non-pregnant and pregnant uterus (Kammerer et al., 2000; Soilleux et al., 2002).

In response to implantation, the uterine lining develops into the decidua, which is maintained by progesterone

(Norwitz et al., 2001). Interglandular tissues increase in quantity, and the cytoplasm of resident stromal cells is distended with glycogen, lipid and vimentin-type intermediate filaments (Fig. 45.1, Zone III). Temporal and spatial expression of growth factors and cytokines (e.g., insulin-like growth factor 1 and its binding protein) suggests that these molecules may influence decidualization (Crossey et al., 2002). Decidual granular leukocytes intermingle with resident maternal cells and invasive fetal cells (Zone III) (Drake et al., 2001; Kamat and Isaacson, 1987; Red-Horse et al., 2001; Starkey et al., 1988). These immune cells are involved in innate pattern recognition, mostly NK cells with some macrophages, dendritic cells and T-lymphocytes. Novel patterns of cytokine/chemokine expression in the decidua, as well as specialized adhesion molecules on uterine vessels (Kruse et al., 1999), probably attract this unusual leukocyte population, which functions in immunity and cytotrophoblast differentiation. Dendritic cell protein ICAM-3-grabbing non-integrin (DC-SIGN+) cells, occasionally found in the endometrium, are abundant in the decidua and associate with NK cells (Kammerer et al., 2003, 1999; Pereira et al., 2003; Soilleux et al., 2002). The unusual immune cell population in the decidua suggests that when macrophage/dendritic cell progenitors (Mφ/DC) latently infected with CMV are attracted to the endometrium and early gestation decidua, CMV could be reactivated in the presence of inflammatory stimuli.

Development of the hemochorial human placenta

The embryo's acquisition of a supply of maternal blood is a critical hurdle in pregnancy maintenance. The mechanics of this process are accomplished by the placenta's specialized epithelial cells, termed cytotrophoblasts. The histology of the maternal-fetal interface is diagrammed in Fig. 45.1. The placenta is composed of individual units termed chorionic villi, each with a connective core that contains fetal blood vessels and numerous macrophages (Hofbauer cells) that often lie under a thick basement membrane (Fig. 45.1, Zone I). Placentation is a stepwise process whereby cytotrophoblast progenitor cells, attached to the basement membrane as a polarized epithelium, leave the membrane to differentiate along one of two independent pathways depending on their location. In floating villi, they fuse to form a multinucleate syncytial covering attached at one end to the tree-like fetal portion of the placenta (Zone I). The rest of the villus floats in a stream of maternal blood, which optimizes exchange of substances between the mother and fetus across the placenta. In the pathway that gives rise to anchoring villi, which attach the placenta to the uterine wall (Zone II), cytotrophoblasts aggregate into cell columns of non-polarized mononuclear cells that attach to and then penetrate the uterine wall. The ends of the columns terminate within the superficial endometrium, where they give rise to invasive cytotrophoblasts. During interstitial invasion a subset of these cells, either individually or in small clusters, comingles with resident decidual, myometrial and immune cells. During endovascular invasion, masses of cytotrophoblasts open the termini of uterine arteries and veins they encounter, then migrate into the vessels, thereby diverting maternal blood flow to the placenta (Zone III). In arterioles, cytotrophoblasts replace the endothelial lining and partially disrupt the muscular wall, whereas in veins, they are confined to the portions of the vessels near the inner surface of the uterus. Together, the two components of cytotrophoblast invasion anchor the placenta to the uterus and permit a steady increase in the supply of maternal blood that is delivered to the developing fetus.

Invasive cytotrophoblasts modulate the expression of stage-specific antigens

During uterine remodeling, cytotrophoblasts switch from an epithelial to a mesenchymal type (Table 45.1). Cytotrophoblasts express novel adhesion molecules and proteinases that enable the cells' attachment and invasion, as well as immune modulating factors that play a role in maternal tolerance of the hemiallogeneic fetus (Cross et al., 1994; Norwitz et al., 2001). Interstitial invasion requires downregulation of integrins characteristic of epithelial cells ($\alpha 6\beta 4$) and novel expression of $\alpha 1\beta 1$, $\alpha 5\beta 1$ and $\alpha V\beta 3$ (Damsky et al., 1994). Endovascular cytotrophoblasts that remodel maternal blood vessels transform their adhesion receptor phenotype to resemble the endothelial cells they replace (Fig. 45.1, site 1) turning on the expression of VE-(endothelial) cadherin, platelet-endothelial adhesion molecule-1 and vascular endothelial adhesion molecule-1 (Damsky and Fisher, 1998; Zhou et al., 1997).

Degradation of the basement membrane and extracellular matrix of the uterine stroma is precisely regulated during placentation (Fisher et al., 1985). Cytotrophoblasts upregulate urokinase-type plasminogen activator (uPA) (Queenan et al., 1987; Solberg et al., 2003), matrix metalloproteinase-9 (MMP-9) (Librach et al., 1991) and inhibitors such as tissue inhibitor of metalloproteinases-3, a likely regulator of proteolytic activity and invasion depth (Bass et al., 1997) (Table 45.1). Molecules that may function in maternal immune tolerance are also produced, such as the non-classical major histocompatibility complex (MHC) class Ib molecule HLA-G (Kovats et al., 1990; McMaster et al., 1995) and interleukin-10 (IL-10) (Roth et al., 1996; Roth and Fisher, 1999). This remarkable transformation, evidenced by novel expression of differentiation molecules and invasiveness, underscores the extraordinary plasticity of cytotrophoblasts.

CMV infects the placenta in vitro and in utero

Potential routes for CMV transmission

The cellular organization of the placenta suggests potential routes by which CMV infection spreads from the uterus, first to the placenta and then to the embryo/fetus (Fig. 45.1) (Fisher et al., 2000; Pereira et al., 2003). One likely site of transmission is within the uterine wall (sites 1 and 2). Interstitial invasive cytotrophoblasts could encounter infected endometrial glands, uterine blood vessels and decidual granular leukocytes. Endovascular cytotrophoblasts could encounter infected endothelial and vascular smooth muscle cells, as well as maternal immune cells. Once cytotrophoblasts within the uterine wall become infected (site 2), CMV might spread in a retrograde manner through the cell columns to the anchoring chorionic villi (site 3). In the villus stromal cores, virus could be transmitted from infected cytotrophoblasts to fibroblasts, fetal macrophages and possibly endothelial cells that line chorionic vessels. This conjecture is based on focal patterns of CMV protein expression in the placenta (Fisher et al., 2000; Muhlemann et al., 1992). Infected Mφ/DC and sloughed endothelial cells seem likely candidates for entering the venous circulation of the placenta and subsequently carrying the infection via the placental circulation to the fetus. Another likely site of transmission is across the syncytiotrophoblast layer that covers floating chorionic villi (site 4). These placental cells, in direct contact with maternal blood, express the neonatal Fc receptor (FcRn), a molecule that facilitates maternal IgG transfer and passive immunization of the fetus (Simister et al., 1996). The syncytium may allow passage of CMV virions complexed with maternal IgG to the underlying layer of cytotrophoblast progenitor cells that could become infected in the presence of virus-binding antibodies with low avidity (Boppana and Britt, 1995; Fisher et al., 2000; Lazzarotto et al., 1997; Pereira et al., 2003; Revello et al., 2002). Accordingly, adaptive and innate immune responses that reduce infectious virions at the uterine–placental interface likely play a central role in preventing transmission.

CMV protein expression in placental cells in chorionic villi infected in vitro and in utero

Clues about potential routes of prenatal CMV infection emerged from a model tissue culture system (Fig. 45.2(a)). Chorionic villi are plated on filters coated with Matrigel, an extracellular matrix, infected with virus and then cultured

Table 45.1. Selected differentiation molecules expressed by placental trophoblasts[a]

	Floating villus		Column CTB		Invasive CTB	
	CTB	STB zone I	Proximal Zone II	Distal	Interstitial Zone III	Endovascular
Receptors (integrins)						
α1[b]	−	−	−	−	+	+
α4[b]	+	−	+	+	+	+
αV[c]	+	−	+	+	+	+
β1[b,d]	−	−	+	+	+	+
β3[c]	−	−	−	+	+	+
β4[b]	+	−	+	+/−	−	−
β5[c]	+	−	+	−	−	−
β6[c,e]	+	−	+	−	−	−
Proteinase and inhibitors						
MMP-9[f]	−	−	+	+	+	+
TIMP-3[f]	−	−	+	+	+	+
uPA[f]	−	−	+	+	+	+
Immune molecules						
HLA-G[g]	−	−	−	+	+	+
IL-10[h]	+	+	+	+	+	−
FcRn[i]	−	+	−	−	−	−

[a]Adapted from (Damsky and Fisher, 1998) and (Zhou et al., 1997) with permission. Abbreviations: CTB, cytotrophoblasts; STB, syncytiotrophoblasts; MMP, metalloproteinase; TIMP, tissue inhibitor of metalloproteinases; uPA, urokinase-type plasminogen activator; IL, interleukin; FcRn, neonatal Fc receptor; −, not expressed; +, expressed.
[b]Published results:(Damsky et al., 1992; Zhou et al., 1993).
[c](Zhou et al., 1997, Maidji et al., 2006).
[d]Detected in second-trimester villus.
[e]Detected at site of column formation in second trimester.
[f]Published results: (Librach et al., 1991).
[g](McMaster et al., 1995).
[h](Roth and Fisher, 1999).
[i](Simister et al., 1996).

from 2 to 4 days. Experiments that used this model revealed an unexpected pattern of CMV infection (Fisher et al., 2000). Briefly, tissue sections of villus explants that were infected for several days were double-stained with anti-cytokeratin to identify trophoblast cells and with a monoclonal antibody to CMV immediate-early (IE) proteins to identify infected cells. Notably, syncytiotrophoblasts that cover the villus surface were not infected and failed to stain for CMV IE proteins, whereas nuclear staining of small, isolated clusters of underlying cytotrophoblast progenitor cells was observed (Fig. 45.1, site 4). In some tissues, CMV IE protein expression was also detected in cytotrophoblasts

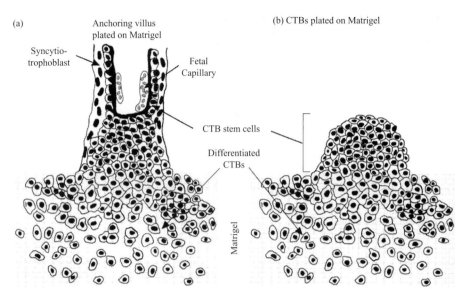

Fig. 45.2. Culture models for studying CMV infection of placental explants and cells. (a) Diagram of an anchoring villus explant attached to a Matrigel substrate via cytotrophoblasts (CTBs) that migrate from the cell columns. (b) Diagram of purified differentiating cytotrophoblasts cultured on Matrigel. The cytotrophoblast progenitor cells aggregate, invade the matrix, and express stage-specific molecules (see Table 45.1). For infection, CMV is added to the medium bathing the explants and purified cytotrophoblasts.

in the cell columns of anchoring villi (Fig. 45.1, site 3). The staining patterns observed when placentas were infected in utero had remarkable similarities to and differences from those observed after infection in vitro. Sometimes, patterns of CMV-infected cells were virtually indistinguishable from those found after infection in vitro; in some locations, isolated clusters of cytotrophoblasts underlying the syncytium were the only cells infected (Fig. 45.3(b)). At other times, nearly all the cytotrophoblast progenitor cells, in highly infected tissues, expressed CMV IE proteins (Fig. 45.3(c), (d)). Comparatively fewer syncytial nuclei stained, but numerous cells within the villus cores stained for viral proteins, including fibroblasts, endothelial cells and macrophages. These studies suggested that in vitro infection is a model for the initial steps in placental infection, whereas in utero infection shows virus transmission from trophoblasts to other cell types in the villus core. The interplay between pathogens and immune responses in other tissues suggest that CMV infection might often occur in the context of the microbial ecology of female reproductive tissues.

Pathogenic microorganisms at the placental–decidual interface

In a study using PCR-based strategies, the presence of viral and bacterial DNA was assessed in biopsy specimens of the decidua and adjacent placentas of 282 healthy pregnancies (McDonagh *et al.*; Pereira *et al.*, 2003). Overall, CMV DNA was detected in 69% of specimens, and CMV with bacteria was detected in 38%. When found in isolation, CMV was detected in 27% of placental samples. Other pathogens included herpes simplex virus type 1 (HSV-1) in 3%; HSV-2 in 9%, and more than one bacterium in 15%. Sixteen percent of placental samples were negative for these pathogens. These findings suggest that early gestation placentas frequently contain DNA from viral and bacterial pathogens.

Detailed analysis of paired first-trimester decidual and placental biopsy specimens from individual pregnancies showed that some pathogens were present in both. CMV DNA was detected in 89% of the decidual samples and 63% of the placentas. When CMV was found in isolation in the decidua (40%), virus was also sometimes present in the placenta (26%). In contrast, when bacterial DNA was detected in the placenta (11%), signals were less frequently found in the decidual samples (6%). Together these results suggest that CMV can be selectively transferred from the decidua, a potential reservoir, to the adjacent placenta. When the effects of gestational age were examined, CMV DNA, with or without other pathogens, was detected in 63% of first-trimester placentas and 74% of second-trimester placentas. Together, samples with both CMV and bacterial DNA increased from 31% in the first trimester to 44% in the second trimester, whereas CMV alone was reduced in the second trimester. Fewer second-trimester placentas were negative for all pathogens. These studies suggested that (a) CMV is commonly present at the uterine-placental

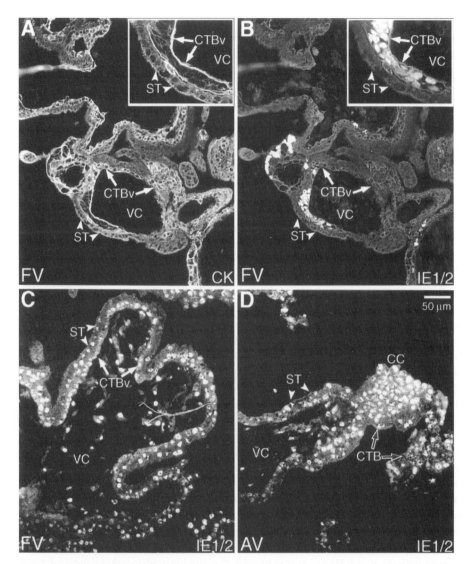

Fig. 45.3. Natural infection of chorionic villi with CMV in utero in cytotrophoblasts and other cells. Both floating villi (FV) (a–c) and anchoring villi (AV) (d) are shown. Tissues were analyzed by using immunolocalization techniques for expression of (a) cytokeratin (CK) and (b, d) CMV IE proteins. (b) In some floating villi, clusters of CMV-infected villous cytotrophoblast progenitors (CTBv) (arrows) underlying the syncytium (ST) (arrowheads) were the only sites of antibody reactivity. Sometimes, numerous cells throughout the villi stained with anti-CMV antibody. (c) Nuclei of syncytiotrophoblasts, villous cytotrophoblasts and stromal components expressed CMV proteins. (d) The same pattern of immunoreactivity was seen in infected anchoring villi. Additionally, cytotrophoblasts in cell columns (CC) stained brightly. VC, villus core.

interface together with pathogenic bacteria, (b) infection tends to increase in the second trimester, and (c) virus is selectively transmitted to the adjacent placenta.

Neutralizing antibodies to CMV gB in placental syncytiotrophoblasts

Development of neutralizing antibodies is delayed when primary CMV infection occurs shortly before or during gestation (Boppana and Britt, 1995; Lazzarotto et al., 1997; Revello et al., 2002), whereas high titers indicate resolution of acute infection and/or reactivation. Antibody responses to CMV in the group of donors from whom paired biopsy specimens were obtained showed that, with one exception, the donors were seropositive with a range of neutralizing activity. Briefly, neutralizing activity in IgG purified from the conditioned medium of biopsy specimens was evaluated. Ten women had low neutralizing titers (0% to 32%), nine had moderate titers (43% to 67%) and four had high titers (70 to 98%).

Some serologic evidence suggests that reinfection with new CMV strains in seropositive women might be associated with symptomatic fetal infection (Boppana et al., 1999). To determine whether multiple strains colonize the placental-decidual interface, a region of the gB gene with characteristic nucleotide differences was sequenced. Sequence analysis of a small number of CMV-positive samples revealed that the gB genotypes were similar to variants in groups 1, 2 and group 3 (Chou and Dennison, 1991). Paired decidua and adjacent placenta from a seropositive donor without detectable neutralizing antibodies contained a mixture of gB genotypes, suggesting that different CMV strains could infect the maternal-fetal interface early in the course of maternal infection.

Patterns of CMV-infected-cell proteins in the decidua and placenta

Decidual biopsy specimens that contained CMV DNA were studied by immunofluorescence confocal microscopy to determine whether viral proteins could be detected (McDonagh et al., 2004; Pereira et al., 2003). Tissue sections of decidual biopsy samples were incubated with a pool of monoclonal antibodies to CMV-infected-cell proteins and to gB, an abundant virion envelope glycoprotein. Staining revealed islands of infected resident uterine and fetal cells, as well as innate immune cells among much larger uninfected areas. Several common staining patterns emerged. In the most highly affected samples, CMV-infected-cell proteins were found in the nuclei and cytoplasm of glandular epithelium (Fig. 45.4(a), *a–c*), vascular endothelium and endovascular cytotrophoblasts (Fig. 45.4(a), *d–f*). Resident decidual cells positive for insulin growth factor binding protein 1 (IGFBP-1) also stained brightly (Fig. 45.4(a), *g–l*). These data indicate that CMV infects a diverse population of maternal cells within the uterine wall and fetal invasive cytotrophoblasts. Innate immune cells showed a staining pattern that was distinctly different from that of CMV-infected cells, suggesting phagocytosis of enveloped virions. Macrophages (CD68+) contained cytoplasmic vesicles that stained strongly for CMV gB (Fig. 45.4(b), *a–c*). Some gB-positive cells also stained for DC-SIGN (Kammerer et al., 2003; Soilleux et al., 2001) (Fig. 45.4(b), *d–f*). NK (CD56+) cells were often dispersed among Mφ/DC that were filled with gB-positive vesicles (Fig. 45.4(b), *g*). Occasionally, striking numbers of NK cells and Mφ/DC intermingled (Fig. 45.4(b), *h* and *i*). Additionally, neutrophils inside uterine blood vessels were found near endothelial cells and decidual cells that expressed CMV-infected-cell proteins, suggesting phagocytosis (Fig. 45.4b, *j–l*). These observations suggested that the uterus serves as a reservoir for CMV virions that could potentially infect the placenta.

Different patterns of CMV infection in the decidua mirrored in the adjacent placenta

Examination of CMV proteins in paired decidual and placental biopsy specimens showed three staining patterns (Pereira et al., 2003). In the first, islands in both decidual and placental compartments stained strongly for CMV-infected-cell proteins. This pattern predominated in samples from donors with low neutralizing titers and a few with intermediate titers and other pathogens. In the decidua, cytokeratin-positive glandular epithelial cells, endovascular cytotrophoblasts in remodeled uterine blood vessels, and interstitial cytotrophoblasts were sometimes positive. Resident decidual cells strongly stained for viral proteins, suggesting that these cells were permissive for viral replication. In the adjacent portions of the placenta, floating villi contained syncytiotrophoblasts and cytotrophoblast progenitor cells expressing CMV-infected-cell proteins that localized to the nuclei and cytoplasm. Abundant vesicles amassed close to the plasma membrane of the villus surface and contained gB. In regions with infected syncytiotrophoblasts, fibroblasts and fetal capillaries in the villus core expressed infected-cell proteins. Invasive cytotrophoblasts in developing cell columns that anchor the placenta to the uterine wall also stained. In contrast, Mφ/DCs within the villus stromal cores contained infected-cell proteins in cytoplasmic vesicles but not in the nuclei, suggesting phagocytosis.

In the second group of paired biopsy specimens, the number of cells that stained for CMV-infected-cell proteins was reduced in the decidua, and occasional focal infection was found in the placenta. This pattern predominated in samples from donors with low to intermediate neutralizing titers, several of which contained other pathogens. In the decidua, CMV replication was detected in some glandular epithelial cells and decidual cells. In the interstitium, Mφ/DCs were abundant throughout, especially near infected glands and blood vessels. These cells contained gB-positive cytoplasmic vesicles but were not infected. Sometimes the adjacent placentas contained small clusters of cytotrophoblast progenitor cells that expressed CMV-infected-cell proteins. Isolated gB-containing vesicles were present in the overlying syncytiotrophoblast layer. In the villus core, Mφ/DCs containing CMV gB-positive vesicles were often observed. In other placental biopsies, only gB-containing vesicles were detected in syncytiotrophoblasts and villus core Mφ/DCs without infection.

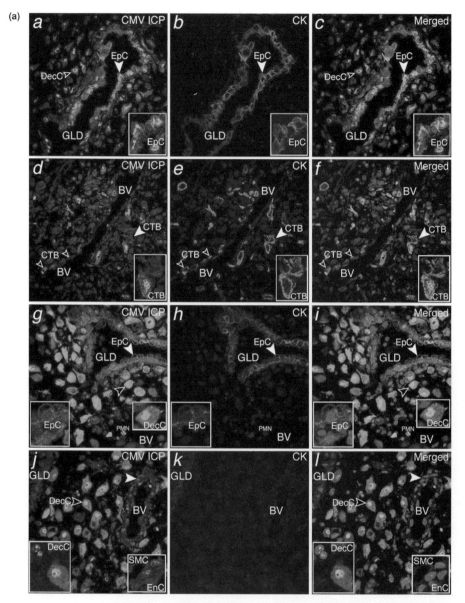

Fig. 45.4. Panel (a): CMV replicates in diverse cell types in uterine decidua. CMV infects endometrial glands (GLD), uterine blood vessels (BV), resident decidual cells (DecC) and cytotrophoblasts (CTB) in the decidua. (*a*)–(*c*), Decidual biopsy specimens stained for CMV-infected-cell proteins (ICP, green) and cytokeratin (CK, red), which identified epithelial cells (EpC). (*d*)–(*i*), CMV-infected interstitial and endovascular CTB and DecC. (*j*)–(*l*), Endothelial cells (EnC) and smooth muscle cells (SMC) of uterine blood vessels (BV) are infected. Panel (b): Abundant innate immune cells infiltrating the decidua contain CMV proteins. (*a*)–(*c*) CMV gB (green), macrophages (Mφ/DC, CD68, red). (*g*)–(*h*) DC-SIGN+ (green) macrophage/dendritic cells (Mφ/DC) take up CMV gB (red). (*g* (and) *h*) CD56+ (green) natural killer (NK) cells target infection sites. (*i*) DC-SIGN+ cells containing gB. (*j*)–(*l*) Neutrophils (PMN) with phagocytosed proteins from virus-infected cells and endothelial cells (EnC) positive for von Willebrand factor (vWF) in blood vessels (BV). "Merged" indicates colocalized proteins (yellow). Large arrowheads indicate area shown in insets. (See color plate section.)

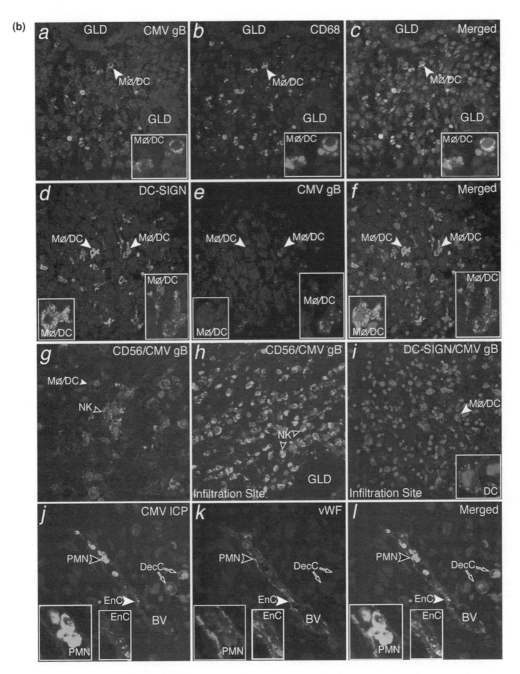

Fig. 45.4. (*cont.*) (See color plate section.)

In the last group of paired biopsy specimens, few cells stained for CMV-infected-cell proteins in the decidua, and none were found in the placenta. This pattern predominated in samples from donors with intermediate to high neutralizing titers, several of which contained other pathogens.

In the decidua, neutrophils with viral proteins were found in uterine blood vessels near infected cells. In the adjacent portions of the placenta, syncytiotrophoblasts contained numerous CMV gB-positive vesicles but were not infected. In villus core Mφ/DCs, gB accumulated in large cytoplasmic vesicles. When placentas were stained for IgG, syncytiotrophoblasts contained many positive vesicles, and gB colocalized with a small subset of them. In villus core Mφ/DCs, some gB-staining vesicles colocalized with the more abundant IgG-positive vesicles. FcRn-positive vesicles at the apical and basolateral membranes suggested IgG transcytosis in syncytiotrophoblasts (Simister and Story, 1997). In some cases, the presence of viral nucleocapsids in syncytiotrophoblasts was confirmed by electron microscopy.

These studies concluded that CMV is commonly present at the maternal-fetal interface, one possible explanation for why pregnant women shed virus from the cervix (Collier et al., 1995; Shen et al., 1993; Stagno et al., 1975). Bacteria were often found in donors with intermediate to high neutralizing titers whose uninfected placentas contained virion proteins suggesting limited CMV replication in the decidua. Reactivation from decidual Mφ/DCs might occur as a consequence of inflammatory responses to pathogenic bacteria and could depend on the number of latently infected Mφ/DCs infiltrating the uterus (Cook et al., 2002; Hahn et al., 1998; Soderberg-Naucler et al., 2001). Placentas from healthy pregnant donors contained isolated areas of infection that were a small part of the whole tissue. Since these tissues were from normal pregnancies, placental infection that leads to fetal transmission likely involves the decidual and placental components that stained for infected-cell proteins, i.e., an exacerbation of the situation found in samples from women with the lowest neutralizing titers and some with intermediate titers as well as bacterial pathogens.

Coordinated immune responses suppressed CMV infection of the placenta in women with intermediate to high neutralizing titers, one explanation for a correlation between high-avidity IgG and protection against vertical transmission (Boppana and Britt, 1995; Revello et al., 2002). The most remarkable result is that women with uncomplicated pregnancies had suppressed infection in the decidua. Virion-IgG complexes may be transported to the placenta without infection, a process that demonstrates the efficacy of innate and adaptive immunity. CMV infection of the decidua is a novel paradigm and further illustrates how this virus utilizes host immunity (Mocarski, 2002) by exploiting maternal hyporesponsiveness.

Analysis of CMV DNA and proteins expressed in placentas from uncomplicated deliveries by PCR and immunohistochemistry showed evidence of transplacental transmission (McDonagh et al., 2006). CMV DNA was detected in 62% of term placentas examined. In biopsy specimens from placentas with high levels of CMV DNA and low maternal neutralizing titers, fetal blood vessels contained leukocytes with viral replication proteins. Some cord blood samples contained CMV DNA, confirming viral replication. In placentas with low levels of viral DNA and high neutralizing titers, villus core macrophages and dendritic cells contained CMV gB, comparable to infection in early gestation, suggesting virion uptake without transmission. Together the results showed that CMV infection spreads from villus cytotrophoblasts to stromal fibroblasts, placental blood vessels and fetal leukocytes in late gestation. Over 5% of uncomplicated deliveries contained CMV replication proteins, suggesting a higher incidence of transplacental transmission and asymptomatic congenital infection than previously thought.

Complexes of IgG and CMV virions transcytosed from maternal circulation across syncytiotrophoblasts to underlying cytotrophoblasts

Immunohistochemical analysis of early gestation biopsy specimens showed an unusual pattern of CMV replication proteins in underlying cytotrophoblast progenitor cells. Whereas syncytiotrophoblasts were spared in placentas with low to moderate CMV neutralizing titers, cytotrophoblasts were infected, suggesting virion transcytosis from maternal blood (Pereira et al., 2003). Early steps of CMV infection and the role of FcRn were examined using the villus explant model (Fig. 45.2(a)) and polarized epithelial cells (Tugizov et al., 1996). The results showed that (i) maternal IgG modulates CMV infection in chorionic villi, (ii) FcRn transcytoses IgG–virion complexes that retain infectivity with low neutralizing antibodies, (iii) villus core macrophages capture transcytosed IgG-virions, (iv) IgG and gB accumulate in caveolae and (v) CMV DNA is present in syncytiotrophoblasts without viral replication. Receptor-mediated transport and caveolar endocytosis explain the infection patterns in villus cytotrophoblasts and CMV virion gB accumulation in vesicular compartments in utero (Pereira et al., 2003). The rapid kinetics of receptor-mediated transport of IgG–virions was similar in syncytiotrophoblasts and polarized T-84 intestinal epithelial cells expressing FcRn: transcytosed immune complexes were detected in villus core macrophages (explants), underlying cytotrophoblasts or the basal medium (cells). In villus explants, IgG–virion transcytosis and macrophage uptake were blocked with trypsin treatment and soluble protein A. The results suggest that CMV virions could disseminate to the placenta by co-opting the receptor-mediated transport pathway for IgG. It was recently reported that passive immunization with hyperimmune IgG at midgestation prevents congenital disease and growth restriction in infected infants of mothers with primary CMV infection (Nigro et al., 2005). This remarkable outcome suggests once CMV replication has been interrupted, functional villi develop that transport neutralizing IgG to the fetus, reducing dissemination.

Receptors for CMV virions are developmentally regulated in cytotrophoblasts

CMV replication in distinct cytotrophoblast populations suggests that virion receptors could be developmentally regulated as these specialized cells proceed along the differentiation pathway from the fetal to the maternal compartment (Fig. 45.1). Function-blocking methods and immunohistochemical analysis were used to correlate infection with expression of CMV receptors in cytotrophoblasts in situ and in vitro (Maidji et al., 2006). In placental villi, syncytiotrophoblasts express a virion receptor, epidermal growth factor receptor (EGFR) (Wang et al., 2003), but lack integrin coreceptors, and endocytosis occurs without replication. IgG–CMV virion complexes transcytosed by FcRn reach underlying cytotrophoblasts (Maidji et al., 2006). Some EGFR-expressing cells selectively initiate expression of a coreceptor, αV integrin (Feire et al., 2004; Wang et al., 2005), and focal infection can occur. In cell columns, proximal cytotrophoblasts lack receptors, and distal cells express integrins α1β1 and αVβ3 but remain uninfected. In the uterine decidua, invasive cytotrophoblasts expressing integrin coreceptors upregulate EGFR, thereby dramatically increasing susceptibility. These findings indicate that virion engagement with receptors in the placenta (i) changes as cytotrophoblasts differentiate and (ii) correlates with spatially distinct sites of CMV replication in maternal and fetal compartments in utero.

CMV infection dysregulates cytotrophoblast differentiation/invasion in vitro

CMV replicates in placental cytotrophoblasts in vitro

Several groups have reported that cytotrophoblasts isolated from early gestation (Fisher et al., 2000; Hemmings et al., 1998) and term placentas (Halwachs-Baumann et al., 1998) are susceptible to CMV infection. A detailed examination of the viral life cycle was done using an in vitro model of progenitor cytotrophoblasts from chorionic villi plated as a monolayer on Matrigel and cultured from 2 to 4 days after infection (see Fig. 45.2(b)) (Fisher et al., 2000; Librach et al., 1991). Under these conditions the cells form aggregates, analogous to cell columns, and differentiate along the invasive pathway. In CMV-infected cells, nuclear staining for IE proteins was detected by 24 hours and cytoplasmic staining for gB was detected by 72 hours in 20 to 40% of the cells. There was an increase in the titers of intracellular and progeny virions released during the culture period, establishing that differentiating cytotrophoblasts are fully permissive for CMV replication.

Investigation of the effects of viral infection in cytotrophoblasts showed considerable changes, evidenced by dysregulated expression of stage-specific adhesion and immune molecules, as well as metalloproteinases and their inhibitors (Fisher et al., 2000; Maidji et al., 2002; Yamamoto-Tabata et al., 2004). Importantly, the cells' central function, invasion, was significantly impaired following infection.

CMV infection in vitro downregulates cytotrophoblast expression of HLA-G

In healthy placentas, the non-classical MHC class Ib molecule HLA-G is expressed in differentiating cytotrophoblasts, particularly cells in anchoring villi with an increasing gradient of expression in the distal columns that is maintained once the cells enter the uterine wall (Kovats et al., 1990; McMaster et al., 1995). Immunolocalization experiments showed that CMV infection of differentiating cytotrophoblasts in vitro downregulates expression of HLA-G (Fisher et al., 2000). At late times when high levels of CMV gB were detected (Fig. 45.5(a)), staining for HLA-G was either greatly reduced or lost (Fig. 45.5(b)). This was in contrast to cells that were not infected with CMV and stained with anti-HLA-G.

Several CMV genes downregulate expression of classical MHC class Ia molecules (for review see Ploegh, 1998). Studied in the context of cytotrophoblasts infected with CMV mutants in which all of the genes known to downregulate cell surface expression of MHC class Ia molecules are deleted, Jones and Muzithras, (1992), showed that HLA-G expression was not rescued (Fisher et al., 2000). Others reported that HLA-G is resistant to the effects of CMV protein US11, which binds to class I heavy chains and mediates their dislocation to the cytosol and subsequent proteasomal degradation (Schust et al., 1998). Subsequent analyses using chimeric molecules of MHC class Ia and Ib showed that the degradation efficiency depended on sequences in the heavy-chain cytosolic tail that HLA-G lacks (Barel et al., 2003). Since the mechanism of HLA-G downregulation does not involve CMV glycoproteins that alter class Ia expression, it is most likely novel.

CMV infection in vitro downregulates α1β1 integrin expression and impairs cytotrophoblast invasion

Congenital CMV infection is associated with abnormal placentation at a morphological level and intrauterine growth restriction (Benirschke et al., 1974), likely related to impaired remodeling of uterine arterioles by invasive

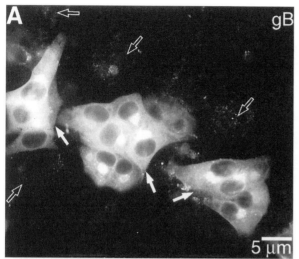
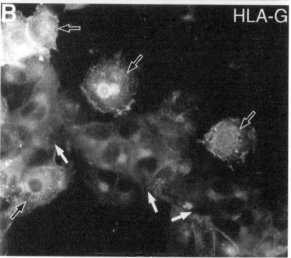

Fig. 45.5. CMV infection impairs cytotrophoblast expression of HLA-G in vitro. Purified cytotrophoblasts were isolated and infected with CMV. At 72 h, the cells were stained for (a) gB and (b) HLA-G expression. Cells that did not express gB (black arrows) expressed HLA-G, and staining for gB (white arrows) was associated with a marked reduction in HLA-G expression.

cytotrophoblasts. This prompted examination of the expression of the laminin/collagen receptor integrin α1β1 in the context of CMV infection. This extracellular matrix receptor is both a stage-specific antigen whose expression is preferentially associated with cytotrophoblasts inside the uterine wall (Damsky et al., 1992) and an adhesion molecule that mediates invasion in vitro (Damsky et al., 1994). Co-localization of CMV gB (Fig. 45.6(a) and (c)) and integrin α1 expression (Fig. 45.6(b) and (d)) showed that cells that did not stain for gB (Fig. 45.6(a)) expressed integrin α1 in a plasma membrane-associated pattern (Fig. 45.6(b)). Diffuse cytoplasmic staining for gB in infected cytotrophoblasts was also correlated with integrin α1 expression (see cell marked with an asterisk in Fig. 45.6(c) and (d)), but accumulation of gB in vesicles (Fig. 45.6(c)) at late times after infection was associated with the absence of staining for integrin α1 (Fig. 45.6(d)). In contrast, immunostaining for another integrin whose expression is upregulated as the cells invade, the fibronectin receptor α5 that functions to inhibit invasion, was not affected.

Flow cytometric analysis and RT-PCR were used to quantify proteins expressed on the surface of freshly isolated cytotrophoblasts from term placentas and changes in differentiating cells infected with VR1814, a pathogenic clinical strain (Tabata et al., 2006). Significant downregulation of HLA-G at the protein level shown by immunohistochemistry was confirmed, and transcription was reduced in infected cells. Likewise, infected cytotrophoblasts significantly dysregulated integrin α1 and α5 proteins. Integrin α9 and VE-cadherin, which promote cell-cell adhesion, were also reduced by infection. Cytotrophoblasts isolated from placentas with CMV DNA and virion gB in syncytiotrophoblasts and in villus core macrophages were uninfected and showed similar expression of the differentiation molecules studied.

The impact of CMV infection on cytotrophoblast invasion was examined using an in vitro assay (see Fig. 45.2(b)) (Fisher et al., 2000). This functional assay tests the ability of isolated cytotrophoblasts plated on the upper surfaces of Matrigel-coated filters to penetrate the surface, pass through pores in the underlying filter, and emerge on the lower surface of the membrane (Damsky et al., 1994; Librach et al., 1991). Invasion is quantified by determining the number of cytokeratin-positive cell processes that emerge through the filter pores. The invasion ability of cells infected with CMV was dramatically impaired, as compared with control uninfected cells, suggesting that functional defects could result from a constellation of virus-induced changes that impair cell–matrix and cell–cell adhesion. Interestingly, the effect on invasion was greater than could be accounted for by the number of CMV-infected cells, suggesting that the presence of infected cells in the invading aggregates influences the behavior of the population as a whole.

CMV infection downregulates MMP activity altering cell-cell and cell–matrix interactions

MMPs are a family of degradative enzymes that remodel the extracellular matrix during many processes, including cell migration, vascularization, and invasion (Chang and

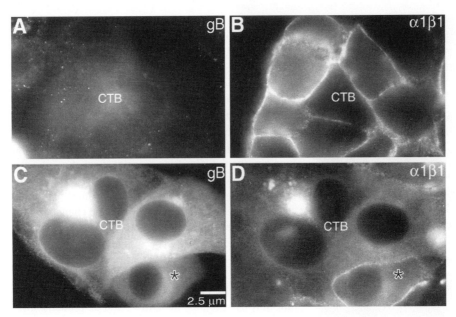

Fig. 45.6. CMV infection in vitro eventually downregulates cytotrophoblast expression of integrin α1. Purified cytotrophoblasts were infected with CMV in vitro. At 72 h, the cells were fixed and stained for expression of gB and integrin α1. Cytotrophoblasts that did not express gB (a) displayed prominent staining for integrin α1 in a plasma membrane-associated pattern (b). Likewise, cells that stained in a diffuse cytoplasmic pattern for gB (c) also reacted with the anti-integrin antibody (d, cell marked with an asterisk). However, when gB was localized in a vesicular pattern, integrin staining was not detected (d).

Werb, 2001). MMPs are highly regulated during translation and post-translationally by activation and secretion. Invasive cytotrophoblasts secrete relatively large amounts of MMP-9 in early gestation, when invasion peaks; later, when invasion is complete, MMP-9 levels fall (Librach et al., 1991). Accordingly, cytotrophoblast invasion is also regulated by factors controlling MMP activation. The inactive proenzyme is activated by cleavage and removal of an inhibitory domain. Activated MMP-9 is absolutely required for invasion, whereas pro-MMP-9 is associated with non-invasive cells (Fisher et al., 1989; Librach et al., 1991).

Examination of cytotrophoblasts and endothelial cells infected with CMV in vitro showed altered MMP protein and activity (Yamamoto-Tabata et al., 2004). Infection with VR1814, an endothelial cell-tropic CMV strain, but not AD169, a laboratory strain, reduced MMP-9 activity, thereby decreasing the cells' capacity to degrade the extracellular matrix. Likewise, MMP-2 activity in uterine microvascular endothelial cells was reduced. Since VR1814-infected endothelial cells transmit infection to cocultured differentiating cytotrophoblasts in vitro (Maidji et al., 2002), infection could undermine contacts between endothelial cells and cytotrophoblasts (Fig. 45.2, site 1). The observation that uterine arterioles are infected by CMV in utero (Pereira et al., 2003) suggests that virus could spread to cytotrophoblasts and in a retrograde direction to the placenta proper (i.e., floating chorionic villi) and to fetal blood vessels in the villus core.

CMV IL-10 dysregulates MMP activity

Several cytokines and growth factors regulate MMP expression and activity. For example, IL-1β is an autocrine stimulator of MMP-9 secretion and cytotrophoblast invasion of Matrigel in vitro (Librach et al., 1994). In contrast, human IL-10 (hIL-10) downregulates these processes and impairs cytotrophoblast invasion (Roth et al., 1996; Roth and Fisher, 1999). Recent reports indicated that CMV IL-10 (cmvIL-10) (Kotenko et al., 2000) binds the hIL-10 receptor 1 (hIL-10R1) with affinity similar to that of natural ligand (Jones et al., 2002) and has comparable immunosuppressive activity (Spencer et al., 2002). Analysis of the cmvIL-10 genes from several strains showed very high sequence conservation, suggesting conserved functions (Kotenko et al., 2000; Spencer et al., 2002). Like other intracellular pathogens that infect macrophages, CMV exploits the IL-10 signaling pathway, expressing an IL10 homologue and upregulating the cell's production of the cytokine (Kotenko et al., 2000; Redpath et al., 2001). Although cmvIL-10 shares only 27% sequence identity with hIL-10, the proteins have essentially identical affinity for the receptor, IL-10R1, and similarly reorganize the cell surface receptor complex (Jones et al., 2002).

Both cytotrophoblasts and endothelial cells express IL-10R1, suggesting possible autocrine and paracrine regulation by its ligand (Cattaruzza et al., 2003; Roth and Fisher, 1999). hIL-10 in cytotrophoblasts' culture medium can suppress allogeneic lymphocyte reactivity (Roth et al., 1996), an important link between immune protection of the fetus and cytotrophoblast invasion of the uterus. Likewise, recombinant cmvIL-10 can inhibit proliferation of mitogen-stimulated peripheral blood mononuclear cells and production of proinflammatory cytokines at a level comparable to that of hIL-10 (Spencer et al., 2002). Together these findings suggest that cmvIL-10 might, like the cellular molecule, impair invasion of differentiating cytotrophoblasts. MMP activity was examined in uterine microvascular endothelial cells and differentiating cytotrophoblasts in vitro treated with purified recombinant cmvIL-10 or hIL-10 (Yamamoto-Tabata et al., 2004). Culture medium and cell lysates of treated endothelial cells contained less MMP activity than untreated contols, suggesting that the viral cytokine inhibits proteinase production in the absence of infection and that cmvIL-10-and hIL-10 have comparable effects. Likewise, levels of MMP-9 activity in differentiating cytotrophoblasts treated with these cytokines were significantly reduced in a dose-dependent fashion, confirming previous results (Roth and Fisher, 1999).

CMV IL-10 impairs endothelial cell migration and cytotrophoblast invasiveness in vitro

Having shown that cmvIL-10 downregulates MMP-2 and MMP-9 activity, the effect of reduced proteinase activity on fibroblast and endothelial cell function was examined in cell wound healing assays. Briefly, subconfluent cells were scratched ("wounded") and then incubated until control cells closed the wound. Infection with VR1814 or treatment with hIL-10 and cmvIL-10 had impaired endothelial cell wound closure but had no inhibitory effect on fibroblast migration. To assess the effect on cytotrophoblasts, the frequency with which the cells passed through narrow pores in a Matrigel-coated filter was quantified. Treatment with cmvIL-10 alone impaired invasion to a level comparable to that of hIL-10-treated cells, and significantly fewer cells traversed the filter pores after treatment with cmvIL-10 as compared with control untreated cells. Together these results indicated that, like hIL-10, cmvIL-10 impairs endothelial cell migration in wound closure assays and cytotrophoblast invasion as previously observed in CMV-infected cells in vitro (Fisher et al., 2000). These studies suggest that CMV exploits an immune mechanism to dysregulate endothelial cell migration and cytotrophoblast invasion (Yamamoto-Tabata et al., 2004).

Concluding remarks

We are just beginning to appreciate how the unusual anatomy of the maternal-fetal interface is advantageous for CMV spread to the placenta and how innate and adaptive immunity often precludes transplacental transmission. These studies open the door to testing a variety of hypotheses regarding CMV infection of placental tissues. Numerous questions and challenges remain. What is the functional significance of the static picture we obtained of immune defenses and viral proteins at the placental-decidual interface? Does coinfection with viruses and pathogenic bacteria in the decidua and adjacent placenta correlate with fetal transmission in early and late gestation? Additionally it will be interesting to decipher the network of cytokines and chemokines that regulates trafficking of immune cells in the infected decidua. Finally, identifying the molecules used for virion attachment and entry into cytotrophoblasts and syncytiotrophoblasts is crucial to the development of therapeutic strategies. One key to the puzzle of resolving infection in utero will be the capacity to gauge the threshold for maternal hyporesponsive. Onset of inflammation could trigger CMV reactivation and processes whereby NK cells, macrophages and dendritic cells control infection in the decidua. We theorize that detailed studies will resolve the serious dichotomy between the devastating consequences of congenital CMV infection and our lack of knowledge, at the molecular level, of the mechanisms involved.

REFERENCES

Ahlfors, K., Ivarsson, S. A., Harris, S. et al. (1984). Congenital cytomegalovirus infection and disease in Sweden and the relative importance of primary and secondary maternal infections. Preliminary findings from a prospective study. Scand. J. Infect. Dis., 16, 129–137.

Barel, M. T., Pizzato, N., Van Leeuwen, D., Bouteiller, P. L., Wiertz, E. J., and Lenfant, F. (2003). Amino acid composition of alpha1/alpha2 domains and cytoplasmic tail of MHC class I molecules determine their susceptibility to human cytomegalovirus US11-mediated down-regulation. Eur. J. Immunol., 33, 1707–1716.

Bass, K. E., Li, H., Hawkes, S. P. et al. (1997). Tissue inhibitor of metalloproteinase-3 expression is upregulated during human cytotrophoblast invasion in vitro. Dev. Genet., 21, 61–67.

Benirschke, K. and Kaufmann, P. (2000). *Pathology of the Human Placenta*. 4th edn. New York: Springer.

Benirschke, K., Mendoza, G. R., and Bazeley, P. L. (1974). Placental and fetal manifestations of cytomegalovirus infection. *Virchow's Arch. B Cell Pathol.*, **16**, 121–139.

Boppana, S. B. and Britt, W. J. (1995). Antiviral antibody responses and intrauterine transmission after primary maternal cytomegalovirus infection. *J. Infect. Dis.*, **171**, 1115–1121.

Boppana, S. B., Fowler, K. B., Britt, W. J., Stagno, S., and Pass, R. F. (1999) Symptomatic congenital cytomegalovirus infection in infants born to mothers with preexisting immunity to cytomegalovirus. *Pediatrics*, **104**, 55–60.

Britt, W. J. (1999). Congenital cytomegalovirus infection. In *Sexually Transmitted Diseases and Adverse Outcomes of Pregnancy*, P. J. Hitchcock, H. T. MacKay, and J. N. Wasserheit, eds., pp. 269–281. Washington, DC: ASM Press.

Bulmer, J. N., Morrison, L., Longfellow, M., Ritson, A., and Pace, D. (1991). Granulated lymphocytes in human endometrium: histochemical and immunohistochemical studies. *Hum. Reprod.*, **6**, 791–798.

Cattaruzza, M., Slodowski, W., Stojakovic, M., Krzesz, R., and Hecker, M. (2003). Interleukin-10 induction of nitric oxide synthase expression attenuates CD40-mediated interleukin-12 synthesis in human endothelial cells. *J. Biol. Chem.*, **11**, 11.

Chang, C. and Werb, Z. (2001). The many faces of metalloproteases: cell growth, invasion, angiogenesis and metastasis. *Trends Cell Biol.*, **11**, S37–S43.

Chou, S. W. and Dennison, K. M. (1991). Analysis of interstrain variation in cytomegalovirus glycoprotein B sequences encoding neutralization-related epitopes. *J. Infect. Dis.*, **163**, 1229–1234.

Collier, A. C., Handsfield, H. H., Ashley, R. *et al.* (1995). Cervical but not urinary excretion of cytomegalovirus is related to sexual activity and contraceptive practices in sexually active women. *J. Infect. Dis.*, **171**, 33–38.

Cook, C. H., Zhang, Y., McGuinness, B. J., Lahm, M. C., Sedmak, D. D., and Ferguson, R. M. (2002). Intra-abdominal bacterial infection reactivates latent pulmonarycytomegalovirus in immunocompetent mice. *J. Infect. Dis.*, **185**, 1395–1400.

Cross, J. C., Werb, Z., and Fisher, S. J. (1994). Implantation and the placenta: key pieces of the development puzzle. *Science*, **266**, 1508–1518.

Crossey, P. A., Pillai, C. C., and Miell, J. P. (2002). Altered placental development and intrauterine growth restriction in IGF binding protein-1 transgenic mice. *J. Clin. Invest.*, **110**, 411–418.

Damsky, C. H. and Fisher, S. J. (1998). Trophoblast pseudovasculogenesis: faking it with endothelial adhesion receptors. *Curr. Opin. Cell Biol.*, **10**, 660–666.

Damsky, C. H., Fitzgerald, M. L., and Fisher, S. J. (1992). Distribution patterns of extracellular matrix components and adhesion receptors are intricately modulated during first trimester cytotrophoblast differentiation along the invasive pathway, in vivo. *J. Clin. Invest.*, **89**, 210–222.

Damsky, C. H., Librach, C., Lim, K. H. *et al.* (1994). Integrin switching regulates normal trophoblast invasion. *Development*, **120**, 3657–3666.

Drake, P. M., Gunn, M. D., Charo, I. F. *et al.* (2001). Human placental cytotrophoblasts attract monocytes and CD56(bright) natural killer cells via the actions of monocyte inflammatory protein 1alpha. *J. Exp. Med.*, **193**, 1199–1212.

Feire, A. L., Koss, H., and Compton, T. (2004). Cellular integrins function as entry receptors for human cytomegalovirus via a highly conserved disintegrin-like domain. *Proc. Natl. Acad. Sci. USA*, **101**, 15470–15475.

Fish, K. N., Soderberg-Naucler, C., Mills, L. K., Stenglein, S., and Nelson, J. A. (1998). Human cytomegalovirus persistently infects aortic endothelial cells. *J. Virol.*, **72**, 5661–5668.

Fisher, S., Genbacev, O., Maidji, E., and Pereira, L. (2000). Human cytomegalovirus infection of placental cytotrophoblasts in vitro and in utero: implications for transmission and pathogenesis. *J. Virol.*, **74**, 6808–6820.

Fisher, S. J., Leitch, M. S., Kantor, M. S. Basbaum, C. B., and Kramer, R. H. (1985). Degradation of extracellular matrix by the trophoblastic cells of first-trimester human placentas. *J. Cell. Biochem.*, **27**, 31–41.

Fisher, S. J., Cui, T. Y., Zhang, L. *et al.* (1989). Adhesive and degradative properties of human placental cytotrophoblast cells in vitro. *J. Cell. Biol.*, **109**, 891–902.

Fowler, K. B. and Pass, R. F. (1991). Sexually transmitted diseases in mothers of neonates with congenital cytomegalovirus infection. *J. Infect. Dis.*, **164**, 259–264.

Fowler, K. B., Stagno, S., and Pass, R. F. (2003). Maternal immunity and prevention of congenital cytomegalovirus infection. *J. Am. Med. Assoc.*, **289**, 1008–1011.

Griffiths, P. D. and Baboonian, C. (1984). A prospective study of primary cytomegalovirus infection during pregnancy: final report. *Br. J. Obstet. Gynaecol.*, **91**, 307–315.

Hahn, G., Jores, R., and Mocarski, E. S. (1998). Cytomegalovirus remains latent in a common precursor of dendritic and myeloid cells. *Proc. Natl. Acad. Sci. USA*, **95**, 3937–3942.

Halwachs-Baumann, G., Wilders-Truschnig, M., Desoye, G. *et al.* (1998). Human trophoblast cells are permissive to the complete replicative cycle of human cytomegalovirus. *J. Virol.*, **72**, 7598–7602.

Hemmings, D. G., Kilani, R., Nykiforuk, C., Preiksaitis, J., and Guilbert, L. J. (1998). Permissive cytomegalovirus infection of primary villous term and first trimester trophoblasts. *J. Virol.* **72**, 4970–4979.

Hoang, V. M., Foulk, R., Clauser, K., Burlingame, A., Gibson, B. W., and Fisher, S. J. (2001). Functional proteomics: examining the effects of hypoxia on the cytotrophoblast protein repertoire. *Biochemistry*, **40**, 4077–4086.

Istas, A. S., Demmler, G. J., Dobbins, J. G., and Stewart, J. A. (1995). Surveillance for congenital cytomegalovirus disease: a report from the National Congenital Cytomegalovirus Disease Registry. *Clin. Infect. Dis.*, **20**, 665–670.

Jones, B. C., Logsdon, N. J., Josephson, K., Cook, J., Barry, P. A., and Walter, M. R. (2002). Crystal structure of human cytomegalovirus IL-10 bound to soluble human IL10R1. *Proc. Natl. Acad. Sci. USA*, **99**, 9404–9409.

Jones, T. R. and Muzithras, V. P. (1992). A cluster of dispensable genes within the human cytomegalovirus genome short component: IRS1, US1 through US5, and the US6 family. *J. Virol.*, **66**, 2541–2546.

Kamat, B. R. and Isaacson, P. G. (1987). The immunocytochemical distribution of leukocytic subpopulations in human endometrium. *Am. J. Pathol.*, **127**, 66–73.

Kammerer, U., Marzusch, K., Krober, S., Ruck, P., Handgretinger, R., and Dietl, J. (1999). A subset of CD56+ large granular lymphocytes in first-trimester human decidua are proliferating cells. *Fertil. Steril.*, **71**, 74–79.

Kammerer, U., Schoppet, M., McLellan, A. D. *et al.* (2000). Human decidua contains potent immunostimulatory CD83(+) dendritic cells. *Am. J. Pathol.*, **157**, 159–169.

Kammerer, U., Eggert, A. O., Kapp, M. *et al.* (2003). Unique appearance of proliferating antigen-presenting cells expressing DC-SIGN (CD209) in the decidua of early human pregnancy. *Am. J. Pathol.*, **162**, 887–896.

King, A., Wellings, V., Gardner, L., and Loke, Y. W. (1989). Immunocytochemical characterization of the unusual large granular lymphocytes in human endometrium throughout the menstrual cycle. *Hum. Immunol.*, **24**, 195–205.

Kondo, K., Xu, J. and Mocarski, E. S. (1996). Human cytomegalovirus latent gene expression in granulocyte-macrophage progenitors in culture and in seropositive individuals. *Proc. Natl Acad. Sci. USA*, **93**, 11137–11142.

Kotenko, S. V., Saccani, S., Izotova, L. S., Mirochnitchenko, O. V., and Pestka, S. (2000). Human cytomegalovirus harbors its own unique IL-10 homolog (cmvIL-10). *Proc. Natl Acad. Sci. USA*, **97**, 1695–1700.

Kovats, S., Main, E. K., Librach, C., Stubblebine, M., Fisher, S. J., and DeMars, R. (1990). A class I antigen, HLA-G, expressed in human trophoblasts. *Science*, **248**, 220–223.

Kruse, A., Hallmann, R., and Butcher, E. C. (1999). Specialized patterns of vascular differentiation antigens in the pregnant mouse uterus and the placenta. *Biol. Reprod.*, **61**, 1393–1401.

Lazzarotto, T., Spezzacatena, P., Pradelli, P., Abate, D. A., Varani, S., and Landini, M. P. (1997). Avidity of immunoglobulin G directed against human cytomegalovirus during primary and secondary infections in immunocompetent and immunocompromised subjects. *Clin. Diag. Lab. Immunol.*, **4**, 469–473.

Lazzarotto, T., Varani, S., Spezzacatena, P. *et al.* (1998). Delayed acquisition of high-avidity anti-cytomegalovirus antibody is correlated with prolonged antigenemia in solid organ transplant recipients. *J. Infect. Dis.*, **178**, 1145–1149.

Librach, C. L., Werb, Z., Fitzgerald, M. L. *et al.* (1991). 92-kD type IV collagenase mediates invasion of human cytotrophoblasts. *J. Cell Biol.*, **113**, 437–449.

Librach, C. L., Feigenbaum, S. L., Bass, K. E. *et al.* (1994). Interleukin-1 beta regulates human cytotrophoblast metalloproteinase activity and invasion in vitro. *J. Biol. Chem.*, **269**, 17125–17131.

Maidji, E., Percivalle, E., Gerna, G., Fisher, S., and Pereira, L. (2002). Transmission of human cytomegalovirus from infected uterine microvascular endothelial cells to differentiating/invasive placental cytotrophoblasts. *Virology*, **304**, 53–69.

Maidji, E., Genbacev, O., Chang, H. T., and Pereira, L. (submitted). Developmental regulation of human cytomegalovirus receptors in cytotrophoblasts correlates with distinct replication sites in the placenta.

Maidji, E., McDonagh, S., Genbacev, O., Tabata, T., and Pereira, L. (2006). Maternal antibodies enhance or prevent cytomegalovirus infection in the placenta by neonatal Fc receptor-mediated transcytosis. *Am. J. Pathol.*, **168**, 1210–1226.

McDonagh, S., Maidji, E., Ma, W., Chang, H.-T., Fisher, S., and Pereira, L., (2004). Viral and bacterial pathogens at the maternal-fetal interface. *J. Infect. Dis.*, **190**, 826–834.

McDonagh, S., Maidji, E., Chang, H.-T., and Pereira, L. (2006). Patterns of human cytomegalovirus infection in term placentas: a preliminary analysis. *J. Clin. Virol.*, **35**, 210–215.

McMaster, M. T., Librach, C. L., Zhou, Y. *et al.* (1995). Human placental HLA-G expression is restricted to differentiated cytotrophoblasts. *J. Immunol.*, **154**, 3771–3778.

Mocarski, E. S. (2002). Immunomodulation by cytomegaloviruses: manipulative strategies beyond evasion. *Trends Microbiol.*, **10**, 332–339.

Muhlemann, K., Miller, R. K., Metlay, L., and Menegus, M. A. (1992). Cytomegalovirus infection of the human placenta: an immunocytochemical study. *Hum. Pathol.*, **23**, 1234–1237.

Nakamura, Y., Sakuma, S., Ohta, Y., Kawano, K., and Hashimoto, T. (1994). Detection of the human cytomegalovirus gene in placental chronic villitis by polymerase chain reaction. *Hum. Pathol.*, **25**, 815–818.

Nigro, G., Adler, S. P., La Torre, R., and Best, A. M. (2005). Passive immunization during pregnancy for congenital cytomegalovirus infection. *N. Engl. J. Med.*, **353**, 1350–1362.

Norwitz, E. R., Schust, D. J., and Fisher, S. J. (2001). Implantation and the survival of early pregnancy. *N. Engl. J. Med.*, **345**, 1400–1408.

Pass, B. F. (2001). Cytomegalovirus. In *Fields Virology*, D. M. Knipe, and P. M. Howley, eds., 4th edn. Vol. 2, pp. 2675–2705. New York: Lippincott-Raven.

Pass, R. F., Little, E. A., Stagno, S., Britt, W. J., and Alford, C. A. (1987). Young children as a probable source of maternal and congenital cytomegalovirus infection. *N. Engl. J. Med.*, **316**, 1366–1370.

Pereira, L., Maidji, E., McDonagh, S., Genbacev, O., and Fisher, S. (2003). Human cytomegalovirus transmission from the uterus to the placenta correlates with the presence of pathogenic bacteria and maternal immunity. *J. Virol*, **77**, 13301–13314.

Ploegh, H. L. (1998). Viral strategies of immune evasion. *Science*, **280**, 248–253.

Queenan, J. T., Kao, L. C., Arboleda, C. E. *et al.* (1987). Regulation of urokinase-type plasminogen activator production by cultured human cytotrophoblasts. *J. Biol. Chem.*, **262**, 10903–10906.

Red-Horse, K., Drake, P. M., Gunn, M. D., and Fisher, S. J. (2001). Chemokine ligand and receptor expression in the pregnant uterus: reciprocal patterns in complementary cell subsets suggest functional roles. *Am. J. Pathol.*, **159**, 2199–2213.

Redpath, S., Ghazal, P., and Gascoigne, N. R. (2001). Hijacking and exploitation of Il-10 by intracellular pathogens. *Trends Microbiol.*, **9**, 86–92.

Revello, M. G., Zavattoni, M., Furione, M., Lilleri, D., Gorini, G., and Gerna, G. (2002). Diagnosis and outcome of preconceptional and periconceptional primary human cytomegalovirus infections. *J. Infect. Dis.*, **186**, 553–557.

Roth, I. and Fisher, S. J. (1999). IL-10 is an autocrine inhibitor of human placental cytotrophoblast MMP-9 production and invasion. *Dev. Biol.*, **205**, 194–204.

Roth, I., Corry, D. B., Locksley, R. M., Abrams, J. S., Litton, M. J., and Fisher, S. J. (1996). Human placental cytotrophoblasts produce the immunosuppressive cytokine interleukin 10. *J. Exp. Med.*, **184**, 539–548.

Schust, D. J., Tortorella, D., Seebach, J., Phan, C., and Ploegh, H. L. (1998). Trophoblast class I major histocompatibility complex (MHC) products are resistant to rapid degradation imposed by the human cytomegalovirus (HCMV) gene products US2 and US11. *J. Exp. Med.*, **188**, 497–503.

Shen, C. Y., Chang, S. F., Yen, M. S. *et al.* (1993). Cytomegalovirus excretion in pregnant and nonpregnant women. *J. Clin. Microbiol.*, **31**, 1635–1636.

Simister, N. E. and Story, C. M. (1997). Human placental Fc receptors and the transmission of antibodies from mother to fetus. *J. Reprod. Immunol.*, **37**, 1–23.

Simister, N. E., Story, C. M., Chen, H. L., and Hunt, J. S. (1996). An IgG-transporting Fc receptor expressed in the syncytiotrophoblast of human placenta. *Eur. J. Immunol.*, **26**, 1527–1531.

Sinzger, C., Müntefering, H., Löning, T., Stöss, H., Plachter, B., and Jahn, G. (1993). Cell types infected in human cytomegalovirus placentitis identified by immunohistochemical double staining. *Virchows Archiv. A Pathol. Anat. Histopathol.*, **423**, 249–256.

Soderberg-Naucler, C., Fish, K. N., and Nelson, J. A. (1997). Reactivation of latent human cytomegalovirus by allogeneic stimulation of blood cells from healthy donors. *Cell*, **91**, 119–126.

Soderberg-Naucler, C., Streblow, D. N., Fish, K. N., Allan-Yorke, J., Smith, P. P., and Nelson, J. A. (2001). Reactivation of latent human cytomegalovirus in CD14(+) monocytes is differentiation dependent. *J. Virol.*, **75**, 7543–7554.

Soilleux, E. J., Morris, L. S., Lee, B. *et al.* (2001). Placental expression of DC-SIGN may mediate intrauterine vertical transmission of HIV. *J. Pathol.*, **195**, 586–592.

Soilleux, E. J., Morris, L. S., Leslie, G. *et al.* (2002). Constitutive and induced expression of DC-SIGN on dendritic cell and macrophage subpopulations in situ and in vitro. *J. Leukoc. Biol.*, **71**, 445–457.

Solberg, H., Rinkenberger, J., Dano, K., Werb, Z., and Lund, L. R. (2003). A functional overlap of plasminogen and MMPs regulates vascularization during placental development. *Development*, **130**, 4439–4450.

Spencer, J. V., Lockridge, K. M., Barry, P. A. *et al.* (2002). Potent immunosuppressive activities of cytomegalovirus-encoded interleukin-10. *J. Virol.*, **76**, 1285–1292.

Stagno, S., Reynolds, D., Tsiantos, A. *et al.* (1975). Cervical cytomegalovirus excretion in pregnant and nonpregnant women: suppression in early gestation. *J. Infect. Dis.*, **131**, 522–527.

Stagno, S., Reynolds, D. W., Pass, R. F., and Alford, C. A. (1980). Breast milk and the risk of cytomegalovirus infection. *N. Engl. J. Med.*, **302**, 1073–1076.

Stagno, S., Pass, R. F., Dworsky, M. E. *et al.* (1982). Congenital cytomegalovirus infection: The relative importance of primary and recurrent maternal infection. *N. Engl. J. Med.*, **306**, 945–949.

Starkey, P. M., Sargent, I. L., and Redman, C. W. (1988). Cell populations in human early pregnancy decidua: characterization and isolation of large granular lymphocytes by flow cytometry. *Immunology*, **65**, 129–134.

Tabata, T., McDonagh, S., Kawakatsu, H., and Pereira, L. (2006). Cytotrophoblasts infected with a pathogenic human cytomegalovirus strain dysregulate cell-matrix and cell-cell adhesion molecules: a quantitative analysis. *Placenta*, July 3. (Epub ahead of print)

Tugizov, S., Maidji, E., and Pereira, L. (1996). Role of apical and basolateral membranes in replication of human cytomegalovirus in polarized retinal pigment epithelial cells. *J. Gen. Virol.*, **77**, 61–74.

Wang, X., Huang, D. Y., Huong, S. M., and Huang, E. S. (2005). Integrin alphavbeta3 is a coreceptor for human cytomegalovirus. *Nat. Med.*, **11**, 515–521.

Wang, X., Huong, S. M., Chiu, M. L., Raab-Traub, N., and Huang, E. S. (2003). Epidermal growth factor receptor is a cellular receptor for human cytomegalovirus. *Nature*, **424**, 456–461.

Yamamoto-Tabata, T., McDonagh, S., Chang, H.-T., Fisher, S., and Pereira, L. (2004). Human cytomegalovirus interleukin-10 downregulates matrix metalloproteinase activity and impairs endothelial cell migration and placental cytotrophoblast invasiveness in vitro. *J. Virol.*, **78**, 2831–2840.

Zhou, Y., Damsky, C. H., Chiu, K., Roberts, J. M., and Fisher, S. J. (1993). Preeclampsia is associated with abnormal expression of adhesion molecules by invasive cytotrophoblasts. *J. Clin. Invest.*, **91**, 950–960.

Zhou, Y., Fisher, S. J., Janatpour, M. *et al.* (1997). Human cytotrophoblasts adopt a vascular phenotype as they differentiate. A strategy for successful endovascular invasion? *J. Clin. Invest.*, **99**, 2139–2151.

Part III

HHV-6A, 6B, and 7

46

HHV-6A, 6B, and 7: pathogenesis, host response, and clinical disease

Yasuko Mori and Koichi Yamanishi

Department of Microbiology, Osaka University Graduate School of Medicine, Japan

Human herpesvirus 6(HHV-6) is a human pathogen of emerging clinical significance. HHV-6 was first isolated from patients with lymphoproliferative disorders in 1986 (Salahuddin *et al.*, 1986). HHV-6 isolates are classified into two groups as variants A(HHV-6A) and variant B(HHV-6B) (Schirmer *et al.*, 1991. The two variants are closely related but show consistent differences in biological, immunological, epidemiological, and molecular properties. HHV-6B is the major causative agent of exanthem subitum (ES) (Yamanishi *et al.*, 1988), but no clear disease has yet been associated with HHV-6A.

Human herpesvirus 7 (HHV-7) was isolated in 1990 from a healthy individual whose cells were stimulated with antibody against CD3 and then incubated with interleukin-2 (Frenkel *et al.*, 1990). This virus is one of the causative agents of ES (Tanaka *et al.*, 1994). Therefore, HHV-6 and HHV-7 are also called Roseolovirus. HHV-6 and HHV-7 are ubiquitous, and more than 90% of adults have antibody to both viruses. These viruses have extensive homology and belong to the β-herpesvirus subfamily.

The genome of HHV-6A is 159 321 bp in size, has a base composition of 43% G + C, and contains 119 open reading frames. The overall structure is 143 kb bounded by 8 kb of direct repeats, DRL (left) and DRR (right), containing 0.35 kb of terminal and junctional arrays of human telomere-like simple repeats (Gompels *et al.*, 1995). A total of 115 potential open reading frames (ORFs) were identified within the 161 573-bp contiguous sequence of the entire HHV-6B genome (HST) (Isegawa *et al.*, 1999). The HHV-6B(Z29) genome is 162 114 bp long and is composed of a 144 528-bp unique segment (U) bracketed by 8793-bp direct repeats (DR). The genomic sequence allows prediction of a total of 119 unique open reading frames (ORFs), 9 of which are present only in HHV-6B. The overall nucleotide sequence identity between HHV-6A and HHV-6B is 90%. The most divergent regions are DR and the right end of the unique region, spanning ORFs U86 to U100. These regions have 85 and 72% nucleotide sequence identity, respectively (Dominguez *et al.*, 1999).

Virus entry and establishment of infection

Cell tropism in vitro

HHV-6A and HHV-6B replicate most efficiently in vitro in peripheral blood mononuclear cells (PBMCs) or cord blood lymphocytes (CBL), and several isolates have been adapted to grow efficiently in continuous T-cell lines. HHV-6 replicates in activated CD4 T lymphocytes in vivo. HHV-6A and HHV-6B differ in their capacities to replicate in specific transformed T-lymphocyte cell lines. Of the two most widely used strains of HHV-6A, strain GS is most commonly propagated in the T-cell line HSB-2 and strain U1102 is usually propagated in J JHAN cells. HHV-6B (Z29 or HST) is grown most often in primary lymphocytes and has been adapted for growth in the Molt-3 or MT-4–T cells line. While T cells are most widely used for propagation of HHV-6A and HHV-6B, cell lines of neural, epithelial, and fibroblastic origin have different levels of permissiveness for HHV-6 growth in vitro. However, none of these cells are in general use for routine propagation of the virus. In patients with dual infection, only HHV-6A persisted in CSF, which suggests that HHV-6A has greater neurotropism (Hall *et al.*, 1998). Furthermore, CD8 T-lymphocytes, gamma/delta T-lymphocytes and natural killer (NK) cells support HHV-6 replication in association with surface expression of CD4 (Lusso *et al.*, 1991a,b, 1995; Hall *et al.*, 1998).

Grivel *et al.* showed that HHV-6A and HHV-6B replicate in human lymphoid tissue, but have significant differences in effects on cellular viability and immunological phenotype (Grivel *et al.*, 2003). There is productive infection of both

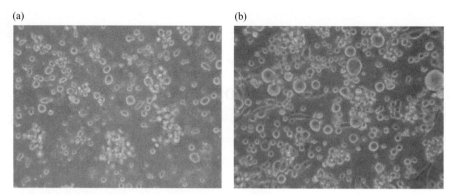

Fig. 46.1. Cytopathic effects of HHV-6A or HHH-7. (a) HSB-2 cells were infected with HHV-6A. (b) SupT1 cells were infected with HHV-7.

CD4+ and CD8+ T-cells, although HHV-6B is markedly less efficient than HHV-6A in targeting CD8+ T-cells. CD46 and CD3 are down-modulated in HHV-6 infected tissues. However CD3 down-modulation is restricted to infected cells, while the loss of CD46 expression is generalized. Thus, the down-modulation of CD46 in HHV-6 negative cells most likely represents an authentic bystander effect. Moreover, HHV-6 infection markedly enhanced the production of CC chemokine RANTES.

In contrast, HHV-7 has a narrow tropism for CD4+ T-cells, associated with infectivity for PHA-stimulated PBMCs, CBLs and in an immature T- cell line SupT1 (Cermelli et al., 1997). Both HHV-6 and HHV-7 induce a cytopathic effect in infected cells which is characterized by ballooning degeneration (Fig. 46.1).

Cell tropism in vivo

The in vivo host tissue range of HHV-6 is broader than its in vitro host range might suggest and includes lymph nodes, lymphocytes, macrophages and monocytes, kidney tubule endothelial cells, salivary glands, and CNS tissues, where viral gene products have been localized to neurons and oligodendrocytes.

HHV-6 genomes and/or antigens are detetable in lymph nodes of patients with sinus histiocytosis with massive lymphadenopathy (SHML) (Levine et al., 1992), tubular epithelial cells, endothelial cells and histiocytes in kidney (Kurata et al., 1990), salivary glands (Fox et al., 1990), and central nervous system (CNS) tissues, where viral gene products have been localized to neurons and oligodendrocytes (Luppi et al., 1994). HHV-6 is also detected in lesions of Langerhans cell histiocytosis in the syndrome of Langerhans cell histiocytosis (Leahy et al., 1993).

HHV-6 was isolated from CD4+ CD8− and CD3+ CD4+ mature T-lymphocytes but could not be isolated from CD4− CD8+, CD4− CD8−, and CD3− T-cells in the peripheral blood of exanthem subitum patients. HHV-6 predominantly infected CD4+ CD8+, CD4+ CD8−, and CD3+ CD4+ cells with mature phenotypes and rarely infected CD4− CD8+ cells from cord blood mononuclear cells, which suggested a predominant tropism of HHV-6 for mature CD4 T-lymphocytes (Takahashi et al., 1989).

So far, two cell types have been recognized as sites of HHV-7 infection in vivo, including CD4+ T-lymphocytes and epithelial cells of salivary glands (Black et al., 1993). HHV-7 is frequently isolated from saliva of healthy adults (Wyatt and Frenkel, 1992). A recent study showed that cells expressing the HHV-7 structural antigen were also detectable in lungs, skin, and mammary glands. Liver, kidney, and tonsils were also positive, although the number of HHV-7-positive cells was low. Large intestine, spleen, and brain were negative for HHV-7 infection (Kempf et al., 1998).

Entry

HHV-6 is characterized by a broad tropism for human cell types but a narrow range of host species. Santoro et al. (1999) identified human CD46 as the cellular receptor for HHV-6. CD46 is a ubiquitous type 1 glycoprotein expressed on the surfaces of all nucleated human cells (Seya et al., 1990). It was originally purified as a complement (C) regulatory protein; it binds C3b and C4b on host cells to allow factor I-mediated inactivation of these C fragments, and it plays an important role in protecting host cells from autologous C protein (Seya et al., 1990). CD46 is also a cellular receptor for measles virus. Evidence for CD46 receptor activity included (i) A selective and progressive down-regulation of the surface membrane expression of CD46 in activated human CD4+ T-cells in the course of HHV-6A and HHV-6B infection, (ii) inhibition of HHV-6 infection and associated cell fusion by Mab against CD46 and by soluble CD46, and (iii) non-human cells being rendered susceptible to HHV-6-mediated membrane fusion and HHV-6 entry by expression of CD46. However, the expression of CD46 was not sufficient for HHV-6 fusion and infection in all human cell types, suggesting either that a specific co-receptor is needed or that some cells express an inhibitor of the CD46 receptor activity. Mori et al. (2002) found that HHV-6A, but not HHV-6B can mediate fusion-from-without (FFWO) in a variety of human cells, including Vero cells which are an old world monkey cell line. Chinese hamster ovary (CHO) cells are highly resistant to infection by HHV-6 and cell-cell fusion induced by HHV-6A. However HHV-6A, but not HHV-6B induced cell–cell fusion in CHO cells expressing human CD46 without virus replication. Thus, the induction of cell- cell- fusion in the target cells by HHV-6A requires human CD46. Thus, HHV-6A mediates syncytia formation in target cells expressing human CD46 without associated virus replication. Human CD46 is composed of four short consensus repeats (SCRs), a Ser/Thr(ST)-rich domain, 13-amino-acid sequence of unknown significance (UK), a transmembrane domain, and a cytoplasmic tail (CYT) (Seya et al., 1990). The SCR2, -3 and - 4 of the CD46 ectodomain were essential for the HHV-6A induced cell-cell fusion. Another report indicates that the SCR domains 2 and 3 are required for HHV-6 receptor activity (Greenstone et al., 2002).

The products encoded by the U100 gene of HHV-6A have been reported to form a complex containing polypeptides. The U100 gene complex is a major component of the HHV-6 virion and a target for virus-neutralizing antibodies. The gene has an intron-exon structure, resulting in a highly spliced mRNA transcript, and is unique to HHV-6 and HHV-7 (Pfeiffer et al., 1995; Skrincosky et al., 2001). U100 gene products of HHV-6A are mainly composed of 80- and 78-kDa glycoproteins and furthermore, the 80-kDa gene product is the third glycoprotein component of the gH-gL complex in HHV-6A infected cells (Mori et al., 2003a,b). Based on these characteristics, U100 gene products were designated as glycoprotein Q(gQ). The gH-gL-gQ complex is identified as a viral ligand for human CD46 (Mori et al., 2003a,b). The gH-gL complex alone or gQ alone in a transient expression system were unable to bind to CD46. The interaction with CD46 might require additional associations or modification in HHV-6 infected cells. Santoro et al. showed that gH of HHV-6 is a ligand for human CD46, however gH alone does not bind to CD46, and the interaction between gH and CD46 requires HHV-6 infection (Santoro et al., 2003). Therefore, to date, whether one glycoprotein of the gH–gL–gQ complex binds to CD46 directly or whether the steric conformation of the complex itself is required for the interaction with CD46 is unknown.

The entry of herpes viruses into cells is a complex process that is still incompletely understood. In several cases, it appears to require not only a cellular receptor to interact with the virus attachment protein but also at least one additional molecule to interact with the virus and facilitate penetration. Studies on other herpesviruses have provided indirect evidence of a role for homologue of the gH-gL and gB molecules in membrane fusion. In HHV-6, specific monoclonal antibodies against glycoprotein H (gH) and glycoprotein B (gB) inhibited virus-induced cell fusion event and infection (Foa Tomasi et al., 1991; Mori et al., 2002). Considering the previous reports, it seems likely that the process involves several steps. First, HHV-6 gH-gL-gQ complex binds to CD46 and at the same time, gB binds to an unknown cellular molecule, thereby triggering fusogenic activity. Subsequently, viral envelope glycoproteins, probably gB and gH-gL-gQ may act to induce envelope–cell or cell–cell fusion. gB or gH or both are candidates for the actual fusogenic glycoprotens. HHV-7 infects CD4+ T-lymphocye in vitro. The glycoprotein CD4, a member of the immunoglobulin superfamily, is a critical component of the receptor for HHV-7 (Lusso et al., 1994). A selective and progressive downregulation of the surface membrane expression of CD4 was observed in human CD4+ T-cells in the course of HHV-7 infection. Various murine monoclonal antibodies (MAbs) to CD4 and the recombinant soluble form of human CD4 caused a dose-dependent inhibition of HHV-7 infection in primary CD4+ T-lymphocytes. Moreover, radiolabeled HHV-7 specifically bound to cervical carcinoma cells (HeLa) expressing human CD4. However, HHV-7 can infect cells that do not express detectable CD4. It is likely that other host molecules act as receptors; the need for multiple sequential receptors to enable cell-to-cell migration of the virus in tissues is a well-documented phenomenon in other herpesviruses.

The human immunodeficiency virus type 1 (HIV-1) co-receptors, CXC-chemokine receptor (CXCR)4 and CC-chemokine receptor(CCR)5, have been studied to determine whether they serve similar functions for HHV-6A, HHV-6B and HHV-7. Cells from individuals lacking CCR5 were able to support growth of all three viruses, and these individuals were seropositive for the viruses, indicating that this molecule is not essential for viral replication. HHV-7 infection also causes a progressive loss of the surface CXCR4 in CD4(+) T-cells, accompanied by a reduced intracellular Ca^{2+} flux and chemotaxis in response to stromal cell-derived factor-1 (SDF-1), the specific CXCR4 ligand. Moreover, CXCR4 is downregulated from the surface of HHV-7-infected T-cells independently of CD4. Because intracellular CXCR4 antigen and mRNA levels are unaffected in productively HHV-7-infected cells, the down-regulation of CXCR4 apparently does not involve a transcriptional block (Secchiero et al., 1998). However, another report demonstrates that CXCR4 is not involved in HHV-7 infection. The natural ligand of CXCR4, SDF-1alpha, was not able to inhibit HHV-7 infection in SupT1 cells or in CD8(+) T-cell-depleted peripheral blood mononuclear cells. Also, a specific CXCR4 antagonist with potent antiviral activity against T-tropic HIV strains (50% inhibitory concentration IC(50), 1 to 10 ng/ml), completely failed to inhibit HHV-7 infection (IC(50), >250 μ/ml) (Zhang et al., 2000). Unlike HIV-1, HHV-6 and HHV-7 infections do not require expression of CXCR4 or CCR5, whereas marked down-regulation of CXCR4 is induced by these viruses (Yasukawa et al., 1999).

Two HHV-7 glycoproteins have been identified as being able to bind the cell surface proteoglycans heparan and heparan sulfate (Secchiero et al., 1997a,b; Skrincosky et al., 2001). They are the virion glycoprotein, gB and spliced glycoprotein encoded by U100. Thus, soluble heparin was found to block HHV-7 infection and syncytium formation in the SupT1 cell line. The CD4 antigen is a critical component of the receptor for the T-lymphotropic HHV-7 suggesting that heparin-like molecules also play an important role in the HHV-7-entry process. As described above, gB is one of the HHV-7 envelope proteins involved in the adsorption of virus-to-cell surface proteoglycans (Secchiero et al., 1997a,b). Analysis of the biochemical properties of recombinant gp65, (U100 gene products), also revealed a specific interaction with heparin and heparan sulfate proteoglycans and not with closely related molecules such as N-acetylheparin and de-N-sulfated heparin, suggesting that HHV-7 gp65 may contribute to viral attachment to cell surface proteoglycans (Skrincosky et al., 2001). The products of U100 are targets for complement-independent neutralization.

Envelope glycoproteins for entry process

The genes U39 and U48 of HHV-6 and HHV-7 encode the conserved surface glycoproteins gB and gH, which contribute to virus-cell fusion.

HHV-6 gH forms complexes with glycoprotein L (gL, encoded by U82), resulting in the formation of a gp100 complex (Liu et al., 1993). Recently, gQ (encoded by U100) was shown to be a third component of gH-gL complex in HHV-6 (Mori et al., 2003a,b). This gQ is unique to the genus of HHV-6 and HHV-7. The gQ gene is subject to differential splicing, and a number of enveloped glycoprotein –encoding genes, gQ genes of HHV-6A and –6B demonstrate only 72.1% sequence identity. This glycoprotein may have a role in the differential consequences of HHV-6A and B infections. Along with gB and gH, gQ contains epitopes recognized by variant specific neutralizing antibodies.

An unusual feature of HHV-6 in comparison to other herpesviruses is the lack of viral glycoproteins in the plasma membrane (Cirone et al., 1994). HSB-2 T-lymphoid cells and human cord blood mononuclear cells infected with HHV-6 reveal the presence, in the cell cytoplasm, of annulate lamellae (AL), which are absent in uninfected cells (Cardinali et al., 1998). Viral glycoproteins are stored in newly formed annulate lamellae, which function as a viral glycoprotein storage compartment and as a putative site of O-glycosylation. It is proposed that, during viral morphogenesis, nucleocapsids released from the nucleus have a primary envelope that lacks glycoproteins but, in the cytoplasm, this is removed and replaced by a secondary envelope containing glycoproteins acquired from the annulate lamella. Further modification of glycoproteins by glycosylation during transit through the Golgi apparatus occurs before mature virions are released.

Spread in host, mechanisms of tissue damage

Growth properties

HHV-6 and HHV-7 replication cycles are approximately 3 days in activated CBLs grown in the presence of IL-2 or PHA. Even in most permissive systems, the infectious yields are relatively low, commonly ranging from 10^3 to 10^5 infectious units per ml. Centrifugal infection increases the infectious titer.

Effects of virus infection on host cells

HHV-6 infection has profound effects on host cells. These lead to the development of the classic cytopathic effect of ballooning and multinucleated giant cells.

In the case of HHV-7, multinucleated giant cells occur, not by fusion of cells into syncytia, but by polyploidization (Secchiero et al., 1998). The giant cells, which represent the hallmark of in vitro HHV-7 infection, arise from single CD4(+) T-cells undergoing a process of polyploidization that is linked to disregulation of cyclin-dependent kinase cdc2 and cyclin B. This leads to an accumulation of cells in the G_2 to M phase of the cell cycle, with nuclei continuing to reproduce in the absence of cell division (Secchiero et al., 1998).

Several cytokines can be induced by HHV-6 and HHV-7 infection. Interferon-alpha, interleukin 1 beta, and tumor necrosis factor are induced by HHV-6 (Kikuta et al., 1990; Flamand et al., 1991). But, exposure of human macrophages to HHV-6 profoundly impairs their ability to produce IL-12 upon stimulation with IFN-gamma and LPS, providing a novel potential mechanism of HHV-6-mediated immunosuppression (Smith et al., 2003). HHV-6 can infect NK cells and T lymphocytes. HHV-6 and HHV-7 induces IL-15 in human PBMC and increases their NK activity (Flamand et al., 1996; Atedzoe et al., 1997; Gosselin et al., 1999). The induction of NK cell activity by HHV-6 is abrogated by monoclonal antibodies to IL-15 but not by mAbs to other cytokines (IFN-alpha, IFN-gamma, TNF-alpha, TNF-beta, IL-2, IL-12). IL-15 protein synthesis is increased in response to HHV-6, and addition of IL-15 to PBMC cultures is found to severely curtail HHV-6 expression. Taken together, the host responds to HHV-6 and HHV-7 infection by up-regulating IL-15 production, which then results in an enhancement of NK cell activity; this, in turn, may play a major role in the control of the viral infection (Flamand et al., 1996; Atedzoe et al., 1997; Gosselin et al., 1999).

HHV-6 affects HIV-1 infection in a coreceptor-dependent manner, suppressing CCR5-tropic but not CXCR4-tropic HIV-1 replication. HHV-6 increases the production of the CCR5 ligand RANTES CC-chemokine, the most potent HIV-inhibitory CC chemokine, and that exogenous RANTES mimics the effects of HHV-6 on HIV-1, providing a mechanism for the selective blockade of CCR5-tropic HIV-1 (Grivel et al., 2001). HHV6 infection induces de novo synthesis of the RANTES in endothelial cells as well (Caruso et al., 2003).

HHV-6A infection induces cell-surface expression of CD4, which then allows infection by HIV-1 of cells such as gamma/delta T cells that were previously refractile to infection (Lusso et al., 1991a,b, 1995; Caruso et al., 2003). HHV-6A, but not HHV-6B or HHV-7, down-regulates cell surface expression of CD3, and HHV-7 predominantly down-regulates CD4 (Furukawa et al., 1994).

HHV-6A, HHV-6B and HHV-7 were evaluated for their effects on in vitro colony formation of hemopoietic progenitor cells derived from CBLs. Formation of both granulocyte/macrophage and erythroid colonies was suppressed after infection with HHV-6B. Although HHV-6A suppressed the formation of erythroid colonies as efficiently as HHV-6B, HHV-6A did not exhibit significant suppressive effect on the formation of granulocyte/macrophage colonies. HHV-7 had no effect on either lineage (Isomura et al., 1997). Furthermore, the suppressive effects of HHV-6 on thrombopoiesis in vitro was evaluated. Using CBLs as the source of hematopoietic progenitors, two types of colonies, megakaryocyte colony-forming units and non-megakaryocyte colony-forming units colonies, were established. HHV-6A and HHV-6B inhibited thrombopoietin-inducible both megakaryocyte and non-megakaryocyte colony formation. In contrast, HHV-7 had no effect on thrombopoietin-inducible- colony formation (Isomura et al., 2000). More differentiated CD34+ cells, which were a major source of hematopoietic progenitor cells, were more susceptible to the effects of HHV-6, indicating that the targets for hematopoietic suppression by HHV-6 are the differentiated cells (Isomura et al., 2003). In contrast, in bone marrow-derived cells, both HHV-6A and HHV-6B suppressed erythroid, granulocyte-macrophage, and multipotential precursors of the granulocyte, erythrocyte, monocyte, and megakaryocyte lineages (Carrigan and Knox, 1995). The mechanisms of cell death in the human CD4+ T-cell line J JHAN mediated by HHV-6 were investigated (Inoue et al., 1997) by transmission electron microscopy infected cells showed characteristics of apoptosis, such as chromatin condensation and fragmentation of nuclei, but few virus particles were detected in apoptotic cells. Two-color flow cytometric analysis revealed that DNA fragmentation was present predominantly in uninfected cells but not in cells that were productively infected with HHV-6 (Inoue et al., 1997). Acute in vitro HHV-7 infection induced (i) the formation of giant multinucleated syncytia, which eventually underwent necrotic lysis, and (ii) single-cell apoptosis. Using electron microscopy analysis, all syncytia contained large amounts of virions and most cells within syncytia them exhibited clear evidence of necrosis, whereas apoptosis was predominantly observed in single cells. Although empty viral capsids could be identified in the cytoplasm of approximately 25% of single cells exhibiting an apoptotic morphology, few mature virions were observed in these cells. Thus, it appears that apoptosis occurred predominantly in uninfected bystander cells but not in productively HHV-7-infected cells (Secchiero et al., 1997a,b). Apoptosis induced by HHV-6 in cord blood mononuclear cells (CBMCs) was also investigated. CBMCs prestimulated with phytohemagglutinin (PHA) were infected with HHV-6 and cultured with interleukin 2 (IL-2) for 5 days. The percentage of the hypodiploid fraction by cell cycle analysis and the percentage of cells showing apoptosis determined by terminal deoxytransferase (TdT)- mediated dUTP nick end-labeling (TUNEL) assay were significantly higher in HHV-6-infected CBMC compared with uninfected CBMC. 7A6 antigen, induced on the mitochondria membrane in apoptotic cells, was mainly expressed in CD4+ cells; 7A6 antigen was also detected in HHV-6-infected cells as determined by expression of gH.

Thus, HHV-6 induces apoptosis in HHV-6-infected CBMCs different from T-cells lines (Ichimi et al., 1999). In order to confirm that apoptosis of CD4+ T lymphocytes also occurs in HHV-6 infection in vivo, apoptosis of lymphocytes isolated from nine patients with exanthem subitum and from an adult patient with severe HHV-6 infection was examined (Yasukawa et al., 1998). PBMCs were cultured for 3 days and apoptosis of lymphocytes was examined by flow cytometry of propidium iodide-stained DNA. The percentages of hypodiploid DNA, indicating apoptosis, in lymphocytes from 10 patients with HHV-6 infection were significantly higher than those from five infant patients with non-infectious diseases and five healthy adults ($P < 0–0002$). DNA fragmentation was also detected in lymphocytes from patients with HHV-6 infection. Apoptosis appears to occur predominantly in CD4+ T-lymphocytes and HHV-6 is isolated from the CD4+ T lymphocyte fraction (Yasukawa et al., 1998).

Accordingly, in CBLs, infected cells are apoptotic, while in transformed cells, infected cells die by necrotic lysis and apoptosis is triggered in non-productively infected cells. The latter observation suggests that the virus may be able to inhibit apoptosis in at least some cells and that its replication might be enhanced by suppression of apoptosis.

To dissect the underlying molecular events, the role of death-inducing ligands belonging to the tumor necrosis factor (TNF) cytokine superfamily was investigated (Secchiero et al., 2001a,b). HHV-7 selectively up-regulated the expression of TNF-related apoptosis-inducing ligand (TRAIL), but not that of CD95 ligand or TNF-alpha in SupT1 or primary activated CD4(+) T-cells. Moreover, in a cell-to-cell-contact assay, HHV-7-infected CD4(+) T-lymphocytes were cytotoxic for bystander uninfected CD4(+) T-cells through the TRAIL pathway. By contrast, HHV-7 infection caused a marked decrease of surface TRAIL-R1, but not of TRAIL-R2, CD95, TNF-R1, or TNF-R2. Of note, the down-regulation of TRAIL-R1 selectively occurred in cells coexpressing HHV-7 antigens that became resistant to TRAIL-mediated cytotoxicity. These data suggest that the TRAIL-mediated induction of T-cell death may represent an important immune evasion mechanism of HHV-7, helping the virus to persist in the host organism throughout its lifetime (Secchiero et al., 2001a,b).

Disease consequences

Clinical features in hosts

Primary infection
Both HHV-6 and HHV-7 are ubiquitous viruses, and infection occurs during infancy. HHV-6B is a causative agent of ES (Yamanishi et al., 1988). In most cases, ES is benign; it is associated with other symptoms including diarrhea, cough, lymph node swelling as bulging fontanel. ES is a common disease of infants all over the world. Typically, the infant gets sudden fever, which lasts for a few days, and a rash appears on the trunk and face and spreads to the lower extremities as the fever subsides. In adults, primary infections can cause mononucleosis like disease and hemophagocytic syndrome (Akashi et al., 1993). HHV-7 can also cause ES and was isolated from PBMCs of a infant with typical ES (Tanaka et al., 1994). The median age of children with primary HHV-7 infection was 26 months, which is significantly older than that of children with primary HHV-6 infection (median, 9 months).

Immune response during primary infection
The early immune response was studied by assessing interferon (IFN) and natural killer cell activity in 13 patients with ES associated with HHV-6 infection during the acute and convalescent phases (Takahashi et al., 1992). Only IFN-alpha was significantly increased in the plasma of patients during the acute febrile phase compared with the convalescent period. The inhibitory effect of IFN-alpha and IFN-beta on HHV-6 replication was demonstrated in vitro with cord blood mononuclear cells. Natural killer cell activity was also significantly augmented in the acute phase, especially in the exanthem period, compared to in the convalescent phase. These results suggest that the enhanced IFN-alpha response and natural killer cell activity in the acute early phase of the disease may play pivotal roles in the recovery from ES.

Other symptoms associated with primary HHV-6 and 7 infection
The primary infection by HHV-6 and HHV-7 can cause a highly febrile illness in childhood, complicated by seizures (Torigoe et al., 1996). Cases of possible HHV-6-associated encephalitis in young children have been reported (Asano et al., 1992). Self-limited involvement of the central nervous system (CNS) is a relatively common complication of primary infection with HHV-6 in normal children. Liver dysfunction (Asano et al., 1990; Tajiri et al., 1990), idiopathic thrombocytopenic purpura (Yoshikawa et al., 1993) are also associated with HHV-6 infection.

Reactivation of HHV-6 and its clinical symptoms
Since HHV-6 and HHV-7 establish latency following primary infection, they are important pathogens in immunocompromised hosts. Reactivation of HHV-6 and HHV-7 ocurres in patients after bone marrow transplantation,

solid organ transplantation such as liver, renal and heart transplantation, and AIDS.

Bone marrow transplantation (BMT)

Asymptomatic HHV-6 reactivations appear to be common following allogeneic BMT (Cone et al., 1999), but HHV-6 reactivation associated with symptoms such as bone marrow suppression, encephalitis (Drobyski et al., 1994; Tsujimura et al., 1998; Rodrigues, 1999), pneumonitis (Cone et al., 1993) and acute graft-versus-host disease (GVHD) in BMT recipients has also been recognized. Idiopathic marrow suppression occurred frequently in patients with concurrent HHV-6 viremia (Drobyski et al., 1993). Infection with HHV-6 has been correlated with the development of skin rashes. HHV-6 DNA was detected in skin and/or rectal biopsies more frequently in allogeneic recipients with severe GVHD (92%) than in those with either moderate (55%) or mild GVHD (22%), suggesting that the presence of HHV-6 DNA in the skin or rectum may be a factor in determining GVHD severity (Appleton et al., 1995).

Solid organ transplantation

HHV-6 infection after liver transplantation is associated with an immunosuppressive state (Singh et al., 1995, 2002a,b). Acute febrile illness characterized by life-threatening thrombocytopenia, progressive encephalopathy and skin rash occurred with invasive HHV-6 infection in a liver transplant recipient (Singh et al., 1995). Prolonged suppression of the HHV-6 memory response, but not overall T-helper cell function was documented and may play a role in the pathogenesis of HHV-6 infection in liver transplant recipients (Singh et al., 2002a,b). The memory response to CMV after liver transplantation was significantly more robust than to HHV-6 (Singh et al., 2002a,b). Griffiths et al. conducted a prospective study of the possible relationship of HHV-6 and HHV-7 infection with clinical symptoms after liver transplantation (Griffiths et al., 1999). Although the virus load for HCMV was significantly greater than that for HHV-6 or HHV-7, HHV-6 and HHV-7 may be the cause of some episodes of hepatitis and pyrexia (Griffiths et al., 1999). HHV-6 and CMV are significantly and independently associated with biopsy-proven graft rejection after liver transplantation (Griffiths et al., 2000).

AIDS

Reactivation of HHV-6 has been reported to be possibly associated with interstitial pneumonia, encephalitis, and retinal disorder in AIDS patients, but specific clinical syndromes associated with reactivation are rare.

The other possible associated diseases

Multiple sclerosis (MS)

Several studies have suggested an association between HHV-6 and MS (Challoner et al., 1995; Soldan et al., 1997). However, negative results were also seen in other reports (Coates and Bell, 1998). There was no significant difference between MS patients and non-MS-patients by staining brains immunocytochemically (Coates and Bell, 1998). Therefore, whether HHV-6 contributes to MS pathogenesis in unclear.

Drug hypersensitivity

Drug-induced hypersensitivity syndrome is characterized by a severe, potentially fatal, multi organ hypersensitivity reaction that usually appears after prolonged exposure to certain drugs. Its delayed onset and clinical resemblance to infectious mononucleosis suggest that underlying viral infections may trigger and activate the disease in susceptible individuals receiving these drugs. Reactivation of HHV-6, possibly in concert with HHV-7 may contribute to the development of a severe drug-induced hypersensitivity syndrome (Suzuki et al., 1998; Tohyama et al., 1998).

REFERENCES

Akashi, K., Eizuru, Y., Sumiyoshi, Y. et al. (1993). Brief report: severe infectious mononucleosis-like syndrome and primary human herpesvirus 6 infection in an adult [see comments]. *N. Engl. J. Med.*, **329**(3), 168–171.

Appleton, A. L., Sviland, L., Peiris, J. S. et al. (1995). Human herpes virus-6 infection in marrow graft recipients: role in pathogenesis of graft-versus-host disease. Newcastle upon Tyne Bone Marrow Transport Group. *Bone Marrow Transpl*, **16**(6), 777–782.

Asano, Y., Yoshikawa, T., Kajita, Y. et al. (1992). Fatal encephalitis/encephalopathy in primary human herpesvirus-6 infection. *Arch. Dis. Child.*, **67**(12), 1484–1485.

Asano, Y., Yoshikawa, T., Suga, S. et al. (1990). Fatal fulminant hepatitis in an infant with human herpesvirus-6 infection [letter]. *Lancet*, **335**(8693), 862–863.

Atedzoe, B. N., Ahmad, A., and Menezes, J. (1997). Enhancement of natural killer cell cytotoxicity by the human herpesvirus-7 via IL-15 induction. *J. Immunol.*, **159**(10), 4966–4972.

Black, J. B., Inoue, N., Kite-Powel, K. et al. (1993). Frequent isolation of human herpesvirus 7 from saliva. *Virus Res.*, **29**(1), 91–98.

Cardinali, G., Gentile, M., Cirone, M. et al. (1998). Viral glycoproteins accumulate in newly formed annulate lamellae following infection of lymphoid cells by human herpesvirus 6. *J. Virol.*, **72**(12), 9738–9746.

Carrigan, D. R. and Knox, K. K. (1995). Bone marrow suppression by human herpesvirus-6: comparison of the A and B variants of the virus [letter; comment]. *Blood*, **86**(2), 835–836.

Caruso, A., Favilli, F., Rotola, A. *et al.* (2003). Human herpesvirus-6 modulates RANTES production in primary human endothelial cell cultures. *J. Med. Virol.*, **70**(3), 451–458.

Cermelli, C., Pietrosemoli, P., Meacci, M. *et al.* (1997). SupT-1: a cell system suitable for an efficient propagation of both HHV-7 and HHV-6 variants A and B. *New Microbiol.*, **20**(3), 187–196.

Challoner, P. B., Smith, K. T., Parker, J. D. *et al.* (1995). Plaque-associated expression of human herpesvirus 6 in multiple sclerosis. *Proc. Natl Acad. Sci. USA*, **92**(16), 7440–7444.

Cirone, M., Campadelli Fiume, G., Foa-Tomasi, L. *et al.* (1994). Human herpesvirus 6 envelope glycoproteins B and H-L complex are undetectable on the plasma membrane of infected lymphocytes. *AIDS Res. Hum. Retroviruses*, **10**(2), 175–179.

Coates, A. R. and Bell, J. (1998). HHV-6 and multiple sclerosis. *Nat. Med.*, **4**(5), 537–538.

Cone, R. W., Hackman, R. C., Huang, M. L. *et al.* (1993). Human herpesvirus 6 in lung tissue from patients with pneumonitis after bone marrow transplantation [see comments]. *N. Engl. J. Med.*, **329**(3), 156–161.

Cone, R. W., Huang, M. L., Corey, L. *et al.* (1999). Human herpesvirus 6 infections after bone marrow transplantation: clinical and virologic manifestations [In Process Citation]. *J. Infect. Dis.*, **179**(2), 311–318.

Dockrell, D. H. (2003). Human herpesvirus 6: molecular biology and clinical features. *J. Med. Microbiol.*, **52**(Pt 1), 5–18.

Dominguez, G., Dambaugh, T. R., Stamey, F. R. *et al.* (1999). Human herpesvirus 6B genome sequence: coding content and comparison with human herpesvirus 6A. *J. Virol.*, **73**(10), 8040–8052.

Drobyski, W. R., Dunne, W. M., Burd, E. M. *et al.* (1993). Human herpesvirus-6 (HHV-6) infection in allogeneic bone marrow transplant recipients: evidence of a marrow-suppressive role for HHV-6 in vivo. *J. Infect. Dis.*, **167**(3), 735–739.

Drobyski, W. R., Knox, K. K., Majewski, D. *et al.* (1994). Brief report: fatal encephalitis due to variant B human herpesvirus-6 infection in a bone marrow-transplant recipient. *N. Engl. J. Med.*, **330**(19), 1356–1360.

Flamand, L., Gosselin, J., and Petlett, P. E. (1991). Human herpesvirus 6 induces interleukin-1 beta and tumor necrosis factor alpha, but not interleukin-6, in peripheral blood mononuclear cell cultures. *J. Virol.*, **65**(9), 5105–5110.

Flamand, L., Stefanescu, I., and Menezes, J. (1996). Human herpesvirus-6 enhances natural killer cell cytotoxicity via IL-15. *J. Clin. Invest.*, **97**(6), 1373–1381.

Foa Tomasi, L., Boscaro, A., di Eaeta, S. *et al.* (1991). Monoclonal antibodies to gp100 inhibit penetration of human herpesvirus 6 and polykaryocyte formation in susceptible cells. *J. Virol.*, **65**(8), 4124–4129.

Fox, J. D., Briggs, M., Ward, P. A. *et al.* (1990). Human herpesvirus 6 in salivary glands [see comments]. *Lancet*, **336**(8715), 590–593.

Frenkel, N., Schirmer, E. C., Wyatt, L. S. *et al.* (1990). Isolation of a new herpesvirus from human CD4+ T cells. *Proc. Natl Acad. Sci. USA*, **87**(2), 748–752.

Furukawa, M., Yasukawa, M., Yakushijin, Y. *et al.* (1994). Distinct effects of human herpesvirus 6 and human herpesvirus 7 on surface molecule expression and function of CD4+ T cells. *J. Immunol.*, **152**(12), 5768–5775.

Gompels, U. A., Nicholas, J., Lawrence, G. *et al.* (1995). The DNA sequence of human herpesvirus-6: structure, coding content, and genome evolution. *Virology*, **209**(1), 29–51.

Gosselin, J., TomoIu, A., Gallo, R. C. *et al.* (1999). Interleukin-15 as an activator of natural killer cell-mediated antiviral response. *Blood*, **94**(12), 4210–4219.

Greenstone, H. L., Santoro, F., Lusso, P. *et al.* (2002). Human herpesvirus 6 and measles virus employ distinct CD46 domains for receptor function. *J. Biol. Chem.*, **277**(42), 39112–39118.

Griffiths, P. D., Ait-Khaled, M., Bearcroft, C. P. *et al.* (1999). Human herpesviruses 6 and 7 as potential pathogens after liver transplant: prospective comparison with the effect of cytomegalovirus. *J. Med. Virol.*, **59**(4), 496–501.

Griffiths, P. D., Clark, D. A., and Emery, V. C. (2000). Beta-herpesviruses in transplant recipients [In Process Citation]. *J. Antimicrob. Chemother.*, **45**(Suppl T3), 29–34.

Grivel, J. C., Ito, Y., Faga, G. *et al.* (2001). Suppression of CCR5- but not CXCR4-tropic HIV-1 in lymphoid tissue by human herpesvirus 6. *Nat. Med.*, **7**(11), 1232–1235.

Grivel, J. C., Santoro, F., Chen, S. *et al.* (2003). Pathogenic effects of human herpesvirus 6 in human lymphoid tissue ex vivo. *J. Virol.*, **77**(15), 8280–8289.

Hall, C. B., Caserta, M. T., Schnabel, K. C. *et al.* (1998). Persistence of human herpesvirus 6 according to site and variant: possible greater neurotropism of variant A. *Clin. Infect. Dis.*, **26**(1), 132–137.

Ichimi, R., Jin-no, T., and Ito, M. (1999). Induction of apoptosis in cord blood lymphocytes by HHV-6 [In Process Citation]. *J. Med. Virol.*, **58**(1), 63–68.

Inoue, Y., Yasukawa, M., and Fugita, S. (1997). Induction of T-cell apoptosis by human herpesvirus 6. *J. Virol.*, **71**(5), 3751–3759.

Isegawa, Y., Mukai, T., Nakano, K. *et al.* (1999). Comparison of the complete DNA sequences of human herpesvirus 6 variants A and B. *J. Virol.*, **73**(10), 8053–8063.

Isomura, H., Yamada, M., Namba, H. *et al.* (1997). Suppressive effects of human herpesvirus 6 on in vitro colony formation of hematopoietic progenitor cells. *J. Med. Virol.*, **52**(4), 406–412.

Isomura, H., Yoshida, M., Namba, H. *et al.* (2000). Suppressive effects of human herpesvirus-6 on thrombopoietin-inducible megakaryocytic colony formation in vitro. *J. Gen. Virol.*, **81**(Pt 3), 663–673.

Isomura, H., Yoshida, M., Namba, H. *et al.* (2003). Interaction of human herpesvirus 6 with human CD34 positive cells. *J. Med. Virol.*, **70**(3), 444–450.

Kempf, W., Adams, V., Mirandola, P. *et al.* (1998). Persistence of human herpesvirus 7 in normal tissues detected by expression of a structural antigen. *J. Infect. Dis.*, **178**(3), 841–845.

Kikuta, H., Nakane, A., Lu, H. *et al.* (1990). Interferon induction by human herpesvirus 6 in human mononuclear cells. *J. Infect. Dis.*, **162**(1), 35–38.

Kurata, T., Iwasaki, T., Sata, T. *et al.* (1990). Viral pathology of human herpesvirus 6 infection. *Adv. Exp. Med. Biol.*, **278**, 39–47.

Leahy, M. A., Krejci, S. M., Friednash, M. *et al.* (1993). Human herpesvirus 6 is present in lesions of Langerhans cell histiocytosis. *J. Invest. Dermatol.*, **101**(5), 642–645.

Levine, P. H., Jahan, N., Murari, P. *et al.* (1992). Detection of human herpesvirus 6 in tissues involved by sinus histiocytosis with massive lymphadenopathy (Rosai–Dorfman disease). *J. Infect. Dis.*, **166**(2), 291–295.

Liu, D. X., Gompels, U. A., Nicholas, J. *et al.* (1993). Identification and expression of the human herpesvirus 6 glycoprotein H and interaction with an accessory 40K glycoprotein. *J. Gen. Virol.*, **74**(Pt 9), 1847–1857.

Luppi, M., Barozzi, P., Maiorana, A. *et al.* (1994). Human herpesvirus 6 infection in normal human brain tissue [letter]. *J. Infect. Dis.*, **169**(4), 943–944.

Lusso, P., Malnati, M., de Mania, A. *et al.* (1991a). Productive infection of CD4+ and CD8+ mature human T cells populations and clones by human herpesvirus 6. Transcriptional downregulation of CD3. *J. Immunol.*, **147**(2), 685–691.

Lusso, P., De Maria, A., Malnati, M. *et al.* (1991a). Induction of CD4 and susceptibility to HIV-1 infection in human CD8+ T lymphocytes by human herpesvirus 6. *Nature*, **349**(6309), 533–535.

Lusso, P., Secchiero, P., Crowley, R. W. *et al.* (1994). CD4 is a critical component of the receptor for human herpesvirus 7: interference with human immunodeficiency virus. *Proc. Natl Acad. Sci. USA*, **91**(9), 3872–3876.

Lusso, P., Garzino-Demo, A., Crowley, R. W. *et al.* (1995). Infection of gamma/delta T lymphocytes by human herpesvirus 6: transcriptional induction of CD4 and susceptibility to HIV infection. *J. Exp. Med.*, **181**(4), 1303–1310.

Mori, Y., Seya, T., Huang, H. L. *et al.* (2002). Human herpesvirus 6 variant A but not variant B induces fusion from without in a variety of human cells through a human herpesvirus 6 entry receptor, CD46. *J. Virol.*, **76**(13), 6750–6761.

Mori, Y., Akkapaiboon, P., Yang, X. *et al.* (2003a). The human herpesvirus 6 U100 gene product is the third component of the gH-gL glycoprotein complex on the viral envelope. *J. Virol.*, **77**(4), 2452–2458.

Mori, Y., Yang, X., Akkapaiboon, P. *et al.* (2003b). Human herpesvirus 6 variant A glycoprotein H-glycoprotein L-glycoprotein Q complex associates with human CD46. *J. Virol.*, **77**(8), 4992–4999.

Pfeiffer, B., Thomson, B., and Chadran, B. (1995). Identification and characterization of a cDNA derived from multiple splicing that encodes envelope glycoprotein gp105 of human herpesvirus 6. *J. Virol.*, **69**(6), 3490–3500.

Rodrigues, G. A. (1999). Human herpes virus 6 fatal encephalitis in a bone marrow recipient. *Scand. J. Infect. Dis.*, **31**, 313–315.

Salahuddin, S. Z., Ablashi, D. V., Maskham, P. D. *et al.* (1986). Isolation of a new virus, HBLV, in patients with lymphoproliferative disorders. *Science*, **234**(4776), 596–601.

Santoro, F., Greenstone, H. L., Insinga, A. *et al.* (2003). Interaction of glycoprotein H of human herpesvirus 6 with the cellular receptor CD46. *J. Biol. Chem.*, **278**(28), 25964–25969.

Santoro, F. M., Kennedy, P. E., Locatelli, G. *et al.* (1999). CD46 is a cellular receptor for human herpesvirus 6 [In process citation]. *Cell*, **99**(7), 817–827.

Schirmer, E. C., Wyatt, L. S., Yamanishi, K. *et al.* (1991). Differentiation between two distinct classes of viruses now classified as human herpesvirus 6. *Proc. Natl Acad. Sci. USA*, **88**(13), 5922–5926.

Secchiero, P., Flamand, L., Gibellini, D. *et al.* (1997a). Human herpesvirus 7 induces CD4(+) T-cell death by two distinct mechanisms: necrotic lysis in productively infected cells and apoptosis in uninfected or nonproductively infected cells. *Blood*, **90**(11), 4502–4512.

Secchiero, P., Sun, D., De Vico, A. L. *et al.* (1997b). Role of the extracellular domain of human herpesvirus 7 glycoprotein B in virus binding to cell surface heparan sulfate proteoglycans. *J. Virol.*, **71**(6), 4571–4580.

Secchiero, P., Bertolaso, L., Casareto, L. *et al.* (1998a). Human herpesvirus 7 infection induces profound cell cycle perturbations coupled to disregulation of cdc2 and cyclin B and polyploidization of CD4(+) T-cells. *Blood*, **92**(5), 1685–1696.

Secchiero, P., Zella, D., Barabitsskaja, O. *et al.* (1998b). Progressive and persistent downregulation of surface CXCR4 in CD4(+) T cells infected with human herpesvirus 7. *Blood*, **92**(12), 4521–4528.

Secchiero, P., Mirandola, P., Zella, D. *et al.* (2001). Human herpesvirus 7 induces the functional up-regulation of tumor necrosis factor-related apoptosis-inducing ligand (TRAIL) coupled to TRAIL-R1 down-modulation in CD4(+) T cells. *Blood*, **98**(8), 2474–24781.

Seya, T., Hara, T., Matsumoto, M. *et al.* (1990). Complement-mediated tumor cell damage induced by antibodies against membrane cofactor protein (MCP, CD46). *J. Exp. Med.*, **172**(6), 1673–1680.

Singh, N., Carrigan, D. R., Gayowski, T. *et al.* (1995). Variant B human herpesvirus-6 associated febrile dermatosis with thrombocytopenia and encephalopathy in a liver transplant recipient [published erratum appears in *Transplantation* 1996 Feb 27;61(4):677]. *Transplantation*, **60**(11), 1355–1357.

Singh, N., Bentlejewski, C., Carrigan, D. R. *et al.* (2002a). Persistent lack of human herpesvirus-6 specific T-helper cell response in liver transplant recipients. *Transpl. Infect. Dis.*, **4**(2), 59–63.

Singh, N., Husain, S., Carrigan, D. R. *et al.* (2002b). Impact of human herpesvirus-6 on the frequency and severity of recurrent hepatitis C virus hepatitis in liver transplant recipients. *Clin. Transpl.*, **16**(2), 92–96.

Skrincosky, D., Hocknell, P., Whetter, L. *et al.* (2001). Identification and analysis of a novel heparin-binding glycoprotein encoded by human herpesvirus 7 [in process citation]. *J. Virol.*, **74**(10), 4530–4540.

Smith, A., Santoro, F., Di Lullo, G. et al. (2003). Selective suppression of IL-12 production by human herpesvirus 6. *Blood.*

Soldan, S. S., Berti, R., Salem, N. et al. (1997). Association of human herpes virus 6 (HHV-6) with multiple sclerosis: increased IgM response to HHV-6 early antigen and detection of serum HHV-6 DNA. *Nat. Med.*, **3**(12), 1394–1397.

Suzuki, Y., Inagi, R., Acono, T. et al. (1998). Human herpesvirus 6 infection as a risk factor for the development of severe drug-induced hypersensitivity syndrome. *Arch. Dermatol.*, **134**(9), 1108–1112.

Tajiri, H., Nose, O., Baba, K. et al. (1990). Human herpesvirus-6 infection with liver injury in neonatal hepatitis [letter]. *Lancet*, **335**(8693), 863.

Takahashi, K., Sonoda, S., Higashi, K. et al. (1989). Predominant CD4 T-lymphocyte tropism of human herpesvirus 6-related virus. *J. Virol.*, **63**(7), 3161–3163.

Takahashi, K., Segal, E., Kondo, T. et al. (1992). Interferon and natural killer cell activity in patients with exanthem subitum. *Pediatr. Infect. Dis. J.*, **11**(5), 369–373.

Tanaka, K., Kondo, T., Torigoe, S. et al. (1994). Human herpesvirus 7: another causal agent for roseola (exanthem subitum). *J. Pediatr.*, **125**(1), 1–5.

Tohyama, M., Yahata, Y., Yasukawa, M. et al. (1998). Severe hypersensitivity syndrome due to sulfasalazine associated with reactivation of human herpesvirus 6. *Arch. Dermatol.*, **134**(9), 1113–1117.

Torigoe, S., Koide, W., Yamada, M. et al. (1996). Human herpesvirus 7 infection associated with central nervous system manifestations. *J. Pediatr.*, **129**(2), 301–305.

Tsujimura, H., Iseki, T., Date, Y. et al. (1998). Human herpesvirus-6 encephalitis after bone marrow transplantation: magnetic resonance imaging could identify the involved sites of encephalitis [letter]. *Eur. J. Haematol.*, **61**(4), 284–285.

Wyatt, L. S. and Frenkel, N. (1992). Human herpesvirus 7 is a constitutive inhabitant of adult human saliva. *J. Virol.*, **66**(5), 3206–3209.

Yamanishi, K., Okuno, T. et al. (1988). Identification of human herpesvirus-6 as a causal agent for exanthem subitum [see comments]. *Lancet*, **1**(8594), 1065–1067.

Yasukawa, M., Inoue, Y., Ohminami, H. et al. (1998). Apoptosis of CD4+ T lymphocytes in human herpesvirus-6 infection. *J. Gen. Virol.*, **79**(Pt 1), 143–147.

Yasukawa, M., Hasegawa, A., Sakai, I. et al. (1999). Down-regulation of CXCR4 by human herpesvirus 6 (HHV-6) and HHV-7. *J. Immunol.*, **162**(9), 5417–5422.

Yoshikawa, T., Asano, Y., Kobayashi, I. et al. (1993). Exacerbation of idiopathic thrombocytopenic purpura by primary human herpesvirus 6 infection. *Pediatr. Infect. Dis. J.*, **12**(5), 409–410.

Zhang, Y., Hatse, S., De Clerq, E. et al. (2000). CXC-chemokine receptor 4 is not a coreceptor for human herpesvirus 7 entry into CD4(+) T cells. *J. Virol.*, **74**(4), 2011–2016.

HHV-6A, 6B, and 7: molecular basis of latency and reactivation

Kazuhiro Kondo[1] and Koichi Yamanishi[2]

[1]Department of Microbiology, The Jikei University School of Medicine, Tokyo, Japan
[2]Department of Microbiology, Osaka University Graduate School of Medicine, Japan

Introduction

The human β-herpesvirus subfamily consists of human cytomegalovirus (HCMV), human herpesvirus 6 (HHV-6), and human herpesvirus 7 (HHV-7). HHV-6 and HHV-7 belong to the Roseolovirus genus of the β-herpesviruses, and the HHV-6 species are divided into two variants: HHV-6A and HHV-6B. These viruses establish a lifelong infection of their host, reactivate frequently, and reactivated viruses are shed into the saliva (Jordan, 1983; Krueger et al., 1990). Some evidence suggests that the molecular mechanisms of viral latency and reactivation are shared among these viruses. HHV-6B is reactivated from latency after coinfection with HHV-7 (Katsafanas et al., 1996), and HCMV disease is frequently associated with concurrent HHV-6 and HHV-7 reactivation in transplant patients (Lautenschlager et al., 2000; Mendez et al., 2001)

The sites of these viruses during latency are not completely defined. For HHV-6B, viral DNA is detected predominantly in the peripheral blood monocytes/macrophages of seropositive healthy adults (Kondo et al., 1991). Furthermore, primary cultured macrophages support latent HHV-6B infection, and viral reactivation is induced in them by treatment with 12-0-tetradecanoylphorbol-13-acetate (TPA) (Kondo et al., 1991). HHV-6B also establishes latency in myeloid cell lines (Yasukawa et al., 1999), and that HHV-6B is detectable in CD34 (+) peripheral blood progenitor cells (Luppi et al., 1999). Therefore, HHV-6B appears to establish latency in hematopoietic progenitor cells.

HHV-6A is detectable in the peripheral blood of seropositive adults (Drobyski et al., 1993); however, a cell population that might harbor latent HHV-6A has not been identified. Unlike HHV-6B, HHV-6A does not establish latency in cultured macrophages (K. Kondo et al., unpublished data).

Some evidence suggests that latent HHV-6 infection in the brain may be involved in the pathology of certain neurological diseases, such as recurrent febrile figures (Hall et al., 1994; Kimberlin and Whitley, 1998; Kondo et al., 1993), multiple sclerosis (MS) (Challoner et al., 1995; Sola et al., 1993) and encephalitis (Caserta et al., 1994). However, the site of HHV-6 latency in the brain has not been identified.

HHV-7 can be reactivated from latently infected peripheral blood mononuclear cells by T-cell activation, and it was first isolated from the purified CD4 (+) T-cells of a healthy individual; however, the range of cell types in which HHV-7 can establish true latency is not clear (Frenkel et al., 1990; Katsafanas et al., 1996). A variety of tissues contain infected cells at a late stage of HHV-7 infection, suggesting that HHV-7 might cause a persistent infection rather than a true latent infection (Kempf et al., 1997a). Since HHV-6B can be recovered after the latently infected cells are superinfected with HHV-7, these viruses may use similar mechanisms to maintain their latency (Katsafanas et al., 1996).

The investigation of latency-associated transcripts is important for understanding the molecular basis of herpesvirus persistence; however, the latency-associated transcripts of HHV-6A and HHV-7 have not yet been identified. In this chapter, we discuss the molecular mechanisms of HHV-6B latency and reactivation that are suggested based on its latency-associated transcripts (Kondo et al., 2002, 2003b).

Latency-associated transcripts of HHV-6

Two types of HHV-6B latency-associated transcripts (H6LTs) have been identified in the gene locus of the immediate early (IE) 1/2 genes (Kondo et al., 2002). They are detected only in latently infected cells in vitro and in vivo. Although they are encoded in the same direction as the immediate early (IE) 1/2 genes and share their protein-coding region with IE1/2, their transcription start sites and exon(s) are different from those of the productive-phase transcripts (Mirandola et al., 1998; Schiewe et al., 1994) (Fig. 47.1). Type I H6LTs originate at the latent start site (LSS) 1, which is located 9.7 kilobases upstream of the IE1/2 start site, and Type II H6LTs originate at LSS2, which is located between exons 2 and 3 of IE1/2 (Fig. 47.1). In addition, novel short ORFs with latency-associated exons are encoded at the 5 proximal region of the H6LTs (ORF99, ORF142, and ORF145 in Fig. 47.1) (Kondo et al., 2002).

The structures of the H6LTs are similar to those of HCMV latency-specific transcripts (Kondo and Mocarski, 1995; Kondo et al., 1996); the latter encode IE1/IE2 ORFs, and short ORFs appear in the latency-specific exon. Furthermore, in the case of the HCMV latent transcripts, the translation of the IE1/IE2 protein is probably prevented by the existence of latency-specific ORFs upstream of the IE1/IE2 ORFs. Similarly, the HHV-6 IE1/IE2 protein is not detectable in latently infected macrophages. These findings suggest that viral replication of HCMV and HHV-6 may be suppressed at the point of translation of the major immediate early proteins during latency. The function of these upstream ORFs is discussed below.

Consistent with these findings, HHV-6 and HCMV exhibit similarities in their latent infections: (i) Both viruses can establish latency in cells of the monocyte/macrophage lineage (Kempf et al., 1997b; Taylor-Wiedeman et al., 1991); (ii) both viruses tend to persist in the latent state but are reactivated frequently, and the reactivated viruses are shed into the saliva (Jordan, 1983; Krueger et al., 1990); (iii) methylation of the immediate-early gene locus is observed similarly in HHV-6 and HCMV, suggesting that the latent viral genome of these two viruses is locally methylated (Gompels et al., 1995; Honess et al., 1989); and (iv) viral reactivation of HHV-6 is associated with HCMV reactivation (DesJardin et al., 1998; Humar et al., 2000).

The HHV-6 late gene U94, which is a homologue of the adeno-associated virus type 2 (AAV-2) rep gene (Rapp et al., 2000; Thomson et al., 1991), has also been reported to be expressed during latency (Rotola et al., 1998). Because other human β-herpesviruses, such as HCMV and human herpesvirus 7, do not encode homologues of U94 in their genomes (Chee et al., 1990; Megaw et al., 1998; Nicholas, 1996) the U94 gene may play some role that is specific to HHV-6. The Rep protein of AAV-2 is a site-specific endonuclease and helicase that is involved in site-specific integration of the viral genome into the host genome. Chromosomally integrated HHV-6 DNA has been observed in lymphomas (Luppi et al., 1993), and the integrated viral DNA is reportedly transmitted stably in the germ line (Daibata et al., 1998). These findings suggest that the U94 gene may relate to HHV-6 integration. However, no evidence has been reported so far to support this possibility.

Gene regulation of latency-associated transcripts

In the gene regulation of the latency-associated transcripts, a similarity between HHV-6 and HCMV has been observed using a recombinant HHV-6 (Kondo et al., 2003b). The recombinant virus has an enhanced green fluorescent protein-puromycin gene cassette containing the CMV major immediate-early promoter (HCMV-MIEP) (Fig. 47.2). Neither viral replication in T-cells nor latency/reactivation in macrophages is impaired in this recombinant virus. During HHV-6 latency, however, no expression of EGFP driven by the HCMV-MIEP is detected (Fig. 47.3(A)).

Gene expression from the HCMV-MIEP was investigated using the 5'-rapid amplification of cDNA ends (RACE) method (Fig. 47.3(B)), which showed the EGFP mRNA is transcribed from the latent infection transcription start sites (LSSs) 1 and 2 of HCMV (Fig. 47.3(C)), which are used to express the latency-associated transcripts of HCMV (Kondo et al., 1996). The finding that the HCMV MIEP showed a latency-associated activity in the context of HHV-6 latency suggested that the transcriptional control of HHV-6 latency may share some common mechanism with that of HCMV latency (Kondo et al., 2003a).

First molecular event of HHV-6 reactivation

To identify the first molecular event of HHV-6 reactivation, the latent infection system of HHV-6 was used. In this system, macrophages are infected with HHV-6B and cultured for 4 weeks. At 4 weeks postinfection, macrophages show no signs of viral replication, such as viral protein expression or infectious virus production. Viral reactivation is induced by treatment with TPA (20 ng/ml) for 7 days (Kondo et al., 1991).

At the early stage of the induction (3 and 5 days after the treatment with TPA), the proportion of cells that express the type I H6LTs significantly increases; however, transcription of productive-phase IE1/IE2 is not detected at days 0, 3, and 5 (Fig. 47.4). At this phase, IE1 protein is detectable in the cells without the production of infectious virus. Because productive-phase IE1 mRNAs are not detectable, the H6LTs, which contain the IE1 ORF (Fig. 47.1), are thought to be translated into IE1 protein at the first stage of viral reactivation. A similar molecular event has been

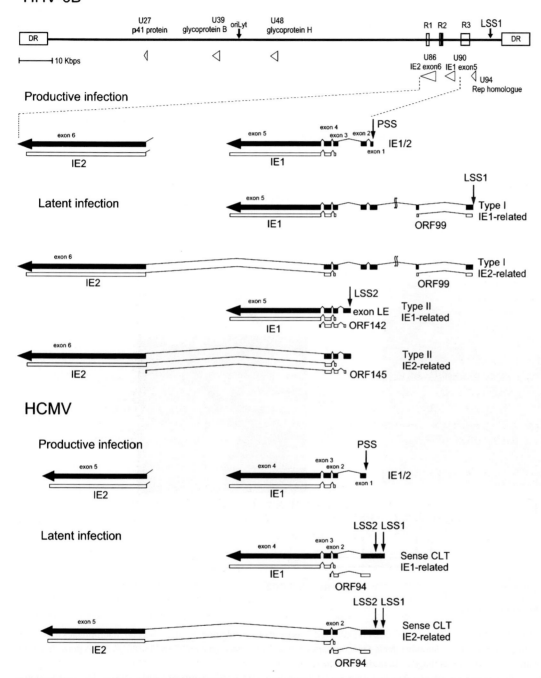

Fig. 47.1. Structures of the HHV-6 and HCMV latency-associated transcripts. Schematic drawings of the H6LT structures are shown. Productive-phase transcripts are also shown. The drawings of the mRNAs are in the same orientation relative to the viral genome. Thin lines represent introns; thick arrows represent exons. All exons and introns are drawn to scale. Latency-associated exons starting from latent start site (LSS) 1 and LSS2 are depicted. The position of the productive start site (PSS) is also shown. In HHV-6, exon 1 of the type I latent transcript is 138-bp longer than that of IE1/2. Two additional exons of the type I latent transcripts are located approximately 7.8 kb and 9.7 kb upstream from the PSS. ORFs of IE1, IE2, and putative latency-associated proteins ORF99, ORF142, and ORF145 are depicted. In HCMV, exon 1 of the cytomegalovirus latency-associated transcript (CLT) is longer than that of IE1/2. Latency-associated exons starting from LSS1 and LSS2 are depicted. ORFs of IE1, IE2, and putative latency-associated proteins ORF94 are depicted.

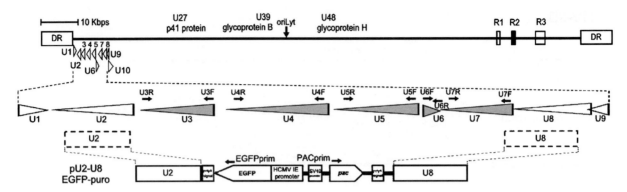

Fig. 47.2. Structure of recombinant HHV-6. At the top is a map of the HHV-6B genome, with the region U1-U9 expanded below. In the middle, shaded arrows show the U3-U7 ORFs that were replaced by the EGFP-puro cassette. The bottom diagram represents the EGFP-puro cassette pU2-U8 EGFP-puro. The open box represents the EGFP gene and human cytomegalovirus major immediate-early promoter. The puromycin-N-acetyl-transferase gene (*pac*) and SV40 early promoter are depicted.

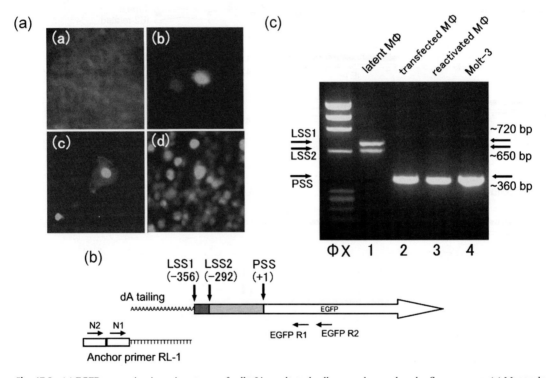

Fig. 47.3. (a) EGFP expression in various types of cells. Live cultured cells were observed under fluorescence. (a) Macrophages that were latently infected with EGFP-HHV-6; (b) latently infected macrophages that were(transfected with plasmid pU2-U8 EGFP-puro shown in Fig. 47.2(c) reactivation-induced macrophages; (d) productively infected Molt-3 cells.
(b) HCMV IE1/IE2 promoter and PCR primers. The EGFP gene and transcription start sites are drawn to scale. The productive infection transcription start site of IE1/IE2 mRNA (PSS indicated as +1) and two latent infection transcription start sites (LSS1 and LSS2: ref. 21) are shown. The locations of the PCR primers are depicted, and a schematic drawing shows the usage of the anchor primer RL-1.
(c) 5'-RACE amplification of the EGFP transcripts. RNA from latently infected macrophages (Mφ) (lane 1), latently infected macrophages that were transfected with plasmid pU2-U8 EGFP-puro shown in Fig. 47.2 (lane 2), reactivation-induced macrophages (lane 3), and productively infected Molt-3 cells (lane 4), was analyzed by the 5'-RACE method. The 5'-end of the transcript initiating at each of PSS (~360 bp), LSS1 (~720 bp), and/or LSS2 (~650 bp) was detected. Hae III-digested φX174 DNA fragments were used as size markers (φX).

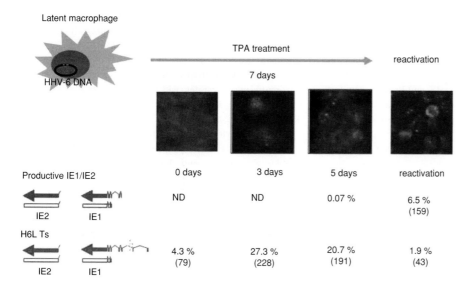

Fig. 47.4. mRNA and protein expression in latently infected macrophages. Latently infected macrophages were treated with TPA for 3, 5, and 7 days (reactivation). Cells were then stained with a mono-specific antibody against IE1. Percentage of H6LT-expressing cells during viral latency and reactivation. The percentages of H6LT-positive cells during viral reactivation were estimated. The copy number of each type of transcript in one H6LT-positive cell is shown in parentheses. The percentage of cells that showed the productive IE1/IE2 is also shown.

observed in transplant patients: approximately two-thirds of reactivation-positive patients express the type I H6LTs 1–3 weeks before the onset of HHV-6 reactivation (Kondo et al., 2003b). This intermediate phase of viral reactivation is different from the complete reactivation phase that is characterized by the expression of productive-phase IE1/IE2 transcripts (Hummel et al., 2001; Soderberg-Naucler et al., 2001), and this intermediate phase seems to be relatively stable (Kondo et al., 2003b).

Transfection of an IE1-expression vector into latent macrophages stimulates HHV-6 reactivation. As described above, H6LTs have latency-associated small ORFs upstream of the IE1/IE2 ORFs (Fig. 47.1). For certain other mRNAs that have small upstream ORFs (uORFs) that restrict the translation of the downstream ORFs, regulation at the translational and mRNA level is important for release from the uORF control (Hoffman et al., 2001; Nomura et al., 2001). An alteration in the regulation of translation as well as the increase in H6LTs might contribute to increased IE1 protein expression and viral reactivation (Kondo et al., 2003b).

Since the reactivation of HHV-6 and HHV-7 is related to graft-versus-host disease in transplant recipients (Yoshikawa et al., 2002) and to drug-induced hypersensitivity syndrome, these viruses might be reactivated by a strong generalized immunological response. However, the trigger that induces viral reactivation has not been identified.

Summary

In the Roseolovirus genus, some of the latency-associated transcripts of HHV-6B have been identified. Since HHV-6B and HCMV have some similarities in their latent transcripts and latent gene regulation, latency-associated transcripts of HHV-6 and HCMV might be involved in mechanizing that are common to β-herpesviruses latency. If so, similar transcripts may be identified in HHV-6A and HHV-7. Investigation of these transcripts should increase our understanding of the molecular bases of Roseolovirus latency and reactivation, about which little is known.

REFERENCES

Caserta, M. T., Hall, C. B., Schnabel, K. et al. (1994). Neuroinvasion and persistence of human herpesvirus 6 in children. *J. Infect. Dis.*, **170**, 1586–1589.

Challoner, P. B., Smith, K. T., Parker, J. D. et al. (1995). Plaque-associated expression of human herpesvirus 6 in multiple sclerosis. *Proc. Natl. Acad. Sci. USA*, **92**, 7440–7444.

Chee, M. S., Bankier, A. T., Beck, S. et al. (1990). Analysis of the protein-coding content of the sequence of human cytomegalovirus strain AD169. *Curr. Top. Microbiol. Immunol.*, **154**, 125–169.

Daibata, M., Taguchi, T., Sawada, T., Taguchi, H., and Miyoshi, I. (1998). Chromosomal transmission of human herpesvirus 6 DNA in acute lymphoblastic leukaemia. *Lancet*, **12**, 543–544.

DesJardin, J. A., Gibbons, L., Cho, E. *et al.* (1998). Human herpesvirus 6 reactivation is associated with cytomegalovirus infection and syndromes in kidney transplant recipients at risk for primary cytomegalovirus infection. *J. Infect. Dis.*, **178**, 1783–1786.

Drobyski, W. R., Eberle, M., Majewski, D., and Baxter-Lowe, L. A. (1993). Prevalence of human herpesvirus 6 variant A and B infections in bone marrow transplant recipients as determined by polymerase chain reaction and sequence-specific oligonucleotide probe hybridization. *J. Clin. Microbiol.*, **31**, 1515–1520.

Frenkel, N., Schirmer, E. C., Wyatt, L. S. *et al.* (1990). Isolation of a new herpesvirus from human CD4+ T cells. *Proc. Natl Acad. Sci. USA*, **278**, 748–752.

Gompels, U. A., Nicholas, J., Lawrence, G. *et al.* (1995). The DNA sequence of human herpesvirus-6: structure, coding content, and genome evolution. *Virology*, **209**, 29–51.

Hall, C. B., Long, C. E., Schnabel, K. C. *et al.* (1994). Human herpesvirus-6 infection in children. A prospective study of complications and reactivation. *N. Engl. J. Med.*, **331**, 432–438.

Hoffmann, B., Valerius, O., Andermann, M., and Braus, G. H. (2001). Transcriptional autoregulation and inhibition of mRNA translation of amino acid regulator gene cpcA of filamentous fungus *Aspergillus nidulans*. *Mol. Biol. Cell*, **12**, 2846–2857.

Honess, R. W., Gompels, U. A., Barrell, B. G. *et al.* (1989). Deviations from expected frequencies of CpG dinucleotides in herpesvirus DNAs may be diagnostic of differences in the states of their latent genomes. *J. Gen. Virol.*, **70**, 837–855.

Humar, A., Malkan, G., Moussa, G., Greig, P. Levy, G., and Mazzulli, T. (2000). Human herpesvirus-6 is associated with cytomegalovirus reactivation in liver transplant recipients. *J. Infect. Dis.*, **181**, 1450–1453.

Hummel, M., Zhang, Z., Yan, S. *et al.* (2001). Allogeneic transplantation induces expression of cytomegalovirus immediate-early genes in vivo: a model for reactivation from latency. *J. Virol.*, **75**, 4814–4822.

Jordan, M. C. (1983). Latent infection and the elusive cytomegalovirus. *Rev. Infect. Dis.*, **5**, 205–215.

Katsafanas, G. C., Schirmer, E. C., Wyatt, L. S., and Frenkel, N. (1996). In vitro activation of human herpesviruses 6 and 7 from latency. *Proc. Natl Acad. Sci. USA*, **93**, 9788–9792.

Kempf, W., Adams, V., Mirandola, P. *et al.* (1997a). Persistence of human herpesvirus 7 in normal tissues detected by expression of a structural antigen. *J. Infect. Dis.*, **71**, 841–845.

Kempf, W., Adams, V., Wey, N. *et al.* (1997b). CD68+ cells of monocyte/macrophage lineage in the environment of AIDS-associated and classic-sporadic Kaposi sarcoma are singly or doubly infected with human herpesviruses 7 and 6B. *Proc. Natl Acad. Sci. USA*, **94**, 7600–7605.

Kimberlin, D. W. and Whitley, R. J. (1998). Human herpesvirus-6: neurologic implications of a newly-described viral pathogen. *J. Neurovirol.*, **4**, 474–485.

Kondo, K. and Mocarski, E. S. (1995). Cytomegalovirus latency and latency-specific transcription in hematopoietic progenitors. *Scand. J. Infect. Dis.* Suppl, **99**, 63–67.

Kondo, K., Kondo, T., Okuno, T., Takahashi, M., and Yamanishi, K. (1991). Latent human herpesvirus 6 infection of human monocytes/macrophages. *J. Gen. Virol.*, **72**, 1401–1408.

Kondo, K., Nagafuji, H., Hata, A., Tomomori, C., and Yamanishi, K. (1993). Association of human herpesvirus 6 infection of the central nervous system with recurrence of febrile convulsions. *J. Infect. Dis.*, **167**, 1197–1200.

Kondo, K., Kaneshima, H., and Mocarski, E. S. (1994). Human cytomegalovirus latent infection of granulocyte-macrophage progenitors. *Proc. Natl Acad. Sci. USA*, **91**, 11879–11883.

Kondo, K., Xu, J., and Mocarski, E. S. (1996). Human cytomegalovirus latent gene expression in granulocyte-macrophage progenitors in culture and in seropositive individuals. *Proc. Natl Acad. Sci. USA*, **93**, 11137–11142.

Kondo, K., Shimada, K., Sashihara, J., Tanaka-Taya, K., and Yamanishi, K. (2002). Identification of human herpesvirus 6 latency-associated transcripts. *J. Virol.*, **76**, 4145–4151.

Kondo, K., Nozaki, H., Shimada, K., and Yamanishi, K. (2003a). Detection of a gene cluster that is dispensable for human herpesvirus 6 replication and latency. *J. Virol.*, **162**, 10719–10724.

Kondo, K., Sashihara, J., and Shimada, K. (2003b). Recognition of a novel stage of beta-herpesvirus latency in human herpesvirus 6. *J. Virol.*, **77**, 2258–2264.

Krueger, G. R., Wassermann, K., De Clerck, L. S. *et al.* (1990). Latent herpesvirus-6 in salivary and bronchial glands [letter; comment]. *Lancet*, **336**, 1255–1256.

Lautenschlager, I., Lappalainen, M., Linnavuori, K., Suni, J., and Hockerstedt, K. (2000). CMV infection is usually associated with concurrent HHV-6 and HHV-7 antigenemia in liver transplant patients. *J. Clin. Virol.*, **13 Suppl 1**, S57-S61.

Luppi, M., Marasca, R., Barozzi, P. *et al.* (1993). Three cases of human herpesvirus-6 latent infection: integration of viral genome in peripheral blood mononuclear cell DNA. *J. Med Virol.*, **40**, 44–52.

Luppi, M., Barozzi, P., Morris, C. *et al.* (1999). Human herpesvirus 6 latently infects early bone marrow progenitors in vivo. *J. Virol.*, **73**, 754–759.

Megaw, A. G., Rapaport, D., Avidor, B., Frenkel, N., and Davison, A. J. (1998). The DNA sequence of the RK strain of human herpesvirus 7. *Virology*, **244**, 119–132.

Mendez, J. C., Dockrell, D. H., Espy, M. J. *et al.* (2001). Human beta-herpesvirus interactions in solid organ transplant recipients. *J. Infect. Dis.*, **183**, 179–184.

Mirandola, P., Menegazzi, P., Merighi, S., Ravaioli, T., Cassai, E., and Di Luca, D. (1998). Temporal mapping of transcripts in herpesvirus 6 variants. *J. Virol.*, **72**, 3837–3844.

Nicholas, J. (1996). Determination and analysis of the complete nucleotide sequence of human herpesvirus 7. *J. Virol.*, **70**, 5975–5989.

Nomura, A., Iwasaki, Y., Saito, M. *et al.* (2001). Involvement of upstream open reading frames in regulation of rat V(1b) vasopressin receptor expression. *Am. J. Physiol. Endocrinol. Metab.*, **280**, E780–E787.

Rapp, J. C., Krug, L. T., Inoue, N., Dambaugh, T. R., and Pellett, P. E. (2000). U94, the human herpesvirus 6 homolog of the parvovirus nonstructural gene, is highly conserved among isolates and is expressed at low mRNA levels as a spliced transcript. *Virology*, **268**, 504–516.

Rotola, A., Ravaioli, T., Gonelli, A., Dewhurst, S., Cassai, E., and Di Luca, D. (1998). U94 of human herpesvirus 6 is expressed in latently infected peripheral blood mononuclear cells and blocks viral gene expression in transformed lymphocytes in culture. *Proc. Natl Acad. Sci. USA*, **95**, 13911–13916.

Schiewe, U., Neipel, F., Schreiner, D., and Fleckenstein, B. (1994). Structure and transcription of an immediate-early region in the human herpesvirus 6 genome. *J. Virol.*, **68**, 2978–2985.

Soderberg-Naucler, C., Streblow, D. N., Fish, K. N., Allan-Yorke, J., Smith, P. P., and Nelson, J. A. (2001). Reactivation of latent human cytomegalovirus in CD14(+) monocytes is differentiation dependent. *J. Virol.*, **75**, 7543–7554.

Sola, P., Merelli, E., Marasca, R. *et al.* (1993). Human herpesvirus 6 and multiple sclerosis: survey of anti-HHV-6 antibodies by immunofluorescence analysis and of viral sequences by polymerase chain reaction. *J. Neurol. Neurosurg. Psychiatry*, **56**, 917–919.

Taylor-Wiedeman, J., Sissons, J. G., Borysiewicz, L. K., and Sinclair, J. H. (1991). Monocytes are a major site of persistence of human cytomegalovirus in peripheral blood mononuclear cells. J. Gen. Virol. **72**, 2059–2064.

Thomson, B. J., Efstathiou, S., and Honess, R. W. (1991). Acquisition of the human adeno-associated virus type-2 rep gene by human herpesvirus type-6. *Nature*, **351**, 78–80.

Yasukawa, M., Ohminami, H., Sada, E. *et al.* (1999). Latent infection and reactivation of human herpesvirus 6 in two novel myeloid cell lines. *Blood*, **93**, 991–999.

Yoshikawa, T., Asano, Y., and Ihira, M. (2002). Human herpesvirus 6 viremia in bone marrow transplant recipients: clinical features and risk factors. *J. Infect. Dis.*, **66**, 847–853.

48

HHV-6A, 6B, and 7: immunobiology and host response

Fu-Zhang Wang and Philip E. Pellett

Molecular Biology Department, Lerner Research Institute, Cleveland Clinic Foundation, OH, USA

Introduction

The discoveries of *Human herpesvirus 6* variant A (HHV-6A), *Human herpesvirus 6* variant B (HHV-6B) and *Human herpesvirus 7* (HHV-7) followed the development of methods for activation and long-term culture of peripheral blood T lymphocytes. Based on their shared biological properties and nucleotide sequences, HHV-6A, HHV-6B, and HHV-7 are classified as members of the roseolovirus genus of the betaherpesvirus subfamily. HHV-6A and HHV-6B are very closely related, with most of their encoded proteins sharing greater than 90% amino acid sequence identity; most HHV-7 protein sequences share 30% to 60% amino acid sequence identity with their HHV-6 counterparts (for review, see Yamanishi et al., 2007 and elsewhere in this volume). Roseoloviruses share many genetic and biologic properties with the more distantly related cytomegaloviruses. All of the roseoloviruses infect T lymphocytes in vivo and in vitro, cause similar damage to infected cells, and have overlapping but distinct disease spectra.

Primary infection with HHV-6B is the major cause of roseola infantum (also known as roseola, exanthem subitum, 3-day-fever, or sixth disease), a febrile rash illness common in early childhood (for review, see Braun *et al.*, 1997; Yamanishi *et al.*, 2007 and elsewhere in this volume); primary HHV-7 infections can also cause roseola, albeit less frequently. Roseoloviruses can affect the central nervous system; patients with HHV-6 primary infection sometimes develop seizures or convulsions. HHV-6A and HHV-6B infect various types of neural cells and in some studies have been associated with demyelinating diseases, including multiple sclerosis (MS) and progressive multifocal leukoencephalopathy (for review see Caserta *et al.*, 2001; Tyler, 2003). HHV-6 associated pneumonia, encephalitis, hepatitis, and hematopoietic stem cell suppression have been observed after stem cell transplantation, more often in association with HHV-6B than HHV-6A (for review see Clark and Griffiths, 2003; Ljungman, 2002; Yoshikawa, 2003). In addition, HHV-6 and HHV-7 immune suppressive activities may also indirectly contribute to fungal, bacterial, or human cytomegalovirus (HCMV) infections (Boeckh and Nichols, 2003; Ljungman, 2002). A role for HHV-6 infections in the progression of HIV disease has been debated (Braun *et al.*, 1997; Caserta *et al.*, 2001; Clark and Griffiths, 2003). Obviously, many questions remain about the pathogenesis of these viruses, with many of these questions revolving around their immunobiology.

Much of our consideration of these viruses, and justification for studying them, is based on their roles as human pathogens. This has led many experiments to be interpreted in the context of how the results might explain a pathogenic outcome that might be considered negative from the perspective of the infected host, that is, how the virus avoids the immune system and how it creates disease. Usually overlooked is the fact that, by far, the most common outcome of infection with these viruses is not disease, but a lifelong dynamic biological interaction between the virus and host that seldom manifests as disease. Thus, while the processes by which the virus evades or otherwise delays immune responses during the early stages of infection, avoids being eliminated during latency, and causes disease are important, it is worth considering that much of the immunobiology of these viruses is likely to involve a highly regulated process of *stimulation* of host responses. This stimulation must be balanced with the immunoevasive tactics to achieve a state that has almost been idealized by the roseoloviruses: healthy infected hosts capable of lifelong transmission.

Cell tropism

In this section we discuss the effects of HHV-6A, HHV-6B, and HHV-7 on cells of the hematopoietic lineage in the context of the immunobiology of these viruses. HHV-6A and HHV-6B have apparently broader host ranges than does HHV-7; this is likely due to their choices of cellular receptors (for review, see Yamanishi et al., 2007). The cellular receptor for both HHV-6A and HHV-6B is CD46, a member of the family of regulators of complement activation, which is expressed on all nucleated cells; co- or alternative receptors remain to be identified. CD4, the marker of helper T lymphocytes, is a critical component of a receptor for HHV-7. As for HSV, CMV, and HHV-8, heparan sulfate-like molecules mediate the initial HHV-7 attachment to target cell surfaces.

In vitro

All three viruses can productively infect primary CD4+ T-lymphocytes; activation of these cells is required for efficient viral replication (Table 48.1). HHV-6A, but not HHV-6B, can also efficiently infect primary CD4−/CD8+ T-lymphocytes (Table 48.1) (Grivel et al., 2003; Lusso et al., 1991a; Takahashi et al., 1989). T-lymphocyte cell lines are widely used for cultivating these viruses: the HSB-2 and J JHAN cell lines for HHV-6A, Molt-3 and MT-4 cells for HHV-6B, and Sup-T1 cells for HHV-7. HHV-6A can also productively infect primary NK cells (Lusso et al., 1993). Both HHV-6A and HHV-6B replicate in human peripheral blood monocyte-derived immature dendritic cells, and in intrathymic T progenitor cells in SCID-Hu mice (Asada et al., 1999; Gobbi et al., 1999; Kakimoto et al., 2002; Kondo et al., 1991). Although HHV-6A can productively infect terminally and incompletely differentiated cells, the virus can enter CD34+ hematopoietic stem cells and express virally encoded genes (including *U16–17* and *U91*), but not produce viral progeny (Isomura et al., 2003; Knox and Carrigan, 1992; Luppi et al., 1999). HHV-6 infection of fresh monocyte/macrophages does not produce virus either, although many of these cells contain viral DNA (Clark, 2000; Kondo et al., 1991); as described below, these represent latent infections (Kondo et al., 2002b).

In addition to cells of the immune system, HHV-6 also replicates in many other cells (summarized in Table 48.1; for review, see Braun et al., 1997; Clark, 2000). Our understanding of the cell tropism of HHV-6A and HHV-6B is complicated by the fact that in the various studies, only one or the other variant was used and end points have differed, from expression of specific virally encoded mRNAs or proteins, to detection of infectious progeny.

In vitro, HHV-7 growth is restricted to activated cord blood lymphocytes, purified T lymphocytes, and CD4+ immature SupT1 cells (for review see Black and Pellett, 1999).

In vivo

An important recent observation based on improved methods for cultivation of monocytes/macrophages was that during the acute phase of primary infection, HHV-6B load (both DNA and virus titer) is nearly one log greater in these cells than in CD4+ T-lymphocytes (Kondo et al., 2002a). This extends earlier work in which HHV-6B was frequently detected in CD4+ T lymphocytes obtained both during the acute phase of primary infection and from healthy adults. During the convalescent phase of primary infection and in healthy adults, HHV-6 DNA is detected primarily in monocytes/macrophages, and phorbol ester treatment induces lytic infection; this confirms that the virus establishes latency in these cells (Kondo et al., 1991, 2002b). Another possible site of HHV-6B persistence is in epithelial cells that line tonsillar crypts (Roush et al., 2001).

Because cells that harbor latent HHV-6 can be induced to the lytic state upon exposure to various activating stimuli, virus activity that could contribute to pathogenesis might be found in association with diverse immune stimulation events. For example, drug hypersensitivity syndrome (DHS), or drug rash with eosinophilia and systemic symptoms, presents as fever, rash, and internal organ lesions. A number of case reports have described active HHV-6 infection during DHS, but the exact role played by the virus is not clear. Two mechanisms of virus involvment have been hypothesized. Some drugs reduce B-cells and cause hypogammaglobulinemia, which has been hypothesized to trigger HHV-6 reactivation (Kano et al., 2004). Alternatively, immune responses to some drugs may activate cells harboring HHV-6, leading to virus reactivation. Cases of DHS have also been linked to EBV and CMV (for review see Wong and Shear, 2004).

Little is known of the in vivo cellular distribution of HHV-6A. It has been infrequently detected in peripheral blood mononuclear cells (PBMC) and in over 50% of lungs (Cone et al., 1996), but the type of cells it inhabits is not known.

HHV-6B and HHV-7 (but not HHV-6A) antigens are frequently detectable in salivary glands (Fox et al., 1990; Kempf et al., 1998), but only HHV-7 has been frequently cultured from saliva (Wyatt and Frenkel, 1992).

HHV-7 has been detected in over 50% of PBMC specimens collected from healthy individuals and from patients prior to bone marrow transplantation. In addition, HHV-7 antigens have been detected in a variety of lymphoid and non-lymphoid cells. The virus may establish latency

Table 48.1. Cell Tropism of HHV-6A and HHV-6B

Cells	Progeny virus[a]	Virus tested		Infected cells (%)	References
		HHV-6A	HHV-6B		
In vitro					
astrocytes	+	+	+		(He et al., 1996)
epidermal cell line	−	NT	+		(Yoshikawa et al., 2003a)
endothelial cells	+	+	NT	1–38	(Caruso et al., 2003; Wu & Shanley, 1998)
CD34 positive stem cells	−	NT	+		(Isomura et al., 2003)
immature thymocytes	−	−	−		(Roffman and Frenkel, 1990)
mature thymocytes	+	−	+		(Roffman and Frenkel, 1990)
thymocytes + anti-CD3	NT	NT	+		(Roffman and Frenkel, 1991)
thymocytes + anti-CD3 + IL2	NT	NT	+		(Roffman and Frenkel, 1991)
CBL	−	−	+	5–77	(Black et al., 1989)
CBL + PHA	+	NT	+		(Black et al., 1989)
CBL + PHA + IL2	+	NT	+		(Black et al., 1989)
CBMC + PHA	NT	NT	+	5–6	(Kikuta et al., 1990a)
CBMC + anti-CD3 + IL2	NT	NT	+	50–90	(Kikuta et al., 1990a)
CBMC + PHA	NT	NT	+	35–56	(Kikuta et al., 1990a)
PBMC	NT	NT	−		(Kikuta et al., 1990a)
PBMC + anti-CD3	NT	NT	+	27–70	(Kikuta et al., 1990a)
PBMC + PHA	NT	NT	−		(Kikuta et al., 1990a)
PBL	1	NT	+	2–15	(Black et al., 1989; Frenkel et al., 1990)
PBL + PHA	5	NT	+		(Frenkel et al., 1990)
PBL + IL2	4	NT	+		(Frenkel et al., 1990)
PBL + IL2 + PHA	5	NT	+		(Frenkel et al., 1990)
CD28 positive T cells	0	NT	+		(Frenkel et al., 1990)
CD28 T cells + PHA	3	NT	+		(Frenkel et al., 1990)
CD28 T cells + IL2	1	NT	+		(Frenkel et al., 1990)
CD28 T cells + PHA + IL2	6	NT	+		(Frenkel et al., 1990)
tonsilar CD4+ T cells	+	+	+		(Grivel et al., 2003)
tonsilar CD8+ T cells	+	+	+	5–20[b]	(Grivel et al., 2003)
NK cells		+	NT		(Lusso et al., 1993)
monocytes	−	+	+		(Burd & Carrigan 1993)
macrophages					
dendritic cells	+	+	+	2	(Asada et al., 1999)
dendritic cells	+	+	+	>90	(Kakimoto et al., 2002)
dendritic cells	+	+	+	30–95	(Hirata et al., 2001)
JJHAN cells	+	+	−	>85	(Wyatt et al., 1990)
HSB-2	+	+	−	28–90	(Ablashi et al., 1991; Wyatt et al., 1990)
Sup T1	+	+	−	>90	(Ablashi et al., 1991)
Molt-3	+	−	+	>90	(Ablashi et al., 1991)
MT-4	+	NT	+		(Asada et al., 1989; Black et al., 1989)
MRC-5 fibroblast	+	+	−		(Robert et al., 1996)
liver cell line	+	+	+	50–90[c]	(Cermelli et al., 1996)
mink lung epithelial cells	+	NT	+		(Simmons et al., 1992)

(cont.)

Table 48.1. (cont.)

Cells	Progeny virus[a]	Virus tested		Infected cells (%)	References
		HHV-6A	HHV-6B		
In vivo (ES patients)					
ES patients					
CD4+ T lymphocytes	+	−	+		(Kondo et al., 2002a; Takahashi et al., 1989; Yasukawa et al., 1998)
CD8+ T lymphocytes	−	−	+		(Yasukawa et al., 1998)
Monocytes/macrophage	+	−	+	0.03–2	(Kondo et al., 2002a)
SCID-hu Thy/Liv mice					
CD4+ T cell progenitors	−	+	+		(Gobbi et al., 1999)
CD3+ cells	+	+	+		(Gobbi et al., 1999)

CBL (umbilical cord blood lymphocytes), CBMC (umbilical cord blood mononuclear cells), PBL (peripheral blood lymphocytes), PBMC (peripheral blood mononuclear cells), NT (not tested)
[a] $\log_{10}$ virus titer per ml of culture supernatant.
[b] 20% of tonsilar CD8+ T cells were infected with HHV-6A compared with 5% with HHV-6B viruses.
[c] 90% cells of a liver cell line were infected with HHV-6A, compared with 50% with HHV-6B viruses.

in CD4+ T-lymphocytes in vivo since it can be activated from PBMC by PHA or anti-CD3 stimulation.

Antigens

Roseolovirus genomes encode about 90 genes. The immunogenicity of individual viral proteins depends on their level of expression, novelty to the host, some aspects of their structure and/or composition, and degree of exposure to the immune system. In addition, adaptive immune effects can target different stages of the viral life cycle. For example, proteins expressed on the virion surface during lytic infection can be targets for neutralizing antibodies, and proteins needed intracellularly for virus replication can be targets of cytotoxic T-lymphocytes (CTL). Important questions relate to what antigens are presented to the immune system during latency, and how this contributes to regulation of latency and reactivation.

HHV-6A and HHV-6B antigens

Latent antigens

Latent transcription has been studied in greatest detail for HHV-6B. Kondo and co-workers identified four species of HHV-6B latency-associated transcripts (H6LTs) that are expressed from the ie1/ie2 region (Kondo et al., 2002b). It remains to be determined whether the proteins encoded by these latent transcript open reading frames are expressed as protein and whether any portion of the immune response is directed at them. The HHV-6 latency transcripts are similar in structure to some CMV latency-associated transcripts that originate from both DNA strands in the ie1/ie2 region (Kondo et al., 1996) and express proteins recognized by sera from healthy CMV seropositive individuals (Landini et al., 2000).

Di Luca and colleagues have identified transcripts from U94, the HHV-6 homologue of adeno-associated virus type 2 rep gene, as the only HHV-6 transcripts detected in PBMC from healthy individuals (Rotola et al., 1998). HHV-6 viral replication was blocked in cells transfected with plasmids encoding U94, further supporting a potential role for this gene during latency. Levels of anti-U94 antibodies in serum from healthy individuals are very low (Caselli et al., 2002; Rapp et al., 2000), but their prevalence and titers are higher in patients with MS (Caselli et al., 2002).

Lytic antigens

Most of the virally encoded proteins are expressed during the lytic cycle of viral replication. Lytic antigens present in purified virion particles or infected cell lysates have been analyzed by immunoprecipitation and/or immunoblot analyses with serum from immunized mice or rabbits, or from infected humans.

HHV-6B virions are composed of more than 29 polypeptides that range in size from 30 to 280 kDa, of which about 25–30 peptides, including 8 glycoproteins, are recognized by positive human sera (Balachandran et al., 1989; Shiraki et al., 1989). Human immune responses to HHV-6B IE antigens were detected by immunofluorescence, although the

Table 48.2. HHV-6 MAbs

Target Protein	Antibody designation	Cross-reactivity HHV-6A	HHV-6B	HHV-7	Neutralization	References	Commercial source
U86 (IE1)	AIE1-32	+	NT	NT	NT	(Mori et al., 2003b)	
U91-86 (IE-2)	P6H8	+	−	NT	NT	(Arsenault et al., 2003)	
U17-16 (IE-B)	B701	+	NT	NT	NT	(Flebbe-Rehwaldt et al., 2000)	
U27, p41	9A5D12	+	+	±	−	(Balachandran et al., 1989; Berneman et al., 1992)	
U27, p41/38	C-5	+	−	±	NT	(Berneman et al., 1992; Iyengar et al., 1991)	Chemicon
U94 (54 kDa)	anti-REP	−	+	NT	NT	(Dhepakson et al., 2002)	
U39 (gB)	6A5H7[a]	+	+	−	NT	(Balachandran et al., 1989; Berneman et al., 1992)	ABI
	OHV1	−	+	NT	−	(Okuno et al., 1992; Takeda et al., 1996)	
	2D9	+	−	−	NT	(Campadelli-Fiume et al., 1993)	
	87-y-13	+	−	NT	+	(Takeda et al., 1996)	
	2D10[a]	+	+	−	+[b]	(Foa-Tomasi et al., 1992)	
U48 (gH)	7A2	+	+	−	−	(Anderson & Gompels 1999; Balachandran et al., 1989)	
	OHV3/9	−	+	NT	+	(Okuno et al., 1990; Takeda et al., 1997)	
	2E4	+	+	−	+	(Foa-Tomasi et al., 1991; Foa-Tomasi et al., 1994; Liu et al., 1993a)	
	1D3	+	+	±	+	(Liu et al., 1993a; Neipel et al., 1992)	
	5E7	+	+	−	+	(Liu et al 1993a; Neipel et al., 1992)	
U100 (gQ)	2D6[a]	+	−	−	+	(Balachandran et al., 1989; Qian et al., 1993)	
	au100–119	+	NT	NT	NT	(Mori et al., 2003a)	
	au100–124	+	NT	NT	NT	(Mori et al., 2003a)	
U11 (p101)	C3108–103	−	+	NT	NT	(Pellett et al., 1993)	Chemicon

NT (not tested)
[a]Several other MAbs to the same protein were described simultaneously, but the relationships among them are not clear.
[b]Neutralization only in the presence of complement.
Many other HHV-6 MAbs have also been produced, but their viral protein targets are not as well characterized.

individual protein targets were not identified (Eizuru and Minamishima, 1992).

Monoclonal antibodies (MAbs)

HHV-6-specific MAbs have been used to identify specific virally-encoded proteins and their functions (Table 48.2). Some of the MAb are variant specific, while others recognize both variants; a few also react with HHV-7 antigens.

Targets of complement independent neutralization

Anti-gB antibodies neutralize HHV-6A and HHV-6B infection and cell fusion (Mori et al., 2002; Santoro et al., 1999; Takeda et al., 1996). The epitope of one neutralizing gB MAb (87-Y-13) is in the vicinity of amino acid 134 (Takeda et al., 1996).

As for other herpesviruses, HHV-6A gH and gL depend on each other for proper processing and expression on the cell surface or viral envelopes. The epitope for the OHV3 MAb to HHV-6B gH maps near amino acid 389 (Takeda et al., 1997). MAb 2E4, 5E7 and 1D3, react with gH from both HHV-6 variants via conformational epitopes that include sequences between amino acids 145 to 230, plus residue 652 (Anderson et al., 1996; Anderson and Gompels, 1999). A complex of gH, gL, and gQ appears to be required for binding to the

Table 48.3. HHV-7 MAbs

Reference	Target Protein	MAb Designation	Cross-reactivity[d]	Commercial source
(Foa-Tomasi et al., 1994)	U14, pp85	3B1[a]	± HHV-6A and -6B	Chemicon
(Takeda et al., 2000)	U14	24G7		
	U27	5H4	+ HHV-6B	
(Skrincosky et al., 2001)	gQ (U100)	19F8[a]		
(Foa-Tomasi et al., 1994)	p121	3H12		
	p51	2C1		
(Nakagawa et al., 1997)	gp78, 110	5E12[b]		
	gp85, 80, 45	5F12[b]		
	52 kDa	16B4		
	40 kDa	7C10[c]	++ HHV-6A and -6B	
	40 kDa	10F1[c]		
	120, 210, 180	5A3	+ HHV-6A and -6B	
	34	2B8		
(Tsukazaki et al., 1998)	125 kDa	IK3[a]		
	p120	IK16		
	p85	IK5[a]		
	50 kDa	IK27		
	125 kDa	IK10	± HHV-6A and -6B	
Okuno T., personal	IFA	KR3		
communication	IFA	KR4		

[a]Two or more MAbs were made for the same protein.
[b]Neutralizing antibody
[c]MAbs recognize two different proteins.
[d]Cross-reactivity: positive by IFA and immune precipitation (++), positive by IFA (+), and weakly positve by IFA (±).
None of these MAbs cross-react with HCMV.

HHV-6 cellular receptor, CD46, since neither the gH-gL complex nor gQ expressed alone binds to CD46 (Mori et al., 2003b; Santoro et al., 2003). MAbs against gH neutralize viral infectivity and block formation of polykaryocytes (Balachandran et al., 1989; Foa-Tomasi et al., 1991; Qian et al., 1993).

Targets for diagnosis
Essentially all individuals positive by immunofluorescence for HHV-6 mount a readily detectable serologic response to the U11 protein, which can be used as a marker of HHV-6 infection with respect to the other human herpesviruses, including HHV-7 (Black et al., 1996b; Neipel et al., 1992; Yamamoto et al., 1990). HHV-6B *U11* (homologous to HCMV *UL32*/pp150) encodes a tegument protein of 101 kDa, which shares 81% amino acid identity with its HHV-6A counterpart (p100) (Neipel et al., 1992; Pellett et al., 1993). U11 antigenic epitopes recognized by human serum have been mapped to near its carboxyl-terminal region, which has only limited sequence similarity and no cross-reactivity with its HCMV counterpart (Neipel et al., 1992). MAb C3108–103 against U11 is HHV-6B specific; the epitope is in the vicinity of amino acid 723 (Pellett et al., 1993).

75% of HHV-6 positive sera reacted with the gH-gL complex expressed in transfected T-lymphocytes, but use of these glycoproteins for diagnosis has not been established (Liu et al., 1993b). An ELISA based on a 110 kDa glycoprotein affinity-purified with monoclonal antibody 2E2 was reactive with 56% to 96% of human sera from different serum donor categories (Iyengar et al., 1991); it is not known which HHV-6 glycoprotein this corresponds to. HHV-6 positive human sera that had high titer by IFA reacted very weakly with bacterially expressed HHV-6 major capsid protein (UL57) in immunoblots (Littler et al., 1990).

Non-structural proteins are also targets of the humoral response. About 10%–30% of human sera react with HHV-6 p41, the DNA polymerase processivity factor encoded by gene *U27*; higher rates of both IgG and IgM reactivity to p41 have been observed in some patient populations (Patnaik et al., 1995; Soldan et al., 1997), but the basis for this is not understood. As mentioned above, responses to undefined HHV-6B IE antigens have been detected by immunofluorescence (Eizuru and Minamishima, 1992).

HHV-7 antigens

About 20 polypeptides were identified in HHV-7 infected cell lysates, seven of which were glycoproteins (Foa-Tomasi et al., 1994; Nakagawa et al., 1997). Two prominent HHV-7 antigens are encoded by the U11 and U14 genes, which encode the tegument proteins, pp89 and pp85, respectively (Stefan et al., 1999).

HHV-7 monoclonal antibodies

Table 48.3 summarizes HHV-7 MAbs that have been generated in several laboratories.

Targets of complement independent neutralization

HHV-7 infection can be neutralized by MAb 5E12 and 5F12, which react with glycoproteins of 78 kDa and 85 kDa, respectively (Nakagawa et al., 1997). HHV-7 gB (U39) and gQ (U100/gp65) bind to heparan sulfate-like molecules on cell surfaces, consistent with a role in viral entry; anti-gp65 antibodies block HHV-7 infectivity (Skrinkosky et al., 2000).

Targets for diagnosis

Although serologic reactivity to intact HHV-7 gB is generally weak, an ELISA based on amino acids 129–152 of gB was both sensitive and specific (Franti et al., 2002). U11/pp89 and U14/pp85 are sensitive and specific serologic markers for HHV-7 (Foa-Tomas: et al., 1994; Stefan et al., 1999), with pp85 being recognized somewhat more frequently than pp89. MAb 5E1, which recognizes U14 (pp85) is a useful marker for HHV-7 since it does not cross-react with HHV-6 antigens and can be used on formalin-fixed, paraffin-embedded tissue (Foa-Tomas: et al., 1996; Kempf et al., 1997).

Immunologic cross-reactivity

The most commonly used serologic methods (e.g., IFA and ELISA) cannot reliably differentiate HHV-6A from HHV-6B infections. There is limited antigenic cross-reactivity between the HHV-6 variants and HHV-7; under the conditions of most assays, this cross-reactivity can occasionally lead to false-positive determinations of an individual's serostatus.

HHV-6A and HHV-6B

A major criterion for defining and distinguishing the HHV-6 variants is their patterns of reactivity with panels of variant-specific MAbs (Table 48.2). Most MAbs generated against one HHV-6 variant react with the other, but some are variant-specific. Similarly, more than 90% of HHV-6-specific CD4+ T lymphocyte clones react with both HHV-6A and HHV-6B (Yasukawa et al., 1993) (the target antigens have not been identified). This is consistent with the extensive amino acid sequence conservation between the viruses (Dominguez et al., 1999). By IFA, 95% of 234 healthy adult Malaysians had similar IgG titers to HHV-6A and HHV-6B (Yadav et al., 1991), as did 80% of 136 healthy adults in the United States (Chandran et al., 1992). The titer differences in some individuals may reflect different responses to unique antigens of either virus, differential responses to common antigens of both viruses, or the nature of primary infection or reactivation. A reliable variant-specific serologic test is needed to better understand the biology of the two variants.

HHV-6 and HHV-7

There is some antigenic cross-reactivity between HHV-6 and HHV-7. Hyperimmune mouse sera against one virus reacts to the other (Black and Pellett, 1999). Adsorption of serum with either HHV-6A or HHV-6B antigens removes about 20–40% of HHV-7 IgG reactivity. Similarly, about 30% of CD4+ T lymphocyte clones that react with both HHV-6A and HHV-6B react with HHV-7 (Yasukawa, et al., 1993), consistent with the level of their amino acid sequence conservation (Dominguez et al., 1999). Some weak or uncertain cross-reactions have also been observed for some MAbs against HHV-6 or HHV-7 (Tables 48.2 and 48.3).

This limited cross-reactivity does not generally lead to HHV-6 seroconversion in individuals naïve for HHV-6 at the time of their primary HHV-7 infection. Anti-HHV-6 IgG titers increased in about 60% of individuals with prior HHV-6 infection, suggesting possible reactivation of HHV-6 by HHV-7, and/or restimulation of reactivity with shared antigens (Caserta et al., 1998; Hall et al., 1994; Huang et al., 1997; Tanaka et al., 1994; Torigoe et al., 1995). Similarly, primary HHV-6 infection does not lead to HHV-7 seroconversion, and HHV-7 primary infection can occur in the presence of high titers of HHV-6 antibodies (Hidaka et al., 1994; Wyatt et al., 1991). However, in HHV-6 naïve individuals, primary HHV-7 infection can transiently induce cross-reactive HHV-6 IgM (213) (Fig. 48.1). In one of two patients who had HHV-7 infections that preceded HHV-6 infection, HHV-7 IgG levels rose slightly after HHV-6 infection (Yoshida et al., 2002b). Simultaneous high-titer increases in HHV-6 and HHV-7 antibody titers in young children are most likely due to dual primary infection rather than cross-reactivity (Ward et al., 2001). Ward and colleagues provide evidence that IFA titers above 32 can be accepted as true positives (Ward et al., 2002).

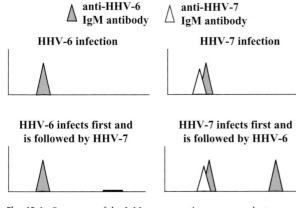

Fig. 48.1. Summary of the IgM cross-reactive responses between HHV-6 and HHV-7. From Yoshida *et al.* (2002a), courtesy of Dr. Mariko Yoshida, with permission from the American Society of Microbiology.

Roseoloviruses and other viruses

About 4% of HHV-6 specific CD4+ T lymphocyte clones responded to HCMV (Yasukawa *et al.*, 1993). HCMV vaccination or natural infection led to 4-fold or greater titer rises to HHV-6, with most of the cross reactivity in this assay being traced to the conserved gB proteins of the two viruses (Adler *et al.*, 1993). Primary infections with HHV-6 or HHV-7 can be clinically misdiagnosed as measles or rubella in children aged younger than 5 years (Black *et al.*, 1996a; Oliveira *et al.*, 2003). To complicate the matter, confirmed infections of measles, HCMV, or EBV have been associated with induction of HHV-6 reactive IgM and significant rises in HHV-6 specific IgG levels, possibly due to reactivation of HHV-6 by the other virus or a more general non-specific immune activation (LaCroix *et al.*, 2000; Linde *et al.*, 1988; Suga *et al.*, 1992a). The cross-reactivity between HCMV and HHV-7 does not confound the results of most serology assays (Black *et al.*, 1996b).

Immune response

In spite of the clear ability of these viruses to infect and kill a variety of immune effector cells both in vitro and in vivo, and to trigger a variety of mechanisms that can be seen as immunoevasive (described below), an immune response sufficient to control the infection develops rapidly following primary HHV-6 and HHV-7 infections. Thus, the likely transient and localized immune evasion or immune manipulation tactics are sufficient to allow establishment of the viral infection (including latency), but in the end have no discernable adverse long-term effects in otherwise healthy hosts. In this section, we describe immunologic outcomes such as antibody titers. In the following section we discuss regulation of these responses.

Immune response after primary infection

Innate immune response

HHV-6 and HHV-7 infections induce production of immune-regulatory chemokines and cytokines (Table 48.4). Among them, regulated upon activation, normal T expressed and secreted (RANTES), a proinflammatory β-chemokine, is known for inducing local responses by selectively attracting monocytes (the target for HHV-6 latency) and lymphocytes (a vehicle for virus spread). Interleukin-1β (IL-1β) enhances inflammatory and interferon-γ (IFN-γ) responses, and is needed for IL-6-dependent, B-lymphocyte immune responses. Both IFN-α and IFN-β inhibit HHV-6 replication in vitro (Takahashi *et al.*, 1992). However, tumor necrosis factor-α (TNF-α), normally an antiviral cytokine, may enhance release of extracellular HHV-6 by stimulating monocyte differentiation (Arena *et al.*, 1997).

HHV-6 and HHV-7 infections also enhance NK cell activity, possibly by inducing IL-15 production, which stimulates the proliferation of T lymphocytes and NK cells (Atedzoe *et al.*, 1997; Flamand *et al.*, 1996). NK cells are very effective in killing autologous HHV-6 infected cells, which may play a major role in controlling viral infection (Malnati *et al.*, 1993).

Antibody response

Given their high seroprevalence in adults, almost all infants have maternal antibodies against these viruses at birth. Antibody titers decline sharply from birth to a nadir at 3 to 6 months of age (Fig. 48.2). HHV-6 seroprevalence increases sharply from 6 months after birth into the second year, when the seroprevalence begins to approximate that in healthy adults; this is the period in which almost all HHV-6B primary infections occur (for review see Braun *et al.*, 1997; Yamanishi *et al.*, 2007). HHV-7 primary infection most often occurs after HHV-6, with seroprevalence not accumulating to adult levels until the early teens (Yamanishi *et al.*, 2007).

IgM antibodies

IgM antibodies develop 5 to 7 days after the onset of clinical symptoms, reach their highest titers in 2–3 weeks and disappear by 2 months post infection. At least one target of the IgM response is the 101K antigen encoded by

Table 48.4. HHV-6A infection and innate immunity

Cells tested	Expression of immunomodulatory protein or gene			References
	Enhanced	Inhibited	Unchanged	
Endothelial cells	IL-8			(Caruso et al., 2002; Caruso et al., 2003)
	MCP-1			
	RANTES			
PBMC	IL-1β			(Flamand et al., 1991)
	IFN-1α			(Kikuta et al., 1990b; Takahashi et al., 1992)
	TNF-α			(Arena et al., 1997)
	IL-10	IL-12		(Arena et al., 1999)
		IFN-γ		
Tonsilar lymphoid tissue[a]	RANTES		MIP-1α	(Grivel et al., 2001; Grivel et al., 2003)
			MIP1-β	
			IL-1α	
			IL-1β	
Tonsilar lymphoid cells			RANTES,	(Grivel et al., 2001)
			MIP-1α	
			MIP-1β	
CD4+ lymphocytes		IL-2		(Flamand et al., 1995)
SupT1	IL-18	IL-10	IL-1	(Mayne et al., 2001)
		IL-14	IL-8	
			IL-12	
			IFN-γ	
Monocytes and lines	IL-10			(Li et al., 1997)
	IL12			
	IL-15			(Arena et al., 2000)
Macrophages		IL-12	RANTES	(Smith et al., 2003)
			TNF-α	
			MIP-1β	
NK cells[b]	IL-15			(Atedzoe et al., 1997; Flamand et al., 1996)

[a]HHV-6B has a similar effect.
[b]HHV-7 has a similar effect.

HHV-6 *U11* (LaCroix et al., 2000). An HHV-6-specific neutralizing IgM response develops after HHV-6 primary infection, regardless of whether it happens before or after HHV-7 infection. In contrast, while HHV-7 primary infection of HHV-6-naïve individuals induces IgM antibodies that can neutralize both HHV-6 and HHV-7, there is no IgM response to either virus when HHV-7 infection follows HHV-6 (Yoshida et al., 2002b) (Fig. 48.1).

IgG antibodies

HHV-6 IgG antibodies usually appear within 10 days to two weeks after the onset of clinical symptoms, increase in avidity over time, and remain at measurable levels for many years (Braun et al., 1997). The initial IgG response is of low avidity. Antibody avidity increases with time, making it a useful marker for identifying recent infections and for discriminating primary infections from reactivations (Ward et al., 1993, 2001). HHV-6-specific IgG4 was detected in all bone marrow transplant recipients whose HHV-6 IgG antibody titers increased by at least 8-fold, whereas in pregnant women and in children less than three years of age, HHV-6-specific IgG4 was never detected (Carricart et al., 2004). The possibility that IgG4 antibodies may be a marker for HHV-6 reactivation warrants further study.

Neutralizing antibodies

HHV-6 neutralizing antibodies are present at the time of birth and during and after the rash period of primary infection, but not during the febrile stage (Asada et al., 1989; Suga et al., 1990; Yoshida et al., 2002b), suggesting that maternal antibodies have the capacity to block viral infection. Additional mechanisms may also contribute to the

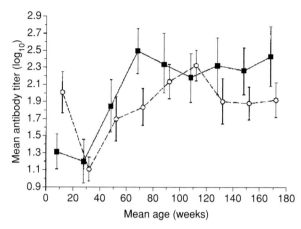

Fig. 48.2. Comparison of the change with age of the geometric mean titers of IgG antibodies to HHV-6 and HHV-7 in children. Geometric mean titers for HHV-6 (black squares) and HHV-7 (open circles) were calculated for 20-week age intervals from birth to 179 weeks. When the titer was <10 it was given a nominal value of 5. Bars represent the mean ± twice the standard error of the mean. The numbers of serum samples tested in each group were as follows: 0 to 19 weeks, 26; 20 to 39 weeks, 36; 40 to 59 weeks, 36; 60 to 79 weeks, 35; 80 to 99 weeks, 31; 100 to 119 weeks, 35; 120 to 139 weeks, 27; 140 to 159 weeks, 24; 160 to 179 weeks, 19. From Ward et al. (2001), courtesy of Dr. Katherine Ward, with permission from the American Society of Microbiology.

resistance to infection early in life, because antibody alone is seldom sufficient to prevent infection, as exemplified by the incomplete protection afforded by transfer of high-titered anti-CMV immunoglobulins to organ transplant recipients. Thus, in immunocompetent infants in the early months after birth, protection from HHV-6 infection and disease is the result of a combination of maternally derived antibodies (initially transplacental, then via mother's milk, some of which are neutralizing), and the child's innate immune functions.

Despite the close genetic and antigenic relationship between HHV-6B and HHV-7, their complement-independent IgG neutralizing antibodies, as detected in vitro, do not cross react with each other; this is a reflection of the differences in the viral ligands that interact with the receptors (CD46 and CD4, respectively) used by these viruses to infect target cells (Lusso et al., 1994; Santoro et al., 1999; Yoshida et al., 2002a, b). This does not exclude the possibility that antibodies against one virus provide some protection against the others in vivo. In contrast to neutralizing IgG, HHV-7 specific IgM antibodies neutralize HHV-6 infection (Yoshida et al., 2002b), but the targets have not been identified.

T lymphocyte response

HCMV nucleocapsid proteins and tegument proteins are better than the membrane glycoproteins at inducing T lymphocyte proliferation (Ljungman et al., 1985). Similarly, neither HHV-6A nor HHV-6B membrane glycoproteins induce T-lymphocyte proliferation in healthy adults; instead, these antigens inhibit T-lymphocyte proliferation to mitogens or antigens (Horvat et al., 1993). Antigen preparations mainly composed of the nucleocapsid proteins and tegument proteins of HHV-6A and HHV-6B induce T-lymphocyte proliferation responses of healthy seropositive children and adults (Soldan et al., 2000; Yakushijin et al., 1991); the response peaks later after primary HHV-6 infection (4 weeks) than for other herpesvirus infections (1 to 2 weeks) (Kumagai et al., 2006). More HHV-6 seropositive, healthy adults responded to HHV-6B antigen than that to HHV-6A antigen.

As with VZV, both HLA dependent and independent cytotoxicity have been observed for HHV-6-specific CD4+ T-lymphocyte clones, suggesting heterogeneous functions of CD4+ T-lymphocytes (Arvin et al., 1991; Yakushijin et al., 1992).

CTLs are a product of the Th1 pathway, which is regulated in part by IL-12. HHV-6 virions are sufficient to inhibit the ability of macrophages to produce IL-12 in response to IFN-gamma or lipopolysaccharide (Smith et al., 2003). Although a CTL response eventually develops, it is easy to imagine that a short deferral in the development of the response helps the infection get established.

Possible role of reactivation

About 5% of healthy adults have anti-HHV-6 IgM antibodies, suggesting periodic reactivation in the absence of clinical sequelae (Balachandra et al., 1989; Ohashi et al., 2002; Suga et al., 1992b). During pregnancy, HHV-6 reactivation, as identified by HHV-6 DNAemia, was associated with higher IgG titers, but had no effect on IgM levels (Dahl et al., 1999).

Immune responses in immunocompromised hosts

Allogeneic bone marrow and blood stem cell transplantation

HHV-6 activity is very common after blood stem cell transplantation (SCT), with HHV-6B being more commonly detected than HHV-6A. HHV-7 activity is not detected as often in PBMC, possibly due to the low CD4+ cell counts after transplantation (Boutolleau et al., 2003; Miyoshi et al., 2001; Wang et al., 1996). Because of their high prevalences, most of the post-transplant activity of these viruses is due to either reactivation or reinfection; primary infections are rare. It is difficult to interpret serological data in these patients because they are often severely immune suppressed and exposed to many blood products. HHV-6 antibody titers do increase (including neutralizing antibodies), but often this is not linked to the presence of viral DNAemia or infectious virus in bodily fluids (Molden et al., 1997; Wilborn et al., 1994; Yoshikawa et al., 1991). Geometric mean antibody titers were significantly higher in recipients without HHV-6 viremia than in those with viremia (Yoshikawa et al., 2002), consistent with a stronger immune response being linked to reduced virus activity. Anti-HHV-7 antibody titer increased in an allogeneic SCT patient with HHV-7-associated meningitis (Yoshikawa et al., 2003b).

After SCT, reconstitution of antigen specific T-lymphocyte responses to HSV, VZV, and CMV do not correlate with the recovery of lymphocyte population levels, nor with the ability to proliferate in response to mitogens. Specific responses develop only after reactivation, reinfection, or vaccination. After allogeneic SCT, more patients showed higher levels of HHV-6B- than HHV-6A-specific T-lymphocyte proliferation responses, in agreement with HHV-6B infection being more common in this setting (Wang et al., 1999). In addition, HHV-6 DNAemia was associated with a lack of HHV-6 specific T lymphocyte responses, regardless of the presence of HHV-6-associated disease, again suggesting a role of immunity in regulating viral activity.

Solid organ transplantation

As with allogeneic SCT, HHV-6B activity is common in the early stages after liver transplantation. Both reactivation and primary infection lead to HHV-6 specific IgM and IgG responses after liver transplantation, but these responses are frequently transient, the instability of the response possibly being due to a lingering immune deficit or other clinical issue (DesJardin et al., 1998; Yoshikawa et al., 2000). Fatal primary HHV-6A infection has been reported in the face of IgM and IgG responses after renal transplantation (Rossi et al., 2001).

HHV-6 specific T-helper lymphocyte proliferation was suppressed after liver transplantation and recovered slower than for HCMV (Singh et al., 2002a). Similar to patients after SCT, HHV-6 specific T lymphocyte responses are weaker in patients with HHV-6 viremia. Nonetheless, responses were normal to the T lymphocyte mitogen, Concanavalin A, suggesting a more specific deficit. Studies on transplanted livers showed that HHV-6 increases vascular expression of adhesion molecules like ICAM-1 and VCAM-1, thus inducing lymphocyte infiltration that may contribute to graft rejection (Lautenschlager et al., 2002).

Multiple sclerosis (MS)

MS is considered to be an autoimmune disease of the central nervous system, in which myelin is destroyed by autoreactive T cells that target certain myelin-specific proteins. The trigger for this activity is not known, but several viruses have been suggested as potential causes or contributors, among them, HHV-6A and HHV-6B. As reviewed in detail elsewhere, experimental approaches to questions of HHV-6 involvement in MS have included (i) PCR analyses of blood, cerebrospinal fluid, and brain tissues, (ii) testing for the presence of viral antigens by immunohistochemistry, (iii) and virus-specific immune responses in blood and intrathecally. The results have been mixed and are difficult to interpret. Thus several studies have noted elevated frequencies of detecting HHV-6 infection in MS patients and in affected brains relative to other neurologic diseases or healthy controls, while others have found no differences. One tenet relating to proof of etiology is consistency of association, which certainly has not been attained with respect to observations among the several groups that have studied this problem. Nonetheless, there has been sufficient consistency of overlapping and complementary data from multiple studies from some research groups and between several groups, to preclude dismissing the possible association. Importantly, studies that have looked the closest at the affected tissues have found some of the strongest associations (Cermelli et al., 2003; Goodman et al., 2003). Thus, we consider this an important area for continued research.

There are several connections to immunobiology. HHV-6 is a constitutive inhabitant of brains, and MS is an inflammatory disease. It is not a stretch to imagine that the immunomodulatory activities of the virus might affect the biology of T-cells in the brain. It is also possible that unusual activity of the virus in the course of the disease might manifest itself in measurable changes in various immune markers. The virus could thus play roles in either as the direct causative agent of the disease or by modulating the course of pre-existing disease. Some recent results consistent with these possibilities are as follows.

(i) In a study that found an association between HHV-6 activity and MS activity, serum IL-12 levels were elevated during the periods of simultaneous disease and virus activity (Chapenko et al., 2003). IL-12 regulates some cytokines and development of Th1 responses. Perplexing in this regard is the contemporaneously published report that HHV-6A markedly suppresses IL-12 expression in macrophages (Smith et al., 2003), the discrepancy possibly being rooted in the differences between the complex in vivo situation and the in vitro purified cell population.

(ii) Cell culture supernatants from HHV-6A- and HHV-6B-infected SupT1 cells induced a non-apoptotic death in cultured primary dendrocytes but not in primary astrocytes (Kong et al., 2003).

(iii) MS patients had somewhat elevated rates of generating T cell lines that were cross-reactive between HHV-6 antigens and myelin basic protein (Cirone et al., 2002). Possibly related to this, a seven amino acid segment of myelin basic protein is identical to a sequence encoded by *U24* (a protein of unknown function) of both HHV-6A and HHV-6B. This sequence is a more frequent target of cross-reactive CD4+ cytotoxic T cells in MS patients than in controls (Tejada-Simon et al., 2003).

(iv) In a study in which HHV-6 DNA was detected more frequently in serum and cerebrospinal fluid of MS patients than controls, MS patients had lower frequencies of T cells that recognize the major HHV-6 antigen (101K or p100, encoded by *U11*), slightly lower IgG titers against 101K, and markedly elevated serum IgM to the same protein (Tejada-Simon et al., 2002). When infected cell lysates were used as the antigens, HHV-6A specific T-lymphocyte proliferation response were detected more often in patients with relapsing-remitting MS than in the healthy controls, with no differences in the frequency of HHV-6B or HHV-7 specific responses (Soldan et al., 2000). Again, these differences were not found in patients who were mainly in the chronic progressive stage (Enbom et al., 1999).

(v) Results of comparisons of serologic responses to the complex array of HHV-6 antigens present in infected cells by immunofluorescence assays have shown little difference between MS cases and controls (Ablashi et al., 1998, 2000; Enbom et al., 1999). Interestingly, differences have consistently been seen in some studies when defined antigens (IgG to U94/rep and IgM to p41/38) have been used (Caselli et al., 2002; Soldan et al., 1997). IgG antibodies against HHV-6 are often detected in cerebral spinal fluids from MS patients, but it is still unclear whether this reflects real viral activity or non-specific immunoactivation (Ablashi et al., 1998; Enbom et al., 1997). No differences were found in HHV-6-specific IgG subclasses in sera from MS patients compared with healthy controls (Enbom et al., 1999).

In sum, the accumulated diverse results suggest that in at least some MS patients, disease activity and progression are somehow connected to HHV-6 activity and immunobiology; the question remains of whether the virus contributes to the disease or is a fuzzy marker for some aspect of the disease process.

Virally mediated immune modulation

HHV-6 affects almost all the components of the immune system, including both innate and adaptive immune functions. Having discussed some of the end points of these functions, we will now discuss the underlying mechanisms. For heuristic reasons, we will trace these effects outward from the effects on infected cells, to the induction and expression of viral and cellular cytokines, and then the responses triggered by these molecules.

Cell surface markers

As summarized in Tables 48.4, 48.5, and 48.6, the roseoloviruses each trigger mechanisms that result in changes in expression of cell surface markers and other immunomodulators, leading to profound effects on immune-related cell functions and the organismal response to the infection.

Effects on specific cell types

NK cells

HHV-6 infects and kills NK cell clones cultured in vitro. In addition, HHV-6 also induces NK cells to express CD4, the helper T lymphocyte surface marker and the major cellular receptor for HIV-1, which can render NK cells permissive to HIV infection; this has led to speculation that HHV-6 not only causes immune suppression but also contributes to AIDS progression (Emery et al., 1999; Lusso et al., 1993). However, HHV-6 infection of PBMC, which include a variety of cell types, results in enhanced NK activity and NK-mediated killing of HHV-6 infected cells (Flamand et al., 1996; Malnati et al., 1993). Thus, virus-mediated killing of NK cells and NK-mediated killing of virus infected cells is regulated in part by the other cells in the system.

Stem cells

Although none of the roseoloviruses kill blood stem cells, they do affect their growth (Table 48.6). In vitro, HHV-7 inhibits the growth of granulocytic/erythroid/monocyte/megakaryocytic progenitors, but not their more differentiated progeny. In contrast, HHV-6 has less effect on the progenitors, but inhibits the growth of the more differentiated progeny (Isomura et al., 1997, 2003; Knox and Carrigan, 1992; Mirandola et al., 2000). Exposure of bone marrow precursors to HHV-6 inhibited their ability to respond to growth factors such as granulocyte-macrophage colony-stimulating factor and interleukin-3, and also reduced the outgrowth of macrophages from bone marrow (Burd and Carrigan, 1993). This may be due to induction of IFN-α by HHV-6 (Knox and Carrigan, 1992). HHV-6 also infects monocytes/macrophages, although these cells are not as prone to develop the typical CPE seen in CD4+ T-cells after HHV-6 infection. Nonetheless, the virus does cause dysfunction of blood monocytes and blocks their differentiation to macrophages (Burd et al.,

Table 48.5. Effects of HHV-6 or HHV-7 infection on cell surface markers related to immune functions

Marker	Cells	Effect	Virus tested	References
CD3	PHA stimulated lymphocytes	R	HHV-6A, -6B	(Lusso et al., 1991b; Yasukawa et al., 1999)
	Tonsilar cells	R	HHV-6A, -6B	(Grivel et al., 2003)
CD4	PHA stimulated lymphocytes	R	HHV-7	(Lusso et al., 1994; Yasukawa et al., 1999)
	PHA stimulated T lymphocytes	NC	HHV-6A, -6B	(Santoro et al., 1999)
	CD8+ lymphocytes	E	HHV-6A	(Lusso et al., 1991a)
	γ/δ T lymphocytes	E	HHV-6A	(Lusso et al., 1995)
	Tonsilar cells	E	HHV-6A, -6B	(Grivel et al., 2003)
	Dendritic cells	NC	HHV-6A, -6B	(Asada et al., 1999)
	NK cell	E	HHV-6A	(Lusso et al., 1993)
CD46	PHA stimulated T lymphocytes	R	HHV-6A, -6B	(Santoro et al., 1999)
	Tonsilar cells	R[a]	HHV-6A, -6B	(Grivel et al., 2003)
	Dendritic cells	NC	HHV-6A, -6B	(Asada et al., 1999)
CD80	Dendritic cells, six dpi	E	HHV-6A, -6B	(Kakimoto et al., 2002)
CD83	two dpi	NC	HHV-6A, -6B	(Hirata et al., 2001)
	six dpi	E	HHV-6A, -6B	(Kakimoto et al., 2002)
CD86	six dpi	E	HHV-6A, -6B	(Kakimoto et al., 2002)
CXCR4	PHA stimulated lymphocytes	R	HHV-6A, -6B, -7	(Cesarman and Knowles, 1999; Yasukawa et al., 1999)
	Tonsilar cells	NC	HHV-6A	(Grivel et al., 2001)
	Dendritic cells	NC	HHV-6A, -6B	(Asada et al., 1999)
CCR5	PHA stimulated lymphocytes	NC	HHV-6A, -6B, -7	(Yasukawa et al., 1999)
	Tonsilar cells	NC	HHV-6A	(Grivel et al., 2001)
	Dendritic cells	NC	HHV-6A, -6B	(Asada et al., 1999)
TNF receptors	J JHAN cells	E	HHV-6A, -6B	(Inoue et al., 1997)
HLA-I	Dendritic cells, two dpi	R	HHV-6A	(Hirata et al., 2001)
	six dpi	E	HHV-6A, -6B	(Kakimoto et al., 2002)
HLA-II	two dpi	NC	HHV-6A, -6B	(Hirata et al., 2001)
	six dpi	E	HHV-6A, -6B	(Kakimoto et al., 2002)
	Epidermal cell line	E	HHV-6B	(Yoshikawa et al., 2003a)
ICAM-1	Epidermal cell line	E	HHV-6B	(Yoshikawa et al., 2003a)

R (reduced expression), E (enhanced expression), NC (no change), dpi (days post infection)
[a]The reduction is greater for HHV-6A than HHV-6B.

1993; Burd and Carrigan, 1993). There is disagreement as to whether HHV-6A or HHV-6B is the more potent inhibitor of hematopoietic stem cell growth (Carrigan, 1995; Isomura et al., 1997, 2003). The mechanism for HHV-7 inhibition of blood stem cells is unknown.

T-lymphocytes

HHV-6 and HHV-7 infected T lymphocytes form balloon-like cells. These cells are usually mono- or binucleated and short-lived (Lusso et al., 1991b). HHV-6A can induce cell fusion via its cellular receptor (CD46) in the absence of viral protein synthesis (Mori et al., 2002; Santoro et al., 1999). HHV-7 infection also induces formation of giant, multi-nucleated CD4+ T-cells, possibly due to polyploidization of infected cells because of interrupted cell cycles (Secchiero et al., 1997, 1998a). HHV-6B infection shuts off host cell DNA synthesis, but stimulates host cell protein synthesis, which possibly also interferes with the cell cycle and creates a proper intracellular milieu for viral replication (Black et al., 1992; Øster et al., 2005). In SCID-Hu thymus/liver mice, HHV-6A and HHV-6B infection affects almost all of the major lymphoid cellular

Table 48.6. Effects of HHV-6 or HHV-7 infection on immune-related cell functions

Function	Cells	Effect	Virus tested	References
Growth	CD34+ stem cells	R	HHV-6B	(Isomura et al., 2003)
	macrophage	R	HHV-6B	(Burd et al., 1993)
Respiratory burst capacity	monocytes	R	HHV-6A, HHV-6B	(Burd and Carrigan, 1993)
Migration	PHA + lymphocytes	R	HHV-7	(Secchiero et al., 1998c)
Survival				
SCID-hu Thy/Liv mice	thymocytes	R	HHV-6A, HHV-6B	(Gobbi et al., 1999)
tonsilar culture	CD4+ lymphocytes	R	HHV-6A, HHV-6B	(Grivel et al., 2003)
	CD8+ lymphocytes	R	HHV-6A, HHV-6B	(Grivel et al., 2003)
Apoptosis				
in vitro	JJHAN cells	15%	HHV-6A, HHV-6B	(Inoue et al., 1997)
	CBL + PHA	0%	HHV-6B	(Ichimi et al., 1999)
	CBL + PHA + IL2	51%	HHV-6B	(Ichimi et al., 1999)
in vivo (ES patients)	CD4+ T lymphocytes	31%		(Takahashi et al., 1989; Yasukawa et al., 1998)
	CD8+ T lymphocytes	11%		(Yasukawa et al., 1998)

R (reduced)

subsets including CD4 and/or CD8 positive T-cells, but most severely depletes CD4 negative and CD8 negative intrathymic T-progenitor cells (Gobbi et al., 1999). HHV-6A replicates in and kills CD4+ and CD8+ T-cells with almost equal efficiency, while HHV-6B predominantly replicates in and depletes CD4+ T-cells (Grivel et al., 2003).

HHV-6A and HHV-6B induce a dramatic and generalized down modulation of the CD46 molecule in both infected and non-infected cells, while CD3 was downmodulated only in infected lymphocytes, with some differences in this activity between HHV-6A and HHV-6B (Furukawa et al., 1994; Grivel et al., 2003). In contrast, CD4 is upregulated after HHV-6A and HHV-6B infection, possibly via direct activation of the CD4 promoter in infected cells (Flamand et al., 1998; Grivel et al., 2003). HHV-6A showed a stronger effect on CD3 expression in CD4+ lymphocytes than HHV-6B, but the two viruses had similar effects on lymphoid tissues cultured ex vitro (Furukawa et al., 1994; Grivel et al., 2003). HHV-7 uses CD4 as its cellular receptor; CD4 but not CD3 expression is reduced after HHV-7 infection (Furukawa et al., 1994; Lusso et al., 1994; Secchiero et al., 1998c). Down modulation of CD46 may lead to spontaneous complement activation and cytotoxicity of the affected cells. CD3 is an important component of the T-cell antigen receptor and is critical for transduction of the T-cell activation signal upon interaction with the antigen peptide-HLA complex. HHV-6 or HHV-7 infected lymphocytes lose their ability to proliferate in response to anti-CD3 antibodies and to kill virus infected cells (Furukawa et al., 1994).

T-cell apoptosis

Like other herpesviruses, HHV-6 and HHV-7 lytic infections lead to host cell death via necrotic lysis (Inoue et al., 1997; Secchiero et al., 1997; Yasukawa et al., 1998). In addition, CD4+ T-lymphocytes die from virus-triggered apoptosis. This induction is dependent on viral replication for HHV-7 and is independent of viral replication for HHV-6 (Inoue et al., 1997; Secchiero et al., 1997). HHV-6-mediated apoptosis is regulated by the Fas–Fas ligand system and the apoptosis induced by HHV-7 seems to be controlled by bcl-2 (Inoue et al., 1997; Secchiero et al., 1997). In support of this, inhibition of the apoptotic pathway by enhanced expression of bcl-2 enhances HHV-7 infection, as observed for other viruses including Epstein–Barr virus (Razvi and Welsh, 1995; Secchiero et al., 1998b). Both HHV-6A and HHV-6B incorporate the important cell regulatory protein, p53, into virion particles; p53 regulates the cell cycle and protects a portion of infected cells from apoptosis (Takemoto et al., 2005, Øster et al., 2005). The basis for the choice between the two distinct fates (necrosis or apoptosis) of infected cells is unknown.

HHV-7 infection also induces tumor necrosis factor-related apoptosis-inducing ligand (TRAIL) production, which provides a trans-acting signal that triggers apoptosis of nearby uninfected cells (Secchiero et al., 2001). Simultaneously, TRAIL receptor 1 (TRAIL-R1) is down modulated in HHV-7 infected T lymphocytes. Thus, the virus triggers the death of nearby cells, which may protect it from the activity of immune effector cells such as NK cells and CTL, while protecting infected cells from similarly triggered death.

Proliferation

HHV-6A and HHV-6B viral envelope proteins inhibit T lymphocyte proliferation induced by phytohemagglutinin (PHA), IL-2, or antigens (Horvat *et al.*, 1993). Interaction of inactivated HHV-6A viral particles with PBMC inhibits proliferation of both CD4+ and CD8+ T lymphocytes and their responses to IL-2. This defect is apparently due to induction of defective IL-2 receptors or defects in IL-2 induced signaling pathway in these cells, as exogenous IL-2 does not correct the HHV-6 induced proliferation defect (Flamand *et al.*, 1995).

Dendritic cells

Dendritic cells are important antigen presenting cells for CD4 and CD8 T lymphocytes. Immature dendritic cells support HHV-6A or HHV-6B replication (Hirata *et al.*, 2001; Kakimoto *et al.*, 2002). Most of the infected cells are not killed, and differentiate into the mature forms, but these cells are functionally deficient and incapable of supporting lymphocyte proliferation (Kakimoto *et al.*, 2002). This is in contrast to HCMV, which selectively infects mature dendritic cells and down-regulates their cellular markers, thus impairing their function.

Histiocytes

Langerhans cell histiocytosis and hemophagocytic histiocytosis are characterized by dysregulated proliferation and migration of histiocytes (tissue macrophages). These diseases can be triggered by other diseases, use of certain drugs, or infections including HSV, HCMV and EBV. Cases of hemophagocytic histiocytosis have been associated with HHV-6 activity following organ transplantation and in previously healthy individuals (Rossi *et al.*, 2001; Tanaka *et al.*, 2002).

Cytokine production

HHV-6A, HHV-6B, and HHV-7 have profound influences on cytokine production by various immune cells (Table 48.4 and Fig. 48.3).

An important issue in the organismal response to infectious agents is the balance between the Th1 and Th2 arms of the immune system. There have been many studies of the effect of HHV-6 infection on the ability of target cells to produce cytokines that affect this balance, with sometimes diametrically opposed results. As discussed in detail by Lusso and colleagues (Smith *et al.*, 2003), this is probably due, at least in part, to the use of different cell types or cell populations in ex vivo conditions that do not fully represent in vivo regulatory circuits. IL-12 plays a pivotal role in

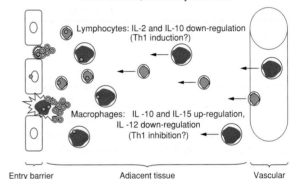

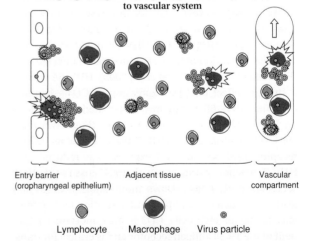

Fig. 48.3. Immunobiological events during early primary HHV-6 infection and establishment of latency. (See color plate section.)

inducing Th1 responses, and IL-10 is one of the key effectors in shifting the balance toward Th2 responses. Under some conditions, HHV-6 infection of PBMC induces IL-10 expression, which inhibits IL-12 production (Arena et al., 1999; Li et al., 1997). Both HHV-6A and HHV-6B infection of monocytes transiently induce low levels of IL-12 production; simultaneously, these same infections substantially restrict the level of IL-12 induction in response to IFN-γ and lipopolysaccharide; the sum is a net reduction in IL-12 production (Li et al., 1997; Smith et al., 2003). From these results, it has been argued that HHV-6 infection might lead to inhibition of Th1-polarized immune responses. This is supported by microarray experiments involving HHV-6B infection of a T cell line that harbors HTLV-1 (Takaku et al., 2005). In contrast, five days after HHV-6 infection, SupT1 cells expressed higher levels of IL-18 and other proinflammatory genes, while the level of IL-12 was unchanged and IL-10 was down-regulated (Mayne et al., 2001). In addition, HHV-6 infection induces proinflammatory chemokines, including RANTES, despite encoding a beta chemokine receptor that down-regulates RANTES transcription (Caruso et al. 2003; Grivel et al., 2001, 2003; Milne et al., 2000). From these data, it has been argued that HHV-6 infection leads to induction of a Th1 response (Mayne et al., 2001). We have summarized these activities in a model of some of the early events following HHV-6 infection (Fig. 48.3).

Interaction of HHV-6A virions with CD4+ T-lymphocytes inhibits IL-2 mRNA synthesis and IL-2 production induced by PHA or OKT3 (Flamand et al., 1995). IL-2 plays a major role in regulating T-lymphocyte and NK cell functions. HHV-6A, HHV-6B, and HHV-7 each downregulates the CXCR4 chemokine receptor leading to loss of response to the CXCR4 specific ligand, stromal cell-derived factor-1 (Hasegawa et al., 2001; Secchiero et al., 1998c; Yasukawa et al., 1999).

Infection of primary astrocytes had only modest effects on expression of inflammatory genes. Interestingly, when the HHV-6A-infected astrocytes were treated with a pro-inflammatory mixture of TNF-α, IL-1β, and IFN-γ, anti-inflammatory genes were strongly induced (Meeuwsen et al., 2005). There was very little overlap between the genes induced by infection of astrocytes vs. the HSB-2 T cell line.

Virally encoded immune modulators

Several herpesviruses, including CMV and HHV-8, encode genes homologous to human cellular chemokines or chemokine receptors, which may play important roles in pathogenesis and immune evasion. *U12* of both HHV-6 and HHV-7 encodes a functional beta-chemokine receptor (Isegawa et al., 1998; Nakano et al., 2003). HHV-6 *U51* encodes a functional chemokine receptor and is expressed in HHV-6 infected human endothelial cells (Caruso et al., 2003; Milne et al., 2000). While the product of *U12* interacts with beta-chemokines (also called CC chemokines) and activates, at least, the calcium-related signaling pathway, expression of HHV-6 U51 suppresses the transcription of RANTES, which recruits T-lymphocytes, NK cells, monocytes and eosinophils to inflammatory sites. Down-regulation of RANTES may compromise the function of these cells, as has been suggested for CMV US28. HHV-6B *U83* encodes a highly active CC chemokine that has been tested against the known chemokine receptors and interacts only with CCR2, a receptor present on macrophages and monocytes (Luttichau et al., 2003; Zou et al., 1999). HHV-6A U83 encodes two different forms of CC chemokines (full length being an agonist and the spliced form being an antagonist) that interact with a wide array of receptors other than CCR2 (Dewin et al., 2006). These activities may contribute to the process by which the virus establishes latency in such cells.

Other immune evasion mechanisms

HHV-6 gB and gH-gL complexes are not detectable on the plasma membrane of infected lymphocytes (Cirone et al., 1994), which may constitute an immune avoidance strategy. It has been reported that HHV-6A down-regulates HLA class I antigen in dendritic cells which may prevent the cells from HLA-I dependent killing, but the opposite was found in another paper (Hirata et al., 2001; Kakimoto et al., 2002).

HHV-7 *U21* encodes a type I membrane protein that binds to class I HLA-1 molecules and reduces their level of cell surface expression by diverting them to lysosomes (Hudson et al., 2001). Unexpectedly, the redirection is not mediated by the cytoplasmic tail of U21, but by its ER-lumenal domain (Hudson et al., 2003). This represents a novel mechanism for lysosomal sorting and for immune evasion.

Clinical significance of immunomodulation

A lot of interest has been concentrated on identifying the pathologic role of these viruses in immunocompromised patients. The rationale is that all the other herpesviruses cause significant diseases in this group of patients. In addition to directly causing pathologic lesions, it is also possible that these three viruses may indirectly contribute to other infectious pathogens by inhibiting the immune system (Griffiths, 2003).

Organ transplantation

HHV-6, but not HHV-7, infection is related to graft rejection in both adult and pediatric liver transplant patients (Feldstein et al., 2003; Griffiths et al., 1999). HHV-6 infection is related to higher CMV viral loads, CMV syndromes and diseases, bacteriemia, fungal disease, and mortality (DesJardin et al., 1998, 2001; Humar et al., 2000, 2002; Rogers et al., 2000). HHV-6 negative patients may experience primary infection, and these patients are more likely to develop fungal infections (Dockrell et al., 1999). In addition, HHV-6 may lead to hepatitis due to hepatitis C virus, and acute liver failure after liver transplantation (Harma et al., 2003; Rogers et al., 2000; Singh et al., 2002b). Similar findings have also been made in lung and heart-lung transplant patients (Jacobs et al., 2003), although HHV-6 infection was associated only with fever in one study of liver transplant recipients (217). After renal transplantation, HHV-7, but not HHV-6 DNAemia is related to graft rejection, higher plasma CMV DNA loads, CMV disease and graft dysfunction (Kidd et al., 2000; Osman et al., 1996; Tong et al., 2000, 2002).

Prophylaxis with valacyclovir or ganciclovir, two effective anti-herpesvirus agents, lead to reduced staphylococcal, candida and other fungal infections after renal and heart transplantation (Lowance et al., 1999; Wagner et al., 1995). In addition to the effects such therapy may have on CMV activity, the effects of this therapy on HHV-6 and HHV-7 may have contributed to the observed benefit. Future work on therapy targeted at roseoloviruses is needed, because these viruses frequently become active earlier than CMV in many patients.

HIV disease

Because of its impact on the immune system, HHV-6 has long been hypothesized to accelerate the progress of HIV infection. HIV disease is more likely to progress in HHV-6 infected infants and active HHV-6A and HHV-6B replication is frequently observed in patients with late stage AIDS (Clark et al., 1996; Emery et al., 1999; Kositanont et al., 1999). While this argues for either or both of the HHV-6 variants being copathogens for HIV, some data runs counter to this. Differences in methods and patient groups may account for some of the disagreement. In several studies there was no relationship between the presence of HHV-6 DNA in saliva or peripheral blood cells, or serological responses and AIDS pathogenesis (for review see Braun et al., 1997).

Future directions

Several areas of roseolovirus immunobiology seem ripe for further study, including (i) events during the earliest stages of primary infection, including identification of the target cells, modulation of immune responses, and establishment of latency, (ii) interactions with innate immune functions, including triggering of innate responses by engagement of receptors such as the Toll-like receptors, (iii) further study of the targets of cellular immunity and the effectiveness of these responses during disease, (iv) the relationship between virus-mediated immune suppression and other infections, (v) the possible contributions of HHV-6 immunomodulation to MS, (vi) interactions of these viruses with the various apoptotic pathways, (vii) the circumstances under which these viruses might affect the balance between the Th1- and Th2-type responses, (viii) mechanisms for modulating HLA-1 expression or activity, and (ix) identification of the mechanisms by which the virus regulates stimulation of immunity. It will be important to extend studies that are done in cultured purified cells to systems that more fully represent the complexity of in vivo regulatory mechanisms.

REFERENCES

Ablashi, D. V., Balachandran, N., Josephs, S. F. et al. (1991). Genomic polymorphism, growth properties, and immunologic variations in human herpesvirus-6 isolates. *Virology*, **184**, 545–552.

Ablashi, D. V., Lapps, W., Kaplan, M., Whitman, J. E., Richert, J. R., and Pearson, G. R. (1998). Human Herpesvirus-6 (HHV-6) infection in multiple sclerosis: a preliminary report. *Mult. Scler.*, **4**(6), 490–496.

Ablashi, D. V., Eastman, H. B., Owen, C. B. et al. (2000). Frequent HHV-6 reactivation in multiple sclerosis (MS) and chronic fatigue syndrome (CFS) patients. *J. Clin. Virol.*, **16**(3), 179–191.

Adler, S. P., McVoy, M., Chou, S., Hempfling, S., Yamanishi, K., and Britt, W. (1993). Antibodies induced by a primary cytomegalovirus infection react with human herpesvirus 6 proteins. *J. Infect. Dis.*, **168**, 1119–1126.

Anderson, R. A. and Gompels, U. A. (1999). N- and C-terminal external domains of human herpesvirus-6 glycoprotein H affect a fusion-associated conformation mediated by glycoprotein L binding the N terminus. *J. Gen. Virol.*, **80**, 1485–1494.

Anderson, R. A., Liu, D. X., and Gompels, U. A. (1996). Definition of a human herpesvirus-6 betaherpesvirus-specific domain in glycoprotein gH that governs interaction with glycoprotein gL: substitution of human cytomegalovirus glycoproteins permits group-specific complex formation. *Virology*, **217**(2), 517–526.

Arena, A., Liberto, M. C., Capozza, A. B., and Foca, A. (1997). Productive HHV-6 infection in differentiated U937 cells: role of TNF alpha in regulation of HHV-6. *New Microbiol.*, **20**(1), 13–20.

Arena, A., Liberto, M. C., Iannello, D., Capozza, A. B., and Foca, A. (1999). Altered cytokine production after human herpes virus type 6 infection. *N. Microbiol.*, **22**(4), 293–300.

Arena, A., Merendino, R. A., Bonina, L., Iannello, D., Stassi, G., and Mastroeni, P. (2000). Role of IL-15 on monocytic resistance to human herpesvirus 6 infection. *N. Microbiol.*, **23**(2), 105–112.

Arsenault, S., Gravel, A., Gosselin, J., and Flamand, L. (2003). Generation and characterization of a monoclonal antibody specific for human herpesvirus 6 variant A immediate-early 2 protein. *J. Clin. Virol.*, **28**(3), 284–290.

Arvin, A., Sharp, M., Smith, S., *et al.* (1991). Equivalent recognition of varicella-zoster virus immediate early protein (IE62) and glycoprotein I by cytotoxic T lymphocytes of either CD4+ or CD8+ phenotype. *J. Immunol.*, **146**, 257–264.

Asada, H., Yalcin, S., Balachandra, K., Higashi, K., and Yamanishi, K. (1989). Establishment of titration system for human herpesvirus 6 and evaluation of neutralizing antibody response to the virus. *J. Clin. Microbiol.*, **27**, 2204–2207.

Asada, H., Klaus-Kovtun, V., Golding, H., Katz, S. I., and Blauvelt, A. (1999). Human herpesvirus 6 infects dendritic cells and suppresses human immunodeficiency virus type 1 replication in coinfected cultures. *J. Virol.*, **73**(5), 4019–4028.

Atedzoe, B. N., Ahmad, A., and Menezes, J. (1997). Enhancement of natural killer cell cytotoxicity by the human herpesvirus-7 via IL-15 induction. *J. Immunol.*, **159**(10), 4966–4972.

Balachandra, K., Ayuthaya, P. I., Auwanit, W. *et al.* (1989). Prevalence of antibody to human herpesvirus 6 in women and children. *Microbiol. Immunol.*, **33**(6), 515–518.

Balachandra, N., Amelse, R. E., Zhou, W. W., and Chang, C. K. (1989). Identification of proteins specific for human herpesvirus 6-infected human T cells. *J. Virol.*, **63**, 2835–2840.

Berneman, Z. N., Ablashi, D. V., Li, G. *et al.* (1992). Human herpesvirus 7 is a T-lymphotropic virus and is related to, but significantly different from, human herpesvirus 6 and human cytomegalovirus. *Proc. Natl Acad. Sci. USA*, **89**(21), 10552–10556.

Black, J. B. and Pellett, P. E. (1999). Human herpesvirus 7. *Rev. Med. Virol.*, **9**, 245–262.

Black, J. B., Sanderlin, K. C., Goldsmith, C. S., Gary, H. E., Lopez, C., and Pellett, P. E. (1989). Growth properties of human herpesvirus-6 strain Z29. *J. Virol. Methods*, **26**, 133–145.

Black, J. B., Lopez, C., and Pellett, P. E. (1992). Induction of host cell protein synthesis by human herpesvirus 6. *Virus Res.*, **22**(1), 13–23.

Black, J. B., Durigon, E., Kite-Powell, K. *et al.* (1996a). Seroconversion to human herpesvirus 6 and human herpesvirus 7 among Brazilian children with clinical diagnoses of measles or rubella. *Clin. Infect. Dis.*, **23**, 1156–1158.

Black, J. B., Schwarz, T. F., Patton, J. L. *et al.* (1996b). Evaluation of immunoassays for detection of antibodies to human herpesvirus 7. *Clin. Diagn. Lab. Immunol.*, **3**, 79–83.

Boeckh, M. and Nichols, W. S. (2003). Immunosuppressive effects of beta-herpesviruses. *Herpes*, **10**(1), 12–16.

Boutolleau, D., Fernandez, C., Andre, E. *et al.* (2003). Human herpesvirus (HHV)-6 and HHV-7: two closely related viruses with different infection profiles in stem cell transplantation recipients. *J. Infect. Dis.*, **187**(2), 179–186.

Braun, D. K., Dominguez, G., and Pellett, P. E. (1997). Human herpesvirus 6. *Clin. Microbiol. Rev.*, **10**, 521–567.

Burd, E. M. and Carrigan, D. R. (1993). Human herpesvirus 6 (HHV-6)-associated dysfunction of blood monocytes. *Virus Res.*, **29**, 79–90.

Burd, E. M., Knox, K. K., and Carrigan D. R. (1993). Human herpesvirus-6-associated suppression of growth factor-induced macrophage maturation in human bone marrow cultures. *Blood*, **81**, 1645–1650.

Campadelli-Fiume, G., Guerrini, S., Liu, X., and Foa-Tomasi, L. (1993). Monoclonal antibodies to glycoprotein B differentiate human herpesvirus 6 into two clusters, variants A and B. *J. Gen. Virol.*, **74**, 2257–2262.

Carricart, S. E., Bustos, D., Biganzoli, P., Nates, S. E., and Pavan, J. V. (2004). Isotype immune response of IgG antibodies at the persistence and reactivation stages of human herpes virus 6 infection. *J. Clin. Virol.*, **31**(4), 266–269.

Carrigan, D. R. (1995). Human herpesvirus-6 and bone marrow transplantation. *Blood*, **85**(1), 294–295.

Caruso, A., Rotola, A., Comar, M. *et al.* (2002). HHV-6 infects human aortic and heart microvascular endothelial cells, increasing their ability to secrete proinflammatory chemokines. *J. Med. Virol.*, **67**(4), 528–533.

Caruso, A., Favilli, F., Rotola, A. *et al.* (2003). Human herpesvirus-6 modulates RANTES production in primary human endothelial cell cultures. *J. Med. Virol.*, **70**(3), 451–458.

Caselli, E., Boni, M., Bracci, A. *et al.* (2002). Detection of antibodies directed against human herpesvirus 6 U94/REP in sera of patients affected by multiple sclerosis. *J. Clin. Microbiol.*, **40**(11), 4131–4137.

Caserta, M. T., Hall, C. B., Schnabel, K., Long, C. E., and D'Heron, N. (1998). Primary human herpesvirus 7 infection: a comparison of human herpesvirus 7 and human herpesvirus 6 infections in children. *J. Pediatr.*, **133**(3), 386–389.

Caserta, M. T., Mock, D. J., and Dewhurst, S. (2001). Human herpesvirus 6. *Clin. Infect. Dis.*, **33**(6), 829–833.

Cermelli, C., Concari, M., Carubbi, F. *et al.* (1996). Growth of human herpesvirus 6 in HEPG2 cells. *Virus Res.*, **45**, 75–85.

Cermelli, C., Berti, R., Soldan, S. S. (2003). *et al.* High frequency of human herpesvirus 6 DNA in multiple sclerosis plaques isolated by laser microdissection. *J. Infect. Dis.*, **187**(9), 1377–1387.

Cesarman, E. and Knowles, D. M. (1999). The role of Kaposi's sarcoma-associated herpesvirus (KSHV/HHV-8) in lymphoproliferative diseases. *Semin. Cancer. Biol.*, **9**(3), 165–174.

Chandran, B., Tirawatnapong, S., Pfeiffer, B. and Ablashi, D. V. (1992). Antigenic relationships among human herpesvirus-6 isolates. *J. Med. Virol.*, **37**(4), 247–254.

Chapenko, S., Millers, A., Nora, Z., Logina, I., Kukaine, R., and Murovska, M. (2003). Correlation between HHV-6 reactivation and multiple sclerosis disease activity. *J. Med. Virol.*, **69**(1), 111–117.

Cirone, M., Campadelli-Fiume, G., Foa-Tomasi, L., Torrisi, M. R., and Faggioni, A. (1994). Human herpesvirus 6 envelope glycoproteins B and H-L complex are undetectable on the plasma membrane of infected lymphocytes. AIDS *Res. Hum. Retroviruses*, **10**(2), 175–179.

Cirone, M., Cuomo, L., Zompetta, C. *et al.* (2002). Human herpesvirus 6 and multiple sclerosis: a study of T cell cross-reactivity to viral and myelin basic protein antigens. *J. Med. Virol.*, **68**(2), 268–272.

Clark, D. A. (2000). Human herpesvirus 6. *Rev. Med. Virol.*, **10**(3), 155–173.

Clark, D. A., and Griffiths, P. D. (2003). Human herpesvirus 6: relevance of infection in the immunocompromised host. *Br. J. Haematol.*, **120**(3), 384–395.

Clark, D. A., Ait-Khaled, M., Wheeler, A. C. *et al.* (1996). Quantification of human herpesvirus 6 in immunocompetent persons and post-mortem tissues from AIDS patients by PCR. *J. Gen. Virol.*, **77**, 2271–2275.

Cone, R. W., Huang, M. L., Hackman, R. C., and Corey, L. (1996). Coinfection with human herpesvirus 6 variants A and B in lung tissue. *J. Clin. Microbiol.*, **34**, 877–881.

Dahl, H., Fjaertoft, G., Norsted, T., Wang, F. Z., Mousavi-Jazi, M., and Linde, A. (1999). Reactivation of human herpesvirus 6 during pregnancy. *J. Infect. Dis.*, **180**(6), 2035–2038.

DesJardin, J. A., Gibbons, L., Cho, E. *et al.* (1998). Human herpesvirus 6 reactivation is associated with cytomegalovirus infection and syndromes in kidney transplant recipients at risk for primary cytomegalovirus infection. *J. Infect. Dis.*, **178**(6), 1783–1786.

DesJardin, J. A., Cho, E., Supran, S., Gibbons, L., Werner, B. G., and Snydman, D. R. (2001). Association of human herpesvirus 6 reactivation with severe cytomegalovirus-associated disease in orthotopic liver transplant recipients. *Clin. Infect. Dis.*, **33**(8), 1358–1362.

Dewin, D. R., Catusse, J., and Gompels, U. A. (2000). Identification and characterization of U83A viral chemokine, a broad and potent beta-chemokine agonist for human CCRs with unique selectivity and inhibition by spliced isoform. *J. Immunol.* **176**(1), 544–556.

Dhepakson, P., Mori, Y., Jiang, Y. B. *et al.* (2002). Human herpesvirus-6 rep/U94 gene product has single-stranded DNA-binding activity. *J. Gen. Virol.*, **83**(4), 847–854.

Dockrell, D. H., Mendez, J. C., Jones, M. *et al.* (1999). Human herpesvirus 6 seronegativity before transplantation predicts the occurrence of fungal infection in liver transplant recipients. *Transplantation*, **67**(3), 399–403.

Dominguez, G., Dambaugh, T. R., Stamey, F. R., Dewhurst, S., Inoue, N., and Pellett, P. E. (1999). Human herpesvirus 6B genome sequence: coding content and comparison with human herpesvirus 6A. *J. Virol.*, **73**, 8040–8052.

Eizuru, Y. and Minamishima, Y. (1992). Evidence for putative immediate early antigens in human herpesvirus 6-infected cells. *J. Gen. Virol.*, **73**, 2161–2165.

Emery, V. C., Atkins, M. C., Bowen, E. F. *et al.* (1999). Interactions between beta-herpesviruses and human immunodeficiency virus in vivo: evidence for increased human immunodeficiency viral load in the presence of human herpesvirus 6. *J. Med. Virol.*, **57**(3), 278–282.

Enbom, M., Martin, C., Fredrikson, S., Jagdahl, L., Dahl, H., and Linde, A. (1997). Intrathecal antibody production to lymphotropic herpesviruses in patients with multiple sclerosis. *Neurol. Infect. Epidemiol.*, **2**, 107–111.

Enbom, M., Wang, F. Z., Fredrickson, S., Martin, C., Dahl, H., and Linde, A. (1999). Similar humoral and cellular immunological reactivities to human herpesvirus 6 in patients with multiple sclerosis and controls. *Clin. Diagn. Lab. Immunol.*, **6**, 545–549.

Feldstein, A. E., Razonable, R. R., Boyce, T. G. *et al.* (2003). Prevalence and clinical significance of human herpesviruses 6 and 7 active infection in pediatric liver transplant patients. *Pediatr. Transpl.*, **7**(2), 125–129.

Flamand, L., Gosselin, J., D'Addario, M. *et al.* (1991). Human herpesvirus 6 induces interleukin-1 beta and tumor necrosis factor alpha, but not interleukin-6, in peripheral blood mononuclear cell cultures. *J. Virol.*, **65**(9), 5105–5110.

Flamand, L., Gosselin, J., Stefanescu, I., Ablashi, D., and Menezes, J. (1995). Immunosuppressive effect of human herpesvirus 6 on T-cell functions: suppression of interleukin-2 synthesis and cell proliferation [published erratum appears in Blood, **86**, 418, 1995]. *Blood*, **85**(5), 1263–1271.

Flamand, L., Stefanescu, I., and Menezes, J. (1996). Human herpesvirus-6 enhances natural killer cell cytotoxicity via IL-15. *J. Clin. Invest.*, **97**, 1373–1381.

Flamand, L., Romerio, F., Reitz, M. S., and Gallo, R. C. (1998). CD4 promoter transactivation by human herpesvirus 6. *J. Virol.*, **72**(11), 8797–8805.

Flebbe-Rehwaldt, L. M., Wood, C., and Chandran, B. (2000). Characterization of transcripts expressed from human herpesvirus 6A strain GS immediate-early region B U16-U17 open reading frames. *J. Virol.*, **74**(23), 11040–11054.

Foa-Tomasi, L., Boscaro, A., Di Gaeta, S., and Campadelli-Fiume, G. (1991). Monoclonal antibodies to gp100 inhibit penetration of human herpesvirus 6 and polykaryocyte formation in susceptible cells. *J. Virol.*, **65**, 4124–4129.

Foa-Tomasi, L., Guerrini, S., Huang, T., and Campadelli-Fiume, G. (1992). Characterization of human herpesvirus-6 (U1102) and (GS) gp112 and identification of the Z29-specified homolog. *Virology*, **191**, 511–516.

Foa-Tomasi, L., Avitabile, E., Ke, L., and Campadelli-Fiume, G. (1994). Polyvalent and monoclonal antibodies identify major immunogenic proteins specific for human herpesvirus 7-infected cells and have weak cross-reactivity with human herpesvirus 6. *J. Gen. Virol.*, **75**, 2719–2727.

Foa-Tomasi, L., Fiorilli, M. P., Avitabile, E., and Campadelli-Fiume, G. (1996). Identification of an 85 kDa phosphoprotein as an immunodominant protein specific for human herpesvirus 7-infected cells. *J. Gen. Virol.*, **77**, 511–518.

Fox, J. D., Briggs, M., Ward, P. A., and Tedder, R. S. (1990). Human herpesvirus 6 in salivary glands. *Lancet*, **336**(8715), 590–593.

Franti, M., Aubin, J. T., Saint-Maur, G. *et al.* (2002). Immune reactivity of human sera to the glycoprotein B of human herpesvirus 7. *J. Clin. Microbiol.*, **40**(1), 44–51.

Frenkel, N., Schirmer, E. C., Katsafanas, G., and June, C. H. (1990). T-cell activation is required for efficient replication of human herpesvirus 6. *J. Virol.*, **64**(9), 4598–4602.

Furukawa, M., Yasukawa, M., Yakushijin, Y., and Fujita S. (1994). Distinct effects of human herpesvirus 6 and human herpesvirus 7 on surface molecule expression and function of CD4+ T cells. *J. Immunol.*, **152**, 5768–5775.

Gobbi, A., Stoddart, C. A., Malnati, M. S. *et al.* (1999). Human herpesvirus 6 (HHV-6) causes severe thymocyte depletion in SCID-hu Thy/Liv mice. *J. Exp. Med.*, **189**(12), 1953–1960.

Goodman, A. D., Mock, D. J., Powers, J. M., Baker, J. V., and Blumberg, B. M. (2003). Human herpesvirus 6 genome and antigen in acute multiple sclerosis lesions. *J. Infect. Dis.*, **187**(9), 1365–1376.

Griffiths, P. D. (2003). The indirect effects of virus infections. *Rev. Med. Virol.*, **13**, 1–3.

Griffiths, P. D., Ait-Khaled, M., Bearcroft, C. P. *et al.* (1999). Human herpesviruses 6 and 7 as potential pathogens after liver transplant: prospective comparison with the effect of cytomegalovirus. *J. Med. Virol.*, **59**(4), 496–501.

Grivel, J. C., Ito, Y., Faga, G. *et al.* (2001). Suppression of CCR5- but not CXCR4-tropic HIV-1 in lymphoid tissue by human herpesvirus 6. *Nat. Med.*, **7**(11), 1232–1235.

Grivel, J. C., Santoro, F., Chen, S. *et al.* (2003). Pathogenic effects of human herpesvirus 6 in human lymphoid tissue ex vivo. *J. Virol.*, **77**(15), 8280–8289.

Hall, C. B., Long, C. E., Schnabel, K. C. *et al.* (1994). Human herpesvirus-6 infection in children. A prospective study of complications and reactivation. *N. Engl. J. Med.*, **331**(7), 432–438.

Harma, M., Hockerstedt, K., and Lautenschlager, I. (2003). Human herpesvirus-6 and acute liver failure. *Transplantation*, **76**(3), 536–539.

Hasegawa, A., Yasukawa, M., Sakai, I., and Fujita, S. (2001). Transcriptional down-regulation of CXC chemokine receptor 4 induced by impaired association of transcription regulator YY1 with c-Myc in human herpesvirus 6-infected cells. *J. Immunol.*, **166**(2), 1125–1131.

He, J., McCarthy, M., Zhou, Y., Chandran, B., and Wood, C. (1996). Infection of primary human fetal astrocytes by human herpesvirus 6. *J. Virol.*, **70**, 1296–1300.

Hidaka, Y., Okada, K., Kusuhara, K., Miyazaki, C., Tokugawa, K., and Ueda, K. (1994). Exanthem subitum and human herpesvirus 7 infection. *Pediatr. Infect. Dis. J.*, **13**(11), 1010–1011.

Hirata, Y., Kondo, K., and Yamanishi, K. (2001). Human herpesvirus 6 downregulates major histocompatibility complex class I in dendritic cells. *J. Med. Virol.*, **65**(3), 576–583.

Horvat, R. T., Parmely, M. J., and Chandran, B. (1993). Human herpesvirus 6 inhibits the proliferative responses of human peripheral blood mononuclear cells. *J. Infect. Dis.*, **167**(6), 1274–1280.

Huang, L. M., Lee, C. Y., Liu, M. Y., and Lee, P. I. (1997). Primary infections of human herpesvirus-7 and human herpesvirus-6: a comparative, longitudinal study up to 6 years of age. *Acta Paediatr.*, **86**, 604–608.

Hudson, A. W., Howley, P. M., and Ploegh, H. L. (2001). A human herpesvirus 7 glycoprotein, U21, diverts major histocompatibility complex class I molecules to lysosomes. *J. Virol.*, **75**(24), 12347–12358.

Hudson, A. W., Blom, D., Howley, P. M., and Ploegh, H. L. (2003). The ER-lumenal domain of the HHV-7 immunoevasin U21 directs class I MHC molecules to lysosomes. *Traffic*, **4**(12), 824–837.

Humar, A., Malkan, G., Moussa, G., Greig, P., Levy, G., and Mazzulli, T. (2000). Human herpesvirus-6 is associated with cytomegalovirus reactivation in liver transplant recipients. *J. Infect. Dis.*, **181**(4), 1450–1453.

Humar, A., Kumar, D., Caliendo, A. M. *et al.* (2002). Clinical impact of human herpesvirus 6 infection after liver transplantation. *Transplantation*, **73**(4), 599–604.

Ichimi, R., Jin-no, T., and Ito, M. (1999). Induction of apoptosis in cord blood lymphocytes by HHV-6. *J. Med. Virol.*, **58**(1), 63–68.

Inoue, Y., Yasukawa, M., and Fujita, S. (1997). Induction of T-cell apoptosis by human herpesvirus 6. *J. Virol.*, **71**, 3751–3759.

Isegawa, Y., Ping, Z., Nakano, K., Sugimoto, N., and Yamanishi, K. (1998). Human herpesvirus 6 open reading frame U12 encodes a functional beta-chemokine receptor. *J. Virol.*, **72**(7), 6104–6112.

Isomura, H., Yamada, M., Yoshida, M. *et al.* (1997). Suppressive effects of human herpesvirus 6 on in vitro colony formation of hematopoietic progenitor cells. *J. Med. Virol.*, **52**(4), 406–412.

Isomura, H., Yoshida, M., Namba, H., and Yamada, M. (2003). Interaction of human herpesvirus 6 with human CD34 positive cells. *J. Med. Virol.*, **70**(3), 444–450.

Iyengar, S., Levine, P. H., Ablashi, D., Neequaye, J., and Pearson, G. R. (1991). Sero-epidemiological investigations on human herpesvirus 6 (HHV-6) infections using a newly developed early antigen assay. *Int. J. Cancer*, **49**, 551–557.

Jacobs, F., Knoop, C., Brancart, F. *et al.* (2003). Human herpesvirus-6 infection after lung and heart–lung transplantation: a prospective longitudinal study. *Transplantation*, **75**(12), 1996–2001.

Kakimoto, M., Hasegawa, A., Fujita, S., and Yasukawa, M. (2002). Phenotypic and functional alterations of dendritic cells induced by human herpesvirus 6 infection. *J. Virol.*, **76**(20), 10338–10345.

Kano, Y., Inaoka, M., and Shiohara, T. (2004). Association between anticonvulsant hypersensitivity syndrome and human herpesvirus 6 reactivation and hypogammaglobulinemia. *Arch. Dermatol.*, **140**(2), 183–188.

Kempf, W., Adams, V., Wey, N. *et al.* (1997). CD68+ cells of monocyte/macrophage lineage in the environment of AIDS-associated and classic-sporadic Kaposi sarcoma are singly or doubly infected with human herpesviruses 7 and 6B. *Proc. Natl Acad. Sci. USA*, **94**, 7600–7605.

Kempf, W., Adams, V., Mirandola, P. *et al.* (1998). Persistence of human herpesvirus 7 in normal tissues detected by expression of a structural antigen. *J. Infect. Dis.*, **178**(3), 841–845.

Kidd, I. M., Clark, D. A., Sabin, C. A. *et al.* (2000). Prospective study of human betaherpesviruses after renal transplantation: association of human herpesvirus 7 and cytomegalovirus co-infection with cytomegalovirus disease and increased rejection. *Transplantation*, **69**(11), 2400–2404.

Kikuta, H., Lu, H., Tomizawa, K., and Matsumoto, S. (1990a). Enhancement of human herpesvirus 6 replication in adult human lymphocytes by monoclonal antibody to CD3. *J. Infect. Dis.*, **161**(6), 1085–1087.

Kikuta, H., Nakane, A., Lu, H., Taguchi, Y., Minagawa, T., and Matsumoto, S. (1990b). Interferon induction by human herpesvirus 6 in human mononuclear cells. *J. Infect. Dis.*, **162**(1), 35–38.

Knox, K. K., and Carrigan, D. R. (1992). In vitro suppression of bone marrow progenitor cell differentiation by human herpesvirus 6 infection. *J. Infect. Dis.*, **165**(5), 925–929.

Kondo, K., Kondo, T., Okuno, T., Takahashi, M., and Yamanishi, K. (1991). Latent human herpesvirus 6 infection of human monocytes/macrophages. *J. Gen. Virol.*, **72**, 1401–1408.

Kondo, K., Xu, J., and Mocarski, E. S. (1996). Human cytomegalovirus latent gene expression in granulocyte-macrophage progenitors in culture and in seropositive individuals. *Proc. Natl Acad. Sci. USA*, **93**(20), 11137–11142.

Kondo, K., Kondo, T., Shimada, K., Amo, K., Miyagawa, H., and Yamanishi, K. (2002a). Strong interaction between human herpesvirus 6 and peripheral blood monocytes/macrophages during acute infection. *J. Med. Virol.*, **67**(3), 364–369.

Kondo, K., Shimada, K., Sashihara, J., Tanaka-Taya, K., and Yamanishi, K. (2002b). Identification of human herpesvirus 6 latency-associated transcripts. *J. Virol.*, **76**(8), 4145–4151.

Kong, H., Baerbig, Q., Duncan, L., Shepel, N., and Mayne, M. (2003). Human herpesvirus type 6 indirectly enhances oligodendrocyte cell death. *J. Neurovirol.* **9**(5), 539–550.

Kositanont, U., Wasi, C., Wanprapar, N. *et al.* (1999). Primary infection of human herpesvirus 6 in children with vertical infection of human immunodeficicncy virus type 1. *J. Infect. Dis.*, **180**, 50–55.

Kumagai, T., Yoshikawa, T., Yoshida, M. *et al.* (2006). Time course characteristics of human herpesvirus 6 specific cellular immune response and natural killer cell activity in patients with exanthema subitum. *J. Med. Virol.*, **78**(6), 792–799.

LaCroix, S., Stewart, J. A., Thouless, M. E., and Black, J. B. (2000). An immunoblot assay for detection of immunoglobulin M antibody to human herpesvirus 6. *Clin. Diagn. Lab. Immunol.*, **7**(5), 823–827.

Landini, M. P., Lazzarotto, T., Xu, J., Geballe, A. P., and Mocarski, E. S. (2000). Humoral immune response to proteins of human cytomegalovirus latency-associated transcripts. *Biol. Blood Marrow Transpl.*, **6**(2), 100–108.

Lautenschlager, I., Harma, M., Hockerstedt, K., Linnavuori, K., Loginov, R., and Taskinen, E. (2002). Human herpesvirus-6 infection is associated with adhesion molecule induction and lymphocyte infiltration in liver allografts. *J. Hepatol.*, **37**(5), 648–654.

Li, C., Goodrich, J. M., and Yang, X. (1997). Interferon-gamma (IFN-gamma) regulates production of IL-10 and IL-12 in human herpesvirus-6 (HHV-6)-infected monocyte/macrophage lineage. *Clin. Exp. Immunol.*, **109**(3), 421–425.

Linde, A., Dahl, H., Wahren, B., Fridell, E., Salahuddin, Z., and Biberfeld, P. (1988). IgG antibodies to human herpesvirus-6 in children and adults and in primary Epstein–Barr virus infections and cytomegalovirus infections. *J. Virol. Methods*, **21**, 117–123.

Littler, E., Lawrence, G., Liu, M. Y., Barrell, B. G., and Arrand, J. R. (1990). Identification, cloning, and expression of the major capsid protein gene of human herpesvirus 6. *J. Virol.*, **64**, 714–722.

Liu, D. X., Gompels, U. A., Foa-Tomasi, L., and Campadelli-Fiume, G. (1993a). Human herpesvirus-6 glycoprotein H and L homologs are components of the GP100 complex and the GH external domain is the target for neutralizing monoclonal antibodies. *Virology*, **197**, 12–22.

Liu, D. X., Gompels, U. A., Nicholas, J., and Lelliott, C. (1993b). Identification and expression of the human herpesvirus 6 glycoprotein H and interaction with an accessory 40K glycoprotein. *J. Gen. Virol.*, **74**, 1847–1857.

Ljungman, P. (2002). Beta-herpesvirus challenges in the transplant recipient. *J. Infect. Dis.*, **186** Suppl. 1, S99–S109.

Ljungman, P., Wahren, B., and Sundqvist, V. A. (1985). Lymphocyte proliferation and IgG production with herpesvirus antigens in solid phase. *J. Virol. Method.*, **12**, 199–208.

Lowance, D., Neumayer, H. H., Legendre, C. M. *et al.* (1999). Valacyclovir for the prevention of cytomegalovirus disease after renal transplantation. International Valacyclovir Cytomegalovirus Prophylaxis Transplantation Study Group. *N. Engl. J. Med.*, **340**(19), 1462–1470.

Luppi, M., Barozzi, P., Morris, C., *et al.* (1999). Human herpesvirus 6 latently infects early bone marrow progenitors in vivo. *J. Virol.*, **73**(1), 754–759.

Lusso, P., De Maria, A., Malnati, M. *et al.* (1991a). Induction of CD4 and susceptibility to HIV-1 infection in human CD8+ T lymphocytes by human herpesvirus 6. *Nature*, **349**(6309), 533–535.

Lusso, P., Malnati, M., De Maria, A. *et al.* (1991b). Productive infection of CD4+ and CD8+ mature human T cell populations and clones by human herpesvirus 6. Transcriptional down-regulation of CD3. *J. Immunol.* **147**, 685–691.

Lusso, P., Malnati, M. S., Garzino-Demo, A., Crowley, R. W., Long, E. O., and Gallo, R. C. (1993). Infection of natural killer cells by human herpesvirus 6. *Nature*, **362**(6419), 458–462.

Lusso, P., Secchiero, P., Crowley, R. W., Garzino-Demo, A., Berneman, Z. N., and Gallo, R. C. (1994). CD4 is a critical component of the receptor for human herpesvirus 7: interference with human immunodeficiency virus. *Proc. Natl Acad. Sci. USA*, **91**, 3872–3876.

Lusso, P., Garzino-Demo, A., Crowley, R. W., and Malnati, M. S. (1995). Infection of gamma/delta T lymphocytes by human herpesvirus 6: transcriptional induction of CD4 and susceptibility to HIV infection. *J. Exp. Med.*, **181**(4), 1303–1310.

Luttichau, H. R., Clark-Lewis, I., Jensen, P. O., Moser, C., Gerstoft, J., and Schwartz, T. W. (2003). A highly selective CCR2 chemokine agonist encoded by human herpesvirus 6. *J. Biol. Chem.*, **278**(13), 10928–10933.

Malnati, M. S., Lusso, P., Ciccone, E., Moretta, A., Moretta, L., and Long, E. O. (1993). Recognition of virus-infected cells by natural killer cell clones is controlled by polymorphic target cell elements. *J. Exp. Med.*, **178**(3), 961–969.

Mayne, M., Cheadle, C., Soldan, S. S. *et al.* (2001). Gene expression profile of herpesvirus-infected T cells obtained using immunomicroarrays: induction of proinflammatory mechanisms. *J. Virol.*, **75**(23), 11641–11650.

Meeuwsen, S., Persoon-Deen, C., Bsibsi, M. *et al.* (2005). Modulation of the cytokine network in human adult astrocytes by human herpesvirus-6A. *J. Neuroimmunol.*, **164**(1–2), 37–47.

Milne, R. S., Mattick, C., Nicholson, L., Devaraj, P., Alcami, A., and Gompels, U. A. (2000). RANTES binding and down-regulation by a novel human herpesvirus-6 beta chemokine receptor. *J. Immunol.*, **164**(5), 2396–2404.

Mirandola, P., Secchiero, P., Pierpaoli, S. *et al.* (2000). Infection of CD34(+) hematopoietic progenitor cells by human herpesvirus 7 (HHV-7). *Blood*, **96**(1), 126–131.

Miyoshi, H., Tanaka-Taya, K., Hara, J. *et al.* (2001). Inverse relationship between human herpesvirus-6 and -7 detection after allogeneic and autologous stem cell transplantation. *Bone Marrow Transpl.*, **27**(10), 1065–1070.

Molden, J., Chang, Y., You, Y., Moore, P. S., and Goldsmith, M. A. (1997). A Kaposi's sarcoma-associated herpesvirus-encoded cytokine homolog (vIL-6) activates signaling through the shared gp130 receptor subunit. *J. Biol. Chem.*, **272**(31), 19625–19631.

Mori, Y., Seya, T., Huang, H. L., Akkapaiboon, P., Dhepakson, P., and Yamanishi, K. (2002). Human herpesvirus 6 variant A but not variant B induces fusion from without in a variety of human cells through a human herpesvirus 6 entry receptor, CD46. *J. Virol.*, **76**(13), 6750–6761.

Mori, Y., Akkapaiboon, P., Yang, X., and Yamanishi, K. (2003a). The human herpesvirus 6 U100 gene product is the third component of the gH-gL glycoprotein complex on the viral envelope. *J. Virol.*, **77**(4), 2452–2458.

Mori, Y., Yang, X., Akkapaiboon, P., Okuno, T., and Yamanishi, K. (2003b). Human herpesvirus 6 variant A glycoprotein H-glycoprotein L-glycoprotein Q complex associates with human CD46. *J. Virol.*, **77**(8), 4992–4999.

Nakagawa, N., Mukai, T., Sakamoto, J. *et al.* (1997). Antigenic analysis of human herpesvirus 7 (HHV-7) and HHV-6 using immune sera and monoclonal antibodies against HHV-7. *J. Gen. Virol.*, **78**, 1131–1137.

Nakano, K., Tadagaki, K., Isegawa, Y., Aye, M. M., Zou, P., and Yamanishi, K. (2003). Human herpesvirus 7 open reading frame U12 encodes a functional beta-chemokine receptor. *J. Virol.*, **77**(14), 8108–8115.

Neipel, F., Ellinger, K., and Fleckenstein, B. (1992). Gene for the major antigenic structural protein (p100) of human herpesvirus 6. *J. Virol.*, **66**, 3918–3924.

Ohashi, M., Yoshikawa, T., Ihira, M. *et al.* (2002). Reactivation of human herpesvirus 6 and 7 in pregnant women. *J. Med. Virol.*, **67**(3), 354–358.

Okuno, T., Sao, H., Asada, H., Shiraki, K., Takahashi, M., and Yamanishi, K. (1990). Analysis of a glycoprotein for human herpesvirus 6 (HHV-6) using monoclonal antibodies. *Virology*, **176**, 625–628.

Okuno, T., Shao, H., Asada, H., Shiraki, K., Takahashi, M., and Yamanishi, K. (1992). Analysis of human herpesvirus 6 glycoproteins recognized by monoclonal antibody OHV1. *J. Gen. Virol.*, **73**, 443–447.

Oliveira, S. A., Turner, D. J., Knowles, W., Nascimento, J. P., Brown, D. W., and Ward, K. N. (2003). Primary human herpesvirus-6 and -7 infections, often coinciding, misdiagnosed as measles in children from a tropical region of Brazil. *Epidemiol. Infect.*, **131**(2), 873–879.

Osman, H. K. E., Peiris, J. S. M., Taylor, C. E., Warwicker, P., Jarrett, R. F., and Madeley, C. R. (1996). "Cytomegalovirus disease" in renal allograft recipients: is human herpesvirus 7 a cofactor for disease progression? *J. Med. Virol.*, **48**, 295–301.

Øster, B., Bundgaard, B., and Hollsberg, P. (2005). Human herpesvirus 6B induces cell cycle arrest concomitant with p53 phosphorylation and accumulation in T cells. *J. Virol.*, **79**(3), 1961–1965.

Patnaik, M., Komaroff, A. L., Conley, E., Ojo-Amaize, E. A., and Peter, J. B. (1995). Prevalence of IgM antibodies to human herpesvirus 6 early antigen (p41/38) in patients with chronic fatigue syndrome. *J. Infect. Dis.*, **172**, 1264–1267.

Pellett, P. E., Sanchez-Martinez, D., Dominguez, G. *et al.* (1993). A strongly immunoreactive virion protein of human herpesvirus 6 variant B strain Z29: identification and characterization of the gene and mapping of a variant-specific monoclonal antibody reactive epitope. *Virology*, **195**(2), 521–531.

Qian, G., Wood, C., and Chandran, B. (1993). Identification and characterization of glycoprotein gH of human herpesvirus-6. *Virology*, **194**(1), 380–386.

Rapp, J. C., Krug, L. T., Inoue, N., Dambaugh, T. R., and Pellett, P. E. (2000). U94, the human herpesvirus 6 homolog of the parvovirus nonstructural gene, is highly conserved among isolates and is expressed at low mRNA levels as a spliced transcript. *Virology*, **268**, 504–516.

Razvi, E. S. and Welsh, R. M. (1995). Apoptosis in viral infections. *Adv. Virus Res.* **45**, 1–60.

Robert, C., Aubin, J. T., Visse, B., Fillet, A. M., Huraux, J. M., and Agut, H. (1996). Difference in permissiveness of human fibroblast cells to variants A and B of human herpesvirus-6. *Res. Virol.*, **147**(4), 219–225.

Roffman, E. and Frenkel, N. (1990). Interleukin-2 inhibits the replication of human herpesvirus-6 in mature thymocytes. *Virology*, **175**(2), 591–594.

Roffman, E. and Frenkel, N. (1991). Replication of human herpesvirus-6 in thymocytes activated by anti-CD3 antibody. *J. Infect. Dis.*, **164**, 617–618.

Rogers, J., Rohal, S., Carrigan, D. R. *et al.* (2000). Human herpesvirus-6 in liver transplant recipients: role in pathogenesis of fungal infections, neurologic complications, and outcome. *Transplantation*, **69**(12), 2566–2573.

Rossi, C., Delforge, M. L., Jacobs, F. *et al.* (2001). Fatal primary infection due to human herpesvirus 6 variant A in a renal transplant recipient. *Transplantation*, **71**(2), 288–292.

Rotola, A., Ravaioli, T., Gonelli, A., Dewhurst, S., Cassai, E., and Di Luca, D. (1998). U94 of human herpesvirus 6 is expressed in latently infected peripheral blood mononuclear cells and blocks viral gene expression in transformed lymphocytes in culture. *Proc. Natl Acad. Sci. USA*, **95**(23), 13911–13916.

Roush, K. S., Domiati-Saad, R. K., Margraf, L. R. *et al.* (2001). Prevalence and cellular reservoir of latent human herpesvirus 6 in tonsillar lymphoid tissue. *Am. J. Clin. Pathol.*, **116**(5), 648–654.

Santoro, F., Kennedy, P. E., Locatelli, G., Malnati, M. S., Berger, E. A., and Lusso, P. (1999). CD46 is a cellular receptor from human herpesvirus 6. *Cell*, **99**, 817–827.

Santoro, F., Greenstone, H. L., Insinga, A. *et al.* (2003). Interaction of glycoprotein H of human herpesvirus 6 with the cellular receptor CD46. *J. Biol. Chem.*, **278**(28), 25964–25969.

Secchiero, P., Flamand, L., Gilbellini, D. *et al.* (1997). Human herpesvirus 7 induces CD4+ T-cell death by two distinct mechanisms: necrotic lysis in productively infected cells and apoptosis in uninfected or nonproductively infected cells. *Blood*, **90**, 4502–4512.

Secchiero, P., Bertolaso, L., Casareto, L. *et al.* (1998a). Human herpesvirus 7 infection induces profound cell cycle perturbations coupled to disregulation of cdc2 and cyclin B and polyploidization of CD4(+) T cells. *Blood*, **92**(5), 1685–1696.

Secchiero, P., Bertolaso, L., Gibellini, D. *et al.* (1998b). Enforced expression of human bcl-2 in CD4+ T cells enhances human herpesvirus 7 replication and induction of cytopathic effects. *Eur. J. Immunol.* **28**(5), 1587–1596.

Secchiero, P., Zella, D., Barabitskaja, O. *et al.* (1998c). Progressive and persistent downregulation of surface CXCR4 in CD4(+) T cells infected with human herpesvirus 7. *Blood*, **92**(12), 4521–4528.

Secchiero, P., Mirandola, P., Zella, D. *et al.* (2001). Human herpesvirus 7 induces the functional up-regulation of tumor necrosis factor-related apoptosis-inducing ligand (TRAIL) coupled to TRAIL-R1 down-modulation in CD4(+) T cells. *Blood*, **98**(8), 2474–2481.

Shiraki, K., Okuno, T., Yamanishi, K., and Takahashi, M. (1989). Virion and nonstructural polypeptides of human herpesvirus-6. *Virus. Res.*, **13**, 173–178.

Simmons, A., Demmrich, Y., La Vista, A., and Smith, K. (1992). Replication of human herpesvirus 6 in epithelial cells in vitro. *J. Infect. Dis.*, **166**(1), 202–205.

Singh, N., Bentlejewski, C., Carrigan, D. R., Gayowski, T., Knox, K. K., and Zeevi, A. (2002a). Persistent lack of human herpesvirus-6 specific T-helper cell response in liver transplant recipients. *Transpl. Infect. Dis.*, **4**(2), 59–63.

Singh, N., Husain, S., Carrigan, D. R. *et al.* (2002b). Impact of human herpesvirus-6 on the frequency and severity of recurrent hepatitis C virus hepatitis in liver transplant recipients. *Clin. Transpl.*, **16**(2), 92–96.

Skrinkosky, D., Hocknell, P., Whetter, L., Secchiero, P., Chandran, B., and Dewhurst, S. (2000). Identification and analysis of a novel heparin-binding glycoprotein encoded by human herpesvirus 7. *J. Virol.*, **74**, 4530–4540.

Skrincosky, D., Willis, R. A., Hocknell, P. K. *et al.* (2001). Epitope mapping of human herpesvirus-7 gp65 using monoclonal antibodies. *Arch. Virol.*, **146**(9), 1705–1722.

Smith, A., Santoro, F., Di Lullo, G., Dagna, L., Verani, A., and Lusso, P. (2003), Selective suppression of IL-12 production by human herpesvirus 6. *Blood*, **102**(8), 2877–2884.

Soldan, S. S., Berti, R., Salem, N. *et al.* (1997), Association of human herpes virus 6 (HHV-6) with multiple sclerosis: increased IgM response to HHV-6 early antigen and detection of serum HHV-6 DNA. *Nat. Med.*, **3**(12), 1394–1397.

Soldan, S. S., Leist, T. P., Juhng, K. N., McFarland, H. F. and Jacobson, S. (2000). Increased lymphoproliferative response to human herpesvirus type 6A variant in multiple sclerosis patients. *Ann. Neurol.*, **47**(3), 306–313.

Stefan, A., De Lillo, M., Frascaroli, G., Secchiero, P., Neipel, F., and Campadelli-Fiume, G. (1999). Development of recombinant diagnostic reagents based on pp85(U14) and p86(U11) proteins to detect the human immune response to human herpesvirus 7 infection. *J. Clin. Microbiol.*, **37**, 3980–3985.

Suga, S., Yoshikawa, T., Asano, Y., Yazaki, T., and Ozaki, T. (1990). Neutralizing antibody assay for human herpesvirus-6. *J. Med. Virol.*, **30**(1), 14–19.

Suga, S., Yoshikawa, T., Asano, Y. *et al.* (1992a). IgM neutralizing antibody responses to human herpesvirus-6 in patients with exanthem subitum or organ transplantation. *Microbiol. Immunol.*, **36**(5), 495–506.

Suga, S., Yoshikawa, T., Asano, Y., Nakashima, T., Kobayashi, I., and Yazaki, T. (1992b). Activation of human herpesvirus-6 in children with acute measles. *J. Med. Virol.*, **38**, 278–282.

Takahashi, K., Sonoda, S., Higashi, K. *et al.* (1989). Predominant CD4 T-lymphocyte tropism of human herpesvirus 6-related virus. *J. Virol.*, **63**, 3161–3163.

Takaku, T., Ohyashiki, J. H., Zhang, Y., and Ohyashiki, K. (2005). Estimating immunoregulatory gene networks in human herpesvirus type 6-infected T cells. *Biochem. Biophys. Res. Commun.*, **336**(2), 469–477.

Takahashi, K., Segal, E., Kondo, T. *et al.* (1992). Interferon and natural killer cell activity in patients with exanthem subitum. *Pediatr. Infect. Dis. J.*, **11**(5), 369–373.

Takeda, K., Okuno, T., Isegawa, Y., and Yamanishi, K. (1996). Identification of a variant A-specific neutralizing epitope on glycoprotein B (gB) of human herpesvirus-6 (HHV-6). *Virology*, **222**, 176–183.

Takeda, K., Haque, M., Sunagawa, T., Okuno, T., Isegawa, Y., and Yamanishi, K. (1997). Identification of a variant B-specific neutralizing epitope on glycoprotein H of human herpesvirus-6. *J. Gen. Virol.*, **78**, 2171–2178.

Takeda, K., Haque, M., Nagoshi, E. *et al.* (2000). Characterization of human herpesvirus 7 U27 gene product and identification of its nuclear localization signal. *Virology*, **272**(2), 394–401.

Takemoto, M., Koike, M., Mori, Y., *et al.* (2005). Human herpesvirus 6 open reading frame U14 protein and cellular p53 interact with each other and are contained in the virion. *J. Virol.*, **79**(20), 13037–13046.

Tanaka, K., Kondo, T., Torigoe, S., Okada, S., Mukai, T., and Yamanishi, K. (1994). Human herpesvirus 7: another causal agent for roseola (exanthem subitum). *J. Pediatr.*, **125**, 1–5.

Tanaka, H., Nishimura, T., Hakui, M., Sugimoto, H., Tanaka-Taya, K., and Yamanishi, K. (2002). Human herpesvirus 6-associated hemophagocytic syndrome in a healthy adult. *Emerg. Infect. Dis.*, **8**(1), 87–88.

Tejada-Simon, M. V., Zang, Y. C., Hong, J., Rivera, V. M., Killian, J. M., and Zhang, J. Z. (2002). Detection of viral DNA and immune responses to the human herpesvirus 6 101-kilodalton virion protein in patients with multiple sclerosis and in controls. *J. Virol.*, **76**(12), 6147–6154.

Tejada-Simon, M. V., Zang, Y. C., Hong, J., Rivera, V. M., and Zhang, J. Z. (2003). Cross-reactivity with myelin basic protein and human herpesvirus-6 in multiple sclerosis. *Ann. Neurol.*, **53**(2), 189–197.

Tong, C. Y., Bakran, A., Williams, H., Cheung, C. Y., and Peiris, J. S. (2000). Association of human herpesvirus 7 with cytomegalovirus disease in renal transplant recipients. *Transplantation*, **70**(1), 213–216.

Tong, C. Y., Bakran, A., Peiris, J. S., Muir, P., and Simon, H. C. (2002). The association of viral infection and chronic allograft nephropathy with graft dysfunction after renal transplantation. *Transplantation*, **74**(4), 576–578.

Torigoe, S., Kumamoto, T., Koide, W., Taya, K., and Yamanishi, K. (1995). Clinical manifestations associated with human herpesvirus 7 infection. *Arch. Dis. Child.*, **72**(6), 518–519.

Tsukazaki, T., Yoshida, M., Namba, H., Yamada, M., Shimizu, N., and Nii, S. (1998). Development of a dot blot neutralizing assay for HHV-6 and HHV-7 using specific monoclonal antibodies. *J. Virol. Methods*, **73**(2), 141–149.

Tyler, K. L. (2003). Human herpesvirus 6 and multiple sclerosis: the continuing conundrum. *J. Infect. Dis.*, **187**(9), 1360–1364.

Wagner, J. A., Ross, H., Gamberg, P., Valantine, H., Merigan, T. C., and Stinson, E. B. (1995). Prophylactic ganciclovir treatment reduces fungal as well as cytomegalovirus infections after heart transplantation. *Transplantation*, **60**, 1473–1477.

Wang, F. Z., Dahl, H., Linde, A., Brytting, M., Ehrnst, A., and Ljungman, P. (1996). Lymphotropic herpesviruses in allogenic bone marrow transplantation. *Blood*, **88**, 3615–3620.

Wang, F. Z., Linde, A., Dahl, H., and Ljungman, P. (1999). Human herpesvirus 6 infection inhibits specific lymphocyte proliferation responses and is related to lymphocytopenia after allogeneic stem cell transplantation. *Bone Marrow Transpl.*, **24**(11), 1201–1206.

Ward, K. N., Gray, J. J., Fotheringham, M. W., and Sheldon, M. J. (1993). IgG antibodies to human herpesvirus-6 in young children: changes in avidity of antibody correlate with time after infection. *J. Med. Virol.*, **39**, 131–138.

Ward, K. N., Turner, D. J., Parada, X. C., and Thiruchelvam, A. D. (2001). Use of immunoglobulin G antibody avidity for differentiation of primary human herpesvirus 6 and 7 infections. *J. Clin. Microbiol.*, **39**(3), 959–963.

Ward, K. N., Couto, P. X., Passas, J., and Thiruchelvam, A. D. (2002). Evaluation of the specificity and sensitivity of indirect immunofluorescence tests for IgG to human herpesviruses-6 and -7. *J. Virol. Methods*, **106**(1), 107–113.

Wilborn, F., Brinkmann, V., Schmidt, C. A., Neipel, F., Gelderblom, H., and Siegert, W. (1994). Herpesvirus type 6 in patients undergoing bone marrow transplantation: serologic features and detection by polymerase chain reaction. *Blood*, **83**(10), 3052–3058.

Wong, G. A. and Shear, N. H. (2004). Is a drug alone sufficient to cause the drug hypersensitivity syndrome? *Arch. Dermatol.*, **140**(2), 226–230.

Wu, C. A. and Shanley, J. D. (1998). Chronic infection of human umbilical vein endothelial cells by human herpesvirus-6. *J. Gen. Virol.*, **79**, 1247–1256.

Wyatt, L. S. and Frenkel, N. (1992). Human herpesvirus 7 is a constitutive inhabitant of adult human saliva. *J. Virol.*, **66**(5), 3206–3209.

Wyatt, L. S., Balachandran, N., and Frenkel, N. (1990). Variations in the replication and antigenic properties of human herpesvirus 6 strains. *J. Infect. Dis.*, **162**(4), 852–857.

Wyatt, L. S., Rodriguez, W. J., Balachandran, N., and Frenkel, N. (1991). Human herpesvirus 7: antigenic properties and prevalence in children and adults. *J. Virol.*, **65**, 6260–6265.

Yadav, M. Umamaheswari, S., and Ablashi, D. (1991). Antibody reactivity with two strains of human herpesvirus-6 in Malaysians. *J. Med. Virol.*, **33**, 236–239.

Yakushijin, Y., Yasukawa, M., and Kobayashi, Y. (1991). T-cell immune response to human herpesvirus-6 in healthy adults. *Microbiol. Immunol.* **35**(8), 655–660.

Yakushijin, Y., Yasukawa, M., and Kobayashi, Y. (1992). Establishment and functional characterization of human herpesvirus 6-specific CD4+ human T-cell clones. *J. Virol.*, **66**(5), 2773–2779.

Yamamoto, M., Black, J. B., Stewart, J. A., Lopez, C., and Pellett, P. E. (1990). Identification of a nucleocapsid protein as a specific serological marker of human herpesvirus 6 infection. *J. Clin. Microbiol.*, **28**(9), 1957–1962.

Yamanishi, K., Mori, Y., and Pellett, P. E. (2007). Human herpesviruses 6 and 7. *In Fields Virology*, 5th edn., Knipe *et al.*, eds., Philadelphia: Lippincott, Williams, & Wilkins, Vol. 2, Chap. 71, in press.

Yasukawa, M., Yakushijin, Y., Furukawa, M., and Fujita, S. (1993). Specificity analysis of human CD4+ T-cell clones directed against human herpesvirus 6 (HHV-6), HHV-7, and human cytomegalovirus. *J. Virol.*, **67**(10), 6259–6264.

Yasukawa, M., Inoue, Y., Ohminami, H., Terada, K., and Fujita, S. (1998). Apoptosis of CD4+ T lymphocytes in human herpesvirus-6 infection. *J. Gen. Virol.*, **79**, 143–147.

Yasukawa, M., Hasegawa, A., Sakai, I. *et al.* (1999). Down-regulation of CXCR4 by human herpesvirus 6 (HHV-6) and HHV-7. *J. Immunol.*, **162**(9), 5417–5422.

Yoshida, M., Torigoe, S., Ikeue, K., and Yamada, M. (2002a). Neutralizing antibody responses to human herpesviruses 6 and 7 do not cross-react with each other, and maternal neutralizing antibodies contribute to sequential infection with these viruses in childhood. *Clin. Diagn. Lab. Immunol.*, **9**(2), 388–393.

Yoshida, M., Torigoe, S., and Yamada, M. (2002b). Elucidation of the cross-reactive immunoglobulin M response to human herpesviruses 6 and 7 on the basis of neutralizing antibodies. *Clin. Diagn. Lab. Immunol.*, **9**(2), 394–402.

Yoshikawa, T. (2003). Human herpesvirus-6 and -7 infections in transplantation. *Pediatr. Transpl.*, **7**(1), 11–17.

Yoshikawa, T., Suga, S., Asano, Y. *et al.* (1991). Human herpesvirus-6 infection in bone marrow transplantation. *Blood*, **78**, 1381–1384.

Yoshikawa, T., Ihira, M., Suzuki, K. *et al.* (2000). Human herpesvirus 6 infection after living related liver transplantation. *J. Med. Virol.*, **62**, 52–59.

Yoshikawa, T., Asano, Y., Ihira, M. *et al.* (2002). Human herpesvirus 6 viremia in bone marrow transplant recipients: clinical features and risk factors. *J. Infect. Dis.*, **185**(7), 847–853.

Yoshikawa, T., Goshima, F., Akimoto, S. *et al.* (2003a). Human herpesvirus 6 infection of human epidermal cell line: pathogenesis of skin manifestations. *J. Med. Virol.*, **71**(1), 62–68.

Yoshikawa, T., Yoshida, J., Hamaguchi, M. *et al.* (2003b). Human herpesvirus 7-associated meningitis and optic neuritis in a patient after allogeneic stem cell transplantation. *J. Med. Virol.*, **70**(3), 440–443.

Zou, P., Isegawa, Y., Nakano, K., Haque, M., Horiguchi, Y., and Yamanishi, K. (1999). Human herpesvirus 6 open reading frame U83 encodes a functional chemokine. *J. Virol.*, **73**(7), 5926–5933.

HHV-6A, 6B, and 7: persistence in the population, epidemiology and transmission

Vincent C. Emery and Duncan A. Clark

Department of Virology, Royal Free and University College Medical School of UCL, London, UK

Introduction

In common with all human herpesviruses, HHV-6 and HHV-7 establish lifelong infection following initial exposure and seroconversion. True latency as exemplified by HSV-1 and VZV, in which the genome is maintained in a transcriptionally restricted state, has not been conclusively shown for HHV-6 or HHV-7. However, the betaherpesviruses may persist in individuals via low grade replication which is continuously suppressed by a functional immune response. In this chapter we will summarize the current understanding of the epidemiology and persistence of HHV-6 and HHV-7 in the human host and its relevance to transmission. In addition, we will highlight a novel form of persistence for HHV-6 which involves integration into host chromosomal DNA.

Persistence of HHV-6 and HHV-7 in individuals

In the case of both HHV-6 and HHV-7, PCR analysis of peripheral blood mononuclear cells (PBMC) shows that a sensitive nested assay and an adequate quantity of input DNA (at least equivalent to approximately 150000 mononuclear cells or 1μg DNA) can detect viral DNA in healthy immunocompetent individuals suggestive of low levels of latent/persisting virus in peripheral blood (Jarrett et al., 1990; Clark et al., 1996; Kidd et al., 1996). In contrast, viral loads are maintained at high levels in saliva of seropositive individuals, particularly in the case of HHV-7 (Kidd et al., 1996; Fujiwara et al., 2000; see Fig. 49.1). Since the salivary glands are a major site of replication following primary infection with both HHV-6 and HHV-7, saliva is likely to be an important fluid mediating transmission of virus within the community. An investigation of separate salivary glands (submandibular, parotid and lip) in multiple patients has revealed that the submandibular gland is most likely to contain HHV-6 (88%) and HHV-7 DNA (100%) compared to the other anatomic salivary glands, 50%–60% of which were infected (Sada et al., 1996).

However, as described in more detail in Chapter 48 HHV-6 and HHV-7 may exist in a true latent state within cells of the lymphoreticular system and in the case of HHV-6, the central nervous system, i.e., exhibiting transcription patterns restricted to specific genomic regions without undergoing full genomic replication (Kondo et al., 2002).

HHV-6 is neurotropic and analysis of postmortem brain tissue by PCR has shown that up to 85% of individuals harbor HHV-6 DNA (Chan et al., 2001). In this study, HHV-6 variant B predominated in the brain although variant A was detected in 27.5% of brains and coinfections were also observed. Whether a latent transcriptionally silent or restricted expression pattern is present in this anatomic site or whether local replication can occur which facilitates viral persistence in the central nervous system, has not been determined. Following primary infection ~29% of children have HHV-6 DNA in the CSF which is consistent with the central nervous system being an important site of latency (Caserta et al., 1994).

Other studies have revealed widespread distribution of HHV-6 and HHV-7 DNA in organs derived from both immunocompetent and immunocompromised hosts (Clark et al., 1996; Emery et al., 1999) with low viral loads detected in most tissues. However, HHV-6 viral loads were significantly increased in autopsy tissues from AIDS patients compared to controls suggesting upregulation of HHV-6 replication in the latter (Clark et al., 1996).

Epidemiology of HHV-6 and HHV-7

Seroepidemiologic studies of HHV-6 and HHV-7 have used indirect immunofluoresence assays and more recently

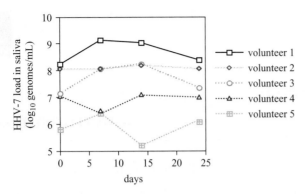

Fig. 49.1. Determination of HHV-7 loads in saliva by quantitative PCR from 5 volunteers showing temporal variation in individuals. Viral loads are expressed as HHV-7 genomes/mL saliva. Adapted from Kidd et al., 1996.

ELISA based assays, with the latter deemed to be more sensitive. Antigenic similarity between HHV-6 and HHV-7 creates the potential problem of cross-reactive HHV-6 and HHV-7 antibodies in human sera (Black et al., 1996). Nevertheless, many studies have consistently shown that HHV-6 and HHV-7 infections are almost universal within the adult population and the viruses have a worldwide distribution. The very close homology between the two HHV-6 variants has hindered attempts to distinguish antibodies to each variant.

Infection with both HHV-6 and HHV-7 occurs early in life. The peak of seroconversion for HHV-7 occurs after 24 months of age (Tanaka-Taya et al., 1996) and is slightly later than seroconversion for HHV-6 which peaks at 13 months (Okuno et al., 1989). Antibody titers are higher in children compared to adults reflecting recent primary infection. Viral loads in blood are also high during this period of acute infection and in the case of HHV-7 can reach 10^7 genomes/μg PBMC DNA. In comparison, HHV-6 loads in blood during primary infection appear to peak at around 10^5 genomes/μg PBMC DNA (Clark et al., 1997; Chiu et al., 1998).

HHV-6 variants A and B

HHV-6 exists as two distinct variants (HHV-6 A and B). Comparative genomic analysis of the prototypes of these variants reveals the number of highly homologous genes but also reveals significant differences in viral proteins (Gompels et al., 1995; Dominguez et al., 1999; Isegawa et al., 1999). At present, the full implications of these differences have not been determined although it is clear that the biological phenotypes can have profound effects. The variants differ with respect to their ability to grow in a range of cell types although both use CD46 as a cellular receptor (Santoro et al., 1999). Interaction with the cellular receptor has been reported to include the participation of the viral glycoproteins gH, gL and gQ (Santoro et al., 2003; Mori et al., 2003). gQ has only 79% amino acid identity between variants which may influence the ability of variants to target different cells. HHV-6 variant A but not variant B has also been shown to induce fusion from without in a variety of human cells mediated through the gB and gH glycoproteins and CD46 (Mori et al., 2002).

A number of PCR systems that allow differentiation between HHV-6 variant A and B have been used extensively in epidemiologic studies. Some of these methods have relied on variant common primers with differentiation of variant type by differences in the presence of restriction endonuclease sites (Dewhurst et al., 1992; Kidd et al., 1998) or hybridization with variant specific probes (Cone et al., 1996). Other studies have used variant specific primers (Chou & Marousek, 1994; Cone et al., 1996).

When the prevalence of each variant is examined at different anatomical sites, HHV-6B is frequently detected in saliva (Aberle et al., 1996; Tanaka-Taya et al., 1996) and it is also the predominant variant in PBMC (Di Luca et al., 1994) and brain tissue (Chan et al., 2001). Co-infection with both variants was found in 22 of 34 lung tissue specimens (Cone et al., 1996) and HHV-6A was more frequently detected in skin biopsies (Di Luca et al., 1996) and CSF (Hall et al., 1998). The absence of HHV-6A in clinical samples most amenable to epidemiologic investigations (blood and saliva) have prevented the true prevalence of this variant from being determined. Although HHV-6B is almost exclusively the cause of febrile illness in young children in the US (Dewhurst et al., 1993), one study has suggested that active HHV-6A infection in young children with febrile illness is more common in Africa (Kasolo et al., 1997).

HHV-6 and HHV-7 genotypes

HHV-6 isolates can clearly be classified as either variant A or variant B, although both are closely related with an overall nucleotide identity of 90%. There is little evidence for HHV-6 intrastrain variation although subgroups within HHV-6B have been suggested by analysis of specific regions of the viral genome (IE-A region and gH) (Chou & Marousek, 1994; Gompels et al., 1993). However, examination of the U94 gene from 13 HHV-6B isolates from the US, Africa and Japan showed 100% amino acid identity (Rapp et al., 2000) suggesting an intolerance of variation in this particular gene. Comparison of the two fully sequenced HHV-7 isolates (RK and JI) shows that intrastrain variation is low although

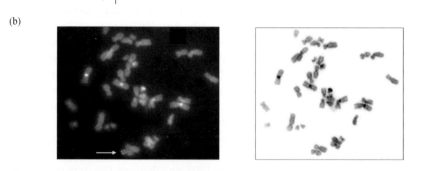

Fig. 49.2. HHV-6 integration into host cell chromosomes. (a) Consistently high viral loads detected in the peripheral blood of an individual at multiple time points by quantitative PCR (adapted from (Clark *et al.*, 1996). (b) FISH analysis using a fluorescently labeled HHV-6 specific probe showing integration of HHV-6 sequences on the short arm of chromosome 11 in V1-LCL (arrowed). (Adapted from Clark *et al.*, 2006.)

more apparent in repeat regions close to either ends of the genome (Megaw *et al.*, 1998). However, analysis of 3 genes encoding the phosphoprotein p100, gB and major capsid protein in 297 people derived from populations in Africa, Asia, Europe and America has suggested the presence of distinct variants (Franti *et al.*, 2001).

HHV-6 integration

An alternative form of HHV-6 persistence characterized by very high viral loads in PBMC and integration of viral sequences into host cell chromosomes is present in a small subset of the population. Luppi *et al.*(1993) first reported three individuals with very high viral loads in PBMC with viral DNA detectable by Southern blotting. Subsequently fluorescent in situ hybridization (FISH) with HHV-6 specific probes identified integrated viral sequences on the short arm of chromosome 17 in all three cases (B cell lymphoma, Hodgkin's disease and a patient with multiple sclerosis) (Torelli *et al.*, 1995). Follow-up studies suggested that the sites of integration were close to or in the telomeres of chromosome 17 (Morris *et al.*, 1999). Of possible relevance, HHV-6 variants have telomere-like repeat sequences in the direct repeat regions that flank the viral genome (Gompels *et al.*, 1995; Dominguez *et al.*, 1999; Isegawa *et al.*, 1999) which may facilitate integration within the telomere. The integrated viral sequences were typed as variant B in all three cases.

More recently, Daibata *et al.* (1998) described a cell line derived from a Burkitt's lymphoma patient with integrated viral sequences (variant B) on chromosome 1q44 and in a follow-up study showed that the asymptomatic husband of this case had integrated virus on chromosome 22q13 (Daibata *et al.*, 1999). Intriguingly, the daughter of this couple had integrated HHV-6 DNA sequences on both chromosomes 1q44 and 22q13 suggesting entry of viral sequences into the germline and chromosomal inheritance. The concept of an "endogenous herpesvirus" is novel and inheritance of viral sequences has only been described for endogenous retroviruses or related genetic elements. In the absence of inheritance, high viral loads found in PBMC may represent integration of viral sequences in a bone marrow progenitor cell which gives rise to a large number of cells/cell types in peripheral blood carrying copies of the viral genome. In the studies by Torelli *et al.* (1995) and Daibata *et al.* (1999), it was suggested that the entire HHV-6 genome was present.

We have also investigated HHV-6 loads in the PBMC of healthy individuals (Clark *et al.*, 1996). Using an input of 1 μg DNA (equivalent to 150000 diploid cells) in a quantitative competitive PCR assay, 9 of 25 blood samples were HHV-6 DNA positive with viral loads in 8 ranging from 5–32 HHV-6 genomes/μg DNA. The remaining person (V1) had a consistent viral load of around 6 $\log_{10}$ genome copies/μg DNA in multiple samples over a ten month period (Clark *et al.*, 1996). An EBV-transformed B-lymphoblastoid cell line was established and FISH analysis using a fluorescently labeled 9 kbp HHV-6 specific probe identified integrated virus close to the end of the short arm of chromosome 11 (Fig. 49.2). The viral sequences were shown to be HHV-6B using variant typing PCR. A more extensive series of individuals with a variety of sites of integration have now been investigated by quantitative PCR showing high viral loads are present in whole blood, serum and hair follicles (Ward et al., 2006). The mean HHV-6 DNA load in whole blood was 7.0 $\log_{10}$ copies/milliliter, in serum it was 5.3 $\log_{10}$ copies/milliliter while in hair follicles it was 4.2 $\log_{10}$ copies/hair follicle.

The expression of HHV-6 genes in vivo in patients with integrated viral sequences has not been studied extensively. Daibata et al. (Daibata et al., 1998) reported the detection of immediate early and late HHV-6 genes in an integrated HHV-6, EBV negative cell line following treatment with TPA (a commonly used stimulator of herpesvirus lytic infection). No non-integrated linear or episomal forms of the HHV-6 genome were detected by Gardella gel analysis suggesting an absence of viral DNA replication (Daibata et al., 1998).

It is important to consider whether integrated HHV-6 is of clinical relevance. Although the biological effects of HHV-6 integration are unknown, integrated virus is a potential confounder in studies investigating HHV-6 disease associations and also in the medical management of infection. There have been a number of false leads and unproven associations between HHV-6 and disease, some of which may have reflected the unrecognized detection of integrated virus and interpreted as a high viral load. To date, there have been no controlled trials of antiviral therapy against HHV-6 infection, but a number of studies have shown the ability of ganciclovir and foscarnet to suppress HHV-6 replication in vitro. This information has been applied clinically to treat suspected cases of HHV-6 disease. From a management perspective, it will be important to differentiate patients with active HHV-6 infection from those patients with integrated HHV-6 to prevent the latter receiving unnecessary exposure to potentially toxic antiviral drugs.

Transmission of HHV-6 and HHV-7

Although primary infection with these viruses usually occurs in early childhood there is evidence that infection with HHV-6 occurs slightly earlier than HHV-7 (Wyatt et al., 1991). Saliva is the most likely vehicle for transmission of both viruses. HHV-6 and HHV-7 DNA can frequently be detected by PCR in the saliva of both adults and children (Jarrett et al., 1990; Kidd et al., 1996; Suga et al., 1995; Tanaka-Taya et al., 1996) and although there are very few HHV-6 isolates derived from saliva, HHV-7 is readily cultured from this source (Wyatt & Frenkel, 1992). Molecular characterization of HHV-6 strains detected within a limited number of families suggest that the virus may be transmitted primarily from mother to child (Yoshikawa et al., 1993; van Loon et al., 1995). For HHV-7, genetic analysis of virus within families also suggests transmission within the family unit from both mothers and fathers (Thawaranantha et al., 2002), and through multigenerational families in the same household (Takahashi et al., 1997).

HHV-6 and HHV-7 have been detected by PCR in 20% and 3% respectively of the cervixes of women in the later stages of pregnancy (Okuno et al., 1995) suggesting the potential for perinatal transmission. This observation is consistent with the identification of active HHV-6 infection during the neonatal period (Hall et al., 1994). PCR analysis of cord blood suggests a prevalence of HHV-6 congenital infection of 1%–2% of births (Aubin et al., 1992; Adams et al., 1998; Dahl et al., 1999) and there are case reports of associated disease (Lanari et al., 2003). HHV-6 reactivation has also been suggested to be more common during pregnancy which may facilitate transmission of virus to the fetus (Dahl et al., 1999). HHV-7, but not HHV-6, was detected in 3 of 29 breast milk samples suggesting that breast feeding may also be a route of transmission for HHV-7 (Fujisaki et al., 1998).

HHV-6 and HHV-7 are now recognized as being common infections in the post-transplant period. In the majority of cases, particularly adults, reactivation of the recipient's virus is the most probable source of active infection. However, transmission from the donor graft is a distinct possibility and has been reported for HHV-6 in a bone marrow transplant recipient (Lau et al., 1998). HHV-6 and HHV-7 DNA have also been detected by PCR in 28% and 50%, respectively, of bone marrow samples from healthy individuals highlighting a possible source of virus for transmission through transplantation (Gautheret-Dejean et al., 2000). There is also evidence suggesting transmission of HHV-6 to infants through living-related liver transplantation from their HHV-6 seropositive mothers (Yoshikawa et al., 2001) and transmission of integrated virus following stem cell transplantation (Clark et al., 2006).

Although HHV-6 and HHV-7 are frequently detected by PCR in PBMC including those of blood donors (Wilborn et al., 1994, 1995), there is no evidence that HHV-6 at least is a cause of post-transfusion hepatitis (Lunel et al., 1991).

Concluding comments

Progress is being made in understanding the persistence of HHV-6 and HHV-7 in the human host and the molecular basis for different forms of persistence. It is clear that both HHV-6 and HHV-7 are well adapted to their human host since even in the developed world seroprevalence rates are almost universal and they are rarely pathogenic in the immunocompetent host.

REFERENCES

Aberle, S. W., Mandl, C. W., Kunz, C., and Popow-Kraupp, T. (1996). Presence of human herpesvirus 6 variants A and B in saliva and peripheral blood mononuclear cells of healthy adults. *J. Clin. Microbiol.*, **34**, 3223–3225.

Adams, O., Krempe, C., Kogler, G., Wernet, P., and Scheid, A. (1998). Congenital infections with human herpesvirus 6. *J. Infect. Dis.*, **178**, 544–546.

Aubin, J. T., Poirel, L., Agut, H. *et al.* (1992). Intrauterine transmission of human herpesvirus 6 [letter]. *Lancet*, **340**, 482–483.

Black, J. B., Schwarz, T. F., Patton, J. L. *et al.* (1996). Evaluation of immunoassays for detection of antibodies to human herpesvirus 7. *Clin. Diag. Lab. Immunol.*, **3**, 79–83.

Caserta, M. T., Hall, C. B., Schnabel, K. *et al.* (1994). Neuroinvasion and persistence of human herpesvirus 6 in children. *Journal of Infectious Diseases*, **170**, 1586–1589.

Chan, P. K., Ng, H. K., Hui, M., and Cheng, A. F. (2001). Prevalence and distribution of human herpesvirus 6 variants A and B in adult human brain. *J. Med. Virol.*, **64**, 42–46.

Chiu, S. S., Cheung, C. Y., Tse, C. Y., and Peiris, M. (1998). Early diagnosis of primary human herpesvirus 6 infection in childhood: serology, polymerase chain reaction, and virus load. *J. Infect. Dis.*, **178**, 1250–1256.

Chou, S. and Marousek, G. I. (1994). Analysis of interstrain variation in a putative immediate-early region of human herpesvirus 6 DNA and definition of variant-specific sequences. *Virology*, **198**, 370–376.

Clark, D. A., Ait-Khaled, M., Wheeler, A. C. *et al.* (1996). Quantification of human herpesvirus 6 in immunocompetent persons and post-mortem tissues from AIDS patients by PCR. *J. Gen. Virol.*, **77**, 2271–2275.

Clark, D. A., Kidd, I. M., and Collingham, K. E. (1997). Diagnosis of primary human herpesvirus 6 and 7 infections in febrile infants by polymerase chain reaction. *Arch. Dis. Child.*, **77**, 42–45.

Clark, D. A., Nacheva, E. P., Leong, H. N. *et al.* (2006). Transmission of integrated human herpesvirus 6 through stem cell transplantation: implications for laboratory diagnosis. *J. Infect. Dis.*, **193**, 912–916.

Cone, R. W., Huang, M. L., Hackman, R. C., and Corey, L. (1996). Coinfection with human herpesvirus 6 variants A and B in lung tissue. *J. Clin. Microbiol.*, **34**, 877–881.

Dahl, H., Fjaertoft, G., Norsted, T., Wang, F. Z., Mousavi-Jazi, M., and Linde, A. (1999). Reactivation of human herpesvirus 6 during pregnancy. *J. Infect. Dis.*, **180**, 2035–2038.

Daibata, M., Taguchi, T., Taguchi, H., and Miyoshi, I. (1998). Integration of human herpesvirus 6 in a Burkitt's lymphoma cell line. *Br. J. Haematol.*, **102**, 1307–1313.

Daibata, M., Taguchi, T., Nemoto, Y., Taguchi, H., and Miyoshi, I. (1999). Inheritance of chromosomally integrated human herpesvirus 6 DNA. *Blood*, **94**, 1545–1549.

Dewhurst, S., Chandran, B., McIntyre, K., Schnabel, K., and Hall, C. B. (1992). Phenotypic and genetic polymorphisms among human herpesvirus-6 isolates from North American infants. *Virology*, **190**, 490–493.

Dewhurst, S., McIntyre, K., Schnabel, K., and Hall, C. B. (1993). Human herpesvirus 6 (HHV-6) variant B accounts for the majority of symptomatic primary HHV-6 infections in a population of U.S. infants. *J. Clin. Microbiol.*, **31**, 416–418.

Di Luca, D., Dolcetti, R., and Mirandola, P. (1994). Human herpesvirus 6: a survey of presence and variant distribution in normal peripheral lymphocytes and lymphoproliferative disorders. *J. Infect. Dis.*, **170**, 211–215.

Di Luca, D., Mirandola, P., Ravaioli, T., Bigoni, B., and Cassai, E. (1996). Distribution of HHV-6 variants in human tissues. [Review] [103 refs]. *Infect. Agents and Dis.*, **5**, 203–214.

Dominguez, G., Dambaugh, T. R., Stamey, F. R., Dewhurst, S., Inoue, N., and Pellett, P. E. (1999). Human herpesvirus 6B genome sequence: coding content and comparison with human herpesvirus 6A. *Journal of Virology*, **73**, 8040–8052.

Emery, V. C., Atkins, M. C., Bowen, E. F. *et al.* (1999). Interactions between beta-herpesviruses and human immunodeficiency virus in vivo: evidence for increased human immunodeficiency viral load in the presence of human herpesvirus 6. *J. Med. Virol.*, **57**, 278–282.

Franti, M., Gessain, A., Darlu, P. *et al.* (2001). Genetic polymorphism of human herpesvirus-7 among human populations. *J. Gen. Virol.*, **82**, 3045–3050.

Fujisaki, H., Tanaka-Taya, K., Tanabe, H. *et al.* (1998). Detection of human herpesvirus 7 (HHV-7) DNA in breast milk by polymerase chain reaction and prevalence of HHV-7 antibody in breast-fed and bottle-fed children. *J. Med. Virol.*, **56**, 275–279.

Fujiwara, N., Namba, H., Ohuchi, R. *et al.* (2000). Monitoring of human herpesvirus-6 and -7 genomes in saliva samples of healthy adults by competitive quantitative PCR. *J. Med. Virol.*, **61**, 208–213.

Gautheret-Dejean, A., Dejean, O., Vastel, L. *et al.* (2000). Human herpesvirus-6 and human herpesvirus-7 in the bone marrow from healthy subjects. *Transplantation*, **69**, 1722–1723.

Gompels, U. A., Carrigan, D. R., Carss, A. L., and Arno, J. (1993). Two groups of human herpesvirus 6 identified by sequence analyses of laboratory strains and variants from Hodgkin's lymphoma and bone marrow transplant patients. *J. Gen. Virol.*, **74**, 613–622.

Gompels, U. A., Nicholas, J., Lawrence, G. *et al.* (1995). The DNA sequence of human herpesvirus-6: structure, coding content, and genome evolution. [Review] [196 refs]. *Virology*, **209**, 29–51.

Hall, C. B., Long, C. E., Schnabel, K. C. *et al.* (1994). Human herpesvirus-6 infection in children. A prospective study of complications and reactivation. *N. Engl. J. Med.*, **331**, 432–438.

Hall, C. B., Caserta, M. T., Schnabel, K. C. *et al.* (1998). Persistence of human herpesvirus 6 according to site and variant: possible greater neurotropism of variant A. *Clin. Infect. Dis.*, **26**, 132–137.

Isegawa, Y., Mukai, T., and Nakano, K. (1999). Comparison of the complete DNA sequences of human herpesvirus 6 variants A and B. *J. Virol.*, **73**, 8053–8063.

Jarrett, R. F., Clark, D. A., Josephs, S. F., and Onions, D. E. (1990). Detection of human herpesvirus-6 DNA in peripheral blood and saliva. *J. Med. Virol.*, **32**, 73–76.

Kasolo, F. C., Mpabalwani, E., and Gompels, U. A. (1997). Infection with AIDS-related herpesviruses in human immunodeficiency virus-negative infants and endemic childhood Kaposi's sarcoma in Africa. *J. Gen. Virol.*, **78**, 847–855.

Kidd, I. M., Clark, D. A., Ait-Khaled, M., Griffiths, P. D., and Emery, V. C. (1996). Measurement of human herpesvirus 7 load in peripheral blood and saliva of healthy subjects by quantitative polymerase chain reaction. *J. Infect. Dis.*, **174**, 396–401.

Kidd, I. M., Clark, D. A., Bremner, J. A., Pillay, D., Griffiths, P. D., and Emery, V. C. (1998). A multiplex PCR assay for the simultaneous detection of human herpesvirus 6 and human herpesvirus 7, with typing of HHV-6 by enzyme cleavage of PCR products. *J. Virol. Methods*, **70**, 29–36.

Kondo, K., Shimada, K., Sashihara, J., Tanaka-Taya, K., and Yamanishi, K. (2002) Identification of human herpesvirus 6 latency-associated transcripts. *J. Virol.*, **76**, 4145–4151.

Lanari, M., Papa, I., Venturi, V. *et al.* (2003). Congenital infection with human herpesvirus 6 variant B associated with neonatal seizures and poor neurological outcome. *J. Med. Virol.*, **70**, 628–632.

Lau, Y. L., Peiris, M., Chan, G. C., Chan, A. C., Chiu, D., and Ha, S. Y. (1998). Primary human herpes virus 6 infection transmitted from donor to recipient through bone marrow infusion. *Bone Marrow Transplantation*, **21**, 1063–1066.

Lunel, F., Agut, H., Robert, C. *et al.* (1991). Is human herpes virus 6 (HHV-6) infection associated with posttransfusion hepatitis? *Transfusion*, **31**, 872.

Luppi, M., Marasca, R., Barozzi, P. *et al.* (1993). Three cases of human herpesvirus-6 latent infection: integration of viral genome in peripheral blood mononuclear cell DNA. *J. Med. Virol.*, **40**, 44–52.

Megaw, A. G., Rapaport, D., Avidor, B., Frenkel, N., and Davison, A. J. (1998). The DNA sequence of the RK strain of human herpesvirus 7. *Virology*, **244**, 119–132.

Mori, Y., Seya, T., Huang, H. L., Akkapaiboon, P., Dhepakson, P., and Yamanishi, K. (2002). Human herpesvirus 6 variant A but not variant B induces fusion from without in a variety of human cells through a human herpesvirus 6 entry receptor, CD46. *J. Virol.*, **76**, 6750–6761.

Mori, Y., Yang, X., Akkapaiboon, P., Okuno, T., and Yamanishi, K. (2003). Human herpesvirus 6 variant A glycoprotein H-glycoprotein L-glycoprotein Q complex associates with human CD46. *J. Virol.*, **77**, 4992–4999.

Morris, C., Luppi, M., McDonald, M., Barozzi, P., and Torelli, G. (1999). Fine mapping of an apparently targeted latent human herpesvirus type 6 integration site in chromosome band 17p13.3. *J. Med. Virol.*, **58**, 69–75.

Okuno, T., Takahashi, K., Balachandra, K. *et al.* (1989). Seroepidemiology of human herpesvirus 6 infection in normal children and adults. *J. Clin. Microbiol.*, **27**, 651–653.

Okuno, T., Oishi, H., Hayashi, K., Nonogaki, M., Tanaka, K., and Yamanishi, K. (1995). Human herpesviruses 6 and 7 in cervixes of pregnant women. *J. Clin. Microbiol.*, **33**, 1968–1970.

Rapp, J. C., Krug, L. T., Inoue, N., Dambaugh, T. R., and Pellett, P. E. (2000). U94, the human herpesvirus 6 homolog of the parvovirus nonstructural gene, is highly conserved among isolates and is expressed at low mRNA levels as a spliced transcript. *Virology*, **268**, 504–516.

Sada, E., Yasukawa, M., Ito, C. *et al.* (1996). Detection of human herpesvirus 6 and human herpesvirus 7 in the submandibular gland, parotid gland, and lip salivary gland by PCR. *J. of Clini. Microbiol.*, **34**, 2320–2321.

Santoro, F., Kennedy, P. E., Locatelli, G., Malnati, M. S., Berger, E. A., and Lusso, P. (1999). CD46 is a cellular receptor for human herpesvirus 6. *Cell*, **99**, 817–827.

Santoro, F., Greenstone, H. L., Insinga, A. *et al.* (2003). Interaction of glycoprotein H of human herpesvirus 6 with the cellular receptor CD46. *J. Biol. Chem.*, **278**, 25964–25969.

Suga, S., Yazaki, T., Kajita, Y., Ozaki, T., and Asano, Y. (1995). Detection of human herpesvirus 6 DNAs in samples from several body sites of patients with exanthem subitum and their mothers by polymerase chain reaction assay. *J. Med. Virol.*, **46**, 52–55.

Takahashi, Y., Yamada, M., Nakamura, J. *et al.* (1997). Transmission of human herpesvirus 7 through multigenerational families in the same household. *Pediatr. Infect. Dis. J.*, **16**, 975–978.

Tanaka-Taya, K., Kondo, T., Mukai, T. *et al.* (1996). Seroepidemiological study of human herpesvirus-6 and -7 in children of different ages and detection of these two viruses in throat swabs by polymerase chain reaction. *J. Med. Virol.*, **48**, 88–94.

Thawaranantha, D., Chimabutra, K., Balachandra, K. *et al.* (2002). Genetic variations of human herpesvirus 7 by analysis of glycoproteins B and H, and R2-repeat regions. *J. Med. Virol.*, **66**, 370–377.

Torelli, G., Barozzi, P., Marasca, R. *et al.* (1995). Targeted integration of human herpesvirus 6 in the p arm of chromosome 17 of human peripheral blood mononuclear cells in vivo. *J. Med. Virol.*, **46**, 178–188.

van Loon, N. M., Gummuluru, S., Sherwood, D. J., Marentes, R., Hall, C. B., and Dewhurst (1995). Direct sequence analysis of human herpesvirus 6 (HHV-6) sequences from infants and comparison of HHV-6 sequences from mother/infant pairs. *Clin. Infect. Dis.*, **21**, 1017–1019.

Ward, K. N., Leong, H. N., Nacheva, E. P. *et al.* (2006). Human herpesvirus 6 chromosomal integration in immunocompetent patients results in high levels of viral DNA in blood, sera, and hair follicles. *J. Clin. Microbiol.*, **44**, 1571–1574.

Wilborn, F., Schmidt, C. A., Zimmermann, R., Brinkmann, V., Neipel, F., and Siegert, W. (1994). Detection of herpesvirus type 6 by polymerase chain reaction in blood donors: random tests and prospective longitudinal studies. *Br. J. Haematol.*, **88**, 187–192.

Wilborn, F., Schmidt, C. A., Lorenz, F. *et al.* (1995). Human herpesvirus type 7 in blood donors: detection by the polymerase chain reaction. *J. Med. Virol.*, **47**, 65–69.

Wyatt, L. S. and Frenkel, N. (1992). Human herpesvirus 7 is a constitutive inhabitant of adult human saliva. *J. Virol.*, **66**, 3206–3209.

Wyatt, L. S., Rodriguez, W. J., Balachandran, N., and Frenkel, N. (1991). Human herpesvirus 7: antigenic properties and prevalence in children and adults. *J. Virol.*, **65**, 6260–6265.

Yoshikawa, T., Asano, Y., Kobayashi, I. *et al.* (1993). Seroepidemiology of human herpesvirus 7 in healthy children and adults in Japan. *J. Med. Virol.*, **41**, 319–323.

Yoshikawa, T., Ihira, M., Suzuki, K. *et al.* (2001). Primary human herpesvirus 6 infection in liver transplant recipients. *J. Pediatr.*, **138**, 921–925.

Part III

Pathogenesis, clinical disease, host response, and epidemiology: gammaherpesviruses

Patrick S. Moore

Clinical and pathological aspects of EBV and KSHV infection

Richard F. Ambinder[1] and Ethel Cesarman[2]

[1]Johns Hopkins School of Medicine Departments of Oncology, Pathology, and Pharmacology Baltimore, MD, USA
[2]Weill Medical College of Cornell University Department of Pathology and Laboratory Medicine New York, NY, USA

The human γ-herpesviruses Epstein–Barr virus (EBV) and Kaposi's sarcoma herpesvirus (KSHV) establish latency in cellular reservoirs that are maintained for the life of the infected individual. Intermittent reactivation leads to infection of new cells within the host and secretion of virions in saliva. Primary infections are usually asymptomatic. However, in immunocompromised patients and in other special but poorly understood circumstances, tumors and other virus-associated diseases may manifest. Both human γ-herpesviruses were first identified in tumors and primary effusion lymphomas are typically dually infected (Cesarman et al., 1995; Chang et al., 1994; Epstein, 2001). For all their similarities, however, there are also striking differences between the viruses. EBV is nearly ubiquitous whereas KSHV is restricted to particular populations. EBV is most commonly associated with B-, T- and NK-cell tumors and epithelial tumors, whereas KSHV is associated with endothelial and B-cell tumors. In this chapter, aspects of virus–disease associations and therapies will be explored.

EBV

Transmission of EBV generally involves oral contact (Cohen, 2000). This might occur through the maternal chewing of food for young infants such as occurs in some cultures, the sharing of eating utensils, or kissing (Niederman et al., 1976). Infection may also occur through genital transmission, blood transfusion, and organ or bone marrow transplantation (Crawford et al., 2002). By adulthood more than 90% of adults show serologic evidence of EBV infection. Primary infection is usually asymptomatic in infancy or childhood, but is commonly associated with the syndrome of infectious mononucleosis when infection first occurs in adolescence or adulthood (Henke et al., 1973). Symptomatic or not, infection is generally lifelong.

Following initial exposure, antibody responses to some latent and lytic antigens persist indefinitely (Henle et al., 1979). Thereafter, infectious virus is shed intermittently in saliva and viral DNA can be detected in peripheral blood mononuclear cells (Ling et al., 2003a,b; Sitki-Green et al., 2004).

Infection in the normal host

Symptomatic infection (infectious mononucleosis also referred to as glandular fever) occurs in less than half of new seroconverters during the late teenage years. The classic manifestations are fever, pharyngitis, cervical lymphadenopathy (often tender), hepatosplenomegaly, malaise and fatigue. The former symptoms and signs usually last one to three weeks, but malaise and fatigue often persist for weeks or months (Rea et al., 2001).

An initial proliferation of EBV-infected B-lymphocytes is followed by the development of NK and T-cell responses (Hislop et al., 2002; Tosato et al., 1979) Laboratory findings include a reactive lymphocytosis (reflecting the proliferation of NK cells and T-cells), hypergammaglobulinemia and the presence of heterophile antibodies (Jenson, 2004). "Monospot" or "slide" tests are in common use and detect antigens on sheep, horse or goat erythrocytes. The appearance of heterophile antibodies appears to reflect broad spectrum B-cell activation rather than cross reaction between erythrocyte antigens and viral antigens. Heterophile antibodies typically persist for several months. Very young patients may not mount heterophile responses. In cases where the diagnosis of primary infection is in doubt, serology to assess the presence of an IgM anti-VCA response is useful. Traditionally determinations of antiviral antibodies have involved immunofluorescence, but now more commonly involve enzyme-linked immunosorbent assays.

The histologic findings in the lymph nodes range from non-specific follicular hyperplasia to a proliferation of large cells resembling lymphoma. In addition, the morphologic features may also resemble those seen in other viral infections, in particular associated with cytomegalovirus, herpes simplex or zoster, or that seen in lymph node draining sites of vaccinations. Lymph nodes from patients with infectious mononucleosis frequently have an immunoblastic proliferation of varying severity, which gives a mottled appearance to a variably expanded paracortex. Plasma cells and plasmacytoid cells are also admixed with immunoblasts and lymphocytes, so there is a polymorphous appearance. Sometimes the immunoblasts form clusters, or even sheets, partially effacing this lymph node, which may be confused with malignant lymphoma (Isaacson et al., 1992).

A multitude of other manifestations are sometimes associated with primary EBV infection. These include: maculopapular rash, particularly common in patients treated with ampicillin; hepatitis; autoimmune hemolytic anemia; genital ulcers; tonsilar enlargement; aplastic anemia; and a variety of neurologic complications including encephalitis, aseptic meningitis, transverse myelitis and others (Ahronheim et al., 1983). Neurologic syndromes may occur in the absence of classic signs, symptoms and laboratory findings described above (Domachowske et al., 1996; Grose et al., 1975; Sumaya, 1987).

In unusual circumstances, primary infection may be fatal. This may occur in the setting of congenital immunodeficiency as elaborated below or it may occur sporadically. Hemophagocytosis is often a prominent feature of fatal infectious mononucleosis (Okano and Gross, 1996).

Therapy

There is no specific therapy for infectious mononucleosis other than supportive care. Antiviral agents such as acyclovir and valacyclovir have been shown to reduce oral viral shedding but not to shorten the course of symptomatic disease (Jenson, 2004; Torre and Tambini, 1999). This lack of clinical efficacy is consistent with the idea that it is the inflammatory response to EBV rather than the destructive effects of the virus per se that are associated with symptoms. In this regard, corticosteroids which have anti-inflammatory properties and are lympholytic have been used to control pharyngitis, lymphadenopathy, splenomegaly and autoimmune manifestations such as severe thrombocytopenia or hemolytic anemia (Roy et al., 2004; Tynell et al., 1996).

Infection in patients with congenital immunodeficiencies

Patients with X-linked agammaglobulinemia lack B cells and seemingly lack the ability to harbor the virus (Faulkner et al., 1999). Neither infectious virus nor viral DNA is detected in either saliva or peripheral blood mononuclear cells. In contrast, various forms of severe combined immunodeficiency (SCID) predispose to fatal infectious mononucleosis, hemophagocytosis, dysgammaglobulinemia and EBV-driven lymphoproliferative diseases (Elenitoba-Johnson and Jaffe, 1997; Filipovich et al., 1994). Whereas SCID patients are vulnerable to many infections and are generally recognized as immunodeficient before primary EBV infection, patients with X-linked lymphoproliferative disease (XLP) often first come to medical attention in association with EBV infection (Seemayer et al., 1995). The genetic defect has been mapped to the SLAM – associated protein (SAP) gene which is expressed on natural killer (NK) cells, CD4+ T-cells and CD8+ T-cells. This molecule is thought to be involved in the coordination of the immune response to EBV and other viral infections (Coffey et al., 1998; Sharifi et al., 2004).

Chronic active EBV

Primary infection that evolves into a severe progressive illness characterized by major organ involvement such as hepatitis, lymphadenitis and hemophagocytosis; extreme elevations of EBV antibody titers; and situations in which EBV is detected by in situ hybridization, immunohistochemistry or PCR (at high copy number) are referred to as chronic active EBV infection (Katano et al., 2004). The disease is much more common in Asia with most reports coming from Japan, Taiwan, Korea and China. Mutations in the SAP gene have not been linked with chronic active EBV infection (Sumazaki et al., 2001). However, in one instance chronic active EBV has been associated with a genetic defect in both alleles of the perforin gene (Katano et al., 2004). Perforin is present in the granules of cytotoxic T-lymphocytes and NK cells and is required for their cytotoxic activity.

Allogeneic transplantation and EBV-specific adoptive T-cell immunotherapy have each been used alone or in combination in the treatment of chronic active EBV infection (Hagihara et al., 2003; Savoldo et al., 2002; Taketani et al., 2002). The experience is limited, however, and reports are mixed.

Infection in HIV patients

Patients with HIV infection typically have increased antibody titers to EBV antigens, increased viral DNA copy number in peripheral blood mononuclear cells and increased viral shedding in oropharyngeal secretions (Ling et al., 2003a,b; Van Baarle et al., 2002). EBV is associated with a variety of malignancies in HIV-infected patients as discussed further below. It is also associated with a benign disorder, oral hairy leukoplakia (Walling et al., 2003). This is a hyperplastic lesion of the oral mucosa, most commonly arising on the lateral aspect of the tongue. Occasionally these raised, white lesions occur in other immunosuppressed populations such as organ transplant recipients. Molecular analysis has revealed that several strains of virus are often present in a single lesion. The lesion is distinctive in that EBER expression is absent and there is high level expression of lytic genes (Cruchley et al., 1997; Gilligan et al., 1990; Webster-Cyriaque et al., 2000). The condition is generally not symptomatic. However, when there are indications for treatment, lesions resolve with acyclovir or valacyclovir therapy (Walling et al., 2003). Therapy is suppressive rather than curative, and recurrence following discontinuation of drug treatment is common.

Other illnesses

A variety of other chronic illnesses have been linked to EBV. In several autoimmune diseases, evidence supporting a link of some sort continues to accrue and the associations are under active investigation. These include systemic lupus erythematosus, multiple sclerosis and rheumatoid arthritis (James et al., 2001; Kang et al., 2004; Levin et al., 2003; Yang et al., 2004). Epitope spreading, cross-reactivity with autoantigens and virus-driven immortalization of autoreactive B cells have all been invoked as mechanisms whereby viral infection might precipitate autoimmunity. The possibility that autoimmunity might lead to increased EBV lytic infection in rheumatoid arthritis has also been considered (Yang et al., 2004). One of the characteristic findings in rheumatoid arthritis is rheumatoid factor, an anti-immunoglobulin autoantibody. Anti-immunoglobulin antibodies lead to lytic activation in latently infected cell lines such as the Akata Burkitt's cell line. Rheumatoid factors from patients' sera have also been found to lead to lytic reactivation.

Chronic fatigue syndrome and lymphoid interstitial pneumonitis are two other illnesses that have been linked to EBV by some investigators. Chronic fatigue syndrome is a poorly understood illness in which patients have chronic fatigue and often sore throat, tender lymphadenopathy, arthralgias, memory loss or headaches (Soto and Straus, 2000; Straus, 1993). These patients often have slightly elevated antibody titers to EBV and other viruses. Lymphoid interstitial pneumonias represent a spectrum of poorly characterized diseases that include idiopathic inflammatory processes and pulmonary lymphoproliferative disorders including malignant lymphomas (Swigris et al., 2002). Lymphoid interstitial pneumonia often occurs in association with other diseases, particularly Sjogren's syndrome and childhood HIV infection. EBV infected lymphocytes are often among the cells in the characteristic infiltrates, particularly in HIV-infected children but the relevance of the virus to the pathogenesis of the process is very uncertain.

EBV-associated tumors

EBV is associated with a variety of malignancies. The association between virus and tumor varies with regard to immunodeficiency, the time between primary infection and tumorigenesis, the importance of geographic factors, the importance of genetic factors, and the malignant tissue itself (lymphoid, epithelial, or smooth muscle) (Fig. 50.1).

The importance of immunodeficiency is illustrated by the observation that organ and hematopoietic stem cell transplant recipients, patients with congenital immunodeficiencies and HIV-infected patients are all at increased risk for EBV-associated B cell malignancies and the much rarer EBV-associated leiomyosarcoma (Knowles, 1999; Loren et al., 2003; McClain et al., 1995). In contrast, no increased risk of EBV-associated nasal lymphoma, nasopharyngeal carcinoma, or gastric carcinoma has been documented in these populations (Filipovich et al., 1994; Grulich et al., 2002; Hsu and Glaser, 2000; Loren et al., 2003; Penn, 1996).

The time between primary infection and malignancy is typically weeks or months in organ transplant recipients, several years in Hodgkin's lymphoma patients, and several decades in nasopharyngeal carcinoma and nasal lymphoma patients (Hjalgrim et al., 2003; Loren et al., 2003; Raab-Traub, 2002). Environmental factors such as exposure to malaria seem to play a role in the pathogenesis of EBV-associated Burkitt's lymphoma in Africa. In regions of Africa where malaria is endemic, Burkitt's lymphoma is a common childhood neoplasm and is uniformly associated with

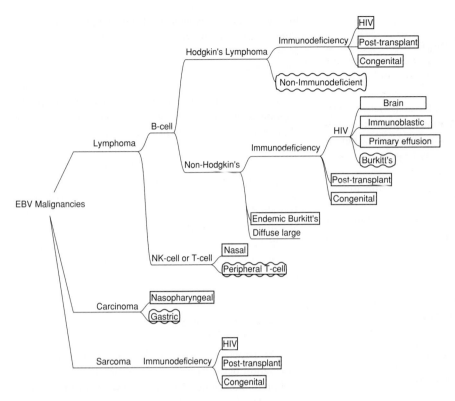

Fig. 50.1. EBV Malignancies. Rectangular boxes indicate malignancies that are almost uniformly associated with EBV. Wavy line boxes indicate malignancies that are associated with EBV in 5%–50% of cases. Blue boxes indicate an association with immunodeficiency.

EBV. In North America and Europe, Burkitt's lymphoma is much less common and is usually not associated with EBV. Populations of African descent in North America seem not to be at increased risk for the tumor (Hsu and Glaser, 2000).

A mix of environmental and genetic factors are implicated in nasopharyngeal carcinoma which is particularly common in Cantonese and Eskimo populations (Yu and Yuan, 2002). In contrast to Burkitt's lymphoma, undifferentiated nasopharyngeal carcinoma is always associated with EBV – even when it occurs in a low risk environment. When high risk Chinese populations emigrate, their risk falls but not to the Caucasian baseline. High risk families are recognized and twin studies confirm a genetic contribution (Jia et al., 2004).

Finally, there is variability in the genetics of the EBV-associated tumors themselves. Burkitt's lymphomas show simple chromosomal translocations that juxtapose immunoglobulin loci, most commonly the heavy-chain locus on chromosome 14, and the c-Myc oncogene. These translocations are recognized as among the defining characteristics of the malignancy. Post transplant lymphoproliferative disorders generally lack karyotypic abnormalities. Hodgkin's lymphoma, primary effusion lymphoma and nasopharyngeal carcinoma show very complex karyotypes.

The determination of EBV association typically involves in situ hybridization for EBER RNA (abundant EBV polymerase III transcripts), or immunohistochemical detection of viral antigens (Ambinder and Mann, 1994). With the exception of peripheral T-cell lymphomas, evidence of viral infection is generally found in most of the tumor cells if any of the tumor cells harbor virus (Anagnostopoulos et al., 1995). This is true at presentation and at relapse, at the primary site and in metastases. In nasopharyngeal carcinoma, several investigators have called attention to heterogeneity in the tumor, with the apparent absence of viral products from sub-populations of cells (Wu et al., 1991; Yao et al., 2000). With the exception of some of the lymphoid proliferations arising in profoundly immunocompromised patients, these tumors are all clonal. Clonality in lymphoid malignancies is readily established by studying antigen receptor rearrangements and in tumors in general by studying a variety of polymorphisms in X chromosomes (where in women, one or the other X will be inactivated). For the EBV-associated malignancies, it is also possible to infer clonality from the study of the viral terminal repeat sequences.

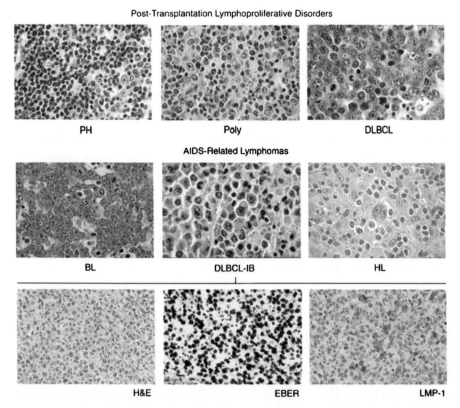

Fig. 50.2. Histopathology of EBV-associated diseases. Top row: Hematoxylin- and eosin- (H&E) stained sections of tissues involved by post-transplantation lymphoproliferative disorders are shown. These include an example of a plasmacytic hyperplasia, showing a majority of mature reactive lymphocytes with some immunoblasts and plasma cells; a polymorphic lymphoproliferative disorder, with a heterogeneous (polymorphic) cell population with atypical immunoblasts; and a diffuse large B-cell lymphoma, or monomorphic PTLD showing sheets of large neoplastic cells (original magnification 630 ×). Middle row: Examples of AIDS-related lymphomas, including: a Burkitt's lymphoma with sheets of medium-sized cells and a "starry sky" pattern due to macrophages with necrotic debris and mitotic figures; a diffuse large B-cell lymphoma with immunoblastic features (large atypical cells with an eccentric nucleus with a central prominent nucleolus and abundant cytoplasm); and an example of a Hodgkin's lymphoma with a classic Reed–Sternberg (original magnification 630 ×). Bottom row: EBV-positive AIDS-related lymphoma, H&E staining shows diffuse infiltration of neoplastic lymphocytes; in situ hybridization for EBER shows dark purple positivity in the majority of the nuclei; and immunohistochemistry for LMP-1 shows cytoplasmic positivity (brown) in many of the tumor cells (original magnification 100 ×).

Burkitt's lymphoma

This is a common childhood neoplasm in areas of Africa that are malarial (Magrath, 1997). The tumor typically arises in the jaw of young boys at the time that adult teeth are erupting. Orbital, abdominal and central nervous system involvement are common. The tumors grow exceedingly rapidly and respond to cytotoxic chemotherapy rapidly. They consist of a diffuse monotonous infiltration of B cells with many mitotic figures, as well as a high rate of spontaneous apoptosis (Fig. 50.2). A "starry sky" pattern is usually present, reflecting the presence of macrophages that have ingested apoptotic tumor cells. Immunophenotypically and genetically all morphologic forms of BL are similar: they express pan B-cell antigens such as CD19 and CD20 and are CD10 and BCL6 positive. Nearly 100% of the cells express the proliferation-associated marker Ki-67 (MIB-1).

In the endemic region, virtually all of the tumors are EBV associated. Studies suggest that antibody titers rise in anticipation of diagnosis. However, serology is not used clinically. The pattern of viral gene expression is very restricted (Niedobitek et al., 1995). Most tumor cells express only latency genes. EBNA1 is expressed but not the other latency nuclear antigens or LMP1. LMP2 mRNA is detected by RT-PCR as well (Tao et al., 1998). Molecular investigation of tumor tissue has shown that the promoters that drive expression of the latency nuclear antigens are densely

CpG methylated (Robertson et al., 1996). In some instances, deletions of latency antigens have been documented (Kelly et al., 2002). Burkitt's lymphoma cell lines are resistant to CD8 T-cell killing in vitro. This reflects their very restricted pattern of viral gene expression, a lack of surface adhesion molecules that facilitate recognition by T-cells, and a failure to process antigens for presentation in MHC class I complex (Moss et al., 1999).

Although there is little doubt that malaria perturbs immune responses, it is not yet clear whether its contribution is mainly as a stimulus to B cell proliferation, as an immunosuppressive factor disrupting T-cell or NK-cell immune surveillance, or perhaps through an entirely different mechanism. Outside the endemic region of Africa, Burkitt's lymphomas are only variably (25%–80%) associated with EBV (Bacchi et al., 1996). The limits of our knowledge are highlighted by the observation that in AIDS patients, the incidence of Burkitt's lymphoma is dramatically increased but these tumors occur in the least immunocompromised AIDS patients (CD4 T-cell >400) and are generally not EBV-associated (Carbone, 2003).

Post transplant lymphoproliferative disorders (PTLD)

Lymphoproliferative diseases arise in approximately 0.5 to 10% of solid organ and bone marrow or hematopoietic stem cell transplant recipients (Swinnen, 2001). The transplanted organ, the immunosuppressive regimen, and previous exposure to EBV are all determinants of risk. In organ transplant recipients tumor typically develops in host B-lymphocytes. The highest risk is associated with bowel transplantation, immunosuppression with OKT3 (a murine monoclonal antibody targeting CD3), and lack of prior exposure to EBV. In bone marrow transplant recipients, tumor typically develops in donor B-lymphocytes and the highest risk is associated with T-cell depletion of the bone marrow graft, high dose immunosuppression (again OKT3) and graft vs. host disease. The recipients' previous exposure to EBV appears to be irrelevant.

Lymphoproliferative diseases in transplant recipients have been classified as plasmacytic hyperplasia, polymorphic B-cell post-transplant lymphoproliferative disease, and monomorphic post-transplant lymphoproliferative disease (Chadburn et al., 1995, 1998; Knowles et al., 1995; Swerdlow, 1997). Histologically, plasmacytic hyperplasia resembles infectious mononucleosis, and is also referred to as infectious mononucleosis-like post-transplant lymphoproliferative disease. The main features are retention of the overall architecture of the tissue and presence of a mixed lymphoid population consisting primarily of lymphocytes, plasmacytoid lymphocytes, plasma cells and scattered immunoblasts; however, little or no cytologic atypia is present. The polymorphic lesions are characterized by destruction of the underlying architecture. These lesions are composed of a polymorphic (or heterogeneous) cell population, and vary from those that show extensive plasmacytic differentiation and minimal cytologic atypia to proliferations that lack plasmacytic differentiation and contain atypical immunoblasts. Individual cell necrosis to large areas of coagulative necrosis may be present. The monomorphic category includes diffuse large B cell lymphoma, Burkitt or Burkitt-like lymphoma, plasma cell myeloma, plasmacytoma and some peripheral T-cell lymphoma. In monomorphic lesions the histologic features are like those seen in immunocompetent individuals, and are classified according to standard criteria most recently described by the World Health Organization (Harris et al., 1997).

EBV is usually associated with B cell lymphoproliferative disease in this setting with the exception of lesions arising several years after transplantation, which are most frequently monomorphic. T-cell lymphomas and Hodgkin's lymphoma in the post-transplant setting are also often EBV associated. As the classification implies these tumors are quite heterogeneous and many different patterns of viral antigen expression are recognized. In most series these tumors are associated almost exclusively type 1 virus (Frank et al., 1995; Tao et al., 2002). Some of these tumors, particularly the plasmacytic hyperplasias and polymorphic B cell post-transplant lymphoproliferative disease, express the full spectrum of antigens expressed by EBV-immortalized lymphoblastoid cell lines. They also express adhesion molecules, class I and class II molecules and are thus particularly susceptible to immune interventions.

The observation that in some cases of post-transplant lymphoma, tumor will regress if immunosuppression is withdrawn or reduced first suggested that lack of immune surveillance plays a critical role in the pathogenesis of these lesions (Porcu et al., 2002; Starzl et al., 1984). This idea was strengthened when it was demonstrated that adoptive cellular immunotherapy was effective in treatment and in the prevention of these tumors, particularly in the bone marrow transplant setting (Papadopoulos et al., 1994; Rooney et al., 1998).

Monitoring viral copy number in peripheral blood mononuclear cells, plasma or whole blood has shown that patients with post-transplant lymphoproliferative disease generally have higher copy numbers – although some patients without tumor also sustain very high viral loads (Rowe et al., 2001; Yang et al., 2000). Several investigators have advocated monitoring viral load as a guide to immunosuppression or to "pre-emptive therapy" (Rowe et al., 2001).

Anti-B cell antibodies have proven very useful in the management of post-transplant lymphoproliferative disease (Gruhn et al., 2003; Yang et al., 2000). A chimeric antibody directed against CD20, rituximab, is widely used in the treatment of B-cell lymphomas in general and is useful in the treatment of post-transplant lymphoma as well. This antibody rapidly depletes B cells in the peripheral blood and thus treatment is virtually always associated with a fall in EBV load as measured in peripheral blood mononuclear cells. However, this fall is independent of tumor response.

AIDS lymphomas

A large fraction of AIDS lymphomas are EBV associated. Brain lymphomas in AIDS patients are virtually always EBV-associated (Camilleri-Broet et al., 1997; MacMahon et al., 1991). Diffuse large B-cell lymphomas with immunoblastic features are also usually EBV-associated (Knowles, 1999).

Many of these tumors express the full spectrum of viral latency genes. In contrast, AIDS Burkitt's lymphoma and primary effusion lymphoma show highly restricted pattern of EBV gene expression (Horenstein et al., 1997). The latter, while usually EBV associated are consistently KSHV associated and are discussed in more detail below. EBV-associated AIDS lymphomas are most common in patients with low CD4 T cell counts. In the case of primary central nervous system lymphomas, CD4 T cell counts were 10/ul in a recent cooperative group study (Ambinder et al., 2003). However, it should be noted that this generalization only applies to non-Hodgkin's lymphomas in HIV patients. Hodgkin's lymphoma typically arises in HIV infected patients with CD4 T cell counts greater than 200 (Glaser et al., 2003). EBV serology has not been found to be useful in identifying patients at risk for lymphoma insofar as virtually all HIV-infected patients with the exception of infants are EBV seropositive. Furthermore, EBV serology has not been helpful in the diagnosis of lymphoma in this setting. Similarly EBV copy number in peripheral blood mononuclear cells is elevated in HIV-infected patients and this elevation is not restricted to those with tumors (Van Baarle et al., 2002). However, detection of viral DNA in cerebrospinal fluid is useful in the differential diagnosis of brain lymphoma in HIV patients (Antinori et al., 1999; De Luca et al., 1995).

Extranodal T/NK cell tumors

These lymphomas are often EBV-associated. They have been classified into nasal, intestinal, and subcutaneous panniculitis-like (Chan et al., 1997; Chiang et al., 1996; Jaffe et al., 1999). Extranodal NK/T-cell lymphomas are characterized histologically by a diffuse lymphomatous infiltrate that is frequently angiocentric and angiodestructive. Coagulative necrosis and mucosal ulceration are common. The degree of association with EBV appears to be determined by both anatomic site and geography. Nasal lymphomas that express CD56 are most common in Asia and are almost always associated with EBV (Cheung et al., 2003). EBV gene expression is similar to that of EBV-associated Hodgkin's lymphoma (EBNA1, LMP1 and LMP2 are expressed but not EBNA2, 3A, 3B, or 3C) (Chiang et al., 1996). The presence of virus helps to distinguish the aggressive NK cell leukemias from more indolent NK lymphoproliferative disease (Gelb et al., 1994).

Nasopharyngeal carcinoma

Most common in Cantonese, nasopharyngeal carcinoma also occurs in Arab, and Eskimo populations (Yu and Yuan, 2002). They typically present in middle age but sometimes occur in adolescents. EBV is consistently associated with the non-keratinizing and undifferentiated subtypes of nasopharyngeal carcinomas. Biopsies show lesions composed of large neoplastic epithelial cells disposed in a syncytium-like array. Abundant, normal appearing lymphocyes are admixed with the epithelial cells, giving rise to the misnomer of lymphoepithelioma. Well-differentiated tumors are often EBV associated as well (Pathmanathan et al., 1995).

Nasopharyngeal carcinoma grows along nerve sheaths and invades the base of the brain and metastasize to lymphatics. Localized tumors are curable with radiation therapy. Metastatic tumors often respond to chemotherapy.

Nasopharyngeal carcinoma expresses a narrow spectrum of viral antigens with EBNA1, LMP2 and sometimes LMP1. NPC is associated with high antibody titers against many EBV antigens including lytic viral antigens (Connolly et al., 2001; Milman et al., 1985). The antibody profile is particularly distinctive because of the presence of IgA antibodies. Antibody titers begin arising years in advance of diagnosis and are sometimes used clinically in the evaluation of patients at high risk (perhaps because of several affected family members).

Viral DNA is present in plasma in patients with nasopharyngeal carcinoma and has emerged as a highly reliable guide to determining prognosis and monitoring therapy (Lin et al., 2004; Lo et al., 2000). This DNA is not encapsidated but is fragmented DNA released from tumor cells undergoing apoptosis (Chan et al., 2003). Spontaneous apoptosis is an ongoing process in most rapidly growing tumors. Radiation and chemotherapy accelerate the process. High levels of viral DNA in plasma at the start of therapy has emerged as the single most important prognostic factor, persistence of high levels in the face of therapy has emerged as a marker of relapse or progression (Chan et al., 2002).

Except in Eskimo populations, these tumors are almost exclusively associated with type 1 virus (Raab-Traub, 2002). A "Chinese strain" has been identified with the number of variations, most notably in the carboxyterminus of the LMP-1 gene where a 30 bp deletion is characteristic.

Adoptive T cell therapy has been explored without much success, perhaps reflecting the very limited antigenic targets (Chua et al., 2001; Moss et al., 1999). There is an interesting preliminary report suggesting the possibility that peptide vaccination is efficacious (Lin et al., 2002). Standard therapy involves external beam radiation often with cytotoxic chemotherapy.

Hodgkin's lymphoma

Approximately one third of Hodgkin's lymphomas are EBV-associated in North America and Western Europe, with a higher fraction in the rest of the world approaching 100% in areas of Africa and Latin America (Ambinder et al., 1993; Chang et al., 1993; Glaser et al., 1997). The tumor usually arises in young adults (15–35 years) with the age incidence curve varying somewhat in different regions of the world. The disease most commonly presents as cervical or supraclavicular lymphadenopathy, may be associated with fevers and night sweats and can often be cured with chemotherapy, radiation therapy or combined modality therapy.

Infectious mononucleosis was recognized as a risk factor long before EBV was recognized as the cause of infectious mononucleosis (Grufferman and Delzell, 1984). A recent study has shown that infectious mononucleosis is associated with an increased incidence of EBV-associated Hodgkin's lymphoma but not other Hodgkin's lymphoma (Hjalgrim et al., 2003). The typical interval between symptomatic primary infection and diagnosis of Hodgkin's lymphoma is 2 to 3 years, but increased risk continues for up to 20 years.

The diagnostic hallmark of Hodgkin's lymphoma is the presence of a minority of neoplastic cells, Reed–Sternberg cells, in a background of non-neoplastic cells. The two major subtypes of Hodgkin's lymphoma are the classical and the lymphocyte predominant forms, but only the former is associated with EBV infection. The histologic subtypes of classical HL are nodular sclerosis, mixed cellularity, lymphocyte rich classical, and lymphocyte depleted. EBV is most frequently associated with the mixed cellularity subtype, and also lymphocyte depleted, especially in the context of HIV infection. While the tumor cells are of B cell origin, B cell antigens like CD20, CD79A and immunoglobulin are frequently negative or weakly expressed. The B cell-specific activator protein (BSAP)/PAX5 can usually be detected by immunohistochemistry. EBV can be detected by in situ hybridization for EBER when present. In these cases, immunohistochemistry can detect expression of LMP-1 and EBNA-1, without EBNA-2.

Although viral antibody titers in patients with newly diagnosed Hodgkin's lymphoma differ from healthy counterparts, the differences are sufficiently small that they have no clinical utility (Chang et al., 2004). Studies are ongoing to determine whether viral DNA in plasma has the same significance in Hodgkin's lymphoma that it does in nasopharyngeal carcinoma.

Gastric cancers

Carcinomas of the stomach, particularly those arising in the gastric antrum carry EBV episomes and express EBNA1 in approximately 10–15% of cases. The incidence of this malignancy varies widely with higher incidences particularly in Japan. However, the percentage of cases associated with virus seems to be relatively constant whether tumors from high or low incidence populations are being studied (Fukayama et al., 1998; Takada, 2000). Although only a minority of these tumors are EBV associated, gastric carcinoma is one of the more common tumors world wide and EBV-associated gastric cancers may well be the most common EBV-associated malignancy when considered globally.

Other EBV-associated tumors

Leiomyosarcomas in the immunocompromised (organ transplant recipients, HIV-infected patients and patients with congenital immunodeficiency) are extraordinarily rare tumors but seem to be commonly EBV-associated (McClain et al., 2000; Reyes et al., 2002; van Gelder et al., 1995). Their pattern of viral gene expression has only had limited study due to their rarity but appears to be distinctive with expression of EBNA-2 but not LMP-1. Lymphomatoid granulomatosis is an EBV-associated B cell lymphoproliferative disease that often involves skin, lungs, brain, kidney and other organs. It is associated with systemic symptoms and areas of necrosis within the tumor. The disease generally arises in older patients. As with leiomyosarcomas the disease is so rare that studies of antigen expression are quite limited. Undifferentiated thymic carcinomas resemble nasopharyngeal carcinomas histologically and are generally EBV-associated.

Breast cancer, hepatocellular cancer, thymoma and other tumors

A multitude of other tumors have been linked with EBV. Breast cancer in particular has received a great deal of attention (Bonnet et al., 1999; Labrecque et al., 1995). Reports suggested that viral nucleic aids and proteins could be found in a large percentage of tumors by Western blot and by in situ hybridization. However, a whole series of studies have either failed to confirm the initial reports or have offered alternate explanations such as cross-reacting antibodies or increased tendency to lytic infection in malignant tissues (Glaser et al., 1998; Huang et al., 2003; Murray et al., 2003). Similarly, there have been reports of EBV in hepatocellular cancer, thymoma and several other malignancies that have not generally been confirmed.

The clinical importance of the viral association

Many of the tumors above are only sometimes associated with EBV, with the determinants of association varying from cofactors such as malaria (Burkitt's lymphoma) to AIDS (brain lymphoma) to other factors (Hodgkin's lymphoma). Although the detection of EBV in the tumor is sometimes useful in helping to establish a diagnosis (as in brain lymphoma in AIDS patients), there are few clinical settings in which the detection of virus per se clearly alters the prognosis or therapy. Evidence has been presented that survival in older patients may be poorer in Hodgkin's lymphoma associated with EBV than in that not associated, but definitive studies in this regard are still lacking and no one has yet advocated different primary therapy for Hodgkin's as a function of EBV status (Clarke et al., 2001). For patients who have failed standard therapies, novel approaches to therapy are being explored. In some instances these approaches involve adoptive immunotherapy, in others activation of viral gene expression. Activation of viral gene expression might lead either to direct cell killing, to expression of dominant viral antigens that might render tumor cells more susceptible to immune surveillance or to sensitization to ganciclovir or similar agents whose cytotoxic activity is dependent on phosphorylation by viral kinases (Chan et al., 2004; Moore et al., 2001; Feng et al., 2004; Ambinder et al., 1996).

KSHV

Endemic in sub-Saharan Africa and in regions near the Mediterranean Sea, KSHV-seropositivity is rare in most parts of the world (Chatlynne et al., 1998; Gao et al., 1996). The virus is transmitted in childhood within families in endemic regions, through sexual contacts in adults in high risk groups (Kedes et al., 1996; Martin et al., 1998; Smith et al., 1999). KSHV is commonly detected in the saliva in seropositives and salivary transmission is likely (Ablashi et al., 2002; Koelle et al., 1997). Some investigators have specifically implicated receptive anal intercourse, oral-genital contact, or oral-anal contact in virus transmission (Dukers et al., 2000; Grulich et al., 1999). Although viral DNA has been detected in seminal fluid, relatively infrequent detection in comparison with saliva and low copy number make the role of seminal fluid in transmission uncertain (Pellett et al., 1999).

Primary KSHV infection

A febrile illness and maculopapular rash may be associated with primary infection in children without immunocompromise (Andreoni et al., 2002). Lymphadenopathy has been associated with seroconversion in men who have sex with men (Casper et al., 2002). Fever, lymphoid hyperplasia, splenomegaly and pancytopenia have been reported in organ transplant recipients (Luppi et al., 2003).

KSHV-associated angioproliferative and lymphoproliferative disorders

The virus was originally discovered in Kaposi's sarcoma (Chang et al., 1994). It is also present in multicentric Castleman's disease and associated plasmablastic lymphoma, and primary effusion lymphoma (PEL).

Kaposi's sarcoma

First described in older men of Mediterranean descent, Kaposi's sarcoma also occurs in regions of Africa where it afflicts children as well as adults, in immunocompromised organ transplant recipients and in HIV-infected individuals. In the latter setting, it is one of the defining illnesses of AIDS and is the most common associated malignancy.

Kaposi's sarcoma lesions often involve the skin or mucous membranes and appear as flat violaceous plaques or nodules. Lesions are generally not painful (except occasionally when they involve the plantar surface of the feet). Skin lesions often appear on the lower legs and it has been hypothesized that this reflects a predilection for relatively hypoxic regions of the body (Haque et al., 2003). Although Kaposi's sarcoma lesions are often disfiguring, and associated edema may be a source of discomfort, they are rarely painful and rarely a cause of death (Fig. 50.3). Lesions commonly involve the gastrointestinal tract and the lungs. The appearance is sufficiently characteristic that

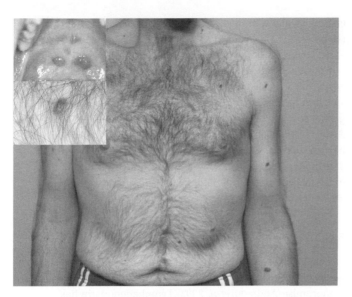

Fig. 50.3. Kaposi's sarcoma. Lesions are often scattered over the trunk and lower extremities. Their appearance is violaceous as a consequence of their neovascularity. The insets show Involvement of the hard palate (top) and a close up of a cutaneous lesion (bottom).

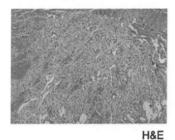 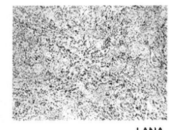

H&E   LANA

Fig. 50.4. Histological section stained with hematoxylin and eosin of a nodular tumor stage lesion of KS. Note the spindle cell proliferation and abundant vasculature. KSHV LANA (ORF-73) expression in KS. Staining with a rat monoclonal antibody revealed LANA positivity (diaminobenzidine, brown) in the nuclei of many spindle cells in a KS lesion. Positivity was also identified in endothelial cells lining the larger vascular spaces that may represent lymphatic vessels (original magnification 100 ×).

biopsy confirmation is not always necessary. Gastrointestinal lesions may be associated with hemorrhage, diarrhea, or obstruction; while pulmonary lesions may lead to fatal respiratory compromise.

The histologic characteristics of the lesions are similar across different affected populations. There are variable mixtures of ectatic, irregularly shaped, round capillary and slit-like endothelial-lined vascular spaces and spindle-shaped cells often with an inflammatory mononuclear cell infiltrate (Fig. 50.4). Red blood cells and hemosiderin pigment are frequently present, often extravasated between the spindle cells. Small granules of intracytoplasmic or extracellular hyalin material may be identified. In early lesions, the spindle cells are low in number compared to the surrounding inflammatory cells. Sometimes the earliest patch and plaque stage lesions are difficult to distinguish from granulation tissue. The spindle cells eventually become the predominant cell population, forming fascicles that compress the vascular slits, and the lesions become progressively nodular (Cockerell, 1991; Lever and Schaumburg-Lever, 1990).

Immunohistochemistry using monoclonal antibodies to LANA, shows that the viral protein is invariably expressed in Kaposi's sarcoma lesions. Nuclear staining with a speckled pattern can be seen in a variable proportion of the spindle cells, endothelial cells lining vascular spaces and in a very small proportion infiltrating CD45+/CD68+ monocytes (Katano et al., 1999; Kellam et al., 1999a,b; Parravicini et al., 2000). Most spindle cells show expression of a restricted set of viral proteins, although a small percentage of cells express lytic antigens (Cannon et al., 1999; Chiou et al., 2002). It has been suggested that these lytic proteins may exert a paracrine effect on surrounding cells.

Spindle cells are thought to originate from circulating peripheral-blood hematopoietic precursor cells (Dupin et al., 1999). In organ transplant recipients, tumor spindle cells may be of donor origin (Barozzi et al., 2003). KS lesions are clonal in at least some instances Rabkin et al., 1997; Gill et al., 1998). There is the possibility that KS begins as a polyclonal inflammatory lesion that sometimes progresses to oligoclonal or monoclonal neoplasia.

Treatment

Asymptomatic lesions do not always require treatment. In AIDS patients, lesions may regress or stabilize with control of HIV (Krown, 2004). Lesions may be treated topically, with a retinoid cream, injections of cytotoxic agents, or irradiation. Disseminated and visceral disease may respond to systemic treatment with alpha interferon or cytotoxic chemotherapy. Liposomal formulations of anthracyclines have proven particularly useful. These agents which are generally not associated with either nausea or alopecia are generally very well tolerated. Paclitaxel is also very active but is often reserved for second-line treatment because of its toxicity profile with severe myalgias and nausea common. There is no established role for antiherpesviral agents such as foscarnate, ganciclovir or cidofovir in the management of KS, although there is an intriguing report that ganciclovir may reduce the incidence of KS in HIV patients being treated for cytomegalovirus retinitis (Robles *et al.*, 1990; Martin *et al.*, 1990).

Castleman's disease and plasmablastic lymphomas

Castleman's disease is a poorly understood atypical lymphoproliferative disorder, usually described as a polyclonal, non-neoplastic condition. Two distinct histopathologic subtypes had been reported before the identification of KSHV. The hyaline vascular type, by far more common, and the plasma cell type.

Castleman's disease can be localized or may be multicentric involving many lymph node groups and spleen. Multicentric Castleman's disease (MCD) is characterized by recurrent fevers, lymphadenopathy, hepatosplenomegaly, autoimmune phenomena and not infrequently progresses to lymphoma or Kaposi's sarcoma, consistent with an association with KSHV infection (Soulier *et al.*, 1995). MCD, also called multicentric angiofollicular hyperplasia, is characterized by a vascular proliferation in the germinal centers, which is reminiscent of KS (Fig. 50.5). In fact, the presence of a lymph node containing both KS and Castleman's disease is not uncommon in HIV-positive patients.

The histologic appearance of Castleman's disease is quite different in the hyaline vascular and plasma cell types. The former is characterized by enlarged lymphoid follicles, small hyalinized germinal centers within an expanded concentric mantle of small lymphocytes, as well as a highly vascularized interfollicular network. In contrast, in the plasma cell type the germinal centers resemble those of follicular hyperplasia, and are composed of a mixture of cleaved and non-cleaved small and large lymphocytes with varying numbers of tingible body macrophages and mitotic figures. The mantle zone is usually intact, and is surrounded by sheets of mature-appearing plasma cells. Transition cases can occur. Both hyaline vascular changes and classic reactive follicles can occur in continuity, both follicle types exhibit the diagnostic onion-skinning of the mantle zones. There is a blurring of the histotypes and these may represent in many cases temporal manifestations of the same disease. Early studies reported the plasma cells to be polytypic in the majority of cases, but in close to 40% of the cases they have been shown to be monotypic, almost always restricted to expression of lambda light chains (Hall *et al.*, 1989).

Since the identification of KSHV in MCD, the understanding of the histology of this disease has changed. While KSHV has been reported in MCD with both hyaline vascular and plasma cell morphology (Larroche *et al.*, 2002), it appears that the majority of cases described in

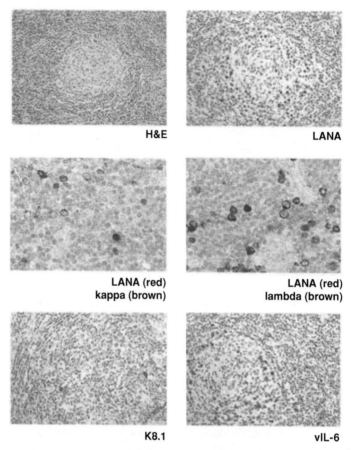

Fig. 50.5. Multicentric Castleman's disease: hematoxylin- and eosin- (H&E) stained section of a lymph node with HIV-associated Castleman's disease showing a single follicle with a large, concentrically arranged mantle zone surrounding a germinal center. The interfollicular area contains a network of small vessels (original magnification 100 ×). Immunohistochemical staining with the following antibodies is shown: LANA (ORF 73), a monoclonal rat antibody was used, showing brown nuclear positivity in cells in the mantle zone (original magnification 100 ×); LANA and kappa, double staining showed nuclear positivity (red staining) in cells that are negative for cytoplasmic kappa (brown staining); LANA and lambda, double staining shows cells that are positive for nuclear LANA (red staining) as well as cytoplasmic lambda (brown staining) (original magnification 400 ×); K8.1, a monoclonal antibody shows cytoplasmic positivity (brown staining) in two cells that are undergoing lytic viral replication (original magnification 100 ×); vIL-6, cytoplasmic staining using a rabbit polyclonal antiserum shows positivity in numerous cells in the mantle zone (original magnification 100 ×).

the literature more closely resemble the plasma cell type of MCD. One report indicates that the KSHV-positive cases showed the highest intensity of angiosclerosis and germinal center and perifollicular vascular proliferation, while plasmacytosis is less pronounced than in the KSHV-negative

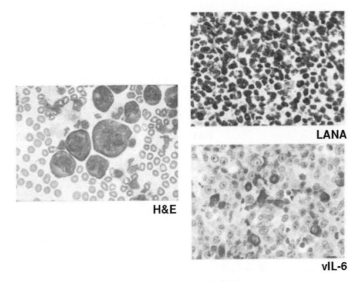

Fig. 50.6. Primary effusion lymphoma: Wright-Giemsa stain air-dried cytocentrifuge preparation of a KSHV-positive primary effusion lymphoma. The tumor cells in this image are considerably larger than normal benign lymphocytes and monocytes. The cells display significant polymorphism and possess moderately abundant basophilic cytoplasm. A prominent, clear perinuclear Golgi zone can be appreciated in several cells. The nuclei vary from large and round to highly irregular, multilobated, and pleomorphic and often contain one or more prominent nucleoli (original magnification 1000 ×). Immunohistochemical staining with the following antibodies is shown: LANA (ORF 73), a monoclonal rat antibody was used, showing brown speckled nuclear positivity in all the neoplastic cells; vIL-6, immunohistochemical staining with a polyclonal rabbit antiserum shows abundant cytoplasmic expression (brown) in many lymphoma cells (original magnification 400 ×).

cases of the plasma cell type (Suda et al., 2001). It now appears that the KSHV-positive cases represent a distinct morphologic variant, resembling more the plasma cell type, but in addition showing the presence of larger cells in the mantle zones, which are approximately twice the size of mantle zone lymphocytes, and characterized by a moderate amount of amphophilic cytoplasm and a large vesicular nucleus containing one or sometimes two prominent nucleoli. These cells have been called plasmablasts, although they frequently have immunoblastic features (Dupin et al., 2000). Expression of IgM can be used to distinguish these plasmablasts from the interfollicular plasma cells that don't express IgM. These cells can be numerous and coalesce.

Immunohistochemistry for KSHV has become a useful diagnostic method for MCD. Monoclonal antibodies to LANA (Dupin et al., 1999) show the presence of KSHV-positive cells, which are the plasmablasts located mostly in the mantle zones of lymph nodes of patients with MCD. These KSHV-infected plasmablasts are B cells that for some unknown reason are monotypic but polyclonal, almost invariably expressing IgMλ (Du et al., 2001). KSHV-positive lymphocytes can also be seen spilling into the germinal centers and in interfollicular areas. One study showed that KSHV-positive endothelial cells can also be found in MCD lymph nodes, in both HIV-positive and -negative patients (Brousset et al., 2001). In addition antibodies to vIL-6 are useful, as this viral protein is also frequently expressed in MCD in scattered plasmablasts surrounding the lymphoid follicles (Cannon et al., 1999a,b; Parravinci et al., 1997; Staskus et al., 1999), and expression of this viral cytokine may confer a worse prognosis (Menke et al., 2002). Lytic antigens are also expressed more frequently in KSHV-infected cells in MCD that in other disorders associated with this virus, suggesting that lytic viral replication may be a feature of MCD (Katano et al., 2000).

Therapy for Castleman's disease remains ill-defined. However, evidence of lytic viral expression has led some to advocate ganciclovir or other antiviral therapy. Indeed, there are small anecdotal reports that indicate responses to ganciclovir (Casper et al., 2004). Other therapies targeting the tissue compartment harboring the virus have also been associated with responses. These include the use of an anti-B-cell antibody rituximab or splenectomy (Corbellino et al., 2001; Lerza et al., 1999; Marcelin et al., 2003).

Primary effusion lymphoma and related lymphomas

Primary effusion lymphomas arise mainly in patients with HIV infection and preferentially involve body cavities and occasionally extranodal sites. These tumors always carry KSHV and are commonly coinfected by EBV. The classical presentation is with signs and symptoms of an effusion in the absence of a tumor mass (Nador et al., 1996). The cells in the effusion are large, have abundant cytoplasm, usually amphophilic to basophilic, and nuclei that range from large, round and regular to highly irregular and pleomorphic, with one or more large prominent nucleoli (Fig. 50.6) (Cesarman et al., 1995). Many cells have plasmacytoid or immunoblastic features. Binucleated or multinucleated cells resemble Reed–Sternberg cells can be seen. Mitotic figures are typically numerous. The immunophenotype is characteristic, as PEL cells express of CD45, CD138 and one or more activation-associated antigens in the frequent absence of B cell-associated antigens and immunoglobulin expression. A B cell origin can be demonstrated by the presence of clonal immunoglobulin gene rearrangements, and the immunoglobulin genes show somatic hypermutation indicating a postgerminal cell stage of differentiation.

Immununohistochemistry shows the presence of LANA and other KSHV proteins in a variable proportion of neoplastic cells, in particular vIL-6. In addition, the majority of PELs are coinfected with EBV, which can be detected by in situ hybridization to EBERs.

Lymphomas containing KSHV can also present as solid tissue masses, usually extranodally, similar to other AIDS-related non-Hodgkin's lymphomas. While some of these lymphomas subsequently develop an effusion, others apparently do not. They usually present as solid extranodal lymphomas and are diagnosed as diffuse large cell, immunoblastic, or anaplastic large cell lymphomas, in which the presence of KSHV in practically all the lymphoma cells could be demonstrated by immunohistochemistry or molecular techniques (Chadburn et al., 2004; Engels et al., 2003). Most of these are immunoblastic in appearance, have a high mitotic rate and variable amounts off apoptotic debris. These lymphomas appear to fall in the spectrum of PEL, as they usually lack expression of B cell antigens and immunoglobulin, they have a similar morphology, and they are frequently co-infected with EBV.

Survival with conventional chemotherapy is dismal, with the reported median survival time less than 6 months (Boulanger, 2005).

Several diseases have been purportedly linked to KSHV. In multiple myeloma patients, the virus was not reported to be in tumor cells but in the associated bone marrow stroma (Rettig et al., 1997; Said et al., 1997). There was the suggestion that production of viral interleukin-6 or cellular interleukin-6 by the stromal cells drove B-cells in the marrow to malignancy. However, many investigators have failed to confirm these findings (Ablashi et al., 2000; Bellos et al., 1999; Brander et al., 2002; Corbellino et al., 1999; Dominici et al., 2000; Drabick et al., 2002; Tarte et al., 1999; Pan et al., 2001). Similarly associations of KSHV with sarcoidosis (Di Alberti et al., 1997) and pulmonary hypertension (Cool et al., 2003) have been reported. Confirmation of a general association with either disease process is lacking (Henke-Gendo et al., 2004; Lebbe et al., 1999; Maeda et al., 2000; Moore, 1998; Regamey et al., 1998; Sugaya et al., 1999).

Conclusions

The human gammaherpesvirus-associated diseases are quite distinct from those associated with other herpesviruses. Rather than tissue destruction in association with lytic infection such as is characteristic of the alpha and beta herpesviruses, the gammaherpesviruses are associated with proliferative diseases and malignancies. The seroprevalence of EBV and KSHV is much more widespread than the associated proliferative diseases. Several of these are most common in immunocompromised patients, but other gammaherpesvirus-associated tumors arise in hosts that are not globally immunocompromised. The host genetic and environmental determinants of disease beyond immunocompromise are poorly understood. Detection of viral nucleic acid or proteins is important in the diagnosis of some of the lymphomas and lymphoproliferative disease. Treatment with virus-specific therapies is still in its infancy. Antivirals that target the viral DNA polymerase such as acyclovir and ganciclovir have very limited if any impact on benign or malignant disease, although there is a hint that these agents may reduce the incidence of tumorigenesis in high risk populations. Two exceptions might be noted: oral hairy leukoplakia clearly responds to antiviral therapy and anecdotal reports suggest that Castleman's disease may also. Adoptive cellular immunotherapies appear to hold promise and have achieved some impressive successes in the bone marrow transplant population in the prevention and treatment of lymphoproliferative disease.

REFERENCES

Ablashi, D. V., Chatlynne, L., Thomas, D. *et al.* (2000). Lack of serologic association of human herpesvirus-8 (KSHV) in patients with monoclonal gammopathy of undetermined significance with and without progression to multiple myeloma. *Blood*, **96**, 2304–2306.

Ablashi, D. V., Chatlynne, L. G., Whitman, J. E., Jr., and Cesarman, E. (2002). Spectrum of Kaposi's sarcoma-associated herpesvirus, or human herpesvirus 8, diseases. *Clin. Microbiol. Rev.*, **15**, 439–464.

Ahronheim, G. A., Auger, F., Joncas, J. H., Ghibu, F., Rivard, G. E., and Raab-Traub, N. (1983). Primary infection by Epstein–Barr virus presenting as aplastic anemia. *N. Engl. J. Med.*, **309**, 313–314.

Ambinder, R. F. and Mann, R. B. (1994). Detection and characterization of Epstein–Barr virus in clinical specimens. *Am. J. Pathol.*, **145**, 239–252.

Ambinder, R. F., Browning, P. J., Lorenzana, I. *et al.* (1993). Epstein–Barr virus and childhood Hodgkin's disease in Honduras and the United States. *Blood*, **81**, 462–467.

Ambinder, R. F., Robertson, K. D., Moore, S. M., and Yang, J. (1996). Epstein–Barr virus as a therapeutic target in Hodgkin's disease and nasopharyngeal carcinoma. *Semin. Cancer Biol.*, **7**, 217–226.

Ambinder, R. F., Lee, S., and Curran, W. J. (2003). Phase II intergroup trial of sequential chemotherapy and radiotherapy for AIDS-related primary central nervous system lymphoma. *Cancer Therapy*, **1**, 215–221.

Anagnostopoulos, I., Hummel, M., and Stein, H. (1995). Frequent presence of latent Epstein–Barr virus infection in peripheral T cell lymphomas. A review. *Leuk. Lymphoma*, **19**, 1–12.

Andreoni, M., Sarmati, L., Nicastri, E. *et al.* (2002). Primary human herpesvirus 8. infection in immunocompetent children. *J. Am. Med. Assoc.*, **287**, 1295–1300.

Antinori, A., De Rossi, G., Ammassari, A. *et al.* (1999). Value of combined approach with thallium-201 single-photon emission computed tomography and Epstein–Barr virus DNA polymerase chain reaction in CSF for the diagnosis of AIDS-related primary CNS lymphoma. *J. Clin. Oncol.*, **17**, 554–560.

Bacchi, M. M., Bacchi, C. E., Alvarenga, M., Miranda, R., Chen, Y. Y., and Weiss, L. M. (1996). Burkitt's lymphoma in Brazil: strong association with Epstein–Barr virus. *Mod. Pathol.*, **9**, 63–67.

Barozzi, P., Luppi, M., Facchetti, F. *et al.* (2003). Post-transplant Kaposi sarcoma originates from the seeding of donor-derived progenitors. *Nat. Med.*, **9**, 554–561.

Bellos, F., Goldschmidt, H., Dorner, M., Ho, A. D., and Moos, M. (1999). Bone marrow derived dendritic cells from patients with multiple myeloma cultured with three distinct protocols do not bear Kaposi's sarcoma associated herpesvirus DNA. *Ann. Oncol.*, **10**, 323–327.

Bonnet, M., Guinebretiere, J. M., Kremmer, E. *et al.* (1999). Detection of Epstein–Barr virus in invasive breast cancers. *J. Natl Cancer Inst.*, **91**, 1376–1381.

Boulanger, E., Gerard, L., Gabarre, J. *et al.* (2005). Prognostic factors and outcome of human herpesvirus 8-associated promary effusion lymphoma in patients with AIDS. *J. Clin. Oncol.*, **23**, 4372–4380.

Brander, C., Raje, N., O'Connor, P. G. *et al.* (2002). Absence of biologically important Kaposi sarcoma-associated herpesvirus gene products and virus-specific cellular immune responses in multiple myeloma. *Blood*, **100**, 698–700.

Brousset, P., Cesarman, E., Meggetto, F., Lamant, L., and Delsol, G. (2001). Colocalization of the viral interleukin-6 with latent nuclear antigen-1 of human herpesvirus-8 in endothelial spindle cells of Kaposi's sarcoma and lymphoid cells of multicentric Castleman's disease. *Hum. Pathol.*, **32**, 95–100.

Camilleri-Broet, S., Davi, F., Feuillard, J. *et al.* (1997). AIDS-related primary brain lymphomas: histopathologic and immunohistochemical study of 51 cases. The French Study Group for HIV-Associated Tumors. *Hum. Pathol.*, **28**, 367–374.

Cannon, J. S., Hamzeh, F., Moore, S., Nicholas, J., and Ambinder, R. F. (1999a). Human herpesvirus 8-encoded thymidine kinase and phosphotransferase homologues confer sensitivity to ganciclovir. *J. Virol.*, **73**, 4786–4793.

Cannon, J. S., Nicholas, J., Orenstein, J. M. *et al.* (1999b). Heterogeneity of viral IL-6 expression in HHV-8-associated diseases. *J. Infect. Dis.*, **180**, 824–828.

Carbone, A. (2003). Emerging pathways in the development of AIDS-related lymphomas. *Lancet Oncol.*, **4**, 22–29.

Casper, C., Wald, A., Pauk, J., Tabet, S. R., Corey, L., and Celum, C. L. (2002). Correlates of prevalent and incident Kaposi's sarcoma-associated herpesvirus infection in men who have sex with men. *J. Infect. Dis.*, **185**, 990–993.

Casper, C., Nichols, W. G., Huang, M. L., Corey, L., and Wald, A. (2004). Remission of HHV-8 and HIV-associated multicentric Castleman disease with ganciclovir treatment. *Blood*, **103**, 1632–1634.

Cesarman, E., Chang, Y., Moore, P. S., Said, J. W., and Knowles, D. M. (1995). Kaposi's sarcoma-associated herpesvirus-like DNA sequences in AIDS-related body-cavity-based lymphomas. *N. Engl. J. Med.*, **332**, 1186–1191.

Chadburn, A., Suciu-Foca, N., Cesarman, E., Reed, E., Michler, R. E., and Knowles, D. M. (1995). Post-transplantation lymphoproliferative disorders arising in solid organ transplant recipients are usually of recipient origin. *Am. J. Pathol.*, **147**, 1862–1870.

Chadburn, A., Chen, J. M., Hsu, D. T. *et al.* (1998). The morphologic and molecular genetic categories of posttransplantation lymphoproliferative disorders are clinically relevant. *Cancer*, **82**, 1978–1987.

Chadburn, A., Hyjek, E., Mathew, S., Cesarman, E., Said, J. and Knowles, D. M. (2004). KSHV-positive solid lymphomas represent an extra-cavitary variant of primary effusion lymphoma. *Am. J. Surg. Pathol.*, **28**, 1401–1416.

Chan, A. T., Lo, Y. M., Zee, B. *et al.* (2002). Plasma Epstein–Barr virus DNA and residual disease after radiotherapy for undifferentiated nasopharyngeal carcinoma. *J. Natl Cancer Inst.*, **94**, 1614–1619.

Chan, A. T., Tao, Q., Robertson, K. D. *et al.* (2004). Azacitidine induces demethylation of the Epstein–Barr virus genome in tumors in patients. *J. Clin. Oncol.*, **22**, 1373–1381.

Chan, J. K., Sin, V. C., Wong *et al.* (1997). Nonnasal lymphoma expressing the natural killer cell marker CD56: a clinicopathologic study of 49 cases of an uncommon aggressive neoplasm. *Blood*, **89**, 4501–4513.

Chan, K. C., Zhang, J., Chan, A. T. *et al.* (2003). Molecular characterization of circulating EBV DNA in the plasma of nasopharyngeal carcinoma and lymphoma patients. *Cancer Res.*, **63**, 2028–2032.

Chang, E. T., Zheng, T., Lennette, E. T. *et al.* (2004). Heterogeneity of risk factors and antibody profiles in Epstein–Barr virus genome-positive and -negative Hodgkin lymphoma. *J. Infect. Dis.*, **189**, 2271–2281.

Chang, K. L., Albujar, P. F., Chen, Y. Y., Johnson, R. M., and Weiss, L. M. (1993). High prevalence of Epstein-Barr virus in the Reed-Sternberg cells of Hodgkin's disease occurring in Peru. *Blood*, **81**, 496–501.

Chang, Y., Cesarman, E., Pessin, M. S. *et al.* (1994). Identification of herpesvirus-like DNA sequences in AIDS-associated Kaposi's sarcoma. *Science*, **266**, 1865–1869.

Chatlynne, L. G., Lapps, W., Handy, M. *et al.* (1998). Detection and titration of human herpesvirus-8-specific antibodies in sera from blood donors, acquired immunodeficiency syndrome patients, and Kaposi's sarcoma patients using a whole virus enzyme-linked immunosorbent assay. *Blood*, **92**, 53–58.

Cheung, M. M., Chan, J. K., and Wong, K. F. (2003). Natural killer cell neoplasms: a distinctive group of highly aggressive lymphomas/leukemias. *Semin. Hematol.*, **40**, 221–232.

Chiang, A. K., Tao, Q., Srivastava, G., and Ho, F. C. (1996). Nasal NK- and T-cell lymphomas share the same type of Epstein–Barr virus latency as nasopharyngeal carcinoma and Hodgkin's disease., *Int. J. Cancer*, **68**, 285–290.

Chiou, C. J., Poole, L. J., Kim, P. S. *et al*. (2002). Patterns of gene expression and a transactivation function exhibited by the vGCR (ORF74) chemokine receptor protein of Kaposi's sarcoma-associated herpesvirus. *J. Virol.*, **76**, 3421–3439.

Chua, D., Huang, J., Zheng, B. *et al*. (2001). Adoptive transfer of autologous Epstein–Barr virus-specific cytotoxic T cells for nasopharyngeal carcinoma. *Int. J. Cancer*, **94**, 73–80.

Clarke, C. A., Glaser, S. A., Dorfman, R. F., *et al*. (2001). Epstein–Barr virus and survival after Hodgkin's disease in a population-based series of women. *Cancer*, **91**, 1579–1587.

Cockerell, C. J. (1991). Histopathological features of Kaposi's sarcoma in HIV infected individuals. *Cancer Surv.*, **10**, 73–89.

Coffey, A. J., Brooksbank, R. A., Brandau, O. *et al*. (1998). Host response to EBV infection in X-linked lymphoproliferative disease results from mutations in an SH2-domain encoding gene. *Nat. Genet.*, **20**, 129–135.

Cohen, J. I. (2000). Epstein–Barr virus infection. *N. Engl. J. Med.*, **343**, 481–492.

Connolly, Y., Littler, E., Sun, N. *et al*. (2001). Antibodies to Epstein-Barr virus thymidine kinase: a characteristic marker for the serological detection of nasopharyngeal carcinoma. *Int. J. Cancer*, **91**, 692–697.

Cool, C. D., Rai, P. R., Yeager, M. E. *et al*. (2003). Expression of human herpesvirus 8 in primary pulmonary hypertension. *N. Engl. J. Med.*, **349**, 1113–1122.

Corbellino, M., Pizzuto, M., Bestetti, G. *et al*. (1999). Absence of Kaposi's sarcoma – associated herpesvirus DNA sequences in multiple myeloma. *Blood*, **93**, 1110–1111.

Corbellino, M., Bestetti, G., Scalamogna, C. *et al*. (2001). Long-term remission of Kaposi sarcoma-associated herpesvirus-related multicentric Castleman disease with anti-CD20 monoclonal antibody therapy. *Blood*, **98**, 3473–3475.

Crawford, D. H., Swerdlow, A. J., Higgins, C. *et al*. (2002). Sexual history and Epstein-Barr virus infection. *J. Infect. Dis.*, **186**, 731–736.

Cruchley, A. T., Murray, P. G., Niedobitek, G., Reynolds, G. M., Williams, D. M., and Young, L. S. (1997). The expression of the Epstein–Barr virus nuclear antigen (EBNA-I) in oral hairy leukoplakia. *Oral Dis.*, **3**(Suppl 1), S177–S179.

De Luca, A., Antinori, A., Cingolani, A. *et al*. (1995). Evaluation of cerebrospinal fluid EBV-DNA and IL-10 as markers for in vivo diagnosis of AIDS-related primary central nervous system lymphoma. *Br. J. Haematol.*, **90**, 844–849.

Di Alberti, L., Piattelli, A., and Artese, L. (1997). Human herpesvirus 8 variants in sarcoid tissues. *Lancet*, **350**, 1655–1661.

Domachowske, J. B., Cunningham, C. K., Cummings, D. L., Crosley, C. J., Hannan, W. P., and Weiner, L. B. (1996). Acute manifestations and neurologic sequelae of Epstein–Barr virus encephalitis in children. *Pediatr. Infect. Dis. J.*, **15**, 871–875.

Dominici, M., Luppi, M., Campioni, D. *et al*. (2000). PCR with degenerate primers for highly conserved DNA polymerase gene of the herpesvirus family shows neither human herpesvirus 8 nor a related variant in bone marrow stromal cells from multiple myeloma patients. *Int. J. Cancer*, **86**, 76–82.

Drabick, J. J., Davis, B. J., Lichy, J. H., Flynn, J. and Byrd, J. C. (2002). Human herpesvirus 8 genome is not found in whole bone marrow core biopsy specimens of patients with plasma cell dyscrasias. *Ann. Hematol.*, **81**, 304–307.

Du, M. Q., Liu, H., Diss, T. C. *et al*. (2001). Kaposi sarcoma-associated herpesvirus infects monotypic (IgM lambda) but polyclonal naive B cells in Castleman disease and associated lymphoproliferative disorders. *Blood*, **97**, 2130–2136.

Dukers, N. H., Renwick, N., Prins, M. *et al*. (2000). Risk factors for human herpesvirus 8 seropositivity and seroconversion in a cohort of homosexual men. *Am. J. Epidemiol.*, **151**, 213–224.

Dupin, N., Fisher, C., Kellam, P. *et al*. (1999). Distribution of human herpesvirus-8 latently infected cells in Kaposi's sarcoma, multicentric Castleman's disease, and primary effusion lymphoma. *Proc. Natl. Acad. Sci. USA*, **96**, 4546–4551.

Dupin, N., Diss, T. L., Kellam, P. *et al*. (2000). HHV-8 is associated with a plasmablastic variant of Castleman disease that is linked to HHV-8-positive plasmablastic lymphoma. *Blood*, **95**, 1406–1412.

Elenitoba-Johnson, K. S. and Jaffe, E. S. (1997). Lymphoproliferative disorders associated with congenital immunodeficiencies. *Semin. Diagn. Pathol.*, **14**, 35–47.

Engels, E. A., Pittaluga, S., Whitby, D. *et al*. (2003). Immunoblastic lymphoma in persons with AIDS-associated Kaposi's sarcoma: a role for Kaposi's sarcoma-associated herpesvirus. *Mod. Pathol.*, **16**, 424–429.

Epstein, M. A. (2001). Reflections on Epstein–Barr virus: some recently resolved old uncertainties. *J. Infect.*, **43**, 111–115.

Faulkner, G. C., Burrows, S. R., Khanna, R., Moss, D. J., Bird, A. G., and Crawford, D. H. (1999). X-Linked agammaglobulinemia patients are not infected with Epstein–Barr virus: implications for the biology of the virus. *J. Virol.*, **73**, 1555–1564.

Feng, W. H., Hong, G., Delecluse, H. J., and Kenney, S. C. (2004). Lytic induction therapy for Epstein–Barr virus positive B-cell lymphomas. *J. Virol.*, **78**, 1839–1902.

Filipovich, A. H., Mathur, A., Kamat, D., Kersey, J. H., and Shapiro, R. S. (1994). Lymphoproliferative disorders and other tumors complicating immunodeficiencies. *Immunodeficiency*, **5**, 91–112.

Frank, D., Cesarman, E., Liu, Y. F., Michler, R. E., and Knowles, D. M. (1995). Posttransplantation lymphoproliferative disorders frequently contain type A and not type B Epstein-Barr virus. *Blood*, **85**, 1396–1403.

Fukayama, M., Chong, J. M., and Kaizaki, Y. (1998). Epstein–Barr virus and gastric carcinoma. *Gastric Cancer*, **1**, 104–114.

Gao, S. J., Kingsley, L., Li, M. *et al*. (1996). KSHV antibodies among Americans, Italians and Ugandans with and without Kaposi's sarcoma. *Nat. Med.*, **2**, 925–928.

Gelb, A. B., van de Rijn, M., Regula, D. P., Jr. *et al*. (1994). Epstein–Barr virus-associated natural killer-large granular lymphocyte leukemia. *Hum. Pathol.*, **25**, 953–960.

Gill, P. S., Tsai, Y. C., Rao, A. P. *et al.* (1998). Evidence for multiclonality in multicentric Kaposi's sarcoma. *Proc. Natl Acad. Sci. USA*, **95**, 8257–8261.

Gilligan, K., Rajadurai, P., Resnick, L., and Raab-Traub, N. (1990). Epstein–Barr virus small nuclear RNAs are not expressed in permissively infected cells in AIDS-associated leukoplakia. *Proc. Natl Acad. Sci. USA*, **87**, 8790–8794.

Glaser, S. L., Lin, R. J., Stewart, S. L. *et al.* (1997). Epstein–Barr virus-associated Hodgkin's disease: epidemiologic characteristics in international data. *Int. J. Cancer*, **70**, 375–382.

Glaser, S. L., Ambinder, R. F., DiGiuseppe, J. A., Horn-Ross, P. L., and Hsu, J. L. (1998). Absence of Epstein–Barr virus EBER-1 transcripts in an epidemiologically diverse group of breast cancers. *Int. J. Cancer*, **75**, 555–558.

Glaser, S. L., Clarke, C. A., Gulley, M. L. *et al.* (2003). Population-based patterns of human immunodeficiency virus-related Hodgkin lymphoma in the Greater San Francisco Bay Area, 1988–1998. *Cancer*, **98**, 300–309.

Grose, C., Henle, W., Henle, G., and Feorino, P. M. (1975). Primary Epstein–Barr-virus infections in acute neurologic diseases. *N. Engl. J. Med.*, **292**, 392–395.

Grufferman, S. and Delzell, E. (1984). Epidemiology of Hodgkin's disease. *Epidemiol. Rev.*, **6**, 76–106.

Gruhn, B., Meerbach, A., Hafer, R., Zell, R., Wutzler, P., and Zintl, F. (2003). Pre-emptive therapy with rituximab for prevention of Epstein–Barr virus-associated lymphoproliferative disease after hematopoietic stem cell transplantation. *Bone Marrow Transpl.*, **31**, 1023–1025.

Grulich, A. E., Olsen, S. J., Luo, K. *et al.* (1999). Kaposi's sarcoma-associated herpesvirus: a sexually transmissible infection? *J. Acquir. Immune Defic. Syndr. Hum. Retrovirol.*, **20**, 387–393.

Grulich, A. E., Li, Y., McDonald, A., Correll, P. K., Law, M. G., and Kaldor, J. M. (2002). Rates of non-AIDS-defining cancers in people with HIV infection before and after AIDS diagnosis. **16**, 1155–1161.

Hagihara, M., Tsuchiya, T., Hyodo, O. *et al.* (2003). Clinical effects of infusing anti-Epstein–Barr virus (EBV)-specific cytotoxic T-lymphocytes into patients with severe chronic active EBV infection. *Int. J. Hematol.*, **78**, 62–68.

Hall, P. A., Donaghy, M., Cotter, F. E., Stansfeld, A. G., and Levison, D. A. (1989). An immunohistological and genotypic study of the plasma cell form of Castleman's disease. *Histopathology*, **14**, 333–346; discussion 429–432.

Haque, M., Davis, D. A., Wang, V., Widmer, I., and Yarchoan, R. (2003). Kaposi's sarcoma-associated herpesvirus (human herpesvirus 8) contains hypoxia response elements: relevance to lytic induction by hypoxia. *J. Virol.*, **77**, 6761–6768.

Harris, N. L., Ferry, J. A., and Swerdlow, S. H. (1997). Posttransplant lymphoproliferative disorders: summary of Society for Hematopathology Workshop. *Semin. Diagn. Pathol.*, **14**, 8–14.

Henke, C. E., Kurland, L. T., and Elveback, L. R. (1973). Infectious mononucleosis in Rochester, Minnesota, 1950 through 1969. *Am. J. Epidemiol.*, **98**, 483–490.

Henke-Gendo, C., Schulz, T. F., and Hoeper, M. M. (2004). HHV-8 in pulmonary hypertension. *N. Engl. J. Med.*, **350**, 194–195; author reply 194–195.

Henle, W., Henle, G., and Lennette, E. T. (1979). The Epstein–Barr virus. *Sci. Am.*, **241**, 48–59.

Hislop, A. D., Annels, N. E., Gudgeon, N. H., Leese, A. M., and Rickinson, A. B. (2002). Epitope-specific evolution of human CD8(+) T cell responses from primary to persistent phases of Epstein–Barr virus infection. *J. Exp. Med.*, **195**, 893–905.

Hjalgrim, H., Askling, J., Rostgaard, K. *et al.* (2003). Characteristics of Hodgkin's lymphoma after infectious mononucleosis. *N. Engl. J. Med.*, **349**, 1324–1332.

Horenstein, M. G., Nador, R. G., Chadburn, A. *et al.* (1997). Epstein–Barr virus latent gene expression in primary effusion lymphomas containing Kaposi's sarcoma-associated herpesvirus/human herpesvirus-8. *Blood*, **90**, 1186–1191.

Hsu, J. L. and Glaser, S. L. (2000). Epstein–Barr virus-associated malignancies: epidemiologic patterns and etiologic implications. *Crit. Rev. Oncol. Hematol.*, **34**, 27–53.

Huang, J., Chen, H., Hutt-Fletcher, L., Ambinder, R. F., and Hayward, S. D. (2003). Lytic viral replication as a contributor to the detection of Epstein–Barr virus in breast cancer. *J. Virol.*, **77**, 13267–13274.

Isaacson, P. G., Schmid, C., Pan, L., Wotherspoon, A. C., and Wright, D. H. (1992). Epstein–Barr virus latent membrane protein expression by Hodgkin and Reed–Sternberg-like cells in acute infectious mononucleosis. *J. Pathol.*, **167**, 267–271.

Jaffe, E. S., Krenacs, L., Kumar, S., Kingma, D. W., and Raffeld, M. (1999). Extranodal peripheral T-cell and NK-cell neoplasms. *Am. J. Clin. Pathol.*, **111**, S46–S55.

James, J. A., Neas, B. R., Moser, K. L. *et al.* (2001). Systemic lupus erythematosus in adults is associated with previous Epstein–Barr virus exposure. *Arthritis Rheum.*, **44**, 1122–1126.

Jenson, H. B. (2004). Virologic diagnosis, viral monitoring, and treatment of Epstein–Barr virus infectious mononucleosis. *Curr. Infect. Dis. Rep.*, **6**, 200–207.

Jia, W. H., Feng, B. J., Xu, Z. L. *et al.* (2004). Familial risk and clustering of nasopharyngeal carcinoma in Guangdong, China. *Cancer*, **101**, 363–369.

Kang, I., Quan, T., Nolasco, H. *et al.* (2004). Defective control of latent Epstein-Barr virus infection in systemic lupus erythematosus. *J. Immunol.*, **172**, 1287–1294.

Katano, H., Sato, Y., Kurata, T., Mori, S., and Sata, T. (1999). High expression of HHV-8-encoded ORF73 protein in spindle-shaped cells of Kaposi's sarcoma. *Am. J. Pathol.*, **155**, 47–52.

Katano, H., Sato, Y., Kurata, T., Mori, S., and Sata, T. (2000). Expression and localization of human herpesvirus 8-encoded proteins in primary effusion lymphoma, Kaposi's sarcoma, and multicentric Castleman's disease. *Virology*, **269**, 335–344.

Katano, H., Ali, M. A., Patera, A. C. *et al.* (2004). Chronic active Epstein-Barr virus infection associated with mutations in perforin that impair its maturation. *Blood*, **103**, 1244–1252.

Kedes, D. H., Operskalski, E., Busch, M., Kohn, R., Flood, J., and Ganem, D. (1996). The seroepidemiology of human herpesvirus 8 (Kaposi's sarcoma-associated herpesvirus): distribution of infection in KS risk groups and evidence for sexual transmission. *Nat. Med.*, **2**, 918–924.

Kellam, P., Bourboulia, D., Dupin, N. (1999). Characterization of monoclonal antibodies raised against the latent nuclear antigen of human herpesvirus 8. *J. Virol.*, **73**, 5149–5155.

Kelly, G., Bell, A., and Rickinson, A. (2002). Epstein–Barr virus-associated Burkitt lymphomagenesis selects for downregulation of the nuclear antigen EBNA2. *Nat. Med.*, **8**, 1098–1104.

Knowles, D. M. (1999). Immunodeficiency-associated lymphoproliferative disorders. *Mod. Pathol.*, **12**, 200–217.

Knowles, D. M., Cesarman, E., Chadburn, A. *et al.* (1995). Correlative morphologic and molecular genetic analysis demonstrates three distinct categories of posttransplantation lymphoproliferative disorders. *Blood*, **85**, 552–565.

Koelle, D. M., Huang, M. L., Chandran, B., Vieira, J., Piepkorn, M., and Corey, L. (1997). Frequent detection of Kaposi's sarcoma-associated herpesvirus (human herpesvirus 8) DNA in saliva of human immunodeficiency virus-infected men: clinical and immunologic correlates. *J. Infect. Dis.*, **176**, 94–102.

Krown, S. E. (2004). Highly active antiretroviral therapy in AIDS-associated Kaposi's sarcoma: implications for the design of therapeutic trials in patients with advanced, symptomatic Kaposi's sarcoma. *J. Clin. Oncol.*, **22**, 399–402.

Labrecque, L. G., Barnes, D. M., Fentiman, I. S., and Griffin, B. E. (1995). Epstein–Barr virus in epithelial cell tumors: a breast cancer study. *Cancer Res.*, **55**, 39–45.

Larroche, C., Cacoub, P., Soulier, J. *et al.* (2002). Castleman's disease and lymphoma: report of eight cases in HIV-negative patients and literature review. *Am. J. Hematol.*, **69**, 119–126.

Lebbe, C., Agbalika, F., Flageul, B. *et al.* (1999). No evidence for a role of human herpesvirus type 8 in sarcoidosis: molecular and serological analysis. *Br. J. Dermatol*, **141**, 492–496.

Lerza, R., Castello, G., Truini, M. *et al.* (1999). Splenectomy induced complete remission in a patient with multicentric Castleman's disease and autoimmune hemolytic anemia. *Ann. Hematol.*, **78**, 193–196.

Lever, W. F. and Schaumburg-Lever, G. (1990). *Histopathology of the Skin*. Philadelphia:Lippincott.

Levin, L. I., Munger, K. L., Rubertone, M. V. *et al.* (2003). Multiple sclerosis and Epstein–Barr virus. *J. Am. Med. Assoc.*, **289**, 1533–1536.

Lin, C. L., Lo, W. F., Lee, T. H. *et al.* (2002). Immunization with Epstein–Barr virus (EBV) peptide-pulsed dendritic cells induces functional CD8+ T-cell immunity and may lead to tumor regression in patients with EBV-positive nasopharyngeal carcinoma. *Cancer Res.*, **62**, 6952–6958.

Lin, J. C., Wang, W. Y., Chen, K. Y., Wei, Y. H., Liang, W. M., Jan, J. S. and Jiang, R. S. (2004). Quantification of plasma Epstein–Barr virus DNA in patients with advanced nasopharyngeal carcinoma. *N. Engl. J. Med.*, **350**, 2461–2470.

Ling, P. D., Lednicky, J. A., Keitel, W. A. *et al.* (2003a). The dynamics of herpesvirus and polyomavirus reactivation and shedding in healthy adults: a 14-month longitudinal study. *J. Infect. Dis.*, **187**, 1571–1580.

Ling, P. D., Vilchez, R. A., Keitel, W. A. *et al.* (2003b). Epstein–Barr virus DNA loads in adult human immunodeficiency virus type 1-infected patients receiving highly active antiretroviral therapy. *Clin. Infect. Dis.*, **37**, 1244–1249.

Lo, Y. M., Chan, A. T., Chan, L. Y. *et al.* (2000). Molecular prognostication of nasopharyngeal carcinoma by quantitative analysis of circulating Epstein–Barr virus DNA. *Cancer Res.*, **60**, 6878–6881.

Loren, A. W., Porter, D. L., Stadtmauer, E. A., and Tsai, D. E. (2003). Post-transplant lymphoproliferative disorder: a review. *Bone Marrow Transpl.*, **31**, 145–155.

Luppi, M., Barozzi, P., Guaraldi, G. *et al.* (2003). Human herpesvirus 8-associated diseases in solid-organ transplantation: importance of viral transmission from the donor. *Clin. Infect. Dis.*, **37**, 606–607; author reply 607.

MacMahon, E. M., Glass, J. D., Hayward, S. D. *et al.* (1991). Epstein–Barr virus in AIDS-related primary central nervous system lymphoma. *Lancet*, **338**, 969–973.

Maeda, H., Niimi, T., Sato, S. *et al.* (2000). Human herpesvirus 8 is not associated with sarcoidosis in Japanese patients. *Chest*, **118**, 923–927.

Magrath, I. T. (1997). Non-Hodgkin's lymphomas: epidemiology and treatment. *Ann. NY Acad. Sci.*, **824**, 91–106.

Marcelin, A. G., Aaron, L., Mateus, C. *et al.* (2003). Rituximab therapy for HIV-associated Castleman disease. *Blood*, **102**, 2786–2788.

Martin, J. N., Ganem, D. E., Osmond, D. H., Page-Shafer, K. A., Macrae, D., and Kedes, D. H. (1998). Sexual transmission and the natural history of human herpesvirus 8 infection. *N. Engl. J. Med.*, **338**, 948–954.

Martin, D. F., Kuppermann, B. D., Wolitz, R. A., Palestine, A. G., Li, H., and Robinson, C. A. (1990). Oral ganciclovir for patients with cytomegalovirus retinitis treated with a ganciclovir implant. Roche Ganciclovir Study Group. *N. Engl. J. Med.*, **340**, 1063–1070.

McClain, K. L., Leach, C. T., Jenson, H. B. *et al.* (1995). Association of Epstein–Barr virus with leiomyosarcomas in children with AIDS. *N. Engl. J. Med.*, **332**, 12–18.

McClain, K. L., Leach, C. T., Jenson, H. B. *et al.* (2000). Molecular and virologic characteristics of lymphoid malignancies in children with AIDS. *J. Acquir. Immune Defic. Syndr.*, **23**, 152–159.

Menke, D. M., Chadbum, A., Cesarman, E. *et al.* (2002). Analysis of the human herpesvirus 8 (HHV-8) genome and HHV-8 vIL-6 expression in archival cases of castleman disease at low risk for HIV infection. *Am. J. Clin. Pathol.*, **117**, 268–275.

Milman, G., Scott, A. L., Cho, M. S. *et al.* (1985). Carboxyl-terminal domain of the Epstein–Barr virus nuclear antigen is highly immunogenic in man. *Proc. Natl. Acad. Sci. USA*, **82**, 6300–6304.

Moore, P. S. (1998). Human herpesvirus 8 variants. *Lancet*, **351**, 679–680.

Moore, S. M., Cannon, J. S., Tanhehco, Y. C., Hamzeh, E. M., and Ambinder, R. F. (2001). Induction of Epstein–Barr virus kinases to sensitize tumor cells to nucleoside analogues. *Antimicrob. Agents Chemother.*, **45**, 2082–2091.

Moss, D. J., Khanna, R., Sherritt, M., Elliott, S. L., and Burrows, S. R. (1999). Developing immunotherapeutic strategies for the control of Epstein–Barr virus-associated malignancies. *J. Acquir. Immune Defic. Syndr.*, **21 Suppl 1**, S80–S83.

Murray, P. G., Lissauer, D., Junying, J. *et al.* (2003). Reactivity with A monoclonal antibody to Epstein–Barr virus (EBV) nuclear antigen 1 defines a subset of aggressive breast cancers in the absence of the EBV genome. *Cancer Res.*, **63**, 2338–2343.

Nador, R. G., Cesarman, E., Chadburn, A. *et al.* (1996). Primary effusion lymphoma: a distinct clinicopathologic entity associated with the Kaposi's sarcoma-associated herpes virus. *Blood*, **88**, 645–656.

Niederman, J. C., Miller, G., Pearson, H. A., Pagano, J. S., and Dowaliby, J. M. (1976). Infectious mononucleosis. Epstein–Barr-virus shedding in saliva and the oropharynx. *N. Engl. J. Med.*, **294**, 1355–1359.

Niedobitek, G., Agathanggelou, A., Rowe, M. *et al.* (1995). Heterogeneous expression of Epstein–Barr virus latent proteins in endemic Burkitt's lymphoma. *Blood*, **86**, 659–665.

Okano, M. and Gross, T. G. (1996). Epstein–Barr virus-associated hemophagocytic syndrome and fatal infectious mononucleosis. *Am. J. Hematol.*, **53**, 111–115.

Pan, L., Milligan, L., Michaeli, J., Cesarman, E., and Knowles, D. M. (2001). Polymerase chain reaction detection of Kaposi's sarcoma-associated herpesvirus-optimized protocols and their application to myeloma. *J. Mol. Diagn*, **3**, 32–38.

Papadopoulos, E. B., Ladanyi, M., Emanuel, D. *et al.* (1994). Infusions of donor leukocytes to treat Epstein–Barr virus-associated lymphoproliferative disorders after allogeneic bone marrow transplantation. *N. Engl. J. Med.*, **330**, 1185–1191.

Parravicini, C., Corbellino, M. *et al.* (1997). Expression of a virus-derived cytokine, KSHV vIL-6, in HIV-seronegative Castleman's disease. *Am. J. Pathol.*, **151**, 1517–1522.

Parravicini, C., Chandran, B., Corbellino, M. *et al.* (2000). Differential viral protein expression in Kaposi's sarcoma-associated herpesvirus-infected diseases: Kaposi's sarcoma, primary effusion lymphoma, and multicentric Castleman's disease. *Am. J. Pathol.*, **156**, 743–749.

Pathmanathan, R., Prasad, U., Chandrika, G., Sadler, R., Flynn, K., and Raab-Traub, N. (1995). Undifferentiated, nonkeratinizing, and squamous cell carcinoma of the nasopharynx. Variants of Epstein–Barr virus-infected neoplasia. *Am. J. Pathol.*, **146**, 1355–1367.

Pellett, P. E., Spira, T. J., Bagasra, O. *et al.* (1999). Multicenter comparison of PCR assays for detection of human herpesvirus 8 DNA in semen. *J. Clin. Microbiol.*, **37**, 1298–1301.

Penn, I. (1996). Cancers in cyclosporine-treated vs azathioprine-treated patients. *Transpl. Proc.*, **28**, 876–878.

Porcu, P., Eisenbeis, C. F., Pelletier, R. P. *et al.* (2002). Successful treatment of posttransplantation lymphoproliferative disorder (PTLD) following renal allografting is associated with sustained CD8(+) T-cell restoration. *Blood*, **100**, 2341–2348.

Raab-Traub, N. (2002). Epstein–Barr virus in the pathogenesis of NPC. *Semin. Cancer Biol.*, **12**, 431–441.

Rabkin, C. S., Janz, S., Lash, A. *et al.* (1997). Monoclonal origin of multicentric Kaposi's sarcoma lesions. *N. Engl. J. Med.*, **336**, 988–993.

Rea, T. D., Russo, J. E., Katon, W., Ashley, R. L., and Buchwald, D. S. (2001). Prospective study of the natural history of infectious mononucleosis caused by Epstein–Barr virus. *J. Am. Board Fam. Pract.*, **14**, 234–242.

Regamey, N., Erb, P., Tamm, M., and Cathomas, G. (1998). Human herpesvirus 8 variants. *Lancet*, **351**, 680.

Rettig, M. B., Ma, H. J., and Vescio, R. A. (1997). Kaposi's sarcoma-associated herpesvirus infection of bone marrow dendritic cells from multiple myeloma patients. *Science*, **276**, 1851–1854.

Reyes, C., Abuzaitoun, O., De Jong, A., Hanson, C., and Langston, C. (2002). Epstein–Barr virus-associated smooth muscle tumors in ataxia-telangiectasia: a case report and review. *Hum. Pathol.*, **33**, 133–136.

Robertson, K. D., Manns, A., Swinnen, L. J., Zong, J. C., Gulley, M. L., and Ambinder, R. F. (1996). CpG methylation of the major Epstein–Barr virus latency promoter in Burkitt's lymphoma and Hodgkin's disease. *Blood*, **88**, 3129–3136.

Robles, R., Lugo, D., Gee, L., and Jacobson, M. A. (1990). Effect of antiviral drugs used to treat cytomegalovirus end-organ disease on subsequent course of previously diagnosed Kaposi's sarcoma in patients with AIDS. *J. Acquir. Immune Defic. Syndr. Hum. Retrovirol.*, **20**, 34–38.

Rooney, C. M., Smith, C. A., Ng, C. Y. *et al.* (1998). Infusion of cytotoxic T cells for the prevention and treatment of Epstein–Barr virus-induced lymphoma in allogeneic transplant recipients. *Blood*, **92**, 1549–1555.

Rowe, D. T., Webber, S., Schauer, E. M., Reyes, J., and Green, M. (2001). Epstein–Barr virus load monitoring: its role in the prevention and management of post-transplant lymphoproliferative disease. *Transpl. Infect. Dis.*, **3**, 79–87.

Roy, M., Bailey, B., Amre, D. K., Girodias, J. B., Bussieres, J. F., and Gaudreault, P. (2004). Dexamethasone for the treatment of sore throat in children with suspected infectious mononucleosis: a randomized, double-blind, placebo-controlled, clinical trial. *Arch. Pediatr. Adolesc. Med.*, **158**, 250–254.

Said, J. W., Rettig, M. R., Heppner, K. *et al.* (1997). Localization of Kaposi's sarcoma-associated herpesvirus in bone marrow biopsy samples from patients with multiple myeloma. *Blood*, **90**, 4278–4282.

Savoldo, B., Huls, M. H., Liu, Z. *et al.* (2002). Autologous Epstein–Barr virus (EBV)-specific cytotoxic T cells for the treatment of persistent active EBV infection. *Blood*, **100**, 4059–4066.

Seemayer, T. A., Gross, T. G., Egeler, R. M. *et al.* (1995). X-linked lymphoproliferative disease: twenty-five years after the discovery. *Pediatr. Res.*, **38**, 471–478.

Sharifi, R., Sinclair, J. C., Gilmour, K. C. *et al.* (2004). SAP mediates specific cytotoxic T-cell functions in X-linked lymphoproliferative disease. *Blood*, **103**, 3821–3827.

Sitki-Green, D. L., Edwards, R. H., Covington, M. M., and Raab-Traub, N. (2004). Biology of Epstein–Barr virus during infectious mononucleosis. *J. Infect. Dis.*, **189**, 483–492.

Smith, N. A., Sabin, C. A., Gopal, R. *et al.* (1999). Serologic evidence of human herpesvirus 8 transmission by homosexual but not heterosexual sex. *J. Infect. Dis.*, **180**, 600–606.

Soto, N. E. and Straus, S. E. (2000). Chronic fatigue syndrome and herpesviruses: the fading evidence. *Herpes*, **7**, 46–50.

Soulier, J., Grollet, L., Oksenhendler, E. *et al.* (1995). Kaposi's sarcoma-associated herpesvirus-like DNA sequences in multicentric Castleman's disease. *Blood*, **86**, 1276–1280.

Starzl, T. E., Nalesnik, M. A., Porter, K. A. *et al.* (1984). Reversibility of lymphomas and lymphoproliferative lesions developing under cyclosporin-steroid therapy. *Lancet*, **1**, 583–587.

Staskus, K. A., Sun, R., Miller, G. *et al.* (1999). Cellular tropism and viral interleukin-6 expression distinguish human herpesvirus 8 involvement in Kaposi's sarcoma, primary effusion lymphoma, and multicentric Castleman's disease. *J. Virol.*, **73**, 4181–4187.

Straus, S. E. (1993). Studies of herpesvirus infection in chronic fatigue syndrome. *Ciba Found. Symp.*, **173**, 132–139; discussion 139–145.

Suda, T., Katano, H., Delsol, G. *et al.* (2001). HHV-8 infection status of AIDS-unrelated and AIDS-associated multicentric Castleman's disease. *Pathol. Int.*, **51**, 671–679.

Sugaya, M., Nakamura, K., Takahiro, W., and Tamaki, K. (1999). Human herpesvirus type 8 is not detected in cutaneous lesions of sarcoidosis. *Br. J. Dermatol.*, **141**, 769.

Sumaya, C. V. (1987). Epstein–Barr virus infections in children. *Curr. Probl. Pediatr.*, **17**, 677–745.

Sumazaki, R., Kanegane, H., Osaki, M. *et al.* (2001). SH2D1A mutations in Japanese males with severe Epstein–Barr virus-associated illnesses. *Blood*, **98**, 1268–1270.

Swerdlow, S. H. (1997). Classification of the posttransplant lymphoproliferative disorders: from the past to the present. *Semin. Diagn. Pathol.*, **14**, 2–7.

Swigris, J. J., Berry, G. J., Raffin, T. A., and Kuschner, W. G. (2002). Lymphoid interstitial pneumonia: a narrative review. *Chest*, **122**, 2150–2164.

Swinnen, L. J. (2001). Organ transplant-related lymphoma. *Curr. Treat. Options Oncol.*, **2**, 301–308.

Takada, K. (2000). Epstein–Barr virus and gastric carcinoma. *Mol Pathol*, **53**, 255–261.

Taketani, T., Kikuchi, A., Inatomi, J. *et al.* (2002). Chronic active Epstein–Barr virus infection (CAEBV) successfully treated with allogeneic peripheral blood stem cell transplantation. *Bone Marrow Transpl.*, **29**, 531–533.

Tao, Q., Robertson, K. D., Manns, A., Hildesheim, A., and Ambinder, R. F. (1998). Epstein–Barr virus (EBV) in endemic Burkitt's lymphoma: molecular analysis of primary tumor tissue. *Blood*, **91**, 1373–1381.

Tao, Q., Yang, J., Huang, H., Swinnen, L. J., and Ambinder, R. F. (2002). Conservation of Epstein–Barr virus cytotoxic T-cell epitopes in posttransplant lymphomas: implications for immune therapy. *Am. J. Pathol.*, **160**, 1839–1845.

Tarte, K., Chang, Y., and Klein, B. (1999). Kaposi's sarcoma-associated herpesvirus and multiple myeloma: lack of criteria for causality. *Blood*, **93**, 3159–3163; discussion 3163–3164.

Torre, D. and Tambini, R. (1999). Acyclovir for treatment of infectious mononucleosis: a meta-analysis. *Scand. J. Infect. Dis.*, **31**, 543–547.

Tosato, G., Magrath, I., Koski, I., Dooley, N., and Blaese, M. (1979). Activation of suppressor T cells during Epstein–Barr-virus-induced infectious mononucleosis. *N. Engl. J. Med.*, **301**, 1133–1137.

Tynell, E., Aurelius, E., Brandell, A. *et al.* (1996). Acyclovir and prednisolone treatment of acute infectious mononucleosis: a multicenter, double-blind, placebo-controlled study. *J. Infect. Dis.*, **174**, 324–331.

Van Baarle, D., Wolthers, K. C., Hovenkamp, E. *et al.*, (2002). Absolute level of Epstein–Barr virus DNA in human immunodeficiency virus type 1 infection is not predictive of AIDS-related non-Hodgkin lymphoma. *J. Infect. Dis.*, **186**, 405–409.

van Gelder, T., Vuzevski, V. D., and Weimar, W. (1995). Epstein–Barr virus in smooth-muscle tumors. *N. Engl. J. Med.*, **332**, 1719.

Walling, D. M., Flaitz, C. M., and Nichols, C. M. (2003). Epstein–Barr virus replication in oral hairy leukoplakia: response, persistence, and resistance to treatment with valacyclovir. *J. Infect. Dis.*, **188**, 883–890.

Webster-Cyriaque, J., Middeldorp, J., and Raab-Traub, N. (2000). Hairy leukoplakia: an unusual combination of transforming and permissive Epstein–Barr virus infections. *J. Virol.*, **74**, 7610–7618.

Wu, T. C., Mann, R. B., Epstein, J. I. *et al.* (1991). Abundant expression of EBER1 small nuclear RNA in nasopharyngeal carcinoma. A morphologically distinctive target for detection of Epstein–Barr virus in formalin-fixed paraffin-embedded carcinoma specimens. *Am. J. Pathol.*, **138**, 1461–1469.

Yang, J., Tao, Q., Flinn, I. W. *et al.* (2000). Characterization of Epstein–Barr virus-infected B cells in patients with posttransplantation lymphoproliferative disease: disappearance after rituximab therapy does not predict clinical response. *Blood*, **96**, 4055–4063.

Yang, L., Hakoda, M., Iwabuchi, K. *et al.* (2004). Rheumatoid factors induce signaling from B cells, leading to epstein–barr virus and B-cell activation. *J. Virol.*, **78**, 9918–9923.

Yao, Y., Minter, H. A., Chen, X., Reynolds, G. M., Bromley, M., and Arrand, J. R. (2000). Heterogeneity of HLA and EBER expression in Epstein–Barr virus-associated nasopharyngeal carcinoma. *Int. J. Cancer*, **88**, 949–955.

Yu, M. C. and Yuan, J. M. (2002). Epidemiology of nasopharyngeal carcinoma. *Semin. Cancer Biol.*, **12**, 421–429.

51

EBV: immunobiology and host response

Denis J. Moss, Scott R. Burrows, and Rajiv Khanna

Infectious Disease and Immunology Division, Queensland Institute of Medical Research and Joint Oncology Program, University of Queensland, Australia

Introduction

The biology and immunology of Epstein–Barr virus (EBV) has continued to fascinate researchers because the lessons learnt provide a platform for understanding the interplay between the biology of this ubiquitous infection, the immune system seeking to restrict its spread and the emergence of a variety of malignancies. As with other gamma herpes viruses, EBV encodes a large set of lytic cycle genes together with a number of latent genes which are associated with expansion of the latent EBV pool in B-lymphocytes. Current evidence suggests that the virus gains entry into the body by infection of B-lymphocytes in the oral cavity via an interaction between the major viral glycoprotein gp340 and the complement receptor CR2 which is expressed on B-cells, although a role for CR2-expressing or non-expressing epithelial and/or T-cells cannot be totally discounted. In either case, evidence suggests that the earliest detectable event following primary infection is the expression of lytic cycle proteins resulting in the release of infectious virus into the oral cavity followed by a generalized seeding of latently infected B-lymphocytes throughout the body. This primary infection results in symptoms of acute infectious mononucleosis (IM) in about 50% of adolescents and is coincident with a marked lymphocytosis (dominated by EBV-specific cytotoxic T-cells) and the appearance of an IgM response to a variety of EBV proteins, most notably the viral capsid antigen, VCA. Current evidence suggests that this cytotoxic T-cell (CTL) response, which includes both CD4+ and CD8+ cells restricts expansion of these latently infected B-cells and results in a long-term carrier state in which there is an equilibrium between the level of secretion of the virus and the number of latently infected B-cells.

Latently infected B cells are of central importance in the overall biology of the virus, and the function of individual latent proteins has been studied in EBV transformed lymphoblastoid cell lines (LCLs). The virus expresses eight EBV latent genes including six nuclear proteins (EBNA1, 2, 3A, 3B, LP and 3C) and two integral membrane proteins (LMP1 and LMP2). Furthermore, virus-infected cells invariably express two small polyadenylated RNAs (EBER-1 and -2) which are often used as a sensitive marker for the presence of EBV within a cell. The nature of the long-term latent infection in vivo has been subject to considerable speculation but is likely to include expression of a limited number of proteins (EBNA1 and LMP1) in a B-cell pool that maintains a phenotype that is poorly recognized by CTL. Thus the virus appears to have evolved so that apart from the clinical effects of IM (which appears to be historically a relatively recent syndrome), most individuals suffer no consequences from carrying a small nucleus of latently infected B-cells which appear to be resistant to CTL recognition and which can, under certain circumstances be reactivated to release relatively low levels of virus into the oral cavity.

The dynamics of the establishment of this small pool of long-lived latently infected B-cells and the CTL response is poorly understood but involves a selection process imposed by the CTL response which recognizes and eliminates B cells with a full complement of latent antigens and a relatively rare differentiation step that permits the emergence of a long-lived memory B cell pool that is resistant to specific lysis and whose phenotype supports the expression of EBNA1 and LMP1. It appears however, that this seemingly elegant balance that ensures the long-term survival of the virus is subject to error on certain occasions resulting in the emergence of EBV-driven B cell malignancies.

These B cell malignancies are classified in terms of the degree of latent antigen expression. Burkitt's lymphoma (BL) is at one end of the spectrum and is characterized by the expression of a single EBV protein (EBNA1 whose phenotype suggests a germinal centre origin (latency 1).

BL cells are well adapted to escape CTL recognition since they have down-regulated expression of class I MHC and of the transporters associated with antigen processing (TAP-1 and/or TAP-2) genes. Furthermore, EBNA1 has a series of glycine-alanine repeat (GAr) sequences that are speculated to exert an inhibitory effect on the endogenous processing of this antigen through class I although it appears this inhibition can be over-ridden in vivo, since both CD4+ and CD8+ EBNA1-specific CTLs have been detected in healthy virus carriers.

Hodgkin's disease (HD) is a second EBV-associated B cell malignancy. In this case, the tumor cell is derived from a post-germinal center B cell and is characterized by expression of EBNA1 and LMP1 and 2 (latency II). It is interesting that the degree of association of HD with EBV is variable according to the histological sub-type ranging from 80% in the case of mixed cellularity to 20% in the case of nodular sclerosing. This difference between histological types presumably reflects the efficiency with which this form of EBV latency has adapted to each of the respective environments associated with these different histological sub-types.

Latency III malignancies have arisen as a result of intense immunosuppression which have prevented the usual efficient culling of B-cells expressing a full spectrum of latent EBV proteins rather than an exploitation of the virus to a new phenotypic niche. These malignancies arise in transplant patients (particularly EBV seronegative graft recipients) and in late stage AIDS patients and in each case the latently-infected B-cell is clearly post-germinal center in origin.

EBV has also adapted to establishing malignancies in a non-B cell environment. Examples of non-B-cell malignancies includes a range of epithelial tumors the clinically most important of which is nasopharyngeal carcinoma (NPC). This malignancy which has a latency II phenotype is most common in south-east Asia, north Africa and Greenland with a low incidence throughout the rest of the world.

The review discusses the role of the EBV-specific CTL response in controlling EBV-infected cells in each of these latency types. Particular attention will be given to newly emerging concepts rather than re-emphasizing historical aspects of EBV immunology which have been well summarized in a series of reviews in the past 10 years (Rickinson and Kieff, 1996; Khanna and Burrows, 2000)

Response during acute infection

The identification of CTL epitopes within EBV proteins was based largely on techniques that favored the definition of CD8+ CTL within EBV latent proteins. In part this has been

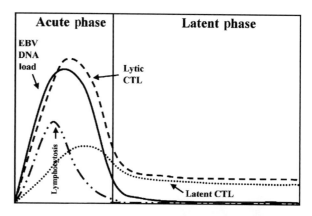

Fig. 51.1. Diagrammatic representation of the dynamics of the activation of a CTL response to EBV lytic and latent proteins in acute primary infection compared to long-term healthy immune individuals. These immune parameters are also shown in relation to EBV viral load and lymphocytosis.

due to an analysis of the CTL response emerging from *in vitro* cultures of PBMC from healthy immune individuals stimulated with autologous LCLs which express EBV latent rather than lytic proteins. In spite of these limitations and the obvious skewing of defined epitopes towards those in latent proteins, a number of lytic cycle epitopes have been defined and have provided a platform for an analysis of the CTL response seen during acute infection and redistribution of this response in healthy individuals although there are certainly indications that the response during acute compared to silent seroconversion may be fundamentally different. The lymphocytosis seen during acute infection can result in a ten fold increase in T-cell numbers and is characterized by cells with an activated phenotype (CD38, HLA DR and CD69) (Callan *et al.*, 1998; Bharadwaj *et al.*, 2001) (Fig. 51.1). These cells also express surface markers with a memory or effector phenotype (i.e., perforin, CD27, CD45RO), lack of expression of CCR7 (Sallusto *et al.*, 1999; Callan *et al.*, 2000; Hislop *et al.*, 2002) and are known to be susceptible to apoptosis after a brief period of in vitro culture (Moss *et al.*, 1985; Bishop *et al.*, 1985). It is not surprising that, during acute infection, which is characterized by high levels of EBV secretion in the oral cavity and high levels of lytic antigen expression in certain lymphoid tissue, the CTL response is directed largely towards lytic proteins. Immediate early gene products in particular have been shown to generate potent responses when visualized by HLA class I tetramer staining of PBMCs from IM patients (Callan *et al.*, 1998; Hislop *et al.*, 2002). Responses to epitopes from the early gene products, such as those derived from BMLF1 and BMRF1 are generally smaller than responses to the immediate early proteins but can still represent up to 12%

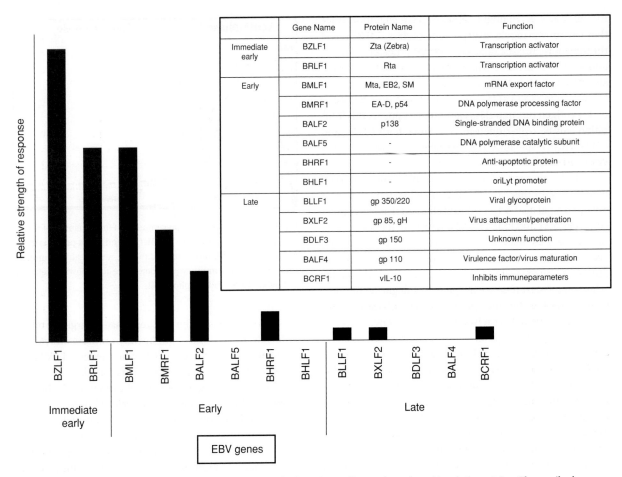

Fig. 51.2. Diagrammatic representation of the relative strength of EBV immediate early, early and late lytic proteins. The ascribed function of each of these proteins is also listed as an insert.

of the CD8+ population (Annels et al., 2000; Callan et al., 1998; Hislop et al., 2002). Current indications are that the response to late cycle lytic proteins is smaller than the response to either the early lytic cycle proteins or to the latent proteins, although it can contribute up to 3% of the CD8+ response during acute infection (Steven et al., 1996; Annels et al., 2000; Hislop et al., 2001). Overall the relative strength of the CTL response between different EBV lytic proteins (shown diagrammatically in Fig. 51.2) raises the possibility that the magnitude of the response is dictated by their order of synthesis. Although there is the general impression that the overall response in acute infection is extremely focused, it needs to be stressed that there are a relatively modest number of lytic cycle epitopes defined and the contribution of CTL reactivity during acute infection within the majority of these proteins is undefined. However, it should be pointed out that recent results have cast some doubt on the in vivo significance of functional significance of the T cell responses to lytic proteins. These reservations are based on the observation that expression of lytic proteins may result in the down-regulation of both class I MHC and TAP proteins (Ressing et al., 2005).

As mentioned previously, much of what is known about the immune parameters established during primary infection has been inferred from individuals undergoing acute IM. A study (Silins et al., 2001) of a small cohort of adolescent EBV-seronegative individuals undergoing asymptomatic primary infection has provided some insight into the immunobiology of the silent primary infection experienced by the majority of individuals. Such individuals did not develop a significant T-cell lymphocytosis in spite of the presence of EBV viral loads comparable to that seen during acute infection raising the possibility that symptomatic seroconversion is associated with the release of cytokines from the activated T-cell expansions rather than developing as a result of virus-induced pathology. These studies reveal a striking difference in the degree of TCR diversity seen in those undergoing symptomatic EBV seroconversion compared to those undergoing silent seroconversion. It appears that an oligoclonal TCR repertoire during primary infection is associated with the appearance of clinical symptoms whereas a polyclonal response predisposes towards silent seroconversion..

Response in healthy virus carriers

As the T-cell lymphocytosis resolves during convalescence, there is a reduction in the number of T-cells with activation markers and the relative contribution of the CTL response directed towards latent and lytic proteins is diminished (Fig. 51.1). Although a wide range of HLA alleles have been shown to present EBV T cell epitopes, in most cases, epitope selection is highly allele specific. There are, however, a number of epitopes that show degeneracy in HLA restriction and are immunogenic in HLA mismatched individuals, thus broadening their potential population coverage if included in a CTL-based EBV vaccine. This includes the PYLFWLAAI epitope from LMP2A that is moderately to strongly immunogenic in HLA A*2301+ individuals and weakly immunogenic in most individuals expressing the more common HLA A*2402 (Burrows et al., 2003). In an earlier example, an EBNA 6 epitope was shown to be presented on three closely related subtypes of the B27 allele (Brooks et al., 1993).

Furthermore, it is clear that the response in healthy immune individuals is not a miniturized version of that seen during acute infection but has been specifically selected to control cell-virus relationships established during long-term latent infection during which the level of EBV secretion is relatively modest and the proportion of latently-infected B cells is less than 1% of that present during acute infection. Analysis of CTL responses using tetramer staining, ELISPOT assays and cytokine production has allowed an estimate of the relative immunodominance in responses in healthy EBV immune individuals. This analysis has revealed that the intensity of the lytic antigen-specific response has waned compared to that seen during acute infection and that the response to latent antigens has increased. It is curious that this increased response is not consistent across all EBV latent proteins but is focused particularly to epitopes within EBNA3A, 3B and 3C with a subdominant response in the case of the two membrane-spanning proteins, LMP1 and 2 and a level of response towards EBNA1 that is controversial (see below). Overall, this relative level of immunodominance within the EBV latent proteins does not appear to be determined by their order of synthesis suggesting that other immunobiological factors are more important. The nuclear location of the EBNA3 proteins ensures their efficient processing and presentation through the endogenous pathway. However, in the case of LMP1 and 2 proteins, evidence suggests that their structure and location frequently favors processing through TAP-independent pathway(s). For example, LMP2 is a membrane-spanning protein with a 119 amino acid cytoplasmic N-terminus domain followed by 12 membrane-spanning segments with minimal, if any projection into the cytoplasm, and a 27 amino acid cytoplasmic C-terminus domain. Several reports (Khanna et al., 1996; Lee et al., 1996) have indicated that many, but not all of the epitopes within LMP2 are TAP-independent and that these epitopes lie within the transmembrane stretches of the protein whereas the TAP-dependent epitopes are markedly less hydrophobic (Lautscham et al., 2003). These observations raise the possibility that processing and presentation by a TAP-independent, proteosome-dependent pathway might be linked either to the transmembrane location of this protein or its extreme hydrophobicity.

Role of CD4+ and CD8+ CTL in control of EBV infection

Under the experimental conditions used for the identification of EBV CTL epitopes, class I-restricted CD8+ CTL effectors have been more commonly recognized than CD4+ effector cells. During IM, expansions of activated CD4+ T-cells are observed; however relatively little is known about their specificity or importance in controlling EBV replication either in terms of provision of direct effector function or as a source of immunological help. Direct ex vivo cytolytic assays from IM patients have demonstrated CD4 T-cell-mediated EBV-specific cytotoxicity, and in one case this response has been mapped to an epitope in BHRF1 (Schmidt and Misko, 1995). Given the importance of CD4+ T-cells in maintaining CD8+ T-cell responses, it will be of great value to further characterize these cells and their target epitopes to define their role in IM.

In healthy immune individuals, CD4+ responses to epitopes from BHRF1, EBNA1 and EBNA3C have been described and cells specific for epitopes derived from these proteins have been found to be cytotoxic effectors and can produce interferon-γ (Schmidt and Misko, 1995; Leen et al., 2001) regardless of the expression of the costimulatory molecules CD27 or CD28. Overall, the hierarchy of CD4+ CTL responses appears to be EBNA3C > EBNA1 > LMP2 >> LMP1 while in contrast the hierarchial

T-helper responses for the same proteins is EBNA1, EBNA3C >> LMP1, LMP2 (Leen et al., 2001). It should be pointed out that the CD4+ assays to detect helper function are based on the release of interferon-gamma and are detecting T-helper activity of a kind thought to reflect CD8 T-cell induction rather than T-cell help associated with a humoral response which would involve analysis for cytokines such as IL-4, IL-5 and IL-13.

The CD4+ and CD8+ CTL response to EBNA1 has received particular attention in recent years. As already mentioned, the pronounced GAr repeat sequences have been reported to inhibit processing and degradation of this protein. Interestingly, most of these CD8+ responses are directed towards epitopes that are COOH-terminal of the GAr domain. The CD8+ response is not derived from full length EBNA1 but from proteins that are prematurely truncated during translation or mal-folded after translation (referred to as defective ribosomal products or DRiPs) (Tellam et al., 2004). These DRiPs are apparently subject to proteosomal- and serine protease- mediated (Voo et al., 2004) degradation and class I presentation. In contrast, it is likely that the CD4 response is derived from full length EBNA1 released from dying cells which is subsequently exogenously processed through the class II pathway.

Role of CTL effector cells in resolution of acute IM

This background information on the CTL responses during primary EBV infection and in healthy immune individuals provides some insight into the protective role of these individual responses in resolution of disease. This issue is of central importance in designing a prophylactic vaccine to prevent the clinical symptoms of IM or a therapeutic vaccine to induce regression of the EBV-associated malignancies. The dynamics of latent compared with a lytic antigen-specific responses in acute EBV infection suggests that the latter strong response is incapable of reducing clinical symptoms and might, be driving symptomology. Generally, waning clinical symptoms are coincident with an increasing latent CTL response (Fig. 51.1). Furthermore, there are several studies that suggest that the induction of a potent CTL response to latent proteins might be the preferred strategy in relation to an IM vaccine and that a response to lytic proteins might be associated with pathology. Firstly, in a detailed study of a patient treated by adoptive immunotherapy of autologous CTL, it was noted that there was a correlation between the induction of a strong latent antigen-specific response and the cessation of disease, while a sustained lytic response was coincident with disease progression (Sherritt et al., 2003). Secondly, a study of HLA identical individuals, one of whom sustained prolonged clinical symptoms from primary EBV infection and the other who recovered after a brief period, has been useful in ascribing the link between the CTL response and the severity of acute symptomology. It was clear that rapid recovery was associated with the induction of a broad latent antigen-specific response and that acute disease corresponded with a sustained and focused lytic-antigen response. Thus, provided that we can assume that the lessons from EBV infection of B lymphocytes in vitro are relevant in vivo and that the initial event in primary infection is contact between the virus and a B lymphocyte, a strong case can be mounted in favor of directing an IM vaccine towards latent rather than lytic proteins. Such a vaccine would restrict the latently-infected B cell pool expansions some of which presumably progress towards expression of lytic proteins which appear to be responsible for the lymphocytosis associated with acute infection.

T-cell receptor usage

It is now clear that acute EBV infection is associated with dramatic perturbations within the peripheral TCR repertoire, particularly within the CD8$^+$ compartment (Callan et al., 1996). Prospective studies on IM patients that have investigated the clonal composition and dynamic regulation of the EBV-specific CTL response have provided an important opportunity to track the developmental process that T-cells undergo from primary to persistent infection (Silins et al., 1996; Callan et al., 1998; Silins et al., 1997). Importantly, these studies have demonstrated different levels of TCR diversity selection depending on the viral epitope that is the target of the response. For example, the TCR repertoire utilized in the response to two HLA-B8-restricted epitopes from the latent antigen EBNA3A (FLRGRAYGL and QAKWRLQTL) was found to be oligoclonal in one IM patient, with preservation of distinct clonotypes into the memory T cell pool (Silins et al., 1996). In contrast, T-cell populations raised against an HLA-B8-binding epitope from the lytic antigen BZLF1 (RAKFKQLL) was highly diverse in several IM patients, with no dramatic signs of repertoire focussing over time (Silins et al., 1997). Studies by Callan et al. have indicated that the larger the CD8$^+$ clonal burst size during IM, the greater the decay observed after symptoms resolve (Callan et al., 2000; Callan, 2003). Thus clonal dominance and immunodominance are less marked in healthy virus carriers than in IM patients. These findings may be related to a limit in the number of cell divisions a T-cell clone can undergo; thus the progeny of clones that have expanded massively during a primary immune response may be more prone to die as a result of senescence (Callan, 2003). Overall, the developing picture in IM is that a broad range of TCRs are selected and maintained within the composite CTL response against natural EBV infection. A relatively diverse T-cell response may be especially important in the quick recovery from IM and the establishment and maintenance of effective lifelong CTL control.

In the persistent virus carrier state, the influence of EBV infection on the peripheral TCR repertoire remains significant but is much less dramatic than during the acute infection. EBV-specific CTL frequencies are surprisingly high in healthy EBV-seropositive individuals, presumably as a consequence of antigen persistence. Since the CTL response to some EBV epitopes is oligoclonal, it was proposed that infection with viruses such as EBV and CMV contribute to the decreasing diversity in the $CD8^+$ T-cell repertoire that occurs with age. Indeed, a report from Silins et al. (1998) supports this contention by demonstrating that the frequently monoclonal response to the EBNA3A epitope FLRGRAYGL is often large enough to dramatically skew the entire TCRBV6 blood repertoire towards oligoclonality.

As in acute IM, EBV-specific $CD8^+$ T cell responses can be either highly focused or restricted in TCR usage depending on the target viral epitope, and it is not clear what controls this variability. For example, a high degree of clonotypic diversity has been shown for the potent CTL response directed towards the HLA B8- and B*4002-binding epitopes from the BZLF1 lytic antigen, with multiple TCRs sharing very few obvious structural features employed in each case (Couedel et al., 1999; Silins et al., 1997). In contrast, a recent analysis of the equally strong response to an HLA B*3501-binding BZLF1 epitope has revealed that a single CTL clonotype often dominates this response in $B3501^+$ individuals (Miles et al., 2005), with almost identical TCRs used by some unrelated individuals (unpublished observation). The basis for the selection of such immunodominant or "public" TCRs is unclear, although it does not appear to be the result of preferential expansion of high avidity TCRs. Other selection pressures may be involved such as cross-reactive stimulation with another foreign epitope or with a positively selecting self-peptide. Another recent proposal based on the crystal structure of an EBV-specific "public" TCR suggests that immunodominant T cell antigen receptors are selected as a result of certain structural properties that may confer better signaling upon ligation (Kjer-Nielsen et al., 2003).

Negative selection pressures can also theoretically limit the diversity of T-cell responses, such as might occur if a viral epitope was highly homologous with a self peptide. However, this is clearly not the explanation for the dominance of the highly conserved TCR structure that is commonly utilized in response to the B8-binding FLRGRAYGL epitope. This TCR can mediate cross-reactive lysis of EBV-positive and EBV-negative target cells expressing the HLA B*4402 alloantigen (Burrows et al., 1994). Not surprisingly, T-cells with this particular TCR are not detected within the EBV-induced memory CTL population in individuals who co-express HLA B8 and B*4402 due to their potential for self-reactivity (Burrows et al., 1995). Interestingly, however, such individuals do still make a response to the FLRGRAYGL–B8 complex through a variety of different TCRs, illustrating the flexibility and reserve strength of the TCR repertoire in the response to a target epitope.

Virus-driven immune modulation

EBV, like many other herpes viruses, has successfully adapted as a persistent infection by developing various strategies to avoid the potentially hostile effects of host immunity. One such adaptive strategy employed by many oncogenic viruses (such as EBV) involves restricted expression of viral genes, thereby minimizing the potential recognition of target antigens (as seen in many EBV-associated malignancies). On the other hand, viruses (including EBV) are also known to interfere more directly with the host immune response by encoding viral genes, that are homologous to cellular effector molecules. Candidate immune evasion strategies against CTL-mediated control have been recognized which act at the level of cytokine regulation and antigen processing and presentation (Cohen, 1999; Khanna et al., 1995; Spriggs et al., 1996). In the last few years, a number of EBV encoded immunomodulators have been identified within the lytic and latent phases of viral infection which may interfere with virus-specific T-cell responses and enhance EBV-infected B-cell proliferation, thus facilitating pathogen dissemination and survival early in the infectious process.

Modulation of the cytokine network

Previous studies have shown that cytokines contribute directly towards the clearance of viral infections. To counter this potential threat, many viruses have evolved to express novel homologues of these cytokines that can act as antagonists. These homologues can be either positive or negative regulators of T cell-mediated immune responses. The EBV encoded, BCRF1 protein expressed during lytic infection exhibits 78% identity to the deduced amino acid sequence of human IL-10 and shares a similar function to its human homologue (Moore et al., 1990). Recombinant BCRF1, like human IL-10 negatively regulates IL-12 which promotes IFN-γ production by T-cells. In addition, BCRF1 also abrogates the inhibitory capacity of T-cells which blocks the outgrowth of EBV-infected B-cells. This effect may be mediated through suppression of T-cell activation-induced IL-2 and IFN-γ production (Bejarano and Massuci, 1998). Apart from its effect on IL-2 and IFN-γ production, it has also been proposed that BCRF1 acts directly on T cells to inhibit co-stimulatory signals mediated via B7 receptors such as CD28 or CTLA-4 (Muller et al., 1998). Since BCRF1 is mainly expressed during the replicative phase of the virus cycle, the role of IL-10 in the modulation of latent infection has remained largely unresolved until recently. Studies carried out by Marshall and colleagues showed that LMP1 preferentially activates regulatory T-cells that secrete IL-10 (Marshall et al., 2003). These IL-10 responses inhibit T cell proliferation and IFN-γ secretion by EBV-specific CD8+ T cells.

Another example of modulation of the cytokine network by EBV comes from studies by Strockbine and colleagues (Strockbine et al., 1998) who have identified a novel EBV-encoded modulator of colony stimulating factor (CSF1). Their studies showed that BARF1 protein, when added into the culture medium, neutralizes the proliferative effects of human CSF-1 which is a pleiotropic cytokine best known for its differentiating effects on macrophages. Thus BARF1 may function to modulate the host immune response to EBV infection by blocking CSF-1 function through inhibition of interferon a (IFN-a) secretion from mononuclear cells (Cohen and Lekstrom, 1999) which is the first cytokine produced in response to virus infection. Recent studies have shown that IFN-a activates the p53 gene in virus-infected cells leading to apoptotic death of infected cells (Takaoka et al., 2003). Based on these studies, we hypothesize that BARF1-mediated blockade of IFN-a would protect EBV-infected cells from death during the early stages of infection thus promoting latent infection. In addition to its potential role in promoting latent infection, the role of BARF1 in modulating innate and adaptive immunity should not be ignored since IFN-a activates NK cells and is necessary for both NK cell blastogenesis and cytotoxicity during herpes virus infections (Brion et al., 1995). Furthermore, preliminary studies carried out in our laboratory have shown that recombinant BARF1 protein can inhibit activation and expansion of memory T-cells from healthy virus carriers (S. Pai and R. Khanna, unpublished observations).

Regulation of antigen processing and presentation

T-cell-mediated immune control of EBV infection can act at either latent or lytic phases. The pattern of viral gene expression at each phase determines the potential target antigens. When considering immune evasion strategies for latent infection, EBNA1 remains one of most comprehensively studied proteins. Levitskaya and colleagues have shown that EBNA1 resists CTL mediated immune recognition through a unique inhibitory mechanism which blocks endogenous processing of CTL epitopes within this antigen (Levitskaya et al., 1995, 1997). It was proposed that this GAr sequence within EBNA1 may influence the folding pattern of this protein and affect its capacity to associate with various components of the ubiquitin/proteasome pathway, including ubiquitin conjugation enzymes and/or regulatory subunits of the proteasome. More recent studies have shown that this inhibitory effect may be overridden in certain types of epithelial cells (Jones et al., 2003). When EBNA1 is expressed in immortalized epithelial cells (SSC12F, SVK), it not only inhibits cell growth but is also endogenously processed through the class I pathway for immune recognition by CD8+ T-cells. On the other hand, neither of these phenomena is observed when EBNA1 is expressed in fully transformed epithelial cells (Hela, Ad/AH).

LMP1 is another latent protein known to modulate the function of immune regulatory proteins in B-cells. This protein has recently been recognized as a functional homologue of human CD40 (Uchida et al., 1999). First evidence for a potential role of EBV latent antigens in the regulation of MHC class I expression came from the observation that LMP1 was capable of reversing down-regulated expression of TAP and HLA class I in BL cells which are characterized by defective antigen processing (Khanna et al., 1995). Recent studies from our laboratory have shown that the c-terminal domain of LMP1 plays an important role in translocating relB from the cytoplasm to the nucleus with a consequent effect on the upregulation of antigen processing genes (Pai and Khanna, 2002). This observation raises the intriguing question of why an EBV protein has evolved with the capacity to up-regulate antigen processing function in the host cells, thereby potentially increasing the chances of its elimination by virus-specific CTLs. A possible explanation is that the virus uses the LMP1 protein to hyper-regulate the antigen processing function of B-cells, and that this not only results in efficient presentation of viral peptides, but also increases the levels of self peptides presented by these cells. Increasing self peptide presentation has two potential consequences (i) these self peptides may compete with viral peptides thus reducing the levels of EBV peptides presented to CTLs thereby allowing immune escape or alternatively (ii) increased self peptide presentation may also contribute towards the development of autoimmune reactivity which is often seen as one of the symptoms in individuals with acute EBV infection. Another plausible hypothesis to explain why EBV modulates antigen processing gene expression via LMP1 involves the long-term host-virus relationship whereby some advantage is gained from deliberately enhancing the chance of EBV-infected B-cells being lyzed by immune surveillance thus protecting the host from an overwhelming infection and maintaining a stable host-virus relationship.

Although much of the emphasis on the immune control of EBV has focused on CD8+ T-cells, recent studies have demonstrated that CD4+ T-cells also play an important role in both primary and latent EBV infection (Precopio et al., 2003). It is not surprising that EBV has evolved immune evasive strategies to counter the potential threat from this effector arm of the immune system. Thus Spriggs and colleagues (Li et al., 1997) have proposed a novel mechanism of blocking peptide presentation through the MHC class II pathway. They showed that, during the late lytic cycle, EBV encodes a type II membrane glycoprotein that specifically binds to the ß chains of MHC class II particularly the HLA DR heterodimer both intracellularly as well as on the cell surface resulting in the retention of MHC class II molecules in the ER thus blocking presentation of class II-restricted T-cell epitopes. Interestingly, subsequent studies have shown that BZLF2 specific antibodies that block the interaction of this protein with MHC class II can also prevent the infection of MHC class II positive B lymphocytes (reviewed in (Spear and Longnecker, 2003). It is possible therefore that BZLF2 plays a dual role, modulating class II-restricted antigen presentation as well facilitating infection of class II positive cells.

T-cell control of EBV-associated malignancies

The EBV-associated malignancies have evolved unique strategies to evade immune recognition allowing them to expand in the face of an existing EBV-specific CTL response (Khanna, 1998; Khanna and Burrows, 2000). Thus, in the case of endemic BL, viral gene expression is restricted to EBNA1 with a phenotype resembling that of resting cells. This combination of properties makes these cells highly resistant to T-cell-mediated immune recognition rendering them incapable of stimulating an EBV or allospecific T-cell response (Rooney et al., 1995). This non-immunogenic phenotype of BL cells is linked to down-regulated expression of MHC class I and TAP-1 and/or TAP-2 genes, whereas expression of the proteasome genes, LMP2 and LMP7 is normal in most cases (Khanna et al., 1994, 1995). It is important to mention here that loss of antigen processing function is not only seen in EBV-positive BL cell lines but also in EBV-negative BL cells. Thus it is likely that the CTL resistant phenotype of BL is a reflection of the nature of the cell type from which the malignant cells are derived. Indeed, Gregory and colleagues have identified normal B-cells which display a phenotype identical to BL cells (Gregory et al., 1987).

While considerable significance has been placed on the apparent loss of MHC class I-molecules in the immune escape of tumor cells, evidence from other human tumors has accumulated that CD4+ T-cells can also play a critical role in immune surveillance (Topalian et al., 1994). Surprisingly, analysis of MHC class II-restricted antigen processing function in TAP-deficient BL cells has revealed that EBV-specific CD4+ CTLs can efficiently recognize these tumor cells (Khanna et al., 1997). Furthermore, in contrast to the consistently low levels of surface MHC class I expression on BL cells, MHC class II expression is normal and quite comparable to that on EBV-transformed normal B-cells. Consistent with these observations, BL cells also show normal levels of the HLA DMB gene product which is an essential component for class II processing. The importance of these studies has been further strengthened by the observation that CD4+ EBNA1-specific CTLs from healthy virus carriers can efficiently recognize not only virus-infected normal B-cells but also BL cells (Munz et al., 2000; Paludan et al., 2002).

In spite of distinct pathologies, NPC and HD share a number of phenotypic features which provide a unique opportunity to study the immune responses to viral antigens expressed in these malignancies. Molecular analysis of fresh biopsies and laboratory-established tumor lines indicate that malignant cells in both NPC and HD express normal levels of HLA class I and TAP1/2 (Khanna et al., 1998; Lee et al., 1998) and express only a limited number of latent proteins (LMP1, LMP2 and EBNA1). A number of studies have shown that, as in the case of healthy virus carriers, the EBV-specific CTL repertoire in HD and NPC patients is strongly focused through the EBNA3A, EBNA3B and EBNA3C proteins and thus have a limited capacity to control these tumors in vivo. Lee and colleagues conducted an exhaustive analysis of EBV-specific T-cell responses in a large panel of HD patients which showed no obvious suppression of the EBV-specific T-cell responses in HD patients when compared to the healthy virus carriers (Lee et al., 1998). These observations were in direct contrast to earlier studies which showed that HD patients often possess a generalized defect in cell-mediated immunity, including impaired responses to mitogens and a decreased capacity of T-cells to respond in a mixed lymphocyte response (Slivnick et al., 1990). Although the precise reason for this loss of T-cell immunity is not known, a recent study by

Marshall and colleagues have shown that the CD4+ T-cell response to the LMP1 protein is dominated by regulatory T-cells which express high levels of IL-10. These responses inhibited T-cell proliferation and INF-γ production by both mitogen and EBV antigens (Marshall et al., 2003). Furthermore, Dukers and colleagues have also shown that LMP1 includes two novel retrovirus homologous sequences within the transmembrane domain which showed strong inhibition of T-cell proliferation and NK cell cytotoxicity (Dukers et al., 2000). These authors proposed that HD or NPC tumor cells may actively secrete LMP1 and thus mediate immunosuppressive effects on tumor infiltrating lymphocytes.

Future prospects for an EBV vaccine

Our understanding of the immune response to EBV appears to be at a point where serious consideration can now be given towards a vaccine to at least some of the EBV-associated diseases. It appears that the best prospects relate to allowing the development of vaccine to prevent the clinical symptoms of IM. As already discussed, a strong argument can be drawn that this vaccine should be directed towards activating a response to epitopes within EBNA3A, 3B and 3C. The hope is that the same vaccine might be effective against the emergence of PTLD in transplant patients. The method of delivering this vaccine is open to question, but given the fact that the recipients of an IM vaccine will be largely healthy adolescents, it is unlikely that a live vaccine delivery system will be used.

As already discussed, the latent antigens expressed in the latency II diseases (NPC and HD) are poorly immunogenic. This consideration, when seen in concert with the fact that these patients are suffering a life-threatening disease means that live vaccine delivery vectors might be acceptable.

There appears to be little prospect for the development of an effective vaccine against latency 1 diseases. This conclusion is based on the relative low frequency of these malignancies and their non-immunogenic phenotype.

REFERENCES

Annels, N. E., Callan, M. F., Tan, L., and Rickinson, A. B. (2000). Changing patterns of dominant TCR usage with maturation of an EBV-specific cytotoxic T cell response. *J. Immunol.*, **165**, 4831–4841.

Bejarano, M. T. and Massuci, M. G. (1998). Interleukin-10 abrogates the inhibition of Epstein–Barr virus-induced B-cell transformation by memory T-cell responses. *Blood*, **92**, 4256–4262.

Bharadwaj, M., Parsons, P. G., and Moss, D. J. (2001). Cost-efficient quantification of enzyme-linked immunospot. *Biotechniques*, **30**, 36–38.

Bishop, C. J., Moss, D. J., Ryan, J. M., and Burrows, S. R. (1985). T lymphocytes in infectious mononucleosis. II. Response in vitro to interleukin-2 and establishment of T-cell lines. *Clin. Exp. Immunol.*, **60**, 70–77.

Brion, A., Cahn, J. Y., Mougin, C. et al. (1995). Herpes virus-related lymphoproliferative disorders following allogeneic bone marrow transplantation: clinical and biological characteristics of six cases. *Nouv. Rev. Fr. Hematol.*, **37**, 289–296.

Brooks, J. M., Murray, R. J., Thomas, W. A., Kurilla, M. G., and Rickinson, A. B. (1993). Different HLA-B27 subtypes present the same immunodominant Epstein–Barr virus peptide. *J. Exp. Med.*, **178**, 879–887.

Burrows, S. R., Khanna, R., Burrows, J. M., and Moss, D. J. (1994). An alloresponse in humans is dominated by cytotoxic T lymphocytes (CTL) cross-reactive with a single Epstein–Barr virus CTL epitope: implications for graft-versus-host disease. *J. Exp. Med.*, **179**, 1155–1161.

Burrows, S. R., Silins, S. L., Moss, D. J., Khanna, R., Misko, I. S., and Argaet, V. P. (1995). T cell receptor repertoire for a viral epitope in humans is diversified by tolerance to a background major histocompatibility complex antigen. *J. Exp. Med.*, **182**, 1703–1715.

Burrows, S. R., Elkington, R. A., Miles, J. J. et al. (2003). Promiscuous CTL recognition of viral epitopes on multiple human leukocyte antigens: biological validation of the proposed HLA A24 supertype. *J. Immunol.*, **171**, 1407–1412.

Callan, M. F. (2003). The evolution of antigen-specific CD8+ T cell responses after natural primary infection of humans with Epstein–Barr virus. *Viral Immunol.*, **16**, 3–16.

Callan, M. F., Steven, N., Krausa, P. et al. (1996). Large clonal expansions of CD8+ T cells in acute infectious mononucleosis. *Nat. Med.*, **2**, 906–911.

Callan, M. F., Tan, L., Annels, N. et al. (1998). Direct visualization of antigen-specific CD8+ T cells during the primary immune response to Epstein–Barr virus In vivo. *J. Exp. Med.* **187**, 1395–1402.

Callan, M. F., Fazou, C., Yang, H. et al. (2000). CD8(+) T-cell selection, function, and death in the primary immuneresponse in vivo. *J. Clin. Invest.*, **106**, 1251–1261.

Cohen, J. I. (1999) The biology of Epstein–Barr virus: lessons learned from the virus and the host. *Curr. Opin. Immunol.*, **11**, 365–370.

Cohen, J. I. and Lekstrom, K. (1999). Epstein–Barr virus BARF1 protein is dispensable for B-cell transformation and inhibits alpha interferon secretion from mononuclear cells. *J. Virol.*, **73**, 7627–7632.

Couedel, C., Bodinier, M., Peyrat, M. A., Bonneville, M., Davodeau, F., and Lang, F. (1999). Selection and long-term persistence of reactive CTL clones during an EBV chronic response are determined by avidity, CD8 variable contribution compensating for differences in TCR affinities. *J. Immunol.*, **162**, 6351–6358.

Dukers, D. F., Meij, P., and Vervoort, M. B. (2000). Direct immunosuppressive effects of EBV-encoded latent membrane protein 1. *J. Immunol.*, **165**, 663–670.

Gregory, C. D., Kirchgens, C., Edwards, C. F. *et al.* (1987). Epstein–Barr virus-transformed human precursor B cell lines: altered growth phenotype of lines with germ-line or rearranged but nonexpressed heavy chain genes. *Eur. J. Immunol.*, **17**, 1199–1207.

Hislop, A. D., Gudgeon, N. H., Callan, M. F. *et al.* (2001). EBV-specific CD8+ T cell memory: relationships between epitope specificity, cell phenotype, and immediate effector function. *J. Immunol.*, **167**, 2019–2029.

Hislop, A. D., Annels, N. E., Gudgeon, N. H., Leese, A. M., and Rickinson, A. B. (2002). Epitope-specific evolution of human CD8(+) T cell responses from primary to persistent phases of Epstein–Barr virus infection. *J. Exp. Med.*, **195**, 893–905.

Jones, R. J., Smith, L. J., Dawson, C. W., Haigh, T., Blake, N. W., and Young, L. S. (2003). Epstein–Barr virus nuclear antigen 1 (EBNA1) induced cytotoxicity in epithelial cells is associated with EBNA1 degradation and processing. *Virology*, **313**, 663–676.

Khanna, R. (1998). Tumour surveillance: missing peptides and MHC molecules. *Immunol. Cell Biol.*, **76**, 20–26.

Khanna, R. and Burrows, S. R. (2000). Role of cytotoxic t lymphocytes in epstein–barr virus-associated diseases. *Annu. Rev. Microbiol.*, **54**, 19–48.

Khanna, R., Burrows, S. R., Argaet, V., and Moss, D. J. (1994). Endoplasmic reticulum signal sequence facilitated transport of peptide epitopes restores immunogenicity of an antigen processing defective tumour cell line. *Int. Immunol.*, **6**, 639–645.

Khanna, R., Rowe, M., Jacob, C. A. *et al.* (1995). Restoration of endogenous antigen processing in Burkitt's lymphoma cells by Epstein–Barr virus latent membrane protein-1: coordinate up-regulation of peptide transporters and HLA-class I antigen expression. *Eur. J. Immunol.*, **25**, 1374–1384.

Khanna, R., Burrows, S. R., Moss, D. J., and Silins, S. L. (1996). Peptide transporter (TAP1 and TAP-2)-independent endogenous processing of Epstein–Barr virus (EBV) latent membrane protein 2A: implications for cytotoxic T-lymphocyte control of EBV-associated malignancies. *J. Virol.*, **70**, 5357–5362.

Khanna, R., Burrows, S. R., Thomson, S. A. *et al.* (1997). Class I processing-defective Burkitt's lymphoma cells are recognized efficiently by CD4+ EBV-specific CTLs. *J. Immunol.*, **158**, 3619–3625.

Khanna, R., Busson, P., Burrows, S.R. *et al.* (1998). Molecular characterization of antigen-processing function in nasopharyngeal carcinoma (NPC): evidence for efficient presentation of Epstein–Barr virus cytotoxic T-cell epitopes by NPC cells. *Cancer Res.*, **58**, 310–314.

Kjer-Nielsen, L., Clements, C. S., Purcell, A. W. *et al.* (2003). A structural basis for the selection of dominant alphabeta T cell receptors in antiviral immunity. *Immunity*, **18**, 53–64.

Lautscham, G., Haigh, T., Mayrhofer, S. *et al.* (2003). Identification of a TAP-independent, immunoproteasome-dependent CD8+ T-cell epitope in Epstein–Barr virus latent membrane protein 2. *J. Virol.*, **77**, 2757–2761.

Lee, S. P., Thomas, W. A., Blake, N. W., and Rickinson, A. B. (1996). Transporter (TAP)-independent processing of a multiple membrane-spanning protein, the Epstein–Barr virus latent membrane protein 2. *Eur. J. Immunol.*, **26**, 1875–1883.

Lee, S. P., Constandinou, C. M., Thomas, W. A. *et al.* (1998). Antigen presenting phenotype of hodgkin reed-sternberg cells: analysis of the HLA class I processing pathway and the effects of interleukin-10 on Epstein–Barr virus-specific cytotoxic T-cell recognition [In Process Citation]. *Blood*, **92**, 1020–1030.

Leen, A., Meij, P., Redchenko, I. *et al.* (2001). Differential immunogenicity of Epstein–Barr virus latent-cycle proteins for human CD4(+) T-helper 1 responses. *J. Virol.*, **75**, 8649–8659.

Levitskaya, J., Coram, M., Levitsky, V. *et al.* (1995). Inhibition of antigen processing by the internal repeat region of the Epstein–Barr virus nuclear antigen-1. *Nature*, **375**, 685–688.

Levitskaya, J., Sharipo, A., Leonchiks, A., Ciechanover, A., and Masucci, M. G. (1997). Inhibition of ubiquitin/proteasome-dependent protein degradation by the Gly-Ala repeat domain of the Epstein–Barr virus nuclear antigen 1. *Proc. Natl Acad. Sci. USA*, **94**, 12616–12621.

Li, Q., Spriggs, M. K., Kovats, S. *et al.* (1997). Epstein–Barr virus uses HLA class II as a cofactor for infection of B lymphocytes. *J. Virol.*, **71**, 4657–4662.

Marshall, N. A., Vickers, M. A., and Barker, R. N. (2003). Regulatory T cells secreting IL10 dominate the immune response to EBV latent membrane protein 1. *J. Immunol.*, **170**, 6183–6189.

Miles, J. J., Elhassen, D., Borg, N. A., *et al.* (2005). CTL recognition of a bulged viral peptide involves biased TCR selection. *J. Immunol.*, **175**, 3826–3834.

Moore, K. W., Vieira, P., Fiorentino, D. F., Trounstine, M. L., Khan, T. A., and Mosmann, T. R. (1990). Homology of cytokine synthesis inhibitory factor (IL-10) to the Epstein–Barr virus gene BCRF1. *Science*, **248**, 1230–1234.

Moss, D. J., Burrows, S. R., Castelino, D. J., Kane, R. G., Pope, J. H., and Rickinson, A. B. (1983). A comparison of Epstein–Barr virus-specific T-cell immunity in malaria-endemic and -nonendemic regions of Papua New Guinea. *Int. J. Cancer*, **31**, 727–732.

Moss, D. J., Bishop, C. J., Burrows, S. R., and Ryan, J. M. (1985). T lymphocytes in infectious mononucleosis. I. T-cell death in vitro. *Clin. Exp. Immunol.*, **60**, 61–69.

Muller, A., Schmitt, L., Raftery, M., and Schönrich, G. (1998). Paralysis of B7 co-stimulation through the effect of viral IL-10 on T cells as a mechanism of local tolerance induction. *Eur. J. Immunol.*, **28**, 3488–3498.

Munz, C., Bickham, K. L., and Subklewe, M. (2000). Human CD4(+) T lymphocytes consistently respond to the latent Epstein–Barr virus nuclear antigen EBNA1. *J. Exp. Med.*, **191**, 1649–1660.

Pai, S. and Khanna, R. (2002). Role of LMP1 in immune control of EBV infection. *Semin. Cancer Biol.*, **11**, 455–460.

Paludan, C., Bickham, K., Nikiforow, S. *et al.* (2002). Epstein–Barr nuclear antigen 1-specific CD4(+) Th1 cells kill Burkitt's lymphoma cells. *J. Immunol.*, **169**, 1593–1603.

Precopio, M. L., Sullivan, J. L., Willard, C., Somasundaran, M., and Luzuriaga, K. (2003). Differential kinetics and specificity of EBV-specific CD4+ and CD8+ T cells during primary infection. *J. Immunol.*, **170**, 2590–2598.

Reedman, B. M., Hilgers, J., Hilgers, F., and Klein, G. (1975). Immunofluorescence and anti-complement immunofluorescence absorption tests for quantitation of Epstein–Barr virus-associated antigens. *Int. J. Cancer*, **15**, 566–571.

Ressing, M. E., Keating, S. E., van Leeuwen, D. *et al.* (2005). Impaired transporter associated with antigen processing-dependent protein transport during productive EBV infection. *J. Immunol.*, **174**, 6829–6838.

Rickinson, A. B. and Kieff, E. (1996). Epstein–Barr virus. In *Fields Virology*. B. N. Fields, D. M. Knipe, and P. M. Howley, eds., pp. 2397–2446. Philadelphia: Lippincott-Raven Publishers.

Rooney, C. M., Smith, C. A., Ng, C. *et al.* (1995). Use of gene-modified virus-specific T lymphocytes to control Epstein-Barr-virus-related lymphoproliferation. *Lancet*, **345**, 9–13.

Sallusto, F., Lenig, D., Forster, R., Lipp, M., and Lanzavecchia, A. (1999). Two subsets of memory T lymphocytes with distinct homing potentials and effector functions. *Nature*, **401**, 708–712.

Schmidt, C. W. and Misko, I. S. (1995). The ecology and pathology of Epstein–Barr virus. *Immunol. Cell Biol.*, **73**, 489–504.

Sherritt, M. A., Bharadwaj, M., Burrows, J. M. *et al.* (2003). Reconstitution of the latent T-lymphocyte response to Epstein–Barr virus is coincident with long-term recovery from posttransplant lymphoma after adoptive immunotherapy. *Transplantation*, **75**, 1556–1560.

Silins, S. L., Cross, S. M., Elliott, S. L. *et al.* (1996). Development of Epstein–Barr virus-specific memory T cell receptor clonotypes in acute infectious mononucleosis. *J. Exp. Med.*, **184**, 1815–1824.

Silins, S. L., Cross, S. M., Elliott, S. L. *et al.* (1997). Selection of a diverse TCR repertoire in response to an Epstein- Barr virus-encoded transactivator protein BZLF1 by CD8+ cytotoxic T lymphocytes during primary and persistent infection. *Int. Immunol.*, **9**, 1745–1755.

Silins, S. L., Cross, S. M., Krauer, K. G., Moss, D. J., Schmidt, C. W., and Misko, I. S. (1998). A functional link for major TCR expansions in healthy adults caused by persistent Epstein–Barr virus infection. *J. Clin. Invest.*, **102**, 1551–1558.

Silins, S. L., Sherritt, M. A., Silleri, J. M. *et al.* (2001). Asymptomatic primary Epstein–Barr virus infection occurs in the absence of blood T-cell repertoire perturbations despite high levels of systemic viral load. *Blood*, **98**, 3739–3744.

Slivnick, D. J., Ellis, T. M., Nawrocki, J. F., and Fisher, R. I. (1990). The impact of Hodgkin's disease on the immune system. *Semin. Oncol*, **17**, 673–682.

Spear, P. G. and Longnecker, R. (2003). Herpesvirus entry: an update. *J. Virol.*, **77**, 10179–10185.

Spriggs, M. K., Armitage, R. J., Comeau, M. R. *et al.* (1996). The extracellular domain of the Epstein–Barr virus BZLF2 protein binds the HLA-DR beta chain and inhibits antigen presentation. *J. Virol.*, **70**, 5557–5563.

Steven, N. M., Leese, A. M., Annels, N. E., Lee, S. P., and Rickinson, A. B. (1996). Epitope focusing in the primary cytotoxic T cell response to Epstein–Barr virus and its relationship to T cell memory. *J. Exp. Med.* **184**, 1801–1813.

Strockbine, L. D., Cohen, J. I., Farrah, T. *et al.* (1998). The Epstein–Barr virus BARF1 gene encodes a novel, soluble colony-stimulating factor-1 receptor. *J. Virol.*, **72**, 4015–4021.

Takaoka, A., Hayakawa, S., Yanai, H. *et al.* (2003). Integration of interferon-alpha/beta signalling to p53 responses in tumour suppression and antiviral defence. *Nature*, **424**, 516–523.

Tellam, J., Connolloy, G., Green, K. J. *et al.* (2004). Endogenous presentation of CD8+ T cell epitopes from Epstein-Barr virus encoded nuclear antigen 1: functional evidence for DriPs as a source of endogenously processed epitopes. *J. Exp. Med.*, **199**, 1421–1431.

Topalian, S. L., Rivoltini, L., Mancini, M., Ng, J., Hartzman, R. J., and Rosenberg, S. A. (1994). Melanoma-specific CD4+ T lymphocytes recognize human melanoma antigens processed and presented by Epstein–Barr virus- transformed B cells. *Int. J. Cancer*, **58**, 69–79.

Uchida, J., Yasui, T., Takaoka-Shichijo, Y. *et al.* (1999). Mimicry of CD40 signals by Epstein–Barr virus LMP1 in B lymphocyte responses. *Science*, **286**, 300–303.

Voo, K. S., Fu, T. Wang, H. Y. *et al.* (2004). Evidence for the presentation of major histocompatibility complex class I restricted Epstein–Barr virus nuclear antigen 1 peptides to CD8+ T lymphocytes. *J. Exp. Med.*, **199**, 459–470.

Yin, Y., Manoury, B., and Fahraeus, R. (2003). Self-inhibition of synthesis and antigen presentation by Epstein–Barr virus-encoded EBNA1. *Science*, **301**, 1371–1374.

52

Immunobiology and host response to KSHV infection

Dimitrios Lagos and Chris Boshoff

Cancer Research UK Viral Oncology Group, Wolfson Institute for Biomedical Research, University College London, London, UK

Introduction

The interplay between malignancy, infection and immunity is best illustrated by the neoplasms related to KSHV (Boshoff and Weiss, 2002): Kaposi sarcoma (KS) is approximately 100 times more common during immunosuppression and can be resolved when iatrogenic immunosuppression is stopped (Euvrard et al., 2003) and during highly active antiretroviral treatment (HAART) of HIV-1 infected individuals (Boshoff and Weiss, 2002). Primary effusion lymphoma (PEL) and plasmablastic multicentric Castleman's disease (MCD) also occur predominantly during immunosuppression. Like other gammaherpesviruses, KSHV persists as a latent episome in B-lymphocytes (Ambroziak et al., 1995; Cesarman et al., 1995; Renne et al., 1996), without provoking host responses that would eliminate infected cells. KSHV acquired a fascinating repertoire of decoys to trick the host immune response enabling establishment of lifelong infection in humans with very few clinical manifestations. When the balance between viral infection and host immunity is disturbed, some of the molecular pathways employed by KSHV to evade host immune responses are directly involved in driving oncogenesis (Moore and Chang, 2003). KSHV is an excellent model to study the coevolution of pathogen attack and mechanisms of host counter attack.

KS is most aggressive in the immunosuppressed and resolves with partial restoration of the immune system (Gill et al., 2002). Since the introduction of HAART, there has also been a dramatic fall in the incidence of KS (Jacobson et al., 1999). Although non-immune mechanisms may contribute to this drop in KS cases and the resolution of established lesions, it is reasonable to propose that immune reconstitution is a major factor in the control of this neoplasm (Box 52.1).

We are only starting to understand how KSHV avoids these host responses, which viral epitopes are targets for adaptive immune responses, and how anti-KSHV immunity is altered during immunosuppression (Table 52.1).

Primary infection

It is thought that KSHV is mainly transmitted by oral exposure to infectious saliva (Pauk et al., 2000), suggesting that mucosal cells are the first port of call. These could be mucosal-associated dendritic cells, macrophages, lymphocytes and/or epithelial cells. KSHV can infect and establish latency in CD34+ hematopoietic progenitors, macrophages and B-lymphocytes in experimental models (Dittmer et al., 1999; Bechtel et al., 2003; Luppi et al., 2005; Wu et al., 2006), but the exact cell type that is predominantly infected at viral exposure is still unknown. KSHV is also present in cells of the endothelial lineage (EC), specifically cells differentiating towards lymphatic endothelium (Dupin et al., 1999; Wang et al., 2004). This microvascular environment is specifically adapted to rapidly eliminate invading pathogens and KSHV must therefore have evolved specific mechanisms to replicate successfully in this niche.

Case reports and epidemiological surveys provide some clues to the consequences of an inadequate immune response to primary KSHV infection: Although primary KSHV infection among immunocompetent individuals can be symptomatic (Andreoni et al., 2002), the development of KSHV-related malignancies is generally associated with immunosuppression. Lymphadenopathy associated with microscopic KS lesions (that is expansion of KSHV-infected EC), occurs in HIV-1 infected individuals, who are thought to be exposed to KSHV for the first time (Oksenhendler et al., 1998). This infers that the lympadenopathic KS seen in African children may also represent primary infection with KSHV, similar to childhood Hodgkin's disease

Box 52.1. Kaposi's sarcoma, immunity and anti-retroviral treatment

For most individuals, living with KSHV is uneventful. However, during immunosuppression the consequences can be severe.

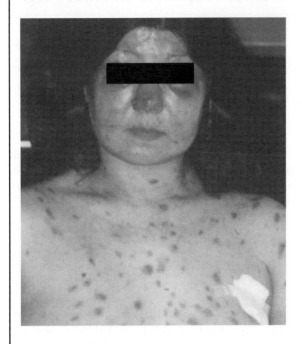

In 1981, Kaposi's sarcoma (KS) became the sentinel of the AIDS epidemic. During the 1980s, prior to the use of any antiretroviral treatment, KS often presented as widespread lesions affecting skin, mucosal surfaces and sometimes internal organs. Periorbital edema was also frequently seen with advanced HIV-1 infection. (Image kindly provided by A. E. Friedman Kien.)

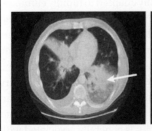 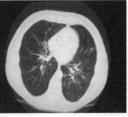

How does HAART prevent KS?

Since the introduction of HAART, the incidence of KS has decreased dramatically, and HAART also leads to rapid KS resolution. The computed tomographic lung scans (Image kindly provided by N. Dupin) show a patient with a large pulmonary KS lesion (left panel) and the improvement in this patient during HAART (right panel). There are several mechanisms by which HAART could lead to KS resolution:

HAART leads to immune reconstitution against KSHV (Wilkinson *et al.*, 2002; Bourboulia *et al.*, 2004). This hypothesis could also explain the resolution of Kaposi's sarcoma in HIV-negative post-organ transplant individuals when immunosuppressive drugs are stopped. Both humoral and cellular immunity might contribute to this.

HIV-1 circulating Tat levels and HIV-1 induced immune activation (including levels of circulating cytokines) are reduced on HAART leading to KS regression (Ensoli *et al.*, 1990; Gallo, 1998). This could explain the often rapid resolution of KS when HAART is initiated, but not the resolution of KS in HIV negative individuals when immunosuppression is stopped (e.g., after an organ transplant). The observation that proangiogenic growth factor (e.g. vascular endothelial growth factor, VEGF) levels decrease during HAART and correlate with KS resolution, supports this theory.

Protease inhibitors (PIs) have a direct anti-spindle cell and/or anti-angiogenic effect (Sgadari *et al.*, 2002) PIs block KS spindle cell growth and angiogenesis in experimental models. Retrospective studies showing that HAART leads to a decreased incidence of Kaposi's sarcoma -and to the resolution of established lesions- were all conducted at a time when PIs were routinely used as part of HAART. However, because of side-effects their use in HAART is now more restricted. Non-PI containing combination anti-retroviral therapy also leads to KS resolution and the incidence of KS remains low in the UK and USA (Gill *et al.*, 2002). However, reports that KS can relapse when a PI-containing regimen is substituted for a non-PI containing regimen (Bani-Sadr *et al.*, 2003) do suggest that PI's directly, or indirectly, play a role in the control of KSHV-infected EC proliferation.

thought to be due to inadequate control of primary EBV infection (Macsween and Crawford, 2003). Furthermore, KS develops more commonly in HIV-1 infected individuals who acquired KSHV after primary HIV-1 infection (Goudsmit *et al.*, 2000), suggesting that an inadequate host response during primary KSHV infection confers the propensity of infected EC to expand, and that EC are one of the first KSHV targets during primary infection. Circulating spindle cells, expressing endothelial and macrophage markers, have been identified from healthy

Table 52.1. Overview of host responses to KSHV infection and future questions

	Cell type	Major findings[a]	Major questions
INNATE IMMUNITY	Dendritic cells	• KSHV infects DC *in vitro* and impairs their antigen presenting properties (Reppocciolo et al., 2006) • Decreased number of pDC in AIDS-KS (Stebbing et al., 2003b) and mDC and pDC in classic KS (Della Bella et al., 2006)	Determine the mechanisms employed by KSHV to regulate DC maturation and function
	Natural Killer cells	• Restoration of NK function correlates with KS resolution on HAART (Sirianni et al., 2002) • KSHV protects KSHV-infected cells from NK cell attack (reviewed in Orange et al., 2002)	Investigate the role of KSHV driven NK cells in control of infection and KS development
	Complement	• Essential for MHV68 control (Kapadia et al. 2002) • KSHV ORF4 is a regulator of complement activation (Spiller et al. 2003)	Determine the role of complement in KSHV infection
ADAPTIVE IMMUNITY	Cytotoxic T cells	• KSHV sepcific CTL epitopes identified[b] • CTL restoration on HAART correlates with viral clearance (Bourboulia et al. 2004)	Determine KSHV specific CTL phenotype and identify further CTL epitopes
	T helper cells	• CD4+ T cells proliferate in response to KSHV (Strickler et al. 1999) • CD4+ T cell count below 200/mm³ is a risk factor for KS development[c]	Determine CD4+ T cell KSHV epitopes and subsets
	B cells	• LANA, K8.1, and ORF65 elicit significant humoral responses[d] • Increase in number of individuals with detectable anti K8.1 responses coincides with plasma KSHV clearance during HAART (Bourboulia et al. 2004) • KSHV neutralizing antibodies reduced in AIDS-KS (Kimball et al. 2004) • Polymorphisms of FCγRIIIA confer protection against KS (Lehrnbecher et al. 2000)	Investigate the neutralizing and effector functions of anti-KSHV antibodies

[a] Key references are given. When more than two references are necessary, they are shown as footnotes.
[b] Osman et al., 1999; Wang et al., 2002; Wang et al., 2002; Wilkinson et al., 2002; Stebbing et al., 2003a; Ribechini et al., 2006
[c] Crowe et al., 1991; Cannon et al., 2003; Engels et al., 2003; Mbulaiteye et al., 2003
[d] Gao et al., 1996; Kedes et al., 1996; Lam et al., 2002; Simpson et al., 1996; Lin et al., 1997

donors and in higher frequency from individuals with KS (Browning et al., 1994). When isolated from the latter group, these spindle cells are infected with KSHV (Sirianni et al., 1997). During HIV-1 infection, all arms of the immune system are affected. Suboptimal NK cell-, humoral- and cellular immune responses may therefore contribute towards the expansion of KSHV-infected EC to precipitate KS, and KSHV-infected plasmablasts to precipitate MCD or PEL.

Innate immunity

The innate arm of the immune system is the first host defence against invading pathogens. The interactions between KSHV and innate immunity are only starting to be explored.

Dendritic cells

Dendritic cells (DC) are professional antigen presenting cells with a pivotal role in the initiation of innate and adaptive immune responses. DC originate from CD34+ haematopoietic stem cells in the bone marrow and differentiate into the myeloid and lymphoid (or plasmacytoid) DC lineages (mDC and pDC respectively). mDC express myeloid lineage markers, remain in the circulation, or differentiate into immature DC (iDC) after migration to skin

(Langerhans cells, CD1a$^+$) and other tissues (interstitial DC, CD1a$^-$). mDC constantly sample their environment and upon foreign antigen encounter they migrate to the lymph nodes where they mature and present antigens to T lymphocytes. In parallel, pDC express lymphoid markers, remain in circulation or cluster around the high endothelial venules of inflamed lymph nodes. These cells migrate into the lymph nodes in response to inflammatory cytokines and they are considered to be the main type I interferon-producing cells during host defence against viral infections. In addition to these typical functions, DC exhibit an extraordinary plasticity and multi-potency in their ability to interact with all cells of the immune system to initiate and orchestrate efficient innate and adaptive immune responses (Bancherau and Steinman, 1998; Patterson, 2000; Shortman and Liu, 2002).

The key role of DC in host responses against viral infections makes them a major target for viral mechanisms to evade host immunity. The development of efficient in vitro iDC generation methods from peripheral blood monocytes (moDC) (Sallusto and Lanzavecchia, 1994) or bone marrow CD34$^+$ stem cells (Caux et al., 1997) has allowed studies of the effects of viruses on DC generation, maturation, and function. Members of the herpesvirus family such as HSV, HHV6, CMV, and EBV use a variety of mechanisms to block DC generation and/or maturation, e.g., CMV directly infects DC and impairs their function and also blocks differentiation of monocytes to DC, whereas EBV induces apoptosis of monocyte DC progenitors (Chapters 31 and 43).

Currently, little is known about the interaction of DC and KSHV. In vitro, although infection of CD34$^+$ hematopoietic progenitors does not affect differentiation to DC (Larcher et al., 2005), KSHV uses the DC-SIGN receptor to directly infect DC resulting in a decrease of their antigen presenting properties (Rappocciolo et al., 2006). In vivo, the importance of DC in the host response to KSHV can be hypothesized based on the high occurrence of KSHV related malignancies in immunosuppressed individuals and the critical role that DC play in the pathogenesis of other herpesviral infections. Moreover, KS occurs at sites rich in DC: Langerhans cells in the skin and interstitial DC in the mucosal surfaces. In the context of HIV-1 infection, the number and function of both DC lineages decrease after primary infection and during high viraemia (Donaghy et al. 2001, 2003). A further reduction in the numbers of pDC has been reported in AIDS-KS in comparison to HIV-1 infected individuals (Stebbing et al., 2003b). Low numbers of both DC subsets (but not CD34$^+$ hematopoietic progenitors) are also reported in classic KS and this decrease correlates with advanced disease (Della Bella et al., 2006). Finally, the number of Langerhans cells is significantly decreased in KS lesions when compared with normal skin, suggesting that KSHV might influence DC maturation or migration (Valcuende-Cavero et al., 1994). However, it is still not clear whether DC are infected by KSHV in vivo and the exact mechanisms that KSHV employs to effect DC maturation and function are yet to be determined.

Natural killer cells

Natural killer (NK) cells are lymphocytes that do not undergo genetic recombination events and thus do not express clonally distributed receptors for antigen. They are found mostly in peripheral blood, spleen, and bone marrow, but can migrate to inflamed tissues in response to various chemoattractants. NK cells mediate direct lysis of target tumor or infected cells by release of perforin and granzymes or by binding to apoptosis inducing receptors on the target cell. Upon activation, NK cells release inflammatory cytokines, which influence the type of adaptive responses. The mechanism of NK function is described by the "missing self" hypothesis (Medzhitov and Janeway, 2002): NK activity is switched off by a set of inhibitory receptors, which are expressed on their cell surface, including killer-cell immunoglobulin-like receptors (KIRs), immunoglobulin-like inhibitory receptors (ILT) and the lectin-like heterodimer CD94-NKG2A. All these receptors are involved in HLA molecule recognition. Each type of KIR is expressed only by a subgroup of NK cells allowing the constant sampling of every single HLA allele. Down-regulation of MHC-I molecules, which occurs in tumor and virally infected cells, results in the withdrawal of the KIR inhibitory signal and subsequent activation of NK cells through a group of receptors termed natural cytotoxicity receptors (NCR) (Medzhitov and Janeway, 2002; Moretta et al., 2002). It has been shown that individuals with decreased or depleted NK activity are prone to HSV, CMV, and EBV infections (Biron et al., 1999). Moreover, herpesviruses evade NK cell-mediated immunity using mechanisms that target every step of NK cell activation (Chapter 31 and Orange et al., 2002).

At least four different mechanisms by which KSHV regulates NK activity can be proposed (for review see Orange et al., 2002): Inhibition of NK activating receptor ICAM-1 by the viral gene K5, selective modulation of MHC-I molecules (HLA-A and HLA-B only) by K5, secretion of viral antagonists (vMIP-I and II) that block chemotactic responses of leukocytes, and decreased number of pDC (see DC section), which are the main type I IFN producers and fundamental for NK function. However, apart from the latter, these mechanisms involve lytic KSHV gene products and do not explain how KSHV latently infected cells that express low levels of MHC-I are protected from NK cells.

There is some evidence for the importance of NK cells in the control of KSHV infection and KS development: first, PEL cell lines are preferentially lyzed by NK cells from healthy blood donors when compared with KSHV$^-$/EBV$^+$ Burkitt lymphoma cell lines. Second, NK cell activity is decreased in individuals with aggressive AIDS-KS in comparison with individuals with indolent classic KS. Finally, NK cell activity is restored within 6 months of HAART in individuals with complete KS resolution and coincides with cell associated KSHV clearance (Sirianni et al., 2002). However, it is still not clear whether NK cell activity is specifically driven by KSHV in infected individuals, as NK cell activity does not differ between HIV-1 infected individuals with and without KS. Further studies should investigate the role of NK cells in the control of KSHV infection and in the pathogenesis of KSHV-related neoplasms.

Complement
Complement activation occurs due to differences in pathogen envelope or membrane composition (alternative pathway), or existence of pathogen specific antibodies (classical pathway) (Walport, 2001a,b). Viruses have evolved evasion mechanisms of complement activity by incorporating complement regulatory proteins into their envelope or by having structural and functional or just functional viral homologues of such regulators (termed regulators of complement activation RCA). The importance of these regulatory homologues was demonstrated in a mouse model of γ-herpesvirus infection. Murine γ-herpesvirus 68 (MHV68) encodes for an RCA, which inhibits complement activation at the level of C3 (the point of convergence of all complement pathways). It was demonstrated that deletion of this protein resulted in decreased virulence and that this was reversed in C3$^-$/C3$^-$ mice. In addition, complement was shown to have a direct effect on viral latency (Kapadia et al., 2002). Furthermore, and similarly to the MHV 68 KSHV encodes for a lytic product (ORF4) that inhibits complement activation at the level of C3 (named KSHV complement control protein, KCP) (Spiller et al., 2003). Based on these observations, it seems reasonable to speculate that KCP plays an important role in the protection of KSHV virions and/or infected cells, against opsonisation, complement mediated virolysis, and humoral immune responses, in particular during cell-to-cell transmission.

Adaptive immunity

T-lymphocytes
T-lymphocytes are in the forefront of the battle of the host's immune system with invading pathogens. Activation of the innate arm of the immune system results in the direct killing of invading pathogens and the initiation and direction of efficient adaptive immune responses, which, if successful, lead to the establishment of immunological memory. Through the MHC machinery CD8+ and CD4+ T-lymphocytes specifically recognize viral peptide antigens, proliferate, and either directly lyze the infected cells (cytotoxic CD8+ T-lymphocytes, CTL) or further orchestrate the adaptive immune response (helper CD4+ T-lymphocytes, Th cells). However, during infection a variety of mechanisms are used by herpesviruses to escape T-cell responses (Ploegh, 1998; Yewdell and Hill, 2002).

Cytotoxic T-lymphocytes
CTL are primed by dendritic cells (DC) and by other professional antigen presenting cells, which present viral antigens through the MHC-I machinery. Following clonal expansion, the primed CTL act against virus by killing infected cells via perforin- and/or Fas-dependent pathways, before new virus particles are made, whereas they also release cytokines and chemokines with antiviral activity.

CTL epitopes
Considering the size of the KSHV genome, only a relatively small number of KSHV specific MHC class I-restricted CTL epitopes have been identified thus far (Fig. 52.1(a)) (Osman et al., 1999; Wang et al., 2000, 2001, 2002; Brander et al., 2001; Micheletti et al., 2002; Wilkinson et al., 2002; Stebbing et al., 2003a; Ribechini et al., 2006). Although the use of these epitopes led to the detection of KSHV-specific CTL responses, these responses are in general weak compared to those seen against other herpesviral antigens. Whether this is due to viral immune escape from CTL, or whether help from autologous antigen presenting cells is necessary for efficient CTL responses (as shown for DC (Wang et al., 2002)) or whether the KSHV genome has just not yet been exhaustively screened for CTL epitopes remains to be elucidated. One difficulty is that in the West, KSHV is predominantly present in HIV-1 infected individuals who exhibit suppressed CTL activity. The majority of CTL epitopes have therefore been identified in HIV-1 infected individuals during HAART, where the immune system is partly restored. Interestingly, T cell responses to LANA and ORF 65 are also detectable, even in KSHV-seronegative HIV-1 infected individuals, implying that KSHV-specific cellular immunity can occur in the absence of antibody responses (Woodberry et al., 2005). However, the peptide epitopes present in these two viral proteins were not identified and it is not clear whether the observed responses were due to CTL or CD4+ cells.

In KSHV, as in other herpesviruses, most of the CTL epitopes have been identified in conserved sites. It was demonstrated that functional CTL epitopes cluster in a

ORF (reference)	Protein product	Expression	Epitope (KSHV strain)	HLA I allele restriction
K1 (Stebbing et al., 2003a)	Transmembrane glycoprotein	Lytic	FRLTERTLF (A)	Cw*3
			FRLTKTIFS (A)	Cw*3
			LRLTQQTFT (C)	Cw*3
			HRQSIWITW (A)	B*2702
			HRQSIWHTL (C)	B*2702
			YPQPVLQTL (C)	B*51
			YPQPVLQHA (A)	B*51
			YPQPVLQRA (A)	B*51
			QPVLQTLCA (A and B)	B*55
			QPVLQTLCG (C)	B*55
ORF 8 (Wang et al., 2002)	Glycoprotein B	Lytic	LMWYELSKI	A*0201
ORF 22 (Micheletti et al., 2002)	Glycoprotein H	Lytic	FLNWQNLLNV	A*0201
K8.1 (Wilkinson et al., 2002)	Glycoprotein gp35-37	Lytic	ELTDALISAFSGSYS	A*0201
			LILYLCVPRCRRKKP	A*0201
ORF26 (Ribechini et al., 2006)	ORF26	Lytic	FQWDSNTQL	A*0201
			IVLESNGFDL	A*0201
			VLDDLSMYL	A*0201
K3 (Ribechini et al., 2006)	vMIR1	Lytic	LPRLTYQEGL	B*7
			GLAAATWVWL	A*0201
K5 (Ribechini et al., 2006)	vMIR2	Lytic	ALYAANNTRV	A*0201
K12 (Brander et al., 2001; Micheletti et al., 2002; Ribechini et al., 2006)	Kaposin A	Latent and induced in lytic	VLLNGWRWRL	A*0201
			VVQELLWFL	A*0201
			LYQRSGDMGL	A*24
			SYSLLTYML	A*24
			YMLAHVTGL	A*0201
			TPRPFPRLEI	B*7

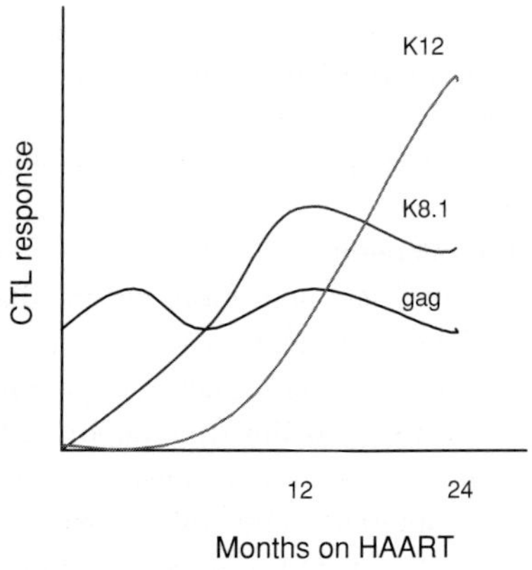

Fig. 52.1. KSHV specific CTL epitopes and CTL recovery during HAART. (a) KSHV specific CTL epitopes: CTL peptide epitopes have been identified in five KSHV encoded proteins. The K1 epitopes all cluster in the most variable region (VR1) and are associated with specific KSHV strains (associated strains are shown in brackets next to the epitopes). No HLA class A epitopes have thus far been identified in K1. K12 (Kaposin A) is the only latent KSHV protein thus far shown to elicit CTL responses. (b) Effects of HAART on the recovery of anti-KSHV CTL responses: CTL activity increases during HAART in HIV-1 infected individuals, with or without KS, against lytic and latent epitopes (K8.1 and K12, epitopes, respectively. HIV-1 gag responses also shown). CTL responses against K12 continue to increase after 12 months on HAART (Bourboulia et al., 2004). These CTL responses could contribute to the observed drop in the incidence of KS in the West since the widespread introduction of HAART. CTL, cytotoxic T-lymphocyte; HAART, highly active anti-retroviral therapy.

positively selected region of the most variable KSHV gene. K1 is a positional homologue of LMP-1 of EBV and contains the two most variable regions (VR1 and VR2) across the entire KSHV genome which are used to classify KSHV into four clades (A, B, C, and D) (Zong et al., 1999). Every viral isolate studied thus far is unique to an infected individual. However, unlike the situation in retroviruses, K1 mutations have not been detected within an infected individual over time. Several, HLA class I restricted epitopes within the VR1 were identified with the use of autologous overlapping peptides corresponding exactly to a patient's own viral sequence (Fig. 52.1(a)). These CTL epitopes are conserved within a specific strain (e.g. A or B), but not between strains. Based on these observations it appears that part of the genetic variability occurring in K1 is driven by a positive selection for CTL recognition, rather than due to CTL escape (Stebbing et al., 2003a). Furthermore, the observed variability does not appear to be due to escape from humoral immunity (a mechanism employed by other viruses such as influenza and HIV-1 where variability in viral surface proteins is driven by escape from humoral immunity resulting a 'antigenic shift'). It seems likely that this selection prevents the complete evasion of all host immune control mechanisms, which would lead to overwhelming viral infection with subsequent death of the host and, therefore, of the virus. It seems that K1, which is an early-lytic product, serves as a "suicide" protein allowing CTL recognition of cells reactivating from latency. Of note, CTL epitopes were also identified in vMIR1 and vMIR2 (Ribechini et al., 2006), two lytic KSHV genes that down-regulate expression of MHC-I and other co-stimulatory proteins (Chapters 31 and 62), whereas vFLIP is able to upregulate expression of MHC-I and ICAM-1 (Lagos et al., unpublihsed data). In addition to K1 recognition by CTL, the above findings reveal two more mechanisms employed by KSHV to regulate immune escape, limit viral dissemination and establish equilibrium in the virus–host co-speciation.

Effects of HAART on CTL

HAART promotes long-term immune reconstitution in patients with and without KS. This reconstitution is also KSHV-specific (Wilkinson et al., 2002; Bourboulia et al., 2004). It has been demonstrated that there is a significant decline of KSHV DNA load in PBMC and plasma during HAART and this correlates with a significant increase of anti-KSHV-specific CD8+ T-cell responses (Bourboulia et al., 2004) (Fig. 52.1(b)). It appears that prolonged HAART (more than 12 months) is necessary for these anti-KSHV effects to be established and maintained in most HIV-1 infected individuals. In individuals with KS, resolution of KS is also associated with significant increases of KSHV specific CD8+ T-cell responses during the first 6–9 months on HAART. Future work has to determine whether other KSHV specific epitopes are able to elicit more potent CD8+ T cell responses and contribute to the restoration of KSHV specific T-cells and whether such responses are stronger and occur earlier than those observed for K8.1 and K12. Moreover, detailed phenotyping of KSHV-specific CD8+ T-cells would give further insight into the anti-KSHV responses in comparison to other viruses that establish persistent infections (Appay et al., 2002).

Helper T-lymphocytes

The final stages of herpesvirus virion assembly occur in endosomal cellular compartments with extensive targeting of viral proteins to endosomes. During this process viral proteins can be efficiently sampled by the MHC-II, leading to the presentation of viral antigens to CD4+ T-lymphocytes.

The association of KS with low CD4+ T-cell count (mainly below 200/mm^3; although on average these values are higher than those associated with other AIDS-associated cancers) (Crowe et al., 1991; Cannon et al., 2003; Engels et al., 2003; Mbulaiteye et al., 2003) and the rapid KS resolution during HAART suggest a potential role for anti-KSHV CD4+ T-cell responses in the control of KSHV infection.

However, although CD4+ T-cell proliferation as a response to KSHV has been reported (Strickler et al., 1999), a correlation between CD4+ T-cell number and KS resolution during HAART has not been observed (Gill et al., 2002). Future studies should determine the KSHV specific CD4+ T-cell epitopes and the patterns of these responses during primary and persistent infection comparing also with other herpesviruses (Amyes et al., 2003).

B-lymphocytes

Antibody responses from B lymphocytes play a major role in anti-viral immunity (Burton, 2002). Antibodies can bind to viral proteins and block viral entry to the host cells (neutralizing antibodies), inhibit release of viral particles from infected cells, or trigger effector functions through their Fc domain causing the lysis of free virions or infected cells by NK cells (antibody-dependent cellular cytotoxicity, ADCC) or by the complement (complement dependent cytotoxicity, CDC).

The importance of humoral immune responses against human herpesviruses has been shown (Chapters 34, 43, 51 and 72). Furthermore, antibody responses against MHV68, in the absence of CD8+ and CD4+ T-cells, can efficiently control MHV 68 replication (Kim et al., 2002).

Antibody responses are recognized and detectable against KSHV latent and lytic proteins. However, the role of these antibodies in controlling KSHV replication or infection remains to be elucidated.

Antibody epitopes and serological assays for anti-KSHV antibody detection

The ORF73 of KSHV encodes for the major latent nuclear antigen of KSHV. More than 70% of infected individuals have detectable anti-LANA antibodies (Gao et al., 1996; Kedes et al., 1996). These humoral immune responses are directed against epitopes in the C-terminus. Detection of anti-LANA antibodies correlates in different populations with the KS burden (Chapter 54), and the detection of anti-LANA antibodies by indirect immunofluorescence is a useful assay for serological surveys (Fig. 52.2(a)). Several studies have suggested that seroconversion and/or a high antibody titer against LANA correlates with risk of KS development in HIV-1 infected individuals (Gao et al., 1996; Sitas et al., 1999; Sitas and Newton, 2001; Ziegler et al., 2003). However, the association between KSHV load in sera or in PBMC and anti-LANA antibody titer is still unclear.

Strong anti-lytic antibody responses are directed against K8.1, which encodes for an envelope glycoprotein that is the positional homologue of EBV gp220/350 (Chandran et al., 1998). Anti-K8.1 antibodies are detectable in approximately 80% of individuals with AIDS-KS and in more than 90% of

(a)

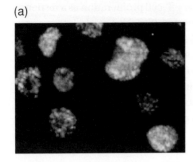

(b)

Assay	Sensitivity	Specificity
Lytic IFA	>95	80-85
LANA IFA	70-90	>95
ORF65 IFA	40	>95
Viral lysate ELISA	85-95	85-90
Recombinant LANA ELISA	60-70	85-90
Recombinant ORF65 ELISA	75-85	85-90
ORF65 peptide epitope ELISA	80-90	85-90
Recombinant K8.1 ELISA	80-95	90-95
K8.1 epitope ELISA	75-95	90-95
MAP K8.1 ELISA	80-95	>95
K8.1 and ORF65 peptide epitope mix ELISA	85-95	90-95
Recombinant K12 ELISA	55	90

Fig. 52.2. Humoral responses to KSHV and reconstitution during HAART (a) Immunofluorescent assay for anti-LANA antibodies: The KSHV LANA elicits antibody responses and is used for serological studies in an indirect IFA. Sera from KSHV infected individuals recognize LANA and a typical nuclear stippling pattern is observed. **(b)** Several KSHV proteins have been shown to elicit potent humoral responses and used in the development of serological assays for the detection of KSHV infection: Sensitivity and specificity of various serological assays as described in comparative studies (see main text) or unpublished results. Sensitivity is calculated based on the assumption that all individuals with KS should be positive for KSHV. In general, assays combining different proteins (e.g. ELISA combining K8.1 and ORF65 epitopes) are more sensitive than single assays. **(c)** The detection of anti-KSHV antibodies in different populations correlated with KS burden: Various serological assays have been employed to conduct KSHV epidemiological. Although the sensitivity and specificity of these assays vary, overall the global seroprevalence correlated with the incidence of KS: White bars correspond to countries with a low KS incidence (mainly AIDS-KS). Light gray to Mediterranean countries where classic KS occurs, and dark grey to Sub-Saharan Africa with a high prevalence of non-HIV-1 (endemic-) and AIDS-KS, West Africa remains a conudrum, because KS is seldom seen, despite a high seroprevalence of KSHV (reviewed in Ablashi *et al.*, 1999; Sarid *et al.*, 1999; Dedicoat and Newton 2002; Dukers and Rezza 2003; Martin 2003; figure courtesy of Dimitra Bourboulia). **(d)** The effect of HAART on anti-KSHV humoral responses: LANA and K8.1 epitopes have been used to assess the effect of HAART on KSHV specific humoral responses (Bourboulia *et al.*, 2004). Reconstitution of humoral immunity during HAART, and in particular an increase number of individuals with detectable anti-K8.1 antibodies, coincides with a reduction of plasma KSHV viraemia. However, the role of these humoral responses in controlling KSHV replication is still not elucidated. LANA latent nuclear antigen; IFA, immunofluorescence; ORF, open reading frame, ELISA, enzyme linked immunosorbent assay; MAP, multiple antigenic peptide

individuals with non-AIDS KS (Fig. 52.2(b)). A K8.1 peptide epitope, with no known sequence similarity to any other pathogen has been used in the form of a multiple antigenic peptide (MAP) for the development of a highly sensitive and specific ELISA to detect KSHV infection (Lam *et al.*, 2002). The sensitivity of this ELISA is improved by combining the K8.1 epitope with a known LANA epitope in a MAP (D.Lagos, unpublished data).

Another lytic antigen that generates humoral responses is the small viral capsid antigen encoded by ORF65 (Simpson *et al.*, 1996; Lin *et al.*, 1997). A combination of an ORF65 peptide epitope with a K8.1 epitope is employed in one of the most sensitive and specific, commercially available assays (Schatz *et al.*, 2001) (Fig. 52.2(b)).

Specific antibody responses among individuals with KS have also been reported against ORF26 and K12, although

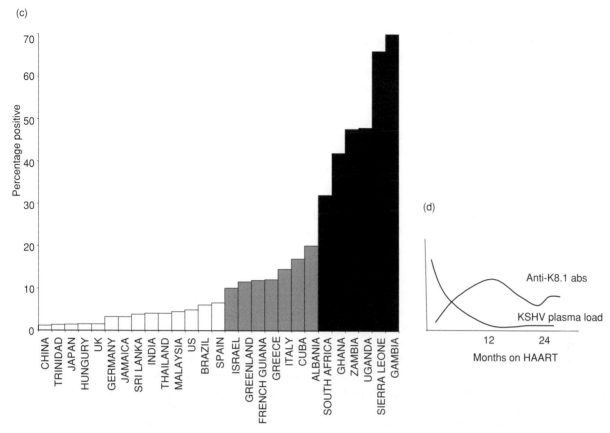

Fig. 52.2. (cont.)

significantly less common than LANA, K8.1, and ORF65 (Schatz et al., 2001).

A variety of serological assays for KSHV detection have been described. These include immunofluorescent assays using PEL cell lines and ELISA using virions, purified recombinant proteins, peptide epitopes, mixtures of peptide epitopes, and multiple antigenic peptide epitopes as antigens. These assays have been successfully used in large epidemiological studies providing insight into KSHV biology, transmission, risk factors for KSHV infection and KS development (Ablashi et al., 1999; Sarid et al., 1999; Dedicoat and Newton, 2002; Dukers and Rezza, 2003; Martin, 2003) (Fig. 52.2(c)). The sensitivity of these assays ranges from less than 80% for individuals with AIDS-KS to more than 90% for HIV-1 negative individuals with KS (Rabkin et al., 1998; Enbom et al., 2000; Spira et al., 2000; Schatz et al., 2001; Dukers and Rezza, 2003; Pellett et al., 2003) (Fig. 52.2(b)). There are some AIDS-KS cases where anti-latent and anti-lytic antibodies are not detectable, but KSHV copies can be detected in plasma and/or PBMCs by quantitative PCR (Lallemand et al., 2000). Whether this is due to low sensitivity of the current serological assays or the defect in the humoral immunity of these individuals remains to be elucidated.

Effects of HAART on humoral responses

Although it is not clear if HAART has any significant effect on anti-LANA antibody titer (Wilkinson et al., 2002; Bourboulia et al., 2004), an increase in the number of individuals with detectable anti-K8.1 antibodies coincides with plasma virus clearance during HAART (Bourboulia et al., 2004) (Fig. 52.2(d)). Based on these results it could be proposed that the humoral arm of the immune system plays an important role in the control of the KSHV replication.

How antibodies contribute to KSHV immunity

It has been shown that sera from KSHV-seropositive individuals can block KSHV infection in vitro (Dialyna et al., 2004; Kimball et al., 2004). Moreover, individuals with AIDS-KS display reduced levels of neutralizing antibodies,

> **Box 52.2. Transmission of cancer, immunity and Kaposi's sarcoma**
>
> Until the end of the eighteenth century, it was believed by many that cancer was a contagious disease. James Nooth, an English surgeon, and Jean Louise Alibert, the founder of the French School of Dermatology and personal physician of King Louis XVIII, were the first to independently challenge this hypothesis: both injected themselves with breast cancer cells, which resulted in short-lived local inflammatory responses, but no tumour establishment. They concluded that cancer was not contagious.
>
> The discovery in 1908 by Peyton Rous that cell-free filtrates from tumors could transmit cancer between Plymouth Rock hens heralded the era of viral oncology and sparked a debate whether viruses were responsible for most cancers. The first evidence that a virus was indeed involved in the pathogenesis of a human cancer only emerged in 1964 with the discovery of Epstein–Barr virus. Two years later Peyton Rous was awarded the Nobel Prize in Physiology of Medicine for his discovery of "tumor inducing viruses."
>
> In the 1950s, selective immunosuppressant drugs were developed and organ transplantation became a life-saving reality. However, the first case of a kidney transplant recipient who developed iatrogenic Kaposi's sarcoma was reported soon afterwards. It was also noticed that Kaposi's sarcoma can disappear when immunosuppression is stopped, linking immunity closely with Kaposi's sarcomagenesis. The transmission of other cancers during organ transplantation, e.g., melanoma, has also been documented.
>
> Until recently, it was widely accepted that iatrogenic Kaposi's sarcoma was due to the loss of immunesurveillance against KSHV: It was thought that KSHV could be transmitted from donor to host, or that immunosuppressive drugs led to the reactivation of KSHV in already infected recipients. The provocative finding in 2003 that certain cases of post-organ transplant Kaposi's sarcoma are due to the transmission of KSHV-infected precancerous cells, revived the debate on the transmission of cancer. Ironically, this is a tumor induced by a virus, where both host cell and pathogen are transmitted simultaneously. These findings infer that KSHV not only infect endothelial cells during periods of immunodeficiency, but that KSHV-infected circulating endothelial cells are present in otherwise healthy individuals. Notably, the concept of cancer cell transmission is further supported by the identification in 2006 of the oldest known somatic mammalian clonal cell population as the causative agent of the canine transmissible venereal tumor.
>
> The wider implications of this are that in populations such as certain sub-Saharan African countries with a large HIV-1 burden where many are immunosuppressed, the transmission of cancer cells between infected individuals, e.g., Kaposi's sarcoma or anogenital cancer may represent a reality. The study of iatrogenic Kaposi's sarcoma would provide further insight into the immunological control of cancer.
>
> **FURTHER READING**
>
> Barozzi, P., Luppi, M., Facchetti, F. et al. (2003). Post-transplant Kaposi's sarcoma originates from the seeding of donor-derived progenitors. *Nat. Med.*, **9**, 554–561.
>
> Birkeland, S. A. and Storm, H. H. (2002). Risk for tumor and other disease transmission by transplantation: a population-based study of unrecognized malignancies and other diseases in organ donors. *Transplantation*, **74**, 1409–1413.
>
> Fitzgerald, P. J. (2000) *From Demons and Evil Spirits to Cancer Genes*. Washington: American Registry of Pathology Publications.

despite the fact that higher total binding antibody levels are observed in this group (Kimball et al., 2004). This implies that the humoral immunity plays a crucial role in the prevention of KS development and that the most immunogenic KSHV antigens are not necessarily the targets of neutralizing antibodies. However, the contribution of KSHV neutralizing antibodies in controlling in vivo infection needs to be addressed further, as the neutralizing titers are low and the specific epitopes not known. K8.1 could be such a neutralizing antibody target as it is directly involved in the process of viral entry into host cells by binding to heparan sulfate (Birkmann et al., 2001; Chapter 23) and reconstitution of anti-K8.1 humoral responses during HAART coincides with virus clearance. Of note, gp 220/350, the EBV positional homologue of K8.1, elicits neutralizing antibody responses and has been investigated as a target for development of an EBV vaccine (Chapter 72). Another candidate for KSHV-specific neutralizing antibodies is glycoprotein B, which is also involved in viral entry (Chapter 23). Rabbit polyclonal antibodies raised against glycoprotein B neutralize infectivity in vitro (Akula et al., 2002). In addition to their neutralizing potential, antibodies can control KSHV infection through their effector functions. It has been reported that the genotype of the low affinity Fc receptor FcγRIIIA can contribute protection or conversely be a risk factor for KS development (Lehrnbecher et al., 2000). This receptor is expressed on the surface of NK cells and could be an important factor influencing ADCC activity. Further studies are necessary to elucidate the role of the humoral immunity in the host defense against KSHV.

Conclusions and future perspectives

Excluding pox viruses, KSHV has pilfered an unprecedented array of cellular genes, mainly to impede the function of host antiviral immune responses. During immunosuppression, both the innate and adaptive anti-KSHV immune responses are hampered, allowing the uncontrolled proliferation of KSHV-infected cells that belong to the B-lymphocyte and EC lineages.

KSHV proteins that elicit humoral and cellular immune responses are being identified and the consequences of immunodeficiency (HIV-1 induced or iatrogenic) and immune-restoration are being elucidated. Such studies will allow the understanding of the anti-KSHV host defence mechanisms and could eventually lead to the generation of an effective vaccine. During the next couple of years, the study of KSHV immunobiology should also provide further insight into tumor and transplant immunology.

REFERENCES

Ablashi, D., Chatlynne, L., Cooper, H. et al. (1999). Seroprevalence of human herpesvirus-8 (HHV-8) in countries of Southeast Asia compared to the USA, the Caribbean and Africa. Br. J. Cancer, **81**, 893–897.

Akula, S. M., Pramod, N. P., Wang, F. Z., and Chandran, B. (2002). Integrin alpha3beta1 (CD 49c/29) is a cellular receptor for Kaposi's sarcoma-associated herpesvirus (KSHV/HHV-8) entry into the target cells. Cell, **108**, 407–419.

Ambroziak, J. A., Blackbourn, D. J., Herndier, B. G. et al. (1995). Herpes-like sequences in HIV-infected and uninfected Kaposi's sarcoma patients. Science, **268**, 582–583.

Amyes, E., Hatton, C., Montamat-Sicotte, D. et al. (2003). Characterization of the CD4+ T cell response to Epstein–Barr virus during primary and persistent infection. J. Exp. Med., **198**, 903–911.

Andreoni, M., Sarmati, L., Nicastri, E. et al. (2002). Primary human herpesvirus 8 infection in immunocompetent children. J. Am. Med. Assoc., **287**, 1295–1300.

Appay, V., Dunbar, P. R., Callan, M. et al. (2002). Memory CD8+ T cells vary in differentiation phenotype in different persistent virus infections. Nat. Med., **8**, 379–385.

Banchereau, J. and Steinman, R. M. (1998). Dendritic cells and the control of immunity. Nature, **392**, 245–252.

Bani-Sadr, F., Fournier, S., and Molina, J. M. (2003). Relapse of Kaposi's sarcoma in HIV-infected patients switching from a protease inhibitor to a non-nucleoside reverse transcriptase inhibitor-based highly active antiretroviral therapy regimen. AIDS, **17**, 1580–1581.

Bechtel, J. T., Liang, Y., Hvidding J., and Ganem, D. (2003). Host range of Kaposi's sarcoma-associated herpesvirus in cultured cells. J. Virol., **77**, 6474–6481.

Birkmann, A., Mahr, K., Ensser, A. et al. (2001). Cell surface heparan sulfate is a receptor for human herpesvirus 8 and interacts with envelope glycoprotein K8.1. J. Virol., **75**, 11583–11593.

Biron, C. A., Nguyen, K. B., Pien, G. C., Cousens, L. P., and Salazar-Mather t5 T. P. (1999). Natural killer cells in antiviral defense: function and regulation by innate cytokines. Annu. Rev. Immunol., **17**, 189–220.

Boshoff, C. and Weiss, R. (2002). AIDS-related malignancies. Nat Rev. Cancer, **2**, 373–382.

Bourboulia, D., Aldam, D. M., Lagos, D. et al. (2004). Short- and long-term effects of highly active antiretroviral therapy on Kaposi sarcoma-associated herpesvirus immune responses and viraemia. AIDS, **18**, 485–493.

Brander, C., O'Connor, P., Suscovich, T. et al. (2001). Definition of an optimal cytotoxic T lymphocyte epitope in the latently expressed Kaposi's sarcoma-associated herpesvirus kaposin protein. J. Infect. Dis., **184**, 119–126.

Browning, P. J., Sechler, J. M., Kaplan, M. et al. (1994). Identification and culture of Kaposi's sarcoma-like spindle cells from the peripheral blood of human immunodeficiency virus-1-infected individuals and normal controls. Blood, **84**, 2711–2720.

Burton, D. R. (2002). Antibodies, viruses and vaccines. Nat. Rev. Immunol., **2**, 706–713.

Cannon, M. J., Dollard, S. C., Black, J. B. et al. (2003). Risk factors for Kaposi's sarcoma in men seropositive for both human herpesvirus 8 and human immunodeficiency virus. AIDS, **17**, 215–222.

Caux, C., Massacrier, C., Vanbervliet, B. et al. (1997). CD34+ hematopoietic progenitors from human cord blood differentiate along two independent dendritic cell pathways in response to granulocyte-macrophage colony-stimulating factor plus tumor necrosis factor alpha: II. Functional analysis. Blood, **90**, 1458–1470.

Cesarman, E., Moore, P. S., Rao, P. H., Inghirami, G., Knowles, D. M., and Chang, Y. (1995). In vitro establishment and characterization of two acquired immunodeficiency syndrome-related lymphoma cell lines (BC-1 and BC-2) containing Kaposi's sarcoma-associated herpesvirus-like (KSHV) DNA sequences. Blood, **86**, 2708–2714.

Chandran, B., Bloomer, C., Chan, S. R., Zhu, L., Goldstein, E., and Horvat, R. (1998). Human herpesvirus-8 ORF K8.1 gene encodes immunogenic glycoproteins generated by spliced transcripts. *Virology*, **249**, 140–149.

Crowe, S. M., Carlin, J. B., Stewart, K. I., Lucas, C. R., and Hoy, J. F. (1991). Predictive value of CD4 lymphocyte numbers for the development of opportunistic infections and malignancies in HIV-infected persons. *J. Acquir. Immune Defic. Syndr.*, **4**, 770–776.

Dedicoat, M. and Newton R. (2002). Review of the distribution of Kaposi's sarcoma-associated herpesvirus (KSHV) in Africa in relation to the incidence of Kaposi's sarcoma. *Br. J. Cancer*, **88**, 1–3.

Della Bella, S., Nicola, S., Brambilla, L. *et al.* (2006). Quantitative and functional defects of dendritic cells in classic Kaposi's sarcoma. *Clin. Immunol.*, **119**, 317–329.

Dialyna, I.A., Graham, D., Rezaee, R. *et al.* (2004). Anti-HHV-8/KSHV antibodies in infected individuals inhibit infection in vitro. *AIDS*, **18**, 1263–1270.

Dittmer, D., Stoddart, C., Renne, R. *et al.* (1999). Experimental transmission of Kaposi's sarcoma-associated herpesvirus (KSHV/HHV-8) to SCID-hu Thy/Liv mice. *J. Exp. Med.*, **190**, 1857–1868.

Donaghy, H., Pozniak, A., Gazzard, B. *et al.* (2001). Loss of blood CD11c(+) myeloid and CD11c(-) plasmacytoid dendritic cells in patients with HIV-1 infection correlates with HIV-1 RNA virus load. *Blood*, **98**, 2574–2576.

Donaghy, H., Gazzard, B., Gotch, F., and Patterson, S. (2003). Dysfunction and infection of freshly isolated blood myeloid and plasmacytoid dendritic cells in patients infected with HIV-1. *Blood*, **101**, 4505–4511.

Dukers, N. H. and Rezza, G. (2003). Human herpesvirus 8 epidemiology: what we do and do not know. *Aids*, **17**, 1717–1730.

Dupin, N., Fisher, C., Kellam, P. *et al.* (1999). Distribution of human herpesvirus-8 latently infected cells in Kaposi's sarcoma, multicentric Castleman's disease, and primary effusion lymphoma. *Proc. Natl Acad. Sci. USA*, **96**, 4546–4551.

Enbom, M., Sheldon, J., Lennette, E. *et al.* (2000). Antibodies to human herpesvirus 8 latent and lytic antigens in blood donors and potential high-risk groups in Sweden: variable frequencies found in a multicenter serological study. *J. Med. Virol.*, **62**, 498–504.

Engels, E. A., Biggar, R. J., Marshall, V. A. *et al.* (2003). Detection and quantification of Kaposi's sarcoma-associated herpesvirus to predict AIDS-associated Kaposi's sarcoma. *AIDS*, **17**, 1847–1851.

Ensoli, B., Barillari, G., Salahuddin, S. Z., Gallo, R. C., and Wong, S. F. (1990). Tat protein of HIV-1 stimulates growth of cells derived from Kaposi's sarcoma lesions of AIDS patients. *Nature*, **345**, 84–86.

Euvrard, S., Kanitakis, J. and Claudy, A. (2003). Skin cancers after organ transplantation. *N. Engl. J. Med.*, **348**, 1681–1691.

Gallo, R. C. (1998). The enigmas of Kaposi's sarcoma. *Science*, **282**, 1837–1839.

Gao, S. J., Kingsley, L., Hoover, D. R. *et al.* (1996). Seroconversion to antibodies against Kaposi's sarcoma-associated herpesvirus-related latent nuclear antigens before the development of Kaposi's sarcoma. *N. Engl. J. Med.*, **335**, 233–241.

Gill, J., Bourboulia, D., Wilkinson, J. *et al.* (2002). Prospective study of the effects of antiretroviral therapy on Kaposi sarcoma-associated herpesvirus infection in patients with and without Kaposi sarcoma. *J. Acquir. Immune Defic. Syndr.*, **31**, 384–390.

Goudsmit, J., Renwick, N., Dukers, N. H. *et al.* (2000). Human herpesvirus 8 infections in the Amsterdam Cohort Studies (1984–1997): analysis of seroconversions to ORF65 and ORF73. *Proc. Natl Acad. Sci. USA*, **97**, 4838–4843.

Jacobson, L. P., Yamashita, T. E., Detels, R. *et al.* (1999). Impact of potent anti-retroviral therapy on the incidence of Kaposi's sarcoma and non-Hodgkin's lymphomas among HIV-1 infected individuals. Multicenter AIDS Cohort Study. *J. Acquir. Immune Defic. Syndr.*, **21**, s34–s41.

Kapadia, S. B., Levine, B., Speck S. H., and t. Virgin, H. W. (2002). Critical role of complement and viral evasion of complement in acute, persistent, and latent gamma-herpesvirus infection. *Immunity*, **17**, 143–155.

Kedes, D. H., Operskalski, E., Busch, M., Kohn, R., Flood J., and Ganem, D. (1996). The seroepidemiology of human herpesvirus 8 (Kaposi's sarcoma-associated herpesvirus): distribution of infection in KS risk groups and evidence for sexual transmission. *Nat. Med.*, **2**, 918–924.

Kim, I. J., Flano, E., Woodland D. L., and Blackman M. A. (2002). Antibody-mediated control of persistent gamma-herpesvirus infection. *J. Immunol.*, **168**, 3958–3964.

Kimball, L. E., Casper, C., Koelle, D. M. *et al.* (2004). Reduced levels of neutralizing antibodies to Kaposi sarcoma-associated herpesvirus in persons with a history of Kaposi sarcoma. *J. Infect. Dis.*, **189**, 2016–2022.

Lallemand, F., Desire, N., Rozenbaum, W., Nicolas J. C., and Marechal V. (2000). Quantitative analysis of human herpesvirus 8 viral load using a real-time PCR assay. *J. Clin. Microbiol.*, **38**, 1404–1408.

Lam, L. L., Pau, C. P., Dollard, S. C., Pellett, P. E., and Spira, T. J. (2002). Highly sensitive assay for human herpesvirus 8 antibodies that uses a multiple antigenic peptide derived from open reading frame K8.1. *J. Clin. Microbiol.*, **40**, 325–329.

Larcher, C., Nguyen, V. A., Furhapter, C. *et al.* (2005). Human herpesvirus-8 infection of umbilical cord-blood-derived CD34+ stem cells enhances the immunostimulatory function of their dendritic cell progeny. *Exp. Dermatol.*, **14**, 41–49.

Lehrnbecher, T. L., Foster, C. B., Zhu, S. *et al.* (2000). Variant genotypes of FcgammaRIIIA influence the development of Kaposi's sarcoma in HIV-infected men. *Blood*, **95**, 2386–2390.

Lin, S. F., Sun, R., Heston, L. *et al.* (1997). Identification, expression, and immunogenicity of Kaposi's sarcoma-associated herpesvirus-encoded small viral capsid antigen. *J. Virol.*, **71**, 3069–3076.

Macsween, K. F. and Crawford, D. H. (2003). Epstein–Barr virus-recent advances. *Lancet Infect. Dis.*, **3**, 131–140.

Martin, J. N. (2003). Diagnosis and epidemiology of human herpesvirus 8 infection. *Semin. Hematol.*, **40**, 133–142.

Mbulaiteye, S. M., Biggar, R. J., Goedert, J. J., and Engels, E. A. (2003). Immune deficiency and risk for malignancy among persons with AIDS. *J. Acquir. Immune Defic. Syndr.*, **32**, 527–533.

Medzhitov, R. and Janeway, C. A. Jr. (2002). Decoding the patterns of self and nonself by the innate immune system. *Science*, **296**, 298–300.

Micheletti, F., Monini, P. Fortini, C. *et al.* (2002). Identification of cytotoxic T-lymphocyte epitopes of human herpesvirus 8. *Immunology*, **106**, 395–403.

Moore, P. S. and Chang Y. (2003). Kaposi's Sarcoma-associated herpesvirus immunoevasion and tumorigenesis: two sides of the same coin? *Annu. Rev. Microbiol.*, **57**, 609–639.

Moretta, A., Bottino, C., Mingari, M. C., Biassoni, and Moretta, L. (2002). What is a natural killer cell? *Nat. Immunol.*, **3**, 6–8.

Murgia, C., Pritchard, J. K., Kim, S. Y. *et al.* (2006). Clonal origin and evolution of a transmissible cancer. *Cell*, **126**, 477–487.

Oksenhendler, E., Cazals-Hatem, D., Schultz, T. F. *et al.* (1998). Transient angiolymphoid hyperplasia and Kaposi's sarcoma after primary infection with human herpesvirus 8 in a patient with human immunodeficiency virus infection. *N. Engl. J. Med.*, **338**, 1585–1591.

Orange, J. S., Fassett, M. S., Koopman, L. A., Boyson, J. E., and Strominger, J. L. (2002). Viral evasion of natural killer cells. *Nature Immunol.*, **3**, 1006–1012.

Osman, M., Kubo, T., Gill, J. *et al.* (1999). Identification of human herpesvirus 8-specific cytotoxic T-cell responses. *J. Virol.*, **73**, 6136–6140.

Patterson, S. (2000). Flexibility and cooperation among dendritic cells. *Nat. Immunol.*, **1**, 273–274.

Pauk, J., Huang, M.-L., Brodie, S. J. *et al.* (2000). Mucosal shedding of human herpesvirus 8 in men. *N. Engl. J. Med.*, **343**, 1369–1377.

Pellett, P. E., Wright, D. J. Engels, E. A. *et al.* (2003). Multicenter comparison of serologic assays and estimation of human herpesvirus 8 seroprevalence among US blood donors. *Transfusion*, **43**, 1260–1268.

Ploegh, H. L. (1998). Viral strategies of immune evasion. *Science*, **280**, 248–253.

Rabkin, C. S., Schulz, T. F., Whitby, D. *et al.* (1998). Interassay correlation of human herpesvirus 8 serologic tests. *J. Infect. Dis.*, **178**, 304–309.

Rappocciolo, G., Jenkins, F.J., Hensler, H.R. *et al.* (2006). DC-SIGN is a receptor for human herpesvirus 8 on dendritic cells and macrophages. *J. Immunol.*, **176**, 1741–1749.

Renne, R., Lagunoff, M., Zhong, W., and Ganem, D. (1996). The size and conformation of Kaposi's sarcoma-associated herpesvirus (human herpesvirus 8) DNA in infected cells and virions. *J. Virol.*, **70**, 8151–8154.

Ribechini, E., Fortini, C., Marastoni, M. *et al.* (2006). Identification of CD8+ T cell epitopes within lytic antigens of human herpes virus 8. *J. Immunol.*, **176**, 923–930.

Sallusto, F. and Lanzavecchia, A. (1994). Efficient presentation of soluble antigen by cultured human dendritic cells is maintained by granulocyte/macrophage colony-stimulating factor plus interleukin 4 and downregulated by tumor necrosis factor alpha. *J. Exp. Med.*, **179**, 1109–1118.

Sarid, R., Olsen, S. J., and Moore, P. S. (1999). Kaposi's sarcoma-associated herpesvirus: epidemiology, virology, and molecular biology. *Adv. Virus Res.*, **52**, 139–232.

Schatz, O., Monini, P., Bugarini, R. *et al.* (2001). Kaposi's sarcoma-associated herpesvirus serology in Europe and Uganda: Multicentre study with multiple and novel assays. *J. Med. Virol.*, **65** 123–132.

Sgadari, C., Barillari, G., Toschi, E. *et al.* (2002). HIV protease inhibitors are potent anti–angiogenic molecules and promote regression of Kaposi sarcoma. *Nature Med.*, **8**, 225–232.

Shortman, K. and Liu, Y. J. (2002). Mouse and human dendritic cell subtypes. *Nat. Rev. Immunol.*, **2**, 151–161.

Simpson, G. R., Schulz, T. F., Whitby, D. *et al.* (1996). Prevalence of Kaposi's sarcoma associated herpesvirus infection measured by antibodies to recombinant capsid protein and latent immunofluorescence antigen. *Lancet*, **348**, 1133–1138.

Sirianni, M. C., Uccini, S., Angeloni, A. Faggioni, A., Cottoni, F., and Ensoli B. (1997). Circulating spindle cells: correlation with human herpesvirus-8 (HHV-8) infection and Kaposi's sarcoma. *Lancet*, **349**, 255.

Sirianni, M. C., Vincenzi, L., Topino, S. *et al.* (2002). NK cell activity controls human herpesvirus 8 latent infection and is restored upon highly active antiretroviral therapy in AIDS patients with regressing Kaposi's sarcoma. *Eur. J. Immunol.*, **32**, 2711–2720.

Sitas, F. and Newton R. (2001). Kaposi's sarcoma in South Africa. *J. Natl Cancer Inst. Monogr.*, 1–4.

Sitas, F., Carrara, H., Beral, V. *et al.* (1999). Antibodies against human herpesvirus 8 in black south African patients with cancer. *N. Engl. J. Med.*, **340**, 1863–1871.

Spiller, O. B., Robinson, M., O'Donnell, E. *et al.* (2003). Complement regulation by Kaposi's sarcoma-associated herpesvirus ORF4 protein. *J. Virol.*, **77**, 592–599.

Spira, T. J., Lam, L., Dollard, S. C. *et al.* (2000). Comparison of serologic assays and PCR for diagnosis of human herpesvirus 8 infection. *J. Clin. Microbiol.*, **38**, 2174–2180.

Stebbing, J., Bourboulia, D., Johnson, M. *et al.* (2003a). KSHV specific CTLs recognize and target Darwinian positively selected autologous K1 epitopes. *J. Virol.*, **77**, 4306–4314.

Stebbing, J., Gazzard, B., Portsmouth, S. *et al.* (2003b). Disease-associated dendritic cells respond to disease-specific antigens through the common heat shock protein receptor. *Blood*, **102**, 1806–1814.

Strickler, H. D., Goedert, J. J. Bethke, F. R. *et al.* (1999). Human Herpesvirus 8 cellular immune responses in homosexual men. *J. Infect. Dis.*, **180**, 1682–1685.

Valcuende-Cavero, F., Febrer-Bosch M. I., and Castells-Rodellas, A. (1994). Langerhans' cells and lymphocytic infiltrate in AIDS-associated Kaposi's sarcoma. An immunohistochemical study. *Acta. Derm. Venereol.*, **74**, 183–187.

Walport, M. J. (2001a). Complement. First of two parts. *N. Engl. J. Med.*, **344**, 1058–1066.

Walport, M. J. (2001b). Complement. Second of two parts. *N. Engl. J. Med.*, **344**, 1140–1144.

Wang, Q. J., Jenkins, F. J., Jacobson, L. P. *et al.* (2000). CD8+ cytotoxic T lymphocyte responses to lytic proteins of human herpes virus 8 in human immunodeficiency virus type 1-infected and-uninfected Individuals. *J. Infect. Dis.*, **182**, 928–932.

Wang, Q. J., Jenkins, F. J., Jacobson, L. P. *et al.* (2001). Primary human herpesvirus 8 infection generates a broadly specific CD8(+) T-cell response to viral lytic cycle proteins. *Blood*, **97**, 2366–2373.

Wang, Q. J., Huang, X. L., Rappocciolo, G. *et al.* (2002). Identification of an HLA A*0201-restricted CD8 (+) T-cell epitope for the glycoprotein B homolog of human herpesvirus 8. *Blood*, **99**, 3360–3366.

Wang, H. S., Trotter M. W., Lagos, D. *et al.* (2004). Kaposi sarcoma herpesvirus-induced cellular reprogramming contributes to the lymphatic endothelial gene expression in Kaposi sarcoma. *Nat. Gen.*, **36**, 687–693

Wilkinson, J., Cope, A., Gill, J. *et al.* (2002). Identification of Kaposi's sarcoma-associated herpesvirus (KSHV)- specific cytotoxic T-lymphocyte epitopes and evaluation of reconstitution of KSHV-specific responses in human immunodeficiency virus type 1-Infected patients receiving highly active antiretroviral therapy. *J. Virol.*, **76**, 2634–2640.

Woodberry, T., Suscovich, T. J., Henry, L. M. *et al.* (2005). Impact of Kaposi sarcoma-associated herpesvirus (KSHV) burden and HIV coinfection on the detection of T cell responses to KSHV ORF73 and ORF65 proteins. *J. Infect. Dis.*, **192**, 622–629.

Wu, W., Vieira, J., Fiore, N. *et al.* (2006). KSHV/HHV-8 infection of human hematopoietic progenitor (CD34+) cells: persistence of infection during hematopoiesis in vitro and in vivo. *Blood*, **108**, 141–151.

Yewdell, J. W. and Hill, A. B. (2002). Viral interference with antigen presentation. *Nat. Immunol.*, **3**, 1019–1025.

Ziegler, J., Newton, R., Bourboulia, D. *et al.* (2003). Risk factors for Kaposi's sarcoma: A case-control study of HIV- seronegative people in Uganda. *Int. J. Cancer*, **103**, 233–240.

Zong, J. C., Ciufo, D. M. Alcendor, D. J. *et al.* (1999). High-level variability in the ORF-K1 membrane protein gene at the left end of the Kaposi's sarcoma-associated herpesvirus genome defines four major virus subtypes and multiple variants or clades in different human populations. *J. Virol.*, **73**, 4156–4170.

53

The epidemiology of EBV and its association with malignant disease

Henrik Hjalgrim, Jeppe Friborg, and Mads Melbye

Department of Epidemiology Research, Statens Serum Institut, Artillerivej 5, 2300 Copenhagen S. Denmark

EPSTEIN-BARR VIRUS EPIDEMIOLOGY

Epidemiology of primary Epstein-Barr virus infection

Epstein-Barr virus (EBV) is an ancient virus, and has probably coevolved with its different hosts over the last 90–100 million years (McGeoch et al., 1995). With the ability to establish lifelong latency and intermittent reactivation after primary infection and with limited clinical symptoms in the majority of infected individuals, EBV has become ubiquitous in all human populations

Age at primary infection

Children in developing countries acquire the infection in the first few years of life, and universal seroconversion is often seen by ages 3–4 years, whereas infection in developed countries often is delayed until adolescence (de The et al., 1975; Haahr et al., 2004; Henle and Henle, 1967; Melbye et al., 1984a,b) (Figure 53.1). In some developed countries a bimodal infection rate, with peaks in children below 5 years and again after 10 years of age, has been described (Edwards and Woodroof, 1979; Henle and Henle, 1967; Lai et al., 1975). Oral EBV excretion between parents and infants, and from intimate partners in adolescence and early adulthood is the likely explanation for the observed bimodality (Crawford et al., 2002; Fleisher et al., 1979).

EBV antibody titers in seropositive individuals vary according to age following a U-shaped pattern, with high titers among infants and in the elderly (above 50 years) (Glaser et al., 1985; Venkitaraman et al., 1985). High antibody titers in infants probably reflect primary infection, whereas in the elderly it may be due to an age-dependent reactivation due to a reduced cellular immune response (Wick and Grubeck-Loebenstein, 1997).

Geographic variation

EBV has been detected in all populations and all areas of the world (IARC, 1997), but with noticeable geographical variation in the distribution of EBV genotypes. Two major types of EBV, type 1 and 2, have been described in humans, varying in the genes that encode some of the nuclear proteins in latently infected cells (Sample et al., 1990). Both types are detected all over the world, with type 1 being the most prevalent. However, in some regions (e.g. central Africa, Papua New Guinea and Alaska) type 2 is more prevalent (Table 53.1) (Gratama and Ernberg, 1995; Zimber et al., 1986). It is assumed that the geographical distribution of the two types in EBV-associated diseases reflects the general prevalence in the areas involved (Gratama and Ernberg, 1995). Thus, there seems to be no clear association between the two types and specific diseases.

In most areas recovery of type 2 is unusual, except in immunodeficient (HIV+ individuals and transplant recipients) carriers. The increased detection in immunodeficent individuals has been explained by an increased exposure to exogenous virus combined with deficient EBV-specific cellular immunity, leading to long-term carriage of multiple EBV genotypes (Gratama and Ernberg, 1995). The frequency of the type 2 genotype in HIV-positive haemophiliacs is comparable to the frequency in healthy individuals, which indicates that the immunodefiency *per se* is not responsible for increased type 2 detection (Yao et al., 1998).

The distribution of specific DNA sequence polymorphisms also shows geographic variation, with the epidemiology of the EBV-encoded oncogene LMP-1 being the most thoroughly studied. Numerous sequence variations have been identified in LMP-1 genes from different EBV isolates, some of which have been associated with an increased risk of nasopharyngeal carcinoma (Jeng et al., 1994).

Table 53.1. Distribution of EBV types 1 and 2 in various clinical conditions and among healthy patients. (Partly reproduced from Gratama and Ernberg, 1995 with permission from Elsevier.)

Country	Patients	N	Type 1 (%)	Type 2 (%)	Both types (%)
China (Hu et al., 1991)	Nasopharyngeal carcinoma	37	86	14	0
Taiwan (Shu et al., 1992)	Nasopharyngeal carcinoma	53	94	4	2
Korea (Kim et al., 2002)	Healthy	26	81	15	4
Japan (Kunimoto et al., 1992)	Healthy	21	95	5	0
USA (Frank et al., 1995)	Post-transplant lymphoproliferative disease	24	100	0	0
USA (Goldschmidts et al., 1992)	HIV-positive	22	55	45	0
Alaska (Abdel-Hamid et al., 1992)	Nasopharyngeal carcinoma	3	0	100	0
Argentina (Correa et al., 2004)	Healthy	183	78	15	7
Brasil (Klumb et al., 2004)	Burkitt's lymphoma	21	86	14	0
Central Africa (Goldschmidts et al., 1992)	Burkitt's lymphoma	16	50	50	0
Papua New Guinea (Aitken et al., 1994)	Burkitt's lymphoma	56	42	53	5
Western Europe (Sandvej et al., 1994)	Hodgkin's disease	55	93	5	1
Australia (Kyaw et al., 1992)	HIV-positive	56	27	30	43
Australia (Kyaw et al., 1992)	Cardiac transplants	18	39	33	28

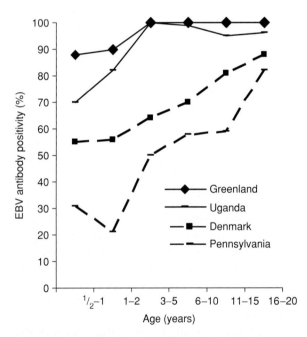

Fig. 53.1. Age-specific distribution of EBV antibody positive individuals in four populations. Reproduced from de The et al., 1975; Henle and Henle, 1967; Melbye et al., 1984.

Studies indicate that LMP-1 sequence variants from nasopharyngeal carcinoma high-incidence areas in Southeast Asia have evolved distinct from LMP-1 variants in nasopharyngeal carcinoma low-incidence areas such as areas of Australia, Papua New Guinea, and Africa (Burrows et al., 2004) suggesting that positive selection pressure on the LMP-1 sequences may enhance the oncogenic potential of virus isolates from nasopharyngeal carcinoma endemic areas.

Sex differences

There is no consistent difference in EBV seroprevalence by sex in children (Golubjatnikov 1973; Lang et al., 1977; Sumaya et al., 1975). In developed countries, this similarity continues into early adolescence, when a higher seroprevalence and an earlier occurrence of infectious mononucleosis among girls indicate earlier exposure to the virus (Crawford et al., 2002).

Generally, antibody titers seem to be higher in females than in males (Biggar et al., 1981; Levine et al., 1982; Wagner et al., 1994). This difference, which also has been observed for other viruses, is in accordance with the notion that women in general mount more vigorous antibody- and cell-mediated immune response following infection or vaccination than men (Beagley and Gockel, 2003).

Socioeconomic factors

Poor socioeconomic conditions have been associated with early primary EBV infection, whereas late primary EBV infection is seen in populations of high socioeconomic status. Based on father's education and the family's living conditions, Henle and colleagues documented a seroprevalence of 60% among young American school children (aged 5 to 10 years) of low socioeconomic status compared to less than 20% in children with high socioeconomic level (Henle et al., 1969). Low income and crowded family conditions have also been found to increase the likelihood of being EBV seropositive in children from other geographical locales, such as Thailand (Mekmullica et al., 2003), Turkey (Ozkan et al., 2003), Ghana (Biggar et al., 1978) and Denmark (Hesse et al., 1983). In an early work by Lang and colleagues (Lang et al., 1977) three genetically different Melanesian populations with differences in living conditions and social patterns were found to have similar patterns of early EBV infection. In all three populations the mothers chew the food before feeding the children. Thus, exposure to saliva either directly or via for example unclean toys are believed to explain differences in socioeconomic conditions. This is in line with the observation that socioeconomic associated differences in sero-prevalence are greatly diminished in age groups who have become sexually active.

Genetic and racial factors

Differences in prevalence and more generally the infection patterns have never been clearly associated with race, but merely seen as differences in socioeconomic, hygienic, and cultural behavior. The high prevalence of EBV infection in populations around the world would indicate that the influence of host-specific characteristics on natural resistance to EBV infection is limited. Yet, the distinct distribution of nasopharyngeal carcinoma (NPC) with high incidence figures observed in Inuits from the Arctic and in South-East Asian populations suggests the existence of a particular immunologic control of EBV in these ethnicities, though the exact mechanism remains to be described (Hildesheim et al., 2002; Yu and Yuan, 2002). Supportive of a genetically determined response to the EBV carrier state is the finding among Greenlandic Inuits of remarkably high titers throughout life of IgG antibodies to EBV-VCA (Melbye et al., 1984a,b).

Transmission

Most frequently, EBV transmission takes place through oropharyngeal secretion. In adolescent and adult cases of IM intimate kissing has been the main route of transmission whereas saliva on, for example, toys and fingers is believed to be major routes of transmission among smaller children. However, 40 years into the discovery of EBV we still need data to better explain the exact determinants of infection. Among EBV seronegative adults, close contact with IM cases (Sawyer et al., 1971), or longer stays together with seropositive persons in a restricted space (Storrie and Sphar, 1976) only infrequently leads to secondary cases. On the contrary, EBV infection frequently takes place among smaller children of low socioeconomic status, in nurseries (Chang et al., 1981) and when sharing a room (Crawford et al., 2002).

Shedding of EBV in saliva among seropositive individuals ranges from 22% to 90% (Apolloni and Sculley, 1994; Haque and Crawford, 1997; Ikuta et al., 2000; Sixbey et al., 1984; Yao et al., 1991). Ling and colleagues observed that shedding of EBV in saliva among adults at any given time over a 12 months period varies between 32% and 73% (Ling et al., 2003). These and other authors were unable to detect any correlation between viral shedding frequency or viral load in saliva and the presence of EBV in PBMCs (Haque and Crawford, 1997; Ling et al., 2003), suggesting that the factors responsible for EBV reactivation in the oropharynx are different from those governing viral load in the blood.

EBV has been detected in cervical secretions in between 8 and 28% of teenage girls and adult women, and in semen samples and samples scraped from the penile sulcus of men (Enbom et al., 2001; Israele et al., 1991; Kapranos et al., 2003; Naher et al., 1992), but evidence on whether EBV is transmitted through genital contact is limited. A recent study found EBV type 2 among homosexual men to be significantly more prevalent than among heterosexual men and to be correlated with the number of sexual partners (van B. D. et al., 2000). However, the exact mode of transmission in these studies remains unknown since it is difficult to distinguish between genital transmission, orogenital contact and kissing.

Transplacental transmission and transmission through breast milk have been reported in rare circumstances, but are considered non-significant modes of transmission (Fleisher and Bologonese, 1984; Kusuhara et al., 1997; Meyohas et al., 1996). EBV may be spread through blood transfusion and as a result of organ transplantation (Alfieri et al., 1996; Scheenstra et al., 2004). One transfusion unit of erythrocytes contains an average of two EBV genomes, in contrast to a whole blood unit which harbored on average 600 to 700 EBV genomes (Wagner et al., 1995). Transmission is of particular concern in association with organ transplantations where primary EBV infection is a major risk factor for post-transplant lymphoproliferative disease (PTLD) (Aguilar et al., 1999; Bodeus et al., 1999; Scheenstra et al., 2004).

EBV viral load epidemiology

During the recent decade, methods for detecting and quantifying cellular and extracellular EBV in peripheral blood have improved significantly. Initially applicable only to small series of patients, modern techniques such as real-time PCR have now made large studies feasible. However, the majority of these have been performed to investigate EBV viral loads in specific diseases, and knowledge on EBV viral load in healthy individuals has mainly been generated from the control groups, rarely selected randomly from the population.

EBV viral load in peripheral blood mononuclear cells (PBMCs) is the combined result of the number of infected B cells and the number of EBV genomes per B-cell. A roughly constant number of infected B cells (1–50 *per* 1,000,000) is present in peripheral blood in the healthy latently infected host, but the number seems to vary considerably between individuals (Khan *et al.*, 1996). Differences in detection methods, sample preparation and measurement units make comparisons of EBV viral loads from different studies difficult. But the EBV viral load appears to be transiently elevated at the time of primary EBV infection (Fan and Gulley, 2001). In general, the viral load observed in PBMCs from healthy individuals is low (<100 DNA genome copies *per* ug DNA) compared to the high EBV loads observed in some EBV-associated diseases (ex. post-transplant lymphoproliferative disease (PTLD)) (Stevens *et al.*, 2002a,b). The low EBV viral loads in most healthy EBV-infected individuals reflect the low frequency of EBV-positive B cells in the circulation, whereas the high EBV loads observed during PTLD and immune suppression are the result of increased numbers of EBV infected B cells (Babcock *et al.*, 1999; Yang *et al.*, 2000), together with an increased number of EBV genomes in some of the infected B cells (Rose *et al.*, 2002). However, EBV viral load in PBMCs in the single healthy individual does not appear to be static. As healthy individuals are followed over time, short episodes of increased viral load can be observed, suggestive of EBV reactivation (Maurmann *et al.*, 2003), and measurement of EBV viral load in PBMCs and plasma seem to detect episodes of EBV reactivation earlier and with greater sensitivity than the traditional serological methods (Figure 53.2). EBV detection in whole blood and serum/plasma is becoming the 'gold standard' and most commonly utilized test, as it is less laborious and more reproducible than PBMCs.

The correlation between EBV viral load in PBMCs and serological response is not obvious (Gartner *et al.*, 2000). Increased anti-p18-VCA, suggestive of lytic viral replication, and decreased anti-EBNA-1 IgG levels has been associated with high EBV loads in HIV carriers (Stevens *et al.*, 2002a,b).

EBV in plasma or serum, which is frequently detected in patients with nasopharyngeal carcinoma or PTLD, is only rarely detected in healthy individuals, although EBV viremia can be detected in association to episodes of EBV reactivation (Lechowicz *et al.*, 2002;).

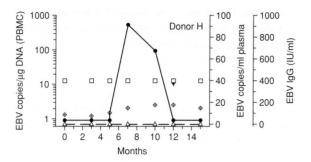

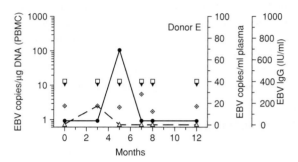

Fig. 53.2. Healthy individuals with serological evidence of EBV reactivation during 15 months of follow-up. -•- viral load (PBMC), -△- Viremia (plasma), ◇ EBV IgG (IU/ml). Partly reproduced from Maurmann *et al.*, 2003.

Infectious mononucleosis

Primary EBV infection is usually considered asymptomatic when occurring in infants and small children, and most of the knowledge on primary infection is derived from studies of adolescent patients with infectious mononucleosis. However, the assumption that primary EBV infection in childhood is always subclinical is probably fallacious, as when looked for, infectious mononucleosis symptoms may also occur in infants in association with primary EBV infection (Chan *et al.*, 2003). Although symptoms may be milder, primary infection in infants is not presumed to be fundamentally different from the characteristic picture of infectious mononucleosis (IARC, 1997).

Primary EBV infection in adolescence causes infectious mononucleosis in more than half of the infected individuals. Symptoms of infectious mononucleosis (glandular fever) commence after an incubation period of 4–7 weeks, and typically (in more than 50%) include fever, lymphadenopathy and pharyngitis (Chang, 1980).

Confirmation of the diagnosis has traditionally been based on the detection of heterophil antibodies, which are present in 86% of adolescents and adults with infectious mononucleosis (Fleisher *et al.*, 1983), but less frequently in acutely infected small children (Chan *et al.*, 1998). However,

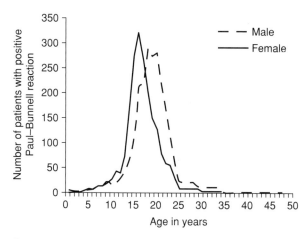

Fig. 53.3. Age-and sex-specific distribution of positive Paul–Bunnell reactions at Statens Serum Institut in Denmark 1965–1969. Reproduced from Rosdahl et al., 1973 with permission from Taylor & Francis Scandinavia.

positive detection of heterophil antibodies can occur in other conditions, including HIV infection, Systemic Lupus Erythematosus, and other viral diseases (Hendry and Longmore, 1993; Horwitz et al., 1979; Macsween and Crawford 2003). Detection of IgM to the viral capsid antigen (VCA) is both more sensitive and specific, and is present at time of onset of clinical symptoms. Both heterophil antibodies and anti-VCA IgM are transient and disappears within months, and detection of EBV-DNA in serum might be useful as a supplement to serology for the diagnosis (Chan et al., 2001).

Epidemiology

The majority of infectious mononucleosis patients are not hospitalized, but reliable data on the population incidence is available from sentinel systems, centralized laboratories or from areas where infectious mononucleosis is a reportable disease. Incidence rates between 60–100 *per* 100,000 person-years in Caucasian populations seem consistent (Evans et al., 1997; Morris and Edmunds, 2002; Rosdahl et al., 1973). In these populations the incidence of infectious mononucleosis increases from the age of 2–4 years to reach a maximum in adolescence and early adulthood, after which the disease incidence decreases, to become rare after 40 years of age (Figure 53.3) (Auwaerter, 1999; Rosdahl et al., 1973). The age-specific distribution of cases reflects the clinical disease ratio of primary EBV infection which is low in children, and may reach 74% among college students (Sawyer et al., 1971). The low incidence among older adults reflects the low number of EBV-uninfected individuals. There seems to be no seasonal variation in incidence rates.

Table 53.2. Factors influencing the development of infectious mononucleosis

EBV immune status
Age at time of infection
IL-10 polymorphisms

The difference in infectious mononucleosis incidence rates between ethnic groups within the same region, probably reflects variation in social and economic factors, influencing age at primary infection (Heath et al., 1972; Melbye et al., 1984a,b), and there is no evidence of racial differences in infectious mononucleosis susceptibility.

Risk factors for infectious mononucleosis

The factors influencing clinical disease are summarized in Table 53.2.

The marked difference in infectious mononucleosis incidence in comparable settings with an equal number of susceptible individuals, indicates that determinants other than immune status and age at infection are involved. As intimate contact appears to account for most cases of infectious mononucleosis (Crawford et al., 2002), age-specific incidence of infectious mononucleosis in otherwise comparable settings can differ due to behavioural differences.

In children, carriage of the ATA haplotype in the promoter of interleukin (IL)-10, is associated with high levels of spontaneous IL-10 and a late age of primary EBV infection. Thus, the ATA haplotype may increase the age at primary infection and perhaps also the risk of symptomatic disease (Helminen et al., 2001).

Studies on HLA-alleles and infectious mononucleosis have produced conflicting results. A higher frequency of HLA-B-3501 among infectious mononucleosis cases compared to controls has been reported, however, the association between infectious mononucleosis, HLA-B-3501 and other HLA-alleles has not been reproduced in other populations (Chang, 1980).

Viral factors, including EBV strain variation, have not been associated with a different ability to cause infectious mononucleosis.

EBV dynamics during infectious mononucleosis

In healthy seropositive individuals EBV DNA in serum is only occasionally detected, but in the acute phase of infectious mononucleosis high loads of EBV DNA in serum is

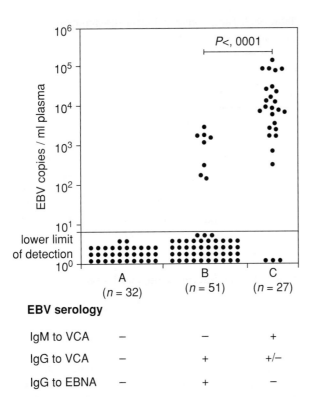

Fig. 53.4. EBV DNA levels in sera from individuals with different EBV-antibody patterns. A: sero-negative, B: sero-positive, C: acute EBV-infection. Reproduced from Berger et al., 2001 with permission from John Wiley & Sons, Inc.

Table 53.3. Proposed guidelines for diagnosing CAEBV (all conditions must be fulfilled). Adapted from Okano et al., 2005 with permission from John Wiley & Sons, Inc.

I. Persistent or recurrent infectious mononucleosis-like symptoms
II. Unusual pattern of anti-EBV antibodies with raised anti-VCA and anti-EA, and/or detection of increased EBV genomes in affected tissue, including the peripheral blood
III. Chronic illness which cannot be explained by other known disease processes at diagnosis*

* EBV-associated diseases such as hemophagocytic lymphohistiocytosis or lymphomas mainly derived from T-cells or NK-cells often develop during the course of illness.

present in most patients (Fig. 53.4) (Berger et al., 2001). The peak in serum viral load is observed in the first seven days of disease, thereafter viral load decreases with resolution of symptoms, although there seem to be considerable inter-individual differences in the decline (Berger et al., 2001). Parallel with the increase in serum viral load, the EBV viral load in peripheral blood mononuclear cells (PBMC) increase to a maximum within the first weeks of the disease, and thereafter declines (Kimura et al., 1999). However, sustained high levels of EBV DNA is found in saliva for at least 6 months after onset of clinical disease, associated with persistent infectivity of saliva (Fafi-Kremer et al., 2005).

Despite the lack of massive expansion in numbers of T lymphocytes in asymptomatic primary EBV infection, both patients with IM and asymptomatic primary infection have similar high EBV viral loads in PBMC. Thus the large T cell expansion seen in IM patients may represent an overreaction, not associated with the control of the primary EBV infection (Silins et al., 2001).

Studies on EBV viral load in primary infection have focused on the time around the infection, and the importance of early versus delayed primary EBV infection on long-term EBV viral load is unknown.

Chronic active EBV infection

Chronic active EBV infection (CAEBV) was first described in the late 1970s, and is characterized by chronic or recurrent infectious mononucleosis-like symptoms and by an unusual pattern of EBV antibodies. Criteria's for diagnosing CAEBV has been suggested earlier, and recently a new set of guidelines has been proposed (Table 53.3) (Okano, et al., 2005; Straus, 1988).

The antibody pattern resembles acute infection and is characterized by high titers of IgG-VCA and IgG-EA, and absence of EBNA antibodies. Patients with CAEBV also have lower frequencies of EBV-specific $CD8^+$ T-cells, compared to infectious mononucleosis patients and healthy individuals (Sugaya et al., 2004). Methods for measuring EBV viral load can be included, as high EBV viral loads in peripheral blood lymphocytes and serum are present (Kimura et al., 2001). There is no known hereditary background, and CAEBV is not associated with mutations in the gene responsible for X-linked lymphoproliferative syndrome (Sumazaki et al., 2001).

CAEBV seem to constitute a disease spectrum with unusual EBV activation, from chronic symptomatic EBV infections with moderately elevated EBV antibodies and a generally good prognosis, to severe chronic active EBV infection with extraordinarily elevated EBV antibodies, clonal expansion of EBV-infected T cells and NK cells, severe clinical and hematological findings, and a generally poor prognosis with high mortality from pancytopenia, lymphoma and hepatic failure (Fig. 53.5) (Kimura et al., 2001; Okano, 2002).

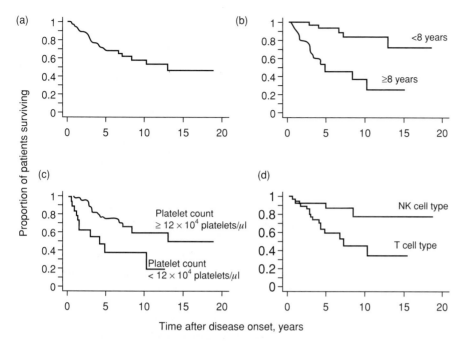

Fig. 53.5. Survival after onset of severe CAEBV. All patients (A), and according to age (B), platelet count (C) and T/NK cell-type of disease (D). Reproduced from (Kimura et al., 2001) with permission from The University of Chicago Press.

Thrombocytopenia and age $> = 8$ years at onset of disease are associated with a poorer outcome (Kimura et al., 2003).

Epidemiology

Studies on CAEBV have been based on case series, and estimates of population incidences are not available. The disease is very rare, and in 2002 a national survey of severe CAEBV in Japan identified 82 patients (Kimura et al., 2003). Mean age at onset of disease in this survey was 11.3 years with men and women equally represented. Many of the studies on CAEBV have originated in Japan, but whether this reflects a true difference in incidence, or an increased awareness is unknown. However, CAEBV in different geographical areas may be of different entities, as CAEBV in Western populations appears to be milder (Savoldo et al., 2002).

X-linked lymphoproliferative syndrome

X-linked lymphoproliferative syndrome (XLP) or Duncan's disease is a rare, primary immunodeficiency that was first described as a familial disorder affecting males with a rapidly fatal course in response to EBV infection (Purtilo et al., 1975). XLP is characterized by three major phenotypes (Table 53.4): fulminant infectious mononucleosis, B cell lymphoma and dysgammaglobulinemia. Occasionally aplastic anemia, vasculitis and pulmonary lymphomatoid granulomatosis are seen (Engel et al., 2003). A patient can develop more than one phenotype.

A lack of immune surveillance of EBV in patients with the infectious mononucleosis phenotype of XLP is assumed, however, the phenotypes with B-cell lymphoma and dysgammaglobulinaemia can be observed in patients with or without signs of previous infection with EBV, suggesting

Table 53.4. Phenotypes of X-linked lymphoproliferative syndrome. Adapted from Engel et al., 2003 with permission from Nature Publishing Group.

Phenotype	Proportion (%)
Fulminant infectious mononucleosis	50
Following infection with Epstein–Barr virus, patients mount a marked polyclonal expansion of B and T cells leading to destruction of the liver and bone marrow	
B-cell lymphoma	30
Extranodal non-Hodgkin's B-cell lymphomas, usually Burkitt's type, most of which involve the ileocecal region of the intestine	
Dysgammaglobulinemia	30
Acquired dysgammaglobulinemia and other abnormalities in immunglobulin synthesis	

Table 53.5. Effect of EBV infection on clinical phenotype in XLP. Adapted from (Sumegi, et al. 2000) with permission from the American Society of Hematology

Phenotype	EBV+ (n = 114)	EBV− (n = 38)	P
Fulminant infectious mononucleosis	70	0	0.0001
Dysgammaglobulinaemia	19	15	0.30
Lymphoproliferative disease	20	21	0.24
Aplastic anemia	5	2	0.03

other antigenic stimuli are also involved in the development of XLP (Table 53.5) (Engel et al., 2003; Sumegi et al., 2000).

Treatment is difficult, haematopoietic stem cell transplantation for fulminant infectious mononucleosis and B-cell lymphomas, and immunoglobulin treatment for agammaglobulinemia has been suggested, but the mortality by the age of 40 years is nearly 100% (Gross et al., 1996; Morra et al., 2001).

The genetic basis for XLP has been identified as an alteration or deletion of the gene SH2D1A, that codes for a cytoplasmatic protein, SAP (SLAM-associated protein, where SLAM is 'signalling lymphocytic activation molecule') (Coffey et al., 1998; Nichols et al., 1998). SAP interacts with several signaling molecules of the SLAM (CD150) family, and is expressed by all T and NK cells. Defective SAP causes selective alterations of the T-/NK-cell function that compromise the ability of these cells to control infection with EBV (Benoit et al., 2000; Engel et al., 2003). Elevated EBV antibody titers are observed in mothers to boys with XLP, although, normal levels of circulating EBV-DNA in XLP patients surviving the initial phase suggest that SAP function is not essential for proper control of EBV replication after primary infection (Sumazaki et al., 2001).

Mutations of SH2D1A are detected in nearly all cases of XLP with a previous family history of XLP, however, mutations of SH2D1A are frequently missing in XLP cases without a family history (Sumegi et al., 2000), although de novo mutations can occur (Sumazaki et al., 2001).

Epidemiology

XLP is estimated to affect approximately 1 in 1,000,000 males (Purtilo et al., 1975). However, this number is likely to be an underestimate, due to the similarity of disease manifestations with other clinically related disorders, such as common variable immunodefiency and the hemophagocytic syndromes (Nichols et al., 2005). The age at onset of clinical disease vary considerably from less than one year to 40 years, with a median of three to eight years (Sumegi et al., 2000). An international XLP registry was established in 1978 and contains over 300 patients from more than 80 families, with up to 17 affected males reported from a single family (Hamilton et al., 1980; Sumegi et al., 2000). XLP patients have been reported from North and South America, Europe and Japan, but it is unknown whether the geographical distribution reflects true differences in incidence or differences in awareness.

Epstein–Barr virus and malignant neoplasms

EBV has been implicated in the development of a wide variety of benign and malignant diseases (Table 53.6). In the following, only the virus' association with malignant diseases will be described. Accordingly, the association between EBV and autoimmune conditions such as multiple sclerosis (Wekerle and Hohlfeld, 2003) or systemic lupus erythematosus (Kang et al., 2004), or immune deficiency-related conditions, such as oral hairy leukoplakia (Niedobitek et al., 1991) and lymphoid interstitial pneumonitis (Swigris et al., 2002) will not be discussed. Focus will be on the main characteristics of EBV-associated cancers and on the evidence linking them with the virus. Nasopharyngeal carcinoma, Burkitt's lymphoma, and Hodgkin's lymphoma will be described in some detail, whereas the association between EBV and other malignant disorders are described more cursorily.

Nasopharyngeal carcinoma

Nasopharyngeal carcinoma is derived from the epithelial lining of the nasopharynx. It typically develops in the lymphoreticular tissue rich area in the fossa of Rosenmüller, and less frequently in the roof and wall of the nasopharynx (IARC, 1997). Histopathologically, two major groups of nasopharyngeal carcinomas are recognized, i.e. keratinizing squamous cell carcinoma (WHO type I), and nonkeratinizing carcinoma, the latter being further split up into differentiated (WHO type II) and undifferentiated carcinomas (WHO type III) (Shanmugaratnam, 1991).

Epidemiology

The occurrence of nasopharyngeal carcinoma is characterized by a remarkable geographical and ethnic variation as reflected in the combined occurrence of all types of cancer in the nusopharynx (Table 53.7). (Yu and Yuan, 2002). The

Table 53.6. Evidence for an association between different types of cancer and EBV. Adapted from Hsu and Glaser, 2000

Malignancy	Lines of evidence
Nasopharyngeal carcinoma	• Elevated anti-EBV antibody titers preceding and at diagnosis • Elevated levels of free EBV DNA at diagnosis • Correlation between anti-EBV antibodies and free virus DNA in plasma, and tumor burden and prognosis • Demonstration of monoclonal EBV in tumor cells
Lymphomas Burkitt's lymphoma variants	• Elevated anti-EBV antibody titers preceding and at diagnosis • Demonstration of monoclonal EBV in tumor cells • Increased occurrence in immune suppressed patients
AIDS associated lymphoma [other than Burkitt' lymphoma	• Increased occurrence compared with general population • Overall risk correlates with immune function • Demonstration of monoclonal EBV in malignant cells
Post-transplant lymphoma	• Increased occurrence compared with general population • Overall risk correlates with immune function • Demonstration of monoclonal EBV in malignant cells
Nasal T/NK lymphoma	• Demonstration of monoclonal EBV in tumor cells
Hodgkin's lymphoma	• Increased risk in infectious mononucleosis patients • Increased risk in immune suppression • Elevated anti-EBV antibody titres preceding and at diagnosis • Demonstration of mononclonal EBV in malignant cells
Gastric adenocarcinoma	• Elevated anti-EBV antibody titers preceding and at diagnosis • Demonstration of monoclonal EBV in tumor cells
Lymphoepithelioma-like carcinoma Leiomyosarcoma	• Demonstration of monoclonal EBV in malignant cells • Increased risk with immunosuppression • Demonstration of mononclonal EBV in malignant cells

tumor is quite rare in most Western countries with incidence rates less than 1 per 100 000 persons per year, as is it indeed in most parts of the world, but high incidence rates are observed in certain ethnic populations in South-East Asia and North Africa and in the circumpolar indigenous populations (Table 53.7). Common to both low-and high incidence areas, nasopharyngeal carcinoma is seen two-to-three times more often in men than in women (Table 53.7). Different age-specific incidence patterns are observed in endemic and non-endemic regions (Parkin *et al.*, 2002; Lee *et al.*, 2003; Yu and Yuan, 2002): In non-endemic regions nasopharyngeal carcinoma occurrence increases continuously with age, whereas in endemic regions the incidence increases with age to peak around the age of 50 years and decrease thereafter. A third bimodal age pattern with a minor incidence peak in adolescents and young adults has been described in some populations with low to intermediate nasopharyngeal carcinoma incidence (Yu and Yuan, 2002; Daoud *et al.*, 2003).

Even within regions where nasopharyngeal carcinoma is endemic considerable variation in disease occurrence can be observed between different ethnic subpopulations. For instance, in the Chinese province of Guangdong the incidence of nasopharyngeal carcinoma is twice as high in Cantonese as in other ethnic groups (Li *et al.*, 1985; Yu *et al.*, 1981; Yu and Yuan, 2002). Familial clustering of nasopharyngeal carcinoma and other cancers is well-established from a plethora of case-reports (Zeng and Jia, 2002). The familial accumulation in turn translates into increased risks for nasopharyngeal carcinomas, e.g., first degree-relatives of Greenlandic Inuits with nasopharyngeal carcinoma have an eight-fold higher risk of the tumor than the general population (Friborg *et al.*, 2005). Epidemiologically, these observations may indicate a genetic predisposition to nasopharyngeal carcinoma, a suspicion that has been supported by genetic studies. Specifically, a meta-analysis of published data for Chinese patients showed increased risk for HLA alleles A2, B14, B46, and decreased

Table 53.7. Incidence rates for nasopharyngeal cancer (all types combined) in different regions. Adapted from Yu and Yuan, 2002 and updated from Parkin, et al., 2002. Data for Greenland from Friborg et al., 2003

Population	Age-standardized (world) incidence rates (per 100,000)		Calendar period
	Males	Females	
Chinese, Hong Kong	21.4	8.3	1993 to 1997
Chinese, Tapei	8.9	3.4	1997
Chinese, Shanghai	4.2	1.5	1993 to 1997
Chinese, Tianjin	1.7	0.5	1993 to 1997
Inuits, Greenland	10.3	8.0	1988 to 1997
Inuits, Athabascans, and Aleuts, Alaska	11.9	5.6	1980 to 1987
Thais, Chiang Mai	3.2	1.3	1993 to 1997
Vietnamese, Hanoi	10.4	4.6	1993 to 1997
Malays, Singapore	6.8	2.0	1993 to 1997
Filipinos, Manila	7.2	2.5	1993 to 1997
Kuwaits, Kuwait	2.6	0.9	1994 to 1997
Algerians, Setif	8.0	2.7	1990 to 1993
Israeli Jews born in Morocco, Algeria or Tunisia	2.8	1.3	1961 to 1981
U.S. Whites (SEER)	0.5	0.2	1993 to 1997

risks for HLA alleles A11, B13 and B22 (Goldsmith et al., 2002). Moreover, susceptibility *loci* have been reported on chromosomes 3 (Xiong et al., 2004), 4 (Feng et al., 2002), 14 [Diehl et al., unpublished observations quoted in (Pickard et al., 2004)] and near the HLA-locus (Lu et al., 1990). Polymorphisms in genes coding for certain enzymes involved in nitrosamine metabolism [Gluthathione S-transferase M1 and cytochrome P450 2E1] also have been reported to correlate with risk for nasopharyngeal carcinoma [reviewed by (Zeng and Jia, 2002; Hildesheim et al., 1997)].

There is good evidence, however, that environmental factors are also significant to the risk of nasopharyngeal carcinoma. Accordingly studies of families emigrating from high to low risk regions have shown that the risk of nasopharyngeal carcinomas decreases between successive generations (IARC, 1997). Among environmental factors, the evidence is particularly strong against certain diets including Cantonese-style salted fish and other preserved foods (for review, see IARC, 1997). Accordingly, a high intake of preserved foods is a common characteristic of the populations where nasopharyngeal carcinoma is endemic, and case-control studies in endemic as well as non-endemic regions have demonstrated an association between intake of such food items and nasopharyngeal carcinoma risk.

Moreover, the risk for nasopharyngeal carcinomas seems to be inversely correlated with the age of first exposure. Consistent with the role of diet, the incidence of nasopharyngeal carcinoma in Hong Kong has decreased over the last decades concomitantly with changes in lifestyle towards a western-world pattern (Lee et al., 2003). Other suggested risk factors have included low socioeconomic status (possibly correlated with high intake of preserved food items), tobacco, and alcohol, and occupational exposure to formaldehyde and wood dust (Hildesheim et al., 2001; IARC, 1997).

It is noteworthy that the association between preserved food and risk for nasopharyngeal carcinoma gains biological plausibility in the context of the familial accumulation of the tumor and its association with EBV. Accordingly, the preserved foods contain carcinogenic nitrosamines, as well as EBV-activating substances (IARC, 1997).

Evidence of association with EBV

Infection with EBV has been implicated in the development of nasopharyngeal carcinoma by several different lines of evidence (Table 53.6). Historically, the first indication was the observation that sera from African and American patients with nasopharyngeal carcihoma were often more positive for precipitating antibodies to antigens prepared from cultured Burkitt's lymphoma cells than controls (Old et al., 1966). This observation has since been confirmed in serological studies showing elevated titers of IgG and in particular IgA antibodies against EBV viral capsid, early and nuclear antigens in nasopharyngeal carcinoma patients data being less compelling for type I than types II and III, manifesting as apparent ethnic variations (IARC, 1997; Raab-Traub, 2000). Antibody titers correlate with stage of disease and has been shown to return to normal levels in long-term disease-free survivors (Yu and Henderson, 2004). More compelling than the sero-prevalence surveys in patients are, however, the results of a prospective study of 9699 persons which showed that presence of IgA anti-EBV viral capsid antigen antibodies or neutralising EBV specific anti-DNase antibodies correlated with subsequent risk for nasopharyngeal carcinoma (Fig. 53.6) (Chien et al., 2001).

The serological findings are corroborated by the demonstration of monoclonal EBV in the malignant nasopharyngeal carcinoma cells (Raab-Traub and Flynn, 1986). This line of evidence is most consistent for nasopharyngeal carcinoma types II and III, but the virus has also been demonstrated in type I carcinomas (Nicholls et al., 1997; Raab-Traub, 2000). Consistent with the assumption of a causal role for the virus in development of the tumor, monoclonal

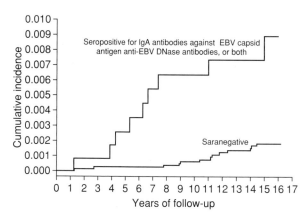

Fig. 53.6. Cumulative incidence of nasopharyngeal carcinoma in persons testing positive or negative for either IgA anti-Epstein–Barr virus viral capsid or neutralizing anti-Epstein–Barr virus DNase antibodies. Reproduced from Chien et al., 2001 with permission from the Massachusetts Medical Society.

EBV has also been demonstrated in pre-invasive dysplastic and carcinoma *in situ* lesions (Pathmanathan et al., 1995) as has the virus been demonstrated in nasopharyngeal carcinoma metastases (Lee et al., 2000).

More recently, the detection and quantification of circulating EBV DNA have attracted interest. In one study, such DNA was demonstrated in 96% of patients with nasopharyngeal carcinoma as compared with only in 7% of controls, and levels of DNA moreover correlated with disease stage (Figure 53.7) (Lo et al., 1999) and, independently hereof, also with prognosis (Lo et al., 2000; Lin et al., 2004).

Tumors of the lymphoid tissues

The tumors of the lymphoid tissues constitute a clinically and epidemiologically heterogeneous group of malignancies with the common characteristic that they are derived from cells belonging to the lymphoid lineage. Three major categories of lymphoid malignancies are recognized today, i.e. B-cell lymphomas, T and NK-cell lymphomas, and Hodgkin's lymphomas (Harris et al., 2001a,b). Within each of these categories, distinct disease entities are recognised based on morphologic, immunophenotypic, genetic and clinical characteristics.

The occurrence of non-Hodgkin's lymphoma generally increases with age and overall lymphomas are more often seen in men than in women with a male : female incidence ratio of 1.5–2:1 (Parkin et al., 2002). Incidence rates vary internationally, age-standardized (world) rates ranging from typically 3–8 and 2–6 per 100 000 Asian men and women to 10–15 and 5–10 per 100 000 in European men and women (IARC, 2002). An as yet unexplained remark-

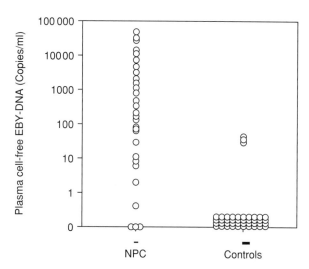

Fig. 53.7. Comparison of plasma cell-free EBV DNA in NPC patients and control subjects. The categories (NPC patients and control subjects) are plotted on the X-axis. The Y-axis denotes the concentration of cell-free EBV DNA (copies of EBV DNA/ml of plasma) detected by the BamHI-W region PCR system. Reproduced from (Lo et al., 1999) with permission from the American Association for Cancer Research.

able increase in the incidence of all types of non-Hodgkin' lymphomas combined was apparent in the latter half of the twentieth century in most regions of the world, amounting to 3%–4% increase annually (Devesa and Fears, 1992). Recent data from Scandinavia suggest that the increase has just as inexplicably begun to subside (Sandin et al., 2006).

Relatively few risk factors have been established for non-Hodgkin's lymphomas (Scherr and Mueller, 1996; Grulich and Vajdic, 2005; Ekstrom-Smedby, 2006). In part, this may reflects that the composite nature of the malignant lymphomas including possible etiological heterogeneity has not always been taken into consideration previously. The most consistently observed risk factor is immune suppression, primary as well as acquired. Other risk factors include familial aggregation (Chang et al., 2005; Goldin et al., 2005), autoimmune conditions (Zintzaras et al., 2005) and exposure to certain hair dyes (Takkouche et al., 2005) and herbicides (Fritschi et al., 2005; Scherr and Mueller, 1996). Several infectious organisms are known or suspected to be etiologically linked to lymphoma development including both bacteria, e.g., *Helicobacter pylori* (Wotherspoon et al., 1991), *Borrelia burgdorferi* (Cerroni et al., 1997), *Campylobacter jejuni* (Lecuit et al., 2004), *Chlamydia psittaci* (Ferreri et al., 2004) and viruses, e.g., human herpesvirus-8 (Cesarman et al., 1995), human T-cell lymphotropic virus type I (Hinuma et al., 1981), hepatis C virus (Pozzato et al., 1994), and EBV (Epstein et al., 1964).

The evidence for an association with EBV infection is the strongest for Burkitt's lymphomas, NK/T-cell lymphomas of the nasal cavity, for malignant lymphomas in immune incompetent patients, and for a subset of Hodgkin's lymphomas. The virus may, however, also be encountered in other types of malignant lymphomas, though less regularly (IARC, 1997). It is noteworthy, therefore, that in a prospective serological investigation elevated IgG ($\geq$ 1:320) and IgM ($\geq$ 1:5) titres of anti-viral capsid antigen antibodies were associated with 2.5-(IgG) and 3.2-fold (IgM) increased risks for non-Hodgkin's lymphoma overall with no apparent difference between different lymphoma subtypes (Mueller et al., 1991).

Burkitt's lymphoma/leukemia
Burkitt's lymphoma is a highly aggressive lymphoma that often presents extranodally or as acute leukemia (Diebold et al., 2001). The presumed cell of origin is a germinal centre B-cell. Based on clinical and epidemiological characteristics, three variants of Burkitt's lymphoma are recognized, i.e., endemic, sporadic, and immunodeficiency-associated Burkitt's lymphoma. Histologically, the tumor is generally characterized by monomorphic cytoarchitecture composed of medium-sized B cells with basophilic cytoplasm and numerous mitotic figures with variations between the tumor variants. A constant feature shared by all Burkitt's lymphoma variants is chromosomal translocations involving the MYC oncogene on chromosome 8 (i.e., either t(8:14), t(2:8) or t(8:22) (Diebold et al., 2001)).

Epidemiology of endemic Burkitt's lymphoma
The endemic variant of Burkitt's lymphoma is primarily a childhood malignancy seen in Papua, New Guinea and in equatorial Africa, where in certain areas it is the most common childhood cancer (van den Bosch, 2004). The tumor occurs two-to-three times as often in boys as in girls and in both genders the incidence of endemic Burkitt's lymphoma peaks at ages 5–9 years (Diebold et al., 2001). Precise incidence rates are difficult to obtain, but data suggest crude incidence rates of 4.6 and 2.9 per 100 000 in Ugandan boys and girls < 15 years (IARC, 2002).

One of the most striking characteristics of endemic Burkitt's lymphoma is the correspondence between its geographical distribution and measures of prevalence of malaria infection, a correlation that is apparent both between and within regions and over time (IARC, 1997). Moreover, the peak ages for endemic Burkitt's lymphoma is also the age interval during which anti-malarial antibodies peak (IARC, 1997). These ecological similarities have been interpreted as reflecting a role for malarial infection in development of endemic Burkitt's lymphoma, as discussed below. Other suspected risk factors, the effects of which are also related to EBV infection, are certain groups of plants used in traditional medicine that may stimulate viral replication. The direct evidence of the role of such is, however, limited (IARC, 1997).

Epidemiology of sporadic Burkitt's lymphoma
Sporadic Burkitt's lymphoma occurs predominantly in children and young adults, and is seen throughout the world (Diebold et al., 2001). The tumor make up a few percent of all lymphomas in industrialized countries, but constitutes up to 50% of all lymphomas in children (Diebold et al., 2001). Like the endemic variant, sporadic Burkitt's lymphoma is seen two-to-three times as often in males as in females. Generally, the incidence of sporadic Burkitt's lymphoma is much lower than that of the endemic variant, e.g., rates of 0.38 and 0.08 per 100 000 are observed in white US boys and girls <15 years (Parkin, 2002). Familial accumulation of the lymphoma has been reported in a few instances, but otherwise few risk factors have been established (IARC, 1997).

Epidemiology of AIDS-related Burkitt's lymphoma
Burkitt's lymphoma frequently is the AIDS defining malignancy in HIV-infected patients (Diebold et al., 2001). The tumor and its association with EBV are described later. Burkitt's lymphoma is also seen in organ transplant recipients.

Evidence of association with EBV
EBV was originally identified in an endemic Burkitt's lymphoma cell culture (Epstein et al., 1964), and of the three lymphoma variants, the endemic type has remained the most strongly associated with the virus. The evidence of an association between Burkitt's lymphoma and EBV includes both serological and molecular biological studies (Table 53.6).

An early classical paper describes a prospective serological investigation set in the Uganda West Nile District, where Burkitt's lymphoma is endemic. Based on an initial collection of blood samples from nearly 42 000 healthy children, children who subsequently developed Burkitt's lymphoma displayed statistically significantly higher titres of antiviral capsid antigen antibodies than their peers, who remained healthy (geometric mean titre 425.5 vs. 125.8). No differences were observed between the two groups of children for anti-early antigen or anti-EBV nuclear antigen antibodies (de-Thé et al., 1978). In a later update of the study, each twofold dilution of antiviral capsid antigen antibody titer was associated with a five-fold in Burkitt's lymphoma risk overall and a nine-fold increased risk of EBV-positive lymphomas (Geser et al., 1982).

Employing different serological techniques, studies have suggested that African Burkitt's lymphoma patients are more often infected with EBV than their peers and also display higher anti-EBV antibody titres (IARC, 1997). Similar patterns have also been observed in sporadic Burkitt's lymphoma patients, in particular children, though with less striking differences vis à vis controls (IARC, 1997).

Large case-series have since the original observation confirmed the presence of EBV in endemic Burkitt's lymphoma cells. Accordingly, virus has been demonstrated in more than 95% of investigated endemic Burkitt's lymphoma cases (IARC, 1997). In contrast, the prevalence of EBV in sporadic Burkitt's lymphoma in general appears to be less than 30% (IARC, 1997; Diebold et al., 2001), albeit with considerable variation in reported estimates ranging between 15 and 88% (Hsu and Glaser, 2000). In AIDS-related Burkitt's lymphoma, the prevalence of EBV is 25 to 50% (Diebold et al., 2001; Raphael et al., 2001).

The mechanism by which EBV contributes to the development of Burkitt's lymphoma is not entirely understood, but the virus's absence in many cases either suggests that it is neither sufficient nor necessary for the tumor to develop or, alternatively, that EBV-positive and -negative tumors are different biological entities (Bellan et al., 2005). For EBV positive tumors, age at infection with the virus and the ability to control infected cells seem critical (Mueller et al., 1996). For endemic Burkitt's lymphoma it has been suggested that early EBV infection may lead to transformation and replication of a large subset of B-lymphocytes. This process in turn may be augmented by recurrent malaria infections that act both as B-cell mitogen and T-cell suppressant. Translocation involving chromosome 8 may then result from the increased cell replication (Klein, 1979; de The, 2000). Some support for the interaction between malaria and EBV comes from studies showing that the number of EBV infected cells is higher during acute malaria than after recovery (Lam et al., 1991) and that the number of EBV infected cells correlate with the intensity of malaria transmission in the area of residence (Moormann et al., 2005). It is noteworthy, however, that in the aforementioned prospective serological investigation, the children who developed endemic Burkitt's lymphoma and children who remained healthy had similar rates of malaria parasitemia before tumor development (de-Thé et al., 1978). Accordingly, other models for the role of EBV in Burkitt's lymphoma development have also been proposed (Hecht and Aster, 2000; van den Bosch, 2004). The occurrence of EBV-positive Burkitt's lymphoma in AIDS patients and in organ transplant recipients would also be consistent with a critical role for immunological control of EBV-infected cells in the lymphoma development, as would an inverse correlation between socioeconomic status and Burkitt's lymphoma occurrence (Hsu and Glaser, 2000).

NK/T-cell lymphomas

EBV is associated with certain types of NK/T-cell lymphomas. These include in particular the extranodal NK/T-cell lymphoma of the nasal type, but also aggressive NK-cell leukemia (Nava and Jaffe, 2005) and possibly angioimmunoblastic T-cell lymphoma (Anagnostopoulos et al., 1992; Chan et al., 1999; Huh et al., 1999; Weiss et al., 1992) and extranodal enteropathy-type T-cell lymphoma (Huh et al., 1999; Quintanilla-Martinez et al., 1997; Zhang et al., 2005). Histologically, extranodal NK/T-cell lymphomas of the nasal type are characterized by a broad morphological spectrum, but an angiodestructive pattern with frequent necrosis and apoptosis is a characteristic finding (Chan et al., 2001; Nava and Jaffe, 2005). As signaled by the name the malignant cells are either of NK-cell (the majority) or T-cell origin. The nasal region is the most frequent site of involvement, but the tumor may also present at other extranodal sites such as skin testis, kidney, upper gastrointestinal tract, and the orbit (Chan et al., 2001; Rizvi et al., 2006).

Epidemiology of mature T- and NK-cell lymphomas

Mature T- and NK-cell tumors are generally rare tumors, and NK/T cell lymphomas of the nasal type even more so. In an international series comprising lymphoma patients from the US, Europe, Asia and South Africa peripheral T-cell lymphoma made up 9.4% of all non-Hodgkin's lymphomas, however, with considerable geographic variation, ranging from 1.5% in Vancouver, Canada to 18.3% in Hong Kong (Rudiger et al., 2002). In the same series, NK/T-cell lymphomas of the nasal type constituted a mere 1.4% of the all investigated lymphomas (Rudiger et al., 2002), all cases except three diagnosed in Hong Kong. Thus, NK/T-cell lymphomas of the nasal type are rare in the Western world, and is more commonly seen in Asia, Mexico and in Central and South America countries (Hsu and Glaser, 2000). In a recent Chinese case series from Hong Kong, NK/T-cell lymphomas of the nasal type made up 6.3% of all non-Hodgkin's lymphomas (Au et al., 2005), and similar proportions have been reported from Peru (Quintanilla-Martinez et al., 1999). Generally, the incidence is held to be higher in men than in women (Hsu and Glaser, 2000). Besides the ethnic variation little is known about risk factors for this small group of lymphomas, but the entity has been described in immune dysfunctional individuals (Stadlmann, 2001).

Evidence of association with EBV

EBV has been incriminated in NK/T-cell lymphoma development exclusively by the demonstration of the virus in the tumor cells (Table 53.6). Accordingly, patient series have shown that the NK/T-cell lymphomas of the nasal type almost invariably (90%) harbor EBV, irrespective of the patient's ethnicity (Chan *et al.*, 2001a,b; Kanavaros *et al.*, 1993; Miyazato *et al.*, 2004; Quintanilla-Martinez *et al.*, 1997); in Asians also when presenting outside the nasal cavity (Chan *et al.*, 1997).

Hodgkin's lymphoma

Hodgkin's lymphoma develops from germinal center B-lymphocytes in the vast majority (> 98%) of all cases, and in rare instances from post-thymic T-cells (Stein *et al.*, 2001). Histologically, the tumor typically contains a small number of malignant cells, which are large mono- and multinucleated cells (Hodgkin's or Reed–Sternberg cells), surrounded by T-lymphocytes in a rosette-like pattern and dispersed in an abundant mixture of reactive inflammatory and accessory cells (Stein, 2001). Based on clinical and biological criteria, two main types of Hodgkin's lymphoma are recognized, i.e., nodular lymphocyte predominant (5%) and classical (95%) Hodgkin's lymphoma, the latter being further divided into four histological subtypes [nodular sclerosing (70%), mixed cellular (20–25%), lymphocyte rich (~ 5%) and lymphocyte depleted (<5%) classical Hodgkin's lymphoma (Stein, 2001).

Epidemiology

Hodgkin's lymphomas constitute 10%–15% of all malignant lymphomas [slighty more when chronic lymphocytic leukemia is disregarded] (Parkin *et al.*, 2002). In Western countries, age-standardized (world) incidence rates are typically in the range of 2–4 per 100 000 in men and 1.5–3 per 100 000 in women, whereas incidence rates < 1 per 100 000 in both men and women are typical for Asia (Parkin *et al.*, 2002). Geographical differences also exist with respect to age-specific incidence rates. In industrialized countries a conspicuous bimodal age distribution with cases accumulating in young adults and the elderly has become one of the lymphomas distinguishing characteristics (Fig. 53.8). In Hodgkin's lymphoma epidemiology literature, this pattern has been referred to as Pattern III, implying the existence of Patterns I and II (Correa and O'Conor, 1971). Of these, Pattern I was seen in developing countries and was characterized by relatively high incidence of Hodgkin's lym-

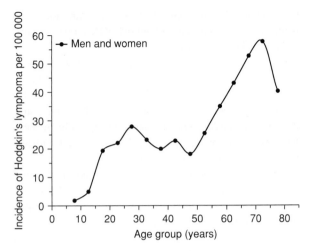

Fig. 53.8. Age-specific incidence of Hodgkin's lymphoma in the white population of Brooklyn, U.S., 1943–52. Reproduced from MacMahon, 1957 with permission from John Wiley & Sons, Inc.

phoma in children, low incidence in the third decade and high incidence in the elderly. Pattern II was perceived as an intermediate between Pattern I and III. A Pattern IV describing a general paucity of Hodgkin's lymphoma in all age groups was also suggested based on data originally reported from Asian countries (Correa and O'Conor, 1971). A more recent survey of register data indicate that, with the possible exception of Asian countries, these archetypical incidence patterns may no longer be as clearly distributed geographically (Macfarlane *et al.*, 1995).

The bi-modal age distribution in Pattern III reflects the age-related distributions of the different subtypes of Hodgkin's lymphoma with the nodular sclerosis subtype making up the bulk of the young adult age peak, and mixed cellularity subtype increasing in frequency with age, but has nevertheless also been used to define epidemiologically (meaningful) disease entities (MacMahon, 1957; MacMahon, 1966). Accordingly, studies of risk factors for Hodgkin's lymphoma have often focused on specific age-groups, i.e., children [<15 years], young adults [15–ca. 44 years], and elderly [≥ca. 45 years], rather than specific Hodgkin's lymphoma subtypes. Presumably reflecting the age distribution of cases, most epidemiological studies have concentrated on Hodgkin's lymphoma in young adults, the risk of which has been associated with an affluent childhood social environment, as measured by long maternal education, small sibling size and housing (Mueller, 1996). In contrast, Hodgkin's lymphoma in children appears to be associated with low socioeconomic status, whereas it plays little if any role for the risk for Hodgkin's lymphoma in the elderly (Mueller, 1996). It has long been suspected that the association with childhood environment in young adults cases reflects a surrogate for loads of infectious diseases in childhood, and that, in young adults, the lymphoma might arise as an untoward reaction to delayed exposure to a common childhood infectious agent (Gutensohn and Cole, 1977). Consistent with this notion, attendance of nursery school or day care for more than 1 year was associated with a reduced risk (odds ratio = 0.64; 95% confidence interval 0.45 to 0.92) for Hodgkin's lymphoma at ages 15–54 years in a recent investigation (Chang et al., 2004). Patients suffering from immune incompetence, whether acquired or inherited, are at increased risk for Hodgkin's lymphoma. In AIDS patients, for instance, the increase in the order of 10-fold (Frisch et al., 2001). Hodgkin's lymphoma is also known to cluster within families suggesting a genetic predisposition to the disease (Goldin et al., 2004). Also, smoking has recently been incriminated in two large case-control studies, suggesting relative risks of around two for current smokers (Briggs et al., 2002; Chang et al., 2004), although previous studies have yielded conflicting results (for review see Briggs et al., 2002). Among investigated occupational exposures, wood working and formaldehyde exposure have frequently been associated with risk for Hodgkin's lymphoma (Mueller, 1996).

Evidence of association with EBV

Epidemiological, serological, and molecular biological studies have all suggested that EBV is involved in the development of at least a proportion of Hodgkin's lymphomas (Table 53.6). Consistent with suspected mechanisms underlying the association with affluence in childhood, history of infectious mononucleosis has been associated with an increased risk for Hodgkin's lymphoma in cohort as well as case-control studies, relative risks typically in the order of two-to-threefold increased (Alexander et al., 2003; Hjalgrim et al., 2000; IARC. 1997). The risk increase seems to be specific to Hodgkin's lymphoma and inversely correlated with time since infectious mononucleosis, in practice restricting it to the young adult age group (Hjalgrim et al., 2000). Serological investigations have also pointed to a role for EBV in Hodgkin's lymphoma pathogenesis. Specifically, though patients with Hodgkin's lymphoma appear not to be more frequently infected with the viruses (as measured by prevalence of antiviral capsid antigen IgG antibodies at diagnosis) than comparable controls, the patients have higher mean titres of these antibodies (IARC, 1997). In case-control studies the patients also demonstrate antibodies against the early antigen complex and at higher titres more often than normal persons (IARC, 1997). Perhaps the most compelling evidence, however, comes from a prospective serological investigation, in

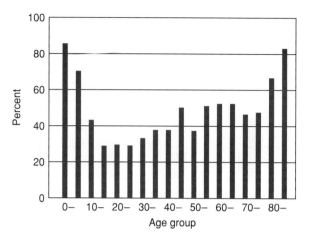

Fig. 53.9. Percentage of Hodgkin's lymphomas positive for EBV by five-year age group (Reproduced from (Glaser et al., 1997)) with permission from John Wiley & Sons, Inc.

which prediagnostic elevated titres of antiviral capsid antigen IgG antibodies (relative risk = 2.6; 90% CI 1.1 to 6.1), anti-diffuse early antigen antibodies (relative risk = 2.6; 90% CI 1.1 to 6.1) and anti-restricted early antigen (1.9; 90% CI 0.90–4.0) were all associated with risk of Hodgkin's lymphoma (adjusted for IgM). In multivariate analyses including all types of anti-EBV antibodies, risk for Hodgkin's lymphoma was associated with high titers of anti-EBV nuclear antigen antibodies (relative risk = 6.7; 90% CI 1.8 to 25) and inversely associated with IgM antibodies (relative risk = 0.07; 90% CI 0.01 to 0.53) (Mueller et al., 1989). The third line of evidence of an association between EBV and Hodgkin's lymphoma is the demonstration of the virus in the malignant cells (Weiss et al., 1987). Importantly, however, the virus is not invariably present in the malignant cells, and the proportion of EBV-positive tumors varies by histological subtype (more common in mixed cellularity than nodular sclerosis Hodgkin's lymphoma), age (less common in young adults than other age groups), sex (more common in men than in women), and geography (more common in developing than developed countries) (Figures 53.9 and 53.10) (Cartwright and Watkins, 2004; Glaser et al., 1997).

The role of EBV in Hodgkin's lymphoma pathogenesis remains uncertain from epidemiological evidence, but there is some evidence to suggest that risk factors may differ between virus-positive and -negative tumors. Accordingly, in some investigations the increased risk for Hodgkin's lymphoma following infectious mononucleosis may be restricted to virus-positive subtypes (Alexander et al., 2000; Hjalgrim et al., 2003), although other investigations have reported no particular predilection for

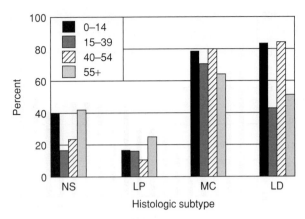

Fig. 53.10. Distribution of EBV positive tumors by histological subtype (Reproduced from (Glaser *et al.*, 1997)) with permission from John Wiley & Sons, Inc.

virus-positive tumors after infectious mononucleosis (Alexander *et al.*, 2003; Sleckman *et al.*, 1998).

It has been speculated that the Hodgkin's lymphoma-mononucleosis association may merely reflect the significance of high socioeconomic status. This speculation is, however, not easily compatible with observations showing that first-degree relatives of mononucleosis patients either have no increased Hodgkin's lymphoma risk (Hjalgrim *et al.*, 2002), or an increased risk for only for virus-positive tumors (Alexander *et al.*, 2003). Also, titres of antiviral capsid antigen antibodies have recently been found to correlate with Hodgkin's lymphoma virus status in both case-control (Alexander *et al.*, 2003; Chang *et al.*, 2004a,b) and prospective studies (Levin *et al.*, 2002). There is also evidence to suggest that smoking is particularly associated with an increased risk for EBV-positive Hodgkin's lymphoma (Briggs *et al.*, 2002; Chang *et al.*, 2004a,b; Glaser *et al.*, 2004), as is low socioeconomic status and race for Hodgkin's lymphoma in childhood (Flavell *et al.*, 2001) and immune-incompetence (Audouin *et al.*, 1992). Finally, inherited susceptibility to EBV-positive Hodgkin's lymphoma has also recently been proposed (Diepstra *et al.*, 2005). None of these different lines of evidence can, however, rule out the simple explanation that the proportion of virus-positive lymphomas merely reflect the number of circulating EBV-infected cells at initiation of lymphoma development (Thorley-Lawson and Gross, 2004).

Lymphoproliferative disease associated with immunodeficiency

The recent WHO classification for tumors of the hematopoietic and lymphatic tissues recognizes four broad clinical settings of immune deficiency that are associated with an increased risk for malignant lymphomas and other lympoproliferative disorders. These are (1) primary immune disorders and deficiencies (Borisch *et al.*, 2001), (2) infection with human immunodeficiency virus (HIV) (Raphael *et al.*, 2001), (3) iatrogenic immune suppression in organ or bone marrow transplant recipients (Harris *et al.*, 2001a,b), and (4) iatrogenic immune suppression associated with methotrexate treatment (Harris and Swerdlow, 2001), typically for auto-immune conditions. With the exception of post-transplant lymphoproliferative disorder, the malignancies observed in these settings are largely similar to sporadic occurring neoplasms.

Primary immune disorders

Primary immune disorders are associated with a substantial risk for malignant disease, reported absolute risks ranging from 12%–25% in patients with Wiskott-Aldrich syndrome, ataxia telangiectasia, and common variable immunodeficiency (Filipovich *et al.*, 1992). Hematopoietic malignancies make up nearly 70% of the observed tumors, clearly different from the normal 8% (Mueller, 1999). Onset of disease is typically in childhood (Borisch *et al.*, 2001). EBV infection plays a significant role in many, though not all, of the malignant lymphomas occurring in patients with primary immune deficiencies (Filipovich *et al.*, 1992) Specifically, loss of immunological control of EBV-infected lymphocytes allows their continued proliferation and malignant transformation, possibly promoted by defective immune regulation and chronic immune stimulation (Filipovich *et al.*, 1992).

Post-transplant lymphoproliferative disease

"Post-transplant lymphoproliferative disorder" (PTLD) in reality defines a spectrum of lymphoid hyperproliferative states that may be observed in solid organ and bone marrow transplant recipients (Loren *et al.*, 2003). PTLDs are most often but not invariably of B-lymphocyte origin, and manifest heterogeneously, possibly reflecting serial development of the disorder (Harris *et al.*, 2001a,b) (Table 53.9). Histologically, it has been suggested that EBV-associated PTLD should include two of the following three features: disruption of underlying architecture by a lymphoproliferative process, presence of monoclonal or polyclonal cell populations, and evidence (typically by *in situ* hybridization for virus-encoded RNA) of EBV in many of the cells (Paya *et al.*, 1999). Although it also includes reactive hyperplasia, the term PTLD is normally used in reference to the malignant end of the PTLD spectrum unless otherwise specified (Green, 2001; Loren *et al.*, 2003).

Table 53.8. Distribution of tumors by primary immunodeficiency syndrome in a combined series of patients with inherited immune deficiencies (Reproduced from Filipovich et al., 1992; Mueller, 1999.) The table is not exhaustive with respect to immune deficiencies carrying increased cancer risk

Immunodeficiency	Total tumors	NHL	Hodgkin's disease	Leukemia	Other tumors
Severe combined immunodeficiency	42	31 (73.8)[a]	4 (9.5)	5 (11.9)	2 (4.8)
Hypogammaglobulinemia	21	7 (33.3)	3 (14.3)	7 (33.3)	4 (19.0)
Common variable immunodeficiency	120	55 (45.8)	8 (6.7)	8 (6.7)	49 (40.8)
IgA deficiency	38	6 (15.8)	3 (7.9)	0 (0)	29 (76.3)
Hyper-UgM syndrome	16	9 (56.3)	4 (25.0)	0 (0)	3 (18.8)
Wiskott-Aldrich syndrome	78	59 (75.6)	3 (3.8)	7 (9.0)	9 (11.5)
Ataxia telangiectasia	150	69 (46.0)	16 (10.7)	32 (21.3)	33 (22.0)
Other immunodeficiencies	25	12 (48.0)	1 (4.0)	4 (16.0)	8 (32.0)
Total immunodeficiency categories	500	252 (50.4)	43 (8.6)	63 (16.0)	142 (28.4)

[a]Percentage of total tumors.
NHL, non-Hodgkin's lymphoma.

Table 53.9. Post-transplant lymphoproliferative disorders (reproduced from Harris et al., 2001 with permission from IARC).

Categories of post-transplant lymphoproliferative diseases (PTLD)

Early lesions
Reactive plasmacytic hyperplasia
Infectious mononucleosis-like
Polymorphic PTLD
Monomorphic PTLD (classified according to the WHO nomenclature)
B-cell neoplasms
Diffuse large B-cell lymphoma (immunoblastic, centroblastic, anaplastic)
Burkitt's/Burkitt's-like lymphoma
Plasma cell myeloma
Plasmacytoma-like lesions
T-cell neoplasms
Peripheral T-cell lymphoma, not otherwise specified
Other types
Hodgkin's lymphoma and Hodgkin's lymphoma-like PTLD

In solid organ transplant recipients, PTLD is typically of recipient origin (>90%), whereas in hematopoietic stem cell transplant recipients it is most often of donor origin (Harris et al., 2001a,b). The organ graft is frequently involved in PTLD (e.g., in 80% of lung transplanted, 33% of liver transplants, and 32% of kidney transplants in children) (Holmes and Sokol, 2002).

Epidemiology The epidemiology of PTLD remains scantily characterized. Occurrence varies by type of transplantation, ranging from a few percent or less in renal transplant recipients to ~20% in recipients of HLA mismatched, T-cell depleted bone marrow, and even 33% of child-recipients of combined liver-kidney transplants (Curtis et al., 1999; Harris et al., 2001a,b; Holmes and Sokol, 2002; Loren et al., 2003).

PTLD may develop as soon as the first week or as late as 9 years after transplantation, but the median latency period is around 6 months in solid organ recipients and 70–90 days in hematopoietic stem cell recipients (Loren et al., 2003). PTLD occurs in all age groups, but is seen in more men than women, which could, however, reflect gender differences in transplantation frequency (Hsu and Glaser, 2000). Inadequate T-cell control of EBV-infected B-lymphocytes is thought to be critical to the development of EBV-positive PTLDs. Consistent with this theory, established risk factors for PTLD include recipient EBV seronegativity (in particular if the donor is EBV-seropositive), primary or reactivated EBV infection following transplantation, high levels of immune suppression (cyclosporine, tacrolimus, antithymocyte globulin, or antilymphocyte antibodies), cytomegalovirus infection, transplanted organ (renal < non-renal) and – less certain – younger age (Aguilar et al., 1999; Loren et al., 2003; Swinnen, 2000).

Evidence of association with EBV The significance of EBV to PTLD development is implied first and foremost by demonstration of the virus in approximately 80% of cases (Harris et al., 2001a,b). EBV-negative PTLDs have been described, and tend to occur with longer latency periods than their virus-positive counterparts (Nalesnik, 2002).

Because early recognition of developing PTLD may affect prognosis, attempts have been made to develop techniques

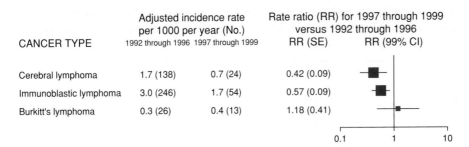

Fig. 53.11. Incidence rates of certain types of non-Hodgkin's lymphoma in 1992 through 1996 (before HAART) and in 1997 through 1999 [after HAART] and rate ratios (RRs) of incidence rates in 1992 through 1996 compared with 1997 through 1999. Reproduced from International Collaboration on HIV and Cancer 2000 with permission from Oxford University Press.

for monitoring EBV infection activity. Decreased anti-EBV nuclear antigen antibody levels have been associated with an increased risk for PTLD (Cen et al., 1993; Riddler et al., 1994). A more useful measure of EBV activity is, however, the assessment of the burden of virus infection in peripheral blood mononuclear cells and serum which, by a wide variety of different assays, have been found to correlate with risk for PTLD (Stevens et al., 2002a,b).

Lymphomas in HIV
EBV infection is involved in different diseases in HIV-infected individuals, in particular malignant lymphomas and leiomyosarcomas.

Malignant lymphoma in people with HIV The risk for malignant lymphomas is increased massively in patients with acquired immune deficiency syndrome (AIDS). Accordingly, aggressive B-cell non-Hodgkin's lymphoma has been an AIDS-defining condition almost since the recognition of the HIV epidemic and is the second most common tumor associated with HIV (Dal Maso and Franceschi, 2003; Lim and Levine, 2005).

The magnitude of reported increases in risk for non-Hodgkin's lymphoma in persons with AIDS have varied somewhat, but generally have been in the order of 100-fold for all types of non-Hodgkin's lymphoma combined in the period before the introduction of Highly Active Anti-Retroviral Therapy (HAART) (Dal Maso and Franceschi, 2003), relative risks possibly being more increased in children (Biggar et al., 2000) and less increased in elderly (Biggar et al., 2004). Particularly elevated relative risks have been reported for high grade diffuse immunoblastic (652-fold increased) and Burkitt's lymphoma (261-fold increased)(Cote et al., 1997). While some uncertainty has existed for Hodgkin's lymphoma, recent data have suggested that the risk for this lymphoma is also increased in HIV-infected persons, although to a much lesser extent, i.e., around 10-fold (Frisch et al., 2001; IARC, 1996).

The risk of non-Hodgkin's lymphoma varies by level of immune suppression as measured by CD4 count and typically is a late manifestation of HIV infection (IARC, 1996). Consistent with this, the introduction of HAART seems to have accompanied by a decrease in AIDS-malignant lymphoma occurrence, notably of the subtypes most strongly associated with EBV (see below) (International Collaboration on HIV and Cancer, 2000; Lim and Levine, 2005) (Fig. 53.11).

In contrast to AIDS-related Kaposi's sarcoma, a human herpesvirus 8-associated malignancy that occurs predominantly in homo- or bisexual men, the occurrence of malignant lymphomas show no predilection for mode of HIV acquisition (IARC, 1996).

HIV itself appears not to be directly involved in the lymphoma development as illustrated by its absence in the malignant cells. Rather, through chronic antigenic stimulation causing B-cell proliferation, and through cytokine dysregulation, the virus may create an environment conducive for the development of malignant lymphomas (Levine, 2000; Knowles, 2001).

The range of different types of malignant lymphomas in HIV-infected persons is wide, but can be categorized according to whether they also occur in immune-competent individuals (Burkitt's lymphoma, diffuse large B-cell lymphoma, extranodal marginal zone lymphoma of mucosa-associated lymphoid tissue type (MALT lymphoma), peripheral T-cell lymphomas and classical Hodgkin's lymphoma), whether they are seen in other immune dysfunctional conditions (polymorphic B-cell lymphoma) or whether they are more specific to HIV infected individuals (primary effusion lymphoma, plasmablastic lymphoma of the oral cavity) (Raphael et al., 2001). However, the various lymphoma subtypes are not equally frequent and a few of these make up the vast majority of cases in AIDS, i.e., Burkitt's lymphoma (50%–60% of all HIV-related lymphomas) and diffuse large B-cell lymphomas (25% of all HIV-related lymphomas many of which present in the central nervous system), primary effusion lymphoma (less than 5% of all HIV-related lymphoma) and plasmablastic lymphoma of the oral cavity (Raphael et al., 2001).

Evidence of association with EBV As for other lymphomas, the primary evidence of EBV involvement in development of HIV-related lymphomas is the demonstration of monoclonal virus in the tumors (Table 53.6). Overall, EBV is present in approximately 60% of HIV-related lymphomas, but the proportion of virus-positive tumors varies considerably with site of presentation and histological subtype. Thus, EBV is almost invariably present in Hodgkin's lymphomas, in (primary) central nervous system lymphomas and in primary effusion lymphomas (so-called PEL), in 80% of diffuse large cell lymphomas with immunoblastic features, in more than 50% of plasmablastic lymphomas of the oral cavity, in 30%–50% of AIDS-related Burkitt's lymphomas, and in 30% of diffuse large B-cell lymphomas of the centroblastic variant (Raphael et al., 2001). As the risk of the various types of non-Hodgkin's lymphoma correlating with level of immune deficiency, a similar correlation arises with respect to prevalence of EBV in the lymphoma (Carbone and Gloghini, 2005).

Gastric carcinoma

Gastric carcinomas are tumors derived from the epithelium of the stomach mucosa with glandular differentiation (Fenoglio-Preiser et al., 2000). Histologically, the tumors either are gland-forming with tubular, acinary, or papillary structures or display a complex mixture of dis-cohesive, isolated cells with variable morphologies, sometimes in combination with glandular, trabecular, or alveolar solid structures (Fenoglio-Preiser et al., 2000). The current WHO classification of tumor of the digestive system distinguishes between tumors occurring at the junction between esophagus and the stomach, many of which would previously have been classified as cancers of the gastric cardia, and gastric cancer differing epidemiologically.

Epidemiology

The incidence of gastric cancer has been decreasing worldwide for several decades (Parkin et al., 2002), yet with an estimated 876 000 incident cases annually it remains the fourth most common cancer worldwide, and because of its relatively poor prognosis the second most common cancer-specific cause of death attributed 647 000 deaths annually (Parkin et al., 2000). There is considerable (more than 10-fold) geographical variation in the incidence of gastric cancer, with high rates in the Andean regions of South America, Eastern Europe, and Eastern Asia, and low rates in Northern Europe, most African countries, and North American whites (Fenoglio-Preiser et al., 2006). For instance, world standardized incidence rates of 6.6 per 100 000 are observed in white American men as compared with rates between 60 and 90 per 100 000 observed in Japanese men (IARC, 2002). Irrespective of this geographical variation, the cancer is twice as common in men as in women (Parkin et al., 2002; Nyren and Adami, 2002). In contrast to decreasing occurrence of gastric cancer, there is evidence to suggest that cancer of the esophageal–gastric junction may be increasing (Newnham et al., 2003; Wijnhoven et al., 2002), although this is still debated (Ekstrom et al., 1999).

Both gastric cancer and cancers of the esophageal–gastric junction are rare before the age of 30 years, but increase with older age (Parkin et al., 2002). Besides age, established risk factors for gastric cancer include familial occurrence, tobacco smoking, certain diets, alcohol, and infection with *Helicobacter pylori* (Nyren and Adami, 2002). With respect to familial occurrence of gastric carcinoma, it has been estimated that familial clustering of gastric cancer occurs in approximately 1% of patients (Shinmura et al., 1999). Increased gastric cancer risk has been described in a number of hereditary conditions, notably the Li–Fraumeni syndrome and hereditary non-polyposis colorectal cancer, but other syndromes may exist (Nyren and Adami, 2002). Familial clustering of gastric cancer may reflect shared genetic or environmental factors, or both. Accordingly, in a study of more than 44 000 Scandinavian twins, compared to men whose twin did not have stomach cancer 7- and 10-fold increased risks for gastric cancer were observed in dizygotic and monozygotic male twins, whose twin had stomach cance. For women, the corresponding relative risk estimates were 6 and 20 respectively (Lichtenstein et al., 2000). This corresponded to inherited factors accounting for 28%, shared environmental factors 10%, and non-shared environmental factors to 62% of the overall gastric cancer risk.

Smoking is associated with stomach cancer risk, in cohort studies amounting to 1.5 to 2-fold increased risk (Tredaniel et al., 1997). Certain dietary items are suspected to be of importance for gastric cancer risk. Accordingly, salt intake and, in some populations, smoked or cured meats have been associated with increased risk of gastric cancer, whereas intake of fresh fruit and vegetables have been associated with a reduced gastric cancer risk (Nyren and Adami, 2002). Finally, several studies have shown that infection with *Helicobacter pylori* carries an increased risk of gastric cancer. Thus, in a Japanese cohort study, 36 cases of gastric carcinoma was observed during follow-up in 1246 *Helicobacter pylori* infected persons compared with no cases among 280 uninfected men (Uemura *et al.*, 2001). Analogously, a meta-analysis of 42 studies showed *Helicobacter pylori* infection to be associated with a two-fold increased risk of gastric cancer (Eslick *et al.*, 1999).

Evidence of an association with EBV

The scientific evidence incriminating EBV in development of gastric carcinoma encompasses the demonstration of monoclonal virus in the malignant cells and aberrant anti-virus antibody patterns before and at diagnosis (Table 53.6).

The first suggestion of an involvement of EBV in gastric carcinoma development came in the early 1990s by the demonstration of the virus in lymphoepithelioma-like carcinomas of the stomach (Burke *et al.*, 1990). Subsequent investigations indicate that the virus is present in the vast majority of this specific subgroup of gastric carcinomas, i.e., 80+% (Fukayama *et al.*, 1998). Importantly, however, the association with EBV is not restricted to lymphoepithelioma-like gastric carcinomas as the virus can also be demonstrated in varying proportions (typically less than 10%) of carcinomas of more common histologies (Fukayama *et al.*, 1998; Imai *et al.*, 1994; Koriyama *et al.*, 2004; Shibata and Weiss, 1992; van Beek *et al.*, 2004).

EBV has also been implicated in gastric carcinoma development by serological studies. Specifically, elevated seroprevalence of anti-viral capsid antigen IgA and IgGy and elevated anti-early antigen antibies and (elevated IgG viral capsid antigen antibody titers) have been described at and before diagnosis of EBV-associated gastric carcinomas (Imai *et al.*, 1994; Levine *et al.*, 1995).

Besides, by histology the proportion of EBV-positive gastric carcinomas appears to vary by gender, age, tumor location, and possibly geography. EBV-positive gastric carcinomas seem to be more common in men than in women. In a large Japanese investigation of 1918 cases, EBV was demonstrated in 83 (6.8%) of 1212 male and in 17 (2.4%) of 706 female cases (Koriyama *et al.*, 2004). Likewise, in a recent Dutch series 38 (11.7%) of 324 gastric carcinomas in men and 3 (1.2%) of 242 carcinoma in women harbored EBV (van Beek *et al.*, 2004), and from smaller US series EBV prevalence of 15%–21% and 3%–5% are reported for gastric carcinomas in men and women, respectively (Shibata, 1998). Overall, the proportion of EBV-positive tumors seems to correlate inversely with age, but the age pattern may differ between gastric carcinoma subtypes (Koriyama *et al.*, 2004; van Beek *et al.*, 2004).

Interestingly, the EBV-positive tumors are not evenly distributed topographically in the stomach. Accordingly, the virus can more often be demonstrated in carcinomas of the cardia and the middle stomach than in the antrum, proportions varying 3–4 fold or more (Koriyama *et al.*, 2004; Takada, 2000; van Beek *et al.*, 2004). Of interest, EBV-positive tumors have been reported to make up a relatively large proportion of gastric carcinomas after partial gastrectomy for non-malignant diseases, published estimates ranging between 27% and 42% (Baas *et al.*, 1998; Chang *et al.*, 2000; Koriyama *et al.*, 2004; Nishikawa *et al.*, 2002; Yamamoto *et al.*, 1994). It has been suggested that this distribution of the EBV-positive tumors reflect that the non-neoplastic mucosa of the proximal stomach may be conditioned to develop EBV-related tumors (Fukayama *et al.*, 1998).

As illustrated in Fig. 53.12 the proportion of EBV-positive gastric carcinomas appears to differ between countries and may even vary within countries (Tashiro *et al.*, 1998). However, so far it has been difficult to define a clear geographic pattern in the distribution of EBV-related gastric carcinomas like those known for nasopharyngeal carcinoma and Burkitt's lymphoma. The precise siginificance of variation in referral patterns, case selection or possible variation in other risk factors for gastric carcinomas is difficult to evaluate in this context (Hsu and Glaser, 2000; Levin and Levine, 1998).

Lymphoepithelioma-like carcinomas may have a better prognosis than other gastric lymphomas, and recently, it has been suggested that other types of EBV-positive gastric carcinomas may also have better prognosis than virus-negative tumors (van Beek *et al.*, 2004).

Given the high incidence of gastric adenocarcinoma worldwide [around 870 000 incident cases annually (Parkin *et al.*, 2001), EBV-related gastric carcinoma, estimated to amount to at least 50 000 cases per year may be the most common of all EBV-associated malignancies (Takada, 2000) (Table 53.10).

Other malignancies associated with EBV infection

EBV has been shown, or is suspected, to be involved in the development of a series of other malignancies, much less frequently occurring than those described in the above sections. These include lymphoepithelioma-like carcinomas and soft tissue sarcomas, for which an association with EBV is compelling, and carcinomas of the breast, thymus, and liver, for which the evidence is less evident.

Lymphoepithelioma-like carcinomas

Lymphoepithelioma-like carcinomas are tumors that morphologically resemble undifferentiated carcinoma of the

Table 53.10. Estimated number of neoplasms associated with EBV (reproduced from Levin and Levine, 1998.)

Malignancy	Estimate of EBV genome positivity	Estimated number of cancers worldwide in 1990	Estimated number of EBV associated neoplasms
Gastric adenocarcinoma	6–12%	876 000	78 840
Nasopharyngeal cancer			
Developed countries	95%	5 500	5 225
Economically developing countries	99%	53 000	52 470
Hodgkin's lymphoma			
Developed countries	30–50%	25 000	10 000
Economically developing countries	60–90%	37 000	27 750
Non-Hodgkin's lymphomas	6–10%	223 000	17 840
Burkitt's lymphoma			
Developed countries	20–30%	600	7 440
Economically developing countries	95%	9 000	8 550
AIDS-related lymphoma	50–90%	9 000	6 300
Smooth muscle sarcomas	Case reports (rare malignancy)		
Lymphoepithelioma like carcinomas of the salivary gland, lung, stomach, thymus	Case reports (rare malignancies)		

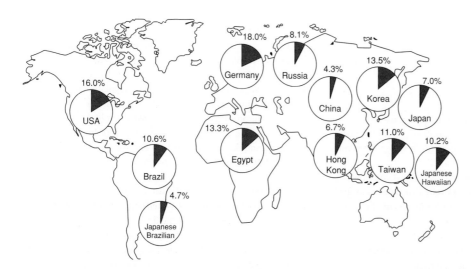

Fig. 53.12. World distribution of proportions of gastric cancers that are EBV-related. Reproduced from Tashiro *et al.*, 1998.

nasopharynx. In addition to the stomach (see above) the tumor has been described in the salivary glands, oral cavity, larynx, thymus, trachea, lungs, breast, uterine cervix, vagina, urinary bladder, skin, stomach (Iezzoni *et al.*, 1995), thyroid (Shek *et al.*, 1996), esophagus (Mori *et al.*, 1994), kidney (Elzevier *et al.*, 2002), ureter (Chalik *et al.*, 1998), and liver (Jeng *et al.*, 2001).

The tumor attracts interest because, in addition to the morphological similarity with nasopharyngeal carcinoma, EBV has been reportedly demonstrated in the malignant cells in some, but not all of the affected organs (Chalik *et al.*, 1998; Elzevier *et al.*, 2002; Iezzoni *et al.*, 1995; Jeng *et al.*, 2001; Mori *et al.*, 1994; Shek *et al.*, 1996).

Also, the prevalence of the virus in the malignant cells follows the same geographical distribution as observed nasopharyngeal carcinoma for salivary gland and lung lymphoepithelial-like carcinomas, being higher in Asian than in Western patients, thereby further underscoring the analogy between the two groups of tumors (Hsu and Glaser, 2000).

Leiomyosarcoma

Leiomyosarcomas are malignant neoplasms of smooth muscle tissues. They are exceedingly rare tumors, occurring at rates around 1 per 100 000, slightly higher in women than in men (Levi *et al.*, 1999; Zahm *et al.*, 1996) The connection with EBV is fairly recent and initially arose from the apparent accumulation in HIV infected children and organ transplant recipients (see for review Jenson, 2000 of cases reported until 1998). Epidemiologically, the association for HIV-infected children has been supported by surveys of cohorts of such children demonstrating excessive occurence of the tumor (Biggar *et al.*, 2000; Granovsky 1998). The conclusive piece of evidence for the association with EBV is, however, the demonstration of the virus in the tumors of immunocompromised hosts (Jenson, 2000).

Other malignancies

In recent years, the involvement of EBV in other malignancies than those discussed above has been debated. These include breast carcinomas (Glaser *et al.*, 2004a,b), hepatocellular carcinoma (Sugawara *et al.*, 1999), and thymomas (Chen, 2002). As yet, however, the evidence for the association with EBV remains controversial.

REFERENCES

Abdel-Hamid, M., Chen, J. J., Constantine, N., Massoud, M., and Raab-Traub, N. (1992). EBV strain variation: geographical distribution and relation to disease state. *Virology*, **190**, 168–175.

Aguilar, L. K., Rooney, C. M., and Heslop, H. E. (1999). Lymphoproliferative disorders involving Epstein-Barr virus after hemopoietic stem cell transplantation. *Curr. Opin. Oncol.*, **11**(2), 96–101.

Aitken, C., Sengupta, S. K., Aedes, C., Moss, D. J., and Sculley, T. B. (1994). Heterogeneity within the Epstein-Barr virus nuclear antigen 2 gene in different strains of Epstein-Barr virus. *J. Gen. Virol.*, **75**(Pt 1):95–100.

Alexander, F. E., Jarrett, R. F., Lawrence, D. *et al.* (2000). Risk factors for Hodgkin's disease by Epstein-Barr virus (EBV) status: prior infection by EBV and other agents. *Br. J. Cancer*, **82**(5), 1117–1121.

Alexander, F. E., Lawrence, D. J., Freeland, J. *et al.* (2003). An epidemiologic study of index and family infectious mononucleosis and adult Hodgkin's disease (HD): evidence for a specific association with EBV+ve HD in young adults. *Int. J. Cancer*, **107**(2), 298–302.

Alfieri, C., Tanner, J., Carpentier, L. *et al.* (1996). Epstein-Barr virus transmission from a blood donor to an organ transplant recipient with recovery of the same virus strain from the recipient's blood and oropharynx. *Blood*, **87**(2), 812–817.

Anagnostopoulos, I., Hummel, M., Finn, T. *et al.* (1992). Heterogeneous Epstein-Barr virus infection patterns in peripheral T-cell lymphoma of angioimmunoblastic lymphadenopathy type. *Blood*, **80**(7), 1804–1812.

Apolloni, A., and Sculley, T. B. (1994). Detection of A-type and B-type Epstein-Barr virus in throat washings and lymphocytes. *Virology*, **202**(2), 978–981.

Au, W. Y., Ma, S. Y., Chim, C. S. *et al.* (2005). Clinicopathologic features and treatment outcome of mature T-cell and natural killer-cell lymphomas diagnosed according to the World Health Organization classification scheme: a single center experience of, 10 years. *Ann. Oncol.*, **16**(2), 206–214.

Audouin, J., Diebold, J., and Pallesen, G. (1992). Frequent expression of Epstein-Barr virus latent membrane protein-1 in tumour cells of Hodgkin's disease in HIV-positive patients. *J. Pathol.*, **167**(4), 381–384.

Auwaerter, P. G. (1999). Infectious mononucleosis in middle age. *JAMA*, **281**(5), 454–459.

Baas, I. O., van Rees, B. P., Musler, A. *et al.* (1998). Helicobacter pylori and Epstein-Barr virus infection and the p53 tumour suppressor pathway in gastric stump cancer compared with carcinoma in the non-operated stomach. *J. Clin. Pathol.*, **51**(9), 662–666.

Babcock, G. J., Decker, L. L., Freeman, R. B., and Thorley-Lawson, D. A. (1999). Epstein-barr virus-infected resting memory B cells, not proliferating lymphoblasts, accumulate in the peripheral blood of immunosuppressed patients. *J. Exp. Med.*, **190**(4), 567–576.

Beagley, K. W., and Gockel, C. M. (2003). Regulation of innate and adaptive immunity by the female sex hormones oestradiol and progesterone. *FEMS Immunol. Med. Microbiol.*, **38**(1), 13–22.

Bellan, C., Lazzi, S., Hummel, M. *et al.* (2005). Immunoglobulin gene analysis reveals 2 distinct cells of origin for EBV-positive and EBV-negative Burkitt lymphomas. *Blood*, **106**(3), 1031–1036.

Benoit, L., Wang, X., Pabst, H. F., Dutz, J., and Tan, R. (2000). Defective NK cell activation in X-linked lymphoproliferative disease. *J. Immunol.*, **165**(7), 3549–3553.

Berger, C., Day, P., Meier, G., Zingg, W., Bossart, W., and Nadal, D. (2001). Dynamics of Epstein-Barr virus DNA levels in serum during EBV-associated disease. *J. Med. Virol.*, **64**(4), 505–512.

Biggar, R. J., Frisch, M., and Goedert, J. J. (2000). Risk of cancer in children with AIDS. AIDS-Cancer Match Registry Study Group. *JAMA*, **284**(2), 205–209.

Biggar, R. J., Gardiner, C., Lennette, E. T., Collins, W. E., Nkrumah, F. K., and Henle, W. (1981). Malaria, sex, and place of residence as factors in antibody response to Epstein-Barr virus in Ghana, West Africa. *Lancet*, **2**(8238), 115–118.

Biggar, R. J., Henle, W., Fleisher, G., Bocker, J., Lennette, E. T., and Henle, G. (1978). Primary Epstein-Barr virus infections in African infants. I. Decline of maternal antibodies and time of infection. *Int. J. Cancer*, **22**(3), 239–243.

Biggar, R. J., Kirby, K. A., Atkinson, J., McNeel, T. S., and Engels, E. (2004). Cancer risk in elderly persons with HIV/AIDS. *J. Acquir. Immune. Defic. Syndr.*, **36**(3), 861–868.

Bodeus, M., Smets, F., Reding, R. et al. (1999). Epstein-Barr virus infection in sixty pediatric liver graft recipients: diagnosis of primary infection and virologic follow-up. *Pediatr. Infect. Dis. J.*, **18**(8), 698–702.

Borisch, B., Raphael, M., Swerdlow, S. H., and Jaffe, E. S. (2001). Lymphoproliferative diseases associated with primary immune disorders. In: Jaffe, E. S., Harris, N. L., Stein, H., Vardiman, J. W., editors. Tumours of Haematopoietic and lymphoid tissues. Lyon: IARC, 257–271.

Briggs, N. C., Hall, H. I., Brann, E. A., Moriarty, C. J., and Levine, R. S. (2002). Cigarette smoking and risk of Hodgkin's disease: a population-based case-control study. *Am. J. Epidemiol.*, **156**(11), 1011–1020.

Burke, A. P., Yen, T. S., Shekitka, K. M., and Sobin, L. H. (1990). Lymphoepithelial carcinoma of the stomach with Epstein-Barr virus demonstrated by polymerase chain reaction. *Mod. Pathol.*, **3**(3), 377–380.

Burrows, J. M., Bromham, L., Woolfit, M. et al. (2004). Selection pressure-driven evolution of the Epstein-Barr virus-encoded oncogene LMP1 in virus isolates from Southeast Asia. *J. Virol.*, **78**(13), 7131–7137.

Carbone, A., and Gloghini, A. (2005). AIDS-related lymphomas: from pathogenesis to pathology. *Br. J. Haematol.*, **130**(5), 662–670.

Cartwright, R. A. and Watkins, G. (2004). Epidemiology of Hodgkin's disease: a review. *Hematol. Oncol.*, **22**(1), 11–26.

Cen, H., Williams, P. A., McWilliams, H. P., Breinig, M. C., Ho, M., and McKnight, J. L. (1993). Evidence for restricted Epstein-Barr virus latent gene expression and anti-EBNA antibody response in solid organ transplant recipients with posttransplant lymphoproliferative disorders. *Blood*, **81**(5), 1393–1403.

Cerroni, L., Zochling, N., Putz, B., and Kerl, H. (1997). Infection by Borrelia burgdorferi and cutaneous B-cell lymphoma. *J. Cutan. Pathol.*, **24**, 457–461.

Cesarman, E., Chang, Y., Moore, P. S., Said, J. W., and Knowles, D. M. (1995). Kaposi's sarcoma-associated Herpesvirus-like DNA sequences in AIDS-related body-cavity-based lymphomas. *N. Engl. J. Med.*, **332**, 1186–1191.

Chalik, Y. N., Wieczorek, R., and Grasso, M. (1998). Lymphoepithelioma-like carcinoma of the ureter. *J. Urol.*, **159**(2), 503–504.

Chan, A. C., Ho, J. W., Chiang, A. K., and Srivastava, G. (1999). Phenotypic and cytotoxic characteristics of peripheral T-cell and NK-cell lymphomas in relation to Epstein-Barr virus association. *Histopathology*, **34**(1), 16–24.

Chan, C. W., Chiang, A. K., Chan, K. H., and Lau, A. S. (2003). Epstein-Barr virus-associated infectious mononucleosis in Chinese children. *Pediatr. Infect. Dis. J.*, **22**(11), 974–978.

Chan, J. K., Sin, V. C., Wong, K. F. et al. (1997). Nonnasal lymphoma expressing the natural killer cell marker CD56: a clinicopathologic study of 49 cases of an uncommon aggressive neoplasm. *Blood*, **89**, 4501–4513.

Chan, J. K.C, Jaffe, E. S., and Ralfkiaer, E. (2001). Ekstranodal, NK/T-cell lymphoma, nasal type. In: Jaffe, E. S., Harris, N. L., Stein, H., Vardiman, J. W., editors. Tumours of haematopoietic and lymphoid tissues. Lyon: IARC, 204–207.

Chan, K. H., Luo, R. X., Chen, H. L., Ng, M. H., Seto, W. H., and Peiris, J. S. (1998). Development and evaluation of an Epstein-Barr virus (EBV) immunoglobulin M enzyme-linked immunosorbent assay based on the 18-kilodalton matrix protein for diagnosis of primary EBV infection. *J. Clin. Microbiol.*, **36**(11), 3359–3361.

Chan, K. H., Ng, M. H., Seto, W. H., and Peiris, J. S. (2001). Epstein-Barr virus (EBV) DNA in sera of patients with primary EBV infection. *J. Clin. Microbiol.*, **39**(11), 4152–4154.

Chang, E. T., Smedby, K. E., Hjalgrim, H. et al. (2005). Family history of hematopoietic malignancy and risk of lymphoma. *J. Natl. Cancer Inst.*, **97**(19), 1466–1474.

Chang, E. T., Zheng, T., Lennette, E. T. et al. (2004). Heterogeneity of risk factors and antibody profiles in epstein-barr virus genome-positive and -negative hodgkin lymphoma. *J. Infect Dis.*, **189**(12), 2271–2281.

Chang, E. T., Zheng, T., Weir, E. G. et al. (2004). Childhood Social Environment and Hodgkin's Lymphoma: New Findings from a Population-Based Case-Control Study. *Cancer Epidemiol Biomarkers Prev.*, **13**(8), 1361–1370.

Chang, M. S., Lee, J. H., Kim, J. P. et al. (2000). Microsatellite instability and Epstein-Barr virus infection in gastric remnant cancers. *Pathol. Int.*, **50**(6), 486–492.

Chang, R. S. (1980). Infectious mononucleosis. Boston: G.K. Hall medical Publishers.

Chang, R. S., Rosen, L., and Kapikian, A. Z. (1981). Epstein-Barr virus infections in a nursery. *Am. J. Epidemiol.*, **113**(1), 22–29.

Chen, P. C., Pan, C. C., Yang, A. H., Wang, L. S., and Chiang, H. (2002). Detection of Epstein-Barr virus genome within thymic epithelial tumours in Taiwanese patients by nested PCR, PCR in situ hybridization, and RNA in situ hybridization. *J. Pathol.*, **197**(5), 684–688.

Chien, Y. C., Chen, J. Y., Liu, M. Y. et al. (2001). Serologic markers of Epstein-Barr virus infection and nasopharyngeal carcinoma in Taiwanese men. *N. Engl. J. Med.*, **345**(26), 1877–1882.

Coffey, A. J., Brooksbank, R. A., Brandau, O. et al. (1998). Host response to EBV infection in X-linked lymphoproliferative disease results from mutations in an SH2-domain encoding gene. *Nat. Genet.*, **20**(2), 129–135.

Correa, P. and O'Conor, G. T. (1971). Epidemiologic patterns of Hodgkin's disease. *Int. J. Cancer*, **8**, 192–201.

Correa, R. M., Fellner, M. D., Alonio, L. V., Durand, K., Teyssie, A. R., and Picconi, M. A. (2004). Epstein-barr virus (EBV) in healthy carriers: Distribution of genotypes and, 30 bp deletion in latent membrane protein-1 (LMP-1) oncogene. *J. Med. Virol.* **73**(4), 583–588.

Cote, T. R., Biggar, R. J., Rosenberg, P. S. et al. (1997). Non-Hodgkin's lymphoma among people with AIDS: incidence, presentation and public health burden. AIDS/Cancer Study Group. *Int. J. Cancer*, **73**, 645–650.

Crawford, D. H., Swerdlow, A. J., Higgins, C. et al. (2002). Sexual history and Epstein-Barr virus infection. *J. Infect Dis.*, **186**(6), 731–736.

Curtis, R. E., Travis, L. B., Rowlings, P. A. et al. (1999). Risk of lymphoproliferative disorders after bone marrow transplantation: a multi-institutional study. *Blood*, **94**(7), 2208–2216.

Dal Maso, L. and Franceschi, S. (2003). Epidemiology of non-Hodgkin lymphomas and other haemolymphopoietic neoplasms in people with AIDS. *Lancet Oncol.*, **4**(2), 110–119.

Daoud, J., Toumi, N., Bouaziz, M. et al. (2003). Nasopharyngeal carcinoma in childhood and adolescence: analysis of a series of 32 patients treated with combined chemotherapy and radiotherapy. *Eur. J. Cancer*, **39**(16), 2349–2354.

de The, G. (2000). Epstein-Barr virus and Burkitt's lymphoma. In: Goedert, J. J., editor. Infectious Causes of Cancer. New Jersey: Humana Press, 77–92.

de The, G., Day, N. E., Geser, A. et al. (1975). Sero-epidemiology of the Epstein-Barr virus: preliminary analysis of an international study – a review. *IARC Sci. Publ.*, (11 Pt 2), 3–16.

de-Thé G., Geser, A., Day, N. E. et al. (1978). Epidemiological evidence for causal relationship between Epstein-Barr virus and Burkitt's lymphoma from Ugandan prospective study. *Nature*, **274**, 756–761.

Devesa, S. S. and Fears, T. (1992). Non-Hodgkin's lymphoma time trends: United States and international data. *Cancer Res.*, **52**, 5432s–5440s.

Diebold, J., Jaffe, E. S., Raphael, M., and Warnke, R. A. (2001). Burkitt lymphoma. In: Jaffe, E. S., Harris, N. L., Stein, H., Vardiman, J. W., editors. Tumours of haematopoietic and lymphoid tissues. Lyon: IARC, 181–184.

Diepstra, A., Niens, M., Vellenga, E. et al. (2005). Association with HLA class I in Epstein-Barr-virus-positive and with HLA class III in Epstein-Barr-virus-negative Hodgkin's lymphoma. *Lancet*, **365**(9478), 2216–2224.

Edwards, J. M., and Woodroof, M. (1979). EB virus-specific IgA in serum of patients with infectious mononucleosis and of healthy people of different ages. *J. Clin. Pathol.*, **32**(10), 1036–1040.

Ekstrom, A. M., Signorello, L. B., Hansson, L. E., Bergstrom, R., Lindgren, A., and Nyren, O. (1999). Evaluating gastric cancer misclassification: a potential explanation for the rise in cardia cancer incidence. *J. Natl. Cancer Inst.*, **91**(9), 786–790.

Ekstrom-Smedby, K. (2006). Epidemiology and etiology of non-Hodgkin lymphoma – a review. *Acta Oncol.*, **45**(3), 258–71.

Elzevier, H. W., Venema, P. L., Kropman, R. F., and Kazzaz, B. A. (2002). Lymphoepithelioma-like carcinoma of the kidney. *J. Urol.*, **167**(5), 2127–2128.

Enbom, M., Strand, A., Falk, K. I., and Linde, A. (2001). Detection of Epstein-Barr virus, but not human herpesvirus 8, DNA in cervical secretions from Swedish women by real-time polymerase chain reaction. *Sex Transm. Dis.*, **28**(5), 300–306.

Engel, P., Eck, M. J., and Terhorst, C. (2003). The SAP and SLAM families in immune responses and X-linked lymphoproliferative disease. *Nat. Rev. Immunol.*, **3**(10), 813–821.

Epstein, M. A., Achong, B. G., and Barr, Y. M. (1964). Virus particles in cultured lymphoblasts from Burkitts lymphoma. *Lancet*, **15**, 702–703.

Eslick, G. D., Lim, L. L., Byles, J. E., Xia, H. H., and Talley, N. J. (1999). Association of Helicobacter pylori infection with gastric carcinoma: a meta-analysis. *Am. J. Gastroenterol.*, **94**(9), 2373–2379.

Evans, A. S., Kaslow, R. A., editors. (1997). Epidemiology and control. In: Viral Infections of Humans. 4. ed. New York: Plenum Medical Book Company.

Fafi-Kremer, S., Morand, P., Brion, J. P. et al. (2005). Long-term shedding of infectious epstein-barr virus after infectious mononucleosis. *J. Infect Dis.*, **191**(6), 985–989.

Fan, H., and Gulley, M. L. (2001). Epstein-Barr viral load measurement as a marker of EBV-related disease. *Mol. Diagn.* **6**(4), 279–289.

Feng, B. J., Huang, W., Shugart, Y. Y. et al. (2002). Genome-wide scan for familial nasopharyngeal carcinoma reveals evidence of linkage to chromosome 4. *Nat. Genet.*, **31**(4), 395–399.

Fenoglio-Preiser, C., Carneiro, F., Correa, P. et al. (2000). Gastric carcinoma. In: Hamilton, S. R., Aaltonen, L. A., editors. Tumours of the Digestive System. Lyon: IARC, 37–68.

Ferreri, A. J., Guidoboni, M., Ponzoni, M. et al. (2004). Evidence for an association between Chlamydia psittaci and ocular adnexal lymphomas. *J. Natl. Cancer Inst.*, **96**(8), 586–594.

Filipovich, A. H., Mathur, A., Kamat, D., and Shapiro, R. S. (1992). Primary immunodeficiencies: genetic risk factors for lymphoma. *Cancer Res.*, **52**, 5465s-5467s.

Flavell, K. J., Biddulph, J. P., Powell, J. E. et al. (2001). South Asian ethnicity and material deprivation increase the risk of Epstein-Barr virus infection in childhood Hodgkin's disease. *Br. J. Cancer*, **85**(3), 350–356.

Fleisher, G., and Bologonese, R. (1984). Infectious mononucleosis during gestation: report of three women and their infants studied prospectively. *Pediatr. Infect Dis.*, **3**(4), 308–311.

Fleisher, G., Henle, W., Henle, G., Lennette, E. T., and Biggar, R. J. (1979). Primary infection with Epstein-Barr virus in infants in the United States: clinical and serologic observations. *J. Infect Dis.*, **139**(5), 553–558.

Fleisher, G. R., Collins, M., and Fager, S. (1983). Limitations of available tests for diagnosis of infectious mononucleosis. *J. Clin. Microbiol.*, **17**(4), 619–624.

Frank, D., Cesarman, E., Liu, Y. F., Michler, R. E., and Knowles, D. M. (1995). Posttransplantation lymphoproliferative disorders frequently contain type A and not type B Epstein-Barr virus. *Blood*, **85**(5), 1396–1403.

Friborg, J., Koch, A., Wohlfarht, J., Storm, H. H., and Melbye, M. (2003). Cancer in Greenlandic Inuit 1973–1997: a cohort study. *Int. J. Cancer*, **107**(6), 1017–1022.

Friborg, J., Wohlfahrt, J., Koch, A., Storm, H., Olsen, O. R., and Melbye, M. (2005). Cancer susceptibility in nasopharyngeal carcinoma families–a population-based cohort study. *Cancer Res.*, **65**(18), 8567–8572.

Frisch, M., Biggar, R. J., Engels, E. A., and Goedert, J. J. (2001). Association of cancer with AIDS-related immunosuppression in adults. *JAMA*, **285**(13), 1736–1745.

Fritschi, L., Benke, G., Hughes, A. M. et al. (2005). Occupational exposure to pesticides and risk of non-Hodgkin's lymphoma. *Am. J. Epidemiol.*, **162**(9), 849–857.

Fukayama, M., Chong, J. M., and Kaizaki, Y. (1998). Epstein-Barr virus and gastric carcinoma. *Gastric Cancer*, **1**(2), 104–114.

Gartner, B. C., Kortmann, K., Schafer, M. *et al.* (2000). No correlation in Epstein-Barr virus reactivation between serological parameters and viral load. *J. Clin. Microbiol.*, **38**(6), 2458.

Geser, A., de The, G., Lenoir, G., Day, N. E., and Williams, E. H. (1982). Final case reporting from the Ugandan prospective study of the relationship between EBV and Burkitt's lymphoma. *Int. J. Cancer*, **29**(4), 397–400.

Glaser, R., Strain, E. C., Tarr, K. L., Holliday, J. E., Donnerberg, R. L., and Kiecolt-Glaser, J. K. (1985). Changes in Epstein-Barr virus antibody titers associated with aging. *Proc. Soc. Exp. Biol. Med.*, **179**(3), 352–355.

Glaser, S. L., Hsu, J. L., and Gulley, M. L. (2004). Epstein-Barr virus and breast cancer: state of the evidence for viral carcinogenesis. *Cancer Epidemiol Biomarkers Prev.*, **13**(5), 688–697.

Glaser, S. L., Keegan, T. H., Clarke, C. A. *et al.* (2004). Smoking and Hodgkin lymphoma risk in women United States. *Cancer Causes Control*, **15**(4), 387–397.

Glaser, S. L., Lin, R. J., Stewart, S. L. *et al.* (1997). Epstein-Barr virus-associated Hodgkin's disease: epidemiologic characteristics in international data. *Int. J. Cancer*, **70**, 375–382.

Goldin, L. R., Landgren, O., McMaster, M. L. *et al.* (2005). Familial aggregation and heterogeneity of non-Hodgkin lymphoma in population-based samples. *Cancer Epidemiol. Biomarkers Prev.*, **14**(10), 2402–2406.

Goldin, L. R., Pfeiffer, R. M., Gridley, G. *et al.* (2004). Familial aggregation of Hodgkin lymphoma and related tumors. *Cancer*, **100**(9), 1902–1908.

Goldschmidts, W. L., Bhatia, K., Johnson, J. F. *et al.* (1992). Epstein-Barr virus genotypes in AIDS-associated lymphomas are similar to those in endemic Burkitt's lymphomas. *Leukemia*, **6**(9), 875–878.

Goldsmith, D. B., West, T. M., and Morton, R. (2002). HLA associations with nasopharyngeal carcinoma in Southern Chinese: a meta-analysis. *Clin. Otolaryngol.*, **27**(1), 61–67.

Golubjatnikov, R., Allen, V. D., Steadman, M., Del Pilar, O. B., and Inhorn, S. L. (1973). Prevalence of antibodies to Epstein-Barr virus, cytomegalovirus and Toxoplasma in a Mexican highland community. *Am. J. Epidemiol.*, **97**(2), 116–124.

Granovsky, M. O., Mueller, B. U., Nicholson, H. S., Rosenberg, P. S., and Rabkin, C. S. (1998). Cancer in human immunodeficiency virus-infected children: a case series from the Children's Cancer Group and the National Cancer Institute. *J. Clin. Oncol.*, **16**(5), 1729–1735.

Gratama, J. W., and Ernberg, I. (1995). Molecular epidemiology of Epstein-Barr virus infection. *Adv Cancer Res.*, **67**, 197–255.

Green, M. (2001). Management of Epstein-Barr virus-induced post-transplant lymphoproliferative disease in recipients of solid organ transplantation. *Am. J. Transplant.*, **1**(2), 103–108.

Gross, T. G., Filipovich, A. H., Conley, M. E. *et al.* (1996). Cure of X-linked lymphoproliferative disease (XLP) with allogeneic hematopoietic stem cell transplantation (HSCT): report from the XLP registry. *Bone Marrow Transplant*, **17**(5), 741–744.

Grülich, A. E. and Vajdic, C. M. (2005). The epidemiology of non-Hodgkin lymphoma. *Pathology*, **37**(6), 409–19.

Gutensohn, N. and Cole, P. (1977). Epidemiology of Hodgkin's disease in the young. *Int. J. Cancer*, **19**, 595–604.

Haahr, S., Plesner, A. M., Vestergaard, B. F., and Hollsberg, P. (2004). A role of late Epstein-Barr virus infection in multiple sclerosis. *Acta. Neurol. Scand.*, **109**(4), 270–275.

Hamilton, J. K., Paquin, L. A., Sullivan, J. L. *et al.* (1980). X-linked lymphoproliferative syndrome registry report. *J. Pediatr.*, **96**(4), 669–673.

Haque, T., and Crawford, D. H. (1997). PCR amplification is more sensitive than tissue culture methods for Epstein-Barr virus detection in clinical material. *J. Gen. Virol.*, **78**(Pt 12), 3357–3360.

Harris, N. L., Jaffe, E. S., Vardiman, J. W. *et al.* (2001). WHO classification of tumours of haematopoietic and lymphoid tissues: Introduction. In: Jaffe, E. S., Harris, N. L., Stein, H., Vardiman, J. W., editors. Tumours of haematopoietic and lymphoid tissues. Lyon: IARC, 12–13.

Harris, N. L., and Swerdlow, S. H. (2001). Methotrexate-associated lymphoproliferative disorders. In: Jaffe, E. S., Harris, N. L., Stein, H., Vardiman, J. W., editors. Tumours of haematopoietic and lymphoid tissues. *Lyon: IARC*, 270–271.

Harris, N. L., Swerdlow, S. H., Frizzera, G., and Knowles, D. M. (2001). Post-transplant lymphoproliferative disorders. In: Jaffe, E. S., Harris, N. L., Stein, H., Vardiman, J. W., editors. Tumours of haematopoietic and lymphoid tissues. *Lyon: IARC*, 264–271.

Heath, C. W., Jr., Brodsky, A. L., and Potolsky, A. I. (1972). Infectious mononucleosis in a general population. *Am. J. Epidemiol.*, **95**(1), 46–52.

Hecht, J. L., and Aster, J. C. (2000). Molecular biology of Burkitt's lymphoma. *J. Clin. Oncol.*, **18**(21), 3707–3721.

Helminen, M. E., Kilpinen, S., Virta, M., and Hurme, M. (2001). Susceptibility to primary Epstein-Barr virus infection is associated with interleukin-10 gene promoter polymorphism. *J. Infect Dis.*, **184**(6), 777–780.

Hendry, B. M., and Longmore, J. M. (1982). Systemic lupus erythematosus presenting as infectious mononucleosis with a false positive monospot test. *Lancet*, 20;**1**(8269), 455.

Henle, G., and Henle, W. (1967). Immunofluorescence, interference, and complement fixation technics in the detection of the herpes-type virus in Burkitt tumor cell lines. *Cancer Res.*, **27**(12), 2442–2446.

Henle, G., Henle, W., Clifford, P. *et al.* (1969). Antibodies to Epstein-Barr virus in Burkitt's lymphoma and control groups. *J. Natl. Cancer Inst.*, **43**(5), 1147–1157.

Hesse, J., Ibsen, K. K., Krabbe, S., and Uldall, P. (1983). Prevalence of antibodies to Epstein-Barr virus (EBV) in childhood and adolescence in Denmark. *Scand J. Infect Dis.*, **15**(4), 335–338.

Hildesheim, A., Anderson, L. M., Chen, C. J. *et al.* (1997). CYP2E1 genetic polymorphisms and risk of nasopharyngeal carcinoma in Taiwan. *J. Natl. Cancer Inst.*, **89**(16), 1207–1212.

Hildesheim, A., Apple, R. J., Chen, C. J. *et al.* (2002). Association of HLA class I and II alleles and extended haplotypes with nasopharyngeal carcinoma in Taiwan. *J. Natl. Cancer Inst.*, **94**(23), 1780–1789.

Hildesheim, A., Dosemeci, M., Chan, C. C. et al. (2001). Occupational exposure to wood, formaldehyde, and solvents and risk of nasopharyngeal carcinoma. *Cancer Epidemiol. Biomarkers Prev.*, **10**(11), 1145–1153.

Hinuma, Y., Nagata, K., Hanaoka, M. et al. (1981). Adult T-cell leukemia: antigen in an ATL cell line and detection of antibodies to the antigen in human sera. *Proc. Natl. Acad. Sci., USA*, **78**(10), 6476–6480.

Hjalgrim, H., Askling, J., Rostgaard, K. et al. (2003). Characteristics of Hodgkin's lymphoma after infectious mononucleosis. *N. Engl. J. Med.*, **349**(14), 1324–1332.

Hjalgrim, H., Askling, J., Sorensen, P. et al. (2000). Risk of Hodgkin's disease and other cancers after infectious mononucleosis. *J. Natl. Cancer Inst.*, **92**(18), 1522–1528.

Hjalgrim, H., Rostgaard, K., Askling, J. et al. (2002). Hematopoietic and lymphatic cancers in relatives of patients with infectious mononucleosis. *J. Natl. Cancer Inst.*, **94**(9), 678–681.

Holmes, R. D., and Sokol, R. J. (2002). Epstein-Barr virus and post-transplant lymphoproliferative disease. *Pediatr Transplant*, **6**(6), 456–464.

Horwitz, C. A., Henle, W., Henle, G., Penn, G., Hoffman, N., and Ward, P. C. (1979). Persistent falsely positive rapid tests for infectious mononucleosis. Report of five cases with four–six-year follow-up data. Am *J. Clin. Pathol.*, **72**(5), 807–811.

Hsu, J. L. and Glaser, S. L. (2000). Epstein-barr virus-associated malignancies: epidemiologic patterns and etiologic implications. *Crit. Rev. Oncol. Hematol.*, **34**(1), 27–53.

Hu, L. F., Zabarovsky, E. R., Chen, F. et al. (1991). Isolation and sequencing of the Epstein-Barr virus BNLF-1 gene (LMP1) from a Chinese nasopharyngeal carcinoma. *J. Gen. Virol.*, **72**(Pt 10), 2399–2409.

Huh, J., Cho, K., Heo, D. S., and Kim, J. E., and Kim, C. W. (1999). Detection of Epstein-Barr virus in Korean peripheral T-cell lymphoma. *Am. J. Hematol.*, **60**(3), 205–214.

IARC. (1996). IARC Monographs on the evaluation of carcinogenic risks to humans: Human immunodeficiency viruses and human T-cell lymphotropic viruses. Lyon: IARC.

IARC. (1997). IARC Monographs on the evaluation of carcinogenic risks to humans: Epstein-Barr virus and Kaposi's sarcoma herpesvirus/herpesvirus 8. LYON: IARC.

Iezzoni, J. C., Gaffey, M. J., and Weiss, L. M. (1995). The role of Epstein-Barr virus in lymphoepithelioma-like carcinomas. *Am. J. Clin. Pathol.*, **103**(3), 308–315.

Ikuta, K., Satoh, Y., Hoshikawa, Y., and Sairenji, T. (2000). Detection of Epstein-Barr virus in salivas and throat washings in healthy adults and children. *Microbes Infect*, **2**(2), 115–120.

Imai, S., Koizumi, S., Sugiura, M. et al. (1994). Gastric carcinoma: monoclonal epithelial malignant cells expressing Epstein-Barr virus latent infection protein. *Proc. Natl. Acad. Sci., USA*, **91**(19), 9131–9135.

International Collaboration on HIV and Cancer. (2000). Highly active antiretroviral therapy and incidence of cancer in human immunodeficiency virus-infected adults. *J. Natl. Cancer Inst.*, **92**(22), 1823–1830.

Israele, V., Shirley, P., and Sixbey, J. W. (1991). Excretion of the Epstein-Barr virus from the genital tract of men. *J. Infect Dis.*, **163**(6), 1341–1343.

Jeng, K. C., Hsu, C. Y., and Liu, M. T., Chung, T. T., and Liu, S. T. (1994). Prevalence of Taiwan variant of Epstein-Barr virus in throat washings from patients with head and neck tumors in Taiwan. *J. Clin. Microbiol.*, **32**(1), 28–31.

Jeng, Y. M., Chen, C. L., and Hsu, H. C. (2001). Lymphoepithelioma-like cholangiocarcinoma: an Epstein-Barr virus-associated tumor. *Am. J. Surg. Pathol.*, **25**(4), 516–520.

Jenson, H. B. (2000). Leiomyoma and Leiomyosarcoma. In: Goedert, J. J., editor. Infectious causes of cancer: Targets for intervention. Totowa, New Jersey: Humana Press, 145–159.

Kanavaros, P., Lescs, M. C., Briere, J. et al. (1993). Nasal T-cell lymphoma: a clinicopathologic entity associated with peculiar phenotype and with Epstein-Barr virus. *Blood*, **81**(10), 2688–2695.

Kang, I., Quan, T., Nolasco, H. et al. (2004). Defective control of latent Epstein-Barr virus infection in systemic lupus erythematosus. *J. Immunol.*, **172**(2), 1287–1294.

Kapranos, N., Petrakou, E., Anastasiadou, C., Kotronias, D. (2003). Detection of herpes simplex virus, cytomegalovirus, and Epstein-Barr virus in the semen of men attending an infertility clinic. Fertil Steril, 79 Suppl **3**, 1566–1570.

Khan, G., Miyashita, E. M., Yang, B., Babcock, G. J., and Thorley-Lawson, D. A. (1996). Is EBV persistence in vivo a model for B cell homeostasis? *Immunity*, **5**(2), 173–179.

Kim, I., Park, E. R., Park, S. H., Lin, Z., and Kim, Y. S. (2002). Characteristics of Epstein-Barr virus isolated from the malignant lymphomas in Korea. *J. Med. Virol.*, **67**(1), 59–66.

Kimura, H., Hoshino, Y., Kanegane, H. et al. (2001). Clinical and virologic characteristics of chronic active Epstein-Barr virus infection. *Blood*, **98**(2), 280–286.

Kimura, H., Morishima, T., Kanegane, H. et al. (2003). Prognostic factors for chronic active Epstein-Barr virus infection. *J. Infect Dis.*, **187**(4), 527–533.

Kimura, H., Morita, M., Yabuta, Y. et al. (1999). Quantitative analysis of Epstein-Barr virus load by using a real-time PCR assay. *J. Clin. Microbiol.*, **37**, 132–136.

Klein, G. (1979). Lymphoma development in mice and humans: diversity of initiation is followed by convergent cytogenetic evolution. *Proc. Natl. Acad. Sci., U S A*, **76**(5), 2442–2446.

Klumb, C. E., Hassan, R., De Oliveira, D. E. et al. (2004). Geographic variation in Epstein-Barr virus-associated Burkitt's lymphoma in children from Brazil. *Int. J. Cancer*, **108**(1), 66–70.

Knowles, D. M. (2001). Biology of non-Hodgkin's lymphoma. *Cancer. Treat. Res.*, **104**, 149–200.

Koriyama, C., Akiba, S., Corvalan, A. et al. (2004). Histology-specific gender, age and tumor-location distributions of Epstein-Barr virus-associated gastric carcinoma in Japan. *Oncol. Rep.*, **12**(3), 543–547.

Kunimoto, M., Tamura, S., Tabata, T., and Yoshie, O. (1992). One-step typing of Epstein-Barr virus by polymerase chain reaction: predominance of type 1 virus in Japan. *J. Gen. Virol.*, **73**(Pt 2), 455–461.

Kusuhara, K., Takabayashi, A., Ueda, K. *et al.* (1997). Breast milk is not a significant source for early Epstein-Barr virus or human herpesvirus 6 infection in infants: a seroepidemiologic study in 2 endemic areas of human T-cell lymphotropic virus type I in Japan. *Microbiol. Immunol.*, **41**(4), 309–312.

Kyaw, M. T., Hurren, L., Evans, L. *et al.* (1992). Expression of B-type Epstein-Barr virus in HIV-infected patients and cardiac transplant recipients. *AIDS Res. Hum. Retroviruses*, **8**(11), 1869–1874.

Lai, P. K., Mackay-Scollay, E. M., and Alpers, M. P. (1975). Epidemiological studies of Epstein-Barr herpesvirus infection in Western Australia. *J. Hyg. (Lond.)*, **74**(3), 329–337.

Lam, K. M., Syed, N., Whittle, H., and Crawford, D. H. (1991). Circulating Epstein-Barr virus-carrying B cells in acute malaria. *Lancet*, **337**(8746), 876–878.

Lang, D. J., Garruto, R. M., and Gajdusek, D. C. (1977). Early acquisition of cytomegalovirus and Epstein-Barr virus antibody in several isolated Melanesian populations. *Am. J. Epidemiol.*, **105**(5), 480–487.

Lechowicz, M. J., Lin, L., and Ambinder, R. F. (2002). Epstein-Barr virus DNA in body fluids. *Curr. Opin. Oncol.*, **14**(5), 533–537.

Lecuit, M., Abachin, E., Martin, A. *et al.* (2004). Immunoproliferative small intestinal disease associated with Campylobacter jejuni. *N. Engl. J. Med.*, **350**(3), 239–248.

Lee, A. W., Foo, W., Mang, O. *et al.* (2003). Changing epidemiology of nasopharyngeal carcinoma in Hong Kong over a 20-year period (1980–99): an encouraging reduction in both incidence and mortality. *Int. J. Cancer*, **103**(5), 680–685.

Lee, W. Y., Hsiao, J. R., Jin, Y. T., and Tsai, S. T. (2000). Epstein-Barr virus detection in neck metastases by in-situ hybridization in fine-needle aspiration cytologic studies: an aid for differentiating the primary site. *Head Neck*, **22**(4), 336–340.

Levi, F., La Vecchia, C., Randimbison, L., and Te, V. C. (1999). Descriptive epidemiology of soft tissue sarcomas in Vaud, Switzerland. *Eur. J. Cancer*, **35**(12), 1711–1716.

Levin, L. I., Lennette, E. T., Ambinder, R., Chang, E. T., Rubertone, M. V., and Mueller, N. (2002). Prediagnostic Epstein-Barr virus serologic patterns in EBV-positive and EBV-negative Hodgkin lymphoma. Presented at the 10th International EBV Symposium, Cairns.

Levin, L. I., and Levine, P. H. (1998). The epidemiology of Epstein-Barr virus-associated human cancers. In: Osato, T., Takada, K., Tokunaga, M., editors. Epstein-Barr virus and human cancer. Tokyo: Japan Scientific Societies Press, 51–74.

Levine, A. (2000). Aids-related lymphoma. In: Goedert, J. J., editor. Infectious causes of cancer: Targets for intervention. Totowa, New Jersey: Humana Press, 129–143.

Levine, P. H., Ebbesen, P., Connelly, R. R., Das, S., Middleton, M., and Mestre, M. (1982). Complement-fixing antibody to Epstein-Barr virus soluble antigen in populations at high and low risk for nasopharyngeal carcinoma. *Int. J. Cancer*, **29**, 265–268.

Levine, P. H., Stemmermann, G., Lennette, E. T., Hildesheim, A., Shibata, D., and Nomura, A. (1995). Elevated antibody titers to Epstein-Barr virus prior to the diagnosis of Epstein-Barr virus-associated gastric adenocarcinoma. *Int. J. Cancer*, **60**(5), 642–644.

Li, C. C., Yu, M. C., and Henderson, B. E. (1985). Some epidemiologic observations of nasopharyngeal carcinoma in Guangdong, People's Republic of China. Natl Cancer Inst Monogr, **69**, 49–52.

Lichtenstein, P., Holm, N. V., Verkasalo, P. K. *et al.* (2000). Environmental and heritable factors in the causation of cancer–analyses of cohorts of twins from Sweden, Denmark, and Finland. *N. Engl. J. Med.*, **343**(2), 78–85.

Lim, S. T., and Levine, A. M. (2005). Recent advances in acquired immunodeficiency syndrome (AIDS)-related lymphoma. *CA Cancer J. Clin.*, **55**(4), 229–241.

Lin, J. C., Wang, W. Y., Chen, K. Y. *et al.* (2004). Quantification of plama Epstein–Barr virus DNA in patients with advanced nasopharyngeal carcinoma. *N. Engl. J. Med.*, **350**(24), 2461–70.

Ling, P. D., Lednicky, J. A., Keitel, W. A. *et al.* (2003). The dynamics of herpesvirus and polyomavirus reactivation and shedding in healthy adults: a 14-month longitudinal study. *J. Infect Dis.*, **187**(10), 1571–1580.

Lo, Y. M., Chan, A. T., Chan, L. Y. *et al.* (2000). Molecular prognostication of nasopharyngeal carcinoma by quantitative analysis of circulating Epstein-Barr virus DNA. *Cancer Res.*, **60**(24), 6878–6881.

Lo, Y. M., Chan, L. Y., Lo, K. W. *et al.* (1999). Quantitative analysis of cell-free Epstein-Barr virus DNA in plasma of patients with nasopharyngeal carcinoma. *Cancer Res.*, **59**(6), 1188–1191.

Loren, A. W., Porter, D. L., Stadtmauer, E. A., and Tsai, D. E. (2003). Post-transplant lymphoproliferative disorder: a review. *Bone Marrow Transplant*, **31**(3), 145–155.

Lu, S. J., Day, N. E., Degos, L. *et al.* (1990). Linkage of a nasopharyngeal carcinoma susceptibility locus to the HLA region. *Nature*, **346**, 470–471.

Macfarlane, G. J., Evstifeeva, T., Boyle, P., and Grufferman, S. (1995). International patterns in the occurrence of Hodgkin's disease in children and young adult males. *Int. J. Cancer*, **61**(2), 165–169.

MacMahon, B. (1957). Epidemiological evidence of the nature of Hodgkin's disease. *Cancer*, **10**(5), 1045–1054.

MacMahon, B. (1966). Epidemiology of Hodgkin's disease. *Cancer Res.*, **26**, 1189–1201.

Macsween, K. F., and Crawford, D. H. (2003). Epstein-Barr virus-recent advances. *Lancet Infect Dis.*, **3**(3), 131–140.

Maurmann, S., Fricke, L., Wagner, H. J. *et al.* (2003). Molecular parameters for precise diagnosis of asymptomatic Epstein-Barr virus reactivation in healthy carriers. *J. Clin. Microbiol.*, **41**(12), 5419–5428.

McGeoch, D. J., Cook, S., Dolan, A., Jamieson, F. E., and Telford, E. A. (1995). Molecular phylogeny and evolutionary timescale for the family of mammalian herpesviruses. *J. Mol. Biol.*, **247**(3), 443–458.

Mekmullica, J., Kritsaneepaiboon, S., and Pancharoen, C. (2003). Risk factors for Epstein-Barr virus infection in Thai infants. *Southeast Asian J. Trop. Med. Public Health*, **34**(2), 395–397.

Melbye, M., Ebbesen, P., and Bennike, T. (1984). Infectious mononucleosis in Greenland: a disease of the non-indigenous population. Scand J. Infect Dis., 16, 9–15.

Melbye, M., Ebbesen, P., Levine, P. H., and Bennike, T. (1984). Early primary infection and high Epstein-Barr virus antibody titers in Greenland Eskimos at high risk for nasopharyngeal carcinoma. Int. J. Cancer, 34, 619–623.

Meyohas, M. C., Marechal, V., Desire, N., Bouillie, J., Frottier, J., and Nicolas, J. C. (1996). Study of mother-to-child Epstein-Barr virus transmission by means of nested PCRs. J. Virol, 70(10), 6816–6819.

Miyazato, H., Nakatsuka, S., Dong, Z. et al. (2004). NK-cell related neoplasms in Osaka, Japan. Am. J. Hematol., 76(3), 230–235.

Moormann, A. M., Chelimo, K., Sumba, O. P. et al. (2005). Exposure to holoendemic malaria results in elevated Epstein-Barr virus loads in children. J. Infect Dis., 191(8), 1233–1238.

Mori, M., Watanabe, M., Tanaka, S., Mimori, K., Kuwano, H., and Sugimachi, K. (1994). Epstein-Barr virus-associated carcinomas of the esophagus and stomach. Arch. Pathol. Lab Med., 118(10), 998–1001.

Morra, M., Howie, D., Grande, M. S. et al. (2001). X-linked lymphoproliferative disease: a progressive immunodeficiency. Annu Rev Immunol, 19, 657–82.

Morris, M. C., and Edmunds, W. J. (2002). The changing epidemiology of infectious mononucleosis? J. Infect, 45(2), 107–109.

Mueller, N. (1999). Overview of the epidemiology of malignancy in immune deficiency. J. Acquir. Immune. Defic. Syndr., 21 Suppl 1, S5–10.

Mueller, N., Evans, A., Harris, N. L. et al. (1989). Hodgkin's disease and Epstein-Barr virus. Altered antibody pattern before diagnosis. N. Engl. J. Med., 320, 689–695.

Mueller, N., Mohar, A., Evans, A. et al. (1991). Epstein-Barr virus antibody patterns preceding the diagnosis of non- Hodgkin's lymphoma. Int. J. Cancer, 49, 387–393.

Mueller, N. E. (1996). Hodgkin's disease. In: Schottenfeld, D., Fraumeni Jr. J., editors. Cancer Epidemiology and Prevention. Oxford: Oxford University Press.

Mueller, N. E., Evans, A. S., and London, W. T. (1996). Viruses. In: Schottenfeld, D., Fraumeni Jr. J., editors. Cancer Epidemiology and Prevention. Oxford: Oxford University Press, 502–531.

Naher, H., Gissmann, L., Freese, U. K., Petzoldt, D., and Helfrich, S. (1992). Subclinical Epstein-Barr virus infection of both the male and female genital tract–indication for sexual transmission. J. Invest Dermatol., 98(5), 791–793.

Nalesnik, M. A. (2002). Clinicopathologic characteristics of post-transplant lymphoproliferative disorders. Recent Results Cancer Res., 159, 9–18.

Nava, V. E. and Jaffe, E. S. (2005). The pathology of NK-cell lymphomas and leukemias. Adv. Anat. Pathol., 12(1), 27–34.

Newnham, A., Quinn, M. J., Babb, P., Kang, J. Y., and Majeed, A. (2003). Trends in the subsite and morphology of oesophageal and Gastric Cancer in England and Wales 1971–1998. Aliment Pharmacol. Ther., 17(5), 665–676.

Nicholls, J. M., Agathanggelou, A., Fung, K., Zeng, X., and Niedobitek, G. (1997). The association of squamous cell carcinomas of the nasopharynx with Epstein-Barr virus shows geographical variation reminiscent of Burkitt's lymphoma. J. Pathol., 183(2), 164–168.

Nichols, K. E., Harkin, D. P., Levitz, S. et al. (1998). Inactivating mutations in an SH2 domain-encoding gene in X-linked lymphoproliferative syndrome. Proc. Natl. Acad. Sci., U S A, 95(23), 13765–13770.

Nichols, K. E., Ma, C. S., Cannons, J. L., Schwartzberg, P. L., and Tangye, S. G. (2005). Molecular and cellular pathogenesis of X-linked lymphoproliferative disease. Immunol. Rev., 203, 180–99.

Niedobitek, G., Young, L. S., Lau, R. et al. (1991). Epstein-Barr virus infection in oral hairy leukoplakia: virus replication in the absence of a detectable latent phase. J. Gen. Virol., 72(Pt 12), 3035–3046.

Nishikawa, J., Yanai, H., Hirano, A. et al. (2002). High prevalence of Epstein-Barr virus in gastric remnant carcinoma after Billroth-II reconstruction. Scand J. Gastroenterol, 37(7), 825–829.

Nyren, O. and Adami, H. O. (2002). Stomach cancer. In: Adami, H. O., Hunter, D., Trichopoulos, D., editors. Textbook of Cancer Epidemiology. New York: Oxford University Press, 162–187.

Okano, M. (2002). Overview and problematic standpoints of severe chronic active Epstein-Barr virus infection syndrome. Crit. Rev. Oncol. Hematol., 44(3), 273–282.

Okano, M., Kawa, K., Kimura, H. et al. (2005). Proposed guidelines for diagnosing chronic active Epstein-Barr virus infection. Am. J. Hematol., 80(1), 64–69.

Old, L. J., Boyse, E. A., and Oettgen, H. P. (1966). Precipitating antibody in human serum to antigen present in cultured Burkitt lymphoma cell. Proc. Natl. Acad. Sci., 56, 1699–1704.

Ozkan, A., Kilic, S. S., Kalkan, A., Ozden, M., Demirdag, K., and Ozdarendeli, A. (2003). Seropositivity of Epstein-Barr virus in Eastern Anatolian Region of Turkey. Asian Pac. J. Allergy Immunol., 21(1), 49–53.

Parkin, D. M., Bray, F., Ferlay, J., and Pisani, P. (2001). Estimating the world cancer burden: Globocan, Int. J. Cancer, 94(2), 153–156.

Parkin, D. M., Whelan, S. L., Ferlay, J., Teppo, L., Thomas, D. B., editors. (2002). Cancer Incidence in Five Continents vol VIII. Lyon, IARC. IARC Scientific Publications No. 155

Pathmanathan, R., Prasad, U., Sadler, R., Flynn, K., and Raab-Traub, N. (1995). Clonal proliferations of cells infected with Epstein-Barr virus in preinvasive lesions related to nasopharyngeal carcinoma [see comments]. N. Engl. J. Med., 333, 693–698.

Paya, C. V., Fung, J. J., Nalesnik, M. A. et al. (1999). Epstein-Barr virus-induced posttransplant lymphoproliferative disorders. ASTS/ASTP EBV-PTLD Task Force and The Mayo Clinic Organized International Consensus Development Meeting. Transplantation, 68(10), 1517–1525.

Pickard, A., Chen, C. J., Diehl, S. R. et al. (2004). Epstein-Barr virus seroreactivity among unaffected individuals within high-risk nasopharyngeal carcinoma families in Taiwan. Int. J. Cancer, 111(1), 117–123.

Pozzato, G., Mazzaro, C., Crovatto, M. et al. (1994). Low-grade malignant lymphoma, hepatitis C virus infection, and mixed cryoglobulinemia. *Blood*, **84**(9), 3047–3053.

Purtilo, D. T., Cassel, C. K., Yang, J. P., and Harper, R. (1975). X-linked recessive progressive combined variable immunodeficiency (Duncan's disease). *Lancet*, **1**(7913), 935–940.

Quintanilla-Martinez, L., Franklin, J. L., Guerrero, I. et al. (1999). Histological and immunophenotypic profile of nasal NK/T cell lymphomas from Peru: high prevalence of p53 overexpression. *Hum. Pathol.*, **30**(7), 849–855.

Quintanilla-Martinez, L., Lome-Maldonado, C., Ott, G. et al. (1997). Primary non-Hodgkin's lymphoma of the intestine: high prevalence of Epstein-Barr virus in Mexican lymphomas as compared with European cases. *Blood*, **89**, 644–651.

Raab-Traub, N. (2000). Epstein-Barr virus and nasopharyngeal carcinoma. In: Goedert, J. J., editor. Infectious causes of cancer: Targets for intervention. Totowa, New Jersey: Humana Press, 93–111.

Raab-Traub, N. and Flynn, K. (1986). The structure of the termini of the Epstein-Barr virus as a marker of clonal cellular proliferation. *Cell*, **47**(6), 883–889.

Raphael, M., Borisch, B., and Jaffe, E. (2001). Lymphomas associated with infection by the human immune deficiency virus (HIV). In: Jaffe, E. S., Harris, N. L., Stein, H., Vardiman, J. W., editors. Tumours of haematopoietic and lymphoid tissues. Lyon: IARC, 260–263.

Riddler, S. A., Breinig, M. C., and McKnight, J. L. (1994). Increased levels of circulating Epstein-Barr virus (EBV)-infected lymphocytes and decreased EBV nuclear antigen antibody responses are associated with the development of posttransplant lymphoproliferative disease in solid-organ transplant recipients. *Blood*, **84**(3), 972–984.

Rizvi, M. A., Evens, A. M., Tallman, M. S., Nelson, B. P., and Rosen, S. T. (2006). T-cell non-Hodgkin's lymphoma. *Blood*, **107**, 1255–1264.

Rosdahl, N., Larsen, S. O., and Thamdrup, A. B. (1973). Infectious mononucleosis in Denmark. Epidemiological observations based on positive Paul-Bunnell reactions from 1940–1969. *Scand J. Infect Dis.*, **5**(3), 163–170.

Rose, C., Green, M., Webber, S. et al. (2002). Detection of Epstein-Barr virus genomes in peripheral blood B cells from solid-organ transplant recipients by fluorescence in situ hybridization. *J. Clin. Microbiol.*, **40**(7), 2533–2544.

Rudiger, T., Weisenburger, D. D., Anderson, J. R. et al. (2002). Peripheral T-cell lymphoma (excluding anaplastic large-cell lymphoma): results from the Non-Hodgkin's Lymphoma Classification Project. *Ann. Oncol.*, **13**(1), 140–149.

Sample, J., Young, L., Martin, B. et al. (1990). Epstein-Barr virus types 1 and 2 differ in their EBNA-3A, EBNA-3B, and EBNA-3C genes. *J. Virol*, **64**(9), 4084–4092.

Sandvej, K., Peh, S. C., Andresen, B. S., and Pallesen, G. (1994). Identification of potential hot spots in the carboxy-terminal part of the Epstein-Barr virus (EBV) BNLF-1 gene in both malignant and benign EBV-associated diseases: high frequency of a 30-bp deletion in Malaysian and Danish peripheral T-cell lymphomas. *Blood*, **84**(12), 4053–4060.

Savoldo, B., Huls, M. H., Liu, Z. et al. (2002). Autologous Epstein-Barr virus (EBV)-specific cytotoxic T cells for the treatment of persistent active EBV infection. *Blood*, **100**(12), 4059–4066.

Sawyer, R. N., Evans, A. S., Niederman, J. C., and McCollum, R. W. (1971). Prospective studies of a group of Yale University freshmen. I. Occurrence of infectious mononucleosis. *J. Infect Dis.*, **123**(3), 263–270.

Scheenstra, R., Verschuuren, E. A., de H. A., et al. (2004). The value of prospective monitoring of Epstein-Barr virus DNA in blood samples of pediatric liver transplant recipients. *Transpl. Infect Dis.*, **6**(1), 15–22.

Scherr, P. A. and Mueller, N. E. (1996). Non-Hodgkin's lymphomas. In: Schottenfeld, D., Fraumeni, J. F., editors. Cancer Epidemiology and Prevention. Oxford New York: Oxford University Press, 920–945.

Shanmugaratnam, K. (1991). Histological Typing of Tumours of the Upper Respiratory Tract and Ear. Berlin: Springer.

Shek, T. W., Luk, I. S., Ng, I. O., and Lo, C. Y. (1996). Lymphoepithelioma-like carcinoma of the thyroid gland: lack of evidence of association with Epstein-Barr virus. *Hum. Pathol.*, **27**(8), 851–853.

Shibata, D. (1998). Epstein-Barr virus-associated *Gastric Cancer* in the United States. In: Osato, T., Takada, K., Tokunaga, M., editors. Epstein-Barr virus and human cancer. Tokyo: Japan Scientific Societies Press, 99–101.

Shibata, D. and Weiss, L. M. (1992). Epstein-Barr virus-associated gastric adenocarcinoma. *Am J. Pathol.*, **140**(4), 769–774.

Shinmura, K., Kohno, T., and Takahashi, M. et al. (1999). Familial *Gastric Cancer*: clinicopathological characteristics, RER phenotype and germline p53 and E-cadherin mutations. *Carcinogenesis*, **20**(6), 1127–1131.

Shu, C. H., Chang, Y. S., Liang, C. L., Liu, S. T., Lin, C. Z., and Chang, P. (1992). Distribution of type A and type B EBV in normal individuals and patients with head and neck carcinomas in Taiwan. *J. Virol. Methods*, **38**(1), 123–130.

Silins, S. L., Sherritt, M. A., and Silleri, J. M. et al. (2001). Asymptomatic primary Epstein-Barr virus infection occurs in the absence of blood T-cell repertoire perturbations despite high levels of systemic viral load. *Blood*, **98**(13), 3739–3744.

Sixbey, J. W., Nedrud, J. G., Raab-Traub, N., Hanes, R. A., and Pagano, J. S. (1984). Epstein-Barr virus replication in oropharyngeal epithelial cells. *N. Engl. J. Med.*, **310**(19), 1225–1230.

Sleckman, B. G., Mauch, P. M., Ambinder, R. F. et al. (1998). Epstein-Barr virus in Hodgkin's disease: correlation of risk factors and disease characteristics with molecular evidence of viral infection. *Cancer Epidemiol Biomarkers Prev*, **7**, 1117–1121.

Smith, J. L., Hodges, E., Quin, C. T., McCarthy, K. P., and Wright, D. H. (2000). Frequent T and B cell oligoclones in histologically and immunophenotypically characterized angioimmunoblastic lymphadenopathy. *Am J. Pathol.*, **156**(2), 661–669.

Stadlmann, S., Fend, F., Moser, P., Obrist, P., Greil, R., and Dirnhofer, S. (2001). Epstein-Barr virus-associated extranodal NK/T-cell lymphoma, nasal type of the hypopharynx, in a renal allograft recipient: case report and review of literature. *Hum. Pathol.*, **32**(11), 1264–1268.

Stein, H. (2001). Hodgkin lymphomas: Introduction. In: Jaffe, E. S., Harris, N. L., Stein, H., Vardiman, J. W., editors. Tumours of haematopoietic and lymphoid tissues. Lyon: IARC, 239.

Stein, H., Delsol, G., Pileri, S. *et al.* (2001). Classical Hodgkin lymphoma. In: Jaffe, E. S., Harris, N. L., Stein, H., Vardiman, J. W., editors. Tumours of haematopoietic and lymphoid tissues. Lyon: IARC, 244–253.

Stein, H., Delsol, G., Pileri, S. *et al.* (2001). Nodular lymphocyte predominant Hodgkin lymphoma. In: Jaffe, E. S., Harris, N. L., Stein, H., Vardiman, J. W., editors. Tumours of haematopoietic and lymphoid tissues. Lyon: IARC, 240–243.

Stevens, S. J., Blank, B. S., Smits, P. H., Meenhorst, P. L., and Middeldorp, J. M. (2002a). High Epstein-Barr virus (EBV) DNA loads in HIV-infected patients: correlation with antiretroviral therapy and quantitative EBV serology. *AIDS*, **16**(7), 993–1001.

Stevens, S. J., Verschuuren, E. A., Verkuijlen, S. A., van den Brule, A. J., Meijer, C. J., and Middeldorp, J. M. (2002b). Role of Epstein-Barr virus DNA load monitoring in prevention and early detection of post-transplant lymphoproliferative disease. *Leuk. Lymphoma.*, **43**(4), 831–840.

Storrie, M. C., Sphar, R. L. (1976). Seroepidemiological studies of polaris Submarine crews. II. Infectious mononucleosis. *Mil. Med.*, **141**(1), 30–32.

Straus, S. E. (1988). The chronic mononucleosis syndrome. *J. Infect Dis.*, **157**(3), 405–412.

Sugawara, Y., Makuuchi, M., Kato, N., Shimotohno, K., and Takada, K. (1999). Enhancement of hepatitis C virus replication by Epstein-Barr virus-encoded nuclear antigen 1. *EMBO J.*, **18**(20), 5755–5760.

Sugaya, N., Kimura, H., Hara, S. *et al.* (2004). Quantitative analysis of Epstein-Barr virus (EBV)-specific CD8+ T cells in patients with chronic active EBV infection. *J. Infect Dis.*, **190**(5), 985–988.

Sumaya, C. V., Henle, W., Henle, G., Smith, M. H., and LeBlanc, D. (1975). Seroepidemiologic study of Epstein-Barr virus infections in a rural community. *J. Infect Dis.*, **131**(4), 403–408.

Sumazaki, R., Kanegane, H., Osaki, M. *et al.* (2001). SH2D1A mutations in Japanese males with severe Epstein-Barr virus–associated illnesses. *Blood*, **98**(4), 1268–1270.

Sumegi, J., Huang, D., Lanyi, A. *et al.* (2000). Correlation of mutations of the SH2D1A gene and epstein-barr virus infection with clinical phenotype and outcome in X-linked lymphoproliferative disease. *Blood*, **96**(9), 3118–3125.

Swigris, J. J., Berry, G. J., Raffin, T. A., and Kuschner, W. G. (2002). Lymphoid interstitial pneumonia: a narrative review. *Chest*, **122**(6), 2150–2164.

Swinnen, L. J. (2000). Posttransplant lymphoproliferative disorders. In: Goedert, J. J., editor. Infectious causes of cancer: Targets for intervention. Totowa, New Jersey: Humana Press, 63–76.

Takada, K. (2000). Epstein-Barr virus and gastric carcinoma. *Mol. Pathol.*, **53**(5), 255–261.

Takkouche, B., Etminan, M., and Montes-Martinez, A. (2005). Personal use of hair dyes and risk of cancer: a meta-analysis. *JAMA*, **293**(20), 2516–2525.

Tashiro, Y., Arikawa, J., Itoh, T., and Tokunaga, M. (1998). Clinicopathological findings of Epstein-Barr virus-related *Gastric Cancer*. In: Osato, T., Takada, K., Tokunaga, M., editors. Epstein-Barr virus and human cancer. Tokyo: Japan Scientific Societies Press, 87–98.

Thorley-Lawson, D. A. and Gross, A. (2004). Persistence of the Epstein-Barr virus and the origins of associated lymphomas. *N. Engl. J. Med.*, **350**(13), 1328–1337.

Tredaniel, J., Boffetta, P., Buiatti, E., Saracci, R., and Hirsch, A. (1997). Tobacco smoking and *Gastric Cancer*: review and meta-analysis. *Int. J. Cancer*, **72**(4), 565–573.

Uemura, N., Okamoto, S., Yamamoto, S. *et al.* (2001). Helicobacter pylori infection and the development of *Gastric Cancer*. *N. Engl. J. Med.*, **345**(11), 784–789.

van Beek, J., zur HA, Klein, K. E. *et al.* (2004). EBV-positive gastric adenocarcinomas: a distinct clinicopathologic entity with a low frequency of lymph node involvement. *J. Clin. Oncol.*, **22**(4), 664–670.

van den Bosch, C. A. (2004). Is endemic Burkitt's lymphoma an alliance between three infections and a tumour promoter? *Lancet Oncol.*, **5**(12), 738–746.

van B. D., Hovenkamp, E., Dukers, N. H. *et al.* (2000). High prevalence of Epstein-Barr virus type 2 among homosexual men is caused by sexual transmission. *J. Infect Dis.*, **181**(6), 2045–2049.

Venkitaraman, A. R., Lenoir, G. M., and John, T. J. (1985). The seroepidemiology of infection due to Epstein-Barr virus in southern India. *J. Med. Virol.*, **15**(1), 11–16.

Wagner, H. J., Hornef, M., Teichert, H. M., Kirchner, H. (1994). Sex difference in the serostatus of adults to the Epstein-Barr virus. *Immunobiology*, **190**(4–5), 424–429.

Wagner, H. J., Kluter, H., Kruse, A., Bucsky, P., Hornef, M., and Kirchner, H. (1995). Determination of the number of Epstein-Barr virus genomes in whole blood and red cell concentrates. *Transfus. Med.*, **5**(4), 297–302.

Weiss, L. M., Jaffe, E. S., Liu, X. F., Chen, Y. Y., Shibata, D., and Medeiros, L. J. (1992). Detection and localization of Epstein-Barr viral genomes in angioimmunoblastic lymphadenopathy and angioimmunoblastic lymphadenopathy-like lymphoma. *Blood*, **79**(7), 1789–1795.

Weiss, L. M., Strickler, J. G., Warnke, R. A., Purtilo, D. T., and Sklar, J. (1987). Epstein-Barr viral DNA in tissues of Hodgkin's disease. *Am J. Pathol.*, **129**(1), 86–91.

Wekerle, H., and Hohlfeld, R. (2003). Molecular mimicry in multiple sclerosis. *N. Engl. J. Med.*, **349**(2), 185–186.

Wick, G., Grubeck-Loebenstein, B. (1997). Primary and secondary alterations of immune reactivity in the elderly: impact of dietary factors and disease. Immunol Rev, **160**, 171–84.

Wijnhoven, B. P., Louwman, M. W., Tilanus, H. W., and Coebergh, J. W. (2002). Increased incidence of adenocarcinomas at the gastro-oesophageal junction in Dutch males since the 1990s. *Eur. J. Gastroenterol. Hepatol.*, **14**(2), 115–122.

Wotherspoon, A. C., Ortiz-Hidalgo, C., Falzon, M. R., and Isaacson, P. G. (1991). Helicobacter pylori-associated gastritis and primary B-cell gastric lymphoma [see comments]. *Lancet*, **338**, 1175–1176.

Xiong, W., Zeng, Z. Y., Xia, J. H. *et al.* (2004). A susceptibility locus at chromosome 3p21 linked to familial nasopharyngeal carcinoma. *Cancer Res.*, **64**(6), 1972–1974.

Yamamoto, N., Tokunaga, M., Uemura, Y. *et al.* (1994). Epstein-Barr virus and gastric remnant cancer. *Cancer*, **74**(3), 805–809.

Yang, J., Tao, Q., Flinn, I. W. *et al.* (2000). Characterization of Epstein-Barr virus-infected B cells in patients with posttransplantation lymphoproliferative disease: disappearance after rituximab therapy does not predict clinical response. *Blood*, **96**(13), 4055–4063.

Yao, Q. Y., Croom-Carter, D. S., Tierney, R. J. *et al.* (1998). Epidemiology of infection with Epstein-Barr virus types 1 and 2: lessons from the study of a T-cell-immunocompromised hemophilic cohort. *J. Virol*, **72**(5), 4352–4363.

Yao, Q. Y., Rowe, M., Martin, B., Young, L. S., and Rickinson, A. B. (1991). The Epstein-Barr virus carrier state: dominance of a single growth-transforming isolate in the blood and in the oropharynx of healthy virus carriers. *J. Gen. Virol.*, **72**(Pt 7), 1579–1590.

Yu, M. C., Henderson, B. E. (1996). Nasopharyngeal cancer. In: Schottenfeld, D., Fraumeni Jr. J., editors. Cancer Epidemiology and Prevention. Oxford: Oxford University Press, 603–618.

Yu, M. C., Ho, J. H., Ross, R. K., and Henderson, B. E. (1981). Nasopharyngeal carcinoma in Chinese—salted fish or inhaled smoke? *Prev. Med.*, **10**(1), 15–24.

Yu, M. C. and Yuan, J. M. (2002). Epidemiology of nasopharyngeal carcinoma. *Semin. Cancer Biol.*, **12**(6), 421–429.

Zahm, S. H., Tucker, M. A., Fraumeni Jr., J. (1996). Soft tissue sarcomas. In: Schottenfeld, D., Fraumeni Jr. J, editors. Cancer Epidemiology and Prevention. Oxford: Oxford University Press, 984–999.

Zeng, Y. X. and Jia, W. H. (2002). Familial nasopharyngeal carcinoma. *Semin. Cancer Biol.*, **12**(6), 443–450.

Zhang, W. Y., Li, G. D., Liu, W. P. *et al.* (2005). Features of intestinal T-cell lymphomas in Chinese population without evidence of celiac disease and their close association with Epstein-Barr virus infection. *Chin. Med. J. (Engl.)*, **118**(18), 1542–1548.

Zimber, U., Adldinger, H. K., Lenoir, G. M. *et al.* (1986). Geographical prevalence of two types of Epstein-Barr virus. *Virology*, **154**(1), 56–66.

Zintzaras, E., Voulgarelis, M., and Moutsopoulos, H. M. (2005). The risk of lymphoma development in autoimmune diseases: a meta-analysis. *Arch. Intern. Med.*, **165**(20), 2337–2344.

54

The epidemiology of KSHV and its association with malignant disease

Jeffrey N. Martin

Department of Epidemiology and Biostatistics, University of California, San Francisco, 185 Berry Street, Suite 5700 San Francisco, CA, USA

Introduction

In 1872, Moritz Kaposi, a Hungarian dermatologist, described six patients with multifocal brown–red or blue–red nodules or plaques on the feet and hands (Kaposi, 1872). Initially called "Idiopathisches multiples Pigmentsarcoma der Haut" (multiple idiopathic sarcoma of the skin) by Kaposi, the condition later became known as Kaposi's sarcoma (KS). Decades later, after the epidemiology of KS began to be investigated, its uneven geographic distribution suggested that exogenous factors were etiologically important. Subsequently, as the AIDS epidemic unfolded in the early 1980s, homosexual men were found to be up to 20 times more likely than other risk groups to develop KS, a markedly disproportionate risk that led to the hypothesis that the exogenous factor was a sexually transmitted infectious agent (Beral et al., 1990). Numerous microbial candidates were proposed (Drew et al., 1982; Huang et al., 1992; Wang et al., 1993) but for none was convincing evidence demonstrated until Kaposi's sarcoma-associated herpesvirus (KSHV), or human herpesvirus 8 (HHV-8), was discovered in 1994 (Table 54.1) (Chang et al., 1994). In a short period following the discovery of KSHV, consensus rapidly developed that it is a necessary, albeit not sufficient, causal agent of KS (Whitby et al., 1995; Gao et al., 1996a,b; Martin et al., 1998; Renwick et al.,1998; O'Brien et al., 1999). This discovery was more than academic in that, because of the AIDS epidemic, KS is now worldwide the fourth most common cancer caused by an infectious agent, following gastric, cervical, and hepatic cancer. Subsequently, it was also determined that KSHV has a potentially causal role in primary effusion lymphoma (PEL) (Cesarman et al., 1995), also known as body cavity-based lymphoma, and multicentric Castleman's disease (Soulier et al., 1995). Now that the clinical importance of KSHV has been established, attention has turned towards unraveling of what is proving to be a complicated epidemiologic profile for the virus.

Diagnosis of KSHV infection

While nucleic acid amplification techniques were originally used to identify the presence of KSHV DNA in KS tissue, when applied to peripheral blood these techniques are much less sensitive as compared to detection of KSHV-specific antibodies. Even among patients with KS, of whom virtually all have detectable KSHV DNA in their KS lesions, only approximately 40 to 60% have detectable KSHV DNA in either plasma or peripheral white blood cells (IARC Working Group, 1997). Among persons without KS, the group for which a diagnostic test for KSHV is most needed, the prevalence of KSHV DNA in blood is much lower, especially in HIV-uninfected populations, and is always less common than the detection of KSHV-specific antibodies. For this reason, there is currently little role for nucleic acid-based testing of peripheral blood in the diagnosis of KSHV infection (Spira et al., 2000). Instead, the primary means of KSHV diagnosis is antibody testing, which is described in detail in Chapter 52. What follows is a brief overview of antibody testing that provides the requisite perspective for which to interpret epidemiologic studies of the distribution and transmission of KSHV infection.

Initial serologic assays for KSHV antibodies

After the finding that DNA from PEL biopsy specimens contains KSHV sequences (Cesarman et al., 1995), the original assays for KSHV antibodies were developed using cell lines obtained from patients with PEL (Miller et al., 1996; Kedes et al., 1996; Gao et al., 1996a,b; Simpson et al., 1996) One of the first platforms were indirect immunofluorescence assays (IFAs) that utilized the cell lines in an

Table 54.1. Original detection of KSHV DNA by polymerase chain reaction in various tissue specimens

Tissue type	No. evaluated	No. (%) positive for KS330
KS, AIDS-related	27	25 (93)
Lymphoma, AIDS-related	27	3 (11)
Lymph nodes, AIDS-related	12	3 (25)
Lymphoma, non-AIDS	29	0
Lymph nodes, non-AIDS	7	0
Vascular tumors, HIV unknown	5	0
Opportunistic infections	13	0
Consecutive surgical biopsies, HIV unknown	49	0

From Chang et al. (1994).

uninduced state where KSHV is primarily in its latent phase. These assays detect antibodies to KSHV latency-associated nuclear antigen (LANA or LNA-1), the product of open reading frame (ORF) 73 (Rainbow et al., 1997; Kedes et al., 1997a,b). Extensive evaluation of these assays determined that anti-LANA seropositivity is found in approximately 80% of persons with KS and less than 5% of non-male-homosexual adults in the USA or Northern Europe (i.e., specificity of at least 95%) (Kedes et al., 1996; Gao et al., 1996a,b; Simpson et al., 1996). Subsequently, it was determined that induction, using phorbol ester, of KSHV into a lytic phase resulted in IFAs with greater, albeit not complete, sensitivity (approximately 95%) in terms of identifying KS patients, while maintaining seropositivity of less than 10% in non-homosexual adults in the USA (Chandran et al., 1998). In an attempt to improve throughput and eliminate the subjective interpretation inherent in IFAs, a variety of other first-generation assays with comparable performance characteristics were developed. These include enzyme immunoassays (EIA) detecting antibodies against (a) bacterially derived recombinant portions of a minor capsid protein (ORF 65) (Simpson et al., 1996), LANA (Renwick et al., 1998), and glycoprotein K8.1 (Raab et al., 1998; Engels et al., 2000); (b) synthetic peptides portions of K8.1 and ORF 65 (Spira et al., 2000; Pau et al., 1998); and (c) whole virus (Chatlynne et al., 2001; Martin et al., 2000).

Methodologic challenges in serologic assay development

Although first-generation antibody assays, particularly those detecting anti-LANA antibodies, have been useful in epidemiologic work, no single first-generation serologic assay has demonstrated very high sensitivity and specificity, and agreement between assays has been suboptimal. In a study of seven first-generation antibody assays examining 143 serum specimens, the percentage of KSHV-seropositive specimens determined by the different assays ranged from 0% to 54% for the subset of specimens from blood donors, 27% to 60% for HIV-infected persons without KS, and 49% to 93% for KS patients (Rabkin et al., 1998). More recently, a comparison of KSHV antibody testing from six laboratories, using newly developed assays or second-generation versions of previously examined assays, found improved agreement when testing serum specimens from persons with KS (all six laboratories found all 21 specimens to be positive) but only modest agreement when evaluating 1000 specimens from blood donors (a low risk group for KSHV infection) (Pellett et al., 2003).

In part, the interassay disagreement that has been observed may be because certain assays target different antibodies for which inherent sensitivity and specificity for KSHV infection may differ (e.g., antibodies against lytic-phase versus latent-phase antigens). In other instances, however, assay calibration (i.e., differentiating positive from negative results) has not been done in a standardized fashion across assays with reference to a wide spectrum of gold standard KSHV-infected (true positive) and KSHV-uninfected (true negative) subjects. Determining assay sensitivity by limiting the true positive reference group to persons with KS, as has been typically done in the initially described assays, may result in estimates of sensitivity that are unrealistically inflated. This is because it is now recognized that, among KSHV-infected persons, antibody titer is highest and therefore easier to detect in KS patients (Gao et al., 1996a,b). One attempt to reduce this "spectrum bias" (Ransohoff and Feinstein, 1978) was by Engels et al., who used diluted serum from KS patients in an attempt to mimic KSHV-infected persons without KS and found rapidly diminishing sensitivity with only minimal dilution (Engels et al., 2000). However, how much dilution is needed to mimic infected but non-diseased persons is not known. Another attempt was the use of homosexual men without KS but who had detectable KSHV in their saliva (Casper et al., 2002a,b). These persons, however, may be enriched for antibody-positivity if the presence of KSHV antigen drives antibody production. Therefore, more work is needed in identifying gold standard KSHV-infected reference subjects without KS for the evaluation of assay sensitivity.

While early serologic investigators at a minimum had the presence of KS as a basis for forming a true positive reference group, assembling a true negative (KSHV-uninfected) reference group has been particularly vexing because of the lack of any analogous gold standard certifying absence of infection. For example, the use of blood donors (Simpson et al., 1996; Pau et al., 1998; Rabkin et al., 1998; Tedeschi et al., 1999) is problematic because they may include men with undisclosed homosexual activity, the primary risk factor for KSHV infection in developed countries (described below). Approaches used in more recent work to optimize the assembly of a true negative reference group have capitalized on what is now known about the epidemiology of KSHV infection and of KS per se. In the USA, for example, this includes the use of virginal women and of young children who are just past the age of harboring maternal antibodies (Martin et al., 2000), HIV-infected hemophiliacs and their female sexual partners, both of whom were known not to subsequently develop KS after a substantial period of observation (Engels et al., 2000), and homosexual women (Casper et al., 2002a,b).

In addition to the uncertainties in assembling the reference populations for assay calibration, other technical differences have likely contributed to poor interassay agreement. For example, the method of cut-off generation for a positive versus negative result has varied considerably. Some investigators have set cut-offs a priori by taking the mean of between 5 and 40 individuals considered to be uninfected and then adding two to five standard deviations (Renwick et al., 1998; Simpson et al., 1996; Pau et al., 1998; Chatlynne et al., 2001; Rabkin et al., 1998; Tedeschi et al., 1999; Davis et al., 1997). The small sample sizes used in these calculations and the wide range of standard deviations employed likely result in substantial variation across assays. An improved approach to cut-off generation has been used in more recent work where receiver-operating characteristic (ROC) curves were described (Engels et al., 2000; Martin et al., 2000; Casper et al., 2002; Corchero et al., 2001; Laney et al., 2006). ROC curves are not dependent upon an a priori cut-off, but instead show the paired sensitivity and specificity estimates associated with various empiric cut-offs. However, what has not yet been performed is an assessment of interassay agreement by having each assay examine sera from a panel of well-conceived true negative and true positive subjects and then compare ROC curves, generated in a standard fashion for each assay. Until this is done, it will not be possible to compare agreement between contemporary assays.

Approaches using a combination of antibody assays

An approach featuring a highly sensitive high-throughput serologic screening assay followed by a more labor-intensive confirmatory assay with both very high sensitivity and specificity, akin to what is done for the diagnosis of HIV infection, cannot yet be performed for KSHV infection because of the lack of a such confirmatory assay. Nonetheless, use of a combination of assays has been investigated in an attempt to improve assay accuracy compared to individual assays used in isolation (Engels et al., 2003; Casper et al., 2002; Laney et al., 2006). In the most comprehensive analysis of assay combinations, joint use of EIAs featuring K8.1, ORF 73, ORF 65, and whole virus lysate antigens and a latent-phase IFA only marginally improved sensitivity (while holding specificity constant) compared to the best performing individual assays (Engels et al., 2000). Rather than parallel use of multiple assays, the same degree of improvement in accuracy can be obtained when assays are used serially, with the use of a high-throughput EIA first, reserving the more time-intensive IFA in an attempt to resolve specimens scoring in the indeterminate range in the EIA (Engels et al., 2000). Not only is this more cost-efficient than simultaneous testing with both assays, the improvement in accuracy can be substantial depending upon the initial EIA used (Casper et al., 2002a,b).

Recently developed eukaryotically derived recombinant antigen-based serologic assays

While the use of induced PEL cell IFAs increases assay sensitivity, the lack of a KSHV-uninfected isogeneic control cell line hinders the discrimination of KSHV-specific antibody binding vs. non-specific binding to cellular components. Furthermore, because PEL cell IFAs express most or all of the KSHV-encoded genes, including those conserved across all herpesviruses, there is the threat of cross-reactivity with other herpesviruses. To address this, Inoue et al. used a mammalian expression system with BHK-21 cells infected with recombinant Semliki Forest virus (SFV) carrying individual KSHV proteins that are unique to KSHV (Inoue et al., 2000). This approach has the advantage of having an isogeneic control, very high antigen expression, and, because it is a mammalian system, protein glycosylation, which may be an important component of epitope antigenicity. To date, separate BHK-21-based IFAs expressing ORF K8.1, ORF 73, and ORF 65 have been established. (Inoue et al., 2000; Quinlivan et al., 2001). Among these, the K8.1SFV IFA has exhibited the best performance. Among 72 KS patients, the K8.1SFV IFA detected antibodies in 94.4%, and among 30 blood donors, 2 (6.7%) were reactive, thus indicating an estimated specificity of at least 93.3%. These approaches will offer greatest utility when they are available in high throughput formats, and in this regard, Laney et al. have recently developed an EIA featuring a baculovirus-insect cell system-derived full length LANA protein as the antigen substrate (Laney et al., 2006).

Seroreversion

Further complicating the interpretation of serologic testing is the phenomenon of a negative result following a positive result, termed seroreversion, noted in longitudinal observation of individual subjects. For example, Quinlivan et al. found that 27 (82%) of 33 subjects who had at least one time point seropositive for antibodies to LANA had at least one subsequent time point exhibiting seroreversion (Quinlivan et al., 2001). This has also been reported by others (Chohan et al., 2004 and Minhas et al., 2006). Whether seroreversion is the result of assay measurement error (i.e., inadequate reproducibility) or whether it reflects true biologic diminution or loss of antibody is not known. In any case, its presence clouds the interpretation of a single seronegative serologic test result in a cross-sectional study.

Differential reactivity to KSHV antigens over time

Related to the idea that biologic phenomena may be responsible for seroreversion is the finding that KSHV-infected persons may develop antibodies to different antigens at different points in time. There are few longitudinal studies available, especially those with adequate lead-in periods that first establish seronegativity, but in work that has been done with antigen-specific assays, it appears that seroconversion to different antigens can occur at different times (Quinlivan et al., 2001; Biggar et al., 2003; Spira et al., 2001). This further highlights how the currently available assays targeting single antigens are likely not optimally sensitive for detecting infection.

Utility of currently available serologic assays

For epidemiologic work where between group comparisons are the primary focus, even using first-generation serologic assays, despite their poor inter-laboratory agreement, has resulted in reproducible and plausible inferences (described below). Use of currently available serologic assays for individual-level diagnosis, however, be it in an epidemiologic study in the determination of seroconversion among individual subjects, or in the clinical setting, requires greater caution. The lack of gold standards in the development of assays, the apparent lack of concurrent high-level sensitivity and specificity among those first-generation assays that have been evaluated most extensively, and the phenomenon of seroreversion make definitive diagnosis of the presence or absence of KSHV infection problematic at an individual level. The only exception is persons who test positive on a very specific assay, such as the anti-LANA IFA (at least as performed in experienced laboratories). Currently, there is no Food and Drug Administration-licensed assay for KSHV antibodies; testing is limited to research laboratories. Clinicians who seek to use the avaible assays should be aware of their pitfalls and knowledgeable about their performance characteristics. Finally, the recent success in developing an essentially 100% sensitive and specific serologic assay for HIV infection, has raised expectations for the serologic detection of all newly described pathogens, including KSHV. Although not directly studied, the sensitivity and specificity of currently available KSHV antibody assays may not appreciably differ from antibody assays for other herpesviruses, none of which by virtue of their earlier discovery was investigated with the serologic expectations of the contemporary era. Whether or not the recently developed eucaryotically-derived recombinant antigen-based assays will demonstrate very high and reproducible specificity and sensitivity upon wide scale testing or whether there exist inherent biologic limitations to the serologic detection of KSHV infection remains to be determined.

Epidemiology of KSHV infection

Prevalence of infection Geographic distribution

Extensive worldwide surveys of KSHV seroprevalence using the same serologic assay and same method of sampling of subjects (e.g., similar age groups) have not been performed. Even with this limitation, three major patterns of seroprevalence have reproducibly emerged: high-level endemic, intermediate-level endemic, and non-endemic. High-level endemic areas are defined by those with seroprevalences between 30% and 70% among general adult populations and are found in many parts of Africa (Olsen et al., 1998; Mayama et al., 1998; Gessain et al., 1999) and the Middle East, e.g., Egypt (Andreoni et al., 1999). As is discussed below, it is the catastrophic intersection between the endemic nature of KSHV and the HIV epidemic in sub-Saharan Africa that has resulted in KS becoming the most common adult malignancy in many areas there (Chokunonga et al., 2000; Wabinga et al., 2000).

However, even within these geographically constrained areas there nonetheless exists important differences in KSHV seroprevalence from region to region. For example, recent work using a standardized approach to antibody testing found considerably higher seroprevalence in Uganda than compared to South Africa (Butler et al., 2006).

Intermediate-level endemic areas feature KSHV seroprevalences between 10 and 25% in the general population and are found primarily in the Mediterranean area (Angeloni et al., 1998; Whitby et al., 1998; Cattani et al., 2003) Again even within this defined geographic area, there is considerable heterogeneity. For example, among blood donors in Italy, prevalence was estimated to be 7.3% in Northern and Central Italy and 24.6% in Southern Italy (Whitby *et al.*, 1998).

Non-endemic areas are those with seroprevalences less than 10% in the general population. These include North America, Central America, South America, Northern Europe, and Asia. In these non-endemic areas, however, certain population groups have seroprevalences that rival those in high and intermediate-level prevalence regions. In particular, it is homosexual men across these non-endemic areas that have consistently been shown to have the highest seroprevalence; between 30% and 60% of HIV-infected homosexual men in these areas and 20% and 30% of HIV-uninfected homosexual men are KSHV-infected (Martin *et al.*, 1998; O'Brien *et al.*, 1999; Kedes *et al.*, 1996; Chandran *et al.*, 1998; Melbye *et al.*, 1998; Dukers *et al.*, 2000). This contrasts with less than 10% prevalence in most reports of women and non-homosexual men in the general population of these areas (Martin *et al.*, 1998; Kedes *et al.*, 1996; Smith *et al.*, 1999; Kedes *et al.*, 1997a,b). Other notable pockets of concentrated prevalence (not all of which have been confirmed by other investigators) in otherwise non-endemic areas include an estimated seroprevalence of 65% among Brazilian Amerindians >30 years of age (Biggar *et al.*, 2000), 33% among adults in Papua New Guinea (Rezza *et al.*, 2001), 20% among adults of the Noir-Marron, an ethnic group of African origin residing in French Guiana (Plancoulaine *et al.*, 2000), and 25% among Hispanic children in South Texas in the USA (Baillargeon *et al.*, 2002). Although considerable work has now firmly established the marked geographic differences in KSHV seroprevalence, it is notable (as will be discussed below) that the explanation for this is unknown. Whether the answer rests in host genetic or behavioral differences, influences from other exogenous environmental influences, or viral variants is unresolved.

Temporal patterns

Studies of genomic strain variability have concluded that KSHV is an ancient human virus, introduced at least tens of thousands of years ago (Hayward, 1999) (and discussed below). Descriptions of KS in the 1800s and the finding of high KSHV seroprevalences in geographically distinct and remote isolated populations (Biggar *et al.*, 2000; Rezza *et al.*, 2001; Whitby *et al.*, 2004) substantiate this. There is, however, debate as to the introduction of KSHV in sentinel populations such as homosexual men in the USA and Northern Europe. Two initial reports hypothesized that an epidemic of KSHV infection in homosexual men took place concurrently with that of HIV infection (O'Brien *et al.*, 1999;

Melbye *et al.*, 1998). This hypothesis was based upon the finding of an initial high incidence of KSHV infection in these studies at the beginning of their observation in 1981 and 1982, respectively. However, a more direct examination of homosexual men in San Francisco as early as 1978, prior to the HIV epidemic, found that seroprevalence was already 24.9% (Osmond *et al.*, 2002). An endemic state of KSHV infection in homosexual men has also been suggested in Denmark in the 1970s, both in a study directly measuring KSHV seroprevalence (Hjalgrim *et al.*, 2001) and in a study of KS which found that never-married men (a crude surrogate for homosexual men) were significantly at risk (Hjalgrim *et al.*, 1996). Therefore, the introduction of KSHV infection appears to have substantially preceded that of HIV, although how long KSHV has been transmitted at high rates among homosexual men is not known.

There is little information on the patterns of KSHV infection in different populations over time. In Africa, among samples collected between 1972 and 1978 in Uganda and Tanzania, the seroprevalence of KSHV infection was similar to that found in the 1980s and 1990s, suggesting there has been little influence from the emerging HIV epidemic (deThe *et al.*, 1999). In homosexual men in developed countries, there had been speculation, based upon the report of either decreased incidence of AIDS-associated KS or a decline in KS as a proportion of new AIDS cases, that the prevalence of KSHV infection had fallen in the late 1980s and early 1990s (Rutherford *et al.*, 1990; Dore *et al.*, 1996; Jones *et al.*, 1999). However, a decline in the overall KS incidence rate could have been caused by reduced HIV transmission alone, resulting in fewer immunocompromised persons available to develop KS. Similarly, a decline in KS as a proportion of new AIDS cases could be caused by a decline in the proportion of new cases occurring in homosexual men since KS is uncommon in risk groups other than homosexual men. Direct examination of KSHV seroprevalence in homosexual men in San Francisco (including both HIV-infected and uninfected men) found a stable prevalence between 26% and 29% in the periods spanning 1978–80, 1984–85, and 1995–96 (Osmond *et al.*, 2002). Similarly, KSHV seroprevalence was stable at approximately 60% in the period spanning 1985 to 1995 among homosexual men in Italy who had recently acquired HIV infection (Rezza *et al.*, 2000a,b).

Genotypic diversity of infection

The entire KSHV genome was sequenced shortly after its detection (Russo *et al.*, 1996; Neipel *et al.*, 1997), and considerable work thereafter has documented extensive genotypic heterogeneity across populations. Initial work examining genotypic diversity focused on segments of ORF 26 and ORF 75, and although there was not extensive overall variation (only 1.5% of nucleotide positions), there was enough clustering to form three distinct but narrow subtypes in the initial 12 specimens examined (Zong et al., 1997). Subsequently, ORF K1, K12, 73, K14.1, and K15 have also been examined in many more specimens, resulting in the finding of significantly more genotypic heterogeneity and a much more complicated interpretation. Of these regions, the far left hand (ORF K1) and right hand (ORF K15) sides of the genome are most interesting. ORF K1 is the most heterogenous, with up to 44% amino acid differences across strains, allowing for the formation of at least five major subtypes and at least 24 subgroups, many of which indicate intertype recombination (Biggar et al., 2000; Nicholas et al., 1998; Zong et al., 1999; Cook et al., 1999; Meng et al., 1999; Zong et al., 2002). This degree of diversity has been seen with relatively few isolates examined thus far (less than 250); as more are sequenced, it is apparent that even more distinct subtypes will be identified (Whitby et al., 2004). ORF K15 features two highly diverged alleles, termed P (for predominant) and M (for minor) corresponding to their prevalence in isolates examined to date, which have only 33% amino acid homology to one another (Poole et al., 1999). The two alleles are so disparate that it has been suggested the minor form was introduced via a recombination event with a related but as yet undocumented primate virus (Poole et al., 1999).

While there is an impressive degree of between-subject genotypic diversity, the data on within-subject heterogeneity are conflicting. The majority of initial reports examining sequence variability within individuals either at one time point with multiple samplings or over time did not find evidence of strain (Meng et al., 1999; Zong et al., 1999; Stebbing et al., 2001; Codish et al., 2000), and even among those that did (Gao et al., 1999; Lacoste et al., 2000a,b), intrahost variability was very low. More recently, however, work examining three different types of oral fluid collection, as well as blood, and using a high-fidelity PCR approach, found that among 24 Malawians, 16 had evidence of strain variability in ORF K1 (Beyari et al., 2003). Seven of the subjects harbored two or more subtypes. The reasons for the discrepancy between this and prior work is not clear, but if these findings are confirmed, they will demand significant caution in performing and interpreting future molecular epidemiology studies, particularly those focusing on interpersonal transmission.

Nomenclature schemes for the genotypic diversity of KSHV are still in evolution and not yet standardized between authors. Based on ORF K1 typing alone, at least three approaches have been proposed. Zong et al. (1997) proposed naming subtypes A–D, with numerical subgroups within subtypes (e.g., A1–A5'). Cook et al. (1999) proposed subtypes A–C with two forms of subgroups, one denoted with numbers (e.g., A3 and A5) and another with superscripts (e.g., A'). Finally, Meng et al. (1999) proposed genotypes I–IV with subtypes (e.g., I–A to I–F). To each of these schemes, a fifth major subtype (termed subtype E) was subsequently described among remote isolated South American populations (Biggar et al., 2000; Whitby et al., 2004). Overall genotypic classification is even more complicated because there is not complete linkage in strain diversity across the genome. For example, diversity in ORF K15, although limited to the P vs. M nomenclature, is largely independent of ORF K1 genotype (Zong et al., 2002; Lacoste et al., 2000a,b). When the internal coding regions (e.g., ORF 26, K12, 73, 75) are also considered, there becomes the need to describe at least three or four segments to fully describe a strain (e.g., as C3/A/A2/M) (Zong et al., 2002).

Despite the complexity in nomenclature, there do appear to be emerging patterns in the geographic distribution of the different subtypes. Following the classification scheme proposed by Zong et al. for ORF K1 (Zong et al., 1997, 2002), it has been observed that B subtypes are found almost exclusively in sub-Saharan Africa, D subtypes in South Asia/Australia/Pacific, and A and C subtypes in the U.S./Europe/North Asia (with a notable exception being the presence of A5 subtypes in Africa). This has led to the speculation that KSHV was present in the origins of modern humans in Africa (B subtype), and that the separation into the three main branches (A/C, B, and D) is explained by isolation and founder effects associated with the original migrations of human out of Africa, first to the Middle East, and then South Asia (D subtype), and later to Europe, North Asia, and the Americas (A and C subtypes) (Hayward, 1999; Zong et al., 2002). Notable examples of this geographic association are seen in immigrants whose KSHV sequences match those of their countries of origin rather than their adopted residence (Zong et al., 2002). The story is not entirely consistent, however, because of the unexpected finding of subtype E in isolated South American populations (Biggar et al., 2000; Whitby et al., 2004). Whereas it would have been expected that novel subtypes in South America would be most closely related to subtypes A and C (or even B), subtype E is most closely related to subtype D. Finally, the finding of M allele types for ORF K15 in ORF K1 A, B, or C strains further complicates the explanation regarding the geographic spread of the virus over time.

Aside from tracing the spread of KSHV over time and across human populations, the other implications of the substantial genotypic diversity are not well understood.

Table 54.2. Current strength of evidence[a] for various routes of KSHV transmission in endemic vs. non-endemic areas

Route of transmission	Endemic areas	Non-endemic areas
Sexual transmission among homosexual men	++	+++
Sexual transmission among heterosexual men and women	++	+
Non-sexual horizontal transmission in childhood	+++	n.s.
Injection drug use	n.s.	+++
Vertical transmission	+	n.s.
Blood transfusion	+++	+
Solid organ transplantation	+++	+++

[a] + denotes weak evidence; ++ denotes moderate evidence; +++ denotes definitive or strong evidence; − denotes presence of studies but no supportive evidence; n.s. denotes not yet studied.

First, while it is likely that the considerable heterogeneity in ORF K1 is providing clues regarding a powerful biological selection process, whether this involves immune evasion or some other mechanism is not known. Second, it is not known whether genotype plays a role in the ease of transmissibility and acquisition of KSHV. For example, it has not been established whether the localization of the B subtype in Africa can explain the high KSHV seroprevalence there compared to other regions. If genotype is important in viral transmission, high transmissibility is likely not limited to subtype B, as E subtypes in remote South American populations are also associated with very high community seroprevalences (Biggar et al., 2000; Whitby et al., 2004). Third, there has thus far been no convincing evidence for the importance of genotype in either the development of KSHV-related disease per se, the type of KSHV-related disease manifestation (KS vs. primary effusion lymphoma vs multicentric Castleman's diseases), or clinical severity once disease occurs. Of these potential questions, data are most abundant, but not yet definitive, on the issue of association with type of disease where work to date finds no correlation (Zong et al., 2002; Lacoste et al., 2000a,b). One report found an association between single nucleotide polymorphisms (SNPs) at nucleotide positions 1032 and 1055 of ORF 26, but this was among many SNPs evaluated and requires confirmation (Endo et al., 2003). The lack of evidence for the importance of genotype in these various questions should not be interpreted as no role for genotype, but rather a lack of definitive data owing primarily to study designs that have focused on convenience samples of virus obtained from diseased patients (most of whom have a poorly characterized clinical course), rather than systematic sampling of asymptomatically-infected individuals (Whitby et al., 2004) and well-characterized diseased individuals. The current inability to detect and sequence KSHV DNA from all KSHV-infected individuals (as defined by antibody-positivity) is a substantial obstacle to addressing these questions.

Routes of transmission

Current knowledge about KSHV transmission can be summarized as follows (Table 54.2). There is definitive evidence that it is transmitted by some form of intimate contact between homosexual men and equally persuasive evidence that it is transmitted in childhood by a horizontal non-sexual route in high-level endemic areas. There is also strong evidence that it is transmitted by infected organs in transplantation, by sharing of equipment among injection drug users, and by transfusion of whole unprocessed blood in high-level endemic areas. What is not known are the specific sexual behaviors that transmit KSHV among homosexual men, the exact means of horizontal spread to children in endemic areas, whether KSHV is transmitted vertically, and whether transmission occurs via transfusion of blood products that have undergone conventional processing techniques.

Transmission in non-endemic areas

Sexual transmission

Initial seroepidemiologic studies postulated that KSHV was sexually transmitted by showing that, other than in KS patients, seroprevalence was highest in homosexual men and other groups at highest risk for sexually transmitted disease (STD). For example, Kedes et al. (1996) using an IFA for antibodies directed against LANA, found among STD clinic clients in San Francisco that 6% of heterosexuals, 13% of HIV-uninfected homosexual men, and 35% of HIV-infected homosexual men were seropositive; seroprevalence in screened blood donors was 1%. Reports of this type, however, describing an association between risk of STD and KSHV seroprevalence, provide only indirect evidence for sexual transmission. More definitive evidence is found in studies with direct measurement of sexual activity, controlled for other potential routes of spread. Among a population-based sample of homosexual men in San Francisco, KSHV seroprevalence increased linearly with the number of male intercourse partners in the previous two years (Fig. 54.1) (Martin et al., 1998). This association was independent of recreational drug use, transfusion history, CD4 lymphocyte count, and HIV serostatus. The strength of this association, confirmed by others (O'Brien et al., 1999;

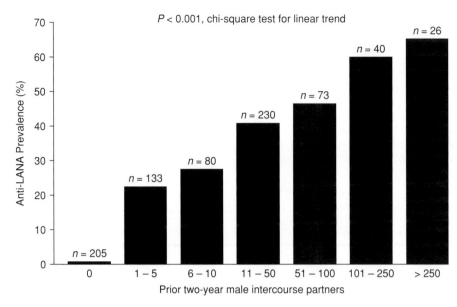

Fig. 54.1. Prevalence of antibodies to KSHV latency-associated nuclear antigen (LANA) by number of prior two-year male intercourse partners among men in San Francisco. Number atop each column signifies number of subjects in each group. From Martin et al., 1998.

Melbye et al., 1998; Dukers et al., 2000; Pauk et al., 2000; Jacobson et al., 2000a,b; Diamond et al., 2001; Casper et al., 2002a,b), leaves little doubt that some form of intimate contact transmits the virus among homosexual men. However, because "sexual partner" is defined broadly in most of these reports to include a variety of practices (e.g., insertive and receptive penile-anal intercourse, penile–oral intercourse, and oral–anal contact), these data alone do not pinpoint the specific route of sexual transmission.

Even prior to the discovery of KSHV, many studies had sought to identify the specific route of transmission for the putative KS agent. Some (Jacobson et al., 1990; Beral et al., 1992; Grulich et al., 1997), but not all (Archibald et al., 1990; Lifson et al., 1990; Page-Bodkin et al., 1992; Elford et al., 1992) found that insertive oral–anal sexual practices ("rimming") were a risk factor for KS and, by extension, were a risk factor for the as-yet-undiscovered KS agent. The discovery of KSHV was hoped to bring clarity to this question, but initial studies among homosexual men have been conflicting, variously reporting the strongest association for penile–anal intercourse, penile–oral intercourse, oral-anal contact, or kissing. To date, at least 8 studies have evaluated specific practices (Table 54.3) (O'Brien et al., 1999; Melbye et al., 1998; Dukers et al., 2000; Pauk et al., 2000; Jacobson et al., 2000a,b; Diamond et al., 2001; Casper et al., 2002a,b; Grulich et al., 1999). For almost all of the acts, at least one study has reported an association. However, for no act have all (or nearly all) studies found an association. Receptive penile-anal intercourse, the act that has attracted the most support, is paradoxically one in which the apparent culprit body fluid, semen, is now known to rarely harbor KSHV (Pauk et al., 2000; Diamond et al., 1997; Koelle et al., 1997).

There are numerous potential biases, reviewed elsewhere (Martin and Osmond, 2000), inherent in the work to date that might explain the inconsistency among studies evaluating specific routes of KSHV sexual transmission. One potential bias is inaccuracy in measuring exposure, in this case the self-report of sexual acts, which is complicated in cross-sectional studies by not knowing the relevant period of exposure to query. A second problem, deficiencies in sensitivity and/or specificity of KSHV serologic assays, particularly with the first-generation assays used to date, results in both misclassification of who is infected and mistaken ascertainment of sexual practices in longitudinal studies by querying for sexual behavior during the incorrect time period. Finally, because sexual acts are correlated in homosexual men, failure to adjust for all of the relevant acts can lead to confounding. In other words, finding an association for a particular act may simply be because that act is correlated with another act that is the true culprit in transmission. All but one (Pauk et al., 2000) of the studies to date were assembled to study HIV infection, and hence in general did not record acts, such as kissing, where saliva is passed. Moreover, no study recorded information on less obvious uses of saliva in various sexual acts such as a lubricant for penile-anal intercourse or when a finger is inserted into an anus (Butler et al., 2003).

Table 54.3. Studies evaluating specific sexual practices as routes of KSHV transmission in homosexual men

		Specific Sexual Practice						
		Penile–anal intercourse		Penile–oral intercourse		Oral-anal contact		
Study	Design	Ins.[a]	Rec.[a]	Ins.	Rec.	Ins.	Rec.	Kissing
Melbye, 1998 (Melbye et al., 1998)	cohort	ne[c]	+[b]	ne	−[b]	−	−	−
O'Brien, 1999 (O'Brien et al., 1999)	cohort	+	+	−	−	+	−	ne
Grulich, 1999 (Grulich et al., 1999)	cross-sectional	−	−	−	−	−	−	ne
Dukers, 2000 (Dukers et al., 2000)	cohort	−	−	+	+	−	−	ne
Jacobson, 2000 (Jacobson et al., 2000)	cohort	ne	+	−	−	ne	ne	ne
Pauk, 2000 (Pauk et al., 2000)	cross-sectional	ne	ne	ne	ne	ne	ne	+
Diamond, 2001 (Diamond et al., 2001)	cross-sectional	−	+	ne	ne	ne	ne	ne
Casper, 2002 (Casper et al., 2002a,b)	cross-sect/cohort	−	−	ne	ne	−	−	ne

[a] "Ins." denotes insertive practice of the act; "Rec." denotes receptive practice of the act
[b] "+" indicates an association was found; "−" indicates no association
[c] "ne" denotes the act was not evaluated

Recording of acts where saliva is exchanged is important because, unlike semen, saliva is now known to be the body fluid that most commonly harbors KSHV (Pauk et al., 2000; Koelle et al., 1997). Careful work from Seattle, for example, found that among KSHV-seropositive homosexual men, 30% of oral samples contained KSHV DNA, vs. 1% of genital and anal samples (Pauk et al., 2000). Therefore, failure to record all of the relevant acts may result both in the inability to find the true culprit act of transmission and the spurious assertion of the importance of a correlated but non-transmitting act.

Recognition that saliva is the body fluid that most commonly harbors KSHV has naturally focused attention on transmission by kissing (Pauk et al., 2000). However, because kissing is common in all population groups, the low prevalence of KSHV in the general population argues against kissing as a dominant route of spread. Indeed, other herpesviruses transmitted by kissing (e.g., EBV) are highly prevalent in the general population. One scenario where kissing could be the major route of spread but still not result in high prevalence in the general population is if KSHV was recently introduced into homosexual men and has not yet spread to others. Data from San Francisco, however, show that KSHV was not recently introduced into homosexual men. Seroprevalence among homosexual men in San Francisco in 1978–80 was estimated to already be high at 28.4% and stable over the next 15 years (26.4% in 1995–96), arguing against kissing as the dominant route of spread. (Osmond et al., 2002).

The most recent US Public Health Service guidelines for the prevention of KSHV infection reflect the uncertainty in the literature about its transmission (US Public Health Service and Infectious Disease Society of America, 2002). They state that the major routes of KSHV transmission appear to be "oral (via) semen, and through blood via needle sharing" and that patients should be counseled that "kissing and sexual intercourse with persons who have high risk of being infected with KSHV (e.g., persons who have KS or who are HIV–infected), might lead to acquisition of the agent that causes KS." Admittedly, this guideline is rated CIII (meaning evidence for efficacy is insufficient), but it poses a quandary for homosexual men, leaving great uncertainty about whether any form of contact is safe.

In contrast to the data for sexual transmission in homosexual men, evidence for sexual transmission in heterosexual men or women is less convincing. In a large study of 2718 STD clinic attendees in London, KSHV seroprevalence in heterosexual men and women was 4.6% compared to 18.5% in (mostly HIV-uninfected) homosexual men (Smith et al., 1999). Among the heterosexual men and women, there was no association between KSHV seropositivity and either number of sexual partners or current or prior history of STDs. Several other studies have found associations between KSHV seropositivity and STD history (either HIV, genital warts, syphilis, gonorrhea, herpes simplex virus 2, or chlamydial infection) among women (Sosa et al., 1998; Tedeschi et al., 2000; Cannon et al., 2001; Greenblatt et al., 2001; Janier et al., 2002; Goedert et al., 2003), but whether this truly represents sexual transmission rather than a surrogate for other types of incompletely controlled for behavior (e.g., injection drug use) is not clear. Among the two studies which best controlled for injection drug use by restricting to those women who denied either injection drug use (Cannon et al., 2001) or who were seronegative for hepatitis C virus infection (Goedert et al., 2003), one study reported an association between STD history and KSHV seropositivity (Cannon et al., 2001) but the other did not (Goedert et al., 2003). To date, although one report found a trend towards higher seropositivity in women with earlier sexual debut (de Sanjose et al., 2002), no study has revealed the same unequivocal direct relationship between KSHV seropositivity and number of sexual partners as seen in homosexual men. Moreover, in what should be the most powerful evaluation of heterosexual transmission among women, a history of sex with male bisexual partners has not been associated with KSHV seropositivity (Cannon, et al., 2001; Greenblatt et al., 2001). Given the scarcity of KSHV in semen, the lack of significant heterosexual transmission of KSHV is not surprising. Finally, given the general uncertainty as to whether heterosexual transmission occurs to any appreciable extent in non-endemic areas, there has been no enlightening work as to which specific sexual practices might be operative.

Injection drug use

The paucity of KS among HIV-infected non-homosexual injection drug users (Beral et al., 1990) led to the prediction that the putative agent of KS would be low among injection drug users. Indeed, KSHV seroprevalence in injection drug users is much lower than in homosexual men (Renwick et al., 1998; Simpson et al., 1996) but whether injection drug use can transmit KSHV to any extent is under active investigation. The strongest evidence comes from Cannon et al. who evaluated women in the US-based HIV Epidemiology Research Study (HERS) (Cannon et al., 2001). Compared to non-users, injection drug users were more likely to be KSHV-infected in a dose-response manner depending on drug use frequency. Furthermore, when restricted to women with low-risk sexual behavior, those who were hepatitis C virus-infected were 20 times more likely to be KSHV-infected. The inference that KSHV can be transmitted through injection drug use has subsequently been supported in at least 3 other studies in women and men (Diamond et al., 2001; Goedert et al., 2003; Atkinson et al., 2003). In contrast, no association for injection drug use was reported among women in the Women's Interagency HIV Study (WIHS), but this cross-sectional analysis evaluated only the prior 6-month injection drug use history and did not evaluate dose-response trends or an association with HCV seropositivity (a better marker of lifetime injection drug use) (Greenblatt et al., 2001). Similarly, no association was found among injection drug users in Baltimore, but again the study lacked accurate measurement of the lifetime magnitude of injection drug use behavior, critical in a population where everyone has practiced at least some of this behavior (Bernstein et al., 2003). Finally, a study of both male and female drug users in Amsterdam also failed to show an association for injection drug use (Renwick et al., 2002), but admittedly lacked adequate statistical power. Taken together, the available data do support that injection drug use can transmit KSHV. Nonetheless, the efficiency of spread by injection drug use (defined as the probability of transmission per each contact with a KSHV-infected person where injection drug use equipment is shared) is likely very low as evidenced by the markedly lower prevalence in injection drug users as compared to homosexual men. This is consistent with the biological data finding KSHV DNA far more commonly in saliva, a body fluid commonly exchanged during male homosexual activity, than in whole blood, the culprit fluid exchanged among injection drug users.

Blood transfusion

The possibility of transmission by blood transfusion was raised by Blackbourn et al. (1997) who recovered KSHV from peripheral blood mononuclear cells from a single blood donor and were able to propagate the virus in previously uninfected target cells. Further concern was introduced with the finding, reviewed above, that injection drug use (i.e., exposure to minute quantities of blood) can apparently transmit KSHV. Confirmation of an actual transmission event in non-endemic areas via blood transfusion, however, has to date not been demonstrated. The most suggestive evidence comes from a study of 284 initially KSHV-seronegative individuals who received a blood transfusion and were followed for 6 months. Two persons developed KSHV seroreactivity by 6 months, compared to no such seroconversions among 75 individuals who did not receive a transfusion (Dollard et al., 2005). If the seroconversions were indeed from the blood transfusion, then the risk of HHV-8 infection per transfused unit was estimated to 0.082% (95% CI, 0.05 to 0.20%). However, because linked donor specimens were not available and the control group was small in number, it is not possible to definitively prove that the seroconversions were due to the transfusion and not from other sources. Two other smaller look-back studies of a total of 32 known KSHV-antibody-positive blood donors and their associated transfusion recipients failed to detect a seroconversion among the recipients (Operskalasi et al., 1997; Engels et al., 1999). Hence while at this time it cannot be definitively proven or disproven if transmission via blood transfusion occurs in non-endemic settings where modern blood-banking techniques are practiced, if transmission does occur efficiency is likely to be low. Other epidemiologic data support this view. For transfusion of non-cellular components (e.g., fresh frozen plasma, cryoprecipitate, or factor concentrates), that the risk from transfusion, at least in non-endemic areas, is very low is substantiated by indirect data in (a) hemophiliacs where KSHV seroprevalence is very low (0% to 3%) (Kedes et al., 1996; Gao et al., 1996a,b; Simpson et al., 1996), and (b) HIV-infected hemophiliacs in the 1980's who had a very low incidence of KS. For transfusion of cellular components (e.g., red blood cells), the low incidence of KS among the initial cohort of persons in the 1980s, other than hemophiliacs, who acquired HIV via blood transfusion similarly argues for a very low risk of transmission (Beral et al., 1990). Both the hemophiliacs and red blood cell transfusion recipients were in many cases infected by blood donations from homosexual men who harbored HIV and likely also had a high prevalence of KSHV infection. That so few developed KS strongly suggests that KSHV is very inefficiently spread via transfusion in non-endemic areas with modern blood-banking practices. As such, there has been to date no forceful movement in the US blood banking community to universally screen for KSHV (Dodd 2005). This stance has been further substantiated by the apparent very low seroprevalence of KSHV infection in individuals who have passed the standard medical and behavioral screening for blood donation. In a study of 1000 representative blood donors, KSHV seroprevalence was estimated to be approximately 3% (Pellett et al., 2003). Among the blood donors found to antibody-positive, no donor had detectable evidence of KSHV DNA upon testing of their whole blood.

That KSHV transmission by injection drug use (where only minute quantities of blood are exchanged) has been established in non-endemic areas but transmission by transfusion (where large quantities are exchanged) has not is seemingly inconsistent. The paradox may be explained by the composition of the material exchanged. In injection drug use, fresh whole blood is exchanged, which is replete with mononuclear cells, the host cells for KSHV when it is present in the circulation. In contrast, mononuclear cells are intentionally (albeit not completely) removed in all forms of blood transfusion in most non-endemic areas. Although elements of blood plasma are exchanged in both injection drug use and transfusion, cell-free KSHV DNA is rarely found in plasma. In addition, it has required the presence of multiply exposed injection drug users (e.g., daily drug use over several decades) to delineate a risk associated with this practice. The only comparably exposed group in non-endemic areas to be examined in transfusion medicine were 19 persons from France with thalessemia or sickle cell disease who received a mean of 326 red blood cell transfusions (Lefrere et al., 1997). No instances of KSHV infection were found in these individuals, but, of note, they received only white-blood-cell-reduced (a more complete technique of white blood cell removal than standard processing) red cells, and they were examined for the presence of KSHV only with PCR techniques, not by antibody testing. In a smaller group ($n = 9$) of patients with sickle cell disease who had over 100 red blood cell transfusions and did have KSHV antibody testing performed, two were seropositive, but the sample size was too small to ascertain whether this was significantly greater than the background seroprevalence in the population (Challine et al., 2001).

Organ transplantation

Several studies have confirmed the ability of KSHV to be transmitted through renal transplantation (Regamey et al., 1998; Diociaiuti et al., 2000; Luppi et al., 2000a,b). The initial sentinel work from Switzerland found that 12% (25/206) of renal transplant recipients negative for antibodies to KSHV prior to surgery seroconverted within one year after transplantation, (Regamey et al., 1998). Two of the 25 developed KS. The inference that most, if not all, of these apparent seroconversions were caused by the allograft was strengthened by finding that serum from five out of six donors to seroconverters was positive for KSHV antibodies compared to nought out of eight donors to nonseroconverters. In addition, transmission through blood products was ruled out in several cases. Subsequently, elegant molecular work performed on eight renal transplant recipients with post-transplant KS determined that, among five patients, individual cells microdissected from KS lesions were of donor origin and were KSHV-infected (Barozzi et al., 2003). This finding not only substantiates the ability of KSHV to be transmitted via renal transplantation but implies that, in at least some cases, the virus is spread not as free virus but instead in a cell-associated form in KS progenitor cells. Finally, although the data are not as conclusive, transmission through liver transplantation has also been reported (Andreoni et al., 2001 and Marcelin et al., 2004). Now that transmission through solid organ transplantation has been confirmed, there are beginning to be calls for routine screening of organ donors and recipients (Moore, 2003; Michaels and Jenkins, 2003). Indeed, it is this setting where there is the most urgent need for the development of commercially available high throughput KSHV diagnostic assays. Difficulties in the assays for KSHV antibodies will make this an imperfect process, but the idea seems most warranted in non-endemic areas where the low prevalence of KSHV infection among donors means that few organs will need to be discarded because of KSHV-seropositivity

Table 54.4. Studies evaluating the association between age and KSHV seroprevalence in pre-pubescent children in Africa, the Middle East, and Italy

Country/population (reference)	Age group	N	Percent KSHV seropositive	
			Anti-latent Antibody	Anti-lytic Antibody
Cameroon	Age 7–12 mo	32		12.5[a]
Clinic patients	Age 13–24 mo	28		14.3
(Gessain et al., 1999)	Age 3–4	36		13.9
	Age 5–8	34		23.5
	Age 9–11	36		25.0
	Age 12–14	28		39.2
	Age 15–20	27		48.0
	Pregnant women	189		54.5
Uganda	Age 0–5	35	20[b]	28[b]
Hospital outpatients	Age 5–9	48	38	42
(Mayama et al., 1998)	Age 20–24	53	36	46
Egypt	Age <1	42	7.1	16.6
Vaccinees	Age 1–3	40	10.0	37.5
(Andreoni et al., 1999)	Age 4–6	40	7.5	45.0
	Age 7–9	38	10.5	57.8
	Age 10–12	36	5.5	52.7
Italy	Age 3–5	90	1.1	
Hospital inpatients	Age 6–10	94	6.3	
(Whitby et al., 2000)	Age 11–15	38	7.8	

[a] an immunofluorescence assay detecting antibodies to both lytic and latent-phase antigens was used.
[b] percentages extrapolated from figure.

and those that are may be able to be given to recipients who are seropositive.

Transmission in endemic areas

Non-sexual horizontal transmission

In high-level endemic areas, such as the Middle East and Africa, an age-dependent increase in KSHV seroprevalence during childhood provides definitve evidence for some form of non-sexual horizontal transmission (Table 54.4). In intermediate-level endemic areas, e.g., the Mediterranean, fewer comparable data exist (Perna et al., 2000; Whitby et al., 2000); although only one report is suggestive of an age-dependent increase in KSHV seroprevalence before puberty (Whitby et al., 2000), this is substantiated by the finding of increased seroprevalence in the children of patients with KS, relative to persons without KS (Angeloni et al., 1998). Indeed, that prevalence at the time of puberty in some high-level endemic areas is nearly that seen in adulthood suggests that non-sexual horizontal transmission is the dominant route of spread; (this, of course, assumes that seroreversion is not common and therefore not masking the occurrence of a continuing high incidence of infection in adulthood). For example, in Cameroon, Gessain et al. demonstrated that after loss of maternal antibody by 6 months of age, there was a monotonic increase in KSHV seroprevalence from 13% in 7- to 24- month olds to 39% in 12- to 14-year-olds (Gessain et al., 1999). There was a similar pattern found among Ugandan children (Mayama et al., 1998). In Egypt, prevalence was 17% in 0- to 1-year-olds ranging to 58% among 7 to 9 years (Andreoni et al., 1999).

That saliva is the body fluid that most commonly harbors KSHV lends the biologic plausibility that some form of non-sexual horizontal transmission is the dominant form of spread in endemic areas. The exact mode of spread, however, is not known. Some of the first reports from sub-Saharan Africa found that maternal KSHV seropositivity was a risk factor for seropositivity among children, leading to the conclusion that mother-to-child spread was the most significant route (Bourboulia et al., 1998; Sitas et al., 1999a,b). These data, however, were not controlled for the family's community of residence (and hence background prevalence of KSHV infection), and did not consider whether this association might be confounded by father-to-child, sibling-to-sibling, or extrafamilial spread. In a cross-sectional study that evaluated all family members, Plancoulaine et al. (2000) found evidence for both mother-to-child and sib-to-sib spread, but not father-to-child or spouse-to-spouse. This, however, was performed in French Guiana, where a seroprevalence of only 15% among persons 15 to 40 years old was reported, even when using a more sensitive induced IFA antibody assay. Whether or not the findings apply to areas with much higher prevalence, such as Africa, is not clear. A similar cross-sectional family study from Israel, where again seroprevalence among adults was only slightly greater than 10%, found a role for mother-to-child spread but did not examine the role of sib-to-sib spread (Davidovici et al., 2001). Most recently, a study of children in a high prevalence area in rural Tanzania found that having a KSHV-seropositive mother, father, or next-older sibling was associated with being KSHV-seropositive and that the magnitude of the risk was about the same across these relatives (Mbulaiteye et al., 2003a,b). Importantly, there was also an age-dependent increase in KSHV seroprevalence among children who did not have a seropositive first-degree relative, suggesting that non-familial transmission also occurs. Transmission emanating from outside of the immediate family has also been reported in initial molecular epidemiologic work performed among family members in Malawi (Cook et al., 2002a, b).

Taken together, these studies suggest that a variety of relationship types (i.e., mother–child, father–child, sib–child, non-family member–child) may be important in KSHV transmission. It is likely that no single relationship type has any universal significance per se in transmitting KSHV but rather that transmission is a product of salivary shedding in the infected individual and as-of-yet undetermined sociocultural practices that promote saliva passage to either interrupted skin or mucosal surfaces in the uninfected child. Some interesting theories have been proposed but for which supportive data are currently lacking. One of the most speculative put forward is the blood-sucking promoter arthropod hypothesis which suggests that the bite of a child by a bloodsucking arthropod triggers two subsequent events: (a) transfer of anti-hemostatic (anticlotting, vasodilators, and anti-platelet agents) and immunodulators from the arthropod to the human skin; and (b) use of saliva by a caregiver to relieave the itch of the bite (Coluzzi et al., 2002, 2003, 2004 and Ascoli et al., 2006). In this theory, the arthropod is not the biological vector for KSHV, but rather a promoter of infection by creating a hospitable microenvironment in the skin for KSHV infection and then facilitating contact with KSHV-containing saliva. As has been the case for horizontal transmission of hepatitis B virus infection in endemic areas, identifying the precise mechanisms by which KSHV is spread to children will be a considerable challenge. The exact mode of spread notwithstanding, why non-sexual horizontal transmission in children is so common in one part of the world but so uncommon in others (e.g., the USA) is not understood. While an association between lower education and KSHV seropositivity in some studies in endemic areas (Sitas et al., 1999a,b; Newton et al., 2003) suggests that region-specific behavioral factors may be important, the role of region-specific differences in host-mediated response to KSHV remains largely unexplored. Although a culprit gene has not yet been identified, segregation analysis in a French Guiana population suggests that a recessive gene controlling susceptibility to KSHV infection may explain the rapidly rising KSHV seroprevalence up to puberty in the population with a subsequent plateau thereafter (Plancoulain et al., 2003).

Sexual transmission

While sexual transmission among homosexual men appears to occur in KSHV-endemic areas just as it does in non-endemic areas (Perna et al., 2000; Rezza et al., 1998), data on heterosexual transmission in endemic areas are conflicting. That sexual transmission may occur is evidenced in some areas where there is a monotonic increase in KSHV seropositivity through adulthood (Olsen et al., 1998; Sitas et al., 1999a,b; Newton et al., 2003; Lavreys et al., 2003) or where risk of KSHV infection among married individuals is associated with KSHV-seropositivity or presence of KS per se in their spouses (Mbulaiteye et al., 2003a,b; Brambilla et al., 2000). Alternatively, these finding might simply be explained by continued non-sexual transmission during adulthood. The best evidence for heterosexual transmission in intermediate-level endemic areas comes from one report from Sicily showing an association between prostitution, STD clinic attendance and KSHV-seropositivity (Perna et al., 2000), although others have not confirmed this (Masini et al., 2000). In high-level endemic areas, the best evidence is from two studies from Cameroon (Bestetti et al., 1998, Rezza et al., 2000a,b), two from Kenya (Lavreys et al., 2003; Baeten et al., 2002), and one from Nigeria (Eltom et al., 2002a,b) each showing a relationship between KSHV-seropositivity and prostitution and/or history of at least one STD. The work from Kenya was also notable for associations between KSHV seropositivity and lack of condom use and lack of circumcision. (Baeten et al., 2002). However, several other studies have found no role for heterosexual transmission (Mayama et al., 1998; Newton et al., 2003; Rezza et al., 1998; Enbom et al., 1999; Wawer *et al.*, 2001; Vitale *et al.*, 2000; Marcelin *et al.*, 2002; Enbom *et al.*, 2002). In particular, there is marked inconsistency in high-level endemic areas between what should be a powerful marker of sexual behavior – HIV infection – and KSHV serostatus with some studies showing an association (Bestetti *et al.*, 1998; Nuvor *et al.*, 2001; Hladik *et al.*, 2003) but others not (Sitas *et al.*, 1999; Rezza *et al.*, 2000; Baeten *et al.*, 2002; Marcelin *et al.*, 2002; He *et al.*, 1998). This is in contrast to the universal association seen between HIV infection and KSHV serostatus in homosexual men in low-level endemic areas (Martin *et al.*, 1998; Renwick *et al.*, 1998; O'Brien *et al.*, 1999). In terms of direct information on number of sexual partners in endemic areas, Sitas *et al.* (1999a,b) found a very small risk associated with lifetime sexual partners but others have not confirmed this (Lavreys *et al.*, 2003; Baeten *et al.*, 2002). Of particular acts examined, the one report that examined kissing did not show an association with KSHV seropositivity (Lavreys *et al.*, 2003).

To date, no longitudinal studies evaluating sexual transmission of KSHV that follow initially seronegative adults have been performed. Given the high prevalence of KSHV infection that is already present by puberty in endemic areas, attempts with cross-sectional studies to assess the role of either current or past sexual behavior in determining KSHV serostatus are methodologically challenging. The expectation of these cross-sectional studies would be associations that are attenuated. Therefore, definitive evidence will likely await longitudinal study.

Vertical transmission
The occurrence of KS in young children, and, in particular, a case report of KS in a 6-day-old child (Gutierrez-Ortega *et al.*, 1989) has suggested that KSHV can be vertically transmitted. Because of the presence of maternal antibody in infants, documentation of vertical transmission relies upon detection of KSHV DNA. Mantina *et al.* (2001) evaluated the newborns of 89 Zambian women who were KSHV-antibody positive. In a blood draw taken at 24 hours of life, 2 of 89 (2.2%) had detectable KSHV DNA in peripheral blood cells by polymerase chain reaction (PCR). Because KSHV DNA sequences could not be detected from the mothers, it cannot be determined whether or not these two cases represent true vertical infection or PCR contamination. Even if they do represent true infection, it would appear that the incidence and efficiency of vertical infection is quite low.

Blood transfusion
Because of the high prevalence of KSHV infection in endemic areas, if transmission via blood transfusion occurred, even if inefficient, it could pose a significant public health concern. A study of Ugandan children with sickle-cell disease found a dose–response relationship between number of transfusions received and KSHV-seropositivity, even after adjustment for age (Mbulaiteye *et al.*, 2003). The overall estimated KSHV transmission risk was 2.6% (95% confidence interval 1.9% to 3.3%) per unit transfusion. If it is assumed that the prevalence of KSHV among donors in Uganda is approximately 50%, then the risk associated with receipt of a transfusion from a KSHV-seropositive donor is 5%. This finding of KSHV transmission via blood transfusion was recently confirmed in a longitudinal study, also conducted in Uganda (Hladik *et al.*, 2006). This work also showed that blood units stored less than 4 days prior to use were associated with a higher risk of KSHV transmission than units stored for more than 4 days. Of note, however, is that in Uganda transfusion recipients are typically given fresh unprocessed whole blood. Whether or not these same per unit risks occur when fractionated blood products (e.g., leukocyte-depleted red blood cells or plasma) are used, as is the case in more developed settings, is not known. The finding of KSHV DNA in the serum of a substantial proportion of blood donors in at least one African population lends credence to the (Enbom *et al.*, 2002) concern.

Disease manifestations

Primary infection syndrome
Very little is known about the clinical manifestations of primary KSHV infection. A major reason for this is the absence of clinically available diagnostic tests that could be used to evaluate large numbers of symptomatic persons. Furthermore, the phenomenon of seroreversion, which occurs with the currently available research-level serologic assays, makes identification of seroconversion uncertain in the absence of long-standing and repeated documentation of seronegativity (as would only be available in a formal cohort study). As such, in adults, all that is known comes from three reports of what are believed to represent primary infection. In the first, an HIV-infected man developed a sudden but transient onset of angiolymphoid hyperplasia with fever, arthralgia, cervical adenopathy, and splenomegaly (Oksenhendler *et al.*, 1998). The second report involved two transplant recipients who each received a kidney from same KSHV-seropositive donor; one recipient developed disseminated KS and the other had fever, splenomegaly, and pancytopenia (Luppi *et al.*, 2000a,b). These reports emphasize the potential severity of primary infection, but because they were identified on the basis of symptoms

they do not indicate what percentage of new infections are associated with clinical symptoms. Moreover, the reports may not represent primary infection in immunocompetent hosts. The third report described five cases of KSHV seroconversion that developed during the longitudinal observation of HIV-uninfected homosexual men (Wang et al., 2001). Four of the five had one or more symptoms of lymphadenopathy, diarrhea, fatigue, or rash. Although the symptoms were self-limiting, their longevity and severity were difficult to ascertain from the retrospective study design. Furthermore, this study reported a KSHV incidence of only 3.7 cases/1000 person–year, which seemingly could not account for the prevalence of 9.2% observed at the beginning of the cohort's observation, raising questions about whether the seroconversions detected represented only the cases that were the most overt immunologically and perhaps clinically. Nonetheless, this 4:1 ratio of symptomatic to asymptomatic infection is intriguing and merits further dedicated prospective study.

In children, a study of 86 one- to four-year olds in Egypt with fever of undetermined origin found six children with KSHV DNA in saliva but without KSHV antibodies, thus presumably representing primary infection (Andreoni et al., 2002). Of the three children for whom a follow-up blood sample was obtained, all developed KSHV antibodies. In addition to fever, five of the six children developed a rash that first appeared on the face and gradually spread to the trunk, arms, and legs. Five of the six also had upper respiratory tract infection symptoms and two had lower respiratory tract infection symptoms. While this report again demonstrates the severity of disease that can occur, its hospital-based sampling precludes an understanding of the overall frequency of symptomatic disease among children with primary infection. There has also been one report of a 1-month-old girl with DiGeorge anomaly, a primary immunodeficiency, who had widespread KSHV dissemination with virus detected in peripheral blood mononuclear cells, bone marrow, spleen, and lymph nodes as well as in endothelial and epithelial cells of the skin, lungs, esophagus, intestine, choroid plexus, and heart (Sanchez-Velasco et al., 2001). She died of multi-organ failure. Of interest from a transmission viewpoint is that there was no evidence of KSHV infection in her mother.

Kaposi's sarcoma

There are four forms of KS, defined on the basis of their epidemiologic context. "Classic" KS is the syndrome originally described by Kaposi (1872), and it has recently been thoroughly reviewed (Iscovich et al., 2002). It is found most frequently in older men (over 50 years) of Mediterranean or Eastern European heritage and is characterized initially by bluish-red painless spots on the feet and lower legs that subsequently progress, if untreated, to form raised, nodular growths that may ulcerate and bleed. In the latter stages of disease, the entire lower extremities as well as the hands and arms may become involved. Although the disease course is typically indolent, internal involvement does occur in approximately 10% of cases.

African or "endemic" KS is most common in sub-Saharan Africa. Even before the AIDS epidemic, portions of sub world Saharan Africa, particularly the Nile-Congo watershed, had among the highest incidences of KS in the world (Davies et al., 1964; Hutt and Burkitt, 1965). In these areas, KS represented 4 to 10% of all adult cancers and was mainly a disease of men aged 30 to 50 years old. Like classic KS, endemic KS manifests primarily as localized plaques and nodules on the feet and lower legs, but visceral involvement is more common than in the classic form.

The third form of KS was described shortly after the advent of solid organ transplantation (Siegel et al., 1969; Penn, 1979), and foreshadowed the powerful influence of immunosuppression on KS development. In this form, called "post-transplant" or "iatrogenic" KS, both disseminated cutaneous involvement and visceral disease are common. As noted earlier, recent work has shown that among cases that develop because of de novo transmission of KSHV, cells within the KS lesions are often of donor origin (Barozzi et al., 2003). This implies that either circulating KSHV-infected spindle-like cells or lymphoid cells trapped in the allograft or endothelial cells (or their precursors) residing in the allograft are the critical transplanted element that leads to KS lesion formation. Interestingly, lesions often diminish with lessening of the immunosuppressive regimen (Penn, 1979), but because this reduction is often accompanied by organ rejection, KS is a feared post-transplant complication. The finding that KS lesions are sometimes of donor cellular origin implies that donor-derived KSHV-specific cytotoxic T-cells could be a useful form of therapy that could obviate the need to lessen immunosuppression.

The fourth form of KS, originally described in young homosexual men, heralded the beginning of the HIV epidemic in 1981 (Fig. 54.2) (Friedman-Kien, 1981; Hymes et al., 1981). "Epidemic" or "AIDS-associated" KS became the most common HIV-associated malignancy, particularly affecting persons who acquired HIV via male homosexual behavior (Beral et al., 1990). Prior to the introduction of effective anti-HIV therapy, HIV-infected homosexual men were estimated to have a 20-fold higher risk of KS development than other HIV transmission risk groups (Beral et al., 1990) a lifetime cumulative incidence of

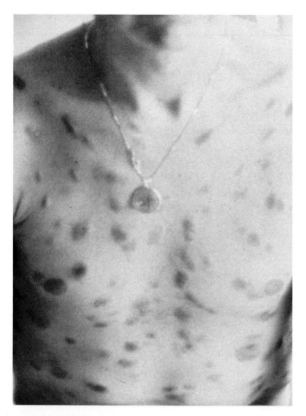

Fig. 54.2. Diffuse cutaneous Kaposi's sarcoma in a homosexual man.

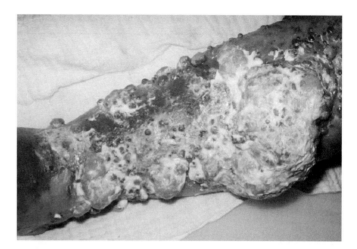

Fig. 54.3. Fulminant nodular Kaposi's sarcoma of the lower extremity in a patient with AIDS.

37% (Hoover *et al.*, 1993). Cutaneous AIDS-related KS, typically the earliest presentation, is often disseminated, cosmetically disfiguring, and complicated by bulky lesions, lymphatic obstruction, and extremity or facial swelling (Fig. 54.3) (Kaplan and Northfelt, 1997). Subsequent visceral manifestations, especially pulmonary and gastrointestinal involvement, are common (Friedman *et al.*, 1985; Mitchell *et al.*, 1992) and convey a poor prognosis. Prior to 1996 (i.e., prior to the era of highly active antiretroviral therapy for HIV and improved chemotherapy for KS), the median survival for HIV-infected persons with visceral involvement was 15 months (Krown *et al.*, 1997). However, even persons with KS confined to the skin and/or lymph nodes also had significant mortality with a median survival of 27 months (Krown *et al.*, 1997). As it has with other complications of HIV infection, the advent of highly active antiretroviral therapy has dramatically altered the prognosis of AIDS-associated KS. In a study of 287 patients with KS from 1990–1999, use of highly active antiretroviral therapy was associated with an 81% reduction in mortality (Tam *et al.*, 2002).

The introduction of potent antiretroviral therapy for HIV infection in the mid-1990s has also led to a dramatic reduction in the incidence of AIDS-associated KS in resource-rich settings (Eltom *et al.*, 2002a,b; Portsmouth *et al.*, 2003). In contrast, in portions of sub-Saharan Africa, where KSHV is endemic and antiretroviral therapy is not widely available, KS is now the most common adult malignancy. For example, in Uganda the incidence of KS has increased more than 20-fold in men between 1964 and 1968 and 1989 and 1991 (Wabinga *et al.*, 1993). A similar situation exists in Zimbabwe, where the HIV epidemic is largely unchecked and where KS is now the most common cancer overall in adults, most common in men (40% of all cancers) and the second most common in women (18% of all cancers) and children (10% of all cancers) (Chokunonga *et al.*, 2000). As is seen in AIDS-associated KS in resource-rich settings, the clinical manifestations of KS in sub-Saharan Africa have also changed. The most common presentations are now more aggressive forms such as lymphadenopathic or visceral KS, for which effective, affordable treatment is generally unavailable (Wabinga *et al.*, 1993; Desmond-Hellmann *et al.*, 1991).

The disproportionate risk of KS among HIV-infected homosexual men led to the hypothesis that a sexually transmitted infectious agent, other than HIV, was etiologically important (Beral *et al.*, 1990). This epidemiologically driven hypothesis re-invigorated an intense laboratory investigation for the causative agent that ultimately resulted in the identification of KSHV (Chang *et al.*, 1994). In a relatively short period of time since the discovery of KSHV, there have been a large number of epidemiologic studies evaluating its causal role in KS (Table 54.5). In the absence of experimental evidence (e.g., Koch's postulates), epidemiologists assess causality using Hill's criteria (Hill, 1965). These

Table 54.5. Studies estimating the association between KSHV infection and AIDS-related Kaposi's sarcoma[a]

Reference	KSHV antigen targeted	Antibody assay format	Association between KSHV and AIDS-KS, point estimate (95% CI)[b]
Case-control studies			
Miller et al., 1996	p40	immunoblot	13.4 (4.5–42)
Miller et al., 1996	lytic cycle	IFA[d]	12.2 (4.1–38)
Gao et al., 1996a,b	LNA[c]	immunoblot	18.9 (5.4–70)
Kedes et al., 1996	LNA	IFA	8.5 (3.1–23)
Gao et al., 1996a,b	LNA	IFA	16.3 (5.3–50)
Simpson et al., 1996	LNA	IFA	10.2 (4.2–25)
Simpson et al., 1996	ORF65	EIA[e]	9.2 (2.7–31)
Lennette et al., 1996	lytic cycle	IFA	1.8 (0.53–5.8)
Lennette et al., 1996	LNA	IFA	4.2 (2.2–8.0)
Longitudinal studies			
Martin et al., 1998	LNA	IFA	2.5 (1.7–3.8)
Renwick et al., 1998[f]	ORF65.2 ORF73	EIA	3.3 (1.9–5.8)
Renwick et al., 1998[g]	ORF65.2 ORF73	EIA	5.2 (2.9–9.3)
O'Brien et al., 1999	LNA	IFA	3.6 (1.7–9.5)

[a]limited to studies which measure KSHV infection by antibody response and either directly control for number of sexual partners or restrict analyses to HIV-infected homosexual men
[b]odds ratios are reported for case-control studies and hazard ratios for longitudinal studies
[c]latent nuclear antigen
[d]immunofluorescence assay
[e]enzyme immunoassay
[f]hazard ratio shown is for KSHV prevalent infection
[g]hazard ratio shown is for KSHV seroconverters.

criteria are discussed in Table 54.6 in order of their importance. The overwhelming assessment of these criteria, coupled with the finding that KSHV is invariably present in KS tumor specimens from all forms of KS throughout the world, is that KSHV is a necessary causal agent of KS. However, because only a small fraction of persons infected with KSHV develop KS, it is concluded that KSHV is a necessary, but not sufficient, causal agent of KS.

Of other potential cofactors operating along with KSHV in the etiology of KS, immunosuppression in general, and HIV infection, in particular, confer the greatest risk. Among HIV-infected persons, the magnitude of immunosuppression, as evidenced by CD4+ T-cell count, is predictive of development of KS (Renwick et al., 1998; Jacobson et al., 2000a,b). Timing of KSHV infection relative to HIV infection may be important as well as the risk of developing KS was significantly greater in one study (Renwick et al., 1998), and of similar magnitude but not statistically significant in a second study (Jacobson et al., 2000a,b), in persons who acquire KSHV after as compared to before HIV infection. Studies of this nature have potential methodologic pitfalls (Cannon and Pellett, 2001), however, and could conceivably be explained by what appears to be KSHV seroconversion actually being KSHV reactivation and reappearance of antibody-positivity. Two potential genetic risk factors have also been described and await confirmation. The FF genotype of the low affinity Fc gamma receptor IIIA is underrepresented in patients with KS, whereas the VF genotype confers greater risk (Lehrnbecher et al., 2000). Homozygosity for allele G at amino acid 174 of the IL6 promoter, associated with increased IL6 production, has been related to the development of KS while homozygosity of allele C appears protective (Foster et al., 2000). However, it is not known whether these genetic factors influence development of KS via pathogenic acceleration among KSHV infected persons or via enhancing the acquisition of KSHV *per se*.

Despite substantial investigation, the identification of cofactors, in addition to KSHV, for development of KS among immunocompetent individuals is largely incomplete. The role of cofactors is particularly evident in Africa, where prior to the AIDS epidemic, there was tremendous heterogeneity in KS incidence; this heterogeneity is not fully explained by underlying geographic differences in KSHV prevalence (Dedicoat and Newton, 2003). The absence of KS among Ethiopian immigrants to Israel compared to Israeli-born residents, despite higher KSHV

Table 54.6. Assessment of the Hill criteria for the role of KSHV infection in the etiology of Kaposi's sarcoma

Criterion	Comment
Temporality	Demonstrating that KSHV infection precedes KS is the *sine qua non* for causality. KSHV infection has been shown to precede KS in several studies (Whitby *et al.*, 1995; Gao *et al.*, 1996; Martin *et al.*, 1998; Renwick *et al.*, 1998; O'Brien *et al.*, 1999; Moore *et al.*, 1996; Lefrere *et al.*, 1996) thus dispelling notions that KS tumors, by being hospitable breeding grounds, result in the subsequent presence of KSHV. Importantly, KSHV infection is temporally associated with KS independent of degree of sexual exposure (Martin *et al.*, 1998) (excluding the possibility that KSHV is just a marker for another as-yet-undiscovered sexually transmitted pathogen) and immunocompromise (Whitby *et al.*, 1995; Gao *et al.*, 1996; Martin *et al.*, 1998; Renwick *et al.*, 1998; O'Brien *et al.*, 1999).
Strength of Association	After adjusting for all known potential confounding factors, statistical associations between a putative cause and disease that maintain a large magnitude are less likely to be explained by unaccounted for confounding factors and hence more likely to be valid associations. In longitudinal studies of KSHV and KS, the relevant association to be evaluated is KS incidence in KSHV-infected persons compared to KSHV-uninfected persons. If it is accepted that KS *per se* does not cause KSHV infection to be detected, associations from case-control studies are also relevant. Of studies of AIDS-related KS that measured KSHV infection by serologic means and directly controlled for number of sexual partners (Martin *et al.*, 1998) or restricted analyses to homosexual men (Gao *et al.*, 1996; Renwick *et al.*, 1998; O'Brien *et al.*, 1999; Miller *et al.*, 1996; Kedes *et al.*, 1996; Gao *et al.*, 1996; Simpson *et al.*, 1996; Lennette *et al.*, 2002) the magnitude of association between KSHV and KS ranges from 2.5 to 5.2 (hazard ratios) in longitudinal studies and 1.8 to 18.9 (odds ratios) in case-control studies.
Consistency	All published epidemiologic reports addressing a possible association between KSHV and, KS, with the exception of one have found a direct association. While it is formally possible that an unrecognized bias in either subject selection or variable measurement could account for the association between KSHV and KS seen in all studies to date, this is improbable because such a bias is unlikely to be consistently present in such a wide array of studies which vary by design, participant selection, and assay formats. Furthermore, the remarkable consistency in results makes chance a very unlikely explanation.
Biologic Plausibility	There are several potential mechanisms by which KSHV may cause, KS, described in Chapter 56.
Dose-Response Relationship	Among HIV and KSHV co-infected homosexual men, this criterion has been satisfied by the finding that detectable peripheral blood mononuclear cell-associated KSHV is associated with the subsequent development of KS (Engels *et al.*, 2003).
Coherence	This criterion implies that a cause-and-effect interpretation for the association in question does not conflict with what is otherwise known about either the disease or the putative causal agent. A causal role for KSHV in KS is compatible with existing knowledge in that the epidemiology of KSHV *per se* matches that long predicted for the agent of KS (e.g., highest prevalences in groups at greatest risk for, KS, and, in developed settings, sexually transmitted).
Analogy	Although a weak criterion, there is analogous evidence for a causal role of KSHV in KS. Two herpesviruses closely related to KSHV, herpesvirus saimiri and Epstein-Barr virus (EBV), are oncogenic.
Specificity	That a single cause must cause a single disease is clearly outdated (Rothman and Greenland, 1998) and likely violated by KSHV which has also at least been associated with primary effusion lymphoma (Cesarman *et al.*, 1995) and multicentric Castleman's disease (Soulier *et al.*, 1995).
Experimental evidence	In SCID mice, injection of KSHV into transplanted human skin results in the formation of lesions that are morphologically and phenotypically consistent with KS (Foreman *et al.*, 2001).

seroprevalence in the Ethiopians, is a well-documented example of some heretofore undiscovered protective factor (Grossman *et al.*, 2002). Studies which have evaluated factors associated with KS that were performed prior to the identification of KSHV have had their interpretations clouded by the possibility that these factors are associated with acquisition of KSHV. This pertains to, for example, genetic studies where in at least some reports an increased risk for classic KS has been observed in persons with HLA DR5 and a protective effect observed for HLA DR3 (Contu *et al.*, 1984). Both male gender and older age have for long been identified as a significant risk factors for KS, and neither can be fully explained by an increased risk for acquisition of KSHV infection. However, mechanistic explanation

Table 54.7. Current strength of evidence* for a causal role of KSHV infection in various diseases

Disease	Strength of evidence
Kaposi's sarcoma	+++
Primary effusion lymphoma	++
Multicentric Castleman's disease	++
Hemophagocytic lymphohistiocytosis	++
Pulmonary hypertension	+
Prostate cancer	+
Amyotrophic lateral sclerosis	+
Multiple myeloma	−
Sarcoidosis	−

+ denotes weak evidence; ++ denotes moderate evidence;
*+++ denotes strong evidence;
− denotes that initial claims have been largely refuted.

for these factors is unknown. Higher levels of immune activation, measured by circulating neopterin and beta-2-microglobulin, have also been associated with classical KS, but it has not been determined whether this is a cause or a consequence of KS (Touloumi et al., 1999). More recent studies that were either limited to participants with KSHV infection or adjusted for KSHV infection are most notable for the absence of demonstrable associations. Nonetheless, two new potential behavioral factors have been identified that require further investigation. In classic KS, smoking was found to be protective; the effect of smoking on inflammatory cytokines was the speculated mechanism (Goedert et al., 2002). In endemic KS, going barefoot more than half the time was a risk factor (Ziegler et al., 2003). It has been suggested that fine soil particles might pass through the skin of barefoot individuals and block the lymphatic system, causing local immunosuppression in the lower limbs and predisposing to the development of KS (Ziegler, 1993).

Other diseases

KSHV also has been associated with primary effusion lymphoma (Cesarman et al., 1995), multicentric Castleman's disease (Soulier et al., 1995), and hemophagocytic lymphohistiocytosis (Fardet et al., 2001) (Table 54.7). The rarity of these disorders will likely preclude their ever being scrutinized with Hill's criteria, as was discussed for KS. Among other diseases that have been hypothesized to be caused by KSHV, multiple myeloma (Rettig et al., 1997) has generated the most interest because of its frequency and clinical severity. From an ecological viewpoint, the association lacks plausibility given that multiple myeloma is not more common in populations in which KSHV prevalence is high. In addition, numerous individual subject-level studies (Parravicini et al., 1997; Masood et al., 1997; Whitby et al., 1997; Ablashi et al., 2000; Brander et al., 2002) have failed to confirm the initial claim. Most recently, claims have also been made for an association between KSHV infection and pulmonary hypertension (Cool et al., 2003), prostate cancer (Hoffman et al., 2004), and amyotrophic lateral sclerosis (Cermelli et al., 2003). The clinical impact of these conditions, especially prostate cancer, is sure to prompt much additional work in the next several years seeking to confirm these associations.

Acknowledgments

Supported in part by the National Institutes of Health (U01 CA78124, R01 CA119903 P30 MH62246, and P30 AI27763) and the University of California Universitywide AIDS Research Program (CC99-SF-001).

REFERENCES

Ablashi, D. V., Chatlynne, L., Thomas, D. et al. (2000). Lack of serologic association of human herpesvirus-8 (KSHV) in patients with monoclonal gammopathy of undetermined significance with and without progression to multiple myeloma. *Blood*, **96**(6), 2304–2306.

Andreoni, M., El-Sawaf, G., Rezza, G. et al. (1999). High seroprevalence of antibodies to human herpesvirus-8 in Egyptian children: evidence of nonsexual transmission. *J. Natl Cancer Inst.*, **91**(5), 465–469.

Andreoni, M., Goletti, D., Pezzotti, P. et al. (2001). Prevalence, incidence and correlates of HHV-8/KSHV infection and Kaposi's sarcoma in renal and liver transplant recipients. *J. Infect.*, **43**(3), 195–199.

Andreoni, M., Sarmati, L., Nicastri, E. et al. (2002). Primary human herpesvirus 8 infection in immunocompetent children. *J. Am. Med. Assoc.*, **287**(10), 1295–1300.

Angeloni, A., Heston, L., Uccini, S. et al. (1998). High prevalence of antibodies to human herpesvirus 8 in relatives of patients with classic Kaposi's sarcoma from Sardinia. *J. Infect. Dis.*, **177**(6), 1715–1718.

Archibald, C. P., Schechter, M. T., Craib, K. J. et al. (1990). Risk factors for Kaposi's sarcoma in the Vancouver Lymphadenopathy-AIDS Study. *J. Acquir. Immune Defic. Syndr.*, **3** Suppl. 1, S18–S23.

Ascoli, V., Facchinelli, L., Valerio, L., Zucchetto, A., Dal Maso, L., and Coluzzi, M. (2006). The distribution of mosquito species in areas with high and low incidence of classic Kaposi's sarcoma and seroprevalence for Kaposi's sarcoma-associated/human herpesvirus 8 (KSHV/HHV-8). 9th International Workshop on KSHV and Related Agents. Hyannis, Massachusetts. July, 12–15.

Atkinson, J., Edlin, B. R., Engels, E. A. *et al.* (2003). Seroprevalence of human herpesvirus 8 among injection drug users in San Francisco. *J. Infect. Dis.*, **187**(6), 974–981.

Baeten, J. M., Chohan, B. H., Lavreys, L. *et al.* (2002). Correlates of human herpesvirus 8 seropositivity among heterosexual men in Kenya. *AIDS*, **16**(15), 2073–2078.

Baillargeon, J., Leach, C. T., Deng, J. H. *et al.* (2002). High prevalence of human herpesvirus 8 (HHV-8) infection in south Texas children. *J. Med. Virol.*, **67**(4), 542–548.

Barozzi, P., Luppi, M., Facchetti, F. *et al.* (2003). Post-transplant Kaposi sarcoma originates from the seeding of donor-derived progenitors. *Nat. Med.*, **9**(5), 554–561.

Beral, V., Peterman, T. A., Berkelman, R. L. *et al.* (1990). Kaposi's sarcoma among persons with AIDS: a sexually transmitted infection? *Lancet*, **335**(8682), 123–128.

Beral, V., Bull, D., Darby, S. *et al.* (1992). Risk of Kaposi's sarcoma and sexual practices associated with faecal contact in homosexual or bisexual men with AIDS. *Lancet*, **339**(8794), 632–635.

Bernstein, K. T., Jacobson, L. P., Jenkins, F. J. *et al.* (2003). Factors associated with human herpesvirus type 8 infection in an injecting drug user cohort. *Sex Transm. Dis.*, **30**(3), 199–204.

Bestetti, G., Renon, G., Mauclere, P. *et al.* (1998). High seroprevalence of human herpesvirus-8 in pregnant women and prostitutes from Cameroon [letter]. *AIDS*, **12**(5), 541–543.

Beyari, M. M., Hodgson, T. A., Cook, R. D. *et al.* (2003). Multiple human herpesvirus-8 infection. *J. Infect. Dis.*, **188**(5), 678–689.

Biggar, R. J., Whitby, D., Marshall, V. *et al.* (2000). Human herpesvirus 8 in Brazilian Amerindians: a hyperendemic population with a new subtype. *J. Infect. Dis.*, **181**(5), 1562–1568.

Biggar, R. J., Engels, E. A., Whitby, D. *et al.* (2003). Antibody reactivity to latent and lytic antigens to human herpesvirus-8 in longitudinally followed homosexual men. *J. Infect. Dis.*, **187**(1), 12–18.

Blackbourn, D. J., Ambroziak, J., Lennette, E. *et al.* (1997). Infectious human herpesvirus 8 in a healthy North American blood donor. *Lancet*, **349**(9052), 609–611.

Bourboulia, D., Whitby, D., Boshoff, C. *et al.* (1998). Serologic evidence for mother-to-child transmission of Kaposi sarcoma-associated herpesvirus infection [letter]. *J. Am. Med. Assoc.*, **280**(1), 31–32.

Brambilla, L., Boneschi, V., Ferrucci, S. *et al.* (2000). Human herpesvirus-8 infection among heterosexual partners of patients with classical Kaposi's sarcoma. *Br. J. Dermatol.*, **143**(5), 1021–1025.

Brander, C., Raje, N., O'Connor, P. G. *et al.* (2002). Absence of biologically important Kaposi sarcoma-associated herpesvirus gene products and virus-specific cellular immune responses in multiple myeloma. *Blood*, **100**(2), 698–700.

Butler, L., Mosam, A., Kiepiela, P., Mzolo, S., Mbisa, G., Whitby, D., Brander, C., Scadden, D., Hladik, W., Dollard, S., and Martin, J. (2006) Lack of age dependence in KSHV seroprevalence among children in a population-based study in South Africa: Evidence for at least two epidemiologic patterns of KSHV transmission in Africa. 9th International Workshop on KSHV and Related Agents. Hyannis Massachusetts. (July), 12–15.

Butler, L. M., Osmond, D. H., Martin, J. N. (2003) Use of saliva as a lubricant in sexual practices among homosexual men: Clues to the route of Kaposi's sarcoma-associated herpesvirus (KSHV) transmission. Seventh International AIDS Malignancy Conference. Bethesda, Maryland. April, 28.

Cannon, M. J. and Pellett, P. E. (2001). Effect of order of infection with human immunodeficiency virus and human herpesvirus 8 on the incidence of Kaposi's sarcoma. [Comment On: *J. Infect. Dis.*, 2000, **181**(6), 1940–9 UI: 20298916]. *J Infect. Dis.*, **183**(8), 1304–1305.

Cannon, M. J., Dollard, S. C., Smith, D. K. *et al.* (2001). Blood-borne and sexual transmission of human herpesvirus 8 in women with or at risk for human immunodeficiency virus infection. HIV Epidemiology Research Study Group. *N. Engl. J. Medi.*, **344**(9), 637–643.

Casper, C., Krantz, E., Taylor, H. *et al.* (2002a). Assessment of a combined testing strategy for detection of antibodies to human herpesvirus 8 (HHV-8) in persons with Kaposi's sarcoma, persons with asymptomatic HHV-8 infection, and persons at low risk for HHV-8 infection. *J. Clin. Microbiol.*, **40**(10), 3822–3825.

Casper, C., Wald, A., Pauk, J. *et al.* (2002b). Correlates of prevalent and incident Kaposi's sarcoma-associated herpesvirus infection in men who have sex with men. *J. Infect. Dis.*, **185**(7), 990–993.

Cattani, P., Cerimele, F., Porta, D. *et al.* (2003). Age-specific seroprevalence of Human Herpesvirus 8 in Mediterranean regions. *Clin. Microbiol. Infect.*, **9**(4), 274–279.

Cermelli, C., Vinceti, M., Beretti, F. *et al.* (2003). Risk of sporadic amyotrophic lateral sclerosis associated with seropositivity for herpesviruses and echovirus-7. *Eur. J. Epidemiol.*, **18**(2), 123–127.

Cesarman, E., Chang, Y., Moore, P. S. *et al.* (1995). Kaposi's sarcoma-associated herpesvirus-like DNA sequences in AIDS-related body-cavity-based lymphomas. *N. Engl. J. Med.*, **332**(18), 1186–1191.

Chandran, B., Smith, M. S., Koelle, D. M. *et al.* (1998). Reactivities of human sera with human herpesvirus-8-infected BCBL-1 cells and identification of HHV-8-specific proteins and glycoproteins and the encoding cDNAs. *Virology*, **243**(1), 208–217.

Chang, Y., Cesarman, E., Pessin, M. S. *et al.* (1994). Identification of herpesvirus-like DNA sequences in AIDS-associated Kaposi's sarcoma. *Science*, **266**(5192), 1865–1869.

Challine, D., Roudot-Thoraval, F., Sarah, T. *et al.* (2001). Seroprevalence of human herpes virus 8 antibody in populations at high or low risk of transfusion, graft, or sexual transmission of viruses. *Transfusion*, **41**(9), 1120–1125.

Chatlynne, L. G., Lapps, W., Handy, M. *et al.* (2001). Detection and titration of human herpesvirus-8-specific antibodies in sera from blood donors, acquired immunodeficiency syndrome patients, and Kaposi's sarcoma patients using a whole virus enzyme-linked immunosorbent assay. *Blood*, **92**(1), 53–58.

Chohan, B. H., Taylor, H., Obrigewitch, R. *et al.* (2004). Human herpesvirus 8 seroconversion in Kenyan women by enzyme-linked immunosorbent assay and immunofluorescence assay. *J. Clin. Virol.*, **30**(2), 137–144.

Chokunonga, E., Levy, L. M., Bassett, M. T. *et al.* (2000). Cancer incidence in the African population of Harare, Zimbabwe: second results from the cancer registry 1993–1995. International *J. Cancer*, **85**(1), 54–59.

Codish, S., Abu-Shakra, M., Ariad, S. *et al.* (2000). Manifestations of three HHV-8-related diseases in an HIV-negative patient: immunoblastic variant multicentric Castleman's disease, primary effusion lymphoma, and Kaposi's sarcoma. *Am. J. Hematol.*, **65**(4), 310–314.

Cook, P. M., Whitby, D., Calabro, M. L. *et al.* (1999). Variability and evolution of Kaposi's sarcoma-associated herpesvirus in Europe and Africa. International Collaborative Group. *AIDS*, **13**(10), 1165–1176.

Cook, R. D., Hodgson, T. A., Molyneux, E. M. *et al.* (2002a). Tracking familial transmission of Kaposi's sarcoma-associated herpesvirus using restriction fragment length polymorphism analysis of latent nuclear antigen. *J. Virol. Methods*, **105**(2), 297–303.

Cook, R. D., Hodgson, T. A., Waugh, A. C. *et al.* (2000b). Mixed patterns of transmission of human herpesvirus-8 (Kaposi's sarcoma-associated herpesvirus) in Malawian families. *J. Gen. Virol.*, **83**(7), 1613–1619.

Coluzzi, M., Manno, D., Guzzinati, S. *et al.* (2002). The blood-sucking arthropod bite as possible cofactor in the transmission of human herpesvirus-8 infection and in the expression of Kaposi's sarcoma disease. *Parassitologia*, **44**(1–2), 123–129.

Coluzzi, M., Calabro, M. L., Manno, D. *et al.* (2003). Reduced seroprevalence of Kaposi's sarcoma-associated herpesvirus (KSHV), human herpesvirus 8 (HHV8), related to suppression of Anopheles density in Italy. *Med. Vet. Entomol.*, **17**(4), 461–464.

Coluzzi, M., Luisella Calabro, M., Manno, D. *et al.* (2004). Saliva and the transmission of human herpesvirus 8: potential role of promoter-arthropod bites. *J. Infect. Dis.*, **190**(1), 199–200.

Contu, L., Cerimele, D., Pintus, A., Cottoni, F., and La Nasa, G. (1984). HLA and Kaposi's sarcoma in Sardinia. *Tissue Antigens*, **23**(4), 240–245.

Cool, C. D., Rai, P. R., Yeager, M. E. *et al.* (2003). Expression of human herpesvirus 8 in primary pulmonary hypertension. *N. Engl. J. Med.*, **349**(12), 1113–1122.

Corchero, J. L., Mar, E. C., Spira, T. J. *et al.* (2001). Comparison of serologic assays for detection of antibodies against human herpesvirus 8. *Clin. Diagn. Lab. Immunol.*, **8**(5)., 913–921.

Davidovici, B., Karakis, I., Bourboulia, D. *et al.* (2001). Seroepidemiology and molecular epidemiology of Kaposi's sarcoma-associated herpesvirus among Jewish population groups in Israel. *J. Nat. Cancer Inst.*, **93**(3), 194–202.

Davies, J. N. P., Elmes, S., and Hutt, M.S.R. (1964). Cancer in an African community, 1897–1956. An analysis of the records of Mengo Hospital, Kampala, Uganda: Part 1. *Br. Med. J.*, **1**, 259–264.

Davis, D. A., Humphrey, R. W., Newcomb, F. M. *et al.* (1997). Detection of serum antibodies to a Kaposi's sarcoma-associated herpesvirus-specific peptide. *J. Infect. Dis.*, **175**(5), 1071–1079.

Dedicoat, M. and Newton, R. (2003). Review of the distribution of Kaposi's sarcoma-associated herpesvirus (KSHV) in Africa in relation to the incidence of Kaposi's sarcoma. *Br. J. Cancer*, **88**(1), 1–3.

de Sanjose, S., Marshall, V., Sola, J. *et al.* (2002). Prevalence of Kaposi's sarcoma-associated herpesvirus infection in sex workers and women from the general population in Spain. *Int. J. Cancer*, **98**(1), 155–158.

DeSantis, S. M., Pau, C. P., Archibald, L. K. *et al.* (2002). Demographic and immune correlates of human herpesvirus 8 seropositivity in Malawi, Africa. *Int. J. Infect. Dis.*, **6**(4), 266–269.

Desmond-Hellmann, S. D., Mbidde, E. K., Kizito, A. *et al.* (1991). The value of a clinical definition for epidemic KS in predicting HIV seropositivity in Africa. *J. Acquir. Immune Defic. Syndr.*, **4**(7), 647–651.

de-Thé, G., Bestetti, G., van Beveren, M. *et al.* (1999). Prevalence of human herpesvirus 8 infection before the acquired immunodeficiency disease syndrome-related epidemic of Kaposi's sarcoma in East Africa. *J. Nat. Cancer Insti.*, **91**(21), 1888–1889.

Diamond, C., Huang, M. L., Kedes, D. H. *et al.* (1997). Absence of detectable human herpesvirus 8 in the semen of human immunodeficiency virus-infected men without Kaposi's sarcoma. *J. Infect. Dis.*, **176**(3), 775–777.

Diamond, C., Thiede, H., Perdue, T. *et al.* (2001). Seroepidemiology of human herpesvirus 8 among young men who have sex with men. The Seattle Young Men's Survey Team. *Sex. Transmi. Dis.*, **28**(3), 176–183.

Diociaiuti, A., Nanni, G., Cattani, P. *et al.* (2000). HHV8 in renal transplant recipients. *Transpl. Int.*, **13** Suppl. 1, S410–S412.

Dollard, S. C., Nelson, K. E., Ness, P. M., Stambolis, V., Kuehnert, M. J., Pellett, P. E., and Cannon, M. J. (2005). Possible transmission of human herpesvirus-8 by blood transfusion in a historical United States cohort. *Transfusion*, **45**(4), 500–503.

Dore, G. J., Li, Y., Grulich, A. E. *et al.* (1996). Declining incidence and later occurrence of Kaposi's sarcoma among persons with AIDS in Australia: the Australian AIDS cohort. *AIDS*, **10**(12), 1401–1406.

Drew, W. L., Conant, M. A., Miner, R. C. *et al.* (1982). Cytomegalovirus and Kaposi's sarcoma in young homosexual men. *Lancet*, **2**(8290), 125–127.

Dukers, N. H., Renwick, N., Prins, M. *et al.* (2000). Risk factors for human herpesvirus 8 seropositivity and seroconversion in a cohort of homosexual men. *Am. J. Epidemiol.*, **151**(3), 213–224.

Elford, J., Tindall, B., and Sharkey T. (1992). Kaposi's sarcoma and insertive rimming [letter]. *Lancet*, **339**(8798), 938.

Eltom, M. A., Jemal, A., Mbulaiteye, S. M. *et al.* (2002a). Trends in Kaposi's sarcoma and non-Hodgkin's lymphoma incidence in the United States from 1973 through 1998. *J. Natl. Cancer Inst.*, **94**(16), 1204–1210.

Eltom, M. A., Mbulaiteye, S. M., Dada, A. J. *et al.* (2002b). Transmission of human herpesvirus 8 by sexual activity among adults in Lagos, Nigeria. *AIDS*, **16**(18), 2473–2478.

Enbom, M., Tolfvenstam, T., Ghebrekidan, H. et al. (1999). Seroprevalence of human herpes virus 8 in different Eritrean population groups. *J. Clin. Virol.*, **14**(3), 167–172.

Enbom, M., Urassa, W., Massambu, C. et al. (2002). Detection of human herpesvirus 8 DNA in serum from blood donors with HHV-8 antibodies indicates possible bloodborne virus transmission. *J. Med. Virol.*, **68**(2), 264–267.

Endo, T., Miura, T., Koibuchi, T. et al. (2003). Molecular analysis of human herpesvirus 8 by using single nucleotide polymorphisms in open reading frame 26. *J. Clin. Microbiol.*, **41**(6), 2492–2497.

Engels, E. A., Eastman, H., Ablashi, D. V., et al. (1999). Risk of transfusion-associated transmission of human herpesvirus 8. *J. Natl. Cancer Inst.*, **91**(20), 1773–1775.

Engels, E. A., Whitby, D., Goebel, P. B. et al. (2000). Identifying human herpesvirus 8 infection: performance characteristics of serologic assays. *J. Acquir. Immune Defic. Syndr.*, **23**(4), 346–354.

Engels, E. A., Biggar, R. J., Marshall, V. A. et al. (2003). Detection and quantification of Kaposi's sarcoma-associated herpesvirus to predict AIDS-associated Kaposi's sarcoma. *AIDS*, **17**(12), 1847–1851.

Fardet, L., Blum, L., Kerob, D. et al. (2001). Human herpesvirus 8 associated hemophagocytic lymphohistiocytosis in human immunodeficiency virus-infected patients. *Clin. Infect. Dis.*, **37**(2), 285–291.

Foreman, K. E., Friborg, J., Chandran, B. et al. (2001). Injection of human herpesvirus-8 in human skin engrafted on SCID mice induces Kaposi's sarcoma-like lesions. *J. Dermatol. Sci.*, **26**(3), 182–193.

Foster, C. B., Lehrnbecher, T., Samuels, S. et al. (2000). An IL6 promoter polymorphism is associated with a lifetime risk of development of Kaposi sarcoma in men infected with human immunodeficiency virus. *Blood*, **96**(7), 2562–2567.

Friedman, S. L., Wright, T. L., and Altman, D. F. (1985). Gastrointestinal Kaposi's sarcoma in patients with acquired immunodeficiency syndrome. Endoscopic and autopsy findings. *Gastroenterology*, **89**(1), 102–108.

Friedman-Kien, A. E. (1981). Disseminated Kaposi's sarcoma syndrome in young homosexual men. *J. Am. Acad. Dermatol.*, **5**(4), 468–471.

Gao, S. J., Kingsley, L., Hoover, D. R. et al. (1996a). Seroconversion to antibodies against Kaposi's sarcoma-associated herpesvirus-related latent nuclear antigens before the development of Kaposi's sarcoma. *N. Engl. J. Med.*, **335**(4), 233–241.

Gao, S. J., Kingsley, L., Li, M. et al. (1996b). KSHV antibodies among Americans, Italians and Ugandans with and without Kaposi's sarcoma. *Nat. Med.*, **2**(8), 925–928.

Gao, S. J., Zhang, Y. J., Deng, J. H. et al. (1999). Molecular polymorphism of Kaposi's sarcoma-associated herpesvirus (Human herpesvirus 8) latent nuclear antigen: evidence for a large repertoire of viral genotypes and dual infection with different viral genotypes. *J. Infect. Dis.*, **180**(5), 1466–1476.

Gessain, A., Mauclere, P., van Beveren, M. et al. (1999). Human herpesvirus 8 primary infection occurs during childhood in Cameroon, Central Africa. *Int. J. Cancer*, **81**(2), 189–192.

Goedert, J. J., Vitale, F., Lauria, C. et al. (2002). Risk factors for classical kaposi's sarcoma. *J. Natl. Cancer Inst.*, **94**(22), 1712–1718.

Goedert, J. J., Charurat, M., Blattner, W. A. et al. (2003). Risk factors for Kaposi's sarcoma-associated herpesvirus infection among HIV-1-infected pregnant women in the USA. *AIDS*, **17**(3), 425–433.

Greenblatt, R. M., Jacobson, L. P., Levine, A. M. et al. (2001). Human herpesvirus 8 infection and Kaposi's sarcoma among human immunodeficiency virus-infected and -uninfected women. *J. Infect. Dis.*, **183**(7), 1130–1134.

Grossman, Z., Iscovich, J., Schwartz, F. et al. (2002). Absence of Kaposi sarcoma among Ethiopian immigrants to Israel despite high seroprevalence of human herpesvirus 8. *Mayo Clin. Proc.*, **77**(9), 905–909.

Grulich, A. E., Kaldor, J. M., Hendry, O. et al. (1997). Risk of Kaposi's sarcoma and oroanal sexual contact. *Am. J. Epidemiol*, **145**(8), 673–679.

Grulich, A. E., Olsen, S. J., Luo, K. et al. (1999). Kaposi's sarcoma-associated herpesvirus: a sexually transmissible infection? *J. Acquir. Immune Defic. Syndr. Hum. Retrovirol.*, **20**(4), 387–393.

Gutierrez-Ortega, P., Hierro-Orozco, S., Sanchez-Cisneros, R. et al. (1989). Kaposi's sarcoma in a 6-day-old infant with human immunodeficiency virus. *Arch. Dermatoll.*, **125**(3), 432–433.

Hayward, G. S. (1999). KSHV strains: the origins and global spread of the virus. *Semin. Cancer Biol.*, **9**(3), 187–199.

He, J., Bhat, G., Kankasa, C. et al. (1998). Seroprevalence of human herpesvirus 8 among Zambian women of childbearing age without Kaposi's sarcoma (KS) and mother–child pairs with KS. *J. Infect. Dis.*, **178**(6), 1787–1790.

Hill, A. B. (1965). The environment and disease: association or causation? *Proc. Roy. Soc. Med.*, **58**, 295–300.

Hjalgrim, H., Melbye, M., Lecker, S. et al. (1996). Epidemiology of classic Kaposi's sarcoma in Denmark between 1970 and 1992. *Cancer*, **77**(7), 1373–1378.

Hjalgrim, H., Lind, I., Rostgaard, K. et al. (2001). Prevalence of human herpesvirus 8 antibodies in young adults in Denmark (1976–1977). *J. Natl. Cancer Inst.*, **93**(20), 1569–1571.

Hladik, W., Dollard, S. C., Downing, R. G. et al. (2003). Kaposi's sarcoma in Uganda: risk factors for human herpesvirus 8 infection among blood donors. *J. Acquir. Immune Defic. Syndr.*, **33**(2), 206–210.

Hladik, W., Dollard, S. C., Mermin, J., Fowlkes, A. L., Dowing, R., Amin, M. M., Banage, F., Nzaro, E., Kataaha, P., Dondero, T. J., Pellett, P. E., and Lackritz, E. M. Transmission of human herpersvirus 8 by blood transfusion. New England Journal of Medicine. In press.

Hoffman, L. J., Bunker, C. H., Pellett, P. E. et al. (2004). Elevated seroprevalence of human herpesvirus 8 among men with prostate cancer. *J. Infect. Dis.*, **189**(1), 15–20.

Hoover, D. R., Black, C., Jacobson, L. P. et al. (1993). Epidemiologic analysis of Kaposi's sarcoma as an early and later AIDS outcome in homosexual men. *Am. J. Epidemiol.*, **138**(4), 266–278.

Huang, Y. Q., Li, J. J., Rush, M. G. *et al.* (1992). HPV-16-related DNA sequences in Kaposi's sarcoma. *Lancet,* **339**(8792), 515–518.

Hutt, M. S. R. and Burkitt, D. (1965). Geographical distribution of cancer in East Africa: A new clinicopathological approach. *Br. Med. J.,* **2**, 719–722.

Hymes, K. B., Cheung, T., Greene, J. B. *et al.* (1981). Kaposi's sarcoma in homosexual men-a report of eight cases. *Lancet,* **2**(8247), 598–600.

IARC Working Group (1997). Kaposi's sarcoma herpesvirus/human herpesvirus 8. *IARC Monogr. Eval. Carcinog. Risks Hum.,* **70**, 375–492.

Inoue, N., Mar, E. C., Dollard, S. C. *et al.* (2000). New immunofluorescence assays for detection of Human herpesvirus 8-specific antibodies. *Clin. Diagn. Lab. Immunol.,* **7**(3), 427–435.

Iscovich, J., Boffetta, P., Franceschi, S. *et al.* (2000). Classic kaposi sarcoma: epidemiology and risk factors. *Cancer,* **88**(3), 500–517.

Jacobson, L. P., Munoz, A., Fox, R. *et al.* (1990). Incidence of Kaposi's sarcoma in a cohort of homosexual men infected with the human immunodeficiency virus type 1. The Multicenter AIDS Cohort Study Group. *J. Acquir. Immune Defic. Syndr.,* **3** Suppl. 1, S24–S31.

Jacobson, L. P., Jenkins, F. J., Springer, G. *et al.* (2000a). Interaction of human immunodeficiency virus type 1 and human herpesvirus type 8 infections on the incidence of Kaposi's sarcoma. *J. Infect. Dis.,* **181**(6), 1940–1949.

Jacobson, L. P., Springer, G., Jenkins, F. J. *et al.* (2000b). Armenian H. HHV-8 infection: Incidence and risk factors in the Multicenter AIDS Cohort Study (MACS). Paper presented at 3rd International Workshop on Kaposi Sarcoma-Associated Herpesviruses and Related Agents: Amherst, MA.

Janier, M., Agbalika, F., de La Salmoniere, P. *et al.* (2002). Human herpesvirus 8 seroprevalence in an STD clinic in Paris: a study of 512 patients. *Sex. Transm. Dis.,* **29**(11), 698–702.

Jones, J. L., Hanson, D. L., Dworkin, M. S. *et al.* (1999). Effect of antiretroviral therapy on recent trends in selected cancers among HIV-infected persons. Adult/Adolescent Spectrum of HIV Disease Project Group. *J. Acquir. Immune Defic. Syndr.,* **21** Suppl. 1, S11–S17.

Kaplan, L. D. and Northfelt D.W. (1997). Malignancies associated with AIDS. In Sande, M. A., Volberding, P. A., eds. *The Medical Management of AIDS.* 5th edn. Philadelphia: W.B. Saunders, p. 41322.

Kaposi, M. (1872). Idiopathisches multiples Pigmentsarcom der Haut. *Arch. Derm. Syph.,* **4**, 2675–2678.

Kedes, D. H., Operskalski, E., Busch, M. *et al.* (1996). The seroepidemiology of human herpesvirus 8 (Kaposi's sarcoma-associated herpesvirus): distribution of infection in KS risk groups and evidence for sexual transmission. *Nat. Med.,* **2**(8), 918–924.

Kedes, D. H., Ganem, D., Ameli, N. *et al.* (1997a). The prevalence of serum antibody to human herpesvirus 8 (Kaposi sarcoma-associated herpesvirus) among HIV-seropositive and high-risk HIV-seronegative women. *J. Am. Med. Assoc.,* **277**(6), 478–481.

Kedes, D. H., Lagunoff, M., Renne, R. *et al.* (1997b). Identification of the gene encoding the major latency-associated nuclear antigen of the Kaposi's sarcoma-associated herpesvirus. *J. Clin. Invest.,* **100**(10), 2606–2610.

Koelle, D. M., Huang, M. L., Chandran, B. *et al.* (1997). Frequent detection of Kaposi's sarcoma-associated herpesvirus (human herpesvirus 8) DNA in saliva of human immunodeficiency virus-infected men: clinical and immunologic correlates. *J. Infect. Dis.,* **176**(1), 94–102.

Krown, S. E., Testa, M. A., and Huang, J. (1997). AIDS-related Kaposi's sarcoma: prospective validation of the AIDS Clinical Trials Group staging classification. AIDS Clinical Trials Group Oncology Committee. *J. Clin. Oncol.,* **15**(9), 3085–3092.

Lacoste, V., Judde, J. G., Briere, J. *et al.* (2000a). Molecular epidemiology of human herpesvirus 8 in africa: both B and A5 K1 genotypes, as well as the M and P genotypes of K14.1/K15 loci, are frequent and widespread. *Virology,* **278**(1), 60–74.

Lacoste, V., Kadyrova, E., Chistiakova, I. *et al.* (2000b). Molecular characterization of Kaposi's sarcoma-associated herpesvirus/human herpesvirus-8 strains from Russia. *J. Gen. Virol.,* **81**(5), 1217–1222.

Lampinen, T. M., Kulasingam, S., Min, J. *et al.* (2000). Detection of Kaposi's sarcoma-associated herpesvirus in oral and genital secretions of Zimbabwean women. *J. Infect. Dis.,* **181**(5), 1785–1790.

Laney, A. S., Peters, J. S., Manzi, S. M., Kingsley, L. A., Chang, Y., and Moore, P. S. Use of a multiantigen detection algorithm for diagnosis of Kaposi's sarcoma-associated herpesvirus infection. *J. Clin. Micro.* In press.

Lavreys, L., Chohan, B., Ashley, R. *et al.* (2003). Human herpesvirus 8: seroprevalence and correlates in prostitutes in mombasa, kenya. *J. Infect. Dis.,* **187**(3), 359–363.

Lefrere, J. J., Meyohas, M. C., Mariotti, M. *et al.* (1996). Detection of human herpesvirus 8 DNA sequences before the appearance of Kaposi's sarcoma in human immunodeficiency virus (HIV)-positive subjects with a known date of HIV seroconversion. *J. Infect. Dis.,* **174**(2), 283–287.

Lefrere, J. J., Mariotti, M., Girot, R. *et al.* (1997). Transfusional risk of HHV-8 infection. *Lancet,* **350**, 217.

Lehrnbecher, T. L., Foster, C. B., Zhu, S. *et al.* (2000). Variant genotypes of FcgammaRIIIA influence the development of Kaposi's sarcoma in HIV-infected men. *Blood,* **95**(7), 2386–2390.

Lennette, E. T., Blackbourn, D. J., and Levy J. A. (1996). Antibodies to human herpesvirus type 8 in the general population and in Kaposi's sarcoma patients. *Lancet,* **348**(9031), 858–861.

Lifson, A. R., Darrow, W. W., Hessol, N. A. *et al.* (1990). Kaposi's sarcoma in a cohort of homosexual and bisexual men. Epidemiology and analysis for cofactors. *Am. J. Epidemiol,* **131**(2), 221–231.

Luppi, M., Barozzi, P., Santagostino, G. *et al.* (2000a). Molecular evidence of organ-related transmission of Kaposi sarcoma-associated herpesvirus or human herpesvirus-8 in transplant patients. *Blood,* **96**(9), 3279–3281.

Luppi, M., Barozzi, P., Schulz, T. F. *et al.* (2000b). Bone marrow failure associated with human herpesvirus 8 infection after transplantation. *N. Engl. J. Med.*, **343**(19), 1378–1385.

Mantina, H., Kankasa, C., Klaskala, W. *et al.* (2001). Vertical transmission of Kaposi's sarcoma-associated herpesvirus. *Int. J. Cancer*, **94**(5), 749–752.

Marcelin, A. G., Grandadam, M., Flandre, P. *et al.* (2002). Kaposi's sarcoma herpesvirus and HIV-1 seroprevalences in prostitutes in Djibouti. *J. Med. Virol.*, **68**(2), 164–167.

Marcelin, A. G., Roque-Afonso, A. M., Hurtova, M., Dupin, N., Tulliez, M., Sebagh, M., Arkoub, Z. A., Guettier, C., Samuel, D., Calvez, V., and Dussaix, F. (2004) Fatal disseminated Kaposi's sarcoma following human herpesvirus 8 primary infections in liver-transplant recipients. Liver Transpl. 10:295–300.

Martin, J. N. and Osmond, D. H. (1999). Kaposi's sarcoma-associated herpesvirus and sexual transmission of cancer risk. *Curr. Opin. Oncol.*, **11**(6), 508–515.

Martin, J. N. and Osmond D. H. (2000). Determining specific sexual practices associated with human herpesvirus 8 transmission. *Am. J. Epidemiol.*, **151**(3), 225–229; discussion 230.

Martin, J. N., Ganem, D. E., Osmond, D. H. *et al.* (1998). Sexual transmission and the natural history of human herpesvirus 8 infection. *N. Engl. J. Med.*, **338**, 948–954.

Martin, J. N., Amad, Z., Cossen, C. *et al.* (2000). Use of epidemiologically well-defined subjects and existing immunofluorescence assays to calibrate a new enzyme immunoassay for human herpesvirus 8 antibodies. *J. Clin. Microbiol.*, **38**(2), 696–701.

Masini, C., Abeni, D. D., Cattaruzza, M. S. *et al.* (2000). Antibodies against human herpesvirus 8 in subjects with non-venereal dermatological conditions. *Br. J. Dermatol.*, **143**(3), 484–490.

Masood, R., Zheng, T., Tulpule, A. *et al.* (1997). Kaposi's sarcoma-associated herpesvirus infection and multiple myeloma. *Science*, **278**(5345), 1970–1971.

Mayama, S., Cuevas, L. E., Sheldon, J. *et al.* (1998). Prevalence and transmission of Kaposi's sarcoma-associated herpesvirus (human herpesvirus 8) in Ugandan children and adolescents. *Int. J. Cancer*, **77**(6), 817–820.

Mbulaiteye, S. M., Biggar, R. J., Bakaki, P. M. *et al.* (2003a). Human herpesvirus 8 infection and transfusion history in children with sickle-cell disease in Uganda. *J. Natl. Cancer Inst.*, **95**(17), 1330–1335.

Mbulaiteye, S. M., Pfeiffer, R. M., Whitby, D. *et al.* (2003b). Human herpesvirus 8 infection within families in rural Tanzania. *J. Infect. Dis.*, **187**(11), 1780–1785.

Melbye, M., Cook, P. M., Hjalgrim, H. *et al.* (1998). Risk factors for Kaposi's-sarcoma-associated herpesvirus (KSHV/HHV-8) seropositivity in a cohort of homosexual men, 1981–1996. *Int. J. Cancer*, **77**(4), 543–548.

Meng, Y. X., Spira, T. J., Bhat, G. J. *et al.* (1999). Individuals from North America, Australasia, and Africa are infected with four different genotypes of human herpesvirus 8. *Virology*, **261**(1), 106–119.

Michaels, M. G., and Jenkins, F. J. (2003). Human herpesvirus 8: is it time for routine surveillance in pediatric solid organ transplant recipients to prevent the development of Kaposi's sarcoma? *Pediatr. Transpl.*, **7**(1), 1–3.

Miller, G., Rigsby, M. O., Heston, L. *et al.* (1996). Antibodies to butyrate-inducible antigens of Kaposi's sarcoma-associated herpesvirus in patients with HIV-1 infection. *N. Engl. J. Med.*, **334**(20), 1292–1297.

Minhas, V., Crabtree, K. L., M'soka, T. J., Phiri, S., Kankasa, C., West, J. T., Mitchell, C. D., and Wood, C. (2006) Early childhood infection by Kaposi's sarcoma-associated herpesvirus in Zambia and he role of HIV-1 as a risk factor. 9th International Workshop on KSHV and Related Agents. Hyannis, Massachusetts. July 12–15.

Mitchell, D. M., McCarty, M., Fleming, J. *et al.* (1992). Bronchopulmonary Kaposi's sarcoma in patients with AIDS. *Thorax*, **47**(9), 726–729.

Moore P. S. (2003). Transplanting cancer: donor-cell transmission of Kaposi sarcoma. *Nat. Med.*, **9**(5), 506–508.

Moore, P. S., Kingsley, L. A., Holmberg, S. D. *et al.* (1996). Kaposi's sarcoma-associated herpesvirus infection prior to onset of Kaposi's sarcoma. *AIDS*, **10**(2), 175–180.

Neipel, F., Albrecht, J. C., and Fleckenstein, B. (1997). Cell-homologous genes in the Kaposi's sarcoma-associated rhadinovirus human herpesvirus 8: determinants of its pathogenicity? *J. Virol.*, **71**(6), 4187–4192.

Newton, R., Ziegler, J., Bourboulia, D. *et al.* (2003). The seroepidemiology of Kaposi's sarcoma-associated herpesvirus (KSHV/HHV-8) in adults with cancer in Uganda. *Int. J. Cancer*, **103**(2), 226–232.

Nicholas, J., Zong, J. C., Alcendor, D. J. *et al.* (1998). Novel organizational features, captured cellular genes, and strain variability within the genome of KSHV/HHV8. *J. Natl Cancer Inst. Monogr*, **23**, 79–88.

Nuvor, S. V., Katano, H., Ampofo, W. K. *et al.* (2001). Higher prevalence of antibodies to human herpesvirus 8 in HIV-infected individuals than in the general population in Ghana, West Africa. *Eur. J. Clin. Microbiol. Infect. Dis.*, **20**(5), 362–364.

O'Brien, T., Kedes, D., Ganem, D. *et al.* (1999). Evidence for concurrent epidemics of human herpesvirus 8 and human immunodeficiency virus type 1 in US homosexual men: rates, risk factors, and relationship to Kaposi's sarcoma. *J. Infect. Dis.*, **180**(4), 1010–1017.

Oksenhendler, E., Cazals-Hatem, D., Schulz, T. F. *et al.* (1998). Transient angiolymphoid hyperplasia and Kaposi's sarcoma after primary infection with human herpesvirus 8 in a patient with human immunodeficiency virus infection. *N. Engl. J. Med.*, **338**(22), 1585–1590.

Olsen, S. J., Chang, Y., Moore, P. S. *et al.* (1998). Increasing Kaposi's sarcoma-associated herpesvirus seroprevalence with age in a highly Kaposi's sarcoma endemic region, Zambia in 1985. *AIDS*, **12**(14), 1921–1925.

Operskalski, E. A., Busch, M. P., Mosley, J. W. *et al.* (1997). Blood donations and viruses. *Lancet*, **349**(9061), 1327.

Osmond, D. H., Buchbinder, S., Cheng, A. *et al.* (2002). Prevalence of Kaposi sarcoma-associated herpesvirus infection in homosexual men at beginning of and during the HIV epidemic. *J. Am. Med. Assoc.*, **287**(2), 221–225.

Page-Bodkin, K., Tappero, J., Samuel, M. *et al.* (1992). Kaposi's sarcoma and faecal-oral exposure [letter]. *Lancet*, **339**(8807), 1490.

Parravicini, C., Lauri, E., Baldini, L. *et al.* (1997). Kaposi's sarcoma-associated herpesvirus infection and multiple myeloma. *Science*, **278**(5345), 1969–1979.

Pau, C. P., Lam, L. L., Spira, T. J. *et al.* (1998). Mapping and serodiagnostic application of a dominant epitope within the human herpesvirus 8 ORF 65-encoded protein. *J. Clin. Microbiol.*, **36**(6), 1574–1577.

Pauk, J., Huang, M. L., Brodie, S. J. *et al.* (2000). Mucosal shedding of human herpesvirus 8 in men. *N. Engl. J. Med.*, **343**(19), 1369–1377.

Pellett, P. E., Wright, D. J., Engels, E. A. *et al.* (2003). Multicenter comparison of serologic assays and estimation of human herpesvirus 8 seroprevalence among US blood donors. *Transfusion*, **43**(9), 1260–1268.

Penn I. (1979). Kaposi's sarcoma in organ transplant recipients: report of 20 cases. *Transplantation*, **27**(1), 8–11.

Perna, A. M., Bonura, F., Vitale, F. *et al.* (2000). Antibodies to human herpes virus type 8 (HHV8) in general population and in individuals at risk for sexually transmitted diseases in Western Sicily. *Int J. Epidemiol.*, **29**(1), 175–179.

Plancoulaine, S., Abel, L., van Beveren, M. *et al.* (2000). Human herpesvirus 8 transmission from mother to child and between siblings in an endemic population. *Lancet*, **356**(9235), 1062–1065.

Plancoulaine, S., Gessain, A., van Beveren, M. *et al.* (2003). Evidence for a recessive major gene predisposing to human herpesvirus 8 (HHV-8) infection in a population in which HHV-8 is endemic. *J. Infect. Dis.*, **187**(12), 1944–1950.

Poole, L. J., Zong, J. C., Ciufo, D. M. *et al.* (1999). Comparison of genetic variability at multiple loci across the genomes of the major subtypes of Kaposi's sarcoma-associated herpesvirus reveals evidence for recombination and for two distinct types of open reading frame K15 alleles at the right-hand end. *J. Virol.*, **73**(8), 6646–6660.

Portsmouth, S., Stebbing, J., Gill, J. *et al.* (2003). A comparison of regimens based on non-nucleoside reverse transcriptase inhibitors or protease inhibitors in preventing Kaposi's sarcoma. *AIDS*, **17**(11), F17–F22.

Quinlivan, E. B., Wang, R. X., Stewart, P. W. *et al.* (2001). Longitudinal seroreactivity to human herpesvirus 8 (KSHV) in the Swiss HIV Cohort 4.7 years before KS. Swiss HIV Cohort Study. *J. Med. Virol.*, **64**(2), 157–166.

Raab, M. S., Albrecht, J. C., Birkmann, A. *et al.* (1998). The immunogenic glycoprotein gp35–37 of human herpesvirus 8 is encoded by open reading frame K8.1. *J. Virol.*, **72**(8), 6725–6731.

Rabkin, C. S., Schulz, T. F., Whitby, D. *et al.* (1998). Interassay correlation of human herpesvirus 8 serologic tests. HHV-8 Interlaboratory Collaborative Group. *J. Infect. Dis.*, **178**(2), 304–309.

Rainbow, L., Platt, G. M., Simpson, G. R. *et al.* (1997). The 222- to 234-kilodalton latent nuclear protein (LNA) of Kaposi's sarcoma-associated herpesvirus (human herpesvirus 8) is encoded by orf73 and is a component of the latency-associated nuclear antigen. *J. Virol.*, **71**(8), 5915–5921.

Ransohoff, D. F., and Feinstein AR. (1978). Problems of spectrum and bias in evaluating the efficacy of diagnostic tests. *N. Engl. J. Med.*, **299**(17), 926–930.

Regamey, N., Tamm, M., Wernli, M. *et al.* (1998). Transmission of human herpesvirus 8 infection from renal-transplant donors to recipients. *N. Engl. J. Med.*, **339**(19), 1358–1363.

Renwick, N., Halaby, T., Weverling, G. J. *et al.* (1998). Seroconversion for human herpesvirus 8 during HIV infection is highly predictive of Kaposi's sarcoma. *AIDS*, **12**, 2481–2488.

Renwick, N., Dukers, N. H., Weverling, G. J. *et al.* (2002). Risk factors for human herpesvirus 8 infection in a cohort of drug users in the Netherlands, 1985–1996. *J. Infect. Dis.*, **185**(12), 1808–1812.

Rettig, M. B., Ma, H. J., Vescio, R. A. *et al.* (1997). Kaposi's sarcoma-associated herpesvirus infection of bone marrow dendritic cells from multiple myeloma patients. *Science*, **276**(5320), 1851–1854.

Rezza, G., Lennette, E. T., Giuliani, M. *et al.* (1998). Prevalence and determinants of anti-lytic and anti-latent antibodies to human herpesvirus-8 among Italian individuals at risk of sexually and parenterally transmitted infections. *Int. J. Cancer*, **77**(3), 361–365.

Rezza, G., Dorrucci, M., Serraino, D. *et al.* (2000a). Incidence of Kaposi's sarcoma and HHV-8 seroprevalence among homosexual men with known dates of HIV seroconversion. Italian Seroconversion Study. *AIDS*, **14**(11), 1647–1653.

Rezza, G., Tchangmena, O. B., Andreoni, M. *et al.* (2000b). Prevalence and risk factors for human herpesvirus 8 infection in northern Cameroon. *Sex. Transm. Dis.*, **27**(3), 159–164.

Rezza, G., Danaya, R. T., Wagner, T. M. *et al.* (2001). Human herpesvirus-8 and other viral infections, Papua New Guinea. *Emerg. Infect. Dis.*, **7**(5), 893–895.

Rothman, K. J. and Greenland, S. (1998). *Causation and Causal Inference. Modern Epidemiology*. Philadelphia, PA: Lippincott-Raven, pp. 7–28.

Russo, J. J., Bohenzky, R. A., Chien, M. C. *et al.* (1996). Nucleotide sequence of the Kaposi sarcoma-associated herpesvirus (HHV8). *Proc. Natl Acad. Sci. USA*, **93**(25), 14862–14867.

Rutherford, G. W., Payne, S. F., and Lemp G.F. (1990). The epidemiology of AIDS-related Kaposi's sarcoma in San Francisco. *J. Acquir. Immune Defic. Syndr.*, **3** Suppl. 1, S4–S7.

Sanchez-Velasco, P., Ocejo-Vinyals, J. G., Flores, R. *et al.* (2001). Simultaneous multiorgan presence of human herpesvirus 8 and restricted lymphotropism of Epstein-Barr virus DNA sequences in a human immunodeficiency virus-negative immunodeficient infant. *J. Infect. Dis.*, **183**(2), 338–342.

Siegel, J. H., Janis, R., Alper, J. C. *et al.* (1969). Disseminated visceral Kaposi's sarcoma. Appearance after human renal homograft operation. *J. Am. Med. Assoc.*, **207**(8), 1493–1496.

Simpson, G. R., Schulz, T. F., Whitby, D. *et al.* (1996). Prevalence of Kaposi's sarcoma associated herpesvirus infection by antibodies to recombinant capsid protein and latent antigen. *Lancet*, **348**(9035), 1133–1138.

Sitas, F., Carrara, H., Beral, V. *et al.* (1999). Antibodies against human herpesvirus 8 in black South African patients with cancer. *N. Engl. J. Med.*, **340**(24), 1863–1871.

Sitas, F., Newton, R., and Boshoff, C. (1999a,b). Increasing probability of mother-to-child transmission of HHV-8 with increasing maternal antibody titer for HHV-8 [letter]. *N. Engl. J. Med.*, **340**(24), 1923.

Smith, N. A., Sabin, C. A., Gopal, R. *et al.* (1999). Serologic evidence of human herpesvirus 8 transmission by homosexual but not heterosexual sex. *J. Infect. Dis.*, **180**(3), 600–606.

Sosa, C., Klaskala, W., Chandran, B. *et al.* (1998). Human herpesvirus 8 as a potential sexually transmitted agent in Honduras. *J. Infect. Dis.*, **178**(2), 547–551.

Soulier, J., Grollet, L., Oksenhendler, E. *et al.* (1995). Kaposi's sarcoma-associated herpesvirus-like DNA sequences in multicentric Castleman's disease. *Blood*, **86**(4), 1276–1280.

Spira, T. J., Lam, L., Dollard, S. C. *et al.* (2000). Comparison of serologic assays and PCR for diagnosis of human herpesvirus 8 infection. *J. Clini. Microbiol.*, **38**(6), 2174–2180.

Spira, T. J., Inoue, N., Corchero, J. *et al.* (2001). Serologic responses to recombinant HHV-8 latent and lytic antigens over time in HIV infected patients. Paper presented at: 8th Conference on Retroviruses and Opportunisitic Infections, Chicago, IL.

Stebbing, J., Wilder, N., Ariad, S. *et al.* (2001). Lack of intra-patient strain variability during infection with Kaposi's sarcoma-associated herpesvirus. *Am. J. Hematol.*, **68**(2), 133–134.

Tam, H. K., Zhang, Z. F., Jacobson, L. P. *et al.* (2002). Effect of highly active antiretroviral therapy on survival among HIV-infected men with Kaposi sarcoma or non-Hodgkin lymphoma. *Int. J. Cancer*, **98**(6), 916–922.

Tedeschi, R., De Paoli, P., Schulz, T. F. *et al.* (1999). Human serum antibodies to a major defined epitope of human herpesvirus 8 small viral capsid antigen. *J. Infect. Dis.*, **179**(4), 1016–1020.

Tedeschi, R., Caggiari, L., Silins, I. *et al.* (2000). Seropositivity to human herpesvirus 8 in relation to sexual history and risk of sexually transmitted infections among women. *Int. J. Cancer*, **87**(2), 232–235.

Touloumi, G., Hatzakis, A., Potouridou, I. *et al.* (1999). The role of immunosuppression and immune-activation in classic Kaposi's sarcoma. *Int. J. Cancer*, **82**(6), 817–821.

US Public Health Service and Infectious Diseases Society of America. (2002). Guidelines for Preventing Opportunistic Infections Among HIV-infected Persons. *Morb. Mortal. Wkly Rep.*, **51**(RR08), 1–46.

Vitale, F., Viviano, E., Perna, A. M. *et al.* (2000). Serological and virological evidence of non-sexual transmission of human herpesvirus type 8 (HHV8). *Epidemiol. Infect.*, **125**(3), 671–675.

Wabinga, H. R., Parkin, D. M., Wabwire-Mangen, F. *et al.* (1993). Cancer in Kampala, Uganda, in 1989–91: changes in incidence in the era of AIDS. *Int. J. Cancer*, **54**(1), 26–36.

Wabinga, H. R., Parkin, D. M., Wabwire-Mangen, F. *et al.* (2000). Trends in cancer incidence in Kyadondo County, Uganda, 1960–1997. *Br. J. Cancer*, **82**(9), 1585–1592.

Wang, Q. J., Jenkins, F. J., Jacobson, L. P. *et al.* (2001). Primary human herpesvirus 8 infection generates a broadly specific CD8(+) T-cell response to viral lytic cycle proteins. *Blood*, **97**(8), 2366–2373.

Wang, R. Y., Shih, J. W., Weiss, S. H. *et al.* (1993). Mycoplasma penetrans infection in male homosexuals with AIDS: high seroprevalence and association with Kaposi's sarcoma. *Clin. Infect. Dis.*, **17**(4), 724–729.

Wawer, M. J., Eng, S. M., Serwadda, D. *et al.* (2001). Prevalence of Kaposi sarcoma-associated herpesvirus compared with selected sexually transmitted diseases in adolescents and young adults in rural Rakai District, Uganda. *Sex. Transm. Dis.*, **28**(2), 77–81.

Whitby, D., Howard, M. R., Tenant-Flowers, M. *et al.* (1995). Detection of Kaposi sarcoma associated herpesvirus in peripheral blood HIV-infected individuals and progression to Kaposi's sarcoma. *Lancet*, **346**(8978), 799–802.

Whitby, D., Boshoff, C., Luppi, M. *et al.* (1997). Kaposi's sarcoma-associated herpesvirus infection and multiple myeloma. *Science*, **278**(5345), 1971–1972.

Whitby, D., Luppi, M., Barozzi, P. *et al.* (1998). Human herpesvirus 8 seroprevalence in blood donors and lymphoma patients from different regions of Italy. *J. Natl Cancer Inst.*, **90**(5), 395–397.

Whitby, D., Luppi, M., Sabin, C. *et al.* (2000). Detection of antibodies to human herpesvirus 8 in Italian children: evidence for horizontal transmission. *Br. J. Cancer*, **82**(3), 702–704.

Whitby, D., Marshall, V. A., Bagni, R. K. *et al.* (2004). Genotypic characterization of Kaposi's sarcoma-associated herpesvirus in asymptomatic infected subjects from isolated populations. *J. Gen. Virol.*, **85**(1), 155–163.

Ziegler J.L. (1993). Endemic Kaposi's sarcoma in Africa and local volcanic soils. *Lancet*, **342**(8883), 1348–1351.

Ziegler, J., Newton, R., Bourboulia, D. *et al.* (2003). Risk factors for Kaposi's sarcoma: a case-control study of HIV-seronegative people in Uganda. *Int. J. Cancer*, **103**(2), 233–240.

Zong, J., Ciufo, D. M., Viscidi, R. *et al.* (2002). Genotypic analysis at multiple loci across Kaposi's sarcoma herpesvirus (KSHV) DNA molecules: clustering patterns, novel variants and chimerism. *J. Clin. Virol.*, **23**(3), 119–148.

Zong, J. C., Metroka, C., Reitz, M. S. *et al.* (1997). Strain variability among Kaposi sarcoma-associated herpesvirus (human herpesvirus 8) genomes: evidence that a large cohort of United States AIDS patients may have been infected by a single common isolate. *J. Virol.*, **71**(3), 250.

Zong, J. C., Ciufo, D. M., Alcendor, D. J. *et al.* (1999). High-level variability in the ORF-K1 membrane protein gene at the left end of the Kaposi's sarcoma-associated herpesvirus genome defines four major virus subtypes and multiple variants or clades in different human populations. *J. Virol.*, **73**(5), 4156–4170.

55

EBV-induced oncogenesis

Nancy Raab-Traub

Department of Microbiology and Immunology, Lineberger Comprehensive Cancer Center, University of North Carolina at Chapel Hill, USA

Introduction

The Epstein–Barr virus (EBV) is a human herpesvirus that is a ubiquitous infectious agent, infecting greater than 90% of the world's population (Henle et al., 1969). The majority of infections occur early in life without significant illness. However, EBV is clearly an important factor in multiple human cancers. This dichotomy raises the question as to what are the unique aspects of infection in those who develop cancers. The study of EBV and its associated tumors points to specific interactions between environmental, genetic, and viral factors.

Many of the malignancies associated with EBV develop in the setting of immunosuppression or have endemic patterns of incidence (Raab-Traub, 1996). EBV has potent growth transforming properties in vitro where it efficiently induces permanent growth of infected lymphocytes (Nilsson et al., 1971). Therefore it is not surprising that EBV is clearly the etiologic factor in post-transplant lymphoma and a subset of AIDS-associated lymphomas.

The endemic patterns of incidence characteristic of many EBV-associated tumors were initially apparent as EBV was originally isolated from samples of African Burkitt's Lymphoma (BL) (Epstein et al., 1964). This childhood tumor develops with high incidence in subequatorial Africa (Burkitt, 1962a). EBV was subsequently identified in nasopharyngeal carcinoma (NPC), a major tumor that occurs with extraordinarily high incidence in the southern Chinese and with elevated incidence in Inuit populations and in Mediterranean Africa (Henle et al., 1978a; Wolf et al., 1973). EBV has also been identified in a subset of T-cell lymphomas that develop with increased frequency in Taiwan and Japan and in parotid gland tumors that occur most frequently among Inuits (Su et al., 1990; Saemundsen et al., 1982).

Finally, there are the more recently identified tumors associated with EBV, a subset of Hodgkin's lymphoma (HL) and gastric carcinoma (Weiss et al., 1989a,b; Shibata et al., 1991). The factors that contribute to the development of these tumors are unknown but the environmental and immune components may be similar to those that contribute to the development of EBV cancers with endemic incidence patterns or due to immune impairment. It is likely that environmental or genetic factors increase infection of distinct susceptible cell populations and activate cellular pathways that are highly synergistic with EBV genes that affect cell growth.

This chapter will review the pathogenesis of EBV infection, the characteristics of EBV-associated tumors, the molecular biology of latent infection, and biochemical properties of EBV genes as they relate to tumor development.

EBV infection in vivo

EBV is the prototype member of the Herpesvirus subfamily, Gammaherpesviridae, and like other herpesviruses, the virus establishes a latent infection with life-long persistence in the infected host (Kieff and Rickinson, 2001). The virus is transmitted by salivary exchange and may initially infect the epithelial cells of the oropharynx, posterior nasopharynx, parotid gland and duct, and possibly tonsilar lymphocytes (Miller et al., 1973; Wolf et al., 1984; Sixbey et al., 1984). Hybridization in situ has detected evidence of EBV DNA in cells lining the parotid duct and EBV DNA and replicative mRNAs have been detected in sloughed oropharyngeal epithelial cells and tonsilar lymphoid cells (Sixbey et al., 1984). Through infection of trafficking lymphocytes, the virus then establishes a

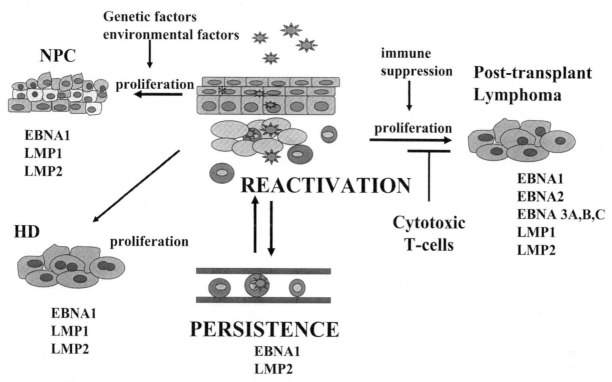

Fig. 55.1. **EBV pathogenesis**. EBV is transmitted by saliva and infects oropharyngeal epithelial cells and lymphocytes. The virus persists in memory B cells that have limited EBV expression, possibly only EBNA1 or LMP2. The virus frequently reactivates from peripheral blood lymphocytes producing virus and may be directly shed from lymphocytes into the nasopharynx or may replicate in mucosal epithelial cells. In combination with possible genetic changes such as the absence of p16 expression, the virus may establish a latent infection in a basal epithelial cell. Additional genetic changes may enable expression of EBNA1, LMP1, and LMP2 which may not be presented by specific HLA types. The viral episome is maintained in the infected epithelial cell which rapidly becomes malignant in nasopharyngeal carcinoma (NPC). Similar events may occur in the development of Hodgkin Disease (HD). In the context of immunosuppression, the virus can reactivate to full latent expression with expression of EBNA2, 2, 3A,3B,3C, LMP1, and LMP2. The transformed cells may develop into post-transplant lymphoma in the absence of cytotoxic T-lymphocytes.

persistent latent infection in bone marrow and peripheral blood memory B-lymphocytes (Fig. 55.1). Virus expression is tightly restricted in latently infected B-lymphocytes with no viral gene expression or with expression limited to the EBV nuclear antigen 1 (EBNA1), and/or latent membrane protein 2 (LMP2) (Babcock *et al.*, 2000a). The state of EBV latency may reactivate and express additional viral genes that induce cell growth, including the other EBNAs and LMP1 and LMP2. The proliferation of the infected lymphocytes is controlled by cytotoxic T-cells (CTLs) that primarily recognize the EBNA2 and EBNA3 proteins (Murray *et al.*, 1990). Therefore in immunosuppressed patients who lack CTL control, EBV-infected B-lymphocytes may proliferate and develop into B-cell lymphomas (Fig. 55.1). EBV infection also may reactivate into replicative infection at mucosal sites and infectious virus is frequently detected in saliva.

The infected peripheral lymphocytes can be explanted in vitro and established as permanent lymphoblastoid cell lines (LCLs). The majority of the infected cells in the cell lines do not produce virus but instead are latently infected and maintain the EBV genome as a multi-copy episome (Rickinson, 2001). In vitro, an occasional cell in some cell lines may reactivate into viral replication and produce infectious virus. The infectious virus produced by cell lines or virus that is present in throat washings will infect primary B-lymphocytes, establish a latent infection, and induce growth transformation.

The ability of the virus to efficiently transform B-cells in culture to immortalized, transformed cells undoubtedly underlies its connection to human cancers. In B-cell lines grown in vitro, the carefully regulated, coordinate expression of multiple viral gene products induces permanent continuous cell growth.

Characteristics of latent infection

DNA structure

The EBV genome that is encapsidated in the virion is a 185 kb double-stranded, linear DNA molecule that is replicated by a virally encoded DNA polymerase (Kieff and Rickinson, 2001). Within latently infected cells, the viral genome is an extrachromosomal episome that is present in multiple copies (Adams and Lindahl, 1975). The episome has a nucleosomal structure and is replicated by the host DNA polymerase (Shaw, 1985; Shaw et al., 1979). The linear viral genome is largely unique DNA interspersed with short direct tandem repeats. At the ends of the viral DNA there are multiple copies of a 500 bp direct tandem repeated sequence (Given et al., 1979). Due to the variable numbers of this terminal repeat (TR) element the terminal restriction enzyme fragments are heterogeneous in size. Identification of the terminal restriction enzyme fragments of linear virion DNA on Southern blots will reveal ladder arrays of heterogeneous DNA fragments that contain different numbers of TR (Fig. 55.2(a)). After entry into the cell, the linear form circularizes through the TR to form viral episomal DNA. The restriction enzyme fragment representing the fused termini of the episomal form of EBV can be distinguished from the terminal restriction fragments of the linear genomes because the fused fragments are larger and contain the unique DNA sequences adjacent to the terminal repeats from both ends of the genome (Raab-Traub and Flynn, 1986). Therefore the fused termini restriction enzyme fragment will hybridize to DNA probes of unique DNA from either end of the linear genome (Fig. 55.2(a)).

Identification of the EBV termini is particularly useful because it permits discrimination between viral replicative and latent states and also is a predictor of the clonality of the viral genome. In the initial studies, a single band representing the EBV fused termini was detected in NPC and in monoclonal lymphomas (Fig. 55.2(b)). The identification of a single band indicated that all of the EBV episomes were identical to one another with regard to number of TR (Raab-Traub and Flynn, 1986). This indicated that the tumors contained a homogeneous clonal population of EBV genomes and suggested by extension cellular monoclonality. This provided the first evidence that NPC like BL is a monoclonal proliferation and revealed that the malignancy had developed from a single EBV-infected cell. The link between the homogeneity of the EBV genome and cellular clonality has been confirmed in multiple studies of lymphoid tumors where clonality can be determined through analysis of the immunoglobulin joining region (Brown et al., 1988).

Most EBV tumors contain a single clonal population of EBV genomes as evidenced by the detection of a single restriction enzyme fragment (Fig. 55.2(b)). Clonal EBV genomes are present in Hodgkin's disease and in many lymphomas that develop in immunosuppressed patients (Weiss et al., 1989a,b). Oral hairy leukoplakia (HLP) is an unusual lesion that may develop on the lateral borders of the tongue in HIV infected or immunosuppressed individuals (Greenspan et al., 1985). It is the only pathologic manifestation of a permissive EBV infection and identification of the EBV termini detects abundant ladder arrays of linear DNA (Fig. 55.2(b)) (Gilligan et al., 1990a).

EBV expression in latent infection

Multiple viral genes are expressed in latently infected lymphocytes maintained in vitro and at least three different patterns of EBV expression have been detected in latently infected cells and tissues (Rowe et al., 1987). In cell lines transformed in vitro and in lymphomas that develop in transplant recipients, six EBNA proteins (EBNA 1, 2, 3A, 3B, 3C, and leader protein, EBNA-LP) are expressed (Rickinson, 2001). These proteins regulate their own expression and also regulate expression of the latent membrane proteins, LMP1 and LMP2 (Wang et al., 1990). In addition, the non-polyadenylated EBER RNAs and rightward transcripts from the BamHI A region are expressed (BARTS) (Brooks et al., 1993). This state of latent infection is termed Type 3 latency. EBV expression is more restricted in other types of latent infections that have been identified in tumors and in peripheral blood lymphocytes. Type 1 latency is the most restricted with expression of EBNA1 and the EBERs and is found in BL. In Type 2 latency found in NPC and HL, EBNA1, LMP1, LMP2, EBERs, and BARTs are expressed. In peripheral blood lymphocytes, EBV may not express any genes or may only express EBNA1 or LMP2. This has been referred to as Type 0 latency (Rickinson, 2001).

The EBNA2 and EBNA3 proteins are the major targets of EBV-specific cytotoxic T lymphocytes (CTL) (Rickinson and Moss, 1997). Expression of these proteins has been detected in tonsillar lymphocytes and during infectious mononucleosis but they have not been detected in latently infected peripheral blood lymphocytes (Babcock and Thorley-Lawson, 2000b). Of the cancers that are associated with EBV, the EBNA2 and 3 proteins are only expressed in lymphomas that develop in immunosuppressed patients such as post-transplant lymphomas (Young et al., 1989). Due to the expression of the EBNA CTL targets, the post-transplant lymphomas can be successfully treated by immune therapy (Rooney et al., 1995) (Fig. 55.1). Reduction

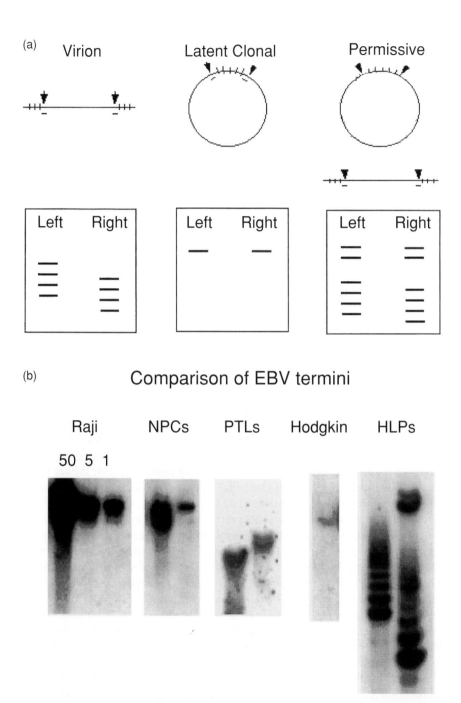

Fig. 55.2. **Identification of the EBV termini identifies episomal and linear viral DNA.** (a) A is present at the termini of the linear DNA. The number of terminal repeats (TR), homologous direct repeat 500 bp sequence, differs between individual DNA molecules such that the terminal restriction enzyme fragments that contain the TR are heterogeneous in size and form a ladder array on gels representing molecules that have differing numbers of the TR element. Upon entry into the cell, the viral DNA circularizes through the TR to form the intracellular, extrachromosomal episome. This circularization produces a fused restriction enzyme fragment that can be identified with DNA probes representing unique DNA adjacent to the TR from either ends of the linear genome. (b) A single fused restriction enzyme fragment representing the EBV episomal DNA is detected in most EBV malignancies including NPC, PTL, and HD. The Raji cell line and dilutions is used for comparison of copy number. HLP represents a permissive infection.

of immunosuppression or infusion of EBV-specific CTLs that recognize the EBNA proteins can result in regression of the EBV-infected lymphoma. In other EBV associated tumors that develop in non-immunosuppressed individuals and in some patients with AIDS, the EBNA2 and 3 proteins are not expressed (Raab-Traub, 1996). The expression of LMP1 and LMP2 independent of transactivation by the EBNA proteins, the major CTL targets, may be one factor that contributes to the development of these tumors.

The EBNA proteins

The EBNA 1 protein is essential for maintenance and replication of the viral episome by the host DNA polymerase during latent infection (Yates et al., 1985). EBNA1 binds to the origin of replication for the plasmid form of the viral genome and is essential for plasmid replication. EBNA1 also binds to cellular chromosomes and mediates equivalent partitioning of the viral genomes to the daughter cells. Although EBNA1 is expressed in all dividing EBV infected cells, the protein is not recognized by CTLs and the latently infected cells can persist in the presence of a functioning immune system (Levitskaya et al., 1995). The lack of CTL recognition of EBNA1 is due to the presence of a large repeated element of glycine and alanine. This sequence apparently spares EBNA1 from proteosomal degradation and presentation by MHC class I molecules (Levitskaya et al., 1997).

The EBNA 2 protein is essential for growth transformation of lymphocytes and is also a transcriptional transactivator (Cohen et al., 1989). EBNA2 interacts with the RBPJk protein to activate gene expression (Grossman et al., 1994; Henkel et al., 1994). RBPJk is the DNA binding protein and transcription factor that is activated by the Notch signaling pathway. Activated Notch has been shown to partially substitute for EBNA2 in transformation (Hofelmayr et al., 2001). EBNA2 also interacts with multiple cellular transcriptional proteins through which it regulates the viral promoters for the latent membrane proteins, LMP1 and LMP2, for the B-cell activation marker, CD23, and the EBV receptor, CD21 (Johannsen et al., 1995). Two types of EBNA2 have been identified, encoded by quite divergent sequences (Dambaugh et al., 1984). The type of EBNA2 gene, EBNA2A or 2B, distinguishes two types of EBV, EBV1 or 2. EBV1 is more prevalent than EBV2 in Western populations, however, EBV2 infection is prevalent in central Africa, in New Guinea, and among Alaskan Eskimos (Zimber et al., 1986). Coinfection with both EBV types is frequently detected in HIV infected patients and has also been detected in normal individuals (Walling et al., 1992). Recent studies indicate that multiple strains are detected in most individuals (Sitki-Green et al., 2003).

The EBNA3 genes are also encoded by divergent sequences that co-segregate with the EBNA2 type (Sample et al., 1990). Thus the sequence type of the EBNA2 and EBNA3 genes define Type 1 and Type 2 of EBV. All of the EBNA3 proteins interact with the cellular RBPJk protein and may modulate transactivation of the LMP1 promoter and other genes by the EBNA2 protein (Robertson et al., 1996).

Latent membrane protein 1

LMP1 is considered the EBV oncogene as it can transform rodent fibroblasts in vitro and is essential for B-cell transformation (Wang et al., 1985). Transgenic mice that express LMP1 in B cells have increased development of B cell lymphomas (Kulwhicit et al., 1998). LMP1 has profound effects on cellular gene expression and induces expression of multiple genes including adhesion molecules, anti-apoptotic functions, growth factors, and growth factor receptors (Wang et al., 1988). The biochemical properties of LMP1 that are in part responsible for these effects on cellular expression are its ability to activate the NFKB transcription factors and to interact with the cellular molecules that mediate signals from the tumor necrosis factor family of receptors (Mosialos et al., 1995). These molecules, entitled TRAFs, form heterotrimeric complexes that transduce signals that depending on the receptor may activate NFKB, induce cellular growth, or induce apoptosis. Thus the activation of the TRAF pathway is likely the key property of LMP1 that mediates its effects on cellular growth regulation.

The LMP1 protein has a short cytoplasmic amino terminus, a six membrane-spanning domain that is responsible for spontaneous aggregation in the plasma membrane, and signaling domains in the carboxyl terminus (Fennewald et al., 1984). The cytoplasmic carboxyl terminus contains two signaling domains, C-terminal activation region 1 (CTAR1) and CTAR2 (Huen et al., 1995). CTAR1 binds TRAFs 1, 2, 3, and 5 while CTAR2 binds the TNF receptor-associated death domain protein (TRADD) and its partner, the TNF receptor-interacting protein (RIP) (Devergne et al., 1996; Izumi et al., 1997). Signaling from these two domains leads to NF-κB activation as well as c-Jun N-terminal kinase (JNK) and p38 mitogen-activated protein kinase (MAPK) activation (Eliopoulos and Young, 1998; Eliopoulos et al., 1999). In reporter assays, LMP1 containing CTAR2 but deleted for CTAR1 (LMP1-CTAR2) induces greater NFκB activity, however electrophoretic mobility shift assays (EMSA) indicate that LMP1 deleted for CTAR2 but containing CTAR1 (LMP1-CTAR1) activates at least 3 heterodimeric forms of NFκB including p50/p50, p50/p52, and p52/p65 dimeric forms (Paine et al., 1995;

Miller et al., 1998). These forms are more abundant than the p50/p65 form that is the predominant form of NFκB activated by CTAR2. EBV containing LMP1-CTAR1 is also capable of transforming lymphocytes (Kaye et al., 1999).

Expression of LMP1 affects different cellular genes in lymphocytes and epithelial cells. In both cell types, NFKB transcription factors are activated although different forms of NFKB are activated in the two cell types. Activation of NFKB increases expression of B-cell activation markers in lymphoid cells, and expression of the A20 gene in both lymphoid and epithelial cells. In epithelial cells, LMP1 activates transcription of the epidermal growth factor receptor (EGFR), which is also detected at high levels in NPC (Miller et al., 1995b). Several studies have shown LMP1-CTAR1 has unique properties including the ability to induce expression of the EGFR, TRAF1, and CD54 (Miller et al., 1997; Devergne et al., 1998). The ability of CTAR1 to activate NFκB p50/p50 homodimers may be responsible for its unique ability to induce EGFR expression. Chromatin precipitation assays of the EGFR promoter in NPC have detected 50/p50 homodimers in a complex with bcl3 (Thornburg et al., 2003). It is presently unknown if EBV infection affects bcl3 activity or if the activation of bcl3 is a unique event in NPC.

Latent membrane protein 2 (LMP2)

The LMP2 proteins, LMP2A and LMP2B, are expressed in transformed lymphocytes and in NPC and HL (Young et al., 1991; Busson et al., 1992). The LMP2 gene contains exons located at both ends of the linear EBV genome and can be only transcribed across the fused termini of the episomal form or in some rare integrated events (Laux et al., 1988; Sample et al., 1989). Two distinct forms of mRNA encodes the 54 kd and 40 kd LMP2A and 2B proteins. The 2.3 kb and 2.0 kb RNAs have different promoters and the two RNAs each have a unique first exon and share exons 2 to 9 (Sample et al., 1989). The first exon of LMP2A (exon 1A) encodes the hydrophilic N-terminus whereas the first exon of the B form (exon 1B) is non-coding.

Genetic studies have revealed that LMP2A and B are not required for EBV dependent-transformation of B-cells, however, LMP2A is an important factor in maintaining EBV in a non-replicative state (Longnecker and Miller, 1990). This is accomplished by its ability to alter signaling from the B-cell receptor (BCR), to keep the infected lymphocytes in a non-activated state and maintain a latent infection in B-cells. LMP2 is an integral membrane protein with 12 transmembrane spanning regions. The amino terminal domain that is unique to LMP2A is cytoplasmic and contains multiple potential protein recognition sequences and signaling domains. The motifs include an immunoreceptor tyrosine-based activation motif (ITAM) with two spaced tyrosine residues. This motif is recognized by the Lyn/Syk kinases to transduce BCR signaling (Miller et al., 1995a). LMP2 also contains a PY motif that interacts with the NEDD4 family of ubiquitin ligases (Longnecker et al., 2000; Ikeda et al., 2001). LMP2 apparently sequesters the lyn kinase within lipid rich rafts and promotes its degradation thus blocking BCR signaling and B-cell activation (Dykstra et al., 2001).

Studies in transgenic mice have revealed that LMP2 also provides a cell survival signal (Caldwell et al., 1998). A recent study, using microarray analysis, revealed that LMP2 interferes with expression of specific transcription factors that regulate B-cell development resulting in enhancement of cellular survival (Portis and Longnecker, 2003). In studies in the HaCat epithelial cell line, LMP2 induced growth in soft agar and inhibited differentiation through activation of PI3 kinase and the Akt kinase (Scholle et al., 2000). LMP2 also activates Akt in lymphocytes (Swart et al., 2000). One target of the activated Akt in epithelial cells is GSK3β, an important component in the Wnt/β-catenin signaling pathway. GSK3β exists in a cytoplasmic complex with APC and Axin and it is within this complex that GSK3β phosphorylates β-catenin leading to ubiquitination and degradation of β-catenin by the proteosome complex. GSK3β is inactivated by phosphorylation by Akt (Chen et al., 2000; Cross et al., 1995). Therefore Akt activation may inhibit phosphorylation of β-catenin resulting in its stabilization. In epithelial cells expression of LMP2 greatly increases the levels of β-catenin and also induces its nuclear translocation (Morrison et al., 2003). This property requires activation of Akt and phosphorylation of GSK3. Activation of β-catenin occurs frequently in the development of carcinoma frequently through genetic mutations and it is likely that activation of this pathway is an important factor in EBV effects on epithelial cell growth.

The powerful effects of LMP2 on epithelial cell growth are also suggested by a recent study that revealed that EBV infected epithelial cell clones rapidly emerged from primary infected cultures (Moody et al., 2003). This growth advantage was linked to those clones that had fewer numbers of TR, a property that resulted in increased expression of LMP2.

EBV-encoded RNAs (EBER)

In EBV infected cells, two small non-polyadenylated RNA molecules designated EBER 1 and EBER 2 are transcribed by RNA polymerase III (Lerner et al., 1981). These 170 bp RNAs are encoded by adjacent sequences that have considerable homology. The EBERs exist as ribonucleoprotein complexes and are the most abundantly expressed viral transcript with 10^5 or 10^6 copies per infected cell (Howe and Steitz, 1986). Genetic studies indicate that EBER expression is not essential for lymphocyte transformation and their function remains obscure (Swaminathan et al., 1991). The Akata BL cell line is unique in that it can be cured of EBV infection. The loss of EBV results in the loss of the ability of Akata cells to form tumors in nude mice (Komano et al., 1998). Expression of EBERS partially revert this loss, potentially through effects on bcl2 (Komano et al., 1999). Similar studies of an EBV infected gastric epithelial cell line have shown that the EBERS induce altered growth properties through induction of expression of IGF1 (Iwakiri et al., 2003).

The extraordinary abundance and stability of the EBER ribonucleoprotein complexes in embedded sections makes in situ detection of EBER expression a useful diagnostic tool to identify EBV-associated diseases (Ambinder and Mann, 1994). However, the EBERs are not expressed at all times in all cells and are not expressed in all examples of EBV infection (Gilligan et al., 1990a; Pathmanathan et al., 1995a). Thus the absence of EBER expression does not necessarily indicate that the lesion does not contain EBV (Niedobitek et al., 1991a,b). The EBERs are not expressed in the differentiated form of NPC or in oral hairy leukoplakia (HLP), a site of EBV replication that contains viral particles, replicative gene products, and linear viral DNA (Gilligan et al., 1990a). The lack of EBER expression in HLP revealed that EBERs were not required for viral replication and indicated that the detection of EBER expression denotes latent EBV infection.

BamHI A transcripts (BARTS)

The BamH A RNAs were initially identified by cDNA cloning of EBV RNAS expressed in NPC (Gilligan et al., 1990b; Hitt et al., 1989). These RNAs are transcribed rightward through the BamHI A fragments (BARts) and are antisense to multiple replicative functions. At least three mRNAs are abundantly expressed in NPC and consistently detected on Northern blots, while in lymphoid cell lines, these RNAs are only detectable by PCR amplification of cDNAs (RT-PCR) (Gilligan et al., 1990b; Brooks et al., 1993; Sadler and Raab-Traub, 1995b).

In NPC the RNAs are also readily detectable by in situ hybridizations and are transcribed in all cells (Gilligan et al., 1990b). The cDNA clones contain distinct exons and patterns of alternate splicing that produce previously unidentified open reading frames (ORFs) (Sadler and Raab-Traub, 1995b). These cDNAs have been detected by RT-PCR in NPC, BL, parotid carcinoma, peripheral blood lymphocytes, and LCL samples. At the 3' end of all of the mRNAs is an ORF that would encode a 174 amino acid (aa) protein, *BamHI A rightward frame 0* or BARF0. This is an unusual ORF with the translational stop codon embedded in the polyadenylation signal (Sadler and Raab-Traub, 1995b).

An alternatively spliced cDNA, RK-BARF0, was identified that extended the BARFO ORF from 174 to 279 codons and would encode a protein of approximately 30 kDa. This splice was detected in the least abundant mRNA. The amino terminus of RK-BARF0 protein contains a highly hydrophobic region that resembles an endoplasmic reticulum targeting signal peptide sequence. In yeast two hybrid studies, RK-BARF0 and BARF0 interacted with the extracellular domain of Notch 3 and Notch 4 (Kusano and Raab-Traub, 2001).

Notch defines a family of transmembrane receptor proteins found in a variety of organisms including mammals. Notch is synthesized in the endoplasmic reticulum (ER), and further processed in the trans-Golgi network (TGN) to produce two fragments which are then linked through disulfide bonds (Blaumueller et al., 1997). After ligand binding, Notch is proteolytically cleaved releaving the carboxy terminal domains. This activated intracellular form of Notch is then thought to activate effector molecules, such as the DNA binding protein, RBP-Jk (Fortini, 1994). Activated Notch and RBP-Jk activate expression of several mammalian genes including erbB2a and NF-κB2 and as previously described, the EBNA2 and EBNA3 proteins interact with RBP-Jk to activate expression of LMP1 (Henkel et al., 1994; Grossman et al., 1994). The direct interaction of RK-BARF0 with Notch induces the proteosomal degradation of Notch. Although the RK-BARF0 protein has not yet been detected, EBV infected cells have very low levels of Notch suggesting that RK-BARF0 may be expressed during EBV infection.

The cDNA representing the most abundant RNA contains the RB2 or A73 ORF (Sadler and Raab-Traub, 1995b). The RB2 ORF is formed from 4 exons and has been shown to interact with the receptor for activated kinases (RACK1) (Smith et al., 2000). The RK103 ORF, also called RPMS1, encodes a potential protein that also interacts with RBP-Jk (Sadler and Raab-Traub, 1995b; Smith et al., 2000). The specific splice that is unique to RPMS1 is also readily detected in peripheral blood lymphocytes (Chen et al., 1999b). Although the protein products for these novel ORFs have not been identified, the intriguing properties of the possible proteins suggests that these complex RNAs may encode additional proteins expressed in latent infection in epithelial cells or in B-lymphocytes in vivo.

Malignancies associated with EBV

The malignancies associated with EBV are distinct cancers that develop in the setting of immunosuppression, occur with endemic patterns of incidence, or are a discrete subset of more common cancers. The most consistent and significant associations include post-transplant lymphoma, African Burkitt's lymphoma, Hodgkin's disease, and nasopharyngeal carcinoma (Raab-Traub, 1996).

Post-transplant lymphoproliferative disease

The ability of EBV to cause cancer is most clearly indicated by the development of B-cell lymphoproliferations in patients who are deficient in T-cell mediated immunity following bone marrow or solid organ transplantation. The majority of cases of post-transplant lymphoma (PTL) are EBV-positive. These proliferations are initially polyclonal but frequently progress to oligoclonal or monoclonal lymphoma and clonal or bi-clonal EBV is readily detected (Fig. 55.2). Depending on the degree or regimen for immunosuppression, PTL develops in 5–15% of cardiac transplants, 10% of heart-lung transplants, in 1 to 3% of renal transplants, and approximately 1 to 2% of bone marrow transplants.

EBV infection in post-transplant lymphoma is an example of Type 3 latency that includes expression of the major CTL targets, the EBNA2 and EBNA3 proteins (Young *et al.*, 1989). In some cases, the disease may regress after reduction in immunosuppressive therapy indicating that the cells are still susceptible to EBV-specific cytotoxic T-cells. Adoptive or prophylactic immunotherapy has also been successful (Rooney *et al.*, 1997). However, there is also variability in EBV gene expression and in the monoclonal, more monomorphic post-transplant lymphomas there may be more restricted Type 1 or 2 latency patterns of viral expression. A recent report described an intriguing case of lymphoma that did not respond to CTL infusion. Subsequent analysis revealed that the EBV strain in the tumor contained a deletion in EBNA3B and that the CTL preparation that had been expanded ex vivo and administered was predominantly directed against EBNA3B (Gottschalk *et al.*, 2001). This provided the first evidence of an EBV escape mutant that evaded immune control due to the deletion of a specific protein. EBNA3B has been shown to not be essential for B-cell immortalization in vitro and its loss would provide an immunoselective advantage in vivo (Tomkinson *et al.*, 1993).

Burkitt's lymphoma

EBV was originally detected in cell lines established from the unusual childhood malignancy, Burkitt's lymphoma (BL) (Epstein *et al.*, 1964). Burkitt's lymphoma was first recognized by a British surgeon working in the colonial office in East Africa (Burkitt, 1962b). He described the clinical and epidemiologic features of this tumor and discovered that the tumor occurred with high incidence in an endemic geographic region that was coincident with the endemic malarial belt of Central and East Africa. Fresh tumor biopsies were sent to Dr. Anthony Epstein in London where he succeeded in establishing cell lines. In some lines, herpesvirus particles were detected by electron microscopy. This virus was subsequently shown to be distinct from other known human herpesviruses and subsequent seroepidemiologic studies revealed that EBV infection was widespread in all populations with the majority of adults having antibodies to the virus (Henle and Henle, 1974).

The early seroepidemiologic studies provided additional evidence that EBV was associated with the cancer. In endemic areas, children become infected with EBV during the first two years of life and endemic BL patients had significantly elevated antibody titers to viral antigens, including the viral capsid antigen (VCA) and early replicative functions (early antigen, EA) (Henle *et al.*, 1971). Prospective epidemiologic studies in Uganda indicated that high EBV VCA antibodies preceded the development of the tumor by months or years.

Characteristics of EBV Infection in BL

Although patients with BL have elevated titers to replicative antigens, EBV gene expression in BL is tightly latent and its expression is very restricted (Rickinson, 2001). Most cells express only EBNA1 and the EBERs. This restricted state of expression is only found in BL and was subsequently termed Type 1 latency. The expression of EBNA1 in the absence of the transcriptional transactivator EBNA2 and EBNA3 proteins reflects the use of an alternate promoter for EBNA1 (Sample *et al.*, 1991). This promoter in the BamHI Q fragment, Qp, is regulated by both IRF and STAT transcription factors (Sample *et al.*, 1992; Chen *et al.*, 1999a). The BARTs have also been detected in BL sample by RT-PCR. Recent studies have indicated that expression in BL may be somewhat heterogeneous with some cells expressing LMP1 and the EBNA proteins that are characteristic of Type 3 latency (Niedobitek *et al.*, 1995). EBV expression in BL also changes in vitro and most BL cell lines reactivate into Type 3 latency with expression of the additional EBNAs and the LMPs. In vitro, this change in expression results in an altered growth pattern with rapid growth of clumped cells and elevated expression of lymphocyte activation molecules, adhesion molecules, and HLA antigens (Rowe *et al.*, 1987).

All of the tumors from the endemic areas contain EBV in all of the malignant cells and each tumor contains a clonal form of the EBV episome indicating that the tumor developed from a single EBV-infected cell (Raab-Traub and Flynn, 1986) (Fig. 55.2).

Contributing factors

The detection of consistent chromosomal rearrangements in many human cancers suggested that these would cause genetic changes that could alter cellular gene's expression or function. BL was one of the first cancers to be shown to have a characteristic chromosomal translocation and these translocations were eventually shown to involve chromosomal rearrangments of the c-myc oncogene with the loci that encode the immunoglobulin heavy and light chains (Dalla-Favera et al., 1982; Magrath, 1990). This rearrangement induced the aberrant activation of the c-myc oncogene, a critical step in the control of cellular proliferation.

Rare childhood lymphomas in Western countries were subsequently shown to resemble Burkitt's lymphoma histologically. These tumors occur 100-fold less frequently than the endemic form but also are marked by the characteristic translocations between c-myc and the immunoglobulin loci. It is intriguing that the sporadic and endemic forms of BL have different breakpoints with regard to c-myc (Pelicci et al., 1986). The endemic form has breakpoints many kb 5′ to c-myc while the breakpoint in the sporadic form usually occurs in the first exon or intron (Magrath, 1990). These differences in the translocation break point may reflect an effect of EBV in the development of the translocation.

Deregulated c-myc expression is found in all forms of BL suggesting that this is an essential step in the development of this lymphoma. As the translocations involve the immunoglobulin loci, it is possible that they occur during variable gene rearrangement or class switching. The cell surface markers, CD10 and CD77, which are characteristic of BL suggest that BL cells may represent a germinal center B-cell (Rickinson, 2001). Germinal centers are greatly expanded in chronic malarial infection and during HIV infection. The elevated titer to EBV replicative antigens that are characteristic of BL suggest that EBV reactivation and replication has occurred. The activation of viral replication and the expansion of germinal centers are likely contributing factors to the increased risk of development of BL in areas of endemic malaria.

AIDS-associated lymphoma

Lymphomas develop in approximately 3% of AIDS patients and the incidence of BL is greatly increased in HIV-infected patients (Ambinder, 2001). Although in HIV infection, many types of lymphoid malignancies may develop, BL tends to develop early in the course of AIDS progression. The tumors resemble classical BL histologically and also possess the characteristic translocations with the chromosomal breakpoints similar to those in the sporadic BL.

Other B-cell malignancies also occur at high incidence in AIDS and approximately 50% of these are EBV-associated. Central nervous system lymphoma is extremely rare in the general population but occurs in 0.5% of patients with AIDS. All of the CNS lymphomas are EBV positive (MacMahon et al., 1992). Possible genetic or environmental factors that contribute to the development of EBV-positive lymphoma or CNS lymphoma have not yet been identified although the effect of HIV infection on the cytokine network may influence lymphoma development. Both IL6 and IL10 are elevated during HIV infection and promote the growth of EBV-infected B cells (Stewart et al., 1994). In addition to the reduced immune control during HIV infection, abnormal synthesis of these cytokines could activate paracrine or autocrine pathways that influence the outgrowth of EBV-infected cells and promote lymphoma development.

Nasopharyngeal carcinoma

Nasopharyngeal carcinoma (NPC) is an epithelial tumor, that similarly to BL, is characterized by marked geographic and population differences in incidence (Raab-Traub, 2002). It develops with high incidence in southern China and southeast Asia where it may represent 20% of all cancer cases, occurring at a rate of $100/10^5$/year in some regions. The tumor also frequently develops in Eskimo populations and occurs with elevated incidence in Mediterranean Africa. The tumor occurs rarely in Caucasian population, however, unlike BL, all cases of NPC that develop in endemic or nonendemic regions contain EBV (Raab-Traub et al., 1987).

Early seroepidemiologic studies revealed that, similar to patients with BL, patients with NPC had elevated antibody titers to the replicative antigens, VCA and EA. However, NPC patients uniquely had elevated IgA antibodies to these antigens. Detection of IgA antibodies to EBV precedes the development of NPC by several years and the levels also correlate with tumor burden and recurrence (Henle and Henle, 1974). These data suggest that EBV reactivation and replication precede the development of NPC while the induction of IgA antibodies indicates that the replication is occurring at mucosal surfaces.

Subsequent studies revealed that viral DNA and the EBV nuclear antigen, EBNA, were detected in the malignant epithelial cells rather than in the abundant infiltrating lymphoid cells (Wolf et al., 1973). This was the first detection of EBV within epithelial cells.

The tumor presents with varying degrees of differentiation and has been classified by the World Health

Organization into three categories (Shanmugaratnam, 1978). Squamous cell carcinomas, WHO1 tumors, are highly differentiated with characteristic epithelial growth patterns and keratin filaments. Non-keratinizing WHO2 carcinomas retain epithelial cell shape and growth patterns. Undifferentiated carcinomas, WHO3, do not produce keratin and lack a distinctive growth pattern. In addition many tumors have mixed degrees of differentiation or may present as WHO3 at the primary site with increased differentiation in metastatic lymph nodes. The WHO2 and WHO3 tumors have elevated IgG and IgA titers to VCA and EA whereas the WHO1 tumors have EBV serologic profiles similar to control populations. This initially suggested that EBV was only associated with the WHO II and III types. However, subsequent studies have also consistently detected EBV in WHO1 tumors from the Orient (Pathmanathan et al., 1995a). However, in other studies, EBV was not detected in WHO1 NPC from some areas (Niedobitek et al., 1991a,b). The consistent detection of EBV in most NPC from both endemic and non-endemic areas suggests that EBV is an essential cofactor in the development of this tumor.

Characteristics of EBV infection in NPC

EBV infection in NPC is primarily latent with expression of replicative antigens in some cells. Identification of the EBV terminal restriction enzyme fragments in NPC revealed that the EBV genomes were homogeneous and clonal with faint ladder arrays representing linear DNA (Fig. 55.2(b)) (Raab-Traub and Flynn, 1986). This confirmed that EBV infection was predominantly latent and suggested that the tumor was also clonal. The detection of linear DNA also indicated that the tumor was likely the site of the antigenic stimulus for the elevated antibody responses to EBV replicative antigens.

Initial studies of viral expression in NPC revealed striking differences in comparison with EBV expression in transformed B cells. The sequences that were subsequently shown to encode EBNA2 and the EBNA3 proteins were not transcribed and there was abundant transcription from the BamHI A and EcoDhet fragments (Raab-Traub et al., 1983). This pattern of expression was subsequently classified Type 2 latency with expression of EBNA1 from the Qp promoter and transcription of LMP1 and LMP2 (Nonkwelo et al., 1996). Two distinct LMP1 mRNAs were identified in NPC and included the standard 2.8 kb mRNA transcribed from the LMP1 EDL1 promoter and a larger 3.7 kb mRNA that initiated within the TR (Gilligan et al., 1990b; Sadler and Raab-Traub, 1995a). This mRNA has been shown to be regulated by SP1 and STAT3 transcription factors (Sadler and Raab-Traub, 1995a; Chen et al., 2001). LMP1 has been suggested to activate STAT signaling and activated nuclear STAT was detected in NPC. This may indicate that LMP1 in NPC is auto-regulated and that perhaps constitutive STAT activation is a factor that leads to tumor development (Chen et al., 2003).

The abundant transcription from the Bam HI A fragment was further characterized and shown to encode a family of 3′ co-terminal, intricately spliced transcripts (BARTs) that contain multiple potential ORFs (Sadler and Raab-Traub, 1995b). The putative protein products of these ORFs have properties that could in part substitute for the EBNA proteins. RK103/RPMS1 interacts with a co-repressor of RBPJk and negatively affects Notch signaling (Zhang et al., 2001). RKBARF0 also increases LMP1 expression and induces Notch degradation (Kusano and Raab-Traub, 2001). Although Notch inhibits differentiation in some cell types, in epithelial cells Notch induces differentiation. The identification of multiple effects on the Notch pathway by the putative BamHI A proteins and the EBNA proteins suggests that EBV usurps this pathway in both lymphoid and epithelial cells.

EBV infection has been shown to be an early event in the development of NPC and has been identified in rare examples of high grade dysplasia and isolated carcinoma in situ (CIS). In an initial survey, the lesions were extremely rare (11/1798 or 0.6%) with coexistent nasopharyngeal intraepithelial neoplasia with invasive cancer in approximately 3% (58/1798). This extreme rarity of lesions without concomitant carcinoma and the development of invasive carcinoma within 1 year indicated a rapid progression of the initiated cell from dysplasia to carcinoma in situ and invasive cancer (Pathmanathan et al., 1995b). Thus the biologic behavior of NPC is quite distinct from that observed in the malignant progression of mammary carcinoma or cervical cancer where intraductal cancer of the breast or carcinoma in situ of the cervix may persist for years. All cells in examples of CIS expressed EBERs and LMP1 revealing that the lesions were homogeneously infected. Clonal EBV episomes were detected without detectable linear forms of the genome indicating that the neoplasias were a predominantly latent infection. The presence of a single clonal form of EBV implies that the hyperplasia or dysplasia represents a focus of EBV-induced cellular proliferation (Pathmanathan et al., 1995b). One extensive study in high-risk Chinese populations revealed that in early dysplasia EBV was present in a subset of cells while EBV infection in high grade dysplasia was homogeneous and uniform. These studies suggest that an early genetic change precedes EBV infection and induces dyplastic growth and that the EBV infected cells apparently overtake the population and the lesion rapidly progress to CIS (Yeung et al., 1993). A genetic factor may also influence the ability of EBV to establish a latent infection in epithelial cells rather than replicate as is believed to occur in normal oropharyngeal cells (Fig. 55.1).

During primary infection and during reactivated infection, oropharyngeal epithelial cells with evidence of viral replication have been detected and are thought to be the source for viral shedding (Sixbey et al., 1984). The high IgA titers to EBV replicative antigens that precede the development of NPC patients to VCA likely reflect increased viral replication and antigenic stimulation. The elevated IgA titers may actually contribute to the development of NPC by enhancing epithelial infection as it has been shown that secretory IgA facilitates entry into epithelial cells (Gan et al., 1997). In the development of NPC, increased viral replication, perhaps at lymphoid/mucosal epithelial interfaces, increases the likelihood of establishing a latent, transforming infection of an epithelial cell that may have already had an initiating genetic change. This establishment of latent infection and expression of critical viral transforming functions in an epithelial cell in combination with genetic changes that may facilitate latent infection or are synergistic with EBV transforming proteins are likely to be critical events that lead to the development of NPC. This process could be influenced by the genetic or environmental factors (Fig. 55.1). However, the viral transforming functions are likely essential to the malignant outgrowth.

Contributing factors

The incidence of NPC is low in Western populations where it is only 0.25% of all cancers occurring with a rate of $0.1/10^5$ per yr. However in contrast to the relationship of EBV to Burkitt's lymphoma, EBV is consistently detected in NPC regardless of geographic distribution or the racial background (Yu and Yuan, 2002). The consistent association with a ubiquitous herpesvirus and the remarkable patterns of incidence suggests that other genetic or environmental factors contribute to tumor development.

Comparisons of EBV infection among Indians and Chinese living in Singapore revealed that both populations were infected with EBV early in life, usually between the ages of 6 to 9 (Shanmugaratnam, 1970). Although the two ethnic groups were living in the same general area of Singapore, the NPC incidence was only high in the Chinese population. Elevated incidence is retained by second generation Chinese in other nonendemic regions but gradually decreases with subsequent generations (Buell, 1974). This continued elevated incidence suggested that environmental contaminants were not likely to be a cofactor but rather that genetic or cultural and dietary differences contributed to the development of this disease. One dietary component that has been suggested is exposure to salted fish at an early age (Ho, 1976; Yu et al., 1986). Tumor promoting compounds have also been identified in food products in other populations with elevated incidence (Poirier et al., 1989).

Extensive surveys for activated oncogenes or tumor suppressor loss did not reveal characteristic translocations, mutations in p53 or Rb alterations, or activating ras mutations (Effert et al., 1992; Sun et al., 1995, 1993). This suggests that viral genes affect these pathways, directly or indirectly, such that there is no selection for mutation in these genes (Fries et al., 1996). However, additional genetic changes could develop during tumor growth and contribute to tumor progression and metastasis.

To identify potential tumor suppressor genes, screening of NPC samples has detected specific loss of of DNA sequences indicated by loss of heterozygosity in PCR screenings. This approach has shown that the p16 cyclin dependent kinase inhibitor at 9p21 and the RASSF1a gene at 3p14 are frequently lost in NPC samples (Lo, 2002).

Studies in vitro have shown that reintroduction of the RASSF1a gene into an NPC cell line inhibited growth (Lo, and Huang 2002). This finding suggests that inactivation of this ras isoform is an important contributor to NPC development. Other studies have shown that p16 is not expressed in NPC due to specific methylation of the promoter. In vitro studies have shown that LMP1 expression induces methylation of the p16 promoter and that LMP1 also induces cytoplasmic translocation of the ets transcription factor that regulates p16 promoter activity (Ohtani et al., 2003). The loss of p16 may be highly synergistic with LMP1 expression in the induction of NPC.

Hodgkin's lymphoma

Hodgkin's lymphoma (HL) is a common malignant lymphoma characterized by the loss of lymph node architecture with the majority of infiltrating cells of a nonmalignant phenotype. The malignant cells are the unusual Hodgkin and Reed–Sternberg (RS) cells that constitute about 2% of the tumor mass (Ambinder et al., 1999). Dependent on the ratio of RS cells and the type of infiltrate, HL is histologically distinguished as lymphocyte-predominant, nodular sclerosing, mixed cellularity, or lymphocyte depleted. EBV is always found in the lymphocyte depleted form, approximately 70% of mixed cellularity, 10%–40% of nodular sclerosing and never in lymphocyte enriched (Chapman and Rickinson, 1998).

The disease occurs world-wide but has higher incidence in higher socio-economic groups in Western populations where it occurs with two peaks at ages 25 to 30 or again later than age 45. It was observed years ago that the profile of the early age onset group was similar to patients who developed infectious mononucleosis, the pathologic manifestation occurring in post-adolescent primary EBV infection. A history of IM was noted to be associated with a 2–4 fold increased risk for HL. Retrospective analyses of the serum repository at Yale revealed that elevated EBV titers preceded the development of HL by 2–3 years (Mueller et al., 1989).

The key finding revealing an etiologic association of EBV with HL was the detection of the viral genome and virally encoded proteins in the RS cells (Weiss et al., 1989a,b). Again, the analysis of the EBV genome revealed that HL had clonal EBV episomes, indicating that HL develops from an EBV-infected cell (Fig. 55.2(b)). Monoclonality has also been revealed by immunoglobulin gene rearrangements and in some cases, T-cell receptor rearrangements. The tumors predominantly have expression of B cell markers although T-cell receptor rearrangement has been detected in some cases (Marafioti et al., 2000).

Transcriptional studies have shown that HL has expression of EBNA1, LMP1, LMP2 and the EBERS, indicative of Type 2 latency (Deacon et al., 1993). Several of the genes known to be activated by LMP1 are expressed in HL and activated NFκB has been found in the RS cells (Hinz et al., 2002). The same forms of activated NFκB have been detected in EBV negative RS cells (Knecht et al., 1999). In the EBV negative examples of HL, mutations have been described within the IκB repressor of NFκB (Emmerich et al., 2003). This finding suggests that activation of NFκB is likely an important factor in the development of HD and that it occurs either via LMP1 expression or by other mechanisms.

Although HL frequently responds well to treatment, new methods of targeting EBV infection have been attempted (Bollard et al., 2004). CTL therapy has had some success and new trials are testing inhibitors of NFκB.

T-cell lymphoma

Although long believed to be B-cell trophic, EBV has been detected in an occasional T-cell lymphoma. A particular type of T-cell lymphoma that usually presents in the nasal cavity, also referred to as midline granuloma, is a common tumor in southeast Asians. The first link to EBV was presented in five Japanese cases, all of which were EBV-positive (Harabuchi et al., 1996). The tumors had various T or NK cell markers suggesting EBV infection of a peculiar undifferentiated cell type.

Peripheral T-cell lymphomas that are EBV-positive have also been described in Taiwanese and Japanese populations. In some cases, EBV was only detected in some cells suggesting that the virus infected the tumor secondarily (Kanegane et al., 1999). However, the proportion of EBV infected cells seems to increase over time with emergence of a clonal EBV-infected population indicating that the virally infected cells have some growth advantage and that the fastest growing clone will eventually predominate.

Rare carcinomas

Other undifferentiated carcinomas that develop in other tissues are also associated with EBV. Clonal EBV episomes have been detected in all samples examined of undifferentiated carcinoma of the parotid gland (Raab-Traub et al., 1991). These studies revealed that carcinoma of the parotid gland is also a clonal proliferation of non-permissively infected epithelial cells. Viral shedding is believed to occur in epithelial cells lining the parotid gland without apparent pathology. The establishment of a latent transforming infection in these cells is apparently a rare occurrence that contributes to the development of this tumor. Undifferentiated carcinoma of the parotid gland is an extremely rare cancer that has been most often detected in Alaskan Inuit populations who also have a high incidence of NPC (Lanier et al., 1991).

EBV infection has also been detected in undifferentiated gastric carcinoma, a rare tumor in both Oriental and Caucasian populations (Shibata et al., 1991). These findings indicate that EBV may gain access to epithelial cells outside the naso/oropharynx and that in some instances when this occurs, it leads to the development of carcinoma.

Contributing factors

Genetic factors

Tumor suppressor inactivation

The development of cancer involves multiple oncogenic events and several possibly contributing genetic components have been identified in EBV associated cancers. Loss of heterozygosity (LOH) is a highly informative approach for detecting allelic deletion of potential tumor suppressor functions. This approach has been used most successfully in solid tumors such as NPC. These studies have determined that the highest frequencies of allelic loss occurred on chromosome 3p and 9p (Huang et al., 1991, 1994; Lo and Huang, 2002). Intensive efforts have localized the region on 3p to 3p21.3. Functional evidence of tumor suppressor function within this region have shown that chromosomal transfer into an NPC cell line abrogated growth. The target gene has been demonstrated to be an allelic form of

RASSF1A, a newly discovered gene that contains a ras association domain (Cheng et al., 1998). Thus RASSF1A may modulate ras function.

The site of LOH at 9p21 spans the cyclin-dependent kinase inhibitors (cdki) p15INK4B and p16INK4A and the negative regulator of p53, p14ARF. Loss of p16 has been shown in NPC samples and transfer of p16 induced growth arrest in the NPC cell line HK1 (Lo et al., 1995). Homozygous deletion and promoter methylation of p14 ARF has also been demonstrated in many NPC tumors. The loss of this locus has been shown to occur early in dysplastic nasopharyngeal cells (Lo and Huang, 2002). The loss of this locus in combination with EBV infection likely contributes to the rapid development of invasive NPC.

Similarly, the promoters for p15 and p16 have been shown to be methylated in Hodgkin's lymphoma suggesting that loss of cdki function is also a contributing factor in EBV-associated lymphoid diseases (Garcia et al., 2003).

EBV strain variation

The elevated incidence of EBV-associated malignancies in specific populations suggests that one possibility for these differences in disease incidence may be difference in prevalence of EBV variants. These strains could possess distinct biologic properties or be less immunogenic. The prevalence of specific strains within a population could contribute to these differences in disease incidence. EBV types 1 and 2 are distinguished by sequence changes in the EBV nuclear antigens 2 and 3 (EBNA 2 and 3) and several variants of EBV have been identified by polymorphisms in the viral genome (Abdel-Hamid et al., 1992; Khanim et al., 1996; Lung et al., 1990). Strain specific changes have also been identified in EBNA1, BZLF1, and LMP1 (Miller et al., 1994; Bhatia et al., 1996; Packham et al., 1993; Edwards et al., 1999). The incidence of BL is high in Papua New Guinea with a frequent occurrence of HLA A11. Multiple A11-restricted epitopes have been identified in EBNA3 and analysis of the EBNA3 sequence in the virus prevalent in this area revealed that it contained changes within key positions in the A11 restricted epitopes. These changes and decreased immune recognition may contribute to the prevalence of a given strain within a population and perhaps to a higher viral burden in A11 individuals which might be possible etiologic factor in the development of BL in this region.

Many of these studies have focused on detecting strains possibly unique to NPC. Analyses of strain variation based on restriction enzyme polymorphisms identified a predominant strain in NPC from Southern China (Lung et al., 1990). Various polymorphisms within restriction sites were identified including a loss of an Xho1 restriction enzyme site within the LMP1 gene (Hu et al., 1991). This polymorphism was also present in all NPC from Alaska and in some of the NPC samples from Caucasian Americans but not in samples of NPC from Mediterranean Europe and Africa (Abdel-Hamid et al., 1992).

Further studies of sequence variation within LMP1 revealed that consistent sequence variation distinguished EBV strains and seven phylogenetically distinct strains of LMP1 have been described that have signature changes in the coding sequence (Edwards et al., 1999). Individual isolates differ by these specific base pair (bp) changes, the presence or absence of a 30 bp deletion, the number of 33bp repeats, and a 15 bp insertion within one of the repeats. Strains with or without the deletion have been detected in approximately equal proportions in the various EBV-associated diseases suggesting that all strains can be pathogenic (Miller et al., 1994; Khanim et al., 1996). However, several studies have suggested that LMP1 with the deletion has enhanced transforming potential in vitro and may be present in more aggressive disease forms (Knecht et al., 1992). One study indicated that the enhanced transforming ability of the Chinese strain in BalbC 3T3 cells was transferred with the carboxy terminus that included the 10 aa acid deletion. Deletion of the 10 aa in the B95 LMP1 resulted in the ability to induce transformation and tumorgenicity while insertion of the 10 aa into the Chinese strain eliminated transformation and tumorigenicity (Li et al., 1996).

Heteroduplex tracking assays (HTA) have been useful for distinguishing viral variants and following HIV strain evolution (Nelson et al., 2000). To identify viral variants within a tissue sample, a specific DNA sequence is amplified from the sample, denatured, and reannealed to a single stranded probe of that region (Fig. 55.3(a)). Homoduplexes migrate faster during agarose electrophoresis while the migration of mismatched heteroduplexes is impaired (Fig. 55.3(b)). In the HTA developed for LMP1, the amplified region spans the 30bp deletion (Sitki-Green et al., 2002). Strains are distinguished using a probe that contains the 30bp from the China2 strain (Ch2) and a probe of the same region that spans the deletion (Med-). Probes from two of the strains have been utilized to clearly identify each variant of the LMP1 types, China 1 (Ch1), Mediterranean with the deletion (Med+), Mediterranean without the deletion (Med-), North Carolina (NC) Alaskan (Al), and the prototype, B95. Each form of LMP1 consistently migrates to the same position when hybridized with each probe (Fig. 55.3(b) & 55.3(c)).

Using this approach, HTA revealed that infection with multiple strains of EBV is a frequent occurrence in patients with HIV and also in healthy, asymptomatic carriers

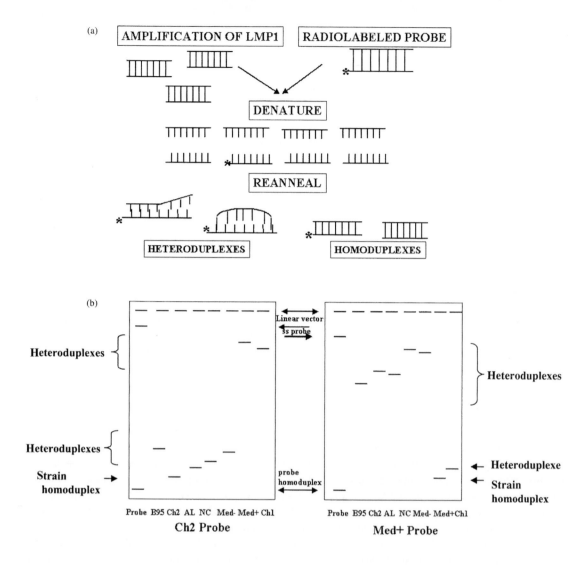

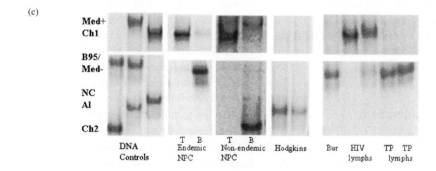

Fig. 55.3. Heteroduplex tracking assay to identify EBV LMP1 variants. (a) HTA analysis is based on the principal that 100% homologous DNA molecules, homoduplexes, will migrate according to size on a polyacrylamide gel, while, heteroduplexes will migrate more slowly because of malformations in the DNA helix corresponding to regions of mismatch. The greater the mismatch of two sequences, the slower the migration of the heteroduplex through a gel matrix. A specific region of LMP1 harboring multiple sequence changes is amplified from each sample, denatured, and hybridized to a single-stranded labeled probe. (b) Diagram of HTA using two probes to form heteroduplexes with each PCR amplified strain that are subjected to electrophoresis through a non-denaturing gel. Distinct migration patterns of heteroduplexes are produced for each strain. (c) HTA analysis reveals single variants in NPC, HD, Burkitt lymphoma (Bur), and HIV and post-transplant (TP) lymphoma samples.

(Sitki-Green et al., 2003). The relative abundance of the strains changes over time with different strains prevalent in the oral cavity than in the peripheral blood at a particular time. HTA analysis of tumor samples has revealed that EBV-associated tumors contain a single strain of EBV while blood and saliva samples usually contain multiple strains of EBV (Fig. 55.3(c)). This provides another perspective of EBV infection in tumors and supports the concept of a homogeneous, clonal infection.

Comparison of the strain prevalence in NPC tumor samples with matching blood samples revealed that the LMP1 variant China1 was almost always in the tumor while other EBV LMP1 variants were present in the blood (Fig. 55.3(c)) (Edwards et al., 2004). In many cases the strain within tumor tissue had changes in the known and computer-predicted HLA restricted epitopes of the HLA type of the patient. Patients with NPC are frequently HLA A2 and A24 and the China 1 strain have been shown to be changed at the strongest A2 epitope. These amino acid substitutions at key positions in these LMP1 epitopes may result in a reduced CTL response that enables immune escape of latently infected cells that express the China 1 LMP1.

The elevated incidence of NPC and BL in restricted populations such as Alaskan Eskimos and Cantonese from Southeastern China may reflect a predominance of a specific MHC type. Higher incidence of a specific MHC haplotype in these populations could have selected for viruses with mutations in putative CTL recognition sequences in LMP-1. The prevalence of such a type in these populations may allow expression of LMP-1 in infected cells to go undetected. Thus a combination of a specific EBV strain in a patient with a particular HLA type could be a contributing factor to tumor development due to decreased immune recognition of a specific LMP1 or perhaps other proteins expressed in the tumor such as LMP2 or the putative BamHI A proteins.

Summary and future considerations

EBV-targeted therapy

The strong association of EBV with major human malignancies provides an opportunity to specifically target EBV or pathways activated by EBV to treat these cancers. A potential vaccine could either protect against infection or possibly eliminate specific pathologic consequences. To prevent viral infection, it would be necessary to completely neutralize EBV at mucosal surfaces through efficient induction of IgA antibodies. This could theoretically be accomplished with a transformation defective EBV that would replicate at mucosal surfaces. Several studies indicate that there are naturally occurring EBV strains that lack the EBNA2 gene and are transformation negative (Sixbey et al., 1991). A genetically engineered strain of EBV that lacked essential transforming proteins yet replicated efficiently at mucosal surfaces might be useful as an attenuated vaccine.

An alternative approach would be a subunit vaccine. The viral glycoprotein gp350, is the most abundant viral glycoprotein and is essential for viral binding and infection. The protective ability of gp350 antibodies has been tested in cotton top marmosets challenged with a lymphoma inducing growth (Finerty et al., 1992). Some protection was provided that seemed to be cell mediated rather than antibody mediated (Wilson et al., 1996). A gp350/vaccinia recombinant was also tested in China in seronegative children. After 1 year, all ten of the control group had seroconverted and had antibodies to VCA, indicating wild-type EBV infection in comparison with the test group where only three had seroconverted (Gu et al., 1995).

A novel approach has developed synthetic peptides representing the predominant CTL epitopes presented by prevalent class I molecules. Expression of a cocktail of EBV epitopes in vaccinia virus indicated that all of the epitopes were processed correctly for the individual HLA classes and that the virus could induce the correct EBV epitope-specific CTLs in vitro (Moss et al., 1996). Many EBV CTL epitopes have been identified and it is possible that an appropriate cocktail could be selected to protect the majority of individuals. It may also be possible to enhance a specific CTL response. In NPC and Hodgkins's disease, the viral proteins which induce the immunodominant CTL response are not expressed. It is possible that the viral expression could be manipulated perhaps through the use of demethylating agents such as azacytidine to induce expression of the viral proteins that would make the cells susceptible to CTL killing (Robertson, 2000). Alternatively, the CTL response to weaker immunogens such as LMP1 or LMP2 could theoretically be enhanced which may enable immune recognition and control of the tumor. Immunotherapy and other approaches to alter EBV expression or induce viral replication are reviewed in other chapters.

The EBV associated cancers are classic examples of the multistep nature of cancer development. The malignancies develop as a combination of a common virus with potent transforming ability, possible immune impairment, increased genetic susceptibility, in part due to HLA type, and genetic changes possibly due to environmental exposure. Potential steps in the pathway to cancer would be some event or exposure that increases the amount of virally infected cells. This might be an increase in viral replication in combination with an expanded population of a specific cell type. Thus in the development of BL or HIV lymphomas, an expansion of germinal center B-cells due to malaria or HIV and their infection by EBV is likely a contributing early event. Important interactions between the intracellular environment and the virus next occur. These include factors that contribute to establishment of a latent, transforming infection rather than a permissive viral replicative infection and the ability to express LMP1 and LMP2 without expression of the CTL targets, EBNA2 and EBNA3. Important contributing factors include activation of STATs, expression of IL6, and lack of p16 expression. The ability of the growing LMP1-expressing cells to evade immune recognition is critical at this point and specific strains of EBV in certain HLA backgrounds would be able to persist. The EBV transforming proteins would take over multiple cellular signal transduction pathways through direct effects and indirect effects on expression of cellular genes. Multiple other genetic changes may occur during this process and have important effects on cell growth. However, the potent effects of EBV on cell gene expression suggest that the latently infected cells would be rapidly growing and quickly invasive. Importantly, this scenario suggests that EBV and expression of viral proteins are essential to the cancer process, to both initiation and progression. The dependence of tumor growth on viral proteins and activation of specific signaling pathways enables targeting of EBV-associated tumors through immunotherapy and specific inhibitors of activated pathways.

REFERENCES

Abdel-Hamid, M., Chen, J. J., Constantine, N. *et al.* (1992). EBV strain variation: geographical distribution and relation to disease state. *Virol.*, **190**, 168–175.

Adams, A. and Lindahl, T. (1975). Intracellular forms of Epstein–Barr virus DNA in Raji cells. *IARC Sci. Publ.*, **11**, 125–132.

Ambinder, R. F., (2001). Epstein–Barr virus associated lymphoproliferations in the AIDS setting. *Eur. J. Cancer*, **37**, 1209–1216.

Ambinder, R. F. and Mann, R. B. (1994). Epstein–Barr-encoded RNA in situ hybridization: diagnostic applications. *Hum. Pathol.*, **25**, 602–605.

Ambinder, R. F., Lemas, M. V., Moore, S. *et al.* (1999). Epstein–Barr virus and lymphoma. *Cancer Treat Res.*, **99**, 27–45.

Babcock, G. J., Hochberg, D., and Thorley-Lawson, A. D., (2000a). The expression pattern of Epstein–Barr virus latent genes in vivo is dependent upon the differentiation stage of the infected B cell. *Immunity*, **13**, 497–506.

Babcock, G. J. and Thorley-Lawson, D. A. (2000b). Tonsillar memory B cells, latently infected with Epstein–Barr virus, express the restricted pattern of latent genes previously found only in Epstein–Barr virus-associated tumors. *Proc. Natl Acad. Sci. USA*, **97**, 12250–12255.

Bhatia, K., Raj, A., Guitierrez, M. I., Judde, J. G. *et al.* (1996). Variation in the sequence of Epstein Barr virus nuclear antigen 1 in normal peripheral blood lymphocytes and in Burkitt's lymphomas. *Oncogene*, **13**, 177–181.

Blaumueller, C. M., Zagouras, P., and Artavanis-Tsakonas, S.(1997). Intracellular cleavage of Notch leads to a heterodimeric receptor on the plasma membrane. *Cell*, **90**, 281–291.

Bollard C. M., S. K., Huls, M. H., Leen, A. *et al.* (2004). The generation and characterization of LMP2-specific CTLs for use as adoptive transfer from patients with relapsed EBV-positive Hodgkin disease. *J. Immunother.*, **27**, 317–327.

Brooks, L. A., Lear, A. L., Young, L. S. *et al.* (1993). Transcripts from the Epstein–Barr virus BamHI A fragment are detectable in all three forms of virus latency. *J. Virol.*, **67**, 3182–3190.

Brown, N. A., Liu, C. R., Wang, Y. F. *et al.* (1988). B-cell lymphoproliferation and lymphomagenesis are associated with clonotypic intracellular terminal regions of the Epstein–Barr virus. *J. Virol.*, **62**, 962–969.

Buell, P., (1974). The effect of migration on the risk of developing nasopharyngeal carcinoma. *Cancer Res.*, **34**, 1189–1191.

Burkitt, D., (1962a). A children's cancer dependent on climatic factors. *Nauchni. Tr. Vissh. Med. Inst. Sofiia*, **194**, 232–234.

Burkitt, D., (1962b). A lymphoma syndrome in African children. *Ann. R. Coll. Surg. Engl.*, **30**, 211–219.

Busson, P., Mccoy, R., Sadler, R. *et al.* (1992). Consistent transcription of the Epstein–Barr virus LMP2 gene in nasopharyngeal carcinoma. *J. Virol.*, **66**, 3257–3262.

Caldwell, R. G., Wilson, J. B., Anderson, S. J. *et al.* (1998). Epstein–Barr virus LMP2A drives B cell development and survival in the absence of normal B cell receptor signals. *Immunity*, **9**, 405–411.

Chapman, A. L. and Rickinson, A. B. (1998). Epstein–Barr virus in Hodgkin's disease. *Ann. Oncol.*, **9** Suppl 5, S5–S16.

Chen, H., Lee, J. M., Wang, Y. *et al.* (1999a). The Epstein–Barr virus latency BamHI-Q promoter is positively regulated by STATs and Zta interference with JAK/STAT activation leads to loss of BamHI-Q promoter activity. *Proc. Natl Acad. Sci. USA*, **96**, 9339–9344.

Chen, H., Smith, P., Ambinder, R. F., and Hayward, S. D. (1999b). Expression of Epstein–Barr virus BamHI-A rightward transcripts in latently infected B cells from peripheral blood. *Blood*, **93**, 3026–3032.

Chen, H., Lee, J. M., Zong, Y. *et al.* (2001). Linkage between STAT regulation and Epstein–Barr virus gene expression in tumors. *J. Virol.*, **75**, 2929–2937.

Chen, H., Cao, L., and Hayward, S. D. (2003). A positive autoregulatory loop of LMP1 expression and STAT activation in epithelial cells latently infected with Epstein–Barr virus. *J. Virol.*, **77**, 4139–4148.

Chen, R. H., Ding, W. V., and Mccormick, F. (2000). Wnt signaling to beta-catenin involves two interactive components. Glycogen synthase kinase-3beta inhibition and activation of protein kinase C. *J. Biol. Chem.*, **275**, 17894–17899.

Cheng, Y., P. N., Lung, M. L., Hampton, G. *et al.* (1998). Functional evidence for a nasopharyngeal carcinoma tumour suppressor gene that maps at chromosome 3p21.3.

Cohen, J. I., Wang, F., Mannick, J., and Kieff, E. (1989). Epstein–Barr virus nuclear protein 2 is a key determinant of lymphocyte transformation. *Proc. Natl Acad. Sci. USA*, **86**, 9558–9562.

Cross, D. A., Alessi, D. R., Cohen, P. *et al.* (1995). Inhibition of glycogen synthase kinase-3 by insulin mediated by protein kinase B. *Nature*, **378**, 785–789.

Dalla-Favera, R., Lombardi, L., Pelicci, P. G. *et al.* (1987). Mechanism of activation and biological role of the c-myc oncogene in B-cell lymphomagenesis. *Ann. N Y Acad. Sci.*, **511**, 207–218.

Dambaugh, T., Hennessy, K., Chamnankit, L. *et al.* (1984). U2 region of Epstein–Barr virus DNA may encode Epstein–Barr nuclear antigen 2. *Proc. Natl Acad. Sci. USA*, **81**, 7632–7636.

Deacon, E. M., Pallesen, G., Niedobitek, G. *et al.* (1993). Epstein–Barr virus and Hodgkin's disease: transcriptional analysis of virus latency in the malignant cells. *J. Exp. Med.*, **177**, 339–349.

Devergne, O., Hatzivassiliou, E., Izumi, K. M. *et al.* (1996). Association of TRAF1, TRAF2, and TRAF3 with an Epstein–Barr virus LMP1 domain important for B-lymphocyte transformation: role in NF-kappaB activation. *Mol. Cell. Biol.*, **16**, 7098–7108.

Devergne, O., Mcfarland, E. C., Mosialos, G. *et al.* (1998). Role of the TRAF binding site and NF-kappaB activation in Epstein–Barr virus latent membrane protein 1-induced cell gene expression. *J. Virol.*, **72**, 7900–7908.

Dykstra, M. L., Longnecker, R., and Pierce, S. K. (2001). Epstein–Barr virus coopts lipid rafts to block the signaling and antigen transport functions of the BCR. *Immunity*, **14**, 57–67.

Edwards, R., Sitki-Green, D., Moore, D. T. *et al.* (2004). Potential selection of LMP1 variants in nasopharyngeal carcinoma. *J. Virol.*, **78**, 868–881.

Edwards, R. H., Seillier-Moiseiwitsch, F., and Raab-Traub, N. (1999). Signature amino acid changes in latent membrane protein 1 distinguish Epstein–Barr virus strains. *Virolo.*, **261**, 79–95.

Effert, P., Mccoy, R., Abdel-Hamid, M., Flynn, K. *et al.* (1992). Alterations of the p53 gene in nasopharyngeal carcinoma. *J.Virol.*, **66**, 3768–3775.

Eliopoulos, A. G. and Young, L. S. (1998). Activation of the cJun N-terminal kinase (JNK) pathway by the Epstein–Barr virus-encoded latent membrane protein 1 (LMP1). *Oncogene*, **16**, 1731–1742.

Eliopoulos, A. G., Gallagher, N. J., Blake, S. M., Dawson, C. W., and Young, L. S. (1999). Activation of the p38 mitogen-activated protein kinase pathway by Epstein–Barr virus-encoded latent membrane protein 1 coregulates interleukin-6 and interleukin-8 production. *J. Biol. Chem.*, **274**, 16085–16096.

Emmerich, F., Theurich, S., Hummel, M. *et al.* (2003). Inactivating I kappa B epsilon mutations in Hodgkin/Reed–Sternberg cells. *J. Pathol.*, **201**, 413–420.

Epstein, M. A., Achong, B. G., and Barr, Y. M. (1964). Virus particles in cultured lymphoblasts from burkitt's lymphoma. *Lancet*, **15**, 702–703.

Fennewald, S., Van Santen, V., and Kieff, E., (1984). Nucleotide sequence of an mRNA transcribed in latent growth-transforming virus infection indicates that it may encode a membrane protein. *J. Virol.*, **51**, 411–419.

Finerty, S., Tarlton, J., Mackett, M. *et al.* (1992). Protective immunization against Epstein–Barr virus-induced disease in cotton-top tamarins using the virus envelope glycoprotein gp340 produced from a bovine papillomavirus expression vector. *J. Gen. Virol.*, **73**, 449–453.

Fortini, M. A. (1994). The suppressor of hairless participates in notch receptor signaling. *Cell*, **79**, 273–282.

Fries, K. L., Miller, W. E., and Raab-Traub, N. (1996). Epstein–Barr virus latent membrane protein 1 blocks p53-mediated apoptosis through the induction of the A20 gene. *J. Virol.*, **70**, 8653–8659.

Gan, Y. J., Chodosh, J., Morgan, A. *et al.* (1997). Epithelial cell polarization is a determinant in the infectious outcome of immunoglobulin A-mediated entry by Epstein–Barr virus. *J. Virol.*, **71**, 519–526.

Garcia, J. F., Camacho, F. I., Morente, M. *et al.* (2003). Hodgkin and Reed–Sternberg cells harbor alterations in the major tumor suppressor pathways and cell-cycle checkpoints: analyses using tissue microarrays. *Blood*, **101**, 681–689.

Gilligan, K., Rajadurai, P., Resnick, L. *et al.* (1990a). Epstein–Barr virus small nuclear RNAs are not expressed in permissively infected cells in Aids-associated leukoplakia. *Proc. Natl Acad. Sci. USA*, **87**, 8790–8794.

Gilligan, K., Sato, H., Rajadurai, P. *et al.* (1990b). Novel transcription from the Epstein–Barr virus terminal EcoRI fragment, DIJhet, in a nasopharyngeal carcinoma. *J. Virol.*, **64**, 4948–4956.

Given, D., Yee, D., Griem, K. *et al.* (1979). DNA of Epstein–Barr virus. V. Direct repeats of the ends of Epstein–Barr virus DNA. *J. Virol.*, **30**, 852–862.

Gottschalk S, N. C., Perez, M., Smith, C. A. *et al.* (2001). An Epstein–Barr virus deletion mutant associated with fatal lymphoproliferative disease unresponsive to therapy with virus-specific CTLs. *Blood*, **97**, 835–843.

Greenspan, J. S., Greenspan, D., Lennette, E. T. *et al.* (1985). Replication of Epstein–Barr virus within the epithelial cells of oral hairy leukoplakia, an Aids-associated lesion. *N. Engl. J. Med.*, **313**, 1564–1571.

Grossman, S. R., Johannsen, E., Tong, X. *et al.* (1994). The Epstein–Barr virus nuclear antigen 2 transactivator is directed to response elements by the J kappa recombination signal binding protein. *Proc. Natl Acad. Sci. USA*, **91**, 7568–7572.

Gu, S. Y., Huang, T. M., Ruan, L. *et al.* (1995). First EBV vaccine trial in humans using recombinant vaccinia virus expressing the major membrane antigen. *Dev. Biol. Stand.*, **84**, 171–177.

Harabuchi, Y., Imai, S., Wakashima, J. *et al.* (1996). Nasal T-cell lymphoma causally associated with Epstein–Barr virus: clinicopathologic, phenotypic, and genotypic studies. *Cancer*, **77**, 2137–2149.

Henkel, T., Ling, P. D., Hayward, S. D. *et al.* (1994). Mediation of Epstein–Barr virus EBNA2 transactivation by recombination signal-binding protein J kappa. *Science*, **265**, 92–95.

Henle, G., and Henle, W. (1976a). Epstein—Barr virus-specific IgA serum antibodies as an outstanding feature of nasopharyngeal carcinoma. *Int. J. Cancer*, **17**, 1–7.

Henle, G., Henle, W., Clifford, P. et al. (1969). Antibodies to Epstein–Barr virus in Burkitt's lymphoma and control groups. *J. Natl Cancer Inst.*, **43**, 1147–1157.

Henle, G., Henle, W., Klein, G. et al. (1971). Antibodies to early Epstein–Barr virus-induced antigens in Burkitt's lymphoma. *J. Natl Cancer Inst.*, **46**, 861–871.

Henle, W., and Henle, G. (1974). Epstein–Barr virus and human malignancies. *Cancer*, **34** (Suppl), 1368–1374.

Henle, W. and Henle, G. (1976b). The sero-epidemiology of Epstein–Barr virus. *Adv. Pathobiol.*, **5**, 5–17.

Hinz, M., Lemke, P., Anagnostopoulos, I., Hacker, C. et al. (2002). Nuclear factor kappaB-dependent gene expression profiling of Hodgkin's disease tumor cells, pathogenetic significance, and link to constitutive signal transducer and activator of transcription 5a activity. *J. Exp. Med.*, **196**, 605–617.

Hitt, M. M., Allday, M. J., Hara, T. et al. (1989). EBV gene expression in an NPC-related tumour. *Embo J.*, **8**, 2639–2651.

Ho, H. C. (1976). Epidemiology of nasopharyngeal carcinoma. In Hirayama, T., ed. *Cancer in Asia*. Baltimore: Univ. Park Press, pp. 49–61.

Hofelmayr, H., Strobl, L. J., Marschall, G. et al. (2001). Activated Notch1 can transiently substitute for EBNA2 in the maintenance of proliferation of LMP1-expressing immortalized B cells. *J. Virol.*, **75**, 2033–2040.

Howe, J. G. and Steitz, J. A., (1986). Localization of Epstein–Barr virus-encoded small RNAs by in situ hybridization. *Proc. Natl Acad. Sci. USA*, **83**, 9006–9010.

Hu, L. F., Zabarovsky, E. R., Chen, F. et al. (1991). Isolation and sequencing of the Epstein–Barr virus BNLF-1 gene (LMP1) from a Chinese nasopharyngeal carcinoma. *J. Gen. Virol.*, **72**, 2399–2409.

Huang, D., L. K., Van Hasselt, A, Woo, J. K. S. et al. (1994). A region of homozygous deletion on chromosome 9p21–22 in primary nasopharyngeal carcinoma. *Cancer Res.*, **54**, 4003–4006.

Huang, D. P., Lo, K. W., Choi, P. H. et al. (1991). Loss of heterozygosity on the short arm of chromosome 3 in nasopharyngeal carcinoma. *Cancer Genet. Cytogenet.*, **54**, 91–99.

Huen, D. S., Henderson, S. A., Croom-Carter, D. et al. (1995). The Epstein–Barr virus latent membrane protein-1 (LMP1) mediates activation of NF-kappa B and cell surface phenotype via two effector regions in its carboxy-terminal cytoplasmic domain. *Oncogene*, **10**, 549–560.

Ikeda, M., Ikeda, A., and Longnecker, R. (2001). PY motifs of Epstein–Barr virus LMP2A regulate protein stability and phosphorylation of LMP2A-associated proteins. *J. Virol.*, **75**, 5711–5718.

Iwakiri, D., Eizuru, Y., Tokunaga, M. et al. (2003). Autocrine growth of Epstein–Barr virus-positive gastric carcinoma cells mediated by an Epstein–Barr virus-encoded small RNA. *Cancer Res.*, **63**, 7062–7067.

Izumi, K. M., and Kieff, E. D. (1997). The Epstein–Barr virus oncogene product latent membrane protein 1 engages the tumor necrosis factor receptor-associated death domain protein to mediate B lymphocyte growth transformation and activate NF-kappaB. *Proc. Natl Acad. Sci. USA*, **94**, 12592–12597.

Johannsen, E., Koh, E., Mosialos, G. et al. (1995). Epstein–Barr virus nuclear protein 2 transactivation of the latent membrane protein 1 promoter is mediated by J kappa and PU.1. *J. Virol.*, **69**, 253–262.

Kanegane, H., Miyawaki, T., Yachie, A. et al. (1999). Development of EBV-positive T-cell lymphoma following infection of peripheral blood T cells with EBV. *Leuk. Lymphoma*, **34**, 603–607.

Kaye, K. M., Izumi, K. M., Li, H. et al. (1999). An Epstein–Barr virus that expresses only the first 231 LMP1 amino acids efficiently initiates primary B-lymphocyte growth transformation. *J. Virol.*, **73**, 10525–10530.

Khanim, F., Yao, Q. Y., Niedobitek, G., Sihota, S. et al. (1996). Analysis of Epstein–Barr virus gene polymorphisms in normal donors and in virus-associated tumors from different geographic locations. *Blood*, **88**, 3491–3501.

Kieff, E. and Rickinson, A. B. (2001). Epstein–Barr virus and its replication. In Fields, B. N., Howley, P. M., Griffin, D. E. et al. (eds.) *Field's Virology*. 4th edn. Philadelphia, PA: Lippincott Williams & Wilkins Publishers.

Knecht, H., Joske, D. J., Bachmann, E. et al. (1992). Significance of the detection of Epstein–Barr virus DNA in lymph nodes in patients with Hodgkin's disease. *Leuk Lymphoma*, **8**, 319–325.

Knecht, H., Berger, C., Mcquain, C., Rothenberger, S. et al. (1999). Latent membrane protein 1 associated signaling pathways are important in tumor cells of Epstein–Barr virus negative Hodgkin's disease. *Oncogene*, **18**, 7161–7167.

Komano, J., Sugiura, M., and Takada, K. (1998). Epstein–Barr virus contributes to the malignant phenotype and to apoptosis resistance in Burkitt's lymphoma cell line Akata. *J. Virol.*, **72**, 9150–9156.

Komano, J., Maruo, S., Kurozumi, K. et al. (1999). Oncogenic role of Epstein–Barr virus-encoded RNAs in Burkitt's lymphoma cell line Akata. *J. Virol.*, **73**, 9827–9831.

Kulwichit, W., Edwards, R. H., Davenport, E. M. et al. (1998). Expression of the Epstein–Barr virus latent membrane protein 1 induces B cell lymphoma in transgenic mice. *Proc. Natl Acad. Sci. USA*, **95**, 11963–11968.

Kusano, S., and Raab-Traub, N. (2001). An Epstein–Barr virus protein interacts with Notch. *J. Virol.*, **15**, 384–395.

Lanier, A. P., Clift, S. R., Bornkamm, G. et al. (1991). Epstein–Barr virus and malignant lymphoepithelial lesions of the salivary gland. *Arctic Med. Res.*, **50**, 55–61.

Laux, G., Perricaudet, M., and Farrell, P. J. (1988). A spliced Epstein–Barr virus gene expressed in immortalized lymphocytes is created by circularization of the linear viral genome. *EMBO J.*, **7**, 769–774.

Lerner, M. R., Andrews, N. C., Miller, G. et al. (1981). Two small RNAs encoded by Epstein–Barr virus and complexed with protein are precipitated by antibodies from patients with systemic lupus erythematosus. *Proc. Natl Acad. Sci. USA*, **78**, 805–809.

Levitskaya, J., Coram, M., Levitsky, V. et al. (1995). Inhibition of antigen processing by the internal repeat region of the Epstein–Barr virus nuclear antigen-1. *Nature*, **375**, 685–688.

Levitskaya, J., Sharipo, A., Leonchiks, A. et al. (1997). Inhibition of ubiquitin/proteasome-dependent protein degradation by the

Gly-Ala repeat domain of the Epstein–Barr virus nuclear antigen 1. *Proc. Natl Acad. Sci. USA*, **94**, 12616–12621.

Li, S. N., Chang, Y. S., and Liu, S. T. (1996). Effect of a 10-amino acid deletion on the oncogenic activity of latent membrane protein 1 of Epstein–Barr virus. *Oncogene*, **12**, 2129–2135.

Lo, K.-W., Huang, D. P., and Lau, K. M. (1995). p16 gene alterations in nasopharyngeal carcinoma. *Cancer Res.*, **55**, 2039–2043.

Lo, K.-W., and Huang, D. P. (2002). Genetic and epigenetic changes in nasopharyngeal carcinoma. *Semin. Cancer Biol.*, **12**, 451–462.

Longnecker, R., and Miller, C. L. (1996). Regulation of Epstein–Barr virus latency by latent membrane protein 2. *Trends Microbiol.*, **4**, 38–42.

Longnecker, R., Merchant, M., Brown, M. E. *et al.* (2000). WW- and SH3-domain interactions with Epstein–Barr virus LMP2A. *Exp. Cell Res.*, **257**, 332–340.

Lung, M. L., Chang, R. S., Huang, M. L. *et al.* (1990). Epstein–Barr virus genotypes associated with nasopharyngeal carcinoma in southern China. *Virology*, **177**, 44–53.

MacMahon, E. M., Glass, J. D., Hayward, S. D. *et al.* (1992). Association of Epstein–Barr virus with primary central nervous system lymphoma in AIDS. *AIDS Res. Hum. Retroviruses*, **8**, 740–742.

Magrath, I., (1990). The pathogenesis of Burkitt's lymphoma. *Adv. Cancer Res.*, **55**, 133–270.

Marafioti, T. H. M., Foss, H. D., Laumen, H. *et al.* (2000). Hodgkin and reed-sternberg cells represent an expansion of a single clone originating from a germinal center B-cell with functional immunoglobulin gene rearrangements but defective immunoglobulin transcription. *Blood*, **95**, 1443–1450.

Miller, C. L., Burkhardt, A. L., Lee, J. H. *et al.* (1995a). Integral membrane protein 2 of Epstein–Barr virus regulates reactivation from latency through dominant negative effects on protein-tyrosine kinases. *Immunity*, **2**, 155–166.

Miller, G., Niederman, J. C., and Andrews, L. L. (1973). Prolonged oropharyngeal excretion of Epstein–Barr virus after infectious mononucleosis. *N. Engl. J. Med.*, **288**, 229–232.

Miller, W. E., Edwards, R. H., Walling, D. M. *et al.* (1994). Sequence variation in the Epstein–Barr virus latent membrane protein 1. *J. Gen. Virol.*, **75**, 2729–2740.

Miller, W. E., Earp, H. S., and Raab-Traub, N. (1995). The Epstein–Barr virus latent membrane protein 1 induces expression of the epidermal growth factor receptor. *J. Virol.*, **69**, 4390–4398.

Miller, W. E., Mosialos, G., Kieff, E. *et al.* (1997). Epstein–Barr virus LMP1 induction of the epidermal growth factor receptor is mediated through a TRAF signaling pathway distinct from NF-kappaB activation. *J. Virol.*, **71**, 586–594.

Miller, W. E., Cheshire, J. L., and Raab-Traub, N. (1998). Interaction of tumor necrosis factor-receptor-associated factor signaling proteins with the latent membrane protein 1 PXQXT motif is essential for induction of epidermal growth factor receptor expression. *Mol. Cell. Biol.*, **18**, 2835–2844.

Moody, C. A., Su, T., and Sixbey, J. W. (2003). Length of Epstein–Barr virus termini as a determinant of epithelial cell clonal emergence. *J. Virol.*, **77**, 8555–8561.

Morrison, J. A., Klingelhutz, A. J., and Raab-Traub, N. (2003). Epstein–Barr virus latent membrane protein 2A activates beta-catenin signaling in epithelial cells. *J. Virol.*, **77**, 12276–12284.

Mosialos, G., Birkenbach, M., Yalamanchili, R. *et al.* (1995). The Epstein–Barr virus transforming protein LMP1 engages signaling proteins for the tumor necrosis factor receptor family. *Cell*, **80**, 389–399.

Moss, D. J., Schmidt, C., Elliott, S. *et al.* (1996). Strategies involved in developing an effective vaccine for EBV-associated diseases. *Adv. Cancer Res.*, **69**, 213–245.

Mueller, N., Evans, A., Harris, N. L. *et al.* (1989). Hodgkin's disease and Epstein–Barr virus. Altered antibody pattern before diagnosis. *N. Engl. J. Med.*, **320**, 689–695.

Murray, R. J., Kurilla, M. G., Griffin, H. M. *et al.* (1990). Human cytotoxic T-cell responses against Epstein–Barr virus nuclear antigens demonstrated by using recombinant vaccinia viruses. *Proc. Natl Acad. Sci. USA*, **87**, 2906–2910.

Nelson, J. A., Bariband, F., Edwards, T., and Swanstrom, R. (2000). Patterns of changes in Human Immunodeficiency Virus type 1 V3 sequence populations late in infection. *J. Virol.*, **74**, 8494–8501.

Niedobitek, G., Hansmann, M. L., Herbst, H. *et al.* (1991a). Epstein–Barr virus and carcinomas: undifferentiated carcinomas but not squamous cell carcinomas of the nasopharynx are regularly associated with the virus. *J. Pathol.*, **165**, 17–24.

Niedobitek, G., Young, L. S., Lau, R. *et al.* (1991b). Epstein–Barr virus infection in oral hairy leukoplakia: virus replication in the absence of a detectable latent phase. *J Gen Virol.*, **72** (12), 3035–3046.

Niedobitek, G., Agathanggelou, A., Rowe, M. *et al.* (1995). Heterogeneous expression of Epstein–Barr virus latent proteins in endemic Burkitt's lymphoma. *Blood*, **86**, 659–665.

Nilsson, K., Klein, G., Henle, W. *et al.* (1971). The establishment of lymphoblastoid lines from adult and fetal human lymphoid tissue and its dependence on EBV. *Int. J. Cancer*, **8**, 443–450.

Nonkwelo, C., Skinner, J., Bell, A. *et al.* (1996). Transcription start sites downstream of the Epstein–Barr virus (EBV) Fp promoter in early-passage Burkitt lymphoma cells define a fourth promoter for expression of the EBV EBNA-1 protein. *J. Virol.*, **70**, 623–627.

Ohtani N, B. P., Gaubatz, S., Sanij, E. *et al.* (2003). Epstein–Barr virus LMP1 blocks p16INK4a-RB pathway by promoting nuclear export of E2F4/5. *J. Cell. Biol.*, **162**, 173–183.

Packham, G., Brimmell, M., Cook, D. *et al.* (1993). Strain variation in Epstein–Barr virus immediate early genes. *Virology*, **192**, 541–550.

Paine, E., Scheinman, R. I., Baldwin, A. S., Jr., and Raab-Traub, N. (1995). Expression of LMP1 in epithelial cells leads to the activation of a select subset of NF-kappa B/Rel family proteins. *J. Virol.*, **69**, 4572–4576.

Pathmanathan, R., Prasad, U., Chandrika *et al.* (1995a). Undifferentiated, nonkeratinizing, and squamous cell carcinoma of the nasopharynx. Variants of Epstein–Barr virus-infected neoplasia. *Am. J. Path.*, **146**, 1355–1367.

Pathmanathan, R., Prasad, U., Sadler, R. et al. (1995b). Clonal proliferations of cells infected with Epstein–Barr virus in preinvasive lesions related to nasopharyngeal carcinoma. *N. Engl. J. Med.*, **333**, 693–698.

Pelicci, P. G., Knowles, D. M. D., Arlin, Z. A. et al. (1986). Multiple monoclonal B cell expansions and c-myc oncogene rearrangements in acquired immune deficiency syndrome-related lymphoproliferative disorders. Implications for lymphomagenesis. *J. Exp. Med.*, **164**, 2049–2060.

Poirier, S., Bouvier, G., Malaveille, C. et al. (1989). Volatile nitrosamine levels and genotoxicity of food samples from high-risk areas for nasopharyngeal carcinoma before and after nitrosation. *Int. J. Cancer*, **44**, 1088–1094.

Portis, T. and Longnecker, R., (2003). Epstein–Barr virus LMP2A interferes with global transcription factor regulation when expressed during B-lymphocyte development. *J. Virol.*, **77**, 105–144.

Raab-Traub, N., (1996). Pathogenesis of Epstein–Barr virus and its associated malignancies. *Semin. Virol.*, **7**, 315–323.

Raab-Traub, N., (2002). Epstein–Barr virus in the pathogenesis of NPC. *Semin. Cancer Biol.*, **12**, 431–441.

Raab-Traub, N., and Flynn, K. (1986). The structure of the termini of the Epstein–Barr virus as a marker of clonal cellular proliferation. *Cell*, **47**, 883–889.

Raab-Traub, N., Hood, R., Yang, C. S. et al. (1983). Epstein–Barr virus transcription in nasopharyngeal carcinoma. *J. Virol.*, **48**, 580–590.

Raab-Traub, N., Flynn, K., Pearson, G. et al. (1987). The differentiated form of nasopharyngeal carcinoma contains Epstein–Barr virus DNA. *Int. J. Cancer*, **39**, 25–29.

Raab-Traub, N., Rajadurai, P., Flynn, K. et al. (1991). Epstein–Barr virus infection in carcinoma of the salivary gland. *J. Virol.*, **65**, 7032–7036.

Rickinson, A. B. and Moss, D. J. (1997). Human cytotoxic T lymphocyte responses to Epstein–Barr virus infection. *Annu. Rev. Immunol.*, **15**, 405–431.

Rickinson, A. A. K. (2001). Epstein–Barr virus. In Fields, B. N., Howley, P. M., Griffin, D. E. et al., eds. *Field's Virology*, 4th edn. Philadelphia, PA: Lippincott Williams and Wilkins.

Robertson, E. S., Lin, J., and Kieff, E. (1996). The amino-terminal domains of Epstein–Barr virus nuclear proteins 3A, 3B, and 3C interact with RBPJ(kappa). *J. Virol.*, **70**, 3068–3074.

Robertson, K. D. (2000). The role of DNA methylation in modulating Epstein–Barr virus gene expression. *Curr. Top. Microbiol. Immunol.*, **249**, 21–34.

Rooney, C. M., Smith, C. A., Ng, C. Y. et al. (1995). Use of gene-modified virus-specific T lymphocytes to control Epstein–Barr-virus-related lymphoproliferation. *Lancet*, **345**, 9–13.

Rooney, C. M., Smith, C. A., and Heslop, H. E. (1997). Control of virus-induced lymphoproliferation: Epstein–Barr virus-induced lymphoproliferation and host immunity. *Mol. Med. Today*, **3**, 24–30.

Rowe, M., Rowe, D. T., Gregory, C. D. et al. (1987). Differences in B cell growth phenotype reflect novel patterns of Epstein–Barr virus latent gene expression in Burkitt's lymphoma cells. *EMBO J.*, **6**, 2743–2751.

Sadler, R. H. and Raab-Traub, N. (1995a). The Epstein–Barr virus 3.5-kilobase latent membrane protein 1 mRNA initiates from a TATA-Less promoter within the first terminal repeat. *J. Virol.*, **69**, 4577–4581.

Sadler, R. H. and Raab-Traub, N. (1995b). Structural analyses of the Epstein–Barr virus BamHI A transcripts. *J. Virol.*, **69**, 1132–1141.

Saemundsen, A. K., Albeck, H., Hansen, J. P. et al. (1982). Epstein–Barr virus in nasopharyngeal and salivary gland carcinomas of Greenland Eskimoes. *Br. J. Cancer*, **46**, 721–728.

Sample, J., Liebowitz, D., and Kieff, E. (1989). Two related Epstein–Barr virus membrane proteins are encoded by separate genes. *J. Virol.*, **63**, 933–937.

Sample, J., Young, L., Martin, B. et al. (1990). Epstein–Barr virus types 1 and 2 differ in their EBNA-3A, EBNA-3B, and EBNA-3C genes. *J. Virol.*, **64**, 4084–4092.

Sample, J., Brooks, L., Sample, C. et al. (1991). Restricted. Epstein–Barr virus protein expression in Burkitt lymphoma is due to a different Epstein–Barr nuclear antigen 1 transcriptional initiation site. *Proc. Natl Acad. Sci. USA*, **88**, 6343–6347.

Sample, J., Henson, E. B., and Sample, C. (1992). The Epstein–Barr virus nuclear protein 1 promoter active in type I latency is autoregulated. *J. Virol.*, **66**, 4654–4661.

Scholle, F., Bendt, K. M., and Raab-Traub, N. (2000). Epstein–Barr virus LMP2A transforms epithelial cells, inhibits cell differentiation, and activates Akt. *J. Virol.*, **74**, 10681–10689.

Shanmugaratnam, K. (1970). A study of nasopharyngeal carcinoma among Singapore Chinese with special reference to migrant status and specific community. *J. Chronic. Dis.*, **23**, 433–441.

Shanmugaratnam, K. (1978). Histological typing of nasopharyngeal carcinoma. *IARC Sci. Publ.*, **20**, 3–12.

Shaw, J. E., (1985). The circular intracellular form of Epstein–Barr virus DNA is amplified by the virus-associated DNA polymerase. *J. Virol.*, **53**, 1012–1015.

Shaw, J. E., Levinger, L. F., and Carter, C. W., Jr. (1979). Nucleosomal structure of Epstein–Barr virus DNA in transformed cell lines. *J. Virol.*, **29**, 657–665.

Shibata, D., Tokunaga, M., Uemura, Y. et al. (1991). Association of Epstein–Barr virus with undifferentiated gastric carcinomas with intense lymphoid infiltration. Lymphoepithelioma-like carcinoma. *Am. J. Pathol.*, **139**, 469–474.

Sitki-Green, D., Edwards, R. H., Webster-Cyriaque, J. et al. (2002). Identification of Epstein–Barr virus strain variants in hairy leukoplakia and peripheral blood by use of a heteroduplex tracking assay. *J. Virol.*, **76**, 9645–9656.

Sitki-Green, D., Covington, M., and Raab-Traub, N. (2003). Compartmentalization and transmission of multiple Epstein–Barr virus strains in asymptomatic carriers. *J. Virol.*, **77**, 1840–1847.

Sixbey, J. W., Nedrud, J. G., Raab-Traub, N. et al. (1984). Epstein–Barr virus replication in oropharyngeal epithelial cells. *N. Engl. J. Med.*, **310**, 1225–1230.

Sixbey, J. W., Shirley, P., Sloas, M. et al. (1991). A transformation-incompetent, nuclear antigen 2-deleted Epstein–Barr virus associated with replicative infection. *J. Infect. Dis.*, **163**, 1008–1015.

Smith, P. R., De Jesus, O., Turner, D. et al. (2000). Structure and coding content of CST (BART) family RNAs of Epstein–Barr virus. *J. Virol.*, **74**, 3082–3092.

Stewart, J. P., Behm, F. G., Arrand, J. R. et al. (1994). Differential expression of viral and human interleukin-10 (IL-10) by primary B cell tumors and B cell lines. *Virology*, **200**, 724–732.

Su, I. J., Lin, K. H., Chen, C. J. et al. (1990). Epstein–Barr virus-associated peripheral T-cell lymphoma of activated CD8 phenotype. *Cancer*, **66**, 2557–2562.

Sun, Y., H. G., and Colburn, N. H. (1993). Nasopharyngeal carcinoma shows no detectable retinoblastoma susceptibility gene alterations. *Oncogene*, **3**, 791–795.

Sun, Y., Hildesheim, A., Lanier, A. E. et al. (1995). No point mutation but decreased expression of the p16/MTS1 tumor suppressor gene in nasopharyngeal carcinomas. *Oncogene*, **10**, 785–788.

Swaminathan, S., Tomkinson, B., and Kieff, E. (1991). Recombinant Epstein–Barr virus with small RNA (EBER) genes deleted transforms lymphocytes and replicates in vitro. *Proc. Natl Acad. Sci. USA*, **88**, 1546–1550.

Swart, R., Ruf, I. K., Sample, J. et al. (2000). Latent membrane protein 2A-mediated effects on the phosphatidylinositol 3-kinase/Akt pathway. *Virol.*, **74**, 10838–10845.

Thornburg, N. J., Pathmanathan, R., and Raab-Traub, N. (2003). Activation of nuclear factor-kappaB p50 homodimer/Bcl-3 complexes in nasopharyngeal carcinoma. *Cancer Res.*, **63**, 8293–8301.

Tomkinson, B., Robertson, E., and Kieff, E. (1993). Epstein–Barr virus nuclear proteins EBNA-3A and EBNA-3C are essential for B-lymphocyte growth transformation. *J. Virol.*, **67**, 2014–2025.

Walling, D. M., Edmiston, S. N., Sixbey, J. W. et al. (1992). Coinfection with multiple strains of the Epstein–Barr virus in human immunodeficiency virus-associated hairy leukoplakia. *Proc. Natl Acad. Sci USA*, **89**, 6560–6564.

Wang, D., Liebowitz, D., and Kieff, E. (1985). An EBV membrane protein expressed in immortalized lymphocytes transforms established rodent cells. *Cell*, **43**, 831–840.

Wang, D., Liebowitz, D., Wang, F. et al. (1988). Epstein–Barr virus latent infection membrane protein alters the human B-lymphocyte phenotype: deletion of the amino terminus abolishes activity. *J. Virol.*, **62**, 4173–4184.

Wang, F., Tsang, S. F., Kurilla, M. G. et al. (1990). Epstein–Barr virus nuclear antigen 2 transactivates latent membrane protein LMP1. *J. Virol.*, **64**, 3407–3416.

Weiss, L. M., Strickler, J. G., Warnke, R. A. et al. (1989a). Epstein–Barr viral DNA in tissues of Hodgkin's disease. *Am. J. Pathol.*, **129**, 86–91.

Weiss, L. M., Movahed, L. A., Warnke, R. A. et al. (1989b). Detection of Epstein–Barr viral genomes in Reed-Sternberg cells of Hodgkin's disease. *N. Engl. J. Med.*, **320**, 502–506.

Wilson, A. D., Shooshstari, M., Finerty, S. et al. (1996). Virus-specific cytotoxic T cell responses are associated with immunity of the cottontop tamarin to Epstein–Barr virus (EBV). *Clin. Exp. Immunol.*, **103**, 199–205.

Wolf, H., Hausen, H. Z., and Becker, V. (1973). EB viral genomes in epithelial nasopharyngeal carcinoma cells. *Nat. New. Biol.*, **244**, 245–247.

Wolf, H., and Haus, M., and Wilmes, E. (1984). Persistence of Epstein–Barr virus in the parotid gland. *J. Virol.*, **51**, 795–798.

Yates, J. L., Warren, N., and Sugden, B. (1985). Stable replication of plasmids derived from Epstein–Barr virus in various mammalian cells. *Nature*, **331**, 812–815.

Yeung, W. M., Zong, Y. S., Chiu, C. T. et al. (1993). Epstein–Barr virus carriage by nasopharyngeal carcinoma in situ. *Int. J. Cancer*, **53**, 746–750.

Young, L., Alfieri, C., Hennessy, K. et al. (1989). Expression of Epstein–Barr virus transformation-associated genes in tissues of patients with EBV lymphoproliferative disease. *N. Engl. J. Med.*, **321**, 1080–1085.

Young, L. S., Deacon, E. M., Rowe, M. et al. (1991). Epstein–Barr virus latent genes in tumour cells of Hodgkin's disease [letter; comment]. *Lancet*, **337**, 1617.

Yu, M. C. and Yuan, J. M. (2002). Epidemiology of nasopharyngeal carcinoma. *Semin. Cancer Biol.*, **12**, 421–429.

Yu, M. C., Ho, J. H., Lai, S. H. et al. (1986). Cantonese-style salted fish as a cause of nasopharyngeal carcinoma: report of a case-control study in Hong Kong. *Cancer Res.*, **46**, 956–961.

Zhang, J., Chen, H., Weinmaster, G. et al. (2001). Epstein–Barr virus BamHi-a rightward transcript-encoded RPMS protein interacts with the CBF1-associated corepressor CIR to negatively regulate the activity of EBNA2 and NotchIC. *J. Virol.*, **75**, 2946–2956.

Zimber, U., Adldinger, H. K., Lenoir, G. M. et al. (1986). Geographical prevalence of two types of Epstein–Barr virus. *Virology*, **154**, 56–66.

KSHV-induced oncogenesis

Don Ganem

Howard Hughes Medical Institute, Departments of Microbiology and Immunology and Medicine, University of California, San Francisco, CA, USA

Human infection by KSHV is associated with the development of at least three proliferative disorders: Kaposi's sarcoma (KS), primary effusion lymphoma (PEL) and a subset of multicentric Castleman's disease (MCD). In keeping with the classification of KSHV as a lymphotropic (γ2) herpesvirus, two of these (PEL and MCD) are primary disorders of the B cell lineage. The third, KS, is a more complex lesion driven by proliferation of cells of endothelial lineage. KSHV is the second human γ-herpesvirus to be linked to neoplasia (EBV being the first). As such, many notions about how KSHV engenders these lesions have been heavily influenced by paradigms derived from the study of EBV-induced malignancies. In EBV, the viral latency program is powerfully immortalizing in vitro, and is thought to be the principal genetic program driving virus-related tumorigenesis. Lytic infection, while presumed important for dissemination of infection to target cells early in infection (and following lytic reactivation at later times), is not thought to play a direct role in the histogenesis of the tumors. As we shall see, although many parallels indeed exist with EBV, the distinctive features of the KSHV-associated diseases makes routine extrapolation from other viral models an enterprise to be undertaken with caution. In this chapter, we will review the biology of the KSHV-associated malignancies and consider the cellular and molecular mechanisms by which KSHV infection contributes to their pathogenesis.

Primary effusion lymphoma (PEL)

PEL is a classical neoplasm involving cells of the B cell lineage (see review by Cesarman, this volume). The malignant cells in PEL are clonal (as judged by VDJ rearrangement; Knowles et al., 1989; Green et al., 1995), fully immortalized, grow readily in culture (Cesarman et al., 1995; Boshoff et al., 1997) and are tumorigenic in nude mice (Picchio et al., 1997). They express few classical B-cell surface markers, but regularly express CD138/syndecan-1 and display somatic hypermutation in Ig and bcl-6 loci, indicating that they are derived from post-germinal center B-cells (Carbone et al., 2001). Consistent with this, transcript profiling suggests that the cells are of plasmablastic lineage (Klein et al., 2003; Jenner et al., 2003). The fact that PEL cells often secrete IL6 and IL10, a feature that is shared with other plasmacyctic neoplasms (Lauta, 2003), also accords with this interpretation.

Virtually all cases of PEL harbor KSHV DNA in every cell; many also display EBV infection as well, though EBV is never found in PEL as the sole pathogen. Where the EBV genome is present, its expression is largely restricted to EBNA 1, EBER RNA and low levels of LMP2a (typical of the so-called Latency I pattern) (Horenstein et al., 1997; Szekely et al., 1998; Schulz, 2001). KSHV infection of PEL cells is predominantly latent, which has made PEL cell lines the most widely studied model for KSHV latency. Most PEL lines also display a small subpopulation of cells staining for markers of lytic reactivation (Staskus et al., 1997; Sturzl et al., 1997). Latently infected PEL cells express at least 5 loci (see below), none of which have been conserved in EBV. Most of these loci were discovered by screening for transcripts or antigens constitutively expressed in PEL cell lines. Their products have been studied intensively for their biochemical and phenotypic properties, usually by overexpression in heterologous cell types. As we shall see, in the aggregate they harbor numerous activities that can deregulate cell growth and augment cell survival, consistent with the notion that KSHV latency drives the generation of PEL. The rarity with which PEL follows KSHV infection, however, also suggests that while viral latency is surely necessary for PEL development, it may not be sufficient for it. Host factors – most likely additional host cell mutations – must also be involved, but the number and identities of these have not been determined. It is known, however, that PEL cells do not harbor rearrangements of MYC or BCL-2 genes. One study reports that cultured PEL cell lines have frequent reduplications of chromosome 7 and 12, as well as abnormalities at 1q21–25 (Gaidano et al., 1999), but the key genes affected by these processes remain to be identified. In addition, two autocrine or paracrine loops involving host genes have been posited to occur in PEL. One report indicates that both HGF (hepatocyte growth factor) and its receptor (c-Met) are expressed in primary PEL tumors and in PEL cell lines (Capello et al., 2000). More widespread has been the recognition that PEL cells usually express the IL6Rα and gp130 chains that mediate responsiveness to IL6, and often secrete human IL6 itself, raising the possibility of an autocrine loop. However, recent studies suggest that it is a viral homologue of IL6 (v-IL6; see below) that actually functions in this role, together with IL10 (Jones et al., 1999).

The KSHV latency program in PEL

Since both KSHV and EBV are lymphotropic herpesviruses linked to B-cell lymphoma, it is natural to imagine that similar mechanisms must underly their oncogenic programs. However, a closer look reveals many phenotypic differences that challenge this assumption. First, while in vitro EBV infection of primary B-cells is strongly immortalizing, there is little evidence that KSHV infection can immortalize lymphocytes on its own. This issue has been most rigorously addressed by Kliche et al. (1998), who showed that under conditions in which EBV efficiently promoted outgrowth of lymphoblastoid cell lines, KSHV failed to do so when the PBMCs were from EBV-negative hosts. Only with B cells from EBV-infected hosts could KSHV infection be linked to B cell outgrowth, and in all cases the resulting LCLs harbored both viral genomes. This would suggest that the KSHV latency program is not strongly immortalizing on its own, and, at least in vitro, either requires one or more cofactors from EBV or acts to stimulate EBV's immortalizing activity. These findings accord well with the finding that most PEL tumors harbor both EBV and KSHV. Nonetheless, it is clear that the *sine qua non* of PEL is KSHV infection, since PEL tumors are not observed in its absence. And since occasional PEL tumors harbor KSHV alone, whatever cofactor(s) are derived from EBV must also be obtainable in some alternative way.

These findings illustrate that KSHV latency must make some genetic contribution to PEL, but do not define the biochemical nature of that contribution or identify the responsible viral gene(s). Two major experimental obstacles have impeded progress on this question. First, KSHV infection of primary B-cells proceeds very inefficiently in vitro, making it difficult to assay biochemical or phenotypic events directly triggered by latency in this lineage. Second, systems for mutating viral genes in the context of the intact KSHV genome are exceedingly inefficient – to date only a few viral genes have been inactivated in this fashion (Delecluse et al., 2001; Xu et al., 2005), though two laboratories have been able to construct genetically marked WT KSHV isolates (Viera et al., 2001; Zhou et al., 2002).

In the absence of such systems, inferences about KSHV's genetic and biochemical contributions to PEL must be derived from studies of the effects of expression of individual latency genes in heterologous cells, usually fibroblasts or other non-lymphoid cells. A previous chapter in this volume described the identification of the viral genes transcribed in latent PEL cell lines; these transcription units and their map positions are pictorially summarized in Fig. 56.1. Here we consider what is known about each of these proteins and how this knowledge might relate to PEL development.

Latency-associated nuclear antigen (LANA)

This large, multifunctional protein is expressed in all latently infected cells in vivo, irrespective of their lineage – it is the universal marker of KSHV latency and is present in KS spindle cells as well as the B-cells of MCD and PEL (Dupin et al., 1999). Studies in Tg mice affirm that its promoter is expressed efficiently in both B-cells and epithelia (Jeong et al., 2002). (Paradoxically, this study failed to demonstrate endothelial expression of LANA, despite its ubiquitous expression in human KS spindle cells. This suggests that either the promoter fragment employed lacked recognition sites for endothelial-specific factors, or there are species differences in LANA gene regulation). The protein has three major domains (Fig. 56.2): a central region composed of variable numbers of highly acidic amino acid repeats, a C-terminal, more basic region involved in DNA binding and oligomerization, and an N-terminal region to which many functions have been ascribed, including chromatin attachment and corepressor recruitment (Krithivas et al., 2000; Piolot et al., 2001; see below). The best-characterized function of LANA is that involved in the establishment and maintenance of the latent viral episome in the nucleus (Ballestas et al., 1999; Cotter and Robertson, 1999). This activity is based upon its ability to (i) bind to sequences in the terminal repeats (TRs) of the genome (Ballestas and Kaye, 2001; Garber et al., 2002); (ii) mediate transient semiconservative DNA replication from TR-containing plasmids (Hu et al., 2002; Lim et al., 2002; Grundhoff and

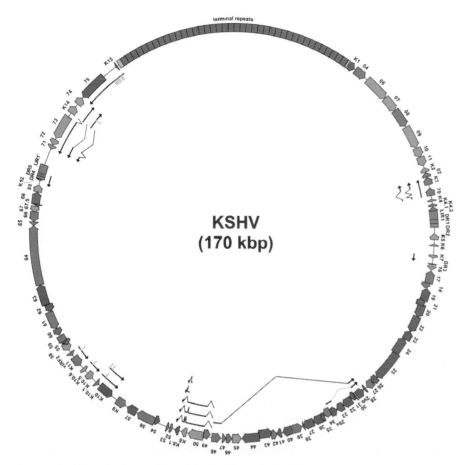

Fig. 56.1. Latency Genes of KSHV. Transcripts of latent genes are depicted as arrows, superimposed on the physical map of the circular, latent viral genome. (See color plate section.)

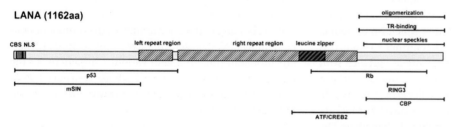

Fig. 56.2. Domain organization of LANA. Regions implicated in binding some of the putative LANA-associated host factors are denoted with lines above or below the name of the corresponding factor. CBS, chromatin binding sequence; NLS, nuclear localization sequence.

Ganem, 2003); and (iii) bind mitotic chromosomes to promote segregation of viral genomes to the progeny of dividing cells (Ballestas *et al.*, 1999; Piolot *et al.*, 2001). However, the story of viral episome maintenance is more complex than this. In many biologically important contexts, while LANA is necessary for plasmid maintenance, it is not always sufficient for it – additional cis-acting epigenetic changes in the viral chromatin appear to be required (Grundhoff and Ganem, 2004). This will be considered more fully in a later section.

Apart from its role in plasmid maintenance, the protein has been suggested to function in several other pathways. Friborg *et al.* (1999) showed that LANA can bind p53, and that cells transfected with LANA displayed reduced activation of p53-dependent reporter genes and increased resistance to p53-dependent programmed cell death triggered by several stimuli. Such an activity could serve to extend the lifespan of a B-cell, though it seems unlikely (by itself) to be able to account for the B-cell proliferation that characterizes PEL. Although direct tests of this have not been carried out in primary B cells, LANA expression can extend the survival of cultured primary endothelial cells, but it does not fully immortalize them (Watanabe et al., 2003). Similarly, we have found that LANA overexpression in Tg mice in several non-lymphoid lineages does not induce either hyperplasia or neoplasia (Grundhoff and Ganem, unpublished data). However, abrogation of p53 activity may produce more dramatic phenotypes in concert with other viral gene products that affect cell proliferation, like the viral cyclin (see below; and Verschuren et al., 2002).

Another reported activity of LANA is binding to the tumor suppressor Rb (Radkov et al., 2000). While it is unclear what fraction of cellular Rb protein is complexed to LANA, that which is bound is inactivated, as judged by the enhanced activity of E2F reporter genes. LANA can also cooperate in 3T3 cell transformation when coexpressed with activated ras genes, an activity that it shares with other DNA tumor virus oncogenes that inactivate Rb. The significance for PEL of this Rb binding, however, has recently been called into question by the finding that many PEL cell lines display loss of the cyclinD-cdk inhibitor p16INK4a (Platt et al., 2002). Since this protein acts to inhibit cellular cyclind/cdk6 from inactivating Rb, its loss should trigger proliferation – but only in cells with functional Rb. Indeed, PEL cell lines remain sensitive to growth inhibition when p16 INK4a expression is restored by transfection. These results imply that despite expression of LANA, Rb function in PEL cells has not been completely inactivated. The fact that one PEL cell line (BC3) has been identified in which Rb protein is missing altogether (Platt et al., 2002) further sustains this impression. As such, these findings are at variance with what is observed in tumors induced by other DNA tumor viruses that strongly inactivate Rb (Kelley et al., 1995; Wrede et al., 1991); in those cases, lesions in Rb and INK4a loci are very uncommon. The partial inhibition of Rb mediated by LANA may provide a selective advantage early in tumorigenesis, but additional lesions in the pathway appear to be required for full oncogenicity.

Another role for LANA in tumorigenesis stems from recent observations that the protein can interact with GSK-3ß, a kinase that phosphorylates and inactivates ß-catenin by targeting it for ubiquitin-mediated proteolysis (Fujimuro et al., 2003). Binding of GSK-3ß relocates the kinase from the cytosol to the nucleus, allowing cellular accumulation of ß-catenin protein, which can then oligomerize with the transcription factor LEF and turn on a proliferative program of gene expression that includes cyclin D, c- myc, and c-jun. In fact, PEL cells display ß-catenin upregulation, and this can be impaired by siRNAs directed against KSHV LANA (Fujimuro et al, 2003). Although the consequences of this for PEL cell growth and survival have not been determined, transient LANA expression in other cell types is associated with enhanced S-phase entry, consistent with the idea that the ß-catenin pathway could be important in KSHV-induced proliferation. And certainly, many other types of cancer are linked to dysregulation of the ß-catenin pathway, including tumors of the colon, esophagus, breast and uterus (Polakis, 2000).

In addition to its effects on ß-catenin/LEF, LANA also can act more directly on the program of host gene expression. Early studies of expression profiling in stably-transfected B cells indicated that many host genes are dysregulated by LANA expression, both positively and negatively (Renne et al., 1996) – though such experiments do not distinguish direct from indirect effects. Other experiments suggest that LANA's principal direct transcriptional activity is repression – for example, LANA will extinguish transcription of reporter genes linked in cis to TR elements containing LANA binding sites; similarly, when LANA is tethered to the DNA binding domain of Gal4, it can repress transcription of GAL4-dependent reporters (Krithivas et al., 2000; Schwam et al., 2000; Garber et al., 2002). This effect is due in part to the recruitment of the mSin3 co-repressor complex via binding to the protein SAP30 (Krithivas et al., 2000). However, it remains unclear how this activity is related – if at all- to oncogenesis (It could, for example, have more to do with the maintenance of viral latency or to the modulation of KSHV chromatin structure.) Similar statements apply to the many other activities described for LANA – such as binding to the nuclear matrix, the bromodomain-containing RING3 protein, me-CpG binding protein 2, heterochromatin protein 1, and various components of the transcription apparatus (Viejo-Borbolla et al., 2003; Platt et al., 1999; Mattsson et al., 2002; Krithivas et al., 2002; Lim et al., 2001, 2003)

v-cyclin

Cotranscribed with LANA from the major latency promoter is a viral homologue of cellular cyclin D. This protein, v-cyclin, is expressed principally from a spliced mRNA from which the upstream LANA gene has been removed (Dittmer et al., 1998; Sarid et al., 1999). V-cyclin is a fully functional cyclin (Chang et al., 1996) in that it can bind to and activate cdk6 (though unlike cellular cyclin D family members, it is much less active on cdk4). The in vitro substrate specificity of v-cyclin/cdk 6 differs substantially from that of host cyclinD/cdk6; allthough both can phosphorylate Rb, the viral cyclin can also trigger cdk6 phosphrylation of p27, histone H1, Id-2 and cdc25a (Godden-Kent et al., 1997; Li et al., 1997). Forced v-cyclin expression can induce S-phase entry in quiescent 3T3 cells, and also overcome an Rb-mediated growth arrest induced by cdk-inhibitors in cultured cells (Swanton et al., 1997). In fact, the v-cyc/cdk6 complex is less sensitive to inhibition by cdk inhibitors like p27, p21 and p16. For p27, at least, this resistance is further accentuated by the fact that the p27 protein is targeted for degradation by dint of its phosphorylation by v-ccylin/cdk6 (Mann et al., 1999; Ellis et al., 1999).

These activities suggest that v-cyclin might promote cellular proliferation in vivo. However, it has been difficult to document such a role for this gene in viral tumorigenesis in vivo, and the study of gene expression in primary PEL tumors turns up numerous discrepancies with the picture painted by studies of v-cyclin biochemistry. For example, despite the fact that v-cyclin expression destabilizes p27 in cultured cells, PEL tumors routinely display abundant p27 expression (Carbone et al., 2000). And the fact that many PEL tumors delete p16INK4a suggests that despite the action of v-cyclin, Rb function is not fully abrogated in latently infected B-cells; further mutational lesions must accumulate in this pathway for full transformation. What v-cyclin does in the economy of the cell prior to the advent of such mutations remains the province of inference, extrapolation, and analogy.

Compounding the dilemma, we lack many experimental tools that are standardly used to approach such problems in other systems. First, there are no animal models of lymphomagenesis by KSHV in which critical notions about v-cyclin's role could be put to the test – for example, via the study of v-cyclin-deficient mutants. Another impediment has been the difficulty in establishing stable cell lines expressing the protein. This is most likely due to the fact that such cells often undergo apoptosis, particularly if they express elevated levels of cdk6 (Ojala et al., 1999). Such problems are not unexpected: apoptosis often follows overexpression of cellular cyclins, and many viral oncogenes that provoke unscheduled DNA synthesis can similarly induce p53 and trigger programmed cell death. V-cyclin- induced apoptosis is also associated with the inactivation of the antiapoptotic factor bcl2 – which, it turns out, is due to its phosphorylation at the hands of vcyclin/cdk6 (Ojala et al., 2000). It is unclear how this problem is mitigated in vivo, but the low levels of v-cyclin protein accumulation in latency likely represent one viral stratagem for doing so. Alternatively, another viral gene product might nullify this apoptotic effect. In this connection it is of interest that Verschuren et al. (2002) have shown that in cultured cells, loss of p53 allowed cells to survive in the presence of elevated levels of v-cyclin. Moreover, when v-cyclin was targeted to the B cell lineage in transgenic mice, lymphomas were observed only when the animals were also p53 -/-. This raises the possibility that the functional inactivation of p53 by LANA expression in KSHV latency (or by v-IRF3; see below) might similarly unmask the oncogenic potential of v-cyclin.

v-FLIP

The third protein encoded by the major latency locus is a viral homologue of the FLICE inhibitory protein, v-FLIP. Transcribed from the same promoter as LANA and v-cyclin, vFLIP is the downstream gene in the spliced, bicstronic mRNA from which v-cyclin is expressed. The failure of attempts to identify moncistronic vFLIP transcripts led to the recognition that an IRES element is embedded within v-cyclin coding sequences (Bieleski and Talbot, 2001; Grundhoff and Ganem, 2001; Low et al., 2001). This implies that both the v-cyclin and LANA mRNAs could template vFLIP translation, though the greater abundance of cyclin mRNA makes it the predominant vFLIP message.

FLIPs as a class are thought to bind adaptor proteins (TRADD and FADD) of the Fas/TNFR signaling pathway via their death effector domains (DEDs) (Thome et al., 1997). This binding impairs the recruitment and activation of caspase 8, leading to blockade of a caspase activation cascade that results in programmed cell death; procaspase 8 can also be directly bound and inhibited. Several other herpesviruses encode v-FLIPs that have been shown to employ this mechanism (Thome et al., 1997). Some papers report that KSHV v-FLIP can function in this fashion (Djerbi et al., 1999, Belanger et al., 2001). However, several laboratories have failed to confirm these findings, and other reports suggest that KSHV v-FLIP can also block cell death via induction of the anti-apoptotic transcription factor NFkB (Chaudhary et al., 1999). vFLIP can be detected in PEL cells complexed with NEMO (or IKKγ) (Liu et al., 2002; Field et al., 2003). This complex activates IKK, leading to phosphorylation of IkB and release of active NFkB. These findings are particularly provocative in view of the observations that (i) PEL cells display high levels of NFkB activity, inhibition of which triggers enhanced cell death (Keller et al., 2000); and (ii) that siRNA-mediated inhibition of v-FLIP in PEL cell lines provokes apoptosis (Guasparri et al., 2004; Godfrey et al., 2005). It thus appears that the major role of v-FLIP in PEL latency in the activation of an anti-apoptotic program, principally through upregulation of NFkB activity. However, KSHV vFLIP also binds to TRAF2 and RIP upstream of IKK, and TRAF binding also results in JNK activation (An et al., 2003) – the roles of these activation events in cell proliferation and survival are not yet understood. Very recently, it has been reported that forced overexpression of KSHV vFLIP in rodent fibroblasts results in classical transformation – growth in soft agar and tumorigenesis in nude mice (Sun et al., 2003). These studies raise the possibility that deregulated vFLIP could contribute to an active proliferative program rather than simply extending cell survival. However, such inferences must be made with caution, since (i) the levels of vFLIP in PEL cells are likely much lower than those achieved in these studies, and (ii) the transforming function of vFLIP occurs in the context of antecedent immortalization, and in cells of heterologous species and cell type.

Finally, other studies (Brown et al., 2003) suggest an additional role for NFkB activation by v-FLIP in KSHV biology. Activation of NFkB inhibits lytic cycle gene expression, and inhibition of NFkB activation promotes lytic reactivation. This implies that apart from its role in cell survival, V-FLIP-mediated NfkB activation may be important for maintaining stable KSHV latency.

K10.5/v-IRF3/LANA2

The KSHV genome harbors at least four genes that encode members of the IRF (interferon regulatory factor) transcription factor family. IRFs are a family of cellular transcription factors, several members of which (esp. IRF3 and IRF 7) are centrally involved in the transcriptional activation of type I interferons – hence their name (Barnes et al., 2002). The KSHV IRF homologues (generically termed v-IRFs) are clustered together in one region of the viral chromosome, suggesting that they arose by duplication of one or more ancestral gene(s) presumably derived from the host genome. Most of the vIRFs are lytic proteins, but one, v-IRF3 (encoded by ORF K10.5), encodes a nuclear protein expressed in latency (Rivas et al., 2001; Lubyova and Pitha, 2000). (For this reason it has also been dubbed LANA-2.) Unlike the LANA/v-cyclin/v-FLIP locus, the vIRF3 gene is not expressed in all latently infected cell types in vivo. Its products are found primarily in latently infected B cells, including PEL cells and cells from MCD, but not in KS spindle cells (Rivas et al., 2001). Like several of its sister vIRFs, vIRF3 expression in mouse fibroblasts inhibits the IRF3/7-mediated induction of the IFN-A4 promoter and impairs the ability of these cells to support IFN induction in response to RNA virus infection – suggesting that vIRF3 can function like a dominant-negative (DN) IRF mutant (Lubyova and Pitha, 2000). However, more recent results in human cells have disputed this simple conclusion, suggesting instead that vIRF3 can actually enhance the binding of IRFs 3 and 7 to the IFN promoters and upregulate IFN release (Lubyova et al., 2003); if so, it is difficult to understand the biological rationale for such an activity, especially since IFNs can be growth-inhibitory in some settings. Easier to relate to the biology of KSHV latency is the observation that vIRF3 protein can also bind and inactivate p53 (Rivas et al., 2001); this activity would be expected to contribute to lifespan prolongation in KSHV-infected B cells, particularly in the context of v-cyclin expression (Verschuren et al., 2002). All of these notions, however, remain to be explicitly tested.

Kaposin

The kaposin locus was initially identified in a screen for genes that are transcibed in uninduced PEL cell cultures (Zhong et al., 1996). In situ hybridization using probes for kaposin mRNA revealed that it is expressed in both uninduced BCBL-1 cells (at a low level) and in variable levels in KS spindle cells lacking markers of lytic reactivation (Staskus et al., 1997; Sturzl et al., 1997). Thus, kaposin transcripts behave as latent mRNAs that, like the LANA/vcyclin/vFLIP mRNAs, can be expressed in both lymphoid and endothelial cells. Recent work from several laboratories has mapped these latent mRNAs and identified their promoter (Li et al., 2002; Pearce et al., 2005; Cai and Cullen, 2006). A second promoter in the kaposin locus is strongly induced during lytic replication (Sadler et al., 1999), owing to the presence of at least one high-affinity binding site for the lytic switch protein RTA (Chang et al., 2002; Song et al., 2003)

Kaposin mRNA encodes at least three proteins via differential initiation of translation (Fig. 56.3(a)) (Sadler et al., 1999). The 3 end of kaposin mRNA bears the coding sequences of ORFK12, initiation at whose AUG directs the synthesis of a 60aa hydrophobic polypeptide known as kaposin A. The protein is found on both the cell surface and on intracellular membranes (Tomkowicz et al., 2002). Interest in this protein was heightened when it was shown that its overexpression in immortalized rodent fibroblasts can trigger morphologic transformation in vitro and tumorigenesis in vivo (Muralidhar et al., 1998). Subsequently it was found that kaposin A can bind cytohesin - 1, a guanine nucleotide exchange factor (GEF) for ARF GTPases and a regulator of integrin-mediated cell adhesion. Binding of kaposin A to cytohesin-1 stimulates GTP binding to ARF1, a process that is implicated in transformation since the transformed phenotype can be reverted by expression of a cytohesin-1 mutant deficient in guanine nucleotide exchange (Kliche et al., 2001). Kaposin A has growth deregulatory potential,

(a)

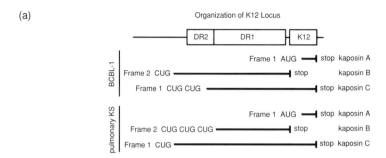

(b)

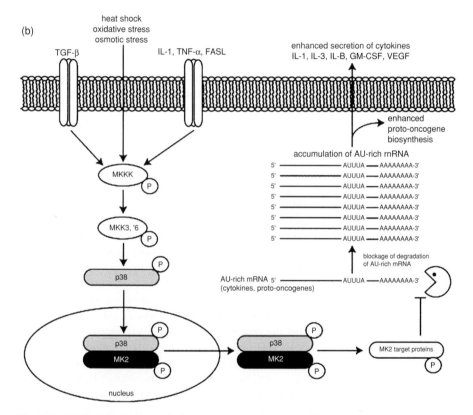

Fig. 56.3. (a) The kaposin locus. Top line, sequence organization of the gene, showing open reading frame (IRF) K12 and the upstream series of tandem direct repeats (DRs) of 23 GC- rich bp. The locus comprises two sets of such Drs(DR1 and DR2) which differ in sequence from each other. Kaposins B and C are derived from translation of the repeats via initiation from CUG codons in different reading frames; kaposin B is encoded solely by the repeats, while kaposin C extends into ORF K12. Sequence differences between different isolates of KSHV result in the production of kaposins B and C from CUGs located at different locations in the locus; shown here to illustrate this is the coding arrangement in KSHV cloned from BCBL-1PEL cells (top), and a primary KS tumor from lung tissue(bottom). (b) Schematic illustration of the p38/MK2 pathway. Activation of p38 via inflammatory or others stresses leads to its nuclear import, where it binds and phoyphorylates MK2 can phosphorylate some nuclear transcription factors. Active MK2-p38 complexes can also be exported from the nucleus to the cytosol, where MK2-p38 complexes can also be exported from the nucleus to the cytosol, where MK@ can phosphorylate additional targets involved in stabilizaton of transcripts bearing AU-rich elements (AREs). Such AREs are typically found in cytokine mRNAs. Kaposin B binds and activates MK2 in a fashion that is independent of upstream inflammatory or oxidative stresses.

especially in cells that have already undergone immortalization. But determination of its role in authentic KSHV tumorigenesis will require examination of its effects in primary cells of lymphoid and endothelial lineage. Such tests should be possible in transgenic mice, though none has yet been reported.

Immediately 5¹ to the K12 open reading frame is a series of tandemly repeated 23-nt GC-rich elements of two families, termed DR (*d*irect *r*epeat) 1 and DR2. Because this region lacks AUG codons, it was initially assumed to be noncoding. However, multiple proteins are produced from this region by initiation at variant CUG codons. (Sadler *et al.*, 1999). One of these, Kaposin B, is encoded predominantly by the repeat sequences; another, kaposin C, expresses the repeats fused in frame to ORF K12, producing a membrane-bound isoform of kaposin B. The functions of kaposins B and C have long been mysterious, but recent findings indicate that they likely function as adapter proteins in signal transduction. Specifically, they bind and activate a kinase, MK2, that is normally a target of p38 phosphorylation (McCormick and Ganem, 2005; Fig 56.3(b) summarizes the key features of the p38-MK2 pathway). The activation mechanism is complex, but appears to require p38, suggesting that kaposin B either increases the sensitivity of MK2 to p38, or decreases the accessibility of p38-phophorylated MK2 to phosphatase action. One result of this activation is the stabilization of mRNAs bearing AU-rich elements in their 3 UTRs (See Fig 56.3(b))– an important result, since such elements are found primarily in the highly regulated transcripts of key cytokines (e.g. IL1,3,4,6, TNF, GM-CSF), growth factors (VEGF) and oncogenes (c-myc). PEL cells are known to produce abundant cytokines (notably IL6, vIL6 and IL10) and many PEL lines are dependent upon one or more of these factors for cell growth or survival in vitro (Aoki *et al.*, 2000; Jones *et al.*, 1999). Cytokines and growth factors also play important roles in KS pathogenesis (see below), and it is likely that kaposin contributes to their production in this disease as well. It is important to point out, however, that post-transcriptional regulation by kaposin is not likely to be the sole modulator of cytokine and growth factor expression in KSHV infection – many of these genes may be controlled transcriptionally as well, by both viral and host factors (see, for example, An *et al.*, 2002).

Latent KSHV miRNAs

Recently it has become clear that in addition to the aforementioned coding RNAs, the latency program of KSHV also generates up to 12 micro RNAs (miRNAs) (Pfeffer *et al.*, 2005; Cai *et al.*, 2005; Samols *et al.*, 2005). These miRNAs are derived primarily from the latent kaposin mRNAs, with all but two emanating from intronic regions of the transcripts (Cai and Ciullen, 2006). (The two encoded in the body of the kaposin mRNA could arise from either latent or lytic kaposin RNAs, but they are only weakly induced during lytic replication.) The function(s) of these miRNAs are not known.

Other KSHV genes and PEL

There is general agreement that the aforementioned genes are *bona fide* products of viral latency. However, there is one viral gene with a likely role in PEL that has not been definitively classified as a latent gene – that for the viral homologue of IL6 (v-IL6). In most cultured PEL cells, this gene is very weakly expressed in the absence of chemical inducers of lytic reactivation, and is strongly upregulated by the latter. This has led most to characterize it as a lytic gene (Nicholas *et al.*, 1997; Staskus *et al.*, 1999; Katano *et al.*, 2000); the low-level expression in the absence of inducers has been ascribed to spontaneous lytic reactivation. However, Parravicini *et al.* (2000) observed by immunohistochemistry on PEL biopsies that a small number of cells in the tumor expressed vIL6 in the absence of another marker of lytic reactivation (vIRF1). They have proposed on this basis that some primary PEL tumor cells can express v-IL6 in the absence of lytic reactivation, though this appears not to be the case for most latently infected PEL cells. Interestingly, when cultured PEL are exposed to IFN-γ, they can express vIL6 without activating any other viral gene (Chatterjee *et al.*, 2002); this lends credence to the idea that the gene can sometimes be expressed outside of the lytic cycle. Whether vIL6 is expressed from a small number of lytically infected cells or is coming from an alternative transcriptional program, there is evidence that its action is important in PEL biology. All PEL cells express the gp130 subunit that allows response to vIL6 (Molden *et al.*, 1997), and in cultured PEL lines, growth can be partially inhibited by anti-vIL6 (but not anti-IL6) antibodies (Jones *et al.*, 1999). (More dramatic inhibition is obtained when both human IL10 and vIL6 are inhibited; Jones *et al.*, 1999.) These results suggest that despite their seeming autonomy, PEL cells do respond to autocrine and paracrine signals, and that these signals can emanate from the host as well as the viral genome.

Multicentric Castleman's disease (MCD)

Castleman's disease is a polyclonal lymphoproliferative lesion that occurs in two histologic types. The first, or "plasma cell variant" is characterized by extensive plasma cell proliferation but preservation of the nodal architecture. The second or "hyaline-vascular" type, displays prominent, abnormal germinal centers and marked, aberrant neoangiogenesis. Clinically, Castleman's disease occurs in two forms, a localized form involving only a single node or node cluster; this form is unlinked to KSHV and can be treated with local excision of the involved tissue. The second form, multicentric Castleman's disease (MCD), is an aggressive systemic illness characterized by fever, weight loss, splenomegaly and diffuse lymphadenopathy. MCD occurs at increased frequency in AIDS patients, and in this context is nearly always linked to KSHV infection (Soulier et al., 1995); histologically, these cases are usually of the plasma cell type. However, MCD does occur rarely in HIV-negative subjects; in this context, only 40–50% of cases show KSHV DNA in the lesions (Soulier et al., 1995; Parravicini et al., 1997). Although polyclonal (Du et al., 2001), MCD is an aggressive disease that is often treated with chemotherapeutic drugs just like a lymphoma. In fact, microscopic foci of clonal plasmablastic lymphoma have been reported to arise within foci of MCD (Dupin et al., 2000; Oksenhendler et al., 2002).

The polyclonality of MCD suggests that the process is being driven by paracrine signaling factors to which a large number of B cells can respond. Consistent with this idea, all forms of MCD appear to be associated with the overproduction of IL6, and there are strong reasons to implicate IL6 signaling in disease pathogenesis. First, IL6 is a known inducer of B cell differentiation, proliferation and survival (Horn et al., 2000). Second, IL6 overproduction in mice leads to an MCD-like illness (Brandt et al., 1990). Third, high levels of circulating IL6 correlate with MCD exacerbations (Oksenhendler et al., 2000). And fourth, administration of neutralizing IL6 mAbs to patients with MCD reverses their fever and other systemic symptoms and ameliorates their splenomegaly (Beck et al., 1994), although this finding has been tested primarily in HIV-negative MCD patients, not all of whom are KSHV-positive.

KSHV infection is localized to the B cells of the "mantle zones" surrounding the germinal centers of MCD (Dupin et al., 1999; Parravicini et al., 2000; Katano et al., 2000). Despite the fact that MCD is a polyclonal lesion, all KSHV-positive cells in the lesion bear lambda light chains, usually on IgM (Du et al., 2001) – the origin of this peculiar finding remains unclear. Many of these cells are latently infected, as judged by the presence of LANA staining – from 10–50% of mantle zone cells (typically around 30%) have been reported to be LANA-positive in various series (Dupin et al., 1999; Parravicini et al., 2000; Katano et al., 2000). In addition to KSHV latency, however, MCD also displays abundant lytic infection. From 5–25% of LANA-positive cells in the mantle zone stain for lytic markers – many more than in PEL or KS (Staskus et al., 1999; Katano et al., 2000, Parravicini et al., 2000). These lytically infected cells stain prominently for v-IL6 – an important finding given the suspected role for IL6 signaling in this disease. (Although IL6 and vIL6 differ in their requirement for IL6Rα, both signal via gp130 and thus induce nearly identical signals in recipient cells (Nicholas 2003).) Clinical evidence also links MCD to lytic KSHV replication. MCD typically occurs in patients with high KSHV loads in the PBMC compartment, a manifestation of extensive lytic growth (Oksenhendler et al., 2000, Grandadam et al., 1997, Boivin et al., 2002). In fact, an MCD-like syndrome has even been seen in primary KSHV infection (Oksenhendler et al., 1998), where lytic infection is typically predominant. (It should be emphasized, however, that most primary infections with KSHV are subclinical and do not engender MCD).

The discovery that vIL6 production is prominent in the expression program of MCD is satisfying, especially given its ability to signal along pathways shared by human IL6 (Nicholas, 2003). Nonetheless, it is clear that human IL6 continues to be overproduced even in KSHV-associated MCD (Oksenhendler et al., 2000), and it is difficult to judge the relative contributions of each of these two proteins to the disease state. Most experts assume that vIL6 is predominant, but there is little direct evidence on either side, and it seems likely that both proteins contribute to the disease. The source of human IL6 in KSHV-linked cases is now starting to become clear. One pathologic study shows that h-IL6-positive cells are found mainly within the follicular centers (Parravicini et al., 1997) – a place with few KSHV-positive cells. This suggests that one source is reactive, uninfected B lymphocytes. However, some mantle-zone cells in that study were also positive, and it has recently been found that lytically infected cells produce high levels of cellular IL6 as well as v-IL6 (Glaunsinger and Ganem, 2004b). Given the extensive amount of lytic replication in MCD, and the correlation of this with both disease progression and circulating human IL6 levels, it is reasonable to suspect that these cells are also contributing to the raised steady-state levels of h-IL6.

Kaposi's sarcoma

The choice of the word sarcoma in the naming of KS is unfortunate, for KS resembles classical sarcomas very little, both in terms of its histology and clinical behavior.

Unlike most classical cancers, which arise as a clonal outgrowth of a single cell type, KS lesions are histologically very complex (Regezi et al., 1993a,b). The main proliferating element is the so-called *spindle cell*, so named after its spindle-like shape. Marker studies indicate that this cell is in the endothelial lineage, though there has been controversy over its exact position in this lineage (Herndier and Ganem, 2001). Some evidence favors it being derived from lymphatic rather than blood vessel endothelium (Beckstead et al., 1985), based upon the expression of markers characteristic of lymphatic endothelium such as VEGF-R3, VEGF-C and podoplanin (Weninger et al., 1999; Skobe et al., 1999; Marchio et al., 1999). However, this conclusion is still inferential, and spindle cells within any given lesion can display variability in the expression of markers (Regezi et al., 1993a,b). Moreover, recent studies show that KSHV infection of vascular epithelial cells can reprogram them to express lymphatic markers (Wang et al., 2004; Hong et al., 2004; Carroll et al., 2004). Irrespective of their precise origin, spindle cells clearly represent the main proliferative element in KS. However, they are not the sole element – all KS lesions also contain (i) variable (but substantial) numbers of infiltrating monocytes, T-cells and plasma cells; and (ii) a profusion of aberrant, slit-like neovascular spaces. These neovascular channels, the most distinctive histologic signature of KS, are only partially lined with KSHV-positive cells (Dupin et al., 1999), lack pericyte or smooth muscle accompaniment, and are prone to leakage and rupture. As a result, KS lesions also often display edema and hemorrhage, giving them a grossly purplish or bruise-like appearance. It is thus useful to think of KS as subsuming three formally separable (but probably interdependent) processes – a *proliferative* component (chiefly involving spindle cells), an *inflammatory* component and an *angiogenic* component. As we shall see, KSHV may make different genetic contributions to each of these components of the disease.

KS can occur in several tissues, but is most commonly localized to the skin, especially in the lower extremities in classical, HIV-negative forms of the disease. In the skin, it involves the dermis, with sparing of the overlying epidermis (Parravicini et al., 2000). Cutaneous involvement, while potentially disfiguring, is not life-threatening. Dermal KS begins as a so-called *patch* lesion, in which spindle cells are clearly demonstrable but are not necessarily the dominant element of the lesion. Inflammatory cells and neovascular elements are prominent at this stage, which can somewhat resemble granulation tissue. Subsequently, the accumulation of spindle cells becomes more apparent, as the lesion progresses through a plaque-like stage to the *nodular* stage, in which masses of spindle cells generate macroscopically visible nodules or masses.

As noted above, the clinical behavior of KS in immunocompetent adult hosts is very indolent- cutaneous KS is typically a disease which people die *with* but not *of*. In fact, spontaneous remissions of classical KS, while not common, are well-documented (However, in immunocompromised hosts – and in young children in KSHV-endemic regions – KS can be more aggressive, involving lymphoreticular structures, the GI tract and the lung.) This indolent behavior suggests that KS is a proliferative state that is on the cusp between the benign and the malignant. Consistent with this inference, analysis of KS clonality has shown that many KS lesions are oligo- or polyclonal (Judde et al., 2000; Gill et al., 1998; Delabesse et al., 1997). While this conclusion has been disputed by some (Rabkin et al., 1997), their own analyses showed evidence of non-clonality in numerous tumors. The heated controversy surrounding KS clonality is misplaced. The pathogenetically important finding is that many macroscopic KS lesions have evidence of oligo- or polyclonality – not that *all* of them do. In any polyclonal process, it is expected that, in some cases, some clones will fare better than others. The instructive feature of the studies of clonality in KS is how different they are from similar studies of classical cancers like breast or colon cancer – in which exceptions to monoclonality are almost never found.

The cell biology of the spindle cell also supports the view that KS is at a (somewhat indistinct) border between hyperplasia and neoplasia. KS spindle cells, unlike many tumor cells, remain highly dependent upon exogenous growth signals when cultured in vitro. Gallo, Ensoli and their colleagues were the first to find methods to reproducibly grow KS spindle cells in culture, and found them to be dependent upon the cytokine-rich conditioned medium of activated T-cells (Caveat: after in vitro culture, the cells produced in this fashion generally lose the viral genome; see below.) (Ensoli et al., 1989, 2001; Miles et al., 1990; Ensoli and Sturzl, 1998). Nor do they display genetic instability, another hallmark of traditional cancers: KS spindle cells are generally diploid, and classical KS lesions do not display microsatellite instability, though some advanced AIDS-KS lesions do (Bedi et al., 1995). Spindle cells also lack classical findings associated with transformation – they do not form foci, grow in soft agar or form tumors in nude mice. However, an interesting phenotype is observed when the cells are injected subcutaneously in nude mice (Salahuddin et al., 1988). They do not grow, but survive for a brief interval – during which slit-like new vessels *of murine origin* appear in the surrounding tissue. When the human implant involutes, these vessels likewise disappear. This suggests a model for KS that involves a complicated paracrine minuet between several partners. In this model, spindle cells require growth factors from their microenvironment (perhaps from infiltrating inflammatory cells) for their proliferation, but also seem to produce angiogenic (and proinflammatory?) substances to recruit the other components of the lesion. In this view, none of the partners in this process is fully autonomous; each depends upon the other (Ensoli and Sturzl, 1998). If correct, this is a very different biology than most classical cancers – so it should not surprise us if the viral contributions to its pathogenesis turn out to differ from those of classical DNA tumor viruses.

KSHV and KS: the big picture

The epidemiology of KSHV strongly points to a critical role for this infection in KS pathogenesis – KSHV DNA is always found in KS tumors, irrespective of whether they derive from classical or AIDS-related KS (Chang et al., 1994; Moore and Chang 1995; Huang et al., 1995; Schulz 1999). At the population level, KSHV infection tracks strongly with KS risk – the prevalence of infection is high in groups in which KS is frequent, and low in those in which it is rare (Kedes et al., 1996; Gao et al., 1996). This statement applies both to risk groups within the USA and to populations around the globe (Schulz, 1999). At the level of individual HIV-infected patients, infection with KSHV preceeds the onset of KS (Moore et al., 1996a,b) and predicts an elevated risk of KS tumorigenesis (Martin et al., 1998).These data, which in the aggregate derive from the study of thousands of subjects, strongly indicate that KSHV infection is the *sine qua non* of KS – without it, clinical KS does not occur. But to say it is necessary for KS development is not to say it is sufficient – indeed, there is strong evidence that it is not. First of all, 2%–7% of the US population has serologic evidence of infection (Schulz, 1999), yet most of these individuals have no measurable risk of developing KS. This indicates that cofactors are clearly required for tumorigenesis. In AIDS-related KS, that cofactor is clearly HIV infection – a fact that is strongly supported by (i) the dramatic reduction in KS incidence that has accompanied reduction of HIV viremia via antiretroviral therapy (Portsmouth et al., 2003; Gates and Kaplan 2002); and (ii) the remission of clinical KS in patients treated with HAART alone (Lebbe et al., 1998; Cattelan et al., 2001; Gill et al., 2002). HIV-1 infection predisposes to KS much more strongly than does HIV-2 infection (Ariyoshi et al., 1998). How HIV infection promotes KS development is still actively debated. Several in vitro studies have suggested that HIV infection can augment KSHV replication in both cell-autonomous and paracrine fashions (Harrington et al., 1997; Varthavaki et al., 1999, 2002; Huang et al., 2001). Secreted HIV tat protein has also been proposed as a growth factor for KS spindle cells, again on the basis of experiments in cultured cells (for review see Barillari and Ensoli, 2002). However, the in vivo importance of these observations remains to be proven. Cell-autonomous mechanisms of KSHV activation, for example, require that cells be dually infected with both HIV and KSHV – which is exceedingly rare in vivo (Staskus et al., 1997). (This caveat does not apply to paracrine mechanisms of activation). The fact that KS is strongly augmented by therapeutic immunosuppression (e.g., with cyclosporin) makes it likely that T cell depletion by HIV is also centrally involved in the amplification of KS risk, e.g., due to the inability to contain KSHV replication.

The identity of the cofactor(s) in classical KS remain unknown. Their characterization is the last remaining Great Unsolved Problem in the human biology of KS, Unfortunately, though – and in marked contrast to AIDS-KS (Beral et al., 1990) – the epidemiology of classical KS has not proffered strong clues to their identity. There are hints, however, that host genetic factors may play a role. Such hints derive from the identification of populations that have a low risk of classical KS despite a high prevalence of KSHV infection. In one such group (Ethiopians), even after the supervention of AIDS KS developed at a 12-fold lower rate than in other AIDS-afflicted groups (Grossman et al., 2002). In such populations whatever host factors are modulating KS risk, they must operate post the acquisition of KSHV.

KSHV gene expression in KS

As noted above, KSHV DNA is present in all KS tumors, irrespective of clinical type or disease stage. Within the tumor, KSHV specifically targets the spindle cell compartment (Boshoff et al., 1995; Staskus et al., 1997; Dupin et al., 1999), with little or no infection of other cell types. (One report suggests that monocytes in the lesions may be infected (Blasig et al., 1997), but this has not been confirmed in other studies (Parravicini et al., 2000; Staskus et al., 1997.) Using known latency genes (as defined by their pattern of expression in PEL cell lines) as probes in *in situ* hybridization studies, it was shown that most KS spindle cells are latently infected; however, a small subpopulation (1%–2%) express markers of lytic infection (Staskus et al., 1997; Dupin et al., 1999; Sturzl et al., 1997, Katano et al., 2000). Several groups have enumerated the latency genes expressed in KS spindle cells in vivo, using immunohistochemistry or *in situ* hybridization on KS biopsies. In general, all of the genes discussed previously in PEL latency are expressed in latently infected spindle cells, save for v-IRF3 (LANA 2) (Rivas et al., 2001). Careful studies (Katano et al.,

2000; Parravicini et al., 2000) also show that, in KS, v-IL6 is produced only in the minor subset of cells that is truly in the lytic cycle – here, there is no suggestion that KS cells can express this gene outside of the lytic cycle.

The discovery that most spindle cells display latent infection is in accord with herpesviral dogma that the latency program drives tumor formation. Consistent with this, examination of early (patch) lesions of KS shows that only 10–30% of spindle-like cells are LANA-positive (Dupin et al., 1999), while in later lesions virtually all such cells are latently infected (Staskus et al., 1997; Dupin et al., 1999). This clearly implies that latently infected cells have a growth (or survival) advantage in vivo. And certainly, many of the in vitro properties of the latency genes are commensurate with this inference. Examples include: the inhibition of p53 and the partial abrogation of Rb by LANA, the induction of NFkB by v-FLIP, the stimulation of cdk6 by v-cyclin, the potentiation of growth deregulation by kaposin A and the upregulation of ß-catenin by LANA. All of these activites could contribute to endothelial cell survival and proliferation, and, as noted earlier, LANA expression can indeed prolong the lifespan of primary endothelial cells in culture (Watanabe et al., 2003). But since most of these activities were discovered in experiments involving overexpression of individual viral proteins in heterologous cell types that were already immortalized, their contributions to the in vivo biology of KS remain to be defined.

Another experimental perspective on this issue comes from examination of cells infected with authentic KSHV. When KSHV virions are applied to most established cell lines, a latent infection results that appears to have no phenotypic consequences (Viera et al., 2001; Lagunoff et al., 2002; Bechtel et al., 2003). However, when KSHV is used to infect *primary endothelial cells*, the situation is dramatically different. In the early days of the culture, there is dramatic lytic replication and fairly efficient spread of infection through the monolayer (Ciufo et al., 2001; Gao et al., 2003; C. Grossman and DG, unpublished data). By 10–14 days, the entire culture is LANA –positive, with most cells being latently infected. These cells also display a dramatic elongation to a spindle morphology (Fig. 56.4) that is remarkably similar to that seen in KS tumors in vivo (Fig. 56.4). Importantly, however, in most experimenters' hands the cells are not immortalized (Gao et al., 2003, Tang et al., 2003; Grossman et al., 2006), though there is one dissenting report (Flore et al., 1998). While they may undergo some prolongation of lifespan, KSHV-infected endothelial cells are not capable of indefinite proliferation – at least not in conventional culture media. The cells fail to grow in soft agar, and no reports of tumorigenesis by KSHV-bearing cells in nude mice have yet appeared. While these results could simply reflect the inadequacy of current culture conditions, they certainly suggest that, at a minimum, the KSHV latency program is much less potent than that of EBV in cell immortalization. This, in turn, raises questions as to whether this more subtle latency phenotype is sufficient to drive KS pathogenesis all by itself.

In fact, independent evidence from clinical studies suggests that lytic replication as well as latency also plays a pivotal role in KS development. Martin et al. (1999) showed that in patients with advanced AIDS, addition of parenteral ganciclovir – a drug that blocks lytic but not latent KSHV infection – resulted in a prompt and dramatic decline in the incidence of new KS tumors. This is a powerful and interesting result because most of these patients have carried HIV and KSHV for many years – therefore, the impact of GCV is not likely to be due simply to the reduction of early dissemination to target cells. Rather, it appears that ongoing lytic replication is continuously necessary throughout the entire natural history of KSHV infection in order to support lesion formation. Consistent with this, patients with KS typically have high levels of KSHV DNA in the circulation (Whitby et al., 1995; Campbell et al., 2000; Quinlivan et al., 2002; Cannon et al., 2003a,b, Engels et al., 2003) – just as do patients with MCD, another disease in which lytic KSHV replication is thought to play an important role.

How might lytic replication contribute to KS tumor development? Here I outline three non-exclusive possibilities. The first derives from the observation that latent KSHV infection is not immortalizing. If spindle cells cannot grow indefinitely, then in order for a tumor mass to expand, KSHV-positive cells that die must be replaced by new latently infected cells. The most obvious source of such cells would be from *de novo* infection of endothelia with virus produced by lytic replication. The second model derives from recent observations of Grundhoff and Ganem (2004), who showed that when cells newly latently infected with KSHV are placed under conditions of rapid proliferation, they rapidly segregate the viral genome. With continued passage, at least in some lines, rare subpopulations can emerge in which latent infection has been stabilized. In such cells, the KSHV genome can be maintained indefinitely as an autonomous episomal replicon – just as it is in PEL cells in vivo. Examination of these rare, stably latent subclones reveals that *cis*-acting, epigenetic changes in the viral chromosome are responsible for stabilization (though the biochemical nature of these epigenetic changes is still unknown). Two lines of evidence support the relevance of these observations to the in vivo situation. First, exactly the same phenomena are observed in primary endothelial cells, which reproduce the main features of KS spindle cell biology (Grundhoff and Ganem, 2004). More importantly,

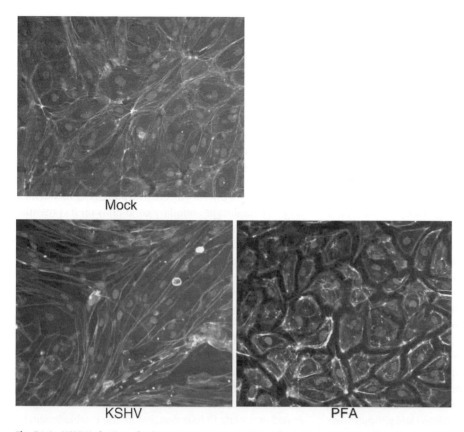

Fig. 56.4. KSHV infection of culture primary endothelial cells results in morphologic changes resembling spindling in vivo. Primary blood endothelial cells were mock infected(top) or infected with KSHV (botttom left); three weeks later, following spread of virus through the culture, the culture was 100% latently infected. Cells were then stained with phalloidin; note extensive spindling of the infected culture.Bottom right: cells were infected with KSHV and immediately carried in Phosphonofomate (PFA), an inhibitor of KSHV replication that blocks spread throught the culture; this blocks widespread establishment of latency and spindling.

when infected KS spindle cells are explanted directly from clinical specimens and placed under conditions favoring their proliferation, they too rapidly – and invariably – segregate their viral episomes (Flamand *et al.*, 1996; Aluigi *et al.*, 1996; Dictor *et al.*, 1996). This instability may be one explanation for the relative clinical indolence of KS, since cells that proliferate aggressively will likely lose their latent infection – and with it their virally endowed growth advantage. Second, it offers another reason why lytic replication is continuously required for KS development – namely, to restore latent infection to spindle cells that have lost their KSHV genomes (or recruit other cells to latency to replace those lost from the latent pool via episome segregation).

The third manner in which lytic KSHV replication may contribute to KS pathogenesis harkens back to the fact that KS is an amalgam of three processes: proliferation, inflammation and angiogensis. Since lytically infected cells die, they cannot contribute importantly to the proliferative component of the disease. However, if lytically infected cells produce paracrine signaling molecules, they could promote both the inflammatory and angiogenic components of the lesion. In fact, examination of the KSHV genome (Russo *et al.*, 1996; Nicholas *et al.*, 1997; Nicholas, 2003) reveals numerous viral genes whose products are secreted signaling molecules – many of which are homoloues of cellular cytokines or chemokines. And interestingly, the majority of these are expressed in the lytic cycle – examples include the three viral CC chemokines and v-IL6. Several of the viral chemokines have been shown to be chemotactic for both Th2 cells (Sozzani *et al.*, 1998; Stine *et al.*, 2000) and endothelial cells (Haque *et al.*, 2001). The former observation suggests that these chemokines may blunt antiviral (and anti-tumor) Th1 responses by favoring Th2 polarization of the local antiviral response – consistent with this, one of these (vCCL2) was shown to extend the survival of cardiac allografts in rodents, in part by impairing CTL infiltration (DeBruyne *et al.*, 2000). The activity on endothelial chemotaxis raises the possibility that KS lesions may be able to recruit more endothelial targets for infection. Endothelial chemotaxis may also relate to observations that application of several viral chemokines to chick chorioallantoic membranes stimulates angiogensis (Boshoff et al., 1997; Stine et al., 2000), though it is also possible that angiogenesis in these models is due to substances released from inflammatory cells recruited by the chemokines). Another lytic protein, v-IL6, in addition to its known roles in B-cell survival, differentiation and proliferation, has also been suggested to affect local angiogenesis (Aoki et al., 1999), perhaps via induction of VEGF production. Recent studies also indicate that vIL6 signaling can block STAT2 phosphorylation by type I IFN signaling, inhibiting both their growth-arresting potential and also their antiviral action (Chatterjee et al., 2002).

Another viral signaling molecule about which much has been written is the viral GPCR homologue (v-GPCR), a member of the chemokine receptor subfamily of the seven transmembrane G protein coupled receptors (Cesarman et al., 1996). Expression of this protein also is restricted to the lytic cycle (Kirshner et al., 1999; Chiou et al., 2002). The protein displays constitutive signaling activity when expressed in the absence of known ligands, though its activity can be further upregulated by chemokines like GRO-α (Arvanitakis et al., 1997; Gershengorn et al., 1998). The resulting singaling activates the MAPK, PI3-kinase and p38 pathways (Sodhi et al., 2000; Smit et al., 2002), as well as activating NFkB activity (Schwarz and Murphy, 2001), and at least in 3T3 cells can stimulate cell proliferation (Bais et al., 1998). In keeping with this broad signaling activity, many host genes are upregulated in response to vGPCR expression in transfected cells (Polson et al., 2002). Among these is VEGF (Bais et al., 1998; Sodhi et al., 2000), a major mediator of angiogenesis and vascular permeability – and a molecule long suspected of a pathogenetic role in KS based on the prominence of neovascularity and edema in affected tissues. In keeping with these in vitro findings, expression of vGPCR in several different cell lineages in transgenic mice produces focal angioproliferative lesions that share some features with KS (Yang et al., 2000; Guo et al., 2003; Montaner et al., 2003). Because this single viral gene product can be linked to both proliferation and angiogenesis, it is seductive to imagine that it is the key player in KS pathogenesis (Montaner et al., 2003).

Several complicating facts, however, must be reckoned with. First, vGPCR is a lytic cycle gene, and there is no evidence that it is expressed in the majority of proliferating, latently infected KS spindle cells (caveat: for a powerful signaling molecule like this, levels below those detectable by in situ hybridization could still be biologically important). If its expression is restricted to lytic infection, then several conclusions follow. First, its cell-autonomous, pro-mitotic activity is likely to be nullified by the direct cytotoxicity resulting from the lytic cycle. Second, it has recently been found that KSHV lytic replication results in a strong block to de novo host gene expression, mediated primarily by virus-induced host mRNA degradation (Glaunsinger and Ganem, 2004a,b). Indeed, in lytically infected endothelial cells in culture, very few of the genes upregulated by vGPCR transfection were found to be expressed – although a limited and transient induction of VEGF-C was observed (Glaunsinger and Ganem, 2004b). It is to be emphasized that these results do not negate a role for vGPCR in KS pathogenesis, but they do place important boundary conditions on its potential roles. For vGPCR to play a role in the proliferative component of the tumor, it will have to be shown that the gene can be expressed outside of the traditional lytic cycle – if not in canonical latency, then in response to some extracellular signal or milieu. While this has not yet been observed, it is not without precedent – recall, for example, that in response to IFN-γ, vIL6 can be expressed by KSHV-positive cells in the absence of any other lyic gene expression (Chatterjee et al., 2002). Even if vGPCR is only expressed in lytic replication, it could still contribute to the angiogenic component of KS, since while the block to host expression is strong, it is not absolute–low levels of host transcripts can still be generated very early in infection, before the establishment of the shutoff. But given the attenuation of its ability to induce VEGF and other genes in this context, it would be predicted that substantial lytic replication would be required to generate KS risk. Interestingly, this is exactly what is observed in vivo – patients with KS generally have very high circulating KSHV loads (Whitby et al., 1995; Campbell et al., 2000; Quinlivan et al., 2002; Cannon et al., 2003a,b, Engels et al., 2003).

Conclusions

The pathogenesis of KSHV-related neoplasms reprises many of the themes struck by other models of herpesviral oncogenesis, but also elaborates variations on them and, more importantly, mandates consideration of entirely new ones. Chief among the latter is the apparent dependence of KS (and likely MCD as well) on continued operation of the lytic cycle. If current notions about this are correct, they have an important potential clinical corollary – namely, that treatment with drugs that block lytic KSHV replication would not only prevent KS development but could potentially arrest or even reverse established KS lesions. Putting this notion into practice, however, may not be simple, as we have no accurate idea of the duration for which such therapy would need to be administered. This would be expected to depend upon the lifespan of latently infected cells, the frequency with which episomes are segregated in vivo, the levels of KSHV production, and the efficiency of *de novo* infection/reinfection – all factors of which we have little quantitative understanding. Therefore, treatment duration will have to be determined empirically, and is almost certain to be many months. This, in turn, will require therapies that are safe, non-toxic and orally bioavailable. Whether currently available drugs meet these criteria is debatable, and less toxic and expensive drugs may well be required. If such can be found, however, it would allow this notion to be put to its definitive test in a clinical trial.

REFERENCES

Aluigi, M. G., Albini, A., Carlone, S. *et al.* (1996). KSHV sequences in biopsies and cultured spindle cells of epidemic, iatrogenic and Mediterranean forms of Kaposi's sarcoma. *Res. Virol.*, **147**(5), 267–275.

An, J., Lichtenstein, A. K., Brent, G., and Rettig, M. B. (2002). The Kaposi sarcoma-associated herpesvirus (KSHV) induces cellular interleukin 6 expression: role of the KSHV latency-associated nuclear antigen and the AP1 response element. *Blood*, **99**(2), 649–654.

An, J., Sun, Y., Sun, R., and Rettig M. B. (2003). Kaposi's sarcoma-associated herpesvirus encoded vFLIP induces cellular IL-6 expression: the role of the NF-kappaB and JNK/AP1 pathways. *Oncogene*, **22**(22), 3371–3385.

Aoki, Y., Jaffe, E. S., Chang, Y. *et al.* (1999). Angiogenesis and hematopoiesis induced by Kaposi's sarcoma-associated herpesvirus-encoded interleukin-6. *Blood*, **93**(12), 4034–4043.

Aoki, Y., Yarchoan, R., Braun, J., Iwamoto, A., and Tosato, G. (2000). Viral and cellular cytokines in AIDS-related malignant lymphomatous effusions. *Blood*, **96**(4), 1599–1601.

Ariyoshi, K., Schim van der Loeff, M., Cook, P. *et al.* (1998). Kaposi's sarcoma in the Gambia, West Africa is less frequent in human immunodeficiency virus type 2 than in human immunodeficiency virus type 1 infection despite a high prevalence of human herpesvirus 8. *J. Hum. Virol.*, **1**(3), 193–199.

Arvanitakis, L., Geras-Raaka, E., Varma, A., Gershengorn, M. C., and Cesarman, E. (1997). Human herpesvirus KSHV encodes a constitutively active G-protein- coupled receptor linked to cell proliferation. *Nature*, **385**, 347–350.

Asou, H., Said, J. W., Yang, R. *et al.* (1998). Mechanisms of growth control of Kaposi's sarcoma-associated herpes virus-associated primary effusion lymphoma cells. *Blood*, **91**, 2475–2481.

Bais, C., Santomasso, B. Coso, O. *et al.* (1998). G-protein-coupled receptor of Kaposi's sarcoma-associated herpesvirus is a viral oncogene and angiogenesis activator. *Nature*, **391**, 86–89.

Ballestas, M. E. and Kaye, K. M. (2001). Kaposi's sarcoma-associated herpesvirus latency-associated nuclear antigen 1 mediates episome persistence through cis-acting terminal repeat (TR) sequence and specifically binds TR DNA. *J. Virol.*, **75**(7), 3250–3258.

Ballestas, M. E., Chatis, P. A., and Kaye, K. M. (1999). Efficient persistence of extrachromosomal KSHV DNA mediated by latency-associated nuclear antigen. *Science*, **284**(5414), 641–644.

Barillari, G. and Ensoli, B. (2002). Angiogenic effects of extracellular human immunodeficiency virus type 1 Tat protein and its role in the pathogenesis of AIDS-associated Kaposi's sarcoma. *Clin. Microbiol. Rev.*, **15**(2), 310–326.

Barnes, B., Lubyova, B., and Pitha, P. M. (2002). On the role of IRF in host defense. *J. Interferon Cytokine Res.*, **22**(1), 59–71.

Bechtel, J. T., Liang, Y., Hvidding, J., and Ganem, D. (2003). Host range of Kaposi's sarcoma-associated herpesvirus in cultured cells. *J. Virol.*, **77**, 6474–6481.

Beck, J. T., Hsu, S. M., Wijdenes, J. *et al.* (1994). Brief report: alleviation of systemic manifestations of Castleman's disease by monoclonal anti-interleukin-6 antibody. *N. Engl. J. Med.*, **330**, 602–605.

Beckstead, J. H., Wood, G. S., and Fletcher, V. (1985). Evidence for the origin of Kaposi's sarcoma from lymphatic endothelium. *Am. J. Pathol.*, **119**(2), 294–300.

Bedi, G. C., Westra, W. H., Farzadegan, H., Pitha, P. M., and Sidransky, D. (1995). Microsatellite instability in primary neoplasms from HIV+ patients. *Nat. Med.*, **1**, 65–68.

Belanger, C., Gravel, A., Tomoiu, A. *et al.* (2001). Human herpesvirus 8 viral FLICE-inhibitory protein inhibits Fas-mediated apoptosis through binding and prevention of procaspase-8 maturation. *J. Hum. Virol.*, **4**, 62–73.

Beral, V., Peterman, T. A., Berkelman, R. L., and Jaffe, H. W. (1990). Kaposi's sarcoma among persons with AIDS: a sexually transmitted infection? [see comments]. *Lancet*, **335**, 123–128.

Bieleski, L. and Talbot, S. J. (2001). Kaposi's sarcoma-associated herpesvirus vCyclin open reading frame contains an internal ribosome entry site. *J. Virol.*, **75**(4), 1864–1869.

Blasig, C., Zietz, C., Haar, B. *et al.* (1997). Monocytes in Kaposi's sarcoma lesions are productively infected by human herpesvirus 8. *J. Virol.*, **71**(10), 7963–7968.

Boivin, G., Cote, S., Cloutier, N., Abed, Y., Maguigad, M., and Routy J. P. (2002). Quantification of human herpesvirus 8 by real-time PCR in blood fractions of AIDS patients with Kaposi's sarcoma and multicentric Castleman's disease. *J. Med. Virol.*, **68**(3), 399–403.

Boshoff, C., Schulz, T. F., Kennedy, M. M. *et al.* (1995). Kaposi's sarcoma-associated herpesvirus infects endothelial and spindle cells. *Nat. Med.*, **1**, 1274–1278.

Boshoff, C., Endo, Y., Collins, P. D. *et al.* (1997). Angiogenic and HIV-inhibitory functions of KSHV-encoded chemokines. *Science*, **278**, 290–294.

Brandt, S. J., Bodine, D. M., Dunbar, C. E., and Nienhuis, A. W. (1990). Dysregulated interleukin 6 expression produces a syndrome resembling Castleman's disease in mice. *J. Clin. Invest.* **86**, 592–599.

Brown, H. J., Song, M. J., Deng, H., Wu, T. T., Cheng, G., and Sun, R. (2003). NF-kappaB inhibits gammaherpesvirus lytic replication. *J. Virol.*, **77**(15), 8532–8540.

Cai, X and Cullen, B. R. (2006). Transcriptional origin of Kaposi's sarcoma-associated herpesvirus microRNAs. *J. Virol.*, **80**(50):2234–2242.

Cai, X., Lu, S., Zhang, Z., Gonzalez, C.M., Damania, B., and Cullen B.R. (2005). Kaposi's sarcoma-associated herpesvirus expresses an array of viral microRNAs in latently infected cells. *Proc. Natl Acad. Sci.*, **102**, 5570–5575.

Campbell, T. B., Borok, M., Gwanzura, L. *et al.* (2000). Relationship of human herpesvirus 8 peripheral blood virus load and Kaposi's sarcoma clinical stage. *AIDS*, **14**(14), 2109–2116.

Cannon, M., Philpott, N. J., and Cesarman, E. (2003a). The Kaposi's sarcoma-associated herpesvirus G protein-coupled receptor has broad signaling effects in primary effusion lymphoma cells. *J. Virol.*, **77**, 57–67.

Cannon, M. J., Dollard, S. C. Black, J. B. *et al.* (2003b). Risk factors for Kaposi's sarcoma in men seropositive for both human herpesvirus 8 and human immunodeficiency virus. *AIDS* **17**, 215–222.

Capello, D, Gaidano, G., Gallicchio, M. *et al.* (2000). The tyrosine kinase receptor met and its ligand HGF are co-expressed and functionally active in HHV8-positive primary effusion lymphoma. *Leukemia* **14**, 285–291.

Carbone, A., Gloghini, A., Bontempo, D. *et al.* (2000). Proliferation in HHV8-positive primary effusion lymphomas is associated with expression of HHV8 cyclin but independent of p27kip1. *Am. J. Pathol.*, **156**, 1209–1215.

Carbone, A., Gloghini, A., Capello, D., and Gaidano, G. (2001). Genetic pathways and histogenetic models of AIDS-related lymphomas. *Eur. J. Cancer*, **37**(10), 1270–1275.

Carroll, P. A., Brezeau, E., and Lagunoff, M. (2004). Kaposi's sarcoma-associated herpesvirus infection of blood endothelial cells induces lymphatic differentiation. *Virology*, **328**(1), 7–18.

Cattelan, A. M., Calabro, M. L., Gasperini, P. *et al.* (2001). Acquired immunodeficiency syndrome-related Kaposi's sarcoma regression after highly active antiretroviral therapy: biologic correlates of clinical outcome. *J. Natl Cancer Inst. Monogr.*, **28**, 44–49.

Cesarman, E., Chang, Y., Moore, P. S., Said, J. W., and Knowles, D. M. (1995). Kaposi's sarcoma-associated herpesvirus-like DNA sequences in AIDS- related body-cavity-based lymphomas. *N. Engl. J. Med.*, **332**, 1186–1191.

Cesarman, E., Nador, R. G., Bai, F. *et al.* (1996). Kaposi's sarcoma-associated herpesvirus contains G protein-coupled receptor and cyclin D homologs which are expressed in Kaposi's sarcoma and malignant lymphoma. *J. Virol.*, **70**(11), 8218–8223.

Cesarman, E., Mesri, E. A., and Gershengorn, M. C. (2000). Viral G protein-coupled receptor and Kaposi's sarcoma: a model of paracrine neoplasia? *J. Exp. Med.* **191**, 417–422.

Chang, P. J., Shedd, D., Gradoville, L. *et al.* (2002). Open reading frame 50 protein of Kaposi's sarcoma-associated herpesvirus directly activates the viral PAN and K12 genes by binding to related response elements. *J. Virol.*, **76**(7), 3168–3178.

Chang, Y., Cesarman, E., Pessin, M. S. *et al.* (1994). Identification of herpesvirus-like DNA sequences in AIDS-associated Kaposi's sarcoma. *Science*, **266**, 1865–1869.

Chang, Y., Moore, P. S., Talbot, S. J. *et al.* (1996). Cyclin encoded by KS herpesvirus. *Nature*, **382**(6590), 410–411.

Chatterjee, M., Osborne, J., Bestetti, G., Chang, Y., and Moore, P. S. (2002). Viral IL-6-induced cell proliferation and immune evasion of interferon activity. *Science*, **298**, 1432–1435.

Chaudhary, P. M., Jasmin, A., Eby, M. T., and Hood, L. (1999). Modulation of the NF-B pathway by virally encoded death effector domains-containing proteins. *Oncogene*, **18**, 5738–5746.

Chiou, C. J., Poole, L. J., Kim, P. S. *et al.* (2002). Patterns of gene expression and a transactivation function exhibited by the vGCR (ORF74) chemokine receptor protein of Kaposi's sarcoma- associated herpesvirus. *J. Virol.*, **76**, 3421–3439.

Ciufo, D. M., Cannon, J. S., Poole, L. J. *et al.* (2001). Spindle cell conversion by Kaposi's sarcoma-associated herpesvirus: formation of colonies and plaques with mixed lytic and latent gene expression in infected primary dermal microvascular endothelial cell cultures. *J. Virol.*, **75**(12), 5614–5626.

Cotter, M. A., 2nd and Robertson, E. S. (1999). The latency-associated nuclear antigen tethers the Kaposi's sarcoma- associated herpesvirus genome to host chromosomes in body cavity-based lymphoma cells. *Virology*, **264**(2), 254–264.

Cotter, M. A., 2nd, Subramanian, C., and Robertson E. S. (2001). The Kaposi's sarcoma-associated herpesvirus latency-associated nuclear antigen binds to specific sequences at the left end of the viral genome through its carboxy-terminus. *Virology*, **291**(2), 241–259.

Davis, M. A., Sturzl, M. A., Blasig, C. *et al.* (1997). Expression of human herpesvirus 8-encoded cyclin D in Kaposi's sarcoma spindle cells [see comments]. *J. Natl Cancer Inst.*, **89**, 1868–1874.

DeBruyne, L. A., Li, K., Bishop, D. K., and Bromberg, J. S. (2000). Gene transfer of virally encoded chemokine antagonists vMIP-II and MC148 prolongs cardiac allograft survival and inhibits donor-specific immunity. *Gene Ther.*, **7**(7), 575–582.

Delabesse, E., Oksenhendler, E., Lebbe, C., Verola, O., Varet, B., and Turhan A.G. (1997). Molecular analysis of clonality in Kaposi's sarcoma. *J. Clin. Pathol.*, **50**(8), 664–668.

Delecluse, H. J., Kost, M., Feederle, R., Wilson, L., and Hammerschmidt, W. (2001). Spontaneous activation of the lytic cycle in cells infected with a recombinant Kaposi's sarcoma-associated virus. *J. Virol.*, **75**(6), 2921–2928.

Deng, H., Chu, J. T., Rettig, M. B., Martinez-Maza, O., and Sun, R. (2002). Rta of the human herpesvirus 8/Kaposi sarcoma-associated herpesvirus up-regulates human interleukin-6 gene expression. *Blood*, **100**, 1919–1921.

Dictor, M., Rambech, E., Way, D., Witte, M., and Bendsoe, N. (1996). Human herpesvirus 8 (Kaposi's sarcoma-associated herpesvirus) DNA in Kaposi's sarcoma lesions, AIDS Kaposi's sarcoma cell lines, endothelial Kaposi's sarcoma simulators, and the skin of immunosuppressed patients. *Am. J. Pathol.*, **148**(6), 2009–2016.

Dittmer, D., Lagunoff, M., Renne, R., Staskus, K., Haase, A., and Ganem, D. (1998). A cluster of latently expressed genes in

Kaposi's sarcoma-associated herpesvirus. *J. Virol.*, **72**, 8309–8315.

Djerbi, M., Screpanti, V., Catrina, A. I., Bogen, B., Biberfeld, P., and Grandien, A. (1999). The inhibitor of death receptor signaling, FLICE-inhibitory protein defines a new class of tumor progression factors. *J. Exp. Med.*, **190**, 1025–1032.

Du, M.Q., Liu, H., Diss, T.C. *et al.* (2001). Kaposi sarcoma-associated herpesvirus infects monotypic (IgM lambda) but polyclonal naive B cells in Castleman disease and associated lymphoproliferative disorders. Blood, **97**(7), 2130–2136.

Dupin, N., Fisher, C., Kellam, P. *et al.* (1999). Distribution of human herpesvirus-8 latently infected cells in Kaposi's sarcoma, multicentric Castleman's disease, and primary effusion lymphoma. *Proc. Natl Acad. Sci. USA*, **96**, 4546–4551.

Dupin, N., Diss, T. L., Kellam, P. *et al.* (2000). HHV-8 is associated with a plasmablastic variant of Castleman's disease that is linked to HHV8-positive plasmablastic lymphoma. *Blood*, **95**, 1406–1412.

Ellis, M., Chew, Y. P., Fallis, L. *et al.* (1999). Degradation of p27(Kip) cdk inhibitor triggered by Kaposi's sarcoma virus cyclin–cdk6 complex. *EMBO J.*, 18: 644–653.

Engels, E. A., Biggar, R. J., Marshall, V. A. *et al.* (2003). Detection and quantification of Kaposi's sarcoma-associated herpesvirus to predict AIDS-associated Kaposi's sarcoma. *AIDS*, **17**(12), 1847–1851.

Ensoli, B. and Sturzl, M. (1998). Kaposi's sarcoma: a result of the interplay among inflammatory cytokines, angiogenic factors and viral agents. *Cytokine Growth Factor Rev.*, **9**(1), 63–83.

Ensoli, B., Nakamura, S., Salahuddin, S. Z. *et al.* (1989). AIDS-Kaposi's sarcoma-derived cells express cytokines with autocrine and paracrine growth effects. *Science*, **243**, 223–226.

Ensoli, B., Sgadari, C., Barillari, G., Sirianni, M. C., Sturzl, M., and Monini, P. (2001). Biology of Kaposi's sarcoma. *Eur. J. Cancer*, **37**, 1251–1269.

Field, N., Low, W., Daniels, M. *et al.* (2003). KSHV vFLIP binds to IKK-gamma to activate IKK. *J. Cell Sci.*, **116**(18), 3721–3728.

Flamand, L., Zeman, R.A., Bryant, J.L., Lunardi-Iskandar, Y., and Gallo, R.C. (1996). Absence of human herpesvirus 8 DNA sequences in neoplastic Kaposi's sarcoma cell lines. *J. Acquir. Immune Defic. Syndr. Hum. Retrovirol.*, **13**(2), 194–197.

Flore, O., Rafii, S., Ely, S., O'Leary, J. J., Hyjek, E. M., and Cesarman, E. (1998). Transformation of primary human endothelial cells by Kaposi's sarcoma-associated herpesvirus. *Nature*, **394**, 588–592.

Friborg, J., Jr., Kong, W., Hottiger, M.O., and Nabel, G.J. (1999). p53 inhibition by the LANA protein of KSHV protects against cell death. *Nature*, **402**(6764), 889–894.

Fujimuro, M., Wu, F.Y., ApRhys, C. et al. (2003). A novel viral mechanism for dysregulation of beta-catenin in Kaposi's sarcoma-associated herpesvirus latency. *Nat. Med.*, **9**(3), 300–306.

Gaidano, G, Capello, D., Cilia, A. M. *et al.* (1999). Genetic characterisation of HHV8/KSHV-positive primary effusion lymphoma reveal frequent mutations of BCL6: impliations for disease pathogenesis and histogenesis. *Genes Chromosomes Cancer*, **24**, 16–23.

Gao, S. J., Kingsley, L., Li, M. *et al.* (1996). KSHV antibodies among Americans, Italians and Ugandans with and without Kaposi's sarcoma. *Nat. Med.*, **2**, 925–928.

Gao, S.J., Deng, J.H., and Zhou, F.C. (2003) Productive lytic replication of a recombinant Kaposi's sarcoma-associated herpesvirus in efficient primary infection of primary human endothelial cells. *J. Virol.*, **77**(18), 9738–9749.

Garber, A.C., Shu, M.A., Hu, J., and Renne, R. (2001). DNA binding and modulation of gene expression by the latency-associated nuclear antigen of Kaposi's sarcoma-associated herpesvirus. *J. Virol.*, **75**(17), 7882–7892.

Garber, A.C., Hu, J., and Renne, R. (2002). Latency-associated nuclear antigen (LANA) cooperatively binds to two sites within the terminal repeat, and both sites contribute to the ability of LANA to suppress transcription and to facilitate DNA replication. *J. Biol. Chem.*, **277**(30), 27401–27411.

Gates, A.E., and Kaplan, L.D. (2002). AIDS malignancies in the era of highly active antiretroviral therapy. *Oncology (Huntingt)*, **16**(5), 657–665.

Gershengorn, M. C., Geras-Raaka, E., Varma, A., and Clark-Lewis, I. (1998). Chemokines activate Kaposi's sarcoma-associated herpesvirus G protein- coupled receptor in mammalian cells in culture. *J. Clin. Invest.*, **102**, 1469–1472.

Gill, J., Bourboulia, D., Wilkinson, J. *et al.* (2002). Prospective study of the effects of antiretroviral therapy on Kaposi sarcoma–associated herpesvirus infection in patients with and without Kaposi sarcoma. *J. Acquir. Immune Defic. Syndr.*, **31**(4), 384–390.

Gill, P.S., Tsai, Y.C., Rao, A.P. *et al.* (1998). Evidence for multiclonality in multicentric Kaposi's sarcoma. *Proc Natl Acad. Sci. USA*, **95**(14), 8257–8261.

Glaunsinger, B. and Ganem, D. (2004). Lytic KSHV infection inhibits host gene expression by accelerating global mRNA turnover. *Molec. Cell.*, **13**, 713–723.

Glaunsinger, B. and Ganem, D. (2004). Highly selective escape from Kaposi's sarcoma associated herpesvirus-mediated most shut-off: implications for the pathogenesis of Kaposi's sarcoma. *J. Exp. Med.*, **200**, 391–398.

Godden-Kent, D., Talbot, S., Boshoff, C. *et al.* (1997). The cyclin encoded by Kaposi's sarcoma-associated herpesvirus stimulates cdk6 to phosphorylate the retinoblastoma protein and histone H1. *J. Virol.*, **71**, 4193–4198.

Godfrey, A., Anderson, J., Papanastasiou A., Takeuchi Y., Boshoff C. (2005). Inhibiting primary effusion lymphoma by lentiviral vectors encoding short hairpin RNA. *Blood*, **105**(6), 2510–2518.

Grandadam, N. Dupin, N., Calvez, V. *et al.* (1997). Exacerbations of clinical symptoms in human immunodeficiency virus type 1-infected patients with multicentric Castleman's disease are associated with a high increase in Kaposi's sarcoma herpesvirus DNA load in peripheral blood mononuclear cells. *J. Infect. Dis.*, **175** 1198–1201.

Green, I., Espiritu, E., Ladanyi, M. *et al.* (1995). Primary lymphomatous effusions in AIDS: A morphological, immunophenotypic, and molecular study. *Modern Pathol.* **8**, 39.

Grossman, Z., Iscovich, J., Schwartz, F. et al. (2002). Absence of Kaposi sarcoma among Ethiopian immigrants to Israel despite high seroprevalence of human herpesvirus 8. *Mayo Clin Proc.*, **77**(9), 905–909.

Grossman, C., Podogrobskina, S., Skobe, M., and Ganem, D. (2006). Activation of NF-κB by the latent v-FLIP gene of KSHV is required for the spindle shape of virus-infected endothelial cells and contributes to their proinflammatory phenotype *J. Virol.*, **80**(14), 7179–7185.

Grundhoff, A. and Ganem, D. (2001). Mechanisms governing expression of the v-FLIP gene of Kaposi's sarcoma-associated herpesvirus. *J. Virol.*, **75**(4), 1857–1863.

Grundhoff, A, and Ganem, D. (2003). The latency-associated nuclear antigen of Kaposi's sarcoma-associated herpesvirus (KSHV) permits replication of terminal repeat-containing plasmids. *J. Virol.*, **77**, 2779–2783.

Grundhoff, A. and Ganem, D. (2004) The inefficient establishment of KSHV latency suggests an additional role for lytic viral replication in KS pathogenesis. *J. Clin. Invest.* **113**, 124–136.

Grundhoff, A., Sullivan, C., and Ganem, D. (2006). A combined computational and microarray-based approach identifies novel microRNAs encoded by human gamma-herpesviruses. *RNA*, **12**, 733–750.

Guasparri, I., Keller, S. A., and Cesarman, E. (2004). KSHV vFLIP is essential for the survival of infected lymphoma cells. *J. Exp. Med.*, **199**(7), 993–1003.

Guo, H. G., Sadowska, M., Reid, W., Tschachler, E., Hayward, G., and Reitz, M. (2003). Kaposi's sarcoma-like tumors in a human herpesvirus 8 ORF74 transgenic mouse. *J. Virol.*, **77**, 2631–2639.

Haque, N.S., Fallon, J.T., Taubman, M.B., and Harpel, P.C. (2001). The chemokine receptor CCR8 mediates human endothelial cell chemotaxis induced by I-309 and Kaposi sarcoma herpesvirus-encoded vMIP-I and by lipoprotein(a)-stimulated endothelial cell conditioned medium. *Blood*, **97**(1), 39–45.

Harrington, W. Jr, Sieczkowski, L., Sosa, C. et al. (1997). Activation of HHV-8 by HIV-1 tat. *Lancet*, **349**(9054), 774–775.

Herndier B. and Ganem, D. (2001). The biology of Kaposi's sarcoma. *Cancer Treat. Res.*, **104**, 89–126.

Hong, Y. K., Foreman, K., Shin, J. W. et al. (2004). Lymphatic reprogramming of blood vascular endothelium by Kaposi sarcoma-associated herpesvirus. *Nat. Genet.*, **36**(7):683–685.

Horenstein, M.G., Nador, R.G., Chadburn, A. *et al.* (1997). Epstein–Barr virus latent gene expression in primary effusion lymphomas containing Kaposi's sarcoma-associated herpesvirus/human herpesvirus-8. *Blood*, **90**(3), 1186–1191.

Horn, F., Henze, C., and Heidrich, K. (2000). Interleukin-6 signal transduction and lymphocyte function. *Immunobiology*, **202**(2), 151–167.

Hu, J., Garber, A.C., and Renne, R. (2002) The latency-associated nuclear antigen of Kaposi's sarcoma-associated herpesvirus supports latent DNA replication in dividing cells. *J. Virol.*, **76**(22), 11677–11687.

Huang, L.M., Chao, M.F., Chen, M.Y. et al. (2001). Reciprocal regulatory interaction between human herpesvirus 8 and human immunodeficiency virus type 1. *J. Biol. Chem.*, **276**(16), 13427–13432.

Huang, Y. Q., Li, J. J., Kaplan, M. H. et al. (1995). Human herpesvirus-like nucleic acid in various forms of Kaposi's sarcoma. *Lancet*, **345**, 759–761.

Jenner, R.G., Maillard, K., Cattini, N. et al. (2003). Kaposi's sarcoma-associated herpesvirus-infected primary effusion lymphoma has a plasma cell gene expression profile. *Proc. Natl Acad Sci USA*, **100**(18), 10399–10404.

Jeong, J.H., Hines-Boykin, R., Ash, J.D., and Dittmer, D.P. (2002). Tissue specificity of the Kaposi's sarcoma-associated herpesvirus latent nuclear antigen (LANA/orf73) promoter in transgenic mice. *J. Virol.*, **76**(21), 11024–11032.

Jones, K.D., Aoki, Y., Chang, Y., Moore, P.S., Yarchoan, R., and Tosato, G. (1999). Involvement of interleukin-10 (IL-10) and viral IL-6 in the spontaneous growth of Kaposi's sarcoma herpesvirus-associated infected primary effusion lymphoma cells. *Blood*, **94**(8), 2871–2879.

Judde, J.G., Lacoste, V., Briere, J. et al. (2000). Monoclonality or oligoclonality of human herpesvirus 8 terminal repeat sequences in Kaposi's sarcoma and other diseases. *J. Natl Cancer Inst.*, **92**(9), 729–736.

Katano, H., Sato, Y., Kurata, T., Mori, S., and Sata, T. (2000). Expression and localization of human herpesvirus 8-encoded proteins in primary effusion lymphoma, Kaposi's sarcoma, and multicentric Castleman's disease. *Virology* **269**, 335–344.

Kedes, D. H., Operskalski, E., Busch, M., Kohn, R., Flood, J., and Ganem, D. (1996). The seroepidemiology of human herpesvirus 8 (Kaposi's sarcoma- associated herpesvirus): distribution of infection in KS risk groups and evidence for sexual transmission. *Nat. Med.* **2**, 918–924.

Keller, S. A., Schattner, E. J., and Cesarman, E. (2000). Inhibition of NF-B induces apoptosis of KSHV-infected primary effusion lymphoma cells. *Blood*, **96**, 2537–2542.

Kelley, M. J., Otterson, G. A., Kaye, F. J., Popescu, N. C., Johnson, B. E., and Dipaolo, J. A. (1995). CDKN2 in HPV-positive and HPV-negative cervical-carcinoma cell lines. *Int. J. Cancer*, **63**(2), 226–230.

Kirshner, J. R., Staskus, K., Haase, A., Lagunoff, M., and Ganem, D. (1999). Expression of the open reading frame 74 (G-protein-coupled receptor) gene of Kaposi's sarcoma (KS)-associated herpesvirus: implications for KS pathogenesis. *J. Virol.*, **73**, 6006–6014.

Kledal, T. N., Rosenkilde, M. M. Coulin, F. et al. (1997). A broad-spectrum chemokine antagonist encoded by Kaposi's sarcoma- associated herpesvirus. *Science*, **277**, 1656–1659.

Klein, U., Gloghini, A., Gaidano, G. et al. (2003). Gene expression profile analysis of AIDS-related primary effusion lymphoma (PEL) suggests a plasmablastic derivation and identifies PEL-specific transcripts. *Blood*, **101**(10), 4115–4121.

Kliche, S., Kremmer, E., Hammerschmidt, W., Koszinowski, U., and Haas, J. (1998). Persistent infection of Epstein-Barr virus-positive B lymphocytes by human herpesvirus 8. *J. Virol.*, **72**(10), 8143–8149.

Kliche, S., Nagel, W., Kremmer, E. et al. (2001). Signaling by human herpesvirus 8 kaposin A through direct membrane recruitment of cytohesin-1. *Mol. Cell.*, **7**(4), 833–843.

Knowles, D. M., Inghirami, G., Ubriaco, A., and Dalla-Favera, R. (1989). Molecular genetic analysis of three AIDS-associated neoplasms of uncertain lineage demonstrates their B-cell derivation and the possible pathogenetic role of the Epstein-Barr virus. *Blood*, **73**, 792.

Krithivas, A., Young, D. B., Liao, G., Greene, D., and Hayward, S. D. (2000). Human herpesvirus 8 LANA interacts with proteins of the mSin3 corepressor complex and negatively regulates Epstein–Barr virus gene expression in dually infected PEL cells. *J. Virol.*, **74**(20), 9637–9645.

Krithivas, A., Fujimuro, M., Weidner, M., Young, D.B., and Hayward, S.D. (2002). Protein interactions targeting the latency-associated nuclear antigen of Kaposi's sarcoma-associated herpesvirus to cell chromosomes. *J. Virol.*, **76**(22), 11596–11604.

Lagunoff, M., Bechtel, J., Venetsanakos, E., *et al.* (2002). De novo infection and serial transmission of Kaposi's sarcoma-associated herpesvirus in cultured endothelial cells. *J. Virol.*, **76**(5), 2440–2448.

Lauta, V.M. (2003) A review of the cytokine network in multiple myeloma: diagnostic, prognostic, and therapeutic implications. *Cancer*, **97**(10), 2440–2452.

Lebbe, C., Blum, L., Pellet, C. *et al.* (1998). Clinical and biological impact of antiretroviral therapy with protease inhibitors on HIV-related Kaposi's sarcoma. *AIDS*, **12**(7), F45–F49.

Leger-Ravet, M. B., Peuchmaur, M., Devergne, O. *et al.* (1991). Interleukin-6 gene expression in Castleman's disease. *Blood*, **78**, 2923–2930.

Li, M., Lee, H., Yoon, D. W. *et al.* (1997). Kaposi's sarcoma-associated herpesvirus encodes a functional cyclin. *J. Virol.*, **71**(3), 1984–1991.

Li, H., Komatsu, T., Dezube, B. J., and Kaye, K. M. (2002). The Kaposi's sarcoma-associated herpesvirus K12 transcript from a primary effusion lymphoma contains complex repeat elements, is spliced, and initiates from a novel promoter. *J. Virol.*, **76**(23), 11880–11888.

Lim, C., Sohn, H., Gwack, Y., and Choe, J. (2000). Latency-associated nuclear antigen of Kaposi's sarcoma-associated herpesvirus (human herpesvirus-8) binds ATF4/CREB2 and inhibits its transcriptional activation activity. *J. Gen. Virol.*, **81**(11), 2645–2652.

Lim, C., Sohn, H., Lee, D., Gwack, Y., and Choe, J. (2002). Functional dissection of latency-associated nuclear antigen 1 of Kaposi's sarcoma-associated herpesvirus involved in latent DNA replication and transcription of terminal repeats of the viral genome. *J. Virol.*, **76**(20), 10320–10331.

Lim, C., Lee, D., Seo, T., Choi, C., and Choe, J. (2003). Latency-associated nuclear antigen of Kaposi's sarcoma-associated herpesvirus functionally interacts with heterochromatin protein 1. *J. Biol. Chem.*, **278**(9), 7397–7405.

Liu, C., Okruzhnov, Y., Li, H., and Nicholas, J. (2001). Human herpesvirus 8 (HHV-8)-encoded cytokines induce expression of and autocrine signaling by vascular endothelial growth factor (VEGF) in HHV-8-infected primary-effusion lymphoma cell lines and mediate VEGF-independent antiapoptotic effects. *J. Virol.*, **75**(22), 10933–10940.

Liu, L., Eby, M. T., Rathore, N., Sinha, S. K., Kumar, A., and Chaudhary, P. M. (2002). The human herpes virus 8-encoded viral FLICE inhibitory protein physically associates with and persistently activates the IB kinase complex. *J. Biol. Chem.*, **277**, 13745–13751.

Low, W., Harries, M., Ye, H., Du, M.Q., Boshoff, C., and Collins, M. (2001). Internal ribosome entry site regulates translation of Kaposi's sarcoma-associated herpesvirus FLICE inhibitory protein. *J. Virol.*, **75**(6), 2938–2945.

Lubyova, B. and Pitha, P.M. (2000). Characterization of a novel human herpesvirus 8-encoded protein, vIRF-3, that shows homology to viral and cellular interferon regulatory factors. *J. Virol.*, **74**(17), 8194–8201.

Lubyova, B., Kellum, M.J., Frisancho, A.J., and Pitha, P.M. (2003). Kaposi's Sarcoma-associated herpesvirus-encoded vIRF-3 stimulates the transcriptional activity of cellular IRF-3 and IRF-7. *J. Biol. Chem.*, Dec 10.

Lukac, D. M., Kirshner, J. R., and Ganem. D. (1999). Transcriptional activation by the product of open reading frame 50 of Kaposi's sarcoma-associated herpesvirus is required for lytic viral reactivation in B cells. *J. Virol.*, **73**, 9348–9361.

McCormick, C. and Ganem, D. (2005). The kaposin B protein of KSHV activates the p38/MK2 pathway and stabilizes cytokine mRNAs. *Science*, **307**, 739–741.

Mann, D. J., Child, E. S., Swanton, C., Laman, H., and Jones, N. (1999). Modulation of p27(Kip1) levels by the cyclin encoded by Kaposi's sarcoma-associated herpesvirus. *EMBO J.*, 18: 654–663.

Marchio, S., Primo, L., Pagano, M. *et al.* (1999). Vascular endothelial growth factor-C stimulates the migration and proliferation of Kaposi's sarcoma cells. *J Biol Chem.*, **274**(39), 27617–27622.

Martin, D. F., Kuppermann, B. D., Wolitz, R. A., Palestine, A. G., Li, H., and Robinson, C. A. (1999). Oral ganciclovir for patients with cytomegalovirus retinitis treated with a ganciclovir implant. Roche Ganciclovir Study Group. *N. Engl. J. Med.*, **340**, 1063–1070.

Martin, J. N., Ganem, D. E., Osmond, D. H., Page-Shafer, K. A., Macrae, D., and Kedes, D.H. (1998). Sexual transmission and the natural history of human herpesvirus 8 infection. *N. Engl. J. Med.*, **338**(14), 948–954.

Mattsson, K., Kiss, C., Platt, G. M. *et al.* (2002). Latent nuclear antigen of Kaposi's sarcoma herpesvirus/human herpesvirus-8 induces and relocates RING3 to nuclear heterochromatin regions. *J. Gen. Virol.*, **83**(1), 179–188.

Miles, S. A., Rezai, A. R., Salazar-Gonzalez, J. F. *et al.* (1990). AIDS Kaposi sarcoma-derived cells produce and respond to interleukin 6. *Proc. Natl Acad. Sci. USA*, **87**, 4068–4072.

Molden, J., Chang, Y., You, Y., Moore, P.S., and Goldsmith, M.A. (1997). A Kaposi's sarcoma-associated herpesvirus-encoded cytokine homolog (vIL-6) activates signaling through the shared gp130 receptor subunit. *J. Biol. Chem.*, **272**(31), 19625–19631.

Montaner, S., Sodhi, A., Molinolo, A. *et al.* (2003). Endothelial infection with KSHV genes in vivo reveals that vGPCR initiates Kaposi's sarcomagenesis and can promote the tumorigenic potential of viral latent genes. *Cancer Cell*, **3**, 23–36.

Moore, P. S. and Chang, Y. (1995). Detection of herpesvirus-like DNA sequences in Kaposi's sarcoma in patients with and without HIV infection. *N. Engl. J. Med.*, **332**, 1181–1185.

Moore, P. S., Boshoff, C., Weiss, R. A., and Chang, Y. (1996a). Molecular mimicry of human cytokine and cytokine response pathway genes by KSHV. *Science*, **274**, 1739–1744.

Moore, P. S., Kingsley, L. A., Holmberg, S. D. *et al.* (1996b). Kaposi's sarcoma-associated herpesvirus infection prior to onset of Kaposi's sarcoma. *AIDS*, **10**, 175–180.

Muralidhar, S., Pumfery, A. M., Hassani, M. *et al.* (1998). Identification of kaposin (ORF K12) as a human herpesvirus 8 (Kaposi's sarcoma associated herpesvirus) transforming gene. *J. Virol.*, **72**, 4980–4988.

Neipel, F., Albrecht, J. C., Ensser, A. *et al.* (1997a). Human herpesvirus 8 encodes a homolog of interleukin-6. *J. Virol.*, **71**, 839–842.

Neipel, F., Albrecht, J. C. and Fleckenstein, B. (1997b). Cell-homologous genes in the Kaposi's sarcoma-associated rhadinovirus human herpesvirus 8: determinants of its pathogenicity? *J. Virol.*, **71**, 4187–4192.

Nicholas, J. (2003). Human herpesvirus-8-encoded signalling ligands and receptors. *J. Biomed. Sci.*, **10**(5), 475–489.

Nicholas, J., Ruvolo, V. R., Burns, W. H. *et al.* (1997). Kaposi's sarcoma-associated human herpesvirus-8 encodes homologues of macrophage inflammatory protein-1 and interleukin-6. *Nat. Med.* 1997; **3**, 287–292.

Ojala, P. M., Tiainen, M., Salven, P. *et al.* (1999). Kaposi's sarcoma-associated herpesvirus-encoded v-cyclin triggers apoptosis in cells with high levels of cyclin-dependent kinase 6. *Cancer Res.*, **59**(19), 4984–4989.

Ojala, P. M., Yamamoto, K., Castanos-Velez, E., Biberfeld, P., Korsmeyer, S. J., and Makela, T.P. (2000). The apoptotic v-cyclin-CDK6 complex phosphorylates and inactivates Bcl-2. *Nat. Cell. Biol.*, **2**(11), 819–825.

Oksenhendler, E., Cazals-Hatem, D., Schulz T. F. *et al.* (1998). Transient angiolymphoid hyperplasia and Kaposi's sarcoma after primary infection with human herpesvirus 8 in a patient with human immunodeficiency virus infection. *N. Engl. J. Med.*, **338**, 1585–1590.

Oksenhendler, E., Carcelain, G., Aoki Y. *et al.* (2000). High levels of human herpesvirus 8 viral load, human interleukin 6, interleukin 10, and c-reactive protein correlate with exacerbation of multicentric Castleman's disease in HIV-infected patients. *Blood*, **96**, 2069–2073.

Oksenhendler, E., Boulanger, E., Galicier, L. *et al.* (2002). High incidence of Kaposi sarcoma-associated herpesvirus-related non-Hodgkin lymphoma in patients with HIV infection and multicentric Castleman disease. *Blood*, **99**(7), 2331–2336.

Parravicini, C., Corbellino, M., Paulli, M., Magrini, U., and Lazzarino, M. (1997). Expression of a virus-derived cytokine, KSHV vIL6, in HIV-seronegative Castleman's disease. *Am. J. Pathol.*, **151**, 1517–1522.

Parravicini, C., Chandran, B., Corbellino M. *et al.* (2000). Differential viral protein expression in Kaposi's sarcoma-associated herpesvirus-infected diseases: Kaposi's sarcoma, primary effusion lymphoma, and multicentric Castleman's disease. *Am. J. Pathol.*, **156**, 743–749.

Pearce, M., Matsumura, S., and Wilson, A. C. (2005). Transcripts encoding K12, v-FLIP, v-cyclin, and the MicroRNA cluster of Kaposi's sarcoma-associated herpesvirus originate from a common promoter. *J. Virol.*, **79**(22), 14457–14454.

Pfeffer, S., Sewer, A., Lagos-Quintana, M., *et al.* (2005). Identification of microRNAs of the herpesvirus family. *Nat. Methods*, **2**(4), 269–276.

Picchio, G. R., Sabbe, R. E., Guliza, R. J., McGrath, M. S., Herndier, B. G., and Mosier, D. E. (1997). The KSHV/HHV8-infected BCBL-1 lymphoma line causes tumors in SCID mice but fails to transmit virus to a human peripheral blood mononuclear cell graft. *Virology*, **238**, 22–29.

Piolot, T., Tramier, M., Coppey, M., Nicolas, J.C., and Marechal, V. (2001). Close but distinct regions of human herpesvirus 8 latency-associated nuclear antigen 1 are responsible for nuclear targeting and binding to human mitotic chromosomes. *J. Virol.*, **75**(8), 3948–3959.

Platt, G., Carbone, A., and Mittnacht, S. (2002). p16INK4a loss and sensitivity in KSHV associated primary effusion lymphoma. *Oncogene*, **21**(12), 1823–1831.

Platt, G.M., Simpson, G.R., Mittnacht, S., and Schulz, T.F. (1999). Latent nuclear antigen of Kaposi's sarcoma-associated herpesvirus interacts with RING3, a homolog of the *Drosophila* female sterile homeotic (fsh) gene. *J. Virol.*, **73**(12), 9789–9795.

Polakis, P. (2000). Wnt signaling and cancer. *Genes Dev.*, **14**, 1837–1851.

Polson, A. G., Wang, D., DeRisi, J., and Ganem, D. (2002). Modulation of host gene expression by the constitutively active G protein-coupled receptor of Kaposi's sarcoma-associated herpesvirus. *Cancer Res.*, **62**, 4525–4530.

Portsmouth, S., Stebbing, J., Gill, J. *et al.* (2003). A comparison of regimens based on non-nucleoside reverse transcriptase inhibitors or protease inhibitors in preventing Kaposi's sarcoma. *AIDS*, **17**(11), F17–F22.

Quinlivan, E.B., Zhang, C., Stewart, P.W., Komoltri, C., Davis, M.G., and Wehbie, R.S. (2002) Elevated virus loads of Kaposi's sarcoma-associated human herpesvirus 8 predict Kaposi's sarcoma disease progression, but elevated levels of human immunodeficiency virus type 1 do not. *J. Infect. Dis.*, **185**(12), 1736–1744.

Rabkin, C., Janz, S., Lash, A. *et al.* (1997). Monoclonal origin of multicentric Kaposi's sarcoma lesions. *N. Engl. J. Med.*, **336**, 988–993.

Radkov, S. A., Kellam, P., and Boshoff, C. (2000). The latent nuclear antigen of Kaposi sarcoma-associated herpesvirus targets the retinoblastoma-E2F pathway and with the oncogene Hras transforms primary rat cells. *Nat. Med.*, **6**(10), 1121–1127.

Regezi, J. A., MacPhail, L.A., Daniels, T.E. *et al.* (1993a). Oral Kaposi's sarcoma: a 10-year retrospective histopathologic study. *J. Oral Pathol. Med.*, **22**(7), 292–297.

Regezi, J.A., MacPhail, L.A., Daniels, T.E., DeSouza, Y.G., Greenspan, J.S., and Greenspan, D. (1993b). Human immunodeficiency virus-associated oral Kaposi's sarcoma. A heterogeneous cell population dominated by spindle-shaped endothelial cells. *Am. J. Pathol.*, **143**(1), 240–249.

Renne, R., Zhong, W., Herndier, B. *et al.* (1996). Lytic growth of Kaposi's sarcoma-associated herpesvirus (human herpesvirus 8) in culture. *Nat. Med.*, **2**, 342–346.

Rivas, C., Thlick, A.E., Parravicini, C., Moore, P.S., and Chang, Y. (2001). Kaposi's sarcoma-associated herpesvirus LANA2 is a B-cell-specific latent viral protein that inhibits p53. *J. Virol.*, **75**(1), 429–438.

Russo, J. J., Bohenzky, R. A., Chien, M. C. *et al.* (1996). Nucleotide sequence of the Kaposi sarcoma-associated herpesvirus (HHV8). *Proc. Natl Acad. Sci. USA*, **93**, 14862–14867.

Sadler, R., Wu, L., Forghani, B. *et al.* (1999). A complex translational program generates multiple novel proteins from the latently expressed kaposin (K12) locus of Kaposi's sarcoma-associated herpesvirus. *J. Virol.*, **73**(7), 5722–5730.

Salahuddin, S.Z., Nakamura, S., Biberfeld, P. *et al.* (1988). Angiogenic properties of Kaposi's sarcoma-derived cells after long-term culture in vitro. *Science*, 1 **242**(4877), 430–433.

Sarid, R., Wiezorek, J. S., Moore, P. S., and Chang Y. (1999). Characterization and cell cycle regulation of the major Kaposi's sarcoma-associated herpesvirus (Human herpesvirus 8) latent genes and their promoter. *J. Virol.*, **73**, 1438–1446.

Samols, M. A., Hu J., Skalsky R. L., and Renne, R. (2005). Cloning and identification of a microRNA cluster within the latency-asssociated region of Kaposi's sarcoma-associated herpesvirus *J. Virol.*, **79**, 9301–9305.

Schulz, T. F. (1999). Epidemiology of Kaposi's sarcoma-associated herpesvirus/human herpesvirus 8. *Adv. Cancer Res.*, **76**, 121–160.

Schulz, T.F. (2001). KSHV/HHV8-associated lymphoproliferations in the AIDS setting. *Eur. J. Cancer*, **37**(10), 1217–1226.

Schwam, D.R., Luciano, R.L., Mahajan, S.S., Wong L., and Wilson, A.C. (2000). Carboxy terminus of human herpesvirus 8 latency-associated nuclear antigen mediates dimerization, transcriptional repression, and targeting to nuclear bodies. *J. Virol.*, **74**(18), 8532–8540.

Schwarz, M. and Murphy, P. M. (2001). Kaposi's sarcoma-associated herpesvirus G protein-coupled receptor constitutively activates NF-kappa B and induces proinflammatory cytokine and chemokine production via a C-terminal signaling determinant. *J. Immunol.*, **167**, 505–513.

Skobe, M., Brown, L.F., Tognazzi, K. *et al.* (1999). Vascular endothelial growth factor-C (VEGF-C) and its receptors KDR and flt-4 are expressed in AIDS-associated Kaposi's sarcoma *J. Invest. Dermatol.*, **113**(6), 1047–1053.

Smit, M. J., Verzijl, D., Casarosa, P., Navis, M., Timmerman, H., and Leurs, R. (2002). Kaposi's sarcoma-associated herpesvirus-encoded G protein-coupled receptor ORF74 constitutively activates p44/p42 MAPK and Akt via G(i) and phospholipase C-dependent signaling pathways. *J. Virol.*, **76**, 1744–1752.

Sodhi, A., Montaner, S., Patel, V. *et al.* (2000). The Kaposi's sarcoma-associated herpes virus G protein-coupled receptor up-regulates vascular endothelial growth factor expression and secretion through mitogen-activated protein kinase and p38 pathways acting on hypoxia-inducible factor 1alpha. *Cancer Res.*, **60**, 4873–4880.

Song, M.J., Deng, H., and Sun, R. (2003). Comparative study of regulation of RTA-responsive genes in Kaposi's sarcoma-associated herpesvirus/human herpesvirus 8. *J. Virol.*, **77**(17), 9451–9462.

Soulier, J., Grollet, L., Oksenhendler, E. *et al.* (1995). Kaposi's sarcoma-associated herpesvirus-like DNA sequences in multicentric Castleman's disease. *Blood*, **86**, 1276–1280.

Sozzani, S., Luini, W., Bianchi, G. *et al.* (1998). The viral chemokine macrophage inflammatory protein-II is a selective Th2 chemoattractant. *Blood*, **92**(11), 4036–4039.

Staskus, K. A., Zhong, W., Gebhard, K. *et al.* (1997). Kaposi's sarcoma-associated herpesvirus gene expression in endothelial (spindle) tumor cells. *J. Virol.*, **71**, 715–719.

Staskus, K. A., Sun, R., Miller, G. *et al.* (1999). Cellular tropism and viral interleukin-6 expression distinguish human herpesvirus 8 involvement in Kaposi's sarcoma, primary effusion lymphoma, and multicentric Castleman's disease. *J. Virol.*, **73**, 4181–4187.

Stine, J.T., Wood, C., Hill, M. *et al.* (2000). KSHV-encoded CC chemokine vMIP-III is a CCR4 agonist, stimulates angiogenesis, and selectively chemoattracts TH2 cells. *Blood*, **95**(4), 1151–1157.

Sturzl, M., Blasig, C., Schreier, A. *et al.* (1997). Expression of HHV-8 latency-associated T0.7 RNA in spindle cells and endothelial cells of AIDS-associated, classical and African Kaposi's sarcoma. *Int. J. Cancer*, **72**, 68–71.

Sun, Q., Zachariah, S., and Chaudhary, P.M. (2003). The human herpes virus 8-encoded viral FLICE-inhibitory protein induces cellular transformation via NF-{kappa}B activation. *J. Biol. Chem.*, **278**(52), 52437–52445.

Swanton, C., Mann, D. J., Fleckenstein, B., Neipel, F., Peters, G., and Jones, N. (1997). Herpes viral cyclin/Cdk6 complexes evade inhibition by CDK inhibitor proteins. *Nature (Lond.)*, **390**, 184–187.

Szekely, L., Chen, F. Teramoto, N. *et al.* (1998). Restricted expression of Epstein-Barr virus (EBV)-encoded, growth transformation-associated antigens in an EBV- and human herpesvirus type 8-carrying body cavity lymphoma line. *J. Gen. Virol.*, **79**, 1445–1452.

Tang, J., Gordon, G.M., Muller, M.G., Dahiya, M., and Foreman, K.E. (2003). Kaposi's sarcoma-associated herpesvirus latency-associated nuclear antigen induces expression of the helix-loop-helix protein Id-1 in human endothelial cells. *J. Virol.*, **77**(10), 5975–5984.

Thome, M., Schneider, P., Hofmann, K. *et al.* (1997). Viral FLICE-inhibitory proteins (FLIPs) prevent apoptosis induced by death receptors. *Nature*, **386**, 517–521.

Tomkowicz, B., Singh, S. P., Cartas, M., and Srinivasan, A. (2002). Human herpesvirus-8 encoded Kaposin: subcellular localization using immunofluorescence and biochemical approaches. *DNA Cell Biol.*, **21**(3), 151–162.

Varthakavi, V., Browning, P.J., and Spearman P. (1999). Human immunodeficiency virus replication in a primary effusion lymphoma cell line stimulates lytic-phase replication of Kaposi's sarcoma-associated herpesvirus. *J. Virol.*, **73**(12), 10329–10338.

Varthakavi, V., Smith, R.M., Deng, H., Sun, R., and Spearman, P. (2002). Human immunodeficiency virus type-1 activates lytic cycle replication of Kaposi's sarcoma-associated herpesvirus through induction of KSHV Rta. *Virology*, **297**(2), 270–280.

Verschuren, E.W., Klefstrom, J., Evan, G.I., and Jones, N. (2002). The oncogenic potential of Kaposi's sarcoma-associated herpesvirus cyclin is exposed by p53 loss in vitro and in vivo. *Cancer Cell*, **2**(3), 229–241.

Viejo-Borbolla, A., Kati, E., Sheldon, J.A. *et al.* (2003). A domain in the C-terminal region of latency-associated nuclear antigen 1 of Kaposi's sarcoma-associated herpesvirus affects transcriptional activation and binding to nuclear heterochromatin. *J. Virol.*, **77**(12), 7093–7100.

Viera, J., O'Hearn, P., Kimball, L., Chandran, B., and Corey, L. (2001). Activation of Kaposi's sarcoma-associated herpesvirus (human herpesvirus 8) lytic replication by human cytomegalovirus. *J. Virol.*, **75**, 1378–1386.

Wang, H. W., Trotter, M. W., Lagos, D. *et al.* (2004). Kaposi sarcoma herpesvirus-induced cellular reprogramming contributes to the lymphatic endothelial gene expression in Kaposi sarcoma. *Nat. Genet.*, **36**(7), 687–693.

Watanabe, T., Sugaya, M., Atkins, A. M. *et al.* (2003). Kaposi's sarcoma-associated herpesvirus latency-associated nuclear antigen prolongs the life span of primary human umbilical vein endothelial cells. *J. Virol.*, **77**, 6188–6196.

Weninger, W., Partanen, T.A., Breiteneder-Geleff, S. *et al.* (1999). Expression of vascular endothelial growth factor receptor-3 and podoplanin suggests a lymphatic endothelial cell origin of Kaposi's sarcoma tumor cells. *Lab. Invest.*, **79**(2), 243–251.

Whitby, D., Howard, M. R., Tenant-Flowers, M. *et al.* (1995). Detection of Kaposi sarcoma associated herpesvirus in peripheral blood of HIV-infected individuals and progression to Kaposi's sarcoma. *Lancet*, **346**, 799–802.

Wrede, D., Tidy, J.A., Crook, T., Lane, D., and Vousden, K.H. (1991) Expression of RB and p53 proteins in HPV-positive and HPV-negative cervical carcinoma cell lines. *Mol. Carcinog.*, **4**(3), 171–175.

Xu, Y., AuCoin, D. P., Huete, A. R., Cei, S. A., Hanson, L. J., and Pari, G. S. (2005). A Kaposi's sarcoma-associated herpesvirus/human herpesvirus 8 ORF50 deletion mutant is defective for reactivation of latent virus and DNA replication. *J. Virol.*, **79**(6), 3479–3487.

Yang, T. Y., Chen, S. C. Leach, M. W. *et al.* (2000). Transgenic expression of the chemokine receptor encoded by human herpesvirus 8 induces an angioproliferative disease resembling Kaposi's sarcoma. *J. Exp. Med.*, **191**, 445–454.

Zhong, W., Wang, H., Herndier, B., and Ganem, D. (1996). Restricted expression of Kaposi sarcoma-associated herpesvirus (human herpesvirus 8) genes in Kaposi sarcoma. *Proc. Natl Acad. Sci. USA*, **93**, 6641–6646.

Zhou, F. C., Zhang, Y. J., Deng, J. H. *et al.* (2002). Efficient infection by a recombinant Kaposi's sarcoma-associated herpesvirus cloned in a bacterial artificial chromosome: application for genetic analysis. *J. Virol.*, **76**, 6185–6196.

Part IV

Non-human primate herpesviruses

Edited by Ann Arvin, Patrick Moore, and Richard Whitley

57

Monkey B virus

Julia Hilliard

Department of Biology, Georgia State University,
Atlanta, GA, USA

Introduction

B virus (Cercopithecine herpesvirus 1, herpesviridae), an alphaherpesvirus endemic in macaque monkeys, has the unique distinction of being the only one of nearly 35 identified non-human primate herpesviruses that is highly pathogenic in humans. B virus has been positively linked with more than two dozen human deaths since the first report describing it in 1933, five of those in the last 12 years, following exposures involving macaques in during acute B virus infection. B virus, unique among the non-human herpesviruses, is included in this volume because it is distinctively neurotropic and neurovirulent in the foreign human host inadvertently exposed by handling macaque monkeys generally used in biomedical research. Untreated B virus infections in humans result in an extremely high mortality rate (~80%) and, consequently, present unique and potentially lethal challenges for individuals handling macaque monkeys or macaque cells and tissues. Infection in humans is associated with breach of primary skin or mucosal defenses and subsequent contamination of the site with virus from a macaque or cells or tissues harvested from this animal. Fomites, contaminated particulates or surfaces, can serve as source of virus as well. In one case, human-to-human transmission was reported and attributed to a shared tube of medication which resulted in contamination at a broken skin site with cream used to treat another patient's bite wound. Later, the same patient autoinoculated one eye during manipulation of a contact lens. In 28 zoonotic cases occurring during the 1980s and 1990s out a total of 46 documented cases confirmed since 1933, 80% have survived infection with the advent of antiviral therapies in contrast to 80% mortality reported in untreated patients. Timely antiviral intervention is an effective means of reducing B virus-associated morbidity and preventing a fatal outcome.

History

The first case to appear in the medical literature was described as follows. A laboratory worker accidentally bitten by a monkey, apparently recovered from the bite, but immediately afterward fell ill of a febrile disease with progressive symptoms of ascending myelitis and died 15 days after the first symptoms of involvement of the central nervous system (CNS). The gross and histological picture included areas of softening in the mid brain and widely diffuse areas of perivascular lymphocytic infiltration. While the brain of this individual was contaminated with a coliform bacterium, it yielded, on rabbit brain passage, a bacteriologically sterile tissue cell culture isolate that killed rabbits with invariably characteristic neurologic symptoms and also caused an exaggerated skin lesion that was subsequently followed by ascending myelitis and death. The virus present in the brains of these animals was thoroughly compared with known strains of herpes viruses by crossed immunity reactions which will be elsewhere described. This agent produced lethargic encephalitis in Cebus but not in rhesus monkeys.

Gay and Holden (1933) reported an ultrafiltrable agent, similar to herpes simplex virus, recovered from this brain tissue as received from Albert Sabin. They initially designated the isolate "W" virus, noting that it caused similar disease in rabbits infected by either intradermal or intracranial routes, but a rhesus macaque exposed to virus showed no illness. Within a year of these first reports by Gay and Holden, Albert Sabin independently reported an ultrafilterable agent that he identified as "B" virus from tissues of this same index patient, naming the virus by using the initial of the last name of the patient. These studies were expanded with the observation that B virus, deadly in this patient, caused disease strikingly different from HSV. Sabin described the case as follows: in 1932, a young physician

(WB) was bitten by a macaque monkey and later developed localized erythema at the site of the animal bite. This apparent localized infection was followed by lymphangitis, lymphadenitis, and ultimately a transverse myelitis, with the demise of WB ascribed to respiratory failure. At the time of WB's death, tissue specimens were obtained for laboratory investigation.

The virus subsequently has been called B virus, herpes B virus, herpesvirus simiae, or Cercopithecine herpesvirus 1. The lethality of B virus infection in rabbits was described by Sabin (1934) who showed that infectivity was independent of route of inoculation. Experimentally infected dogs, mice, and guinea pigs, on the other hand, showed no susceptibility regardless of route of infection. Both Gay and Holden, as well as Sabin, observed that B virus induced immunological reactions in an infected host similar to HSV-1. The virus was noted also to share similarity with pseudorabies as well as with other viruses, including SA8 and two additional herpes non-human primate alpha-herpesviruses recently described, HPV-2, originally described as SA8 (Simian Agent 8)(Eberle et al., 1995) and Langur herpesvirus (J. Hilliard, unpublished data).

Twelve fatalities were identified by 1959 along with five survivors. Detection of antibodies in humans, in the absence of clinical symptoms but with a history of working with macaques, is unreliable; however, these tests early antibody could not discriminate between antibodies induced by HSV types 1 and 2 vs. B virus. Subsequently, with the development of more precise tests, Freifeld et al. (1995) observed a high risk population ($n = 325$) that antibodies were rarely, if ever, present in the absence of a history of clinical symptoms. Following another fatal case, however, antibodies were found to be present in at least two coworkers and one additional individual with no previous history of HSV 1 or 2 (J. Hilliard, unpublished data). Two of the three reported a significant illness, describing symptoms commensurate with early stages of B virus infection nearly a decade earlier but with full recovery. These observations suggest B virus may reactivate and be responsible for maintenance of high antibody titers long after acute illness; however, there are too few cases to suggest with certainty that B virus reactivates in humans who survive acute disease.

Distribution in nature

All species of macaques appear to serve as the natural hosts of B virus. There are, in general, genotypic differences associated with B virus depending on the species of macaques from which it was isolated. There is an absence of strong evidence to suggest that there is a difference in the pathogenesic mechanisms of these different genotypes when they infect humans. The macaque host is found most often in the Asian wilds, but colonies of these animals have been exported to a number of other regions, for example, the Isle of Mauritius and Gibralter. B virus can also infect humans (1987, 1987, 1989; Benson et al., 1989; Artenstein et al., 1991), as well as other species of monkeys housed next to macaques (Loomis et al., 1981; Wilson et al., 1990). Other vertebrate species can be infected, including other non-human primates, but in such cases the infected animal serves as a foreign host and frequently succumbs to infection. N/P B virus transmission results from direct contact, whether from animal to animal, animal to person, person to person, or contaminated object to animal or person. There has been only one recognized case of human-to-human transmission observed in 1987 (Palmer, 1987; Weigler, 1992; Weigler et al., 1993).

B virus is highly prevalent in host natural performed reservoirs. Estimations of prevalence have been by a variety of investigators and techniques for both wild and captive macaque populations (Shah and Southwick, 1965; DiGiacomo and Shah, 1972; Kessler and Hilliard, 1990; Weigler, 1992; Freifeld et al., 1995; Sato et al., 1998). Transmission of infection correlates with onset of sexual activity, facilitating transmission of the virus among animals within a group (Weigler et al., 1995). Crowding of animals during transportation seems to accelerate the spread of infection within a community (Keeble et al., 1958; Keeble, 1960). A number of captive colonies worldwide are attempting to define and breed macaques free of B virus, but generally, due to the nature of the virus, antibodies are usually the only measure of prior infection. Investigators will be challenged greatly as they try to eliminate a virus that has coevolved with this host for nearly 30 million years!

As would be expected of an alphaherpesvirus infection in the natural host results is frequently associated with mild clinical signs, if any. B virus infection, however, can have serious consequences under certain immunosuppressive conditions, as observed by a number of investigators and reported by Chellman and colleagues (Chellman et al., 1992). Under these conditions, virus shedding from mucosal membranes can be documented easily by virus isolation in cell culture. In most infected animals, persistent, high antibodies throughout the lifetime of the host provide supportive evidence that B virus, as with HSV, reactivates periodically. N/P Virus can be reactivated in vitro (Boulter, 1975; Vizoso, 1975) from ganglia harvested from asymptomatic seropositve animals. In healthy animals, virus reactivation can be documented by recovery of virus from mucosal samples; however, virus is excreted for only short periods of time (Weigler et al., 1993; J. Hilliard, unpublished data). Collectively, these observations are not surprising in view of data derived from other alpha herpes viruses.

The virus

Isolation and growth properties of B virus

In 2003, the Department of Justice listed B virus as a Select Agent when it is outside of the natural host further restricting work with this virus, a potential tactical agent of terrorism. Because the agent is capable of causing death in up to 80% of untreated cases, the Center for Disease Control and Prevention (CDC) has undertaken the responsibility of defining agent summary statements for work performed with B virus. Isolation of virus is recommended in BL-3 containment laboratories while growth and propagation is strictly confined to BL-4 maximum containment facilities. Obviously, early work with this agent was done under far less stringent containment.

As noted, B virus was initially isolated from rabbit brain homogenates following fatal zoonotic infections. Within a decade after its discovery, chorioallantoic membranes or embryonated eggs were used for growth and propagation of B virus. By 1954, B virus was reported isolated from primary rhesus kidney tissue used for polio vaccine production. Virus was also noted to be present in rhesus central nervous system tissue. Shortly thereafter, monkey kidney and chick embryo were found to support in vitro replication of virus. In B cells, virus induces syncytial cells uniquely characteristic of this agent.

Following virus isolation, B virus was found to be relatively stable in cell culture media stored at 4 °C. Long-term storage, however, required −80 °C, not −20 °C. These observations have been important for optimizing recoverability of virus from clinical samples to better understand the agent from both the macaque host and others, including humans.

B virus replicates to high titer in cell lines derived from Old World monkeys, particularly in Vero cells derived from African green monkey and vervet kidney cells. Rabbit kidney cells, BSC-1, and LLC-RK also support replication of B virus. Vero cells are an optimal cell line for isolation of virus from clinical specimens. Infected cells balloon, fusing into polykaryocytes that expand outwardly as more cells become infected. Eosinophilic, intranuclear inclusions (Cowdry type A bodies) are observed following fixation and staining of infected monolayers of cells, but inclusions are neither always observed in infected animals nor in some humans with zoonotic infection. As a result, intranuclear inclusion bodies should not be relied upon as a diagnostic marker. In the event this agent is inadvertently isolated in a BL-2 laboratory, cultures should be sealed and forwarded to a registered specialty laboratory that can handle this select agent safely and in accordance with federal guidelines.

In culture, B virus grows with kinetics similar to HSV (Weigler et al., 1993). Virus particles adsorb to cells, resulting in fusion and virus penetration of susceptible cells with suitable receptors. The nature of the cell receptors will be discussed in further detail later. Early in infection (3–4 hours), virus activity eclipses, but cellular responses can be detected by preliminary microarray analysis within the first hour post infection (Zao et al., unpublished data). Although host cell machinery is halted once virus enters the cell, innate immune responses of the cell post infection work presumably to counteract the virus. This, too, will be discussed in more detail later in this chapter. By 4 hours postinfection, DNA synthesis increases dramatically as does synthesis of polypeptides (Hilliard et al., 1987). Morphogenesis of the the virus is also similar to that of HSV, as shown by electron microscopy studies during the time course of infection (Ruebner et al., 1975). Within 6–10 hours after infection, infectious virions are detectable. By 24–28 hours postinfection, intracellular and extracellular virus levels plateau. Similar to HSV, B virus expresses sequential classes of proteins, i.e., immediate early, early, and late proteins (Hilliard et al., 1987). Homologous glycoproteins, as well as structural proteins, are encoded by the B virus genome (Slomka et al., 1995). Previous studies have characterized the antigenic relatedness of many of these proteins to those from HSV types 1 and 2, and to other non human primate alphaherpesviruses (Eberle et al., 1989; Hilliard et al., 1989).

The B virus genome

Two complete B virus genome sequences derived from cynomologus and rhesus monkeys, respectively (Harrington et al., 1992; Perelygina et al., 2003) have been published along with a number of partial sequence analyses (Bennett et al., 1992; Killeen et al., 1992). The total genome length has been calculated to be 156 789 base pairs for rhesus derived B virus and x bp for cynomolgus derived B virus.

B virus contains a double-stranded DNA genome of approximately 162 kbp. One strain of virus originating from a cynomologus monkey has been mapped and subcloned by Harrington et al. The genome contains two unique regions (Ul and Us) flanked by a pair of inverted repeats, two of which are at the termini and two internally located, an arrangement allowing four sequence-orientation isomeric forms. The overall size of the genome is slightly larger than HSV-1 (152 kbp) and HSV-2 (155 kbp). The guanosine:cytosine content of the DNA was calculated to be 75% based on the buoyant density of viral DNA. Eberle et al. published data which established the presence in B virus of gene homology to HSV-1 and HSV-2, gB, gC, gD, gE, and gG. Further examination of the sequences of the nine major glycoproteins demonstrated that the 75% of the GC content was conserved within most glycoproteins. Harrington et al. showed that the location of genes within the Ul regions of HSV and B virus were collinear; one gene rearrangement was described in an isolate which originated in a cynomolgus macaque. Homologues of HSV Us9 and Us10 genes were noted to be located upstream of the Us glycoprotein gene cluster in contrast to the downstream location of these genes in HSV Us region. This rearrangement was affirmed according to hybridization data and the proposed physical map of Harrington et al. Sequence analysis (unpublished) of the prototype strain (E2490) which originated from a rhesus macaque, however, illustrates that B virus DNA is colinear in these same regions with the HSV-1 genomic arrangement (L. Perelygina et al., 2000, unpublished data).

To date, sequences for only a few B virus genes have been submitted to GeneBank, i.e., homologues of gB, gD, gC, gG, gJ, and gI, largely covering the sequence of the Us region. Nonetheless, with a number of laboratories engaged in the sequencing of this virus, the majority of the genome sequence will be accomplished likely within a short time. Each of the glycoproteins for which sequence information is available, except gG, has about 50% identity with HSV, slightly higher for HSV-2 than HSV-1. B virus gG is a homologue of HSV-2 gG and is closer in size to gG-2 (699 kbp) than gG-1 (238 kbp). Glycoprotein sequences demonstrated that all cysteines are conserved as are the majority of glycosylation sites. This conservation suggests that B virus glycoproteins have similar secondary structure to that characterized in HSV. Sequence analyses from these laboratories also suggest that B virus and HSV types 1 and 2 probably evolved from a common ancestor. Using restriction length polymorphisms (RLPs), as a guide, several investigators have shown intrastrain variation among both human and non human primate derived isolates, the significance of which remains to be studied. Eberle et al. postulated the possible existence of B virus isolates, which vary with respect to pathogeneicity for non-macaque species, based on the existence of three distinct B virus genotypes found during phylogenetic analyses; however, this postulate must be examined in a suitable animal model. In zoonotic infections, unfortunately little is usually known about the species of most source animals, but where data are actually available many rhesus macaques have been identified targeting this species as the harbinger of a unique, highly pathogenic strain that can cause zoonoses. Published case summaries that implicate other macaque species and in one case a baboon, are difficult, if not impossible to confirm.

Synthesis of viral proteins

Approximately 23 major polypeptides have been identified by electrophoresis in denaturing polyacrylamide gels (Fig. 57.3), but over 50 different polypeptides have been identified by immunoblot analysis. Each has been assigned an infected cell polypeptide number as an initial reference point. The number may be an underestimate of the total produced, but it serves as a basis for comparison in ongoing studies. Molecular weight of these infected-cell polypeptides ranged from about 10 000–250 000 Daltons. Over 75% of the expected coding capacity of the viral DNA was accounted for by these infected cell polypeptides. At least nine bands from electrophoresed infected cell polypeptides containing viral glycoproteins have been thus far identified. Many of these glycoproteins have been cloned and sequenced by two groups. The proteins encoded were mapped to genes by the Us region which was largely colinear to the HSV glycoproteins gD, gI, gJ, and gG, as previously described. Sequence analysis of selected genes show that B virus is most closely related to herpesvirus papio 2 (HVP-2). Although there are protein homologues in herpesviruses of New World monkeys, very little, if any, cross-reactivity exists between B virus and the New World monkey herpesviiruses.

The kinetics of synthesis of the proteins and glycoproteins in infected cells in culture were found to have a course similar to that observed for HSV, although infectious virus was detectable slightly earlier, appearing 6 hours post-infection Both host cell DNA and protein synthesis appeared curtailed during the first 4 hours postinfection. As for glycoproteins, only glucosamine and some mannose were incorporated during the infection in vitro. B virus polypeptides/glycoproteins can be grouped into classes that differ in their relative rates of synthesis at different times throughout the virus replication cycle, as is characteristic of alpha herpesviruses.

Pathology and pathogenesis

During the course of B virus infection, some factors are observed not only in the natural host, but also in the experimentally infected host and the infected human as a result of zoonotic exposure. Those common factors will be discussed initially, then specific details for each of these host groups will be provided. First, there are various outcomes in infected hosts and evidence can be deduced from the literature that route of infection may play an important role. Specific details are lacking, but some observations can be made. The route of inoculation predicts differences in the time course of infection and spread through the central nervous system and visceral organs, e.g., spleen, adrenal, kidney, and in some cases even heart. Routes of infection are unique to each of the categories of hosts: natural, experimentally infected, and human zoonotic infections. For example, venereal transmission of the virus is common in macaque hosts, whereas intranasal virus can be experimentally delivered to a rabbit, or in the case of zoonotic exposure to a human by accidental aerosolization. However, these routes share one common feature, namely the involvement of mucosal membranes.

The cells that come into contact with the virus initially are another important factor to the permissiveness of the infection. For example, nasal mucosa has been found to be a less ideal site for virus replication than lung. However, nasal mucosa is not entirely resistant since increasing titers of virus can be isolated from these sites. Another important consideration in B virus pathogenesis is the dose of the virus initially introduced. The role of dose remains a challenging issue for study. Both dose and route of inoculation are important factors with respect to the onset of disease. For example, a far greater quantity of virus is required to infect rabbits by aerosolization than by an intradermal route of inoculation, although practically it remains unconfirmed whether these routes and doses parallel human versus non-human primate studies. Also, dose may be an important factor in contributing to associated morbidity and mortality. The commonality of each exposure route is generally a mucous membrane. Another common feature of natural, experimental, or zoonotic infection is that B virus can be found in the CNS shortly after the onset of acute infection. But where this virus goes and what it does differs widely in a natural infection versus an infection of a susceptible foreign host, the latter often succumbing to respiratory failure after neurologic deterioration.

The natural host

The macaque, the natural host of B virus, typically suffers little to no morbidity as a consequence of infection. Exceptions appear rarely and seem to involve specific accompanying factors, e.g., immunosuppression. Typically, once a macaque becomes infected following exposure of mucous membranes to virus, infection is relatively self-limiting. The virus may replicate at the site of inoculation and induce a localized erythema. There is also evidence of a limited focal infection of liver and kidney in some macaques. Virus travels via the peripheral nerves subserving the site of inoculation to associated dorsal route ganglia. Latent infection can then be established in the ganglia, with intermittent reactivation of the virus throughout the life of the macaque. In rare cases, viremia has been observed. Virus was also recovered from urine as well as multiple organs. Reactivation from latency has been observed in the natural host as judged by rising antibody titers as well as from recovery of virus by co-cultivation of sensory ganglia with cell monolayers.

During active replication of B virus in the natural host, isolation of virus can be readily accomplished from buccal, conjunctival, or genital mucosa swabs, predictable sites from which an alphaherpesvirus may be recovered during an active infection. The frequency of active infections within a seropositive group of macaques has been observed to be quite low, with relatively brief periods of excretion of virus from mucosal sites. Mucosal ulcers extend down to the papillary layer of the dermis. Two distinct zones have been described, namely a central area of necrosis and a surrounding zone of ballooning degeneration. Around the lesion, "normal" epithelium exists. An eosinophilic polymorphonuclear infiltration characterizes the histopathology of the lesion. Postmortem examination of monkey tissues from animals euthanatized at the time of active virus shedding shows histological evidence of perivascular cuffing of immune infiltrates in sections of spinal cord. Similar examinations of latently infected, healthy animals show no indication of virus from peripheral sites, but virus was recovered from sensory ganglia.

Experimental infections

Rabbits, mice, rats, guinea pigs and chickens have been experimental hosts of B virus as previously mentioned. Disease is not a uniform consequence following inoculation of B virus into mice and guinea pigs; however, several strains of B virus have increased virulence for the mouse. One strain, identified as E2490 was avirulent for white rats and chickens; nonetheless antibody developed after infection. Cotton rats infected by either intraperitoneal, subcutaneous, or intracerebral routes succumbed to infection with selected strains. Rats showed typical hind leg paralysis secondary to transverse meyelitis similar to symptoms in the rabbit. Reagan and colleagues selected, by serial passage human isolates of B virus, strains capable of infecting mice, hamster, and white chicks. With respect to experimental infections, a review of the literature suggests that the rabbit is perhaps the most useful small animal model since virus replicates in rabbits to high titers, making it a particularly good model for testing antiviral agents.

Using the rabbit, as well as the mouse model, investigators have shown that virus dose was important depending on the route of inoculation. Experimentally infected animals given low doses of intradermal virus developed only erythema that disappeared within a few days and was not associated with further apparent symptoms. In contrast, animals receiving a larger dose developed a necrotic lesion that was generally followed by CNS invasion. B virus subsequently appeared in the regional lymph nodes late after infection. These nodes drained the area of initial infection and with time, necrosis of the infected nodes occurred, as seen upon post mortem. In the CNS focal lesions were seen in pons, medulla, and spinal cord. Spread was most often facilitated by travel through the peripheral nerves, but in rare cases hematogenous route of spread in experimentally as well as inadvertently infected hosts has been described.

Cervical spinal cord and medulla oblongata were the primary sites for virus recovery post mortem. With time post infection, virus was found in olfactory regions of the brain, which may have been due to movement of the virus centripetally through the nerves innervating nasal mucosa. Perivascular cuffing and glial infiltration were characteristic histopathology findings upon examination of brain tissue. Hepatic congestion was accompanied by infiltration of polymorphonuclear and mononuclear cells seen in the periportal areas of the liver. Scattered necrotic foci can be found throughout the lobes of the liver. The presence of inclusions was seen mainly in the regions of inflammation, around pyknotic or karyorrhetic hepatocytes. When lesions were present on skin in the foreign host, the depth of the involved tissue was significantly thicker than that found on mucous membranes, explaining perhaps the reason B virus was recovered weeks or months later from these sites in foreign hosts.

Development of animal models for studies of B virus have been limited by the lack of antiviral drugs or a protective vaccine designed specifically to treat or prevent this infection since there is grave concern for individuals about actively working with this neurovirulent virus should an accident occur even when BL-4 laboratories are available and appropriate protocols are in place.

Human infection

Human infection with B virus generally occurs through an occupational exposure to a macaque shedding virus at a site which comes into contact with broken skin or mucosal membranes. Several cases where no monkey contact occurred in years suggested that virus could be reactivated. Review of all confirmed cases of B virus in humans can be summarized as follows.

The most striking characteristic of human B virus infection is the involvement of the patient's CNS as a target of infection, specifically the upper spinal cord and lower brain.

These areas are the principal sites for virus replication as observed with clinical, laboratory, and post-mortem data, but initially the infected individual generally experiences a flu-like syndrome followed by numbness or parathesias around the site of inoculation. An ascending myelitis occurs during the final stages of the infection in humans, resulting ultimately in respiratory failure. Virus can be recovered at skin sites of inoculation for extended periods of time and viral DNA can be detected generally in cerebrospinal fluid by the time neurological symptoms are experienced. Antibodies can also be detected in the CSF. Generally, death is associated with respiratory complications. Cutaneous lesions, from which B virus can be isolated, sometimes develop late in infection. Edema and degeneration of motor neurons are prominent. Even with advancing disease Cowdry type A eosinophilic intranuclear inclusions can be found in only a few cases, and certainly not uniformly. Gliosis and astrocytosis are late histopathologic findings, thus, there can be evidence of myelitis, encephalomyelitis, or encephalitis, or combinations of each of these conditions.

Pathogenesis of B virus infection has been studied for each of the reported fatal cases and in some surviving cases. With fatal disease, generally, CNS lesions are localized within the upper cervical spinal cord, sometimes extending into the medulla and pons. In some cases hemorrhagic infarcts can be visualized in these areas, whereas in other cases damage appears minimal in spite of the fact that the patient generally succumbs after prolonged ventilatory support. In some cases, patients are alert, but paralyzed and in other cases patients remain in a comatose state which results in respiratory failure. Survivors have varying degrees of morbidity, seen, ranging from little-to-no sequelae to more severe, incapacitating sequelae. Some survivors experience slow progressive neurologic decline, whereas others report few if any effects long term. Several survivors have subsequently given birth to healthy babies with no ill effects for either the mother or infant. Monitoring of the vaginal canal for virus shedding in these individuals prior to delivery has been negative. In several reports, the ocular effects of B virus infection have been reported. Histopathological examination of the patient's eye revealed a multifocal necrotizing retinitis associated with a vitritis, optic neuritis, and prominent panuveitis. A "herpes-like" virus was identified in the involved retina by electron microscopy in one case. Post mortem vitreous cultures taken from both eyes and retina have been positive for B virus. Thus, B virus can produce infection and destruction of retinal tissue similar to that of other herpesviruses. Ophthalmic zoster-like symptoms have been reported as well and in one particular case, reactivation of latent infection was speculated to have occurred.

To summarize human pathogenesis, the tissues and organs that become infected by B virus vary in some cases perhaps according to the route of infection. If skin is the primary site of infection, the virus usually, but not always replicates in the skin leading in some cases to localized erythema. Knowledge of the site of initial replication is useful for the development of guidelines for disease prevention and also for retrieval of a virus isolate that then allows unequivocal diagnosis. Subsequently, lymphangitis and lymph node involvement are observed. Viremia has not been proven to occur in humans, although with the application of more sensitive assays, e.g., polymerase chain reaction, further insights may be uncovered. With lymphatic involvement, the virus can spread abdominal viscera, where it has been isolated previously. Nevertheless, spread via neuronal routes is the fundamental route of transmission of the virus, as it is with HSV given the involvement of the spinal cord and CNS. Visceral organs, including heart, liver, spleen, lungs, kidneys, and adrenals demonstrate congestion and focal necrosis with variations in the extent of involvement from patient to patient. Recent human cases failed to demonstrate necrosis, but virus was isolated from adrenal, kidney, lung, and liver tissue collected at autopsy. In cases where B virus infection is suspected, medical personnel should follow published guidelines at the time of injury or observation of symptoms of possible infection.

Latency

A characteristic of all herpesviruses is the ability to become latent and reactivate when provoked with the proper stimulus. B virus is no exception. Reactivated infection has been described in both populations of macaques from the wild and captive established colonies. Unequivocal evidence of latent infection caused by B virus in macaques came with studies on frequency of recovery of B virus in monkey kidney cell culture systems. Wood and Shimada obtained six isolates from 650 pools of monkey kidneys, suggesting at least 1% of macaque kidneys contain latent virus that can be reactivated by culturing the cells. Virus was also isolated from rhesus tissues by Boulter and colleagues as well as by cocultivation from a variety of neuronal tissues including gasserian ganglia, trigeminal ganglia, dorsal route ganglia, and spinal cord. Latent virus was also isolated by cocultivation of tissues from experimentally infected rabbits, further supporting the rabbit as a potentially good animal model for B virus infections. Latency likely occurs in human infection as cutaneous recurrences have been documented and there are cases where an individual has not been in contact with macaques for years or even decades but antibodies exist at high levels.

As in HSV infections in humans, a prominent factor associated with reactivation of B virus in the macaque appears to be stress, particularly that associated with the capture and shipment of animals from the wild to captivity. Shedding of virus following reactivation also occurs with illness and during the breeding season of the natural host. No information is yet available on the state of the viral DNA during latency or on the molecular or biochemical events associated with the establishment and reactivation of latent virus.

Epidemiology

Animals

The majority of adult macaques and a very few younger animals in the wild have been reported to be seropositive for antibodies B virus. However, colonies of animals exist in the wild that have been found to be largely seronegative, but each of these colonies was established apart from original natural habitats to meet escalating needs of the scientific community and thus, the epidemiological pattern of virus infection was modified by human intervention. The high seroprevalence in macaques in the wild, the highly infectious nature within captive colonies, and low morbidity in this host confirmed the macaque as the natural host. More recent studies indicate that animals became infected at a higher incidence at the onset of puberty. The increased incidence appears to be associated with sexual transmission within the colony. Infants and juveniles have been reported to demonstrate a very low incidence of infection as judged by the low prevalence of B virus antibodies. Since antibody levels may reflect presence of maternal antibody in animals in contact with dams, it is of importance that both age groups are virus positive, suggesting transmission other than sexual activity occurs.

No particular species of macaque appears to be excluded as a natural host for B virus infection, although there is minimal data available from certain species and absent in the case of others. Although presence of antibodies has been confirmed in the majority of the different species of macaques, there has been speculation that virus isolated from certain species is less neurovirulent or less neurotropic than virus shed by rhesus macaques. Differences in the restriction endonuclease profiles of the different isolates from different macaque species have been reported, but the lack of available data on the types of macaques involved with each of the documented human cases has not permitted rigorous evaluation of this hypothesis.

Virus shedding during either primary or recurrent infections has been noted to occur at unpredictable frequency with widely variable duration. Analysis of available data indicates that macaques shed virus for a longer duration during primary infection, and for short periods, even hours following reactivation. Levels of shed virus, as measured from mucosal swabs range from 10^2–10^3 pfu/ml in one diagnostic laboratory.

Humans

B virus is an infection that humans rarely contract, but when they do, nearly 80% of untreated cases result in fatality. Epidemiological analysis indicates B virus is usually acquired via zoonotic transmission from either a macaque or infected cells or tissues from the animal. There is, however, one documented case of transmission from human-to-human as previously described, supporting the assumption that B virus can be transmitted similarly to HSV-1 or HSV-2, through mucosal contact with virus which is sometimes present in secretions or wound sites. A recent fatal case which resulted from exposure of ocular membranes to virus from a monkey in the process of being transported refocused attention on an earlier report implicating this type of transmission in the epidemiological analysis of zoonotic transmission of the virus. Current analyses of cases suggest categorization of risk levels with regard to the severity of injury is not useful. The low incidence of B virus infection in humans makes it difficult to reach statistical conclusions, but analysis of cases occurring during the last decade support the fact that first aid of injured or contaminated sites plays a major role in infection control. Only minimal disruption of the protective skin layer or instillation directly to a mucosal membrane can result in initiation of infection when the site is exposed to viable virus. The level of virus needed to initiate an infection in humans remains unknown. Where data are available, rhesus macaques were most frequently implicated as the source of infectious virus in reported human cases, but alone this is insufficient to conclude that the rhesus is uniquely important in the establishment of zoonotic infections. Other species of macaques and even a baboon have been linked to fatal zoonotic infections.

The incidence of zoonotic infections has been correlated retrospectively with periods of increased usage of macaques particularly in biomedical research. Evaluation of past cases underscores that transmission of the virus is often associated with no more than a superficial scratch or puncture, suggesting that once virus gains entry into a host, the ability to initiate disease is perhaps dose independent, at least in some cases. However, this point remains unsubstantiated. Dose and route of entry are topics that require further study to clarify importance in zoonotic infection. Likewise, incidence and prevalence of zoonotic infections must be estimated cautiously since little data regarding the virus source is available from clinically recognized cases.

Host immune responses

Antibodies specific for B virus have been studied in both the natural and the foreign hosts by a wide variety of methods, including serum neutralization with or without complement, competitive RIA, multiple types of ELISA including competition ELISA, and western blot. Limited serial observations have been available from both the natural or foreign host, but comparison of available data have been useful in that relatively consistent responses are induced in both hosts. The time course over which antibodies develop has been measured in wild macaques, captive colony populations, individually imported animals, experimentally infected macaques, zoonotically infected humans, and even in vaccine trial recipients. The ELISA methodologies provide a rapid diagnostic tool with increased sensitivities of detection, and enhanced specificity when competition protocols are utilized. The antibodies which develop in response to herpes B virus infection in both humans and non-human primates are capable of neutralizing HSV-1 and HSV-2, as well as non human primate alpha herpesviruses. The HSV antibodies are not able to neutralize B virus, indicating the presence of virus specific antigens unique to B virus. Sequence data have been useful in confirming the existence of virus specific epitopes.

The humoral immune responses which develop after a B virus infection either in the susceptible host, either natural or foreign, had characteristic patterns of viral antigen recognition throughout the course of infection. The glycoproteins induced antibodies early in the course of infection. Antibodies began to appear within 7–10 days after the infection and consisted of IgM. Within 14–21 days after the onset of acute infection, IgG antibodies were present. In rare cases, the infected host remained persistently antibody negative in spite of virus isolation. The pattern of the immune response was altered in the cases of humans who have had a previous infection with HSV-1 or HSV-2, since viral antigens that are shared among the three viruses induce an anamnestic response toward shared protein or glycoprotein sequences. Neutralizing antibodies develop in both the natural and foreign host, but at significantly lower levels than the foreign host. The nature and specificity of the humoral responses make it possible to design enhanced serological testing strategies to rapidly identify detectable antibodies and will provide the basis for future diagnostic strategies.

Clinical Manifestations of disease

Observation of the clinical pattern of disease is important for rapid diagnosis of B virus infection in both macaques and humans. In the natural host, recognition of early infection allows removal of infected monkeys from captive colonies that are being established as B virus-free. In B virus-free colonies, it is important to remove seropositive animals and isolate animals with equivocal results to prevent infection of other colony members, or in seropositive colonies to minimize risk to humans who have to handle them. Macaques are not treated with antivirals since the prevalence of infection is generally cost prohibitive. In the case of humans, early recognition of disease facilitates treatment with antivirals, principally nucleoside analogues, a course which appears to significantly lower the morbidity and mortality. Notably, immunosuppression, e.g., administration of corticosteroids, is often associated with reactivated mild disease in the natural host, whereas other agents appear to be capable of facilitating systemic B virus dissemination, culminating in death.

Humans exposed to herpes B virus demonstrate clinically variable signs of infection. Most often, illness after exposure to viable virus is apparent within days to weeks, but in some cases there appears to be a delay in development of acute disease. The reasons for this delay are unknown and, though rare, delays may even range from months to years, making diagnosis difficult. Once symptoms appear, the clinical progression is associated with relatively consistent symptoms, including flu-like illness, lymphadenitis, fever, headache, vomiting, myalgia, cramping, meningeal irritation, stiff neck, limb paresthesias, urinary retention with an ascending paralysis culminating in inability of the patient to maintain respiration, requiring ventilatory support. Cranial nerve signs, e.g., nystagmus and diplopia are also common to most published cases. Sinusitis and conjunctivitis have been observed in some. The array of symptoms may be related to the dose of virus with which the individual was infected or the route of inoculation. Summary descriptions of human cases can be found in two comprehensive reviews.

A summary of reported cases indicates that the highest percentage of deaths post infection occur within weeks postonset. In some cases however life was prolonged artificially for months or years. Incubation times from identifiable exposures to onset of clinical symptoms ranges from days to years, but the majority of cases occur within days to months. Virus has been recovered from throat, buccal, and conjunctival sites, as well as from lesions, vesicles, or injury sites as late as weeks to months post infection. The majority of clinical cases are associated with bites (50%), with fomites (8%) saliva (<5%), and aerosols described as other modes of exposure (10%).

Diagnosis

Non-human primates

B virus infection in macaques is identified by either virus isolation or the presence of specific antibodies or both. The neutralization assay dominated as a diagnostic tool in macaques and humans for many decades. The time required for the results of this test was often a drawback. The dot-blot, RIA, ELISA, and western blots were subsequently developed. Three of these techniques rely on the use of monoclonal antibodies. Each of these tests can be accomplished in less than a day, and are available through commercial laboratories as well as through a national resource laboratory subsidized through NIH's National Center for Research Resources. All of these assays utilize B virus infected cells for antibody detection, making them more effective than other types of assays which rely on HSV-1. This is a particularly important point with respect to diagnostic tools utilized to recognize early laboratory signs of infection for the establishment of B virus-free colonies. Currently, there are no diagnostic serologic tools to identify infected macaques that lack detectable antibodies; however, there are some promising assays being developed for diagnosis of HSV-2 infections in humans that may be adapted for identification of B virus infection in macaques. When selecting an assay for detection of antibodies, the sensitivity and specificity of the test for a specific species of macaque should be known and considered in the final evaluation of the results. Tests dependent on monoclonal antibodies or recombinant reagents should have defined sensitivity and specificity for each macaque species to be tested. Finally, evaluation of a macaque is optimal when analysis is performed on multiple samples collected at different times, especially in cases when the antibody titer is low (<1:50). A constellation of different tests at numerous time points may be necessary in some cases to correctly determine the status of an animal with low antibody titers, particularly when such an animal is housed in a B virus-free colony.

Virus isolation is the gold standard for diagnosis of infected macaques. Unfortunately, virus isolation is not a particularly sensitive diagnostic tool, with the possibility of many false negatives. Nonetheless, standard cell culture for virus isolation is still a valuable tool for the colony manager and for the veterinarian. Virus positive cultures can be easily recognized with the unique cytopathic effect produced by B virus, but unequivocal confirmation of the identification requires either electrophoretic analysis of infected cell polypeptides or restriction endonuclease digested DNA. More recently, several PCR reactions have been described which can be used to verify the identity of the virus; however, this diagnostic tool is costly for colony management. Nonetheless, when a possible zoonotic infection must be confirmed, PCR may be beneficial for identification of B virus in macaques.

Other species of monkeys become infected infrequently with B virus. These are usually animals that have been co-housed or housed in close proximity to B virus infected macaques at some time. Since many, if not all non human primates harbor indigenous alpha herpesviruses, the important diagnostic point is to differentiate specific antibodies from cross-reactive ones. Euthanasia is generally advised in the case of a B virus infection in a non-macaque monkey since it is likely that the animal will succumb and, in the meantime, would pose a great risk to anyone attempting to treat the infection. B virus has been identified in the patas monkey, colobus monkey, and Debrazza and Thompson *et al.* (in press). In each case, there was a major concern for the people responsible for care of the animal, particularly since these animals often have severe morbidity and are shedding virus. Currently, the most effective assay for diagnosis of B virus in a non macaque monkey would be a competition ELISA to facilitate discrimination between specific and cross-reactive antibodies similar to the challenge faced when diagnosing infection in humans.

Humans

The evaluation of clinical symptoms associated with an antibody or virus positive case is the gold standard for diagnosis of B virus infection in an exposed individual. Both serological and virological techniques are available for diagnosis of B virus infected humans. The CDC has published specified guidelines for recognition and treatment of such infections. In the case of a suspected infection, several emergency resources are available. Contact with the CDC or the laboratories recommended in the CDC guidelines can expedite laboratory support for the clinician suspecting an infection. Generally, a rise in B virus specific antibodies over several days during acute infection can be used to the etiologic agent. However, in other cases, data are equivocal and decisions with regard to the patient must be based on a complex decision table collectively using all diagnostic tools, including clinical symptoms. Virus isolation is again the gold standard for diagnosis, however virus isolation is frequently not possible even under the best of circumstances. Serological diagnosis of B virus in humans is a complex task when an individual with a suspect infection has detectable antibodies as a result of a previous HSV-1 or HSV-2 infection. As discussed in a previous section, significant cross-reactivity exists among these viruses. In the absence of these cross-reactive antibodies, diagnosis is rapid and straightforward, with confirmation using the neutralization assay and/or western blot. This was not the case prior to the development of rapid diagnostic competitive ELISAs and RIAs. The diagnostic tests for humans are performed currently by only a few facilities that have been licensed and have access to BL-4 containment laboratories for the preparation of B virus antigen.

Virus identification can be accomplished by isolation using conventional cell culture, and in clinical emergencies with PCR. The identity of isolates should be confirmed by electrophoretic analysis of infected cell polypeptides or restriction endonuclease digested DNA. The application of PCR is most helpful in the symptomatic patient if virus cannot be recovered. PCR is also a useful tool for monitoring the efficacy of antiviral interventions.

Control of B virus infection

Multiple levels of prevention can be used to prevent B virus infection in both humans and non-human primates, ranging from attempts to eliminate virus to designing methods to work safely in environments where there is increased risk for contracting this agent. The CDC has published detailed guidelines for maximizing protection for individuals working with macaque monkeys. Further, the NIH's National Center for Research Resources has funded the development of B virus-free colonies for NIH-funded research involving these animals in attempt to ultimately eliminate this virus from colonies used for biomedical research. Nonetheless, B virus infected monkeys are plentiful and require attentive handling adhering to strict guidelines, including barrier precautions.

When B virus is present, it can be inactivated with either heat or formaldehyde. Other inactivators include detergents and bleach. Individuals who work in a decontaminated area should still be alert to injury prevention. Minimizing fomites, however, decreases worker risk and reduces virus spread among animals. One B virus infection in a human was acquired from a cage after sustaining a scratch, underscoring that surface decontamination is important in infection control.

As early as the 1930s, attempts were made to identify an effective vaccine for protection of individuals who could be exposed to this virus while working with macaques or their cells or tissues. Limited vaccine trials were performed in human volunteers and although short-term antibody was induce, it was observed to wane quickly and the vaccine was not pursued further at that time. Recently, a recombinant vaccine was tested and found to induce antibodies in macaques, but the duration of antibodies and protection remain to be studied.

Antiviral therapy has been recognized as an effective prevention of infection progression in humans and animal trials as well, when administered sufficiently early after exposure. Acyclovir and the related family of nucleoside analogues were noted to be effective when given in high doses, e.g., acyclovir at 10–15 mg/kg three times daily for 14–21 days. Efficacy of therapy in cases of infection in humans has been monitored by inhibition of peripheral virus shedding in some cases and by reduction in CSF antibodies or viral DNA load in others. Ganciclovir has a greater efficacy in vitro and thus was used in all proven cases since 1989 with success. Interestingly, prior to 1987, in at least five retrospectively recognized cases, individuals fared well in the absence of antiviral therapy, but overall, the use of acyclovir and ganciclovir remains the recommended therapy by CDC. Generally, antiviral therapy is reserved for human with a clinically apparent infection, however it is also used by an increasing number of facilities for post-injury prophylaxis or after laboratory results indicate an animal may have been actively infected around the time of the exposure. Postinjury prophylaxis has been performed with famciclovir or valcyclovir, as well, both in that have demonstrated efficacy in vitro. Recommendations and guidelines have been published by the CDC, as discussed previously and can be readily accessed. Only a handful of physicians have had experience in the treatment of B virus zoonosis and their participation and expertise were important in the development of the CDC guidelines.

Finally, with respect to prevention, the value of wound cleansing following a potential exposure due to a bite, scratch, splash, or other suspicious injuries is very mandatory. Guidelines for wound cleaning are described in detail in the CDC Guidelines. Every institution working with macaques should have an injury protocol with immediate availability of first aid, a secondary care plan, and last but not least an infectious disease specialist who is a member of the institution's prevention and care response team.

Conclusions

B virus is usually a rapidly advancing, devastating disease which can be interrupted with effective use of antiviral therapies if deployed sufficiently soon after infection. The guidelines for treatment and prevention are widely published and can be rapidly accessed either through CDC or the diagnostic resource using the world wide web address www.gsu.edu/bvirus. Diagnostic techniques are rapidly improving to support clinical diagnosis and information regarding sample collection and evaluation is available at any time to clinical care centers in case of emergencies.

With the newer diagnostic techniques, sensitivity of detection is improving and the barriers posed by the high degree of cross-reactivity among this family of viruses are rapidly being diminished.

Because of the risk of human disease, precautionary methods must be followed in the workplace. Proper attention to the details of housing, management, handling of macaque monkeys, and organized exposure response measures using the CDC guidelines can minimize B virus zoonotic infections. Rapid identification of infection is essential for early inititation of antiviral drug therapy which can prevent further mortality associated with this very interesting alphaherpesvirus.

REFERENCES

Anon. (1987). B-virus infection in humans–Pensacola, Florida. *Morb. Mortal. Wkly Rep.*, **36**(19), 289–290, 295–296.

Anon. (1987). Leads from the MMWR. B-virus infection in humans–Pensacola, Florida. *J. Am. Med. Assoc.*, **257**(23), 3192–3193, 3198.

Anon. (1989). B virus infections in humans – Michigan. *Morb. Mortal. Wkly Rep.*, **38**(26), 453–454.

Artenstein, A. W., Hicks, C. B., Goodwin, B. S. Jr. et al. (1991). Human infection with B virus following a needlestick injury. *Rev. Infect. Dis.*, **13**(2), 288–291.

Bennett, A. M., Harrington, L., and Kelly, D. C. et al. (1992). Nucleotide sequence analysis of genes encoding glycoproteins D and J in simian herpes B virus. *J. Gen. Virol.*, **73**(11), 2963–2967.

Benson, P. M., Malane, S. L., Banks, R. et al. (1989). B virus (Herpesvirus simiae) and human infection. *Arch. Dermatol.*, **125**(9), 1247–1248.

Boulter, E. A. (1975). The isolation of monkey B virus (Herpesvirus simiae) from the trigeminal ganglia of a healthy seropositive rhesus monkey. *J. Biol. Stand.*, **3**(3), 279–280.

Chellman, G. J., Lukas, V. S., Eugui, E. M. et al. (1992). Activation of B virus (Herpesvirus simiae) in chronically immunosuppressed cynomolgus monkeys. *Lab. Anim. Sci.*, **42**(2), 146–151.

DiGiacomo, R. F. and Shah, K. V. (1972). Virtual absence of infection with Herpesvirus simiae in colony-reared rhesus monkeys (Macaca mulatta), with a literature review on antibody prevalence in natural and laboratory rhesus populations. *Lab. Anim. Sci.*, **22**(1), 61–67.

Eberle, R., Black, D., and Hilliard, J. K. (1989). Relatedness of glycoproteins expressed on the surface of simian herpes-virus virions and infected cells to specific HSV glycoproteins. *Arch. Virol.*, **109**(3–4), 233–252.

Eberle, R., Black, D. H., Lipper, S. et al. (1995). Herpesvirus papio 2, an SA8-like alpha-herpesvirus of baboons. *Arch. Virol.*, **140**(3), 529–545.

Freifeld, A. G., Hilliard, J., Southers, J. et al. (1995). A controlled seroprevalence survey of primate handlers for evidence of asymptomatic herpes B virus infection. *J. Infect. Dis.*, **171**(4), 1031–1034.

Gay, F. P. and Holden, M. (1933). Isolation of herpes virus from several cases of epidemic encephalitis. *Proc. Soc. Exp. Biol. Med.*, **30**, 1051–1053.

Harrington, L., Wall, L. V., and Kelly, D. C. et al. (1992). Molecular cloning and physical mapping of the genome of simian herpes B virus and comparison of genome organization with that of herpes simplex virus type 1. *J. Gen. Virol.*, **73**(5), 1217–1226.

Hilliard, J. K., Eberle, R., Lipper, S. L. et al. (1987). Herpesvirus simiae (B virus): replication of the virus and identification of viral polypeptides in infected cells. *Arch. Virol.*, **93**(3–4), 185–198.

Hilliard, J. K., Black, D., and Eberle, R. (1989). Simian alphaherpesviruses and their relation to the human herpes simplex viruses. *Arch. Virol.*, **109**(1–2), 83–102.

Keeble, S. A. (1960). B virus infection in monkeys. *Ann. NY Acad. Sci.*, **85**, 960–969.

Keeble, S. A., Christofinis, G. J., and wood, W. et al. (1958). Natural B virus infection in rhesus monkeys. *J. Path. Bacteriol.*, **76**, 189–199.

Kessler, M. J. and Hilliard, J. K. (1990). Seroprevalence of B virus (Herpesvirus simiae) antibodies in a naturally formed group of rhesus macaques. *J. Med. Primatol.*, **19**(2), 155–160.

Killeen, A. M., Harrington, L., Wall, L. V. et al. (1992). Nucleotide sequence analysis of a homologue of herpes simplex virus type 1 gene US9 found in the genome of simian herpes B virus. *J. Gen. Virol.*, **73**(1), 195–199.

Loomis, M. R., O'Neill, T., Bush, M. et al. (1981). Fatal herpesvirus infection in patas monkeys and a black and white colobus monkey. *J. Am. Vet. Med. Assoc.*, **179**, 1236–1239.

Palmer, A. E. (1987). B virus, Herpesvirus simiae: historical perspective. *J. Med. Primatol.*, **16**(2), 99–130.

Perelygina, L., Zhu, L., Zurkuhlen, H. et al. (2003). Complete sequence and comparative analysis of the genome of herpes B virus (cercopithicine herepsvirus 1) from a rhesus monkey. *J. Virol.*, **77**(11), 6167–6177.

Ruebner, B. H., Kevereux, D., Rorvik, M. et al. (1975). Ultrastructure of Herpesvirus simiae (Herpes B ivurs). *Exp. Mol. Pathol.*, **22**(3), 317–325.

Sabin, A. B. (1934). Studies on the B virus. II. Properties of the virus and pathogenesis of the experimental disease in rabbits. *Br. J. Exp. Pathol.*, **15**, 268–279.

Sato, H., Arikawa, J., Fururya, M. et al. (1998). Prevalence of herpes B virus antibody in nonhuman primates reared at the National University of Japan. *Exp. Anim.*, **47**(3), 199–202.

Shah, K. V. and Southwick, C. H. (1965). Prevalence of antibodies to certain viruses in sera of free-living rhesus and of captive monkeys. *Ind. J. Med. Res.*, **53**, 488–500.

Slomka, M. J., Harrington, L., Arnold, C. et al. (1995). Complete nucleotide sequence of the herpesvirus simiae glycoprotein G gene and its expression as an immunogenic fusion protein in bacteria. *J. Gen. Virol.*, **76**(9), 2161–2168.

Vizoso, A. D. (1975). Recovery of herpes simiae (B virus) from both primary and latent infections in rhesus monkeys. *Br. J. Exp. Pathol.*, **56**(6), 485–488.

Weigler, B. J. (1992). Biology of B virus in macaque and human hosts: a review. *Clin. Infect. Dis.*, **14**(2), 555–567.

Weigler, B. J., Hird, D. W., Hilliard, J. K. et al. (1993). Epidemiology of cercopithecine herpesvirus 1 (B virus) infection and shedding in a large breeding cohort of rhesus macaques. *J. Infect. Dis.*, **167**(2), 257–263.

Weigler, B. J., Scinicariello, F., and Hilliard, J. K. (1995). Risk of venereal B virus (cercopithecine herpesvirus 1) transmission in rhesus monkeys using molecular epidemiology. *J. Infect. Dis.*, **171**(5), 1139–1143.

Wilson, R. B., Holscher, M. A., Chang, T. et al. (1990). Fatal herpesvirus simiae (B virus) infection in a patas monkey (*Erythrocebus patas*). *J. Vet. Diagn. Invest.*, **2**(3), 242–244.

Simian varicella virus

Ravi Mahalingam[1] and Donald H. Gilden[1,2]

Departments of Neurology[1] and Microbiology[2], University of Colorado Health Sciences Center, Denver, CO, USA

Introduction

After primary infection (chickenpox) in children, varicella zoster virus (VZV) becomes latent in cranial, dorsal root and autonomic ganglia along the entire neuraxis and may reactivate decades later to produce zoster. The incidence of zoster and its attendant neurological complications is related to a natural decline in cell-mediated immunity (CMI) to VZV that occurs with aging, and which also develops in immunocompromised organ transplant recipients, and patients with cancer or AIDS. Yet the mechanism of reactivation and the cascade of events that are precipitated by impaired CMI to VZV are still unknown. To study such events require an animal model of varicella. While experimental animal models of latency and pathogenesis exist for closely related viruses such as herpes simplex types 1 and 2, VZV causes disease exclusively in humans. Thus, lack of a good animal model has hampered the studies of varicella latency and pathogenesis. Several attempts to produce disease by experimental inoculation of animals have led to seroconversion without clinical symptoms (Takahashi et al., 1975; Myers et al., 1980, 1985; Matsunaga et al., 1982; Wroblewska et al., 1982; Walz-Cicconi et al., 1986). Subcutaneous inoculation of the Oka VZV (vaccine strain) into the breast of a chimpanzee has been shown to produce viremia and mild rash restricted to the site of inoculation (Cohen et al., 1996). VZV DNA was detected in blood mononuclear cells (MNCs) of the chimpanzee during the 10-day incubation period. Mild varicella was observed resembling the low-level infection seen in some children vaccinated with VZV, but latency was not studied.

In contrast, simian varicella virus (SVV) causes a natural varicella-like disease of non-human primates. Herein, we describe the biology of SVV, its close similarity to VZV, and its usefulness as a model to study VZV pathogenesis and latency.

Simian varicella virus (SVV) is an alphaherpesvirus that infects Old World monkeys and causes a naturally occurring exanthematous disease similar to human varicella (White et al., 2001). Epidemic outbreaks in African green or vervet (*Cercopithicus aethiops*), Patas (*Erythocebus patas*), and various species of macaque (*Macaca sp.*) monkeys were first reported in the 1960s and 1970s at five primate centers in both the USA and UK. Virus isolated during these outbreaks was shown to be very similar to VZV in terms of its tissue culture characteristics (Soike et al., 1984a). Clinical (Padovan and Cantrell, 1986; Myers and Connelly, 1992) (Fig. 58.1), immunological (Felsenfeld and Schmidt, 1977,1979) and pathological (Wenner et al., 1977; Padovan and Cantrell, 1986; Dueland et al., 1992) changes produced by SVV infection of primates are similar to those in human varicella. Like VZV, primary SVV infection causes viremia, and infectious virus can be recovered from blood MNCs (Clarkson et al., 1967; Wolf et al., 1974; Soike et al., 1984a). Occasionally, rash becomes hemorrhagic and disseminated (Soike, 1992). Like disseminated varicella in immunosuppressed patients, lung and liver are the most severely affected organs (Roberts et al., 1984). Histological examination of skin and viscera reveals foci of hemorrhagic necrosis, inflammation and eosinophilic intranuclear inclusions (Clarkson et al., 1967; Wolf et al., 1974). Like VZV, SVV becomes latent in ganglia at multiple levels of the neuraxis (Mahalingam et al., 2002).

SVV reactivation has been observed in infected monkeys exposed to social and environmental stress (Soike et al., 1984a). Both the 1968 and 1974 outbreaks of varicella in *Erythrocebus patas* monkeys at the Tulane National Primate Research Center, Covington, LA, were attributed to reactivation of SVV (Soike, 1992). SVV reactivation often appears as a whole-body rash in contrast to VZV reactivation in humans (zoster) which is generally localized to 1–3 dermatomes. Zoster in monkeys is often obscured by fur

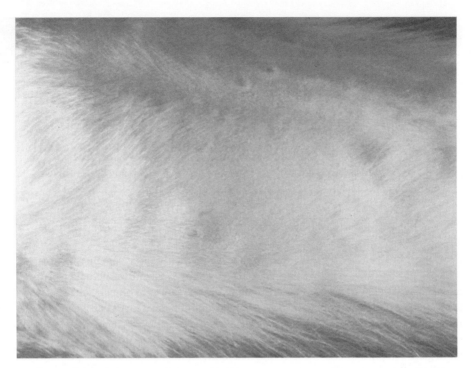

Fig. 58.1. Vesicular rash on the abdomen of an African green monkey infected with simian varicella virus. (Reprinted with permission of *Ann. NY Acad. Sci.*)

and the duration of rash is generally less than one week. SVV has been isolated from skin vesicles after reactivation (Fig. 58.2) (Soike *et al.*, 1984a). Identical restriction enzyme profiles have been detected in the genomes of SVV isolated from primary infection and reactivation in the same monkey (Gray and Gusick, 1996). Neither VZV nor SVV has been isolated from blood of otherwise healthy, asymptomatic immunocompetent humans or primates.

Similarities between SVV and VZV

SVV and VZV encode antigenically related polypeptides, and SVV-specific antibodies cross-react with human VZV in serum neutralization and complement fixation tests (Felsenfeld and Schmidt, 1979; Soike *et al.*, 1987; Fletcher and Gray, 1992). Although VZV does not cause disease in non-human primates, it has been used to immunize and protect monkeys from SVV infection (Felsenfeld and Schmidt, 1979). To date, there is no evidence that SVV can infect or cause disease in humans. It seems likely that humans exposed to VZV are protected against SVV infection since nearly all adults in North America are VZV-seropositive and since VZV can protect monkeys from SVV infection.

Simian varicella virus genome

SVV is an enveloped, double-stranded DNA virus. The SVV genome is colinear (Pumphrey and Gray, 1992; White *et al.*, 1997) with that of VZV, sharing similarities in size and structure. The two virus genomes share 70–75% DNA homology (Davison and Scott, 1986; Gray and Oakes, 1984; Clarke *et al*, 1992; Gray *et al.*, 1992). The entire SVV genome has been sequenced, and analysis showed that SVV DNA is 124 784 bp in size, 100 bp shorter than VZV DNA, and its G+C content is 40.4% (Gray *et al.*, 2001, unpublished observations). The left end of the SVV genome contains a small segment (665 bp) that consists of 506 bp of unique sequences flanked on either side by 79 bp inverted repeats; part of this inverted repeat sequence (64 bp) is present at the junction of the long and short segments of the SVV genome. The unique short (U_S) component composed of a 4909-bp region bracketed by 7557-bp inverted repeats (IR_S). The entire short segment of the SVV genome ($U_S+IR_S+TR_S$) is 147 bp longer than its VZV counterpart. However, the unique short segment (U_S) is slightly shorter than that of VZV.

There are a total of 74 methionine-initiated open reading frames (ORFs) (Fig. 58.3). This includes 71 distinct SVV genes since 3 ORFs (69, 70 and 71) are duplicated within the repeat regions. The gene organizations of the SVV and VZV genomes are similar if not identical. Of the 70 unique SVV ORFs, 68 share extensive homology with the corresponding VZV genes (Gray et al., 2001). Several SVV genes, including thymidine kinase (Pumphrey and Gray, 1996), uracil DNA glycosylase (Ashburn and Gray, 1999), glycoproteins E (Gray et al., 2001), B (Pumphrey and Gray, 1994), L and H (Ashburn and Gray, 2002) and C (Gray and Byrne, 2003), have been characterized either at the level of RNA or protein and shown to be very similar to their VZV counterparts.

A detailed comparison of the SVV and VZV sequences revealed several important differences at the leftward end (Fig. 58.4): (i) the left end of the SVV genome contains a 660 bp segment that consists of 506 bp of unique sequence flanked on either side by 79 bp inverted segments; (ii) an 879-bp ORF A and a 420 bp ORF (LE) in SVV that are absent in VZV. ORFA has 42% amino acid identity to SVV ORF 4 and 49% to VZV ORF 4; (iii) a 342-bp ORF B in SVV with 35% amino acid identity to a 387-bp ORF located to the left of ORF 1 on the VZV genome; and (iv) a 303-bp ORF in SVV with 27% amino acid identity to VZV ORF 1. No homologue of VZV ORF 2 was detected. Further, all of the known strains of SVV lack a VZV ORF 2 homologue (Mahalingam et al., 2000). Transcripts specific for ORFs A and B have been detected in SVV-infected cells in culture and in acutely infected monkey ganglia. In vitro transcription-translation followed by immunoprecipitation of SVV ORF A showed that it encodes a 35-kD protein (Mahalingam et al., 2000). Thus, the only major difference between SVV and VZV DNA is in the leftward terminus, possibly underlying the species specificity of SVV infection for monkeys.

The U_S of both VZV and SVV DNA invert, resulting in two major isomers of the virus DNA. A small (88-bp) repeat DNA segment brackets the U_L of VZV DNA. Like VZV, ~5% of SVV DNA molecules have an inverted U_L segment in productively infected cells. Further, the SVV genome exists either as circles or concatemers in SVV-infected cells (Clarke et al., 1995), as also shown for VZV (Kinchington et al., 1985). Like VZV, SVV and transfected SVV DNA produce a cytopathic effect in tissue culture, characterized by the formation of syncytia preceding cell lysis, a low virus titer and cell-associated virus (Soike et al., 1984b; Soike, 1992; Clarke et al., 1992).

SVV pathogenesis

Experimental inoculation of SVV in African green monkeys has generated two models of varicella infection. Intratracheal inoculation of 10^4 pfu of SVV into monkeys results in vesicular skin rash at 7–10 days post-infection (p.i.)

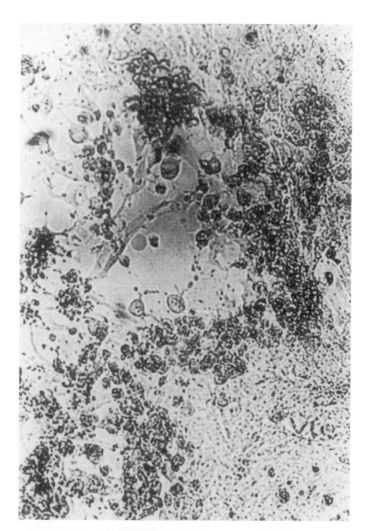

Fig. 58.2. Viral cytopathic effect resulting from infection of Vero (African green monkey kidney) cells using reactivated simian varicella virus isolated from monkeys. (Reprinted with permission of *Ann. NY Acad. Sci.*)

(Figs. 58.1 and 58.5). Viremia can be detected as early as 3 days p.i., peaking at ~5 days p.i., and disappearing by 11 days p.i., indicating hematogenous spread of the virus throughout the body. Hepatitis and pneumonia have been detected at the peak of rash, as suggested in Fig. 58.5. Induction of antibody responses by 12 days p.i correlates with the resolution of rash (Wenner et al., 1977; Iltis et al., 1982; Soike et al., 1984a; Dueland et al., 1992; Gray et al., 1998; Gray, 2003). The time course and route of spread of SVV to ganglia in monkeys after intratracheal or intravenous inoculation was determined by analyzing DNA extracted from monkey tissues 5–60 days later (Mahalingam et al., 2001). SVV DNA was detected in

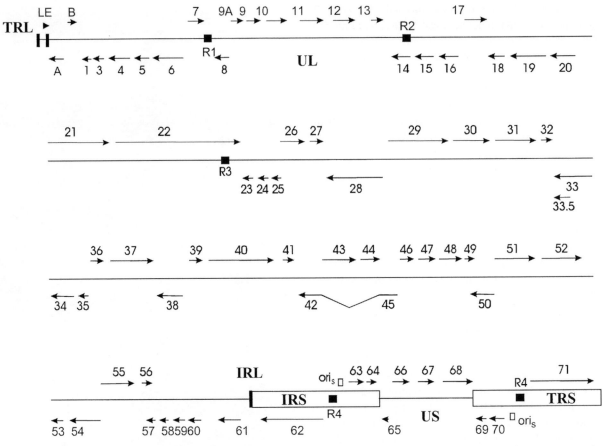

Fig. 58.3. Complete genome map of SVV. The unique long segment (UL) of the genome is flanked by 64-bp of inverted repeats (TRL and IRL). The left end of the SVV genome contains 665 bp segment that contains 506 bp of unique sequence flanked on either side by 79 bp inverted repeats; part of this inverted repeat sequence (64 bp) is present at the junction of the long and short segments (IR$_L$) of the virus genome. The unique short segment (US) is flanked by 7557-bp of inverted repeats (IRS and TRS). Arrows indicate the direction and location of the 73 SVV ORFS corresponding to the nomenclature conventions of VZV. Black boxes indicate the repeated sequences (R1, R2, R3, and R4). The putative origins of DNA replication (ori$_s$) are shown. (Reprinted with permission of Virology.)

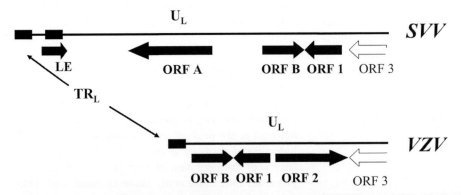

Fig. 58.4. Sequence organization at the leftward end of the SVV and VZV genomes. TR$_L$ indicates the 64- and 80-bp of terminal repeat sequences located at the leftward end of the SVV and VZV genomes, respectively. U$_L$ indicates the leftmost parts of the unique long regions of the virus genomes. SVV ORFs within the 3600-bp SVV EcoRI-I fragment and homologous to the VZV ORFs are shown. ORF B was assigned based on amino acid sequence similarity between SVV and VZV sequences upstream of ORF 1. ORFs LE and A are present in SVV but not in VZV, whereas ORF 2 is present only in VZV. (Reprinted with permission of *Virology*.)

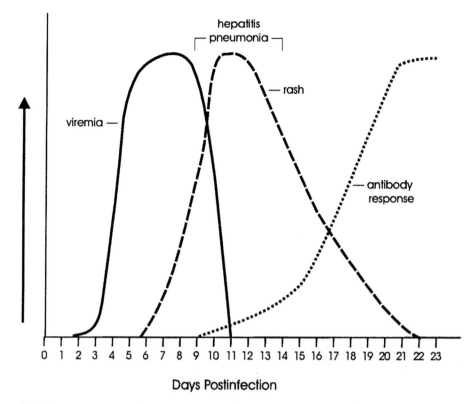

Fig. 58.5. Summary of the clinical course and pathogenesis of experimental SVV infection in monkeys. (Reprinted with permission of *J. Med. Primatol.*)

ganglia of monkeys sacrificed 6–7 days later (before rash). Intravenous inoculation produced more SVV DNA-positive ganglia (63%) than after intratracheal inoculation (13%), pointing to the role of hematogenous spread in ganglionic infection. Like other organs, monkey ganglia become infected with SVV before the appearance of rash (Mahalingam *et al.*, 2001). SVV-specific antigens and nucleic acids have been detected in liver, lung, spleen, adrenal gland, kidney, lymph node, bone marrow, and in ganglia at all levels of the neuraxis (Wenner *et al.*, 1977; Roberts *et al.*, 1984; Padovan and Cantrell, 1986; Dueland *et al.*, 1992; Gray *et al.*, 2002).

Further, experimental intratracheal inoculation of SVV in monkeys results in the persistence of virus DNA for months to years in several tissues, including ganglia, liver and blood MNCs (White *et al.*, 2002a). SVV DNA representing multiple regions of the viral genome has been detected in blood MNCs of SVV-infected monkeys at 7 days and 10 months p.i. (White *et al.*, 2002b), suggesting the presence of most if not all of the virus genome. SVV-infected monkeys that were sacrificed at 10 months p.i., had viremia during acute varicella and SVV may have persisted in blood MNCs.

It is also possible that MNCs were being infected while trafficking through tissue where SVV DNA continued to be expressed. Multiple SVV-specific transcripts, including late transcripts, were detected in ganglia from these monkeys (Table 58.1), indicating viral DNA replication and possible assembly of infectious viral particles (White *et al.*, 2002a). Vero cells that were cocultivated with blood MNCs 14 months after intratracheal inoculation did not develop a cytopathic effect, and SVV DNA could not be detected after three subcultivations of Vero cells in tissue culture (White *et al.*, 2002b). It is not clear whether these results represent persistence of the SVV genome as a result of infection of MNCs during acute varicella, or an ongoing abortive infection of MNCs, but the latter appears more likely. In vitro attempts by several laboratories to infect MNCs with VZV have yielded mixed results, but suggest that these cells are only semipermissive for VZV (Arbeit *et al.*, 1982; Gilden *et al.*, 1987; Koropchak *et al.*, 1989; Soong *et al.*, 2000; Zerboni *et al.*, 2000). In all studies, VZV-specific DNA and proteins were detected in T and B cells, monocytes and macrophages, but infectious VZV was recovered primarily from T lymphocytes (Arbeit *et al.*, 1982; Koropchak *et al.*,

Table 58.1. Detection of SVV-specific transcripts in ganglia, lung or liver of virus-infected adult African green monkeys

ORF	Ganglia (months p.i.)				Lung (months p.i.)				Liver (months p.i.)			
	2	5	10	12	2	5	10	12	2	5	10	12
IE 4	3/3[a]	3/3	3/3	1/1	nd[b]	nd	2/2	0/1	nd	nd	0/1	0/1
IE 62	3/3	3/3	2/3	1/1	nd	nd	0/2	nd	nd	nd	0/1	nd
IE 63	3/3	3/3	3/3	1/1	0/3	0/3	2/2	nd	1/2	1/3	1/1	nd
E 21	2/3	3/3	3/3	1/1	nd	nd	2/2	nd	nd	nd	1/1	nd
E 28	2/3	3/3	3/3	1/1	0/3	0/3	0/2	0/1	1/2	1/3	0/1	0/1
E 29	3/3	3/3	3/3	1/1	0/3	0/3	2/2	0/1	1/2	1/3	1/1	0/1
L 40	0/3	3/3	3/3	1/1	0/3	0/3	0/2	0/1	1/2	1/3	0/1	0/1

[a] number of animals positive/number analyzed.
[b] nd = not done.
IE – immediate-early; E – Early; L – late
Reprinted with permission of *J. Neurovirol.*

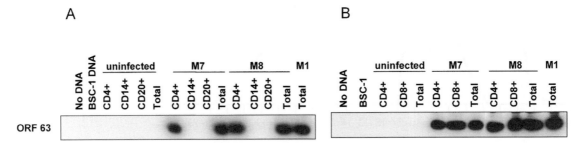

Fig. 58.6. Detection of SVV ORF 63-specific DNA in peripheral blood MNC subpopulations of SVV-infected adult African green monkeys. MNCs from an uninfected monkey and two SVV-infected monkeys (M7 and M8) at 14 months (a) and 23 months (b) after intratracheal inoculation with SVV were sorted by flow cytometry using (a) anti-CD4, anti-CD14 and anti-CD20 monoclonal antibodies and (b) anti-CD4 and anti-CD8 monoclonal antibodies. MNC DNA from the acutely infected monkey (M1) was used as a positive control. DNA extracted from the MNC populations was analyzed by nested PCR followed by Southern blot hybridization. SVV DNA was detected exclusively in CD4+ and CD8+ cells. (Modified and reprinted with permission of *Virology.*)

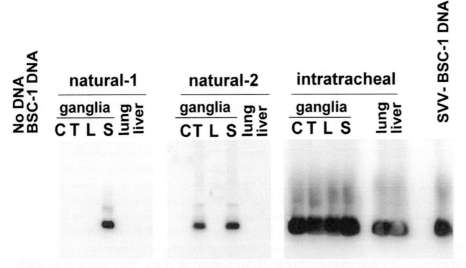

Fig. 58.7. Detection of SVV DNA in ganglia from monkeys naturally infected with SVV. DNA extracted from pooled cervical (C), thoracic (T), lumbar (L), and sacral (S) ganglia, lung and liver from two monkeys (natural-1 and -2) exposed to an intratracheally infected monkey (intratracheal) was analyzed by nested PCR using primers and probes specific for SVV ORF 63. DNA was omitted in one of the reactions (No DNA). DNA from uninfected (BSC-1 DNA) and SVV-infected BSC-1 cells in culture (SVV-BSC-1 DNA) was used as a negative and positive control, respectively. (Modified and reprinted with permission of *J. Virol.*)

1989; Soong et al., 2000). At 14 months p.i., SVV-specific DNA was detected in CD4+ and CD8+ cells, but not in CD14+ or CD20+ cells (Fig. 58.6) (White et al., 2002b). Detection of SVV DNA in blood MNCs likely reflects infection acquired while trafficking through tissue where SVV DNA persists.

The second model of SVV infection in African green monkeys is the simulated natural infection in which SVV-seronegative monkeys are exposed to monkeys previously inoculated intratracheally with SVV (Mahalingam et al., 2002). As noted, monkeys given SVV by intra-tracheal inoculation develop a diffuse rash by 10–12 days after inoculation, and a mild rash also develops at 10–14 days in monkeys caged with the experimentally infected monkeys. SVV DNA is detectable in skin scrapings of the naturally infected monkeys, indicating that the disease is caused by SVV, although SVV DNA is detected only occasionally in the blood MNCs of these monkeys. Six to 8 weeks after the resolution of rash, SVV DNA is detected in multiple ganglia along the neuraxis but not in lung or liver (Fig. 58.7), indicating that latent infection is restricted to ganglia. This monkey model of SVV infection will, for the first time, allow analysis of the extent to which SVV is transcribed during latency and can also be used to dissect, at the molecular level, the cascade of cellular and immune factors in the reactivation process. This is important since VZV reactivation in elderly and immunocompromised individuals produces serious, often chronic and sometimes fatal neurological disease.

Acknowledgments

This work was supported in part by Public Health Service grants NS 32623 and AG 06127 from the National Institutes of Health. We thank Marina Hoffman for editorial review and Cathy Allen for preparing the manuscript.

REFERENCES

Annunziato, P., LaRussa, P., Lee, P. et al. (1998). Evidence of latent varicella-zoster virus in rat dorsal root ganglia. *J. Infect. Dis.*, **178** (Suppl. 1), S48–S51.

Arbeit, R. D., Zaia, J. A., Valerio, M. A., and Levin, M. J. (1982). Infection of human peripheral blood mononuclear cells by varicella-zoster virus. *Intervirology*, **18**, 56–65.

Ashburn, C. V. and Gray, W. L. (1999). Identification and characterization of the simian varicella virus uracil DNA glycosylase. *Arch. Virol.*, **144**, 2161–2172.

Ashburn, C. V. and Gray, W. L. (2002). Expression of the simian varicella virus glycoprotein L and H. *Arch. Virol.*, **147**, 335–348.

Clarke, P., Rabkin, S. D., Inman, M. V. et al. (1992). Molecular analysis of simian varicella virus DNA. *Virology*, **190**, 597–605.

Clarke, P., Beer, T., and Gilden, D. H. (1995). Configuration and terminal sequences of the simian varicella virus genome. *Virology*, **207**, 154–159.

Clarkson, M. J., Thorpe, E., and McCarthy, K. (1967). A virus disease of captive vervet monkeys (*Cercopithecus aethiops*) caused by a new herpesvirus. *Arch. Gesamte Virusforsch.*, **22**, 219–234.

Cohen, J. I., Moskal, T., Shapiro, M., and Purcell, R. H. (1996). Varicella in chimpanzees. *J. Med. Virol.*, **50**, 289–292.

Davison, A. J. and Scott, J. E. (1986). The complete DNA sequence of varicella-zoster virus. *J. Gen. Virol.*, **67**, 1759–1816.

Dueland, A. N., Martin, J. R., Devlin, M. E. et al. (1992). Acute simian varicella infection. Clinical, laboratory, pathologic, and virologic features. *Lab. Invest.*, **66**, 762–773.

Felsenfeld, A. D. and Schmidt, N. J. (1977). Antigenic relationship among several simian varicella-like viruses and varicella-zoster virus. *Infect. Immun.*, **15**, 807–812.

Felsenfeld, A. D. and Schmidt, N. J. (1979). Varicella-zoster virus immunizes patas monkeys against simian varicella-like disease. *J. Gen. Virol.*, **42**, 171–178.

Fletcher, T. M. and Gray, W. L. (1992). Simian varicella virus: characterization of virion and infected cell polypeptides and the antigenic cross-reactivity with varicella-zoster virus. *J. Gen. Virol.*, **73**, 1209–1215.

Gilden, D. H., Hayward, A. R., Krupp, J., Hunter-Laszlo, M., Huff, J. C., and Vafai, A. (1987). Varicella-zoster virus infection of human mononuclear cells. *Virus Res.*, **7**, 117–129.

Gray, W. L. (2003). Pathogenesis of simian varicella virus. *J. Med Virol.*, **70** (Suppl. 1), S4–S8.

Gray, W. L. and Byrne, B. H. (2003) Characterization of simian varicella virus glycoprotein C, which is nonessential for *in vitro* replication. *Arch. Virol.*, **148**, 537–545.

Gray, W. L. and Gusick, N. J. (1996). Viral isolates derived from simian varicella epizootics are genetically related but are distinct from other primate herpesviruses. *Virology*, **224**, 161–166.

Gray, W. L. and Oakes, J. E. (1984). Simian varicella virus DNA shares homology with human varicella-zoster virus DNA. *Virology*, **136**, 241–246.

Gray, W. L., Pumphrey, C. Y., Ruyechan, W. T., and Fletcher, T. M. (1992). The simian varicella virus and varicella zoster virus genomes are similar in size and structure. *Virology*, **186**, 562–572.

Gray, W. L., Williams, R. J., Chang, R., and Soike, K. F. (1998). Experimental simian varicella virus infection of St. Kitts vervet monkeys. *J. Med. Primatol.*, **27**, 177–183.

Gray, W. L., Starnes, B., White, M. W., and Mahalingam, R. (2001). The DNA sequence of the simian varicella virus genome. *Virology*, **284**, 123–130.

Gray, W. L., Mullis, L., and Soike, K. F. (2002). Viral gene expression during acute simian varicella virus infection. *J. Gen. Virol.*, **83**, 841–846.

Iltis, J. P., Arrons, M. C., Castellano, G. A. et al. (1982). Simian varicella virus (delta herpesvirus) infection of patas monkeys leading to pneumonia and encephalitis. *Proc. Soc. Exp. Biol. Med.*, **169**, 266–279.

Kinchington, P. R., Reinhold, W. C., Casey, T. A., Straus, S. E., Hay, J., and Ruyechan, W. T. (1985). Inversion and circularization of the varicella-zoster virus genome. *J. Virol.*, **56**, 194–200.

Koropchak, C. M., Solem, S. M., Diaz, P. S., and Arvin, A. M. (1989). Investigation of varicella-zoster virus infection of lymphocytes by in situ hybridization. *J. Virol.*, **63**, 2392–2395.

Mahalingam, R., White, T., Wellish, M., Gilden, D. H., Soike, K., and Gray, W. L. (2000). Sequence analysis of the leftward end of simian varicella virus (EcoRI-I fragment) reveals the presence of an 8-bp repeat flanking the unique long segment and an 881-bp open-reading frame that is absent in the varicella zoster virus genome. *Virology*, **274**, 420–428.

Mahalingam, R., Wellish, M., Soike, K., White, T., Kleinschmidt-DeMasters, B. K., and Gilden, D. H. (2001). Simian varicella virus infects ganglia before rash in experimentally infected monkeys. *Virology*, **279**, 339–342.

Mahalingam, R., Traina-Dorge, V., Wellish, M., Smith, J., and Gilden, D. H. (2002). Naturally acquired simian varicella virus infection in African green monkeys. *J. Virol.*, **76**, 8548–8550.

Matsunaga, Y., Yamanishi, K., and Takahashi, M. (1982). Experimental infection and immune response of guinea pigs with varicella-zoster virus. *Infect. Immun.*, **37**, 407–412.

Myers, M. G. and Connelly, B. L. (1992). Animal models of varicella. *J. Infect. Dis.*, **166**(Suppl. 1), 548–550.

Myers, M. G., Duer, H. L., and Hausler, C. K. (1980). Experimental infection of guinea pigs with varicella-zoster virus. *J. Infect. Dis.*, **142**, 414–420.

Myers, M. G., Stanberry, L. R., and Edmond, B. J. (1985). Varicella-zoster virus infection of strain 2 guinea pigs. *J. Infect. Dis.*, **151**, 106–113.

Padovan, D. and Cantrell, C. A. (1986). Varicella-like herpesvirus infection of nonhuman primates. *Lab. Anim. Sci.*, **36**, 7–13.

Pumphrey, C. Y. and Gray, W. L. (1992). The genomes of simian varicella virus and varicella zoster virus are colinear. *Virus Res.*, **26**, 255–266.

Pumphrey, C. Y. and Gray, W. L. (1994). DNA sequence and transcriptional analysis of the simian varicella virus glycoprotein B gene. *J. Gen. Virol.*, **75**, 3219–3227.

Pumphrey, C. Y. and Gray, W. L. (1996). Identification and analysis of the simian varicella virus thymidine kinase gene. *Arch. Virol.*, **151**, 43–55.

Roberts, E. D., Baskin, G. B., Soike, K., and Gibson, S. V. (1984). Pathologic changes of experimental simian varicella (Delta herpesvirus) infection in African green monkeys (*Cercopithecus aethiops*). *Am. J. Vet. Res.*, **45**, 523–530.

Soike, K. F. (1992). Simian varicella virus infection in African and Asian monkeys. The potential for development of antivirals for animal diseases. *Ann. NY Acad. Sci.*, **653**, 323–333.

Soike, K. F., Rangan, S. R., and Gerone, P. J. (1984a). Viral disease models in primates. *Adv. Vet. Sci. Comp. Med.*, **28**, 151–199.

Soike, K. F., Baskin, G., Cantrell, C., and Gerone, P. (1984b). Investigation of antiviral activity of 1-beta-D-arabinofuranosylthymine (ara-T) and 1-beta-D-arabinofuranosyl-E-5-(2-bromovinyl) uracil (BV-ara-U) in monkeys infected with simian varicella virus. *Antiviral Res.*, **4**, 245–257.

Soike, K. F., Keller, P. M., and Ellis, R. W. (1987). Immunization of monkeys with varicella-zoster virus glycoprotein antigens and their response to challenge with simian varicella virus. *J. Med. Virol.*, **22**, 307–313.

Soong, W., Schultz, J. C., Patera, A. C., Sommer, M. H., and Cohen, J. I. (2000). Infection of human T lymphocytes with varicella-zoster virus: an analysis with viral mutants and clinical isolates. *J. Virol.*, **74**, 1864–1870.

Takahashi, M., Okuno, Y., Otsuka, T., Osame, J., and Takamizawa, A. (1975). Development of a live attenuated varicella vaccine. *Biken. J.*, **18**, 25–33.

Walz-Cicconi, M. A., Rose, R. M., Dammin, G. J., and Weller, T. H. (1986). Inoculation of guinea pigs with varicella-zoster virus via the respiratory route. *Arch. Virol.*, **88**, 265–277.

Wenner, H. A., Abel, D., Barrick, S., and Seshumurty, P. (1977). Clinical and pathogenetic studies of Medical Lake macaque virus infections in cynomolgus monkeys (simian varicella). *J. Infect. Dis.*, **135**, 611–622.

White, T. M., Mahalingam, R., Kolhatkar, G., and Gilden, D. H. (1997). Identification of simian varicella virus homologues of varicella zoster virus genes. *Virus Genes*, **15**, 265–269.

White, T. M., Gilden, D. H., and Mahalingam, R. (2001). An animal model of varicella virus infection. *Brain Pathol.*, **11**, 475–479.

White, T. M., Mahalingam, R., Traina-Dorge, V., and Gilden, D. H. (2002a). Simian varicella virus DNA is present and transcribed months after experimental infection of adult African green monkeys. *J. Neurovirol.*, **8**, 191–203.

White, T. M., Mahalingam, R., Traina-Dorge, V., and Gilden, D. H. (2002b). Persistence of simian varicella virus DNA in CD4(+) and CD8(+) blood mononuclear cells for years after intratracheal inoculation of African green monkeys. *Virology*, **303**, 192–198.

Wolf, R. H., Smetana, H. F., Allen, W. P., and Felsenfeld, A. D. (1974). Pathology and clinical history of Delta herpesvirus infection in patas monkeys. *Lab. Anim. Sci.*, **24**, 218–221.

Wroblewska, Z., Devlin, M., Reilly, K., van Trieste, H., Wellish, M., and Gilden, D. H. (1982). The production of varicella zoster virus antiserum in laboratory animals. Brief report. *Arch. Virol.*, **74**, 233–238.

Zerboni, L., Sommer, M., Ware, C. F., and Arvin, A. M. (2000). Varicella-zoster virus infection of a human CD4-positive T-cell line. *Virology*, **270**, 278–285.

59

Primate betaherpesviruses

Peter A. Barry[1,2,3] and W. L. William Chang[1]

[1]Center for Comparative Medicine,
[2]Department of Pathology and Laboratory Medicine,
[3]California National Primate Research Center, University of California, Davis, CA, USA

The last few years have witnessed significant expansion of the simian cytomegalovirus (CMV) model of human CMV (HCMV) infection. Progress in the utilization of the simian CMV models has been highlighted by a better understanding of natural history, development of species-specific reagents and techniques, sequencing of several viral genomes, and generation of a bacterial artificial chromosome (BAC) containing a full-length CMV genome. This work has demonstrated that, not only is there strong conservation of genomic organization and coding content, but also that the simian CMV exhibit significant parallels to HCMV in the course of viral infection in both immunocompetent hosts and those without a fully functional immune system. A wide range of experimental approaches into the molecular biology of HCMV, mechanisms of HCMV persistence and pathogenesis, and the design of novel treatment and prevention strategies are now possible in different non-human primate (NHP) models.

Characterization of simian betaherpesviruses has been restricted almost exclusively to CMV. The single report that is consistent with the existence of human herpesvirus (HHV)-6/7-like viruses in non-human primates (NHP) is based on the amplification of a short DNA sequence with nucleic and amino acid homologies to DNA polymerase of HHV-6 and 7 (Lacoste et al., 2000). In contrast, CMV has been isolated from multiple genera and species of old and new world NHP. Each simian species probably harbors its own variant of CMV that has co-evolved with its host during primate evolution. For this review, relevant examples are included from different NHP CMV to describe a monolithic simian CMV phenotype. However, comparative studies between different NHP CMV are extremely limited. There are likely to be important and, as yet, undiscovered variations between the different CMV isolates.

Natural history

Historical evidence of CMV in NHP

The earliest observations of CMV infection in NHP during the first part of the twentieth century were remarkable for their prescient descriptions of CMV–host relationships based entirely on microscopic characterization of the protozoan-like (cytomegalic) cells that had been previously noted in infant humans (Ribbert, 1904; Goodpasture and Talbot, 1921) and guinea pigs (Jackson, 1920). The first published report of NHP CMV occurred three years after Cole and Kuttner discovered that the salivary gland agent of guinea pigs was viral (filterable) in origin (Cole and Kuttner, 1926). In 1929, Stewart and Rhoads (Stewart and Rhoads, 1929) detected CMV cytopathology in tissues from the nasal passages of rhesus macaques (*Macaca mulatta*) acutely infected with poliomyelitis virus (PV). Although there was no PV-associated histopathology, they observed an "intracellular lesion [that] consisted of an acidophilic degeneration of the nuclear chromatin leading to the appearance strongly suggesting inclusion bodies." They also noted that "the lesion is not constant in all monkeys," but did recognize the lesion in the majority of monkeys examined. The lesions were frequently unaccompanied by any signs of a host inflammatory response. Covell extended these findings in 1931 by broadening the tissue distribution of the inclusion-bearing cells and articulating the low pathogenic potential of the probable virus. "I have encountered similar inclusions, not only in the situation mentioned by Stewart and Rhoads but, in addition, in the epithelial cells of the trachea, lungs and bile ducts. [That] such inclusions unaccompanied by symptoms in an animal like the monkey [are] caused by some virus of low virulence is a fair assumption." In 1935, Cowdry and

Scott made the seminal discovery that CMV could establish latency and reactivate from it. They observed that treatment of monkeys with irradiated ergosterol resulted in development of a large number of inclusions in the multiple tissues that were not seen in untreated animals. While it was concluded that ergosterol did not directly cause inclusion formation, the authors suggested that the treatment "may have activated or intensified a process already latent in the kidneys." Since the inclusions had the histological features of those described in humans and other species, they raised the "possibility of a virus being present in the kidney without any attention being called to it by any clinically recognizable symptoms of disease." The authors also concluded that "[the] association between persistence of inclusions and presence of active virus may be stressed."

Taken together, the earliest descriptions of the cytomegalic cells in NHP portrayed the probable virus as a ubiquitous infectious agent with low pathogenic potential that could establish persistent infections, reactivate from a latent state, and remain undetected in apparently healthy hosts. It was not until the first isolation of CMV from an African green monkey (AGM) (*Cercopithecine aethiops*) in 1962 (Black *et al.*, 1963), by one of the groups that had first isolated HCMV in 1956, that reagents became available to explore in detail the natural history and molecular biology of simian CMV.

Seroprevalence

Simian CMV has been described as "adventitious contaminants" during culture of primary simian cells (Smith *et al.*, 1969), a fact that is not surprising given the seroprevalence of CMV in colony-reared animals. Like HCMV, simian CMV is ubiquitous in NHP populations (Black *et al.*, 1963; Swack and Hsiung, 1982; Swack *et al.*, 1971; Andrade *et al.*, 2003; Eizuru *et al.*, 1989; Minamishima *et al.*, 1971; Kessler *et al.*, 1989; Blewett *et al.*, 2001, 2003). In breeding colonies of rhesus macaques, 50% of infants are seropositive by 6 months of age, and almost 100% are seropositive by 1 year of age (Vogel *et al.*, 1994). Similarly high rates of infection have been reported in NHP trapped in the wild, including AGM, rhesus and Japanese (*Macaca fuscata*) macaques, drill monkeys (*Mandrillus leucophaeus*), baboons (*Papio* sp.), and marmosets (*Callithrix jacchus*) (Eizuru *et al.*, 1989; Minamishima *et al.*, 1971; Blewett *et al.*, 2001, 2003; Nigida *et al.*, 1979; Ohtaki *et al.*, 1986; Jones-Engel *et al.*, 2006). The routes of transmission are not known. Virus is probably transmitted horizontally from mother to infant via breast milk and saliva, similar to identified modes in humans (Alford and Britt, 1993). Virus is also excreted in urine, adding another potential route of spread of the virus to naïve cohorts. There are no immunological or virological data indicating vertical transmission, although low rates cannot be excluded (Vogel *et al.*, 1994). Furthermore, there are no reports of spontaneously aborted monkey fetuses or neonates exhibiting histopathologic or clinical sequelae consistent with transplacental CMV infection. Rhesus macaques reach sexual maturity between 2.5 and 3 years, and virtually all breeding-age females are seropositive for rhesus CMV (RhCMV). Based on congenital HCMV infection rates in seropositive humans (Fowler *et al.*, 2003), transplacental transmission of CMV in NHP is likely to be rare ($\leq 1\%$).

The degree of CMV seroprevalence dramatically changes if animals are reared in smaller cohorts physically separated from seropositive animals. Efforts are underway at the National Primate Research Centers in the United States to develop breeding populations of macaques that are specific pathogen free (SPF) for herpes B virus (*Cercopithecine herpesvirus* 1), an alphaherpesvirus genetically related to herpes simplex virus (HSV) (Huff and Barry, 2003). SPF re-derivation involves separating the infant from the dam at birth, and hand rearing in a nursery. One offshoot of this program has been the recognition that the vast majority of infants are also seronegative for RhCMV and other endemic infectious agents. As long as the seronegative animals are segregated from CMV-infected monkeys, the animals remain CMV-free well past the age of sexual maturity (Minamishima *et al.*, 1971; Nigida *et al.*, 1979).

Multiple strains of CMV are present within each colony for each NHP species. Analyses of independent primary CMV isolates from naturally infected rhesus and Japanese macaques, AGM, and chimpanzee (*Pan troglodytes*) have shown that each isolate possesses distinct restriction fragment profiles (Eizuru *et al.*, 1989; Swinkels *et al.*, 1984; Alcendor *et al.*, 1993). Multiple strains have probably been introduced into each breeding facility by the importation of animals from different locations around the world and the occasional relocation of monkeys between breeding facilities.

Infection in immunocompetent hosts

Pathogenesis

Primary infection of healthy immunocompetent NHP, either by natural routes of exposure or experimental inoculation, does not result in overt clinical signs of disease. Since infection can naturally occur within the first months of life, simian CMV has low pathogenic potential, even in infants. Transient hematological changes, such as lymphocytosis, monocytosis, and, neutrophilia, are observed in some rhesus macaques following intravenous inoculation, but not orally inoculated monkeys (Lockridge et al., 1999). Mononucleosis is an uncommon but clinically important outcome of primary HCMV infection (Alford and Britt, 1993) that has not been associated with CMV infection in non-human primates. Recurrent infection is similarly unremarkable in terms of clinical outcomes. As noted above, the earliest postmortem descriptions of CMV in monkeys revealed that a large percentage of healthy animals had cytomegalic cells in the absence of overt disease (Stewart and Rhoads, 1929). The presence of the inclusion-bearing cells is now the exception. In recent years, inclusions have been rarely observed in tissues of immunocompetent monkeys. The reasons for this apparent change in frequency are not known, but may be related to improvements in colony management practices that may have reduced stresses in the animals. There is only a single description of recurrent CMV disease in NHP not associated with immunodeficiency or immunosuppression. Eight of 12 chimps euthanized in 1955 for a variety of clinical conditions were found to have characteristic CMV inclusions in the parotid and submaxillary glands (Vogel and Pinkerton, 1955). Three of the eight were further found to have CMV inclusions associated with focal to extensive areas of inflammation and necrosis in the adrenal cortex. One chimp also had a prominent myocarditis together with numerous cytomegalic cells. Although there was no evidence of immune suppression in these chimps, many were infected with *Mycobacterium tuberculosis* and enteric bacteria, which may have sapped their immune vigor, resulting in activation of CCMV.

Viral dynamics of primary infection

Since seroconversion begins long before the age of sexual maturity, primary infection most likely occurs via the oral mucosa following ingestion of virus-positive breast milk or saliva. The general course of primary infection involves rapid bloodstream dissemination from the site of infection to multiple tissues throughout the body. In monkeys naturally exposed to RhCMV, viral DNA can be PCR amplified from plasma coincident with the earliest detection of antiviral antibodies (these authors, unpublished). Although the time of exposure to virus can never be precisely defined in natural infections, the kinetics of CMV DNA in blood in relation to host immune responses suggest that spread of the virus through the blood is a normal component of early infection. This pattern of detection of viral DNA in plasma is recapitulated in experimental infections. Animals inoculated either intravenously (IV) or orally with RhCMV usually develop peak copy numbers of viral genomes in plasma at 7 days post inoculation, coincident with the development of anti-RhCMV IgM (Lockridge et al., 1999). Monkeys inoculated IV with 10^5 to 10^6 plaque forming units (PFU) of RhCMV characteristically reach approximately 10^4 and 10^6 genome equivalents per milliliter of plasma within 5 and 7 days, respectively (Sequar et al., 2002; Chang and Barry, 2003). Plasma CMV DNA levels decline after 7 days, although the rate of decline is variable between monkeys. Some become CMV DNA negative by 3 weeks post-inoculation, while others exhibit a more gradual decline with low copy numbers (1000/ml of plasma) present out to as long as 11 weeks. After its initial clearance, viral DNA is rarely detected in plasma. The presence of viral DNA or virus in the blood is not always observed with other forms of inoculation. Intraperitoneal injection of AGMCMV into rhesus macaques did not result in viremia, although the animals remained viuric for over two years (Swack and Hsiung, 1982). Similarly, subcutaneous inoculation of RhCMV efficiently results in systemic spread of virus, but RhCMV DNA is frequently undetectable in plasma (these authors, unpublished).

By the time CMV DNA is first amplified from plasma, the virus has probably disseminated throughout the body. RhCMV DNA can be detected in oral and genital swabs within two weeks of IV inoculation (these authors, unpublished) and in multiple tissues by 2 weeks (Lockridge et al., 1999). Viral DNA is usually detectable in the spleen and frequently from axillary and inguinal lymph nodes, kidney, bone marrow, and liver (Lockridge et al., 1999; Sequar et al., 2002). In addition, the parotid and submandibular glands appear to be preferred sites after natural exposure to virus (unpublished). In acutely infected animals, lymphofollicular hyperplasia and neutrophilic splenitis are the most prominent histopathological changes observed in IV and orally inoculated animals (Lockridge et al., 1999). Although no cytomegalic cells have been observed following experimental inoculation, cells expressing the viral immediate-early 1 (IE1) protein have been observed in the spleen of IV-inoculated monkeys (Lockridge et al., 1999; Chang and Barry, 2003). The vast majority of antigen-positive cells following acute infection are localized to the perifollicular regions, with lower numbers of IE1-positive cells observed within the germinal centers or in the red pulp. The location of IE1-positive cells within the spleen changes over time such that, by 6 months, the majority of staining cells is within the red pulp.

Immunological parameters of primary infection

The development of viral-specific immune responses is rapid and increases in intensity as viral plasma DNA loads decrease (Lockridge et al., 1999). Antibodies to IgM become detectable 1 to 2 weeks post-inoculation (p.i.) and usually become undetectable by 4 to 8 weeks. Anti-CMV IgG develop 2 to 5 weeks p.i. and continue to increase for a period of 3 to 6 months. Neutralizing antibody titers follow the same kinetics as CMV-specific responses. Affinity maturation of antiviral IgG, measured as an increase in avidity, continues for a period of at least 6 months, even if antibody titers reached a plateau 3 months earlier. Antiviral antibodies are directed against multiple viral structural and non-structural antigens, although each monkey develops a distinct pattern of reactivity on western blots. Antibodies develop to glycoprotein B (gB) (Yue et al., 2003) and the RhCMV equivalents of phosphoproteins (pp) 28, 65, and 150 (Yue et al., 2006), as well as to other structural and non-structural proteins soon after infection (Vogel et al., 1994). The region of RhCMV gB corresponding to the AD-1 region of HCMV gB is highly conserved and especially immunogenic (Kropff and Mach, 1997; Kravitz et al., 1997), and can be neutralized by monoclonal antibodies specific to the AD-1 region of HCMV gB (Kropff and Mach, 1997). Analysis of gB-specific and neutralizing titers in rhesus macaques indicates that gB encodes a large proportion of neutralizing epitopes, but not all (Yue et al., 2003). The NHP CMV encode all of the counterparts of the HCMV envelope glycoproteins (Davison et al., 2003; Hansen et al., 2003; Rivailler et al., 2006), and some of these, such as gH and the gM/gN complex, may represent additional targets of neutralizing antibodies, similar to HCMV (Mach et al., 2000; Urban et al., 1996).

Cellular immune responses to total RhCMV antigens and to the IE 1 and 2, and pp65 proteins of RhCMV are detected as early as 2 weeks following experimental CMV infection in rhesus macaques and generally precede the onset of antibody responses (A. Kaur, unpublished data). The magnitude of the CMV-specific cellular immune responses increases with time and by 6 months to 1 year have reached levels comparable to those seen in naturally infected macaques. Cytolytic and cytokine-secreting CD8[+] T-lymphocytes specific to RhCMV IE1, IE2, and pp65 and the CMV-encoded interleukin-10 (cmvIL-10) are readily detected in long-term CMV-infected rhesus macaques (Kaur et al., 2003; Pitcher et al., 2002). A. Kaur, unpublished data). In addition, CD8[+] T lymphocyte-mediated cytolytic activity to an unidentified early protein presented by rhesus CMV-infected fibroblasts is detected in CMV-seropositive macaques (Kaur et al., 1996). Although robust CD4[+] T lymphocyte responses to total RhCMV antigens are detected in the majority of CMV-seropositive macaques (Kaur et al., 2002), the immunodominant target specificity of this response has not yet been determined.

Virological and immunological parameters of chronic infection

Two salient features characterize the persistent phase of infection: chronic viral shedding and stability of the antiviral immune responses. It has long been recognized that healthy, infected monkeys can remain viuric for many years following primary infection (Swack and Hsiung, 1982; Asher et al., 1974). In a cross-sectional survey of three subspecies of colony-reared and wild-caught baboons, baboon CMV (BaCMV) was isolated from approximately 50% of the animals (Blewett et al., 2001), a detection rate that is similar to colony-reared rhesus macaques (these authors, unpublished). For BaCMV, virus was isolated almost exclusively from saliva and throat swabs and only rarely from genital swabs or urine. Molecular techniques for the detection of RhCMV DNA have yielded similar results. In a longitudinal study involving repeated sampling, some monkeys had amplifiable RhCMV DNA in oral and/or genital fluids at multiple timepoints over a 30-day period (Huff et al., 2003). A cross-sectional analysis of adult males indicated that approximately 50% were DNA-positive at any one time. In contrast to the clearance of CMV DNA from the blood within a few weeks, the presence of infectious virus and/or viral DNA in mucosal fluids demonstrates that there is active and ongoing virus replication at mucosal surfaces, probably for the life of the infected host.

Active viral gene expression at mucosal surfaces does not necessarily engender phenotypic changes or inflammatory responses at the site of infection. Antigen-positive cells can be detected occasionally by immunohistochemistry in tissues such as the spleen (Lockridge et al., 1999) and salivary glands (these authors, unpublished data). What is especially noteworthy is that the tissues are frequently histologically normal, without any cellular infiltrate in response to viral antigen production. The level of viral replication is sufficient, presumably, to enable horizontal transmission to naïve cohorts, while at the same time minimizing tissue destruction and host immune responses. At the level of the infected host, therefore, it can be stated that CMV is a persistent virus because of the chronic, ongoing production of viral antigens and progeny virions. At the cellular level, however, CMV can clearly establish, maintain, and recrudesce from a quiescent state. Based on the high frequency of animals that shed virus and the social dynamics of NHP populations, seropositive animals should be regularly challenged with heterotypic strains of virus that may be immunologically distinct from the variant associated with primary infection. It is unknown whether prior immune responses restrict subsequent challenge following natural exposure. Seropositive monkeys can be reinfected following experimental RhCMV inoculation with as little as 100 plaque forming units of a subsequent prolonged viuria of the challenge virus (L. Picker and J. Nelson, unpublished data).

The relatively constant exposure to CMV antigens (endogenous and exogenous) probably explains the pattern of antiviral immune responses observed in long-term infected monkeys. End-point IgG titers to total viral antigen preparations hover around the plateau level achieved at the end of the primary infection (Yue et al., 2003; Baroncelli et al., 1997). Although there can be a wide range of antiviral/neutralizing antibody titers and avidity indices observed amongst infected animals, only minor fluctuations occur over time within any one monkey. However, different results can be observed if antibody responses to individual viral antigens are assayed longitudinally. While antibody responses to gB usually parallel those to total RhCMV antigens, a minority of monkeys exhibit changes in gB reactivity while total antibody responses remain unchanged (Yue et al., 2003). Cellular responses to RhCMV antigens also appear to be relatively stable over time. In one study, the frequency of $CD4^+$ T-cells secreting IFN-γ following stimulation with RhCMV antigens remained within a twofold range over a 6-month period (Kaur et al., 2002). Similar to antibody titers, a wide range of CMV-specific $CD4^+$ responses occurs within a cohort of infected monkeys.

The stability of the virus-host relationship, exemplified by the absence of disease, places a relatively high immunological burden upon the infected host. One study of healthy, CMV-positive rhesus macaques observed that 0.16%–5.8% of total $CD4^+$ T-lymphocytes were CMV-specific (Kaur et al., 2002). In a cross-sectional analysis of eight healthy CMV-seropositive macaques, 0.4% to 8% of peripheral $CD8^+$ T-lymphocytes were specific for CMV antigens (A. Kaur, unpublished data). Comparably high frequencies of CMV-specific memory T-cells have been observed in persistently HCMV-infected humans (Kern et al., 2002; Gillespie et al., 2000; Sylwester et al., 2005). In contrast to humans, however, IE1 but not pp65, appears to be the dominant protein recognized by CMV-specific $CD8^+$ T-lymphocytes in rhesus macaques (A. Kaur, unpublished data).

Infection in non-immunocompetent hosts

Retroviral-induced immunodeficiency

The first published descriptions of fulminant CMV disease in NHP were in the context of rhesus macaques naturally coinfected with the immunosuppressive simian type D retrovirus (SRV). Beginning in the late 1960s and occurring through the early 1980s, periodic outbreaks of an acquired immunodeficiency disease were observed in macaque species housed at the California and New England Primate Centers (Henrickson et al., 1984; London et al., 1983; Henrickson et al., 1983; Letvin et al., 1983a,b; Osborn et al., 1984; King et al., 1983). The disease was characterized by persistent lymphadenopathy, severe wasting, chronic diarrhea, high morbidity and mortality, and multiple opportunistic infections, including activated CMV. Because of the strong immunological and pathological similarities between immunodeficient macaques and the emerging human AIDS, intense efforts were initiated to isolate the etiological agent of the so-called simian AIDS (SAIDS). The great majority of the SAIDS cases were due to the spread of SRV from healthy carriers that were unknowingly infected with this immunodeficiency-inducing virus. Subsequently, simian immunodeficiency virus (SIV) was isolated at the New England Primate Center from a few immunodeficient rhesus macaques that were free of SRV (Gardner et al., 1994).

The presence of cytomegalic cells containing cytoplasmic and/or intranuclear inclusions in tissues from immunodeficient monkeys, often associated with tissue necrosis and neutrophilic infiltration, bore almost all of the hallmarks of CMV disease in human AIDS patients. The incidence of CMV disease in monkeys with SAIDS caused by SIV or SRV can be variable, but upwards of one-third to one-half of CMV seropositive animals exhibit evidence of CMV activation at necropsy (Kaur et al., 2003; Osborn et al., 1984; King et al., 1983; Kuhn et al., 1999; Baskin et al., 1988). As with HCMV, simian CMV can produce end-organ disease in different tissues, including central and peripheral nervous system, lung, lymph nodes, liver, gastrointestinal tract, and arteries (Baskin, 1987). Depending on the thoroughness of sampling, CMV pathology can be detected within multiple tissues of an animal or may be limited to just a single site. To date, CMV retinitis has not been reported in a SAIDS monkey. A single published report describes the electron micrographic detection of herpesvirus-like particles within the eyes of two SIV-infected, RhCMV seropositive macaques (Conway et al., 1990). The reasons for the absence of detectable CMV retinitis in monkeys are not known. They may be related to the relatively rapid onset of SAIDS (within 1–2 years of SIV or SRV inoculation) and the frequent early termination of experiments to spare the animals excess pain and suffering.

The activation of RhCMV infection during SAIDS pathogenesis is similar to that of HCMV during human AIDS and stands in marked contrast to the status of the virus during persistent infection in immunocompetent hosts. In addition to the increased frequency of cytomegalic cells, other changes include an increased frequency of detectable viral DNA in blood, elevated genome copy numbers in tissues, and declining measures of anti-CMV immune functions, such as CTL activity, cytokine secretion, and neutralizing antibody titers (Sequar et al., 2002; Kaur et al., 2003). The magnitude and timing of the changes can be used to predict those animals most at-risk for developing RhCMV disease. The kinetics of these perturbations are variable, dependent, in part, on the relative timing of CMV and SIV infection.

If SIV infection occurs during the primary phase of RhCMV infection, the onset of RhCMV disease and SAIDS is both accelerated and more severe, compared to older monkeys that are persistently infected with RhCMV at the time of SIV infection (Sequar et al., 2002). Five juvenile rhesus macaques inoculated with SIV two to four weeks after RhCMV infection (either experimental or natural exposure) died with SAIDS or with early lymphoid depletion within 10–25 weeks of SIV inoculation. Three of the monkeys required euthanasia between 10 to 15 weeks post-SIV and died with histological evidence of RhCMV disease in multiple tissues. Compared to controls infected with only RhCMV, all five coinfected animals had elevated RhCMV genome copy numbers in plasma and tissues at the time of necropsy. A different pattern of RhCMV infection emerges when the time interval between RhCMV and SIV infection is increased. When monkeys persistently infected with RhCMV are inoculated with SIV, the range in the time of death post-SIV is greatly extended (10 ->72 weeks) (Sequar et al., 2002; Kaur et al., 2003). One study observed that SIV-positive monkeys with histologically confirmed RhCMV disease have significantly shorter median time of death (17 weeks) than monkeys without RhCMV disease (57 weeks) (Kaur et al., 2003). The same study also noted significant associations between the potential for RhCMV disease and changes in virological and immunological markers of RhCMV infection. Monkeys that had multi-organ disease due to reactivated RhCMV had large increases in RhCMV plasma DNAemia and lower neutralizing antibody titers at death, compared to the monkeys without histological evidence of RhCMV disease. In addition, there were significant reductions over time in RhCMV-specific $CD4^+$ and $CD8^+$ T lymphocytes in those animals with RhCMV sequelae. The declines in immune competence in these monkeys appear to have been specific to RhCMV. No significant correlations were observed between changes in anti-RhCMV antibodies and those specific to the rhesus rhadinovirus and lymphocryptovirus (related to the human herpesviruses, human herpesvirus 8 and Epstein–Barr virus -EBV, respectively) (Kaur et al., 2003).

A second study has also observed that specific changes in parameters of RhCMV infection can be used to predict the occurrence of RhCMV disease in SIV-infected monkeys. Four of five animals with RhCMV sequelae exhibited at least two of the following characteristics prior to death: (a) either a failure to develop an increase in anti-RhCMV antibody avidity or a decline in avidity over time, (b) a progressive decline in anti-RhCMV antibody titers, and/or (c) prolonged detection of RhCMV DNA in plasma (Sequar et al., 2002). Immunodeficient monkeys without RhCMV disease had no more than one of these characteristics.

Many papers published since the advent of HIV and AIDS have speculated on the role of HCMV in augmenting HIV pathogenesis (Drew et al., 1985; Robain et al., 2001; Peterman et al., 1985; Webster, 1991). Studies of RhCMV and SIV coinfection are consistent with the notion that activated RhCMV can enhance progression to SAIDS (Sequar et al., 2002; Kaur et al., 2003). Rigorous experiments demonstrating a causal effect of RhCMV on SIV pathogenesis are still required. One study has noted a possible direct effect of CMV on HIV-1 infection in chimpanzees (Castro et al., 1992). Two chimps seropositive for chimpanzee CMV (CCMV) were infected with HIV-1. PBMC cultures had been persistently negative for isolation of HIV over a 3–4-year period. After intrarectal and/or intravenous inoculation with CCMV-infected human fibroblasts, HIV was recovered from the PBMC from both chimps. One was positive for HIV isolation six times over a 12-month period, and HIV was recovered once from PBMC from the other chimp. Two chimps similarly treated with uninfected fibroblasts did not reactivate HIV.

Transplantation

The onset of CMV sequelae in NHP is not limited to immunodeficiency but can also be a factor in another clinically relevant parallel of HCMV pathobiology. CMV disease has been observed in immunosuppressed NHP receiving either allografts or xenografts, although the number of published descriptions is limited to date. The frequency of activated CMV appears to be related to the intensity of the immunosuppression regime. Xenograft recipients, such as either rhesus- or pig-to-baboon, that undergo treatments designed to prevent acute rejection (e.g., anti-thymocytic globulin – ATG) can develop CMV histopathology similar to HCMV disease in human allograft recipients, including pneumonitis and vasculopathies (Teranishi et al., 2003; Mueller et al., 2002; Ghanekar et al.,

2002). Prophylactic antiviral therapies common in human transplant recipients are not routinely employed in NHP studies. In the case of the pig-to-baboon xenograft, viral histopathology occurred only in the species-appropriate tissues; no cross-species disease was observed (Mueller et al., 2002). The mechanisms of CMV reactivation in these studies are poorly defined, primarily because the studies were not designed initially to identify causal relationships to transplant-associated CMV disease. A potential association with recipient CMV serostatus was noted in one rhesus-to-rhesus renal allograft study (Pearson et al., 2002). When monkeys were treated with antibodies to block the CD40/CD40 ligand signaling pathway, disseminated CMV disease was seen only in the CMV seronegative recipients ($n = 3$, seropositive donor), but not in 15 seropositive recipients.

Two early studies provide intriguing hints of potential stimuli for triggering reactivation of CMV. In the first study, CMV seropositive cynomolgus macaques were treated with a regimen of three immunosuppressive agents (ATG, cyclophosphamide, and cortisone acetate) given multiple times over 18 days (Ohtaki et al., 1986). With this treatment protocol, 2 of 6 monkeys exhibited only a limited number of cytomegalic cells following necropsy 21 days after initiation of immunosuppression. If the animals were infected with varicella zoster virus (VZV) 3 days after the first immunosuppressive injection, 100% of the monkeys ($n = 11$) developed severe and systemic reactivation of CMV, similar in pathology to HCMV disease in human transplant recipients. CMV inclusions were observed in multiple tissues, and 50% of the animals developed pneumonia. Other tissues demonstrated evidence of CMV vasculitis, consistent with a critical role of the endothelium in simian CMV reactivation. None of the animals exhibited evidence of VZV disease. Similar rates of CMV reactivation were observed when immunosuppressed monkeys were injected with formalin-inactivated VZV, demonstrating that active VZV replication was not essential for the development of CMV lesions (Ohtaki et al., 1988).

The utility of NHP as experimental models to study transplantation-associated CMV disease remains to be determined, based on the fact that the frequency of CMV disease in allograft and xenograft recipients is unknown. There are multiple examples in the literature of long-term studies of simian xenografts (>300 days post-transplant) occurring in the absence of clinical or histopathological evidence of reactivated CMV. Based on the transplant literature, it appears that the incidence of CMV disease in NHP is lower than in human allograft recipients. Whether this is due to sampling error or differences in reactivation potential following immunosuppression is unknown.

Immunosuppression associated with measles virus

CMV activation and disease can also be observed following viral, non-iatrogenic immunosuppression. Macaques are highly susceptible to infection by measles virus, a paramyxovirus that can induce temporary immunosuppression in non-SIV/SRV-infected monkeys (McChesney et al., 1997; Willy et al., 1999). Measles virus pathogenesis in NHP is similar to infection in humans, ranging from subclinical, to mild (skin rash), to fatal infection. Disseminated CMV infection (lung, lymph node, and stomach) has been detected in Japanese macaques that died of measles virus infection (Choi et al., 1999).

Fetal Infection

RhCMV can cause a range of developmental and growth defects in rhesus macaque fetuses similar to those observed in human infants congenitally infected with HCMV. However, the published studies of CMV-induced fetal disease in rhesus macaques required direct inoculation of fetuses with virus in utero. Until transmission across the placenta can be demonstrated (either natural or experimental), fetal infection in NHP should be viewed as a model of intrauterine pathogenesis. Taking advantage of timed matings in NHP, it is possible to establish the time of conception to within two days (Tarantal, 1990; Tarantal and Hendrickx, 1988a,b). Using ultrasound guidance, needles can be directed through the abdominal wall of the dam to deliver virus to precise locations within the developing fetus at defined stages of gestation. Growth and developmental outcomes can be prospectively monitored by ultrasound, and fetal samples (blood, amniotic fluid, and tissue) can be obtained by needle biopsy (Tarantal, 1990; Tarantal and Hendrickx, 1988a,b).

Inoculation of rhesus macaque fetuses with RhCMV has been done via the intra-amniotic (IA), intracranial (IC), and IP routes from late in the first trimester through mid-gestation (Tarantal et al., 1998; London et al., 1986; Chang et al., 2002). Severe developmental anomalies were observed in approximately 50% of inoculated fetuses, independent of the route of inoculation. Some fetuses, however, are developmentally normal even with inoculating titers as high as 10^6 PFU delivered in the late first trimester (Barry et al., 2006). The developing CNS appears to be especially sensitive to CMV disease, with a spectrum of developmental abnormalities ranging from focal lesions to severe bilateral anomalies (Tarantal et al., 1998; London et al., 1986; Chang et al., 2002). These include microcephaly, lissencephaly, ventricular dilatation, leptomeningitis, encephalitis, and periventricular calcifications, all hallmarks of congenital HCMV infections. Some of the neuropathological changes, especially lissencephaly and microcephaly, are consistent with early insults to CNS development (Barkovich and Lindan, 1994; Hayward et al., 1991; Twickler et al., 1993). The periventricular zones and the choroid plexus are early targets for RhCMV infection following IC inoculation of RhCMV (Chang et al., 2002). The systemic distribution of RhCMV-infected cells soon after IC inoculation supports the hypothesis that RhCMV readily crosses the blood–cerebrospinal fluid barrier to sites of susceptible neuronal stem cells and protoneurons. The cortical malformations observed in the inoculated fetuses may have resulted from an early cytopathic effect that initiated a cascade of defects in proliferation, migration, and organization.

Although RhCMV histopathology was limited to just the brain in one study (London et al., 1986), other sequelae have usually been observed, including intrauterine growth retardation and systemic RhCMV disease (Tarantal et al., 1998; Chang et al., 2002; Barry et al., 2006). Placental abnormalities (deciduitis, infarction, calcification, and lymphocytic infiltration) have been seen in some inoculated fetuses (London et al., 1986).

Molecular biology

As more simian CMV sequences have become available on GenBank, it is now possible to extend the comparisons of their coding content and genetic organization with that of HCMV to include simian–simian analyses. In general, the strong parallels between the natural histories of the primate CMV are reciprocated at the structural and genomic levels, although important interspecies differences exist. An overarching issue in comparing CMV genomes is the consideration of what factors have driven adaptation of a CMV species to its particular host. Since viruses are obligate intracellular pathogens, CMV evolution is driven by virus–host interactions. Commonalities amongst and distinctions between primate CMV can be viewed as a reflection of the similarities and variations of selective pressures between the different but closely related primate hosts.

For any genetic element to be fixed within the population of any CMV species, it must have conferred a selective advantage during evolution from a progenitor CMV. This is equally applicable to both coding and non-coding portions of the genome. Regions of cross-species sequence identity, therefore, represent those domains where significant sequence divergence would produce a selective disadvantage. Conversely, highly divergent domains can be considered as focal points for evolutionary adaptation necessary to maintain optimal replication of the virus during host speciation. What might distinguish the macro- and microselective pressures between hosts is essentially unknown. Comparisons of CMV natural histories indicate that genetic changes have not come at the expense of altering the unifying concept of the CMV-host relationship. That is, CMV is a virus with low pathogenic potential that establishes a lifelong persistence in an immunocompetent host.

Virion structure

The basis for inclusion in the *Herpesviridae* family is the structural conservation of a linear double-stranded DNA genome packaged within an icosadeltahedral capsid (100 to 110 nm in diameter) composed of 162 capsomers. The nucleocapsid is surrounded in turn by a featureless tegument and a viral glycoprotein-studded envelope (Roizman and Pellet, 2001). By definition, the simian CMV adhere to this rule, and they exhibit little structural distinction from HCMV (Fig. 59.1). Mature virus particles and distinct capsid forms are observed by electron micrograph in infected cells. The variant capsid structures include the A (empty capsid, no DNA), B (scaffolding proteins but no DNA), and C (mature capsids containing DNA) forms characteristic of HCMV and HSV (Blewett et al., 2001, 2003; Lee et al., 1988). The RhCMV virion is identical in size to that of HCMV (220–230 nm), whereas those of BaCMV and drill CMV are slightly smaller (140–230 nm) (Blewett et al., 2001, 2003). The range in sizes of these latter two simian CMV species is apparently due to variability in the size of the envelope. Similarly, the B-capsid form of AGMCMV is almost identical in size (inner radius = 49.5 nm) with that of HCMV (50 nm). Density mapping of the AGMCMV B-capsid demonstrates that the architecture (i.e., T = 16 triangulation geometry, capsomer shape, and intercapsomer triplexes) is strongly conserved with other herpesviruses (Trus et al., 1999; Butcher et al., 1998; Chen et al., 1999). Some distinctions in structure have been observed between the cytoplasmic forms of the B capsid of AGMCMV and HCMV, although the differences may have resulted from the loss of some protein constituents during purification (Trus et al., 1999; Chen et al., 1999).

Genome coding content

The genomes of the RhCMV (Hansen et al., 2003; Rivailler et al., 2006) and CCMV (Davison et al., 2003) genomes have been fully sequenced and described in the literature, as have selected regions of the AGMCMV genome. A partially completed sequence of BaCMV has been deposited on GenBank (AC090446), although there has been no published analysis of it, yet. There has been strong conservation of coding content, nucleotide and amino acid sequences,

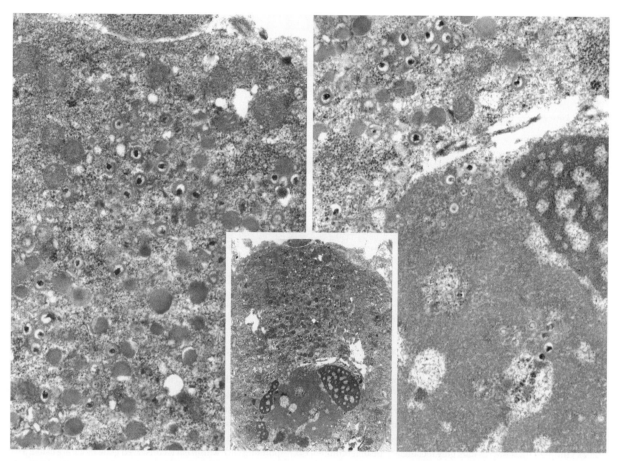

Fig. 59.1. Electron micrographs of RhCMV virions in a cochlear cell of a rhesus macaque fetus. A rhesus macaque fetus was inoculated intracranially with RhCMV strain 68–1, and the cochlea was removed and processed for electron microscopy 25 days later (S. Tinling, A. Tarantal, P. Barry, unpublished). A low magnification (center) and two high magnification (right and left) images of a cytomegalic cell of unknown type are presented illustrating nuclear and cytoplasmic forms of the RhCMV capsid and virion, respectively.

and linear genetic order amongst the primate CMV following the divergence and speciation of their hosts. Noted distinctions are observed, however, between the primate CMV. These include the selective addition (or loss) of genes within one CMV genome relative to the others, and the high rate of interspecific (but not necessarily intraspecific) sequence variation of some viral proteins that bind to highly conserved cellular proteins.

The coding content of HCMV is still open to debate 13 years after the original analysis of the AD169 sequence predicted 208 ORF (Chee et al., 1990). One recent study compared potential ORF of HCMV and CCMV reasoning that legitimate coding regions would likely have been conserved between viruses isolated from the two most closely related primate hosts. This led to the recognition of 145 ORF in the tissue culture adapted AD169 strain of HCMV, 164–167 in wild-type HCMV, and 165 in a CCMV strain that was isolated from an adult chimp (Davison et al., 2003). A subsequent study, using an algorithm that evaluates coding potential by looking for pattern relationships of HCMV amino acid sequences to the Swiss-Prot/TrEMBL database of proteins (Murphy et al., 2003a), predicted that AD169 encodes 192 proteins. Finally, comparisons of clinical isolates of HCMV with each other and with tissue culture adapted strains have led to the conclusion that there are 252 ORF in clinical isolates, almost 30 of which have not been described before (Murphy et al., 2003b).

The vast majority of ORF in HCMV have counterparts in the CCMV and RhCMV genomes. Two RhCMV genomes have been sequenced and annotated. One sequence (GenBank accession number AY186194) was derived from purified virion DNA of a low passage strain (68-1, available from ATCC) that had been cultured on primary rhesus fibroblasts (Hansen et al., 2003). The other sequence (GenBank

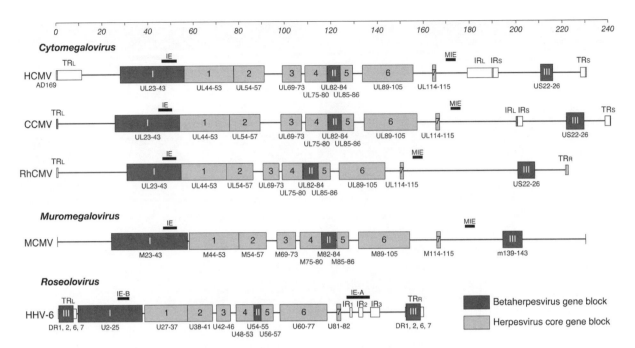

Fig. 59.2. Schematic illustration of the genome structure and gene arrangement of representative viruses comprising the Subfamily *Betaherpesvirinae* and two non-human primate CMV. The size scale at the top is shown in kbp. The horizontal lines represent unique regions of the viral genomes. Open rectangles represent reiterated sequences in the viral genomes. TRL, IRL, IRS, and TRS denote terminal or internal inverted repeats flanking the UL and US components, respectively. For RhCMV and HHV-6, TRL and TRR denote terminal direct repeats at the left and right termini of the viral genomes, respectively. Filled rectangles represent sequence blocks consisting of genes in similar orientation and/or encoding homologous amino acid sequences. The sequence blocks of conserved core genes among the herpesvirus family (block 1 though 7, shown as light grey rectangles) and conserved genes found only in betaherpesvirus subfamily (block I through III, shown as dark grey rectangles) are diagrammed. Corresponding ORF within each conserved gene block are listed. The locations of two complex IE loci within each viral genome are marked with black bars. Gene nomenclature and location are from the following references: HCMV AD169 (Davison *et al.*, 2003; Chee *et al.*, 1990), CCMV (Davison *et al.*, 2003), MCMV (Rawlinson *et al.*, 1996), and HHV-6 (Gompels *et al.*, 1995). The nomenclature for RhCMV genes (Hansen *et al.*, 2003) is based on the layout shown in Fig. 59.3(b).

accession number DQ120516) corresponds to a RhCMV (strain 180.92) isolated from an SIV-infected macaque that had been passaged six times in human fibroblasts and seven times on rhesus fibroblasts (Rivailler *et al.*, 2006).

The 68-1 strain, first isolated in 1968 (Asher *et al.*, 1974), contains a 221 459 bp genome that potentially encodes 230 ORF of 100 or more contiguous amino acids, each of which possesses a translation initiation codon (Hansen *et al.*, 2003). Some of the RhCMV ORF have no apparent equivalent in the HCMV and CCMV genomes, and it is not known whether they represent expressed genes. The total of 230 RhCMV genes should be considered provisional at this point in time and subject to reinterpretation with subsequent analysis. The 180.92 strain genome (215,678 bp) potentially encodes 258 ORF and includes 8 additional ORF not found in 68-1 and 34 ORF that were not listed in the characterization of 68-1 (Rivailler *et al.*, 2006). The 180.92 strain lacks 10 ORF that are present within the 68-1 genome.

Expression analysis has not been performed to determine whether the potential ORF are, in fact, expressed. Whatever the final tally, it is evident that evolution of RhCMV in its rhesus host has resulted in coding capacity not found in either HCMV or CCMV (described below).

Importantly, the sequences of both the 68-1 and 180.92 genomes are consistent with the interpretation that there have been deletions and rearrangements during in vitro passage. Comparison of the 180.92 sequence with that of 68-1 (Rivailler *et al.*, 2006) led to the recognition that there is a discontinuity between the genomes within the portion of the genome corresponding to the ULb′ region of HCMV. ULb′ represents a labile region of the HCMV genome that is deleted and rearranged during tissue culture adaptation, such that the intact sequence is found in clinical isolates of HCMV and not in strains that have undergone extensive passage in vitro. The fact that there is the same lability within the corresponding region of the RhCMV genome indicates that deletion and rearrangement can occur within a limited number of serial passages in tissue culture.

Genome structures

A hallmark of herpesvirus genomes is the conservation of its sequence organization. Based on the copy number, location, and orientation of repeat elements, herpesviral genomes can be grouped into six classes, designed A to F (Roizman and Pellet, 2001). Three types of genome structure have been identified in the members of *Betaherpesvirinae* (Fig. 59.2). HCMV and CCMV possess a complex type E genome, consisting of two unique components (UL and US), each flanked by inverted repeats RL and RS, respectively (Davison et al., 2003). The size of CCMV repeat elements flanking the UL component (TRL and IRL) is considerably smaller than the AD169 and Towne strains of HCMV, but is similar to those of Toledo and low-passage clinical isolates (Prichard et al., 2001). The RhCMV, AGMCMV, and BaCMV genomes each consist of one unique sequence with no internal repeat elements subdividing the genomes into two components (type F genome) (Chang and Barry, 2003; Hansen et al., 2003; Hayward et al., 1984; Rivailler et al., 2006) (E. Blewett, unpublished data). The RhCMV genome contains a 750-bp sequence element from the left end of the genome variably repeated ($0 - \geq 4$) at the right end of the genome (predominantly one or two copies) (Chang and Barry, 2003), similar to the termini of the guinea pig CMV (GPCMV) genome (McVoy et al., 1997). The RhCMV genome does not undergo genome inversion at the junction between the UL and US genes (Chang and Barry, 2003).

Gene arrangements

Based on the completely sequenced betaherpesvirus genomes (Davison et al., 2003; Hansen et al., 2003; Chee et al., 1990; Nicholas, 1996; Cha et al., 1996; Gompels et al., 1995; Rawlinson et al., 1996; Vink et al., 2000), there are several fundamental principles of betaherpesvirus genetic architecture (Fig. 59.2). These relate to the extent of genetic conservation amongst the herpesvirus family members. Primate CMV genes can be grouped into those present (a) in all herpesviruses, (b) only in betaherpesviruses, and (c) only in primate CMV. Genes in CCMV have been named based on their sequence and positional homology with HCMV (Fig. 59.3(a)) (Davison et al., 2003). Both murine and rat CMV (MCMV and RCMV, respectively) exhibit a simple genome structure (type F) with ORF colinear only to the UL region of HCMV genome (Fig. 59.2). The nomenclature for MCMV and RCMV ORF numbers them from the left to the right end of the genome (Rawlinson et al., 1996; Vink et al., 2000). The numbers of the homologous ORF are arranged to be congruent with the HCMV numbering system for the UL region. ORF with sequence homology to HCMV ORF are indicated by uppercase prefixes (M or R), whereas those not conserved in HCMV genome are designated with lowercase prefixes. As described by Hansen et al. (2003), RhCMV genes are sequentially numbered beginning at the first ORF at the left end of the genome. To emphasize the higher level of genomic colinearity between members of Genus *Cytomegalovirus* for this review, RhCMV ORF are designated according to their HCMV homologues (Fig. 59.2 and 59.3(b)). The original designations (Hansen et al., 2003) are also presented in Fig. 59.3(b).

The core genes inherited from the herpesvirus family progenitor are located within seven core-gene blocks in the central region of the viral genome (Fig. 59.2) (Roizman and Pellet, 2001). Core genes include those encoding proteins involved in nucleic acid metabolism, DNA replication, and virion structure and maturation (Table 59.1). Sequence analysis of the 68-1 strain of RhCMV did not identify a full-length UL71 gene due to the presence of an apparent single base insertion (Hansen et al., 2003). However, a highly conserved UL71 ORF is present within BaCMV (AC090446; E. Blewett, unpublished data) and the 180.92 RhCMV isolate (Rivailler et al., 2006), although both predicted peptides are shorter than the UL71 of either HCMV or CCMV. The UL22-33 block of genes was originally considered to be betaherpesvirus-specific (Roizman and Pellet, 2001). Analysis of the HCMV and CCMV genomes has led to the recognition that the UL22 ORF does not represent a true gene (Davison et al., 2003). With more betaherpesvirus sequences now available, betaherpesvirus-specific gene blocks (beta-blocks) can now be expanded to include UL23-43 (block I), UL82-84 (block II), and US22-26 (block III) (Fig. 59.2). These gene clusters are retained in the viral genomes across all three genera of *Betaherpesvirinae* with identical order and polarity along with the core-gene blocks, except that beta-block III is within the direct repeat regions of HHV6/7 and at the left end of the tupaia herpesvirus genome (Bahr and Darai, 2001). Included within these are three unique gene families (UL25, UL82, and US22) and one G-protein coupled receptor (UL33) that have no counterparts in the genomes of alpha- or gammaherpesviruses. In addition to the seven pan-herpesviral core gene blocks and three beta-blocks, two complex IE loci are positionally preserved within the betaherpesviral genomes with high similarity in both structures and splicing patterns (Davison et al., 2003; Nicholas, 1996; Rawlinson et al., 1996; Colberg-Poley et al., 1992; Chang et al., 1995; Barry et al., 1996; Nicholas, 1994; McCormick et al., 2003; Schiewe et al., 1994) (Fig. 59.2).

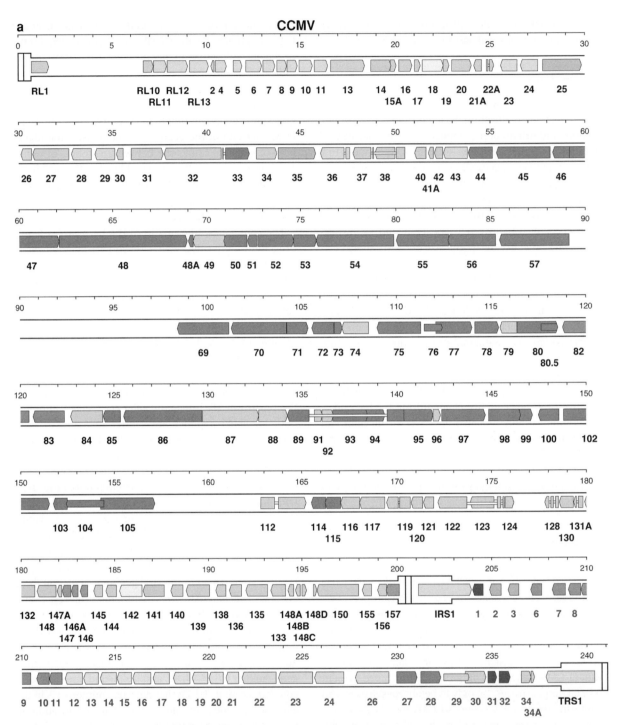

Fig. 59.3. Layout of the genes in the (a) CCMV and (b) RhCMV genomes. The size scales are in kbp. Reiterated sequences (TRL, IRL, IRS, and TRS of CCMV; TRL and TRR of RhCMV) are shown in a thicker format than the unique components of the viral genomes. Colored arrows with gene nomenclature listed below denote the order, orientation, and gene family (grouped according to the key) of predicted protein-coding regions within each viral genome. Narrow white bars represent introns connecting the coding exons. The prefixes of genes corresponding to those in HCMV UL region (shown in black text) and US (shown in blue text) have been omitted. Genes corresponding to those in HCMV AD169 RL and RS regions are given their full nomenclature. Colors differentiate between conserved core genes in the Family *Herpesviridae* with subsets of non-core genes, grouped into unique gene families, conserved in Subfamily *Betaherpesvirinae*, or Genus *Cytomegalovirus*. The nomenclature system for HCMV and CCMV genes is applied to the homologous genes within the RhCMV genome. The RhCMV ORF originally described in Hansen *et al.*, 2003 are listed within each colored arrow. RhCMV ORF with no apparent HCMV homologue are not listed in this figure and can be found in the original manuscript. (a) modified with permission from reference (Davison *et al.*, 2003) (copyright 2003, The Society for General Microbiology).

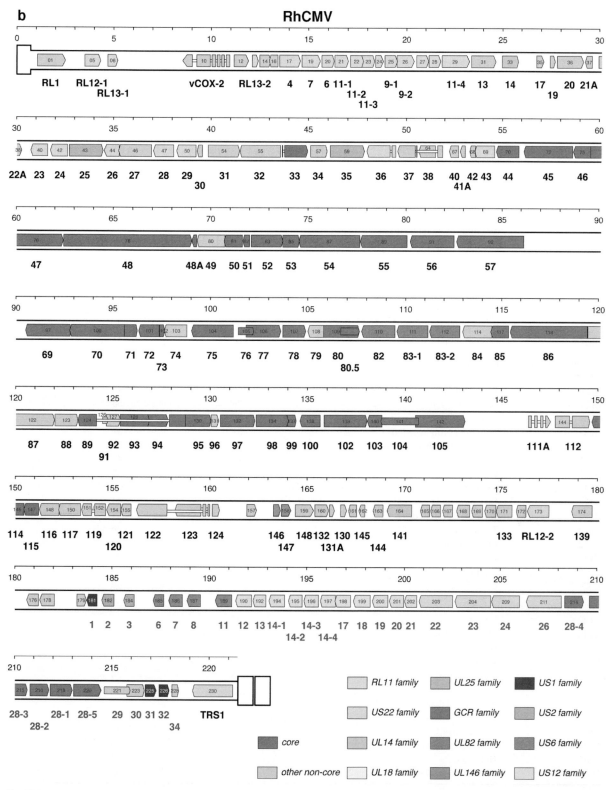

Fig. 59.3. (cont.)

Table 59.1. Primate CMV protein identities

ORF	Gene product/function	Identity (%) CCMV/HCMV	Identity (%) RhCMV/HCMV
Herpesvirus core proteins			
UL44	DNA polymerase processivity factor	90	79
UL45	Ribonucleotide reductase	71	59
UL48	Large tegument protein	54	44
UL48A	Smallest tegument protein	63	69
UL54	DNA polymerase	82	74
UL55	Glycoprotein B	76	62
UL56	Transport/capsid assembly	87	82
UL57	Single strand DNA binding protein	77	72
UL70	Helicase/primase component	79	71
UL72	dUTPase	73	61
UL73	Glycoprotein N	52	46
UL75	Glycoprotein H	64	50
UL78	G protein-coupled receptor	60	33
UL80	Assemblin (proteinase)	81	73
UL80.5	Assembly protein precursor	63	50
UL85	Minor capsid protein	86	76
UL86	Major capsid protein	89	78
UL97	Phosphotransferase	71	61
UL98	DNase/exonuclease	87	72
UL99	Tegument protein pp28	50	33
UL100	Glycoprotein M	66	51
UL114	Uracil N-glycosylase	83	70
UL115	Glycoprotein L	66	51
Betaherpesvirus-specific proteins			
TRS-1	Tegument protein	63	41
UL25	Tegument protein	60	43
UL27	Unknown	76	58
UL30	Unknown	45	32
UL32	Tegument protein pp150	51	37
UL33	G protein-coupled receptor	71	59
UL36	vMIA	76	48
UL37	vICA	51	32
UL40	NK inhibitor?	52	29
UL74	Glycoprotein O	51	44
UL82	Tegument protein pp71	68	44
UL83	Tegument protein pp65	74	36/42[a]
UL122	Immediate-early 2	72	48
UL123	Immediate-early 1	71	27
US22	Tegument protein	80	47
US24	US22 family	85	66
Primate CMV specific proteins			
UL4	Unknown	25	27
UL18	MHC class I homologue	52	[b]
UL21A	Unknown	69	39
UL111A	vIL-10	[b]	27
UL146	α-chemokine	25	30
US1	Unknown	70	56
US2	Accelerated degradation of MHC class I and II	62	33
US3	Accelerated degradation of MHC class I and II	52	24
US6	Inhibition of TAP	40	26
US11	MHC class I downregulation	47	29
US12	Unknown	58	34
US28/28-5	β-chemokine receptor	71	39

[a] UL83–1 and UL83–2, respectively.
[b] UL18 and 111A homologues not present in RhCMV and CCMV, respectively.

Accession numbers for amino acid identities: BK000394 (HCMV AD169), AF480884 (CCMV), and AY186194 (RhCMV). Amino identities were determined using the GAP program (Scoring Matrix: Blosum62, Gap creation penalty: 8, Gap extension penalty: 2) of SeqWeb® (version 2, San Diego, CA).

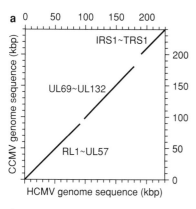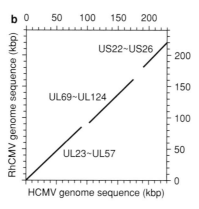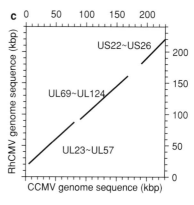

Fig. 59.4. Matrix plot demonstration of the sequence colinearity between (a) HCMV and CCMV, and (b) HCMV and RhCMV (Strain 68–1). The diagrams were computed and plotted using the Compare program (moving window: 30, stringency: 24) of SeqWeb® (version 2, San Diego, CA). The corresponding ORF within the colinear regions of each plot are indicated. The comparison of the HCMV and CCMV genomes using the same criteria has been published previously (Davison et al., 2003). GenBank accession numbers of the genome sequences used for comparison are BK000394 (HCMV AD169), AF480884 (CCMV), and AY186194 (RhCMV).

The conserved gene blocks comprise more than 80% of the total genome content of HHV-6 and HHV-7. The other two betaherpesvirus subgroups are distinguished from HHV-6/7 by larger genome sizes resulting from the presence of highly divergent genes, including tandemly arrayed, genus-specific, gene families. The HCMV genome contains the RL11 family at the left end of the genome and the US2, US6, US12 families near the right end, all of which are present in CCMV and RhCMV (Fig 59.3(a) and 59.3(b)). These families are not present in rodent CMV.

Genomic DNA sequences

Phylogenetic analysis of mammalian and avian herpesviruses based on the sequences of several core-genes, including gB and DNA polymerase, demonstrate that CCMV is the closest known relative of HCMV (McGeoch et al., 2000). Although RhCMV and AGMCMV branch away from the consensus sequence of HCMV and CCMV, these primate CMV cluster into a distinct sublineage among the betaherpesvirus subfamily, taxonomically equivalent to Genus *Cytomegalovirus* (van Regenmortel et al., 2000). Co-speciation of virus and host has been a prominent feature in herpesvirus evolution (McGeoch et al., 1995). The evolutionary branching points that separate the Old from New World primate CMV, and HCMV from CCMV are congruent with the dates of divergence of their hosts (23.3 million years or 5.5 million years ago, respectively) (McGeoch et al., 2000). The DNA sequences of HCMV and CCMV are closely colinear throughout the entire viral genome except for three regions (Fig. 59.4(a)). Regions of divergence include the RL11 gene family locus (7–16 kbp in CCMV) and the origin of DNA replication (*ori*Lyt, 90–98 kbp in CCMV). The largest distinct difference of their sequence organization (180–200 kbp region of CCMV) corresponds to the 19 kbp region that is missing from the AD169 genome but is present in Toledo and clinical isolates (ULb′) (Davison et al., 2003; Cha et al., 1996). The genome sequence of RhCMV exhibits a greater level of sequence discontinuity from HCMV than does CCMV (Figs. 59.4(b)). The colinear relationship of RhCMV to both HCMV and CCMV is largely retained in the central portion of their genomes where the conserved seven core-gene blocks, two beta-gene blocks, and the major immediate-early (MIE) locus are located (Fig. 59.4(b) and 59.4(c)). Sequence discrepancies are found at the *ori*Lyt region (87–90 kbp in RhCMV), the ULb′ region, and the left terminus of the genome. The region of the AGMCMV genome encoding *ori*Lyt (Anders and Punturieri, 1991) is strongly conserved with *ori*Lyt of RhCMV. The sequence from 161 kbp to the right end of the RhCMV genome is no longer colinear to HCMV (Fig. 59.4(b)) or CCMV (Fig. 59.4(c)), except the third beta-gene block comprising the US22-26 ORF. The lack of colinearity in the matrix plots is probably the result of the different copy numbers of ORF belonging to US6, US14, and GCR gene families within this region of RhCMV (Fig. 59.3).

A common feature of the genome in all betaherpesviruses is the absence of any functional coding regions between UL105 and the UL111A ORF. The latter ORF is found only in primate CMV except CCMV (discussed below). As large a genome as CMV possesses, there are relatively few non-coding areas of the genome, outside of the region between UL57 and UL69, which contains *ori*Lyt. The presence of a 3–4 kbp stretch without apparent coding function begs the question of what function it might serve in the CMV genome, as well as all betaherpesviral genomes. No site-directed mutational analyses have been reported for this portion of the genome, and the area is intact in tissue culture-adapted strains that have deleted other portions of the genome (Cha *et al.*, 1996). Preliminary evidence has been reported that this region of the HCMV genome may represent a stable intron of an unidentified viral transcript (Murphy *et al.*, 2003a, b).

Herpesvirus core proteins

As would be expected for proteins present in all herpesviruses, the core proteins constitute some of the most conserved ORF between HCMV and simian CMV (Table 59.1). Sequence identities of most core proteins are 60%–90% for CCMV/HCMV alignments and 50%–82% for RhCMV/HCMV alignments. The proteins involved in nucleic acid metabolism, DNA replication, and genome packaging are especially conserved when comparing either CCMV or RhCMV with HCMV. The functional importance of the high sequence identity in these proteins is emphasized by in vitro studies evaluating susceptibility to anti-HCMV drugs. RhCMV and HCMV are comparably inhibited by the currently approved compounds ganciclovir, foscarnet (Swanson *et al.*, 1998), and cidofovir, and to benzimidizole nucleosides (North *et al.*, 2004). These drugs are known to target the HCMV DNA polymerase (pUL54), phosphotransferase (pUL97), transport/capsid assembly protein (pUL56), and the DNA packaging protein (pUL89) (Krosky *et al.*, 1998; Underwood *et al.*, 1998; Emery, 2001).

Consistent with the conservation of capsid structure, there is strong sequence conservation of the proteins involved in capsid assembly, particularly for the minor (pUL85) and major (pUL86) capsid proteins mCP and MCP, respectively), and the mCP-binding protein (pUL46). The fourth capsid protein, the small capsid protein (pUL48A), is the most divergent of the group. pUL48A, which has been localized to the hexon tip (Chen *et al.*, 1999), is one of the rare exceptions to the rule that CCMV proteins are more conserved with their HCMV homologues than are those of RhCMV (Table 59.1). The two regions of pUL48A that are the most conserved in any comparison of HCMV, CCMV, and RhCMV (75% identity), corresponding to amino acids 13-31 and 43-75 of HCMV, are involved in binding to the major capsid protein (MCP) of HCMV (Lai and Britt, 2003).

There are five viral proteins, encoded by UL32, 80, 80.5, 82, and 99, that are known to be intimately associated with the capsid either during assembly or within the mature virion, three of which are encoded by core gene members. These include the assemblin maturational proteinase (pUL80) and the capsid assembly protein precursor (pAP) (pUL80.5), both of which are only transiently present within the immature capsid (Chan *et al.*, 2002; Wood *et al.*, 1997), and the tegument phosphoprotein pp28 (ppUL99) (Gibson, 1996). Whereas the proteinase domain of pUL80 is uniformly conserved, the pAP portion exhibits considerably more heterogeneity (Table 59.1). Extensive work with AGMCMV has mapped functional domains within these two proteins. Amino acids involved in the active site and proteolytic cleavage site of assemblin (Welch *et al.*, 1991), and the self-interaction of pAP and binding to MCP (Wood *et al.*, 1997) are the most conserved between simian CMV (AGMCMV, CCMV, and RhCMV) and HCMV. pp28 is the most divergent of all the core proteins with only 50 (CCMV/HCMV) and 33% (RhCMV/HCMV) amino acid identities (Table 59.1). There is only 18% identity between the pp28 proteins of CCMV and RhCMV (not shown). Conserved amino acids in pp28 are predominantly confined to the amino terminal one-third of the protein, suggesting that these may represent the domains that interact with capsid proteins.

Betaherpesvirus-specific proteins

The betaherpesvirus-specific proteins (beta-proteins) have diverged between species to a greater extent than have the core proteins. The CCMV betaherpesvirus proteins are 45%–85% identical with their HCMV equivalents (Table 59.1), which is less than the range of core protein identities (60%–90%). The same proteins of RhCMV have retained 27%–69% amino acid identities with the corresponding HCMV proteins, considerably lower than observed for the core proteins (50%–82%). Sequence variability appears to be limited to comparisons between species and is not a common theme for comparisons of an ORF between isolates of the same species. Some of the RhCMV ORF that are especially divergent from their HCMV counterparts, such as pUL37, ppUL83, and pUL123, are highly conserved between different RhCMV isolates. All three ORF exhibit >97% identity when comparing primary RhCMV isolates with strain 68-1 (these authors, unpublished data). The absence of intraspecies variation and the presence of profound interspecies divergence are consistent with the hypothesis that there were intense selective pressures on these proteins during adaptation to the host. One possible interpretation of the greater divergence of RhCMV beta-proteins versus those of CCMV is that this group of proteins may interact with cellular proteins to a greater extent than the core proteins. According to this scenario, as the cellular proteins diverged in sequence following the ape/monkey split, there was a compensatory evolution of viral proteins to maintain the putative interactions.

Some of the monkey beta-proteins are almost unrecognizable from their HCMV counterparts. The UL40 protein of HCMV has been implicated in modulation of natural killer (NK) cell activity by virtue of a nine amino acid sequence in its leader peptide that is also found in the leader peptide of most HLA-C molecules (Cerboni et al., 2001). The nonamer peptide of HLA-C is bound by the non-classical, MHC class I protein, HLA-E, in a TAP-dependent fashion. This complex can activate inhibitory receptors on NK cells. Evidence has been presented that the HCMV-derived peptide of UL40 may function via a similar mechanism, although the issue is not resolved (Cerboni et al., 2001). The RhCMV UL40 protein is only 29% identical to HCMV UL40, and BLASTP searches with it fail to identify its positional homologue within HCMV. However, RhCMV UL40 contains a nonamer sequence within the predicted leader peptide (VMAPRTLLL) that matches that found in the UL40 protein of the AD169 strain and clinical isolates of HCMV (VMAPRTLIL), and CCMV (TMAPKTLLI). One possible implication of the apparent conservation of the UL40 nonamer within the primate CMV UL40 is that dramatic sequence shifts within certain ORF during co-speciation of CMV with its host may not preclude strong functional homology.

Gene duplication events have helped shape the genomes of betaherpesviruses, in general, and CMV, in particular. There are three gene families (UL25, UL82, and US22) within all betaherpesviruses, and 11 unique gene families have been described for HCMV (Davison et al., 2003; Hansen et al., 2003; Chee et al., 1990; Nicholas, 1996; Gompels et al., 1995; Rawlinson et al., 1996; Vink et al., 2000). The HCMV gene families have been conserved both in number and genomic location in both RhCMV and CCMV with one notable exception. The UL82 family is within beta-block II and is comprised of the upper and lower matrix proteins, pp71 (ppUL82) and pp65 (ppUL83), and pUL84. Both RhCMV and BaCMV have a tandem duplication of the UL83 ORF, as opposed to the single UL83 locus found in HCMV and CCMV. This gene duplication produces in a small gap in the matrix plot of the two-dimensional comparison between the RhCMV and either HCMV or CCMV (Fig. 59.4(b) and 59.4(c), around 110–113 kbp in RhCMV). The two RhCMV UL83 ORF are 41% identical at the amino acid level. While the function of pUL83-1 has not been analyzed, pUL83-2 localizes to the nucleus (Yue et al., 2006) and has slightly higher sequence identity to HCMV UL83 than does the RhCMV UL83-1 ORF (42 vs. 36%). In addition, pUL83-2 elicits stronger cellular responses than pUL83-1 (L. Picker, unpublished). The UL83 duplication in monkey CMV bears some resemblance to the situation in murine CMV (MCMV) in which both M83 and M84 loci have sequence homology with HCMV UL83. Although M83 is analogous in position and homologous in sequence to the UL83 gene of HCMV, it also has homology to HCMV pp71 (UL82) (Morello et al., 1999; Cranmer et al., 1996). While the M84 protein is not present within the virion, it, too, has homology with HCMV pUL84, a regulatory protein with incompletely defined functions (Lischka et al., 2003). M84 is considered the MCMV homologue of HCMV pp65 (UL83).

The simian CMV contain two loci found in all other betaherpesviruses that are usually expressed with immediate-early (IE) kinetics, UL36 and 37, and the MIE region coding for IE1 and IE2 (UL123 and 122, respectively) (Fig. 59.3). UL36 and 37 of HCMV code for the viral inhibitor of caspase-8-induced apoptosis (vICA) and viral mitochondrial inhibitor of apoptosis (vMIA), respectively. Both functions are conserved in the RhCMV homologues, although vMIA of RhCMV and HCMV have retained only 32% amino acid identity (McCormick et al., 2003). Interestingly, a naturally occurring RhCMV variant without vICA activity does not impair growth, persistence, or pathogenesis in vivo (Chang and Barry, 2003; Chang et al., 2002; McCormick et al., 2003). Unlike the UL36 and 37 genes in all other betaherpesviruses, which are expressed with IE kinetics, the RhCMV UL36 and 37 genes are transcribed with delayed-early kinetics (McCormick et al., 2003).

The organization, splicing patterns, and strong transcriptional activity of the AGMCMV and RhCMV MIE region (Alcendor et al., 1993; Chang et al., 1990, 1995; Barry et al., 1996; Jeang et al., 1982, 1984, 1987) are similar to those found in HCMV (Stenberg et al., 1989). While the overall structure of the MIE locus is conserved in the betaherpesviruses, there has been significant sequence divergence of the IE coding region in monkey CMV. The IE1 proteins of RhCMV and AGMCMV are only 27%–29% identical with HCMV IE1, the least of all beta-protein comparisons, and only 40% identical with each other (Chang et al., 1995; Barry et al., 1996). In contrast, the IE2 proteins of both monkey CMV are approximately 49% identical with HCMV IE2 and 65% identical to each other (Chang et al., 1995; Barry et al., 1996). The prominent divergence of monkey CMV IE1 is further emphasized by the strong conservation of the CCMV

IE1 and IE2 ORF with those of HCMV (71 and 72%, respectively), suggesting that the monkey CMV IE1 sequence was especially labile during adaptation to a monkey host.

Primate CMV-specific proteins

Primate CMV contain numerous ORF not found in other betaherpesviruses, some of which are restricted to a subset of the primate CMV members. These are largely clustered at either end of the UL portion of the viral chromosome and within the US region, with the exception of the CMV interleukin-10 (cmvIL-10) homologue encoded by UL111A. There are several notable features about these ORF besides their restriction to primate CMV. For the most part, those found within UL are some of the most variable in pair-wise alignments between any two primate CMV. Sequence identities range between 25 and 65% for CCMV/HCMV and <29%–39% for RhCMV/HCMV. The left end of UL in RhCMV is so divergent that either the putative ORF within this region (Hansen et al., 2003; Rivailler et al., 2006) are unique to the monkey lineage of CMV and/or only have vestigial homology to their HCMV counterpart, similar to that proposed for UL40. Several of the RhCMV ORF in this region are present within BaCMV, and the DNA sequence of the left end of the RhCMV genome does not align with the corresponding regions of HCMV and CCMV (Fig. 59.4(b) and 59.4(c)).

The right end of UL also has sequence discontinuity between the primate CMV, especially when RhCMV is compared to either HCMV or CCMV. This appears to be the result of a variety of factors including high sequence diversity and the loss of gene colinearity. This same region (UL/b') has either been deleted or undergone rearrangement in tissue culture-adapted strains of HCMV (Cha et al., 1996). The linear order of genes is distinct for each primate CMV (Fig. 59.3). A likely arrangement of ORF within ULb' has been proposed for RhCMV (Rivailler et al., 2006), and sequence homologues to HCMV UL128, 130, 131A, 132, 148 – 144, and 141 are present within either or both of RhCMV strains 68-1 and 180.92. There are no sequence homologues within RhCMV for HCMV UL140 – 157, although there is a large number of uncharacterized ORF within this region of the RhCMV genome that could possibly be functional homologues. For examples, there are some potential structural similarities between the rh174 ORF of RhCMV with the UL139 ORF of HCMV (these authors, unpublished data). The proposed arrangement of genes within RhCMV ULb' has been confirmed by sequence amplification of the corresponding region of the RhCMV genome from RhCMV circulating in rhesus macaque populations, with one notable exception. PCR amplification of DNA purified from buccal swabs of naturally infected rhesus macaques has identified an additional 1.5 kb of ULb' DNA present within wild-type RhCMV not present within either 68-1 or 180.92 (these authors, unpublished data). UL128. The lack of UL128 in RhCMV is intriguing since UL128 has been identified also in the closely related Colburn stain of AGMCMV, albeit with a premature stop codon within the first exon like that in CCMV (Davison et al., 2003; Akter et al., 2003). Some of the genes within the UL/b' region of simian CMV, such as UL146, have radically diverged from their HCMV homologue to a point of barely detectable homology.

A RhCMV version of the HCMV pUL146 α-chemokine has been identified (accession number AY183378; M. Penfold, unpublished data) based on conservation of a short amino acid sequence (ELRCXC) that is both critical for neutrophil activation by cellular CXC chemokines and present in almost all clinical isolates of HCMV (Prichard et al., 2001). Apart from this motif, however, the remainder of the protein has little identity with HCMV or CCMV pUL146 (30 and 25% amino acid identities, respectively). Notably, the sequence of pUL146 of HCMV is extremely variable (50% divergence) between different clinical isolates (Prichard et al., 2001). UL146 is one of a few HCMV genes with a high degree of intra-species sequence polymorphism (20–50%). Others include UL73 (gN), UL74 (gO), UL144 (TNF receptor), UL4, and UL11 (Rasmussen et al., 2003 and references therein). In contrast, primary isolates of RhCMV from the California National Primate Research Center exhibit 99% identity for pUL146 (these authors, unpublished data).

These ORF appear to be the exceptional sites for genetic heterogeneity between HCMV isolates since most other genes that have been analyzed are considerably more conserved. For example, the US9 and US28 coding regions in clinical isolates of HCMV are >96% identical with the sequences of AD169 (Rasmussen et al., 2003). Therefore, the profound sequence divergence in most of the primate CMV-specific proteins must have occurred during co-speciation with the host following radiation of the primates. The US28 and UL111A ORF, which encode a viral β-chemokine receptor and cmvIL-10 (Lockridge et al., 2000; Kotenko et al., 2000), respectively, are illustrative for the extent of sequence divergence that can occur without loss of functional activity.

RhCMV, BaCMV, and AGMCMV (strain 9610, accession numbers AY340790–340794) (Sahagun-Ruiz et al., 2004) each contain a tandem array of five genes that are homologous to HCMV US28 by position and sequence. The five

RhCMV US28 proteins have a range of identities with HCMV pUS28 (24–39%) that is comparable to the identities between HCMV pUS27 and pUS28 (31%) and between themselves (21%–41%). Of the five, only one (RhCMV US28-5) binds the membrane-bound chemokine, fractalkine (FKN), and multiple β-chemokines with similar binding affinities as HCMV pUS28 (Penfold et al., 2003). Moreover, functional RhCMV US28-5 has been localized to the mature virion, like HCMV US28 (Penfold et al., 2003). Based on the low homology between RhCMV pUS28-5 and HCMV pUS28 (39% identity), it is reasonable to speculate that evolution of the primate US28 coding regions has been driven by maintenance of a high affinity for the host's chemokines. However, it appears that the US28 chemokine receptors have diverged to a much greater extent than might be predicted by the rate of divergence of cellular ligands. The human and rhesus macaque FKN proteins are 93% identical, indicating that US28 evolution was not proportionate to the rate of change of this particular cellular ligand. The evolutionary pressures that have driven the rate of change of pUS28 sequences may be especially complicated since pUS28 binds to multiple cellular ligands (Penfold et al., 2003).

Similarly, cmvIL-10 proteins encoded by RhCMV and HCMV are as divergent from each other (27% identical) as they are from their host species' cellular IL-10 (cIL-10) (Lockridge et al., 2000). The divergence of cmvIL-10 is distinct from viral IL-10 encoded by EBV (ebvIL-10), which is 90% identical to cIL-10. The sequence of cmvIL-10 is stable amongst multiple clinical isolates of HCMV (Hector and Davison, 2003) and RhCMV (these authors, unpublished data), indicating that sequence variation occurs between species, not within species. cmvIL-10 functions through the IL-10 receptor (Kotenko et al., 2000; Jones et al., 2002; Spencer et al., 2002), binding with an affinity almost identical to that of cIL-10 (Jones et al., 2002). As with pUS28, it appears that the cmvIL-10 proteins have diverged to a much greater extent than might be predicted by the rate of divergence of cIL-10 receptors. Although there is no available monkey IL-10 receptor sequence to enable a rhesus/human comparison, rhesus dendritic cells (DC) respond as well as human DC to recombinant human cIL-10 (these authors, unpublished data), suggesting a strong conservation of the IL-10 receptor between humans and rhesus macaques. Transduction of cIL-10 by a progenitor primate CMV and subsequent genetic drift in sequence could impart new functions to the viral IL-10, although this presents something of a conundrum for the virus. On one hand, genetic drift in a transduced cellular gene can result in the acquisition of novel functions. On the other, this could result in the conversion of a non-immunogenic "self" protein into a highly immunogenic "non-self" protein. The crystal structure of the cmvIL-10 homodimer bound to the high affinity IL-10 receptor is similar to that of cIL-10 and the receptor (Jones et al., 2002). Distinctions in quaternary structures between these two complexes suggest potential differences in downstream signaling pathways, although it has not yet been determined what functional phenotype separates cmvIL-10 from cIL-10 (Kotenko et al., 2000; Jones et al., 2002; Spencer et al., 2002).

The UL111A locus of primate CMV is in a state of genetic flux. The structure of the cIL-10 gene consists of five exons/four introns. The monkey UL111A genes (RhCMV, AGMCMV, and BaCMV) have lost the intron between exons 4 and 5 (126), while the HCMV UL111A has further lost the intron between exons 3 and 4 (Lockridge et al., 2000; Kotenko et al., 2000). In contrast, the ebvIL-10 gene has no introns. CCMV has no UL111A ORF (Davison et al., 2003), similar to the rodent CMV genomes. It may be that CCMV, like murine CMV, up-regulates expression of cellular IL-10 following infection of cells (Redpath et al., 1999), obviating the need to both encode its own IL-10 function and maintain the integrity of the UL111A gene.

The absence of UL111A in CCMV (and rodent CMV) serves as an important reminder that while the primate CMV share an overwhelming repertoire of genes and similarities in natural history, each species has adapted to its niche in its own unique way, jettisoning, transducing, or modifying coding capacity and regulatory regions as selective pressures dictated. In some cases, this meant having to evolve independent mechanisms for similar virus/host scenarios, as may be the case for activation of IL-10 through expression in the context of either the viral or host genome. Another potential example of this is provided by the apparent importance of cyclooxygenase 2 (COX-2) in the CMV life cycle.

Infection of human fibroblasts with HCMV alters the level of more than 250 cellular genes prior to replication of the viral genome, including COX-2 (Zhu et al., 1998). The function of elevated COX-2 remains to be determined, but the constellation of cellular genes whose expression levels are temporally changed along with COX-2 point to a need for the virus to regulate intracellular and extracellular inflammatory responses. Indeed, HCMV infection of fibroblasts is severely attenuated in the presence of COX-2 inhibitors (Zhu et al., 2002). RhCMV does not increase cellular COX-2 levels (J. Nelson, unpublished data), but it may have come up with its own solution to the regulation of COX-2. RhCMV encodes a multiply spliced COX-2 homologue at the left end of UL that is approximately 75% identical with the cellular COX-2 protein (Hansen et al., 2003).

Deletion of RhCMV COX-2 does not impair growth in fibroblasts but does inhibit replication in endothelial cells (J. Nelson, unpublished data). Assuming retention of function, transduction of cellular COX-2 by monkey CMV would appear to be an example of convergent evolution whereby the virus is better able to control its own destiny by modulating host inflammatory processes. Although the mechanism may differ from that employed by HCMV, the net effect is probably the same.

Summary

In sum, the simian CMV are an important primate complement to the other animal models of HCMV. Progress in characterizing them at the molecular and biological levels facilitates new avenues of inquiry into the mechanisms of HCMV persistence and pathogenesis. It is now possible to define the role of specific gene products in CMV natural history by applying the same DNA modification tools elegantly used for genetic engineering of bacterial artificial chromosomes containing the genomes for HCMV, MCMV, RCMV, and GPCMV. The full-length RhCMV genome has been cloned into a BAC (Chang et al., 2003), enabling the efficient and accurate introduction of any site-directed mutation into the viral genome. In addition, novel vaccine and chemotherapeutic intervention strategies can be tested in primate hosts that closely approximate the human condition.

Acknowledgments

The authors would like to thank Meghan Eberhardt, Jennifer Huff, Glenn Jackson, Jennifer Johnson, Rachel Kravitz, Kristen Lockridge, Getachew Sequar, Yujuan Yue, and Shan Shan Zhou for their contributions. The authors would also like to thank Kristina Abel, James Carlson, Amitinder Kaur, Lisa Strelow, and Kate Wasson for their critical reading of the material, and Earl Blewett, Laurie Brignolo, Don Canfield, Amitinder Kaur, Andrew Lackner, Jay Nelson, Louis Picker, Mark Penfold, P. Rivailler, Meredith Simon, Abigail Spinner, Ross Tarara, Steve Tinling, and F. Wang for sharing unpublished data. P.A.B would also like to express his deepest appreciation to Pam, Amelia, and Watson for their support and patience.

REFERENCES

Akter, P., Cunningham, C., McSharry, B. P. *et al.* (2003). Two novel spliced genes in human cytomegalovirus. *J. Gen. Virol.*, **84**(5), 1117–1122.

Alcendor, D. J., Barry, P. A., Pratt-Lowe, E., and Luciw, P. A. (1993). Analysis of the rhesus cytomegalovirus immediate-early gene promoter. *Virology*, **194**, 815–821.

Alford, C. A. and Britt, W. J. (1993). Cytomegalovirus. In *The Human Herpesviruses*, ed. B. Roizman, B. J. Whitley, and C. Lopez, pp. 227–255. New York: Raven Press.

Anders, D. G. and Punturieri, S. M. (1991). Multicomponent origin of cytomegalovirus lytic-phase DNA replication. *J. Virol.*, **65**(2), 931–937.

Andrade, M. R., Yee, J., Barry, P. A. *et al.* (2003). Prevalence of antibodies to selected viruses in a long–term closed breeding colony of rhesus macaques (*Macaca mulatta*) in Brazil. *Am. J. Primatol.*, **59**, 123–128.

Asher, D. M., Gibbs, J. C. J., Lang, D. J., Gadjusek, D. C., and Chanock, R. M. (1974). Persistent shedding of cytomegalovirus in the urine of healthy rhesus monkeys. *Proc. Soc. Exp. Biol. Med.*, **145**, 794–801.

Bahr, U. and Darai, G. (2001). Analysis and characterization of the complete genome of tupaia (tree shrew) herpesvirus. *J. Virol.*, **75**(10), 4854–4870.

Barkovich, A. J. and Lindan, C. E. (1994). Congenital cytomegalovirus infection of the brain: imaging analysis and embryologic considerations. *Am. J. Neuroradiol.*, **15**, 703–715.

Baroncelli, S., Barry, P. A., Capitanio, J. P., Lerche, N. W., Otsyula, M., and Mendoza, S. P. (1997). Cytomegalovirus and simian immunodeficiency virus coinfection: longitudinal study of antibody responses and disease progression. *J. AIDS*, **15**, 5–15.

Barry, P. A., Alcendor, D. J., Power, M. D., Kerr, H., and Luciw, P. A. (1996). Nucleotide sequence and molecular analysis of the rhesus cytomegalovirus immediate-early gene and the UL121-117 open reading frames. *Virology*, **215**, 61–72.

Barry, P. A., Lockridge, K. M., Salamat, S. *et al.* (2006). Nonhuman primate models of intrauterine cytomegalovirus infection. *ILAR J.*, **47**, 49-64.

Baskin, G. B. (1987). Disseminated cytomegalovirus infection in immunodeficient rhesus macaques. *Am. J. Path.*, **129**, 345–352.

Baskin, G. B., Murphey-Corb, M., Watson, E. A., and Martin, L. N. (1988). Necropsy findings in rhesus monkeys experimentally infected with cultured simian immunodeficiency virus (SIV)/delta. *Vet. Pathol.*, **25**(6), 456–467.

Black, P. H., Hartley, J. W., and Rowe, W. P. (1963). Isolation of a cytomegalovirus from African Green Monkey (28115). *Proc. Soc. Exp. Biol. Med.*, **112**, 601–605.

Blewett, E. L., Lewis, J., Gadsby, E. L., Neubauer, S. R., and Eberle, R. (2003). Isolation of cytomegalovirus and foamy virus from the drill monkey (*Mandrillus leucophaeus*) and prevalence of antibodies to these viruses amongst wild-born and captive-bred individuals. *Arch. Virol.*, **148**(3), 423–433.

Blewett, E. L., White, G., Saliki, J. T., and Eberle, R. (2001). Isolation and characterization of an endogenous cytomegalovirus (BaCMV) from baboons. *Arch. Virol.*, **146**(9), 1723–1738.

Butcher, S. J., Aitken, J., Mitchell, J., Gowen, B., and Dargan, D. J. (1998). Structure of the human cytomegalovirus B capsid by electron cryomicroscopy and image reconstruction. *J. Struct. Biol.*, **124**(1), 70–76.

Castro, B. A., Homsy, J., Lennette, E., Murthy, K. K., Eichberg, J. W., and Levy, J. A. (1992). HIV-1 expression in chimpanzees can be activated by CD8+ cell depletion or CMV infection. *Clin. Immunol. Immunopathol.*, **65**(3), 227–233.

Cerboni, C., Mousavi-Jazi, M., Wakiguchi, H., Carbone, E., Karre, K., and Soderstrom, K. (2001). Synergistic effect of IFN-gamma and human cytomegalovirus protein UL40 in the HLA-E-dependent protection from NK cell-mediated cytotoxicity. *Eur. J. Immunol.*, **31**(10), 2926–2935.

Cha, T., Tom, E., Kemble, G., Duke, G., Mocarski, E., and Spaete, R. (1996). Human cytomegalovirus clinical isolates carry at least 19 genes not found in laboratory strains. *J. Virol.*, **70**(1), 78–83.

Chan, C. K., Brignole, E. J., and Gibson, W. (2002). Cytomegalovirus assemblin (pUL80a): cleavage at internal site not essential for virus growth; proteinase absent from virions. *J. Virol.*, **76**(17), 8667–8674.

Chang, W. L. and Barry, P. A. (2003). Cloning of the full-length rhesus cytomegalovirus genome as an infectious and self-excisable bacterial artificial chromosome for analysis of viral pathogenesis. *J. Virol.*, **77**(9), 5073–5083.

Chang, W. L., Tarantal, A. F., Zhou, S. S., Borowsky, A. D., and Barry, P. A. (2002). A recombinant rhesus cytomegalovirus expressing enhanced green fluorescent protein retains the wild-type phenotype and pathogenicity in fetal macaques. *J. Virol.*, **76**(18), 9493–9504.

Chang, Y.-N., Crawford, S., Stall, J., Rawlins, D. R., Jeang, K.-T., and Hayward, G. S. (1990). The palindromic series I repeats in the simian cytomegalovirus immediate-early promoter behave as both strong basal enhancers and cyclic AMP response elements. *J. Virol.*, **64**, 264–277.

Chang, Y.-N., Jeang, K.-T., Lietman, T., and Hayward, G. S. (1995). Structural organization of the spliced immediate-early gene complex that encodes the major acidic nuclear (IE1) and transactivator (IE2) proteins of African green monkey cytomegalovirus. *J. Biomed. Sci.*, **2**, 105–130.

Chee, M. S., Bankier, A. T., Beck, S. *et al.* (1990). Analysis of the protein-coding content of the sequence of human cytomegalovirus strain AD169. *Curr. Topics Microbiol. Immunol.*, **154**, 125–169.

Chen, D. H., Jiang, H., Lee, M., Liu, F., and Zhou, Z. H. (1999). Three-dimensional visualization of tegument/capsid interactions in the intact human cytomegalovirus. *Virology*, **260**(1), 10–16.

Choi, Y. K., Simon, M. A., Kim, D. Y. *et al.* (1999). Fatal measles virus infection in Japanese macaques (*Macaca fuscata*). *Vet Pathol.*, **36**(6), 594–600.

Colberg-Poley, A. M., Santomenna, L. D., Harlow, P. P., Benfield, P. A., and Tenney, D. J. (1992). Human cytomegalovirus US3 and UL36-38 immediate-early proteins regulate gene expression. *J. Virol.*, **66**(1), 95–105.

Cole, R. and Kuttner, A. G. (1926). A filterable virus present in the submaxillary glands of guinea pigs. *J. Exp. Med.*, **44**, 855–873.

Conway, M. D., Didier, P., Fairburn, B. *et al.* (1990). Ocular manifestation of simian immunodeficiency syndrome (SAIDS). *Curr. Eye. Res.*, **9**, 759–770.

Cranmer, L. D., Clark, C. L., Morello, C. S., Farrell, H. E., Rawlinson, W. D., and Spector, D. H. (1996). Identification, analysis, and evolutionary relationships of the putative murine cytomegalovirus homologs of the human cytomegalovirus UL82 (pp71) and UL83 (pp65) matrix phosphoproteins. *J. Virol.*, **70**(11), 7929–7939.

Davison, A. J., Dolan, A., Akter, P. *et al.* (2003). The human cytomegalovirus genome revisited: comparison with the chimpanzee cytomegalovirus genome. *J. Gen. Virol.*, **84**(1), 17–28.

Drew, W. L., Mills, J., Levy, J. *et al.* (1985). Cytomegalovirus infection and abnormal T-lymphocyte subset ratios in homosexual men. *Ann. Intern. Med.*, **103**(1), 61–63.

Eizuru, Y., Tsuchiya, K., Mori, R., and Minamishima, Y. (1989). Immunological and molecular comparisons of simian cytomegaloviruses isolated from African green monkey (*Ceropithicus aethiops*) and Japanese macaque (*Macaca fuscata*). *Arch. Virol.*, **107**, 65–75.

Emery, V. C. (2001). Progress in understanding cytomegalovirus drug resistance. *J. Clin. Virol.*, **21**(3), 223–228.

Fowler, K. B., Stagno, S., and Pass, R. F. (2003). Maternal immunity and prevention of congenital cytomegalovirus infection. *J. Am. Med. Assoc.*, **289**(8), 1008–1011.

Gardner, M. B., Endres, M., and Barry, P. A. (1994). The Simian retroviruses: SIV and SRV. In *The Retroviridae*, ed. J. Levy, pp. 133–276. New York: Plenum Press.

Ghanekar, A., Lajoie, G., Luo, Y. *et al.* (2002). Improvement in rejection of human decay accelerating factor transgenic pig-to-primate renal xenografts with administration of rabbit antithymocyte serum. *Transplantation*, **74**(1), 28–35.

Gibson, W. (1996). Structure and assembly of the virion. *Intervirology*, **39**(5–6), 389–400.

Gillespie, G. M., Wills, M. R., Appay, V. *et al.* (2000). Functional heterogeneity and high frequencies of cytomegalovirus-specific CD8(+) T lymphocytes in healthy seropositive donors. *J. Virol.*, **74**(17), 8140–8150.

Gompels, U. A., Nicholas, J., Lawrence, G. *et al.* (1995). The DNA sequence of human herpesvirus-6: structure, coding content, and genome evolution. *Virology*, **209**(1), 29–51.

Goodpasture, E. W. and Talbot, F. W. (1921). Concerning the nature of "protozoan–like" cells in certain lesions of infancy. *Am. J. Dis. Child.*, **21**, 415–421.

Hansen, S. G., Strelow, L. I., Franchi, D. C., Anders, D. G., and Wong, S. W. (2003). Complete sequence and genomic analysis of rhesus cytomegalovirus. *J. Virol.*, **77**, 6620–6636.

Hayward, G. S., Ambinder, R., Ciufo, D., Hayward, S. D., and LaFemina, R. L. (1984). Structural organization of human herpesvirus DNA molecules. *J. Invest. Dermatol.*, **83**(1 Suppl.), 29s–41s.

Hayward, J. C., Titelbaum, D. S., Clancy, R. R., and Zimmerman, R. A. (1991). Lissencephaly–pachygyria associated with congenital cytomegalovirus infection. *J. Child Neurol.*, **6**, 109–114.

Hector, R. and Davison, A. J. (2003). In *9th International Cytomegalovirus Workshop*, May 20–25, Maastricht, the Netherlands.

Henrickson, R. V., Maul, D. H., Osborn, K. G. *et al*. (1983). Epidemic of acquired immunodeficiency in rhesus monkeys. *Lancet*, **1**(8321), 388–390.

Henrickson, R. V., Maul, D. H., Lerche, N. W. *et al*. (1984). Clinical features of simian acquired immunodeficiency syndrome (SAIDS) in rhesus monkeys. *Lab. Anim. Sci.*, **34**(2), 140–145.

Huff, J. E., Eberle, R., Capitanio, J., Zhou, S.-S., and Barry, P. A. (2003). Differential detection of B virus and rhesus cytomegalovirus in rhesus macaques. *J. Gen. Virol.*, **84**, 83–92.

Huff, J. L. and Barry, P. A. (2003). B-virus (Cercopithecine herpesvirus 1) infection in humans and macaques: potential for zoonotic disease. *Emerg. Infect. Dis.*, **9**(2), 246–250.

Jackson, L. (1920). An intracellular protozoan parasite of the ducts of the salivary glands of the guinea pig. *J. Infect. Dis.*, **26**, 347–350.

Jeang, K.-T., Cho, M.-S., and Hayward, G. S. (1984). Abundant constitutive expression of the immediate-early 94K protein from cytomegalovirus (Colburn) in a DNA-transfected mouse cell line. *Mol. Cell. Biol.*, **4**, 2214–2223.

Jeang, K. T., Chin, G., and Hayward, G. S. (1982). Characterization of cytomegalovirus immediate-early genes. I. Nonpermissive rodent cells overproduce the IE94K protein form CMV (Colburn). *Virology*, **121**, 393–403.

Jeang, K.-T., Rawlins, D. R., Rosenfeld, P. J., Shero, J. D., Kelly, T. J., and Hayward, G. S. (1987). Multiple tandemly repeated binding sites for cellular nuclear factor 1 that surround the major immediate-early promoters of simian and human cytomegalovirus. *J. Virol.*, **61**, 1559–1570.

Jones, B. C., Logsdon, N. J., Josephson, K., Cook, J., Barry, P. A., and Walter, M. R. (2002). Crystal structure of human cytomegalovirus IL-10 bound to soluble human IL-10R1. *Proc. Natl Acad. Sci. USA*, **99**(14), 9404–9409.

Jones-Engel, L., Engel, G. A., Heidrich, J. *et al*. (2006). Temple monkeys and health implications of commensalism, Kathmandu, Nepal. *Emerg. Infect. Dis.*, **12**, 900–906.

Kaur, A., Daniel, M. D., Hempel, D., Lee-Parritz, D., Hirsch, M. S., and Johnson, R. P. (1996). Cytotoxic T-lymphocyte responses to cytomegalovirus in normal and simian immunodeficiency virus-infected macaques. *J. Virol.*, **70**, 7725–7733.

Kaur, A., Hale, C. L., Noren, B., Kassis, N., Simon, M. A., and Johnson, R. P. (2002). Decreased frequency of cytomegalovirus (CMV)-specific CD4+ T lymphocytes in simian immunodeficiency virus-infected rhesus macaques: inverse relationship with CMV viremia. *J. Virol.*, **76**(8), 3646–3658.

Kaur, A., Kassis, N., Hale, C. L. *et al*. (2003). Direct relationship between suppression of virus-specific immunity and emergence of cytomegalovirus disease in simian AIDS. *J. Virol.*, **77**(10), 5749–5758.

Kern, F., Bunde, T., Faulhaber, N. *et al*. (2002). Cytomegalovirus (CMV) phosphoprotein 65 makes a large contribution to shaping the T cell repertoire in CMV-exposed individuals. *J. Infect. Dis.*, **185**(12), 1709–1716.

Kessler, M. J., London, W. T., Madden, D. L. *et al*. (1989). Serological survey for viral diseases in the Cayo Santiago rhesus macaque population. *Puerto Rican Health Sci. J.*, **8**, 95–97.

King, N. W., Hunt, R. D., and Letvin, N. L. (1983). Histopathologic changes in macaques with an acquired immunodeficiency syndrome (AIDS). *Am. J. Pathol.*, **113**(3), 382–388.

Kotenko, S. V., Saccani, S., Izotova, L. S., Mirochnitchenko, O. V., and Pestka, S. (2000). Human cytomegalovirus harbors its own unique IL-10 homolog (cmvIL-10). *Proc. Natl Acad. Sci. USA*, **97**(4), 1695–1700.

Kravitz, R. H., Sciabica, K. S., Cho, K., Luciw, P. A., and Barry, P. A. (1997). Cloning and characterization of the rhesus cytomegalovirus glycoprotein B. *J. Gen. Virol.*, **78**, 2009–2013.

Kropff, B. and Mach, M. (1997). Identification of the gene coding for rhesus cytomegalovirus glycoprotein B and immunological analysis of the protein. *J. Gen. Virol.*, **78**, 1999–2007.

Krosky, P. M, Underwood, M. R., Turk, S. R. *et al*. (1998). Resistance of human cytomegalovirus to benzimidazole ribonucleosides maps to two open reading frames: UL89 and UL56. *J. Virol.*, **72**(6), 4721–4728.

Kuhn, E. M., Stolte, N., Matz-Rensing, K. *et al*. (1999). Immunohistochemical studies of productive rhesus cytomegalovirus infection in rhesus monkeys (*Macaca mulatta*) infected with simian immunodeficiency virus. *Vet. Pathol.*, **36**(1), 51–56.

Lacoste, V., Mauclere, P., Dubreuil, G. *et al*. (2000). Simian homologues of human gamma-2 and betaherpesviruses in mandrill and drill monkeys. *J. Virol.*, **74**(24), 11993–11999.

Lai, L. and Britt, W. J. (2003). The interaction between the major capsid protein and the smallest capsid protein of human cytomegalovirus is dependent on two linear sequences in the smallest capsid protein. *J. Virol.*, **77**(4), 2730–2735.

Lee, J. Y., Irmiere, A., and Gibson, W. (1988). Primate cytomegalovirus assembly: evidence that DNA packaging occurs subsequent to B capsid assembly. *Virology*, **167**(1), 87–96.

Letvin, N. L., Eaton, K. A., Aldrich, W. R. *et al*. (1983a). Acquired immunodeficiency syndrome in a colony of macaque monkeys. *Proc. Natl Acad. Sci. USA*, **80**(9), 2718–2722.

Letvin, N. L., Aldrich, W. R., King, N. W., Blake, B. J., Daniel, M. D., and Hunt, R. D. (1983b). Experimental transmission of macaque AIDS by means of inoculation of macaque lymphoma tissue. *Lancet*, **2**(8350), 599–602.

Lischka, P., Sorg, G., Kann, M., Winkler, M., and Stamminger, T. (2003). A nonconventional nuclear localization signal within the UL84 protein of human cytomegalovirus mediates nuclear import via the importin alpha/beta pathway. *J. Virol.*, **77**(6), 3734–3748.

Lockridge, K. M., Sequar, G., Zhou, S. S., Yue, Y., Mandell, C. M., and Barry, P. A. (1999). Pathogenesis of experimental rhesus cytomegalovirus infection. *J. Virol.*, **73**, 9576–9583.

Lockridge, K. M., Zhou, S. S., Kravitz, R. H. *et al*. (2000). Primate cytomegaloviruses encode and express an IL-10-like protein. *Virology*, **268**(2), 272–280.

London, W. T., Sever, J. L., Madden, D. L. *et al*. (1983). Experimental transmission of simian acquired immunodeficiency syndrome (SAIDS) and Kaposi-like skin lesions. *Lancet*, **2**(8355), 869–873.

London, W. T., Martinez, A. J., Houff, S. A. et al. (1986). Experimental congenital disease with simian cytomegalovirus in rhesus monkeys. *Teratology*, **33**, 323–331.

Mach, M., Kropff, B., Dal Monte, P., and Britt, W. (2000). Complex formation by human cytomegalovirus glycoproteins M (gpUL100) and N (gpUL73). *J. Virol.*, **74**(24), 11881–11892.

McChesney, M. B., Miller, C. J., Rota, P. A. et al. (1997). Experimental measles. I. Pathogenesis in the normal and the immunized host. *Virology*, **233**(1), 74–84.

McCormick, A. L., Skaletskaya, A., Barry P. A., Mocarski, E. S., and Goldmacher, V. S. (2003). Differential function and expression of the viral inhibitor of caspase 8-induced apoptosis (vICA) and the viral mitochondria-localized inhibitor of apoptosis (vMIA) cell death suppressors conserved in primate and rodent cytomegaloviruses. *Virology, in press*.

McGeoch, D. J., Cook, S., Dolan, A., Jamieson, F. E., and Telford, E. A. (1995). Molecular phylogeny and evolutionary timescale for the family of mammalian herpesviruses. *J. Mol. Biol.*, **247**(3), 443–458.

McGeoch, D. J., Dolan, A., and Ralph, A. C. (2000). Toward a comprehensive phylogeny for mammalian and avian herpesviruses. *J. Virol.*, **74**(22), 10401–10406.

McVoy, M. A., Nixon, D. E., and Adler, S. P. (1997). Circularization and cleavage of guinea pig cytomegalovirus genomes. *J. Virol.*, **71**(6), 4209–4217.

Minamishima, Y., Graham, B. J., and Benyesh-Melnick, M. (1971). Neutralizing antibodies to cytomegaloviruses in normal simian and human sera. *Infect. Immun.*, **4**(4), 368–373.

Morello, C. S., Cranmer, L. D., and Spector, D. H. (1999). In vivo replication, latency, and immunogenicity of murine cytomegalovirus mutants with deletions in the M83 and M84 genes, the putative homologs of human cytomegalovirus pp65 (UL83). *J. Virol.*, **73**(9), 7678–7693.

Mueller, N. J., Barth, R. N., Yamamoto, S. et al. (2002). Activation of cytomegalovirus in pig-to-primate organ xenotransplantation. *J. Virol.*, **76**(10), 4734–4740.

Murphy, E., Rigoutsos, I., Shibuya, T., and Shenk, T. E. (2003a). Reevaluation of human cytomegalovirus coding potential. *Proc. Natl Acad. Sci. USA, in press*.

Murphy, E., Yu, D., Grimwood, J. et al. (2003b). Coding potential of laboratory and clinical strains of human cytomegalovirus. *Proc. Natl Acad. Sci. USA, in press*.

Nicholas, J. (1994). Nucleotide sequence analysis of a 21-kbp region of the genome of human herpesvirus-6 containing homologues of human cytomegalovirus major immediate-early and replication genes. *Virology*, **204**(2), 738–750.

Nicholas, J. (1996). Determination and analysis of the complete nucleotide sequence of human herpesvirus 7. *J. Virol.*, **70**(9), 5975–5989.

Nigida, S. M., Falk, L. A., Wolfe, L. G., and Deinhardt, F. (1979). Isolation of a cytomegalovirus from salivary glands of white-lipped marmosets (*Saguinus fuscicollis*). *Lab. Anim. Sci.*, **29**(1), 53–60.

North, T. W., Sequar, G., Townsend, L. B. et al. (2004). Rhesus cytomegalovirus is similar to human cytomegalovirus in susceptibility to benzimidizole nucleosides. *Antimicrob. Agents Chemother.*, **48**, 2760–2765.

Ohtaki, S., Kodama, H., Hondo, R., and Kurata, T. (1986). Activation of cytomegalovirus infection in immunosuppressed cynomolgus monkeys inoculated with varicella-zoster virus. *Acta Patholog. Jpn.*, **36**, 1553–1563.

Ohtaki, S., Hondo, R., Kodama, H., and Kurata, T. (1988). Experimental activation of latent cytomegalovirus infection of the captive bred (F1) cynomolgous monkeys by live or killed varicella-zoster virus inoculated under immunosuppression. *Acta Pathol. Jpn.*, **38**, 967–978.

Osborn, K. G., Prahalada, S., Lowenstine, L. J., Gardner, M. B., Maul, D. H., and Henrickson, R. V. (1984). The pathology of an epizootic of acquired immunodeficiency in rhesus macaques. *Am. J. Pathol.*, **114**, 94–103.

Pearson, T. C., Trambley, J., Odom, K. et al. (2002). Anti-CD40 therapy extends renal allograft survival in rhesus macaques. *Transplantation*, **74**(7), 933–940.

Penfold, M. E., Schmidt, T. L., Dairaghi, D. J., Barry, P. A., and Schall, T. J. (2003). Characterization of the rhesus cytomegalovirus US28 locus. *J. Virol.*, **77**(19), 10404–10413.

Peterman, T. A., Drotman, D. P., and Curran, J. W. (1985). Epidemiology of the acquired immunodeficiency syndrome (AIDS). *Epidemiol. Rev.*, **7**, 1–21.

Pitcher, C. J., Hagen, S. I., Walker, J. M. et al. (2002). Development and homeostasis of T cell memory in rhesus macaque. *J. Immunol.*, **168**(1), 29–43.

Prichard, M. N., Penfold, M. E., Duke, G. M., Spaete, R. R., and Kemble, G. W. (2001). A review of genetic differences between limited and extensively passaged human cytomegalovirus strains. *Rev. Med. Virol.*, **11**(3), 191–200.

Rasmussen, L., Geissler, A., and Winters, M. (2003). Inter- and intragenic variations complicate the molecular epidemiology of human cytomegalovirus. *J. Infect. Dis.*, 2003, **187**(5), 809–819.

Rawlinson, W. D., Farrell, H. E., and Barrell, B. G. (1996). Analysis of the complete DNA sequence of murine cytomegalovirus. *J. Virol.*, **70**(12), 8833–8849.

Redpath, S., Angulo, A., Gascoigne, N. R., and Ghazal, P. (1999). Murine cytomegalovirus infection down-regulates MHC class II expression on macrophages by induction of IL-10. *J. Immunol.*, **162**(11), 6701–6707.

Ribbert, D. (1904). Uber protozoenartige zellen in der niere eines syphilitischen neugoborenen und in der parotis von kindern. *Zentralbl. Allg. Pathol.*, **15**, 945–948.

Rivailler, P., Kaur, A., Johnson, R. P. et al. (2006). Genomic sequence of rhesus cytomegalovirus 180.92: insights into the coding potential of rhesus cytomegalovirus. *J. Virol.*, **80**, 4179–4182.

Robain, M., Boufassa, F., Hubert, J. B., Persoz, A., Burgard, M., and Meyer, L. (2001). Cytomegalovirus seroconversion as a cofactor for progression to AIDS. *AIDS*, **15**(2), 251–256.

Roizman, B. and Pellet, P. E. (2001). The Family *Herpesviridae*: A brief introduction. In *Field's Virology*, 4th edn. ed. D. M. Knipe and P. M. Howley, pp. 2381–2397. Philadelphia: Lippincott Williams & Wilkins.

Sahagun-Ruiz, A., Sierra-Honigmann, A. M., Krause, P. et al. (2004). Simian cytomegalovirus encodes five rapidly evolving chemokine receptor homologues. *Virus Genes*, **28**, 71–83.

Schiewe, U., Neipel, F., Schreiner, D., and Fleckenstein, B. (1994). Structure and transcription of an immediate-early region in the human herpesvirus 6 genome. *J. Virol.*, **68**(5), 2978–2985.

Sequar, G., Britt, W. J., Lakeman, F. D. et al. (2002). Experimental coinfection of rhesus macaques with rhesus cytomegalovirus and simian immunodeficiency virus: pathogenesis. *J Virol.*, **76**(15), 7661–7671.

Smith, K. O., Thiel, J. F., Newman, J. T. et al. (1969). Cytomegaloviruses as common adventitious contaminants in primary African green monkey kidney cell cultures. *J. Natl Cancer Inst.*, **42**(3), 489–496.

Spencer, J. V., Lockridge, K. M., Barry, P. A. et al. (2002). Potent immunosuppressive activities of cytomegalovirus- encoded interleukin-10. *J. Virol.*, **76**(3), 1285–1292.

Stenberg, R. M., Depto, A. S., Fortney, J., and Nelson, J. A. (1989). Regulated expression of early and late RNAs and proteins from the human cytomegalovirus immediate-early gene region. *J. Virol.*, **63**, 2699–2708.

Stewart, F. W. and Rhoads, C. P. (1929). Lesions in nasal mucous membranes of monkeys with acute poliomyelitis. *Proc. Soc. Exp. Biol. Med.*, **26**, 664–665.

Swack, N. S. and Hsiung, G. D. (1982). Natural and experimental simian cytomegalovirus infections at a primate center. *J. Med. Primatol.*, **11**, 169–177.

Swack, N. S., Liu, O. C., and Hsiung, G. D.(1971). Cytomegalovirus infections of monkeys and baboons. *Am. J. Epidemiol.*, **94**, 397–402.

Swanson, R., Bergquam, E., and Wong, S. W. (1998). Characterization of rhesus cytomegalovirus genes associated with anti-viral susceptibility. *Virology*, **240**(2), 338–348.

Swinkels, B. W., Geelen, J. L., Wertheim-van Dillen, P., van Es, A. A., and van der Noordaa, J. (1984). Initial characterization of four cytomegalovirus strains isolated from chimpanzees. Brief report. *Arch. Virol.*, **82**(1–2), 125–128.

Sylwester, A. W., Mitchell, B. L., Edgar, J. B. et al. (2005). Broadly targeted human cytomegalovirus-specific CD4+ and CD8+ T cells dominate the memory compartments of exposed subjects. *J. Exp. Med.*, **202**, 673–685.

Tarantal, A. F. (1990). Interventional ultrasound in pregnant macaques: embryonic/fetal applications. *J. Med. Primatol.*, **19**(1), 47–58.

Tarantal, A. F. and Hendrickx, A. G. (1988a). Use of ultrasound for early pregnancy detection in the rhesus and cynomolgus macaque (*Macaca mulatta* and *Macaca fascicularis*). *J. Med. Primatol.*, **17**(2), 105–112.

Tarantal, A. F. and Hendrickx, A. G. (1988b). The use of ultrasonography for evaluating pregnancy in macaques. In *Nonhuman Primates – Developmental Biology and Toxicology*, ed. D. Newbert, H.-J. Merker, and A. G. Hendrickx, pp. 91–99. Berlin: Ueberreuter Wissenschaft.

Tarantal, A. F., Salamat, S., Britt, W. J., Luciw, P. A., Hendrickx, A. G., and Barry, P. A. (1998). Neuropathogenesis induced by rhesus cytomegalovirus in fetal rhesus monkeys (*Macaca mulatta*). *J. Infect. Dis.*, **177**, 446–450.

Teranishi, K., Alwayn, I. P., Buhler, L. et al. (2003). Depletion of anti-Gal antibodies by the intravenous infusion of Gal type 2 and 6 glycoconjugates in baboons. *Xenotransplantation* **10**(4), 357–367.

Trus, B. L., Gibson, W., Cheng, N., and Steven, A. C. (1999). Capsid structure of simian cytomegalovirus from cryoelectron microscopy: evidence for tegument attachment sites. *J. Virol.*, **73**(3), 2181–2192.

Twickler, D. M., Perlman, J., and Maberry, M. C. (1993). Congenital cytomegalovirus infection presenting as cerebral ventriculomegaly on antenatal sonography. *Am. J. Perinatol.*, **10**, 404–406.

Underwood, M. R., Harvey, R. J., Stanat, S. C. et al. (1998). Inhibition of human cytomegalovirus DNA maturation by a benzimidazole ribonucleoside is mediated through the UL89 gene product. *J. Virol.*, **72**(1), 717–725.

Urban, M., Klein, M., Britt, W. J., Hassfurther, E., and Mach, M. (1996). Glycoprotein H of human cytomegalovirus is a major antigen for the neutralizing humoral immune response. *J. Gen. Virol.*, **77**, 1537–1547.

van Regenmortel, M. H. V., Fauquet, C. M., Bishop, D. H. L. et al. (2000). Seventh Report of the International Committee on Taxonomy of Viruses. http://www.virustaxonomyonline.com/virtax/lpext.dll?f=templates&fn =main-h.htm.

Vink, C., Beuken, E., and Bruggeman, C. A. (2000). Complete DNA sequence of the rat cytomegalovirus genome. *J Virol.*, **74**(16), 7656–7665.

Vogel, F. S. and Pinkerton, H. (1955). Spontaneous salivary gland disease virus in chimpanzees. *Arch. Pathol.*, **60**, 281–285.

Vogel, P., Weigler, B. J., Kerr, H., Hendrickx, A., and Barry, P. A. (1994). Seroepidemiologic studies of cytomegalovirus infection in a breeding population of rhesus macaques. *Lab. Anim. Sci.*, **44**, 25–30.

Webster, A. (1991). Cytomegalovirus as a possible cofactor in HIV disease progression. *J. AIDS*, **4**(Suppl. 1), S47–S52.

Welch, A. R., Woods, A. S., McNally, L. M., Cotter, R. J., and Gibson, W. (1991). A herpesvirus maturational proteinase, assemblin: identification of its gene, putative active site domain, and cleavage site. *Proc. Natl Acad. Sci. USA*, **88**(23), 10792–10796.

Willy, M. E., Woodward, R. A., Thornton, V. B. et al. (1999). Management of a measles outbreak among Old World nonhuman primates. *Lab. Anim. Sci.*, **49**(1), 42–48.

Wood, L. J., Baxter, M. K., Plafker, S. M., and Gibson, W. (1997). Human cytomegalovirus capsid assembly protein precursor (pUL80.5) interacts with itself and with the major capsid protein (pUL86) through two different domains. *J. Virol.*, **71**(1), 179–190.

Yue, Y., Zhou, S. S., and Barry, P. A. (2003). Antibody responses to rhesus cytomegalovirus glycoprotein B in naturally infected rhesus macaques. *J. Gen. Virol.*, in press.

Yue, Y., Kaur, A., Zhou, S. S. *et al.* (2006). Characterization and immunological analysis of the rhesus cytomegalovirus homologue (Rh112) of the human cytomegalovirus UL83 lower matrix phosphoprotein (pp. 65). *J. Gen. Virol.*, **87**, 777–787.

Zhu, H., Cong, J. P., Mamtora, G., Gingeras, T., and Shenk, T. (1998). Cellular gene expression altered by human cytomegalovirus: global monitoring with oligonucleotide arrays. *Proc. Natl Acad. Sci. USA*, **95**(24), 14470–14475.

Zhu, H., Cong, J. P., Yu, D., Bresnahan, W. A., and Shenk, T. E. (2002). Inhibition of cyclooxygenase 2 blocks human cytomegalovirus replication. *Proc. Natl Acad. Sci. USA*, **99**(6), 3932–3937.

60

Gammaherpesviruses of New World primates

Bernhard Fleckenstein and Armin Ensser

Institut für Klinische und Molekulare Virologie Erlangen, Germany

Introduction

Numerous Gamma-herpesviruses, a large subfamily of the herpes group, have limited pathogenic potential upon primary infection of their natural host. They are most relevant however as tumor viruses of the hematopoietic system and form an important chapter of viral oncology. The prototype of the genus lymphocryptovirus (γ1-herpesvirus), Epstein-Barr Virus (EBV), was the first clearly identified human herpesvirus. EBV causes lymphomas of B-cell origin and other lymphoproliferative syndromes, nasopharyngeal carcinomas and, possibly, gastric cancer. The second known genus of gamma-herpesviruses, rhadinoviruses or γ2-herpesviruses, is biologically and molecularly distinct. The prototypic members of this group, termed Herpesvirus (H.) saimiri (HVS) and H. ateles (HVA), were detected as T-lymphotropic tumor viruses in neotropical primates and raised primary interest from the fact that they cause fulminant T-cell lymphomas in numerous primates as well as in rabbits, although no exact correlates of these tumors exist in human pathology. This led to the identification of novel viral membrane-associated T-cell oncoproteins, termed Stp and Tip. These are small adaptor molecules that efficiently act on T-lymphocyte signaling. The viruses have been used as expression vectors in T-lymphocytes and allow to study mechanisms of episomal persistence in components of the T-cell system. Later on it became clear that certain strains of HVS can transform human T-lymphocytes to continuous growth in an antigen- and mitogen-independent fashion, providing for the first time a reliable means of human T-lymphocyte immortalization in cell culture. Additional interest in the γ2-herpesviruses arose when the Kaposi-sarcoma-associated Human Herpesvirus 8 (KSHV/HHV8) was identified as the first human pathogenic rhadinovirus. However, in view of the complex biology of Kaposi's Sarcoma or other neoplastic diseases such as body cavity-based B-cell lymphomas and multifocal Castleman's Disease, it is by far less clear which KSHV/HHV8 genes encode the relevant oncoproteins of KSHV/HHV-8. In this chapter, we wanted to focus mostly on the basic biology and gene expression profiles of HVS and HVA, on the viral mechanisms of oncogenic transformation, and possible applications of these viruses as T-cell vectors and in cell-based immunotherapy.

Herpesvirus saimiri

Natural occurrence and pathology

The rhadinovirus (γ2-herpesvirus) Herpesvirus saimiri (HVS) is regularly found in squirrel monkeys (*Saimiri sciureus*), whose natural habitat are South American rainforests. Squirrel monkeys are usually infected via saliva within the first two years of life. The virus does not cause disease or tumors and establishes lifelong persistence in the species (Melendez et al., 1968). In other New World primate species such as tamarins (*Saguinus (S.) spp.*), common marmosets (*Callithrix (C.) jacchus*) or owl monkeys (*Aotus trivirgatus*), the infection with HVS causes acute peripheral T-cell lymphoma within less than two months after experimental infection (Melendez et al., 1969; Wright et al., 1976; for review see Fleckenstein and Desrosiers, 1982). The experimental infection is usually performed intramuscularly or intravenously. Intramuscular injection of purified virion DNA also causes disease in susceptible primates (Fleckenstein et al., 1978b). HVS strains were classified into the three subgroups A, B and C depending on the pathogenic properties and on the sequence divergence in the left-terminal non-repetitive genomic region (Desrosiers and Falk, 1982; Medveczky et al., 1989; Medveczky et al., 1984). The major representative strains are A11 (Falk et al., 1972) for subgroup A, B-S295C (Melendez et al., 1968) and B-SMHI (Daniel et al., 1975) for subgroup B, and C488 (Biesinger et al., 1990) and C484 (Medveczky et al., 1984) for subgroup C. Viruses of subgroup B are considered to be less oncogenic, subgroup C strains have the strongest oncogenic properties. Tamarins are susceptible to viruses of all subgroups, while subgroup B viruses were reported as not being able to cause disease in adult common marmosets (reviewed in Fickenscher and Fleckenstein, 2002). The parental strain C488 as well as various viral deletion mutants cause acute peripheral T-cell lymphoma within only a few weeks in common marmosets or in cottontop tamarins (*S. oedipus*) (Duboise et al., 1998a; Ensser et al., 2001; Glykofrydes et al., 2000; Duboise et al., 1998b; Knappe et al., 1998a,b). Remarkably, high intravenous doses of HVS strain C488 can induce a similar fulminant disease in Old World monkeys such as rhesus and cynomolgus monkeys (*Macaca (M.) mulatta, M. fascicularis*). The pathological findings in macaques were similar to those in New World primates, and the disease in cynomolgus monkeys was designated as a pleomorphic peripheral T-cell lymphoma or alternatively as a pleomorphic T-lymphoproliferative disorder (Alexander et al., 1997; Knappe et al., 2000a). Whereas HVS infection or pathogenicity has not been reported in rodents, a non-permissive infection and tumor induction was described in New Zealand white rabbits, although with variable efficiency (Ablashi et al., 1985; Medveczky et al., 1989). HVS can be isolated from peripheral blood cells of persistently infected squirrel monkeys, or from leukemic animals, presumably from infected T cells, by co-cultivation with permissive owl monkey kidney (OMK) cells (Falk et al., 1972). HVS replicates productively and induces cell lysis of OMK cells (Daniel et al., 1976). A series of transformed T-cell lines were derived from leukemias or tumors of virus-infected tamarins and could be cultivated continuously for several years (reviewed in Fleckenstein and Desrosiers, 1982). While virus particles were found initially in most cases, virus production was frequently lost after prolonged culture. The episomal DNA is heavily methylated in such cell lines (Desrosiers et al., 1979), and some of these cell lines carried rearrangements or large deletions in the episomal HVS genomes (Kaschka-Dierich et al., 1982). Marmoset and tamarin T-cells can be transformed by HVS to stable T-cell lines in vitro and are designated as semi-permissive, since virus particles are released, although to lower titers than from OMK cells (Desrosiers et al., 1986; Kiyotaki et al., 1986; Schirm et al., 1984; Szomolanyi et al., 1987).

Genome structure and replication

HVS is the prototype of the subfamily *rhadinovirus* (g2-herpesviruses) (Roizman et al., 1992). The term "rhadino" viruses uses the ancient Greek word "ραδινοσ" for fragile (Roizman et al., 1992), because the genomic viral DNA splits upon isopyknic centrifugation into two classes of highly different density, the L-DNA containing the viral protein-coding genes (low density, low G+C content) and the terminal non-coding repetitive H-DNA (high density, high G+C content). The intact rhadinoviral so-called M-genome has intermediate density in CsCl gradients (M-DNA). Two strains of HVS, #A11 and the highly oncogenic subgroup C strain #C488 were sequenced (Albrecht et al., 1992a; Ensser et al., 2003). In the case of HVS A11, the H-DNA contains multiple tandem repeats of 1444 bp with 70.8% G+C, whereas the long unique L-DNA has 112 930 bp with 34.5% G+C (Albrecht et al., 1992a; Fleckenstein and Desrosiers, 1982). The size of the total M-DNA genome is variable due to different numbers of H-DNA segments attached to both ends of the linear virion genome. In strain C488, the L-DNA comprises 113027 bp, and it is flanked by two distinct repeat units of 1318 and 1458 bp. The shorter unit is a subset of the longer repeat unit of which 140 bp are deleted. The size of the packaged C488 M-genome is approx. 155 kbp, ranging from 130–160 kbp due to variable numbers of terminal H-DNA segments (Ensser et al., 2003). The HVS L-DNA genomes contain at least 76 to 77 open reading frames and 5 to 7 U-RNAs (Albrecht et al., 1992a; Hör et al., 2001; Ensser et al., 2003). These are the gene blocks of typical herpesvirus genes which are highly conserved between herpesvirus families (Gompels et al., 1988; Albrecht and Fleckenstein, 1990). Flanking or interspersed are genes which do not usually occur in other herpesviruses families, among these are transforming oncogenes and viral homologues of cellular genes which will be described below. While most genes are well conserved between different HVS strains, there is extensive sequence variation at the so-called left end of the HVS L-DNA and in the region of the R transactivator gene *orf50* and the glycoprotein gene *orf51* (Biesinger et al., 1990; Thurau et al., 2000; Hör et al., 2001; Ensser et al., 2003). The genome structures of HVS and KSHV/HHV-8 are compared in Fig. 60.1. Not much is known about the replication mechanisms of rhadinoviruses in general or of HVS in particular. The HVS A11 origin of lytic replication was mapped to the untranslated region upstream of the thymidylate synthase gene (Lang and Fleckenstein, 1990; Schofield, 1994). A putative origin in the left-terminal region of the L-DNA was described to mediate plasmid maintenance in strain C484 (Kung and Medveczky, 1996) that is neither conserved between different HVS strains, nor is it required for viral replication or episomal persistence in strain C488 or C484 (Ensser et al., 1999; Medveczky et al., 1989). In transformed human T cells, HVS persists as stable non-integrated episomes at high copy number (Biesinger et al., 1992). There are no indications yet for the genetic correlate of a plasmid-like origin of replication and of the viral factors involved. In contrast to herpes simplex virus, the infection of tissue culture cells by HVS is asynchronous (Randall et al., 1985). Therefore, the classification of HVS genes to the immediate-early (IE) phase of infection has been difficult and was mostly based on experiments using cycloheximide to inhibit viral protein synthesis. The IE gene *ie57* codes for a nuclear phosphoprotein of 52 kDa (Nicholas et al., 1988; Randall et al., 1984) with structural and functional homology with ICP27/IE63 of herpes simplex virus and EBV BMLF1. Correspondingly, IE57 stimulates the expression of unspliced and represses the expression of spliced transcripts (Whitehouse et al., 1998). IE57 further redistributes nuclear components of the splicing machinery (Cooper et al., 1999) and is involved in nuclear RNA export (Goodwin et al., 1999). Thus, the *ie57* post-transcriptional regulator appears to be the sole regulatory viral IE gene. A strong viral transactivator function was mapped to the delayed-early gene *orf50* (Nicholas et al., 1991), the homologue to the R transactivator of EBV. Due to differential splicing and promoter usage, the gene codes for a larger protein ORF 50A and for a smaller C-terminal variant ORF 50B. The transactivation domain resides in the C-terminus of the ORF 50 proteins and binds to the TATA-binding protein in the basal transcription complex. Post-transcriptional inhibition of spliced *orf50A* transcripts by the IE57 can not have functional relevance in this context, suggesting that orf50 exerts the dominant function for regulation of replication, at least in HVS strain C488. While *ie57* is highly conserved between subgroup A and C, the genomic *orf50* region encoding this major viral transactivator was found to be strongly divergent (Thurau et al., 2000; Ensser et al., 2003). Neither HVS nor HVA encode a homologue to the bZip/Zta of EBV or KSHV (Sinclair, 2003). The HVS ORF73 protein of strain A11 and C488 localizes to the host cell nucleus, and like the latent nuclear antigen LANA of KSHV, it can associate with host cell chromosomal DNA (Hall et al., 2000; Schäfer et al., 2003). The A11 ORF73 is highly expressed in HVS-infected human epithelial cancer cell lines, it can associate with the cellular p32, thereby coactivating heterologous as well as its own promoter (Hall et al., 2002). A11 ORF73 further binds to GSK-3ß, which is involved in *WNT*-signaling and possibly contributes to oncogenic transformation (Fujimuro and Hayward, 2003). Although not detectable by Northern blotting from C488-transformed human T-cells (Fickenscher et al., 1996), transcripts of this gene are found by RT-PCR. The HVS C488 orf73 gene product can downregulate the orf50A and B promoters and prevents the ORF50 mediated activation of viral replication gene promoters, and it can block the initiation of the lytic replication cascade. This suggests that HVS ORF73 can control the transition between rhadinoviral latency and lytic replication (Schäfer et al., 2003).

Rhadinoviruses like HVS and KSHV contain several intronless viral genes that are homologous to cellular genes; it might be speculated on a role for reverse transcription in this context. While a few of these likely captured cellular gene homologs are unique to specific viruses, some are common to several rhadinoviruses (Fig. 60.1) or to γ-herpesviruses including EBV. This may suggest that the uptake of cellular genes is a rather infrequent event during herpesvirus evolution. Most of these cellular homologues can be categorized into two major groups: (I) genes related to nucleotide metabolism or cellular growth control, and (II) genes that modulate innate or adaptive immune functions (discussed below). HVS homologues to enzymes of the nucleotide metabolism include a dihydrofolate reductase (*orf2*, DHFR) and a functional thymidylate synthase (*orf70*, TS). Both *orf3* and *orf75* encode large tegument proteins, which share local homology to formylglycineamide ribotide amidotransferase (FGARAT) (summarized in Ensser et al., 2003). The functions of these enzymes may possibly augment the free nucleotide pool and could thus facilitate DNA synthesis and virus replication. *Orf2* and the adjacently located viral U-RNA genes are dispensable for virus replication and T-cell transformation (Ensser et al., 1999). HVS *orf72* codes for a functional viral cyclin D that is expressed in semipermissive HVS-transformed marmoset T-cells and is resistant to cyclin-dependent kinase inhibitors $p16^{Ink4a}$, $p21^{Cip1}$ and $p27^{Kip1}$. This deregulation pushes the cell cycle towards the S phase, thereby supporting virus replication in permissive cells (Nicholas et al., 1992; Jung et al., 1994; Swanton et al., 1997). Although enhanced replication might secondarily promote transformation or tumor induction, the viral cyclin seems to provide only auxiliary functions, since it is not required for replication, T-cell transformation and lymphomagenesis (Ensser et al., 2001).

Immunomodulatory proteins
Rhadinoviruses target various host mechanisms involved in pathogen elimination, both in the innate and adaptive immune system. Two HVS genes are functional regulators of the complement system; the *orf4* codes for a complement control protein homologue (CCPH), which inhibits C3 convertase, an enzyme involved in the initiation of early steps in

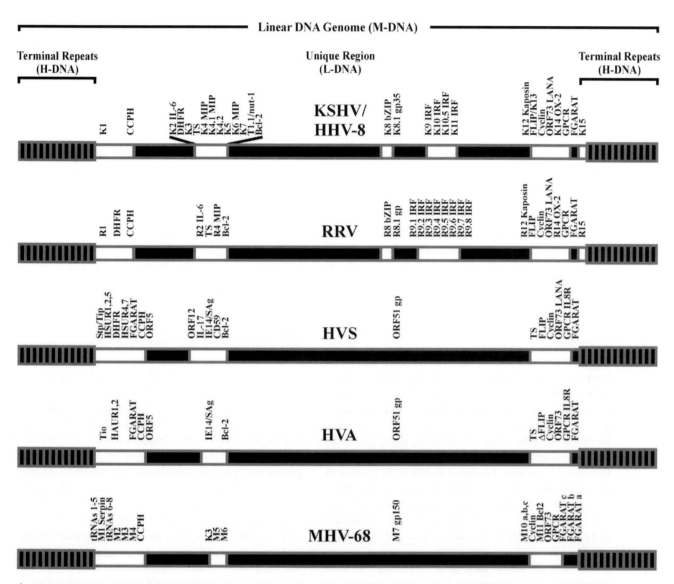

Fig. 60.1. Genome structure of selected rhadinoviruses. The genome structures of the rhadinoviruses KSHV/HHV-8 (Russo *et al.*, 1996; Neipel *et al.*, 1997), rhesus rhadinovirus (RRV; Alexander *et al.*, 2000; Searles *et al.*, 1999), herpesvirus saimiri (HVS; Albrecht *et al.*, 1992a; Ensser *et al.*, 2003), herpesvirus ateles (HVA; Albrecht, 2000), murine herpesvirus 68 (MHV-68; Virgin *et al.*, 1997) are shown with special respect to variable areas harboring non-conserved genes or genes with homology to cellular counterparts (white boxes). Conserved genomic regions of virus genes with typical herpesvirus functions are shown in black. Abbreviations are: bZIP, basic-leucine zipper protein. CCPH, complement control protein homologue. DHFR, dihydrofolate reductase. FGARAT, formylglycineamide ribotide amidotransferase. FLIP, FLICE inhibitory protein. gp, glycoprotein. GPCR, G-protein coupled receptor. HSUR or HAUR, HVS or HVA-encoded URNA. IRF, interferon regulatory factor. MIP, macrophage-inflammatory protein. SAg, superantigen homologue. Stp, saimiri transformation-associated protein. Tio, two-in-one-protein. Tip, tyrosine kinase-interacting protein. TS, thymidylate synthase.

complement activation (Albrecht and Fleckenstein, 1992; Fodor *et al.*, 1995). *Orf15* is a viral variant of CD59, which prevents the insertion of the membrane attack complex formed by C8 and C9, and thus blocks the terminal complement cascade (Albrecht *et al.*, 1992b; Rother *et al.*, 1994). T-cell stimulatory functions have been described for cellular CD59 via CD2 (Korty *et al.*, 1991; Deckert *et al.*, 1995), but functional data are not available for the viral CD59. The orf12 has homology to the K3 and K5 genes of KSHV (Coscoy and Ganem, 2000; Ishido *et al.*, 2000a,b; Means *et al.*, 2002), but is dispensable for replication and human T-cell transformation in vitro (Knappe *et al.*, 1998a).

Several rhadinoviral ORFs encode potent inhibitors of cell death or apoptosis, such as *orf16* and *orf71*. The ORF16 is a viral Bcl-2 homologue (Bellows *et al.*, 2000; Derfuss *et al.*, 1998; Nava *et al.*, 1997). Both Bcl-XL and viral Bcl-2 inhibit cell death induced by either cell-autonomous (independent of death receptors) or receptor-mediated mechanisms, depending on the cell type studied. The ORF71, a viral FLICE (FADD-like interleukin 1-converting enzyme (ICE)-like protease) inhibitory protein (vFLIP), interacts with cellular FADD (Fas-associated protein with death domains) and FLICE via homophilic interaction of their respective death-effector domains, therefore blocks formation of the death-signal-induced signaling complex, and consequently prevents caspase 8 (FLICE) activation. Although the vFLIP inhibited death-receptor-dependent apoptosis and partially protected permissive OMK cells from Fas-dependent apoptosis at a late stage of infection (Thome *et al.*, 1997), the vFLIP was dispensable for virus replication to high virus titers, T-cell transformation and lymphoma induction (Glykofrydes *et al.*, 2000).

The HVS gene *orf13* led to the discovery of its cellular homologue ctla-8 (Rouvier *et al.*, 1993) that codes for IL-17, a CD4+ T-cell specific cytokine. The viral IL-17 is functionally not distinguishable from its cellular counterpart that is capable of supporting T-cell proliferation (Yao *et al.*, 1995; Fossiez *et al.*, 1998). However, deletions of the HVS C488 *orf13/vIL-17* had no phenotype with regard to virus replication and oncogenicity (Knappe *et al.*, 1998a). In contrast to the vIL17 that is unique to HVS, G-protein coupled receptors (GPCR) are found in most rhadinoviruses. The HVS *orf74* encodes a viral IL-8 receptor (IL-8R) that is classified to the low-affinity B type of IL-8R (Ahuja and Murphy, 1993; Murphy, 1994; Nicholas *et al.*, 1992).

The viral immediate early gene *orf14/vSag* has local homology to the superantigen (Sag) of mouse mammary tumor virus (MMTV) and to murine *mls* superantigens (Thomson and Nicholas, 1991). Although recombinant viral IE14/vSag protein bound to MHC class II molecules and stimulated T-cell proliferation, there is no evidence of a selective advantage for specific Vb families that would be typical for superantigens, neither after stimulation of human T-cells with IE14/vSag in vitro (Yao *et al.*, 1996; Duboise *et al.*, 1998a), nor after infection and transformation with HVS (Knappe *et al.*, 1997). The HVS C488 ie14/vsag (Thomson and Nicholas, 1991) is dispensable for viral replication but its role in the transformation of human and simian T-cells in vitro or pathogenicity has remained controversial (Knappe *et al.*, 1997, 1998b; Duboise *et al.*, 1998a). Like other rhadinoviruses, HVS has acquired a series of cellular genes, but most if not all of these genes are dispensable for virus replication, T-cell transformation in culture, and pathogenesis in susceptible New World primates. Similar to KSHV infected B-cell lines, many of the cell-homologous viral genes are only expressed during lytic virus replication, but not in transformed human lymphocytes (Fickenscher *et al.*, 1996; Knappe *et al.*, 1997).

Oncogenesis

The major factors responsible for induction of T-cell leukemia and T-cell transformation in vitro reside in the variable region at the left end of the HVS L-DNA (Koomey *et al.*, 1984; Desrosiers *et al.*, 1985a; Desrosiers *et al.*, 1986; Murthy *et al.*, 1989; Chou *et al.*, 1995; Duboise *et al.*, 1998b). In subgroup A and B strains there is only one gene at this position, termed stpA or stpB (saimiri trans-formation associated protein of subgroup A or B strains) (Murthy *et al.*, 1989; Hör *et al.*, 2001). At the homologous location, the virus strains of subgroup C carry two open reading frames, that were later termed *stpC* (saimiri transformation-associated protein of subgroup C strains) and *tip* (tyrosine kinase interacting protein) (Biesinger *et al.*, 1990; Jung and Desrosiers, 1991; Biesinger *et al.*, 1995) (Fig. 60.2). The closely related HVA encodes the protein Tio at the homologous genomic position (Albrecht *et al.*, 1999). StpA and B share limited sequence homology with StpC, but are structurally unrelated to Tip (Fig. 60.2). While not required for viral replication, deletion of either *stpC* or *tip* abolishes the transformation by HVS in vitro and pathogenicity in vivo (Duboise *et al.*, 1996, 1998b; Knappe *et al.*, 1997; Medveczky *et al.*, 1993). Both *stpC* and *tip* genes are transcribed into a single bicistronic mRNA from a common promoter directed toward the left genomic end of the L-DNA, where *tip* is situated downstream of *stpC*. The transcription of *stpC/tip* is regulated similarly to cellular IE genes in human T-cells and no obvious viral factors seem to be involved. In C488-transformed human T-cells, *stpC* and *tip* are the only constitutively transcribed viral genes. (Biesinger *et al.*, 1995; Fickenscher *et al.*, 1996; Fickenscher *et al.*, 1997). The StpC protein is a 102 aa perinuclear membrane-associated phosphoprotein with a predicted molecular mass of approximately 10 kDa but migrates with an apparent molecular mass of 20 kDa. The N-terminus of StpC consists of 17 mostly charged amino acids. The C-terminus is a hydrophobic region, which probably serves as an anchor to perinuclear membranes. In between are 18 collagen tripeptide repeats (GPX)n, which may mediate multimerization of the protein (Fig. 60.2) (Biesinger *et al.*, 1990; Fickenscher *et al.*, 1997; Jung and Desrosiers, 1991, 1992, 1994). *stpA* of strain A11 and *stpC* of strain C488 transfected rodent fibroblasts formed foci in vitro and induced tumors in nude mice (Jung *et al.*,

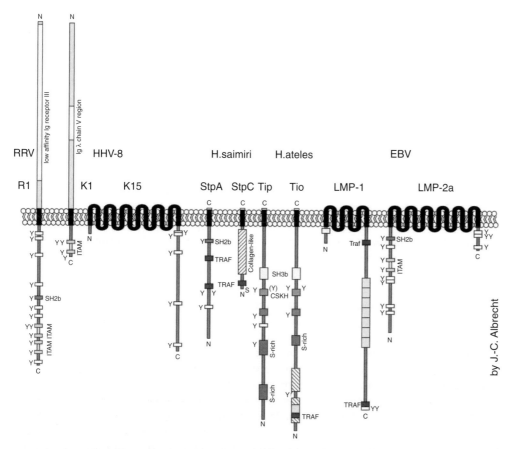

Fig. 60.2. Structural diversity of the major gammaherpesvirus signaling proteins. The HVS oncoproteins Stp, Tip, or HVA Tio, the KSHV K1 and K15, RRV R1 proteins are shown along with the EBV LMP1, LMP2a. CSKH, C-terminal Src kinase homology region. ITAM, immunoreceptor tyrosine-containing activation motif. SH3b, domain interacting with src-family kinase SH3 domain. SH2b, domain interacting with src-family kinase SH2 domain. S-rich, Serine rich motif. TRAF, potential binding site for TNF-R associated factors. Y and YY, tyrosine and double-tyrosine residues, putative signaling motifs. Black, Transmembrane domain. N or C, amino- or carboxyterminus of the protein, respectively.

1991). *stpA* transgenic mice developed polyclonal peripheral T-cell lymphoma, while an *stpC* transgene induced epithelial tumors (Kretschmer *et al.*, 1996; Murphy *et al.*, 1994). StpA was reported to bind to and to be phosphorylated by the non-receptor tyrosine kinase Src (Lee *et al.*, 1997). The non-transforming StpB also associates with Src (Choi *et al.*, 2000). StpC was shown to interact with the small G-protein Ras and stimulated mitogen activated protein (MAP) kinase activity (Jung and Desrosiers, 1995). Both proteins StpA and StpC interact with TNF-associated factors (TRAFs) leading to nuclear factor kappa B (NFkB) activation (Lee *et al.*, 1999; Sorokina *et al.*, 2004). Tip was first observed as a 40 kD phosphoprotein that coprecipitated with the T-cell-specific non-receptor tyrosine kinase p56[lck] in C488-transformed T-cells and was only detectable by a phosphotransferase assay. The protein was thus named tyrosine kinase interacting protein (Tip) and could be identified as the gene product of the leftmost C488 reading frame (Biesinger *et al.*, 1995). Tip of HVS strain C488 has 256 aa and a predicted molecular mass of 29 kD. Considerable interstrain variation of the *tip* genes has been observed (Greve *et al.*, 2001; Ensser *et al.*, 2003), but the common denominators are a N-terminal glutamate-rich region, which is duplicated in some strains, followed by one or two serine-rich regions, a bipartite kinase interacting domain, and a C-terminal hydrophobic domain which anchors the molecule at the inside of the plasma membrane. The kinase interacting domain consists of nine amino acids with homology to the C-terminal regulatory regions of various Src kinases (CSKH), and a proline-rich SH3-domain-binding sequence (SH3B); both motifs are required for the interaction with the kinase (Fig. 60.2) (Biesinger *et al.*,

1995; Jung et al., 1995a; Heck et al., 2006). Several tyrosine residues, three of which are conserved between all strains investigated, are a substrate for the tyrosine kinase Lck. The phosphorylated tyrosine residue 127 of Tip (pY127) was identified by biophysical binding analyses as a potential third Lck interaction site at the Lck-SH2 domain (Bauer et al., 2004). Y127 is the major tyrosine phosphorylation site of Tip, but this does not enhance Lck binding in T cells. Recombinant virus expressing mutations in Tip show that the strong Lck binding mediated by cooperation of both SH3B and CSKH motifs is essential for transformation of human T cells by herpesvirus saimiri C488, whereas the Y127 of Tip was particularly required for transformation in the absence of exogenous interleukin-2, suggesting its involvement in cytokine signaling pathways (Heck et al., 2006). Tip binding to Lck modulates the kinase activity: (Fickenscher et al., 1997; Hartley et al., 1999; Lund et al., 1997a; Wiese et al., 1996). When compared with their non-infected parental clones, HVS C488-transformed human T-cell clones had increased basal levels of tyrosine phosphorylation (Wiese et al., 1996). Dependent on the presence of both the CSKH or SH3B motifs, Tip could activate Lck even when the regulatory tyrosines Y394 and Y505 of Lck had been mutated, suggesting a novel mechanism of Lck activation (Hartley et al., 1999), which may result in an altered substrate specificity of the kinase contributing to the abrogation of ZAP70 phosphorylation (Cho et al., 2004). This dysregulation may further link Tip-bound Lck to alternative downstream effectors. Since constitutively active Lck mutants have an oncogenic potential, stimulation of Lck signaling by Tip would contribute to the activated phenotype of HVS-transformed T-cells and to the transformation process, whereby Tip and StpC would act in synergy.

In addition to Lck, phosphorylated signal transducer and activator of transcription (STAT) factors 1 and 3 were immunoprecipitated with Lck and Tip-C484 (Lund et al., 1997b). The implication of Y114 with constitutive active STATs, especially STAT3, and the role of STATs in growth regulation and oncogenesis in multiple cell types (Bowman et al., 2000; Bromberg et al., 2000) suggested a central role for Tip-induced STAT activity in viral T-cell transformation. However, recombinant herpesvirus saimiri C488 expressing Tip with a tyrosine-to-phenylalanine mutation at position 114 was able to transform primary human T-lymphocytes in the absence of STAT1 or STAT3 activation (Heck et al., 2005). Thus, the essential function of Tip in lymphocyte transformation does not rely on Lck-mediated STAT1 or 3 phosphorylation. When Tip was highly expressed in stable tip-transfected Jurkat T-cells, low basal levels of tyrosine phosphorylation, impaired response to T-cell-receptor activation, and downregulation of CD3 and CD4 were observed. Tip further partially reversed the transformed phenotype of fibroblasts, which had lost contact inhibition after transfection with a constitutively active mutant of Lck. These effects were even more pronounced when Tip Tyrosine 114 was mutated in position 114 to Serine (Y114S) to enhance its binding to Lck (Guo et al., 1997; Jung et al., 1995b). Enhanced binding and activation of Lck by Tip carrying a Y114S might provide an explanation for the increased transformation efficiency, however, there were no differences in Lck binding for Tip Y114F (Heck et al., 2006) and a Tip Y114 phosphopeptide exhibits no significant affinity for the SH2 domain of Lck (Bauer et al., 2004).

The activation of Lck and the inhibition of T-cell signaling by Tip may be two different aspects of the same function, since the activation of Lck by Tip might trigger negative feedback mechanisms in stably transfected Jurkat cells expressing high levels of Tip, such as apoptosis (Hasham and Tsygankov, 2004). Another possible reason for this are the low expression levels of Tip in such HVS-transformed primary human and simian T-cells, while p56^{lck} is abundantly expressed; any possible changes in the Lck enzymatic activity after binding of Tip may be masked by the excess free Lck. Tip function has evolved in the context of the natural infection of squirrel monkeys, where uncontrolled T-cell transformation seems not to occur. A better understanding of HVS biology in squirrel monkeys could help to elucidate this problem (Greve et al., 2001).

A cellular Tip-associated protein of 65 kDa termed Tap could contribute to T-cell activation by Tip (Yoon et al., 1997), although Tap is an RNA export factor that has no known T-cell-specific functions as yet (Grüter et al., 1998). Coexpression of Tip and a recently identified lysosomal WD-repeat protein p80 at high levels in 293 and Jurkat cells induced enlarged endosomal vesicles and recruited Lck and TCR complex into these vesicles for trafficking or degradation. Since Tip is constitutively present in lipid rafts, it was also found that Tip can recruit p80 into lipid rafts; the C-terminus of Tip seems to interact with Lck to recruit TCR complex to lipid rafts, and TCR and Lck then may interact with p80 to initiate the aggregation and internalization of the lipid raft domain and thereby downregulate the TCR complex (Park et al., 2002, 2003). The lipid raft association of Tip is essential for the TCR and CD4 downregulation but not for the inhibition of TCR signal transduction and the activation of STAT3 transcription factor (Cho et al., 2006).

Growth transformation of human T-cells

Rapidly proliferating T-lymphoblastic tumor cell lines such as Jurkat (Schneider et al., 1977) are frequently used as a cellular and biochemical model for primary human T-cells, although they display a strongly altered phenotype with respect to signal transduction, gene regulation and proliferation control. On the other hand, primary human T-cell culture is laborious and requires repeated stimulation with a mitogen or specific antigen in the presence of accessory cells expressing the appropriate MHC restriction elements. Since they are limited in their natural life span, it is rarely possible to grow primary T-lymphocytes to large numbers. A practical method of T-cell transformation became available through the observation that HVS strain C488 stimulated human T-lymphocytes to stable antigen-independent growth in culture (Biesinger et al., 1992). These growth-transformed human T-cells retained many essential T-cell functions including the MHC-restricted antigen- specific reactivity of their parental T-cell clones (Bröker et al., 1993; De Carli et al., 1993; Weber et al., 1993), they are not tumorigenic in nude or SCID mice, but could induce xenogenic graft-versus-host disiease similar as primary human T-cells (Huppes et al., 1994). These observations have opened up a novel research direction which links T-cell biology, signal transduction pathways and transforming viral functions. Although HVS-transformed Old and New World monkey T-lymphocytes produce infectious viral particles in many cases, it was not possible to isolate virus from transformed human T-cell cultures (Biesinger et al., 1992). Although the formal proof that the virus can never be reactivated from transformed human T-lymphocytes is difficult, neither treatment with phorbol esters or nucleoside analogues, nor other drugs that can cause reactivation of other viruses such as EBV or KSHV, nor specific or non-specific stimulation of the T-cells could induce virion production (Fickenscher et al., 1996). StpC and Tip are the only viral proteins which have been regularly demonstrated in HVS-transformed human T-cells. The non-coding viral U-RNA genes (HSUR, HVS URNA) were abundantly expressed in a similar way to the EBER RNAs of EBV, but deletion of all HSUR did not influence virus replication or T-cell transformation (Ensser et al., 1999). While the viral gene *stpC/tip* was strongly and inducibly transcribed into a bicistronic message (Fickenscher et al., 1996; Medveczky et al., 1993), other viral transcription was rarely detected. The gene *ie14/vsag* was abundantly transcribed for a few hours only after of stimulation of transformed human T-cells with phorbol ester, and the IE gene *ie57*, the early gene *orf50*, and the viral thymidylate synthase gene were found transcribed at extremely low abundance or only after additional T-cell stimulation (Knappe et al., 1997; Thurau et al., 2000). These findings argue for a strong block of virus replication in C488-transformed human T-cells that is downstream of the expression of the regulatory genes *orf50* and *ie57*.

The transformation procedure and the specific properties of HVS-transformed T-cells have been comprehensively reviewed (Fickenscher and Fleckenstein, 2001; Ensser et al., 2002; Fickenscher and Fleckenstein, 2002; Ensser and Fleckenstein, 2004). Briefly, the infection of peripheral blood mononuclear cells, cord blood cells, thymocytes, or established T-cell clones by HVS C488 results in T-cell lines that continuously grow without restimulation with antigen or mitogen and do not require the presence of feeder or antigen presenting cells. The morphology of such lines resembles the irregular shape of T blasts, they carry non-integrated viral episomes in high copy number, and have a normal karyotype (Troidl et al., 1994). The HVS strain C488 is commonly used for the targeted transformation of human T cells; other subgroup C virus strains were able to transform human T-cells, but to a varying extent (Fickenscher et al., 1997). The surface phenotype of the transformed T-lymphocytes resembles mature, activated T cells, that are CD4+CD8− or CD4−CD8+ T cells and carry ab- or gd-type T-cell receptors; transformation of established T-cell clones demonstrated that the phenotype and HLA-restriction of the parental T-cells is conserved. If transformed by the same virus strain, ab and gd-clones were similar with respect to viral persistence, virus gene expression, proliferation and Th1-type cytokine production. The phenotype of HVS-transformed T-cells is remarkably stable for many months in culture, a significant technical advance over immortalization of human T-cells by the hybridoma technique or infection with HTLV-1 (Biesinger et al., 1992; reviewed in Fickenscher and Fleckenstein, 2002). While many normal T-cell functions are preserved, a few specific cellular and biochemical features are changed in comparison with their parental cells. This relates to the hyper-responsiveness to CD2 ligation (Meuer et al., 1984; Mittrücker et al., 1992). Second, the protein tyrosine kinase $p53/56^{lyn}$ is expressed and enzymatically active in HVS transformed T-cells (Fickenscher et al., 1997; Wiese et al., 1996). Third, HVS-transformation shifts the range of cytokines secreted by stimulated T-cells towards a Th1 profile: IL-4 and IL-5 production is diminished and secretion of IL-2 and IFN-g is increased in comparison with parental cells. (Bröker et al., 1993; De Carli et al., 1993; Weber et al., 1993). A novel IL-10-like cellular gene is specifically overexpressed in HVS-transformed T-cells, termed *ak155* or IL-26 (Knappe et al.,

2000b). Whereas IL-26 receptors have not been found on T-cells, this cytokine induces STAT activation in epithelial cells (Hör et al., 2004). Thus, it is unlikely that IL-26 contributes to HVS-mediated T cell-transformation. However, this cytokine may be involved in the lymphocyte-epithelium interaction which is typical for various gamma herpesviruses.

T-cell transformation by HVS C488 was used to study T cells from primary human immunodeficiencies, and in many cases has been the only way to cultivate and amplify the patients' cells for further research. HVS transformed T-cell lines were established from patients with a variety of genetic T-cell defects (reviewed in Fickenscher and Fleckenstein 2001). HVS-transformed human CD4+ T-cells provide a productive system for T-lymphotropic viruses such as HHV-6 (F. Neipel and B. Fleckenstein, unpublished data) and human immunodeficiency virus (HIV) (Nick et al., 1993).

Vectors for gene therapy

Both oncogenic and non-transforming HVS variants have been used as eukaryotic expression vectors. HVS vectors were used to define the transforming functions of the HTLV-1 X region and the *stpC* oncogene was successfully substituted by cellular *ras* (Guo et al., 1998), by the K1 gene of KSHV/HHV-8 (Lee et al., 1998), or by R1 of rhesus monkey rhadinovirus (RRV) (Fig. 60.2) (Damania et al., 1999), in deletion mutants which still contained the *tip* gene. HVS has been used as a vector for growth hormone, for secreted alkaline phosphatase, anti-inflammatory cytokines and for green fluorescent protein (Desrosiers et al., 1985b, 1996; Hoggard et al., 2004; Stevenson et al., 1999; Wieser et al., 2005). A non-transforming replication-competent HVS vector expressing the bovine growth hormone in persistently infected simian T cells produced high amounts of the circulating bovine hormone in experimentally infected New World primates (Desrosiers et al., 1985b, 1986). This suggested that episomally persisting, non-integrating HVS vectors could be used for therapy of hereditary genetic disorders, like cytokine receptor deficiencies (Altare et al., 2001). HVS-vectors efficiently transduce human mesenchymal cells including bone marrow stromal cells (Frolova-Jones et al., 2000) or haematopoietic precursors (Doody et al., 2004); infection of human hematopoietic progenitor cells is somewhat less efficient and with a tendency towards partially differentiated cells (Stevenson et al., 1999). Limited replication of HVS replication was observed in certain human cell types (Daniel et al., 1975; Simmer et al., 1991; Stevenson et al., 1999). Although totipotent mouse embryonic stem (ES) cells were infected under drug selection with rather stable transgene expression (Stevenson et al., 2000a), the infection of differentiated murine or rat cells is mostly inefficient.

The behavior of HVS C488 in various Old World monkey systems is of interest although macaque T-cell lines were shown to shed low amounts of virus particles in many cases (Alexander et al., 1997; Knappe et al., 2000a), reinfusion of autologous transformed T cells into the donor macaques did not induce disease, the infused T-cells persisted for extended periods, and the animals were protected against tumor induction by challenge with the HVS C488 virus (Knappe et al., 2000a). Conversely an attempt to improve the biological safety of HVS vectors by inserting the prodrug activating thymidine kinase gene of herpes simplex virus looked promising in vitro (Hiller et al., 2000b), but failed in vivo: the recombinant HVS-TK viruses not only showed no response to the administration of ganciclovir but induced tumors even more rapidly than the wild-type HVS control (Hiller et al., 2000a). Nevertheless, since gene transfer into primary human T-cells by transfection or retroviral transduction methods remains difficult, the maintained functional phenotype of HVS-transformed T lymphocytes supports the use of HVS-vectors for human T-cells (reviewed in Fickenscher and Fleckenstein, 2002). Transformation-competent HVS-vectors might be valuable for the targeted amplification of functional human T-cells, or even for therapeutic redirection of human T-cell antigen specificity, as a tool for experimental cancer therapy applications.

Herpesvirus ateles

Natural occurrence and pathology

Herpesvirus ateles can be isolated at a high rate from spider monkeys (*Ateles (A.) spp.*) (for review see Fleckenstein and Desrosiers, 1982). Isolate #810 from *A. geoffroyii* (Melendez et al., 1972) is officially classified as ateline herpesvirus type 2, whereas isolate #73 and related strains (#87, 93, 94) from *A. paniscus* were designated as ateline herpesvirus type 3 (Falk et al., 1974). HVA replicates in OMK cells (Daniel et al., 1976), but remains mostly cell-associated with syncytia formation. As a result, supernatants of such cultures have lower and unstable HVA titers. Like HVS, HVA is not pathogenic in its natural host, but causes acute T-cell lymphoma in various New World primate species including tamarins (*Saguinus oedipus*) and owl monkeys (*Aotus trivirgatus*) (Hunt et al., 1972). The pathological changes are similar to those observed after HVS infection. In addition, HVA transforms T-cells of certain New World monkey species such as cotton-top tamarins in culture,

Table 60.1. Gammherpesviruses

Designation, Abbreviation	Host	Associated pathogenicity
Rhadinovirus species		
Kaposi's sarcoma associated herpesvirus, KSHV	Human	Kaposi's sarcoma, multicentric Castleman's disease, primary effusion lymphoma
Retroperitoneal fibromatosis-associated herpesvirus, RFHV, MnRhRV	Rhesus monkey	Retroperitoneal fibromatosis?
Rhesus monkey rhadinovirus, RRV	Rhesus monkey	B-cell hyperplasia?
Herpesvirus saimiri, HVS[a].	Squirrel monkey	T-cell lymphoma in other neotropical monkeys
Herpesvirus ateles, HVA	Spider monkey	T-cell lymphoma in other neotropical monkeys
Alcelaphine herpesvirus 1, AHV-1	Wildebeest	Malignant catarrhal fever in cattle
Alcelaphine herpesvirus 2, AHV-2	Hartebeest, Topi	
Ovine herpesvirus 2, OHV-2	Sheep	Malignant catarrhal fever in cattle and deer
Caprine herpesvirus 2	Goat	Chronic disease in deer?
Bovine herpesvirus 4, BHV-4	Cattle	None reported
Equine herpesvirus 2 and 5, EHV-2, -5	Horse	Mononucleosis in horses?
Porcine lymphotropic herpesviruses, PLHV-1/2	Pig	None reported
Herpesvirus sylvilagus	Cottontail rabbit	Mononucleosis in rabbits?
Murine gammaherpesvirus 68, MHV-68	Wood mouse, Bank vole	Mononucleosis in mice
Lymphocryptovirus Species		
Epstein–Barr Virus, EBV, HHV-4[a]	Human	B-cell lymphoma; NPC; Hodgkin's disease, other
Chimpanzee LCV, Herpesvirus pan	Chimpanzee	
Baboon LCV, Herpesvirus papio	Baboon	Spontaneous B-cell lymphoma (and in immunosuppressed animals)
Rhesus LCV, Cercopethine HV 15	Rhesus Monkey, Macaca mulatta	Spontaneous B-cell lymphoma (and in immunosuppressed animals)
cynomolgus LCVs (HVMF1, Cyno-EBV, Si-IIA-EBV)	Cynomolgus sp, Macaca fascicularis	Spontaneous B-cell lymphoma (and in immunosuppressed animals)
Marmoset LCV, CalHV3	Common marmoset	Spontaneous B-cell lymphoma
SmiLHV1	Gold-handed tamarin	Unknown
SscLHV1	Squirrel monkey	Unknown
PpiLHV1	White-faced saki	Unknown

[a]Type species

yielding cytotoxic T-cell lines (Falk et al., 1978; reviewed in Fleckenstein and Desrosiers, 1982). Human T-cells have not been susceptible to transformation with various HVA strains.

Genome structure and replication

HVA strain #73 has a similar genome structure as HVS (Albrecht, 2000; Fleckenstein et al., 1978a)(Fig. 60.1). The long unique L-DNA containing all the virus genes has 108 409 bp with 36.6% G+C, and the terminal repetitive H-DNA without coding capacity contains multiple tandem repeats of 1582 bp with 77.1% G+C. The HVA genome contains 73 ORFs and only two genes for U-RNA like transcripts (Albrecht, 2000; Albrecht et al., 1999). While the viral SAG, Cyclin, GPCR homologues of HVS are conserved in HVA, it does not encode homologues to the ORF12, vIL17, vCD59 nor vFLIP (Fig. 60.1). The impression is rather convincing that HVA resembles an ancient variant of HVS which has either collected a smaller set of cell-homologous genes or has secondarily lost several genes.

Oncogenesis

In HVA strain #73, a spliced gene with two exons was detected in the left-terminal L- to H-DNA transition region. The derived viral protein shares local sequence homology with StpC and Tip of HVS and was therefore termed Tio ("two in one," Fig. 60.2). Tio is expressed in HVA-transformed simian T cells. After cotransfection, Tio bound to and was phosphorylated by the Src kinases Lck or Src (Albrecht et al., 1999). Human T-cells can be successfully transformed by recombinant HVS C488 in which the StpC and Tip genes were replaced by either the HVA #73 region containing the promoter and both exons of Tio, or a cDNA of Tio transcribed from a heterologous promoter; thus, Tio can substitute for both StpC and Tip in human T-cell transformation (Albrecht et al., 2004). Tyrosine phosphorylation of Tio is required for transformation of human T-cells in the context of a recombinant HVS genome (Albrecht et al., 2005), and it has been found that Tio induces NFkB signaling through direct interaction with TRAF6 (Heinemann et al., 2006).

Lymphocryptoviruses of New World primates

Gammaherpesviruses that are closely related to EBV were recognized in several species of Old World primates from the mid-70s. Until recently the paradigm was that the lymphocryptoviruses (LCV) are restricted to Old World primates including humans (Wang et al., 2001). However, a virus was isolated from common marmosets, both from healthy animals and animals with spontaneous B-cell lymphomas (Ramer et al., 2000; Cho et al., 2001); Related LCV have also been detected in several other New World primate species (de Thoisy et al., 2003; Table 60.1). This marmoset LCV (CalHV3) clearly had a EBV-like genome structure, yet several Old World primate LCV specific genes (Rivailler et al., 2002b) were absent in this isolate (Rivailler et al., 2002a). Namely, strong divergences were found in the LMP1 and 2, and the EBNA-LP, -2, and -3, and the marmoset LCV does not have homologues to BCRF1/vIL10, BARF1/CSF-1R, BARF0, EBERs, and several other EBV genes of unknown function. Also, the organization of the putative marmoset LCV OriP-region is clearly distinct from the Old World primate LCV; the *family of repeats* are a succession of two different and diverged repeat subunits, and it lacks the *dyad symmetry* elements (Rivailler et al., 2002a). In-vitro transformation of B-cells by human and simian OWP-LCV seems to be mostly restricted to the natural host or closely related species (Moghaddam et al., 1998). However, experimental T-cell tumors can be induced in rabbits following infection by Cynomolgus (Cyno-EBV) and Baboon (HVP) -LCV (Hayashi et al., 2001).

Conclusions

The γ-herpesvirus subgroups *Lymphocryptovirus* and *Rhadinovirus* occur in New World as well as Old World primates including humans. Several members of both virus subgroups are closely related to viral oncogenesis, though the simian viruses do not generally provide an uncomplicated model for multifaceted human diseases. Kaposi's sarcoma is a complex entity that may be caused by the direct transforming action of viral oncogenes as well as a chronic inflammatory reaction, which may be amended or modulated by KSHV-encoded or -induced cytokines and/or angiogenic factors. No comparable animal model could be based on the use of the KSHV-related primate γ2-herpesviruses. Although a comparable virus-associated acute peripheral pleomorphic T-cell lymphoma is not known yet in humans, Herpesvirus saimiri can serve as an experimental model for general tumor development in humans. The ability of certain HVS-strains to transform human T lymphocytes to provides a promising tool for laboratory studies in T-cell immunology, including inherited and acquired immunodeficiency. Stp, Tip and Tio represent new classes of membrane-bound viral oncoproteins, most likely as small adaptor polypeptides that proficiently dominate T-cell signaling. Recombinant rhadinoviruses can deliver foreign genes into primary human mesenchymal cells and T-lymphocytes; this may prepare the ground for future therapeutic applications of persisting rhadinoviral vectors in adoptive immunotherapy.

Acknowledgments

Original work included in this review article was supported by the Deutsche Forschungsgemeinschaft (Sonderforschungsbereich 466 and 643), the Wilhelm Sander-Stiftung, the Federal Ministry of Education and Research (BMBF) and the Interdisciplinary Center for Clinical Research (IZKF) at the University of Erlangen-Nuremberg.

REFERENCES

Ablashi, D. V., Schirm, S., Fleckenstein, B. *et al.* (1985). Herpesvirus saimiri-induced lymphoblastoid rabbit cell line: growth characteristics, virus persistence, and oncogenic properties. *J. Virol.*, **55**, 623–633.

Ahuja, S. K. and Murphy, P. M. (1993). Molecular piracy of mammalian interleukin-8 receptor type B by herpesvirus saimiri. *J. Biol. Chem.*, **268**, 20691–20694.

Albrecht, J. C., Müller-Fleckenstein, I., Schmidt, M., Fleckenstein, B. and Biesinger, B. (2005). Tyrosine phosphorylation of the Tio oncoprotein is essential for transformation of primary human T cells. *J. Virol.*, **79**, 10507–10513.

Albrecht, J. C., Biesinger, B., Müller-Fleckenstein, I., Lengenfelder, D., Schmidt, M., Fleckenstein, B., and Ensser, A. (2004). Herpesvirus ateles Tio can replace herpesvirus saimiri StpC and Tip oncoproteins in growth transformation of monkey and human T cells. *J. Virol.*, **78**, 9814–9819.

Albrecht, J. C. (2000). Primary structure of the herpesvirus ateles genome. *J. Virol.*, **74**, 1033–1037.

Albrecht, J. C. and Fleckenstein, B. (1990). Structural organization of the conserved gene block of Herpesvirus saimiri coding for DNA polymerase, glycoprotein B, and major DNA binding protein. *Virology*, **174**, 533–542.

Albrecht, J. C. and Fleckenstein, B. (1992). New member of the multigene family of complement control proteins in herpesvirus saimiri. *J. Virol.*, **66**, 3937–3940.

Albrecht, J. C., Nicholas, J., Biller, D. *et al.* (1992a). Primary structure of the herpesvirus saimiri genome. *J. Virol.*, **66**, 5047–5058.

Albrecht, J. C., Nicholas, J., Cameron, K. R., Newman, C., Fleckenstein, B., and Honess, R. W. (1992b). Herpesvirus saimiri has a gene specifying a homologue of the cellular membrane glycoprotein CD59. *Virology*, **190**, 527–530.

Albrecht, J. C., Friedrich, U., and Kardinal, C. (1999). Herpesvirus ateles gene product Tio interacts with nonreceptor protein tyrosine kinases. *J. Virol.*, **73**, 4631–4639.

Alexander, L., Du, Z., Rosenzweig, M., Jung, J. U., and Desrosiers, R. C. (1997). A role for natural simian immunodeficiency virus and human immunodeficiency virus type 1 nef alleles in lymphocyte activation. *J. Virol.*, **71**, 6094–6099.

Alexander, L., Denekamp, L., Knapp, A., Auerbach, M. R., Damania, B., and Desrosiers, R. C. (2000). The primary sequence of rhesus monkey rhadinovirus isolate 26–95: sequence similarities to Kaposi's sarcoma-associated herpesvirus and rhesus monkey rhadinovirus isolate 17577. *J. Virol.*, **74**, 3388–3398.

Altare, F., Ensser, A. *et al.* (2001). Interleukin-12 receptor beta1 deficiency in a patient with abdominal tuberculosis. *J. Infect. Dis.*, **184**, 231–236.

Bauer, F., Hofinger, E., Hoffmann, S., Rösch, P., Schweimer, K., and Sticht, H. (2004). Characterization of LcK-binding elements in the herpesviral regulatory Tip protein. *Biochemistry*, **43**, 14932–14939.

Bellows, D. S., Chau, B. N., Lee, P., Lazebnik, Y., Burns, W. H., and Hardwick, J. M. (2000). Antiapoptotic herpesvirus Bcl-2 homologs escape caspase-mediated conversion to proapoptotic proteins. *J. Virol.*, **74**, 5024–5031.

Biesinger, B., Trimble, J. J., Desrosiers, R. C., and Fleckenstein, B. (1990). The divergence between two oncogenic herpesvirus saimiri strains in a genomic region related to the transforming phenotype. *Virology*, **176**, 505–514.

Biesinger, B., Müller-Fleckenstein, I., Simmer, B. *et al.* (1992). Stable growth transformation of human T lymphocytes by herpesvirus saimiri. *Proc. Natl. Acad. Sci. USA*, **89**, 3116–3119.

Biesinger, B., Tsyganov, A. Y., Fickenscher, H. *et al.* (1995). The product of the herpesvirus saimiri open reading frame 1 (tip) interacts with T cell-specific kinase p56^{lck} in transformed cells. *J. Biol. Chem.*, **270**, 4729–4734.

Bowman, T., Garcia, R., Turkson, J., and Jove, R. (2000). STATs In oncogenesis. *Oncogene*, **19**, 2474–2488.

Bromberg, J. and Darnell, J. E. Jr. (2000). The role of STATs in transcriptional control and their impact on cellular function. *Oncogene*, **19**, 2468–2473.

Bröker, B. M., Kraft, M. S., Klauenberg, U. *et al.* (1997). Activation induces apoptosis in Herpesvirus saimiri-transformed T cells independent of CD95 (Fas, APO-1). *Eur. J. Immunol.*, **27**, 2774–2780.

Cho, Y., Ramer, J., Rivailler, P., Quink, C., Garber, R. L., Beier, D. R., and Wang, F. (2001). An Epstein–Barr-related herpesvirus from marmoset lymphomas. *Proc. Natl Acad. Sci. USA*, **98**, 1224–1229.

Cho, N. H., Feng, P., Lee, S. H., Lee, B. S., Liang, X., Chang, H., and Jung, J. U. (2004). Inhibition of T cell receptor signal transduction by tyrosine kinase-interacting protein of Herpesvirus saimiri. *J Exp. Med.*, **200**, 681–687.

Cho, N. H., Kingston, D., Chang, H., Kwon, E. K., Kim, J. M., Lee, J. H., Chu, H., Choi, M. S., Kim, I. S., and Jung, J. U. (2006). Association of herpesvirus saimiri tip with lipid raft is essential for downregulation of T-cell receptor and CD4 coreceptor. *J. Virol.*, **80**, 108–118.

Choi, J. K., Ishido, S., and Jung, J. U. (2000). The collagen repeat sequence is a determinant of the degree of herpesvirus saimiri STP transforming activity. *J. Virol.*, **74**, 8102–8110.

Chou, C. S., Medveczky, M. M., Geck, P., Vercelli, D., and Medveczky, P. G. (1995). Expression of IL-2 and IL-4 in T lymphocytes transformed by herpesvirus saimiri. *Virology*, **208**, 418–426.

Cooper, M., Goodwin, D. J., Hall, K. T. *et al.* (1999). The gene product encoded by ORF 57 of herpesvirus saimiri regulates the redistribution of the splicing factor SC-35. *J. Gen. Virol.*, **80**, 1311–1316.

Coscoy, L. and Ganem, D. (2000). Kaposi's sarcoma-associated herpesvirus encodes two proteins that block cell surface display of MHC class I chains by enhancing their endocytosis. *Proc. Natl Acad. Sci. USA*, **97**, 8051–8056.

Damania, B., Li, M., Choi, J. K., Alexander, L., Jung, J. U., and Desrosiers, R. C. (1999). Identification of the R1 oncogene and its protein product from the rhadinovirus of rhesus monkeys. *J. Virol.*, **73**, 5123–5131.

Daniel, M. D., Silva, D., Jackman, D. *et al.* (1975). Reactivation of squirrel monkey heart isolate (Herpesvirus saimiri strain) from latently infected human cell cultures and induction of malignant lymphoma in marmoset monkeys. *Bibl. Haematol.*, 392–395.

Daniel, M. D., Silva, D., and Ma, N. (1976). Establishment of owl monkey kidney 210 cell line for virological studies. *In Vitro*, **12**, 290.

De Carli, M., Berthold, S., Fickenscher, H. *et al.* (1993). Immortalization with herpesvirus saimiri modulates the cytokine secretion profile of established Th1 and Th2 human T cell clones. *J. Immunol.*, **151**, 5022–5030.

de Thoisy, B., Pouliquen, J. F., Lacoste, V., Gessain, A., and Kazanji, M. (2003). Novel gamma-1 herpesviruses identified in free-ranging new world monkeys (golden-handed tamarin

(*Saguinus midas*), squirrel monkey (*Saimiri sciureus*), and white-faced saki (*Pithecia pithecia*)) in French Guiana. *J. Virol.*, **77**, 9099–9105.

Deckert, M., Ticchioni, M., Mari, B., Mary, D., and Bernard, A. (1995). The glycosylphosphatidylinositol-anchored CD59 protein stimulates both T cell receptor zeta/ZAP-70-dependent and -independent signaling pathways in T cells. *Eur. J. Immunol.*, **25**, 1815–1822.

Derfuss, T., Fickenscher, H., Kraft, M. S. *et al.* (1998). Antiapoptotic activity of the herpesvirus saimiri-encoded Bcl-2 homolog: stabilization of mitochondria and inhibition of caspase-3-like activity. *J. Virol.*, **72**, 5897–5904.

Desrosiers, R. C. and Falk, L. A. (1982). Herpesvirus saimiri strain variability. *J. Virol.*, **43**, 352–356.

Desrosiers, R. C., Mulder, C., and Fleckenstein, B. (1979). Methylation of herpesvirus saimiri DNA in lymphoid tumor cell lines. *Proc. Natl Acad. Sci. USA*, **76**, 3839–3843.

Desrosiers, R. C., Bakker, A., Kamine, J., Falk, L. A., Hunt, R. D., and King, N. W. (1985a). A region of the herpesvirus saimiri genome required for oncogenicity. *Science*, **228**, 184–187.

Desrosiers, R. C., Kamine, J., Bakker, A. *et al.* (1985b). Synthesis of bovine growth hormone in primates by using a herpesvirus vector. *Mol. Cell Biol*, **5**, 2796–2803.

Desrosiers, R. C., Silva, D. P., Waldron, L. M., and Letvin, N. L. (1986). Nononcogenic deletion mutants of herpesvirus saimiri are defective for in vitro immortalization. *J. Virol.*, **57**, 701–705.

Doody, G. M., Leek, J. P., Bali, A. K., Ensser, A., Markham, A. F., and de Wynter, E. A. (2005). Marker gene transfer into human haemopoietic cells using a herpesvirus saimiri-based vector. *Gene Ther.*, **12**, 373–379.

Duboise, S. M., Guo, J., Desrosiers, R. C., and Jung, J. U. (1996). Use of virion DNA as a cloning vector for the construction of mutant and recombinant herpesviruses. *Proc. Natl Acad. Sci. USA*, **93**, 11389–11394.

Duboise, S. M., Guo, J., Czajak, S. *et al.* (1998a). A role for herpesvirus saimiri orf14 in transformation and persistent infection. *J. Virol.*, **72**, 6770–6776.

Duboise, S. M., Guo, J., Czajak, S., Desrosiers, R. C., and Jung, J. U. (1998b). STP and Tip are essential for herpesvirus saimiri oncogenicity. *J. Virol.*, **72**, 1308–1313.

Ensser, A. (2006). Transformation by herpesviruses: focus on T-cells. *Future Virology*, **1**, 109–121.

Ensser, A. and Fleckenstein, B. (2005). T-Cell Transformation and Oncogenesis by gamma-2-Herpesviruses. *Adv. Cancer. Res.*, **63**, 91–128.

Ensser, A. and Fleckenstein, B. (2004). Herpesvirus saimiri transformation of human T Lymphocytes. In *Current Protocols in Immunology*. New York: Current protocols, John Wiley & Sons, Inc., p. 7.21.1–7.21.10.

Ensser, A., Pfinder, A., Müller-Fleckenstein, I., and Fleckenstein, B. (1999). The URNA genes of herpesvirus saimiri (strain C488) are dispensable for transformation of human T cells in vitro. *J. Virol.*, **73**, 10551–10555.

Ensser, A., Glykofrydes, D., Niphuis, H. *et al.* (2001). Independence of herpesvirus-induced T cell lymphoma from viral cyclin D homologue. *J. Exp. Med.*, **193**, 637–642.

Ensser, A., Neipel, F., and Fickenscher, H. (2002). Rhadinovirus pathogenesis. In Bogner, E. and Holzenburg, A. eds *Structure–Function Relationships of Human Pathogenic Viruses*, New York: Kluwer Academic Publishers / Plenum Publishers, pp. 349–429.

Ensser, A., Thurau, M., Wittmann, S., and Fickenscher, H. (2003). The primary structure of the herpesvirus saimiri strain C488 genome. *Virology*, **314**, 471–487.

Falk, L. A., Wolfe, L. G., and Deinhardt, F. (1972). Isolation of herpesvirus saimiri from blood of squirrel monkeys (*Saimiri sciureus*). *J. Natl Cancer Inst.*, **48**, 1499–1505.

Falk, L. A., Nigida, S. M., Deinhardt, F., *et al.* (1974). Herpesvirus ateles: properties of an oncogenic herpesvirus isolated from circulating lymphocytes of spider monkeys (Ateles sp.). *Int. J. Cancer*, **14**, 473–482.

Falk, L. A., Johnson, D., and Deinhardt, F. (1978). Transformation of marmoset lymphocytes in vitro with Herpesvirus ateles. *Int. J. Cancer*, **21**, 652–657.

Fickenscher, H. and Fleckenstein, B. (2001). Herpesvirus saimiri. *Phil. Trans. Roy. Soc. Lond B Biol. Sci.*, **356**, 545–567.

Fickenscher, H. and Fleckenstein, B. (2002). Growth-transformation of human T cells. *Meth. Microbiology* **32**, 657–692.

Fickenscher, H., Biesinger, B., Knappe, A., Wittmann, S., and Fleckenstein, B. (1996). Regulation of the herpesvirus saimiri oncogene stpC, similar to that of T-cell activation genes, in growth-transformed human T lymphocytes. *J. Virol.*, **70**, 6012–6019.

Fickenscher, H., Bökel, C., Knappe, A. *et al.* (1997). Functional phenotype of transformed human alphabeta and gammadelta T cells determined by different subgroup C strains of herpesvirus saimiri. *J. Virol.*, **71**, 2252–2263.

Fleckenstein, B. and Desrosiers, R. C. (1982). Herpesvirus saimiri and herpesvirus ateles. In B. Roizman, ed. *The Herpesviruses*, Vol. 1, New York, London: Plenum Press, pp. 253–332.

Fleckenstein, B., Bornkamm, G. W., Mulder, C. *et al.* (1978a). Herpesvirus ateles DNA and its homology with Herpesvirus saimiri nucleic acid. *J. Virol.*, **25**, 361–373.

Fleckenstein, B., Daniel, M. D., Hunt, R. D., Werner, J., Falk, L. A., and Mulder, C. (1978b). Tumour induction with DNA of oncogenic primate herpesviruses. *Nature*, **274**, 57–59.

Fodor, W. L., Rollins, S. A., Bianco Caron, S. *et al.* (1995). The complement control protein homolog of herpesvirus saimiri regulates serum complement by inhibiting C3 convertase activity. *J. Virol.*, **69**, 3889–3892.

Fossiez, F., Banchereau, J., Murray, R., Van, K. C., Garrone, P., and Lebecque, S. (1998). Interleukin-17. *Int. Rev. Immunol.*, **16**, 541–551.

Frolova-Jones, E. A., Ensser, A., Stevenson, A. J., Kinsey, S. E., and Meredith, D. M. (2000). Stable marker gene transfer into human bone marrow stromal cells and their progenitors using novel herpesvirus saimiri-based vectors. *J. Hematother. Stem Cell Res.*, **9**, 573–581.

Fujimuro, M. and Hayward, S. D. (2003). The latency-associated nuclear antigen of Kaposi's sarcoma-associated herpesvirus manipulates the activity of glycogen synthase kinase-3beta. *J. Virol.*, **77**, 8019–8030.

Glykofrydes, D., Niphuis, H., Kuhn, E. M. et al. (2000). Herpesvirus saimiri vFLIP provides an antiapoptotic function but is not essential for viral replication, transformation, or pathogenicity. *J. Virol.*, **74**, 11919–11927.

Gompels, U. A., Craxton, M. A., and Honess, R. W. (1988). Conservation of gene organization in the lymphotropic herpesviruses herpesvirus saimiri and Epstein–Barr virus. *J. Virol.*, **62**, 757–767.

Goodwin, D. J., Hall, K. T., Stevenson, A. J., Markham, A. F., and Whitehouse, A. (1999). The open reading frame 57 gene product of herpesvirus saimiri shuttles between the nucleus and cytoplasm and is involved in viral RNA nuclear export. *J. Virol.*, **73**, 10519–10524.

Grassmann, R., Dengler, C., Müller-Fleckenstein, I. et al. (1989). Transformation to continuous growth of primary human T lymphocytes by human T-cell leukemia virus type I X-region genes transduced by a Herpesvirus saimiri vector. *Proc. Natl Acad. Sci. USA*, **86**, 3351–3355.

Grassmann, R., Berchtold, S., Radant, I. et al. (1992). Role of human T-cell leukemia virus type 1 X region proteins in immortalization of primary human lymphocytes in culture. *J. Virol.*, **66**, 4570–4575.

Greve, T., Tamguney, G., Fleischer, B., Fickenscher, H., and Bröker, B. M. (2001). Downregulation of p56(lck) tyrosine kinase activity in T cells of squirrel monkeys (*Saimiri sciureus*) correlates with the nontransforming and apathogenic properties of herpesvirus saimiri in its natural host. *J. Virol.*, **75**, 9252–9261.

Grüter, P., Tabernero, C., von Kobbe, C. et al. (1998). TAP, the human homolog of Mex67p, mediates CTE-dependent RNA export from the nucleus. *Mol. Cell*, **1**, 649–659.

Guo, J., Duboise, M., Lee, H. et al. (1997). Enhanced downregulation of Lck-mediated signal transduction by a Y114 mutation of herpesvirus saimiri tip. *J. Virol.*, **71**, 7092–7096.

Guo, J., Williams, K., Duboise, S. M., Alexander, L., Veazey, R., and Jung, J. U. (1998). Substitution of ras for the herpesvirus saimiri STP oncogene in lymphocyte transformation. *J. Virol.*, **72**, 3698–3704.

Hall, K. T., Giles, M. S., Calderwood, M. A., Goodwin, D. J., Matthews, D. A., and Whitehouse, A. (2002). The Herpesvirus Saimiri open reading frame 73 gene product interacts with the cellular protein p32. *J. Virol.*, **76**, 11612–11622.

Hall, K. T., Giles, M. S., Goodwin, D. J. et al. (2000). Analysis of gene expression in a human cell line stably transduced with herpesvirus saimiri. *J. Virol.*, **74**, 7331–7337.

Hartley, D. A., Hurley, T. R., Hardwick, J. S., Lund, T. C., Medveczky, P. G., and Sefton, B. M. (1999). Activation of the lck tyrosine-protein kinase by the binding of the tip protein of herpesvirus saimiri in the absence of regulatory tyrosine phosphorylation. *J. Biol. Chem.*, **274**, 20056–20059.

Hasham, M. G. and Tsygankov, A. Y. (2004). Tip, and Lck-interacting protein of Herpesvirus saimiri, causes Fas-and Lck-dependent apoptosis of T lymphocytes. *Virology*, **320**, 313–329.

Hayashi, K., Ohara, N., Teramoto, N. et al. (2001). An animal model for human EBV-associated hemophagocytic syndrome: herpesvirus papio frequently induces fatal lymphoproliferative disorders with hemophagocytic syndrome in rabbits. *Am. J. Pathol.*, **158**, 1533–1542.

Heck, E., Lengenfelder, D., Schmidt, M., Müller-Fleckenstein, I., Fleckenstein, B., Biesinger, B., and Ensser, A. (2005). T Cell Growth Transformation by Herpesvirus saimiri is independent of STAT3, Activation. *J. Virol.*, **79**, 5713–5720.

Heck, E., Friedrich, U., Gack, M. U., Lengenfelder, D., Schmidt, M., Müller-Fleckenstein, I., Fleckenstein, B., Ensser, A., and Biesinger, B. (2006). Growth Transformation of Human T-cells by Herpesvirus saimiri Requires Multiple Tip-Lck Interaction Motifs. *J. Virol.*, **80**, 9934–9942.

Heinemann, S., Biesinger, B., Fleckenstein, B., and Albrecht, J. C. (2006). NFkappaB signaling is induced by the oncoprotein Tio through direct interaction with TRAF6. *J. Biol. Chem.*, **281**, 8565–8572.

Hiller, C., Tamguney, G., Stolte, N. et al. (2000a). Herpesvirus saimiri pathogenicity enhanced by thymidine kinase of herpes simplex virus. *Virology*, **278**, 445–455.

Hiller, C., Wittmann, S., Slavin, S., and Fickenscher, H. (2000b). Functional long-term thymidine kinase suicide gene expression in human T cells using a herpesvirus saimiri vector. *Gene Ther.*, **7**, 664–674.

Hoge, A. T., Hendrickson, S. B., and Burns, W. H. (2000). Murine gammaherpesvirus 68 cyclin D homologue is required for efficient reactivation from latency. *J. Virol.*, **74**, 7016–7023.

Hoggarth, J. H., Jones, E., Ensser, A., and Meredith, D. M. (2004). Functional expression of thymidine kinase in human leukaemic and colorectal cells, delivered as EGFP fusion protein by herpesvirus saimiri-based vector. *Cancer Gene Ther.*, **11**, 613–624.

Hör, S., Pirzer, H., Dumoutier, L., Bauer, F., Wittmann, S., Sticht, H., Renaud, J. C., De Waal, M. R., and Fickenscher, H. (2004). The T-cell lymphokine interleukin-26 targets epithelial cells through the interleukin-20 receptor 1 and interleukin-10 receptor 2 chains. *J. Biol. Chem.*, **279**, 33343–33351.

Hör, S., Ensser, A., Reiss, C., Ballmer-Hofer, K., and Biesinger, B. (2001). Herpesvirus saimiri protein StpB associates with cellular Src. *J. Gen. Virol.* **82**, 339–344.

Hunt, R. D., Melendez, L. V., Garcia, F. G., and Trum, B. F. (1972). Pathologic features of Herpesvirus ateles lymphoma in cotton-topped marmosets (*Saguinus oedipus*). *J. Natl Cancer Inst.*, **49**, 1631–1639.

Huppes, W., Fickenscher, H., 't Hart, B. A., and Fleckenstein, B. (1994). Cytokine dependence of human to mouse graft-versus-host disease. *Scand. J. Immunol.*, **40**, 26–36.

Ishido, S., Choi, J. K., Lee, B. S. et al. (2000a). Inhibition of natural killer cell-mediated cytotoxicity by Kaposi's sarcoma-associated herpesvirus K5 protein. *Immunity*, **13**, 365–374.

Ishido, S., Wang, C., Lee, B. S., Cohen, G. B., and Jung, J. U. (2000b). Downregulation of major histocompatibility complex class I molecules by Kaposi's sarcoma-associated herpesvirus K3 and K5 proteins. *J. Virol.*, **74**, 5300–5309.

Jung, J. U. and Desrosiers, R. C. (1991). Identification and characterization of the herpesvirus saimiri oncoprotein STP-C488. *J. Virol.*, **65**, 6953–6960.

Jung, J. U. and Desrosiers, R. C. (1992). Herpesvirus saimiri oncogene STP-C488 encodes a phosphoprotein. *J. Virol.*, **66**, 1777–1780.

Jung, J. U. and Desrosiers, R. C. (1994). Distinct functional domains of STP-C488 of herpesvirus saimiri. *Virology*, **204**, 751–758.

Jung, J. U. and Desrosiers, R. C. (1995). Association of the viral oncoprotein STP-C488 with cellular ras. *Mol. Cell Biol*, **15**, 6506–6512.

Jung, J. U., Trimble, J. J., King, N. W., Biesinger, B., Fleckenstein, B. W., and Desrosiers, R. C. (1991). Identification of transforming genes of subgroup A and C strains of herpesvirus saimiri. *Proc. Natl Acad. Sci. USA*, **88**, 7051–7055.

Jung, J. U., Stager, M., and Desrosiers, R. C. (1994). Virus-encoded cyclin. *Mol. Cell Biol.*, **14**, 7235–7244.

Jung, J. U., Lang, S. M., Friedrich, U. *et al.* (1995a). Identification of Lck-binding elements in tip of herpesvirus saimiri. *J. Biol. Chem.*, **270**, 20660–20667.

Jung, J. U., Lang, S. M., Jun, T., Roberts, T. M., Veillette, A., and Desrosiers, R. C. (1995b). Downregulation of Lck-mediated signal transduction by tip of herpesvirus saimiri. *J. Virol.*, **69**, 7814–7822.

Kaschka-Dierich, C., Werner, F. J., Bauer, I., and Fleckenstein, B. (1982). Structure of nonintegrated, circular Herpesvirus saimiri and Herpesvirus ateles genomes in tumor cell lines and in vitro- transformed cells. *J. Virol.*, **44**, 295–310.

Kiyotaki, M., Desrosiers, R. C., and Letvin, N. L. (1986). Herpesvirus saimiri strain 11 immortalizes a restricted marmoset T8 lymphocyte subpopulation in vitro. *J. Exp. Med.*, **164**, 926–931.

Knappe, A., Hiller, C., Thurau, M. *et al.* (1997). The superantigen-homologous viral immediate-early gene ie14/vsag in herpesvirus saimiri-transformed human T cells. *J. Virol.*, **71**, 9124–9133.

Knappe, A., Hiller, C., Niphuis, H. *et al.* (1998a). The interleukin-17 gene of herpesvirus saimiri. *J. Virol.*, **72**, 5797–5801.

Knappe, A., Thurau, M., Niphuis, H. *et al.* (1998b). T-cell lymphoma caused by herpesvirus saimiri C488 independently of ie14/vsag, a viral gene with superantigen homology. *J. Virol.*, **72**, 3469–3471.

Knappe, A., Feldmann, G., Dittmer, U. *et al.* (2000a). Herpesvirus saimiri-transformed macaque T cells are tolerated and do not cause lymphoma after autologous reinfusion. *Blood*, **95**, 3256–3261.

Knappe, A., Hör, S., Wittmann, S., and Fickenscher, H. (2000b). Induction of a novel cellular homolog of interleukin-10, AK155, by transformation of T lymphocytes with herpesvirus saimiri. *J. Virol.*, **74**, 3881–3887.

Koomey, J. M., Mulder, C., Burghoff, R. L., Fleckenstein, B., and Desrosiers, R. C. (1984). Deletion of DNA sequence in a nononcogenic variant of Herpesvirus saimiri. *J. Virol.*, **50**, 662–665.

Korty, P. E., Brando, C., and Shevach, E. M. (1991). CD59 functions as a signal-transducing molecule for human T cell activation. *J. Immunol.*, **146**, 4092–4098.

Kretschmer, C., Murphy, C., Biesinger, B. *et al.* (1996). A herpes saimiri oncogene causing peripheral T-cell lymphoma in transgenic mice. *Oncogene*, **12**, 1609–1616.

Kung, S. H. and Medveczky, P. G. (1996). Identification of a herpesvirus saimiri cis-acting DNA fragment that permits stable replication of episomes in transformed T-cells. *J. Virol.*, **70**, 1738–1744.

Lang, G. and Fleckenstein, B. (1990). Trans-activation of the thymidylate synthase promoter of herpesvirus saimiri. *J. Virol.*, **64**, 5333–5341.

Lee, H., Trimble, J. J., Yoon, D. W., Regier, D., Desrosiers, R. C., and Jung, J. U. (1997). Genetic variation of herpesvirus saimiri subgroup A transforming protein and its association with cellular src. *J. Virol.*, **71**, 3817–3825.

Lee, H., Veazey, R., Williams, K. *et al.* (1998). Deregulation of cell growth by the K1 gene of Kaposi's sarcoma-associated herpesvirus. *Nat. Med.* **4**, 435–440.

Lee, H., Choi, J. K., Li, M., Kaye, K., Kieff, E., and Jung, J. U. (1999). Role of cellular tumor necrosis factor receptor-associated factors in NF-kappaB activation and lymphocyte transformation by herpesvirus saimiri STP. *J. Virol.*, **73**, 3913–3919.

Lund, T., Medveczky, M. M., and Medveczky, P. G. (1997a). Herpesvirus saimiri Tip-484 membrane protein markedly increases p56^{lck} activity in T cells. *J. Virol.*, **71**, 378–382.

Lund, T. C., Garcia, R., Medveczky, M. M., Jove, R., and Medveczky, P. G. (1997b). Activation of STAT transcription factors by herpesvirus saimiri Tip-484 requires p56^{lck}. *J. Virol.*, **71**, 6677–6682.

Means, R. E., Ishido, S., Alvarez, X., and Jung, J. U. (2002). Multiple endocytic trafficking pathways of MHC class I molecules induced by a Herpesvirus protein. *EMBO. J.*, **21**, 1638–1649.

Medveczky, M. M., Szomolanyi, E., Hesselton, R., DeGrand, D., Geck, P., and Medveczky, P. G. (1989). Herpesvirus saimiri strains from three DNA subgroups have different oncogenic potentials in New Zealand white rabbits. *J. Virol.*, **63**, 3601–3611.

Medveczky, M. M., Geck, P., Sullivan, J. L., Serbousek, D., Djeu, J. Y., and Medveczky, P. G. (1993). IL-2 independent growth and cytotoxicity of herpesvirus saimiri-infected human CD8 cells and involvement of two open reading frame sequences of the virus. *Virology*, **196**, 402–412.

Medveczky, P., Szomolanyi, E., Desrosiers, R. C., and Mulder, C. (1984). Classification of herpesvirus saimiri into three groups based on extreme variation in a DNA region required for oncogenicity. *J. Virol.*, **52**, 938–944.

Melendez, L. V., Daniel, M. D., Hunt, R. D., and Garcia, F. G. (1968). An apparently new herpesvirus from primary kidney cultures of the squirrel monkey (*Saimiri sciureus*). *Lab. Anim. Care*, **18**, 374–381.

Melendez, L. V., Hunt, R. D., King, N. W. *et al.* (1972). Herpesvirus ateles, a new lymphoma virus of monkeys. *Nature New Biol.*, **235**, 182–184.

Meuer, S. C., Hussey, R. E., Fabbi, M. et al. (1984). An alternative pathway of T-cell activation: a functional role for the 50 kd T11 sheep erythrocyte receptor protein. *Cell*, **36**, 897–906.

Mittrücker, H. W., Müller-Fleckenstein, I., Fleckenstein, B., and Fleischer, B. (1992). CD2-mediated autocrine growth of herpes virus saimiri-transformed human T lymphocytes. *J. Exp. Med.*, **176**, 909–913.

Moghaddam, A., Koch, J., Annis, B., and Wang, F. (1998). Infection of human B lymphocytes with lymphocryptoviruses related to Epstein–Barr virus. *J. Virol.*, **72**, 3205–3212.

Murphy, C., Kretschmer, C., Biesinger, B. et al. (1994). Epithelial tumours induced by a herpesvirus oncogene in transgenic mice. *Oncogene*, **9**, 221–226.

Murphy, P. M. (1994). The molecular biology of leukocyte chemoattractant receptors. *Annu. Rev. Immunol.*, **12**, 593–633.

Murthy, S. C., Trimble, J. J., and Desrosiers, R. C. (1989). Deletion mutants of herpesvirus saimiri define an open reading frame necessary for transformation. *J. Virol.*, **63**, 3307–3314.

Nava, V. E., Cheng, E. H. Y., Veliuona, M. et al. (1997). Herpesvirus saimiri encodes a functional homolog of the human bcl-2 oncogene. *J. Virol.*, **71**, 4118–4122.

Neipel, F., Albrecht, J. C., and Fleckenstein, B. (1997). Cell-homologous genes in the Kaposi's sarcoma associated rhadinovirus human herpesvirus 8: determinants of its pathogenicity? *J. Virol.*, **71**, 4187–4192.

Nicholas, J., Gompels, U. A., Craxton, M. A., and Honess, R. W. (1988). Conservation of sequence and function between the product of the 52-kilodalton immediate-early gene of herpesvirus saimiri and the BMLF1-encoded transcriptional effector (EB2) of Epstein–Barr virus. *J. Virol.*, **62**, 3250–3257.

Nicholas, J., Coles, L. S., Newman, C., and Honess, R. W. (1991). Regulation of the herpesvirus saimiri (HVS) delayed-early 110-kilodalton promoter by HVS immediate-early gene products and a homolog of the Epstein–Barr virus R trans activator. *J. Virol.*, **65**, 2457–2466.

Nicholas, J., Cameron, K. R., and Honess, R. W. (1992). Herpesvirus saimiri encodes homologues of G protein-coupled receptors and cyclins. *Nature*, **355**, 362–365.

Nick, S., Fickenscher, H., Biesinger, B., Born, G., Jahn, G., and Fleckenstein, B. (1993). Herpesvirus saimiri transformed human T cell lines: a permissive system for human immunodeficiency viruses. *Virology*, **194**, 875–877.

Park, J., Lee, B. S., Choi, J. K., Means, R. E., Choe, J., and Jung, J. U. (2002). Herpesviral protein targets a cellular WD repeat endosomal protein to downregulate T lymphocyte receptor expression. *Immunity.*, **17**, 221–233.

Park, J., Cho, N. H., Choi, J. K., Feng, P., Choe, J., and Jung, J. U. (2003). Distinct roles of cellular Lck and p80 proteins in herpesvirus saimiri Tip function on lipid rafts. *J. Virol.*, **77**, 9041–9051.

Ramer, J. C., Garber, R. L., Steele, K. E., Boyson, J. F., O'Rourke, C., and Thomson, J. A. (2000). Fatal lymphoproliferative disease associated with a novel gammaherpesvirus in a captive population of common marmosets. *Comp. Med.*, **50**, 59–68.

Randall, R. E., Newman, C., and Honess, R. W. (1984). A single major immediate-early virus gene product is synthesized in cells productively infected with herpesvirus saimiri. *J. Gen. Virol.*, **65**, 1215–1219.

Randall, R. E., Newman, C., and Honess, R. W. (1985). Asynchronous expression of the immediate-early protein of herpesvirus saimiri in populations of productively infected cells. *J. Gen. Virol.*, **66**, 2199–2213.

Rivailler, P., Cho, Y. G., and Wang, F. (2002a). Complete genomic sequence of an Epstein–Barr virus-related herpesvirus naturally infecting a new world primate: a defining point in the evolution of oncogenic lymphocryptoviruses. *J. Virol.*, **76**, 12055–12068.

Rivailler, P., Jiang, H., Cho, Y. G., Quink, C., and Wang, F. (2002b). Complete nucleotide sequence of the rhesus lymphocryptovirus: genetic validation for an Epstein–Barr virus animal model. *J. Virol.*, **76**, 421–426.

Roizman, B., Desrosiers, R. C., Fleckenstein, B., Lopez, C., Minson, A. C., and Studdert, M. J. (1992). The family Herpesviridae: an update. The Herpesvirus Study Group of the International Committee on Taxonomy of Viruses. *Arch. Virol.*, **123**, 425–449.

Rother, R. P., Rollins, S. A., Fodor, W. L. et al. (1994). Inhibition of complement-mediated cytolysis by the terminal complement inhibitor of herpesvirus saimiri. *J. Virol.*, **68**, 730–737.

Rouvier, E., Luciani, M. F., Mattei, M. G., Denizot, F., and Golstein, P. (1993). CTLA-8, cloned from an activated T cell, bearing AU-rich messenger RNA instability sequences, and homologous to a herpesvirus saimiri gene. *J. Immunol.*, **150**, 5445–5456.

Russo, J. J., Bohenzky, R. A., Chien, M.-C. et al. (1996). Nucleotide sequence of the Kaposi's sarcoma associated herpesvirus (HHV8). *Proc. Natl Acad. Sci. USA*, **93**, 14862–14867.

Schäfer, A., Lengenfelder, D., Grillhösl, C., Wieser, C., Fleckenstein, B., and Ensser, A. (2003). The latency-associated nuclear antigen homolog of herpesvirus saimiri inhibits lytic virus replication. *J. Virol.*, **77**, 5911–5925.

Schirm, S., Müller, I., Desrosiers, R. C., and Fleckenstein, B. (1984). Herpesvirus saimiri DNA in a lymphoid cell line established by in vitro transformation. *J. Virol.*, **49**, 938–946.

Schneider, U., Schwenk, H. U., and Bornkamm, G. (1977). Characterization of EBV-genome negative "null" and "T" cell lines derived from children with acute lymphoblastic leukemia and leukemic transformed non-Hodgkin lymphoma. *Int. J. Cancer*, **19**, 621–626.

Schofield, A. (1994). Investigations of the origins of replication of herpesvirus saimiri. *Open University*, 1–220.

Schweimer, K., Hoffmann, S., Bauer, F. et al. (2002). Structural investigation of the binding of a herpesviral protein to the SH3 domain of tyrosine kinase Lck. *Biochemistry*, **41**, 5120–5130.

Searles, R. P., Bergquam, E. P., Axthelm, M. K., and Wong, S. W. (1999). Sequence and genomic analysis of a Rhesus macaque rhadinovirus with similarity to Kaposi's sarcoma-associated herpesvirus/human herpesvirus 8. *J. Virol.*, **73**, 3040–3053.

Simmer, B., Alt, M., Buckreus, I. et al. (1991). Persistence of selectable herpesvirus saimiri in various human haematopoietic and epithelial cell lines. *J. Gen. Virol.*, **72**, 1953–1958.

Sinclair, A. J. (2003). bZIP proteins of human gammaherpesviruses. *J. Gen. Virol.*, **84**, 1941–1949.

Sorokina, E. M., Merlo, J. J., Jr., and Tsygankov, A. Y. (2004). Molecular mechanisms of the effect of Herpesvirus saimiri protein StpC on the signaling pathway leading to NF-kappa B activation. *J. Biol. Chem.* **279**, 13469–13477.

Stevenson, A. J., Cooper, M., Griffiths, J. C. et al. (1999). Assessment of Herpesvirus saimiri as a potential human gene therapy vector. *J. Med. Virol.*, **57**, 269–277.

Stevenson, A. J., Clarke, D., Meredith, D. M., Kinsey, S. E., Whitehouse, A., and Bonifer, C. (2000a). Herpesvirus saimiri-based gene delivery vectors maintain heterologous expression throughout mouse embryonic stem cell differentiation in vitro. *Gene Ther.*, **7**, 464–471.

Stevenson, A. J., Giles, M. S., Hall, K. T. et al. (2000b). Specific oncolytic activity of herpesvirus saimiri in pancreatic cancer cells. *Br. J. Cancer*, **83**, 329–332.

Swanton, C., Mann, D. J., Fleckenstein, B., Neipel, F., Peters, G., and Jones, N. (1997). Herpes viral cyclin/Cdk6 complexes evade inhibition by CDK inhibitor proteins. *Nature*, **390**, 184–187.

Szomolanyi, E., Medveczky, P., and Mulder, C. (1987). In vitro immortalization of marmoset cells with three subgroups of herpesvirus saimiri. *J. Virol.*, **61**, 3485–3490.

Thome, M., Schneider, P., Hofmann, K. et al. (1997). Viral FLICE-inhibitory proteins (FLIPs) prevent apoptosis induced by death receptors. *Nature*, **386**, 517–521.

Thomson, B. J. and Nicholas, J. (1991). Superantigen function. *Nature*, **351**, 530.

Thurau, M., Whitehouse, A., Wittmann, S., Meredith, D., and Fickenscher, H. (2000). Distinct transcriptional and functional properties of the R transactivator gene orf50 of the transforming herpesvirus saimiri strain C488. *Virology*, **268**, 167–177.

Troidl, B., Simmer, B., Fickenscher, H. et al. (1994). Karyotypic characterization of human T-cell lines immortalized by Herpesvirus saimiri. *Int. J. Cancer*, **56**, 433–438.

Virgin, H. W., Latreille, P., Wamsley, P. et al. (1997). Complete sequence and genomic analysis of murine gammaherpesvirus 68. *J. Virol.*, **71**, 5894–5904.

Wang, F., Rivailler, P., Rao, P., and Cho, Y. (2001). Simian homologues of Epstein–Barr virus. *Phil. Trans. Roy. Soc. Lond B Biol. Sci.*, **356**, 489–497.

Weber, F., Meinl, E., Drexler, K. et al. (1993). Transformation of human T-cell clones by Herpesvirus saimiri: intact antigen recognition by autonomously growing myelin basic protein-specific T cells. *Proc. Natl Acad. Sci. USA*, **90**, 11049–11053.

Whitehouse, A., Cooper, M., and Meredith, D. M. (1998). The immediate-early gene product encoded by open reading frame 57 of herpesvirus saimiri modulates gene expression at a post-transcriptional level. *J. Virol.*, **72**, 857–861.

Wiese, N., Tsygankov, A. Y., Klauenberg, U., Bolen, J. B., Fleischer, B., and Bröker, B. M. (1996). Selective activation of T cell kinase p56^{lck} by Herpesvirus saimiri protein tip. *J. Biol. Chem.*, **271**, 847–852.

Wieser, C., Stumpf, D., Grillhösl, C., Lengenfelder, D., Gay, S., Fleckenstein, B., and Ensser, A. (2005). Regulated and constitutive expression of anti-inflamatory cytokines by non-transforming Herpesvirus saimiri vectors. *Gene Ther.*, **12**, 396–406.

Wright, J., Falk, L. A., Collins, D., and Deinhardt, F. (1976). Mononuclear cell fraction carrying Herpesvirus saimiri in persistently infected squirrel monkeys. *J. Natl Cancer Inst.*, **57**, 959–962.

Yao, Z. B., Fanslow, W. C., Seldin, M. F. et al. (1995). Herpesvirus saimiri encodes a new cytokine, IL-17, which binds to a novel cytokine receptor. *Immunity*, **3**, 811–821.

Yao, Z. B., Maraskovsky, E., Spriggs, M. K., Cohen, J. I., Armitage, R. J., and Alderson, M. R. (1996). Herpesvirus saimiri open reading frame 14, a protein encoded by a T-lymphotropic herpesvirus, binds to MHC class-II molecules and stimulates T-cell proliferation. *J. Immunol.*, **156**, 3260–3266.

Yoon, D. W., Lee, H., Seol, W., DeMaria, M., Rosenzweig, M., and Jung, J. U. (1997). Tap: a novel cellular protein that interacts with tip of herpesvirus saimiri and induces lymphocyte aggregation. *Immunity*, **6**, 571–582.

61

EBV and KSHV – related herpesviruses in non-human primates

Blossom Damania

Lineberger Comprehensive Cancer Center, Department of Microbiology and Immunology, University of North Carolina, NC, USA

Introduction

Herpesviruses can be found in primates throughout the animal kingdom. In the animal kingdom, the order of primates is classified into two suborders, the Prosimians and the Anthropoids (Fig. 61.1(a)). Prosimians are the earliest and most primitive of primates and are comprised of lemurs, lorises and tarsiers. Tarsiers share characteristics that are intermediate between the prosimians and the anthropoids, and hence are sometimes considered a third suborder. The Anthropoids are classified into platyrrhines (flat nosed) and catarrhines (downward pointing nose).

The platyrrhines are New World monkeys found exclusively in Mexico and Central and South America. This group includes tamarins, common marmosets, squirrel monkeys and spider monkeys. Evolution of the platyrrhines has been a subject of intense debate. Most believe that the origin and early diversification of platyrrhines occurred on the African continent. It is thought that the platyrrhines then crossed the Atlantic Ocean to the Americas at a time when sea levels were lower and the ocean ridges in the Atlantic were likely exposed as islands, creating pathways that were conducive to platyrrhine migration.

The catarrhines are sub-divided into Cercopithecoids or Old World monkeys (with tails) and Hominids (no tails) (Fig. 61.1(b)). Old World monkeys are found in both Africa and Asia. The rhesus monkey (*Macaca mulatta*) and the cynomolgus monkey (*Macaca fascicularis*) are examples of Old World primates found in Asia, while African green monkeys and baboons are Old World primates found exclusively in Africa. The Hominids include apes like chimpanzees, gibbons, gorillas, orangutans, and humans. Hominids are divided into three groups: the *pongidae* (orangutans) and the *hylabatidae* (gibbons) that live in Asia, and the *panidae*, including gorillas and chimpanzees, that live in Africa. The divergence of the platyrrhines and the catarrhines is thought to have occurred 35 million years ago and the divergence of the cercopithecoids from the hominoids is thought to have occurred about 25 million years ago. These estimates are based on paleontological fossil records, as well as sequence comparisons of mitochondrial genes (Schrago and Russo, 2003; Stewart and Disotell, 1998).

Nomenclature

A wide body of literature has identified the presence of the gammaherpesvirinae throughout the animal kingdom (Fig. 61.1). These viruses include members of both the lymphocryptovirus (LCV) and rhadinovirus sub-families of the gammaherpesvirinae. The name Lymphocrypto is derived from the Latin word *lympha* meaning "water" and the Greek word *kryptos* meaning "concealed," and the name Rhadino is derived from the Greek adjective *rhadinos*, meaning slender (ICTV website). Many of these non-human primate gammaherpesviruses are distinctly related to the human lymphocryptovirus, Epstein–Barr virus (EBV/HHV-4) and the human rhadinovirus, Kaposi's sarcoma-associated herpesvirus (KSHV/HHV-8).

The nomenclature used for the primate herpesviruses can be quite obscure. Names such as Herpesvirus papio and Herpesvirus pan are not specific since they do not clearly designate which herpesvirus is being identified. To clarify this, the International Committee on the Taxonomy of Viruses (ICTV) has suggested a defined nomenclature system which uses the family or sub-family of the natural host followed by the sequential number in order of discovery (ICTV website). Examples of this nomenclature system are *Cercopithecine herpesvirus* 17 which refers to the 17th herpesvirus found in rhesus macaques (also known as rhesus monkey rhadinovirus (RRV)), while *Cercopithecine herpesvirus* 15 refers to the 15th herpesvirus found in rhesus

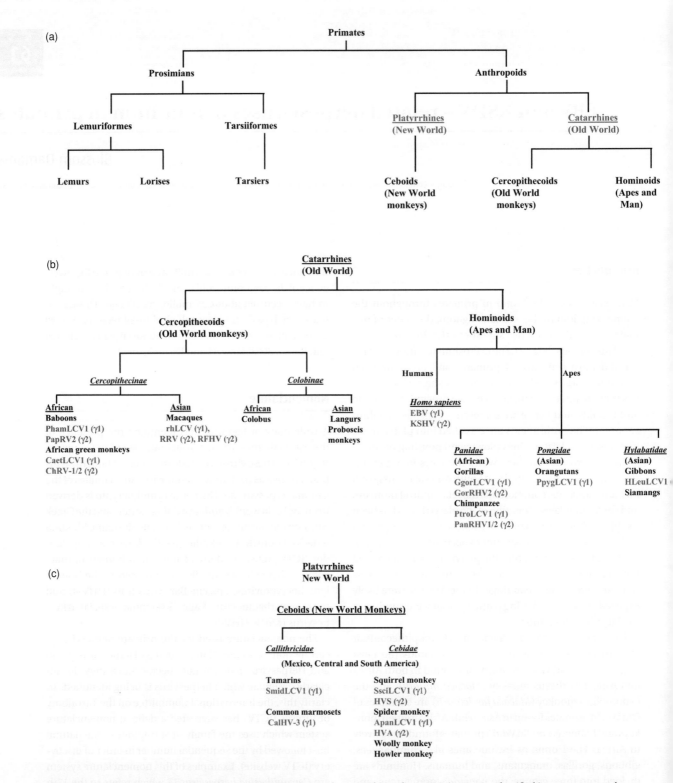

Fig. 61.1. Classification of primates and gammaherpesviruses in the Animal Kingdom. (a) Primates are classified into two groups; the Prosimians and the Anthropoids. (b) Classification of the Catarrhines or Old World Primates. The gammaherpesviruses found in the different primate species are shown in gray. (c) Classification of the Platyrrhines or New World Primates. The gammaherpesviruses found in the different primate species are shown in gray.

macaques also referred to as rhesus EBV. In order to facilitate recognition and easy usage, several investigators have combined the host species and virus for vernacular usage, e.g., baboon LCV. Further, due to the identification of multiple isolates of primate rhadinoviruses, some investigators have further chosen to numerically identify the lineage. For example, *Papio anubis* RV2 or PapRV2 is the alternate name for one of two rhadinoviruses found in baboons, whereas ChRV1 is the name of one of two rhadinoviruses found in African Green monkeys (Whitby *et al.*, 2003; Greensill *et al.*, 2000b) (Table 61.1).

Evolution of New and Old World Lymphocryptoviruses

The platyrrhines diverged from the catarrhines around 35 million years ago, and hence parallel the divergence of the New World and Old World lymphocryptoviruses. Thus, the rhesus LCV and human EBV genomes are more closely related to each other than the common marmoset LCV genome. However, it is clearly evident that both these viruses evolved from a common ancestral viral genome since many genes are conserved between these different lymphocryptoviruses. For example, several essential genes like EBV nuclear antigen 1 (EBNA-1), which is required for episome maintenance, and BZLF1 and BRLF1, which are required for viral replication, are conserved between the Old and New World lymphocryptoviruses and speak to the importance of their functions in the viral lifecycle (Tables 61.2 and 61.3). Other genes like the colony-stimulating factor 1 receptor (CF1R) homologue and the interleukin 10 (IL-10) homologue are present in only the Old World lymphocryptoviruses like EBV and rhesus LCV, but are absent from the New World lymphocryptovirus genome (Tables 61.2 and 61.3). This suggests that these two genes were captured by rhesus LCV or an ancestral virus after the divergence of the New and Old World LCV, and were selected for and retained by the human virus because they provide a biological advantage during the viral lifecycle.

Lymphocryptoviruses of Old World Monkeys

There are several lymphocryptoviruses that have been identified in both Old and New World monkeys (Table 61.1). Similar to their human counterpart, EBV, all these viruses are capable of immortalizing B cells in vitro. These viruses manifest both persistent infection and B-cell lymphomagenesis raising the speculation that a biological selection for these two characteristic properties of lymphocryptoviruses has existed throughout evolution. The first clue that Old World primates were indeed infected with EBV-related viruses came from studies demonstrating that the serum of several Old World primates exhibited antibody cross-reactivity against human EBV (Dunkel *et al.*, 1972; Kalter *et al.*, 1972; Naito *et al.*, 1971; Levy *et al.*, 1971; Landon and Malan, 1971). Lymphocryptoviruses were identified in baboons, common marmosets, gorillas and orangutans, and several LCV cell lines containing these viruses have been established in vitro (Rabin *et al.*, 1977a,b; Neubauer *et al.*, 1979; Rasheed *et al.*, 1977). Interestingly, viruses from these cell lines were shown to immortalize both autologous B cells, as well as B cells from closely related species (Falk *et al.*, 1977; Ishida and Yamamoto, 1987; Neubauer *et al.*, 1979; Rabin *et al.*, 1977a,b; Rangan *et al.*, 1986). Further, analysis of the restriction digestion patterns of the lymphocryptovirus herpesvirus papio (HVPapio) from baboons revealed that the viral genome was organized in a collinear fashion with human EBV and that the genomes shared 40% homology (Heller *et al.*, 1981; Heller and Kieff, 1981). To date, multiple lymphocryptoviruses have been identified from different Old World primates such as chimpanzees (Landon *et al.*, 1968), baboons (Vasiljeva *et al.*, 1974), African green monkeys (Bocker *et al.*, 1980), orangutans (Rasheed *et al.*, 1977) and gorillas (Neubauer *et al.*, 1979).

Other studies give credence to the close similarity between the simian and human lymphocryptoviruses. For example, rhesus macaques contain two rhesus lymphocryptoviruses (Type 1 and Type 2) similar to the situation in humans (Cho *et al.*, 1999). In the human population, there are two types of EBV isolates, EBV-1 and EBV-2 that can be distinguished by genetic polymorphisms in the EBNA genes (Dambaugh *et al.*, 1980, 1984, 1986; Zimber *et al.*, 1986; Rowe *et al.*, 1989; Rowe and Clarke, 1989; Sample *et al.*, 1990). EBV-1 is more efficient in B cell immortalization than EBV-2 (Rickinson *et al.*, 1987; Cohen *et al.*, 1989). The two types of rhesus LCVs have similar genetic polymorphisms as seen in the human isolates, and share the same biological properties (Cho *et al.*, 1999). Thus, both the human and non-human primate lymphocryptoviruses share similar genomic organizations and biological properties, which suggests that they arose from the same ancestral lymphocryptovirus and that there exists a similar selection pressure for the evolution of two different LCVs in both humans and macaques.

The rhesus LCV genome

The complete rhesus LCV (type 1) genome has been cloned and sequenced (Rivailler *et al.*, 2002b). Rhesus LCV encodes

Table 61.1. Nomenclature of primate gammaherpesviruses

Species	Full Virus Name	Other Name	ICTV	Abbreviation	Reference
Old World Primates		**Lymphocryptoviruses**			
Chimpanzee	*Pan troglodytes* LCV1	Herpesvirus pan	*Pongine herpesvirus 1*	PtroLCV1	Greensill *et al.*, 2000a,b
Bonobo	*Pan paniscus* LCV1			PpanLCV1	Ehlers *et al.*, 2003
Gorilla	*Gorilla gorilla* LCV1	Gorilla herpesvirus	*Pongine herpesvirus 3*	GgorLCV1	Ehlers *et al.*, 2003
Gorilla	*Gorilla gorilla* LCV2	Gorilla herpesvirus	*Pongine herpesvirus 3*	GgorLCV2	Ehlers *et al.*, 2003
Orangutan	*Pongo pygmaeus* LCV1	Orangutan herpesvirus	*Pongine herpesvirus 2*	PpygLCV1	Ehlers *et al.*, 2003
White-cheeked gibbon	*Hylobates leucogenys* LCV1			HleuLCV1	Ehlers *et al.*, 2003
White-handed gibbon	*Hylobates lar* LCV1			HlarLCV1	Ehlers *et al.*, 2003
Hanuman langur	*Semnopithecus entellus* LCV1			SentLCV1	Ehlers *et al.*, 2003
Hamadryas baboon	*Papio hamadryas* LCV1	Herpesvirus papio	*Cercopithecine herpesvirus 12*	PhamLCV1	Ehlers *et al.*, 2003
Hamadryas baboon	*Papio hamadryas* LCV2	Herpesvirus papio	*Cercopithecine herpesvirus 12*	PhamLCV2	Ehlers *et al.*, 2003
Mandrill	*Mandrillus sphinx* LCV1			MsphLCV1	Ehlers *et al.*, 2003
Mandrill	*Mandrillus sphinx* LCV2			MsphLCV2	Ehlers *et al.*, 2003
Black and White colobus	*Colobus guereza* LCV1			CgueLCV1	Ehlers *et al.*, 2003
Western red colobus	*Piliocolobus badius* LCV1			PbadLCV1	Ehlers *et al.*, 2003
Black mangabey	*Cercocebus aterrimus* LCV1			CateLCV1	Ehlers *et al.*, 2003
Rhesus macaque	*Macaca mulatta* LCV1	Rhesus EBV	*Cercopithecine herpesvirus 15*	MmuLCV1	Franken *et al.*, 1996
Cynomolgus macaque	*Macaca fascicularis* LCV1			MfasLCV1	Ehlers *et al.*, 2003
Japanese macaque	*Macaca fuscata* LCV1			MfusLCV1	Ehlers *et al.*, 2003
Japanese macaque	*Macaca fuscata* LCV2			MfusLCV2	Ehlers *et al.*, 2003
Wanderoo	*Macaca silenus* LCV1			MsilLCV1	Ehlers *et al.*, 2003
Magot	*Macaca sylvanus* LCV1			MsylLCV1	Ehlers *et al.*, 2003
Tibet macaque	*Macaca tibetana* LCV1			MtibLCV1	Ehlers *et al.*, 2003
Patas monkey	*Erythrocebus patas* LCV1			EpatLCV1	Ehlers *et al.*, 2003
African green monkey	*Chlorocebus aethiops* LCV	African green monkey EBV-like virus	*Cercopithecine herpesvirus 14*	CaetLCV1	Bocker *et al.*, 1980
New World Primates					
Common squirrel monkey	*Saimiri sciureus* LCV1			SsciLCV1	Ehlers *et al.*, 2003
Common squirrel monkey	*Saimiri sciureus* LCV2			SsciLCV2	Ehlers *et al.*, 2003
Saki	*Pithecia pithecia* LCV1			PpitLCV1	Ehlers *et al.*, 2003
White-fronted capuchin	*Cebus albifrons* LCV1			CalbLCV1	Ehlers *et al.*, 2003
Black spider monkey	*Ateles paniscus* LCV1			ApanLCV1	Ehlers *et al.*, 2003
Black-penciled marmoset	*Callithrix penicillata* LCV1			CpenLCV1	Ehlers *et al.*, 2003
Common marmoset	*Callithrix jacchus* LCV1	Marmoset LCV		CjacLCV1/ CalHV3	Cho *et al.*, 2001
Red-handed tamarin	*Saguinus midas* LCV1			SmidLCV1	Ehlers *et al.*, 2003
		Rhadinoviruses			
Old World Primates					
Chimpanzee	*Pan troglodytes* RV1			PanRHV1a/ PtRV1	Greensill *et al.*, 2000a,b
Chimpanzee	*Pan troglodytes* RV1			PanRHV1b	Greensill *et al.*, 2000a,b
Chimpanzee	*Pan troglodytes* RV2	Pan Rhadino-herpesvirus 2		PanRHV2	Greensill *et al.*, 2000a,b

(cont.)

Table 61.1. (cont.)

Species	Full Virus Name	Other Name	ICTV	Abbreviation	Reference
Gorilla	*Gorilla gorilla* RV1			GorRHV1	Lacoste *et al.*, 2000a,b
Baboon	*Papio anubis* RV2			PapRV2	Whitby *et al.*, 2003
Mandrill	*Mandrillus sphinx* RHV1			MndRHV1	Lacoste *et al.*, 2000a,b
Mandrill	*Mandrillus sphinx* RHV2			MndRHV2	Lacoste *et al.*, 2000a,b
Rhesus macaque	*Macaca mulatta* RV1	Retroperitoneal fibromatosis herpesvirus		MmuRV1/ RFHVMm	Rose *et al.*, 1997
Rhesus macaque	*Macaca mulatta* RV2	Rhesus monkey rhadinovirus	*Cercopithecine herpesvirus 17*	RRV/MmuRV2	Desrosiers *et al.*, 1997
Cynomolgus macaque	*Macaca fascicularis* RV2			MGVMf	Rose *et al.*, 2003
Pig-tailed macaque	*Macaca nemestrina* RV1			MneRV1/ RFHVMn	Rose *et al.*, 1997
Pig-tailed macaque	*Macaca nemestrina* RV2			MneRRV/ MneRV2	Schultz *et al.*, 2000
African green monkey	*Chlorocebus aethiops* RV1	Chlorocebus rhadinovirus 1		ChRV1	Greensill *et al.*, 2000a,b
African green monkey	*Chlorocebus aethiops* RV2	Chlorocebus rhadinovirus 2		ChRV2	Greensill *et al.*, 2000a,b
New World Primates					
Common squirrel monkey	*Saimiri sciureus* RV	Herpesvirus saimiri	*Saimiriine herpesvirus 2*	HVS/SaHV-2	Albrecht and Fleckenstein., 1990
Spider monkey	*Ateles paniscus* RV	Herpesvirus ateles 3	*Ateline herpesvirus 3*	HVA3	Albrecht and Fleckenstein., 2000

In order to achieve consistency, the full virus name indicates first the species in which the virus was found, and then the virus itself; RV = rhadinovirus and LCV = lymphocryptovirus. Lineages 1 and 2 are also indicated. The other name and abbreviation refers to the name and abbreviations assigned by different laboratories who found the same or similar virus.

Table 61.2. A comparison of proteins encoded by the rhesus and human lymphocryptoviruses

Rhesus LCV	% aa similarity to EBV	Function
LMP1	32.4	Transforming protein
LMP2A	57	Signal modulator
EBER-1	–	Small RNA
EBER-2	–	Small RNA
EBNA-1	46.3	Episomal maintenance
EBNA-2	29.8	Nuclear protein
EBNA-3A	29.4	Nuclear protein
EBNA-3B	30.5	Nuclear protein
EBNA-3C	31.2	Nuclear protein
BCRF1	84.1	IL-10 homologue
BARF1	75	CF1R homologue
BHRF1	72.8	Bcl-2 homologue
BALF1	84.1	Bcl-2 homologue
BZLF1	71.3	Transcription factor
BRLF1	76.3	Transcription factor
BALF5	94.8	DNA polymerase

eighty open reading frames (ORFs) and each ORF shares homology to a corresponding gene in human EBV. The average gene homology between EBV and rhesus LCV is 75.6% (Rivailler *et al.*, 2002b). Each ORF is located at an equivalent position in the viral genome (Rivailler *et al.*, 2002b). Many of the latent and lytic genes of rhesus LCV are conserved with those of human EBV. Latent genes include those of the EBV nuclear antigens, EBNA-1, 2, 3A, 3B, 3C, the EBV-encoded small RNAs (EBERs) and the latent membrane proteins LMP1, 2A and 2B (Rivailler *et al.*, 1999, 2002b; Blake *et al.*, 1999; Cho *et al.* 1999; Franken *et al.*, 1996; Jiang *et al.*, 2000; Peng *et al.*, 2000). Both the rhesus LCV and human EBV genomes have four homologues of cellular genes: CSF1R (BARF1), two bcl-2 homologues (BHRF1 and BALF1) and an IL-10 homologue (BCRF1) (Rivailler *et al.*, 2002b). Interestingly, although the bcl-2 homologues are conserved between the Old and New World lymphocryptoviruses (Tables 61.2 and 61.3), the IL-10 homologue and the colony-stimulating factor 1 receptor were recently acquired genes, and are not present in an LCV genome isolated from a

Table 61.3. A comparison of proteins encoded by the human and marmoset lymphocryptoviruses

Marmoset LCV	% aa similarity to EBV	Function	Positional homologue in EBV
C1	–	Unique gene (Transforming gene)	LMP-1
C2	–	Unique gene	BILF2
C3	–	Unique gene	EBNA-3
C4	–	Unique gene	BHLF1
C5	–	Unique gene	EBNA-2
C6	–	Unique gene	none
C7	–	Unique gene	LMP-2
ORF39 (EBNA-1)	36.0	Episomal maintenance	EBNA-1
ORF 64 (BHRF1)	20.5	Bcl-2 homologue	BHRF1
ORF 1 (BALF1)	27.6	Bcl-2 homologue	BALF1
ORF 43 (BZLF1)	29.0	Transcription factor	BZLF1
ORF 42 (BRLF1)	39.0	Transcription factor	BRLF1
ORF 5 (BALF5)	73.5	DNA polymerase	BALF5

common marmoset (Rivailler *et al.*, 2002b) (Tables 61.2 and 61.3). Table 61.2 shows a list of important genes encoded by rhesus LCV and their function.

Latency, immune-modulatory and transforming genes of rhesus LCV

Epstein–Barr virus nuclear antigen-1 (EBNA-1)

The latency gene, EBV EBNA-1 is a critical gene required for establishment and maintenance of the viral genome in the latent state. Both baboon LCV (*Cercopithecine herpesvirus 12* or herpesvirus papio) and rhesus LCV (*Cercopithecine herpesvirus 15*) encode homologues of EBV EBNA-1 that are highly conserved (Blake *et al.*, 1999; Yates *et al.*, 1996). The same is true for the EBNA-1 protein from a lymphocryptovirus infecting cynomolgus monkeys (Ohara *et al.*, 2000). Interestingly, these simian viral EBNA-1 proteins are slightly smaller than the human viral protein due to differences in the glycine-alanine (GAR) repeat domain. The baboon and rhesus LCV EBNA-1 proteins can both function to support EBV ori-P-dependent plasmid replication and maintenance, similar to EBV EBNA-1 (Marechal *et al.*, 1999; Ruf *et al.*, 1999). In addition, the molecular mechanisms governing latent gene expression such as the EBNA-1 and EBNA-2 transcripts are also conserved among the primate LCVs (Ruf *et al.*, 1999; Fuentes-Panana *et al.*, 1999).

However, one difference between these proteins is that, although the EBV EBNA-1 protein can inhibit antigen presentation to escape CTL surveillance (Levitskaya *et al.*, 1995), this immunomodulatory function is not conserved in the rhesus LCV EBNA-1 protein (Blake *et al.*, 1999) using in vitro assays. However, in naturally and experimentally infected rhesus macaques, the LCV EBNA-1 protein appeared to play a role in immune evasion in vivo (Fogg *et al.*, 2005).

Epstein–Barr virus nuclear antigen-2 (EBNA-2)

Despite the fact that the EBNA-2 protein in the rhesus and baboon LCVs show only limited homology to each other and to human EBV, their functional characteristics such as their interactions with the transcription factor RBP-Jk have been retained (Ling *et al.*, 1993; Ling and Hayward, 1995; Cho *et al.*, 1999; Peng *et al.*, 2000). The polyproline repeat in the rhesus and baboon EBNA-2 proteins is shorter than the EBV EBNA-2 protein (Peng *et al.*, 2000). However, since this region appears to be dispensable for transactivation and B cell immortalization (Yalamanchili *et al.*, 1994) the significance of this divergence may be minimal. As mentioned above, genetic polymorphisms in the EBNA-2 genes have suggested the presence of two types of LCVs in rhesus macaques, similar to the situation in humans.

Epstein–Barr virus nuclear antigen- 3A,3B,3C (EBNA-3A, 3B, 3C)

The rhesus LCV latency-associated genes, EBNA-3A, 3B and 3C, show loose homology to human EBV EBNA-3A, 3B and 3C genes. Again, despite the limited conservation in sequence among these proteins, the interaction with RBP-Jk has been retained (Dalbies-Tran *et al.*, 2001; Zhao *et al.*, 2003; Jiang *et al.*, 2000). Further, the transactivation function of EBNA-3C has also been conserved between the rhesus, baboon and human viral proteins, and all three proteins can interact with the Spi proteins (Zhao *et al.*, 2003). Both non-human primate 3C proteins can support transcriptional activation mediated by the Spi proteins in the presence of EBNA-2 (Zhao *et al.*, 2003). Despite these similarities, gene replacement studies demonstrated that the rhesus LCV EBNA-3 genes were unable to functionally substitute for the EBV EBNA-3 genes in the EBV genome, for immortalization of human B-cells (Jiang *et al.*, 2000). However, the ability of this recombinant virus to immortalize rhesus B cells was not tested.

EBV latent membrane protein (LMP-1)

The EBV-encoded latent membrane protein 1 (LMP1) structurally and functionally resembles a constitutively active TNF family receptor. LMP1 aggregates in the plasma membrane and can activate a multitude of signaling pathways in the cell resulting in cell proliferation and transformation. Sequence analysis of the LMP-1 proteins from baboons (*Cercopithicine herpesvirus 12* or herpesvirus papio) and rhesus monkeys (*Cercopithicine herpesvirus 15*) showed that although the transmembrane domains of these proteins are conserved with that of EBV LMP-1, there is great divergence within the carboxy-terminal cytoplasmic domains of these proteins (Franken *et al.*, 1996). The C-terminal domain of EBV LMP1 has been shown to be essential for B-cell immortalization and interaction with members of the tumor necrosis factor receptor family. A comparative study of the simian LMP-1 proteins with EBV LMP-1 showed that the simian LCV LMP-1 proteins could induce NF-kB activity, bind tumor necrosis factor associated factor −3 (TRAF3) and induce ICAM1 expression (Franken *et al.*, 1996). This is likely through the multiple TRAF3 binding sites (PXQXT/S) that are contained within the simian LCV LMP1 C-terminal domain (Franken *et al.*, 1996). A similar study performed with an LCV LMP1 protein from cynomolgus monkeys (*Macaca fascicularis*) shows that this simian LMP1 protein also contains two PXQXT/S motifs and retains its ability to activate the NF-kB pathway (Faucher *et al.*, 2002). It has recently been reported that the transmembrane domain of EBV LMP1, specifically FWLY (amino acids 38–41), is critical for signal transduction which includes raft localization of the viral protein, TRAF3 interaction and NF-kB activation (Yasui *et al.*, 2004). Although the identical FWLY motif is not present in either the baboon or rhesus LCV LMP-1 proteins, the simian LMP-1 viral proteins may contain motifs that are functionally similar to FWLY, since they can activate NF-kB. Further, Eliopoulos and Young (1998) have reported that LMP1 homologues from the baboon and rhesus EBV are also capable of activating the c-Jun N-terminal kinase (JNK) pathway (Eliopoulos and Young, 1998). Thus, activation of the NF-kB and JNK pathways by the primate LMP1 proteins is an important function that has been conserved throughout evolution.

EBV latent membrane protein-2 (LMP-2)

The LMP2A homologues in the baboon and rhesus LCV genomes show homology to EBV LMP2 and contain an immunoreceptor tyrosine based activation motif (ITAM) (Franken *et al.*, 1996; Rivailler *et al.*, 1999). All three primate LCV LMP2A proteins contain 12 transmembrane domains, and although the amino acids in the cytoplasmic domain are quite different, the ITAM and proline-rich domains are well conserved. These conserved motifs/domains in EBV LMP2A have been shown to be required for interaction with protein tyrosine kinases (Portis *et al.*, 2002) and are essential for LMP2A function. Moreover, the rhesus LCV LMP2B gene is located at an equivalent genomic position as EBV LMP2B, and the EBNA-2 responsiveness and the bidirectional nature of the LMP1-LMP2B promoter is conserved between the rhesus and human lymphocryptoviruses (Rivailler *et al.*, 1999).

Rhesus LCV as an animal model system for EBV

Historically, several investigators attempted and failed to infect Old World primates such as baboons and rhesus macaques with human EBV (Frank *et al.*, 1976; Gerber *et al.*, 1969; Levine *et al.*, 1980). This failure to establish EBV infection in Old World primates may be due to the route of inoculation used in these studies, pre-existing antibody cross-reactivity due to natural LCV infection in the primates, or the utilization of non-transforming deletion mutants of EBV, namely P3HR1 (Levine *et al.*, 1980). It is also possible that there is a species restriction imposed on EBV infection of non-human primates, since LCVs tend to be competent for immortalization of B-cells from the same or closely related species, but immortalization potential varies for B-cells from a more divergent species. For example, Moghaddam *et al.* (1998) found that rhesus LCV did not immortalize human B cells, and human EBV could not immortalize rhesus monkey B cells (Moghaddam *et al.*, 1998). Further, since the rhesus LCV was able to infect human B cells, the species restriction was after virus penetration (Moghaddam *et al.*, 1998). Rhesus and baboon LCVs have been reported to be incapable of immortalizing human B-cells (Falk *et al.*, 1977), although other reports suggest that this is possible at a much lower frequency (Rabin *et al.*, 1977a; Gerber *et al.*, 1977). In a similar manner, EBV has been shown to immortalize B cells from chimpanzees, which are more closely related to humans, and chimpanzee LCV can immortalize human B-cells (Gerber et al., 1977; Ishida and Yamamoto, 1987). Likewise, baboon LCV can immortalize B-cells from gibbons, rhesus and cynomolgus macaques (Gerber et al., 1977).

In light of the fact that human EBV fails to establish long-term infection in rhesus macaques, rhesus LCV serves as a valuable animal model to study EBV pathogenesis since successful experimental infection of naïve rhesus macaques with rhesus LCV has been previously reported (Moghaddam et al., 1997). Naïve rhesus macaques were orally infected with rhesus LCV and this resulted in an acute and persistent LCV infection, which closely resembled that seen with primary EBV infection of humans. Initial viral load peaked between 4 to 21 days and declined to almost undetectable levels over a 3-month period (Rao et al., 2000). Immune activation was evidenced three days after oral inoculation by the presence of T-cells expressing IL-2, IL-10 and gamma interferon. Activated CTL activity against LCV infected cells was observed in the first few weeks post-infection similar to what has been described for infectious mononucleosis patients in the human population (Wang, 2001). In addition, antibody responses against EBNA-2 and viral capsid antigens develop within 2 weeks post-inoculation (Moghaddam et al., 1997; Mohle et al., 1997; Rao et al., 2000). Persistent viral infection could be detected in the oropharynx of infected animals by PCR (Cho et al., 1999; Moghaddam et al., 1997; Mohle et al., 1997; Rao et al., 2000) and in B-cells, and a percentage of these infected B cells were immortalized and could be grown in tissue culture (Moghaddam et al., 1997; Mohle et al., 1997). Persistent infection as measured by RT-PCR of the rhesus LCV EBER genes in peripheral blood mononuclear cells (PBMCs) was detected three years post-infection (Rao et al., 2000). Thus, clinically speaking, primary, acute and persistent infection of macaques with rhesus LCV appears to closely mimic EBV infection of humans, further validating the use of rhesus LCV as an animal model system to study EBV pathogenesis.

The potential to use the rhesus LCV animal model system to study EBV-associated tumorigenesis is the subject of current and future investigation. Rivailler et al. reported that four immunosuppressed macaques infected orally with LCV failed to debelop lymphoproliferative disease. However, intravenous inoculation of autologous LCV immortalized B cells in four SHIV89.6P-infected animals resulted in one severely immunosuppressed animal developing an aggressive monoclonal LCV-positive lymphoma (Rivailler et al., 2004). Feichtinger et al. (1992a,b) have shown that when cynomolgus monkeys naturally infected with LCV were infected with simian immunodeficiency virus (SIV), malignant B cell lymphomas containing DNA which cross-hybridized with human EBV were detected. In another study, squamous epithelial proliferative lesions in SIV-infected rhesus monkeys were also shown to contain EBV-like sequences by immunohistochemistry and in situ hybridization (Baskin et al., 1995). A study on SIV-infected monkeys at the Tulane Primate Center showed that SIV-infected macaques have a higher rhesus LCV load in PBMCs than uninfected animals, but that the virus load varies widely among animals during disease progression (Habis et al., 2000).

The current availability of the genomic sequence of rhesus LCV will facilitate the construction of recombinant LCVs that can be tested in rhesus macaques. Such studies will provide an understanding of the contribution of individual genes to the life cycle of these lymphocryptoviruses and serve to verify rhesus LCV as a tractable system to model EBV pathogenesis.

Other lymphocryptoviruses in Old World primates

A recent study by Ehlers et al. (2003) has identified the presence of novel lymphocryptoviruses in several species including baboons, chimpanzees, and gorillas (Table 61.1). Interestingly, this group found evidence for a second lymphocryptovirus in gorillas, baboons, mandrills and Japanese macaques (Fig. 61.2). Together these data raise the possibility that another yet to be discovered human lymphocryptovirus, different from the type 1 and 2 human EBV strains, may exist in the human population. This theme will be revisited when discussing the family of primate rhadinoviruses.

Lymphocryptoviruses of New World monkeys

Early serological studies had indicated that there was no evidence for the presence of lymphocryptoviruses in New World primates since there was no antibody cross-reactivity with human EBV from sera of New World monkeys (Frank et al., 1976). However, Ramer et al. (2000) recently reported the identification of novel viral DNA sequences from common marmoset monkeys (*Callithrix jaccus*) afflicted with spontaneous B-cell lymphomas. These sequences were most closely related to EBV and suggested the presence of a novel lymphocryptovirus in New World primates. Subsequently, the first EBV-related herpesvirus in New World primates was cloned from common marmoset monkeys (Cho et al., 2001; Jenson et al., 2002). This virus was formally named Callitrichine herpesvirus

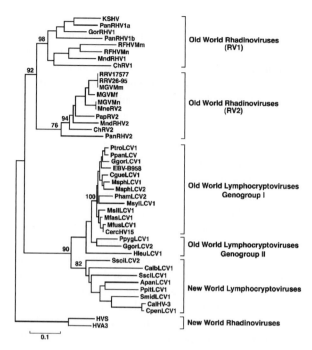

Fig. 61.2. Phylogenetic analysis of the gammaherpesviruses. Forty-four DNA polymerase nucleotide sequences (400bp) were aligned using the Clustal W matrix and edited in GeneDoc (v.2.6) to remove gaps. The tree was rooted using the New World Rhadinoviruses, HVS and HVA3 as the Outgroup. The Neighbor-Joining tree was constructed in Mega 2.1 from pairwise sequence distances calculated using the Kimura 2-parameter (K80) method. Bootstrap values were determined by 100 replica samplings. Sequences included in the phylogenetic analysis: KSHV (U75698); PanRHV1a (*Pan troglodytes*, AF250879); GorRHV1 (*Gorilla gorilla*, AF250886); PanRHV1b (*Pan troglodytes*, AF250882); RFHVMm (*Macaca mulatta*, AF005479); MndRHV1 (*Mandrillus sphinx*, AF282943); ChRV1 (*Chlorocebus aethiops*, AJ251573); RRV17577 (*Macaca mulatta*, AF083501); RRV26-95 (AF029302); MGVMm (*Macaca mulatta*, AF159033); MGVMf (*Macaca fascicularis*, AF159032); MGVMn (*Macaca nemestrina*, AF159031); MneRV2 (*Macaca nemestrina*, AF204167); PapRV2 (*Papio anubis*, AY270026); MndRHV2 (*Mandrillus sphinx*, AF282939); ChRV2 (*Chlorocebus aethiops*, AJ251574); PanRHV2 (*Pan troglodytes*, AF346490); PtroLCV1 (*Pan troglodytes*, AF534226); PpanLCV1 (*Pan paniscus*, AF534220); GgorLCV1 (*Gorilla gorilla*, AF534225); EBV-B95.8 (V01555); CgueLCV1 (*Colobus guereza*, AF534219); MsphLCV1 (*Mandrillus sphinx*, AF534227); MsphLCV2 (*Mandrillus sphinx*, AY174066); PhamLCV2 (*Papio hamadryas*, AF534229); MsylLCV1 (*Macaca sylvanus*, AY172956); MsilLCV1 (*Macaca silenus*, AF534222); MfasLCV1 (*Macaca fascicularis*, AF534221); MfusLCV1 (*Macaca fuscata*, AF534224); CercHV-15 (*Cercopithicine*, AY037858); PpygLCV1 (*Pongo pygamaeus*, AY129398); GgorLCV2 (*Gorilla gorilla*, AY129395); HleuLCV1 (*Hylobates leucogenys*, AY174068); SsciLCV2 (*Saimiri sciureus*, AY139024); CalbLCV1 (*Cebus albifrons*, AY139027); SsciLCV1 (*Saimiri sciureus*, AY172953); ApanLCV1

3 or CalHV3. A closely related virus to CalHV3 was also seen in squirrel monkeys (*Saimiri scireus*) (Cho et al., 2001). Sequencing of the CalHV3 or marmoset LCV DNA revealed that the genomic organization was similar to that of EBV (Rivailler et al., 2002a). Sequence analysis of the 73 open-reading frames (ORFs) revealed that although many genes showed high homology to genes in EBV, there were some striking differences between the two genomes as well.

The marmoset LCV (CalHV3) genome

The marmoset LCV genome is composed of approximately 160 000 nucleotides. Of the 73 ORFs found in the marmoset LCV genome, 59 of these share homology to genes found in all herpesviruses. Six additional genes encoded by ORFs 1,6,39,43,44 and 45 show homology to EBV BALF1, BILF1, EBNA-1, BZLF1, BZLF2 and gp350, respectively (Rivailler et al., 2002a). The eight other marmoset ORFs show no sequence relatedness to either cellular or viral genes and were named C0 through C7 (Table 61.3). Based on their genomic position only, C0, C1,C2, C3,C4, C5 and C7 are in the equivalent genomic locations as EBV EBNA-LP, LMP1, BILF-2, EBNA-3, BHLF1, EBNA-2 and LMP2, respectively. In addition to encoding unique genes, there are also eleven EBV genes that are not present in marmoset LCV. These include the EBERs, BARF0, BCRF1, BARF1, and BDLF3 (Rivailler et al., 2002a).

CalHV3 C1

C1 is a positional homologue of EBV LMP1. Although it shares no homology with LMP1 at the amino acid level and does not contain the PXQXT/S motifs that are contained in the C-terminus of the rhesus LCV and human EBV, C1 is a functional homologue of LMP1. It can transform rodent fibroblasts in vitro and can also induce NF-kB activity to similar levels as LMP1. Hence, C1 can interact with the TRAFs through an alternative TRAF binding motif (Wang et al., 2001).

CalHV3 ORF39 (EBNA-1)

The CalHV3 EBNA-1 protein shows homology to EBV EBNA-1 in the C-terminal domain and the GR-rich

---

Fig. 61.2. (*cont.*) (*Ateles paniscus*, AY139028); PpitLCV1 (*Pithecia pithecia*, AY139025); SmidLCV1 (AY166693); CalHV-3 (*Cercopithicine*, AY049065); CpenLCV1 (*Callithrix penicillata*, AY139026); HVS (*Saimiri*, M31122); HVA3 (*Ateline*, AF083424). We thank R.K. Bagni and D. Whitby for help with the construction of the phylogenetic tree.

domains, which in EBV EBNA-1, are required for episomal maintenance (Wang et al., 2001). However, the CalHV3 EBNA-1 homolog does not contain the Gly-Ala repeat region, which has previously been shown to be involved in immune-modulation (Levitskaya et al., 1995).

CalHV3 C5

CalHV3 C5 is a positional homologue of EBNA-2 and shares no relatedness at the amino acid level. However like EBV EBNA-2, the C5 protein has a cluster of C-terminal acidic residues that may be important for transcriptional transactivation (Rivailler et al., 2002a). Unlike the EBV and rhesus LCV EBNA-2, C5 is missing the polyproline repeat, which is present in EBV EBNA-2 (Yalamanchili et al., 1996).

CalHV3 C7

C7 is a positional homologue of EBV LMP2. Similar to LMP2, it contains 12 transmembrane domains but a shorter N-terminus and a longer C-terminus (Rivailler et al., 2002a). The latter contains five tyrosine residues, three of which may serve as part of Src-homology-2 (SH2) binding motifs (Rivailler et al., 2002a).

New World primates as an animal model system for EBV

Historically, an extensive body of work has been published on using New World primates as an animal model system to study EBV (Shope et al., 1973; Miller et al., 1972, 1973). EBV readily infects and immortalizes B-cells from common marmosets (Desgranges et al., 1976; Rabin et al., 1977b). In fact one of the most widely used EBV-infected cell lines, B95-8, is a marmoset B-cell line infected with human EBV (Miller et al., 1972). New World monkey species, including the cotton-top tamarin (*Sanguinus oedipus*), and owl monkey (*Aotus trivirgatus*) develop B-cell lymphomas upon infection with EBV (Cleary et al., 1985; Johnson et al., 1983; Epstein et al., 1973a,b; Miller et al., 1977; Werner et al., 1975). Some publications suggest that common marmosets (*Callithrix jacchus*) also develop lymphoproliferative disease when infected with EBV DNA, and that lymphosarcomas in these animals contain EBV DNA (Falk et al., 1976). Conversely, others have reported no substantial evidence of lymphoproliferative disease or lymphoma in EBV-infected common marmosets (de-The et al., 1980; Ablashi et al., 1978). Infection of common marmosets is thought to serve as a model for primary and persistent EBV infection (Wedderburn et al., 1984).

Inconsistency in the induction of tumors by EBV in common marmosets, suggests that the cotton top tamarin is a more susceptible animal model for EBV oncogenesis. However, the cotton top tamarin was declared endangered in 1973 following the exportation of twenty to forty thousand tamarins from Colombia to the United States for use in biomedical research related to colonic adenocarcinoma (Hernandez-Camacho, 1976; Clapp et al., 1982). Hence, their potential value as an animal model for EBV pathogenesis is limited due to their unavailability as well as the expense of the monkeys.

A comprehensive study on lymphocryptoviruses (LCV) that infect New and Old World primates has identified the presence of many lymphocryptoviruses from a multitude of primates (Ehlers et al., 2003; de Thoisy et al., 2003) (Table 61.1). These studies were done using degenerate PCR and revealed that some New and Old World monkeys are infected with two different lymphocryptoviruses, denoted as LCV1 and LCV2 (Table 61.1). In each primate species examined, one LCV virus was more closely related to human EBV and grouped in the same genogroup as EBV (Fig. 61.2), while the viruses that were less closely related to EBV all grouped together in a second lymphocryptovirus genogroup (Ehlers et al., 2003) (Fig. 61.2).

Evolution of New and Old World rhadinoviruses

The Old World rhadinoviruses like RRV, RFHV and KSHV share more sequence relatedness amongst each other than with the New World rhadinovirus, HVS (see chapter on *Herpesvirus saimiri*), exemplifying the split of the platyrrhines and catarrhines 35 million years ago. Similar to the situation for the divergence of the lymphocryptoviruses, the rhadinoviral genomes of Old and New World primates both retain key viral genes such as Orf73 or Latency associated nuclear antigen (LANA), which is required for episomal maintenance of the viral genome, and Orf50/Rta which is required for viral replication. However, other proteins like viral interleukin 6 (vIL-6), macrophage inflammatory proteins (MIPs I, II and III), and the viral interferon regulatory factors (vIRFs) are only encoded by the Old World rhadinoviral genomes, RRV and KSHV, but are not present in the HVS genome, suggesting that these genes are more recent acquisitions in the rhadinovirus family, occurring after the split of the Old and New World primates. These proteins likely play key roles in the escape from immune surveillance and survival of the rhadinoviruses in their host species, and thus have been retained by KSHV, the most recent addition to the rhadinovirus evolutionary tree.

Rhadinoviruses of Old World primates

A wide body of literature supports the prevailing view that rhadinoviruses can be found throughout the animal kingdom in both Old and New World primates (Fig. 61.1). Rhadinoviruses that infect New World monkeys include herpesvirus saimiri (HVS) whose natural host is the squirrel monkey and herpesvirus ateles (HVA), which infects spider monkeys (Table 61.1) (Melendez et al., 1969, 1972). Rhadinoviruses that infect Old World monkeys include rhesus monkey rhadinovirus (RRV) and retroperitoneal fibromatosis herpesvirus (RFHV) (Rose et al., 1997; Desrosiers et al., 1997).

Phylogenetic analysis

Among Old World primates, rhesus monkey rhadinovirus (RRV) and closely related viruses like RFHV, are gamma-2 herpesviruses of the macaque genus (Rose et al., 1997; Desrosiers et al., 1997). The similarity between the genomes of RRV and KSHV is high and all of the open reading frames (ORFs) in RRV have at least one homologue in KSHV (Alexander et al., 2000; Searles et al., 1999). RRV replicates lytically in cell culture and multiple isolates have been obtained independently by different laboratories (Desrosiers et al., 1997; Searles et al., 1999). The genomes of these isolates have been fully sequenced (Alexander et al., 2000; Searles et al., 1999). Rhadinoviruses closely related to RRV have been cultured from other macaque species, specifically *Macaca nemestrina* and *Macaca fascicularis* (Auerbach et al., 2000; Mansfield et al., 1999).

Short stretches of related but phylogenetically distinct sequences have also been amplified from *Macaca mulatta* and *Macaca nemestrina* (Bosch et al., 1999; Strand et al., 2000; Schultz et al., 2000). The putative viruses represented by these sequences, named retroperitoneal fibromatosis herpesvirus *macaca mulatta* and *macaca nemestrina* (RFHVMm and RFHVMn, respectively), have been difficult to culture and lack information on genomic organization and sequence relatedness of the complete viral genome. Short stretches of related sequence have also been amplified from African green monkeys (*Chlorocebus aethiops*). In one particular study on rates of infection, 6 of 68 monkeys were found to be infected with *Chlorocebus aethiops* rhadinovirus 1 (ChRV1) while 22 of 68 monkeys were positive for *Chlorocebus aethiops* rhadinovirus 2 (ChRV2) (Greensill et al., 2000b). Thus, the putative viruses represented by these sequences fall into two distinct phylogenetic groupings RV1 and RV2 (Fig. 61.2), neither of which have yet been successfully cultured in vitro (Greensill et al., 2000b). In these studies, PCR products of the DNA polymerase genes from ChRV1, ChRV2, RFHVMm, and RFHVMn were amplified (Rose et al., 1997; Bosch et al., 1999; Strand et al., 2000; Schultz et al., 2000).

The above phylogenetic studies suggested the presence of at least two distinct lineages of KSHV-like rhadinoviruses in primates. One lineage contains KSHV, RFHVMm, RFHVMn, and ChRV1, and the other contains RRV, ChRV2 and *Macaca nemestrina* rhadinovirus type 2 (MneRV2). Short stretches of rhadinovirus sequences have since been amplified from chimpanzees, gorillas and mandrills (Lacoste et al., 2000a,b; 2001; Greensill et al., 2002a). Similar to the two distinct rhadinoviruses found in rhesus macaques and African green monkeys, both mandrills and chimpanzees also contain two gamma-2 herpesviruses, MndRHV1 and MndRHV2 for mandrills and PtRV-1 or PanRHV1a/1b and PanRHV2 for chimpanzees (Greensill et al., 2000a; Lacoste et al., 2000a,b) (Table 61.1, Fig. 61.2).

Retroperitoneal fibromatosis herpesviruses: RFHVMm and RFHVMn

Sequence from the RFHVMm and RFHVMn viruses were amplified from macaques (*Macaca mulatta* and *Macaca nemestrina*) affected with retroperitoneal fibromatosis (RF) (Rose et al., 1997). RF is a vascular fibroproliferative disease that resembles Kaposi's sarcoma (KS) morphologically and histologically (Rose et al., 1997). Nine of 40 *Macaca nemestrina* monkeys with retroperitoneal fibromatosis were positive for RFHvMn by PCR, while two out of two *Macaca mulatta* monkeys with RF were positive for RFHvMm. Two of two unaffected *Macaca nemestrina* monkeys were negative for RFHvMn by PCR (Rose et al., 1997). As described above, phylogenetic analysis demonstrated that these two viruses clustered with KSHV in the RV1 genogroup, while RRV and MneRV2 cluster in a RV2 genogroup. This classification was originally based on the sequence of the viral DNA polymerase gene. To date, only a 7.7 kb fragment of the RFHVMm genomic sequence has been cloned (Rose et al., 2003). This segment of the viral genome codes for glycoprotein B (gB), ORF 9, ORF10, vIL6, vDHFR, K3 and viral thymidylate synthase (TS). These genes are organized in a similar linear fashion as the corresponding homologs in KSHV. However, RFHVMm and RFHVMn are missing ORF11. Analysis of the amino acid similarity between the RFHVMm/RFHVMn and KSHV proteins indicated that RFHVMm and RFHVMn are most closely related to KSHV than any other virus, thus supporting their grouping in the RV1 lineage (Rose et al., 2003). Further comparisons and evolutionary

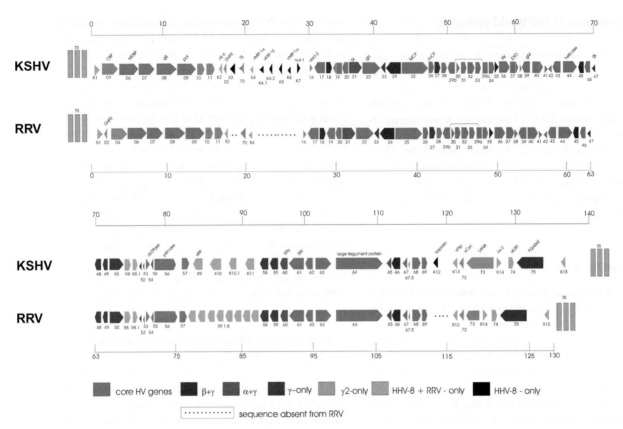

Fig. 61.3. Alignment of the KSHV and RRV genomes. The different colors signify ORFs contained in KSHV and RRV 26–95 that are conserved in the indicated herpesvirus subfamilies or subgroups. The square side of the symbol signifies the 5′ end and the pointed side of the symbol signifies the 3′ end of the depicted ORFs. The ORFs are not drawn to scale. (Taken from Alexander et al., 2000, with permission from the *Journal of Virology*.) (See color plate section.)

analyses await sequencing of the complete RFHVMm and RFHVMn genomes. The RFHVs are currently being amplified from paraffin-embedded or frozen retroperitoneal fibromatosis tumor samples, and are not widely prevalent in the macaque populations housed in most US primate centers.

Rhesus monkey rhadinovirus (RRV)

Greater than 90% of adult macaques at the New England Regional Primate Center (NERPRC) are seropositive for RRV (Mansfield *et al.*, 1999; Desrosiers *et al.*, 1997). A similar frequency of infected macaques was also found at the Oregon Regional Primate Research Center (Wong *et al.*, 1999). Thus, RRV appears to be a natural infectious agent of macaques. However, newborn macaques can be raised free of RRV by hand-rearing (Mansfield *et al.*, 1999). RRV isolated from one species can readily infect macaques of another species upon experimental inoculation (Mansfield *et al.*, 1999). Although gB sequences of RRV isolates from three different macaque species, *Macaca mulatta*, *Macaca nemestrina* and *Macaca fascicularis* were all closely related, they clustered according to species of origin (Auerbach *et al.*, 2000). A limited study of R1 sequences of RRV from three different species did not reveal a clustering according to species of origin (Damania *et al.*, 1999).

Genomic organization of RRV

Two complete RRV genomes have been sequenced at the Oregon Regional Primate Research Center (ORPRC) and the NERPRC. RRV strain 26–95 from NERPRC and RRV strain 17577 from ORPRC are very similar both in sequence

Table 61.4. A comparison of proteins encoded by the human and macaque rhadinoviruses

RRV (strain 26–95)	% aa similarity to KSHV	Function	Positional homologue in KSHV
R1	33.0%	Unique gene (Transforming gene)	K1
R2/ vIL-6	30.6%	IL-6 homologue	vIL-6
R4/vMIP	42.4%	MIP homologue	vMIP I,II,III
Orf16	58.0%	Bcl-2 homologue	vBcl-2
Orf50/Rta	55.0%	Transcription factor	Orf50/Rta
R8	53.0%	Replication protein	K8/bZip
R8.1	43.0%	Glycoprotein	K8.1
R9.1	60.6%	IRF homologue	vIRF
R13	40.1%	FLIP homologue	vFLIP/Orf71
Orf72	50.2%	Cyclin homologue	vCyclin/Orf72
Orf73	24.9%	Episome maintenance	LANA/Orf73
Orf74	54.7%	G-protein coupled receptor	vGPCR/Orf74
R14	37.6%	N-CAM Ox-2 homologue	K14

and genomic organization (Searles et al., 1999; Alexander et al., 2000). Only four of the 84 ORFs exhibited less than 95% sequence identity at the amino acid level (Alexander, 2000). The primary sequence of the long unique region (LUR) of RRV2695 consists of 130 733 base pairs that contain 84 open reading frames (Fig. 61.3). The overall organization of the RRV genome was found to be very similar to that of human KSHV (Alexander et al., 2000). BLAST search analysis revealed that in almost all cases, RRV coding sequences have greater degrees of similarity to corresponding KSHV sequences than to any other herpesvirus (Table 61.4). All of the ORFs present in KSHV have at least one homologue in RRV except KSHV K3 and K5, K7 (nut-1), and K12 (Kaposin). RRV contains one macrophage inflammatory gene (MIP-1) and eight interferon regulatory factor (vIRF) homologues compared to three MIP-1/vCCLs and four vIRF genes in KSHV. All homologues are correspondingly located in KSHV and RRV with the exception of DHFR. The location of the DHFR gene in KSHV is different from that in RRV and HVS, suggesting that KSHV may have rearranged or reacquired the DHFR gene during the course of evolution from an Old World rhadinovirus to the human rhadinovirus or that RRV acquired the DHFR gene after divergence from KSHV (Fig. 61.3). Only four of the corresponding ORFs between RRV strain 26–95 and RRV strain 17577 exhibit less than 95% sequence identity: these include the glycoproteins H and L genes, uracil DNA glycosidase, and a tegument protein (ORF 67). Analysis of the two genomes indicate that RRV26–95 and RRV17577 are clearly independent isolates of the same virus species and both are closely related in structural organization and overall sequence to KSHV (Searles et al., 1999; Alexander et al., 2000). In addition to homology between the KSHV and RRV ORFs, there is also similarity with respect to the splicing patterns of viral genes. For example, the RRV Orf50, R8 and R8.1 polycistronic transcript is spliced in the same manner as the transcript encoding the corresponding genes in KSHV, (DeWire et al., 2002; Lin et al., 2002) and the LANA, vCyclin, vFLIP transcripts are likewise spliced in a similar fashion (DeWire et al., 2002).

RRV R1

The first open reading frame of RRV encodes for a gene named R1, which is located at an equivalent position in the genome as the K1 gene of KSHV (Damania et al., 1999). Analogous to KSHV K1, R1 is also a transforming gene (Damania et al., 1999). R1 can transform rodent fibroblasts and functionally substitute for STP-C of HVS in immortalizing common marmoset PBMCs to IL-2 independent growth in vitro (Damania et al., 1999). Injection of R1-expressing rodent fibroblasts into nude mice resulted in the formation of multifocal and disseminated tumors in these mice (Damania et al., 1999). Although R1 shows limited sequence homology to K1, the amino-terminal extracellular domains of both K1 and R1 closely resemble members of the immunoglobulin receptor superfamily and exhibit 40% similarity to each other at the amino acid level (Damania et al., 1999; Lee et al., 1998). However, the cytoplasmic tail of R1 is significantly longer than that of K1 and contains several potential SH2 binding motifs, which function as ITAMs to elicit B-cell activation (Damania et al., 2000).

RRV vIL6

KSHV, RRV and RFHV are the only herpesviruses that encode for a viral interleukin 6 homologue (vIL6). RRV vIL-6 has been shown to functionally stimulate the IL-6 receptor/gp130 pathway (Kaleeba *et al.*, 1999). The IL-6R-binding residues in the KSHV and RRV vIL-6 proteins are conserved suggesting that RRV vIL-6 may also bind gp130 in the absence of IL-6R, similar to KSHV vIL-6 (Kaleeba *et al.*, 1999).

RRV vGPCR

KSHV and RRV contain genes for a viral G-protein coupled receptors (vGPCR) that shows homology to the cellular GPCR, IL-8 receptor. Like KSHV vGPCR (for review see Moore and Chang, 2003), RRV vGPCR can transform NIH3T3 fibroblasts in vitro, and stimulate an increased secretion of vascular endothelial growth factor from these cells. RRV vGPCR has been shown to activate the ERK1/2 (p44/42) mitogen-activated protein kinase signaling pathway (Estep *et al.*, 2003). These results suggest that RRV vGPCR, like KSHV vGPCR, may play a role in viral pathogenesis in vivo. The RRV vGPCR transcript is bicistronically expressed with RRV R 15 (Pratt *et al.*, 2005). RRV R15 encodes a viral CD200 protein which shares homology with human and KSHV CD200 proteins (Langlais *et al.*, 2006).

RRV Orf50/Rta and RRV R8

The KSHV Orf50/Rta transactivator is encoded by a polycistronic transcript, which also contains the multiply spliced KSHV K8 and K8.1 genes. Analogous to the situation with KSHV, the homologous genes in RRV, Orf50/Rta, R8 and R8.1, respectively, are also encoded by a polycistronic, spliced transcript (DeWire *et al.*, 2002; Lin *et al.*, 2002). The KSHV Orf50 mRNA has a small 5′ exon, followed by a larger second exon encoding the remainder of the Orf50 sequence (Zhu *et al.*, 1999). Similarly in RRV, the Orf50 mRNA has a small upstream exon followed by a larger second exon (DeWire *et al.*, 2002; Lin *et al.*, 2002). In contrast, the gamma-1 herpesvirus, EBV, encodes an Orf50 homolog, BRLF1, whose cDNA is identical to the genomic ORF (Manet *et al.*, 1989). The RRV Orf50 protein is localized to the nucleus and functions as a transcriptional activator (DeWire *et al.*, 2002). A striking observation is that the KSHV Orf50 protein can activate certain RRV promoters, while the RRV Orf50 protein can also activate a subset of KSHV promoters, suggesting that there is a conservation in protein function of the Orf50/Rta transactivators of these rhadinoviruses (DeWire *et al.*, 2002; Damania, 2004).

Unrecognizable from the RRV genomic sequence alone, two other spliced genes of RRV include the R8 and R8.1 genes. The R8 protein is localized in the nucleus and shows 39% identity and 53% similarity at the amino acid level to the K8/bZip protein of KSHV. The R8.1 protein is localized in the cytoplasm and shows 26% identity and 43 % similarity at the amino acid level. The R8.1 protein has two potential glycosylation sites (NXS/T) (DeWire *et al.*, 2002).

RRV LANA

RRV also encodes a latency-associated nuclear antigen (R-LANA). Similar to KSHV LANA, R-LANA exhibits a nuclear speckled localization and possesses the ability to homodimerize. R-LANA can inhibit viral lytic replication by repressing the transactivation function of RRV Orf50/Rta. The mechanism for this repression involves the recruitment of histone deacetylase complexes since R-LANA's ability to repress RRV Orf50 transactivation was reversed by the addition of the HDAC inhibitor trichostatin A (TSA) and TSA could significantly reactivate RRV from latently infected cells (Dewire and Damania, 2005).

RRV transcription program

The overall transcription profile of the RRV lytic cycle is very similar to that of KSHV. The immediate early genes expressed during the RRV lifecycle are Orf50 and Orf57, similar to the case seen with KSHV reactivation. Consistent with the KSHV transcriptome, early genes transcribed by RRV include vIL6, DNA polymerase, and R1 (DeWire *et al.*, 2002; Dittmer *et al.*, 2005). An exception to this pattern is the cluster of genes classically defined as latent in KSHV, i.e., Orf73 (LANA), vCyclin, and vFLIP, which are expressed as delayed early genes during the RRV lytic cycle (DeWire *et al.*, 2002). Late transcripts include those of RRV vIRF-1, Orf62, Orf65, and gB genes (DeWire *et al.*, 2002; Dittmer *et al.*, 2005).

RRV capsid structure

As with other herpesviruses, RRV lytic infection of rhesus fibroblasts leads to the synthesis of three distinct intranuclear capsid species. A and B capsids do not contain viral genomes, while C capsids do contain the viral genome at their center and are considered infectious. There are multiple similarities in capsid structure and assembly between KSHV and RRV. Both viruses make all three types of intranuclear capsids (A, B and C) during lytic infection, and the three RRV capsid species are similar in structure to KSHV as measured by transmission electron microscopy (TEM) (O'Connor *et al.*, 2003). In addition, both the RRV and KSHV virions assemble with similar slow kinetics and the capsids possess a highly conserved protein composition (O'Connor *et al.*, 2003). Both the RRV and KSHV capsid proteins include the major capsid protein (MCP) encoded by ORF25, components of the triplex, TRI-1 and TRI-2, encoded by RRV ORFs 62 and 26 respectively, RRV SCIP encoded by ORF65, and RRV SCAF encoded by ORF 17.5 (O'Connor et al., 2003). All five RRV capsid proteins demonstrate similarity to their KSHV homologues at the amino acid level (O'Connor et al., 2003; Alexander et al., 2000; Searles et al., 1999). However, one difference between these viruses is the efficiency of capsid assembly. As opposed to the inefficiency of KSHV maturation following reactivation from latently infected B-cell lines (Nealon et al., 2001), de novo RRV infection results in the release of much higher levels of infectious virions with genome-containing C capsids at their center and a lower amount of the incomplete A and B capsids which do not contain viral genomes (O'Connor et al., 2003). This discrepancy may explain the reason why RRV can be grown to high titers ($\sim 10^6$ pfu/ml) (DeWire et al., 2003) in vitro relative to KSHV, since only virions containing intact viral genomes (i.e. C capsids) are infectious (O'Connor et al., 2003). Three-dimensional structure comparisons of the RRV capsid structure by electron cryomicroscopy have shown that the A capsid is empty and its penton channels are open, the B-capsid contains a scaffolding core and its penton channels are closed, and the C-capsid contains a DNA genome closely packed as regularly spaced density shells (25 Å apart), and its penton channels are open (Yu et al., 2003). The RRV A capsid reconstruction was achieved at 15-Å resolution (Fig. 61.4), which is the best, achieved for any gammaherpesvirus to date. The best resolution for the KSHV capsid was achieved at 24-Å and both capsids appeared almost identical (Yu et al., 2003; Wu et al., 2000). Further, although the RRV capsid showed overall structural similarities to alpha and betaherpesvirus capsids, there were prominent differences in the Ta triplex and SCIP structures suggesting that SCIP and triplex, together with tegument and envelope proteins, confer structural, and potentially functional, specificity to alpha-, beta- and gamma-herpesviruses (Yu et al., 2003) (Fig. 61.4). Thus, this study validates the use of RRV as a model system for the study of KSHV and other gammaherpesviruses, since the latter appear significantly different from the alpha and beta herpesviruses, despite the fact that the individual structural proteins of all three groups of herpesviruses share a high degree of homology.

RRV pathogenesis

Wong et al. (1999) at the ORPRC experimentally inoculated rhesus macaques with RRV (strain 17577) with and without SIVmac239 co-infection to determine whether RRV played a role in the development of lymphoproliferative disease. In contrast to two control animals inoculated with SIV-

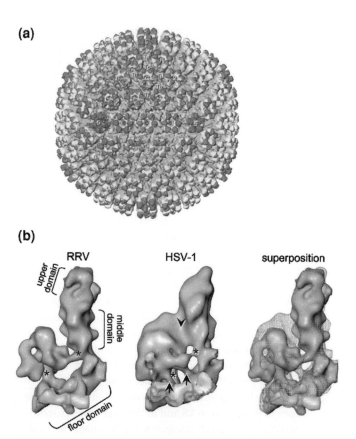

Fig. 61.4. Structural similarity between the KSHV and RRV capsids. (a) The RRV A capsid structure at 15 Angstrom resolution. (b) Structural difference between the gammaherpesvirus RRV and alphaherpsvirus HSV-1 capsids. The figure represents one penton sub-unit and one triplex (Ta) that was computationally extracted from the RRV A capsid taken at 15 Angstroms shown in panel A, and an HSV-1 capsid map filtered to the same resolution. The RRV and HSV-1 Ta triplex interacts with MCP through the leg connected to the MCP floor domain, as well as through a small link to the MCP middle domain (indicated by asterisks). The differences between the RRV and HSV-1 capsids are indicated by an arrowhead and arrows, and represent interactions that are present in HSV-1 but missing in RRV.
(Taken from Yu et al., 2003, with permission from the *Journal of Virology*.)

mac239 or RRV alone, two of two animals coinfected with SIVmac239 and RRV17577 developed hyperplastic lymphoproliferative disease resembling the multicentric plasma cell variant of Castleman's disease, characterized by persistent angiofollicular lymphadenopathy, hepatomegaly, splenomegaly and hypergammaglobulinemia. Hypergammaglobulinemia was associated with severe immune-mediated hemolytic anemia in one RRV17577/SIV-infected macaque. Thus, experimental RRV17577 infection of

SIV-infected rhesus macaques was associated with the hyperplastic B cell lymphoproliferative manifestations analogous to those seen in individuals infected with KSHV. Mansfield et al. (1999) at the NERPRC have also performed co-infections using RRV (strain 26–95) and SIV mac239. Experimental infection of macaques was associated with a lymphadenopathy that was characterized by paracortical hyperplasia and vascular hypertrophy/hyperplasia that subsequently was replaced by marked follicular hyperplasia. In the most severe cases, this follicular hyperplasia destroyed the medullary sinuses and completely effaced the normal lymph node architecture. Similar changes have been found in KSHV infected, HIV-negative human patients with histologic features of angioimmunoblastic lymphadenopathy and reactive lympadenopathy. B-cell proliferation is a feature common to multicentric Castleman's disease and angioimmunoblastic lymphadenopathy (Mansfield et al., 1999). However, 12 weeks post-RRV infection, these pathologies appeared to be resolved. Thus, the immune system in these macaques was able to halt the progression of the hyperplasia. In addition, Mansfield et al. (1999) observed that three of four monkeys co-infected with RRV and SIV developed an arteriopathy. This arteriopathy was similar to the vascular endothelial lesion seen in patients with KS and to the large vessel arteritis in MHV68 infected mice. Despite some drawbacks to the RRV model system, a large number of critical questions can still be addressed using this system of experimental infection.

RRV as an animal model system for KSHV

Since its discovery in 1994, studies to identify a KSHV lytic culture system have been intense. Although lytic systems for KSHV have been developed in several laboratories using reactivated B-cells, 293 cells and de novo infection of endothelial cell lines (Renne et al., 1998; Lagunoff et al., 2002; Poole et al., 2002; Cannon et al., 2000, Sun et al., 1998; Moses et al., 1999; Foreman et al., 1997), these systems yield low quantities of virus resulting in limited replication and serial transmission. The lack of a traditional permissive system for KSHV limits the ability to study the temporal order of events of the full virus life cycle. There have been two KSHV bacterial artificial chromosomes (BAC) constructed to date (Zhou et al., 2002; Delecluse et al., 2001). However, methods to analyze properties of recombinant KSHVs are limited. In contrast, RRV can be grown to high titers ($\sim 1 \times 10^6$ pfu/ml) in rhesus fibroblasts (RhFs) (DeWire et al., 2003) and both plaque assays and real-time PCR assays to measure RRV replication have been devised (DeWire et al., 2003). In addition, RRV can be used as a genetic system to create recombinant RRVs as exemplified by the construction of a recombinant RRV virus expressing green fluorescent protein (RRV-GFP)(DeWire et al., 2003). An infectious RRV model system has been developed such that naïve RRV-negative rhesus macaques inoculated with RRV demonstrate persistent viral infection (Mansfield et al., 1999). Use of the rhesus virus can help address a large number of critical questions. These include the ability to define the relative importance and contribution of individual genes to the establishment of primary infection, dissemination, persistence, tropism, pathologic manifestations and immune avoidance strategies.

At the present time, RRV is the closest simian KSHV homologue that can be grown lytically and has a genetic system to analyze viral gene function. The transcription program of RRV resembles that of KSHV (DeWire et al., 2002), the capsid structure and assembly of RRV and KSHV virions are very homologous (O'Connor et al., 2003; Yu et al., 2003) and a method to generate RRV recombinant viruses has been established (DeWire et al., 2003). Thus, the biological properties of RRV, the ability to construct recombinant RRVs and the ability to generate persistent RRV infection in naïve rhesus macaques experimentally infected with RRV, makes RRV a tractable model to study the KSHV lifecycle in vitro and in vivo.

Conclusions

The presence of gammaherpesviruses in most primates tested to date alludes to the fact that these viruses evolved with their host species. They share similarity in genomic sequence, organization and biological properties. Current evidence indicates that there are two distinct lineages of primate rhadinoviruses and lymphocryptoviruses, both of which are evolutionarily related to KSHV. This suggests that the gammaherpesviruses have diversified from a common ancestor in a manner mediating co-speciation of herpesviruses with their host species. As this theme is conserved for all gammaherpesviruses of Old World Primates including the great apes, it raises the possibility that viruses belonging to a second major phylogenetic grouping of lymphocryptoviruses and rhadinoviruses may be found in humans. The evidence suggests the possible existence of a novel genogroup 2 human lymphocryptovirus which include viruses like GgorLCV2 and PpygLCV1 (Ehlers et al., 2003), and a novel human rhadinovirus belonging to the RV2 genogroup, which include viruses like RRV and Pan-RHV2 (Lacoste et al., 2000a, 2001).

The non-human primate viruses provide a means to model human infection in an experimental setting that would not be possible in humans. While use of the simian viruses as animal models for human EBV and KSHV are still in the early developmental stage, they will likely prove useful for studying the pathogenesis, prevention, and treatment of gammaherpesvirus infections.

Acknowledgments

We would like to thank C.C. Tomlinson, S.M. DeWire, C. Gonzalez and D. Dittmer for proof-reading of the manuscript.

REFERENCES

Ablashi, D. V., Pearson, G., Rabin, H. et al. (1978). Experimental infection of Callithrix jacchus marmosets with Herpesvirus ateles, Herpesvirus saimiri, and Epstein Barr virus. Biomedicine, 29, 7–10.

Albrecht, J. C. (2000). Primary structure of the Herpesvirus ateles genome. J. Virol., 74, 1033–1037.

Albrecht, J. C. and Fleckenstein, B. (1990). Structural organization of the conserved gene block of Herpesvirus Saimiri coding for DNA polymerase, glycoprotein B, and major DNA binding protein. Virology, 174, 533–542.

Alexander, L., Denenkamp, L., Knapp, A. et al. (2000). The primary sequence of rhesus rhadinovirus isolate 26–95: sequence similarities to Kaposi's sarcoma herpesvirus and rhesus rhadinovirus isolate 17577. J. Virol., 74, 3388–3398.

Auerbach, M. R., Czajak, S. C., Johnson, W. E., Desrosiers, R. C., and Alexander. L. (2000). Species specificity of macaque rhadinovirus glycoprotein B sequences. J. Virol., 74, 584–590.

Baskin, G. B., Roberts, E. D., Kuebler, D. et al. (1995). Squamous epithelial proliferative lesions associated with rhesus Epstein–Barr virus in simian immunodeficiency virus-infected rhesus monkeys. J. Infect. Dis., 172, 535–539.

Blake, N. W., Moghaddam, A., Rao, P. et al. (1999). Inhibition of antigen presentation by the glycine/alanine repeat domain is not conserved in simian homologues of Epstein–Barr virus nuclear antigen 1. J. Virol., 73, 7381–7389.

Blake, N. W., Moghaddam, A., Rao, P. et al., (1999). Inhibition of antigen presentation by the glycine/alanine repeat domain is not conserved in simian homologues of Epstein-Barr virus nuclear antigen 1. J. Virol., 73, 7381–7389.

Bocker, J. F., Tiedemann, K. H., Bornkamm, G. W., and zur H. Hausen, H. (1980). Characterization of an EBV-like virus from African green monkey lymphoblasts. Virology, 101, 291–295.

Bosch, M. L., Harper, E., Schmidt, A. et al. (1999). Activation in vivo of retroperitoneal fibromatosis-associated herpesvirus, a simian homologue of human herpesvirus-8. J. Gen. Virol., 80, 467–475.

Cannon, J. S., Ciufo, D., Hawkins, A. L. et al. (2000). A new primary effusion lymphoma-derived cell line yields a highly infectious Kaposi's sarcoma herpesvirus-containing supernatant. J. Virol., 74, 10187–10193.

Cho, Y., Ramer, J., Rivailler, P. et al. (2001). An Epstein–Barr-related herpesvirus from marmoset lymphomas. Proc. Natl Acad. Sci. USA, 98, 1224–1229.

Cho, Y. G., Gordadze, A. V., Ling, P. D., and Wang, F. (1999). Evolution of two types of rhesus lymphocryptovirus similar to type 1 and type 2 Epstein–Barr virus. J. Virol., 73, 9206–9212.

Clapp, N. K., Littlefield, L. G., and Lushbaugh, C. C. (1982). Colon carcinoma in subhuman primates. Gastroenterology, 83, 519.

Cleary, M. L., Epstein, M. A., Finerty, S. et al. (1985). Individual tumors of multifocal EB virus-induced malignant lymphomas in tamarins arise from different B-cell clones. Science, 228, 722–724.

Cohen, J. I., Wang, F., Mannick, J., and Kieff, E. (1989). Epstein–Barr virus nuclear protein 2 is a key determinant of lymphocyte transformation. Proc. Natl Acad. Sci. USA, 86, 9558–9562.

Dalbies-Tran, R., Stigger-Rosser, E., Dotson, T., and Sample, C. E. (2001). Amino acids of Epstein–Barr virus nuclear antigen 3A essential for repression of Jkappa-mediated transcription and their evolutionary conservation. J. Virol., 75, 90–99.

Damania, B., Li, M., Choi, J. K., Alexander, L., Jung, J. U., and Desrosiers, R. C. (1999). Identification of the R1 oncogene and its protein product from the Rhadinovirus of Rhesus monkeys. J. Virol., 73, 5123–5131.

Damania, B., DeMaria, M., Jung, J. U., and Desrosiers, R. C. (2000). Activation of lymphocyte signaling by the R1 protein of rhesus monkey rhadinovirus. J. Virol., 74, 2721–2730.

Damania, B. J. J., Bowser, B. S., DeWire, S. M., Staudt, M., and Dittmer, D. P. (2004). Comparison of the Rta/Orf50 transactivator proteins of gamma-2 herpesviruses. J. Virol., 78(10), 5491–5499.

Dambaugh, T., Raab-Traub, N., Heller, M. et al. (1980). Variations among isolates of Epstein–Barr virus. Ann. N Y Acad. Sci., 354, 309–325.

Dambaugh, T., Hennessy, K., Chamnankit, L., and Kieff, E. (1984). U2 region of Epstein–Barr virus DNA may encode Epstein–Barr nuclear antigen 2. Proc. Natl Acad. Sci. USA, 81, 7632–7636.

Dambaugh, T., Wang, F., Hennessy, K., Woodland, E., Rickinson, A., and Kieff, E. (1986). Expression of the Epstein-Barr virus nuclear protein 2 in rodent cells. J. Virol., 59, 453–462.

de Thoisy, B., Pouliquen, J. F., Lacoste, V., Gessain, A., and Kazanji, M. (2003). Novel gamma-1 herpesviruses identified in free-ranging new world monkeys (golden-handed tamarin (Saguinus midas), squirrel monkey (Saimiri sciureus), and white-faced saki (Pithecia pithecia) in French Guiana. J. Virol., 77, 9099–9105.

Delecluse, H. J., Kost, M., Feederle, R., Wilson, L., and W. Hammerschmidt (2001). Spontaneous activation of the lytic cycle in cells infected with a recombinant Kaposi's sarcoma-associated virus. J. Virol., 75, 2921–2928.

Desgranges, C., Lenoir, G., de-The, G., Seigneurin, J. M., Hilgers, J., and Dubouch, P. (1976). In vitro transforming activity of EBV.

I-Establishment and properties of two EBV strains (M81 and M72) produced by immortalized *Callithrix jacchus* lymphocytes. *Biomedicine*, **25**, 349–352.

Desrosiers, R. C., Sasseville, V. G., Czajak, S. C. et al. (1997). A herpesvirus of rhesus monkeys related to the human Kaposi's sarcoma-associated herpesvirus. *J. Virol.*, **71**, 9764–9769.

de-The, G., Dubouch, P., Fontaine, C. et al. (1980). Natural antibodies to EBV-VCA antigens in common marmosets (*Callithrix jacchus*) and response after EBV inoculation. *Intervirology*, **14**, 284–291.

DeWire, S. M., McVoy, M. A., and Damania, B. (2002). Kinetics of expression of rhesus monkey rhadinovirus (RRV) and identification and characterization of a polycistronic transcript encoding the RRV Orf50/Rta, RRV R8, and R8.1 genes. *J. Virol.*, **76**, 9819–9831.

DeWire, S. M., Money, E. S., Krall, S. P., and Damania, B. (2003). Rhesus monkey rhadinovirus (RRV): construction of a RRV-GFP recombinant virus and development of assays to assess viral replication. *Virology*, **312**, 122–134.

Dewire, S. M., and Damania, B. (2005). The latency-associated nuclear antigen of rhesus monkey rhadinovirus inhibits viral replication through repression of Orf50/Rta transcriptional activation. *J. Virol.*, **79**, 3127–3138.

Dittmer, D., Stoddart, C., and Renne, R. (1999). Experimental transmission of Kaposi's sarcoma-associated herpesvirus (KSHV/HHV-8) to SCID-hu Thy/Liv mice. *J. Exp. Med.*, **190**, 1857–1868.

Dittmer, D. P., Gonzalez, C. M., Vahrson, W., De Wire, S. M., Hines-Boykin, R., and Damania, B. (2005). Whole-genome transcription profiling of rhesus monkey rhadinovirus. *J. Virol.* **79**(13), 8637–8650.

Dunkel, V. C., Pry, T. W. Henle, G., and Henle, W. (1972). Immunofluorescence tests for antibodies to Epstein–Barr virus with sera of lower primates. *J. Natl Cancer Inst.*, **49**, 435–440.

Ehlers, B., Ochs, A., Leendertz, F., Goltz, M., Boesch, C., and Matz-Rensing, K. (2003). Novel simian homologues of Epstein–Barr virus. *J. Virol.*, **77**, 10695–10699.

Eliopoulos, A. G. and Young, L. S. (1998). Activation of the cJun N-terminal kinase (JNK) pathway by the Epstein–Barr virus-encoded latent membrane protein 1 (LMP1). *Oncogene*, **16**, 1731–1742.

Epstein, M. A., Hunt, R. D., and Rabin, H. (1973a). Pilot experiments with EB virus in owl monkeys (*Aotus trivirgatus*). I: Reticuloproliferative disease in an inoculated animal. *Int. J. Cancer*, **12**, 309–318.

Epstein, M. A., Rabin, H., Ball, G., Rickinson, A. B., Jarvis, J., and Melendez, L. V. (1973b). Pilot experiments with EB virus in owl monkeys (*Aotus trivirgatus*). II. EB virus in a cell line from an animal with reticuloproliferative disease. *Int. J. Cancer*, **12**, 319–332.

Estep, R. D., Axthelm, M. K., and Wong, S. W., (2003). A G protein-coupled receptor encoded by rhesus rhadinovirus is similar to ORF74 of Kaposi's sarcoma-associated herpesvirus. *J. Virol.*, **77**, 1738–1746.

Falk, L., Deinhardt, F., Wolfe, L., Johnson, D., Hilgers, J., and de-The, G. (1976). Epstein–Barr virus: experimental infection of *Callithrix jacchus* marmosets. *Int. J. Cancer*, **17**, 785–788.

Falk, L. A., Henle, G., Henle, W., Deinhardt, F., and Schudel, A. (1977). Transformation of lymphocytes by Herpesvirus papio. *Int. J. Cancer*, **20**, 219–226.

Faucher, S., Dimock, K., and Wright, K. E. (2002). Characterization of the Cyno-EBV LMP1 homologue and comparison with LMP1s of EBV and other EBV-like viruses. *Virus Res.*, **90**, 63–75.

Feichtinger, H., Kaaya, E., Putkonen, P. et al. (1992a). Malignant lymphoma associated with human AIDS and with SIV-induced immunodeficiency in macaques. *AIDS Res. Hum. Retroviruses*, **8**, 339–348.

Feichtinger, H., Li, S. L., Kaaya, E. et al. (1992b). A monkey model for Epstein–Barr virus-associated lymphomagenesis in human acquired immunodeficiency syndrome. *J. Exp. Med.*, **176**, 281–286.

Fogg, M. H., Kaur, A., Cho, Y. G., and Wang, F. (2005). The CD8+ T-cell response to an Epstein-Barr virus-related gammaherpesvirus infecting rhesus macaques provides evidence for immune evasion by the EBNA-1 homologue. *J. Virol.* **79**, 12681–12691.

Foreman, K. E., Bacon, P. E., Hsi, E. D., and Nickoloff, B. J. (1997). In situ polymerase chain reaction-based localization studies support role of human herpesvirus-8 as the cause of two AIDS-related neoplasms: Kaposi's sarcoma and body cavity lymphoma. *J. Clin. Invest.*, **99**, 2971–2978.

Frank, A., Andiman, W. A., and Miller, G. (1976). Epstein–Barr virus and nonhuman primates: natural and experimental infection. *Adv. Cancer Res.*, **23**, 171–201.

Franken, M., Devergne, O., Rosenzweig, M., Annis, B., Kieff, E., and Wang, F. (1996). Comparative analysis identifies conserved tumor necrosis factor receptor-associated factor 3 binding sites in the human and simian Epstein–Barr virus oncogene LMP1. *J. Virol.*, **70**, 7819–7826.

Fuentes-Panana, E. M., Swaminathan, S., and Ling, P. D. (1999). Transcriptional activation signals found in the Epstein–Barr virus (EBV) latency C promoter are conserved in the latency C promoter sequences from baboon and Rhesus monkey EBV-like lymphocryptoviruses (cercopithicine herpesviruses 12 and 15). *J. Virol.*, **73**, 826–833.

Gerber, P., Branch, J. W., and Rosenblum, E. N. (1969). Attempts to transmit infectious mononucleosis to rhesus monkeys and marmosets and to isolate herpes-like virus. *Proc. Soc. Exp. Biol. Med.*, **130**, 14–19.

Gerber, P., Kalter, S. S., Schidlovsky, G., Peterson, W. D. Jr., and Daniel, M. D. (1977). Biologic and antigenic characteristics of Epstein–Barr virus-related Herpesviruses of chimpanzees and baboons. *Int. J. Cancer*, **20**, 448–459.

Greensill, J., Sheldon, J. A., Murthy, K. K., Bessonette, J. S., Beer, B. E., and Schulz, T. F. (2000a). A chimpanzee rhadinovirus sequence related to Kaposi's sarcoma-associated herpesvirus/human herpesvirus 8: increased detection after HIV-1 infection in the absence of disease. *AIDS*, **14**, F129–135.

Greensill, J., Sheldon, J. A., and Renwick, N. M. (2000b). Two distinct gamma-2 herpesviruses in African green monkeys: a second gamma-2 herpesvirus lineage among old world primates? *J. Virol.*, **74**, 1572–1577.

Habis, A., Baskin, G., Simpson, L., Fortgang, I., Murphey-Corb, M., and Levy, L. S. (2000). Rhesus lymphocryptovirus infection during the progression of SAIDS and SAIDS-associated lymphoma in the rhesus macaque. *AIDS Res. Hum. Retroviruses*, **16**, 163–171.

Heller, M. and Kieff, E. (1981). Colinearity between the DNAs of Epstein–Barr virus and herpesvirus papio. *J. Virol.*, **37**, 821–826.

Heller, M., Gerber, P., and Kieff, E. (1981). Herpesvirus papio DNA is similar in organization to Epstein–Barr virus DNA. *J. Virol.*, **37**, 698–709.

Hernandez-Camacho, J. C. R. (1976). The nonhuman primates of Colombia. In Thorington, R. W., Jr. and Heltne, P. G. eds. *Neotropical Primates: Field Studies and Conservation.* Washington, DC: National Academy of Sciences.

ICTV. Website: http://www.ncbi.nlm.nih.gov/ICTVdb/Ictv/fs_herpe.htm. International Committee on the Taxonomy of Viruses.

Ishida, T. and Yamamoto. K. (1987). Survey of nonhuman primates for antibodies reactive with Epstein–Barr virus (EBV) antigens and susceptibility of their lymphocytes for immortalization with EBV. *J. Med. Primatol.*, **16**, 359–371.

Jenson, H. B., Ench, Y., Zhang, Y. S., Gao, J., Arrand, J. R., and Mackett, M. (2002). Characterization of an Epstein–Barr virus-related gammaherpesvirus from common marmoset (*Callithrix jacchus*). *J. Gen. Virol.*, **83**, 1621–1633.

Jiang, H., Cho, Y. G., and Wang. F. (2000). Structural, functional, and genetic comparisons of Epstein–Barr virus nuclear antigen 3A, 3B, and 3C homologues encoded by the rhesus lymphocryptovirus. *J. Virol.*, **74**, 5921–5932.

Johnson, D. R., Wolfe, L. G., Levan, G., Klein, G., Ernberg, I., and Aman, P. (1983). Epstein–Barr virus (EBV)-induced lymphoproliferative disease in cotton-topped marmosets. *Int. J. Cancer*, **31**, 91–97.

Kaleeba, J. A., Bergquam, E. P., and Wong. S. W. (1999). A rhesus macaque rhadinovirus related to Kaposi's sarcoma-associated herpesvirus/human herpesvirus 8 encodes a functional homologue of interleukin-6. *J. Virol.*, **73**, 6177–6181.

Kalter, S. S., Heberling, R. L., and Ratner, J. J. (1972). EBV antibody in sera of non-human primates. *Nature*, **238**, 353–354.

Lacoste, V., Mauclere, P., Dubreuil, G., Lewis, J., Georges-Courbot, M. C., and Gessain, A. (2000a). KSHV-like herpesviruses in chimps and gorillas. *Nature*, **407**, 151–152.

Lacoste, V., Mauclere, P., and Dubreuil, G. (2000b). Simian homologues of human gamma-2 and betaherpesviruses in mandrill and drill monkeys. *J. Virol.*, **74**, 11993–11999.

Lacoste, V., Mauclere, P., Dubreuil, G., Lewis, J., Georges-Courbot M. C., and Gessain, A. (2001). A novel gamma 2-herpesvirus of the Rhadinovirus 2 lineage in chimpanzees. *Genome Res.*, **11**, 1511–1519.

Lagunoff, M., Bechtel, J., Venetsanakos, E., *et al.* (2002). De novo infection and serial transmission of Kaposi's sarcoma-associated herpesvirus in cultured endothelial cells. *J. Virol.*, **76**, 2440–2448.

Landon, J. C. and Malan, L. B. (1971). Seroepidemiologic studies of Epstein–Barr virus antibody in monkeys. *J. Natl Cancer Inst.*, **46**, 881–884.

Landon, J. C., Ellis, L. B., Zeve, V. H., and Fabrizio, D. P. (1968). Herpes-type virus in cultured leukocytes from chimpanzees. *J. Natl Cancer Inst.*, **40**, 181–192.

Langlais, C. L., Jones, J. M., Estep, R. D., and Wong, S. W. (2006). Rhesus rhadinovirus R15 encodes a functional homologue of human CD200. *J. Virol.*, **80**, 3098–3103.

Lee, H., Veazey, R., Williams, K. *et al.* (1998). Deregulation of cell growth by the K1 gene of Kaposi's sarcoma- associated herpesvirus. *Nat. Med.*, **4**, 435–440.

Levine, P. H., Leiseca, S. A., Hewetson, J. F. *et al.* (1980). Infection of rhesus monkeys and chimpanzees with Epstein–Barr virus. *Arch. Virol.*, **66**, 341–351.

Levitskaya, J., Coram, M., Levitsky, V. *et al.* (1995). Inhibition of antigen processing by the internal repeat region of the Epstein–Barr virus nuclear antigen-1. *Nature*, **375**, 685–688.

Levitskaya, J., Coram, M., Levitsky, V. *et al.*, (1995). Inhibition of antigen processing by the internal repeat region of the Epstein–Barr virus nuclear antigen-1. *Nature*, **375**, 685–688.

Levy, J. A., Levy, S. B., Hirshaut, Y., Kafuko, G., and Prince, A. (1971). Presence of EBV antibodies in sera from wild chimpanzees. *Nature*, **233**, 559–560.

Lin, S. F., Robinson, D. R., Oh, J., Jung, J. U., Luciw, P. A., and Kung, H. J. (2002). Identification of the bZIP and Rta homologues in the genome of rhesus monkey rhadinovirus. *Virology*, **298**, 181–188.

Ling, P. D. and Hayward, S. D. (1995). Contribution of conserved amino acids in mediating the interaction between EBNA2 and CBF1/RBPJk. *J. Virol.*, **69**, 1944–1950.

Ling, P. D., Ryon, J. J., and Hayward, S. D. (1993). EBNA-2 of herpesvirus papio diverges significantly from the type A and type B EBNA-2 proteins of Epstein–Barr virus but retains an efficient transactivation domain with a conserved hydrophobic motif. *J. Virol.*, **67**, 2990–3003.

Manet, E., Gruffat, H., and Trescol-Biemont, M. C. (1989). Epstein–Barr virus bicistronic mRNAs generated by facultative splicing code for two transcriptional trans-activators. *EMBO J.*, **8**, 1819–1826.

Mansfield, K., Westmoreland, S. V., DeBakker, C. D. *et al.* (1999). Experimental infection of rhesus and pig-tailed macaques with macaque rhadinoviruses. *J. Virol.*, **73**, 10320–10328.

Marechal, V., Dehee, A., Chikhi-Brachet, R. Piolot, T., Coppey-Moisan, M., and Nicolas, J. C. (1999). Mapping EBNA-1 domains involved in binding to metaphase chromosomes. *J. Virol.*, **73**, 4385–4392.

Melendez, L. V., Daniel, M. D., Garcia, F. G., Fraser, C. E., Hunt, R. D., and King, N. W. (1969). Herpesvirus saimiri. I. Further characterization studies of a new virus from the squirrel monkey. *Lab. Anim. Care*, **19**, 372–377.

Melendez, L. V., Hunt, R. D., King, N. W. et al. (1972). Herpesvirus ateles, a new lymphoma virus of monkeys. *Nat. New Biol.*, **235**, 182–184.

Miller, G., Niederman, J. C., and Stitt, D. A. (1972). Infectious mononucleosis: appearance of neutralizing antibody to Epstein–Barr virus measured by inhibition of formation of lymphoblastoid cell lines. *J. Infect. Dis.*, **125**, 403–406.

Miller, G., Shope, T., Coope, D. et al. (1977). Lymphoma in cotton-top marmosets after inoculation with Epstein–Barr virus: tumor incidence, histologic spectrum antibody responses, demonstration of viral DNA, and characterization of viruses. *J. Exp. Med.*, **145**, 948–967.

Moghaddam, A., Rosenzweig, M., Lee-Parritz, D., Annis, B., Johnson, R. P., and Wang, F. (1997). An animal model for acute and persistent Epstein–Barr virus infection. *Science*, **276**, 2030–2033.

Moghaddam, A., Koch, J., Annis, B., and Wang, F. (1998). Infection of human B lymphocytes with lymphocryptoviruses related to Epstein–Barr virus. *J. Virol.*, **72**, 3205–3212.

Mohle, R., Green, D., Moore, M. A., Nachman, R. L., and Rafii, S. (1997). Constitutive production and thrombin-induced release of vascular endothelial growth factor by human megakaryocytes and platelets. *Proc. Natl Acad. Sci. USA*, **94**, 663–668.

Moore, P. S. and Chang, Y. (2003). Kaposi's sarcoma-associated herpesvirus immunoevasion and tumorigenesis: two sides of the same coin? *Annu. Rev. Microbiol.*, **57**, 609–639.

Moses, A. V., Fish, K. N., Ruhl, R. et al. (1999). Long-term infection and transformation of dermal microvascular endothelial cells by human herpesvirus 8. *J. Virol.*, **73**, 6892–6902.

Naito, M., Ono, K., Doi, T., Kato, S., and Tanabe, S. (1971). Antibodies in human and monkey sera to herpes-type virus from a chicken with Marek's disease and to EB virus detected by the immunofluorescence test. *Biken J.*, **14**, 161–166.

Nealon, K., Newcomb, W. W., Pray, T. R., Craik, C. S., Brown, J. C., and Kedes, D. H. (2001). Lytic replication of Kaposi's sarcoma-associated herpesvirus results in the formation of multiple capsid species: isolation and molecular characterization of A, B, and C capsids from a gammaherpesvirus. *J. Virol.*, **75**, 2866–2878.

Neubauer, R. H., Rabin, H., Strnad, B. C., Nonoyama, M., and Nelson-Rees, W. A. (1979). Establishment of a lymphoblastoid cell line and isolation of an Epstein–Barr-related virus of gorilla origin. *J. Virol.*, **31**, 845–848.

O'Connor, C. M., Damania, B., and Kedes, D. H. (2003). De novo infection with rhesus monkey rhadinovirus leads to the accumulation of multiple intranuclear capsid species during lytic replication but favors the release of genome-containing virions. *J. Virol.*, **77**, 13439–13447.

Ohara, N., Hayashi, K., Teramoto, N. et al. (2000). Sequence analysis and variation of EBNA-1 in Epstein–Barr virus-related herpesvirus of cynomolgus monkey. *Intervirology*, **43**, 102–106.

Peng, R., Gordadze, A. V., Fuentes Panana, E. M. et al. (2000). Sequence and functional analysis of EBNA-LP and EBNA2 proteins from nonhuman primate lymphocryptoviruses. *J. Virol.*, **74**, 379–389.

Poole, L. J., Yu, Y., Kim, P. S., Zheng, Q. Z., Pevsner, J., and Hayward, G. S. (2002). Altered patterns of cellular gene expression in dermal microvascular endothelial cells infected with Kaposi's sarcoma-associated herpesvirus. *J. Virol.*, **76**, 3395–3420.

Portis, T., Cooper, L., Dennis, P., and Longnecker, R. (2002). The LMP2A signalosome – a therapeutic target for Epstein–Barr virus latency and associated disease. *Front Biosci.*, **7**, d414–d426.

Pratt, C. L., Estep, R. D., and Wong, S. W. (2005). Splicing of rhesus rhadinovirus R15 and ORF74 bicistronic transcripts during lytic infection and analysis of effects on production of vCD200 and vGPCR. *J. Virol.*, **79**, 3878–3882.

Rabin, H., Neubauer, R. H., Hopkins, R. F., 3rd, Dzhikidze, E. K., Shevtsova, Z. V., and Lapin, B. A. (1977a). Transforming activity and antigenicity of an Epstein–Barr-like virus from lymphoblastoid cell lines of baboons with lymphoid disease. *Intervirology*, **8**, 240–249.

Rabin, H., Neubauer, R. H., Hopkins, R. F., and Levy, B. M. (1977b). Characterization of lymphoid cell lines established from multiple Epstein–Barr virus (EBV)-induced lymphomas in a cotton-topped marmoset. *Int. J. Cancer*, **20**, 44–50.

Ramer, J. C., Garber, R. L., Steele, K. E., Boyson, J. F., O'Rourke, C., and Thomson, J. A. (2000). Fatal lymphoproliferative disease associated with a novel gammaherpesvirus in a captive population of common marmosets. *Comp. Med.*, **50**, 59–68.

Rangan, S. R., Martin, L. N., Bozelka, B. E., Wang, N., and Gormus, B. J. (1986). Epstein–Barr virus-related herpesvirus from a rhesus monkey (*Macaca mulatta*) with malignant lymphoma. *Int. J. Cancer*, **38**, 425–432.

Rao, P., Jiang, H., and Wang, F. (2000). Cloning of the rhesus lymphocryptovirus viral capsid antigen and Epstein–Barr virus-encoded small RNA homologues and use in diagnosis of acute and persistent infections. *J. Clin. Microbiol.*, **38**, 3219–3925.

Rasheed, S., Rongey, R. W., Bruszweski, J. et al. (1977). Establishment of a cell line with associated Epstein–Barr-like virus from a leukemic orangutan. *Science*, **198**, 407–409.

Renne, R., Blackbourn, D., Whitby, D., Levy, J., and Ganem, D. (1998). Limited transmission of Kaposi's sarcoma-associated herpesvirus in cultured cells. *J. Virol.*, **72**, 5182–5188.

Renne, R., Dittmer, D., Kedes, D. et al. (2004). Experimental transmission of Kaposi's sarcoma-associated herpesvirus (KSHV/HHV-8) to SIV-positive and SIV-negative rhesus macaques. *J. Med. Primatol.*, **33**, 1–9.

Rickinson, A. B., Young, L. S., and Rowe, M. (1987). Influence of the Epstein–Barr virus nuclear antigen EBNA 2 on the growth phenotype of virus-transformed B cells. *J. Virol.*, **61**, 1310–1317.

Rivailler, P., Quink, C., and Wang, F. (1999). Strong selective pressure for evolution of an Epstein–Barr virus LMP2B homologue in the rhesus lymphocryptovirus. *J. Virol.*, **73**, 8867–8872.

Rivailler, P., Cho, Y. G., and Wang, F. (2002). Complete genomic sequence of an Epstein–Barr virus-related herpesvirus naturally infecting a new world primate: a defining point in the evolution of oncogenic lymphocryptoviruses. *J. Virol.*, **76**, 12055–12068.

Rivailler, P., Jiang, H., Cho, Y. G., Quink, C., and Wang, F. (2002). Complete nucleotide sequence of the rhesus lymphocryptovirus: genetic validation for an Epstein–Barr virus animal model. *J. Virol.*, **76**, 421–426.

Rivailler, P., Carville, A., Kaur, A. et al., (2004). Experimental rhesus lymphocryptovirus infection in immunosuppressed macaques: an animal model for Epstein-Barr virus pathogenesis in the immunosuppressed host. *Blood*, **104**, 1482–1489.

Rose, T. M., Strand, K. B., Schultz, E. R. et al. (1997). Identification of two homologs of the Kaposi's sarcoma-associated herpesvirus (human herpesvirus 8) in retroperitoneal fibromatosis of different macaque species. *J. Virol.*, **71**, 4138–4144.

Rose, T. M., Ryan, J. T., Schultz, E. R., Raden, B. W., and Tsai, C. C. (2003). Analysis of 4.3 kilobases of divergent locus B of macaque retroperitoneal fibromatosis-associated herpesvirus reveals a close similarity in gene sequence and genome organization to Kaposi's sarcoma-associated herpesvirus. *J. Virol.*, **77**, 5084–5097.

Rowe, D. T. and Clarke, J. R. (1989). The type-specific epitopes of the Epstein–Barr virus nuclear antigen 2 are near the carboxy terminus of the protein. *J. Gen. Virol.*, **70**(Pt 5), 1217–1229.

Rowe, M., Young, L. S., Cadwallader, K., Petti, L. Kieff, E., and Rickinson, A. B. (1989). Distinction between Epstein–Barr virus type A (EBNA 2A) and type B (EBNA 2B) isolates extends to the EBNA 3 family of nuclear proteins. *J. Virol.*, **63**, 1031–1039.

Ruf, I. K., Moghaddam, A., Wang, F., and Sample, J. (1999). Mechanisms that regulate Epstein–Barr virus EBNA-1 gene transcription during restricted latency are conserved among lymphocryptoviruses of Old World primates. *J. Virol.*, **73**, 1980–1989.

Sample, J., Young, L., Martin, B., Chatman, T. Kieff, E., and Rickinson, A. (1990). Epstein–Barr virus types 1 and 2 differ in their EBNA-3A, EBNA-3B, and EBNA-3C genes. *J. Virol.*, **64**, 4084–4092.

Schrago, C. G. and Russo, C. A. (2003). Timing the origin of new world monkeys. *Mol. Biol. Evol.*, **20**, 1620–1625.

Schultz, E. R., Rankin, G. W. Jr., Blanc, M. P., Raden, B. W., Tsai, C. C., and Rose, T. M. (2000). Characterization of two divergent lineages of macaque rhadinoviruses related to Kaposi's sarcoma-associated herpesvirus. *J. Virol.*, **74**, 4919–4928.

Searles, R. P., Bergquam, E. P., Axthelm, M. K., and Wong, S. W. (1999). Sequence and genomic analysis of a rhesus macaque rhadinovirus with similarity to Kaposi's sarcoma-associated herpesvirus/human herpesvirus 8. *J. Virol.*, **73**, 3040–3053.

Shope, T., Dechairo, D., and Miller, G. (1973). Malignant lymphoma in cottontop marmosets after inoculation with Epstein–Barr virus. *Proc. Natl Acad. Sci. USA*, **70**, 2487–2491.

Stewart, C. B. and Disotell, T. R. (1998). Primate evolution – in and out of Africa. *Curr. Biol.*, **8**, R582–R588.

Strand, K., Harper, E., Thormahlen, S. et al. (2000). Two distinct lineages of macaque gamma herpesviruses related to the Kaposi's sarcoma associated herpesvirus. *J. Clin. Virol.*, **16**, 253–269.

Sun, R., Lin, S. F., Gradoville, L., Yuan, Y., Zhu, F., and Miller, G. (1998). A viral gene that activates lytic cycle expression of Kaposi's sarcoma- associated herpesvirus. *Proc. Natl Acad. Sci. USA*, **95**, 10866–10871.

Vasiljeva, V. A., Markarjan, D. S., Lapin, B. A. et al. (1974). Establishment of continuous cell lines from leukocytes culture of a hamadryas baboon with leukosis-reticulosis. *Neoplasma*, **21**, 537–544.

Wang, F. (2001). A new animal model for Epstein–Barr virus pathogenesis. *Curr. Top. Microbiol. Immunol.*, **258**, 201–219.

Wang, F., Rivailler, P., Rao, P., and Cho, Y. (2001). Simian homologues of Epstein–Barr virus. *Phil. Trans. R. Soc. Lond. B Biol. Sci.*, **356**, 489–497.

Wedderburn, N., Edwards, J. M., Desgranges, C., Fontaine, C., Cohen, B., and de The G. (1984). Infectious mononucleosis-like response in common marmosets infected with Epstein–Barr virus. *J. Infect. Dis.*, **150**, 878–882.

Werner, J., Wolf, H., Apodaca, J., and zur Hausen, H. (1975). Lymphoproliferative disease in a cotton-top marmoset after inoculation with infectious mononucleosis-derived Epstein–Barr virus. *Int. J. Cancer*, **15**, 1000–1008.

Whitby, D., Stossel, A., Gamache, C., et al. (2003). Novel Kaposi's sarcoma-associated herpesvirus homolog in baboons. *J. Virol.*, **77**, 8159–8165.

Wong, S. W., Bergquam, E. P., Swanson, R. M. et al. (1999). Induction of B cell hyperplasia in simian immunodeficiency virus-infected rhesus macaques with the simian homologue of Kaposi's sarcoma- associated herpesvirus. *J. Exp. Med.*, **190**, 827–840.

Wu, L., Lo, P., Yu, X., Stoops, J. K., Forghani, B., and Zhou, Z. H. (2000). Three-dimensional structure of the human herpesvirus 8 capsid. *J. Virol.*, **74**, 9646–9654.

Yalamanchili, R., Tong, X., Grossman, S., Johannsen, E., Mosialos, G., and Kieff, E. (1994). Genetic and biochemical evidence that EBNA 2 interaction with a 63-kDa cellular GTG-binding protein is essential for B lymphocyte growth transformation by EBV. *Virology*, **204**, 634–641.

Yalamanchili, R., Harada, S., and Kieff, E. (1996). The N-terminal half of EBNA2, except for seven prolines, is not essential for primary B-lymphocyte growth transformation. *J. Virol.*, **70**, 2468–2473.

Yasui, T., Luftig, M., Soni, V., and Kieff, E. (2004). Latent infection membrane protein transmembrane FWLY is critical for intermolecular interaction, raft localization, and signaling. *Proc. Natl Acad. Sci. USA*, **101**, 278–283.

Yates, J. L., Camiolo, S. M., Ali, S., and Ying, A. (1996). Comparison of the EBNA1 proteins of Epstein–Barr virus and herpesvirus papio in sequence and function. *Virology*, **222**, 1–13.

Yu, X. K., O'Connor, C. M., Atanasov, I., Damania, B., Kedes, D. H., and Zhou, Z. H. (2003). Three-dimensional structures of the A, B, and C capsids of rhesus monkey rhadinovirus: insights into gammaherpesvirus capsid assembly, maturation, and DNA packaging. *J. Virol.*, **77**, 13182–13193.

Zhao, B., Dalbies-Tran, R., Jiang, H. *et al.* (2003). Transcriptional regulatory properties of Epstein–Barr virus nuclear antigen 3C are conserved in simian lymphocryptoviruses. *J. Virol.*, **77**, 5639–5648.

Zhou, F. C., Zhang, Y. J., Deng, J. H. *et al.* (2002). Efficient infection by a recombinant Kaposi's sarcoma-associated herpesvirus cloned in a bacterial artificial chromosome: application for genetic analysis. *J. Virol.*, **76**, 6185–6196.

Zhu, F. X., Cusano, T., and Yuan. Y. (1999). Identification of the immediate-early transcripts of Kaposi's sarcoma- associated herpesvirus. *J. Virol.*, **73**, 5556–5567.

Zimber, U., Adldinger, H. K., Lenoir, G. M. *et al.* (1986). Geographical prevalence of two types of Epstein–Barr virus. *Virology*, **154**, 56–66.

Part V

Subversion of adaptive immunity

Edited by Richard Whitley and Ann Arvin

Herpesvirus evasion of T-cell immunity

Benjamin E. Gewurz[1], Jatin M. Vyas[2], and Hidde L. Ploegh[1]

[1]Department of Pathology, Harvard Medical School, Boston, MA, USA
[2]Division of Infectious Disease, Department of Medicine, Massachusetts General Hospital, Boston, MA, USA

The multiple layers of the human immune response present a challenge to viruses, which must survive and multiply within a host for a sufficient period of time to allow successful transmission to susceptible individuals. Given the large proteomes and comparatively low polymerase error rate of human herpesviruses, antiviral immunity at first glance appear to have the upper hand. Nonetheless, herpesviruses manage prolonged incubation periods following initial infection, with systemic dissemination and prolonged secretion, often from multiple sites. In contrast to the similarly large poxviruses, the ability to subsequently establish persistent infection is a hallmark of the human herpesviruses. To enable this lifestyle, the herpesviruses devote a significant proportion of their genome coding capacity to the expression of immuno-evasins, a collection of molecules that disrupt normal immune physiology. Each human herpesvirus studied has evolved elegant cell biological solutions to problems posed by the immune response.

Innate immunity, an evolutionarily conserved and relatively non-specific system of pattern recognition molecules hardwired in the genome, cytokines such as interferons, phagocytes and natural killer (NK) cells, represents the first line deployed against microbial invaders, including herpesviruses (Janeway and Medzhitov, 2002). The clonal expansion of B- and T- lymphocytes that bear antigen-specific receptors for viral epitopes underlies the adaptive antiviral immune response, laying the groundwork for a highly pathogen-specific defense. Such specificity comes at a price – lymphocyte proliferation requires time to unfold, and innate immunity, in particular NK-cell activity, limits the initial herpesvirus spread. Indeed, NK cell immune deficiencies result in dramatic infection by several herpesviruses (McClain *et al.*, 1988; Biron *et al.*, 1989). There is significant cross-talk between the innate and adaptive systems, and preliminary pathogen recognition by the innate immune system directly contributes to the development of adaptive immunity. Further, the eventual adaptive response utilizes branches of the innate system for crucial effector function (Medzhitov and Janeway, 1999).

Innate and adaptive immunity act in concert to allow recovery from acute herpesvirus infection. Adaptive immunity then allows for lifelong immunological memory, affording both control of persistent herpesvirus infection and protection against reinfection. Once present, virus-specific CD4+ T-lymphocytes then coordinate the adaptive antiviral response, directing the production of virus-specific immunoglobulin by B-lymphocytes, the antiviral activity of CD8+ T-lymphocytes and NK cells, and further stimulating the activity of phagocytic cells.

Through millennia of coevolution, herpesviruses have largely reached a state of equilibrium with their human hosts. At the cost of a large proportion of their coding capacity, herpesviruses perturb adaptive immunity to achieve persistent infection, in general with remarkably little collateral damage to their hosts. However, lapses in T-cell immunity, such as by immunosuppressive agents or by coinfection with other pathogens such as Human Immunodeficiency Virus, can lead to significant herpesvirus-associated pathology.

Human herpesvirus genome size and polymerase fidelity place constraints on epitope mutation, and generally do not allow for antigenic variation as a means to avoid T-cell immunity. Herpesviruses therefore, have devised a range of mechanisms to subvert adaptive immunity. Generalized T-cell immuno-evasion strategies shared by herpesviruses include latency, restriction of viral gene expression to immunoprivileged sites such as the CNS, interference with complement, cytokines, NK-cell function, and apoptosis,

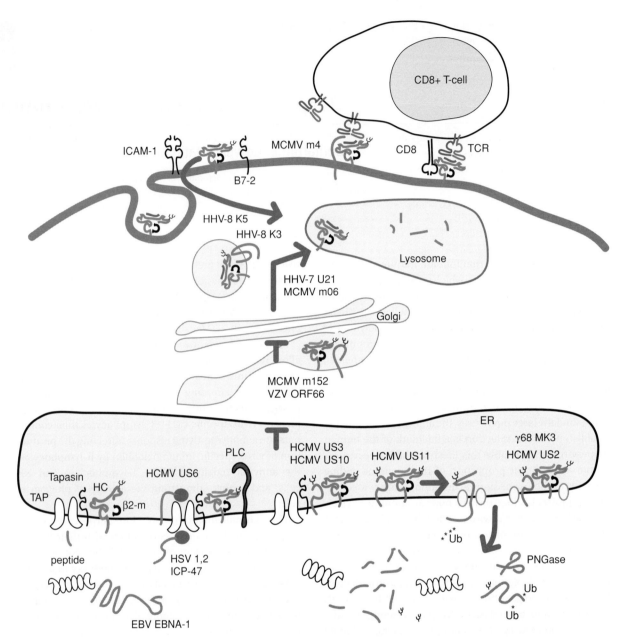

Fig. 62.1. Herpesvirus immunoevasins that directly interfere with class I MHC molecule biosynthesis. Class I MHC molecules are assembled from free HC and β-2 microglobulin within the ER, along with antigenic peptide. Peptides are produces by cytosolic proteasome degradation. The EBV EBNA-1 GAr domain interferes with proteasomal degradation in-*cis*. Tapasin and the PLC facilitate loading of peptide cargo onto empty class I MHC molecules. HSV-1,2 ICP47 and HCMV US6 block TAP peptide transport, while HCMV US3 inhibits tapasin and retains class I complexes in the ER. Following receipt of peptide, the loaded class I MHC molecules travel through the secretory pathway to the cell surface. HCMV US10 delays transport of class II molecules from the ER, while VZV ORF66 and MCMV m152 retain class I MHC in the Golgi complex. HCMV US2, US11 and MHV-68 MK3 dislocate class I molecules via an unidentified ER membrane pore to the cytosol. The dislocated class I MHC heavy chains are ubiquitinated (Ub) and deglycosylated by cellular PNGase prior to proteasomal cleavage. HHV-7 U21, MCMV m6 and HHV-8 K3 redirect class I molecules from the secretory to the endolysosomal pathway for degradation. HHV-8 K5 likewise targets class I MHC, B7-2 and ICAM-1 molecules to the endolysosomal pathway for destruction. MCMV m4 disrupts recognition of cell surface-disposed class I MHC molecules by CD8+ T-cells. (See color plate section.)

all of which are reviewed in detail in other chapters. This section will highlight the cell biology that underlies herpesvirus evasion of T-cell immunity.

Disruption of class I MHC antigen presentation

Presentation of virus-derived antigenic peptides by major histocompatibility (MHC) class I molecules plays a key role in the clearance of many viruses from the body. Viral proteins expressed in the cytosol may be targeted for degradation and presented by class I MHC, alerting CD8+ T-cells to the presence of an intracellular viral pathogen. CD8+ lymphocytes bear the T-cell receptor (TCR), which recognizes peptides in an MHC-restricted fashion. Recognition of peptide cargo derived from foreign proteins alerts the CD8+ T-cell, and in the proper context stimulates cytotoxic T-cell (CTL) mediated lysis of the infected target cell. Though sacrificing the host cell, lysis ultimately limits the spread of the viral pathogen (Heemels and Ploegh, 1995). Interference with the class I pathway appears to be a central mechanism of immuno-evasion of persistent viruses, herpesviruses in particular (Tortorella et al., 2000). All human herpesviruses examined thus far employ strategies to perturb class I MHC antigen presentation to CD8+ T-cells (Fig. 62.1, Table 62.1).

Class I MHC molecules are heterotrimeric complexes that consist of a heavy chain, light chain and antigenic peptide (Heemels and Ploegh, 1995). The class I MHC heavy chain is a 43-kDa polymorphic type I membrane glycoprotein that binds antigenic peptide cargo, generally of 8–10 residues in length. The heavy chain α1 and α2 domains form the peptide-binding groove, consisting of two antiparallel α-helices and an eight-stranded β-sheet (Bjorkman et al., 1987). The class I MHC light chain, or β-2 microglobulin, is an invariant 12-kDa protein of the immunoglobulin (Ig) fold family.

Class I MHC peptide ligands are primarily generated in the cytosol by the 26S proteasome, a barrel-shaped multicatalytic threonine protease complex whose 20S core is composed of α and β subunits. The β subunits, x, y and z, contain the protease active sites with tryptic, chymotryptic and caspase-like protease activities, respectively (Voges et al., 1999). Upon Interferon-γ (IFN-γ) stimulation, LMP-2, LMP-7 and MECL-1 replace the x, y, and z subunits, respectively, giving rise to the immunoproteasome. IFN-γ also induces expression of the 11S proteasome regulator PA28αβ. The mammalian MHC complex encodes the LMP2 and LMP7 subunits (Brown et al., 1991). While the proteasome and immunoproteasome have substrate specificity, the immunoproteasome may generate peptides with motifs suitable for class I MHC presentation at higher frequency (Nazif and Bogyo, 2001).

Interference with proteasomal proteolysis

Both human CMV (HCMV) and murine CMV (MCMV) can disrupt immunoproteasome formation (Khan et al., 2004). MCMV appears to achieve this phenotype via its M27 gene-product. M27 targets STAT2, a key molecule in the IFN-γ signal transduction pathway, for degradation by the ubiquitin-proteasome pathway. Deletion of M27 restores fibroblast immunoproteasome formation and enhances sensitivity to IFN-γ in cell culture (Khan et al., 2004). MCMV mutants that lack functional M27 activity are attenuated in growth and virulence (Abenes et al, 2001), a phenotype that is partially restored in IFN-γ receptor knockout mice (Zimmermann, 2005). M27 is conserved in all γ-herpsevirinae; the homologous HCMV UL27 remains poorly characterized, though HCMV UL27 deletion mutants likewise display attenuated growth in culture and in vivo (Prichard et al., 2006).

EBV and CMV encode factors that disrupt proteasomal proteolysis of specific substrates. Vigorous CD8+ T-cell responses can be detected against all EBV nuclear antigens, except EBNA-1, which eludes T-cell recognition (Khanna et al., 1995). EBNA-1 is essential for viral genome persistence during cell division and is a major protein expressed during latency (Lee et al., 2004). Although EBNA-1 specific CD8+ T-cells can be isolated from peripheral blood of EBV-infected individuals, they are less abundant than T-cells specific for other EBV nuclear antigens. Further, EBNA-1-specific T-cells generally fail to be activated during EBV infection (Khanna et al., 1995; Blake et al., 1997). This stealth behavior has been attributed to the unusually long EBNA-1 half-life, enabled by the presence of its internal Gly–Ala repeat domain (GAr). The GAr domain is reported to act as a cis-inibitor of ubiquitin-proteasomal proteolosis in B cells, and thereby prevents the introduction of EBNA peptides into the class I pathway. The GAr domain is both necessary and sufficient for altering protein half-life, and cytosolic fusion proteins that harbor GAr motifs gain resistance to proteasomal proteolysis (Dantuma et al., 2002). For instance, fusion of a 200-residue or even 17-residue Gly–Ala repeat to EBNA-4 confers resistance to proteasome degradation and results in reduced antigen presentation of EBNA-4 epitopes (Dantuma et al. 2002). Several mechanisms have been proposed to explain the inhibitory function of the GAr domain, for instance the formation of tightly-folded beta-sheet structures that resist disassembly and/or interactions with the ubiquitin-proteasomal pathway. GAr also reduce the rate of EBNA-1

Table 62.1. Human herpesvirus immuno-evasins of adaptive T-cell immunity discussed in the chapter

Virus	Immuno-evasin	Putative mechanism
HSV 1/2		
	ICP47	Blocks TAP peptide transport
	Unknown	CD83 internalization and inhibition of DC function.
	Unknown	Inhibition of DC cell maturation
	US1	Kinase activity inhibits CD4+ T-cell activation by B cells
	US3	Kinase activity inactivates (stuns) CTLs in trans
	Unknown	Intracellular redistribution of class II MHC molecules
VZV		
	?ORF66	Retains class I in the Golgi complex
	Unknown	Inhibition of DC function, down-regulation of multiple surface proteins
	Unknown	Reduction of cell surface ICAM-1 (CD54)
	Unknown	Inhibition of Jak/STAT expression, disruption of IFN-γ signaling
EBV		
	EBNA-1	Gly-Ala repeat domain blocks proteasomes in cis
	BCRF1	IL-10 homologue, down-regulates class I expression
	General	Anchor residue mutations prevent epitope presentation by subset of class I alleles (epitope loss)
	Gp25-gp42-gp85	Inhibits DC maturation
	Unknown	Inhibition of monocyte phagocytic function
	LMP-2A	Activates env superantigen, may dysregulate CD4+ T cell responses
	gp42	Inhibits class II MHC recognition by CD4+ T-cells
CMV		
	Pp65 (UL83	Kinase activity blocks proteasomal proteolysis of IE-1
	US2	Targets folded class I and class II molecules for proteasome degradation
	US3	Inhibits tapasin, retains folded class I and class II molecules in the ER
	US6	Blocks TAP peptide transport
	US8	Binds free class I heavy chains, function unknown
	US10	Delays egress of folded class I molecules from ER
	US11	Targets class I heavy chains for proteasome degradation via a Derlin-1 pathway
	UL18	class II homologue, binds to LIR-1 (ILT-2) inhibitory receptor on APCs, lymphocytes
	UL111A	IL-10 homologue, downregulates class I expression
	UL111.5A	IL-10 homologue, expressed during latency
	M27, ?UL27	Targets STAT2 for degradation, impairs immunoprotasome formation
	Unknown	Interference with DC activity and expression of multiple DC surface proteins, including CD83
	UL20	TCR-γ chain homologue, function unknown
	Unknown	Targets Jak1 for proteasomal degradation, disrupts IFN-γ upregulation of class II MHC expression
	Unknown	Alters trafficking of class II MHC molecules
HHV-6		
	Unknown	Down-regulation of TCR/CD3 expression
HHV-7		
	U21	Targets class I for lysosomal degradation
HHV-8		
	K3/MIR1	Induces rapid internalization of cell surface class I
	K5/MIR2	Induces rapid internalization of cell surface class I, ICAM-1, and B7-2, and PE-CAM

translation (Dantuma et al., 2002). Nonetheless, EBNA-1 peptides can circumvent GAr blockade at a low level via defective ribosomal products (DriPs), misfolded polypeptides that result from errors in translation or folding. DriPs are rapidly degraded and may contribute a significant percentage of all peptides to the class II pathway. Thus, DriPs that do not contain functional GAr sequences should be susceptible to proteasomal degradation, and CD8+ T-cell recognition of EBNA-1 derived peptides have now been described (Lee et al., 2004; Tellam et al., 2004; Voo et al., 2004).

The HCMV matrix phosphoprotein 65 (pp65) can disrupt antigen presentation of epitopes derived from immediate-early protein 1 (IE1) in trans. The pp65 kinase can phosphorylate IE1, and through an unknown mechanism, prevent the proteasomal degradation of IE1 (Gilbert et al., 1996).

Interference with peptide transport

Empty class I MHC molecules receive their peptide cargo shortly after assembly in the endoplasmic reticulum (ER). Empty class I molecules are generally short-lived, and are either retained within the ER or dissociate (Heemels and Ploegh, 1995). Thus, antigenic peptides must be pumped across the ER membrane to reach nascent class I complexes, and this process represents a key control point in the class I MHC biosynthetic pathway. Peptide transport is accomplished by a dedicated MHC-encoded ATP-binding cassette (ABC) family member, the transporter associated with antigen presentation (TAP) (Neefjes et al., 1993). TAP molecules are heterodimers formed by the association of TAP-1 and TAP-2 subunits, which together comprise the peptide-binding site. Peptide substrates, optimally 8–12 residues in length, interact with TAP in two distinct phases: ATP-independent binding; subsequent ATP-dependent peptide transport versus rapid dissociation from TAP (Heemels and Ploegh, 1995).

Several human herpesviruses have convergently evolved polypeptides that inhibit TAP peptide transport. HSV-1 and HSV-2 encode a cytosolic 9-kDa (88 residues HSV-1; 86 residues HSV-2) immediate early gene product, called infected-cell protein 47 (ICP47) (York et al., 1994; Hill et al., 1995). The HSV-1 and HSV-2 ICP47 molecules demonstrate 47% amino acid sequence identity and appear to utilize the same mechanism. ICP47 of both HSVs binds to TAP with high affinity ($K_D = 50$ nM) at a site that overlaps the peptide binding site of both TAP subunits, and functions as a competitive inhibitor of TAP-peptide interactions (Ahn et al., 1997; Tomazin et al., 1998; Pfander et al., 1999). 100- to 1000-fold molar excess of peptide is required to overcome ICP47 inhibition of TAP peptide-transport (Tomazin et al., 1998). ICP47 functions in a species-specific fashion and inhibits human, but not murine, TAP. Residues 3–34 of ICP47 are sufficient to inhibit TAP transport, even when a synthetic 32-mer is added to permeablized cells (Galocha et al., 1997; Neumann et al., 1997; Tomazin et al., 1998).

Preliminary nuclear magnetic resonance structural characterization suggests that ICP47 undergoes a conformational change from an unstructured state in solution to the formation of a helix-turn-helix motif in the presence of a lipid environment (Pfander et al., 1999). The lipid environment greatly increases binding affinity of ICP47 with TAP, where ICP47's amino-terminal helix serves as a membrane anchor (Aisenbray, 2006). How ICP47 itself avoids transport and ATP-induced dissociation remains unclear, but it may rely on interactions outside the TAP peptide binding site to stabilize its cytosolic localization (Galocha et al., 1997). Further understanding of ICP47 function requires structural analysis of the TAP-ICP47 complex.

Apparently despite 100-fold lower affinity for murine TAP, ICP47 deletion mutants nonetheless exhibit reduced neurovirulence in a murine infection model, a phenotype that required the presence of CD8+ T-cells (Goldsmith et al., 1998). Akin to its use by HSV, ICP47 may also at some point be used in clinical applications. Indeed, several groups have explored ICP47 immuno-evasion in applications ranging from gene therapy to xenotransplantation (Berger et al., 2000; Crew and Phanavanh, 2003; Radosevich et al., 2003).

HCMV likewise disrupts TAP transport, though by a distinct approach. The HCMV US genome region encodes a cluster of immuno-evasins that comprise the US2, US6 and US11 glycoprotein families (the US2–US11 gene products) (Britt and Mach, 1996). At least six of these ten gene-products are now known to interact with the class I MHC biosynthetic pathway. HCMV US6 is a 21-kD ER-resident type I integral membrane glycoprotein that is expressed during the late phase of viral infection. US6 interferes with TAP by binding with micromolar affinity to the ER-lumenal face of the transporter. The ER-lumen domain of US6 is necessary and necessary for TAP inhibition (Ahn et al., 1997; Kyritsis et al., 2001). US6 does not appear to function as a competitive inhibitor of TAP peptide transport, and US6 neither influences the amount of peptides that bind to TAP nor the TAP-peptide affinity (Kyritsis et al., 2001). Rather, US6 reduces TAP1 affinity for ATP and may thereby cut off the energy source for peptide transport (Hewitt et al., 2001).

How do interactions with the ER lumen between US6 and TAP influence the cytosolic nucleotide-binding domain? Though presently awaiting experimental confirmation, US6 likely induces a conformational rearrangement that is transmitted to the TAP cytoplasmic ATP-binding site (Hewitt et al., 2001; Kyritsis et al., 2001). Indeed, US6 affects the conformational stability of TAP. In the presence of either US6 or ATP, TAP remains stable at 37 °C, whereas the isolated heterodimer would normally dissociate (Hewitt et al., 2001). Taken together, US6 appears to either lock TAP in a conformational intermediate of its catalytic cycle, or may induce an aberrant conformation. Similarly, recombinant HSV engineered to express other class I MHC immunoevasins cause increased viral burden in the CNS (Orr, 1995). Additional herpesvirinae-encoded TAP inhibitors have recently been discovered, including Epstein–Barr BNLF2a (Ressing, 2005 and Wiertz, E.J., personal communication).

Herpesviruses encode multiple cytokines (virokines) that alter antiviral immunity (reviewed in other chapters). Both EBV and CMV encode homologues of interleukin-10 (IL-10) that retain some, but not all IL-10 functions. Both EBV and CMV IL-10 suppress class I surface levels *in vitro*, including via downmodulation of TAP1 expression and therefore ER peptide transport (Zeidler *et al.*, 1997; Spencer *et al.*, 2002; Jenkins *et al.*, 2004).

Interference with ER chaperones required for class I biosynthesis

Class I MHC molecules are assembled in a multistep process. ER chaperones, including the lectins calreticulin and calnexin, and the thioreductase ERp57 facilitate folding of nascent class I molecules (Cresswell, 2000). The heavy chain/β-2 microglobulin heterodimer is then recruited to the peptide loading complex (PLC), a multiprotein assembly that that includes TAP and facilitates peptide loading (Cresswell, 2000). The ER-resident molecule tapasin is uniquely dedicated to class I molecule assembly. Tapasin tethers empty class I molecules to TAP and also possesses peptide exchange activity, optimizing the class I peptide repertoire by selecting for high affinity class I-peptide complexes (Momburg and Tan, 2002).

The human cytomegalovirus has evolved a mechanism to subvert the interaction between tapasin and empty class I molecules that await peptide cargo. US3, expressed during the immediate-early period of HCMV infection, is 23-kDa type I integral membrane capable of oligomerization (Jones *et al.*, 1996; Misaghi *et al.*, 2004). US3 binds directly to both class I molecules and tapasin, and causes ER-retention of class I via two mechanisms. First, the US3 ER lumenal domain contains a retention sequence that is distinct from the canonical KDEL or KKXX ER-retention motifs. The US3 residues Ser-58, Glu-63, and Lys-64 are required for ER-retention and may interact with an ER-resident protein, such as tapasin (Lee *et al.*, 2003; Misaghi *et al.*, 2004). US3 may retain class I molecules in the ER via direct association, in effect physically preventing class I molecules from traveling along the secretory pathway to the cell surface (Lee *et al.*, 2003; Misaghi, *et al.*, 2004). Interestingly, both the US3 ER-lumenal and transmembrane domains are required to bind class I molecules, and the affinity of class II binding appears to correlate with the extent of ER retention for certain alleles (Lee *et al.*, 2000; Park *et al.*, 2004). NMR structural analysis and comparison with the homologous CMV US2 gene-product (see below) suggests that the US3 ER-lumenal domain forms an Ig-like fold. Though Ig-like folds underlie many protein–protein interactions, even when present at high concentrations, the US3 ER-lumenal domain by itself does not appear to interact with class I with any measurable affinity in vitro or in vivo (Lee *et al.*, 2000; Misaghi *et al.*, 2004). Thus, the transmembrane domain does not appear to simply increase US3 local concentration by confining it to the plane of the ER membrane. Although the structural mechanism by which both the soluble and transmembrane domains are required for class I binding remains unclear, interactions within the lipid bilayer underlie the activity of several herpesvirus class I immuno-evasins.

US3 has a short half-life and associates with class I molecules only transiently. Perhaps the dominant mechanism of US3 function instead results from its direct inhibition of tapasin-dependent peptide loading (Park *et al.*, 2004). Reminiscent of US6 activity, US3 may induce a conformational change in tapasin and thereby alter tapasin-induced peptide loading and exchange activity. A subset of class I alleles do not require tapasin for peptide loading and surface expression, and these class II molecules largely escape US3-mediated ER retention (Park *et al.*, 2004). An alternatively spliced form of US3 lacking the transmembrane domain can associate with tapasin, but not class I MHC molecules, and acts as an endogenous dominant negative inhibitor of US3 function (Shin, 2006). The truncated US3 isoform may modulate US3 function across different cell types or different stages of infection, though the role of truncated US3 isoforms during infection awaits further characterization.

Perhaps US3 evolved dual mechanisms for class I retention to cope with the extensive heavy chain sequence and structural polymorphism present in a given outbred human population. Though no other human herpesviruses are known to inhibit ER chaperones, the murine herpesvirus γ-68 K3 gene product and adenovirus E19 likewise exploit tapasin to interfere with class I molecule assembly (Bennett *et al.*, 1999; Lybarger *et al.*, 2003).

Destruction of class I molecules via proteasomal proteolysis

Herpesviruses appear to have studied cellular pathways that control protein turnover and craftily manipulate multiple such pathways to reduce the abundance of the class I MHC molecule on the cell surface. One such pathway, utilized by HCMV and murine γ-herpesvirus-68, requires proteasomal proteolysis itself to break down newly synthesized class II molecules.

During the early period of HCMV infection, the ER-resident US2 and US11 gene-products are expressed with β, or delayed early kinetics. US2 and US11 independently bind to class I molecules undergoing assembly and rapidly target their ER dislocation, the rapid transfer from the ER to the cytosol. Once in the cytosol, class I heavy chains are deglycosylated by a cellular N-glycanase and then degraded. Via emerging pathways that resemble cellular quality control pathways, US2 and US11 trick the cell into recognizing nascent class I molecules as misfolded proteins and selectively accelerate the rate constant of the dislocation reaction (Wiertz et al., 1996a,b).

US2 is a 199-residue type I integral membrane protein, with an amino-terminal ER-lumenal domain comprised of an Ig-like fold, a single transmembrane domain, and a short carboxyterminal cytoplasmic tail (Gewurz et al., 2001a). Although it targets a population of newly synthesized ER-resident class all I molecules for degradation, US2 recognizes a class I surface that apparently arises late in the biosynthesis and assembly of class I molecules in the ER (Gewurz et al., 2001a). SiRNA-mediated knockdown of β2-microglobulin light chain expression blocks US2 association with and the dislocation of class I MHC molecules (Blom et al., 2004). Recombinant US2 likewise associates with the folded class I, and not with the free class I heavy chains in vitro (Gewurz et al., 2001b). Interactions between the US2 and class I ER-lumenal domains are required for subsequent removal of class I molecules from the ER: mutation of a single class I residue at the US2-binding site abrogates dislocation (Gewurz et al., 2001a).

US2 associates with the class I MHC heavy chain at the junction between the peptide-binding cleft and the α3 domain. The class I binding surface recognized by US2 has several important properties. US2 chooses a relatively conserved surface on the highly polymorphic class I molecule, allowing it to interact with many class I alleles (Gewurz et al., 2001a, b). The sequence of class I peptide cargo does not influence US2 binding, and US2 likely also binds with empty class I molecules awaiting receipt of peptide, as would be the case when US2 and US6 are coexpressed (Gewurz et al., 2001a, b). Further, the proposed binding surface for the peptide-loading complex maps to a face of the class I MHC molecule opposite that of the US2 binding site. Thus, US2 should have access to class I even when associated with the multisubunit PLC, and so diminishes the probability of class I molecule escape from the ER.

NK-cells scan for the loss of class I surface expression, providing an important back-up function, as cells without class I MHC are no longer recognized by CD8+ T-cells. Upon recognition of cells that have lost surface expression of class I molecules, in particular the HLA-C, -E and -G locus products, NK cytotoxic activity is stimulated (Lanier, 2003). In contrast, NK cell inhibitory receptors specific for these class I loci restrain NK-cell activity against host cells with surface disposed class I MHC molecules. Interestingly, the US2 ER-lumenal domain dictates binding to class I molecules in a locus-specific fashion (Gewurz et al., 2001b). US2, and perhaps by a similar mechanism US11, downregulates HLA-A and HLA-B, but not HLA-C, HLA-E molecules (Schust et al., 1998; Furman et al., 2000; Barel et al., 2003). Such locus specificity may allow HCMV to selectively diminish antigen presentation to CD8+ T-cells, which rely heavily on HLA-A and HLA-B products, whereas NK-cell inhibitory receptors predominantly recognize HLA-C, HLA-E and HLA-G molecules. Further highlighting this dichotomy, the signal peptide of HCMV UL40 supplies a peptide ligand for HLA-E in a TAP-independent fashion, assuring that loaded HLA-E complexes can travel to the cell surface even during the expression of US2, US6 or US11 (Tomasec et al., 2000).

US2 association does not significantly alter the conformation of the class I molecule (Gewurz, et al., 2001a). How then does US2 initiate the dislocation of class I molecules from the ER? Though important molecular details of the US2 pathway remain to be elucidated, it appears likely that US2 recruits cellular factors following association with class I MHC. The US2 Ig-like fold has multiple additional binding surfaces that could associate with additional ER-resident proteins, for example the loops between its beta-strands that by analogy mediate immunoglobulin and TCR binding to antigens (CDR loops) (Gewurz et al., 2001a). Alternatively, the US2 cytoplasmic tail is required for dislocation and may also interact with cytosolic or membrane proteins (Furman et al., 2002). The intramembrane-cleaving protease, signal peptide peptidase associates with US2 and is required for dislocation of the class I MHC complex from the ER (Loureiro, 2006).

US2 triggers the mono-, di- and triubiquitination of folded molecules (Furman et al., 2003). However, removal of all lysine residues from the class I cytoplasmic tail does not prevent dislocation (ubiquitination is not thought to occur in the oxidizing environment of the ER) (Furman et al., 2003). A ubiquitin-independent step must therefore initiate dislocation, with ubiquitin attachment occurring either on the class I cytoplasmic tail, or on an ER-lumenal lysine residue following dislocation. Alternatively, ubiquitination of cellular machinery involved in assembly of the dislocation complex may be required to initiate class I MHC removal from the ER. Recombinant class I MHC molecules that lack lysine residues continue to be dislocated by US11, but not US2, even though CMV immuno-evasins require the activity of cellular E1 ubiquitin activating enzymes for US2-mediated dislocation (Hassink, 2006). Once in the cytosol, class I molecules are deglycosylated by cellular enzyme peptide: N-glycanase (PNGase or PNG1) (Blom et al., 2004). N-glycanase cleaves the β-aspartyl-glucosamine bond of glycans attached to Asn residues. The products of the N-glycanase reaction are a free oligosaccharide and a peptide containing an Asp residue at the site of hydrolysis (formerly an Asn). The class I heavy chain is then rapidly degraded by the proteasome. Deglycosylation precedes proteasomal degradation, as siRNA-mediated knock-down of PNGase expression in US2+ cells results in the accumulation of glycosylated class I heavy chains in the cytosol (Blom et al., 2004).

US2 binds to the folded class I complex with micromolar affinity, and the recombinant US2-HLA-A2 complex is sufficiently stable to survive consecutive size exclusion and ion exchange chromatography steps. The stability of the complex raises the question of whether it must be disassembled prior to exit from the ER (Gewurz et al., 2001a, b). If so, dissociation would require ER machinery that has yet to be identified. Rather, experimental evidence increasingly suggests that US2 dislocates intact class I MHC molecules. Chimeric class I MHC molecules bearing an ER-lumenal green fluorescence protein (GFP) undergo US2- and US11-mediated ER dislocation (as evidenced by the Asn-to-Asp sequence conversion that accompanies PNGase-mediated removal of the N-linked glycan, previously attached in the ER) (Fiebiger et al., 2002). Fluorescent, deglycosylated intermediates can be recovered from the cytosol and imply that the GFP moiety traversed the membrane in a folded state. Likewise, chimeric class I MHC molecules with an appended ER-lumenal dihydrofolate reductase (DHFR) domain, a tightly folded moiety of considerable size, undergo dislocation by US2 and US11. Again, deglycosylated class I heavy chains with a folded DHFR can be retrieved from the cytosol (Tirosh et al., 2003).

Which ER membrane pore might accommodate a complex of folded molecules? Preliminary experiments implicated the Sec61 pore in ER dislocation, a membrane complex that allows insertion of secretory and membrane proteins into the ER during their biosynthesis (Wiertz et al., 1996a,b). However, it has been difficult to identify a complex between Sec61 and proteins undergoing dislocation. Importantly, the glycosylated US2–class I complex would not likely be accommodated by the Sec61 translocon, given the strict upper limit of the pore diameter suggested by the structure of the analogous archea SecY complex. Physiological measurements of the Sec61 translocon itself also suggest that a folded US2-class I complex would not be allowed through (Hamman et al., 1997; Van den Berg et al., 2004). By analogy with the US11 pathway (see below), an unidentified pore most likely accommodates the US2–class II MHC complex.

US11 is a 215-residue ER-resident glycoprotein that is homologous with US2. US11 likewise directs the degradation of class I MHC heavy chains within minutes of their synthesis (Wiertz et al., 1996a,b). US11 induces the expression of X-box binding protein 1 (XBP-1), a key transcription factor that regulates the unfolded protein response (UPR) pathway. XBP-1 expression coincides with that of US11 in human cytomegalovirus infected foreskin fibroblasts, and the UPR appears to facilitate US11-medicated degradation of class I MHC (Tirosh, 2005). In the presence of US11, polyubiquitinated conjugates are affixed to class II heavy chains, in a fashion that appears to be independent of their tertiary structure. Whereas US2 causes addition of 1–3 ubiquitin moieties only to folded class II molecules, US11 attacks unfolded class I heavy chains and folded class I molecules alike. Ubiquitination is required for the US11 ER dislocation reaction (Kikkert et al., 2001; Shamu et al., 2001; Furman et al., 2003). Cells that express both US11 and a temperature-sensitive mutant of the E1 ubiquitin-activating enzyme demonstrate normal US11-mediated degradation of class I molecules at permissive temperatures. However, upon shift to non-permissive temperatures, the class I heavy chains remain within the ER (Kikkert et al., 2001). Isopeptide linkage between the ε-amino group of target proteins and ubiquitin residue 48 slates multiple proteins for proteasomal destruction, and likewise appears required for extraction of the class I heavy chain from the ER membrane in the US11 pathway (Flierman et al., 2003; Varadan et al., 2004). US11 may direct the ubiquitin-conjugating enzyme E2-25K, perhaps along with the E3 ligases MARCHVII/axotrophin or gp78, to attach polyubiquitin conjugates to class I MHC (Flierman, 2006).

Whereas the US11 cytoplasmic tail is dispensable for its function, the US11 transmembrane domain plays an active role in dislocation (Furman et al., 2002; Lilley et al., 2003). US11 Gln-192 is required for interactions with host proteins within the plane of the membrane, in particular Derlin-1 (Lilley and Ploegh, 2004). Derlin-1 is a recently identified homologue of yeast Der1p, an ER membrane protein that is required for the degradation of a subset of misfolded yeast ER proteins (Knop et al., 1996). A Derlin-1 dominant-negative mutant prevents US11-, but not US2-mediated class I dislocation (Lilley and Ploegh, 2004). The integral membrane protein VIMP associates with Derlin-1 and recruits a complex of cytosolic proteins, the cytosolic p97 ATPase (also known as VCP, or CDC48 in yeast) and its cofactor complex Ufd1-Npl4 (Ye et al., 2001, 2004). A complex containing US11, ubiquitinated class I heavy chain, Derlin-1, VIMP, and p97 has been detected (Ye et al., 2004; Lilley, 2005). Further, p97 activity is required for US11-mediated heavy chain retro-translocation (Ye et al., 2001, 2004). The P97–Ufd1–Npl4 complex recognizes proteins undergoing ER retro-translocation and provides the driving force for protein movement into the cytosol (Ye et al., 2001). Thus, P97 captures MHC heavy chains marked by US11 for disposal, and following poly-ubiquitination, extracts them from the ER membrane. The multiple membrane spanning Derlin-1 interacts with class I heavy chains both before and immediately after dislocation to the cytosol. Perhaps in concert with accessory proteins, Derlin-1 may comprise the exit channel utilized by the US11 pathway (Lilley and Ploegh, 2004; Ye et al., 2004). A dominant negative Derlin-1 mutant blocks US11-, but not US2-dependent degradation of class I molecules (Lilley and Ploegh, 2004).

The apparent redundancy of US2 and US11 appears to contradict the general parsimony of viral genomes brought about by selective pressure. Yet, US2 and US11 are present in the genomes of multiple clinical HCMV isolates (Erica Mayer, Rebecca Tirabassi and Hidde Ploegh, data unpublished). Retention of both US2 and US11 may benefit CMV in several fashions. The two immuno-evasins utilize distinct dislocation pathways, and perhaps maximize the number of complexes that can be extruded during a given time. Since US2 and US11 recognize distinct intermediates in class I assembly, perhaps US2 serves an editing function and catches proteins missed by US11 (it is known whether for example US11 can bind to class I molecules occupied by PLC). Alternatively, either pathway may be preferred in a given cell type, a notion that is supported by experimental data from HCMV infection of human dendritic cells and from analogous MCMV inhibitors of class I (Hengel et al., 2000; Rehm et al., 2002). Finally, the distinct US2 and US11 binding sites on class I allow US2 and US11 to target distinct subsets of class I alleles and thereby counter class I polymorphism (Machold et al., 1997; Gewurz et al., 2001a,b; Barel et al., 2003). The MCMV immuno-evasins likewise bind class I molecules in an allele-specific fashion and cooperatively prevent antigen presentation to a variety of CTL clones (Kavanagh et al., 2001a,b).

The murine γ-herpesvirus-68 evolved a distinct pathway for proteasomal proteolysis of ER-resident class I molecules. The MK3 locus encodes an E3 ubiquitin ligase that directs the ubiquitination of the class I MHC cytosolic tail. MK3 forms a multiprotein complex with class I molecules, tapasin and TAP, and targets properly folded class II molecules during the peptide loading stage (Lybarger et al., 2003). Association with tapasin/TAP appears to determine the class I allele-specificity (Wang et al., 2004). Although initially characterized as a member of the plant homeodomain/leukemia-associated protein (PHD/LAP) family, a recent solution structure of the MK3 cytosolic domain reveals it to be a variant member of the RING domain family (Dodd et al., 2004). RING motifs are 8 kDa zinc-binding domains that serve as adaptors for E2 ligases. RING domains do not generally possess their own enzymatic function, but instead provide substrate selectivity by directing E2 ubiquitin ligase activity (Freemont, 2000). The MK3 ring domain associates with cellular ubiquitin-conjugating enzymes UBCH5A-C and UBCH13, which have previously been shown to function in concert with cellular RING domain proteins. MK3 ubiquitination of the class I MHC molecule stimulates its removal from the ER (Bartee et al., 2004). Akin to US11, MK3 requires the cellular proteins Derlin-1 and AAA-ATPase p97 for dislocation (Wang, 2006).

Disruption of the class I secretory pathway

Following receipt of peptide cargo, stable class II complexes exit the ER and traverse the Golgi en route to the cell surface. Herpesviruses once again a specific step in class I molecule biosynthesis, interfering with export of class I molecules. The HCMV US10 gene-product encodes a type I integral membrane glycoprotein that associates with class I molecules and delays egress of the class I MHC molecules from the ER (Furman et al., 2002). The mechanism of US10 action remains uncertain. While US10 expression does not appear to alter the kinetics of class II MHC molecule degradation by US2 or US11, perhaps US10 serves to retard class I molecule egress from the ER and thereby minimize the probability that class I molecules escape US2/11 mediated degradation. For instance, at the onset of the early period of viral infection, US2 and US11 likely encounter a large population of class I molecules retained by US3 during the IE period.

HCMV US8 encodes a 26-kDa type I membrane glycoprotein that partially co-localizes with markers of the endolysosomal pathway. Although US8 associates with free class I MHC heavy chains within the ER, the significance of US8 association has not been fully elucidated: US8 expression does not appear to alter the maturation of class I products in cellular transfectants (Tirabassi and Ploegh, 2002). It remains possible that US8 exerts its effect on class II trafficking in concert with other CMV immuno-evasins. Indeed, such cooperative activity has been observed with the MCMV class II inhibitors m4 and m152 (Kavanagh et al., 2001a,b). The MCMV m152 gene-product (gp40) blocks the export of class I from an ER-Golgi intermediate compartment (ERGIC) (Ziegler et al., 2000). Although the mechanism remains to be fully defined, m152-mediated class I molecule retention does not require the m152 cytoplasmic tail or transmembrane domains. Further, class I molecules continue to be retained in the secretory pathway after the complex dissociates (Ziegler et al., 2000). The m4 gene-product forms biochemically distinct complexes with differential stabilities with class I molecules in the presence and absence of m152 (Kavanagh et al., 2001a,b).

Cell surface expression of class I molecules is reduced upon VZV infection, an effect that has been observed in both human T-cells in the SCID-hu thymus/liver mouse model and in skin biopsy specimens (Abendroth et al., 2001a,b; Nikkels et al., 2004). Microscopic and biochemical experiments demonstrate the accumulation of class I MHC molecules in the Golgi compartment in VZV-infected cells (Abendroth et al., 2001a,b). The ORF66 gene-product is expressed during the early period of virus infection and serves to retain class I molecules in the Golgi complex. Cellular transfectants that express ORF66 demonstrate reduced cell surface expression of class I MHC (Abendroth et al., 2001a,b). The molecular mechanism by which VZV halts class I in the Golgi has yet to be fully elucidated. The UL49.5 gene-product of several varicelloviruses including bovine herpesvirus I, pseudorabies virus, and equine herpesvirus 1, though not of varicella zoster, blocks the TAP peptide transporter through conformational arrest and subsequent proteasomal degradation (Koopers-Lalic, 2005).

Rerouting of class I molecules from the Golgi to the endolysosomal pathway

The human herpesvirus 7 (HHV-7) interferes with the class I MHC antigen presentation via the U21 gene product. U21 is a 55-kDa integral membrane glycoprotein that associates tightly with folded class I molecules within the ER, shortly after class I molecule biosynthesis (Hudson et al., 2001). Although the molecular affinity remains unknown, U21 association with multiple class I alleles appears strong and survives treatment with .01% SDS in cellular extracts (Hudson et al., 2001). The complex travels at least as far as the trans-Golgi network, where U21 diverts class I to the endolysosomal pathway. class I molecules are then degraded by lysosomal proteases.

MCMV employs a similar strategy via its m6 gene product. M6 is a type I ER-resident integral membrane glycoprotein that likewise associates with class I molecules within the ER and redirects them for lysosomal destruction. M6 utilizes a dileucine sorting signal within its cytoplasmic tail to achieve relocalization to lysosomes (Reusch et al., 1999). Surprisingly, although the U21 cytoplasmic tail can likewise utilize a dileucine-like sorting motif to mediate its own intracellular sequestration, U21's cytoplasmic domain is dispensable for its function. U21 truncation mutants that lack cytoplasmic tails continue to target class I MHC molecules to lysosomes (Hudson et al., 2003). Perhaps the U21 cytoplasmic tail is required for other U21 functions, for instance retrieval of surface-disposed class I molecules?

Akin to most herpesvirus immuno-evasins of the class I pathway, U21 demonstrates no significant homology with cellular proteins. Even HHV-6 U21, with its 50% amino acid similarity to HHV-7 U21, does not appear to interact with class I MHC molecules (Hudson et al., 2001). The function of HHV-6 U21 remains to be determined.

Retrieval of cell surface class I molecules

HHV-8 relies upon two type III integral membrane proteins to perturb the class I MHC pathway during the early lytic cycle of viral replication, K3 and K5 (also called MIR-1 and MIR-2, for modulator of immune recognition) (Coscoy and Ganem, 2003). K3 and K5 function independently and utilize interactions within the lipid bilayer to recognize their targets, highlighting the skilled manipulation of cell biology co-opted by herpesviruses to subvert class I (Ishido et al., 2000; Sanchez et al., 2002). Additional cellular cofactors may be involved K3/5 recognition of class I MHC.

K3 and K5 share approximately 40% amino acid identity and are predicted to have cytoplasmic amino- and carboxy-terminal domains, two transmembrane domains, and a short ER lumenal domain (Coscoy and Ganem, 2003). Though initially characterized as a PHD/LAP domain, it appears likely that K3/K5 instead contain a variant RING domain (Scheel and Hofmann, 2003; Bartee et al., 2004; Dodd et al., 2004). Surprisingly, although they are homologous to the γ-herpesvirus 68 MK3 gene product that targets class I for ER dislocation, K3/5 instead re-route mature class I molecules to the endolysosomal pathway. Inhibition of lysosomal acidification by chloroquin or bafilomycin prevents class II molecule degradation (Fruh et al., 2002). Covalent attachment of short-ubiquitin chains can mediate multiple intracellular trafficking processes, such as endocytosis and sorting to multi-vesicular bodies (MVB). Thus, K3 and K5 appear to function as E3 ligases and thereby initiate internalization of cell surface-disposed (or perhaps recycling) class I molecules to MVBs (Coscoy and Ganem, 2003). The K5 RING domain promotes ubiquitin transfer in an ATP- and E2-dependent reaction in vitro (Coscoy et al., 2001). Disruption of the K3 RING domain prevents class I molecule internalization, even though association with class I still takes place (Hewitt et al., 2002).

The majority of K3 and K5 molecules localize to the ER. Nonetheless, class II molecules exit the ER apparently unscathed and reach the plasma membrane with normal kinetics in the presence of K3 and K5 (Coscoy and Ganem, 2003). Perhaps ubiquitination of class I cytoplasmic tails might occur while the molecules are still in the ER and thereby mark them for eventual plasma membrane internalization. Alternatively, the minority of K3 and K5 that travels along the secretory pathway may be the active population. The available experimental evidence favors the latter model (Hewitt et al., 2002; Coscoy and Ganem, 2003).

Ubiquitination of the conserved class I MHC cytoplasmic tail Lys-340 residue provides an internalization signal (Hewitt et al., 2002). Interestingly, in an apparently novel enzymatic reaction, K3 can catalyze ubiquitination of cysteine residues via thiolester bond formation. class I MHC molecules that lack lysine residues in their cytoplasmic tails undergo cysteine-ubiquitination, which is sufficient to target class I for endocytosis and degradation (Cadwell, 2005). Sorting of ubiquitinated surface membrane proteins to MVB requires the activity of multiple cellular proteins, including dynamin and tumor susceptibility gene-101 (TSG101) (Hewitt et al., 2002; Coscoy and Ganem, 2003). SiRNA-mediated knockdown of TSG101 expression prevents K3- and K5-mediated endocytosis of class I MHC molecules.

K3 subsequently directs the internalized class I molecules to lysosomes, perhaps via the concerted action of two distinct sorting motifs: a YXXφ motif (where Y represents tyrosine; X signifies any residue; φ signifies a hydrophobic residue) and a diacidic cluster region. YXXφ motifs are recognized by the adaptor protein (AP) complexes AP-1, AP-2 and AP-3, and direct trafficking into clathrin coated vesicles (Owen and Evans, 1998). The K3 Y_{152}AAV motif directs class I molecules to the *trans*-Golgi network via AP-1. The K3 diacidic cluster motif subsequently targets class I to the lysosomal compartment (Means et al., 2002). Acid cluster dileucine motifs sort proteins from the trans-Golgi network to lysosomes via cargo proteins, including the so called Golgi-localized, γ-ear-containing, ARF-binding proteins (GGAs) (Takatsu et al., 2001).

Proteasome activity also plays a key role in K3-mediated sorting of class II to the endocytic compartment, and small molecule proteasome inhibitors prevent K3-mediated delivery of class I MHC molecules to the dense endosomal compartment (Lorenzo et al., 2002). Proteasome inhibition does not appear to increase cell surface expression of class I, however. Thus, the specific mechanistic role of the proteasome in the K3 pathway remains to be determined. Once within the endosomal compartment, cysteine protease activity removes the class I cytoplasmic tail, and an aspartyl protease subsequently cleaves class I within the plane of the membrane, liberating a soluble class I MHC molecule (Lorenzo et al., 2002).

Poxviruses and several other herpesviruses also encode an immuno-evasin of the K3 family that likewise target class I molecules, suggesting a common evolutionary origin. These unrelated viruses appear to have acquired K3 and K5 from the mammalian MARCH family, a group of 9 subcellular integral membrane proteins that target glycoproteins for lysosomal destruction (Bartee et al., 2004). Like K3 and K5, MARCH IV and MARCH IX possess ubiquitin-ligase activity against the class I cytoplasmic tail and stimulate endocytosis (Bartee et al., 2004). MARCH proteins may participate in the regulation of endogenous class I surface expression, perhaps in a fashion analogous to regulation of growth factor receptors endocytosis by E3 ligases (Hicke, 2001). Interestingly, the extreme constraints on the retroviral genome may have forced HIV-1 to convergently evolve a unique approach for class I MHC inhibition via its Nef gene-product, which has no homology to MARCH proteins. Nef is a cytosolic protein that appears to promote endocytosis of class I molecules by a distinct pathway that involves cellular phosphofurin acidic cluster sorting protein-1 (PACS-1) (Piguet et al., 2000).

K3 and K5 are adjacent in the HHV-8 genome and likely arose via gene duplication. Once again, why does a herpesvirus retain homologous factors with apparently overlapping function and kinetics? As with HCMV, K3 and K5 may counteract allelic variation (albeit less prevalent among class I cytoplasmic tails) and may function to varying degrees among various cell types. Indeed, K5 significantly downmodulates HLA-A and HLA-B locus products, whereas K3 downregulates HLA-A, -B, -C and -E molecules (Ishido et al., 2000). Further, K5 targets additional proteins for endocytosis, and additional K3 targets may likewise exist. Studies of the MARCH family reveal an analogous an functional division: several MARCH proteins have a spectrum similar to K3, while a second subset more closely resemble K5 target specificity (Bartee, et al., 2004). Indeed, the RING domain of K3 can be replaced with the corresponding domain of a cellular MARCH homologue without altering K3 function (Goto et al., 2003).

Interference with class I molecules at the cell surface

The cell surface itself represents the final compartment for the inhibition of class I MHC display of antigenic peptides. Though no examples of physical interference with TCR recognition of class I/peptide complex are yet known among the human herpesviruses, MCMV m4 appears to do so. The m4 gene-product encodes a 34-kDa type I integral membrane glycoprotein (gp34) that initially associates with folded class II molecules within the ER. The m4-class II complex is then exported to the cell surface. Where M4 may sterically hinder TCR association the class I MHC–peptide complex. m4 thereby blocks antigen presentation at the cell surface to $K^{(b)}$-restricted clones (Kavanagh et al., 2001a,b). Cell tropism has been observed for m4 function, with greater inhibitory function present in macrophages than in fibroblasts (LoPiccolo et al., 2003), and macrophage infection with MCMV deletion mutants suggest synergistic function between its three class I immuno-evasins (LoPiccolo et al., 2003).

Interference with the immunological synapse

T-cells form stable associations with antigen presenting cells (APCs) known as the immunological synapse to facilitate cell signaling. Intracellular adhesion molecule-1 (ICAM-1, or CD54) is a member of the Ig-superfamily and plays a key role in stable synapse formation, binding tightly to its T cell counter-receptor, LFA-1. ICAM-1 represents another cellular target of K5 and, like class I, is re-routed for lysosomal degradation, apparently by the same pathway (Ishido et al., 2000; Coscoy et al., 2001). Reduction of ICAM-1 cell surface expression has been observed on infected keratinocytes from skin biopsy specimen of VZV-infected patients (Nikkels et al., 2004). HHV-8 infection also leads to the downregulation of PE-CAM (CD31) surface expression, and may even occur during the latent stage of infection (Tomescu et al., 2003).

Interference with costimulation

Interactions between numerous cell surface receptors tightly regulate the context of T-cell activation to restrain the production of T-cell toxins. Along with recognition of an MHC–peptide complex, initial T-cell activation requires simultaneous, costimulatory signals from the APC. Interactions between costimulatory molecules and their counter-receptors present an additional step in T-cell activation that herpesviruses disrupt.

Professional APCs express the costimulatory molecules B7-1 and B7-2, which independently can provide an important second signal for T-cell activation. HHV-8 K5 and murine-γ68 MK3 perturb this control point of adaptive immunity. Both K5 and MK3 target B7-2 molecules for degradation, apparently by the same pathways utilized for class I degradation (Ishido et al., 2000; Coscoy et al., 2001; Wang et al., 2004). Although B7-1 and B7-2 are both functionally and structurally similar, B7-1 lacks cytoplasmic tail lysines and escapes both K5 and MK3. Introduction of lysines into the B7-1 cytoplasmic tail confers susceptibility to K5-mediated degradation (Coscoy et al., 2001). Why should two herpesviruses destroy B7-2 and not B7-1? Perhaps such selectivity helps the virus to strike a balance with the host. For example, mice deficient in both B7 molecules have a more profound immunodeficiency than those lacking B7-2 alone (Borriello et al., 1997). Inhibition of just B7-2 may enable the establishment of persistent infection but limit damage to its host. Indeed, MCMV encodes a class I-like molecule that likewise may function to reduce host damage. The m157 gene-product encodes a class I-like NK-cell ligand that allows control of MCMV acute infection. Strains whose NK cells fail to recognize this CMV-encoded ligand do not survive acute infection, whereas persistent infection is established only in strains whose NK cells control acute viremia (Arase et al., 2002; Bubic et al., 2004).

Though at first glance downmodulation of B7-2 appears unique to gamma-herpesviruses, the targeting of B7 molecules was most likely usurped from the mammalian genome. Several MARCH proteins, including MARCH I, MARCH II and MARCH VIII (c-MIR) likewise target B7-2, apparently by the same pathway (Goto et al., 2003; Bartee et al., 2004). Further, a subset of MARCH proteins (IV and IX) target class II, whereas others (I and VIII) target both B7-2 and class II, reminiscent of K3 and K5, respectively (Bartee et al., 2004). The K5 gene-product targets PE-CAM for lysosomal degradation, apparently via the same pathway described previously for disposal of class I MHC molecules by K5 (Mansouri, 2006).

Interference with APC function

Dendritic cells (DCs) are professional antigen-presenting cells that play a crucial role in stimulation of adaptive T-cell responses. Multiple members of the human herpesvirus family decrease the capacity of DC to stimulate T-cells.

HCMV infects a subset of DCs and disrupts their activity. HCMV-infected DCs demonstrate reduced capability to stimulate T cell proliferation and cytotoxicity, a phenotype that has been attributed to pleiotropic effects on the DC. These include reduced surface expression of multiple proteins (including class I MHC and II, B7-1 and B7-2 and CD40) as well as reduced capacity to secrete stimulatory cytokines and a functional unresponsiveness to maturation stimuli (Hertel et al., 2003). Monocyte-derived DCs infected with HCMV do not migrate toward several lymphoid chemokines, potentially delaying the kinetics of primary CD8+ T-cell activation (Moutaftsi et al., 2004). Functional paralysis of multiple DC functions has likewise been observed following MCMV infection of DCs (Andrews et al., 2001). Further, VZV infection of mature dendritic cells causes downregulation of a similar subset of cell surface molecules (Morrow et al., 2003). Infection of DCs can even facilitate VZV dissemination and support infection of T-cells themselves (Abendroth et al., 2001). VZV-infected T-lymphocytes play an important role in supporting persistent viremia.

HSV-1 can infect immature DCs and inhibit their maturation (Kobelt et al., 2003). EBV infection of monocytes can similarly prevent their development into dendritic cells, an activity that is observed even with UV-inactivated virion. The trimolecular gp25-gp42-gp85 complex appears to exert this inhibitory activity via interactions with class II MHC at the monocyte membrane (Li et al., 2002). EBV-infected monocytes also demonstrate significantly reduced phagocytic activity, though the mechanism remains incompletely understood (Savard et al., 2000).

HSV also interferes with DC function by perturbing CD83, a 45-kD cell surface adhesion molecule important for DC interaction with T-cells. Within hours after HSV infection, CD83 cell surface expression is significantly reduced, a phenotype that has been attributed to re-routing of CD83 molecules to the endolysosomal pathway. The molecular mechanism, including the responsible HSV factor(s), remains to be determined (Kruse et al., 2000). However, a similar reduction in DC CD83 surface disposition during CMV infection has been attributed to TGF-β expression by HCMV-infected fibroblasts (Arrode et al., 2002).

HSV-1 infection of B cells strongly inhibits their ability to stimulate CD4+ T-cells (Barcy and Corey, 2001). The immediate-early HSV US1 gene-product ICP22 is both necessary and sufficient for this phenotype, by an unknown mechanism.

Stunning of Cytotoxic T-cell activity

HSV-1 infection of target cells appears to exert an inhibitory effect *in trans* on CTLs. Inactivated, or stunned, CTL are transiently incapable of cytokine synthesis or cytotoxic granule release in response to TCR ligation (Sloan et al., 2003). The phenomenon requires close cell–cell contact between CTL and the HSV-infected target cell (Sloan et al., 2003), and HSV penetration into T-cells.

Though no *de novo* viral transcription or translation is required, the TCR signal transduction cascade is inhibited at the level of the linker for activation of T cells (LAT). Through an uncharacterized mechanism, HSV infection reduces LAT phosphoryation (Sloan, 2006).

CTL escape mutants

EBV, like other herpesviruses, is a genetically stable virus. Nonetheless, mutations occur at low frequency, and may allow EBV to adapt to populations where a particular class I MHC allele or haplotype prevails. For example, mutations that affect class I binding (anchor residues) are regularly detected in HLA-A11 epitopes of South East Asia EBV isolates, where greater than 50% of the population expresses HLA-A11. In contrast, HLA-A11 epitope loss is much less common in central African isolates, where HLA-A11 is absent (de Campos-Lima et al., 1993).

Ligation of inhibitory receptors

HCMV and MCMV each encode a viral class I MHC molecule homologue. The HCMV UL18 molecule forms a complex with β2-microglobulin and peptide, and is exported to the cell surface. Interestingly, UL18 is resistant to the activity of the HCMV class I immuno-evasins (Park et al., 2002). Rather than presenting antigenic peptide to CD8+ T-cells, UL18 binds tightly to LIR-1 (ILT2, or CD85), an inhibitory receptor expressed on monocytes, dendritic cells and lymphocytes (Willcox et al., 2003). UL18 binds to LIR1 with >1000-fold higher affinity than the association between class I MHC and LIR1 (Willcox et al., 2003). Though it is not yet clear to what extent UL18 modifies lymphocyte function, the widespread expression pattern of LIR-1 suggests that UL18 may potentially alter multiple steps in T-cell activation.

Inhibition of T-cell receptor signaling

Several herpesviruses alter the interaction between APC and T-cells from within T-lymphocytes. The lymphotropic HHV-6A has been reported to reduce expression of the TCR/CD3 complex on the transcriptional level, with transcriptional downregulation of multiple components of the T-cell receptor signaling apparatus. An HHV-6 factor expressed during the late stage of virus infection has been implicated (Lusso et al., 1991). HCMV UL20 encodes a protein with amino acid sequence similarity to both the constant and variable regions of the T-cell receptor γ chain (Beck and Barrell, 1991). Further studies are required to elucidate the role of the putative HCMV TCR γ homologue.

Though not yet observed among the lymphotropic human herpesviruses, the Herpesvirus saimiri (HVS) interferes with downstream components of the TCR signal transduction pathway. The HVS Tip (tyrosine kinase–interacting protein) gene-product interferes with early signaling events of the TCR signal transduction pathway (Cho et al., 2004). Tip constitutively localizes to lipid rafts, where it binds to the SH3 domain of Lck, a member of the Src tyrosine kinase family. Tip interacts also with endosomal protein 80 and induces endosomal vesicle formation, thus sequestering Lck. Tip may also interfere with T-cell signaling by promoting the internalization of lipid rafts (Cho et al., 2004b).

Erroneous T-cell activation

EBV infection transactivates the env gene, a superantigen encoded by the human endogenous retrovirus HERV-K18. LMP-2 activity is sufficient for env induction at the transcriptional level (Sutkowski *et al.*, 2001). Env preferentially activates the TCR Vβ13 subset of CD4+ T-cells (Sutkowski *et al.*, 2001). While it remains to be determined if env transactivation supports EBV immuno-evasion or is incidental, it is noteworthy that superantigen activity can deregulate the establishment of specific immunity. In a more direct fashion, MCMV primes the development of CD8+ T-cells specific for virus epitopes that are not presented in relevant tissues, where they are hidden by immuno-evasin activity (Holtappels *et al.*, 2004).

Disruption of class II MHC antigen presentation

The class II MHC antigen presentation pathway presents antigenic peptides derived from the extracellular compartment to CD4+ T-cells. Whereas class II MHC molecules are expressed by most nucleated cells, class II expression is largely restricted to APC, such as DC, monocyte/macrophages, and B-cells, though immune cytokines can induce class II expression on a variety of other cell types. APC deliver pathogens (or material derived from pathogens) via phagocytosis or receptor-medicated endocytosis into the endolysosomal pathway for destruction (Denzin and Cresswell, 1995).

Class II MHC molecules are heterotrimeric complexes that contain the class II α and β chains, and an antigenic peptide. There are three class II loci: DP, DQ and DR. The class II αβ heterodimer undergoes folding within the ER and associates with an accessory protein called the invariant chain (Ii). Ii prevents class II peptide loading within the ER, and by virtue of a dileucine motif within its cytoplasmic tail, shuttles the nascent class II molecules through the TGN to the lysosomal compartments (Wubbolts and Neefjes, 1999). Ii is degraded within the lysosomal compartment, where the class II molecules encounter peptide-fragments produced by lysosomal proteolysis of internalized material. The MHC-encoded HLA-DM molecule then catalyzes exchange of the class II-bound Ii peptide called CLIP with higher affinity, lysosomally-derived peptide ligands. Peptide-loaded class II molecules are exported to the cell surface for antigen presentation to CD4+ T-cells. Not surprisingly, herpesviruses manipulate antigen presentation by the class II MHC pathway as well.

Interference with class II expression

The expression of class II MHC molecules is under the control of both constitutive and inducible elements (Boss 1997). Class II is constitutively expressed on APCs, activated T-cells, and thymic epithelial cells, whereas a subset of cells upregulate class II MHC expression in an IFN-γ dependent fashion. In response to IFN-γ, the Jak/STAT signaling pathway is activated and translates the IFN-γ signal into transcriptional responses. Stat1α activity upregulates expression of the class II transcriptional activator CIITA, which in turn drives the expression of class II molecules (Boss, 1997). Fibroblasts, endothelial and epithelial cells all upregulate CIITA in response to IFN-γ (Boss, 1997).

HCMV interferes with the IFN-γ pathway of class II upregulation by several distinct mechanisms. During the immediate-early and early phases of virus infection, an HCMV factor targets JAK1 to the proteasome (Miller *et al.*, 1998). MCMV also interferes with IFN-γ upregulation of class II transcription, though apparently does not involve STAT1α perturbation (Heise *et al.*, 1998). Also, as mentioned earlier, MCMV M27 targets STAT2 for protosomal degradation. VZV also interferes with Jak/STAT signaling, apparently by the inhibition of Jak/STAT2 protein synthesis (Abendroth and Arvin, 2001).

Manipulation of class II molecules

The HLA-DR-α and HLA-DM-α molecules are targeted for proteasomal degradation in cells that are engineered to overexpress HCMV US2 (Tomazin, *et al.*, 1999). US3 has also been shown to interact with class II molecules and to retain them in the ER (Chevalier and Johnson, 2003). The observation that HLA-DRα and HLA-DMα are targeted for degradation by US2 is not readily explained by the structural data from the US2-HLA-A2 complex, as the class I binding surface recognized by US2 is not conserved on class II molecules (Gewurz *et al.*, 2001). Thus, it appears likely that a different US2 binding site is required for the downmodulation of class II MHC molecules. Likewise, though tapasin plays a key role in US3 interactions with class I molecules, tapasin is not known to interact with class II MHC complexes. Perhaps US3 might interact with the invariant chain in an analogous fashion in its class II pathway? Alternatively, US3 may also use a different mechanism altogether to retain class II molecules in the ER. In any case, it will be interesting to determine whether US2 and US3 alter the class II pathway in HCMV-infected cells.

HCMV has also been reported to alter trafficking of class II molecules within infected cells, causing the retention of vesicles bearing class II molecules in an aberrant perinuclear distribution (Cebulla *et al.*, 2002). A similar effect of HCMV has been observed in latently infected cells, where a block in protein trafficking causes the accumulation of class II molecules in intracellular vesicles. The responsible HCMV factor(s) have not been identified, but do not involve the US2–11 gene products (Slobedman *et al.*, 2002). Murine infection models demonstrate HSV-mediated intracellular redistribution of class II MHC molecules within the CNS (Lewandowski et al., 1993). Further studies are required to better define the biology underlying this observation.

The EBV BZLF2 gene-product (gp42) is a 42-kDA type II integral membrane glycoprotein that binds to class II MHC molecules. BZLF2 has been reported to interfere with CD4+ T-cell activation (Spriggs et al., 1996). Gp42 is known to associate with class II MHC molecules to facilitate EBV entry into B cells. The molecular structure of the gp42–class II MHC complex has been determined, and gp42 belongs to the C-type lectin family and has homology with a family of human NK-cell receptors that bind to class II MHC (Mullen et al., 2002).

gp42 occurs in two forms, including a soluble form generated by proteolytic cleavage within the ER. Soluble gp42 is secreted, and may inhibit cell surface class II MHC recognition by CD4+ T-cells. Secreted gp42 was detected during EBV lytic replication (Ressing, 2005).

Conclusions

Selective pressure exerted by adaptive immunity has led herpesviruses to convergently evolve a surprising number of immuno-evasins that specifically dysregulate T-cell responses. Even so, numerous herpesvirus gene-products have yet to be ascribed functions, in particular factors required for growth in vivo but dispensable for growth in cell culture. Further mechanisms of T-cell evasion by herpesviruses are sure to be discovered. Multiple herpesvirus-encoded micro-RNAs have been discovered, and may well serve as immunoevasins, as has been described for other viruses (Sullivan, 2005). With the set of immuno-evasins better defined, an ongoing challenge will be to define the specific role of T-cell immuno-evasins during the various stages of the herpesvirus lifecycle. An enhanced understanding of how herpesviruses solve the immunological puzzles faced during primary infection, dissemination, establishment of latency, reactivation, and sporadic shedding will be a challenging, though important endeavor. Such knowledge should directly lead to the development of novel antiviral agents, vaccines, gene therapy, and permit the application of immuno-evasins themselves to immunological disease states outside of viral biology.

Acknowledgments

We would like to acknowledge Amy Hudson for help with the figure.

REFERENCES

Abendroth, A. and Arvin, A. M. (2001). Immune evasion as a pathogenic mechanism of varicella zoster virus. Semin. Immunol., 13(1), 27–39.

Abendroth, A., Lin, I., Slobedman, B. et al. (2001a). Varicella-zoster virus retains major histocompatibility complex class II proteins in the Golgi compartment of infected cells. J. Virol., 75(10), 4878–4888.

Abendroth, A., Morrow, G., Cunningham, A. L. et al. (2001b). Varicella-zoster virus infection of human dendritic cells and transmission to T cells: implications for virus dissemination in the host. J. Virol., 75(13), 6183–6192.

Abenes, G., Lee, M., Haghjoo, E. et al. (2001). Murine cytomegalovirus open reading frame M27 plays an important role in growth and virulence in mice. J. Virol., 75(4), 1697–1707.

Ahn, K., Gruhler, A., Galocha, B. et al. (1997). The ER-luminal domain of the HCMV glycoprotein US6 inhibits peptide translocation by TAP. Immunity, 6(5), 613–621.

Aisenbrey, C., Sizun, C., Koch, J. et al. (2006). Structure and dynamics of membrane-associated ICP47, a viral inhibitor of the MHC I antigen processing machinery. J. Biol. Chem. Epub.

Andrews, D. M., Andoniou, C. E., Granucci, F. et al. (2001). Infection of dendritic cells by murine cytomegalovirus induces functional paralysis. Nat. Immunol., 2(11), 1077–1084.

Arase, H., Mocarski, E. S., Campbell, A. E. et al. (2002). Direct recognition of cytomegalovirus by activating and inhibitory NK cell receptors. Science, 296(5571), 1323–1326.

Arrode, G., Boccaccio, C., Abasrado, J. P. et al. (2002). Cross-presentation of human cytomegalovirus pp65 (UL83) to CD8+ T cells is regulated by virus-induced, soluble-mediator-dependent maturation of dendritic cells. J. Virol., 76(1), 142–150.

Barcy, S. and Corey, L. (2001). Herpes simplex inhibits the capacity of lymphoblastoid B cell lines to stimulate CD4+ T cells. J. Immunol., 166(10), 6242–6249.

Barel, M. T., Ressing, M., Pizzato, N. et al. (2003). Human cytomegalovirus-encoded US2 differentially affects surface expression of class II MHC locus products and targets membrane-bound, but not soluble HLA-G1 for degradation. J. Immunol., 171(12), 6757–6765.

Bartee, E., Mansouri, M., Hovey Nerenburg, B. T. et al. (2004). Downregulation of major histocompatibility complex class II by human ubiquitin ligases related to viral immune evasion proteins. J. Virol., 78(3), 1109–1120.

Beck, S. and Barrell, B. (1991). An HCMV reading frame which has similarity with both the V and C regions of the TCR gamma chain. DNA Seq, 2(1), 33–38.

Bennett, E. M., Bennink, J. R., Yewdell, J. W. et al. (1999). Cutting edge: adenovirus E19 has two mechanisms for affecting class II MHC expression. J. Immunol., 162(9), 5049–5052.

Berger, C., Xuereb, S., Johnson, D. C. et al. (2000). Expression of herpes simplex virus ICP47 and human cytomegalovirus US11 prevents recognition of transgene products by CD8(+) cytotoxic T lymphocytes. J. Virol., 74(10), 4465–4473.

Biron, C. A., Byron, K. S., and Sullivan, J. L. (1989). Severe herpesvirus infections in an adolescent without natural killer cells. *N. Engl. J. Med.*, **320**(26), 1731–1735.

Bjorkman, P. J., Saper, M. A., Samraoni, B. et al. (1987). Structure of the human class II histocompatibility antigen, HLA-A2. *Nature*, **329**(6139), 506–512.

Blake, N., Lee, S., Redchenko, I. et al. (1997). Human CD8+ T cell responses to EBV EBNA1: HLA class II presentation of the (Gly-Ala)-containing protein requires exogenous processing. *Immunity*, **7**(6), 791–802.

Blom, D., Hirsch, C., Stern, P. et al. (2004). A glycosylated type I membrane protein becomes cytosolic when peptide: N-glycanase is compromised. *EMBO. J.*, **23**(3), 650–658.

Borriello, F., Sethna, M. P., Boyd, S. D. et al. (1997). B7-1 and B7-2 have overlapping, critical roles in immunoglobulin class switching and germinal center formation. *Immunity*, **6**(3), 303–313.

Boss, J. M. (1997). Regulation of transcription of class II MHC genes. *Curr. Opin. Immunol.*, **9**(1), 107–113.

Britt, W. J. and Mach, M. (1996). Human cytomegalovirus glycoproteins. *Intervirology*, **39**(5–6), 401–412.

Brown, M. G., Driscoll, J., and Monaco, J. J. (1991). Structural and serological similarity of MHC-linked LMP and proteasome (multicatalytic proteinase) complexes. *Nature*, **353**(6342), 355–357.

Bubic, I., Wagner, M., Krmpotic, A. et al. (2004). Gain of virulence caused by loss of a gene in murine cytomegalovirus. *J. Virol.*, **78**(14), 7536–7544.

Cadwell, K. and Coscoy, L. (2005). Ubiquitination on nonlysine residues by a viral E3 ubiquitin ligase. *Science* **309**(5731), 127–130.

Cebulla, C. M., Miller, D. M., Zhang, Y. et al. (2002). Human cytomegalovirus disrupts constitutive class II MHC expression. *J. Immunol.*, **169**(1), 167–176.

Chevalier, M. S. and Johnson, D. C. (2003). Human cytomegalovirus US3 chimeras containing US2 cytosolic residues acquire major histocompatibility class II and II protein degradation properties. *J. Virol.*, **77**(8), 4731–4738.

Cho, N. H., Feng, P., Lee, S. H. et al. (2004a). Inhibition of T cell receptor signal transduction by tyrosine kinase-interacting protein of Herpesvirus saimiri. *J. Exp. Med.*, **200**(5), 681–687.

Cho, N. H., Wingston, D., Chang, N. et al. (2004b). Association of herpesvirus Saimiri Tip is essential for downregulation of T-cell receptor and CD4 coreceptor. *J. Urol.*, **80**(1), 108–118.

Coscoy, L. and Ganem, D. (2003). PHD domains and E3 ubiquitin ligases: viruses make the connection. *Trends Cell Biol.*, **13**(1), 7–12.

Coscoy, L., Sanchez, D. J., and Ganem, D. (2001). A novel class of herpesvirus-encoded membrane-bound E3 ubiquitin ligases regulates endocytosis of proteins involved in immune recognition. *J. Cell. Biol.*, **155**(7), 1265–1273.

Cresswell, P. (2000). Intracellular surveillance: controlling the assembly of MHC class I-peptide complexes. *Traffic*, **1**(4), 301–305.

Crew, M. D. and Phanavanh, B. (2003). Exploiting virus stealth technology for xenotransplantation: reduced human T cell responses to porcine cells expressing herpes simplex virus ICP47. *Xenotransplantation*, **10**(1), 50–59.

Dantuma, N. P., Sharipo, A., and Masucci, M.G. (2002). Avoiding proteasomal processing: the case of EBNA1. *Curr. Top. Microbiol. Immunol.*, **269**, 23–36.

de Campos-Lima, P. O., Gavioli, R., Zhang, Q. J. et al. (1993). HLA-A11 epitope loss isolates of Epstein–Barr virus from a highly A11+ population. *Science*, **260**(5104), 98–100.

Denzin, L. K. and Cresswell, P. (1995). HLA-DM induces CLIP dissociation from class II MHC alpha beta dimers and facilitates peptide loading. *Cell*, **82**(1), 155–165.

Dodd, R. B., Allen, M. D., Brown, S. E. et al. (2004). Solution structure of the kaposi's sarcoma-associated herpesvirus K3 N-terminal domain reveals a novel E2-binding C4HC3-type RING domain. *J. Biol. Chem.*

Fiebiger, E., Story, C., Ploegh, H. L. et al. (2002). Visualization of the ER-to-cytosol dislocation reaction of a type I membrane protein. *EMBO. J.*, **21**(5), 1041–1053.

Flierman, D., Ye, Y., Dai, M. et al. (2003). Polyubiquitin serves as a recognition signal, rather than a ratcheting molecule, during retrotranslocation of proteins across the endoplasmic reticulum membrane. *J. Biol. Chem.*, **278**(37), 34774–34782.

Flierman, D., Coleman, C. S., Pickart, C. M. et al. (2006). E2-25K mediates US11-triggered retro-translocation of class II MHC heavy chains in a permeabilized cell system. *Proc Natl Acad Sci* **103**(31), 11589–11594.

Freemont, P. S. (2000). RING for destruction? *Curr. Biol.*, **10**(2), R84–R87.

Fruh, K., Bartee, E., Gouveia, K. et al. (2002). Immune evasion by a novel family of viral PHD/LAP-finger proteins of gamma-2 herpesviruses and poxviruses. *Virus Res.*, **88**(1–2), 55–69.

Furman, M. H., Ploegh, H. L., and Schust, D. J. (2000). Can viruses help us to understand and classify the class II MHC molecules at the maternal-fetal interface? *Hum. Immunol.*, **61**(11), 1169–1176.

Furman, M. H., Ploegh, H. L., and Tortorella, D. (2002). Membrane-specific, host-derived factors are required for US2- and US11-mediated degradation of major histocompatibility complex class II molecules. *J. Biol. Chem.*, **277**(5), 3258–3267.

Furman, M. H., Loureiro, J., Ploegh, H. L. et al. (2003). Ubiquitinylation of the cytosolic domain of a type I membrane protein is not required to initiate its dislocation from the endoplasmic reticulum. *J. Biol. Chem.*, **278**(37), 34804–34811.

Galocha, B., Hill, A., Barnett, B.C. et al. (1997). The active site of ICP47, a herpes simplex virus-encoded inhibitor of the major histocompatibility complex (MHC)-encoded peptide transporter associated with antigen processing (TAP), maps to the NH2-terminal 35 residues. *J. Exp. Med.*, **185**(9), 1565–1572.

Gewurz, B. E., Gaudet, R., Tortorella, D. et al. (2001a). Antigen presentation subverted: Structure of the human cytomegalovirus protein US2 bound to the class II molecule HLA-A2. *Proc. Natl Acad. Sci. USA*, **98**(12), 6794–6799.

Gewurz, B. E., Wang, E. W., Tortorella, D. et al. (2001b). Human cytomegalovirus US2 endoplasmic reticulum-lumenal domain dictates association with major histocompatibility complex class II in a locus-specific manner. *J. Virol.*, **75**(11), 5197–5204.

Gilbert, M. J., Riddell, S. R., Plachter, B. *et al.* (1996). Cytomegalovirus selectively blocks antigen processing and presentation of its immediate-early gene product. *Nature*, **383**(6602), 720–722.

Goldsmith, K., Chen, W., Johnson, D.C. *et al.* (1998). Infected cell protein (ICP)47 enhances herpes simplex virus neurovirulence by blocking the CD8+ T cell response. *J. Exp. Med.*, **187**(3), 341–348.

Goto, E., Ishido, S., Ohgimoto, S. *et al.* (2003). c-MIR, a human E3 ubiquitin ligase, is a functional homolog of herpesvirus proteins MIR1 and MIR2 and has similar activity. *J. Biol. Chem.*, **278**(17), 14657–14668.

Hamman, B. D., Chen, J. C., Johnson, E. E. *et al.* (1997). The aqueous pore through the translocon has a diameter of 40–60 A during cotranslational protein translocation at the ER membrane. *Cell*, **89**(4), 535–544.

Hassink, G. C., Barel, M. T., Van Voorden, S. B. *et al.* (2006). Ubiquitination of class II MHC heavy chains is essential for dislocation by human cytomegalovirus-encoded US2 but not US11. *J. Biol Chem.* July, 2006 (in press, epublication)

Heemels, M. T. and Ploegh, H. (1995). Generation, translocation, and presentation of MHC class I-restricted peptides. *Annu. Rev. Biochem.*, **64**, 463–491.

Heise, M. T., Connick, M., and Virgin, H. W. 4th (1998). Murine cytomegalovirus inhibits interferon gamma-induced antigen presentation to CD4 T cells by macrophages via regulation of expression of major histocompatibility complex class II-associated genes. *J. Exp. Med.*, **187**(7), 1037–1046.

Hengel, H., Reusch, U., Geginat, G. *et al.* (2000). Macrophages escape inhibition of major histocompatibility complex class I-dependent antigen presentation by cytomegalovirus. *J. Virol.*, **74**(17), 7861–7868.

Hertel, L., Lacaille, V. G., Strobl, H. *et al.* (2003). Susceptibility of immature and mature Langerhans cell-type dendritic cells to infection and immunomodulation by human cytomegalovirus. *J. Virol.*, **77**(13), 7563–7574.

Hewitt, E. W., Gupta, S. S., Mufti, D. *et al.* (2001). The human cytomegalovirus gene product US6 inhibits ATP binding by TAP. *EMBO J.*, **20**(3), 387–396.

Hewitt, E. W., Duncan, L., Mufti, D. *et al.* (2002). Ubiquitylation of class II MHC by the K3 viral protein signals internalization and TSG101-dependent degradation. *EMBO J.*, **21**(10), 2418–2429.

Hicke, L. (2001). A new ticket for entry into budding vesicles-ubiquitin. *Cell*, **106**(5), 527–530.

Hill, A., Jugovic, P. *et al.* (1995). Herpes simplex virus turns off the TAP to evade host immunity. *Nature*, **375**(6530), 411–415.

Holtappels, R., Podlech, J., York, I. *et al.* (2004). Cytomegalovirus misleads its host by priming of CD8 T cells specific for an epitope not presented in infected tissues. *J. Exp. Med.*, **199**(1), 131–136.

Hudson, A. W., Howley, P. M., and Ploegh, H. L. (2001). A human herpesvirus 7 glycoprotein, U21, diverts major histocompatibility complex class II molecules to lysosomes. *J. Virol.*, **75**(24), 12347–12358.

Hudson, A. W., Blom, D., Howley, P. M. *et al.* (2003). The ER-lumenal domain of the HHV-7 immunoevasin U21 directs class II MHC molecules to lysosomes. *Traffic*, **4**(12), 824–837.

Ishido, S., Choi, J. K., Lee, B. S. *et al.* (2000). Inhibition of natural killer cell-mediated cytotoxicity by Kaposi's sarcoma-associated herpesvirus K5 protein. *Immunity*, **13**(3), 365–374.

Janeway, C. A., Jr. and Medzhitov, R. (2002). Innate immune recognition. *Annu. Rev. Immunol.*, **20**, 197–216.

Jenkins, C., Abendroth, A., and Slobedman, B. (2004). A novel viral transcript with homology to human interleukin-10 is expressed during latent human cytomegalovirus infection. *J. Virol.*, **78**(3), 1440–1447.

Jones, T. R., Wiertz, E. J., Sun, L. *et al.* (1996). Human cytomegalovirus US3 impairs transport and maturation of major histocompatibility complex class II heavy chains. *Proc. Natl Acad. Sci. USA*, **93**(21), 11327–11333.

Kavanagh, D. G., Gold, M. C., Wagner, M. *et al.* (2001a). The multiple immune-evasion genes of murine cytomegalovirus are not redundant: m4 and m152 inhibit antigen presentation in a complementary and cooperative fashion. *J. Exp. Med.*, **194**(7), 967–978.

Kavanagh, D. G., Koszinowski, U. H., and Hill, A. B. (2001b). The murine cytomegalovirus immune evasion protein m4/gp34 forms biochemically distinct complexes with class I MHC at the cell surface and in a pre-Golgi compartment. *J. Immunol.*, **167**(7), 3894–3902.

Khan, S., Zimmermann, A., Bassler, M. *et al.* (2004). A cytomegalovirus inhibitor of gamma interferon signaling controls immunoproteasome induction. *J. Virol.*, **78**(4), 1831–1842.

Khanna, R., Burrows, S. R., Steigerwald-Mullen, P. M. *et al.* (1995). Isolation of cytotoxic T lymphocytes from healthy seropositive individuals specific for peptide epitopes from Epstein–Barr virus nuclear antigen 1: implications for viral persistence and tumor surveillance. *Virology*, **214**(2), 633–637.

Kikkert, M., Hassink, G., Barel, M. *et al.* (2001). Ubiquitination is essential for human cytomegalovirus US11-mediated dislocation of class I MHC molecules from the endoplasmic reticulum to the cytosol. *Biochem. J.*, **358**(2), 369–377.

Knop, M., Finger, A., Brawn, T. *et al.* (1996). Der1, a novel protein specifically required for endoplasmic reticulum degradation in yeast. *EMBO. J.*, **15**(4), 753–763.

Kobelt, D., Lechmann, M., and Steinkasserer, A. (2003). The interaction between dendritic cells and herpes simplex virus-1. *Curr. Top. Microbiol. Immunol.*, **276**, 145–161.

Koopers-Lalic, D., Reits, E. A., Ressing, M. E. *et al.* (2005). Varicelloviruses avoid T cell recognition by UL49.5-mediated inactivation of the transporter associated with antigen processing. *Proc. Natl. Acad. Sci.* **102**(14): 5144–9.

Kruse, M., Rosorius, O., Kratzer, F. *et al.* (2000). Mature dendritic cells infected with herpes simplex virus type 1 exhibit inhibited T-cell stimulatory capacity. *J. Virol.*, **74**(15), 7127–7136.

Kyritsis, C., Gorbulev, S., Hutschenreiter, S. *et al.* (2001). Molecular mechanism and structural aspects of transporter associated with antigen processing inhibition by the cytomegalovirus protein US6. *J. Biol. Chem.*, **276**(51), 48031–48039.

Lanier, L. L. (2003). Natural killer cell receptor signaling. *Curr. Opin. Immunol.*, **15**(3), 308–314.

Lee, S., Park, B., and Ahn, K. (2003). Determinant for endoplasmic reticulum retention in the luminal domain of the human cytomegalovirus US3 glycoprotein. *J. Virol.*, **77**(3), 2147–2156.

Lee, S., Yoon, J., Park, B. *et al.* (2000). Structural and functional dissection of human cytomegalovirus US3 in binding major histocompatibility complex class II molecules. *J. Virol.*, **74**(23), 11262–11269.

Lee, S. P., Brooks, J. M., Al-Jarrah, H. *et al.* (2004). CD8 T cell recognition of endogenously expressed Epstein–Barr virus nuclear antigen 1. *J. Exp. Med.*, **199**(10), 1409–1420.

Lewandowski, G. A., Lo, D., and Bloom, F. E. *et al.* (1993). Interference with major histocompatibility complex class II-restricted antigen presentation in the brain by herpes simplex virus type 1: a possible mechanism of evasion of the immune response. *Proc. Natl Acad. Sci. USA*, **90**(5), 2005–2009.

Li, L., Liu, D., Fletcher, L. *et al.* (2002). Epstein–Barr virus inhibits the development of dendritic cells by promoting apoptosis of their monocyte precursors in the presence of granulocyte macrophage-colony-stimulating factor and interleukin-4. *Blood*, **99**(10), 3725–3734.

Lilley, B. N. and Ploegh, H. L. (2004). A membrane protein required for dislocation of misfolded proteins from the ER. *Nature*, **429**(6994), 834–840.

Lilley, B. N. and Ploegh, H. L. (2005). Multiprotein complexes that link dislocation, ubiquitination, and extraction of misfolded proteins from the endoplasmic reticulum membrane. *Proc. Natl Acad. Sci.*, **102**(40), 14296–14301.

Lilley, B. N., Tortorella, D., and Ploegh, H. L. (2003). Dislocation of a type I membrane protein requires interactions between membrane-spanning segments within the lipid bilayer. *Mol. Biol. Cell.*, **14**(9), 3690–3698.

LoPiccolo, D. M., Gold, M. C., Kavanaugh, G. D. *et al.* (2003). Effective inhibition of K(b)- and D(b)-restricted antigen presentation in primary macrophages by murine cytomegalovirus. *J. Virol.*, **77**(1), 301–308.

Lorenzo, M. E., Jung, J. U., and Ploegh, H. L. (2002). Kaposi's sarcoma-associated herpesvirus K3 utilizes the ubiquitin–proteasome system in routing class major histocompatibility complexes to late endocytic compartments. *J. Virol.*, **76**(11), 5522–5531.

Loureiro, J., Lilley, B. N., Spooner, E. *et al.* (2006). Signal peptide peptidase is required for dislocation from the endoplasmic reticulum. *Nature* **441**(7095), 894–897.

Lusso, P., Malnati, M., De Maria, A. *et al.* (1991). Productive infection of CD4+ and CD8+ mature human T cell populations and clones by human herpesvirus 6. Transcriptional down-regulation of CD3. *J. Immunol.*, **147**(2), 685–691.

Lybarger, L., Wang, X., Harris, M. R. *et al.* (2003). Virus subversion of the class II MHC peptide-loading complex. *Immunity*, **18**(1), 121–130.

Machold, R. P., Wiertz, E. J., Jones, T. R. *et al.* (1997). The HCMV gene products US11 and US2 differ in their ability to attack allelic forms of murine major histocompatibility complex (MHC) class II heavy chains. *J. Exp. Med.*, **185**(2), 363–366.

Mansouri, M., Douglas, J., and Rose, P. P. (2006). Kaposi's sarcoma herpesvirus K5 eliminates CD31/PECAM from endothelial cells. *Blood* in press e-publication.

McClain, K., Gehrz, R., Grierson, H. *et al.* (1988). Virus-associated histiocytic proliferations in children. Frequent association with Epstein–Barr virus and congenital or acquired immunodeficiencies. *Am. J. Pediatr. Hematol. Oncol.*, **10**(3), 196–205.

Means, R. E., Ishido, S., Alvarez, X. *et al.* (2002). Multiple endocytic trafficking pathways of class II MHC molecules induced by a Herpesvirus protein. *EMBO J.*, **21**(7), 1638–1649.

Medzhitov, R. and Janeway, C. A. Jr. (1999). Innate immune induction of the adaptive immune response. *Cold Spring Harb. Symp. Quant. Biol.*, **64**, 429–435.

Miller, D. M., Rahill, B. M., Boss, J. M. *et al.* (1998). Human cytomegalovirus inhibits major histocompatibility complex class II expression by disruption of the Jak/Stat pathway. *J. Exp. Med.*, **187**(5), 675–683.

Misaghi, S., Sun, Z. Y., Stern, P. *et al.* (2004). Structural and functional analysis of human cytomegalovirus US3 protein. *J. Virol.*, **78**(1), 413–423.

Momburg, F. and Tan, P. (2002). Tapasin-the keystone of the loading complex optimizing peptide binding by class I MHC molecules in the endoplasmic reticulum. *Mol. Immunol.*, **39**(3–4), 217–233.

Morrow, G., Slobedman, B., Cunningham, A. L. *et al.* (2003). Varicella-zoster virus productively infects mature dendritic cells and alters their immune function. *J. Virol.*, **77**(8), 4950–4959.

Moutaftsi, M., Brennan, P., Spector, S. A. *et al.* (2004). Impaired lymphoid chemokine-mediated migration due to a block on the chemokine receptor switch in human cytomegalovirus-infected dendritic cells. *J. Virol.*, **78**(6), 3046–3054.

Mullen, M. M., Haan, K. M., Longnecker, R. *et al.* (2002). Structure of the Epstein–Barr virus gp42 protein bound to the class II MHC receptor HLA-DR1. *Mol. Cell.*, **9**(2), 375–385.

Nazif, T. and Bogyo, M. (2001). Global analysis of proteasomal substrate specificity using positional-scanning libraries of covalent inhibitors. *Proc. Natl Acad. Sci. USA*, **98**(6), 2967–3972.

Neefjes, J. J., Momburg, F., and Hammerling, G. J. (1993). Selective and ATP-dependent translocation of peptides by the MHC-encoded transporter. *Science*, **261**(5122), 769–771.

Neumann, L., Kraas, W., Uebel, S. *et al.* (1997). The active domain of the herpes simplex virus protein ICP47: a potent inhibitor of the transporter associated with antigen processing. *J. Mol. Biol.*, **272**(4), 484–492.

Nikkels, A. F., Sadzot-Delvaux, C., and Pierard, G. E. (2004). Absence of intercellular adhesion molecule 1 expression in varicella zoster virus-infected keratinocytes during herpes zoster: another immune evasion strategy? *Am. J. Dermatopathol.*, **26**(1), 27–32.

Orr, M. T., Edelmann, K. H, Vieira, J. *et al.* (2005). Inhibition of class II MHC Is a Virulence Factor in Herpes Simplex Virus Infection of Mice. *PLOS Pathogens*, **1**(1), 62-71.

Owen, D. J. and Evans, P. R. (1998). A structural explanation for the recognition of tyrosine-based endocytotic signals. *Science*, **282**(5392), 1327–1332.

Park, B., Oh, H., Lee, S. *et al.* (2002). The class II MHC homolog of human cytomegalovirus is resistant to down-regulation mediated by the unique short region protein (US)2, US3, US6, and US11 gene products. *J. Immunol.*, **168**(7), 3464–3469.

Park, B., Kim, Y., Shin, J. *et al.* (2004). Human cytomegalovirus inhibits tapasin-dependent peptide loading and optimization of the class II MHC peptide cargo for immune evasion. *Immunity*, **20**(1), 71–85.

Pfander, R., Neumann, L., Zweckstetter, M. *et al.* (1999). Structure of the active domain of the herpes simplex virus protein ICP47 in water/sodium dodecyl sulfate solution determined by nuclear magnetic resonance spectroscopy. *Biochemistry*, **38**(41), 13692–13698.

Piguet, V., Wan, L., Borel, C. *et al.* (2000). HIV-1 Nef protein binds to the cellular protein PACS-1 to downregulate class II major histocompatibility complexes. *Nat. Cell. Biol.*, **2**(3), 163–167.

Prichard, M. N., Quenelle, D. C., Bidanset, D. J. *et al.* (2006). Human cytomegalovirus UL27 is not required for viral replication in human tissue implanted in SCID mice. *Virology J*, **3**, 18-20.

Radosevich, T. J., Seregina, T., Link, C. J. *et al.* (2003). Effective suppression of class II major histocompatibility complex expression by the US11 or ICP47 genes can be limited by cell type or interferon-gamma exposure. *Hum. Gene. Ther.*, **14**(18), 1765–1775.

Rehm, A., Engelsberg, A., Tortorella, D. *et al.* (2002). Human cytomegalovirus gene products US2 and US11 differ in their ability to attack major histocompatibility class II heavy chains in dendritic cells. *J. Virol.*, **76**(10), 5043–5050.

Ressing, M. E., Keating, S. E., van Leeuwen, D. *et al.* (2005.) Impaired transporter associated with antigen processing-dependent peptide transport during productive EBV infection. *J. Immunol.*, **174**(11), 6829–6838.

Ressing, M. E., van Leeuwen, D., Verreck, F. A. (2005). Epstein-Barr virus gp42 is posttranslationally modified to produce soluble gp42 that mediates HLA class II immune evasion. *J. Virol.*, **79**(2), 841–52.

Reusch, U., Muranyi, W., Lucin, P. *et al.* (1999). A cytomegalovirus glycoprotein re-routes class II MHC complexes to lysosomes for degradation. *EMBO J.*, **18**(4), 1081–1091.

Sanchez, D. J., Coscoy, L., and Ganem, D. (2002). Functional organization of MIR2, a novel viral regulator of selective endocytosis. *J. Biol. Chem.*, **277**(8), 6124–6130.

Savard, M., Belanger, C., Tardif, M. *et al.* (2000). Infection of primary human monocytes by Epstein–Barr virus. *J. Virol.*, **74**(6), 2612–2619.

Scheel, H. and Hofmann, K. (2003). No evidence for PHD fingers as ubiquitin ligases. *Trends Cell. Biol.*, **13**(6), 285–287; author reply 287–288.

Schust, D. J., Tortorella, D., and Ploegh, H. L. (1998). Trophoblast class II major histocompatibility complex (MHC) products are resistant to rapid degradation imposed by the human cytomegalovirus (HCMV) gene products US2 and US11. *J. Exp. Med.*, **188**(3), 497–503.

Shamu, C. E., Flierman, D., Ploegh, H. L. *et al.* (2001). Polyubiquitination is required for US11-dependent movement of class II MHC heavy chain from endoplasmic reticulum into cytosol. *Mol. Biol. Cell.*, **12**(8), 2546–2555.

Shin, J., Park, B. Lee, S. *et al.* (2006). A short isoform of human cytomegalovirus US3 functions as a dominant negative inhibitor of the full-length form. *J. Vir.* **80**(11), 5397–5404.

Sloan, D. D., Zahariadis, G., Posavad, C. M. *et al.* (2003). CTL are inactivated by herpes simplex virus-infected cells expressing a viral protein kinase. *J. Immunol.*, **171**(12), 6733–6741.

Sloan, D. D., Han, J. Y., Sandifer, T. K. *et al.* (2006). Inhibition of TCR signaling by herpes simplex virus. *J. Immunol.*, **176**(3), 1825–1833.

Slobedman, B., Mocarski, E. S., Arvin, A. *et al.* (2002). Latent cytomegalovirus down-regulates major histocompatibility complex class II expression on myeloid progenitors. *Blood*, **100**(8), 2867–2873.

Spencer, J. V., Lockridge, K. M., Barry, P. A. *et al.* (2002). Potent immunosuppressive activities of cytomegalovirus-encoded interleukin-10. *J. Virol.*, **76**(3), 1285–1292.

Spriggs, M. K., Armitage, R. J., Comeau, M. R. *et al.* (1996). The extracellular domain of the Epstein–Barr virus BZLF2 protein binds the HLA-DR beta chain and inhibits antigen presentation. *J. Virol.*, **70**(8), 5557–5563.

Sullivan, C. S., Grundhoff, A. T., Tevethia, S. *et al.* (2005). SV40-encoded microRNAs regulate viral gene expression and reduce susceptibility to cytotoxic T cells. *Nature*, **432**(7042), 682–686.

Sutkowski, N., Conrad, B., Thorky-Lawson, D. A. *et al.* (2001). Epstein–Barr virus transactivates the human endogenous retrovirus HERV-K18 that encodes a superantigen. *Immunity*, **15**(4), 579–589.

Takatsu, H., Katoh, Y., Shiba, Y. *et al.* (2001). Golgi-localizing, gamma-adaptin ear homology domain, ADP-ribosylation factor-binding (GGA) proteins interact with acidic dileucine sequences within the cytoplasmic domains of sorting receptors through their Vps27p/Hrs/STAM (VHS) domains. *J. Biol. Chem.*, **276**(30), 28541–28545.

Tellam, J., Connolly, G., Green, K. J. *et al.* (2004). Endogenous presentation of CD8+ T cell epitopes from Epstein–Barr virus-encoded nuclear antigen 1. *J. Exp. Med.*, **199**(10), 1421–1431.

Tirabassi, R. S. and Ploegh, H. L. (2002). The human cytomegalovirus US8 glycoprotein binds to major histocompatibility complex class II products. *J. Virol.*, **76**(13), 6832–6835.

Tirosh, B., M. Furman, H., Tortorella, D. *et al.* (2003). Protein unfolding is not a prerequisite for endoplasmic reticulum-to-cytosol dislocation. *J. Biol. Chem.*, **278**(9), 6664–6672.

Tirosh, B., Iwakoshi, N. N., Lilley B. N. et al. (2005). Human cytomegalovirus protein US11 provokes an unfolded protein response that may facilitate the degradation of class II major histocompatibility complex products. *J. Virol.*, **79**(5), 2768–2779.

Tomasec, P., Braud, V. M., Rikards, C. et al. (2000). Surface expression of HLA-E, an inhibitor of natural killer cells, enhanced by human cytomegalovirus gpUL40. *Science*, **287**(5455), 1031.

Tomazin, R., van Schoot, N. E., Goldsmith, K. et al. (1998). Herpes simplex virus type 2 ICP47 inhibits human TAP but not mouse TAP. *J. Virol.*, **72**(3), 2560–2563.

Tomazin, R., Boname, J., Hegde, N. R. et al. (1999). Cytomegalovirus US2 destroys two components of the class II MHC pathway, preventing recognition by CD4+ T cells. *Nat. Med.*, **5**(9), 1039–1043.

Tomescu, C., Law, W. K., and Keles, D. H. (2003). Surface downregulation of major histocompatibility complex class II, PE-CAM, and ICAM-1 following de novo infection of endothelial cells with Kaposi's sarcoma-associated herpesvirus. *J. Virol.*, **77**(17), 9669–9684.

Tortorella, D., Gewurz, B. E., Furman, M. H. et al. (2000). Viral subversion of the immune system. *Annu. Rev. Immunol.*, **18**, 861–926.

Van den Berg, B., Clemons, W. M., Jr., Collinson, I. et al. (2004). X-ray structure of a protein-conducting channel. *Nature*, **427**(6969), 36–44.

Varadan, R., Assfalg, M., Haririnia, A. et al. (2004). Solution conformation of Lys63-linked di-ubiquitin chain provides clues to functional diversity of polyubiquitin signaling. *J. Biol. Chem.*, **279**(8), 7055–7063.

Voges, D., Zwickl, P., and Braumeister, W. (1999). The 26S proteasome: a molecular machine designed for controlled proteolysis. *Annu. Rev. Biochem.*, **68**, 1015–1068.

Voo, K. S., Fu, T., Wang, H. Y. et al. (2004). Evidence for the presentation of major histocompatibility complex class I-restricted Epstein–Barr virus nuclear antigen 1 peptides to CD8+ T lymphocytes. *J. Exp. Med.*, **199**(4), 459–470.

Wang, X., Lybarger, L., Connors, R. et al. (2004). Model for the interaction of gammaherpesvirus 68 RING-CH finger protein mK3 with major histocompatibility complex class II and the peptide-loading complex. *J. Virol.*, **78**(16), 8673–8686.

Wang, X., Ye, Y., Lencer, W. et al. (2006). The viral E3 ubiquitin ligase mK3 uses the Derlin/p97 endoplasmic reticulum-associated degradation pathway to mediate down-regulation of major histocompatibility complex class II proteins. *J. Biol. Chem.*, **281**(13), 8636–8644.

Wiertz, E. J., Jones, T. R., Sun, L. et al. (1996a). The human cytomegalovirus US11 gene product dislocates class II MHC heavy chains from the endoplasmic reticulum to the cytosol. *Cell*, **84**(5), 769–779.

Wiertz, E. J., Tortorella, D., Bogya, M. et al. (1996b). Sec61-mediated transfer of a membrane protein from the endoplasmic reticulum to the proteasome for destruction. *Nature*, **384**(6608), 432–438.

Willcox, B. E., Thomas, L. M., and Bjorkman, P. J. (2003). Crystal structure of HLA-A2 bound to LIR-1, a host and viral major histocompatibility complex receptor. *Nat. Immunol.*, **4**(9), 913–919.

Wubbolts, R. and Neefjes, J. (1999). Intracellular transport and peptide loading of class II MHC molecules: regulation by chaperones and motors. *Immunol. Rev.*, **172**, 189–208.

Ye, Y., Meyer, H. H., and Rapoport, T. A. (2001). The AAA ATPase Cdc48/p97 and its partners transport proteins from the ER into the cytosol. *Nature*, **414**(6864), 652–656.

Ye, Y., Shibata, Y., Yun, C. et al. (2004). A membrane protein complex mediates retro-translocation from the ER lumen into the cytosol. *Nature*, **429**(6994), 841–847.

York, I. A., Roop, C., Andrew, D. W. et al. (1994). A cytosolic herpes simplex virus protein inhibits antigen presentation to CD8+ T lymphocytes. *Cell*, **77**(4), 525–535.

Zeidler, R., Eissner, G., Meissner, P. et al. (1997). Downregulation of TAP1 in B lymphocytes by cellular and Epstein–Barr virus-encoded interleukin-10. *Blood*, **90**(6), 2390–2397.

Ziegler, H., Muranyi, W., Burgert, H. G. et al. (2000). The luminal part of the murine cytomegalovirus glycoprotein gp40 catalyzes the retention of class II MHC molecules. *EMBO. J.*, **19**(5), 870–881.

Zimmermann, A., Trilling, M., Wagner, M. et al. (2005). A cytomegaloviral protein reveals a dual role for STAT2 in IFN-γ signaling and antiviral responses. *J. Exp. Med.*, **201**(10), 1543–1553.

Subversion of innate and adaptive immunity: immune evasion from antibody and complement

Lauren M. Hook and Harvey M. Friedman

Department of Medicine, University of Pennsylvania School of Medicine, PA, USA

Many herpesviruses encode immune evasion molecules that interfere with activities mediated by antibody and complement, suggesting the importance of antibody and complement in host defense against herpes infections. How does this observation reconcile with the clinical findings that severe infections develop mostly in subjects with T-cell deficiencies, such as transplant recipients or those with advanced HIV infection? An explanation that we favor is that T-cells assume a pivotal role in host defense partly because herpesviruses are very effective at limiting the activities of antibody and complement. Support for this hypothesis comes from experimental studies using mutant HSV-1 strains defective in antibody and complement immune evasion that demonstrate a marked increased in effectiveness of antibody and complement in host defense against the mutant viruses (Lubinski et al., 2002).

Newborns lack mature T-cell repertoires and generally have low serum complement levels; therefore, observations in human newborns provide opportunities to assess the contributions of antibodies independent of T-cells and perhaps complement in host defense against herpesviruses. The severity of HSV and CMV infection in the fetus and newborn are greatly reduced when the infection in the mother is recurrent rather than primary. In recurrent infection, antibodies pass transplacentally to the fetus and protect against the infection. Passive transfer of VZV antibodies from mother to fetus protects the newborn from severe chickenpox when exposed days to weeks after delivery. Similarly, treating newborns with varicella zoster immune globulin greatly reduces the severity of infection in infants born too soon after onset of chickenpox in their mothers to benefit from passive transfer of maternal antibodies. Therefore, lacking mature T-cells, newborns rely on passive transfer of maternal IgG antibodies to modify disease severity, suggesting that antibodies are partially effective against herpesviruses. The immune evasion strategies of herpesviruses target the IgG Fc domain, but do not inhibit neutralizing activities mediated by the IgG Fab domain, which likely accounts for the partial protection provided by antibodies.

Role of the herpesvirus IgG Fc receptor in immune evasion

Introduction

Herpesviruses encode glycoproteins that bind the Fc domain of IgG, referred to as viral IgG Fc receptors (vFcγR). Table 63.1 lists the human herpesviruses that encode vFcγRs and the genes involved. Non-human herpesviruses, pseudorabies virus (PRV) and murine cytomegalovirus (MCMV), also express vFcγRs, suggesting that vFcγRs fulfill important roles in pathogenesis (Favoreel et al., 1997; Thale et al., 1994). FcγRs are detected on many microorganisms, including staphylococci (protein A), streptococci (protein G), schistosomes, trypanosomes, hepatitis C virus (core protein), and coronaviruses (S peplomer protein). FcγRs are also detected on mammalian cells (cFcγRs) and regulate B-cell activation, phagocytosis (engulfing particles ≥ 1 μM), endocytosis, antibody-dependent cellular cytotoxicity (ADCC), and release of inflammatory mediators (Raghavan and Bjorkman, 1996). Below, we discuss the structure and function of vFcγRs and consider similarities with cFcγRs.

The IgG Fc domain mediates important antibody effector activities, including C1q binding, interacting with cFcγR on NK cells to trigger ADCC, phagocytosis and release of cytokines and proinflammatory molecules from

Table 63.1. IgG Fc receptors encoded by human herpes viruses

Virus	Gene	Protein	Comments
HSV-1, HSV-2	U_S8	gE	Low affinity FcγR; homology with domain 2 of human FcγRII (Dubin et al., 1994)
HSV-1, HSV-2	U_S8, U_S7	gE-gI complex	gE-gI forms a higher affinity FcγR than gE alone (Dubin et al., 1990).
CMV	U_L118, U_L119	gp68	Homology with domain 3 of FcγR1 (Atalay et al., 2002)
CMV	TRL11, IRL11	gp34	Homology with FcγRII/III domain 2 (Atalay et al., 2002)
VZV	ORF68	gE	VZV gE amino acids 328–500 shares homology with HSV-1 gE 211–381 (region involved in Fc binding) (Litwin et al., 1992)

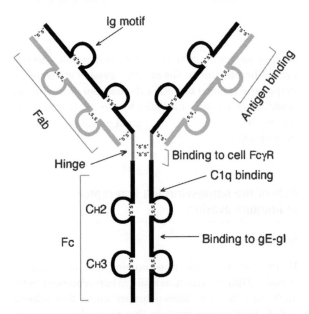

Fig. 63.1. Schematic drawing of the IgG molecule. Four immunoglobulin motifs are shown on the IgG heavy chains (black) and two on the IgG light chains (grey). Sites of interaction are shown between the IgG Fc domain and FcγRs on mammalian cells, C1q and HSV-1 gE-gI.

granulocytes and macrophages. Figure 63.1 depicts an IgG molecule with its Fc domain showing the regions involved in C1q binding and interaction with cFcγRs or the HSV-1 vFcγR (gE-gI).

IgG Fc receptors on mammalian cells

Specific cellular Fc receptors interact with each of the immunoglobulin classes, IgA, IgD, IgE, IgG and IgM. However, only IgG Fc receptors have been detected on human herpesviruses; therefore, the discussion below focuses on cFcγRs.

Three classes of cFcγRs are present on mammalian cells, including FcγRI (CD64), FcγRII (CD32) and FcγRIII

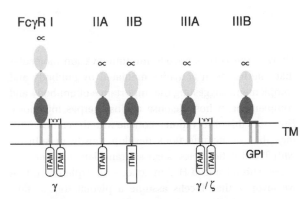

Fig. 63.2. Schematic drawing of cellular FcγRs. The FcγRs contain an α chain that has two or three Ig superfamily motifs (shown as ovals). The motif closest to the cell membrane (dark grey) functions as the IgG Fc binding domain. FcγR1 has two γ chains that contain ITAM (immunoreceptor tyrosine-based activation motif) sequences. FcγRII has two isoforms, IIA and IIB. IIA has an ITAM, while IIB has an ITIM (immunoreceptor tyrosine-based inhibitory motif) that inhibits activation signals. FcγRIII has two isoforms, IIIA that has ITAMs and IIIB that has glycophosphatidyl inositol (GPI) linkage.

(CD16) (Fig. 63.2) (Raghavan and Bjorkman, 1996). FcγRI is detected on granulocytes (neutrophils, eosinophils and mast cells), monocytes and macrophages, and is a heterodimer consisting of one α-chain and two γ-chains. The α-chain contains three extracellular Ig-like domains. The membrane proximal domain is the region primarily involved in Fc binding activity. The γ-chains are linked by a disulfide bond and are necessary for cell signaling events and for expression of the α chain at the cell surface. The γ-chains contain amino acid sequences, referred to as ITAMs (immunoreceptor tyrosine-based activation motifs) that become phosphorylated at tyrosine positions upon cross-linking of the FcγR. The ITAMs trigger intracellular signaling events that are initiated by src family protein tyrosine kinases and that induce phagocytosis and endocytosis. FcγRI binds single IgG molecules (monomeric IgG) with high affinity ($2 \times 10^9 - 5 \times 10^9$ M^{-1}). IgG complexes are required for efficient triggering of FcγRII and FcγRIII since these receptors bind monomeric IgG with low affinity ($\sim 10^6$ M^{-1}).

FcγRII has two human isoforms, IIA and IIB. Both contain a single α-chain with two Ig-like extracellular domains. The membrane proximal domain is involved in Fc binding activity. The cytoplasmic domain of FcγRIIA contains an ITAM motif, while IIB has an ITIM motif (immunoreceptor tyrosine-based inhibitory motif) that inhibits cell activation. Receptors with ITIMs are found on neutrophils, macrophages, mast cells and B cells and contain sequences that are phosphorylated at a tyrosine position upon receptor cross-linking leading to inhibition of activation signals (Ravetch and Bolland, 2001).

FcγRIII in involved in ADCC (NK cell-mediated), phagocytosis and endocytosis. This receptor has two isoforms, IIIA with a polypeptide chain anchor, and IIIB with a glycophosphatidyl inositol (GPI) linkage. FcγRIIIA contains an α chain with two Ig-like extracellular domains, and a γ- or ζ-chain that contains ITAMs. FcγRIIIB has only an α-chain with two extracellular Ig-like motifs. IgG Fc interacts with the membrane proximal Ig-like domains of both FcγRIII isotypes. FcγRIIIA is found on macrophages, mast cells and as the only FcγR on NK cells, where it mediates ADCC, while IIIB is detected on neutrophils.

Herpes simplex virus FcγR

Both HSV-1 and HSV-2 encode vFcγRs, although considerably more is known about the structure and functions of the HSV-1 FcγR, which is discussed below.

gE and gI structure

Glycoproteins gE and gI form a heterodimeric complex that contains one molecule each of gE and gI and that functions as an FcγR (Chapman et al., 1999; Johnson et al., 1988). HSV-1 gE strain 17 has a molecular mass of $\sim$80 kDa and is a 550 amino acid type 1 transmembrane glycoprotein, although strain NS, used extensively in the authors' laboratory, encodes two additional amino acids, glycine and glutamine, at positions 186 and 187 respectively (Lin et al., 2004). The NS strain gE ectodomain includes 421 amino acids with a predicted signal sequence from amino acids 1–23, two N-linked glycosylation sites, a transmembrane domain (422–446), and a large cytoplasmic tail (447–552) that undergoes serine phosphorylation (Edson et al., 1987).

HSV-1 strain 17 gI has a molecular mass of $\sim$70 kD and contains 390 amino acids. Sequences of strains KOS and NS differ from strain 17 in that a 7-amino acid repeat at position 225–231 in strain 17 is absent in KOS and NS (H. M. Friedman, unpublished observations). HSV-1 strain NS gI has a predicted signal sequence from amino acid 1–20, three N-linked glycosylation sites, a transmembrane domain (267–287), and a large cytoplasmic tail (288–383).

Glycoprotein gE binds Fc in the absence of gI, while gI cannot bind Fc without gE. The gE-gI complex binds Fc with higher affinity than gE alone (Bell et al., 1990; Dubin et al., 1990). IgG monomers bind to the gE–gI complex with an affinity of $0.4 \times 10^7 - 2 \times 10^7$ M^{-1}, while gE binds IgG aggregates, but not IgG monomers (Chapman et al., 1999; Dubin et al., 1990). Approximately 4×10^6 vFcγR binding sites are present on HSV-1 infected cells in vitro, which exceeds the number of cFcγR detected on human leukocytes by $\sim$100-fold (Johansson and Blomberg, 1990). The HSV-1 FcγR binds human IgG4 with higher affinity than IgG1 or IgG2, while IgG3 fails to bind (Johansson et al., 1984). A substitution of arginine for histidine at IgG4 Fc amino acid 435 abolishes Fc binding to gE-gI, which is consistent with the observation that most human IgG3 allotypes contain an arginine at Fc position 435 (Chapman et al., 1999). IgG subclass concentrations in serum are age dependent, but in general, IgG1 is most abundant, followed by IgG2, with considerably lower concentrations of IgG3 and IgG4. IgG1 and IgG3 are potent activators of complement, while IgG2 is slightly less so, and IgG1 binds to FcγRIIIA on NK cells to mediate ADCC (Ghirlando et al., 1995). Therefore, by interacting with IgG1 and IgG2, the vFcγR is binding the two most abundant IgG subclasses and potentially interfering with complement activation and ADCC mediated by these subclasses.

Mapping studies have determined that gE amino acids 24–211 are required to form a complex with gI, while gI amino acids 43–192 interact with gE (Basu et al., 1995; Rizvi and Raghavan, 2001). Two approaches were used to define regions on gE involved in Fc binding. Fragments of gE DNA were fused to HSV-1 gD DNA and expressed in mammalian cells. The smallest gE fragment to retain FcγR activity included gE amino acids 183–402 (sequences based on strain 17) (Dubin et al., 1994). Linker insertion mutagenesis was used as a second approach to evaluate gE domains involved in FcγR activity. Four amino acid inserts at each of ten positions between gE amino acids 235–380 eliminated IgG Fc binding. Therefore, the results of the two approaches were complementary, establishing the gE domain between amino acids 183 and 402 as sufficient for Fc binding, while mutations between amino acids 235 and 380 resulted in loss of function. The crystal structure has been solved for

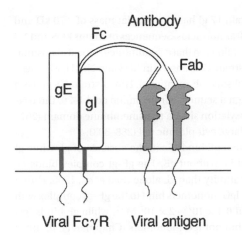

Fig. 63.3. Schematic drawing of antibody bipolar bridging. The IgG Fab domains bind to the viral antigen and the Fc domain of the same antibody molecule binds to the vFcγR (gE-gI).

the interaction of the IgG Fc fragment with a soluble form of cFcγRIII (Sondermann et al., 2000). Five contact sites were identified on the cFcγR over a linear range of 73 amino acids, suggesting that the much broader linear range of gE mutations that resulted in loss of function likely reflect changes in conformation and contact sites. This conclusion is supported by a low-resolution crystal structure of the gE–gI/Fc complex that was solved at 5 Å (Sprague et al., 2006). The crystal structure was verified by a theoretical prediction model of gE–Fc interaction that was based on the crystal structure of the gE C-terminal ectodomain (CgE amino acids 213–390) solved at 1.78 Å. The gE–gI/Fc crystal structure demonstrates that two gE-gI molecules interact with one Fc dimer and predicts that Fc interfaces with gE amino acids 225, 245–247, 249–250, 256, 258, 311, 316, 318–322, 324 and 338–342. Loss of Fc binding when gE is mutated at other sites likely occurs because of changes in gE conformation.

The HSV-1 FcγR and immune evasion

An IgG antibody molecule that is directed against HSV-1 can bind by its Fab domain to viral antigens on the virion or infected cell while the Fc domain of the same antibody molecule binds to the vFcγR (Fig. 63.3) (Frank and Friedman, 1989). Antibody bipolar bridging is used to describe this form of antibody binding, which requires considerable flexibility of the IgG molecule at the hinge region. Studies of the dynamic conformations of IgG in solution and bound to receptors confirm IgG has the flexibility to mediate bridging (Zheng et al., 1992). The crystal structure of the gE–gI/Fc complex is also compatible with antibody bipolar bridging (Sprague et al., 2006). Antibody bridging is postulated to be an important immune evasion strategy, since the vFcγR binds the Fc domain of antibody molecules that are targeting the virus. The affinity of the HSV-1 FcγR for Fc is ∼100-fold lower than that of cFcγR1; therefore, binding of monomeric, non-immune IgG is limited. The IgG Fab domain binds with high affinity to the target antigen, which anchors the IgG Fc domain onto the virion or infected cell surface. The vFcγR is then able to bind the IgG Fc domain to block its activities.

Figure 63.1 shows the regions on Fc that interact with host and viral proteins. The region on IgG that binds to cFcγRs is located at the lower portion of the hinge region and the upper margin of the C_H2 domain (Sondermann et al., 2000). The IgG Fc C_H2 domain interacts with C1q to initiate complement activation, while the C_H2–C_H3 interface of the Fc domain binds to gE–gI, which is similar to the site of interaction between protein A and Fc (Johansson et al., 1989; Miletic and Frank, 1995). Despite the distance between domains on Fc involved in binding to gE–gI, C1q and cFcγRs, the HSV-1 FcγR is effective at blocking functions mediated by these regions of the Fc molecule (Dubin et al., 1991).

Studies were performed to assess the role of the vFcγR in pathogenesis. A mutant HSV-1 strain was produced by introducing 4 amino acids at gE position 339 (based on the sequence of strain 17). The mutant virus expressed gE and gI at the infected cell surface, but failed to bind IgG Fc measured by rosetting assays using IgG-coated erythrocytes and by flow cytometry using biotin-labeled non-immune human IgG (Nagashunmugam et al., 1998). Wild-type, gE mutant and gE-restored viruses were injected into the murine flank to assess the contribution of the vFcγR to virulence. The Fc domain of murine IgG does not bind to the HSV-1 FcγR; therefore, the three virus strains were expected to cause similar disease in mice, which was the observed result (Johansson et al., 1985; Nagashunmugam et al., 1998). Human IgG does bind to the HSV-1 FcγR; therefore, passive transfer of HSV antibodies was predicted to be more active against the vFcγR defective strain than against wild-type or restored virus. When infection was performed one day following passive transfer of HSV IgG antibodies, approximately 100-fold higher titers of gE mutant virus were required to cause the same level of disease as wild-type or restored virus. Passive transfer of non-immune human IgG or murine HSV IgG antibodies showed no differences among the various strains. Therefore, these in vivo studies define a contribution of the vFcγR to pathogenesis that depends upon the ability of the virus to block activities mediated by the IgG Fc domain. Synergy between gC and gE in mediating immune evasion was demonstrated in vitro and in vivo using an HSV-1 mutant virus defective in C3b and IgG Fc binding (Lubinski et al., 2002). Glycoproteins gC and gE interfere with complement activation at different steps in the cascade, which likely contributes to the synergy.

Additional mechanisms have been proposed for vFcγR-mediated immune evasion. The vFcγR promotes capping of viral antigens on the surface of infected cells in response to human HSV antibodies (Rizvi and Raghavan, 2003). The antibodies promote virus spread cell-to-cell when gE is expressed on the cell surface, which suggests that when antibodies are present, gE enables the virus to remain intracellular to avoid neutralization. In separate studies, the binding of Fc to gE-gI was noted to be pH dependent (Sprague et al., 2004). Binding of Fc occurs at an affinity of $2 \times 10^7 - 3 \times 10^7$ M^{-1} at pH 7.4, which is the pH at the cell surface. In contrast, no binding occurred at pH 6.0. Based on antibody internalization studies described below, the results suggest that the vFcγR may internalize IgG and then dissociate within acidic intracellular compartments promoting degradation of antibodies. The crystal structure of the gE–gI/Fc interaction predicts that histidines at gE position 247 and Fc positions 310 and 435 are likely involved in Fc dissociation from gE at acidic pH (Sprague et al., 2006).

Human CMV FcγR

Cells infected with human CMV (HCMV) express $\sim 10^6$ IgG Fc receptors per cell that have an association constant of 2×10^8 M^{-1} (Antonsson and Johansson, 2001). Two HCMV vFcγRs have been reported (Atalay et al., 2002; Lilley et al., 2001). The first is a 234-amino acid type 1 transmembrane glycoprotein that migrates with an apparent molecular mass of 34 kDa (gp34) and has three potential N-linked glycosylation sites in the ectodomain (Lilley et al., 2001). The glycoprotein is encoded by TRL11 and IRL11, which are identical copies of a gene found in the terminal and internal repeats of the HCMV DNA long fragment. The cytoplasmic tail of gp34 has 31 amino acids and contains a conserved dileucine motif that is postulated to participate in IgG endocytosis. Sequence similarities were detected between gp34 and domain 2 of cFcγRII and III (Atalay et al., 2002). The other HCMV FcγR is encoded by the UL119–118 open reading frame that produces a 347 amino acid type 1 transmembrane glycoprotein with a molecular mass of 68 kDa (gp68) (Atalay et al., 2002). The glycoprotein has 12 potential N-linked sites and an immunoglobulin supergene family-like variable domain that shares sequence homology with cFcγRI domain 3 (Atalay et al., 2002). The cytoplasmic tail has a possible modified ITIM-like motif (WSYKRL) that may be involved in cell signaling events. The lack of laboratory animal models for HCMV has hampered attempts to define the role of the HCMV FcγRs in pathogenesis.

Varicella zoster FcγR

The VZV US8 gene encodes gE, which functions as an FcγR on infected human cells (Litwin et al., 1992). Glycoprotein gE is a 623-amino acid type 1 transmembrane glycoprotein that has a signal sequence of 24 amino acids, a 544-amino acid extracellular domain with three predicted N-linked glycosylation sites, a 17-amino acid transmembrane domain and a 62 amino acid cytoplasmic tail. Binding of IgG Fc to gE initiates endocytosis, unloading the IgG cargo in lysosomal vesicles and subsequent recycling of gE to the cell surface (Olson and Grose, 1997). Endocytosis requires the gE cytoplasmic tail, and is mediated by tyrosine phosphorylation of a YAGL endocytosis motif (Olson and Grose, 1997). VZV gE shares sequence similarities with HSV gE, but not with cFcγRs (Litwin et al., 1992). Similar to HCMV, the in vivo relevance of the VZV FcγR in immune evasion has not been determined because of the lack of animal models.

vFcγRs on non-human mammalian herpesviruses

Murine CMV

The m138 (fcr-1) gene of MCMV encodes a vFcγR that has a molecular mass of 88 kDa and is a 569 amino acid type 1 transmembrane glycoprotein. The protein has a predicted signal sequence of 17 amino acids, a transmembrane domain from amino acids 535–552, 10 potential N-linked glycosylation sites, and a 17 amino acid cytoplasmic tail (Thale et al., 1994). Studies were performed to assess the function of the vFcγR in its natural host by preparing a mutant virus deficient in the fcr-1 gene and a revertant strain (Crnkovic-Mertens et al., 1998). The fcr-1 deficient strain showed normal replication kinetics in vitro, but significantly reduced replication in vivo. To determine if the reduced replication in vivo was caused by increased susceptibility to antibody, mutant and revertant strains were injected into B cell deficient mice. The expectation was that the two strains would have similar replication patterns in antibody deficient mice; however, this did not occur, suggesting that the vFcR had little or no role in pathogenesis. While this conclusion is potentially correct, other explanations are also possible. For example, to demonstrate a role for the HSV-1 FcγR in pathogenesis, small deletions were made in gE to abolish Fc binding without interfering with virus spread, another activity mediated by gE (Nagashunmugam et al., 1998). A similar approach may be required to assess the potential role of the MCMV vFcγR in pathogenesis.

Pseudorabies virus

PRV gE and gI form a molecular complex that functions as a vFcγR (Favoreel et al., 1997). PRV US8 encodes gE, a 62 kD type 1 transmembrane glycoprotein containing 577 amino acids, including an extracellular domain of 428 amino acids, a transmembrane domain of 26 amino acids, and a cytoplasmic tail of 123 amino acids (Klupp et al., 2004). PRV US7 encodes gI, which is a type 1 transmembrane glycoprotein containing 366 amino acids, including an extracellular domain of 285 amino acids, a transmembrane domain from amino acid 286–308, and a cytoplasmic tail of 58 amino acids (Klupp et al., 2004).

Studies performed in swine kidney cells demonstrate that PRV-specific antibodies induce capping of viral glycoproteins followed by their extrusion from the cell surface (Favoreel et al., 1997). Phosphorylation of two tyrosine motifs in the gE cytoplasmic tail are required for glycoprotein capping (Favoreel et al., 1999). Studies of PRV in swine monocytes, which are infected by PRV during natural infection, demonstrate that antibodies induce endocytosis of viral glycoproteins with co-internalization of MHC class I proteins (Favoreel et al., 2003). Endocytosis removes viral glycoproteins from the cell surface and reduces the effectiveness of antibody dependent complement lysis of infected cells. Endocytosis is not uniquely mediated by gE-gI, but the vFcγR contributes to this activity (Van de Walle et al., 2003).

Summary of vFcγR studies

Activities mediated by the vFcγRs of human and non-human herpesviruses can be summarized as follows. First, antibody bipolar bridging is an important mechanism used by vFcγRs to protect the virus and infected cell against activities mediated by the IgG Fc domain, including complement activation and ADCC. Second, some vFcγRs mediate antibody capping, while others promote antibody internalization. In acidic intracellular compartments, antibodies may dissociate from the vFcγR and degrade, while the vFcγR recycles to the cell surface. Third, potential ITIM motifs have been noted on some vFcγRs that may regulate responses to antibody. Fourth, the HSV-1 FcγR is a virulence factor, reducing the effectiveness of antibodies in vivo.

Role of the herpesvirus complement receptors in immune evasion

Introduction

The complement system plays an important role in both the innate and adaptive immune responses to viral infection. Activation of complement early following viral infection relies on the presence of highly specific recognition proteins, which have evolved to recognize and bind pathogen associated molecular patterns (PAMPs). These pattern recognition proteins include natural antibodies (IgM), C1q, C-reactive protein, mannan-binding lectin, and ficolins H and L. IgG and IgM antibodies are able to trigger the activation of complement following induction of specific humoral immune responses.

Complement is activated by one of three different pathways: classical, mannan-binding lectin (MBL), or alternative (Fig. 63.4). The classical complement pathway was the first pathway to be identified, and is normally considered to be antibody-dependent. Activation of the classical pathway occurs when the first component of the pathway, C1, binds the Fc region of either natural antibody or specific IgG antibody in complex with viral antigen. The classical pathway is also triggered in an antibody-independent manner when C1 binds directly to virions or infected cells.

Activation of the MBL pathway is antibody-independent and occurs when one of the C-type lectins, MBL, ficolin H, or ficolin L recognizes carbohydrate structures on the surface of pathogens. The alternative complement pathway was originally described as the antibody-independent pathway (the MBL pathway was identified much later). Activation of the alternative pathway is spontaneous as a continued low-level release of the internal thioester bond of C3 allows it to bind to a wide range of "foreign" sites. The diversity of serum recognition proteins able to recognize and activate complement allows the complement system to protect against a wide variety of microbial pathogens.

Recently a fourth pathway for complement activation was described that involves SIGN-R1, a C-type lectin detected on marginal-zone macrophages in the spleen. The unique feature of this pathway is that SIGN-R1 binds C1q and activates the classical complement pathway in the absence of immunoglobulins. SIGN-R1 also binds the capsular polysaccharide of S. pneumoniae, and perhaps carbohydrates on other microbial pathogens, leading to C3 deposition on the organism and enhanced innate resistance to infection (Kang et al., 2006).

Activation of the complement cascade leads to numerous effector functions that result in neutralization and elimination of virus, thereby limiting spread, infection and disease. These include neturalization of viral particles, phagocytosis of complement-opsonized virus and virus-infected cells, direct lysis of virus and infected cells by the formation of pores known as the membrane attack complex, induction of inflammation, and enhancement of the adaptive immune response.

Regulation of complement

Given the complexity of the complement system, with over 30 complement proteins involved in activating the three divergent complement pathways, proper control is imperative. Regulation of the complement systems is necessary to prevent inappropriate activation and injury to bystander cells. Therefore, complement is tightly regulated by proteins present in serum and expressed on the surface of cells. These complement regulatory proteins include C1 inhibitor, CD59, and a class of proteins referred to as regulators of complement activation (RCA). RCA proteins include secreted plasma factor H, C4-binding protein and membrane bound complement regulatory proteins 1, 2, 3 (CR1, CR2, CR3), membrane cofactor protein (MCP) and decay accelerating factor (DAF) (Carroll, 2000; Da Costa et al., 1999; Spear et al., 1995; Spiller et al., 1997). Both CR2 and DAF are GPI-linked.

RCA proteins are homologous in structure, characterized by the presence of motifs known as short consensus repeats (SCRs). SCR motifs contain approximately 58 to 66 amino acids, with four conserved cysteine residues disulfide linked (cys 1 to 3, and cys 2 to 4) and several hydrophobic residues. SCR motifs are highly conserved, sharing 30%–40% amino acid identity. However, the number of SCRs contained within RCA proteins is highly variable, for example, both MCP and DAF contain four SCRs, while CR1 contains 30.

As the complement system plays an important role in host defense against viral infection, not surprisingly, viruses have evolved numerous mechanisms to control complement. Strategies employed by viruses fall into three categories: (1) viral proteins which are homologous to mammalian complement regulatory proteins; (2) viral proteins which have no sequence homology, but which share functional characteristics with complement regulatory proteins; and (3) viruses that incorporate host complement regulatory proteins into their envelope during viral maturation and egress.

Strategies employed by human herpesviruses to evade complement immunity

Viral proteins homologous to human complement regulatory proteins: Kaposi's sarcoma associated herpesvirus complement control protein

Sequencing of the Kaposi's sarcoma associated herpesvirus (KSHV) genome indicated that one gene, KSHV open reading frame 4 (ORF4), encoded a protein displaying a high degree of homology to many complement regulatory proteins, including RCA proteins DAF and MCP (Neipel et al., 1997; Russo et al., 1996). The KSHV ORF4 was predicted to encode a protein of 550 amino acids residues, with the first 270 amino acids forming four SCRs sharing 24.7% identity with DAF (Spiller et al., 2003b).

Characterization of transcripts produced by KSHV ORF4 indicated that three transcripts were produced, one full length, and two smaller, alternatively spliced forms (Spiller et al., 2003b). All three protein isoforms contained the four amino-terminal SCRs and transmembrane regions, not a GPI anchor present in DAF, and collectively, are referred to as KSHV complement control protein (KCP) or kaposica (Mullick et al., 2003; Spiller et al., 2003b).

Functional studies indicated that all three forms prevented C3 deposition on cell surfaces (Spiller et al., 2003b). Addition of a soluble form of each KCP isoform accelerated the decay of the classical pathway C3-convertase (Spiller et al., 2003a). All three forms of soluble KCP also accelerated the decay of the alternative pathway C3-convertase; however, they were 1000-fold less efficient than DAF, indicating that KCP mainly affects the classical pathway C3-convertase.

KCP acts as a cofactor for factor I (fI) mediated cleavage and inactivation of C3b and C4b (Mullick et al., 2003; Spiller et al., 2003a). KCP results in fI mediated cleavage of C4b to C4d, when both soluble and cell bound. KCP also acts as a cofactor for fI mediated cleavage of C3b to iC3b, and induces cleavage of iC3b to C3d, the only viral protein shown to date to do so. Binding affinity of KCP is higher for C4b than C3b, which may explain differences in the ability of KCP to degrade the classical and alternative pathway C3-convertases.

Viral proteins with no sequence homology, yet functional similarities with human complement regulatory proteins

HSV-1 and HSV-2 glycoprotein gC

HSV-1 and HSV-2 encode gC, a viral complement control protein that inhibits complement activation by

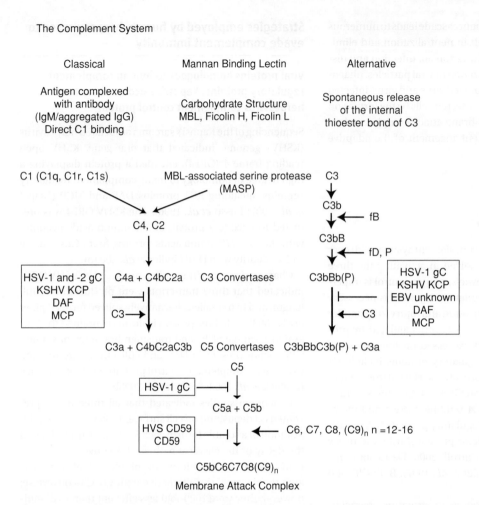

Fig. 63.4. Sites of interaction between herpesviruses and the complement cascade. The boxed type identifies the sites in the complement cascade inhibited by viral proteins or by host-derived cellular proteins captured by viruses.

binding C3b (Friedman et al., 1984; Kostavasili et al., 1997). gC of HSV-1 (gC-1) was the first complement control protein identified, and has been extensively characterized. Both gC-1 and gC-2 are rarely absent from clinical isolates, underscoring their importance *in vivo*. Moreover, gC is well conserved among members of the alpha-herpesvirus family, with homologues present in VZV, PRV, bovine herpesvirus 1 (BHV-1), and equine herpesviruses 1 and 4 (EHV-1, EHV-4). Despite this high degree of sequence conservation among alphaherpesviruses, gC displays little sequence homology with known complement regulatory proteins.

gC-1 and gC-2 are encoded by the UL44 gene and are type I membrane glycoproteins of 511 and 480 amino acids respectively, which are expressed on virions and infected cells. Both are highly glycosylated with 9 and 7 N-linked glycosylation sites respectively (Rux et al., 1996). gC-1 also contains several O-linked glycosylation sites, localized to the amino terminus of the protein; gC-2, however, is not O-linked glycosylated. gC-1 and gC-2 share eight highly conserved cysteines, the disulfide bonding pattern of which has been determined for gC-1, and is likely similar for gC-2 and the gC homologues from other herpesviruses (Rux et al., 1996).

gC of both HSV-1 and HSV-2 binds C3b in a purified form and when expressed on the surface of transfected cells (Eisenberg et al., 1987; Tal-Singer et al., 1991). However, only HSV-1 infected cells express gC that is able to bind C3b (Friedman et al., 1984). Cells infected with HSV-2 display no C3b receptor activity (Friedman, 1986; Friedman et al., 1984). Lack of binding to C3b appears unrelated to affinity of gC-2 for C3b, as optical biosensor technology indicates that gC-2 has a tenfold higher affinity for C3b compared with gC-1 (Rux et al., 2002). One possible explanation may be that other host cell membrane components or viral glycoproteins expressed on the HSV-2 infected cell surface may interfere with the ability of gC-2 to bind C3b.

Both gC-1 and gC-2 bind C3 and its activation products C3b, iC3b and C3c (Kostavasili et al., 1997; Tal-Singer et al., 1991). This binding is mediated by C3b regions, which are well conserved in both glycoproteins. Four regions in gC-1 and three in gC-2 were identified by site-directed and linker insertion mutagenesis, with binding phenotypes confirmed in rosetting assays using C3b-coated sheep erythrocytes (Hung et al., 1992; Seidel-Dugan et al., 1990).

Functional studies indicate that gC-1 prevents complement-mediated neutralization of HSV-1 by binding C3b, thereby inhibiting activation of the classical complement pathway (Friedman et al., 1996; Harris et al., 1990). Evidence suggests that gC-2 may function in a similar manner (Gerber et al., 1995). Neutralization of HSV-1 in the absence of gC-1 is mediated by a C5 dependent mechanism that does not require viral lysis, aggregation, or prevention of viral attachment (Friedman et al., 2000). Complement likely interferes with HSV infection at a stage following viral attachment, for example, during virus entry or uncoating (Friedman et al., 2000).

gC-1 also prevents complement-mediated cell lysis of HSV-1 infected cells by accelerating the decay of the alternative pathway C3 convertase, C3bBb (Fries et al., 1986; Harris et al., 1990). The half-life of the C3bBb complex is extended three- to four-fold by the binding of properdin to C3b in the convertase. gC-1 contains a properdin interacting domain, localized to the amino-terminus, which interferes with the binding of properdin to C3b, destabilizing the C3 convertase (Hung et al., 1994; Kostavasili et al., 1997). By interfering with properdin's ability to bind C3b, gC-1 prevents activation of the alternative complement pathway. This prevents lysis of HSV-1 infected cells.

gC-1 also contains a C5 interacting domain which prevents C5 from binding C3b (Fries et al., 1986). gC-1 thus interferes with activation of both the classical and alternative complement pathways, limiting neutralization of both virus and lysis of virus-infected cells. While both gC of HSV-1 and HSV-2 prevent complement-mediated neutralization of HSV virions, differences do exist. Only gC-1 is able to disrupt the activation of alternative pathway C3 convertase (Fries et al., 1986; Kostavasili et al., 1997). Moreover, the region of gC-1 important in blocking the binding of C5 and properdin to C3b is absent in gC-2.

Studies comparing the importance of both complement interacting domains of gC-1 were evaluated both in vitro and in an in vivo model of HSV pathogenesis (Lubinski et al., 1999). Complement neutralization experiments performed with a low passage clinical isolate that had been mutated within the C3 binding domain, the C5 and properdin blocking domain, or both, indicated that while both domains were important, elimination of the C3 binding domains significantly diminished the ability of gC to modulate complement (Lubinski et al., 1999). Similar results were seen in vivo in a murine model of HSV pathogenesis. HSV-1 was mutated in the C5 and properdin blocking, the C3 binding, or both domains (double mutant). Each mutant virus was significantly more attenuated than the wild type HSV-1 virus (Lubinski et al., 1999). That the C3 binding domain mutant was as attenuated as the gC double mutant indicated that the C3 domain is more important than the C5 and properdin in modulating complement activity.

EBV complement regulatory activity: unidentified protein

In addition to gC of HSV-1 and HSV-2, evidence suggests that Epstein–Barr virus (EBV) encodes a complement regulatory protein displaying no sequence homology with known human complement regulatory proteins. EBV virions derived from either marmoset or human B lymphoblastoid cells maintains complement regulatory activities (Mold et al., 1988). Incubation of purified EBV with immune human serum resulted in the cleavage of C3 into the inactive C3c. In addition, EBV functions as a cofactor for the Factor I mediated cleavage of C3b and iC3b and C4b and iC4b. No degradation occurred in the absence of Factor I. EBV accelerates the decay of the alternative, but not the classical C3 convertase. The EBV envelope protein responsible for this complement regulatory activity remains unknown. No virally encoded proteins with homology to known complement regulatory proteins have been identified; therefore, cellular proteins incorporated into the virion are possibly mediating this effect.

Viruses that incorporate human complement regulatory proteins into their envelope during viral maturation and egress: human CMV

HCMV-infected cells remain susceptible to antibody-mediated complement cytolysis for only a brief time following acute infection, suggesting that the cells are protected from complement lysis. Analyses of the complete genomic sequence of HCMV revealed no homologues of known complement regulatory proteins, and HCMV does not appear to encode a C3 binding protein (Smiley and Friedman, 1985). It was hypothesized that HCMV may alter the expression of host-encoded complement regulatory proteins in order to interfere with complement (Spiller et al., 1996). Candidates included DAF, MCP, and CD59, since each are expressed on uninfected cells that are permissive to infection by HCMV.

Studies examining the cell surface expression of both DAF and MCP by HCMV infected human foreskin fibroblasts indicated that levels were enhanced at 24, 48, and 72 hours post infection compared with mock-infected controls. Maximal expression was seen 72 hours post infection with a 3.4-fold and 8-fold increase in MCP and DAF respectfully. Expression of CD59, however, remained relatively stable (Spiller et al., 1996).

Incubation of HCMV virions with complement alone consumed complement activity and resulted in C3 deposition on the surface of the virion, yet resulted in negligible amounts of C9 deposition and no loss of viral infectivity (Spiller et al., 1997). These data suggest that HCMV is able to regulate complement and accomplishes this by interfering with the complement system upstream of C9 activation. Studies examining the expression of MCP, DAF, and CD59 on HCMV virions produced in human foreskin fibroblasts indicated that the three complement regulators were captured by the virion during egress and maturation (Spear et al., 1995; Spiller et al., 1997).

The mechanism by which MCP, DAF, and CD59 become incorporated within the HCMV virion remains unknown. Incorporation could represent a passive capture of upregulated plasma membrane proteins, as levels of both DAF and CD59 are increased during HCMV infection and are readily incorporated into foreign membranes (Spiller et al., 1996). Moreover, the distribution of both DAF and CD59 expressed on the surface of the virion correlates roughly with levels of each detected on the surface of the host derived cells, indicating that virions may obtain the host cell derived complement regulatory proteins in a passive manner (Spear et al., 1995). Incorporation, however, could be an immune evasion strategy adopted by HCMV, in order to protect virions and virus infected cells from complement-mediated neutralization. Treatment of HCMV virus with an anti-DAF antibody, not anti-CD59, reduced HCMV infectious titer in the presence of complement, indicating that DAF interferes with complement-mediated neutralization of HCMV virus (Spear et al., 1995).

Strategies employed by non-human mammalian herpesviruses to evade complement immunity

Viral proteins homologous to mammalian complement regulatory proteins

Murine Gammaherpesvirus 68: MHV-68 RCA

Murine Gammaherpesvirus 68 (γHV68) gene 4 product is a complement regulatory protein, with significant homology to both virally encoded and cellular proteins, including the herpesvirus saimiri complement control protein homologue (CCPH), DAF, and MCP (Virgin et al., 1997). γHV68 ORF 4 includes four regions with homology to SCRs of RCA complement regulatory proteins. γHV68 gene 4, named γHV68 RCA, produces a 5.2 kb bicistronic mRNA of the late kinetic class, encoding multiple γHV68 RCA proteins, including both plasma membrane bound and soluble forms (Kapadia et al., 1999).

Functional studies indicate that γHV68 RCA interferes with both murine and human complement activation, resulting in a decrease in C3b deposition (Kapadia et al., 1999). γHV68 RCA was found to prevent activation of both the classical and alternative complement pathways (Kapadia et al., 1999).

The γHV68 RCA contributes to virulence in mice, as γHV68 virus mutated within the RCA protein was more attenuated during both acute and persistent γHV68 infection when compared with wild type or marker rescued virus (Kapadia et al., 2002). γHV68 RCA accomplishes this by interfering with the complement system, as the virulent phenotype of the γHV68 RCA protein mutant virus was restored in mice lacking C3. Interestingly, γHV68 RCA was not involved in evading C3 mediated innate immunity during latent infection.

Herpesvirus saimiri (HVS): complement control protein homologue (CCPH)

While determining the nucleotide sequence of genes within the vicinity of STP-A and STP-C (saimiri transformation associated protein of subgroup A and C), a gene was detected that encodes a protein displaying a significant degree of homology to the RCA protein family (Albrecht and Fleckenstein, 1992; Albrecht et al., 1992a). This protein, named complement control protein homologue (CCPH), is encoded by HVS 04, and contains four SCRs within its N-terminal domain (amino acids 21–265), seven potential amino-linked glycosylation sites, and a transmembrane domain.

HVS 04 was found to encode two transcripts, one full length, and one smaller, alternatively spliced form. The unspliced transcript encodes a membrane-bound glycoprotein (mCCPH) of 65–75 kD, similar to the membrane-bound RCAs MCP, DAF, CR1, and CR2. Splicing produced a secreted glycoprotein (sCCPH) of 47–53 kD, like the soluble complement inhibitors C4-binding protein and Factor H. Functional studies indicated a role for CCPH in complement regulation. Cells stably transfected with mCCPH were approximately two times more resistant to complement mediated cell lysis, with levels similar when compared with DAF as a control (Fodor et al., 1995).

HVS: CD59

In addition to HVS CCPH, sequence analyses of the HVS genome indicated the presence of a second gene, HVS 15 that encodes a protein sharing significant homology with the complement regulatory protein CD59 (Albrecht et al., 1992b). The HVS 15 ORF consists of 363 nucleotides, sharing 64% sequence identity with human CD59 cDNA and was predicted to encode a protein of 121 amino acids with 48% identity to human CD59. Both HVSCD59 and CD59 have hydrophobic carboxyl-terminal sequences, which for CD59, is replaced by a GPI anchor. Additional studies confirmed that HVS 15 protein product was also a GPI linked membrane glycoprotein (Rother et al., 1994). The overall structure of both HVS 15 and CD59 were expected to be very similar as the proteins shared amino acid identities and a single N-linked glycosylation site, and all cysteines were highly conserved.

Expression of either HVSCD59 or squirrel monkey CD59 (SMCD59), the natural host of HVS, on the surface of Balb/3T3 cells rendered the cells resistant to complement-mediated cell lysis by human serum (Rother et al., 1994). However, only HVSCD59 expressing cells were protected from challenge with rat serum, indicating that HVSCD59 is less species specific than either human or SMCD59. Protection occurred following C3b deposition, suggesting that HVSCD59 prevents complete formation and function of the membrane attack complex (Rother et al., 1994). It was hypothesized that the location of the N-linked glycosylation site was responsible for the less species restrictive phenotype of HVSCD59, as the N-linked glycosylation of human CD59 appears necessary for its function.

Viral proteins with no sequence homology, yet functional similarities with mammalian complement regulatory proteins, and that incorporate host complement regulatory proteins: PRV gC and unknown host cell derived complement regulatory protein(s)

Pseudorabies virus (PRV) is protected from complement-mediated innate immunity by the presence of at least two proteins able to interfere with complement, gC and one or more host cell derived complement regulatory proteins. PRV gC shares homology with gC from other members of the alpha-herpesvirus family, and like HSV-1 gC, mediates viral attachment and facilitates immune evasion by binding C3. Neutralization experiments comparing PRV-CPK, a virus containing both gC and host cell derived complement regulatory proteins, and PRV-ΔgC-CPK which expresses the host cell derived complement regulatory proteins, yet lacks gC were performed (Maeda et al., 2002). The PRV virus lacking gC was more readily neutralized by swine serum than the wild type virus, suggesting that gC protects PRV from complement-mediated neutralization.

Pseudorabies virus (PRV) in which gC was deleted was propagated on either swine kidney derived CPK or rabbit kidney derived RK13 cells and then tested for susceptibility to complement-mediated virus neutralization using either swine or rabbit serum as the source of complement (Maeda et al., 2002). Results indicated that the gC deletion mutant grown in the CPK porcine cells was protected from neutralization mediated by swine serum. However, PRV derived from the RK13 rabbit cells was susceptible, suggesting that in the absence of gC, PRV was protected by at least one additional complement regulatory protein. No known homologues of complement regulatory proteins exist within the PRV genome; therefore, a host cell derived complement regulatory protein likely confers protection. Additional studies indicated that while the greatest level of protection was obtained when both gC and the cell derived factor(s) were coexpressed, the cell derived factor(s) afforded the most protection.

Summary of viral complement regulatory proteins

The complement system is an early innate defense able to thwart viral infection. Viruses have evolved numerous mechanisms to interfere with complement that are summarized in Fig. 63.4. Strategies reflect those used by the host to regulate and control complement activation and include encoding complement regulatory proteins that can be secreted or expressed on the surface of virions and infected cells or up-regulating and incorporating the host's own complement regulatory proteins on infected cells and within virions. Expression of complement control proteins by viruses can impart the capacity for increased infection and spread, resulting in greater virulence.

REFERENCES

Albrecht, J. C. and Fleckenstein, B. (1992). New member of the multigene family of complement control proteins in herpesvirus saimiri. *J. Virol.*, **66**(6), 3937–3940.

Albrecht, J. C., Nicholas, J., Biller, D. *et al.* (1992a). Primary structure of the herpesvirus saimiri genome. *J. Virol.*, **66**(8), 5047–5058.

Albrecht, J. C., Nicholas, J., Cameron, K. R., Newman, C., Fleckenstein, B., and Honess, R. W. (1992b). Herpesvirus saimiri has a gene specifying a homologue of the cellular membrane glycoprotein CD59. *Virology*, **190**(1), 527–530.

Antonsson, A. and Johansson, P. J. (2001). Binding of human and animal immunoglobulins to the IgG Fc receptor induced by human cytomegalovirus. *J. Gen. Virol.*, **82**(5), 1137–1145.

Atalay, R., Zimmermann, A., Wagner, M. *et al.* (2002). Identification and expression of human cytomegalovirus transcription units coding for two distinct Fcgamma receptor homologs. *J. Virol.*, **76**(17), 8596–8608.

Basu, S., Dubin, G., Basu, M., Nguyen, V., and Friedman, H. M. (1995). Characterization of regions of herpes simplex virus type 1 glycoprotein E involved in binding the Fc domain of monomeric IgG and in forming a complex with glycoprotein I. *J. Immunol.*, **154**(1), 260–267.

Bell, S., Cranage, M., Borysiewicz, L., and Minson, T. (1990). Induction of immunoglobulin G Fc receptors by recombinant vaccinia viruses expressing glycoproteins E and I of herpes simplex virus type 1. *J. Virol.*, **64**(5), 2181–2186.

Carroll, M. C. (2000). The role of complement in B cell activation and tolerance. *Adv. Immunol.*, **74**, 61–88.

Chapman, T. L., You, I., Joseph, I. M., Bjorkman, P. J., Morrison, S. L., and Raghavan, M. (1999). Characterization of the interaction between the herpes simplex virus type I Fc receptor and immunoglobulin G. *J. Biol. Chem.*, **274**(11), 6911–6919.

Crnkovic-Mertens, I., Messerle, M., Milotic, I. *et al.* (1998). Virus attenuation after deletion of the cytomegalovirus Fc receptor gene is not due to antibody control. *J. Virol.*, **72**(2), 1377–1382.

Da Costa, X. J., Brockman, M. A., Alicot, E. *et al.* (1999). Humoral response to herpes simplex virus is complement-dependent. *Proc. Natl Acad. Sci. USA*, **96**(22), 12708–12712.

Dubin, G., Frank, I., and Friedman, H. M. (1990). Herpes simplex virus type 1 encodes two Fc receptors which have different binding characteristics for monomeric immunoglobulin G (IgG) and IgG complexes. *J. Virol.*, **64**(6), 2725–2731.

Dubin, G., Socolof, E., Frank, I., and Friedman, H. M. (1991). Herpes simplex virus type 1 Fc receptor protects infected cells from antibody-dependent cellular cytotoxicity. *J. Virol.*, **65**(12), 7046–7050.

Dubin, G., Basu, S., Mallory, D. L., Basu, M., Tal-Singer, R., and Friedman, H. M. (1994). Characterization of domains of herpes simplex virus type 1 glycoprotein E involved in Fc binding activity for immunoglobulin G aggregates. *J. Virol.*, **68**(4), 2478–2485.

Edson, C. M., Hosler, B. A., and Waters, D. J. (1987). Varicella-zoster virus gpI and herpes simplex virus gE: phosphorylation and Fc binding. *Virology*, **161**(2), 599–602.

Eisenberg, R. J., Ponce de Leon, M., Friedman, H. M. *et al.* (1987). Complement component C3b binds directly to purified glycoprotein C of herpes simplex virus types 1 and 2. *Microb. Path.*, **3**(6), 423–435.

Favoreel, H. W., Nauwynck, H. J., Van Oostveldt, P., Mettenleiter, T. C., and Pensaert, M. B. (1997). Antibody-induced and cytoskeleton-mediated redistribution and shedding of viral glycoproteins, expressed on pseudorabies virus-infected cells. *J. Virol.*, **71**(11), 8254–8261.

Favoreel, H. W., Nauwynck, H. J., and Pensaert, M. B. (1999). Role of the cytoplasmic tail of gE in antibody-induced redistribution of viral glycoproteins expressed on pseudorabies-virus-infected cells. *Virology*, **259**(1), 141–147.

Favoreel, H. W., Nauwynck, H. J., Halewyck, H. M., Van Oostveldt, P., Mettenleiter, T. C., and Pensaert, M. B. (2003). Antibody-induced endocytosis of viral glycoproteins and major histocompatibility complex class I on pseudorabies virus-infected monocytes. *J. Gen. Virol.*, **80**(5), 1283–1291.

Fodor, W. L., Rollins, S. A., Bianco-Caron, S. *et al.* (1995). The complement control protein homolog of herpesvirus saimiri regulates serum complement by inhibiting C3 convertase activity. *J. Virol.*, **69**(6), 3889–3892.

Frank, I. and Friedman, H. M. (1989). A novel function of the herpes simplex virus type 1 Fc receptor: participation in bipolar bridging of antiviral immunoglobulin G. *J. Virol.*, **63**(11), 4479–4488.

Friedman, H. M. (1986). Laboratory diagnosis of herpes viruses in the immunocompromised host. *Adv. Exp. Med. Biol.*, **202**, 83–93.

Friedman, H. M., Cohen, G. H., Eisenberg, R. J., Seidel, C. A., and Cines, D. B. (1984). Glycoprotein C of herpes simplex virus 1 acts as a receptor for the C3b complement component on infected cells. *Nature*, **309**(5969), 633–635.

Friedman, H. M., Wang, L., Fishman, N. O. *et al.* (1996). Immune evasion properties of herpes simplex virus type 1 glycoprotein gC. *J. Virol.*, **70**(7), 4253–4260.

Friedman, H. M., Wang, L., Pangburn, M. K., Lambris, J. D., and Lubinski, J. (2000). Novel mechanism of antibody-independent complement neutralization of herpes simplex virus type 1. *J. Immunol.*, **165**(8), 4528–4536.

Fries, L. F., Friedman, H. M., Cohen, G. H., Eisenberg, R. J., Hammer, C. H., and Frank, M. M. (1986). Glycoprotein C of herpes simplex virus 1 is an inhibitor of the complement cascade. *J. Immunol.*, **137**(5), 1636–1641.

Gerber, S. I., Belval, B. J., and Herold, B. C. (1995). Differences in the role of glycoprotein C of HSV-1 and HSV-2 in viral binding may contribute to serotype differences in cell tropism. *Virology*, **214**(1), 29–39.

Ghirlando, R., Keown, M. B., Mackay, G. A., Lewis, M. S., Unkeless, J. C., and Gould, H. J. (1995). Stoichiometry and thermodynamics of the interaction between the Fc fragment of human IgG1 and its low-affinity receptor Fc gamma RIII. *Biochemistry*, **34**(41), 13320–13327.

Harris, S. L., Frank, I., Yee, A., Cohen, G. H., Eisenberg, R. J., and Friedman, H. M. (1990). Glycoprotein C of herpes simplex virus type 1 prevents complement-mediated cell lysis and virus neutralization. *J. Infect. Dis.*, **162**(2), 331–337.

Hung, S. L., Srinivasan, S., Friedman, H. M., Eisenberg, R. J., and Cohen, G. H. (1992). Structural basis of C3b binding by glycoprotein C of herpes simplex virus. *J. Virol.*, **66**(7), 4013–4027.

Hung, S. L., Peng, C., Kostavasili, I. *et al.* (1994). The interaction of glycoprotein C of herpes simplex virus types 1 and 2 with the alternative complement pathway. *Virology*, **203**(2), 299–312.

Johansson, P. J. and Blomberg, J. (1990). Characterization of herpes simplex virus type 1-induced Fc receptor in its interaction with rabbit immunoglobulin G (IgG). *Apmis*, **98**(8), 685–694.

Johansson, P. J., Hallberg, T., Oxelius, V. A., Grubb, A., and Blomberg, J. (1984). Human immunoglobulin class and subclass specificity of Fc receptors induced by herpes simplex virus type 1. *J. Virol.*, **50**(3), 796–804.

Johansson, P. J., Myhre, E. B., and Blomberg, J. (1985). Specificity of Fc receptors induced by herpes simplex virus type 1: comparison of immunoglobulin G from different animal species. *J. Virol.*, **56**(2), 489–494.

Johansson, P. J. H., Nardells, F. A., Sjoquist, J., Schroder, A. K., and Christensen, P. (1989). Herpes simplex type 1-induced Fc receptor binds to the Cgamma2-Cgamma3 interface region of IgG in the area that binds staphylococcal protein A. *Immunology*, **66**, 8–13.

Johnson, D. C., Frame, M. C., Ligas, M. W., Cross, A. M., and Stow, N. D. (1988). Herpes simplex virus immunoglobulin G Fc receptor activity depends on a complex of two viral glycoproteins, gE and gI. *J. Virol.*, **62**(4), 1347–1354.

Kang, Y-S., Do, Y., Lee, H-K. *et al.* (2006). A dominant complement fixation pathway for pneumococcal polysaccharides initiated by SIGN-R1 interacting with C1q. *Cell*, **125**(1); 46–58.

Kapadia, S. B., Levine, B., Speck, S. H., and Virgin, H. W. t. (2002). Critical role of complement and viral evasion of complement in acute, persistent, and latent gamma-herpesvirus infection. *Immunity*, **17**(2), 143–155.

Kapadia, S. B., Molina, H., van Berkel, V., Speck, S. H., and Virgin, H. W. T. (1999). Murine gammaherpesvirus 68 encodes a functional regulator of complement activation. *J. Virol.*, **73**(9), 7658–7670.

Klupp, B. G., Hengartner, C. J., Mettenleiter, T. C., and Enquist, L. W. (2004). Complete, annotated sequence of the pseudorabies virus genome.[erratum appears in *J. Virol.* 2004 Feb;78(4):2166]. *J. Virol.*, **78**(1), 424–440.

Kostavasili, I., Sahu, A., Friedman, H. M., Eisenberg, R. J., Cohen, G. H., and Lambris, J. D. (1997). Mechanism of complement inactivation by glycoprotein C of herpes simplex virus. *J. Immunol.*, **158**(4), 1763–1771.

Lilley, B. N., Ploegh, H. L., and Tirabassi, R. S. (2001). Human cytomegalovirus open reading frame TRL11/IRL11 encodes an immunoglobulin G Fc-binding protein. *J. Virol.*, **75**(22), 11218–11221.

Lin, X., Lubinski, J. M., and Friedman, H. M. (2004). Immunization strategies to block the herpes simplex virus type 1 immunoglobulin G Fc receptor. *J. Virol.*, **78**(5), 2562–2571.

Litwin, V., Jackson, W., and Grose, C. (1992). Receptor properties of two varicella-zoster virus glycoproteins, gpI and gpIV, homologous to herpes simplex virus gE and gI. *J. Virol.*, **66**(6), 3643–3651.

Lubinski, J., Wang, L., Mastellos, D., Sahu, A., Lambris, J. D., and Friedman, H. M. (1999). In vivo role of complement-interacting domains of herpes simplex virus type 1 glycoprotein gC. *J. Exp. Med.*, **190**(11), 1637–1646.

Lubinski, J. M., Jiang, M., Hook, L. *et al.* (2002). Herpes simplex virus type 1 evades the effects of antibody and complement in vivo. *J. Virol.*, **76**(18), 9232–9241.

Maeda, K., Hayashi, S., Tanioka, Y., Matsumoto, Y., and Otsuka, H. (2002). Pseudorabies virus (PRV) is protected from complement attack by cellular factors and glycoprotein C (gC). *Virus Res.*, **84**(1–2), 79–87.

Miletic, V. D. and Frank, M. M. (1995). Complement-immunoglobulin interactions. *Curr. Opin. Immunol.*, **7**(1), 41–47.

Mold, C., Bradt, B. M., Nemerow, G. R., and Cooper, N. R. (1988). Epstein-Barr virus regulates activation and processing of the third component of complement. *J. Exp. Med.*, **168**(3), 949–969.

Mullick, J., Bernet, J., Singh, A. K., Lambris, J. D., and Sahu, A. (2003). Kaposi's sarcoma-associated herpesvirus (human herpesvirus 8) open reading frame 4 protein (kaposica) is a functional homolog of complement control proteins. *J. Virol.*, **77**(6), 3878–3881.

Nagashunmugam, T., Lubinski, J., Wang, L. *et al.* (1998). In vivo immune evasion mediated by the herpes simplex virus type 1 immunoglobulin G Fc receptor. *J. Virol.*, **72**(7), 5351–5359.

Neipel, F., Albrecht, J. C., and Fleckenstein, B. (1997). Cell-homologous genes in the Kaposi's sarcoma-associated rhadinovirus human herpesvirus 8: determinants of its pathogenicity? *J. Virol.*, **71**(6), 4187–4192.

Olson, J. K. and Grose, C. (1997). Endocytosis and recycling of varicella-zoster virus Fc receptor glycoprotein gE: internalization mediated by a YXXL motif in the cytoplasmic tail. *J. Virol.*, **71**(5), 4042–4054.

Raghavan, M. and Bjorkman, P. J. (1996). Fc receptors and their interactions with immunoglobulins. *Ann. Rev. Cell Dev. Biol.*, **12**, 181–220.

Ravetch, J. V. and Bolland, S. (2001). IgG Fc receptors. *Ann. Rev. Immunol.*, **19**, 275–290.

Rizvi, S. M. and Raghavan, M. (2001). An N-terminal domain of herpes simplex virus type Ig E is capable of forming stable complexes with gI. *J. Virol.*, **75**(23), 11897–11901.

Rizvi, S. M. and Raghavan, M. (2003). Responses of herpes simplex virus type 1-infected cells to the presence of extracellular antibodies: gE-dependent glycoprotein capping and enhancement in cell-to-cell spread. *J. Virol.*, **77**(1), 701–708.

Rother, R. P., Rollins, S. A., Fodor, W. L. *et al.* (1994). Inhibition of complement-mediated cytolysis by the terminal complement inhibitor of herpesvirus saimiri. *J. Virology*, **68**(2), 730–737.

Russo, J. J., Bohenzky, R. A., Chien, M. C. *et al.* (1996). Nucleotide sequence of the Kaposi sarcoma-associated herpesvirus (HHV8). *Proc. Natl. Acad. Sci. USA*, **93**(25), 14862–14867.

Rux, A. H., Moore, W. T., Lambris, J. D. *et al.* (1996). Disulfide bond structure determination and biochemical analysis of glycoprotein C from herpes simplex virus. *J. Virol.*, **70**(8), 5455–5465.

Rux, A. H., Lou, H., Lambris, J. D., Friedman, H. M., Eisenberg, R. J., and Cohen, G. H. (2002). Kinetic analysis of glycoprotein C of herpes simplex virus types 1 and 2 binding to heparin, heparan sulfate, and complement component C3b. *Virology*, **294**(2), 324–332.

Seidel-Dugan, C., Ponce de Leon, M., Friedman, H. M., Eisenberg, R. J., and Cohen, G. H. (1990). Identification of C3b-binding regions on herpes simplex virus type 2 glycoprotein C. *J. Virol.*, **64**(5), 1897–1906.

Smiley, M. L. and Friedman, H. M. (1985). Binding of complement component C3b to glycoprotein C is modulated by sialic acid on herpes simplex virus type 1-infected cells. *J. Virol.*, **55**(3), 857–861.

Sondermann, P., Huber, R., Oosthuizen, V., and Jacob, U. (2000). The 3.2-A crystal structure of the human IgG1 Fc fragment-Fc gammaRIII complex. *Nature*, **406**(6793), 267–273.

Spear, G. T., Lurain, N. S., Parker, C. J., Ghassemi, M., Payne, G. H., and Saifuddin, M. (1995). Host cell-derived complement control proteins CD55 and CD59 are incorporated into the virions of two unrelated enveloped viruses. Human T cell leukemia/lymphoma virus type I (HTLV-I) and human cytomegalovirus (HCMV). *J. Immunol.*, **155**(9), 4376–4381.

Spiller, O. B., Morgan, B. P., Tufaro, F., and Devine, D. V. (1996). Altered expression of host-encoded complement regulators on human cytomegalovirus-infected cells. *Eur. J. Immunol.*, **26**(7), 1532–1538.

Spiller, O. B., Hanna, S. M., Devine, D. V., and Tufaro, F. (1997). Neutralization of cytomegalovirus virions: the role of complement. *J. Infect. Dis.*, **176**(2), 339–347.

Spiller, O. B., Blackbourn, D. J., Mark, L., Proctor, D. G., and Blom, A. M. (2003a). Functional activity of the complement regulator encoded by Kaposi's sarcoma-associated herpesvirus. *J. Biol. Chem.*, **278**(11), 9283–9289.

Spiller, O. B., Robinson, M., and O'Donnell, E. (2003b). Complement regulation by Kaposi's sarcoma-associated herpesvirus ORF4 protein. *J. Virol.*, **77**(1), 592–599.

Sprague, E. R., Martin, W. L., and Bjorkman, P. J. (2004). pH dependence and stoichiometry of binding to the Fc region of IgG by the herpes simplex virus Fc receptor gE-gI. *J. Biol. Chem.*, **279**(14), 14184–14193.

Sprague, E. R., Wang, C., Baker, D., and Bjorkman, P. J. (2006). Crystal structure of the HSV-1 Fc receptor bound to Fc reveals a mechanism for antibody bipolar bridging. *PloS. Biol.*, **4**(6); e148. DOI: 10.1371/journal.pbio.0040148.

Tal-Singer, R., Seidel-Dugan, C., Fries, L. *et al.* (1991). Herpes simplex virus glycoprotein C is a receptor for complement component iC3b. *J. Infect. Dis.*, **164**(4), 750–753.

Thale, R., Lucin, P., Schneider, K., Eggers, M., and Koszinowski, U. H. (1994). Identification and expression of a murine cytomegalovirus early gene coding for an Fc receptor. *J. Virol.*, **68**(12), 7757–7765.

Van de Walle, G. R., Favoreel, H. W., Nauwynck, H. J., and Pensaert, M. B. (2003). Antibody-induced internalization of viral glycoproteins and gE-gI Fc receptor activity protect pseudorabies virus-infected monocytes from efficient complement-mediated lysis. *J. Gen. Virol.*, **84**(4), 939–947.

Virgin, H. W. T., Latreille, P., Wamsley, P. *et al.* (1997). Complete sequence and genomic analysis of murine gammaherpesvirus 68. *J. Virol.*, **71**(8), 5894–5904.

Zheng, Y., Shopes, B., Holowka, D., and Baird, B. (1992). Dynamic conformations compared for IgE and IgG1 in solution and bound to receptors. *Biochemistry*, **31**(33), 7446–7456.

Part VI

Antiviral therapy

Edited by Ann Arvin and Richard Whitley

64

Antiviral therapy of HSV-1 and -2

David W. Kimberlin and Richard J. Whitley

Department of Pediatrics, University of Alabama at Birmingham, AL, USA

Introduction

The discovery of effective antiviral agents has been facilitated by advances in the fields of molecular biology and virology. In the pre-antiviral era, the widely held belief was that any therapeutically meaningful interference with viral replication would destroy the host cell upon which viral replication was dependent. A growing understanding of host cell–virus interactions and viral replication, however, has led to the development of safe and effective antivirals. These agents act by impeding entry of viruses into host cells; interfering with viral assembly, release, or de-aggregation; inhibiting transcription or replication of the viral genome; or interrupting viral protein synthesis.

Antiviral agents can be used to treat disease (a therapeutic strategy), to prevent infection (a prophylactic strategy), or to prevent disease (a preemptive strategy). Prophylaxis refers to the administration of an agent to patients at risk of contracting infection (e.g., acyclovir given to HSV-seropositive renal transplant recipients). Pre-emptive treatment refers to the administration of a drug after there is evidence of infection, but before there is evidence of disease (e.g., ganciclovir given to bone marrow transplant recipients with positive CMV culture, but no symptoms of infection).

The effectiveness of antiviral therapy sometimes is limited by the development of antiviral resistance. Antiviral drug resistance has increased in parallel with the expanded use of, and indications for, antiviral therapy. Resistance most commonly occurs in patients with chronic and/or progressive infections who have been exposed to prolonged or repeated courses of therapy. An impaired host immune system which cannot fully contribute to suppressing viral replication, thus leaving to antiviral agent(s) as the sole defense against ongoing viral disease, also predisposes to the development of antiviral resistance, as does administration of the antiviral agent at doses which produce subtherapeutic drug concentrations relative to that needed for virocidal or virostatic activity. In general, antiviral resistance should be suspected if the clinical response to therapy is less than that anticipated on the basis of prior experience (Kimberlin et al., 1995b).

There are a number of antiviral medications with activity against HSV-1 and HSV-2. With the exception of foscarnet and cidofovir, all are nucleoside analogues. While three of these medications (acyclovir, famciclovir, and valaciclovir) are used to treat the overwhelming majority of cases of HSV-1 and HSV-2, the other medications reviewed in this chapter (cidofovir, foscarnet, ganciclovir, and valganciclovir) also have activity against the alpha herpesviruses and are indicated in certain circumstances, such as the treatment of some acyclovir-resistant HSV isolates. Discussion in this chapter of the efficacies of these first-line and second-line drugs will be limited to their use as second-line agents for HSV-1 and HSV-2 infections. Antiviral treatment of VZV and CMV can be found in Chapters 70 and 71, respectively.

First-line antiviral agents for HSV-1 and HSV-2 infections

Acyclovir

Acyclovir is in many regards the prototypic antiviral agent. The notable safety profile of acyclovir relates to its initial activation by the viral-induced enzyme thymidine kinase. Acyclovir is most active against HSV; activity against VZV also is substantial but approximately ten-fold less. Epstein Barr virus (EBV) is only moderately susceptible to acyclovir because EBV has minimal thymidine kinase activity. Activity against CMV is poor because CMV does not have a unique thymidine kinase, and CMV DNA polymerase is poorly inhibited by acyclovir triphosphate. Acyclovir is the most frequently prescribed antiviral agent. It has been available for clinical use for over two decades and has demonstrated remarkable safety and efficacy against mild to severe infections caused by HSV and VZV in both normal and immunocompromised patients.

Mechanism of action and pharmacokinetics

Acyclovir is a deoxyguanosine analogue with an acyclic side chain that lacks the 3′-hydoxyl group of natural nucleosides (Wagstaff et al., 1994). Following preferential uptake by infected cells, acyclovir is monophosphorylated by virus-encoded thymidine kinase; host cell thymidine kinase is approximately 1 millionfold less capable of converting acyclovir to its monophosphate derivative. Subsequent diphosphorylation and triphosphorylation are catalyzed by host cell enzymes, resulting in acyclovir triphosphate concentrations that are 40 to 100 times higher in HSV-infected cells than in uninfected cells (Elion, 1982). Acyclovir triphosphate prevents viral DNA synthesis by inhibiting the viral DNA polymerase. In vitro, acyclovir triphosphate competes with deoxyguanosine triphosphate as a substrate for viral DNA polymerase. Because acyclovir triphosphate lacks the 3′-hydroxyl group required to elongate the DNA chain, the growing chain of DNA is terminated. In the presence of the deoxynucleoside triphosphate complementary to the next template position, the viral DNA polymerase is functionally inactivated (Reardon and Spector, 1989). In addition, acyclovir triphosphate is a much better substrate for the viral polymerase than for cellular DNA polymerase α, resulting in little incorporation of acyclovir into cellular DNA.

The oral bioavailability of acyclovir is poor, with only 15%–30% of the oral formulations being absorbed. Following a 200 mg dose, a peak concentration of about 0.5 μg/ml is attained at approximately 1.5 to 2.5 hours (Wagstaff et al., 1994). Higher doses of acyclovir result in higher serum concentrations. Food does not substantially alter extent of absorption. After intravenous doses of 2.5 to 15 mg/kg, steady-state concentrations of acyclovir range from 6.7 to 20.6 μg/ml. Acyclovir is widely distributed; high concentrations are attained in kidneys, lung, liver, heart, and skin vesicles; concentrations in the cerebrospinal fluid (CSF) are about 50% of those in the plasma (Wagstaff et al., 1994). Acyclovir crosses the placenta and accumulates in breast milk. Protein binding ranges from 9% to 33% and less than 20% of drug is metabolized to biologically inactive metabolites.

In the absence of compromised renal function, the half-life of acyclovir is 2 to 3 hours in older children and adults and 2.5 to 5 hours in neonates with normal creatinine clearance. More than 60% of administered drug is excreted in the urine (Wagstaff et al., 1994). Elimination is prolonged in patients with renal dysfunction; the half-life is approximately 20 hours in persons with end-stage renal disease, necessitating dose modifications for those with creatinine clearance less than 50 ml/min per 1.73 m^2 (Laskin et al., 1982). Acyclovir is effectively removed by hemodialysis but not by continuous ambulatory peritoneal dialysis (Krasny et al., 1982).

Antiviral therapy

Clinical efficacy in HSV-1 and HSV-2 infections
Genital herpes

For the treatment of first episode genital herpes, the dose of oral acyclovir is 200 mg orally five times per day, or 400 mg orally three times per day (Table 64.1). Neither higher doses of oral acyclovir nor the addition of topical acyclovir provide added benefit (Wald et al., 1994). Duration of therapy in first episode disease is 7–10 days (Anonymous, 2002). Acyclovir therapy for the treatment of first episode genital herpes reduces the duration of viral shedding by about a week, time to healing of lesions by approximately four days, and time to complete resolution of signs and symptoms by approximately two days (Bryson et al., 1983; Mertz et al., 1984) (Table 64.2).

For the episodic treatment of recurrent genital herpes, dosing options for acyclovir include 200 mg orally five times per day, or 800 mg orally two times per day, administered for 5 days (Anonymous, 2002) (Table 64.1). Topical acyclovir provides no clinical benefit in the episodic management of recurrences and is not recommended (Corey et al., 1982; Luby et al., 1984). A recent study indicates that 2 days of oral acyclovir therapy (800 mg three times per day) is also efficacious in the episodic treatment of genital HSV recurrences (Wald et al., 2002). When started within 24 hours of the onset of a genital herpes recurrence, oral acyclovir reduces the duration of viral shedding by approximately two days, time to healing by just over a day, and time to complete resolution of signs and symptoms by approximately a day (Tyring et al., 1998) (Table 64.2). Episodic treatment does not reduce the length of time to subsequent recurrence (Nilsen et al., 1982; Reichman et al., 1984; Ruhnek-Forsbeck et al., 1985).

In addition to the treatment of an active genital herpes infection, acyclovir has been effectively used to prevent recurrences of genital herpes. The most frequent indication for suppressive acyclovir therapy is in patients with frequently recurrent genital infections, in whom chronic

Table 64.1. Therapeutic management of genital herpes[a]

	First clinical episode (treat orally for 7–10 days[b])	Episodic recurrent infection[e] (treat orally for 5 days)	Oral suppressive therapy	Episodic recurrent infection in HIV-infected persons (treat orally for 5–10 days)	Oral suppressive therapy in HIV-infected persons	Advantages	Disadvantages[f]
Acyclovir	200 mg 5×/day *or* 400 mg 3×/day	200 mg 5×/day *or* 800 mg 2×/day	400 mg 2×/day	200 mg 5×/day *or* 400 mg 3×/day	400–800 mg 2×/day or 3×/day	Less expensive; Smaller tablets; Liquid formulation available	Less convenient dosing regimens
Valaciclovir	1000 mg/ 2×/day	500 mg 2×/day[c] *or* 1000 mg 1×/day	500 mg 1×/day[d] *or* 1000 mg 1×/day	1000 mg 2×/day	500 mg 2×/day	More convenient dosing regimens	More expensive; Larger caplet
Famciclovir	250 mg 3×/day	125 mg 2×/day	250 mg 2×/day	500 mg 2×/day	500 mg 2×/day	More convenient dosing regimens; Smaller tablet	More expensive

[a] Modified from Reference (Anonymous, 2002).
[b] The range of duration of therapy relates to differences in treatment durations in the original clinical studies. If the shorter course of therapy is initially prescribed, the patient should be reevaluated toward the end of treatment and therapy should be continued if new lesions continue to form, if complications develop, or if systemic signs and symptoms have not abated.
[c] Three-day course of therapy also acceptable
[d] For patients with ≤9 recurrences/year
[e] When started within 24 hours of the recurrence
[f] Allergic and other adverse reactions to acyclovir, valaciclovir, and famciclovir are rare.

Table 64.2. Efficacies of acyclovir, valaciclovir, and famciclovir in the treatment of genital HSV disease

	First episode genital herpes	Episodic treatment of genital herpes recurrences	Suppressive therapy for genital herpes
Acyclovir	2-day decrease in time to complete resolution of signs and symptoms (vs. placebo) (Mertz et al., 1984)	1.1-day decrease in time to complete resolution of signs and symptoms (vs. placebo) (Tyring et al., 1998)	After 1 year of therapy, 44% of acyclovir recipients were recurrence-free, vs. 2% of placebo recipients (Mertz et al., 1988b)
	4-day decrease in time to healing of lesions (vs. placebo) (Mertz et al., 1984)	1.2-day decrease in time to healing of lesions (vs. placebo) (Tyring et al., 1998)	After 4 months (120 days) of therapy, 71% of acyclovir recipients were recurrence-free, vs. 6% of placebo recipients (Douglas et al., 1984)
	7-day decrease in duration of viral shedding (vs. placebo) (Mertz et al., 1984)	2.0-day decrease in duration of viral shedding (vs. placebo) (Tyring et al., 1998)	80–94% reduction in days with subclinical shedding (vs. placebo) (Wald et al., 1997; Wald et al., 1996)
Valaciclovir	Compared with acyclovir, no difference in time to healing of lesions, duration of symptoms, and duration of viral shedding (Fife et al., 1997)	1.9-day decrease in time to complete resolution of signs and symptoms (vs. placebo) (Spruance et al., 1996)	After 16 weeks (112 days) of therapy, 69% of valaciclovir recipients were recurrence-free, vs. 9.5% of placebo recipients (Patel et al., 1997)
		1.9-day decrease in time to healing of lesions (vs. placebo) (Spruance et al., 1996)	Compared with acyclovir, no difference in effectiveness (Reitano et al., 1998)
		2.0-day decrease in duration of viral shedding (vs. placebo) (Spruance et al., 1996)	81% reduction in days with subclinical shedding (vs. placebo) (Wald et al., 1998)
		Compared with acyclovir, no difference in time to healing of lesions, duration of symptoms, and duration of viral shedding (Bodsworth et al., 1997; Tyring et al., 1998)	Compared with acyclovir, no difference in reduction of subclinical shedding (Wald et al., 1998)
Famciclovir	Compared with acyclovir, no difference in time to healing of lesions, duration of symptoms, and duration of viral shedding (Loveless et al., 1995)	0.5-day decrease in duration of signs and symptoms (vs. placebo) (Sacks et al., 1996a)	After 4 months (120 days) of therapy, 78% of famciclovir recipients were recurrence-free, vs. 42% of placebo recipients (Mertz et al., 1997b)
		1.0-day decrease in time to healing of lesions (vs. placebo) (Sacks et al., 1996a)	87% reduction in days with subclinical shedding (vs. placebo) (Sacks et al., 1997)
		1.6-day decrease in duration of viral shedding (vs. placebo) (Sacks et al., 1996a)	
		Compared with acyclovir, no difference in time to healing of lesions, duration of symptoms, and duration of viral shedding (Chosidow et al., 2001)	

suppressive acyclovir therapy reduces the frequency of recurrences by approximately 75% (Douglas et al., 1984; Mertz et al., 1988a; Mertz et al., 1988b; Mindel et al., 1988; Straus et al., 1984) (Table 64.2). One quarter to one-third of patients on suppressive therapy experience no further recurrences while taking acyclovir. Daily administration of acyclovir maintains a high degree of efficacy and little toxicity, even after more than 5 years of continuous suppressive therapy (Goldberg et al., 1993). Suppressive therapy reduces the frequency of asymptomatic shedding of HSV in the genital tract by more than 80% (Wald et al., 1997; Wald et al., 1996) (Table 64.2). The acyclovir dose when used as suppressive therapy is 400 mg administered twice daily (Table 64.1).

The historic rationale for episodic treatment of genital herpes was that, in many patients, the frequency and/or severity of clinical recurrences made treatment of the recurrences desirable, but they were not sufficiently frequent or annoying to warrant daily suppressive therapy. Advances in recent years in our understanding of asymptomatic viral shedding have begun to shift our therapeutic management away from episodic treatment and toward suppressive therapy (Kimberlin and Rouse, 2004). The current rationale for suppressive treatment is as follows: (1) most persons with first episode genital herpes are at risk of frequent recurrences over the next few years (Benedetti et al., 1994); (2) 70%–80% of patients receiving suppressive therapy remain recurrence-free at 4 months (Table 64.2), vs. 5%–10% of persons receiving placebo (Douglas et al., 1984; Mertz et al., 1988b; Mertz et al., 1997b; Patel et al., 1997; Reitano et al., 1998); (3) days with subclinical (asymptomatic) shedding are reduced by 80%–95% compared with placebo (Table 64.2) (Sacks et al., 1997; Wald et al., 1997; Wald et al., 1998; Wald et al., 1996); (4) suppressive therapy reduces the risk of HSV transmission to uninfected partners (Corey et al., 2004); (5) quality of life often is improved in patients with frequent recurrences who receive suppressive compared with episodic treatment (Alexander and Naisbett, 2002); and (6) suppressive therapy is safe (Douglas et al., 1984; Mertz et al., 1997b; Patel et al., 1997; Reitano et al., 1998).

HSV gingivostomatitis and recurrent herpes labialis

Treatment of primary gingivostomatitis in pediatric patients using oral acyclovir decreases time to cessation of symptoms by 30%–50%, and time to lesion healing by 20%–25% (Aoki et al., 1993). Compared with patients receiving placebo, subjects treated with oral acyclovir at 600 mg/m^2 per dose administered four times per day for 10 days experienced cessation of drooling in 4 days (vs. 8 days in placebo recipients) and resolution of gum swelling in 5 days (vs. 7 days in placebo recipients). Intraoral lesions in acyclovir recipients healed at 6 days (vs. 8 days in placebo recipients), and extraoral lesions healed in 7 days (vs. 9 days in placebo recipients) (Aoki et al., 1993).

Oral acyclovir has a more modest effect in the treatment of recurrent herpes labialis (Raborn et al., 1988; Raborn et al., 1987), and treatment of these patients should be individualized (Kimberlin and Prober, 2003). In general, therapeutic benefit is enhanced if treatment is initiated as soon as possible after onset of symptoms, preferably within 24 to 48 hours of onset of the recurrence. Among patients who start treatment in the prodrome or erythema lesion stage, acyclovir therapy (400 mg five times a day for 5 days) reduces the duration of pain by approximately one-third, and the healing time to loss of crust by approximately one-fourth (Spruance et al., 1990). Topical acyclovir cream may also modestly decrease the duration of a clinical recurrence of herpes labialis by approximately half a day (approximately $4\frac{1}{2}$ days for topical acyclovir recipients, compared with approximately 5 days for placebo recipients) (Spruance et al., 2002), although benefit of topical acyclovir is not conferred by acyclovir ointment, which has a polyethylene glycol base (Shaw et al., 1985; Spruance et al., 1984).

Prophylactic acyclovir also has been used to prevent reactivation of herpes labialis following exposure to ultraviolet radiation, facial surgery, or exposure to sun and wind while skiing (Gold and Corey, 1987; Spruance et al., 1991; Spruance et al., 1988). Topical acyclovir cream also is effective in preventing recurrent herpes labialis in skiers (Raborn et al., 1997) and in persons with a history of frequent recurrences of herpes labialis (Gibson et al., 1986). Long-term suppressive therapy reduces the number of recurrences of oral infection in those with histories of frequent recurrences (Rooney et al., 1993). In one study of 400 mg of oral acyclovir administered twice daily for 4 months, clinical recurrences were reduced by more than half, and culture-confirmed recurrences were reduced by more than two-thirds (Rooney et al., 1993).

Herpes simplex encephalitis (HSE)

For herpes simplex encephalitis, intravenous acyclovir should be administered at 30 mg/kg per day for 14–21 days for the treatment of HSE (Whitley et al., 1986). Some experts recommend higher dosages of intravenous acyclovir be considered (45–60 mg/kg per day), although neurotoxicity can be a limiting factor in increasing the dose in larger children and adults. In untreated patients, mortality from HSE exceeds 70%, and only 2.5% of survivors return to normal neurologic function. Even with appropriate administration of antiviral therapy, substantial mortality and morbidity from HSE remain (Skoldenberg et al., 1984), with 19% of patients dying and 62% of survivors having residual neurologic sequelae (Whitley et al., 1986). Patients with a Glasgow coma score of less than 6, those older than 30 years, and those with encephalitis for longer than 4 days have a poorer outcome (Whitley et al., 1986).

Neonatal HSV

For neonatal HSV disease, intravenous acyclovir at 60 mg/kg per day delivered in three divided daily doses is currently recommended (American Academy of Pediatrics, 2003; Kimberlin et al., 2001a). The dosing interval of intravenous acyclovir may need to be increased in premature infants, based upon their creatinine clearance (Englund et al., 1991). Duration of therapy is 21 days for patients with disseminated or CNS neonatal HSV disease, and 14 days for patients with HSV infection limited to the SEM (American Academy of Pediatrics, 2003). The primary apparent

Table 64.3. Mortality and morbidity outcomes among 295 infants with neonatal HSV infection, evaluated by the National Institutes of Allergy and Infectious Diseases' Collaborative Antiviral Study Group between 1974 and 1997[a]

Extent of disease	Treatment			
	Placebo (Whitley et al., 1980a)	Vidarabine (Whitley et al., 1991a)	Acyclovir (Whitley et al., 1991a) 30 mg/kg per day	Acyclovir (Kimberlin et al., 2001a) 60 mg/kg per day
Disseminated disease	$n = 13$	$n = 28$	$n = 18$	$n = 34$
Dead	11 (85%)	14 (50%)	11 (61%)	10 (29%)
Alive	2 (15%)	14 (50%)	7 (39%)	24 (71%)
Normal	1 (50%)	7 (50%)	3 (43%)	15 (63%)
Abnormal	1 (50%)	5 (36%)	2 (29%)	3 (13%)
Unknown	0 (0%)	2 (14%)	2 (29%)	6 (25%)
Central nervous system infection	$n = 6$	$n = 36$	$n = 35$	$n = 23$
Dead	3 (50%)	5 (14%)	5 (14%)	1 (4%)
Alive	3 (50%)	31 (86%)	30 (86%)	22 (96%)
Normal	1 (33%)	13 (42%)	8 (27%)	4 (18%)
Abnormal	2 (67%)	17 (55%)	20 (67%)	9 (41%)
Unknown	0 (0%)	1 (3%)	2 (7%)	9 (41%)
Skin, eye, or mouth infection	$n = 8$	$n = 31$	$n = 54$	$n = 9$
Dead	0 (0%)	0 (0%)	0 (0%)	0 (0%)
Alive	8 (100%)	31 (100%)	54 (100%)	9 (100%)
Normal	5 (62%)	22 (71%)	45 (83%)	2 (22%)
Abnormal	3 (38%)	3 (10%)	1 (2%)	0 (0%)
Unknown	0 (0%)	6 (19%)	8 (15%)	7 (78%)

[a] Adapted from Kimberlin (2001).

toxicity associated with the use of this dose of intravenous acyclovir is neutropenia, with approximately one-fifth of patients with localized HSV disease (CNS or SEM) developing an absolute neutrophil count (ANC) of $\leq 1000/\mu l$ (Kimberlin et al., 2001a). Although the neutropenia resolves either during continuation of intravenous acyclovir or following its cessation, it is prudent to monitor neutrophil counts at least twice weekly throughout the course of intravenous acyclovir therapy, with consideration being given to decreasing the dose of acyclovir or administering granulocyte colony stimulating factor (GCSF) if the ANC remains below $500/\mu L$ for a prolonged period of time (Kimberlin et al., 2001a). All patients with CNS HSV involvement should have a repeat lumbar puncture at the end of intravenous acyclovir therapy to determine that the specimen is PCR-negative in a reliable laboratory, and to document the end-of-therapy CSF indices (Kimberlin et al., 2001b). Those persons who remain PCR-positive should continue to receive intravenous antiviral therapy until PCR-negativity is achieved (Kimberlin et al., 1996b; Kimberlin et al., 2001b).

In the pre-antiviral era, 85% of patients with disseminated neonatal HSV disease died by one year of age, as did 50% of patients with CNS neonatal HSV disease (Whitley et al., 1980a) (Table 64.3). Evaluations of two different doses of vidarabine and of a lower dose of acyclovir (30 mg/kg/day for 10 days) documented that both of these antiviral drugs reduce mortality to comparable degrees (Whitley et al., 1991a; Whitley et al., 1980a; Whitley et al., 1983), with mortality rates at 1 year from disseminated disease decreasing to 54% and from CNS disease decreasing to 14% (Whitley et al., 1991a) (Table 64.3). Despite its lack of therapeutic superiority, the lower dose of acyclovir quickly supplanted vidarabine as the treatment of choice for neonatal HSV disease due to its favorable safety profile and its ease of administration. Unlike acyclovir, vidarabine had to be administered over prolonged infusion times and in large volumes of fluid.

With utilization of a higher dose of acyclovir (60 mg/kg per day for 21 days), 12 month mortality is further reduced to 29% for disseminated neonatal HSV disease and to 4% for CNS HSV disease (Kimberlin et al., 2001a) (Figs. 64.1 and

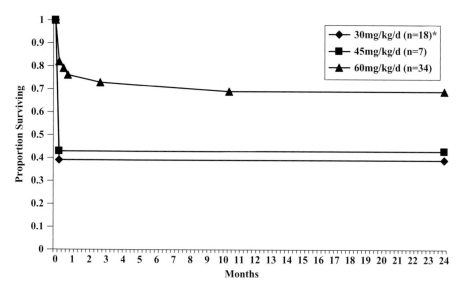

Fig. 64.1. Mortality in patients with disseminated neonatal HSV disease. (From Kimberlin et al., 2001a.)

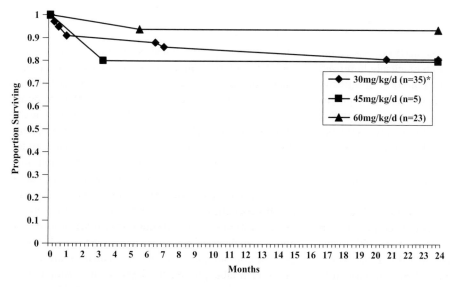

Fig. 64.2. Mortality in patients with CNS neonatal HSV disease. (From Kimberlin et al., 2001a.)

64.2). Differences in mortality at 24 months among patients treated with the higher dose of acyclovir and the lower dose of acyclovir are statistically significant after stratification for disease category (CNS vs. disseminated) (Kimberlin et al., 2001a). Lethargy and severe hepatitis are associated with mortality among patients with disseminated disease, as are prematurity and seizures in patients with CNS disease (Kimberlin et al., 2001b).

Improvements in morbidity rates with antiviral therapies have not been as dramatic as with mortality. In the pre-antiviral era, 50% of survivors of disseminated neonatal HSV infections were developing normally at 12 months of age (Whitley et al., 1980a) (Table 64.3). With utilization of the higher dose of acyclovir for 21 days, this percentage has increased to 83% (Kimberlin et al., 2001a) (Fig. 64.3). In the case of CNS neonatal HSV disease, 33% of patients in the pre-antiviral era were developing normally at 12 months of age (Whitley et al., 1980a) (Table 64.3), while 31% of higher dose acyclovir recipients develop normally at 12 months today (Kimberlin et al., 2001a) (Fig. 64.3). While

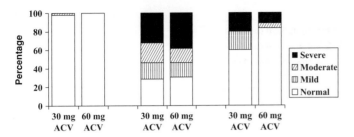

Fig. 64.3. Morbidity among patients with known outcomes after 12 months of life. (From Kimberlin et al., 2001a.)

these differences are not dramatic, it is important to note that as more neonates survive neonatal HSV disease based upon the mortality data presented above, the total numbers of patients who subsequently develop normally is higher today even while the percentages of survivors with normal development are not dramatically different. Seizures at or before the time of initiation of antiviral therapy are associated with increased risk of morbidity both in patients with CNS disease and in patients with disseminated infection (Kimberlin et al., 2001b).

Unlike disseminated or CNS neonatal HSV disease, morbidity following SEM disease has dramatically improved during the antiviral era. Prior to utilization of antiviral therapies, 38% of SEM patients experienced developmental difficulties at 12 months of age (Whitley et al., 1980a) (Table 64.3). With vidarabine and lower dose acyclovir, these percentages were reduced to 12% and 2%, respectively (Whitley et al., 1991a). In the high-dose acyclovir study, no SEM patients developed neurologic sequelae at 12 months of life (Kimberlin et al., 2001a) (Fig. 64.3).

In the pre-antiviral era, 70% of neonates with disease initially limited to skin vesicles experienced progression of disease to involvement of the CNS or visceral organs (Whitley et al., 1980b). It is likely that the initial reduction in morbidity among patients with SEM disease from 38% (Whitley et al., 1980a) to 2–12% (Whitley et al., 1991a) resulted from antiviral therapy impeding this progression to CNS or disseminated disease categories, each of which carries a higher risk of neurologic sequelae (Whitley et al., 1988). The continued reduction in morbidity among patients with SEM disease seen in the recently completed high-dose acyclovir study might relate to a redefinition of what constitutes SEM vs. CNS involvement. Prior to the application of PCR technology to neonatal HSV disease, patients were classified as having SEM disease if they had no overt laboratory or clinical evidence of viral dissemination to the viscera and/or CNS. The lack of CNS involvement was manifest by no CNS symptomatology (seizures, abnormal neuroimaging studies, abnormal electroencephalograms,

etc.) and normal CSF indices. As discussed above, however, PCR analysis of CSF specimens from neonates classified by these criteria as having SEM disease revealed that approximately one-quarter (7 of 29, or 24%) of these infants actually had HSV DNA present in their CSF during the acute disease course (Kimberlin et al., 1996b). One of these seven patients subsequently developed significant neurologic impairment by age 12 months. Thus, it is possible that at least some of the SEM patients in the earlier studies who subsequently developed neurologic impairment actually had subclinical CNS disease, which could only be detected by means of the powerful investigative tool provided by PCR beginning in the 1990s. These data have resulted in a revised classification of CNS disease, such that a positive CSF PCR result is now sufficient to classify a patient as having CNS HSV infection.

Another possible explanation for the neurologic impairment previously experienced by some infants with SEM disease could be that, while low level viremia from the cutaneous lesions results in seeding of the CNS, initial damage to brain tissue during the acute illness does not occur either due to a host response to infection or due to antiviral therapy. Subclinical reactivation of virus within the CNS, with or without a clinical cutaneous recurrence, might then produce neurologic impairment, as has been suggested (Kimberlin, 2001; Whitley et al., 1991b). Supporting this hypothesis, HSV DNA has been detected in the CSF of an SEM infant at the time of a cutaneous recurrence (Kimberlin et al., 1996a). Randomized, controlled studies of long-term suppressive oral acyclovir therapy following the acute neonatal disease are currently being conducted by the NIAID Collaborative Antiviral Study Group to evaluate this hypothesis. At the current time, however, no evidence exists to suggest that suppressive oral acyclovir therapy is beneficial in preventing neurologic complications. Furthermore, almost half of infants receiving oral acyclovir in an open-label phase I/II investigation developed neutropenia while on therapy (Kimberlin et al., 1996a), raising substantial questions about the safety of such a therapeutic approach outside of the strictly monitored confines of a clinical investigation.

HSV disease in the immunocompromised host

Acyclovir also is indicated for the treatment of disseminated HSV infections in otherwise normal hosts, including pregnant women, and mucocutaneous HSV infections in immunocompromised hosts (Kimberlin and Prober, 2003). Similarly, HSV infections of the lip, mouth, skin, perianal area, or genitals may be much more severe in immunocompromised patients than in normal hosts, with HSV lesions tending to be more invasive, slower to heal, and associated with prolonged viral shedding. Intravenous acyclovir therapy is very beneficial in such patients (Wade et al., 1982). Immunocompromised patients receiving acyclovir have a shorter duration of viral shedding and more rapid healing of lesions than patients receiving placebo (Meyers et al., 1982). Oral acyclovir therapy is also very effective in immunocompromised patients (Shepp et al., 1985).

Acyclovir prophylaxis of HSV infections is of clinical value in severely immunocompromised patients, especially those undergoing induction chemotherapy or transplantation. Intravenous or oral administration of acyclovir reduces the incidence of symptomatic HSV infection from about 70% to 5%–20% (Saral et al., 1981). A sequential regimen of intravenous acyclovir followed by oral acyclovir for 3 to 6 months can virtually eliminate symptomatic HSV infections in organ transplant recipients. A variety of oral dosing regimens, ranging from 200 mg 3 times daily to 800 mg twice daily, have been used successfully. Among bone marrow transplant recipients and patients with AIDS, acyclovir-resistant HSV isolates have been identified more frequently after therapeutic acyclovir administration than during prophylaxis (Wade et al., 1983).

HSV keratitis or keratoconjunctivitis
Topical therapy with acyclovir for HSV ocular infections is effective, but probably not superior to trifluridine (Hovding, 1989). Long-term suppressive therapy reduces the number of recurrences of ocular infection in those with histories of frequent recurrences (Herpetic Eye Disease Study Group, 1998, 2000).

Challenges for achieving clinical benefit, including adverse drug effects

Perhaps the most prominent challenge impacting clinical benefit of acyclovir therapy relates to the timing of drug initiation following onset of disease symptoms. In the case of life-threatening HSV disease, consideration of HSV as a possible cause of the illness is needed in order to then initiate acyclovir therapy. In the case of less severe but still consequential infections, such as primary genital herpes, the patient must present to medical attention, be correctly diagnosed, and then started on antiviral therapy as quickly as possible to achieve maximal benefit.

Acyclovir is a safe drug which is generally very well tolerated. Oral acyclovir sometimes causes mild gastrointestinal upset, rash, and headache. If it extravasates, intravenous acyclovir can cause severe inflammation, phlebitis, and sometimes a vesicular eruption leading to cutaneous necrosis at the injection site. If given by rapid intravenous infusion or to poorly hydrated patients or those with pre-existing renal compromise, intravenous acyclovir can cause reversible nephrotoxicity due to the formation of acyclovir crystals precipitating in renal tubules and causing an obstructive nephropathy. Administration of acyclovir by the intravenous route occasionally is associated with rash, sweating, nausea, headache, hematuria, and hypotension. High doses of intravenous acyclovir (60 mg/kg per day) in neonates and prolonged use of oral acyclovir following neonatal disease have been associated with neutropenia (Kimberlin et al., 1996a, 2001b).

The most serious side effect of acyclovir is neurotoxicity, which usually occurs in subjects with compromised renal function who attain high serum concentrations of drug (Revankar et al., 1995). Neurotoxicity is manifest as lethargy, confusion, hallucinations, tremors, myoclonus, seizures, extrapyramidal signs, and changes in state of consciousness, developing within the first few days of initiating therapy. These signs and symptoms usually resolve spontaneously within several days of discontinuing acyclovir.

Although acyclovir is mutagenic at high concentrations in some in vitro assays, it is not teratogenic in animals. Limited human data suggest that acyclovir use in pregnant women is not associated with congenital defects or other adverse pregnancy outcomes (Reiff-Eldridge et al., 2000).

The likelihood of renal toxicity of acyclovir is increased when administered with nephrotoxic drugs such as cyclosporine or amphotericin B. Somnolence and lethargy may occur in subjects being treated with both zidovudine and acyclovir. Concomitant administration of probenicid prolongs acyclovir's half-life, whereas acyclovir can decrease the clearance and prolong the half-life of drugs such as methotrexate that are eliminated by active renal secretion.

Clinical indications

Acyclovir is licensed in the United States for the treatment of initial episodes and management of recurrent episodes of genital herpes, for the treatment of chickenpox, and for the treatment of acute herpes zoster infections. It is also indicated for the treatment of neonatal HSV disease, herpes simplex encephalitis, mucocutaneous and viscerally disseminated herpes infections in immunocompromised hosts, and the treatment of chickenpox in the normal host.

Antiviral resistance

Resistance of HSV to acyclovir has become an important clinical problem, especially among immunocompromised patients exposed to long-term therapy (Englund et al., 1990). Viral resistance to acyclovir usually results from mutations in the viral TK gene although mutations in the viral DNA polymerase gene also occur rarely. Resistant isolates can cause severe, progressive, debilitating mucosal disease and, rarely, visceral dissemination (Field and Biron, 1994; Lyall et al., 1994). Isolates of HSV resistant to acyclovir also have been reported in normal hosts, most commonly in patients with frequently recurrent genital infection who have been treated with chronic acyclovir (Morfin and Thouvenot, 2003).

Famciclovir/penciclovir

Famciclovir is the inactive diacetyl ester prodrug of penciclovir, an acyclic nucleoside analogue. Following oral ingestion and systemic absorption, famciclovir is rapidly deacetylated and oxidized to form the active parent drug penciclovir.

Mechanism of action and pharmacokinetics

In cells which are infected with HSV, the viral thymidine kinase (TK) phosphorylates penciclovir to its monophosphate derivative, which in turn is converted to the active penciclovir triphosphate by cellular kinases. Penciclovir triphosphate inhibits viral DNA polymerase by competing with deoxyguanosine triphosphate for incorporation into the growing DNA strand. While penciclovir triphosphate is neither an obligate DNA chain terminator nor an inactivator of the DNA polymerase, once incorporated penciclovir triphosphate does retard the rate of subsequent nucleotide incorporation. Penciclovir is approximately 100-fold less potent than acyclovir in inhibiting herpesvirus DNA polymerase activity. By virtue of its high intracellular concentrations and long intracellular half-life (7 to 20 hours), though, it remains an effective antiviral agent.

The bioavailability of penciclovir following oral administration of famciclovir is about 70%. Peak concentrations of drug after intravenous administration of 10 mg/kg are approximately six-fold higher than those attained after oral doses of 250 mg. Food delays absorption but does not affect the final plasma drug concentration. Following oral administration, little or no famciclovir is detected in plasma or urine. The plasma half-life of penciclovir is about 2.5 hours, and almost three-quarters is recovered unchanged in the urine. Measurable penciclovir concentrations are not detectable in plasma or urine following topical administration of penciclovir cream. A 12-hour dosing interval is recommended for those with creatinine clearances between 30 and 50 ml/min per 1.73 m^2, and a 24-hour interval for those with creatinine clearances less than 30 ml/min per 1.73 m^2 (Boike et al., 1994).

Antiviral therapy

Penciclovir's (and thus famciclovir's) spectrum of activity against herpesviruses is similar to that of acyclovir. In addition to HSV, penciclovir has demonstrable *in vitro* activity against VZV, EBV, and hepatitis B virus (HBV).

Clinical efficacy in HSV-1 and HSV-2 infections

Genital herpes

In the episodic treatment of genital herpes, famciclovir reduces time to healing, time to cessation of viral shedding, and durations of lesion edema, vesicles, ulcers, and crusts when compared with placebo (Sacks et al., 1996b). Times to cessation of all symptoms and of moderate to severe lesion tenderness, pain, and burning are also reduced (Sacks et al., 1996b). For suppression of genital HSV recurrences, famciclovir delays the time to the first recurrence of genital herpes when compared with placebo (Diaz-Mitoma et al., 1998; Mertz et al., 1997a). Dosing and anticipated benefits of treatment of primary and recurrent genital herpes, and of suppressive therapy, are shown in Tables 64.1 and 64.2, respectively.

Recurrent herpes labialis

Topical penciclovir (Denavir) for the treatment of recurrent herpes labialis reduces time to healing and duration of pain by about half a day (Boon et al., 2000). Topical penciclovir cream decreases the time to lesion healing by approximately 1 to 2 days when compared with placebo (Boon et al., 2000; Spruance et al., 1997), and is equally effective as topical acyclovir cream (Lin et al., 2002). Additional benefit is noted in a reduction in lesion area; faster loss of lesion-associated symptoms; and reductions in daily assessments of pain, itching, burning, and tenderness (Boon et al., 2000). Faster healing and pain resolution occurs both among patients who first apply penciclovir cream in the prodrome and erythema stages and among those who start treatment in the papule and vesicle lesion stages (Spruance et al., 1997). Application of medicine should begin as early as possible, preferably during the prodromal phase, and should be continued every 2 hours during waking hours for 4 days. (Diaz-Mitoma et al., 1998; Mertz et al., 1997a)

Challenges for achieving clinical benefit, including adverse drug effects

Famciclovir is as well tolerated as acyclovir. Complaints of nausea, diarrhea, and headache occurred in clinical trials, but at frequencies similar to those reported by placebo recipients. No clinically significant drug interactions have been reported to date, although concentrations of famciclovir among volunteers increase by about 20% in patients receiving concomitant cimetidine or theophylline administration.

Clinical indications

Famciclovir was approved by the FDA for the treatment of acute herpes zoster in 1994, and subsequently was approved for the treatment and suppression of genital HSV disease in immunocompetent patients. Famciclovir is also approved for the treatment of recurrent mucocutaneous HSV disease in HIV-infected patients. Topical penciclovir is approved for the treatment of recurrent herpes labialis in adults.

Dosage regimens

For the episodic treatment of recurrent genital HSV disease, the dosage of famciclovir is 125 mg twice daily, administered for 5 days (Table 64.1). The recommended dose for suppression of genital HSV is 250 mg twice daily for up to 1 year (Table 64.1). Note that the lack of harmonization of treatment regimens resulted from different doses of famciclovir being studied in the clinical trials; this produced the unusual dosage recommendation of decreasing the suppression dose to treat a genital HSV recurrence. The safety and efficacy of famciclovir therapy beyond 1 year of treatment have not been established. For recurrent orolabial or genital HSV infection in HIV-infected patients, the recommended dose is 500 mg twice daily for 7 days.

Application of topical penciclovir to recurrent herpes labialis lesions should begin as early as possible, preferably during the prodromal phase, and should be continued every 2 hours during waking hours for 4 days.

Dose reduction of famciclovir is recommended for patients with compromised renal function. A 12-hour dosing interval is recommended for persons with creatinine clearances between 30 and 50 ml/min per 1.73 m^2, and a 24-hour interval for those with creatinine clearances less than 30 ml/min per 1.73 m^2 (Boike et al., 1994).

The safety and efficacy of famciclovir and topical penciclovir in children have not been established. No liquid or suspension formulation exists currently.

Antiviral resistance

Because penciclovir, like acyclovir, must be activated by the viral encoded TK enzyme, TK-deficient viral strains are resistant to both acyclovir and penciclovir. Strains of HSV whose resistance to acyclovir is conferred by alteration of the TK enzyme or by DNA polymerase mutations may remain sensitive to penciclovir (Kimberlin et al., 1995a).

Valaciclovir

Valaciclovir is the L-valyl ester of acyclovir that is rapidly converted to acyclovir after oral administration by first-pass metabolism in the liver (Jacobson, 1993). Licensed in 1995, it has a safety and efficacy profile similar to which of acyclovir but offers potential pharmacokinetic advantages.

Mechanism of action and pharmacokinetics

As a prodrug of acyclovir, valaciclovir has the same mechanism of action, antiviral spectrum, and resistance profiles as those of its parent drug, acyclovir. Following oral administration of valaciclovir, rapid and complete conversion to acyclovir occurs with first-pass intestinal and hepatic metabolism. The bioavailability of valaciclovir exceeds 50%, which is three to five times greater than that of acyclovir (Soul-Lawton et al., 1995). Peak serum concentrations, attained about 1.5 hours after a dose, are proportional to the amount of drug administered; they range from 0.8 to 8.5 µg/ml for doses of 100 to 2000 mg (Weller et al., 1993). The area under the drug concentration time curve approximates that seen after intravenous acyclovir. All other pharmacokinetic characteristics are similar to those of acyclovir (Nadal et al., 2002).

Antiviral therapy

Acyclovir is most active in vitro against HSV, with activity against VZV being about tenfold less. Although EBV has only minimal thymidine kinase activity, EBV DNA polymerase is susceptible to inhibition by acyclovir triphosphate and thus EBV is moderately susceptible to acyclovir in vitro. Activity against CMV is limited by CMV's lack of a gene for thymidine kinase; furthermore, CMV DNA polymerase is poorly inhibited by acyclovir triphosphate.

Clinical efficacy in HSV-1 and HSV-2 infections

Genital herpes

Valaciclovir treatment of first-episode genital HSV is as effective as acyclovir therapy, while at the same time providing a more favorable dosing schedule compared with acyclovir (Fife et al., 1997) (Tables 64.1 and 64.2). In the treatment of recurrent genital HSV, valaciclovir decreases the duration of lesions, the duration of pain, and the duration of viral shedding when compared to placebo (Spruance et al., 1996). Valaciclovir also is as effective as acyclovir for the episodic treatment of recurrent genital HSV, again providing a more favorable dosing schedule compared with acyclovir (Tyring et al., 1998) (Tables 64.1 and 64.2). It should be administered for 3 to 5 days when administered as episodic treatment (Anonymous, 2002; Leone et al., 2002). Valaciclovir is also effective in suppressing recurrences of genital HSV when administered as once-daily suppressive therapy (Reitano et al., 1998). Valaciclovir has recently demonstrated efficacy in the suppression of recurrent herpes labialis with 500 mg once-daily (Baker et al., 2000).

Recurrent herpes labialis
Valaciclovir administered at high doses for short periods of time (2 grams orally twice a day for 1 day) reduces the time to lesion healing and time to cessation of pain and/or discomfort compared to placebo, with the overall duration of the episode being decreased by approximately one day (Spruance et al., 2003). However, early valaciclovir treatment does not appear to increase the likelihood that a clinical recurrence will be aborted prior to cold sore lesion development (Chosidow et al., 2003; Spruance et al., 2003).

Valaciclovir administered as a 500 mg dose once daily is effective in suppressing recurrences of herpes labialis, with almost two-thirds of treated patients remaining recurrence-free during four months of suppressive therapy compared with approximately one-third of placebo recipients (Baker and Eisen, 2003; Baker et al., 2000).

Herpes simplex encephalitis
Herpes simplex encephalitis is managed acutely with intravenous acyclovir, as discussed above. A randomized, controlled trial of long-term suppressive oral valaciclovir therapy following the treatment of the acute HSE disease is currently being conducted by the NIAID Collaborative Antiviral Study Group. This study will determine whether subclinical reactivation of HSV within the brain contributes to the neurologic impairment experienced by many HSE survivors. At the current time, however, no evidence exists to suggest that suppressive oral valaciclovir therapy is beneficial in preventing neurologic complications.

Challenges for achieving clinical benefit, including adverse drug effects
The profiles of adverse effects and potential drug interactions observed with valaciclovir therapy are the same as those observed with acyclovir treatment. Neurotoxicity has not been reported in humans to date, although it has been observed in animal models (Jacobson, 1993). Manifestations resembling thrombotic microangiopathy have been described in patients with advanced HIV disease receiving very high doses of valaciclovir (8 grams per day), but the multitude of other medications being administered to such patients makes the establishment of a causal relationship to valaciclovir difficult (Bell et al., 1997). Although causation has not been established, use of valaciclovir at such high doses should involve evaluation of potential risks and benefits.

A limited number of adverse drug interactions with acyclovir have been reported. Subjects being treated with both zidovudine and acyclovir can develop severe somnolence and lethargy. The likelihood of renal toxicity is increased when acyclovir is administered with nephrotoxic drugs such as cyclosporine and amphotericin B. Concomitant administration of probenicid decreases renal clearance of acyclovir and prolongs its half-life; conversely, acyclovir can decrease the clearance of drugs such as methotrexate that are eliminated by active renal secretion.

Clinical indications
Valaciclovir is indicated for the treatment of herpes zoster, and for the treatment or suppression of genital herpes. Although data from controlled clinical trials are limited, because of greater bioavailability, valaciclovir may be advantageous in treating infections caused by viruses relatively less sensitive to acyclovir than HSV (e.g., VZV and CMV).

Dosage regimens
Adult treatment doses for HSV-1 and HSV-2 infections are: 1) 1 gram orally twice daily for 7–10 days for first episode genital herpes (Table 64.1, 64.2) 500 mg orally twice daily for 3–5 days for episodic treatment of recurrent genital HSV disease (Table 64.1); and 64.3) 1 gram orally once daily for suppression of recurrent genital HSV (Table 64.1). Suppression of recurrent oral herpes infections has been accomplished with single daily doses of 500 mg.

Valaciclovir dosages in children are not yet established. A valaciclovir oral suspension has recently been formulated and is undergoing Phase I evaluation in infants and children.

With decreasing creatinine clearance, the dosing interval should be spread. With significant renal impairment, the dose should also be reduced in half. Acyclovir is removed during hemodialysis, and therefore an extra dose of valaciclovir should be administered following completion of hemodialysis. Supplemental doses of valaciclovir are not required following chronic ambulatory peritoneal dialysis (CAPD) and continuous arteriovenous hemofiltration/dialysis (CAVHD).

Antiviral resistance

HSV resistance to acyclovir can result from mutations in either the viral TK gene or the viral DNA polymerase gene. Although these acyclovir-resistant isolates exhibit diminished virulence in animal models, among HIV-infected patients they can cause severe, progressive, debilitating mucosal disease and (rarely) visceral dissemination (Gateley et al., 1990). Acyclovir-resistant strains of HSV also have been recovered from cancer chemotherapy patients, bone marrow and solid organ transplant recipients, children with congenital immunodeficiency syndromes, and neonates (Kimberlin et al., 1996a). Although it is uncommon, genital herpes caused by acyclovir-resistant isolates has also been reported in immunocompetent hosts who usually have received chronic acyclovir therapy (Kost et al., 1993).

Second-line antiviral agents for HSV-1 and HSV-2 infections cidofovir

Cidofovir was first approved for use in the United States for the therapy of AIDS-associated retinitis caused by CMV, and this remains the main indication for this antiviral agent. With a mechanism of action independent of viral TK activity, however, cidofovir can have a role in the management of HSV-1 and HSV-2 infections which are acyclovir resistant, as described below.

Mechanism of action and pharmacokinetics

Cidofovir is a novel acyclic phosphonate nucleotide analogue. In its native form, cidofovir already has a single phosphate group attached, and thus viral enzymes are not required for initial phosphorylation of drug. In this regard, it is dissimilar to the nucleoside analogues such as acyclovir and ganciclovir. Cellular kinases sequentially attach two additional phosphate groups, converting cidofovir to its active diphosphate form.

Cidofovir has a mechanism of action which is similar to other nucleoside analogues. The active cidofovir diphosphate serves as a competitive inhibitor of DNA polymerase (Ho et al., 1992). While cidofovir is taken up by both virally infected and uninfected cells, the active form of the drug exhibits a 25- to 50-fold greater affinity for the viral DNA polymerase as compared to the cellular DNA polymerase, thereby selectively inhibiting viral replication (Ho et al., 1992). Incorporation of cidofovir into the growing viral DNA chain results in reductions in the rate of viral DNA synthesis.

Only 2%–26% of cidofovir is absorbed after oral administration, requiring that cidofovir be administered intravenously in the clinical management of patients. The plasma half-life of cidofovir is 2.6 hours, but active intracellular metabolites of cidofovir have half-lives of 17 to 48 hours (Cundy et al., 1995). Ninety percent of the drug is excreted in the urine, primarily by renal tubular secretion (Lalezari et al., 1995).

Antiviral therapy

While primarily a CMV drug, cidofovir has demonstrable activity against HSV as well. Due to its unique phosphorylation requirements for activation, the drug usually maintains activity against acyclovir- and foscarnet-resistant HSV isolates (Safrin et al., 1999). Although cidofovir is less potent in vitro against HSV than is acyclovir, its favorable pharmacokinetic profile increases its anti-HSV activity. Cidofovir also has demonstrated in vitro activity against varicella-zoster virus, Epstein–Barr virus, human herpesvirus-6, human herpesvirus-8, polyomaviruses, adenovirus, and human papillomavirus (HPV).

Clinical efficacy in HSV-1 and HSV-2 infections

The primary use for cidofovir at the current time is for the management of CMV retinitis in patients with acquired immunodeficiency syndrome (AIDS) (Lalezari et al., 1997; Studies of Ocular Complications of AIDS Research Group in collaboration with the AIDS Clinical Trials Group, 1997). However, cidofovir has been utilized successfully in the management of disease caused by acyclovir-resistant HSV isolates (Lalezari et al., 1994). Due in part to its toxicity profile (described below), cidofovir does not have a role in antiviral prophylaxis of herpesvirus infections.

The safety and efficacy of cidofovir in children have not been studied. Due to the risk of long-term carcinogenicity and reproductive toxicity, the use of cidofovir in children warrants caution.

Challenges for achieving clinical benefit, including adverse drug effects

The principle adverse event associated with systemic administration of cidofovir is nephrotoxicity. Cidofovir concentrates in renal cells in amounts 100 times greater than is seen in other tissues, producing severe proximal convoluted tubule nephrotoxicity when concomitant hydration and administration of probenecid are not employed (Cundy et al., 1995; Lalezari et al., 1995). When present, renal toxicity manifests as proteinuria and glycosuria. In order to decrease the potential for nephrotoxicity, aggressive intravenous prehydration and coadministration of probenecid are required with each cidofovir dose. Within 48 hours prior to delivery of each dose of cidofovir, serum creatinine and urine protein must be determined, with adjustment in dose as indicated. Due to its potential for nephrotoxicity, cidofovir should not be administered concomitantly with other potentially nephrotoxic agents (e.g., intravenous aminoglycosides (e.g., tobramycin, gentamicin, and amikacin), amphotericin B, foscarnet, intravenous pentamidine, vancomycin, and non-steroidal anti-inflammatory agents).

Cidofovir's potential for nephrotoxicity, neutropenia, ocular hypotony, and metabolic acidosis are judged significant enough to warrant warning statements from the FDA in the package insert. Cidofovir is carcinogenic, teratogenic, and causes hypospermia in animal studies.

Clinical indications

Cidofovir is licensed for the treatment of CMV retinitis in AIDS patients. The safety and efficacy of cidofovir for the treatment of other CMV infections, including those in non-HIV-infected individuals, or of resistant HSV infections has not been established.

Dosage regimens

Due to poor oral bioavailability (2%–26%), cidofovir can only be administered intravenously or topically. The recommended induction dose of cidofovir for patients with a serum creatinine of ≤ 1.5 mg/dl, a calculated creatinine clearance >55 ml/min, and a urine protein <100 mg/dl (equivalent to <2 + proteinuria) is 5 mg/kg body weight administered once weekly for two consecutive weeks. The recommended maintenance dose of cidofovir is 5 mg/kg body weight administered once every 2 weeks. Aggressive intravenous prehydration and coadministration of probenecid are required with each cidofovir dose. Cidofovir must not be administered intraocularly due to the potential for ocular hypotony.

Cidofovir is contraindicated in patients with serum creatinine >1.5 mg/dL, calculated creatinine clearance ≤ 55 ml/min, or urine protein ≥ 100 mg/dl (equivalent to $\geq 2+$ proteinuria). The maintenance dose of cidofovir must be reduced from 5 mg/kg to 3 mg/kg for an increase in serum creatinine of 0.3–0.4 mg/dl above baseline. Cidofovir therapy must be discontinued if serum creatinine increases ≥ 0.5 mg/dl above baseline.

Foscarnet

Foscarnet is an organic analogue of inorganic pyrophosphate, with the chemical name of phosphonoformic acid (PFA). As such, it is the only antiherpes drug that is not a nucleoside or nucleotide analogue. It has the potential to chelate divalent metal ions, such as calcium and magnesium, to form stable coordination compounds. It is not a first-line drug but is useful for the treatment of infections caused by resistant herpes viruses.

Mechanism of action and pharmacokinetics

Foscarnet directly inhibits DNA polymerase by blocking the pyrophosphate binding site and preventing cleavage of pyrophosphate from deoxynucleotide triphosphates (Wagstaff and Bryson, 1994). It is a non-competitive inhibitor of viral DNA polymerases or HIV reverse transcriptase, and is not incorporated into the growing viral DNA chain. It is approximately 100-fold more active against viral enzymes than host cellular enzymes.

Foscarnet is poorly absorbed after oral administration, with a bioavailability of only about 20%, thereby limiting foscarnet's delivery to the intravenous route. Maximum serum concentration attained after a dose of 60 mg/kg is approximately 500 μmol/l (Wagstaff and Bryson, 1994). Data are limited regarding tissue distribution, but CSF concentrations are about two-thirds of those in serum. Eighty percent of an administered dose of foscarnet is eliminated unchanged in the urine; half-life is 48 hours, and dosage adjustments are necessary even in the presence of minimal degrees of renal dysfunction. Hemodialysis efficiently eliminates foscarnet and therefore an extra dose of drug is recommended after a 3-hour dialysis run (MacGregor et al., 1991). There are no pharmacokinetic data for foscarnet in neonates.

Antiviral therapy

Foscarnet inhibits all known human herpesviruses, including acyclovir-resistant HSV and VZV strains and most ganciclovir-resistant CMV isolates. It also is active against HIV. While the drug concentrations required for inhibition of viral replication vary markedly, they generally range from 10 to 130 μM for HSV, 100 to 300 μM for CMV, and 10 to 25 μM for HIV.

Clinical efficacy in HSV-1 and HSV-2 infections

While primarily a CMV drug, foscarnet has demonstrable activity against HSV as well, and infections caused by acyclovir-resistant strains of HSV have been successfully controlled with foscarnet (Safrin et al., 1991a; Safrin et al., 1991b).

The safety and efficacy of foscarnet in the pediatric population has not been established. Potential exists for deposition of foscarnet in the developing teeth and bone of children. Therefore, administration of foscarnet to pediatric patients should be undertaken only after careful evaluation and only if the potential benefits for treatment outweigh the potential risks.

Challenges for achieving clinical benefit, including adverse drug effects

The most common adverse effects of foscarnet are nephrotoxicity and metabolic derangements. Evidence of nephrotoxicity includes azotemia, proteinuria, acute tubular necrosis, crystalluria, and interstitial nephritis (Studies of Ocular Complications of AIDS Research Group in collaboration with the AIDS Clinical Trials Group, 1992). Serum creatinine concentrations increase in up to 50% of patients, usually during the second week of therapy. Fortunately, renal function returns to normal within two to four weeks of discontinuing therapy in most affected patients. Pre-existing renal disease, concurrent use of other nephrotoxic drugs, dehydration, rapid injection of large doses, or continuous intravenous infusion of drug are risk factors for developing renal dysfunction (Deray et al., 1989).

Metabolic disturbances associated with foscarnet therapy include symptomatic hypo- and hypercalcemia and hypo- and hyperphosphatemia (Markham and Faulds, 1994). Hypocalcemia is due to direct chelation of ionized calcium by the drug, and patients can have such symptoms as paresthesias, tetany, seizures, and arrythmias. Metabolic disturbances can be minimized if foscarnet is administered by slow infusion, with rates not exceeding 1 mg/kg per min. Common central nervous system (CNS) symptoms associated with foscarnet therapy are headache, tremor, irritability, seizures, and hallucinations. Fever, nausea, vomiting, abnormal serum hepatic enzymes, anemia, granulocytopenia, and genital ulcerations also have been reported. The genital ulcerations appear to be associated with high urinary concentrations of drug.

Concomitant use of amphotericin B, cyclosporine, gentamicin, and other nephrotoxic drugs increases the likelihood of renal dysfunction associated with foscarnet therapy. Co-administration of pentamidine increases the risk of hypocalcemia. Anemia and neutropenia are more common when patients also are receiving zidovudine. No drug–drug interactions are known to exist with the concomitant use of foscarnet and ganciclovir.

Foscarnet's major toxicity of renal impairment is judged significant enough to warrant warning statements from the FDA in the package insert. Serum creatinine should be monitored frequently, and adequate hydration with foscarnet administration is imperative. Elevations in serum creatinine are usually, but not always, reversible following discontinuation or dose adjustment of foscarnet. Patients receiving foscarnet must also be monitored for development of mineral and electrolyte abnormalities that might result in seizures, including hypocalcemia, hypophosphatemia, hyperphosphatemia, hypomagnesemia, and hypokalemia.

Clinical indications

Foscarnet is indicated for the treatment of acyclovir-resistant mucocutaneous HSV infections in immunocompromised patients, and is the drug of choice for both HSV and VZV infections caused by acyclovir-resistant strains. Foscarnet also is indicated for the treatment of CMV retinitis in patients with AIDS.

Dosage regimens

When used for the treatment of acyclovir-resistant strains of HSV, foscarnet should be administered at 120 mg/kg per day in three divided doses. In patients with AIDS, foscarnet therapy should be initiated within 7 to 10 days of suspicion of infection caused by acyclovir-resistant HSV or VZV. Therapy should be continued until lesions have resolved.

The degree of dose reduction is proportional to reduction in creatinine clearance; when creatinine clearance is 50% of normal, the dose should be reduced by about 50%. Detailed tables of dosage adjustments are available in the foscarnet package insert.

Antiviral resistance

Foscarnet does not require activation by viral kinases, including thymidine kinase, and therefore is active in vitro against HSV TK-deficient mutants. Resistance occurs as a result of DNA polymerase mutations (Kimberlin et al., 1995a). Strains of CMV, HSV, and VZV with three- to five-fold reduced sensitivity to foscarnet have been reported (Kimberlin et al., 1995b; Safrin et al., 1994; Snoeck et al., 1994). These isolates may respond to therapy with acyclovir (Safrin et al., 1994) or cidofovir (Snoeck et al., 1994). Conversely, infections caused by acyclovir-resistant strains of HSV and VZV have been successfully controlled with foscarnet (Safrin et al., 1991a; Safrin et al., 1991b).

Ganciclovir

Ganciclovir is a nucleoside analogue that differs from acyclovir by having an extra hydroxymethyl group on the acyclic side chain.

Mechanism of action and pharmacokinetics

As with acyclovir and penciclovir, the first step in ganciclovir phosphorylation is carried out by a virus-encoded enzyme, and the final steps by cellular enzymes. Ganciclovir triphosphate is a competitive inhibitor of herpesviral DNA polymerases, resulting in cessation of DNA chain elongation (Markham and Faulds, 1994). Ganciclovir triphosphate also has some activity against cellular DNA polymerases, and this potential for incorporation into cellular DNA accounts for ganciclovir's significant toxicities. Ganciclovir has similar activity to acyclovir against HSV-1, HSV-2, and VZV but, in contrast with acyclovir, its greatest activity is against CMV.

Peak serum concentrations of ganciclovir after 5 mg/kg of intravenously-administered drug range from 8 to 11 μg/ml. Concentrations of ganciclovir in the central nervous system range from 24% to 70% of those in the plasma, with brain concentrations of approximately 38% of plasma levels (Fletcher et al., 1986). Most of an administered dose of ganciclovir is eliminated unchanged in the urine, with an elimination half-life of 2 to 3 hours. Intracellular ganciclovir triphosphate has a half-life of more than 24 hours.

Oral bioavailability of ganciclovir is poor, with less than 10% of drug being absorbed following oral administration (Frenkel et al., 2000; Jacobson et al., 1987; Markham and Faulds, 1994). Despite this, an oral dose of 1000 mg of ganciclovir produces a peak plasma concentration of 1 μg/ml. Intravitreal drug concentrations achieved during intravenous induction therapy also average 1 μg/ml, while subretinal concentrations are comparable to those achieved in plasma (Kuppermann et al., 1993).

The pharmacokinetic of intravenous ganciclovir in the neonatal population are similar to those of adults (Trang et al., 1993). Following intravenous administration of 6 mg/kg of ganciclovir, peak concentrations of 7.0 μg/ml are achieved. The mean elimination half-life is 2.4 hours.

Dose reduction, proportional to the degree of reduction in creatinine clearance, is necessary for persons with impaired renal function. A supplemental dose is recommended after dialysis because it is efficiently removed by hemodialysis (Swan et al., 1991).

Antiviral therapy

Ganciclovir's greatest in vitro activity is against CMV, although it is also as active as acyclovir against HSV-1 and HSV-2 and almost as active against VZV.

Challenges for achieving clinical benefit, including adverse drug effects

Myelosuppression is the most common adverse effect of ganciclovir; dose-related neutropenia (less than 1000 WBC/μl) is the most consistent hematologic disturbance, with an incidence of about 40% of ganciclovir-treated patients (Markham and Faulds, 1994). Neutropenia is dose limiting in about 15% of subjects, and is reversible upon cessation of drug. Neutropenia is less frequent following oral administration of ganciclovir (Drew et al., 1995). Hematopoietic growth factors may be useful in preventing or managing neutropenia. Thrombocytopenia (less than 50 000 platelets/μl) occurs in approximately 20% of treated patients, while anemia in about 2% of ganciclovir recipients. Due to its marrow suppressive effects, ganciclovir should not be administered if the absolute neutrophil count is less than 500 cells/μl or if the platelet count is less than 25 000 cells/μL.

Two to 5% of ganciclovir recipients experience headache, confusion, altered mental status, hallucinations, nightmares, anxiety, ataxia, tremors, seizures, fever, rash, and abnormal levels of serum hepatic enzymes, either singly or in some combination (Markham and Faulds, 1994). Intraocular injection of ganciclovir can cause transient increases in intraocular pressure with associated intense pain and amaurosis lasting up to 30 minutes.

Since both zidovudine and ganciclovir have the potential to cause neutropenia and anemia, some patients may not tolerate concomitant therapy with these drugs at full dosage. Renal clearance of ganciclovir decreases in the presence of probenicid. Generalized seizures have been reported in patients who received ganciclovir and imipenem-cilastatin, and these drugs should not be used concomitantly unless the potential benefits outweigh the risks.

In preclinical test systems, ganciclovir is mutagenic, carcinogenic, and teratogenic. Additionally, it causes irreversible reproductive toxicity in animal models. The use of ganciclovir in the pediatric population warrants extreme caution due to this potential for long-term carcinogenicity and reproductive toxicity. Administration of ganciclovir to pediatric patients should be undertaken only after careful evaluation and only if the potential benefits of treatment outweigh the potential risks.

Clinical indications

Ganciclovir is indicated for the treatment and prevention of CMV infections in immunocompromised patients. Its role in the treatment of HSV-1 or HSV-2 infections is limited to unique situations in which coverage of these viruses in addition to CMV is desirable.

Dosage regimens

The usual therapeutic and prophylactic dose of ganciclovir is 10 mg/kg per day, given by intravenous infusion twice a day for 2 to 3 weeks. For continued suppressive therapy to prevent relapse of infection or for long-term prophylaxis, either of the following may be used: (1) 5 mg/kg as a single daily dose each day of the week; or (2) 6 mg/kg administered 5 days a week. Despite the absence of data, utilization of intravenous ganciclovir is largely being supplanted by oral valganciclovir in clinical practice.

Dose reduction, roughly proportional to the degree of reduction in creatinine clearance, is necessary in persons with impaired renal function (Spector et al., 1995; Swan et al., 1991). When creatinine clearance is between 50 and 79 ml/min per 1.73 m^2, half of the usual dose should be given every 12 hours. This same dose should be given every 24 hours if creatinine clearance is between 25 and 49 ml/min per 1.73 m^2. Twenty-five percent of the usual dose should be given every 24 hours if creatinine clearance is less than 25 ml/min per 1.73 m^2. Because ganciclovir is efficiently removed by hemodialysis, a supplemental dose is recommended after dialysis (Swan et al., 1991).

Antiviral resistance

Strains of HSV that are resistant to acyclovir because of TK deficiency also are much less sensitive to ganciclovir. DNA polymerase HSV mutants that are ganciclovir-resistant have been generated in vitro but are not yet a clinical problem.

Valganciclovir

Valganciclovir was approved by the FDA in March, 2001. Because it is well absorbed after oral administration, it may represent a favorable option to intravenously-administered ganciclovir for the treatment and suppression of CMV infections in immunocompromised hosts.

Mechanism of action and pharmacokinetics

Valganciclovir is an L-valine ester prodrug of ganciclovir and as such has the same mechanism of action, antiviral spectrum, and potential for development of resistance as ganciclovir (Cocohoba and McNicholl, 2002). Valganciclovir is rapidly converted to ganciclovir, with a mean plasma half-life of about 30 minutes (Jung and Dorr, 1999). The absolute bioavailability of valganciclovir exceeds 60% and actually is enhanced by about 30% with concomitant administration of food (Brown et al., 1999). The area under the curve of ganciclovir after oral administration of valganciclovir is one-third to one-half of that attained after intravenous administration of ganciclovir. Patients with impaired renal function require dosage reduction that is roughly proportional to their reduction in creatinine clearance (Cocohoba and McNicholl, 2002).

Antiviral therapy

Valganciclovir provides a more tolerable means by which ganciclovir can be delivered to the body than does intravenous ganciclovir. Studies of this drug to date have not included investigations of use for HSV infections.

Challenges for achieving clinical benefit, including adverse drug effects

Based upon data from 370 subjects participating in clinical trials, the most common side effects associated with valganciclovir therapy include diarrhea (41%), nausea (30%), neutropenia (27%), anemia (26%), and headache (22%) (Cocohoba and McNicholl, 2002).

Clinical indications

Valganciclovir has similar indications to ganciclovir. However, based upon limited controlled trials published to date, it currently is approved for the induction and maintenance therapy of CMV retinitis (Martin et al., 2002).

Dosage regimens

The recommended dose of valganciclovir for induction therapy is 900 mg twice daily for 2 weeks. The recommended dose for maintenance therapy is 900 mg once daily.

Antiviral resistance

Resistance mechanisms are identical between ganciclovir and valganciclovir. Since selective pressure resulting from exposure to lower concentrations of drug appears to increase the likelihood of resistance developing among CMV isolates (Drew et al., 1999), it is likely that the higher serum and tissue concentrations of ganciclovir achieved with administration of valganciclovir will produce less emergence of resistance when compared to oral ganciclovir. Whether or not this is seen in the clinical setting requires completion of Phase IV trials.

REFERENCES

Alexander, L. and Naisbett, B. (2002). Patient and physician partnerships in managing genital herpes. *J. Infect. Dis.*, **186**, S57–65.

American Academy of Pediatrics (2003). Herpes simplex. In *2003 Red Book: Report of the Committee on Infectious Diseases*, ed. Pickering, L. K. American Academy of Pediatrics, Elk Grove Village, IL, pp. 344–353.

Anonymous (2002). Sexually transmitted diseases treatment guidelines 2002. *Morb. Mortal. Wkly Rep.*, **51**, RR-6, 12–17.

Aoki, F. Y., Law, B. J., Hammond, G. W. *et al.* and The Acyclovir-Gingivostomatitis Research Group (1993). Acyclovir (ACV) suspension for treatment of acute herpes simplex virus (HSV) gingivostomatitis in children: a placebo(PL) controlled, double blind trial. 33rd Interscience Conference on Antimicrobial Agents and Chemotherapy. New Orleans, LA, p. 399, Abstract #1530.

Baker, D. and Eisen, D. (2003). Valacyclovir for prevention of recurrent herpes labialis: 2 double-blind, placebo-controlled studies. *Cutis*, **71**, 239–242.

Baker, D. A., Deeter, R. G., Redder, K., and Phillips, J. A. (2000). Valacyclovir effective for suppression of recurrent HSV-1 herpes labialis. 40th Interscience Conference on Antimicrobial Agents and Chemotherapy. Toronto, Ontario, Canada, p. 263, Abstract #464.

Bell, W. R., Chulay, J. D., and Feinberg, J. E. (1997). Manifestations resembling thrombotic microangiopathy in patients with advanced human immunodeficiency virus (HIV) disease in a cytomegalovirus prophylaxis trial (ACTG 204). *Medicine*, **76**, 369–380.

Benedetti, J., Corey, L., and Ashley, R. (1994). Recurrence rates in genital herpes after symptomatic first-episode infection. *Ann. Intern. Med.*, **121**, 847–854.

Bodsworth, N. J., Crooks, R. J., Borelli, S. *et al.* and the International Valaciclovir HSV Study Group (1997). Valaciclovir versus aciclovir in patient initiated treatment of recurrent genital herpes: a randomised, double blind clinical trial. *Genitourin. Med.*, **73**, 110–116.

Boike, S. C., Pue, M. A., Freed, M. I. *et al.* (1994). Pharmacokinetics of famciclovir in subjects with varying degrees of renal impairment. *Clin. Pharmacol. Ther.*, **55**, 418–426.

Boon, R., Goodman, J. J., Martinez, J., Marks, G. L., Gamble, M., and Welch, C. (2000). Penciclovir cream for the treatment of sunlight-induced herpes simplex labialis: a randomized, double-blind, placebo-controlled trial. Penciclovir Cream Herpes Labialis Study Group. *Clin. Ther.*, **22**, 76–90.

Brown, F., Banken, L., Saywell, K., and Arum, I. (1999). Pharmacokinetics of valganciclovir and ganciclovir following multiple oral dosages of valganciclovir in HIV- and CMV-seropositive volunteers. *Clin. Pharmacokinet.*, **37**, 167–176.

Bryson, Y. J., Dillon, M., Lovett, M. *et al.* (1983). Treatment of first episodes of genital herpes simplex virus infection with oral acyclovir. A randomized double-blind controlled trial in normal subjects. *N. Engl. J. Med.*, **308**, 916–921.

Chosidow, O., Drouault, Y., Leconte-Veyriac, F. *et al.* (2001). Famciclovir vs. aciclovir in immunocompetent patients with recurrent genital herpes infections: a parallel-groups, randomized, double-blind clinical trial. *Br. J. Dermatol.*, **144**, 818–824.

Chosidow, O., Drouault, Y., Garraffo, R., Veyssier, P., and Valaciclovir Herpes Facialis Study, G. (2003). Valaciclovir as a single dose during prodrome of herpes facialis: a pilot randomized double-blind clinical trial. *Br. J. Dermatol.*, **148**, 142–146.

Cocohoba, J. M. and McNicholl, I. R. (2002). Valganciclovir: an advance in cytomegalovirus therapeutics. *Ann. Pharmacother.*, **36**, 1075–1079.

Corey, L., Nahmias, A. J., Guinan, M. E., Benedetti, J. K., Critchlow, C. W., and Holmes, K. K. (1982). A trial of topical acyclovir in genital herpes simplex virus infections. *N. Engl. J. Med.*, **306**, 1313–1319.

Corey, L., Wald, A., Patel, R. *et al.* and the Valacyclovir HSV Transmission Study Group (2004). Once-daily valacyclovir to reduce the risk of transmission of genital herpes. *N. Engl. J. Med.*, **350**, 11–20.

Cundy, K. C., Petty, B. G., Flaherty, J. *et al.* (1995). Clinical pharmacokinetics of cidofovir in human immunodeficiency virus-infected patients. *Antimicrob. Agents Chemother.*, **39**, 1247–1252.

Deray, G., Martinez, F., Katlama, C. *et al.* (1989). Foscarnet nephrotoxicity: mechanism, incidence and prevention. *Am. J. Nephrol.*, **9**, 316–321.

Diaz-Mitoma, F., Sibbald, R. G., Shafran, S. D., Boon, R., Saltzman, R. L., and the Collaborative Famciclovir Genital Herpes Research Group (1998). Oral famciclovir for the suppression of recurrent genital herpes: a randomized controlled trial. *J. Am. Med. Assoc.*, **280**, 887–892.

Douglas, J. M., Critchlow, C., Benedetti, J. *et al.* (1984). A double-blind study of oral acyclovir for suppression of recurrences of genital herpes simplex virus infection. *N. Engl. J. Med.*, **310**, 1551–1556.

Drew, W. L., Ives, D., Lalezari, J. P. *et al.* and the Syntex Cooperative Oral Ganciclovir Study Group (1995). Oral ganciclovir as maintenance treatment for cytomegalovirus retinitis in patients with AIDS. *N. Engl. J. Med.*, **333**, 615–620.

Drew, W. L., Stempien, M. J., Andrews, J. *et al.* (1999). Cytomegalovirus (CMV) resistance in patients with CMV retinitis and AIDS treated with oral or intravenous ganciclovir. *J. Infect. Dis.*, **179**, 1352–1355.

Elion, G. B. (1982). Mechanism of action and selectivity of acyclovir. *Am. J. Med.*, **73**, 7–13.

Englund, J. A., Zimmerman, M. E., Swierkosz, E. M., Goodman, J. L., Scholl, D. R., and Balfour, H. H., Jr. (1990). Herpes simplex virus resistant to acyclovir. A study in a tertiary care center. *Ann. Intern. Med.*, **112**, 416–422.

Englund, J. A., Fletcher, C. V., and Balfour, H. H., Jr. (1991). Acyclovir therapy in neonates. *J. Pediatr.*, **119**, 129–135.

Field, A. K. and Biron, K. K. (1994). The end of innocence revisited: resistance of herpesviruses to antiviral drugs. *Clin. Microbiol. Rev.*, **7**, 1–13.

Fife, K. H., Barbarash, R. A., Rudolph, T., Degregorio, B., Roth, R., and the Valaciclovir International Herpes Simplex Virus Study Group (1997). Valaciclovir versus acyclovir in the treatment of first-episode genital herpes infection. Results of an international, multicenter, double-blind, randomized clinical trial. *Sexually Transm. Dis.*, **24**, 481–486.

Fletcher, C., Sawchuk, R., Chinnock, B., de Miranda, P., and Balfour, H. H., Jr. (1986). Human pharmacokinetics of the antiviral drug DHPG. *Clin. Pharmacol. Ther.*, **40**, 281–286.

Frenkel, L. M., Capparelli, E. V., Dankner, W. M. *et al.* and The Pediatric AIDS Clinical Trials Group (2000). Oral ganciclovir in children: pharmacokinetics, safety, tolerance, and antiviral effects. *J. Infect. Dis.*, **182**, 1616–1624.

Gateley, A., Gander, R. M., Johnson, P. C., Kit, S., Otsuka, H., and Kohl, S. (1990). Herpes simplex virus type 2 meningoencephalitis resistant to acyclovir in a patient with AIDS. *J. Infect. Dis.*, **161**, 711–715.

Gibson, J. R., Klaber, M. R., Harvey, S. G., Tosti, A., Jones, D., and Yeo, J. M. (1986). Prophylaxis against herpes labialis with acyclovir cream – a placebo-controlled study. *Dermatologica*, **172**, 104–107.

Gold, D. and Corey, L. (1987). Acyclovir prophylaxis for herpes simplex virus infection. *Antimicrob. Agents Chemother.*, **31**, 361–367.

Goldberg, L. H., Kaufman, R., Kurtz, T. O. *et al.* (1993). Long-term suppression of recurrent genital herpes with acyclovir. A 5-year benchmark. Acyclovir Study Group. *Arch. Dermatol.*, **129**, 582–587.

Herpetic Eye Disease Study Group (1998). Acyclovir for the prevention of recurrent herpes simplex virus eye disease. *N. Engl. J. Med.*, **339**, 300–306.

Herpetic Eye Disease Study Group (2000). Oral acyclovir for herpes simplex virus eye disease: effect on prevention of epithelial keratitis and stromal keratitis. *Arch. Ophthalmol.*, **118**, 1030–1036.

Ho, H. T., Woods, K. L., Bronson, J. J., De Boeck, H., Martin, J. C., and Hitchcock, M. J. (1992). Intracellular metabolism of the antiherpes agent (S)-1-[3-hydroxy-2-(phosphonylmethoxy)-propyl]cytosine. *Mol. Pharmacol.*, **41**, 197–202.

Hovding, G. (1989). A comparison between acyclovir and trifluorothymidine ophthalmic ointment in the treatment of epithelial dendritic keratitis. A double blind, randomized parallel group trial. *Acta Ophthalmol.*, **67**, 51–54.

Jacobson, M. A. (1993). Valaciclovir (BW256U87): the L-valyl ester of acyclovir. *J. Med. Virol.*, **Suppl**, 150–153.

Jacobson, M. A., de Miranda, P., Cederberg, D. M. *et al.* (1987). Human pharmacokinetics and tolerance of oral ganciclovir. *Antimicrob. Agents Chemother.*, **31**, 1251–1254.

Jung, D. and Dorr, A. (1999). Single-dose pharmacokinetics of valganciclovir in HIV- and CMV-seropositive subjects. *J. Clin. Pharmacol.*, **39**, 800–804.

Kimberlin, D. W. (2001). Advances in the treatment of neonatal herpes simplex infections. *Rev. Med. Virol.*, **11**, 157–163.

Kimberlin, D. W. and Prober, C. G. (2003). Antiviral agents. In *Principles and Practice of Pediatric Infectious Diseases*, ed. Long, S. S., Pickering, L. K., and Prober, C. G. Philadelphia: Churchill Livingstone, pp. 1527–1547.

Kimberlin, D. W. and Rouse, D. J. (2004). Genital herpes. *N. Engl. J. Med.*, **350**(19), 1970–1977.

Kimberlin, D. W., Coen, D. M., Biron, K. K. *et al.* (1995a). Molecular mechanisms of antiviral resistance. *Antiviral Res.*, **26**, 369–401.

Kimberlin, D. W., Crumpacker, C. S., Straus, S. E. *et al.* (1995b). Antiviral resistance in clinical practice. *Antiviral Res.*, **26**, 423–438.

Kimberlin, D., Powell, D., Gruber, W. *et al.* and The National Institute of Allergy and Infectious Diseases Collaborative Antiviral Study Group (1996a). Administration of oral acyclovir suppressive therapy after neonatal herpes simplex virus disease limited to the skin, eyes and mouth: results of a phase I/II trial. *Pediatr. Infect. Dis. J.*, **15**, 247–254.

Kimberlin, D. W., Lakeman, F. D., Arvin, A. M. *et al.* and The National Institute of Allergy and Infectious Diseases Collaborative Antiviral Study Group (1996b). Application of the polymerase chain reaction to the diagnosis and management of neonatal herpes simplex virus disease. *J. Infect. Dis.*, **174**, 1162–1167.

Kimberlin, D. W., Lin, C. Y., Jacobs, R. F. *et al.* and The National Institute of Allergy and Infectious Diseases Collaborative Antiviral Study Group (2001a). Safety and efficacy of high-dose intravenous acyclovir in the management of neonatal herpes simplex virus infections. *Pediatrics*, **108**, 230–238.

Kimberlin, D. W., Lin, C. Y., Jacobs, R. F. *et al.* and The National Institute of Allergy and Infectious Diseases Collaborative Antiviral Study Group (2001b). Natural history of neonatal herpes simplex virus infections in the acyclovir era. *Pediatrics*, **108**, 223–229.

Kost, R. G., Hill, E. L., Tigges, M., and Straus, S. E. (1993). Brief report: recurrent acyclovir-resistant genital herpes in an immunocompetent patient. *N. Engl. J. Med.*, **329**, 1777–1782.

Krasny, H. C., Liao, S. H., de Miranda, P., Laskin, O. L., Whelton, A., and Lietman, P. S. (1982). Influence of hemodialysis on acyclovir pharmacokinetics in patients with chronic renal failure. *Am. J. Med.*, **73**, 202–204.

Kuppermann, B. D., Quiceno, J. I., Flores-Aguilar, M. *et al.* (1993). Intravitreal ganciclovir concentration after intravenous administration in AIDS patients with cytomegalovirus retinitis: implications for therapy. *J. Infect. Dis.*, **168**, 1506–1509.

Lalezari, J. P., Drew, W. L., Glutzer, E. *et al.* (1994). Treatment with intravenous (S)-1-[3-hydroxy-2-(phosphonylmethoxy)propyl]-cytosine of acyclovir-resistant mucocutaneous infection with herpes simplex virus in a patient with AIDS. *J. Infect. Dis.*, **170**, 570–572.

Lalezari, J. P., Drew, W. L., Glutzer, E. *et al.* (1995). (S)-1-[3-hydroxy-2-(phosphonylmethoxy)propyl]cytosine (cidofovir): results of a phase I/II study of a novel antiviral nucleotide analogue. *J. Infect. Dis.*, **171**, 788–796.

Lalezari, J. P., Stagg, R. J., Kuppermann, B. D. *et al.* (1997). Intravenous cidofovir for peripheral cytomegalovirus retinitis in patients with AIDS. A randomized, controlled trial. *Ann. Intern. Med.*, **126**, 257–263.

Laskin, O. L., Longstreth, J. A., Whelton, A. *et al.* (1982). Effect of renal failure on the pharmacokinetics of acyclovir. *Am. J. Med.*, **73**, 197–201.

Leone, P. A., Trottier, S., and Miller, J. M. (2002). Valacyclovir for episodic treatment of genital herpes: a shorter 3-day treatment course compared with 5-day treatment. *Clin. Infect. Dis.*, **34**, 958–962.

Lin, L., Chen, X. S., Cui, P. G. *et al.* and Topical Penciclovir Clinical Study, G. (2002). Topical application of penciclovir cream for the treatment of herpes simplex facialis/labialis: a randomized, double-blind, multicentre, aciclovir-controlled trial. *J. Dermatol. Treatm.*, **13**, 67–72.

Loveless, M., Harris, W., and Sacks, S. (1995). Treatment of first episode genital herpes with famciclovir. *35th Interscience Conference on Antimicrobial Agents and Chemotherapy.* San Francisco, CA; Abstract H12, Abstract H12.

Luby, J. P., Gnann, J. W., Jr., Alexander, W. J. *et al.* (1984). A collaborative study of patient-initiated treatment of recurrent genital herpes with topical acyclovir or placebo. *J. Infect. Dis.*, **150**, 1–6.

Lyall, E. G., Ogilvie, M. M., Smith, N. M., and Burns, S. (1994). Acyclovir resistant varicella zoster and HIV infection. *Arch. Dis. Child.*, **70**, 133–135.

MacGregor, R. R., Graziani, A. L., Weiss, R., Grunwald, J. E., and Gambertoglio, J. G. (1991). Successful foscarnet therapy for cytomegalovirus retinitis in an AIDS patient undergoing hemodialysis: rationale for empiric dosing and plasma level monitoring. *J. Infect. Dis.*, **164**, 785–787.

Markham, A. and Faulds, D. (1994). Ganciclovir. an update of its therapeutic use in cytomegalovirus infection. *Drugs*, **48**, 455–484.

Martin, D. F., Sierra-Madero, J., Walmsley, S. *et al.* and the Valganciclovir Study Group (2002). A controlled trial of valganciclovir as induction therapy for cytomegalovirus retinitis. *N. Engl. J. Med.*, **346**, 1119–1126.

Mertz, G. J., Critchlow, C. W., Benedetti, J. *et al.* (1984). Double-blind placebo-controlled trial of oral acyclovir in first-episode genital herpes simplex virus infection. *J. Am. Med. Assoc.*, **252**, 1147–1151.

Mertz, G. J., Eron, L., Kaufman, R. *et al.* (1988a). Prolonged continuous versus intermittent oral acyclovir treatment in normal adults with frequently recurring genital herpes simplex virus infection. *Am. J. Med.*, **85**, 14–19.

Mertz, G. J., Jones, C. C., Mills, J. *et al.* (1988b). Long-term acyclovir suppression of frequently recurring genital herpes simplex virus infection. A multicenter double-blind trial. *J. Am. Med. Assoc.*, **260**, 201–206.

Mertz, G. J., Loveless, M. O., Levin, M. J. *et al.* and the Collaborative Famciclovir Genital Herpes Research Group (1997a). Oral famciclovir for suppression of recurrent genital herpes simplex virus infection in women. A multicenter, double-blind, placebo-controlled trial. *Arch. Intern. Med.*, **157**, 343–349.

Mertz, G. J., Loveless, M. O., Levin, M. J. *et al.* and the Collaborative Famciclovir Genital Herpes Research Group (1997b). Oral famciclovir for suppression of recurrent genital herpes simplex virus infection in women. A multicenter, double-blind, placebo-controlled trial. *Arch. Intern. Med.*, **157**, 343–349.

Meyers, J. D., Wade, J. C., Mitchell, C. D. *et al.* (1982). Multicenter collaborative trial of intravenous acyclovir for treatment of mucocutaneous herpes simplex virus infection in the immunocompromised host. *Am. J. Med.*, **73**, 229–235.

Mindel, A., Faherty, A., Carney, O., Patou, G., Freris, M., and Williams, P. (1988). Dosage and safety of long-term suppressive acyclovir therapy for recurrent genital herpes. *Lancet.*, **1**, 926–928.

Morfin, F. and Thouvenot, D. (2003). Herpes simplex virus resistance to antiviral drugs. *J. Clin. Virol.*, **26**, 29–37.

Nadal, D., Leverger, G., Sokal, E. M. *et al.* (2002). An investigation of the steady-state pharmacokinetics of oral valacyclovir in immunocompromised children. *J. Infect. Dis.*, **186**, S123–S130.

Nilsen, A. E., Aasen, T., Halsos, A. M. *et al.* (1982). Efficacy of oral acyclovir in the treatment of initial and recurrent genital herpes. *Lancet*, **2**, 571–573.

Patel, R., Bodsworth, N. J., Woolley, P. *et al.* and the International Valaciclovir HSV Study Group (1997). Valaciclovir for the suppression of recurrent genital HSV infection: a placebo controlled study of once daily therapy. *Genitourin. Med.*, **73**, 105–109.

Raborn, G. W., McGaw, W. T., Grace, M., Tyrrell, L. D., and Samuels, S. M. (1987). Oral acyclovir and herpes labialis: a randomized, double-blind, placebo-controlled study. *J. Am. Dent. Assoc.*, **115**, 38–42.

Raborn, G. W., McGaw, W. T., Grace, M., and Percy, J. (1988). Treatment of herpes labialis with acyclovir. Review of three clinical trials. *Am. J. Med.*, **85**, 39–42.

Raborn, G. W., Martel, A. Y., Grace, M. G., and McGaw, W. T. (1997). Herpes labialis in skiers: randomized clinical trial of acyclovir cream versus placebo. *Oral Surg., Oral Med., Oral Pathol., Oral Radiol. Endodontics*, **84**, 641–645.

Reardon, J. E. and Spector, T. (1989). Herpes simplex virus type 1 DNA polymerase. Mechanism of inhibition by acyclovir triphosphate. *J. Biol. Chem.*, **264**, 7405–7411.

Reichman, R. C., Badger, G. J., Mertz, G. J. *et al.* (1984). Treatment of recurrent genital herpes simplex infections with oral acyclovir. A controlled trial. *Jama.*, **251**, 2103–2107.

Reiff-Eldridge, R., Heffner, C. R., Ephross, S. A., Tennis, P. S., White, A. D., and Andrews, E. B. (2000). Monitoring pregnancy outcomes after prenatal drug exposure through prospective pregnancy registries: a pharmaceutical company commitment. *Am. J. Obstet. Gyn.*, **182**, 159–163.

Reitano, M., Tyring, S., Lang, W. *et al.* and the International Valaciclovir HSV Study Group (1998). Valaciclovir for the suppression of recurrent genital herpes simplex virus infection: a large-scale dose range-finding study. *J. Infect. Dis.*, **178**, 603–610.

Revankar, S. G., Applegate, A. L., and Markovitz, D. M. (1995). Delirium associated with acyclovir treatment in a patient with renal failure. *Clin. Infect. Dis.*, **21**, 435–436.

Rooney, J. F., Straus, S. E., Mannix, M. L. *et al.* (1993). Oral acyclovir to suppress frequently recurrent herpes labialis. A double-blind, placebo-controlled trial. *Ann. Intern. Med.*, **118**, 268–272.

Ruhnek-Forsbeck, M., Sandstrom, E., Andersson, B. *et al.* (1985). Treatment of recurrent genital herpes simplex infections with oral acyclovir. *J. Antimicrob. Chemother.*, **16**, 621–628.

Sacks, S. L., Aoki, F. Y., Diaz-Mitoma, F., Sellors, J., and Shafran, S. D. (1996a). Patient-initiated, twice-daily oral famciclovir for early recurrent genital herpes. A randomized, double-blind multicenter trial. Canadian Famciclovir Study Group. *J. Am. Med. Assoc.*, **276**, 44–49.

Sacks, S. L., Aoki, F. Y., Diaz-Mitoma, F., Sellors, J., Shafran, S. D., and the Canadian Famciclovir Study Group (1996b).

Patient-initiated, twice-daily oral famciclovir for early recurrent genital herpes. A randomized, double-blind multicenter trial. *J. Am. Med. Assoc.*, **276**, 44–49.

Sacks, S. L., Hughes, A., Rennie, B., and Boon, R. (1997). Famciclovir for suppression of asymptomatic and symptomatic recurrent genital herpes shedding: a randomized, double-blind, double-dummy, parallel-group, placebo-controlled trial. *37th Interscience Conference on Antimicrobial Agents and Chemotherapy.* Toronto, Ontario, Canada; Abstract H-73.

Safrin, S., Berger, T. G., Gilson, I. *et al.* (1991a). Foscarnet therapy in five patients with AIDS and acyclovir-resistant varicella-zoster virus infection. *Ann. of Inter. Medi..*, **115**, 19–21.

Safrin, S., Crumpacker, C., Chatis, P. *et al.* and The AIDS Clinical Trials Group (1991b). A controlled trial comparing foscarnet with vidarabine for acyclovir-resistant mucocutaneous herpes simplex in the acquired immunodeficiency syndrome. *N. Engl. J. Med.*, **325**, 551–555.

Safrin, S., Kemmerly, S., Plotkin, B. *et al.* (1994). Foscarnet-resistant herpes simplex virus infection in patients with AIDS. *J. Infect. Dis.*, **169**, 193–196.

Safrin, S., Cherrington, J., and Jaffe, H. S. (1999). Cidofovir. Review of current and potential clinical uses. *Adv. Expe. Med. Biol.*, **458**, 111–120.

Saral, R., Burns, W. H., Laskin, O. L., Santos, G. W., and Lietman, P. S. (1981). Acyclovir prophylaxis of herpes-simplex-virus infections. *N. Engl. J. Med.*, **305**, 63–67.

Shaw, M., King, M., Best, J. M., Banatvala, J. E., Gibson, J. R., and Klaber, M. R. (1985). Failure of acyclovir cream in treatment of recurrent herpes labialis. *Bri. Med. J. Clini. Res.*, **291**, 7–9.

Shepp, D. H., Newton, B. A., Dandliker, P. S., Flournoy, N., and Meyers, J. D. (1985). Oral acyclovir therapy for mucocutaneous herpes simplex virus infections in immunocompromised marrow transplant recipients. *Ann. Inter. Med.*, **102**, 783–785.

Skoldenberg, B., Forsgren, M., Alestig, K. *et al.* (1984). Acyclovir versus vidarabine in herpes simplex encephalitis. Randomised multicentre study in consecutive Swedish patients. *Lancet.*, **2**, 707–711.

Snoeck, R., Andrei, G., Gerard, M. *et al.* (1994). Successful treatment of progressive mucocutaneous infection due to acyclovir- and foscarnet-resistant herpes simplex virus with (S)-1-(3-hydroxy-2-phosphonylmethoxypropyl)cytosine (HPMPC). *Clin. Infect. Dis.*, **18**, 570–578.

Soul-Lawton, J., Seaber, E., On, N., Wootton, R., Rolan, P., and Posner, J. (1995). Absolute bioavailability and metabolic disposition of valaciclovir, the L-valyl ester of acyclovir, following oral administration to humans. *Antimicrob. Agents Chemother.*, **39**, 2759–2764.

Spector, S. A., Hsia, K., Wolf, D., Shinkai, M., and Smith, I. (1995). Molecular detection of human cytomegalovirus and determination of genotypic ganciclovir resistance in clinical specimens. *Clin. Infect. Dis.*, **21**, S170–S173.

Spruance, S. L., Crumpacker, C. S., Schnipper, L. E. *et al.* (1984). Early, patient-initiated treatment of herpes labialis with topical 10% acyclovir. *Antimicrob. Agents Chemother.*, **25**, 553–555.

Spruance, S. L., Hamill, M. L., Hoge, W. S., Davis, L. G., and Mills, J. (1988). Acyclovir prevents reactivation of herpes simplex labialis in skiers. *J. Am. Med. Assoc.*, **260**, 1597–1599.

Spruance, S. L., Stewart, J. C., Rowe, N. H., McKeough, M. B., Wenerstrom, G., and Freeman, D. J. (1990). Treatment of recurrent herpes simplex labialis with oral acyclovir. *J. Infect. Dis.*, **161**, 185–190.

Spruance, S. L., Freeman, D. J., Stewart, J. C. *et al.* (1991). The natural history of ultraviolet radiation-induced herpes simplex labialis and response to therapy with peroral and topical formulations of acyclovir. *J. Infect. Dis.*, **163**, 728–734.

Spruance, S. L., Tyring, S. K., DeGregorio, B., Miller, C., Beutner, K., and the Valaciclovir HSV Study Group (1996). A large-scale, placebo-controlled, dose-ranging trial of peroral valaciclovir for episodic treatment of recurrent herpes genitalis. *Arch. Intern. Med.*, **156**, 1729–1735.

Spruance, S. L., Rea, T. L., Thoming, C., Tucker, R., Saltzman, R., and Boon, R. (1997). Penciclovir cream for the treatment of herpes simplex labialis. A randomized, multicenter, double-blind, placebo-controlled trial. Topical Penciclovir Collaborative Study Group. *J. Am. Med. Assoc.*, **277**, 1374–1379.

Spruance, S. L., Nett, R., Marbury, T., Wolff, R., Johnson, J., and Spaulding, T. (2002). Acyclovir cream for treatment of herpes simplex labialis: results of two randomized, double-blind, vehicle-controlled, multicenter clinical trials. *Antimicrob. Agents Chemother.*, **46**, 2238–2243.

Spruance, S. L., Jones, T. M., Blatter, M. M. *et al.* (2003). High-dose, short-duration, early valacyclovir therapy for episodic treatment of cold sores: results of two randomized, placebo-controlled, multicenter studies. *Antimicrob. Agents Chemother.*, **47**, 1072–1080.

Straus, S. E., Takiff, H. E., Seidlin, M. *et al.* (1984). Suppression of frequently recurring genital herpes. A placebo-controlled double-blind trial of oral acyclovir. *N. Engl. J. Med.*, **310**, 1545–1550.

Studies of Ocular Complications of AIDS Research Group in collaboration with the AIDS Clinical Trials Group (1992). Mortality in patients with the acquired immunodeficiency syndrome treated with either foscarnet or ganciclovir for cytomegalovirus retinitis. *N. Engl. J. Med.*, **326**, 213–220.

Studies of Ocular Complications of AIDS Research Group in collaboration with the AIDS Clinical Trials Group (1997). Parenteral cidofovir for cytomegalovirus retinitis in patients with AIDS: the HPMPC peripheral cytomegalovirus retinitis trial. A randomized, controlled trial. *Ann. Intern. Med.*, **126**, 264–274.

Swan, S. K., Munar, M. Y., Wigger, M. A., and Bennett, W. M. (1991). Pharmacokinetics of ganciclovir in a patient undergoing hemodialysis. *Am. J. Kidney Dis.*, **17**, 69–72.

Trang, J. M., Kidd, L., Gruber, W. *et al.* and the National Institute of Allergy and Infectious Diseases Collaborative Antiviral Study Group (1993). Linear single-dose pharmacokinetics of ganciclovir in newborns with congenital cytomegalovirus infections. *Clin. Pharmacol. Ther.*, **53**, 15–21.

Tyring, S. K., Douglas, J. M., Jr., Corey, L., Spruance, S. L., Esmann, J., and the Valaciclovir International Study Group (1998). A randomized, placebo-controlled comparison of oral valacyclovir and acyclovir in immunocompetent patients with recurrent genital herpes infections. *Arch. Dermatol.*, **134**, 185–191.

Wade, J. C., Newton, B., McLaren, C., Flournoy, N., Keeney, R. E., and Meyers, J. D. (1982). Intravenous acyclovir to treat mucocutaneous herpes simplex virus infection after marrow transplantation: a double-blind trial. *Ann. Intern. Med.*, **96**, 265–269.

Wade, J. C., McLaren, C., and Meyers, J. D. (1983). Frequency and significance of acyclovir-resistant herpes simplex virus isolated from marrow transplant patients receiving multiple courses of treatment with acyclovir. *J. Infect. Dis.*, **148**, 1077–1082.

Wagstaff, A. J. and Bryson, H. M. (1994). Foscarnet. A reappraisal of its antiviral activity, pharmacokinetic properties and therapeutic use in immunocompromised patients with viral infections. *Drugs*, **48**, 199–226.

Wagstaff, A. J., Faulds, D., and Goa, K. L. (1994). Aciclovir. A reappraisal of its antiviral activity, pharmacokinetic properties and therapeutic efficacy. *Drugs*, **47**, 153–205.

Wald, A., Benedetti, J., Davis, G., Remington, M., Winter, C., and Corey, L. (1994). A randomized, double-blind, comparative trial comparing high- and standard-dose oral acyclovir for first-episode genital herpes infections. *Antimicrob. Agents Chemother.*, **38**, 174–176.

Wald, A., Zeh, J., Barnum, G., Davis, L. G., and Corey, L. (1996). Suppression of subclinical shedding of herpes simplex virus type 2 with acyclovir. *Ann. Intern. Med.*, **124**, 8–15.

Wald, A., Corey, L., Cone, R., Hobson, A., Davis, G., and Zeh, J. (1997). Frequent genital herpes simplex virus 2 shedding in immunocompetent women. Effect of acyclovir treatment. *J. Clin. Investig.*, **99**, 1092–1097.

Wald, A., Warren, T., Hu, H. *et al.* (1998). Suppression of subclinical shedding of herpes simplex virus type 2 in the genital tract with valaciclovir. *38th Interscience Conference on Antimicrobial Agents and Chemotherapy*. San Diego, California; Abstract H-82.

Wald, A., Carrell, D., Remington, M., Kexel, E., Zeh, J., and Corey, L. (2002). Two-day regimen of acyclovir for treatment of recurrent genital herpes simplex virus type 2 infection. *Clin. Infect. Dis.*, **34**, 944–948.

Weller, S., Blum, M. R., Doucette, M. *et al.* (1993). Pharmacokinetics of the acyclovir pro-drug valaciclovir after escalating single- and multiple-dose administration to normal volunteers. *Clin. Pharmacol. Ther.*, **54**, 595–605.

Whitley, R. J., Nahmias, A. J., Soong, S. J., Galasso, G. G., Fleming, C. L., and Alford, C. A. (1980a). Vidarabine therapy of neonatal herpes simplex virus infection. *Pediatrics*, **66**, 495–501.

Whitley, R. J., Nahmias, A. J., Visintine, A. M., Fleming, C. L., and Alford, C. A. (1980b). The natural history of herpes simplex virus infection of mother and newborn. *Pediatrics*, **66**, 489–494.

Whitley, R. J., Yeager, A., Kartus, P. *et al.* (1983). Neonatal herpes simplex virus infection: follow-up evaluation of vidarabine therapy. *Pediatrics*, **72**, 778–785.

Whitley, R. J., Alford, C. A., Hirsch, M. S. *et al.* (1986). Vidarabine versus acyclovir therapy in herpes simplex encephalitis. *N. Engl. J. Med.*, **314**, 144–149.

Whitley, R. J., Corey, L., Arvin, A. *et al.* (1988). Changing presentation of herpes simplex virus infection in neonates. *J. Infect. Dis.*, **158**, 109–116.

Whitley, R. J., Arvin, A., Prober, C. *et al.* and The National Institute of Allergy and Infectious Diseases Collaborative Antiviral Study Group (1991a). A controlled trial comparing vidarabine with acyclovir in neonatal herpes simplex virus infection. *N. Engl. J. Med.*, **324**, 444–449.

Whitley, R. J., Arvin, A., Prober, C. *et al.* and The National Institute of Allergy and Infectious Diseases Collaborative Antiviral Study Group (1991b). Predictors of morbidity and mortality in neonates with herpes simplex virus infections. *N. Engl. J. Med.*, **324**, 450–454.

Antiviral therapy of varicella-zoster virus infections

John W. Gnann, Jr.

Departments of Medicine, Pediatrics and Microbiology, Division of Infectious Diseases,
University of Alabama at Birmingham and the Birmingham VA Medical Center Birmingham, AL, USA

Introduction

Primary infection caused by varicella-zoster virus (VZV) is manifest by varicella (chickenpox), while reactivation of latent virus causes herpes zoster (shingles). In immunocompetent children, varicella is usually not a serious disease, but can cause severe morbidity and mortality in adults and in immunocompromised individuals. Similarly, herpes zoster is associated with much greater morbidity in patients with impaired cell-mediated immune responses. In addition, herpes zoster can cause prolonged pain (postherpetic neuralgia) that can be very difficult to manage, particularly in older individuals. The outcomes of varicella and herpes zoster, especially in immunocompromised patients, have been dramatically improved by the development of safe and effective antiviral drugs with potent activity against VZV. Early drugs with modest efficacy and substantial toxicity (e.g., interferon, vidarabine, etc.) have been replaced by antiviral agents with enhanced *in vitro* activity, improved pharmacokinetic properties, and excellent safety profiles.

Diagnosis

Most experienced physicians will be able to make an accurate clinical diagnosis of chickenpox based on the distinctive appearance of the skin lesions (Fig. 65.1(a)). The clinical syndrome of a child with mild constitutional symptoms, the typical diffuse vesicular rash, and no prior history of chickenpox is strongly suggestive of the diagnosis, especially if there has been exposure to VZV within the previous two weeks. However, in countries where the incidence of varicella is dramatically declining (such as the United States), younger physicians will have fewer opportunities to see patients with chickenpox and may feel less confident with the clinical diagnosis. In addition, a variety of atypical presentations may occur in immunocompromised patients that will require laboratory confirmation. The classical dermatomal presentation of herpes zoster is also highly distinctive and readily lends itself to clinical diagnosis, although the diagnosis may be obscure initially in patients who present with dermatomal neuralgic pain prior to the onset of skin lesions (Fig. 65.1(b)).

Culture for VZV is performed by inoculating vesicular fluid onto monolayers of human fetal diploid kidney or lung cells. Unlike HSV, VZV is labile and every effort should be made to minimize the time spent in specimen transport and storage. Ideally, fluid should be aspirated from clear vesicles using a tuberculin syringe containing 0.2 ml of viral transport medium, inoculated directly into tissue culture at the bedside (or taken immediately to the laboratory), and then incubated at 36 °C in 5% CO_2 atmosphere. If no vesicles or pustules are available for aspiration, the clinician should carefully remove overlying debris or crusts from the freshest lesions available, swab the underlying ulcers, and place the swab directly into viral transport medium for rapid delivery on ice to the laboratory. Characteristic cytopathic effects are usually evident in tissue culture in 3–7 days, although cultures should be held for 14 days before they are declared negative. The culture process can be accelerated by using centrifugation cultures in shell vials. Identification of the viral isolate is confirmed by staining the monolayer with VZV-specific monoclonal antibodies. In general, viral culture for VZV is highly specific but slow, insensitive, and expensive.

Since VZV is not shed asymptomatically, demonstration of VZV virions, antigens, or nucleic acids in body fluids or tissues (other than sensory ganglia) is diagnostic of active infection. Visualization of multinucleated giant cells or herpesvirus virions in tissues by histopathology or electron microscopy does not distinguish between VZV

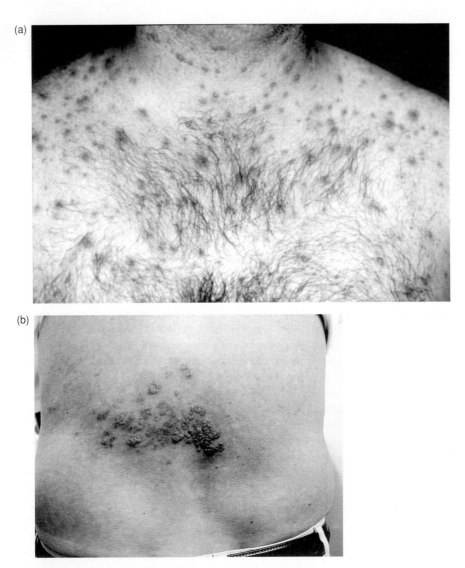

Fig. 65.1. Clinical appearance of varicella and herpes zoster. (a) Typical generalized vesicular rash of chickenpox in an adult. (b) Typical dermatomal papulo-vesicular rash of shingles in an adult. (See color plate section.)

and herpes simplex virus (HSV). Immunohistochemical staining of viral antigens can provide a more specific diagnosis. Direct fluorescent antigen (DFA) staining using fluorescein-conjugated monoclonal antibodies to detect VZV glycoproteins in infected epithelial cells is especially helpful for making a rapid diagnosis when the clinical presentation is atypical. To perform the DFA assay, epithelial cells are scraped from the base of a vesicle or ulcer with a scalpel blade, smeared on a glass slide, fixed with cold acetone, stained with fluoroescein-conjugated monoclonal antibodies, and then examined using a fluorescence microscope. By using virus-specific monoclonal antibodies, HSV can be readily distinguished from VZV, making DFA staining a much more powerful technique then a simple Tzanck preparation. DFA is also more sensitive than virus culture, especially in later stages of VZV infection when virus isolation becomes more difficult. In a population of 92 HIV-infected adults with suspected herpes zoster, DFA and viral culture were positive in 85 of 92 (92%) and 60 of 92 (65%) patients, respectively (Dahl *et al.*, 1997).

Using the polymerase chain reaction (PCR) to detect VZV nucleic acids in clinical specimens is an important diagnostic method (Stranska *et al.*, 2004). PCR overcomes the difficulties inherent in culturing labile VZV and has been used successfully to detect viral DNA in cerebrospinal fluid (CSF) from patients with VZV encephalitis and in ocular fluids and tissues from cases of VZV retinitis. Diagnosing VZV infection of the central nervous system (CNS) can be difficult, especially when there are no concomitant cutaneous lesions. Examination of the CSF usually reveals a moderate lymphocytic pleocytosis, normal to moderately elevated protein, and normal glucose. The PCR for VZV DNA in CSF should be positive in more than 75% of cases. In one series of 34 HIV-infected patients with VZV neurologic complications, the mean CSF white blood cell count was 126/mm^3, the mean protein concentration was 230 mg/dl, and the PCR was positive for VZV in all cases (De La Blanchardiere et al., 2000).

Serologic techniques can be used to determine susceptibility to VZV infection and to document rising antibody titers following varicella. Serum IgG becomes detectable several days after the onset of varicella and titers peak after 2 to 3 weeks, so routine serologic testing provides only a retrospective diagnosis. Acute infection can be confirmed by VZV-specific serum IgM titers, but antigen detection techniques are usually faster and more reliable. Patients with herpes zoster are VZV-seropositive at the time of disease onset, but most show a significant rise in antibody titer during the convalescent phase. A variety of methods have been used to detect VZV antibodies, but many laboratories have adopted an enzyme-linked immunosorbent assay (ELISA) or a latex agglutination (LA) assay for VZV serodiagnosis. The ELISA is capable of detecting IgG or IgM responses, is a reliable indicator of immune status following natural infection, and is readily automated. However, the ELISA may not be sufficiently sensitive to detect vaccine-induced immunity. The LA assay is rapid, simple, inexpensive and highly sensitive, but cannot be automated or used to detect IgM.

Drugs with activity against VZV

Acyclovir and valacyclovir

Acyclovir, an acyclic analogue of guanosine, is a selective inhibitor of VZV and HSV replication (Whitley and Gnann, 1992). The drug is converted to acyclovir monophosphate by virus-encoded thymidine kinase (TK), a reaction that does not occur to any significant extent in uninfected cells. Cellular enzymes catalyze the subsequent diphosphorylation and triphosphorylation steps which yield high concentrations of acyclovir triphosphate in VZV-infected cells. Acyclovir triphosphate inhibits viral DNA synthesis by competing with deoxyguanosine triphosphate as a substrate for viral DNA polymerase. Incorporation of acyclovir triphosphate into viral DNA results in obligate chain termination since the molecule lacks the 3-hydroxyl group required for further DNA chain elongation. Viral DNA polymerase is tightly associated with the terminated DNA chain and is functionally inactivated. Viral DNA polymerase has a much higher affinity for acyclovir triphosphate than does cellular DNA polymerase, resulting in little incorporation of acyclovir triphosphate into cellular DNA. The median inhibitory concentration of acyclovir necessary to reduce VZV plaque counts by 50% (IC50) is approximately 3 µg/ml.

After oral administration, acyclovir is slowly and incompletely absorbed with bioavailability of about 15–30%. Following oral administration of multiple doses of 200 mg or 800 mg of acyclovir, mean plasma peak concentrations at steady state are approximately 0.6 and 1.6 µg/ml, respectively. Plasma protein binding is less than 20%. Acyclovir penetrates well into most tissues, including the CNS. About 85% of an administered acyclovir dose is excreted unchanged in the urine via glomerular filtration and tubular secretion. The terminal plasma half-life of acyclovir is 2–3 hours in adults and 3–4 hours in neonates with normal renal function, but is extended to about 20 hours in anuric patients.

Valacyclovir is an orally administered prodrug of acyclovir that overcomes the problem of poor oral bioavailability and exhibits improved pharmacokinetic properties (Acosta and Fletcher, 1997). Valacyclovir, the L-valine ester of acyclovir, is well absorbed from the gastrointestinal tract via a stereospecific transporter and undergoes essentially complete first pass conversion in the gut and liver to yield acyclovir and L-valine. Using this prodrug formulation, the bioavailability of acyclovir is increased to about 54%, yielding peak plasma acyclovir concentrations that are three- to fivefold higher than those achieved with oral administration of the parent compound. Oral valacyclovir doses of 500 mg or 1000 mg produce peak plasma acyclovir concentrations of 3–4 and 5–6 µg/ml, respectively. Following administration of valacyclovir at a dose of 2 g orally four times daily, plasma acyclovir area-under-the-curve (AUC) values approximate those produced by acyclovir given intravenously at a dose of 10 mg/kg every 8 hours. Acyclovir AUC values after oral valacyclovir dosing are slightly higher in elderly individuals when compared with younger control groups, presumably due to declines in creatinine clearance associated with aging.

Acyclovir is cleared primarily by renal mechanisms so dosage modification for both acyclovir and valacyclovir are required for patients with significant renal dysfunction. The mean elimination half-life of acyclovir after a single 1 gram dose of valacyclovir is about 14 hours in patients with end-stage renal disease. Acyclovir is readily removed by hemodialysis, but not by peritoneal dialysis. No specific dosage modification for these drugs is required for patients with hepatic insufficiency. Acyclovir and valacyclovir are not approved for use in pregnancy, but have been widely use to treat serious HSV and VZV infections in pregnant women without evidence of maternal or fetal toxicity (Reiff-Eldridge et al., 2000).

Acyclovir is an extremely safe and well-tolerated drug. Local inflammation and phlebitis may occur following extravasation of intravenous acyclovir. Renal dysfunction resulting from accumulation of acyclovir crystals in the kidney has been observed following rapid intravenous infusion of large doses of acyclovir, but is uncommon and usually reversible. Acyclovir-related neurotoxicity (including agitation, hallucinations, disorientation, tremors, and mild clonous) has been reported, most often in elderly patients with underlying CNS abnormalities and renal insufficiency (Hellden et al., 2003). Oral acyclovir therapy is rarely associated with either neurotoxicity or nephrotoxocity. Studies of patients receiving long-term acyclovir for chronic suppression of genital herpes have revealed no cumulative toxicity (Tyring et al., 2002).

At standard doses, valacyclovir is also a very safe and well-tolerated drug (Acosta and Fletcher 1997). A syndrome of thrombotic microangiopathy (characterized by fever, microangiopathic hemolytic anemia, thrombocytopenia, and renal dysfunction) was observed in AIDS patients receiving high dose valacyclovir (8 grams per day) in a clinical trial. However, this syndrome has not been observed in immunocompetent patients receiving valacyclovir at standard doses (up to 3 grams per day). There is no contraindication to using valacyclovir at approved doses in HIV-infected patients. Clinically significant interactions between acyclovir or valacyclovir and other drugs are extremely uncommon.

Acyclovir is available in topical, oral, and intravenous formulations. The dermatologic preparation consists of 5% acyclovir in a cream or polyethylene glycol ointment base. Topical acyclovir is intended for treatment of minor mucocutaneous HSV infections and plays no role in treatment of VZV. Oral acyclovir preparations include a 200 mg capsule, 400 and 800 mg tablets, and a liquid suspension (200 mg per 5 ml). Acyclovir sodium for intravenous infusion is supplied as a sterile water-soluble powder that must be reconstituted and diluted to a concentration of 50 mg/ml. The approved dose of oral acyclovir for chickenpox is 200 mg/kg (up to a maximum of 800 mg) 4–5 times daily for 5 days. Adults with herpes zoster can be treated with oral acyclovir at a dose of 800 mg five times daily. The recommended dose of intravenous acyclovir for VZV infections is 10 mg/kg every 8 hours, although higher doses (12–15 mg/kg) are sometimes used for life-threatening infections, especially in immunocompromised patients. Dosage reduction is required in patients with renal insufficiency. Valacyclovir is available as 500 mg and 1000 mg tablets. The recommended dose for immunocompetent adults with varicella or herpes zoster is 1000 mg three times daily for 7 days. Because a suspension formulation of valacyclovir is not available, clinical experience with this drug in children with chickenpox is limited.

Penciclovir and famciclovir

Penciclovir is an acyclic guanine derivative that resembles acyclovir in chemical structure, mechanism of action, and spectrum of antiviral activity (Perry and Wagstaff, 1995). Like acyclovir, penciclovir is first monophosphorylated by viral TK, then further modified to the triphosphate form by cellular enzymes. Penciclovir triphosphate blocks viral DNA synthesis through competitive inhibition of viral DNA polymerase. Unlike acyclovir triphosphate, penciclovir triphosphate is not an obligate chain terminator and can be incorporated into the extending DNA chain. Intracellular concentrations of penciclovir triphosphate are higher then those seen with acyclovir triphosphate. In VZV infected cells, the half-life values for penciclovir triphosphate and acyclovir triphosphate are 7 hours and 1 hour, respectively. However, this potential advantage is offset by the lower affinity of penciclovir triphosphate for viral DNA polymerase. The median IC50 of penciclovir for VZV in MRC-5 cells is 4.0 μg/ml. Because penciclovir is very poorly absorbed, famciclovir (the diacetyl ester of 6-deoxy-penciclovir) was developed as the oral formulation. The first acetyl side chain of famciclovir is cleaved by esterases found in the intestinal wall and the second acetyl group is removed on first pass through the liver. Oxidation catalyzed by aldehyde oxidase occurs at the six position, yielding penciclovir.

When administered as the famciclovir prodrug, the bioavailability of penciclovir is about 77%. Following a single oral dose of 250 mg or 500 mg of famciclovir, peak plasma penciclovir concentrations of 1.9 and 3.5 μg/ml are achieved at 1 hour. The pharmacokinetics of penciclovir are linear and dose dependent over a famciclovir dosing range of 125–750 mg. Penciclovir is not metabolized, but is eliminated unchanged in urine, with an elimination half-life of about 2 hours after intravenous administration. Penciclovir for intravenous administration has not been commercially marketed. Famciclovir is available as 125 mg, 250 mg, and 500 mg tablets. In the United States, the recommended dose of famciclovir for uncomplicated herpes zoster is 500 mg three times daily. Famciclovir doses of 250 mg three times daily and 750 mg once daily are approved for treatment of shingles in some countries and appear to be comparable with respect to cutaneous healing of herpes zoster (Shafran et al., 2004). Adjustment of the famciclovir dose is required in patients with creatinine clearance of <60 ml/min. The adverse effects most frequently reported by patients participating in clinical trials of famciclovir were headache and nausea, although these symptoms did not differ significantly between famciclovir and placebo recipients.

Other drugs

Brivudin

Brivudin (bromovinyl deoxyuridine) is a highly potent thymidine nucleoside analogue with selective activity against HSV-1 and VZV (Keam et al., 2004). The mechanism of action of brivudin appears to be inhibition of the viral DNA polymerase. The drug is well-absorbed after oral administration and has a favorable pharmacokinetic profile which permits once-daily dosing. Brivudin is generally well-tolerated; nausea is the most frequently reported adverse event. Because of concerns about the safety profile of the drug, commercial development of brivudin was halted in the United States. The drug is available in several countries as a 125 mg tablet and as a 0.1% ointment for ophthalmologic use.

Foscarnet

Foscarnet (phosphonoformic acid) is a pyrophosphate analogue that functions as an inhibitor of viral DNA polymerase by blocking the pyrophosphate binding site (Wagstaff and Bryson, 1994). Unlike the nucleoside analogues discussed above, foscarnet does not require intracellular activation by TK, therefore, TK-deficient HSV and VZV isolates that are resistant to acyclovir and related drugs remain susceptible to foscarnet. Foscarnet is administered only by the intravenous route and 80%–90% of an administrated dose is excreted unchanged in the urine. The appropriate dose of foscarnet for treatment of acyclovir-resistant VZV infections has not been assessed systematically, but doses ranging from 40 mg/kg every 8 hours to 100 mg/kg every 12 hours have been used successfully. The most important adverse effect associated with foscarnet therapy is nephrotoxicity. Dose limiting renal toxicity was noted in 15%–20% of patients treated with foscarnet for CMV retinitis. Loading the patient with intravenous saline prior to foscarnet infusion can help reduce the risk of nephrotoxicity. Foscarnet can also induce a variety of electrolyte and metabolic abnormalities, most notably hypocalcemia. Foscarnet-induced electrolyte disturbances can predispose the patient to cardiac arrhythmias, tetany, altered mental status, or seizures. To avoid serious adverse effects that can result from bolus infusion, foscarnet must be administered with an infusion pump over a duration of at least one hour. Serum creatinine levels should be checked at least three times weekly in patients receiving foscarnet and the dosage adjusted according to the manufacturer's guidelines.

Vidarabine

Vidarabine (adenine arabinoside) was the first intravenous antiviral drug accepted for widespread clinical use and was shown to be effective for VZV infections in immunocompromised patients. Vidarabine has now been replaced by more effective and less toxic antiviral drugs.

Interferon

Administration of alpha-interferon to immunocompromised patients with herpes zoster reduces the risk of viral dissemination, but has little impact on dermatomal rash healing or pain. Interferon therapy was associated with significant adverse events and has been supplanted by more specific antiviral drugs.

Clinical indications for therapy

Varicella

Children

In healthy children, varicella is associated with low rates of morbidity and mortality. For most children, supportive care alone is sufficient. Astringent soaks, antipruritics, and antipyretics (preferably acetaminophen) improve comfort. Trimming the fingernails closely helps prevent bacterial superinfections caused by scratching. If bacterial cellulitis (especially caused by group A streptococcus) develops, antibiotics may be required.

Oral acyclovir has been evaluated for treatment of uncomplicated varicella in immunocompetent children (Balfour et al., 1990; Dunkle et al., 1991). Acyclovir therapy, initiated within 24 hours of the onset of rash, resulted in shorter duration of fever, fewer skin lesions, and accelerated lesion healing. Overall, oral acyclovir was well tolerated and reduced the duration of symptomatic illness by about 24 hours. The populations studied in these clinical trials were not significantly large to assess the impact of acyclovir therapy on the incidence of varicella complications. Unlike acyclovir, valacyclovir and famciclovir are not available as suspension formulations and have not been evaluated extensively for treatment of varicella in small children. Some pediatricians still view antiviral therapy as optional for otherwise healthy children with chickenpox. Since the introduction of the varicella vaccine in the United

Table 65.1. Antiviral therapy for VZV infections

	Drug	Dose[a]	Major toxicities
Immunocompetent patients			
Varicella	Acyclovir	20 mg/kg (800 mg max.) po 5 times daily × 5 d. In adults, famciclovir and valacyclovir will also likely be effective.	None; minor nausea or headache
Herpes zoster	Acyclovir	800 mg po 5 times daily × 7–10 d	As above
	Valacyclovir	1000 mg po every 8 h × 7 d	None; minor nausea or headache
	Famciclovir	500 mg po every 8 h × 7 d	None; minor nausea or headache
	Brivudin[b]	125 mg po once daily × 7 d	Potentially lethal interaction with fluoropyrimidines (e.g., 5-fluorouracil)
Immunocompromised patients			
Varicella	Acyclovir	10–15 mg/kg (or 500 mg /m^2) intravenously every 8 h for ≥7 d	Nephrotoxicity (rare); CNS disturbances (rare)
Herpes zoster	Acyclovir	IV therapy (as above). Mild to moderately immunocompromised patients (including most AIDS patients) can be treated with oral therapy.	As above
Disseminated VZV syndromes (e.g., encephalitis, pneumonitis)	Acyclovir	IV therapy (as above)	As above
Infection caused by acyclovir-resistant VZV	Foscarnet	60–90 mg/kg intravenously every 12 h until healed (≥10 d)	Nephrotoxicity (common): electrolyte disturbances (common), seizures, arrhythmias, anemia, genital ulcers

[a] Doses given are for adults with normal renal function.
[b] Not licensed in the United States.

States in 1995, the incidence of chickenpox has declined dramatically, reducing the need for antiviral options in this population.

Adults

Immunocompetent adolescents and adults with varicella can be seriously ill, with high fever, hundreds of cutaneous lesions, incapacitating constitutional symptoms, and a higher risk of complications (especially pneumonitis). Since they are likely to miss at least seven days of school or work, interventions that will reduce the duration of the acute illness are warranted. In a placebo-controlled trial of therapy for 148 adults with varicella, acyclovir (800 mg orally five times daily) was shown to reduce the duration of new lesion formation, reduce the maximum number of lesions, accelerate cutaneous healing, and shorten the duration of fever (Wallace *et al.*, 1992). Similarly, a study of acyclovir treatment in otherwise healthy adolescents demonstrated shorter duration of new lesion formation and of constitutional symptoms, including fever (Balfour *et al.*, 1992). In these studies, the benefit of acyclovir therapy was minimal when treatment was initiated later than 24 hours after rash onset. Overall, acyclovir reduced the duration of illness by about two days. Valacyclovir and famciclovir are also likely to be effective in this setting, but data from controlled clinical trials are lacking. While antiviral therapy is considered optional for healthy children with varicella, the higher potential for morbidity clearly favors treatment in adolescents and adults (Table 65.1). Available data are insufficient to determine whether acyclovir therapy reduces the risk of complications such as pneumonitis or encephalitis.

In immunocompetent patients, visceral dissemination of varicella most often involves the CNS (presenting as cerebellar ataxia, encephalitis, transverse myelitis, or stroke syndromes) or the lungs (viral pneumonitis) (Gnann, 2002). No controlled studies of antiviral therapy for these complications of varicella have been performed. However, information derived from clinical experience and case reports suggests that intravenous acyclovir (10–15 mg/kg every 8 hours) may be beneficial (Haake *et al.*, 1990; Wilkins *et al.*, 1998) (Table 65.1).

The decision whether to initiate antiviral therapy in a patient with chickenpox will hinge on the patients age, underlying medical conditions, and the risk of complications (Arvin, 2002). In general, young children (under age

12 years) are at lower risk for complications than are adolescents or adults. An exception may be secondary pediatric cases in a household, who tend to have more severe disease than the index case. Benefits of antiviral therapy are minimal for healthy children presenting with greater than 24 hours of illness. Because of the greater risk of complications, antiviral therapy is appropriate for adolescents and adults with chickenpox, probably even for those presenting 48–72 hours into the course of illness. Immunocompromised patients with varicella are at significant risk for viral dissemination and visceral involvement and should always receive antiviral therapy.

Pregnant women
Although based more on case reports than on prospectively acquired data, the evidence that varicella in pregnancy is associated with enhanced morbidity is compelling (Nathwani et al., 1998). Women who contract varicella while pregnant have an estimated 10% risk for developing severe VZV pneumonitis. Aggressive antiviral therapy is recommended for a pregnant woman with varicella who develops any evidence of pulmonary involvement, including cough, shortness of breath, or abnormal chest radiograph. Data from clinical trials are lacking, but several case series have reported clinical improvement in pregnant women with varicella pneumonia who were treated with intravenous acyclovir. Although acyclovir is not approved for use during pregnancy for any indication, no fetal toxicity attributable to acyclovir has been demonstrated and the risk-benefit ratio clearly supports the use of acyclovir in the setting of maternal varicella pneumonia (Reiff-Eldridge et al., 2000). Many experts favor antiviral therapy (with acyclovir or valacyclovir) for all pregnant women with chickenpox in an effort to reduce maternal morbidity. No data are available to indicate whether treating the mother will alter the risk of the rare fetal varicella syndrome (Harger et al., 2002).

Immunocompromised patients
The availability of safe and effective antiviral drugs has greatly reduced the high mortality rate previously associated with varicella in immunocompromised patients. Populations at high risk include organ transplant recipients, patients with cancer (especially hematologic malignancies), and other patients receiving immunosuppressive medications (including corticosteroids). Because of the high frequency of visceral involvement in immunocompromised children (or adults) with chickenpox, antiviral therapy is mandatory (Nyerges et al., 1988). A small placebo-controlled trial of intravenous acyclovir in immunocompromised children with varicella demonstrated a dramatic reduction in the frequency of VZV pneumonitis from 27% to 0% (Prober et al., 1982). Therapy with intravenous acyclovir (10 mg/kg or 500 mg/m^2 every 8 hours for 7–10 days) should be initiated at the first sign of infection. A switch to oral antiviral therapy (acyclovir, valacyclovir, or famciclovir) can be considered when the patient is afebrile and new lesion formation has ceased. When feasible, the dosage of immunosuppressive medications should be temporarily reduced in immunosuppressed patients with varicella. Despite the lack of data from large-scale controlled trials, the safety and efficacy of intravenous acyclovir have led to its acceptance as the drug of choice for varicella in severely immunocompromised patients (Table 65.1). Oral antiviral therapy may be efficacious in modestly immunocompromised patients (e.g., those with solid tumor malignancies or a low-dose corticosteroids), but prospectively acquired data are limited. In a retrospective review of 14 pediatric heart transplant recipients with varicella, half received intravenous acyclovir and half received oral valacyclovir; all patients recovered without serious complications (Dodd et al., 2001).

Patients with HIV infection
Varicella does not appear to be unusually severe in most HIV-seropositive children, although some investigators have reported a longer duration of new lesion formation and higher median lesion counts. A variety of varicella complications in HIV-infected children have been reported (including DIC, pneumonitis, hepatitis, and encephalitis), although reliable incidence figures are not available. Deaths attributable to chickenpox in children with HIV infection are rare and are usually due to pneumonitis. No controlled prospective studies of antiviral therapy for chickenpox in HIV-infected children have been reported, so recommendations must be derived from anecdotal experience. Most clinicians prescribe oral antiviral therapy, reserving intravenous acyclovir for patients with unusually severe or complicated infections (Gershon et al., 1997).

Herpes zoster

Immunocompetent adults
The goals of therapy for herpes zoster in immunocompetent adults are to accelerate the events of cutaneous healing, reduce the severity of acute neuritis, and most importantly, to reduce the incidence, severity, and duration of chronic pain (Gnann and Whitley, 2002). Even without antiviral therapy, the cutaneous lesions of herpes zoster almost always resolve within a month. However, chronic pain (postherpetic neuralgia) can persist for months or even years and is the most significant manifestation of herpes zoster in the normal host (Johnson, 2002). Three oral

antiviral drugs are currently approved in the United States for treatment of herpes zoster. Acyclovir, valacyclovir, and famciclovir have been demonstrated to reduce the duration of viral shedding, promote resolution of skin lesions, and limit the duration of pain when antiviral therapy is initiated within 72 hours of lesion onset (Table 65.1).

In placebo-controlled trials, oral acyclovir (800 mg five times daily for 7 days) was shown to accelerate cutaneous healing and to reduce the severity of acute neuritis in immunocompetent adults with herpes zoster (McKendrick et al., 1986; Huff et al., 1988; Wood et al., 1988; Morton and Thomson, 1989). Overall, acyclovir therapy reduced the duration of new vesicle formation by about 1.5 days and the time to 50% lesion healing by about 2.5 days. These clinical trials with acyclovir showed variable benefit for reduction of the frequency and duration of postherpetic neuralgia (PHN), partially due to limitations in study design and population size. Data from these studies were reexamined in another analysis which demonstrated that acyclovir was significantly superior to placebo for reducing the duration of "zoster associated pain," defined as the continuum of pain measured from initial onset until final resolution (Wood et al., 1996). Among patients ≥50 years of age, the median time to resolution of pain was 41 days and 101 days and the proportion with persistent pain at 6 months was 15% and 35% in the acyclovir and placebo treatment groups, respectively. Intravenous acyclovir is also effective in this setting, but is impractical for outpatient management of most patients with shingles. Extending oral acyclovir therapy beyond 7 days does not produce any additional benefit (Wood et al., 1994).

Valacyclovir (1000 mg three times daily for 7 days) was compared with oral acyclovir in a study of 1141 immunocompromised patients over 50 years of age with herpes zoster (Beutner et al., 1995). When initiated within 72 hours of lesion onset, the two drugs were equivalent for accelerating the events of cutaneous healing, but valacyclovir was superior to acyclovir in shortening the median time to resolution of zoster associated pain (38 days vs. 51 days; $P = 0.001$). The proportion of patients still experiencing pain at six months was 25.7% in the acyclovir treatment group and 19.3% in the valacyclovir groups (P = 0.02). Extending valacyclovir therapy to 14 days did not result in any additional benefit.

In a controlled trial conducted in 419 immunocompetent patients presenting within 24 hours of lesion onset, famciclovir (500 mg three times daily) was significantly superior to placebo in reducing the duration of viral shedding, limiting the duration of lesion formation, and accelerating the events of cutaneous healing (Tyring et al., 1995). In a subset of shingles patients ≥50 years of age who had persistent pain after skin healing ($n = 170$), the median duration of PHN was reduced from 163 days to 63 days ($P = 0.004$) in the placebo and famciclovir treatment Groups, respectively. In a study comparing famciclovir and acyclovir, the two drugs were shown to have similar efficacy for herpes zoster (Degreef and the Famciclovir Herpes Zoster Study Group, 1994).

Valacyclovir and famciclovir were compared for treatment of herpes zoster in immunocompetent patients in a randomized clinical trial. In this population of 597 patients ≥50 years of age enrolled within 72 hours of rash onset, the two drugs were shown to be therapeutically equivalent, both in terms of cutaneous healing and pain resolution (Tyring et al., 2000). At six months after onset of shingles, 19% of patients in each treatment group still reported pain. Acyclovir, valacyclovir, and famciclovir are all well tolerated and appear to be approximately comparable in clinical efficacy for managing herpes zoster in the immunocompetent host. Because their improved pharmacokinetic properties allow simpler dosing regimens, valacyclovir and famciclovir are preferred over acyclovir for this indication. Comparative drug cost is also a legitimate variable in selecting an antiviral drug for treatment of herpes zoster.

Brivudin (125 mg once daily × 7 days) was compared with acyclovir (800 mg 5 times daily × 7 days) in a study of 1227 immunocompetent adults with herpes zoster. Brivudin was judged to be superior to acyclovir for reducing the time to cessation of new vesicle formation and equivalent to acyclovir in terms of cutaneous healing and acute pain alleviation (Wassilew and Wutzler, 2003a,b). In a follow-up survey of subjects ≥50 years old, the incidence of PHN was lower in brivudin recipients (32.7%) than in acyclovir recipients (43.5%) (Wassilew and Wutzler, 2003a,b). Brivudin is commercially available in several European Union countries, but has not been approved in the United Kingdom or the United States because of concerns about potential drug-related toxicities (Gross et al., 2003).

Certain characteristics have been defined which identify immunocompetent patients at highest risk for complications of shingles and thus most likely to benefit from antiviral therapy. Careful studies have clearly showed that older age, greater skin surface area involved with herpes zoster, and severity of pain at time of clinical presentation are all predictors of more severe and long lasting pain (Wood et al., 1996; Dworkin et al., 1998; Harrison et al., 1999; Whitley et al., 1999; Nagasako et al., 2002). Patients meeting these criteria should be targeted for therapy with antiviral drugs and potent analgesics. Conversely, patients under 50 years of age are at lower risk for severe or prolonged pain and an argument could be made that antiviral therapy in this group is optional. Available efficacy data from published studies relate to patients who present within 72 hours of lesion onset, although patients frequently present for medical care beyond that window (Wood et al., 1998). The presence of new vesicles correlates with recent viral replication and may be a marker for patients who would benefit from antiviral therapy, even beyond 72 hours. In addition, patients presenting with the high-risk characteristics cited above should be considered for antiviral treatment, even when presenting beyond 72 hours after lesion onset. However, patients whose lesions that have all begun to crust are unlikely to derive benefit from antiviral therapy.

Adding corticosteroids to antiviral therapy in patients with acute herpes zoster has been suggested as a way to reduce pain. A study conducted in the United Kingdom compared acyclovir with and without prednisolone in 400 immunocompetent patients over 18 years of age (Wood et al., 1994). Another clinical trial, conducted in the United States, enrolled 208 patients over 50 years of age into a four-armed study (acyclovir plus placebo, prednisone plus placebo, acyclovir plus prednisone, placebo plus placebo) (Whitley et al., 1996). Both studies targeted patients within 72 hours of the appearance of lesions. Both of these studies demonstrated that corticosteroid therapy led to a reduction of pain during the acute phase of herpes zoster, but neither showed any reduction in the risk of postherpetic neuralgia (Wood et al., 1994; Whitley et al., 1996). Addition of corticosteroids to antiviral therapy for treatment of herpes zoster in selected older adults may result in improvements in quality of life measurements such as reduction in time to uninterrupted sleep, reduction in time to return to usual activities, and reduction in analgesic use (Whitley et al., 1996). In the American trial cited above, prednisone was given for three weeks (60 mg daily for 7 days, 30 mg daily for 7 days, and 15 mg daily for 7 days), although it is possible that shorter courses of prednisone are also effective. Corticosteroid therapy can have significant adverse effects and should not be used in patients at risk for steroid toxicity (e.g., patients with diabetes mellitus, gastritis, etc.). Although only the combination of corticosteroids plus acyclovir has been studied, combination therapy using valacyclovir or famciclovir is assumed to be equally effective. Use of corticosteroids for herpes zoster without concomitant antiviral therapy is not recommended. Furthermore, use of corticosteroids in immunocompromised patients with herpes zoster has not been evaluated and is not recommended.

Symptomatic measures should be suggested to keep the patient with herpes zoster more comfortable. Patients should keep the cutaneous lesions clean and dry to reduce the risk of bacterial superinfection. Patients may wash the skin lesions with soap and water in the shower and then carefully pat the skin dry with a clean towel. Some patients find warm or cool astringent soaks (e.g., Domeboro® solution) to be soothing. A sterile non-occlusive, non-adherent dressing placed over the involved skin will protect the lesions from contact with clothing, which may be especially helpful for patients with increased skin sensitivity (i.e., allodynia). There is no role for topical creams or ointments (including topical acyclovir or penciclovir) in management of herpes zoster. The acute pain of shingles can be very severe and should not be underestimated by the clinician. The pain may be disproportionate to the rash; that is, patients with limited skin involvement can still have severe neuralgic pain. Pain is the most important symptom of herpes zoster and should be aggressively managed. In patients with severe neuralgic pain, sympathetic nerve blocks can provide rapid, but temporary relief (Opstelten et al., 2004). Short-acting narcotic analgesics given on a scheduled (rather than as-needed) basis should be prescribed. Some models used to explain the pathogenesis of PHN suggests that early attenuation of acute pain will reduce the degree of nociceptive input that reaches the spinal cord neurons and prevent the initiation of central mechanisms of chronic pain, thereby reducing the risk of PHN (Dworkin et al., 2000).

Medical management of established PHN is complex and often requires a multifaceted approach (Dworkin and Schmader, 2003; Johnson and Dworkin, 2003). Opioid analgesics are the mainstay of therapy during the acute phases of neuralgic pain (Table 65.2). A clinical trial with controlled-release oxycodone for patients with PHN demonstrated a significant level of pain reduction (67% of those receiving oxycodone versus 11% receiving placebo) as measured by visual analogue scale (Watson and Babul, 1998). Long-acting opioid preparations (oral or transdermal) are preferable to short-acting analgesics for management of chronic PHN. Several randomized, controlled clinical trials have shown tricyclic antidepressants (including amitriptyline, nortriptyline and desipramine) to be effective in reducing the pain of PHN, either as a single agent or in combination with other drugs (Raja et al., 2002; Bowsher, 2003). Because tricyclic antidepressants are frequently associated with sedation and anticholinergic side effects, treatment should begin with a relatively low dose at bedtime, with a gradual increase in dosage as required and tolerated. Nortriptyline is as efficacious as amitriptyline for PHN, but nortriptyline is associated with fewer adverse effects in elderly patients (Watson et al., 1998). In two clinical trial, the anticonvulsant gabapentin was shown to significantly reduce established PHN when

Table 65.2. Management of postherpetic neuralgia

Drug	Dosing	Comments	Adverse effects
Opioid analgesics	Varies with drug	Begin with short-acting drug at morphine oral equianalgesic dose of 5–15 mg every 4 hr. After 2 wk, convert to equianalgesic does of long-acting drug[a]	Sedation, nausea, constipation, dizziness, dependence, abuse, overdose
Gabapentin[b]	Begin with 100 mg po every 8 hr	Titrate dose up by 300 mg/d (in divided doses) to target dose of 1800–3600 mg/d, as tolerated	Somnolence, dizziness, ataxia, peripheral edema
Tricyclic antidepressants	Nortriptyline 25 mg po at bedtime	Titrate dose up to 75–150 mg/d, as necessary. Amitriptyline also effective but may cause more adverse effects in elderly patients. Desipramine is option if nortriptyline causes excess sedation	Sedation, confusion, anticholinergic effects (dry mouth, blurred vision, constipation, urinary retention)
Lidocaine (5%) patch	Apply to painful area; up to 3 patches can be used at a time for a maximum of 12 hr daily	Apply only to healed, intact skin. Patches may be cut to size. Especially helpful for allodynia. Benefit apparent within 2 weeks.	Localized skin irritation only. Systemic toxicity from cutaneous absorption of lidocaine is very rare.

[a] Options for long-acting opioid analgesics include: controlled-release morphine, controlled-release oxycodone, transdermal fentanyl, levorphanol, methadone.
[b] Pregabalin is available as an alternative to gabapentin.
(Modified with permission from Gnann and Whitley, *N. Engl. J. Med.*, 2002.)

used alone or in combination with other modalities (Rowbotham *et al.*, 1998; Rice and Maton, 2001). For treatment of PHN, physicians should initiate gabapentin at a low dose of 100 mg three times daily and escalate (in increments of 100 mg t.i.d.) as required, watching for adverse effects such as somnolence, dizziness, and ataxia. Total daily doses of 1800–3600 mg may be required (Stacey and Glanzman, 2003). Pregabalin has also been shown to be effective and well-tolerated in studies of patients with PHN and is likely to replace gabapentin for this indication (Dworkin *et al.*, 2003; Sabatowski *et al.*, 2004). The adverse effects of these medications can be additive (such as sedation due to opioid analgesics, tricyclic antidepressants, and gabapentin), especially in elderly patients (Schmader, 2001). Local transdermal administration of lidocaine via patches has been shown to significantly reduce PHN in two controlled trials (Davies and Galer, 2004). Topical treatments should only be used on intact healed skin. Topical application of capsaicin cream can provide relief of PHN for some patients, but the local stinging and burning associated with capsaicin may be intolerable for many individuals. In a controlled clinical trial of 277 patients with intractable PHN, intrathecal injection of 60 mg of methylprednisolone acetate once weekly for 4 weeks resulted in significant pain reduction, but these results require confirmation (Kotani *et al.*, 2000). There is no evidence that prolonged administration of antiviral drugs has any benefit for treatment of established PHN (Acosta and Balfour, 2001).

Herpes zoster ophthalmicus

Special emphasis should be given to patients presenting with herpes zoster involving the first division of the trigeminal nerve because of the potential for sight-threatening ocular complications. The ophthalmic division of the trigeminal nerve is the cranial nerve most frequently affected by herpes zoster. Without antiviral therapy, 50% of patients with herpes zoster ophthalmicus (HZO) will develop significant ocular complications (which can include neurotrophic keratopathy, episcleritis, iritis, epithelial or stromal keratitis, etc.) (Liesegang, 1999). Controlled prospective clinical trials clearly demonstrated that oral acyclovir therapy reduced the frequency of serious late ocular inflammatory complications of HZO from about 50%–60% to 20%–30% (Cobo *et al.*, 1986; Harding and Porter, 1991; Herbort *et al.*, 1991; Hoang-Xuan *et al.*, 1992; Beutner *et al.*, 1995). A clinical trial comparing the efficacy of valacyclovir and acyclovir for HZO demonstrated the two drugs to be comparable (Colin *et al.*, 2000). Similarly, a controlled study comparing acyclovir and famciclovir in 454 patients with HZO found that the prevalence of severe and non-severe ocular manifestations (58%) was the same for both treatment groups (Tyring et al., 2001a,b). Some experts favor intravenous acyclovir as initial therapy for patients (especially immunocompromised patients) with severe HZO. Systemic antiviral therapy has largely replaced topical antiviral preparations for treatment of the ocular complications of HZO. Systemic or topical corticosteroids may be indicated for some of the ocular inflammatory phenomena that accompany HZO (e.g., uveitis), but should only be administered under the supervision of an experienced ophthalmologist (Liesegang, 1999). Available data strongly support the routine and early use of systemic antiviral therapy in all patients with HZO in an effort to reduce the risk of ocular complications (Severson et al., 2003; Zaal et al., 2003).

Immunocompromised patients

Patients with disorders of cell-mediated immunity are at increased risk for development of herpes zoster. In this population, those patients with the greatest degree of immunosuppression (such as hematopoietic stem-cell transplant (HSCT) recipients or patients with lymphoproliferative malignancies) are at highest risk for VZV dissemination and visceral organ involvement. Clinical trials with intravenous acyclovir for localized or disseminated herpes zoster in immunocompromised patients clearly demonstrated that treatment resulted in more rapid virus clearance and halted disease progression (Serota et al., 1982; Balfour et al., 1983). Subsequent studies in HSCT recipients have demonstrated that acyclovir, in addition to promoting faster disease resolution, is highly effective at preventing VZV dissemination (Meyers et al., 1984; Shepp et al., 1986). Because most VZV-related fatalities result from disseminated infection, the ability to prevent dissemination has markedly reduced the herpes zoster mortality rate in immunocompromised patients. In addition, intravenous acyclovir is considered the drug of choice for treating dissemination when it occurs, although efficacy data from prospective studies are limited (Balfour et al., 1983; Whitley et al., 1992). The recommended dose of intravenous acyclovir for herpes zoster in severely immunocompromised patients is 10–15 mg/kg (or 500 mg/m^2) every 8 hours (Table 65.1). When the infection is under control, therapy can be switched from intravenous acyclovir to an oral antiviral drug for the remainder of the course of treatment. Patients should be treated until healing is complete or for a minimum of 10–14 days (whichever is longer) to reduce the risk of relapsing disease.

Treating shingles in immunocompromised patients on an outpatient basis with oral antiviral drugs is an attractive approach, although supporting data are limited. One small study randomized 27 allogenic HSCT recipients with herpes zoster to either oral or intravenous acyclovir. No VZV dissemination occurred in either group, and no differences in healing or clinical outcome were apparent (Ljungman et al., 1989). Published data from clinical trials with famciclovir and valacyclovir for herpes zoster in immunocompromised patients remain limited, but a growing body of clinical experience suggests that these drugs are safe and effective in this setting (Tyring et al., 2001a,b). For less severely immunosuppressed patients, oral therapy with acyclovir (800 mg five times daily), valacyclovir (1000 mg three times daily), or famciclovir (500 mg three times daily), coupled with close clinical observation, is a reasonable option. Because of the risk of ocular involvement, intravenous acyclovir plus evaluation by an ophthalmologist are recommended for highly immunocompromised patients who present with HZO.

HIV-seropositive patients

The incidence of herpes zoster is about 15-fold higher in HIV-seropositive men than in age-matched controls. Shingles in this population is associated with higher rates of CNS complications, necrotizing retinitis, and recurrent episodes. Prospectively acquired data to guide clinicians when selecting antiviral therapy for herpes zoster in HIV-seropositive patients are currently limited. Nearly 300 HIV-infected patients with shingles were enrolled in controlled studies comparing orally administered acyclovir with the investigational antiviral drug sorivudine. Overall, the time to cessation of new vesicle formation, total crusting, and resolution of zoster-associated pain were 3–4 days, 7–8 days, and about 60 days, respectively (Bodsworth et al., 1997; Gnann et al., 1998). These studies confirm the efficacy and safety of oral antiviral therapy for herpes zoster in patients with HIV infection. Valacyclovir and famciclovir have not been systematically evaluated as treatments for herpes zoster in HIV-infected patients, although anecdotal clinical experience suggests therapeutic benefit. Long term administration of antiherpes virus drugs to prevent recurrences of herpes zoster in patients with AIDS is not routinely recommended. Because of the documented risk of relapsing infection, VZV disease in HIV-seropositive patients should be treated until all lesions are completely resolved, which is often longer than the standard 7–10-day course. What impact anti-VZV therapy may have on the risk of subsequent complications such as CNS infection or retinitis is unknown. Adjunctive therapy of herpes zoster with corticosteroids has not been evaluated in HIV-infected patients and is not currently recommended.

On the basis of clinical experience, most physicians select intravenous acyclovir as the drug of choice to treat severe or complicated herpes zoster in HIV-infected patients. The literature contains numerous case reports documenting successful therapy of neurologic complications with intravenous acyclovir (Poscher, 1994; Lionnet et al., 1996). Some experts have recommended intravenous acyclovir for initial therapy of HZO in HIV-infected patients, although oral therapy appears adequate in most cases.

A syndrome of herpetic retinal necrosis can occur as a late complication of herpes zoster in either immunocompetent or immunocompromised patients, but is seen with the greatest frequency in patients with AIDS. Responses to intravenous acyclovir or ganciclovir have been inconsistent and disappointing. Several case reports have documented preservation of vision in patients treated with a combination of intravenous ganciclovir plus foscarnet, with or without intravitreal ganciclovir (Galindez et al., 1996). The optimal duration of induction therapy and options for long-term maintenance therapy for acute retinal necrosis in HIV-seropositive patients have not been established (Ormerod et al., 1998). When VZV retinitis occurs in immunocompetent patients, the clinical outcome is clearly improved by acyclovir therapy and the prognosis is better. In this population, a suggested treatment regimen based on clinical experience is intravenous acyclovir (10–15 mg/kg every 8 hours) for 10–14 days, followed by oral valacyclovir 1 gram po three times a day for 4–6 weeks (Palay et al., 1991).

Clinical indications for prophylaxis

Varicella

Immunocompetent patients

Administration of varicella vaccine within the first few days after exposure to VZV will produce a protective (or partially protective) immune response in VZV seronegative individuals (Watson et al., 2000). About half of patients receiving post-exposure immunization may still develop some signs and symptoms of chickenpox, but the disease manifestations are usually very mild. Postexposure vaccination appears to be more effective and less expensive than pre-emptive therapy with antiviral drugs. This approach may be useful for managing VZV exposures that occur in a family, in the workplace, or in a medical care setting.

Pregnant women

Advisory committees have recommended administration of varicella-zoster immune globulin (VZIG) to VZV-susceptible pregnant women who have been exposed to varicella (Centers for Disease Control and Prevention, 1996). For maximal efficacy, VZIG must be administered as soon as possible after exposure (within 96 hours). VZIG (as available in the United States) is administered by deep intramuscular injection at a dose of 125 units/10 kg of body weight, to a maximum of 625 units. Intravenous immunoglobulin also contains substantial titers of VZV-specific IgG and may be substituted if VZIG is not available. Unfortunately, in this time-critical scenario, the true VZV serologic status of a pregnant woman with a negative history of varicella is often not known. The clinician may be faced with a decision to initiate passive immunoprophylaxis empirically or to wait for the results of serologic testing. The ideal time to determine VZV serologic status is before pregnancy, when vaccination can be offered to women who are confirmed to be seronegative (Glantz and Mushlin, 1998). Varicella vaccination of pregnant women is not currently recommended because of the theoretical risk of the live virus vaccine for both the fetus and the mother. Prophylactic (or pre-emptive) therapy with acyclovir for a pregnant woman after VZV exposure may be effective, but is an unproven approach.

Immunocompromised (including HIV-seropositive) patients

VZV-seronegative immunocompromised patients with a defined close exposure to either chickenpox or herpes zoster should receive VZIG to provide passive immunity (Zaia et al., 1983). In most cases, VZIG administration will not prevent infection in the susceptible host, but it will significantly reduce the severity of the resultant illness. Placebo-controlled trials in immunocompromised children have demonstrated that VZIG ameliorates the severity of chickenpox and that it significantly reduces the risk of disseminated infection. A single treatment reduces the risk of disseminated infection by about 75% and provides four weeks of passive immunity. VZIG must be administered within 96 hours of exposure at the dose described above. VZIG is not useful for the treatment of established varicella or herpes zoster. The efficacy of VZIG prophylaxis in HIV-seropositive children or adults has not been evaluated prospectively.

Prophylactic administration of acyclovir following VZV exposure has been studied to a limited extent in susceptible immunocompetent patients, but not in immunocompromised individuals. In studies of healthy children conducted in Japan, varicella developed in 16% of the children prophylactically treated with acyclovir and in 100% of children in the control group (Asano et al., 1993) About 80% of children prophylactically treated with acyclovir subsequently seroconverted, indicating VZV infection without significant disease (Suga et al., 1993). However, additional data are required before this approach of preemptive antiviral chemotherapy can be routinely recommended in either immunocompetent or immunocompromised populations. A suggested (but unvalidated) regimen is acyclovir 200 mg orally four or five times daily for 21 days beginning five days after VZV exposure.

Concerns about the use of the live, attenuated VZV$_{oka}$ vaccine in immunocompromised patients have focused on the potential for the vaccine virus to cause disease and on the possibility that immunocompromised patients will fail to mount a protective immune response. Limited experience with the vaccine in leukemic children and renal transplant recipients have demonstrated that it can be used safely in highly selected populations (Arbeter et al., 1990; Furth and Fivush, 2002).

Herpes zoster

Immunocompetent patients

There are no circumstances that warrant antiviral chemotherapy to try to prevent herpes zoster in immunocompetent individuals. A live-virus vaccine has proven to be effective for preventing herpes zoster and reducing PHN (Oxman et al., 2005). A randomized, double-blind, placebo-controlled clinical trial enrolling 38,546 adults (age 60 and over) was conducted to evaluate the live attenuated Oka/Merck VZV vaccine. The primary endpoint was "herpes zoster burden of illness," a composite score capturing zoster incidence, duration, and severity of total pain and discomfort. Compared with placebo, the vaccine reduced the zoster burden of illness by 61.1%, reduced the incidence of herpes zoster by 51.3%, and reduced the incidence of PHN by 66.5% ($P < 0.001$ for all comparisons). The vaccine was associated with mild reactogenicity (local erythema or tenderness) in 48.3% of recipients, but was otherwise well tolerated. The herpes zoster vaccine was approved for use in the United States in 2006 for immunocompetent adults 60 years of age and over.

Immunocompromised patients

Drug regimens designed to prevent HSV recurrences in immunocompromised patients undergoing cancer chemotherapy or organ transplantation will also effectively prevent herpes zoster (Ljungman, 2001). Combined results from two placebo-controlled trials of long-term (6 months) acyclovir prophylaxis in HSCT recipients demonstrated herpes zoster in 11 (18%) of 62 placebo recipients and in none of the 62 acyclovir treated patients (Lundgren et al., 1985; Perren et al., 1988). Interestingly, the incidence of zoster increased dramatically after the discontinuation of prophylaxis such that, 12 months after transplantation, the cumulative number of herpes zoster cases was virtually identical between the acyclovir and placebo groups. Nonetheless, acyclovir prophylaxis effectively prevents herpes zoster during the early post-transplant period when patients are most severely immunosuppressed and thus have the highest risk for VZV-related complications. Although transplant specialists almost universally recommend 3–6 months of acyclovir prophylaxis, no consensus currently exists regarding the relative merits of longer term prophylaxis. Development of a heat-inactivated VZV vaccine for use in immunocompromised patients is an area of active investigation (Hata et al., 2002).

HIV-seropositive patients

Antiviral chemoprophylaxis for prevention of herpes zoster in patients with AIDS is not routinely recommended. A significant number of HIV-seropositive patients take suppressive antiviral drugs to prevent genital HSV reactivations, which may also prevent herpes zoster. In patients with multiple recurrent episodes of herpes zoster, chemoprophylaxis could be considered (e.g., valacyclovir 1 gram orally twice a day or famciclovir 500 mg orally twice a day), although this approach is unvalidated.

Drug-resistant varicella-zoster virus

Since first reported in 1988, multiple isolates of acyclovir-resistant VZV have been recovered from immunocompromised patients, usually HIV-infected individuals with very low CD4+ T-lymphocyte counts. The mechanism of resistance is based on the deletion or truncation of the gene expressing thymidine kinase. Most isolates resistant to acyclovir are also resistant to valacyclovir, famciclovir, penciclovir, and ganciclovir, all of which depend on viral TK for activation. A strong association exists between acyclovir-resistant VZV and the presence of atypical skin lesions (Boivin et al., 1994; Levin et al., 2003a,b). One report described four HIV-seropositive adults undergoing chronic suppressive acyclovir therapy who developed disseminated hyperkeratotic papules that failed to respond to acyclovir (Jacobson et al., 1990). In vitro susceptibility testing confirmed that the VZV isolates were acyclovir-resistant with a mean IC50 for acyclovir of 20 μg/ml, compared with 0.75 μg/ml for the reference strain (VZV$_{oka}$). Although the mechanisms that lead to the development of acyclovir resistance are incompletely understood, clinical data indicate that many cases are associated with inadequate dosing of acyclovir for either acute therapy or long-term suppression, possibly allowing for selection of TK-deficient mutants. Clinicians using acyclovir or related drugs for treatment of varicella or herpes zoster in AIDS patients should utilize the full therapeutic dose and continue therapy until all VZV lesions have completely resolved (Jacobson et al., 1990).

The drug of choice for treatment of acyclovir-resistant VZV disease is foscarnet, an inhibitor of viral DNA polymerase that is not dependent on TK for activation (Breton et al., 1998) (Table 65.1). In a series of 13 patients with AIDS and acyclovir-resistant VZV infections treated with intravenous foscarnet, 10 patients (77%) had complete lesion healing after a mean of 17.8 days of therapy (Breton et al., 1998). Most cases of disease caused by acyclovir-resistant VZV have been limited to cutaneous involvement, although a few instances of visceral infection caused by acyclovir-resistant VZV have been reported, including cases of retinal necrosis and meningoradiculitis.

Fortunately, VZV isolates resistant to both acyclovir and foscarnet have been encountered infrequently. The molecular biology of these duly-resistant isolates has not been fully explored, but a mutation in the viral DNA polymerase can account for both acyclovir and foscarnet resistance. Cidofovir would likely retain activity against these isolates and would become the drug of choice for patients with disease caused by dually-resistant VZV.

REFERENCES

Acosta, E. P. and Balfour, H. H., Jr. (2001). Acyclovir for treatment of postherpetic neuralgia: efficacy and pharmacokinetics. *Antimicrob. Agents Chemother.*, **45**, 2771–2774.

Acosta, E. P. and Fletcher, C. V. (1997). Valacyclovir. *Ann. Pharmacother.*, **31**, 185–191.

Arbeter, A. M., Granowetter, L., Starr, S. E. et al. (1990). Immunization of children with acute lymphoblastic leukemia with live attenuated varicella vaccine without complete suspension of chemotherapy. *Pediatrics*, **85**, 338–344.

Arvin, A. M. (2002). Antiviral therapy for varicella and herpes zoster. *Semin. Pediatr. Infect. Dis.*, **13**, 12–21.

Asano, Y., Yoshikawa, T., Suga, S. et al. (1993). Postexposure prophylaxis of varicella in family contacts by oral acyclovir. *Pediatrics*, **92**, 219–222.

Balfour, H. H., Bean, B., Laskin, O. L. et al. (1983). Acyclovir halts progression of herpes zoster in immunocompromised patients. *N. Engl. J. Med.*, **308**, 1448–1453.

Balfour, H. H., Kelly, J. M., Suarez, C. S. et al. (1990). Acyclovir treatment of varicella in otherwise healthy children. *J. Pediatr.*, **116**, 633–639.

Balfour, H. H., Jr., Rotbart, H. A., Feldman, S. et al. (1992). Acyclovir treatment of varicella in otherwise healthy adolescents. The Collaborative Acyclovir Varicella Study Group. *J. Pediatr.*, **120** (4, Part 1), 627–633.

Beutner, K. R., Friedman, D. J., Forszpaniak, C. et al. (1995). Valaciclovir compared with acyclovir for improved therapy for herpes zoster in immunocompetent adults. *Antimicrob. Agents Chemother.*, **39**, 1546–1553.

Bodsworth, N. J., Boag, F., Burdge, D. et al. (1997). Evaluation of sorivudine (BV-araU) versus acyclovir in the treatment of acute localized herpes zoster in human immunodeficiency virus-infected adults. *J. Infect. Dis.*, **176**, 103–111.

Boivin, G., Edelman, C. K., Pedneault, L. et al. (1994). Phenotypic and genotypic characterization of acyclovir-resistant varicella zoster viruses isolated from persons with AIDS. *J. Infect. Dis.*, **170**, 68–75.

Bowsher, D. (2003). Factors influencing the features of postherpetic neuralgia and outcome when treated with tricyclics. *Eur. J. Pain*, **7**, 1–7.

Breton, G., Fillet, A. M., Katlama, C. et al. (1998). Acyclovir-resistant herpes zoster in human immunodeficiency virus-infected patients: results of foscarnet therapy. *Clin. Infect. Dis.*, **27**, 1525–1527.

Centers for Disease Control and Prevention (1996). Prevention of varicella: recommendations of the Advisory Committee on Immunization Practices (ACIP). *Morb. Mortal. Weekly Rep.*, **45**, 1–36.

Cobo, L. M., Foulks, G. N., Liesgang, T. et al. (1986). Oral acyclovir in the treatment of acute herpes zoster ophthalmicus. *Ophthalmology*, **93**, 763–770.

Colin, J., Prisant, O., Cochener, B. et al. (2000). Comparison of the efficacy and safety of valaciclovir and acyclovir for the treatment of herpes zoster ophthalmicus. *Ophthalmology*, **107**, 1507–1511.

Dahl, H., Marcoccia, J., and Linde, A. (1997). Antigen detection: the method of choice in comparison with virus isolation and serology for laboratory diagnosis of herpes zoster in human immunodeficiency virus-infected patient. *J. Clin. Microbiol.*, **35**, 345–349.

Davies, P. S. and Galer, B. S. (2004). Review of lidocaine patch 5% studies in the treatment of postherpetic neuralgia. *Drugs*, **64**, 937–947.

De La Blanchardiere, A., Rozenberg, F., Caumes, E. et al. (2000). Neurological complications of varicella-zoster virus infection in adults with human immunodeficiency virus infection. *Scand. J. Infect. Dis.*, **32**, 263–269.

Degreef, H. and the Famciclovir Herpes Zoster Study Group (1994). Famciclovir, a new oral antiherpes drug: results of the first controlled clinical study demonstrating its efficacy and safety in the treatment of uncomplicated herpes zoster in immunocompetent patient. *Int. J. Antimicrob. Agents*, **4**, 241–246.

Dodd, D. A., Burger, J., Edwards, K. M. et al. (2001). Varicella in a pediatric heart transplant population on nonsteroid maintenance immunosuppression. *Pediatrics*, **108**, E80.

Dunkle, L. M., Arvin, A. M., Whitley, R. J. et al. (1991). A controlled trial of acyclovir for chickenpox in normal children. *N. Engl. J. Med.*, **325**, 1539–1544.

Dworkin, R. H. and Schmader, K. E. (2003). Treatment and prevention of postherpetic neuralgia. *Clin. Infect. Dis.*, **36**, 877–882.

Dworkin, R. H., Boon, R. J., Griffin, D. R. et al. (1998). Postherpetic neuralgia: impact of famciclovir, age, rash severity, and acute pain in herpes zoster patients. *J. Infect. Dis.*, **178** (Suppl. 1), S76–S80.

Dworkin, R. H., Perkins, F. M., and Nagasako, E. M. (2000). Prospects for the prevention of postherpetic neuralgia in herpes zoster patients. *Clin. J. Pain*, **16** (Suppl. 2), S90–100.

Dworkin, R. H., Corbin, A. E., Young, J. P., Jr. et al. (2003). Pregabalin for the treatment of postherpetic neuralgia: a randomized, placebo-controlled trial. *Neurology*, **60**, 1274–1283.

Furth, S. L. and Fivush, B. A. (2002). Varicella vaccination in pediatric kidney transplant candidates. *Pediatr. Transpl.*, **6**, 97–100.

Galindez, O. A., Sabates, N. R., Whitacre, M. W. et al. (1996). Rapidly progressive outer retinal necrosis caused by varicella zoster virus in a patient infected with human immunodeficiency virus. *Clin. Infect. Dis.*, **22**, 149–151.

Gershon, A. A., Mervish, N., LaRussa, P. et al. (1997). Varicella-zoster virus infection in children with underlying human immunodeficiency virus infection. *J. Infect. Dis.*, **176**, 1496–1500.

Glantz, J. C. and Mushlin, A. I. (1998). Cost-effectiveness of routine antenatal varicella screening. *Obstet. Gynecol.*, **91**, 519–528.

Gnann, J. W., Jr. (2002). Varicella-zoster virus: atypical presentations and unusual complications. *J. Infect. Dis.*, **186** (Suppl. 1), S91–S98.

Gnann, J. W., Jr. and Whitley, R. J. (2002). Clinical practice. Herpes zoster. *N. Engl. J. Med.*, **347**, 340–346.

Gnann, J. W., Crumpacker, C. S., Lalezari, J. P. et al. (1998). Sorivudine versus acyclovir for treatment of dermatomal herpes zoster in human immunodeficiency virus-infected patients: results from a randomized, controlled clinical trial. *Antimicrob. Agents Chemother.*, **42**, 1139–1145.

Gross, G., Schofer, H., Wassilew, S. et al. (2003). Herpes zoster guideline of the German Dermatology Society (DDG). *J. Clin. Virol.*, **26**, 277–289; discussion 291–293.

Haake, D. A., Zakowski, P. C., Haake, D. L. et al. (1990). Early treatment with acyclovir for varicella pneumonia in otherwise healthy adults: retrospective controlled study and review. *Rev. Infect. Dis.*, **12**, 788–798.

Harding, S. P. and Porter, S. M. (1991). Oral acyclovir in herpes zoster ophthalmicus. *Curr. Eye Res.*, **10** (Suppl.), 177–182.

Harger, J. H., Ernest, J. M., Thurnau, G. R. et al. (2002). Frequency of congenital varicella syndrome in a prospective cohort of 347 pregnant women. *Obstet. Gynecol.*, **100**, 260–265.

Harrison, R. A., Soong, S., Weiss, H. L. et al. (1999). A mixed model for factors predictive of pain in AIDS patients with herpes zoster. *J. Pain Symptom Managem.*, **17**, 410–417.

Hata, A., Asanuma, H., Rinki, M. et al. (2002). Use of an inactivated varicella vaccine in recipients of hematopoietic-cell transplants. *N. Engl. J. Med.*, **347**, 26–34.

Hellden, A., Odar-Cederlof, I., Diener, P. et al. (2003). High serum concentrations of the acyclovir main metabolite 9-carboxymethoxymethylguanine in renal failure patients with acyclovir-related neuropsychiatric side effects: an observational study. *Nephrol. Dial. Transpl.*, **18**, 1135–1141.

Herbort, C. P., Buechi, E. R., Piguet, B. et al. (1991). High dose oral acyclovir in acute herpes zoster ophthalmicus: the end of the corticosteroid era. *Curr. Eye Res.*, **10** (Suppl.), 171–175.

Hoang-Xuan, T., Buchi, E. R., Herbot, C. P. et al. (1992). Oral acyclovir for herpes zoster ophthalmicus. *Ophthalmology*, **99**, 1062–1071.

Huff, J. C., Bean, B., Balfour, H. H. et al. (1988). Therapy of herpes zoster with oral acyclovir. *Am. J. Med.*, **85** (Suppl. 2A), 84–88.

Jacobson, M. A., Berger, T. G., Fikrig, S. et al. (1990). Acyclovir-resistant varicella zoster virus infection after chronic oral acyclovir therapy in patients with the acquired immunodeficiency syndrome (AIDS). *Ann. Intern. Med.*, **112**, 187–191.

Johnson, R. W. (2002). Consequences and management of pain in herpes zoster. *J. Infect. Dis.*, **186** (Suppl. 1), S83–S90.

Johnson, R. W. and Dworkin, R. H. (2003). Treatment of herpes zoster and postherpetic neuralgia. *Br. Med. J.*, **326**, 748–750.

Keam, S. J., Chapman, T. M., and Figgitt, D. P. (2004). Brivudin (bromovinyl deoxyuridine). *Drugs*, **64**, 2091–2097.

Kotani, N., Kushikata, T., Hashimoto, H. et al. (2000). Intrathecal methylprednisolone for intractable postherpetic neuralgia. *N. Engl. J. Med.*, **343**, 1514–1519.

Levin, M. J., Dahl, K. M., Weinberg, A. et al. (2003a). Development of resistance to acyclovir during chronic infection with the Oka vaccine strain of varicella-zoster virus, in an immunosuppressed child. *J. Infect. Dis.*, **188**, 954–959.

Levin, M. J., Smith, J. G., Kaufhold, R. M. et al. (2003b). Decline in varicella-zoster virus (VZV)-specific cell-mediated immunity with increasing age and boosting with a high-hose VZV vaccine. *J. Infect. Dis.*, **188**, 1336–1344.

Liesegang, T. J. (1999). Varicella zoster viral disease. *Mayo Clin. Proc.*, **74**, 983–998.

Lionnet, F., Pulik, M., Genet, P. et al. (1996). Myelitis due to varicella-zoster virus in 2 patients with AIDS: successful treatment with acyclovir. *Clin. Infect. Dis.*, **22**, 138–140.

Ljungman, P. (2001). Prophylaxis against herpesvirus infections in transplant recipients. *Drugs*, **61**, 187–196.

Ljungman, P., Lonnqvist, B., Ringden, O. et al. (1989). A randomized trial of oral versus intravenous acyclovir for treatment of herpes zoster in bone marrow transplant recipients. *Bone Marrow Transpl.*, **4**, 613–615.

Lundgren, G., Wilecek, H., Lönnqvist, B. et al. (1985). Acyclovir prophylaxis in bone marrow transplant recipients. *Scand. J. Infect. Dis.*, **47** (Suppl. 7), 137–144.

McKendrick, M. W., McGill, J. I., White, J. E. et al. (1986). Oral acyclovir in acute herpes zoster. *Br. Med. J.*, **293**, 1529–1532.

Meyers, J. D., Wade, J. C., Shepp, D. H. et al. (1984). Acyclovir treatment of varicella-zoster virus infection in the compromised host. *Transplantation*, **37**, 571–574.

Morton, P. and Thomson, A. N. (1989). Oral acyclovir in the treatment of herpes zoster in general practice. *N Z Med. J.*, **102**, 93–95.

Nagasako, E. M., Johnson, R. W., Griffin, D. R. et al. (2002). Rash severity in herpes zoster: correlates and relationship to postherpetic neuralgia. *J. Am. Acad. Dermatol.*, **46**, 834–839.

Nathwani, D., Maclean, A., Conway, S. *et al.* (1998). Varicella infections in pregnancy and the newborn. A review prepared for the UK Advisory Group on Chickenpox on behalf of the British Society for the Study of Infection. *J. Infect.*, **36** (Suppl. 1), 59–71.

Nyerges, G., Meszner, Z., Gyarmati, E. *et al.* (1988). Acyclovir prevents dissemination of varicella in immunocompromised children. *J. Infect. Dis.*, **157**, 309–313.

Opstelten, W., van Wijck, A. J., and Stolker, R. J. (2004). Interventions to prevent postherpetic neuralgia: cutaneous and percutaneous techniques. *Pain*, **107**, 202–206.

Ormerod, L. D., Larkin, J. A., Margo, C. A. *et al.* (1998). Rapidly progressive herpetic retinal necrosis: a blinding disease characteristic of advanced AIDS. *Clin. Infect. Dis.*, **26**, 34–45.

Oxman, M. N. *et al.* (2005). A vaccine to prevent herpes zoster and postherpetic neuralgia in older adults. *N. Engl. J. Med.*, **352**, 2271–2284.

Palay, D. A., Sternberg, P., Jr., Davis, J. *et al.* (1991). Decrease in the risk of bilateral acute retinal necrosis by acyclovir therapy. *Am. J. Ophthalmol.*, **112**, 250–255.

Perren, T. J., Powles, R. L., Easton, D. *et al.* (1988). Prevention of herpes zoster in patients by long-term oral acyclovir after allogenic bone marrow transplantation. *Am. J. Med.*, **85** (Suppl. 2A), 99–101.

Perry, C. M. and Wagstaff, A. J. (1995). Famciclovir: a review of its pharmacological properties and therapeutic efficacy in herpesvirus infections. *Drugs*, **50**, 396–415.

Poscher, M. E. (1994). Successful treatment of varicella-zoster virus meningoencephalitis in patients with AIDS: report of 4 cases and review. *AIDS*, **8**, 1115–1117.

Prober, C. G., Kirk, L. E., and Keeney, R. E. (1982). Acyclovir therapy of chickenpox in immunocompromised children: a collaborative study. *J. Pediatr.*, **101**, 622–625.

Raja, S. N., Haythornthwaite, J. A., Pappagallo, M. *et al.* (2002). Opioids versus antidepressants in postherpetic neuralgia: a randomized, placebo-controlled trial. *Neurology*, **59**, 1015–1021.

Reiff-Eldridge, R., Heffner, C. R., Ephross, S. A. *et al.* (2000). Monitoring pregnancy outcomes after prenatal drug exposure through prospective pregnancy registries: a pharmaceutical company commitment. *Am. J. Obstet. Gynecol.*, **182**, 159–163.

Rice, A. S. and Maton, S. (2001). Gabapentin in postherpetic neuralgia: a randomized, double blind, placebo controlled study. *Pain*, **94**, 215–224.

Rowbotham, M., Harden, N., Stacey, B. *et al.* (1998). Gabapentin for the treatment of postherpetic neuralgia: a randomized controlled trial. *J. Am. Med. Assoc.*, **280**, 1837–1842.

Sabatowski, R., Galvez, R., Cherry, D. A. *et al.* (2004). Pregabalin reduces pain and improves sleep and mood disturbances in patients with post-herpetic neuralgia: results of a randomized, placebo-controlled clinical trial. *Pain*, **109**, 26–35.

Schmader, K. (2001). Herpes zoster in older adults. *Clin. Infect. Dis.*, **32**, 1481–1486.

Serota, F. T., Starr, S. E., Bryan, C. K. *et al.* (1982). Acyclovir treatment of herpes zoster infections: use in children undergoing bone marrow transplantation. *J. Am. Med. Assoc.*, **247**, 2132–2135.

Severson, E. A., Baratz, K. H., Hodge, D. O. *et al.* (2003). Herpes zoster ophthalmicus in Olmsted County, Minnesota: have systemic antivirals made a difference? *Arch. Ophthalmol.*, **121**, 386–390.

Shafran, S. D., Tyring, S. K., Ashton, R. *et al.* (2004). Once, twice, or three times daily famciclovir compared with aciclovir for the oral treatment of herpes zoster in immunocompetent adults: a randomized, multicenter, double-blind clinical trial. *J. Clin. Virol.*, **29**, 248–253.

Shepp, D. H., Dandliker, P. S., and Meyers, J. D. (1986). Treatment of varicella-zoster infection in severely immunocompromised patients: a randomized comparison of acyclovir and vidarabine. *N. Engl. J. Med.*, **314**, 208–212.

Stacey, B. R. and Glanzman, R. L. (2003). Use of gabapentin for postherpetic neuralgia: results of two randomized, placebo-controlled studies. *Clin. Ther.*, **25**, 2597–2608.

Stranska, R., Schuurman, R., de Vos, M. *et al.* (2004). Routine use of a highly automated and internally controlled real-time PCR assay for the diagnosis of herpes simplex and varicella-zoster virus infections. *J. Clin. Virol.*, **30**, 39–44.

Suga, S., Yoshikawa, T., Ozaki, T. *et al.* (1993). Effect of oral acyclovir against primary and secondary viraemia in incubation period of varicella. *Arch. Dis. Child.*, **69**, 639–642.

Tyring, S., Barbarash, R. A., Nahlik, J. E. *et al.* (1995). Famciclovir for the treatment of acute herpes zoster: effects on acute disease and post-herpetic neuralgia: a randomized, double-blind, placebo-controlled trial. *Ann. Int. Med.*, **123**, 89–96.

Tyring, S. K., Beutner, K. R., Tucker, B. A. *et al.* (2000). Antiviral therapy for herpes zoster: randomized, controlled clinical trial of valacyclovir and famciclovir therapy in immunocompetent patients 50 years and older. *Arch. Fam. Med.*, **9**, 863–869.

Tyring, S., Belanger, R., Bezwoda, W. *et al.* (2001a). A randomized, double-blind trial of famciclovir versus acyclovir for the treatment of localized dermatomal herpes zoster in immunocompromised patients. *Cancer Invest.*, **19**, 13–22.

Tyring, S., Engst, R., Corriveau, C. *et al.* (2001b). Famciclovir for ophthalmic zoster: a randomised aciclovir controlled study. *Br. J. Ophthalmol.*, **85**, 576–581.

Tyring, S. K., Baker, D., and Snowden, W. (2002). Valacyclovir for herpes simplex virus infection: long-term safety and sustained efficacy after 20 years' experience with acyclovir. *J. Infect. Dis.*, **186** (Suppl. 1), S40–S46.

Wagstaff, A. J. and Bryson, H. M. (1994). Foscarnet: a reappraisal of its antiviral activity, pharmacokinetic properties and therapeutic use in immunocompromised patients with viral infections. *Drugs*, **48**, 199–226.

Wallace, M. R., Bowler, W. A., and Murray, N. B. (1992). Treatment of adult varicella with oral acyclovir. *Ann. Intern. Med.*, **117**, 358–363.

Wassilew, S. W. and Wutzler, P. (2003a). Oral brivudin in comparison with acyclovir for improved therapy of herpes zoster in immunocompetent patients: results of a randomized, double-blind, multicentered study. *Antiviral Res.*, **59**, 49–56.

Wassilew, S. W. and Wutzler, P. (2003b). Oral brivudin in comparison with acyclovir for herpes zoster: a survey study on postherpetic neuralgia. *Antiviral Res.*, **59**, 57–60.

Watson, B., Seward, J., Yang, A. *et al.* (2000). Postexposure effectiveness of varicella vaccine. *Pediatrics*, **105**, 84–88.

Watson, C. P. and Babul, N. (1998). Efficacy of oxycodone in neuropathic pain: a randomized trial in postherpetic neuralgia. *Neurology*, **50**, 1837–1841.

Watson, C. P., Vernich, L., Chipman, M. *et al.* (1998). Nortriptyline versus amitriptyline in postherpetic neuralgia: a randomized trial. *Neurology*, **51**, 1166–1171.

Whitley, R. J. and Gnann, J. W. (1992). Acyclovir: a decade later. *N. Engl. J. Med.*, **327**, 782–789.

Whitley, R. J., Gnann, J. W., Hinthorn, D. *et al.* (1992). Disseminated herpes zoster in the immunocompromised host: a comparative trial of acyclovir and vidarabine. *J. Infect. Dis.*, **165**, 450–455.

Whitley, R. J., Weiss, H., Gnann, J. W. *et al.* (1996). Acyclovir with and without prednisone for the treatment of herpes zoster. A randomized, placebo-controlled trial. The National Institute of Allergy and Infectious Diseases Collaborative Antiviral Study Group. *Ann. Intern. Med.*, **125**, 376–383.

Whitley, R. J., Weiss, H. L., Soong, S. J. *et al.* (1999). Herpes zoster: risk categories for persistent pain. *J. Infect. Dis.*, **179**, 9–15.

Wilkins, E. G., Leen, C. L., McKendrick, M. W. *et al.* (1998). Management of chickenpox in the adult. A review prepared for the UK Advisory Group on Chickenpox on behalf of the British Society for the Study of Infection. *J. Infect.*, **36** (Suppl. 1), 49–58.

Wood, M. J., Ogan, P. H., McKendrick, M. W. *et al.* (1988). Efficacy of oral acyclovir treatment of acute herpes zoster. *Am. J. Med.*, **85** (Suppl. 2A), 79–83.

Wood, M. J., Johnson, R. W., McKendrick, M. W. *et al.* (1994). A randomized trial of acyclovir for 7 days or 21 days with and without prednisolone for treatment of acute herpes zoster. *N. Engl. J. Med.*, **330**, 896–900.

Wood, M. J., Kay, R., Dworkin, R. H. *et al.* (1996). Oral acyclovir therapy accelerates pain resolution in patients with herpes zoster: a meta-analysis of placebo-controlled trials. *Clin. Infect. Dis.*, **22**, 341–347.

Wood, M. J., Shukla, S., Fiddian, A. P. *et al.* (1998). Treatment of acute herpes zoster: effect of early (<48 h) versus late (48–72 h) therapy with acyclovir and valaciclovir on prolonged pain. *J. Infect. Dis.*, **178** (Suppl. 1), S81–S84.

Zaal, M. J., Volker-Dieben, H. J., and D'Amaro, J. (2003). Visual prognosis in immunocompetent patients with herpes zoster ophthalmicus. *Acta Ophthalmol. Scand.*, **81**, 216–220.

Zaia, J. A., Levin, M. J., Preblud, S. R. *et al.* (1983). Evaluation of varicella-zoster immune globulin: protection of immunosuppressed children after household exposure to varicella. *J. Infect. Dis.*, **147**, 737–743.

Antiviral therapy for human cytomegalovirus

Paul D. Griffiths[1] and Michael Boeckh[2]

[1]Royal Free and University College Medical School, London, UK
[2]Program in Infectious Diseases, Fred Hutchinson Cancer Research Center, Seattle, WA, USA

Introduction

The remit of this chapter is to summarize what is known about licensed antiviral drugs for CMV. In summary, we do not possess a single anti-CMV drug, which is potent and safe enough to be given to all individuals infected with this virus. What follows therefore, is the evidence-base for prescribing the existing compounds with the objective of maximizing therapeutic efficacy and cost-effectiveness while minimizing toxicity.

Licensed drugs and mechanism of action

Nucleosides

Ganciclovir (GCV) and acyclovir (ACV) are related nucleosides (see Fig. 66.1) which are anabolized by a common cellular pathway. After activation, they are competitive inhibitors of CMV encoded DNA polymerase. In cells infected with CMV, the first stage of phosphorylation is achieved by the UL97 protein kinase. Once GCV is monophosphorylated within the virus-infected cell, it is charged and so unable to diffuse out of the cell. A concentration gradient is thereby formed across the plasma membrane, aiding diffusion of more GCV into the infected cell. Cellular enzymes convert GCV monophosphate to the triphosphate. GCV triphosphate is a potent inhibitor of CMV DNA polymerase and has a long intracellular half-life. Selectivity for virus-infected cells is achieved both by UL97 activation and because GCV triphosphate is a better inhibitor of CMV-encoded DNA polymerase than cellular DNA polymerase.

Ganciclovir possesses a free hydroxyl at a position equivalent to the 3' of the open sugar ring and so can allow DNA elongation. This means that it is not an obligate chain terminator, although chain termination usually occurs after incorporation of one or more molecules. The ability to allow chain elongation is theoretically undesirable because it might occur in uninfected cells leading to a mutagenic event in cellular DNA; GCV in particular is oncogenic at low dosages in rodents due to this incorporation into cellular DNA.

ACV can also be activated by UL97 (Talarico et al., 1999) and acyclovir triphosphate is a potent inhibitor of CMV DNA polymerase (Mar et al., 1985) so that this compound can also inhibit CMV. Acyclovir triphosphate is an obligate chain terminator and also a suicide inhibitor of herpesvirus DNA polymerase (Furman et al., 1984). In combination, these characteristics potently inhibit CMV replication. However, the intracellular half-life of ACV-triphosphate is significantly shorter than that of GCV-triphosphate so that high drug levels and frequent dosing are needed for ACV to control CMV replication in vivo (Lowance et al., 1999). Selectivity for virus-infected cells is achieved by UL97 activation and because ACV triphosphate is a better inhibitor of CMV-encoded DNA polymerase than cellular DNA polymerase.

The oral absorption of GCV is poor while that of ACV is better but also variable between individuals. Oral bioavailability of these compounds has been improved via esters which are absorbed and then cleaved in the intestinal wall and/or liver to release free compound. Valganciclovir is the valine ester of GCV. Valaciclovir is the valine ester of ACV.

Nucleotides

Cidofovir (CDV) is a nucleotide. These compounds are phosphonates, structurally equivalent to the nucleoside monophosphate but without the charge which would prevent the molecule crossing the plasma membrane. Cidofovir bypasses the UL97 step and is converted to the diphosphate (equivalent to the nucleoside triphosphate; see

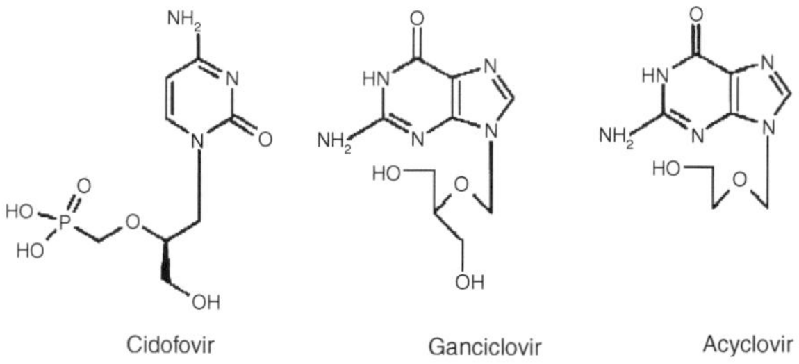

Fig. 66.1. Chemical structures of licensed antiviral drugs with activity against CMV in vivo.

Fig. 66.2) by cellular enzymes. The selectivity of CDV resides in the preferential inhibition of CMV DNA polymerase rather than cellular DNA polymerase by CDV diphosphate.

Foscarnet

Pyrophosphate is eliminated when a phosphodiester bond is formed as a natural nucleoside triphosphate and is incorporated into a growing DNA chain. Foscarnet is structurally analogous to pyrophosphate and inhibits CMV DNA polymerase by binding to the enzymic site for pyrophosphate. Since pyrophosphate is one of the products of DNA enzyme activity, foscarnet is a product inhibitor, not a substrate inhibitor, and so does not compete with the natural nucleotides.

Fomivirsen

Molecules complementary (antisense) to mRNA bind mRNA to prevent expression of the encoded gene. For CMV, the antisense molecule fomivirsen binds to the major immediate-early transactivator gene. The half-life of this compound is long because it contains modified nucleosides such as phosphorothioates (substitution of sulfur into the phosphodiester background) and/or modified sugar residues, which are not readily degraded by host cell enzymes. In contrast to the other compounds mentioned above, fomvirsen is administered intravitreally only to the end-organ involved with CMV retinitis and so does not affect systemic CMV.

Clinical efficacy; challenges for achieving clinical benefit

Opportunistic infection with CMV occurs when a patient is immunocompromised because the immune system is immature (fetus/neonate), dysregulated (engrafting hematopoietic stem cell transplant), suppressed pharma-

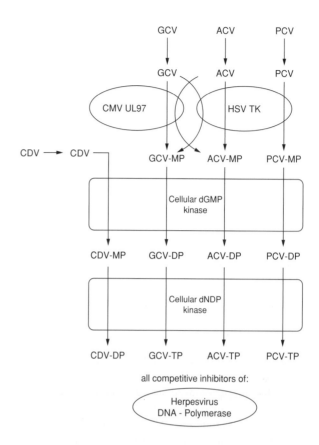

Enzymes encoded by herpesviruses are shown as ovals.
Enzymes encoded by mammalian cells are shown as rectangles.

ACV = acyclovir
GCV = ganciclovir
PCV = penciclovir
MP = monophosphate
DP = diphosphate
TP = triphosphate

CDV = cidofovir
TK = thymidine kinase
UL97 = 97th gene in unique long region

Fig. 66.2. Anabolism of anti-viral drugs to make active forms.

cologically (solid organ transplant recipient) or suppressed by HIV infection (AIDS). The clinical benefits of treatment must therefore be seen in the context of these complex medical cases and require a detailed understanding of disease pathogenesis in each of the patient groups. Specifically, there is evidence (Rubin, 1991) that CMV has "direct effects" (where the virus can be seen histologically in the affected end-organ) and "indirect effects" where the virus is statistically associated with and may trigger conditions such as graft rejection, accelerated atherosclerosis, an immunosuppressive syndrome and death (not attributable to CMV end-organ disease). Antiviral treatment has the potential of inhibiting both direct and indirect effects but

Table 66.1. CMV diseases in the immunocompromised

Symptoms	Solid T_x	BMT/SCT_x	AIDS
Direct effects			
Fever/hepatitis	+++	+	+
Gastrointestinal	++	++	+
Retinitis	+	+	+++
Pneumonitis	+	+++	
Myelosuppression		+	
Encephalopathy		+	+
Polyradiculopathy			+
Addisonian			+
Indirect effects			
Immunosuppression	+	+	
Rejection/GvHD	+	?	
Atherosclerosis	+		
Death		+	+

Table 66.2. Implications of the CMV viral load results from 1975

CMV is a systemic infection

Sampling of urine can provide a paradigm of CMV replication in inaccessible target organs

There may be a threshold value of viral load above which disease becomes common

Antiviral therapy may have clinical benefits even if it cannot completely stop virus replication

A short duration of therapy may provide clinical benefit, even though virus excretion continues for years

Pathogenesis

Viremia and viral load

Most CMV end-organ disease in the immunocompromised is caused by viremic spread to multiple organs (Table 66.1). The risk of CMV disease correlates strongly with high CMV viral loads as first described in 1975 by Stagno and colleagues (Stagno et al., 1975). They compared viruria in neonates with symptomatic congenital, asymptomatic congenital, or perinatal infection. The group with CMV disease had, on average, one log higher viruria than those with asymptomatic congenital infection, who in turn had an average one log higher viruria than those with perinatal infection (see Fig. 66.3). This observation has a series of implications for understanding pathogenesis and for focussing antiviral therapy (see Table 66.2). For example, the results suggested that there might be a threshold viral load above which CMV disease became common. This possibility has been investigated using

carefully controlled clinical trials are required to prove this definitively.

All seropositive individuals should be assumed to possess latent CMV capable of reactivation. Thus, if they become immunocompromised, CMV frequently reactivates from latency and may cause disease (reactivation infection). In addition, organs harvested from a seropositive individual may transmit virus (Grundy et al., 1988), irrespective of whether the recipient is seronegative (primary infection) or seropositive (reinfection).

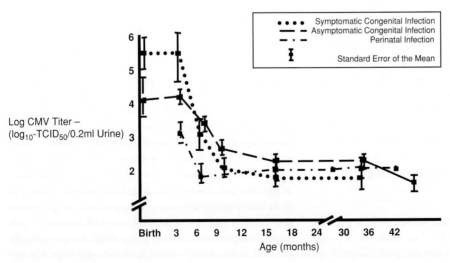

Fig. 66.3. CMV load From Stagno *et al.*, 1975.

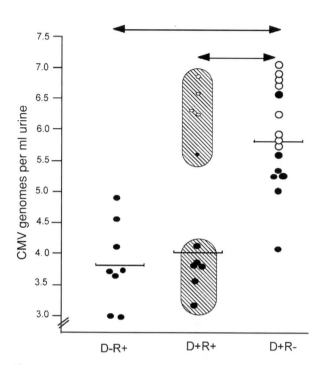

Fig. 66.4. Inter-relationships between peak CMV viral load, donor recipient serostatus and CMV disease in 35 patients with active CMV infection after renal transplantation. (Reprinted with permission from Cope, 1997b)

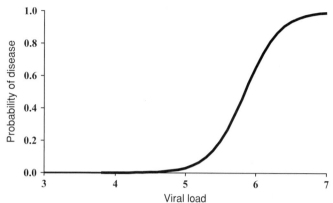

Fig. 66.5. The threshold concept From Cope, 1997b

quantitative-competitive PCR (QCPCR), which showed that, after renal transplant, a significant correlation is apparent (Cope et al., 1997b) between the median values of maximum viruria post-transplant and the presence of CMV disease (see Fig. 66.4). The same is true when viral load is measured in blood (Hassan-Walker et al., 1999) from renal transplant, liver transplant, and stem cell transplant patients, with CMV viral loads in the blood significantly greater in patients with CMV disease in each case (Cope et al., 1997a,b; Gor et al., 1998).

Donor/recipient serostatus at the time of transplant also identifies (Betts et al., 1977) patients at risk of CMV disease (e.g. see Fig. 66.4). For recipients of solid organs, highest risk groups are D+R− (ie donor seropositive, recipient seronegative), followed by D+R+, then D−R+. These groups represent primary infection, reinfection plus reactivation and reactivation infections, respectively. For stem cell transplant recipients, the highest risk is D−R+, followed by D+R+, then D+R−. These groups correspond to reactivation, reactivation in the presence of marrow from immune donors and possible transmission of virus from donor marrow, respectively. In addition, multiple studies in all transplant patient groups identified viremia as a risk factor for CMV disease (Meyers et al., 1990). Multivariate statistical analyses showed that for all patient populations, high viral load remained a risk factor for CMV disease after viremia and donor/recipient serostatus had been controlled statistically. In contrast, donor/recipient serostatus and viremia were no longer statistically significant once viral load had been controlled (Cope et al., 1997a,b; Gor et al., 1998). Thus, high viral load is the major determinant of CMV disease and the classically defined risk factors of donor/recipient serostatus and viremia are markers of CMV disease because of their association with high viral load. In addition, the relationship between increasing viral load and disease is non-linear, with a threshold value above which CMV disease is much more common (Cope et al., 1997a,b) (Fig. 66.5). This finding implies (Table 66.2) that potent prevention of disease could be achieved if drugs were deployed to prevent viral load exceeding critical values.

Serial measurements of viremia in several groups of immunocompromised patients demonstrated that CMV replicates with rapid dynamics, approximating to a doubling time (viral load increasing) or half-life (viral load decreasing) of one day (Emery et al., 1999). The half-life is even shorter among patients experiencing primary infection (Emery et al., 2002). This means that its reputation as a "slowly growing" virus is undeserved and that drugs of high potency are required to interfere with its replication. Thus, viral load measurements explain much of the pathogenesis of CMV disease and are important for understanding disease processes, for targeting the deployment of antiviral drugs, for measuring the success of antiviral therapy and for predicting the development of resistance (see later).

Disease processes within infected organs

Direct effects

Much of the end-organ disease caused by CMV can be attributed to *lysis*, i.e., destruction of cells as a direct result of virus replication. This can literally be seen clearly in the special case of the retinal cells destroyed by CMV (i.e. retinitis) but similar processes probably account for hearing loss, hepatitis, adrenalitis, gastrointestinal tract ulceration, encephalitis, and polyradiculopathy. In all of these cases, CMV can be seen histopathologically in biopsies, can be cultured from biopsies (showing productive replication) and responds to antiviral therapy. In contrast, some other diseases associated with CMV may be triggered by the virus, but may be caused by immune responses.

CMV pneumonitis appears typically in the second month post stem cell transplant after patients have had CMV viremia and asymptomatic CMV lung infection as shown by bronchial lavage at day 35 (Schmidt *et al.*, 1991). Thus, marrow engraftment, often associated with GvHD, represents a risk factor for CMV pneumonitis, implying that an aberrant immune response may contribute to disease (for review, see Grundy *et al.*, 1987). However, CMV can also occur before engraftment. Once established, CMV pneumonitis responds very poorly to ganciclovir alone, but the addition of immunoglobulin may give an improved response rate (Ljungman *et al.*, 1992). A cytokine-driven disease caused by abnormal cell-mediated effectors is suspected and, if correct, could explain why CMV pneumonitis is uncommon in AIDS patients with low CD4 counts. An alternative hypothesis is that the pulmonary toxicity of chemotherapy and/or irradiation causes damage which predisposes to viral pneumonia when viral replication occurs in the lung following transplantation (Schmidt *et al.*, 1991). A corollary to the former hypothesis (Grundy *et al.*, 1987) was that restoration of the immune deficit in AIDS patients with anti-retroviral medication, might trigger CMV pneumonitis. Although we are unaware of any such cases of CMV pneumonitis in AIDS patients given HAART, an inflammatory response to CMV is commonly seen in the *eye*, with corresponding increased levels of patient morbidity (Karavellas *et al.*, 1999).

Indirect effects

CMV is associated with an increased incidence of acute graft rejection. The presumed pathogenesis involves CMV infection of the transplanted organ acting like a transplantation antigen, marking the organ for immune attack. Evidence for CMV playing this pathogenic role includes statistical association (Grattan *et al.*, 1989), detection of CMV in organs undergoing rejection, apparent response of late rejection to ganciclovir therapy in an uncontrolled study (Reinke *et al.*, 1994), and a significant reduction in biopsy-proven acute graft rejection among patients randomized to high-dose valaciclovir in a placebo-controlled trial of prophylaxis after renal transplant (Lowance *et al.*, 1999).

CMV is also associated with accelerated atherosclerosis after heart transplantation (Grattan *et al.*, 1989). CMV persists in monocytes/macrophages that could be attracted to sites of graft atheroma, either bringing CMV to that site or facilitating the formation of foam cells laden with oxidized lipids (Guetta *et al.*, 1997). CMV major immediate-early protein binds p53 in arterial smooth muscle cells (Speir *et al.*, 1994) suggesting that CMV could reduce apoptosis leading to proliferation of such cells. The US28 gene of CMV encodes a chemokine receptor which, once transferred experimentally to smooth muscle cells, confers the ability to migrate towards a source of chemokines. Thus, CMV infection might stimulate chemotactic mobility of these cells towards a site of inflammation (Streblow *et al.*, 1999). Finally, CMV stimulates the formation of reactive oxidized intermediates and could contribute further to the progression of atherosclerosis (Speir *et al.*, 1996). Irrespective of the mechanism(s), follow-up of heart allograft patients who took part in a placebo-controlled trial of GCV reported reduced accelerated atherosclerosis among those allocated the drug (Valantine *et al.*, 1999), so replicating in humans what had previously been shown with rat CMV in rats (Lemstrom *et al.*, 1997).

CMV infection is associated with an increased incidence of bacterial or fungal superinfection (Falagas *et al.*, 1996; Nichols *et al.*, 2002) follow-up of the heart allograft patients mentioned above demonstrated reduced fungal infection in those randomized to receive GCV (Wagner *et al.*, 1995). This implies that CMV is functionally immunosuppressive and possible mechanisms have been reviewed recently (Boeckh and Nichols, 2003). If CMV does contribute to the net level of immuosuppression, this could explain why it is associated with EBV-induced lymphoproliferative disease. It could also explain why AIDS patients with first episode CMV retinitis have a significantly higher mortality rate if their CMV viral load in blood is above the median of the whole group of patients (Bowen *et al.*, 1996) and why the death rate (in the pre-HAART era) was associated more strongly with CMV viral load than with HIV viral load (Spector *et al.*, 1999). Recent results show that this same effect is still present in the era of HAART (Deayton *et al.*, 2004).

Clinical manifestations of CMV end-organ disease

The major clinical manifestations of CMV disease in different groups of immunocompromised patients are summarized in Table 66.1. These should be defined with reference to the criteria laid down at the International CMV Workshop (Ljungman *et al.*, 2002) which include: compatible clinical features plus signs of end-organ dysfunction plus demonstration of CMV in the affected organ (exception retina). In particular, diseases should be described in terms of the body system affected and the term "CMV syndrome" should be avoided.

Fever/leukopenia

CMV viremia is often associated with prolonged spiking fever (e.g. >38 °C on two consecutive days), with or without leukopenia. These constitutional symptoms may resolve spontaneously or may lead to end-organ disease. Other causes of fever (e.g., bacteremia) and leukopenia (e.g., doses of immunosuppressive drugs) must be excluded. CMV-related marrow graft failure has been described as a rare complication after stem cell transplant.

Hepatitis

Transaminases may be raised (e.g., >2.5 × upper limit of normal), with or without alkaline phosphatase representing an obstructive component. Hyperbilirubinemia may be present but frank jaundice is uncommon. Hepatitis usually resolves spontaneously but may herald other end-organ disease. It is predominantly seen in solid organ transplant recipients, with a predeliction to liver transplantation.

Gastrointestinal disease

CMV may involve the gastrointestinal tract anywhere from the mouth to the anus. The presentation is usually with pain, often accompanied by fever. Esophagitis, odynophagia and abdominal pain mimicking perforation indicate involvement of the esophagus/colon, respectively. Endoscopy reveals mucosal ulcerations, with or without *Candida* superinfection. The ulcers respond slowly to anti-CMV treatment and may perforate and/or hemorrhage.

Retinitis

This can occur in any immunocompromised patient but is most common in AIDS. Symptoms, if present, include "floaters," flashing lights, and/or loss of central vision. Small peripheral lesions may be unnoticed by the patient; lesions involving the macula may be imminently sight-threatening and demand immediate treatment. Involvement of a large proportion of the retina interrupts retinal/scleral attachment and represents a risk factor for retinal detachment. Before the availability of HAART, most patients had progression of retinitis and the goal of treatment was to preserve vision (for review,

see Jacobson, 1997). Treatment with HAART may be followed by vitritis (see Pathogenesis section), with paradoxical impaired vision despite better control of retinitis. Retinitis is also seen in the neonates born with symptomatic congenital CMV infection and rarely in transplant recipients (Crippa *et al.*, 2001).

Encephalitis

In AIDS patients, CMV reaches the brain by one of two routes; extension of a neighboring endotheliitis or via the choroid plexus. In the former case, the encephalitis follows a subacute course, difficult to distinguish from HIV dementia. In the latter, necrotizing ventricular encephalitis produces cranial nerve defects, nystagmus and ventriculomegaly (reviewed in Griffiths and McLaughlin, 1997). In both cases, response to treatment is poor. Encephalitis is a rare complication in stem cell transplant recipients.

Polyradiculopathy

An AIDS patient with a very low CD4 count presents with subacute weakness of the lower limbs, with or without bladder paralysis. Lumbar puncture reveals abundant polymorphonuclear leukocytes in the CSF. Immediate treatment is indicated but the clinical response is poor.

Pneumonitis

Most cases occur after stem cell transplantation with or without concurrent graft versus host disease (see Pathogenesis section). There is rapid onset of dyspnea plus hypoxia. Chest X-ray may be relatively clear initially but progresses to show interstitial infiltrates. Co-infection with aspergillus is common in stem cell transplant recipients. There is a high mortality, with poor response to treatment (Ljungman *et al.*, 1992).

Hearing loss

This may be apparent at birth in neonates born with symptomatic congenital CMV infection. It is also clear that hearing may be normal at birth but may deteriorate months or years later, irrespective of whether symptoms were present at birth. The hearing loss may be bilateral or unilateral.

Laboratory diagnosis

Detection of viremia

This can be performed by any published method which has been shown to provide a good positive predictive value for CMV disease, e.g. 50%–60% for the patient population to

Table 66.3. Strategies for chemotherapy of CMV

Term used	When drug given	Risk of disease	Acceptable toxicity	Treatment decision prompted by:
True prophylaxis	Before active infection	Low	None	Clinician
Delayed prophylaxis	Before active infection but after rejection	Medium	Low	Clinician
Suppression	After peripheral detection of virus	Medium	Low	Laboratory
Pre-emptive therapy	After systemic detection of virus	High	Medium	Laboratory
Treatment	Once disease apparent	Established	High	Both

be followed. Thus, the rapid diagnostic techniques using cell culture amplification testing of virus (termed DEAFF testing in Europe (Griffiths et al., 1984) and shell-vial in the USA (Gleaves et al., 1984) are no longer sufficiently sensitive and should be replaced with newer methods. Examples include PCR in whole blood (Kidd et al., 1993), PCR in plasma (Spector et al., 1992), ultrasensitive quantitative plasma PCR assays (Boeckh et al., 1996) and antigenemia (The et al., 1990). Recent results demonstrate that PCR from whole blood is superior to either PCR in plasma or peripheral blood leukocytes (Razonable et al., 2002) and has the advantage of not requiring separation of blood specimens with the attendant risks of contamination and mis-labeling. A randomized trial has shown PCR to be superior to conventional cell culture for deciding when to initiate pre-emptive therapy (Einsele et al., 1995). Laboratory protocols differ and it is important that all aspects of each method are followed in detail including sample processing and virus detection. These have been optimized to avoid the detection of latent virus while providing good sensitivity for predicting disease **not** necessarily the highest sensitivity for detecting asymptomatic infection (see Fig. 66.5). Thus, it is not possible to "mix and match" different aspects of PCR protocols.

CNS involvement

PCR of CSF is the method of choice for diagnosing CMV CNS infection (Shinkai et al., 1995).

DEAFF/Shell vial

This method is still sufficiently sensitive and robust to diagnose CMV lung infection using bronchoalveolar lavage fluid. Cells from this fluid can also be cytocentrifuged and stained with monoclonal antibodies but this approach, while more rapid, lacks sensitivity compared to DEAFF/shell vial amplification. The assay is also very well suited to detect CMV in biopsy specimens (e.g., lung, gastrointestinal tissue).

Histopathology

This is performed on tissue biopsies to detect classic Cowdry type A intranuclear "Owl's eye" inclusion bodies. It is insensitive and so has a high specificity for disease (Mattes et al., 2000).

Cell culture

This is performed on tissue biopsies after tissue is minced and inoculated directly on to cells. It is slow but sensitive.

Serology

Many enzyme immunoassays are commercially available for the detection of CMV IgG antibodies pre-transplant in both donor and recipient. Serologic testing has no role to play post-transplant.

Clinical indications for antiviral prophylaxis and dosage regimens

Management

The principles of managing CMV infection and disease in the immunocompromised host are to anticipate their development, to define policies for monitoring patients routinely for the presence of viremia according to their baseline risk of CMV disease, and to enhance surveillance if patients develop a condition likely to increase their risk of CMV disease. Using the principles of evidence-based medicine, the patient will then be offered prophylaxis or pre-emptive therapy based upon an assessment of their individualized risk of disease, together with data from controlled clinical trials in the same patient group supporting the efficacy and safety of possible antiviral interventions.

Strategies for deploying antiviral agents

Different strategies have been devised for controlling CMV disease based on the efficacies and toxicities of the drugs available at present (summarized in Table 66.3).

True prophylaxis

This strategy should be followed where baseline risk of disease is high, the chance of severe disease is also high and where at least one double-blind, randomized, placebo-controlled trial supports the efficacy and safety of prophylaxis in the target population. The drug is given from the time of transplant onwards (or from the time of engraftment in the case of GCV in stem cell transplants) and continued for the duration studied in the controlled clinical trial which provided evidence for its use. This is termed "true prophylaxis" because, from a virologic perspective, it administers the drug before there is active virus replication. By giving the drug early, prophylaxis may provide clinical benefits even if the drug has relatively low antiviral potency.

Delayed prophylaxis

At baseline, a decision was made that true prophylaxis was not indicated. However, the patient's situation has changed eg because augmented immunosuppression is required to control an episode of graft rejection and so it is decided to start prophylaxis now (Hibberd et al., 1995). This is still termed "prophylaxis" because the drug is given before there is active virus replication and a drug with relatively low potency may be used.

Suppression

Some laboratories monitor weekly samples of urine and/or saliva from transplant patients and process them by a method shown to provide a moderate positive predictive value for CMV disease, e.g., 30% (Kidd et al., 1993). If CMV is detected, an antiviral drug is given with the intention of suppressing virus replication below the level needed to cause viremia. A drug with moderate potency is required to keep CMV suppressed.

Pre-emptive therapy

This term describes intervention when the results of laboratory tests indicate that a patient is at imminent risk of CMV disease (Rubin, 1991). Nowadays it refers to detection of viremia in any immunocompromised patient but in the past was also used when asymptomatic lung infection was detected after stem cell transplantation (Schmidt et al., 1991). In the first example, the patient should be monitored by collecting weekly samples of blood processed by laboratory methods known to provide a high positive predictive value for CMV disease, e.g., 50%–60% (Kidd et al., 1993). The objective is to give an antiviral drug with the intention of halting CMV viremia before it reaches the high viral loads required to cause disease. A drug with high potency is therefore required.

Decision-points for starting pre-emptive therapy must be based upon the results of clinicopathologic studies with the assay under evaluation. Examples include qualitative detection of viremia by PCR or antigenemia where the assay level of detection has been shown to be associated with a high risk of disease, or two consecutive samples PCR-positive. Alternatively, if samples are processed by real-time quantitative PCR, then any value above a pre-determined cut-off should trigger antiviral intervention. The results of viral dynamic assessments can also be applied to this problem; patients at risk of disease can be identified by the absolute value of viral load found in the first PCR-positive sample, coupled with an assessment of individual viral dynamics by calculating the rate of increase from the last PCR-negative sample (Emery et al., 2000). All of these approaches work well in clinical practice and comparative studies are required to determine if any one of them is superior to the others.

The treatment of neonates born with symptomatic congenital CMV infection also fits into this category because the objective is to prevent new end-organ damage.

Treatment of established disease

When a patient meets the case definition of CMV disease because he/she has compatible symptoms and signs, together with detection of CMV in the affected organ, a highly potent drug is required which will penetrate the affected organ and resolve the disease, including any immunopathologic components.

Results of double-blind, randomized, placebo-controlled trials

Results of published trials of licensed drugs defined according to these criteria are given in Table 66.4. It will be seen that the most potent drug *in vitro*, ganciclovir, has been subjected to several such clinical trials while foscarnet and cidofovir have not. Other agents such as interferon-alpha, acyclovir, valaciclovir and immunoglobulin, have also been evaluated although they were traditionally not thought to have useful anti-CMV activity.

For the endpoint of CMV infection, Table 66.4 shows that, in addition to ganciclovir (Balfour et al., 1989; Cheeseman et al., 1979; Lui et al., 1992), interferon alpha (Cheeseman et al., 1979; Lui et al., 1992; Ljungman et al., 1992) and acyclovir (Lowance et al., 1999; Balfour et al., 1989; Prentice et al., 1994) have activity against CMV in vivo. The only two studies not to show an effect were the two studies of

Table 66.4. Double-blind, placebo-controlled, randomized trials of CMV

Strategy	Drug	Significantly reduced CMV infection/disease/indirect effects			
		Bone marrow	Renal	Heart	Liver
Treatment	GCV	Reed (1990)			
Pre-emptive	GCV				Paya
Suppressive	GCV	**Goodrich** (1991)			
Prophylaxis	Interferon		Cheeseman (1979)		
			Hirsch (1983)		
			Lui (1992)		
	ACV	*Prentice* (1993)	Balfour (1989)		
	VACV		**Lowance** (1999)		
	Ig		(Metselaar) (1989)		SNYDMAN (1993)
	GCV	Winston (1993)		**Merigan** (1992)	Gane (1997)
		Goodrich (1993)		Macdonald (1995)	

Font used for name of first author indicates significant benefit for the following endpoints:
Plain = reduced infection.
Italics = reduced infection plus reduced disease.
Plain Bold = reduced infection plus reduced disease plus reduced indirect effects.
Italics Bold = reduced infection plus reduced indirect effects.
Capitals = reduced disease.
Name in brackets – no effect.

immunoglobulin (Metselaar et al., 1989; Snydman et al., 1993). This implies that, if immunoglobulin has a role in the prophylaxis of CMV disease, it may not work by inhibiting CMV replication.

For the endpoint of CMV disease, Table 66.4 shows that ganciclovir failed to demonstrate a significantly better resolution of established CMV disease than placebo (Reed et al., 1990). Part of this disappointing outcome may be attributed to the low dose (2.5 mg/kg t.i.d.) and/or short duration used (14 days) to treat gastrointestinal disease in stem cell transplant patients (Reed et al., 1990). Nevertheless, it illustrates the difficulty of treating established CMV disease and so argues that the other strategies, which aim to prevent CMV disease, should always be pursued in preference to waiting for disease to present. Ganciclovir did reduce CMV disease when used in the suppressive mode for stem cell transplant patients (Goodrich et al., 1991). It also had a significant benefit when used in one (Goodrich et al., 1993) of two trials of prophylaxis after stem cell transplant; the second study (Winston et al., 1993) showed a strong trend in favor of GCV which just failed to reach conventional statistical significance. Ganciclovir also significantly reduced CMV disease following prophylaxis given orally to liver transplant patients (Gane et al., 1997) and intravenously to heart transplant patients (Macdonald et al., 1995; Merigan et al., 1992). However, benefit after heart transplant was evident only in the low risk group, with no effect in the D+R− group of one study (Merigan et al., 1992), whereas the opposite outcome was seen in a second (Macdonald et al., 1995). This difference might result from the longer treatment course in the latter study, together with a design difference such that patients experiencing rejection were given additional doses of GCV. Prophylactic ACV significantly reduced CMV disease after renal transplant (Balfour et al., 1989), as did prophylactic valaciclovir (Lowance et al., 1999). In a prophylaxis trial after stem cell transplantation, acyclovir significantly decreased CMV viremia and showed a non-significant trend towards reduced CMV disease (Prentice et al., 1994). A trial of immunoglobulin prophylaxis showed reduced "CMV syndrome" in liver transplant recipients despite having no significant effect on CMV infection (Snydman et al., 1993). Sub-group analysis showed an effect on CMV-associated fungal superinfection (part of the pre-defined "CMV syndrome") so it remains possible that the immunoglobulin predominantly reduces fungal rather than CMV infection. CMV-specific immune globulin and a gH monoclonal antibody were ineffective in stem cell tranplant recipients (Boeckh et al., 2001; Bowden et al., 1991).

Table 66.4 also summarizes the impact of these drugs on the indirect effects of CMV infection. The number of deaths in the solid organ transplant populations is too low to provide the statistical power to address this endpoint. After stem cell transplant, GCV significantly improved survival when used suppressively (Goodrich et al., 1991). However, when used prophylactically, no effect was seen (Goodrich et al., 1993; Winston et al., 1993). This was not a problem of small sample size and neither study demonstrated even a trend in favor of ganciclovir. The most likely explanations are that (i) some patients with viremia still received pre-emptive therapy (Goodrich et al., 1993) so reducing CMV-induced mortality in both arms (ii) neutropenia induced by prophylactic GCV predisposed patients to succumb to bacterial or fungal superinfections, so mitigating the potential benefits of this drug. Overall, these studies indicate that GCV is too toxic a compound to be used for prophylaxis after stem cell transplant, although it is literally life-saving when used in a suppressive mode (Goodrich et al., 1991). This illustrates that, in prophylaxis, all patients are exposed to side-effects and that suppression or preemptive therapy, by limiting the number of patients exposed to the drug, can produce an enhanced therapeutic ratio. In contrast, ACV prophylaxis after stem cell transplant produced a survival benefit (Prentice et al., 1994), presumably because its more modest efficacy was not offset by serious toxicity. After renal transplant, VACV produced a marked reduction in biopsy-proven acute graft rejection corresponding to a 50% decrease in incidence among seronegative recipients at risk of primary infection (Lowance et al., 1999). The effects in seropositive recipients were smaller, implying that CMV (rather than another herpesvirus susceptible to the drug) is responsible for this indirect effect and that most CMV-induced graft rejection occurs in the subset of patients with primary infection. Following heart transplantation, GCV significantly reduced fungal infections (Wagner et al., 1995) and accelerated atherosclerosis (Valantine et al., 1999).

Table 66.5 summarizes randomized studies which compared two anti-CMV strategies. Boeckh et al. (1996) compared antigenemia-guided preemptive therapy with ganciclovir prophylaxis at engraftment and found a higher CMV disease rate at day 100 with pre-emptive therapy; however, there was no statistically significant difference at day 400 between the two groups. Invasive bacterial and fungal infections were more common with GCV prophylaxis, resulting in similar mortality rates at day 400 (Boeckh et al., 1996). Humar et al. compared GCV based on a surveillance BAL at day 35 with antigenemia-guided preemptive therapy and found these two strategies equivalent in a small randomized trial (Humar et al., 2001). Reusser et al. compared foscarnet with GCV for preemptive therapy in stem cell transplant recipients (Reusser et al., 2002). Survival without CMV disease was similar between the groups, however, GCV caused more neutropenia. Foscarnet was associated with more electrolyte imbalances but renal insufficiency was no different between the two groups. One trial by Winston et al. compared valacyclovir with ganciclovir prophylaxis in stem cell transplant recipients. The incidence of CMV disease was similar in both groups, however, the trial was not large enough to make meaningful conclusions (Winston et al., 2003). Another small trial by Winston et al. compared sequential intravenous and oral ganciclovir with intravenous ganciclovir for 3 months in D+/R− liver transplant recipients (Winston and Busuttil, 2004). The incidence of CMV disease was not statistically different between the groups.

In liver transplant patients, prophylaxis with GCV is superior to prophylaxis with ACV (Winston et al., 1995).

Table 66.5. List of randomized trials of two strategies (for results see text; includes open-label trials)

Strategy	Drug	Bone marrow	Renal	Heart	Liver
Prophylaxis vs. Prophylaxis	ACV / GCV				Winston et al., 1995
Pre-emptive vs. Prophylaxis	GCV / GCV	Boeckh et al., 1996			
Suppression vs. Pre-emptive	GCV / GCV	Humar et al., 2001			
Preemptive vs. Pre-emptive	FSC / GCV	Reusser et al., 2002			
Prophylaxis vs. Prophylaxis	GCV / V-ACV	Winston et al., 2003			
Prophylaxis vs. Prophylaxis	GCV (oral) / GCV (iv)				Winston and Busuttil 2004
Prophylaxis vs. Prophylaxis	GCV (oral) / V-GCV		Paya et al., 2004	Paya et al., 2004	Paya et al., 2004

A large randomized double-blind trial of valganciclovir versus oral GCV in D+/R− solid organ transplant recipients showed similar rates of CMV disease with the two compounds (Paya et al., 2004). Neutropenia was observed more frequently with valganciclovir. In another randomized trial in AIDS patients with CMV retinitis valganciclovir showed similar activity to intravenous ganciclovir for treatment of retinitis (Martin et al., 2002).

Additional randomized trials compared different methods of detecting CMV in blood for preemptive therapy and found equivalence between antigenemia and pp67 mRNA (Gerna et al., 2003a,b) and IE mRNA (Gerna et al., 2003a,b). An earlier randomized trial by Einsele et al. established that PCR-based detection by CMV viremia is superior to culture-based detection of viremia for initiation of preemptive therapy (Einsele et al., 1995). A comparison of ganciclovir plus foscarnet (each at half dose) compared to full dose ganciclovir showed that these two drugs are not synergistic in humans when used for pre-emptive therapy (Mattes, 2004).

Aspects of CMV management in HIV-infected individuals

The introduction of highly active antiretroviral therapy (HAART) for HIV has dramatically changed the

Table 66.6. Relative merits of prophylaxis vs. pre-emptive therapy

Proposed advantages of prophylaxis
Proven benefit controlled clinical trials
- *CMV disease*
- *indirect effects*

Avoids complicated logistical problems
- *real-time laboratory assays*
- *organization of sample collection*
- *geographical location*

Protects against HSV, VZV

Overall, may be more cost-effective
- *costs of laboratory tests*
- *indirect effects CMV*
- *other herpesviruses*

Proposed advantages of pre-emptive therapy
Target resources on patients most at need (financial, skill)

Treat when viral load lower
- *shorter treatment*
- *reduced recurrences*
- *reduced resistance?*

Allows low level stimulation of immunity
- *reduces late-onset disease?*

Protects patients non-compliant with prophylaxis

It is possible that PET may also reduce indirect effects

From Snydman, 2006, Singh, 2006.

significance of CMV in HIV-infected individuals. There is now good evidence that in patients with CMV retinitis who have a sustained response to HAART, CMV viremia disappears promptly (Deayton et al., 1999) and maintenance treatment can be discontinued without relapse of retinitis. Several groups have reported HAART-naïve patients with good CD4 (>150/μl) and HIV virologic responses (Lin et al., 2002) to therapy who have been able to stop anti-CMV maintenance medications completely without disease progression (Whitcup et al., 1999). Thus, intravenous or oral therapy (i.e., Valganciclovir (Martin et al., 2002) can be used until the anticipated return of the patient's CMV-specific immunity. CMV disease can still occur within 4 months of HAART initiation despite adequate suppression of HIV replication (Jacobson et al., 1997). Some patients also develop immune recovery vitritis when HAART is initiated at the time of CMV retinitis (Karavellas et al., 1999; Whitcup et al., 1999). Alternatives to intravenous and oral antivirals for the treatment of CMV retinitis are available. In the current era, intraocular implants are used primarily in salvage regimens (disease progression with first-line agents) or in patients for whom immunologic recovery with HAART is not anticipated.

Conclusions

1. Decisions about which drugs to recommend for particular treatment strategies must draw upon evidence-based medicine provided by the results of controlled clinical trials. Decisions must consider toxicity as well as efficacy.
2. For stem cell transplant patients, prophylaxis with ACV (Prentice et al., 1994) or VACV (Lowance et al., 1999) is recommended; however, virologic monitoring and pre-emptive therapy are still required to allow GCV to be administered (Goodrich et al., 1991). Since the latter study showed that, of the samples of urine, saliva, and blood processed, only blood provided prognostic value, this conclusion probably applies to pre-emptive therapy as well.
3. The toxicity problems of GCV apply specifically to the stem cell transplant population where GCV and VACV have been shown to be equally potent in practice (Winston et al., 2003). A head-to-head comparison of low dose GCV versus ACV for prophylaxis after liver transplant shows that GCV is superior (Winston et al., 1995).
4. Prophylaxis and pre-emptive therapy are both effective strategies for preventing CMV disease. Their relative merits are hotly debated (see Table 66.6).
5. Similar data from AIDS patients cannot be presented because, remarkably, no trials have been designed based on these virologic criteria. Two trials (Feinberg et al., 1998; Spector et al., 1996) have been conducted of clinical prophylaxis but these are not the same as true prophylaxis because, at the time of randomization, although no patients had CMV disease, some of them would be expected to have asymptomatic infection. Indeed, the subsequent virologic studies show that oral GCV had its greatest effect when given to the subset receiving true prophylaxis and had little effect in the subset receiving pre-emptive therapy (Spector et al., 1998). In contrast, the virologic studies of VACV demonstrated that this drug had its greatest effect when given for pre-emptive therapy (Griffiths et al., 1998). This might be thought to imply that VACV is more potent in vivo than oral GCV but a randomized head-to-head comparison would be needed to test this possibility. Such a trial is unlikely to be conducted because the high dose of VACV chosen (2 g q.i.d.) was poorly tolerated by the AIDS patients (Feinberg et al., 1998), although the same dose was safe when studied in renal transplant patients

(Lowance et al., 1999). Furthermore, the incidence of CMV disease in the current era of HIV management has declined due to immune reconstitution following initiation of HAART.

6. The ACV and VACV studies do show that potent inhibition of CMV DNA polymerase by ACV-TP triphosphate can have clinical utility under some circumstances. In the renal transplant study, the authors provide evidence that plasma levels of ACV were higher than expected because of poor renal clearance, but were still lower than would be required to inhibit CMV based on in vitro data (Fletcher et al., 1991), which demonstrates clearly that the IC50 levels produced by fibroblast cell cultures are misleadingly high.

7. Although the incidence of CMV end-organ disease has been dramatically reduced in both transplant and HIV patients, the indirect effects of CMV remain important. Recent data in unrelated donor or T-cell depleted stem cell transplant recipients demonstrate that preemptive therapy alone, although quite effective in reducing the risk of CMV disease, has not eliminated the survival disadvantage associated with CMV seropositivity (Boeckh and Nichols, 2004). In AIDS patients, CMV viremia remains an important factor for poor outcome in the era of highly-active antiretroviral therapy (Deayton et al., 2004). Indeed, once CMV viremia was accounted for in multivariable models, HIV viral load was no longer associated significantly with death (Deayton et al., 2004).

8. In the case of neonates born with symptomatic CMV infection with CNS involvement, a study by Kimberlin et al. (2003) shows that the proportion who develop progressive hearing loss can be decreased by a six week course of GCV at 6 mg/kg i.v. bid. Although this study was not placebo-controlled (due to the ethical problems of administering an intravenous placebo to neonates), the results of this seminal study are included here because they are clinically important and entirely consistent with the pathogenetic implications of neonatal viral load (see Fig. 66.3 and Table 66.2).

Resistance

Resistance to GCV maps to two genetic loci, UL97 and DNA polymerase. In general, changes in UL97 are common and confer low level resistance while changes in DNA polymerase are rare but some of them confer cross-resistance to other antiviral drugs.

Methods used to define resistance

It is important to note that both UL97 and DNA polymerase are large genes in which spontaneous polymorphisms exist. It is not therefore possible to sequence the gene from a patient, find a genetic change compared to the standard laboratory strain, AD169, and then conclude that resistance has developed. A mutation identified in a patient sample must be examined by marker transfer (site-directed mutagenesis) before it can be concluded that the mutation is responsible for conferring resistance. In the process of marker transfer, the genetic sequence is altered in a laboratory-adapted strain and it is proven that this change confers resistance to the antiviral drug by analyzing the phenotype in plaque reduction tests. To demonstrate that no additional changes have been introduced by mistake, the resistant strain should then be back-mutated to the wild type and it should be proven that sensitivity to the antiviral drug has returned. Given the slow evolution of cytopathic effect in vitro, these experiments are time-consuming, inefficient and expensive. In addition, the requirement for selection by means of ganciclovir is undesireable because it offers the potential of introducing additional changes at the in vitro passage level. However, recent technical changes have made ganciclovir selection now no longer necessary so it should become easier in the future for marker transfer experiments to be performed. These technical advantages include a particular strain that has been developed with a novel restriction enzyme site, the ability to use cosmid clones of the genome to reconstitute infectious viruses and the recent cloning of CMV as a bacterial artificial chromosome (Adler et al., 2003; Chou et al., 2002). All of the mutations described in the sections which follow have been identified in clinical samples and proven by marker transfer experiments to confer resistance.

Gene UL 97

Gene UL97 produces a serine/threonine kinase enzyme which is essential for virus replication. Through studies with a gene deleted virus, and with an experimental drug (maribavir) which inhibits gene UL97, it was shown that UL97 is important for nuclear egress (Krosky et al., 2003). It has also recently been shown that UL97 phosphorylates elongation factor 1 delta at codon serine 133. This is exactly the biochemical change made by the cellular CDC2 plus cyclin B when they prepare the nuclear envelope for dissolution just prior to mitosis. It is therefore tempting to suggest that UL97 mimics this cellular pathway to prepare the cell to release into the cytoplasm virions synthesized in the nucleus (Kawaguchi and Kato, 2003).

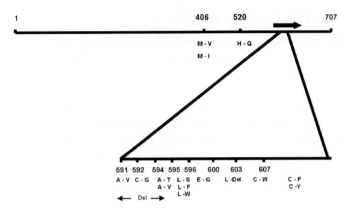

Fig. 66.6. UL97 mutations conferring GCV resistance. (From Chen, 2002.)

Figure 66.6 shows the mutations which confer ganciclovir resistance in gene UL97. Many of these individual mutations have been transferred to recombinant vaccinia viruses and shown to significantly reduce phosphorylation of ganciclovir compared to wild-type. However, the reductions in phosphorylation are rather low (e.g., 10% reduction for the deletion of 590–593). If CMV replication continues in the presence of ganciclovir then additional mutations can occur in UL97 which do not themselves confer resistance but act to partially restore the efficiency of the enzyme. For example, by transferring the individual mutations into recombinant vaccinia viruses, Chou and colleagues were able to show that D605E compensates for an A594P mutation (Chou et al., 2000).

When these UL97 mutants are propagated in vitro they appear to have identical replication kinetics in one step growth curves (Chou et al., 2002). This makes it very difficult to identify the true significance of these mutations in vivo and represents one of many deficiencies of studying this virus in fibroblasts (for review, see Griffiths, 2002). Fortunately, the high rate of replication demonstrated in patients explains how CMV variants resistant to GCV can evolve, and provides a basis for calculating their relative fitness compared to wild type (Emery et al., 1999). These mathematical modelling techniques can also be used to explain and predict the circumstances under which resistant strains become prominent (Emery and Griffiths, 2000). In summary, short courses of GCV are unlikely to select resistant strains, but long or repeated courses, especially with oral GCV, provide ideal opportunities for resistant strains to flourish. They also demonstrate why resistant strains are cultured infrequently in practice; the process of incubating mixed populations of strains for 3–4 weeks in cell cultures lacking GCV allows the wild-type virus to out-compete the mutant strain, leading to the incorrect conclusion that resistance is not present in vivo.

Gene UL54 (DNA polymerase)

Fig. 66.7 shows a schematic representation of the DNA polymerase gene showing the important catalytic sites and areas where resistance to ganciclovir or foscarnet or cidofovir have been mapped. In contrast to the finding with UL97 mutants, changes in UL54 often confer a growth disadvantage upon virus replication in vitro (Chou et al., 2003) which may help explain the infrequency of their detection in patients.

Although the three-dimensional structure of CMV DNA polymerase is not known, important insights into its mechanism of action can be gleaned by comparison with the known structures of related enzymes (Chou et al., 2003). Changes at the exonuclease site (Fig. 66.7) probably facilitate pyrophosphorolysis (i.e., the reverse reaction of DNA polymerization) which results in the excision of an incorporated drug moiety. Changes in region V interfere with the normal function of "thumb" (GCV/CDV cross-resistance) and "fingers" pyrophosphate exchange and acceptance of the incoming nucleotide (GCV/Foscarnet cross-resistance). Changes at other regions of the enzyme may reflect subtle conformational effects on these or other functions of the enzyme. At least one such change can confer hypersensitivity to foscarnet, a phenomenon which was first described for HSV but which is now frequently encountered in HIV.

Patterns of cross-resistance

Given the structural similarity of, GCV and ACV (Fig. 66.1), it would be expected that virus resistant to one compound exhibits cross-resistance to the other. This is difficult to prove because fibroblast cell cultures do not demonstrate the sensitivity of CMV to ACV, let alone its resistance. In practice, GCV has been used so widely that the small number of resistant strains available for study have been selected through the use of this drug and all of these viruses should be assumed to exhibit cross-resistance to ACV.

If strains of CMV resistant to GCV due to mutations in UL97 are encountered in clinical practice and alternative treatment is required then foscarnet is the first choice. Cidofovir is an alternative which, by bypassing UL97, has the advantage of avoiding the genetic change commonly selected for under GCV pressure (Safrin et al., 1997).

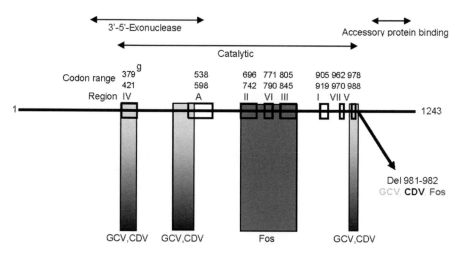

Fig. 66.7. Mutations in CMV DNA polymerase which confer antiviral resistance. (From Chou, 2002, 2003.)

If resistance to GCV has been acquired through mutations in UL54 then precise details of the genetic changes are required. Many of the changes confer cross-resistance to cidofovir (see Fig. 66.7) so this drug is not usually indicated. Foscarnet remains the drug of choice for UL54 mutants; although one particular mutant exhibits low-level cross-resistance to ganciclovir, cidofovir and foscarnet.

Recognition of resistance in clinical practice

The early studies of CMV in AIDS patients receiving chronic GCV therapy were important because they provided laboratory strains to allow a definition of biochemical resistance in vitro (Drew et al., 1991; Erice et al., 1989). However, they underestimated the incidence of resistance because viruses from samples of urine or blood were propagated in cell cultures in vitro. Most such clinical samples contain mixed populations of wild-type and resistant strains of CMV. As explained earlier, the UL97 mutants have decreased fitness in the absence of GCV (Emery et al., 1999). As a result, they are readily out-competed by wild strains in the laboratory, especially given the requirement for serial passage in vitro in order to provide high titer inocula for the plaque reduction test. This problem can be bypassed by either collecting samples from patients with CMV end-organ disease, which are less likely to contain mixed populations of virus, or by using molecular techniques to detect genetic markers of resistance directly in the patient samples without passage in vitro.

Bowen et al. used a point mutation assay and sequencing to identify GCV resistance in 10/45 (22%) AIDS patients with CMV retinitis (Bowen et al., 1998). Limaye and colleagues (Limaye et al., 2000) examined blood isolates from 25 cases of CMV disease in recipients of solid organ

Table 66.7. Management algorithm for suspected resistant CMV

When to suspect drug resistance
1. Drug-naïve patient:
   - If viremia fails to disappear with preemptive therapy
     - culture-positive > 3 weeks
     - increasing antigenemia levels > 2 weeks
     - increasing PCR levels > 2 week
   - If viremia appears during prophylaxis
     - Any culture positivity
     - Increasing level for > 2 weeks

Diagnostic

Obtain blood PCR or DNA from site and sequence UL97 (UL54)

Drug therapy:
- *Check compliance/dose/schedule*
- *swap to alternative antiviral agent*

General
- Reduction of immunosuppression if feasible (in severe cases or resistant CMV disease "sacrificing" the transplanted organ may be considered or necessary)

If toxicity appears:
- *GCV/foscarnet each at half-dose*
- Novel compounds needed

transplants and found GCV resistance in 5 (20%). Liu et al. (2000) showed that virtually all CMV DNA extracts from the eyes of untreated AIDS patients had wild type UL97 sequences, consistent with the concept that UL97 mutants have impaired fitness in the absence of GCV. Hu et al. (2002) identified 13 (15%) UL97 mutations in vitreus samples from 87 AIDS patients and found the same mutations in the blood of 11 of these patients, showing that changes in blood strains frequently mirror those in the eye. Boivan et al used restriction fragment length polymorphisms and direct sequencing of UL97 to detect resistant strains in approximately 12% of AIDS patients receiving valganciclovir and showed that UL97 sequencing directly from the blood correlated well with disease progression (Boivin et al., 2001). They also showed UL97 sequence discordance when the same samples were passed in cell culture, consistent with the concept that cell cultures preferentially select wild type isolates during passage in vitro (Gilbert and Boivin, 2003).

It should now be clear that resistance to GCV has been underestimated in the past. New drugs targeted at different CMV genes are required (see Chapter 68) and randomized controlled trials are essential to define their efficacy.

The basic principles to help avoid the development of resistance are to reduce CMV replication in the presence of drug (i.e., treat with potent compounds and adequate doses for a short time and then stop therapy) and to treat promptly at an early stage (when the virus load is low) (Table 66.7). Serially monitored patients with increasing viral loads over several weeks are at high risk of having drug resistance, especially after prolonged prior exposure to the drug. Ideally, treated patients should be followed with serial quantitative measures of CMV viral load to demonstrate when CMV replication has been controlled and so optimize when treatment can be stopped (or an alternative antiviral drug used). Randomized controlled clinical trials are required to determine whether such individualization of therapy duration confers advantages over prescription of a course of standard length.

REFERENCES

Adler, H., Messerle, M., and Koszinowski, U. H. (2003). Cloning of herpesviral genomes as bacterial artificial chromosomes. *Rev. Med. Virol.*, **13**(2), 111–121.

Balfour, H. H., Jr., Chace, B. A., Stapleton, J. T., Simmons, R. L., and Fryd, D. S. (1989). A randomized, placebo-controlled trial of oral acyclovir for the prevention of cytomegalovirus disease in recipients of renal allografts. *N. Engl. J. Med.*, **320**(21), 1381–1387.

Betts, R. F., Freeman, R. B., Douglas, R. G., Jr., and Talley, T. E. (1977). Clinical manifestations of renal allograft derived primary cytomegalovirus infection. *Am. J. Dis. Child.*, **131**(7), 759–763.

Boeckh, M. and Nichols, W. G. (2003). Immunosuppressive effects of beta-herpesviruses. *Herpes*, **10**(1), 12–16.

Boeckh, M. and Nichols, W. G. (2004). The impact of cytomegalovirus serostatus of donor and recipient before hematopoietic stem cell transplantation in the era of antiviral prophylaxis and preemptive therapy. *Blood*, **103**(6), 2003–2008.

Boeckh, M., Gooley, T. A., Myerson, D., Cunningham, T., Schoch, G., and Bowden, R. A. (1996). Cytomegalovirus pp65 antigenemia-guided early treatment with ganciclovir versus ganciclovir at engraftment after allogeneic marrow transplantation: a randomized double-blind study. *Blood*, **88**(10), 4063–4071.

Boeckh, M., Bowden, R. A., Storer, B. et al. (2001). Randomized, placebo-controlled, double-blind study of a cytomegalovirus-specific monoclonal antibody (MSL-109) for prevention of cytomegalovirus infection after allogeneic hematopoietic stem cell transplantation. *Biol. Blood Marrow Transpl.*, **7**(6), 343–351.

Boivin, G., Gilbert, C., Gaudreau, A., Greenfield, I., Sudlow, R., and Roberts, N. A. (2001). Rate of emergence of cytomegalovirus (CMV) mutations in leukocytes of patients with acquired immunodeficiency syndrome who are receiving valganciclovir as induction and maintenance therapy for CMV retinitis. *J. Infect. Dis.*, **184**(12), 1598–1602.

Bowden, R. A., Fisher, L. D., Rogers, K., Cays, M., and Meyers, J. D. (1991). Cytomegalovirus (CMV)-specific intravenous immunoglobulin for the prevention of primary CMV infection and disease after marrow transplant. *J. Infect. Dis.*, **164**(3), 483–487.

Bowen, E. F., Wilson, P., Cope, A. et al. (1996). Cytomegalovirus retinitis in AIDS patients: influence of cytomegaloviral load on response to ganciclovir, time to recurrence and survival. *AIDS*, **10**(13), 1515–1520.

Bowen, E. F., Emery, V. C., Wilson, P. et al. (1998). Cytomegalovirus polymerase chain reaction viraemia in patients receiving ganciclovir maintenance therapy for retinitis. *AIDS*, **12**(6), 605–611.

Cheeseman, S. H., Rubin, R. H., Stewart, J. A. et al. (1979). Controlled clinical trial of prophylactic human-leukocyte interferon in renal transplantation. Effects on cytomegalovirus and herpes simplex virus infections. *N. Engl. J. Med.*, **300**(24), 1345–1349.

Chou, S., Miner, R. C., and Drew, W. L. (2000). A deletion mutation in region V of the cytomegalovirus DNA polymerase sequence confers multidrug resistance. *J. Infect. Dis.*, **182**(6), 1765–1768.

Chou, S., Waldemar, R. H., Senters, A. E. et al. (2002). Cytomegalovirus UL97 phosphotransferase mutations that affect susceptibility to ganciclovir. *J. Infect. Dis.*, **185**(2), 162–169.

Chou, S., Lurain, N. S., Thompson, K. D., Miner, R. C., and Drew, W. L. (2003). Viral DNA polymerase mutations associated with drug resistance in human cytomegalovirus. *J. Infect. Dis.*, **188**(1), 32–39.

Cope, A. V., Sabin, C., Burroughs, A., Rolles, K., Griffiths, P. D., and Emery, V. C. (1997a). Interrelationships among quantity of human cytomegalovirus (HCMV) DNA in blood, donor-recipient serostatus, and administration of methylprednisolone as risk factors for HCMV disease following liver transplantation. *J. Infect. Dis.*, **176**(6), 1484–1490.

Cope, A. V., Sweny, P., Sabin, C., Rees, L., Griffiths, P. D., and Emery, V. C. (1997b). Quantity of cytomegalovirus viruria is a major risk factor for cytomegalovirus disease after renal transplantation. *J. Med. Virol.*, **52**(2), 200–205.

Crippa, F., Corey, L., Chuang, E. L., Sale, G., and Boeckh M. (2001). Virological, clinical, and ophthalmologic features of cytomegalovirus retinitis after hematopoietic stem cell transplantation. *Clin. Infect. Dis.*, **32**(2), 214–219.

Deayton, J., Mocroft, A., Wilson, P., Emery, V. C., Johnson, M. A., and Griffiths, P. D. (1999). Loss of cytomegalovirus (CMV) viraemia following highly active antiretroviral therapy in the absence of specific anti-CMV therapy. *AIDS*, **13**(10), 1203–1206.

Deayton, J. R., Sabin, C., Johnson, M. A., Emery, V. C., Wilson, P., and Griffiths, P. D. (2004). Cytomegalovirus viraemia remains an important risk factor for disease progression and death in HIV-infected patients receiving highly active antiretroviral therapy. *Lancet*, **363**(9427), 2116–2121.

De Clercq, E., Naesens, L., De Bolle, L., Schols, D,, Zhang, Y., and Neyts, J. (2001). Antiviral agents active against human herpesviruses HHV-6, HHV-7 and HHV-8. *Rev. Med. Virol.*, **11**(6), 381–395.

Drew, W. L., Miner, R. C., Busch, D. F. *et al.* (1991). Prevalence of resistance in patients receiving ganciclovir for serious cytomegalovirus infection. *J. Infect. Dis.*, **163**(4), 716–719.

Einsele, H., Ehninger, G., Hebart, H. *et al.* (1995). Polymerase chain reaction monitoring reduces the incidence of cytomegalovirus disease and the duration and side effects of antiviral therapy after bone marrow transplantation. *Blood*, **86**(7), 2815–2820.

Emery, V. C. and Griffiths, P. D. (2000). Prediction of cytomegalovirus load and resistance patterns after antiviral chemotherapy. *Proc. Natl Acad. Sci. USA*, **97**(14), 8039–8044.

Emery, V. C., Cope, A. V., Bowen, E. F., Gor, D., and Griffiths, P. D. (1999). The dynamics of human cytomegalovirus replication in vivo. *J. Exp. Med.*, **190**(2), 177–182.

Emery, V. C., Sabin, C. A., Cope, A. V., Gor, D., Hassan-Walker, A. F., and Griffiths, P. D. (2000). Application of viral-load kinetics to identify patients who develop cytomegalovirus disease after transplantation. *Lancet*, **355**(9220), 2032–2036.

Emery, V. C., Hassan-Walker, A. F., Burroughs, A. K., and Griffiths, P. D. (2002). Human cytomegalovirus (HCMV) replication dynamics in HCMV-naive and -experienced immunocompromised hosts. *J. Infect. Dis.*, **185**(12), 1723–1728.

Erice, A., Chou, S., Biron, K. K., Stanat, S. C., Balfour, H. H., Jr., and Jordan, M. C. (1989). Progressive disease due to ganciclovir-resistant cytomegalovirus in immunocompromised patients. *N. Engl. J. Med.*, **320**(5), 289–293.

Falagas, M. E., Snydman, D. R., Griffith, J., and Werner, B. G. (1996). Exposure to cytomegalovirus from the donated organ is a risk factor for bacteremia in orthotopic liver transplant recipients. Boston Center for Liver Transplantation CMVIG Study Group. *Clin. Infect. Dis.*, **23**(3), 468–474.

Feinberg, J. E., Hurwitz, S., Cooper, D. *et al.* (1998). A randomized, double-blind trial of valaciclovir prophylaxis for cytomegalovirus disease in patients with advanced human immunodeficiency virus infection. AIDS Clinical Trials Group Protocol 204/Glaxo Wellcome 123-014 International CMV Prophylaxis Study Group. *J. Infect. Dis.*, **177**(1), 48–56.

Fletcher, C. V., Englund, J. A., Edelman, C. K., Gross, C. R., Dunn, D. L., and Balfour, H. H. (1991). Jr. Pharmacologic basis for high-dose oral acyclovir prophylaxis of cytomegalovirus disease in renal allograft recipients. *Antimicrob. Agents Chemother.*, **35**(5), 938–943.

Furman, P. A., St. Clair, M. H., and Spector, T. (1984). Acyclovir triphosphate is a suicide inactivator of the herpes simplex virus DNA polymerase. *J. Biol. Chem.*, **259**(15), 9575–9579.

Gane, E., Saliba, F., Valdecasas, G. J. *et al.* (1997). Randomised trial of efficacy and safety of oral ganciclovir in the prevention of cytomegalovirus disease in liver-transplant recipients. The Oral Ganciclovir International Transplantation Study Group [corrected]. *Lancet*, **350**(9093), 1729–1733.

Gerna, G., Baldanti, F., Lilleri, D. *et al.* (2003a). Human cytomegalovirus pp67 mRNAemia versus pp65 antigenemia for guiding preemptive therapy in heart and lung transplant recipients: a prospective, randomized, controlled, open-label trial. *Transplantation*, **75**(7), 1012–1019.

Gerna, G., Lilleri, D., Baldanti, F. *et al.* (2003b). Human cytomegalovirus immediate-early mRNAemia versus pp65 antigenemia for guiding pre-emptive therapy in children and young adults undergoing hematopoietic stem cell transplantation: a prospective, randomized, open-label trial. *Blood*, **101**(12), 5053–5060.

Gilbert, C. and Boivin, G. (2003). Discordant phenotypes and genotypes of cytomegalovirus (CMV) in patients with AIDS and relapsing CMV retinitis. *AIDS*, **17**(3), 337–341.

Gleaves, C. A., Smith, T. F., Shuster, E. A., and Pearson, G. R. (1984). Rapid detection of cytomegalovirus in MRC-5 cells inoculated with urine specimens by using low-speed centrifugation and monoclonal antibody to an early antigen. *J. Clin. Microbiol.*, **19**(6), 917–919.

Goodrich, J. M., Mori, M., Gleaves, C. A. *et al.* (1991). Early treatment with ganciclovir to prevent cytomegalovirus disease after allogeneic bone marrow transplantation. *N. Engl. J. Med.*, **325**(23), 1601–1607.

Goodrich, J. M., Bowden, R. A., Fisher, L., Keller, C., Schoch, G., and Meyers, J. D. (1993). Ganciclovir prophylaxis to prevent cytomegalovirus disease after allogeneic marrow transplant. *Ann. Intern. Med.*, **118**(3), 173–178.

Gor, D., Sabin, C., Prentice, H. G. *et al.* (1998). Longitudinal fluctuations in cytomegalovirus load in bone marrow transplant patients: relationship between peak virus load, donor/recipient serostatus, acute GVHD and CMV disease. *Bone Marrow Transpl.*, **21**(6), 597–605.

Grattan, M. T., Moreno-Cabral, C. E., Starnes, V. A., Oyer, P. E., Stinson, E. B., and Shumway, N. E. (1989). Cytomegalovirus infection is associated with cardiac allograft rejection and atherosclerosis. *J. Am. Med. Assoc.*, **261**(24), 3561–3566.

Griffiths, P. D. (2002). The 2001 Garrod lecture. The treatment of cytomegalovirus infection. *J. Antimicrob. Chemother.*, **49**(2), 243–253.

Griffiths, P. D. and McLaughlin, J. E. (1997). Cytomegalovirus. *Infect. Centr. Nerv. Syst.*, 107–115.

Griffiths, P. D., Panjwani, D. D., Stirk, P. R. et al. (1984). Rapid diagnosis of cytomegalovirus infection in immunocompromised patients by detection of early antigen fluorescent foci. *Lancet*, **2**(8414), 1242–1245.

Griffiths, P. D., Feinberg, J. E., Fry, J. et al. (1998). The effect of valaciclovir on cytomegalovirus viremia and viruria detected by polymerase chain reaction in patients with advanced human immunodeficiency virus disease. AIDS Clinical Trials Group Protocol 204/Glaxo Wellcome 123-014 International CMV Prophylaxis Study Group. *J. Infect. Dis.*, **177**(1), 57–64.

Grundy, J. E., Shanley, J. D., and Griffiths, P. D. (1987). Is cytomegalovirus interstitial pneumonitis in transplant recipients an immunopathological condition? *Lancet*, **2**(8566), 996–999.

Grundy, J. E., Lui, S. F., Super, M. et al. (1988). Symptomatic cytomegalovirus infection in seropositive kidney recipients: reinfection with donor virus rather than reactivation of recipient virus. *Lancet*, **2**(8603), 132–135.

Guetta, E., Guetta, V., Shibutani, T., and Epstein, S. E. (1997). Monocytes harboring cytomegalovirus: interactions with endothelial cells, smooth muscle cells, and oxidized low-density lipoprotein. Possible mechanisms for activating virus delivered by monocytes to sites of vascular injury. *Circ. Res.*, **81**(1), 8–16.

Hassan-Walker, A. F., Kidd, I. M., Sabin, C., Sweny, P., Griffiths, P. D., and Emery, V. C. (1999). Quantity of human cytomegalovirus (CMV) DNAemia as a risk factor for CMV disease in renal allograft recipients: relationship with donor/recipient CMV serostatus, receipt of augmented methylprednisolone and antithymocyte globulin (ATG). *J. Med. Virol.*, **58**(2), 182–187.

Hibberd, P. L., Tolkoff-Rubin, N. E., Conti, D. et al. (1995). Preemptive ganciclovir therapy to prevent cytomegalovirus disease in cytomegalovirus antibody-positive renal transplant recipients. A randomized controlled trial. *Ann. Intern. Med.*, **123**(1), 18–26.

Hirsch, M. S., Schooley, R. T., Cosimi, A. B., et al. (1983). Effects of interferon-alpha on cytomegalovirus reactivation syndromes in renal-transplant recipients. *N. Engl. J. Med.*, **308**(25), 1489–1493.

Hu, H., Jabs, D. A., Forman, M. S. et al. (2002). Comparison of cytomegalovirus (CMV) UL97 gene sequences in the blood and vitreous of patients with acquired immunodeficiency syndrome and CMV retinitis. *J. Infect. Dis.*, **185**(7), 861–867.

Humar, A., Lipton, J., Welsh, S., Moussa, G., Messner, H., and Mazzulli, T. (2001). A randomised trial comparing cytomegalovirus antigenemia assay vs screening bronchoscopy for the early detection and prevention of disease in allogeneic bone marrow and peripheral blood stem cell transplant recipients. *Bone Marrow Transpl.*, **28**(5), 485–490.

Jacobson, M. A. (1997). Treatment of cytomegalovirus retinitis in patients with the acquired immunodeficiency syndrome. *N. Engl. J. Med.*, **337**(2), 105–114.

Jacobson, M. A., Zegans, M., Pavan, P. R. et al. (1997). Cytomegalovirus retinitis after initiation of highly active antiretroviral therapy. *Lancet*, **349**(9063), 1443–1445.

Karavellas, M. P., Plummer, D. J., Macdonald, J. C. et al. (1999). Incidence of immune recovery vitritis in cytomegalovirus retinitis patients following institution of successful highly active antiretroviral therapy. *J. Infect. Dis.*, **179**(3), 697–700.

Kawaguchi, Y. and Kato, K. (2003). Protein kinases conserved in herpesviruses potentially share a function mimicking the cellular protein kinase cdc2. *Rev. Med. Virol.*, **13**(5), 331–340.

Kidd, I. M., Fox, J. C., Pillay, D., Charman, H., Griffiths, P. D., and Emery, V. C. (1993). Provision of prognostic information in immunocompromised patients by routine application of the polymerase chain reaction for cytomegalovirus. *Transplantation*, **56**(4), 867–871.

Kimberlin, D. W., Lin, C. Y., Sanchez, P. J. et al. (2003). Effect of ganciclovir therapy on hearing in symptomatic congenital cytomegalovirus disease involving the central nervous system: a randomized, controlled trial. *J. Pediatr.*, **143**(1), 16–25.

Krosky, P. M., Baek, M. C., and Coen, D. M. (2003). The human cytomegalovirus UL97 protein kinase, an antiviral drug target, is required at the stage of nuclear egress. *J. Virol.*, **77**(2), 905–914.

Lemstrom, K., Sihvola, R., Bruggeman, C., Hayry, P., and Koskinen, P. (1997). Cytomegalovirus infection-enhanced cardiac allograft vasculopathy is abolished by DHPG prophylaxis in the rat. *Circulation*, **95**(12), 2614–2616.

Limaye, A. P., Corey, L., Koelle, D. M., Davis, C. L., and Boeckh, M. (2000). Emergence of ganciclovir-resistant cytomegalovirus disease among recipients of solid-organ transplants. *Lancet*, **356**(9230), 645–649.

Lin, D. Y., Warren, J. F., Lazzeroni, L. C., Wolitz, R. A., and Mansour, S. E. (2002). Cytomegalovirus retinitis after initiation of highly active antiretroviral therapy in HIV infected patients: natural history and clinical predictors. *Retina*, **22**(3), 268–277.

Liu, W., Shum, C., Martin, D. F., Kuppermann, B. D., Hall, A. J., and Margolis, T. P. (2000). Prevalence of antiviral drug resistance in untreated patients with cytomegalovirus retinitis. *J. Infect. Dis.*, **182**(4), 1234–1238.

Ljungman, P., Engelhard, D., Link, H. et al. (1992). Treatment of interstitial pneumonitis due to cytomegalovirus with ganciclovir and intravenous immune globulin: experience of European Bone Marrow Transplant Group. *Clin. Infect. Dis.*, **14**(4), 831–835.

Ljungman, P., Griffiths, P., and Paya, C. (2002). Definitions of cytomegalovirus infection and disease in transplant recipients. *Clin. Infect. Dis.*, **34**(8), 1094–1097.

Lowance, D., Neumayer, H. H., Legendre, C. M. et al. (1999). Valacyclovir for the prevention of cytomegalovirus disease after renal transplantation. International Valacyclovir Cytomegalovirus Prophylaxis Transplantation Study Group. *N. Engl. J. Med.*, **340**(19), 1462–1470.

Lui, S. F., Ali, A. A., Grundy, J. E., Fernando, O. N., Griffiths, P. D., and Sweny, P. (1992). Double-blind, placebo-controlled trial of human lymphoblastoid interferon prophylaxis of cytomegalovirus infection in renal transplant recipients. *Nephrol. Dial. Transpl.*, **7**(12), 1230–1237.

Macdonald, P. S., Keogh, A. M., Marshman, D. *et al.* (1995). A double-blind placebo-controlled trial of low-dose ganciclovir to prevent cytomegalovirus disease after heart transplantation. *J. Heart Lung Transpl.*, **14**(1 Pt 1), 32–38.

Mar, E. C., Huang, E. S., Cheng, Y. C., and Chiou, J. F. (1985). Inhibition of cellular DNA polymerase alpha and human cytomegalovirus-induced DNA polymerase by the triphosphates of 9-(2-hydroxyethoxymethyl)guanine and 9-(1,3-dihydroxy-2-propoxymethyl)guanine. *J. Virol.*, **53**(3), 776–780.

Martin, D. F., Sierra-Madero, J., Walmsley, S. *et al.* (2002). A controlled trial of valganciclovir as induction therapy for cytomegalovirus retinitis. *N. Engl. J. Med.*, **346**(15), 1119–1126.

Mattes, F. M., McLaughlin, J. E., Emery, V. C., Clark, D. A., and Griffiths, P. D. (2000). Histopathological detection of owl's eye inclusions is still specific for cytomegalovirus in the era of human herpesviruses 6 and 7. *J. Clin. Pathol.*, **53**(8), 612–614.

Mattes, F. M., Hainsworth, E. G., Geretti, A. M., *et al.* (2004). A randomized, controlled trial comparing ganciclovir to ganciclovir plus foscarnet (each at half dose) for preemptive therapy of cytomegalovirus infection in transplant recipients. *J. Infect. Dis.*, **189**(8), 1355–1361.

Merigan, T. C., Renlund, D. G., Keay, S. *et al.* (1992). A controlled trial of ganciclovir to prevent cytomegalovirus disease after heart transplantation. *N. Engl. J. Med.*, **326**(18), 1182–1186.

Metselaar, H. J., Rothbarth, P. H., Brouwer, R. M., Wenting, G. J., Jeekel, J., and Weimar, W. (1989). Prevention of cytomegalovirus-related death by passive immunization. A double-blind placebo-controlled study in kidney transplant recipients treated for rejection. *Transplantation*, **48**(2), 264–266.

Meyers, J. D., Ljungman, P., and Fisher, L. D. (1990). Cytomegalovirus excretion as a predictor of cytomegalovirus disease after marrow transplantation: importance of cytomegalovirus viremia. *J. Infect. Dis.*, **162**(2), 373–380.

Nichols, W. G., Corey, L., Gooley, T., Davis, C., and Boeckh, M. (2002). High risk of death due to bacterial and fungal infection among cytomegalovirus (CMV)-seronegative recipients of stem cell transplants from seropositive donors: evidence for indirect effects of primary CMV infection. *J. Infect. Dis.*, **185**(3), 273–282.

Paya, C., Humar, A., Dominguez, E. *et al.* (2004). Efficacy and safety of valganciclovir vs. oral ganciclovir for prevention of cytomegalovirus disease in solid organ transplant recipients. *Am. J. Transpl.*, **4**(4), 611–620.

Paya, C. V., Wilson, J. A., Espy, M. J., *et al.* (2002). Preemptive use of oral ganciclovir to prevent cytomegalovirus infection in liver transplant patients: a randomized, placebo-controlled trial. *J. Infect. Dis.*, **185**(7), 854–860.

Prentice, H. G., Gluckman, E., Powles, R. L. *et al.* (1994). Impact of long-term acyclovir on cytomegalovirus infection and survival after allogeneic bone marrow transplantation. European Acyclovir for CMV Prophylaxis Study Group. *Lancet*, **343**(8900), 749–753.

Razonable, R. R., Brown, R. A., Wilson, J. *et al.* (2002). The clinical use of various blood compartments for cytomegalovirus (CMV) DNA quantitation in transplant recipients with CMV disease. *Transplantation*, **73**(6), 968–973.

Reed, E. C., Wolford, J. L., Kopecky, K. J. *et al.* (1990). Ganciclovir for the treatment of cytomegalovirus gastroenteritis in bone marrow transplant patients. A randomized, placebo-controlled trial. *Ann. Intern. Med.*, **112**(7), 505–510.

Reinke, P., Fietze, E., Ode-Hakim, S. *et al.* (1994). Late-acute renal allograft rejection and symptomless cytomegalovirus infection. *Lancet*, **344**(8939–8940), 1737–1738.

Reusser, P., Einsele, H., Lee, J. *et al.* (2002). Randomized multicenter trial of foscarnet versus ganciclovir for preemptive therapy of cytomegalovirus infection after allogeneic stem cell transplantation. *Blood*, **99**(4), 1159–1164.

Rubin, R. H. (1991). Preemptive therapy in immunocompromised hosts. *N. Engl. J. Med.*, **324**(15), 1057–1059.

Safrin, S., Cherrington, J., and Jaffe, H. S. (1997). Clinical uses of cidofovir. *Rev. Med. Virol.*, **7**(3), 145–156.

Schmidt, G. M., Horak, D. A., Niland, J. C., Duncan, S. R., Forman, S. J., and Zaia, J. A. (1991). A randomized, controlled trial of prophylactic ganciclovir for cytomegalovirus pulmonary infection in recipients of allogeneic bone marrow transplants; The City of Hope-Stanford-Syntex CMV Study Group. *N. Engl. J. Med.*, **324**(15), 1005–1011.

Shinkai, M. and Spector, S. A. (1995). Quantitation of human cytomegalovirus (HCMV) DNA in cerebrospinal fluid by competitive PCR in AIDS patients with different HCMV central nervous system diseases. *Scand. J. Infect. Dis.*, **27**(6), 559–561.

Singh, N. (2006). Antiviral drugs for cytomegalovirus in transplant recipients: advantages of preemptive therapy. *Rev. Med. Virol.*, **16**(5), 281–287.

Snydman, D. R., Werner, B. G., Dougherty, N. N. *et al.* (1993). Cytomegalovirus immune globulin prophylaxis in liver transplantation. A randomized, double-blind, placebo-controlled trial. The Boston Center for Liver Transplantation CMVIG Study Group. *Ann. Intern. Med.*, **119**(10), 984–991.

Snydman, D. R. (2006). The case for cytomegalovirus prophylaxis in solid organ transplantation. *Rev. Med. Virol.* **16**(5), 289–295.

Spector, S. A., Merrill, R., Wolf, D., and Dankner, W. M. (1992). Detection of human cytomegalovirus in plasma of AIDS patients during acute visceral disease by DNA amplification. *J. Clin. Microbiol.*, **30**(9), 2359–2365.

Spector, S. A., McKinley, G. F., Lalezari, J. P. *et al.* (1996). Oral ganciclovir for the prevention of cytomegalovirus disease in persons with AIDS. Roche Cooperative Oral Ganciclovir Study Group. *N. Engl. J. Med.*, **334**(23), 1491–1497.

Spector, S. A., Wong, R., Hsia, K., Pilcher, M., and Stempien, M. J. (1998). Plasma cytomegalovirus (CMV) DNA load predicts CMV disease and survival in AIDS patients. *J. Clin. Invest.*, **101**(2), 497–502.

Spector, S. A., Hsia, K., Crager, M., Pilcher, M., Cabral, S., and Stempien, M. J. (1999). Cytomegalovirus (CMV) DNA load is an independent predictor of CMV disease and survival in advanced AIDS. *J. Virol.*, **73**(8), 7027–7030.

Speir, E., Modali, R., Huang, E. S. *et al.* (1994). Potential role of human cytomegalovirus and p53 interaction in coronary restenosis. *Science*, **265**(5170), 391–394.

Speir, E., Shibutani, T., Yu, Z. X., Ferrans, V., and Epstein, S. E. (1996). Role of reactive oxygen intermediates in cytomegalovirus gene expression and in the response of human smooth muscle cells to viral infection. *Circ. Res.*, **79**(6), 1143–1152.

Stagno, S., Reynolds, D. W., Tsiantos, A., Fuccillo, D. A., Long, W., and Alford, C. A. (1975). Comparative serial virologic and serologic studies of symptomatic and subclinical congenitally and natally acquired cytomegalovirus infections. *J. Infect. Dis.*, **132**(5), 568–577.

Streblow, D. N., Soderberg-Naucler, C., Vieira, J. *et al.* (1999). The human cytomegalovirus chemokine receptor US28 mediates vascular smooth muscle cell migration. *Cell*, **99**(5), 511–520.

Talarico, C. L., Burnette, T. C., Miller, W. H. *et al.* (1999). Acyclovir is phosphorylated by the human cytomegalovirus UL97 protein. *Antimicrob. Agents Chemother.*, **43**(8), 1941–1946.

The, T. H., van der, B. W., van den Berg, A. P., van der Giessen, M. *et al.* (1990). Cytomegalovirus antigenemia. *Rev. Infect. Dis.*, **12** Suppl. 7, S734–S744.

Valantine, H. A., Gao, S. Z., Menon, S. G. *et al.* (1999). Impact of prophylactic immediate posttransplant ganciclovir on development of transplant atherosclerosis: a post hoc analysis of a randomized, placebo-controlled study. *Circulation*, **100**(1), 61–66.

Wagner, J. A., Ross, H., Hunt, S. *et al.* (1995). Prophylactic ganciclovir treatment reduces fungal as well as cytomegalovirus infections after heart transplantation. *Transplantation*, **60**(12), 1473–1477.

Whitcup, S. M., Fortin, E., Lindblad, A. S. *et al.* (1999). Discontinuation of anticytomegalovirus therapy in patients with HIV infection and cytomegalovirus retinitis. *J. Am. Med. Assoc.*, **282**(17), 1633–1637.

Winston, D. J. and Busuttil, R. W. (2004). Randomized controlled trial of sequential intravenous and oral ganciclovir versus prolonged intravenous ganciclovir for long-term prophylaxis of cytomegalovirus disease in high-risk cytomegalovirus-seronegative liver transplant recipients with cytomegalovirus-seropositive donors. *Transplantation*, **77**(2), 305–308.

Winston, D. J., Ho, W. G., Bartoni, K. *et al.* (1993). Ganciclovir prophylaxis of cytomegalovirus infection and disease in allogeneic bone marrow transplant recipients. Results of a placebo-controlled double-blind trial. *Ann. Intern. Med.*, **118**(3), 179–184.

Winston, D. J., Wirin, D., Shaked, A., and Busuttil, R. W. (1995). Randomised comparison of ganciclovir and high-dose acyclovir for long-term cytomegalovirus prophylaxis in liver-transplant recipients. *Lancet*, **346**(8967), 69–74.

Winston, D. J., Yeager, A. M., Chandrasekar, P. H., Snydman, D. R., Petersen, F. B., and Territo, M. C. (2003). Randomized comparison of oral valacyclovir and intravenous ganciclovir for prevention of cytomegalovirus disease after allogeneic bone marrow transplantation. *Clin. Infect. Dis.*, **36**(6), 749–758.

New approaches to antiviral drug discovery (genomics/proteomics)

Mark N. Prichard

Department of Pediatrics, University of Alabama at Birmingham, Birmingham, AL, USA

Introduction

Discovery of antiviral drugs has always been an opportunistic endeavor. Small molecules in general and nucleoside analogues in particular have led investigators to discover uncharacterized viral gene products that could be exploited for the purpose of antiviral chemotherapy. Great strides have also been made in understanding fundamental events in the viral replication cycle including the binding of viral glycoproteins to cellular receptors, viral regulatory proteins that control expression of viral and cellular gene expression, viral genes that affect the synthesis and packaging of the viral genome, and viral factors that subvert the host immune response (Whitley and Roizman, 2001). Many of the viral genes that contribute to these processes are known and for some of them, the precise function is understood at the molecular level. For these targets it is comparatively simple to reduce the essential function to a biochemical assay, such as a polymerase or protease assay for use in a high throughput screen in order to identify small molecule inhibitors of enzyme function (Liu and Roizman, 1993). This approach has facilitated the proactive and rational search for specific enzyme inhibitors and has led to the development of effective antiviral therapies. Although this approach is effective, it requires well-characterized targets with a defined biochemical function, and can be applied only to a very small proportion of the essential viral gene products. At present, the best targets for antiviral chemotherapy likely remain undescribed and unutilized.

The development of new classes of antiviral drugs is limited by our understanding of biology. More often than not, it is unclear which viral gene products contribute to essential functions. Less clear still is the precise function or functions that the constituent proteins perform such that the biochemical activity can not be modeled in vitro. Thus, the challenge and rate-limiting step in this process is to identify the functions of gene products that are required for viral replication and to define precisely the molecular mechanisms involved with these processes.

Advances in genomics and associated technologies are offering new opportunities to investigators to answer such questions. This endeavor is driving technological developments in bioinformatics, genetics and laboratory automation and promises to generate a host of new resources that can be brought to bear on all fields of biology (Collins et al., 2003). Advances in molecular virology will help drive this effort and will also benefit tremendously as virus–host interactions are defined in more detail and on a grander scale. Genomics, proteomics and related technologies can also be applied specifically to the discovery and development of antiviral therapies. Techniques and approaches that are particularly suited to this task are discussed and early experiments in this arena will be described.

Development of bioinformatics and computational tools

The emerging and evolving fields of genomics and proteomics are changing the way that biological research is conducted and technologies associated with these efforts can be applied effectively to the study of viral biology. The development of these fields is driven in part by the technological advances that produce genomic sequences more efficiently every year (Venter et al., 2003). Significant technological advances in chemistry, biotechnology, and bioinformatics are also major drivers in this field and each of these efforts has produced tremendous new resources and even greater quantities of raw data. Perhaps the most defining characteristic of these emerging fields of research is the tremendous size and complexity of the data sets they generate. Significant computational resources are required to manage the volumes of data, manipulate it, and parse it into databases that can be queried by researchers. This process requires training in computer science and mathematics. Investigators who specialize in these fields will contribute greatly to any future drug discovery projects using these new technologies. Bioinformatics resources are also required to analyze the data, identify patterns and display the patterns in a way that can be interpreted by investigators in the field. Data that is processed in this manner is designed to help investigators understand the problem at hand and can help them make hypotheses. Inferences drawn from these efforts need to be tested and confirmed in the laboratory, but the process helps to focus valuable research time on prioritized compounds or genes.

The application of computational methods to the study of herpesviruses biology is particularly intriguing. Large DNA viruses present a unique set of well characterized genomes that are comparatively well studied and characterized (Davison et al., 2002). New tools developed by scientists in bioinformatics can be applied to these genomes to test their ability to predict the organization of viral genes, their global coding capacity and the function of viral proteins (Novotny et al., 2001; Rigoutsos et al., 2003). Laboratory confirmation of transcriptional patterns and gene expression and gene function is essential to this process, particularly early on when the bioinformatics algorithms are being tested on these genomes. The genetic tractability of herpesviruses and availability of genome wide methods to test these hypotheses make this an ideal system to validate new approaches to study biological processes (Stingley et al., 2000). Communication and cooperation between the specialists in bioinformatics and bench level virologists is essential and will facilitate the incremental improvement of algorithms predictive of biological structure and function. The iterative process of algorithm refinement and biological confirmation will lead to computational approaches that are increasingly predictive of viral biology.

Studying new methods in bioinformatics in herpesviruses presents certain virus specific problems. Even within the alphaherpesviruses, the variation in G + C content will present a codon bias that must be taken into consideration. The genomic organization of 3′ coterminal transcription units as well as readthrough of certain stop codons will complicate the computational analysis as well as laboratory characterization of gene expression. Indeed, this is true in other viruses, such as SV40 where algorithms trained on mammalian genomes fail in many cased because of conservative assumptions about splicing sites and polyadenylation signals. Nevertheless, the genomics studies at the level of herpesviruses will be particularly instructive and will guide efforts to define and interpret sequences from more complex genomes, such as the human genome.

Data relevant to the discovery of new drugs tend to be concentrated at the intersection of large data sets. Databases that contain information related to biological function, chemical structure, and the biologic activity of small molecules all can contribute to the search for new lead compounds. The nature of this problem is inherently complex and databases will be required to handle the volumes of data. In the near term, computational methods can suggest aspects of viral replication that might be targeted specifically by small molecule inhibitors. Similarly, these methods may identify small molecules with well described biological effects that could be used to probe cellular functions that may be required by the virus. In the long term, computational approaches have the potential to link databases containing information on chemical structure, protein structure, biochemical activity, and biologic activity of small molecules. It may eventually be possible to mine existing data in a meaningful way to suggest chemical classes that might be used to inhibit known biochemical activities.

Impact of genomics and related fields on herpesvirus research

The scientific landscape has changed dramatically in the last 15 years with the completion of the DNA sequence for the genomes of all eight known human herpesviruses (Baer et al., 1984; Chee et al., 1990; Davison and Scott, 1986; Dolan et al., 1998; Gompels et al., 1995; McGeoch et al., 1988, 1991; Pfeiffer et al., 1995; Russo et al., 1996). This is a very significant step in the path towards understanding the biology of herpesvirus infections. These and other resources in the publicly available databases are tremendously valuable to scientists studying herpesvirus infections and provide a map and common reference points to help scientists describe precisely viral transcripts and open reading frames (ORFs). Genomic sequences can also be used to compare genomic organization among all the herpesviruses, and represents a starting point in the path towards the identifying evolutionary relationships in this virus family. Importantly, the nucleotide sequences in the databases are not static. Sequence data are inherently noisy and most genomic sequences in GenBank have mistakes that need to be corrected when they are identified, especially in information-dense viral genomes. Annotations of viral genomes are conducted with the best tools available at the time of submission, but they become outdated as gene prediction algorithms improve and as experiments in the laboratory identify new genes (Cha et al., 1996). Since the annotation process is evolving, scientists should expect to find inconsistencies among the annotations of different genomes, as the terminology used to describe gene function is continually evolving (Ashburner et al., 2000). Thus, prototype viral genomes will need to be updated and reannotated in an iterative process, particularly as new strains and viruses are sequenced (Davison et al., 2003). Versioning of genomes and annotations is becoming more important when comparing sequences and annotations due to the continual annotation process, analogous to the versioning of software and human genome release versions in NCBI.

Genomics studies in herpesviruses initially focused on defining the structure and coding capacity of each of the viral genomes and comparing them with annotated sequences of related viruses. The DNA sequence and structure of the genomes is comparatively simple to define, yet even for these simple organisms it is not possible to predict with any certainty which, if any genes will be expressed in the context of an infection. Depending on the algorithms used, different numbers of ORFs will identified and laboratory experimentation is required to confirm which ORFs are actually expressed in the context of a viral infection (Davison et al., 2003; Rigoutsos et al., 2003). As synthesized microarrays become less expensive, oligonucleotide probes which hybridize to putative exons and splice junctions can be used for confirming the expression of predicted transcripts and splice variants in a bulk fashion (Shoemaker et al., 2001). Continued experimentation and consistent reannotation among the submitted sequences will help define how these viruses, and indeed their human host use DNA to regulate and code for all the required functions. As this knowledge base expands, relationships among all the herpesviruses will crystallize and molecular evolutionary patterns will start to emerge.

The viral proteome represents all of the proteins expressed by the virus and reflects both the processing of RNA transcripts as well as the post-translational processing that occurs. Proteomics methods have the potential to be particularly powerful because it can distinguish the modification of viral gene products during the course of viral infection and can help characterize how proteolysis, glycosylation and phosphorylation impact viral replication. At one level, mass spectrometry and protein microsequencing can be used to identify sets of viral proteins involved in a particular biologic process (Greco et al., 2001). Genome wide searches using algorithms to predict protein structure or identify conserved motifs can also be used to generate hypotheses regarding protein function (Oien et al., 2002). Yeast two-hybrid studies provide an experimental approach for the study protein-protein interactions among viral and cellular proteins and will help to provide information about functional complexes in an infected cell. Efforts underway to construct protein-protein interaction maps have the potential to help understand which gene products cooperate in biological processes.

The emerging field of chemical genetics will also likely impact the discovery of antiviral therapies and could be one of the most useful tools (Strausberg and Schreiber, 2003). Genes can be classified in orthologous groups (Tatusov et al., 1997) and small molecules can be classified into families based on the chemical structure. Genetics can be used to characterize the phenotype associated with a particular gene, and in an analogous manner the biological effect of a drug, or chemotype, can be associated with small molecules. Relating chemotypes and genotypes can help identify the molecular targets and pathways affected by groups of compounds. This information can be used to infer the mechanism of action of candidate molecules by comparing the chemotype with existing phenotypes associated with viruses containing mutations in different pathways. This process might also be particularly useful in identifying cellular response patterns associated with drug toxicity that could be used to eliminate lead compounds early in the discovery process (Waring et al., 2002).

New resources for use in drug discovery

Genomics and proteomics are promising new fields with lofty goals, but can they provide immediate utility to efforts currently underway to identify new classes of antiviral drugs? At present, the impact of these fields is most apparent in the widespread use of data and tools provided by the publicly available databases. The GenBank, EMBL, and DDBJ nucleotide databases provided freely on the web are a tremendous resource to everyone and most researchers use the databases or related tools on a regular basis. The National Center for Biotechnology Information (http://www.ncbi.nlm.nih.gov/) and the European Bioinformatics Institute (http://www.ebi.ac.uk/services/index.html) websites in particular provide access, to basic tools and services that are used in laboratories every day. These tools include nucleotide and protein database searching tools, genome maps, structural databases and pattern recognition tools. The STDGEN database provided by Los Alamos National Laboratories (http://www.stdgen.lanl.gov/) is a wonderful resource that provides specific genomic and proteomic information on herpesviruses and contains BLAST search results with links to other viral orthologues and conserved orthologous groups. Tools provided by these organizations are continually upgraded and new tools appear on a regular basis. Thus, a review of the available tools will be quickly outdated and can not substitute for a trip to the web sites listed in this text.

A number of new material resources have also been created through the automation of laboratory procedures. Microarrays of several different types are commercially available for characterizing changing transcription patterns in infected cells (Browne et al., 2001). Herpesvirus specific microarrays have also been constructed and can rapidly assess viral transcript changes in response to stimuli (Stingley et al., 2000). Expression clone libraries have been produced in efforts designed to assay gene function and virus knockout libraries have been assembled by a number of investigators. Each of the resources described here has the potential to be used in a genome wide search to identify viral genes that are important in the replication process.

Application of new technologies to cell-based antiviral assays

New tools and resources described herein, have the potential to be extremely useful in the drug discovery process and some strategies are currently in use. Many of the new strategies are unproven, and as such, are high risk activities that are used sparingly in the industrial setting. Nevertheless, high risk–high reward strategies have their place in the discovery process, particularly in the search for new classes of antivirals. The specific application of new technologies and resources to conventional screening and development activities has the potential to make an immediate and positive impact on the drug discovery process.

Cell-based screens for small molecules with antiviral activity have been utilized for all of the herpesviruses. Historically, most approved therapies for herpesvirus infections resulted from this approach to antiviral discovery, but continued screening of the same libraries with very similar assays is not likely to identify new lead compounds. It is possible to change the assays to bias the hit compounds away from molecules already identified in previous screens and towards molecules with different mechanisms of action. For example, screening recombinant viruses that lack the thymidine kinase (in herpes simplex virus (HSV)), or recombinant viruses lacking the UL97 kinase (in cytomegalovirus (CMV)) will identify small molecules and nucleosides that do not require phosphorylation to be active. Lead compounds identified in these particular screens would also be candidates for the treatment of drug resistant infections. Genetically sensitized viruses, like the recombinants described above, might react more strongly to weakly active compounds and could unmask these molecules in existing chemical libraries. Candidate molecules with unusual mechanisms of action or good pharmacologic properties could then be selected for chemical modification to improve the antiviral activity.

As an alternative to the conventional endpoint of cytopathic effect inhibition, the affect of small molecules on viral transcriptional patterns could be monitored to reveal molecules with unusual mechanisms of action. Microarray technologies would be particularly useful in this regard, but it limits the number of compounds that could be examined in detail. In essence, this approach has already been validated through the characterization of gamma or late viral transcripts by treatment with phosphonoacetic acid (Stingley et al., 2000). The cellular transcriptional response to small molecules could also be monitored simultaneously to measure changes in the host response to infection induced by the small molecules (Browne et al., 2001; Fruh et al., 2001). Microarrays can also help identify the mechanisms of transformation in infected cells and could potentially lead to better therapies for virus induced malignancies (Moses et al., 2002). Potential toxicities could also be identified at an early stage by monitoring the induction of cellular genes associated with the response to toxic compounds (Waring et al., 2002). Data generated by such an approach could also be queried at a later date using chemical genetics techniques to classify and cluster the chemotypes of molecules in the library.

Application of new technologies to biochemical assays

Biochemical screening assays will likely derive the greatest benefit from genomics and proteomics technologies. The increased characterization of viral gene products will likely identify additional biochemical activities that can be converted rapidly into small molecule screens. Homology searching algorithms also play a major role because of their ability to extend knowledge from one herpesvirus to related viruses. BLAST searches with a known gene can identify orthologues in other herpesviruses and related genes (paralogues) within the same virus in an effort to identify viral proteins with a similar biochemical activity (Davison et al., 2002). For example, an orthologue of the HSV protease was identified in CMV and a similar biochemical assay could be used for both to screen for inhibitors of this biochemical activity (Jarvest et al., 1999; Pinto et al., 1999).

Many viral gene products have no known function, yet possess characteristic motifs that could potentially be used in biochemical screens (Rigoutsos et al., 2003). Hypotheses generated by searches such as these could be tested in the laboratory and if confirmed could be used in a biochemical screen. For instance, nucleotide binding motifs in poorly characterized genes could be used to identify nucleosides that bind to these sites with high affinity. Similarly, a structural search revealed that *UL57* in CMV appears to be related at a structural level to some endonucleases (Novotny et al., 2001). If this activity were confirmed in the laboratory, a biochemical screen could be used to identify specific inhibitors of this activity and might be effective in inhibiting viral replication given that this gene is known to be essential for viral replication.

Biochemical assays based on protein-protein interactions are capable of identifying molecules with antiviral activity. Information garnered from proteomics methods or yeast-two hybrids could be used to devise a rapid assay for protein–protein interactions that are presumed to be important for viral replication. Screening of small molecule libraries or peptide libraries could identify specific inhibitors that also possess antiviral activity (Liuzzi et al., 1994). This same strategy could be employed to identify inhibitors that disrupt the interaction of viral and cellular proteins that appear to be important viral replication. If fact, it may be possible to perform the high throughput screen directly in yeast if the interaction was originally defined in this system.

The best characterized molecular targets have had their crystal structures determined. Given these data, it is possible to recrystallize these molecules with known inhibitors to identify protein binding sites or to dock small molecules *in silico* to identify molecules in improved binding affinities to the active site (Stoll et al., 2003). This approach is particularly useful in lead optimization and medicinal chemistry efforts to increase potency. For any of the technologies discussed here, their greatest utility is generating testable hypotheses that could identify new and unexploited targets for antiviral therapy.

Application of new technologies to functional assays

Genetic approaches can identify gene products that are essential for viral replication, but without a biochemical assay, it is not possible to screen for inhibitors of these molecules. Functional genomics approaches can be employed to try to identify surrogate phenotypes for interesting genes. With these sorts of assays, the surrogate assays do not necessarily measure the relevant functional aspect of the gene in question. Any inhibitors identified from screens based on surrogate assays need to be validated in secondary assays (Tugendreich et al., 2001). Although surrogate approaches are high risk high reward propositions, they are particularly useful for screening ion channels or other molecules that require an intact membrane for activity (Hahnberger et al., 1996).

Application of new technologies to characterize mechanism of action and spectrum of activity

New technological developments also impact how researchers conduct preclinical studies on compounds with antiviral activity. Mechanism of action studies still involve the isolation of drug resistant viruses, but genomic sequencing of drug resistant viruses can be faster than conducting conventional marker transfer studies to identify the molecular targets of investigational drugs (S.W. Chou, pers. commun.). Direct sequencing is also cost effective in identifying resistance mutations in clinical isolates where the mechanisms of drug resistance are well characterized (Lurain et al., 2001).

Genomics approaches can also be used to help predict the spectrum of activity of a compound if the mechanism of action is known. Homology searches can be used to identify gene families common to a wide variety of organisms and are called clusters of orthologous groups (COGs) (Tatusov et al., 1997). This process was also conducted for all sequenced herpesviruses and a set of viral COGs was assembled (Montague and Hutchison, 2000). In addition to helping define orthologues in this group of viruses, the COGs can also be used to construct genome-wide phylogenetic trees, that closely match trees constructed using the highly conserved core genes (Davison et al., 2002). COGs can also be clustered based on the viruses in which they appear, and can help to define a theoretical spectrum of activity for antiviral drugs based on the conservation of the molecular targets. A comparison of the predicted drug efficacy (shaded area) is compared with antiviral activity reported in the literature (+ or −) in Table 67.1. A number of interesting disparities are immediately apparent. Penciclovir did not appear to be active against EBV, and neither acyclovir nor penciclovir exhibited significant antiviral activity against HHV8, despite the fact that they possess relatively well conserved thymidine kinases. These results are explained in part by apparent low activity of the HHV8 thymidine kinase and narrow substrate specificity (Gustafson et al., 2000). The activity of ganciclovir in viruses without TK orthologues can be explained

Table 67.1. Predicted spectrum of activity based on molecular target conservation

Drug	Molecular target	COG #(43) (Identity)	HSV1	HSV2	VZV	EBV	HHV8	CMV	HHV6A	HHV6B
Acyclovir	Thymidine kinase[a] (15, 23)	COG97 (18.9%)	+ (23)	+ (23)	+ (4)	+ (12)	− (31)	− (29)	− (37)	− (37)
Penciclovir	Thymidine kinase[a] (22)	COG97 (18.9%)	+ (6)	+ (6)	+ (6)	− (37)	− (37)	− (6)	− (37)	− (37)
Ganciclovir	Thymidine kinase[a] (15, 23)	COG97[a] (18.9%)	+ (39)	+ (39)	+ (14)	+ (39)	+ (31, 42)	+ (39)	+ (37)	+ (37)
	Protein kinase[a] (34, 55)	COG60[a] (17.2%)								
Foscarnet	DNA polymerase (10)	COG51 (27.6%)	+ (62)	+ (32)	+ (2)	+ (16)	+ (37)	+ (37, 62)	+ (37)	+ (37)
Cidofovir	DNA polymerase (20)	COG51 (27.6%)	+ (20)	+ (20)	+ (20)	+ (20)	+ (37)	+ (20)	+ (37)	+ (37)
4-oxo-dihydro-quinolines	DNA polymerase (46)	COG51 (27.1)	+ (57)	+ (57)	+ (57)	+ (57)	+ (57)	+ (57)	− (57)	− (57)
BDCRB	Terminase (UL89) (60)	COG59 (22.8%)	− (58)	− (58)	− (65)	− (58)	− (65)	+ (58)	− (65)	− (65)
	Terminase (UL56) (33)	COG93 (20.5%)								
maribavir	UL97 (5)	COG60 (17.2%)	− (65, 66)	− (65, 66)	− (65)	+ (66)	− (65)	+ (66)	− (65)	− (65)

[a] The molecular target is the polymerase (COG51), but the compounds derive most of their selectivity at the level of phosphorylation by the COGs shown.

by the alternative phosphorylation by *UL97* protein kinase in cytomegalovirus and related orthologues in the other β herpesviruses (Littler *et al.*, 1992; Sullivan *et al.*, 1992). The high degree of conservation among the herpesviruses in the DNA polymerase is very predictive for broad efficacy of foscarnet, cidofovir, and the 4-oxoquinoline derivatives. The exception is the reduced susceptibility of HHV6A,B, that can be explained by an unusual V823A polymorphism in the active site of these viruses. Of interest, both of the benzimidazole analogs (maribavir and BDCRB) exhibit a very limited spectrum of activity, which is not predicted given the well conserved molecular target, particularly with BDCRB. Like other computational methods described herein, their greatest utility of this approach is generating a hypothesis to be tested in the laboratory. Future mechanism of action studies for this series of compounds will be needed to explain the limited spectrum of activity for this series of compounds.

Conclusions

As genomics and related technologies develop, they will be applied to the study of herpesvirus biology and to the discovery of new antiviral drugs to treat these infections. Initial reports have provided indications that these strategies may be particularly useful in this family of viruses. These approaches hold promise and will likely make substantial contributions to the field as the technologies mature.

Acknowledgment

I thank David Shivak for his helpful comments and his critical reading of the manuscript.

REFERENCES

Ashburner, M., Ball, C. A., Blake, J. A. *et al.* (2000). Gene ontology: tool for the unification of biology. The Gene Ontology Consortium. *Nat. Genet.*, **25**, 25–29.

Baba, M., Konno, K., Shigeta, S., and De Clercq E. (1986). Inhibitory effects of selected antiviral compounds on newly isolated clinical varicella-zoster virus strains. *Tohoku J. Exp. Med.*, **148**, 275–283.

Baer, R., Bankier, A. T., Biggin, M. D. *et al.* (1984). DNA sequence and expression of the B95–8 Epstein-Barr virus genome. *Nature*, **310**, 207–211.

Biron, K. K. and Elion, G. B. (1980). In vitro susceptibility of varicella-zoster virus to acyclovir. *Antimicrob. Agents Chemother.*, **18**, 443–447.

Biron, K. K., Harvey, R. J., Chamberlain, S. C. et al. (2002). Potent and selective inhibition of human cytomegalovirus replication by 1263W94, a benzimidazole L-riboside with a unique mode of action. *Antimicrob. Agents Chemother.*, **46**, 2365–2372.

Boyd, M. R., Bacon, T. H., Sutton, D., and Cole, M. (1987). Antiherpesvirus activity of 9-(4-hydroxy-3-hydroxy-methylbut-1-yl)guanine (BRL 39123) in cell culture. *Antimicrob. Agents Chemother.*, **31**, 1238–1242.

Browne, E. P., Wing, B., Coleman, D., and Shenk, T. (2001). Altered cellular mRNA levels in human cytomegalovirus-infected fibroblasts: viral block to the accumulation of antiviral mRNAs. *J. Virol.*, **75**, 12319–12330.

Cha, T. A., Tom, E., Kemble, G. W., Duke, G. M., Mocarski, E. S., and Spaete, R. R. (1996). Human cytomegalovirus clinical isolates carry at least 19 genes not found in laboratory strains. *J. Virol.*, **70**, 78–83.

Chee, M. S., Bankier, A. T., Beck, S. et al. (1990). Analysis of the protein-coding content of the sequence of human cytomegalovirus strain AD169. *Curr. Top. Microbiol. Immunol.*, **154**, 125–169.

Cheng, Y. C., Grill, S., Derse, D., et al. (1981). Mode of action of phosphonoformate as an anti-herpes simplex virus agent. *Biochim. Biophys. Acta*, **652**, 90–98.

Colby, B. M., Shaw, J. E., Elion, G. B., and Pagano, J. S. (1980). Effect of acyclovir [9-(2-hydroxyethoxymethyl)guanine] on Epstein–Barr virus DNA replication. *J. Virol.*, **34**, 560–568.

Collins, F. S., Green, E. D., Guttmacher, A. E., and Guyer, M. S. (2003). A vision for the future of genomics research. *Nature*, **422**, 835–847.

Collins, P. and Oliver, N. M. (1985). Comparison of the in vitro and in vivo antiherpes virus activities of the acyclic nucleosides, acyclovir (Zovirax) and 9-[(2-hydroxy-1-hydroxymethylethoxy)methyl]guanine (BWB759U). *Antiviral Res.*, **5**, 145–156.

Darby, G., Larder, B. A., Bastow, K. F., and Field, H. J. (1980). Sensitivity of viruses to phosphorylated 9-(2-hydroxyethoxymethyl)guanine revealed in TK-transformed cells. *J. Gen. Virol.*, **48**, 451–454.

Datta, A. K. and Hood. R. E. (1981). Mechanism of inhibition of Epstein–Barr virus replication by phosphonoformic acid. *Virology*, **114**, 52–59.

Davison, A. J. and Scott, J. E. (1986). The complete DNA sequence of varicella-zoster virus. *J. Gen. Virol.*, **67**(9), 1759–1816.

Davison, A. J., Dargan, D. J., and Stow, N. D. (2002). Fundamental and accessory systems in herpesviruses. *Antiviral Res.*, **56**, 1–11.

Davison, A. J., Dolan, A., Akter, P. et al. (2003). The human cytomegalovirus genome revisited: comparison with the chimpanzee cytomegalovirus genome. *J. Gen. Virol.*, **84**, 17–28.

De Clercq, E., Sakuma, T., Baba, M. et al. (1987). Antiviral activity of phosphonylmethoxyalkyl derivatives of purine and pyrimidines. *Antiviral Res.*, **8**, 261–272.

Dolan, A., Jamieson, F. E., Cunningham, C., Barnett B. C., and McGeoch, D. J. (1998). The genome sequence of herpes simplex virus type 2. *J. Virol.*, **72**, 2010–21.

Earnshaw, D. L., Bacon, T. H., Darlison, S. J., Edmonds, K., Perkins, R. M., and Vere Hodge, R. A. (1992). Mode of antiviral action of penciclovir in MRC-5 cells infected with herpes simplex virus type 1 (HSV-1), HSV-2, and varicella-zoster virus. *Antimicrob. Agents Chemother.*, **36**, 2747–2757.

Elion, G. B. (1982). Mechanism of action and selectivity of acyclovir. *Am. J. Med.*, **73**, 7–13.

Fruh, K., Simmen, K., Luukkonen, B. G., Bell, Y. C., and Ghazal, P. (2001). Virogenomics: a novel approach to antiviral drug discovery. *Drug Discov. Today*, **6**, 621–627.

Gompels, U. A., Nicholas, J., Lawrence, G. et al. (1995). The DNA sequence of human herpesvirus-6: structure, coding content, and genome evolution. *Virology*, **209**, 29–51.

Greco, A., Bienvenut, W., Sanchez, J. C. et al. (2001). Identification of ribosome-associated viral and cellular basic proteins during the course of infection with herpes simplex virus type 1. *Proteomics*, **1**, 545–549.

Gustafson, E. A., Schinazi, R. F., and Fingeroth, J. D. (2000). Human herpesvirus 8 open reading frame 21 is a thymidine and thymidylate kinase of narrow substrate specificity that efficiently phosphorylates zidovudine but not ganciclovir. *J. Virol.*, **74**, 684–692.

Hahnenberger, K. M., Krystal, M., Esposito, K., Tang, W., and Kurtz, S. (1996). Use of microphysiometry for analysis of heterologous ion channels expressed in yeast. *Nat. Biotechnol.*, **14**, 880–883.

Harmenberg, J., Wahren, B., and Oberg, B. (1980). Influence of cells and virus multiplicity on the inhibition of herpesviruses with acycloguanosine. *Intervirology*, **14**, 239–244.

Jarvest, R. L., Pinto, I. L., Ashman, S. M. et al. (1999). Inhibition of herpes proteases and antiviral activity of 2-substituted thieno[2,3-d]oxazinones. *Bioorg. Med. Chem. Lett.*, **9**, 443–448.

Kedes, D. H. and Ganem, D. (1997). Sensitivity of Kaposi's sarcoma-associated herpesvirus replication to antiviral drugs. Implications for potential therapy. *J. Clin. Invest.*, **99**, 2082–2086.

Kern, E. R., Richards, J. T., Overall, J. C. Jr., and Glasgow, L. A. (1981). A comparison of phosphonoacetic acid and phosphonoformic acid activity in genital herpes simplex virus type 1 and type 2 infections of mice. *Antiviral Res.*, **1**, 225–235.

Krosky, P. M., Underwood, M. R., Turk, S. R. et al. (1998). Resistance of human cytomegalovirus to benzimidazole ribonucleosides maps to two open reading frames: UL89 and UL56. *J. Virol.*, **72**, 4721–4728.

Littler, E., Stuart, A. D., and Chee, M. S. (1992). Human cytomegalovirus UL97 open reading frame encodes a protein that phosphorylates the antiviral nucleoside analogue ganciclovir. *Nature*, **358**, 160–162.

Liu, F., and Roizman, B. (1993). Characterization of the protease and other products of amino-terminus-proximal cleavage of the herpes simplex virus 1 UL26 protein. *J. Virol.*, **67**, 1300–1309.

Liuzzi, M., Deziel, R., Moss, N. et al. (1994). A potent peptidomimetic inhibitor of HSV ribonucleotide reductase with antiviral activity in vivo. *Nature*, **372**, 695–698.

Long, M. C., Bidanset, D. J., Williams, S. L., Kushner, N. L. and Kern, E. R. (2003). Determination of antiviral efficacy against lymphotropic herpesviruses utilizing flow cytometry. *Antiviral Res.*, **58**, 149–157.

Lurain, N. S., Weinberg, A., Crumpacker, C. S., and Chou, S. (2001). Sequencing of cytomegalovirus UL97 gene for genotypic antiviral resistance testing. *Antimicrob. Agents Chemother.*, **45**, 2775–2780.

Martin, J. C., Dvorak, C. A., Smee, D. F., Matthews, T. R., and Verheyden, J. P. (1983). 9-[(1,3-Dihydroxy-2-propoxy)-methyl]guanine: a new potent and selective antiherpes agent. *J. Med. Chem.*, **26**, 759–761.

McGeoch, D. J., Dalrymple, M. A., Davison, A. J. *et al.* (1988). The complete DNA sequence of the long unique region in the genome of herpes simplex virus type 1. *J. Gen. Virol.*, **69**(7), 1531–1574.

McGeoch, D. J., Cunningham, C., McIntyre, G., and Dolan, A. (1991). Comparative sequence analysis of the long repeat regions and adjoining parts of the long unique regions in the genomes of herpes simplex viruses types 1 and 2. *J. Gen. Virol.*, **72**(12), 3057–3075.

Medveczky, M. M., Horvath, E., Lund, T., and Medveczky, P. G. (1997). In vitro antiviral drug sensitivity of the Kaposi's sarcoma-associated herpesvirus. *AIDS*, **11**, 1327–1332.

Montague, M. G. and Hutchison, C. A., 3rd. (2000). Gene content phylogeny of herpesviruses. *Proc. Natl Acad. Sci. USA*, **97**, 5334–5339.

Moses, A. V., Jarvis, M. A., Raggo, C. *et al.* (2002). A functional genomics approach to Kaposi's sarcoma. *Ann. NY Acad. Sci.*, **975**, 180–191.

Novotny, J., Rigoutsos, I., Coleman, D., and Shenk, T. (2001). In silico structural and functional analysis of the human cytomegalovirus (HHV5) genome. *J. Mol. Biol.*, **310**, 1151–1166.

Oien, N. L., Brideau, R. J., Hopkins, T. A. *et al.* (2002). Broad-spectrum antiherpes activities of 4-hydroxyquinoline carboxamides, a novel class of herpesvirus polymerase inhibitors. *Antimicrob. Agents Chemother.*, **46**, 724–730.

Pfeiffer, B., Thomson, B., and Chandran, B. (1995). Identification and characterization of a cDNA derived from multiple splicing that encodes envelope glycoprotein gp105 of human herpesvirus 6. *J. Virol.*, **69**, 3490–3500.

Pinto, I. L., Jarvest, R. L., Clarke, B. (1999). Inhibition of human cytomegalovirus protease by enedione derivatives of thieno[2,3-d]oxazinones through a novel dual acylation/alkylation mechanism. *Bioorg. Med. Chem. Lett.*, **9**, 449–452.

Rigoutsos, I., Novotny, J., Huynh, T. *et al.* (2003). In silico pattern-based analysis of the human cytomegalovirus genome. *J. Virol.*, **77**, 4326–4344.

Russo, J. J., Bohenzky, R. A., Chien, M. C. *et al.* (1996). Nucleotide sequence of the Kaposi sarcoma-associated herpesvirus (HHV8). *Proc. Natl Acad. Sci. USA*, **93**, 14862–14867.

Shoemaker, D. D., Schadt, E. E., Armour, C. D. *et al.* (2001). Experimental annotation of the human genome using microarray technology. *Nature*, **409**, 922–927.

Stingley, S. W., Ramirez, J. J., Aguilar, S. A. *et al.* (2000). Global analysis of herpes simplex virus type 1 transcription using an oligonucleotide-based DNA microarray. *J. Virol.*, **74**, 9916–9927.

Stoll, V., Stewart, K. D., Maring, C. J. *et al.* (2003). Influenza neuraminidase inhibitors: structure-based design of a novel inhibitor series. *Biochemistry*, **42**, 718–727.

Strausberg, R. L. and Schreiber, S. L. (2003). From knowing to controlling: a path from genomics to drugs using small molecule probes. *Science*, **300**, 294–295.

Sullivan, V., Talarico, C. L., Stanat, S. C., Davis, M., Coen, D. M., and Biron, K. K. (1992). A protein kinase homologue controls phosphorylation of ganciclovir in human cytomegalovirus-infected cells. *Nature*, **358**, 162–164.

Tatusov, R. L., Koonin, E. V., and Lipman. D. J. (1997). A genomic perspective on protein families. *Science*, **278**, 631–637.

Thomsen, D. R., Oien, N. L., Hopkins, T. A. *et al.* (2003). Amino acid changes within conserved region III of the herpes simplex virus and human cytomegalovirus DNA polymerases confer resistance to 4-oxo-dihydroquinolines, a novel class of herpesvirus antiviral agents. *J. Virol.*, **77**, 1868–1876.

Townsend, L. B., Devivar, R. V., Turk, S. R., Nassiri, M. R., and Drach, J. C. (1995). Design, synthesis, and antiviral activity of certain 2,5,6-trihalo-1-(beta-D-ribofuranosyl)benzimidazoles. *J. Med. Chem.*, **38**, 4098–4105.

Tugendreich, S., Perkins, E., Couto, J. *et al.* (2001). A streamlined process to phenotypically profile heterologous cDNAs in parallel using yeast cell-based assays. *Genome Res.*, **11**, 1899–1912.

Underwood, M. R., Harvey, R. J., Stanat, S. C. *et al.* (1998). Inhibition of human cytomegalovirus DNA maturation by a benzimidazole ribonucleoside is mediated through the UL89 gene product. *J. Virol.*, **72**, 717–725.

Venter, J. C., Levy, S., Stockwell, T., Remington, K., and Halpern, A. (2003). Massive parallelism, randomness and genomic advances. *Nat. Genet.*, **33**(Suppl), 219–227.

Wahren, B. and Oberg. B. (1980). Inhibition of cytomegalovirus late antigens by phosphonoformate. *Intervirology*, **12**, 335–339.

Waring, J. F., Gum, R., Morfitt, D. *et al.* (2002). Identifying toxic mechanisms using DNA microarrays: evidence that an experimental inhibitor of cell adhesion molecule expression signals through the aryl hydrocarbon nuclear receptor. *Toxicology*, **181–182**, 537–550.

Whitley, R. J. and Roizman, B. (2001). Herpes simplex virus infections. *Lancet*, **357**, 1513–1518.

Williams, S. L., Hartline, C. B., Kushner, N. L. *et al.* (2003). In vitro activities of benzimidazole D- and L-ribonucleosides against herpesviruses. *Antimicrob. Agents Chemother.*, **47**, 2186–2192.

Zacny, V. L., Gershburg, E., Davis, M. G., Biron, K. K., and Pagano, J. S. (1999). Inhibition of Epstein–Barr virus replication by a benzimidazole L-riboside: novel antiviral mechanism of 5, 6-dichloro-2-(isopropylamino)-1-beta-L-ribofuranosyl-1H-benzimidazole. *J. Virol.*, **73**, 7271–7277.

68

Candidate anti-herpesviral drugs; mechanisms of action and resistance

Karen K. Biron

Clinical Virology, GlaxoSmithKline, Research Triangle Park, NC, USA

Research into the molecular biology of herpes replication in recent years has revealed novel targets for drug development (Fig. 68.1). The characterization and functional assay of these targets have been facilitated by advancements in gene expression, protein purification, proteonomics, bioinformatics, and efficient robotic screening technologies. The pipeline for new herpes drugs has been expanding as drug candidates have evolved more rapidly due to improvements in chemical synthesis (i.e., combinatorial and parallel synthesis methods), and with aids for drug design (X-ray crystallography, in silico computer modeling tools, as well as chemoinformatics). Many new herpes inhibitors have been reported, and most of these possess novel modes of actions. Several have entered clinical evaluation, with some later discontinued because of safety issues. This chapter will describe promising drug candidates in early development that appear to act at individual steps of the viral replication cycle, and focus on those that have the most potential for success (Table 68.1).

The chemotherapy of herpes infections was markedly advanced by the discovery of the first, highly selective antiherpetic agent, acyclovir (ACV, Zovirax®; [9-(2-hydroxyethoxymethyl)guanine]) (Elion et al., 1977). Since the introduction of this agent, there has been only incremental progress in new drug approvals for the myriad of diseases caused by this family of diverse pathogens. The drugs approved since the introduction of ACV include valacyclovir (VACV, Valtrex®, the L-valine ester prodrug of ACV, penciclovir (PCV; [9-(4-hydroxy-3-hydroxymethylbutyl-1-yl) guanine]), a related nucleoside analogue with a similar basis for drug action against HSV and VZV, and its prodrug, famciclovir (FCV, Famvir®). More efficacious treatment of CMV disease was achieved with yet another guanosine analogue ganciclovir (GCV, Cymevene®, Cytovene®; 9-(1,3-dihydroxy- 2-propoxymethyl)guanine), and its recently approved prodrug, valganciclovir (Valcyte®; L-Valine, 2-[(2-amino-1,6-dihydro-6- oxo-9H-purin-9-yl)methoxy]-3-hydroxypropyl ester, monohydrochloride),. The treatment of ocular CMV infections was advanced by the antisense agent ISIS 2922 (formivirsen, Vitravene®). Broad-spectrum antiherpetics include the pyrophosphate analogue foscarnet (PFA, Foscavir®; trisodium phosphonoformate, phosphonoformic acid) and the nucleotide analogue cidofovir (CDV, HPMPC, Vistide®; (S)-1-(3-hydroxy-2-phosphonylmethoxypropyl)cytosine).

Although these agents have proven efficacious in the prophylaxis and treatment of herpes infections, there remains a need for drugs with higher potency, more rapid and durable antiviral action, more convenient dosing regimens, and importantly, fewer and less severe side effects. Because these systemic drugs ultimately target the viral DNA polymerase, and the nucleoside analogs are viral TK-dependent, cross-resistance can occur (Erice, 1999). New drugs with novel mechanisms of actions would provide valuable alternatives. Ideally, the new drug would eliminate the latent reservoir; a challenging goal since the herpesviruses have evolved complex strategies to persist under the reach of host defense mechanisms.

The drug development process: an overview

The scientific literature abounds with reports of the in vitro anti-herpetic activities of diverse organic molecules and biological products, and in many cases, the selectivity index (SI; the ratio of cellular toxicity to antiviral potency in vitro) appears promising (Snoeck et al., 2002). However, the demonstration of in vitro activity is only the first step in the long and arduous journey from the laboratory bench into the clinic (Scolnick et al., 2001). Other considerations, particularly absorption, distribution, metabolism and excretion (ADME) parameters are

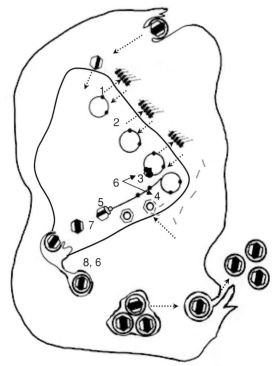

Fig. 68.1. Herpesvirus replication cycle illustrating precedented and novel drug targets (numbered) and their general stage of function in the viral replication cycle. (Adapted from Roizman et al., 1993.)

key to success. Lipinski's rule-of-five analysis (Lipinski et al., 2001) which established guidelines regarding structural properties most often associated with viable drug candidates has been embraced by the pharmaceutical industry.

The discovery and development process is slow and costly. The industry average to bring a new drug to market was estimated at over $500 million dollars for drugs introduced in 1990 and is undoubtedly higher today (Boston Consulting; Pharmaceutical R&D Costs, 1993). The time from synthesis of a new drug to regulatory approval has grown to over 14 years from an average of 8 years in the 1960s, according to analyses by the Tufts Center for the Study of Drug Development. Figure 68.2 provides a schematic review of some of the major preclinical development activities generally required to advance a drug to approval.

Historically, anti-infectives have been discovered through the screening of compound libraries directly against the replicating organism. This classic approach was used in the discovery of all the currently approved systemic antiherpetics. ACV, which was originally synthesized to potentiate the anticancer activity of the nucleoside analogue, cytosine arabinoside (Ara C), by inhibition of adenosine deaminase (the enzyme responsible for its metabolic breakdown), emerged as a potent antiherpetic during random screening in herpes simplex virus (HSV)-infected cells (Elion et al., 1977).

Screening of diverse chemical libraries in virally-infected cell cultures, although less efficient than individual enzyme or target-based screens (discussed below), provides the opportunity to identify new viral targets. Active inhibitors can then serve as laboratory tools to probe the biology of viral replicative events. The mechanisms of novel action are defined by identifying changes in the phenotype of infected, treated cells, often aided by time of inhibitor addition and withdrawal experiments. Antiviral selectivity is indicated by the ability of the virus to develop resistance to escape drug inhibition, and genetic mapping of resistance mutations identifies the viral target(s).

A second approach to the discovery of new inhibitors consists of direct screening of compounds against a catalytic enzyme or other biological function. Often screening and inhibitor optimization may be directed by structural

Table 68.1. New anti-herpes inhibitors in the discovery and development pipeline

Drug/ compound class/ chemical structure	Virus/ antiviral activity per status (early 2004)	Mechanism of action (MOA)/target gene(s)	Key reference(s)
Inhibitors of early replication events			
PD146626 (benzothiophene)	• HSV-1, IC$_{50}$ 0 ~ 0.1 µM • Cytotoxicity ≥1.0 µM (HFF) • early preclinical	• MOA unknown; MOI-dependent in vitro activity • blocks IE (VP16 and ICP0) gene expression • cell target likely no resistant virus	Boulware et al., 2001 Hamilton et al., 2002
CMV423 (tetrahydroindolizine derivative)	• CMV, HHV-6, HHV-7 • IC$_{50}$ range CMV: 0.005–0.05 µM (at low MOI) • IC$_{50}$ range HHV-6: 0.1–0.3 µM • activity cell-type dependent for HHV-6 • Preclinical	• MOA unknown; MOI-dependent in vitro activity • cell target likely: no resistant virus • host tyrosine kinase may be involved • blocks early event prior to viral DNA synthesis	Snoeck et al., 2002 DeBolle et al., 2004 Cirone et al., 1996
828, 951, and 1028 non-nucleoside pyrrolo[2,3-*d*]pyrimidines 951	• CMV • all three compounds comparable to GCV (IC$_{50}$ 0.4–1.0 µM) • early preclinical	• MOA unknown; MOI-dependent in vitro activity • blocks early event prior to viral DNA synthesis	Jacobson et al., 1999
Inhibitors of herpes DNA polymerase			
Lobucavir (LBV) (cyclobutyl guanosine analogue)	• VZV, CMV, HBV • clinical anti-CMV activity demonstrated in HIV-infected subjects • development terminated 2002.	• phosphorylated by cellular enzymes • triphosphate a potent inhibitor of CMV DNA polymerase (limits chain extension) • target gene: pol	Tenney et al., 1997 Dunkle, 1996 *Lalezari et al., 1997*

Omaciclovir (H2G)
Carbocyclic guanosine analogue
 	
Prodrug MIV-606
 	
H2G
	• VZV, HSV-1 and 2, EBV
	• More potent vs VZV than ACV
	• efficacy demonstrated in simian VZV infection in African green monkeys
	• resistance profile similar to ACV for TK- mutants
	• phase II clinical studies
		• MOA similar to ACV:
		  – substrate for VZV & HSV 1 & 2 TK
		  – competitive inhibitor of viral DNA polymerase
		• MOA differences from ACV:
		  – not an obligate chain terminator, but limits chain extension
		  – substrate for mitochondrial TK
		  – longer intracellular t$_{1/2}$ of H2G-TP
		• resistance mutations:
		  – VZV TK frameshift mutations:
		  – dels A76, G805, or A806 produce truncated polypeptide
		  – cross resistant to ACV
			Abele et al., 1991
			Soike et al., 1993
			Lowe et al., 1995
			Ng et al., 2001

(cont.)

Table 68.1. (cont.)

Drug/ compound class/ chemical structure	Virus/ antiviral activity per status (early 2004)	Mechanism of action (MOA)/target gene(s)	Key reference(s)
Alkoxyalky ester of CDV (nucleotide analogue)	• broad spectrum antiviral • herpes activity IC$_{50}$ range 0.5–30.0 μM • potential therapeutic for smallpox, rescue of herpes-resistant infections in immunocompromised • accelerated development through Phase I for smallpox	• nucleotide monophosphate, further phosphorylated by cell enzymes • competitive inhibitor of viral DNA synthesis • single point mutations in pol confer CDV-resistance	Ciesla *et al.*, 2003 De Clercq, 2002 Safrin *et al.*, 1997 Neyts *et al.*, 2004 Aldeon *et al.*, 2003 Painter and Hostetier, 2004 Kern *et al.*, 2004a

A-5021
Guanosine analogue
	• HSV-1 & 2; IC$_{50}$ range 0.013–0.15ug/ml
	• VZV IC50 ∼ 0.77 ug/ml
	• more potent vs HSV-1 than ACV in vitro and in animal models
		• MOA similar to ACV:
		  – substrate for VZV & HSV 1 & 2 TK
		  – competitive inhibitor of viral DNA polymerase
		  – longer intracellular t$_{1/2}$ of A-5021-TP vs ACV-TP
		  – not a chain terminator, but limits chain extension
		• resistance profile similar to ACV for TK mutants
			Ono *et al.*, 1998
			Iwayama *et al.*, 1998
			Iwayama *et al.*, 1999

BCNAs
bicyclic pyrimidine nucleoside analogues
	• VZV
	• highly potent at sub-nanomolar concentrations IC50 1nM10–μM
		• MOA not fully elucidated:
		  – substrate for VZV TK
		  – TK- deficient VZV also resistant to BCNAs
		  – no triphosphate detected in VZV-infected cells
			Balzarini and McGuigan, 2002
			DeClercq, 2003a,b
			McGuigan *et al.*, 2003
			Sienaert *et al.*, 2002
			Balzanini *et al.*, 2002

PNU-183792 non-nucleoside (4-oxo-DHQs) naphthalene carboxamide	• VZV, HSV, CMV, HHV8, EBV • CMV IC$_{50}$ ∼ 0.95 μM; comparable to GCV • HSV-1 & 2,VZV, HHV8 IC50 ∼3.5 μM • EBV IC50 0.17 μM • no detectable cross-resistance with approved antivirals	• inhibitor of viral DNA polymerase • competitive inhibition with the binding of natural substrate (dTTP) to the polymerase enzyme, with a low level affinity for the enzyme substrate complex that was not defined	Vaillancourt *et al.*, 2000 Oien *et al.*, 2002 Thomsen *et al.*, 2003 Wathen, 2002
Inhibitors of herpes helicase-primase			
T157602 2-aminothiazole	• HSV • IC$_{90}$ = 3 μM	• Inhibits viral DNA synthesis • stabilizes the helicase-primase complex trapping the enzyme on the DNA substrate, and blocking all activities of the complex.	Spector *et al.*, 1998

(cont.)

Table 68.1. (*cont.*)

Drug/ compound class/ chemical structure	Virus/ antiviral activity per status (early 2004)	Mechanism of action (MOA)/target gene(s)	Key reference(s)
BILS 179 BS thiazolylphenyl containing compounds	• HSV • 10-15 times more active than ACV in vitro (EC$_{50s}$ 27nM- 100nM) • Efficacy studies in animals demonstrated comparable &/or superior efficacy to ACV	• stabilizes the helicase-primase complex and DNA substrate, imposing a physical constraint both to enzyme progression (DNA-unwinding reaction), and primase catalytic activity • Resistance mutations in UL5 • Rapid selection of stable, pathogenic phenotype	Crute *et al.*, 2002 Kleyman *et al.*, 2003a,b Liuzzi *et al.*, 2004
BAY 57-1293 triazole urea compounds	• HSV IC$_{50}$ 20 nM • ~100-fold more sensitive that ACV against HSV	• inhibits viral DNA synthesis • novel mode of action inhibits the ATPase activity of the viral helicase-primase complex in a dose-dependent manner (IC$_{50}$ of 30 nM). • Resistance mutations in UL5, UL52	Kleymann *et al.*, 2002 Kleymann, 2003a Betz *et al.*, 2002
Compound 9	• CMV IC50 0.039 μM • Range of analogs 0.4 → 10 μM • Leads comparable to CDV, GCV in potency	• Inhibits viral DNA synthesis • Target; UL70 component of helicase-primase complex, based on co-IP. • Irreversible covalent binding proposed; no viral resistance genetics confirmation yet reported	Cushing *et al.*, 2006

Inhibitors of the portal protein of HSV/ viral DNA packaging

Drug/ compound class/ chemical structure	Virus/ antiviral activity per status (early 2004)	Mechanism of action (MOA)/target gene(s)	Key reference(s)
WAY 150138 benzamide thiourea compounds	• alpha herpes viruses	• inhibitor of viral DNA cleavage & packaging • target gene: HSV UL6 • resistance mutations UL6 – Glu121Asp, Ala618Val, Gln621Arg	van Zeijl *et al.*, 2000, Visalli and van Zeijl, 2003 Newcomb and Brown, 2002
Comp I N-methylbenzyl-N'-arylthiourea analogues	• VZV (IC$_{50s}$ 0.1 to 0.6 μM)	• VZV DNA cleavage and packaging is restricted via inhibition of the ORF54 gene • ORF54 resistance in 2 isolates due to changes in codons 324 & 408 in 1 isolate and codon Gly407Asp in another isolate	Visalli *et al.*, 2003 van Zeijl *et al.*, 2000 Akanitapichat and Bastow, 2002)

Hydroxyacridone derivative(s)
 	
5-chloro-1,3-dihydroxyacridone
	• HSV IC$_{50}$ ~10 μM
	• hCMV IC$_{50}$ <10 μM (multiple derivatives)
	• early preclinical
		• MOA unknown, selectivity questionable
		• diverse phenotype in treated, HSV-infected cells; reduction in:
		  – viral DNA packaging
		  – production of B capsids
		  – infectious virions
			Akanitapichat and Bastow, 2002
			Lowden and Bastow, 2003

(*cont.*)

Table 68.1. (*cont.*)

Drug/ compound class/ chemical structure	Virus/ antiviral activity per status (early 2004)	Mechanism of action (MOA)/target gene(s)	Key reference(s)
Inhibitors of the CMV terminase complex			
BAY 38-4766	• CMV • IC$_{50}$ ~1 µM • Anti CMV activity comparable to GCV in hollow fiber mouse model	• novel, late-stage inhibition of UL89 and UL56 gene products (2 subunits of the CMV terminase) • reduction in viral DNA packaging • resistance mutations in UL89, UL56	Buerger *et al.*, 2001 Reefschlaeger *et al.*, 2001 McSharry *et al.*, 2001a,b

TCRB & BDCRB benzimidazole ribosides	• CMV
	• IC$_{50}$ < 3 µM
		• inhibits viral DNA cleavage and packaging
		• target genes: UL89, UL56
		• resistance mutations:
		  – pUL89: Asp344Glu, Ala355Thr
		  – pUL56: Gln204Arg
			Townsend *et al.*, 1995
			Underwood *et al.*, 1998
			Krosky *et al.*, 1998

GW275175X B-D-ribopyranosyl derivative of BDCRB	• hCMV; IC$_{50}$ range 0.16-2.03 µM • antiviral activity similar to GCV in vitro • not active vs animal CMV; SCID hu efficacy model tested • Phase I single-dose study completed	• inhibits viral DNA cleavage and packaging • target genes UL89, UL56 • mutations conferring cross resistance: – UL89: Asp344Glu, Ala 355Thr UL56: Gln204Arg	Underwood *et al.*, 2003 Williams *et al.*, 2003 Krosky *et al.*, 1998
Inhibitors of the CMV UL97 protein kinase			
Indole carbazoles	• hCMV; IC$_{50}$ range 0.009–0.4 µM	• inhibits pUL97autophosphorylation and pUL97-dependent GCV phosphorylation • target gene UL97	Zimmermann *et al.*, 2000 Marschall *et al.*, 2001 Slater *et al.*, 1999

Maribavir, 1263W94	• CMV, IC$_{50}$ values are assay, cell-type dependent, and range from 0.08–26 µM
	• generally 3–10-fold more potent than GCV
	• EBV; IC$_{50}$ values for lytic viral DNA synthesis reduction 0.2–17 µM
		• inhibits viral DNA synthesis and nucleocapsid maturation/egress
		• target genes/resistance mutations
		  – UL97: Leu397Arg (AD169)
		  – UL27 gene: Leu335Pro (Towne), Arg233Ser (AD169), Ala406Val, Cys415 stop (AD169), Trp362Arg (AD169)
			Biron *et al.*, 2002
			Komazin *et al.*, 2003
			Chou *et al.*, 2004
			Lalezari *et al.*, 2002
			Williams *et al.*, 2003
			Ma *et al.*, 2006

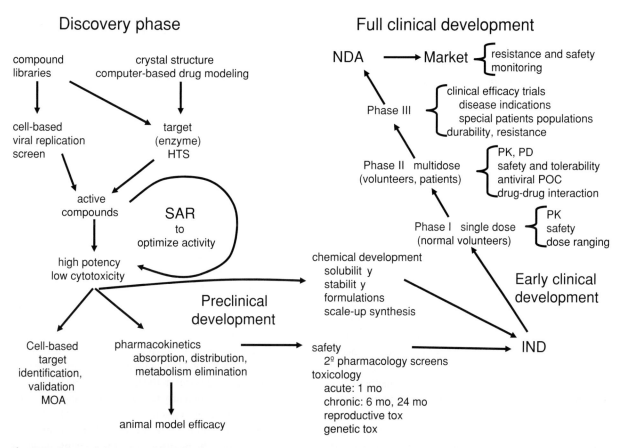

Fig. 68.2. Schematic overview of drug development process.

modeling. This approach is highly efficient, and has been particularly successful in the human immunodeficiency virus (HIV) arena, producing candidates or approved drugs targeting HIV entry, fusion, genetic integration, protease, and the HIV reverse transcriptase. Significant efforts to identify herpes protease inhibitors have not been successful to date, but direct screening of herpes DNA polymerases and the helicase-primases have produced exciting drug candidates with strong development potential.

A few principles emerge from the collective experiences in the field of antiviral drug discovery. The ideal target will be unique to the virus, or sufficiently distinct from the host cell counterparts to allow preferential inhibition, and will be essential for viral replication (in vitro for assay purposes) and for disease pathogenesis in the host. The genetic barrier to resistance will be high, and drug-resistant variants will pay a penalty in replication competence or tissue tropism. In the case of the alpha herpesviruses, drug-resistant variants will lack the ability to reactivate from latency.

An active antiviral compound must have other attributes in order to progress successfully through the drug development process. The chemical and pharmaceutical development criteria of cost-effective manufacturing, product stability, good solubility, oral bioavailability, and acceptable protein binding preclude development of high molecular weight compounds, or complex biological products, except as topical or injectable formulations. For the well-defined catalytic sites of many target enzymes, small molecule inhibitors (≤ 600 Da MW) can provide the ideal "fit." However, for the less well-defined catalytic sites of some enzymes, or the broad surfaces of protein–protein interactions (Tsai et al., 1997), larger MW inhibitors, such as protein mimetics, may be required. Protein-protein interactions comprise many opportunities for antiviral intervention, but from a pharmaceutical perspective, these remain challenging targets (Arkim and Wells, 2004).

Host cell targets as an approach to virus inhibition

Drugs that target host cellular functions have been considered as potential antiviral agents (Shugar, 1999) and the herpes virus literature documents the antiherpes activity of a variety of host cell kinase inhibitors, such as roscovitin and inhibitors of p38 and cdk-E (Schang, 2002; Schang et al., 2002; Chang, 2003). Investigators have looked at the effects of various antimetabolites on the ability of host cells to support viral replication. Although these are useful probes for discerning the contributions of host functions to viral growth, none have yet been shown to have clinical development potential as systemic therapies for the herpes diseases.

Reveratrol, a natural plant phytoalexin, was recently shown to inhibit HSV 1 and 2 replication early in the infection cycle by inhibition of ICP-4 (Docherty et al., 1999). The mechanism may not directly involve a virus target, but could have application as a topical agent similar to the anti-inflammatory effect of n-docosanol 10% cream (Abreva®). One category of host targets which may be fruitful for the development of novel therapeutics that deserves mention here are immune response modulators. The herpes viruses have developed multiple ways to evade the host's innate immunity and to block antigen presentation required for the adaptive immune responses. Thus, agents which protect or augment host defense mechanisms by interfering with viral immune evasion functions may provide additional tools in disease management. Such agents could complement antiviral drugs and may potentiate vaccine efficacy (Miller et al., 2002). For example, Imiquimod, an immune response modifier approved for the topical treatment of external genital and perianal warts, has recently been shown to be an agonist to the toll-like receptor 7 (TLR-7) (Hemmi et al., 2002). The related analog, resiquimod, has also been shown to have immunomodulatory properties and efficacy as a topical therapeutic agent in genital HSV-2 infections models (Bernstein et al., 2001; Miller et al., 2002). TRL-7 may be involved in the induction of cytokines, especially alpha interferon, and other antiviral effector molecules which may enhance cell mediated immunity (Wang et al., 2005). Moreover, Imiquimod has also been shown to have potent adjuvant/priming properties in several vaccine models (Rechtsteiner et al., 2005; Thomsen et al., 2004). Several candidate TLR agonists, plus other immunomodulatory agents are in development for various viral diseases, but will not be discussed further.

Antiviral targets in early replication events

In principle, an inhibitor that blocks the very earliest steps in the invasion of a cell by a virus should effectively restrict the spread of infection and could also serve as a prophylactic agent. However, inhibition of herpes viral attachment and uncoating may not be feasible, since there are no unique, restrictive mechanisms for herpes entry that could be exhaustively (and presumably safely) disabled.

This is in contrast to the prospects for the antagonist of the CCR5 host receptor element required for HIV infection (Baba et al., 1999), the recently approved HIV fusion inhibitor (LaBranchea et al., 2001) in HIV infection, and the rhinovirus uncoating blocker (Diana et al., 1987).

Immediate early gene (IE) expression or the transactivation functions of their products could after the earliest replication events for intervention, and their inhibition should effectively restrict productive viral infections and potentially decrease reactivation from latency. However, since the transcription of viral genes and the viral-mediated transactivation intimately involve host transcriptional machinery and factors, selectively would be difficult to attain.

Three or four series of compounds with designated early modes of action have emerged from cell-based screening programs. Time-of-addition studies or quantitation of viral transcription and translation indicated that these classes of compounds acted after the adsorption phase of HSV or CMV infection but before viral DNA synthesis. Two striking features of their mechanism of action (MOA) were common to these agents: their in vitro potency was compromised by increased multiplicity of infection (MOI), and the investigators were unable to select resistant viruses, despite repeated attempts to passage virus in the presence of the inhibitors. These features, particularly the latter, are consistent with inhibition of a cellular target. In the case of CMV423 (see below), the inhibition of a host protein kinase is demonstrated. Although the in vitro SIs for these agents indicate at least a preferential inhibition of viral growth, drug development potential of these compounds is doubtful. They will be briefly described.

PD146626

The activity of the benzothiophene class was identified in a random compound screening program. The lead compound, PD146626 (9-(methyloxy)-3,4-dihydro[1]benzothieno[2,3-f][1,4]thiazepin-5(2H)-one), was shown to inhibit HSV type 1 (HSV-1) replication by blocking immediate early viral gene expression, specifically VP16 and ICP0 expression. However, viruses deleted for the VP16 and ICP0 loci ("knock-out" viruses) lacked resistance to PD146626, and the compound showed apparent anti-viral activity against CMV, which lacks VP16 and ICP0 homologues. Moreover, PD146626 could exert this inhibitory effect in cells pretreated before viral infection, or in cells treated with only short exposures (up to 2 hours) during viral infection. Thus, PD146626 apparently targets a cellular function critical for the expression of HSV-1 immediate early genes (Boulware et al., 2001). Extensive SAR studies that focused on stereospecific substitution on the diazepine ring and optimal nitrogen substitution achieved striking improvements as evidenced by a 2-log enhancement in potency and a 3-log improvement in therapeutic index. However, in vivo efficacy could not be determined due to metabolic issues, and thus the safety consequences of this inhibitory mechanism remains to be determined (Hamilton et al., 2002).

Non-nucleoside pyrrolopyrimidines 828, 951, and 1028
Three structurally distinct analogues in a series of non-nucleoside pyrrolo[2,3-D]pyrimidines emerged from a cell-based screening program (Jacobson et al., 1999). At low MOIs compounds 828, 951, and 1028 all showed potency comparable to that of GCV. One of these compounds, 828, was tested for toxicity and shown to be less toxic against human bone marrow progenitor cells than GCV, a key improvement.

CMV423
Perhaps the best-studied agent with activity early in the herpes life cycle is CMV423, 2-chloro-3-pyridin-3-yl-5,6,7,8- tetrahydroindolizine-1-carboxamide. This tetrahydroindolizine derivative is active against CMV, HHV-6, and HHV-7 at low concentrations, but shows only modest activity against HSV-1 and -2 and none against varicella-zoster virus (VZV) (Snoeck et al., 2002; De Bolle, 2004). The synergistic activity against CMV observed when CMV423 was combined with GCV, PFA, or CDV suggested that CMV423 was inhibiting a different step in viral replication, most likely an earlier one, than these DNA polymerase inhibitors. A series of studies aimed at defining the point of inhibition, using the low multiplicity of infection (MOI) multi-cycle format and probing for the expression of the IE (immediate early) and E (early) antigens showed transient reductions in the levels of IE antigen detectable on days 1 and again on days 4 and 5, in concert with first- and second- round of viral replication. Interestingly, CMV423 was able to block substantial expression of IE antigen at the viral input of 0.1 PFU/cell, an MOI at which antiviral activity is lost, indicating that low IE expression is sufficient to overcome the block to replication. This result suggests that any drug directed against the CMV IE gene would have to be almost 100% effective to produce the desired virus suppression.

Further work on the mechanism of inhibition of human herpesvirus (HHV)-6 replication again pointed to a cell target, as inhibition occurred in a cell-line dependent fashion (De Bolle et al., 2004). The molecular target in HHV-6 is most likely a different early event, occurring before viral DNA synthesis but after IE antigen production. Based on the similarity of the action of herbimycin, which is known to inhibit cellular tyrosine kinase activity through binding to heat shock protein (Cirone et al., 1996) and to block infection of human T lymphoid cells by HHV-6, the antiviral action of CMV423 is likely to be mediated through inhibition of a host cell tyrosine kinase. Preclinical safety and pharmacokinetic studies on this interesting inhibitor continue (Aventis, data on file; Bournique et al., 2001). The clinical relevance of the MOI-dependence, and the safety margin with host inhibitory mechanisms, remain to be determined.

ISIS 13312
One very specific and clinically validated inhibitor of CMV IE gene expression is the approved anti-sense agent formivirsen (ISIS 2922, Vitravene®). Its utility is greatly limited due to the need for monthly intravitreal injections, and the occurrence of adverse ocular reactions. ISIS 13312, an analogue of ISIS 2922, has been shown to have a longer half-life than ISIS 2922 (approximately 2 months in monkey retina) and could provide the advantage of less frequent dosing (Henry et al., 2001). However, ISIS 13312 is not currently in clinical development.

Antiviral targets in the herpesvirus DNA replication complex

The six or seven essential proteins that comprise the herpes viral DNA replication machinery offer several attractive enzyme targets for drug development, as well as some of the more challenging protein-protein interactions (Matthews et al., 1993; Anders and McCue, 1996; Loregian and Coen, 2006). These components of the HSV replication machinery include the single-stranded DNA binding protein (ICP8, pUL29), the polymerase accessory factor (pUL42), the helicase-primase complex (pUL5, pUL8, pUL 52) and the viral DNA polymerase (pUL30). HSV requires an origin-binding protein specifically (pUL9). These proteins work in concert, are co-localized within specific intranuclear structures, and are found in association with other viral and host proteins involved in the replication cycle events. In principle, points of antiviral intervention could include those that affect protein recruitment and transport (post-translational modification), the sequentially–ordered protein–protein binding events in replisome assembly, and the individual catalytic functions of the enzymes involved in the DNA synthetic process.

The direct inhibition of the DNA polymerase function through nucleoside/nucleotide substrate analogues or pyrophosphate mimics, such as seen with the ACV, GCV, and PFA, is a clinically-validated approach. Discovery efforts continue to exploit this well-validated target, usually in concert with the viral encoded nucleoside kinase for added selectivity in the monophosphorylation step (or also including thymidylate kinase activity). Successful inhibition of the HIV RT through non-catalytic mechanisms (non-nucleotide reverse transcriptase inhibitors such as nevarapine and efaverenz) have prompted the search for similar agents in herpes discovery screening programs. Representatives in both these categories are in advanced preclinical or early clinical testing. Also in the pipeline are agents that interfere with the function of the helicase primase complex (Fig. 68.3).

Herpesvirus DNA polymerase inhibitors

The herpes virus DNA polymerase is a multifunctional enzyme that possesses both a deoxynucleotide polymerizing activity and a 3′–5′ exonuclease proofreading function, and the structure of the herpes virus replicating complex has been modeled (Franklin et al., 2001). The polymerase polypeptide shares regions of sequence similarity with the catalytic subunits of other alpha – like DNA polymerases of eukaryotes (Braithwaite and Ito, 1991). The conserved regions involved in substrate recognition within the polymerase have been determined by comparative modeling with the Klenow polymerase, and by genetic analysis of mutants resistant to nucleoside/nucleotide analogs (Gibbs et al., 1998; Larder et al., 1987). These regions (I, II, III, V, VII and the delta *region C) are non-contiguous, indicating the broad areas of contact across the polymerase polypeptide during the catalytic polymerization process. The ability of an inhibitor to interfere with correct folding through binding outside of the catalytic sites could impair enzyme function, although mutational escape may be more feasible, based on precedence in the HIV NNRTI series (Spence et al., 1995).

Nucleoside/nucleotide analogue inhibitors

The apparent tolerance of the herpes DNA polymerases for modified acyclic and carbocyclic sugar moieties, exemplified by ACV, GCV, and PCV, drove additional exploration in the purine nucleoside series during the late 1980s and the early 1990s. The discovery of oxetanocins with the structural characteristic of two hydroxymethyl groups located on a rigid 4-membered ring led to the synthesis and antiviral evaluation of a number of related compounds and investigation of their antiviral properties (Sakuma et al., 1991; Sekiyama et al., 1998). Compounds in the oxytanocin series of base analogues, characterized by a carbocyclic sugar moiety, were investigated and showed broad-spectrum activity against the herpesviruses.

Lobucavir

Lobucavir, (R)-9-[4-hydroxy-2-(hydroxymethyl)butyl] guanine], (LBV, cygalovir, BMS 180194), a cyclobutyl analogue of guanine arose from the oxytanocin series and was advanced through early clinical evaluations (Yang et al., 1996a, b). The ultimate outcome serves to illustrate the risks associated with the discovery and development process.

LBV has antiviral activity against HIV, hepatitis B virus, and most herpesviruses, and the triphosphate of LBV is a potent inhibitor of hCMV DNA polymerase in vitro. However, Tenney et al. (1997) showed that this nucleoside analogue is phosphorylated intracellularly to its triphosphate form in both infected and uninfected cells, with phosphorylated metabolite levels only two- to three-fold higher in CMV-infected cells compared to uninfected cells. The lack of selective anabolism in virally infected cells (a factor contributing to the broad antiviral activity) provides the potential for substrate utilization by host cell DNA polymerases with corresponding safety risks.

LBV was advanced to the clinic. Preliminary human data showed a dose-related anti-CMV effect (Dunkle, 1996). A clinical study in HIV- and CMV-co-infected patients demonstrated a 50% reduction in CMV viruria and a greater than 1 log reduction in HIV viral load from semen at the highest dose. Side effects were dose-related, and included mild to moderate diarrhea and nausea in 10%–20%, and 7%–12% of recipients respectively (Lalezari et al., 1997).

Despite promising early clinical results, an international Phase III study of LBV as therapy for hepatitis B was suspended in February 1999 due to safety concerns. Toxicologic studies in rodents had suggested increased incidence of stomach, vaginal and cervical cancers with long-term exposure.

Omaciclovir H2G and its pro-drug

Another carbocyclic guanosine analogue, H2G, (R)-9-[4-hydroxy-2-(hydroxymethyl)butyl]guanine (omaciclovir), was shown to be a potent broad-spectrum antiherpes agent especially active against VZV (Abele et al., 1991). The MOA is similar to that of ACV, with less selectivity as a substrate for TK. Resistance mechanisms at the TK locus overlap with those of ACV (Ng et al., 2001). H2G is not an obligate chain terminator, although once incorporated, H2G-MP will only support limited chain elongation (Lowe et al., 1995). The triphosphate of H2G has a considerably longer intracellular half-life in infected cells than does ACV-triphosphate (Lowe et al., 1995), a feature that could provide dosing advantages over VACV if clinically validated. Preclinical efficacy studies in the simian varicella model indicated superior potency over ACV (Soike et al., 1993). However, species-specific differences in metabolism of ACV make such comparisons misleading. ACV oral bioavailability is lower in monkeys than in humans, and the higher aldehyde oxidase levels in monkeys result in faster metabolic clearance in monkeys than in humans, dogs, and rodents (de Miranda and Burnette 1994; de Miranda and Good, 1992).

MIV-606

(ABT-606; [L-valine-(2-hydroxy-4-hydroxymethyl-butylyl) guanine]) is a prodrug of H2G that significantly enhances its oral bioavailability. MIV-606 is quickly converted to H2G, with undetectable concentration of parent prodrug MIV-606 (Medivir AB, Huddinge Sweden, unpublished data). – Three phase I studies with a total of more than 100 volunteers, including subjects 65 years of age and older, demonstrated that MIV-606 was safe and well tolerated after multiple dosing up to total daily doses of 1500 mg.

A phase II study comparing 250, 500, and 750 mg twice daily of MIV-606 with 800 mg five times a day of ACV in zoster patients has also been completed. Trial results suggested equivalent or superior efficacy of MIV-606, compared to ACV, at significantly lower doses. If this claim can translate into an improved therapeutic effect of MIV-606 at a more convenient dose, it could provide enough improvement over current therapies to justify further development. Availability of MIV-606 could potentially lead to much wider treatment of zoster, and the broad spectrum of action could benefit patients with compromised immune function, such as transplant recipients, cancer patients, and AIDS patients (Medivir AB, Huddinge Sweden, unpublished data).

Alkoxyalkyl esters of cidofovir (CDV)

CDV is a nucleotide (monophosphate) analog with broad spectrum anti-herpes activity that is licensed for the intravenous treatment of CMV retinitis in HIV-infected patients. CDV is phosphorylated by cellular enzymes, and the CDV-diphosphate (DP) is a competitive inhibitor of viral DNA polymerase (Safrin *et al.*, 1997). Mechanistically, CDV-DP inhibits many viral DNA polymerases, and recent studies document activity against pox viral infections (Neyts *et al.*, 2004; De Clercq, 2002). In CMV, resistance to CDV can arise from single point mutations in the polymerase locus, usually mapping to the exonuclease functional domains (Chou *et al.*, 2003).

CDV exhibits a number of drawbacks that greatly limit its utility as an anti-herpetic agent. Oral bioavailability is low (<5%) requiring IV administration, usually on a weekly or semi-weekly basis, and dose-dependent nephrology may require pre-hydration, dose reduction and/or co-treatment with probenecid. Other safety liabilities were documented in preclinical toxicology studies Vistide® [package insert], Gilead Sciences, 1999.

Prodrug strategies, accelerated by the threats of bioterrorism, have been employed to increase oral bioavailability and improve the safety profile of CDV (Huggins *et al.*, 2002). The basic prodrug design exploited a natural fatty acid (lysophosphatidylcholine) molecule as carrier to facilitate drug absorption in the gastrointestinal tract. The lipid ester conjugates were much more active in vitro (EC_{50} values at least 100-fold lower) than CDV or cyclic CDV against a range of herpes viruses, including strains of HSV, VZV, CMV, EBV, HHV-6, and HHV-8. SAR of the ether lipid ester analogs defined a 20 atom optimum for alkyl chain length, and explored the nature of the linker group (Williams-Aziz *et al.*, 2005). Consistent with the observed increase in antiviral potency of the 1-O-hexadecyloxypropyl conjugate of CDV in cell culture, studies with radiolabelled compound confirmed increased cell penetration (10–20 fold) and higher intracellular levels (100-fold) of the active antiviral form CDV-DP than those measured in cells treated with CDV parent drug (Aldern *et al.*, 2003).

These lipid carrier prodrugs showed significant advantages over CDV in several in vivo models of murine and human CMV (Bidanset *et al.*, 2004; Kern *et al.*, 2004a; Wan *et al.*, 2005; Kern *et al.*, 2004b). Higher levels of protection were also achieved with the CDV oral prodrugs in a lethal cowpox challenge model (Huggins, 2002). Studies evaluating the oral bioavailability and tissue distribution of ^{14}C-labeled hexadecyloxypropyl-cidofovir (HDP-CDV), octadecyloxyethyl-cidofovir (ODP-CDV), and oleyloxypropyl-cidofovir (OLP-CDV) in female NIH Swiss mice demonstrated that these alkoxyalkyl esters are highly orally bioavailable (88–97%) and do not concentrate in the kidney (Ciesla *et al.*, 2003). Thus these compounds may avoid the dose-limiting toxicity of CDV, if these results translate into the clinic.

The lead compound, CMX001, will be progressed through phase I safety and pharmacokinetic studies in humans for potential use as a smallpox treatment or vaccine rescue (Painter and Hostetler, 2004). Such a therapeutic could also provide a safer salvage therapy for ACV or GCV resistant viruses in immunocompromised patients with life-threatening herpes infections.

This prodrug strategy was successfully applied to another nucleotide phosphonate 9-(S)-(3-Hydroxy-2-phosphonomethoxypropyl)adenine [(S)-HPMPA] with a similar enhancement of in vitro antiviral potency (Beadle *et al.*, 2006).

A-5021

Armed with structure activity relationship (SAR) clues from the crystal structure of the HSV-1 TK complexed with GCV (Brown *et al.*, 1995), and substrate potency comparisons with ACV, PCV, H2G and the oxytanocins, the scientists at Ajinomoto set out to design a novel series of nucleoside analogues. Extensive exploration of the side chain conformation and enantiomeric specificity in the oxytanocin series lead to the identification of potent activity in a compound with a cyclopropyl sugar (Sekiyama et al., 1998). The lead molecule in this series, **A-5021**, (1'S,2'R)-9-{[1',2'-bis(hydroxymethyl)cycloprop-1'-yl]methyl}guanine, showed superior in vitro potency over the gold standards ACV or PCV against HSV-1 and VZV in vitro; however, the difference for HSV-2 was only marginal (Iwayama et al., 1998). The compound was also active against EBV and HHV-6, but not HHV-8 (Neyts et al., 2001). Since HSV-2 infection remains the most prevalent disease worldwide, A-5021 must show other development advantages over ACV, VACV and FCV to warrant the time and development investment for the genital herpes indications.

The mechanism of action of A-5021 was investigated (Ono et al., 1998) and found to be qualitatively similar to that of ACV and PCV. A-5021 is anabolized to the monophosphate by the herpes TK enzymes and to the diphosphate by GMP kinase, as is ACV-MP. Levels of A-5021 triphosphate accumulating in HSV-1 or VZV-infected cells were higher than those for ACV-TP, but were roughly comparable to PCV-TP levels. The intracellular half life of A-5021-TP was longer than that of ACV-TP, but somewhat shorter than that of PCV-TP. However, ACV-TP had the most potency at the level of HSV DNA polymerase inhibition, with A-5021-TP intermediate in potency. Incorporation studies showed A-5201-MP could be incorporated into a growing DNA chain, although subsequent chain elongation was inefficient. The anti-HSV-1 and -2 activities were shown to be potentiated in vitro by the immunosuppressive agent mycophenolate mofetil, a finding consistent with the mechanism of competitive inhibition of GTP incorporation, since this agent is known to cause a reduction in cell dGTP pools (Neyts and De Clercq, 2001). A disadvantage of A-5021 is the likely cross-resistance with the most prevalent phenotype of ACV-resistant HSV, the TK-deficient phenotype.

A series of in vitro and in vivo studies suggested potential advantages of A-5021 over ACV for infections mediated by HSV-1. A-5021 exhibited more prolonged antiviral action than did ACV after short exposure of infected cells in vitro. This superior potency and durability carried over into several animal models of HSV-1 infection (Iwayama et al., 1999). In a comparison using once-a-day oral administration with equivalent 25 mg doses, A-5021 demonstrated advantages over ACV in reducing the severity in HSV-1 cutaneous lesions. While the oral bioavailability and AUC of A-5021 is approximately half that of ACV, the superior in vitro potency and the prolonged effect contributed to better efficacy in this cutaneous HSV-1 murine infection model. When initiation of therapy by the intravenous route (100 mg/kg) was delayed to day 4 postinfection, A-5021 again was more effective in diminishing disease spread than ACV or PCV.

A-5021 treatment also resulted in a complete survival of mice infected intracerebrally with HSV-1 after IV dosing with 25 mg/kg A-5021 TID, compared to only 50% survival at 100 mg/kg IV ACV TID dosing (Iwayama et al., 1999). The levels of A-5021 in the brain were not presented. Higher uptake of antiviral agent into the infected organ could be a major factor in the superior efficacy of A-5021 in this model, and a clear advantage of A-5021 over ACV, which has limited ability to penetrate the blood-brain barrier (de Miranda and Good, 1982).

In another variation of time of addition and withdrawal treatments in the animal model, high dose intrapertional (ip) infection of SCID mice was followed by once daily subcutaneous treatment (50 mg/kg). After 4 days of treatment, initiated at 1 hour, or 1 or 2 days post-infection, the delay in mortality and ultimate number of survivors was far greater in the A-5021 treated groups than in the ACV-treated groups (Neyts et al., 2001). No pharmacokinetic information was provided to allow comparisons of actual systemic exposures.

In contrast to the superior performance of A-5021 against the gold standard of ACV in all the HSV-1 infection models, the efficacy of A-5021 was not distinguished from that of PCV in a model of systemic infection with HSV-2 (Iwayama et al., 1999).

A-5021 has entered clinical development. It remains to be seen if the advantages in potency and duration of antiviral effects seen in cell culture and animal models will translate into superior efficacy in the various HSV and VZV disease indications. The ophthalmic use for herpetic keratitis is under development. Another proposed clinical application would be its use in gene therapy approaches to cancer, utilizing the HSV-1 TK vectors, since A-5021 is less cytotoxic than GCV, which is currently used (Hasegawa et al., 2000).

BCNA compounds

A new structural class of bicyclic furo pyrimidines (BCNAs) have recently been discovered that demonstrate both highly specific and selective anti-VZV in vitro activity (Balzarini and McGuigan, 2002; McGuigan et al., 2003; De Clercq, 2003a,b). The starting point for these compounds was BVDU, ((E)-5-(2-bromovinyl)-2'-deoxyuridine), which was established in the early 1980s as having good antiviral activity but low selectivity. The BCNAs are characterized by a long alkyl or alkylaryl side-chain at the base moiety that may be responsible for both their antiviral properties and their lipophilic properties. The compounds are highly potent at sub-nanomolar concentrations, and cytotoxicity has not been observed at high micromolar concentrations.

The MOA has not been fully elucidated, but the compounds lose their antiviral activity against TK-deficient VZV strains, demonstrating that phosphorylation by the VZV-encoded TK is essential. Kinetic studies with purified enzymes revealed that the compounds were indeed a substrate for VZV TK, which is able to phosphorylate the BCNA compounds to both their corresponding 5'-mono and -diphosphate derivatives; a factor in their anti-VZV selectivity. Another indication of the unusual selectivity of this class of nucleoside analogs was the lack of substrate recognition by cellular kinases which contribute to the anabolism of other pyrimidine analogs; the cytosolic or mitochondrial TKs, cyrosolic dTMP kinase, and most striking, nucleoside diphosphate kinase, the host enzyme which converts BVDU-DP to the active triphosphate form. Consistent with this observation, no 5-triphosphate of BCNA could be detected in VZV-infected cells (Sienaert et al., 2002). Information on the inhibitory effects of BCNA anabolites on the VZV DNA polymerase is not yet available.

There is no clear cut correlation between their affinity for VZV TK and the antiviral potency of the compounds, indicating that an additional SAR is likely (Balzarini and McGuigan, 2002). The closely related Simian varicella virus (SVV) is not sensitive to BCNA although in vitro studies indicate that SVV TK is able to phosphorylate BCNAs. Unfortunately this precludes the utility of the SVV animal model in the therapeutic development of BCNAs (Sienaert et al., 2004).

The BCNAs are highly stable and not liable to breakdown by nucleoside/nucleobase catabolic enzymes (Balzarini et al., 2002). The fact that they are not susceptible to degradation by thymidine phosphorylase and that they do not inhibit dihydropyrimidine dehydrogenase are key improvements over BVDU. Further clinical development is anticipated.

Non-nucleotide inhibitors
PNU-26730
In an effort to identify non-substrate inhibitors of the herpes polymerase with broad-spectrum activity, Pharmacia researchers set up herpes polymerase-based screens and tested 80 000 representatives of different compound diversity. Selectivity was achieved by secondary evaluation of hits against the mammalian DNA polymerases alpha, gamma and delta. The systematic discovery program identified the activity of the naphthalene carboxamide series, exemplified by the initial active compound, PNU-26730 (Vaillancourt et al., 2000). Further optimization in this series led to a quinolone ring substitution and the 4-hydroxyquinoline-3-carboxamides series. Increased potency against the CMV, HSV-1 and VZV DNA polymerases was achieved by adding substitutions at the 6 position on the quinolone ring yielding the 4-oxo-dihydroquinolines (4-oxo-DHQs) series of compounds. These compounds, represented by PNU-182171 and PNU-183792, were also more active than the initial lead and the gold standard ACV against VZV and CMV, but showed no enhanced activity against HSV-1 or 2. These 4-oxo-DHQs were not active against other RNA and DNA virus tested: vaccinia, SV-40, adenovirus, HBV, influenza A, coxsackie B or VSV. (Brideau et al., 2002; Knechtel et al., 2002; Wathen, 2002).

PNU-183792
One of the 4-oxo-DHQ compounds, PNU-183792 (N-(4-cholorobenzyl)-1-methyl-6-(4-morpholinylmethyl)-4-oxo-1,4 dihydro-3-quinolinecarboxamide) was selected for additional investigations. Efficacy studies in a murine model of lethal MCMV infection showed antiviral activity similar to GCV when treatment was initiated up to 24 hours post infection, but was less efficacious at comparable doses given 48 hours postinfection (Brideau et al., 2002). Other properties required for a drug candidate were demonstrated: for example, PNU-183792 was orally bioavailable in dogs and rodents, achieving concentrations above the IC_{50}, with reasonable rates of clearance and a half life of 3 hours in dogs. The important measure of available drug levels is at the intracellular site of action, and although this information was not published for PNU-183792, it is likely to be similar to the actual plasma concentrations. Nucleoside and nucleotide analogues may have an advantage over non-nucleoside inhibitors of DNA polymerase in this regard, as the $t_{1/2}$ of the triphosphate active form anabolized within the cell compartment can exceed plasma levels of unchanged drug.

The strong correlation between polymerase inhibition and viral replication inhibition in the analogue series supports inhibition of viral DNA polymerase as the MOA (Fig. 68.3). Further mechanistic studies into the nature of the polymerase inhibition showed competition with the binding of natural substrate (dTTP) to the polymerase enzyme, with a low-level affinity for the enzyme substrate complex that was not defined. Points of drug interaction with target protein were characterized by resistant virus bearing point mutation(s) in the DNA polymerase gene (Oien et al., 2002; Thomsen et al., 2003).

This promising class of compounds will be active against the drug-resistant TK variants of HSV and VZV, and the current in vitro profile shows activity against clinically relevant HSV and CMV polymerase mutants (Thomsen et al., 2003). This profile is consistent with this class of compounds interacting at a different molecular site in the polymerase polypeptide.

Information on the current development status is limited since Pharmacia was purchased by Pfizer. The selectivity screens have reduced the likelihood of mechanism-based toxicity within the series leads; and the safety profile will be defined by full in vivo toxiologic studies. Other key questions with this type of molecule and the nature of the MOA will be potency compared to valacyclovir or famciclovir, durability of action (related to frequency of dosing), and the ease of viral escape (resistance).

Herpes helicase-primase inhibitors

Efforts to identify drugs targeting other components of the DNA replication complex have focused on another enzyme, the helicase-primase (Hall and Matson, 1999). In the herpesviruses, the helicase-primase complex consists of 3 proteins that associate as a trimeric complex to carry out the essential tasks of unwinding the dsDNA in the 5′ to 3′ direction, RNA polymerase activity and ssDNA-stimulated ATPase activities (Crute and Lehman, 1991; Parry et al., 1993). In HSV, these are the gene products of UL5, UL8, and UL52 ORFs. The drug candidates recently identified from screens targeting helicase-primase represent the next generation, and an exciting new class of antiviral agents. The major unknowns with this MOA include the ease of emergence of resistance in the clinic, and the pathogenicity (including reactivation) and transmission of potential of resistant virus.

T157602

The scientists at Tularik Inc. screened a library of >190,000 samples consisting of small organic molecules and natural products, using a novel filtration assay for the detection of the helicase DNA unwinding activity (Sivaraja et al., 1998). The most active selective compound was a 2-aminothiazole compound, T157602 (Spector et al., 1998). Preliminary MOA studies suggested that T157602 stabilized the helicase-primase complex, effectively trapping the enzyme on the DNA substrate and blocking all 3 activities of the complex (Fig. 68.3). The compound was a reversible inhibitor ($IC_{50} = 5$ μM), of the helicase activity of the HSV UL5/8/52 complex, but was less active against other helicases, and could also interfere with primase activity at higher concentrations ($IC_{50} = 20$ μM).

Strains of HSV-1 and HSV-2 resistant to T157602 that were selected in the laboratory carried individual point mutations in the UL5 viral gene that resulted in amino acid substitutions in the corresponding UL5 protein. Marker transfer studies confirmed the role of these genetic changes in the resistance phenotype, both at the level of the UL5 enzyme subunit and of mutant virus. Animal-model efficacy studies were not reported for this series.

In vitro cytotoxic studies revealed no apparent cellular toxicities at concentrations exceeding 100 μM, indicating a therapeutic window greater than 30-fold. However, as of 2003, the 2-aminothiazole compounds are no longer included in the Tularik development pipeline, suggesting safety deficiencies arose during the phase I/II clinical studies.

BILS 179 BS

Related compounds with more potent helicase-primase activity emerged from enzyme-based screens at Boehringer Ingelheim (Crute et al., 2002) and cell-based viral replication screens at Bayer AG (Kleymann et al., 2002). The thiazolylphenyl-containing compounds represented by BILS 179 BS inhibited all three enzyme activities of the HSV helicase-primase complex at 100 nM or lower concentrations. The antiviral activity was specific for HSV, with no activity against VZV, and human or murine CMV. Preliminary data suggest that the mechanism of inhibition involves a stabilization of the interaction between the enzyme complex and the DNA substrate, most likely by imposing a physical constraint both to enzyme progression through the DNA-unwinding reaction and to primase catalytic activity (Fig. 68.3).

Resistant viruses were selected by serial passage in BILS 179 BS for more definitive MOA studies. Helicase-primase purified from cells infected with these resistant viruses demonstrated decreased inhibition in an in vitro DNA-dependent ATPase assay that corresponded with antiviral activity. Single base pair mutations clustered in the N-terminus of the UL5 gene that resulted in single amino acid changes in the UL5 protein were identified by marker transfer and DNA sequence analysis. These results were consistent with helicase-primase inhibitor activity mediated through specific interaction with the UL5 protein (Liuzzi et al., 2004).

BILS 179 BS was 10–15 times more active than ACV in vitro ($EC_{50}s$ 27 nM–100 nM). Cytotoxicity effects were somewhat dependent on cell type, and additional experiments are needed to better clarify the cytotoxicity profile of these compounds. Efficacy studies were conducted

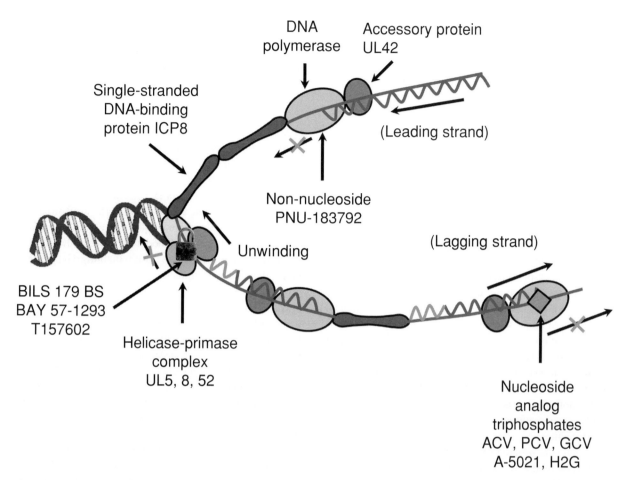

Fig. 68.3. HSV DNA replication targets. (Adapted from Crumpacker and Schaffer, 2002.)

in murine models of primary cutaneous and genital disease, using ACV as the treatment comparator (Crute *et al.*, 2002). In the cutaneous model of progressive zosterform disease (hairless SKH-1 mouse infected with HSV-1 strain KOS), BILS 179 BS demonstrated comparable efficacy to ACV when treatment was initiated 3 hours post infection (1 × or 4 × daily). However, BILS 179 BS was superior to ACV when treatment frequency was reduced, or when initial treatment was delayed by 65 hours.

Comparable results were evident in the genital disease model (Swiss Webster mice vaginally infected with HSV-2 strain HG-52). Efficacy was based on a composite disease severity scoring system that included mortality. Again, BILS 179 BS had similar efficacy to ACV when treatment was initiated at 3 hours (1 × or 4 × daily), and superior efficacy when treatment frequency was reduced or when initial treatment was delayed by 65 hours. Actual drug exposures were not reported for these studies; however, BILS 179 BS was reportedly bioavailable, and on a weight-dosing basis, BILS 179

BS showed superior activity to ACV. Disappointing findings from a drug development perspective included the identification of pre-existing resistant variants within the wild type virus population, and rapid selection of highly resistant growth-competent viruses in vitro that maintained a stable drug-resistant phenotype in the absence of drug. Of more clinical relevance was the demonstration that two resistant strains studied were fully competent for disease pathogenesis (by cutaneous or intracerebral routes in mice), and for reactivation from latency in an ocular infection model (Liuzzi *et al.*, 2004). By contrast, ACV-resistant strains of HSV were generally less virulent in various infection models. This safety feature is based on the biology of HSV, and the mechanism of action of the drug ((Elion *et al.*, 1977). ACV resistant clinical isolates are generally TK-deficient, and as a consequence less pathogenic in the immune competent population and less competent for reactivation from latency (recurrences are ACV-susceptible). The potential for transmission of drug-resistant strains into the general population is a public health consideration and requires careful monitoring (Shin et al., 2001; Bacon et al., 2003). The clinical development timetable for this compound is unknown at this time (mid 2006).

BAY 57-1293

The Bayer discovery program used a fluorometric high-throughput screening assay that identified inhibition in any target essential for viral replication in cell culture. Over 400,000 compounds were tested at 10 μM, and several compound classes with activity were identified (Kleymann, 2003 a,b). The triazole urea class of analogues was selected for additional study. Profiling and modeling techniques were employed, and optimization to improve the solubility led to the 2-pyridyl substituent in the para position of the phenyl ring in the lead compound to create BAY 57-1293 (N-[5-(aminosulfonyl)-4-methyl-1,3-thiazol-2-yl]-N-methyl-2-[4-(2-pyridinyl)phenyl]acetamide). BAY 57-1293 inhibited the replication of HSV type 1 and 2 in Vero cells (IC_{50} of 20nM) with a selectivity index of 2,500; ACV had an IC_{50} of 1 μM and a selectivity index of 250 under comparable conditions. There was no appreciable activity against VZV or CMV. BAY 57-1293 was equally active against ACV-resistant TK or polymerase mutants, and the activity was irrespective of cell type (Kleymann et al., 2002). The in vitro replication block was reversible upon drug removal, and significant activity was still demonstrated when added late post infection.

Researchers selected virus resistant to each of the three analogues in the series. Resistance resulted from point mutations in UL5 (present in all six resistant strains), or in one case, a UL5 mutation together with a point mutation in UL52. These mutations in UL5 were clustered between nucleotides 1045 to 1077, a region that corresponds to the amino acids from 349 to 359 involved in the alpha helicase region that is most homologous across the herpesviridae (Kleymann et al., 2002). BAY 57-1293 inhibits the ATPase activity of the viral helicase-primase complex in a dose-dependent manner (IC_{50} of 30 nM).

The treatment potential of BAY57-1293 was investigated in several cutaneous and systemic animal models of disease (Betz et al., 2002). The activities of orally administered BAY 57-1293 for the treatment of acute HSV-1 and HSV-2 infections were assessed in a widely-used murine lethal challenge model of disseminated herpes. Mice were infected intranasally and treated, starting 6 hours later for 5 consecutive days, three times a day. BAY 57-1293 and comparator drugs (ACV, GCV, VACV, FCV, Brivudin) were tested in escalating doses, and ED50 (dose at which 50% of the infected animals survive) values calculated. With an ED_{50} of 0.5 mg/kg of body weight TID against HSV-1 and HSV-2, BAY 57-1293 was the most potent compound tested.

Comparable values for ACV were 22 and 16 mg/kg of body weight. No toxic side effects of BAY 57-1293 treatment were apparent in the mice upon gross inspection, and the highest dose tested (60 mg/kg TID) appeared to be well tolerated. Comparable results were shown in a rat lethal challenge model.

In the cutaneous zosterform model, oral treatment of HSV-2 established by dermal scarification was delayed until establishment of disease (day 3) and then animals were treated for 5 days TID with 15 and 60 mg of BAY 57-1293 per kg and 60 and 240 mg of VACV per kg. The lower dose of BAY 57-1293 was statistically more efficacious than the highest dose of VACV used ($P < 0.011$), based on a compiled disease severity score.

In the guinea pig vaginal model of HSV-2 genital herpes, delayed treatment with BAY 57-1293 (20 mg/kg 2 × daily orally; days 4–14 post infection) rapidly shut down disease progression. VACV at 7.5 × higher dose levels produced only a weak response. Benefit in terms of time to healing was clearly superior in the BAY 57-1293 treatment group. Perhaps the most promising results observed in the animal studies were the observation that acute treatment in this model could reduce the number of subsequent recurrences. This latter outcome may reflect the more potent and rapid shut down of the virus feeding the latency reservoir, and illustrates the importance of rapid diagnosis and treatment of the primary infection.

In these studies, the actual drug exposures (PK parameters) for BAY 57-1293 and comparators were not reported (Betz et al., 2002) making it difficult to compare potencies. However, the PK for single 1 mg/kg dose in female BALB/C mice indicated high oral bioavailability C_{max} 4.4 μM after 1 hour, and relatively slow elimination from the plasma ($T_{max} = 1$ hr; $t\frac{1}{2}$ 6 hours). Oral bioavailability >60% and an elimination half-life of >6 hours has also been observed in rats and dogs. Plasma concentrations with these properties would exceed 0.025 μM at 24 hours post dose. Under the conditions used in the cutaneous efficacy model studies with 15 and 60 mg doses administered 3 times daily, one would expect significant accumulations of drug levels above IC_{90} over the 5-day course of treatment; providing extended antiviral cover in the post-dosing period (Kleymann et al., 2002). BAY 57-1293 shows the potential for once daily dosing, a convenience important for chronic suppression. From a pharmaceutical manufacturing perspective, such potency has advantages in smaller pill size and burden (number of pills per dose), resulting in economic savings in the amount of drug substance.

The long duration of drug exposure can offer advantages in terms of efficiency in reduced frequency of dosing, but must be balanced by an excellent safety profile to avoid undesired consequences of toxic build up. Early toxicology studies indicated that once-daily dosing of dogs with 30, 100, and 300 mg/kg of BAY57-1293 for 28 days was well tolerated. The identical dosing protocol in rats, however, resulted in a dose-dependent transitional hyperplasia of the urinary bladder epithelium (Kleymann et al., 2002). Based on a structural similarity to the diuretic drug, Diamox® (acetylzolamide), the Bayer toxicologists hypothesized that inhibition of the carbonic anhydrase enzymes led to bladder hyperplasia. Sulfonamides with broad inhibitory activity against the carbonic anhydrases of rats, dogs, and humans, only cause this bladder hyperplasia in the rodents. The in vitro inhibition of a carbonic anhydrase standard assay by BAY57-1293 occurs at 2 μM; 100-fold above the viral inhibitory concentration. Extended toxicologic evaluations will be required to further clarify this observation. The overall preclinical profile of this compound would support clinical development, and the evidence of superior potency and more rapid onset of action, and durability compared to the gold standard therapy, make it one of the most promising agents in the development pipeline (2004).

A novel series of inhibitors of the CMV helicase primase function was identified in a cell-based viral replication (single cycle) assay (Cushing et al., 2006). The imidazolylpyrimidine core scaffold was substituted extensively at the 2-, 4-, 5-, and 6 positions to produce an active series of analogs with in vitro potencies ranging from 0.04–0.30 μM. The SAR revealed the importance of the imidazole/nitro group dyad, and the nature of the substituents at the 4 position. The chemical features were consistent with a mechanism of action involving a covalent binding to a target protein. Irreversible binding to the UL70 component of the CMV helicase primase complex (UL102, UL105, UL70) was demonstrated by co-immunoprecipitation of UL70 bound to radiolabeled inhibitor (Cushing et al., 2006). Resistance selection is not yet reported for these new inhibitors. Two compounds provide excellent starting points for the further optimization for the necessary properties of a viable drug candidate.

Inhibitors of DNA processing and packaging

After herpesvirus DNA replication, the concatemeric product is packaged into preformed capsids and cut into unit-length genomes by site-specific cleavage. At least seven HSV proteins have been identified as participants in this process; pUL6, pUL15, pUL17, pUL25, pUL28, pUL32 and pUL33 (Beard et al., 2002) and many of these have been confirmed as essential for viral replication. By analogy with DNA bacteriophage packaging and processing, a terminase complex binds to the capsid portal, trims the concatemeric DNA at a specific sequence with unique structural features (Adelman et al., 2004), translocates the DNA into the capsid and finally cleaves the DNA at a repeat of the specific sequence. The HSV pUL6 protein has been shown to form the capsid portal (Newcomb et al., 2001, 2003). A variety of evidence indicates that the pUL15 and pUL28 proteins form the terminase complex that cleaves the HSV DNA at the sequence before and after packaging (Beard et al., 2002; White et al., 2003; Przech et al., 2003). The packaging genes are well-conserved among the herpesviruses; for example at least six of the seven HSV genes have close homologues in CMV. Of the terminase components CMV pUL89, pUL56 and pUL104 are the homologues of HSV pUL15, pUL28 and UL6 (Fig. 68.4). Biochemical and structural studies of the hCMV pUL89 and pUL56 suggest that the pUL56 binds to the viral DNA, while pUL89 mediates DNA cleavage via an ATP-dependent-nuclease activity (Bogner et al., 1998; Scheffczik et al., 2002; Scholg et al., 2003). Since the processing and packaging of concatemeric DNA has no exact counterpart in the human cell this target presents the possibility of discovering very selective antiviral agents.

Inhibitors of the portal protein of HSV

WAY 150138

Activity of the thiourea class of compounds emerged from cell-based replication screens, revealing a striking degree of specificity within the alpha herpesviruses, but no activity across other human herpesviruses (Visalli and van Zeijl, 2003). Minor structural changes in the main scaffold resulted in >10-fold shifts in activity between HSV and VZV, and the lead HSV compound, WAY 150138, (benzamide, N-[3-chloro-4-[[[(5-chloro-2,4-dimethoxyphenyl)amino]thioxomethyl] amino]phenyl]-2-fluoro-). Identification of the portal protein as the molecular target was made by the generation and mapping of laboratory-derived resistant mutants (van Zeijl et al., 2000; Visalli and van Zeijl, 2003). The portal proteins of HSV-1 and HSV-2 share 86% amino acid identity or similarity, while VZV (pUL54) and human CMV (pUL104) portal proteins share only 44% and 27% identity/similarity, respectively. Although these homologues share a high degree of functional homology, and strong overall amino acid identity in conserved domains, no broad spectrum inhibitors have yet been identified.

The individual mutations identified in the HSV-1 strains resistant to WAY-150138 suggested points of interaction with the compound resulted from the folding of the UL6 protein in its active 3- dimensional conformation. A

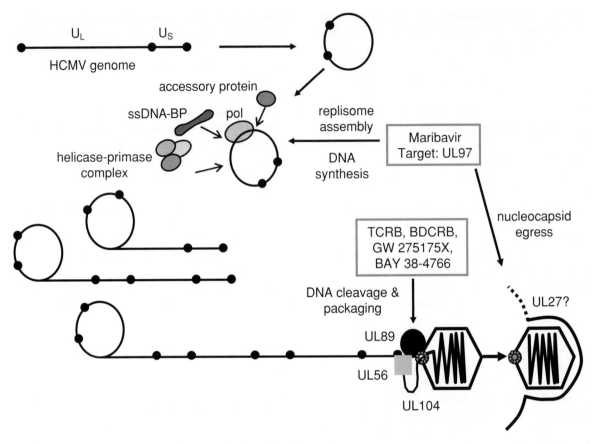

Fig. 68.4. Inhibitors of CMV DNA replisome, packaging, and nucleocapsid egress.

crystal structural model for the portal protein to aid in understanding the mechanism of UL6 binding and in further drug design was not available. Research on this class of portal protein inhibitors continues. No information is currently published on the other preclinical properties of these compounds that would indicate their potential as herpes simplex therapeutics.

Comp I

Subsequent screening of related compounds in the thiourea series revealed that a small chemical modification (addition of a spacer, -HC(CH3)-, between the aryl ring and the thiourea nitrogen) yielded compounds active against VZV, but with loss of activity against HSV. Three *N*-methylbenzyl-*N'*-arylthiourea analogues (Comp I, Comp II, and Comp III) were selected for further study.

A number of MOA studies were conducted confirming that VZV DNA cleavage and packaging is inhibited by these thiourea compounds via inhibition of the ORF54 gene (Visalli *et al.*, 2003). Resistant viral isolates were found to possess mutations in the VZV ORF54 gene, the homologue of HSV UL6, similar to the mechanism of WAY-150138 (van Zeijl *et al.*, 2000; Newcomb and Brown, 2002). As expected, treatment of wild-type virus with the inhibitor resulted in the absence of DNA-containing capsids, and restriction in the spread of infectious VZV to adjacent uninfected cells.

Current marketed VZV antivirals all target the DNA polymerase, and virus resistant to these new thiourea compounds are not cross-resistant to the approved drugs. Thus, targeted inhibition of the VZV ORF54 protein may prove to be a productive approach in identifying new agents to complement existing antivirals in the treatment of VZV infections.

Dihydroxyacridone series

The dihydroxyacridone series was investigated in order to target a MOA other than viral DNA polymerase (Akanitapichat *et al.*, 2000). Initial attempts focused on analogues with functional groups at the 5, 6, or 8 positions. The 5-Cl congener (5-chloro-1,3-dihydroxyacridone) was determined to be the most selective inhibitor of HSV and was selected for additional study. Mechanistic studies suggested that HSV replication was blocked after DNA and late protein synthesis. Further studies (Akanitapichat and

Bastow, 2002) indicated that maturation of replicating DNA and late virion production were inhibited in the same dose-dependent manner, resulting in a two- to three-fold reduction in the production of B capsids. Of interest was the inability to isolate resistant virus, although these attempts were limited, attempts to isolate resistant virus were unsuccessful.

Additional chemical elaboration and parallel synthesis of compounds in this series (Lowden and Bastow, 2003) identified compounds that were active against CMV (ED_{50} value of 1.4 μM at low MOI) and some that were active against both CMV and HSV. At least one compound in this series inhibited cell replication (mean $CC_{50}s = 33$ μM), but did not have antiviral activity. Preliminary mechanistic studies indicated the likelihood of diverse MOAs. While this has some appeal, more extensive work may be needed to determine the real selectivity and safety of this series of compounds.

Inhibitors of the CMV terminase complex

TCRB and BDCRB

The first selective inhibitors of the hCMV terminase complex, TCRB (2,5,6-trichloro-1-ß-D-ribofuranosyl benzimidazole) and its analogue BDCRB (1-(ß-D-ribofuranosyl)-2-bromo-5,6-dichlorobenzimidazole) arose serendipitously from a chemistry effort to modify the broad spectrum transcriptional inhibitor DRB into an anti-tumor agent (Townsend and Revenkar, 1970). The antiviral activity was uncovered during subsequent screening for antiviral activity in the series (Townsend et al., 1995). In contrast to the action of GCV, viral DNA synthesis was unaffected in a single round of replication. The phenotype of infected, treated cells was consistent with a block in the viral DNA cleavage and packaging (Fig. 68.4).

Genetic mapping studies of the BDCRB and TCRB-resistant mutants of Towne and AD169 strains confirmed the interaction of these inhibitors with two subunits of the terminase complex (Krosky et al., 1998; Underwood et al., 1998). Specific point mutations were identified in the UL89 gene, which encodes the small subunit required for the nuclease cleavage of the precursor viral DNA into unit genome lengths (Bogner, 2002). A mutation was also selected in the UL56 gene, which encodes the large subunit responsible for sequence-specific DNA binding to the pac motifs, and ATP-dependent translocation of the viral DNA into the preformed capsids for final cleavage and packaging.

Precisely how two unrelated compound series, the β-D-ribosyl benzimidazoles and the sulfonamides, block DNA processing and packaging is not currently understood. The exact binding sites for BDCRB and BAY 38-4766 on the terminase subunits are apparently different, based on lack of cross-resistance (Evers et al., 2004). Their binding could disrupt protein-protein interaction via allosteric mechanisms, or could directly interfere with enzymatic activity. The genome maturation process is complex, and occurs at the viral replication center sites, where viral and cellular transcriptional and DNA replication machinery also assemble (Dittmer et al., 2005; McVoy and Nixon, 2005; Thoma et al., 2006). BDCRB treatment of CMV-infected cells resulted in a major block to correct unit genome cleavage, and also allowed a minor level of monomer plus larger than unit product genomes resulting from skipped cleavages (McVoy and Nixon, 2005). This inhibitor also may directly interfere with the interaction of the pUL56 and the portal protein pUL104, as evidenced by the ability of BDCRB to block their co-immunoprecipitation from CMV-infected cells (Dittmer et al., 2005). Consistent with a direct interaction of the pUL56 terminase subunit with the portal protein, resistance modifications in UL89 and UL56 to BDCRB, TCRB and BAY 38-4766 were accompanied by a compensatory change in UL104, which alone did not confer resistance (Buerger et al., 2001; Reefschlaeger et al., 2001; Komazin et al., 2004). These interesting inhibitors continue to help elucidate the genome maturation events.

These two lead benzimidazole ribosides showed potent, selective activity for human CMV. However, pharmacokinetic studies indicated metabolic lability of the glycosidic bond between the base and the sugar moieties (Good et al., 1994). Recently, the identification of two cellular enzymes that catalyze the cleavage of the glycosidic bonds of BDCRB and TCRB were reported (Lorenzi et al., 2006). An active chemical program was undertaken to stabilize this linkage (Townsend et al., 1999; Chulay et al., 1999). The results of this effort were fruitful; yielding two clinical candidates, GW275175X, an inhibitor of the hCMV DNA terminase process packaging, and BW1263W94 (maribavir), an inhibitor of the pUL97 protein kinase (information as of 2003). The application of amino acid esters as pro drugs of BDCRB has also been successful, identifying L-Asp-BDCRB as a potential candidate for further development (Lorenzi et al., 2005).

GW275175X

A benzimidazole with a pyranosyl sugar moiety selected for further development was **GW275175X** (2-bromo-5,6-dichloro-1-ß-D-ribopyranosyl-1-H-benzimidazole), a compound whose antiviral activity is specific for hCMV; there was no in vitro inhibition of HSV-types 1 or 2, VZV, or other DNA and RNA viruses tested (Williams et al., 2003; Underwood et al., 2004). MOA studies (Underwood et al., 2004) supported inhibition of viral cleavage and packaging, consistent with the mechanism of BRCRB. As expected, virus with the BDCRB- and TCRB-resistant mutations in

UL89 were cross resistant to GW275175X. One notable aspect of the MOA is the rapid reversibility of the BDCRB or GW275175X block in infected cell culture, with resumption of viral DNA concatamer processing and restoration of the rate of viral yield production occurring within 8–10 hours following drug washout (Underwood et al., 2004).

A battery of preclinical toxicology testing sufficient to support initial Phase I studies in humans (GSK, data on file) was completed for GW275175X. No significant adverse activity in in vivo assays designed to predict effects on metabolic parameters were exhibited. Other in vitro assessments of GW275175X were encouraging; pharmacology screens, and in vitro and in vivo mutagenecity tests were clean, and liver enzyme studies were clean. GW275175X was evaluated for toxicity in rodents (28-day acute, 6-month chronic) and primates (28-day acute). Systemic exposures at the various doses ranged from 60- to100-fold the in vitro IC_{50} for CMV inhibition. Importantly, penetration into the CNS and vitreous humor in primates was good, ranging from approximately 2 × the IC_{50} at 50 mg/kg/day to 8X the IC_{50} at 200 mg/kg per day. These characteristics would be important for treatment of congenital and ocular CMV disease.

Based on the overall preclinical properties and safety profile, GW275175X was progressed into Phase I single-escalating dose (100–1600 mg) studies. No drug-related or clinically significant changes from baseline were seen in vital signs, ECG, or clinical laboratory values, and all adverse events were considered mild. The pharmacokinetic profile indicated several advantages of this benzimidazole ribose over the parent BDCRB and the analogue, maribavir, including better CNS penetration, longer plasma half-life, and reduced serum protein binding.

While the overall preclinical and initial phase I data encouraged further clinical development, this compound was not advanced due to the sponsor's decision to progress the other anti-CMV agent from the benzimidazole riboside series (1263W94, maribavir) instead.

BAY 38–4766

The non-nucleosidic BAY 38–4766, 3-hydroxy-2,2-dimethyl-N-[4([[5-(dimethylamino)-1-naphthyl]sulfonyl]amino)-phenyl]propanamide compound emerged from a cell-based discovery program as the lead highly selective inhibitor of human, monkey and rodent CMV. Resistance to this drug was genetically mapped to the UL89 and the UL56 ORFs, indicating that this class of compound also targeted the hCMV terminase complex (Reefschlaeger et al., 2001; Buerger et al., 2001). The drug susceptibilities of 36 hCMV clinical isolates to the BAY 38–4766 and GCV were evaluated in two different phenotypic assays. All isolates including those resistant to GCV were inhibited by at least 50% at a concentration of approximately 1 μM of BAY-38–4776 (McSharry et al., 2001a,b). Antiviral activity comparable to GCV was demonstrated in a hollow-fiber model where hCMV-infected human cells entrapped in hollow fibers were transplanted into immunodeficient mice (Weber et al., 2001). Viruses resistant to BAY 38–4766 are not cross resistant to current marketed CMV drugs GCV, CDV or PFA.

A favorable pharmacokinetic profile has been demonstrated in humans for the initial lead compound in this series. A phase I study in healthy male subjects after single oral doses of BAY 38–4776 (100 to 2000 mg) indicated that the drug was well tolerated with no adverse events or changes in vital signs or lab parameters. The C_{max}s ranged from 0.33 mg/l (100 mg dose) to 4.2 mg/l (2000 mg/l dose) and occurred within 0.5 to 5 hours. After C_{max} concentrations were reached, drug was eliminated from plasma, with a $t_{1/2}$ of 3 to 5 hours reaching a terminal half life of 12–16 hours. The increases in AUC and C_{max} were dose dependent (Nagelschmitz et al., 1999).

As of 2004, work continued to advance a compound from this interesting series into full clinical development.

Protease inhibitors

Impressive success in the development of protease inhibitors (PIs) in the treatment of HIV infection has not been paralleled in the herpesviruses. The PIs for HIV infection were introduced in 1996 and quickly set a new standard of care, dramatically extending the life of patients with HIV infection. Success in the design of therapeutic agents targeting the HIV protease is partly attributed to the well-defined structural features of the catalytic site in this aspartyl protease (Supuran et al., 2003). In contrast, the herpes proteases belong to the serine protease family, and are characterized by a distinctive catalytic triad of his, his, ser within the less tractable active site. The cleavage sites are unique and highly conserved across the herpesviruses. The herpes proteases comprise the N-terminal sequence of the capsid scaffold protein. After completion of capsid assembly, auto cleavage by the protease releases the scaffold, permitting DNA packaging (Gibson et al., 1994).

The herpes protease is essential for the production of infectious virus, and therefore represents a valid target. The quest for inhibitors of these proteases was facilitated by the development of efficient enzyme-based screens and wide-ranging X-ray crystallographic structure and catalytic site features that became available in the mid-1990s (Borthwick et al., 1998; Holwerda, 1997; Qiu and Abdelmeguid, 1999; Waxman and Darke, 2000). Figure 68.5 illustrates the appli-

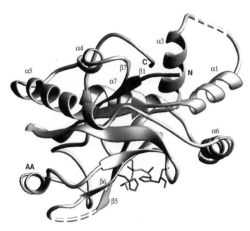

Fig. 68.5. The HSV-2 protease monomer. Two disordered surface loops are shown as dashed lines (N-terminal residues 1–16 are disordered). The two histidines in the active site are shown in red, one on the β6 and the other on the hairpin turn between β2 and β3, while the inhibitor diisopropyl phosphate covalently bound to the catalytic serine is in green on β5. (Reprinted with permission from Hoog et al., 1997.)

cation of X-ray crystallographic structural information to the design and optimization of enzyme inhibitors (Hoog et al., 1997), a tool used successfully in the HIV aspartyl PI discovery programs (Erickson et al., 1990).

Several major pharmaceutical companies took up this quest, and several mechanism-based peptide and heterocyclic inhibitors of either the reversible or irreversible type were identified (Borthwick, 2005). However, these were not always active in virally-infected cells, and none have been progressed into clinical development to date. Any inhibitor would have to be capable of uptake not only into cells, but also into the capsid structure within the nucleus of the infected cells. This nucleocapsid barrier may contribute to the poor antiviral activity reported for compounds that are potent inhibitors of the enzyme assay in vitro (Borthwick, 2005). The protease as a target remains to be successfully exploited.

Inhibitors of the CMV UL97 encoded protein kinase

The CMV-encoded UL97 protein kinase has several features that make it highly attractive as a chemotherapeutic target. It belongs to a family of serine-threonine protein kinases highly conserved across all mammalian herpesviruses, suggesting its potential as a broad spectrum target (Chee et al., 1989; Smith and Smith, 1989). The pUL97 shares structural features with aminoglycoside phosphotransferases; bacterial enzymes known to phosphorylate sugar-containing moieties, which may account for its fortuitous ability to monophosphorylate GCV and ACV (Littler et al., 1992; Sullivan et al., 1992; Talarico et al., 1999; Zimmerman et al., 1997; Michel and Mertens, 2004). This nucleoside phosphotransferase (ACV, GCV) activity has also been reported for the EBV homologue BGLF4 (Zacny et al., 1999), but not for the alphaherpes virus kinase homologues. Importantly, the pUL97 differs from a prototypic serine-threonine protein kinase biochemically (high pH and NaCl optima) and substrate motif specificity (He et al., 1997; Baek et al., 2002).

The study of the replication functions of these herpes protein kinases is complicated by the fact that they are not absolutely essential for growth in cultured cells. Null mutants of the protein kinases of HSV-1, VZV, and CMV have shown variable phenotypes in different cell types, under different culture conditions, complicating MOA studies and predictably, quantitative drug inhibition studies (Moffat et al., 1998; Chou et al., 2006). Studies into the function of the HSV-1 pUL13 and the VZV gene 47 homologues indicate multiple activities throughout the virus replication cycle. These include regulatory roles in early gene expression, indirect effects on host gene expression, late protein post-translational modifications associated with virion maturation, and contributions to tissue-specific pathogenesis. (Purves et al., 1993; Kato et al., 2001; Kenyon et al., 2001; Coulter et al., 1993; Overton et al., 1994; Ng et al., 1994; Michel et al., 1999; Kawaguchi et al., 1999; Moffat et al., 1998; Pritchard et al., 1999; Wolf et al., 2001; Krosky et al., 2003b; Marschall et al., 2005; Hu and Cohen, 2005).

Therefore, inhibition of such a target could cumulatively penalize viral replication. These proteins undoubtedly play essential roles in disease pathogenesis (Moffat et al., 1998). In the case of the human CMV pUL97, the high degree of interstrain sequence conservation (Lurain et al., 2001) coupled with the observations that there are no null mutants of the CMV pUL97 in clinical strains would argue that this is an ideal target. Two series of unrelated compounds are potent inhibitors of the CMV pUL97, and their MOA studies have extended our current knowledge of pUL97 function. Proof of concept for one of these has been achieved in the clinic.

Indolocarbazoles

Indolocarbazoles have been investigated as potential antiviral agents based on the fact that they are competitive inhibitors of the ATP binding sites of kinases in the protein kinase C family (Zimmerman et al., 2000; Marschall et al., 2001). A series of indolocarbazoles was recently analyzed and three (Go6976, K252a, K352c) were established to be highly effective inhibitors (IC$_{50}$s ranging from 0.009 to 0.4 μM) of both GCV-sensitive and -resistant hCMV, with little effect against HSV. Cytotoxicity assays in proliferating cells reportedly indicated that the effective antiviral concentration of these compounds was significantly lower than those affecting cellular functioning. However, attempts to select resistant virus under the selective pressure of increasing concentrations of drug indicated that resistance was lost or restricted to low-level replication at higher drug concentrations, hinting that cellular functions may be involved (Kawaguchi and Kato, 2003). Alternative explanations include the possibility that resistance to Go6976 results in severe growth impairment, which could be established by the replication competence of a virus strain with deleted target. Growth impairment (1–2 logs titer reduction) has been reported for the deleted UL97 hCMV (Prichard et al., 1999; Wolf et al., 2001). Efforts to elucidate the exact MOA of the indolcarbazoles have focused on the hCMV pUL97 protein kinase. Indolcarbazoles with anti-CMV activity inhibited pUL97 protein kinase autophosphorylation in vitro, and mutant virus encoding a non-functional pUL97 (catalytic site mutant) deletion was completely insensitive to the indocarbazoles (Marschall et al., 2001).

A series of symmetrical indolocarbazoles were independently synthesized to investigate SARs against a range of herpesviruses (Slater et al., 1999). Several novel and potent inhibitors of hCMV were identified, although none were progressed to clinical development. Many of these had reasonable SIs in the normal diploid fibroblasts used for CMV activity, yet they were extremely toxic to human marrow stem cell differentiation. The development potential of this indolocarbazole class of compounds is unknown based on currently available information, which does not address pharmacokinetics and safety properties.

Recently a series of quinazolines with anti-CMV activity was shown to act through inhibition of the pUL97 (Herget et al., 2004). Limited testing against cell protein Kinases indicated viral PK selectivity, although they also block host EGFR. The series appears promising, based on available data.

Maribavir
BW1263W94 1-(β-L-ribofuranosyl)-2-isopropylamino-5,6-dichlorobenzimidazole (maribavir), was derivatized from the original benzimidazole BDCRB and TCRB (Townsend et al., 1995) as part of efforts to stabilize their metabolically labile glycosidic linkage and improve oral bioavailability (Chulay et al., 1999; Townsend et al., 1995, 1999). The precedence of flipping the sugar conformation to the L or unnatural biologic form had been established in the nucleoside analog inhibitors of HIV RT as a way of reducing mechanism-based toxicity and rapid metabolic clear-

ance. The potency of the β-L-BDCRB was amplified by various substitutions for the halogen in the 2-position of the benzimidazole base. The resulting development candidate BW1263W94 showed potent activity for CMV and EBV, but no other viruses, including the various animal CMV strains tested (Kern et al., 2004). An unexpected finding was the change in the MOA: maribavir no longer exerted significant inhibition of viral DNA processing and packaging. Instead, maribavir strongly reduced viral DNA synthesis in the quiescent MRC-5 lung fibroblasts used in this study. The mechanism was not mediated through a substrate analog inhibition of the CMV DNA polymerase. Maribavir was not phosphorylated in infected cells, nor did the compound itself or any of its synthetic phosphorylated derivatives inhibit the CMV DNA polymerase (Biron et al., 2002).

The discovery that maribavir was a selective inhibitor of the pUL97 came simultaneously from 2 independent approaches: selection and genetic mapping of a resistant virus strain, and fortuitously, from a broad protein kinase-inhibitor screening effort (Biron et al., 2002). Resistant virus selected with a related analog in the series encoded a Leu397Arg amino acid substitution in pUL97, which conferred a 20- to 200-fold less sensitive phenotype to maribavir. This resistant virus remained susceptible to BDCRB and other approved anti-CMV drugs, including GCV, and was fully competent for in vitro growth. Supporting evidence for the pUL97 as the target was provided by studies with the pUL97 enzyme: the wild type pUL97-catalyzed phosphorylation of histone 2b was inhibited by maribavir (IC50 = 2 nM) while pUL97 with the Leu397Arg mutation was not (IC50 > 1000 nM). A second resistance mutation in the UL97 ORF was selected in the laboratory in the context of a clinical strain following serial passage in increasing concentrations of drug. The resulting point mutation encoded a Thr409Met change, which is also located close to the ATP-binding domain, and far upstream of the GCV resistance mutations which map to the substrate binding domain (Chou, 2006; Chou et al., 2002). The resulting resistance phenotype was intermediate relative to that of the Leu397Arg mutation in AD169, conferring 80-fold vs. 200-fold increase (Biron et al., 2002; Chou, 2006). Maribavir maintains activity against all GCV resistant UL97 mutants identified to date, indicating that the interactions of these two drugs with the protein kinase are distinct (McSharry et al., 2001; Biron et al., 2002).

Reduction in viral DNA synthesis by maribavir may be a consequence of inadequate or improper phosphorylation of pUL44 by the pUL97 kinase. The pUL97 carries a NLS, and locates to the nucleus during the replication cycle (Michel et al., 1996). A direct interaction with, and phosphorylation by, pUL97 of the pUL44, the DNA processivity factor, has been reported (Krosky et al., 2003; Marshall et al., 2003). This interaction was linked to the co-localization of pUL44 and pUL97 in the replication complexes (Marshall et al., 2003).

The pUL97 has been shown to exert its major effects late in CMV replication (Wolf et al., 2001; Krosky et al., 2003a) based on studies with the RCΔ97 (Prichard et al., 1999). Consistent with studies of UL97 null virus, maribavir treatment of CMV-infected foreskin fibroblasts (HFF) also resulted in an increase of type A empty capsids (Wolf et al., 2001) or type C DNA filled capsids (Krosky et al., 2003a). These empty and precursor capsids accumulated in the nucleus of infected HFF cells at late times in the replication cycle, after infection with RCΔ97, or in wild-type infected cells treated with maribavir. "Studies with HSV (Kato et al., 2006; Simpson-Holley et al., 2004) and with the CMV UL97 deficient virus (Wolf et al., 2001; Krosky et al., 2003a) have suggested a role for these viral protein kinases in nucleocapsid egress. The large nucleocapsids cannot exit through the nuclear membrane, which is composed of a tight structural matrix of proteins called lamins, without disassembly of lamin subunits in order to relax and open the junctions. Cellular p32 protein is reported to recruit pUL97 to the lamin B receptor, where it is hypothesized that pUL97 phosphorylates specific lamin components, resulting in their redistribution (Marschall et al., 2005). Thus the viral protein kinase regulates a host protein substrate during virion maturation. The block of the CMV UL97 kinase activity by maribavir results in nuclear retention and accumulation of nucleocapsids (Wolf et al., 2001; Krosky et al., 2003a).

A second genotype has been associated with maribavir resistance following laboratory passage of both laboratory and clinical strains of CMV (Chou et al., 2004; Komazin et al., 2003; Chou, 2006). Mutations in the UL27 ORF, encoding changes of Arg233Ser, Ala269Thr, Leu335Phe, Leu335Pro, Trp362Arg, or Ala406Val-415stop, are reported to confer only a modest level of maribavir resistance (twofold–5-fold increase in IC50s). Little is known about the function of pUL27 at this time. However, the UL27 homolog of mCMV, known as M27, was shown by mutagenesis studies to be non-essential for growth in culture, but was required for virulence and mortality in vivo (Abenes et al., 2001). The CMV UL27 (1824 bp ORF, 608 amino acids) is transcribed as an early-late gene (Stamminger et al., May 2002; Chou et al., 2004), and has been shown to be nonessential for growth in vitro. The pUL27 encodes a nuclear localization signal (NLS); deletional mutagenesis resulted in cytoplasmic retention and a one-half log reduction in viral titers (Chou et al., 2004).

Viral encapsidation and nuclear egress involve the action of a number of viral gene products (Mettenleiter, 2002),

and the pUL97 clearly plays a role in the process. Data are accumulating which point to a role of the UL97 protein kinase action in CMV virion morphogenesis, perhaps by directing the normal intranuclear and intracytoplasmic distribution of viral proteins required for virion assembly and intracellular movement during the sequential steps of primary envelopment, tegumentation, translocation and final particle maturation (Azzeh et al., 2006; Chou et al., 2004; Prichard et al., 2005). The pp65 antigen, product of the UL83 ORF, is phosphorylated by the pUL97 in transiently co-transfected cells, and its phosphorylation in cells infected with wild-type AD169 is blocked by maribavir, but pp65 phosphorylation is not blocked in cell infected with the maribavir-resistant strain Leu397Arg (Sethna, GSK data on file). Consistent with these findings, the intranuclear distribution of pp65 is altered in cells infected with the UL97 deficient strain, or in cells infected with wild type virus and treated with maribavir (Pritchard et al., 2005). The pUL27 contains several proposed pUL97 substrate motifs (Baek et al., 2002; Chou et al., 2004). The elucidation of the role of pUL27 in the maribavir-resistant phenotype awaits further investigation on its function.

As maribavir progresses in clinical development, it will be important to understand the basis for drug resistance and its correlation with clinical outcome. The UL27 genetic changes that conferred resistance to maribavir resulted in only a low-grade resistance (three- to four-fold elevated IC50s) compared to the highly resistant phenotype of the L397RpUL97 strain. The gene sequence in 16 clinical isolates was 96% conserved, with no changes at the locations of the four UL27 maribavir resistance mutations noted. From a clinical perspective, the UL27 gene appears more tolerant of mutations than the UL97 gene (98% gene conservation; Lurain et al., 2001), and the resulting levels of maribavir resistance may not preclude drug efficacy. It remains to be seen whether the prolonged drug selection pressure of prophylactic or suppressive regimens results in the accumulation of additional and multiple mutations in the UL27 and UL97 target genes, and potentially in as yet unidentified maribavir targets or UL97 substrates.

Preclinical toxicology testing of maribavir has been comprehensive, with overall results establishing a good safety profile (Koszalka et al., 2002). These results contrast favorably with results of preclinical testing of GCV and CDV, both of which have a litany of toxicologic and tolerability concerns.

The pharmacokinetic profile of maribavir in rodents and primates demonstrated excellent oral bioavailability, although drug levels in the brain, cerebrospinal fluid, and vitreous humor of cynomolgus monkeys were low. Maribavir is highly bound to human plasma proteins, principally the albumin fraction; however, the binding is reversible in vitro. The impact of this property on efficacious dosing regimens remains to be determined.

Maribavir has successfully completed a series of Phase I–II clinical trials (Wang et al., 2003; Lu and Thomas, 2004). In Phase I studies in healthy volunteers and HIV-infected subjects, single oral doses of 50 to 1600 mg produced similar dose-proportional pharmacokinetics. Maribavir was rapidly absorbed following oral administration with Cmaxs occurring within 1 to 3 hours. Absorption was at least 30% to 40%, and drug was eliminated from plasma with a t1/2 of 3 to 5 hours. The plasma and urinary excretion profiles indicated that the drug was extensively metabolized, with the major metabolite identified as the N-dealkylated analogue, which did not show anti-viral activity in vitro.

A pilot study was conducted in HIV patients ($n=8$) with CMV retinitis, in order to measure the steady state pharmacokinetics in ocular tissues following 8 days of oral dosing. Antiviral drug levels were achieved in ocular tissues, although substantially lower than those found in plasma. This result indicates a potential for drug efficacy in CNS infections in congenital disease. As expected, blood CMV DNA levels in those viremic retinitis patients responded with a viral load drop. Additional Phase 1 studies included the important drug–drug interaction study using the drug cocktail approach to identify liver cytochrome P-450 enzymes capable of metabolizing maribavir, or being inhibited by maribavir (Ma et al., 2006).

No safety concerns of note were observed in these studies; however, mild to moderate taste disturbance and headache were reported in 80% and 53% of the subjects, respectively (Wang et al., 2003; Lu and Thomas, 2004). The taste disturbance was presumed to be due to secretion of drug or its principal metabolite metabolite into the salivary glands after systematic absorption and while not a safety concern, could have implications for adherence.

A subsequent phase I/II clinical trial was conducted to further determine the pharmacokinetics of maribavir and to monitor asymptomatic CMV shedding in semen in HIV-infected men (Lalezari et al., 2002). Six dosage regimens (100, 200, or 400 mg three times a day, or 600, 900, or 1200 mg twice a day) or a placebo were evaluated for 28 days. In that proof of concept study, potent anti-CMV activity (2.9 to 3.7 $\log_{10}$ reductions in PFU/ml in semen) was established at all doses. The reductions in CMV titers for all regimens compared well with results reported for the approved doses of CDV (5 mg/kg) in a comparable trial (Lalezari et al., 1995). Maribavir was reasonably well tolerated and safe with taste disturbance again the most frequently reported adverse event. Other adverse events reported by a higher percentage of subjects receiving maribavir than placebo included diarrhea, nausea, rash, pruritus, and fever.

Maribavir has recently demonstrated prophylactic efficacy in a Phase II randomized, double-blind, placebo-controlled trial in allogenic stem cell transplant patients ($N=111$). Doses of 100 mg BID, 400 mg QD, and 400 mg BID for 12 weeks all reduced the rate of CMV reactivation; preemptive therapy was required for 15%, 30%, and 15% of the respective maribavir doses, relative to 57% for placebo recipients (ViroPharma Inc. press release March 29, 2006). The overall safety profile of maribavir in the 12 week study recapitulates earlier clinical results. The durability of the anti-viral effects and incidence of resistance is under study.

Maribavir is clearly the most advanced new anti herpes drug in the clinical development pipeline. Based on urgent medical need and the favorable development characteristics of maribavir, the FDA has granted Fast Track Status for the prevention of CMV infections in allogenic bone marrow and solid organ transplant patients (ViroPharma Inc. press release Feb. 7, 2005).

Antivirals with activity against EBV, HHV-6, HHV-7, and HHV-8

While anti-viral drug development efforts continue for HSV_1 VZV, and CMV utilizing both old and new targets, lack of progress against EBV virus is notable. There are several reasons for this. Primary EBV infection is generally subclinical in immunocompetent individuals. However, it may cause infectious mononucleosis (generally a benign and self-limiting disease) but the window of opportunity for antiviral treatment during the clinical course is short. The lytic EBV manifestation of oral hairy leukoplakia in immunocompromised patients responds to therapy with ACV. EBV-associated lymphoproliferative diseases, Burkitt's lymphoma and nasopharyngeal carcinoma, all of which may develop without obvious preceding immunodeficiency, remains a major unmet medical need. Latent EBV infection is considered either the etiologic agent for these conditions or a major contributing factor. (Thorley-Lawson and Gross, 2004).

From a drug development perspective; it is not yet clear what EBV or (host) functions to target; and the value of a viral replication inhibitor is unknown (Okano, 2003). The L-benzimidazole riboside, maribavir, which is in clinical developments for CMV disease, also shows activity against EBV in vitro, apparently by blocking both the appearance of linear forms of newly synthesized EBV DNA and the accumulation of the early antigen EA-D (Zacny et al., 1999).

While the exact mechanism is unclear, it may be involve the EBV protein kinase, BGLF4, a close homolog of the hCMV UL97. This viral protein autophosphorylates, and has also been reported to phosphorylate the analogous DNA polymerase processivity factor, EA-D (Chen et al., 2000). In lytically infected Akata cells, the level of hyperphosphorylated EA-D was reduced by maribavir treatment, similar to the impact of maribavir treatment on the hCMV pUL44. However, direct inhibition of the phosphorylation of EA-D has not been demonstrated, and maribavir did not block the phosphorylation of EA-D by EBV protein kinase in transient co-expression assays with these two viral genes (Gershburg and Pagano, 2002). Therefore the phenotype of maribavir-treated Alcata cells is consistent with inhibition of BGLF4 function; thus mechanism studies must be addressed within the context of the infected cell. While much remains to be determined regarding maribavir's mechanism of action against EBV, it should be considered a viable candidate for further study.

Information on the incidence of EBV-associated lymphomas in transplant patients treated prophylatically for CMV infections with maribavir may yield insights into the relationship of lytic replication to the post transplant lymphoproliferative diseases (Razonable et al., 2005).

Research targeted at developing antivirals against human herpesvirus type 6 (HHV-6), type 7 (HHV-7) and type 8 (HHV-8) has been limited. A new series of arylsulfone derivatives have been shown to have in vitro activity against HHV-6 and HHV-7, as well as CMV. While work with this series of compounds is preliminary, a new MOA of indirect inhibition of viral DNA synthesis may be involved (Naesens et al., 2006; Razonable et al., 2005). Both HHV-6 and HHV-7 have an extremely high prevalence rate of about 95% in the US, but in the vast majority of cases their presence is associated with mild self-limiting symptoms, usually fever and rash, where treatment isn warranted. Infection with HHV-8 is more serious since reactivation is in the form of Kaposi's sarcoma (Ablashi, 2002). Immune preservation or reconstitution in AIDS patients by highly active anti-retroviral therapy (HAART) has reduced the incidence of Kaposis, indicting the protective effects of the functional immune system in this infection.

A systematic approach to identifying antivirals against HHV-6, HHV-7 and HHV-8 has been completed (de Clercq et al., 2001b). Approved antivirals (ACV, VACV, PCV, FCV, GCV, PFA, CDV, and brivudin) and investigational compounds (Lobucavir, H2G, A-5021, D/L-cyclohexenyl G and S2242) with demonstrated activity against herpesviruses were evaluated in appropriate in vitro systems. The most potent compounds with the highest antiviral selectivity index were: (i) for HHV-6; PFA, S2242, A-5021 and CDV; (ii) for HHV-7; S2242, CDV and PFA; and (iii) for HHV-8; S2242, CDV and GCV.

Conclusions

The pipeline is indeed rich with new antiherpes agents. Many of these act by novel, and as yet unvalidated mechanisms of action from a therapeutic viewpoint. Their successful performance in the clinic will increase our understanding of the role of these new targets in viral disease.

For the two HSV helicase-primase inhibitors, a critical development milestone will be the human safety data for the thiazole class of compounds, the ease of viral escape (resistance), and the pathogenecity and transmissibility of mutant virus. The hCMV terminase inhibitor candidates start with the advantage of a highly selective and clearly essential target. However, it remains to be seen whether there are unanticipated (non-mechanism-based) toxicities in human studies with the two chemical series of inhibitors. Positive efficacy results in the Phase III clinical studies of the candidate CMV drug, maribavir, would provide target validation for the first inhibitor of a viral protein kinase.

As these drug candidates achieve regulatory approval, and with their expanded clinical use, the impact of drug potency and MOA on the emergence of resistance in the population will become the focus of studies. Resistance to the currently licensed antivirals (ACV, PCV, and their prodrugs) is low at <1.07 based on HSV isolates, a figure that has remained relatively constant since these drugs have been on the market, in spite of their widespread use (Bacon et al., 2003). The vast majority of ACV-resistant HSV (TK-deficient) viruses are not capable of reactivating after latency, losing the transmission opportunity, and thus the presence of ACV-resistant virus in the overall population is acceptable. In an immunocompromised patient, the risk of developing resistance is much greater than in an immunocompetent individual, and clinical outcome becomes the critical issue. The availability of rescue therapies with novel MOAs will help fill this medical need.

REFERENCES

Abele, G., Cox, S., Bergman, S. et al. (1991). Antiviral activity against VZV and HSV type 1 and type 2 of the (+) and (−) enantiomers of (R,S)-9-[4-hydroxy-2-(hydroxymethyl) butyl] guanine, in comparison to other closely related acyclic nucleosides. Antivir. Chem. Chemother., **2**, 163–169.

Abenes, G., Lee, M., Haghjoo, E., Tong, T., Zhan, X., and Liu, F. (2001). Murine cytomegalovirus open reading frame M27 plays an important role in growth and virulence in mice. *J. Virol.*, **75**, 1697–1707.

Ablashi, D. V., Chatlynne, L. G., Whitman, J. E., Jr., and Cesarman, E. (2002). Spectrum of Kaposi's sarcoma-associated herpesvirus, or human herpesvirus 8, diseases. *Clin. Microbiol. Rev.*, **15**, 439–464.

Akanitapichat, P. and Bastow, K. F. (2002). The antiviral agent 5-chloro-1,3-dihydroxyacridone interferes with assembly and maturation of herpes simplex virus. *Antiviral Res.*, **53**, 113–126.

Akanitapichat, P., Lowden, C. T., and Bastow, K. F. (2000).1,3-dihydroxyacridone derivatives as inhibitors of herpes virus replication. *Antiviral Res.*, **45**, 123–134.

Aldern, K. A., Ciesla, S. L., Winegarden, K. L., and Hostetler, K. Y. (2003). Increased antiviral activity of 1-O-hexadecyloxypropyl-[2-(14)C]cidofovir in MRC-5 human lung fibroblasts is explained by unique cellular uptake and metabolism. *Mol. Pharmacol.*, **63**, 678–681.

Arkin, M. R. and Wells, J. A. (2004). Small-molecule inhibitors of protein-protein interactions: progressing towards the dream. *Nat. Rev. Drug Discov.*, **3**, 301–317.

Azzeh, M., Honigman, A., Taraboulos, A., Rouvinski, A., and Wolf, D. G. (2006). Structural changes in human cytomegalovirus cytoplasmic assembly sites in the absence of UL97 kinase activity. *Virology*, in press.

Baba, M., Nishimura, O., Kanzaki, N. *et al.* (1999). A small-molecule, nonpeptide CCR5 antagonist with highly potent and selective anti-HIV-1 activity. *Proc. Natl Acad Sci. USA*, **96**, 5698–5703.

Bacon, T. H., Levin, M. J., Leary, J. J., Sarisky, R. T., and Sutton, D. (2003). Herpes simplex virus resistance to acyclovir and penciclovir after two decades of antiviral therapy. *Clin. Microbiol. Rev.*, **16**, 114–128.

Baek, M. C., Krosky, P. M., He, Z., and Coen, D. M. (2002). Specific phosphorylation of exogenous protein and peptide substrates by the human cytomegalovirus UL97 protein kinase. Importance of the P+5 position. *J. Biol. Chem.*, **277**, 29593–29599.

Balzarini, J. and McGuigan, C. (2002). Bicyclic pyrimidine nucleoside analogues (BCNAs) as highly selective and potent inhibitors of varicella-zoster virus replication. *J. Antimicrob. Chemother.*, **50**, 5–9.

Balzarini, J., Sienaert, R., Liekens, S. *et al.* (2002). Lack of susceptibility of bicyclic nucleoside analogs, highly potent inhibitors of varicella-zoster virus, to the catabolic action of thymidine phosphorylase and dihydropyrimidine dehydrogenase. *Mol. Pharmacol.*, **61**, 1140–1145.

Beadle, J. R., Wan, W .B., Ciesla, S. L. *et al.* (2006). Synthesis and antiviral evaluation of alkoxyalkyl derivatives of 9-(S)-(3-hydroxy-2-phosphonomethoxypropyl)adenine against cytomegalovirus and orthopoxviruses. *J. Med. Chem.*, **49**, 2010–2015.

Beard, P. M., Taus, N. S., and Baines, J. D. (2002). DNA cleavage and packaging proteins encoded by genes U(L)28, U(L)15, and U(L)33 of herpes simplex virus type 1 form a complex in infected cells. *J. Virol.*, **76**, 4785–4791.

Bernstein, D. I., Harrison, C. J., Tomai, M. A., and Miller, R. L. (2001). Daily or weekly therapy with resiquimod (R-848) reduces genital recurrences in herpes simplex virus-infected guinea pigs during and after treatment. *J. Infect. Dis.*, **183**, 844–849.

Betz, U. A., Fischer, R., Kleymann, G., Hendrix, M., and Rubsamen-Waigmann, H. (2002). Potent in vivo antiviral activity of the herpes simplex virus primase-helicase inhibitor BAY 57-1293. *Antimicrob. Agents Chemother.*, **46**, 1766–1772.

Bidanset, D. J., Beadle, J. R., Wan, W. B., Hostetler, K. Y., and Kern, E. R. (2004). Oral activity of ether lipid ester prodrugs of cidofovir against experimental human cytomegalovirus infection. *J. Infect. Dis.*, **190**, 499–503.

Biron, K. K., Harvey, R. J., Chamberlain, S. C. *et al.* (2002). Potent and selective inhibition of human cytomegalovirus replication by 1263W94, a benzimidazole L-riboside with a unique mode of action. *Antimicrob.Agents Chemother.*, **46**, 2365–2372.

Bogner, E., Radsak, K., and Stinski, M. F. (1998). The gene product of human cytomegalovirus open reading frame UL56 binds the pac motif and has specific nuclease activity. *J. Virol.*, **72**, 2259–2264.

Bogner, E. (2002). Human cytomegalovirus terminase as a target for antiviral chemotherapy. *Rev. Med. Virol.*, **12**, 115–127.

Borthwick, A. D. (2005). Design of translactam HCMV protease inhibitors as potent antivirals. *Med. Res. Rev.*, **25**, 427–452.

Borthwick, A. D., Weingarten, G., Haley, T. M. *et al.* (1998). Design and synthesis of monocyclic beta-lactams as mechanism-based inhibitors of human cytomegalovirus protease. *Bioorg. Med. Chem. Lett.*, **8**, 365–370.

Boston Consulting Group analysis based on DiMasi, J. A. *et al.* (1993). As quoted by The Office of Technology Assessment in Pharmaceutical Research and Development: Cost, Risks, Rewards.

Boulware, S. L., Bronstein, J. C., Nordby, E. C., and Weber, P. C. (2001). Identification and characterization of a benzothiophene inhibitor of herpes simplex virus type 1 replication which acts at the immediate early stage of infection. *Antiviral Res.*, **51**, 111–125.

Bournique, B., Lambert, N., Boukaiba, R., and Martinet, M. (2001). In vitro metabolism and drug interaction potential of a new highly potent anti-cytomegalovirus molecule, CMV423 (2-chloro 3-pyridine 3-yl 5,6,7,8-tetrahydroindolizine I-carboxamide). *Br. J. Clin. Pharmacol.*, **52**, 53–63.

Braithwaite, D. K. and Ito, J. (1993). Compilation, alignment, and phylogenetic relationships of DNA polymerases. *Nucl. Acids Res.*, **21**, 787–802.

Brideau, R. J., Knechtel, M. L., Huang, A. *et al.* (2002). Broad-spectrum antiviral activity of PNU-183792, a 4-oxo-dihydroquinoline, against human and animal herpesviruses. *Antiviral Res.*, **54**, 19–28.

Brown, D. G., Visse, R., Sandhu, G. *et al.* (1995).Crystal structures of the thymidine kinase from herpes simplex virus type-1 in complex with deoxythymidine and ganciclovir. *Nat. Struct. Biol.*, **2**, 876–881.

Buerger, I., Reefschlaeger, J., Bender, W. *et al.* (2001). A novel non-nucleoside inhibitor specifically targets cytomegalovirus DNA maturation via the UL89 and UL56 gene products. *J. Virol.*, **75**, 9077–9086.

Buerger, I., Reefschlaeger, J., Bender, W. (2001). A novel nonnucleoside inhibitor specifically targets cytomegalovirus DNA maturation via the UL89 and UL56 gene products. *J. Virol.*, **75**, 9077–9086.

Chee, M. S., Lawrence, G. L., and Barrell, B. G. (1989). Alpha-, beta- and gammaherpesviruses encode a putative phosphotransferase. *J. Gen. Virol.*, **70**(5), 1151–1160.

Chou, S. (2006). UL27 and UL97 resistance mutations selected after passage of clinical CMV isolates under maribavir. 31st International Herpesvirus Workshop. 31st International Herpesvirus Workshop [Seattle, WA July 22-28; Oral Presentation 10.13].

Chou, S., Lurain, N. S., Thompson, K. D., Miner, R. C., and Drew, W. L. (2003). Viral DNA polymerase mutations associated with drug resistance in human cytomegalovirus. *J. Infect. Dis.*, **188**, 32–39.

Chou, S., Marousek, G. I., Senters, A. E., Davis, M. G., and Biron, K. K. (2004). Mutations in the human cytomegalovirus UL27 gene that confer resistance to maribavir. *J. Virol.*, **78**, 7124–7130.

Chulay, J., Biron, K., Wang L. *et al.* (1999). Development of novel benzimidazole riboside compounds for treatment of cytomegalovirus disease. *Adv. Exp. Med Biol.*, **458**, 129–134.

Ciesla, S. L., Trahan, J., Wan, W. B. *et al.* (2003). Esterification of cidofovir with alkoxyalkanols increases oral bioavailability and diminishes drug accumulation in kidney. *Antiviral Res.*, **59**, 163–171.

Cirone, M., Zompetta, C., Tarasi, D., Frati, L., and Faggioni, A. (1996). Infection of human T lymphoid cells by human herpesvirus 6 is blocked by two unrelated protein tyrosine kinase inhibitors, biochanin A and herbimycin. *AIDS Res. Hum. Retroviruses*, **12**, 1629–1634.

Crumpacker, C. S. and Schaffer, P. A. (2002). New anti-HSV therapeutics target the helicase-primase complex. *Nat. Med.*, **8**, 327–328.

Crute, J. J. and Lehman, I. R. (1991). Herpes simplex virus-1 helicase-primase. Physical and catalytic properties. *J. Biol. Chem.*, **266**, 4484–4488.

Crute, J. J., Grygon, C. A., Hargrave, K. D. *et al.* (2002). Herpes simplex virus helicase-primase inhibitors are active in animal models of human disease. *Nat. Med.*, **8**, 386–391.

De Bolle, L., Andrei, G., Snoeck, R. *et al.* (2004). Potent, selective and cell-mediated inhibition of human herpesvirus 6 at an early stage of viral replication by the non-nucleoside compound CMV423. *Biochem. Pharmacol.*, **67**, 325–336.

De Clercq, E. (2002). Cidofovir in the therapy and short-term prophylaxis of poxvirus infections. *Trends Pharmacol. Sci.*, **23**, 456–458.

De Clercq, E. (2003a). Highly potent and selective inhibition of varicella-zoster virus replication by bicyclic furo[2,3-d]pyrimidine nucleoside analogues. *Med. Res. Rev.*, **23**, 253–274.

De Clercq, E. (2003b). New inhibitors of human cytomegalovirus (HCMV) on the horizon. *J. Antimicrob. Chemother.*, **51**, 1079–1083.

De Miranda, P. and Burnette, T. C. (1994). Metabolic fate and pharmacokinetics of the acyclovir prodrug valaciclovir in cynomolgus monkeys. *Drug Metab. Dispos.*, **22**, 55–59.

De Miranda, P. and Good, S. S. (1992). Species differences in the metabolism and disposition of antiviral analogues. *Antiviral Chem. Chemo.*, **3**, 1–8.

Diana, G. D., Oglesby, R. C., Akullian, V. *et al.* (1987). Structure-activity studies of 5-[[4-(4,5-dihydro-2-oxazolyl) phenoxy]alkyl]-3-methylisoxazoles: inhibitors of picornavirus uncoating. *J. Med. Chem.*, **30**, 383–388.

Dittmer, A., Drach, J. C., Townsend, L., Fischer, A., and Bogner, E. (2005). Interaction of the putative human cytomegalovirus portal protein pUL104 with the large terminase subunit pUL56 and its inhibition by benzimidazole-D-ribonucleosides. *J. Virol.*, **79**, 14660–14667.

Docherty, J. J., Fu, M. M., Stiffler, B. S., Limperos, R. J., Pokabla, C. M., and DeLucia, A. L. (1999). Resveratrol inhibition of herpes simplex virus replication. *Antiviral Res.*, **43**, 145–155.

Dunkle, L. M. (1996). Lobucavir: a promising broad-spectrum antiviral agent. **Eleventh** *International Conference on AIDS*, Vancouver, abstract Th.B.943.

Elion, G. B., Furman, P. A., Fyfe, J. A., de Miranda, P., Beauchamp, L., and Schaeffer, H. J. (1977). Selectivity of action of an antiherpetic agent, 9-(2-hydroxyethoxymethyl) guanine. *Proc. Natl Acad. Sci. USA*, **74**, 5716–5720.

Erickson, J., Neidhart, D. J., VanDrie, J. *et al.* (1990). Design, activity, and 2.8 A crystal structure of a C2 symmetric inhibitor complexed to HIV-1 protease. *Science*, **249**, 527–533.

Evers, D. L., Komazin, G., Ptak, R. G. *et al.* (2004). Inhibition of human cytomegalovirus replication by benzimidazole nucleosides involves three distinct mechanisms. *Antimicrob. Agents Chemother.*, **48**, 3918–3927.

Franklin, M. C., Wang, J., and Steitz, T. A. (2001). Structure of the replicating complex of a pol alpha family DNA polymerase. *Cell*, **105**, 657–667.

Gershburg, E. and Pagano, J. S. (2002). Phosphorylation of the Epstein–Barr virus (EBV) DNA polymerase processivity factor EA-D by the EBV-encoded protein kinase and effects of the L-riboside benzimidazole 1263W94. *J. Virol.*, **76**, 998–1003.

Gibson, W., Welch, A. R., and Hall, W. R. T. (1994). Assembling a herpesvirus serine maturational proteinase and a new molecular target for antivirals. *Perspect Drug Discov Design*, **2**, 413–416.

Good, S. S., Owens, B. S., Townsend, L. B., and Drach, J. C. (1994). The disposition in rats and monkeys of 2-bromo-5,6,-dichloro-1-(beta-ribofuranosyl)benzimididazole (BDCRB) and its 2,5,6-trichloro congener (TCRB). *Antivir. Res.*, **23**, 103.

Hall, M. C. and Matson, S. W. (1999). Helicase motifs: the engine that powers DNA unwinding. *Mol. Microbiol.*, **34**, 867–877.

Hamilton, H. W., Nishiguchi, G., Hagen, S. E. *et al.* (2002). Novel benzthiodiazepinones as antiherpetic agents: SAR improvement of therapeutic index by alterations of the seven-membered ring. *Bioorg. Med Chem. Lett.*, **12**, 2981–2983.

Hasegawa, Y., Nishiyama, Y., Imaizumi, K. *et al.* (2000). Avoidance of bone marrow suppression using A-5021 as a nucleoside analog for retrovirus-mediated herpes simplex virus type I thymidine kinase gene therapy. *Cancer Gene Ther.*, **7**, 557–562.

He, Z., He, Y. S., Kim, Y. *et al.* (1997). The human cytomegalovirus UL97 protein is a protein kinase that autophosphorylates on serines and threonines. *J. Virol.*, **71**, 405–411.

Hemmi, H., Kaisho, T., Takeuchi, O. *et al.* (2002). Small antiviral compounds activate immune cells via the TLR7 MyD88-dependent signaling pathway. *Nat. Immunol.*, **3**, 196–200.

Henry, S. P., Miner, R. C., Drew, W. L. *et al.* (2001). Antiviral activity and ocular kinetics of antisense oligonucleotides designed to inhibit CMV replication. *Invest. Ophthalmol. Vis. Sci.*, **42**, 2646–2651.

Herget, T., Freitag, M., Morbitzer, M., Kupfer, R., Stamminger, T., and Marschall, M. (2004). Novel chemical class of pUL97 protein kinase-specific inhibitors with strong anticytomegaloviral activity. *Antimicrob. Agents Chemother.*, **48**, 4154–4162.

Holwerda, B. C. (1997). Herpesvirus proteases: targets for novel antiviral drugs. *Antiviral Res.*, **35**, 1–21.

Hoog, S. S., Smith, W. W., Qiu, X. *et al.* (1997). Active site cavity of herpesvirus proteases revealed by the crystal structure of herpes simplex virus protease/inhibitor complex. *Biochemistry*, **56**, 14023–14029.

Hu, H. and Cohen, J. I. (2005). Varicella-zoster virus open reading frame 47 (ORF47) protein is critical for virus replication in dendritic cells and for spread to other cells. *Virology*, **337**, 304–311.

Huggins, J. W., Baker, R. O., Beadle, J. R., and Hostetler, K. Y. (2002). Orally active ether lipid prodrugs of cidofovir for the treatment of smallpox. *Antivir. Res.*, **53**, A66, 104.

Iwayama, S., Ono, N., Ohmura, Y. *et al.* (1998). Antiherpesvirus activities of (1'S,2'R)-9-[[1',2'-bis(hydroxymethyl)cycloprop-1'-yl]methyl]guanine (A-5021) in cell culture. *Antimicrob. Agents Chemother.*, **42**, 1666–1670.

Iwayama, S., Ohmura, Y., Suzuki, K. *et al.* (1999). Evaluation of anti-herpesvirus activity of (1'S,2'R)-9-[[1',2'-bis(hydroxymethyl)cycloprop-1'-yl]methyl]-guanine (A-5021) in mice. *Antiviral Res.*, **42**, 139–148.

Jacobson, J. G., Renau, T. E., Nassiri, M. R. *et al.* (1999). Non-nucleoside pyrrolopyrimidines with a unique mechanism of action against human cytomegalovirus. *Antimicrob. Agents Chemother.*, **43**, 1888–1894.

Kato, A., Yamamoto, M., Ohno, T. *et al.* (2006). Herpes simplex virus 1-encoded protein kinase UL13 phosphorylates viral Us3 protein kinase and regulates nuclear localization of viral envelopment factors UL34 and UL31. *J. Virol.*, **80**, 1476–1486.

Kawaguchi, Y. and Kato, K. (2003). Protein kinases conserved in herpesviruses potentially share a function mimicking the cellular protein kinase cdc2. *Rev. Med. Virol.*, **13**, 331–340.

Kern, E. R. (2003). In vitro activity of potential anti-proxvirus agents. *Antiviral Res.*, **57**, 35–40.

Kern, E. R., Collins, D. J., Wan, W. B., Beadle, J. R., Hostetler, K. Y., and Quenelle, D. C. (2004a). Oral treatment of murine cytomegalovirus infections with ether lipid esters of cidofovir. *Antimicrob. Agents Chemother.*, **48**, 3516–3522.

Kleymann, G. (2003a). Novel agents and strategies to treat herpes simplex virus infections. *Expert. Opin. Investig. Drugs*, 12, 165–183.

Kleymann, G. (2003b). Helicase-primase inhibitors. *Drugs of the Future*, **28**, 257–265.

Kleymann, G., Fischer, R., Betz, U. A. *et al.* (2002). New helicase-primase inhibitors as drug candidates for the treatment of herpes simplex disease. *Nat. Med.*, **8**, 392–398.

Knechtel, M. L., Huang, A., Vaillancourt, V. A., and Brideau, R. J. (2002). Inhibition of clinical isolates of human cytomegalovirus and varicella zoster virus by PNU-183792, a 4-oxo-dihydroquinoline. *J. Med. Virol.*, **68**, 234–236.

Komatsu, T., Ballestras, M. E., Barbera, A. J., Kelly-Clarke, B., and Kaye, K. M. (2004). KSHV LA NA-1 binds DNA as an oligomer and residues N-terminal to the oligomerization domain are essential for DNA replication and episome persistence. *Virology*, **319**, 225–236.

Koszalka, G. W., Johnson, N. W., Good, S. S. (2002). Preclinicat and toxicology studies of 1263W94, a potent and selective inhibitor of human cytomegalovirus replication. *Antimicrob. Agents Chemother*, **46**, 2373–2380.

Komazin, G., Ptak, R. G., Emmer, B. T., Townsend, L. B, and Drach, J. C. (2003). Resistance of human cytomegalovirus to the benzimidazole L-ribonucleoside maribavir maps to UL27. *J Virol.*, **77**, 11499–11506.

Komazin, G., Townsend, L. B., and Drach, J. C. (2004). Role of a mutation in human cytomegalovirus gene UL104 in resistance to benzimidazole ribonucleosides. *J. Virol.*, **78**, 710–715.

Krosky, P. M., Baek, M. C., Jahng, W. J. *et al.* (2003b). The human cytomegalovirus UL44 protein is a substrate for the UL97 protein kinase. *J. Virol.*, **77**, 7720–7727.

Krosky, P. M., Baek, M. C., and Coen, D. M. (2003a). The human cytomegalovirus UL97 protein kinase, an antiviral drug target, is required at the stage of nuclear egress. *J. Virol.*, **77**, 905–914.

Krosky, P. M., Underwood, M. R., Turk, S.R. *et al.* (1998). Resistance of human cytomegalovirus to benzimidazole ribonucleosides maps to two open reading frames: UL89 and UL56. *J. Virol.*, **72**, 4721-4728.

LaBranche, C. C., Galasso, G., Moore, J. P., Bolognesi, D. P., Hirsch, M. S., and Hammer, S. M. (2001). HIV fusion and its inhibition. *Antiviral Res.*, **50**, 95–115.

Lalezari, J. P. (1997). New treatment options for CMV retinitis in AIDS. *Adv. Nurse Pract.*, **5**, 45–9.

Lalezari, J. P., Drew, W. L., Glutzer, E. *et al.* (1995). (S)-1[3-hydroxy-2-(phosphonylmethoxy)propyl] cytosine (cidofovir): results of a phase I/II study of a novel antiviral nucleotide analogue. *J. Infect. Dis.*, **171**, 788–796.

Lalezari, J. P., Aberg, J. A., Wang, L. H. *et al.* (2002). Phase I dose escalation trial evaluating the pharmacokinetics, anti-human cytomegalovirus (HCMV) activity, and safety of 1263W94 in human immunodeficiency virus-infected men with asymptomatic HCMV shedding. *Antimicrob. Agents Chemother.*, **46**, 2969–2976.

Lipinski, C. A., Lombardo, F., Dominy, B. W., and Feeney, P. J. (2001). Experimental and computational approaches to estimate solubility and permeability in drug discovery and development settings. *Adv. Drug Deliv. Rev.*, **46**, 3–26

Littler, E., Stuart, A. D., and Chee, M. S. (1992). Human cytomegalovirus UL97 open reading frame encodes a protein that phosphorylates the antiviral nucleoside analogue ganciclovir. *Nature*, **358**, 160–162.

Liuzzi, M., Kibler, P., Bousquet, C. et al. (2004). Isolation and characterization of herpes simplex virus type 1 resistant to aminothiazolylphenyl-based inhibitors of the viral helicase-primase. *Antiviral Res.*, **64**, 161–170.

Loregian, A., and Coen, D. M. (2006). Selective anti-cytomegalovirus compounds discoverd by screening for inhibitors of subunit interactions of the viral polymerase, *Chem. Biol.*, **13**, 191–200.

Lorenzi, P. L., Landowski, C. P., Brancale, A. et al. (2006). N-methylpurine DNA glycosylase and 8-oxoguanine dna glycosylase metabolize the antiviral nucleoside 2-bromo-5,6-dichloro-1-(beta-D-ribofuranosyl)benzimidazole. *Drug Metab. Dispos.*, **34**, 1070–1077.

Lorenzi, P. L., Landowski, C. P., Song, X. et al. (2005). Amino acid ester prodrugs of 2-bromo-5,6-dichloro-1-(beta-D-ribofuranosyl)benzimidazole enhance metabolic stability in vitro and in vivo. *J. Pharmacol. Exp. Ther.*, **314**, 883–890.

Lowden, C. T. and Bastow, K. F. (2003). Cell culture replication of herpes simplex virus and, or human cytomegalovirus is inhibited by 3,7-dialkoxylated, 1-hydroxyacridone derivatives. *Antiviral Res.*, **59**, 143–154.

Lowe, D. M., Alderton, W. K., Ellis M. R. et al. (1995). Mode of action of (R)-9-[4-hydroxy-2-(hydroxymethyl)butyl]guanine against herpesviruses. *Antimicrob. Agents Chemother.*, **39**, 1802–1808.

Lu, H. and Thomas, S. (2004). Maribavir (ViroPharma). *Curr. Opin. Investig. Drugs*, **5**, 898–906.

Lurain, N. S., Weinberg, A., Crumpacker, C. S., and Chou S. (2001). Sequencing of cytomegalovirus UL97 gene for genotypic antiviral resistance testing. *Antimicrob. Agents Chemother.*, **45**, 2775–2780.

Ma, J. D., Nafziger, A. N., Villano, S. A., and J. S., Jr. (2006). Maribavir pharmacokinetics and the effects of multiple-dose maribavir on cytochrome P450 (CYP) 1A2, CYP 2C9, CYP 2C19, CYP 2D6, CYP 3A, N-acetyltransferase-2, and xanthine oxidase activities in healthy adults. *Antimicrob. Agents Chemother.*, **50**, 1130–1135.

Marschall, M., Stein-Gerlach, M., Freitage, M., Kupfer, R., van Den, BM., and Stamminger, T. (2001). Inhibitors of human cytomegalovirus replication drastically reduce the activity of the viral protein kinase pUL97. *J.Gen. Virol.*, **82**, 1439–1450.

Marschall, M., Freitag, M., Suchy, P. et al. (2003). The protein kinase pUL97 of human cytomegalovirus interacts with and phosphorylates the DNA polymerase processivity factor pUL44. *Virology*, **311**, 60–71.

Marschall, M., Marzi, A., aus dem, S. P., et al., (2005). Cellular p32 recruits cytomegalovirus kinase pUL97 to redistribute the nuclear lamina. *J. Biol. Chem.*, **280**, 33357–33367.

Matthews, J. T., Terry, B. J., and Field, A. K. (1993). The structure and function of the HSV DNA replication proteins: defining novel antiviral targets. *Antiviral Res.*, **20**, 89–114.

McGuigan, C., Jukes, A., Blewett, S. et al. (2003). Halophenyl furanopyrimidines as potent and selective anti-VZV agents. *Antivir. Chem. Chemother.*, **14**, 165–170.

McSharry, J. J., McDonough, A., Olson, B. et al. (2001a). Susceptibilities of human cytomegalovirus clinical isolates to BAY38-4766, BAY43-9695, and ganciclovir. *Antimicrob. Agents Chemother.*, **45**, 2925–2927.

McSharry, J. J., McDonough, A., Olson, B., Talarico, C., Davis, M., and Biron, K. K. (2001b). Inhibition of ganciclovir-susceptible and -resistant human cytomegalovirus clinical isolates by the benzimidazole L-riboside 1263W94. *Clin. Diagn. Lab. Immunol.*, **8**, 1279–1281.

McVoy, M. A. and Nixon, D. E. (2005). Impact of 2-bromo-5,6-dichloro-1-beta-D-ribofuranosyl benzimidazole riboside and inhibitors of DNA, RNA, and protein synthesis on human cytomegalovirus genome maturation. *J. Virol.*, **79**, 11115–11127.

Mettenleiter, T. C. (2002). Herpesvirus assembly and egress. *J Virol.*, **76**, 1537–1547.

Michel, D., Pavic, I., Zimmermann, A. et al. (1996). The UL97 gene product of human cytomegalovirus is an early-late protein with a nuclear localization but is not a nucleoside kinase. *J. Virol.*, **70**, 6340–6346.

Miller, R. L., Tomai, M. A., Harrison, C. J., and Bernstein, D. I. (2002). Immunomodulation as a treatment strategy for genital herpes: review of the evidence. *Int. Immunopharmacol.*, **2**, 443-451.

Moffat, J. F., Zerboni, L., Sommer, M. H. et al. (1998). The ORF47 and ORF66 putative protein kinases of varicella-zoster virus determine tropism for human T cells and skin in the SCID-hu mouse. *Proc. Natl Acad. Sci. USA*, **95**, 11969–11974.

Nagelschmitz, J., Moeller, J. G., Stass, H. H., Wadel, C., and Kuhlmann, J. (1999). Safety, tolerability, and pharmacokinetics of single oral doses of BAY 38-4766 – a novel nonnucleosidic inhibitor of human cytomegalovirus (HCMV) replication – in healthy male subjects. In *Program and Abstracts of the* **Thirty-ninth** *Interscience Conference on Antimicrob Agents and Chemother*, San Francisco, CA, Abstract 945, 322.

Naesens, L., Stephens, C. E., Andrei, G. et al. (2006). Antiviral properties of new arylsulfone derivatives with activity against human betaherpesviruses. *Antiviral Res.*, in press.

Newcomb, W. W. and Brown, J. C. (2002). Inhibition of herpes simplex virus replication by WAY-150138: assembly of capsids depleted of the portal and terminase proteins involved in DNA encapsidation. *J Virol.*, **76**, 10084–10088.

Newcomb, W. W., Juhas, R. M., Thomsen, D. R. et al. (2001). The UL6 gene product forms the portal for entry of DNA into the herpes simplex virus capsid. *J. Virol.*, **75**, 10923–10932.

Newcomb, W. W., Juhas, R. M., Thomsen, D. R. et al. (2001). The UL6 gene product forms the portal for entry of DNA into the herpes simplex virus capsid. *J. Virol.*, **75**, 10923–10932.

Newcomb, W. W., Thomsen, D. R., Homa, F. L., and Brown, J. C. (2003). Assembly of the herpes simplex virus capsid: identification of soluble scaffold-portal complexes and their role in formation of portal-containing capsids. *J. Virol.*, **77**, 9862–9871.

Neyts, J. and De Clercq, E. (2001). The anti-herpesvirus activity of (1′S,2′R)-9-[[1′,2′-bis(hydroxymethyl)-cycloprop-1′-yl]methyl]guanine is markedly potentiated by the immunosuppressive agent mycophenolate mofetil. *Antiviral Res.*, **49**, 121–127.

Neyts, J., Naesens, L., Ying, C., De Bolle, L., and De Clercq, E. (2001). Anti-herpesvirus activity of (1′S,2′R)-9-[[1′,2′-bis(hydroxymethyl)-cycloprop-1′-yl]methyl] x guanine (A-5021) in vitro and in vivo. *Antiviral Res.*, **49**, 115–120.

Neyts, J., Leyssen, P., Verbeken, E., and De Clercq, E. (2004). Efficacy of cidofovir in a murine model of disseminated progressive vaccinia. *Antimicrob. Agents Chemother.*, **48**, 2267–2273.

Ng, T. I., Shi, Y., Huffaker, H. J. et al. (2001). Selection and characterization of varicella-zoster virus variants resistant to (R)-9-[4-hydroxy-2-(hydroxymethyl)butyl]guanine. *Antimicrob. Agents Chemother.*, **45**, 1629–1636.

Oien, N. L., Brideau, R. J., Hopkins, T. A. et al. (2002). Broad-spectrum antiherpes activities of 4-hydroxyquinoline carboxamides, a novel class of herpesvirus polymerase inhibitors. *Antimicrob. Agents Chemother.*, **46**, 724–730.

Okano, M. (2003). The evolving therapeutic approaches for Epstein-Barr virus infection in immunocompetent and immunocompromised individuals. *Curr. Drug Targets. Immune. Endocr. Metabol. Disord.*, **3**, 137–142.

Ono, N., Iwayama, S., Suzuki, K. et al. (1998). Mode of action of (1′S,2′R)-9-[[1′,2′-bis(hydroxymethyl) cycloprop-1′-yl]methyl]guanine (A-5021) against herpes simplex virus type 1 and type 2 and varicella-zoster virus. *Antimicrob. Agents Chemother.*, **42**, 2095–2102.

Painter, G. R. and Hostetler, K.Y. (2004). Design and development of oral drugs for the prophylaxis and treatment of smallpox infection. *Trends Biotechnol.*, **22**, 423–427.

Prichard, M. N., Britt, W. J., Daily, S. L., Hartline, C. B., and Kern, E. R. (2005). Human cytomegalovirus UL97 Kinase is required for the normal intranuclear distribution of pp65 and virion morphogenesis. *J. Virol.*, **79**, 15494–15502.

Prichard, M. N., Gao, N., Jairath, S. et al. (1999). A recombinant human cytomegalovirus with a large deletion in UL97 has a severe replication deficiency. *J. Virol.*, **73**, 5663–5670.

Przech, A. J., Yu, D., and Weller, S. K. (2003). Point mutations in exon I of the herpes simplex virus putative terminase subunit, UL15, indicate that the most conserved residues are essential for cleavage and packaging. *J. Virol.*, **77**, 9613–9621.

Qiu, X. Y. and Abdelmeguid, S. S. (1999). Human herpes proteases In Dunn, B. M., ed. *Proteases of Infectious Agents*. San Diego: Academic Press, 93–115.

Razonable, R. R., Brown, R. A., Humar, A., Covington, E., Alecock, E., and Paya, C. V. (2005). Herpesvirus infections in solid organ transplant patients at high risk of primary cytomegalovirus disease. *J. Infect. Dis.*, **192**, 1331–1339.

Rechtsteiner, G., Warger, T., Osterloh, P., Schild, H., and Radsak, M. P. (2005). Cutting edge: priming of CTL by transcutaneous peptide immunization with imiquimod. *J. Immunol.* **174**, 2476–2480.

Reefschlaeger, J., Bender, W., Hallenberger, S. et al. (2001). Novel non-nucleoside inhibitors of cytomegaloviruses (BAY 38-4766): in vitro and in vivo antiviral activity and mechanism of action. *J. Antimicrob. Chemother.*, **48**, 757–767.

Roizman, B., Whitley, R. J., and Lopez, C., eds. (1993). *The Human Herpesvirses*. New York, NY: Raven Press.

Safrin, S., Cherrington, J., and Jaffe, H. S. (1997). Clinical uses of cidofovir. *Rev. Med. Virol.*, 7, 145–156.

Sakuma, T., Saijo, M., Suzutani, T. et al. (1991). Antiviral activity of oxetanocins against varicella-zoster virus. *Antimicrob. Agents Chemother.*, **35**, 1512–1514.

Schang, L. M. (2002). Cyclin-dependent kinases as cellular targets for antiviral drugs. *J. Antimicrob. Chemother.*, **50**, 779–792.

Schang, L. M., Bantly, A., Knockaert, M. et al. (2002). Pharmacological cyclin-dependent kinase inhibitors inhibit replication of wild-type and drug-resistant strains of herpes simplex virus and human immunodeficiency virus type 1 by targeting cellular, not viral, proteins. *J. Virol.*, **76**, 7874–7882.

Scheffczik, H., Savva, C. G., Holzenburg, A., Kolesnikova, L., and Bogner, E. (2002). The terminase subunits pUL56 and pUL89 of human cytomegalovirus are DNA-metabolizing proteins with toroidal structure. *Nucl. Acids Res.*, **30**, 1695–1703.

Scolnick, E. M., Richards, F. M., Eisenberg, D. S., and Kim, P. S., eds. (2001). *Drug Discovery and Design* (Advances in Protein Chemistry) **51**, Academic Press.

Sekiyama, T., Hatsuya, S., Tanaka, Y. et al. (1998). Synthesis and antiviral activity of novel acyclic nucleosides: discovery of a cyclopropyl nucleoside with potent inhibitory activity against herpesviruses. *J. Med. Chem.*, **41**, 1284–1298.

Shin, Y. K., Cai, G. Y., Weinberg, A., Leary, J. J., and Levin, M. J. (2001). Frequency of acyclovir-resistant herpes simplex virus in clinical specimens and laboratory isolates. *J. Clin. Microbiol.*, **39**, 913–917.

Shugar, D. (1999). Viral and host-cell protein kinases: enticing antiviral targets and relevance of nucleoside, and viral thymidine, kinases. *Pharmacol. Ther.*, **82**, 315–335.

Sienaert, R., Andrei, G., Snoeck, R., De Clercq, E., McGuigan, C., and Balzarini, J. (2004). Inactivity of the bicyclic pyrimidine nucleoside analogues against simian varicella virus (SVV) does not correlate with their substrate activity for SVV-encoded thymidine kinase. *Biochem. Biophys. Res. Commun.*, **315**, 877–883.

Sienaert, R., Naesens, L., Brancale, A., De Clercq, E., McGuigan, C., and Balzarini, J. (2002). Specific recognition of the bicyclic pyrimidine nucleoside analogs, a new class of highly potent and selective inhibitors of varicella-zoster virus (VZV), by the VZV-encoded thymidine kinase. *Mol. Pharmacol.*, **61**, 249–254.

Simpson-Holley, M., Baines, J., Roller, R., and Knipe, D. M. (2004). Herpes simplex virus 1 U(L)31 and U(L)34 gene products promote the late maturation of viral replication compartments to the nuclear periphery. *J. Virol.*, **78**, 5591–5600.

Slater, M. J., Cockerill, S., Baxter, R. et al. (1999). Indolocarbazoles: potent, selective inhibitors of human cytomegalovirus replication. *Bioorg. Med. Chem.*, **7**, 1067–1074.

Smith, R. F. and Smith, T. F. (1989). Identification of new protein kinase-related genes in three herpesviruses, herpes simplex virus, varicella-zoster virus, and Epstein–Barr virus. *J. Virol.*, **63**, 450–455.

Snoeck, R., Andrei, G., Bodaghi, B. *et al.* (2002). 2-Chloro-3-pyridin-3-yl-5,6,7,8-tetrahydroindolizine-1-carboxamide (CMV423), a new lead compound for the treatment of human cytomegalovirus infections. *Antiviral Res.*, **55**, 413–424.

Soike, K. F., Bohm, R., Huang, J. L., and, Oberg, B. (1993). Efficacy of (-)-9-[4-hydroxy-2-(hydroxymethyl)butyl]guanine in African green monkeys infected with simian varicella virus. *Antimicrob. Agents Chemother.*, **37**, 1370–1372.

Spector, F. C., Liang, L., Giordano, H., Sivaraja, M., and Peterson, M. G. (1998). Inhibition of herpes simplex virus replication by a 2-amino thiazole via interactions with the helicase component of the UL5-UL8-UL52 complex. *J. Virol.*, **72**, 6979–6987.

Spence, R. A., Kati, W. M., Anderson, K. S., and Johnson, K. A. (1995). Mechanism of inhibition of HIV-1 reverse transcriptase by nonnucleoside inhibitors. *Science*, **267**, 988–993.

Stamminger, T., Gstaiger, M., Weinzierl, K., Lorz, K., Winkler, M., and Schaffner, W. (2002). Open reading frame UL26 of human cytomegalovirus encodes a novel tegument protein that contains a strong transcriptional activation domain. *J. Virol.*, **76**, 4836–4847.

Sullivan, V., Talarico, C. L., Stanat, S. C., Davis, M., Coen, D. M., and Biron, K. K. (1992). A protein kinase homologue controls phosphorylation of ganciclovir in human cytomegalovirus-infected cells. *Nature*, **359**, 85.

Supuran, C. T., Casini, A., and Scozzafava, A. (2003). Protease inhibitors of the sulfonamide type: anticancer, antiinflammatory, and antiviral agents. *Med. Res. Rev.*, **23**, 535–558.

Talarico, C. L., Burnette, T. C., Miller, W. H. *et al.* (1999). Acyclovir is phosphorylated by the human cytomegalovirus UL97 protein. *Antimicrob. Agents Chemother.*, **43**, 1941–1946.

Tenney, D. J., Yamanaka, G., Voss, S. M. *et al.* (1997). Lobucavir is phosphorylated in human cytomegalovirus-infected and -uninfected cells and inhibits the viral DNA polymerase. *Antimicrob. Agents Chemother.*, **41**, 2680–2685.

Thoma, C., Borst, E., Messerle, M., Rieger, M., Hwang, J. S. and Bogner, E. (2006). Identification of the interaction domain of the small terminase subunit pUL89 with the large subunit pUL56 of human cytomegalovirus. *Biochemistry*, **45**, 8855–8863.

Thomsen, D. R., Oien, N. L., Hopkins, T. A. *et al.* (2003). Amino acid changes within conserved region III of the herpes simplex virus and human cytomegalovirus DNA polymerases confer resistance to 4-oxo-dihydroquinolines, a novel class of herpesvirus antiviral agents. *J. Virol.*, **77**, 1868–1876.

Thomsen, L. L., Topley, P., Daly, M. G., Brett, S. J., and Tite, J. P. (2004). Imiquimod and resiquimod in a mouse model: adjuvants for DNA vaccination by particle-mediated immunotherapeutic delivery. *Vaccine*, **22**, 1799–1809.

Townsend, L. B. and Revankar, G. R. (1970). Benzimidazole nucleosides, nucleotides, and related derivatives. *Chem. Rev.*, **70**, 389–438.

Townsend, L. B., Devivar, R. V., Turk, S. R., Nassiri, M. R., and Drach, J. C. (1995). Design, synthesis, and antiviral activity of certain 2,5,6-trihalo-l-(beta-D-ribofuranosyl)benzimidazoles. *J. Med. Chem.*, **38**, 4098–4105.

Townsend, L. B., Gudmundsson, K. S., Daluge, S. M. *et al.* (1999). Studies designed to increase the stability and antiviral activity (HCMV) of the active benzimidazole nucleoside, TCRB. *Nucleosides Nucleotides*, **18**, 509–519.

Tsai, C. J., Lin, S. L., Wolfson, H. J., and Nussinov, R. (1997). Studies of protein-protein interfaces: a statistical analysis of the hydrophobic effect. *Protein Sci.*, **6**, 53–64.

Underwood, M. R., Harvey, R. J., Stanat, S. C. *et al.* (1998). Inhibition of human cytomegalovirus DNA maturation by a benzimidazole ribonucleoside is mediated through the UL89 gene product. *J. Virol.*, **72**, 717–725.

Vaillancourt, V. A., Cudahy, M. M., Staley, S. A. *et al.* (2000). Naphthalene carboxamides as inhibitors of human cytomegalovirus DNA polymerase. *Bioorg. Med. Chem. Lett.*, **10**, 2079–2081.

Van Zeijl, M., Fairhurst, J., Baum, E. Z., Sun, L., and Jones, T. R. (1997). The human cytomegalovirus UL97 protein is phosphorylated and a component of virions. *Virology*, **231**, 72–80.

van Zeijl, M., Fairhurst, J., Jones, T. R. *et al.* (2000). Novel class of thiourea compounds that inhibit herpes simplex virus type 1 DNA cleavage and encapsidation: resistance maps to the UL6 gene. *J. Virol.*, **74**, 9054–9061.

Visalli, R. J. and van Zeijl, M. (2003). DNA encapsidation as a target for antiherpesvirus drug therapy. *Antiviral Res.*, **59**, 73–87.

Visalli, R. J., Fairhurst, J., Srinivas, S. *et al.* (2003). Identification of small molecule compounds that selectively inhibit varicella-zoster virus replication. *J. Virol.*, **77**, 2349–2358.

Wang, L. H., Peck, R. W., Yin, Y., Allanson, J., Wiggs, R., and Wire, M. W. (2003). Phase I safety and pharmacokinetic trials of 1263W94, a novel oral anti-human cytomegalovirus agent, in healthy and human immunodeficiency virus-infected subject. *Antimicrob. Agents Chemother.*, **47**, 1334–1342.

Wan, W. B., Beadle, J. R., Hartline, C. *et al.* (2005). Comparison of the antiviral activities of alkoxyalkyl and alkyl esters of cidofovir against human and murine cytomegalovirus replication in vitro. *Antimicrob. Agents. Chemother.*, **49**, 656–662.

Wathen, M. W. (2002). Non-nucleoside inhibitors of herpesviruses. *Rev. Med. Virol.*, **12**, 167–178.

Waxman, L. and Darke, P. L. (2000). The herpesvirus proteases as targets for antiviral chemotherapy. *Antivir. Chem. Chemother.*, **11**, 1–22.

Wang, Y., Abel, K., Lantz, K., Krieg, A. M., McChesney, M. B., and Miller, C. J. (2005). The Toll-like receptor 7 (TLR7) agonist, imiquimod, and the TLR9 agonist, CpG ODN, induce antiviral cytokines and chemokines but do not prevent vaginal transmission of simian immunodeficiency virus when applied intravaginally to rhesus macaques. *J. Virol.*, **79**, 14355–14370.

Weber, O., Bender, W., Eckenberg, P. *et al.* (2001). Inhibition of murine cytomegalovirus and human cytomegalovirus by a novel non-nucleosidic compound in vivo. *Antiviral Res.*, **49**, 179–189.

White, C. A., Stow, N. D., Patel, A. H., Hughes, M., and Preston, V. G. (2003). Herpes simplex virus type 1 portal protein UL6 interacts with the putative terminase subunits UL15 and UL28. *J Virol.*, **77**, 6351–6358.

Williams, S. L., Hartline, C. B., Kushner, N. L. *et al.* (2003). In vitro activities of benzimidazole D- and L-ribonucleosides against herpesviruses. *Antimicrob. Agents Chemother.*, **47**, 2186–2192.

Williams-Aziz, S. L., Hartline, C. B., Harden, E. A. *et al.* (2005). Comparative activities of lipid esters of cidofovir and cyclic cidofovir against replication of herpesviruses in vitro. *Antimicrob. Agents Chemother.*, **49**, 3724–3733.

Wolf, D. G., Courcelle, C. T., Prichard, M. N., and Mocarski, E. S. (2001). Distinct and separate roles for herpesvirus-conserved UL97 kinase in cytomegalovirus DNA synthesis and encapsidation. *Proc. Natl Acad. Sci. USA*, **98**, 1895–1900.

Wolf, D. G., Courcelle, C. T., Prichard, M. N., and Mocarski, E. S. (2001). Distinct and separate roles for herpesvirus-conserved UL97 kinase in cytomegalovirus DNA synthesis and encapsidation. *Proc. Natl Acad. Sci. U.S.A*, **98**, 1895–1900.

Zacny, V. L., Gershburg, E., Davis, M. G., Biron, K. K., and Pagano, J. S. (1999). Inhibition of Epstein-Barr virus replication by a benzimidazole L-riboside: novel antiviral mechanism of 5,6-dichloro-2-(isopropylamino)-1-beta-L-ribofuranosyl-1H-benzimidazole. *J Virol.*, **73**, 7271–7277.

Zimmermann, A., Wilts, H., Lenhardt, M., Hahn, M., and Mertens, T. (2000). *Fifteenth International Conference on Antiviral Res.* Indolocarbazoles exhibit strong antiviral activity against human cytomegalovirus and are potent inhibitors of the pUL97 protein kinase. *Antiviral Res.*, **48**, 49–60.

Part VII

Vaccines and immunotherapy

Edited by Ann Arvin and Koichi Yamanishi

Herpes simplex vaccines

George Kemble and Richard Spaete

MedImmune Vaccines, Inc., Mountain View, CA, USA

Introduction

Genital herpes, caused by both herpes simplex virus (HSV) types 1 and 2, can result in painful vesicular and ulcerative lesions on the genitalia and the genital tract, and may cause both urologic and neurologic problems. Following primary infection, HSV establishes a latent infection in the local ganglia and can reactivate on multiple occasions with manifestations ranging from asymptomatic viral shedding to painful recurrences of genital or orofacial lesions (Whitley, 2001). HSV-2 is the predominant etiologic agent of genital herpes and data from the second and third National Health and Nutrition Examination Surveys, spanning 1976 to 1994, demonstrated that the prevalence of HSV-2 infection increased by 30% since the late 1970's with the highest rates in teenagers and young adults (Fleming et al., 1997). It is estimated that more than 1.6 million individuals are infected annually with HSV-2 in the USA (Armstrong et al., 2001). From the perspective of vaccine development, however, genital herpes caused by HSV-1 cannot be overlooked. Although genital herpes caused by HSV-1 is generally less severe than HSV-2, HSV-1 is ubiquitous, infects a larger portion of the population than HSV-2, and the percentage of HSV-1 positive cultures isolated from individuals presenting with genital herpes appears to be increasing (Ribes et al., 2001).

In addition to the pain and potential complications (e.g. psychological distress), that genital herpes causes in the infected individual, it is also responsible for increasing the risk of sexual transmission of HIV (Holmberg et al., 1988). Shedding infectious virus during birth may infect the newborn and cause neonatal herpes (Wald et al., 1995). Neonatal herpes caused by either HSV-1 or HSV-2, although relatively rare, can result in disseminated and/or central nervous system infections resulting in death or significant developmental impairments (Kimberlin et al., 2001). The risk of neonatal herpes can be significantly reduced by Cesarean delivery when active lesions are detected immediately prior to birth; however in contrast to HIV transmission, subclinical shedding of infectious virus from the mother's genital tract during birth can cause neonatal herpes (Brown et al., 2003). Despite the advances made in antiviral therapy over the past 20 years, genital herpes and neonatal herpes remain significant public health problems. Antiviral drugs can reduce the frequency of viral shedding and severity of symptoms associated with genital herpes and when given promptly can reduce some of the poor outcomes of neonatal herpes (Stanberry et al., 1999; Kimberlin et al., 2001). However, like many antiviral therapies, the effectiveness of the drug is limited by the development of viral resistance as well as delays in initiating treatment. Unfortunately, the awareness of neonatal herpes for acutely ill infants is low and the characteristic skin vesicles pathogonomonic for neonatal herpes do not occur in more than 30% of patients; both of these factors have contributed to the lack of progress in shortening the critical interval between diagnosis and treatment (Kimberlin et al., 2001).

Cesarean delivery in high risk situations and antiviral treatment can reduce the total number of neonatal herpes cases; however, the frequency of inapparent genital lesions during delivery and the inability to quickly and specifically deliver antiviral therapy to many infected newborns combine to create an unacceptable burden of neonatal herpes cases (Stratton et al., 2000). Moreover, infected women who do not have a history of genital lesions would not be targeted for antiviral prophylaxis, yet may excrete the virus. A vaccine approach that aims at reducing the overall burden of genital herpes and reducing the likelihood of viral transmission during birth should provide the largest public health benefit.

The feasibility of a vaccine approach is predicated on evidence that an immune response can positively modify the resulting disease. Specifically for neonatal herpes, maternal serostatus and the timing of infection relative to delivery has an impact on the frequency of neonatal herpes infections. Neonatal herpes occurred at a lower rate in neonates born to women who seroconverted prior to delivery than in neonates whose mothers did not seroconvert, demonstrating that the maternal immune status could impact the resulting disease (Brown et al., 1997; Brown et al., 2003). The mechanism of immune protection of the child remains unclear but transplacental transfer of maternal antibodies to HSV is likely to be important. In addition, serologic status also appears to have an impact on acquisition and/or outcome of infection with the heterologous virus type. Several studies have indicated that preexisting immunity to HSV-1, which is generally acquired early in life, can influence the outcome of HSV-2 infection at a later age (reviewed in Whitley, 2001). Individuals who were HSV-1 seropositive were not protected from acquiring HSV-2, but were approximately three times less likely to report a history of genital herpes than those who were HSV-1 seronegative (Langenberg et al., 1999; Xu et al., 2002). These data indicated that immunity elicited by prior infection with HSV-1 modified the disease due to the ensuing HSV-2 infection. Limited data suggests that the immune response elicited by HSV-2 infection may be even more robust than that elicited by a HSV-1 infection. Pregnant women with antibodies to HSV-2 were not infected with HSV-1 in contrast to women with no prior immunity (Stanberry et al., 2002). Many of the vaccines in this review are derived from the antigens of HSV-2. These vaccines are expected to induce type specific immunity to the etiologic agent that is presumed to cause more significant disease as well as provide cross-protective immunity to HSV-1. Specific vaccines to prevent HSV-1 orofacial lesions have not been targets of significant development activity.

Notwithstanding widespread agreement that a vaccine will be the most cost effective way to reduce the morbidity associated with HSV infections (Arvin and Prober, 1997), no licensed vaccine is currently available to address the problems presented by these viruses. Development of herpesvirus vaccines present special hurdles associated with the complex replication cycles and propensity of these viruses to establish lifelong infections. Since much of the HSV disease burden is due to recurrent infection, a therapeutic as well as a prophylactic vaccine is needed. In addition, this family of viruses has also evolved mechanisms to counteract the immune response of the host. These cautions, however, are mitigated by the successful introduction of effective herpes vaccines such as Varivax® for the prevention of chicken pox and veterinary vaccines for Aujeszky's disease and Marek's disease, caused by alpha-herpesviruses of pigs and chickens, respectively. This chapter will attempt to summarize the key steps and the more recent milestones in developing an effective vaccine for the prevention of disease caused by HSV-1 and -2.

History of HSV vaccine development

The history of HSV vaccine trials in humans is fast approaching the century mark with the ultimate goal of an efficacious vaccine still elusive. In the early to middle decades of the twentieth century, experimentalists used infectious wild-type viruses isolated from active lesions or passaged through animals to immunize individuals with the hope of having an impact on recurrent herpes. These approaches were later displaced by vaccine strategies using inactivated virus or glycoprotein extracts. An excellent status report of previous vaccine development efforts that surveys the foundation of HSV vaccine strategies and that informs present day efforts is provided in a comprehensive review of a decade ago (Burke, 1993). For a variety of reasons including cost of clinical trials and difficulties in measuring clinical endpoints, many of these HSV vaccine candidates were not evaluated in rigorous placebo controlled, blinded, studies. Much more recently, Chiron Corporation and GlaxoSmithKline have sponsored double blind placebo controlled trials of two subunit vaccines that have put earlier basic and preclinical research vaccine concepts to the ultimate test. Other vaccine concepts need to be tested with similar rigor in clinical trials.

Development of live, attenuated vaccines

Live attenuated vaccines have many clear advantages as vaccine strategies. In principle, they can present the full range of all viral antigens to the immune system of the host, stimulating both the humoral and cell-mediated adaptive immune responses as well as innate immunity. This is an important consideration in rationalizing approaches to a vaccine because laboratory-based correlates of immune protection are not yet defined for the herpes simplex viruses. Generally, live vaccines evoke a longer-lived immune response than that elicited by other vaccine strategies. Additionally, powerful molecular tools exist for engineering recombinant vaccine viruses that can be employed to incorporate particular features designed to achieve the appropriate balance between attenuation and immunogenicity.

Developing a live, attenuated vaccine for HSV presents various challenges. HSV has evolved several mechanisms to evade the host immune response, including functions that interfere with the production of interferon and products that inhibit the presentation of viral antigens to the host immune system (Johnson and Hill, 1998; Barcy and Corey, 2001; Lorenzo et al., 2001; Leib, 2002; Hegde et al., 2003). The advantage of removing these immune response modifiers has yet to be addressed in clinical trials. Removal could potentially increase the immunogenicity of the vaccine but it could also possibly create a scenario where superinfection or revaccination leads to significant reactogenicity. Another challenge to live vaccine approaches for HSV prevention is neurotropism. HSV establishes latent infections in sensory ganglia and can on rare occasion invade the central nervous system to cause encephalitis (Whitley, 2001). The optimal properties for a live, attenuated HSV vaccine candidate would remove the pathogenic signatures from the virus such that vaccination would not elicit any of the pain or ulcerative lesions typical of natural infection yet enable sufficient levels of replication in the host to elicit a vigorous immune response. In addition, the neurovirulence of the vaccine would need to be eliminated, although its propensity to establish a latent infection might be left intact. The ability of the vaccine to establish a latent infection could be viewed as a positive characteristic, since subclinical reactivation could restimulate the immune system, creating a more durable and effective immune response. However, delivering a vaccine that will establish a latent infection carries with it the concern that reactivation could result in transmission or disease at a time when the individual has become immunosuppressed due to infection or chemotherapy. In addition to these biological traits, any live HSV vaccine must be genetically stable and be able to be produced at sufficient quantities for effective administration.

Among the first live, attenuated HSV vaccines that were specifically manipulated to attempt to meet the above criteria were made by recombinant techniques. One of the viruses R7020 was constructed by replacing an approximately 14.5 kbp deletion extending from the α27 gene (UL54) in the unique long segment of the genome across the internal inverted repeats of HSV-1 with a fragment of HSV-2 encoding at least the gG glycoprotein (Meignier et al., 1988). This construct was significantly attenuated in small animal models as well as in an exquisitely HSV sensitive nonhuman primate model (Aotus trivirgatus), and the neuroattenuation was genetically stable following serial passage through mouse brains (Meignier et al., 1988, 1990). R7020 had a reduced propensity for establishing a latent infection and provided protection from direct challenge in animals. R7020 was evaluated in Phase 1 human trials. This construct was favored over a related tk negative construct (denoted R7017), since R7020 retained the tk gene and, therefore, retained sensitivity to available antiviral drugs such as acyclovir. Unfortunately, despite the promising immunogenicity results from the animal studies, the vaccine was poorly immunogenic in humans even given two doses of 10^5 PFU each and it was concluded that this vaccine was overly attenuated (Cadoz et al., 1992). Although further development of these constructs as vaccines for immunocompetent individuals was aborted, they are still being evaluated as potential oncolytic agents for various cancer indications (for review see Varghese and Rabkin, 2002).

The next iteration of live attenuated HSV vaccines were developed based on the identification of a neurovirulence determinant identified as the $\gamma_1 34.5$ gene. Removal of this gene, which is present in two copies in the genome of HSV, attenuated the neurovirulence of HSV-1 to a much greater extent than deletions of other specific genes that had been previously tested and did not significantly reduce the ability to replicate in cells that could be considered for vaccine production (Chou et al., 1990; Whitley et al., 1993). Experiments in small animal models demonstrated that this construct abolished the ability of the virus to migrate to and replicate in the central nervous system of mice and guinea pigs. An HSV-2 derivative of this construct denoted RAV 9395 was generated in which both copies of the $\gamma_1 34.5$ gene were deleted as well as the ORFs antisense to the $\gamma_1 34.5$ gene and the adjacent UL55 and UL56 ORFs. Since RAV 9395 was constructed from HSV-2, it was expected to elicit a more relevant immune response than the corresponding HSV-1 construct. RAV 9395 was tested in the guinea pig model of genital herpes and was shown to be attenuated and immunogenic. Following challenge of animals with the wild-type HSV-2 strain, animals previously vaccinated with 10^4–10^5 PFU of RAV 9395 were significantly protected from clinical disease compared to controls, and recurring lesions caused by the wild-type strain were reduced. Whether this was due to an inability to establish a latent infection in the dorsal root ganglia or a diminished ability to reactivate from this site is unclear (Spector et al., 1998). The $\gamma_1 34.5$ mutants were also characterized by their inability to grow in certain cell types in vitro, particularly those derived from nervous tissue. This characteristic, however, was not genetically stable in the HSV-1 background and could be reverted upon serial passage in these cells types (Mohr et al., 2001). Further development of this or any recombinant based on deletion of the $\gamma_1 34.5$ genes will require an analysis of the potential consequences of this instability, such as identifying compensatory mutations after serial passage and their effect(s) on attenuation. Recently, a vaccine candidate lacking both copies of $\gamma_1 34.5$ as well as UL55, UL56 and the US10-12 region of HSV-2 (G) was shown to be genetically stable; this vaccine candidate remained highly attenuated following 9 serial passages in the CNS of mice. This highly attenuated candidate protected guinea pigs from disease following challenge with the wild type virus (Prichard et al., 2005).

Another set of approaches for making live, attenuated vaccines are based upon deletions or modifications to the viral genome that limit the replication of the virus except in specialized cell lines and have been denoted DISC, for disabled infectious single cycle mutants. In principle, a gene required for replication of HSV DNA or to produce infectious virus is removed from the genome and infectious virus is recovered on a cell line that provides the function in trans. Blocking different points in the replication cycle can alter the quantity and types of viral proteins expressed in a nonpermissive infected cells (Farrell et al., 1994; Da Costa et al., 1997). Vaccine candidates with deletions of the gH, ICP8, ICP27 and ICP10 encoded functions have been constructed and tested. Recombinant HSV-2 viruses lacking the PK domain of ICP10 (the ribonucleotide reductase) have been tested in guinea pigs with favorable results. Exploration of the immune response in mice clearly demonstrated a Th1 type response characterized by development of both CD4+ Th1 and CD8+ CTLs with antiviral activity (Gyotoku et al., 2002). Newer forms of DISC vaccines have been constructed in which two genes have been deleted and have been tested in mice. These modified vaccine elicited an immune response yet had significantly reduced quantities of latent viral DNA in the murine host (Da Costa et al., 1999).

Preclinical evaluations of HSV-1 and -2 constructs lacking gH were tested in the guinea pig model and protected the animals in both prophylactic and therapeutic settings (McLean et al., 1994; Boursnell et al., 1997). A gH deleted HSV-2 strain HG52 was tested in a Phase 1 clinical trial to evaluate safety in HSV-2 seropositive and seronegative volunteers under the sponsorship of Cantab Pharmaceuticals. On the basis of acceptable safety and immunogenicity data reported for the prophylactic vaccine candidate, 485 patients were enrolled and vaccinated in a double-blind, placebo controlled Phase 2 trial of the DISC vaccine for the treatment of recurrent genital herpes. The results of this study have not yet been reported. The development of the prophylactic vaccine appears to have been discontinued.

Several of the DISC strategies are being exploited in the field of vectored vaccines. Nef antigens of simian immunodeficiency virus (SIV) were introduced into an HSV-1 mutant lacking ICP27. This replication incompetent vector elicited both cellular and humoral immune responses to HSV and SIV in rhesus monkeys and protected the animals following challenge 5 months post-vaccination (Murphy et al., 2000). Many of the DISC viruses are being considered as potential vectors for use in gene therapy as well (reviewed in Rees et al., 2002).

Subunit vaccines

Inactivated virus, glycoprotein extracts and recombinant subunit vaccines do not have several of the concerns associated with the development of live, attenuated vaccines such as neurotropism, transmission, or reactivation at a later time. Along with fewer safety concerns, a strength of these approaches is the ability to generate a well-defined biological product that can preserve conformational epitopes vital to eliciting an authentic immune response. A major consideration when choosing a subunit approach is the inclusion of an approvable adjuvant/antigen delivery system capable of eliciting both an antibody and a CTL response in humans.

Among the limitations of the subunit approach are the relatively narrow range of epitopes to which the immune system is exposed and the manner in which they elicit an immune response. Immunity generated to a specific target antigen may differ depending on how it is presented to the immune system and can also be affected by the HLA repertoire of the vaccinated individual. Strain variation coupled with HLA variability in an outbred population might influence the efficacy of the subunit protein vaccine in different subpopulations. The route of antigen presentation is another factor that must be considered, since an antigen introduced parenterally may elicit a different immune response than one that is expressed from a virally infected cell.

Many different inactivated HSV or glycoprotein preparations have been tested over the past several decades. Claims of positive benefit have resulted in use on a relatively large scale in some countries. Most of these claims, however, have not been substantiated by data from prospective, double-blind, placebo controlled clinical trials to establish safety and efficacy. Two recombinant subunit vaccine candidates, developed independently by Chiron and GlaxoSmithKline, are notable exceptions to this criticism. Both of these vaccines have been evaluated in relatively large, double-blind, placebo controlled trials to evaluate their impact on the occurrence of genital herpes disease or the prevention of new HSV-2 infection. The results of these studies will be described in more detail.

The Chiron subunit vaccine was made by expressing recombinant forms of two major surface glycoproteins of HSV-2, gB_2 and gD_2 lacking the carboxy-terminal regions, in Chinese hamster ovary (CHO) cells. The choice of

Table 69.1. Evaluation of recombinant subunit vaccine studies

	Dose (μg)	Regimen	Population	N	Vaccine effect reductions[a]	Comments
gB$_2$/gD$_2$/MF59						
	10	4 × 1 wk	guinea pig	15	Incidence, severity and mortality	Recurrence of challenge not reported
	30	0,1,6 mo	HSV-2$^-$ Monogamous	531	No reduction in acquisition or severity	Transient reduction of acquisition in females only for the first 150 days of the trial
			HSV-2$^-$ STD clinic	1862		
gD$_2$/ASO4						
	5	0,1,3 mo	guinea pig	15	Viral shedding, disease severity and recurrence	Incidence not reduced Mortality decreased
	20	0,1,6 mo	HSV-1$^-$ / HSV-2$^-$	847	Genital herpes disease in HSV-1$^-$/HSV-2$^-$ females only	Efficacy against genital herpes disease was not demonstrated in whole population or other subpopulations. Evidence of a trend toward prevention of infection in HSV-1$^-$/HSV2$^-$ females
			HSV-1$^±$ / HSV-2$^-$	1867		

[a] Observations with reported statistical significance.

these particular subunits relied on much basic research developed over the years that identified these glycoproteins as important stimulators of potent humoral and cellular responses (reviewed in Spear, 1985). These purified subunits were combined with the adjuvant MF59, a 5% squalene oil-in-water emulsion, to make the vaccine. The gD$_2$ subunit combined with MF59 was evaluated in the guinea pig model for its ability to protect the animals from a challenge with HSV-2. Animals that received 4 weekly doses of the vaccine developed significant serum IgG, as well as salivary, vaginal, and nasal IgA responses against HSV. Following intravaginal challenge with a lethal dose of HSV-2, vaccinated animals were significantly protected as measured by an decrease in disease incidence, severity and mortality (O'Hagan et al., 1999).

A large clinical trial of the combination gB$_2$ and gD$_2$ subunit vaccine was conducted that evaluated the ability of this vaccine to prevent HSV-2 infection. The vaccine contained 30μg each of gB$_2$ and gD$_2$ combined with MF59 and given intramuscularly at 0, 1 and 6 months to adults who where seronegative for HSV-2 and were either attending an STD clinic or had a monogamous partner who was infected with HSV-2. The participants were followed for one year and acquisition of HSV-2 was measured by isolation of the virus in culture or seroconversion to HSV-2 proteins other than gB$_2$ or gD$_2$ (Corey et al., 1999). Despite high titer HSV antibody responses, this vaccine had no impact on the overall frequency of acquisition of infection and did not modify the disease. The only difference between vaccine and placebo groups was a transient reduction in HSV acquisition in female subjects during the initial 150 days of the trial. The lack of impact on disease severity contrasted to an earlier study of this vaccine for a therapeutic indication. In the prior study, 212 adults with recurrent genital herpes were enrolled in a double-blind study and monitored for the number and frequency of recurrences as well as the duration and severity of each episode. As in the prophylactic trial, the number or frequency of recurrences was unchanged, however, the severity and duration of the first confirmed recurrence post vaccination was reduced significantly. (Straus et al., 1997). The reason for these differences between the prophylactic and therapeutic trials is not clear but may relate to the difference between the natural history of a recurrent lesion that occurs when the host has immunity and a primary lesion in an individual who is immunologically naïve.

Another HSV subunit vaccine is under development by GlaxoSmithKline in which a purified carboxy-terminal truncated gD$_2$ expressed in CHO cells was formulated with the ASO4 adjuvant, containing aluminum hydroxide and 3-O-deacylated monophosphoryl lipid A (3-MPL). This vaccine was also evaluated in the guinea pig model. The vaccine was formulated by adding 5μg of gD2 to ASO4 and injected subcutaneously into the animals at 0, 1 and 3 months followed by an intravaginal challenge with HSV-2 two weeks later. Vaccination did not alter the incidence of infection, but it did reduce the titer of shed virus as well as the severity of the lesions and mortality. Recurrent lesions due to the challenge virus were also reduced when the number of episodes of recurrence was compared to controls (Bourne et al., 2003).

This HSV vaccine was tested in a large double-blind randomized clinical trial to assess its ability to reduce the occurrence of genital herpes disease. Adults who were seronegative for HSV-2 were enrolled, vaccinated with 20 μg of gD_2 combined with alum and 3-MPL at 0, 1 and 3 months and monitored for the acquisition of genital herpes disease. The primary analyses did not show a vaccine effect. There was no reduction in the acquisition of genital herpes disease in HSV-2 seronegative adults who had received vaccine. However, post hoc analyses demonstrated that the vaccine significantly protected HSV-1 seronegative / HSV-2 seronegative women from acquiring genital herpes caused by HSV-2 (Stanberry et al., 2002). In addition, although it did not reach statistical significance, there was a trend toward a reduction in HSV-2 infection in this same group.

Many of the differences between the results of the gD2/gB2/MF59 and gD2/ASO4 vaccine trials are enigmatic. Both vaccines protected guinea pigs from direct challenge with a high titered inoculum of HSV-2 indicating that these subunit compositions evoked similar immune responses in this animal model. Immunization of human subjects with gD2/gB2/MF59 resulted in the production of neutralizing antibodies as well as memory CD4+ T cells specific for the antigens in the vaccine (Langenberg et al., 1995). However recent studies suggest that this vaccine may have induced only low levels of antibodies that mediate antibody-dependent cellular cytotoxicity in humans (Kohl et al., 2000). The gD2/ASO4 vaccine also elicited high levels of neutralizing antibodies in humans as well as gD specific lymphoproliferation and interferon γ (Stanberry et al., 2002). These adaptive immune responses, however, were not different between the groups protected from acquisition of genital herpes and those that were not. The reason for the efficacy of this vaccine in women and not men as well as the lack of effect in females who were HSV-1 seropositive will require additional studies; there is no obvious explanation for these differences. The positive results in HSV-1 seronegative/HSV-2 seronegative women in this trial have prompted GlaxoSmithKline Biologicals in conjunction with the National Institute of Allergy and Infectious Diseases to initiate a pivotal Phase 3 efficacy trial in 7,550 women who are seronegative to both HSV 1 and HSV 2.

Other approaches to vaccination

Many options for the development of prophylactic HSV vaccines are currently being explored in preclinical studies and several have progressed to immunogenicity studies in the guinea pig model of HSV. DNA vaccines that expressed either a full length or secreted, carboxy-terminal truncated form of gD2 reduced the lesion severity and number of recurrent lesions following challenge (Strasser et al., 2000). Other more novel approaches such as ISCOMS (immunostimulating complex particles) made from detergent extracted preparations of virions have been tested in guinea pigs (Simms et al., 2000), and attenuated Salmonella vaccines harboring a gD plasmid have been evaluated in rodents and shown to protect the animals following challenge (Flo et al., 2001). Peptide vaccines are being evaluated based on the identification of immunologically dominant epitopes, but to date most have not developed past studies in the mouse model (Gierynska et al., 2002; BenMohamed et al., 2003). Approaches using chimeric DNA vaccines combining viral glycoprotein epitopes, protein fusions of viral glycoproteins with bacterial open reading frames, or with chemokines are being tested in mice. Alternative adjuvants such as CpG molecules are being added to formulations of peptide and DNA vaccines. Vectored approaches using other viruses offer other vaccine strategies. For example, VZV has been used as a vector to express HSV gD, and has been shown to protect against experimental HSV challenge in a guinea pig model (Heineman et al., 1995). Further development of these new approaches as well as new ideas should continue to be advanced with time.

Conclusions

The goal of a safe, efficacious HSV vaccine has several components. Clearly the most easily measured benefit is to reduce the rate of acquistition of genital herpes disease. Reduction of the incidence of this disease or reduction of viral shedding from infected individuals should have a direct impact on the number of neonatal herpes cases every year as well as on the sexual transmission of HIV. The two most recent large clinical trials of subunit vaccine candidates have highlighted some of the issues that may need to be addressed during the development of a successful HSV vaccine. Gender differences influenced the vaccine efficacy as did the preexisting HSV-1 serological status. The mechanisms of these interactions are not understood at this point and the influence of these differences on other vaccine strategies cannot be predicted. Further studies to understand how these factors affect vaccine efficacy should be done. In addition, genital herpes caused by HSV-1 appears to be increasing and HSV-1 can also cause severe neonatal herpes. A successful vaccine should confer immunity to both etiologic agents. Ultimately, the role of gender, pre-existing immunity, and effectiveness for preventing both HSV-1 and HSV-2 disease and the impact on public health will be needed to evaluate HSV vaccine candidates.

Animal studies and serological assays as measures of the immune response may not be sufficient to completely predict the functional behavior and immunogenicity of a vaccine in humans. The immunogenicity of R7020, was poor in humans and the gD2/gB2/MF59 vaccine, while stimulating robust neutralizing antibodies was unable to protect individuals from acquisition of HSV-2 despite the promising immunogenicity and protection in mice and guinea pigs. These results highlight the need to further explore the mechanisms of functional immunity in humans at a fundamental and detailed level in order to define informative surrogate markers for the clinical development of an HSV vaccine candidate. In addition, the efficacy trials of the subunit vaccines confirmed that prevention of infection is a difficult endpoint to achieve and may misdirect the effort away from relieving the burden of disease associated with genital herpes. The potential for transmission of herpes during birth as a consequence of asymptomatic viral shedding despite vaccine induced immunity will have to be considered to predict the impact of candidate vaccines on neonatal herpes.

Although a specific vaccine and immunization strategy have not yet been identified for HSV, the overall progress made by the field has brought an increased understanding of the complexity of HSV-1 and HSV-2 disease and elucidated many issues that can now be addressed. A vaccine for human papilloma virus (HPV), another sexually transmitted disease, has recently been shown to have positive results in Phase 2 clinical trials (Koutsky et al., 2002; Galloway, 2003). These virus-like particle vaccines have provided significant immunity to prevent establishment of a persistent infection. Adding an HSV vaccine to an armamentarium of STD vaccines would provide a major positive impact on public health throughout the world.

REFERENCES

Armstrong, G. L., Schillinger, J., Markowitz, L. et al. (2001). Incidence of herpes simplex virus type 2 infection in the United States.' Am. J. Epidemiol., 153(9), 912–920.

Arvin, A. M. and Prober, C. G. (1997). Herpes simplex virus Type 2 – a persistent problem. N. Engl. J. Med., 337, 1158–1159.

Barcy, S. and Corey, L. (2001). Herpes simplex inhibits the capacity of lymphoblastoid B cell lines to stimulate CD4+ T cells. J. Immunol., 166(10): 6242–6249.

BenMohamed, L., Bertrand, G., McNamara, C. D. et al. (2003). Identification of novel immunodominant CD4+ Th1-type T-cell peptide epitopes from herpes simplex virus glycoprotein D that confer protective immunity. J. Virol., 77(17), 9463–9473.

Bourne, N., Bravo, F. J., Francotte, M. et al. (2003). Herpes simplex virus (HSV) type 2 glycoprotein D subunit vaccines and protection against genital HSV-1 or HSV-2 disease in guinea pigs. J. Infect. Dis., 187(4), 542–549.

Boursnell, M. E., Entwisle, C., Blakeley, D. et al. (1997). A genetically inactivated herpes simplex virus type 2 (HSV-2) vaccine provides effective protection against primary and recurrent HSV-2 disease. J. Infect. Dis., 175(1), 16–25.

Brown, Z. A., Selke, S., Zeh, J. et al. (1997). The acquisition of herpes simplex virus during pregnancy. N. Engl. J. Med., 337(8), 509–515.

Brown, Z. A., Wald, A., Morrow, R. A., Selke, S., Zeh, J., and Corey, L. (2003). Effect of serologic status and cesarean delivery on transmission rates of herpes simplex virus from mother to infant. J. Am. Med. Assoc., 289(2), 203–209.

Burke, R. L. (1993). Current status of HSV vaccine development. In The Human Herpesviruses. R. J. W. a. C. L. B. Roizman. New York, Raven Press, pp. 367–379.

Cadoz, M., Micoud, M., Mallaret, M. et al. (1992). Phase 1 trial of R7020: a live attenuated recombinant herpes simplex (HSV) candidate vaccine. ICAAC Washington DC (Abstract).

Chou, J., Kern, E. R., Whitley, R. J., and Roizman, B. (1990). Mapping of herpes simplex virus-1 neurovirulence to gamma 134.5, a gene nonessential for growth in culture. Science, 250(4985), 1262–1266.

Corey, L., Langenberg, A. G., Ashley, R. et al. (1999). Recombinant glycoprotein vaccine for the prevention of genital HSV-2 infection: two randomized controlled trials. Chiron HSV Vaccine Study Group. J. Am. Med. Assoc., 282(4), 331–340.

Da Costa, X. J., Bourne, N., Stanberry, L. R., and Knipe, D. M. (1997). Construction and characterization of a replication-defective herpes simplex virus 2 ICP8 mutant strain and its use in immunization studies in a guinea pig model of genital disease. Virology, 232(1), 1–12.

Da Costa, X. J., Jones, C. A., and Knipe, D. M. (1999). Immunization against genital herpes with a vaccine virus that has defects in productive and latent infection. Proc. Natl Acad. Sci. USA, 96(12), 6994–6998.

Farrell, H. E., McLean, C. S., Harley, C., Efstathiou, S., Inglis, S., and Minson A. C. (1994). Vaccine potential of a herpes simplex virus type 1 mutant with an essential glycoprotein deleted. J. Virol., 68(2), 927–932.

Fleming, D. T., McQuillan, G. M., Johnson, R. E. et al. (1997). Herpes simplex virus type 2 in the United States, 1976 to 1994. N. Engl. J. Med., 337(16), 1105–1111.

Flo, J., Tisminetzky, S., and Baralle, F. (2001). Oral transgene vaccination mediated by attenuated Salmonellae is an effective method to prevent Herpes simplex virus-2 induced disease in mice. *Vaccine*, **19**(13–14), 1772–1782.

Galloway, D. A. (2003). Papillomavirus vaccines in clinical trials. *Lancet. Infect. Dis.*, **3**(8), 469–475.

Gierynska, M., Kumaraguru, U., Eo, S. K., Lee, S., Krieg, A., and Rouse, B. T. (2002). Induction of CD8 T-cell-specific systemic and mucosal immunity against herpes simplex virus with CpG-peptide complexes. *J. Virol.*, **76**(13), 6568–6576.

Gyotoku, T., Ono, F., and Aurelian, L. (2002). Development of HSV-specific CD4+ Th1 responses and CD8+ cytotoxic T lymphocytes with antiviral activity by vaccination with the HSV-2 mutant ICP10DeltaPK. *Vaccine*, **20**(21–22), 2796–2807.

Hegde, N. R., Chevalier, M. S., and Johnson, D. C. (2003). Viral inhibition of MHC class II antigen presentation. *Trends Immunol.*, **24**(5), 278–285.

Heineman, T. C., Connelly, B. L., Bourne, N., Stanberry, L. R., and Cohen, J. (1995). Immunization with recombinant varicella-zoster virus expressing herpes simplex virus type 2 glycoprotein D reduces the severity of genital herpes in guinea pigs. *J. Virol.*, **69**(12), 8109–8113.

Holmberg, S. D., Stewart, J. A., Gerber, A. R. *et al.* (1988). Prior herpes simplex virus type 2 infection as a risk factor for HIV infection. *J. Am. Med. Assoc.*, **259**(7), 1048–1050.

Johnson, D. C. and Hill, A. B. (1998). Herpesvirus evasion of the immune system. *Curr. Top. Microbiol. Immunol.*, **232**, 149–177.

Kimberlin, D. W., Lin, C. Y., Jacobs, R. F. *et al.* (2001). Natural history of neonatal herpes simplex virus infections in the acyclovir era. *Pediatrics*, **108**(2), 223–229.

Kohl, S., Charlebois, E. D., Sigouroudinia, M. *et al.* (2000). Limited antibody-dependent cellular cytotoxicity antibody response induced by a herpes simplex virus type 2 subunit vaccine., *J. Infect. Dis.*, **181**(1), 335–339.

Koutsky, L. A., Ault, K. A., Wheeler, C. M. *et al.* (2002). A controlled trial of a human papillomavirus type 16 vaccine. *N. Engl. J. Med.*, **347**(21), 1645–1651.

Langenberg, A. G., Burke, R. L., Adair, S. F. *et al.* (1995). A recombinant glycoprotein vaccine for herpes simplex virus type 2: safety and immunogenicity [corrected]. *Ann. Intern. Med.*, **122**(12), 889–898.

Langenberg, A. G., Corey, L., Ashley, R. L., Leong, W. P., and Straus, S. E. (1999). A prospective study of new infections with herpes simplex virus type 1 and type 2. Chiron HSV Vaccine Study Group. *N. Engl. J. Med.*, **341**(19), 1432–1438.

Leib, D. A. (2002). Counteraction of interferon-induced antiviral responses by herpes simplex viruses. *Curr. Top. Microbiol. Immunol.*, **269**, 171–185.

Lorenzo, M. E., Ploegh, H. L., and Tirabassi, R. S. (2001). Viral immune evasion strategies and the underlying cell biology. *Semin. Immunol.*, **13**(1), 1–9.

McLean, C. S., Erturk, M., Jennings, R. *et al.* (1994). Protective vaccination against primary and recurrent disease caused by herpes simplex virus (HSV) type 2 using a genetically disabled HSV-1. *J. Infect. Dis.*, **170**(5), 1100–1109.

Meignier, B., Longnecker, R., and Roizman, B. (1988). In vivo behavior of genetically engineered herpes simplex viruses R7017 and R7020: construction and evaluation in rodents. *J. Infect. Dis.*, **158**(3), 602–614.

Meignier, B., Martin, B., Whitley, R. J., and Roizman, B. (1990). In vivo behavior of genetically engineered herpes simplex viruses R7017 and R7020. II. Studies in immunocompetent and immunosuppressed owl monkeys (*Aotus trivirgatus*). *J. Infect. Dis.*, **162**(2), 313–321.

Mohr, I., Sternberg, D., Ward, S., Leib, D., Mulvey, M., and Gluzman, Y. (2001). A herpes simplex virus type 1 gamma34.5 second-site suppressor mutant that exhibits enhanced growth in cultured glioblastoma cells is severely attenuated in animals. *J. Virol.*, **75**(11), 5189–5196.

Murphy, C. G., Lucas, W. T., Means, R. E. *et al.* (2000). Vaccine protection against simian immunodeficiency virus by recombinant strains of herpes simplex virus. *J. Virol.*, **74**(17), 7745–7754.

O'Hagan, D., Goldbeck, C., Ugozzoli, M., Ott, G., and Burke, R. L. (1999). Intranasal immunization with recombinant gD2 reduces disease severity and mortality following genital challenge with herpes simplex virus type 2 in guinea pigs. *Vaccine*, **17**(18), 2229–2236.

Prichard, M. N., Kaiwar, R., Jackman, W. T. *et al.* (2005). Evaluation of AD472, a live attenuated recombinant herpes simplex virus type 2 vaccine in guinea pigs. *Vaccine*, **23**, 5424–5431.

Rees, R. C., McArdle, S., Mian, S. *et al.* (2002). Disabled infectious single cycle-herpes simplex virus (DISC-HSV) as a vector for immunogene therapy of cancer. *Curr. Opin. Mol. Ther.*, **4**(1), 49–53.

Ribes, J. A., Steele, A. D., Seabolt, J. P., and Baker, D. J. (2001). Six-year study of the incidence of herpes in genital and nongenital cultures in a central Kentucky medical center patient population. *J. Clin. Microbiol.*, **39**(9), 3321–3325.

Simms, J. R., Heath, A. W., and Jennings, R. (2000). Use of herpes simplex virus (HSV) type 1 ISCOMS 703 vaccine for prophylactic and therapeutic treatment of primary and recurrent HSV-2 infection in guinea pigs. *J. Infect. Dis.*, **181**(4), 1240–1248.

Spear, P. (1985). Glycoproteins specified by Herpes simplex viruses. In Roizman, B., ed. *The Herpesviruses*. New York: Plenum, **3**, 315–356.

Spector, F. C., Kern, E. R., Palmer, J. *et al.* (1998). Evaluation of a live attenuated recombinant virus RAV 9395 as a herpes simplex virus type 2 vaccine in guinea pigs. *J. Infect. Dis.*, **177**(5), 1143–1154.

Stanberry, L., Cunningham, A., Mertz, G. (1999). New developments in the epidemiology, natural history and management of genital herpes. *Antiviral Res.*, **42**(1), 1–14.

Stanberry, L. R., Spruance, S. L., Cunningham, A. L. *et al.* (2002). Glycoprotein-D-adjuvant vaccine to prevent genital herpes. *N. Engl. J. Med.*, **347**(21), 1652–1661.

Strasser, J. E., Arnold, R. L., Pachuk, C., Higgins, T. J., and Bernstein, D. I. (2000). Herpes simplex virus DNA vaccine efficacy: effect of glycoprotein D plasmid constructs. *J. Infect. Dis.*, **182**(5), 1304–1310.

Stratton, K., Durch, J., and Lawrence, R. eds. (2000). *Vaccines for the 21st Century. A Tool for Decision Making.* Washington, DC: National Academy Press.

Straus, S. E., Wald, A., Kost, R. G. *et al.* (1997). Immunotherapy of recurrent genital herpes with recombinant herpes simplex virus type 2 glycoproteins D and B: results of a placebo-controlled vaccine trial. *J. Infect. Dis.*, **176**(5), 1129–1134.

Varghese, S. and Rabkin, S. D. (2002). Oncolytic herpes simplex virus vectors for cancer virotherapy. *Cancer Gene Ther.*, **9**(12), 967–978.

Wald, A., Zeh, J., Selke, S., Ashley, R. L., and Corey, L. (1995). Virologic characteristics of subclinical and symptomatic genital herpes infections. *N. Engl. J. Med.*, **333**(12), 770–775.

Whitley, R. J. (2001). Herpes simplex viruses. In Knipe, D. M. and Howley, P. M., eds. *Fields Virology, 4th edn.* Lippincott, Williams & Wilkins, **2**.

Whitley, R. J., Kern, E. R., Chatterjee, S., Chou, J., and B. Roizman (1993). Replication, establishment of latency, and induced reactivation of herpes simplex virus gamma 1 34.5 deletion mutants in rodent models. *J. Clin. Invest.*, **91**(6), 2837–2843.

Xu, F., Schillinger, J. A., Sternberg, M. R. *et al.* (2002). Seroprevalence and coinfection with herpes simplex virus type 1 and type 2 in the United States, 1988–1994. *J. Infect. Dis.*, **185**(8), 1019–1024.

70

Varicella-zoster vaccine

Anne A. Gershon

Department of Pediatrics, Columbia University College of Physicians and Surgeons,
New York, NY, USA

Varicella vaccines: background

A live attenuated varicella vaccine, the Oka strain, was developed by Takahashi and his colleagues in Japan the early 1970s (Takahashi et al., 1974). This vaccine is now being adminstered to varicella-susceptible healthy children and adults in many countries; it is produced by at least 3 manufacturers worldwide (Merck and Co., Glaxo SmithKline, and Biken Institute/Aventis Pasteur). Although the vaccine was developed in Japan, the largest experience with it comes from the United States, where the Merck formulation was licensed for routine use in healthy susceptible individuals over the age of 1 year in 1995 (Centers for Disease Control, 1996). In both pre- and postlicensure studies (Gershon et al., 1984a, b; White, 1997; Sharrar et al., 2000) the vaccine was demonstrated to be extremely safe. Adverse effects in healthy persons are few and quite transient: a sore arm after the injection in 20%–25%, and a very minor rash resembling mild varicella in about 5%, usually appearing a month after immunization (White, 1997). A small proportion of vaccinees (15%) may also experience mild fever. It takes about a week to demonstrate antibodies to varicella-zoster virus (VZV) after immunization, but protection often results even after an exposure has occurred. As a result of widespread immunization of children, the epidemiology of varicella has begun to change in the United States, with a reported marked decline in incidence in sentinel areas, where active surveillance for the disease is being carried out (Seward et al., 2002). Vaccination is now being explored for the possibility of its preventing or modifying zoster. In a very real sense, the development of live varicella vaccine paved the way for the development of other vaccines against herpesviruses.

A number of possible misconceptions concerning varicella and varicella vaccine are listed in Table 70.1. This manuscript will discuss these misconceptions in the framework of the history of development of the live vaccine and its record regarding safety and efficacy of prevention, with regard to varicella as well as zoster.

History of development of the live attenuated vaccine

In 1974, when the first publication concerning the Oka varicella vaccine appeared, there was considerable controversy concerning whether use of a vaccine against a herpesvirus was likely to be safe and could possibly be effective. In Japan, the strategy used was first to vaccinate healthy children and then to gradually try to immunize safely immunocompromised children, progressing from the mildly to the severely immunocompromised. This possibly protective approach was taken because at that time, many young children were surviving cancer only to die of varicella. In studies in Japan, involving less than 200 healthy and immunocompromised children, it was found that the Oka strain appeared to be safe, although more needed to be learned about its efficacy. Because immunocompromised children in the Untied States were similarly faced with the possibility of surviving malignancy but not surviving chickenpox, interest in the Oka strain began to increase during the decade of the 1970s. While vaccine use remained controversial in the United States, most experts in the field believed that the risk-benefit ratio had become, by the late 1970s, appropriate to explore the safety and efficacy of varicella vaccine in children with underlying acute lymphoblastic leukemia in remission, because they had a 7% mortality from varicella (Feldman et al., 1975). Studies showed that the vaccine could be used safely in these high-risk children, although some developed fairly extensive vaccine-associated rashes that required treatment with antiviral drugs (Gershon, 1995). Importantly, the vaccine

Table 70.1. Misconceptions concerning varicella vaccine and its use

---
Varicella and zoster are invariably mild diseases.
The vaccine is not very efficacious.
Zoster will become epidemic with widespread vaccination.
Varicella will cause more disease in older age groups if vaccine is given routinely to children.
The vaccine is too expensive to use.
The vaccine is not safe.

---

proved to be highly protective against varicella, despite the weakened immune systems of these children. Because of the high-risk nature of varicella in children with malignancies, it was not possible to conduct a controlled efficacy study. Vaccine efficacy, however, could be tested because of the high clinical attack rate of varicella in susceptible children following a household exposure to VZV (Gershon et al., 1984a,b). As data regarding the clinical efficacy of the vaccine began to emerge, significant interest developed in determining if the vaccine would prove safe and effective in healthy children, thus eventually eliminating much of the necessity to immunize immunocompromised children.

Virology of the attenuated Oka strain of VZV

The original virus was isolated from a 3-year-old, otherwise healthy Japanese boy with varicella. To prepare the seed lot, the virus was passaged 11 times at 34 °C in human embryonic fibroblasts, 12 times at 37 °C in guinea pig fibroblasts, and 5 times in human diploid fibroblasts (WI-38 and MRC-5 cells) at 37 °C. (Takahashi et al., 1974) Additional passages were carried out by the manufacturers to prepare the vaccine to be marketed. Because VZV is so strongly cell-associated, the final product had to be sonicated and clarified by centrifugation to produce live cell-free virus.

Fortunately, it was possible soon after the vaccine was developed, to be able to distinguish between the wild type virus and the Oka strain, which made possible the reliable analysis of clinical information following vaccination. Initially it was necessary to propagate VZV from a rash or other body tissue or fluid in order to identify whether the vaccine type virus was implicated when a complication of vaccination was suspected (Gelb, et al., 1987). Eventually, however, it became possible to distinguish between vaccine and wild type VZV using polymerase chain reaction (PCR) without having to resort to virus isolation. (LaRussa et al., 1992; Gomi et al., 2000, 2001; Loparev et al., 2000a, b) A number of mutations have been found to be present in the Oka vaccine strain that are not present in the parental Oka virus (Gomi et al., 2000, 2001; Loparev, et al., 2000a, b). Although it is known that most of the mutations in the vaccine strain are in open reading frame (ORF) 62, exactly which mutations are associated with attenuation have not yet been identified. The Oka strain replicates less efficiently in human skin than does wild type VZV, as studied in the SCID-hu mouse model (Moffat et al., 1998).

Based on the vast quantity of clinical experience with the live VZV vaccine, there is overwhelming clinical evidence that the vaccine virus is attenuated. Both the incidence and severity of rash following vaccination compared to natural infection are decreased by a factor of about 20, whether vaccination is given by injection or inhalation (Bogger-Goren et al., 1982; Gershon, 2001). Transmission of the Oka strain from healthy vaccinees with rash to other susceptibles is extremely rare and has been reported only on 4 occasions (LaRussa et al., 1997; Salzman et al., 1997; Sharrar et al., 2000). This is in marked contrast to the extraordinarily high degree of contagion of the wild type virus in which roughly 90% of susceptibles develop clinical varicella after family exposures (Ross et al., 1962). Finally contact cases of Oka varicella, which occur with some frequency after vaccinating leukemic children as well as rarely from healthy populations, are extremely mild or subclinical (Tsolia et al., 1990; Sharrar et al., 2000). Transmission has only occurred when the vaccinee has manifested a rash due to the Oka strain, and there has been no clinical evidence of reversion of the vaccine strain to virulence.

Safety of the varicella vaccine for healthy individuals

With any preventive medical intervention that is to be used widely on a routine basis, particularly in children, safety is the major concern. Live varicella vaccine has proven to be extremely safe when given to susceptible children, as indicated by extensive pre- and postmarketing studies in the United States. Prior to licensure over 9000 healthy children and 2000 adults were safely immunized in clinical trials (Gershon, 1995; White, 1997). Adverse effects were minor and transient.

A post-marketing safety study of the vaccine was begun at its licensure in 1995, by investigators at Merck and Company and at Columbia University (Sharrar et al., 2000). Medical providers and consumers were asked on a voluntary basis, to submit information on possible adverse reactions to the vaccine they observed. In addition to clinical information, samples of rashes and other possibly involved fluids and tissues were submitted to analyze first for VZV by PCR, and then to distinguish between the two types of virus if VZV was identified (LaRussa et al., 1992). Although these data were collected passively, and the information therefore is necessarily incomplete, important data emerged from the study. It was crucial to be able to distinguish between vaccine and wild-type viruses because the temporal relationship of vaccination and development of rash and other symptoms would seem to implicate the vaccine virus without laboratory identification. Had it not been possible to distinguish between the two viruses, many adverse events would have erroneously been attributed to the vaccine type virus.

In the first 4 years after licensure, over 16 million doses of varicella vaccine were distributed in the United States. In the postmarketing study covering this period, rash was the most frequently reported adverse event, and almost all rashes consisting of more than 50 skin lesions were found to be caused by the wild type virus. There were fewer than five patients with more than 200 skin lesions shown to be caused by the Oka strain; this is below the average number seen in children experiencing natural varicella. There were 19 reports of encephalitis and 24 reports of ataxia during the year following vaccination, but the Oka strain of virus was not implicated in any of these illnesses. Wild-type VZV was, however, implicated in one patient with ataxia and one with encephalitis. Although there have been many reported fatalities due to wild type VZV, there have been no reports of fatal VZV infection caused by the Oka strain (Sharrar et al., 2000).

A handful of serious disseminated infections have been reported in children who were thought to be immunologically normal when vaccinated, but were eventually identified as immunodeficient. The varicella vaccine virus remains sensitive to acyclovir and other antiviral drugs. All of these children received antiviral therapy and recovered from the VZV infection. These include one child each with human immunodeficiency virus (HIV) infection and essentially no CD4 lymphocytes (Kramer et al., 2001), asthma and high dose steroids (Sharrar et al., 2000), adenosine deaminase (ADA) deficiency with immunodeficiency (Ghaffar et al., 2000), neuroblastoma diagnosed and treated right after vaccination (Levin, 2003), and a deficiency in natural killer cells (Levy et al., 2003).

Zoster has been reported after vaccination but infrequently. In the first 4 years after licensure, the Oka strain was identified in 22 patients and wild type VZV in 10 with zoster (Sharrar et al., 2000). To date, after distribution of over 40 million doses in the United States, there have been less than 50 reported cases of zoster shown to be due to the Oka strain (Galea et al., 2002).

Immunogenicity of varicella vaccine in healthy children and adolescents

In prelicensure studies, children under 12 years of age had a seroconversion rate of 97% after one dose of vaccine, as determined by the exquisitely sensitive glycoprotein immunosorbent assay (ELISA) 6 weeks after immunization. This test is not available on a commercial basis. Adolescents and adults had a seroconversion rate of 82% after one dose of vaccine, which rose to 99% after 2 doses (Provost et al., 1991; Gershon, 1995). A seroconversion rate of 91.5% was noted after one dose of vaccine, using an immune adherence antibody assay (IAHA), in 2565 Japanese children immunized between 1987–1993 (Asano, 1996). Unfortunately, commercially available ELISAs are neither sensitive nor specific enough to detect reliably antibodies after VZV immunization (Saiman, et al., 2001). There were a number of reports of failure to seroconvert (using a commercial ELISA test) in healthy children and adults in the Merck-Columbia post-licensure study (Sharrar et al., 2000). Most of these probably represent a failure of the test used rather than of the vaccine itself. The most sensitive and reliable method to measure antibodies to VZV, the fluorescent antibody to membrane antigen test (FAMA), is not amenable to performance on a large scale, and therefore remains a research tool (Williams et al., 1974; Gershon, 1995). In studies in leukemic children, this assay indicated a seroconversion rate of 82% after one dose of vaccine and 95% after two doses (Gershon et al., 1996). A convenient test that is sensitive and specific to reliably measure VZV antibody titers on a large scale basis continues to be sorely needed.

Efficacy and post-licensure effectiveness of varicella vaccine

Early studies in vaccinated leukemic children who were in remission from their illness and usually received two doses of varicella vaccine indicated not only that the vaccine was safe but also that it was highly protective against varicella (Gershon et al., 1984a,b). About 85% of vaccinated leukemic children were completely protected against varicella after household exposure and those who developed breakthrough infection had mild disease requiring no antiviral therapy. In contrast, one would expect that, in varicella-susceptibles, about 90% would become obviously infected following a household exposure to the virus (Ross et al., 1962). Early studies in healthy children indicated a similar degree of protection against household exposure, following 1 dose of vaccine, with breakthrough disease in about 15% (White, 1996).

Two double blind placebo-controlled studies of varicella vaccine in healthy children were performed, involving a total of about 1500 children. Both indicated that the vaccine provided protection of about 90% (Weibel et al., 1984; 1985; Varis and Vesikari, 1996). In these studies, higher doses of vaccine (10 000–17 000 plaque forming units-pfu) were associated with better protection than lower doses (1000 pfu). Many different doses of varicella vaccine have been studied in various clinical trials. The currently licensed Merck vaccine contains about 3000 pfu per dose, and the Glaxo SmithKline (GSK) vaccine contains about 10 000 pfu at the time of release, which prior to expiration date falls to about 3000 pfu. The Merck vaccine is lyophilized and frozen, while the GSK product is lyophilized and stored in the refrigerator (Gershon et al., 2002). No direct comparison of efficacy of these vaccines has been performed, and therefore it is assumed that they are similar in efficacy. Clearly both are highly efficacious.

A postlicensure case-control effectiveness study involving PCR-proven cases of varicella in otherwise healthy children examined the performance of varicella vaccine in clinical practice in New Haven, CT. This study indicated that the vaccine in the US is about 85% effective in preventing all varicella, and virtually 100% protective against severe varicella in otherwise healthy children (Vazquez et al., 2001). There were 202 children with varicella and 389 matched controls. Of these, 23% with varicella and 61% of controls had been vaccinated (vaccine effectiveness 85%). Of 56 vaccinated children with varicella, 86% had only mild disease; in contrast 48% of the 187 unvaccinated children had mild varicella. Studying the vaccine as it is used in clinical practice is especially significant because the vaccine itself is labile and loses potency if it is not stored properly, as indicated in the package insert, lyophilized and frozen.

Perhaps the best indication of the effectiveness of varicella vaccine, however, is the reported dramatic decline in the disease since 1995. This has been observed in sentinel areas of the USA (Seward et al., 2002). Varicella is often mild and uncomplicated in otherwise healthy children, but it may unpredictably be associated with significant morbidity and even mortality. In the United States, in the pre-vaccine era, there were about 100 annual deaths from varicella and and 11 000 hospitalizations. Most reported deaths from varicella occurred in otherwise healthy individuals. Beginning in 1995, active surveillance of varicella in three sentinel counties in Texas, California, and Pennsylvania, was carried out by investigators at the Centers for Disease Control (CDC). Vaccination coverage in the year 2000 in the sentinel counties in children aged 19 to 35 years of age ranged from 73.6% to 83.8%. For the period of study, the number of cases of varicella and hospitalizations decreased sharply, with a reduction ranging between 71%–84% in the 3 counties. Hospitalizations for varicella per 100 000 persons decreased from 2.7–4.2 in 1995–1998 to 0.6 in 1999 and 1.5 in 2000. The long-standing recognized seasonality of varicella with increases in incidence of disease in winter and early spring also disappeared after 2000. The decrease in varicella occurred in individuals of all age groups including infants too young to be immunized and also adults, who were less likely to be immunized than children, indicating that herd immunity had developed (Seward et al., 2002) (see figure in Seward chapter).

A prospective study of the incidence of varicella in 11 day-care centers in North Carolina between 1995–1999, indicated a similar decrease in the incidence of varicella due to vaccination. A case control analysis of this population indicated vaccine effectiveness of 83% (Clements et al., 1999). In a further analysis of this population, the rate of varicella vaccine coverage increased from 4.4% in 1995 to 63.1% in 1999. The incidence of varicella per 1000 person–months fell from 16.74 in July 1996 to 1.53 cases in December 1999. Because the decrease in varicella disease exceeded the increase in vaccination rate over the period studied, the investigators proposed that herd immunity had occurred (Clements, et al., 2001).

Considerations of vaccine use

In the United States, contraindications to varicella vaccine include pregnancy, allergy to vaccine components, and immunodeficiency. It is recommended that children receiving doses of steroids of over 2 mg/kg per day of prednisone or its equivalent NOT be immunized unless this medication can be discontinued for at least 3 months before vaccination. There are currently no programs for immunization of children with underlying leukemia because of potential safety concerns. On the other hand, studies of children with infection with human immunodeficiency virus (HIV) have indicated that it is safe to immunize them as long as their CD4 lymphocytes exceed 25% of their total lymphocytes in their peripheral blood. Two doses of vaccine are given to HIV-infected children, 4–8 weeks apart (Levin et al., 2001). The CDC has supported this recommendation (Centers for Disease Control 1999). Children undergoing renal transplantation have been safely immunized in French studies. These children have had protection against varicella and also have had a decreased incidence of zoster, compared to similar children who experienced natural varicella (Broyer and Boudailliez, 1985a, b; Broyer et al., 1997).

Because transmission of the vaccine virus to others is rare, healthy persons who have close contact with susceptible individuals who are at high risk to develop severe varicella are recommended to be immunized. This includes, for example, healthy children whose pregnant mothers are susceptible to varicella, and children whose varicella-susceptible siblings have malignant diseases for which they are being treated.

While the major thrust of vaccine use in the United States is in young children who have not been exposed to the virus, the vaccine often provides protection to susceptibles who have already been exposed. That post-exposure vaccination can be successful was best demonstrated in studies in Japan in the 1970s and 1980s (Asano et al., 1977, 1982). In these studies, family members who were exposed to varicella were immunized within 3 days and the disease was largely prevented. Vaccination was also used successfully to control an outbreak of varicella in a shelter for homeless families that was experiencing an epidemic of chickenpox (Watson et al., 2000).

The vaccine has been shown to be cost effective in a number of studies in the United States and abroad (Lieu et al., 1994; Beutels et al., 1996; Burnham et al., 1998; Coudeville et al., 1999; Diez Domingo et al., 1999; Brisson and Edmunds, 2002). In general this is a vaccine that is geared for use in developed countries, where it is not uncommon for children to be cared for out of the home as both parents are employed, or in single parent households where there is only one breadwinner.

Persistent questions regarding varicella vaccine

While ideally a vaccine should induce protection of close to 100% against a given disease, breakthrough cases of chickenpox have consistently been reported despite the administration of varicella vaccine, an observation first made in the early clinical trials involving leukemic children (Gershon et al., 1984a, b). The rate at which breakthrough varicella has occurred has varied from study to study. There are a myriad of possible explanations for the phenomenon. One obvious one is that not even natural varicella induces total immunity in every individual. Second cases of natural varicella are well recognized to occur (Gershon et al., 1984a, b; Junker et al., 1989, 1991). It is unrealistic to expect a viral vaccine to provide better protection than the natural illness itself. Another indication that complete immunity to VZV may never be quite achievable is the existence of zoster, which is due to reactivation of latent VZV in persons with partial immunity. Unless a vaccine that does not induce latent infection is developed and widely used, herd immunity will be required to control diseases due to VZV in addition to personal immunity from the vaccine itself.

There is now general agreement that varicella vaccine is both safe and effective. A number of important questions about the vaccine have been raised recently. None of these uncertainties preclude the use of varicella vaccine, but all need further exploration. The remainder of this chapter will address these issues.

Does immunity to varicella wane with time after immunization?

There are two types of vaccine failure, which have been termed primary and secondary. Primary vaccine failure, commonly called a "no take," is said to occur when there is no measurable immune response to a vaccine that was administered and the person remains susceptible to the immunizing product. Persons who received varicella vaccine and developed full blown infections which are severe have probably experienced this phenomenon. In the Merck-Columbia postmarketing study, there were 11 reports of severe varicella despite immunization (Sharrar et al., 2000). How often primary vaccine failure occurs is unknown, but it should be recalled that even with the very sensitive gp ELISA antibody test, the seroconversion rate in healthy children was 97%, not 100%. Considering that about 4 million children are immunized annually in the United States, there would be expected to be over 100 000 children annually who might have primary vaccine failure. This might be true for other vaccines as well and underscores the need for strong herd immunity in protection against infections after vaccination.

Secondary vaccine failure is said to occur when an immune response brought about by vaccination decreases with time, leaving the vaccinee with varying degrees of susceptibility to the disease. At present, there is little evidence for secondary vaccine failure due to waning of immunity to VZV after immunization of healthy children, but subtle degrees of waning immunity may be difficult to identify. An extremely high degree of persistence of antibodies and cellular immunity to VZV have been reported for as long as 20 years after vaccination, in Japanese and American studies (Asano et al., 1994; Arvin and Gershon, 1996; Ampofo et al., 2002). Moreover, studies in over 400 vaccinated adults indicate that there is no increase in the incidence or severity of breakthrough varicella with time, with up to 20 years of follow-up (Ampofo *et al.*, 2002). Were immunity to be waning, one would expect that breakthrough disease would become more frequent and more severe with time after vaccination, but this has not been observed.

Nevertheless there are hints that the current vaccine strategy in the U.S. may need some adjustment to provide better protection, especially to young children. It is disquieting that about 10% of children may develop a modified form of varicella despite vaccination, and in some studies the rate has been even higher. In four studies, the breakthrough rate of varicella in children followed for up to 10 years after immunization, ranged between 18%–34% (Clements *et al.*, 1995, 1999; Johnson *et al.*, 1997; Takayama *et al.*, 1997). This breakthrough varicella may occur months to years after immunization, and it is caused by wild type VZV (LaRussa *et al.*, 2000). It may be so mild that it is misdiagnosed clinically as insect bites or hives. It occurs mainly in individuals who have low VZV antibody levels following immunization.

A number of outbreaks of varicella in vaccinated young children have been reported in the United States (Dworkin *et al.*, 2002; Galil *et al.*, 2002a, b; Gershon, 2002). Some of these cases may have resulted from secondary vaccine failure. In addition, there are other possibilities to explain these outbreaks. The vaccine is labile, and improper storage may account for primary vaccine failure in some children. Children with asthma may have less ability to mount a protective immune response, possibly related to medications such as steroids (Izurieta *et al.*, 1997; Shapiro and LaRussa, 1997). Currently, a CDC study to examine the seroconversion rate to VZV in vaccinated asthmatic children, as determined by FAMA, is underway in the United States, which should provide an answer to this question. In two reports, children vaccinated when they were less than 15 months old had higher rates of breakthrough varicella than those immunized when they were older (Dworkin *et al.*, 2002; Galil *et al.*, 2002a, b). When varicella vaccine is administered with an interval of less than one month after another live vaccine has been given, the incidence of breakthrough varicella increases (Centers for Disease Control, 2001) (Table 70.2).

One report of an outbreak of chickenpox in a day-care center in New Hampshire, in which the rate of vaccination in attendees was high is especially compelling with regard to the possibility of secondary vaccine failure (Galil *et al.*, 2002a, b). In this outbreak, the effectiveness of the vaccine was only 44%, much lower than in any previous report. In this study, 25/88 (28.4%) of children developed varicella in a 6-week period. It seems likely that the index case, whose varicella was quite extensive, had experienced primary vaccine failure. In the other involved children, the

Table 70.2. Factors associated with vaccine failure/breakthrough disease

Improper storage of vaccine
<14 months old when immunized
Asthma
<30 days between MMR and varicella vaccine
>30 months since immunization
Low vaccine dosage

Table 70.3. Factors associated with successful vaccination

High vaccine dosage (over 10 000 pfu)
Two doses of vaccine, which provide higher antibody titers which in turn correlate with better protection

only factor that was associated with vaccine failure was an interval of greater than 3 years since vaccination. However, the children involved were very young, and it may be that the age at vaccination combined with the interval of time after immunization also played a role in predisposing them to breakthrough varicella. Continued investigations will be necessary to further understand whether waning immunity is a significant factor in breakthrough disease and how frequently it might occur, but it seems to be a real possibility. A follow up of the study conducted in private practices in New Haven has indicated that vaccine efficacy decreases with time, from 97% in year 1 to 72% in year 6 (Vazquez *et al.*, 2003), which confirms and extends the above observations of Galil *et al.* (2002a, b).

It may be that a second dose of varicella vaccine given routinely will alleviate potential problems of primary and secondary vaccine failure (Gershon, 2002). (Table 70.3) One possible way in which this could be accomplished in a practical manner is to administer routinely two doses of vaccine as measles, mumps, rubella, varicella (MMRV). Developing an immunogenic formulation of the varicella component of MMRV has proven to be a difficult task. Even a formulation of very high titered VZV (40 000 pfu) did not produce significantly higher titers of VZV antibodies, although it appeared to be safe (Shinefield, *et al.*, 2002). However, MMR and varicella vaccine may be administered safely together, and many children receive the two vaccine formulations at the same time although in separate syringes at different body sites (White, 1996).

It should be emphasized that breakthrough varicella is almost always a mild infection. Reports of varicella of normal severity in vaccines are few and probably represent mostly episodes of primary vaccine failure (Sharrar *et al.*,

Table 70.4. A comparison of the reported percentage of immunocompromised patients developing zoster who were vaccinated and those who experienced natural infection

Underlying diagnosis	Interval of observation in years	Vaccinees N (%)	Natural varicella N (%)	Reference
Leukemia	6	(6)	(19)	Takahashi et al., 1990
Leukemia	6	34 (0)	73 (21)	Brunell et al., 1986
Leukemia	10	96 (4)	96 (16)	Hardy et al. 1991
Renal transplantation	10	212 (7)	415 (13)	Broyer et al., 1997

2000). Zoster may be more of a concern although it appears that zoster is more common after natural than vaccine infection (see below). If skin lesions of varicella predispose to latency, as has been suggested by experimental evidence (Chen et al., 2003), then it would be important to try to prevent breakthrough infection in order to minimize the chance of developing zoster.

Varicella-susceptible adults may be safely immunized against varicella. Two doses are utilized, 4–8 weeks apart. Adults manifest lower seroconversion rates after one dose of vaccine than children, and therefore two doses are routinely administered. As in children, adverse effects are minimal and protection is high (Gershon, et al., 1988; 1990; Ampofo et al., 2002).

Serologic testing following immunization is usually discouraged because VZV antibody tests are both insensitive and results may be non-specific. Whether adults with no history of varicella should have serologic testing prior to immunization or simply be given two doses of vaccine if they have no history of past varicella remains moot. Inadvertent administration of vaccine to persons with immunity to varicella is not harmful (Gershon et al., 2002).

Zoster: effects and potential effects on its incidence in the vaccine era

Although use of varicella vaccine is now contraindicated in immunocompromised individuals, early vaccine studies often involved these children because they were at high risk of developing severe varicella. (Table 70.4) In these vaccinees, the incidence of zoster was shown to be lower than after natural infection (Hardy et al., 1991; Arvin and Gershon, 1996). Thus, there is every reason to predict that vaccination would also be protective against zoster in healthy children. Although the data are of necessity not controlled, the existing information since 1995 to the present strongly suggests that this is the case. Although healthy vaccinees have developed zoster, less than 50 known cases have been reported after distribution of over 40 million doses of vaccine between 1995 and 2002 (White, 1996; Sharrar et al., 2000; Galea et al., 2002). The rate of zoster after vaccination is roughly 20 times less the expected rate for that age group (Gershon et al., 2002).

Recently several studies have addressed the question of whether exposure to varicella is protective against zoster, because it is known that zoster is associated with a low cell-mediated immune response to VZV. It was found that in vaccinated leukemic children, both household exposure and additional doses of varicella vaccine correlated with greater protection against zoster than a single dose of vaccine alone (Gershon et al., 1996a, b). A case-control study has shown that following natural varicella, there is a lower incidence of zoster in individuals who have exposures to children with VZV infections in comparison to those who do not (Thomas et al., 2002). Based on such data, using computer modeling, a theoretical calculation of the incidence of zoster in a highly vaccinated population has been made. This model predicts an epidemic of zoster with accompanying significant mortality in countries where varicella vaccination is routine (Brisson et al., 2002). These observations, even though theoretical, have led to reluctance to use varicella vaccine routinely in some countries. It is therefore important to put the possibility into perspective.

The reported incidence of zoster in healthy individuals aged 40–50 in developed countries ranges between 2–4 cases per 1000 person–years of observation (Hope-Simpson, 1965; Donahue et al., 1995). It was calculated that the rate of zoster would double in countries where routine vaccination is being carried out (Brisson et al., 2002). This would lead to an incidence of 4–8 cases per 1000 person–years of observation in this age group. The incidence of zoster per 1000 person–years of observation in other high risk groups has been reported to be as follows: vaccinated leukemics 8, unvaccinated leukemics 25, adults with AIDS 50, children with AIDS 300 (Gershon et al., 1996a, b). Thus the projected increase in the incidence of zoster based on computer modeling might double but even this is unlikely to represent an epidemic. Moreover, the mortality of zoster appears to be less than that from varicella, the primary infection, and thus the validity of an increasing incidence of zoster leading to significantly increased mortality must be questioned (Feldman et al., 1973; 1975; Whitley et al. 1982a,b; Shepp et al., 1988). Finally, as yet, no actual increase in the incidence of zoster has been observed in the United States although the CDC is collecting epidemiologic data on the issue. Should an increase in zoster be recognized, however, it can logically be approached by immunization to prevent zoster, as described below.

Vaccination to prevent zoster in the elderly

It is estimated that about 20% of individuals who have had natural varicella will develop zoster during their lifetime, usually if they become immunocompromised or elderly. After age 50, the incidence of zoster climbs steadily with each advancing decade. While mortality from zoster is rare, morbidity from this infection remains a significant medical problem. The risk of developing the severe and painful complication of post-herpetic neuralgia (PHN) also increases with increasing age. It has been recognized for years that zoster occurs when the cell-mediated immune (CMI) response falls to below a critical level, and with advancing age, fewer and fewer people maintain a positive CMI response to VZV, although their antibody titers remain intact or may even increase (Arvin et al., 1978; Berger et al., 1981; Gershon and Steinberg, 1981; Burke et al., 1982; Hardy et al., 1991).

In attempts to explore whether vaccination may be used to boost immunity to VZV and possibly be used to prevent zoster, at least 8 clinical trials have been performed by investigators in the United States and Europe. These trials have determined that it is possible to boost CMI responses safely in many, although not all, elderly subjects. Varying doses of vaccine from roughly 1000 to 12 000 pfu have been employed. Some of these studies employed controls and others did not; in each, the subjects and medical personnel was aware of whom had received which vaccine. While no firm conclusions can be made from these studies, it appeared that vaccination seemed to modify zoster. All observed cases of zoster were mild in these otherwise healthy adults (Levin, 2001).

Based on these apparently successful open label studies, a large double blind placebo controlled study of immunization of healthy individuals over the age of 60 is currently being carried out. This study has now enrolled approximately 30 000 subjects and the observational period is still in progress. After a 3-year follow-up interval, the code will be broken and the data will be analyzed. At present, no results from this study are available, but there should be some published information by 2005. The vaccine employed is the live attenuated product, at a dose of about 20 000 pfu, which is roughly ten times the dose that is administered to healthy children (Levin, 2001) (see update below).

Use of inactivated varicella vaccine in patients at high risk to develop zoster

As in the studies described above to try to prevent zoster in elderly individuals, these studies were undertaken to try to boost the CMI response to VZV in highly immunocompromised patients who are at even greater risk to develop zoster than elderly patients. Because of the possibility of inducing another serious VZV infection with the live vaccine itself, however, an inactivated formulation of the vaccine was utilized. In an early controlled study, three doses of heat-inactivated vaccine were administered to a heterogeneous group of 75 patients; the incidence of zoster remained unchanged but the illness appeared to have been modified (Redman et al., 1997). In a second, more successful clinical trial, 4 doses were employed, including one given a month before transplantation, and the subject population was more homogeneous and included only patients with lymphoma who had undergone autologous stem cell transplantation (Hata et al., 2002). A dose of 6115 pfu of heat-inactivated VZV was administered, which was well tolerated although induration, erythema, or pain occurred after 10% of the doses. The rate of zoster was significantly decreased in vaccines compared to controls. Zoster occurred in 17/56 (30%) of the evaluable unvaccinated control patients and in only 7/53 (13%) vaccinees. Protection correlated with reconstitution of CD4 T-cell immunity to VZV. Because all the patients who developed zoster received antiviral therapy for their illness, it was not possible to compare the severity of zoster in the vaccines and controls. While this vaccine remains experimental, it holds promise for eventual prevention of zoster in immunocompromised patients. It also suggests an approach that might successfully prevent infections with other herpesviruses in the immunocompromised (Hata et al., 2002).

Recent developments

There are two recent changes in policy with regard to recommendations for VZV vaccine use in the United States. They involve a CDC mandated second dose of varicella vaccine for all children, and the use of the newly licensed by the FDA of combined measles-mumps-rubella-varicella (MMRV) vaccine. An additional development concerns vaccination of healthy older adults against zoster. Recently it was demonstrated that zoster can be prevented by immunization of healthy individuals over the age of 60 years with a different formulation of the Oka vaccine VZV strain that contains over 10 times the dose of virus as the monovalent varicella vaccine.

As has been mentioned, by 2002, numerous outbreaks of varicella were being observed in immunized children in day care facilities and schools in the United States. Vaccine efficacy rates were calculated to vary from 85% to as low as 44%.(Galil et al., 2002b) One study showed that it appeared that the vaccine failure rate after 1 dose of vaccine might be as high as 20%, which alone could account for apparent breakthrough disease. In 2006, a study of the seroconversion against VZV of 16 month old children vaccinated in a practice setting at Vanderbilt University in 2004, indicated a seroconversion rate of 76% (FAMA $\geq$ 1:4) 16 weeks after 1 dose of Varivax (Michalek, Gershon et al., personal communication). As part of a study conducted by Merck study (Kuter et al., 2004), roughly 1000 children received a second dose of varicella vaccine 3 months after the first dose. A similar number of children were followed for the same interval but received only 1 dose of vaccine. In these children who received 2 doses, the seroconversion rate 6 weeks after the second dose increased to 99.5%, and the geometric mean titer (GMT) to 141.5, indicating a marked booster response after the second dose. In this study, the gp ELISA assay was used to assess humoral immunity. In October, 2006, the FDA approved the use of the combined vaccine MMRV for use in the United States. Marked boosting of humoral immunity following a second dose of MMRV was also observed (Shinefield et al., 2005a,b). Boosting against VZV was about 10 times greater than boosting against the MMR components, in which it was only about 2 times greater. Importantly, as part of the Merck study (Kuter et al., 2004), protection against varicella over 10 years of follow up was significantly higher after 2 doses of vaccine than 1 dose, 94% vs 98% respectively.

Due to the costs, inconvenience, and transmission of wild-type VZV associated with the numerous outbreaks of varicella, as well as the consistently observed boosting of both humoral and cell mediated immunity after a second dose of vaccine, the ACIP mandated a second routine dose of varicella vaccine for infants and children, with catch up programs, in June 2006. For harmonization with MMR vaccine, MMRV will usually be given at 12–15 months of age with a second dose at 4–6 years of age. Details concerning this recommendation should become available on the CDC website in the near future. As yet this information is unpublished.

Without a second dose of vaccine it was predicted that there would be an accumulation of vaccinated children destined to become varicella-susceptible young adults, potentially at high risk to develop severe varicella. This would especially be liable to occur in the setting of less opportunity for boosting of immunity due to less exposure to cases of varicella. In addition, it had been found by the CDC that outbreak control with a second dose was expensive and almost impossible to implement. While it is uncertain that there will be complete protection against varicella after 2 routine doses of varicella vaccine, it is projected that the numbers of breakthrough cases will decrease significantly, with a subsequent decrease in transmission of the virus, and a decrease in outbreaks.

Monovalent varicella vaccine contains a dose of about 1350 plaque forming units (pfu) of virus, but MMRV contains about ten times this amount. The increased dose of varicella vaccine in MMRV was required in order to reach an acceptable seroconversion against VZV. It is hypothesized that the measles component in MMRV may suppress the immune response to VZV. This dose of virus in MMRV is similar to the dose of vaccine used to prevent zoster.

In 2005, it was shown in a double-blind placebo-controlled study that vaccination of healthy adults over age 60 years resulted in significant protection against zoster and that in preventing zoster, postherpetic neuralgia was also prevented (Oxman et al., 2005). In vaccinees aged 60–69 years, the vaccine was 64% effective in protection against zoster. Although the vaccine was less effective in preventing zoster in vaccinees aged 70–79 years (41%), it was 55% protective against PHN in this age group. Many questions about the use of this vaccine remain, such as the duration of immunity, but thus far the vaccine appears to be safe and effective when used in this manner. Currently the decisions are being made as to exactly how this vaccine should be used in the elderly population; the outcome should be known in the fall of 2006 (see CDC website for further information).

Conclusions

Despite the controversial introduction, varicella vaccines represent the first truly successful preventive measure against VZV. Although the approach of routine vaccine regimens for children may require some adjustment, the vaccine safely prevents most cases of clinical varicella, which saves lives, hospitalizations, and resources. Recipients of live vaccine are also at decreased risk to develop zoster. The promise of prevention of zoster in individuals who already have latent infection with the wild type virus due to past natural infection with VZV is a potential goal that is likely to be accomplished with either live or inactivated vaccine or both. A new era in herpesvirus virology is well underway.

REFERENCES

Ampofo, K., Saiman, L., La Russa, P., Steinberg, S., Annunziato, P., and Gershon, A. (2002). Persistence of immunity to live attenuated varicella vaccine in healthy adults. *Clin. Infect. Dis.*, **34**(6), 774–779.

Arvin, A. and Gershon, A. (1996). Live attenuated varicella vaccine. *Annu. Rev. Microbiol.*, **50**, 59–100.

Arvin, A. M., Pollard, R. B., Rasmussen, L., and Metigan, T. (1978). Selective impairment in lymphocyte reactivity to varicella-zoster antigen among untreated lymphoma patients. *J. Infect. Dis.*, **137**, 531–540.

Asano, Y. (1996). Varicella vaccine: the Japanese experience. *J. Infect. Dis.*, **174**, S310–S313.

Asano, Y., Nakayama, H., Yasaki, T. *et al.* (1977). Protection against varicella in family contacts by immediate inoculation with live varicella vaccine. *Pediatrics*, **59**, 3–7.

Asano, Y., Hirose, S., Iwayama, S., Miyata, Yazaki, T., and Takahashi, M. (1982). Protective effect of immediate inoculation of a live varicella vaccine in household contacts in relation to the viral dose and interval between exposure and vaccination. *Biken J.*, **25**, 43–45.

Asano, Y., Suga, S., Yoshikawa, T. *et al.* (1994). Experience and reason: twenty year follow up of protective immunity of the Oka live varicella vaccine. *Pediatrics*, **94**, 524–526.

Berger, R., Florent, G., and Just, M. (1981). 'Decrease of the lymphoproliferative response to varicella-zoster virus antigen in the aged. *Infect. Immunol.*, **32**, 24–27.

Beutels, P., Clara, R., Tormans, G., Vandoorsalaer, E., and Van Damme, P. (1996). Costs and benefits of routine varicella vaccination in German children. *J. Infect. Dis.*, **174**, S335–S341.

Bogger-Goren, S., Baba, K., Husley, P., Yabuuchi, H., Takahashi, M., and Ogra, P. (1982). Antibody response to varicella-zoster virus after natural or vaccine-induced infection. *J. Infect. Dis.*, **146**, 260–265.

Brisson, M. and Edmunds, W. J. (2002). The cost-effectiveness of varicella vaccination in Canada. *Vaccine*, **20**(7–8), 1113–1125.

Brisson, M., Gay, N., Do, W. J., and Andrews, N. J. (2002). Exposure to varicella boosts immunity to herpes-zoster: implications for mass vaccination against chickenpox. *Vaccine*, **20**, 2500–2507.

Broyer, M. and Boudailliez, B. (1985a). Prevention of varicella infection in renal transplanted children by previous immunization with a live attenuated varicella vaccine. *Transpl. Proc.*, **17**, 151–152.

Broyer, M. and Boudailliez, B. (1985b). Varicella vaccine in children with chronic renal insufficiency. *Postgrad. Med J.*, **61 (S4)**, 103–106.

Broyer, M., Tete, M. T., Guest, G., Gugnadoux, M. F., and Rouzioux, C. (1997). Varicella and zoster in children after kidney transplantation: long term results of vaccination. *Pediatrics*, **99**, 35–39.

Burke, B. L., Steele, R., W., Beard, O. W., Woods, J. S., Cain, T. D., and Marmer, D. J. (1982). Immune responses to varicella-zoster in the aged. *Arch. Intern. Med.*, **142**, 291–293.

Burnham, B. R., Wells, T. S., and Riddle, J. R. (1998). A cost–benefit analysis of a routine varicella vaccination program for United States Air Force Academy cadets. *Milit. Med.* **163**(9), 631–634.

Centers for Disease Control (1996). Prevention of varicella: Recommendations of the Advisory Committee on Immunization Practices (ACIP). *Morb. Mortal. Wkly Rep.*, **45**, 1–36.

Centers for Disease Control (1999). Prevention of varicella. Update. *Morb. Mortal. Wkly. Rep.*, **48**, 1–6.

Centers for Disease Control (2001). Simultaneous administration of varicella vaccine and other recommended childhood vaccines – United States, 1995–1999. *Morb. Mortal. Wkly. Rep.*, **50**, 1058–1061.

Chen, J., Gershon, A., Silverstein, S. J., Li, Z. S., Lung, P., and Gershon, M. D. (2003). Latent and lytic infection of isolated guinea pig enteric and dorsal root ganglia by varicella zoster virus. *J. Med. Virol.*, **70**, S71–S78.

Clements, D., Moreira, S. P., Coplan, P., Bland, C., and Walter, E. (1999). Postlicensure study of varicella vaccine effectiveness in a day-care setting. *Pediatr. Infect. Dis. J.*, **18**, 1047–1050.

Clements, D. A., Armstrong, C. B., Ursano, A. M., Moggio, M., Walter, E. B., and Wilfert, C. M (1995). Over five-year follow-up of Oka/Merck varicella vaccine recipients in 465 infants and adolescents. *Pediatr. Infect. Dis. J.*, **14**, 874–879.

Clements, D. A., Zaref, J. I., Bland, C. L., Walter, E. B., and Coplan, P. (2001). Partial uptake of varicella vaccine and the epidemiological effect on varicella disease in 11 day-care centers in North Carolina. *Arch. Pediatr. Adolesc. Med.*, **155**, 433–461.

Coudeville, L., Paree, F., Lebrun, T., and Sally, J. (1999). The value of varicella vaccination in healthy children: cost–benefit analysis of the situation in France. *Vaccine*, **17**(2), 142–151.

Diez Domingo, J., Ridao, M., Latour, J., Ballester, A., and Morant, A. (1999). A cost benefit analysis of routine varicella vaccination in Spain. *Vaccine*, **17**(11–12), 1306–1311.

Donahue, J. G., Choo, P. W., Manson, J. E., and Platt, R. (1995). The incidence of herpes zoster. *Arch. Intern. Med.*, **155**(15), 1605–1609.

Dworkin, M. S., Jennings, C. E., Thomas-Roth, J., (Lang, J. E., Stukenberg, C., and Lumpkin, J R.) (2002). An outbreak of varicella among children attending preschool and elementary school in Illinois. *Clin. Infect. Dis.*, **35**, 102–104.

Feldman, S., Hughes, W. T., and Kim, H. Y. (1973). Herpes zoster in children with cancer. *Am. J. Dis. Child.*, **126**, 178–184.

Feldman, S., Hughes, W., and Daniel, C., (1975). Varicella in children with cancer: 77 cases. *Pediatrics*, **80**, 388–397.

Galea, S., Sweet, A., Gershon, A., *et al.* (2002). *The Postmarketing Safety Review of Reports of Herpes Zoster after the Administration of VARIVAXR [Varicella Virus Vaccine Live (OKA/MERCK)*. Fifth Annual Conference on Vaccine Research, Baltimore, MD.

Galil, K., Fair, E., Mountcastle, N., Britz, P., and Seward, J. (2002a). Younger age at vaccination may increase risk of varicella vaccine failure. *J. Infect. Dis.*, **186**, 102–105.

Galil, K., Lee, B., Strine, T. *et al.* (2002b). Outbreak of varicella at a day-care center despite vaccination. *N. Engl. J. Med.*, **347**, 1909–1915.

Gelb, L. D., Dohner, D. E., Gershon, A. *et al.* (1987). Molecular epidemiology of live, attenuated varicella virus vaccine in children and in normal adults. *J. Infect. Dis.* **155**, 633–640.

Gershon, A. (1995). Varicella-zoster virus: prospects for control. *Adv. Pediatr. Infect. Dis.*, **10**, 93–124.

Gershon, A. (2002). Varicella vaccine: are two doses better than one? *N. Engl. J. Med.*, **347**, 1962–1963.

Gershon, A. and Steinberg, S. (1981). Antibody responses to varicella-zoster virus and the role of antibody in host defense. *Am. J. Med. Sci.*, **282**, 12–17.

Gershon, A., LaRussa, P., and Steinberg, S. (1996a). Varicella vaccine: use in immunocompromised patients. *Infectious Disease Clinics of North America*, ed. R. E. J. White. Philadelphia: W. B. Saunders, **10**, 583–594.

Gershon, A., LaRussa, P., Steinberg, S., Lo, S. H., Murevish, N., and Meier, P. (1996b). The protective effect of immunologic boosting against zoster: an analysis in leukemic children who were vaccinated against chickenpox. *J. Infect. Dis.*, **173**, 450–453.

Gershon, A., Takahashi, M., and Seward, J. (2002). Live attenuated varicella vaccine. In *Vaccines*, ed. S. Plotkin and W. Orenstein, 4th edn, pp. 783–823. Philadelphia: W.B. Saunders.

Gershon, A. A. (2001). Live-attenuated varicella vaccine. *Infect. Dis. Clin. N. Amer.*, **15**, 65–81.

Gershon, A. A., Steinberg, S., Gelb, L. *et al.* (1984a). Clinical reinfection with varicella-zoster virus. *J. Infect. Dis.*, **149**, 137–142.

Gershon, A. A., Steinberg, S., Gelb, L. *et al.* (1984b). Live attenuated varicella vaccine: efficacy for children with leukemia in remission. *J. Am. Med. Assoc*, **252**, 355–362.

Gershon, A. A., Steinberg, S., La Russa, P. *et al.* (1988). Immunization of healthy adults with live attenuated varicella vaccine. *J. Infect. Dis.*, **158**, 132–137.

Gershon, A. A., Steinberg, S., Gelb, L. *et al.* (1990). Live attenuated varicella vaccine: protection in healthy adults in comparison to leukemic children. *J. Infect. Dis.*, **161**, 661–666.

Ghaffar, F., Carrick, K., Rogers, B. B., Margraf, L. R., Krisher, K., and Ramillo, O. (2000). Disseminated infection with varicella-zoster virus vaccine strain presenting as hepatitis in la child with adenosine deaminase deficiency. *Pediatr. Infect. Dis. J.*, **19**, 764–765.

Gomi, Y., Imagawa, T., Takahashi, M., and Yamanishi, K. (2000). Oka varicella vaccine is distinguishable from its parental virus in DNA sequence of open reading frame 62 and its transactivation activity. *J. Med. Virol.* **61**, 497–503.

Gomi, Y., Imagawa, T., Takahashi, M., and Yamanish, K. (2001). Comparison of DNA sequence and transactivation activity of open reading frame 62 of Oka varicella vaccine and its parental viruses. *Arch. Virol.*, **S17**, 49–56.

Hardy, I. B., Gershon, A., Steinberg, S. *et al.* (1991). The incidence of zoster after immunization with live attenuated varicella vaccine. A study in children with leukemia. *N. Engl. J. Med.*, **325**, 1545–1550.

Hata, A., Asanuma, H., Rinki, M. *et al.* (2002). Use of an inactivated varicella vaccine in recipients of hematopoietic- cell transplants. *N. Engl. J. Med.*, **347**(1), 26–34.

Hope-Simpson, R. E. (1965). The nature of herpes zoster: a long term study and a new hypothesis. *Proc. Roy. Soc. Med.*, **58**, 9–20.

Izurieta, H., Strebel, P., and Blake, P. (1997). Post-licensure effectiveness of varicella vaccine during an outbreak in a child care center. *J. Am. Med. Assoc.*, **278**, 1495–1498.

Johnson, C., Stancin, T., Fattlar, D., Rome, L. P., and Kumar, M. L. (1997). A long-term prospective study of varicella vaccine in healthy children. *Pediatrics*, **100**, 761–766.

Junker, A. K., Angus, E., and Thomas, E. (1991). Recurrent varicella-zoster virus infections in apparently immunocompetent children. *Pediatr. Infect. Dis. J.*, **10**, 569–575.

Junker, K., Avnstorp, C., Neilsen, C., and Hansen, N. (1989). Reinfection with varicella-zoster virus in immunocompromised patients. *Curr. Probl. Dermatol.*, **18**, 152–157.

Kramer, J. M., LaRussa, P., Tsai, W. C. *et al.* (2001). Disseminated vaccine strain varicella as the acquired immunodeficiency syndrome-defining illness in a previously undiagnosed child. *Pediatrics*, **108**(2), E39.

Kuter, B., Matthews, H., Shinefield, H. *et al.* (2004). Ten year follow-up of healthy children who received one or two injections of varicella vaccine. *Pediatr. Infect. Dis. J.* **23**(2), 132–137.

LaRussa, P., Lungu, O., Gershon, A., Steinberg, S., and Silverstein, S. (1992). Restriction fragment length polymorphism of polymerase chain reaction products from vaccine and wild-type varicella-zoster virus isolates. *J. Virol.*, **66**, 1016–1020.

LaRussa, P., Steinberg, S. *et al.* (1997). Transmission of vaccine strain varicella-zoster virus from a healthy adult with vaccine-associated rash to susceptible household contacts. *J. Infect. Dis.*, **176**, 1072–1075.

LaRussa, P., Steinberg, S., Merwice, F., and Gershon, A. (2000). Viral strain identification in varicella vaccinees with disseminated rashes. *Pediatr. Infect. Dis. J.*, **19**, 1037–1039.

Levin, M. J. (2001). Use of varicella vaccines to prevent herpes zoster in older individuals. *Arch. Virol. Suppl.* **17**, 151–160.

Levin, M. J. (2003). Development of acyclovir resistance during chronic Oka strain varicella-zoster virus infection in an immunocompromised child. *J. Infect. Dis.*, **188**, 954–959.

Levin, M. J., Gershon, A. A., Weinberg, A. *et al.* (2001). Immunization of HIV-infected children with varicella vaccine. *J. Pediatr.*, **139**(2), 305–310.

Levy, O., Orange, J. S., Hibberd, P. *et al.* (2003). Disseminated varicella infection due to vaccine (Oka) strain varicella-zoster virus in a patient with a novel deficiency in natural killer cells. *J. Infect. Dis.*, **188**, 948–953.

Lieu, T., Cochi, S., Black, S. *et al.* (1994). Cost-effectiveness of a routine varicella vaccination program for U.S. children. *J. Am. Med. Assoc.*, **271**, 375–381.

Loparev, V. N., Argaw, T., Krause, P., Takayama, M., and Schmid, S. (2000a). Improved identification and differentiation of varicella-zoster virus (VZV) wild type strains and an attenuated varicella vaccine strain using a VZV open reading frame 62-based PCR. *J. Clin. Micro.*, **38**, 3156–3160.

Loparev, V. N., McCaustland, K., Holloway, B., Krause, P. R., Takayama, M., and Schmid, S. (2000). Rapid genotyping of varicella-zoster virus vaccine and wild type strains with fluorophore-labeled hybridization probes. *J. Clin. Micro.*, **38**, 4315–4319.

Moffat, J. F., Zerboni, L., Kinchington, P., Grose, C., Kaneshima, H., and Arvin, A. (1998). Attenuation of the vaccine Oka strain of varicella-zoster virus and role of glycoprotein C in alpha-herpesvirus virulence demonstrated in the SCID-hu mouse. *J. Virol.*, **72**, 965–974.

Oxman, M. N., Levin, M. J., Johnson, G. R. *et al.* (2005). A vaccine to prevent herpes zoster and postherpetic neuralgia in older adults. *N. Engl. J. Med.*, **352**(22), 2271–2284.

Provost, P. J., Krah, D. L., Kuter, B. J. *et al.* (1991). Antibody assays suitable for assessing immune responses to live varicella vaccine. *Vaccine*, **9**, 111–116.

Redman, R., Nader, S., Zerboni, L. *et al.* (1997). Early reconstitution of immunity and decreased severity of herpes zoster in bone marrow transplant recipients immunized with inactivated varicella vaccine. *J. Infect. Dis.*, **176**, 578–585.

Ross, A. H., Lencher, E., and Reitman, G. (1962). Modification of chickenpox in family contacts by administration of gamma globulin. *N. Engl. J. Med.*, **267**, 369–376.

Saiman, L., LaRussa, P., Steinberg, S. *et al.* (2001). Persistence of immunity to varicella-zoster virus vaccination among health care workers. *Inf. Cont. Hosp. Epidemiol.*, **22**, 279–283.

Salzman, M. B., Sharrar, R., Steinberg, S., and LaRussa, P. (1997). Transmission of varicella-vaccine virus from a healthy 12 month old child to his pregnant mother. *J. Pediatr.*, **131**, 151–154.

Seward, J. F., Watson, B. M., Peterson, C. L. *et al.* (2002). Varicella disease after introduction of varicella vaccine in the United States, 1995–2000. *J. Am. Med. Assoc.*, **287**(5), 606–611.

Shapiro, E. and LaRussa, P. (1997). Vaccination for varicella – just do it. *J. Am. Med. Assoc.*, **278**, 1529–1530.

Sharrar, R. G., LaRussa, P., Galea, S. *et al.* (2000). The postmarketing safety profile of varicella vaccine. *Vaccine*, **19**, 916–923.

Shepp, D., Dandliker, P., and Meyers, J. (1988). Current therapy of varicella zoster virus infection in immunocompromised patients. *Am. J. Med.*, **85 (S2A)**, 96–98.

Shinefield, H., Black, S., Staehle, B. *et al.* (2002). Vaccination with measles, mumps, and rubella vaccine and varicella vaccine: safety, tolerability, immunogenicity, persistence of antibody, and duration of protection against varicella in healthy children. *Pediatr. Infect. Dis. J.*, **21**, 555–561.

Shinefield, H., Williams, W. R., Marchant, C. *et al.* (2005a). Dose–response study of a quadrivalent measles, mumps, rubella and varicella vaccine in healthy children. *Pediatr. Infect. Dis. J.*, **24**(8), 670–675.

Shinefield, H., Black, S., Digilio, L. *et al.* (2005b). Evaluation of a quadrivalent measles, mumps, rubella and varicella vaccine in healthy children. *Pediatr. Infect. Dis. J.*, **24**(8), 665–669.

Takahashi, M., Otsuka, T., Okuno, Y., Asano, T., Yazahi, T., and Isomura, S. (1974). Live vaccine used to prevent the spread of varicella in children in hospital. *Lancet*, **2**, 1288–1290.

Takayama, N., Minamitani, M., and Takayama, M. (1997). HIgh incidence of breakthrough varicella observed in healthy Japanese lchildren immunized with live varicella vaccine (Oka strain). *Acta Paediatr. Jpn.*, **39**, 663–668.

Thomas, S., Wheeler, J., and Hall, A. J. (2002). Contacts with varicella or with children and protection against herpes zoster in adults: a case-control study. *Lancet*, **360**, 678–682.

Tsolia, M., Gershon, A., Steinberg, S., and Gelb, L. (1990). Live attenuated varicella vaccine: evidence that the virus is attenuated and the importance of skin lesions in transmission of varicella-zoster virus. *J. Pediatr.*, **116**, 184–189.

Varis, T. and Vesikari, T. (1996). Efficacy of high titer live attenuated varicella vaccine in healthy young children. *J. Infect. Dis.*, **174**, S330–S334.

Vazquez, M., LaRussa, P., Gershon, A., Steinberg, S., Freudigman, K., and Shapiro, E. (2001). The effectiveness of the varicella vaccine in clinical practice. *N. Engl. J. Med.*, **344**, 955–960.

Vazquez, M., LaRussa, P., Gershon, A., *et al.* (2003). Effectiveness of varicella vaccine after 8 years. Infectious Disease Society of America 41 St Annual Meeting, San Diego, CA.

Watson, B., Seward, J., Yang, A. *et al.* (2000). Post exposure effectiveness of varicella vaccine. *Pediatrics*, **105**, 84–88.

Weibel, R., Neff, B. J., Kuter, B. J. *et al.* (1984). Live attenuated varicella virus vaccine: efficacy trial in healthy children. *N. Engl. J. Med.*, **310**, 1409–1415.

Weibel, R., Kuter, B. J., Neff, B. *et al.* (1985). Live Oka/Merck varicella vaccine in healthy children: further clinical and laboratory assessment. *J. Am. Med. Assoc.* **245**, 2435–2439.

White, C. J. (1996). Clinical trials of varicella vaccine in healthy children. *Infect. Dis. Clin. N. Amer.*, **10**, 595–608.

White, C. J. (1997). Varicella-zoster virus vaccine. *Clin. Infect. Dis.*, **24**, 753–763.

Whitley, R., Hilty, M., Haynes, R. *et al.* (1982). Vidarabine therapy of varicella in immunosuppressed patients. *J. Pediatr.*, **101**(1), 125–131.

Whitley, R., Soong, S., Dolin, R. *et al.* (1982). Early vidarabine to control the complications of herpes zoster in immunosuppressed patients. *N. Engl. J. Med.*, **307**, 971–975.

Williams, V., Gershon, A., and Brunell, P. (1974). Serologic response to varicella-zoster membrane antigens measured by indirect immunofluorescence. *J. Infect. Dis.*, **130**, 669–672.

71

Human cytomegalovirus vaccines

Thomas C. Heineman

Division of Infectious Diseases and Immunology
Saint Louis University School of Medicine, Missouri, USA

Efforts to develop a human cytomegalovirus (HCMV) vaccine began more than 30 years ago in response to then recent reports that HCMV was capable of causing severe congenital disease. During the intervening years, our understanding of HCMV biology and immunology has increased dramatically. That knowledge, coupled with the introduction of several new vaccine methodologies, opened the door to an impressive expansion of HCMV vaccine research, particularly during the past decade. This chapter focuses on the principles underlying HCMV vaccine development and on the vaccine approaches that are currently under investigation.

Cytomegalovirus and human disease

The manifestations of HCMV infection vary with the age and immunocompetence of the host. In both adults and children, HCMV infection is usually asymptomatic. On rare occasions, otherwise healthy adults with primary HCMV infection will experience an infectious mononucleosis-like syndrome, with prolonged fever and mild hepatitis (Cohen and Corey, 1985). However, HCMV can cause serious morbidity and mortality when the host is unable to mount an adequate immune response or when infection is acquired in utero.

Congenital HCMV infection occurs in about 1% of children born in the USA, resulting in approximately 40 000 new infections each year (Pass and Burke, 2002; Plotkin, 1999). More than 90% of infected infants are asymptomatic at birth, and most will escape serious consequences of HCMV infection. However, even among initially asymptomatic children, 5%–15% will eventually develop sequelae of infection including hearing loss, mental retardation, chorioretinitis or cerebral palsy (Fowler et al., 1992; Revello and Gerna, 2002; Pass and Burke, 2002; Stagno et al., 1982, 1986). Children born with symptomatic HCMV disease have a substantially worse prognosis. Approximately 10% will die, and most of the survivors will display profound deficits as the result of central nervous system damage (Istas et al., 1995; Pass and Burke, 2002). All together, 4000 to 8000 children in the USA develop HCMV-related neurological disease each year, making HCMV the leading infectious cause of congenital mental retardation and deafness (Fowler et al., 1992; Plotkin, 1999).

Despite the availability of antiviral therapy, HCMV disease also remains a feared complication in persons undergoing immunosuppressive therapy for malignancies or organ transplantation, and in persons with AIDS. In these individuals, who have severely impaired cellular immunity, HCMV can affect almost any organ system, and it commonly causes pneumonia, retinitis, hepatitis and ulcerative lesions of the gastrointestinal tract (Pass, 2001). For example, HCMV causes symptomatic illness in 35%, and death in 2% of all renal transplant recipients (Adler, 1996). In hematopoietic stem cell transplant (HSCT) recipients, the most common disease manifestation of HCMV infection is interstitial pneumonia (Leather and Wingard, 2001). Historically, this disease typically occurs during the first 100 days following transplantation. However, late-onset HCMV pneumonia is becoming more common due to the use of HCMV antiviral prophylaxis or pre-emptive therapy during the first 3 months following HSCT (Boeckh et al., 1996; Leather and Wingard, 2001).

The case for a cytomegalovirus vaccine

Recognition of HCMV disease as a major public health problem has grown in the medical and scientific communities, if not among the general public. HCMV infection causes more CNS disease than did either *Hemophilus influenzae* b or congenital rubella prior to their near eradication in the USA through vaccination (Pass and Burke, 2002). Moreover, it has been observed that HCMV infection now causes as many cases of mental retardation as the common genetic syndromes, trisomy 21 and fragile X chromosome (Plotkin, 1999). The disease burden associated with cytomegalovirus infection is estimated to cost the US healthcare system at least 4 billion dollars annually, with the majority of the cost attributable to long-term sequelae experienced by individuals who acquire congenital HCMV disease. These data placed HCMV in the highest priority grouping of vaccine targets in a recent Institute of Medicine report (Stratton *et al.*, 2000).

One alternative to vaccination, prevention of HCMV infection through public health measures, is complicated by the high prevalence of HCMV, its persistence following primary infection, its many avenues of transmission (including blood, urine, saliva, semen, breast milk, donated organs) and its propensity to be shed for long periods of time following primary infection, especially by children (Pass, 2001). Of particular relevance, non-pregnant women evaluated in a randomized, controlled trial who were given explicit instructions on methods to avoid HCMV infection nonetheless acquired HCMV infection at rates equivalent to women who received no counseling (Adler *et al.*, 1996).

The successful prevention and treatment of HCMV disease in immunocompromised patients has greatly improved in recent years due to continuing refinements in prophylactic and preemptive therapy for high risk individuals as well as an expanding arsenal of antiviral agents. Despite this, as many as 50% of solid organ transplant recipients develop symptomatic HCMV disease resulting in significant morbidity (Fishman and Rubin, 1998; Patel and Paya, 1997; Sia and Patel, 2000; Simon and Levin, 2003), and even with optimal therapy, mortality from HCMV pneumonia in hematopoietic stem cell transplant recipients may exceed 40% (Leather and Wingard, 2001). Recent data also suggest that antiviral therapy offers some benefit to newborns with HCMV disease (Michaels *et al.*, 2003; Kimberlin *et al.*, 2003). However, treatment alone will undoubtedly benefit only a minority of infants with congenital HCMV disease. Indeed, most infants who ultimately develop sequelae of HCMV infection are asymptomatic at birth and, thus, would not be considered for treatment (Griffiths, 2002). Also, treatment requires long-term antiviral therapy, which carries a substantial risk of complications, and treatment after birth is unlikely to repair organ damage, especially to the central nervous system, that occurred in utero (Kimberlin *et al.*, 2003; Michaels *et al.*, 2003). For all these reasons, then, a vaccine that prevents infection with HCMV, or at least mitigates its effects in vulnerable persons, is essential for eradicating the often devastating disease caused by HCMV.

Natural immunity confers protection

When considering the feasibility and design of an HCMV vaccine, it is important to first establish that natural immunity prevents disease. This issue is complicated for HCMV because virus capable of causing disease may arrive through three distinct avenues: primary infection, reactivation of virus already residing within the host, or reinfection of a previously infected individual with a different strain of HCMV. Data directly addressing the protective efficacy of pre-existing immunity in healthy adults is sparse. However, compelling evidence that previous infection prevents reinfection comes from a study of mothers of children shedding HCMV (Adler *et al.*, 1995). During the course of this study, 9 of 19 (47%) seronegative women developed primary infection, whereas only 3 of 42 (7%) seropositive women showed evidence of new HCMV infection, indicating 85% protection attributable to prior immunity (Plotkin, 2002). In addition, healthy adults with pre-existing immunity to HCMV were significantly protected from HCMV disease compared to seronegative individuals when challenged with the non-attenuated Toledo strain of HCMV (Plotkin *et al.*, 1989; Quinnan *et al.*, 1984). In this case, seropositive persons were also protected from HCMV infection, albeit to a lesser degree.

Since the primary goal of HCMV vaccination is to prevent congenital HCMV disease, the protection offered by preconceptual maternal immunity should predict the potential value of vaccination in this setting. Preconceptual immunity could protect newborns by preventing transmission of the virus to the fetus or by mitigating the effects of infection. Data indicate that maternal immunity to HCMV prior to conception provides both of these elements of protection. Primary infection during pregnancy results in transmission of HCMV to the fetus 15%–40% of the time, whereas women with preexisting immunity transmit HCMV only about 1%–2% of the time (Stagno *et al.*, 1982; Plotkin, 2002). In accordance with these data, a recent study showed that women who have naturally acquired immunity to HCMV prior to conception are 69% less likely to give birth to an infant with congenital HCMV infection than women who are initially seronegative (Fowler *et al.*, 2003). Moreover, congenital HCMV infections in infants born to women with HCMV immunity at the time of conception are considerably less likely to cause symptomatic disease at birth (Fowler *et al.*, 1992; Stagno *et al.*,

1982, 1997). In general, these children also have both fewer and less severe sequelae of HCMV infection, even when considering that adverse outcomes, such as hearing loss and mental retardation, may become apparent only months or years later (Fowler *et al.*, 1992). Maternal immunity prior to conception, however, does not confer complete protection against HCMV transmission to the fetus. Of note, a recent report concluded that while the severity of hearing loss in HCMV congenitally infected children was less if their mothers had preexisting immunity, the incidence of hearing loss was unaffected by maternal serostatus (Ross *et al.*, 2006). Indeed, in populations with high rates of HCMV seropositivity the majority of HCMV infections may occur in infants born to seropositive mothers even given the relatively low risk of transmission (Demmler, 1991; Pass and Burke, 2002; Stagno *et al.*, 1977; Schopfer *et al.*, 1978; Plotkin, 2002; Boppana *et al.*, 2001). Many of these infections presumably occur through the transmission of reactivated maternal virus, although a significant proportion undoubtedly arise from reinfection of the mother with a different strain of HCMV followed by transmission of the new virus to the fetus (Marshall and Plotkin, 1993; Boeckh *et al.*, 1996; Stagno *et al.*, 1982; Boppana *et al.*, 2001). In addition, symptomatic HCMV disease has been well documented in children born to mothers with preconceptual immunity to HCMV (Boppana *et al.*, 1999, 2001; Schopfer *et al.*, 1978; Ahlfors *et al.*, 1999; Morris *et al.*, 1994).

In conclusion, prior immunity to HCMV provides substantial protection against HCMV infection and disease, with the degree of protection estimated to be between 70% and 90% (Adler *et al.*, 1995; Fowler *et al.*, 2003; Plotkin, 2002). This conclusion engenders optimism that vaccination of seronegative girls prior to pregnancy may prevent a substantial proportion of cases of congenital HCMV disease and the attendant early and late sequelae. Moreover, vaccination may ultimately reduce asymptomatic infection and shedding by young children, which would lessen the reservoir of virus available to infect the fetuses of other mothers (Adler, 1988; Pass *et al.*, 1986). Indeed, it has been calculated that a vaccine that is only 60% effective against primary infection would be sufficient to eradicate HCMV from a given community within a developed country (Griffiths *et al.*, 2001).

Immunology of HCMV protection

Both neutralizing antibodies and cell-mediated immunity contribute to protection against HCMV disease (Table 71.1; for review see Gonczol and Plotkin, 2001; Plotkin, 2002; Pass and Burke, 2002). The importance of antibodies in preventing HCMV disease was first suggested by the observation that serious HCMV disease in newborn blood transfusion recipients was less frequent in infants born to seropositive mothers (Yeager *et al.*, 1981). This protection was presumably due to antibodies that had been transferred from the mother to the infant prior to birth. The protective benefit of HCMV antibodies in neonates was reinforced by subsequent data showing that passively administered antibodies, in the form of HCMV immune globulin, protected premature infants from HCMV disease (Snydman *et al.*, 1995). In addition, a nonrandomized study suggested that administration of HCMV-specific hyperimmune globulin to pregnant women may be effective in the treatment and prevention of congenital HCMV infection (Nigro *et al.*, 2005). HCMV immune globulin also appears to offer renal, liver, heart and bone marrow transplant recipients some protection from the most severe effects of HCMV disease (Snydman, 1993; Falagas *et al.*, 1997; Valantine, 1995; Bowden *et al.*, 1986; Glowacki and Smaill, 1994; Messori *et al.*, 1994). Protective levels of antibodies have not been established, but some evidence suggests that higher levels of neutralizing antibodies correlate with a lower risk for reinfection (Adler *et al.*, 1995). Regardless of the clinical setting, however, antibodies alone offer only partial protection and appear to be more effective in mitigating serious HCMV disease than in preventing infection.

Analysis of the HCMV genomic sequence suggests that is capable of encoding in excess of 60 glycoproteins, although how many are actually expressed is unknown (Chee *et al.*,

Table 71.1. Known targets of human immune responses to HCMV

HCMV gene product	Immune response
Glycoproteins	
gB	Major target of neutralizing antibodies; target of CTLs[a]
gH	Important target of neutralizing antibodies; target of CTLs
gM-gN	Target of antibody responses
US2, US3, US6, UL18	Targets of CTLs
Non-structural proteins	
pp65	Major target of CTLs; target of antibody responses
IE1	Important target of CTLs; target of antibody responses
pp150, pp28	Target of CTLs and antibody responses
pp50	Target of CTLs
pp71, pp52	Targets of antibody responses

[a] Cytotoxic T-lymphocytes.

1990; Cha et al., 1996; Davison et al., 2003). Most HCMV neutralizing antibodies, however, appear to recognize a tiny subset of these proteins, namely, glycoprotein B (gB), glycoprotein H (gH) and the glycoprotein M-N (gM-gN) complex (Britt et al., 1990; Kari and Gehrz, 1990; Mach et al., 2000; Marshall et al., 1992, 1994; Rasmussen et al., 1991; Urban et al., 1996).

Glycoprotein B is the most abundant membrane protein in the HCMV envelope (Britt and Mach, 1996). It is highly conserved among all mammalian herpesviruses, and participates in several facets of the virus life cycle including entry and cell–cell spread (Bolds et al., 1996; Compton et al., 1993; Navarro et al., 1993). Recently, it was shown that HCMV entry into cells is mediated by gB binding to the cellular epidermal growth factor receptor (Wang et al., 2003). HCMV gB, like the gB homologues in other herpesviruses, is a large type I membrane protein (for review see Britt and Mach, 1996; Spaete, 1994). It is cleaved by a host cell protease into two peptides, which remain disulfide-linked. Glycoprotein B is modified by N- and O-glycosylation and forms homodimers in both virions and infected cells (Mocarski and Courcelle, 2001). Glycoprotein B appears to be the most immunogenic HCMV protein. Almost all persons develop antibodies to gB following HCMV infection, and gB-specific antibodies account for 40%–70% of the total HCMV neutralizing activity in HCMV seropositive individuals (Britt et al., 1990; Cremer et al., 1985; Kniess et al., 1991; Marshall et al., 1992). Glycoprotein B contains two well-characterized major antigenic domains, AD-1 and AD-2, that are capable of inducing neutralizing antibodies during infection (Britt et al., 1988; Kniess et al., 1991; Marshall et al., 2000; Meyer et al., 1992; Wagner et al., 1992). The antibody response after natural infection is directed most frequently to AD-1, which is highly conserved in clinical isolates (Schoppel et al., 1996; Wada et al., 1997; Chou and Dennison, 1991). However, 11% of HCMV seropositive persons lacked antibodies to linear epitopes on either AD-1 or AD-2, but had neutralizing activity suggesting that for some individuals, different epitopes in gB or epitopes in other HCMV proteins may be more important in the generation of virus neutralizing responses (Marshall et al., 2000).

Glycoprotein H is a relatively abundant component of the virion envelope and is also conserved among the mammalian herpesviruses, although it is much more divergent than gB (Mocarski and Courcelle, 2001). HCMV gH has been shown to participate in membrane fusion, and it may play role in virus entry at a step following attachment (Britt and Mach, 1996; Mocarski and Courcelle, 2001; Keay and Baldwin, 1991; Rasmussen et al., 1984). Glycoprotein H is also an important target of host immune responses, and almost all persons infected with HCMV develop gH-specific antibodies (Urban et al., 1996). In some cases, gH may be the dominant target of neutralizing antibodies as it has been shown to account for 0–58% of the total virus neutralizing activity in persons with a past history of HCMV infection (Urban et al., 1996). Like gB, antigenic domains have been identified in gH (Simpson et al., 1993). Interestingly, HIV-infected persons with CD4 counts less than 100 cells/mm^3 who had histories of past HCMV infections rarely had detectable gH antibody titers compared to persons with higher CD4 counts, while gB titers were unaffected by the CD4 count (Rasmussen et al., 1994). Given that HIV-infected persons with CD4 counts less than 100 cells/mm^3 are at high risk for retinitis due to reactivated HCMV, this finding raises the possibility that gH antibodies may be necessary for containing reactivated virus in some settings.

Recently, the gM-gN complex was recognized as an important target of antibody responses in seropositive adults (Kari and Gehrz, 1990; Mach et al., 2000). Sera from HCMV-infected adults failed to recognize gM or gN when they were expressed alone; however, sera from 62% of previously infected individuals reacted with the gM–gN complex. The importance of gM–gN antibodies in preventing HCMV disease is unknown. A possible link between gM–gN antibodies and human disease, however, was suggested by the observation that the 14 of 16 congenitally infected infants lacked detectable antibodies against this complex, whereas most adults in the same study had gM–gN antibodies (Mach et al., 2000).

In addition to gB, gH and gM–gN, antibodies to several non-envelope HCMV proteins, including pp65, IE1, pp150, pp28, pp71 and pp52, are commonly detected in seropositive people (Pass and Burke, 2002). It remains to be determined whether these antibodies contribute to protection against HCMV infection and disease.

The pivotal role for cell-mediated immunity in the control of HCMV infection is underscored by the fact that virtually all cases of severe HCMV disease not associated with congenital infection occur in persons with profoundly impaired cellular immunity, and the severity of HCMV disease typically correlates with the degree of immunosuppression. Specifically, HLA-restricted CD8$^+$ cytotoxic T lymphocyte (CTL) responses are crucial for the control of HCMV disease in immunocompromised persons (Quinnan et al., 1982; Li et al., 1994; Reusser et al., 1991). Allogeneic marrow transplant recipients are at high risk for HCMV disease until their CD8$^+$ CTLs return. The fundamental importance of CTL responses in controlling HCMV disease was directly assessed by an adoptive transfer study in which marrow transplant recipients received serial transfusions of HCMV-specific CTLs (Walter et al., 1995). None of the 14 very high-risk patients in this study developed HCMV

Table 71.2. Status of HCMV vaccines currently being tested

Vaccine	Stage of testing			
	Preclinical	Human trials		
		Safety	Immunogenicity	Efficacy
Towne vaccine	+	+	+	+
gB subunit vaccines	+	+	+	+[a]
ALVAC-based vaccines	+	+	+	−
Towne/Toledo chimeric vaccines	+	+	−	−
DNA vaccines	+	−	−	−
Peptide vaccines	+	−	−	−
Dense body vaccines	+	−	−	−

[a] This study is ongoing, and no efficacy data are yet available.

viremia or disease. Therefore, considerable effort has been devoted in recent years to identifying the HCMV targets of CTL responses since the induction of such responses may be imperative for the success of an HCMV vaccine. This work led to the discovery that the tegument protein pp65 is the dominant target of virus-specific CTLs. In persons with past HCMV infection, approximately 70–90% of all CTLs that recognize HCMV-infected cells are specific for this protein (Boppana and Britt, 1996; Kern *et al.*, 2002; McLaughlin-Taylor *et al.*, 1994; Wills *et al.*, 1996). Recently, specific peptides derived from the pp65 sequence have been identified that are able to induce HCMV-specific CTL in an HLA-A24-restricted manner (Akiyama *et al.*, 2002; Masuoka *et al.*, 2001).

While it is striking that a single protein induces so much of the CTL response directed against such a complex virus, other HCMV proteins have also been shown to contain CTL epitopes. Most notable among these are the HCMV immediate-early protein, IE1, and the tegument protein, pp150, which in some individuals appears to induce CTL responses with similar precursor frequencies to pp65 (Kern *et al.*, 2000; Gyulai *et al.*, 2000; La Rosa *et al.*, 2005). Like pp65, IE1- and pp150 derived peptides that induce CTL in an HLA-restricted manner have been identified (Frankenberg *et al.*, 2002; La Rosa *et al.*, 2005). In addition, other HCMV antigens that are capable of inducing CTL responses including gB, gH, pp150, pp28, pp50, US2, US3, US6, and US18 (Boppana and Britt, 1996; Gyulai *et al.*, 2000; Elkington *et al.*, 2003).

The effectiveness of an HCMV vaccine is likely to be enhanced by, and may absolutely require, the induction of HCMV-specific CTL responses. Such responses would be expected following inoculation with live attenuated vaccines. However, other vaccine approaches, such as vectored vaccines and DNA vaccines, as discussed below, may require the inclusion of specific CTL epitopes to achieve similar results. Moreover, multiple CTL epitopes may need to be included to ensure maximal coverage in the community at large.

Vaccine development

HCMV has been the target of active vaccine development efforts since the 1970s. Early work focused on the development of live-attenuated vaccines, which have now been tested in numerous human trials and, as a family, continue to show considerable promise. With advances in molecular techniques, and rapidly expanding knowledge of HCMV biology and immunology, several other approaches are currently being applied to the development of safe and effective HCMV vaccines (Table 71.2).

Replicating vaccines

The first HCMV vaccine tested in humans was AD169, a laboratory-adapted strain of HCMV made by passaging virus isolated from human adenoidal tissue a total of 54 times in four different cultured human fibroblast cell lines (Elek and Stern, 1974). A lysate containing infectious virus derived from sonicated AD169-infected cells was administered to HCMV seronegative adults. Twenty-five of 26 volunteers (96%) who received 10 000 plaque forming units (pfu) of virus subcutaneously seroconverted. The vaccine was safe and well tolerated with 12 of 26 recipients exhibiting minor local reactions and one person developing lymphadenopathy and lymphocytosis. None of the vaccinees excreted virus based on cultures of throat washings and urine. Two vaccinees tested a year later showed no reduction in antibody titers. However, evaluation of some of these subjects 8 years later revealed that only half had detectable HCMV antibody or lymphocyte transformation responses (Stern, 1984).

A second clinical trial of AD169 was conducted a few years after the first (Neff et al., 1979). The virus used in this trial was passaged an additional five times and prepared as a filtered sonicate of infected cells. Twenty-four adult men were vaccinated subcutaneously, and all 20 of the initially seronegative individuals developed antibodies to HCMV by one month following vaccination. One year later, immune adherence antibodies had declined slightly while complement-fixing antibodies had declined significantly. Participants with pre-existing immunity to HCMV exhibited no antibody response to vaccination. The vaccine virus could not be detected in leukocytes, urine or throat specimens from the vaccinated seronegative persons and was not transmitted to any of the 10 seronegative contacts of the vaccine recipients, which was taken as evidence for lack of contagiousness of the vaccine virus. AD169 was not pursued further as a vaccine candidate. Instead, attention turned to the HCMV Towne strain as a potential live attenuated vaccine, and Towne remains today the best-studied HCMV vaccine candidate.

The Towne strain of HCMV was isolated in 1970 from the urine of a 2-month old infant with congenital disease, then passaged 125 times exclusively in WI-38 human diploid fibroblasts, including three clonings (Plotkin et al., 1975). It was characterized in 1975 prior to its use in clinical trials and was shown to possess several characteristics that distinguished it from native HCMV indicating that it had been altered by cell culture passage. These included increased production of cell-free virus, thermostability and trypsin resistance. In addition, safety tests in various animals and cell lines showed the virus stocks to be free of adventitious agents.

In the first published human trial describing Towne vaccination, all 10 seronegative adults inoculated intramuscularly seroconverted within four weeks while 11 seronegative adults inoculated both intranasally and orally failed to seroconvert (Just et al., 1975). Five persons with pre-existing immunity to HCMV were vaccinated with Towne and showed no increase in antibody titers. None of the participants had systemic symptoms or atypical lymphocytosis; however, 7 of the original 10 seronegative vaccinees developed mild local reactions beginning 14–16 days following vaccination and lasting about a week. As with the AD169, Towne could not be isolated from the leukocytes or urine of any vaccinee, suggesting that Towne is attenuated and unable to persist in vaccinated persons.

A second early trial with Towne largely reinforced the findings from the first trial (Plotkin et al., 1976). Once again, persons inoculated intranasally failed to seroconvert whereas all seronegative volunteers who were vaccinated subcutaneously acquired HCMV-specific antibodies, and no excretion of vaccine virus from these individuals could be documented. In contrast to the earlier study, however, all 4 seronegative participants in this trial acquired complement-fixing antibodies compared to 1 of 10 in the first trial. Also, both initially seropositive vaccinees developed IgM antibodies, raising the possibility that Towne may reinfect persons who had previously been infected with native HCMV.

Subsequent human trials with Towne confirmed its ability to elicit both binding and neutralizing antibodies, and demonstrated that Towne-induced antibodies have similar specificities to the antibodies arising from natural HCMV infection (Gonczol et al., 1989). Early studies showed that both binding and neutralizing antibody titers in response to Towne vaccination were substantially lower than those following natural infection (Gonczol et al., 1989; Adler et al., 1995). However, a more recent study showed that a new lot of Towne vaccine induced titers of neutralizing antibodies comparable to those induced by natural infection and that the response was dose dependent (Adler et al., 1998). In this study, as in earlier trials, the level of Towne-induced antibodies waned over the course of a year, while those in naturally seropositive women remained stable.

The ability of Towne to induce cellular immune responses is well documented. Towne vaccination of healthy seronegative adults uniformly results in HCMV-specific lymphocyte responses, a surrogate for CD4+ cell activation, which persist for at least 10 months (Gehrz et al., 1980; Starr et al., 1981; Fleisher et al., 1982; Plotkin et al., 1989; Adler et al., 1995, 1998). In addition, Towne consistently elicits HCMV-specific CD8+ CTL responses in immunocompetent individuals (Quinnan et al., 1984; Adler et al., 1998).

Towne has also been tested in a series of studies in prospective kidney transplant recipients, a population that is at high risk for HCMV disease following transplantation (Glazer et al., 1979; Marker et al., 1981; Starr et al., 1981; Plotkin et al., 1984, 1991, 1994; Brayman et al., 1988; Balfour, 1991). Most renal transplant candidates developed humoral and cellular immune responses following Towne vaccination. The responses, however, tended to be delayed or diminished when compared to those of healthy vaccinees (Starr et al., 1981; Plotkin et al., 1984, 1991). Three controlled trials have been conducted in which renal transplant candidates received either Towne vaccine or a placebo (Balfour, 1991; Plotkin et al., 1991, 1994). Each of

Table 71.3. Protective efficacy of Towne vaccination in seronegative renal transplant recipients who received kidneys from seropositive donors

Trial	n (vaccine/ placebo)	All HCMV disease		Severe HCMV disease		% reduction of all disease	% reduction of severe disease
		Vaccine	Placebo	Vaccine	Placebo		
Plotkin et al., 1991	67 (36/31)	14 (39%)	17 (55%)	2 (6%)	11 (35%)	46%	83%
Balfour 1991	35 (21/14)	8 (38%)	6 (43%)	2 (10%)	5 (36%)	12%	72%
Plotkin et al., 1994	61 (37/24)	14 (38%)	14 (59%)	0 (0%)	4 (17%)	36%	100%
All	163 (94/69)	36 (38%)	37 (54%)	4 (4%)	20 (29%)	30%	86%

these trials yielded similar results (Table 71.3). Vaccination with Towne failed to prevent HCMV infection following transplantation, and while the incidence of total HCMV disease was decreased, this effect did not achieve statistical significance. However, in the highest risk population, namely HCMV seronegative persons who received a kidney from a seropositive donor, the incidence of severe HCMV disease was reduced by 72%–100%, a degree of protection comparable to that stimulated by natural infection (Plotkin et al., 1991).

The efficacy of Towne vaccination was also assessed in a controlled challenge study. In that study, seronegative adults were vaccinated with Towne and challenged with the non-attenuated, low-passage Toledo strain of HCMV (Plotkin et al., 1989). The ability of Toledo to cause disease was confirmed when all 6 seronegative, unvaccinated persons challenged subcutaneously with 10 or 100 pfu of Toledo developed clinical symptoms of HCMV disease as well as evidence of infection based positive viral cultures from their blood, urine and/or saliva. Twelve adults who had been vaccinated with Towne 1 year earlier were challenged with Toledo. All 5 who were challenged with 10 pfu of Toledo were protected from infection and disease. However, of the 7 Towne-vaccinated persons who were challenged with 100 pfu of Toledo, most (4/7) showed evidence of infection based on virus culture, one had clinical illness and 3 had laboratory abnormalities suggestive of HCMV infection. In contrast, naturally seropositive persons were protected from challenge with 100 pfu of Toledo; however, 5/5 seropositive individuals challenged with 1000 pfu of Toledo exhibited clinical disease, laboratory abnormalities and/or positive HCMV cultures. Therefore, in this small study, Towne appeared to afford some protection against HCMV infection and disease, but less than natural infection. This study and an earlier challenge study in seropositive, unvaccinated individuals (Quinnan et al., 1984) provided valuable information not only on the protective efficacy of Towne relative to natural infection, but also on the dose dependence and natural history of HCMV disease in immunocompetent adults. However, challenge studies with HCMV may no longer be possible given contemporary regulatory standards designed to ensure volunteer safety.

To assess the protective efficacy of Towne in a more natural setting, a placebo-controlled study was performed in seronegative women with children in daycare. This was, in effect, a challenge study as the parents of children in daycare are at high risk for HCMV infection (Pass et al., 1986). In this population, Towne vaccination failed to protect women from HCMV infection, while natural infection was highly protective against re-infection with HCMV (Adler et al., 1995).

Towne remains the only HCMV vaccine candidate that has completed efficacy testing in any human population. In the final estimation, Towne vaccination induces both humoral and cellular immunity, and it is capable of providing some protection against HCMV disease in certain settings. However, it is clearly less protective than natural infection, particularly in its ability to prevent infection with native HCMV, which may be critical for preventing congenital disease. In an effort to enhance the immunogenicity of Towne, the co-administration of recombinant human IL-12 with Towne was evaluated in a recent clinical trial (Jacobson et al., 2006). This combination proved to be well tolerated and resulted in enhanced HCMV-specific antibody and T cell responses.

The nature of the deficit in Towne's ability to stimulate protective immunity is unknown, but it has been suggested that the lower neutralizing antibody titers induced by Towne compared to natural infection may be at fault (Wang et al., 1996). Regardless, the experience with Towne suggested that it is overly attenuated and prompted researchers to pursue less attenuated live vaccines that will, ideally, retain the excellent safety and tolerability profiles of Towne.

The high level of attenuation exhibited by Towne is presumably due to genetic mutations introduced during its extensive passage in cultured cells (Huang et al., 1980; Prichard et al., 2001). Furthermore, recent data indicate

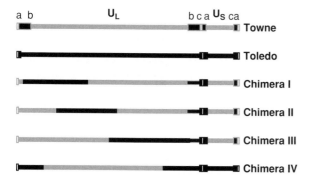

Fig. 71.1. Genomic structures of the two parental strains and four chimeras. The specific regions of each chimera's genome derived from Towne(▬) and Toledo(▬) are shown. The UL/b' region(▬) of Toledo is marked(courtesy of George Kemble)

that HCMV Towne contains numerous mutations throughout in its genome when compared to the non-attenuated Toledo strain of HCMV (G. Kemble, personal communication, 2003); however, the specific mutations causing attenuation are not known. In an effort to produce a vaccine that is intermediate in attenuation between HCMV Towne and wild-type virus, genetic recombinants were constructed in which regions from the HCMV Toledo genome were substituted for the corresponding regions of the Towne genome using cosmid-based mutagenesis (Kemble et al., 1996). Four independent chimeric viruses (referred to as Chimeras I–IV) were produced in which every region of the Towne genome was replaced sequentially by Toledo sequences (Fig. 71.1). Each of the four chimeric vaccine candidates made using this approach contains the UL/b region of the HCMV genome. This region, which is predicted to encode 19 proteins, is universally found in the genomes of circulating HCMV isolates but is not present in it entirety in many HCMV strains that have undergone extensive passage in cell culture, such as AD169 (Cha et al., 1996). It was hypothesized that by using this approach, one or more of the Towne/Toledo recombinants would contain some, but not all, of the mutations that confer attenuation on Towne. This, in turn, should result in a chimeric virus that is attenuated relative to Toledo, but less attenuated than Towne.

The four Towne/Toledo recombinant viruses were evaluated in a recently completed double-blinded, placebo controlled clinical trial (Heineman et al., 2003). The study was designed to determine whether the vaccine candidates are safe and well tolerated, whether they are attenuated relative to Toledo and whether they are shed in the blood, urine or saliva of vaccinees. Healthy HCMV seropositive adults each received a single dose of 1000 pfu of one of the four investigational vaccines or an inactive placebo. Participants were evaluated weekly for 8 weeks, then less frequently for the remainder of a year, for clinical or laboratory evidence of HCMV infection and disease. All four vaccine candidates were safe and well-tolerated although as a group they produced more local reactogenicity than the placebo. As predicted, each of the Towne/Toledo chimeric vaccine candidates was attenuated relative to Toledo based on comparison to the previous Toledo challenge data discussed above (Quinnan et al., 1984; Plotkin et al., 1989). This attenuation was evident from the paucity of laboratory abnormalities suggestive of HCMV infection in the recipients of the chimeric vaccine candidates in contrast to those noted in HCMV seropositive persons who had received the same dose of Toledo (Table 71.4). However, the degree of attenuation of the four Towne/Toledo chimeras relative to each other could not be discerned from this initial trial. Like Towne, none of the vaccine candidates was cultured from the blood, urine or saliva of any vaccinee or any of their close contacts suggesting that systemic infection did not occur in this population. Immunogenicity data from this trial are pending. Future studies are planned to address the safety and immunogenicity of these vaccine candidates in seronegative persons, who comprise the target population for vaccination.

Table 71.4. Towne/Toledo chimeric vaccine candidates are attenuated relative to Toledo in natural seropositives inoculated with 1000 pfu

Vaccine	Laboratory abnormalities[a]	Virus isolated
Chimera I	0/5	0/5
Chimera II	1/5[c]	0/5
Chimera III	0/5	0/5
Chimera IV	1/5[d]	0/5
Chimeras I-IV	**2/20**	**0/20**
Placebo	1/5[c]	0/5
HCMV Toledo[b]	**5/5**	**2/5**

[a] Defined as elevated aspartate aminotransferase (AST) or atypical lymphocytosis.
[b] From Plotkin, et al., 1989.
[c] Elevated AST. In the case of Chimera II, the volunteer had an elevated AST prior to vaccination.
[d] Atypical lymphocytosis of 9% at week 8 after vaccination only.

Subunit vaccines

Subunit vaccines, in which a single or a few specific proteins are used in combination with an adjuvant to stimulate protective immunity, are attractive for several reasons. Most importantly, they are not infectious and contain no genetic material thus eliminating some safety concerns. Also, using modern molecular genetic methods, large amounts of the vaccine antigens can be produced easily and cheaply. Finally, subunit vaccines for numerous infectious diseases have been studied extensively in animals and, in some cases, have progressed to human trials. Of particular relevance, recent data suggest that a subunit vaccine derived from a single herpes simplex virus (HSV) type 2 protein may protect seronegative women from disease caused by primary HSV infection (Stanberry et al., 2002).

As discussed above, HCMV gB is both highly immunogenic and highly conserved between HCMV isolates. For these reasons, and because it is the best studied HCMV glycoprotein, gB has been the primary antigen used in most HCMV subunit vaccine studies. Glycoprotein B used in vaccine studies has been modified to facilitate its purification. To that end, its hydrophobic transmembrane domain has been removed, and it has been mutated to eliminate its internal proteolytic cleavage site. Thus, the form of gB used in human trials is expressed in Chinese hamster ovary cells and is purified as an excreted protein consisting of a single 807 amino acid peptide (Pass et al., 1999).

The choice of vaccine adjuvants has considerable impact on the immunogenicity of subunit vaccines. In the human trials reported to date, HCMV gB has been combined with either aluminum hydroxide (alum), the adjuvant used in the licensed hepatitis B vaccines, or MF59, a proprietary oil-in-water emulsion of squalene (Chiron Vaccines, Emeryville California) (Ott et al., 1995). MF59 was previously shown to induce higher antibody titers than alum when combined with a variety of viral antigens (McElrath, 1995). Accordingly, virtually all healthy seronegative adults inoculated at 0, 1 and 6 months with HCMV gB combined with MF59 developed levels of binding and neutralizing antibodies comparable to those induced by natural infection, whereas persons vaccinated similarly with gB/alum produced significantly lower titers of gB-specific antibodies (Pass et al., 1999). Also, IgG and IgA antibodies to gB were present in the saliva or nasal washes of most gB/MF59 recipients (Wang et al., 1996). Dose comparison studies demonstrated that low doses of gB (5 μg) combined with MF59 elicited antibody responses similar to those observed with higher doses (30 or 100 μg) (Pass et al., 1999; Frey et al., 1999). Toddlers who received three 20 μg doses of gB/MF59 developed mean gB binding and neutralizing antibody titers six-fold higher than were observed in earlier adult studies (Mitchell et al., 2002). Following vaccination with gB/MF59, neutralizing antibody titers waned rapidly, and it was suggested that insufficient CD4$^+$ responses might have contributed to this decline. Nonetheless, neutralizing antibody titers rebounded dramatically after an additional dose of vaccine (Plotkin, 2001; Pass and Burke, 2002). Vaccination with gB/MF59 also induced strong lymphocyte proliferative responses to both gB and HCMV, and these declined little during the year following vaccination (Pass and Burke, 2002). The HCMV subunit vaccines caused more injection site pain than placebo; however, both were generally well tolerated.

The studies described above laid the groundwork for efficacy trials of the gB/MF59 subunit vaccine. Currently, the ability of gB/MF59 to prevent congenital HCMV infection in the children of healthy seronegative women is being assessed in a double-blinded, placebo controlled trial (R. Pass, personal communication, 2006). In addition, a study is being planned to determine whether gB/MF59 vaccination protects adolescents from HCMV infection, a population that may ultimately be targeted for vaccination (D. Bernstein, personal communication, 2003). While HCMV subunit vaccines have thus far focused on the use of gB as the immunogen, future subunit vaccines may include gH, gM-gN, and perhaps other HCMV antigens.

Vectored vaccines

A number of viruses have been utilized as vectors to express potential vaccine antigens. Of these, the attenuated ALVAC strain of canarypox has been most extensively employed as a vector for the delivery of HCMV antigens (Baxby and Paoletti, 1992; Tartaglia et al., 1992; Plotkin et al., 1995). The ALVAC genome will accommodate the insertion of large exogenous DNA fragments providing great flexibility in the choice of antigen genes or combinations of genes. While it can infect human cells and express foreign antigens, its own genome is not replicated and progeny virions are not produced, thus reducing the risk of vaccine-associated complications. Most importantly from the perspective of vaccine efficacy, foreign antigens expressed by ALVAC are transported and processed authentically within cells allowing their presentation in the context of MHC class I molecules. This, in turn, may facilitate the stimulation of CTL responses that mimic those of natural infection (Pialoux et al., 1995; Clements-Mann et al., 1998; Taylor et al., 1995; Plotkin et al., 1995).

Because of its preeminence as target for neutralizing immunity, gB was the first HCMV antigen chosen for expression by ALVAC. Studies in mice and guinea pigs showed that two doses of ALVAC-gB induced neutralizing antibodies and also high levels of HCMV-specific CD8$^+$ CTL responses (Gonczol et al., 1995). UV-inactivated ALVAC-gB failed to induce CTLs indicating that de novo synthesis of gB was required. In addition, prior vaccinia virus exposure did not inhibit the gB-specific immunity induced by ALVAC-gB in mice, addressing an issue that may become more important if vaccinia vaccination rates increase in response to bioterrorism concerns. The promise of the initial animal studies, however, was not fully realized in early human trials. Even after three doses of ALVAC-gB, seronegative adults failed to develop significant HCMV neutralizing antibody titers perhaps reflecting low levels of antigen production (Adler et al., 1999).

ALVAC-gB proved far more successful when it was used to "prime" the immune system in so-called prime-boost vaccination strategies. HCMV seronegative adults who were primed with two doses of ALVAC-gB at days 0 and 30, then boosted with a single dose of Towne at day 90 developed binding and neutralizing antibody titers at least as high as naturally seropositive individuals (Adler et al., 1999). Similarly, individuals primed with two doses of ALVAC-gB, then boosted with gB/MF59 subunit vaccine developed high antibody titers and lymphoproliferative anti-HCMV responses. These humoral and cellular responses, however, were not significantly different from those elicited by three doses of gB/MF59 alone, thus demonstrating no clear benefit to priming with ALVAC-gB (Bernstein et al., 2002).

The greatest value of canarypox-based vaccines may derive from their ability to stimulate specific CTL responses. ALVAC expressing pp65, an abundant tegument protein that is a major CTL target in naturally HCMV seropositive persons, induced CD8$^+$ CTL responses in all seronegative persons tested (Berencsi et al., 2001). The CTL responses were detected after two doses of ALVAC-pp65 and were present at frequencies comparable to those seen in naturally seropositive individuals. Ultimately, canarypox-based vaccines that express both CTL and neutralizing antibody targets, such as pp65 and gB, may be used in prime-boost vaccination protocols. For example, two doses of an ALVAC-based vaccine may be followed by a boost with a subunit or live-attenuated vaccine, to confer high levels of both cellular and humoral immunity.

Peptide vaccines

The development of peptide vaccines for HCMV represents an effort to directly stimulate a protective CTL response. Toward this end, a 9 amino acid minimal cytotoxic epitope derived from HCMV pp65 was identified and lipidated at its amino terminus to allow its administration without an adjuvant (Diamond et al., 1997; Martinon et al., 1992). HLA A2.1 transgenic mice immunized with this peptide, in combination with the PADRE pan-HLA-DR T-helper epitope, developed HCMV-specific CTL. Subsequent studies showed that linking the HCMV pp65 epitope directly to the PADRE epitope in the same peptide elicited vigorous HCMV-specific CTL responses in HLA transgenic mice when delivered either subcutaneously or intranasally (La Rosa et al., 2002). In either case, the response was significantly enhanced by the co-administration of CpG-containing single stranded DNA, which enhances the immune response and biases it in the direction of Th1 activity (Klinman, 2003). A repertoire of HCMV epitopes specific for different HLA alleles has been defined that should provide 90% coverage to the Caucasian population, although the derivation of four or more additional CTL epitopes would be needed to attain 90% coverage for African Americans or Asians (Longmate et al., 2001). Peptide vaccination may have its primary utility in therapeutic rather than prophylactic vaccination as HLA allele-specific peptides may be limited in their ability to elicit immunity in the population at large (Gonczol and Plotkin, 2001). To that end, the HCMV-pp65-specific memory CTL response could be amplified in a hematopoietic stem cell donor prior to transplantation by administration of a peptide vaccine, thereby providing protection against HCMV disease in the recipient (La Rosa et al., 2002).

DNA vaccines

The initially surprising discovery that direct injection of purified DNA encoding specific antigens can induce protective immunity led to the development of DNA vaccination strategies for many pathogens including HCMV (Wolff et al., 1990; Ulmer et al., 1993). In this approach, as with live attenuated and vectored vaccines, HCMV antigens are synthesized and processed using authentic cellular pathways thus allowing their expression in the context of MHC class I molecules (Tang et al., 1992; Ulmer et al., 1993; Raz et al., 1994). This approach, therefore, has the potential to induce both humoral and cellular immunity to HCMV. While DNA vaccines for HCMV have yet to be studied in humans, compelling data, some of which is discussed below, has been generated in animal models.

The first DNA vaccine for HCMV consisted of a plasmid containing the gene for pp65 (Pande et al., 1995). Most of the mice injected intramuscularly with this plasmid developed antibodies to pp65 confirming that vaccination with HCMV DNA was capable of eliciting an antigen-specific immune response. The protective efficacy of DNA vaccination was subsequently demonstrated in mice (Gonzales Armas et al., 1996). After inoculation with the murine CMV

(MCMV) pp89 gene, the major target for CD8+ T-cells (Reddehase and Koszinowski 1984; Holtappels et al., 1998), mice exhibited 45% protection against lethal challenge as well as significantly lower viral titers in the spleen and salivary glands. A DNA vaccine expressing a different MCMV antigen, M84, which is homologous to HCMV pp65, also afforded some protection to mice. Coimmunization with both pp89 and M84 DNA vaccines provided the best protection suggesting that the most successful DNA vaccines may express multiple antigens (Morello et al., 2000; Ye et al., 2002).

Considerable evidence suggests that both humoral and cell-mediated immunity participate in the control of HCMV disease. Accordingly, DNA vaccines expressing gB were tested in mice and shown to elicit neutralizing antibodies (Hwang et al., 1999). Therefore, a second generation of HCMV DNA vaccines was designed to stimulate both neutralizing antibodies to HCMV and HCMV-specific CTL responses. These vaccines consisted of a cocktail of plasmids encoding pp65, to stimulate CTL responses, and gB, to induce neutralizing antibodies (Endresz et al., 1999; Schleiss et al., 2000). After three immunizations, all mice developed gB- and pp65-specific antibodies, and about 60% developed pp65-specific CTL responses. Similarly, guinea pigs also developed antibodies to both antigens.

Recently, various innovative methods to enhance immune responses have been applied to HCMV DNA vaccines. Aluminum salts, which are licensed for use as adjuvants in humans, and CpG oligodeoxynucleotides have both been shown to enhance antibody responses to DNA vaccines (Ulmer et al., 1999; Klinman et al., 2000). A DNA vaccine containing the HCMV gB gene and administered with aluminum phosphate gel elicited significantly higher antibody responses in mice than the gB gene without aluminum phosphate gel, although no difference was seen in neutralizing antibody titers (Temperton, 2002; Temperton et al., 2003). However, the addition of CpG oligodeoxynucleotides to aluminum phosphate gel enhanced the ability of the gB gene to stimulate neutralizing antibodies. Using a related approach, several laboratories have shown that coinoculation of animals with genes encoding immunostimulatory molecules in addition to viral antigens can provide enhanced protection against disease (Tsuji et al., 1997; Xiang and Ertl, 1995; Cull et al., 2002). Applying this approach, mice coimmunized with the MCMV gB and type I interferon genes exhibited enhanced protection against MCMV challenge when compared to mice that received the MCMV gB gene alone (Cull et al., 2002). It is interesting to note that DNA vaccination with type I interferons alone also reduce the level of MCMV infection (Yeow et al., 1998; Cull et al., 2002; Bartlett et al., 2002). Recently, the use of full-length murine and guinea pig CMVs cloned as bacterial artificial chromosomes (BACs) have been used as DNA vaccines. In principle, BAC vaccines would deliver the full complement of viral genes thereby inducing a wide range of antiviral immune responses (Cicin-Sain et al., 2003; Schleiss et al., 2006). Preconceptual maternal immunization of guinea pigs with a replication-disable guinea pig CMV BAC significantly protected their offspring against congenital CMV disease (Schleiss et al., 2006).

DNA vaccines for HCMV are still in their infancy, and safety issues stemming from the inoculation of exogenous DNA still need to be resolved. Nonetheless, this approach is remarkably versatile and may ultimately have an important place in HCMV vaccine development.

Subviral particles

Upon infection with HCMV, cultured fibroblasts release not only infectious virions but also non-infectious particles (Craighead et al., 1972; Fiala et al., 1976; Sarov and Abady, 1975). These non-infectious particles may be either dense bodies, which are enveloped structures consisting of viral tegument proteins and glycoproteins but lacking a capsid, or non-infectious enveloped particles (NIEPs), which are similar to normal virions except for the absence of DNA and the presence of an additional polypeptide. Glycoprotein B and the tegument protein pp65 are major constituents of dense bodies, and sera from HCMV seropositive individuals react with these particles (Baldick and Shenk, 1996; Forghani and Schmidt, 1980; Gibson and Irmiere, 1984; Irmiere and Gibson, 1983; Roby and Gibson, 1986). For this reason, dense bodies have long been considered as possible HCMV vaccines (Bia et al., 1980; Fiala et al., 1976; Gibson and Irmiere, 1984; Sarov et al., 1975; Stinski, 1976). More recent studies showed that dense bodies enter cells efficiently, presumably through the interaction of envelope glycoproteins with cellular receptors, thus mimicking normal infection (Pepperl et al., 2000; Schmolke et al., 1995; Topilko and Michelson, 1994). Mice transgenic for human HLA-A2 were immunized with dense bodies without an adjuvant. After only a single inoculation, the mice developed high virus neutralization titers, and those that received three doses retained substantial virus neutralizing activity for at least a year (Pepperl et al., 2000). The immunized mice developed antibodies to gB, gH, pp65, pp150 and several unidentified proteins. Given the importance of cellular immunity in controlling HCMV disease, it is significant to note that the immunized mice also developed high levels of HCMV-specific CTLs despite the absence of HCMV protein synthesis. Recently, it was shown that genetically modified dense bodies containing foreign proteins could be generated (Pepperl-Klindworth et al., 2002). In light of this, it may be possible to produce dense body-based vaccines that are modified to improve their HCMV immunogenicity through the inclusion or enhanced expression of specific antigens. Dense body technology therefore, represents another innovative approach to HCMV vaccine development that deserves continued exploration.

Challenges for HCMV vaccine development

Species-specificity of HCMV

HCMV has a very limited host range, and no practical animal model for HCMV infection has been identified (Mocarski and Courcelle, 2001). While the CMVs of certain other animal species are well studied and very useful for addressing many aspects of vaccine development, they are genetically distinct from HCMV and may not behave identically during natural infection. Thus, for any new HCMV vaccine candidate initial safety and efficacy data can be derived from animal studies using analogous vaccines made from animal CMVs. However, this data will need to be interpreted cautiously, and valid safety and efficacy data will require human trials. Moreover, the species specificity of HCMV is an impediment for testing live, presumably attenuated vaccine candidates. Without the ability to assess HCMV virulence in an animal model, attenuation can only be confirmed through human trials. While this was accomplished for the Towne/Toledo chimeric vaccine candidates described above, it undoubtedly complicates vaccine development efforts.

Efficacy testing

The primary goal of HCMV vaccination is the prevention of congenital disease. However, given that the incidence of HCMV disease is about 0.1% of all births, a prospective trial to assess vaccine efficacy against HCMV disease would require tens of thousands of participants and a lengthy follow-up period to ensure that late sequelae of CMV infection, such as hearing and intelligence deficits, are not missed. However, an efficacy trial to determine the ability of a vaccine to protect newborns from HCMV infection could be done with a manageable number of subjects. Assuming a fetal infection rate of 1%, vaccine efficacy of 80% and a 2-year follow-up period, such a trial would require fewer than 5000 participants (Plotkin, 1999). Moreover, surrogate endpoints for vaccine efficacy could be tested initially to exclude less promising vaccine candidates from future large trials. For example, the ability of a vaccine to prevent infection in seronegative mothers with children in daycare would require less than 200 participants, given the high incidence of HCMV infection in that population (Plotkin, 1999).

When to vaccinate

To prevent congenital disease, HCMV vaccination should be administered to women prior to their becoming pregnant, and it has been proposed that vaccination of girls between the ages of 11 and 13 would be appropriate (Plotkin, 1999). However, the persistence of the immune response would need to be determined before a final schedule could be recommended. If a vaccine induced long-lived immunity, early childhood vaccination should be considered. If, however, immunity is less durable, later vaccination or regular boosters may be appropriate.

Summary

At present, vaccination remains the best hope for preventing most cases of congenital HCMV disease. Several new HCMV vaccination strategies have emerged in the past decade that take advantage of our current understanding of the host immune response to HCMV infection. Moreover, some older approaches, such as live attenuated vaccines, are being readdressed using modern molecular genetic approaches to enhance protective efficacy. More than ever, the development of a safe and effective HCMV vaccine seems to be an achievable goal. The most important scientific challenge that remains is to refine our understanding of the immunology of HCMV disease protection in order to rationally design vaccines that are both safe and effective. In addition, agreement must be reached within the medical and scientific communities on the best approaches for efficacy testing of new HCMV vaccines before the large trials necessary for licensure can be conducted.

REFERENCES

Adler, S. P. (1988). Molecular epidemiology of cytomegalovirus: viral transmission among children attending a day care center, their parents, and caretakers. *J. Pediatr.*, **112**, 366–372.

Adler, S. P. (1996). Current prospects for immunization against cytomegaloviral disease. *Infect. Agents. Dis.*, **5**, 29–35.

Adler, S. P., Starr, S. E., Plotkin, S. A. *et al.* (1995). Immunity induced by primary human cytomegalovirus infection protects against secondary infection among women of childbearing age. *J. Infect. Dis.*, **171**, 26–32.

Adler, S. P., Finney, J. W., Manganello, A. M., and Best, A. M. (1996). Prevention of child-to-mother transmision of cytomegalovirus by changing behaviors: a randomized controlled trial. *Pediatr. Infect. Dis. J.*, **15**, 240–246.

Adler, S. P., Hempfling, S. H., Starr, S. E., Plotkin, S. A., and Riddell, S. (1998). Safety and immunogenicity of the Towne strain cytomegalovirus vaccine. *Pediatr. Infect. Dis. J.*, **17**, 200–206.

Adler, S. P., Plotkin, S. A., Gonczol, E. *et al.* (1999). A canarypox vector expressing cytomegalovirus (CMV) glycoprotein B primes for antibody responses to a live attenuated CMV vaccine (Towne). *J. Infect. Dis.*, **180**, 843–846.

Ahlfors, K., Ivarsson, S. A., and Harris, S. (1999). Report on a long-term study of maternal and congenital cytomegalovirus infection in Sweden. Review of prospective studies available in the literature. *Scand. J. Infect. Dis.*, **31**, 443–457.

Akiyama, Y., Maruyama, K., Mochizuki, T., Sasaki, K., Takaue, Y., and Yamaguchi, K. (2002). Identification of HLA-A24-restricted CTL epitope encoded by the matrix protein pp65 of human cytomegalovirus. *Immunol. Lett.*, **83**, 21–30.

Baldick, C. J. Jr. and Shenk, T. (1996). Proteins associated with purified human cytomegalovirus particles. *J. Virol.*, **70**, 6097–6105.

Balfour, H. H. (1991). Prevention of cytomegalovirus disease in renal allograft recipients. *Scand. J. Infect. Dis.*, **78**, 88–93.

Bartlett, E. J., Cull, V. S., Brekalo, N. L., Lenzo, J. C., and James, C. M. (2002). Synergy of type I interferon-A6 and interferon-B naked DNA immunotherapy for cytomegalovirus infection. *Immunol. Cell Biol.*, **80**, 425–435.

Baxby, D. and Paoletti, E. (1992). Potential use of non-replicating vectors as recombinant vaccines. *Vaccine*, **10**, 8–9.

Berencsi, K., Gyulai, Z., Gonczol, E. *et al.* (2001). A canarypox vector-expressing cytomegalovirus (CMV) phosphoprotein 65 induces long-lasting cytotoxic T cell responses in human CMV-seronegative subjects. *J. Infect. Dis.*, **183**, 1171–1179.

Bernstein, D. I., Schleiss, M. R., Berencsi, K. *et al.* (2002). Effect of previous or simultaneous immunization with canarypox expressing cytomegalovirus (CMV) glycoprotein B (gB) on response to subunit gB vaccine plus MF59 in healthy CMV-seronegative adults. *J. Infect. Dis.*, **185**, 686–690.

Bia, F. J., Griffith, B. P., Tarsio, M., and Hsiung, G. D. (1980). Vaccination for the prevention of maternal and fetal infection with guinea pig cytomegalovirus. *J. Infect. Dis.*, **142**, 732–738.

Boeckh, M., Gooley, T. A., Myerson, D., Cunningham, T., Schoch, G., and Bowden, R. A. (1996). Cytomegalovirus pp65 antigenemia-guided early treatment with ganciclovir versus ganciclovir at engraftment after allogeneic marrow transplantation: a randomized double-blind study. *Blood*, **88**, 4063–4071.

Bolds, S., Ohlin, M., Garten, W., and Radsak, K. (1996). Structural domains involved in human cytomegalovirus glycoprotein B-mediated cell-cell fusion. *J. Gen. Virol.*, **77**, 2297–2302.

Boppana, S. B. and Britt, W. J. (1996). Recognition of human cytomegalovirus gene products by HCMV-specific cytotoxic T cells. *Virology*, **222**, 293–296.

Boppana, S. B., Fowler, K. B., Britt, W. J., Stagno, S., and Pass, R. F. (1999). Symptomatic congenital cytomegalovirus infection in infants born to mothers with preexisting immunity to cytomegalovirus. *Pediatrics*, **104**, 55–60.

Boppana, S. B., Rivera, L. B., Fowler, K. B., Mach, M., and Britt, W. J. (2001). Intrauterine transmission of cytomegalovirus to infants of women with preconceptional immunity. *N. Engl. J. Med.*, **344**, 1366–1371.

Bowden, R. A., Sayers, M., Flournoy, N. *et al.* (1986). Cytomegalovirus immune globulin and seronegative blood products to prevent primary cytomegalovirus infection after marrow transplantation. *N. Engl. J. Med.*, **314**, 1006–1010.

Brayman, K. L., Dafoe, D. C., Smythe, W. R. *et al.* (1988). Prophylaxis of serious cytomegalovirus infection in renal transplant candidates using live human cytomegalovirus vaccine. *Arch. Surg.*, **123**, 1502–1508.

Britt, W. J. and Mach, M. (1996). Human cytomegalovirus glycoproteins. *Intervirology*, **39**, 401–412.

Britt, W. J., Vugler, L., and Stephens, E. B. (1988). Induction of complement-dependent and -independent neutralizing antibodies by recombinant-derived human cytomegalovirus gp55–116 (gB). *J. Virol.*, **62**, 3309–3318.

Britt, W. J., Vugler, L., Butfiloski, E. J., and Stephens, E. B. (1990). Cell surface expression of human cytomegalovirus (HCMV) gp55–116 (gB): Use of HCMV-recombinant vaccinia virus-infected cells in analysis of the human neutralizing antibody response. *J. Virol.*, **64**, 1079–1085.

Cha, T. A., Tom, E., and Kemble, G. W. (1996). Human cytomegalovirus clinical isolates carry at least 19 genes not found in laboratory strains. *J. Virol.*, **70**, 78–83.

Chee, M. S., Bankier, A. T., Beck, S. *et al.* (1990). Analysis of the protein-coding content of the sequence of human cytomegalovirus strain AD169. *Curr. Top. Microbiol. Immunol.*, **154**, 125–169.

Chou, S. W. and Dennison, K. M. (1991). Analysis of interstrain variation in cytomegalovirus glycoprotein B sequences encoding neutralization-related epitopes. *J. Infect. Dis.*, **163**, 1229–1234.

Clements-Mann, M. L., Weinhold, K., Matthews, T. J. *et al.* and NIAID AIDS Vaccine Evaluation Group (1998). Immune responses to human immuodeficiency virus (HIV) type 1 induced by canarypox expressing HIV-1MN gp 120, HIV-1SF2 recombinant gp120, or both vaccines in seronegative adults. *J. Infect. Dis.*, **177**, 1230–1240.

Cohen, J. I. and Corey, G. R. (1985). Cytomegalovirus infection in the normal host. *Medicine*, 100–114.

Compton, T., Nowlin, D. M., and Cooper, N. R. (1993). Initiation of human cytomegalovirus infection requires initial interaction with cell surface heparin sulfate. *Virology*, **193**, 834–841.

Craighead, J. E., Kanich, R. E., and lmeida, J. D. (1972). Nonviral microbodies with viral antigenicity produced in cytomegalovirus-infected cells. *J. Virol.*, **10**, 766–775.

Cremer, N. E., Cossen, C. K., Shell, G. R., and Pereira, L. (1985). Antibody response to cytomegalovirus polypeptides captured by monoclonal antibodies on the solid phase in enzyme immunoassays. *J. Clin. Microbiol.*, **21**, 517–521.

Cull, V. S., Broomfield, S., Bartlett, E. M., Brekalo, N. L., and James, C. M. (2002). Coimmunisation with type I IFN genes enhances protective immunity against cytomegalovirus and myocarditis in gB DNA-vaccinated mice. *Gene Ther.*, **9**, 1369–1378.

Davison, A. J., Dolan, A., Akter, P. et al. (2003). The human cytomegalovirus genome revisited: comparison with the chimpanzee cytomegalovirus genome. *J. Gen. Virol.*, **84**, 17–28.

Demmler, G. J. (1991). Infectious Diseases Society of America and Centers for Disease Control. Summary of a workshop on surveillance for congenital cytomegalovirus disease. *Rev. Infect. Dis.*, **13**, 329

Diamond, D. J., York, J., Sun, J. Y., Wright, C. L., and Forman, S. J. (1997). Development of a candidate HLA A* 0201 restricted peptide-based vaccine against human cytomegalovirus infection. *Blood*, **90**, 1751–1767.

Elek, S. D. and Stern, H. (1974). Development of a vaccine against mental retardation cased by cytomegalovirus infection in utero. *Lancet*, **1**, 1–15.

Elkington, R., Walker, S., Crough, T. et al. (2003). *Ex vivo* profiling of CD8+ -T-cell responses to human cytomegalovirus reveals broad and multispecific reactivities in healthy virus carriers. *J. Virol.*, **77**, 5226–5240.

Endresz, V., Kari, L., Berencsi, K. et al. (1999). Induction of human cytomegalovirus (HCMV)-glycoprotein B (gB)-specific neutralizing antibody and phosphoprotein 65 (pp65)-specific cytotoxic T lymphocyte responses by naked DNA immunization. *Vaccine*, **17**, 50–58.

Falagas, M. E., Snydman, D. R., Rathazer, R. et al. and The Boston Center for Liver Transplantation CMVIG Study Group (1997). Cytomegalovirus immune globulin (CMVIG) prophylaxis is associated wth increased survival after orthotopic liver transplantation. *Clin. Transpl.*, **11**, 432–437.

Fiala, M., Honess, R. W., Heiner, D. C. et al. (1976). Cytomegalovirus, proteins. I. Polypeptides of virions and dense bodies. *J. Virol.*, **19**, 243–254.

Fishman, J. A. and Rubin, R. H. (1998). Infection in organ-transplant recipients. *N. Engl. J. Med.*, **338**, 1741–1751.

Fleisher, G. R., Starr, S. E., Friedman, H. M., and Plotkin, S. A. (1982). Vaccination of pediatric nurses with live attenuated cytomegalovirus. *Am. J. Dis. Child.*, **136**, 294–296.

Forghani, B. and Schmidt, N. J. (1980). Humoral immune response to virions and dense bodies of human cytomegalovirus determined by enzyme immunofluorescence assay. *J. Med. Virol.*, **6**, 119–127.

Fowler, K. B., Stagno, S., Pass, R. F., Britt, W. J., Boll, T. J., and Alford, C. A. (1992). The outcome of congenital cytomegalovirus infection in relation to maternal antibody status. *N. Engl. J. Med.*, **326**, 663–667.

Fowler, K. B., Stagno, S., and Pass, R. F. (2003). Maternal immunity and prevention of congenital cytomegalovirus infection. *J. Am. Med. Assoc.*, **289**, 1008–1011.

Frankenberg, N., Pepperl-Klindworth, S., Meyer, R. G., and Plachter, B. (2002). Identification of a conserved HLA-A-2 restricted decapeptide from the IE1 protein (pUL123) of human cytomegalovirus. *Virology*, **295**, 208–216.

Frey, S. E., Harrison, C., Pass, R. F. et al. (1999). Effects of antigen dose and immunization regimens on antibody responses to a cytomegalovirus glycoprotein B subunit vaccine. *J. Infect. Dis.*, **180**, 1700–1703.

Gehrz, R. C., Christianson, W. R., Linner, K. M., Groth, K. E., and Balfour, Jr. H. H. (1980). Cytomegalovirus Vaccine: Specific humoral and cellular immune responses in human volunteers. *Arch. Intern. Med.*, **140**, 936–939.

Gibson, W. and Irmiere, A. (1984). Selection of particles and proteins for use as human cytomegalovirus subunit vaccines. *Birth Defects*, **20**, 305–324.

Glazer, J. P., Friedman, H. M., Grossman, R. A., et al. (1979). Live cytomegalovirus vaccination of renal transplant candidates. *Ann. Intern. Med.*, **91**, 676–683.

Glowacki, L. S. and Smaill, F. M. (1994). Use of immune globulin to prevent symptomatic cytomegalovirus disease in transplant recipients: a meta-analysis. *Transplant*, **8**, 10–18.

Gonczol, E. and Plotkin, S. (2001). Development of a cytomegalovirus vaccine: lessons from recent clinical trials. *Expert. Opin. Biol. Ther.*, **1**, 401–412.

Gonczol, E., Lanacone, J., Furlini, G., Ho, W. Q., and Plotkin, S. A. (1989). Humoral immune response to cytomegalovirus Towne vaccine strain and to Toledo low-passage strain. *J. Infect. Dis.*, **159**, 851–859.

Gonczol, E., Berencsi, K., Pincus, S. et al. Plotkin, S. A. (1995). Preclinical evaluation of an ALVAC (canarypox)-human cytomegalovirus glycoprotein B vaccine candidate. *Vaccine*, **13**, 1080–1085.

Gonzales Armas, J. C., Morello, C. S., Cranmer, L. D., and Spector, D. H. (1996). DNA immunization confers protection against murine cytomegalovirus infection. *J. Virol.*, **70**, 7921–7928.

Griffiths, P. D. (2002). Strategies to prevent CMV infection in the neonate. *Semin. Neonatol.*, **7**, 293–299.

Griffiths, P. D., McLean, A., and Emery, V. C. (2001). Encouraging prospects for immunization against primary cytomegalovirus infection. *Vaccine*, **19**, 1356–1362.

Gyulai, Z., Endresz, V., Burian, K. et al. (2000). Cytotoxic T lymphocyte (CTL) responses to human cytomegalovirus pp65, IE1-exon4, gB, pp150, and pp28 in healthy individuals; reevaluation of prevalence of IE1-specific CTLs. *J. Infect. Dis.*, **181**, 1537–1546.

Heineman, T. C., Schleiss, M., Bernstein, D., Fast, P., Spaete, R., and Kemble, G. (2003). Safety results from a phase 1 study of four live, recombinant HCMV Towne/Toledo chimeric vaccines. *9th International Cytomegalovirus Workshop and 1st International Betaherpesvirus Workshop, Maastricht, the Netherlands.* (Abstract)

Holtappels, R., Podlech, J., Geginat, G., Steffens, H. P., Thomas, D., and Reddehase, M. J. (1998). Control of murine cytomegalovirus in the lungs; relative but not absolute immunodominance of the immediate-early 1 nonapeptide during the antiviral cytolytic T-lymphocyte response in pulmonary infiltrates. *J. Virol.*, **72**, 7201–7212.

Huang, E. S., Houng, S. M., Tegtmeier, G. E., and Alford C. (1980). Cytomegalovirus: Genetic variation of viral genomes. *Ann. N. Y. Acad. Sci.*, **354**, 332–346.

Hwang, E. S., Park, J. W., Kim, D. J., Park, C. G., and Cha, C. Y. (1999). Induction of neutralizing antibody against human cytomegalovirus (HCMV) with DNA-mediated immunization of HCMV glycoprotein B in mice. *Micro. Immunol.*, **43**, 307–310.

Irmiere, A. and Gibson, W. (1983). Isolation and characterization of a non-infectious viron-like particle released from cells infected with human strains of cytomegalovirus. *Virology*, **130**, 118–133.

Istas, A. S., Demmler, G. J., Dobbins, J. G., and Stewart, J. A. (1995). Surveillance for congenital cytomegalovirus disease: a report from the National Congenital Cytomegalovirus Disease Registry. *Clin. Infect. Dis.*, **20**, 665–670.

Jacobson, M. A., Sinclair, E., Bredt, B. et al. (2006). Safety and immunogenicity of Towne cytomegalovirus vaccine with or without adjuvant recombinant interleukin-12. *Vaccine*, **24**, 5311–5319.

Just, M., Buergin-Wolff, A., Emoedi, G., and Hernandez, R. (1975). Immunisation trials with live attenuated cytomegalovirus TOWNE 125. *Infections*, **3**, 111–114.

Kari, B. and Gehrz, R. (1990). Analysis of human antibody responses to human cytomegalovirus envelope glycoproteins found in two families of disulfide linked glycoprotein complexes designated gC-I and gC-II. *Arch. Virol.*, **114**, 213–228.

Keay, S. and Baldwin, B. (1991). Anti-idiotype antibodies that mimic gp86 of human cytomegalovirus inhibit viral fusion but not attachment. *J. Virol.*, **65**, 5124–5128.

Kemble, G., Duke, G., and Winter, R. (1996). Defined large-scale alteration of the human cytomegalovirus genome constructed by cotransfection of overlapping cosmids. *J. Virol.*, **70**, 2044–2048.

Kern, F., Faulhaber, N., Frommel, C. et al. (2000). Analysis of CD8 T cell reactivity to cytomegalovirus using protein-spanning pools of overlapping pentadecapeptides. *Eur. J. Immunol.*, **30**, 1676–1682.

Kern, F., Bunde, T., Faulhaber, N. et al. (2002). Cytomegalovirus (CMV) phosphoprotein 65 makes a large contribution to shaping the T cell repertoire in CMV-exposed individuals. *J. Infect. Dis.*, **185**, 1709–1716.

Kimberlin, D. W., Lin, C. Y., Sanchez, P. J. et al. and the National Institute of Allergy and Infectious Diseases Collaborative Antiviral Study Group (2003). Effect of ganciclovir therapy on hearing in symptomatic congenital cytomegalovirus disease involving the central nervous system: a randomized, controlled trial. *J. Pediatr.*, **143**, 16–25.

Klinman, D. M. (2003). CpG DNA as a vaccine adjuvant. *Expert Rev. Vaccines*, **2**, 305–315.

Klinman, D. M., Ishii, K. J., and Verthelyi, D. (2000). CpG DNA augments the immunogenicity of plasmid DNA vaccines. *Curr. Top Microbiol. Immunol.*, **247**, 131–142.

Kniess, N., Mach, M., Fay, J., and Britt, W. J. (1991). Distribution of linear antigenic sites on glycoprotein gp55 of human cytomegaloviurs. *J. Virol.*, **65**, 138–146.

Koff, R. S. (2001). Hepatitis vaccine. *Infect. Dis. Clin. North Am.*, **15**, 83–95.

La Rosa, C., Wang, Z., Brewer, J. C. et al. (2002). Preclinical development of an adjuvant-free peptide vaccine with activity against CMV pp65 in HLA transgenic mice. *Blood*, **100**, 3681–3689.

La Rosa, C., Wang, Z., Lacey, S. F. et al. (2005). Characterization of host immunity to cytomegalovirus pp150 (UL32). *Hum. Immunol.*, **66**, 116–126.

Leather, H. L. and Wingard, J. R. (2001). Infections following hematopoietic stem cell transplantation. In Davis, C., ed. *Infectious Disease Clinics of North America. Infections in the Compromised Host.* Philadelphia: W. B. Saunders Company, pp. 483–520.

Li, C. R., Greenberg, P. D., Gilbert, M. J., Goodrich, J. M. and Riddell, S. R. (1994). Recovery of HLA-restricted cytomegalovirus (CMV)-specific T-cell responses after allogeneic bone marrow transplant: correlation with CMV disease and effect of ganciclovir prophylaxis. *Blood*, **83**, 1971–1979.

Longmate, J., York, J., LaRosa, C. et al. (2001). Population coverage by HLA class-I restricted cytotoxic T-lymphocyte epitopes. *Immunogenetics*, **52**, 165–173.

Mach, M., Kropff, B., Dal Monte, P., and Britt, W. (2000). Complex formation by human cytomegalovirus glycoproteins M (gpUL100) and N (gpUL73). *J. Virol.*, **74**, 11881–11892.

Marker, S. C., Simmons, R. L., and Balfour, Jr. H. H. (1981). Cytomegalovirus vaccine in renal allograft recipients. *Transpl. Proc.*, **13**, 117–119.

Marshall, G. S. and Plotkin, S. A. (1993). Cytomegalovirus Vaccines. In Roizman, B., Whitley, R. J., and Lopez, C., (eds.) *The Human Herpesviruses.*, New York: Raven Press, Ltd., pp. 381.

Marshall, G. S., Rabalais, G. P., Stout, G. G., and Waldeyer, S. L. (1992). Antibodies to recombinant-derived glycoprotein B after natural human cytomegalovirus infection correlate with neutralizing activity. *J. Infect. Dis.*, **165**, 381–384.

Marshall, G. S., Stout, G. G., Knights, M. E. et al. (1994). Ontogeny of glycoprotein gB-specific antibody and neutralizing activity during natural cytomegalovirus infection. *J. Med. Virol.*, 77–83.

Marshall, G. S., Li, M., Stout, G. G. et al. (2000). Antibodies to the major linear neutralizing domains of cytomegalovirus glycoprotein B among natural seropositives and CMV subunit vaccine recipients. *Viral Immunol.*, **13**, 329–341.

Martinon, F., Gras-Masse, H., Boutillon, C. et al. (1992). Immunization of mice with lipopeptides bypasses the prerequisite for adjuvant immune response of BALB/c mice to human immunodeficiency virus envelope glycoprotein. *J. Immunol.*, **149**, 3416–3422.

Masuoka, M., Yoshimuta, T., Hamada, M. et al. (2001). Identification of the HLA-A24 peptide within cytomegalovirus protein pp65 recognized by CMV-specific cytotoxic T lymphocytes. *Viral Immunol.*, **14**, 369–377.

McElrath, M. J. (1995). Selection of potent immunological adjuvants for vaccine construction. *Semin. Cancer Biol.*, **6**, 375–385.

McLaughlin-Taylor, E., Pande, H., Forman, S. J. et al. (1994). Identification of the major late human cytomegalovirus matrix protein pp65 as a target for CD8+ virus-specific cytotoxic T lymphocytes. *J. Med. Virol.*, **43**, 103–110.

Messori, A., Rampazzo, R., Scroccaro, G., and Martini, N. (1994). Efficacy of hyperimmune anti-cytomegalovirus immunoglobulins for the prevention of cytomegalovirus infection in recipients of allogeneic bone marrow transplantation: a meta-analysis. *Bone Marrow Transpl.*, **13**, 163–167.

Meyer, H., Sundqvist, V. A., Pereia, L., and Mach, M. (1992). Glycoprotein gp116 of human cytomegalovirus contains epitopes for strain-common and strain-specific antibodies. *J. Gen. Virol.*, **73**, 2375–2383.

Michaels, M. G., Greenberg, D. P., Sabo, D. L., and Wald, E. R. (2003). Treatment of children with congenital cytomegalovirus infection with ganciclovir. *Pediatr. Infect. Dis. J.*, **22**, 504–509.

Mitchell, D. K., Holmes, S. J., Burke, R. L., Duliege, A. M., and Adler, S. P. (2002). Immunogenicity of a recombinant human cytomegalovirus gB vaccine in seronegative toddlers. *Pediatr. Infect. Dis. J.*, **21**, 133–138.

Mocarski, E. S. and Courcelle, C. T. (2001). Cytomegaloviruses and their replication. In Knipe, M. D. and Howley, P. M. (eds.) *Fields Virology*, 4th, edn. pp. 2629–2673. Philadelphia: Lippincott Williams & Wilkins

Morello, C. S., Ye, M., and Spector, D. H. (2000). Suppression of murine cytomegalovirus (MCMV) replication with DNA vaccine encoding MCMC M84 (A homolog of human cytomegalovirus pp65). *J. Virol.*, **74**, 3696–3708.

Morris, D. J., Sims, D., Chiswick, M., Das, V. K., and Newton, V. E. (1994). Symptomatic congenital cytomegalovirus infection after maternal recurrent infection. *Pediatr. Infect. Dis. J.*, **13**, 61–64.

Navarro, D., Paz, P., Tugizov, S., Topp, K., La Vail, J., and Pereira, L. (1993). Glycoprotein B of human cytomegalovirus promotes virion penetration into cells, transmission of infection from cell to cell, and fusion of infected cells. *Virology*, **197**, 143–158.

Neff, B. J., Weibel, R. E., Buynak, E. B., McAllen, A. A., and Hillman, M. R. (1979). Clinical and laboratory studies of live cytomegalovirus vaccine Ad-169. *Proc. Soc. Exp. Biol. Med.*, **160**, 32–37.

Nigro, G., Adler, S. P., La Torre, R., and Best, A. M. (2005). Passive immunization during pregnancy for congenital cytomegalovirus infection. *N. Engl. J. Med.*, **353**, 1350–1362.

Ott, G., Barchfeld, G. L., and Van Nest, G. (1995). Enhancement of humoral response against human influenza vaccine with the simple submicron oil/water emulsion adjuvant MF59. *Vaccine*, **13**, 1557–1562.

Pande, H., Campo, K., and Tanamachi, B. (1995). Direct DNA immunization of mice with plasmid DNA encoding the tegument protein pp65 (ppUL83) of human cytomegalovirus induces high levels of circulating antibody to the encoded protein. *Scand. J. Infect. Dis.[Suppl.]*, **99**, 117–120.

Pass, R. F. (2001). Cytomegalovirus. In D. M. Knipe and P. M. Howley (eds.) *Fields Virology*, 4th, edn. pp. 2675–2705. Philadelphia, PA: Lippincott Williams & Wilkins, pp. 2675–2705.

Pass, R. F. and Burke, R. L. (2002). Development of cytomegalovirus vaccines: prospects for prevention of congenital CMV infection. *Semin. Pediatric. Infect. Dis.*, **13**, 196–204.

Pass, R. F., Hutto, C., Ricks, R., and Cloud, G. A. (1986). Increased rate of cytomegalovirus infection among parents of children attending day-care centers. *N. Engl. J. Med.*, **314**, 1414–1418.

Pass, R. F., Duliege, A. M., Sekulovich, R., Percell, S., Britt, W., and Burke, R. L. (1999). A subunit cytomegalovirus vaccine based on recombinant envelope glycoprotein B and a new adjuvant. *J. Infect. Dis.*, **180**, 970–975.

Patel, R. and Paya, C. V. (1997). Infections in solid-organ transplant recipients. *Clin. Microbiol. Rev.*, **10**, 86–124.

Pepperl-Klindworth, S., Frenkenberg, N., and Plachter, B. (2002). Development of novel vaccine strategies against human cytomegalovirus infection based on subviral particles. *J. Clin. Virol.*, **25**, S75–S85.

Pepperl, S., Munster, J., Mach, M., Harris, J. R., and Plachter, B. (2000). Dense bodies of human cytomegalovirus induce both humoral and cellular immune responses in the absence of viral gene expression. *J. Virol.*, **74**, 6132–6146.

Pialoux, G., Excler, J. L., Riviere, Y. *et al.* The AGIS Group, and and L'Agence Nationale De Recherche Sur Le Sida (1995). A prime-boost approach to HIV preventive vaccine using a recombinant canarypox virus expressing glycoprotein 160 (MN) followed by a recombinant glycoprotein 160 (MN/LAI). *AIDS, Res. Hum. Retroviruses.*, **11**, 381.

Plotkin, S. A. (1999). Vaccination against cytomegalovirus, the changeling demon. *Pediatr. Infect. Dis. J.*, **18**, 313–316.

Plotkin, S. A. (2001). Vaccination against cytomegalovirus. *Arch. Virol. Supplementum*, 121–134.

Plotkin, S. A. (2002). Is there a formula for an effective CMV vaccine? *J. Clin. Virol.*, **25**, S13–S21.

Plotkin, S. A., Furukawa, T., Zygraich, N., and Huygelen, C. (1975). Candidate cytomegalovirus strain for human vaccination. *Infect. Immun.*, **12**, 521–527.

Plotkin, S. A., Farquhar, J. and Horberger, E. (1976). Clinical trials of immunization with the Towne 125 strain of human cytomegalovirus. *J. Infect. Dis.*, **134**, 470–475.

Plotkin, S. A., Smiley, M. L., Friedman, H. M. *et al.* (1984). Towne-vaccine-induced prevention of cytomegalovirus disease after renal transplants. *Lancet*, **1**, 528–530.

Plotkin, S. A., Starr, S. E., Friedman, H. M., Gonczol, E., and Weibel, R. E. (1989). Protective effects of Towne cytomegalovirus vaccine against low-passage cytomegalovirus administered as a challenge. *J. Infect. Dis.*, **159**, 860–865.

Plotkin, S. A., Starr, S. E., Friedman, H. M. *et al.* (1991). Effect of Towne live virus vaccine on cytomegalovirus disease after renal transplant. A controlled trial. *Ann. Intern. Med.*, **114**, 525–531.

Plotkin, S. A., Higgins, R., and Kurtz, J. B. (1994). Multicenter trial of Towne strain attenuated virus vaccine in seronegative renal transplant recipients. *Transplantation*, **58**, 1176–1178.

Plotkin, S. A., Cadoz, M., Meignier, B. *et al.* (1995). The safety and use of canarypox vectored vaccine. *Dev. Biol. Stand.*, **84**, 165–170.

Prichard, M. N., Penfold, M. E., Duke, G. M., Spaete, R. R., and Kemble, G. W. (2001). A review of genetic differences between limited and extensively passaged human cytomegalovirus strains. *Rev. Med. Virol.*, **11**, 191–200.

Quinnan, G. V., Kirmani, N., Rook, A. H. et al. (1982). Cytotoxic T cells in cytomegalovirus infection. HLA-restricted T-lymphocyte and non T-lymphocyte cytotoxic responses correlate with recovery from cytomegalovirus infection in bone marrow transplant recipients. *N. Engl. J. Med.*, **307**, 6–19.

Quinnan, G. V., Delery, M. R. A., Frederick, W. R. et al. (1984). Comparative virulence and immunogenicity of the Towne strain and a nonattenuated strain of cytomegalovirus. *Ann. Intern. Med.*, **101**, 478–483.

Rasmussen, L., Matkin, C., Spaete, R., Pachl, C., and Merigan, T. C. (1991). Antibody response to human cytomegalovirus glycoproteins gB and gH after natural infection in humans. *J. Infect. Dis.*, **164**, 835–842.

Rasmussen, L., Morris, S., Wolitz, R. et al. (1994). Deficiency in antibody response to human cytomegalovirus glycoprotein gH in human immunodeficiency virus-infected patients at risk for cytomegalovirus retinitis. *J. Infect. Dis.*, **170**, 673–677.

Rasmussen, L. E., Nelson, R. M., Kelsall, D. C., and Merigan, T. C. (1984). Murine monoclonal antibody to a single protein neutralizes the infectivity of human cytomegalovirus. *Proc. Natl Acad. Sci. USA*, **81**, 876–880.

Raz, E., Carson, D. A., Parker, S. E. et al. (1994). Intradermal gene immunization: the possible role of DNA uptake in the induction of cellular immunity to viruses. *Proc. Natl Acad. Sci. USA*, **91**, 9519–9523.

Reddehase, M. J. and Koszinowski, U. H. (1984). Significance of herpesvirus immediate early gene expression in cellular immunity to cytomegalovirus infection. *Nature*, **312**, 367–371.

Reusser, P., Riddell, S. R., Meyers, J. D., and Greenberg, P. D. (1991). Cytotoxic T lymphocyte response to cytomegalovirus following allogeneic bone marrow transplantation: pattern of recovery and correlation with cytomegalovirus and disease. *Blood*, **78**, 1373–1380.

Revello, M. G. and Gerna, G. (2002). Diagnosis and management of human cytomegalovirus infection in the mother, fetus and newborn infant. *Clin. Microbiol. Rev.*, **15**, 680–715.

Roby, C. and Gibson, W. (1986). Characterization of phosphoproteins and protein kinase activity of virions, noninfectious enveloped particles, and dense bodies of human cytomegalovirus. *J. Virol.*, **59**, 714–727.

Ross, S. A., Fowler, K. B., Ashrith, G. et al. (2006). Hearing loss in children with congenital cytomegalovirus infection born to mothers with preexisting immunity. *J. Pediatr.*, **148**, 332–336.

Sarov, I., and and Abady, I. (1975). The morphogenesis of human cytomegalovirus; isolation and polypeptide characterization of cytomegalovirions and dense bodies. *Virology*, **66**, 464–473.

Schleiss, M. R., Bourne, N., Jensen, N. J., Bravo, F., and Bernstein, D. I. (2000). Immunogenicity evaluation of DNA vaccine that target guinea pig cytomegalovirus proteins glycoprotein B and UL83. *Viral Immunol.*, **13**, 155–167.

Schleiss, M. R., Stroup, G., Pogorzelski, K., and McGregor, A. (2006). Protection against congenital cytomegalovirus (CMV) disease, conferred by a replication-disabled, bacterial artificial chromosome (BAC)-based DNA vaccine. *Vaccine*, **24**, 6175–6186.

Schmolke, S., Drescher, P., Jahn, G., and Plachter, B. (1995). Nuclear targeting of the tegument protein pp65 (UL83) of human cytomegalovirus: an unusual bipartite nuclear localization signal functions with other portions of the protein to mediate its efficient nuclear transport. *J. Virol.*, **69**, 1071–1078.

Schopfer, K., Lauber, E., and Krech, U. (1978). Congenital cytomegalovirus infection in newborn infants of mothers infected before pregnancy. *Arch. Dis. Child.*, **53**, 536–539.

Schoppel, K., Hassfurhter, E., Britt, W. J., Ohlin, M., Borrebaeck, C. A., and Mach, M. (1996). Antibodies specific for the antigenic domain 1 (AD-1) of glycoprotein B (gpUL55) of human cytomegalovirus bind to different substructures. *Virology*, **216**, 133–145.

Sia, I. G. and Patel, R. (2000). New strategies for prevention and therapy of cytomegalovirus infection and disease in solid-organ transplant recipients. *Clin. Microbiol. Rev.*, **13**, 83–121.

Simon, D. M., M. P. and Levin, S. M. (2003). Infectious Complications of solid organ transplantations. In Burke, A. Cunha, M. D. and Guest Editor, eds. *Infectious Disease Clinics of North America: Infections in the Compromised Host*, Philadelphia, PA: W. B. Saunders Company, pp. 521–549.

Simpson, J. A., Chow, J. C., Baker, J. et al. (1993). Neutralizing monoclonal antibodies that distinguish three antigenic sites on human cytomegalovirus glycoprotein H have conformationally distinct binding sites. *J. Virol.*, **67**, 489–496.

Snydman, D. R. (1993). Review of the efficacy of cytomegalovirus immune globulin in the prophylaxis of CMV disease in renal transplant recipients. *Transpl. Proc.*, **25**, 25–26.

Snydman, D. R., Werner, B. G., Meissner, H. C. et al. (1995). Use of cytomegalovirus immunoglobulin in multiple transfused premature neonates. *Pediatr. Infect. Dis.*, **14**, 34–40.

Spaete, R. R. (1994). A recombinant subunit vaccine approach to HCMV vaccine development. *Transplant Proc.*, **23**, 90–96.

Stagno, S., Reynolds, D. W., Huang, E. S., Thames, S. D., Smith, R. J., and Alford, C. A. (1977). Congenital cytomegalovirus infection. *N. Engl. J. Med.*, **296**, 1254–1258.

Stagno, S., Pass, R. F., Dworsky, M. E. et al. (1982). Congenital cytomegalovirus infection. The relative importance of primary and recurrent maternal infection. *N. Engl. J. Med.*, **306**, 945–949.

Stagno, S., Pass, R. F., Cloud, G. et al. (1986). Primary cytomegalovirus infection in pregnancy. Incidence, transmission to fetus, and clinical outcome. *J. Am. Med. Assoc.*, **256**, 1904–1908.

Stagno, S., Reynolds, D. W., and Huang, E. S. (1997). Congenital cytomegalovirus infection. *N. Engl. J. Med.*, **296**, 1254–1258.

Stanberry, L. A., Spruance, S. L., Cunningham, A. L. and For the GlaxoSmithKline Herpes Vaccine Efficacy Study Group. (2002). Glycoprotein-D-adjuvant vaccine to prevent genital herpes. *N. Engl. J. Med.*, **347**, 1652–1660.

Starr, S. E., Glazer, J. P., Friedman, H. M., Farquhar, J. D. and Plotkin, S. A. (1981). Specific cellular and humoral immunity after immunization with live Towne strain cytomegalovirus vaccine. *J. Infect. Dis.*, **143**, 585–589.

Stern, H. (1984). Live cytomegalovirus vaccination of healthy volunteers: Eight-year follow-studies. *Birth Defects: Original Article Series*, **20**, 263–269.

Stinski, M. F. (1976). Humans cytomegalovirus: glycoproteins associated with virions and dense bodies. *J. Virol.*, **19**, 594–609.

Stratton, K. R., Durch, J., and Lawrence, R. S., eds. (2000). *Vaccines for the 21st century: A Tool for Decision making*. Washington, D. C.: National Academy Press.

Tang, D. C., DeVitt, M., and Johnston, S. A. (1992). Genetic immunization is a simple method for eliciting an immune response. *Nature*, **356**, 152–154.

Tartaglia, J., Perkus, M. E., Taylor, J. *et al.* (1992). NYVAC: a highly attenuated strain of vaccinia virus. *Virology*, **188**, 217–232.

Taylor, J., Meignier, B., Tartaglia, J., Languest, B., VanderHoeven, J., and Franchini, G. (1995). Biological and immunogenic properties of a canarypox-rabies recombinant, ALVAC-RG (vCP65) in non-avian species. *Vaccine*, **13**, 539–549.

Temperton, N. J. (2002). DNA vaccines against cytomegalovirus: current progress. *Int. J. Antimicrob. Agents*, **19**, 169–172.

Temperton, N. J., Quenelle, D. C., Lawson, K. M. *et al.* (2003). Enhancement of humoral immune responses to a human cytomegalovirus DNA vaccine: Adjuvant effects of aluminum phosphate and CpG oligodeoxynucleotides. *J. Med. Virol.*, **70**, 86–90.

Topilko, A., and Michelson, S. (1994). Hyperimmediate entry of human cytomegalovirus virions and dense bodies into human fibroblasts. *Res. Virol.*, **145**, 75–82.

Tsuji, T., Hamajima, K, Fukushima, J. *et al.* (1997). Enhancement of cell-mediated immunity against HIV-1 induced by coinoculation of plasmid-encoded HIV-1 antigen with plasmid expressing IL-12. *J. Immunol.*, **158**, 4008–4013.

Ulmer, J. B., Donnelly, J. J., Parker, S. E. *et al.* (1993). Heterologous protection against influenza by infection of DNA encoding a viral protein. *Science*, **259**, 1745–1749.

Ulmer, J. B., DeWitt, C. M., Chastain, M. *et al.* (1999). Enhancement of DNA vaccine potency using conventional aluminum adjuvants. *Vaccine*, **18**, 18–28.

Urban, M., Klein, M., Britt, W. J., Hassfurther, E., and Mach, M. (1996). Glycoprotein H of human cytomegalovirus is a major antigen for the neutralizing humoral immune response. *J. Gen. Virol.*, **77**, 1537–1547.

Valantine, H. A. (1995). Prevention and treatment of cytomegalovirus disease in thoracic organ transplant patients: evidence for a beneficial effect of hyperimmune globulin. *Transpl. Proc.*, **27 (Suppl 1)**, 49–57.

Wada, K., Mizuno, S., Ohta, H. and Nishiyama, Y. (1997). Immune response to neutralizing epitope on human cytomegalovirus glycoprotein B in Japanese: correlation of serologic respone with HLA-type. *Microbiol. Immunol.*, **41**, 841–845.

Wagner, B., Kroff, B., Kalbacher, H. *et al.* (1992). A continuous sequence of more than 70 amino acids is essential for antibody binding to the dominant antigenic site of glycoprotein gp58 of human cytomegalovirus. *J. Virol.*, **66**, 5290–5297.

Walter, E. A., Greenberg, P. D., Gilbert, M. J. *et al.* (1995). Reconstitution of cellular immunity against cytomegalovirus in recipients of allogeneic bone marrow by transfer of T-cell clones from the donor. *N. Engl. J. Med.*, **16**, 1038–1044.

Wang, J. B., Adler, S. P., Hempfling, S., Burke, R. L., Duliege, A. M., and Plotkin, S. A. (1996). Mucosal antibodies to human cytomegalovirus glycoprotein B occur following both natural infection and immunization with human cytomegalovirus vaccines. *J. Infect. Dis.*, **174**, 387–392.

Wang, X., Huong, S. M., Chiu, M. L., Raab-Traub, N., and Huang, E. S. (2003). Epidermal growth factor receptor is a cellular receptor for human cytomegalovirus. *Nature*, **424**, 456–461.

Wills, M. R., Carmichael, A. J., Mynard, K. *et al.* (1996). The human cytotoxic T-lymphocyte (CTL) response to cytomegalovirus is dominated by structural protein pp65: frequency, specificity, and T-cell receptor usage of pp65-specific CTL. *J. Virol.*, **70**, 7569–7579.

Wolff, J. A., Malone, R. W., Williams, P. *et al.* (1990). Direct gene transfer into mouse muscle *in vivo*., *Science*, **247**, 1465–1468.

Xiang, Z. and Ertl, H. C. (1995). Manipulation of the immune response to a plasmid-encoded viral antigen by coinoculaton with plasmids expressing cytokines. *Immunity*, **2**, 129–135.

Ye, M., Morello, C. S. and Spector, D. H. (2002). Strong CD8 T-cell responses following coimmunization with plasmids expressing the dominant pp89 and subdominant M84 antigens of murine cytomegalovirus correlate with long-term protection against subsequent viral challenge. *J. Virol.*, **76**, 2100–2112.

Yeager, A. S., Grumet, F. C., Hafleigh, E. B., Arvin, A. M., Bradley, J. S., and Prober, C. G. (1981). Prevention of transfusion-acquired cytomegalovirus infections in newborn infants. *J. Pediatr.*, **98**, 281–287.

Yeow, W. S., Lawson, C. M., and Beilharz, M. W. (1998). Antiviral activities of individual murine IFN-α subtypes *in vivo*. Intramuscular injection of IFN expression constructs reduces cytomegalovirus replication. *J. Immunol.*, **160**, 2932–2939.

Epstein–Barr virus vaccines

Andrew J. Morgan[1] and Rajiv Khanna[2]

[1]Division of Virology, Department of Cellular and Molecular Medicine, School of Medical Sciences, University of Bristol, UK
[2]Tumour Immunology Laboratory, Division of Infectious Diseases and Immunology, Queensland Institute for Medical Research, Herston, Australia

Introduction

Primates and their γ-herpesviruses enjoy a largely peaceful coexistence where a balance of power has been reached over evolutionary time. Coevolution probably began before primate speciation and has allowed these viruses to develop sophisticated systems for the evasion of host immune responses. As a consequence, herpesvirus vaccines have been especially difficult to design because of viral latency, persistence, and immune modulation. Epstein–Barr virus (EBV) persists for the life of the individual in the face of a range of antibody responses, some of which are virus-neutralizing in vitro and a multitude of cell-mediated responses, including viral-specific CD8+ T-cells, CD4+ T-cells and NK cells. At least 95% of the adult population is infected with EBV and, for the vast majority, there are no clinical consequences whatsoever and an asymptomatic carrier state is maintained. It is not clear whether advantages are conferred to humans by lifelong EBV infection, but it is possible that some immunological effects, such as bias of the T-cell receptor repertoire are provided on a population-wide basis. Whether unselective mass vaccination of healthy individuals to prevent or modify EBV infection may cause more problems than it would solve must be considered.

M.A. Epstein first put forward ideas on the development of EBV vaccines in 1976. These original proposals were based on the notion that vaccination might prevent EBV infection and break the link in the complex chains of events that lead to EBV-associated disease. Since that time, a better understanding of EBV biology has led to the elaboration of more sophisticated vaccination strategies. Presently, it seems most unlikely that vaccination of any kind will achieve sterilizing immunity against herpesviruses. The murine γ-herpesvirus, MHV68, establishes the same steady-state levels of lytic and latent infection whatever the route of infection or dose. It may be that a single virus particle successfully infecting a single target cell will be enough to establish persistent infection in a susceptible subject (Tibbetts, 2003). The goal of EBV vaccination is the prevention of disease and not of infection. Vaccination that could modify infection, or at least the subsequent immunological status of the infected person with respect to EBV, may prevent or minimize disease. It should be noted that EBV will not have evolved to evade vaccine-induced immune responses where they are qualitatively and/or quantitatively different from naturally occurring immune responses. An important precedent for herpesvirus vaccination is the attenuated varicella zoster virus (VZV) Oka strain vaccine that may not prevent infection but is able to prevent disease. More recently, the concept of therapeutic vaccination to treat EBV-associated tumors themselves has begun to emerge (Khanna et al., 2001; Ong et al., 2003; Khanna et al., 2005).

An understanding of the life cycle and cellular habitats of EBV should be an essential prerequisite in the rational design of EBV vaccines. Unfortunately, the biology of EBV in vivo remains poorly understood and the various approaches to EBV vaccine design discussed below are, of necessity, based on a number of unproven assumptions. EBV is an orally transmitted infection and is able to infect B-cells travelling in the circulation in the oropharynx or resident in lymphoid tissue in this region. The point of infection is presumed to be the oropharyngeal epithelium but the identity of the primary target cell is not clear. It has not been possible to convincingly demonstrate the presence of EBV in oropharyngeal epithelial cells in vivo. Nevertheless, it has been shown recently, using polarized tongue and orophayngeal epithelial cells in vitro, that EBV-infected donor cells in saliva are very efficient at infecting recipient epithelial cells at their apical surface by cell–cell contact. However, these same epithelial cells are refractory to infection with free virus at their apical surface. It is also shown that neighboring epithelial cells are infected by cell–cell transmission and free virus is produced at both the apical and basolateral epithelial surfaces (Tugizov et al., 2003). Presumably, it is the latter cell-free virus that subsequently infects B-cells circulating within the oropharyngeal epithelium and oropharyngeal lymphoid tissues.

EBV infects and transforms B-cells in vitro and six EBV nuclear antigens, EBNAs 1 to 6 and two viral latent membrane-proteins, LMP1 and 2, expressed in the transformed B-cells are responsible for their changed growth and phenotype. These latency antigens potentially offer a range of targets for vaccine-induced cell-mediated immune responses. Healthy seropositive individuals carry CD8+ T-cells that are specific for epitopes in the latent antigens, in particular EBNA3, 4 and 6. However, EBV gene expression in infected B-cells in vivo is quite different and the growth-transformed phenotype has only been detected in the B-cell follicles of tonsils while in peripheral blood, EBV is detected only in a very small number of resting memory B-cells when EBV gene expression is restricted to LMP2 or does not occur at all (Thorley-Lawson, 2001).

A normal healthy immune response appears to be essential in maintaining the asymptomatic carrier-state as demonstrated by the occurrence of post-transplant lymphoproliferative disease (PTLD) in immunosuppressed organ transplant recipients and Non-Hodgkin's B-cell lymphomas in AIDS patients whose immune systems are seriously impaired. This strongly indicates that some aspects of EBV infection are under immune control and that vaccine-induced immune responses may be able to regulate primary infection and/or modify subsequent persistent infection. Most primary infections occur in the first few years in life and any prophylactic vaccine to control EBV diseases must allow for this. It would be a daunting task to deliver an EBV vaccine to large populations in Africa and China where primary infection occurs soon after birth.

Each EBV-associated disease probably arises for a complex set of different reasons and each may require a different vaccination strategy. Present approaches can be divided into those that seek to prevent or modify infection and those that might be used therapeutically to direct existing or de novo immune responses against the EBV-associated tumors. The therapeutic approach may prove to be particularly difficult, as, despite extensive efforts over a number of years, no tumors to date have consistently been controlled in humans by vaccine-induced immune responses. Modification of EBV infection may yet prove to be the correct approach and an interesting parallel may be drawn with a recent trial of a human papillomavirus (HPV) virus-like particle vaccine. In a trial involving 2392 young women, no cases of HPV 16 infection or cervical intraepithelial neoplasia were detected in vaccinated women in contrast to the control group (Koutsky et al., 2002). Immunotherapeutic approaches to the treatment of cervical carcinoma have so far been unsuccessful. The logistics and costs associated with mass HPV vaccination of populations at risk will probably exceed those likely to be incurred with a prophylactic EBV vaccine and would at least set an important precedent if adopted as a public health measure.

Infection by more than one strain of EBV in both healthy and immunocompromised individuals appears to be unexceptional (Walling et al., 2003). This raises difficult questions about the induction of immunity by EBV infection itself and about what vaccine-induced immune responses could realistically be expected to achieve. Infection by more than one strain simultaneously from one donor would not rule out the presence of subsequent virus-induced protective immune responses. However, if a second strain were able to infect an individual following an earlier infection with another strain, then it would suggest that the second EBV strain is able to evade the broad spectrum of humoral and cellular immune responses induced by the first EBV infection. A precedent for this situation has been found earlier with cytomegalovirus (Bale et al., 1996). Another consequence of the existence of several strains of EBV is that strain differences will have to be incorporated into any prophylactic or therapeutic vaccine formulations that contain elements that differ between strains.

Since EBV infection is almost completely non-permissive in vitro, it is still not technically feasible to produce EBV itself on a large enough scale to support even a small vaccine trial where killed or attenuated forms could be used. Moreover, since EBV has been formally classified as a Grade I carcinogen (Ablashi et al., 1997), and a number of its genes can independently transform certain cell types, the use of killed, attenuated or recombinant EBV vaccines can probably be ruled out for the time being. The possible composition of an EBV vaccine must be restricted to viral components that are non-transforming, however, this need not exclude non-transforming derivatives of viral transforming gene products such as synthetic peptides.

EBV causes infectious mononucleosis (IM), post-transplant lymphoproliferative disease (PTLD) and is associated with undifferentiated nasopharyngeal carcinoma (NPC), certain types of Hodgkin's lymphoma (HL), certain T-cell lymphomas, a subset of gastric carcinomas, and endemic Burkitt's lymphoma (BL). It is conceivable that a prophylactic vaccine or a postinfection vaccine that could modify but not prevent EBV infection could reduce the incidence of all diseases associated with EBV. The fact that increased antibody levels against virus capsid antigen

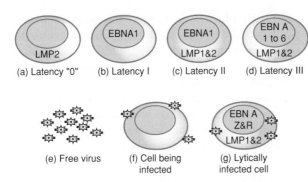

Fig. 72.1. Potential targets for EBV vaccine-induced immune responses.

In addition to the virus itself there are at least six different potential cellular targets for vaccine-induced immune responses. (**a**) Resting memory B-cells in which only LMP2 transcripts have been detected (Latence 0). These cells are few in number, there being only ~1 per 10^6 B-cells in the peripheral circulation, and are probably immunologically invisible; (**b**) BL cells are the only known example where EBNA1 is the sole EBV product and is usually referred to as Latency I. EBNA1 is not presented in an MHC class I context but is probably presented in a MHC class II context to CD4+ T-cell; (**c**) Infected B-cells in the default program where EBNA1, LMP1 and LMP2 are expressed. It has been hypothesized that this program allows for the differentiation of infected B-lymphoblasts into memory cells and provides signals necessary to maintain the infected blast cell against a background of immunological signals that would normally promote either proliferation or apoptosis. This program is often referred to as Latency II and the same or similar EBV latency gene expression profile is found in NPC and HD tumor cells; (**d**) All EBV latency genes are expressed and the cell is activated to become a proliferating lymphoblast and is referred to as being in the growth program or Latency III. This latency type is found in PTLD and some BL and could represent a good target for vaccine-induced immune responses through the EBNA3 family of products. (**e**) Free virus found in the oropharynx and at the basolateral face of the oropharyngeal epithelium may be subject to control by virus-neutralizing antibodies; (**f**) B-cells in the process of being infected may be the subject of antibody and cell-mediated control; (**g**) A small minority of infected B-cells will enter the lytic cycle and are potential targets for both cell-mediated and humoral responses.

(VCA) are prognostic for both BL and NPC suggests that immune intervention prior to the onset of disease could be beneficial. The success of such approaches will depend on whether the apparent reactivation of EBV is associated with the cause of NPC or is simply a consequence of tumor development.

Figure 72.1 illustrates the possible targets for vaccine-induced immune responses. These include free virus itself that might be susceptible to inactivation by vaccine-induced circulating or mucosal neutralizing antibodies. Naturally occurring virus-neutralizing antibodies are generated mainly against the major envelope glycoprotein, gp350 and much early work in EBV vaccine development focused on producing recombinant forms of this molecule (Morgan, 1992). Gp350 is also a target for cell-mediated responses (Khanna et al., 1999a,b,c; Wilson et al., 1999; Adhikary et al., 2006). Other lytic cycle products such as gp85, gp42, the gB homologue and the products of the BZLF1, BMRF1, BDLF3 and BILF2 open reading frames have not been investigated in the context of vaccine development. CD8+ T-cell responses against BZLF1 predominate in healthy seropositives and vaccine-induced immune responses against BZLF1 in EBV seronegatives might have a role to play. It is not known how many EBV-infected B-cells enter the lytic cycle or the location of the cells that do. Very few B-cells infected and transformed with EBV in vitro enter the lytic cycle, being less than 5%. Since free virus is shed in the oropharynx, it is assumed that epithelial cells and/or B-cells in this region are responsible and might therefore be regulated by immune responses. It must be assumed for the time being that vaccine-induced immune responses against lytic cycle products would act on these cells and/or the virus they produce. The increased oral shedding of EBV in immunosuppressed patients is consistent with this view (Preiksaitis et al., 1992). Current strategies to control EBV disease by vaccination are described below, while adoptive T-cell immunotherapy for these diseases is described elsewhere in this volume.

Vaccines to prevent infectious mononucleosis

In the wealthier Western societies primary EBV infection is often delayed until adolescence whereupon it gives rise to IM in 30% and 50% of individuals. It is still an open question as to why the remaining 50% to 70% of individuals become infected without symptoms or disease. However, it has been found that asymptomatic individuals display broad expansions of their TcR repertoire, while acute IM donors show oligoclonal expansion of TcR families (Silins et al., 2001). Perhaps of even greater interest is the small minority who apparently never become infected. A higher production of IFNα and IL-6 and a greater number of monocytes were detected in cultures of peripheral blood lymphocytes from EBV-seronegative adults (Jabs et al., 1996). The genetic and immunological differences between EBV seropositives and seronegatives remains obscure but would be informative as far as vaccine design is concerned. Since these immunological parameters are unknown, a vaccine cannot be designed on an entirely rational basis. IM almost always resolves itself over a relatively short time and is only very rarely fatal. The question arises as to whether large-scale vaccination of otherwise healthy children is justified when set against the actual risks of illness and its socio-economic consequences.

Which stages in the process and maintenance of EBV infection are susceptible to control by vaccination? What target antigens need to be recognized by vaccine-induced immune responses to prevent IM? The differentiation pathways of EBV-infected cells, the types of B-cell that are infected and the EBV proteins expressed in vivo have been tentatively identified and include a memory B-cell that may only express LMP2, a proliferating and activated B-cell expressing the full panel of EBV latent genes in the growth program or Latency III, and B-cells in Latency II which may subsequently generate the memory reservoir B-cells (Thorley-Lawson, 2001). Cells in Latency III have only been found in the germinal center of lymphoid follicles and these are regions in which cytotoxic T-cells (CTL) are poorly represented probably because EBV-specific CD8 T-cells lack homing receptors for lymphoid infection sites (Chen et al., 2001). CD4+ T-cells are detectable at low frequency within B-cell follicles and may, therefore, interact directly with EBV-infected B-cells at this site. It is possible that CD4+ T-cells primed by gp350 or latency antigen vaccination would become reactivated on viral challenge (Adhikary et al., 2006). Such cells could influence the course of IM by inducing apoptosis of EBV-infected B-cells within infected lymph nodes and by down regulating the large monoclonal or oligoclonal populations of CD8+ T-cells that account for much of the lymphocytosis that is symptomatic of IM.

Prophylactic EBV vaccine development has focused on the gp350 and EBNA3 antigens. Systemic virus neutralizing antibodies can be easily induced by vaccination with gp350 and an appropriate adjuvant and, while epithelial cell infection may be unaffected, it is conceivable that free virus liberated on the basolateral surface of infected oropharyngeal epithelium could be neutralized and minimize transmission to circulating naïve B-cells. While infection itself will not be prevented, the effective virus dose at the B-cell level would be greatly diminished. The induction of mucosal immune responses in the orapharynx may prove to be more effective and the oral/nasal administration of gp350 in conjunction with mucosal adjuvants such as Iscoms (Wilson et al., 1999), cholera toxin B-subunit or the E.coli heat labile enterotoxin B-subunit, EtxB (Williams et al., 1999), should be investigated. However, there is some evidence that mucosal IgA specific for gp350 actually enhances infection of certain epithelial cells in vitro (Gan et al., 1997).

The strategy would be to prevent or modify primary EBV infection by vaccination of children before primary infection. The disease itself is caused by excessive CD8+ T-cell responses to EBV infection, and in particular, to EBV lytic antigens. Any vaccine that could allow a more rigorous control of the primary infection phase may therefore prevent the disease or reduce its severity. Other explanations for the pathogenesis of IM, unconnected to the dose of virus at primary infection, are possible and include differences in NK and CD4+ T-cell responses (Wilson & Morgan, 2002), expansion of a CD28 subset of CD4+ T-cells (Uda et al., 2002) and autoimmune responses (McClain et al., 2003). Until these issues are better understood, it will be difficult to take account of them.

Gp350

The major EBV envelope glycoprotein, gp350, binds to the CR2 complement receptor on B-cells and is consistent with it being a target for neutralizing antibodies. Following attachment the virus infects the target cell through envelope fusion events involving other EBV envelope glycoproteins gp85, gp42 and gp25 (Borza & Hutt-Fletcher, 2002). More recent work has shown that gp350 is not an absolute requirement for EBV infection to take place. A recombinant EBV in which the gp350 gene had been deleted was able infect a range of B-cell lines and epithelial cells, albeit at a lower efficiency (Janz et al., 2000). The early observation that serum EBV neutralizing antibodies largely recognized the major viral envelope glycoprotein, gp350 set the scene for subsequent work over a number of years involving a New World primate, the cottontop tamarin (*Saguinus oedipus Oedipus*). Oligoclonal B-cell lymphomas closely resembling those seen in post-transplant lymphoproliferative disease (PTLD) can be routinely induced in these animals by injection of EBV. The characterization and purification of tractable quantities of the gp350 viral envelope glycoprotein from both natural sources and by recombinant DNA methods was carried out. Recombinant gp350 in combination with adjuvants or when expressed in vaccinia or adenovirus vectors, induced protective immunity in cottontop tamarins susceptible to EBV-induced B-cell lymphoma. Protective immunity was not dependent on the induction of gp350-specific neutralizing antibodies but was achieved through cell-mediated immune responses (Morgan, 1992). Gp350 vaccine formulations have since been shown to induce CTL responses as well as neutralizing antibody (Khanna et al., 1999c, Wilson et al., 1996). The mechanism of protection in this animal model is unknown. Did the protective responses induced in the tamarin act on the virus or on tumor cells? Since the tumor cells have a Latency III phenotype and do not express gp350, the induced immune responses were probably able to reduce the effective virus dose on challenge since the induction of tumors by EBV is dose dependent. Derivatives of the gp350 vaccines described above (Jackman et al., 1999) have been evaluated in human trials (Denis, 2005). The results of these trials strongly indicate that gp350 vaccination of seronegative young adults prevents IM but does not prevent EBV infection. Surprisingly, little attention has been placed on developing DNA vaccines coding for gp350. Immunization of mice with such a vector gave rise to antibodies to gp350, antibody-dependent cellular cytotoxicity (ADCC) and gp350-specific CTLs (Jung et al., 2001).

The cottontop tamarin has a number of shortcomings as a model of EBV infection and disease. This species is not infected by the oral route and does not sustain a persistent infection. A further complication is that the tamarin has an unusually restricted histocompatibility complex polymorphism and only expresses the alleles G, F, and E, associated primarily with NK cell function (Cadavid et al., 1999). Moreover, contrary to earlier beliefs, tamarins and marmosets have been found to carry their own resident γ-herpesviruses (de Thoisy et al., 2003).

A recombinant derivative of the Chinese vaccinia Tien Tan strain expressing gp350 was used to vaccinate a small group of both seronegative and seropositive children in Southern China. Antibody levels to gp350 were raised in seropositive subjects and were induced in those who were seronegative at the beginning of the trial. Six out of nine vaccinated children who were seronegative for EBV at the time of vaccination remained seronegative for at least three years after vaccination (Gu et al., 1995). The particular vaccinia recombinant used in this trial would not be currently acceptable for large-scale use on safety grounds. The Modified Vaccinia Ankara (MVA) strain would provide an acceptable alternative vector (Stittelaar et al., 2001).

Some development work has been carried out on the generation of a recombinant varicella zoster virus (VZV) vaccine vector for the delivery of EBV genes and VZV recombinants were produced which are able to express EBV gp350 (Lowe et al., 1987). It may be timely to explore this option further given the success of the Oka VZV vaccine strain and its incorporation into national vaccine programs in the USA, Japan and elsewhere.

A murine γ-herpesvirus (MHV 68) is increasingly being used to model EBV biology and this virus induces a mononucleosis-like syndrome in mice (Blackman et al., 2000). Vaccination studies have been carried out using this model and the MHV 68 major envelope glycoprotein gp150, an analogue of EBV gp350 (Stewart et al., 1996) was incorporated into a recombinant vaccinia virus vector and used to vaccinate mice prior to intranasal challenge with MHV 68. Virus-neutralizing antibodies were induced and the mononucleosis-like syndrome normally caused by MHV 68 was almost completely eliminated. MHV 68 latency was established in the vaccinated mice nevertheless (Stewart et al., 1999). These results are a cause for some optimism in that appropriately administered EBV gp350 could prevent IM even if the establishment of latent, persistent EBV infection was unaffected.

EBNA3

Another approach using synthetic peptides based on the EBNA3 latent antigen, to induce cell-mediated immune responses, was developed in parallel and has also been the subject of small-scale human trials (Khanna et al., 1999a,b,c). This approach utilizes latent antigen epitopes restricted through common MHC class I alleles to induce CD8+ T-cell responses in the vaccinee. Strong support for this approach came from the demonstration that autologous CD8+ T-cells against EBNA3, propagated ex vivo and introduced into immunosuppressed patients at high risk of PTLD, were able to prevent PTLD and in some cases cause PTLD to regress (Gottschalk et al., 2002). In other words, CTLs specific for some EBV latent antigens can control the propagation of EBV-infected B-cell tumors in vivo. A Phase I human trial has been carried out to establish whether an EBNA 3 synthetic peptide, FLRGRAYGL, incorporated into a water-in-oil emulsion adjuvant, can be safely used to induce epitope-specific CTL responses (Moss et al., 1998). Ultimately, a collection of epitopes will be used to span the majority of HLA types and encompass strain variation in target populations. Similar strategies may be adopted with peptide epitopes from lytic cycle antigens such as gp350 and BZLF1. Until it is known which T-cell specificities are important in protecting against IM, there may be a case for constructing an epitope vaccine using epitopes from both lytic and latent antigens. Vaccination with a latency antigen inserted into a DNA plasmid expression vector has been tested in the MHV 68 murine γ-herpesvirus model using the M2 latency-associated gene. M2 DNA vaccination had no effect on virus replication in the lung but did reduce the latently infected cell burden in the early, but not the later, stages of infection (Usherwood et al., 2001).

One serious hurdle for peptide-based vaccines is the relatively large number of epitopes that would need to be incorporated into a single vaccine so that it could be delivered to a wide range of individuals with different HLA types. A vaccine formulation with so many components may face difficulties with regulatory approval. This problem can be overcome using polyepitope constructs (Thomson et al., 1996). The polyepitope corresponds to the linking of minimalized CTL epitopes within a single coding sequence as a "string of beads" and has been shown to be highly efficient in inducing protective CTL responses when delivered as part of a live viral vector or a recombinant DNA plasmid (Thomson et al., 1998, 1996). Gp350 subunit vaccines avoid these problems since all possible epitopes are contained within the whole protein and sequence variation between different EBV isolates appears to be minimal. To what extent do CTLs reactivated from memory T-cells by autologous LCLs and assayed against peptide-coated targets, or targets infected with vaccinia recombinants, reflect in vivo CTL activities? The therapeutic effects on PTLD, of EBV-specific CTLs grown ex vivo, support the view that CTLs of one or other latent antigen are responsible for these effects (Sherritt et al., 2003). Which cell types and which antigen specificities are responsible for the beneficial effects of infusion of ex vivo grown T-cells, is not yet clear.

Vaccines to prevent post-transplant lymphoproliferation disease

Approximately 10% of seronegative children receiving solid organ transplants develop PTLD during the first year after transplant. The five-year survival of patients who develop PTLD is poor being only 35% for renal transplant recipients and 26% for heart transplant recipients. The risk of developing significant morbidity or PTLD following primary EBV infection in non-immune transplant recipients is about 20 times greater than in seropositive transplant recipients. Pediatric transplant patients are much more likely to be seronegative than adult patients since EBV infection increases with increasing age. Primary EBV infection occurs in about 70% of all seronegative recipients during the first 6 months following transplantation. This is the period during which the most intensive immunosuppression occurs. Immunization of seronegative patients before transplantation provides a realistic opportunity to test whether the presence of antibody to EBV or residual EBV-specific T-cell responses still active during immunosuppression will protect against infection, spread or pathogenic effects of EBV following transplantation.

Therapeutic vaccines to prevent Hodgkin's disease and nasopharygeal carcinoma

Of the interventions designed to treat human malignancies, immunotherapy with CTL is increasingly being recognized as potentially the most efficient strategy with minimal side effects (Savoldo et al., 2000; Bollard et al., 2004; Straathof et al., 2005). The key factors in the development of a CTL-based therapeutic strategy are the characterization of therapeutic immune correlates, and the delineation of the specific portions of the tumor-associated antigens that elicit these responses. $CD8^+$ CTLs are considered important for protection against various virus-associated malignancies and have emerged as the major element in the immune control of malignant cells (Khanna et al., 1999b). Indeed, a number of studies have recently been published, which have shown that adoptive immunotherapy can be successfully used to reverse the outgrowth of polyclonal B-cell lymphomas in transplant patients (Khanna et al., 1999a,b,c; Rooney et al., 2002).

Approximately half of HD cases involve EBV-positive tumor cells while all cases of undifferentiated NPC are EBV positive. Prophylactic vaccination of seronegative children or seropositive adults could lead to the reduction or elimination in the incidence of HD and NPC. However, the logistics, potential costs, and timescale of such a program may be disproportionate when seen in the context of other health priorities such as hepatitis, cervical carcinoma, malaria, HIV and others.

Despite being quite different cell types and at different locations, HD and NPC tumor cells express the EBV latent antigens, EBNA1, LMP1 and LMP2 and these are potential targets for the immune system. It is, therefore, surprising that the immune system is not able to kill these cells and indicates that viral immune evasion mechanisms are operating. One aspect of this phenomenon is already partly understood in so far as EBNA1 includes a glycine-alanine repeat (GAr) domain that not only may block its proteasomal degradation but also inhibits EBNA1 mRNA translation in cis (Yin et al., 2003). Whether EBNA1 is degraded and processed in an MHC class I pathway in epithelial cells seems to depend on the type of epithelial cell. When EBNA1 is artificially expressed in epithelial cells of squamous origin, it appears to both inhibit growth and be degraded in a way that renders the cells targets for HLA-matched EBNA1-specific CTLs. Neither of these phenomena were observed when EBNA1 was expressed in epithelial cells of glandular origin (Jones et al., 2003). Despite the presence of significant numbers of EBNA1-specific T-cells generated by cross-priming (Blake et al., 2000), NPC and HD cells are not effectively targeted. More recent studies have shown that epitopes from EBNA1 can be endogenously processed and presented on the cell surface. These epitopes are primarily derived from newly synthesized protein as defective ribosomal products (Tellam et al., 2004). LMP1 and LMP2 are potential targets and CTLs specific for epitopes in these proteins are found in the circulation, albeit at relatively low levels and CTL responses to LMP epitopes are said to be subdominant in relation to CTL responses to epitopes in EBNA3 and in BZLF1. T-cell responses and antibody responses against LMP1 have been difficult to detect in humans (Khanna et al., 1998a; Meij et al., 2002). Both LMP1 and LMP2 may interfere with their own MHC class I presentation and may be poor targets and/or weak inducers of CTLs (Dukers et al., 2000; Ong et al., 2003). LMP1 and LMP2 have a plethora of effects on the biochemistry of EBV-infected cells some of which could impact on antigenic processing and presentation as well as on cell growth and differentiation (Dawson et al., 2003; Portis and Longnecker, 2003). Another important observation in regard to CTL recognition of LMP1 and LMP2 is that the majority of the T-cell epitopes from these proteins are processed through a TAP-independent pathway (Khanna et al., 1996; Lee et al., 1996). TAP-deficient LCLs expressing LMP proteins are more efficiently recognized by LMP-specific CTLs than TAP-positive LCLs. These observations suggest that in the absence of TAP, ER generated LMP epitopes are presented more efficiently. On the other hand, presentation of these epitopes may be significantly reduced if TAP is expressed, as the peptides originating from the cytoplasmic compartment compete with ER generated LMP epitopes. It is therefore tempting to speculate that LMP-positive NPC and HD cells may have evolved to maintain TAP expression which limits the presentation of CTL epitopes from LMP1 and LMP2 and thus allows these tumors to escape CTL recognition in vivo.

Broadly speaking, two types of approach to therapeutic vaccination to treat NPC, HD and BL can be adopted. First, specific enhancement of effector cell responses to EBV proteins expressed in these cancers and secondly, enhancement of the presentation of the antigens in question by the tumor cells themselves. CTLs specific for LMP2 are detected in the circulation of NPC patients but are not found in the tumor lymphocyte infiltrate. NPC and HD cells also appear to have a normal MHC class I presentation pathway, at least in terms of MHC class I and TAP expression (Khanna et al., 1998b; Lee et al., 1998). Since both these cancers express identical viral proteins, it is anticipated that common immunotherapeutic protocols may be developed. It is important to remember that even if antigen presentation is unimpeded and specific CTLs are present at the tumor site in sufficient numbers, numerous other mechanisms, not necessarily related to EBV products, may prevent tumors cells being removed by the immune system (Gandhi et al., 2006). There are many elements of the CTL recognition and target cell destruction process that have not yet been evaluated for NPC and HD tumor cells. These could include the expression of coreceptors and adhesion molecules, production of cytokines that provide an inappropriate milieu for CTLs, production of T-cell inhibitory receptors such as Fas, altered proteasome function and other tumor cell-specific factors.

Recent studies on HL patients have indicated that regulatory T-cells and LAG-3 play a pivotal role in suppressing EBV-specific T cell immunity (Gandhi et al., 2006.)

LMP polyepitope vaccines

Although adoptive transfer of EBV-specific T cells has recently been tested for the treatment of relapsed HD, only a limited long-term therapeutic benefit was observed (Roskrow et al., 1998). One of the major limiting factors in the development of an efficient therapeutic strategy is the viral antigens expressed in these malignancies are not only poorly immunogenic but also in some cases have the potential to initiate an independent neoplastic process in normal cells. Thus a strategy which can overcome both these potential limitations is likely to provide a safe and long-term therapeutic benefit to cancer patients.

One such strategy involves the delivery of immunogenic determinants from LMP1 and LMP2 as a polyepitope vaccine. Indeed, initial studies from one of our laboratories have shown that multiple HLA class-I-restricted LMP1 CTL epitopes, when used as a polyepitope vaccine in a poxvirus vector, efficiently induced a strong CTL response and this response could reverse the outgrowth of LMP1-expressing tumors in HLA-A2 K^b mice (Duraiswamy et al., 2003b, 2004). A polyepitope-based vaccine for HD and NPC has a number of advantages over the traditionally proposed vaccines, which are based on full-length LMP antigens. Previous studies from our laboratory have indicated that polyepitope proteins are extremely unstable within the cytoplasm and may be rapidly degraded as a result of their limited secondary and tertiary structure. In contrast, full-length LMP antigens are unlikely to be degraded rapidly and may initiate various intracellular signalling events leading to the development of secondary cancers at the site of injection. Another important advantage includes the ability of a polyepitope vaccine to induce long-term protective CTL responses against a large number of CTL epitopes using a relatively small construct without any obvious need for a cognate help. Finally, the polyepitope-based vaccine is also likely to overcome any potential problem with the prevalence of LMP1 genetic variants in different ethnic groups of the world (Duraiswamy et al., 2003a).

Although the poxvirus polyepitope vaccine vector provides long-lived expression of encoded epitopes, there are concerns in terms of its safety profile with adverse side effects including postvaccine encephalitis when used in humans. Moreover, the poxvirus-based LMP1-polyepitope vaccine contained only HLA A2-restricted epitopes and the

HLA A2 allele is carried by only about 55% of the individuals in most populations. If a CTL-based therapy for NPC and HD is to be applicable to a significant number of patients, the target population must be presented through HLA alleles present at high frequency in the patient population. In this context, in addition to LMP1, LMP2-specific responses restricted through A11, A24 and B40 are of particular interest because these alleles are very common in the Southern Chinese population (A11, 56%; A24, 27%; B40, 28%), particularly where NPC is endemic. To overcome these potential limitations, a novel approach has been devised of activating LMP-specific CTL responses with a replication-incompetent adenovirus encoding multiple epitopes from LMP1 and LMP2 (Duraiswamy et al., 2004). This replication-incompetent adenovirus vaccine contains both LMP1 and LMP2 epitopes restricted through HLA alleles common in different ethnic groups including NPC endemic regions (HLA A2, A11, A23, A24, A27, B40 and B57). It has been estimated that these optimally selected MHC class I-restricted epitopes would include more than 90% of the Asian, African and Caucasian populations. Attractive features of adenovirus-based vaccines are their well-characterized genetic arrangement and function, as well as their extensive and safe usage in North American army recruits without inducing adverse side effects (Imler, 1995). Adenovirus-based vectors are being increasingly recognized for high efficiency and low toxicity and have been used in multiple human gene therapy clinical trials and preclinical vaccine applications. These vectors are also increasingly being used for cancer immunotherapy (Kusumoto et al., 2001). Two of the most promising recent reports were studies in non-human primate models of the Ebola virus and HIV (Shiver et al., 2002; Sullivan et al., 2000). In each study, an immunization regimen that included priming with plasmid DNA followed by boosting with adenovirus vector particles showed the induction of effective CTL responses when compared with the plasmid DNA alone (Sullivan et al., 2000). This new polyepitope vaccine is based on an E1/E3-deleted recombinant adenovirus comprising a chimeric Ad5/F35 vector that has been engineered to substitute the shorter-shafted fiber protein from Ad35 strain. This expression system provides an advantage over previous Ad5 vectors with respect to efficiency of expression of recombinant protein in hematopoietic stem cells and dendritic cells (Yotnda et al., 2001). Our studies with the Ad5F35 LMP polyepitope vaccine have shown that each of the epitopes in this vaccine is not only efficiently processed endogenously by the human cells but also recalls memory CTL responses specific for LMP antigens in healthy virus carriers and HD patients. Furthermore, the adenoviral polyepitope vaccine is capable of inducing a primary T-cell response, which was shown to be therapeutic in a tumour challenge system (Smith et al., 2006).

Altered antigen processing of LMPs using bacterial toxins

Since NPC is an epithelial tumor at a mucosal surface, the question of whether mucosal vaccine adjuvants might have a role to play in their treatment has been considered. One such adjuvant that has reached an advanced stage of development is the cholera toxin-like E. coli heat labile enterotoxin B-subunit (EtxB) (Williams et al., 1999). Bacterial protein toxins are molecules that combine unique cell binding with efficient cytosolic delivery properties. Toxoid derivatives of the adenylate cyclase toxin of Bordetella pertussis, pertussis toxin, anthrax toxin, and Shiga toxin B subunit have been investigated as potential vehicles for delivery of exogenous peptides or proteins into the MHC class I presentation pathway (de Haan and Hirst, 2002). Recent work has established that EtxB possesses important features that makes it uniquely placed to be used as a delivery vehicle for MHC class I-restricted T-cell responses (De Haan et al., 2002).

LMP-1 and LMP-2 are colocalized within plasma membrane GM_1-rich lipid rafts in LCLs (Higuchi et al., 2001). LMP1 can be ubiquitinated and degraded through a proteasome pathway (Aviel et al., 2000) while the LMP2 intracellular N-terminal polypeptide binds Nedd4-like ubiquitin ligases and is also subject to proteasomal processing (Ikeda et al., 2002). MHC class I-restricted antigen presentation of LMP2 is unusual as some, but not all, epitopes are presented independently of TAP (Khanna et al., 1996; Lee et al., 1996). It is unclear at present why LMPs are not always effectively presented to CTL by LCLs in the absence of peptide epitope pre-sensitization or LMP2 expression by recombinant vaccinia. However, it has been shown that the treatment of EBV-positive LCLs with EtxB results in colocalization, capping and internalisation of LMP1 and 2. EtxB itself binds the ganglioside, GM_1, at the plasma membrane, enters the cell by endocytosis, and then the trans-Golgi network or endoplasmic reticulum by retrograde trafficking. LCLs treated with EtxB show a greatly increased susceptibility to killing by LMP1 and LMP2-specific CTLs (Ong et al., 2003). The mechanism by which EtxB causes this enhancement of antigen presentation by LCLs requires further investigation but these results indicate that EtxB interferes with the normal distribution and pathways of LMP turnover (Ong et al., 2003). The possibility therefore exists that EtxB could serve both as a mucosal adjuvant in the conventional sense by enhancing mucosal immune responses in the nasopharynx and also by enhancing the presentation of LMP1 and LMP2 in NPC tumor cells in vivo. Further work is needed to establish whether EtxB can enhance the CTL killing of EBV-infected epithelial cells expressing LMP1 and/or LMP2 as it does for LCLs. To this end, it has recently been shown in one of the authors' laboratories that EtxB enhances the killing by LMP2-specific CTLs of H103 oral epithelial carcinoma cells expressing LMP2 (O. Salim, A. D. Wilson and A. J. Morgan, unpublished data).

One explanation for the failure of the immune system to kill HD and NPC tumor cells is that expression levels of the main potential immunological target, LMP2, are too low. Indeed, the unequivocal detection of LMP2 protein as opposed to RNA transcript in NPC cells has yet to be achieved. An EBV-transformed LCL, stably transfected with a plasmid expressing LMP2A under the control of an ecdysone analogue Ponasterone A (No et al., 1996), has been created in one of our laboratories. Following exposure to Ponasterone A, the level of LMP2A was increased ten fold and was localized in the plasma membrane. Increased LMP2A expression resulted in the up-regulation of LMP1 expression, and had a blocking effect on the EBV spontaneous lytic cycle by down-regulating the expression of both the BZLF1 and BRLF1 genes. In normal LCL, LMP2 is not efficiently processed or presented to CTLs by MHC class I (Dukers et al., 2000; Ong et al., 2003). The tenfold increase in LMP2A expression induced by Ponasterone A did not result in any increase in lysis by an MHC class I restricted LMP2A specific CTL line. Susceptibility to CTL lysis was enhanced by treatment with EtxB but the enhancement was only marginally higher in the Ponasterone A-induced targets compared to the controls with normal levels of LMP2 (G. Patsos, A.D. Wilson, and A.J. Morgan, unpublished data). These data suggest that LMP2 processing and presentation is impaired in some way and that access to different, more efficient presentation pathways, will render LMP2-expressing cells more susceptible to specific CTLs.

Therapeutic vaccines for Burkitt's lymphoma

Whether prophylactic vaccination with EBV gp350 or latent antigen polyepitope formulations would prevent or reduce the incidence of endemic BL remains an open question. Raised levels of antibody against VCA are prognostic for BL and it has been suggested that control of EBV replication by vaccination before primary infection or before ant-VCA levels rise may have a protective effect. The prospect of devising a therapeutic vaccine for BL is rather problematical because of the absence of MHC class I-mediated antigen targets. Endemic BL cells were thought to express EBNA1 only but it has recently been found that three out of fifteen EBV-positive endemic BLs tested also expressed a truncated EBNA LP, EBNA3a, 3b and 3c (Kelly et al., 2002). Although CTLs specific for the EBNA3 family may be abundant in these patients, it has been argued that the absence of LMP1 expression in the tumor cells does not allow the up regulation of antigen processing machinery. LMP1 may upregulate antigen-presenting functions in B-cells through an NF-κB pathway (Pai et al., 2002).

The restriction of EBV gene expression to EBNA1 and a consistent loss of antigen processing function through the MHC class I pathway in BL cells, severely restricts the potential use of antigen-specific immunotherapeutic strategies. However, recent studies have provided some promising alternative therapeutic strategies for these malignancies. One such strategy involves targeting the tumor cells through virus-specific CD4+ CTLs. Previous studies from one of our laboratories have shown that BL cell lines displaying antigen processing defects through the MHC class I pathway are efficiently recognized by EBV-specific CD4+ CTLs. Furthermore, these tumor cells also express normal levels of all the essential components involved in the processing of T-cell epitopes through the MHC class II pathway. The importance of these studies has been further strengthened by the observation that CD4+ EBNA1-specific CTLs from healthy virus carriers can efficiently recognize virus-infected normal B-cells as well as BL cells expressing EBNA1 only (Munz et al., 2000; Paludan et al., 2002). These observations demonstrate that it may be possible to target EBNA1 through the MHC class II pathway (Paludan et al., 2005). It raises the possibility that a vaccine based on EBNA1 that induces a strong CD4 T cell response may provide therapeutic benefit to BL patients.

One attractive way to deliver EBNA1 through the MHC class II pathway is to enable this antigen to gain access to endosomal or lysosomal compartments. There are two major pathways by which antigens are targeted to these compartments. The traditional pathway involves the phagocytosis or endocytosis of exogenous antigens, followed by degradation by acid proteases in the endosomal or lysosomal compartments. On the other hand, MHC class II-restricted presentation of endogenously synthesized proteins mainly involves membrane antigens that are thought to enter the endosomal or lysosomal pathway by internalization from the cell surface. The lysosome-associated membrane protein (LAMP-1) and the invariant chain are transmembrane proteins, which are predominantly localized in the lysosomes and endosomes, respectively. The cytoplasmic domains of these proteins contain specific targeting or address signals that mediate their translocation to the specific compartments. Previous studies from one of our laboratories have shown that these targeting signal sequences can be utilized to direct multiple MHC class II-restricted CTL epitopes into the endosomal and lysosomal compartments (Thomson et al., 1998). This approach not only preferentially translocates the polyepitope protein to these compartments but also enhances endogenous presentation of CTL epitopes. Furthermore, this strategy was successfully used to activate a virus-specific memory CTL response from peripheral blood lymphocytes. Endosome/lysosome-targeted EBNA1 is currently being tested as a therapeutic vaccine in a non-immunogenic murine B cell tumor model in which the tumor cells express EBNA1. If this vaccine strategy is successful in reversing the outgrowth of these tumor cells, it is possible that an EBNA1 vaccine may not only be applicable to BL but also against other EBV-associated malignancies such as HD and NPC.

Another interesting strategy involves treatment of the BL cells with soluble CD40 ligand (CD40L) (Khanna et al., 1997). This treatment is highly effective in reversing the down-regulated expression of antigen processing genes involved in MHC class I-restricted presentation. Moreover, CD40L-treated BL cells regain susceptibility to EBV-specific CTL-mediated lysis. These data suggest that direct infusion of soluble CD40L at tumor sites or cytokine-mediated induction of CD40 ligand on bystander lymphocytes should be considered as an alternative approach to restoring immunogenicity of malignant cells. Taken together, these preclinical studies provide an important platform for the development of a therapeutic strategy for BL based on a combination of EBNA1 vaccination and CD40L injection.

Recently, a novel approach to override the GAr-mediated proteosomal block on EBNA1 by specifically targeting this antigen for rapid degradation by a process of cotranslational ubiquitination combined with N-end rule targeting, has been explored (Tellam et al., 2001). These studies showed that enhanced intracellular degradation of EBNA1 was coincident with an induction of a very strong EBNA1-specific CTL response, and restored the endogenous processing of MHC class I-restricted CTL epitopes within EBNA1 for immune recognition by EBV-specific CTLs. It has also been shown recently that EBNA1 can be degraded in some epithelial cells of squamous origin and these cells are subsequently susceptible to MHC class I-restricted, EBNA1-specific CTLs (Jones et al., 2003). These observations raise the possibility of developing therapeutic strategies to modulate the stability of EBNA1 in normal and malignant cells. These schemes may involve treatment of virus-infected cells with synthetic or biological mediators capable of enhancing stable ubiquitination and rapid intracellular degradation of EBNA1 in vivo. Because the substrate specificity of the ubiquitin-proteasome pathway is conferred by the E3 ubiquitin-protein ligases, then one approach may involve manipulation of the ubiquitin-dependent proteolytic machinery by targeting specific E3 ubiquitin-protein ligases to direct the degradation of otherwise stable cellular proteins, such as EBNA1. Potentially, this engineered proteolysis system could be utilized as a therapeutic method to counteract the proteasomal block conferred on EBNA1 through the *cis*-acting inhibitory GAr domain.

The MHV 68 model of γ-herpesvirus infection has indicted a role for CD4+ T-cells in both the control of infection (Hogan et al., 2001) and in the control of tumor cells expressing MHV 68 antigens. When MHV 68-infected S11 cells were injected subcutaneously into nude mice, adoptively transferred lymphocytes caused the regression of S11 tumors and CD4+ T-cells were most effective in preventing tumor formation. CD4+ T-cells were also present in the regressing tumors (Robertson et al., 2001).

Conclusions

The limitations imposed on EBV vaccine design include (1) the behavior of EBV in vivo is poorly understood such that the anatomical location of infected cells, the site at which they become infected, and the site at which new virus is produced, are not known with confidence; (2) the correlates of immune protection against, or modification of, in vivo EBV infection are unknown; (3) killed or attenuated variants of EBV cannot be used as vaccines because of the oncogenic potential of the virus and a number of its components; (4) the virus infection persists for life in the face of humoral and cell mediated immune responses; (5) although numerically very significant, only a very small proportion of the infected population will develop disease. Despite the fact that recent human trials have indicated that gp350 vaccination can prevent IM, but not EBV infection, in seronegative young adults (Denis, 2005), the immunological basis for this is remains unclear. Until further human trials have taken place it is unlikely that any correlates of protective immunity against either infection or disease will become known with only limited information coming from animal models of related viruses. It is impossible to say at this stage what effects gp350 vaccine-induced mucosal or systemic immune responses might have on primary EBV infection or existing EBV infection. Once latency has been established, will immune responses in the vaccinee be more effective in preventing EBV disease than in a normal unvaccinated seropositive? Large scale and unselective prophylactic mass vaccination are presently impractical given current public health priorities and may even be unwise. Unless a clear benefit of such vaccination in a sizeable population can be demonstrated, such as in young seronegative adults in Western countries, resources will inevitably be focussed on therapeutic strategies for those who have already developed disease. Our increased knowledge of the antigen presentation and processing pathways of the main EBV-associated tumours, NPC and HD, has given rise to rational and novel immunotherapeutic strategies based on the enhancement of either LMP-specific CTLs or enhancement of LMP antigen presentation in the tumours themselves. Until recently, there were no immunotherapeutic strategies for treating endemic BL but the induction of appropriate CD4+ T-cells by vaccination may offer a way forward. The conducting of properly controlled human trials to evaluate the options set out above is clearly the first priority and little further progress can be expected until they take place.

REFERENCES

Ablashi, D., Bornkamm, G.W., Boshoff, C. *et al.* (1997). Epstein–Barr virus and Kaposi's sarcoma herpesvirus/human herpesvirus. In *IARC Monographs on the evaluation of carcinogenic risks to humans*, Lyon: IARC, pp. 497.

Adhikary, D., Behrends, V., Mossman, A., Wilter, K., Bornkamm, G. W., and Mautner, J. (2006). Control of Epstein–Barr virus infection in vitro by T helper cells specific for virion glycoproteins. *J. Exp. Med.*, **203**, 805–808.

Aviel, S., Winberg, G., Massucci, M., and Ciechanover, A. (2000). Degradation of the Epstein–Barr virus latent membrane protein 1 (LMP1) by the ubiquitin-proteasome pathway. Targeting via ubiquitination of the N-terminal residue. *J. Biol. Chem.*, **275**, 23491–23499.

Bale, J. F., Jr., Petheram, S. J., Souza, I. E., and Murph, J. R. (1996). Cytomegalovirus reinfection in young children. *J. Pediatr.*, **128**, 347–352.

Blackman, M. A., Flano, E., Usherwood, E., and Woodland, D. L. (2000). Murine gamma-herpesvirus-68: a mouse model for infectious mononucleosis? *Mol. Med. Today*, **6**, 488–490.

Blake, N., Haigh, T., Shaka'a, G., Croom-Carter, D., and Rickinson, A. (2000). The importance of exogenous antigen in priming the human CD8+ T cell response: lessons from the EBV nuclear antigen EBNA1. *J. Immunol.*, **165**, 7078–7087.

Bollard, C. M., Aguilar, L., Straathof, K. C. *et al.* (2004). Cytotoxic T lymphocyte therapy for Epstein–Barr virus+ Hodgkin's disease. *J. Exp. Med.*, **200**(12), 1623–1633.

Borza, C. M. and Hutt-Fletcher, L. M. (2002). Alternate replication in B cells and epithelial cells switches tropism of Epstein–Barr virus. *Nat. Med.* **8**, 594–599.

Cadavid, L. F., Mejia, B. E., and Watkins, D. I. (1999). MHC class I genes in a New World primate, the cotton-top tamarin (*Saguinus oedipus*), have evolved by an active process of loci turnover. *Immunogenetics*, **49**, 196–205.

Chen, G., Shankar, P., Lange, C. *et al.* (2001). CD8 T cells specific for human immunodeficiency virus, Epstein–Barr virus, and cytomegalovirus lack molecules for homing to lymphoid sites of infection. *Blood*, **98**, 156–164.

Dawson, C. W., Tramountanis, G., Eliopoulos, A. G., and Young, L. S. (2003). Epstein–Barr virus latent membrane protein 1 (LMP1) activates the phosphatidylinositol 3-kinase/Akt pathway to promote cell survival and induce actin filament remodeling. *J. Biol. Chem.*, **278**, 3694–3704.

de Haan, L., and Hirst, T. R. (2002). Bacterial toxins as versatile delivery vehicles. *Curr. Opin. Drug Discov. Devel.*, **5**, 269–278.

de Haan, L., Hearn, A. R., Rivett, A. J., and Hirst, T. R. (2002). Enhanced delivery of exogenous peptides into the class I antigen processing and presentation pathway. *Infect. Immun.*, **70**, 3249–3258.

de Thoisy, B., Pouliquen, J. F., Lacoste, V., Gessain, A., and Kazanji, M. (2003). Novel gamma-1 herpesviruses identified in free-ranging new world monkeys (golden-handed tamarin (*Saguinus midas*), squirrel monkey (*Saimiri sciureus*), and white-faced saki (*Pithecia pithecia*), in French Guiana. *J. Virol.*, **77**, 9099–9105.

Denis, M. J. (2005). The invention relates to the use of an EBV membrane antigen or derivative thereof in combination with a suitable adjuvant in the manufacture of a vaccine for the prevention of infectious mononucleosis (IM), and to vaccine compositions suitable for prevention of IM. United States Patent Application # 20050053623. http://www.uspto.gov/patft/index.html

Dukers, D. F., Meij, P., Vervoort, M. B. *et al.* (2000). Direct immunosuppressive effects of EBV-encoded latent membrane protein 1. *J. Immunol.*, **165**, 663–670.

Duraiswamy, J., Burrows, J. M., Bharadwaj, M. *et al.* (2003a). Ex vivo analysis of T-cell responses to Epstein–Barr virus-encoded oncogene latent membrane protein 1 reveals highly conserved epitope sequences in virus isolates from diverse geographic regions. *J. Virol.*, **77**, 7401–7410.

Duraiswamy, J., Sherritt, M., Thomson, S. *et al.* (2003b). Therapeutic LMP1 polyepitope vaccine for EBV-associated Hodgkin disease and nasopharyngeal carcinoma. *Blood*, **101**, 3150–3156.

Duraiswamy, J., Bharadwaj, M., Tellam, J., *et al.* (2004). Induction of therapeutic T-cell responses to subdominant tumor-associated viral oncogene after immunization with replication-incompetent polyepitope adenovirus vaccine. *Cancer Res.*, **64**(4), 1483–1489.

Gan, Y. J., Chodosh, J., Morgan, A., and Sixbey, J. W. (1997). Epithelial cell polarization is a determinant in the infectious outcome of immunoglobulin A-mediated entry by Epstein–Barr virus. *J. Virol.*, **71**, 519–526.

Gandhi, M. K., Lambley, E., Duraiswamy, J. *et al.* (2006). Expression of LAG-3 by tumor-infiltrating lymphocytes is co-incident with the suppression of latent membrane antigen-specific CD8+

T-cell function in Hodgkin lymphoma patients. *Blood*, [Epub ahead of print].

Gottschalk, S., Heslop, H. E., and Roon, C. M. (2002). Treatment of Epstein–Barr virus-associated malignancies with specific T cells. *Adv. Cancer Res.*, **84**, 175–201.

Gu, S. Y., Huang, T. M., Ruan, L. *et al.* (1995). First EBV vaccine trial in humans using recombinant vaccinia virus expressing the major membrane antigen. *Dev. Biol. Stand.*, **84**, 171–177.

Higuchi, M., Izumi, K. M., and Kieff, E. (2001). Epstein–Barr virus latent-infection membrane proteins are palmitoylated and raft-associated: protein 1 binds to the cytoskeleton through TNF receptor cytoplasmic factors. *Proc. Natl Acad. Sci. USA*, **98**, 4675–4680.

Hogan, R. J., Zhong, W., Usherwood, E. J., Cookenham, T., Roberts, A. D., and Woodland, D. L. (2001). Protection from respiratory virus infections can be mediated by antigen-specific CD4(+) T cells that persist in the lungs. *J. Exp. Med.*, **193**, 981–986.

Ikeda, M., Ikeda, A., and Longnecker, R. (2002). Lysine-independent ubiquitination of Epstein-Barr virus LMP2A. *Virology*, **300**, 153–159.

Imler, J. L. (1995). Adenovirus vectors as recombinant viral vaccines. *Vaccine*, **13**, 1143–1151.

Jabs, W. J., Wagner, H. J., Neustock, P., Kluter, H., and Kirchner, H. (1996). Immunologic properties of Epstein–Barr virus-seronegative adults. *J. Infect. Dis.*, **173**, 1248–1251.

Jackman, W. T., Mann, K. A., Hoffmann, H. J., and Spaete, R. R. (1999). Expression of Epstein–Barr virus gp350 as a single chain glycoprotein for an EBV subunit vaccine. *Vaccine*, **17**, 660–668.

Janz, A., Oezel, M., Kurzeder, C. *et al.* (2000). Infectious Epstein–Barr virus lacking major glycoprotein BLLF1 (gp350/220) demonstrates the existence of additional viral ligands. *J. Virol.*, **74**, 10142–10152.

Jones, R. J., Smith, L. J., Dawson, C. W., Haigh, T., Blake, N. W., and Young, L. S. (2003). Epstein–Barr virus nuclear antigen 1 (EBNA1) induced cytotoxicity in epithelial cells is associated with EBNA1 degradation and processing. *Virology*, **313**, 663–676.

Jung, S., Chung, Y. K., Chang, S. H. *et al.* (2001). DNA-mediated immunization of glycoprotein 350 of Epstein-Barr virus induces the effective humoral and cellular immune responses against the antigen. *Mol. Cells*, **12**, 41–49.

Kelly, G., Bell, A., and Rickinson, A. (2002). Epstein–Barr virus-associated Burkitt lymphomagenesis selects for downregulation of the nuclear antigen EBNA2. *Nat. Med.*, **8**, 1098–1104.

Khanna, R., Burrows, S. R., Moss, D. J., and Silins, S. L. (1996). Peptide transporter (TAP-1 and TAP-2)-independent endogenous processing of Epstein–Barr virus (EBV) latent membrane protein 2A: implications for cytotoxic T-lymphocyte control of EBV-associated malignancies. *J. Virol.*, **70**, 5357–5362.

Khanna, R., Cooper, L., Kienzle, N., Moss, D. J., Burrows, S. R., and Khanna, K. K. (1997). Engagement of CD40 antigen with soluble CD40 ligand up-regulates peptide transporter expression and restores endogenous processing function in Burkitt's lymphoma cells. *J. Immunol.*, **159**, 5782–5785.

Khanna, R., Burrows, S. R., Nicholls, J., and Poulsen, L. M. (1998a). Identification of cytotoxic T cell epitopes within Epstein–Barr virus (EBV) oncogene latent membrane protein 1 (LMP1): evidence for HLA A2 supertype-restricted immune recognition of EBV-infected cells by LMP1-specific cytotoxic T lymphocytes. *Eur. J. Immunol.*, **28**, 451–458.

Khanna, R., Busson, P., Burrows, S. R. *et al.* (1998b). Molecular characterization of antigen-processing function in nasopharyngeal carcinoma (NPC): evidence for efficient presentation of Epstein–Barr virus cytotoxic T-cell epitopes by NPC cells. *Cancer Res.*, **58**, 310–314.

Khanna, R., Bell, S., Sherritt, M. *et al.* (1999a). Activation and adoptive transfer of Epstein–Barr virus-specific cytotoxic T cells in solid organ transplant patients with posttransplant lymphoproliferative disease. *Proc. Natl Acad. Sci. USA*, **96**, 10391–10396.

Khanna, R., Moss, D. J., and Burrows, S. R. (1999b). Vaccine strategies against Epstein–Barr virus-associated diseases: lessons from studies on cytotoxic T-cell-mediated immune regulation. *Immunol. Rev.*, **170**, 49–64.

Khanna, R., Sherritt, M., and Burrows, S. R. (1999c). EBV structural antigens, gp350 and gp85, as targets for ex vivo virus-specific CTL during acute infectious mononucleosis: potential use of gp350/gp85 CTL epitopes for vaccine design. *J. Immunol.*, **162**, 3063–3069.

Khanna, R., Tellam, J., Duraiswamy, J., and Cooper, L. (2001). Immunotherapeutic strategies for EBV-associated malignancies. *Trends Mol. Med.*, **7**, 270–276.

Khanna, R., Moss, D. J., and Gandhi, M. (2005). Application of emerging immunotherapeutic strategies for Epstein–Barr virus-associated malignancies. *Nat. Clin. Pract. Oncol.*, **2**, 138–149.

Koutsky, L. A., Ault, K. A., Wheeler, C. M. *et al.* (2002). A controlled trial of a human papillomavirus type 16 vaccine. *N. Engl. J. Med.*, **347**, 1645–1651.

Kusumoto, M., Umeda, S., Ikubo, A. *et al.* (2001). Phase 1 clinical trial of irradiated autologous melanoma cells adenovirally transduced with human GM-CSF gene. *Cancer Immunol. Immunother.*, **50**, 373–381.

Lee, S. P., Thomas, W. A., Blake, N. W., and Rickinson, A. B. (1996). Transporter (TAP)-independent processing of a multiple membrane-spanning protein, the Epstein–Barr virus latent membrane protein 2. *Eur. J. Immunol.*, **26**, 1875–1883.

Lee, S. P., Constandinou, C. M., Thomas, W. A. *et al.* (1998). Antigen presenting phenotype of Hodgkin Reed–Sternberg cells: analysis of the HLA class I processing pathway and the effects of interleukin-10 on Epstein–Barr virus-specific cytotoxic T-cell recognition. *Blood*, **92**, 1020–1030.

Lowe, R. S., Keller, P. M., Keech, B. J. *et al.* (1987). Varicella-zoster virus as a live vector for the expression of foreign genes. *Proc. Natl Acad. Sci. USA*, **84**, 3896–3900.

McClain, M. T., Rapp, E. C., Harley, J. B., and James, J. A. (2003). Infectious mononucleosis patients temporarily recognize a unique, cross-reactive epitope of Epstein–Barr virus nuclear antigen-1. *J. Med. Virol.*, **70**, 253–257.

Meij, P., Vervoort, M. B., Bloemena, E. et al. (2002). Antibody responses to Epstein–Barr virus-encoded latent membrane protein-1 (LMP1) and expression of LMP1 in juvenile Hodgkin's disease. *J. Med. Virol.*, **68**, 370–377.

Morgan, A. J. (1992). Epstein–Barr virus vaccines. *Vaccine*, **10**, 563–571.

Moss, D. J., Suhrbier, A., and Elliott, S. L. (1998). Candidate vaccines for Epstein–Barr virus. *Br. Med. J.*, **317**, 423–424.

Munz, C., Bickham, K. L., Subklewe, M. et al. (2000). Human CD4(+) T lymphocytes consistently respond to the latent Epstein–Barr virus nuclear antigen EBNA1. *J. Exp. Med.*, **191**, 1649–1660.

No, D., Yao, T. P., and Evans, R. M. (1996). Ecdysone-inducible gene expression in mammalian cells and transgenic mice. *Proc. Natl Acad. Sci. USA*, **93**, 3346–3351.

Ong, K. W., Wilson, A. D., Hirst, T. R., and Morgan, A. J. (2003). The B subunit of *Escherichia coli* heat-labile enterotoxin enhances CD8(+) cytotoxic-T-lymphocyte killing of Epstein–Barr virus-infected cell Lines. *J. Virol.*, **77**, 4298–4305.

Pai, S., O'Sullivan, B. J., Cooper, L., Thomas, R., and Khanna, R. (2002). RelB nuclear translocation mediated by C-terminal activator regions of Epstein–Barr virus-encoded latent membrane protein 1 and its effect on antigen-presenting function in B cells. *J. Virol.*, **76**, 1914–1921.

Paludan, C., Bickham, K., Nikiforow, S. et al. (2002). Epstein–Barr nuclear antigen 1-specific CD4(+) Th1 cells kill Burkitt's lymphoma cells. *J. Immunol.*, **169**, 1593–1603.

Paludan, C., Schmid, D., Landthaler, M. et al. (2005). Endogenous MHC class II processing of a viral nuclear antigen after autophagy. *Science*, **307**(5709), 593–596.

Portis, T., and Longnecker, R. (2003). Epstein–Barr virus LMP2A interferes with global transcription factor regulation when expressed during B-lymphocyte development. *J. Virol.*, **77**, 105–114.

Preiksaitis, J. K., Diaz-Mitoma, F., Mirzayans, F., Roberts, S., and Tyrrell, D. (1992). Quantitative oropharyngeal Epstein–Barr virus shedding in renal and cardiac transplant recipients: relationship to immunosuppressive therapy, serologic responses, and the risk of posttransplant lymphoproliferative disorder. *J. Infect. Dis.*, **166**, 986–994.

Robertson, K. A., Usherwood, E. J., and Nash, A. A. (2001). Regression of a murine gammaherpesvirus 68-positive b-cell lymphoma mediated by CD4 T lymphocytes. *J. Virol.*, **75**, 3480–3482.

Rooney, C. M., Bollard, C., Huls, M. H. et al. (2002). Immunotherapy for Hodgkin's disease. *Ann. Hematol.*, **81 Suppl 2**, S39–42.

Roskrow, M. A., Rooney, C. M., Heslop, H. E. et al. (1998). Administration of neomycin resistance gene marked EBV specific cytotoxic T-lymphocytes to patients with relapsed EBV-positive Hodgkin disease. *Hum. Gene Ther.*, **9**, 1237–1250.

Savoldo, B., Heslop, H. E., and Rooney, C. M. (2000). The use of cytotoxic t cells for the prevention and treatment of Epstein–Barr virus induced lymphoma in transplant recipients. *Leuk. Lymphoma*, **39**, 455–464.

Sherritt, M. A., Bharadwaj, M., Burrows, J. M. et al. (2003). Reconstitution of the latent T-lymphocyte response to Epstein–Barr virus is coincident with long-term recovery from posttransplant lymphoma after adoptive immunotherapy. *Transplantation*, **75**, 1556–1560.

Shiver, J. W., Fu, T. M., Chen, L. et al. (2002). Replication-incompetent adenoviral vaccine vector elicits effective anti-immunodeficiency-virus immunity. *Nature*, **415**, 331–335.

Silins, S. L., Sherritt, M. A., Silleri, J. M. et al. (2001). Asymptomatic primary Epstein–Barr virus infection occurs in the absence of blood T-cell repertoire perturbations despite high levels of systemic viral load. *Blood*, **98**, 3739–3744.

Smith, C., Cooper, L., Burgess, M. et al. (2006). Functional Reversion of Antigen-specific CD8+ T cells from patients with Hodgkin Lymphoma following in vitro stimulation with recombinant polyepitope. *J. Immunol.*, **177**(7), 4897–4906.

Stewart, J. P., Janjua, N. J., Pepper, S. D. et al. (1996). Identification and characterization of murine gammaherpesvirus 68 gp150: a virion membrane glycoprotein. *J. Virol.*, **70**, 3528–3535.

Stewart, J. P., Micali, N., Usherwood, E. J., Bonina, L., and Nash, A. A. (1999). Murine gamma-herpesvirus 68 glycoprotein 150 protects against virus-induced mononucleosis: a model system for gamma-herpesvirus vaccination. *Vaccine*, **17**, 152–157.

Stittelaar, K. J., Kuiken, T., de Swart, R. L. et al. (2001). Safety of modified vaccinia virus Ankara (MVA) in immune-suppressed macaques. *Vaccine*, **19**, 3700–3709.

Straathof, K. C., Bollard, C. M., Popat, U. et al. (2005). Treatment of nasopharyngeal carcinoma with Epstein–Barr virus-specfic T lymphocytes. *Blood*, **105**(5), 1898–1904.

Sullivan, N. J., Sanchez, A., Rollin, P. E., Yang, Z. Y., and Nabel, G. J. (2000). Development of a preventive vaccine for Ebola virus infection in primates. *Nature*, **408**, 605–609.

Tellam, J., Sherritt, M., Thomson, S. et al. (2001). Targeting of EBNA1 for rapid intracellular degradation overrides the inhibitory effects of the Gly–Ala repeat domain and restores CD8+ T cell recognition. *J. Biol. Chem.*, **276**, 33353–33360.

Tellam, J., Connolly, G., Green, K. J. et al. (2004). Endogenous presentation of CD8+ T cell epitopes from Epstein–Barr-virus-encoded nuclear antigen 1. *J. Exp. Med.*, **199**(10), 1421–1431.

Thomson, S. A., Elliott, S. L., Sherritt, M. A. et al. (1996). Recombinant polyepitope vaccines for the delivery of multiple CD8 cytotoxic T cell epitopes. *J. Immunol.*, **157**, 822–826.

Thomson, S. A., Burrows, S. R., Misko, I. S., Moss, D. J., Coupar, B. E., and Khanna, R. (1998). Targeting a polyepitope protein incorporating multiple class II-restricted viral epitopes to the secretory/endocytic pathway facilitates immune recognition by CD4+ cytotoxic T lymphocytes: a novel approach to vaccine design. *J. Virol.*, **72**, 2246–2252.

Thorley-Lawson, A. D. (2001). Epstein–Barr virus: exploiting the immune system. *Nat. Rev. Immunol.*, **1**, 75–82.

Tibbetts, S. A., L. J., Van Berkel, V., McClellan, J. S., Jacoby, M. A., Kapadia, S. B., Speck, S. H., Virgin, H. W. 4th. (2003). Establishment and maintenance of gammaherpesvirus latency are independent of infective dose and route of infection. *J. Virol.* **77**, 7696–7701.

Tugizov, S. M., Berline, J. W., and Palefsky, J. M. (2003). Epstein–Barr virus infection of polarized tongue and nasopharyngeal epithelial cells. *Nat. Med.*, **9**, 307–314.

Uda, H., Mima, T., Yamaguchi, N. *et al.* (2002). Expansion of a CD28-intermediate subset among CD8 T cells in patients with infectious mononucleosis. *J. Virol.*, **76**, 6602–6608.

Usherwood, E. J., Ward, K. A., Blackman, M. A., Stewart, J. P., and Woodland, D. L. (2001). Latent antigen vaccination in a model gammaherpesvirus infection. *J. Virol.*, **75**, 8283–8288.

Walling, D. M., Brown, A. L., Etienne, W., Keitel, W. A., and Ling, P. D. (2003). Multiple Epstein–Barr virus infections in healthy individuals. *J. Virol.*, **77**, 6546–6550.

Williams, N. A., Hirst, T. R., and Nashar, T. O. (1999). Immune modulation by the cholera-like enterotoxins: from adjuvant to therapeutic. *Immunol. Today*, **20**, 95–101.

Wilson, A. D., and Morgan, A. J. (2002). Primary immune responses by cord blood CD4(+) T cells and NK cells inhibit Epstein–Barr virus B-cell transformation in vitro. *J. Virol.*, **76**, 5071–5081.

Wilson, A. D., Shooshstari, M., Finerty, S., Watkins, P., and Morgan, A. J. (1996). Virus-specific cytotoxic T cell responses are associated with immunity of the cottontop tamarin to Epstein–Barr virus (EBV). *Clin. Exp. Immunol.*, **103**, 199–205.

Wilson, A. D., Lovgren-Bengtsson, K., Villacres-Ericsson, M., Morein, B., and Morgan, A. J. (1999). The major Epstein–Barr virus (EBV) envelope glycoprotein gp340 when incorporated into Iscoms primes cytotoxic T-cell responses directed against EBV lymphoblastoid cell lines. *Vaccine*, **17**, 1282–1290.

Yin, Y., Manoury, B., and Fåhraeus, R. (2003). Self-inhibition of synthesis and antigen presentation by Epstein–Barr virus-encoded EBNA1. *Science*, **301**, 1371–1374.

Yotnda, P., Onishi, H., Heslop, H. E. *et al.* (2001). Efficient infection of primitive hematopoietic stem cells by modified adenovirus. *Gene Ther.*, **8**, 930–937.

73

DNA vaccines for human herpesviruses

Thomas G. Evans and Mary Wloch

Vical Incorporated, San Diego, CA, USA

General design of DNA vaccines

DNA vaccines are circular, double-stranded plasmid DNA (pDNA) molecules, which are capable of initiating the expression of protein antigens of interest when introduced into cells. For this purpose, the pDNA contains an eukaryotic expression cassette consisting of a transcriptional promoter, a protein coding sequence derived from the target antigen gene, and a transcriptional terminator (Fig. 73.1). Although many different promoters have been investigated, none have been shown to be clearly superior to the constitutive CMV IE promoter. DNA vaccines can consist of single genes on one plasmid, multiple genes on one plasmid, multiple plasmids, or a combination of the above. In bicistronic or tricistronic constructs, internal ribosomal entry sites (IRES) or equivalent sequences, dual or triple promoters, or cleavable linkage regions in fusion proteins can be used for expression of multiple genes. Upon transfer into cells, the pDNA enters the nucleus and transcribes a messenger RNA (mRNA) encoding the antigen of interest. The antigen can be identical to the wild-type protein of the pathogen, or can be genetically modified to improve immunogenicity and/or reduce toxicity to the host. The pDNA may also contain an antibiotic resistance gene and a bacterial origin of replication for growth and propagation in E. coli. Constructs using selection elements for bacterial replication other than antibiotic elements have also been utilized.

For vaccination, the purified pDNA is reconstituted in aqueous vehicles, or formulated and injected. A variety of delivery routes have been used, including intramuscular, intradermal, subcutaneous, transcutaneous, and mucosal (Ulmer, 2001). In the mouse, the route of delivery (e.g., intradermal versus intramuscular) may affect the antibody levels as well as the production of antigen specific Th1-like or Th2-like cytokines (Feltquate et al., 1997). DNA vaccines, in which de novo production of the relevant immunogen is achieved without the use of live agents, combine some of the positive aspects of immune stimulation inherent in live-attenuated vaccines, such as enhanced cellular immune responses, with the safety and defined antigenicity of recombinant subunit vaccines. Furthermore, pDNAs expressing different antigens can easily be co-administered in a single formulation, enabling multivalent vaccines to be designed and tested with relative ease.

Mechanism of action

To develop rational approaches for enhancing DNA vaccine potency, an understanding of the mechanism of action of DNA vaccines is essential. The mechanism by which immune responses are initiated after intramuscular DNA vaccination has been a subject of debate for many years. Early discussions centered around three possible mechanisms: direct transfection of APCs, transfer of antigen from transfected muscles to APCs, or direct T cell priming by transfected myocytes (Padoll and Beckerleg, 1995). Data from experiments in which transfected myoblasts from $H-2^k$ mice were transplanted into naïve $H-2^d \times H-2^k$ mice indicated that transgene encoded antigen could be transferred from the transfected myoblasts to host APC for generation of an antigen specific immune response (Ulmer et al., 1996). Additional reports from experiments in which chimeric mice were used to characterize the role of bone marrow-derived APCs in priming immune responses after intramuscular DNA vaccination supported the hypothesis that antigen produced by muscle cells is transferred to APCs for initiation of antigen specific immune responses (Doe et al., 1996; Corr et al., 1996). While these experiments ruled out a major role for direct T-cell priming by muscle cells, and indicated that antigen could be transferred to bone marrow-derived APC for T-cell priming, other experiments suggested that muscle expression is not critical for the generation of antigen specific immune responses after intramuscular DNA vaccination. Experiments in which injected muscles were removed within 1 to 10 minutes after injection, without diminishing the resulting B- and T-cell immune responses, argued for direct APC transfection (Torres et al., 1997). A more recent study suggested that both mechanisms, direct transfection of bone marrow derived APC and cross-priming with antigen produced by muscle cells, are involved, and that cross-priming by antigen transfer is the predominant mechanism (Corr et al., 1999). Increased local inflammatory responses with a resultant increase in APC migration to the muscle may play as great a role in cross-priming as the actual expression of gene product in the muscle. Furthermore, much of the pDNA injected into the muscle may be transported directly to the lymph nodes via the lymphatics, and thus the studies of Torres et al. may involve mechanisms other than direct APC transfection (Mena et al., 2001).

The role of dermal cell expression of DNA vaccine-encoded antigens after intradermal or gene gun vaccination is still unclear. Direct transfection of APCs upon dermal injections of DNA vaccines may play a more extensive role in the induction of immune responses to DNA vaccination than the cross-priming that occurs in muscle cells. APCs such as Langerhans cells and macrophages are more numerous in the dermis and direct transfection of these cells has been shown after intradermal DNA vaccination and DNA vaccination by gene gun (Raz et al., 1994). However, ablation of transfected dermal tissue within 24 hours of gene gun inoculation greatly diminished the antigen specific antibody response and precluded the generation of antigen specific CTL, suggesting a role for transfected dermal cells, other than migrating APCs, in the generation of an immune response after gene gun vaccination.

It is now generally believed that multiple mechanisms: cross-priming of APCs in the muscle or skin, direct transfection of APCs transiting the tissues, and uptake of pDNA by cells in the lymphatics or lymph nodes, are involved in immune response induction after DNA vaccination. However, in all of these cases, there is reason to believe that improved transfection of APCs, facilitated by the appropriate signals to allow for increased antigen or pDNA uptake, maturation, and migration to the local lymph tissues, will be critical in improving responses to DNA vaccines.

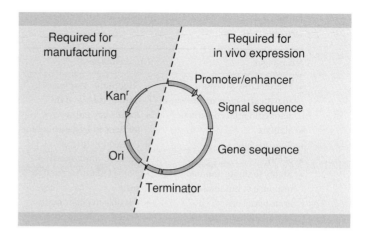

Fig. 73.1. Basic technology: plasmid DNA.

DNA vaccines: advantages and disadvantages

DNA vaccines have many advantages over other platforms, with the result that these products are used extensively as vaccine research tools. Many of these same advantages may facilitate development of therapeutic or prophylactic vaccination for herpesvirus infections (Table 73.1). In general, because gene constructs are easily modified, a very large number of differing constructs and combinations of immunogen genes can be rapidly developed and tested, which is not feasible with recombinant proteins. Injection of DNA can be readily used to investigate the function or protective effect of specific genes, combinations of genes, or effect of gene modifications. The combination of predictive algorithms for MHC Class I and II epitopes, combined with DNA vaccination in transgenic mice, has proven to be a powerful approach in antigen discovery for vaccination strategies targeting T-cell immunity.

In order to increase safety, target immunogens can be genetically modified to specifically, stably and uniformly remove biologically active regions of the proteins. For example, kinase or transactivating activity of key herpesvirus proteins can be removed, and yet the genes that contain the key T-cell or B-cell epitopes, regions, or exons of the gene can be retained. The effect of using a secretory leader or removal of transmembrane and cytoplasmic sequences can also be readily evaluated. Furthermore, the effect of glycosylation sites, minor amino acid changes, or the effects of combination genes that may form neutralization complexes (such as the gH/gL/gO complex in CMV, gH/gL complex in HSV, or gE/gI complex in VZV) can be much more quickly investigated, than when using techniques that apply recombinant protein or viral vectors.

Table 73.1. DNA vaccination approaches for herpes viruses

Advantages	Disadvantages
• Manufacture process and analytical testing are the same across different constructs • Stability • Time to clinic • Safety • Ability to titrate immune response to humoral or T-cell arms based on formulations/adjuvants • Ease of multivalent approaches • Ability to modify or detoxify the genes of interest • Lack of prior immunity or immune responses to the plasmid backbone	• Suboptimal responses in human trials to date • Regulatory pathway influenced by gene therapy • Population fear of "genetic" immunization • Not yet manufactured to scale • Possible need for more than a single injection to induce responses in humans

Herpesvirus subgroup	Virus	Tumor association
alpha	HSV-1	none
	HSV-2	none
	VZV	none
beta	CMV	none
	HHV-6	none
	HHV-7	none
gamma	EBV	Burkitts lymphoma, Gastric carcinoma, Nasopharyngeal carcinoma, Hodgkin's disease, Post-transplant lymphoproliferative disease, T-cell lymphoma, Leiomyosarcoma
	HHV-8	Kaposi sarcoma of HIV positive and negative patients, body cavity lymphoma, Castleman's disease

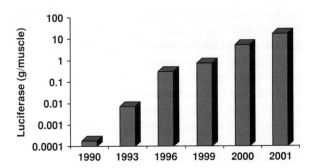

Fig. 73.2. Increase in the expression of the luciferase gene in vivo in muscle over the past decade (Vical in house data)

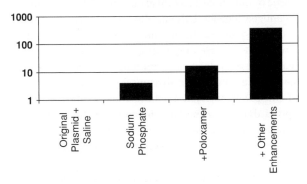

Fig. 73.3. Improvements in T-cell responses by formulation and delivery mechanism

In the past decade, improvements in both plasmid design and formulations have led to approximately a 5-log increase in expression in muscle of the reporter gene, luciferase. The last log of this increase has been achieved using electroporation, which is being studied in man (Fig. 73.2). However, it is important to realize that *in vitro* or *in vivo* expression of the gene construct does not strictly equate with immunologic response to the DNA vaccine.

For the administration of plasmid DNA, both in animals and humans, a range of suitable DNA formulations have been established that can enhance either humoral or cellular immune memory to provide appropriate immune responses for protection against the target pathogen. For example, the use of cationic lipids such as Vaxfectin drives a stronger humoral response than is achieved with unformulated pDNA, (Hartikka et al., 2001), whereas formulation of DNA vaccines with poloxamers tends to enhance T cell responses but has less of an effect on B cell responses (Shiver et al., 2002) (Fig. 73.3).

Thus, a single plasmid DNA vaccine can be used in animal models to define potential correlates of protection by simply changing the DNA vaccine formulation or route of administration. As an example, in the influenza murine model, the use of pDNA encoding NP is protective when given intramuscularly and generates CD8+ T-cell responses, (Ulmer et al., 1993) but is less effective when given intradermally by the gene gun route which generated greater antibody responses (Robinson et al., 1997).

Unlike genetic vaccines that use viral or bacterial vectors to deliver DNA encoded antigens, with DNA vaccines there are no problems with pre-existing or induced immunity to the DNA vaccines that could blunt or abrogate the desired immune response. Thus, repeated boosting over many years appears feasible, if necessary. In this regard, DNA vaccines may also be superior to the use of HSV or CMV as homologous or carrier vaccine vectors to induce an immune response to a subdominant, but possibly more protective antigen.

A major advantage of DNA vaccines or DNA immunotherapeutics is that they are well tolerated and have been demonstrated to be safe in animals and in over 1000 humans. There has been persistent concern in the use of DNA vaccines with the potential for integration into the cellular DNA, but no published preclinical animal studies or human trials have demonstrated integration. In the preclinical studies published to date, the rate of integration has been shown to be at least 1000-fold lower than the risk posed by spontaneous mutations in the human genome (Martin et al., 1999; Ledwith et al., 2000).

DNA vaccines with many different antigen configurations can be produced with the same manufacturing platform, greatly simplifying the production process. Likewise, analytical testing of the plasmid varies little from one DNA vaccine to another, and downstream processing is relatively straightforward. Therefore, the time required to move from concept to animal testing and to the clinic is markedly shortened. Multiple plasmids can be processed in the same facility, and then combined in a final vaccine formulation. Properly formulated DNA vaccines can be stored in liquid form at refrigerated or room temperature for many years. Lastly, DNA vaccines do not require the handling of the pathogen or any mammalian cell substrates (with the associated risk of adventitious agents) at any point in the manufacturing process.

At present, the disadvantages of a DNA vaccine approach are similar to those of many emerging, disruptive technologies. The greatest criticism is the lack of substantive data in humans (see discussion below). The regulatory hurdles surrounding DNA have been originally placed nearly on level with those of gene therapy, and are only now beginning to be adjusted for the safety profile and knowledge of the technology that has emerged in the past decade. In addition, there will be a need to overcome the general fear in the public that this is not a "DNA altering" technology. Lastly, although DNA vaccines will eventually be quite inexpensive to produce, the technology is only now beginning to achieve the efficiencies of scale (such as in line fermentation, lysis, and column purification) that will drive down the costs of manufacture.

Standard DNA technology involves selecting individual genes and cloning them into a vector. A unique method of using DNA for herpesvirus vaccine studies is to inject the DNA as a provirus, which has been modified to remove only one or a few genes. This is now feasible with the advent of recombinant bacmid (bacterial artificial chromosome) technology, which allows for an infective proviral DNA construct to be made using *E. coli*. (Hahn et al., 2003; Suter et al., 1999). Such an approach has focused on removal of the immune evasion genes, to both decrease virulence and promote a greater immune response to the defective virus. Unfortunately, the bacmid can usually only be propagated as a single plasmid per single bacterium, and thus the yield from a fermentation is quite low. In general, the bacmid is then often propagated as a defective virus using a classic CMV-competent or trans-supplying cell line, and results in a replication defective virus for use in the vaccine trials. Although the injection of the bacmid into the host would likely result in some degree of defective virion production, the regulatory and safety hurdles surrounding such an approach would not be trivial.

Features of pDNA constructs especially conducive to herpesvirus vaccine development

As reviewed in previous chapters, there is minimal data that true sterilizing immunity to herpesvirus infections can be easily achieved through any present vaccine strategy. It may be a more realistic goal to limit the initial viral spread and thereby reduce the number of initially infected neurons (for HSV and VZV), or to limit the extent of reactivation of virus (EBV and CMV). Whether control of viral replication can best be achieved by use of a vaccine designed to induce antibody or T-cell-based immunity may depend on the clinical setting. As discussed below, prevention of CMV maternal-fetal transmission may be mostly antibody mediated, whereas prevention of CMV disease following infection in the hematopoietic cell transplant patient appears to be mostly T cell mediated. Nevertheless, most vaccine approaches to herpesvirus infections may require a greater degree of T-cell-mediated immunity than an approach to some other acute viral infections. The result of the HSV subunit trials has shown that adjuvants that bias toward a Th1 response may play a role in protective efficacy (Koelle and Corey, 2003).

DNA vaccines administered intramuscularly have been shown to induce balanced B- and T-cell responses, and will elicit CD8+ T-cell responses, which protein subunit vaccines, in general, cannot (Ulmer, 2001). Recent studies in macaques have shown that the T-cell responses induced by plasmid vaccination tend to be evenly balanced between CD4+ and CD8+ T-cells, whereas responses to adenovirus vectors are generally skewed toward CD8+ T-cell responses (Casimiro et al., 2003). A balanced T-cell response may be important in Herpesvirus infections, in which the role of CD4+ T-cells as well as CD8+ T-cells has been implicated in protection (Koelle and Corey, 2003).

In addition, as demonstrated in prime-boost experiments, DNA vaccines may be superior to other vaccine modalities in promoting long-term memory (McShane, 2002). This priming of memory responses may lead to a greater degree of recall responses, both T-cell and antibody, upon boosting by natural primary infection or viral reactivation. For example, monkeys that were immunized with a candidate authrax DNA vaccine were protected from a fatal challenge and manifested a rapid and rigorous recall response, despite a lack of protection neutralizing antibody at the time of challenge of viral data (Letvin et al., 2006). It is not presently known whether this long-term T-cell memory response may be more critical in vaccine induced protection than the present focus on increasing the number of antigen specific effector cells quantified shortly after vaccination at the peak of the response.

DNA vaccines also have an advantage over the use of conventional live attenuated herpesvirus vaccines, such as the CMV Towne strain vaccine, in that they can be designed to encode relevant antigens without including the multiple immune evasion genes carried by human herpesviruses (Mocarski, 2002). In natural infection, many of these immune evasion gene products are designed to downregulate the T-cell response, and thus avoid recognition and lytic or non-lytic removal by $CD4^+$, $CD8^+$ or NK positive T-cells. Because immune evasion gene products may preclude responses to antigens produced during late infection, the antigens likely to be efficiently recognized by T-cells are those produced early in the infection process such as those encoded by immediate early genes. In addition, preformed structural proteins carried in by the virus may access the Class I pathway directly following infection of the cell or the Class II pathway as exogenous antigen (Tabi et al., 2001; McLaughlin-Taylor et al., 1994) and result in T-cell responses.

Additionally, the amount of early antigen proteins made by conventional live attenuated vaccines may be small as compared to the physical mass of structural proteins, and thus the immune response may be skewed in part by attenuated or vectored vaccines to these late gene products that are not as well presented on the infected cell surface during natural infection. By using DNA vaccines that can promote the production of early antigen gene products in mass equivalent to those of the structural genes, T-cells can potentially be "taught" to recognize and destroy infected cells at an early stage by focusing the immune response on viral proteins that are expressed early in infection, before the Class I or Class II presentation is down-regulated by the ongoing natural infection.

Likewise, the antigens and epitopes recognized in chronic herpesvirus infection, during which the virus is continually replicating and shedding structural genes, may not be equivalent to those that would be recognized during acute infection or during initial reactivation. That is, the focus on the T cell epitopes that are dominant during ongoing chronic infection and therefore easily identified, as has also occurred in the HIV vaccine arena, may not be predictive of the epitopes that are important in actual virus control (Letvin et al., 2006). Identification and measurement of the specific immune effectors that limit viral replication after acute infection or reactivation may be much more useful for predicting prophylactic vaccine outcome.

Animal and human experience with DNA vaccines

Many of the studies in larger animal models with DNA vaccines have focused on using this technology to induce cytotoxic T-cells (CTL). Several studies have demonstrated induction of strong CTL responses by parenteral immunization of primates with DNA encoding SIV and/or HIV proteins. In addition, DNA vaccines have been used successfully as priming vaccines in non-human primate models of prime-boost vaccination. Notably, Robinson et al. demonstrated that priming with a DNA vaccine containing genes encoding antigen from non-infectious SHIV 89.6, followed by a boost with recombinant modified vaccinia Ankara (MVA) encoding SHIV 89.6 genes, protected 24 of 24 macaques from disease progression following intrarectal challenge with the homologous virus (Amara et al., 2002). Merck and the NIH have used DNA alone or formulated with poloxamers or alum, and then boosted with adenovirus, to protect macaques from SIV challenge (Shiver et al., 2002).

In humans, the immune responses to date have been less robust. In a clinical trial conducted by Hoffman et al. a malaria DNA vaccine induced $CD4^+$ or $CD8^+$ T-cell responses in all subjects; however; the responses were not of large magnitude (Wang et al., 2001). In the Merck trials of over 300 subjects to date, approximately 37% of subjects have had measurable gamma interferon positive ELISPOT responses after three or four vaccinations with 5 mg of formulated (aluminum or the poloxamer CRL 1005) or unformulated DNA encoding HIV Gag. (Emini, 2003 Keystone meeting). Although the frequency of response was not 100%, the number of spots induced were similar to the number of T cell responses (both $CD4^+$ and $CD8^+$ T cells) reported by Merck after use of a live attenuated varicella vaccine in the elderly (about 100 spots/million T cells) (Caufield, ICAAC, 2003).

The low response rate in humans to the HIV gag DNA vaccine have been due to the inherently poor immunogenicity of the Gag antigen. This can be hypothesized due to the fact that canarypox vectors encoding Gag have induced CTL responses in about one third of subjects (Belshe et al., 2001) whereas the same vector encoding CMV pp65 induced CTL responses in 100% of naïve subjects (Berencsi et al., 2001). Similarly, DNA vaccines encoding highly immunogenic antigens such as CMV pp65 may be more effective in inducing robust T cell responses in humans than those reported for the HIV gag DNA vaccine. However, initial data from a bivalent pp65, gB DNA vaccine formulated in the poloxamer CRLI005 also appeared to have an approximate 41% response rate (unpublished viral data.)

While it is well known that DNA vaccination stimulates $CD4^+$ and $CD8^+$ T-cell immune responses in the vaccinated host, the ability to generate a protective humoral response is not as well characterized, especially in humans. Reasonable, but not robust, vaccine-induced antibody levels have been measured in clinical trials of hepatitis B vaccine administered by gene gun (Roy et al., 2000; Letvin et al., 2006). In a recent malaria vaccine trial, DNA immunization primed for increase antibody responses following experimental challenge (S. Hoffman, personal communication). A single dose of DNA, given by electroporation or in an antibody-inducing formulation, is able to protect cats and dogs from rabies challenge for up to one year (Osorio et al., 1999). A DNA vaccine given intramuscularly has generated protective levels of antibody and protected horses from encephalitic West Nile Virus challenge (Davis et al., 2001). In addition, DNA has protected non-human primates from challenge with malaria, influenza, and herpes viruses (Ulmer, 2001). Two vaccines based on induction of antibody are now licensed in animals – a hemorrhagic necrosis virus vaccine for Salmon and a WUV vaccine for horses (Ulmer et al., 2006).

Improving DNA vaccine potency

There are several possible approaches to increasing the potency of DNA vaccines. First, modification of the plasmid DNA vector to increase expression levels has resulted in increased immunogenicity in vivo (Fig. 73.2) (Hartikka et al., 2001; Norman et al., 1997). Changing the nucleotide sequence of certain genes to better reflect preferential codon usage in mammalian cells can result in markedly higher levels of expression in eukaryotic cells in vitro and, when incorporated into a DNA vaccine vector, can increase immunogenicity substantially (Andre et al., 1998; Uchijima et al., 1998).

Another general approach to improving DNA vaccines involves adjuvants. Adjuvants can include proteins, small molecule compounds or DNA plasmids encoding immunomodulating proteins, such as cytokines, chemokines and costimulatory molecules. The specific examples are too numerous to list here, but are reviewed elsewhere (Sasaki et al., 1998; Ulmer et al., 2006). We and others have shown that simple mixtures of DNA vaccines with adjuvants are sometimes effective, but appropriate formulation may be required. For example, certain aluminum gels, such as aluminum phosphate, when mixed with DNA vaccines, enhance antibody responses, (Ulmer et al., 1999) while others, such as aluminum hydroxide, inhibit responses as a consequence of electrostatic interaction between the negatively charged DNA and positively charged adjuvant. This detrimental effect can be overcome with appropriate formulation to prevent such binding. We have assessed the effects of cationic lipids, and shown them to enhance the B-cell response without down-regulating the T-cell induction (Hartikka et al., 2001). On the other hand, in our laboratories and others the use of poloxamers has led to an increase in T-cell responses with no detrimental effect on antibodies (Fig. 73.3).

DNA vaccines for specific human herpesviruses
Cytomegalovirus

Genes of interest

The immune response to CMV during acute or chronic infection has been determined by the study of acute and chronic infection in animal models and in man. Antibody appears critical in the prevention of maternal-fetal transmission, and is primarily directed to the envelope glycoproteins, especially gB (Plotkin, 1999). The control of CMV infection in transplant recipients and HIV-infected persons is associated with preserved cellular immune responses, including $CD4^+$, $CD8^+$, and NK T-cells. The $CD8^+$ T cell responses are directed primarily at the immediate early (IE) genes of CMV and at the abundant tegument protein pp65. Approximately 92% of persons have $CD8^+$ responses to pp65 and another 76% to exon 4 of IE1 (Gyulai et al., 2000; Wills et al., 1996). In addition, another one-third of infected individuals have CTL responses to gB. Although pp150 responses have been noted, the degree of these responses are not of the magnitude of those induced by pp65 or IE1.

Almost all infected persons have $CD4^+$ responses to CMV, although the antigen and epitope mapping is not as fully investigated as those for $CD8^+$ T-cells (Kern et al., 2002).

The use of DNA to protect in the maternal fetal situation would likely rely on greater antibody induction, although whether antibodies to gB are sufficient is still debated. An advantage of a DNA approach would be to use polycistronic constructs, such as those encoding the gH/gL/gO or gM/gN complexes or individual envelope proteins, to elicit antibodies that neutralize via fusion inhibition or other mechanisms.

Animal studies

The plasmid DNA approach to CMV disease has already been validated in a series of recent animal studies. Almost all of these studies have concentrated on the use of gB, the pp65 homologues, or IE1, and in each case have needed to use the species specific strains for the source of the encoded gene (Hwang et al., 1999; Morello et al., 2000; Schleiss et al., 2000; Endresz et al., 1999, 2001). pDNA vaccines encoding murine CMV IE1 and pp65 homologues have elicited immunity associated with 100–1000-fold reduction in viral titers in a mouse model of CMV infection (Ye et al., 2002). In the guinea pig model of maternal-fetal transmission of CMV, DNA encoding gB, but not the pp65 homologue, was capable of partial protection of the newborn pup (Schleiss et al., 2000). (Schleiss, 2004). In addition, the use of pDNA encoding a secreted, transmembrane deleted, form of the gB protein has been shown to elicit higher antibody titers than full length gB in the murine model. (Endresz et al., 2001).

Human trials

Vical Inc. of San Diego moved a poloxamer-formulated bivalent CMV DNA vaccine encoding gB and pp65 into human clinical trials in 2003. The gB gene can be truncated to remove the transmembrane and cytoplasmic domain, thus allowing for greater secretion. The pp65 construct may need modification to remove a published putative kinase encoding region (Gallez-Hawkins et al., 2002). The IE1 constructs being considered for a trivalent vaccine can be engineered to remove both the potential transactivation regions and other biologic activities. A trivalent product that includes the IE1 gene is now in late preclinical development.

The bivalent gB/pp65 vaccine has been tested in both rabbits and mice, and was found to be highly immunogenic for the production of both antibodies (gB) and T cells (pp65). The majority of the vaccine-induced T cell responses in BALB/c mice, as measured in a gamma interferon ELISPOT assay using overlapping peptides encoding the entirety of pp65, are found in the amino terminal half of the protein. The frequency of spot forming cells in mice is higher than that seen with influenza NP, IE1, or similar antigens, when administered on a similar schedule at a similar dose. Studies with the murine pp65 homologue, hCMV pp65, and NP have all shown an improved T cell response using the poloxamer CRL1005. In studies in seropositive, non-vaccinated humans, the gamma interferon positive T cell responses to chronic infection, which may not mirror responses to vaccination, are found to be more frequent in the C-terminal region of the protein, as in contrast to the vaccine induced responses in mice.

Phase 1 studies of this vaccine revealed that three doses of up to 5 mg total DNA induced T cell responses in approximately half of vaccinated individuals. This vaccine has now moved into a Phase 2 study, in which the clinical endpoint is the prevention in CMV seropositive stem cell transplant recipients of detectable CMV viremias after vaccinations of both the donor and the recipient.

Herpes simplex virus 1 and 2

Genes of interest

There appear to be two different approaches to using DNA vaccines in HSV, which may be independently moved forward, or possibly combined. The first would be to increase the antibody response to gB, and/ or gD, or to the gH/gL complex by the use of DNA-augmented by adjuvants, formulations, or cytokines. The second would be to limit viral growth by the recognition and destruction of cells that are in the earliest phases of replication, and prior to the numerous HSV-directed immune evasion mechanisms. In such a scenario, the DNA vaccine would be focused on the early antigens, and those most carefully scrutinized include ICP4, ICP0, and ICP27. ICP 47, which blocks antigen presentation to $CD8^+$ T cells, would be another early antigen for vaccine inclusion, but some biologic modification may be necessary. Other proteins of interest include those that are more abundantly expressed in later stages of virion formation, including the structural proteins VP5, VP13/14, VP16 and VP22.

Animal studies

The concept of direct DNA vaccination for HSV was investigated by a number of different investigators shortly after the discovery of the DNA vaccines (Wolff et al., 1990). In 1994, Rouse et al. showed that an in vitro model of DNA transfection could be used to generate gB or ICP27-specific CTL from splenocytes (Rouse et al., 1994). Initial reports of low level antibody production and partial protection in mice using gD constructs, (Ghiasi et al., 1995), were followed by more impressive mouse or guinea pig studies using both gB and gD (Bourne et al., 1996a,b; Kriesel et al., 1996; McClements et al., 1996, 1997). The versatility of the DNA approach has been used to study most of the putative targets of neutralization, including gB, gC, gD, gH/gL or combinations of these (Nass et al., 1998; Cha et al., 2002; Lee et al., 2002). Protection in some experiments using the recurrent zosterform model of HSV appeared to be mediated by T-cells to either gB or ICP27 (Manickan et al., 1995a,b).

Whether these models could be used to predict the need for mucosal versus systemic immunization is not known; however, some studies take advantage of the availability of the DNA constructs in the relapsing guinea pig or acute murine HSV models to test such concepts (Shroff et al., 1999; Eo et al., 2001). In addition, as the results from protection were almost never 100% in early studies, HSV DNA vaccine models have been used extensively to study improvements to the technology, include the use of plasmid or gene modification, (Higgins et al., 2000) alphavirus replicons, (Hariharan et al., 1998) adjuvants, (Bernstein et al., 1999) and cytokine, chemokine or co-stimulatory enhancements (Sin et al., 1998, 1999b; Flo et al., 2000; Sin et al., 2000a,b; Harle et al., 2001; Sin et al., 2001). As in other vaccine systems, the highest titers are often achieved by using a prime-boost approach of initial DNA vaccination, followed by another modality (protein, another vector, or killed virus) (McShane, 2002; Sin et al., 1999a). A DNA prime followed by an inactivated virion was capable of inducing a 4 log reduction in virus shedding in calves that were challenged with bovine herpesvirus-1 (Toussant et al., 2005).

Human trials

No trials of candidate HSV DNA vaccines have been reported in humans despite extensive preclinical work. The relative success of the GlaxoSmithKline vaccine, which used an MPL-based adjuvant to promote a greater T-cell response with Th1 bias, may lead to renewed interest in this approach. Encouraging trial results using replication-defective viruses, such as the DICS-virus, would also be likely to speed the movement of plasmid-based products into humans. Trials of DNA vaccines encoding the early antigens of HSV for use in the therapeutic setting have been planned using gene gun technology, but whether those trials will move forward is not known.

Varicella-zoster virus

Genes of interest

The transmembrane glycoprotein gE, and to a lesser extent gB, contain the major neutralizing antibody targets after VZV natural infection or OKA vaccination. Mapping of CTL targets indicates that immediate early antigens, along with gE, are common (Arvin et al., 2002). The most extensively studied, and first likely target for DNA vaccination is IE62 (Abendroth et al., 1999). There are several biological activities associated with IE62 that may need to be deleted from a vaccine candidate in an attempt to decrease potential transactivation. Other genes that have been suggested to be used as CTL targets in VZV vaccines include IE63 and the thymidine kinase. IE63 is expressed during latency in seropositive subjects, and thus inclusion of this gene in a DNA vaccine may raise concerns about immunopathology (Debrus et al., 1995).

Animal studies

As has been found in CMV and HSV, attempts to augment the generation of a B-cell response have used secreted forms of surface glycoproteins; for example, by removing the transmembrane portions of gE. Publications using a 1.8 kb secreted gE plasmid construct made in the vector pRC/CMV have demonstrated that secreted-gE is expressed very poorly in vitro and elicits suboptimal immunogenicity in mice or guinea pigs (Massaer et al., 1999; Hasan et al., 2002). Normally the glycoprotein gE forms a heterodimer with gI, with gI providing chaperone activity that modulates the trafficking of the gE-gI heterodimer through the golgi and ultimately to display on the cell surface. The lack of gI chaperoning activity may explain the low titers seen in these DNA vaccination studies when injecting the gE plasmid alone. Other studies have shown improvement in titers of gE when administered intradermally by gene gun, although this approach again favored a Th2 bias (Stasikova et al., 2003).

Human trials

No VZV DNA vaccine has moved into the clinic, although the clearest indication would be for use in the immunocompromised setting, in which the use of the licensed live-attenuated vaccine is either contraindicated or not recommended. A bivalent or trivalent vaccine using gE and early antigens formulated in a way to bias toward T-cell over antibody responses is presently a favored approach.

Epstein–Barr virus

Genes of interest

Studies of $CD8^+$ T-cell immune response to EBV have shown that there is often a massive proliferation of T-cells that are narrowly focused on either one or a few MHC

Class I-restricted epitopes (Rickinson et al., 2001). The T-cell response is needed to prevent unchecked viral-driven B cell proliferation. In T-cell deficiency, the emergence of certain EBV-related tumors occurs (for review see elsewhere in this volume), and little role has been observed for antibody-mediated control.

Nonetheless, an antibody-based approach has been used to attempt to prevent or control primary infection, with the majority of investigations focused on the major surface glycoprotein gp350, using Type 1 strains that are most prevalent in Western populations. Little work has been accomplished with other potentially important surface glycoproteins.

For T-cell response induction, initial studies focused on the key early and latency antigens, EBNA1, EBNA2, and LMP1. During the acute infection, T-cells are also rapidly expanded to the lytic antigens, particularly BZLF1, BRLF1 and BMLF1. $CD8^+$ T cell epitopes to most of these genes have been mapped to the HLA-allele for which they are restricted (Rickinson et al., 2001). In persistent infection there is a change in the hierarchy of the genes recognized, with greater responses focused on EBNA3A, EBNA3B, EBNA3C, and LMP2. Since the responses to EBV appear to be narrowly focused, and yet to cover a broad array of HLA haplotypes, this virus may represent an ideal situation to use DNA vaccines based on the polytope approach (Thomson et al., 1998). In such a model, which has been moved to human clinical trials in the HIV vaccine field, multiple epitopes, or epitope dense regions are linked in a plasmid construct using designs that optimize proteosomal cleavage and class I presentation (Livingston et al., 2001). The use of a helper epitope is often employed to improve $CD4^+$ responses and enhance $CD8^+$ T-cell memory.

As with other herpesviruses, it will be necessary to study and potentially modify biologically active elements that may appear to pose safety risk, especially for a known carcinogenic virus. Removal of immune evasion elements could be accomplished for EBNA1 removal of the glycine-arginine repeat (Gar) site responsible for preventing the protein from undergoing degradation by the protesosome (and thus lack of presentation to the Class I system) (Koelle and Corey, 2003).

Animal studies

Studies using DNA vaccines have been quite limited in EBV. A vaccine based on a few HLA-restricted CTL epitopes has been evaluated in mice, but no human studies have been published (Thomson et al., 1998). Studies in mice have shown the expected immunogenicity using DNA constructs encoding gp350 (Jung et al., 2001).

Human trials

No trials of DNA vaccines have been undertaken in EBV.

Summary

DNA vaccination, as with any new emerging technology, has passed through a series of unreasonable positive expectations, and has suffered at the hands of poorly defined negative criticisms. Although no definitive human efficacy data exist, however, the technology is only a little more than a decade old. The results in human trials to date have been encouraging, but suboptimal, and may have suffered form use of first generation vectors, lack of formulations, and poorly selected immunogens and disease states. Human herpesvirus diseases represent a frontier in which this technology is likely to prove whether it can live up to its enormous promise and potential. If initial trials in CMV or HSV show promise in the coming two years, renewed enthusiasm for moving this approach into humans with the remaining herpesviruses should follow.

REFERENCES

Abendroth, A., Slobedman, B., Springer, M. L., Blau, H. M., and Arvin, A. M. (1999). Analysis, of immune responses to varicella zoster viral proteins induced by DNA vaccination. *Antiviral Res.*, **44**, 179–192.

Andre, S., Seed, B., Eberle, J., Schraut, W., Bultmann, A., and Haas, J. (1998). Increased immune response elicited by DNA vaccination with a synthetic gp120 sequence with optimized codon usage. *J. Virol.*, **72**, 1497–1503.

Amara, R. R., Villinger, F., Altman, J. D. et al. (2002). Control of a mucosal challenge and prevention of AIDS by a multiprotein DNA/MVA vaccine. *Vaccine*, **20**, 1949–1955.

Arvin, A. M., Sharp, M., Moir, M. et al. (2002). Memory cytotoxic T cell responses to viral tegument and regulatory proteins encoded by open reading frames 4, 10, 29, and 62 of varicella-zoster virus. *Viral Immunol.*, **15**, 507–516.

Belshe, R. B., Stevens, C., Gorse, G. J. et al. (2001). Safety and immunogenicity of a canarypox-vectored human immunodeficiency virus Type 1 vaccine with or without gp120: a phase 2 study in higher- and lower-risk volunteers. *J. Infect. Dis.*, **183**, 1343–1352.

Berencsi, K., Gyulai, Z., Gonczol, E. et al. (2001). A canarypox vector-expressing cytomegalovirus (CMV) phosphoprotein 65 induces long-lasting cytotoxic T cell responses in human CMV- seronegative subjects. *J. Infect. Dis.*, **183**, 1171–1179.

Bernstein, D. I., Tepe, E. R., Mester, J. C., Arnold, R. L., Stanberry, L. R., and Higgins, T. (1999). Effects of DNA immunization formulated with bupivacaine in murine and guinea pig models of genital herpes simplex virus infection. *Vaccine*, **17**, 1964–1969.

Bourne, N., Milligan, G. N., Schleiss, M. R., Bernstein, D. I., and Stanberry, L. R. (1996a). DNA immunization confers protective immunity on mice challenged intravaginally with herpes simplex virus type 2. *Vaccine*, **14**, 1230–1234.

Bourne, N., Stanberry, L. R., Bernstein, D. I., and Lew, D. (1996b). DNA immunization against experimental genital herpes simplex virus infection. *J. Infect. Dis.*, **173**, 800–807.

Casimiro, D. R., Chen, L., Fu, T. M. *et al.* (2003). Comparative immunogenicity in rhesus monkeys of DNA plasmid, recombinant vaccinia virus, and replication-defective adenovirus vectors expressing a human immunodeficiency virus type 1 gag gene. *J. Virol.*, **77**, 6305–6313.

Cha, S. C., Kim, Y. S., Cho, J. K. *et al.* (2002). Enhanced protection against HSV lethal challenges in mice by immunization with a combined HSV-1 glycoprotein B:H:L gene DNAs. *Virus Res.*, **86**, 21–31.

Corr, M., Lee, D. J., Carson, D. A., and Tighe, H. (1996). Gene vaccination with naked plasmid DNA: mechanism of CTL priming. *J. Exp. Med.*, **184**, 1555–1560.

Corr, M., von Damm, A., Lee, D. J., and Tighe, H. (1999). In vivo priming by DNA injection occurs predominantly by antigen transfer. *J. Immunol.*, **163**, 4721–4727.

Davis, B. S., Chang, G. J., Cropp, B. *et al.* (2001). West Nile virus recombinant DNA vaccine protects mouse and horse from virus challenge and expresses in vitro a noninfectious recombinant antigen that can be used in enzyme-linked immunosorbent assays. *J. Virol.*, **75**, 4040–4047.

Debrus, S., Sadzot-Delvaux, C., Nikkels, A. F., Piette, J., and Rentier, B. (1995). Varicella-zoster virus gene 63 encodes an immediate-early protein that is abundantly expressed during latency. *J. Virol.*, **69**, 3240–3245.

Doe, B., Selby, M., Barnett, S., Baenziger, J., and Walker, C. M. (1996). Induction of cytotoxic T lymphocytes by intramuscular immunization with plasmid DNA is facilitated by bone marrow-derived cells. *Proc. Natl Acad. Sci. USA*, **93**, 8578–8583.

Endresz, V., Kari, L., Berencsi, K. *et al.* (1999). Induction of human cytomegalovirus (HCMV)-glycoprotein B (gB)-specific neutralizing antibody and phosphoprotein 65 (pp65)-specific cytotoxic T lymphocyte responses by naked DNA immunization. *Vaccine*, **17**, 50–58.

Endresz, V., Burian, K., Berencsi, K. *et al.* (2001). Optimization of DNA immunization against human cytomegalovirus. *Vaccine*, **19**, 3972–3980.

Eo, S. K., Gierynska, M., Kamar, A. A., and Rouse, B. T. (2001). Prime-boost immunization with DNA vaccine: mucosal route of administration changes the rules. *J. Immunol.*, **166**, 5473–5479.

Feltquate, D. M., Heaney, S., Webster, R. G., and Robinson, H. L. (1997). Different T helper cell types and antibody isotypes generated by saline and gene gun DNA immunization. *J. Immunol.*, **158**, 2278–2284.

Flo, J., Beatriz Perez, A., Tisminetzky, S., and Baralle, F. (2000). Superiority of intramuscular route and full length glycoprotein D for DNA vaccination against herpes simplex 2. Enhancement of protection by the co-delivery of the GM-CSF gene. *Vaccine*, **18**, 3242–3253.

Gallez-Hawkins, G., Lomeli, N. A., X, L. L. *et al.* (2002). Kinase-deficient CMVpp65 triggers a CMVpp65 specific T-cell immune response in HLA-A*0201.Kb transgenic mice after DNA immunization. *Scand. J. Immunol.*, **55**, 592–598.

Ghiasi, H., Cai, S., Slanina, S., Nesburn, A. B., and Wechsler, S. L. (1995). Vaccination of mice with herpes simplex virus type 1 glycoprotein D DNA produces low levels of protection against lethal HSV-1 challenge. *Antiviral Res.* **28**, 147–157.

Gyulai, Z., Endresz, V., Burian, K. *et al.* (2000). Cytotoxic T lymphocyte (CTL) responses to human cytomegalovirus pp65, IE1-Exon4, gB, pp150, and pp28 in healthy individuals: reevaluation of prevalence of IE1-specific CTLs. *J. Infect. Dis.*, **181**, 1537–1546.

Hahn, G., Jarosch, M., Wang, J. B., Berbes, C., and McVoy, M. A. (2003). Tn7-mediated introduction of DNA sequences into bacmid-cloned cytomegalovirus genomes for rapid recombinant virus construction. *J. Virol. Methods*, **107**, 185–194.

Hariharan, M. J., Driver, D. A., Townsend, K. *et al.* (1998). DNA immunization against herpes simplex virus: enhanced efficacy using a Sindbis virus-based vector. *J. Virol.*, **72**, 950–958.

Harle, P., Noisakran, S., and Carr, D. J. (2001). The application of a plasmid DNA encoding IFN-alpha 1 postinfection enhances cumulative survival of herpes simplex virus type 2 vaginally infected mice. *J. Immunol.* **166**, 1803–1812.

Hartikka, J., Bozoukova, V., Ferrari, M. *et al.* (2001). Vaxfectin enhances the humoral immune response to plasmid DNA-encoded antigens. *Vaccine*, **19**, 1911–1923.

Hasan, U. A., Harper, D. R., Wren, B. W., and Morrow, W. J. (2002). Immunization with a DNA vaccine expressing a truncated form of varicella zoster virus glycoprotein E. *Vaccine*, **20**, 1308–1315.

Higgins, T. J., Herold, K. M., Arnold, R. L., McElhiney, S. P., Shroff, K. E., and Pachuk, C. J. (2000). Plasmid DNA-expressed secreted and nonsecreted forms of herpes simplex virus glycoprotein D2 induce different types of immune responses. *J. Infect. Dis.*, **182**, 1311–1320.

Hwang, E. S., Kwon, K. B., Park, J. W., Kim, D. J., Park, C. G., and Cha, C. Y. (1999). Induction of neutralizing antibody against human cytomegalovirus (HCMV) with DNA-mediated immunization of HCMV glycoprotein B in mice. *Microbiol. Immunol.*, **43**, 307–310.

Jung, S., Chung, Y. K., Chang, S. H. *et al.* (2001). DNA-mediated immunization of glycoprotein 350 of Epstein–Barr virus induces the effective humoral and cellular immune responses against the antigen. *Mol. Cells*, **12**, 41–49.

Kern, F., Bunde, T., Faulhaber, N. et al. (2002). Cytomegalovirus (CMV) phosphoprotein 65 makes a large contribution to shaping the T cell repertoire in CMV-exposed individuals. *J. Infect. Dis.*, **185**, 1709–1716.

Koelle, D. M., and Corey, L. (2003). Recent progress in herpes simplex virus immunobiology and vaccine research. *Clin. Microbiol.*, **16**, 96–113.

Kriesel, J. D., Spruance, S. L., Daynes, R. A., and Araneo, B. A. (1996). Nucleic acid vaccine encoding gD2 protects mice from herpes simplex virus type 2 disease. *J. Infect. Dis.*, **173**, 536–541.

Ledwith, B. J., Manam, S., Troilo, P. J. et al. (2000). Plasmid DNA vaccines: investigation of integration into host cellular DNA following intramuscular injection in mice. *Intervirology*, **43**, 258–272.

Lee, H. H., Cha, S. C., Jang, D. J. et al. (2002). Immunization with combined HSV-2 glycoproteins B2 : D2 gene DNAs: protection against lethal intravaginal challenges in mice. *Virus Genes*, **25**, 179–188.

Letvin, N. L., Mascola, J. R., Sun, V. et al. (2006). Preserved CD4+ central memory T cells and survival in vaccinated SIV-challenged monkeys. *Science*, **312**.

Livingston, B. D., Newman, M., Crimi, C., McKinney, D., Chesnut, R., and Sette, A. (2001). Optimization of epitope processing enhances immunogenicity of multiepitope DNA vaccines. *Vaccine*, **19**, 4652–4660.

Manickan, E., Rouse, R. J., Yu, Z., Wire, W. S., and Rouse, B. T. (1995a). Genetic immunization against herpes simplex virus. Protection is mediated by CD4+ T lymphocytes. *J. Immunol.*, **155**, 259–265.

Manickan, E., Yu, Z., Rouse, R. J., Wire, W. S., and Rouse, B. T. (1995b). Induction of protective immunity against herpes simplex virus with DNA encoding the immediate early protein ICP 27. *Viral Immunol.*, **8**, 53–61.

Martin, T., Parker, S. E., Hedstrom, R. et al. (1999). Plasmid DNA malaria vaccine: the potential for genomic integration after intramuscular injection. *Hum. Gene. Ther.*, **10**, 759–768.

Massaer, M., Haumont, M., Garcia, L. et al. (1999). Differential neutralizing antibody responses to varicella-zoster virus glycoproteins B and E following naked DNA immunization. *Viral Immunol.*, **12**, 227–236.

McClements, W. L., Armstrong, M. E., Keys, R. D., and Liu, M. A. (1996). Immunization with DNA vaccines encoding glycoprotein D or glycoprotein B, alone or in combination, induces protective immunity in animal models of herpes simplex virus-2 disease. *Proc. Natl Acad. Sci. USA*, **93**, 11414–11420.

McClements, W. L., Armstrong, M. E., Keys, R. D., and Liu, M. A. (1997). The prophylactic effect of immunization with DNA encoding herpes simplex virus glycoproteins on HSV-induced disease in guinea pigs. *Vaccine*, **15**, 857–860.

McLaughlin-Taylor, E., Pande, H., Forman, S. J. et al. (1994). Identification of the major late human cytomegalovirus matrix protein pp65 as a target antigen for CD8+ virus-specific cytotoxic T lymphocytes. *J. Med. Virol.* **43**, 103–110.

McShane H. (2002). Prime-boost immunization strategies for infectious diseases. *Curr. Opin. Mol. Ther.*, **4**, 23–27.

Mena, A., Andrew, M. E., and Coupar, B. E. (2001). Rapid dissemination of intramuscularly inoculated DNA vaccines. *Immunol. Cell Biol.*, **79**, 87–89.

Mocarski, E. S., Jr. (2002). Immunomodulation by cytomegaloviruses: manipulative strategies beyond evasion. *Trends Microbiol.*, **10**, 332–339.

Morello, C. S., Cranmer, L. D., and Spector, D. H. (2000). Suppression of murine cytomegalovirus (MCMV) replication with a DNA vaccine encoding MCMV M84 (a homolog of human cytomegalovirus pp65). *J. Virol.*, **74**, 3696–3708.

Nass, P. H., Elkins, K. L., and Weir, J. P. (1998). Antibody response and protective capacity of plasmid vaccines expressing three different herpes simplex virus glycoproteins. *J. Infect. Dis.*, **178**, 611–617.

Norman, J. A., Hobart, P., Manthorpe, M., Felgner, P., and Wheeler, C. (1997). Development of improved vectors for DNA-based immunization and other gene therapy applications. *Vaccine*, **15**, 801–803.

Osorio, J. E., Tomlinson, C. C., Frank, R. S. et al. (1999). Immunization of dogs and cats with a DNA vaccine against rabies virus. *Vaccine*, **17**, 1109–1116.

Padoll, D. M. and Beckerleg, A. M. (1995). Exposing the immunology of naked DNA vaccines. *Immunity*, **3**, 165–169.

Plotkin, S. A. (1999). Vaccination against cytomegalovirus, the changeling demon. *Pediatr. Infect. Dis. J.*, **18**, 313–325; quiz 326.

Raz, E., Carson, D. A., Parker, S. E. et al. (1994). Intradermal gene immunization: the possible role of DNA uptake in the induction of cellular immunity to viruses. *Proc. Natl Acad. Sci. USA*, **91**, 9519–9523.

Rickinson, A. B., and Kieff, E. (2001). Epstein–Barr virus. In Knipe, D. M., and Howley, P. M. eds. *Fields Virology*. Philadelphia: Lippincott Williams and Wilkins, pp. 2575–2628.

Robinson, H. L., Boyle, C. A., Feltquate, D. M., Morin, M. J., Santoro, J. C., and Webster, R. G. (1997). DNA immunization for influenza virus: studies using hemagglutinin- and nucleoprotein-expressing DNAs. *J. Infect. Dis.*, **176**, Suppl. 1, S50–S55.

Rouse, R. J., Nair, S. K., Lydy, S. L., Bowen, J. C., and Rouse, B. T. (1994). Induction in vitro of primary cytotoxic T-lymphocyte responses with DNA encoding herpes simplex virus proteins. *J. Virol.*, **68**, 5685–5689.

Roy, M. J., Wu, M. S., Barr, L. J. et al. (2000). Induction of antigen-specific CD8+ T cells, T helper cells, and protective levels of antibody in humans by particle-mediated administration of a hepatitis B virus DNA vaccine. *Vaccine*, **19**, 764–778.

Sasaki, S., Tsuji, T., Asakura, Y., Fukushima, J., and Okuda, K. (1998). The search for a potent DNA vaccine against AIDS: the enhancement of immunogenicity by chemical and genetic adjuvants. *Anticancer Res.*, **18**, 3907–3915.

Schleiss, M. R., Bourne, N., Jensen, N. J., Bravo, F., and Bernstein, D. I. (2000). Immunogenicity evaluation of DNA vaccines that target guinea pig cytomegalovirus proteins glycoprotein B and UL83. *Viral Immunol.*, **13**, 155–167.

Schleiss, M. R., Bowne, N., Stroup, G., Bravo, F. J., Jensen, N. J., and Bernstein, D. I. (2004). Protection against congenital megalovirus infection and disease in guinea pigs, conferred by a purified recombinant glycoprotein B vaccine. *J. Infect. Dis.*, **189**(8), 1374–1381.

Shiver, J. W., Fu, T. M., Chen, L. *et al.* (2002). Replication-incompetent adenoviral vaccine vector elicits effective anti-immunodeficiency-virus immunity. *Nature*, **415**, 331–335.

Shroff, K. E., Marcucci-Borges, L. A., de Bruin, S. J. *et al.* (1999). Induction of HSV-gD2 specific CD4(+) cells in Peyer's patches and mucosal antibody responses in mice following DNA immunization by both parenteral and mucosal administration. *Vaccine*, **18**, 222–230.

Sin, J. I., Kim, J. J., Ugen, K. E., Ciccarelli, R. B., Higgins, T. J., and Weiner, D. B. (1998). Enhancement of protective humoral (Th2) and cell-mediated (Th1) immune responses against herpes simplex virus-2 through co-delivery of granulocyte–macrophage colony-stimulating factor expression cassettes. *Eur. J. Immunol.*, **28**, 3530–3540.

Sin, J. I., Bagarazzi, M., Pachuk, C., and Weiner, D. B. (1999a). DNA priming-protein boosting enhances both antigen-specific antibody and Th1-type cellular immune responses in a murine herpes simplex virus-2 gD vaccine model. *DNA Cell Biol.*, **18**, 771–779.

Sin, J. I., Kim, J. J., Arnold, R. L. *et al.* (1999b). IL-12 gene as a DNA vaccine adjuvant in a herpes mouse model: IL-12 enhances Th1-type CD4+ T cell-mediated protective immunity against herpes simplex virus-2 challenge. *J. Immunol.*, **162**, 2912–2921.

Sin, J. I., Kim, J. J., Pachuk, C., Satishchandran, C., and Weiner, D. B. (2000a). DNA vaccines encoding interleukin-8 and RANTES enhance antigen-specific Th1-type CD4(+) T-cell-mediated protective immunity against herpes simplex virus type 2 in vivo. *J. Virol.*, **74**, 11173–11180.

Sin, J. I., Kim, J., Dang, K. *et al.* (2000b). LFA-3 plasmid DNA enhances Ag-specific humoral- and cellular-mediated protective immunity against herpes simplex virus-2 in vivo: involvement of CD4+ T cells in protection. *Cell Immunol.*, **203**, 19–28.

Sin, J. I., Kim, J. J., Zhang, D., and Weiner, D. B. (2001). Modulation of cellular responses by plasmid CD40L: CD40L plasmid vectors enhance antigen-specific helper T cell type 1 CD4+ T cell-mediated protective immunity against herpes simplex virus type 2 in vivo. *Hum. Gene. Ther.*, **12**, 1091–2002.

Stasikova, J., Kutinova, L., Smahel, M., and Nemeckova, S. (2003). Immunization with Varicella-zoster virus glycoprotein E expressing vectors: comparison of antibody response to DNA vaccine and recombinant vaccinia virus. *Acta Virol.*, **47**, 1–10.

Suter, M., Lew, A. M., Grob, P. *et al.* (1999). BAC-VAC, a novel generation of (DNA) vaccines: a bacterial artificial chromosome (BAC) containing a replication-competent, packaging-defective virus genome induces protective immunity against herpes simplex virus 1. *Proc. Natl Acad. Sci. USA*, **96**, 12697–12702.

Tabi, Z., Moutaftsi, M., and Borysiewicz, L. K. (2001). Human cytomegalovirus pp65- and immediate early 1 antigen-specific HLA class I-restricted cytotoxic T cell responses induced by cross- presentation of viral antigens. *J. Immunol.*, **166**, 5695–5703.

Thomson, S. A., Sherritt, M. A., Medveczky, J. *et al.* (1998). Delivery of multiple CD8 cytotoxic T cell epitopes by DNA vaccination. *J. Immunol.*, **160**, 1717–1723.

Torres, C. A., Iwasaki, A., Barber, B. H., and Robinson, H. L. (1997). Differential dependence on target site tissue for gene gun and intramuscular DNA immunizations. *J. Immunol.*, **158**, 4529–4532.

Toussaint, J. F., Letellier, C., Paquet, D., Dispas, M., and Kerkhofs, P. (2005). Prime-boost strategies combining DNA and inactivated vaccines confer high immunity and protection in cattle against bovine herpesvirus-1. *Vaccine*, **23**, 5073–5081.

Uchijima, M., Yoshida, A., Nagata, T., and Koide, Y. (1998). Optimization of codon usage of plasmid DNA vaccine is required for the effective MHC class I-restricted T cell responses against an intracellular bacterium. *J. Immunol.*, **161**, 5594–5599.

Ulmer, J. B. (2001). An update on the state of the art of DNA vaccines. *Curr. Opin. Drug Discov. Devel.*, **4**, 192–197.

Ulmer, J. B., Donnelly, J. J., Parker, S. E. *et al.* (1993). Heterologous protection against influenza by injection of DNA encoding a viral protein. *Science*, **259**, 1745–1749.

Ulmer, J. B., Deck, R. R., Dewitt, C. M., Donnhly, J. I., and Liu, M. A. (1996). Generation of MHC class I-restricted cytotoxic T lymphocytes by expression of a viral protein in muscle cells: antigen presentation by non-muscle cells. *Immunology*, **89**, 59–67.

Ulmer, J. B., DeWitt, C. M., Chastain, M. *et al.* (1999). Enhancement of DNA vaccine potency using conventional aluminum adjuvants. *Vaccine*, **18**, 18–28.

Ulmer, J. B., Wahren, B., and Liu, M. A. (2006). Gene-based vaccines recent technical and clinical advances. *Trends in Molec. Med.*, **12**(8).

Wang, R., Epstein, J., Baraceros, F. M. *et al.* (2001). Induction of CD4(+) T cell-dependent CD8(+) type 1 responses in humans by a malaria DNA vaccine. *Proc. Natl Acad. Sci. USA*, **98**, 10817–10822.

Wills, M. R., Carmichael, A. J., Mynard, K. *et al.* (1996). The human cytotoxic T-lymphocyte (CTL) response to cytomegalovirus is dominated by structural protein pp65: frequency, specificity, and T-cell receptor usage of pp65-specific CTL. *J. Virol.*, **70**, 7569–7579.

Wolff, J. A., Malone, R. W., Williams, P. *et al.* (1990). Direct gene transfer into mouse muscle in vivo. *Science*, **247**, 1465–1468.

Ye, M., Morello, C. S., and Spector, D. H. (2002). CD8 T-cell responses following coimmunization with plasmids expressing the dominant pp89 and subdominant M84 antigens of murine cytomegalovirus correlate with long-term protection against subsequent viral challenge. *J. Virol.*, **76**, 2100–2112.

74

Adoptive immunotherapy for herpesviruses

Ann M. Leen, Uluhan Sili, Catherine M. Bollard, and Cliona M. Rooney

Center for Cell and Gene Therapy, Baylor College of Medicine, Houston, TX, USA

Introduction

Herpesvirus infections rarely cause significant problems in the immunocompetent human host. However, in the immunosuppressed, for example, recipients of hematopoietic stem cell transplants (HSCT) (Rooney et al., 1998), solid organ transplants (SOT), or human immunodeficiency virus (HIV)-infected individuals, viral infections/reactivations are common and are associated with considerable morbidity and mortality. The resultant uncontrolled infections correlate with a lack of cellular immunity against viral antigens (Weinberg et al., 2001). While effective antiviral drugs are available for the treatment of some herpesvirus infections, adoptive immunotherapy, which is the artificial reconstitution of virus-specific T-cells with in vitro expanded cytotoxic T-lymphocytes (CTLs), for the prophylaxis and/or treatment of herpesviruses is an attractive option. The γ-herpesvirus, Epstein–Barr virus (EBV) is also associated with a heterogeneous range of malignancies and diseases that occur in apparently immunocompetent individuals and since these malignancies also express "foreign" viral antigenic targets they may also be good candidates for immunotherapy (Rickinson and Kieff, 2001). The advances in such adoptive immunotherapeutic approaches will be discussed in this chapter.

Therapy for herpesvirus-related infections and diseases

Infectious complications relating to herpes simplex virus (HSV), varicella zoster virus (VZV) (Asanuma et al., 2000), Kaposi's sarcoma virus (KSV) (Wang et al., 2000), human herpesvirus (HHV)-6, -7 (Clark, 2002; Clark et al., 2003; Clark and Griffiths, 2003), cytomegalovirus (CMV) (Michaelides et al., 2002) and EBV (Heslop et al., 1994) are common in immunocompromised individuals. In particular, during allogeneic HSCT and SOT, conditioning regimens involving a combination of immunosuppressive drugs and radiation therapy eliminate the recipient immune system. T-cell depletion, delayed T-cell recovery in vivo, and prolonged immunosuppressive treatments are all associated with a significant risk of herpesvirus reactivations post-transplant. In the HSCT setting, immune recovery occurs after engraftment and expansion of the recipient immune system, in vivo (Weinberg et al., 2001). However, following SOT the patient remains in an immunosuppressed state lifelong, and thus the recipient immune system can never achieve its full potential. Treatments for herpesvirus infections include vaccination approaches, which aim to evoke an immune response by administration of an immunogen, as a peptide or DNA, directly into patients. However, in the immunocompromised host, vaccines may not function optimally. Anti-viral drugs, such as acyclovir and ganciclovir inhibit productive virus replication in vivo, and can effectively control α- and β-herpesvirus infections, in which disease is associated with the lytic life cycle. However in the case of CMV, antiviral drugs appear to alter subsequent reactivations such that antiviral T-cells recover less effectively, leading to a late, chronic CMV-reactivation, particularly in association with chronic graft vs. host disease (GvHD) (Junghanss et al., 2002; Nguyen et al., 1999). In addition, drug resistant escape mutants have been reported (Springer et al., 2005; Razonable and Paya, 2003).

Most antiherpes viral agents are prodrugs that are activated by lytic cycle kinases, and thus have limited efficacy against γ-herpesviruses, such as EBV, whose pathology is associated with its latent cycle. EBV-associated lymphoproliferative disease (LPD) in which virus-transformed

Table 74.1. Human herpesviruses

Herpesvirus subgroup	Virus	Tumor association
alpha	HSV-1	none
	HSV-2	none
	VZV	none
beta	CMV	none
	HHV-6	none
	HHV-7	none,
gamma	EBV	Burkitt's lymphoma, Gastric carcinoma, Nasopharyngeal carcinoma, Hodgkin's disease, Post-transplant lymphoproliferative disease, T-cell lymphoma, Leiomyosarcoma
	HHV-8	Kaposi sarcoma of HIV positive and negative patients, body cavity lymphoma, Castleman's disease

B-cells proliferate in an uncontrolled manner, has emerged as a significant complication of both HSCT (d'Amore et al., 1991) and SOT (Straathof et al., 2002; Savoldo et al., 2001). EBV is also linked with a number of tumors that are not associated with iatrogenic or intrinsic immunosuppression including Hodgkin's disease (HD), nasopharyngeal carcinoma (NPC), and Burkitt's lymphoma (BL). (Rickinson and Kieff, 2001.) A recent advance in the treatment of EBV-LPD in HSCT recipients has been the humanized anti-B cell monoclonal antibody, rituximab, designed for the treatment of follicular lymphoma, but which has proved effective for the treatment of EBV positive B-cell lymphomas (Kuehnle et al., 2000). However, rituximab has little efficacy against HD, which rarely express CD20, or NPC (Table 74.1).

The potential for using in vitro expanded virus-specific CTLs as either prophylaxis or treatment for viral infections/reactivations stemmed from the observation that viral reactivations post-transplant were clearly associated with the lack of recovery of virus-specific T-cells. Donor leukocyte infusions (DLIs) had therapeutic benefits for the treatment of EBV positive lymphomas occurring after HSCT (Papadopoulos et al., 1994). However, GvHD resulting from the presence of alloreative T cells was a common side effect, and a pure population of virus-specific cells was predicted to be safer and therapeutically beneficial. Since CMV- and EBV-associated diseases remain potentially fatal complications in the immunosuppressed these viruses have been the focus of adoptive immunotherapy approaches. A variety of strategies have been developed, some of which have been translated into the clinic and assessed for safety and efficacy and a number of these will now be reviewed.

Cytomegalovirus

As many as 80% of healthy individuals show evidence of past CMV exposure and persisting humoral and cellular immunity. The virus remains latent in cells of the myeloid lineage but reactivation from their resting state occurs sporadically, (Mocarski and Courcelle, 2001; Pass, 2001). Analysis of the T cell immune response to individual CMV proteins has indicated that there is a hierarchy of immunodominance, i.e. certain proteins tend to be strong targets of T-cell immunity while other proteins are subdominant. In the case of CMV the bulk of the CD8+ T cell immune response is directed against two immunodominant proteins, pp65 and IE (Bunde et al., 2005; Kern et al., 2000). pp65 is a matrix protein produced during the late phase, and it is thought that during primary infection, the initial viral input dominates the immune response, since the presentation of subsequently expressed viral proteins to the immune response is inhibited. Conversely, reactivation of virus from a resting state may result in the formation of T-cell memory dominated by the immediate early (IE) protein, which is transcribed prior to the initiation of viral immune evasion strategies. Thus IE may also be an important target for CTL infusions.

Epstein–Barr virus

The γ-herpesvirus, EBV, establishes latent infections in target B-lymphocytes, (Rickinson and Kieff, 2001; Rickinson and Moss, 1997)). In type III latency the eight virally encoded latent cycle proteins; nuclear antigens EBNAs 1, 2, 3A, 3B, 3C, -LP and latent membrane proteins LMPs 1 and 2, along with two small non-polyadenylated RNAs (or EBERs) and the BamHI A RNAs cause continuous B-cell proliferation resulting in EBV-transformed lymphoblastoid cell lines (LCLs). Latency types I and II demonstrate a more restricted pattern of latent gene expression. Latency II was first described in EBV-positive Hodgkin's disease where the EBERs, the BamHI A RNAs, EBNA1, and LMP1 and 2 are expressed. EBV-associated nasopharyngeal carcinoma (NPC) also expresses a latency II pattern of gene expression. Latency I was first described in EBV-positive Burkitt's lymphoma (BL) lines, which express EBERs, the BamHI A RNAs, and EBNA1 (Rickinson and Kieff, 2001). Note that EBNA1 is the only viral protein expressed in all the different forms of malignancy-associated latency, and in each type of latency a different transcriptional promoter is used for EBNA1 expression (Amyes et al., 2003). This protein is absolutely required for episomal maintenance of the viral genome. However, in a cell, which is not cycling, it is thought

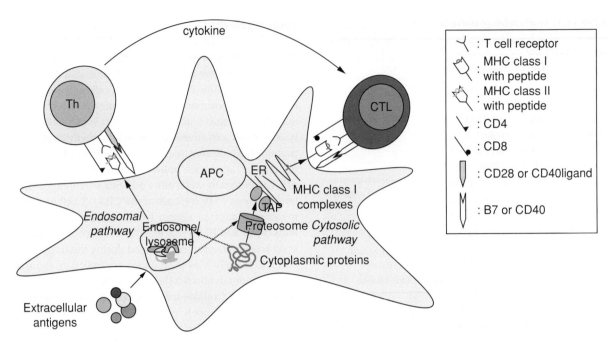

Fig. 74.1. Generation of cell-mediated immune response. (See color plate section.)

that virus persists without the expression of EBNA1, and only LMP2 can be detected in EBV-infected resting B-cells (type 0 latency) (Qu and Rowe, 1992; Tierney et al., 1994; Miyashita et al., 1997).

Initial work identifying the targets of the strong specific memory T-cell response in healthy seropositive donors demonstrated the dominance of reactivities against early lytic cycle proteins and the latent antigens EBNA3A, -B, and –C in the majority of individuals tested, restricted through a wide range of MHC class I alleles. LMP2 is also a common target for specific T-cells but reactivity is generally weak and of low frequency, when compared to that of the immunodominant antigens. In contrast, only rare reactivities specific for epitopes derived from EBNA1, EBNA2, EBNA-LP, and LMP1 have been identified (Rickinson and Moss, 1997). Memory T-cells specific for the latency-associated antigens persist throughout the lifetime of the normal healthy host and the frequency of CTL precursors directed against different viral epitopes remains relatively stable within an individual (Hislop et al., 2002; Amyes et al., 2003).

T-cell activation

The design of successful immunological strategies to treat human virus-associated diseases and malignancies requires an understanding of the effector processes that control viral infection and the mechanisms viruses use to evade such responses.

Virus-specific CD4+ Th cells and CD8+ CTLs mediate the effector mechanisms necessary to resolve acute infection as well as providing immune memory, which protects against re-exposure to acute virus infection and controls the reactivation of latent viruses (Abbas et al., 1996). CD8+ CTLs recognize virus-infected cells through interaction of their T-cell receptor with virus-derived peptides bound to the major histocompatibility complex (MHC) class I molecule of the infected cell. Viral proteins endogenously synthesized in the infected cell are degraded into short antigenic peptides by the cellular antigen-processing machinery, carried to the cell surface by MHC molecules, where they are presented to T-cells circulating through lymphoid tissues. These peptides are generally 8–10 amino acids long, generated within cells by a cytoplasmic proteolytic complex known as the proteosome and then transported into the endoplasmic reticulum by TAP (transporters associated with antigen processing), where they are complexed with MHC class I molecules for cell surface presentation (Jondal et al., 1996; Pamer and Cresswell, 1998). Since virtually all nucleated cells express MHC class I, any virus-derived protein may be presented by MHC class I molecules and should be susceptible to subsequent recognition by specific CD8+ T-cells. A role for CD8-mediated viral control has clearly been documented in animal models, further supported by the identification of a number of mechanisms whereby viruses have evolved ways of evading the MHC class I antigen presentation pathway (McMichael, 1998) (Fig. 74.1).

For activating (priming) naïve CTL precursors, antigenic peptides must be presented by professional APCs, which also provide the necessary co-stimulatory signals (i.e., interaction of B7 or CD40 on APC with CD28 or CD40L on T-cells, respectively) (Sigal et al., 1999). If the T-cell receptor is engaged without costimulatory signals, T-lymphocytes can become anergized. However, activated CTLs do not need costimulatory molecules to exert their effector functions, namely, cytolysis or induction of apoptosis of the target cell. Importantly, target cells frequently do not express co-stimulatory molecules. CMV and EBV are interesting exceptions in which latency occurs in professional APCs.

CD4+ T-cells play a role in antibody responses and also recognize antigens that are phagocytosed from an exogenous source, and processed and presented in the context of MHC class II molecules. Only APCs that are MHC class II-positive can activate CD4+ T-cell precursors. CD4+ T-cells also play a role in anti-viral immunity; activated Th cells produce a variety of cytokines including IL-2, IFN-γ, and TNF-α, which have direct anti-viral activity. Simultaneously, these activated T-cells also serve to condition APCs to activate virus-specific CTLs. When the infected cell is MHC class II positive, CD4+ T-cells can also be cytolytic to the target cells and this function has been clearly demonstrated for herpesvirus infections including CMV, EBV, HSV, and VZV (Lanzavecchia, 1996; Borysiewicz and Sissons, 1994).

Strategies for producing T-cells for adoptive immunotherapy

The generation of virus-specific CTLs or T-cell clones for adoptive immunotherapy is an attractive alternative to anti-viral drug therapy as infused CTLs have the potential to persist in vivo without related toxicity. Prior to using in vitro expanded CTLs for infusion purposes the cells must fulfil a number of requirements.
 (i) All cell preparation must be carried out under good manufacturing practices (GMP).
 (ii) CTL lines or T cell clones must be virus-specific and lack reactivity with recipient alloantigens or self-antigens.
 (iii) CTL lines/clones should include both specific CD4+ and CD8+ T-cells.
 (iv) Cells for infusion must be present in sufficient quantities for safety testing and infusion.

To meet these requirements the choice of antigen and APC to be used for activation and expansion purposes must be carefully chosen, and immunological and virological monitoring of patients post-infusion is desirable to demonstrate the safety and efficacy of T-cell therapy. Since immunodominant T-cell target antigens and sources of APCs have already been identified for both CMV and EBV, and related infections constitute a significant problem in the immunocompromised human host, initial adoptive immunotherapeutic strategies focused on these two herpesviruses.

Adoptive immunotherapy for cytomegalovirus

A number of factors are predictive of CMV infection post-HSCT transplant including:
 (i) receiving a graft from an HLA-mismatched or unrelated donor,
 (ii) recipient CMV seropositivity coupled with donor CMV-negativity,
 (iii) the use of submyeloablative or reduced intensity, highly immunosuppressive conditioning regimens.

It has been shown that recovery of CD8+, CMV-specific CTLs in the early post-transplantation period inversely correlates with the development of CMV-related disease, and it has been reported that, in up to 65% of patients, CMV-specific CTLs do not develop during this period, leaving this cohort at high risk of virus-related complications (Pass, 2001). In a pioneering study by Walter and colleagues, CD8+ CMV-specific T cell clones were isolated and expanded from the blood of bone marrow donors and administered to 14 patients prophylactically at weekly intervals in doses escalating from 3.3×10^6/kg to 1×10^9/kg, beginning 30–40 days post-transplant (Walter et al., 1995). The infused clones were reactive against CMV virion proteins, including the immunodominant T-cell target, pp65. Careful monitoring of the status of CMV-specific immunity pre-infusion indicated that 11 of the 14 donors lacked any evidence of anti-viral activity pre-infusion, while after the first infusion responses were detected in all donors. The magnitude of these responses increased with successive injections but specific CD8+ T-cell immunity did not persist in patients who did not have a concurrent recovery of CD4+ T-cells, highlighting the importance of Th cells in the maintenance of anti-viral activity *in vivo*. In a number of infused recipients the authors could directly correlate CMV T-cell immunity and the persistence (for up to 12 weeks) of transferred T-cells by following rearranged Vα and Vβ genes for the T-cell receptor (TCR) as molecular markers. Neither CMV viremia nor disease developed in any of the treated patients (Walter et al., 1995).

A second CMV immunotherapy trial was published by Einsele and colleagues in 2002 (Einsele et al., 2002). Polyclonal CMV-specific CTL lines were infused into eight HSCT recipients who had persisting or recurring CMV infection despite the prolonged use of anti-viral medications. Donors were CMV sero-positive and included HLA-matched siblings, HLA-matched unrelated donors, or HLA mismatched related or unrelated donors. At the time of the first CTL infusion, seven of the eight patients treated were still receiving some form of immunosuppression as prophylaxis for GvHD.

Polyclonal CTL lines were prepared by stimulating PBMCs with CMV lysate, which is a source of multiple CMV antigens that could be phagocytosed and presented by peripheral blood monocytes. The CTLs were expanded using autologous, irradiated PBMC feeder cells to present CMV lysate, and IL-2. A total T-cell dose of $1 \times 10^7/m^2$ was administered without toxicity. In all cases the lines were predominantly CD4+ and CMV specificity was confirmed prior to infusion using proliferation assays. The advantage of this method is that CTL lines containing both CD4+ and CD8+ T-cells with a broad range of antigen and epitope specificities could be induced and infused. The efficacy of CTL infusions was assessed using immunological assays to measure the functional capabilities of PBMCs drawn from patients at two-weekly intervals postinfusion and viral load was assessed using quantitative or semi-quantitative PCR analysis.

Following T-cell therapy, six of the eight patients, all of whom lacked anti-CMV reactivity before adoptive transfer, responded in vitro to CMV protein and had no detectable levels of CMV in PBMCs. Viral load as determined by quantitative PCR showed significant reductions following therapy in 7/7 evaluable patients. This reduction in viral load was persistent in five, and transient in two patients. Two patients who did get a CMV reactivation received a course of intense immunosuppression for GvHD around the time of T-cell therapy. Immunological monitoring supported the assertion that infusion of virus-specific CD4+ T-cell lines hastened the *in vivo* recovery of virus-specific CD8+ T-cells, as significant expansions of peptide-specific CD8+ T-cells, detectable by tetramer, were discernible within 2 months of therapy.

This trial confirmed the efficacy of T-cell therapy, either as prophylaxis or treatment, for CMV infection and disease post-HSCT. It also provided a simple and rapid means to reconstitute long-term CD4 and CD8 CMV-specific immunity using CTL doses >2 logs lower than that used in the previous study.

Despite the positive outcome of both these trials there were also some associated difficulties. In the case of Walter and colleagues the methodology used for CTL clone generation required a skin biopsy for the generation of dermal fibroblasts for use as APCs. In addition, live virus was used to stimulate specific CD8+ T-cell reactivity. From a therapeutic point of view, each T-cell clone can only be specific for one epitope peptide from one antigen. Therefore the breadth of reactivities generated for infusion may be lacking in some donors depending on the number of different clones infused, and the paucity of CD4+ cells probably affected the persistence of these cells in vivo. Finally, from a practical point of view the generation of large numbers of specific T-cell clones for infusion is time consuming, technically difficult, and expensive.

In the second study, CTL lines could be generated for only 68% of patients, suggesting that CMV CTL generation using PBMCs pulsed with CMV lysate may be a suboptimal production method. Further optimization, perhaps by using professional APCs, may improve the overall percentage of successful lines generated. Both studies reported poor results achieved in patients receiving immunosuppressive therapy to counteract GvHD, illustrating one potential barrier to effective immunotherapy for HSCT recipients in the early post-transplant period.

Adoptive immunotherapy for EBV post-transplant lymphoproliferation disease

The majority of EBV-PTLD in HSCT recipients are of donor B-cell origin. Malignant B-cells usually express the complete panel of latent viral antigens, as well as abundant co-stimulatory molecules. Thus, they are highly immunogenic, and in healthy individuals are eliminated by circulating EBV-specific CTL. The incidence of EBV lymphoproliferation in high-risk patients, i.e. those receiving a T-cell depleted transplant from an unrelated donor or an HLA-mismatched, related donor, ranges from 1% to 25% (Curtis *et al.*, 1999). By contrast, removal of B-cells from the graft decreases the incidence to less than 2%, suggesting that uncontrolled EBV-driven lymphoproliferation may be favored when the ratio of T-: B-cells is severely disrupted (Hale and Waldmann, 1998). An increase in EBV DNA in peripheral blood, measured by quantitative real time PCR is used to predict the development of EBV-LPD, with several studies confirming that EBV load correlates with an increased risk of LPD (Rooney *et al.*, 1995a,b; Stevens *et al.*, 2001; van Esser *et al.*, 2002; Wagner *et al.*, 2003).

EBV-associated PTLD is a good target for immunotherapy since most donors are seropositive, and EBV-specific CTLs can readily be reactivated from PBMC using LCLs as APCs for stimulation and expansion. LCLs are easily made by infecting donor PBMCs with a laboratory strain of EBV, resulting in the outgrowth of B-cell lines expressing target antigens identical to those expressed in LPD. Since 1993, our group has infused over 60 stem cell recipients with donor-derived EBV-specific T-cell lines. $2 \times 10^7 CTL/m^2$, was established as a safe and efficacious dose for both prophylaxis and treatment (Rooney et al., 1995a,b 1998a,b). In each case the CTL lines were polyclonal, with CD4:CD8 ratios ranging from 2:98 to 98:2. The first 26 patients enrolled in this study received CTLs which were genetically marked with a retroviral vector containing the neomycin resistance gene (neo), allowing the collection of data about the persistence and localization of infused cells in vivo. In addition, 6 patients received virus-specific CTL after the onset of lymphoma.

None of the patients treated with EBV-specific CTL as prophylaxis developed PTLD, in contrast with an incidence of 11.5% in a historical untreated control group (Heslop and Rooney, 1997). At study entry 9 patients had elevated EBV–DNA levels, which is highly predictive of the development of LPD. Analysis of EBV-DNA levels postinfusion showed direct evidence of anti-viral activity as DNA levels decreased by up to four logs within 1–3 weeks of the first T-cell infusion. In patients who received marked cells, specific CTLs could be detected for up to 78 months post CTL (Rooney et al., 1998a,b).

Although CTL had proven effective at decreasing viral load, it was uncertain whether infusions of T-cells could be successful in treating an already established lymphoma. We treated a total of six patients with evident lymphoma and in five of the six patients complete remission was achieved. In the remaining patient, comprehensive in vitro characterization revealed the increased dominance of a virus deletion mutant after CTL infusion (Gottschalk et al., 2001). The donor CTL line generated by co-culture of donor PBMCs with an LCL generated using the B95-8 virus strain revealed epitope reactivity directed predominantly against the immunodominant EBNA3B antigen, and specifically against two immunodominant epitope peptides within this antigen; namely AVFDRKSDAK (AVF), aa 399–408 and IVTDFSVIK (IVT), aa 416–424, both recognized in the context of the HLA A*11 allele (Gottschalk et al., 2001). Sequence analysis of the resident patient tumor revealed two resident viruses. One harbored a deletion in the EBNA3B gene, which removed the AVF and IVT peptide sequences. Since the virus with the wild type EBNA3B could no longer be detected after CTL infusion, the CTL line had reduced ability to recognize the mutant virus. This is a concern for all adoptive immunotherapy protocols as this case illustrates that, even in a polyclonal system, a mutation in a tumor-specific antigen can ultimately result in tumor escape.

In total over 160 patients received CTLs, most as prophylaxis and 6 as treatment for established lymphoma. In one patient who received CTL for treatment of bulky nasopharyngeal disease, the infusion caused an inflammatory response which required mechanical ventilation. However the child made a full recovery and achieved complete remission (Straathof et al., 2005). The authors were unsuccessful in generating a CTL line for two eligible patients whose donors were EBV-seronegative. An additional problem with CTL use is that the total time for LCL and CTL production and testing is approximately 12 weeks, while the aggressiveness of this lymphoma means that CTL should be administered prophylactically for high-risk patients. Despite this, in the absence of effective antiviral agents, adoptive immunotherapy was an attractive alternative as EBV-specific CTLs are safe and effective at controlling and treating EBV in high-risk patients post-transplant. More recently, monoclonal anti-B-cell antibodies such as rituximab demonstrated overall response rates of 69%–100% when used as a treatment for LPD post HSCT (Kuehnle et al., 2000). Since rituximab is now widely available, it has now largely replaced CTL as the preferred treatment of EBV after HSCT. In the 6 months usually required for B cell recovery after treatment, endogenous antiviral immunity recovers and is able to control EBV when it reappears.

Adoptive immunotherapy for EBV post-solid organ transplant

Although it has been shown that adoptive immunotherapy is an effective treatment of EBV-LPD in the HSCT recipient, the optimal treatment for patients receiving solid organ transplants has yet to be established. In this cohort, LPD is usually of recipient origin, thus the preparation of EBV-specific CTLs requires the use of autologous or HLA-matched cells. Autologous EBV-specific CTL can be generated from the peripheral blood of SOT patients prior to transplant (Haque et al., 1998), but a number of groups have also reported the successful generation of virus-specific CTL lines from patients receiving immunosuppression, including those with overt lymphoma, showing that EBV-specific CTL persist, but are unable to function in vivo (Straathof et al., 2002; Savoldo et al., 2001; Khanna et al., 1999; Comoli et al., 2002). Ten SOT patients with high viral load received autologous EBV-specific CTLs and eight showed a subsequent normalization of EBV–DNA levels and an increase in virus-specific CTL precursors (Haque et al., 1998; Comoli et al., 2002). Until recently, the persistence of infused CTL had not been examined (Savoldo et al., 2001; Comoli et al., 2002). Savoldo and colleagues have investigated the in-vivo safety, efficacy and persistence of autologous EBV CTL for the treatment of SOT recipients at high-risk for EBV-associated PTLD (Savoldo et al., 2006). Twelve SOT recipients at high risk for PTLD, or with active disease, received autologous CTL infusion without toxicity. Real-time PCR monitoring of EBV-DNA showed a transient increase in plasma EBV-DNA suggestive of lysis of EBV-infected cells, although there was no consistent decrease in virus load in peripheral blood mononuclear cells. Interferon-γ Elispot assay and tetramer analysis showed an increase in the frequency of EBV-responsive T cells, which returned to pre-infusion levels after 2–6 months. None of the treated patients developed PTLD. One patient with liver PTLD showed a complete response, and one with ocular disease had a partial response stable for over one year (Savoldo et al., 2006). These data are consistent with an expansion and persistence of adoptively transferred EBV-CTL, that is limited in the presence of continued immunosuppression, but that nonetheless produced clinically useful anti-viral activity.

Adoptive transfer of EBV-specific CTL for Hodgkin's lymphoma

Having shown that EBV infected cells, which express a wide range of EBV encoded antigens, are susceptible to immunotherapy our group is now evaluating if the malignant cells of Hodgkin's disease, which express a more restricted pattern of antigens, are also targets for this approach. In a Phase I dose escalation study we have evaluated the use of autologous EBV-specific CTL for patients with EBV-positive Hodgkin's disease (Roskrow et al., 1998). We treated eight patients with relapsed Hodgkin disease with two infusions ($2 \times 10^7/m^2$–$1.2 \times 10^8/m^2$) of EBV-specific CTL. In seven of these patients the CTL were retrovirally marked. Increases in anti-viral immunity, and decreases in virus load demonstrated the in vivo biological activity of the infused CTL and gene-marked T cells could be detected for up to 9 months. Trafficking to tumor sites was demonstrated in two patients by in situ hybridization to the neo marker gene in mediastinal tumor tissue and by PCR in a malignant pleural effusion. Further, partial tumor responses were observed. However, no patient with bulky disease was cured. In a second group, treated with CTL as adjuvant therapy after autologous stem cell rescue, four of five patients remain in remission over 24 months after CTL infusion, including one patient who had residual disease after HSCT and prior to CTL infusion.

Although these results have been promising the antiviral responses were transient, and no patient with aggressive relapsed Hodgkin's disease has been cured. This may be due to a lack of specificity of the EBV-specific CTL for the subdominant LMP1 and LMP2 antigens present on the Hodgkin's tumor. Using dendritic cells transduced with LMP2 to stimulate and expand the CTL, LMP2-specific CTL have been generated that have an increased cytolytic activity to LMP2 positive targets in vitro when compared to EBV-CTL (Gahn et al., 2001; Rooney et al., 2002; Bollard et al., 2004). A clinical trial using LMP2-specific CTL for the treatment of Hodgkin's and non-Hodgkin's lymphoma expressing a type II latency has recently begun.

Adoptive transfer of EBV-specific CTL for nasopharyngeal carcinoma

Nasopharyngeal carcinoma is a malignant disease with a variable range of incidence depending on age, geographical location, race, and EBV exposure. It has an annual incidence of nearly 1 case per 100 000 children <21 yrs in the USA (Niedobitek, 2000). The non-keratinizing NPCs are uniformly associated with EBV. Despite the good overall survival rates, particularly in children, current NPC treatment regimens including radiotherapy and chemotherapy are still far from ideal. Follow-up reports have shown increased risks for treatment-related morbidity and mortality (Pao et al., 1989). Late medical complications after treatment for NPC include growth hormone deficiency, hypothyroidism, pulmonary fibrosis, and secondary malignancies. It is therefore, desirable to develop novel therapies that could improve disease free survival in relapsed/refractory patients and which might ultimately reduce the incidence of long-term treatment related complications in all patients.

Chua et al., treated four patients with advanced nasopharyngeal carcinoma with 5×10^7–3×10^8 autologous EBV CTL (Chua et al., 2001). Although it was difficult to confirm improved tumor control in these patients who had significantly bulky disease, the treatment was safe and elevations in CTL precursor frequency were seen. In 3 patients, host surveillance of EBV replication was restored resulting in a reduction in the plasma EBV burden. Straathof and colleagues have treated 10 patients with advanced NPC with autologous CTLs. All patients tolerated the CTLs, although one developed increased swelling at the site of pre-existing disease. At 19 to 27 months after infusion, 4 patients treated in remission from locally advanced disease remain disease free. Of 6 patients with refractory disease prior to treatment, 2 had complete responses, and remain in remission over 11 to 23 months after treatment; 1 had a partial remission that persisted for 12 months; 1 has had stable disease for more than 14 months; and 2 had no response. These results demonstrate that administration of EBV-specific CTLs to patients with advanced NPC is feasible, appears to be safe, and can be associated with significant antitumor activity (Straathof et al., 2005).

For EBV+ve tumors, such as HD and NPC, which arise in patients with an intact immune system, approaches that overcome immune evasion strategies used by these immunogenic tumors may be required. Further improvements in the *in vivo* function and persistence of CTL may require genetic modification of CTL lines to provide resistance to tumor-derived immunosuppressive chemokines and cytokines (Bollard et al., 2002; Foster and Rooney, 2006). Alternatively, modifications to the host or tumor environment may be sufficient (Dudley et al., 2002).

Multivirus-specific CTL lines

Since both EBV and CMV reactivations are common side effects post-transplant, some groups have considered generating bi-virus specific CTLs for infusion purposes (Sun et al., 1999, 2000). Lucas and colleagues carried out a phase I/II clinical protocol for the generation and infusion of EBV and CMV-specific CTL, initiated by culturing donor-derived PBMC with irradiated donor-derived LCL transduced with a retrovirus expressing pp65 (Lucas et al., 2000). Two further stimulations with the transduced LCL were performed before assessing the CMV and EBV-specific cytolytic activity of the line. Clinical data is not yet available from this study. Our group has also generated multivirus-specific CTL lines for therapeutic purposes by genetically modifying APCs to enable production of CD4$^+$ and CD8$^+$ T lymphocytes specific for CMV, EBV, and multiple serotypes of adenovirus from a single cell culture. Eleven multivirus-specific CTL lines were administered as prophyaxis or treatment to immunocompromised patients. In all cases the single T lymphocyte line was able to expand in vivo into multiple discrete virus-specific populations that could supply clinically measurable antiviral activity, and all patients with evidence of active CMV, EBV or adenoviral infection had a relatively rapid reduction in viral titer and resolution of disease symptoms, which coincided with the expansion of virus-specific CTL. Therefore, we can conclude that monoculture-derived multispecific CTL could provide a safe and efficient means to restore virus-specific immunity in the immunocompromised host (Leen et al., 2006b).

CMV and EBV immunotherapy in HIV positive individuals

Adoptive immunotherapy approaches have been applied to the treatment of acquired immunodeficiency syndrome (AIDS) where pathogenicity is synonymous with the depletion of CD4+ T-lymphocytes, and the consequent increased susceptibility to infections, either from *de novo* exposure or reactivation of latent viruses such as EBV (Riddell et al., 1996). To date, no group has targeted the herpesvirus infections/reactivations that occur as a result of HIV-induced immunosuppression. Brodie and colleagues have assessed the safety and efficacy of expanding and transferring up to 3.3×10^9 cells/m^2 autologous HIV-1 specific, Gag-specific CD8+ T-cell clones to HIV-infected individuals, and reported the accumulation of the transferred cells at sites adjacent to HIV-infected cells in the lymph nodes (Brodie et al., 1999; Brodie et al., 2000). In addition, levels of circulating productively infected CD4+ T-cells transiently decreased. However within 7 days of infusion the percentage of productively infected cells had returned to pre-infusion levels, suggesting that adoptive immunotherapy may not be efficacious in this patient cohort. Since the advent of highly active antiretroviral therapy (HAART) the incidence of EBV+ve CNS lymphomas has decreased. Strangely and perhaps controversially however, the incidence of other EBV+ve lymphomas has not (Levine et al., 2001). Since the overall health and life expectancy of patients with HIV has improved with HAART, the potential for adoptive transfer of herpesvirus-specific T-cells in these patients should perhaps be revisited.

Alternative approaches for activating virus-specific CTLs

In the outlined adoptive immunotherapy approaches there are a number of differences in terms of the phenotype of the infused cells, the choice of antigen for activation, the APC utilized to stimulate T-cells, the CTL expansion methods, and also the numbers of cells that are infused. The relative advantages and disadvantages of these methods, as well as alternative approaches which may be attempted in future studies, will be discussed.

Clones vs. polyclonal lines

The original Riddell CMV immunotherapy protocol, which proved efficacious in vivo, relied on the infusion of large numbers (3.3×10^6 cells/kg to 1×10^9 cells/kg) of CD8+ T-cell clones (Walter et al., 1995). In contrast, infusion of smaller numbers (1×10^7–2×10^7/m^2) of polyclonal, virus-specific CD4+ and CD8+ CTL lines proved efficacious in the context of CMV and EBV prophylaxis and/or treatment in the transplant and tumor setting, suggesting that a mixed population of CD4+ and CD8+ T-cells rather than

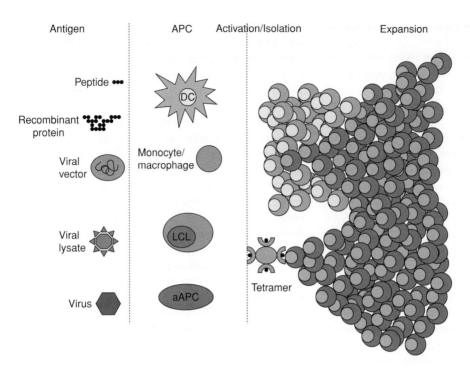

Fig. 74.2. Generation of antigen-specific T-cells.

the quantity of cells is the important factor for infusion purposes in situations where the recipient immune system has been depleted (Einsele *et al.*, 2002; Rooney *et al.*, 1995a,b; Peggs *et al.*, 2003).

Antigen

There are a number of options when choosing a source of antigen to stimulate an immune response. Riddell and colleagues used live CMV, (Walter *et al.*, 1995) and Einsele *et al.* utilized CMV lysate to stimulate CMV-specific immunity, (Einsele *et al.*, 2002) while Rooney and colleagues used an EBV-transformed B-cell line expressing EBV lytic and latent antigens to stimulate an immune response (Rooney *et al.*, 1995a,b). Alternative sources of antigen, which have been investigated in *in vitro* studies, include live or inactivated virus, recombinant protein, replication-defective viral vectors expressing one or more immunodominant T cell target antigens (Bonini *et al.*, 2001), or antigenic peptides (Fig. 74.2) (Foster *et al.*, 2003; Szmania *et al.*, 2001). Since the recipients of adoptively transferred T-cells are profoundly immunosuppressed, the use of live/attenuated virus is unwise, but replication incompetent viral vectors expressing a transgene may offer the ideal antigen source, capable of stimulating both CD4+ and CD8+ T cell simultaneously.

APC

The choice of APC for activation of an immune response may differ from that chosen to expand cells to the numbers necessary for infusion and GMP testing. In the case of EBV, LCLs provide an excellent APC with which to stimulate and expand polyclonal EBV-specific T-cells. However, when one considers the treatment of other EBV-associated malignancies such as Hodgkin's disease or NPC where gene expression is limited to the sub-dominant T-cell target antigens LMP1 (Gottschalk *et al.*, 2003), LMP2, and EBNA1, the use of LCLs is problematic since reactivity to early lytic cycle antigens and the immunodominant EBNA3 proteins is preferentially expanded (Rooney *et al.*, 2002; Gottschalk *et al.*, 2003; Rooney *et al.*, 1998, 2001). Thus, transducing LCLs, activated monocytes, or DCs with a viral vector which over-expresses the tumor-associated antigens may be advantageous for the simulation and expansion of a CTL line with more focused reactivity (Keever-Taylor *et al.*, 2001; Leen *et al.*, 2006a). In the case of CMV, where there is a distinct lack of an ideal APC, a number of groups have relied on the generation of DCs, which are then pulsed with CMV lysate or epitope peptide (Szmania *et al.*, 2001), or transduced with vectors expressing immunodominant T-cell antigens (Bonini *et al.*, 2001; Keever-Taylor *et al.*, 2001), as a means to stimulate reactivity (Fig. 74.2). However, although DCs are the most potent APCs available, their inability to proliferate in vitro means that large blood volumes are required to produce sufficient DC for CTL expansion, therefore DC numbers are limiting, and DC generation is time consuming.

Selection of specific T-cells

More recently, tetramer technology has facilitated the isolation of antigen-specific T-cells directly from peripheral blood (Fig. 74.2). Tetramers consist of four biotin-labeled HLA molecules bound together with streptavidin (Altman et al., 2001) and labeled with fluorochrome. Each HLA molecule is associated with a peptide epitope that binds to peptide-specific CTLs, which can then be directly visualized and isolated by fluorescence-activated cell-sorting (FACS). Once isolated, these cells can either be infused immediately or expanded ex vivo. This method precludes the carry-over of contaminating alloreactive T-cells, which could potentially induce GvHD in vivo. Cobbold and colleagues have recently used this approach to select CMV-specific T cells for the treatment of HSCT patients. CMV-specific $CD8^+$ T cells were isolated from the blood of stem cell transplant donors using HLA-peptide tetramers followed by selection with magnetic beads. The selected cells were infused directly into nine patients within 4 hours of selection. The cell dose was lower than those infused in conventional immunotherapeutic strategies (medium cell dosage was $8.6 \times 10(3)/kg$), however CMV-specific $CD8^+$ T cells became detectable in all patients within 10 days of infusion, and TCR clonotype analysis showed persistence of infused cells in two patients studied. CMV viremia was reduced in every case and eight patients cleared the infection, including one patient who had a prolonged history of CMV infection that was refractory to antiviral therapy. This novel approach to adoptive transfer has considerable potential for antigen-specific T cell therapy (Cobbold et al., 2005). However, each tetramer is specific for only one epitope limiting the repertoire of infused T-cells and, as yet, there are limited HLA class II tetramers available. Thus infused CTL lines may not persist in vivo due to lack of CD4+ help, and can be made only for patients with specific HLA phenotypes.

CTL expansion

The ideal immunotherapy protocol requires the generation of polyclonal virus-specific CD4+ and CD8+ T-cells in the shortest time possible. As cells are activated they begin to expand and through subsequent rounds of expansion, more and more APCs are needed for restimulation purposes. In particular, the need to expand large numbers of virus-specific CTLs for infusion post-SOT is a persistent problem. The number of APCs required for such protocols is frequently a limiting factor. Vaz-Santiago and colleagues tried to circumvent this problem by using PBMCs pulsed with a soluble recombinant chimeric protein, IE1-pp65, to activate and expand memory CD4+ and CD8+ CMV-specific T-cells but while CMV-specific T-cells could be activated, the problems associated with the expansion of sufficient numbers of cells for infusion and testing purposes were not dealt with in this study (Vaz-Santiago et al., 2002). Sili and colleagues have addressed this issue by utilizing Ad5f35pp65-transduced DCs to activate specific T-cells and then successfully expanded the stimulated population using autologous LCLs transduced with the Ad5f35pp65 vector, without loss of CMV specificity (Sili et al., 2003). Alternative expansion programs rely on the use of activated B and T cells, or the use of artificial APCs (aAPCs) (Melenhorst et al., 2006; Coughlin et al., 2004; Mans et al., 2003), but to date success has been limited by the loss of antigen specificity over time. An emerging option for both the activation and the expansion of virus-specific T-cells from a mixed PBMC population lies with the development of novel aAPCs based on the use of an antigen-HLA-epitope peptide complex coupled with a co-stimulatory molecule. Oelke and colleagues have recently pioneered such an approach by immobilizing a dimeric HLA immunoglobulin (HLA-Ig) onto beads together with CD28-specific antibody; the HLA molecules is then loaded with a known epitope peptide and used to activate and expand antigen-specific T cells from peripheral blood (Oelke et al., 2003). Resultant CTL lines were compared with those attained by conventional DC stimulation, and aAPC-based CTL activation was found to be equivalent or even better than DC-induced activation, with no appreciable loss in antigen specificity or growth rate detected over time. Thus, future immunotherapy trials may adopt such HLA-based aAPCs as being more cost effective than current methods of CTL generation and expansion. In addition, aAPCs can be prepared in bulk in advance and stored for use at a later date without loss of function, thus a more standardized approach to the generation of CTL lines for immunotherapy purposes is available. However, this method is limited by the requirement for specific peptides for folding into the HLA molecule, which also restricts the breadth of the CTL repertoire.

Regulation

The final barrier to initiating an adoptive immunotherapy trial for the prophylaxis and/or treatment of herpesvirus infections in the human host relates to the extensive regulations and time consuming applications which must be submitted to a number of regulatory agencies including the Internal Review Board (IRB), Recombinant DNA Advisory committee (RAC), and Food and Drug Administration (FDA) prior to initiation of any novel immunotherapy protocols. Few Institutions have the infrastructure and facilities required to fulfill all of these regulatory requirements. In addition, each reagent needed for the generation of a CTL line must be available as a clinical grade product, necessitating extensive and expensive analysis and testing. To date, for example, not all the components needed for the generation of mature monocyte-derived DCs are obtainable as clinical grade products due to the high costs of quality assurance and control costs which must be undertaken before a product is certified for human use.

Conclusions and future considerations

Herpesviruses are a significant cause of morbidity and mortality in immunocompromised individuals. Adoptive transfer of virus-specific CTLs has proven safe and effective at preventing and treating such infections in a number of instances, but there is room for improvement in the activation and expansion protocols utilized to allow the generation of virus-specific CTL lines in the shortest time possible. The major criticism of many immunotherapeutic approaches discussed is that they rely on the presence of a seropositive donor, from which specific T-cells can be activated and expanded. Thus, extension of this work to include seronegative SOT recipients or stem cell donors will increase the scope of this treatment to include all patients at risk of developing an infection or having a viral reactivation post-transplant (Savoldo et al., 2002; Park et al., 2006). New and more sensitive techniques to accurately monitor viral loads and thus predict viral reactivations in vivo have also been developed and used to predict EBV and CMV infections in immunocompromised individuals, allowing pre-emptive treatment, and monitoring of the efficacy post-treatment (Rooney et al., 1995a; Wagner et al., 2003b). In the future such monitoring may be extended to cover all herpesviruses, thereby utilizing a rational approach to the treatment of resultant infections either using adoptive immunotherapy or conventional antiviral reagents.

REFERENCES

Abbas, A. K., Murphy, K. M., and Sher, A. (1996). Functional diversity of helper T lymphocytes. *Nature*, **383**, 787–793.

Altman, J. D., Moss, P. A., Goulder, P. J. et al. (2001). Phenotypic analysis of antigen-specific T lymphocytes. *Science*, **274**, 94–96.

Amyes, E., Hatton, C., Montamat-Sicotte, D., et al. (2003). Characterization of the CD4$^+$ T cell response to Epstein–Barr virus during primary and persistent infection. *J. Exp. Med.*, **198**(6), 903–911.

Asanuma, H., Sharp, M., Maecker, H. T., Maino, V. C., and Arvin, A. M. (2000). Frequencies of memory T cells specific for varicella-zoster virus, herpes simplex virus, and cytomegalovirus by intracellular detection of cytokine expression. *J. Infect. Dis.*, **181**, 859–866.

Bollard, C. M., Rossig, C., Calonge, M. J. et al. (2002). Adapting a transforming growth factor beta-related tumor protection strategy to enhance antitumor immunity. *Blood*, **99**, 3179–3187.

Bollard, C. M., Aguilar, L., Straathof, K. C. et al. (2004). Cytotoxic T lymphocyte therapy for Epstein–Barr virus$^+$ Hodgkin's disease. *J. Exp. Med.*, **200**(12), 1623–1633.

Bonini, C., Lee, S. P., Riddell, S. R., and Greenberg, P. D. (2001). Targeting antigen in mature dendritic cells for simultaneous stimulation of CD4+ and CD8+ T cells. *J. Immunol.*, **166**, 5250–5257.

Borysiewicz, L. K. and Sissons, J. G. (1994). Cytotoxic T cells and human herpes virus infections. *Curr. Top. Microbiol. Immunol.*, **189**, 123–150.

Brodie, S. J., Lewinsohn, D. A., Patterson, B. K. et al. (1999). In vivo migration and function of transferred HIV-1-specific cytotoxic T cells. *Nat. Med.*, **5**, 34–41.

Brodie, S. J., Patterson, B. K., Lewinsohn, D. A. et al. (2000). HIV-specific cytotoxic T lymphocytes traffic to lymph nodes and localize at sites of HIV replication and cell death. *J. Clin. Invest.*, **105**, 1407–1417.

Bunde, T., Kirchner, A., Hoffmeister, B. et al. (2005). Protection from cytomegalovirus after transplantation is correlated with immediate early 1-specific CD8 T cells. *J. Exp. Med.*, **201**(7), 1031–1036.

Chua, D., Huang, J., Zheng, B. et al. (2001). Adoptive transfer of autologous Epstein-Barr virus-specific cytotoxic T cells for nasopharyngeal carcinoma. *Int. J. Cancer*, **94**, 73–80.

Clark, D. A. (2002). Human herpesvirus 6 and human herpesvirus 7: emerging pathogens in transplant patients. *Int. J. Hematol.*, **76** Suppl. **2**, 246–252.

Clark, D. A. and Griffiths, P. D. (2003). Human herpesvirus 6: relevance of infection in the immunocompromised host. *Br. J. Haematol.*, **120**, 384–395.

Clark, D. A., Emery, V. C., and Griffiths, P. D. (2003). Cytomegalovirus, human herpesvirus-6, and human herpesvirus-7 in hematological patients. *Semin. Hematol.*, **40**, 154–162.

Cobbold, M., Khan, N., Pourgheysari, B. et al. (2006). Adoptive transfer of cytomegalovirus-specific CTL to stem cell transplant patients after selection by HLA-peptide tetramers. *J. Exp. Med.* **202**(3), 379–386.

Comoli, P., Labirio, M., Basso, S. et al. (2002). Infusion of autologous Epstein–Barr virus (EBV)-specific cytotoxic T cells for prevention of EBV-related lymphoproliferative disorder in solid organ transplant recipients with evidence of active virus replication. *Blood*, **99**, 2592–2598.

Coughlin, C. M., Vance, B. A., Grupp, S. A., and Vonderheide, R. H. (2004). RNA-transfected CD40-activated B cells induce functional T-cell responses against viral and tumor antigen targets: implications for pediatric immunotherapy **103**(6), 2046–2054.

Curtis, R. E., Travis, L. B., Rowlings, P. A. *et al.* (1999). Risk of lymphoproliferative disorders after bone marrow transplantation: a multi-institutional study. *Blood*, **94**, 2208–2216.

d'Amore, E. S., Manivel, J. C., Gajl-Peczalska, K. J. *et al.* (1991). B-cell lymphoproliferative disorders after bone marrow transplant. An analysis of ten cases with emphasis on Epstein–Barr virus detection by in situ hybridization. *Cancer*, **68**, 1285–1295.

Dudley, M. E., Wunderlich, J. R., Robbins, P. F. *et al.* (2002). Cancer regression and autoimmunity in patients after clonal repopulation with antitumor lymphocytes. *Science*, **298**, 850–854.

Einsele, H., Roosnek, E., Rufer, N., *et al.* (2002). Infusion of cytomegalovirus (CMV)-specific T cells for the treatment of CMV infection not responding to antiviral chemotherapy. *Blood*, **99**, 3916–3922.

Foster, A. E. and Rooney, C. M. (2006). Improving T cell therapy for cancer, in press. *Expert Opin. Biol. Their.* **6**(3), 215–229.

Foster, A. E., Gottlieb, D. J., Marangolo, M. *et al.* (2003). Rapid, large-scale generation of highly pure cytomegalovirus-specific cytotoxic T cells for adoptive immunotherapy. *J. Hematother. Stem Cell Res.*, **12**, 93–105.

Gahn, B., Siller-Lopez, F., Pirooz, A. D. *et al.* (2001). Adenoviral gene transfer into dendritic cells efficiently amplifies the immune response to LMP2A antigen: a potential treatment strategy for Epstein–Barr virus–positive Hodgkin's lymphoma. *Int. J. Cancer*, **93**, 706–713.

Gottschalk, S., Ng, C. Y., Perez, M., *et al.* (2001). An Epstein–Barr virus deletion mutant associated with fatal lymphoproliferative disease unresponsive to therapy with virus-specific CTLs. *Blood*, **97**, 835–843.

Gottschalk, S., Edwards, O. L., Sili, U. *et al.* (2003). Generating CTLs against the subdominant Epstein–Barr virus LMP1 antigen for the adoptive immunotherapy of EBV-associated malignancies. *Blood*, **101**, 1905–1912.

Hale, G. and Waldmann, H. (1998). Risks of developing Epstein–Barr virus-related lymphoproliferative disorders after T-cell-depleted marrow transplants. CAMPATH Users. *Blood*, **91**, 3079–3083.

Haque, T., Amlot, P. L., Helling, N. *et al.* (1998). Reconstitution of EBV-specific T cell immunity in solid organ transplant recipients. *J. Immunol.*, **160**, 6204–6209.

Heslop, H. E. and Rooney, C. M. (1997). Adoptive cellular immunotherapy for EBV lymphoproliferative disease. *Immunol. Rev.*, **157**, 217–222.

Heslop, H. E., Li, C., Krance, R. A., Loftin, S. K., and Rooney, C. M. (1994). Epstein–Barr infection after bone marrow transplantation. *Blood*, **83**, 1706–1708.

Hislop, A. D., Annels, N. E., Gudgeon, N. H., Leese, A. M., and Rickinson, A. B. (2002). Epitope-specific evolution of human CD8(+) T cell responses from primary to persistent phases of Epstein–Barr virus infection. *J. Exp. Med.*, **195**, 893–905.

Jondal, M., Schirmbeck, R., and Reimann, J. (1996). MHC class I-restricted CTL responses to exogenous antigens. *Immunity*, **5**, 295–302.

Junghanss, C., Boeckh, M., Carter, R. A. *et al.* (2002). Incidence and outcome of cytomegalovirus infections following nonmyeloablative compared with myeloablative allogeneic stem cell transplantation, a matched control study. *Blood*, **99**, 1978–1985.

Keever-Taylor, C. A., Margolis, D., Konings, S. *et al.* (2001). Cytomegalovirus-specific cytolytic T-cell lines and clones generated against adenovirus-pp65-infected dendritic cells. *Biol. Blood Marrow Transpl.*, **7**, 247–256.

Kern, F., Faulhaber, N., Frommel, C. *et al.* (2000). Analysis of CD8 T cell reactivity to cytomegalovirus using protein-spanning pools of overlapping. *Eur. J. Immunol.* **30**(6), 1676–1682.

Khanna, R., Bell, S., Sherritt, M. *et al.* (1999). Activation and adoptive transfer of Epstein–Barr virus-specific cytotoxic T cells in solid organ transplant patients with posttransplant lymphoproliferative disease. *Proc. Natl Acad. Sci. USA*, **96**, 10391–10396.

Kuehnle, I., Huls, M. H., Liu, Z. *et al.* (2000). CD20 monoclonal antibody (rituximab) for therapy of Epstein–Barr virus lymphoma after hemopoietic stem-cell transplantation. *Blood*, **95**, 1502–1505.

Lanzavecchia, A. (1996). Mechanisms of antigen uptake for presentation. *Curr. Opin. Immunol.*, **8**, 348–354.

Leen, A., Ratnayake, M., Foster, A., Ahmed, N., Rooney, C. M. and Gottschalk, S. (2006a). Contact activated Monocytes: efficient antigen presenting cells for the stimulation of antigen-specific T cells. *J. Immunother.* (in press)

Leen, M., Myers, G. D., Sili, U. *et al.* (2006b). Monoculture-derived T lymphocytes specific for multiple viruses expand and produce clinically relevant effects in immunocompromised patients. *Nature Med., Nat. Med.*, **12**(10), 1160–1166.

Levine, A. M., Seneviratne, L., and Tulpule, A. (2001). Incidence and management of AIDS-related lymphoma. *Oncology (Huntingt)*, **15**, 629–639.

Li, H. and Minarovits (2003). Host cell-dependent expression of latent Epstein-Barr virus genomes: regulation by DNA methylation. *J. Adv. Cancer Res.* **89**, 133–156.

Lucas, K. G., Sun, Q., Burton, R. L. *et al.* (2000). A phase I–II trial to examine the toxicity of CMV- and EBV-specific cytotoxic T lymphocytes when used for prophylaxis against EBV and CMV disease in recipients of CD34-selected/T cell-depleted stem cell transplants. *Hum Gene Ther.*, **11**, 1453–1463.

Maus, M. V., Thomas, A. K., Leonard, D. G. *et al.* (2002). Ex vivo expansion of polyclonal and antigen-specific cytotoxic T lymphocytes by artificial APCs expressing ligands for the T-cell receptor, CD28 and 4–1BB. *Nat. Biotechnol.*, **20**, 143–148.

McMichael, A. (1998). T cell responses and viral escape. *Cell*, **93**, 673–676.

Melenhorst, J. J., Solomon, S. R., Shenoy, A. et al. (2006). Robust expansion of viral antigen-specific CD4+ and CD8+ T cells for adoptive T cell therapy using gene-modified activated T cells as antigen presenting cells. *J. Immunother.*, **29**(4), 436–443.

Michaelides, A., Glare, E. M., Spelman, D. W. et al. (2002). beta-Herpesvirus (human cytomegalovirus and human herpesvirus 6) reactivation in at-risk lung transplant recipients and in human immunodeficiency virus-infected patients. *J. Infect. Dis.*, **186**, 173–180.

Miyashita, E. M., Yang, B., Babcock, G. J., and Thorley-Lawson, D.A. (1997). Identification of the site of Epstein–Barr virus persistence in vivo as a resting B cell. *J. Virol.*, **71**, 4882–4891.

Mocarski, E. S. and Courcelle, C. (2001). Cytomegaloviruses and their replication. In Knipe, D. M. and Howley, P. M. eds. *Fields Virology*. Philadelphia: Lippincott Williams & Wilkins, pp. 2629–2673.

Nguyen, Q., Champlin, R., Giralt, S. et al. (1999). Late cytomegalovirus pneumonia in adult allogeneic blood and marrow transplant recipients. *Clin. Infect. Dis.*, **28**, 618–623.

Niedobitek, G. (2000). Epstein–Barr virus infection in the pathogenesis of nasopharyngeal carcinoma. *Mol. Pathol.*, **53**, 248–254.

Oelke, M., Maus, M. V., Didiano, D. et al. (2003). Ex vivo induction and expansion of antigen-specific cytotoxic T cells by HLA-Ig-coated artificial antigen-presenting cells. *Nat. Med.*, **9**, 619–624.

Pamer, E. and Cresswell, P. (1998). Mechanisms of MHC class I–restricted antigen processing. *Annu. Rev. Immunol.*, **16**, 323–358.

Pao, W. J., Hustu, H. O., Douglass, E. C., Beckford, N. S., and Kun, L. E. (1989). Pediatric nasopharyngeal carcinoma: long term follow-up of 29 patients. *Int. J. Radiat. Oncol. Biol. Phys.*, **17**, 299–305.

Papadopoulos, E. B., Ladanyi, M., Emanuel, D. et al. (1994). Infusions of donor leukocytes to treat Epstein–Barr virus-associated lymphoproliferative disorders after allogeneic bone marrow transplantation. *N. Engl. J. Med.*, **330**, 1185–1191.

Park, K. D., Marti, L., Kurtzberg, J. and Szabolcs, P. (2006). In vitro priming and expansion of cytomegalovirus-specific Th1 and Tc1 T cells from naive cord blood lymphocytes. *Blood*, **108**(5), 1770–1773.

Pass, R. (2001). Cytomegalovirus. In Knipe, D. M. and Howley, P. M. eds. *Fields Virology*. Philadelphia: Lippincott Williams & Wilkins, pp. 2675–2705.

Peggs, K. S., Verfuerth, S., Pizzey, A. et al. (2003). Adoptive cellular therapy for early cytomegalovirus infection after allogeneic stem-cell transplantation with virus-specific T-cell lines. *Lancet*, **362**, 1375–1377.

Qu, L. and Rowe, D. T. (1992). Epstein–Barr virus latent gene expression in uncultured peripheral blood lymphocytes. *J. Virol.*, **66**, 3715–3724.

Razonable, R. R. and Paya, C. V. et al. (2003). Herpesvirus infections in transplant recipients: current challenges in the clinical management of cytomegalovirus and Epstein–Barr virus infections. *Herpes.*, **10**(3), 60–65.

Rickinson, A. B. and Kieff, E. (2001). Epstein–Barr virus. In Knipe, D. M. and Howley, P. M., eds. *Fields Virology*. Philadelphia, PA: Lippincott Williams + Wilkins, pp. 2575–2628.

Rickinson, A. B. and Moss, D. J. (1997). Human cytotoxic T lymphocyte responses to Epstein–Barr virus infection. *Annu. Rev. Immunol.*, **15**, 405–431.

Riddell, S. R., Elliott, M., Lewinsohn, D. A. et al. (1996). T-cell mediated rejection of gene-modified HIV-specific cytotoxic T lymphocytes in HIV-infected patients. *Nat. Med.* **2**, 216–223.

Rooney, C. M., Loftin, S. K., Holladay, M. S. et al. (1995a). Early identification of Epstein-Barr virus-associated post-transplantation lymphoproliferative disease. *Br. J. Haematol.*, **89**, 98–103.

Rooney, C. M., Smith, C. A., Ng, C. Y. et al. (1995b). Use of gene-modified virus-specific T lymphocytes to control Epstein–Barr-virus-related lymphoproliferation. *Lancet*, **345**, 9–13.

Rooney, C. M., Roskrow, M. A., Suzuki, N. et al. (1998a). Treatment of relapsed Hodgkin's disease using EBV-specific cytotoxic T cells. *Ann. Oncol.*, **9**, Suppl 5, S129–S132.

Rooney, C. M., Smith, C. A., Ng, C. Y. et al. (1998b). Infusion of cytotoxic T cells for the prevention and treatment of Epstein–Barr virus-induced lymphoma in allogeneic transplant recipients. *Blood*, **92**, 1549–1555.

Rooney, C. M., Aguilar, L. K., Huls, M. H., Brenner, M. K., and Heslop, H. E. (2001). Adoptive immunotherapy of EBV-associated malignancies with EBV-specific cytotoxic T-cell lines. *Curr. Top. Microbiol. Immunol.*, **258**, 221–229.

Rooney, C. M., Bollard, C., Huls, M. H. et al. (2002). Immunotherapy for Hodgkin's disease. *Ann. Hematol.*, **81** Suppl 2, S39–S42.

Roskrow, M. A., Suzuki, N., Gan, Y. et al. (1998). Epstein–Barr virus (EBV)-specific cytotoxic T lymphocytes for the treatment of patients with EBV-positive relapsed Hodgkin's disease. *Blood*, **91**, 2925–2934.

Savoldo, B., Goss, J. A., Hammer, M. M. et al. (2006). Treatment of solid organ transplant recipients with autologous Epstein–Barr virus-specific cytotoxic T lymphocytes (CTL). *Blood.*, Epub ahead of print.

Savoldo, B., Goss, J., Liu, Z. et al. (2001). Generation of autologous Epstein-Barr virus-specific cytotoxic T cells for adoptive immunotherapy in solid organ transplant recipients. *Transplantation*, **72**, 1078–1086.

Savoldo, B., Cubbage, M. L., Durett, A. G. et al. (2002). Generation of EBV-specific CD4+ cytotoxic T cells from virus naive individuals. *J. Immunol.*, **168**, 909–918.

Sigal, L. J., Crotty, S., Andino, R., and Rock, K. L. (1999). Cytotoxic T-cell immunity to virus-infected non-haematopoietic cells requires presentation of exogenous antigen. *Nature*, **398**, 77–80.

Sili, U., Huls, M. H., Davis, A. R. et al. (2003). Large-scale expansion of dendritic cell-primed polyclonal human cytotoxic T-lymphocyte lines using lymphoblastoid cell lines for adoptive immunotherapy. *J. Immunother.*, **26**, 241–256.

Springer, K. L., Chou, S., Li, S. et al. (2005). How evolution of mutations conferring drug resistance affects viral dynamics and clinical outcomes of cytomegalovirus-infected hematopoietic cell transplant recipients. *J. Clin. Microbiol.*, **43**(1), 208–213.

Stevens, S. J., Verschuuren, E. A., Pronk, I. *et al.* (2001). Frequent monitoring of Epstein–Barr virus DNA load in unfractionated whole blood is essential for early detection of posttransplant lymphoproliferative disease in high-risk patients. *Blood,* **97,** 1165–1171.

Straathof, K. C., Savoldo, B., Heslop, H. E., and Rooney, C. M. (2002). Immunotherapy for post-transplant lymphoproliferative disease. *Br. J. Haematol.,* **118,** 728–740.

Straathof, K. C., Bollard, C. M., Popat, U. *et al.* (2005). Treatment of nasopharyngeal carcinoma with Epstein–Barr virus specific T lymphocytes. *Blood,* **105**(5), 1898–1904.

Sun, Q., Pollok, K. E., Burton, R. L. *et al.* (1999). Simultaneous ex vivo expansion of cytomegalovirus and Epstein–Barr virus-specific cytotoxic T lymphocytes using B-lymphoblastoid cell lines expressing cytomegalovirus pp65. *Blood,* **94,** 3242–3250.

Sun, Q., Burton, R. L., Dai, L. J., Britt, W. J., and Lucas, K. G. (2000). B lymphoblastoid cell lines as efficient APC to elicit CD8+ T cell responses against a cytomegalovirus antigen. *J. Immunol.,* **165,** 4105–4111.

Szmania, S., Galloway, A., Bruorton, M. *et al.* (2001). Isolation and expansion of cytomegalovirus-specific cytotoxic T lymphocytes to clinical scale from a single blood draw using dendritic cells and HLA-tetramers. *Blood,* **98,** 505–512.

Tierney, R. J., Steven, N., Young, L. S., and Rickinson, A. B. (1994). Epstein–Barr virus latency in blood mononuclear cells: analysis of viral gene transcription during primary infection and in the carrier state. *J. Virol.,* **68,** 7374–7385.

van Esser, J. W., Niesters, H. G., van der, H. B. *et al.* (2002). Prevention of Epstein–Barr virus-lymphoproliferative disease by molecular monitoring and preemptive rituximab in high-risk patients after allogeneic stem cell transplantation. *Blood,* **99,** 4364–4369.

Vaz-Santiago, J., Lule, J., Rohrlich, P. *et al.* (2002). IE1-pp65 recombinant protein from human CMV combined with a nanoparticulate carrier, SMBV, as a potential source for the development of anti-human CMV adoptive immunotherapy. *Cytotherapy,* **4,** 11–19.

Wagner, H. J., Sili, U., Gahn, B. *et al.* (2003). Expansion of EBV latent membrane protein 2a specific cytotoxic T cells for the adoptive immunotherapy of EBV latency type 2 malignancies: influence of recombinant IL12 and IL15. *Cytotherapy,* **5,** 231–240.

Walter, E. A., Greenberg, P. D., Gilbert, M. J. *et al.* (1995). Reconstitution of cellular immunity against cytomegalovirus in recipients of allogeneic bone marrow by transfer of T-cell clones from the donor. *N. Engl. J. Med.,* **333,** 1038–1044.

Wang, Q. J., Jenkins, F. J., Jacobson, L. P. *et al.* (2000). CD8+ cytotoxic T lymphocyte responses to lytic proteins of human herpes virus 8 in human immunodeficiency virus type 1-infected and -uninfected individuals. *J. Infect. Dis.,* **182,** 928–932.

Weinberg, K., Blazar, B. R., Wagner, J. E. *et al.* (2001). Factors affecting thymic function after allogeneic hematopoietic stem cell transplantation. *Blood,* **97,** 1458–1466.

75

Immunotherapy of HSV infections – antibody delivery

David W. Kimberlin

Division of Pediatric Infectious Diseases, The University of Alabama at Birmingham, AL, USA

Passive immunization involves utilizing polyclonal or monoclonal antibodies as a form of immunotherapy. Antibodies can mediate their effects through several mechanisms, including opsonization and C-mediated lysis, but in particular antibody-dependent cell-mediated cytolysis (ADCC) and neutralization. Antibody immunotherapy has been demonstrated to be efficacious for the treatment and prevention of infection or disease caused by viruses other than herpes simplex virus (HSV) (Abzug et al., 1995; Reed et al., 1988; Feltes et al., 2003; Saez-Llorens et al., 1998; Subramanian et al., 1998; The IMpact-RSV Study Group, 1998). While intriguing data exist in animal models suggesting that such a therapeutic intervention may also be of benefit in the management of HSV infections, to date no controlled studies have demonstrated the benefit of such an approach in humans. This chapter explores the potential of such an approach in people, as well as the limitations in current knowledge.

Immune responses following HSV infection

Host resistance to HSV infections includes non-specific mechanisms such as interferons, neutrophils, complement, macrophages, and natural killer cells, as well as specific mechanisms including humoral (antibody) immunity, T-cell-mediated immunity (such as cytotoxic T-cells and T-helper activity), and cytokine release. The relative importance of these various mechanisms is different for initial vs. recurrent HSV disease. Animal studies suggest that activated macrophages, interferons, and, to a lesser extent, natural killer cells are important in limiting initial HSV infection, whereas humoral immunity and cell-mediated immunity are important in controlling both initial and recurrent infections. Adoptive transfer studies suggest that either virus-specific antibody or lymphocytes can protect animals against initial HSV infection (as discussed below), but several lines of evidence suggest that cell mediated immunity responses play the central role in controlling recurrent HSV infections (Koelle et al., 2000; Posavad et al., 1996, 1997, 2000; Stanberry et al., 2000). Mucocutaneous herpes is more severe in patients with impaired or defective cell mediated immunity (Posavad et al., 1997; Whitley et al., 1998), but not in patients with agammaglobulinemia.

Following acquisition of HSV-1 or HSV-2, IgM antibodies appear transiently and are followed by production of IgG and IgA antibodies which persist over time. Both neutralizing antibodies and antibody-dependent cellular cytotoxic (ADCC) antibodies generally appear between 2 weeks and 6 weeks following infection and persist for the lifetime of the host. The host response to virus-specific infected cell polypeptides and the development of neutralizing antibodies have been defined through immunoblot and immunoprecipitation assays (Bernstein et al., 1985; Eberle et al., 1981). Following infection, antibodies directed against glycoprotein (g)B, gC, gD, gE, gG1, gG2, and ICP-4 appear sequentially. Of note, the intensity of host antibody responses to virus-specific polypeptides and high concentrations of neutralizing antibodies are not protective against HSV recurrences.

Neonates

The host responses of neonates with HSV disease differ from those of older children and adults. Infected neonates will produce HSV-specific IgM antibodies (as detected by immunofluorescence) within three weeks of acquisition of the viral infection. HSV-specific IgM concentrations increase rapidly during the first 2 to 3 months, and in some infants may be detectable for as long as one year following

Table 75.1. Protective effect of neutralizing antibody in prevention of neonatal HSV disease

Neutralizing antibody titer (cord blood or 2 weeks of life)	Exposed during delivery but uninfected ($n=33$)	Exposed during delivery and infected ($n=29$)
<1:5	0 (0%)	12 (41%) $P<0.00001$
1:5 to 1:20	7 (21%)	15 (52%)
>1:20	26 (79%)	2 (7%) $P<0.0002$

From Prober et al. (1987).

neonatal infection. HSV IgG antibodies also appear by 3–4 weeks in most infants. The viral surface glycoproteins gB and gD are the most reactive immunodeterminants (Sullender et al., 1987) and, indeed, account for the majority of neutralizing antibodies.

Human studies suggesting of protection by HSV antibodies

Adults

Type-specific antibodies against one type of HSV may have limited ability to protect against acquisition of the other HSV type. For example, pre-existing antibody directed against HSV-1 correlates with protection against acquisition of genital HSV-2 infection (Breinig et al., 1990; Cowan et al., 1994; Eberhart-Phillips et al., 1998; Fleming et al., 1997; Gibson et al., 1990; Johnson et al., 1989; Mertz et al., 1992; Nahmias et al., 1990; Rosenthal et al., 1997). The influence of pre-existing type-specific HSV-1 antibodies on acquisition of HSV-2 infection can also be inferred from recent successes, although somewhat limited, in HSV vaccine development. A candidate HSV-2 glycoprotein D subunit vaccine adjuvanted with alum combined with 3-deacylated monophosphoryl lipid A (MPL) has recently demonstrated promising results. In two large Phase III studies, the vaccine has been demonstrated to be safe and, in a subset of volunteers, effective in preventing HSV-1 or -2 genital herpes disease (vaccine efficacy ∼75%) and HSV-2 infection (vaccine efficacy ∼40%) (Stanberry et al., 2002). In both studies, efficacy was limited to women who were HSV-1 and -2 seronegative prior to vaccination. There was no evidence of vaccine efficacy in men or in women who were HSV 1+/2- prior to vaccination.

While there is some degree of cross-protection conferred by pre-existing HSV-1 antibody on the acquisition of HSV-2 infection, the protection is incomplete. Similarly, vaccines have been developed which generate robust humoral responses yet fail to protect against HSV-2 infection (Stanberry et al., 2000). As such, it is difficult to envision a circumstance whereby passive antibody immunotherapy will play a role in the management of genital HSV infection and disease.

Neonates

Both maternal antibody status (Brown et al., 2003; Prober et al., 1987; Yeager and Arvin, 1984; Yeager et al., 1980) and type of maternal infection (primary vs. recurrent) (Brown et al., 1987, 1991, 2003; Corey and Wald, 1999; Nahmias et al., 1971) influence transmission of HSV from mother to baby. Neonates with higher neutralizing antibody titers acquired transplacentally are less likely to become infected with HSV following perinatal exposure of passage through an infected birth canal (Prober et al., 1987), illustrating the protective effects of preexisting antibody in preventing neonatal HSV disease (Table 75.1). Additionally, infants born to mothers who have a first episode of genital HSV infection near term are at much greater risk of developing neonatal herpes than are those whose mothers have recurrent genital herpes (Brown et al., 1987, 1991, 2003; Corey and Wald, 1999; Nahmias et al., 1971). This increased risk, however, is not solely due to lower concentrations of transplacentally passaged HSV-specific antibody, since women with first episode disease also shed virus for a longer period of time and in higher quantities. The largest assessment of the influence of type of maternal infection on likelihood of neonatal transmission involved almost 40,000 women without clinical evidence of genital HSV infection who were cultured within 48 hours of delivery (Fig. 75.1). Of these, 121 women were identified who both were asymptomatically shedding HSV and for whom sera were available for serologic analysis. In this large trial, 57% of babies delivered to women with first episode primary infection developed neonatal HSV disease, compared with 25% of babies delivered to women with first episode non-primary

Table 75.2. Protective effect of neutralizing antibody in limiting extent of neonatal HSV disease

Neutralizing antibody titer (1 week of life)	Extent of disease		
	SEM ($n=17$)	CNS ($n=19$)	Disseminated ($n=11$)
<1:5	6 (35%)	2 (11%)	8 (73%) $P<0.01$
1:5 to 1:20	8 (47%)	15 (78%)	3 (27%)
>1:20	3 (18%)	2 (11%)	0 (0%)

From Sullender et al. (1987).

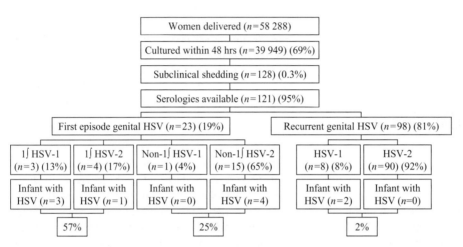

Fig. 75.1. Type of maternal infection and risk of HSV transmission to the neonate. (Data from Brown et al., 2003.)

infection and 2% of babies delivered to women with recurrent HSV disease (Brown et al., 2003).

Among HSV-infected neonates, anti-HSV neutralizing antibody titers have been shown to correlate with the extent of the disease (Sullender et al., 1987), with babies with higher neutralizing antibody titers being more likely to have localized disease (and less likely to have disseminated disease) once they are infected (Table 75.2). Similarly, high maternal or neonatal anti-HSV ADCC antibody levels or high neonatal antiviral neutralizing levels are each independently associated with an absence of disseminated HSV infection (Kohl et al., 1989) (Table 75.3).

Animal models of antibody immunotherapy in HSV infection and disease

The natural immune responses to HSV infection, both humoral and cellular, are strongly directed against the surface glycoproteins gB and gD, and both human and humanized antibodies directed against gB and gD have been shown to be beneficial as prophylactic and therapeutic agents in animal models of HSV infection (Baron et al., 1976; Bravo et al., 1996; Kern et al., 1992; Lake et al., 1992). In models of disease prevention, administration of polyclonal or monoclonal neutralizing antibodies prior to infection with HSV confers significant protection in mice. Similarly, administration of antibodies as late as 72 hours after infection dramatically decreases mortality as well as the quantity of virus detected in organs such as the brain and lungs (Kern et al., 1992). In a murine model of neonatal HSV disease with a high challenge dose, protection was highly associated with ADCC activity (Kohl et al., 1990). In a low dose challenge model, neutralizing activity of antibody alone was associated with protection in vivo (Kohl et al., 1990). In a guinea pig model of neonatal HSV, combination therapy with passive anti-HSV antibody and acyclovir was effective even when administered on day 3 post-infection, reducing mortality from 82% to 44%. Acyclovir alone was effective only when begun on day 0, and antibody alone

Table 75.3. Protective effect of neutralizing and ADCC antibody in limiting extent of neonatal HSV disease

Neonatal ADCC	Neonatal neutralizing antibody titer		
	<1:5 ($n=15$)	1:5 to 1:20 ($n=25$)	>1:20 ($n=6$)
SEM			
$1:10^4$ to $1:10^6$	2	6	3
0 to $1:10^3$	4	2	2
CNS			
$1:10^4$ to $1:10^6$	2	5	0
0 to $1:10^3$	0	9	0
Disseminated			
$1:10^4$ to $1:10^6$	0	0	0
0 to $1:10^3$	7	3	1

From Kohl et al. (1989).

was effective when begun on or before day 2 (Bravo et al., 1996). Also in guinea pigs, administration of HSV-specific antibody protects the sacral ganglia from HSV infection resulting from vaginal challenge (Bourne and Stanberry, 1993), suggesting a role for antibody in protecting the neuron early in primary HSV infection, possibly by blocking infection of the sensory nerve ending or alternatively by acting at the level of the ganglia (Stanberry et al., 2000).

Limitations of antibody immunotherapy

As noted above, prospects for passive antibody immunotherapy for genital HSV infection and disease seem remote. However, the protection against infection and amelioration of disease severity afforded by neutralizing and ADCC antibodies in neonatal HSV may portend a future role for this manifestation of HSV infection. While antibody therapy offers promise for improving neonatal HSV disease prevention and outcome, studies in humans have yet to be performed. In addition, an HSV hyperimmune globulin preparation does not exist, and the amount of anti-HSV antibodies present in conventional intravenous gammaglobulin (IVIG) preparations is low and variable, such that unacceptable large volumes would need to be injected to potentially confer protective immunity. For these reasons, use of IVIG in the management of neonates with HSV disease cannot be recommended at this time.

The development of human and humanized monoclonal antibodies obviates the current problems with pooled IVIG preparations, and may allow for the systematic evaluation of the therapeutic benefit of passive immunization in neonatal HSV disease. Human monoclonal antibodies offer further potential advantages over murine and chimeric antibodies such as longer circulating half life and reduced or possibly undetectable immunogenicity. At least two human monoclonal antibodies exist which could one day be evaluated in neonatal HSV disease.

HSV 863 is an HSV gD group Ib human monoclonal antibody of IgG1gamma isotype. In vitro studies showed that HSV 863 reacts with all of the 99 strains of HSV-1 and HSV-2 tested. It has potent neutralizing activity in the absence of complement, with an IC_{50} range of 0.05–0.35 µg/ml, with IVIG being approximately 128 to 256 times less potent. The neutralization IC_{50} for HSV 863 in the presence of complement was identical. HSV 863 confers a marked dose-dependent increase in ADCC activity, with maximal ADCC efficacy being achieved with concentrations of HSV 863 as low as 1 µg/ml with HSV-1 and 5 µg/ml with HSV-2. The half life of this monoclonal antibody is approximately 19 days in monkeys, with no apparent side effects, toxicity or immunogenicity following single or multiple dose administration. In vivo, using a neonatal HSV model, HSV 863 proved effective both prophylactically and therapeutically. When administered prior to virus challenge, the ED_{50} was 1–8 mg/kg for protection against a $10 \times LD_{50}$ challenge with HSV-1 or HSV-2. The antibody was protective in dose of 30 mg/kg up to 2 days after viral challenge and up to 72 hours post-infection when administered in dose of 90 mg/kg. In combination treatment with acyclovir, there were indications of additive effects, but no interference. HSV 863 at 10 mg/kg given 72 hours after infection was 90% protective, and doses of 1.5 to 15 mg/kg reduced both skin lesion severity and abundance in a murine model of cutaneous HSV disease. In a murine ascending myelitis model, treatment with HSV 863 or acyclovir substantially reduced the extent of detectable latent ganglionic infection, especially when given prophylactically 24 hours prior to HSV inoculation. Production of this product, though, is currently on hold pending discussions with potential manufacturers of commercial-grade product.

HX-8 is a human monoclonal antibody which binds HSV-1 and -2. It is produced by Epicyte Pharmaceutical in genetically modified corn and neutralizes both HSV-1 and HSV-2. It is currently being developed as a topical human antibody, but to date has not been tested in humans.

Summary

The immunobiology of HSV infections is complex. Cell mediated and humoral immunities are both important in the immunologic response to HSV infection, but millennia of evolution have provided the virus with the means by which to evade even the intact immune system, both maintaining latency and allowing for intermittent reactivation of disease. These facts likely limit the utility of passive antibody immunotherapy in the management of genital HSV infection. However, evidence for protection against infection and amelioration of disease severity afforded by neutralizing and ADCC antibodies in neonatal HSV may portend a future role for this manifestation of HSV infection. While antibody therapy offers promise for improving neonatal HSV disease prevention and outcome, studies in humans have yet to be performed.

REFERENCES

Abzug, M. J., Keyserling, H. L., Lee, M. L., Levin, M. J., and Rotbart, H. A. (1995). Neonatal enterovirus infection: virology, serology, and effects of intravenous immune globulin. *Clin. Infect. Dis.*, **20**, 1201–1206.

Baron, S., Worthington, M. G., Williams, J., and Gaines, J. W. (1976). Postexposure serum prophylaxis of neonatal herpes simplex virus infection of mice. *Nature*, **261**, 505–506.

Bernstein, D. I., Garratty, E., Lovett, M. A., and Bryson, Y. J. (1985). Comparison of Western Blot Analysis to microneutralization for the detection of type-specific herpes simplex virus antibodies. *J. Med. Virol.*, **15**, 223–230.

Bourne, N. and Stanberry, L. R. (1993). Modification of primary and recurrent genital herpes in guinea pigs by passive immunoprophylaxis [abstract 156]. *Antiviral Res.*, **20** (Suppl. 1), 127.

Bravo, F. J., Bourne, N., Harrison, C. J. et al. (1996). Effect of antibody alone and combined with acyclovir on neonatal herpes simplex virus infection in guinea pigs. *J. Infect. Dis.*, **173**, 1–6.

Breinig, M. K., Kingsley, L. A., Armstrong, J. A., Freeman, D. J., and Ho, M. (1990). Epidemiology of genital herpes in Pittsburg: serologic, sexual, and racial correlates of apparent and inapparent herpes simplex infections. *J. Infect. Dis.*, **162**, 299–305.

Brown, Z. A., Vontver, L. A., and Benedetti, J. (1987). Effects on infants of a first episode of genital herpes during pregnancy. *N. Engl. J. Med.*, **317**, 1246–1251.

Brown, Z. A., Benedetti, J., Ashley, R. et al. (1991). Neonatal herpes simplex virus infection in relation to asymptomatic maternal infection at the time of labor. *N. Engl. J. Med.*, **324**, 1247–1252.

Brown, Z. A., Wald, A., Morrow, R. A., Selke, S., Zeh, J., and Corey, L. (2003). Effect of serologic status and cesarean delivery on transmission rates of herpes simplex virus from mother to infant. *J. Am. Med. Assoc.*, **289**, 203–209.

Corey, L. and Wald, A. (1999). Genital herpes. In Holmes, K. K., Sparling, P. F., Mardh, P. A. et al. eds. *Sexually Transmitted Diseases*. McGraw-Hill, New York, pp. 285–312.

Cowan, F. M., Johnson, A. M., Ashley, R., Corey, L., and Mindel, A. (1994). Antibody to herpes simplex virus type 2 as serological marker of sexual lifestyle in populations. *Br. Med. J.*, **309**, 1325–1329.

Eberhart-Phillips, J., Dickson, N. P., Paul, C. et al. (1998). Herpes simplex type 2 infection in a cohort aged 21 years. *Sex. Transm. Infect.*, **74**, 216–218.

Eberle, R., Russell, R. G., and Rouse, B. T. (1981). Cell-mediated immunity to herpes simplex virus: recognition of type-specific and type-common surface antigens by cytotoxic T cell populations. *Infect. Immun.*, **34**, 795–803.

Feltes, T. F., Cabalka, A. K., Meissner, H. C. et al., and the Cardiac Synagis Study Group (2003). Palivizumab prophylaxis reduces hospitalization due to respiratory syncytial virus in young children with hemodynamically significant congenital heart disease. *J. Pediatr.*, **143**, 532–540.

Fleming, D. T., McQuillan, G. M., Johnson, R. E. et al. (1997). Herpes simplex virus type 2 in the United States, 1976 to 1994. *N. Engl. J. Med.*, **337**, 1105–1111.

Gibson, J. J., Hornung, C. A., Alexander, G. R., Lee, F. K., Potts, W. A., and Nahmias, A. J. (1990). A cross-sectional study of herpes simplex virus types 1 and 2 in college students: occurrence and determinants of infection. *J. Infect. Dis.*, **162**, 306–312

Johnson, R. E., Nahmias, A. J., Magder, L. S., Lee, F. K., Brooks, C. A., and Snowden, C. B. (1989). A seroepidemiologic survey of the prevalence of herpes simplex virus type 2 infection in the United States. *N. Engl. J. Med.*, **321**, 7–12.

Kern, E. R., Vogt, P. E., Co, M. S., Kohl, S., and Whitley, R. J. (1992). Treatment of herpes simplex virus type 2 infections in mice with murine and humanized monoclonal antibodies (MABS). International Society for Antiviral Research. Vancouver, BC, Canada, Abstract No. 125.

Koelle, D. M., Schomogyi, M., and Corey, L. (2000). Antigen-specific T cells localize to the uterine cervix in women with genital herpes simplex virus type 2 infection. *J. Infect. Dis.*, **182**, 662–670.

Kohl, S., West, M. S., Prober, C. G., Sullender, W. M., Loo, L. S., and Arvin, A. M. (1989). Neonatal antibody-dependent cellular cytotoxic antibody levels are associated with the clinical presentation of neonatal herpes simplex virus infection. *J. Infect. Dis.*, **160**, 770–776.

Kohl, S., Strynadka, N. C., Hodges, R. S., and Pereira, L. (1990). Analysis of the role of antibody-dependent cellular cytotoxic antibody activity in murine neonatal herpes simplex virus infection with antibodies to synthetic peptides of glycoprotein D and monoclonal antibodies to glycoprotein B. *J. Clin. Invest.*, **86**, 273–278.

Lake, P., Alonso, P., Subramanyam, J., and Nottage, B. (1992). SDZ HSV 863: A human monoclonal antibody to HSV 1 and HSV 2 (gD Ib) which attenuates acute infection, neurogenic cutaneous lesion formation and the establishment of viral latency. International Society for Antiviral Research. Vancouver, BC, Canada.

Mertz, G. J., Benedetti, J., Ashley, R., Selke, S. A., and Corey, L. (1992). Risk factors for the sexual transmission of genital herpes. *Ann. Intern. Med.*, **116**, 197–202.

Nahmias, A. J., Josey, W. E., Naib, Z. M., Freeman, M. G., Fernandez, R. J., and Wheeler, J. H. (1971). Perinatal risk associated with maternal genital herpes simplex virus infection. *Am. J. Obstet. Gynecol.*, **110**, 825–837.

Nahmias, A. J., Lee, F. K., and Beckman-Nahmias, S. (1990). Seroepidemiological and sociological patterns of herpes simplex virus infection in the world. Scand. Infect. Dis, **69 (Suppl)**, 19–36

Posavad, C. M., Koelle, D. M., and Corey L. (1996). High frequency of CD8+ cytotoxic T-lymphocyte precursors specific for herpes simplex viruses in persons with genital herpes. *J. Virol.*, **70**, 8165–8168.

Posavad, C. M., Koelle, D. M., Shaughnessy, M. F., and Corey, L. (1997). Severe genital herpes infections in HIV-infected individuals with impaired herpes simplex virus-specific CD8+ cytotoxic T lymphocyte responses. *Proc. Natl Acad. Sci. USA*, **94**, 10289–10294.

Posavad, C. M., Huang, M. L., Barcy, S., Koelle, D. M., and Corey L. (2000). Long term persistence of herpes simplex virus-specific CD8+ CTL in persons with frequently recurring genital herpes. *J. Immunol.*, **165**, 1146–1152.

Prober, C. G., Sullender, W. M., Yasukawa, L. L., Au, D. S., Yeager, A. S., and Arvin, A. M. (1987). Low risk of herpes simplex virus infections in neonates exposed to the virus at the time of vaginal delivery to mothers with recurrent genital herpes simplex virus infections. *N. Engl. J. Med.*, **316**, 240–244.

Reed, E. C., Bowden, R. A., Dandliker, P. S., Lilleby, K. E., and Meyers, J. D. (1988). Treatment of cytomegalovirus pneumonia with ganciclovir and intravenous cytomegalovirus immunoglobulin in patients with bone marrow transplants. *Ann. Intern. Med.*, **109**, 783–788.

Rosenthal, S. L., Stanberry, L. R., Biro, F. M. *et al.* (1997). Seroprevalence of herpes simplex virus types 1 and 2 and cytomegalovirus in adolescents. *Clin. Infect. Dis.*, **24**, 135–139.

Saez-Llorens, X., Castano, E., Null, D. *et al.* (1998). Safety and pharmacokinetics of an intramuscular humanized monoclonal antibody to respiratory syncytial virus in premature infants and infants with bronchopulmonary dysplasia. The MEDI-493 Study Group. *Pediatr. Infect. Dis. J.*, **17**, 787–791.

Stanberry, L. R., Cunningham, A. L., Mindel, A. *et al.* (2000). Prospects for control of herpes simplex virus disease through immunizations. *Clin. Infect. Dis.*, **30**, 549–566.

Stanberry, L. R., Spruance, S. L., Cunningham, A. L. *et al.* and The GlaxoSmithKline Herpes Vaccine Efficacy Study Group (2002). Glycoprotein-D-adjuvant vaccine to prevent genital herpes. *N. Engl. J. Med.*, **347**, 1652–1661.

Subramanian, K. N., Weisman, L. E., Rhodes, T. *et al.* (1998). Safety, tolerance and pharmacokinetics of a humanized monoclonal antibody to respiratory syncytial virus in premature infants and infants with bronchopulmonary dysplasia. MEDI-493 Study Group. *Pediatr. Infect. Dis. J.*, **17**, 110–115.

Sullender, W. M., Miller, J. L., Yasukawa, L. L. *et al.* (1987). Humoral and cell-mediated immunity in neonates with herpes simplex virus infection. *J. Infect. Dis.*, **155**, 28–37.

The IMpact-RSV Study Group (1998). Palivizumab, a humanized respiratory syncytial virus monoclonal antibody, reduces hospitalization from respiratory syncytial virus infection in high-risk infants. *Pediatrics*, **102**, 531–537.

Whitley, R. J., Kimberlin, D. W., and Roizman, B. (1998). Herpes simplex viruses. *Clin. Infect. Dis.*, **26**, 541–553.

Yeager, A. S. and Arvin, A. M. (1984). Reasons for the absence of a history of recurrent genital infections in mothers of neonates infected with herpes simplex virus. *Pediatrics*, **73**, 188–193.

Yeager, A. S., Arvin, A. M., Urbani, L. J., and Kemp, J. A., 3rd (1980). Relationship of antibody to outcome in neonatal herpes simplex virus infections. *Infect. Immun.*, **29**, 532–538.

Part VIII

Herpesviruses as Therapeutic Agents

Edited by Richard Whitley and Bernard Roizman

76

Herpesviruses as therapeutic agents

Frank Tufaro and James M. Markert

University of British Columbia, British Columbia, Canada
Department of Surgery, Brain Tumor Research Laboratories, The University of Alabama at Birmingham, Birmingham, AL, USA

Introduction

After more than a decade of intensive research and development efforts, the translation of promising viral-based gene therapies from the research lab to the clinic is both promising and unexpectedly challenging. Many of the same properties that make viral vectors attractive candidates to deliver genes for therapeutic purposes also impede the path to successful clinical development.

Vectors for clinical use must be manufactured in relatively high yields such that hundreds of thousands or even millions of "doses" can be generated in a safe and cost-effective manner. Moreover, the resulting vector must exhibit genetic as well as structural stability, withstand storage at various temperatures for up to several years, and cause little or no toxicity in animals, and ultimately in humans.

Herpes simplex viruses (HSV), while widespread in nature, have not been tested in human clinical studies as often as several other commonly used vectors, such as adenovirus, adeno-associated viruses (AAV), and retroviruses. In many ways however, HSV is emerging as a viable therapeutic platform and several clinical studies are either ongoing or planned for the very near future. The reason for this increased focus on HSV is due in part attributable to the unique properties that make HSV a stable and potentially potent vector for controlled gene delivery. In addition, the increasing experience with replication-competent vectors in human clinical studies has made it more familiar with clinicians.

Properties of therapeutic HSV vectors

Therapeutic HSV can be characterized as replication-competent or replication-defective. Replication competent vectors, such as the oncolytic vectors described in this chapter, are usually deleted for "non-essential" viral genes to render the vector less "toxic" as measured by the ability to cause disease in susceptible animal models. These vectors are often referred to as "replication-attenuated." If they are designed to treat cancer, they are "oncolytic" in the sense that they are at least partially replication competent in tumor cells, and largely replication defective in surrounding tissue.

This differential permissiveness has been shown in several studies to be due to the unique environment of the tumor cell vs. the "normal" surrounding cell. For example, HSV-1 mutants such as G207 are now being tested in clinical trials for anti-cancer activity. R3616, which is similar to G207, is an HSV-1 mutant that is deleted for the viral anti-PKR gene, $\gamma_1 34.5$. The R3616 mutant infects *ras*-transformed but not untransformed cells, which suggests that the Ras-signaling pathway compensates for the loss of the virus' own anti-PKR mechanism (Farassati *et al.*, 2001). HSV-1, therefore, predominantly uses the host anti-PKR mechanism to infect transformed cells and its selectiveness for transformed cells makes it a good candidate for an anti-cancer therapeutic.

Replication defective HSV vectors are deleted for one or more genes that are known to be essential for viral replication in otherwise permissive cells. As a result, defective vectors can only be manufactured using cell lines that are modified to contain the complementing viral genes. These vectors often exhibit reduced toxicity in non-complementing cells compared to wild-type virus, and appear to be largely non-toxic when administered to animals. Although many different replication defective HSV vectors have been generated, only a few of them represent viable candidates for clinical development, and none have been tested in humans to date.

Properties of non-replicating HSV vectors for therapeutic use

There are two basic approaches to generating replication defective HSV vectors: amplicons and whole genome vectors.

Plasmid-based amplicon vectors

Amplicons, first described over 20 years ago (Spaete and Frenkel, 1982), are defective HSV particles produced from plasmids containing the gene of interest, an origin of replication and a packaging signal. Plasmids are incapable of replicating without HSV helper functions, either in the form of helper virus, or resident on cosmids or bacterial artificial chromosomes. The resulting vectors contain multiple copies of the therapeutic gene, and are capable of infecting cells via the HSV entry pathway. Despite the potential safety advantages of such a system, in practice it is relatively difficult to generate high titer stocks devoid of helper virus. Although advances in generating helper-free stocks have helped somewhat (Fraefel et al., 1996), this is offset at least in part by an increase in the complexity of manufacturing. Moreover, the plasmid sequences transferred into cells by amplicons are not HSV genomes, so consistent, regulated expression has been difficult to achieve in animals. Amplicon vectors are unique in their ability to deliver up to 153 kb of heterologous DNA into a wide range of mammalian cells (Wade-Martins et al., 2001).

In an attempt to extend the stability and duration of expression from amplicon vectors, and thus improve potential usefulness in gene therapy, hybrid amplicons consisting of elements of the AAV genome were constructed and tested for their ability to direct stable gene transduction by site-specific integration (Wang et al., 2002). The vector constructs, which contained the AAV inverted terminal repeats and the Rep gene were packaged as amplicons and compared to a standard amplicon vector in cell culture. Interestingly, the hybrid vectors improved the stable transduction frequency compared with controls, and the transgene was integrated into the host cell chromosome. The ability of the HSV amplicon construct to integrate into the host cell chromosome may hold promise for further improvements in long-term gene expression in situations where long-term gene expression is a priority.

Another approach for improving the efficiency of HSV-derived amplicon vectors has been to re-target the amplicon to make it more cell-type specific by reducing its ability to attach to all but the target cells. Grandi et al. (2004) have developed a method to re-target amplicon vectors by replacing the gC heparan sulfate binding domain with a model ligand, in this instance the hexameric histidine tag. They demonstrated enhanced binding of modified virus to receptor-positive cells with no loss of infectivity. This approach holds promise for reducing the dose required for adequate therapeutic effect. This would also have the potential to improve the prospect for the manufacture of clinical supplies. These and other enhancements will first require optimization in animal models prior to their inclusion in HSV therapeutics intended for human use.

Replication defective whole genome vectors

The second vector type is represented by HSV genomes deleted for essential genes. To grow these viruses, cell lines approved for clinical manufacturing are modified to contain the viral gene or genes required to complement the defect in the defective vector. Deletion of one or other of the essential immediate-early genes (ICP4, ICP27) results in a virus that cannot replicate (DeLuca et al., 1985; McCarthy et al., 1989; Samaniego et al., 1997, 1998; Wu et al., 1996), except in cells that complement the null mutations by providing ICP4 or ICP27 in trans (DeLuca et al., 1985; Samaniego et al., 1998; Wu et al., 1996). In practice, the only potentially clinically useful vector strains have two or more deletions to reduce the potential that a recombination event with the viral gene resident in the complementing cell will lead to a replication competent contaminant during manufacturing. Multiply deleted vectors cannot replicate in non-complementing cells and do not express early or late genes. These vectors can also contain additional defects in viral genes that lead to desirable properties such as increased yield, reduced cytotoxicity, genome stability or altered immune response.

Another approach for increasing the yield of non-replicating vectors is by modifying the complementing cells. For example, complementing cell lines can be made to express the complementing sequences only upon HSV infection, thereby reducing cytotoxicity and enabling robust replication and high yields during manufacture. Viruses generated in this manner can be designed to be relatively non-toxic, especially in neuronally- derived cell types (Palmer et al., 2000; Lilley et al., 2001).

Use of HSV vectors to modify the nervous system

Herpes simplex virus vectors are particularly well suited for the delivery of genes to neurons. In natural infections, the wild-type virus particle targets with high efficiency from peripheral inoculation to the nucleus of sensory neurons in the dorsal root ganglion. Once in the nucleus, the viral genomes establish latency, in which they persist for the life of the host as intranuclear episomal elements. Although wild-type virus may be reactivated from latency, recombinant vectors that are entirely replication defective retain the ability to establish a persistent state in neurons, but are unable to replicate (or reactivate) in the nervous system.

Most viral gene expression is attenuated as the virus enters latency and is tightly regulated. Fortunately, the virus does express the LAT transcripts, which indicates that there is no absolute block to HSV-based gene expression in the neuron following the establishment of latency. Chimeric promoter constructs containing the LAT promoter enhancer region can confer long-term activity on otherwise silenced exogenous promoters (Palmer et al., 2000; Lilley et al., 2001). Vectors in which the LAT promoter is made to control exogenous gene expression have also been shown to express foreign genes in mouse dorsal root ganglia (DRG) for months following footpad inoculation (Marshall et al., 2000). These vectors allow long term expression in dorsal root ganglia and the CNS of animal models. They also retain the ability to be transported via the axon to distant sites, a feature that may be useful for targeted delivery to the peripheral or central nervous system in the clinical setting.

Peripheral nervous system (PNS)

Latency of wild-type HSV occurs in the sensory ganglia of peripheral nerves and long-term expression of transgenes from HSV vector has proved feasible in the PNS (Goins et al., 1999). Expression of NGF and other neurotrophic factors using the LAP2 and heterologous promoters to drive expression has persisted long enough to demonstrate the therapeutic potential of such constructs in the clinical setting for the treatment of neuropathy (Chattopadhyay et al., 2002, 2003; Goss et al., 2002a,b). Expression of enkephalin peptides from defective HSV vector backbones has also been demonstrated in animal models of chronic pain suggesting that as little as several weeks of gene expression might provide therapeutic benefit (Goss et al., 2001, 2002a, b; Hao et al., 2003).

Central nervous system (CNS)

It would normally be expected that infection of the CNS with HSV would cause encephalitis, by contrast with the latent infection established in the PNS. It has been demonstrated quite convincingly, however, that even replication competent HSV constructs such as the oncolytic vectors G207 and strain 1716 can be delivered safely to the human brain for the treatment of malignant glioma. Therefore it would be expected that replication defective HSV should be non-toxic following CNS delivery. In fact, this has been demonstrated in animals for certain HSV recombinants with multiple IE gene deletions (Krisky et al., 1998), or with IE gene deletions (ICP4, 27) coupled with inactivating mutations in ICP34.5/open-reading frame P and VP16 (Lilley et al., 2001). Vectors such as these would be highly appropriate vehicles to arm with therapeutic genes either to preserve or modify neuronal function or to destroy tumor cells. These vectors express minimal levels of any of the IE genes in non-complementing cells and transgene expression can be maintained for extended periods with promoter systems containing LAT promoter elements (Palmer et al., 2000).

Additionally, HSV-based vectors allow highly effective gene delivery both to cultured neurons and to the CNS in animal models. Moreover, these vectors are efficiently transported from the site of inoculation to connected sites within the CNS and less so within the PNS. This has been demonstrated by gene delivery to both the striatum and substantia nigra following striatal inoculation, to the spinal cord, spinal ganglia, and brainstem following spinal cord infection, and to retinal ganglia neurons following injection in the superior colliculus and thalamus (Lilley et al., 2001).

In a comprehensive study of vector delivery, Palmer et al. (2000) have identified combinations of deletions from the HSV genome that allow efficient gene delivery to spinal dorsal root ganglia (DRGs) following peripheral inoculation into the footpad or sciatic nerve of mice. This showed that LAT promoter elements can confer long term expression in the context of different exogenous promoters, and that partial replication-competence may be more efficient for gene delivery following footpad or nerve injection. The efficiency of retrograde transport and subsequent gene expression following footpad or sciatic nerve inoculation was determined to be dose dependent, and not as efficient as with replication competent vectors. This may be due to the need to penetrate a barrier of accessory cells or otherwise increase the relative amount of vector available at the site of inoculation.

These unique viruses show an encouraging lack of toxicity following injection as well as relatively long-term expression: capabilities that have important implications for therapeutic uses where target neurons are in regions of the nervous system that are relatively inaccessible by normal therapeutic techniques. These target cells might include the dopaminergic neurons of the substantia nigra that are affected in Parkinson's disease (Yamada et al., 1999), the retinal ganglion cells, or delivery to the DRG for the treatment of pain, or to repair the spinal cord or nerves.

Malignant glioma

Malignant glioma is a malignancy of the CNS that can be treated by surgery, radiation, and chemotherapy. To date, only replication competent HSV has been tested in clinical studies with some success to treat refractory disease. Replication defective vector candidates have also been designed to arm the HSV vector in such a way to provide a more potent antitumor effect than has been demonstrated so far with the replication-attenuated vectors.

Interestingly, the TK gene of HSV has been introduced into a variety of non-HSV vectors and tested for its ability to kill tumor cells in the presence of ganciclovir, but never in the HSV vector itself. Candidate HSV vectors have been generated that are equipped with additional genes that might be useful to treat brain tumors. For example, connexin 43, which is the major component of astrocyte gap junctions, has been introduced into an HSV vector to increase the formation of intercellular junctions in a manner that may potentiate HSV/tk-based cancer treatment by promoting the transfer of activated ganciclovir from cell to cell (Sanson *et al.*, 2002). Likewise, inclusion of antitumor factors such as the cytokine TNF alpha appear to provide added benefit if expressed in high concentrations in the tumor and surrounding tissue from an HSV vector backbone (Moriuchi *et al.*, 1998).

Additional work has been performed in an attempt to regulate vector-directed gene expression such that it is either naturally activated in the tumor cell environment or induced at will through the use of exogenous inducers. In this regard, HSV-1 amplicon vectors that are regulated by the cell cycle have been developed to generate glioma-specific HSV amplicon therapeutics (Ho *et al.*, 2004). The design of one such construct is based on the observation that cell cycle dependent factor CDF-1 appears to be specifically expressed during the G(0)/G(1) phase of the cell cycle and its binding site is located within the cyclin A promoter. In non-dividing cells, transactivation of a cyclin A promoter via the interaction of a Gal4/NF-YA fusion protein with Gal4-binding sites is prevented by the presence of CDF-1, which acts as a repressor. By contrast, in proliferating cells such as those in actively growing tumor, CDF-1 is presumably absent and transactivation occurs. These regulatory elements have been incorporated, along with tissue-specific elements such as the GFAP enhancer, into HSV amplicon vectors to target expression to a specific group of cells. This construct has been shown to exhibit both cell-type specific and cell cycle dependent transgene expression in glioma-bearing animals. These vector properties, if active in animal models of disease, would reduce the need for targeting at the level of cell attachment and entry, and may represent an important step in developing a vector that can be delivered systemically or locoregionally to target the maximum number of tumor cells in the context of metastatic disease.

Another approach to gene regulation adapted to the HSV system that is not limited to glioma therapy, is the tetracycline-inducible gene expression system. Of the known eukaryotic regulatory systems, the tet-inducible system is perhaps the most widely used because of its tight regulation and the availability of tetracycline, which is suitable for human clinical use. These constructs contain a tetracycline response element (TRE) linked to a promoter such as the heterologous promoter CMV, or the HSV ICP0 promoter (Schmeisser *et al.*, 2002). Studies have demonstrated that these constructs result in tetracycline inducible gene expression that is not cell type specific, and are capable of inducible expression for several days in irreversibly differentiated NT2 cells, which is a neuronally committed human teratocarcinoma cell line that differentiates into neuron-like hNT cells following treatment with retinoic acid. The ability to turn gene expression on and off following intratumoral or systemic delivery of an HSV-based cancer therapeutic could allow for the inclusion of increasingly potent and potentially toxic gene products into HSV vectors to enhance antitumor efficacy.

Towards optimizing HSV vectors for therapeutic use

One of the most difficult problems in developing safe and efficient viral therapeutics is to determine the optimal dose of vector that will be effective in humans. In an effort to address this problem, the HSV TK gene has been shown to function as a useful marker gene for the direct in vivo localization of TK expression by positron emission tomography (PET). Several double and triple HSV amplicon vector constructs expressing HSV-1 TK, green fluorescent proteins, and *E. coli* cytosine deaminase have been generated and tested by injecting between 10^7 and 10^8 transducing units into subcutaneously Gli36dEGFR gliomas in nude mice. All amplicon vector constructs mediated GFP expression and sensitized the cells toward ganciclovir and 5-fluro-cytosine mediated cell killing in a drug-dose dependent manner (Jacobs *et al.*, 2003.). Moreover, functional proportional coexpression of the PET marker gene TK and the linked therapeutic E. coli CD gene was observed. TK expression could be imaged by PET in vivo even with apparent suboptimal transduction and gene expression. This raises the exciting possibility that the expression of HSV TK from therapeutic HSV vectors could serve as a useful marker for non-invasive imaging of vector distribution following administration. This would be extremely useful in Phase I and Phase II clinical trials and could provide a powerful means for optimizing dose, formulation, and the rate and mode of delivery.

Non-replicating vectors: current trends

No replication-defective HSV vector has yet been tested in human clinical studies for the treatment of disease. This is somewhat surprising given that replication competent vectors were first introduced into humans in 1998 for the treatment of malignant glioma. It is likely that this situation will change now that the clinical experience with replication competent HSV has been largely positive. Replication defective HSV vectors have many desirable qualities for use as therapeutics. They can be engineered to express several genes at once, manufactured in complementing cell lines that have the potential to yield more replication-defective virus than the replication-attenuated vectors already in use, and they do not replicate following administration to the patient. Thus, the effective dose cannot increase following administration. In this way, replication-defective vectors are more "drug-like" than are the replication competent vectors. The possibility to equip the vector with potentially toxic gene products for cancer therapy or to effect long term gene expression in the nervous system for the treatment of pain, neuropathy or CNS disease will provide the motivation to move these novel therapeutics from the research laboratory to the clinic.

Oncolytic HSV

Introduction

The original genetically engineered viruses examined as antitumor oncolytic agents studied as it was already a well-studied, non-integrating, neurotropic virus with oncolytic were HSV-1 mutants utilized in a preclinical models of human glioma (Markert et al., 1992; Martuza et al., 1991). HSV-1 was properties whose essential and non-essential genes have been identified (Fig. 76.1(a)). Deletion of the neurovirulence genes from an oncolytic HSV vector can effectively produce selective targeting of tumor cells for oncolysis. It has been estimated that 30 kilobase-pairs of the HSV genome could be replaced with foreign DNA while maintaining virus replication. Clinically utilized anti-viral drug regimens already exist to interrupt HSV infection, which adds a margin of safety to its clinical use as an oncolytic agent.

The first engineered replication-competent HSV-1-derivative examined for oncolytic effects was *dl*sptk, a thymidine kinase deletion mutant (Martuza et al., 1991). As a result of this mutation, *dl*sptk can only replicate in mitotically-active cells that can supply both thymidine kinase and pools of available nucleotides necessary for viral DNA replication. Efficacy was demonstrated in multiple animal models of glioma and other nervous system tumors (Martuza et al., 1991; Markert et al., 1993). However, clinical studies were not pursued with *dl*sptk because (i) evidence of low-level encephalitis was seen on histological examination of treated mice, and (ii) its tk mutation made it resistant to, the major antivirals in use for HSV infection, acyclovir and ganciclovir. Other HSV-1 vectors studied with markedly decreased virulence in the normal CNS but capable of oncolysis include R3616 (which contains a one kilobase deletion in both copies of the $\gamma_1 34.5$ gene locus) (Chou et al., 1990; Chou and Roizman, 1992)(Fig. 76.1(b)) and hrR3 (which contains a disabling *lacZ* insertion into the $U_L 39$ locus) (Goldstein and Weller, 1988) (Fig. 76.1(c)).

The two $\gamma_1 34.5$ gene copies that are deleted in R3616 are located in the inverted repeat regions flanking the Unique Long (U_L) segment of the HSV-1 genome, and encode a 263 amino acid protein with dual functions. First, $\gamma_1 34.5$ is responsible for the neurovirulence properties of HSV-1. Second, the $\gamma_1 34.5$ gene product (ICP34.5) subverts a major response of the host cell to HSV infection. Upon viral infection, double-stranded RNA is produced, and a stress response occurs in the host cell. Protein kinase R (PKR) is activated, shutting down translation in the infected cell as an antiviral protective mechanism by phosphorylating and inactivating eukaryotic initiation factor-2α (eIF-2α). ICP34.5 recruits protein phosphatase-1a in order to dephosphorylate eIF-2α and allow protein synthesis and viral replication to proceed (He et al., 1997). Studies have demonstrated that HSV-1 mutants lacking functional ICP34.5 activity produce a lytic infection only in cells with defective PKR pathways (Chou et al., 1990; Chou and Roizman, 1992). Over expression of Ras appears to allow $\Delta\gamma_1 34.5$ HSV-1 replication in tumor cells due to a defective PKR pathway (Farassati et al., 2001). R3616 produced no neurovirulence or encephalitis but maintained antiglioma activity in nude mouse models (Markert et al., 1993).

$U_L 39$ encodes the large subunit of the enzyme ribonucleotide reductase (ICP6) which HSV utilizes for nucleotide synthesis after infection of post-mitotic cells, such as neurons, which would otherwise not support the HSV

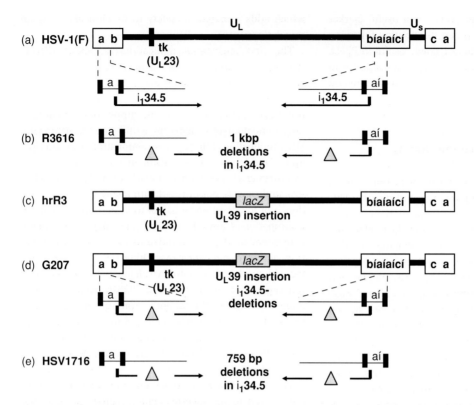

Fig. 76.1. The wild-type herpes simplex virus type 1 genome consists of two major adjacent segments (the Unique long and Unique short segments), each flanked by inverted repeats. The $\gamma_1 34.5$ genes are located in the inverted repeats flanking the UL segment. 1b. The R3616 HSV-1 mutant possesses a 1 kilo-basepair deletion in both copies of the $\gamma_1 34.5$ gene.1c. hrR3 contains a *lacZ* insertion in the UL39 locus, inactivating the ICP6 (ribonucleotide reductase) gene product.1d. G207 was constructed to possess both the *lacZ* insertion inactivating the UL39 locus and deletions in both genes $\gamma_1 34.5$.1e. HSV1716 is similar to R3616 in that too contains deletions in both copies of the $\gamma_1 34.5$ gene, inactivating the ICP34.5 protein.(62)

replication cycle. Dividing cells however, can provide cellular ribonucleotide reductase *in trans* obviating the need for the viral protein (Goldstein and Weller, 1988). The oncolytic HSV-1 hrR3 has a *lacZ* insertional mutation in $U_L 39$ renders the viral ribonucleotide reductase nonfunctional. As a result, the virus produces a lytic infection only in dividing cells, including those found in neoplasms, such as malignant glioma (Mineta *et al.*, 1994). A potential additional benefit is that the ribonucleotide reductase-deficient virus is hypersensitive to the anti-viral effects of acyclovir and ganciclovir (Coen *et al.*, 1989)

Oncolytic HSV in malignant glioma

To decrease the possibility of recombination to wild-type virus and further increase the safety of oncolytic HSV-1, a new mutant, G207, was constructed. This virus is a double mutant with deletions in both copies of the $\gamma_1 34.5$ gene locus as well as a *lacZ* insertion into the $U_L 39$ locus (Mineta *et al.*, 1995) (Fig. 76.1(d)). G207 retains susceptibility to standard anti-HSV therapies such as acyclovir, since the thymidine kinase gene is intact; due to the inactivation of $U_L 39$, G207 is in fact modestly hypersensitive to acyclovir (Coen *et al.*, 1989; Mineta *et al.*, 1995).

G207 was shown to produce antiglioma effects in multiple preclinical glioma models (Mineta *et al.*, 1995), and was shown to be safe for inoculation at high titers in mice and subsequently in non-human primates (New World owl monkeys *Aotus nancymae*) (Hunter *et al.*, 1999). Of 16 *Aotus*, 13 received intracerebral inoculations of either 1×10^7 or 1×10^9 pfu of G207, two received vehicle and one received 1×10^3 pfu of the wild-type parent HSV-1(F). None of the G207-inoculated animals died due to virus-induced complications (three died from non-neurologic reasons), whereas the control HSV-1(F)-infected monkey succumbed quickly to HSV encephalitis as expected (Hunter *et al.*, 1999). Although no clinical signs of HSV-incited illness were evident in the G207 administered animals, increased levels of anti-HSV antibodies were reported.

Based on these safety and efficacy reports, G207 was moved into a Phase I clinical trial (Markert *et al.*, 2000a,b). Twenty-one patients with recurrence or progression of malignant glioma after standard therapy were enrolled. All patients had to have undergone prior external beam radiotherapy (minimal dose 5000 cGy) in addition to either craniotomy and surgical debulking (seventeen patients) or biopsy alone (four patients). Ten patients also had been given one or more chemotherapeutics. A Karnofsky performance score of ≥70 were required for entry. Primary tumor histologies included fifteen glioblastomas, one gliosarcoma, four anaplastic astrocytomas, and one anaplastic mixed glioma.

This dose-escalation study was intended to determine the maximally tolerated dose (MTD) and any dose-limiting toxicities of G207. Patients were allocated to cohorts by dose level (three patients per cohort); a standard dose escalation scheme using half-log increments was used, with a maximal achievable dose of 3×10^9 pfu established as the ultimate upper limit of G207 to potentially be administered. A waiting period of 10 days between each patient within a cohort and of 28 days between each cohort was included to monitor signs of acute toxicity and/or the development of encephalitis. All patients were given one intratumoral injection into the enhancing portion of the tumor (according to MRI or CT scan), except those treated at the highest dose level. All patients treated with this dose, 3×10^9 pfu, had their tumors stereotactically inoculated in five different enhancing tumor loci as demonstrated by pre-operative imaging studies.

The results demonstrate the safety of G207 administration. An MTD was not established, as even with inoculation of 3×10^9 pfu, there were no definitive dose limiting toxicities, nor any requirement for the use of anti-viral drugs. In the few post-treatment histologic specimens available for review due to subsequent biopsy, tumor resection, or autopsy, there was no evidence of encephalitis (determined by H&E staining) or major inflammatory changes observed. Of the nineteen patients who underwent serologic testing, five were seronegative prior to treatment with G207. Of these five, one patient (treated at the highest dose level) seroconverted after inoculation. Thus, the virus was shown to be extremely well tolerated, even at very high doses.

While efficacy was not the primary endpoint of this study, certain findings support the antiglioma effects of G207 in this trial. Efficacy endpoints of average time to progression by MRI was 116 days and overall median survival of 190 days were only modestly above average in this dose escalation study of patient with recurrent tumors. However, eight of twenty patients revealed reduced enhancement volumes of their tumors at one month after treatment, suggesting that treatment at higher doses and perhaps under a different dosing regimen might improve the response to G207 therapy.

In an effort to gain additional data regarding G207 in the treatment of human glioma, a follow-up Phase Ib study was developed. Objectives of the Phase Ib study include validating the safety and tolerability (MTD) of G207 administration via divided escalating doses given both intratumorally and into functional brain adjacent to the resected tumor. This trial was also designed to evaluate the ability of G207 to replicate within the tumor post-inoculation, define the characteristics of G207 replication in these patients (e.g., virus shedding and reactivation, immunogenicity, impact of cell-mediated immune responses), as well as determine the mean time to disease progression and overall survival. Enrollment in this study has been completed, and data analysis is in progress.

A third study of G207 in patients with malignant brain tumors is scheduled to begin at the University of Alabama, Birmingham in January, 2005. This study will examine the effects of post-inoculation radiation on G207 treatment. The study is based on extensive preclinical data which demonstrates that a single fraction of radiation, when administered approximately 24 hours after G207, increases the replication and spread of viral infection within brain tumors as well as many other neoplasms.

Almost simultaneously with the Phase I trials of G207, HSV1716, derived from the parent wild-type strain HSV-1 17+, also underwent clinical trials to evaluate its toxicity in patients with recurrent malignant glioma (Rampling *et al.*, 2000). This single-mutant replication-selective virus has a genetically engineered deletion of 759 base-pairs within both copies of the $\gamma_1 34.5$ gene (Fig. 76.1(e)). HSV1716 was demonstrated to be avirulent in SCID mice, and therefore safe enough to pursue as a possible oncolytic vector therapy candidate in 1994 (Valyi-Nagi *et al.*, 1994). Moreover, efficacy studies in animal models supported utilizing HSV1716 as a possible novel treatment approach to malignant gliomas. Based on preclinical safety and efficacy profiles, HSV1716 was pursued as an anti-glioma agent for humans. Safety and toxicity of HSV1716 administration to patients was first examined in a study that enrolled nine total patients, eight of whom were diagnosed with GBM and one with anaplastic astrocytoma (Rampling *et al.*, 2000). All patients had been treated with prior radiotherapy, and had a KPS of at least 60. In addition, all subjects had also undergone previous surgery and six had received chemotherapy at the time of enrollment. Immunohistochemistry of injected regions when available showed no signs of immunoreactivity for

HSV-1, and the only HSV seronegative patient in the trial did not demonstrate seroconversion. No maximum tolerated dose was established because at the highest dose tested, 1×10^5 pfu, HSV1716 was well tolerated, with no evidence of encephalitis.

A second clinical trial examining HSV1716 suggested that replication occurs in at least some of the high-grade gliomas treated with intratumoral injection (Papanastassiou et al., 2002). Twelve patients with KPS between 60 and 90 were enrolled in this study; eleven GBM patients and one anaplastic astrocytoma patient. Of the GBM patients, there was one newly diagnosed patient; the remaining patients were treated at tumor recurrences. Eleven patients had prior surgery, ten patients had prior radiation therapy, and three had been given some previous chemotherapy. For this trial, all the enrollees were inoculated with 1×10^5 pfu HSV1716 intratumorally, and then underwent surgical resections four to nine days afterwards. Again, no acute toxicity was observed, nor was virus administration responsible for any adverse events. Unlike the first study, both seronegative patients became seropositive by the end of the study. In two patients, HSV1716 was recovered from the resected tumors, but semiquantitative PCR detection methods identified the virus within the tumor tissue of ten patients. The results from the two patients supported the possibility of HSV1716 replication within the tumor. The authors concluded that HSV1716 could feasibly replicate in situ within tumors without toxicity in patients with malignant glioma.

Recently, it was reported that tumor tissue from one of the patients inoculated intratumorally with HSV1716 was cultured in vitro and tested for the presence of that virus (Harland et al., 2002). Though none was found, when the cells were re-infected in vitro, a small fraction was found to not undergo lysis. These cells – which themselves began to proliferate – continued to shed HSV716 at low levels. The authors concluded that this suggested the possibility that, in vivo, a similar persistence of HSV may occur, allowing the virus to continue killing tumor cells over extended periods of time. Further studies of HSV1716's efficacy and safety are ongoing. The virus will be injected into the surrounding brain tissue around the tumors after surgical resection, similar to the Phase Ib trial in progress with G207.

In a recently reported study aimed at examining the safety of HSV1716 inoculation into the brain surrounding the enhancing tumor, twelve patients with newly-diagnosed or recurrent malignant glioma underwent resection followed by inoculation of 10^5 pfu of HSV1716 into the tumor bed. No dose limiting toxicities were observed. Three patients remain alive and clinically stable at 15, 18 and 22 months postsurgery and HSV1716 injection (Harrow et al., 2004).

Oncolytic HSV for Non-CNS malignancies

While the concept of genetically engineered oncolytic HSV-1 was originally developed for the treatment of malignant glioma and other CNS tumors, it was soon explored in preclinical models of other difficult to treat tumors, that developed outside the CNS, including neurofibrosarcomas, melanoma, and non-small cell lung carcinoma, as well as cancer of the breast, liver, pancreas, ovary, head and neck, gallbladder, bladder, prostate, stomach, and colon. Of these, HSV1716 has been studied clinically in patients with melanoma, and NV1020 in patient with colorectal metastases to the liver.

HSV1716: melanoma

Genetically-engineered HSV has been demonstrated to be effective as an oncolytic agent against melanoma in a wide variety of preclinical studies (Miller et al., 2001; Miller and Fraser, 2000; Randazzo et al., 1997; Toda et al., 1999) To explore the possible use of HSV in the treatment of metastatic melanoma (Mackie et al., 2001) performed a pilot study in which five patients with stage 4 melanoma underwent inoculation of HSV1716 into subcutaneous melanoma nodules. Two patients received a single injection of 10^3 pfu of 1716, two received two injections, and one received four injections. Flattening of injected nodules was seen in a single patient, and follow-up biopsies demonstrated tumor necrosis in patient receiving multiple injections; no necrosis was seen in control nodules treated with saline. Immunohistochemical staining was positive for the HSV UL42, a 65 kD DNA-binding protein which is essential for HSV DNA replication and virus growth. Patients tolerated the treatment well, and no change in IgG and IgM titers to HSV were seen. No evidence of response was seen in non-treated lesions, however. Further studies of HSV in melanoma have not yet been reported.

NV1020: colorectal metastases

The third conditionally replication competent HSV-1 to be tested in clinical trials as an oncolytic virus was actually the first such HSV ever to be studied in humans. NV1020 is a purified, mapped form of the virus R7020, which was initially tested in humans as a vaccine against wild-type HSV-1 and 2. R7020 is a genetically engineered virus initially engineered as a candidate for prophylactic immunization against HSV-1 and HSV-2 infection (Meignier,

1991) NV1020 was constructed with a deletion of a 15 kbp region encompasses the UL56 gene and the internal inverted long repeat, extending to the promoter regulatory elements of the ICP 4 gene of the HSV-1 viral genome and includes one copy of the $\gamma_1 34.5$ gene. Additionally, a 700 base pair deletion of the native thymidine kinase gene is present that also presents expression of the overlapping transcripts of the UL24 region. Because it was originally designed as a vaccine, a 5.2 kb fragment of the HSV-2 DNA encoding HSV-2 glycoproteins G, D, I and a portion of E is included, as well as a copy of the HSV-1 thymidine kinase gene under the $\alpha 4$ promoter. This maintains sensitivity to antiviral agents such as acyclovir. The virus was extensively tested for genetic stability, with no increase in virulence after nine passages in mouse brain. It has been tested for virulence in mice, guinea pigs, rabbits and the sensitive primate species, *Aotus nancymae* (Meignier, 1991; Meignier et al., 1988, 1990). It has been demonstrated to be safe in *Aotus* at doses up to 10^7 pfu by a variety of routes, including intravenous, oral, subcutaneous, and intramuscular. It retains toxicity when administered intracranially, likely due to the retention of an intact copy of the $\gamma_1 34.5$ gene.

Safety has been demonstrated in humans at doses up to 10^8 pfu when administered peripherally in the vaccine trial, and while the virus retained immunogenicity in humans, two doses were required to induce antibody formation. R7020 has been examined as a candidate antitumor agent for a variety of non-CNS tumors in a variety of preclinical models, including hepatoma, colorectal carcinoma, head and neck epithelial squamous cell carcinoma and prostate adenocarcinoma xenografts.

A Phase I study of NV1020 has been conducted in patients with colorectal carcinoma metastatic to the liver. NV1020 was delivered via percutaneous hepatic artery infusion in patients with hepatic metastatic colorectal. Three days after infusion, patients underwent surgery for placement of a hepatic infusion pump; at that time, both tumors and non-malignant liver were biopsied. Patients were observed for 28 days before starting regional chemotherapy. Preliminary results presented at the American Society of Clinical Oncology showed no dose limiting toxicities in the first nine patients, treated at three dose levels (1.3×10^6, 10^7, 1.3×10^7 pfu). Some patients did develop fever, nausea, and headache. Viral DNA but not infectious virus was demonstrated by PCR examination of the hepatic venous outflow. Virus was demonstrated by immunohistochemistry in tumor tissue but not normal liver, and all patients demonstrated a decrease in CEA, a marker for colorectal cancer, over a 28-day period (Fong et al., 2002). A report on the complete trial of all twelve patients treated up to a dose of 1×10^8 pfu is expected shortly. A Phase I//II trial is under way which is designed to examine safety and tolerability of NV1020 in this setting, as well as possible synergies with chemotherapy.

HSV and other cancers

While trials have been opened for patients with other cancers including mesothelioma and head and neck cancers, results remain unpublished at the time of this writing.

Oncolytic HSV: current directions

The potential of HSV used alone as an oncolytic virus is clearly illustrated through these trials (Table 76.1). However, it is likely that recalcitrant tumors such as malignant glioma may require a multi-pronged approach for successful treatment. The proven safety of these engineered viruses permits us to consider the use of HSV-1 mutants that serve not only to kill tumors via infecting, replicating and lyzing them, but also by functioning as vectors to deliver anti-tumor genes. Preclinical studies using engineered HSV-1 mutants in combination with standard treatment modalities are promising. The enhancement of anti-tumor activity of G207 or other HSV-1 mutants (4009, 7020, 3616) with low-dose and high-dose irradiation has been shown in models of malignant glioma as well as other tumors, including hepatoma, radioresistant squamous cell carcinoma (Advani et al., 1998; Bradley et al., 1999), and cervical cancer (Blank et al., 1999). Combination therapy administering both the $\gamma_1 34.5$-deletion mutant R3616 followed by ionizing radiation to mice with human U87 malignant glioma xenografts showed significant growth delay of flank tumors and extended survival of animals with intracranial tumors over the use of either treatment alone (Bradley et al., 1999). These findings have also been demonstrated in intracranial U87 tumors treated with G207 followed by treatment with or without radiation (Markert et al., 2000a,b). In at least some models, this interaction is not simply additive but appears synergistic, possibly due to enhanced viral replication and better dissemination of the virus allowing greater reduction of tumor volume after combination therapy. Increased efficacy has been shown when HSV-1 has been given in conjunction with chemotherapeutic agents, although the purported mechanisms of this increased efficacy vary (Chahlavi et al., 1999).

The demonstrated safety and promise demonstrated by the mutant viruses G207, HSV1716, and NV1020 warrants the further investigation of novel HSV-1 gene therapy vectors. Transgene expression of interleukins or cytokines to enhance immune response against neoplastic cells,

Table 76.1. HSV for the oncolytic viral treatment of tumors

VIRUS	Tumor-selective virus-derivative	Engineered mutation(s) to target tumors	Clinical trials	Tumors targeted
Herpes simplex virus-1	G207	1. Deletion of both $\gamma_1 34.5$ copies 2. *LacZ* insertion in UL39 (ICP6-inactivation)	Phase I, IB completed Phase I XRT trial approved	Glioma
	HSV1716	1. Deletion of both $g_1 34.5$ copies	3 Phase I studies, pilot completed	Glioma, melanoma
	NV1020	1. Deletion, 15 kbp region (UL56 gene to internal ILR) 2. Insertion of HSV-2 gG, gD, gI, partial gE 3. Insertion of HSV-1 tk under alpha-4 4. 700 kbp deletion of UL23-UL24	Phase I completed, Phase I/II underway	Colorectal metastases

anti-angiogenic factors to impede growth of vascular supplies to tumors, or suicide genes to augment the cytotoxic effects of chemotherapeutic agents are all possibilities under study that may demonstrate improved efficacy against human malignancies. Thus, the use of HSV as a portion of a multi-modality treatment regimen involving radiation, chemotherapy and gene therapy, as well possibly oncolytic viral therapy, may hold an important place in the future treatment of patients suffering from these conditions.

REFERENCES

Advani, S. J., Sibley, G., Song, P. Y. *et al.* (1998). Enhancement of replication of genetically engineered herpes simplex virus by ionizing radiation: a new paradigm for destruction of therapeutically intractable tumors. *Gene Ther.*, **5**, 160–165.

Blank, S. V., Rubin, S. C., Coukos, G., Amin, K. M., Albelda, S. M., and Molnar-Kimber, K. L. (1999). Replication-selective herpes simplex virus type 1 mutant therapy of cervical cancer is enhanced by low-dose radiation. *Hum. Gene Ther.*, **13**, 627–639.

Bradley, J. D., Kataoka, Y., Advani, S. *et al.* (1999). Ionizing radiation improves survival in mice bearing intracranial high-grade gliomas injected with genetically modified herpes simplex virus. *Clin. Cancer Res.*, **5**, 1517–1522.

Chahlavi, A., Todo, T., Martuza, R. L., and Rabkin, S. D. (1999). Replication-competent herpes simpelx virus vector G207 and cisplatin combination therapy for head and neck squamous cell carcinoma. *Neoplasia*, **1**, 162–169.

Chattopadhyay, M., Wolfe, D., Huang, S. *et al.* (2002). In vivo gene therapy for pyridoxine-induced neuropathy by herpes simplex virus-mediated gene transfer of neurotrophin-3. *Ann. Neurol.*, **51**, 19–27.

Chattopadhyay, M., Goss, J., Lacomis, D. *et al.* (2003). Protective effect of HSV-mediated gene transfer of nerve growth factor in pyridoxine neuropathy demonstrates functional activity of trkA receptors in large sensory neurons of adult animals. *Eur. J. Neurosci.*, **17**, 732–740.

Chou, J. and Roizman, B. (1992). The gamma 1(34.5) gene of herpes simplex virus 1 precludes neuroblastoma cells from triggering total shutoff of protein synthesis characteristic of programed cell death in neuronal cells. *Proc. Natl Acad. Sci. USA*, **89**, 3266–3270.

Chou, J., Kern, E. R., Whitley, R. J., and Roizman, B. (1990). Mapping of herpes simplex virus-1 neurovirulence to gamma 134.5, a gene nonessential for growth in culture. *Science*, **250**, 1262–1266.

Coen, D. M., Goldstein, D. J., and Weller, S. K. (1989) Herpes simplex virus ribonucleotide reductase mutants are hypersensitive to acyclovir. *Antimicrob. Agents Chemother.*, **33**, 1395–1399 (Erratum appears in *Antimicrob. Agents Chemother.*, **33**, 1827).

DeLuca, N. A., McCarthy, A. M., and Schaffer, P. A. (1985). Isolation and characterization of deletion mutants of herpes simplex virus type 1 in the gene encoding immediate-early regulatory protein ICP4. *J. Virol.*, **56**, 558–570.

Farassati, F., Yang, A. D., and Lee, P. W. (2001). Oncogenes in Ras signalling pathway dictate host-cell permissiveness to herpes simplex virus 1. *Nat. Cell. Biol.*, **3**, 745–750.

Fong, Y., Kermeny, N., Jarnagin, W. *et al.* (2002). Phase I study of a replication-competent herpes simplex oncolytic virus for treatment of hepatic colorectal metastases. *ASCO Annual Meeting.* Orlando, FL, May 18–21.

Fraefel, C., Song, S., Lim, F. *et al.* (1996). Helper virus-free transfer of herpes simplex virus type 1 plasmid vectors into neural cells. *J. Virol.*, **70**, 7190–7197.

Goins, W. F., Lee, K. A., Cavalcoli, J. D. *et al.* (1999). Herpes simplex virus type 1 vector-mediated expression of nerve growth factor protects dorsal root ganglion neurons from peroxide toxicity. *J. Virol.*, **73**, 519–532.

Goldstein, D. J. and Weller S. K. (1988). Factor(s) present in herpes simplex virus type 1-infected cells can compensate for the loss of the large subunit of the viral ribonucleotide reductase: characterization of an ICP6 deletion mutant. *Virology*, **166**, 41–51.

Goss, J. R., Mata, M., Goins, W. F., Wu, H. H., Glorioso, J. C., and Fink, D. J. (2001). Antinociceptive effect of a genomic herpes simplex virus-based vector expressing human proenkephalin in rat dorsal root ganglion. *Gene Ther.*, **8**, 551–556.

Goss, J. R., Harley, C. F., Mata, M. et al. (2002a). Herpes vector-mediated expression of proenkephalin reduces bone cancer pain. *Ann. Neurol.*, **52**, 662–665.

Goss, J. R., Goins, W. F., Lacomis, D., Mata, M., Glorioso, J. C., and Fink, D. J. (2002b). Herpes simplex-mediated gene transfer of nerve growth factor protects against peripheral neuropathy in streptozotocin-induced diabetes in the mouse. *Diabetes*, **51**, 2227–2232.

Grandi, P., Spear, M., Breakefield, X. O., and Wang, S. (2004). Targeting HSV amplicon vectors. *Methods*, **33**, 179–186.

Hao, S., Mata, M., Goins, W., Glorioso, J. C., and Fink, D. J. (2003). Transgene-mediated enkephalin release enhances the effect of morphine and evades tolerance to produce a sustained antiallodynic effect in neuropathic pain. *Pain*, **102**, 135–142.

Harland, J., Papanastassiou, V., and Brown, S. M. (2002). HSV1716 persistence in primary human glioma cells in vitro. *Gene Ther.*, **9**, 1194–1198.

Harrow, S., Papanastassiou, V., Harland, J. et al. (2004). HSV 1716 injection into the brain adjacent to tumour following surgical resection of high-grade glioma: safety data and long-term survival. *Gene Ther.*, **11**, 1648–1658.

He, B., Gross, M., and Roizman, B. (1997). The gamma(1)34.5 protein of herpes simplex virus 1 complexes with protein phosphatase 1alpha to dephosphorylate the alpha subunit of the eukaryotic translation initiation factor 2 and preclude the shutoff of protein synthesis by double-stranded RNA-activated protein kinase. *Proc. Natl Acad. Sci. USA*, **94**, 843–848.

Ho, I. A., Hui, K. M., and Lam, P. Y. (2004). Glioma-specific and cell cycle-regulated herpes simplex virus type 1 amplicon viral vector. *Hum. Gene Ther.*, **15**, 495–508.

Hunter, L. D., Martuza, R. L., Feigenbaum, F. et al. (1999). Attenuated, replication-competent herpes simplex virus type 1 mutant G207: safety evaluation of intracerebral injection in nonhuman primates. *J. Virol.*, **73**, 6319–6326.

Jacobs, A. H., Winkeler, A., Hartung, M. et al. (2003). Improved herpes simplex virus type 1 amplicon vectors for proportional coexpression of positron emission tomography marker and therapeutic genes. *Hum. Gene Ther.*, **14**, 277–297.

Krisky, D. M., Wolfe, D., Goins, W. F., et al. (1998). Deletion of multiple immediate-early genes from herpes simplex virus reduces cytotoxicity and permits long-term gene expression in neurons. *Gene Ther.*, **5**, 1593–1603.

Lilley, C. E., Groutsi, F., Han, Z. et al. (2001). Multiple immediate-early gene-deficient herpes simplex virus vectors allowing efficient gene delivery to neurons in culture and widespread gene delivery to the central nervous system in vivo. *J. Virol.*, **75**, 4343–4356.

McCarthy, A. M., McMahan, L., and Schaffer, P. A. (1989). Herpes simplex virus type 1 ICP27 deletion mutants exhibit altered patterns of transcription and are DNA deficient. *J. Virol.*, **63**, 18–27.

MacKie, R. M., Stewart, B., and Brown, S. M. (2001). Intralesional injection of herpes simplex virus 1716 in metastatic melanoma. *Lancet*, **357**, 525–526.

Marconi, P., Krisky, D., Oligino, T. et al. (1996). Replication-defective herpes simplex virus vectors for gene transfer in vivo. *Proc. Natl Acad. Sci. USA*, **93**, 11319–11320.

Markert, J. M., Coen, D. M., Malick, A., Mineta, T., and Martuza, R. L. (1992). Expanded spectrum of viral therapy in the treatment of nervous system tumors. *J. Neurosurg.* **77**, 590–594.

Markert, J. M., Malick, A., Coen, D. M., and Martuza, R. L. (1993). Reduction and elimination of encephalitis in an experimental glioma therapy model with attenuated herpes simplex mutants that retain susceptibility to acyclovir. *Neurosurgery*, **32**, 597–603.

Markert, J. M., Gillespie, G. Y., Weichselbaum, R. R., Roizman, B., and Whitley, R. J. (2000a). Genetically engineered HSV in the treatment of glioma: a review. *Rev. Med. Virol.*, **10**, 17–30.

Markert, J. M., Medlock, M. D., Rabkin, S. D. et al. (2000b). Conditionally replicating herpes simplex, virus., mutant, G207 for the treatment of malignant glioma: results of a phase I trial. *Gene Ther.*, **7**, 867–874.

Marshall, K. R., Lachmann, R. H., Efstathiou, S., Rinaldi, A., and Preston, C. M. (2000). Long-term transgene expression in mice infected with a herpes simplex virus type 1 mutant severely impaired for immediate-early gene expression. *J. Virol.*, **74**, 956–964.

Martuza, R. L., Malick, A., Markert, J. M., Ruffner, K. L., and Coen, D. M. (1991). Experimental therapy of human glioma by means of a genetically engineered virus mutant. *Science*, **252**, 854–856.

Meignier, B. (1991). Genetically engineered attenuated herpes simplex viruses. *Rev. Infect. Dis.*, **13** Suppl 11, S895–S897.

Meignier, B., Longnecker, R., and Roizman, B. (1988). In vivo behavior of genetically engineered herpes simplex viruses R7017 and R7020: construction and evaluation in rodents. *J. Infect. Dis.*, **158**, 602–614.

Meignier, B., Martin, B., Whitley, R. J., and Roizman, B. (1990). In vivo behavior of genetically engineered herpes simplex viruses R7017 and R7020. II. Studies in immunocompetent and immunosuppressed owl monkeys (*Aotus trivirgatus*). *J. Infect. Dis.*, **162**, 313–321.

Miller, C. G. and Fraser, N. W. (2000). Role of the immune response during neuro-attenuated herpes simplex virus-mediated tumor destruction in a murine intracranial melanoma model. *Cancer Res.*, **60**, 5714–5722.

Miller, C. G., Krummenacher, C., Eisenberg, R. J., Cohen, G. H., and Fraser, N. W. (2001). Development of a syngenic murine B16 cell line-derived melanoma susceptible to destruction by neuroattenuated HSV-1. *Mol. Ther.*, **3**, 160–168.

Mineta, T., Rabkin, S. D., and Martuza, R. L. (1994). Treatment of malignant gliomas using ganciclovir-hypersensitive, ribonucleotide reductase-deficient herpes simplex viral mutant. *Cancer Res.*, **54**, 3963–3966.

Mineta, T., Rabkin, S. D., Yazaki, T., Hunter, W. D., and Martuza, R. L. (1995). Attenuated multi-mutated herpes simplex virus-1 for the treatment of malignant gliomas. *Nat. Med.*, **1**, 938–943.

Moriuchi, S., Oligino, T., Krisky, D. et al. (1998). Enhanced tumor cell killing in the presence of ganciclovir by herpes simplex virus type 1 vector-directed coexpression of human tumor necrosis factor-alpha and herpes simplex virus thymidine kinase. *Cancer Resi.*, **58**, 5731–5737.

Palmer, J. A., Branston, R. H., Lilley, C. E., *et al*. (2000). Development and optimization of herpes simplex virus vectors for multiple long-term gene delivery to the peripheral nervous system. *J. Virol.*, **74**, 5604–5618.

Papanastassiou, V., Rampling, R., Fraser, M. *et al*. (2002). The potential for efficacy of the modified (ICP 34.5(-)) herpes simplex virus HSV1716 following intratumoural injection into human malignant glioma: a proof of principle study. *Gene Ther.*, **9**, 398–406.

Rampling, R., Cruickshank, G., Papanastassiou, V. *et al*. (2000). Toxicity evaluation of replication-competent herpes simplex virus (ICP 34.5 null mutant 1716) in patients with recurrent malignant glioma. [see comment]. *Gene Ther.*, **7**, 859–866.

Randazzo, B. P., Bhat, M. G., Kesari, S., Fraser, N. W., and Brown, S. M. (1997). Treatment of experimental subcutaneous human melanoma with a replication-restricted herpes simplex virus mutant. *J. Invest. Dermatol.*, **108**, 933–937.

Samaniego, L. A., Webb, A. L., and DeLuca, N. A. (1995). Functional interactions between herpes simplex virus immediate-early proteins during infection: gene expression as a consequence of ICP27 and different domains of ICP4. *J. Virol.*, **69**, 5705–5715.

Samaniego, L. A., Wu, N., and DeLuca, N. A. (1997). The herpes simplex virus immediate-early protein ICP0 affects transcription from the viral genome and infected-cell survival in the absence of ICP4 and ICP27. *J. Virol.*, **71**, 4614–4625.

Samaniego, L. A., Neiderhiser, L., and DeLuca, N. A. (1998). Persistence and expression of the herpes simplex virus genome in the absence of immediate-early proteins. *J. Virol.*, **72**, 3307–3320.

Sanson, M., Marcaud, V., Robin, E., Valery, C., Sturtz, F., and Zalc, B. (2002). Connexin 43-mediated bystander effect in two rat glioma cell models. *Cancer Gene Ther.*, **9**, 149–155.

Schmeisser, F., Donohue, M., and Weir, J. P. (2002). Tetracycline-regulated gene expression in replication-incompetent herpes simplex virus vectors. *Hum. Gene Ther.*, **13**, 2113–2124.

Shah, A. C., Benos, D., Gillespie, G. Y., and Markert, J. M. Oncolytic viruses: clinical applications as vectors for the treatment of malignant gliomas. *J. Neurooncol.*, **65**, 203–226.

Spaete, R. R. and Frenkel, N. (1982). The herpes simplex virus amplicon: a new eucaryotic defective-virus cloning-amplifying vector. *Cell*, **30**, 295–304.

Toda, M., Rabkin, S. D., Kojima, H., and Martuza, R. L. (1999). Herpes simplex virus as an in situ cancer vaccine for the induction of specific anti-tumor immunity. *Hum. Gene Ther.*, **10**, 385–393.

Valyi-Nagy, T., Fareed, M. U., O'Keefe, J. S. *et al*. (1994). The herpes simplex virus type 1 strain 17+ gamma 34.5 deletion mutant 1716 is avirulent in SCID mice. *J. Gen. Virol.*, **75**, 2059–2063.

Wade-Martins, R., Smith, E. R., Tyminski, E., Chiocca, E. A., and Saeki, Y. (2001). An infectious transfer and expression system for genomic DNA loci in human and mouse cells. *Nat. Biotechnol.*, **19**, 1067–1070.

Wang, Y., Camp, S. M., Niwano, M. *et al*. (2002). Herpes simplex virus type 1/adeno-associated virus rep(+) hybrid amplicon vector improves the stability of transgene expression in human cells by site-specific integration. *J. Virol.*, **76**, 7150–7162.

Wu, N., Watkins, S. C., Schaffer, P. A., and DeLuca, N. A. (1996). Prolonged gene expression and cell survival after infection by a herpes simplex virus mutant defective in the immediate-early genes encoding ICP4, ICP27, and ICP22. *J. Virol.*, **70**, 6358–6369.

Yamada, M., Oligino, T., Mata, M., Goss, J., Glorioso, J., and Fink, D. J. (1999). Herpes simplex virus vector-mediated expression of Bcl-2 prevents 6-hydroxydopamine-induced degeneration of neurons in the substantia nigra in vivo. *Proc. Natl Acad. Sci. USA*, **96**, 4078–4083.

Index

A-5021 1229–1230
A-capsids 30, 189, 450
Achong, Bert 344
actin-related protein (ARP) 39–40
acute retinal necrosis (ARN) 643, 649, 660
  mouse model 650
acyclovir 663
  adverse effects 1161, 1178
    neurotoxicity 1161
  B virus treatment 1041
  clinical indications 1161
  EBV treatment 420, 421
  HCMV treatment 1192
  HSV treatment 663, 664, 1153–1162
    genital herpes 1154–1156, 1157
    gingivostomatitis 1157
    herpes simplex encephalitis (HSE) 1157
    immunocompromised hosts 1160–1161
    neonatal HSV 1157–1160
    resistance 1161–1162, 1164–1165
    severe infection 664–666
  mechanism of action 1154, 1177
  pharmacokinetics 1154, 1177–1178
  timing of drug initiation 1161
  VZV treatment 1177–1178
    adults 1180
    children 1179
    herpes zoster 1182, 1185
    immunocompromised hosts 1181, 1185
    pregnant women 1181
    resistance 1187–1188
  see also valaciclovir
AD169 vaccine 1278–1279
adhesion molecules, HCMV infection effects 767
adoptive immunotherapy *see* immunotherapy
African green monkey cytomegalovirus *see* simian cytomegalovirus

AIDS
  HCMV disease and 795
  HHV-6 reactivation 839
  HSV interactions 661–662
  immunoblastic lymphomas and 525
  Kaposi's sarcoma and 347, 434, 435–436, 974–975, 976, 1017
  lymphomas, EBV association 891, 994
    AIDS-related Burkitt lymphoma
    malignant lymphoma
  simian AIDS (SAIDS) 1055–1056
    CMV infection relationships 1055–1056
  see also human immunodeficiency virus (HIV)
AL-RNA 82
alkaline nuclease 73
alkoxyalkyl esters of cidofovir 1165–1166
Allo-MDM model, HCMV growth 770–773
allograft transplantation, HCMV transmission 806
  infection establishment
  see also transplantation
α0 RL2 gene 71
α3ß1 integrin 369
α4 RS1 gene 80
α22 gene 80
α27 gene 79
α47 gene 82
α-TIF protein 78
αX RNA 82
alphaherpesviruses 61
  DNA replication 138–142
    cell cycle and 141
    location of 139
    maturation and packaging 141
    origins of 138–139
    proteins involved 139–141
    recombination 141–142
  egress from host cell 151–159
  evolutionary relationships 16
  gene products and functions 70–82, 164
  genome comparisons 19–20, 61–64
    L component genes unique to HSV 65–66
    S component genes unique to HSV 66–67
    VZV genes that are absent from HSV genomes 64–65
  genome structure 138
  latency 142
  RNA processing 131–133
  transcription initiation 128–131
    role of IE proteins 129
    TATA box-containing promoters 128–131
    viral transcription factors 128–129
  see also B virus; herpes simplex viruses (HSV); simian varicella virus (SVV); varicella zoster virus (VZV)
ALVAC vectored HCMV vaccine 1282–1283
amplicon vectors 1342
annexin II 232
annotation 14–15

anti-host strategies 165, 170
  blocking of interferon pathways to host defense 168
  blocking of pro-apoptotic cellular functions 168–169, 327
  mRNA degradation in infected cells 166–167
  protein degradation in infected cells 167–168
  suppression of NF-(K)B activation 165–166
  see also specific viruses
antibody responses 921
  B virus 1038–1039
  evasion of 624, 1137
  see also FcγR
  HCMV 781–782, 1276–1277
    in placental syncytiotrophoblasts 819–820
  HHV-6/HHV-7 857–859
    IgG 858
    IgM 857–858
    neutralizing antibodies 858–859
  HSV 624, 1332–1333
    evasion 624
    human studies suggesting protection 1333–1334, 1335
    neonates 624, 1332–1334
  immunotherapy approaches 1332
    animal models 1334–1335
    limitations 1335
  KSHV 921–925
    anti-KSHV antibody detection 921–923
    differential response over time 963
    functions 923–925
    HAART effects 923
  neonates 624, 1137, 1332–1334
  simian CMV 1054, 1055
  VZV 708
    during reactivation 709
antigen presentation 1130
  disruption of 1119, 1128–1129
    by EBV 911
    by HHV-7 1126
  see also MHC functions, modulation of
  DNA vaccine mechanisms of action 1306–1307
  see also dendritic cells (DC)
antigens
  HHV-6 853–855
    complement-independent neutralization targets 854–855
    diagnostic targets 855
    latent antigens 853
    lytic antigens 853–854
    monoclonal antibody studies 854
  HHV-7 856
    complement-independent neutralization targets 856
    diagnostic targets 856
    monoclonal antibody studies 855, 856
  see also antigen presentation

antiviral agents 1153, 1219
  development 1221–1224
    approaches 70, 1219, 1242
    biochemical assays 1214–1215
    bioinformatics and computational tools 1211–1212
    cell based antiviral assays 1214
    DNA replication complex as target 1227–1235
    early replication events as targets 1226–1227
    functional assays 1215
    genomics impact on research 1212–1213
    host cell targets 1225–1226
    mechanism of action studies 1215
    new resources 1213–1214
    process 1219–1225
    spectrum of activity studies 1215–1216
  DNA polymerase inhibitors 1228–1232
  DNA processing and packaging inhibitors 1235
    portal protein inhibitors 1235–1237
    protease inhibitors 1238–1239
    terminase complex inhibitors 1236–1238
    UL97 encoded protein kinase inhibitors 1239
  helicase-primase inhibitors 1232–1235
  resistance 1153
    acyclovir 1161–1162, 1164–1165, 1187–1188
    famciclovir/penciclovir 1163
    foscarnet 1167
    ganciclovir 1169, 1204–1206
    valganciclovir 1169
  see also specific agents and viruses
apoptosis 168, 327–328
  apoptotic signaling 548
    extrinsic pathway 548
    inhibition of extrinsic signaling 551–552
    intrinsic pathway 548
  induction of 326
    HHV-6/HHV-7 837–838
  inhibition/evasion of 266, 327–328, 330–331
    alteration of extrinsic pathways 331–332, 551–552
    blocking of pro-apoptotic cellular functions 168
    EBV
    HCMV cellular tropism and 774
    herpesvirus saimiri 1079–1080
    HHV-6/HHV-7 863
    in Burkitt's lymphoma 525–526
    KSHV 445, 548–552, 1011–1012
    mitochondrial anti-apoptotic proteins 551–552
    vICA 330
    vMIA 328–330
artificial insemination of donor semen, HCMV transmission 807
assembly see virion assembly
assembly protein (AP) 54
  precursor (pAP) 54
ATF/CREB site 275, 282, 283–284
  EBV lytic induction 407–408

atherosclerosis, HCMV and 1196
attachment to host cell 50
  gammaherpesviruses 364–366
  HCMV, induction of physiological changes 265
  HSV 94–95
autoimmune disease 642
  EBV and 345
  see also immunopathology

B7 molecules 1128
B cell receptor, lytic EBV infection induction 404
B cells 921
  activation
    as EBV target cells 360, 904, 1293
      EBV persistence 472–474
      penetration mechanisms 366–369
      viral exploitation of regulatory mechanisms 518–519
    as KSHV target cells 360–361
      role as reservoirs for viral amplification 437
    KSHV response 921–925
      anti-KSHV antibody detection 921–923
      functions 923–925
      HAART effects 923
  response evasion
B virus 1033–1034, 1041
  control of infection 1040–1041
    antiviral therapy 1041
    prevention 1040–1041
    vaccine development 1041
  diagnosis 1039–1040
    animals 1039–1040
    humans 1040
  disease manifestations 1039
  distribution in nature 1032–1033
  epidemiology 1037–1038
    animals 1037–1038
    humans 1038
  genome 1033–1034
    sequence analysis 1034
  growth properties 1033
  history 1031–1032
  immune responses 1038–1039
  isolation 1033
  latency 1037
    reactivation 1037
  pathogenesis 1034–1037
    experimental infections 1035–1036
    human infection 1036–1037
    natural host 1035
  pathogenicity in humans 1031
  transmission 1035
  vaccination 1041
B-capsids 30, 189, 450

baboon lymphocryptovirus
   EBNA-1 homologues 1098
   EBNA-2 homologues 1098
   LMP-1 1099
   LMP-2 1099
   see also lymphocryptoviruses
BALF1 471
   gene product 470
BamHI A transcripts (BARTS) 992, 995
BARF0 ORF 992
BARF1 gene product 418, 470–471, 910
Barr, Yvonne 344
BART genes 478–479
BAY 38-4766 1238
BAY 57-1293 1234–1235
Bcl-2-related proteins
   EBV 470
   KSHV 551–552
Bcl-3 protein 610
BCNA compounds 1230–1231
BCRF1 protein 909–910
BDCRB 1237
benign meningitis 659
β_2 microglobulin (β_2m) 232
βX RNA 82
betaherpesviruses 177
   capsid assembly 218, 312
      protein interactions and 312–314
   cell cycle dysregulation 253–254, 326–327
   DNA encapsidation 218, 314–315
   DNA synthesis 217, 295
      initiation mechanism 301
      rolling circle versus linear model 295–296
   entry into host cells 214–216
   envelope glycoproteins 192, 214, 234–236
   gene expression regulation 216–217, 241
      factors stimulating IE gene expression 252–253
      late genes 302–305
      MIE transcriptional enhancers 243–246
      silencing of IE genes 246–247
   gene products 205–211
   genes 178–188, 204–213
      core genes 204–211, 213
      gene capture 187–188
      gene duplication 186–187, 1067
      gene families 187, 205–211, 212–213, 1067
      gene function 188, 204–212
      genetic content 178–186
      IE genes 242–243, 252–253
      MIE genes 248–249
      sequences 178
   genome structure 177–178, 189–191
   host response modulation 324–332
      apoptosis suppression 327–328, 330–332
      impact on host cell cycle 326–327
      interferon regulated factor 3 (IRF-3) modulation 325

      interferon response gene activation 325
      NF-(K)B activation 325
   latency 219, 843
   nucleotide metabolism 217–218
   proteins encoded 179–183
      structural proteins 213–214
   reactivation from latent state 843
   replication 204–212, 217, 295–296
      origins 299–302
      regulation 216–217, 241
   replication proteins 296–299
      DNA polymerase and accessory protein 297–298
      helicase-primase complex 296–297
      IE2 299
      origin binding proteins 299
      single-stranded DNA binding protein 298
      UL84 298–299
   RNA molecules 192
   tegument assembly 315–319
   virion structure 188–192
      capsid 191, 213
      tegument 191–192, 213
   see also cytomegaloviruses; roseoloviruses; specific viruses
BGLF4 kinase 418
BHLF1 promoter 467–469
BHRF1 gene 414
   gene product 418, 470
BILS 179 BS 1232–1234
biochemical assays 1214–1215
bioinformatics 1211–1212
biological criteria 7, 27
blastogenic responses to HSV infection 594
bleeding complications, VZV 685
blood transfusion
   HCMV transmission 805–806
      infection establishment
   KSHV transmission 969–970, 973
BMLF1 gene product 470
BMRF1 gene 414
BMRF1 protein 417
BMRF2 protein 472
bone marrow transplant (BMT)
   CMV pneumonitis and 788–789
   HCMV immune response and 783
   herpes zoster epidemiology and 726
   HHV-6 reactivation 839
   HHV-6/HHV-7 immune responses and 859–860
   see also immunocompromised hosts; transplantation
breast cancer 893
breast milk, HCMV transmission 796–797
brivudin 1179
   VZV treatment 1179
      herpes zoster 1182
BRLF1 gene 404, 405–406, 467
   promoter 406
      regulation 408–409, 410–411, 414–415

BRLF1 protein (Rta) 410, 467
   activation of cellular fatty acid synthase gene 416
   cell cycle effects 416
   early lytic gene regulation 417
   late gene expression and 419–420
   role in lytic induction 414–415
   see also Rta viral lytic switch protein
BRLF1-knockout virus 415–416
BRRF1 gene product 417
Burkitt, Denis 342–344
Burkitt's lymphoma (BL) 342–345, 525–526, 887–888, 889–890, 904–905, 993–994
   contributing factors 994
   EBV gene expression in 993–994
   epidemiology
      AIDS-related BL
      endemic BL
      sporadic BL
   evidence of association with EBV
   T cell control of 911
   therapeutic vaccine development 1300–1301
butyrate, lytic EBV gene transcription induction 409
BW1263W94
BZLF1 gene 404, 405–406, 467
   autoregulation 408
   promoter 406, 408
      activating factors 406–408, 414–415
      negative regulatory elements 408
BZLF1 protein (ZEBRA) 410, 467, 469
   activation of cellular genes 411
   activation of methylated ZRE motifs 411
   cell cycle effects 412
   dispersion of PML bodies 413
   early lytic gene regulation 417
   effects on host cell environment 412
   effects on p53 412–413
   immune response modulation 413–414
   replication function 411
   transcriptional effects 410–411
BZLF1-knockout virus 411–412

C1 protein 1101
C5 protein 1102
C7 protein 1102
C-capsids 30, 189, 450
C/EBP binding motifs 446–448
   C/EBPα 440–441
cancer
   HCMV infection and
   transmission of 924
   see also specific types of cancer; tumor induction
candidate drugs see antiviral agents
capsid 188–192
   assembly 31, 53–54, 268, 311
      betaherpesviruses 218, 312
      protein interactions and 312–314

      maturation 314–315
   protein composition 48, 213, 313
   structure 31–34, 48–49
      betaherpesviruses 191, 213, 1058
      gammaherpesviruses 351, 362, 450
      rhesus rhadinovirus 1106–1107
capsid transport nuclear protein (CTNP) 54
capsid transport tegument protein (CTTP) 54
capsid-like structures 30
captured genes 17
carcinoma see specific carcinomas
case fatality rate (CFR), VZV 718–719
Castleman's disease 895–896, 1014
   multicentric (MCD) 349, 895–896, 1014–1015
      KSHV gene expression patterns 496–497
   therapy 896
vCCL proteins 547
   HSV responses 628
CD4+ receptor 835–836
CD4+ T lymphocytes see T helper cells (CD4+)
CD8+ T lymphocytes see cytotoxic T lymphocytes (CD8+)
CD13 protein 232, 790
CD14+ monocytes, HCMV latency 769
CD33+ GM-Ps, HCMV latency 773
CD34+ hematopoietic progenitors, HCMV latency 773
CD40L, Burkitt's lymphoma therapy 1301
CD46 receptor 834–835
   downmodulation of 863
CD59 complement regulatory protein, HVS 1146–1147
CD83 molecule 1129
cdc34 degradation 167–168
cdk induction 253–254, 268
   reactivation from latency and 610–611
cell cycle 541
   DNA replication and 141
   dysregulation by betaherpesviruses 253–254, 326–327
   dysregulation by EBV
      BRLF1 416
      BZLF1 412
   dysregulation by KSHV 541–548
      during latency 541–546
      during lytic replication 445
      KSHV mitogenic signaling proteins 546–548
   HCF-1 protein role 119
   see also apoptosis
cell tropism
   HCMV 231–232
      determinants of endothelial cell tropism 767–768
      determinants of myeloid lineage cell tropism 773–774
      role of apoptotic inhibitors 774
   HHV-6 834, 850–853
      in vitro 833–834
   HHV-7 834, 850–853
      in vitro 834
   VZV 679–680

cell-to-cell spread 157
    gE-gI role 157, 158
    US9 protein role 157
    VZV 158
central nervous system infections *see* nervous system disease
cerebellar ataxia, VZV and 684–685
Chang, Yuan 347–348
chemokines
    HSV response 628
    MCK-1
    MCK-2
    response evasion
    vCXCL1
chickenpox *see* varicella zoster virus (VZV)
chorionic villi, HCMV protein expression 817–818
chromatin organization, latent genome 381
chronic active EBV infection (CAEBV) 886
    epidemiology
chronic fatigue syndrome 887
cidofovir (CDV)
    adverse effects 1165–1166
    alkoxyalkyl esters of 1229–1243
    clinical indications 1166
    HCMV treatment 1192–1193
    HSV treatment 1165–1166
        clinical efficacy 1165
        dosage regimens 1166
    mechanism of action 1165
    pharmacokinetics 1165
class A genomes 13
class B genomes 13
class C genomes 13
class D genomes 13
class E genomes 13–14
class F genomes 14
classification 3–6, 8
    biological criteria 7, 27
    genomic criteria 7
    morphological criteria 3–7, 27
    serological criteria 7
    species definition 7–8
CMV423 1227
CMV *see* cytomegaloviruses
CMV latency-associated transcripts (CLTs) 773
CMV pneumonitis 788–789, 1196, 1197
CMV retinitis 643, 789, 1197
cold sores 657
colorectal metastasis management 1348–1349
Comp I 1236–1237
Comp II 1236–1237
Comp III 1236–1237
complement receptors
    type 2 (CR2) 364–365
        signal transduction 364–365
    viral, role in immune evasion 1142–1143

complement response 1142–1143
  activation 1142–1143
  evasion of 1137, 1142–1147
    deregulation 919, 1078–1079
    EBV complement regulatory activity 1145
    HCMV 1145–1146
    HSV glycoprotein gC 1143–1145
    HVS CD59 1146–1147
    HVS complement control protein homologue (CCPH) 1146
    KSHV complement control protein 1143
    MHV-68 RCA 1146
    pseudorabies virus (PRV) 1147
  regulation of 1143
  to HSV 625
  to KSHV 919
computational tools 1211–1212
concanavalin A-MDM (Con A-MDM), HCMV growth and 594
congenital infection
  congenital varicella syndrome 715
  HCMV 796, 814
  simian CMV 1057–1058
  see also neonatal infection
core functions 44–48, 56
  capsid assembly 53–54
  DNA synthesis 52–53
  entry into host cells 50–51, 93
    attachment 50, 94–95
    fusion 50–51, 100–103
    intracellular transport 51, 103–104
    site of entry 100
    viral DNA release 51
  gene expression regulation 51–52
  maturation 55–56
  structural proteins 48–50
  see also specific functions
core genes 16–17, 18–19
  betaherpesviruses 204–211, 213
corticosteroid treatment, herpes zoster 1183
CpG ODN, effect on HSV response 628
CR2 *see* complement receptors
cutaneous infections
  HSV 597, 658–659
    suppression 664
    treatment of recurrent disease 664
  VZV 675
    glycoprotein functions 679–680
    herpes zoster dermatomal distribution 722
    lesion characteristics 683–684
    pathogenesis evaluation 675–676
    primary infection clinical pattern 683–684
    regulatory proteins 680–683
    SCIDhu model 677–679
    secondary bacterial infection 684
    see also varicella zoster virus (VZV)

cutaneous lymphocyte-associated antigen (CLA) 620–621
vCXCL1 chemokine
CXCR4 receptor 835–836
vCYC protein (K cyclin) 492, 496, 529, 544–546
   role in cell transformation 545–546
cyclin-dependent kinases (CDKs), VZV effects on 676–677
cyclins 541
   infection effects 327
     cyclin A inhibition 268
     induction 253–254, 268
     VZV 676–677
   K cyclin (vCYC) 492, 496, 529, 544–546
     role in cell transformation 545–546
   KSHV v-cyclin functions 1010–1011
cyclooxygenase-2 (COX-2) 252, 1069–1070
cytokines
   HCMV infection and 767, 769–770
     reactivation from latency 770–773
   HHV-6/HHV-7 infection and 836–837, 857
     response modulation 864–865
   KSHV-associated disease and 356
   response evasion by gammaherpesviruses
     cytokine network modulation by EBV 909–910
   see also specific cytokines
cytomegalic inclusion disease (CID) of the newborn 795
cytomegaloviruses (CMV) 795
   CMV pneumonitis 788–789, 1196, 1197
   CMV retinitis 643, 789
   envelope proteins 235
   gene function 188
   genome comparisons 204
   genome structures 177–178
   non-human primate (NHP) CMVs 1051
     historical evidence of 1051–1052
     see also simian cytomegalovirus
   replication
     initiation of DNA synthesis 301
     origin 299–301
   T cell response evasion 1119
   tegument structure 38
   see also betaherpesviruses; *specific cytomegaloviruses*
cytoplasmic egress facilitator (CEF) proteins 56
cytoplasmic egress tegument protein (CETP) 56
cytotoxic T lymphocytes (CD8+) 919
   EBV response 907
     during acute infection 905–907
     in healthy virus carriers 907–908
     receptor usage 908–909
     role in infectious mononucleosis resolution 908
   HAART effects on 921
   HCMV response 782–785, 1277–1278
     T cell clonal composition 783–784
     T cell phenotypic analysis 784
   HSV responses 618–621
     CD8 epitopes 620
     populations of HSV-specific CD8+ cells 620
     T-cell co-stimulation 623–624
   immunotherapy approaches 1000, 1297–1300, 1320–1321
     adoptive immunotherapy 1321–1322, 1323–1325
     bi-virus specific CTL lines 1325
     CTL activation approaches 1325–1328
   KSHV CTL epitopes 919–921
   response evasion
     CTL escape mutants 1129
     EBV 910
     HCMV 784–785
     HSV-1 1129
     KSHV
   simian CMV response 1054, 1055
   see also T lymphocytes
cytotrophoblasts, HCMV infection and 816–817
   HLA-G expression downregulation 824
   impact on cytotrophoblast invasion 825, 827
   MMP dysregulation 825–827
     vIL-10 effects 826–827
   viral replication *in vitro* 824

databases 1213–1214
decidual infection, HCMV 820–823
deenvelopment-reenvelopment pathway *see* egress from host cell
dendritic cells (DC) 704, 917–918
   antigen presentation function, interference with 1128–1129
   HCMV infection of 788, 1128
   HHV-6 modulation of 864
   HSV interactions 616–618, 1128–1129
   in stromal keratitis 646
   KSHV response 918
   plasmacytoid (pDC) 625–627
   T-cell response initiation 705
   VZV interactions 700, 704–706
     immune evasion strategy 706, 1128
dense bodies (DB) 28–30
deoxyuridine triphosphatase (DUT) 53, 140–141
dihydroxyacridone series 1236–1238
DISC vaccines 1256
disciform keratitis (DK) 644
   see also keratitis
DNA
   encapsidation 54–55, 218, 314–315
   release into host cell 51
   synthesis
     betaherpesviruses 217, 295
     initiation mechanism 301
     proteins involved 139–141, 217
     see also replication
   see also genome

DNA helicase–primase complex   140, 296–297, 449
  inhibitors of   1232–1235
    BAY 57-1293   1234–1235
    BILS 179 BS   1232–1234
    T157602   1232
DNA polymerase   140, 297–298, 1228
  accessory protein   297–298
  HCMV drug resistance and   1204
  inhibitors of   1228–1232
    non-nucleotide inhibitors   1231–1232
    nucleoside/nucleotide analogue inhibitors   1228–1231
  KSHV   449–450
  regulatory sequences   282
DNA polymerase processivity factor   283, 449–450
DNA tumor viruses   516–517
DNA vaccines
  advantages of   1307–1308, 1309
  animal and human experience with   1310–1311
  disadvantages of   1308, 1309
  EBV   1313–1314
    animal studies   1314
    genes of interest   1313–1314
  general design   1306
  HCMV   1283–1284, 1311–1312
    animal studies   1312
    genes of interest   1311–1312
    human trials   1312
  HSV   1312–1313
    animal studies   1312–1313
    genes of interest   1312
    human trials   1313
  improving potency   1311
    adjuvants   1311
  mechanism of action   1306–1307
  plasmid DNA construct features   1309–1310
  VZV   1313
    animal studies   1313
    genes of interest   1313
    human trials   1313
drug development *see* antiviral agents
drug hypersensitivity, HHV-6/HHV-7 and   839, 851
Duncan's disease *see* X-linked lymphoproliferative syndrome (XLP)
duplicated genes   17–19
  betaherpesviruses   186–187, 1067

E-selectin   620
EA complex   469
early (E) genes   264, 282, 283–284
  EBV lytic genes   404
    products   417–418, 467, 469
    regulation   417
  functions of   267–269
    cell preparation for viral DNA replication   268–269
    direct involvement in viral replication   267–268
    modulation of host immune responses   269

HCMV   264–279
  functions   267–269
  identification of   264–265
  virus-mediated changes prior to expression   265–266
KSHV   506–508
transactivating functions of IE proteins   269–272
  assays   271
  mutational analysis   271–272
transcription initiation   128–129
transcription regulation
  HHV-6   280–283
  UL4 gene   277–279
  UL54 gene   275–277
  UL112–113 genes   273–275
see also immediate early (IE) genes
EB1 protein *see* BZLF1 protein (ZEBRA)
EB2   470
EBNA1   380–381, 476–520, 990
  CalHV3 ORF39 homologue   1101–1102
  cellular proteins that interact with   386
  comparison with LANA   393
  cytotoxic T cell response evasion   910, 1119–1120
  expression in Burkitt's lymphoma   993
  GAr domain   1119–1120
  gene function   476
  homologs in old world monkeys   1098
  OriP binding role in latency   381–382, 519–520
  plasmid segregation mechanisms   388
  properties   384–386, 519–520
    C-terminal DNA binding domain   384–385
    metaphase chromosome attachment   385
    N-terminal domain linking activity   385
    proteosome inhibition by GA repeats   386, 1119–1120
    transcription regulation   385–386
  therapeutic vaccine development   1300–1301
EBNA2   476, 519, 520–521, 988, 990
  homologs in old world monkeys   1098
  protein interactions   520–521
EBNA3 family   476–477, 521–522
  EBNA3   519, 521–522, 988, 990
  EBNA4   519, 521
  EBNA6   519, 521, 522
  expression in post transplant lymphoproliferative disease   993
  homologs in old world monkeys   1098–1099
  prophylactic vaccine development   1296–1297
EBNA5 (EBNA-LP)   477, 519, 521
EBP2, EBNA1 interaction   386
EBV-encoded RNAs (EBERs)   478, 991–992
EBV-induced EBI-3 gene
EBV-induced EBI-3 protein
Eddy, Bernice   515
egress from host cell   151–157
  alphaherpesviruses   151–159
  cell-to-cell spread   157

gE-gI role   157
US9 protein role   157
deenvelopment-reenvelopment pathway model   152, 154–157
   evidence and arguments against   156–157
   evidence and arguments for   154–156
EBV   420
nuclear egress   55–56
   betaherpesviruses   315–318
single envelopment pathway model   151–154
   evidence and arguments against   153–154
   evidence and arguments for   152–153
VZV   158–159
encephalitis
HCMV   1197
HSV   591–592, 597–598, 643, 650, 659
   treatment   1157, 1164
VZV   684–685
endocytosis, entry into host cell   50–51
endothelial cells
as site of KSHV latency   437
HCMV infection
   aortic macrovascular ECs (AEC)   766–767
   apoptotic inhibitor role   774
   as site of persistence   765–768, 774–775
   brain microvascular ECs (BMVEC)   766–767
   determinants of EC tropism   767–768
   MMP dysregulation   826, 827
   spread within host
KSHV gene expression in culture   494
enhancer core complex assembly   118–120
entry into host cells   50–51
alphaherpesviruses   93–105
attachment   50, 94–95, 364–366
betaherpesviruses   214–216, 231–232, 234–236
entry activated cell signaling   233
fusion *see* membrane fusion
gammaherpesviruses   362–370, 374
   cell surface signaling   370–373
innate immunity activation   234
   coordination of   236
intracellular transport   51, 103–104, 373
   mechanisms   103–104, 214–216
receptors
   CD4   835–836
   CD46   834–835
   gD receptor interactions   95–100
   integrins   233–234
   receptor preference and usage   99
site of entry   100
viral DNA release   51
see also specific viruses
envelope   38–39
assembly   39
protein composition   50, 93–94
   betaherpesviruses   192, 214, 234–236

   gammaherpesviruses   362–364
   HCMV   192, 214, 319
envelopment pathways *see* egress from host cell
envelopment process   55–56, 145, 311–312
betaherpesviruses   218–219, 318
   HCMV   315, 320
budding from nuclear membrane   146–147
gK role   147
model   148
UL11 protein role   147
UL31/UL34 protein complex role   145–146
US3 protein role   147
epidemiology *see specific viruses*
epidermal growth factor receptor (EGFR)   232–233
epithelial cell infection
EBV   474
KSHV, gene expression in culture   494
Epstein, Anthony   344
Epstein-Barr nuclear antigen *see* EBNA
Epstein-Barr virus (EBV)   342, 351–356, 517, 518–529, 904–905, 986
activation of lytic infection   404–409
   as EBV-positive tumor treatment strategy   421
   by TPA and butyrate   409
   BZLF1 gene autoregulation   408
   future research issues   421–422
   initial steps   406
   lytic viral gene cascade   404, 467–472
   negative regulatory elements   408
   organization of IE gene region   405–406
   Rp regulation   408–409
   stimuli   404–405, 409
   Zp promoter activating factors   406–408
   see also BRLF1 protein; BZLF1 protein
assembly   420
capsid structure   362
chronic active EBV   886
   epidemiology
co-evolution with host   1292
discovery of   342–344
disease consequences   344–345, 346, 351–356, 885–887
   chronic active EBV   886
   HIV patients   887
   immunocompromised hosts   886
   primary infection in normal host   885–886
   therapy   886
   see also tumor induction (below)
early lytic gene products   417–418, 467, 469
   host response modulators   418
   replication proteins   417, 469–470
   SM protein   418
   transcription factors   417
   viral kinase   418
egress from host cell   420

Epstein-Barr virus (EBV) (cont.)
  entry into host cell 1292–1293
    attachment 364–365, 374
    cell surface signaling 370–371
    penetration 366–369
    structural proteins involved 363
  envelope glycoproteins 351
  epidemiology
    age at primary infection
    genetic and racial factors
    geographic variation
    primary infection
    sex differences
    socioeconomic factors
    viral load
  gene content 352–353, 463
  gene expression and regulation
    during latency 380, 464–465
    early lytic genes 404
    in Burkitt's lymphoma 993–994
    in nasopharyngeal carcinoma 527, 995
    in post transplant lymphoproliferative disease 993
    late genes 419–420, 469, 471–472
    lytic cycle gene products 469–472
  genome comparisons 350
  genome structure 361–362, 461–462, 988
  glycoproteins 351, 471–472
  host response
    during acute infection 905–907
    in healthy virus carriers 907–908, 1293
    role in infectious mononucleosis resolution 908
    role of CD4+ and CD8+ T lymphocytes 907
    T cell receptor usage 908–909
  host response evasion 909–911
    antigen processing and presentation regulation 911
    apoptosis responses
    B cell responses
    complement regulatory protein 1145
    cytokine network modulation 909–910
    cytotoxic T cell responses 910, 1119–1120, 1129
    erroneous T cell activation 1129–1130
    interferon responses
    interleukin responses
    MHC class II function 1131
    monocyte function 1128–1129
    natural killer (NK) cell responses
    T helper cell responses
  IE proteins 410–416
    see also BRLF1 protein; BZLF1 protein
  immunopathology and 345
  infection by multiple strains 1293
  infection course 986–987
  intracellular transport 373
  late proteins 420, 471–472
  latency 345–347, 379–388, 461, 462–465, 904, 986–987, 988–992
    alternative forms of 465–467, 479
    chromatin organization 381
    DNA methylation 381–382
    DNA structure 988
    episomal latent genome properties 380–381, 988
    factors influencing stringency 409
    gene expression 380, 464–465, 988–992
    gene functions 475–479
    persistence in vivo 472–474
    see also EBNA1; origin of plasmid replication (OriP)
  life cycle 345–347
  membrane proteins 363–472
  monocyte infection
  neutrophil infection
  new world primates as animal model system 1098, 1102
  non-Hodgkin lymphoma
  pathogenesis of lytic infection 403–404
  phylogenetic relationships 349–350
  plasmid segregation mechanisms 388
  replication 418–419
    BZLF1 role 411
    latent phase 387–388
    lytic replication 418–419, 467–472
    replication proteins 417, 469–470
  rhesus lymphocryptovirus as animal model system 1097, 1099–1100
  strain variation 474–475
  structural proteins 472
  target cells 360
  tegument proteins 362
  transmission 885
  treatment
    adoptive immunotherapy 1323–1325
    antiviral drug development 1242
    immunotherapy 1000, 1297–1300, 1319–1320
    of lytic infection 420–421, 886
  tumor induction 342, 518–529, 530, 887–893, 904–905, 986–987
    Burkitt's lymphoma (BL) 525–526, 887–888, 889–890, 993–994
    clinical importance 893
    clonality and 988
    determination of EBV association 888
    EBV-targeted therapy 1000–1001
    exploitation of B-cell regulatory mechanisms 518–519
    gastric cancers 892, 997
    genetic factors 997–1000
    HIV/AIDS lymphomas 891, 994
    Hodgkins' lymphoma (HL) 526–527, 892, 996–997
    immune surveillance and 528–529, 890
    immunoblastic lymphomas 525
    immunocompromised hosts
    leiomyosarcomas 892
    lymphoepithelioma-like carcinomas
    lymphomatoid granulomatosis 892

molecular interactions 517
nasopharyngeal carcinoma 527, 888, 891–892, 994–996
NK/T cell tumors 891, 997
post transplant lymphoproliferative disorders (PTLD) 890–891, 993
strain variation and 998–1000
T cell control of 911–912
viral growth transformation proteins 519–522
viral latent membrane proteins (LMPs) 522–525
vaccine development 345, 1000, 1292–1294, 1301–1302
Burkitt's lymphoma 1300–1301
DNA vaccines 1313–1314
future prospects 912
Hodgkins disease prevention 1297–1300
infectious mononucleosis prevention 1294–1297
nasopharygeal carcinoma prevention 1297–1300
post-transplant lymphoproliferative disease prevention 1297
see also gammaherpesviruses
ER chaperones, interference with 1122
erythema multiforme 659
ethnic factors see racial factors
evolution
co-evolution with host 7, 16
genome comparisons 15–20
alphaherpesviruses 16, 19–20, 61–64
betaherpesviruses 178–188, 204–213
gammaherpesviruses 350–351
mammalian herpesvirus group 16–19
three major groups 15–16
herpesvirus-common core functions 44–48
lymphocryptoviruses 1095
rhadinoviruses 1102
exanthem subitum (ES) 838
extracellular-signal-regulated kinase (ERK) 372
MAPK/ERK pathway 252, 278–279
eye disease see acute retinal necrosis (ARN); keratitis; ocular disease; uveitis

FAK 371
famciclovir 664
clinical indications 1163
HSV treatment 1162–1163
dosage regimens 1163
genital herpes 1156, 1162
herpes labialis 1162
resistance 1163
mechanism of action 1162
pharmacokinetics 1162
side effects 1162–1163
VZV treatment 1178–1179
herpes zoster 1182
fatty acid synthase (FAS) gene activation 416
FcγR 1137–1138, 1142
Fc receptors on mammalian cells 1138–1139

FcγRI 1138–1139
FcγRII 1139
FcγRIII 1139
HCMV FcγR 1141
HSV FcγR 1139–1141
gE and gI structure 1139–1140
immune evasion mechanisms 1140–1141
MCMV FcγR 1141–1142
pseudorabies virus FcγR 1142
VZV FcγR 1141
fetal infection, simian CMV 1057–1058
see also congenital infection
fever
glandular see infectious mononucleosis
HCMV infection and 1197
malignant catarrhal (MCF)
fever blisters 657
vFLIP protein 492, 496, 497–498
functions 1011–1012
apoptosis inhibition 551, 1011–1012, 1080
fomivirsen, HCMV treatment 1193
foscarnet
adverse effects 1167, 1179
clinical indications 1167
HCMV treatment 1193
HSV treatment 1166–1167
clinical efficacy 1166–1167
dosage regimens 1167
resistance 1167
Kaposi's sarcoma treatment 435
lytic EBV infection treatment 420–421
mechanism of action 1166
pharmacokinetics 1166
VZV treatment 1179
functional assays 1215
fusion see membrane fusion

G207 treatment 1346–1347
G-protein-coupled receptors (GPCRs) 253
vGPCR protein 546, 1020, 1106
GABP transcription factors 120–121
γ1 34.5 gene 71
γ1 34.5 protein 65, 71
gammaherpesviruses 341–342, 351, 1085
capsid structure 351
diseases associated 897
entry into host cells
attachment 364–366
cell surface signaling 370–373
penetration 366–370
structural proteins involved 362–364
envelope glycoproteins 351, 362–364, 367–369
genome comparisons 350–351
genome structure 341
latency 342, 379–380

gammaherpesviruses (*cont.*)
    establishment of 379–380
    gene expression 380
    sites of 437–438
  non-human primates 1076, 1108–1109
    nomenclature 1093–1095, 1096
    see also herpesvirus saimiri (HVS); lymphocryptoviruses; rhadinoviruses
  phylogenetic relationships 349–350
  replication 341–342
  tumor induction 342
  see also Epstein-Barr virus (EBV); Kaposi's sarcoma-associated herpesvirus (KSHV); lymphocryptoviruses; rhadinoviruses
ganciclovir 664
  adverse effects 1168
  B virus therapy 1041
  clinical indications 1168
  dosage regimens 1168–1169
  EBV-positive tumor management 421
  HCMV treatment 1192
    resistance 1204–1206
  HSV treatment 1167–1169
    resistance 1169
  Kaposi's sarcoma treatment 435
  lytic EBV infection treatment 420, 421
  mechanisms of action 1167–1168
  pharmacokinetics 1168
ganglionitis 643, 650–651
gastric cancers 892, 997
  epidemiology
  evidence of association with EBV
gene capture, betaherpesviruses 187–188
gene content 14–15
  alphaherpesviruses 19–20, 163, 164
  betaherpesviruses 178–186, 204–213, 241
    core genes 204–211, 213
    gene families 187, 212–213
    IE genes 242–243
    MIE genes 248–249
  captured genes 17
  core genes 16–17, 18–19, 204–211, 213
  duplicated genes 17–19, 186–187, 1067
  gammaherpesviruses
    EBV 352–353
    KSHV 354–355
gene expression 14–15
  during latency 380
    EBV 380, 464–465, 988–992
    KSHV 380, 492, 497–498
    VZV 691–692
    see also latency-associated transcripts (LATs)
  EBV lytic genes 404
    early gene regulation 417
    late gene regulation 419–420
  KSHV 490, 494

    in culture 490–494
    in Kaposi's sarcoma 495–496, 894, 1017–1020
    latent genes 497–498
    lytic genes, kinetic classification 438–439
    multicentric Castleman's disease 496–497
    primary effusion lymphomas 496
    regulation 497–508
  regulation 51–52, 133–134
    betaherpesviruses 216–217, 241, 252–253
    early EBV lytic genes 417
    HHV-6 latency-associated transcripts 844
    host gene expression 324
    KSHV 497–508
    see also early (E) genes; immediate early (IE) genes; late (L) genes
  splicing 15
  transcription initiation 128–131
    MIE transcriptional enhancers 243–246
    role of viral IE proteins 129
    TATA box-containing promoters 128–131
    viral transcription factors 128–129
  see also transcription
gene functions
  alphaherpesviruses 70–82, 164
  betaherpesviruses 188, 204–212
  EBV latent genes 475–479
  modulation of host immune responses 269
  replication 70, 204–212, 267–268, 296
gene products 70–82
  betaherpesviruses 205–211
  functions, drug development and 1211
  herpesvirus-common gene products 44–45, 48
  see also gene expression; proteins
gene therapy *see* viral vectors
genital HCMV infection 800–801
genital HSV infection 596–597, 657–658, 1253
  antibody responses 624
  primary infection 596–597
  reactivation 597, 658
  treatment 665, 1155, 1156
    acyclovir 1154–1157
    famciclovir 1162
    valaciclovir 1163–1164
genome 10, 163–164
  classes of 13–14
    class A 13
    class B 13
    class C 13
    class D 13
    class E 13–14
    class F 14
  comparisons and evolution 15–20
    alphaherpesviruses 19–20, 61–64, 1033–1034, 1045
    betaherpesviruses 178–188, 204–213
    gammaherpesviruses 350–351

lymphocryptoviruses 1095
mammalian herpesvirus group 16–19
gene content 14–15, 163, 164, 178–186
packaging 34–35, 54–55, 1235
inhibitors of 1235
release into host nucleus 51
sequences 11–12, 14
alphaherpesviruses 61
betaherpesviruses 178
structure *see* genome structure
see also specific viruses
genome structure 10–14, 34–35
alphaherpesviruses 138
betaherpesviruses 177–178, 189–191, 1061
gammaherpesviruses 341
rhadinoviruses 1077
repeats 10–13, 164
segment inversion 13
see also specific viruses
genomic criteria 7
genomics
bioinformatics and computational tools 1211–1212
databases 1213–1214
impact on herpesvirus research 1212–1213
see also antiviral agents
genotypic diversity, KSHV 964–966
geographic distribution of subtypes 965
gingivostomatitis treatment 1157
glandular fever *see* infectious mononucleosis
glanulocyte-macrophage progenitors (GM-Ps), HCMV latency 773
glycogen synthase kinase 3ß (GSK-3ß) 544, 991
LANA interaction 1010
glycoprotein B (gB)
alphaherpesviruses 76
role in egress from host cell 158
role in membrane fusion 100, 101–102, 104–105
VZV 104–105
betaherpesviruses 214, 235, 236
HCMV 1277
gammaherpesviruses
EBV 367, 471–472
KSHV 369
glycoprotein C (gC) 78
attachment to host cell 94–95
role in complement response evasion
HSV 1143–1145
pseudorabies virus 1147
VZV 679
glycoprotein D (gD) 67, 81, 95–96
crystal structure 95
implications for envelopment pathway 155–156
interferon response and 626
receptors 96–99
animal orthologues 99

receptor preference and usage 99
role in membrane fusion 100
role in blocking apoptosis 169
glycoprotein E (gE) 81
HSV 1139–1140
role in cell-to-cell spread 157, 158
VZV 679–680
role in egress from host cell 158–159
role in membrane fusion 104–105
glycoprotein G (gG) 66–67, 81
glycoprotein gp42 367–369, 471
glycoprotein gp60 472
glycoprotein gp110 471–472
glycoprotein gp150 472
glycoprotein gp350/220 364–365, 370–371, 471
prophylactic EBV vaccine development 1295–1296
glycoprotein gpK8.1 365–366, 369, 500
anti-K8.1 antibodies 921–922
glycoprotein H (gH) 75
HCMV 1277
role in entry into host cell 235–236
alphaherpesviruses 100–101, 104–105
EBV 367–368, 471
KSHV 369
VZV 104–105
structural features
glycoprotein I (gI) 81
HSV 1139–1140
role in cell-to-cell spread 157
VZV 158, 680
glycoprotein J (gJ) 67, 81
role in blocking apoptosis 169
glycoprotein K (gK) 79
negative control of membrane fusion 103
role in envelopment 147
glycoprotein K8.1 500
glycoprotein L (gL) 71
role in membrane fusion
alphaherpesviruses 100, 101
EBV 367–368, 471
KSHV 369
glycoprotein M (gM) 73, 471, 1277
glycoprotein N (gN) 79, 471, 1277
glycoprotein Q (gQ) 836
glycoproteins 38, 93–94
B virus 1034
betaherpesvirus envelope glycoproteins 192, 214, 234–236
HCMV 192, 214, 319
HHV-6 836
HHV-7 836
trafficking 319–320
complexes 192
gCI 192
gCII 192
gCIII 192

glycoproteins (cont.)
   gammaherpesviruses
      EBV 351, 471–472
      envelope glycoproteins 351, 362–364, 367–369
      KSHV 450
   implications for envelopment pathway 152–153, 155
   role in entry into host cell 50–51, 93
      betaherpesviruses 214, 234–236, 836
      gammaherpesviruses 367–369
   VZV, role in T-cell and skin tropism 679–680
   see also specific glycoproteins
vGPCR protein 546, 1020, 1106
Gross, Ludwik 515
GSJ-3ß see glycogen synthase kinase 3ß (GSK-3ß)
Guillain-Barre' syndrome (GBS), CMV and 789
GW275175X 1237–1238

H2G 1228–1229
HAART (highly-active anti-retroviral therapy)
   effects on cytotoxic T lymphocytes 921
   effects on humoral responses 923
   HCMV infection and 1201–1202
   Kaposi's sarcoma and 435–436, 916
HAUSP/USP7, EBNA1 interaction 386
HCF see host cell factor
hearing loss, HCMV and 1197
helicase-primase complex see DNA helicase–primase complex
hemophagocytic lymphohistiocytosis (HL) 434
Henle, Gertrude & Werner 344–345
heparin binding domain (HBD) 365
heparin sulfate 50
   HHV-7 interactions 836
   KSHV interaction 365, 366
   modified 98–99
heparin sulfate proteoglycans (HSPGs) 232, 235
hepatitis
   HCMV and 1197
   VZV and 684
herpes B virus see B virus
herpes labialis 596
   primary infection 596
   reactivation 596
   treatment
      acyclovir 1157
      famciclovir 1162
      valaciclovir 1164
herpes simplex encephalitis (HSE) 591–592, 597–598, 643, 650, 659
   treatment
      acyclovir 1157
      valaciclovir 1164
herpes simplex virus type 1 (HSV-1)
   acute retinal necrosis (ARN) 649–650
   capsid structure 32, 33–34
   cutaneous infections 597
   encephalitis 597–598, 650, 659
   epidemiology 656
   genome comparisons 61–64
   genome structure and packaging 34–35
   host response evasion
      dendritic cell infection 1128–1129
      FcγR role 1139–1141
      glycoprotein gC role in complement evasion 1143–1145
      stunning of cytotoxic T cell activity 1129
   infection sites 596
   latency-associated transcripts (LATs) 604
   orolabial infection 596, 657
      primary infection 596
      reactivation 596
      treatment 665, 1157, 1162, 1164
   RNA processing 131–132
   tegument
      composition 35
      structure 36–38
   transcription initiation 128–131
      role of IE proteins 129–131
      viral transcription factors 128–129
   transmission 589
   treatment see herpes simplex viruses
   see also alphaherpesviruses; herpes simplex viruses (HSV)
herpes simplex virus type 2 (HSV-2)
   acute retinal necrosis 649–650
   CNS infection 659
   epidemiology 656–657
      HIV interactions 656–657, 661–662
   genital infection 658
   genome comparisons 61–64
   herpetic whitlow 597, 659, 665
   host response evasion 1143–1145
   infection sites 596
   transmission 589
      dynamics 663
      viral shedding 662
   see also alphaherpesviruses; herpes simplex viruses (HSV)
herpes simplex viruses (HSV)
   as therapeutic vectors 1341
      nervous system modification 1342–1344
      non-replicating vectors 1341, 1342, 1344–1345
      optimization for therapeutic use 1344–1345
      replication-competent vectors 1341
      see also oncolytic HSV
   cell-to-cell spread 157
      gE-gI role 157
      US9 protein role 157
   compromised host infections 598–599
   cutaneous infections 597, 658–659
      recurrent disease treatment 664
      suppression 664
   disease spectrum 657
   disseminated HSV 660
   egress from host cell 152–157

deenvelopment-reenvelopment pathway model 154–157
single envelopment pathway model 152–154
entry into host cell 93
   attachment 94–95
   gD receptor interactions 95–100
   site of entry 100
genital infection *see* genital HSV infection
genome comparisons 61–64
   L component genes unique to HSV 65–66
   S component genes unique to HSV 66–67
host response 592–596, 630, 1332–1333
   antibody responses 624, 1332–1334
   CD4 T helper cell responses 621–623
   CD8+ cytotoxic T-cell responses 618–621
   chemokines 628
   dendritic cell interactions 616–618
   disease consequences and 596
   immunomodulators and 628
   innate immunity 624–628
   natural killer (NK) cells 628–629
   newborns 594–596, 624, 1332–1334
   NKT cells 629
   stress effects 630
   T-cell co-stimulation 623–624
   TCRγ cells 629–630
host response evasion 165
   dendritic cell function 1128–1129
   TAP peptide transport inhibition 1121
   see also anti-host strategies
IE (immediate early) gene regulation 112
   ancillary factors 120
   blocking in latency establishment 606–607
   enhancer core complex assembly 112–120
   multiple regulatory domains 112
immunocompromised hosts 661–662
   treatment 665
immunopathology and 642–643, 651
infection, definitions of 589
latency 590–591, 602
   establishment 606–608
   latency-associated transcripts (LATs) 604–606
   latent genome characteristics 602–603
   maintenance of 608–609
   model systems 602–603
   reactivation from 122–123, 609–612
   T-cell responses 618–619
membrane proteins 93–94
neonatal infection 598, 660–661, 1253
   outcomes 1158
   transmission during delivery 660–661, 1253
   treatment 665, 1157–1160
nervous system disease 597–598, 650–651, 659
   encephalitis 591–592, 597–598, 643, 650, 659
   ganglionitis 643, 650–651
   treatment 665, 1157, 1164

ocular disease 659–660
   acute retinal necrosis 649, 660
   keratoconjunctivitis 597
   stromal keratitis (SK) 644–645
   treatment 665, 1161
   uveitis 649
oncolytic *see* oncolytic HSV
pathogenesis 589
   host response impact 592–596
   unique biological properties influencing 589–591
pathology 591
   CNS disease 591–592
receptors 97
replication of *see* replication
transmission 589
   during childbirth 660–661
   dynamics 663
   sexual, reduction strategy 664
   viral shedding 662
treatment 663–664, 665
   acyclovir 663, 664, 1153–1162
   antibody immunotherapy 1332, 1334–1335
   cidofovir 1165–1166
   famciclovir/penciclovir 1162–1163
   foscarnet 1166–1167
   ganciclovir 1167–1169
   portal protein inhibitors 1235–1237
   severe infection 664–666
   valaciclovir 663–664, 1163–1165
   valganciclovir 1169
vaccination 1253–1254, 1257, 1258–1259
   DNA vaccines 1312–1313
   history of vaccine development 1254
   live attenuated vaccines 1254–1256
   subunit vaccines 1256–1258
see also alphaherpesviruses; herpes simplex virus type 1 (HSV-1); herpes simplex virus type 2 (HSV-2)
herpes zoster
   complications 726–727
   epidemiology 721–729
      age of varicella infection and 723, 725
      age specificity 722–724
      deaths 727–728
      exposure to varicella and 725
      hospitalizations 727
      immunocompetence and 725–726
      methodological issues 721–722
      racial differences 724–725
      seasonality and clustering 722
      secular trends 722
      sex differences 724
      stress and 725
   prophylaxis 1187
      elderly patients 1269
   transmissibility 714

herpes zoster (cont.)
    treatment 1181–1186
        herpes zoster ophthalmicus 1184–1185
        immunocompetent adults 1181–1184
        immunocompromised patients 1185
        postherpetic neuralgia 1183–1184
        with HIV 1185–1186
        see also antiviral agents
    vaccination impact 728–729, 1268–1269
        elderly patients 1269
        inactivated varicella vaccine 1269
        prevention 729
        vaccinated children 729
        zoster following vaccination 1264, 1268–1269
    see also varicella zoster virus (VZV)
Herpesviridae composition 15
herpesvirus ateles (HVA) 1084–1086
    genome structure 1085
    natural occurrence 1084
    oncogenesis 1085–1086
    pathology 1084–1085
herpesvirus saimiri (HVS) 528, 1076–1084
    gene therapy vectors 1084
    genome structure 1077
    host response evasion 1129–1130
        CD59 1146–1147
        complement control protein homologue (CCPH) 1146
        immunomodulatory proteins 1078–1080
    oncogenesis 1080–1082
        growth transformation of human T cells 1083–1084
    pathology 1076–1077
    replication 1077–1078
herpesvirus-common gene products 44–45, 48
    see also core functions
herpetic stromal keratitis (HSK) see stromal keratitis
herpetic whitlow 597, 659
    treatment 665
heteroduplex tracking assays (HTA) 998–1000
HHV-6 see human herpesvirus 6
HHV-7 see human herpesvirus 7
histiocytosis 864
histone acetyltransferases (HAT) 550
histone deacetylase (HDAC) inhibition 409, 444
HIV see human immunodeficiency virus
Hodgkin Reed-Sternberg (HRS) cells 526–527
Hodgkins lymphoma (HL) 526–527, 892, 905, 996–997
    adoptive immunotherapy 1324
    epidemiology
    evidence for association with EBV
    infectious mononucleosis as risk factor 892
    prophylactic vaccine development 1297–1300
    T cell control of 911–912
homosexual men, KSHV transmission 966–968
hospitalizations, VZV 719
    herpes zoster 727

host cell factor (HCF) 607, 610, 696
    HCF-1 118
        functions 118–120
        role in cell cycle 119
        role in HSV IE enhancer core complex assembly 118–120
        role in latency-reactivation 122–123
host proteins, viral constituents 39–40
    envelope 38–39
host range 7
host relationships 7
    co-evolution 7, 16
    see also anti-host strategies; entry into host cells
host response
    impact on HSV disease 592–596
    modulation of 324–332
        EBV 413–414, 418
        HHV-6/HHV-7 861–866
        impact on host cell cycle 326–327
        rhadinoviruses 1078–1080
        VZV 700–702
        see also MHC functions, modulation of
    see also apoptosis; immune response; specific viruses
HSV863 1335
HSV1716 1347–1348
    melanoma management 1348
human cytomegalovirus (HCMV) 311
    animal models of infection 241
    capsid assembly 312
        protein interactions and 312–314
    capsid structure 32–34, 191, 312
        protein composition 213
    cell cycle dysregulation 253–254, 326–327
    cellular tropism 231–232
        determinants of endothelial cell tropism 767–768
        determinants of myeloid lineage cell tropism 773–774
        role of apoptotic inhibitors 774
    congenital infection 796, 814
    diagnosis 1197–1198
        cell culture 1198
        CNS involvement 1198
        DEAFF/shell vial 1198
        histopathology 1198
        serology 1198
        viremia detection 1197–1198
    disease spectrum 795, 1196–1197, 1274
        chronic infection and
        encephalitis 1197
        fever/leukopenia 1197
        gastrointestinal disease 1197
        hearing loss 1197
        hepatitis 1197
        immunocompromised patients 1194
        pneumonitis 788–789, 1196, 1197
        polyradiculopathy 1197
        retinitis 643, 789, 1197

DNA encapsidation 218, 314–315
DNA synthesis 217
   DNA polymerase and accessory protein 297–298
   helicase-primase complex 296–297
   single-stranded DNA binding protein 298
drug resistance 1203–1206
   cross-resistance patterns 1204–1205
   management algorithm 1205
   methods to define resistance 1203
   recognition of in clinical practice 1205–1206
   UL54 gene 1204
   UL97 gene 1203–1204
entry into host cells 214–216, 231–232
   cellular receptors 232–234
   entry activated cell signaling 233
   envelope glycoprotein roles 234–236
   innate immunity activation 234, 236
envelope glycoproteins 192, 214, 319
   roles in entry into host cell 234–236
   trafficking 319–320
envelopment 315, 320
epidemiology 795–796
   exposure
   see also transmission (below)
gene content 178–186, 241, 311, 1059
   analysis 14
   core genes 204–211, 213
   gene families 187, 205–211, 212–213, 1067
   genes involved in spread within host
   IE genes 242–243, 248–249
   see also early genes
gene expression regulation 216–217, 241
   early genes 265–266, 269–279
   factors stimulating IE gene expression 252–253
   host gene expression 324
   late genes 303–305
   MIE transcriptional enhancers 243–246
   reactivation of IE genes 247–248
   silencing of IE genes 246–247
genetic variation 188
genome comparisons 178–188, 204–213
   gene capture 187–188
   gene duplication 186–187
   gene function 188
genome structure and packaging 34–35, 189–191
histopathology
host cell range 264
host response 780, 781–788, 1276–1278
   animal models 781
   antibody response 781–782, 1276–1277
   CD4+ T cell response 785–786
   CD8+ cytotoxic T cell response 782–785, 1277–1278
   evasion 784–785, 787–788
   immunocompromised hosts 788–790
   immunosuppression by virus 788
   innate immunity 786–788
   protection by natural immunity 1275–1276
host response modulation 324–332
   apoptosis suppression 327–332
   complement response 1145–1146
   FcγR role 1141
   host cell cycle 326–327
   host gene expression 324
   interferon regulated factor 3 (IRF-3) modulation 325
   MHC class I functions 1122–1125, 1128, 1129
   MHC class II functions 1130–1131
   NF-(K)B activation 325
   peptide transport interference 1121
   proteasomal proteolysis 1119, 1120–1121
   tapasin interference 1122
   vICA 330
   vMIA 328–330
host specificity 1285
immunopathology 788–789
   CMV pneumonitis 788–789, 1196
   CMV retinitis 789
   immune recovery vitritis 789
   inflammatory demyelinating neuropathy 789
   transplant rejection and 789–790
infection establishment
   following community exposure
   transfusion and allograft acquired infection
latency 219
   in myeloid lineage cells 768–775
   sites of 765, 774–775, 780–781
latency-associated transcripts 844
management strategies 1198
   resistant CMV 1205
   with HIV 1201–1202
maturation 218–219
multiple infections
nuclear egress 317–318
pathogenesis
   acute infection
   chronic infections
   direct viral effects 1196
   immunocompromised hosts
   indirect viral effects 1196
   viral load and 1194–1195
perinatal infection 796
persistence 765
   in endothelial cells 765–768, 774–775
   sites of 765, 774–775
placental infection 814, 817–823, 827
   antibodies to CMV in syncytiotrophoblasts 819–820
   CMV protein expression 817–818, 820
   cytotrophoblast HLA-G expression downregulation 824
   cytotrophoblast invasion and 825, 827
   decidual infection relationship 820–823
   integrin expression downregulation 824–825

human cytomegalovirus (HCMV) (cont.)
   MMP dysregulation 825–827
   potential transmission routes 817
   presence at placental-decidual interface 818–819
   replication in cytotrophoblasts *in vitro* 824
   vIL-10 effects 826–827
  prophylaxis 1199, 1202
   delayed 1199
  proteins encoded 179–183
   MIE protein functions 249–252
   structural proteins 213–214
  reactivation from latent state
   Allo-MDM system 770–773
   following transplants 772–773
   sites of 780–781
  reinfection
  replication 217, 296
   disease and
   genes involved in spread within host
   origin 299–301
   regulation 241
   see also persistence
  sources of
  spread within host
   cell-associated spread
   following community exposure
   role of viral genes
   transfusion and allograft acquired infection
  tegument
   assembly 315–318
   composition 35–36, 213–214
   protein distribution 315, 316
   structure 38, 191–192
  transmission 796
   artificial insemination and 807
   breast milk 796–797
   by transfusion 805–806
   child-to-child transmission 797–799
   child-to-parent transmission 799–800
   perinatal acquisition 796–797
   sexual transmission 796, 800–802
   sources in hospitalized patients 797
   sources in the community 797
   to child care providers 802–803, 804
   to healthcare workers 803–805, 806
   transplacental transmission 817
   transplantation and 806–807
   young children as source 797–800
  treatment 1192–1193, 1199, 1202–1203
   fomivirsen 1193
   foscarnet 1193
   immunotherapy 1319, 1321–1322
   nucleosides 1192
   nucleotides 1192–1193
   pre-emptive therapy 1199, 1202
   randomized, controlled trial results 1199–1201
   suppression 1199
   terminase complex inhibitors 1236–1238
   UL97 encoded protein kinase inhibitors 1239
   see also antiviral agents; drug resistance (above)
  treatment challenges 1193–1194
   direct viral effects 1196
   indirect viral effects 1196
   viremia and viral load 1194–1195
   see also drug resistance (above)
  vaccination 1274, 1278–1285
   case for 1274–1275
   DNA vaccines 1283–1284, 1311–1312
   efficacy testing 1285
   host specificity and 1285
   peptide vaccines 1283
   protection by natural immunity 1275–1276
   replicating vaccines 1278–1281
   subunit vaccines 1281–1282
   subviral particles 1284–1285
   vectored vaccines 1282–1283
   when to vaccinate 1285
  see also betaherpesviruses; cytomegaloviruses
human herpesvirus 6 (HHV-6) 279, 280, 833
  antigens 853–855
   complement-independent neutralization targets 854–855
   diagnostic targets 855
   latent antigens 853
   lytic antigens 853–854
   monoclonal antibody studies 854
  cell tropism 850–853
   in vitro 833–834, 851
   in vivo 834, 851
  disease consequences 838–839, 850
   drug hypersensitivity 839
   multiple sclerosis association 839, 860–861
   primary infection 838
   reactivation 838–839
  early promoters, cis-acting sequences 282–283
   DNA polymerase processivity factor (U27) 283
   DNA polymerase (U38) 282
  entry into host cell 834–835
   envelope glycoproteins involved 836
  epidemiology 875–876
  future research 866
  gene content 178–186
   gene families 187
  genome 833
   comparisons 178–187
   gene duplication 186–187
  genotypes 876–877
  growth properties 836
  HHV-6A 833, 843, 850–853, 876
  HHV-6B 833, 843, 850–853, 876

HIV interactions 837, 866
immune response 857–860
   antibody response 857–859
   immunocompromised hosts 859–860
   innate response 857, 858
   primary infection 838, 857–859
   role of reactivation 859
   T lymphocyte response 859, 860
immune response modulation 861–866
   cell surface markers 861, 862
   clinical significance 865–866
   cytokine production 864–865
   dendritic cells 864
   histiocytes 864
   natural killer cells 861
   stem cells 861–862
   T cell receptor signaling inhibition 1129
   T lymphocytes 861, 862–863, 864
   virally encoded immune modulators 865
immunologic cross-reactivity 856–857
infection effect on host cells 836–838
integration 877–878
late gene expression 305
latency-associated transcripts (LATs) 843–844, 853
   gene regulation of 844
latency/persistence 219, 843, 875
   latent antigens 853
proteins encoded 179–183
reactivation from latency 838–839
   AIDS and 839
   first molecular event 844–847
   following bone marrow transplantation 839
   following organ transplantation 839
   immune response 859
regulatory gene products 280–283
   IE-A 281
   IE-B 281–282
   U94 282
replication origins 301–302
transcriptional enhancers 243–245
transmission 878
treatment
see also betaherpesviruses; roseoloviruses
human herpesvirus 7 (HHV-7) 280, 795, 850
antigens 856
   complement-independent neutralization targets 856
   diagnostic targets 856
   monoclonal antibody studies 855, 856
cell tropism 850–853
   in vitro 834, 851
   in vivo 834, 851–853
disease consequences 838–839, 850
   primary infection 838
entry into host cell 835–836
   glycoproteins involved 836
epidemiology 875–876
genotypes 876–877
growth properties 836
host cell modulation 327
immune response 857
   antibody response 857–859
   immunocompromised hosts 859–860
   innate response 857
   primary infection 857–859
   virally encoded immune modulators 865
immune response modulation 863
   cell surface markers 861, 862
   clinical significance 866
   cytokine production 864–865
   MHC class I antigen presentation 1126
   stem cells 861, 862–863
   T lymphocytes 861, 862–863, 864
immunologic cross-reactivity 856–857
infection effects on host cells 836–837
late gene expression 305
latency/persistence 843, 875
replication origins 301–302
transmission 878
treatment
see also betaherpesviruses; roseoloviruses
human herpesvirus 8 (HHV-8) *see* Kaposi's sarcoma-associated herpesvirus (KSHV)
human immunodeficiency virus (HIV)
EBV infection and 887
   immunotherapy 1325
   lymphomas induced 891
HCMV infection and
   CMV retinitis 789
   immunotherapy 1325
   management strategies 1201–1202
herpes zoster epidemiology and 726
HHV-6 interactions 837, 866
HSV interactions 661–662
   HSV-2 656–657, 661–662
KSHV and 347, 349
   anti-retroviral treatment effects 435–436, 916
   Kaposi's sarcoma relationships 976, 1017
membrane fusion 366
VZV prophylaxis 1186–1187
VZV treatment 1181
   herpes zoster 1185–1186
see also AIDS; HAART (highly-active anti-retroviral therapy); immunocompromised hosts
human leukocyte antigen (HLA)
HCMV downregulation of in cytotrophoblasts 824
HSV infection and 594
HVEM (herpes virus entry mediator) 95, 98
animal orthologues 99
as HSV receptor 98, 99
gD interaction 98

vIAP (inhibitor of apoptosis) protein 552
vICA 330
ICER (inducible cAMP early repressors) 611
ICP0 protein 71, 129–130
   role in cell cycle arrest 141
   role in cellular protein degradation 167–168
   role in reactivation from latency 609
     ICP0 promoter 610
   role in viral replication 164
ICP4 (infected cell polypeptide 4) 80, 128–129
ICP5 protein 75
ICP8 protein 76
   role in DNA synthesis 139–140
ICP22 protein 80, 130–131
   role in viral replication 164–165
ICP27 protein 79, 131–132
   role in cell cycle 141–142
   role in cellular protein synthesis shutoff 166
ICP47 protein 82, 1121
IE genes *see* immediate early (IE) genes
IE proteins 133–134
   EBV 410–416
     see also BRLF1 protein; BZLF1 protein
   IE1 216, 248–250, 844–847
   IE2 216, 248–249, 250–252, 299
     role in DNA replication 299
     role in late gene expression 304–305
     UL84 interaction 217, 298
   IE4 132–133
   IE14/vSag 1080
   IE38 249–250
   IE61 130
   IE62 129, 681
   IE63 131, 681
   IE72 249, 250, 266, 270–271
     mutational analysis 272
   IE86 250–252, 266, 270–271
     mutational analysis 271–272
   role in induced gene expression 129, 269–273
     expression assays 271
     mutational analysis 271–272
IE-A locus 242
   HHV-6 281
IE-B locus 242–243
   HHV-6 281–282
IEX-1 protein shutoff in infected cells 166
IgG Fc receptors 1137–1138
   on mammalian cells 1138–1139
   role in immune evasion 1137–1139
   see also FcγR
immediate early (IE) genes 128
   antiviral targets 1226–1227
   betaherpesviruses 242–243, 1067–1068
     factors simulating expression 252–253
     IE1 248–249, 281, 844–847, 1067–1068

     IE2 248–249, 281, 844–847, 1067–1068
     IE-A locus 242, 281
     IE-B locus 242–243, 281–282
     reactivation of 247–248
     silencing of 246–247
     transcriptional enhancers 243–245
   EBV lytic genes 467
     organization of IE gene region 405–406
     stimuli 404–405
     see also BRLF1 gene; BZLF1 gene
   HSV
     ancillary factors 120
     blocking in latency establishment 606–607, 608
     enhancer core complex assembly 112–120
     reactivation from latent state 122–123
   IE57 gene 1078, 1083
   IE62 gene 122
   KHSV IE gene expression 498–500
     activation 506–508
     kinetic classification 438–439
   regulation 112, 243–245
     future studies 123–124
     HSV 122–123, 606–607
     KSHV 506–508
     multiple levels 122
     multiple regulatory domains 112
     VZV 121–122
   see also IE proteins; major immediate early (MIE) genes
immune recovery vitritis 789
immune response 642, 1117–1119
   adaptive responses 1117
     stromal keratitis 647–649
     see also antibody responses
   innate responses 1117
     activation during viral entry 234
     coordination of activation during entry 236
     stromal keratitis 645–647
   modulation/evasion of 1117–1119
     betaherpesviruses 324–332
     early gene functions 269
     rhadinoviruses 1078–1080
     see also complement response; FcγR; MHC functions, modulation of
   role in reactivation from latency 436–437
   tumorigenesis protection
   see also host response; *specific viruses*
immunoblastic lymphomas 525
immunocompromised hosts 1318
   EBV infection 886
     lymphoproliferative disease and
     primary immune disorders
   HCMV infection 788–790
   HHV-6/HHV-7 responses 859–860
   HSV infection 661–662
     treatment 665, 1160–1161

infectious complications of immunosuppression 1318
    therapy 1318–1319
  Kaposi's sarcoma 435–436, 915, 924
  KSHV primary infection consequences 915–917
  simian CMV infection 1055–1058
    fetal infection 1057–1058
    measles virus-associated immunosuppression 1057
    retroviral-induced immunodeficiency 1055–1056
    transplantation 1057
  VZV infection 685–686
    herpes zoster epidemiology and 725–726
    prophylaxis 1186–1187
    treatment 1181, 1185–1186
immunodeficiency see immunocompromised hosts
immunoglobulins
  IgG Fc receptors 1137–1138
    on mammalian cells 1138–1139
    role in immune evasion 1137–1139
    see also FcγR
  see also antibody responses
immunological synapse, interference with 1128
immunopathology 642–643
  HCMV 788–789
    CMV pneumonitis 788–789, 1196
    CMV retinitis 789
    immune recovery vitritis 789
    inflammatory demyelinating neuropathy 789
    transplant rejection and 789–790
  HSV 642–643, 651
    acute retinal necrosis (ARN) 649
    keratitis 643–649
    nervous system disease 650–651
    uveitis 649
immunosuppression
  by HCMV 788
  HSV reactivation and 661–662
    treatment 665
  infectious complications of 1318
  simian retroviral-induced, non-human primates 1055–1056
immunosuppression 1055–1056
  see also immunocompromised hosts
immunotherapy
  adoptive immunotherapy 1321–1322
    EBV post-solid organ transplant 1323–1324
    EBV post-transplant lymphoproliferation disease 1323
    HCMV 1321–1322
    Hodgkin lymphoma 1324
    nasopharyngeal carcinoma 1324–1325
    T cell production 1321
  antibody immunotherapy 1332
    animal models 1334–1335
    limitations of 1335
  bi-virus specific CTL lines 1325

  EBV 1000, 1297–1300, 1319–1320, 1325
  future considerations 1328
  HCMV 1319, 1325
  in HIV positive patients 1325
  infectious complications in immunocompromised patients 1318–1319
  T cell activation 1320–1321, 1325–1328
    antigen 1326
    antigen-presenting cell 1326–1327
    clones vs. polyclonal lines 1325–1326
    CTL expansion 1327
    regulation 1327–1328
    selection of specific T cells 1327
indolocarbazoles 1239–1240
infected-cell protein 47 see ICP47 protein
infectious epithelial keratitis (IEK) 643–644
  see also keratitis
infectious mononucleosis (IM) 345, 403, 885–886
  as risk factor for Hodgkin's lymphoma 892
  cytotoxic T cell response role in resolution 908
  EBV dynamics
  epidemiology
  prophylactic vaccination 1294–1297
    EBNA3 1296–1297
    gp350 1295–1296
  risk factors
  therapy 886
  transmission
  see also Epstein-Barr virus (EBV)
inflammation
  HCMV and
  HSV and 642–643, 651
  see also immunopathology; nervous system disease; ocular disease
inflammatory demyelinating neuropathy, CMV and 789
injection drug use, KSHV transmission 969
inner nuclear membrane (INM) 144–145
integration, HHV-6 877–878
integrins 233–234
  α1ß1 integrin, downregulation by HCMV 824–825
  α3ß1 integrin 369
  interactions during host cell entry 367–369, 371–373
  RGD integrin-binding motif 369
intercellular adhesion molecule 1 (ICAM-1), HCMV and 767
interferon regulated factors (IRF) 1012
  IRF-3 modulation 325
  natural interferon producing cells (NIPCs) 625–627
  vIRF locus 500–502
  vIRF-1 550
  vIRF-2
  vIRF-3 (LANA2) 550, 1012
interferon response gene activation 325
interferon-stimulated genes (ISG), HSV 625

interferons
  blocking of host defense pathways 168
  HSV responses 625–627
    role in latency 618
  IFN-α
    HHV-6 response 838
    VZV responses 677–678, 707, 709
  IFN-γ, HCMV latency and 769–770
    reactivation 771
  in stromal keratitis 646–647
  MHC class II upregulation 1130
  response activation
  response evasion 625
    EBV
    HSV 625
    KSHV
  VZV treatment 1179
interleukins
  IL-1 646
  IL-6 646
    in multicentric Castleman's disease 1015
  IL-8 1080
  IL-10
    HSV responses 628
  IL-12
    HHV-6/multiple sclerosis relationship 860
    HSV responses 627
    in stromal keratitis 646–647
    response modulation by HHV-6 864–865
  IL-15
    HSV responses 627
  IL-17 1080
  IL-18
    HSV responses 627
  response evasion
  stromal keratitis and 646
  vIL-6 547–548, 1014, 1020
    rhesus rhadinovirus 1105–1106
  vIL-10 420, 472, 1069
    MMP dysregulation 826–827
    peptide transport interference 1122
    role in placental infection 827
  see also cytokines
International Committee on Taxonomy of
    Viruses 3
intracellular adhesion molecule-1 (ICAM-1) 1128
IRS1 protein 216, 243, 272–273
  interferon response and 326
ISIS 13312 1227

K1 gene 502, 503
  heterogeneity 965
K1 protein 508, 524–525, 546–547
K3 protein 1126–1127
K5 protein 1126–1127, 1128
K7 protein (vIAP) 552

K8 protein *see* KbZIP
K8.1 gene 365–366, 500
K8.1 glycoprotein 365–366, 369, 500
  anti-K8.1 antibodies 921–922
K10 gene 501
K12 gene 503
K15 gene 502–503
  heterogeneity 965
K15 proteins 503, 524–525
K cyclin (vCYC) 492, 496, 529, 544–546
  role in cell transformation 545–546
Kaposi, Moritz 347, 960
kaposica protein (KCP) 505, 1143
kaposin locus 503–505, 1012–1014
Kaposi's sarcoma (KS) 347–348, 349, 356, 893–895, 924, 960,
    974–978, 1015–1020
  clonality 1016
  dendritic cells and 918
  forms of 974, 975
    African/endemic 974
    classic 974
    epidemic/AIDS-associated 974–975, 976, 1017
    post-transplant/iatrogenic 974
  immunocompetence relationship 435–436, 915, 917–924
    HIV and 976, 1017
  KSHV gene expression 495–496, 894, 1017–1020
    latent infection 1017–1018
    lytic replication 1018–1020
  KSHV role 1017
    Hill criteria 977
  lytic reactivation role in development 434, 546
  natural killer cells and 918–919
  spindle cells 1016
    cell biology 1016–1017
  treatment 435, 894–895
    HAART 435–436, 916
Kaposi's sarcoma-associated herpesvirus (KSHV) 342, 356, 529,
    960
  apoptosis inhibition 445, 548–552
    extrinsic signaling inhibition 551–552
    p53 inhibition 548–551
  capsid structure 33–34, 351, 362, 450
  cell cycle regulation 541–548
    during latency 541–546
    during lytic replication 445
    KSHV mitogenic signaling proteins 546–548
  diagnosis 960
    approaches using assay combinations 962
    differential antibody response over time 963
    initial serologic assays 960–961
    methodological challenges 961–962
    recently developed assays 962
    seroreversion 963
    utility of currently available assays 963
  discovery of 347–348, 960, 961
  disease consequences 348–349, 351, 356, 978

cytokine model 356
immunocompetence and 915–917
oncogenic transformation model 356
primary infection 893, 973–974
see also tumor induction (below)
entry into host cell
attachment 365–366, 374
penetration 369–370
signaling 371–373
structural proteins involved 363, 364
envelope glycoproteins 351
epidemiology 963–964
geographic distribution 963–964
temporal patterns 964
gene content 354–355
gene expression 490, 494
during latency 380, 492, 497–498
early genes 506–508
IE genes 498–500, 506–508
in culture 490–494
in Kaposi's sarcoma 495–496, 894, 1017–1020
multicentric Castleman's disease 496–497
primary effusion lymphomas 496
gene expression regulation 497–508
splicing 497–506
genome comparisons 350–351
genome structure 361
genotypic diversity of infection 964–966
geographic distribution of subtypes 965
host response 917–925
B lymphocytes 921–925
complement 919
cytotoxic T lymphocytes 919–921
dendritic cells 918
differential antibody response over time 963
helper T lymphocytes 921
natural killer cells 918–919
host response evasion
apoptosis responses
B cell responses
complement control protein (KCP) 505, 1143
complement deregulation 1143
cytotoxic T cell responses
interferon responses
interleukin and chemokine responses
natural killer (NK) cell responses 918
retrieval of cell surface MHC class I molecules 1126–1127
T helper cell responses
intracellular transport 373
late genes 450
latency 348, 361, 379–380, 388–393
cell cycle dysregulation during 541–546
DNA replication and segregation 390–393
episomal genomes in latency 388–389
establishment of 379–380
gene expression 380

in primary effusion lymphoma (PEL) 438, 1008–1014
sites of 437–438
see also latency-associated nuclear antigen (LANA)
life cycle 348
lytic reactivation 434
accessory factors 448–450
apoptosis and 445
effects on host cell cycle 445
immunocompetence relationship 435–436
kinetic classification of lytic gene expression 438–439
pathogenic significance 434–435
PEL cell model 438
regulation of 442–450, 508
reservoirs for viral amplification 437–438
Rta lytic switch protein 439
phylogenetic relationships 349–350
primary infection 915–917
regulatory gene functions 540
rhesus rhadinovirus as animal model system 1105, 1108
see also rhesus monkey rhadinovirus
structure 450
target cells 360–361
tegument proteins 450
transmission 893
blood transfusion 969–970, 973
endemic areas 971
injection drug use 969
non-endemic areas 966–971
non-sexual horizontal transmission 971–972
organ transplantation 970–971
routes of 966
sexual transmission 966–969, 972–973
vertical transmission 973
treatment
tumor induction 342, 529, 530, 893–897, 1007
Castleman's disease 349, 496–497, 895–896, 1014–1015
double EBV/KSHV carrying PEL cells 529–530
primary effusion lymphoma (PEL) 348, 349, 496, 896–897, 1007–1014
treatment approach 1020–1021
see also Kaposi's sarcoma
see also gammaherpesviruses
KbZIP protein 442–500, 508
as origin binding protein 445–446
effects on host cell cycle 445, 547–548
p53 inhibition 550
kelch domain 118
keratitis 643–649, 659
disciform (DK) 644
infectious epithelial (IEK) 643–644
stromal (SK) 623, 643, 644–645, 655
animal models 645
innate reactions 645–647
treatment 665
acyclovir 1161

keratoconjunctivitis 597
  treatment 1161
KIE-2 protein
KIS protein *see* K1 protein
KSHV-gB amino acid 366

lamins 144–145, 317
LANA *see* latency-associated nuclear antigen (LANA)
Langerhans cell histiocytosis 864
LAT promoter element (LAP1) 604
  see also latency-associated transcripts (LATs)
late (L) genes 302
  expression regulation
    betaherpesviruses 302–305
    EBV 419–420, 469, 471–472
  gene products 420, 471–472
  KSHV 450
  transcription initiation 128–129
latency 434
  alphaherpesviruses 142
  betaherpesviruses 219, 843
  gammaherpesviruses 342, 379–380
    alternative forms of 465–467
    establishment of 379–380
    gene expression 380, 464–465, 492, 497–498
    PEL cell model 438
    sites of 437–438
  latent phase replication 302
  see also persistence; reactivation from latent state; *specific viruses*
latency-associated nuclear antigen (LANA) 380–390, 1008
  anti-LANA antibody detection 921, 961
  comparison with EBNA1 393
  DNA binding motif and domain 391–392
    DS-like element identification 391–392
    terminal repeat functions as plasmid origin 392
  expression in primary effusion lymphoma (PEL) 1008–1010
  functions 1008–1010
  LANA1 529, 544
    cell cycle dysregulation 544
    expression patterns 496
    p53 inhibition 550
  LANA2 (vIRF-3) 550, 1012
  modular domain structure 389–390
  role in episomal maintenance 390–393, 1008–1009
    episomal segregation 390–391
    trans-requirements for 392–393
    transcriptional regulation and signaling properties 390
  see also Kaposi's sarcoma-associated herpesvirus (KSHV)
latency-associated transcripts (LATs) 66, 82, 591
  CMV LATs (CLTs) 773
  HCMV 844
  HHV-6 843–844, 853
    gene regulation of 844
  HSV 604–606
    major ORFs 606
    promoter 604
    role in latency establishment 607–608
    role in reactivation from latency 611–612
    structure 604
  VZV 691, 692–693, 695
    activities related to cellular proteins 696
    functions 693
    localization related to latency 695–696
latent membrane proteins (LMPs) 518–519, 522–525
  LMP1 477–478, 518, 522, 523, 990–991
    apoptosis inhibition
    CTAR1/CTAR2 domains 990–991
    lymphocryptoviruses of old world monkeys 1099
    nasopharyngeal carcinoma and 527, 995, 998
    protein interactions 523
    role in host response evasion 910–911
  LMP2 907, 991
    LMP2a 478, 518–519, 522, 991
    LMP2b 478, 522, 524, 991
    lymphocryptoviruses of old world monkeys 1099
    modulation of cellular signaling 524–525
  prophylactic EBV vaccine development 1298–1299
    altered antigen processing using bacterial toxins 1299–1300
Lck tyrosine kinase 1082
leiomyosarcomas 892
leukopenia, HCMV infection and 1197
LMPs *see* latent membrane proteins
lobucavir (LBV) 1228
loss of heterozygosity (LOH) approach 997–998
Luman protein 610
lymphoblastoid cell line (LCL) 462–465
lymphocryptoviruses (LCV) 1085, 1086, 1096
  evolution 1095
  of new world monkeys 1100–1102
    as animal model system for EBV 1102
    see also marmoset lymphocryptovirus (CalHV3)
  of old world monkeys 1095–1100
    EBNA-1 homologues 1098
    EBNA-2 homologues 1098
    EBNA-3 family homologues 1098–1099
    LMP-1 proteins 1099
    LMP-2 proteins 1099
  see also gammaherpesviruses; rhesus lymphocryptovirus
lymphoepithelioma-like carcinomas
lymphoid interstitial pneumonias 887
lymphomas
  EBV-associated
    evidence of association with EBV
    in AIDS 891, 994
    T/NK cell tumors 891, 997
  immunoblastic 525
  KSHV-associated 897
    primary effusion (PEL) 348, 349, 496, 896–897
  non-Hodgkin

plasmablastic *see* Castleman's disease
  see also Burkitt's lymphoma (BL); Hodgkins lymphoma (HL)
lymphomatoid granulomatosis 892
lymphoproliferative disorders
  gammaherpesviruses and 342
  post transplant *see* post transplant lymphoproliferative disorders (PTLD)
  X-linked lymphoproliferative syndrome (XLP)
    epidemiology
lytic replication
  EBV 418–419, 467–472
    activation of 404–409
    early lytic gene products 417–418
    early lytic gene regulation 417
    IE protein functions 410–416
    late gene regulation 419–420
    late viral proteins 420
    treatment of lytic infection 420–421
    viral assembly and egress 420
    viral replication 418–419
  goals of 434
  KSHV 434
    effects on host cell cycle 445
    in Kaposi's sarcoma 1018–1020
    kinetic classification of lytic gene expression 438–439
    regulation of 446–450, 508
    viral enzymes and accessory factors 448–450
  see also reactivation from latent state

M140 gene 773–774
M141 gene 773–774
macrophages
  HCMV latency 769
  HCMV spread within host
  role in stromal keratitis 646
major capsid protein (MCP) 48
  HCMV 314
  see also capsid
major histocompatibility complex (MHC) *see* MHC functions, modulation of
major immediate early (MIE) genes
  betaherpesviruses 248–249, 1067
    functions of gene products 249–252
    reactivation of 247–248
    silencing of 246–247
    transcriptional enhancers 243–246
  see also immediate early (IE) genes
major latency locus
malignant catarrhal fever (MCF)
malignant glioma
  oncolytic HSV and 1346–1348
  therapeutic HSV vector application 1344
MAPK *see* mitogen activated protein kinase (MAPK) pathway
MARCH proteins 1127, 1128
Marek's disease herpesvirus (MDHV)

maribavir
  mechanisms of action
marmoset lymphocryptovirus (CalHV3) 1100–1101
  as animal model system for EBV 1098, 1102
  C1 protein 1101
  C5 protein 1102
  C7 protein 1102
  genome 1101
  ORF39 (EBNA-1) 1101–1102
  see also lymphocryptoviruses
matrix metalloproteinases (MMPs), dysregulation by HCMV 825–826
  role in placental infection 827
  vIL-10 effects 826–827
maturation 55–56, 218–219
  capsid 314–315
  viral DNA 141
MCK-1 chemokine
MCK-2 chemokine
measles virus, non-human primates 1057
MEF2D transcription factor 407
melanoma management 1348
membrane fusion 50–51, 100–103, 236
  cell-cell fusion assay 100
  gammaherpesviruses 366–370
  glycoprotein roles 23 100–102, 367–369
    gB role 100, 101–102, 104–105, 367, 369
    gD-receptor interaction role 100
    gE role VZV 104
    gH role 100–101, 367–368, 369
    gL role 100, 101, 367–368, 369
    gp42 role 367–369
  negative control of 102–103
    gB role 102, 104–105
    gK role 103
    in VZV 104–105
    UL20 protein role 103
membrane proteins
  alphaherpesviruses 93–94
  EBV 363–472
  KSHV 450
    expression patterns 502–503
    terminal membrane proteins (TMP) 503
  see also envelope; *specific proteins*
meningitis, benign 659
MHC functions, modulation of 269
  MHC class I 1119
    APC function interference 1128–1129
    by HCMV 787, 824
    by VZV 700–702
    costimulation interference 1128
    CTL escape mutants 1129
    destruction of class I molecules 1122–1125
    ER chaperones 1122
    erroneous T cell activation 1129

MHC functions, modulation of (*cont.*)
  immunological synapse interference 1128
  inhibitory receptor ligation 1129
  interference with class I molecules at cell surface 1127
  peptide transport interference 1121–1122
  proteasomal proteolysis 1119–1121, 1122–1125
  rerouting of class I molecules 1126
  retrieval of cell surface class I molecules 1126–1127
  secretory pathway disruption 1125–1126
  stunning of CTL activity 1129
  T cell receptor signaling inhibition 1129
 MHC class II 1130–1131
  by EBV 911
  by HMCV 789–790
  by VZV 702–704
  interference with class II expression 1130
  manipulation of class II molecules 1130–1131
vMIA 328–330
microarray technologies 1214
MIE genes *see* major immediate early (MIE) genes
vMIP proteins 515
mitogen activated protein kinase (MAPK) pathway 371
 MAPK/ERK pathway 252, 278–279
MIV-606 1229
MK3 1125, 1128
modified heparin sulphate 98–99
Mollaret's meningitis 659
monkey B virus *see* B virus
monocyte-derived macrophages (MDM), HCMV latency and 769
 apoptotic inhibitor role 774
 growth in Allo-MDM 770–773
 growth in Con A-MDM 769–770
Moore, Patrick 347–348
morphological criteria 3–7, 27
 see also virion structures
mortality, VZV 718–719
 herpes zoster 727–728
mouse mammary tumor virus (MMTV) 515
mRNA export factor 470
mRNAs 39
 degradation of in infected cells 166–167
 export to cytoplasm 131
multicentric Castleman's disease (MCD) 349, 1014–1015
 KSHV gene expression patterns 496–497
multifunctional regulator of expression (MRE) 51–52
multiple myeloma 349, 897
multiple sclerosis, HHV-6 association 839, 860–861
murine cytomegalovirus (MCMV) 781
 FcγR 1141–1142
 host response evasion 1125, 1126, 1128
 see also cytomegaloviruses (CMV)
murine gammaherpesvirus-68 (MHV-68)
 host response evasion 1125
  complement response 1146

 model for immune control of lytic reactivation 436–437
 molecular biology
 pathology
 vaccination studies 1296
murine leukemia virus 515

nasopharyngeal carcinoma (NPC) 527, 888, 891–892, 994–996
 characteristics of EBV infection 995–996
 contributing factors 996
 epidemiology
  geographical variation
  racial variation
 evidence for association with EBV
 prophylactic vaccine development 1297–1300
 risk factors
 T cell control of 911–912
 therapy 892
  adoptive immunotherapy 1324–1325
 tumor suppressor inactivation 997–998
 viral expression in NPC cells 527, 995
 viral strain and 998–1000
natural interferon producing cells (NIPCs) 625–627
natural killer (NK) cells 918–919
 cell surface receptors 787
 HCMV response 786–788
 HHV-6/HHV-7 response 857
  viral modulation of 861
 HSV responses 628–629
  NKT cells 629
 KSHV response 918–919
 response evasion
  EBV
  HCMV 787–788
  HSHV
  KSHV 918
NC7 capsid protein 77
ND10 (nuclear domain 10) 265–266
 importance in viral replication 139
 PML protein 168
 role in IE gene transcription 265–266
 see also PML (promyelocytic leukemia) bodies
nectins 96–98
 animal orthologues 99
 nectin1 95–96, 97
  expression in host tissues 97, 99
  functional domain 97
  gD interaction 97
 nectin2 97–98
neonatal infection
 antibody responses 624, 1137
 HCMV, cytomegalic inclusion disease (CID) 795
 HSV 598, 660–661, 1253
  antibody responses 624, 1332–1334
  disseminated infection 598

immune response characteristics 594–596, 1332–1333
    outcomes 1158
    transmission during delivery 660–661, 1253
    treatment 665, 1157–1160
  VZV 686, 715
  see also congenital infection
nervous system disease
  B virus
    HCMV 1197
  HSV and 597–598, 650–651, 659
    ganglionitis 643, 650–651
    herpes simplex encephalitis (HSE) 591–592, 597–598, 643, 650, 659
    neonates 598, 1157–1160
    treatment 665, 1157, 1164
  therapeutic HSV vector applications 1342–1344
    central nervous system 1343
    malignant glioma 1344
    peripheral nervous system 1343
  VZV
    cerebellar ataxia 684–685
    encephalitis 684–685
neurovirulence 590
neutrophils
  polymorphonuclear neutrophils (PMN)
    stromal keratitis response 645–646
  role in HSV response 625
newborns *see* neonatal infection
NF-(K)B activation 165–166, 325, 370
  BZLF1 effects 414
  EBV 990–991
  KSHV 443, 551, 1011–1012
NK cell lymphomas 891
  epidemiology
  evidence of association with EBV
NK cells *see* natural killer (NK) cells
NKT cells, HSV responses 629
non-Hodgkin lymphoma
non-human primates (NHP) 1093
  cytomegaloviruses (CMVs) 1051
    historical evidence of 1051–1052
    see also simian cytomegalovirus
  gammaherpesviruses 1076, 1108–1109
    nomenclature 1093–1095, 1096
    see also herpesvirus saimiri (HVS); lymphocryptoviruses; rhadinoviruses
non-nucleoside pyrrolopyrimidines 1227
noninfectious enveloped particles (NIEP) 28–30
Notch proteins 992
nuclear domain 10 *see* ND10
nuclear egress 55–56
  betaherpesviruses 315–318
nuclear egress lamina protein (NELP) 55
nuclear egress membrane protein (NEMP) 55
nuclear envelope 144–145

nuclear factor of activated T-cells (NFAT) 443–444
nuclear lamina 144–145
nuclear membrane
  budding from 146–147
  envelopment at 145
    model 148
  inner nuclear membrane (INM) 144–145
  outer nuclear membrane (ONM) 144
nucleocapsid
  envelopment *see* envelopment process
  intracellular transport in host cells 51, 103–104
    mechanisms 103–104, 214–216
  see also capsid
nucleosome organization, EBV 381
nucleotide metabolism 53
  betaherpesviruses 217–218
NV1020 1348–1349

OBPs *see* origin binding proteins (OBPs)
Oct-1 protein 113–116
  diverse interactions 113–116
  latency establishment and 607
Oct-2 protein 696
ocular disease
  B virus 1036–1037
  herpes zoster ophthalmicus treatment 1184–1185
  HSV 643, 659–660
    treatment 665, 1161
  see also acute retinal necrosis (ARN); keratitis; uveitis
Oka varicella vaccine 1262
  history of development 1262–1263
  safety 1263–1264
  virology of attenuated Oka strain 1263
oncogenesis *see* tumor induction
oncolytic HSV 1345–1350
  current directions 1349–1350
  in malignant glioma 1346–1348
  in non-CNS malignancies 1348–1349
    colorectal metastases 1348–1349
    melanoma 1348
open reading frames (ORFs) 70–82
  functions 70–82
  gene content analysis 14, 163
  HSV latency-associated transcripts (LATs) 606
  ORF1 64, 82
  ORF2 64
    HCMV 279
    VZV 82
  ORF4 505, 693, 1143
  ORF10 122, 696
  ORF13 64–65, 82
  ORF21 693, 695
  ORF29 693, 695, 696
  ORF32 65, 82

open reading frames (ORFs) (cont.)
  ORF39 1101–1102
  ORF40 505–506
  ORF41 505–506
  ORF47 682–683
  ORF50 440, 492
    as origin-binding protein 445–446
    expression patterns 498, 506–507
    rhesus rhadinovirus 1106
  ORF57 65
    KSHV 506
    VZV 82
  ORF62 693, 695–696
  ORF63 692–693, 695
  ORF64 681
  ORF66 683, 693, 1126
  ORF73 1078
  ORF-O 65, 71
  ORF-P 65, 71
  ORF-S/L 65, 82
  ORFK1 502
    heterogeneity 965
    promoter 502
  ORFK3 506
  ORFK9 500
  ORFK10 501
  ORFK10.5 501
  ORFK11 501–502
  ORFK15 502–503
    heterogeneity 965
  ori_{Lyt} ORFs 301
  see also genomics; specific genes
oral hairy leukoplakia 887, 988
ORFs see open reading frames
organ transplantation see transplantation
origin binding proteins (OBPs) 299
  KSHV 445–446
  OBP-1/Kid, OriP interaction 386–387
origin of plasmid replication (OriP)
  cellular proteins that interact with 386–387
  DNA replication mechanism 387
  molecular biology 382–384
  plasmid segregation mechanisms 388
  role in EBV latency 381
    EBNA1 binding effects 381–382
  see also Epstein-Barr virus (EBV)
origin of replication sequences (ori) 138–139
  betaherpesviruses 299–302
  herpesvirus saimiri 1077–1078
  latent phase replication 302
  roseolovirus 301–302
  see also ori_{Lyt}
ori_{Lyt} 52
  betaherpesviruses 296
  cytomegalovirus 299–301

    open reading frames and transcripts 301
    structure 300
  EBV 467–469
  KSHV 446
    binding proteins 445–446
  roseoloviruses 301–302
ORI(S) RNA 82
orolabial infection, HSV-1 596, 657
  primary infection 596
  reactivation 596
  treatment 665, 1157, 1162, 1164
outer nuclear membrane (ONM) 144
Ox2 protein

p27 protein, v-cyclin interaction 1010
p38 MAPK pathway 252, 278–279
p53 tumor suppressor protein 252, 548–550
  BZLF1 effects on 412–413
  inactivation by tumor viruses 517, 530
    Burkitt's lymphoma and 526
    KSHV (HHV-8) 529, 548–551
  infection effects on 327
  LANA interaction 1009–1010
p72 regulatory protein 331
p86 regulatory protein 326–327, 331
PAF (primase-associated factor) 505–506
parotid gland carcinoma 997
pathogenesis see specific viruses
PD146626 1226–1227
penciclovir
  herpes labialis treatment 1162
  VZV treatment 1178
  see also famciclovir
peptide transport, interference with 1121–1122
persistence
  EBV 472–474
  HCMV 765
    sites of 765
  HHV-6/HHV-7 875
  simian CMV 1054–1055
PGC coactivator 121
pharyngitis, HSV infection and 596
phosphatidylinositol 3-kinase (PI3K) pathway 252
phospholipids, implications for envelopment pathway
  153–154
PI 3-K 371–373
placenta
  development in early gestation 814–816
    cytotrophoblast functions 816–817
    diverse cell types in the uterus 814–816
    hemochorial human placenta 816
  HCMV infection 814, 817–823, 827
    antibodies to CMV in syncytiotrophoblasts 819–820
    CMV protein expression patterns 817–818, 820
    decidual infection relationship 820–823

down regulation of cytotrophoblast HLA-G expression 824
impact on cytotrophoblast invasion 825, 827
integrin expression downregulation 824–825
MMP dysregulation 825–827
potential transmission routes 817
presence at placental-decidual interface 818–819
replication in cytotrophoblasts *in vitro* 824
vIL-10 effects 826–827
pathogenic microorganisms at placental-decidual interface 818–819
PML (promyelocytic leukemia) bodies
BZLF1 dispersion of 413
PML protein 168
see also ND10
pneumonia, varicella 684
immunocompromised hosts 685
pneumonitis, CMV 788–789, 1196, 1197
PNU-26730 1231
PNU-182171 1231
PNU-183792 1231–1232
polyamines 39
polymerase accessory protein 297–298
polymorphonuclear neutrophils (PMN)
HMCV spread within host
stromal keratitis response 645–646
polyoma virus 515
polyradiculopathy 1197
post transplant lymphoproliferative disorders (PTLD) 890–891, 993
adoptive immunotherapy 1323
EBV gene expression 993
epidemiology
evidence of association with EBV
management 890–891
prophylactic vaccine development 1297
postherpetic neuralgia (PHN) 726
management 1183–1184
POU proteins 113, 607
Oct-1 113–116
pp28 protein 318–319, 1066
pp65 DNA vaccine 1283–1284
pp65 protein 782–783
PR protease (assemblin) 218
precursor of assembly protein (pAP) 54
pregnancy, VZV infection 686
prophylaxis 1186
treatment 1181
primary effusion lymphoma (PEL) 348, 349, 896–897, 1007–1014
EBV co-infection 529–530, 1007
KSHV gene expression patterns 496
KSHV latency program 1008–1014
kaposin 1012–1014
LANA 1008–1010
v-cyclin 1010–1011

v-FLIP 1011–1012
vIRF3/LANA2 1012
PEL cell model
double EBV/KSHV carrying PEL cells 529–530
KSHV gene expression 490–494
KSHV latency and reactivation 438
primary pulmonary hypertension (PPH) 349
primates *see* non-human primates
programmed cell death *see* apoptosis
promoters
HSV latency-associated transcripts (LATs) 604
ICP0, role in reactivation from latency 610
late genes 302–304
ORFK1 502
TATA box 128–131
viral transcription factors 128–129
see also gene expression
promyelocytic leukemia *see* PML (promyelocytic leukemia) bodies
protease inhibitors 1238–1239
proteasomal proteolysis
destruction of MHC class I molecules 1122–1125
interference with 1119–1121
protein kinase C (PKC), role in lytic reactivation 443
protein-linking integrin-associated protein and cytoskeleton 1 (PLIC1)
proteins 179–183
B virus 1034
functions, expression of 163
herpesvirus-common gene products 44–45, 48
see also core functions
major virion proteins 29
structural proteins 48–50
betaherpesviruses 213–214
capsid 48–49, 313
envelope 50, 93–94
tegument 49, 362, 450
see also envelope; gene products; host proteins; membrane proteins; *specific proteins*
proteomics
bioinformatics and computational tools 1211–1212
databases 1213–1214
pseudorabies virus (PRV)
complement response evasion 1147
FcγR 1142
pyrimidine deoxynucleoside kinase 140

R1 gene 1105
R8 protein 1106
R8.1 protein 1106
R7020 vaccine 1255
racial factors
EBV epidemiology
VZV epidemiology 724–725
RAP *see* KbZIP protein
RAV 9395 1255

Rb pathway inactivation by tumor viruses   517, 530
   Burkitt's lymphoma and   526
   KSHV (HHV-8)   529, 544
      LANA role   1010
RBP-Jk DNA binding protein   440, 507–508, 992
reactivation from latent state
   betaherpesviruses   843
      IE genes   247–248
   immune control of   435–436
      model   436–437
   see also lytic replication; specific viruses
recombination   53, 141–142
regulators of complement activation (RCA)   1143
   MHV-68 RCA   1146
renal transplantation
   KSHV transmission   970–971
   see also transplantation
replication   48, 52–53, 138–142
   alphaherpesviruses   138–142
   antiviral targets
      DNA replication complex   1227–1235
      early replication events   1226–1227
   betaherpesviruses   204–212, 216–217, 295–296
      replication origins   299–302
      replication proteins   296–299
      rolling circle versus linear model   295–296
   cell cycle and   141
   cell preparation for   268–269
   DNA encapsidation   54–55
      betaherpesviruses   218, 314–315
   DNA maturation and packaging   141, 218–219, 1235
   gammaherpesviruses   341–342
      rhadinoviruses   1077–1078
      see also lytic replication
   gene functions   70, 204–212, 296
      early genes   267–268
   initiation of DNA synthesis   301
   late gene expression and   304
   latent phase   302
   location of DNA synthesis   139
   mobilization of cellular proteins   164–165
   origins of (ori)   138–139
      betaherpesviruses   299–302
      see also ori_{Lyt}
   OriP DNA replication mechanism   387
   proteins involved in DNA synthesis   139–141, 217
   recombination   53, 141–142
   regulation   51–52
      betaherpesviruses   216–217, 241
   strategies   163
      see also anti-host strategies
   see also lytic replication; persistence; specific viruses
retinitis
   CMV   643, 789, 1197
   HSV   643

retinoblastoma (Rb) protein (pRB1)   541
   see also Rb pathway inactivation by tumor viruses
retroperitoneal fibromatosis (RF)   350
   rhadinoviruses from   1103–1104
      phylogenetic analysis   1103
RGD integrin-binding motif   369
rhadinoviruses   341, 1076, 1085, 1086, 1096
   evolution   1102
   from mice and other mammals
   from old world primates   1086–1108
      phylogenetic analysis   1103
   from retroperitoneal fibrosis (RF)   1103–1104
   genome structure   1077
   immunomodulatory proteins   1078–1080
   replication   1077–1078
   see also gammaherpesviruses; specific viruses
rhesus cytomegalovirus (RhCMV) see simian cytomegalovirus
rhesus lymphocryptovirus (LCV)
   as animal model system for EBV   1097, 1099–1100
   EBNA-1 homologues   1098
   EBNA-2 homologues   1098
   EBNA-3 family homologues   1098–1099
   genome   1095
   LMP-1   1099
   LMP-2   1099
   see also lymphocryptoviruses
rhesus monkey rhadinovirus (RRV)   350, 1086–1108
   as animal model for KSHV   1105, 1108
   capsid structure   1106–1107
   genome structure   1104–1105
   natural occurrence
   Orf50/Rta   1106
   pathogenesis   1107–1108
   phylogenetic analysis   1103
   R1 gene   1105
   R8 protein   1106
   R8.1 protein   1106
   transcription program   1106
   vGPCR   1106
   vIL-6   1105–1106
   see also rhadinoviruses
rheumatoid arthritis   887
rheumatoid factor   887
ribonucleotide reductase (RR1)   53, 140, 330–331
RK-BARF0   992
RL10 protein   192
RNA
   alphaherpesviruses
      processing   131–133
      synthesis initiation   128–131
   betaherpesviruses   192
   EBV-encoded RNAs (EBERs)   478, 991–992
   virus-associated (vRNAs)   301
   see also mRNAs
RNA tumor viruses   515–516

class I 516
class II 516
roseoloviruses 850
   antigens 853–856
   future research 866
   genetic analysis 212
   genome comparisons 204
   immunologic cross-reactivity 856–857
   origin binding proteins 299
   replication origins 301–302
   see also betaherpesviruses; human herpesvirus 6 (HHV-6); human herpesvirus 7 (HHV-7)
Rous, Peyton 514, 924
RPMS1 ORF 992
Rta viral lytic switch protein
   EBV 467
      see also BRLF1 protein
   KSHV 439–500, 506–508
      apoptosis and 445
      as origin-binding protein 445–446
      p53 inhibition 550
      regulatory functions 506–508
   rhesus rhadinovirus 1106

Sabin, Albert 1031–1032
saimiri transformation-associated proteins (Stp) 1080–1081, 1083
sarcoidosis 349
SCIDhu model 677–679
segment inversion 13
   class D genomes 13
   class E genomes 13
serological criteria 7
seroreversion 963
sex differences
   EBV epidemiology
   VZV epidemiology 724
sexual transmission
   HCMV 796, 800–802
   KSHV 966–969, 972–973
   see also genital HSV infection
SFp32,EBNA1 interaction 386
shingles *see* herpes zoster; varicella zoster virus (VZV)
Shope, Richard 514–515
signaling
   apoptotic signaling 548
      extrinsic pathway 548
      inhibition of extrinsic signaling 551–552
      intrinsic pathway 548
   during entry into host 370–373
   entry activated cell signaling 233
   KSHV mitogenic signaling proteins 546–548
   LANA signaling properties 390
   modulation of by LMP2 524–525
simian AIDS (SAIDS) 1055–1056
   CMV infection relationships 1055–1056

simian cytomegalovirus 1051, 1070
   infection in immunocompetent hosts 1052–1055
      chronic infection 1054–1055
      immune responses 1053–1054, 1055
      pathogenesis 1052–1053
      primary infection dynamics 1053
   infection in immunocompromised hosts 1055–1058
      fetal infection 1057–1058
      measles virus-associated immunosuppression 1057
      retroviral-induced immunodeficiency 1055–1056
      transplantation 1056–1057
   molecular biology 1058–1070
      betaherpesvirus-specific proteins 1064, 1066–1068
      gene arrangements 1061–1065
      genome coding content 1058
      genome structures 1061
      genomic DNA sequences 1065–1066
      herpesvirus core proteins 1064, 1066
      primate CMV-specific proteins 1064, 1068–1070
      tegument structure 38
   multiple strains 1052
   seroprevalence 1052
   virion structure 1058
simian immunodeficiency virus (SIV) 1055–1056
   CMV infection relationships 1055–1056
simian varicella virus (SVV) 691, 1043–1044
   comparisons with VZV 1044, 1045
   genome 1044–1045
   pathogenesis 1045–1049
   reactivation from latency 1043–1044
single-stranded DNA binding protein (SSB) 298, 449
skin eye and mouth (SEM) disease, neonates 598, 661
skin infections *see* cutaneous infections
SM gene 414
SM protein 418
small capsid protein (SCP) 48–49, 314
small replicator transcript 301
Sp1 transcription factor 120
species definition 7–8
spermidine 39
spermine 39
spindle cells 1016
   cell biology 1016–1017
   KSHV latent infection in 1017–1018
splicing 15
stem cell transplantation (SCT)
   HHV-6/HHV-7 response and 859–860
   see also immunocompromised hosts; transplantation
Stewart, Sarah 515
stomach carcinoma *see* gastric cancers
Stp (saimiri transformaton-associated proteins) 1080–1081, 1083
stress
   herpes zoster epidemiology and 725
   HSV response and 630

stromal keratitis (SK) 623, 643, 644–645, 655
  adaptive immunity 647–649
  animal models 645
  innate reactions 645–647
    polymorphonuclear neutrophil (PMN) response 645–646
structures *see* virion structures
syncytiotrophoblasts, antibody response to HCMV 819–820

T0.7 transcript 492–493, 495, 503
T1.1 transcript 492–493, 495–496
T157602 1232
T cell lymphomas 891, 997
  epidemiology
  evidence of association with EBV
T cells *see* T lymphocytes
T helper cells (CD4+) 497–498, 921
  EBV response 907
  HCMV response 785–786
  HSV responses 621–623
    T-cell co-stimulation 623–624
  immunotherapy approaches 1321
  in stromal keratitis 647–649
  KSHV response 921
  response evasion
    EBV 911
    KSHV
  simian CMV response 1055
  see also T lymphocytes
T lymphocytes 919
  EBV responses 907
    malignancy control 911–912
    receptor usage 908–909
  growth transformation of 1083–1084
  HCMV response 782–785
  HHV-6/HHV-7 response 859
    immunocompromised hosts 860
    multiple sclerosis relationships 861
    viral modulation of 861, 862–863, 864
  immunotherapy approaches 1320–1321
    adoptive immunotherapy 1321
    CTL activation approaches 1325–1328
  in stromal keratitis 647–649
  infection by HHV-6 833–834, 861, 862–863
  infection by HHV-7 834, 861, 862–863
  infection by VZV 675, 700
    glycoprotein functions 679–680
    modulation of MHC class I expression 701
    pathogenesis evaluation 675–676
    regulatory proteins 680–683
    SCIDhu model 677
    transmission to T-cells 704–705
  response evasion 1120
    CTL escape mutants 1129
    erroneous T cell activation 1129
    inhibition of T cell receptor signaling 1129
    stunning of CTL activity 1129
    see also MHC functions, modulation of
  TCRγ cells, HSV responses 629–630
  VZV responses 707–708
    during latency 708
    during reactivation 709
  see also cytotoxic T lymphocytes (CD8+); T helper cells (CD4+)
tapasin, interference with 1122
TATA box 128–131
taxonomy 3, 4–6
  see also classification
TCRB 1237
TCRγ cells, HSV responses 629–630
tegument 154
  assembly 154–155
    betaherpesviruses 315–318
    implications for envelopment pathway 154–155
    protein trafficking and incorporation 318–319
  composition 35–36, 49, 213
  structure 36–38
    betaherpesviruses 191–192, 213
    EBV 362
    KSHV 450
TER heterodimeric terminase 54
terminal membrane proteins (TMP) 503
therapeutic vectors *see* viral vectors
thrombocytopenia, VZV and 685
Tio protein 1085–1086
Tip (tyrosine kinase interacting protein) 1080, 1081–1082, 1083
TLRs *see* toll like receptors (TLRs)
TNFRs (tumor necrosis factor receptors) 97
toll like receptors (TLRs) 234
  TLR9 626
Towne vaccination 1279–1281
TPA, lytic gene induction
  EBV 409
  KSHV 442–443, 444
transcription
  alphaherpesviruses 128–131
    role of IE proteins 129
    TATA box-containing promoters 128–131
    viral transcription factors 128–129
  betaherpesviruses
    MIE transcriptional enhancers 243–246
    reactivation of IE genes 247–248
  EBNA1 regulatory properties 385–386
  LANA regulatory properties 390
  rhesus rhadinovirus 1106
  see also early (E) genes; gene expression; immediate early (IE) genes; latency-associated transcripts (LATs)
transfusion *see* blood transfusion
transmission *see specific viruses*
transplant rejection, CMV and 789–790
transplant vasculopathies, HCMV and 790
transplantation

EBV infection, adoptive immunotherapy 1323–1324
HCMV transmission 625, 806–807
   graft rejection and 1196
HHV-6 reactivation 839
HHV-6/HHV-7 immune responses and 859–860
   clinical significance of immunomodulation 866
KSHV transmission 970–971
simian CMV infection and 1056–1057
see also allograft transplantation; bone marrow transplant (BMT); immunocompromised hosts; post transplant lymphoproliferative disorders (PTLD)
transporter associated with antigen presentation (TAP) proteins 1121–1122
TRF1/2,OriP interaction 387
TRS1 protein 216, 243, 272–273
   interferon response and 326
tumor induction
   herpesvirus ateles 1085–1086
   herpesvirus saimiri 1080–1082
   history 514–515
   immune surveillance and 527–529, 890
   viral strategy as risk factor 514
   virus-host cell interactions carrying risk 514, 517
   see also DNA tumor viruses; Epstein-Barr virus (EBV); Kaposi's sarcoma-associated herpesvirus (KSHV); RNA tumor viruses
tumor necrosis factor alpha (TNF-alpha)
   HCMV latency and 769–770
   HSV responses 627
   inhibition by BZLF1 413–414
tumor progression 515
tumor suppressor inactivation 997–998
   see also p53 tumor suppressor protein
tumor viruses *see* DNA tumor viruses; RNA tumor viruses; *specific viruses*
tyrosine kinase interacting protein (TIP) 1080, 1081–1082, 1083

U11 protein 855
U12 gene 865
U21 gene 865
U21 protein 1126
U27 283
U38 282
U51 gene 865
U94 gene 282, 844
U94 transcripts 853
UL1 gene 71
UL1.5 gene 65
UL2 gene 72
UL3 gene 72
UL4 gene 72
   expression regulation 277–279
UL5 gene 72
UL5 protein 140
UL6 gene 72
UL6 protein
   molecular mimicry 648
UL7 gene 72
UL8 gene 72
UL8.5 gene 65, 73
UL9 gene 73
UL9.5 gene 73
UL10 gene 73
UL11 gene 73
UL11 protein 147
UL12 gene 73, 140
UL12 protein 140
UL12.5 gene 74
UL13 gene 74
UL13 protein kinase 130
   role in viral replication 164–165
UL14 gene 74
UL15 gene 74
UL15.5 gene 66, 74
UL16 gene 74
UL17 gene 74
UL18 gene 74
UL18 molecule 1129
UL19 gene 75
UL20 gene 75
UL20 protein 103
   negative control of membrane fusion 103
UL20.5 gene 66, 75
UL21 gene 75
UL22 gene 75
UL23 gene 75
UL24 gene 75
UL25 gene 76
UL26 gene 76
UL26.5 gene 76
UL27 gene 76
   maribavir resistance and
UL27.5 gene 66, 76
UL28 gene 76
UL29 gene 76
UL30 gene 76
UL31 gene 76
UL31 protein 145–147, 148
   implications for envelopment pathway 153
UL31/UL34 protein complex 145–146, 148
UL32 gene 76
UL32 protein 38
UL33 gene 77
UL34 gene 77, 217
UL34 protein 146–147, 148
   implications for envelopment pathway 153
   phosphorylation by US3 147
UL35 gene 77

UL36 gene 77, 774, 1067
UL36 protein 216
   apoptosis suppression 327–328, 330
   implications for envelopment pathway 154
   role in replication 273, 299
UL37 gene 77, 1067
UL37 proteins 216–217
   apoptosis suppression 327–330
   implications for envelopment pathway 154
   role in replication 273, 299
UL37x1/vMIA gene 774
UL38 gene 77
UL38 protein 273, 299
UL39 gene 77
UL40 gene 77
UL40 protein 1067
UL41 gene 77
UL41 protein
   mRNA degradation in infected cells 166–167
UL42 gene 77
UL43 gene 77
UL43.5 gene 66, 78
UL44 gene 78
UL44 protein 297–298
UL45 gene 78
UL46 gene 78
UL47 gene 78
UL48 gene 78
UL48A protein 1066
UL49 gene 78
UL49.5 gene 79
UL50 gene 79
UL51 gene 79
UL52 gene 79
UL52 polypeptide 142
UL53 gene 79
UL54 gene 79
   expression regulation 275–277
   HCMV drug resistance and 1204
UL54 protein 297–298
UL55 gene 79
UL56 gene 66, 80
UL57 protein 298
UL59 ORF 301
UL69 gene 216
UL69 protein 253
   host cell modulation 326–327
UL70 protein 296–297
UL80a protein 314
UL80.5 protein 314
UL82 gene 216
UL82 protein 253
   host cell modulation 326–327
UL83 gene 1067
UL83 protein 35–36

UL84 protein 217, 298–299
   IE2 interaction 217, 298
UL97 gene 1203–1204
   encoded protein kinase inhibitors 1239
UL99 gene 303
UL99 protein 318–319
UL100 gene products 835, 836
UL102 protein 296–297
UL105 protein 296–297
UL111A gene 1069
UL112 gene
   transcription regulation 273–275
UL112 protein 217
UL113 gene
   transcription regulation 273–275
UL113 protein 217
UL144 gene 331
UL146 protein 1068
uracil DNA glycosidase (UNG) 53, 72
uracil N-glycosylase 140
US1 gene 66, 80
US1.5 gene 80
US2 gene 66, 80
US2 protein 1122–1124, 1125, 1130
US3 gene 80, 243, 273
US3 protein 147, 1130
   role in blocking apoptosis 169
   tapasin interference 1122
US4 gene 66–67, 81
US5 gene 67, 81
US6 gene 67, 81
US6 protein 1121
US7 gene 81
US8 gene 81, 1125
US8.5 gene 67, 81
US9 gene 81
US9 protein
   role in cell-to-cell spread 157
US10 gene 81
US10 protein 1125
US11 gene 67, 81
US11 protein 1124–1125
US12 gene 67, 82
US22 gene family 212–213
US28 protein 1068–1069
uveitis 643, 649
   rabbit model 649

vaccination *see* DNA vaccines; *specific viruses*
valaciclovir
   adverse effects 1164, 1178
   clinical indications 1164
   HSV treatment 663–664, 1163–1165
      dosage regimens 1164
      genital herpes 1156, 1163–1164

    herpes labialis 1164
    herpes simplex encephalitis 1164
    resistance 1164–1165
    transmission reduction 664
  pharmacokinetics 1163, 1177
  VZV treatment 1177, 1178
    herpes zoster 1182
valganciclovir
  adverse effects 1169
  clinical indications 1169
  dosage regimens 1169
  HSV treatment 1169
  mechanism of action 1169
  pharmacokinetics 1169
  resistance 1169
varicella (chickenpox) *see* varicella zoster virus (VZV)
varicella zoster virus (VZV) 675, 1175
  comparisons with simian varicella virus (SVV) 1044, 1045
  congenital varicella syndrome 715
  cutaneous infection 675
    glycoprotein functions 679–680
    lesion characteristics 683–684
    mechanisms 677–679
    primary infection clinical pattern 683–684
    secondary bacterial infection 684
  dendritic cell (DC) interactions 700, 704–706
    immune evasion strategy 706
  diagnosis 1175–1177
    culture 1175
    direct fluorescent antigen (DFA) staining 1176
    polymerase chain reaction (PCR) 1176–1177
    serological techniques 1177
  disseminated infection 685
  drug resistance 1187–1188
  egress from host cell 158–159
  entry into host cell 104–105
    gE role 104
  epidemiology 713
    age specificity 715–717, 722–724
    climate and 715, 717
    complications 726–727
    congenital varicella syndrome 715
    deaths 718–719, 727–728
    dermatomal distribution 722
    hospitalizations 719, 727
    immunocompetence and 725–726
    periodicity and seasonality 714, 721–722
    pre-vaccine era 713–719
    racial differences 724–725
    secular trends 722
    sex differences 724
    stress and 725
    urban/rural setting relationship 717
    vaccination impact 719–721, 728–729
    varicella 713–721

  genome comparisons 61–64
    genes that are absent from HSV genomes 64–65
  glycoprotein functions 679–680
    glycoprotein C 679
    glycoprotein E 104–105, 158–159, 679–680
    glycoprotein I 158, 680
  host response 678–679, 707
    during latency 708
    during primary infection 707–708
    during reactivation 709
    interferon-a response 677–678, 707, 709
    persistence of VZV-specific memory 708
    T-cell responses 707–708
  host response evasion 700
    downmodulation of cell-surface MHC class I expression 700–702
    during dendritic cell infection 706, 1128
    FcγR role 1141
    inhibition of MHC class II upregulation 702–704
    MHC class I secretory pathway disruption 1126
  IE gene expression regulation 121–122
  latency 689
    comparison with other alphaherpesviruses 694–695
    establishment of 693
    future directions 696
    immunity during 708
    models 690–691, 693–694, 695–696
    proteins expressed 692–693, 695–696
    site of 689, 690
    transcripts expressed 691–692
    viral DNA load 689–690
  pathogenesis 1043
    evaluation 675–676
    lack of animal model 1043
    SCIDhu model 677–679
  primary infection clinical pattern 683–685
    CNS disease 684–685
    hepatitis 684
    immunocompromised hosts 685–686
    in pregnancy 686
    neonates 686
    thrombocytopenia 685
    varicella pneumonia 684, 685
  prophylaxis 1186–1187
    herpes zoster 1187
    immunocompetent patients 1186, 1187
    immunocompromised patients 1186–1187
    pregnant women 1186
    varicella 1186–1187
    with HIV infection 1187
    see also vaccination (below)
  reactivation from latency 694, 1043
  regulatory protein functions 680–683
    IE62 protein 681
    IE63 protein 681

varicella zoster virus (VZV) (*cont.*)
    ORF47 protein 682–683
    ORF64 protein 681
    ORF66 protein 683
  replication effects on host cyclins 676–677
  RNA processing 132–133
  T-cell infection 675, 677, 700
    glycoprotein functions 679–680
    transmission to T-cells 702–704
  transcription initiation 128–131
    role of IE proteins 130, 131
    viral transcription factors 129
  transmission 713–714
  treatment 1177–1180, 1186
    acyclovir 1177–1178
    brivudin 1179
    children 1179–1180
    drug resistance 1187–1188
    famciclovir 1178–1179
    foscarnet 1179
    herpes zoster 1181–1186
    immunocompetent adults 1180–1184
    immunocompromised patients 1181, 1185
    interferon 1179
    penciclovir 1178
    pregnant women 1181
    valacyclovir 1177, 1178
    varicella 1179–1181
    vidarabine 1179
    with HIV 1181, 1185–1186
    see also antiviral agents
  vaccination 1186–1187, 1262
    considerations of use 1265–1266
    DNA vaccines 1313
    duration of immunity 1266–1268
    efficacy and effectiveness 1264–1265
    elderly patients 1269
    epidemiological impact 719–721, 728–729
    herpes zoster 728–729, 1187
    immunogenicity in healthy children and adolescents 1264
    inactivated varicella vaccine 1269
    live attenuated vaccine development 1262–1263
    misconceptions 1263
    questions 1266
    safety 1263–1264
    varicella 1186–1187
    virology of attenuated Oka strain 1263
    zoster and 1264, 1268–1269
    vaccine failure 1263, 1266–1268
  see also alphaherpesviruses
vascular disease, HCMV and
vectors *see* viral vectors

vidarabine, VZV treatment 1179
VIP protein 502
viral vectors 1341
  herpesvirus saimiri as gene therapy vector 1084
  HSV 1341
    amplicons 1342
    nervous system modification 1342–1344
    optimization for therapeutic use 1344–1345
    replication-competent vectors 1341
    replication-defective vectors 1341, 1342, 1344–1345
    see also oncolytic HSV
virion assembly 27–28, 311–312
  capsid assembly 31, 53–54, 268, 311
    betaherpesviruses 218, 312–314
  EBV 420
  envelope assembly 39
  tegument assembly 154–155
virion structures 27, 30
  betaherpesviruses 188–192
    simian CMV 1058
  capsid 31–34, 48–49, 191
  envelope 38–39
  genome 10–14, 34–35, 138, 189–191
  KSHV 450
  tegument 35–38, 191–192
  see also specific structures
VP1–3 protein 37–38
VP1/2 protein 77
VP5 protein 31–32
VP11/12 tegument protein 78
VP13/14 tegument protein 78
VP16 protein 78
  latency establishment and 606–607
  role in HSV IE enhancer core complex assembly 116–117
  structure 116–117
  transcription activation (TA) domain 117
VP19C capsid protein 77
VP22 protein 78
VP23 protein 32, 74
VP26 protein 77
VPK (viral serine-threonine protein kinase) 49

WAY-150138 1235–1236

X-linked lymphoproliferative syndrome (XLP)
  epidemiology
  genetic basis

ZEBRA protein *see* BZLF1 protein
ZI motifs 406–407
ZII motif 407
zoster *see* herpes zoster; varicella zoster virus (VZV)
Zta protein *see* BZLF1 protein (ZEBRA)